Volume **II**

Principles and
Practice of
EMERGENCY
MEDICINE

Principles and Practice of

EMERGENCY MEDICINE

Editor-in-Chief

George R. Schwartz, M.D., F.A.C.E.P.
Emergency Medicine, Santa Fe, New Mexico
Visiting Associate Professor of Emergency
Medicine, Medical College of Pennsylvania,
Philadelphia, Pennsylvania
Past Associate Professor and Director, Department of
Emergency Medicine, University of New
Mexico Medical School,
Albuquerque, New Mexico

Editors

C. Gene Cayten, M.D., M.P.H., F.A.C.S.
Director, Institute for Trauma and
Emergency Care, Professor of Surgery
and Preventive and Community Medicine,
New York Medical College, Valhalla,
New York
Director of Surgery, Our Lady of Mercy Medical Center,
Bronx, New York

Thom A. Mayer, M.D., F.A.C.E.P.
Chairman, Department of Emergency
Medicine, Fairfax Hospital,
Falls Church, Virginia
Associate Professor of Emergency Medicine and
Pediatrics, Georgetown University
and George Washington University
Schools of Medicine, Washington, D.C.

Mary Anne Mangelsen, M.D., Ph.D., F.A.C.P.
Chairman and Medical Director, Department
of Emergency Medicine, W.A. Foote Memorial
Hospital, Jackson, Michigan
Clinical Instructor, Emergency Services, University of Michigan,
Ann Arbor, Michigan

Barbara K. Hanke, M.D., F.A.C.E.P.
Staff Emergency Physician,
St. Vincent Hospital, Santa Fe, New Mexico
Clinical Assistant Professor of Medicine, University of California
San Francisco; Valley Medical Center,
Fresno, California

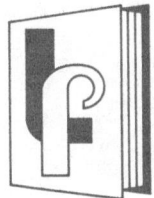

Volume II
Third Edition

Lea & Febiger   1992   Philadelphia/London

Lea & Febiger
Box 3024
200 Chester Field Parkway
Malvern, Pennsylvania 19355-9725
U.S.A.
(215) 251-2230

Executive Editor—Carroll C. Cann
Manuscript Editor—Jessica Howie Martin
Production Manager—Thomas J. Colaiezzi

Library of Congress Cataloging-in-Publication Data
Principles and practice of emergency medicine / George R. Schwartz . . .
[et al.].—3rd ed.
     p.   cm.
   Includes index.
   ISBN 0–8121–1373–X
   1. Emergency medicine.   I. Schwartz, George R.
   [DNLM: 1. Critical Care. 2. Emergencies. 3. Emergency Medicine.
WB   105 P957]
RC86.7.P74   1992
616.02'5—dc20
DNLM/DLC
for Library of Congress   91–44532
                                                                CIP

Reprints of chapters may be purchased from Lea & Febiger in
quantities of 100 or more. Contact Sally Grande in the Sales Department.

PRINTED IN THE UNITED STATES OF AMERICA

Print number: 5   4   3   2   1

Dedications

George R. Schwartz, M.D.: To Emergency Medicine physicians, whose care has made the world a better and safer place; to my late father, Milton Schwartz, whose gifts I appreciate more and more; and to Kathleen, whose light shines on everything I do.

C. Gene Cayten, M.D.: To Marianna, Carasandra, and Christopher for their love and support.

Mary Anne Mangelsen, M.D.: In fierce praise of the healing world, past, present, and to come; to Leif (genes, but oh, so much more).

Thom Mayer, M.D.: To my wife Maureen and our sons, Josh, Kevin, and Gregory, whose love and support sustain me in all things.

Barbara K. Hanke, M.D.: To my son, Austin, some of whose milestones I probably missed while working arduously on this book, and to Rod, who gave me moral support tempered only by a needed sense of reality.

Preface

The third edition of *Principles and Practice of Emergency Medicine* has been designed to add to the Second Edition and to further broaden and deepen the authoritative scope of the textbook. *Clinical usefulness has been a key component in this edition.*

We have also made significant changes in the Third Edition to reflect the growth and development of the field of Emergency Medicine. Almost every section has undergone major revision, with a focus toward making it thorough and clinically applicable. We have amplified the Resuscitation chapter and included special considerations of brain death and organ retrieval, as well as ethical issues. In our evaluation and management of selected presentations, we have attempted to expand the range to make the book more clinically useful by including special conditions such as pelvic pain in women, dysphagia, fever, and sepsis. Part III, which deals with procedures, diagnostic tools, and techniques, has been expanded significantly because of the growth in imaging techniques of use to the emergency physician. We have focused on tests and procedures that are the most useful in the Emergency Department, and explored their limitations and complications. We have added substantially to the chapters on management of wounds and removal of foreign bodies from the eye, ear, and nose; and concomitantly, increased attention has been paid to local anesthesia. The section on pain management in the Emergency Department has been enlarged. In the section on trauma, we have attempted to identify the areas of traumatology of most use in emergency medicine, and have added areas of increased depth concerning traumatology and trauma systems, as well as prehospital management of trauma. We have also attempted to provide a breakdown in general considerations involving epidemiology in the general approach and specific management issues and presentations in emergency situations. We have provided special considerations of trauma in pregnancy, trauma in the elderly, and pediatric trauma because of the need for special attention in these groups.

The section dealing with nontraumatic organ system emergencies (clinical emergency medicine) has been expanded greatly. The increased depth of this area, along with the increasing subdivision of chapters, should render it far easier to access clinically relevant material in the acute emergency situation. *The hallmark of this section is clinical usefulness.*

For ease of use, we have established a new form for most chapters that includes careful attention to a capsule at the beginning and a specific order, including pathophysiology, management, and clinical pitfalls. Prehospital management has been an area of increased focus as well. Because of today's litigious climate, we have added "medicolegal pearls" when appropriate. In the acute situation, it is helpful to access additional help, and we have included national contacts or ways to access more information. In this edition, we have also added an enlarged section on obstetric and gynecologic emergencies. The sections on pediatric and geriatric emergencies have also been broadened. In the section on psychiatric and behavioral emergencies, we have attempted to increase the patient-oriented approach to expedite the care of acutely disturbed psychiatric patients by emergency and acute care physicians.

The area of environmental emergencies has been emphasized, and special new sections on wilderness and travel medicine, as well as diseases of travellers, help to round out the additions to the section.

The discussion of toxicology has been expanded and reflects the increasing depth and subspecialization in this area. A symptom-oriented approach has been used when possible.

In Part XII, we have produced a comprehensive overview of Emergency Medical Service (EMS) systems. We have emphasized the "operational" approach and how to implement the most effective system, including ground and air transport and disaster planning, with special attention to the evaluation of the system. In Section II of Part XII, we have expanded the foreign models so that our system can be compared with those of other countries. In other editions, other countries were featured. Also added is a special chapter concerning EMS and terrorism.

Part XIII is a completely new section involving Emergency Department management, focusing on administrative issues of critical importance in maintaining and managing an effective Emergency Department.

The final medicolegal section (Part XIV) has been planned and edited to provide up-to-date medicolegal guidance, particularly in our specialty, in which litigation has increased and there is currently far more attention to the standard of emergency care. With the growth of our specialty, consideration of quality, legal liability, Emergency Department risk management, hospital responsibility, and avoiding errors has become essential.

The Index has been an area of increased focus. Particularly in a book that is both comprehensive and designed for Emergency Department use, information must be readily retrievable. To that end, we have enlarged the Index and cross-referenced it extensively to make it most useful in the acute care situation. The Table of Contents has also been expanded and subdivided to enhance access.

This edition shows the meticulous care of the editors in organizing information in the most readily accessible form. To this end, we have included as many photographs, illustrations, tables, and charts as possible, and information for ready reference. Whenever possible, we have included laboratory testing and appropriate normal values.

As the field of emergency medicine has grown, we have developed an expanded cadre of enthusiastic practitioners of the art and specialty of emergency medicine who have contributed to this work. We have well over 300 contributors, a vast majority of them practitioners of emergency medicine. One advantage of this is that we are getting a "hands-on" approach whenever possible. At the same time, emergency medicine is built on a foundation that includes the entire critical care medicine continuum, from scene to outcome, and this requires sophisticated input from other specialty areas as well. The editors have been privileged to work with a diverse and talented group of contributors. This interaction has allowed us to bring an expanded, comprehensive, and authoritative textbook to aid the practitioner in the care of patients.

Santa Fe, New Mexico   George R. Schwartz, M.D.
Valhalla, New York   C. Gene Cayten, M.D.
Jackson, Michigan   Mary Anne Mangelsen, M.D.
Falls Church, Virginia   Thom A. Mayer, M.D.
Santa Fe, New Mexico   Barbara K. Hanke, M.D.

Acknowledgments

The preparation of a work of this size and scope requires the deep commitment of many people working in diverse roles and with varied responsibilities. In such a tremendous effort, it is difficult to single out individuals because so many are involved. Yet there are some who deserve special recognition.

Carroll Cann, our editor, has been enormously helpful in many ways, from steering the last edition to completion to easing the transition from W.B. Saunders Company to the highly dedicated team at Lea & Febiger. Words are insufficient to indicate all he has done. Christian C.F. "Kit" Spahr, Jr. died recently at a young age, but his enthusiasm and welcome as we moved to his company will long be remembered. We would also like to thank Tom Colaiezzi, who supervised the production of this major revision and greatly expanded edition. He has overseen the many changes we have made to a more useful format and, in addition, has created a new design. We have the entire team at Lea & Febiger to thank for rapid production and creative promotion.

Dr. George Schwartz would like to thank particularly the following: Kathleen, his wife and partner, who helped in more ways than can be enumerated—from muse to disciplinarian, she has kept this project moving; Dr. Barbara Hanke, whose organizational abilities were vital as the work expanded and who unflinchingly took on extra duties when the need presented; Mrs. Beatrice Schwartz-Hertzberg, who has helped in every way possible and has been a continuous influence to maintain quality; Ruth, Rebekah, Rachel, Moses, and Abigail, who have provided the family environment, love, and inspiration; and the hundreds of contributors who took to their task with relish and are the backbone of this work.

Dr. Gene Cayten would like to acknowledge "the Fellows and staff of the Institute for Trauma and Emergency Medical Care at New York Medical College. These Fellows and staff have made my work on this text possible through their collaboration and support. I am especially appreciative of Dr. Louis L. R. del Guercio's support for our endeavors in trauma and emergency care at New York Medical College."

Dr. Mary Anne Mangelsen would like to raise hands in commendation to her family in and out of medicine, especially to Leif, Pat, Marci, Becky, Barbara, and her JCES colleagues who provided the cheer and support that formed the critical milieu for this work.

Dr. Thom Mayer would like to extend his deepest gratitude to his colleagues and friends at Fairfax Hospital, Department of Emergency Medicine, and to his family, whose combined encouragement has made his contribution to this work possible.

Dr. Barbara Hanke would like to thank "Jane Knowles for her expert library and reference research, and George Schwartz, quite simply, for sharing his wisdom and experience. I also appreciate all the authors who took time away from their families to help in this endeavor. Dr. Patricia S. Bailey and Dr. Robert K. Knopp are also fondly remembered as guides and mentors in my practice of emergency medicine."

Contributors

JOSE A. ACOSTA, M.D.
Chief Resident, Department of Surgery, University of New Mexico School of Medicine, Albuquerque, New Mexico

STEPHEN L. ADAMS, M.D., F.A.C.P., F.A.C.E.P.
Associate Chief, Section of Emergency Medicine, Northwestern University Medical School. Associate Director, Emergency Medical Services, Northwestern Memorial Hospital. Project Medical Director, Chicago Central Mobile Intensive Care Program, Department of Emergency Services, Northwestern Memorial Hospital, Chicago, Illinois

NANAKRAM R. AGARWAL, M.D., M.P.H., F.R.C.S., F.A.C.S.
Associate Professor of Surgery, New York Medical College. Chief, Surgical Intensive Care Unit, Our Lady of Mercy Medical Center, Bronx, New York

RICHARD V. AGHABABIAN, M.D.
Division Director, Division of Emergency Medicine and Associate Professor of Medicine, Department of Medicine, University of Massachusetts Medical School, Worcester, Massachusetts

JAMES W. ALBERS, M.D., Ph.D.
Professor of Neurology and Director, Neuromuscular Section, Department of Neurology, University of Michigan Medical Center, Ann Arbor, Michigan

MAURICE ALBIN, M.D.
Professor of Anesthesiology, University of Texas, San Antonio, Texas

MICHAEL F. ALTIERI, M.D., F.A.A.P.
Section of Pediatric Emergency Medicine, Fairfax Hospital, Falls Church, Virginia. Associate Professor of Pediatrics in Emergency Medicine, George Washington University School of Medicine, Washington, D.C.

JAMES T. AMSTERDAM, D.M.D., M.D.
Professor of Emergency Medicine, University of Cincinnati, Poland, Ohio. Chairman, Department of Emergency Medicine, Western Reserve Care System, Northside Medical Center, Youngstown, Ohio

ELLEN E. ANDERSON, M.D.
Formerly Surgical Associate, Medical College of Pennsylvania. Currently Missionary Physician in Africa.

GAIL V. ANDERSON, M.D., F.A.C.E.P.
Assistant Professor, Department of Community Health, Division of Emergency Medicine, Grady Memorial Hospital, Atlanta, Georgia

WILLIAM McD. ANDERSON, M.D.
Assistant Professor of Medicine, Physiology, and Biophysics, Louisiana State University School of Medicine. Chief, Section of Pulmonary and Critical Care Medicine and Director of Medical Intensive Care Unit, Veterans Administration Medical Center, Shreveport, Louisiana

REBECCA A.H. ANWAR, Ph.D.
Associate Professor of Emergency Medicine, Department of Emergency Medicine, Medical College of Pennsylvania, Philadelphia, Pennsylvania

KENT F. ARGUBRIGHT, M.D.
Assistant Professor, Department of Obstetrics/Gynecology, Division of Maternal-Fetal Medicine and Department of Pediatrics, University of New Mexico School of Medicine. Staff Physician, University of New Mexico Hospital, Albuquerque, New Mexico

LYNN AUGENSTEIN, M.D., F.A.C.E.P.
Assistant Professor of Emergency Medicine, University of Florida Health Science Center, Jacksonville, Florida

ELLIS D. AVNER, M.D.
Professor of Pediatrics, Director, Division of Nephrology, Children's Hospital and Medical Center, University of Washington Medical School, Seattle, Washington

MARTIN E. BACON, M.D.
National Naval Medical Center, Department of Cardiology, Bethesda, Maryland

WADIE F. BAHOU, M.D.
Assistant Professor of Medicine, Division of Hematology, State University of New York, Health Sciences Center, Stony Brook, New York

DAVID BALDWIN, JR., M.D.
Assistant Director, Section of Endocrinology and Metabolism, Rush-Presbyterian St. Luke's Medical Center, Chicago, Illnois

NICHOLAS BALSANO, M.D., F.A.C.S.
Associate Clinical Professor of Surgery, New York Medical College. Associate Director of Surgery, Our Lady of Mercy Medical Center, Bronx, New York

STEVEN R. BENNETT, M.D.
Fellow, Vitreoretinal Service, The Eye Institute, Medical College of Wisconsin, Milwaukee, Wisconsin

THEODORE BENZER, M.D.
New York University School of Medicine. Associate Director, Emergency Medical Services, Bellevue and New York University Hospital Centers, New York, New York

GARRETT E. BERGMAN, M.D.
Professor of Pediatrics, The Medical College of Pennsylvania. Associate Staff, St. Christopher's Hospital for Children, Philadelphia, Pennsylvania

JAMES L. BERNAT, M.D.
Professor of Clinical Medicine (Neurology), Dartmouth Medical School, Hanover, New Hampshire. Chief, Neurology Section, Veterans Administration Medical Center, White River Junction, Vermont

EDGAR B. BILLOWITZ, M.D., F.A.C.E.P.
Staff Emergency Physician, St. Vincent Hospital, Santa Fe, New Mexico

NICHOLAS G. BIRCHER, M.D.
International Resuscitation Research Institute, University of Pittsburgh Medical Center, Pittsburgh, Pennsylvania

ELLEN B. BISHOP, M.D.
The Medical College of Pennsylvania. St. Christopher's Hospital for Children, Philadelphia, Pennsylvania

JAMES C. BLANKENSHIP, M.D.
Clinical Assistant Professor, Thomas Jefferson University, Philadelphia, Pennsylvania. Geisinger Medical Center, Danville, Pennsylvania

THOMAS P. BLECK, M.D., F.A.C.E.P.
Assistant Professor, Health and Science Center, Department of Neurology, University of Virginia Medical Center, Charlottesville, Virginia

ANDREW BLITZER, D.D.S., M.D.
Professor of Clinical Otolaryngology, Department of Otolaryngology, Columbia University. Director, Division of Head and Neck Surgery, Columbia-Presbyterian Medical Center, New York, New York

PAULA L. BOCKENSTEDT, M.D.
Hematology/Oncology Division, University of Michigan, Ann Arbor, Michigan

ROBERT BOLTE, M.D., F.A.A.P.
Director of Emergency Department, Primary Children's Medical Center, Salt Lake City, Utah

MICHAEL J. BONO, M.D., F.A.C.E.P.
Assistant Professor of Emergency Medicine and Associate Program Director, Emergency Medicine Residency Program, Eastern Virginia Graduate School of Medicine, Norfolk, Virginia

WILLIAM F. BOUZARTH, M.D., F.A.C.S. (Deceased)
Professor of Neurological Surgery, The Medical College of Pennsylvania. Staff Physician, Hospital of the Medical College of Pennsylvania, Philadelphia, Pennsylvania

JAMES K. BOUZOUKIS, M.D., F.A.C.S., F.A.C.E.P.
Director of Emergency Medicine, Residency Training Program, Medical Center of Delaware, Wilmington, Delaware

DAVID M. BOWLING, M.D.
Clinical Fellow in Otolaryngology, Harvard Medical School. Resident in Otolaryngology, Massachusetts Eye and Ear Infirmary, Boston, Massachusetts

EDWARD L. BRADLEY, III
Department of Surgery, New York University School of Medicine, New York, New York

DANIEL BRANDES, M.D.
Instructor, Emergency Medicine, College of Osteopathic Medicine of the Pacific, Pomona, California. Director of Emergency Services, Greater El Monte Community Hospital, South El Monte, California

ROBERT R. BRINSON, M.D.
Gastroenterologist, Montgomery Internal Medicine Residency Program. Clinical Assistant Professor, University of Alabama, Birmingham School of Medicine, Montgomery, Alabama

MARK B. BROMBERG, M.D., Ph.D.
Assistant Professor of Neurology, Department of Neurology, University of Michigan Medical Center, Ann Arbor, Michigan

DAVID BROOKE, M.D., F.A.C.E.P.
Chairman, Department of Emergency Medicine, Lakeland Regional Medical Center, Lakeland, Florida

MARC D. BROWN, M.D.
Assistant Professor of Dermatology, Director of Mohs Surgery Unit, University of Rochester, Rochester, New York

DOUGLAS D. BRUNETTE, M.D.
Department of Emergency Medicine, Hennepin County Medical Center, Minneapolis, Minnesota

ARON S. BUCHMAN, M.D.
Assistant Professor of Neurological Sciences, Rush Medical College, Chicago, Illinois

PAUL I. BULAT, M.D., F.A.C.E.P.
Instructor in Medicine, Division of Emergency Medicine, The University of Massachusetts Medical School. Director of Emergency Services, St. Luke's Hospital of New Bedford, Inc., New Bedford, Massachusetts

RICHARD E. BURNEY, M.D.
Chief, Emergency Services, Department of Surgery, University of Michigan Hospitals. Associate Professor of Surgery, University of Michigan, Ann Arbor, Michigan

CHARLES B. CAIRNS, M.D.
E.M. Foundation Scholar, UCLA School of Medicine, Department of Emergency Medicine, Harbor-University of California at Los Angeles Medical Center, Torrance, California

JEFFREY P. CALLEN, M.D.
Associate Professor of Medicine; Chief, Residency Program, University of Kentucky, Louisville, Kentucky

RUSSELL J. CARLISLE, M.D., F.A.C.E.P.
Emergency Staff Physician, St. Francis Medical Center, Lynwood, California. Assistant Clinical Professor, Department of Family Medicine, University of Southern California School of Medicine, Los Angeles, California

THOMAS R. CARRACIO, Pharm. D., D.A.B.A.T.
Assistant Professor of Emergency Medicine, State University of New York at Stony Brook. Visiting Assistant Clinical Professor of Pharmacology and Toxicology, New York College of Osteopathic Medicine, Old Westbury, New York Clinical Coordinator, Nassau County Medical Center. Long Island Regional Poison Control Center, East Meadow, New York

ROSANNE CARRERO, M.D.
Assistant Medical Director, EMS; Attending Physician, St. Joseph Hospital, Bellingham, Washington, and Ketchikan General Hospital, Ketchikan, Alaska

C. GENE CAYTEN, M.D., M.P.H., F.A.C.S.
Director, Institute for Trauma and Emergency Care, Professor of Surgery and Preventive and Community Medicine, New York Medical College, Valhalla, New York. Director of Surgery, Our Lady of Mercy Medical Center, Bronx, New York

RICHARD E. CHAISSON, M.D.
Director, AIDS Service, Johns Hopkins Hospital, Baltimore, Maryland

ROBERT S. CHARLES, M.D.
Department of Urology, Temple University. The Medical College of Pennsylvania, Philadelphia, Pennsylvania

CLARK CHIPMAN, M.D., F.A.C.E.P.
Chief, Emergency Services, Emmanuel Hospital. Professor, Health Science Center. Clinical Associate, University of Oregon, Portland, Oregon.

NANCY CLARK, M.D.
Emergency Physician, Department of Emergency Medicine, Northwestern Memorial Hospital, Chicago, Illinois

JOHN R. CLARKE, M.D., F.A.C.S.
Professor of Surgery, Director of Trauma Center, The Medical College of Pennsylvania, Philadelphia, Pennsylvania

R. CARTER CLEMENTS, M.D.
President-Elect, Department of Emergency Medicine, Highland General Hospital, Oakland, California

ARNOLD M. COHN, M.D.
Professor, Department of Otolaryngology, Wayne State University, Detroit, Michigan

STEPHEN A. COLUCCIELLO, M.D., F.A.C.E.P.
Attending Physician, Emergency Department, Broward General Medical Center, Fort Lauderdale, Florida

PATRICK CONNELL, M.D.
Acting Chairman, Department of Emergency Medicine, Highland General Hospital, Oakland, California

ERRIKOS CONSTANT, M.D., D.D.S., F.A.C.S.
Clinical Associate Professor of Surgery, College of Human Medicine, Michigan State University, East Lansing. Staff Surgeon (Plastic Surgery), Sparrow Hospital, St. Lawrence Hospital, and Ingram Medical Center, Lansing, Michigan

FRANCIS L. COUNSELMAN, M.D., F.A.C.E.P.
Assistant Professor and Associate Director, Division of Emergency Medicine, Eastern Virginia Graduate School of Medicine, Norfolk, Virginia

GERARD R. COX, M.D.
Attending Physician, Naval Hospital, Portsmouth, Virginia. Clinical Instructor of Military and Emergency Medicine, Uniformed Services. University of the Health Sciences, Bethesda, Maryland

MARILYN K. CROGHAN, M.D.
Department of Radiation Oncology, University of Arizona College of Medicine, Tucson, Arizona

RITA K. CYDULKA, M.D., F.A.C.E.P.
Attending Physician, MetroHealth Medical Center Emergency Department. Senior Instructor, Department of Surgery, Case Western Reserve University School of Medicine, Cleveland, Ohio

CHRISTOS S. DAGADAKIS, M.D., M.P.H.
Director of Emergency Psychiatry; Lecturer, Department of Psychiatry and Behavioral Sciences, University of Washington School of Medicine. Harborview Medical Center, Seattle, Washington

ROBERT H. DAILEY, M.D.
Consultant in Emergency Medicine, Clinical Professor of Medicine, University of California/San Francisco. Staff Emergency Physician, Merritt Hospital, Oakland, California

LAWRENCE DALL, M.D.
Associate Professor of Medicine, Chief, Section of Infectious Diseases, School of Medicine, University of Missouri/Kansas City, Kansas City, Missouri

JAMIE DANANBERG, M.D.
Department of Endocrinology and Metabolism, University of Michigan Hospitals, Ann Arbor, Michigan. Emergency Physician, W.A. Foote Memorial Hospital, Jackson, Michigan

ROBERT C. DAUSER, M.D.
Assistant Professor, University of Michigan, Ann Arbor, Michigan

STEVEN J. DAVIDSON, M.D., M.B.A., F.A.C.E.P.
Professor of Emergency Medicine, Head, Pre-hospital Care, Medical College of Pennsylvania, Philadelphia, Pennsylvania

RALPH K. DELLA RATTA, M.D.
Attending Physician, Division of General Internal Medicine, Winthrop University Hospital. Instructor of Medicine, State University of New York at Stony Brook, Mineola, Long Island, New York

GERALD B. DEMAREST, M.D.
Associate Professor of Surgery and Director, Burn and Trauma Service, University of New Mexico Medical Center, Albuquerque, New Mexico

JEFFREY DEMBO, D.D.S., M.S.
Assistant Professor of Oral and Maxillofacial Surgery, University of Kentucky College of Dentistry, Lexington, Kentucky

WILLIAM E. DeMUTH, JR., M.D.
Professor of Surgery Emeritus, College of Medicine, Pennsylvania State University. Attending Surgeon, Carlisle Hospital, Carlisle, Pennsylvania

MERLE L. DIAMOND, M.D., F.A.C.E.P.
Internal Medicine, Diamond Headache Clinic, Chicago, Illinois

SEYMOUR DIAMOND, M.D.
Director, Diamond Headache Clinic, Adjunct Professor of Pharmacology, The Chicago Medical School. Clinical Associate, Department of Medicine, University of Chicago, Chicago, Illinois

ALAN R. DIMICK, M.D.
Associate Professor of Surgery; Director, Burn Center, University of Alabama, Birmingham, Alabama

CONSTANCE J. DOYLE, M.D., F.A.C.E.P.
Senior Attending Physician, W.A. Foote Memorial Hospital, Jackson, Michigan. Clinical Instructor, Department of Surgery, University of Michigan, Ann Arbor, Michigan.

STEPHEN J. DRESNICK, M.D.
President, The Sterling Group, Miami, Florida

BASIM A. DUBAYBO, M.D.
Assistant Professor of Medicine, Division of Pulmonary and Critical Care Medicine, Wayne State University School of Medicine, Detroit, Michigan. Staff Physician, Veterans Administration Medical Center, Allen Park, Michigan

NICHOLAS DUFEU, M.D.
Anesthesia and Intensive Care Specialist, SAMU 94, Hôpital Henri Mondor, Paris, France

JOHN D. DUNN, M.D., F.A.C.E.P.
Director, Emergency Medicine, Brownwood Regional Medical Center, Brownwood, Texas

MICHAEL S. EASTON, M.D.
Assistant Professor and Research Psychiatrist, Rush Medical University. Director, Rush Chemical Dependency Program, Department of Psychiatry, Rush-Presbyterian-St. Luke's Medical Center, Chicago, Illinois

FREDERIC E. ECKHAUSER, M.D.
Chief, Division of Gastrointestinal Surgery, Professor of Surgery, University of Michigan Medical Center, Ann Arbor, Michigan

DENNIS R. EHRHARDT, M.D.
Medical Director, Clinical Laboratory, St. Vincent Hospital, Santa Fe, New Mexico

FRANK EHRLICH, M.D., F.A.C.S.
Clinical Professor of Surgery, University of Pennsylvania. Deputy Director Department of Surgery, Graduate Hospital, Philadelphia, Pennsylvania

MICKEY S. EISENBERG, M.D., Ph.D.
Professor of Medicine, Director of Emergency Medicine Services, University of Washington Medical Center, Seattle, Washington

DEMETRIUS ELLIS, M.D.
Professor of Pediatrics, Director of Pediatric Nephrology, University of Pittsburgh School of Medicine. Director, Division of Pediatric Nephrology, Children's Hospital of Pittsburgh, Pittsburgh, Pennsylvania

JOHN I. ELLIS, M.D.
Emergency Medicine, Department and Faculty (TBA), Highland General Hospital, San Francisco, California

CHARLES L. EMERMAN, M.D., F.A.C.E.P.
Chairman, Department of Emergency Medicine, MetroHealth Medical Center, Cleveland, Ohio

DAVID K. ENGLISH, M.D.
Assistant Chief, Department of Emergency Medicine, Highland General Hospital, Oakland, California. Instructor in Medicine, University of California at San Francisco School of Medicine, San Francisco, California

ALAN EPSTEIN, M.D.
Associate Professor of Medicine, Rush Presbyterian-St. Luke's Medical Center, Hinsdale, Illinois

MICHAEL E. ERVIN, M.D.
Director, Emergency and Trauma Center, Miami Valley Hospital, Dayton, Ohio

DONALD FALACE, D.M.D.
Professor and Director, Dental Emergency Clinic, Department of Oral Health Science, University of Kentucky College of Dentistry, Lexington, Kentucky

BEVERLY FAUMAN, M.D.
Department of Psychiatry, University of Maryland School of Medicine, Baltimore, Maryland

DAVID V. FELICIANO, M.D., F.A.C.S.
Professor of Surgery, Emory University School of Medicine. Chief of Trauma and Tumor Services, Grady Memorial Hospital, Atlanta, Georgia

NEIL A. FENSKE, M.D., F.A.C.E.P.
Professor of Medicine, Director, Division of Dermatology, Department of Internal Medicine. Professor of Pathology, Department of Pathology, University of South Florida College of Medicine. Chief, Dermatology Section, H. Lee Moffitt Cancer Center and Research Institute, Tampa, Florida

ALAN I. FIELDS, M.D.
Department of Respiratory Care Services, Children's National Medical Center, Washington, D.C.

PAULA FINK, M.D.
Emergency Department, Minneapolis Children's Medical Center, South Minneapolis, Minnesota

NEAL FLOMENBAUM, M.D., F.A.C.P., F.A.C.E.P.
Clinical Associate Professor of Medicine, State University of New York Health Science Center at Brooklyn. Chairman, Emergency Medicine, Long Island College Hospital, Brooklyn, New York. Chief Medical Consultant, New York City Poison Control Center.

JOSEPH F. FOWLER, JR., M.D.
Assistant Professor of Dermatology, University of Louisville School of Medicine, Louisville, Kentucky

SCOTT B. FREEMAN, M.D., F.A.C.E.P.
Residency Director and Assistant Professor, Section of Emergency Medicine, Wayne State University. Detroit Receiving Hospital and University Health Center Emergency Department, Detroit, Michigan

FREDERICK G. FREITAG, D.O.
Associate Director, Diamond Headache Clinic. Visiting Lecturer, Chicago College of Osteopathic Medicine. Clinical Associate, Department of Medicine, University of Chicago, Chicago, Illinois

ARNOLD P. FRIEDMAN, M.D.
Adjunct Professor of Neurology, University of Arizona Medical School, Tucson, Arizona

STUART R. FRITZ, M.D.
Emergency Physicians Professional Association, Minneapolis, Minnesota. Clinical Instructor, Department of Family Practice, University of Minnesota, Minneapolis, Minnesota

SHERYL G.A. GABRAM, M.D., F.A.C.S.
Assistant Professor, University of Connecticut School of Medicine. Medical Director, Life Star Helicopter Program. Assistant Director of Trauma Program, Hartford Hospital, Hartford, Connecticut

DONALD S. GANN, M.D. F.A.C.S.
Professor and Associate Chairman, Department of Surgery, University of Maryland School of Medicine, Baltimore, Maryland

LUCILLE GANS, M.D.
Division of Emergency Medicine, University of Massachusetts Medical School, Worcester, Massachusetts

JORGE M. GARCIA, M.D.
Associate Clinical Professor of Surgery, George Washington University. Chief, Cardiac Division, Washington Hospital Center, Washington, D.C.

RALPH R. GARRAMONE, M.D.
EMS/Trauma Fellow, Hartford Hospital, Hartford, Connecticut

JAMES G. GARRICK, M.D.
Director, Center for Sports Medicine, St. Francis Memorial Hospital, San Francisco, California

SALLY S. GARRIGAN, M.S.W.
Good Samaritan Hospital and Medical Center, Portland, Oregon

CLOYD B. GATRELL, M.D.
HHC-8 Infantry Division, Division Surgeon, Department of the Army, Feilbingert, Germany

ROBIN GAUPP, M.D.
Attending Radiology Physician, St. Vincent Hospital, Santa Fe, New Mexico

THOMAS A. GENNARELLI, M.D., F.A.C.S.
Professor of Neurosurgery of the University of Pennsylvania. Vice Chairman, Department of Neurosurgery, Hospital of the University of Pennsylvania, Philadelphia, Pennsylvania

STEVEN E. GENTRY, M.D.
Assistant Professor of Medicine, University of Pittsburgh School of Medicine. Assistant Head, Pulmonary Unit, Montefiore Hospital, Pittsburgh, Pennsylvania

JAMES E. GEORGE, M.D., J.D., F.A.C.E.P.
Emergency Physician, Underwood Memorial Hospital; President, Emergency Physician Associates, P.A.; Partner, Law Firm of George and Korin, Woodbury, New Jersey

JAMES E. GERACE, M.D.
Chief, Pulmonary Medicine, and Chief of Staff, Phoenix Memorial Hospital, Phoenix, Arizona

WILLIAM S. GILMER, M.D.
Department of Psychiatry, Rush Presbyterian-St. Luke's Medical Center, Chicago, Illinois

DAVID GINSBURG, M.D.
Associate Professor, Hematology/Oncology Division, University of Michigan, Ann Arbor, Michigan

AARON E. GLATT, M.D., F.A.C.P.
Assistant Chief, Division of Infectious Diseases, Nassau County Medical Center, East Meadow, New York. Assistant Professor of Medicine, State University of New York at Stony Brook, Stony Brook, New York.

LEWIS GOLDFRANK, M.D., F.A.C.E.P.
Associate Professor of Clinical Medicine, New York University School of Medicine. Director of Emergency Medical Services, Bellevue and New York University Medical Centers, New York, New York

LEON GOLDMAN, M.D.
Professor Emeritus in Dermatology, University of Cincinnati College of Medicine; Consulting Dermatologist, University Hospital and Children's Hospital; Director, Laser Laboratory and Laser Treatment Center, Jewish Hospital, Cincinnati, Ohio

H. WARREN GOLDMAN, Ph.D., M.D.
Associate Professor and Chief of Neurosurgery, The Medical College of Pennsylvania. Staff Physician, The Medical College Hospital, Philadelphia, Pennsylvania

JAMES J. GORDON, M.D.
Fellow, Infectious Diseases, University of Michigan Medical School, Ann Arbor, Michigan. Director, Infectious Diseases, McLaren Hospital, Flint, Michigan

THOMAS GOUGE, M.D.
Associate Professor of Clinical Surgery, Department of Surgery, New York University School of Medicine, New York, New York

GARY J. GRAD, M.D.
Clinical Assistant Professor, Department of Psychiatry, Cornell University Medical College. Lecturer in Psychiatry, Columbia College of Physicians and Surgeons. Senior Assistant Attending Psychiatrist, North Shore University Hospital, New York, New York

BARBARA H. GREENE, M.D.
Associate Professor of Medicine, Emory University, Medical Director, Walk-In Clinic, Grady Memorial Hospital, Atlanta, Georgia

RUTH ANN GREENFIELD, M.D.
Duke University Medical Center. Associate Professor in Medicine, Electrophysiology and Cardiology, Durham, North Carolina

DAVID GREGORY, M.D.
Captain, United States Public Health Service. Senior Consultant in Infectious Disease, by Indian Health Service, Santa Fe Indian Hospital, Santa Fe, New Mexico

CINDY L. GRINES, M.D.
Cardiology Department, William Beaumont Hospital, Royal Oak, Michigan. Assistant Professor of Medicine, Director, Acute Interventional Cardiology, Division of Cardiology, University of Kentucky College of Medicine, Lexington, Kentucky

M. V. GRINIOV, M.D.
Professor and Director, I.I. Djanelidze Research Institute of First Aid, Budapeshtskag, Leningrad, U.S.S.R.

CHARLES M. GRUDEM, M.D.
Medical Director, Spine Care Center, Fairview Southdale Hospital Diplomate, American Board of Emergency Medicine (ABEM). Fellow, North American Spine Society. Founder and President, Industrial Medical Services, Golden Valley, Minnesota

KATHLEEN HANDAL, M.D., F.A.C.E.P.
Attending Physician, Emergency Medicine, John C. Lincoln Medical Center, Phoenix, Arizona. Consultant, International Emergency Medical Systems

BARBARA K. HANKE, M.D., F.A.C.E.P.
Staff Emergency Physician, St. Vincent Hospital, Santa Fe, New Mexico. Clinical Assistant Professor of Medicine, University of California, San Francisco; Valley Medical Center, Fresno, California

CHERIE A. HARGIS, M.D.
Department of Emergency Medicine, Highland General Hospital, Oakland, California

HOWARD O. HAVERTY, M.D.
Section of Gastroenterology, Medical College of Georgia, Augusta, Georgia

PHILIP L. HENNEMAN, M.D., F.A.C.E.P.
Assistant Professor of Medicine, UCLA School of Medicine. Director, Adult Emergency Department, Department of Emergency Medicine, Harbor-UCLA Medical Center, Torrance, California

GREGORY P. HESS, M.D.
Assistant Professor of Emergency Medicine, Georgetown Medical Center. Liaison for the President's Council on Competitiveness. Advisor to U.S.D.A., E.P.A., and F.D.A., Washington, D.C.

STEPHEN D. HIGGINS, M.D.
Assistant Clinical Professor, Obstetrics and Gynecology, Harbor-UCLA Medical Center. Director of Emergency Services, St. Francis Medical Center, Lynwood, California

MARY ANN HOWLAND, Pharm.D.
Associate Professor of Clinical Pharmacy, St. John's University, Jamaica, New York; Consultant, Poison Control Center, New York, New York

JOSEPH C. HOWTON, M.D.
Assistant Chief, Department of Emergency Medicine, Highland General Hospital, Oakland, California. Assistant Clinical Professor of Medicine, University of California at San Francisco School of Medicine, San Francisco, California

PHILIPPE HROUDA, Ph.D., M.D.
Hôpital Henri Mondor, Paris, France

J. STEPHEN HUFF, M.D., F.A.C.E.P
Associate Residency Director, Division of Emergency Medicine, Eastern Virginia Graduate School of Medicine, Norfolk, Virginia

STEVE HULSEY, M.D.
Senior Resident, Department of Emergency Medicine, UCSF School of Medicine, Highland Hospital, Oakland, California

H. RANGE HUTSON, M.D.
Instructor, Division of Emergency Medicine, Department of Medicine, University of Tennessee, Memphis, Tennessee

KENNETH V. ISERSON, M.D., M.B.A., F.A.C.E.P.
Medical Director, Southern Arizona Rescue Association. Associate Professor of Surgery and Residency Director, Emergency Medicine, University of Arizona College of Medicine, Tucson, Arizona

TSGUHARU ISHIDA, M.D., Ph.D.
Associate Professor, Division of E.M. and C.C.M., Hyogo College of Medicine, Hyogo, Japan

RAO R. IVATURY, M.D., F.A.C.S.
Associate Professor of Surgery, New York Medical College. Chief of Trauma, Co-Director of SICU, Lincoln Hospital, Bronx, New York

JOHN R. JACOBS, M.D.
Associate Professor, Department of Otolaryngology, Wayne State University Medical School, Detroit, Michigan

LENWORTH M. JACOBS, M.D.
Professor of Surgery, University of Connecticut School of Medicine, Director, Department of EMS/Trauma, Hartford Hospital, Hartford, Connecticut

SHELDON JACOBSON, M.D., F.A.C.E.P.
Emergency Medicine Medical Director, Hospital of the University of Pennsylvania, Philadelphia, Pennsylvania

TIMOTHY G. JANS, M.D.
Assistant Professor, Department of Emergency Medicine, Pulmonary/Critical Care Division, Department of Medicine, Wright State University School of Medicine, Dayton, Ohio

JOHN B. JEFFERS, M.D.
Director, Emergency Services, Wills Eye Hospital, Philadelphia, Pennsylvania

MARK T. JOBE, M.D.
Clinical Instructor, Campbell Clinic, Hand Surgery, Memphis, Tennessee

LOREN JOHNSON, M.D.
Staff Emergency Physician, Sutter Community Hospital, Sacramento, California

JAMES H. JONES, M.D., F.A.C.E.P.
Assistant Clinical Professor of Emergency Medicine, Indiana University School of Medicine. Medical Director, Emergency Medical Services, Methodist Hospital of Indiana, Indianapolis, Indiana

E. JEFF JUSTIS, JR., M.D., F.A.C.S.
Clinical Associate Professor, Department of Orthopedics, University of Tennessee, Memphis. Attending Orthopedic Surgeon, Campbell Clinic, Memphis, Tennessee

LESTER J. KARAFIN, M.D.
Professor of Surgery and Chief, Section of Urology, The Medical College of Pennsylvania. Professor of Urology, Temple University, Philadelphia, Pennsylvania

DOROTHY KARANDANIS, M.D.
Associate Professor of Medicine, Emory University School of Medicine. Director, Medical Clinic, Grady Memorial Hospital, Atlanta, Georgia

WAYNE J. KATON, M.D.
Professor and Chief, Consultation/Liaison Service, Department of Psychiatry, University of Washington Medical School, Seattle, Washington

CAROL A. KAUFFMAN, M.D.
Professor of Medicine, University of Michigan Medical School. Chief, Section of Infectious Diseases, Veterans Administration Medical Center, Ann Arbor, Michigan

BALKRISHENA KAUL, Ph.D.
Adjunct Professor, Department of Clinical Pharmacy; Director, Toxicology and RIA Laboratories, New York City Department of Health, New York, New York

GABOR D. KELEN, M.D., F.A.C.E.P.
Associate Professor of Emergency Medicine, Director of Research, Johns Hopkins University School of Medicine, Baltimore, Maryland

ARTHUR L. KELLERMAN, M.D., M.P.H.
Associate Professor and Chief, Division of Emergency Medicine, Department of Internal Medicine, University of Tennessee, Memphis. Director of Emergency Department, Regional Medical Center, Memphis, Tennessee

KATHLEEN KELLY, M.D.
Fairfax Hospital, Falls Church, Virginia. Assistant Professor, Emergency Medicine, Georgetown University School of Medicine, Washington, D.C.

KEVIN M. KELLY, M.D., Ph.D.
Attending Physician, Emergency Medicine, W.A. Foote Memorial Hospital, Jackson, Michigan. Assistant Professor, Department of Neurology, University of Michigan Medical Center, Ann Arbor, Michigan

A. RICHARD KENDALL, M.D., F.A.C.S.
Professor of Urology, Temple University School of Medicine, Philadelphia, Pennsylvania

MORTON J. KERN, M.D.
Assistant Professor of Medicine, Cardiac Catheterization Laboratory, St. Louis, Missouri

JOHN KETTLEY, M.S.W., A.C.S.W.
Senior Social Worker and Program Coordinator of Psychiatric Emergency Services, Department of Psychiatry, University of Michigan Hospital, Ann Arbor, Michigan

MARTIN R. KLEMPERER, M.D.
Director, Bone Marrow Transplant Unit, All Children's Hospital, St. Petersburg, Florida

NATHAN S. KLINE, M.D.
Department of Psychiatry, Albert Einstein College of Medicine, Yeshiva University, Bronx, New York

JAMES A. KNOL, M.D.
Assistant Professor of Surgery, Division of Gastroenterologic Surgery, Department of Surgery, University Medical Center, University of Michigan, Ann Arbor, Michigan

KRISTI KOENIG, M.D.
Assistant Adjunct Professor, Assistant Pre-Hospital Corr., Emergency Medicine, University of California Ervine Hospital, Orange, California

SHARON KOLBER, M.D.
Emergency Medicine Resident, University of New Mexico School of Medicine, Albuquerque, New Mexico

BARBARA S. KOPPEL, M.D.
Associate Professor of Neurology, New York Medical College, Valhalla, New York. Attending Neurologist, Metropolitan Hospital Center, New York, New York

MARK J. KOTAPKA, M.D.
Department of Neurosurgery, Hospital of the University of Pennsylvania, Philadelphia, Pennsylvania

MICHAEL KOZMINSKI, M.D.
St. Joseph Urological Associates, Inc., St. Joseph, Missouri

DAVID A. KRAMER, M.D., F.A.C.E.P.
Residency Director, Division of Emergency Medicine, Northwestern University Medical School, Chicago, Illinois

MITCHELL KRUCOFF, M.D., F.A.C.C.
Duke University Medical Center, Durham, North Carolina

ALEXANDER KUEHL, M.D., M.P.H., F.A.C.S.
Assistant Professor of Clinical Surgery and Public Health. Former Director for the Emergency Medical Program, New York, New York; Director, Emergency Medicine, New York Hospital-Cornell Medical Center, New York

KEN KULIG, M.D., F.A.C.E.P.
Medical Director, Rocky Mountain Poison Center. Director, Clinical Toxicology Center, Denver General Hospital. University of Colorado Health Services, Denver, Colorado

CAROL L. KULP-SHORTEN, M.D.
Private Practice, Dermatology, Louisville, Kentucky

GRANT La FARGE, M.D., F.A.C.C., F.A.C.P.
Clinical Professor of Medicine, University of New Mexico. Staff Cardiologist, St. Vincent Hospital, Santa Fe, New Mexico

F. LaLANDE-MEARY, M.D.
Vanves, Paris, France

PATRICIA L. LAMB, M.D.
Attending Staff Physician, W.A. Foote Memorial Hospital, Jackson, Michigan. Clinical Instructor, University of Michigan, Emergency Services, Ann Arbor, Michigan

STEPHEN F. LARSON, M.D.
Alameda County Health Care Services. Highland General Hospital, Oakland, California

BEN LERMAN, M.D.
Assistant Chief, Emergency Medicine, Highland General Hospital, San Francisco, California

DAVID G. LEVINE, M.D.
Assistant Clinical Professor of Psychiatry, School of Medicine, University of California, San Francisco. Director, Psychiatric Services, Marin General Hospital, Marin County, California

LAWRENCE M. LEWIS, M.D., F.A.C.E.P.
Associate Professor of Surgery and Medicine, Division of Emergency Medicine, St. Louis University Hospital, St. Louis, Missouri

ROBERT D. LIBKE, M.D.
Valley Medical Center, Department of Internal Medicine, Fresno, California

MICHAEL P. LILLY, M.D.
Brown University, Division of Biology and Medicine, Rhode Island Hospital, Providence, Rhode Island

JEAN-PIERRE LINDENMAYER, M.D.
Assistant Clinical Professor, Department of Psychiatry, Albert Einstein College of Medicine, Yeshiva University. Director, Bronx Psychiatry Center, Bronx, New York

JOSEPH LINDSAY, JR., M.D.
Director, Section of Cardiology, Washington Hospital Center. Professor of Medicine, George Washington University School of Medicine, Washington, D.C.

MARKUS D.W. LIPP, M.D.
Anesthetist, Clinic of Anesthesiology, University of Mainz, Mainz, Germany

GEORGE I. LITMAN, M.D.
Professor of Medicine, Chairman, Subcouncil of Cardiology, Northeastern Ohio Universities, College of Medicine, Chairman, Department of Medical Education, Chief of Cardiology, Akron General Medical Center, Akron, Ohio

EMILY JEAN LUCID, M.D.
Associate Professor and Chairman of Emergency Medicine, Medical College of Pennsylvania, Allegheny Campus. Director, Division of Emergency Medicine, Allegheny General Hospital, Pittsburgh, Pennsylvania

MILTON N. LURIA, M.D.
Professor of Medicine and Health Services, University of Rochester, School of Medicine and Dentistry. Physician, Strong Memorial Hospital; Consultant, The Genesee Hospital, Rochester, New York

ROBERT C. LUTEN, M.D.
Pediatric Emergency Medicine, University Medical Center, Jacksonville, Florida

CARLOS E. MAAS, M.D.
Senior Fellow, Division of Pulmonary and Critical Care Medicine, Detroit, Michigan. Sleep Disorders Fellow, Neurology Section, Veterans Administration Medical Center, Allen Park, Michigan

WILLIAM MacAUSLAND, M.D.
Faulkner Hospital, Jamaica Plain, Massachusetts

TIMOTHY MacCLEAN, M.D.
Associate Chairman, Emergency Service and Acute Care, U.S.A.F., Medical Center, Wright-Patterson Air Force Base, Ohio

JOHN F. MADDEN, M.D.
Hahnemann Hospital, Philadelphia, Pennsylvania

JOHN C. MAINO II, M.D., F.A.C.E.P.
Project Medical Director, Jackson County, Michigan. Vice Chairman and Assistant Medical Director, Emergency Department, W.A. Foote Memorial Hospital, Jackson, Michigan

ROLAND D. MAIURO, Ph.D.
Department of Psychiatry and Behavioral Sciences, University of Washington School of Medicine, Harbor View Medical Center, Seattle, Washington

MARY ANNE MANGELSEN, M.D., Ph.D., F.A.C.P.
Chairman and Medical Director, Department of Emergency Medicine, W.A. Foote Memorial Hospital, Jackson, Michigan. Clinical Instructor, Emergency Services, University of Michigan, Ann Arbor, Michigan

JOHN R. MANGIARDI, M.D.
Chief, Neurosurgery, Lincoln Hill Hospital, New York, New York

KARL G. MANGOLD, M.D.
Clinical Instructor, University of California, San Francisco; Past President, American College of Emergency Physicians. Partner, The Fischer-Mangold Group, Pleasanton, California. Director, Department of Emergency Medicine, Vesper Memorial Hospital, San Leandro, California

BENEDICT S. MANISCALCO, M.D.
Assistant Clinical Professor of Medicine (Cardiology), University of South Florida College of Medicine. Director of Cardiology, St. Joseph's Hospital, Tampa, Florida

STEPHEN J. MARKS, M.D.
Assistant Professor of Neurology, New York Medical College, Valhalla, New York

GARY J. MARTIN, M.D., F.A.C.E.P., F.A.C.C.
Chief, Section of General Internal Medicine, Northwestern University Medical School, Chicago, Illinois

JEAN T. MARTIN, M.D.
Staff Physician of Emergency Medicine, Walter Reed Army Medical Center, Silver Spring, Maryland

RONALD E. MASON, M.D.
Chief Medical Resident, Montgomery Internal Medicine Residency Program. Instructor in Medicine, University of Alabama, School of Medicine, Birmingham, Alabama

KENNETH L. MATTOX, M.D.
Professor of Surgery, Baylor College of Medicine. Director, Surgical Emergency Services, Ben Taub General Hospital, Houston, Texas

MARK A. MAULDIN, M.D., Capt., M.C., U.S.A.
7th Medical Command, General Hospital A.P.O., New York, New York

DANIEL L. MAXWELL, M.D., Lt. Cdr., M.C., U.S.N.R.
Chief and Administrative Fellow, Division of Pulmonary and Critical Care Medicine, Wayne State University, Detroit, Michigan

THOM A. MAYER, M.D., F.A.C.E.P.
Chairman, Department of Emergency Medicine, Fairfax Hospital, Falls Church, Virginia. Clinical Associate Professor of Emergency Medicine and Pediatrics, Georgetown University School of Medicine, Washington, D.C.

JAMES McCARTY, M.D.
Pediatric Infectious Diseases, Valley Children's Hospital, Fresno, California

MARK McCLUNG, M.D.
Fellow, Forensic Psychiatry, Department of Psychiatry, Rush Presbyterian-St. Luke's Medical Center, Chicago, Illinois

RAJALAXMI McKENNA, M.D.
Associate Professor of Medicine, Unit Director, Platelet Function, Radiohematology, and Venous Thrombosis Diagnostic Laboratories, Rush Presbyterian-St. Luke's Medical Center, Chicago, Illinois

SUSAN V. McLEER, M.D.
Director, Emergency Services, Professor and Vice Chairman, Department of Psychiatry, Medical College of Pennsylvania, Philadelphia, Pennsylvania

DAVID B. McMICKEN, M.D., F.A.C.E.P.
The Medical Group, Inc., Columbus, Georgia

NORMAN E. McSWAIN, JR., M.D.
Professor, Department of Surgery, Tulane University School of Medicine, New Orleans, Louisiana

LEONARDO MENDEZ, M.D.
Fellow in Hepatology, Veterans Administration Medical Center, Miami, Florida

CRAIG S. MILLER, D.M.D., M.S.
Assistant Professor and Assistant Director, Dental Emergency Clinic, Department of Oral Health Science, University of Kentucky College of Dentistry, Lexington, Kentucky

VAN H. MILLER, M.D.
Emergency Physician, Emergency Medicine, St. Francis Medical Center, Lynwood, California

JOHN A. MILTON, M.D.
Wills Eye Hospital, Philadelphia, Pennsylvania

HOWARD C. MOFENSON, M.D., F.A.A.P., F.A.A.C.T.
Professor of Pediatric and Emergency Medicine, State University of New York at Stony Brook. Mercer County Medical Center, East Meadow, New York

WILLIAM W. MONTGOMERY, M.D.
Professor of Otolaryngology, Harvard Medical School, Surgeon in Otolaryngology, Massachusetts Eye and Ear Infirmary, Boston, Massachusetts

FRANKLIN G. MOSER, M.D.
Chief of Neuroradiology, Lemex Hill Hospital, New York, New York

LAWRENCE MOTTLEY, M.D.
Medical Director/EMS, New York City Health and Hospital Corporation, Maspeth, New York

MICHAEL W. MULHOLLAND, M.D.
University of Michigan Medical Center, Ann Arbor, Michigan

JANE G. MURPHY, M.D., Ph.D.
Research Director, New York Medical College, Valhalla, New York

KENNETH A. MURPHY, JR., Pharm.D.
Pharmacy Clinical Coordinator, W.A. Foote Memorial Hospital. Adjunct Assistant Professor, Ferris State University College of Pharmacy. Clinical Assistant Professor, University of Michigan College of Pharmacy, Jackson, Michigan

HENRY W. MURRAY, M.D.
Associate Professor of Medicine; Chief, Division of Infectious Diseases, The New York Hospital-Cornell Medical Center, New York, New York

ABDOLLAH B. NAFICY, M.D.
Fellow of Infectious Diseases, The New York Hospital-Cornell Medical Center, New York, New York

VENKAT NARAYAN, M.D.
Associate Clinical Professor, Department of Surgery, University of New Mexico School of Medicine, Albuquerque, New Mexico. Staff Neurosurgeon, St. Vincent Hospital, Santa Fe, New Mexico

CHARLES W. NEEDHAM, M.D., F.A.C.S.
Staff Neurosurgeon, Norwalk Hospital, Norwalk, and Greenwich Hospital, Greenwich, Connecticut

EDWARD NEWTON, M.D.
Assistant Professor, University of Southern California School of Medicine, South Pasadena, California

GARY G. NICHOLAS, M.D., F.A.C.S.
Clinical Professor of Surgery, Hahneman University, Philadelphia. Assistant Chairman, Department of Surgery, Program Director Residency in General Surgery, Lehigh Valley Hospital Center, Allentown, Pennsylvania

JAMES T. NIEMANN, M.D.
Associate Professor of Medicine, UCLA School of Medicine. Director of Research, University of Emergency Medicine, Harbor-UCLA Medical Center, Torrance, California

ERIC K. NOJI, M.D., F.A.C.E.P.
Department of Emergency Medicine, The Johns Hopkins Hospital and School of Medicine, Baltimore, Maryland

ROBERT A. NOZIK, M.D.
Clinical Professor of Ophthalmology, Proctor Foundation for Research in Ophthalmology, University of California, San Francisco, San Francisco, California

HAROLD OSBORN, M.D., F.A.C.E.P.
Associate Professor of Medicine, New York Medical College, Valhalla, New York

H. F. OXER, M.D.
Medical Director, St. John Ambulance Association, W.A., Belmont, West Australia

JOHN J. PAHIRA, M.D.
Associate Professor of Surgery/Urology and Director, Center for Kidney Stone Disease, Georgetown University Hospital and Medical Center, Washington, D.C.

EDDY D. PALMER, M.S., M.D.
Attending Staff, Hackettstown Community Hospital, Hackettstown, New Jersey

DONALD R. PAUGH, M.D.
Division of Surgery, Department of Otolaryngology, University of Michigan, Wenatchee, Washington

JOHN A. PAYNE, M.D.
Associate Professor of Medicine, Rush Medical College. Digestive Disease Associates, Limited, Hinsdale, Illinois

ANTHONY C. PEARSON, M.D.
Assistant Professor of Medicine, St. Louis University Medical Center, Cardiology, St. Louis, Missouri

LEONARD F. PELTIER, M.D., Ph.D.
Professor of Surgery, University of Arizona. Head, Section of Orthopedic Surgery, University Medical Center, Tucson, Arizona

PAUL E. PEPE, M.D., F.A.C.P., F.C.C.P., F.A.C.E.P., F.C.C.M.
Associate Professor, Departments of Surgery, Pediatrics, and Medicine, Baylor College of Medicine and the Harris County Hospital District Emergency-Trauma Center. Director, City of Houston Emergency Medical Services. President, National Association of Emergency Medical Services Physicians, Houston, Texas

MARK A. PEPPERCORN, M.D.
Harvard Digestive Diseases Center, Harvard-Thorndike Laboratory, Charles A. Dana Research Institute. Division of Gastroenterology, Harvard Medical School and Beth Israel Hospital, Boston, Massachusetts

LAURA PETERSON, M.D.
Division of Emergency Medicine, University of Massachusetts Medical School, Worcester, Massachusetts

MYRON B. PETERSON, M.D., Ph.D.
Director, Pediatric Critical Care Services, New England Medical Center Hospitals, Boston, Massachusetts

CARL J. POST, Ph.D.
Associate Professor of Health Science, New York Medical College. Graduate School of Health Science, Valhalla, New York

JOHN E. PRESCOTT, M.D., F.A.C.E.P.
Assistant Administrative Director, Cape Fear Valley Medical Center, Fayetteville, North Carolina

DENNIS P. PRICE, M.D.
Attending Physician, Emergency Department, Bellevue Hospital Center, Emergency Medical Services, New York, New York. Staff Physician, The Medical Center at Princeton, Princeton, New Jersey

ROBERT R. PROULX, M.D.
Assistant Professor, University of Southern California School of Medicine, Los Angeles, California. Staff, St. Joseph Medical Center, Burbank, California. Voluntary Attending Assistant Professor, University of Southern California—Los Angeles County Hospital, Los Angeles, California

JOHN J. PURCELL, JR., M.D.
Associate Clinical Professor of Ophthalmology, St. Louis University School of Medicine. Director, Department of Ophthalmology, St. Mary's Health Center, St. Louis, Missouri

HARRIS RABINOVITCH, M.D.
Director of Education, Associate Professor, Medical College of Pennsylvania, Philadelphia, Pennsylvania

THEODORE RABINOVITCH, M.D., F.R.C.S.C.
Proctor Foundation, San Francisco, California

ERIC C. RACKOW, M.D., F.A.C.P.
Professor and Vice Chairman, Department of Medicine, New York Medical College. Chairman, Department of Medicine, St. Vincent's Hospital and Medical Center, New York, New York

PRAKASHCHANDRA M. RAO, M.D., F.R.C.S. (C), F.A.C.S.
Associate Professor of Clinical Surgery, New York Medical College. Chief of Head and Neck Surgery, Chief of Surgical Endoscopy, Lincoln Medical and Mental Health Center, Bronx, New York

STEVEN A. RAPER, M.D.
Assistant Professor of Surgery, University of Michigan Medical Center, Ann Arbor, Michigan

MARSHA D. RAPPLEY, M.D.
Assistant Professor, Michigan State University Department of Pediatrics, Lansing, Michigan

SUSHMA REDDY, M.D.
Assistant Professor of Medicine, Division of Endocrinology and Hypertension, Harper and Grace Hospitals. Wayne State University School of Medicine, Detroit, Michigan

BRUCE M. REINOEHL, M.D., F.A.C.E.P.
Sparrow Hospital, Emergency Department, Dewitt, Michigan

EARL J. REISDORFF, M.D., F.A.C.E.P.
Associate Professor, College of Human Medicine, Michigan State University. Assistant Residency Director—Education, Emergency Medicine Residency—Lansing, Michigan State University, Lansing, Michigan

KAREN RHEUBAN, M.D.
Associate Professor of Pediatrics, University of Virginia Medical Center, Charlottesville, Virginia

JONATHAN E. RHOADS, JR., M.D., F.A.C.S.
Clinical Professor of Surgery, University of Pennsylvania. Chairman, Department of Surgery, York Hospital, York, Pennsylvania

RONALD L. RHULE, D.O., F.A.C.O.E.P.
Diplomat, American Osteopathic Board of Emergency Medicine. Associate Clinical Professor, Internal Medicine, Michigan State University College of Human Medicine. Assistant Director, Military Affairs, M.S.U. Emergency Medicine Residency Program, Sparrow Hospital, Lansing, Michigan

CHARLES A. RILEY, M.D.
Associate Clinical Professor of Medicine, University of New Mexico School of Medicine, Albuquerque, New Mexico. Staff Physician, St. Vincent Hospital, Santa Fe, New Mexico

JUDY RIZZO, M.S., R.N., C.N.S.
Psychiatric Emergency Service, Department of Psychiatry, University of Michigan Hospital, Ann Arbor, Michigan

JAMES R. ROBERTS, M.D.
Professor of Emergency Medicine, Medical College of Pennsylvania. Chairman, Department of Emergency Medicine, Mercy Catholic Medical Center, Philadelphia, Pennsylvania

MONT R. ROBERTS, M.D., F.A.C.E.P.
Emergency Department, Sparrow Hospital, East Lansing, Michigan

DONALD A. ROMIG, M.D.
Associate Clinical Professor of Medicine, University of New Mexico School of Medicine, Albuquerque, New Mexico. Staff Physician, St. Vincent Hospital, Santa Fe, New Mexico

MARTHA ROPER, M.D.
Division of Acute Care Clinic, Emergency Medicine, Highland General Hospital, Oakland, California

JOSEPH ROSENBLUM, M.D.
Consulting Cardiologist, San Francisco Heart Institute, Seton Medical Center. Associate Clinical Professor, University of California, San Francisco, Daly City, California

MONICA ANN ROSENTHAL, M.D., F.A.C.E.P.
Assistant Chief, Emergency Medicine, Highland General Hospital. Assistant Clinical Professor of Medicine, University of California at San Francisco, Oakland, California

BRUCE R. ROTHWELL, D.M.D., M.S.D.
Director, Hospital Dentistry, University of Washington Medical Center. Associate Professor, Hospital Dentistry and Department of Oral and Maxillofacial Surgery, School of Dentistry, University of Washington, Seattle, Washington

JOHN M. ROSSI, M.D.
Emergency Department, Hennepin County Hospital and Medical Center, Minneapolis, Minnesota

GEORGE J. RUBEIZ, M.D.
Fellow, Division of Pulmonary/Critical Care Medicine, Wayne State University School of Medicine, Detroit, Michigan

WALLACE RUBIN, M.D.
Clinical Professor, Department of Otorhinolaryngology and Biocommunication, Louisiana State University, New Orleans, Louisiana

BRENT RUOFF, M.D.
Assistant Professor of Medicine, Division of Cardiology, Department of Internal Medicine, Department of Surgery/Emergency/Trauma Division, St. Louis University, St. Louis, Missouri

ROBERT A. RUSNAK, M.D.
Associate Physician, Department of Emergency Medicine, Hennepin County Medical Center, Minneapolis, Minnesota

THOMAS D. SABIN, M.D.
Associate Clinical Professor of Medicine, Boston University, Framingham, Massachusetts

PETER SAFAR, M.D.
Distinguished Services Professor and Director, Resuscitation Research Center, University of Pittsburgh Medical Center, Pittsburgh, Pennsylvania

ARTHUR P. SAFRAN, M.D.
Associate Clinical Professor of Medicine, Neurology, Boston University, Framingham, Massachusetts

STEVEN A. SAHN, M.D.
Professor of Medicine, Director, Division of Pulmonary and Critical Care Medicine, Medical University of South Carolina. Director and Attending Physician, Medical Intensive Care Unit, Medical University Hospital, Medical University of South Carolina, Charleston, South Carolina

DOUGLAS M. SALYARDS, M.D.
Emergency Department, W.A. Foote Memorial Hospital, Jackson, Michigan

JOEL R. SAPER, M.D., F.A.C.P.
Director, Michigan Head Pain and Neurological Institute, Ann Arbor, Michigan. Clinical Professor of Medicine (Neurology), Michigan State University, East Lansing, Michigan

KARIN H. SATRA, M.D.
Private Practice. Department of Dermatology, Columbia College of Physicians and Surgeons, New York, New York

MICHAEL R. SAYRE, M.D.
Assistant Professor of Emergency Medicine, Medical College of Pennsylvania, Allegheny Campus. Attending Physician, Emergency Medicine, Allegheny General Hospital, Pittsburgh, Pennsylvania

MARIE D. SCHAFLE, M.D.
Center for Sports Medicine, Saint Francis Memorial Hospital, San Francisco, California

EUGENE R. SCHIFF, M.D.
Professor of Medicine, Chief, Division of Hepatology, Center for Liver Diseases, University of Miami, School of Medicine, Miami, Florida

SANDRA M. SCHNEIDER, M.D., F.A.C.E.P.
Associate Professor of Medicine, University of Pittsburgh School of Medicine. Head, Emergency Medical Services Unit, Montefiore Hospital, Pittsburgh, Pennsylvania

JOHN M. SCHOFFSTALL, M.D.
Assistant Professor, Department of Emergency Medicine, Medical College of Pennsylvania, Philadelphia, Pennsylvania

KATHLEEN S. SCHRANK, M.D.
Associate Professor of Clinical Medicine, University of Miami School of Medicine. Medical Director, Jackson Memorial Hospital Emergency Care Center, Miami, Florida

BERNARD M. SCHUMAN, M.D.
Professor of Medicine, Section of Gastroenterology, Medical College of Georgia, Augusta, Georgia

DANIEL P. SCHUSTER, M.D.
Pulmonary Division, Director, M.I.C.U./R.I.C.U., Washington University Medical Center, St. Louis, Missouri

STEVEN D. SCHWAITZBERG, M.D.
Director, Surgical Intensive Care Unit, New England Medical Center Hospitals, Boston, Massachusetts

GEORGE R. SCHWARTZ, M.D., F.A.C.E.P.
Emergency Medicine, Santa Fe, New Mexico. Visiting Associate Professor of Emergency Medicine, Medical College of Pennsylvania, Philadelphia, Pennsylvania. Past Associate Professor and Director, Department of Emergency Medicine, University of New Mexico Medical School, Santa Fe, New Mexico

JOSEPH A. SCHWARTZ, M.D.
Assistant Professor, Department of Psychiatry. Director of Psychiatric Emergency Services, University of Michigan Hospital, Ann Arbor, Michigan

T. DUNCAN SELLERS, M.D., F.A.C.C.
Geisinger Medical Center, Danville, Pennsylvania

PAUL N. SEWARD, M.D., F.A.C.E.P., F.A.A.P.
Chairman, Department of Emergency Medicine, University Hospital, Augusta, Georgia

RAJESH SHAH, M.D.
Ambulatory Care Department, W.A. Foote Memorial Hospital, Jackson, Michigan

SID SHAH, M.D.
Attending Physician, Emergency Department, W.A. Foote Memorial Hospital, Jackson, Michigan

ARTHUR SHAPIRO, M.D.
Clinical Professor of Obstetrics and Gynecology, University of Miami School of Medicine, Miami, Florida

SANJIV SHARMA, M.D.
Pulmonary Fellow, Division of Pulmonary Disease, Nassau County Medical Center, East Meadow, New York

DANIEL J. SHEA, M.D., F.A.C.E.P.
Assistant Professor of Medicine, Division of Emergency Medicine, The University of Massachusetts Medical School. Associate Director of Emergency Services, St. Luke's Hospital of New Bedford, Inc., New Bedford, Massachusetts

PHILIP D. SHENEFELT, M.D.
Assistant Professor of Medicine, Division of Dermatology and Cutaneous Surgery. Department of Internal Medicine, University of South Florida College of Medicine. Assistant Chief, Dermatology Section, James A. Haley Veterans Hospital, Tampa, Florida

SUZANNE M. SHEPHERD, M.D.
Department of Emergency Medicine, Georgetown University Medical Center, Washington, D.C.

HARVEY SILVERMAN, M.D.
Adjunct Assistant Professor of Clinical Medicine, Dartmouth Medical School. Emergency Physician, Catholic Medical Center, Manchester, New Hampshire

MARK E. SILVERMAN, M.D.
Professor of Medicine (Cardiology), Emory University School of Medicine, Atlanta, Georgia

DAVID P. SIMMONS, M.D.
Clinical Instructor in Orthopaedic Surgery, Harvard Medical School. Assistant Orthopaedic Surgeon, Massachusetts General Hospital. Active Staff, Faulkner Hospital. Active Staff, New England Deaconess Hospital, Boston, Massachusetts

HOWARD M. SIMONS, M.D.
Clinical Associate Professor of Dermatology, University of Pennsylvania Medical School, Philadelphia, Pennsylvania. Chief of Dermatology, Abington Memorial Hospital, Abington, Pennsylvania

JEFFREY SIPSEY, M.D.
Los Angeles County Department of Health Sciences, Emergency Medical Services, Medical Alert Center, Los Angeles, California

MORTON S. SKORODIN, M.D.
Associate Professor of Medicine, Staff Physician, Ambulatory Care and Medical Services, Edward Hines, Jr. Veterans Hospital. Stritch School of Medicine, Loyola University of Chicago, Chicago, Illinois

JOHN E. SMIALEK, M.D.
Associate Professor and Head, Forensic Pathology, University of Maryland, School of Medicine. Associate Professor, Department of Pathology, Johns Hopkins University School of Medicine. Chief Medical Examiner, State of Maryland

MARTIN J. SMILKSTEIN, M.D., F.A.C.E.P., D.A.B.M.T.
Assistant Professor of Emergency Medicine, Director, Medical Toxicology Fellowship Program, Oregon Health Sciences University, Portland, Oregon

MICHAEL C. SMITH, M.D.
Attending Neurologist, Assistant Professor, Department of Neurosciences, Rush Memorial College, Rush Presbyterian-St. Luke's Medical Center, Chicago, Illinois

RONALD K. SMITH, D.O.
Director, Emergency Medical Services, University of Pittsburgh, Westmoreland Hospital, Greensburg, Pennsylvania

JOHN SOMBERG, M.D.
Assistant Professor of Medicine and Pharmacology; Chief, Division of Clinical Pharmacology, The Chicago Medical School, North Chicago, Illinois

STEVEN B. SORIN, M.D.
Chief, Section of Rheumatology, Department of Medicine, Mount Sinai Medical Center. Assistant Professor, Case Western Reserve University School of Medicine, Cleveland, Ohio

STEVEN M. SORNSIN, M.D., F.A.C.E.P.
Associate Chief, Department of Emergency Medicine. Emergency Medicine Residency Program, Highland General Hospital, Oakland, California

JAMES R. SOWERS, M.D.
Professor of Medicine and Physiology. Director, Endocrinology and Hypertension Division, Harper and Grace Hospitals, Wayne State University School of Medicine, Detroit, Michigan

GEORGE L. SPAETH, M.D., F.A.C.S.
Professor of Ophthalmology, Jefferson Medical College. Director of Glaucoma Services, Wills Eye Hospital, Philadelphia, Pennsylvania

DANIEL SPITZER, M.D.
Department of Neurosurgery, Lenox Hill Hospital, New York, New York

RICHARD STEINMARK, M.D.
Division of Emergency Medicine, Northwestern University Medical School, Chicago, Illinois

JOSEPH E. STEINMETZ, M.D.
Division of Cardiology, College of Medicine, University of Kentucky Medical Center, Lexington, Kentucky

RONALD D. STEWART, M.D., F.A.C.E.P., F.R.C.P.(C)
Associate Professor of Surgery/EM, University of Toronto, Toronto, Ontario, Canada

ERIC STIRLING, M.D.
Acting Chief, Department of Emergency Medicine, Highland General Hospital, Oakland, California

JOHN H. STONE, M.D.
Professor of Medicine (Cardiology) and Community Health (Emergency Medicine), Emory University School of Medicine. Chief of General Surgery, University of Maryland Hospital, Baltimore, Maryland

JACK L. STOUT, M.D.
President, Emergency Consulting, Fairfax, Virginia

MICHAEL J. SULLIVAN, M.D.
University of Michigan Department of Otorhinolaryngology. Department of Emergency Medicine, W.A. Foote Memorial Hospital, Ann Arbor, Michigan

PANAGIOTIS N. SYMBAS, M.D.
Professor of Surgery, Division of Thoracic and Cardiovascular Surgery, Emory University School of Medicine. Director, Thoracic and Cardiovascular Surgery, Grady Memorial Hospital; Consultant, Veterans Administration Medical Center, and associated hospitals, Atlanta, Georgia

JAMES V. TALANO, M.D.
Director, Cardiology Graphics, Northwestern Memorial Hospital, Chicago, Illinois

SATYANARAYANA TATINENI, M.D.
Division of Cardiology, Department of Internal Medicine, Department of Surgery/Emergency/Trauma Division, St. Louis University, St. Louis, Missouri

STEVEN A. TELIAN, M.D.
University of Michigan, W. A. Foote Memorial Hospital, Ann Arbor, Michigan

SUMNER E. THOMPSON, M.D.
Associate Professor of Medicine, Emory University School of Medicine, Atlanta, Georgia

CHRISTOPHER TRUSS, M.D.
Associate Professor of Medicine, Division of Gastroenterology, University of Alabama, Birmingham, Alabama

JAMES R. TRYON, M.D., F.A.C.E.P.
Director, Department of Emergency Medicine, Presbyterian Health Care Services, Albuquerque, New Mexico

J. N. TSIBIN, M.D.
Chief, FMS System, Moscow, Russia

ALAN J. TUCHMAN, M.D.
York Medical College, Lincoln Hospital, Bronx, New York

JAMES R. UNGAR, M.D., F.A.C.E.P.
Emergency Physician, Mercy Hospital, Bakersfield, California

AUDREY URBANO-BROWN, M.D., F.A.C.E.P.
Assistant Clinical Professor of Emergency Medicine, University of New Mexico School of Medicine. Staff Emergency Physician, St. Joseph Hospital, Albuquerque, New Mexico

PHILIPPE D. VAILLANCOURT, M.D.
Department of Neurology, Kaiser Foundation Hospital, San Rafael, California

TERENCE D. VALENZUELA, M.D., F.A.C.E.P.
Section of Emergency Medicine, Department of Surgery, University of Arizona College of Medicine, Tucson, Arizona

MICHAEL VANDORMAEL, M.D.
Professor of Medicine, Division of Cardiology, Hôpital de la Citadelle, Liege, Belgium

JONATHAN VARGAS, M.D., F.A.C.E.P.
Assistant Professor of Emergency Medicine, Residency Program Director, Emergency Medicine Residency Program, Eastern Virginia Graduate School of Medicine, Norfolk General Hospital, Norfolk, Virginia

DAVID L. VESELY, M.D., Ph.D.
Professor of Medicine, Physiology, and Biophysics, Veterans Hospital, Tampa, Florida

ELLIOTT P. VICHINSKY, M.D.
Associate Director, Hematology/Oncology Department, Childrens Hospital Medical Center, Oakland, California

RAYMOND N. VITULLO, M.D.
Associate Professor of Medicine, Clinical Cardiac Electrophysiology, Duke University Medical Center, Durham, North Carolina

GEORGE R. VOELZ, M.D.
Assistant Division Leader, Health Programs, Health Safety and Environment Division, Los Alamos National Laboratory, University of California, Los Alamos, New Mexico

STEPHANIE VON AMMON CAVANAUGH, M.D.
Associate Professor of Psychiatry; Chief, Psychiatric Consultation and Liaison Service, Rush Medical College, Rush Presbyterian-St. Luke's Hospital, Chicago, Illinois

RUSSELL G. WAGNER, M.D.
Acting Medical Director, Emergency Department, University of Alabama/Birmingham, Birmingham, Alabama

KRISTI WATTERBERG, M.D.
Assistant Professor, Department of Pediatrics, Division of Neonatology, University of New Mexico School of Medicine, Newborn Intensive Care Unit, University of New Mexico Hospital, Albuquerque, New Mexico

MARVIN A. WAYNE, M.D., F.A.C.E.P.
Medical Director, Emergency Medical Services, Bellingham, Washington. Attending Physician, Emergency Department, St. Joseph Hospital, Bellingham, Washington

ARTHUR W. WEAVER, M.D.
Professor of Surgery, Department of Surgery, Wayne State University, Detroit, Michigan

MAX HARRY WEIL, M.D.
Professor and Chairman, Department of Medicine, Professor of Physiology and Biophysics, Chief, Division of Cardiology, Chicago Medical School. Attending Physician, North Chicago Veterans Administration Medical Center and St. Mary of Nazareth Hospital Center, Chicago, Illinois

SCOTT S. WEISSMAN, M.D.
Associate Clinical Director, The New York Eye and Ear Infirmary. Attending Physician, Department of Ophthalmology, Manhattan Eye, Ear and Throat Hospital, New York, New York

NANETTE K. WENGER, M.D.
Professor of Medicine, Emory University School of Medicine, Director, Cardiac Clinics, Atlanta, Georgia

HOWARD A. WERMAN, M.D.
Division of Emergency Medicine, Ohio State University, Columbus, Ohio

MARK D. WESTFALL, M.D.
Department of Emergency Medicine, Northwestern Memorial Hospital, Chicago, Illinois

J. MARCUS WHARTON, M.D.
Duke University Medical Center, Durham, North Carolina

STEPHEN J. WHEELER, M.D.
Highland General Hospital, Department of Emergency Medicine, Oakland, California

ROBERT R. WHIPKEY, M.D., F.A.C.E.P.
Chairman, Department of Emergency Medicine, Westmoreland Hospital, Greensburg, Pennsylvania

ROBERT L. WHIPPLE, III, M.D.
Clinical Assistant Professor of Medicine (Cardiology), Emory University, School of Medicine, Atlanta, Georgia

MICHAEL E. WHITING, M.D.
Department of Emergency Medicine, Highland General Hospital, Oakland, California

MELVIN D. WICHTER, M.D.
Associate Professor, Department of Neurosciences, Rush Medical College. Chairman, Department of Neurology, Christ Medical Center, Oak Lawn, Illinois

JOHN G. WIEGENSTEIN, M.D.
Professor, Section of Emergency Medicine, Michigan State University. Director, Ingham Medical Center, Lansing, Michigan

EDWARD J. WING, M.D.
Associate Professor of Medicine, University of Pittsburgh School of Medicine, Assistant Head Physician, Infectious Disease Unit, Montefiore Hospital, Pittsburgh, Pennsylvania

ALAN WINKELSTEIN, M.D.
Professor of Medicine, University of Pittsburgh School of Medicine. Head Physician, Clinical Immunology Unit, Montefiore Hospital, Pittsburgh, Pennsylvania

JOHN S. WITHERS, M.D.
Emergency Medicine, Grady Memorial Hospital and Emory University School of Medicine, Atlanta, Georgia

CONSTANCE B. WOFSY, M.D.
AIDS Activities Division, San Francisco General Hospital and University of California, San Francisco, California

CHRISTOPHER K. WUERKER, M.D.
Emergency Medicine, Highland Hospital, Oakland, California

DON YEALY, M.D.
Resuscitation Research Center, University of Pittsburgh, Pittsburgh, Pennsylvania

GARY P. YOUNG, M.D.
Chief, Emergency Medical Section, Portland Veterans Affairs Medical Center. Assistant Professor, Emergency Medicine and Internal Medicine, Oregon Health Sciences University, Portland, Oregon

MICHAEL ZEVITZ, M.D.
Assistant Director of Cardiology, Mount Sinai Hospital, Chicago, Illinois

DAVID N. ZULL, M.D.
Residency Director, Emergency Medicine/Internal Medicine Training Program, Northwestern University Medical Hospital. Associate Chief of Medicine, Northwestern Memorial Hospital, Chicago, Illinois

LESLIE ZUN, M.D.
Northwestern Memorial Hospital, Chicago, Illinois

Contents

Part IV
TRAUMA

Part V
NONTRAUMATIC ORGAN SYSTEM EMERGENCIES

Volume II

Part VI
OBSTETRIC AND GYNECOLOGIC EMERGENCIES

Part VII
PEDIATRIC EMERGENCIES

59

Overview of Pediatric Emergency Medicine

Part VIII
GERIATRIC EMERGENCIES

Part IX

PSYCHIATRIC AND BEHAVIORAL EMERGENCIES

61 Psychiatric and Behavioral Emergencies

62 Clinical Evaluation of Psychiatric and Behavioral Emergencies

Part X

ENVIRONMENTAL EMERGENCIES

Introduction: Maturation of Emergency Medicine

"In the first place, in the physician or surgeon no quality takes rank with imperturbability. . . . Imperturbability means coolness and presence of mind under all circumstances, calmness amid storm, clearness of judgment in the moments of grave peril, immobility, impassiveness, or to use an old expressive word, phlegm."

William Osler, M.D. from "Aequanimitas," 1889, Philadelphia, Pennsylvania

The first and second editions of *Principles and Practice of Emergency Medicine* (PPEM) were designed to provide sound knowledge and techniques to aid in the care of patients, to cover the critical care medicine continuum—from scene to outcome—and to focus on the early diagnosis and management of the acutely ill and injured by the myriad components of the Emergency Medical Services (EMS) system.

The fact that the book has been widely used internationally indicates that, despite differences in EMS delivery systems from country to country, we have been able to serve the needs of physicians and other medical personnel worldwide who require information about acute medical problems.

Emergency medicine, as we know it today, has been built upon the work of many physicians, researchers, scholars, and administrators who developed Emergency Departments, intensive and critical care units, and EMS delivery systems. The modern era of resuscitation started in the 1950s with institution of emergency respiratory resuscitation, followed by cardiac resuscitation, cardiac intensive care, and modern life support for polytrauma.

No matter how sophisticated or advanced any of the components of EMS may be, however, the overall effectiveness of the system still depends on the strength of the weakest link. The patient who lies unattended in the field may be doomed regardless of the caliber of the emergency or intensive care unit. The experience and skill of the rescue squad and its organizational placement, supervision, and support represent critical links. The receiving hospital must be geared into the EMS system in a predescribed way, and must have physicians, nurses, team, facilities, and communications in place and ready to respond. From this perspective of the importance of continuity, *Principles and Practice of Emergency Medicine* has maintained the broad view of the practice of emergency medicine, including a detailed examination of EMS systems in the United States and abroad, as well as the administrative components of the system.

EMERGENCY MEDICINE AS A SPECIALTY

When the Introduction for the first edition of PPEM was written in 1978, Emergency Medicine had not yet become a specialty within the American

medical care system. That introductory chapter traced the historical origins of
the growth of the specialty of Emergency Medicine while also detailing societal changes and needs that encouraged its development. The conclusion
stated:

> Emergency Medicine is developing as a specialty because of evolutionary
> changes in American medicine and profound changes in our society. There has
> been no great leap in scientific understanding or technologic development, but
> changes have reached a sufficiently high level so that the Emergency Depart-
> ment can offer special advantages for sick and injured patients. What has be-
> come evident is a great need for physicians to perform suitable tests and proce-
> dures that will facilitate rapid diagnosis and improve on-the-spot treatment.
> Those in the discipline are working to develop new tests and to stimulate clinical
> research that will increase diagnostic accuracy. Suitable standards, long overdue,
> are being developed now with care and sophistication.

The status of emergency medicine as a field of special interest, its potential
for development, and its prestige as an academic discipline were enhanced
greatly with formation of the American College of Emergency Physicians and
the University Association for Emergency Medicine (now Society of Academic
Emergency Medicine, SAEM) and initial publication of the *Annals of Emergency
Medicine* in 1972. Emergency medicine as one of the board-certified specialties
of American medicine became a realty when the American Board of Emergency Medicine was created in 1976 and was designated a member of the
American Board of Medical Specialties in 1979.

More than a decade has passed since the prized specialty designation was
won, and another milestone was passed in 1990 with acceptance of Emergency Medicine as a primary board within the American specialty system.
The past decade has witnessed tremendous growth in residency training programs and the development of specialty journals and books addressing the
needs of physicians who treat acute medical problems, written by practitioners and educators who have developed depth within the field of emergency
medicine.

The training of emergency medical practitioners has resulted in demonstration of enhanced capability on a daily basis, with demonstrable improvements
in patient care. Reputations are always built upon quality.

Yet, despite enormous progress, emergency medicine as a separate discipline is still largely underdeveloped in many medical schools, particularly in
the Northeastern portion of the United States, which had previously been
seen as offering medical leadership, but which have adhered to outmoded
ways of practice.

Even in medical centers and schools with separate Emergency Medicine Departments, faculty emergency physicians are not generally on a par with
other faculty. There may be academic departments, but there are few endowed "chairs." Faculty rank is also not common at the higher levels.

The other clinical departments of Medicine, Surgery, and Pediatrics are not
anxious to take the clinical resources of the Academic Health Services Center
from the education of their own residents. Similarly, curriculum time for
medical student education is still limited and funding for research in emergency medicine is scarce, particularly at the "basic" research or "bench" level.
Valuable facilities, such as the Resuscitation Research Institute in Pittsburgh,
providing such needed basic research, are not given high priority by granting
agencies.

The results of fending off and avoiding the specialty of Emergency Medicine for more than a decade are now being seen dramatically in several large
cities where a systemic pattern of inattention has resulted in inconsistent, and
in some instances negligent, patient care. In the next decade we will witness
attempts to catch up rapidly by major institutions who are now suffering the
consequences of public and professional shame as well as litigation.

EMERGENCY MEDICINE MULTIHOSPITAL GROUPS

A unique development in emergency medicine has been the multihospital group. In the Introduction to the first edition of *Principles and Practice of Emergency Medicine*, it was pointed out that such large groups offered increased physician security, a means of advancement within a system, and the possibility of special educational and research services. The Introduction to the second edition followed the multihospital trend and indicated that there would be rapid growth followed eventually by a countertrend toward decentralization. This latter movement has not yet occurred.

Review of the large groups currently operating shows competition among groups for lucrative hospital contracts, and a movement toward quantity of contracts with increases in size. Intergroup competition has also become sharp. The aspects of little administrative burden for the practicing emergency physician, along with good wages and overall job security within a group (i.e., if the group loses a contract with a hospital and a physician can move to another of the group's contract hospitals), has resulted in strengthening of the larger groups. Some of these have also moved into staffing other health facilities, such as military hospitals and jails.

One danger of large group management practices is that maintenance of the hospital contract becomes paramount, leading to timidity in dealing with the hospital administrators and staffing discussions based less on quality than on avoidance of any controversy or even occasional necessary conflict.

EMERGENCY MEDICINE IN THE MARKETPLACE

When a new arrangement, structure, practitioner, or system evolves that meets patient needs more effectively, and when full-time dedication to this new system results in a better outcome, it is an effective "product." Such a "product" will eventually find its way into the overall matrix of available human services. In this way, emergency medicine in its development can be likened to a new and useful technology. In this context, let us examine some overlapping stages of entry of a new "product" into society.

1. *Creative process*—"Idea soup" or the "aha" stage, leading to conceptual blueprints (e.g., emergency medicine in the late 1950s and early 1960s).
2. *Reduction to practice*—The concept becomes real and organized. It "works" and it fills a need (late 1960s, early 1970s—the "Alexandria" plan, the "Pontiac" plan).
3. *Entry into the marketplace*—Reactions are generally hostile, with the vigor of hostility depending on the perceived threat to the status quo. Also, the fact that it is different becomes a problem. When something is new, people wonder how it will fit inside the old form. Most do not yet perceive that many other changes will be needed (e.g., major structural changes in Emergency Departments and EMS systems). Power and economics are seen as threatened (mid-late 1970s).
4. *Phases of endorsement*—Emergence of "champions" who help the pioneers by lending credibility to the new "product," the new practitioner, for example Emergency Medicine Certification 1979, Residency Programs, Academic Departments (1980s).
5. *Acknowledgment phase*—Wide use—a "star" is born. We are currently entering this phase. Utility is demonstrated and expanded.
6. *Stage of invisibility*—Taken for granted, completely incorporated into the

fabric of professional society with a clearly defined role, as if it had always been.

Emergency medicine is entering the phase of acknowledgment, although the exact location of our movement depends on the individual's vantage point. Although the specialty is secure, the exact role is sometimes uncertain as we cross into other specialty "boundaries." Such boundaries are not rigid, and time has demonstrated their fluidity.

The significance of seeing the maturation of emergency medicine in this context allows us also to focus on the important issues of each stage in terms of the cutting edge of the field, as well as in lagging regions.

The "acknowledgment" phase means that we no longer have to proclaim our presence and our territory: instead the need is to practice, research, and expand the usefulness of the clinical specialty.

Those not on the "cutting edge" might still have to fight the battles begun in the 1970s to gain acceptance and, in some university situations, to gain minimal recognition.

FUTURE TRENDS IN EMERGENCY MEDICINE

Much of the logic concerning future developments and trends has been extrapolative in nature. That is, the future projection is seen as an extrapolation from the past. This type of thought can be misleading. A transportation planner in 1880 produced a complex sketch of future transportation systems in the United States for the year 1980—a 100-year projection. He created an elegant network of railroad tracks with minilines, "feeder" lines, and every imaginable pattern of railroad vehicles. He even designed futuristic aerodynamic railroad cars. The planner, however, overlooked the development of the automobile and the airplane. Similarly, emergency medicine will not continue in a straight extrapolated pattern. As in any new field, some early directions can be misleading (e.g., witness the rapid expansion and contraction of urgent care centers in some areas). Also, unexpected events can lead to dramatic and unanticipated—even paradigm—changes.

One striking example of the need for new equipment is the protective garb worn and the precautions taken against AIDS. As medical students in the 1960s and 1970s can attest, they frequently found themselves with blood or secretions from patients on their hands or clothing. The days when such contamination was considered "casual" are now gone. This major change in practice represents the sort of change that cannot be foreseen through simple extrapolative reasoning.

Extrapolative reasoning demonstrates advances in the use of technology in diagnosing patients and one can reliably predict the more extensive use of MRI scans and likely "PET" scans (positive emission tomography). Similarly, the growth of the elderly population (e.g., people over 100—centenarians are the most rapidly growing age group in America) will require increased focus on this group, who have particular needs for home health care and other nonhospital treatment. Use of communication by computers as well as fax machines is increasing the ability to pass information from patients to physicians as well as interphysician transfers. Increasing roles for EMS personnel have been seen over the past decade and will continue to grow as medicine is brought more to the field. In the past decade we witnessed in-field intubation and defibrillation becoming standard techniques. In the next decade we will see further extensions, as exemplified by the recent debate over the use of succinylcholine in the field.

Other changes and advances will also come through medications developed by biogenetics. The rapid use and acceptance of erythropoietin is an example.

Advances to increase speed of diagnosis are also expected with more rapid toxicology screens and other diagnostic tests.

CONCLUSION

The Introduction to the first edition of this book was termed "development;" the second was termed "progress." With this third edition of *Principles and Practice of Emergency Medicine*, we are viewing a markedly changed and still dynamic landscape. This Introduction is subtitled "Maturation of Emergency Medicine." The most suitable definition of maturation is "to advance toward ripening." Indeed, the rapid movement to higher standards of care and the increased and gratifying organization of professionally run emergency departments and EMS systems with concomitant benefits to patients are clearly manifest. This textbook, edited and written primarily by emergency physicians, bears witness to the growing expertise within the emergency medicine community. Increased subspecialization is a maturational movement toward depth and specificity. There is still much to do to expand the usefulness of emergency medicine in practice and research.

As to ripening, the third edition of *Principles and Practice in Emergency Medicine* represents a prolific harvest of knowledge covering the broad range of the specialty area of Emergency Medicine.

George R. Schwartz, M.D.

Volume **II**

GASTROINTESTINAL EMERGENCIES

ESOPHAGEAL EMERGENCIES

Sid Shah

CAPSULE

Esophageal emergencies present a difficult diagnostic challenge to the emergency physician. Symptoms such as chest pain may suggest either an esophageal or a cardiac pathology. A hypovolemic patient may present with a massive variceal hemorrhage or more subtle blood loss from esophagitis. Wheezing, cough, and aspiration pneumonia may be caused by reflux and regurgitation of gastric contents, the so-called pulmonary manifestations of esophageal disease. Distal esophageal lacerations and incarcerated paraesophageal hernias often mimic an acute abdomen.

CLINICAL EVALUATION

The following are major presenting symptoms of esophageal pathology in the emergency department (ED).

Hemorrhage from esophageal pathology accounts for approximately 25% of all causes of upper gastrointestinal bleeding. The three major esophageal entities responsible for the bleeding are esophageal varices (14%), erosive esophagitis (6%), and Mallory-Weiss tears (5%).[1] Mallory-Weiss tears most often present with postemetic hematemesis. Patients with occult bleeding may present with hematemesis, hematochezia, melena, and symptoms of blood loss such as dizziness, postural hypotension, dyspnea, and shock.

Dysphagia commonly indicates esophageal disease (see also Chap. 24). Characteristics of dysphagia such as onset, relationship to the type of bolus and temperature of the bolus generally allow distinction between mechanical dysphagia such as stricture, tumor, or foreign body and motor dysphagia such as achalasia or systemic diseases.

Odynophagia indicating an inflamed mucosal surface may be caused by reflux esophagitis. The patient describes a dull substernal ache intensified by swallowing fluids.

Heartburn, an extremely common symptom, is usually not described as a pain but rather an uncomfortable sensation located below the sternum and tending to move up into the midchest and neck, waxing and waning in intensity. Heartburn usually occurs after meals and is aggravated by recumbency or heavy lifting and alleviated by antacids. Heartburn is caused by the effect of acid or alkali reflux on the altered esophageal mucosa.

Chest pain of esophageal origin may be indistinguishable from that of angina pectoris.[2] Both types of pain tend to be retrosternal and often last for just a few minutes. Both can radiate into the neck and arms, although radiation to the left arm may be more characteristic of cardiac pain. Radiation of pain to the abdomen is more characteristic of an esophageal disorder. Esophageal pain is frequently alleviated by antacids, but some of the cardiac medications, such as nitroglycerin, also relieve esophageal pain. And for unknown reasons, antacids dampen pain in about 10% of patients with cardiac pain.[3] Associated symptoms such as dysphagia, heartburn, and regurgitation are commonly present with chest pain of esophageal origin. Severe chest pain radiating between the shoulder blades and associated with emesis may be caused by Boerhaave's syndrome. Chest pain in the presence of recent esophageal instrumentation may suggest traumatic esophageal perforation.

Regurgitation is an unequivocal symptom of esophageal reflux. It is retrograde propulsion of fluid into the mouth, usually at night or on bending over. Nocturnal wheezing and frequent coughing spells raise the possibility of gastroesophageal reflux. Regurgitation is usually caused by stomach or duodenal contents leaking through an incompetent lower esophageal sphincter.

Water brash is a less common symptom of esophageal reflux than heartburn and regurgitation. It refers to the sudden filling of the mouth with a clear, slightly salty fluid that comes in extremely large quantities.

The fluid appears to be secreted by the salivary glands and should not be confused with regurgitation of gastric or duodenal contents.

HISTORY AND PHYSICAL EXAMINATION

Past history should include inquiring about cirrhosis, alcohol abuse, cancer, coagulopathies, connective tissue disorders, drug ingestion, and frequent drug use.

A set of vital signs must include heart and respiratory rates and orthostatic blood pressures.

Oropharynx and nares should be checked for dried blood. A white rim of dried antacid around the mouth may suggest frequent episodes of heartburn.

Skin examination reveals many important clues. Telangiectases on lips, mouth, palms, and soles may represent Weber-Osler-Rendu syndrome associated with mucosal telangiectasia. Bullous eruptions after mild trauma may suggest epidermolysis bullosa dystrophica, which is associated with esophageal stricture. Stigmata of cirrhosis or evidence of underlying malignancy (acanthosis nigricans) may be found.

Lymphadenopathy may suggest either malignancy or infection. Chest auscultation may reveal crackles and wheezes, which may be the pulmonary manifestations of regurgitation and reflux. The presence of subcutaneous emphysema after forced emesis or esophageal instrumentation indicates esophageal perforation. The abdomen should be noted for fullness, tenderness, spider angiomata, presence of free fluid, and any organomegaly. Examination of the rectum and stool for occult blood should be performed routinely.

DIAGNOSTIC MEASURES

A chest x ray is helpful when pulmonary manifestations of esophageal disease are suspected. Presence of pneumonitis and occasionally pleural effusion aid in the diagnosis of esophageal reflux disease. Mediastinal air and pleural effusions are seen on chest x ray in the presence of esophageal rupture. The presence of gastric loculus in the chest cavity has long been interpreted by radiologists as the presence of hiatus hernia.

Esophagography establishes the existence of an esophageal hiatal hernia in most cases. It is of limited use in establishing a diagnosis of gastroesophageal reflux disease, although it helps in detecting certain complications of gastroesophageal reflux such as a stricture or an ulcer. There is some controversy as to the ideal contrast medium for esophagogram in someone suspected of having a perforated esophagus. Some prefer to use barium for better discrimination, whereas others prefer a water-soluble contrast dye such as gastrograffin to minimize tissue reaction. In an emergency situation, gastrograffin can be used initially, and if this does not allow recognition of the perforation, barium can then be used for a better resolution.

Endoscopy has been advocated as the procedure of choice in the initial evaluation of upper gastrointestinal blood loss. Endoscopic examination of the esophagus is the most effective method of identifying mucosal changes in the lower esophagus suggestive of gastroesophageal reflux disease. Histologic confirmation of reflux and other clinical entities such as Barrett's esophagus is usually made by mucosal biopsy through an endoscopic examination.

Esophageal manometry studies indicate a potential for reflux if lower esophageal sphincter hypotension is demonstrated. Esophageal manometry is also performed to exclude an underlying esophageal motility disorder and assess the adequacy of esophageal peristalsis.

Esophageal pH monitoring for 12 to 24 hours in ambulatory patients has been shown to be an accurate test for detecting gastroesophageal reflux. The primary use of prolonged pH monitoring is to evaluate patients with atypical symptoms or an incomplete response to therapy.[4-6]

Provocative tests have been devised in an effort to provoke esophageal pain. The intravenous administration of edrophonium (Tensilon) causes an increase in the amplitude and duration of peristaltic contractions triggered by swallowing. The test provokes chest pain only in patients with motility disorders, not in normal subjects.[3] Although in esophageal acid perfusion the **Bernstein test** infrequently precipitates esophageal motor dysfunction, it is useful for duplicating pain caused by gastroesophageal reflux.[6]

DIFFERENTIAL DIAGNOSIS AND MANAGEMENT

ESOPHAGEAL VARICES

Esophageal varices result from portal hypertension caused by many diseases. The most common cause of portal hypertension in the Western countries is alcoholic cirrhosis. The triggering factor that leads a varix to bleed is unclear, but reflux esophagitis and the presence of ascites do not appear to be important. There is poor correlation between the actual pressure in the portal system and the propensity of a varix to bleed. Although variceal bleeding is usually suspected in a cirrhotic patient, other nonvariceal causes such as gastritis and ulcers actually account for up to 30% of bleeding lesions in these patients.[7] Bleeding varices may present as hematemesis, hematochezia, melena, or any combination of these. Bleeding may stop spontaneously, recur, or progress to shock. Variceal bleeding stops spontaneously in about 60% of patients, but it is not possible to predict which patients will continue to bleed and will require further emergency therapy.[8]

HEMODYNAMIC STABILIZATION

All patients with suspected variceal bleeding require hospitalization. Unless expert gastroenterologists are at hand, after initial stabilization, patients should be transferred to a center where advanced treatment facilities are available, because rebleeding is common and subsequent management is complicated by impaired synthesis of coagulation factors and thrombocytopenia.

Initial consideration in massive variceal bleeding is prevention of exsanguination. Central venous access is recommended by some as a means to measure central venous pressure in addition to providing vascular access. In a rapidly deteriorating situation, unmatched 0 negative blood can be transfused with fresh frozen plasma. Blood samples should be drawn for type and cross match, complete blood count, platelet count, measurement of blood urea nitrogen (BUN), serum creatinine, electrolytes, prothrombin time and partial thromboplastin time and liver enzyme studies.

After hemodynamic stabilization is achieved, emergency endoscopy is mandatory to confirm that the patient is bleeding from the varices. Large endoscopes permit reasonable aspiration of liquid blood.

PHARMACOLOGIC THERAPY

Vasopressin and nitroglycerin infusion is frequently used when variceal bleeding is first suspected. Therapy may be continued after the diagnosis has been confirmed endoscopically.[8] The effectiveness of vasopressin remains unproved despite a number of controlled trials, but it appears to have an overall efficacy of approximately 50%.[9] It should be used with caution in patients with cardiac ischemia and those with significant peripheral vascular disease. The combination of nitroglycerin and vasopressin has been shown to reduce the side effects caused by the use of vasopressin alone and to potentiate the hemodynamic effects in the portal bed.[10]

The recommended dose of vasopressin is 1 U/minute for 20 minutes followed by 0.4 to 0.6 U/minute depending on the clinical response.[11] Nitroglycerin can be administered intravenously, sublingually, or transdermally. The current recommendation[11] for the use of nitroglycerine is an intravenous infusion beginning at 40 µg/minute, gradually increased every 20 minutes to a maximum dose of 300 µ/minute as long as systemic arterial blood pressure remains over 100 mm Hg.

BALLOON TAMPONADE

Although the Sengstaken-Blakemore tube arrests variceal bleeding in about 90% of cases,[11,12] its use is considered a temporary measure. It allows time for resuscitation and planning further management as rebleeding occurs in up to 60% of patients after the tube is removed.[12]

The Sengstaken-Blakemore rubber tube is designed with two balloons, the gastric and the esophageal. It is introduced by the oral route or the nares with both balloons deflated. Its position in the stomach should be confirmed radiologically before inflation of the gastric balloon with about 150 cc of air. The tube is then pulled out until resistance is encountered and then held securely at that level. In this position, the tube should tamponade the afferent venous supply to the esophageal varices. The esophageal balloon is inflated if bleeding persists for 15 to 20 minutes after the inflation of the gastric balloon. This balloon is inflated using a blood pressure cuff to 40 45 mm of Hg. The Blakemore tube also has a channel to irrigate and suction the stomach.

ENDOSCOPIC INJECTION SCLEROTHERAPY

Varices may be injected with a sclerosing solution during endoscopy. This has become a popular and effective method of arresting acute bleeding. Emergency sclerotherapy can be used as the first intervention during diagnostic endoscopy or can be delayed until after the variceal hemorrhage has been controlled by conservative measures with or without the use of pharmacologic agents or balloon tamponade.[7] Sclerosing agents act by causing rapid thrombosis secondary to intimal damage to the vein. Fibrosis and obliteration of the vein subsequently follow. Sodium tetradecyl is the most widely used agent in this country. Sclerotherapy is the emergency treatment of choice for variceal bleeding at most institutions in the U.S.

PORTACAVAL SHUNT SURGERY

This is aimed at portal decompression and is achieved by various operative procedures, all of which create a large connection between the high pressure portal and low pressure systemic venous system. Nonselective shunts such as portacaval anastomoses decompress the entire portal system. These are generally used in emergent situations. More selective shunts that decompress only the varices are an elective procedure. Emergency shunt surgery carries with it almost a 50% mortality rate and is infrequently undertaken.

OTHER PROCEDURES

Procedures such as percutaneous transhepatic obliteration of varices are performed at very few institutions. Laser coagulation, electrocautery, and endoscopic elastic banding of varices have yet to be proven effective in controlled trials.[8]

ESOPHAGEAL LACERATION AND PERFORATION

Postemetic injury can be responsible for either mucosal tears, as in Mallory-Weiss syndrome, or esophageal rupture, as in Boarhaave's syndrome.

Vomiting is associated with rapid changes of intrathoracic and intra-abdominal pressures. A rapid downward thrust of the diaphragm associated with abdominal wall contractions increases gastric and esophageal pressures. If the upper end of the esophagus does not relax immediately to allow emesis, the rapid rise in esophageal pressure can cause rupture at the posterolateral aspect of the distal esophagus, its weakest point.

Mallory-Weiss tears usually reflect arterial bleeding from an acute laceration of gastroesophageal mucosa. Although, in a typical case, persistent retching and forceful vomiting are followed by emesis of bright red blood, retching is not always implicated in Mallory-Weiss tears. The amount of blood loss is generally small, but occasionally massive hemorrhage may follow a particularly large tear. Most bleeding episodes cease spontaneously and rebleeding is unusual. Management follows general guidelines for upper gastrointestinal hemorrhage.

Classic **esophageal rupture,** as described by **Boarhaave,** follows a heavy meal and vomiting in an otherwise healthy man. A gravely ill-appearing patient complains of severe mid or lower chest pain radiating to back and between the scapulae, accompanied by cyanosis, dyspnea, and diaphoresis. Signs of mediastinal air take a few hours to appear. Subcutaneous emphysema or palpable crepitus may be evident on the chest wall, neck, or supraclavicular fossae.

Traumatic esophageal perforation is far more common than postemetic injuries. Clinical signs are similar to those caused by postemetic perforation. The esophagus can be traumatized by ingestion of foreign bodies including chemicals and corrosives, erosion from cancer, and instrumentation such as endoscopy and esophageal obturator airway placement. Vigorous suctioning at birth or attempts to feed by nasogastric tube may cause esophageal perforation in the newborn. Blunt trauma causing esophageal rupture is generally accompanied by massive chest and abdominal injuries. Penetrating chest or upper abdominal wounds can cause an isolated esophageal perforation, although this is infrequent. Occult perforation of the esophagus should be suspected in any patient with chest pain and a feeling of a "stuck" foreign body.

The diagnosis of perforation is generally suspected from a careful history and a physical examination. A pleural effusion and mediastinal air may be seen on a chest radiograph. Widening of the mediastinum with blurring of its contours may also be seen. Confirmation of esophageal perforation is made with a swallow of radiopaque contrast material. Iatrogenic perforation after instrumentation is usually easily recognized. Spontaneous perforations after vomiting are more often confused with other clinical conditions. Approximately 25% of patients with esophageal perforations undergo laparotomy with the mistaken diagnosis of perforated viscus. The management is usually surgical. The possibility of improving outcome correlates directly with early diagnosis and intervention.

GASTROESOPHAGEAL REFLUX DISEASE

Heartburn affects an estimated 10% to 20% of Americans and is one of the most common complaints encountered in clinical practice today.[13] The triad of heartburn, dyspepsia, and regurgitation is the hallmark of gastroesophageal (GE) reflux disease. Frequently, patients present to the ED with complaints related to complications of GE reflux rather than with classic symptoms of the disease itself.

Atypical reflux may be responsible for chronic or recurrent hoarseness. Pulmonary symptoms such as wheezing and recurrent pneumonia may occur especially in children. Nocturnal wheezing may be related to recumbency.

The pathogenesis of the gastroesophageal reflux disease may be a mechanically defective lower esophageal sphincter and an incompetent antireflux barrier caused by delayed gastric emptying.

Major complications of gastroesophageal reflux are upper gastrointestinal bleeding, stricture formation, and Barrett's esophagus. Occasionally, GE reflux remains entirely silent until a major complication presents, such as bleeding.

Bleeding from gastroesophageal reflux accounts for 6 to 7% of all cases of UGI hemorrhage.[14] Chronic esophagitis leads to disruption of the mucosal surface and exposure of the papillary pegs of submucosa which contain blood vessels. Ulceration may expose larger vessels including arterioles in the submucosa. The situation may be aggravated by vasculitis as in scleroderma, coagulopathies, superimposed infection or drugs such as nonsteroidal anti-inflammatory agents.

Esophageal ulcer is an uncommon complication of gastroesophageal reflux disease. It usually presents as continuous, intense chest pain and dysphagia. Infrequently, this can lead to massive hematemesis. A deep ulcer can involve the muscular layer of the esophagus and may cause perforation. **Strictures** are found only in about half of the patients with dysphagia and may be entirely asymptomatic. Pathogenesis of strictures can be explained by recurrent episodes of mucosal and submucosal inflammation caused by chronic reflux of gastric contents in the esophagus with subsequent healing and scar formation. The most common form of stricture is located at or just above the esophagogastric junction. The diagnosis is made by barium esophagography or endoscopy. About half of all strictures occur in conjunction with Barrett's esophagus.

Barrett's esophagus is generally a disease of elderly white men with a history of heavy smoking and alcohol use. It is complicated by an increased incidence of cancer. Signs and symptoms of heartburn and regurgitation are more common in patients with benign disease than in those with malignant disease.

Avoiding citrus fruits, fatty or tomato-based foods, chocolates, nuts, caffeinated beverages, and eating at least three small meals ameliorates symptoms of gastroesophageal reflux. Other recommended life style modifications are losing weight, regular physical exercise, smoking cessation, and sleeping with the head of the bed elevated. Histamine blockers decrease the gastric acid without affecting lower esophageal sphincter motility and are widely used for severe symptoms of gastroesophageal reflux.

ESOPHAGEAL HIATUS HERNIA

A hiatus hernia is not an illness but an anatomic condition. Frequently there is difficulty in setting up a criterion for its presence. Both the exact location of the diaphragmatic opening and the junction between the esophagus and the stomach must be located precisely before a hernia can be defined, and finding both sites can be difficult. The diagnosis is usually made by radiologic studies.

The two types of esophageal hiatus hernias are the sliding and the paraesophageal hernia.

Sliding esophageal hiatus hernia is the most common variety. The esophagogastric junction and portions of the proximal part of the stomach "slide" through the esophageal hiatus into the posterior mediastinum. Such herniations are known to move in and out of the thorax with changes in intrathoracic and intraabdominal pressures. Most of these hernias occur in adults, although this type does occur in children and may even be present at birth.

Although clinical findings may suggest esophageal hernia, the diagnosis must be confirmed by objective evidence of gastroesophageal reflux because the majority of sliding hiatal hernias are asymptomatic. Classic symptoms of gastroesophageal reflux such as substernal chest pain, heartburn, and regurgitation are more likely to occur or become exacerbated in a slouched position or when one is bending at the waist. Constricting garments accentuate the discomfort. Recumbency often aggravates the symptoms. Occasionally pulmonary symptoms caused by nocturnal aspiration of gastric contents dominate the clinical picture.

Paraesophageal hiatus hernia is a rare, life-threatening condition that occurs in about 5% of patients with hernias through the esophageal hiatus.[15] This type of hernia is characterized by displacement of a portion of stomach into the thorax through the gas-

troesophageal hiatus alongside the esophagus. The esophagogastric junction is in its normal position and the fundus of the stomach may move up into the thorax anterior and lateral to the body of the esophagus. A paraesophageal hiatus hernia tends to enlarge with time, and in some patients the entire stomach protrudes into the thorax, occasionally along with other viscera.

Unlike sliding hiatal hernia, in which symptoms are primarily the result of deranged physiology, symptoms of a paraesophageal hernia are mechanical. The patient may be asymptomatic, and diagnosis is usually suspected from routine chest x rays. The most common symptom is epigastric or substernal chest pain. Some patients have vague symptoms such as postprandial indigestion, substernal fullness, nausea, or occasional retching. Symptoms of esophageal reflux are generally absent. Rarely, the stomach may rotate counterclockwise within the thorax, causing incarceration, strangulation, and perforation. A patient with incarcerated paraesophageal hernia may present to the emergency department as one with an acute abdomen. Incarceration is said to occur in about 30% of patients with paraesophageal hernias,[16] although others[17] doubt if the incidence is that high. Mortality rate reaches almost 50% when intervention is initiated at this stage of the disease.[18]

ESOPHAGEAL MOTILITY DISORDERS

Patients presenting to the ED with chest pain or dysphagia frequently have underlying esophageal motility disorders. Although specific diagnoses cannot be made without special studies such as esophageal manometry, an understanding of these disorders is important to the ED evaluation of these common symptoms.

ACHALASIA

Achalasia is characterized by abnormal peristalsis in the body of the esophagus and failure of lower esophageal sphincter (LES) to relax normally in response to swallowing. Over time, this loss of propulsive peristaltic movement and failure of relaxation of the LES leads to dilation of the distal esophagus. Most of the cases of achalasia are primary or idiopathic, although the condition may be encountered secondarily in Chagas disease, amyloidosis, diffuse esophageal leiomyomatosis, and intestinal pseudo-obstruction.

Dysphagia and regurgitation are the most common symptoms of achalasia. They are less frequently encountered with chest pain than other esophageal disorders.[3]

NUTCRACKER ESOPHAGUS

This is the term used for the esophageal motility disorder characterized by manometric findings of high-amplitude peristaltic contractions.[19] The precise pathophysiology remains undetermined, but one theory holds that the nutcracker esophagus may be a manometric marker for a more diffuse disorder of the esophagus or the gastrointestinal tract that is similar to irritable bowel syndrome.[20] High-amplitude manometric peristaltic contractions are a common finding in patients undergoing evaluation for noncardiac chest pain, and occur more commonly than diffuse spasm.

SCLERODERMA AND OTHER CONNECTIVE TISSUE DISORDERS

Scleroderma is associated with the most pronounced abnormality of esophageal motor function. Occasionally, patients with systemic lupus erythematosus, rheumatoid arthritis, and primary Sjogren's syndrome and polymyositis show involvement of the lower esophageal sphincter and the lower two thirds of the esophagus.

The motility disorder ranges from decreased amplitude of the peristaltic waves to complete absence of esophageal response to a swallow. Classically, dysphagia and heartburn are most frequently encountered. Symptoms correlate poorly with objective esophageal motility tests.

DIFFUSE ESOPHAGEAL SPASM (DES)

DES is marked by bouts of chest pain caused by intermittent high-amplitude simultaneous nonperistaltic contractions in the distal esophagus. Intermittent chest pain and some degree of dysphagia with solids and liquids are the major symptoms. Richter et al.[2] documented this condition in only 2% of patients evaluated for noncardiac chest pain. Both the nutcracker esophagus and the nonspecific esophageal motility disorders have been found to be associated with noncardiac chest pain about four times more frequently.

NONSPECIFIC ESOPHAGEAL MOTILITY DYSFUNCTION

A significant number of patients undergoing manometric examination for evaluation of noncardiac chest pain demonstrate various nonspecific abnormalities of esophageal contractions and the lower esophageal sphincter. Castell and Richter refer to the condition as nonspecific motility disorder, and in their experience, it was diagnosed in 36% of all patients with esophageal motility disorders.[2,3]

Patients with known esophageal motility disorders who present to the ED with exacerbation of their symptoms frequently find relief from nitrates or calcium channel blockers such as nifedipine. Stress frequently triggers an exacerbation of esophageal motility disorder symptoms. In these patients, abundant reassurance and occasional use of anxiolytic medications are generally effective.

REFERENCES

1. Gardner, B., and Richardson, J.D.: Gastrointestinal bleeding. *In* Polk, H.C., Stone, H.H., and Gardner, B. Basic Surgery. Edited by Norwalk, CT, Appleton-Century-Croft, 1983.
2. Richter, J.E., Bradley, L.A., and Castell, D.O.: Esophageal chest pain; current controversies in pathogenesis, diagnosis and therapy. Ann. Intern. Med. 110:66, 1989.
3. Castell, D.O.: Chest pain from the esophagus. *In* Issues in Critical Care: Selected Readings from Emergency Medicine. Edited by Atkins, H. New York; Cahners Publishing Company, 1989.
4. Castell, D.O., and Holtz, A.; Gastroesophageal reflux. Postgrad. Med. 86:141, 1989.
5. Kouchman, J.A., Wiener, G.J., Wu, W.C., et al.: Reflux laryngitis and its sequelae. J. Voice 2:78, 1988.
6. Marshall, J.B.: Diagnosis of esophageal motility disorders. Postgrad. Med. 87:81, 1990.
7. Terblanche, J., Yakoob, H.I., Bornman, P.C., et al.: Acute bleeding varices; a five year prospective evaluation of tamponade and sclerotherapy. Ann. Surg. 194:521, 1981.
8. Terblanche, J., Burroughs, A.K., and Hobbs, K.E.F.: Controversies in the management of bleeding esophageal varices. N. Engl. J. Med. 320:1393, 1989.
9. Hussey, K.P.: Vasopressin therapy for upper gastrointestinal tract hemorrhage: Has its efficacy been proven? Arch. Intern. Med. 145:1263, 1985.
10. Groszmann, R.J., Kravetz, D., Bosch, J., et al.: Nitroglycerine improves the hempdynamic response to vasopressin in portal hypertension. Hepatology 2:757, 1982.
11. Galambos, M.R., and Galambos, J.T.: How to cope with bleeding esophageal varices. J. Crit. Illness 5:603, 1990.
12. Novis, B.H., Duys, P., Barbezat, G.O., et al.: Fiberoptic endoscopy and the use of Sengstaken tube in acute gastrointestinal hemorrhage in patients with portal hypertension and varices. Gut 17:258, 1976.
13. Marshall, J.: Gastroesophageal reflux. A problem oriented symposium. Postgrad. Med. 85:910, 1989.
14. Silverstein, F.E., Gilbert, D.A., Tedesco, F.J., et al.: The national ASGE survey on upper gastrointestinal bleeding. II. Clinical Prognostic factors. Gastrointest. Endosc. 27:80, 1981. III. Endoscopy in upper gastrointestinal bleeding. Gastrointest. Endosc. 27:94, 1981.
15. Ozdemir, I.A., Burke, W.A., and Ikins, P.M.: Paraesophageal hernia: A life threatening disease. Ann. Thorac. Surg. 16:547, 1973.
16. Hill, L.D., and Tobias, J.A.: Paraesophageal hernia. Arch. Surg. 96:735, 1968.
17. Ellis, F.H., Jr.: Diaphragmatic hiatal hernias. Postgrad. Med. 88:113, 1990.
18. Hill, L.D.: Incarcerated paraesophageal hernia: a surgical emergency. Am. J. Surg. 126:280, 1973.
19. Castell, D.O.: The nutcracker esophagus and other primary esophageal motility disorders. *In* Dalton, J.E., and Dalton, C.B. Esophageal Motility Testing. Edited by Castell, D.O., Richter, New York, Elsevier Science Publishing Co., 1987, pp. 130–42.
20. Nelson, J.B., and Castell, D.O. Esophageal motility disorders. Dis. Mon. 34:297, 1988.

FOREIGN BODY INGESTION

Airway obstruction: emergency measures

Suspect perforation: surgical consultation

Directly visualized: removal with Magill forceps

LOCATION BY X RAY

— **Impacted in esophagus**

Button battery: emergent endoscopy

Mild symptoms: observation for several hours

Failure to progress:

Unable to locate per x ray: contrast study
Endoscopic removal: secure airway in a child

Evaluation for pathophysiology that led to
impaction and assessment of mucosal damage

Postremoval impaction treated as potential perforation

— **Identified in stomach**

Symptomatic: endoscopy

Asymptomatic: serial films, q 3–4 days

Fails to pass pylorus after 7 days: endoscopy

— **Identified in lower GI tract**

Symptomatic: surgical consultation

Asymptomatic: serial films, q 7 days
stools for occult blood for sharp objects

SWALLOWED FOREIGN BODIES

Marsha D. Rappley and Sid Shah

CAPSULE

Foreign bodies of the upper gastrointestinal tract are responsible for acute morbidity; a chronic, often undiagnosed morbidity; and approximately 1500 deaths in the United States each year. Of these bodies, 80% to 90% pass spontaneously, but 10% to 20% require endoscopic removal and 1% require surgical removal.[1]

INTRODUCTION

The esophagus has the least distensible lumen of the gastrointestinal tract. Esophageal foreign bodies are most frequently lodged in three areas of anatomic narrowing, as illustrated in Figure 49-1: (1) the cervical esophagus at C6 or the cricopharyngeus, (2) the cross-

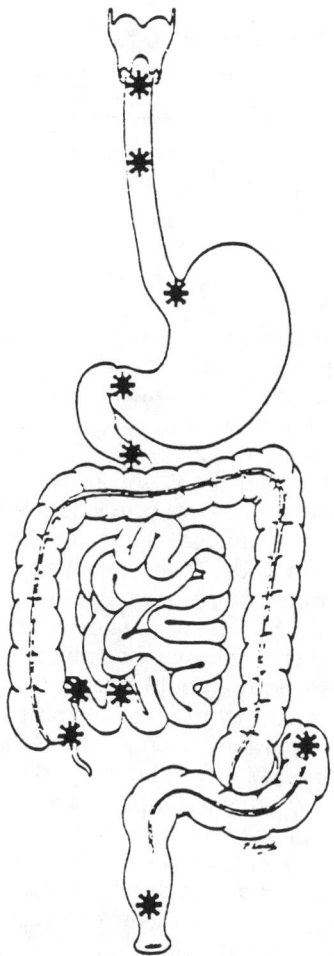

FIG. 49-1. Anatomic areas in the alimentary canal where foreign objects may arrest after ingestion. (With permission from Hamilton, J.K., and Potter, D.E.: Foreign bodies in the gut. In *Gastrointestinal Disease, Pathophysiology, Diagnosis, Management.* Fourth Edition. Edited by Sleisenger, M.H. and Fordham, J.S. Philadelphia, W.B. Saunders, 1989, p. 211).

ever, have been noted to become impacted, causing extensive damage to the mucosal wall.[3] Button batteries that become impacted in the esophagus represent a true emergency because they can cause rapid liquification necrosis of the mucosa from their strong alkaline content.[1,4] It may be difficult to distinguish a battery from a coin if the history is not helpful. An anterior projection of the battery in x ray reveals the bilaminar structure as a double density; the lateral projection reveals a step-off junction. The coin on lateral image has a sharper edge.

It is axiomatic that, in children, one foreign body suggests the presence of another. Seventeen percent of children have had one or more ingestions.[2,5] Lodgement of a foreign body may suggest an underlying anatomic anomaly. Half of these children have significant medical or social risk factors such as esophageal anomaly or disease, mental retardation, hyperactivity, child abuse, or a chaotic and unsupervised family life.[2]

Patients under 40 years are more likely to have a true foreign body; those over 60 are more likely to have a food bolus impaction as a foreign body.[2] The elderly are particularly at risk because of dental prostheses, which reduce palatal sensation. Alcohol may have the same effect and also decrease the gag reflex. Retarded persons may ingest inappropriate objects. Foreign bodies are not uncommon among prisoners seeking secondary gain.

Meat boluses and bones are the most frequent offenders. Ominous sharp objects include toothpicks and bones, the two items most often requiring surgical removal, as well as nails, needles, safety pins, and dental prostheses. Anhydrous pills, gelatin capsules, and enteric-coated tablets are also a problem in adults, with occasional development of pill bezoars in the stomach that must be removed to avoid breakup and absorption. The most common drugs associated with esophageal mucosal injury in patients under 40 years are antibiotics. For those over 40 years, the drugs most often involved are KCl, quinidine, and indomethacin.[3,6]

ing of the aortic arch; and (3) the gastroesophageal sphincter.

Three groups of patients are at risk for esophageal foreign body: pediatric, geriatric, and those impaired cognitively or functionally, such as alcoholics or the mentally ill.

Children represent 80% of cases of esophageal foreign bodies. The peak age is 38 months and the range is from 3 months to adolescence.[1,2] Infants swallow items that have been placed in their mouths, most often by siblings. The risk increases with developmental competency, increased mobility from crawling to walking, and the sensorimotor-oral stage of exploration.

Coins are the most frequent offenders cited by all authors. Bones, buttons, marbles, button batteries, and straight pins follow in frequency.[2] Small food items such as peanuts that pose a risk if aspirated into the airway do not generally cause a problem in the esophagus. Vitamins and other anhydrous pills, how-

CLINICAL PRESENTATION

Clinical presentation may be only a history of ingestion. One third of patients may be asymptomatic. It cannot be overstated that a positive history of foreign body ingestion in a child should not be dismissed.[5] Symptoms may include choking, gagging, or vomiting at the time of ingestion, refusal to take foods, drooling, respiratory stridor, or wheezing and complaint of pain with localization in older children. Less than 20% have an abnormal physical examination.[2,15] The examination should include palpation for subcutaneous emphysema in addition to scrutiny of the head, neck, chest, and abdomen. Direct and indirect laryngoscopy may help to locate the foreign body. Diagnostic studies include chest x ray in posterior-anterior and lateral views that give adequate visualization of the neck soft tissues, the esophagus, and the stomach bubble. See Table 49-1 for indications for x ray.[7,8] If the object is suspected to be sharp or large, stool should be checked for blood. It may be necessary to locate an area of impaction with water-soluble contrast media or a barium-soaked pledget, but there is a risk in using these procedures in the presence of perforation or obstruction.

MANAGEMENT

Eighty percent of foreign bodies pass uneventfully into the gastrointestinal (GI) tract.[1] Management of an obstructed airway is discussed elsewhere in the text. If the child is breathing comfortably and able to talk without difficulty and the suspected object is smooth rather than sharp, the child can be observed for several hours after ingestion. A soft catheter may be used to suction oral secretions, minimizing the risk of aspiration.

Major complications may ensue after 24 hours, making endoscopic removal much more difficult. These include erosion of the mucosa so that the foreign body must be dissected from the esophageal wall. The erosion can lead to perforation with resulting mediastinitis, tracheoesophageal fistula, or a potentially fatal aortoesophageal fistula. Tracheal compression, aspiration of secretions, atelectasis from airway obstruction, pleural effusion, pneumothorax, lung abscess, and sepsis are additional complications of retained foreign bodies.

FOREIGN BODY REMOVAL

Removal of the esophageal foreign body has been controversial. Currently, many authors do not recommend removal with a Fogarty or Foley catheter under fluoroscopy because the airway cannot be adequately safeguarded in a child.[1,2,5,9] Friedman categorically states that "esophageal foreign bodies should be removed under general anesthesia with a secured airway."[5] This is because the dislodged foreign body can possibly obstruct the laryngeal outlet. Catheter removal is contraindicated in cases of anatomic abnormality, a retained foreign body, a sharp, radiolucent, or unknown foreign body, or an uncooperative patient. Endoscopic removal provides the advantage of an assessment of mucosal injury and the presence of another foreign body. The drawback of endoscopy, however, is that it has required general anesthesia in children. With the advent of shorter-acting anesthetics, however, this risk may be substantially less.

The foreign body should not be pushed into the stomach because this may cause compression of the trachea or perforation. Agents such as diazepam (Valium) and meperidine must be avoided because of their sedative effect, which compromises the airway and the handling of secretions. Anticholinergics decrease secretions but increase the risk of gastric outlet obstruction. Proteolytic enzymatic degradation of a meat bolus has been complicated by degradation of the partially eroded mucosal wall. Administration of glucagon to relax esophageal smooth muscle, although it is usually effective, has been complicated by vomiting, which further compromises the airway.

If the foreign body is passed into the stomach, an abdominal film can be obtained at 3- to 4-day intervals until the object passes the pylorus. If it does not pass the gastric outlet in 7 days, or if symptoms arise, endoscopic removal may be considered. Although it usually takes a benign course thereafter, the foreign body may yet lodge in the lower gut because of anatomic configurations, as illustrated in Figure 49-1. Perforation may manifest as an acute abdomen with pain and fever or as an obstructed bowel with vomiting and distention. Stools should be followed for occult blood in all ingestions of sharp objects.

Fifty percent of children are seen within 3 days of an ingestion, but as many as 20% may not come to medical attention for more than 1 month.[5] They may present with chronic respiratory symptoms, recurrent or migrating pneumonia, or failure to thrive. They may be worked up for cystic fibrosis, allergy, asthma, immunodeficiency syndromes, or mucociliary dysfunction. The long-term complications are related to poor nutritional intake, formation of granulation tissue, and chronic infection.

Less than 1% of all foreign bodies cause perforation,

but for sharp objects the incidence is 15% to 35%.[1] Common sites of impaction or perforation are illustrated in Figure 49-1. The flow of the object is influenced by its size and shape as well as any gut pathology such as Meckel's diverticulum or hernia. Objects usually pass in 48 to 72 hours; the range is up to 14 days. Surgery is indicated for symptoms or if the object fails to progress.

A relatively recent phenomenon is the "body packer" or "mule" who transports cocaine by ingesting grape-sized packets containing 3 to 7 g each. Caruana et al. studied 50 patients imprisoned for this offense and reported ingestions of 54 to 182 packets. Because 1 to 3 g of cocaine can be fatal, with seizures, delirium, and cardiovascular collapse, surgical removal of packets has been the treatment of choice. The above series, however, documented conservative management with the patient receiving nothing by mouth except mineral oil. Venous access was maintained at all times. Packets were passed in an average of 28 hours. Emergency surgery was required in three cases for bowel obstruction. There were no ruptured packets in this series. The authors speculate that this is because the packages appeared to be a manufactured product and not the finger cots or condoms frequently used in the past, which were more subject to rupture.[10]

REFERENCES

1. Webb, W.: Management of foreign bodies of the upper gastrointestinal tract. Gastroenterology 94:204, 1988.
2. Taylor, R.B. Esophageal foreign bodies. Emerg. Med. Clin. North Am. 5:301, 1987.
3. Perry, P.A., Dean, B.S., and Krenzelok, E.P.: Drug induced esophageal injury. Clin. Toxicol. 27:281, 1989.
4. Litovic, T.L. Battery ingestions: Product accessibility and clinical course. Pediatrics 75:469, 1985.
5. Friedman, E.M.: Foreign bodies in the pediatric aerodigestive tract. Ped. Ann. 17:642, 1988.
6. Roach, J.: Anhydrous pill ingestion: A new cause of esophageal obstruction. Ann. Emerg. Med. 16:913, 1987.
7. Savitt, D.L., and Wason, S. Delayed diagnosis of coin ingestion in children. Ann. Emerg. Med. 6:378, 1988.
8. Hodge, D. III: Coin ingestion: Does every child need a radiograph? Ann. Emerg. Med. 14:443, 1985.
9. Krome, R.L.: Swallowed foreign bodies. In Emergency Medicine, a comprehensive study guide. Edited by Tintinalli, J.E., Krome, R.I., and Ruiz, E. New York. McGraw-Hill, 1988.
10. Caruana, D., Weinbach, B., Goerg, D., and Gardner, L.B.: Cocaine-packet ingestion. Ann. Emerg. Med. 100:73, 1984.
11. Hamilton, J.K. and Polter, D.E.: Foreign Bodies in the gut. In Gastrointestinal Disease, Pathophysiology, Diagnosis Management; Third Edition. Edited by Sleisenger, M.H., and Fordtran, J.S. Philadelphia, W.B. Saunders, 1983.

ACUTE GASTROENTERITIS

Christopher Truss

CAPSULE

Acute gastroenteritis is a poor term because current use tends to identify the condition as an infectious disease and at the same time apply the term to all cases of acute onset nausea and vomiting, with or without diarrhea. I use the term for the symptom complex of vomiting, diarrhea, or both. The cause is usually infectious, but certain other diseases can present with these symptoms, and one must be alert to clues that an "acute gastroenteritis" might in fact be a drug toxicity, increased intracranial pressure, or an abdominal catastrophe. The diarrhea component of this syndrome is particularly important because it solidifies the impression that the syndrome is caused by an infection.

INTRODUCTION

Acute gastroenteritis that includes a component of diarrhea, with or without vomiting, is most often caused by infection and can be approached as such by categorizing it as a dysentery or nondysentery on the basis of the presence of leukocytes in the stool. Fever is often associated with viral or bacterial infections and less frequently with parasites or noninfectious causes of gastroenteritis. Initial triage involves deciding whether the problem is a self-limited infection, a more severe life-threatening infection, or a nongastrointestinal problem mimicking gastroenteritis. It is impossible to make an accurate diagnosis of cause on presentation of acute gastroenteritis, and therefore initial diagnosis is based on a knowledge of epidemiology and patterns of presentation as well as a thorough history and physical examination.

The history should be taken with particular attention to recent ingestions of potential poisons. In children, the information must come from the parent and is not as reliable as in adults. Any history of recent medication changes or antibiotic usage should be noted. The review of systems should focus on neurology as well as gastroenterology. The physical examination should include a search for signs of dehydration, which is the most common complication of infectious gastroenteritis. The examination, however, must also be performed with a differential of the noninfectious causes of vomiting in mind. Abdominal examination to exclude appendicitis, obstruction, perforation, or peritonitis should be done because all these conditions can have atypical presentations that might initially suggest gastroenteritis. Neurologic examination to exclude increased intracranial pressure or cerebellar dysfunction should be done. If diarrhea is part of the symptom complex, stool microscopy or proctoscopic examination may be helpful.

PATHOPHYSIOLOGY

The invasive infections probably cause diarrhea by denuding absorptive epithelium, and the subsequent malabsorption of nutrients leads to osmotic diarrhea. At least some enterotoxins work by activating cyclic AMP in the mucosa, enhancing secretion and overwhelming fluid absorptive functions in the distal bowel. For most infections, the pathophysiology is unknown.

CLINICAL PRESENTATION AND EPIDEMIOLOGY

Infectious gastroenteritis may be caused by viruses, bacteria, or parasites. Viruses cause acute gastroenteritis only. Bacteria, whether invasive or toxigenic, usually cause only acute diarrheas. The parasites are more commonly diagnosed during chronic diarrheas. In approaching acute diarrhea, it is important to look for features of dysentery which are pus or blood in the diarrheal stool. Dysentery is caused by microbial invasion of the mucosa, and the more distal its site in the GI tract, the more likely the patient is to have bloody or purulent diarrhea.

VIRAL GASTROENTERITIS

The viruses are not routinely cultured, and specific diagnosis is rarely made outside research institutions.

Two viruses, Norwalk and rotavirus, are responsible for most gastroenteritis. Norwalk virus is the predominant agent causing diarrhea in infants and young children. It usually lasts only 24 to 48 hours. Rotavirus is probably the most common cause of viral gastroenteritis. It tends to last for a week and often causes low-grade fever. Management is symptomatic to control vomiting and diarrhea and correct dehydration. Gastroenteritis caused by these viruses is an acute, self-limited illness and the agents cannot be distinguished clinically.

BACTERIAL GASTROENTERITIS

Bacterial gastroenteritis tends to be a diarrheal illness without as much vomiting as may be seen in viral gastroenteritis or in food poisoning. Because the bacteria invade the mucosa, they produce an inflammatory reaction, resulting in exudate and a purulent diarrhea or dysentery. There may or may not be bleeding. The volume of diarrhea is unpredictable and can lead to dehydration particularly if accompanied by high fever.

Only a few bacteria can be cultured or diagnosed by current clinical laboratory techniques, and many of the bacterial agents listed in treatises are not relevant to most practicing physicians because they are not seen in the United States, or because they cannot be cultured and the diarrhea is self-limited. Bacillary dysentery in the USA is usually caused by Campylobacter jejuni, Salmonella species, and Shigella species. Yersinia causes disease, but much less frequently than the first three.[1,2] These same organisms are responsible for most acute bacterial diarrhea in all developed countries. In comparable studies of adults with acute diarrhea from Switzerland (119 patients), San Francisco (113 patients), and New Zealand (60 patients) the number of proven cases of infectious diarrhea has ranged from 38% to 50%[2-4] and the remainder are culture-negative. The largest portion of these diagnosed infections are bacillary dysenteries caused by Campylobacter jejuni (12 to 25%), Shigella sp. (up to 16%), and Salmonella sp. (2 to 12%). In the two studies that did not exclude cases with recent antibiotic exposure, Clostridium difficile-induced pseudomembranous colitis was the next most common cause of bacterial diarrhea after the three bacillary dysenteries, accounting for about 5% of acute diarrheas. There were one or two cases of Giardia lamblia infection in each series but no cases of amoebic dysentery in San Francisco or Switzerland and only one in New Zealand. Two cases of Yersinia were diagnosed in the San Francisco study, but none in the other two, and only two Vibrio infections seen, both in New Zealand. Thus a quick review of three areas of the "developed" world suggests that our diagnostic efforts need to focus on only a handful of "treatable" infectious causes of acute diarrhea. Many of the undiagnosed cases in these series are probably viral, but these are of short duration and cannot be diagnosed by readily available techniques. Routine stool culture, now available in most hospitals, can detect only C. jejuni, Shigella and Salmonella, and a few can culture for Yersinia. The other bacteria listed in reviews usually cannot be cultured and many are not found in the USA, e.g., *Vibrio cholera* or enterotoxigenic *E. coli*.[2]

The usual course of bacillary dysentery lasts less than 1 week and is associated with fever, blood, or pus in the stool. If these signs are present, the yield on stool culture may approach 80%.[2] By the time the culture is positive, however, most cases will have resolved. The clinical characteristics of Salmonella, Shigella, and Campylobacter are similar and cannot be used to distinguish one from the other.[5] Clinical syndromes range from simple diarrhea to enteric fever secondary to severe dysentery.

Yersinia infections are most often caused by enterocolitica and are increasing in prevalence.[6] The clinical syndromes range from diarrhea and pain to enterocolitis with ulceration in the small and large intestine. Rarely, infection mimics appendicitis or ileitis and will cause mesenteric adenitis. The diarrhea tends to last longer than 2 weeks in more than half of patients but is usually self-limited.

PARASITIC GASTROENTERITIS

Parasites cause a disproportionate amount of chronic infectious diarrhea compared to the bacteria and viruses. In most areas of the United States, there are only 2 or 3 offending parasites, and the more exotic organisms may not be recognized by inexperienced technician. Local laboratories in smaller hospitals often have experience with only a few such as Giardia lamblia, Entamoeba histolytica, or Strongyloides stercoralis.[7] The key to diagnosis is to suspect parasites and be aware of those that local laboratories commonly detect. We do not have reliable tests to exclude parasitic infestations, and therapeutic trials of reliable and safe antimicrobials are part of the diagnostic evaluation of chronic diarrhea.

The most common parasites which cause diarrhea are the protozoans, G. lamblia and E. histolytica. Intestinal helminths, except for S. stercoralis, do not cause as much diarrhea as the protozoans. Of these three parasitic infestations, amebiasis is not common and is usually limited to the southwest or is found in patients with a history of travel to endemic areas. By contrast, giardiasis is ubiquitous in this country and, contrary to textbook lore, the patient rarely gives a history of travel or drinking contaminated water.[8]

Giardia lamblia is currently the most common parasite in the United States causing gastroenteritis. This appears to be true for all areas of the country, whether rural or urban.[7,8] It is not related to socioeconomic conditions or racial groups and probably has little to do with sanitation except for infants in day care centers. It dominates other parasites statistically and accounts for 50 to 97% of all parasites isolated in most areas of the U.S.A. G. lamblia is probably self-limited in many cases that go unrecognized. It can cause chronic diarrhea and is the main organism that should be considered when chronic diarrhea is evaluated. In one prospective series of chronic diarrhea, G. lamblia was thought to be the cause in 24% of cases.[9] Giardiasis symptoms appear to evolve as the infection becomes chronic, with diarrhea becoming slightly less prominent and abdominal pain, flatulence, bloating, and nausea or anorexia becoming more bothersome. Chronic infestation can cause significant weight loss, not clearly caused by malabsorption in all cases, but possibly secondary to profound anorexia.

Strongyloides stercoralis is not uncommon in most areas of the United States. As a helminth, it usually induces eosinophilia. Diarrhea is a common presenting symptom, but in many cases there are upper intestinal symptoms of epigastric pain, anorexia, nausea, and bloating.[10] These worms may burrow into the intestinal wall and cause visceral larvae migrans with cough, wheezing, or rash. The rash may be urticaria.[1] An overwhelming dissemination can occur in immunosuppressed patients on steroids. Diagnosis can be made on stool examination or intestinal biopsy. The stool may contain Charcot-Leyden crystals, which are degenerated eosinophils.

Entamoeba histolytica causes amebic dysentery. This is a colitis with blood, pus, and occasional ulceration of the colonic epithelium. Most cases, however, are nondysenteric and produce watery diarrhea only. Both types are usually self-limited but can be chronic or life-threatening. Eosinophilia is unusual, but in colitis cases the patient has fever and leukocytosis. Endemic areas tend to be the southwestern U.S.A., Mexico, and Latin America.

Blastocystis hominis has recently been classified as a pathogen causing a giardiasis-like syndrome. It may also occur in asymptomatic people. This organism has not been well studied, but may be fairly common.

Cryptosporidium should be mentioned only because it is found in AIDS patients. In normal people, it produces a short infection with diarrhea. It is difficult to diagnose, and there is no effective treatment for it. In patients with AIDs, the diarrhea may be chronic and debilitating.

CLOSTRIDIUM DIFFICILE GASTROENTERITIS

Clostridium difficile is a bacterium that colonizes the colon but is kept suppressed by the normal flora unless the latter is destroyed by broad-spectrum antimicrobials. A toxin produced by proliferating C. difficile can induce mild diarrhea or an inflammatory pseudomembranous colitis (PMC). Less severe diarrhea may also occur. Recent prospective data shows that up to 75% of patients admitted to hospitals may become colonized by C. difficile, and about $\frac{1}{3}$ of those subsequently exposed to antibiotics develop diarrhea.[11] C. difficile probably accounts for 50% of antibiotic-related diarrhea, the rest being caused by nonspecific alteration of colonic flora or overgrowth of Candida albicans. Pseudomembranous colitis may present as only mild limited antibiotic-related diarrhea or as a severe colitis with fever, abdominal pain, toxic megacolon, perforation, or shock. The key to diagnosis is the finding of dysentery following the use of antimicrobials.

TRAVELER'S DIARRHEA

Traveler's diarrhea is a separate entity that encompasses all of the previously mentioned causes as well as agents not endemic to the United States. Most cases are bacterial and resolve without treatment, but the vomiting and diarrhea may be severe enough to cause dehydration. Enterotoxigenic Escherichia coli may be responsible for half of all cases and cause a watery diarrhea that usually lasts 4 days.[12] Salmonella and Shigella tend to produce dysentery, but this is probably much less common than was once suspected. Because antibiotic prophylaxis can reduce the rate of diarrhea by 90% in prospective studies, it is probably fair to assume that most traveler's diarrhea is caused by bacterial pathogens. Amebic dysentery is rare.

Traveler's diarrhea usually occurs in a visitor from a "developed" country going to a less developed country. The more primitive the sewage disposal system, the more likely there is to be fecal contamination of food and water. The attack rate of traveler's diarrhea is 25 to 50%, depending on the traveler's origin and the country which he or she visits.

FOOD POISONING

Bacteria can also cause food poisoning, the three most common organisms being Salmonella sp., Staphylococcus aureus, and Clostridium perfringens.[13] In practice, a specific diagnosis is rarely made because the symptoms are short-lived and the food is usually not available for culture when the patient becomes symptomatic. The diagnosis is suspected by history, and management is similar to that for viral gastroenteritis. Salmonella always leads the list of agents but may be over-represented because it can be cultured from the stool. The usual course of disease lasts only 24 to 48 hours and may be seen as dysentery. There are suggestive patterns for each organism, such as short incubation of 7 hours and profuse vomiting for Staphylococcus and Bacillus cereus. The former is usually associated with meats and the latter, which is rare in the U.S.A., with rice. Salmonella poisoning has been acquired from so many sources (milk, poultry, pork, marijuana, pet turtles) that a history is rarely of any use. C. perfringens is associated with meat or fish; it causes diarrhea without fever, which runs its course in 24 hours. The Vibrio species include the agent of epidemic cholera, Vibrio cholerae, but this is rarely seen in the United States. Other Vibrio species include V. parahaemolyticus and V. non-01 cholerae, which are found in Gulf Coast waters and cause occasional gastroenteritis. These cases are rare (3 in 10 years in one medical center), and unless a specific history of shellfish ingestion is obtained, these organisms can probably be ignored.[14] They can be detected on routine stool examinations or by specialized techniques. Treatment of all bacterial food poisoning is symptomatic.

DIAGNOSTIC TESTING

Microscopic examination of stool for leukocytes and blood is useful for classifying a case of diarrhea as dysentery or not. A drop of feces is mixed with saline on a slide or a swab is immersed in a cup of saline and then touched to a slide. No staining is necessary. More than one or two leukocytes per high-power field is significant.

Stool cultures should not be sent in all cases of gastroenteritis because the yield is low and the effect on management small. When cultures are limited to cases of dysentery, the yield approaches 80%.[2] Cultures for bacterial pathogens were positive in 81% if blood and leukocytes were present in the stool. Culture-proven cases of Campylobacter jejuni had fecal leukocytes in 79% of cases and blood in the stool in 90%. Shigella had fecal leukocytes in 95% and blood in 84%. In contrast, only 56% of parasitic cases had fecal leukocytes and only 33% had blood. In a series from Boston, the best predictor of positive cultures was a combination of fever, duration of illness longer than 24 hours, and blood in the stool or abdominal pain with nausea and vomiting.[15] Positive culture results, however, affected treatment in less than 5% of cases and there was no value to repeated stool cultures over a series of days. This lack of impact of a positive diagnosis in bacillary dysentery is probably caused by the self-limited nature of these infections.

In cases of suspected pseudomembranous colitis, the stool should be checked for white blood cells (WBCs) and a specimen sent for Clostridium difficile toxin and/or culture. If a proctoscopic examination is done, the rectum should be abnormal with at least erythema and edema; often pseudomembranes are seen.

Multiple stool examinations should be done when searching for parasitic infections, and traditionally, three specimens collected on separate days are sent for microscopy. The proctoscopic examination is usually not used except by gastroenterologists and then is usually reserved for chronic cases of diarrhea.

Examination of gastric aspirates is of little benefit except in cases of bleeding or poisoning. Barium studies are of no use. Electrolytes and complete blood counts are used to asses hydration but contribute little to specific diagnosis. These tests occasionally suggest a noninfectious cause of vomiting and diarrhea such as pancreatitis, hepatitis, or diabetic ketoacidosis.

MANAGEMENT AND INDICATIONS FOR ADMISSIONS

SYMPTOMATIC THERAPY

Therapy should be directed at maintaining proper hydration and electrolyte balance, which are usually a problem only in infants, the elderly, or those with intractable vomiting as part of their gastroenteritis. Pediatricians have various diets, some with interesting names such as the "brat diet" (*b*ananas, *r*ice, *a*pplesauce, and *t*oast) that ensure that the child will be well hydrated and provided with glucose and electrolytes. The basis of diet therapy for diarrhea is to reduce agents that stimulate motility, avoid complex and poorly absorbed carbohydrates, and provide adequate water and electrolytes. Caffeine-containing products such as coffee and colas should be avoided. Poorly absorbed carbohydrates include lactose products (milk, cheese, ice cream) and fructose sweeteners (many soft drink beverages). Milk products such as yogurt should also be avoided because the lactose degradation is variable. Certain fruits, such as grapes and prunes, contain poorly absorbed sugars including sorbitol and xylitol. Many peoples regard fruit juice as a staple of diarrhea therapy, and I think that simply making them aware that it might exacerbate the problem is better than absolute prohibition. Simple sugar, glucose, is easily absorbed, facilitates absorption of electrolytes, and can be obtained in a variety of products, including honey. Heavy meals with a large fat content may exacerbate diarrhea by stimulating motility reflexes, and therefore multiple small meals should be encouraged. Vomiting or inability to eat and drink because of dehydration and obtundation are indications for intervention with drugs or intravenous fluids. For adults, antiemetics by suppository are usually adequate. For young children, I would not allow unsupervised use of suppositories longer than one day. If the diarrhea and vomiting are not reduced or signs of dehydration develop, close observation in hospital may be indicated. Elderly or malnourished individuals may also develop more severe problems because of inability to use oral therapy to maintain fluid and electrolyte balance during gastroenteritis.

The use of antiperistaltic drugs is controversial if the patient has a dysentery (see section on Pitfalls), but if the patient does not have fever or bloody, purulent diarrhea, loperamide is recommended to decrease frequency of stools. Loperamide is now available over the counter and should be taken on a regular schedule of every 8 to 12 hours as needed.

SPECIFIC THERAPY (see also Table 49-2)

Patients with fever, bloody diarrhea, and early signs of dehydration require further evaluation. Most of them have a bacillary dysentery caused by Campylobacter jejuni, Salmonella sp., or Shigella sp. if they have not had prior antibiotics. The finding of WBCs in the stool confirms the impression of dysentery and should lead to an initial stool culture. If a patient has had exposure to antibiotics, a stool specimen should be sent for C. difficile toxin. If the patient is suspected of having pseudomembranous colitis, a proctoscopic examination can be diagnostic and initial therapy can be started with metronidazole 250 mg three times a day. If bacillary dysentery is suspected and the patient is severely ill, a broad-spectrum agent such as ciprofloxacin, 500 mg twice a day, or trimethoprim-sulfamethoxazole (TMP-SMX) twice a day can be started. In most cases, by the time the stool culture is reported, the symptoms are resolving and antibiotics can be discontinued. On the other hand, if the patient is still ill, more specific therapy can be used. Erythromycin, for C. jejuni and culture sensitivity for enteric fever from salmonellosis or shigellosis should probably guide therapy if the patient is not responding to TMP-SMX or ampicillin. Yersinia sp. are usually sensitive to TMP-SMX.

PSEUDOMEMBRANOUS COLITIS AND ANTIBIOTIC-RELATED DIARRHEA

Pseudomembranous colitis (PMC) must be treated because it is potentially fatal. The first step in treating PMC is to discontinue the offending antibiotic if the patient is still receiving it. Metronidazole, 250 mg three times a day, or vancomycin, 125 mg three times a day, is given for 10 days to kill the Clostridiom difficile. Vancomycin is expensive, tastes bad, and cannot be given IV, whereas metronidazole is effective orally or intravenously.[16] The initial use of vancomycin for this disorder was based on the erroneous assumption that it was caused by Staphylococcus aureus. PMC has a relapse rate of about 15% with both antimicrobials, and therefore patient follow-up is important. Cholestyramine, 4 g four times a day, has long been useful and works by binding toxin and allowing the natural regrowth of the colonic flora to suppress the C. difficile. I think that this drug is most useful in patients with mild disease or relapse. Relapses can often be multiple and may require a prolonged tapering dose of suppressive drugs.[17]

Antibiotic-related diarrhea that is not due to C. difficile usually resolves within 1 week of discontinuing antibiotics. If the diarrhea has not resolved, I have found that the use of nystatin, 500,000 units orally four times a day, combined with *lactobacillus* powder

TABLE 49-2. SPECIFIC THERAPY FOR GASTROENTERITIS

Infection	Clinical Picture	Treatment
Unknown	Dysentery	If severe, ciprofloxacin, 500 mg bid for 5 days
Campylobacter jejuni	Dysentery	If severe, erythromycin, 250 mg qid
Salmonella species	Dysentery	If severe, TMP/SMX, 160/800 mg bid for 14 days
Shigella species	Dysentery	If severe, TMP/SMX, 160/800 mg bid for 5 days
Yersinia species	Diarrhea, dysentery, colitis pseudoappendicitis	TMP/SMX, 160/800 mg bid for 5 days
Clostridium difficile	Pseudomembranous colitis; antibiotic diarrhea	Metronidazole, 250 mg qid for 10 days
Norwalk virus	Nonspecific gastroenteritis	Symptomatic
Rotavirus	Nonspecific gastroenteritis	Symptomatic
Giardia lamblia	Nonspecific gastroenteritis, tends to be prolonged	Metronidazole, 250 mg tid for 7 days; furazolidone in children (8 mg/kg/day, divided qid)
Strongyloides stercoralis	Nonspecific gastroenteritis and eosinophilia	Thiabendazole, 22 mg/kg bid for 2 days
Blastocystis hominis	Nonspecific gastroenteritis	Metronidazole, 250 mg tid for 7 days
Entamoeba histolytica	Diarrhea or dysentery	Metronidazole, 750 mg tid for 10 days
Cryptosporidium	Debilitating diarrhea in AIDS	No treatment
Traveler's diarrhea		Symptomatic, TMP/SMZ 160/800 mg bid for 3 days

twice a day, is useful. Symptoms can be safely suppressed with loperamide.

PITFALLS

Antibiotics for bacterial diarrheas are routinely used only for C. difficile-induced PMC. Reports of prolongation or induction of the carrier state have caused concern about treating salmonellosis with antibiotics.[18] Nevertheless, treatment is recommended when the patient is severely ill with "enteric fever" and possible bacteremia.

A tradition has developed not to treat dysentery with antimotility drugs for fear of exacerbating the infection. This has been reported in controlled trials of shigellosis to prolong fever and prevent clearance of the organism.[19] Most patients with dysentery, however, are never seen by physicians and are undoubtedly self-medicated with opiate-like drugs such as paregoric and loperamide without evidence of any problem. I reserve use of these agents for cases of dysentery in which the frequency of loose stools is intolerable and diet therapy is not effective.

One of the major pitfalls of diagnosing "gastroenteritis" in the acutely vomiting patient is the failure to recognize other more serious problems such as a central neurologic cause. Increased intracranial pressure as a cause of intractable vomiting should be considered in cases of "gastroenteritis" without diarrhea. Other more obvious clues include headache, altered mental status, focal neurologic signs, and nuchal rigidity. Patients with fever, vomiting, and headache might have meningitis. Those with dizziness or vertigo associated with vomiting might have cerebellar lesions. In all these instances, the absence of diarrhea should lead the physician to a closer neurologic examination and to order additional tests as needed.

Addisonian crisis may present as "gastroenteritis" with nausea and vomiting and/or diarrhea. Diabetic ketoacidosis or hepatitis is occasionally first misdiagnosed as gastroenteritis.

REFERENCES

1. Blaser, M.J.: Infectious diarrheas: Acute, chronic, and iatrogenic. Ann. Intern. Med. *105*:785, 1986.
2. Siegel, D.: Predictive value of stool examination in acute diarrhea. Arch. Pathol. Lab. Med. *111*:715, 1987.
3. Loosli, J., Gyr, H., Stalder, G.A., et al.: Etiology of acute infectious diarrhea in a highly industrialized area of Switzerland. Gastroenterology *88*:75, 1985.
4. Chancellor, A.M., and Ellis-Pegler, R.B.: A clinical and aetiological study of adult patients hospitalised for acute diarrheal disease. N.Z. Med. J. *95*:154, 1982.
5. Blaser, M.J., Wells, J.G., Feldman, R.A., et al.: Campylobacter

enteritis in the United States: A multicenter study. Ann. Intern. Med. *98:*360, 1983.

6. Cover, T.L., and Aber, R.C. *Yersinia enterocolitica.* N. Engl. J. Med. *321:*16, 1989.

7. Pearson, R., Coleman, S., and Truss, C.: Giardiasis in Alabama. Ala. J. Med. Sci. *25:*137, 1988.

8. Carr, M.F., Ma, J., and Green, P.H.R.: *Giardia lamblia* in patients undergoing endoscopy: Lack of evidence for a role in nonulcer dyspepsia. Gastroenterology *95:*972, 1988.

9. Bolin, T.D., Davis, A.E., and Duncombe, V.M.: A prospective study of persistent diarrhoea. Aust. N.Z. J. Med. *12:*22, 1982.

10. Milder, J.E., Walzer, P.D., Kilgore, G., et al.: Clinical features of *Strongyloides stercoralis* infection in an endemic area of the United States. Gastroenterology *80:*1481, 1981.

11. McFarland, L.V., Mulligan, M.E., Kwok, R.Y.Y., and Stam W.E.: Nosocomial acquisition of *Clostridium Difficile* infection. N. Engl. J. Med. *320:*204, 1989.

12. NIH Consensus Conference. Travelers' diarrhea. JAMA *253:*2700, 1985.

13. Snydman, D.R.: Bacterial Food Poisoning. *In* Infectious Diarrhea. Edited by Gorbach, S.L. Boston, Blackwell Scientific Publications, 1986, pp. 201–218.

14. Bonner, J.R., Coker, A.S., Berryman, C.R., and Pollock, H.M.: Spectrum of *Vibrio* infection in a Gulf Coast community. Ann. Intern. Med. *99:*464, 1983.

15. Koplan, J.P., Fineberg, H.V., et al.: Value of stool cultures. Lancet *1:*413, 1980.

16. Teasley, D.G., Olson, M.M., Gerhard, R.L., et al.: Prospective randomized trial of metronidazole versus vancomycin for *Clostridium difficile* associated diarrhea and colitis. Lancet *2:*1043, 1983.

17. Tedesco, F.J.: Treatment of recurrent antibiotic-associated pseudomembranous colitis. Am. J. Gastroenterol. *88:*220, 1982.

18. Rosenthal, S.J.: Exacerbation of salmonella enteritis due to ampicillin. N. Engl. J. Med. *280:*147, 1969.

19. DuPont, H.L., and Hornick, R.B.: Adverse effect of lomotil therapy in shigellosis. JAMA *226:*1525, 1973.

APPENDICITIS

John R. Clarke and John M. Schoffstall

CAPSULE

Appendicitis is a common cause of acute abdominal pain. The optimal treatment of appendicitis is appendectomy, before perforation if possible. Optimal treatment requires recognition of appendicitis in the inflammatory stage and differentiation from causes of acute right lower abdominal pain not requiring surgical treatment, particularly mesenteric adenitis, gastroenteritis, right-sided salpingitis, mittelschmerz, and ruptured corpus luteum. Appendicitis is thought to start with occlusion of the appendiceal lumen, followed by invasion of colonic bacteria through the wall of the appendix, then ischemic necrosis, and finally perforation. The classic findings of acute appendicitis are a vague midabdominal pain subsequently localizing to the right lower abdomen, signs of peritonitis localized over the appendix, and mild systemic findings of infection.

Management of patients with pain over the appendix is based on the probability of appendicitis and the risks of unnecessary appendectomy versus perforation of the inflamed appendix because of delay in treatment. The risks of perforation are greater and therefore the threshold for operation is lower in extremely young and old patients and those with other medical conditions, including pregnancy. The initial management decisions are consultation for possible surgery, discharge with close follow-up,

and additional testing to further clarify ambiguous presentations. Analgesics and antibiotics should be deferred until observation is terminated and treatment for a specific condition has begun. Laxatives, cathartics, and enemas should be avoided in patients who may have appendicitis.

INTRODUCTION

Appendicitis is a common cause of acute abdominal pain and a common reason for emergency abdominal surgery.[1,2] Recognition of acute appendicitis, which is appendicitis in the inflammatory phase before perforation, produces the best results. The diagnosis is still made by collecting and integrating all relative information from the history and physical examination.[2] Subsequent diagnostic procedures invariably prove to be adjuvant rather than definitive. Other conditions not requiring surgery may have the same clinical appearance as appendicitis, making an appendectomy potentially unnecessary. Delays in the removal of inflamed appendices, however, may result in perforation with substantially greater risk to the patient. Therefore, the error of treating nonsurgical conditions as appendicitis can be acceptable.

This chapter reviews the accepted causes and stages of appendicitis. The relationship of the presentation to the stage of disease, the location of the appendix, and the patient's age and sex are discussed. In particular, the relationship of perforation and the patient's age are explored. The physician's management conundrum, the trade-off between the possibility of an unnecessary operation and an avoidable perforation, is examined. The roles of adjuvant diagnostic tests and pharmacological treatments are mentioned.

PATHOPHYSIOLOGY AND ANATOMY

Appendicitis is felt to result typically from obstruction of its lumen by either hyperplastic lymphoid tissue, commonly seen in younger patients, or an appendiceal fecalith.[3] Edema of the occluded segment of appendix over a few hours leads to loss of mucosal integrity and invasion of colonic bacteria across the bowel wall. The edema and inflammation can lead to vascular compromise, often manifest as a small elliptical infarct on the antimesenteric border of the occluded segment. Occasionally the entire inflamed segment becomes gangrenous. Perforation occurs within one or more days with disruption of the ischemic wall of the appendix. Generally, bacause of the obstruction of the lumen proximally, the amount of leakage and contamination is minimal. Usually, the contamination is contained by surrounding loops of bowel and the omentum to form a phlegmon and, if untreated, a localized absess. Often in children and occasionally in adults, as a result of either failure of the bowel and omentum to contain the contamination or free egress of colonic contents, generalized peritonitis develops, frequently accompanied by the septic shock syndrome.

The exact anatomic location of the body and the tip of the appendix, relative to its origin at the base of the cecum, is variable (Fig. 49–2). Most commonly, it lies free-floating in the right lower quadrant of the abdominal cavity. The tip of the appendix may also lie in the true pelvis or may not lie in the peritoneal cavity at all, but in a retroperitoneal position in the right flank behind the cecum. Occasionally, the appendix may be extremely long with its tip extended into the right upper or left lower quadrant.

The clinical manifestation of appendicitis depends on the stage of the disease and the specific anatomic location of the appendix. Early appendicitis is perceived as a visceral discomfort of the intestinal tract with a vague midabdominal pain and signs of gastrointestinal disturbance such as anorexia, nausea, and/or vomiting. With the development of inflammation of the serosal surface of the appendix, signs of peritoneal irritation are localized over the anatomic position of the appendix—classically, the anterior peritoneal surface of the right lower quadrant of the abdomen, occasionally the pelvis for appendices lying

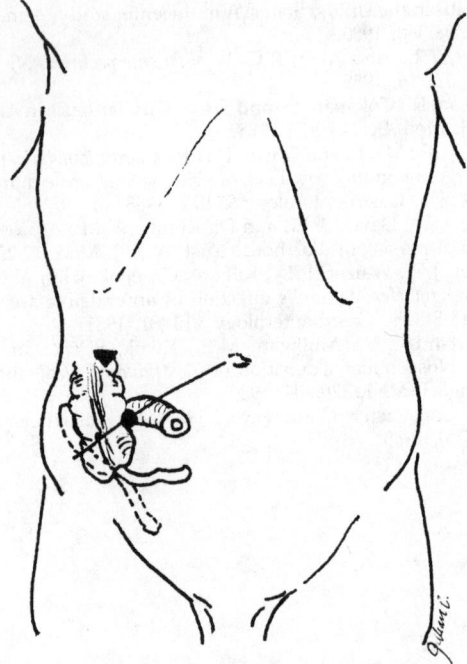

FIG. 49-2. Important anatomic locations of the appendix. The classic clinical location of maximum tenderness, McBurney's point, is identified by the circle. The triangle marks a typical location in a woman 5 months pregnant.

in the pelvis or the right flank for retrocecal appendices.

CLINICAL PRESENTATION AND EXAMINATION

The general topic of evaluating patients with acute abdominal pain is addressed elsewhere. The specific assessment of patients for appendicitis and confounding clinical conditions is described here in detail because of the reliance on the clinical findings to make the diagnosis.

APPENDICITIS

Appendicitis is most common in adolescents and young adults between the ages of 10 and 30.[2,4] The classical presentation of appendicitis, occurring in fewer than half of the patients with the disease and some without it, begins with a vague pain originating from the appendix, usually perceived by the patient in the periumbilical region, but occasionally in the epigastric region. A colicky pain may be superimposed, producing a pain that waxes and wanes but never goes away entirely (unlike classic colic). The pain is accompanied by gastrointestinal symptoms, specifically anorexia, nausea, and, less frequently, vomiting. The anorexia and nausea may precede the pain by a brief interval, but pain is the predominant symptom. Typically, the vomiting is not extensive in amount or duration. The patient may have constipation, leading to ill-advised considerations to stimulate a bowel movement, or may have a mild diarrhea as a result of irritation from an inflammatory focus. The diarrhea is not a dramatic symptom in appendicitis as it is in some infections. Most patients have no change in their bowel habits.

A full-thickness inflammation of the appendix leads to inflammation and irritation of the surrounding structures. The pain changes from vague midabdominal to more specific, anatomically adjacent to the appendix. The classic location of the inflamed appendix and its maximal tenderness is over McBurney's point, 1½ to 2 inches cephalad and medial to the anterior iliac spine on a line toward the umbilicus (see Fig. 49–2).[5] In the uncommon event that the tip of a fully inflamed appendix touches the bladder, urinary symptoms of urgency and frequency may develop in addition to suprapubic tenderness. An inflamed appendix situated below the pelvic brim may produce tenderness only on the right side of a rectal or pelvic examination. Because the cecum lies between a retrocecal appendix and the parietal peritoneum, the tenderness from inflammation of a retrocecal appendix is diffuse over the right flank.

The manifestation of a peritoneal irritation is supported not only by tenderness in the area of palpation, but also by spasm of the overlying muscle (guarding) and rebound tenderness. When examining the patient for signs of peritoneal irritation, the physician should try to gauge the magnitude of the inflammation by identifying how little, not how much, manipulation is necessary to elicit findings. In addition, the physician who starts with a gentle examination indicates to patients that they need not guard themselves against unexpected or unnecessary discomfort, yielding a more reliable examination.

The author's procedure is to start the examination by asking the patient to put one finger on the point of maximum tenderness and to press until he or she begins to sense pain. In doing so, the patient indicates the location of the tenderness. The number of fingers actually used gives an indication of the diffuseness or exactness of the location. The amount of pressure is, in general, inversely proportional to the amount of discomfort.

Patients with significant peritoneal irritation experience discomfort with any movement. This finding may be discovered during the history if the patient indicates that bumps during transport to the hospital aggravated the pain. Patients with lower abdominal peritonitis often walk with a characteristic shuffle: bent over, holding the stomach, and sliding their feet to avoid excessive movement of the abdominal contents. A child who is active and can jump up and down on request rarely has an inflamed appendix. Patients may

be observed lying motionless on the bed, usually on their side, curled in a fetal position or with the right hip flexed. The reluctance to move may be obvious during the examination.

Peritoneal irritation can also be elicited during the examination. We start by jiggling the bed slightly, then, as necessary, proceed to jiggling the patient, jarring the patient by pounding once on the bottom of the heel, and asking him or her to cough. Patients with significant peritonitis may volunteer that they do not want to cough, because they know it will produce pain. During the examination, attention is focused on the patient's face to look for signs of discomfort, such as grimacing.

Palpation of the abdomen is begun distant from the point of maximum tenderness. We usually begin in the left lower quadrant and proceed counterclockwise, ending in the right lower quadrant. We start with a light, almost percussive palpation, and proceed with increasingly deeper palpation, stopping when tenderness and muscle spasm are evident.

Focusing particularly on the point of maximum tenderness, the degree of resistance caused by muscle spasm is noted. A careful examination distinguishes between a tenseness of the abdominal muscle in anticipation of an unpleasant sensation and a reflex tenseness that guards against pressure and deformation of the area surrounding the inflammation. Guarding is even more remarkable if the examination is done with the legs flexed rather than straight. Tenderness anatomically confined to a single muscle such as the rectus abdominus and/or aggravated by tensing the abdominal wall when lifting the head suggests that the tenderness is in the abdominal wall itself, possibly the result of bleeding or injury. Appendicitis without generalized peritonitis usually does not cause board-like rigidity.

Rebound tenderness is considered specific for peritonitis rather than other causes of abdominal tenderness. Tenderness resulting from pressure alone is relieved by the release of pressure. In contrast, movement of the abdominal contents on rapid relief of abdominal wall pressure exacerbates the discomfort experienced by a patient with peritonitis. We perform rebound tenderness tests by pressing on the point of maximum tenderness until the patient experiences pain, maintaining steady pressure until the pain eases and then releasing the pressure quickly while looking for an indication of discomfort on the patient's face. Rovsing's sign is pain over the appendix elicited by pressure over the left lower quadrant.

Other signs have been described to elicit tenderness reactions in parts of the peritoneal cavity not available to direct palpation. The rectal or pelvic examination frequently produces tenderness on the right side. Other signs are found less frequently. The psoas sign elicits irritation when an inflamed appendix lies against the posterior peritoneum over the ileoposoas muscle. We elicit this sign by turning patients onto their left side with their right hip up and then passively extending the thigh, looking for evidence of abdominal discomfort. This sign can also be elicited in a supine patient by active flexion of the hip against resistance. If the inflamed appendix lies over the obturator internus muscle in the pelvis, tenderness may be elicited by passive internal rotation of the flexed right hip—the obturator sign.

Bowel sounds are often present, the silent abdomen being the more common after perforation.

Typically, acute appendicitis produces a mild rise in temperature (99 to 100.4°F or 37.2 to 38°C), if any.

PERFORATED APPENDIX

The typical presentation of a perforated appendix is usually distinguishable from that of acute appendicitis. The distinguishing characteristics are a more diffuse peritonitis or an inflammatory mass and obvious systemic signs of bacterial infection.

If the appendix has perforated, the abdomen is almost always quiet, except in rare instances in which a localized inflammatory mass produces obstruction of the small intestine. A mass may be appreciated in the right lower abdomen on either abdominal palpation or rectal examination. The mass may be a phlegmon consisting of small bowel and omentum attempting to contain the perforation, or a mature abscess. If the perforation is not contained, the extent of the peritonitis is indicated by the extent of peritoneal irritation across the abdomen. Patients with perforated appendices usually have fevers and white blood cell counts consistent with systemic responses to bacterial infection, although in extreme instances patients may be hypothermic and/or have depleted their white cells. Findings of septic shock may be present.

DIFFERENTIAL DIAGNOSIS

The essence of diagnosis in patients who might have appendicitis is distinguishing between acute appendicitis and diseases with similar clinical presentations that do not require laparotomy. If an appendix is already perforated, the need for laparotomy is usually obvious. Other surgically treated conditions that are sometimes confused with appendicitis, such as perforated ulcer, acute cholecystitis, Meckel's diverticulitis, diverticulitis coli, perforated colon cancer, ruptured ectopic pregnancy, ruptured tubo-ovarian abscess, and adnexal (ovarian) torsion, incur no major penalty for being misdiagnosed as appendicitis. Our experience, supported by others, is that if the diagnosis of appendicitis is a serious consideration, fewer than 5% of patients ultimately prove to have other surgical conditions.[6]

The important disgnoses to distinguish from acute appendicitis are mesenteric adenitis and other self-limited causes of abdominal pain not requiring rapid surgical treatment: gastroenteritis, mittelschmerz, ruptured corpus luteum, and salpingitis. For these diagnoses, the physician faces the errors of subjecting the patient to an unnecessary appendectomy on the one hand or allowing the patient to develop an avoidable perforation on the other.

MESENTERIC ADENITIS

Because mesenteric adenitis is only diagnosed pathologically when operating for appendicitis, the presentation obviously mimics appendicitis. The disease seems confined to younger patients with active lymphoid tissue. A history of a preceding upper respiratory infection can sometimes be elicited, although it is important to keep in mind that lymphoid hyperplasia producing obstruction of the appendix is also sometimes provoked by a previous viral illness. Occasionally, patients will have other evidence of viral infection; lymphadenopathy may be palpated in the usual node-bearing regions or the patient may have a lymphocytosis.[7]

GASTROENTERITIS

Distinguishing characteristics of patients with gastroenteritis may include the concurrent presence of similar problems in other members of the family, vomiting and/or diarrhea as the predominant symptoms, the development of pain after the onset of vomiting, and the presence of hyperactive bowel sounds. In our experience, the most difficult cases to distinguish are those with tenderness in the right lower quadrant. Our impression is that the tenderness found in gastroenteritis is slightly more diffuse and is probably the result of distention and irritation of the cecum. Guarding and rebound tenderness are not impressive.

In women of childbearing age, appendicitis may be difficult to distinguish from diseases of the right tube and ovary. Evaluation of the female organs by a pelvic examination is necessary for an adequate appraisal of the patient's condition. As a generalization, in the gynecologic alternatives, the gastrointestinal symptoms are less impressive and signs of peritoneal irritation can be found bilaterally.

MITTELSCHMERZ

Pain associated with rupture of the graafian follicle at ovulation is called mittelschmerz. When ovulation occurs from the right ovary, the condition may be confused with appendicitis. In our experience, confusion usually arises in the young adolescent who has not experienced this pain before. By definition, mittelschmerz occurs in the middle of the menstrual cycle.

The pain develops quickly in the right lower quadrant with no gastrointestinal symptoms or systemic signs of infection. Vaginal spotting may occur from the decline of estrogen. The rupture of a graafian follicle is usually a self-limited condition that dissipates during a short observation period.

RUPTURE OF A CORPUS LUTEUM

Rupture of a corpus luteum occurs near the end of the menstrual cycle. Again, the onset is sudden. It is sometimes associated with exercise or intercourse. The peritoneal irritation is caused by bleeding rather than inflammation. It spreads with the blood, becoming bilateral and occasionally generalized. Blood may be detected if a culdocentesis is done, but unlike an ectopic pregnancy, the pregnancy test is negative. If the bleeding stops before the patient becomes hypovolemic, the condition can be managed nonoperatively. Systemic manifestations are those of hypovolemia, not sepsis. Patients with persistent bleeding to the point of hypovolemia require emergency surgery; such patients are not confused with those having appendicitis.

SALPINGITIS

Salpingitis may be confused with appendicitis if it involves predominantly the right tube. Many such instances are in fact tubovarian abscesses. Although inflammation of the right tube may be difficult to distinguish from inflammation of the neighboring appendix, there are some characteristic differences.[8] Typically, salpingitis occurs around the time of menses. Because the patient's first attack of salpingitis is likely to spread throughout the pelvis, the patient with infection focused in one area has usually had previous episodes. Obvious fever (100 to 102°F or 38 to 39°C) is usually present. Confusion with appendicitis usually occurs after the patient develops gastrointestinal symptoms, but these symptoms usually start late, after the serosa of the small bowel becomes irritated by the pelvic peritonitis, and are mild relative to the pain and tenderness. Despite the unilateral predominance, most patients have some suggestion of bilateral tenderness. Purulent discharge from the os is a helpful finding, but may not be dramatic in patients with an isolated pyosalpinx. The absence of intracellular gram-negative diplococci does not rule out salpingitis. Chlamydia is a frequent cause of salpingitis, particularly the milder salpingitis that is more often confused with appendicitis. Additionally, secondary infection may have become established. Tenderness on motion of the cervix suggests adnexal disease, but can be found in patients with appendicitis when the appendix lies adjacent to the adnexal structures.

Other diseases that have occasionally been cited as mimicking appendicitis are listed in Table 49–3.

TABLE 49-3. DISEASES THAT HAVE SOMETIMES BEEN CONFUSED WITH APPENDICITIS AND ARE NOT MENTIONED IN THE TEXT

Black widow spider bite	Pancreatitis
Endometriosis	Pleuritis
Enteric duplications	Pneumonia
Epididymitis	Porphyria
Epiploic appendage infarction	Primary peritonitis
Foreign body perforation of the bowel	Rectus hematoma
Henoch-Schönlein purpura	Regional enteritis
Incarcerated hernia	Renal colic
Intestinal obstruction	Sickle cell disease
Intussusception	Testicular torsion
Myocardial infarction	Typhoid fever
Omental infarction	Volvulus
	Yersinia enterocolitis

HIGH-RISK CLINICAL SITUATIONS

PREGNANCY

Appendicitis occurs as frequently in the pregnant as in the nonpregnant woman, and with about equal frequency in each trimester.[9] The features of appendicitis in pregnancy are similar to those found in women who are not pregnant.[10] The emergency physician must not be misled by the presence of the pregnancy into ignoring signs and symptoms that would not be ignored in the nonpregnant patient. Two factors make the diagnosis of appendicitis more difficult in pregnancy. First, the appendix is lifted cephalad and pushed laterally and posteriorly by the gravid uterus in the second and third trimesters, and may cause right flank or right upper quadrant pain mimicking pyelonephritis or cholecystitis, both of which are common in pregnancy (see Fig. 49–2). Irritation of the anterior parietal peritoneum may not be present if a large uterus lies between the inflamed appendix and the anterior abdominal wall. Second, some findings occur in both appendicitis and pregnancy. Nausea and vomiting are common in early pregnancy. The physiologic leukocytosis of pregnancy may mimic the leukocytosis of the acute inflammatory response, although it does not have the relative increase in granulocytes and immature cells.

APPENDICITIS IN CHILDREN AND THE ELDERLY

Appendicitis is less common in preschool children and the elderly than in adolescents and young adults. The rapid rate of perforation of acute appendicitis at the extremes of age, however makes it even more important to recognize.[11]

In the very young, diagnosis is hampered by the lack of symptoms and confusion with common gastrointestinal infections. Reluctance to extend the right hip is an infrequent clue that the problem is located in the right iliac fossa.[12]

Although appendicitis is uncommon in the elderly, it represents a substantial cause of acute abdominal pain.[13] The same findings occur in the elderly with appendicitis as in younger patients, but often in a milder form.[14] The findings in an elderly patient therefore seem less impressive than in a younger patient with the same disease. In the elderly, the differential diagnosis must be expanded to consider diverticulitis, carcinoma with obstruction and/or perforation, leaking aortic aneurysm, and mesenteric ischemia.

IMMUNOCOMPROMISED PATIENTS

Patients who are immunocompromised because of chronic steroid therapy, chemotherapy, or disease represent a diagnostic challenge. These patients may be unable to mount a competent immune response, and the usual signs of infection such as fever and elevated leukocyte counts may be late in appearing. The differential diagnoses are also much broader. They vary with the specific co-morbid disease.[15,16] Appendicitis is not common in these patients, with the possible exception of children with leukemia.[16,17] When it occurs, it is frequently advanced, with gangrene and perforation.[16]

Diabetes is associated not only with an altered immune response, but with both somatic and visceral sensory neuropathy. It has been suggested that diabetic patients with appendicitis present with pain that is atypical or unusually mild for their degree of illness.[18] Diabetic patients may have a higher probability of perforation as well as a greater risk from septic complications once the appendix has perforated. Uncontrolled diabetic ketoacidosis can cause abdominal pain and can also result from appendicitis or other

causes of peritonitis. The physician must sometimes consider whether the abdominal pain is the cause or the result of the ketoacidosis, although this dilemma usually occurs with peritonitis, not early acute appendicitis.

The acquired immune deficiency syndrome (AIDS) has dramatically changed the practice of emergency medicine in many areas. Abdominal pain is common in these patients, and the causes are various; most do not require operation.[19] Appendicitis appears to be as common as in other populations, and operation is the usual treatment.[20] Too few cases have been reported to assess how its presentation in AIDS patients differs from that in others.

THE CLINICAL DECISION

The optimal treatment of appendicitis requires appendectomy before perforation, if possible. Patients with other diseases, particularly those associated with inflammation in the right lower quadrant of the abdomen, can have signs, symptoms, and laboratory findings identical to those of patients with appendicitis. Even characteristic findings on imaging studies, such as appendiceal fecaliths, do not guarantee the presence of appendicitis. At best, the diagnosis is an estimate of the probability of appendicitis in a group with similar findings. Both subjective estimates and mathematical models require adjustments for the prevalence or prior expectation of appendicitis versus the alternatives, such as gastroenteritis and salpingitis, and adjustments for the stage of the disease at the time of the examination.[2,21]

Assuming that the clinician recognizes the possibility of appendicitis, the clinical decision is whether the patient, who might have appendicitis or might not, should have an appendectomy or be treated non-

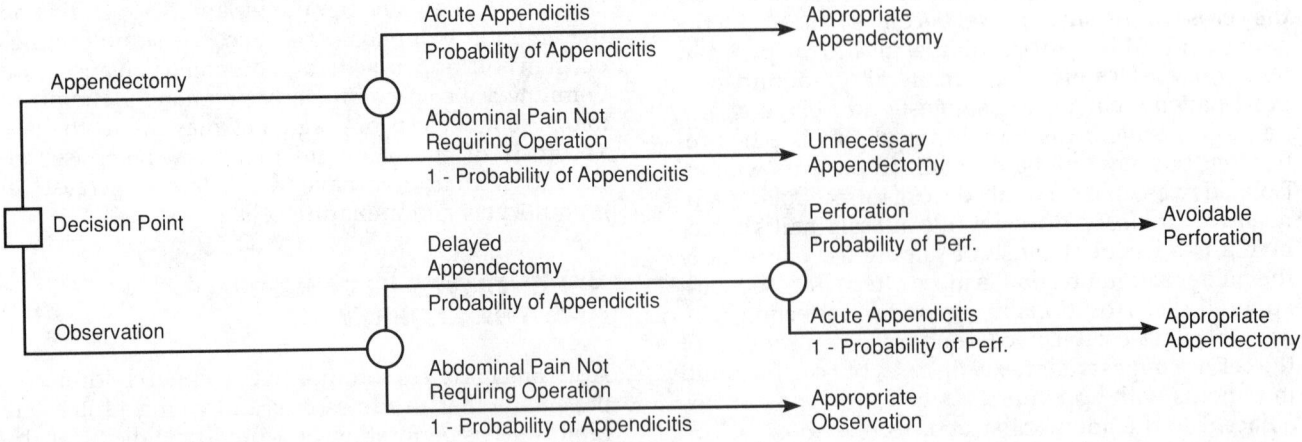

FIG. 49-3. The clinical dilemma represented as a decision tree. The path taken at the circular node is unknown at the time that the decision must be made and is represented by a probability.

operatively (Fig. 49–3). If appendectomy is chosen, it may turn out to be appropriate or, in retrospect, unnecessary if the patient does not have a surgical disease. If the patient is managed nonoperatively instead, the assumption is that patients with conditions not requiring surgery will improve.

If the patient has a disease requiring surgery and surgery is delayed, the condition may deteriorate. For most surgically treated conditions, including perforated appendicitis, the state of the disease is obvious from the clinical state of the patient as monitored during observation. A notable exception is appendicitis, when the silent perforation of an inflamed appendix increases the patient's risk without dramatic heralding signs. (The transient diminution of pain with perforation is perhaps more commonly described than observed.)

The emphasis on removing an appendix when it is inflamed is to avoid the more serious problem of perforated appendix. Delay increases the possibility that acute appendicitis may convert to a perforated appendix, with a dramatic increase in morbidity and mortality rates. Therefore, the trade-off decision is between unnecessarily treating self-limited and nonsurgical conditions with appendectomy or missing opportunities to treat acute appendicitis before it perforates.[22] For the surgeon, this decision is between operating and observing the patient. The decision depends on the relative probabilities of appendicitis and perforation and the relative risks of an avoidable perforation and an unnecessary appendectomy.[2,1]

For the emergency physician, the decision is between calling a surgical consultation and discharging the patient with close outpatient followup. Obviously, the threshold probability of appendicitis that should provoke the emergency physician to call for a surgical consultation is lower than the probability of appendicitis that should provoke a surgeon to perform an appendectomy, because the disadvantages of inappropriate surgical consultation are less than the disadvantages of unnecessary appendectomy and the increased risk of perforation during outpatient observation is, by necessity, greater than that during a more intense observation in the hospital.

The probability that the patient will perforate during a period of observation depends, of course, on how long the patient has had the pain. To an even greater extent, it depends on the age of the patient.[11] For given durations of pain, the lowest perforation rates occur in young adults, but the rates dramatically increase in the very young and the elderly (Table 49–4). For instance, only one in eight 20 year-olds with early appendicitis have a perforation the next day, but over half of 5-year-olds and over two-thirds of 60-year-olds develop a perforation within 24 hours. Because the rate of perforation is higher at the extremes of age, the probability of an avoidable perforation during a period of observation is also higher. Therefore, the threshold probability of appendicitis that activates an interest in surgical treatment should be lower in these patients to maintain the balance between the numbers of overreactions and avoidable delays.

In a pregnant patient, the trade-off remains one between the hazards of unnecessary appendectomy

TABLE 49-4. AVERAGE HOURLY PERFORATION RATES AND OVERALL PROBABILITIES OF PERFORATION ESTIMATED FOR INFLAMED APPENDICES DURING 12-HOUR OBSERVATION PERIODS*

| Age in years | Duration of pain at the start of the observation period | | | |
	12 hrs	24 hrs	36 hrs	48 hrs
5	2.9 %/hr. (0.35)	2.6 %/hr. (0.32)	2.1 %/hr. (0.26)	1.7 %/hr. (0.20)
10	0.9 %/hr. (0.11)	1.1 %/hr. (0.13)	1.0 %/hr. (0.12)	0.9 %/hr. (0.11)
20	0.5 %/hr. (0.06)	0.6 %/hr. (0.07)	0.6 %/hr. (0.07)	0.6 %/hr. (0.07)
30	0.7 %/hr. (0.08)	0.8 %/hr. (0.09)	0.8 %/hr. (0.09)	0.7 %/hr. (0.08)
40	1.2 %/hr. (0.15)	1.4 %/hr. (0.16)	1.3 %/hr. (0.15)	1.1 %/hr. (0.13)
50	2.5 %/hr. (0.29)	2.3 %/hr. (0.28)	1.9 %/hr. (0.23)	1.6 %/hr. (0.19)
60	4.1 %/hr. (0.49)	3.3 %/hr. (0.39)	2.5 %/hr. (0.30)	1.9 %/hr. (0.23)
70	5.3 %/hr. (0.63)	3.8 %/hr. (0.46)	2.8 %/hr. (0.33)	2.0 %/hr. (0.24)

* Based on the patient's age and the duration of pain at the start and end of the observation period as described by Koepsell et al.[11] and Clarke.[22] The overall probability of perforation is the estimated probability that an appendix that is inflamed at the start of the period will be perforated at the end. For two 12-hour periods, the probability equals $P1 + [(1 - P1) \times P2]$.

and the hazards of avoidable perforation. Both the mother and the fetus must be considered. For the mother, the risks of unnecessary appendectomy are comparable to those of a nonpregnant woman. There is a risk of increased fetal loss with laparotomy. Perforation is of even greater concern for the mother during the later stages of pregnancy, but the stresses of perforation increases fetal loss throughout all stages of pregnancy.[23] Overall, as with the extremely young and elderly, pregnancy should make the physician more likely to recommend appendectomy rather than more hesitant.

Ancillary tests should be done only if any of the possible results would change the probability of appendicitis enough to change the choice of management.

ANCILLARY DIAGNOSTIC TESTS

Because there are essentially no definitive diagnostic tests for appendicitis, the diagnosis remains one based on consideration of all the results of the clinical investigation. The results of diagnostic tests are no more important than any finding from the history or physical examination. The role of diagnostic tests in cases that remain ambiguous after the bedside examination is based on three strategies: (1) to confirm the presence of a bacterial infection, (2) to exclude diagnoses other than appendicitis from the differential list, and (3) to attempt to image an inflamed appendix.[24]

The results of the white blood cell (WBC) count may affect the estimated probability of appendicitis, but are no more influential than any other diagnostic finding.[25] Classically, patients have WBC counts between 12,000 and 18,000 per mm_3 with acute appendicitis and 15,000 to 25,000 with perforated appendicitis. WBC counts, however, can be normal or even low. An increased percentage of granulocytes (over 75%) and a shift to immature band forms are also typical, but not pathognomonic. The findings themselves are indicative only of a response to bacterial infection, not to appendicitis per se, and are abnormal with other conditions also. Patients having none of these findings are less likely to have appendicitis.

The urinalysis may be helpful in diagnosing urinary tract diseases. An inflamed appendix lying near the urinary tract may result in red and/or white cells in the urine, but not in large amounts.[26] Bacteria should not be expected in patients with appendicitis, assuming that the specimen has not been contaminated by vaginal or other exogenous organisms.

The visualization of an appendiceal fecalith helps document the presence of cause of obstruction and inflammation of the appendix (Fig. 49–4). Most fecaliths, however, are not radiopaque. The likelihood of discovering a radiopaque fecalith even in patients

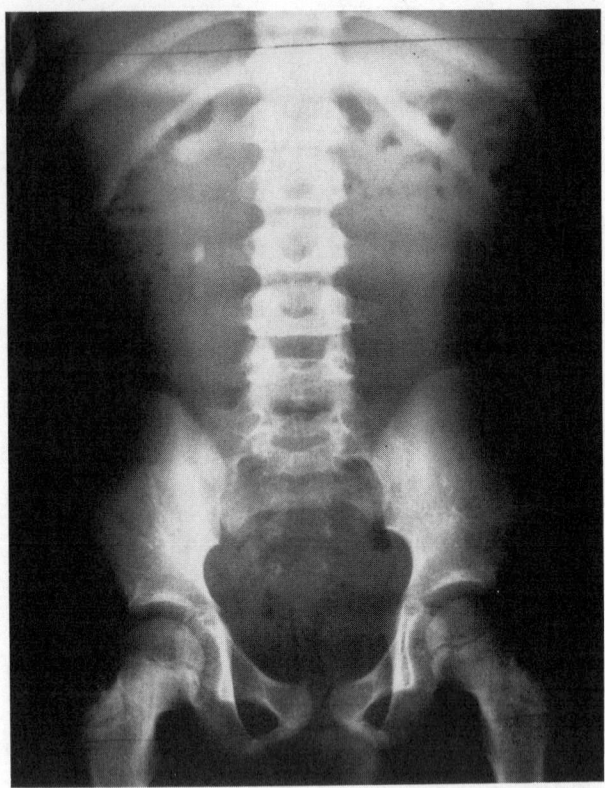

FIG. 49-4. Multiple radiopaque fecaliths in the appendix of an 8 year-old child with acute appendicitis. The oval appearance of the fecaliths is typical. The classic lamination cannot be appreciated. One fecalith is the norm; two are seen occasionally. The usual position is over the right ilium. Appendiceal fecaliths can be in the vicinity of, and be confused with, stones in the right ureter or, as in this case, the gallbladder.

with appendicitis is too low to justify routine use of abdominal roentgenograms to find them.[27] If abdominal roentgenograms are obtained in the evaluation of a patient with abdominal pain, the most common finding associated with appendicitis is local ileus in the right lower quadrant. A soft tissue density in the right lower quadrant, obliteration of either the right flank stripe or psoas shadow, or lumbar scoliosis caused by muscle spasm related to a local inflammatory process are also sometimes seen.[28] None of these findings is specific for appendicitis. Intraperitoneal air is unusual with perforated appendices, unlike perforations of other parts of the gastrointestinal tract, probably because of the proximal obstruction of the small lumen.[29] The greatest usefulness of abdominal roentgenograms is in confirming other suspected conditions.[30]

Many imaging techniques have been used over the years to try to diagnose appendicitis.

Barium enema has been recommended for the diagnosis of appendicitis, perhaps more by radiologists than by surgeons.[30,31] In principle, an appendix that fills to the tip is said to be normal; one that does not is suspected of being obstructed. Between 5 and 10% of normal appendices do not fill completely, however, and cases of appendices that filled "completely" yet proved to be perforated have been reported.[32,33] A barium enema would not usually be part of the emergency center evaluation.[31]

Several of the newer imaging techniques have been proposed as potentially helpful in diagnosing appendicitis, including ultrasound, computed tomography (CT), and the technetium-99m-albumin-colloid leukocyte (TAC) scan. Like its predecessors and no doubt its successors, the TAC scan is not useful in emergency center management of patients with abdominal pain. It does not discriminate well between inflammations of the appendix and the adjacent adnexal structures and it takes too long (up to 5 hours).[34] CT is poor at diagnosing the unruptured appendix and is not helpful in making a disposition in the emergency center.[35] The patient whose phlegmon or periappendiceal abscess is well delineated by CT will have a clinical examination that clearly warrants surgical evaluation.

Ultrasound shows more promise as a technique to improve emergency center diagnosis (Fig. 49–5). Experience with this test has accumulated in recent years, and criteria for diagnosis are evolving.[36–38] Ultrasound has the advantages of being rapid, noninvasive, and capable of being done at the bedside. Its disadvantages are its dependence on the technique of the operator and the current inexperience of most emergency physicians with the modality. Sometimes its use is thwarted by the presence of overlying bowel gas. The reported accuracy of this test varies among investigators, depending in part on the patient population studied, the diameter of the appendix considered to indicate abnormality, and the ultrasonic equipment used; the best results have been obtained with high frequency (5 to 7.5 mHz) probes. Although its role has not been fully defined, it appears that ultrasound may be useful in excluding appendicitis in the patient with abdominal pain without peritoneal signs. In these cases, its specificity has been reported to be between 95 and 100%.[36–38] It may also be useful to identify other sources of pathology such as ileitis, mesenteric adenitis, perforated viscous, and gynecologic complaints.[36,39] Its greatest usefulness is probably in women of child-bearing years because of its ability to also evaluate the gynecologic alternatives. Ultrasound is a tool with potentially wide applicability in emergency medicine beyond the diagnosis of appendicitis, and waits only for emergency physicians to gain more confidence in its use.

MANAGEMENT

The diagnosis of appendicitis is based primarily on information from the history and physical examination. After assessment of this information, the physician should estimate the probability that the patient has appendicitis. Considering the probability that an inflamed appendix would perforate and the relative risk of unnecessary appendectomy and avoidable perforation, the physician should decide whether the probability of appendicitis is low enough to justify sending the patient home for followup 12 to 24 hours later, high enough to justify surgical attention, or at an intermediate level where the results of further tests and a repeat follow-up examination would influence the probability enough to affect the final decision. Ancillary tests take time, particularly in a busy emergency center. The extra time may elicit further information, but may add to the delay in removing an inflamed appendix.

Until a decision is made to treat the patient for appendicitis or another disease, medication that might influence the patient's clinical appearance during observation should not be given.

Analgesics should be deferred until after a decision is made to treat the patient for a specific condition. Antibiotics should not be given until the decision is made to treat the patient for a condition that requires antibiotics. Antimetics are generally not necessary because vomiting is not the major component of the disease. For the rare patient with persistent vomiting, decompression of the stomach with a nasogastric tube is more appropriate. Laxatives, cathartics, and enemas should not be given to patients in whom the diagnosis of appendicitis is being considered. Patients should not be given anything by mouth during the period of intense observation, but should be given intravenous fluids to maintain or restore their fluid balance.

It may be necessary to reduce the fever and attendent high oxygen consumption, before the induction of anesthesia, with antipyretics and other means, but this should be a problem only with the more obvious perforated appendix.

Once the decision is made to do an appendectomy, antibiotics may be given as prophylactic adjuvant therapy. The incidence of septic complications is reduced in patients with gangrenous and perforated appendices receiving antibiotic prophylaxis prior to appendectomy.[40] Our practice is to give patients a single dose of antibiotics to have prophylactic levels at the time of operation and to continue usage if the appendix is gangrenous or perforated at exploration. The antibiotic agent chosen should be one with good activity against the anaerobes and gram-negative aerobes that populate the gut, particularly Bacteroides fragilis and enterococci.[40,41]

PITFALLS

Appendicitis is a common cause of abdominal pain. Even though it is less common in the very young and elderly, it should be thought of as a cause of acute abdominal pain in

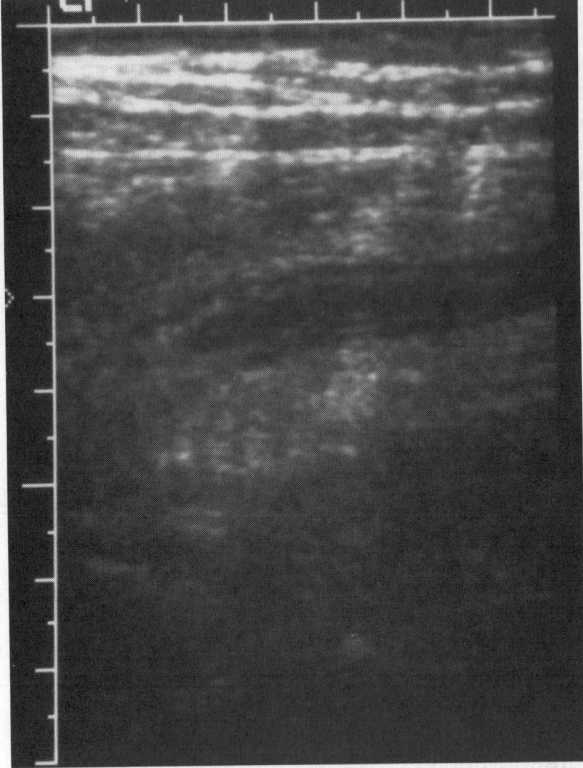

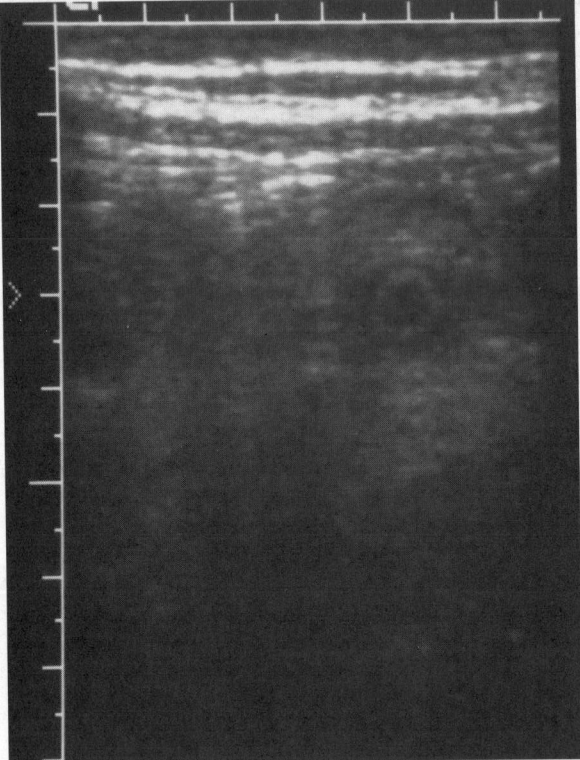

FIG. 49-5. An appendix that can be visualized by ultrasound usually leads to a diagnosis of appendicitis on laparotomy. Radiologists appreciate that the larger the diameter of the appendix, the more likely it is to be diseased. This inflamed appendix was captured on both longitudinal (A) and transverse (B) views. The characteristic bullseye or target image is seen on the latter.

these age groups. It occurs with its usual frequency in women who are pregnant and people with AIDS. It may be the source of uncontrolled diabetic ketoacidosis with sepsis.

Atypical presentations of this common condition are hardly rare. The elderly may have attenuated findings. Women in childbearing years need a pelvic examination to make an accurate assessment. Signs of local peritonitis in a pregnant patient may be moved or covered by a large uterus. Patients taking corticosteroids may not exhibit findings that require an inflammatory response.

No findings or tests are pathognomonic. Ancillary diagnostic tests may add delay rather than influence opinion.

Higher rates of perforation in the very young and elderly mandate more aggressive, not less aggressive, management of possible appendicitis in the extremes of age. The greater consequences of perforation during pregnancy also dictate relatively more emphasis on avoiding a perforation.

Obervation of the patient with possible appendicitis should not be confounded by the administration of analgesics, antibiotics, or laxatives, enemas, or cathartics.

MEDICOLEGAL PEARLS

The decision to implement surgical treatment or to observe a patient with possible appendicitis is a trade-off decision. The legal liability seems greatest when the appendix is found perforated after a period of nonoperative management.[42] The alternative is to advise too many unnecessary appendectomies. In the author's opinion, the best legal protection for physicians is (1) to carefully document all the clinical findings that influenced the decision, (2) for each alternative management option, to indicate an assessment of the relative likelihood and probable consequences of each possible outcome that might occur, and (3) to ensure followup within a time appropriate for the rate at which the appendix might perforate, if it is inflamed.

HORIZONS

Appendicitis is decreasing in incidence for obscure reasons that may relate to diet, and the risks of a perforated appendix are decreasing as our ability to treat septic patients improves.[43]

Attempts to see signs of inflammation localized to the appendix on imaging studies have historically had more promise than accuracy. Newer ultrasonographic devices currently offer the most potential. Experimental work has documented that the tissue characteristics of the inflamed appendix can be distinguished from those of the normal appendix using nuclear magnetic resonance.[44] Because the normal appendix can be imaged by magnetic resonance imaging, MRI may provide an accurate, if not practical, image that is not particularly dependent on technique.[45]

Accurate assessment of the probability of appendicitis and the appropriate use of the above and other ancillary tests may be refined by the use of computers to aid in the probabilistic weighing of signs, symptoms, and test results.[2,21]

REFERENCES

1. Brewer, R.J., Golden, G.T., Hitch, D. et al.: Abdominal pain: an analysis of 1,000 consecutive cases in a university hospital emergency room. Am. J. Surg. 131:219, 1976.
2. de Dombal, F.T.: Diagnosis of acute abdominal pain. Edinburgh, Churchill Livingston, 1980.
3. Wangensteen, O.H., and Dennis, C.: Experimental proof of the obstructive origin of appendicitis in man. Ann. Surg. 110:629, 1939.
4. Lewis, F.R., Holcroft, J.W., Boey, J., et al.: Appendicitis: A critical review of diagnosis and treatment in 1,000 cases. Arch. Surg. 110:677, 1975.
5. McBurney, C.: Experience with early operative interference in cases of disease of the veriform appendix. N.Y. Med. J. 50:676, 1889.
6. Lau, W.Y., Fan, S.T., Yiu, T.F. et al.: Negative findings at appendectomy. Am. J. Surg. 148:375, 1984.
7. McDonald, J.C.: Nonspecific mesenteric lymphadenitis. Surg. Gynecol. Obstet. 116:409, 1963.
8. Bongard, F., Landers, D.V., and Lewis, F.: Differential diagnosis of appendicitis and pelvic inflammatory disease. Am. J. Surg. 150:90, 1985.
9. Cunningham, F.G., and McCubbin, J.G.: Appendicitis complicating pregnancy. Obstet. Gynecol. 45:415, 1975.
10. Brant, H.A.: Acute appendicitis in pregnancy. Obstet. Gynecol. 29:130, 1967.
11. Koepsell, T.D., Inui, T.S., and Farewell, V.T.: Factors affecting perforation in acute appendicitis. Surg. Gynecol. Obstet. 153:508, 1981.
12. Daehlin, L.: Acute appendicitis during the first three years of life. Acta. Chir. Scand. 148:291, 1982.
13. Ludbrook, J., and Spears, G.F.S.: The risk of developing appendicitis. Br. J. Surg. 52:856, 1968.
14. Burns, R.P., Cochran, J.L., Russell, W.L., et al.: Appendicitis in mature patients. Ann. Surg. 201:695, 1985.
15. McKenna, R.J., and Bodey, G.P.: "Surgical Considerations in the immunocompromised cancer patient. In Fundamentals of Surgical Oncology. Edited by McKenna, R.J., and Murphy, G.P. New York, Macmillan Publishing Company, pp. 114—1496, 1986.
16. Nylander, W.A.: The acute abdomen in the immunocompromised host. Surg. Clin. North Am. 68:457, 1988.
17. Ver Steeg, K., LaSalle, A., Ratner, I.: Appendicitis in acute leukemia. Arch. Surg. 114:632, 1979.
18. Latchaw, L.A., and Nguyen, L.: Acute appendicitis in diabetic children. Am. J. Dis. Child. 142:1019, 1988.
19. Barone, J.E., Gingold, B.S., Nealon, T.F., et al.: Abdominal pain in patients with acquired immune deficiency syndrome. Ann. Surg. 204:619, 1986.
20. LaRaja, R.D., Rothenberg, R.E., Odom, J.W., et al.: The incidence of intra-abdominal surgery in acquired immunodeficiency syndrome: a statistical review of 904 patients. Surgery 105:175, 1989.
21. Adams, I.D., Chan, M., Clifford, P.C., et al.: Computer aided diagnosis of acute abdominal pain: A multicentre study. Br. Med. J. 293:800, 1986.
22. Clarke, J.R.: A concise model for the managment of possible appendicitis. Med. Decis. Making 4:331, 1984.
23. Masters, K., Levine, B.A., Gaskill, H.V., et al.: Diagnosing appendicitis during pregnancy. Am. J. Surg. 148:768, 1984.
24. Hoffmann, J., Rasmussen, O.O.: Aids in the diagnosis of acute appendicitis. Br. J. Surg. 76:774, 1989.
25. English, D.C., Allen, W., Coppola, E., et al.: Excessive dependence of the leukocyte cue in diagnosing appendicitis. Am. Surg. 43:399, 1977.
26. Kretchmar, L.H., McDonald, D.F.: The urine sediment in acute appendicitis. Arch. Surg. 87:209, 1963.
27. Field, S., Guy, P.J., Upsdell, S.M., et al.: The erect abdominal radiograph in the acute adbomen: Should its routine use be abandoned? Br. Med. J. 290:1934, 1985.
28. Eisenberg, R.L., Heineken, P., Hedgcock, M.W., et al.: Evaluation of plain abdominal radiographs in the diagnosis of abdominal pain. Ann. Surg. 197:464, 1983.
29. Chavez, C.M., and Morgan, B.D.: Acute appendicitis with pneumoperitoneum: Radiographic diagnosis and report of five cases. Am. Surg. 32:604, 1966.
30. Campbell, J.P.M., and Gunn, A.A.: Plain abdominal radiographs and acute abdominal pain. Br. J. Surg. 75:554, 1988.
31. Smith, D.E., Kirchmer, N.A., and Stewart, D.R.: Use of the barium enema in the diagnosis of acute appendicitis and its complications. Am. J. Surg. 38:829, 1979.
32. Dietz, W.W.: Fallacy of the roengenologically negative appendix. JAMA 208:1495, 1969.
33. Sakover, R.P., and del Fava, R.L.: Frequency of visualization of the normal appendix with the barium enema examination. Am. J. Roentgenol. 121:312, 1974.
34. Henneman, P.L., Marcus, C.S., Butler, J.A., et al.: Appendicitis: Evaluation by TC-99m leukocyte scan. Ann. Emerg. Med. 17:111, 1988.
35. Balthazar, E.J., Megibow, A.J., Hulnick, D., et al.: CT of appendicitis, 147:705, 1986.
36. Jeffrey, R.B., Laing, F.C., and Townsend, R.R.: Acute appendicitis: Sonographic criteria based on 250 cases. Radiology 167:327, 1988.
37. Puylaert, J.B.C.M., Rutgers, P.H., Lalisang, R.I., et al.: A prospective study of ultrasonography in the diagnosis of appendicitis. N. Engl. J. Med. 317:666, 1987.
38. Schwerk, W.B., Wichtrup, B., Ruschoff, J., et al.: Acute and perforated appendicitis: current experience with ultrasound-aided diagnosis. World J. Surg. 14:271, 1990.
39. Gaensler, E.H.L., Jeffrey, R. B., Laing, F.C., et al.: Sonography in patients with suspected acute appendicitis: value in establishing alternative diagnoses. Am. J. Roentgenol. 152:49, 1989.
40. Bauer, T., Vennits, B., Holm, B., et al.: Antibiotic prophylaxis in acute nonperforated appendicitis. Ann. Surg. 209:307, 1989.
41. Levin, S., and Goodman, L.J.: Selected overview of nongynecologic surgical intra-abdominal infections: prophylaxis and therapy. Am. J. Med. 79:146, 1985.
42. Trautlein, J.J., Lambert, R., and Miller, J.: Malpractice in the emergency room: a critical review of undiagnosed appendicitis cases and legal actions. Qual. Assur. Util. Rev. 2:54, 1987.
43. Noer, I.: Decreasing incidence of acute appendicitis. Acta Chir. Scand. 141:431, 1975.
44. Jacobs, D.O., Settle, R.G., Clarke, J.R., et al.: Identification of human appendicitis by in vitro nuclear magnetic resonance. J. Surg. Research 48:107, 1990.
45. Kressel, H.Y., Axel, L., Thickman, D., et al.: NMR imgaing of the abdomen at 0.12 T. Am. J. Roentgenol. 141:1179, 1983.

PERFORATED VISCUS

James K. Bouzoukis

CAPSULE

Perforated viscus is a life-threatening emergency. Perforations can occur at any level of the gastrointestinal tract and in any age group, from the fetus in utero to patients over 100 years. Pneumoperitoneum, the radiologic hallmark of a perforated viscus, is not universally present; at times, it may be from extraperitoneal causes. Not all patients can perceive pain, the cardinal symptom of peritonitis. Likewise, the signs of peritonitis present in varying stages and degrees, depending on the patient's age and debility. Emergency physicians must learn to recognize the risk factors for perforation and the various clinical stages of peritonitis. Because mortality rate is directly related to delays in stabilization and definitive therapy (surgery), one must have a high index of suspicion for, and agressively manage, any patient whose differential diagnosis includes perforated intra-abdominal viscus.

INTRODUCTION

The three categories of life-threatening surgical emergencies that involve the gastrointestinal (GI) tract are uncontrollable hemorrhage, obstruction, and perforation.

Uncontrollable GI hemorrhage is not usually associated with pain, but does manifest itself with signs and symptoms of hypovolemic shock. Indeed, patients usually present with some form of overt blood loss, usually hematemesis or hematochezia. The one notable exception to this presentation pattern involves the older, sedentary patient with a hypotonic megacolon into which a significant amount of blood may accumulate before it is excreted. These patients do have signs and symptoms of hypovolemic shock, including a positive tilt test. Although emergent surgery is not always necessary, early surgical consultation is mandatory.

Bowel obstruction, the second surgical GI emergency, invariably presents with abdominal pain and vomiting; neurologically compromised patients may not be able to perceive pain, however. The physiologic derangements from bowel obstruction include significant fluid loss, both intraluminally from sequestering

and externally from vomiting with resultant dehydration, hypovolemic shock, and electrolyte imbalance; and bowel perforation with resultant peritonitis, septic shock, and death. Failure to decompress and surgically relieve bowel obstruction expeditiously results in the third and potentially most devastating of the surgical GI tract emergencies, the perforated viscus.

Perforated viscus is the ultimate complication of bowel obstruction, significantly raising the morbidity and mortality rates of this condition. The mortality rate of patients presenting with peritonitis from perforation of the small or large bowel approximates 50%. In addition, when perforation is associated with bleeding peptic ulcers, as has been reported to have occurred with 9.9% of patients undergoing emergent surgery for uncontrollable bleeding from peptic ulcers, the mortality rate also approaches 50%. On the other hand, a perforation may be spontaneously confined by the body's defenses, obviating the need for surgery or a prolonged hospital stay.

The potential for death from a perforated viscus cannot be ignored. This condition represents a surgical emergency that must be diagnosed and referred to the surgeon for definitive treatment as soon as possible.

PATHOPHYSIOLOGY AND ANATOMY

Considering the amount of stress to which the GI tract is subjected and which it endures during one's lifetime, it is indeed a remarkably durable structure. Considering the numerous and varied factors that potentially predispose to viscus perforation (Table 49–5), it is remarkable that we do not encounter a significantly higher number of bowel perforations than actually occur. Yet, in a recent review of the British and Scandinavian surgical literature, it was noted that intestinal perforation accounted for less than 5% of the final diagnoses of adult patients who had been hospitalized with acute abdominal pain.

ANATOMIC CONSIDERATIONS

To understand better the various mechanisms for intestinal perforation, one needs to consider the anatomy and physiology of the GI tract. In essence, the GI tract is a muscular, tubular structure into which all ingested foodstuff and other foreign bodies must en-

TABLE 49-5. FACTORS PREDISPOSING TO VISCUS PERFORATION

DRUG THERAPY
  Corticosteroids
  NSAIDs
    Neonates and fetuses in utero
    Elderly
  Cocaine (orally, intranasally)
  Chemotherapeutic agents
  Immunosuppressive therapy
  Interleukin-2
  Enteric-coated KCL
  Ferrous sulfate
  Mannitol (oral)
  Bicarbonate of soda
  Tolazoline (priscoline)
IATROGENIC PROCEDURES
  Endoscopic procedures
    Gastroscopy (esophago/gastroscopy)
    Duodenoscopy
    Sigmoidoscopy (rigid or flexible scope)
    Colonoscopy
      Intracolonic biopsy/polypectomy
      Laparoscopy
      Retrograde cholangiography
  Intraluminal devices
    Biliary endoprosthesis
    Linton-Nachlas balloon tube
  Barium enema
  V-P shunt catheter
  Lumbar discectomy
  Percutaneous nephrolithotomy
  S/P intra-abdominal operative trauma
INFLAMMATORY/METABOLIC
  Peptic ulcer disease
  Crohn's disease
  Ulcerative colitis
  Aortointestinal fistula
  Eosinophilic granuloma
INTRA-ABDOMINAL INFECTIONS
  Ascaris lumbricoides
  Cytomegalovirus
  Necrotizing enterocolitis
  Streptococcus enteriditis—group D
  Typhoid enteritis
  Yersinia enterocolitis
  Pelvic abscess
MALIGNANCIES
  Intrinsic
    Primary carcinoma of:
      Colon
      Stomach
      Small intestine

  Small bowel lymphoma
  Extrinsic
    Carcinoma of:
      Ovary
      Cervix
      Uterus
    Hodgkin's lymphoma
  Metastatic
    Lung carcinoma
MECHANICAL
  Congenital
    Idiopathic perforations of neonates
    Intestinal tract (prematurity and postnatal distress)
    Stomach, small intestine, and/or colon
  Diverticulosis
    Marfan's syndrome
    Ehlers-Danlos syndrome
    Polycystic kidney disease
  Herniae (strangulated)
  Meconium ileus
  Megacolon
  Acquired
    Diverticulosis
    Gallstone perforations
    Mechanical ventilation
    Megacolon (elderly)
    Strangulated intestine
      Adhesive bands
      Closed loop obstruction
      Intussusception
      Pseudo-obstruction of colon
      Volvulus
  Ingested
    Dental metals
    Dose blister packs
    Fishbones
    Pins
    Toothpicks
    Trichobezoars
    Scybalous feces (stercoral ulcers)
VASCULAR COMPROMISE
  Acute mesenteric insufficiency
    Embolic arterial occlusion
    Mesenteric artery thrombosis
    Mesenteric vein thrombosis
    Nonocclusive disease
  Cocaine abuse
  Necrotizing enterocolitis
  Polyarteritis nodosa
  Systemic lupus erythematosus

ter, undergo mechanical and chemical (enzymatic) digestion, absorption, and metabolic assimilation, all while being mechanically propelled and ultimately excreted. In addition to digesting and metabolizing pounds of solid food each day, the jejunum, ileum, and colon may have to absorb passively up to 9000 mL of water provided by exogenous and upper intestinal sources.

The gastrointestinal tract generically consists of the following structures: mucosa, submucosa, inner circular layer of muscles, outer longitudinal layer of muscles, and an investing serosa.

The mucosa is where virtually all of the metabolic action takes place. The mucosal villi result in an an-anatomic configuration that enables the mucosa to have an extensive surface area over which absorption and assimilation can take place. Mucosal cells are among the most rapidly proliferating groups of cells in the body; it has been estimated that these cells reproduce themselves every 48 hours, thus necessitating a continuous, large supply of blood, nutriments, and energy. The intestinal lymph follicles that react to infection and/or inflammation are situated in the mucosa throughout the GI tract, but tend to be more

TABLE 49-6. RISK FACTORS FOR PERFORATED VISCUS

History of peptic ulcer disease (cigarette smokers)
NSAID therapy (neonates and elderly)
Immunocompromised patients
    Long-term steroid therapy
    Chemotherapy
Acquired megacolon (nursing home/institutionalized patients)
Recent GI instrumentation
    BE in the elderly
Ingestion of sharp-tipped foreign bodies

concentrated in the distal ileum. Surrounding the mucosa are the submucosal structures, which contain a rich plexus of blood vessels necessary to supply the metabolically hyperactive mucosal cells. The presence of these vessels and connective tissue makes the submucosal layer the anatomically strongest layer (from a surgical standpoint) of the intestinal wall. The muscle walls surround these mucosal structures with two layers of muscles: the inner-circular layer, which exists as a well developed muscular layer throughout the intestinal tract, and the outer longitudinal layer, which is better developed in the more muscular small bowel than it is in the more distended large bowel, where it exists as isolated bands situated along the circumference of the circular muscle layer.

The entire intestinal tract is surrounded by a layer of mesothelium which, in essence, is the visceral peritoneum. That portion investing bowel is referred to as its serosa, and it is in continuity with the meso of the intestinal tract, between whose layers course the neurovascular supply to the gut.

All blood vessels to the intra-abdominal intestinal tract are branches of the celiac, superior mesenteric, and inferior mesenteric branches of the abdominal aorta, which course along the mesothelium of the bowel. The intestinal branches pass within the serosal layer and penetrate through the muscular wall to the submucosal layer, where a rich vascular plexus is formed, providing nutrient branches to all components of the intestinal wall. The autonomic nerves, which accompany the mesenteric vessels, form their myenteric plexuses, providing motor and sensory function to the bowel. The perception of visceral pain is caused only by stretching (traction, torsion, and distention) or ischemia of these nerve endings.

The final anatomic considerations that serve to explain certain of the causes of viscus perforation are the relative mobility and immobility of different segments of the intestinal tract. The duodenum, which is adherent to the posterior abdominal wall by its short, broad meso, has minimal mobility and hence is subject to perforation by ingested long, sharp objects that cannot negotiate its rather sharp curves. Sharp objects, such as toothpicks and pins, have been known to penetrate into the right kidney through the posterior wall of the duodenum. One consolation of posterior

fixation with a short, wide mesothelium is that posterior perforations are walled off by the subjacent structures and are not likely to cause disseminated peritonitis. The remainder of the small bowel and much of the colon, on the other hand, have a relatively elongated, narrow mesothelium, which results in more bowel motion and mobility. Such an anatomic arrangement, however, enables the bowel to twist on itself (its own mesothelium) or adhesive bands resulting in volvulus, internal herniation, or intussusception.

PATHOPHYSIOLOGY OF PERFORATION

Table 49–6 summarizes most of the known risk factors associated with viscus perforation. Although these factors may appear varied and unrelated, the underlying cause of perforation appears to be the result of either (a) mechanical disruption secondary to direct trauma or from a pre-existing mechanical weakness or (b) loss of blood supply to the intestinal wall from either direct occlusion of the blood supply to the intestine or an indirect compromise of blood supply secondary to inflammatory and mechanical factors.

Whenever mechanical obstruction of the bowel occurs, there is initially a reflex increase of intraluminal fluid secretion and a decrease of fluid absorption by the more distal, distending bowel. In addition, there is an increase of intraluminal gas that is derived predominantly by swallowed air and, to a lesser extent, from gas-forming bacteria, particularly in the colon. Significant gaseous distention of the bowel occurs in adults being ventilated by bag-mask and in infants and children in whom noncuffed endotracheal tubes are used for ventilation unless there is adequate decompression of the stomach by means of nasogastric tubes. Laplace's law states that in a tubular structure, wall tension is the product of the intraluminal pressure times the radius (or diameter) times π. Thus, in the case of a distal obstruction of the colon that has a competent ileocecal valve, tension is proportionally greater (intramural pressure) on the wall of the cecum, which is normally two to three times greater in diameter, than that of the more distal colon, even though the intraluminal pressure of this segment of bowel is the same throughout. Because wall tension exceeds venous pressure, interstitial edema increases and fluid absorption from the lumen decreases further. As intraluminal pressure and wall tension exceed capillary perfusion pressure, tissue hypoxia, cellular death, focal gangrene, and perforation occur. In bowel obstruction, the larger the diameter of the obstructed bowel, the greater the risk of perforation. In cases of strangulation obstruction in which there is a sudden occlusion of the blood supply to the bowel, perforation is obviously related to ischemia and not to the degree of bowel distension.

Diverticula, which can occur in any part of the GI tract, represent a greater risk for perforation because their stomas are more easily occluded and their limited blood supply more easily compromised by either internal or external pressures. The diverticula that occur in the colon of adults are actually pseudodiverticula. They represent subserosal protrusion of mucosa and submucosa that have herniated through the muscle layers of the intestinal wall, probably along the course of penetrating blood vessels. Indeed, these blood vessels become included in the diverticular pouch and are susceptible to erosion (lower GI hemorrhage) or occlusion (perforation of "tics"). Almost 50% of Americans and Western Europeans over age 60 are found to have colonic diverticula, and this appears to be associated with the low roughage in the Western dietary habits. (In third-world countries, there is a significantly lower incidence of colonic diverticula, but this incidence is increasing in their urban population, for whom there is less dietary fiber.) In the pediatric population, diverticulosis is associated with Marfan's and Ehlers-Danlos syndromes. Over 80% of patients with polycystic kidney disease have diverticulosis and hence represent a definite risk for intestinal perforation.

It is known that certain prostaglandins (E and A) not only inhibit pepsin formation and gastric acid secretion but also enhance mucus secretion in both the stomach and the small intestine. It is small wonder, therefore, that use of nonsteroidal anti-inflammatory drugs (NSAIDs), including aspirin, and corticosteroids, all of which inhibit prostaglandin formation, can be associated with increased incidence of peptic ulcer formation and perforation. The incidence of peptic ulcer perforation with the use of NSAIDs appears to be greater at the extremes of life. Fetal bowel perforation has been associated with maternal use of these drugs, and neonatal bowel perforation has been associated with the use of intravenous indomethacin for the treatment of patent ductus arteriosus. Furthermore, an increasing incidence of upper GI hemorrhage and perforations is associated with the use of NSAIDs by patients over 75 years. (Fig. 49–6). (Presumably, this is related to older patients' impaired ability to regenerate mucosa being eroded by the effects of these drugs.)

Likewise, it should be noted that any drugs, treatment regimens, or extended periods of high stress (e.g., extensive burns, major surgery) that interfere with the body's ability to regenerate intestinal mucosa cause an increased incidence of intestinal ulceration and perforation. In an 11-year review from the Sloan-Kettering Institute, there were 31 episodes of "spontaneous" bowel perforation in 30 patients receiving therapy for various malignancies. Seventy-seven percent of these patients had been on corticosteroids alone or in combination with other drugs; 23% of the patients were on chemotherapy alone. Forty-five percent of the perforations involved the small bowel and 55% involved the large bowel; of these, only 52% had malignancy at the perforation site. The operative mortality for these patients was 53%.

Finally, it should be pointed out that, because of the rich lymphatic supply in the deep mucosal layers, particularly of the terminal ileum, any infectious, inflammatory, or neoplastic process that causes destruction or proliferation of intestinal lymphatic tissue can result in compromise of the intramural blood supply

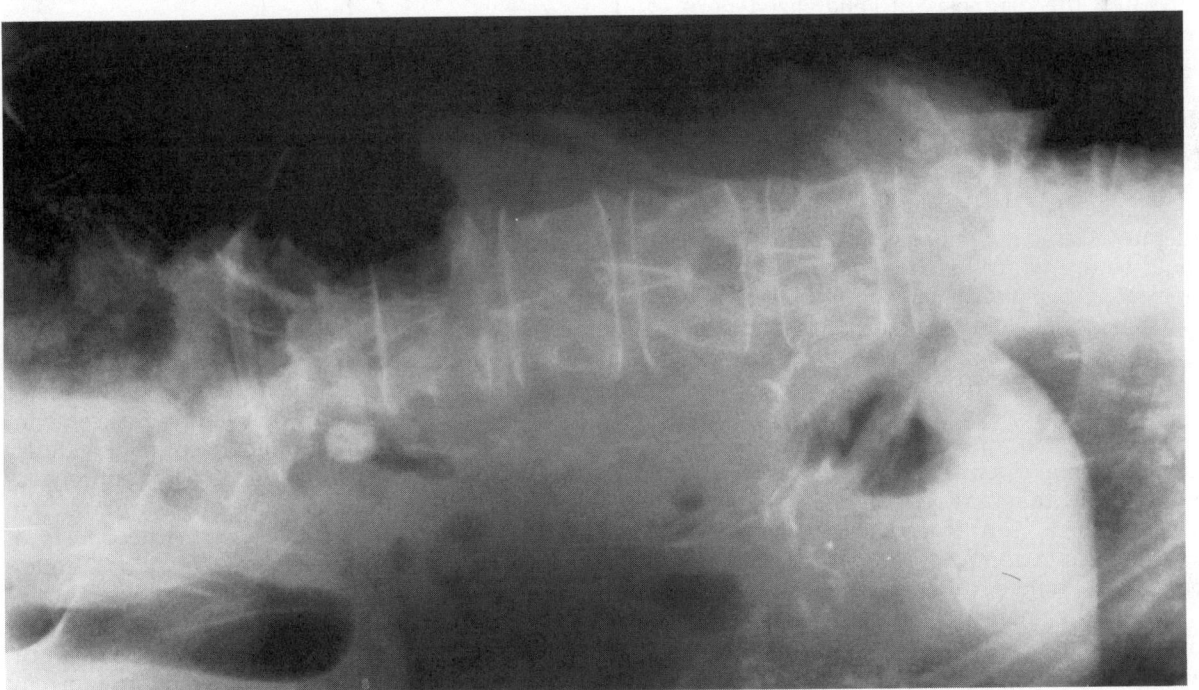

FIG. 49-6.   An 84-year-old woman on NSAIDs for arthritis presented after 2 days of abdominal pain, anorexia, and vomiting. Lateral decubitus film, taken because the patient could not be positioned upright, reveals a massive amount of free air.

and cause bowel perforation. Such may be the mechanism of perforation for the intestinal infections listed in Table 49–5, particularly typhoid enteritis. Further, it has been reported that anywhere from one half to two thirds of all cases of small bowel lymphoma present as small bowel perforations.

PREHOSPITAL ASSESSMENT AND STABILIZATION

The prehospital assessment and stabilization of a patient with a perforated viscus depend on the cause, age, and location of the perforation, as well as the age and debility of the patient. With confined perforations or during the early stages of a free perforation, patients may only have vague and not apparently life-threatening signs or symptoms. Such patients are usually transported to the Emergency Department (ED) by either private automobile or basic life support (BLS) transport. It then becomes a challenge to the triage nurse and the emergency physician to determine if these patients with vague, nonspecific abdominal complaints may have a life-threatening problem.

Patients who mainfest overt signs of peritonitis caused by either chemical irritation (as occurs with a perforated peptic ulcer) or bacterial proliferation may be in extreme distress, manifesting early signs of shock. Although the diagnosis of generalized peritonitis secondary to perforated viscus may not be readily apparent to the first responders, it should be obvious that these patients are experiencing some intra-abdominal catastrophe for which expeditious treatment is appropriate. These patients should be assessed and initially stabilized by paramedics if they are available. An IV should be established using a moderate to large bore needle, and blood specimens should be drawn for hematologic assessments including clotting functions, chemistries, and type and crossmatch. Crystalloid solution such as lactated Ringer's solution should be administered at the rate of approximately 150 to 200 mL per hour to these patients, who are invariably tachycardic and tachypneic from their peritonitis. If the patient manifests signs of shock such as a narrowed pulse pressure or actual hypotension, then a fluid challenge of 250 to 500 mL (20 mL per kg for the pediatric patient) followed by a more rapid administration of fluid (200 to 250 mL per hour) should be initiated while the patient is transported to the nearest, most appropriate ED.

To patients who have a more severe peritonitis and are tachypneic and tachycardic, it is appropriate to administer supplemental oxygen while they are en route to the hospital. Oxygen therapy should definitely be continued as part of the treatment of impending shock.

It is neither necessary nor appropriate for prehospital personnel to administer parenteral narcotics unless the transport time will exceed 20 minutes. Not only may the administration of narcotics obfuscate the physical findings and hence delay the diagnosis of peritonitis, but there is also a good chance that the patient may begin vomiting, and it would not be known if the vomiting were a side effect of the drug or caused by underlying disease process. Furthermore, narcotics can compound the effects of hypovolemic and/or septic shock.

Prehospital use of narcotics, therefore, should be restricted and used only for patients with severe abdominal pain who are not mainfesting signs of shock and whose transport time will be greater than 20 minutes. In such cases, base control physicians may order paramedics to administer small doses of meperidine intravenously only after they have documented the patient's vital signs and have assessed carefully and documented the physical examination of the patient's abdomen, including the status of guarding, rebound tenderness, and presence of bowel sounds. Under no circumstance should patients presenting with signs and symptoms of an acute abdomen be given anything by mouth. In addition, the use of Nitronox is contraindicated because the inhaled or ingested nitrogen worsens the ileus that invariably occurs with bowel obstruction or perforated viscus.

CLINICAL PRESENTATION AND EXAMINATION

The cardinal symptom of patients presenting with perforated viscus is pain. Even though it is not universally present, pain is by far the most important and constant of all symptoms. Its onset may be sudden or gradual and its intensity varies considerably, depending on the cause and location of the perforation. Pain from a perforated peptic ulcer, which occurs most commonly in men in their third through sixth decade of life, is typically explosive in onset and of extreme intensity. Pain from the perforated viscus of an elderly, feeble patient may be barely perceived or entirely absent. Infants, at the other extreme of life, cannot complain of pain but obviously react to the effects of peritoneal irritation. Finally, one should mention those patients who have cord lesions proximal to T-6 and are hence incapable of perceiving the painful stimulus from peritoneal irritation. Shoulder pain referred from peritoneal irritation of the diaphragm may be the only form of pain perceived by these unfortunate patients.

Chemical peritonitis as occurs from a perforated ulcer or gall bladder is extremely irritating and highly symptomatic. On the other hand, spillage from the more distal small bowel and large bowel is not, per se, irritating, and the pain of peritonitis may not develop until the secondary bacterial infection begins to proliferate some time later. Visceral pain from distention of an obstructed loop of bowel may actually be relieved by the perforation and decompression of the distended bowel, which creates a lucid interval between the pain from visceral peritoneal stimulation and that from parietal peritonitis which occurs with the subsequent infection. In spite of all these variations and nuances, however, the patient presenting to the ED with a perforated viscus invariably complains of pain, and it behooves the emergency physician to keep in mind the rare exceptions when a perforated viscus is not initially manifested by pain.

Syncope or near-syncope may occur at the time of initial perforation and has been described as being the initial stage of peritoneal shock. More typically, it is associated with the sudden pain that occurs at the time of perforation of a peptic ulcer and is not caused by hypotension or significant hypovolemia. In the more advanced and late stages of peritonitis, syncope is definitely related to the hypovolemia and hypotension that occurs.

Vomiting is an inconsistent finding with perforated viscus and early peritonitis. Patients whose perforation is confined and does not result in generalized peritonitis may not vomit at all during the course of their illness. When vomiting does occur, it has invariably been preceded by the pain of peritonitis. Initially, vomiting may be slight, but as the peritonitis advances, it becomes persistent and more profuse as the spreading peritonitis causes a paralytic ileus.

Unless the patient has a pre-existing infection or malignancy, or is suffering from one of the collagen diseases, the temperature may not be elevated during the early stages of perforation. At times, during the early stages of an acutely perforated ulcer, the temperature may be subnormal. As secondary peritonitis develops and progresses, patients invariably become febrile. In cases of fulminating peritonitis or the advanced stages of sepsis secondary to peritonitis, the temperature may be subnormal, a grave prognostic sign.

The pulse rate is initially raised, reflecting sympathetic response to the onset of peritonitis. Initially, the pulse rate varies with the symptomatic effects of the perforation. Ultimately, a persistent and progressive tachycardia reflects the progression of hypovolemia and sepsis.

With peritonitis, the respiratory rate is invariably elevated. Because motion aggravates the pain of peritonitis, patients limit the depth of respiration, and breathing becomes more shallow and rapid. The patient reflexly minimizes the diaphragmatic component of respiration. With more advanced stages of peritonitis, tachypnea occurs to compensate for the metabolic acidosis secondary to the intra-abdominal sepsis.

Physical examination of the patient with a perforated viscus, like the symptoms, varies according to the cause and anatomic location of the perforation. It does not require much acumen to diagnose a perforated peptic ulcer in a young man complaining of severe abdominal pain, lying motionless on the stretcher, whose abdomen is as rigid as the proverbial board. More challenging is the infant or the elderly patient whose signs and symptoms are not so obvious. The clinician, therefore, should remember the basics and systematically examine each patient who may have a perforated viscus.

Examination of any patient presenting with abdominal pain begins with an assessment of the throat, lungs, and heart, a point that should be emphasized but need not be belabored. The examination of the abdomen itself begins with inspection of the patient as a whole as well as of the abdomen. In actuality, this part of the examination begins when the history taking is begun and one observes whether the patient appears pale, episodically grimaces with the colicky pain of bowel obstruction, or lies motionless to avoid exacerbating the pain of peritonitis. These patients lie still with their thighs flexed in an effort to relieve tension on the abdominal wall. At this time, one should notice the rapid, shallow respirations that are predominantly thoracic and create minimal motion of the abdomen. Normally, the abdomen is flat or scaphoid and should not become distended until the latter stages of peritonitis develop along with its adynamic ileus and peritoneal fluid accumulation. Patients with large bowel obstruction, with or without perforation, invariably present with a markedly distended and tympanitic abdomen.

One should always auscultate the abdomen before proceeding to palpation with the fingers for two good reasons: (1) manual palpation of the abdomen can stimulate reflex peristaltic activity that might not otherwise have been present in a setting of adynamic ileus, and (2) patients usually remain more relaxed when the doctor presumes to listen for bowel sounds by gently applying the stethoscope than when he or she begins to palpate manually and potentially aggravate pre-existing pain. With earlier localized peritonitis, bowel sounds remain present, though hypoactive, particularly in parts of the abdomen away from the site of inflammation. To diagnose absent bowel sounds, one should listen continuously for 2 or more minutes. Failure to hear peristaltic activity during 30 to 60 seconds certainly suggests abnormally decreased activity, and one does not have to satisfy the purist by listening for at least 2 minutes. After having established whether peristalsis is present, one should use the diaphragm of the stethoscope to palpate the patient's abdomen gently and thus establish whether involuntary guarding or rebound tenderness is present.

In spite of the useful information that can be obtained by listening and palpating with a stethoscope, one should proceed to the next step of the examination, which is manual palpation of the abdomen. This is the one phase of the physical examination that can establish definitively whether peritonitis is present. It is important, therefore, that the patient be placed in an optimally relaxed supine position with the head flat or on a small pillow and the hips flexed to almost 90 degrees. The patient's hands should be placed flat alongside the torso or folded across the anterior chest. Every precaution should be taken to have the patient as relaxed as possible for the examination. The examiner, in turn, should have washed his hands in warm water before the examination so as not to elicit reflex guarding with the placement of cold fingers (or stethoscope). Palpation should begin in a quadrant of the abdomen where the patient has not been experiencing any pain and should be performed with the flat rather than the probing tips of one's fingers. In determining whether peritoneal irritation truly exists, it is important to be able to elicit involuntary guarding. Tenderness is commonly encountered in patients with abdominal complaints, but abdominal rigidity as mainfested by involuntary guarding is specific for parietal peritoneal irritation. The guarding may be localized or generalized depending on the extent of the peritonitis. Other signs that are characteristic of confined perforation (or localized visceral inflammation) include focal rebound tenderness and referred rebound tenderness that occurs at the site of inflammation but is elicited when one suddenly releases the abdominal wall at a locus distant from that site. One should recognize that guarding, which is reflex muscle spasm, occurs in varying degrees and depends on such variables as the degree of noxious irritation of the peritoneum, muscularity of the abdominal wall, and oversedation with muscle relaxants or narcotics. For this reason, the patient with a perforated peptic ulcer presents with "board-like" abdominal rigidity. These perforations usually occur in relatively young, muscular men, and acid is extremely irritating to the peritoneum. On the other hand, an elderly patient with relatively poor muscle tone exhibits much less abdominal rigidity.

Percussion of the abdominal wall should produce a generalized tympanitic effect because of the underlying distended loops of bowel associated with adynamic ileus. This phase of the examination can be diagnostic when one is able to percuss an area of tympany overlying what would normally be liver dullness, if sufficient free air from a perforated ulcer is overlying the anterior surface of the liver.

DIFFERENTIAL DIAGNOSIS

Patients presenting to the ED with perforated viscus invariably have signs and symptoms suggesting an acute intra-abdominal problem. Unless frank signs of peritoneal irritation are present or definitive diagnostic studies (described subsequently) confirm the presence of perforation, one cannot, with any high degree of certainty, distinguish among the various causes of an acute "surgical" abdomen. Indeed, if one can establish with a high degree of certainty that the patient needs surgical intervention, it is not imperative that an otherwise precise diagnosis be made. Thus, it matters not whether the surgeon explores an abdomen that contains gross contamination from a leaking perforated viscus or whether there is a viscus on the verge of perforating because of mechanical distension and/or compromised blood supply.

The signs and symptoms of secondary peritonitis should be known to all practicing clinicians (Table 49–7). Yet there are situations, particularly in debilitated patients, infants and elderly patients, in which some of these findings are not so obvious or discernable, and this makes the diagnosis less obvious. Chapter 14 discusses the various causes of abdominal pain, including the diffuse type. Table 49–8 lists certain of those causes that might mimic some of the findings of secondary peritonitis but for which surgical intervention is definitely not indicated. A careful history and physical examination and appropriate laboratory and x ray studies should enable one to distinguish between the surgical and nonsurgical causes of abdominal pain.

The earlier, focal signs of peritoneal irritation from viscus perforation are related to the anatomic location of the perforation. Thus, any perforation involving a

TABLE 49-7. ACUTE SECONDARY PERITONITIS— SIGNS AND SYMPTOMS

Continuous abdominal pain
Muscle guarding (involuntary)
Spreading tenderness
Absent (minimal) bowel sounds
Vomiting (after onset of pain)
Tachypnea (shallow, thoracic)
Tachycardia
Fever (may be hypothermic)

TABLE 49-8. GENERAL ABDOMINAL PAIN— NONSURGICAL CAUSES

Pancreatitis
Primary peritonitis
Lobar pneumonia
Sickle cell crisis
Tabetic crisis (tertiary syphilis)
Diabetic ketoacidosis
Leukemia
Black widow spider bite
Acute intermittent porphyria
Gastroenteritis

segment of the foregut (esophagogastric junction to the ligament of Trietz) presents initially with epigastric pain; lesions involving the midgut (ligament of Trietz to the midtransverse colon) are referred to the paraumbilical area; and lesions of the hindgut (midtransverse colon to the rectum) are referred to the left lower abdomen. As long as these perforations remain localized and are confined by either omentum, the mesentery of the bowel, or adjacent structures, diffuse peritonitis does not occur. In such situations, exact diagnosis by the emergency physician may be virtually impossible. The consolation is that in the absence of spreading peritonitis, emergent surgery is not necessary. These patients, as a rule, have persistent symptoms of pain that do not respond to sedatives or intestinal antispasmotics, indicating a need for more definitive evaluation by an appropriate specialist.

Peptic ulcers are by far the most common cause of intestinal perforation. Forty to 50% of all nonpostoperative causes of secondary peritonitis are from perforated ulcers. Most ulcers perforate freely into the peritoneal cavity, causing a sudden severe peritoneal reaction from the leaking acidic gastric juices. In certain cases, the leaking fluid may course along the right lateral gutter of the ascending colon down to the right lower quadrant, where localized peritoneal reaction may mimic appendicitis. In a woman, one should consider also the possibility of right tubo-ovarian lesions. Posterior penetrating ulcers confined by the head of the pancreas not only mimic pancreatitis or cholecystitis, but cause a secondary, associated pancreatitis. Furthermore, any time a patient presents with epigastric pain, one must rule out the possibility of an acute myocardial infarction.

INITIAL STABILIZATION

Any patient presenting with signs and symptoms of peritoneal irritation must be treated expeditiously and vigorously as if he has a life-threatening emergency. Indeed, if the patient does have peritonitis secondary to a perforated viscus, he or she does have a life-threatening emergency for which the rise in mortality rate is directly related to the delay in therapy. Regardless of its cause, once intestinal perforation has occurred, certain predictable physiologic changes will follow, and if these changes are not controlled or reversed, the patient will die.

In certain cases, the body's defenses confine the perforation, and this may obviate the need for emergent surgical intervention. Certain perforations may be confined by the intestine's mesothelium, the omentum, or adjacent intra-abdominal structures, as occurs with Crohn's disease, in which fistula formation rather than free peritoneal perforation is more likely to occur. Nevertheless, unless the patients become pain-free and show no signs of peritoneal irritation, they should be treated vigorously as in a case of spreading peritonitis.

The peritoneal cavity is richly supplied with blood vessels and lymphatics and has a surface area estimated to be between 1.5 and 2 m², almost equal to the skin surface area. Thus, when the peritoneum is irritated by the escaping fluid of a perforated viscus, it may cause a significant inflammatory reaction that can result in a major translocation of extracellular body fluid into the peritoneal cavity while its rich lymphatic system rapidly absorbs and disseminates systemically the bacterial contamination that has occured. The peritoneal cavity further produces a protein-rich exudate that adheres to the serosal surface of the intestines causing a decrease in their motility and in effect producing a measure of mechanical obstruction that contributes to the inhibition of peristalsis, ultimately resulting in an adynamic ileus. The intestinal absorption becomes impaired long before its secretions cease, and thus there is a significant sequestration of intestinal fluid within the aperistaltic intestines. Indeed, it has been shown that, in the early phases of bowel obstruction and peritonitis, an actual increase in the secretion of fluid within the intestinal lumen is presumably caused by a local prostaglandin release stimulated by the bowel distention itself. Thus, the patient loses significant amounts of fluids to the peritoneal cavity, the bowel lumen, and the bowel wall itself, which becomes edematous. Furthermore, the patient has lost considerable fluid from vomiting and is obviously unable to replace any of the fluid lost by oral intake. As the peritonitis progresses, fluid losses lead to a significant hypovolemia that ultimately results in shock and death.

Patients with peritonitis, therefore, must be treated aggressively with fluid therapy as part of their initial assessment and stabilization. Initial replacement fluid should be an isotonic solution, preferably lactated Ringer's. The initial volume of replacement fluid depends on the patient's state of hydration and is guided by such parameters as pulse rate, pulse pressure, urine output, and blood pressure. Patients who appear to be significantly volume-depleted as manifested by a narrow pulse pressure or hypotension should be given fluid loads of 500 cc over a 20-minute interval. The fluid load for a dehydrated pediatric patient is 20 cc per kg. Elderly patients or those with significant cardiac disease should be monitored initially with central venous pressure determinations to avoid fluid overloading. If initial fluid requirements in an adult appear to exceed 2L, one may supplement the crystalloid fluid replacement with colloids. In all cases of fluid replacement therapy, multiple vitamins can be added to the first liter of fluid infused and to at least every third liter thereafter.

NASOGASTRIC TUBES

One cannot overemphasize the importance of passing a nasogastric (NG) tube into all patients with an acute "surgical" abdomen. Years ago, before nasogastric tubes were routinely used, patients died from "acute gastric dilation." Failure to pass an NG tube in a patient with an acute abdomen can literally result in "killing your patient with kindness." There are three pertinent reasons why an NG tube should be passed in all patients with signs of peritoneal irritation:

1. A properly functioning NG tube actually stops the leakage from a perforated gastric or duodenal ulcer. Cases have been documented in which premature removal of an NG tube resulted in recurrence of leakage through a previously effective omental seal.
2. When the antrum of the stomach is decompressed and gastric and pancreatico-biliary secretions are aspirated, there is a significant decrease in the stimulation of further biliary and pancreatic secreations, which is essential to putting the gastrointestinal tract "at rest."
3. Swallowed air is by far the main source of gas in intestinal and colonic distention. It has been clearly demonstrated in the surgical literature dating back to 1939 that swallowed air is the key factor responsible for intestinal distention, which further compounds the body's fluid and electrolyte problem by stimulating secretion and interfering with absorption of intestinal juices.

Nasogastric decompression is essential in the management of any acute abdomen, but especially perforated viscus. The emergency physician must be proficient in the passage of NG tubes, knowing how to decongest the nasal mucosa, anesthetize the nasopharynx, and properly position the patient's head and neck for successful passage of the tube while causing minimal discomfort to the patient.

ANTIBIOTIC TREATMENT

The intestinal tract contains a plethora of bacteria and other infectious organisms. A significant portion of the weight of one's feces is made up of viable bacteria. Bacteriologically, the stomach and proximal duodenum are relatively clean. The peritonitis from a perforated peptic ulcer is initially caused by chemical irritation; secondary bacterial infection is usually caused by staphylococcus, streptococcus, or both, and usually takes 24 to 48 hours to develop. The small intestine contains a mixture of bacteria, predominantly Escherichia coli, Streptococcus faecalis, and other gram-negative rods. Anaerobes become more prevalent in the distal small bowel and totally predominate in the large bowel. In a recent review of 71 cases of gangrenous and perforated appendicitis with peritonitis, more than 55 different species of bacteria were isolated, and most were anaerobic. Thus is it a virtual certainty that bacterial inoculation of the peritoneum will occur as a result of a perforated viscus. Animal experimental and human clinical studies have demonstrated that bacteria injected into the peritoneum rapidly appear in the thoracic lymph and thence in the blood stream.

It is impossible to sterilize the intestinal tract or provide antibiotic therapy that will be effective against all intestinal bacteria. Nevertheless, in the face of peritonitis secondary to a perforated viscus, parenteral antibiotic therapy should be initiated as soon as possible to complement the body's own immune system, which otherwise would become overwhelmed by infection (see Sepsis, Chaps. 15 and 60). There is no need to wait for cultures to be obtained. The bacterial inoculation has already occurred; the sooner therapy is started, the better the outcome will be.

Recommended antibiotic treatment during initial stabilization includes either a 2 g loading dose of cefoxitin or a combination of gentamicin (1.5 to 2 mg per kg), ampicillin (1 g), and metronidazole (500 mg) or clindamycin (600 mg).

The initial assessment and stabilization of a patient with spreading peritonitis from a perforated viscus should be initiated before any lab results are known or x rays taken. Likewise, STAT surgical consultation should be obtained at this time. The diagnosis of peritonitis is clinical. Considering that at least 25% of the x rays do not reveal free air initially, one should not hesitate to arrange for the definitive therapy that these patients need. On the other hand, one should not delay in instituting the stabilization procedures outlined above because of the misguided notion that the surgeon will be in shortly to take care of this obviously surgical case. Aggressive efforts must be made to restore a patient's fluid volume and initiate antibiotic therapy for impending sepsis before a general anesthetic is administered, to reduce the operative mortality rate.

It is also important to realize that, because of the abdominal pain and guarding, ventilation is compromised, and in a patient whose metabolic needs for oxygen are greater than normal. Supplemental oxygen in these cases is best administered by mask; patients in such distress tend to gasp through their mouths. The presence of a nasogastric tube further forces them to mouth-breathe.

Finally, in the initial stabilization of a patient with peritonitis, one has to consider the judicious and appropriate use of sedation. For decades, there has been a general misconception that analgesics should be withheld from a patient with acute abdominal pain because their administration would obfuscate the signs of peritonitis and delay unnecessarily the surgeon's decision to operate. There is some truth to this reasoning, but it is not universally true. Injudicious use of narcotics can and does obscure the signs and symptoms of early stages of peritonitis, but the patients are usually not severely symptomatic and certainly should await the surgeon's arrival and assessment before any sedation is administered. On the other hand, the diagnosis of full-blown peritonitis with extensive, generalized rigidity and totally absent bowel sounds will not be confused by the judicious administration of small, intravenous doses of narcotics that can be titrated to meet the patient's needs. Once the surgeon has made a decision to operate, appro-

TABLE 49-9. INITIAL STABILIZATION
Correct hypovolemia
Crystalloid solution with multivitamins (MVI)
Colloid
Nasogastric tube to intermittent suction
Supplemental O$_2$
Foley catheter (I and O)
CVP monitoring (cardiac and elderly patients)
Antibiotics
STAT surgical consult
Sedation

TABLE 49-10. LABORATORY STUDIES/PROCEDURES FOR PERFORATED VISCUS PATIENTS
CBC
BS, SMA-6 (Na, K, Cl, CO$_2$, BUN, Cr)
Amylase, lipase, alkaline, phosphatase, AST, ALT
Type and Hold/Crossmatch; PT, PTT
Urinalysis
Chest x ray
ECG
ABG
Pregnancy test
Obstruction series (lateral decubitus vs. upright)
Diagnostic peritoneal lavage
Computed tomogram of abdomen

priate preoperative sedation should be administered (Table 49–9).

LABORATORY AND OTHER PROCEDURES

It is mandatory that a certain minimum number of laboratory studies and other procedures be performed in any patients in whom presenting signs and symptoms suggest a perforated viscus (Table 49–10). As part of the initial stabilization that has to be administered for these patients, blood specimens can be drawn for appropriate studies while IV lines are being established to initiate fluid replacement and, perhaps, antibiotic therapy. Likewise, while a Foley catheter is being inserted to monitor the patient's urine output, a specimen should be obtained for basic urinalysis and, if necessary, culture and sensitivity. An emergent ECG can be obtained while IVs are being started; pulse oximetry should be used to monitor the oxygen saturation of more critically ill patients; and, if the patient's condition permits, a portable upright chest x ray should be taken shortly after the patient's arrival in the ED. These procedures and maneuvers enable the medical team to obtain minimal basic information necessary to monitor any patient about to undergo emergency laparotomy.

A complete blood count is essential to detect any associated anemia and to measure the degree of an inflammatory response being triggered by the secondary infection. Blood sugar and electrolyte tests are likewise necessary to monitor the extent of pre-existing fluid and electrolyte imbalance and its subsequent correction with replacement therapy. Screening pancreatic, biliary, and hepatic baseline enzyme determinations are important to exclude potential nonsurgical conditions with a clinical presentation that could mimic that of an acute surgical abdomen. The initial treatment of choice for acute pancreatitis or hepatitis is not emergency laparotomy.

An initial ECG can be helpful in determining the cause of upper abdominal pain, particularly in ruling out the possibility of acute myocardial infarction or pericarditis. For patients who have an obvious surgical abdomen along with coexisting coronary artery disease, serial ECGs are needed to monitor the postoperative course and recovery of these patients. Ischemic changes on the ECG should not, per se, deter emergency laparotomy if it is truly indicated. The mortality rate from peritonitis caused by a persistently leaking perforated viscus is virtually 100%.

Routine diagnostic radiographic studies, ordinarily performed in the radiology department, are contraindicated if they are not essential to the clinical diagnosis and interfere with and delay the transfer of the patient to the operating room where definitive treatment will be administered. The admission portable chest x ray, however, is indicated and should be done even while the patient is being hydrated in preparation for surgery. If at all possible, the patient should be propped up because a portable, supine x ray is of little value. Such a preliminary x ray is useful to detect conditions such as a thoracic aortic aneurysm or a lower lobar pneumonia, either of which could contribute to the signs and symptoms of the patient's "acute abdomen." Furthermore, a preoperative chest x ray is always essential to the anesthesiologist, who must be aware of any intrathoracic conditions that could compromise adequate ventilation of the patient.

The most specific noninvasive confirmation of the presence of a perforated viscus is the x ray demonstration of a pneumoperitoneum. Whenever possible and whenever the patient's condition permits, a concentrated effort should be made to demonstrate the presence of free air in the peritoneal cavity. Even though air is normally distributed throughout the entire course of the gastrointestinal tract, it is usually only from perforations of the stomach, duodenum, or colon that enough air is present and concentrated to create a detectible pneumoperitoneum on an x ray. Thus, perforations of the small bowel, unless the result of obstruction/distention, do not demonstrate free air. Rarely is free air associated with a ruptured appendix, the cause of which is intraluminal obstruction.

By far the most common sources of pneumoperitoneum are perforated gastric and/or duodenal ulcers and, to a lesser extent, perforated colonic diverticula. Even perforated peptic ulcers do not demonstrate free air at all times. Various studies in the surgical literature reveal that approximately 25% of perforated peptic ulcers do not demonstrate free air. One definitive study of this subject revealed that, within the first 8 hours, only 50 to 60% of perforated ulcers were found to have free air. Of patients whose perforations had occurred more than 8 hours before to evaluation, 85% demonstrated free air. Furthermore, it has been documented that air from a pre-existing pneumomediastinum may dissect inferiorly into the peritoneal cavity, creating a secondary pneumoperitoneum. Thus, not all cases of perforated viscus result in a pneumoperitoneum, nor are all cases of pneumoperitoneum the result of a perforated intraperitoneal viscus.

When obtaining abdominal x rays as part of the assessment of an acute abdomen, it is imperative to obtain a full, properly done obstruction series and not to rely on the incomplete information provided by a simple flat plate. For patients who are unable to be placed in an upright position, a left lateral decubitus view should be obtained. To increase the yield of seeing free air on this view, the patient should be placed and kept in this position (left side down) for at least 10 minutes before being sent to the x ray suite. The left-side-down view is preferred because from this position air initially trapped in the lesser sac can exit by way of the foramen of Winslow and be seen contrasted against the liver shadow. In general, it is easier to detect air contrasted against the liver shadow than that contrasted against the splenic flexure of the opposite side. The upright view of the abdomen must include the lower thorax and a full view of both hemidiaphragms (Fig. 49–7). Ideally, the patient should be placed in an upright position and the x ray beam should be focused at right angles to the level of the diaphragms. If a tangential view is erroneously taken, smaller amounts of free air are not seen.

When free air is not seen on these traditional x rays, the diagnosis is still in doubt, and the patient's condition permits, other steps can be taken to establish more definitively the diagnosis of perforated viscus. One maneuver is to instill approximately 50 cc of water-soluble contrast material into the stomach by means of the NG tube, place the patient in a right lateral decubitus position for 5 to 10 minutes, and then repeat the obstruction series. This procedure could outline an intramural defect if the leak has sealed or define the perforation site if the leak persists. (A recent, unpublished report by one of our radiologists reveals that combining CT with contrast radiography significantly increases the yield of diagnosing perforating peptic ulcers compared to conventional radiography by demonstrating extraluminal fluid, air, and/or contrast.)

Other x ray findings that might indirectly suggest the presence of a perforated viscus include the loss of a psoas muscle outline, suggesting a retroperitoneal perforation with associated bleeding, and the presence of air in the superior mesenteric and portal veins associated with mesenteric vascular occlusion and bowel necrosis. At no time should an emergent barium enema be performed as part of the diagnostic work-up of a perforated viscus. Barium causes an intense chemical peritonitis and can result in extensive adhesions and bowel obstruction.

Diagnostic peritoneal lavage, if needed, would have a close to 100% specificity but a considerably lower sensitivity for the more difficult diagnostic challenges of perforated viscus. Certainly the presence of intestinal matter, including bile, and a white blood cell count of greater than 500 per mm^3 is highly suggestive of the diagnosis. Recent studies have indicated that the presence of low levels of amylase (20 to 30 i.u.) obtained from peritoneal fluid in the absence of clinical pancreatitis is an even more sensitive determinant for the presence of a perforated intestine. Then, too, diagnostic peritoneal lavage is the only reliable method for establishing the diagnosis of primary peritonitis, which is caused by the hematogenous spread of Staphylococcus and Streptococcus rather than the multivaried flora of bacteria found with a perforated viscus.

MANAGEMENT AND INDICATIONS FOR HOSPITALIZATION

When it comes to disposition of patients who may have a perforated intra-abdominal viscus, there are few options, if any. After the likelihood of the diagnosis has been established by a careful history and physical examination, initial stabilization as outlined in Table 49–9 must be aggressively implemented, including a STAT surgical consultation. Perforated viscus is a potentially life-threatening incident. Although not all cases must undergo a definitive surgical procedure, such a decision can be made only by a qualified surgeon. In the management of these types of cases, it is the emergency physician's responsibility to initiate stabilization and refer appropriately for hospitalization or direct admission to the operating room.

Perforated viscus can manifest itself in various ways, and the emergency physician's responsibility is to recognize the variations. At one extreme is the patient presenting in septic shock with the signs and symptoms of peripheral vascular collapse and decreased vital organ perfusion. Here, more than ever, one must adhere to the ABCs of resuscitation, ensuring adequate airway, ventilation, and oxygenation combined with restoration of adequate circulating volume. An obtunded patient in these circumstances may not be able to provide the classic historical clues needed to diagnose a perforated viscus, but a careful physical examination would reveal definite signs of an intra-abdominal catastrophe. The distended ab-

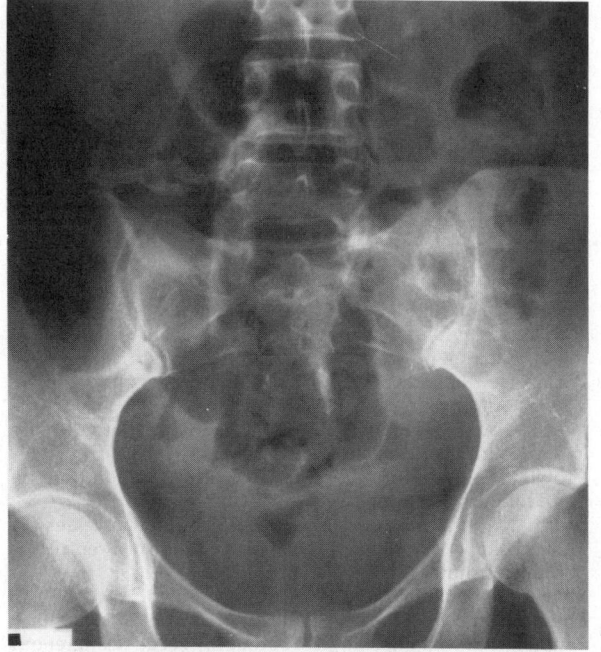

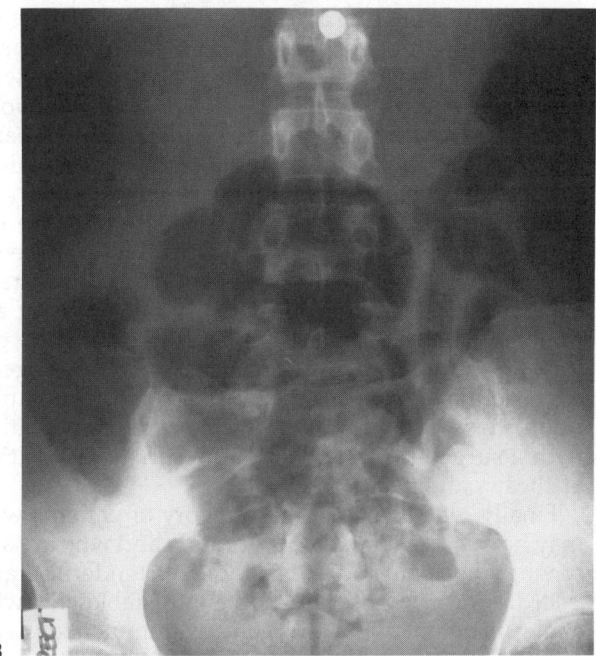

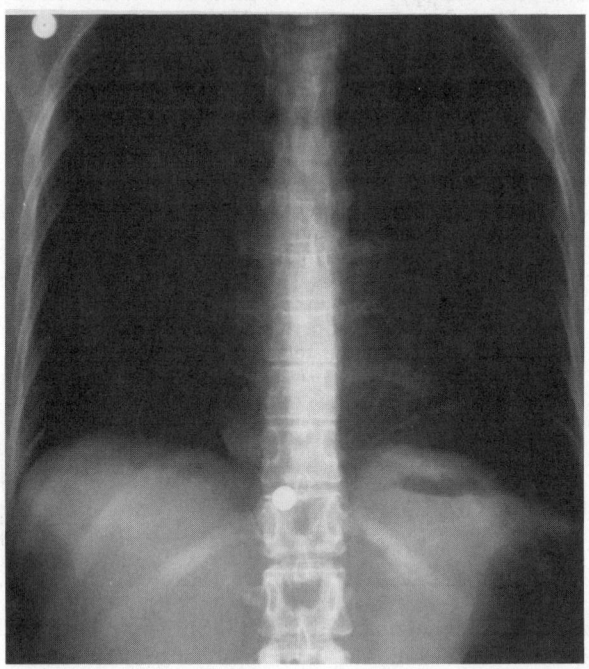

FIG. 49-7. A 37-year-old woman smoker with previous peptic ulcer history presented with a perforated peptic ulcer. Free air is barely noticeable on preliminary supine and upright x rays of the abdomen (A and B) that did not include the lower portion of the chest (C), where extensive free air under both diaphragms is evident.

domen with varying degrees of involuntary rigidity and absent bowel sounds is not likely to be a reflex reaction to sepsis from other sources. Initial baseline chest x ray and urinalysis may or may not exclude these more common sources. Keeping in mind that older, debilitated patients may have concomitant life-threatening problems, one should vigorously pursue ruling out the possibility of a perforated viscus even if pneumonia or pyuria may be present as long as the patient displays signs of peritoneal irritation. In these cases, if an obstructive series of the abdomen fails to

reveal free air, one should perform a diagnostic peritoneal lavage using the Seldinger technique to introduce a tapered tip catheter with multiple perforations for the procedure. Intra-abdominal infection must be drained surgically and the leaking segment of bowel repaired or diverted from the peritoneal cavity. The timing of surgery for these patients is crucial and can be made only in consultation with the operating surgeon. There is no question that vigorous preoperative resuscitation with fluids and antibiotics improves somewhat the dismal prognosis for these patients, who must be automatically admitted to either the operating room or the surgical intensive care unit.

The next category of patients includes those with signs and symptoms of dehydration and hypovolemia, who may or may not have had abdominal pain, but who have findings suggestive of secondary peritonitis. Once again, as long as the possibility of perforated viscus exists, these patients must be expeditiously referred to and admitted by the surgeon. If signs, symptoms, and diagnostic procedures have excluded the likelihood of nonsurgical causes of abdominal pain (see Table 49–8), but rather point to potentially surgically correctable lesions, the surgeon need not have a precise diagnosis to justify operating upon these patients. Once again, early consultation with a surgeon is needed for appropriate disposition of these patients.

Finally, one comes to the category of patients who may have had a confined perforation and who are still having some pain and exhibit localized tenderness and guarding, but whose vital signs are stable and who clinically do not appear to be in any imminent danger. As long as the possibility of a perforated viscus exists (even though it may have spontaneously sealed itself) the management, referral, and disposition of these patients cannot be compromised. These patients still have a potentially life-threatening problem, and until more definitive in-hospital diagnostic procedures rule out this possibility, they must be treated as such. Intravenous access must be established and maintenance fluids administered if there is no need for volume replacement. If bowel sounds are present and the patient is not vomiting, one might defer passing an NG tube, but the patient must be kept strictly from receiving anything by mouth. These patients, although they may appear almost well enough to go home, should be hospitalized or held over for close follow-up evaluations.

REFERENCES

1. Scholz, T.D., and McGuiness, G.A.: Localized intestinal perforation following intravenous indomethacin for patent ductus arteriosis. J. Pediatr. Gastroenterol. Nutr. 7:5, 1988.
2. Lauber, J.S., Abrams, H.L., and Ray, M.C.: Silent bowel perforation during corticosteroid treatment for pemphigus vulgaris. Cutis 43:1, 1988.
3. Von Muhlendahl, K.E.: Perforating gastric ulceration during tolazoline therapy for persistent foetal circulation. Z. Kinderchir. 43:1, 1988.
4. Smedley, F., Hickrsh, T., Taube, M., et al.: Perforated duodenal ulcer and cigarette smoking. J. R. Soc. Med. 81:2, 1988.
5. Dasmahapatra, K.S., Suval, W., and Machiedo, G.W.: Unsuspected perforation in bleeding duodenal ulcers. Am. Surg. 54:1, 1988.
6. Ben-Zvi, J.S., and Daniel, S.J.: Painless gastric perforation in a patient with multiple sclerosis. Am. J. Gastroenterol. 83:9, 1988.
7. Meier, D.E., Imediegwu, O.O., and Tarpley, J.L.: Perforated typhoid enteritis: Operative experience with 108 cases. Am. J. Surg. 157:4, 1989.
8. Lalla, R., Enquist, I., Oloumi, M., et al.: Stercoraceous perforation of the right colon. South. Med. J. 82:1, 1989.
9. Schwartzentruber, D., Lotze, M.T., and Rosenburg, S.A.: Colonic perforation. An unusual complication of therapy with high-dose interleukin-2. Cancer 62:11, 1988.
10. Deakin, M.: Small bowel perforation associated with an excessive dose of slow release diclofenac sodium. Br. Med. J. (Clin. Res.) 297:6646, 1988.
11. Moses, F.M.: Colonic perforation due to oral mannitol. JAMA 260:5, 1988.
12. Gould, J., Tram, J.S., Dan, S.J., et al.: Duodenal perforation as a delayed complication of placement by a biliary endoprosthesis. Radiology 167:2, 1988.
13. Borzotta, A.P., and Groff, D.B.: Gastrointestinal perforation in infants. Am. J. Surg. 155:3, 1988.
14. Paraskeviades, E.C., and Ghauss, M.I.: Ascaris lumbricoides and intestinal perforation. Br. J. Surg. 75:1, 1988.
15. Crowley, L.V., and Bretzke, M.L.: Bowel perforation from ingested unit dose blister-pak. Am. J. Gastroenterol. 83:9, 1988.
16. Sharma, B.S., and Kak, V.K.: Multiple subdural abscesses following colonic perforation—A rare complication of a ventricular peritoneal shunt. Pediatr. Radiol. 18:5, 1988.
17. Bohnen, J., Boulauger, M., Meakins, J.L., and McLean, A.P.H.: Prognosis in generalized peritonitis. Arch. Surg. 118:285, 1983.
18. Bennion, R.S., Thompson, J.E., Baron, E.J., et al.: Gangrenous and perforated appendicitis with peritonitis. Clinical Therapeutics, Vol 12, Suppl. B, Excerpta Medica, 1990.
19. Roberts, J.R.: NSAIDs: GI toxicity. Emerg. Med. News 12:3, 1990.
20. Antimicrobial prophylaxis in surgery. In The Medical Letter on Drugs and Therapeutics 31:806. Edited by Abramowicz, M.: New Rochelle, NY, The Medical Letter, Inc., December 1, 1989.
21. Zamir, O., Shapira, S.C., Udassin, R., et al.: Gastrointestinal perforations in the neonatal period. Am. J. Perinatol. 5:2, 1998.
22. Torosian, M.H., and Turnbull, A.D.: Emergency laparotomy for spontaneous intestinal and colonic perforations in cancer patients receiving corticosteroids and chemotherapy. J. Clin. Oncol. 6:2, 1988.
23. Guess, H.A., West, R., Strand, L.M., et al.: Fatal upper gastrointestinal hemorrhage or perforation among users and nonusers of nonsteroidal anti-inflammatory drugs in Saskatchewan, Canada. J. Clin. Epidemiol. 41:1, 1988.

BIBLIOGRAPHY

Jones, P.F.: Emergency Abdominal Surgery in Infancy, Childhood and Adult Life. 2nd Ed. Oxford, Blackwell Scientific Publications, 1987.

Moody, F.G., Carey, L.C., Jones, R.S., et al. (eds.): Surgical Treatment of Digestive Disease. Chicago, Year Book Publishers, Inc., 1986.

Rubenstein, E., and Federman, D.D. (eds.): Scientific American Medicine, New York, Scientific American, Inc., 1990.

Sabistan, D.C. (ed.): Textbook of Surgery. 13th Ed. Philadelphia, W.B. Saunders Co., 1986.

Schwartz, S.I., and Ellis, H. (eds.): Maingot's Abdominal Operations. 8th Ed. Norwalk, Appleton-Century-Crofts, 1985.

Schwartz, S.I., Shires, G.T., and Spencer, F.C. (eds.): Principles of Surgery. 5th Ed. New York, McGraw-Hill, 1989.

ALIMENTARY TRACT OBSTRUCTION

Edward L. Bradley, III

CAPSULE

Alimentary tract obstruction remains a frequent cause of morbidity and mortality. Although precise data are not available, it has been estimated that one of every five emergency surgical admissions is necessitated by some form of alimentary tract obstruction. It is true that patient response depends on the cause and nature of the obstruction, but for one specific area, intestinal obstruction, the mortality rate approximates 10%. Because there were approximately 3 million emergency surgical admissions in the United States in 1978, it follows that 60,000 people may have died from the effects of alimentary tract obstruction. This mortality rate is excessive. With widespread and proper application of *presently existing* knowledge, this figure could probably be halved.

INTRODUCTION

Alimentary tract obstruction can be best defined as an intrinsic or extrinsic failure of the normal caudad progression of intraluminal contents.

Such a situation has several possible complications. Most apparent is the effect on normal nutrition, which, if permitted to continue, would lead eventually to inanition. Less obvious are the development of dehydration and the threat of alimentary tract perforation with attendant sepsis. These complications are discussed in more detail in the section of this chapter dealing with pathophysiology. If abdominal distention is a feature of the obstruction, the resultant expansion in volume of the abdominal contents takes place at the expense of pulmonary volume and expansion. This causes a decrease in alveolar ventilation and a corresponding increase in unoxygenated blood. Remote effects may occur in other organ systems, initiated by the fall in arterial oxygenation. Finally, in situations characterized by distention and vomiting, the threat of pulmonary aspiration of regurgitated intestinal contents is ever present.

CAUSES

By far the most common cause of alimentary tract obstruction is the temporary cessation of intestinal activity immediately following abdominal surgery, so-called "paralytic ileus." Fortunately, this process is self-limiting. Mechanical obstruction represents the second most common cause of intestinal obstruction. Conditions resulting in mechanical obstruction include adhesions (40%), carcinoma (20%), and incarcerated hernia (10%), with the remainder (30%) divided among the many causes listed in Table 49-11. Because the most effective therapy requires a preliminary diagnosis of the cause of any given obstruction, consideration of the frequency of occurrence should be of therapeutic value. "Common things occur commonly."

PATHOPHYSIOLOGY

Although not all sections of the alimentary tract respond to obstruction in an identical manner, certain physiologic truths can be appreciated from a discussion in general terms.

As noted, alimentary tract obstruction exists when luminal contents fail to progress. Because intraluminal progression of intestinal contents is basically caused by an integrated and coordinated contraction of smooth muscle in the intestinal wall (peristalsis), obstruction could conceivably be produced by either physical obturation to the passage of intestinal contents or the absence of effective peristalsis. The former condition, referred to as *mechanical* obstruction, and the latter state of functional obstruction, called *paralytic ileus*, arise from two completely different causes, but many similar effects may be produced.

The alimentary tract secretes more than 8000 mL of fluid into the lumen daily. Little more than 200 to 400 mL can be recovered in the feces; the efficiency of the resorption mechanism can be easily appreciated. Increases in intraluminal fluid volume occur in intestinal obstruction. The question regarding whether alimentary tract secretions in obstruction actually are increased or whether absorption is decreased has not been resolved. Experimental evidence supporting each theory is available, and, in the author's opinion,

TABLE 49-11. CAUSES OF ALIMENTARY TRACT OBSTRUCTION

Mechanical Causes	Esophagus	Stomach	Duodenum	Small Bowel	Colon
Congenital	Atresia Stenosis	Pyloric stenosis	Atresia Stenosis Duodenal web Annular pancreas Congenital band	Atresia Stenosis External hernia	Atresia Stenosis Meconium ileus Imperforate anus Hirschsprung's disease
Inflammatory	Stricture	Stricture	Stricture	Adhesions Regional enteritis Abscess Stricture	Granulomatous colitis Ulcerative colitis Diverticulitis Abscess Stricture
Neoplastic	Carcinoma Leiomyoma	Carcinoma Lymphoma Sarcoma Polyps	Carcinoma Polyps	Carcinoma Lymphoma Sarcoma Leiomyoma Carcinoid	Carcinoma Sarcoma Lymphoma
Miscellaneous	Foreign body Achalasia	Foreign body Paraesophageal hernia Volvulus	Foreign body Hematoma Superior mesenteric artery syndrome	Foreign body Hematoma Worms Gallstone Bezoars Intussusception Hernia Volvulus	Foreign body Endometriosis Fecal impaction Intussusception Volvulus

Paralytic ileus
Conduction defects: Na$^+$ and K$^+$ abnormalities, as in depletion states and diabetic ketoacidosis
Peristaltic defects: Abnormalities in muscular contraction, as in mesenteric vascular disease and porphyria
Neural irritative states: Overbalanced sympathetic stimulation, as in local or general toxicity and retroperitoneal injuries

the two positions are not mutually exclusive. Regardless of the actual mechanism involved, the amount of intestinal fluid residing in the alimentary tract in a given obstruction will be determined by the site of the obstruction. If the site is distal, a large amount of fluid accumulates above the obstruction. With more proximal obstructions, there is proportionally less intraluminal fluid, as bowel secretion and absorption occur distal to the obstruction in a normal fashion.

If normal absorption of alimentary tract secretions cannot take place, the extracellular fluid secreted into the lumen is functionally lost to the body. Deficits in extracellular fluid volume can be replaced only by borrowing from the intracellular space. This situation becomes aggravated when repeated episodes of vomiting are a prominent feature of the obstruction. Clearly, the net result is profound dehydration, with the attendant abnormalities in all cellular and subcellular systems dependent on solvent transport. Therefore, in addition to obstruction to the flow of intestinal contents resulting in a loss of nutrition, alimentary tract obstruction *invariably produces some degree of dehydration*. This development is of great consequence because the seriousness of the situation has now undergone escalation. It is possible for the human organism to take no external nutrition whatever for periods lasting months, with survival being based on the conversion of stored fat and protein to energy

equivalents. In contrast, underlining the importance of fluid homeostasis, is the observation that few would survive 2 weeks of total fluid deprivation. Persistent extracellular fluid deficits lead to hypotension and shock. Coronary, carotid, and renal thromboses are frequent sequelae of this development in the older age group.

If this were the only problems arising from alimentary tract obstruction, the situation would be sufficiently severe. Another process occurs, however, that by itself places the patient at greatest risk of death: The intestinal tract becomes *distended*. Although simple distention at first may seem innocuous, closer examination reveals the true scope of this complication.

First, distention increases tension in the wall of the ailmentary tract simply by an increase in the radius, pressure remaining constant. This relationship for tubular structures is known as *Laplace's Law* and is illustrated in Figure 49-8. As a corollary, one might expect that, because the cecum has the largest radius in the intestinal tract, rupture from the increased pressure would occur most commonly in this location. The general concept of stress and strain in the wall of the alimentary tract as a direct result of distention, leading to tensions exceeding the yield point and subsequently the cohesive forces of the intestinal wall, with resultant rupture, is worthy of consideration.

Second, the immediate antecedent cause of disten-

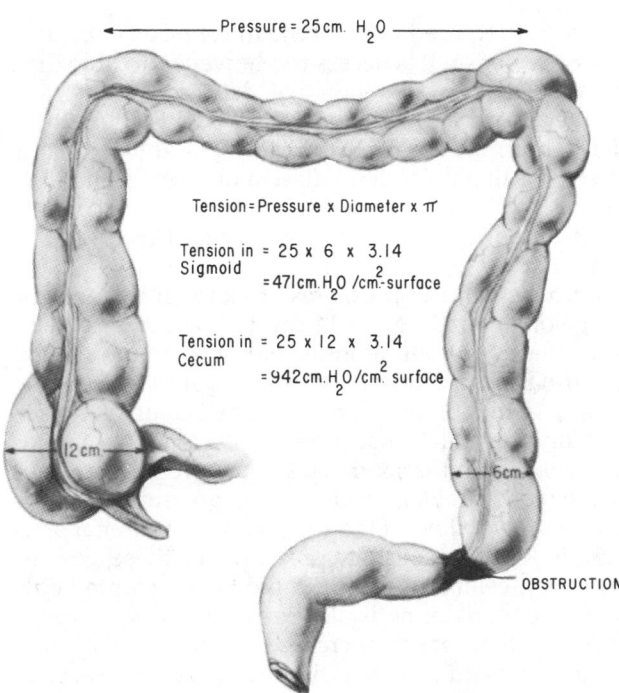

FIG. 49-8. A physical analysis of obstruction relating wall tension to the degree of distention. (From Schwartz, S.I., et al. (eds.): Principles of Surgery. Copyright © 1969 by McGraw-Hill, Inc. Used by permission of the McGraw-Hill Book Co.)

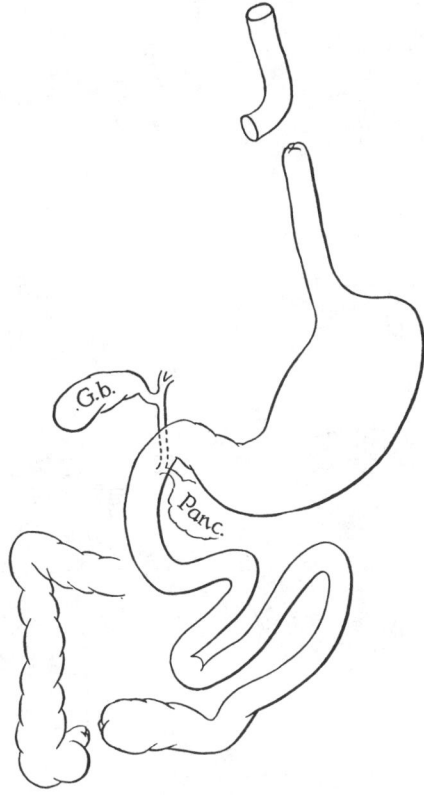

FIG. 49-9. An experimental preparation to investigate the origin of the intestinal gas and the mechanism of distention in intestinal obstruction. In dogs subject to ileal obstruction, if an end cervical esophagostomy prevented air swallowing, little gas, fluid, or distention was present in the obstructed bowel. This work clearly demonstrated that swallowed air was responsible for intestinal distention and that, in the absence of distention, the obstructed gut effectively reabsorbs digestive juices. (With permission from Wangensteen, O.H., and Rea, C.E.: Surgery 5:329, 1939.)

tion is an increase of intraluminal pressure. What is the origin of this excessive pressure? Theoretically, it could have come from increased intraluminal secretion, from gases liberated by the action of bacteria on stagnant intestinal contents, or from swallowed atmospheric air. Wangensteen and Rea[1] designed a simple experiment to test the hypothesis that intestinal gas was primarily the result of swallowed atmospheric gases (Fig. 49-9). Not only was this confirmed by the experiment, but, with the absence of intestinal distention in the group with cervical esophagostomies, it was clearly demonstrated that, whatever abnormalities in intestinal fluid secretion and absorption take place in obstruction, they cannot *in and of themselves* produce increased intestinal pressure with subsequent distention. Therefore, the primary cause of intestinal distention is swallowed air.

What are the dangers of increased intraluminal pressure? We have already discussed the increase in wall tension resulting from pressure-induced distention. If we consider for a moment the final distribution of blood supply to the intestine (Fig. 49-10), it should be clear that intramural blood is vulnerable to increases in intraluminal pressure. Although I am unaware of any studies measuring pressures in venules, capillaries, and arterioles in the bowel wall, it is reasonable to assume that values for these vessels are similar to those of venules, capillaries, and arterioles elsewhere in the body. Under these anatomic circumstances, if

intraluminal pressure exceeded venular pressure, we could expect an increase in capillary pressure. Such increases in capillary pressure would result in Starling disequilibrium, to the extent that there would be not only a net increase in extracellular fluid loss from the capillary into the bowel wall, resulting in thickening and edema, but also intraluminal weeping from mucosal capillaries. Because a new capillary exchange equilibrium would then be achieved at a higher pressure, reabsorption at the venular terminal would be diminished. Concurrent with the increase in transcapillary fluid loss into the extravascular spaces, lymphatic flow would increase. Eventually this cycle, if unchecked, would result in reduced arterial inflow, reduced tissue oxygenation, anaerobic cellular metabolism, and tissue acidosis, culminating in the confluent cell death known as necrosis. Such a scenario for perforation of the alimentary tract has been developed solely from distention and an increase in intraluminal pressure exceeding venular pressure. Clearly, any physical factors acting to reduce blood supply in a more abrupt fashion, such as acute vascular occlusion from thrombosis or volvulus, could promote

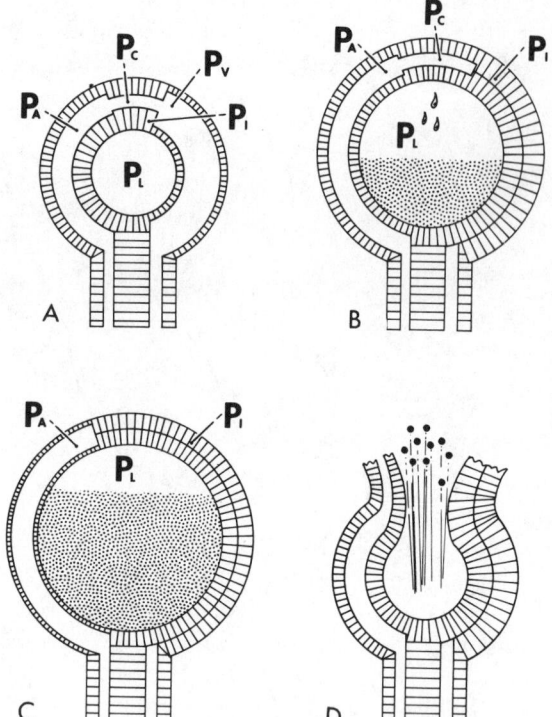

FIG. 49-10.   Diagrammatic representation of the effects of increased intraluminal pressure on the intramural blood flow in a cross section of intestinal wall. P_L = intraluminal pressure, P_I = interstitial pressure, P_V = pressure in venule, P_C = capillary pressure, P_A = arteriolar pressure.

A. Normal conditions: $P_L < P_I < P_V < P_C < P_A$.

B. Increased intaluminal pressure secondary to obstruction: $P_L > P_I > P_V$ but $< P_C < P_A$. Because interstitial pressure exceeds venular pressure, venule closes. Shift in Starling equilibrium results in marked outflow of fluid from capillary.

C. Continued increase in intraluminal pressure: $P_L > P_I > P_V > P_C < P_A$. Both venule and capillary now collapsed by surrounding pressure, resulting in a loss of aerobic cellular perfusion and nutrition.

D. Perforation resulting from cellular necrosis when anaerobic metabolism could no longer maintain viability of interstitial wall.

the preceding change of events in a matter of hours. It is the increase in intraluminal pressure manifested by distention that causes the primary danger in alimentary tract obstruction. When distention can be decompressed by vomiting or other means, as in high jejunal or gastric outlet obstruction, perforation is extremely rare.

Do the pressures in the alimentary tract support these concepts? In fact, little work has been done to support or deny the aforementioned suppositions. The bursting strength of the normal human intestine has ranged from 80 to 260 mm Hg, being in the lower end of this range for colon and higher for small bowel. In the few instances in which intraluminal pressures have been measured proximal to obstructions, small bowel pressures have ranged from 10 to 14 cm H_2O, and colon pressures from 12 to 52 cm H_2O. All these pressures increased with either peristalsis or respiration, but in no case have they approached those

pressures required to burst the intestine as a result of pressure per se. It is necessary, however, to note that, because these were operative data, a Valsalva maneuver, such as might be produced by attempts at defecation, was not performed. It is interesting to speculate that a sudden Valsalva maneuver might increase intraluminal pressure into the region of danger from bursting, particularly with regard to colon distentions.

Because venular pressures are known to be in the range of 10 mm. Hg. ($\sim$ 14 cm. H_2O), it can easily be appreciated that intraluminal pressures in mechanical intestinal obstruction may exceed venular pressure, setting in motion the aforementioned chain of events. Sustained intraluminal pressure becomes an important concept in that, if the sustained pressure exceeds the systolic capillary and venular pressure, necrosis must surely follow. If the sustained intraluminal pressure is less than systolic pressures in these vessels, however, cellular nutrition could be interrupted only during periods of peristalsis when intraluminal pressures are temporarily increased. In this set of circumstances, it is unlikely that tissue necrosis could occur. Because the pressure values measured in paralytic ileus are correspondingly lower, intramural vascular obstruction and subsequent necrosis should be less common if considered solely on a basis of pressure. That perforation rarely occurs in paralytic ileus is amply supported by clinical experience.

We might, therefore, view the range of intraluminal pressures in obstruction affecting intramural blood flow as a continuum—that is, the greater the intraluminal pressure, the less the intramural blood flow and the greater the likelihood of tissue necrosis and perforation. Of course, any factors negatively affecting intramural blood flow, in addition to increased intraluminal pressure, serve only to hasten necrosis and promote earlier perforation. This situation occurs when the mesenteric blood flow is compromised, resulting in strangulated obstruction. Because the time course preceding perforation is greatly shortened by the addition of extrinsic vascular obstruction to the simple obstruction, the course of therapy must also be accelerated when strangulated obstruction is suspected.

Although the concept of such a continuum is valuable from the standpoint of understanding pathophysiology, in a practical sense the actual measurement of intraluminal pressure is both risky and unnecessary. It is sufficient to recognize that distention is present, because fortunately the degree of distention is a reasonably direct function of the magnitude of intraluminal pressure. Clinically, we may infer that the more distention is present proximal to an obstruction, the more likely perforation is to occur, and, therefore, the more urgent decompression has become.

Another particularly virulent form of intestinal obstruction has been referred to as the "closed-loop" obstruction. This situation exists when neither entrance nor exit of intestinal contents is possible from a segment of bowel. Often, such a closed-loop obstruction is also strangulated, as in volvulus or strangulated inguinal hernia, but strangulation is not a prerequisite. An example of a closed-loop obstruction without strangulation is a distal colon obstruction in the presence of a competent ileocecal valve. The added virulence of this form of obstruction is caused primarily by the inherent toxicity of the entrapped intraluminal fluid. Extensive animal experimentation has shown that this intraluminal fluid contains products of bacterial origin that have profound vasodepressive effects. These observations have clear therapeutic implications.

CLINICAL MANIFESTATIONS

Signs and symptoms of alimentary tract obstruction depend to a great degree on the site, nature, and duration of the obstruction.

HISTORICAL FEATURES

In the more distal lesions, the most common complaint is distention. This becomes more prominent as the site of obstruction progresses distally from the upper jejunum. In more proximal lesions, clinically evident distention is not a common feature. Its lack can be attributed to both the small volume of bowel proximal to the lesion and the ability to decompress very proximal lesions by vomiting. With proximal obstruction, however, protracted and projectile vomiting is characteristic. In contrast, as the obstruction progresses distally, vomiting becomes less prominent. The nature of the vomitus, however, becomes more characteristic. Regurgitated ileal contents have a distinctly fecal odor, and vomitus of this type is referred to as feculent vomitus.

Another major feature of the history is the presence of irregular bowel function. With complete obstruction, one would not expect continued passage of feces, and this is generally the case. It is possible, however, to evacuate bowel contents distal to the obstruction and thus appear to have a normal bowel movement after complete obstruction has occurred. Clearly, then, the only circumstance in which the presence of bowel movements effectively can dismiss the diagnosis of complete obstruction is that of *continued* fecal passage. Obstruction and continued fecal passage can continue to coexist in only one situation, a high-grade incomplete or partial intestinal obstruction. The most common example of this is partial colonic obstruction from fecal impaction.

A third major determinant found in the history consists of the existence and nature of associated pain. Characteristically, the pain is associated with the major peristaltic wave and therefore intermittent. Because the major peristaltic wave in the small bowel occurs every 2 to 3 minutes, and in the colon at intervals of 15 to 20 minutes, this feature can often be used to localize the site of obstruction. The pain is usually described as dull and cramping, rising slowly in a crescendo pattern, reaching a maximum lasting around 30 seconds, and gradually receding. The cause of the pain is not known. The strong association with peristalsis, however, suggests that forced distention may be an important factor. It is of significant clinical importance to realize that, because *episodic* pain is associated with intestinal peristalsis, it is not expected to occur in any primary aperistaltic condition.

PHYSICAL FEATURES

Many physical signs are of value in the diagnosis and initial management of alimentary tract obstruction, but two are of paramount importance: (1) the character of the bowel sounds and (2) the presence or absence of abdominal tenderness.

Although the exact causation of bowel sounds as yet is only suspected, it is well known that they do not occur in the absence of peristalsis. Therefore, a failure to detect bowel sounds after listening for several minutes allows a working diagnosis of paralytic ileus. This in itself does not discriminate among the various causes of paralytic ileus. If bowel sounds *are* present, however, their character is of importance. Bowel sounds in mechanical intestinal obstruction are characteristic and frequently pathognomonic in a setting suggesting obstruction. They have been described as high-pitched, rushing, and continuous. No amount of verbal description can equal the experience of actually hearing such sounds. In my opinion, of equal importance to the character of the bowel sounds is the temporal relationship of the abdominal pain to the peristaltic wave that produces them. Cramping abdominal pain coexisting with the characteristic bowel sounds and ceasing when the overactive peristaltic activity ceases is the foundation upon which the diagnosis of mechanical obstruction is made.

Determination of abdominal tenderness is the second major consideration in the physical examination. Uncomplicated alimentary tract obstruction rarely results in other than mild tenderness to palpation. More severe tenderness, particularly in conjunction with rebound tenderness, means parietal peritonitis. This development, in a setting of obstruction, means that either perforation has already occurred or gangrenous bowel is present. This is a physical sign of the utmost importance because the development of bowel necrosis necessarily accelerates the surgical program.

Other physical findings are frequently of value in either assisting in the establishment of the diagnosis or helping define the pathologic stage of the obstruction.

Abdominal distention has been felt to be a sine qua non of obstruction. Although distention is a common finding in intestinal obstruction, as already mentioned, a high obstruction is not associated with abdominal distention. Therefore, the absence of distention does not obviate the presence of obstruction.

Similar comments may be made with regard to the percussion note. If the bowel is distended with air, the characteristic percussion note may be elicited. An additional consideration is that the bowel may contain more fluid than air, making percussive resonance less likely.

Some have set great store by the presence or absence of feces in the rectum on digital examination. As noted, bowel evacuation may or may not take place distal to a complete obstruction, and therefore this sign is of little prognostic significance.

Because postoperative adhesions are the most common cause of mechanical obstruction, the finding of an abdominal scar in a setting suggesting obstruction is of some help in suggesting the diagnosis and in defining the possible cause of the obstruction. Also, because the second most common cause is incarcerated hernia, an examination of the inguinal and femoral regions should be part of every examination with the possible diagnosis of obstruction. This is particularly true when there have been no previous abdominal surgical procedures.

DIAGNOSIS

In the overwhelming majority of instances, the diagnosis of alimentary tract obstruction is obvious from the history and physical examination. Occasionally, further diagnostic studies seem necessary.

No characteristic changes of obstruction are reflected by examination of the patient's blood. Generally, whole blood and serum examinations reveal only some degree of nonspecific dehydration. In one specific instance, however, WBC evaluation may prove beneficial. In instances in which impending or actual necrosis or inflammatory bowel disease is suspected, marked elevations in WBC count are noted frequently. In conjunction with fever and moderate abdominal tenderness, the cause of the alimentary tract obstruction can be strongly suspected. Such suspicions have far-reaching implications for management, as is discussed subsequently.

By far the most helpful adjunct in diagnosis and management is the abdominal radiograph. Plain films of the abdomen taken with the patient in the recumbent and upright or lateral decubitus positions support the clinical diagnosis, frequently can distinguish be-

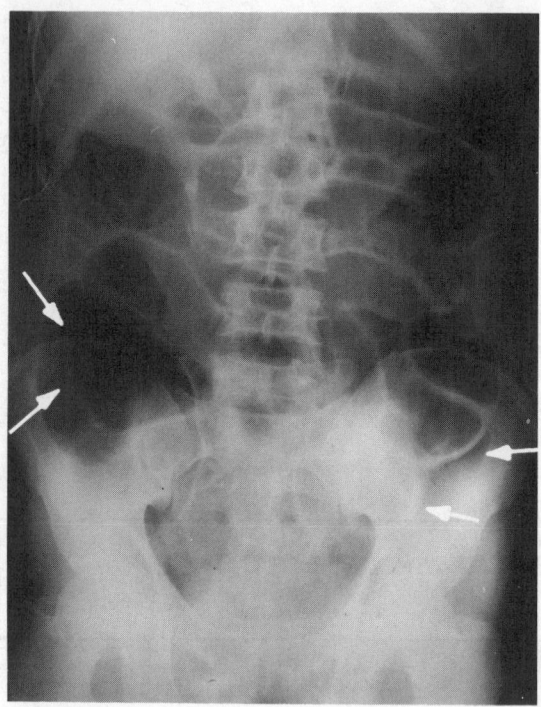

FIG. 49-11. Plain abdominal film of patient with paralytic ileus. Arrows denote the presence of gas in an undistended colon.

tween mechanical and paralytic obstruction, and often suggest the anatomic site of the obstruction (Figs. 49-11 and 49-12). When the plain film suggests that the obstruction is in the colon, many feel that a cautious barium enema for confirmation is in order.

Occasionally, in high mechanical obstruction or other exceptionally rare instances, an upper gastrointestinal series with small bowel follow-through may be required to confirm a clinical diagnosis.

MANAGEMENT

In our discussion of pathophysiology, we have emphasized the major determinants of morbidity and mortality associated with alimentary tract obstruction: extracellular fluid loss with dehydration and increases in intraluminal pressure secondary to air swallowing, ultimately leading to necrosis and perforation. It is clear, therefore, in which directions the primary therapeutic efforts should initially be directed.

Before 1930, the surgical mortality rate for acute obstruction was in the range of 30%. At the present time, it is 5 to 10%. Improved anesthesia, the liberal use of antibiotics and improved techniques in surgery and in patient monitoring all may have improved over the past 40 years, but the primary reason for the re-

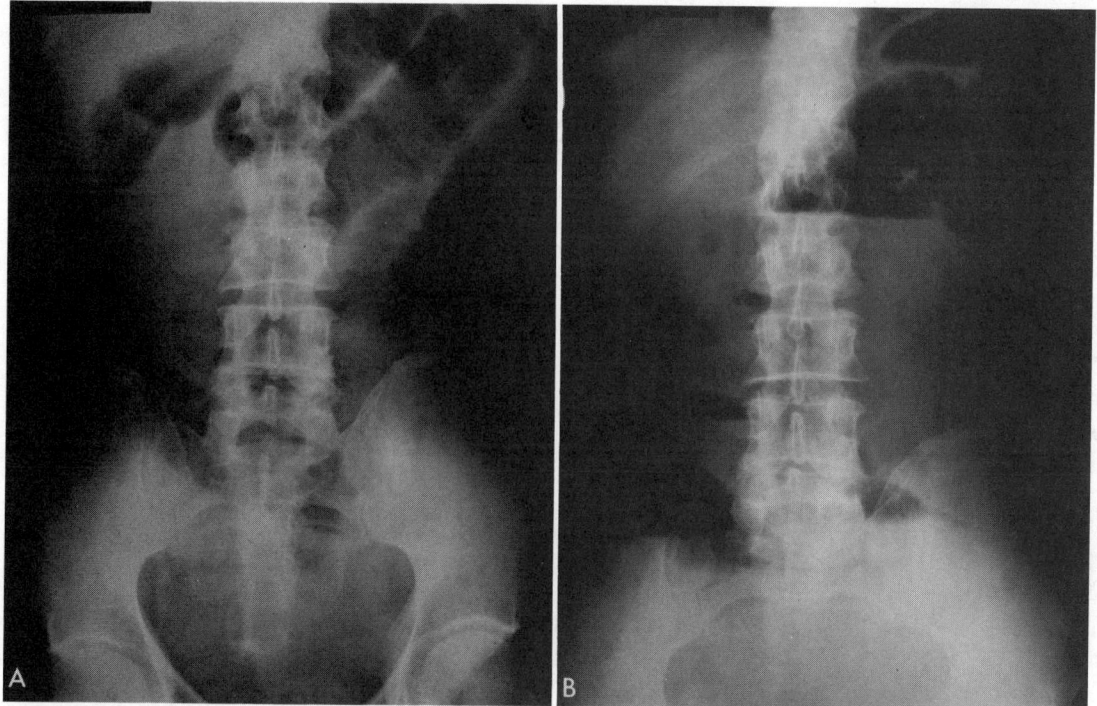

FIG. 49-12.   A. Plain abdominal film of a patient with mechanical small intestinal obstruction. Note the absence of colonic gas. B. Upright abdominal film of the same patient showing air-fluid levels in multiple loops of bowel. By themselves, air-fluid levels are not diagnostic of mechanical obstruction.

duction in mortality rate has been an appreciation of the necessity for preoperative rehydration. Because intraluminal fluid sequestration is an almost invariable process accompanying distention, for the reasons discussed (the so-called "third space" type of fluid loss), it follows that all patients with alimentary tract obstruction regardless of cause are dehydrated, differing only with respect to the degree of dehydration.

A primary effort, therefore, should be directed at rehydration. Because the patient has lost extracellular fluid, the composition of the replacement fluids should closely approximate extracellular fluid. At the present time, this may best be accomplished by the intravenous administration of Ringer's lactate solution in 5% dextrose and water. Potassium supplements should be added as required. Although no precise determinants are available of the total amount of replacement fluid to be given or of the rate of replacement, a few clinical guidelines may be of value. In instances of dehydration, a central venous pressure (CVP) monitoring line is of great assistance. Venous pressure values, particularly when taken in conjunction with hourly urine volumes and pulse and blood pressure information, provide a clinically reliable indication of hydration. As initial goals for the rate and volume of fluid administration, a CVP of >5 and <12 cm. H_2O, hourly urine output exceeding 30 cc/h, pulse <120, and satisfactory blood pressure should be achieved. Generally, this can be accomplished within 5 to 6 hours unless dehydration is particularly severe.

Second, as noted, it is of paramount importance to prevent the further intestinal accumulation of swallowed air. Intestinal intubation can effectively prevent continued aerophagic distention, permitting gradual intestinal absorption of gas already present in the intestine. It can serve no useful purpose to debate the efficiency of short versus long intestinal tubes in the absence of reliable quantitative data, and it is sufficient for our purpose to state that nasogastric tube decompression is eminently satisfactory. Appropriate placement and continued patency are clear prerequisites for the proper function of any decompressing tube.

After intestinal intubation and fluid replacement have been started, further studies can be carried out to determine the probable cause of the obstruction. Isolating the probable cause will determine whether future therapy will include surgery.

The basic distinction to be made is whether the obstruction has been produced by mechanical factors requiring surgical correction or is a manifestation of primary paralytic ileus and will resolve spontaneously. A most important observation in this regard is the presence of abdominal tenderness. Under this circumstance, in a setting of mechanical obstruction, impending or actual intestinal necrosis has complicated the picture. All therapeutic measures must be accelerated greatly if the patient is to survive. In this specific instance, surgical treatment should be regarded as an emergency.

Uncomplicated mechanical intestinal obstruction merely represents an urgent surgical situation, to be

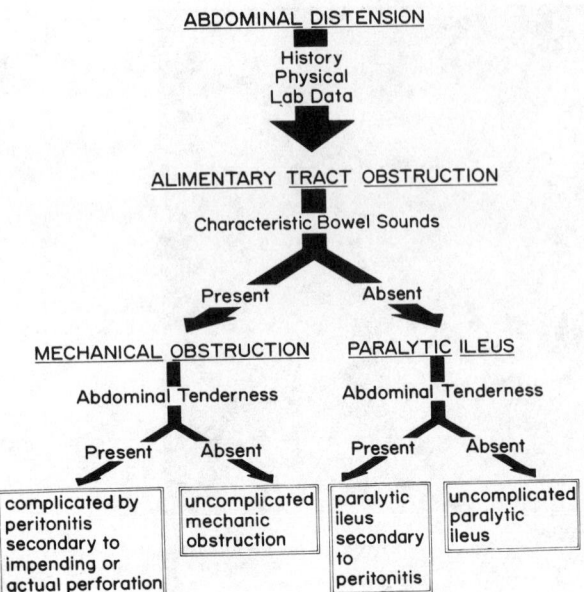

FIG. 49-13. Logic flow diagram emphasizing the clinical importance of abdominal tenderness in alimentary tract obstruction.

undertaken when the patient has been rehydrated and is in a more stable condition. Abdominal tenderness in a setting of paralytic ileus usually means that the ileus is secondary to an inflammatory process, such as appendicitis or cholecystitis. Thus, the therapeutic focus should properly be directed to that required by the inflammatory focus itself, since the resultant paralytic ileus is a secondary self-limiting phenomenon. These principles are expressed in the logic flow diagram shown in Figure 49-13.

SPECIFIC OBSTRUCTIONS

The general principles underlying diagnosis and management of most causes of obstruction have been discussed in the previous section, but certain representative obstructions are either compellingly urgent, sufficiently common, or seemingly divergent from basic principles to warrant individual attention.

ACUTE ESOPHAGEAL OBSTRUCTION

The diagnosis and management of chronic esophageal obstruction only infrequently confronts the emergency physician. On such rare occasions, the history of dysphagia is sufficiently characteristic to enable proper steps to be taken.

Conversely, acute esophageal obstruction is a frequent occurrence in emergency practice. Almost all

these instances result from foreign body ingestion. An ingestion history usually can be obtained from adults, but the diagnosis in children may be more difficult. One particularly helpful sign in children is excessive drooling. Frequently, the patient complains of a sensation of the object "sticking" at a certain highly specific level. A history of foreign body ingestion and subsequent substernal pain, frequently radiating to the neck, should suggest esophageal perforation. In conjunction with cervical subcutaneous emphysema and constitutional reactions, the diagnosis of perforation may be made. More commonly, however, the patient describes a "feeling" that a foreign body is lodged in the esophagus. If the object is metallic, a chest film will establish whether a foreign body is present and, if so, its exact location. As a *general* rule, any foreign body with no sharp or protruding edges that reaches the stomach safely traverses the intestinal tract. If the object is not metallic, esophagoscopy may be the only safe diagnostic alternative. In my opinion, the low incidence of morbidity of diagnosis and therapy with fiberoptic esophagoscopy is far less significant than the morbidity associated with previous suggestions, such as those advocating the blind forcing of a suspected foreign body down the esophagus and into the stomach by further ingestion or other mechanisms. Some reports of foreign body passage through the use of IV glucagon, however, make this one possible alternative treatment, particularly with lodgment of food material in the esophagus.

One particularly urgent form of acute esophageal obstruction is that produced by a lodgment of food in the esophagus at the level of the larynx, producing esophageal *and* laryngeal obstruction. This condition has properly been called the "café coronary." In the most severe form, the patient may have been calmly eating (usually meat) when he suddenly turned blue and became unconscious. Alcohol intake is a common historical finding. Because this situation is not unlike the sequence of events following an acute myocardial infarction, an initiating esophageal obstruction might not be considered. The association with eating, however, should alert the informed physician. An additional helpful feature is that these patients cannot speak. Marked stridor and dyspnea with retractions might substantiate the diagnosis. If the patient is maintaining some respiratory exchange, it is best to let his or her own protective mechanisms dislodge the obstruction. In the absence of effective respiration, urgent removal of the offending plug is necessary. This occasionally can be accomplished by fingers alone. Although rarely at hand under these conditions, a laryngoscope, if immediately available, should be used. In the absence of a laryngoscope, the Heimlich maneuver should be used. Grasping the affected person from behind, the operator places the fist of one hand in the other hand and rapidly squeezes the patient in the subxiphoid area. This maneuver produces a rapid increase in intrathoracic pressure, which may be sufficient to expel the foreign body. Should this maneuver fail to restore gas exchange, cricothyrotomy should not be delayed.

ACUTE GASTRIC DILATION

Mechanical gastric outlet obstruction producing chronic gastric dilation can have various causes. Acute massive gastric dilation, however, can occur in the absence of mechanical factors, presumably as a result of paralytic gastric ileus secondary to overactive sympathetic nervous stimulation. Acute gastric dilation is seen commonly in debilitated patients with nasogastric tubes who are receiving nasal oxygen. Instances of gastric distention leading to bursting have occurred when nasal oxygen has been inadvertently connected to the nasogastric tube. Episodes of acute gastric dilation also occur frequently in diabetic patients.

Whatever the underlying cause, marked gastric distention occurs, and 4 to 5 liters of extracellular fluid may accumulate. Distention of such a degree may produce interference with pulmonary and cardiac function through elevation of the diaphragm. In addition, such marked and rapid fluid losses may produce dehydration and hypovolemia. Vomiting with massive aspiration is a common sequela. The diagnosis in the described patients may be suspected if there are epigastric distention and tympany, repeated episodes of emesis, frequent singultus, and tachycardia. Untreated acute gastric dilation may be fatal. Adequate nasogastric tube drainage and rehydration remain the mainstays of therapy.

EXTERNAL INCARCERATED HERNIA

Because external incarcerated hernias may be the most frequent causes of alimentary tract obstruction in emergency practice, and because their management initially may differ from our general therapeutic principles, a brief discussion seems warranted.

By definition, an incarcerated hernia is an irreducible protrusion of abdominal contents beyond the usual confines of the abdominal cavity, without, however, any compromise of the blood supply to the herniated tissue. In contrast, a strangulated hernia exists when the aforementioned conditions are met, but blood supply is insufficient to maintain viability. The clinical distinction between incarceration and strangulation is not always as simple as the difference in terms might suggest. Because each strangulated hernia must first pass through a stage of incarceration in its temporal course, at many points in the continuum of development, distinction may be difficult. Generally, the development of necrosis is heralded by local tenderness, inflammation, fever, and an elevated WBC. It is of the utmost importance to distinguish between these two types of irreducible hernias be-

cause the advent of necrosis accelerates greatly our mode of therapy.

Three of the most common areas of hernia incarceration are the inguinal, femoral, and umbilical regions. Usually, the patient gives a history of noticing the hernia for several years. On this occasion, however, the previously reducible hernia cannot be replaced. If none of the signs of actual or impending necrosis is present, manipulative reduction of the hernia may be attempted. Such manipulation, particularly if improperly performed, may result in several complications. If necrosis of the hernial sac contents is not recognized before reduction, generalized peritonitis will result when the necrotic material is returned to the abdominal cavity. Second, it is possible to rupture the incarcerated bowel if undue force is applied in an attempt to reduce the hernia. A third possible complication of incarcerated hernia reduction is that of a reduction en masse, in which the incarcerated mass of tissue is returned to the abdominal cavity but is not released from constriction (Fig. 49-14). Because of these potential complications, any patient undergoing successful hernia reduction should be followed continuously in a controlled environment until it can be established that none of these potential complications has developed. Surgical repair of the successfully reduced incarcerated hernia should be undertaken at the earliest convenient time to prevent a recurrence.

Failure to reduce the incarceration is an indication for urgent surgical repair in an effort to prevent the development of strangulation and subsequent necro-

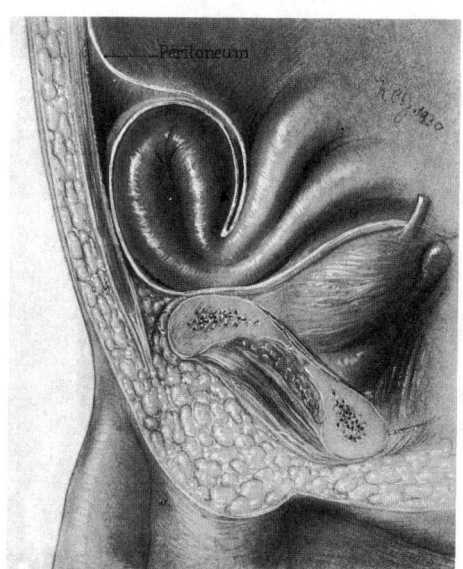

FIG. 49-14. *En masse reduction of an inguinal hernia. In this complication, the entire hernia sac and its contents are "reduced" back within the abdomen. The intestinal component of the hernia, however, is not reduced from the sac. If sufficient constriction is present at the neck of the hernia sac, necrosis of intestine still confirmed within the hernia sac can occur. (With permission from Pearse, H.E., Jr.: Strangulated hernia reduced en masse. Surg. Gynecol. Obstet., 53:822, 1931.)*

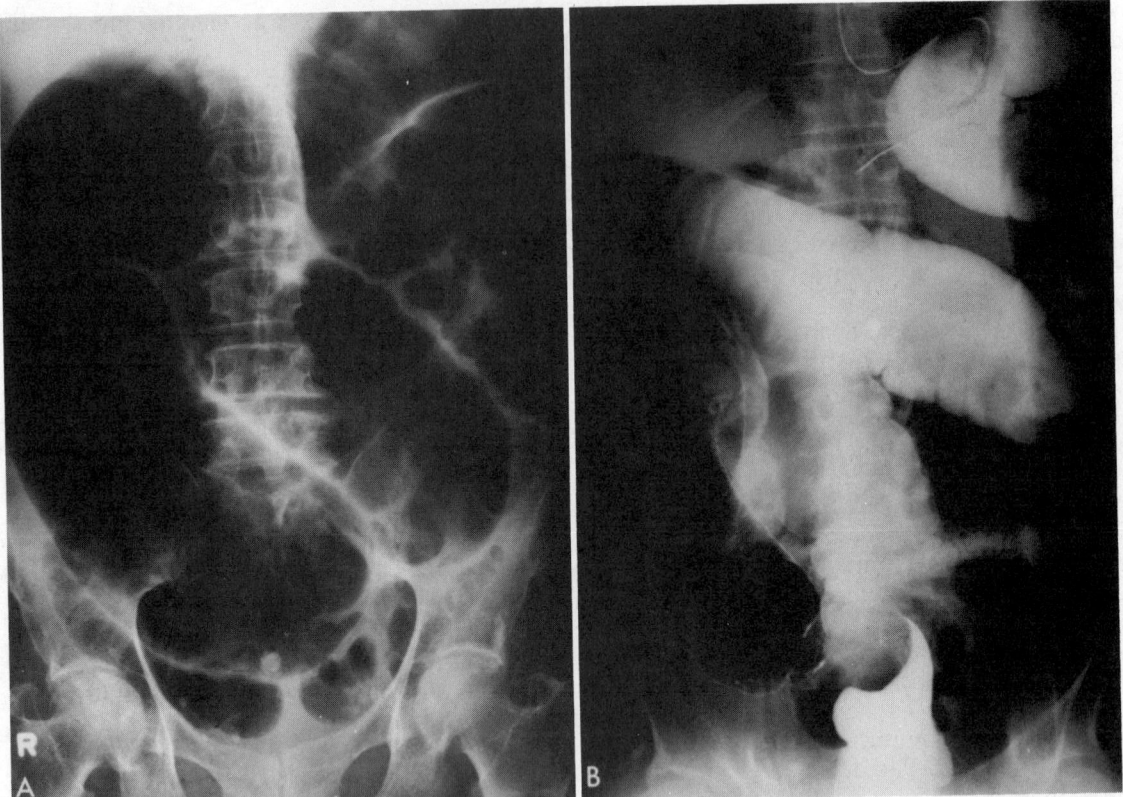

FIG. 49-15. A. Plain abdominal film of a patient with sigmoid volvulus. Note the large gas filled loop of sigmoid pointing toward the right upper quadrant. B. Barium enema x-ray on this same patient. Some barium has passed the area of twisting into the proximal colon. The tapering sigmoid at the point of twist has been referred to as a "parrot's beak."

sis. Preparations are similar to those general principles of management previously discussed.

RECTOSIGMOID OBSTRUCTION

Obstructions localized to the distal colon and rectum require that the emergency physician be familiar with several specialized forms of management peculiar to this region.

One of the basic dissimilarities in the pathophysiology of mechanical colonic obstruction, when compared with mechanical obstruction at other sites, is whether or not the ileocecal valve is functionally competent. In the 30% of patients in whom this valve is competent, distention is limited exclusively to the colon when a distal obstruction exists. Accumulated gases and subsequent distention cannot be "decompressed" back into the small bowel; a closed-loop obstruction exists. Should the abdominal film suggest a closed-loop obstruction, haste in operative decompression is urgent. If, as is usual, the ileocecal valve is not competent, the abdominal film will suggest a rather generalized dilation of both small and large bowel. This situation allows more time for rehydration, gastric decompression, and delineation of the obstruction.

The technique of proctosigmoidoscopy is an indispensable aid in the diagnosis and management of rectosigmoid obstructions. Most of the common causes of acute obstruction in this region, fecal impaction, carcinoma, inflammatory colon diseases, volvulus, and foreign bodies, are easily recognizable when seen through the sigmoidoscope. Occasionally, its use permits non-operative decompression of sigmoid volvulus.

The diagnosis of volvulus can frequently be suspected by careful examination of the abdominal films (Fig. 49-15). A cautious barium enema may reveal the characteristic "parrot's beak." When performing sigmoidoscopy on such patients, the physician finds that a most valuable piece of equipment is a bronchoscopy shield. If the operator is able to decompress the twisted sigmoid by *gentle* manipulation of the sigmoidoscope, the rapid colonic decompression through the sigmoidoscope will amply justify the use of the shield. If decompression can be obtained with the sigmoidoscope, a large red rubber catheter should be placed in the rectosigmoid area to prevent recurrent intestinal torsion in the post-decompression period. Following nonoperative decompression, strong consideration should be given to elective sigmoid resection in good risk patients because the recurrence rate is exceptionally high.

It should be clear that no sigmoidoscopic attempt to reduce a sigmoid volvulus should be made if there is any question of the viability of the involved colon. Nonoperative detorsion of necrotic colon results in death. In general, if sigmoidoscopic detorsion has failed, it is unwise to persist in any further nonoperative attempts, because volvulus represents a classic example of strangulation obstruction.

REFERENCE

1. Wangensteen, O.H., and Rea, C.E.: The distention factor in simple intestinal obstruction. An experimental study with exclusion of swallowed air by cervical esophagostomy. Surgery 5:327, 1939.

BIBLIOGRAPHY

Barnett, W.O., and Hardy, J.D.: Observations concerning the peritoneal fluid in strangulated intestinal obstruction: the effects of removal from the peritoneal cavity. Surgery 43:440, 1958.

Caesar, R.: The acute geriatric abdomen. *In* Geriatric Emergency Medicine. Edited by Bosker, G., Schwartz, G.R., Jones, J.S., and Sequeira, M. St. Louis, C.V. Mosby Co., 1990.

Cohn, I., Jr.: Strangulation obstruction: collective review. Surg. Gynecol. Obstet. *103*:105, 1956.

Cokkins, A.J.: The Management of Abdominal Operations. 2nd ed. London, Lewis, 1957.

Drucker, W.R., and Wright, H.K.: Physiology and pathophysiology of gastrointestinal fluids. Curr. Probl. Surg. May, 1964.

Maingot, R.: Abdominal Operations. 5th ed. New York, Appleton-Century-Crofts, Inc., 1969.

Mucha, P.: Small intestinal obstruction. Surg. Clin. North Am. *67*:597, 1987.

Noer, R.J., and Derr, J.W.: Effect of distention on intestinal revascularization. Arch. Surg. *59*:542, 1949.

Phillips, S.L., and Burns, G.P.: Abdominal disease in the aged. Med. Clin. North Am. *22*:1213, 1988.

Shields, R.: The absorption and secretion of fluid and electrolytes by the obstructed bowel. Br. J. Surg. *52*:774, 1965.

Sperling, L.: Mechanics of simple obstruction: an experimental study. Arch. Surg. *36*:778, 1938.

Van Zwalenburg, C.: Strangulation resulting from strangulation of hollow viscera. Ann. Surg. *46*:780, 1907.

Wangensteen, O.H.: Intestinal Obstructions. 3rd ed. Springfield, Ill., Charles C Thomas, 1955.

Welch, C.E.: Intestinal Obstruction. Chicago, Ill., Year Book Medical Publishers, Inc., 1958.

INTRA-ABDOMINAL INFECTIONS

Abdollah B. Naficy and Henry W. Murray

CAPSULE

Intra-abdominal bacterial infection usually presents as one of three syndromes: (a) spontaneous bacterial peritonitis, which typically occurs in patients with pre-existing ascites; (b) secondary peritonitis resulting from an identifiable preceding cause such as a perforated organ; or (c) intra-abdominal abscess, which now most commonly occurs as a postoperative complication. Polymicrobial infection with both gram-negative aerobic enteric bacilli (e.g., Escherichia coli) and anaerobes (e.g., Bacteroides fragilis) is regularly present except in spontaneous bacterial peritonitis, which is most often caused by a single isolate such as E. coli or Streptococcus pneumoniae. Although the diagnosis of secondary peritonitis or intra-abdominal abscess is usually apparent clinically, occasionally paracentesis or laparotomy may be initially required to confirm the diagnosis. The diagnosis of intra-abdominal abscess has clearly been facilitated by ultrasonography, computed tomography, and radionuclide scanning. Percutaneous guided-needle aspiration can be used to confirm the diagnosis and at the same time provide successful drainage in selected cases. Treatment consists of prompt and adequate drainage combined with effective antimicrobial therapy.

PATHOPHYSIOLOGY

Primary peritonitis is defined as diffuse peritoneal inflammation of microbial origin with no apparent intra-abdominal source of infection. Possible pathogenetic

TABLE 49-11A. CONDITIONS THAT MAY LEAD TO SECONDARY PERITONITIS

ORGAN PERFORATION
    With inflammation (appendicitis, diverticulitis, cholecystitis)
    With ulceration (peptic, typhoid, amebic, tuberculous, cytomegalovirus)
    Post-traumatic instrumentation
    Neoplastic
ORGAN INFARCTION
    Mesenteric vascular occlusion
    Intestinal obstruction
    Intestinal strangulation
POSTSURGICAL
    Operative contamination
    Anastomotic leakage
PANCREATITIS
PENETRATING OR BLUNT TRAUMA
PERITONEAL DIALYSIS
RUPTURE OF AN INTRAPERITONEAL OR VISCERAL ABSCESS

mechanisms include direct hematogenous or lymphatic spread to the peritoneum, bacteria traversing the intact intestinal wall, or organisms ascending the female genital tract. Predisposing factors in children include the nephrotic syndrome and postnecrotic cirrhosis.[1,2] Among adult patients, those with ascites resulting from cirrhosis are most susceptible to spontaneous bacterial peritonitis. In such patients, direct hematogenous spread from an extraperitoneal suppurative focus to pre-existing ascites appears to be the likely mechanism of infection.[3]

In contrast, in secondary bacterial peritonitis, predisposing intraperitoneal conditions can usually be readily identified. Any one of a number of intra-abdominal events may lead to secondary peritonitis (Table 49-11A). Most intra-abdominal abscesses seen today are postoperative complications, usually following gastroduodenal or biliary tract surgery with direct contamination or postoperative leakage of an anastomosis.

Bacterial peritonitis may also complicate antecedent chemical peritonitis initiated, for example, by leakage of gastric, biliary, or pancreatic secretions into the peritoneal cavity. Experimental evidence indicates that suppurative peritonitis cannot be induced by injection of bacteria alone, but instead requires the presence of other factors such as irritating chemical adjuvants, blood (free hemoglobin), and different types of bacteria (bacterial synergism).[4] In areas of peritoneal inflammation, there is release of exudative fluid with a high protein and fibrinogen content and influx of inflammatory phagocytic leukocytes. Such areas may become localized as paralyzed intestinal loops adhere in the fibrinous exudate to the adjacent omentum and mesentery. If localization is not rapidly accomplished or fails to develop, patients are at risk for diffuse suppurative peritonitis or multifocal intraperitoneal infection with abscess formation. In these latter patients,

many of whom are bacteremic, shifts of fluid into the peritoneal cavity and bowel lumen coupled with endotoxemia often leads to intravascular depletion with hypotension, tachycardia, cutaneous vasoconstriction, capillary leakage, hemoconcentration, and lactic acidosis.

In some instances, spontaneous resolution of intraperitoneal infection may occur after minor bacterial contamination and appropriate local and systemic host defense responses. Otherwise, especially in the setting of particularly virulent bacteria, pre-existing debilitating disease, or malnourishment, diffuse peritonitis is favored with hemodynamic collapse and death. Incomplete resolution usually leads to abscess formation within dependent recesses in the peritoneal cavity; visceral abscesses may also develop secondarily. Encapsulated strains of Bacteroides fragilis appear to be protected from phagocytosis, and the capsular polysaccharide of this bacterium represents a virulence factor because it can, by itself, induce abscess formation.[5]

MICROBIOLOGY

The empty motile stomach with secretions of an acid pH normally contains few microorganisms ($<10^3$ colony-forming units [CFU] per mL). The bacteria present are mostly derived from the normal oral flora. Descending the gastrointestinal tract, colony counts gradually increase until they reach the distal ileum and colon, where dramatically high levels of up to 10^{11} CFU per mL of feces are found. In the colon, the ratio of anaerobes to aerobes is approximately 1000:1.[6] It is this distribution of bacteria that contributes to the increased morbidity and mortality from sepsis associated with perforations of the colon compared to perforations of the upper gastrointestinal tract. The relative numbers and sensitivity patterns of the gastrointestinal tract's microflora may be altered by hospitalization, achlorhydria, antacids, prior antibiotic therapy, intestinal hemorrhage, and stasis or obstruction.

Escherichia coli, Streptococcus pneumoniae, and group A streptococci are the most frequent isolates in *primary (spontaneous) bacterial peritonitis*. Because by definition the bowel is intact in primary bacterial peritonitis, it is not surprising that anaerobes play a particularly minor role in this setting and represent less than 10% of all isolates.[7] Mycobacterium tuberculosis and fungal infections occasionally cause primary peritonitis as a result of hematogenous implantation.

In *secondary bacterial peritonitis* and intra-abdominal abscess, anaerobes are virtually always present. These infections are also invariably polymicrobial, and a broad spectrum of both anaerobes and aerobes derived from the intestinal lumen can be isolated from clinical

TABLE 49-12. BACTERIA COMMONLY ISOLATED IN SECONDARY PERITONITIS AND INTRA-ABDOMINAL ABSCESS

Aerobes	Anaerobes
Escherichia coli	Bacteroides fragilis
Klebsiella species	Clostridium species
Proteus species	Peptostreptococci
Enterobacter species	Eubacterium species
Pseudomonas species	Fusobacterium species
Enterococci	Bacteroides melaninogenicus

specimens. The commonest organisms isolated are listed in Table 49-12. Occasionally, infections in adjacent foci caused by organisms such as *Staphylococcus aureus, Neisseria gonorrhoeae,* and *M. tuberculosis* may spread and cause secondary peritonitis. Peritoneal dialysis directly predisposes to secondary peritonitis most often caused by Candida species and staphylococci.

CLINICAL MANIFESTATIONS

Abdominal pain is invariably present in peritonitis. Although pain can initially be localized and suggest the original source of infection, there is often progressive extension of infection resulting in diffuse pain that is exacerbated by any kind of movement including respiration. Other variable symptoms include fever, chills, anorexia, nausea, vomiting, and abdominal distention.

The patient with bacterial peritonitis is usually febrile, tachycardic, and lying supine with knees flexed and shallow respirations to minimize the abdominal pain. There is generalized abdominal tenderness with rebound tenderness indicating involvement of the parietal peritoneum. Guarding and reflex muscular spasm lead to a rigid abdominal wall; this finding may be masked in patients receiving steroid therapy or those in shock. Bowel sounds are diminished or absent. Rectal and pelvic examinations may reveal an area of maximal tenderness or a fluid collection or mass. If there is overwhelming sepsis or inadequate response to therapy, hypotension, hypothermia, oliguria, and delirium may all be present.

In certain patients, the clinical presentation may be atypical or subtle. Cirrhotic patients with spontaneous bacterial peritonitis usually have pre-existing ascites and may present insidiously with low-grade fever alone or worsening of liver disease. With gonococcal (Fitz-Hugh-Curtis syndrome) or chlamydial perihepatitis, there is right upper quadrant pain that may be referred to the right shoulder and accompanied by a friction rub over the liver. Pelvic examination may

reveal adnexal tenderness. Primary tuberculous peritonitis usually has a subacute onset with fever, night sweats, malaise, anorexia, weight loss, and increasing abdominal distention. Extraperitoneal presentations of intra-abdominal infection include empyema of the chest or a suppurative mass in the thigh or flank.

With early localization of peritoneal inflammation, pain and tenderness may become focal and less intense with a concomitant decrease in fever. With the development of intra-abdominal abscess, however, fever returns and localizing symptoms intensify. Occasionally, especially in the elderly, low-grade fever, malaise, anorexia, and weight loss may be the only manifestations; previous or partial antibiotic therapy may also predispose to chronicity.

DIAGNOSIS

Nonspecific laboratory findings include peripheral blood leukocytosis with a left shift on the differential count. An increased hematocrit and blood urea nitrogen result from hemoconcentration. Blood cultures may yield the putative organisms. Paracentesis can be of diagnostic value, especially with primary bacterial peritonitis. In the latter instance, the leukocyte count of the peritoneal fluid is invariably greater than 300 per mm^3 and a predominance of granulocytes is found.[3] If no fluid is aspirated, peritoneal lavage using Ringer's lactate solution can be performed. Any fluid obtained should be examined for gross appearance, cell count with differential, total protein and amylase content, and bacteriologic smears and cultures. Gram-stained smears of ascitic fluid are negative for bacteria in most cases of spontaneous bacterial peritonitis.

Occasionally, *laparoscopy or laparotomy may* be required to exclude a primary intra-abdominal source of peritoneal inflammation. This is especially true in children, in whom it may be otherwise impossible to differentiate between primary bacterial peritonitis and acute appendicitis. With tuberculous peritonitis, multiple nodules may be observed over the peritoneal surface, a biopsy of which confirms the diagnosis.

Abdominal roentgenograms typically demonstrate an ileus pattern with distended loops of bowel. Other possible findings include free air indicating a perforated viscus, obliteration of the peritoneal fat lines and psoas shadows, or in the case of an intra-abdominal abscess, a soft tissue density, extraluminal gas, or organ displacement. Contrast studies by either oral or rectal administration may be useful in confirming the extraluminal location of any air or demonstrating suspected perforation or anastomotic leaks from the gastrointestinal tract. Chest roentgenograms may reveal an elevated diaphragm or a pleural effusion if a subphrenic abscess is present. A *radionuclide scan* of the lungs and liver may show displacement of the indented liver from the right lung base by a subphrenic abscess.

Abdominal ultrasonography is a readily available and noninvasive method for evaluating the presence of an abscess. The latter usually appears as a fluid collection with a slightly irregular wall (Fig. 49-16). Overlying bowel gas and postoperative changes may interfere with interpretation. Taylor et al. reported a sensitivity of 93.3% and a specificity of 98.6% in the diagnosis of abdominal and pelvic abscesses using ultrasonography alone.[8]

Computed tomography (CT) is also useful in identifying an intra-abdominal abscess. Contrast material can be given parenterally to enhance the surrounding capsule and enterally to distinguish loops of bowel from the abscess cavity (Fig. 49-17). The presence of metallic clips or residual barium can diminish accuracy. Using CT in the diagnosis of abdominal and pelvic abscesses, Koehler and Moss reported a sensitivity of 99% and a specificity of 84%.[9]

Gallium-67 scanning locates an abdominal abscess as an area of increased uptake (Figure 49-18) with a sensitivity of 80 to 90%. The specificity of this technique, however, is significantly reduced by excretion of gallium into the intestinal tract (which also adds delay of 48 to 72 hours for optimal scanning) and by uptake in neoplasms or other inflammatory tissue such as normal postoperative sites.

Although technically more difficult, *indium-labeled leukocyte scans* are highly sensitive (86%) and appear more specific (95%) than gallium scans in the detection of abdominal abscesses.[10] Indium-labeled white blood cells are not excreted by the kidneys or intestine, and there is significantly less uptake at postoperative sites than with gallium scanning.

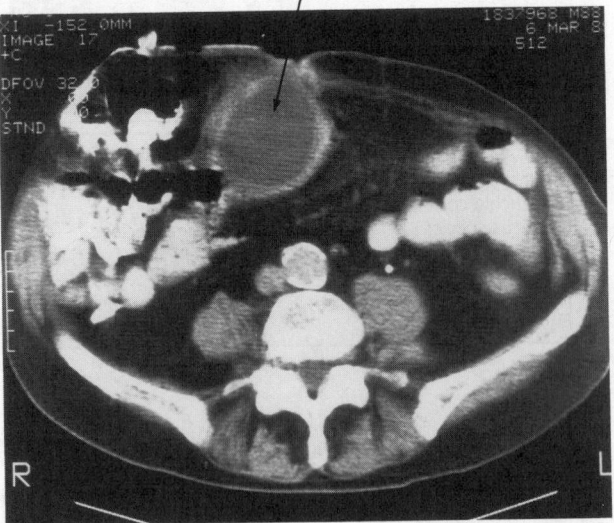

FIG. 49-17. Computed tomograph with contrast demonstrating a ring-enhancing intra-abdominal abscess (arrow) in a patient with Crohn's disease and a colostomy. (Courtesy of Dr. J. Mahal, New York Hospital.)

The initial investigative procedure after conventional radiographic studies in the presence of localized clinical findings should include ultrasonography and/or CT. The latter is preferable in obese patients or those who have had recent surgery. CT appears more accurate for evaluating areas other than the right upper quadrant or pelvis where ultrasound demonstrates equal sensitivity. During either study, definitive diagnosis may be made by guided percutaneous needle aspiration; CT usually provides greater precision for small, deeply seated, or intraperitoneal collections. In the absence of clinical localizing features and if the patient is not critically ill, a radionuclide scan may be

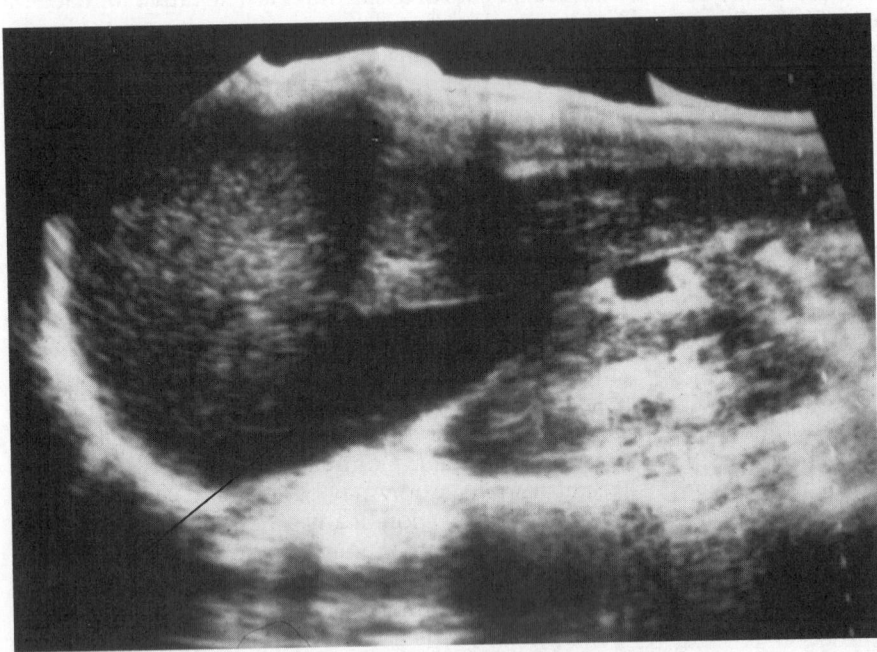

FIG. 49-16. A subhepatic abscess (arrow) which developed after cholecystectomy, diagnosed by ultrasound examination (longitudinal scan). (Courtesy of Dr. W. Rubenstein, New York Hospital.)

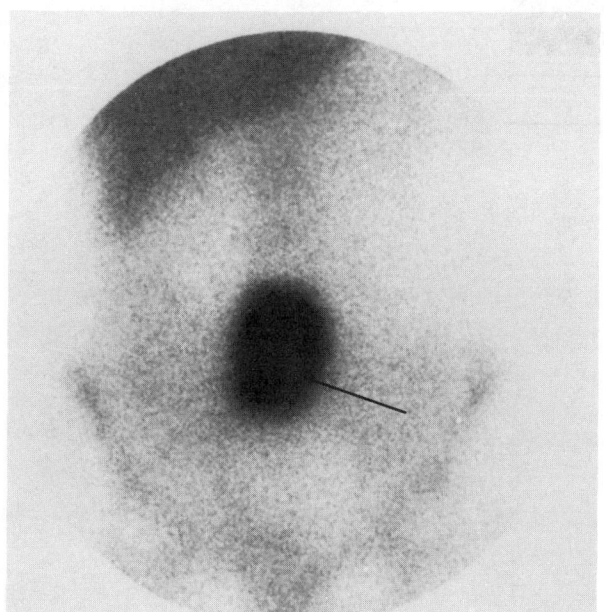

FIG. 49-18. Gallium-67 scan of the abdomen demonstrating a large oval area of intense radioactivity in the mid-lower abdomen (arrow). A pelvic abscess was found at laparotomy. (Courtesy of Dr. S. Sarkar, New York Hospital.)

considered initially. A localized area of increased uptake can then be further evaluated using ultrasound or CT.

TREATMENT

Initial therapy includes withholding anything by mouth, nasogastric intubation and suctioning, intravenous fluid and electrolyte replacement, hemodynamic and respiratory support, and the rapid institution of empiric antimicrobial therapy after blood cultures have been drawn. Increased metabolic demands may necessitate the provision of total parenteral nutrition. Prompt surgical drainage and effective antibiotic therapy to prevent further local bacterial invasion or septicemia are the cornerstones of treatment.

Surgery is required to prevent continuing peritoneal contamination; remove purulent collections, necrotic tissue and foreign material; and allow peritoneal lavage. In the absence of abscess formation, operation is usually not required for peritonitis secondary to pelvic inflammatory disease or in primary bacterial peritonitis.

Recently, in patients with intra-abdominal abscess, there has been a trend to attempt to avoid conventional surgical drainage by first attempting percutaneous catheter drainage guided by sonography or CT. This procedure should be limited to discretely loculated, adequately liquified collections that are safely accessible without traversing intervening bowel, blood vessels, or sterile cavities. Surgical backup must be readily available. In selected cases and experienced hands, success rates of approximately 85% are comparable to traditional operative drainage results. The overall complication rate is about 10%, and includes peritoneal spillage, septicemia, hemorrhage, and fistula formation.[11] In patients who are not satisfactory surgical risks, percutaneous drainage is probably the best alternative.

ANTIBIOTIC THERAPY

Parenteral antibiotics should be started as soon as the diagnosis is considered and after smears and cultures of readily accessible materials are obtained. There is no evidence that supplemental peritoneal irrigation with antibiotics improves outcome. The choice of optimal empiric antibiotic therapy can be made only with a complete understanding of the broad spectrum of potential infecting microorganisms as described earlier, local microbial sensitivity patterns, and the differential toxicities of the wide array of antibacterial agents now available. (See Chap. 50). Cost factors and hospital formulary limitations may also restrict the clinician's choices of therapy.

Empiric antibiotic treatment must be active against both aerobic enteric gram-negative bacilli and anaerobes, especially the Bacteroides fragilis group (Table 49-13). Traditional therapy has been a combination of an aminoglycoside plus either clindamycin or metronidazole. The combination of aztreonam and clindamycin appears to be an effective alternative that can avoid the potential nephrotoxicity and ototoxicity of the aminoglycosides.[12] Third-generation cephalosporins (e.g., cefotaxime, ceftriaxone, or ceftazidime) that demonstrate broad activity against aerobic bowel flora may also substitute for the aminoglycosides. The latter three agents, however, exert little activity against anaerobes, and therefore should not be used alone. If Pseudomonas aeruginosa is a suspected pathogen (e.g., a hospital-acquired infection), ceftazidime is the appropriate third-generation cephalosporin to use. In uncomplicated community-acquired intra-abdominal infection, monotherapy with cefoxitin,[13] piperacillin, ticarcillin-calvulanic acid, or ampicillin-sulbactam[14] is probably as effective as traditional therapy, with less toxicity. Imipenem-cilastatin has the broadest coverage of any single antimicrobial agent, and is as effective as therapy with clindamycin plus an aminoglycoside, even in complicated cases.[15] Agents that exert little or no antianaerobic activity, including first-generation cephalosporins and the newer quinolones, should never be used alone in intra-abdominal infections.

Although enterococci are isolated from approximately 20% of intra-abdominal infections, virtually all patients are adequately treated with antibiotic regi-

TABLE 49-13. EMPIRIC ANTIBIOTIC THERAPY FOR INTRA-ABDOMINAL INFECTIONS

Antibiotic	Dosage*
Traditional combination therapy	
Clindamycin	900 mg IV q8h
plus	
gentamicin†	2 mg/kg IV loading, then 1.5 mg/ kg IV q8h
Alternatives to clindamycin	
Metronidazole	1 g IV loading, then 500 mg IV q6h
Cefoxitin	2 g IV q6h
Ampicillin–sulbactam	3 g IV q6h
Alternatives to gentamicin	
Aztreonam	2 g IV q8h
Cefotaxime	2 g IV q8h
Ceftriaxone	1 g IV q12h
Ceftazidime	2 g IV q8h
Monotherapy in selected cases (see text)	
Cefoxitin	2 g IV q6h
Piperacillin	3 g IV q4h
Imipenem–cilastatin	500 mg IV q6h
Ticarcillin–clavulanic acid	3.1 g IV q4h
Ampicillin–sulbactam	3 g IV q6h

* Adult doses for serious infection provided normal hepatic and renal function.
† Other aminoglycosides (tobramycin or amikacin) may be used.

mens that lack specific activity against enterococci. Reports of enterococcal septicemia in patients who are chronically ill, malnourished, immunosuppressed, on broad-spectrum antibiotics, or have indwelling foreign bodies (e.g., intravenous or dialysis catheters) also make it prudent to add early empiric therapy with antienterococcal agents (e.g., ampicillin, piperacillin, or vancomycin) in these selected patients.[16]

The parenteral antibiotic regimen chosen should be continued for approximately 2 weeks after successful drainage, and can be modified according to the clinical response and culture results.

Bacterial peritonitis complicating chronic peritoneal dialysis is often initially treated with a 2-week course of broad-spectrum intraperitoneal antibiotics (e.g., vancomycin and tobramycin) coupled with an increased frequency of exchanges for one to two days. In severe infections or if the clinical response is poor, the dialysis catheter should be removed and parenteral antibiotics administered.

PROGNOSIS

Spontaneous bacterial peritonitis in patients with an underlying debilitating illness (e.g., cirrhosis and ascites) carries a high mortality (>50%) despite antibiotic therapy. Otherwise, survival is good (>90%). Similarly, the prognosis in secondary peritonitis depends largely on the underlying clinical condition of the pa-

tient. The primary etiologic process, degree of peritoneal contamination, duration of infection before appropriate therapy, and effectiveness of drainage are also important determinants of outcome. The mortality of untreated secondary bacterial peritonitis or intra-abdominal abscess approaches 100%.

REFERENCES

1. Speck, W.T., Dresdale, S.S., and McMillan, R.W.: Primary peritonitis and the nephrotic syndrome. Am. J. Surg. *127*:267, 1974.
2. McDougal, W.S., Izant, R.J., Zollinger, R.M. Jr.: Primary peritonitis in infancy and childhood. Ann. Surg. *181*:310, 1975.
3. Conn, H.O.: Spontaneous bacterial peritonitis in cirrhosis, multiple revisitations. Gastroenterology *70*:455, 1976.
4. Levison, M.E., and Bush, L.M.: Peritonitis and other intraabdominal infections. *In* Principles and Practice of Infectious Diseases. Edited by Mandell, G.L., Douglas, R.G. Jr., and Bennet, J.E. New York, Churchill Livingstone, 1990, p. 636.
5. Onderdonk, A.B., Kasper, D.L., Cisneros, R.L., et al.: The capsular polysaccharide of *Bacteroides fragilis* as a virulence factor: Comparison of the pathogenic potential of encapsulated and unencapsulated strains. J. Infect. Dis. *136*:82, 1977.
6. Nichols, R.L.: Intraabdominal infections: An overview. Rev. Infect. Dis. *7*(Suppl 4):S709, 1985.
7. Targan, S.R., Chow, A.W., Guze, L.B.: Role of anaerobic bacteria in spontaneous peritonitis of cirrhosis: Report of two cases and review of the literature. Am. J. Med. *62*:397, 1977.
8. Taylor, K.J.W., Sullivan, D.C., Wasson, J.F.McI., et al.: Ultrasound and gallium for the diagnosis of abdominal and pelvic abscesses. Gastrointest. Radiol. *3*:281, 1978.
9. Koehler, P.R., and Moss, A.A.: Diagnosis of intraabdominal and pelvic abscesses by computerized tomography. JAMA *244*:49, 1980.
10. Knochel, J.Q., Koehler, P.R., Lee, T.G., et al.: Diagnosis of

abdominal abscesses with computed tomography, ultrasound, and ¹¹¹In leukocyte scans. Radiology *137*:425, 1980.

11. Jeffrey, R.B., Jr.: Percutaneous drainage of abdominal abscesses: The role of the radiologist. *In* New surgical and medical approaches in infectious diseases. Edited by Root, R.K., Trunkey, D.D., and Sande, M.A. New York, Churchill Livingstone, 1987, p. 133.

12. Birolini, D., Moraes, M.F., and de Souza, O.S.: Aztreonam plus clindamycin vs. tobramycin plus clindamycin for the treatment of intraabdominal infections. Rev. Infect. Dis. *7*(Suppl 4)S724, 1985.

13. Drusano, G.L., Warren, J.W., Saah, A.J., et al.: A prospective randomized controlled trial of cefoxitin versus clindamycin-aminoglycoside in mixed anaerobic-aerobic infections. Surg. Gynecol. Obstet. *154*:715, 1982.

14. Kager, L., Malmborg, A.S., Nord, C.E., et al.: A randomized controlled trial of ampicillin plus sulbactam vs. gentamicin plus clindamycin in the treatment of intraabdominal infections: A preliminary report. Rev. Infect. Dis. *8*(Suppl 5):S583, 1986.

15. Kager, L., and Nord, C.E.: Imipenem-cilastatin in the treatment of intraabdominal infections: A review of worldwide experience. Rev. Infect. Dis *7*(Suppl 3):S518, 1985.

16. Dougherty, S.H.: Role of enterococcus in intraabdominal sepsis. Am. J. Surg. *148*:308, 1984.

SELECTED READINGS

Jeffrey, R.B., Jr.: Percutaneous drainage of abdominal abscesses: The role of the radiologist. *In* New surgical and medical approaches in infectious diseases. Edited by Root, R.K., Trunkey, D.D., and Sande, M.A. New York, Churchill Livingstone, 1987, p. 133.

Levison, M.E., and Bush, L.M.: Peritonitis and other intraabdominal infections. *In* Principles and Practice of Infectious Diseases. Edited by Mandell, G.L., Douglas, R.G. Jr., and Bennet, J.E. New York, Churchill Livingstone, 1990, p. 636.

GASTRITIS AND PEPTIC ULCER DISEASE

Michael W. Mulholland and Frederic E. Eckhauser

CAPSULE

Despite the remarkable advances in elucidation of the pathophysiology of acute gastritis and chronic peptic ulcer and in pharmacology that have occurred in the past decade, these disease remain major public health problems. The diseases may present as pain, or with complicating hemorrhage, perforation, or obstruction. A large number of acute and chronic gastrointestinal processes must be distinguished from gastritis or peptic ulcer. Therapeutic choices are varied. Definitive diagnosis must be vigorously pursued so that specific and effective treatment may be rendered.

PATHOPHYSIOLOGY

Acute gastritis and chronic peptic ulcer share many clinical and therapeutic characteristics. It is important to recognize, however, that important differences in pathophysiology and therapy also exist. The term acute gastritis encompasses many disease processes characterized by inflammation and/or superficial ulceration limited to the mucosal layer of the stomach. These mucosal lesions, which may result from a number of noxious stimuli, reflect the loss of mucosal resistance to the injurious effects of gastric acid and pepsin. Factors that cause gastritis experimentally have variously been noted to increase mucosal permeability to luminal acid, decrease mucosal nutrient blood flow, be associated with abnormalities of mucosal prostaglandin production, or decrease mucosal bicarbonate production. The net result of these changes is a decreased ability of the gastric mucosa to withstand acid-peptic digestion and to efficiently repair mucosal loss.

When viewed endoscopically, the gastric mucosa in patients with acute gastritis is edematous and friable, with superficial ulceration and often hemorrhage. In contrast to chronic peptic ulceration, ulcers found in association with acute gastritis do not penetrate beyond the muscularis mucosae, and histologically, submucosal fibrosis is absent in areas of ulceration. Although ulcers may be noted in any region of the stomach, lesions are often most prominent in the acid-secreting fundus. The endoscopic appearance of gastritis may thus closely resemble the findings in severely ill hospitalized patients with "stress" gastritis. In most ambulatory patients, acute gastritis occurs in response to ingestion of some readily identified noxious agent. The most common offenders are alcohol and medications such as aspirin and nonsteroidal anti-inflammatory compounds. Occasionally, patients

Acute Gastritis
Increased mucosal permeability
Decreased mucosal blood flow
Decreased mucosal prostaglandin production
Decreased mucosal bicarbonate secretion

Chronic Peptic Ulceration
Acid secretory abnormalities
    Increased basal secretion
    Increased meal response
    Increased peak secretory capacity
Gastric emptying abnormalities
    Accelerated emptying of liquids
Decreased mucosal prostanoid synthesis

who have had prior gastric surgery may develop gastritis secondary to the effects of intestinal contents refluxed into the stomach.

The pathogenesis of chronic ulceration is distinct from that of acute gastritis.[1] Yet, although physiologic abnormalities have been demonstrated in patients with peptic ulcer, no single defect has been shown to be causative, reflecting both the complexity and the heterogeneity of the disease process (Table 49-14). Patients with peptic ulcer have, on the average, increased secretion of gastric acid. Duodenal ulcer patients demonstrate increased secretion of basal acid. As a group, duodenal ulcer patients demonstrate a greater and more prolonged acid secretory response to a meal. Peak acid secretory responses to stimulants such as histamine or pentagastrin may be increased. A considerable overlap in acid secretory responsiveness, however, exists between ulcer patients and normal people, and most patients with duodenal ulcer fall within the range of normal values. Disturbances in gastric emptying that have been demonstrated in some patients include accelerated emptying of acidic gastric contents into the duodenum occurs following a meal; duodenal acidification fails to inhibit gastric emptying appropriately. The total acid exposure of the duodenal mucosa after a meal has been postulated as increased relative to normal individuals through this mechanism.

Increasing attention has recently been given to potential abnormalities of mucosal defense in patients with peptic ulceration. Gastric mucosal production of prostaglandin E_2 has been reported as decreased in patients with active disease, with prostanoid synthesis increased in healing ulcers treated with cimetidine. In both animals and humans, prostaglandins have been demonstrated to decrease acid secretion and accelerate healing of established duodenal ulcers. Another postulated protective factor is bicarbonate secretion by duodenal and gastric mucosal cells. Because bicarbonate is secreted beneath a mucous gel layer, even a small amount of mucosal bicarbonate secretion might be potentially capable of maintaining neutrality in proximity to the mucosal cell surface. Abnormalities in the protective effects of mucosally produced bicarbonate have been postulated but not yet proven.

CLINICAL PRESENTATION

Both acute gastritis and chronic peptic ulceration must be included in the differential diagnosis of any patient presenting with acute upper abdominal pain. In acute gastritis and uncomplicated chronic peptic ulceration, the pain is typically moderate to severe and localized to the epigastrium. The pain accompanying duodenal ulceration may also be sensed to the right of the midline, and is steady and gnawing or burning in nature. Classically, patients with peptic ulceration are awakened by pain in the morning and obtain relief by ingesting food. Ingestion of antacids produces prompt relief of painful symptoms. Radiation of pain and referred pain are unusual in gastritis and uncomplicated peptic ulceration. Narcotic analgesia is not usually necessary for pain relief, and a requirement for narcotic medication should place the diagnosis of uncomplicated peptic ulceration in question.

A prior history of peptic ulceration should be sought. Patients should be questioned closely about medication use, with emphasis on use of drugs containing nonsteroidal anti-inflammatory compounds or aspirin products. A history of cigarette smoking is important because smoking significantly increases the risk of peptic ulceration or its recurrence after treatment. Most patients with gastritis or uncomplicated peptic ulceration have a paucity of findings on physical examination. Abdominal tenderness may be present in the upper abdomen but is not pronounced. Guarding and rebound are not expected.

COMPLICATIONS

BLEEDING

Both acute gastritis and chronic peptic ulceration may be complicated by hemorrhage. Although most bleeding is occult, rapid and life-threatening hemorrhage may also occur. Significant acute gastrointestinal hemorrhage may occur in patients with acute gastritis, but massive bleeding is more common in patients with chronic duodenal ulceration secondary to erosion into major vessels deep to the submucosa such as the pancreaticoduodenal artery. Hematemesis and melena are dramatic, easily recognized signs of hemorrhage.

Acute hemorrhage is often heralded by syncope. Fatigue secondary to anemia is a common and sometimes ignored symptom of occult hemorrhage. The initial gastritis or peptic ulceration should include guaiac testing of the stool to detect occult hemorrhage. The initial examination and management of patients with upper gastrointestinal hemorrhage is detailed elsewhere in this chapter.

PERFORATION

Chronic peptic ulceration, and less commonly acute gastric injury induced by nonsteroidal anti-inflammatory agents, may be complicated by perforation. Pain is the cardinal symptom. Most patients can clearly identify the time of perforation by the accompanying increase in pain and changes in its characteristics. Symptoms are most commonly confined to the upper quadrants, although localization of pain depends on the portion of the parietal peritoneum in contact with gastric contents. For example, leakage of gastric contents along the right paracolic gutter may cause pain to be most intense in the right lower quadrant, mimicking acute appendicitis. Contact of the diaphragm with gastric contents may cause referral of pain to the scapular region. Perforation into the retroperitoneum or the lesser sac may produce referral of pain to the back in the region of L_1. The pain of perforation is severe and stady, reaches maximal intensity rapidly, and almost always requires narcotic analgesia for relief.

Patients with acute gastric or duodenal perforation usually lie still, often with legs drawn up, to minimize movement of the inflamed peritoneum. The patient usually appears acutely ill, with an anxious facial expression and sweating. Fever is common. Respirations are usually shallow and intercostal. The abdominal examination reveals muscular rigidity, and attempts to palpate deeply are resisted. Bowel sounds may be normal to hyperactive initially, but quickly become hypoactive and then absent. Occasionally, the hepatic dullness to percussion is lost because of gas between the right hemidiaphragm and the liver. Perforation posteriorly into the lesser sac or into the retroperitoneum from the second portion of the duodenum may produce substantially fewer physical findings at first because of the lack of contact of the somatically innervated parietal peritoneum with irritating gastric contents.

OBSTRUCTION

Gastric outlet obstruction may occur as a complication of chronic peptic ulcer disease but not in association with acute gastritis. Peptic ulcers located in the first portion of the duodenum or the pyloric channel may cause obstruction, either as a long-term consequence of the cicatrization that develops as ulcers intermittently recur and heal, or acutely because of the edema surrounding the area of ulceration. Obstruction may occur insidiously so that patients may have advanced disease before seeking medical attention. The affected individual usually complains of intermittent regurgitation of gastric contents, a sensation of epigastric fullness, and weight loss. Pain is not a prominent feature of gastric obstruction, and colic such as that occurring with small bowel obstruction is rare.

Physical examination of patients with gastric outlet obstruction most commonly demonstrates signs of dehydration and, if long-standing, weight loss. A fullness in the epigastrium may be appreciated occasionally, representing the distended stomach. Epigastric tympany occurs as a result of air accumulation within the obstructed stomach.

DIFFERENTIAL DIAGNOSIS

The differential diagnoses to be considered in patients with suspected acute gastritis or chronic peptic ulcer disease may be conveniently categorized by the clinical presentation: pain, hemorrhage, perforation, or obstruction (Table 49-15).

For patients presenting with epigastric pain, the

TABLE 49-15. DIFFERENTIAL DIAGNOSIS FOR GASTRITIS AND PEPTIC ULCER

Presentation as Epigastric Pain

Gastric ulcer	Esophageal spasm
Gastric neoplasm	Esophageal reflux
Biliary colic	Myocardial ischemia
Cholecystitis	Lower lobe pneumonitis
Acute hepatitis	Acute pancreatitis
Hepatic neoplasm	
Hepatic congestion	

Presentation with Acute Hemorrhage

Esophageal ulceration	Duodenal neoplasm
Esophagitis	Pancreatic neoplasm
Mallory-Weiss tear	
Esophageal varices	
Gastric varices	
Gastric ulcer	
Gastric neoplasm	
Angiodysplasia	

Presentation with Perforation

Gastric ulcer	Small intestinal foreign body
Gastric neoplasm	Inflammatory bowel disease
	Small intestinal neoplasm
Colonic neoplasm	
Colonic diverticulitis	
Colonic obstruction	

Presentation with Obstruction

Gastric neoplasm	Autonomic nervous dys-
Duodenal neoplasm	function
Pancreatic neoplasm	Gastric bezoar
Pancreatic pseudocyst	Ingested foreign body

differential diagnosis is broad and includes disease processes that are both intrinsic and extrinsic to the peritoneal cavity. Gastric tumors, both benign and malignant, may present with pain identical to that of peptic ulceration. Calculous biliary disease must often be distinguished from gastritis or peptic ulcer. Biliary colic is frequently sensed in the epigastrium. Migration of the pain to the right upper quadrant, a clear association of painful symptoms with ingestion of a fatty meal, and a failure of antacids to relieve symptoms help to distinguish calculous biliary disease from peptic ulceration. Pancreatitis usually presents with epigastric pain, often with radiation to the back in the region of the upper lumbar vertebrae. Acute hepatitis, hepatic congestion secondary to right heart failure, or hepatic tumors may occasionally be confused with gastritis or peptic ulceration. Esophageal dysmotility, myocardial infarction, and lower lobe pneumonia are examples of extra-abdominal processes that may be present with epigastric pain. In most instances, a thorough history, physical examination, and selected laboratory tests limit the possibilities.

Acute upper gastrointestinal hemorrhage may be caused by several lesions that must be distinguished from gastritis or peptic ulceration so that specific and effective therapy may be provided. Esophageal causes of acute bleeding include esophagitis, esophageal ulcers, Mallory-Weiss tears, and esophageal varices. Gastric lesions to be considered include both benign and malignant gastric ulcers, gastric varices, and angiodysplastic lesions in addition to gastritis or peptic ulceration. Occasionally, intrinsic duodenal tumors or pancreatic neoplasms involving the duodenum may cause acute hemorrhage. A complete consideration of upper gastrointestinal hemorrhage may be found elsewhere in this chapter.

Perforation of any portion of the gastrointestinal tract may produce symptoms and physical findings similar to those noted with perforation caused by peptic ulcer. Both benign and malignant gastric lesions may cause full-thickness injury and thus perforation. Intrinsic small intestinal lesions rarely cause free perforation into the peritoneal cavity; contained perforation with abscess formation is more common. Small intestinal lesions caused by an ingested foreign body (e.g., bone fragment or toothpick), small intestinal neoplasm, and Crohn's disease must be considered. Colonic pathology may frequently present with signs of free perforation that cannot be easily distinguished from those caused by gastric perforation. The most common disease processes include colonic diverticulitis, colonic neoplasm, and distal colonic obstruction with secondary cecal perforation.

Gastric outlet obstruction mimicking that caused by peptic ulceration may be caused by gastric, duodenal, or pancreatic neoplasms that involve the distal stomach or duodenum. Pancreatic pseudocysts located in the region of the pancreatic head may compress the duodenum and cause gastric obstruction. Occasionally, functional derangements of gastric emptying may be confused with anatomic obstruction. The most frequent cause of functional gastroparesis is autonomic nervous dysfunction secondary to diabetes mellitus. Both anatomic obstruction and functional derangements may cause malnutrition, gastric dilation, and epigastric fullness.

DIAGNOSTIC PROCEDURES

When patients present for evaluation of mild abdominal pain with no evidence for acute hemorrhage, perforation, or obstruction, the initial evaluation may often consist of only guaiac testing of the stool for the presence of occult blood and determination of the hematocrit to rule out anemia. In mildly symptomatic patients, if the initial evaluation does not suggest complicated disease, presumptive treatment followed by elective endoscopic evaluation is appropriate. Moderate to severe epigastric pain demands a more thorough initial evaluation and may include complete blood count with differential white blood cell determination, measurement of serum electrolytes, urinalysis, determination of liver function tests and amylase, and selected abdominal radiographs. X-rays should include views of the chest as well as supine and upright films of the abdomen. Anemia may be caused by gastritis or peptic ulcer, either acutely or secondary to chronic occult blood loss. Microcytosis and hypochromia suggest chronicity. Electrolyte abnormalities are prominent in patients with gastric outlet obstruction. Vomiting of gastric secretions rich in hydrogen and chloride ions produce a hypochloremic alkalosis. Renal compensatory mechanisms to conserve hydrogen ions in exchange for potassium result in secondary hypokalemia. Urinalysis and determination of bilirubin, liver enzymes, and amylase are used primarily to exclude nongastric disease processes that may cause confusion with gastritis or peptic ulceration. It is important to realize, however, that amylase values may be elevated in patients with duodenal perforation, presumably from absorption of amylase from the peritoneal cavity.

Abdominal radiographs are most helpful in patients in whom perforation or obstruction is suspected. Pneumoperitoneum is present in 75% of patients with perforated duodenal ulcer. Small amounts of air may not be visualized unless the patient has remained in an upright position for an adequate period of time; 3 minutes is recommended. If the patient is not able to tolerate an upright posture, decubitus films (left side down) are helpful. Perforation into the lesser sac may not be accompanied by subdiaphragmatic air. A characteristic pattern of gas within the lesser sac may, however, be recognized. Gastric outlet obstruction is reflected on plain abdominal films by gastric distention and abnormally large air-fluid levels within the stomach.

ENDOSCOPY

While these tests are helpful in evaluating patients with suspected gastritis or peptic ulceration, a definitive diagnosis should be sought in most cases using upper gastrointestinal endoscopy. An exception to this statement exists for patients with suspected perforation; endoscopic examination with the attendant insufflation of air is contraindicated in cases of perforation. Endoscopy permits evaluation of the esophagus and duodenum in addition to the stomach. Anatomic abnormalities may be identified. Biopsy for histologic examination is possible. In selected circumstances, therapeutic intervention is possible, for example electrocautery of bleeding lesions. Upper gastrointestinal endoscopy is currently considered the "gold standard" for evaluation of suspected gastritis or peptic ulceration.

CONTRAST RADIOGRAPHY

Contrast radiographs have a limited role in the evaluation of patients with gastritis or peptic ulceration. Although singe-contrast studies reliably demonstrate chronic peptic ulcers, they are less sensitive when superficial ulcers are present. Double-contrast examinations greatly enhance diagnostic capability by coating the mucosal surfaces, but are not as useful as endoscopic examination. Of course, mucosal inflammation without ulceration is not demonstrable on contrast radiographs and biopsy is not possible. Contrast studies have no place in the evaluation of acute hemorrhage. The contrast agent coats the mucosal surfaces, hampering subsequent endoscopic evaluation and rendering angiographic studies impossible. Occasionally, patients without radiographic evidence of pneumoperitoneum in whom perforation is suspected may benefit from contrast studies using a water-soluble agent. Extravasation of contrast demonstrates the perforation. In these circumstances, barium should not be used as the contrast agent because this substance is a potent adjuvant for bacterial infection of the peritoneum.

MANAGEMENT

When patients that are evaluated in an Emergency Department (ED) setting appear by history to have uncomplicated acute gastritis or chronic peptic ulcer disease, it may be appropriate to begin initial treatment empirically. Medical treatment must not be continued, however, without making a definitive diag-

nosis. This usually involves elective upper gastrointestinal endoscopy.

The first priority in the treatment of acute gastritis is to identify and discontinue offending agents such as alcohol, NSAIDS, aspirin, and caffeine. In mild cases, withdrawal of noxious stimuli may be sufficient to ensure healing. Active treatment usually consists of measures to inhibit or neutralize gastric acid secretion or measures to provide a "cytoprotective" coating to the stomach. Because they provide greater convenience for the patient than antacids, orally administered H_2-receptor antagonists are commonly administered to inhibit acid secretion and to promote healing of ulcerations. Table 49-16 lists currently available H_2-receptor antagonists commonly used in the treatment of acute gastritis. Sucralfate, a basic aluminum salt of sulfated sucrose, has also been used to treat uncomplicated acute gastritis. In the acidic environment of the stomach, sucralfate adheres to ulcerated mucosa to form a protective barrier. Although the mechanism of action of sucralfate has not been completely defined, this coating is believed to protect the injured mucosa from continuing exposure to acid and pepsin. Sucralfate has been reported to protect against gastric mucosal injury caused by aspirin, ethanol, or concentrated acid or alkali.

Treatment of an uncomplicated peptic ulcer is based upon the dictum "no acid, no ulcer." It is appropriate to begin outpatient treatment of peptic ulcer with an orally administered H_2 receptor antagonist.[2,3] Dosage schedules and reported healing rates for the three clinically available agents, cimetidine, ranitidine, and famotidine are listed in Table 49-16. Although any of the three H_2 receptor antagonists might have advantages for individual patients, when administered at dosages that produce equivalent suppression of acid secretion, the agents usually exhibit similar efficacy. The choice among the drugs is usually arbitrary from a therapeutic standpoint. Significant side effects are not common with any of the listed H_2 receptor antagonists, and usually respond promptly to reduction in dosage. Their safety record is excellent.

TABLE 49-16. USE OF H_2 RECEPTOR ANTAGONISTS IN ACUTE ULCERATION

Agent	Healing Rates (%)
Cimetidine	
300 mg qid	60–80% at 4 weeks, 85–95% at 8 weeks
400 mg hs	80–90% at 8 weeks
Ranitidine	
150 mg bid	85–95% at 8 weeks
300 mg hs	90% at 4 weeks
Famotidine	
20 mg bid	90–95% at 8 weeks
40 mg bid	90% at 8 weeks
40 mg hs	95% at 4 weeks

Sucralfate has also been used as a single agent for initial treatment of peptic ulcer. Healing of duodenal ulcers is produced in 50 to 70% of treated patients at 4 weeks. Side effects are infrequent and mild with the use of sucralfate, occurring in less than 5% of treated cases. No systemic absorption has been noted. This safety factor makes sucralfate attractive for long-term maintenance therapy.

HEMORRHAGE

Acute hemorrhage from gastritis or peptic ulceration represents a medical emergency requiring in-hospital treatment. The first priority is restoration of intravascular volume, with restitution of the oxygen-carrying capacity of the blood. Coagulation defects, if present, must be corrected. Identification of the site and source of blood loss by endoscopic means should be obtained emergently so that specific therapy can be administered. In favorable circumstances, transendoscopic control of hemorrhage can be attempted, either as definitive treatment or, more commonly, as a temporizing measure. Continued and uncontrolled hemorrhage is an indication for surgical intervention.[4] Operative therapy for hemorrhage has two goals: control of the bleeding vessel and permanent reduction in gastric acid secretory capacity. In many cases, these goals can be achieved by oversewing of the bleeding pancreaticoduodenal artery and performance of a vagotomy and gastric drainage procedure.

OBSTRUCTION

The initial treatment of gastric outlet obstruction consists of relief of gastric distention by nasogastric intubation and correction of electrolyte imbalances. Gastric outlet obstruction caused by edema surrounding active ulceration is usually relieved promptly when nasogastric decompression is combined with effective acid suppression. If the stenosis is caused by chronic cicatrization, however, none of the currently available agents can be expected to be of benefit. Pyloric stenosis is a firm indication for operative intervention, and operative treatment should be delayed only long enough to correct coexisting nutritional deficits.

PERFORATION

Perforation remains a strong indication for definitive anti-ulcer surgery in patients with historical or anatomic evidence of chronic peptic ulceration.[5,6] Patients with perforation should be prepared for operation by restoration of intravascular fluid deficits caused by peritoneal inflammation. Nasogastric suction should be instituted. Broad-spectrum antibiotics, effective against polymicrobial enteric flora, should be provided. Operative goals include closure of the perforation, peritoneal debridement, and when appropriate, provision of permanent reduction in acid secretion.

REFERENCES

1. Brooks, F.P.: The pathophysiology of peptic ulcer disease. Dig. Dis. Sci. 30:15S, 1985.
2. Debas, H.T., and Mulholland, M.W.: Drug therapy in peptic ulcer disease. Curr. Prob. Surg. 26:1, 1989.
3. Bertaccini, G., and Coruzzi, G.: Pharmacology of the treatment of peptic ulcer disease. Dig. Dis. Sci. 30:43S, 1985.
4. Hunt, P.S.: Surgical management of bleeding chronic peptic ulcer: A 10-year prospective study. Ann. Surg. 199:44, 1984.
5. Boey, J., Wong, J., and Ong, G.B.: A prospective study of operative risk factors in perforated duodenal ulcers. Ann. Surg. 195:265, 1982.
6. Boey, J., Lee, N.W., Koo, J., et al.: Immediate definitive surgery for perforated duodenal ulcers: A prospective controlled trial. Ann. Surg. 196:338, 1982.

GASTROINTESTINAL BLEEDING

GENERAL PRESENTATION

Eddy D. Palmer

CAPSULE

Arrival of a patient with gastrointestinal bleeding at the emergency department (ED) calls for joint diagnostic and therapeutic efforts by several people. A predesigned plan of action is required if confusion is to be avoided. It should be remembered, however, that no patient requires more careful individualization than does the gastrointestinal bleeder. It is therefore unrealistic to set rigid rules for managing *all* emergencies of this category. The emergency physician has some or all of these immediate responsibilities:

1. Determine whether there has been bleeding.
2. Determine whether there is active bleeding now.
3. Determine whether the bleeding source lies in the upper gastrointestinal tract (proximal to the duodenojejunal junction) or more distally, or both, as the first step in identifying the responsible lesion.
4. Evaluate the patient's background medical status on which the bleeding has been superimposed.
5. Judge the amount of blood lost and the patient's physiologic response.
6. Begin blood replacement.
7. Initiate efforts to stop the bleeding.
8. Initiate or arrange for immediate endoscopic and radiologic efforts to identify the bleeding source.

How far the emergency physician goes with these responsibilities depends on the problem at hand. Whether he or she will call in certain specialists—a gastroenterologist and a radiologist for emergency diagnostic study and a surgeon to share observation of the patient—depends on the initial overview of the problem.

SUBJECTIVE ASSESSMENT

The history of hematemesis, hematochezia, or melena may be clear-cut and reliable. The doctor may witness them, or the patient's clothing may show fresh stains. About one of five patients brought to the emergency department because of supposed gastrointestinal bleeding, however, is found not to have bled but to have misinterpreted something seen in the vomitus or stool as blood. Nongastrointestinal blood that may enter and then be ejected from the gastrointestinal tract may arise from the nose, tracheopulmonary tract, or, for nurslings, from the mother's nipples. Ingestion of blood for fraudulent purposes has become rare. It is often necessary to test specimens of questionable composition for blood.

Estimation of the amount of blood lost from reports of stool and vomitus volume is likely to be wholly unreliable. It must be recalled that a person may exsanguinate into his gastrointestinal tract with no external show of blood. Blood in the stomach quickly becomes diluted, however, and, when it stimulates rapid passage through the tract, becomes grossly diluted. A little blood goes a long way when splashed about clothing, floor, and walls, and estimates of its volume are usually exaggerated.

The bleeder's sudden hypovolemia, hypotension, and anemia, plus the emotional repercussions of a sudden personal catastrophe, must necessarily have a deleterious influence on any underlying medical problem that may be present. It is essential that all information the patient or family may have about the past medical history be obtained early in the assessment. Unfortunately, shock, language problems, and intoxication often interfere with this essential communication. The background medical problems (Table 49-17) that must be of the greatest concern are coronary artery disease, borderline cerebroarterial disease, chronic renal disease, cirrhosis, emphysema, other pulmonary insufficiency problems, and diabetes. Often, of course, the chronic disease has not been previously recognized and comes to light now as a disastrous complication of the bleeding.

OBJECTIVE ASSESSMENT

Assessing the severity and consequences of the hemorrhage at the moment of admission to the ED is an immediate responsibility of the emergency physician. These matters, plus the principles of shock management and resuscitation, are dealt with elsewhere in this chapter, and only the points pertinent to the special problem at hand will be discussed here.

The clinical effects of the bleeding depend on both the amount of blood lost and the rapidity of the bleeding. In the initial stages, the latter is more important than the former. A healthy adult can lose 500 mL of blood quickly, e.g., by blood donation, without feeling any adverse effects. However, the sudden loss of 2000 mL may kill. Approximately 10% of unattended adults who lose half their circulating volume over a 12-hour period die by the time the 50% mark is reached. About one third of people in this country who faint from gastrointestinal bleeding do so in the bathroom, where they are locked in. They may not receive attention for some time.

Often the exact duration of the bleeding is not determinable, so that the first hematocrit and hemoglobin level tests may or may not reflect dilution from spontaneous efforts at volume restoration. In addition, one can seldom be sure that there was no anemia or polycythemia at the time when the bleeding began. For these reasons especially, it is essential that immediate evaluation and evaluation throughout the

emergency be based primarily on the vital signs and their variations. There can be little doubt that insufficient advantage is taken of the help the vital signs can give, owing to the inexplicable habit of relying primarily on laboratory reports.

The patient's general appearance on admission—pallor, sweating, shock—gives essential information about his or her response to the bleeding but does not permit a reliable estimate of the amount of blood lost. A helpful bedside means of judging the loss is examination of the color of the palmar creases when the fingers are forcibly extended. If there is no anemia, an intense red color is seen, even when the patient is in shock. When the circulating hemoglobin level drops below one half of normal, the creases do not turn red upon this maneuver.

Tests of cardiovascular stability (e.g., the well-known tilt test) are found useful by some clinicians, but they cannot be recommended with enthusiasm because they give information only about that moment. The need is for a sign to indicate quickly a sudden rebleed or a sudden failure of the patient's homeostatic protection. The tilt test cannot readily be repeated at frequent intervals. Recording the blood pressure, pulse rate, and respiratory rate every 15 minutes at the start and later every 30 minutes provides reliable information on what the bleeding is doing to the patient.

In most cases it is possible to determine whether the bleeding source is in the upper or lower gastrointestinal tract and whether the bleeding is still active when the patient is first examined, although the information may be somewhat indirect. Witnessing hematemesis answers both of these questions in a reasonable fashion. Although the stomach may retain blood for a considerable period after bleeding has actually stopped and later eject it, this is not often the case. The rule is for the upper gastrointestinal tract to react with irritability and hyperactivity when it fills with blood, so that it quickly empties itself after bleeding has stopped.

For all patients suspected of gastrointestinal bleeding, if hematemesis has not been witnessed or otherwise proved, a nasogastric tube should be passed for sampling of the gastric contents for blood. The ordinary nasogastric tube is much too narrow for evacuating the stomach of blood and clots; the purpose is simply to indicate whether this is upper gastrointestinal bleeding and whether any blood encountered is abundant and fresh or old and remaining only in traces.

If there has been no hematemesis and the gastric drainage contains no blood, but melena or hematochezia is active and vital signs suggest continued bleeding, assumption of middle or lower gastrointestinal bleeding is proper. When the bleeding source is in the jejunum, ileum, or cecum, it is usually difficult to know quickly when the bleeding stops and when it begins again. Changes in the vital signs are most useful.

TABLE 49-17. CAUSES OF UPPER GASTROINTESTINAL HEMORRHAGE IN 1526 ADULT GENERAL HOSPITAL PATIENTS

Bleeding Source	No. Patients	Average Transfusion Requirement Per Bleed (ml)
Duodenal ulcer	402	2275
Esophageal varices	277	3530
Erosive gastritis	213	3510
Gastric ulcer	188	3200
Erosive esophagitis	96	2940
Mallory-Weiss syndrome	92	2220
Stomal ulcer	43	3210
Multiple sources	22	2240
Other lesion	82	—
Undetermined or wrong	111	—

The manner by which blood reaches the outside proves unreliable when judging its point of origin, and the clinician must be cautious not to place much diagnostic value on the appearances of vomitus and stool. One is never justified in guessing a venous source from the color of vomitus or gastric aspirate because of the rapidity with which bright red blood may turn dark in the stomach. Conversion to hematin occurs quickly in the presence of the stomach's hydrochloric acid, and black hematemesis may occur soon after blood has entered the stomach.

The change that blood produces in the appearance of the stool depends on the amount and rapidity of the bleeding, the location of the bleeding source, and the speed of intestinal transit. Grossly bloody stools are seen in upper gastrointestinal bleeding, when blood loss is quick and massive and transit time is rapid. Blood from the distal duodenum or jejunum must be retained in the tract for at least 8 hours to turn black. A black stool may be produced when gross bleeding arises from the ileum or below, but this is rare. Dark red is the rule. Whatever the source, for a black stool to be created, there must be a rapid loss of at least 100 mL of blood.

Gross bleeding from the right colon usually produces dark red stools. Blood from the left colon and sigmoid is ordinarily passed quickly and sometimes appears unaltered. Because it is likely to stimulate diarrhea, it sometimes seems more thoroughly mixed with feces than one might guess it would be.

Accurate assessment of the bleeding demands serial determinations of hemoglobin and hematocrit. It is a responsibility of the emergency physician to arrange for immediate determinations at the time blood is drawn for typing and cross-matching, even though he or she must interpret the initial report with great caution. In cases of massive bleeding there may not be sufficient time to wait for a cross-match. In such cases, type-specific blood is preferable.

Because of the possibility of unrecognized underlying disease, a series of screening chemical tests should be drawn at the same time. A minimum series of tests might be a glucose level, urea nitrogen, creatinine, bilirubin, calcium, potassium, sodium, chloride, and sedimentation rate.

Acute myocardial infarction is a complication in from 1 to 2% of patients who have a gross gastrointestinal bleed. Therefore, electrocardiographic study is a routine requirement early in the course, with the supposition that it will be repeated in 24 hours.

During initial assessment, it is essential that the doctor keep in mind that a small proportion of gastric and duodenal ulcers that bleed perforate at the same time.

UPPER GASTROINTESTINAL BLEEDING

Frederic E. Eckhauser, Steven E. Raper, and James A. Knol

CAPSULE

Acute upper gastrointestinal hemorrhage is a continuing cause of significant morbidity and mortality. These patients must be approached with a comprehensive plan in mind for diagnosis and treatment. The critical elements of such a management scheme include resuscitation and stabilization, nasogastric intubation to confirm the diagnosis and evacuate particulate debris and blood clot from the stomach, early endoscopy and/or angiography to identify the source of bleeding, conservative measures to control bleeding including endoscopic and angiographic techniques, and surgical intervention if necessary. Treatment must be individualized on the basis of the patient's age and general condition, the extent and rate of bleeding, the presence of associated illnesses, transfusion difficulties, the lesion responsible for bleeding, and the patient's response to therapy. Despite improvements in our understanding of the pathophysiology responsible for gastrointestinal hemorrhage, considerable disagreement exists about alternative approaches to the management of these often complex patients. Advances in blood component therapy and new special procedures for diagnosing and managing hemorrhage have helped to reduce patient mortality; however, there is no substitute for mature clinical judgment and sound reasoning. The goals of this chapter are to review the various causes of upper gastrointestinal hemorrhage and to formulate a stepwise, logical approach to the diagnosis and treatment of these patients.

INTRODUCTION

Acute gastrointestinal hemorrhage is a common clinical problem accounting for 1 to 2% of all medical and surgical hospital admissions in the United States.[1] The overall risk of gastrointestinal bleeding correlates with a variety of geographic, seasonal, socioeconomic, and psychologic factors as well as age, and may vary significantly from one institution to another because of differences in patient populations.

The mortality rate from acute gastrointestinal hemorrhage varies from 8 to 10% and has remained relatively constant over the past several decades despite advances in intensive care unit support and the development of new therapeutic modalities.[2] This dichotomy may partly reflect changes over time in the population at risk. Advancing age appears to be an unequivocal risk factor that is independent of other variables.[3] Although age per se does not seem to influence the severity of the initial bleeding episode or the likelihood of recurrent bleeding, the risk of dying varies with age. This may reflect the fact that older patients are more likely to suffer from associated diseases that adversely influence outcome. The observation that nearly half of patients presenting with acute gastrointestinal bleeding are over 60 may partly explain why the benefits of advanced technology have not resulted in the expected improvement in patient survival.

The causes of upper gastrointestinal bleeding are diverse and frequently require individualized treatment. Effective treatment for bleeding esophageal varices may not be appropriate for a bleeding gastric or duodenal ulcer. To improve patient outcome and reduce morbidity resulting from misdirected intervention, physicians must become conversant with current technology related to resuscitation, diagnosis of the site of bleeding, and treatment alternatives, both nonoperative and operative. These components form the basis of effective and safe patient management and will be the subject of this review.

PATHOPHYSIOLOGY

Few conditions in medicine evoke a more vigorous visceral response in clinicians or demand more prompt recognition and treatment than gastrointestinal hemorrhage. Hemorrhage initiates a series of circulatory, metabolic, and neuroendocrine responses aimed at preserving tissue perfusion and delivery of oxygen and energy substrates. The response is graded according to the severity of acute blood loss and the availability of normal compensatory mechanisms.

The initial response to blood loss is contraction of the venous compartment. This compensatory mechanism effectively buffers a blood loss of about 10% of normal blood volume. At the same time, net movement of protein-free fluid from the interstitial space into the vascular space occurs. This is mediated primarily by a reduction in capillary pressure. Complete restitution of blood volume requires translocation of plasma protein from the interstitium to the capillary space. The endocrine and metabolic responses to mild blood loss are negligible.

More significant degrees of blood loss (15 to 20%) are accompanied by enhanced sympathetic activity with arteriolar vasoconstriction in the skin, splanchnic bed, and muscle. Regardless of the severity of initial hemorrhage, cerebral and coronary vessels always dilate. Sympathetic stimulation of the heart increases heart rate and contractility, resulting in increased cardiac output. Significant tachycardia is generally not seen in humans unless blood loss exceeds 10% of blood volume. Aldosterone and antidiuretic hormone or vasopressin are released, resulting in salt and water retention. Increased glycolysis and lipolysis result in hyperglycemia and elevated circulating levels of free fatty acids. Inadequate capillary perfusion and hypoxemia may activate anaerobic pathways, resulting in a slight increase in lactate production. Patients with this degree of blood loss are marginally compensated and may experience thirst, apprehension, weakness, and orthostatic hypotension.

If blood loss continues, cardiac output and renal blood flow decrease, causing profound hypotension and significant oliguria. Because coronary perfusion occurs primarily during diastole, prolonged tachycardia impairs myocardial blood flow, leading to impaired contractility and irritability. Anaerobic transformation of pyruvate to lactate results in severe metabolic acidosis which ultimately interferes with critical cell membrane functions. Cerebral hypoxia from decreased perfusion causes the patient to become obtunded and eventually lose consciousness. Ultimately, normal compensatory mechanisms are exceeded and coronary perfusion falls below the critical value needed to maintain cardiac output. At this point, restitution of circulatory and metabolic homeostasis may be impossible and death may be inevitable.

INITIAL TREATMENT AND RESUSCITATION

Initial treatment can be subdivided into resuscitation (Table 49-17A) and stabilization phases. The acuity of intervention necessary should be determined chiefly by the volume of gastrointestinal hemorrhage and the patient's hemodynamic status. If the patient is hypotensive while supine and the neck veins are flat, one must assume that significant hypovolemia is present. The most appropriate route of venous access for volume restoration is dictated by the condition of the patient and the availability of skilled personnel. Several peripheral intravenous catheters should be inserted using sterile technique. If the patient is profoundly hypovolemic, percutaneous peripheral access may be impossible. In this situation, saphenous cutdown or central venous catheterization should be considered. The chief goal is to insert large-bore catheters with high flow capacity. Extremely high crystalloid flow rates of approximately 150 mL per minute with 1 meter gravity and up to 400 mL per minute with 200 mm Hg pressure can be achieved through short 14-gauge catheters.[3] Placement of a 10-gauge catheter into the greater saphenous vein permits high-pressure infusion of up to 1500 mL per minute of crystalloid or up to 1200 mL per minute of blood. At the same time as catheters are being inserted, blood should be obtained for determination of hematocrit, type, cross-matching, and measurement of other important but less critical indicators of hepatic and renal function.

If possible, a central venous catheter[4] should be inserted during the resuscitation phase to monitor the response to volume replacement. A left atrial catheter would be ideal but is impractical in the Emergency Department (ED) setting. In elderly patients or in patients with a past history of congestive heart failure, chronic obstructive pulmonary disease or renal failure, however, invasive monitoring with a Swan-Ganz catheter to measure pulmonary artery wedge pressure may guard against fluid overload. Serial measurements of central venous oxygen saturation can also provide important information about the circulatory status and the response to therapy. Mixed venous oxygen values in the range of 25 to 40 torr indicate circulatory insufficiency and the need for more intensive treatment.

A Foley catheter should be inserted into the urinary bladder for serial measurements of urine output and specific gravity. Hourly urine volumes of >0.5 mL/kg indicate adequate renal perfusion. Decreased urine volume with increased specific gravity >1.030 and osmolality >700 mOsm/L usually indicate hypovolemia. A nasogastric tube of adequate size (18 Fr) should be inserted to evacuate stomach contents and minimize the risk of vomiting and aspiration. It may also be useful to determine if the source of bleeding is from the upper gastrointestinal tract and to assess the presence and rate of continuing blood loss.

Early resuscitation should consist primarily of infusion of balanced salt or crystalloid solutions. Changes in blood pressure, pulse rate, and general patient appearance provide the most practical guides to monitor the adequacy of early volume restitution. As a general rule, blood should be added to the resuscitation formula when the volume of crystalloid infused exceeds 50 mL/kg body weight. The hematocrit should be maintained at or slightly above 30% to optimize viscosity and hemoglobin-carrying capacity. Higher hematocrit values, however, may be nec-

TABLE 49-17A. INITIAL RESUSCITATION: CRITICAL MEASUREMENTS FOR PATIENTS WITH SIGNIFICANT HYPOVOLEMIA AND SHOCK

	Normal Values
Arterial blood pressure	120/80
Pulse rate	80/min
Urine volume	50 mL/hr
Central venous pressure	5 cm water
Arterial pO$_2$	100 mm Hg
pCO$_2$	40 mm Hg
pH	7.4
SvO$_2$	0.68–0.77
Hematocrit	35–45%

Additional studies requiring placement of a Swan-Ganz catheter include cardiac index (3.2 L/min/m^2), pulmonary artery wedge pressure (3–12 mm Hg), and systemic vascular resistance (2000 dynes/sec/cm^{-5}/m^2).

essary in elderly patients and selected patients with chronic pulmonary or coronary artery disease. In the absence of blood dyscrasias or pre-existing clotting or platelet abnormalities, whole blood or blood component therapy may not be necessary in patients with mild or moderate blood loss.

In addition to improvement in cardiovascular parameters such as pulse and blood pressure, indicators of improving circulatory status include return of color and warmth to the extremities and normalization of capillary refilling time. As hypoxia resolves, the patient's level of consciousness generally improves. Once the patient's clinical condition has been stabilized, efforts should be made to establish the site of upper gastrointestinal bleeding.

CLINICAL EVALUATION (Fig. 49-19)

The causes of upper gastrointestinal bleeding are diverse. According to an extensive survey of 2225 patients performed by the American Society for Gastrointestinal Endoscopy, six entities account for nearly 90% of all bleeding episodes.[5] These conditions are listed in Table 49-18. In many instances, important clues can be identified by obtaining a careful history and performing a thorough physical examination. Hematemesis or vomiting of bright red blood identifies the site of bleeding as proximal to the ligament of Treitz. Melena or passage of tarry, black stools resulting from enzymatic degradation of intraluminal blood, is usually associated with a proximal source of bleeding. Factors such as slow bleeding from a more distal source or delayed intestinal transit, however, may produce melena and therefore limit the reliability of this finding.

A history of chronic drug or alcohol ingestion, previous ulcer disease, or an episode of retching and

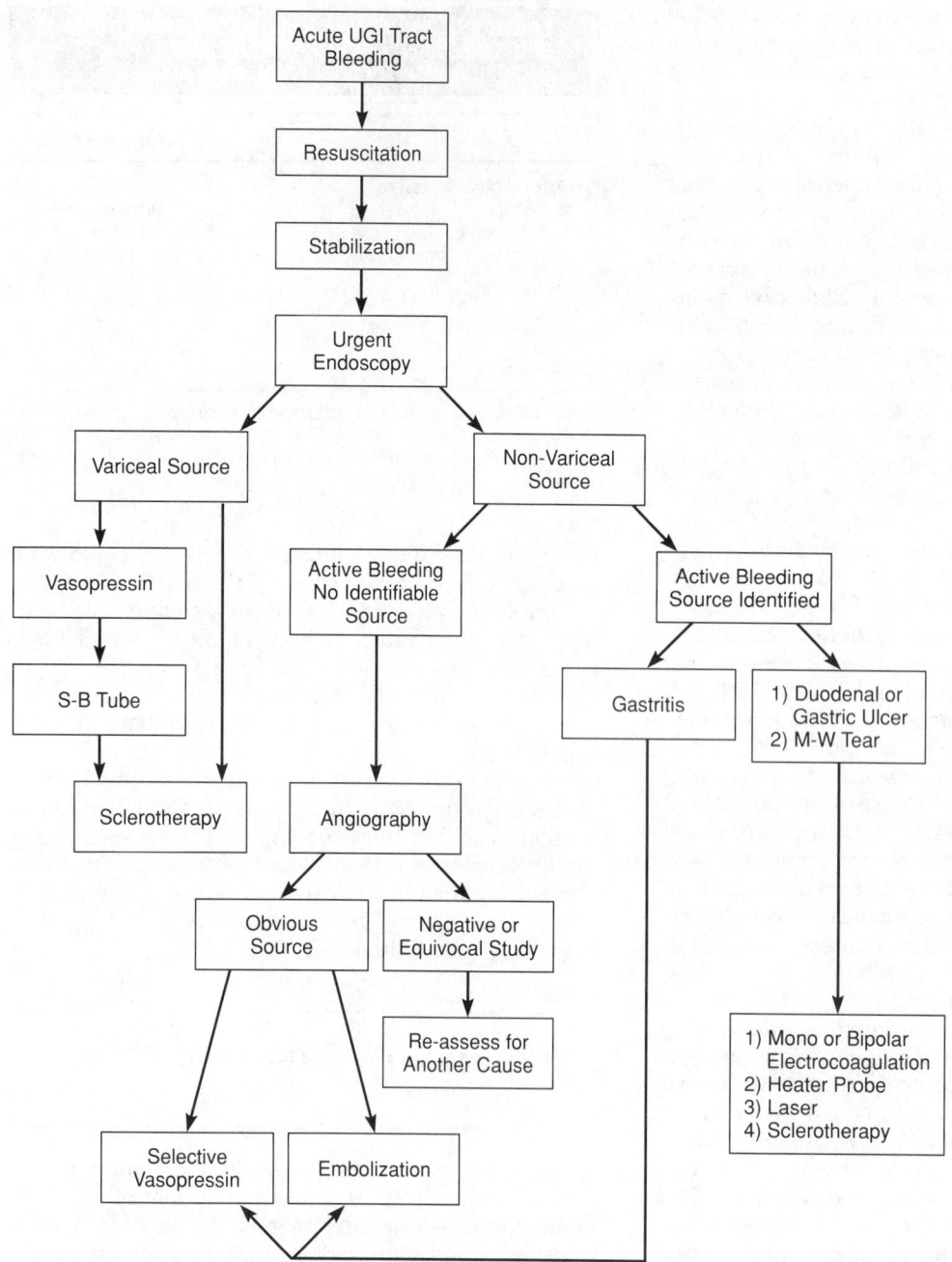

FIG. 49-19. Algorithm for evaluation and management of upper gastrointestinal bleeding.

TABLE 49-18. CAUSES OF UPPER GASTROINTESTINAL TRACT BLEEDING*

Duodenal ulcer	24%
Acute gastritis	20%
Gastric ulcer	15%
Esophageal varices	14%
Esophagitis	6%
Mallory-Weiss tear	5%

* With permission from Gardner, B., and Richardson, J.D.: Gastrointestinal Bleeding. In Basic Surgery. Edited by Polk, H.C., Stone, H.H., and Gardner, B. Norwalk, CT, Appleton-Century-Crofts, 1983.

vomiting that preceded the onset of bleeding may provide important information regarding the source of bleeding. Drugs such as aspirin, steroids, and nonsteroidal anti-inflammatory agents (e.g., phenylbutazone and indomethacin) disrupt the gastric mucosal barrier and cause erosive gastritis and stress ulcerations. Trauma, shock, and sepsis can also contribute to the formation of these lesions. Chronic alcohol ingestion is most commonly associated with bleeding from esophageal or gastric varices but frequently originates from nonvariceal sources such as acute erosive gastritis or peptic ulcers. The Mallory-Weiss syndrome results from a linear tear in the lining of the distal esophagus or proximal stomach near the esophagogastric junction. The tear is usually partial-thickness and may extend for several centimeters. In most patients, an episode of forceful retching precedes the onset of bleeding. Fortunately, the bleeding associated with this condition is frequently self-limited and therefore does not require surgical intervention.

A careful physical examination is essential to identify findings that might alter the diagnosis, and should be conducted once the patient's condition has been stabilized. Clinical findings such as spider angiomata, palmar erythema, gynecomastia, jaundice, muscle wasting, and ascites indicate the presence of chronic liver disease. Splenomegaly, distention of abdominal wall veins, and a venous hum heard over the umbilical area indicate a high likelihood of portal hypertension. Palpation of a mass in the epigastrium suggest the possibility of a gastric cancer, although these lesions rarely cause massive bleeding. The nose and oropharynx should be inspected carefully for potential bleeding sites, especially if additional diagnostic studies fail to demonstrate an obvious source in the esophagus, stomach or duodenum. This is particularly true in patients with hereditary telangiectasia (Osler-Weber-Rendu disease) in whom there may be associated platelet dysfunction. Rarely, patients with other hematologic or connective tissue disorders such as von Willebrand's disease and Ehlers-Danlos syndrome respectively, may present with gastrointestinal bleeding. In general, patients with underlying hematologic disorders are not at risk of "spontaneous" bleeding unless clotting parameters are markedly abnormal and the platelet count is less than $10,000/mm^3$.[6] The risk of bleeding from a pre-existing lesion appears to be higher in these patients than in the normal population, however, even if coagulation parameters are only moderately abnormal.

Nasogastric (NG) intubation should be standard practice in any patient with upper gastrointestinal bleeding and is important for several reasons. An episode of vomiting does not ensure complete evacuation of the stomach and places the patient at continued risk for aspiration. The type of tube used during the evaluation and early treatment phase should be determined by the composition of the stomach contents. Aspiration of "coffee-ground" material containing a minimal amount of particulate debris can be accomplished easily with an 18Fr sump nasogastric tube. A large-bore tube such as a levacuator tube is useful if the initial aspirate contains recently ingested food or gross blood clots. The stomach should be irrigated with 60 to 100 mL aliquots of normal saline or tap water until the effluent is clear of blood clots or debris. Nasogastric intubation and evacuation of the stomach allows one to determine if bleeding has ceased and, in the event of continued bleeding, makes it easy to estimate the rate of continued blood loss. Evacuation of the stomach may also facilitate local hemostasis by diluting the acid-pepsin content of the stomach and

eliminating fibrinolysins that have accumulated in the process of normal clot formation and breakdown. The use of a cold lavage solution has the theoretic benefit of causing local vasoconstriction, but there is little objective data to support its routine use.

When confronted with a patient who presents with upper GI hemorrhage in the ED, it is incumbent on the examining physician to establish early risk and management guidelines. In this setting, several clinical prognostic factors may be useful to determine which patients are at increased risk of death or may need emergency surgical intervention.[5] Frank hematemesis or the passage of maroon-colored stools, along with physical evidence of hemodynamic instability such as postural hypotension or frank shock, are associated with increased risk of death and/or the need for early surgical intervention. Other findings that indicate high risk include an abdominal mass, ascites, congestive heart failure, hepatosplenomegaly and jaundice. The color of the nasogastric aspirate and the stool can also be useful as important predictors of outcome. Continued evidence of red blood in the nasogastric lavage despite continued irrigation with cold or room-temperature saline is evidence of fairly rapid bleeding that may require early endoscopy for diagnosis and possible therapy. Passage of maroon-colored stools in the presence of a demonstrable upper GI source of bleeding indicates rapid intestinal transit but is also associated with brisk bleeding regardless of the source. Findings of red blood in the nasogastric lavage and maroon-colored stools are associated with nearly a fourfold increase in mortality compared to patients with clear or coffee-ground NG aspirates and normal stool color.[5]

DIAGNOSIS OF THE SOURCE

For many years, the treatment of upper gastrointestinal bleeding was based primarily on a clinical diagnosis and the results of a barium contrast examination. Unfortunately, these methods are inaccurate for diagnosing gross lesions such as ulcers or carcinomas in up to 50% of patients, and are virtually useless for identifying mucosal lesions such as gastritis and esophagitis or the source of bleeding when more than one potential bleeding site exists.[7]

More recently, clinicians have placed a greater emphasis on special diagnostic procedures including fiberoptic endoscopy, radionuclide scintigraphy, and angiography (Table 49-19). The need for and timing of these procedures remains controversial, however. This is partly because bleeding stops spontaneously in most patients.[8] Further, even in the best of hands, the potential complications resulting from such procedures may largely offset any benefits.

TABLE 49-19. ENDOSCOPIC TECHNIQUES AVAILABLE FOR OBTAINING GI HEMOSTASIS

Modality	Portability	Expense	Efficacy Nonvariceal	Efficacy Variceal	Potential Drawbacks
MPE	Good	Low	Good	Poor	Depth of injury unpredictable
BPE*	Good	Low	Good	Poor	
HP*	Good	Low	Good	Poor	
Laser	Poor	High	Good	Poor	Labor intensive
Injection Tx†	Good	Low	Variable	Good	10–15% risk of serious complications§

MPE = Monopolar electrocoagulation, BPE = bipolar electrocoagulation, HP = heater probe.
* Equivalent hemostatic efficacy for nonvariceal sources of hemorrhage.
† Sclerosants include absolute alcohol and hypertonic saline with epinephrine.
§ Complications include late stricture formation with dysphagia, perforation with mediastinitis, and 35 to 50% incidence of variceal rebleeding until varix obliteration is complete.

ENDOSCOPY

Several studies, including a randomized, controlled trial published by Peterson et al. in 1981, have demonstrated that routine endoscopy for early diagnosis does not alter outcome in patients with upper gastrointestinal tract bleeding.[9] Allan and Dykes compared routine versus selective endoscopy to determine if early endoscopy conferred any therapeutic benefit in patients with acute upper GI tract bleeding.[10] Following barium contrast examination patients were randomized to undergo selective endoscopy based on certain clinical indications including a history of recent aspirin or alcohol ingestion, severe bleeding with no radiologic abnormality, suspicion of a tumor, or a hiatus hernia noted on the x-ray study. Although a definitive diagnosis was made more frequently in patients undergoing routine endoscopy, there was no therapeutic benefit in terms of duration of hospital stay or frequency of surgical intervention.

Other investigators strongly advocate early endoscopy for diagnosis and therapy in patients with upper gastrointestinal bleeding. In 1978, Himal et al. published the results of a retrospective review of 630 patients admitted with acute upper GI bleeding.[11] Reduced mortality correlated with age <60, blood requirement <10 units, and early identification of the site of bleeding. Using these risk criteria, the authors further showed in a subset of 334 patients that aggressive surgical management combined with early endoscopy led to a threefold decrease in mortality from bleeding gastric ulcers and a twofold decrease in mortality from bleeding of all types. These studies do not provide unequivocal evidence that early endoscopy to determine the source of bleeding improves therapy and reduces mortality. They suggest, however, that early indentification of the bleeding source may be important in selected patients who present with massive hemorrhage and are therefore more likely to require surgery, and in patients with a history of previous hemorrhage in whom up to 40% may be bleeding from a different site.[12]

While the efficacy of "early" endoscopy in improving survival among patients with acute upper gastrointestinal tract bleeding may be debatable, there is little doubt concerning its diagnostic accuracy compared to that of other techniques. Conventional barium contrast examinations have inherent limitations. A clot in the stomach may confuse interpretation of the study. Although such studies may define the presence of a "potential" bleeding source such as esophageal varices or a peptic ulcer, there is no assurance that the lesion identified is the source of bleeding. The usefulness of barium studies is further limited by the identification of more than one potential bleeding source and the presence of superficial mucosal lesions such as erosive gastritis or stress ulcers that may be virtually undetectable. The diagnostic accuracy of fiberoptic endoscopy varies from 90 to 95%.[13] Endoscopy is clearly superior to conventional barium studies for diagnosing the site(s) of bleeding and is now considered the initial diagnostic procedure of choice by many authors.[13,14]

The risks of endoscopy for gastrointestinal hemorrhage are frequently overexaggerated. Several large series have reported extremely low complication and death rates of approximately 0.5% and 0.01% respectively.[15] The more common complications include perforation of the esophagus, stomach, or duodenum; oversedation of the patient resulting in respiratory and central nervous system depression; aspiration pneumonia; cardiac arrythmias; and bleeding caused by local trauma or dislodgement of a clot. Many, if not all, of these complications can be minimized by careful patient observation, evacuation of residual clot and debris from the stomach "before" the procedure, proper positioning of the patient on his or her side rather than back, passage of the endoscope under direct vision rather than blindly, and gentle manipulation of the endoscope during the examination.

RADIONUCLIDE SCINTIGRAPHY

Radioisotopic imaging with either technetium sulfur colloid (TSC) or pertechnetate-labelled red cells (TP) is an effective modality for detecting gastrointestinal bleeding. This technique is noninvasive, has relatively few associated risks, and is accurate, with bleeding rates as low as 0.1 mL/min. It may be particularly valuable for assessing areas of the gastrointestinal tract that are not accessible with conventional endoscopes and in patients with intermittent bleeding. It localizes bleeding to a general region, however, and therefore is not useful for determining the actual site of bleeding. Because most of upper gastrointestinal bleeding originates proximal to the ligament of Treitz and therefore can be evaluated with fiberoptic endoscopy, radionuclide scanning plays a limited role in the initial assessment of these patients.

ANGIOGRAPHY

Angiography has assumed a selective role in the evaluation of patients with upper gastrointestinal hemorrhage. It is particularly useful in patients with severe hemorrhage in whom endoscopy is not technically feasible or fails to localize the site of bleeding. Currently, the percutaneous catheterization technique introduced by Seldinger in the mid-1950s is favored. With this approach, the celiac and superior mesenteric arteries are selectively catheterized. Extravasation of dye indicates active bleeding of at least 0.5 mL/min.[16] If the bleeding site cannot be demonstrated, subselective studies of the left gastric, gastroduodenal, and splenic arteries are performed. Failure to demonstrate bleeding after these maneuvers usually indicates that the bleeding is mucosal or venous in origin or that the rate of bleeding has decreased below a critical value.

Angiography may be most useful to identify "uncommon" causes of upper gastrointestinal hemorrhage such as hematobilia or hemosuccus pancreaticus.[17] Hepatic tumors, trauma, or arteriovenous malformations may cause bleeding into the biliary tree. The clinical manifestations of this condition include recurrent biliary colic, jaundice, and evidence of gastrointestinal hemorrhage. Conventional endoscopy may demonstrate bleeding from the papilla of Vater, but if the hemorrhage is brisk or intermittent, no specific source may be identifiable. Gastrointestinal bleeding associated with pancreatitis can be severe and frequently originates from rupture of visceral artery aneurysms adjacent to the pancreas into the lumen of the gastrointestinal tract.[18] The pathogenesis of this condition involves pancreatic inflammation with activation of proteolytic pancreatic enzymes and aneurysmal dilatation of medium-sized peripancreatic arteries. The arteries most commonly involved in decreasing order of frequency include the splenic, gastroduodenal, superior or inferior pancreaticoduo-

denal, and left gastric, and occasionally the hepatic artery. Patients characteristically present with episodic upper abdominal or right upper quadrant pain, the presence on physical examination of a pulsatile abdominal mass accompanied by a bruit, and premonitory upper gastrointestinal hemorrhage.[18] Delineation of the specific site of bleeding may be extremely difficult, if not impossible, with conventional radiography or fiberoptic endoscopy. In this setting angiography may be crucial for accurately identifying the source of bleeding. In patients who are not suitable candidates for surgery, angiography may be a useful therapeutic technique for transcatheter embolization and obliteration of the bleeding aneurysm. Angiography may also be useful to demonstrate bleeding from an aortoenteric (usually duodenal) fistula occuring after aortic reconstructive surgery.

NONOPERATIVE MANAGEMENT OF UPPER GASTROINTESTINAL HEMORRHAGE

The decision to operate on a patient with acute upper gastrointestinal hemorrhage is influenced by various factors including the extent and rate of bleeding, the age of the patient, the existence of associated conditions such as vascular disease and hypertension, transfusion difficulties, and the pathologic entity responsible for bleeding. The natural history of the condition(s) responsible for acute bleeding, including the risk of rebleeding, must be weighed in the decision as to whether to operate early rather than later. For the patient who presents in the ED with frank shock and exsanguinating hemorrhage (>50 mL/min), the need for urgent surgery is obvious. In this setting, any delay in definitive treatment is poorly tolerated and might result in loss of life. Because bleeding stops spontaneously in nearly 80% of patients, however, surgery can usually be deferred until efforts at resuscitation and diagnosis have been completed. The need for urgent surgical intervention has also been reduced by the development of endoscopic and angiographic techniques to control gastrointestinal hemorrhage (Table 49-20).

TABLE 49-20. DIAGNOSIS OF UPPER GASTROINTESTINAL BLEEDING*

Endoscopy
Visceral angiography
Radionuclide scintigraphy
Barium contrast examinations

* In order of decreasing usefulness.

Numerous pharmacologic agents have been used in an effort to stop or control upper GI hemorrhage. The list of drugs includes H2-receptor antagonists and various peptide hormones such as vasopressin and somatostatin. Vasopressin may be especially useful in patients with a history of variceal bleeding or physical findings compatible with chronic liver disease in whom the likelihood of a variceal source is high. Treatment should be initiated with an IV bolus of 20 U over a 20-minute period followed by continuous infusion of 40 to 60 U per hour until finite endpoints are reached. These include marked reduction or cessation in bleeding or the development of adverse effects such as severe hypertension, bradycardia and/or cardiac arrhythmias. The cardiac effects of vasopressin are a manifestation of coronary vasoconstriction and can be partly offset by simultaneous administration of a vasodilator such as nitroglycerin or nitroprusside. Vasopressin should never be administered without ECG monitoring and may be contraindicated in patients with a history of angina pectoris or a previous myocardial infarction. It should be kept in mind that vasopressin therapy alone rarely achieves permanent hemostasis. Vasopressin administration can be resumed in the event of rebleeding, but the success rate falls off dramatically and other measures should be instituted. Somatostatin, a regulatory neuropeptide, may also be useful for temporary control of variceal hemorrhage and is associated with fewer side effects than vasopressin. Regardless of which agent is used, temporary control of upper GI hemorrhage provides a window during which expedient endoscopy should be performed in a relatively blood-free field to document the source of bleeding and treat the lesion with a variety of techniques including topical hemostatic agents or tissue adhesives, injection sclerotherapy and thermal, electrical, or laser coagulation.

THERAPEUTIC ENDOSCOPY AND ANGIOGRAPHY

Fiberoptic endoscopy permits visual inspection of the mucosal lining of the upper gastrointestinal tract from the level of the oropharynx to the mid or distal duodenum. Despite evidence that endoscopy is highly accurate in identifying potential or actual sources of hemorrhage, the effect of early diagnosis on patient mortality remains controversial. Much of this information, however, was gathered before the development of instruments and techniques for endoscopic hemostasis. The most commonly used devices for thermal treatment of upper gastrointestinal bleeding include YAG and argon lasers, the heater probe and mono and bipolar electrocoagulation.[19]

Monopolar electrosurgery delivers high-frequency electrical current by means of a connecting element directly to tissue. The major disadvantage of this system is that direct tissue contact is required; therefore, a non-stick element cannot be utilized and the coagulum formed by electrocautery can be dislodged when the heating element is withdrawn from the point of contact. This may result in a high incidence of rebleeding.

Bipolar electrosugery uses two probes in direct contact with tissue. Electrical current applied to the tissue is confined close to the electrode tip. It is safer than the monopolar technique because deep, penetrating burns are not produced. As tissue dessication occurs, however, tissue conductivity changes and the amount of energy delivered locally also decreases. This may result in energy levels that are insufficient to produce the desired hemostatic effect.

Lasers impart light energy of a predetermined wavelength that propagates into tissue until it is absorbed by tissue pigments. The lasers used most commonly for endoscopic hemostasis are the argon laser and the neodynium-yttrium-aluminum-garnet (Nd:YAG) laser. The latter has a greater depth of penetration (2 to 4 mm). Lasers achieve hemostasis by raising tissue temperatures. If one is not careful, tissue temperatures can be raised too rapidly, causing vaporization rather than coagulation.

A heater probe transmits heat energy directly to tissue by thermal conduction. The contact time between the electrode tip and the tissue and the amount of energy delivered determines the depth of coagulation. The risk of deep injury is less than with mono and bipolar electrocautery because the operator can program the analog computer linked to the probe to deliver a predetermined amount of energy to the tissue. The maximum depth of injury using the heater probe is approximately 3 mm, even with extended contact times. The probe tips are also insulated with a nonstick Teflon coating that prevents adherence to the coagulated surface. Like the contact laser tip and the monopolar and bipolar thermal cautery systems, the heater probe can be used to tamponade the bleeding vessel. This not only coapts the walls but temporarily stops the flow of blood through the vessel, resulting in a better tissue weld.

The next several sections attempt to summarize the efficacy and safety of the various devices available for endoscopic therapy of upper gastrointestinal bleeding.

MONOPOLAR AND BIPOLAR ELECTROCOAGULATION AND HEATER PROBE

Monopolar units are readily available. The results in human studies for control of nonvariceal sources of bleeding are encouraging. Initial and overall hemostasis rates of 91% and 97% have been reported in some series.[20] Unfortunately, early studies did not evaluate the need for retreatment in patients with different levels of risk. More recent studies of ulcer patients with a visible vessel, an endoscopic stigma that indicates a high likelihood of rebleeding, suggested that recurrent hemorrhage and the need for surgery were markedly reduced among patients treated by electrocoagulation compared to controls receiving medical therapy alone.[21]

One of the major concerns with monopolar electrocoagulation is that the depth of injury is difficult to control. Although perforation resulting from transmural necrosis is a potential complication of this technique, the actual risk demonstrated in studies performed in the United States appears to be low.

The major advantage of the heater probe and bipolar electrocoagulation techniques compared to monopolar electrocoagulation is that the depth of injury and hence the risk of perforation are markedly reduced.

Despite the attractiveness of the heater probe and bipolar electrocautery (both are light, relatively inexpensive, and portable), most of the available efficacy data have been derived from nonrandom, uncontrolled trials. One randomized, controlled multicenter California study of patients with severe ulcer hemorrhage, however, demonstrated a "trend" toward improved hemostasis and reduced hospital mortality in patients treated with heater probe or bipolar electocautery (BICAP) compared to control patients receiving only medical management.[22,23] There were no apparent differences in efficacy or outcome between the two endoscopic techniques.

LASERS

Compared to electrical and thermal techniques for endoscopic hemostasis, the major limitations of laser therapy include lack of portability, expense, and potential for a higher complication rate. The efficacy and saftey of laser therapy for gastrointestinal hemorrhage have been evaluated in many controlled trials, and the conclusions were recently summarized in an excellent review article by Fleischer in 1983.[24]

Regardless of inconsistencies in the stratification and reporting of data, most argon and Nd:YAG laser studies in patients with hemorrhage from peptic ulcers *suggest* decreased rebleeding, improved mortality, and lower treatment costs in laser-treated patients compared to controls. Because lasers are expensive and nonportable, other hemostatic devices such as BICAP and heater probe have achieved greater popularity and more widespread use. Additional randomized, controlled trials will be necessary to better assess the relative merits of these endoscopic treatment modalities in patients with different causes of upper gastrointestinal bleeding.

INJECTION SCLEROTHERAPY

Interest has been renewed in endoscopic injection therapy for variceal and nonvariceal sources of upper gastrointestinal bleeding. The technique is attractive because it is simple and inexpensive. For nonvariceal causes, there is controversy regarding safety and efficacy of absolute alcohol compared to other sclerosant solutions. Absolute alcohol is effective because it dehydrates and fixes the bleeding vessel and surrounding tissues. Other sclerosant solutions such as hypertonic epinephrine solution (HSE) have been used in place of absolute alcohol with comparable hemostatic effects and no difference in the incidence of complications or rebleeding.[25,26]

Regardless of the choice of sclerosant solution, the technique of sclerotherapy is fairly standard. A sclerotherapy device consisting of a retractable 23-gauge needle inside a transparent plastic sheath is introduced through the biopsy channel of any standard endoscope. Small-volume injections should be used to avoid problems with ulceration and perforation. Any overlying clot should be evacuated to insure that bleeding has been effectively controlled.

Injection sclerotherapy (IS) has also been used extensively for bleeding esophageal varices. Numerous studies have proved that sclerotherapy is effective in controlling acute variceal hemorrhage in most cases, and at least one randomized study has concluded that IS is superior to medical therapy and balloon tamponade in this situation.[26] Most of the randomized trials available for analysis have demonstrated that sclerotherapy also effectively reduces the frequency of variceal rebleeding and several have demonstrated a reduction in late mortality from rebleeding, especially after complete obliteration had been achieved. In poor-risk cirrhotics with bleeding esophageal varices, the extent of hepatic dysfunction based on assessment of albumin, bilirubin, the presence of ascites and encephalopathy, and the overall nutritional status of the patient, may be a more important determinant of survival than the technique(s) used to achieve hemostasis.

Sclerotherapy is an attractive alternative to surgical intervention, particularly in patients with marginal hepatic reserve. One must keep in mind, however, that sclerotherapy may cause significant complications in 10% to 15% of patients.[26] The most troublesome complications include dysphagia, aspiration pneumonia, and perforation with mediastinitis. The incidence of complications depends less on the sclerosant used than on the skill and judgment of the endoscopist. Esophageal ulceration is thought by many to be an anticipated side effect of sclerotherapy rather than a complication. Deep ulcers, which usually result from direct intramural injections or large-volume intravariceal injections with significant local extravasation, however, are largely preventable with experience and patience. Uncooperative patients and active bleeding may limit the effectiveness of sclerotherapy for acute hemorrhage and contribute to procedure-related complications.

HORIZONS

The evaluation and management of patients with acute upper gastrointestinal bleeding continues to challenge the ingenuity and judgment of physicians responsible for their care. Initial resuscitation to restore intravascular volume and normalize cardiovascular and hemodynamic parameters must be aggressive and undertaken without delay. Once the patient has been stablized, early endoscopy should be considered. While there are little data to indicate that early endoscopy improves survival, much of this evidence was gathered before techniques for achieving endoscopic hemostasis became available. In addition to identifying the lesion responsible for bleeding, endoscopy may also demonstrate unsuspected pathology and alter the proposed treatment plan. One major advantage of early endoscopy is that definitive treatment can be instituted without delay.

Many therapeutic alternatives are available, including argon and Nd:YAG lasers, monopolar and bipolar electrocautery, heater probe, and injection sclerotherapy. If endoscopic approaches fail to demonstrate the site of bleeding or achieve hemostasis, angiographic techniques are available. These modalities are not mutually exclusive but should be viewed as complementary. The controversy surrounding these techniques will be answered only by carefully planned, randomized, controlled trials. Until then, the selection of one versus another will be dictated by many factors, including availability of devices and skilled operators, cost, patient acceptance, and issues related to efficacy and safety.

REFERENCES

1. Palmer, E.D.: Upper gastrointestinal hemorrhage. JAMA *231*:853, 1975.
2. Bogoch, A.: Hematemesis and melena. Part I. Etiology and medical aspects. *In* Gastroenterology, vol. 1. Edited by Bockus, H.L. Philadelphia, PA, W.B. Saunders Co., 1974.
3. Allan, R., and Dykes, P.: A study of the factors influencing mortality rates from gastrointestinal hemorrhage. Q. J. Med. *45*:533, 1976.
4. Mateer, J.R., Thompson, B.M., and Aprahamian, C., et al.: Rapid fluid resuscitation with central venous catheters. Ann. Emerg. Med. *12*:149, 1983.
5. Silverstein, F.E., Gilbert, D.A., Tedesco, F.J., et al.: The national ASGE survey on upper gastrointestinal bleeding. Parts 1–3. Gastrointest. Endosc. *27*:73, 1981.
6. Coon, W.W.: Drug-related and hematological disorders asso-ciated with gastrointestinal bleeding. *In* Gastrointestinal Hemorrhage. Edited by Fiddian-Green, R.G., and Turcotte, J.G. New York, Grune and Stratton, 1980.
7. Chandler, G.N., Walls, W.D., and Glanville, J.N.: Hematemesis and melena. *In* Modern Topics in Gastrointestinal Endoscopy. Edited by Schiller, K.F.R., and Salmon, P.R. London, Heinemann, 1976.
8. Steer, M.L., and Silen, W.: Diagnostic procedures in gastrointestinal hemorrhage. N. Engl. J. Med. *309*:646, 1983.
9. Peterson, W.L., et al.: Routine early endoscopy in upper gastrointestinal tract bleeding: A randomized, controlled trial. N. Engl. J. Med. *304*:925, 1981.
10. Allan, R., and Dykes, P.: A comparison of routine and selective endoscopy in the management of acute gastrointestinal hemorrhage. Gastrointest. Endosc. *20*:154, 1974.
11. Himal, H.S., Perrault, C., and Mzabi, R.: Upper gastrointestinal hemorrhage. Surgery *84*:448, 1978.
12. Palmer, E.D.: Upper Gastrointestinal Hemorrhage. Springfield, Charles C Thomas, 1970.
13. Stevenson, G.W., Cox, R.R., and Roberts, C.J.: Prospective comparison of double-contrast barium meal examination and fiberoptic endoscopy in acute upper gastrointestinal hemorrhage. Br. Med. J. *2*:723, 1976.
14. Dronfield, M.W., McIllmurray, M.B., Ferguson, R., et al.: A prospective, randomized study of endoscopy and radiology in acute upper-gastrointestinal-tract bleeding. Lancet *1*:1167, 1977.
15. Silvis, S.E., Nebel, O., Rogers, G., et al.: Endoscopic complications. JAMA *235*:928, 1976.
16. Nusbaum, M., and Baum, S.: Radiographic demonstration of unknown sites of gastrointestinal bleeding. Surg. Forum *14*:374, 1963.
17. Koehler, P.R., Nelson, J.A., and Berenson, M.M.: Massive extra-enteric gastrointestinal bleeding: Angiographic diagnosis. Radiology *119*:41, 1976.
18. Eckhauser, F.E., Stanley, J.C., Zelenock, G.B., et al.: Gastroduodenal and pancreaticoduodenal artery aneurysms: a complication of pancreatitis causing spontaneous gastrointestinal hemorrhage. Surgery *88*:335, 1980.
19. Johnston, J.: Endoscopic thermal treatment of upper gastrointestinal bleeding: overview and guidelines. Endosc. Rev. *2*:12, 1985.
20. Gaisford, W.D.: Endoscopic electrohemostasis of active upper gastrointestinal bleeding. Am. J. Surg. *137*:47, 1979.
21. Papp, J.P.: Endoscopic electrocoagulation in the management of upper gastrointestinal tract bleeding. Surg. Clin. North Am. *62*:797, 1982.
22. Jensen, D.M.: Natural history of ulcer bleeding, techniques and controlled trial results with BICAP and heater probe. *In* GI Hemostasis and Tumor Palliation. Edited by Jensen, D.M. Los Angeles, Center for Ulcer Research and Education (CURE), 1987, p.7.
23. Jensen, D.M.: Ibid, p. 9.
24. Fleischer, D.: Endoscopic laser therapy for upper gastrointestinal tract disease. Surv. Dig. Dis. *1*:42, 1983.
25. Sugawa, C., Fujita, Y., Ikeda, T., et al.: Endoscopic hemostasis of bleeding of the upper gastrointestinal tract by local injection of 98% dehydrated alcohol. Surg. Gynecol. Obstet. *162*:159, 1986.
26. Barsoum, M.S., Bolous, F.I., El-Rooby, A.A., et al.: Tamponade and injection sclerotherapy in the management of bleeding esophageal varices. Br. J. Surg. *69*:76, 1982.

LOWER GASTROINTESTINAL BLEEDING

Gail V. Anderson and John S. Withers

CAPSULE

Bleeding from the lower gastrointestinal tract can range from benign to catastrophic. All rectal bleeding should be investigated, even though most hemorrhagic episodes cease spontaneously. The challenge in the emergency department (ED) is to quickly sort out patients who need immediate and aggressive therapy from those that can be worked up in a clinic or outpatient setting. Immediate stabilization, including the administration of blood products as necessary, and timely consultation are essentials of an effective management strategy for life-threatening hemorrhage. Appropriate physical examination and passage of a nasogastric tube help to determine whether the source of bleeding is from the upper or lower gastrointestinal tract. The emergency physician should be aware of the various age-related causes of rectal bleeding and the diagnostic modalities available, including endoscopic and radiologic studies. Many of these studies are obtained by the consultant, who most often should be a surgeon. Most patients do not require operative intervention. Definitive therapy includes intra-arterial vasopressin infusion, embolization, and segmental bowel resection when the hemorrhage cannot be controlled.

ANATOMY AND PATHOPHYSIOLOGY

The lower segment of the gastrointestinal tract is divided from the upper by the ligament of Treitz. Mesenteric arteries supply the small and large bowel. In the rectal region there is additional input from the internal iliac artery.

The appearance of bleeding from the rectum or blood in the stool is largely affected by the rate and site of blood loss. The passage of fresh, bright red blood (hematochezia) usually indicates a distal small bowel or colonic bleeding source; however, 10 to 15% of patients with vigorous hematochezia actually have a more proximal source.[1] In fact, as much as one third of rectal bleeding in the elderly patient can be traced to the upper gastrointestinal tract.[2] In the adult, hematochezia emanating from an upper tract source indicates significant blood loss, usually 500 to 1000 mL.[3]

Intraluminal blood that has undergone significant degradation from contact with gastric juice assumes a spectrum of darker color ranging from maroon to black. The passage of a dark, tarry stool (melena) usually signifies a proximal lesion and/or delayed gastrointestinal transit time. Studies have shown that melenic stools can be produced by 60 to 200 mL of blood.[4,5] In a clinical setting, however, melena suggests much greater blood loss in the adult patient. One study showed an 11 A.M. circadian peak for onset of acute lower gastrointestinal bleeding.[11]

PREHOSPITAL ASSESSMENT AND STABILIZATION

Evaluating and securing the patient's airway, ventilation, and circulatory status is of utmost importance. Persons who have significant rectal bleeding are often lethargic, and therefore at risk for aspiration. As mentioned previously, patients with a history of hematochezia or melena can have an upper gastrointestinal bleeding source. Because swallowed blood is a gastric mucosal irritant that may induce vomiting, steps should be taken to protect the airway in the patient with decreased responsiveness. The patient should be placed on his or her side and suction made readily available. Endotracheal intubation should be performed if an adequate airway cannot be maintained. Oxygen should be administered by nasal canula at 3 to 4 L per minute to the asymptomatic patient. High-flow oxygen is indicated for patients with altered mental status or vital sign abnormalities. Cardiac monitor leads should be attached to the patient. At least one large-bore (16 gauge or greater) intravenous line should be initiated and a second started if the patient demonstrates hypotension, tachycardia, or altered mental status. Hypovolemia should be treated with crystalloid infusion and Medical Antishock Trouser (MAST) application if hypotension persists.

CLINICAL PRESENTATION AND EXAMINATION

Patients with rectal bleeding may range from being asymptomatic to being grossly unstable, with hematochezia or melena. Several bleeding patterns are possible: chronic, low grade; acute, massive; and intermittent, sometimes massive. Patients can have altered mental status secondary to poor cerebral perfusion from acute or chronic blood loss. Although most commonly seen in upper tract hemorrhage, proximal lower tract bleeding can produce altered mental status secondary to encephalopathy in patients with liver disease. Patients with pre-existing medical problems may complain of exacerbation of such problems from blood loss, e.g., chest pain in patients with coronary artery disease. Any history of prior bleeding

TABLE 49-21. COMMON AGE-RELATED CAUSES OF LOWER GASTROINTESTINAL BLEEDING*

Neonates (0–30 days)
  Upper gastrointestinal bleeding
  Anal fissure
  Milk allergy
  Necrotizing enterocolitis
  Midgut volvulus
  Anorectal trauma
  Swallowed maternal blood
Infants (30 days–1 year)
  Upper gastrointestinal bleeding
  Anal fissure
  Milk allergy
  Meckel's diverticulum
  Intussusception
  Infectious diarrhea
  Anorectal trauma
Children and Adolescents
  Upper gastrointestinal bleeding
  Intussusception
  Anal fissure
  Meckel's diverticulum
  Infectious diarrhea
  Colonic polyps
  Hemorrhoids
  Inflammatory bowel disease
Adults
  Upper gastrointestinal bleeding
  Angiodysplasia (vascular ectasia)
  Diverticula
  Hemorrhoids
  Anal fissure
  Carcinoma
  Polyps
  Ischemic bowel
  Inflammatory bowel disease
  Infectious diarrhea
  Foreign body

* Adapted with permission from Mork, V.G., and Anderson, G.V., Jr.: Lower gastrointestinal bleeding. *In* Principles and Practice of Emergency Medicine. 2nd ed. Edited by Schwartz, G.R. Safar, P., Stone, J.H., et al. Philadelphia, W.B. Saunders Co., 1986, p. 1040.

episodes, blood dyscrasias, cancer, or use of anticoagulant medication should be elicited.

Vital signs can be helpful or misleading. Orthostatic changes in heart rate and blood pressure need to be noted. Tachycardia is the usual response in children experiencing intravascular volume depletion. Young, previously healthy adults can compensate for intravascular volume loss, with a smaller increase in heart rate caused by greater endogenous catecholamine release and increased systematic vascular resistance. Therefore, not until a larger percentage of the total blood volume is lost does such a patient show hypotension, marked tachycardia, or altered mental status. The elderly can be the most difficult group of patients in whom to interpret vital signs. The elderly adult with atherosclerotic disease may have mild orthostatic changes with aging. Similarly, the elderly patient taking β blocker medication may not show the expected compensatory rise in heart rate with depleted intravascular volume.

A thorough abdominal examination should be performed. Distention, tenderness, or masses suggest ischemia, perforation, obstruction, or malignancy. The anus should be inspected and the rectum digitally palpated for masses. Any stool should be evaluated for gross or occult blood. Additionally, the skin and mucous membranes should be examined for signs of inadequate perfusion or cyanosis. Other cutaneous findings may be vascular malformations, such as the telangiectasia of Osler-Weber-Rendu syndrome, or petechial/purpuric lesions indicative of vasculitis, platelet dysfunction, or thrombocytopenia.

DIFFERENTIAL DIAGNOSIS

The causes of lower gastrointestinal bleeding are numerous. Hemorrhoids and anal fissures account for most of the benign sources. It is important to note that the presence of hemorrhoids does not eliminate the possibility of other coexistent conditions, e.g., carcinoma, as a cause of bleeding from the rectum. Cytomegalovirus bowel ulceration has recently been implicated as a cause in renal transplant recipients[6] and in patients infected with human immunodeficiency virus (HIV).[7,8] In patients over 60 years old, vascular ectasias are now thought to be a major cause of lower gastrointestinal bleeding.[9] Many of these causes, including the most common, are listed in Table 49-21.

INITIAL STABILIZATION

The severity of the bleeding and the condition of the patient dictate the course of stabilization. If not already accomplished, the steps previously outlined under Prehospital Assessment and Stabilization should be initiated and the patient quickly reassessed for signs of hypovolemia.

The hypotensive, massively bleeding patient needs aggressive fluid resuscitation with crystalloid solution. A blood sample should be immediately sent for type and crossmatch. Insertion of a Foley catheter to monitor urine output can provide indirect assessment of intravascular volume. Cross-matched blood should be transfused when available, but the profoundly hemorrhaging patient may require administration of O-negative or type-specific blood. A central venous line may aid the assessment of the initial resuscitative effort, but placement of such a line must not delay patient stabilization. As the patient's condition becomes stable, care must be taken, particularly in the elderly or very young, not to overload the cardiovascular system with fluid.

LABORATORY PROCEDURES AND OTHER STUDIES

BLOOD

Initial blood studies include a complete blood count, a platelet count, and levels of serum electrolytes, glucose, creatinine, and BUN. Coagulation studies should also be sent. If platelet dysfunction is suspected, i.e., in a patient on chronic aspirin therapy, a bleeding time should be ordered. If the patient is in stable condition and the history and physical examination suggest significant bleeding, a blood sample should be sent for typing. As outlined above, fully cross-matched blood products should be ordered for the unstable or severely hemorrhaging patient.

PROCEDURES

Nasogastric intubation and aspiration help to determine the existence of an upper gastrointestinal source of bleeding. Gastric contents should be inspected for frank or occult blood. Traumatic nasogastric intubation can cause blood to appear in gastric aspirate. Also, about 1% of patients with rectal bleeding and blood-free gastric aspirate have a duodenal bleeding source.[10] If an upper tract bleeding source has been excluded, anoscopy should be performed to identify any anal pathology. If no bleeding site is detected in the patient with evidence of significant blood loss, immediate proctosigmoidoscopy should be arranged. Delay in seeking surgical consultation should be avoided.

OTHER STUDIES

If the origin of the acute hemorrhage remains undetermined, the next step is generally angiography or radionuclide imaging. A sensitivity of 65% for localizing bleeding with contrast arteriography among patients requiring emergency resection has been reported.[7] Canalization of the bleeding segment also allows infusion of vasoactive substances or selective embolization. In a study in which vasopressin was infused, bleeding ceased in approximately 90% of patients; however, 50% of patients rebled after vasopressin infusion was terminated.[11] Embolization can also be attempted once the bleeding site is found angiographically. It is usually reserved for vasopressin infusion failures and patients at poor surgical risk.

Radionuclide imaging is widely used and involves the infusion of technetium-99m (Tc-99), as either a sulfur colloid mixture or labelled red blood cells (RBCs). The sulfur colloid technique is the most sensitive modality available, detecting bleeding rates as slow as 1 mL per minute. Tc-99 sulfur colloid, however, has a half-life of 2 minutes and, with intermittent gastrointestinal hemorrhage, bleeding sites can potentially be missed. In comparison, Tc-99-tagged RBCs have an intravascular half-life of approximately 6 hours. Thus, the likelihood of detecting intermittent bleeding is increased. With sequential imaging, diagnostic sensitivity and specificity of greater than 90% have been reported.[10] In another study, however, accuracy was seen in little more than 50% of patients.[12]

Colonoscopy is not the diagnostic modality of choice in acute, massive bleeding and should be reserved for cases when bleeding has slowed or ceased and adequate bowel preparation has been accomplished. Likewise, barium enema, which interferes with subsequent angiography or colonoscopy, is usually reserved for patients in whom hemorrhage has stopped.

MANAGEMENT AND INDICATIONS FOR ADMISSION

A definite diagnosis may not be possible in the ED. Only stable patients with occult bleeding, however, should be considered for outpatient work-up. Prompt surgical consultation should be obtained for all others.

While the arrival of the consultant is awaited, the patient's hemodynamic condition should be closely monitored. In the elderly, the cardiac status merits careful scrutiny, and ECG evaluation is indicated.

The severity of the bleeding dictates which diagnostic steps are to be taken by the consultant. If the bleeding site cannot be identified or massive hemorrhage persists, partial bowel resection or total colectomy may be required.

- The presence of external hemorrhoids does not rule out other abnormalities.
- Failure to perform a rectal evaluation may unduly delay detection of a carcinoma within reach of the examining finger or anoscope.
- Development of hypovolemic shock in the elderly patient can be insidious.
- Failure to appreciate the severity of blood loss may result in unanticipated cardiac arrest.

REFERENCES

1. Cello, J.P.: Diagnosis and management of lower gastrointestinal tract hemorrhage—Medical staff conference, University of California, San Francisco. West. J. Med. *143*:80, 1985.
2. Rosen, A.M., Fleischer, D.E.: Lower GI bleeding: Updated diagnosis and management. Geriatrics *44*:49, 1989.
3. Schaffner, J.A.: Acute gastrointestinal bleeding. J. Int. Care Med. *1*:289, 1986.
4. Daniel, A., Jr., Egan, S.: Quantity of blood required to produce tarry stool. JAMA *113*:2232, 1939.
5. Schiff, L., Stevens, R.J., Shapiro, N., and Goodman, S.: Observation on the oral administration of citrated blood in man. Am. J. Med. Sci. *203*:409, 1942.
6. Cho, S., Tisnado, J., Liu, C., et al.: Bleeding CMV ulcers of the colon. Am. J. Roentgenol. *136*:1213, 1981.
7. Leitman, I.M., Paull, D.E., and Shires, G.T.: Evaluation and management of massive lower gastrointestinal hemorrhage. Ann. Surg. *209*:175, 1989.
8. Ferguson, C.M.: Surgical complications of human immunodeficiency virus infections. Am. Surg. *54*:4, 1988.
9. Boley, S.J., DiBase, A., Brandt, L.J., et al.: Lower intestinal bleeding in the elderly. Am. J. Surg. *137*:57, 1979.
10. Petter, G.D., and Sellin, J.H.: Lower gastrointestinal bleeding. Gastroenterol. Clin. North Am. *17*:341, 1988.
11. Ergun, G.A.: Circadian periodicity of the time of onset of acute lower gastrointestinal bleeding. Prog. Clin. Biol. Res. *341B*:221, 1990.
12. Bentley, D.E., and Richardson, J.D.: The role of tagged red blood cell imaging in the localization of gastrointestinal bleeding. Arch. Surg. *126*:821, 1991.

CROHN'S DISEASE AND ULCERATIVE COLITIS

Mark A. Peppercorn

CAPSULE

Crohn's disease and ulcerative colitis are the idiopathic inflammatory bowel diseases. Both disorders occur equally often in men and women, and have their peak onset between ages 15 and 40 years, but may affect children and the elderly. They are more common in the developed areas of the world such as the United States and northern Europe, occurring more in Caucasians than in people of color and more in Jews than in nonJews. Neither Crohn's disease nor ulcerative colitis, however, has any geographic, racial, ethnic, or socioeconomic boundaries. Ten to 25% of patients have a close relative with inflammatory bowel disease (IBD). In most patients, these disorders are chronic, with a clinical picture characterized by mild intermittent exacerbations of disease activity controlled by medication. Some, however, present in an acute fashion with fulminant symptoms requiring hospitalization and immediate attention. Although medical therapy for such patients may induce a remission, some need surgical intervention. Therefore, close cooperation between the medical and surgical teams from the onset of hospitalization is required. Although many acute presentations of Crohn's disease and ulcerative colitis are similar, these disorders are generally discussed separately throughout the chapter.

PATHOPHYSIOLOGY

CROHN'S DISEASE

Although various causes have been proposed for both Crohn's disease and ulcerative colitis, the cause and pathogenesis of these disorders remain unknown. Most recent attention regarding Crohn's disease has focused on an infectious cause and disturbances of the immune system. The isolation from certain Crohn's disease patients of an atypical Mycobacterium has rekindled interest in the infectious origin of the disorder.[1] The inability to isolate the organism from many patients and recent immunohistochemical studies, however, have shed doubt on this etiologic conception. Although much investigation into immune system abnormalities has been done, as yet there is no unifying concept of how immunologic abnormalities lead to Crohn's disease.[2] Recent attention has focused on abnormal antigen processing by colonic epithelial cells, leading to an overreactive response by helper T lymphocytes. Successful therapy with agents that modulate T lymphocytes has lent credence to this hypothesis.

The clinical presentations and complications of Crohn's disease can be predicted by an understanding of the anatomic distribution and pathology of the process. Crohn's disease may involve any portion of the gastrointestinal tract from the mouth to the perianal area. Approximately 20% of patients have colonic disease alone, often with sparing of the rectum, and a predominance of right colonic involvement (Crohn's colitis). One third of patients have disease limited to the small intestine, most commonly the distal ileum (Crohn's ileitis). The remaining half of patients have both small-bowel and large-bowel disease (Crohn's ileocolitis). Perianal lesions are present in up to one third of patients, and 5 to 10% of patients have involvement of the mouth, esophagus, gastroduodenum, and/or proximal small intestine, usually in conjunction with disease in the ileum, colon, or both.

In regard to pathology, Crohn's disease is characterized by transmural inflammation involving all layers of the bowel, with involvement of adjacent fat and lymph nodes. The aphthous ulcer, the earliest visible gross mucosal lesion, is associated with submucosal edema and may enlarge and become confluent, giving rise to a cobblestone appearance. The mucosal and submucosal changes can gradually extend to the serosa, with the appearance of granulomas, edema, and inflammatory cells and sinus tracts focally through all the bowel layers. Fibrosis may eventually lead to luminal narrowing and stricturing.

The variable anatomic distribution of Crohn's disease leads to diverse clinical presentations, with the major manifestation of the disorder being dictated by whether involvement is most prominent in the upper GI tract, distal small bowel, colon, or perianal area.[3] In regard to pathophysiology, diarrhea is a result of impaired sodium and water absorption because of the mucosal and submucosal alterations. When this process affects the distal ileum, bile salts are malabsorbed, further promoting diarrhea by impaired colonic water and electrolyte absorption. When the mucosal ulceration extends to superficial blood vessels, hemorrhage may occur; the progression of sinus tracts through the serosa leads to fistulization into adjacent tissue or organs, with resulting extraluminal drainage and infection. Finally, the fibrosing process that leads to stricture formation manifests itself as episodes of bowel obstruction.

ULCERATIVE COLITIS

Unlike Crohn's disease, ulcerative colitis involves only the colon, although the degree of involvement may vary from a process limited to the rectum or rectosigmoid to total colonic involvement. The inflammatory process, which involves the colon in a contiguous fashion, is usually confined to the mucosa and submucosa.[4] The disruption of the normal colonic architecture by crypt cell necrosis and acute and chronic inflammatory cells leads to diminished water and sodium absorption, promoting diarrhea, and the weeping of protein into the gut lumen produces hypoalbuminemia. Bleeding often leads to anemia and is occasionally massive, resulting from the ulcerative process and destroying the mucosa in highly vascularized areas. Repair of the inflammatory process causes deposition of granulation tissue in ulcerated areas, collagen deposits in the lamina propria, and hypertrophy of the muscularis mucosa. The latter may lead to spasm, contributing to painful contractions experienced by patients and to a reversible area of stricturing.

CLINICAL PRESENTATION (Table 49-22)

CROHN'S DISEASE

ORAL LESIONS

As noted, various urgent clinical scenarios may arise from the geographic variability of the inflammatory

TABLE 49-22. EMERGENCY PRESENTATIONS OF IBD

Crohn's Disease
  Gastroduodenal obstruction
  Small-bowel obstruction
  Localized peritonitis
  Hemorrhage
  Fulminant colitis ± toxic megacolon
Ulcerative Colitis
  Fulminant colitis ± toxic megacolon
  Hemorrhage
  Perforation
Extraintestinal Complications
  Enterovesical fistula
  Hydronephrosis
  Renal stones
  Gallstones
  Pancreatitis
  Uveitis and episcleritis
  Erythema nodosum and pyoderma gangrenosum
  Arthritis
  Sclerosing cholangitis
  Vascular thrombosis

process in Crohn's disease. Oral manifestations include mass lesions, fissures, and ulceration, varying in size from tiny aphthous ulcers (canker sores) to large confluent lesions.[5] At times, the oral lesions can be so disabling that emergency therapy is required.

GASTRODUODENAL DISEASE

Patients with involvement of the gastroduodenal area may present with a picture identical to that of acute peptic ulcer disease with disabling epigastric pain.[6] More typically, after a history of several weeks of postprandial discomfort, easy satiety, and intermittent vomiting suggesting partial obstruction, the patient with gastroduodenal Crohn's disease may present with frank high-grade gastric outlet obstruction. Massive upper gastrointestinal (GI) hemorrhage secondary to gastroduodenal Crohn's disease is rare, and differentiation from a bleeding peptic ulcer may be impossible. Finally, an uncommon complication of Crohn's disease involving the ampulla of Vater is recurrent episodes of acute pancreatitis.

ILEITIS

The typical presentation of Crohn's disease involving the small intestine is that of recurring and progressive episodes of right lower quadrant pain and diarrhea. Occasionally associated with vomiting and at times with fever and progressive weight loss, these symptoms usually occur in a subacute fashion not requiring emergency measures. Many patients have progressive symptoms and eventually present in an urgent fashion with intestinal obstruction, sudden severe crampy abdominal pain, distention, vomiting, and either increased watery stools or dramatic decrease in stool and gas output. At times, frank intestinal obstruction may be the initial manifestation of Crohn's disease, although usually, in retrospect, a history of episodes of intestinal upset can be obtained. Most often seen as a result of ileal stenosis, intestinal obstruction may be caused by proximal small-bowel or colonic disease as well.

Just as the fibrosing nature of Crohn's disease often leads to progressive bowel obstruction, so too may the tendency for sinus tracts and fistulae lead to an urgent presentation of acute localized peritonitis with unrelenting abdominal pain, fever, and chills, often in association with a palpable mass on physical exam. As with obstruction, this presentation is most typical of progressive ileal disease but can occur with colonic Crohn's disease or when the proximal small bowel is involved. As with obstruction, the initial manifestation of Crohn's disease may be that of acute localized peritonitis. This is a much less common presentation in Crohn's disease, usually occurring from secondary rupture of an abscess into the free peritoneum or from free perforation of the intestine proximal to an area of stenosis in the absence of an abscess.

COLITIS

At times, the typical manifestation of diarrhea, abdominal pain and fever does not present in a subacute or chronic fashion but occurs in a fulminant manner and is occasionally associated with massive hemorrhage. This urgent presentation is more often seen when the colon is involved than in isolated small-bowel Crohn's disease. Fulminant Crohn's colitis may be associated with progressive colonic dilatation and a picture of toxic megacolon identical to that seen in ulcerative colitis (see subsequent text).

PERINEAL DISEASE

Perirectal disease, presenting with drainage and painful, tender perianal swellings from a combination of perianal fistulae and abscesses, may dominate the clinical picture for many patients and demand urgent intervention.

OTHER PRESENTATIONS

Several urgent presentations can be viewed as complications of Crohn's disease arising from the distribution of the disease and/or its pathophysiologic consequences. Urologic complications include recurrent episodes of cystitis secondary to enterovesical fistulae, obstructive hydronephrosis at times with pyelonephritis secondary to ureteral entrapment by extension of ileal or sigmoid disease into the surrounding mesentery and retroperitoneum, and acute renal colic secondary to uric acid stones related to chronic dehydration and acidosis or calcium oxalate stones related to steatorrhea and increased colonic absorption of oxalate. Acute biliary colic, cholangitis, and cholecystitis may all be seen in the context of ileal Crohn's disease because of an increased lithogenicity of bile related to impaired ileal absorption of bile acids.

ULCERATIVE COLITIS

As with Crohn's disease, the clinical picture of ulcerative colitis varies and usually depends on the anatomic extent of the disease process. Patients with disease limited to the rectum or rectosigmoid often have limited intermittent rectal bleeding with mild diarrhea or even constipation. Patients with more extensive disease involving the left colon may present with more disabling symptoms. They may have up to 10 loose bloody stools a day, mild anemia not requiring transfusion, low-grade fever, and abdominal cramping, but maintain nutrition and show no appreciable weight loss. In a few patients with ulcerative colitis, the process extends into the transverse colon and may involve the entire bowel to the cecum. In some of these patients, the inflammation extends through the muscularis to the serosa, with resultant loss of motor tone. These patients often present in an acutely ill fashion,

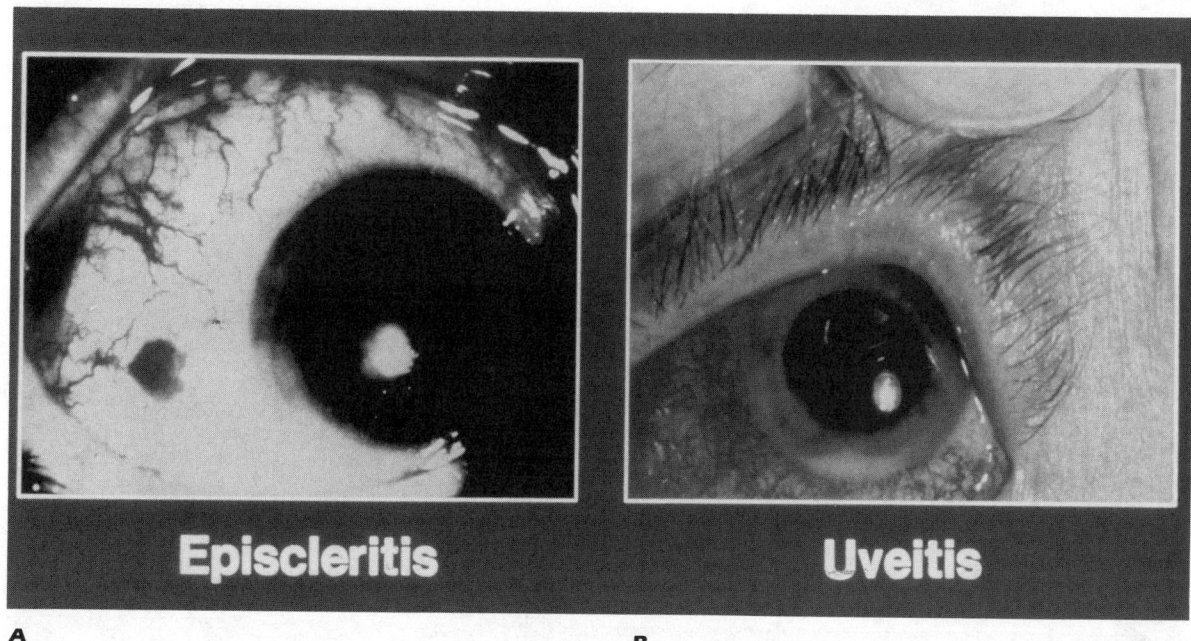

FIG. 49-20. A. Patient with ulcerative colitis and episcleritis with injected ciliary vessels. B. Patient with uveitis. (With permission from the Clinical Teaching Project, Unit I, American Gastroenterology Association, Miller-Fenwick, Inc.)

require urgent intervention, and constitute the most common emergency presentation of ulcerative colitis, which is fulminant disease with possible associated toxic megacolon. Patients with fulminant ulcerative colitis have frequent bloody stools, severe abdominal pain, and rapid weight loss from diminished intake and a catabolic state. Evidence of dehydration, tachycardia, high fever, and abdominal tenderness are all often part of the clinical picture. These patients are clearly toxic but may not have actual colonic dilation. In a subset of these acutely ill patients, however, the colon may dilate progressively as it loses its tone, leading to the picture of toxic megacolon with abdominal distention, a tender tympanitic abdomen with diminished bowel sounds, and an actual diminution in stool output. Such patients are at risk for the most dreaded complication of fulminant ulcerative colitis, perforation. Although perforation may be masked by high-dose steroid treatment, it must be considered in any patient with severe colitis who suddenly deteriorates, with increased abdominal pain, distention, fever, possible shoulder pain, and increased fever with tachycardia. Bleeding requiring blood transfusion is often seen in fulminant colitis. Massive life-threatening hemorrhage requiring urgent surgical intervention is unusual, however.

EXTRAINTESTINAL COMPLICATIONS

Processes affecting organ systems outside the GI tract are associated with both Crohn's disease and ulcer-

ative colitis, and most often occur when there is colonic disease activity. These disorders may in themselves dominate the clinical picture and require urgent attention.

An acute, painful red eye may be a result of either episcleritis or uveitis[7] (Fig. 49-20). Erythema nodosum, presenting as painful, tender red subcutaneous nodules on the extensor surfaces of the arms and legs, usually heralds the onset of increased bowel activity, whereas pyoderma gangrenosum resulting in progressive necrosis of the dermis with deep ulceration correlates with disease in only about 50% of patients[8,9] (Fig. 49-21). Arthritis involving the peripheral joints is a common manifestation of IBD and, although it tends to parallel disease activity, may antedate it. The arthritis is usually migratory and monoarticular and may present in an acute manner with evidence of synovitis.[10] Sclerosing cholangitis, more common in ulcerative colitis than Crohn's disease, usually presents initially with silent elevations of alkaline phosphatase and subsequent progressive hepatic damage leading to jaundice. At times, however, the presentation may be characterized by recurrent attacks of abdominal pain, fever, and leukocytosis, resembling cholangitis secondary to common-duct stones with bacterial infection.[11] Finally, these disorders may predispose to a hypercoagulable state manifested by deep venous thrombosis with possible pulmonary embolism and, less commonly, by arterial thromboses involving the large cranial vessels, retina, glans penis, or vessels to multiple organs in a picture resembling periarteritis nodosum.[12]

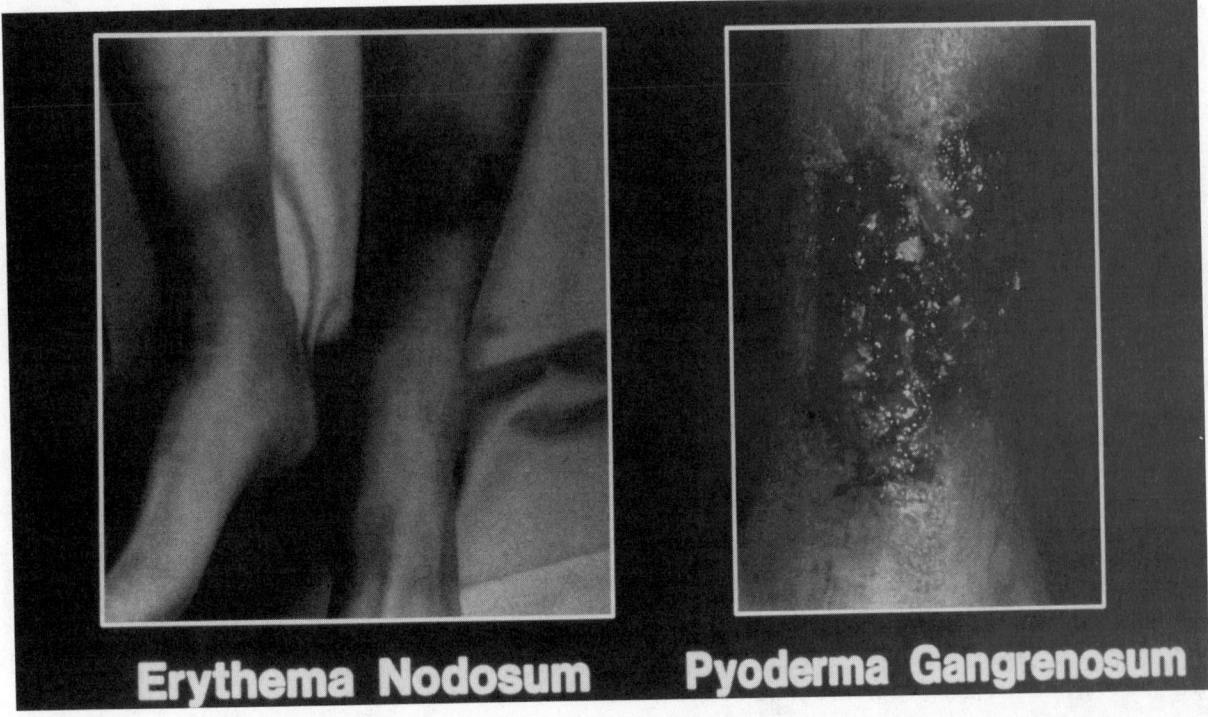

A   **B**

FIG. 49-21. A. Typical tender red nodules of erythema nodosum which usually occur on the extensor surfaces. B. Ulcerating lesion of pyoderma gangrenosum. (With permission from the Clinical Teaching Project, Unit I, American Gastroenterology Association, Miller-Fenwick, Inc.)

DIFFERENTIAL DIAGNOSIS

CROHN'S DISEASE

Crohn's disease involving the mouth can be confused at times with oral candidiasis, herpes simplex lesions, and neoplastic growths. The major confusion in gastroduodenal Crohn's disease is with peptic ulcer disease, although sarcoidosis, tuberculosis, syphilis, cytomegalovirus, granulomatous gastritis, and both lymphoma and adenocarcinoma have to be considered, depending on the clinical picture. When Crohn's disease of the small bowel presents subacutely, differentiation without appropriate x-ray studies from the irritable bowel syndrome, lactose intolerance, and chronic infections such as Giardia may be difficult. Once an abnormality is seen on x ray, other conditions which have to be considered include lymphoma, tuberculosis, carcinoid, Yersinia infection, cytomegalovirus, amebiasis, endometriosis, and chronic ischemia. The latter may be particularly difficult to differentiate from Crohn's disease in the elderly. Presentations with acute localized peritonitis may be impossible on clinical rounds to distinguish from appendicitis, diverticulitis, or perforated malignancy (Table 49-23).

ULCERATIVE COLITIS

When patients present with new-onset severe colitis, the differentiation has to be made between the two forms of IBD, Crohn's disease and ulcerative colitis, and infectious causes or intestinal ischemia. When the patient with known pre-existing IBD presents in a fulminant fashion, superimposed infection has to be excluded. The infections to be considered include Salmonella, Shigella, Campylobacter, Aeromonas hydrophila, hemorrhagic Escherichia coli, cytomegalovirus, and amebiasis. Several of the bacterial infections have been associated with severe colitis, in conjunction with hemolysis and renal failure (the hemolytic uremic syndrome). Ischemic colitis tends to occur in older patients with underlying heart disease. A vascular cause should also be considered in any patient with known underlying vasculitis or associated skin and joint manifestations suggesting a vasculitis (e.g., systemic lupus erythematosus, periarteritis nodosum, Henoch-Schönlein purpura) and in women on birth control pills. Differentiation of Crohn's disease from ulcerative colitis may be difficult, but the presence of perianal lesions, rectum-sparing small-bowel involvement, known fistulae and focality of inflammation, with or without granulomas on biopsy, all suggest the former.[13] When either Crohn's disease or ulcerative colitis presents with massive hemorrhage, other common processes, including diverticulosis, arteriovenous malformations, and neoplastic lesions, must be excluded (Table 49-24).

INITIAL EVALUATION AND STABILIZATION

In patients with known or possible IBD presenting in an urgent fashion, the history and examination should be focused on several key areas. In addition to the presenting complaint, a detailed history should seek a prior known history of Crohn's disease or ulcerative colitis and a family history of inflammatory bowel disease. The possibility of an infectious cause should be sought by eliciting a travel history, known infectious exposures, sexual preference, or known underlying immunocompromised status. A history of prior medications, associated cardiovascular renal disease, and menstrual irregularities should also be sought. Physical examination should focus initially on establishing the volume status of the patient with postural blood pressure and pulse as well as temperature. A careful examination of the abdomen, rectum, perineum, and a pelvic examination in women is mandatory, seeking evidence of abdominal distention, cough, and percussion tenderness suggesting peritoneal irritation, evidence of any mass lesion, obvious blood in the stool, and perineal lesions. Findings of wasting and edema should suggest a chronic process underlying the acute presentation.

Early laboratory tests should include a CBC with differential, sedimentation rate, BUN, glucose, and electrolytes. In the patient with obvious bleeding, a clot should be sent to the blood bank for typing, and clotting parameters including prothrombin time, partial thromboplastin time, platelet count and, when appropriate, bleeding time should be obtained. In the patient with diarrhea, stool samples should be sent for bacterial pathogens, ova, and parasites, and Clostridium difficile toxin if there has been recent antibiotic usage. Blood cultures should be obtained in febrile patients. An upright chest film and flat plate of the abdomen with upright films, looking for evidence of perforation, colonic dilation, or intestinal obstruction, is almost always indicated in the acutely ill patient (Table 49-25).

Patients who show evidence of severe colitis (or ileitis) with signs of toxicity, a picture of intestinal obstruction, evidence of significant hemorrhage, or findings of localized peritonitis all require admission to the hospital. Initial therapeutic efforts are directed at restoring the volume status with intravenous fluids and electrolytes and, when appropriate, packed red blood cells. For patients with obvious obstruction or megacolon, nasogastric suction should be instituted. In the toxic patient with either localized peritonitis or fulminant colitis, once cultures are obtained, broad-

TABLE 49-23. DIFFERENTIAL DIAGNOSIS OF EMERGENCY PRESENTATIONS: CROHN'S DISEASE

Gastroduodenal Obstruction
  Sarcoidosis
  Tuberculosis
  Syphilis
  Cytomegalovirus
  Granulomatous gastritis
  Lymphoma
  Adenocarcinoma
Small Bowel Obstruction
  Lymphoma
  Tuberculosis
  Yersinia
  Carcinoid
  Cytomegalovirus
  Amebiasis
  Endometriosis
  Ischemia
Localized Peritonitis
  Appendicitis
  Diverticulitis
  Perforated carcinoma
Fulminant Colitis

TABLE 49-24. DIFFERENTIAL DIAGNOSIS OF EMERGENCY PRESENTATIONS: ULCERATIVE COLITIS

Fulminant Colitis
  Crohn's disease
  Salmonella
  Shigella
  Campylobacter
  Aeromonas hydrophila
  Hemorrhagic Escherichia coli
  Cytomegalovirus
  Amebiasis
  Ischemia
  Vasculitis
Hemorrhage
  Arteriovenous malformations
  Diverticula
  Neoplastic lesions

TABLE 49-25. INITIAL EVALUATION

History
Physical examination
Laboratory tests
  CBC and differential
  Sedimentation rate
  BUN, glucose, electrolytes
  Pro time, PTT, bleeding time
Type and crossmatch
Stool for bacterial culture, ova and parasites, Clostridium difficile toxin
Blood cultures
Chest x ray and abdominal flat plate

spectrum antibiotics (e.g., ampicillin or a cephalosporin, an aminoglycoside and metronidazole) may be considered as part of the initial urgent therapy. Patients who enter the hospital already on corticosteroids need an increase in the steroid level to stress doses (e.g., 300 mg in 24 hours of hydrocortisone, 48 mg in 24 hours of methylprednisolone, 60 mg in 24 hours of prednisolone). Surgical consultation at the time of admission should be obtained for any patient with evidence of obstruction, localized peritonitis, or fulminant colitis.

PROCEDURES

GASTRIC OUTLET OBSTRUCTION

For patients with Crohn's disease of the gastroduodenal area, a prior *upper GI barium study* showing a narrowed antrum and/or postbulbar stricturing is often diagnostic (Fig. 49-22). *Endoscopy* may be useful, as well, and reveal typical focal ulcers with granulomas on biopsy. Often, however, the endoscopic picture is nonspecific. In the patient presenting with acute gastric outlet obstruction secondary to Crohn's disease, an initial *flat plate of the abdomen* is usually diagnostic, showing evidence of gastric dilation. A barium x ray after a period of nasogastric suction may be useful in documenting continuation or relief of the obstruction.

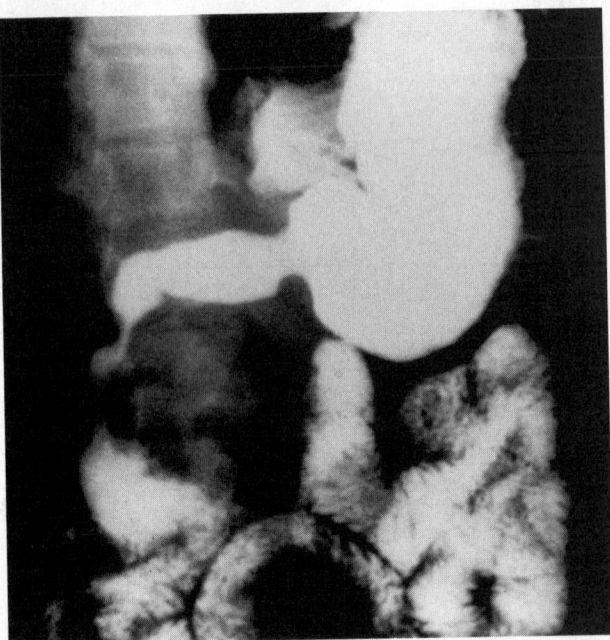

FIG. 49-22. Gastroduodenal Crohn's disease with antral narrowing and postbulbar duodenal strictures. (With permission from the Clinical Teaching Project, Unit I, American Gastroenterology Association, Miller-Fenwick, Inc.)

Endoscopy is generally not indicated in this setting, but should be done in patients who present with upper gastrointestinal bleeding.

SMALL BOWEL OBSTRUCTION

In patients with Crohn's disease involving the more distal small intestine, a *small bowel x ray* may have already been obtained, showing the characteristic abnormalities of segmental narrowing, ulceration and cobblestoning, often with sinus tracts, which usually distinguish Crohn's disease from the other conditions noted above (Fig. 49-23). In the patient whose presentation of Crohn's disease is small-bowel obstruction, a *flat plate x ray of the abdomen with upright films* shows dilated loops of small bowel with air-fluid levels. In patients without prior diagnosis, a small bowel x ray, obtained once the obstruction is relieved, should be diagnostic. On occasion, patients will be operated on when the diagnosis is not suspected and the diagnosis made at laparotomy.

LOCALIZED PERITONITIS

The diagnosis at operation may also be the case for the Crohn's disease patient whose initial presentation is an acute appendicitis-like one. For the patient with known Crohn's disease who presents with localized peritonitis, an *abdominal CT scan* can be useful in distinguishing a frank abscess from an inflammatory mass without abscess.[14]

FULMINANT COLITIS

In patients with Crohn's colitis, the diagnosis has usually been established by *rigid sigmoidoscopy* or *flexible sigmoidoscopy*, in conjunction with an *air contrast barium enema*, or by *colonoscopy*, which is particularly useful at detecting the subtle changes in the more proximal colon often missed on a barium examination. For patients with ulcerative colitis, which always involves the rectum, a *rigid sigmoidoscopy* showing the typical signs of diffuse inflammation may be all that is necessary to make the diagnosis, with *flexible sigmoidoscopy*, *colonoscopy* and *barium enema* used subsequently to establish the extent of disease. For patients presenting with new-onset severe colitis or known colitis involving the rectum, whether it is Crohn's disease or ulcerative colitis but recently in remission, a limited rigid sigmoidoscopy or gentle flexible sigmoidoscopy to confirm the colitic process should be done and can be performed safely. The more extensive colonoscopic procedure and barium enema should be avoided, however, because not only do they not contribute information necessary to the management of such patients, they are uncomfortable and may exacerbate the symptoms and lead to toxic megacolon or even perforation. A *flat plate of the abdomen* should be obtained

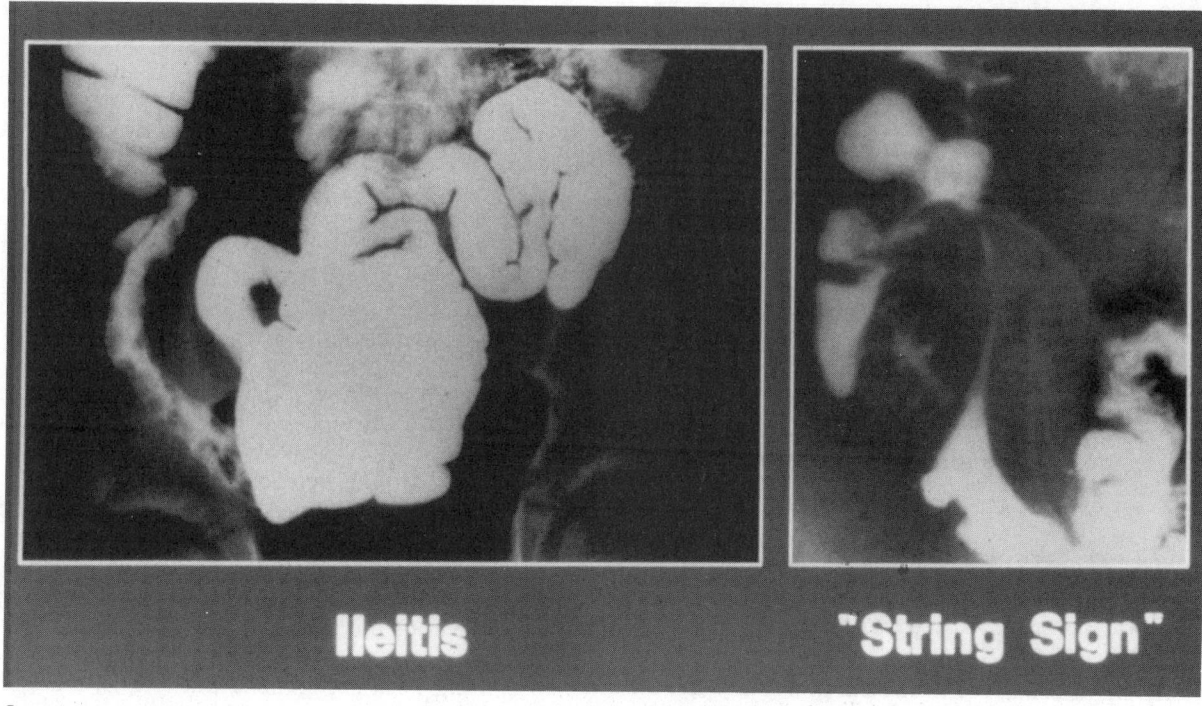

FIG. 49-23. *Small bowel x ray of Crohn's ileitis, with A showing nodularity, ulceration, narrowing and irregularity with separation of bowel loops, B showing severe narrowing caused by stricture and spasm. (With permission from the Clinical Teaching Project, Unit I, American Gastroenterology Association, Miller-Fenwick, Inc.)*

urgently and may show an abnormal gas pattern with ragged, irregular-appearing mucosa. In the most severe cases of toxic megacolon, the x ray may show dilation of the entire colon or a segment, most commonly the transverse colon (Fig. 49-24). An upright chest x ray should be obtained to rule out air under the diaphragm, a sign of intestinal perforation. For patients with toxic colitis and evidence of colonic distention, frequent flat plates are mandatory, because surgery may be indicated in patients with progressive colonic distention and no clinical improvement.

MANAGEMENT

CROHN'S DISEASE (Table 49-26)

INTESTINAL AND GASTRODUODENAL OBSTRUCTION

Most intestinal obstruction from Crohn's disease is partial, although often high grade, and the risks of strangulation small. Therefore, urgent surgery is usually not required. Treatment with intravenous fluids and nasogastric suction should be instituted. In the patient already on oral corticosteroids, intravenous hydrocortisone, methylprednisolone, or prednisolone

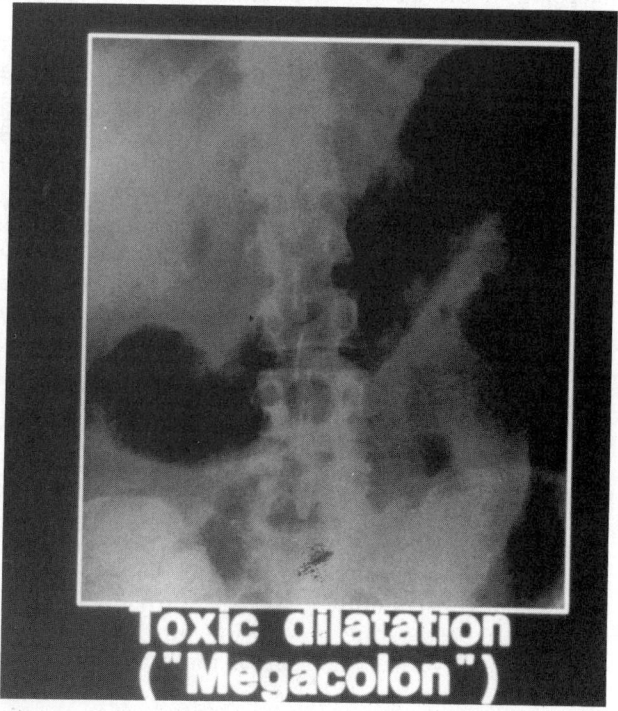

FIG. 49-24. *A dilated, ahaustral transverse colon in a patient with fulminant colitis. Pseudopolyps and submucosal edema project as soft-tissue densities into the lumen. (With permission from the Clinical Teaching Project, Unit I, American Gastroenterology Association, Miller-Fenwick, Inc.)*

TABLE 49-26. MANAGEMENT OF EMERGENCY PRESENTATIONS: CROHN'S DISEASE

Gastroduodenal and Intestinal Obstruction
- Nasogastric suction
- Intravenous fluids
- Intravenous corticosteroids (hydrocortisone 100 mg Q8°, methylprednisolone 16 mg Q8°, or prednisolone 20 mg Q8°)
- Gastrojejunostomy and selective vagotomy (gastroduodenal obstruction) or intestinal resection (small-bowel obstruction) if no response

Localized Peritonitis
- NPO
- Intravenous fluids
- Parenteral antibiotics (ampicillin or a cephalosporin plus gentamicin and metronidazole)
- Stress doses of steroids if already on steroids
- ? parenteral corticosteroids if no abscess on CT scan
- Drainage of abscess and intestinal resection if abscess on CT scan

Fulminant Colitis (see Table 49-27)

Perianal Disease
- Sitz baths
- Oral antibiotics (e.g., cephalosporin)
- Surgical drainage
- Metronidazole or ciprofloxacin

---

should be given at a dose of 300 mg in 24 hours, 48 mg in 24 hours, or 60 mg in 24 hours, respectively, in divided doses to help decrease any inflammation contributing to the obstruction. Intravenous corticosteroids should also be considered in patients not on steroids who are not felt to have an extraluminal complication of their disease.

Most patients respond to nonoperative therapy and can be gradually fed, initally with clear liquids and subsequently with a low-residue diet, and switched to oral steroid medication, usually an initial dose of prednisone at 40 to 60 mg per day with subsequent gradual tapering. For those not responding to an initial trial of medical therapy, resection of the involved intestine is required. Surgery should also be considered before nutritional depletion and/or perforation occur in the patient who continues to have symptoms of partial obstruction or who, after an initial episode of obstruction, has an early rehospitalization.

For patients who present with gastric outlet obstruction from gastroduodenal Crohn's disease, inital management is similar to that of intestinal obstruction, with intravenous fluids and nasogastric suction. H_2 receptor blockers and intravenous corticosteroids should be used as well. For patients who do not respond or subsequently have uncontrollable symptoms, a bypass of the obstruction by gastrojejunostomy with selective vagotomy is indicated.[15]

LOCALIZED PERITONITIS

In the patient with known Crohn's disease who presents with localized peritonitis, it should be assumed that a microperforation has occurred. Intravenous fluids, bowel rest, nasogastric suction if there is a component of obstruction, and broad-spectrum antibiotics (e.g., ampicillin or a cephalosporin plus an aminoglycoside and metronidazole) should be instituted. In patients on corticosteroids, it may be necessary to increase the dose somewhat to cover the stress of the acute episode. The use of corticosteroids initially in this setting in the patient not already on steroids is controversial and has never been subjected to careful study. Because of the risk of promoting the development of large intra-abdominal abscesses with possible secondary perforation, I favor withholding steroids in this setting and observing the clinical response. In the patient who has not responded and in whom a CT scan shows no obvious abscess, parenteral corticosteroids can be cautiously introduced.

If the CT scan shows an abscess, early percutaneous drainage of such abscesses can be carried out, although the risk of an enterocutaneous fistula is high. It is preferable to perform a definitive operation with removal of the abscess, resection of the involved intestine, and a primary anastomosis. For those presenting with generalized peritonitis, emergency surgery is required, with either resection of the involved intestine with closure of the intestine or diversion of intestinal contents and drainage of a ruptured abscess when that situation is encountered.

FULMINANT COLITIS

Fulminant colitis, with and without toxic megacolon, demands urgent attention with hydration, bowel rest, intravenous fluids, parenteral corticosteriods, and antibiotics. This condition is more common in ulcerative colitis than Crohn's disease and is discussed in detail below.

PERIANAL DISEASE

Although some perianal abscesses may resolve with sitz baths and oral antibiotics, most require external drainage under anesthesia, with subsequent careful follow-up to prevent premature closure of the wound.[16] Perianal disease usually occurs in the setting of active intestinal disease, which needs to be treated concurrently with available medications, including sulfasalazine, corticosteroids, and/or metronidazole. The latter, given in high doses of 1 to 2 g per day, may be especially useful for refractory perianal sepsis.[17] Ciprofloxacin has recently been found similarly useful.

ULCERATIVE COLITIS (Table 49-27)

FULMINANT COLITIS

Patients who present with fulminant ulcerative colitis (or Crohn's colitis) need careful observation by both medical and surgical teams. Therapies used to treat diarrhea and pain, such as diphenoxylate with atropine and loperamide, as well as meperidine and anticholinergic agents, should be avoided because of the risk of ileus and colonic dilation. Initial therapy consists of total bowel rest and total parenteral nutrition. The latter can be given initially through a large-bore peripheral line, but if the patient does not improve quickly, a central line is needed. When evidence of colonic dilation is present, bowel decompression is indicated. This can be accomplished most often with the use of a nasogastric tube and a rectal tube. In addition, patients should be instructed to roll onto their abdomens for 10 to 15 minutes every 2 to 3 hours, so that air that accumulates in the transverse colon when the patient is supine will redistribute throughout the colon and hopefully be expelled.[18]

The primary therapy in patients with fulminant ulcerative colitis or Crohn's colitis is that of parenteral corticoids. In patients who have recently been on oral steroids, intravenous hydrocortisone, prednisolone, or methylprednisolone should be used. The latter two agents may be preferable because they are less salt-retaining and more potassium-sparing. Hydrocortisone (300 mg in 24 hours), prednisolone (60 to 80 mg in 24 hours) or methylprednisolone (48 to 60 mg in 24 hours) can be given, either as a continuous infusion or in bolus fashion every 6 to 8 hours.[19] It is not clear that giving the medication by constant infusion is more effective than giving it by the intermittent bolus route. Brief pulses of extremely high doses of corticosteroid (e.g., 300 mg of prednisolone) have been advocated, although there is no proof of the effectiveness of this type of treatment. In patients with ulcerative colitis who are not on recent oral steroids, there is evidence that corticotropin (ACTH) given at 120 U over 24 hours by constant infusion may be more useful than continuous doses of hydrocortisone.[20] Although this form of therapy has been utilized in Crohn's disease also, there are no data regarding its improved efficacy over standard corticosteroid preparations. Fifty to 75% of patients treated with one of these modalities can avoid surgery.

In the toxic patient with high fever, abdominal tenderness, and evidence of leukocytosis, and in the patient with toxic megacolon, parenteral antibiotics should be instituted at the time of admission. As with localized peritonitis in Crohn's disease, ampicillin or a cephalosporin plus gentamicin and metronidazole provide the needed broad coverage. In patients with severe colitis who are less toxic, with no evidence of colonic dilation, antibiotics can be withheld and the response to bowel rest and corticosteroids observed. If, however, such patients develop fever and increasing leukocytosis with band forms on steroids, antibiotics should be initiated. Sulfasalazine, a mainstay of therapy in mild to moderate ulcerative colitis and Crohn's disease, has not been formally evaluated in patients with fulminant colitis. Early addition of this agent to patients with severe disease who are not re-

---

TABLE 49-27. MANAGEMENT OF EMERGENCY PRESENTATIONS: ULCERATIVE COLITIS

Fulminant Colitis
- NPO
- Nasogastric suction, rectal tube, and turning patient if colon is dilated
- Total parenteral nutrition
- Blood transfusion for massive hemorrhage
- Intravenous corticosteroids (hydrocortisone 300 mg in 24 hours, methylprednisolone 48–60 mg in 24 hours, prednisolone 60–80 mg in 24 hours in continuous or divided doses (if already on steroids)
- Corticotropin (ACTH) 120 U in 24 hours as continuous drip (if not already on steroids)
- Parenteral antibiotics (ampicillin or cephalosporin plus gentamicin and metronidazole)
- Early colectomy (48–72 hours) if no response

---

sponding fully to initial management with bowel rest, TPN, and steroids should be considered. There is no information about the possible efficacy of mesalamine (5-aminosalicylate), the new agent based on sulfasalazine's structure, in severe disease. The immunosuppressive drugs, such as azathioprine and 6-mercaptopurine, have not proven useful when subjected to study in acute, severe attacks of inflammatory bowel disease, but there is recent evidence that the use of continuous-infusion cyclosporine in the setting of severe fulminant colitis may reverse the process and prevent colectomy.

For patients not responding to the maximal medical regimen outlined above who continue to appear toxic, with abdominal tenderness, tachycardia, fever, and multiple bloody stools, with or without evidence of colonic dilatation, operation should be considered within 48 to 72 hours. Colonic resection also becomes a major consideration in the patient who becomes less toxic but continues to be seriously ill, with frequent loose, bloody stools and mild cramping, after a period of 2 weeks. Once the decision for surgery has been made, the procedure of choice depends on the total clinical picture, operative findings, and the wishes of the patient after an informed discussion about surgical alternatives. Most patients with fulminant colitis are severely debilitated and are best treated with a subtotal colectomy, ileostomy, and exteriorization of the rectosigmoid as a mucous fistula.[16] This approach leaves open the option of a future ileoanal anastomosis with ileal pouch for those patients with ulcerative colitis. Moreover, for the patients with Crohn's disease with rectal sparing or minimal rectal involvement, a subsequent ileorectal anastomosis can be carried out. On occasion, however, patients undergoing subtotal colectomy have massive hemorrhage from the remaining rectosigmoid segment, requiring emergency resection and resulting in a total proctocolectomy. For patients who are not as severely debilitated but have rectal disease, who are not judged to be candidates for a future ileal anastomosis with pouch or reanastomosis in the case of Crohn's disease, a total proctocolectomy as the initial procedure can be done. In patients who have suffered a perforation, emergency colectomy is clearly indicated, although even with immediate surgery, a mortality as high as 50% can be expected. In the same manner, urgent surgery may be required for the patient who is bleeding massively or whose blood replacement equals or exceeds 2 units a day for two to three consecutive days. In the massively bleeding patient, sigmoidoscopy should be performed to exclude a locally treatable bleeding point in the rectum and to decide whether total proctocolectomy is indicated. In the severely bleeding patient whose rectum does not appear to be the site of major bleeding, a subtotal colectomy can be carried out.

EXTRAINTESTINAL COMPLICATIONS

Cystitis secondary to an enterovesical fistula usually responds to appropriate antibiotic administration determined by urine culture. Pyelonephritis is rarely associated with this complication. Many patients can be handled nonsurgically by treating the underlying bowel disease, and 6-mercaptopurine may be especially useful in treating such fistulae. Ureteral obstruction secondary to an inflammatory mass calls for resection of the involved intestine and ureterolysis. Renal colic is managed in the usual fashion with fluids and analgesics. Stones should be recovered and analyzed to provide guidance for subsequent dietary and medical therapy.

The indications for cholecystectomy in Crohn's patients with biliary colic are similar for other patients with symptomatic gallstones. Episcleritis, erythema nodosum, and peripheral arthritis all tend to follow the clinical course of the underlying bowel disease and usually respond to treatment with corticosteroids, sulfasalazine, metronidazole, or immunosuppressive agents directed at the Crohn's disease or ulcerative colitis. Uveitis and pyoderma gangrenosum, on the other hand, often run a course independent of the intestinal inflammation but typically respond to topical and/or systemic steroids. Other modalities that may be useful in pyoderma gangrenosum include dapsone and topical cromoglycate. In patients with sclerosing cholangitis presenting with fever, chills, and leukocytosis, a secondary bacterial infection should be assumed and parenteral antibiotics given. Methotrexate and ursodeoxycholic acid may be of benefit in the more indolent form of sclerosing cholangitis. In the patient with deep venous thrombosis, the use of intravenous heparin may precipitate massive intestinal hemorrhage, necessitating vena caval interruption. If heparin is tolerated without significant intestinal bleeding, a 7- to 10-day course should be completed, with gradual institution of Coumadin, which can then be continued on a longer-term basis for 3 to 6 months, depending on the degree of intestinal activity.

MEDICOLEGAL PEARLS

- Involve the surgeon early in any patient with intestinal obstruction, localized peritonitis, or fulminant colitis.
- In fulminant colitis, avoid antidiarrheals, narcotic analgesics, and anticholinergic agents because of the risk of ileus and megacolon.
- Avoid colonoscopy and barium enema in the setting of fulminant colitis because of the risk of exacerbating the disease and/or perforation.
- Fever with high-dose corticosteroids suggests possible bacterial infection and is an indication for blood cultures, possible abdominal CT scan, and institution of antibiotics.
- Localized peritonitis in the setting of Crohn's disease usually means a microperforation with secondary bacterial infection and requires antibiotic therapy. Use of corticosteroids in this setting is controversial and should be approached cautiously because of the risk of increasing localized sepsis.

NATIONAL CONTACTS

National Foundation for Ileitis and Colitis: (212) 685-3440

REFERENCES

1. Chiodini, R.J., et al.: Possible role of mycobacteria in inflammatory bowel disease, I. An unclassified mycobacterium species isolated from patients with Crohn's disease. Dig. Dis. Sci. 29:1073, 1984.
2. Jewell, D.P.: Future directions for immunological research. In Inflammatory Bowel Disease—1986. Edited by Rachmilewitz, D. The Netherlands, Martinus Nijkoff, 1986.
3. Farmer, R.G., Hawk, W.A., and Turnbull, R.B.: Clinical patterns in Crohn's disease. A statistical study of 615 patients. Gastroenterology 68:627, 1975.
4. Mottet, N.K.: Histopathologic spectrum of regional enteritis and ulcerative colitis. Philadelphia, W.B. Saunders Co., 1971.
5. Basu, M.K., et al.: Oral manifestations of Crohn's disease. Gut 16:249, 1975.
6. Nugent, F.W., Richmond, M., and Park, S.K.: Crohn's disease of the duodenum. Gut 18:115, 1977.
7. Pitrello, E.A., McKinley, M., and Traniole, F.J. Ocular manifestations of inflammatory bowel disease. Ann. Ophthalmol. 14:356, 1982.
8. Basler, R.: Ulcerative colitis and the skin. Med. Clin. North Am. 64:941, 1980.
9. Thornton, J.R., et al.: Pyoderma gangrenosum and ulcerative colitis. Gut 2:247, 1980.
10. McEwen, C., Linng, C., and Kirsner, J.B.: Arthritis accompanying ulcerative colitis. Am. J. Med. 33:923, 1962.
11. Schrumpf, R.G., et al.: Sclerosing cholangitis in ulcerative colitis. Scand. J. Gastroenterol. 17:33, 1982.
12. Yassinger, S., et al.: Association of inflammatory bowel disease and large vascular lesions. Gastroenterology 71:844, 1978.

13. Kirsner, J.B.: Problems in the differentiation of ulcerative colitis and Crohn's disease of the colon: The need for repeated diagnostic evaluation. Gastroenterology *68*:187, 1975.
14. Goldberg, H.I., et al.: Computed tomography in the evaluation of Crohn's disease. Am. J. Roentgenol. *140*:277, 1983.
15. Fielding, J.F., et al.: Crohn's disease of the stomach and duodenum. Gut *11*:1001, 1970.
16. Glotzer, D.J., and Silen, W.: Indications for operation in inflammatory bowel disease. *In* Inflammatory Bowel Disease. Ed. 2. Edited by Kirsner, J.B., and Shorter, R.G. Philadelphia, Lea & Febiger, 1980.
17. Brandt, L.J., et al.: Metronidazole for Crohn's disease. A follow-up study. Gastroenterology *83*:383, 1982.
18. Present, D.H., et al.: The medical management of toxic megacolon: Techniques of decompression with favorable long-term follow-up. Gastroenterology *80*:1255, 1981.
19. Truelove, S.C., and Witts, L.J.: Cortisone and corticotropin in ulcerative colitis. Br. Med. J. *1*:387, 1959.
20. Meyers, S., et al.: Corticotropin versus hydrocortisone in the treatment of ulcerative colitis: A prospective, randomized double-blind clinical trial. Gastroenterology *85*:351, 1983.

BIBLIOGRAPHY

Aufses, A.H.: Crohn's disease: Surgical treatment. *In* Current Therapy in Gastroenterology and Liver Disease. Ed. 2. Edited by Bayless, T.M. Toronto, Philadelphia, B.C. Decker, Inc., 1986.

Farmer, R.G., Hawk, W.A., and Turnbull, R.B.: Clinical patterns in Crohn's disease. A statistical study of 615 patients. Gastroenterology *68*:627, 1975.

Kirsner, J.B.: Problems in the differentiation of ulcerative colitis and Crohn's disease of the colon: The need for repeated diagnostic evaluation. Gastroenterology *68*:187, 1975.

Mendeloff, A.L.: The epidemiology of idiopathic inflammatory bowel disease. *In* Inflammatory Bowel Disease. Ed. 2. Edited by Kirsner, J.B., and Shorter, R.G. Philadelphia, Lea and Febiger, 1980.

Richert, R.: The important "imposters" in the differential diagnosis of inflammatory bowel disease. J. Clin. Gastroenterol. *6*:153, 1984.

Sacher, D.B., Auslander, M.O., and Walfish, J.S.: Aetiological theories of inflammatory bowel disease. Clin. Gastroenterol. *9*:231, 1980.

Sack, D.M., and Peppercorn, M.A.: Drug therapy of inflammatory bowel disease. Pharmacotherapy *3*:158, 1983.

COLONIC DIVERTICULAR DISEASE*

C. Gene Cayten

CAPSULE

Colonic diverticular disease may present to the emergency physician as mild abdominal pain, an acute abdomen, or massive lower gastrointestinal bleeding. The latter two presentations require expeditious resuscitation and early surgical consultation. Because of the differential diagnosis, it may not be possible nor is it essential to establish a specific diagnosis in the Emergency Department (ED).

INTRODUCTION

The prevalence of diverticular disease has increased with the advancing age of the population. The incidence increases from 5% in the fifth decade to 50% in the ninth decade. It is estimated that, in the population over age 60, the prevalence of diverticulosis is more than 30%.[1] The disease also has widely differing prevalence rates in various geographical areas and ethnic groups.[2,3] It has rapidly increased among Western nations. A dramatic increase has also been described in Japanese immigrants to Hawaii and in urban South African blacks.[3] Vegetarian Westerners, however, have reduced incidence.[4] Earlier in this century, a greater incidence was noted in men compared with women. Recent studies show no sex predilection.

* Based in part on the Chapter "Diverticular Disease" by C. Gene Cayten in *The Clinical Practice of Emergency Medicine*, Edited by Harwood-Nuss, A. Philadelphia, J.B. Lippincott, 1989.

PATHOPHYSIOLOGY

The common causative factor in the development of diverticulosis appears to be a reduction in dietary fiber content.[5] The pathophysiology is related to a pressure gradient between the colonic lumen and the serosa in areas of relative weakness in the bowel wall.[2] High intraluminal pressure can develop within short segments of the colon. According to LaPlace's law of pressures within a cylinder, pressure equals tension divided by radius. Accordingly, the descending and sigmoid colon, which have narrow lumens, have the greatest intraluminal pressures. This pressure causes herniation of diverticula at the points where the intramural vessels penetrate the circular muscle layer, usually between the mesenteric and antimesenteric taenia. Increased fiber intake enlarges the lumen size because of stool bulk, thereby decreasing the intraluminal pressure. This pathophysiology does not appear to explain the predominance of right-sided diverticular disease in the Orient.[3] In the U.S., right-sided diverticula are usually true diverticula, including all layers of the wall. They are generally considered congenital.

PREHOSPITAL ASSESSMENT AND STABILIZATION

Diverticular disease can present as an acute abdomen or massive lower gastrointestinal (GI) bleeding. In both cases, a specific diagnosis is not needed, although starting an intravenous line could be beneficial, particularly if the patient is in shock or if the transport time to the hospital is prolonged. Generally, the intravenous line should be started en route so that prehospital time is not prolonged. Oxygen should also be administered.[5]

CLINICAL PRESENTATION AND EXAMINATION

Most people with diverticulosis remain asymptomatic throughout their lives.[2] Some develop only recurrent left lower quadrant abdominal pain secondary to circular muscle hypertrophy (myochosis). Relatively few develop diverticulitis. Studies of patients with diverticulosis followed for 5 years show an incidence of diverticulitis in 10 to 15%; one series followed for a mean of 15 years yielded a 25% incidence.[1] The longer a patient has diverticulosis, the greater the probability

of complications, primarily diverticulitis and bleeding.[6] Diverticulitis results from inflammation of diverticula with either microperforation or macroperforation (abscess, fistula, peritonitis, or obstruction). Of patients over age 60 with diverticulosis, about one third develop diverticulitis and about one third of these have persistent symptoms and further complications. There is no relationship between the number and size of diverticula and symptoms and the incidence of complications or the probability of recurrent disease.

Massive bleeding occurs in 5 to 25% of patients with diverticulosis (Fig. 49-25). The bleeding comes from an arterial lesion in the vasa recta, characterized by eccentric internal thickening, altered internal elastic lamina, and focal alteration of the media.[7] A disproportionately high tendency (50 to 80%) exists for right colon diverticular hemorrhage. This might be explained by the fact that right-sided diverticula have wider necks and domes. The vasa recta are thus exposed over a greater length of the injurious factor arising from the colon.[7] The bleeding that occurs from diverticulosis stops spontaneously in approximately 70% of patients.[8]

Patients with diverticulosis present to the emergency physician with three common patterns: (1) mild left lower quadrant pain; (2) acute left lower quadrant pain, tenderness, and fever; and (3) massive lower gastrointestinal (GI) bleeding.

MILD LEFT LOWER QUADRANT PAIN (SYMPTOMATIC DIVERTICULOSIS)

Diverticulosis most frequently presents with left lower abdominal pain, but in most cases it is totally asymptomatic. The pain is usually dull, but sometimes it is crampy and intermittent. There is a controversy as to whether symptomatic diverticulosis is secondary to concomitant irritable bowel syndrome caused by the diverticulosis itself.[6,8] Mild diverticular symptoms can be caused by increased intracolonic pressure and circular muscle hypertrophy. Thompson depicts the coexistence of irritable bowel syndrome (IBS) and diverticula in Figure 49-26.[6]

ACUTE LEFT LOWER QUADRANT PAIN, TENDERNESS, AND FEVER (ACUTE DIVERTICULITIS)

Patients with acute diverticulitis present with acute left lower quadrant pain with or without a mass, tenderness, and rebound associated with fever, chills, and leukocytosis. Diarrhea and/or constipation, anorexia, nausea and vomiting may also occur. Occasionally the pain and tenderness occur in the left upper quadrant. In taking a history, questions should focus on GI symptoms, previous similar attacks, previous diagnostic studies, and change in bowel habits. The duration of the attack, characteristics of the pain, and history of the fever should also be elicited. With diverticulitis, the pain may be intermittent, crampy, and associated with nausea and vomiting. The physical examination should take careful note of the patient's temperature, pulse rate, and blood pressure. Signs of peritonitis and the presence of a mass on pelvic and rectal examinations are important to note. In rare cases, tenderness may be found only on rectal examination. Palpation may reveal the outline of the sigmoid colon as a rope-like mass. If the mass is large, fixed, and tender, diverticulitis is likely, although a perforated carcinoma is also possible.

Abdominal x rays (flat and upright) should be performed to look for a mass in the left lower quadrant as well as for free air. An ileus pattern is frequently seen, although evidence of partial small or large bowel obstruction is not uncommon. A complete blood count should be requested with a differential white blood cell (WBC) count. Leukocytosis with a left shift is compatible with the diagnosis of diverticulitis; however, elderly and immune compromised patients may not show such a response. Hackford et al. found that 64% of patients with diverticulitis have normal WBC counts.[9] Approximately 2 to 4% of patients with diverticulitis develop colovesical fistula.

Patients may present with a picture of a ruptured viscus with diffuse tenderness, rebound, guarding, and diminished or absent bowel sounds. Generalized abdominal pain is more commonly found in immunocompromised patients. Rarely, diverticulitis may present with signs of fistulization such as pneumaturia and draining infections of the lower abdomen or the medial aspect of the upper thigh. Colovesical fistulas usually present with dysuria. Fecaluria or pneumaturia is diagnostic.

MASSIVE LOWER GASTROINTESTINAL BLEEDING (DIVERTICULOSIS)

Patients with diverticulosis may present with painless, massive rectal bleeding. Such bleeding is characteristically sudden, often profuse from the onset, and more frequent in older people. The blood is usually bright or dark red. Hypotension is not commonly found when the patient first presents.

The history should focus on the onset, color, amount, and frequency of bloody bowel movements. A history of previous attacks, bleeding tendencies, and bowel habits is important. Many patients with massive rectal bleeding have had a previous episode, suggesting diverticulitis.

Hemodynamic instability should be assessed (blood pressure, pulse, and orthostatic changes). Abdominal and rectal examinations are particularly critical. The abdominal examination should focus on areas of tenderness and the presence or absence of a mass. The rectum should be palpated for masses and the color of the blood in the rectal vault examined. Tenderness should increase the suspicion of nondiverticular causes of bleeding such as ulcerative or ischemic colitis. A mass could represent a carcinoma.

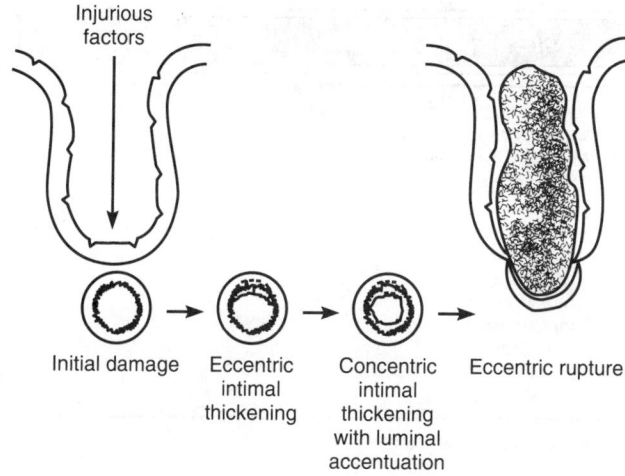

FIG. 49-25. *Proposed pathogenesis of bleeding colonic diverticulosis.*

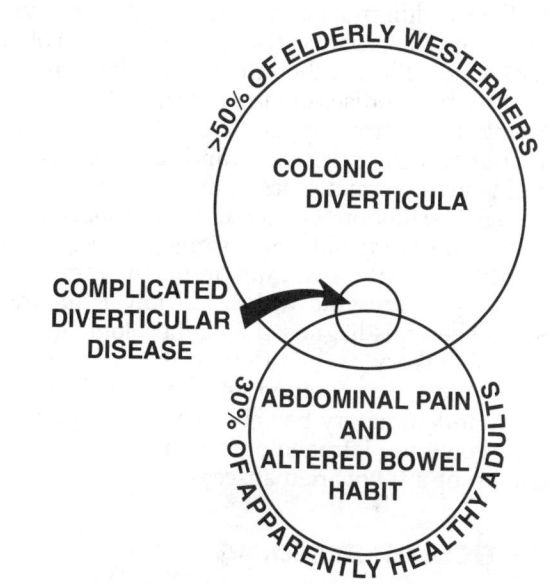

FIG. 49-26. *Schematic representation of the relationship of IBS, uncomplicated diverticular disease, and complicated diverticular disease.*

DIFFERENTIAL DIAGNOSIS

DIVERTICULOSIS

When diverticulosis presents as a mild, sometimes colicky left lower quadrant pain, it must be differentiated from irritable bowel syndrome, Crohn disease, and colon cancer. Diverticulosis can coexist with any of these conditions.[2] For example, Teaque et al. found that, in a group of 40 patients with diverticular disease who had persistent rectal bleeding, 20% had concomitant cancer.[10]

TABLE 49-28. CAUSES OF LOWER GI BLEEDING*

Diverticulosis
Angiodysplasia
Colorectal carcinoma
Colonic polyps
Colitis
   ischemic
   ulcerative
   granulomatous
   radiation
   infections
Rectal ulcer
Trauma
Coagulopathy

* Excludes anal pathology.

ACUTE DIVERTICULITIS

Acute diverticulitis must be distinguished from severe presentations of Crohn's disease, ulcerative colitis, and ischemic colitis, although diverticulitis and inflammatory bowel disease may coexist.[2] It must also be distinguished from appendicitis. Although acute diverticulitis is usually left-sided and appendicitis usually right-sided, certain cases of appendicitis present with left lower abdominal pain, as well as cases of solitary cecal diverticulitis and sigmoid diverticulitis adherent to the right lower quadrant. In women, diverticulitis that presents with a left lower quadrant mass has been misdiagnosed as gynecologic mass.[11] High fever, leukocytosis, and left lower quadrant mass should suggest a perforation and abscess. This may be due to inflammatory bowel disease, colon cancer, sigmoid volvulus, iatrogenic perforation of the rectosigmoid, or a tuboovarian abscess.

DIVERTICULAR BLEEDING

Diverticular bleeding should be distinguished from other causes of profuse lower GI bleeding, such as angiodysplasia, ischemic colitis, and, occasionally, ulcerative colitis and colon or rectal cancer (Table 49-28). It is most difficult to distinguish between diverticular bleeding and angiodysplasia; however, the evaluation and the medical and surgical therapy are similar.

MANAGEMENT AND INDICATIONS FOR HOSPITALIZATION

DIVERTICULOSIS

For the patient with left lower quadrant pain, minimal or no tenderness and with no mass, fever, or leukocytosis, symptomatic therapy with a mild sedative anticholinergic preparation can be recommended. A high-fiber diet and a follow-up flexible sigmoidoscopy should also be recommended.

DIVERTICULITIS

Most patients in whom the diagnosis of diverticulitis is made require hospitalization and IV antibiotics. For the patient in whom the diagnosis of severe diverticulitis is highly probable, an intravenous line should be started, a nasogastric (NG) tube inserted, specimens for blood and urine cultures collected and sent to the laboratory, and a surgical consultation requested. Baseline blood tests and type and hold should also be performed. Abdominal x rays should be obtained to detect free air, signs of abscess, and/or air in the urinary bladder. Sigmoidoscopy and barium enema are generally contraindicated in acute diverticulitis. Sigmoidoscopy is painful, and a barium enema could cause severe peritonitis if there is a perforation or if one develops as a result of the examination. Barium enema and sigmoidoscopy are generally deferred until the diverticulitis has responded to medical therapy. When the diagnosis is in doubt, a CT scan with oral and rectal water soluble contrast is generally more sensitive and specific for diverticulitis and its complications than barium enema.[12,13] CT findings consistent with diverticulitis include bowel wall thickening (≥ 4 mm) and/or mesenteric or fascial soft tissue stranding.[12] Pericolic fluid or gas is considered diagnostic of diverticular abscess.

Analgesics should be avoided until a surgical consultation has been obtained. Morphine and many of its analogues may even cause an exacerbation of diverticulitis by increasing segmental contraction of the colon.

After surgical consultation indicating the high likelihood of diverticulitis, intravenous antibiotics consisting of either an aminoglycoside (gentamicin or tobramycin, 5 mg per kg per day) and clindamycin or cefoxitin (4 g to 6 g daily every 6 hours) should be initiated.[11] The most common organisms are Bacteroides fragilis, Escherichia coli, and Enterococcus. If appendicitis cannot be ruled out, the surgeon may suggest holding off on the initiation of antibiotics.

DIVERTICULAR BLEEDING

For the patient with massive lower GI bleeding, two large-bore intravenous lines (16 gauge or larger) should be inserted. A specimen should be drawn and sent for type and crossmatch for 4 to 6 units of blood. Other baseline blood studies including CBC, electrolytes, and coagulation studies should also be requested. A Foley catheter should be placed. Lactated Ringer's should then be infused at a rate depending on the patient's vital signs and cardiac status. If the patient is not stabilized after 2 L of crystalloid infusion, a central venous line should be inserted and blood given. Among easily measured parameters, hourly urine output is the most reliable measure of the adequacy of resuscitation.[14] Elderly patients with associated cardiac disease should have ECG monitoring to pick up early signs of myocardial ischemia. Oxygen should be administered to all rapidly bleeding patients.

An NG tube should be inserted to help to rule out upper GI bleeding. Upper endoscopy may be needed in some cases to rule out an upper GI source. Flexible sigmoidoscopy should rule out a rectal or rectosigmoid carcinoma.

An aggressive attempt to determine the site of bleeding should be made because such information could reduce the extent of surgical resection if it becomes necessary. If the patient is bleeding at a rate of more than 0.5 mL per minute, it is likely to show up on mesenteric angiography. If a bleeding point is found, intra-arterial vasopressin can be administered. Slower bleeding (0.1 mL per minute) can be picked up using technetium-labeled red blood cell infusion scans.

In a patient in whom the presumptive diagnosis of massive bleeding from diverticulosis or angiodysplasia exists, an intravenous infusion of vasopressin (0.1 to 0.4 units per minute) can be initiated. Most consider such infusions contraindicated in presence of coronary artery disease. Patients with massive lower GI bleeding require an early surgical consultation and admission to an intensive care unit.

PITFALLS

Although less frequently encountered in patients under age 40, diverticulosis is relatively more likely to be complicated and require surgery in younger patients than in older patients.[14]

In women, diverticulitis presenting with a left lower quadrant mass is frequently misdiagnosed as a gynecologic mass.[4]

Even with complicated diverticulitis, the WBC count may be within normal limits, particularly in elderly patients.

Barium enema and sigmoidoscopic examinations using air insufflation may cause perforation and peritonitis in patients who present with acute diverticulitis.

Abdominal tenderness secondary to diverticulitis is less likely to be localized to the left lower quadrant in immunocompromised patients; it is more likely to be generalized.

REFERENCES

1. Chappuis, C.W., and Cohn, I.: Acute colonic diverticulitis. Surg. Clin. North Am. *68*:301, 1988.
2. Almy, T.P., and Howell, D.A.: Diverticular disease of the colon. N. Engl. J. Med. *302*:324, 1980.
3. Mendeloff, A.I.: Thoughts on the epidemiology of diverticular disease. Clin. Gastroenterol. *15*:855, 1986.
4. Gear, J.S.S., Wane, A., Fursdom, P. et al.: Symptomless diverticular disease and intake of dietary fibre. Lancet 511, 1979.
5. Boskers, C., Almy, T., Cello, J.P., et al.: Diverticular disease changing concepts. Updates in Geriatric Emergency Medicine.
6. Thompson, W.G., and Patel, D.G.: Clinical picture of diverticular disease of the colon. Clin. Gastroenterol. *15*:903, 1986.
7. Meyers, M.D., Alonso, D.R., Gray, G.F., and Baer, J.W.: Pathogenesis of bleeding colonic diverticulosis. Gastroenterology 71:577, 1976.
8. Otte, J.O., Larsen, L., and Andersen, J.R.: Irritable bowel syndrome and symptomatic diverticular disease—different disease. Am. J. Gastroenterol. *81*:529, 1986.
9. Hackford, A.W., Schoetz, D.J., Coller, J.A., et al.: Surgical management of complicated diverticulitis. Dis. Colon Rectum 28:317, 1985.
10. Teague, R.H., Thornton, J.R., Manning, A.P., et al.: Colonoscopy for investigation of unexplained rectal bleeding. Lancet i:1350, 1978.
11. Walker, J.D., Gray, L.A., Sr., and Polk, H.C., Jr.: Diverticulitis in women: Unappreciated clinical presentation. Ann. Surg. 185:402, 1977.
12. Johnson, C.D., Baker, M.E., and Rice, R.P.: Diagnosis of acute colonic diverticulitis: Comparision of barium enema and CT. Am. J. Radiol. *148*:541, March, 1987.
13. Labs, J.D., Sarry, M.G., Fishman, E.K., et al.: Complications of acute diverticulitis of the colon: Improved early diagnosis with computerized tomography. Am. J. Surg. *155*:331, 1988.
14. Bauchman, T.G., and Bulkley, G.B.: Current management of patients with lower gastrointestinal bleeding. Surg. Clin. North Am. *67*:651, 1987.

BIBLIOGRAPHY

Eusebio, E.B., and Eisenburg, M.M.: Natural history of diverticular disease of colon in young patients. Am. J. Surg. *125*:308, 1973.

Freischlag, J., Bennion, R.S., and Thompson, J.: Dis. Colon Rectum *29*:639, 1986.

Haubrich, W.S.: Diverticular and diverticular disease of the colon. *In* Bockus' Gastroenterology. Philadelphia, W.B. Saunders, 1985.

Horner, J.L.: Natural history of diverticulosis of the colon. Am. J. Dig. Dis. *3*:343, 1958.

McConnell, D.B., Sasaki, T.M., and Vetto, R.M.: Experience with colovesical fistula. Am. J. Surg. *140*:80, 1980.

ACUTE GALLBLADDER DISEASE

Richard E. Burney

CAPSULE

Acute gallbladder disease is one of the most common causes of acute, persistent upper abdominal pain in patients seen in the emergency department (ED). Its presentation can vary from a simple, self-limited episode of severe pain (biliary colic) to life-threatening sepsis and its pathophysiology from temporary occlusion of the cystic duct to gangrenous cholecystitis or suppurative cholangitis. Its manifestations may be limited to the gallbladder alone, or may involve the entire hepatobiliary tree and pancreas. Symptoms may range from pain only to those associated with septic shock without an obvious source. Acute gallbladder disease should be considered in any patient with one or more episodes of upper right or epigastric abdominal pain lasting hours or more before subsiding, in any patient with abdominal pain and hyperamylasemia, and in any patient with upper abdominal pain or tenderness and signs of sepsis or toxicity. Ultrasonography and cholescintigraphy are the diagnostic procedures of choice. Operation is the definitive form of treatment for patients with acute inflammation of the gallbladder or complications of gallstones.

ANATOMY AND PATHOPHYSIOLOGY

The gallbladder is a pear-shaped, saccular structure densely adherent to the inferior aspect of the liver at approximately the junction of the right and left lobes. It arises from the midportion of the common bile duct and extends in an oblique outward direction. It varies in length from 7 to 10 cm, but usually does not extend above the liver margin unless it is distended or inflamed. The fundus and body of the gallbladder normally contain 30 to 50 mL of bile. The gallbladder cavity communicates with the common bile duct through the narrow cystic duct, the lumen of which has numerous partially-occluding spiral valves. The gallbladder stores and concentrates bile. When stimulated by cholecystokinin, it empties by muscular contraction. Gallbladder bile joins common hepatic duct bile and enters the duodenum after passing through the common bile duct and the ampulla of Vater.

Gallstones are formed through the precipitation of saturated bile salts in the gallbladder. Cholesterol stones are most common in the United States, but bilirubin stones also occur, particularly in patients with alcoholic cirrhosis or hemolytic disorders. Gallstone disease tends to be familial, but the likelihood of developing gallstones is also increased by medications or conditions that affect bile salt metabolism or reabsorption such as pregnancy, use of birth control pills, ileal resection, and agents used to lower blood cholesterol. Most of the symptoms of gallbladder disease result from obstruction by gallstones or sludge-like precipitate at the mouth of the cystic or common bile ducts, and the subsequent inflammation, edema, or ischemia that can accompany this.

Biliary colic is the term commonly given to episodes of uncomplicated pain associated with gallstones. It is thought to occur as a result of distention of the gallbladder associated with a stone obstructing passage of bile through the cystic duct. Symptoms persist until the stone is passed or sufficient distention occurs to allow the stone to fall back into the lumen of the gallbladder.

Transient obstruction of the cystic duct is not necessarily accompanied by inflammation. Transient obstruction of the common bile duct by a stone obstructing the ampulla of Vater occurs also,[1] and can cause similar abdominal pain, as well as other complications such as acute pancreatitis.

Acute cholecystitis is characterized by inflammation and edema of the gallbladder. In most instances, the underlying cause is a stone obstructing or impacted in the cystic duct. Bacterial infection is not a common cause, although it can be a complicating factor. Gallstones are usually present in patients with acute cholecystitis; when the disease occurs in the apparent absence of stones, it is called acalculous cholecystitis.

Acute cholecystitis may be self-limited and subside over several days, or may progress to ischemia and necrosis of the gallbladder wall. In some cases, continuing, subacute inflammation may persist for weeks without progression to necrosis or perforation. When inflammation progresses, gangrenous necrosis of the gallbladder wall can lead to free perforation and peritonitis.

In some instances of persistent inflammation, adjacent structures such as the omentum and colon become adherent to the gallbladder and tend to protect against free perforation. On rare occasions, large stones may erode through the gallbladder wall into the adjacent intestine, causing a cholecystoenteric fistula. If such a stone obstructs the intestine, the resulting picture of intestinal obstruction is called gallstone ileus.[2]

Acute pancreatitis, obstructive jaundice, and acute cholangitis may all be caused by obstruction of the common bile duct at the ampulla of Vater. Either transient or persistent obstruction of the pancreatic duct at the ampulla can induce acute pancreatitis that can vary in severity from mild hyperamylasemia to severe hemorrhagic necrosis or pseudocyst formation. A common channel of pancreatic and common bile ducts at the ampulla of Vater increases the risk of pancreatitis.[3] Simple obstructive jaundice occurs when bile flow is retarded, but there is no accompanying inflammation. Acute cholangitis is inflammation of the biliary tree related to obstruction of the common bile duct.[4] Bacterial infection (suppurative cholangitis) aggravates this disease process and appears to be more common when pigment stones are present in the bile duct.[5]

CLINICAL PRESENTATION

As should be evident from the foregoing discussion, gallbladder disease can have many presentations, depending on the stage and severity of the disease.

HISTORY TAKING IN ACUTE GALLBLADDER DISEASE

A careful history, looking specifically for previous episodes of biliary pain and risk factors for gallstone formation, is frequently the key to interpreting other clinical findings. Questions directed at obtaining detailed information on the onset and character of pain, its location and radiation, the frequency and duration of episodes, and associated symptoms are helpful in differentiating biliary pain from other gastrointestinal complaints. The duration and character of pain are particularly important because biliary pain is rarely if ever sharp, stabbing, or of brief duration. Risk factors should be identified, particularly a family history of gallstone disease, pregnancy, or oral contraceptive use; but also diets and drugs aimed at lowering blood cholesterol and surgical procedures that may have reduced bile salt reabsorption. Risk factors for pigment stones include oriental heritage, chronic hemolysis for any reason, alcoholic cirrhosis, and previous biliary infection.[6]

Although the clinician is dealing with a continuum of pathophysiologic changes, gallbladder disease is most likely to present to the ED at one of several stages: transient obstruction of the cystic or common ducts

(biliary colic), biliary pancreatitis, and acute cholecystitis. Subacute cholecystitis and acute cholangitis are less common.

BILIARY COLIC

Biliary colic in its most common form is severe pain of acute onset, felt in the right upper quadrant of the abdomen or epigastrium. The onset of pain is most often in the late evening or at bedtime, possibly as a result of the shift in location of stones on assuming a supine position. Radiation to the right side of the costal margin or right scapular area is frequently described. The pain is steady, persistent, and distressing, lasting as long as 3 to 5 hours before gradually subsiding. It is not relieved by changes in position or by common over-the-counter medications. It is difficult to differentiate clinically between colic of gallbladder and bile duct origins. A negative ultrasound examination does not rule out the possibility of biliary colic because typical symptoms can occur in the apparent absence of stones.

BILIARY PANCREATITIS

The sudden onset of apparent biliary colic or mid-abdominal pain, with or without radiation to the back, accompanied by hyperamylasemia, makes the diagnosis one of biliary pancreatitis. It is sometimes but not always accompanied by vomiting. Identification of hyperamylasemia is critical because the symptoms and signs can be highly variable. The magnitude of the amylase elevation can be surprisingly high and may seem out of proportion to the other clinical findings. The actual extent of pancreatitis can vary from mild to hemorrhagic.

ACUTE CHOLECYSTITIS

When pain consistent with biliary colic lasts more than 6 hours, the diagnosis of acute cholecystitis must be entertained. Tenderness in the region of the gallbladder is usually present, but need not be dramatic in the early stages of the disease when only mild inflammation is present. Gentle pressure applied in the right upper quadrant may prevent taking a deep breath because of the pain elicited as the tender gallbladder descends toward the examiner's hand, a finding known as Murphy's sign. Other symptoms and signs such as fever and anorexia may be useful when present, but are highly variable and nonspecific.

Fever and leukocytosis are systemic signs that should suggest the possibility of advanced disease, with transmural inflammation. A visible or palpable mass in the right upper quadrant signifies an inflamed, distended gallbladder with adherent omentum, and is usually associated with transmural inflammation or necrosis. Air in the gallbladder wall from invasive bacterial infection, or emphysematous cholecystitis, is a particularly severe form of acute cholecystitis,[7] felt to be more likely in diabetics. Both age and obesity tend to obscure the diagnosis of acute cholecystitis by diminishing the apparent severity of acute signs and symptoms.

OTHER PRESENTATIONS

Subacute cholecystitis is characterized by the persistence of right upper quadrant pain, sometimes with frequent exacerbations or attacks, for days or weeks after an acute episode. Food intake may be reduced, but weight loss is not a prominent feature. There is mild right upper quadrant tenderness. The gallbladder is frequently contracted and thick-walled as a result of the chronic inflammation and may be hard to localize radiographically.

Fever, chills, and obvious jaundice are more characteristic of acute cholangitis than acute cholecystitis. Signs of systemic toxicity are more frequently present as well.

The most uncommon presentation of gallbladder disease is gallstone ileus, gastrointestinal obstruction caused by impaction of a large gallstone in the jejunum or ileum. This condition occurs mainly in elderly women, frequently with a history of prior biliary symptoms.[2] Air in the biliary tree from the underlying cholecystoenteric fistula, an ectopic intra-abdominal stone that changes position, and distended loops of bowel typical of obstruction are together diagnostic of this condition.

DIFFERENTIAL DIAGNOSIS

The differential diagnosis of midepigastric and right upper quadrant abdominal pain is broad (see Table 49-29). The most common condition that must be considered is peptic ulcer disease. The gallbladder and duodenum lie against one another, and inflammation in one can be indistinguishable from inflammation in the other, although one would expect a different pattern of pain in relation to meals.

A less common condition, but one that can mimic acute cholecystitis, is Fitz-Hugh-Curtis syndrome or gonococcal perihepatitis. This occurs in a small percentage of women with pyosalpinx in whom the bacterial infection spreads up the right abdominal gutter to the perihepatic spaces. The right upper quadrant pain may take precedence over the pelvic disease, but signs and symptoms of current or recent pelvic inflammatory disease are usually present.

TABLE 49-29. DIFFERENTIAL DIAGNOSIS IN PATIENTS WITH SUSPECTED ACUTE GALLBLADDER DISEASE

Acute appendicitis
Acute gastroenteritis
Acute hepatitis
Acute myocardial infarction
Fitz-Hugh-Curtis syndrome (suppurative perihepatitis)
Herpes zoster
Malignancy
 Gallbladder
 Pancreas
 Metastatic
Peptic ulcer
Pneumonia
Renal colic/pyelonephritis

Renal colic can be similar in acuteness of onset, but the pain is more commonly in the right flank and radiates downward rather than to the right or upward toward the shoulder. Urinalysis can usually differentiate between this and pyelonephritis and acute gallbladder disease.

Acute gastroenteritis may also have a presentation similar to that of biliary tract disease. Nausea and vomiting are usually more prominent features of gastroenteritis, and abdominal tenderness is rare. Nevertheless, these two conditions can be difficult to differentiate without further testing and follow-up. Acute hepatitis can also mimic biliary tract disease. A history of exposure and prodromal symptoms, and the findings of jaundice and altered synthetic liver function confirm the diagnosis of hepatitis.

Right upper quadrant pain can be seen in patients with herpes zoster. The pain can be severe, but is not usually as acute and disabling. When vesicles are present, the diagnosis is straightforward, but before their appearance differentiation can be difficult. Cancer of the gallbladder is rare, but also mimics the more common benign gallbladder diseases, particularly subacute cholecystitis. It occurs in elderly persons, most commonly those with longstanding gallstones. Cancer of the pancreas can also cause right upper quadrant pain that can be difficult to differentiate from acute gallbladder disease. Weight loss is the best clue to the presence of malignancy.

Acute inflammation in the pleural or pericardial cavity can be mistaken for biliary tract disease. Patients with right lower lobe pneumonia can present with fever, leukocytosis, and apparent right upper quadrant abdominal pain. A chest film is diagnostic. Acute myocardial infarction causing epigastric discomfort and nausea can also be confused with acute gallbladder disease.

Finally, acute appendicitis can mimic acute cholecystitis, particularly in the early stage of the disease when epigastric pain is the chief symptom and before localization in the right lower quadrant is evident.

PROCEDURES

RADIOGRAPHIC PROCEDURES

Plain radiographs, ultrasound examination, and hepatic scintigraphy are the imaging procedures that are most useful in the emergency diagnosis of acute gallbladder disease. Oral cholecystography and endoscopic retrograde cholangiopancreatography are also helpful, but are not first-line procedures in the emergency setting.[8]

Plain abdominal radiographs will demonstrate gallbladder disease only when calcified stones are present (in approximately 15% of patients), the gallbladder wall is calcified, or air is present in the wall or lumen of the gallbladder. They can be helpful in ruling out other intra-abdominal processes, such as perforated ulcer, in patients with severe abdominal pain and tenderness, but may be safely omitted in other patients.

Ultrasound examination is the initial examination of choice for imaging the gallbladder in the emergency setting. It has the advantages of being simple, rapid, painless, noninvasive, and safe in pregnancy, and is usually readily available. Ultrasonography is highly accurate in determining the presence of stones or sludge in the gallbladder. Ultrasound can also give accurate information about the size of the gallbladder and bile ducts, and can detect abnormalities in the abdominal wall or liver that might be confused with gallbladder disease. Localization of tenderness by ultrasound probe over the gallbladder, known as the sonographic Murphy's sign, is sometimes helpful in differentiating gallbladder from nonspecific right upper quadrant pain.

Ultrasound can provide indirect evidence of inflammation or complications of acute cholecystitis. It can be used to detect pericholecystic fluid, which is associated with inflammation of the gallbladder, and can detect larger perihapatic fluid collections that might suggest perforation or abscess formation. In the absence of stones, a thickened gallbladder wall (more than 3.5 mm), or pericholecystic fluid detected by ultrasound are signs that have been found in association with acalculous cholecystitis.[9]

Ultrasonography is sensitive in detecting anatomic abnormalities, particularly stones or sludge, and is helpful when these are found. It is less helpful when negative. It does not have high enough specificity to be used as the sole procedure to rule out acute gallbladder disease in patients with characteristic symptoms. Moreover, it cannot be relied on to rule out acute inflammation, whether or not stones are present.

Cholescintigraphy using 99m-technetium-labeled iminodiacetic acid analogues is used to support the diagnosis of acute cholecystitis.[10] Pharmaceutical agents based on this molecule are rapidly excreted in the bile after intravenous injection, and can be used to identify abnormalities in bile flow. Visualization of the gallbladder confirms patency of the cystic duct and, with rare exceptions, rules out acute cholecystitis. The converse is not always true, however, and both false negative and false positive tests can occur (i.e., visualization of an inflamed gallbladder, failure to visualize a noninflamed gallbladder). Morphine administered in conjunction with cholescintigraphy has been reported to reduce the incidence of false positive tests, presumably by raising biliary pressures.[11,12]

Oral cholecystography is not often ordered in the ED because it does not give rapid results. It requires the overnight intestinal absorption of tablets containing contrast material and may require one or two days to complete. Nevertheless, it remains a highly accurate study for detecting gallbladder disease, and should be considered in patients with typical symptoms of biliary colic but negative ultrasound examination.

Endoscopic retrograde cholangiopancreatography is also a procedure not commonly considered in the emergency diagnosis of biliary tract disease, but it has been used successfully to detect gallstones in patients with typical biliary symptoms and negative ultrasonic as well as normal oral cholecystographic studies.[13]

LABORATORY STUDIES

The combined blood count and differential; liver function tests; and bilirubin, amylase; and lipase are all helpful determinants in patients suspected of having acute gallbladder disease, but are rarely specific or diagnostic.

The white blood cell (WBC) count is expected to be normal in the absence of inflammation, as in biliary colic, but is also frequently normal in patients with substantial inflammation. An elevated WBC count and a left shift in the differential in conjunction with other evidence of biliary disease are signs of transmural inflammation of the gallbladder or cholangitis and demand prompt surgical attention.

Abnormal liver function tests call attention to the liver and biliary tree, but the patterns of abnormality are frequently nonspecific. Transient cystic duct obstruction (biliary colic) should not be expected to lead to abnormalities in LFTs. Abnormal LFTs suggest that the pathophysiologic process involves inflammation or extension beyond the gallbladder. Transient elevations of bilirubin or alkaline phosphatase are presumptive evidence that a stone has passed from the common duct. These are helpful when identified, but are not always detected. Marked elevations of bilirubin and alkaline phosphatase, with relatively normal transaminase values, suggest common duct obstruction. An elevated bilirubin level does not always denote common duct disease, however. Acute cholecystitis can cause elevations of the total bilirubin to 2.5 mg/dL (I have seen levels as high as 4 mg/dL in extremely ill patients in the presence of a normal common bile duct). Transaminase levels may be mildly abnormal in acute cholecystitis, but marked transaminase elevations should suggest hepatitis, not gallbladder disease.

Elevations of amylase or lipase in patients with symptoms of biliary disease, and without other factors predisposing to pancreatic disease, suggest the diagnosis of biliary pancreatitis. Extremely high levels of amylase, five to ten times normal and out of proportion to clinical symptoms, are sometimes seen.

MANAGEMENT AND INDICATIONS FOR ADMISSION

The treatment of gallbladder disease remains predominantly surgical. The physician evaluating a patient with suspected acute gallbladder disease must address these questions: Are the symptoms most likely to be caused by gallbladder disease? If so, can the problem be managed on an outpatient basis, or will the patient require admission or emergency operation?

These questions are most easily answered in the patient with an exacerbation of episodic symptoms who can give a clear history of previous episodes of pain consistent with biliary colic. If gallstones can be demonstrated by ultrasound examination, and the pain subsides (biliary colic usually lasts from three to five hours), outpatient follow-up is the most appropriate course of action, assuming that there are no signs of systemic illness. If gallstones are not demonstrated, but the history strongly suggests biliary symptoms, follow-up examination and additional diagnostic tests, such as oral cholecystography, may be warranted.

In any such patient, the amylase should be checked before discharge from the ED. Biliary pancreatitis is considered a strong indication for admission and operation, because it is correctable by cholecystectomy and evacuation of stones from the common duct (when still present). The risks associated with recurrent pancreatitis are high if this is not done relatively promptly.

Special consideration should be given to patients with frequent attacks (more than once a week) or progressively frequent and severe attacks of biliary colic. Even though acute cholecystitis is not yet present, admission and operation may be the best course of treatment. These symptoms are disabling, and clearly indicate the need for urgent cholecystectomy. Diabetic patients should also receive special attention because of their potential metabolic complications and the persistent clinical impression that they are at higher risk if they develop acute cholecystitis.

If pain persists beyond 6 hours, acute cholecystitis must be considered, particularly if there is localized right upper quadrant tenderness. Fever need not be present, nor is an abnormal WBC count always seen. If gallstones have not been previously demonstrated, ultrasound examination should be done. If gallstones have been previously demonstrated, cholescintigraphy may help to confirm the diagnosis of acute cholecystitis if the gallbladder is not visualized. Even if gallstones are not found by ultrasound, cholescintigraphy visualizing the gallbladder may be useful in ruling out acute cholecystitis in patients with typical symptoms and findings. (Most false negative examinations occur on chronically ill patients in an intensive care unit setting.) If the picture is unclear, before the final decision to admit or discharge is made, surgical consultation may be indicated also.

Patients with fever and other signs of systemic illness usually require admission to the hospital. In these patients, the chief questions are the extent of disease and the timing of the operation. The demonstration of a mass in the right upper quadrant or exquisite tenderness and guarding on physical examination should prompt immediate surgical consultation. In younger women, a history of pelvic infection should be sought and pelvic examination carried out to rule out Fitz-Hugh-Curtis syndrome.

Prompt, if not emergent, cholecystectomy is the preferred treatment for patients with acute cholecystitis.[14] Emergency management consists of admission, hydration, and preparation for the operation. Antimicrobials should be administered as perioperative adjunctive therapy. In pregnant patients, cholecystectomy is safest in the second trimester. Medical management is preferred in the first and third trimesters because of the risk of spontaneous abortion or premature labor.[15]

If there is evidence of acute cholangitis with high fever, chills, and obvious jaundice, the bile duct must be decompressed expeditiously. This can be done in several ways, including endoscopic retrograde cholangiography, percutaneous transhepatic cholangiography, and surgery. In all cases, admission, blood cultures, intravenous hydration, careful monitoring for sepsis, and broad-spectrum antimicrobial coverage should accompany emergency biliary drainage.[16] Sepsis from biliary tract infection is particularly serious in the elderly, who require rapid treatment. (See Sepsis in the Elderly, Chap. 60).

PITFALLS

The chief pitfalls in dealing with acute gallbladder diseases are failure to consider biliary pancreatitis and in the difficulty in recognizing the gallbladder as a cause of symptoms in a patient with an apparently normal ultrasound examination. The first is remedied by always obtaining an amylase and lipase in patients with acute abdominal pain and by remembering that one of the chief causes of acute pancreatitis is gallstones. In regard to the second, one must remember that, despite the excellence of the available imaging modalities, the diagnosis of acute gallbladder disease must sometimes depend on the history and physical examination. A high index of suspicion should prompt surgical consultation even if initial imaging studies appear nondiagnostic.

HORIZONS

For the forseeable future, patients with symptomatic gallstones will require hospitalization for treatment. Much work has been done on the nonsurgical treatment of gallstones during the past two decades, including novel methods of dissolving stones or breaking them up by lithotripsy so that they will pass spontaneously.[17,18] The number of patients eligible for such treatments is small, however, and none of these methods has been shown to be of any value in the symptomatic patient likely to be seen in the ED.

Elective and even emergency cholecystectomy in the nonseptic patient carries little morbidity, and hospital stays have been reduced to 2 to 5 days. Nevertheless, innovations designed to replace standard surgical approaches have been proposed. Percutaneous drainage of the acutely inflamed gallbladder, analogous to drainage of the dilated, obstructed bile duct, is technically feasible if the gallbladder lies adjacent to the abdominal wall. The uninflamed gallbladder containing very small stones can be removed with only laparascopic instruments. These are primarily technical surgical considerations that do not affect the emergency evaluation of patients.

An imaging or diagnostic procedure with better sensitivity and specificity for biliary disease than those currently available is hard to envision, but clearly a possibility, considering the progress that has been made since the days when intravenous cholangiography was the only available test for acute cholecystitis. Until a new procedure is discovered, the diagnosis of acute gallbladder disease in the emergency setting will remain an interesting clinical challenge.

REFERENCES

1. Sullivan, F.J., et al.: Cholangiographic manifestations of acute biliary colic. N. Engl. J. Med. *288*:33, 1973.
2. Moss, J.R., et al.: Gallstone ileus. Am. Surg. *53*:424, 1987.
3. Oria, A., et al.: Risk factors for acute pancreatitis in patients with migrating gallstones. Arch. Surg. *124*:1295, 1989.
4. Boey, J.H., and Way, L.W.: Acute cholangitis. Ann. Surg. *191*:264, 1980.
5. Smith, A.L., et al.: Gallstone disease: The clinical manifestations of infectious stones. Arch. Surg. *124*:629, 1989.
6. Bennion, L.J., and Grundy, S.M.: Risk factors for the development of cholelithiasis in man. N. Engl. J. Med. *299*:1161 and 1221, 1978.
7. Yeatmen, T.J.: Emphysematous cholecystitis: An insidious variant of acute cholecystitis. Am. J. Emerg. Med. *4*:163, 1986.
8. Marton, K.I., and Doubilet, P.: How to image the gallbladder in suspected cholecystitis. Ann. Intern. Med. *1*:722, 1988.
9. Fink-Bennett, D., et al.: The sensitivity of hepatobiliary imaging and real-time ultrasonography in the detection of acute cholecystitis. Arch. Surg. *120*:904, 1985.
10. Weissman, H.S., et al.: Rapid and accurate diagnosis of acute cholecystitis with 99mTC-HIDA cholescintigraphy. Am. J. Roentgenol. *132*:523, 1979.
11. Kim, E.E., et al.: Morphine-augmented cholescintigraphy in the diagnosis of acute cholecystitis. Am. J. Roentgenol. *147*:1177, 1986.
12. Flancbaum, L., et al.: Use of cholescintigraphy with morphine in critically ill patients with suspected cholecystitis. Surgery *106*:668, 1989.
13. Venu, R.P., et al.: Endoscopic retrograde cholangiopancreatography: Diagnosis of cholelithiasis in patient with normal gallbladder x-ray and ultrasound studies. JAMA *249*:758, 1983.
14. Jarvinen, H.J., and Hastbacka, J.: Early cholecystectomy for acute cholecystitis: A prospective randomized study. Ann. Surg. *191*:501, 1980.
15. Landers, D., et al.: Acute cholecystitis in pregnancy. Obstet. Gynecol. *69*:131, 1987.
16. Muller, E.L., et al.: Antibiotics in infections of the biliary tract. Surg. Gynecol. Obstet. *165*:285, 1987.
17. Thistle, J.L., et al.: Dissolution of cholesterol gallbladder stones by methyl tert-butyl ether administered by percutaneous transhepatic catheter. N. Engl. J. Med. *320*:633, 1989.
18. Magnuson, T.H., et al.: How many Americans will be eligible for biliary lithotripsy? Arch. Surg. *124*:195, 1989.

LIVER DISEASE

John A. Payne and Alan Epstein

CAPSULE

Liver disease is often subtle in its appearance and progression until liver reserves are exhausted and drastic measures such as liver transplantation must be attempted to reclaim health. The economics of health care, disenfranchising large segments of our population from ready access to frequent medical evaluations, and the resistance of patients to seeking health evaluation except in emergent situations, places a burden upon the emergency physician to be alert to hepatic abnormalities and arrange for proper follow-up. Fortunately, routine blood tests and radiologic examinations are available to assist in the identification of patients at risk and direct subsequent evaluation in a successful fashion. Advances in our understanding of acute and chronic liver diseases allow more effective identification and treatment. It is hoped that this chapter will provide a framework for the busy emergency physician to deal successfully with the challenge of the patient with liver disease.

INTRODUCTION

Emergency care of the patient with liver disease depends on a careful, directed history and physical examination to suggest a diagnosis, and the corroboration of the diagnosis by laboratory testing.

The rapid assessment of the presence and severity of liver disease is greatly aided by a wide variety of biochemical and radiologic tests readily available to the emergency physician. The proper selection of tests is guided by the patient's history and examination, and the test results must be interpreted in the clinical setting. It is useful to group these commonly ordered tests as indicators of liver cell integrity, cholestasis, or liver function. Radiologic tests offer visual methods of determining the size and shape of the liver and biliary tree.

Loss of liver cell integrity is indicated by the rise in serum transaminases (SGOT, SGPT) and lactate dehydrogenase (LDH). Membrane injury allows the leakage of these enzymes into the circulation. The liver fraction of LDH is only 10% of the normal total level of LDH and has the shortest half-life, approximately 6 hours, so that substantial increases in LDH caused by liver damage are invariably associated with large increases in SGOT and SGPT. Isolated elevations in LDH with normal levels of transaminases probably reflect hemolysis, seen often with chronic liver disease. The transaminases are cleared within 48 hours after release from the hepatocyte; continued persistence indicates ongoing liver injury. In alcoholic liver disease, impaired metabolism limits the production of SGPT and preferential damage of mitochondria enhances the release of SGOT, producing the typical profile of mildly elevated SGOT (<200 IU/L) and normal SGPT seen in alcoholic hepatitis. Massive (>1000 IU/L) elevations of the transaminases can be seen in hepatic ischemia, toxic or viral hepatitis; prompt resolution is most often associated with an isolated hypoxic or toxic episode. Transient, sometimes surprising elevations of the transaminases can be seen associated with acute cholangitis or obstruction of the common bile duct by gallstones.

Cholestasis is the impairment of bile flow; lesions from the hepatocyte to the ampulla of Vater may produce obstruction or reduction of bile secretion. Provided that the hepatocytes "upstream" from the obstruction are metabolically active, they respond by generating excess canalicular membranes, containing alkaline phosphatase, 5' nucleotidase, and leucine aminopeptidase. The excess membrane-bound and free enzymes are regurgitated into the blood stream, causing serum levels to rise. The highest levels are seen when granulomas or metastases initially infiltrate the liver diffusely, distorting the biliary channels without damage to hepatocyte function. With progressive damage and metabolic compromise, the apparent improvement in cholestatic enzymes shown by falling levels actually reflects liver failure. Bile salts are produced in the liver and undergo 10 to 15 enterohepatic cycles per day. Elevated levels are seen in cholestasis, provided that terminal ileal absorption is normal. The poor specificity of this group of tests is caused by the many factors that influence bile salt levels.

Liver function is reflected by the serum levels of bilirubin, albumin, cholesterol, coagulation factors, and bile salts. Newer assays to detect true conjugated and unconjugated bilirubin levels have shown that the traditional bilirubin assays (van den Bergh) are only approximate at best and poorly reflect the distribution between conjugated and unconjugated bilirubin, although the total level is reliable. With these new assays, the level of conjugated bilirubin is low, and any elevation indicates liver injury with a greater sensitivity than serum enzyme levels. An additional fraction, delta bilirubin, is conjugated bilirubin covalently bound to plasma proteins. The disappearance of this fraction from the plasma depends on catabolism of the protein(s) that carry it, so that icterus may persist for weeks after bile flow has been re-established. In the presence of total biliary obstruction, the serum bilirubin rises about 3 mg% per day, because of the daily production of pigment from senescent red blood cells. Faster rates of rise indicate concomitant hemolysis. Chronic hemolysis from artificial heart valves often produces an elevated LDH and bilirubin without evidence of liver injury. Excess conjugated bilirubin is rapidly cleared by the kidneys, so that bilirubinuria may be the first sign of acute liver disease. High levels of bilirubin are seen in the combined presence of liver disease, hemolysis, and renal failure, such as occurs in advanced sickle cell disease, and may exceed 80 mg%.

The serum albumin level is controlled by liver metabolism. The plasma half-life is 3 weeks, so that low levels are a useful indicator of disease chronicity. Poor nutrition may also lower albumin levels. The serum cholesterol is likewise closely maintained by hepatic metabolism. Low cholesterol may indicate severe metabolic impairment; high cholesterol may be the result of long-standing cholestasis. Consideration of these factors may help to put the patient's history in context.

The prothrombin time is a measure of several liver-produced coagulation factors, and is sensitive to fat malabsorption because of the dependence of these factors on vitamin K for activation. In severe acute hepatitis, a response to vitamin K that suggests vitamin malabsorption may actually indicate loss of liver parenchyma and vitamin K stores. It is therefore prudent to administer vitamin K in any patient with a prolonged prothrombin time because liver regeneration may be substantially underestimated if the unsupplemented prothrombin time is used as an indicator. With the increasing use of home parenteral nutrition, acquired vitamin K deficiency may be seen in outpatients who have broad-spectrum antibiotic coverage and inadvertent omission of vitamin K from the parenteral solutions.

Radiologic tests, such as plain films of the abdomen, abdominal ultrasound, and biliary excretion scan, are indispensable aids for the ED evaluation. Most commonly used in patients with abdominal pain, these examinations can identify the presence of gallstones within the gallbladder (abdominal ultrasound) and cystic duct obstruction (biliary scan) with great reliability. These tests are unsatisfactory for the evaluation of common bile duct stones because of a high rate of falsely negative examinations from the echogenic confluence of distal bile duct, pancreatic duct, and duodenum; and the relative ease with which a radioactive tracer may slip past a partial obstruction, producing an apparently normal excretory pattern. In-

trahepatic air may be biliary (acute cholangitis), portal venous (bowel infarction) or within an abscess. A clinical setting of acute pancreatitis often justifies an emergency endoscopic retrograde cholangiopancreatogram and papillotomy to remove an obstructing gallstone.

PATHOPHYSIOLOGY AND ANATOMY

VIRAL HEPATITIS

Acute viral hepatitis is the result of liver injury caused by a virus (hepatitis D) or the immune response to the presence of the virus within the liver (hepatitis A and B).

Best understood is the pathogenesis of hepatitis B. Hepatocyte injury is produced by sensitized T-cells, which recognize a viral antigen. HBeAg or HBcAg, on the surface of an infected cell, in close relation to the native HLA class I antigen. Alpha and beta interferon assist the recognition and elimination of infected hepatocytes by increasing the density of HLA antigen on the hepatocyte surface, and by impairing viral reproduction within the cells. The use of interferon therefore produces an increase in serum transaminases as the infected liver cells are destroyed, with subsequent elimination of the virus. In patients with widespread infection, the simultaneous destruction of the infected cells may threaten survival because of the sudden loss of liver function. Transmission of HBV is predicted by circulating HBV DNA; less sensitive, but also helpful, is the identification of HBeAg.

In hepatitis A, the pathogenetic process appears to be antibody-mediated cytolysis of infected hepatocytes. Specific antibody to the hepatitis A virus capsid binds to the virus on the surface of infected cells; subsequent binding by complement components leads to cell destruction. It appears likely that natural killer cells also play a role in the destructive process. For both hepatitis A and B, the use of corticosteroids suppresses acute liver injury, at the cost of permitting viral proliferation to proceed unopposed. When immunosuppression is subsequently reduced, the increased number of infected cells provides a larger target population for destruction, and the risk of liver failure is ultimately increased.

In contrast, hepatitis D is a cytopathic virus that produces cell death directly. This virus is incomplete and requires the presence of HBsAg for transmission. HDV always occurs coincident with, or superimposed on, hepatitis B infection. The direct cytotoxicity of the HDV serves to reduce HBV viral expression, although rarely to the point where diagnostic tests are invalidated.

Hepatitis C is the newest hepatotrophic virus to be described.[1] It is an RNA virus in the flavivirus or togavirus family that appears to account for most, if not all, parenterally transmitted non-A, non-B viral hepatitis. Early observations suggest that anti-HCV develops slowly in the months after acute infection. When the antibody assay becomes more widely available, the many pressing questions regarding the epidemiology, transmission, and natural history of this virus in epidemic and sporadic non-A, non-B viral hepatitis will be rapidly answered.

Infectious mononucleosis is caused by the Epstein-Barr virus, a ubiquitous virus that commonly infects the liver as part of a systemic illness, but infrequently causes clinically significant liver injury. The mechanism of cell injury is unknown, but is undoubtedly related to direct cytopathic effects as well as the complex immune response to the infection. Immunocompromised patients are most susceptible to severe illness, and the disease may represent a reactivation of a prior infection in such cases. The usual patient has fever, sore throat, and lymphadenopathy, with minor elevations of the serum transaminases. Approximately 10% of patients have jaundice from hemolysis as well as liver injury.

Similarly, Herpes simplex may cause a syndrome of hepatitis as part of a systemic illness, typically in an immunocompromised host. Cell death is probably caused by direct cytotoxicity of the virus; reduction in immune suppression and antiviral therapy are both important for treatment.

Rarely, fulminant hepatitis has been described for each of these agents. Fulminant hepatitis is defined as the onset of hepatic encephalopathy caused by liver damage to a previously normal liver, occurring within 8 weeks of clinical illness. Older patients are susceptible to a syndrome of subfulminant hepatitis, wherein the development of encephalopathy may be delayed for up to 6 months. In each instance, the destruction of liver tissue exceeds the liver's capacity to regenerate, with the accumulation of toxins that cause encephalopathy. If the patient can be supported through the crisis, full regeneration of the liver is the expected outcome, with little residual scarring. The success of liver transplantation in treatment of the syndrome is established, and is worthwhile once the patient reaches a state of hepatic coma.

Infectious agents including cytomegalovirus, adenovirus, coxsackievirus, mycoplasma, and Legionella may cause low-grade elevations in serum transaminases, but generally do not cause severe liver disease.

SEE ALSO ADDENDA ON HEPATITIS AT END OF BOOK

ALCOHOLIC LIVER DISEASE

Alcoholic liver disease occurs when the metabolism of alcohol to acetaldehyde exceeds the ability of the liver to clear the acetaldehyde. Acetaldehyde is a toxic substance that impairs mitochondrial function. The toxicity of acetaldehyde may be potentiated by vitamin deficiencies and immunologic injury as well. Disturbances in lipid, protein, and carbohydrate metabolism accompany the mitochondrial damage to produce the full-blown picture of severe alcoholic hepatitis. A consistent change that is evident even in the absence of inflammation is the enlargement of individual hepatocytes throughout the liver from retained fat and protein. Many of these effects are readily reversible with abstinence, but chronic alcohol ingestion appears to promote fibrogenesis by the fat-storing cells of the liver (Ito cells), and in the presence of hepatic inflammation of any cause leads to the earlier development of portal hypertension and cirrhosis.

The characteristic pattern of serum transaminases (mild to moderate elevation of the SGOT with a normal SGPT) becomes obscured as the disease process becomes chronic and circulatory changes caused by fibrosis contribute to hepatic injury. Chronic alcoholics are often exposed to viral hepatitis or other causes of liver disease, and facile attribution of all liver test abnormalities to alcoholic liver disease in an alcoholic is wrong as much as 50% of the time.

PORTAL HYPERTENSION

Portal hypertension is the increase in pressure in the splanchnic bed that occurs with progressive hepatic scarring. The belief that this process was a "passive" process produced by obstruction to portal blood flow has given way to the notion that potent vasoactive substances, normally cleared by the intact liver, are free to circulate and produce diffuse vasodilation and increased blood flow in the cirrhotic state.[2] The consequence of the vasodilation is the general release of epinephrine and renin to maintain vascular tone. The renal vessels are particularly sensitive to the adrenergic vasoconstriction, and become dependent upon local vasodilation by prostaglandins to maintain renal perfusion. Any cirrhotic is therefore at risk for abrupt renal shutdown and ischemia from the ill-advised use of aspirin or other nonsteroidal anti-inflammatory drugs. When the reactive vasoconstriction becomes sufficiently intense to overwhelm the local renal prostaglandin production, the "hepatorenal syndrome" becomes manifest, with profound oliguria and sodium retention. There may be some opportunity to expand the plasma volume and obtain a short reprieve, perhaps with a peritoneovenous shunt, but liver transplantation is required to significantly improve survival.

Ascites occurs because of avid sodium (and water) retention and overflow of lymph from the hyperdynamic splanchnic and hepatic vascular beds into the abdomen. To the extent that sodium balance can be reduced with dietary restriction and diuretics, the patient can be maintained in a "compensated" state at the expense of reduced renal perfusion. Paracentesis has become the preferred method of treatment of large-volume ascites, but has the risk of depleting opsonins such as complement and fibronectin from the ascitic pool. Should the total protein concentration in ascites drop below 1.0 g/L, depletion of these important proteins becomes assured, and spontaneous bacterial peritonitis is virtually certain to occur. Because depletion of these proteins from the ascitic pool is associated with advanced liver disease, the 1-year mortality following the first bout of spontaneous bacterial peritonitis is a startling 70%.

Bleeding from esophageal and rectal varices is a consequence of the same general vasodilation. When the vessels beneath the mucosa develop sufficient flow to cause dilation, the wall tension increases geometrically as the vessel diameter increases, until the vessel bursts. In all probability, the hemorrhage associated with portal hypertensive gastropathy is caused by the same general process. Ironically, once variceal hemorrhage has occurred, vigorous restitution of blood volume may serve only to ensure a second hemorrhage unless other measures can alter the splanchnic hemodynamics.

Hepatic coma is the result of inefficient clearance of toxins by the liver. The identification of a single agent to account for the entire spectrum of neurologic changes has been elusive, and it seems most likely that several toxins may be active synergistically. Effective measures to reduce plasma ammonia levels also ameliorate the elevations of GABA, aromatic amino acids, and endogenous opioids that may play a contributory role. Recent reports have shown that a benzodiazepine antagonist, flumezanil, can reverse nearly all measured aspects of hepatic encephalopathy for a short time.[3]

DRUG-INDUCED LIVER DISEASE

The liver is a common target for drug toxicity by virtue of its pivotal role in the metabolism and elimination of the vast majority of pharmaceutical agents. The polymorphic genetic control of drug metabolism and the varied immune response to free and bound drug metabolites account for the highly unpredictable responses to most drugs. In contrast, a few drugs, such as acetaminophen, reproducibly and predictably cause liver disease when hepatic compensatory mechanisms are overwhelmed. The liver often responds to a new drug with minor degrees of inflammation that resolve spontaneously despite continued use of the drug. Compulsive elimination of any drug that produces a minor elevation in liver transaminases unnecessarily restricts important therapeutic options.

Unexpected drug toxicity may result from the addition of "innocuous" medicine, such as phenobarbital-containing intestinal antispasmodics, to a regimen that includes isoniazid; the induction of hepatic microsomal enzymes by the barbiturate may then alter a tolerated level of isoniazid metabolites to a toxic one. The most commonly encountered inducer of hepatic enzymes is alcohol, and changes in patterns of drinking might precipitate a drug reaction in a previously stable patient.

Serious hepatotoxicity is associated with jaundice, systemic symptoms, or both, often attributed to a concomitant viral illness. When a hepatotoxic drug is continued in such a circumstance, the mortality rate is directly related to the duration of continued drug ingestion. Persistent hepatic inflammation after discontinuation of a drug may be caused by continued mobilization of the drug from tissue stores or persistent immune attack on altered tissue antigens. Unless structural damage has occurred, e.g., chlorpromazine-induced cholangitis, the effects of drug toxicity are usually eliminated within 6 to 8 weeks. Persistent inflammation beyond this period is usually from another cause.

Acetaminophen toxicity is commonly encountered in the ED. A small amount of acetaminophen is converted to a free radical metabolite capable of binding indiscriminately to cellular proteins. Production of this free radical is increased by substances that induce microsomal enzymes, such as alcohol and barbiturates; its removal depends on the presence of sufficient glutathione within the hepatocyte to harmlessly bind and eliminate the free radicals. Chronically malnourished alcoholic patients are at double jeopardy because the enzyme induction by the alcohol is coupled with the depletion of glutathione by the malnutrition. Significant hepatotoxicity has been documented at modest levels of acetaminophen ingestion (5 to 10 g) under these circumstances. If the patient is seen within 4 hours of ingestion, gastric aspiration and lavage may be helpful. Once the drug enters the intestine, however, successful treatment of acetaminophen toxicity depends on flooding the hepatocyte with sufficient free-radical scavengers, such as N-acetyl cysteine, to prevent the irreversible nonspecific binding to tissue macromolecules that leads to cell death. If the antidote is not administered within 12 hours, the effectiveness is markedly diminished because the macromolecular binding has already occurred. Given the imprecision of the time of ingestion and the variable times for gastric emptying and drug absorption, administration of the antidote within the first 24 hours is usually advised in the hope that some benefit will be obtained. A useful nomogram (Fig. 49-27) has been developed to predict patients at risk for serious liver damage, based on time since ingestion and serum level of acetaminophen. Prescott has detailed a therapeutic regimen, outlined in Table 49-30.[4] In addition to the pharmacologic aspects of the case, attention should be given to the psychiatric needs of the patient.

Reye's syndrome may arguably be classified as hepatotoxic reaction to aspirin ingested at the time of a viral infection by children or young adults. The onset of the syndrome is usually when an otherwise typical viral syndrome is resolving, with symptomatic use of customary doses of aspirin. The patient develops a change in mental status, often progressing to coma, accompanied by hypoglycemia, hyperammonemia,

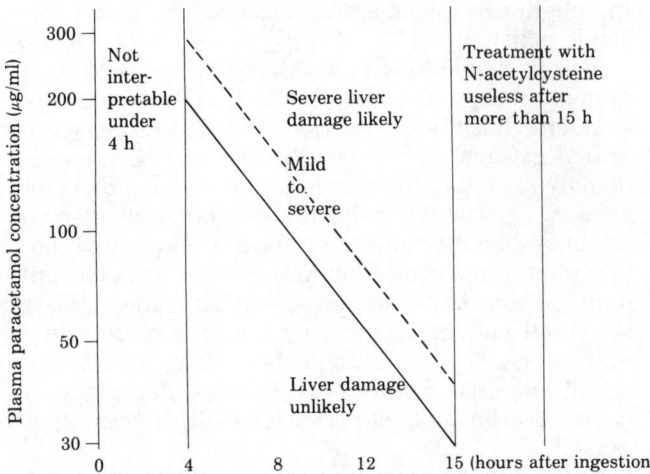

FIG. 49-27. Relationship between plasma concentration time after acetaminophen overdosage and liver damage. Treatment with N-acetylcysteine according to the regimen shown in Table 1 is indicated above the solid line joining 200 µg/mL at 4 hours and 30 µg at 15 hours. Treatment is indicated for up to 24 hours after ingestion because of uncertainties regarding the time of ingestion and rate of absorption. (With permission from Stricker, B.H., and Spoelstra, P.: Drug-induced Hepatic Injury. Amsterdam, Elsevier, 1985, pp. 51–54.)

and severe fatty metamorphosis of the liver. The central nervous system damage is caused by cerebral edema rather than hyperammonemia, and can be treated with hyperventilation, dehydrating agents such as high-dose mannitol, and barbiturate-induced coma until the liver toxicity has resolved. If cerebral function can be preserved, total recovery is common.

IMMUNE-MEDIATED LIVER DISEASE

Autoimmune chronic active hepatitis is a poorly characterized disease that is important because of its usually excellent response to immune suppression with corticosteroids. Patients usually have strongly positive titers of smooth muscle or antinuclear antibody, together with an elevated gamma globulin fraction. Au-

toantibodies to several other intracellular proteins have been found in these patients as well, and seem to be a manifestation of a global defect in the suppressor limb of the humoral immune response. Other causes of chronic liver disease must be excluded because the presence of autoantibodies may be a nonspecific reaction to liver injury. Most patients present with minor symptoms and modest elevations in serum transaminases; a daily dose of 10 mg of prednisone often returns the transaminases and gamma globulin fraction to normal within a few weeks to months. Occasionally patients present with a severe or fulminant hepatitis, requiring high-dose corticosteroids with azathioprine for control; some of these patients come to liver transplantation before the hepatic inflammation can be satisfactorily suppressed. Once the disease activity is controlled, lifelong immune suppression is the rule, although typically at modest levels.

Primary biliary cirrhosis is an autoimmune disorder that occurs rarely in men, and is associated with high levels of antimitochondrial antibody. The antibody is directed against one of several enzyme proteins located in the wall of mitochondria. Efforts to link the autoantibody to the pathogenesis of the disease, which is a chronic, nonsuppurative destructive cholangitis, have so far been unsuccessful. Small bile ducts within the liver parenchyma are destroyed by a local granulomatous inflammatory process. Liver cells and bile ductules above the destroyed ducts respond with a number of changes, most notably an increase in serum alkaline phosphatase. With progressive involvement of the liver, bile secretion becomes progressively impaired until frank jaundice can be noted. A formula, using patient age, total bilirubin, serum albumin, prothrombin time, and degree of edema, is useful in estimating the optimal time for liver transplantation for these patients.[5] Treatment is directed against the effects of chronic cholestasis, including pruritus, bone disease, and vitamin and zinc malabsorption. Recent short-term studies have suggested that low-dose colchicine (0.6 mg bid) and ursodeoxycholic acid (8 to 10 mg per kg per day) ameliorate the early stages of the disease. Whether more toxic treatments such as methotrexate and cyclosporin are also helpful remains to be seen.

Sclerosing cholangitis is a rare disorder often associated with inflammatory bowel disease. The disease is an indolent inflammation of the bile ducts that ultimately causes occlusion of the lumen. Surprisingly extensive disease can be present in an asymptomatic patient with normal chemistries. The immune basis of the disease is suspected, rather than proven, especially because of the clinical setting. These patients usually do not have autoantibody markers. Endoscopic dilation of dominant strictures, a task requiring considerable skill and diligence, may maintain a patient in remission for years. Colchicine and ursodeoxycholic acid may also offer some early palliation in this condition. Generally, once jaundice becomes

N-acetylcysteine Dose (mg/kg)*	Volume of 5% Dextrose†	Duration of Infusion
150	200	15 min
50	500	4 hr
100	1000	16 hr

TABLE 49-30. REGIMEN OF INTRAVENOUSLY ADMINISTERED N-ACETYLCYSTEINE

* Total dose 300 mg/kg in 20 h 15 min.
† Reduced in proportion to body weight in children. 150 mg/kg/15 min is followed by 50 mg/kg/4 h and subsequently 100 mg/kg/16 h.
(With permission from Stricker, B.H., and Spoelstra, P.: Drug-induced Hepatic Injury. Amsterdam, Elsevier, 1985, pp. 51–54.)

overt, or a sequence of recurrent cholangitis and sepsis becomes established, liver transplantation is required.

Granulomatous liver disease is seen in various disorders, including drug toxicity, sarcoidosis, tuberculosis, and other infectious agents. Generally, the liver involvement is important for the evaluation and diagnosis of the patient, but rarely becomes clinically significant. Occasionally a patient has major infiltration of the liver with granulomata to the extent that portal hypertension becomes apparent with full-blown complications of ascites, variceal hemorrhage, and hepatic encephalopathy. Corticosteroids are often administered to reduce the hepatic swelling, but have no proven effect.

METABOLIC LIVER DISEASE

Genetic liver disease is important because of its insidious presentation and the disastrous consequences of failing to recognize and treat the condition promptly. An exceptional ED physician can establish a diagnosis in the brief evaluation period available to him or her. It is important for the ED physician to consider these disorders whenever unexpected elevations in serum transaminases are encountered, and at least alert the patient or his or her primary physician attending to the need for follow-up.

The most notorious of these conditions is Wilson's disease, an inability to excrete copper normally into the bile. Wilson's disease should be considered in any patient with liver disease under age 35. The inexorable accumulation of copper in the liver produces liver inflammation that can mimic a range of lesions, from fulminant hepatitis to chronic persistent hepatitis and cirrhosis. A shift of copper from the engorged liver to the plasma can induce hemolysis. If the process escapes detection, neurologic disease eventually occurs; the range of neurologic expression is also varied, most often with disturbances of gait and station, motor neuron function, and psychological impairment. In younger patients, before central nervous system deposition of copper has produced the characteristic Kayser-Fleischer ring, the diagnosis is most often suggested by the finding of a low serum ceruloplasmin. An elevation of ceruloplasmin into the normal range can be stimulated by active hepatic inflammation and birth control pills, and is seen in 5% of patients with established disease. Supportive data from marked urinary secretion of copper and a serum level of copper that is inappropriate for the measured ceruloplasmin should lead to a diagnostic liver biopsy with an aliquot sent for hepatic copper concentration. Treatment with penicillamine arrests the disease and reverses some of the tissue damage, but must be continued faithfully. Cessation of penicillamine therapy may result in the loss of immune tolerance of this highly immunogenic drug, so that the patient cannot resume the medication; in this way fatal loss of control has occurred.

Idiopathic hemochromatosis is generally present in men between 40 and 60 with tender hepatomegaly and vague systemic complaints that may include arthritis, change in skin pigmentation, congestive heart failure, diabetes mellitus, and impotence. The disease is seen in women, but not until 15 to 20 years after menopause, unless iron supplements have been taken. The serum markers of iron overload, serum iron, total iron-binding capacity, and ferritin may be elevated nonspecifically in any hepatic inflammation, and lead to diagnostic confusion unless the iron content of the liver is determined. HLA phenotyping can be used to discover family members with presymptomatic disease and is useful in sorting out primary from secondary causes of iron overload. Phlebotomy with vitamin supplementation generally arrests the disease.

Alpha-one antitrypsin (A1At) deficiency is caused by transmission of genes that produce an abnormal A1At molecule. Detection of the abnormality is accomplished by measuring the total A1At activity in the serum, or more specifically, identifying the A1At phenotype by electrophoresis. The physiologic role of A1At is to limit the activity of proteases at the site of inflammation. Loss of this suppression is associated with emphysema, neonatal hepatitis, childhood and adult cirrhosis, and hepatoma. The importance of this defense mechanism is established in the pulmonary parenchyma, and replacement therapy has been developed. The relationship between A1At deficiency and liver disease is well established but affects only a few patients with the genotypes at risk, so that replacement therapy is not currently recommended for liver disease. Patients who develop debilitating liver disease are currently treated by liver transplantation.

LIVER DISEASE IN PREGNANCY

The pregnant patient with liver disease presents a particular challenge because successful management may require urgent delivery, sometimes before all pertinent data can be obtained. The patient in the first two trimesters can be considered in much the same way as the nonpregnant patient. Viral hepatitis and gallstones are commonly encountered and evaluated with the usual serologic and ultrasonic tests.* In the third trimester, abdominal pain, elevated transaminases, thrombocytopenia, and even jaundice may be caused by acute fatty liver of pregnancy or pre-eclampsia, conditions that may progress to a fatal outcome for the mother and fetus unless delivery is accomplished promptly. Acute fatty liver of pregnancy is characterized histologically by micro- and macrovesicular fat in the liver. Similar histology is seen in Reye's syndrome and tetracycline, valproic acid, and salicylate toxicity. There is a paucity of inflammation, and serum transaminase elevations are usually only mildly elevated, but there are profound metabolic dis-

---

* See Addendum 1.

turbances with hypoglycemia, hypoprothrombinemia, and hyperammonemia. Restoration of normal function is usually achieved within 48 hours of delivery.

Pre-eclampsia has become recognized as a syndrome of diffuse intravascular coagulopathy. Hypertension is caused by renal involvement, and headaches and stroke may result from central nervous system coagulopathy. The liver is virtually always involved, but is often clinically silent despite widespread deposition of fibrin clots in the hepatic sinusoids. When the coagulopathy is extensive enough to overwhelm the hepatic collateral circulation, microinfarcts develop in the parenchyma. With progression, these coalesce and may lead to rupture of the capsule or infarction of major portions of the liver. Abdominal ultrasound or computerized axial tomography of the liver (with shielding of the fetus) are helpful diagnostic maneuvers.

Systemic lupus erythematosis (SLE) and thrombotic thrombocytopenic purpura are also seen in women of child-bearing age, and should be considered in the differential diagnosis. SLE is suggested by the abnormal consumption of complement. High-dose corticosteroid therapy may be required to control these conditions; delivery does not affect the course of the illness.

VASCULAR LIVER DISEASE

Perfusion of the liver is assured by pressure transmitted by the hepatic arterial supply. When cardiac output is marginal, as in patients with significant cardiomyopathy, a brief hypotensive episode may trigger a surprisingly brisk elevation in serum transaminases, even to the extent that fulminant hepatitis is considered. Unless the hypotension is maintained, the serum transaminases falls by approximately 50% per day until the baseline levels are reached. In the presence of underlying hepatic fibrosis, jaundice may become apparent. Hepatic hypotension often creates a localized coagulopathy, with a fall in coagulation factor levels and a prolongation of prothrombin time that appears disproportionate to other aspects of liver function. Complete recovery should ensue if cardiac function is restored, but repeated episodes lead to cardiac fibrosis.

The Budd-Chiari syndrome is created by occlusion of the hepatic veins by thrombus, tumor, membranous web, or other structure. Constrictive pericarditis may imitate all of the features of the Budd-Chiari syndrome and may require cardiac catheterization to identify the true cause. The onset may be subtle when intrahepatic veins are sequentially obstructed, and resemble the clinical features of decompensated cirrhosis, or florid when a coagulopathy abruptly occludes a major part of hepatic outflow, producing a swollen, tender liver and the rapid, relentless accumulation of protein-rich ascites. The hepatic veins can be evaluated by abdominal ultrasound, computerized tomography (CT) scan, or magnetic resonance imaging (MRI) tech-

niques. Angiography is usually avoided because of the significant risk of acute tubular necrosis caused by intravascular fluid shifts and the hypertonic contrast material.

Portal vein thrombosis is usually well tolerated initially, with few clinical symptoms, unless the thrombus is caused by an intra-abdominal septic process such as diverticulitis. The long-term sequelae, however, include liver atrophy and intractable bleeding from esophageal varices. Loss of the portal vein enormously complicates liver transplantation because of the dependence of the new liver on portal blood for survival. Abdominal ultrasound examination usually identifies a patent portal vein with the use of a Doppler imaging device.

Veno-occlusive disease (VOD) is an unusual reaction to toxins contained in bush tea, a concoction favored by folk healers from the Caribbean. (This potion is also available in "health food" stores, and a careful history of the patient's travels and use of such materials should be obtained.) The major cause of VOD is the potent chemotherapy required for bone marrow transplantation. Elimination of the offending toxins is essential to arrest progression of the process. Treatment is directed at controlling ascites by diuretics and salt restriction.

MASS LESIONS

Space-occupying lesions of the liver may grow asymptomatically to substantial volume unless the growth is rapid, causing painful distention of the liver capsule, or associated with systemic toxicity, as may occur with hepatic abscesses. Often the development of an abscess is insidious, without fever and chills; patients lose weight and energy inexplicably, and appear as if they suffered from advanced malignancy. Hepatic imaging with ultrasound or CT scan usually identifies the lesions accurately, based on the characteristics of the cystic contents. Drainage and/or resection is usually required for successful treatment, although long-term antibiotic treatment may suffice occasionally in high-risk patients.

Benign cysts of the liver are usually incidental findings. Cystadenocarcinomas are sufficiently rare that compulsive diagnostic aspiration of an asymptomatic cyst is unnecessary if the cyst size remains stable over a 6- to 12-month period and the wall of the cyst remains thin. Rarely, polycystic disease so involves the parenchyma that portal hypertension, intestinal compression from hepatomegaly, or both become significant factors. Echinococcal cysts must be removed *en bloc* to avoid contamination of the abdomen with the highly allergenic cyst fluid and attendant risk of anaphylactic shock.

NEOPLASMS

Hepatic neoplasms, including benign adenomas and malignant hepatocellular or cholangiolar adenocarcinomas, may cause local and systemic effects. Local pain is the result of rapid tumor growth, producing liver capsule distention or erosion of the tumor through the capsule with consequent irritation of the adjacent peritoneal or pleural mesothelium. Rupture of highly vascular lesions may occur with severe abdominal pain and shock from hypovolemia. A history of prolonged use of birth control pills raises the possibility of a ruptured hepatic adenoma in a woman with sudden onset of severe intra-abdominal pain.

Systemic effects from metabolically active hepatocellular carcinomas may include hypoglycemia, hypercalcemia, and polycythemia. Abnormal variants of plasma proteins produced by hepatocytes can be seen, but are usually of little clinical significance. The tendency of the hepatocellular carcinomas to invade the hepatic and portal veins may cause vascular occlusion and a dramatic change in clinical status. Rarely, the replacement of hepatic parenchyma by tumor is so extensive that the clinical presentation mimics fulminant hepatic failure.

PREHOSPITAL ASSESSMENT AND STABILIZATION

MENTAL STATUS

Disorientation and coma in the patient with acute liver disease are often caused by hypoglycemia or cerebral edema; in patients with chronic liver disease, hepatic encephalopathy is the usual culprit. For the acute situation, a trial of hypertonic glucose (50% solution) is indicated. If no response is observed, care should be taken to minimize the administration of free water (intravenous glucose solutions) because of the likelihood of aggravating cerebral edema. Prompt transfer to the hospital and monitoring of plasma glucose levels are mandatory.

The patient with chronic liver disease who becomes disoriented is usually experiencing a complication of portal hypertension. Occult sepsis or gastrointestinal hemorrhage must be considered, and a large-bore intravenous line inserted to establish vascular access on the way to the hospital.

CARDIOPULMONARY STATUS

A patient with chronic liver disease may suffer cardiopulmonary compromise because of tremendous expansion of the abdomen with uncontrolled ascites. The rapid accumulation of ascites compresses the pulmonary bases and the right ventricle, leading to decreased cardiac output and significant ventilation and perfusion defects. Removal of 1 or 2 L of ascites often induces a marked diuresis by improving cardiac output and renal perfusion. A second complication of marked ascites is the sudden rupture of the dia-

phragm, either from trauma or as a spontaneous event, which decompresses the abdomen rapidly and produces a unilateral hydrothorax. Although a chest tube may be required to maintain adequate ventilation in the acute situation, patients usually require diuresis, portacaval shunt, or liver transplantation to correct the problem.

GASTROINTESTINAL HEMORRHAGE

Upper gastrointestinal hemorrhage in the patient with portal hypertension may be caused by esophageal or gastric varices or portal hypertensive gastropathy, or the usual differential of bleeding lesions. Rectal varices may also bleed with impressive hematochezia, and if the patient has had prior abdominal surgery, collaterals can develop along the anastamosis. Hemorrhage from these lesions may be controlled by intravenous pitressin, but often requires surgical decompression of the portal system for control. Establishment of intravenous access and colloid replacement are the essential initial steps in management.

CLINICAL PRESENTATION AND EXAMINATION

SIGNS OF LIVER DISEASE

The cutaneous changes of chronic liver disease include palmar erythema, spider telangiectasias, and "paper money skin." These lesions are caused by unmetabolized estrogens and may be particularly florid in chronic alcoholics because of the feminizing effects of alcohol. Tattoos are frequently administered with unsterile needles and associated with drug abuse, increasing the likelihood of coincidental viral hepatitis B, C, and D. Excoriations attest to the severity and duration of pruritus. Xanthomata and pigmentation of the skin suggest primary biliary cirrhosis; telangiectasias of the fingertips invite a search for cutaneous changes of scleroderma and calcinosis. Terry's nails may indicate the sudden development of malignancy or severe protein deficiency. Clubbing may herald the development of hepatoma.

When telangiectasias extend onto the lips and the oral and buccal mucosa, the syndrome of hereditary hemorrhagic telangiectasias (Osler-Weber-Rendu syndrome), associated with cirrhosis in half of the cases, must be considered. Patients with cutaneous lesions of herpes and liver inflammation must be considered for potentially massive hepatic necrosis from disseminated herpes infection. Pyoderma gangrenosum and erythema marginatum are seen with inflammatory bowel disease and may indicate the presence of associated sclerosing cholangitis.

Examination of the eyes may reveal chemosis and conjunctivitis caused by the sicca syndrome. Scleral icterus and the Kayser-Fleischer ring should be sought. Nasal erythema and inflammation may accompany chronic drug abuse. Parotid swelling may indicate chronic alcoholism or the sicca syndrome. Central cyanosis of the lips and buccal membranes may reflect advanced right-to-left shunting from advanced cirrhosis. Thyromegaly may suggest a history of thyroiditis, which may be associated with autoimmune chronic active hepatitis. Flaring of the costal margins and flattening of the diaphragm might suggest lung disease due to A1At. A pericardial rub can be part of the prodrome of acute viral hepatitis B.

Abdominal examination may reveal a prominent pattern of venous collaterals or, less commonly, a caput medusae. The liver edge should be palpated to ascertain tenderness and degree of firmness. Primary biliary cirrhosis and hemachromatosis are often associated with unexpected liver tenderness, more commonly seen in alcoholic liver disease and rapidly expanding metastatic or primary carcinoma. A distinction between gallbladder and hepatic tenderness can often be made by palpating along the entire costal margin. The presence of hepatic rubs indicates hepatic capsule irritation from penetrating malignancy or subjacent hepatic abscess. Ascites, hepatojugular reflux, and a pulsatile liver edge may suggest tricuspid valve insufficiency.

DIFFERENTIAL DIAGNOSIS

ACUTE ONSET OF JAUNDICE*

The acute onset of jaundice is indicated by the presence of bilirubinuria, often preceding the detection of sceral icterus by days. If there has been a period of protracted, nonicteric cholestasis, as may occur with stricture or malignant obstruction of the common bile duct, pruritus is the presenting symptom. Examination of the liver, pancreas, and biliary tree with abdominal ultrasound should be the initial procedure in the investigation of jaundice. If no structural lesions can be demonstrated, a panel of blood tests can be obtained to define the most likely causes of parenchymal liver disease. One should include markers of chronic disease in this panel, especially if examination discloses hepatosplenomegaly, ascites, or cutaneous changes of liver disease, because patient recall may be imprecise.[6]

Viral hepatitis and autoimmune chronic active hepatitis may present at any age.† Alcoholic liver disease

---

* See Addendum 2

† See Addendum 3 for types of hepatitis.

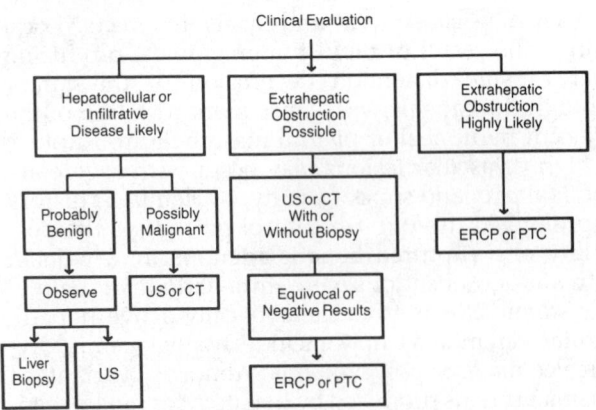

FIG. 49-28. An algorithm for diagnostic evaluation of jaundice. CT = computed tomography, ERCP = endoscopic retrograde cholangiopancreatography, PTC = percutaneous transhepatic cholangiography, US = ultrasonography.

usually occurs in chronic alcoholics, but relatively few chronic alcoholics have liver disease. Wilson's disease and alpha₁ antitrypsin deficiency are considerations in children and young adults; hemachromatosis and primary biliary cirrhosis are possibilities in middle-aged men and women, respectively. Sclerosing cholangiitis and granulomatous disease require ERCP and liver biopsy for definitive diagnosis (Fig. 49-28).[7]

ACUTE ONSET OF ASCITES

Patients complain of early satiety, abdominal bloating, abdominal pain, frequent bowel movements, and weight gain with the onset of ascites. If peripheral edema accompanies these symptoms, a renal, pericardial, or cardiac cause should be sought; if no edema is present, hepatic, pancreatic, infectious, or malignant sources are more likely. If the ascites has become massive, obstruction to venous return from the legs can cause significant pretibial edema from any cause. Paracentesis for diagnostic purposes, with a small-gauge needle, can be done safely without regard for the patient's coagulation status. The ascitic fluid should be assayed for total protein, LDH, amylase, red and white blood cells, and a specimen sent for cell block and aerobic and anaerobic cultures as a minimum. The cultures are best obtained by inoculating aerobic and anaerobic blood culture media in a sterile fashion at the bedside. Grossly turbid fluid should be analyzed for cholesterol and triglycerides, and an aliquot should be allowed to stand to check for separation of chylomicra, which indicates chylous ascites.

ACUTE ONSET OF GASTROINTESTINAL HEMORRHAGE

Gastrointestinal hemorrhage in the patient with liver disease may be massive or subtle. With established esophageal varices, the bleeding site is of gastric or duodenal origin in approximately half of the cases, so that upper endoscopy is essential to establish the cause and institute appropriate therapy. Esophageal varices bleed when the intraluminal pressure exceeds the tensile strength of the variceal wall. Endoscopic indicators of a tendency to bleed include large size, bluish discoloration, visible cherry-red marks, or vessels in the wall of the varix. Endoscopic sclerosis of esophageal varices can often control the acute hemorrhage, but does not improve survival. Gastric varices and portal hypertensive gastropathy do not respond to sclerotherapy or to measures designed to suppress gastric acid production and are strong indications for rapid surgical decompression of the portal system. Similarly, local measures to control bleeding rectal varices are likely to be disastrous. Peptic ulcer disease and Mallory-Weiss tears are also seen in the cirrhotic patient.

ACUTE CHANGE IN MENTAL STATUS

Patients with fulminant hepatic failure have an altered mental status because of hypoglycemia, cerebral edema, and, infrequently, portal-systemic encephalopathy. Hypoglycemia occurs early and is usually the easiest to treat once it is recognized. Cerebral edema is invariably present when the patient becomes comatose, whether responsive to deep pain or not. Focal, fixed neurologic findings should suggest the possibility of intracerebral hemorrhage.

Patients with chronic liver disease and altered mental status, on the other hand, are usually afflicted with portal-systemic encephalopathy. The emphasis in this situation is to identify precipitating causes and correct them, permitting the patient to return to baseline. Hypokalemia, sepsis, dehydration, gastrointestinal bleeding, constipation, and oversedation with medications are common precipitating factors. When these are not apparent, one must consider the occult growth of hepatocellular carcinoma.

HEPATOMEGALY

Asymptomatic hepatomegaly occurs when the enlargement occurs at a slow pace, allowing painless distention of the liver capsule. Typical examples include amyloidosis, fatty liver, polycystic liver disease, echinococcal cyst, and giant cavernous hemangioma of the liver. Tender hepatomegaly is seen in alcoholic hepatitis, acute congestive heart failure, hemochromatosis, primary biliary cirrhosis, acute biliary obstruction (especially with suppurative cholangitis), rapidly enlarging hepatic abscess, or rapidly growing malignancies.

INITIAL STABILIZATION

FULMINANT HEPATIC FAILURE

The patient with fulminant hepatitis has, by definition, acute encephalopathy. Initial stabilization includes measures to combat hypoglycemia, establish intravenous access, and identify the causative agent. Blood and urine cultures should be sent, and baseline chemistries, coagulation tests, and blood cell counts obtained. Patients often require fresh-frozen plasma for replacement of coagulation and opsonin deficiencies, and a clot should be sent to the blood bank for type and crossmatch. If the prothrombin time permits, a Swan-Ganz catheter should be placed to allow accurate monitoring of the patient's state of hydration. Diuretics may be used to achieve a pulmonary wedge pressure in the range of 8 to 10 mm Hg. Fresh-frozen plasma should be used in preference to other volume replacement because of the coagulation and complement factors and opsonins, which can be critical in antimicrobial defense. A Foley catheter should be placed to closely monitor urine output. Measures to evaluate the patient for liver transplantation should be promptly begun.

If the patient has adequate renal function, with a serum creatinine less than 2 g/dL and urine output in excess of 10 cc per hour, and the patient is in Stage III hepatic coma (responsive to deep pain) or Stage IV coma (unresponsive to noxious stimuli), a bolus of intravenous mannitol, 250 mg/kg, should be given rapidly. Patients with renal failure may tolerate a single dose of mannitol, but will surely develop congestive heart failure with repeated doses. The patient's head should remain elevated at a 30-degree angle and care taken to prevent compression of cerebral venous outflow. Controlled hyperventilation and high-dose barbiturates also reduce cerebral edema, but are perhaps best used with a central nervous system pressure monitor and the advice and direction of a competent neurologist. High-dose corticosteroids have no benefit in this setting.

The diagnostic evaluation is dictated by the clinical situation, but often includes a blood and urine screen for acetaminophen and other medications; viral markers for HAV, HBV, HDV, Herpes simplex and Epstein-Barr viruses; ceruloplasmin, serum, and urine copper in patients under 35; and smooth-muscle and antinuclear antibodies. It is often useful to reserve one or two tubes of serum for specific analyses for diseases that are not considered initially.

Rapid transfer of the patient to an intensive care bed is indicated so that serial monitoring of neurologic findings, vital signs, pulmonary wedge pressures, intake and output, blood glucose, coagulation status, and acid-base balance can be established.

HEPATIC ENCEPHALOPATHY

Hepatic encephalopathy generally occurs when metabolic stress surpasses the patient's capacity to detoxify ammonia, aromatic amino acids, and other contributing factors. A review of the patient's medications may reveal inappropriate use of lactulose, neomycin, sedatives, or kaliuretic diuretics. Dietary review may disclose a recent excessive intake of protein, particularly red meat. Dehydration, renal failure, or both, particularly with hypokalemia, can precipitate encephalopathy. Examination of the upper and lower gastrointestinal tract with rectal examination and placement of a nasogastric tube may disclose occult gastrointestinal hemorrhage. If the foregoing measures are unrevealing, one must search diligently for occult sepsis or malignancy. Sepsis may often produce a paradoxic fall in core temperature. If ascites is present, paracentesis for diagnostic purposes is mandatory. The yield of positive cultures is maximized by inoculating blood culture media with ascitic fluid at the bedside.

TOXIC INGESTION

Management of toxic ingestion begins with a careful history and blood and urine screens to identify the toxic agent(s). The pathophysiology and management of acetaminophen toxicity have been discussed previously. Gastric lavage, gastrointestinal purging, forced diuresis, and dialysis may be useful in certain situations.

LABORATORY AND OTHER PROCEDURES

INITIAL BLOOD WORK

Most patients are satisfactorily triaged with a standard chemistry screen. Acute liver injury should be evaluated with IgM antibodies to HAV and anti-HBc, HBsAg, and anti-HCV. If the HBsAg is positive, anti-HDV should be checked. HBV DNA will probably replace HBeAg as a marker for infectivity and may replace the IgM anti-HBc assay as well. The antibody to hepatitis C may remain undetectable for several months after the onset of disease, and a notation to ensure proper follow-up should be made. If the liver disease is severe, a prothrombin time is needed to assess hepatic reserve.

If findings of chronic liver disease are present, tests for autoantibodies, iron overload, Wilson's disease, and A1At may be useful in addition to HBV and HCV markers.*

---

* See Addendum 4 for blood work in hepatitis.

PARACENTESIS

Early paracentesis is indicated for every patient with ascites. The cell count, protein content, bacterial cultures, amylase, lipids, and cell block provide information crucial to patient management. Large-volume paracentesis can be performed on an outpatient basis, but should probably be reserved for inpatients unless the patient is reliable and has ready access to the hospital in the event of a hypotensive reaction.

RADIOLOGIC EVALUATION

Abdominal ultrasound is an excellent screening procedure for patients with abdominal pain, hepatomegaly, or jaundice. A plain film of the abdomen may disclose air in the biliary tree or the portal venous system, and is a useful screening test as well.

ENDOSCOPY

Urgent endoscopy is indicated for any patient with upper gastrointestinal bleeding and liver disease. The need for accurate diagnosis to direct therapy is obvious, and radiologic studies cannot provide enough information or the opportunity for therapeutic intervention. The blind use of a Sengstaaken-Blakemore tube or intravenous pitressin is unsupportable because of the frequency of serious side effects and the common occurrence of gastric or duodenal lesions, which delay treatment.

The gratifying success of emergency endoscopic papillotomy in the relief of sepsis and pain in patients with gallstone pancreatitis make this a procedure to be considered by the ED physician.

MANAGEMENT AND INDICATIONS FOR ADMISSION

ACUTE HEPATITIS

Patients with acute hepatitis require admission if there is evidence of encephalopathy, ascites, or renal failure. Relative indications for admission include the patient who lives alone without access to supervision or who cannot maintain bed rest and food and water intake at home.* An inability to detect the liver by percussion or a prolonged prothrombin time is evidence for significant liver injury, and patients should probably be admitted for observation. Pregnant patients should be admitted for rapid, thorough evaluation.

Patients who are not admitted should be monitored with serial transaminases, bilirubin, prothrombin time, blood urea nitrogen (BUN), creatinine, and

---

* See Addendum 5.

physical examination at least weekly until symptoms subside and the chemistries show a sustained trend toward improvement. Preliminary data suggest that a rise in serum HBV DNA during the acute phase of hepatitis may predict which patients will develop chronic hepatitis B and therefore be candidates for antiviral therapy.

CHRONIC HEPATITIS AND CIRRHOSIS

Most patients with chronic liver disease do not require admission unless there is a sudden deterioration in clinical status. One must consider the development of hepatocellular carcinoma or occult sepsis in such patients. Specific evaluations for new-onset ascites and encephalopathy have been previously discussed.

ALCOHOLIC LIVER DISEASE

Chronic alcoholics with jaundice, fever, and altered mental status require admission. Chronic alcoholic patients with abnormal serum transaminases should be referred for appropriate outpatient workup.

PITFALLS

Errors in patient management, often derived from dearly held myths that defy logical correction, include the following:

1. All alcoholics, i.e., all who ingest alcohol and have abnormal serum transaminases, have alcoholic liver disease. *In fact,* treatable liver disease unrelated to alcohol use is present in a significant minority of patients with apparent alcoholic liver disease.
2. Passage of a nasogastric tube in a patient with esophageal varices precipitates variceal hemorrhage. *In fact,* short-term placement of a nasogastric tube for diagnostic or therapeutic purposes is well tolerated. Long-term placement may occasionally lead to pressure necrosis and hemorrhage from varices.
3. Hepatic encephalopathy is responsible for the delirium and coma of fulminant hepatitis. *In fact,* hypoglycemia is an important, easily treatable factor in acute hepatic encephalopathy. Most mental change is caused by cerebral edema, with protein intolerance playing an insignificant role in the acute situation.

For various reasons, inexperienced ED physicians may be reluctant to perform paracentesis to evaluate ascites. These reasons usually have little validity. It is especially important to obtain ascitic fluid in patients with fever.

In the management of patients with bleeding lesions from portal hypertension, one should remember that the bleeding is initiated by increased intravascular pressure. Excessive volume replacement may be the most important cause of rebleeding in patients with bleeding varices. The lack of direct methods of measuring portal pressure hinders the scientific management of such situations.

Contacts of hepatitis patients may need treatment or immunoprophylaxis.

HORIZONS

TESTING FOR HEPATITIS C

The most important diagnostic test to become available in the near future is the serologic test for hepatitis C. The hepatitis C virus has been linked to the vast majority of post-transfusion hepatitis and sporadic, community-acquired hepatitis currently labelled non-A, non-B viral hepatitis. Early data suggest that this virus is present in low titer and a poor stimulant of antibody production, so that detectable antibody may not be measurable for several months after the onset of hepatitis. Disappearance of detectable antibody seems to correlate with clearance of the infection; persistence of the antibody indicates ongoing hepatitis. The risk to family members and sexual partners of patients with HCV remains to be established.

ANTIVIRAL TREATMENT FOR VIRAL HEPATITIS

Experimental evidence continues to accrue to support the use of alpha-interferon to treat chronic hepatitis B and C. Patients with high levels of HBV DNA, low levels of serum transaminase activity, and positive tests for AIDS are relatively resistant to interferon therapy, but approximately half of treated patients without these characteristics respond with clearance of the HBV virus. The use of interferon for acute viral hepatitis or decompensated chronic hepatitis B is not yet recommended. Optimal treatment regimens for HCV have not yet been established, and the mode of action is not understood, but these should be defined in the near future.

HBV-DNA TESTING

Assays have now been developed, and should be commercially available in the near future, to detect as few as 40 to 50 copies of HBV DNA in a sample of serum. Such exquisite sensitivity may alter some of the traditional views of the carrier state, the relation of hepatitis B and hepatocellular carcinoma, and the risk of person-to-person transmission. It is likely that the availability of such a test would pre-empt the current diagnostic use of anti-HBc and HBeAg.

PHARMACOLOGIC TREATMENT OF PORTAL HYPERTENSION

The use of vasoactive drugs with relative specificity for the splanchnic bed has led to the investigation of beta blockers, in conjunction with nitroglycerin, as a means to reduce portal blood flow and the risk of hemorrhage from esophageal varices. Presently, there are no easy, reliable means of adjusting drug dosage to a suitable level, and the abrupt cessation of beta blockade has been associated with a "rebound" effect, precipitating variceal hemorrhage in a controlled patient. Furthermore, the long-term effect of decreased portal blood flow on residual liver function seems certain to limit the appeal of this option. Hopefully, research will define ways to surmount these problems.

TREATMENT OF CHOLESTATIC LIVER DISEASE

There is great interest in the use of ursodeoxycholic acid and colchicine in the amelioration of the parenchymal effects of chronic bile duct injury. Early data suggest that hepatocyte injury may be reduced for several years, even though the primary disease is not affected. Methotrexate may prove helpful for patients with immunologic bile duct injury.

NATIONAL CONTACTS

1. American Liver Foundation, 1425 Pompton Avenue, Cedar Grove, NJ 07009. The American Liver Foundation, with 25 chapters nationwide, is a voluntary health agency dedicated to fighting all liver diseases through research, education, and patient self-help groups.

2. The Interferon Reimbursement Information Service (IRIS) is a service provided under a grant from Schering Corporation. IRIS gathers and maintains information on the reimbursement policies of insurers on a state-by-state as well as a national basis. It can be reached by calling 1-800-521-7157.

REFERENCES

1. Choo, Q.-L., Kuo, G., Weiner, A.J., et al.: Isolation of a cDNA clone derived from a blood-borne non-A, non-B viral hepatitis genome. Science 244:359, 1989.
2. Schrier, R.W., Arroyo, V., Bernardi, M., et al.: Peripheral arterial vasodilation hypothesis: A proposal for the initiation of renal sodium and water retention in cirrhosis. Hepatology 8:1151, 1988.
3. Bansky, G., Meier, P.J., Riederer, E., et al.: Effects of the benzodiazepine receptor antagonist flumazenil in hepatic encephalopathy in humans. Gastroenterology 97:744, 1989.
4. Stricker, B.H.C., and Spoelstra, P.: Drug-induced Hepatic Injury. Amsterdam, Elsevier, 1985, pp. 51–54.
5. Dickson, E.R., Grambsch, P.M., Fleming, T.R., et al.: Prognosis in primary biliary cirrhosis: Model for decision making. Hepatology 10:1, 1989.
6. Frank, B.B., and Members of the Patient Care Committee of the American Gastroenterological Association: Clinical evaluation of jaundice. JAMA 262:3031, 1989.

SEE ADDENDUM 6 FOR BIBLIOGRAPHY

PANCREATIC DISEASE

Howard O. Haverty and Bernard M. Schuman

CAPSULE

The acute clinical presentation of pancreatitis is almost always in the setting of recent alcohol intake or gallstone disease (Tables 49-31 and 49-32). Severe upper abdominal pain, the predominant feature of the presentation, usually radiates to the back and is paradoxically unassociated with peritoneal signs. Serum amylase elevation is often found but occurs in other disorders as well. The absence of amylase elevation does not exclude pancreatitis. Hypotension, hypovolemia, hypocalcemia, respiratory failure, and collections of pleural or abdominal fluid require early medical evaluation and intervention necessitating hospital admission. Chronic pancreatitis and carcinoma of the pancreas are also discussed.

ACUTE PANCREATITIS

ANATOMY AND PATHOPHYSIOLOGY

ANATOMY

The pancreas is an elongated, flattened gland approximately 12 to 15 cm long.[1] It weighs between 70 and 110 g. Its head is cradled by the medial border of the first, second, and third portions of the duodenum. The neck, body, and tail extend obliquely to the left upper quadrant nearly to the hilus of the spleen. The head of the pancreas rests posteriorly on the inferior vena cava and right renal vein. The neck is continuous with the head and merges with the body. The anterior surface is covered with peritoneum.

There is one major duct (duct of Wirsung), which

begins in the tail and extends through the midgland to the head, where it divides as a "Y." One branch extends downward to join with the common bile duct just before its entrance into the duodenum, called the ampulla of Vater. In about 5% of people, these two ducts enter separately into the duodenum. The sphincter of Oddi surrounds the common bile duct and major pancreatic duct at the entrance to the duodenum.

The accessory pancreatic duct is the second branch of the "Y" and travels through the posterior aspect of the pancreas to enter the duodenum approximately 2.5 cm above and posterior to the ampulla of Vater.

The arterial blood supply to the pancreas comes from the pancreaticoduodenal artery and splenic artery. The veins empty into the portal, splenic, and superior mesenteric veins. Lymph drainage is directed into the pancreaticosplenic nodes, pyloric nodes, and lumbar celiac nodes around the superior mesenteric and celiac arteries. The nerves are derived from the vagus nerve and splanchnic plexus.[2]

Mention should be made of the congenital anomaly of pancreas division, the failure of the dorsal and ventral pancreatic ducts to fuse in the head. This congenital anomaly has been associated with acute pancreatitis.[3]

PATHOPHYSIOLOGY

Because the pancreas is located in a retroperitoneal space without a capsule, peripancreatic inflammation spreads freely. The pancreas undergoes autodigestion by proteolytic enzymes. Current hypotheses as to the events initiating the pancreatitis are obstruction to secretion, reflux of duodenal contents, bile reflux, and intracellular protease activation.[4] The systemic manifestations can be explained by other ongoing processes. The elaboration of bradykinin, for example, causes vasodilation, increase in vascular permeability, pain, and leukocyte accumulation. Hypocalcemia related to fat necrosis,[5] hyperglycemia resulting from injury of pancreatic B-islet cells, and subclinical disseminated intravascular coagulation may occur. Hypoxia and adult respiratory distress syndrome (ARDS) are commonplace in severe disease.[6] Altered renal function with azotemia progresses from hypovolemia and increased renal vascular resistance.[7]

CLINICAL PRESENTATION

A quick assessment of the clinical severity of the patient's illness is essential. The presence of confusion, shortness of breath, hypotension, or vomiting of blood requires immediate attention and stabilization (e.g., intravenous fluids, nasogastric tube, blood type and crossmatch, antibiotics) before further history is taken. Once the patient's stability is attained, important historical features need exploration. These include prior episodes of "gallstone attacks," alcohol consumption,

TABLE 49-31. CAUSES OF ACUTE PANCREATITIS

Most Common
  Ethanol abuse
Common
  Biliary tract disease
  Drug use (azathiaprine, estrogens, corticosteroids, thiazides)
  Endoscopic retrograde cholangiopancreatography (ERCP)
  Hyperlipidemia (Type I, IV, V)
  Hypercalcemia (especially from hyperparathyroid and multiple myeloma states)
  Peptic ulcer disease
  Surgery
  Trauma
Uncommon
  Carcinoma of the pancreas (primary or metastatic)
  Hereditary pancreatitis
  Infectious agents
  Methyl alcohol poisoning
  Pancreas divisum
  Pregnancy (third trimester)
  Scorpion bites
  Vascular factors
Rare
  Cardiopulmonary bypass surgery
  Ductal obstruction by tumor
  Hypotensive shock
  Infection with Campylobacter, Legionella, or Mycoplasma
  Kawasaki disease
  Transplantation (especially renal)
  Upper gastrointestinal endoscopy

TABLE 49-32. DRUGS ASSOCIATED WITH ACUTE PANCREATITIS[22]

Definite Association
  Azathioprine
  Chlorothiazide and hydrochlorothiazide
  Estrogen
  Furosemide
  Sulfonamide
  Tetracycline
Probable Association
  L-Asparaginase
  Iatrogenic hypercalcemia
  Chlorthalidone
  Corticosteroids
  Ethacrynic acid
Insufficient Data
  Phenformin
  Procainamide

a medication list, and recent invasive procedures or operations (ERCP, EGD, coronary bypass, or other intraabdominal surgery). Acute ulcer disease may be suggested by a history of previous ulcer disease, "coffee ground" emesis, hematemesis, or NSAID or ASA use. A family history of hyperlipidemia and/or pancreatitis suggests a hereditary pancreatitis. Features of systemic lupus erythematosus (SLE) or other vascular disease may indicate multiple organ system involvement.

The pain of pancreatitis is steady and boring, located in or just to the left of the epigastrium and radiating through to the back at the level of T 10 to T 12. It may be worsened by lying supine, and the patient may often be found curled up, knees to chest. The patient is also likely to be vomiting. He or she may become dizzy on sitting up as a result of hypovolemia. If the patient complains of shortness of breath, fever, dizziness, or muscular spasms, severe disease should be suspected and prompt admission to an intensive care unit should be arranged after emergency department (ED) stabilization.

PHYSICAL EXAMINATION

The patient may enter the ED clutching his or her abdomen, complaining of or even moaning from abdominal pain. The odor of alcohol may be detected on the breath. He or she may be anxious, confused, or delirious and tremulous from alcohol withdrawal. Patients with severe pancreatitis have a rapid pulse, low blood pressure, shortness of breath, and fever, but the vital signs can be normal in milder cases. The skin and sclerae may have an icteric tinge from bile duct obstruction or hemolysis. Examination of the lungs may reveal basilar rales, but dullness on percussion of the lung base, especially on the left side, suggests pleural effusion, a common accompaniment. The cardiac examination reflects the tachycardia. Supine and standing blood pressures should be taken. A 20 mm Hg drop in the systolic pressure or an increase of 20 beats per minute of the pulse by tilt test indicates volume depletion.

The abdominal examination is usually unrevealing. If inspection of the abdomen reveals a blue-brown discoloration to the flank (Grey-Turner's sign) or periumbilical area (Cullen's sign), peripancreatic bleeding and severe pancreatitis should be suspected. Epigastric tenderness may be present, but rebound tenderness or abdominal wall rigidity means that the pancreatitis has been complicated by peritonitis (Table 49-33).

TABLE 49-33. PHYSICAL EXAMINATION FINDINGS

Vital Signs:	BP ↓, P ↑, R ↑, T ↑, orthostatic "Tilt"
General:	Confusion, disorientation, anxious facies, smell of alcohol, yellow skin
HEENT:	Scleral icterus
Neck:	Flat neck veins
Heart:	Rapid rate
Lungs:	Rales, dullness to percussion, left base
Abdomen:	Abdominal distention with diminished bowel sounds, blue-brown discoloration of flank and periumbilical regions
Rectal:	Negative stool for occult blood
Extremities:	Spasm of muscles (tetany)
Neurologic:	Anxiety, tremulousness, disorientation, and delirium

DIFFERENTIAL DIAGNOSIS

Acute abdominal pain can be a frustrating puzzle to unravel in the ED. The pain of acute cholecystitis tends to localize more to the right upper quadrant and radiate to the right infrascapular area. Acute cholecystitis, however, can be confirmed early with a high degree of confidence by a biliary technetium 99 HIDA scan if no isotope appears in the gallbladder in 60 minutes.

In the postcholecystectomy patient, choledocholithiasis may present with right upper quadrant pain, hyperamylasemia, and vomiting. The serum bilirubin, AST, alkaline phosphatase, and GGT are usually elevated. Identification of this condition is important because nonoperative management with ERCP and endoscopic sphincterotomy may avert a catastrophic illness if symptoms do not subside in 24 to 48 hours.[8,9] An elective cholecystectomy in the patient with a gallbladder in situ should follow at a subsequent hospital admission, however.

The perforated ulcer presents more abruptly, shows distinct peritoneal signs, and is confirmed by intraperitoneal air on the abdominal films.

Mesenteric thrombosis, usually causing steady, diffuse midabdominal pain, should be considered in the elderly patient. Myocardial infarction can usually be excluded by ECG. Acute appendicitis can mimic any acute intra-abdominal process. CT scan can be useful in demonstrating pancreatic inflammatory masses.[23]

PROCEDURES

The presentation of the patient dictates the essential interventional maneuvers. A hypotensive patient requires two large-bore intravenous catheters (16 or 18 gauge). More stable patients may receive the usual 18 or 20 gauge angiocatheters. One should choose fluid replacement and electrolyte replacement according to deficiencies dictated by the blood pressure and blood chemistries. In the patient whose volume status is not predictable, a CVP is required (e.g., in the elderly patient with heart or lung disease). It is not unusual to replace 3 to 4 L in the first 8 hours. Normal saline or lactated Ringer's solution should be given with appropriate electrolyte replacement.

When the volume of urine output cannot be measured dependably, a Foley catheter should be placed. If the patient is nauseated or has an ileus or intractable vomiting, a nasogastric tube should be placed for low intermittent suction but is otherwise not needed. If it becomes important to assess for bleeding from ulcer disease, however, nasogastric suction should be instituted. Laboratory studies are drawn for electrolytes (standard chemistry profile for Na^+, K^+, Cl^-, HCO_3^-, Mg^{++}, Ca^{++}, phosphorus), glucose, serum lipase, amylase, BUN, creatinine, bilirubin, alkaline phosphatase, GGT, AST, ALT, and LDH. A hemogram with Hb, Hct, and platelets should also be done. PH and blood gas determinations for patients who are tachypneic are also indicated.

LABORATORY TESTS

The serum amylase is by far the most common laboratory test used for the diagnosis of acute pancreatitis. A value three to four times the upper limit of normal has reasonable diagnostic dependability (sensitivity 84%, specificity 48%).[10] The magnitude of the elevation has no correlation to the severity of the disease; 10% of cases with lethal pancreatitis have normal amylase values.[11] The amylase-creatinine clearance ratio may be used to exclude macroamylasemia:

Amylase-Creatinine Ratio

$$= 100 \times \frac{\text{Amylase (urine)}}{\text{Amylase (serum)}} \times \frac{\text{Creatinine (serum)}}{\text{Creatinine (urine)}}$$

Values over 5% are considered abnormal and consistent with pancreatitis, although not diagnostic. Values less than 5% in the presence of an elevated serum amylase are consistent with macroamylasemia. Serum lipase activity is elevated in 87% of patients with acute pancreatitis.[12] Hypocalcemia may appear 2 to 3 days after the onset of the pancreatitis. Levels below 8 mg/dL signify a poor prognosis. Hyperglycemia greater than 200 mg/dL reflects pancreatic dysfunction and is also a poor prognostic sign. Moderate hypoproteinemia and hypoalbuminemia are common. Serum aspartate aminotransferase (AST) may be 15 times normal, but may reflect alcoholic liver disease or common bile duct obstruction rather than acute pancreatitis. High alanine aminotransferase (ALT) and alkaline phosphatase should raise the suspicion of biliary tract disease, especially with bilirubin values over 2.5 mg/dL. Leukocytosis on admission may be followed by a dropping hematocrit. Hypoxia may mark the onset of adult respiratory distress syndrome (ARDS).

MANAGEMENT

The differentiation between mild to moderate and severe pancreatitis requires sound judgment. Fever, hypovolemia, hypoxia, hypocalcemia, leucocytosis, declining hematocrit, and rising BUN all portend an ominous outcome (Table 49-34).

Once initial assessment and resuscitation have been accomplished, imaging studies should be ordered and reviewed while the patient is still in the ED.

Scout films of the abdomen may reveal a sentinel loop (distended small bowel loop near the pancreas) or paralytic ileus, both of which should be managed by nasogastric suction. Diffuse pancreatic calcifications indicate chronic pancreatitis and right upper quadrant calcifications frequently represent gallstones. If free air is found on the abdominal upright film, perforation is the cause, not pancreatitis. "Thumbprinting" of a segment of distended intestine points to mesenteric infarction.

TABLE 49-34. RANSON'S CRITERIA FOR PREDICTING THE SEVERITY OF PANCREATITIS	
At admission:	Age over 55 years
	WBC > 16,000
	Blood glucose over 200
	Serum LDH > 350 IU/liter
	AST > 250 units/liter
During initial 48 hours:	Hematocrit drop > 10
	BUN rise of > 5 mg/dL
	Arterial PO_2 < 60 mm Hg
	Base deficit > 4 mEq/L
	Serum Ca^{++} < 8 mg/dL
	Fluid sequestration of > 6 liters

Pulmonary edema without cardiomegaly, when noted on the chest x ray, raises the suspicion of ARDS. A left pleural effusion is a characteristic consequence of acute pancreatitis. Ultrasound of the abdomen to evaluate the pancreas, common bile duct diameter, and liver is essential and should be done within 24 hours after hospital admission, the sooner the better. A CT scan of the abdomen is useful to define pseudocyst, phlegmon, or abscess, but this study depends on the hospital course. The patient with acute pancreatitis and gallstones should be followed closely, and if the pancreatitis progresses, assessment for common bile duct stones should be carried out and consideration for endoscopic sphincterotomy given if ductal stones are likely. Similarly, the pancreatitis patient with a history of trauma to his abdomen, such as might occur in a motor vehicle accident, may be spared a negative exploratory laparotomy if ERCP is done to exclude pancreatic duct rupture.[13] Antibiotics, usually given, have not been proven to prevent subsequent infection.

COMPLICATIONS

Major complications of acute pancreatitis include shock, ARDS, renal insufficiency from acute tubular necrosis, pseudocysts (a collection of fluid within or adjacent to the pancreas, expanding into the lesser omental sac and pararenal space), phlegmon (an ill-defined mass of inflamed peripancreatic tissue), and abscess. Patients with acute pancreatitis are also at increased risk for ulcer disease and its complications of perforation, obstruction, and bleeding. Possible infective organisms are Escherichia coli (22%), enterococcus (17%), and Klebsiella (6%).[23]

PROGNOSTIC INDICATORS

Ranson's criteria for predicting the severity of acute pancreatitis have been generally accepted (Table 49-34). The presence of four or more of these criteria considerably increases the risk of mortality.

CHRONIC PANCREATITIS

Over 90% of adult cases of chronic pancreatitis are caused by alcohol (Table 49-35).[4] Acute exacerbations of pain occur in a setting of chronic pain leading to repetitive ED visits for analgesics. Exocrine and endocrine pancreatic insufficiency can lead to complications from diabetes and malnutrition. Medical treatment is supportive, providing analgesic and replacement (insulin, pancreatin, vitamins) therapy. Surgery may become necessary for intractable pain. Abstinence from alcohol is essential to the success of either medical or surgical treatment.

ANATOMY AND PATHOPHYSIOLOGY

The Marseille revised classification[14] defines chronic pancreatitis as recurrent or persisting abdominal pain (although it may be present without pain) in a person with evidence of exocrine or endocrine insufficiency. Dilation of the pancreatic duct associated with strictures and intraductal protein plugs or calculi may oc-

TABLE 49-35. CAUSES OF CHRONIC PANCREATITIS

Ethanol
Gallstone disease (rare)
Trauma (usually focal)
Hereditary pancreatitis
Pancreas divisum
Hyperparathyroidism
Hyperlipidemia: Type I, IV, V

cur. The gland is frequently calcified, and pseudocysts may develop and then wax or wane.

CLINICAL PRESENTATION

The course of chronic pancreatitis may be insidious and the initial presentation of the patient to the ED physician may appear as hyperglycemia (endocrine insufficiency), diarrhea (exocrine insufficiency), or jaundice (common bile duct obstruction). Pain is absent in 10 to 15% of patients with alcohol-related chronic pancreatitis.

The pain of chronic pancreatitis is boring, dull, and steady. Originating in the epigastrium, it often radiates to the back, and leaning forward lessens its intensity.

Weight loss and steatorrhea are not unusual. Although polyuria and polydipsia are typical, ketoacidosis is uncommon.

PHYSICAL EXAMINATION

Although evidence of poor nutrition may be appreciated and discomfort on palpation of the epigastrium noted, physical findings are otherwise meager. Scleral icterus and a large pseudocyst are occasionally encountered.

LABORATORY TESTS

Blood tests are generally not helpful in the diagnosis of chronic pancreatitis. Routine CBC is usually normal, but fasting glucose, serum bilirubin and alkaline phosphatase may be elevated. Microscopic examination of the feces for fat with Sudan staining may be positive.

DIFFERENTIAL DIAGNOSIS

The clinical presentation of malnutrition, abdominal pain, hyperglycemia, and steatorrhea in the presence of pancreatic calcifications on the scout film is not easily confused with other disease states. This combination of signs and symptoms or components thereof should raise the suspicion of chronic pancreatitis to almost a certainty. It is the early stage of chronic pancreatitis where these features are subtle or lacking that defies diagnosis and so makes one hesitant to respond to urgent requests for a "pain shot."

MANAGEMENT

IMAGING STUDIES

A scout film of the abdomen may provide an important clue to an ongoing pancreatic process when calcifications overlying the pancreatic bed are detected. Ultrasound remains the early study of choice for evaluation of the pancreas. It is particularly useful to identify pseudocysts. The CT scan, although it is the gold standard for examination of the complications of peripancreatic inflammation, pseudocysts, phlegmon, and abscess, is ordinarily not as readily available to the ED physician at the time of the patient's presentation with acute abdominal pain.

An ERCP is often definitive in confirming the diagnosis of chronic pancreatitis. The typical chronically inflamed gland reveals a dilated main duct, sometimes containing multiple strictures that create what has been described as a "chain of lakes." A normal study, however, does not exclude the diagnosis. Obviously, this study is done electively during a quiescent state and is usually indicated only before planned surgical intervention.

TREATMENT

The pain of chronic pancreatitis should initially be treated with non-narcotic analgesics. Narcotics, however, frequently become necessary. After several ED visits by a patient, referral should be made for specialized procedures reserved for recalcitrant disease. Celiac plexus destruction of the innervation to the pancreas by alcohol injection under radiologic guidance[15] has been invoked but is not altogether a satisfactory or long-lasting approach to the pain problem. The use of pancreatic enzyme supplementation for the relief of pain has been shown to be most effective in women with idiopathic pancreatitis[16] and in patients with chronic pancreatitis and normal fecal fat excretion.[17]

When encapsulated enteric-coated microspheres of pancreatin are used, two or three capsules may be needed to suppress endogenous pancreatic secretion, but with uncoated pancreatin, the dose requirement may be as high as eight tablets three or four times daily. An H_2 receptor antagonist (e.g., cimetidine) can be used to prevent the inactivation of enzymes by hydrochloric acid and improve efficacy.[18]

Surgical management may become necessary for intractable pain. The longitudinal pancreaticojejunostomy to drain the dilated pancreatic duct has been helpful in some patients.

COMPLICATIONS

The major complications of chronic pancreatitis include pseudocyst formation, pancreatic ascites, common bile duct stenosis from intrapancreatic common bile duct narrowing as a result of pancreatic inflammation, portal and splenic vein thrombosis, and peptic ulcer disease.

CARCINOMA OF THE PANCREAS

Nearly all patients with pancreatic carcinoma are over age 50. The cancer is a moderately well differentiated mucinous adenocarcinoma[19] that develops insidiously and is usually fatal. The presenting complaints are nonspecific and include weight loss, anorexia, and abdominal pain. Early diagnosis is imperative for improving length of survival and quality of life.

PATHOPHYSIOLOGY AND ANATOMY

The cause of pancreatic cancer has been ascribed to cigarette smoking, dietary agents, diabetes mellitus, and chronic pancreatitis. The pancreas is in close proximity to the common bile duct, porta hepatis, duodenum, and stomach, and it is not surprising that this organ, when attacked by cancer, induces clinical features that reflect encroachment on these structures. It is common, therefore, to see jaundice and gastroduodenal obstruction, which lead to patients' complaints of weight loss, anorexia, and vomiting. Jaundice is seen in 50% of patients.[19]

CLINICAL PRESENTATION AND PHYSICAL EVALUATION

The patient may present to the ED because of vomiting but relate a history of vague, nonspecific complaints of weight loss, anorexia, diarrhea, or weakness. He or she may also present with new onset of pruritus and yellow sclerae and skin. Some patients develop an aversion for meat and a metallic taste in the mouth. Rarely, a patient may have become alarmed by feeling a lump in his right upper quadrant or midepigastrium (the cancer per se or the Courvoisier sign of a distended gallbladder). Severe back pain may be the only or predominant symptom. Less common manifestations are acute pancreatitis, depression, new-onset diabetes, or migratory thrombophlebitis.

DIAGNOSIS

Initial laboratory studies may show a normocytic normochronic anemia. Hyperbilirubinemia and an alkaline phosphatase elevation to 5 times normal makes bile duct obstruction likely.

The imaging study of choice is the CT scan, which reveals a pancreatic mass with asymmetry and loss of tissue fat planes between the pancreas and retroperitoneal structures. There may be common bile duct and intrahepatic bile duct dilatation as well. Metastases may also be noted in the liver and retroperitoneum.

MANAGEMENT

For the patient with vomiting and evidence of gastric retention by the finding of a succussion splash, further evaluation is obviously needed. Hospital admission for rehydration, nasogastric suction, and subsequent radiologic and endoscopic study is required. In patients who are found to have unresectable pancreatic tumors, fine needle aspiration of the pancreas is done to confirm pancreatic carcinoma. Patients who need palliation for gastric outlet or duodenal obstruction should be referred to surgery. Fewer than 10% of patients have lesions that are potentially curable by surgery. Chemotherapy and radiation therapy are presently also of little help.

REFERENCES

1. Basmajian, J.V.: Grant's Method of Anatomy. 10th Edition. Baltimore, Williams and Wilkins Co., 1980.
2. Moore, K.L.: Clinically Oriented Anatomy. Baltimore, Williams and Wilkins Co., 1980.
3. Cotton, P.B.: Congenital anomaly of pancreas divisum as cause of obstructive pain and pancreatitis. Gut 21:105, 1980.
4. Sleisenger, M.H., and Fordtran, J.S.: Gastrointestinal Disease: Pathophysiology, diagnosis, management. 4th Edition. Philadelphia, W.B. Saunders Co.
5. Stewart, A.F., Longo, W., Kreutter, D., Jacob, B., and Burtis, W.J.: Hypocalcemia associated with calcium soap formation in patients with pancreatic fistula. N. Engl. J. Med. 315:496, 1986.
6. Murphy, D., Pack, A.I., and Imrie, C.W.: The mechanism of arterial hypoxia occurring in acute pancreatitis. Q.J. Med. 194:151, 1980.
7. Werner, M.H., Hayes, D.F., Lucas, C.E., and Rosenberg, I.K.: Renal vasoconstriction in association with acute pancreatitis. Am. J. Surg. 127:185, 1974.
8. Goodman, A.J., Neoptolemos, J.P., Carr-Locke, D.L., et al.: Detection of gallstones after acute pancreatitis. Gut 26:125, 1985.
9. Safrany, L., and Cotton, P.B.: A preliminary report: Urgent duodenoscopic sphincterotomy for acute gallstone pancreatitis. Surgery 89:424, 1981.
10. Lin, X.Z., Wang, S.S., Tsai, Y.T., et al.: Serum amylase, iso-amylase, and lipase in the acute abdomen. Their diagnostic value for acute pancreatitis. J. Clin. Gastroenterol. 7:47, 1989.
11. Peterson, L.M., and Brooks, J.R.: Lethal pancreatitis: A diagnostic dilemma. Am. J. Surg. 137:491, 1979.
12. Eckfeldt, J.H., Kolers, J.C., Elson, M.K., et al.: Serum tests for pancreatitis in patients with abdominal pain. Arch. Pathol. Lab. Med. 109:316, 1985.
13. Barkin, J.S., Ferstenberg, R.M., Panullo, W., and Manten, H.D.: Endoscopic retrograde cholangiopancreatography in pancreatic trauma. Gastrointest. Endosc. 34:102, 1988.
14. Singer, M.V., Gyr, K., and Sarles, H.: Revised classifications of pancreatitis. Gastroenterology 89:683, 1985.
15. Bell, S.N., Cole, R., and Roberts-Thomson, I.C.: Coeliac plexus block for control of pain in chronic pancreatitis. Br. Med. J. 281:1604, 1980.
16. Isakson, G., and Ihse, I.: Pain reduction by oral pancreatic enzyme preparation in chronic pancreatitis. Dig. Dis. Sci. 28:97, 1983.
17. Slaff, J., Jacobson, D., Tillman, C.R., et al.: Protease specific suppression of pancreatic exocrine secretion. Gastroenterology 87:44, 1984.
18. Regan, P.T., Malagelada, J.R., DiMagno, E.P., et al.: Comparative effects of antacids, cimetidine, and enteric coating on the therapeutic response to oral enzymes in severe pancreatic insufficiency. N. Engl. J. Med. 297:854, 1977.
19. Kissane, J.M.: Carcinoma of the exocrine pancreas: Pathologic aspects. J. Surg. Oncol. 7:167, 1975.
20. Andrew-Sandberg, A., and Ihse, I.: Factors influencing survival after total pancreatectomy in patients with pancreatic cancer. Ann. Surg. 198:605, 1983.
21. Appelquist, P., Viren, M., Minkkinen, J., et al.: Operative finding, treatment, and prognosis of carcinoma of the pancreas: An analysis of 267 cases. J. Surg. Oncol. 23:143, 1983.
22. Mallory, A., and Kern, F.: Drug induced pancreatitis: A critical review. Gastroenterology 78:813, 1980.
23. Klar, E., and Warshaw, A.L.: Infection after acute pancreatitis. In Infectious Diseases. Edited by Gorbach, S.L., et al. Philadelphia, W.B. Saunders Co., 1992.

BIBLIOGRAPHY

Block, S., Buchler, M., Bittner, R., et al.: Sepsis indicators in acute pancreatitis. Pancreas 2:499, 1987.

Frey, C.F., Gerzof, S.G., Greenberger, N.J., and Vennes, J.D.: Progress in acute pancreatitis. Patient Care, p. 38, March 15, 1989.

Hodgdon, A.K., and Wolfson, A.B.: Pancreatitis. Emerg. Med. Clin. North Am. 8:873, 1990.

ANORECTAL DISORDERS

Monica Ann Rosenthal

CAPSULE

Anorectal complaints are among the common causes of visits to emergency departments (EDs) and ambulatory care centers. Every emergency physician should therefore have a solid understanding of the pathophysiology and management of anorectal disease. Symptoms of anorectal disorders may include pain, pruritus, swelling, and bleeding. Thorough questioning by the clinician regarding these symptoms can often suggest a precise diagnosis. With careful examination by visual inspection, digital palpation, and anoscopy, most anorectal conditions can be satisfactorily diagnosed and managed by emergency physicians.

HISTORY AND PHYSICAL EXAMINATION

The taking of a carefully focused history is extremely important in patients with anorectal disease. Past history of gastrointestinal diseases, diabetes, or bleeding disorders should be documented. Pertinent questions regarding the acute complaint must include the consistency and frequency of the patient's stools and recent changes in bowel habits. Incontinence of stool, liquids, or flatus must be inquired about because many patients do not volunteer such information. A nonjudgmental sexual history should be obtained from every patient and should include specific questioning about anal penetration. Tetanus immunization status should be ascertained because Clostridium tetani is a frequent colonist of the human colon.

Physical examination of the anus and rectum begins with a careful examination of the abdomen. The patient should then be placed in either the lateral decubitus or knee-chest position and the anal area inspected with the patient both relaxed and straining. Palpation—internally, externally, and bidigitally—must be performed in every patient to arrive at an accurate diagnosis. Most patients can tolerate a careful examination done with gentleness and reassurance. Patients who are unable to tolerate adequate examination because of pain or extreme modesty may require sedation or local or even general anesthesia.

Internal inspection with anoscopy should be performed in all cases of bleeding or pruritus and, ideally, should constitute part of the physical examination in every patient with an anorectal complaint.

ANATOMY AND PHYSIOLOGY (FIG. 49-29)

Although they are continuous structures, the rectum and anus develop separately in the embryo and therefore have differing innervation and vascular supply. This fact is significant in understanding anorectal pathology.

The rectum, a 12-cm long structure, is the continuation of the sigmoid colon. It nestles into the concavity of the sacrum and is tethered in position by the puborectalis sling and the rectourethralis muscle. Arterial supply to the rectum is by way of the superior and middle rectal arteries, which are respective branches of the inferior mesenteric and internal iliac arteries. Venous drainage follows the same route, creating an anastomosis between the portal and systemic venous systems. True varices[1] may be found in the rectum in patients with portal hypertension. These are distinct from hemorrhoids,[2] which are felt to be symptomatic engorgement and prolapse of cushions of submucosal vascular tissue and are unrelated to degree of portal pressure. The rectum, like the colon, is lined with reddish columnar epithelium. Innervation of this tissue is autonomic, and therefore lesions of the rectum are generally painless. Deep perirectal abscesses often produce only vague pain or a sensation of pressure. Lymphatic drainage from the rectum follows the vascular supply, with the majority of the rectum draining to mesenteric lymph nodes and thus providing no external clues to deep suppurative processes.

The anal canal is approximately 4 cm long and is angled with its axis toward the umbilicus. The 80-degree angle between the major axes of the anus and the rectum, a hurdle in proctoscopy, contributes to fecal continence. Vascular supply to the anus is by way of the inferior rectal artery and veins, branches of the internal pudendal vessels. Lymphatic drainage is to the inguinal nodes. Two centimeters from the external anal opening is a structure called the dentate or pectinate line. This line is identifiable as a demarcation between the red mucosal lining of the rectum

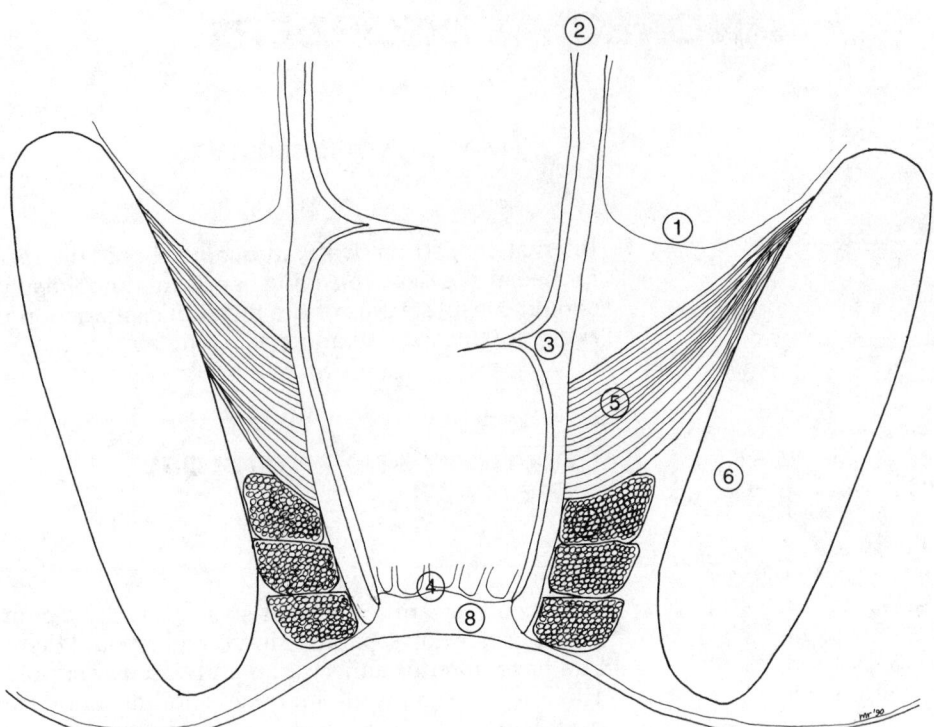

FIG. 49-29. Anatomy of the rectum and anus, coronal cross section. 1 = peritoneal reflection, 2 = rectal mucosa, 3 = internal sphincter, 4 = dentate line, 5 = levator ani, 6 = ischium, 7 = external sphincter, 8 = anoderm.

and the paler squamous epithelium of the anal canal. The dentate line is also marked by valvelike mucosal flaps, which mark the openings of the anal crypts. Anal mucosa, or anoderm, is exquisitely sensitive, being able to discriminate between solids, liquids, and gas. Lesions distal to the dentate line thus generally produce pronounced pain and tenderness.

The contents of the pelvis are supported up from the perineum by a fan-shaped group of three muscles collectively called the levator ani. This muscle group attaches to the pelvic bones and the coccyx. The medial portion of the levator ani is the puborectalis muscle, which forms a sling around the upper rectum and suspends it from the pubis and the coccyx.

The autonomically innervated circular muscle of the colon continues through the rectum and anus as the internal sphincter muscle. Its distal edge is palpable near the external anal opening at the inner edge of the intersphincteric groove. Surgical disruption of a significant portion of the internal sphincter is associated with incontinence.

The external sphincter is a contiguous group of three striated muscles that loop around the anus and attach to the coccyx and to the perineal body and bulbocavernosus muscles. The superiormost portion of the external sphincter is fused with the puborectalis sling and suspends the anal canal within the pelvis, forming the anorectal angle. Weakness or division of the suspensory mechanism at this point produces incontinence and possible rectal prolapse.

HEMORRHOIDS

It is estimated that 50% of persons living in the Western world develop some manifestation of hemorrhoidal symptoms by the age of 50.[3] Despite this, the cause and optimal management of hemorrhoids remains controversial. Theorists have long held that straining and constipation cause patients to develop symptomatic hemorrhoids. This concept, however, has not been upheld in more recent studies of hemorrhoid sufferers.[4,5] Certainly diet and possibly heredity play a role in the development of symptomatic hemorrhoids. But whether hemorrhoids develop because of degeneration of anchoring connective tissue or mechanical stress remains unclear.

External hemorrhoids are subcutaneous masses of vascular tissue visible at the anal verge. They are covered with anoderm and hence are sensitive, but are rarely symptomatic unless they are thrombosed. They do not extend proximal to the dentate line. Thrombosed external hemorrhoids cause exquisite pain. They are readily identifiable as small doughy ovoid masses centered at the anal verge and bluish-black in color. If untreated, they either rupture spontaneously with clot extrusion and a small amount of bleeding, or progressively scar and become resorbed, leaving behind a skin tag of redundant anoderm. The pain of thrombosed external hemorrhoids is caused by distention of the anoderm. If the patient presents within 24 to 36 hours of clot formation, marked relief can be achieved in the ED by incision and drainage or excision of the hemorrhoid under local anesthesia (Fig. 49-30). After that time, removal of the clot or hemorrhoid can become difficult because of scarring, and may result in bleeding. Most thrombosed external hemorrhoids more than 48 hours old resolve spontaneously. Supportive care, whether or not the hemorrhoid has been surgically treated, consists of bulk stool softeners such as psyllium preparations, and frequent sitz baths in plain warm water to facilitate hygiene and reduce inflammation. Popular salves containing local anesthetics and steroid-containing suppositories may produce hypersensitivity reactions or promote infection and therefore should be avoided. Patients frequently insist on using some topical preparation, and should be strongly advised to use only emollient or mildly astringent products such as witch hazel.

Internal hemorrhoids are now felt to be variants on normal anatomic structures present from birth.[4] Submucosal arteriovenous cushions lie within the anal canal in the left lateral, right anterior, and right posterior positions. These cushions normally fill the anal canal, contributing to fecal continence. In hemorrhoidal disease, the mucosa becomes redundant and causes progressive prolapse of the vascular cushion.

Internal hemorrhoids become symptomatic when they prolapse, bleed, or thrombose. Pain is produced by irritation of the anoderm surrounding the prolapsing hemorrhoid. Bleeding internal hemorrhoids are painless and not palpable on digital examination. Rectal pain without visible prolapse, and palpable masses within the rectum should suggest a different diagnosis.

Prolapse of internal hemorrhoids is separated into four grades. Grade I hemorrhoids are visibly prominent on anoscopy but do not extend beyond the dentate line. Grade II hemorrhoids prolapse externally with straining, but reduce sponaneously. They are not evident unless the examiner asks the patient to bear down. Grade III hemorrhoids require manual reduction and frequently cause pruritus and mucoid staining of underclothes. Grade IV hemorrhoids are irreducible and may become thrombosed or gangrenous. Prolapsed internal hemorrhoids can be recognized from external hemorrhoids by their arrangement in the left lateral, right anterior, or right posterior segments of the anal verge, and by the fact that they are covered with reddish mucosa extending above the dentate line.

Patients with grade IV prolapsing internal hemorrhoids require surgical hemorrhoidectomy[4] and may require hospitalization if the hemorrhoids are thrombosed or gangrenous. Patients with symptomatic prolapse grades I through III can be treated as outpatients with a wide variety of nonoperative methods[5] including rubber-band ligation, injection sclerotherapy, cryotherapy, infrared or laser photocoagulation, or

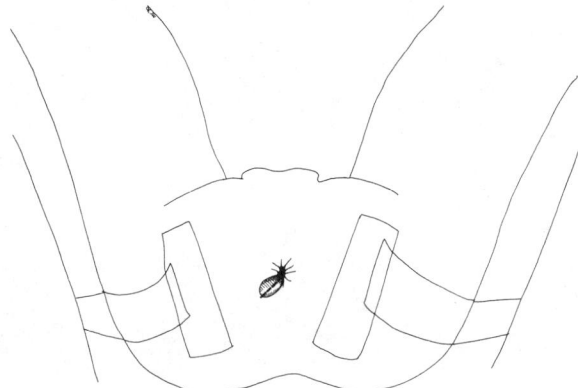

FIG. 49-30.   Excision of thrombosed external hemorrhoid.

bipolar diathermy. All these measures function by causing scarring, which serves to fix the redundant mucosa to the underlying muscle of the rectal wall. All patients with symptomatic prolapsing hemorrhoids benefit from supportive measures as previously described, although such measures may not prevent worsening of the prolapse with time, and they certainly do not lessen the redundancy of the tissues.

Bleeding caused by internal hemorrhoids may or may not be associated with prolapse. The bleeding is painless and is generally limited in amount, unless the patient has a coagulopathy or a large arteriole has been eroded. Most patients report bright red blood, which drips into the toilet bowl after defecation. Proctoscopy reveals bleeding from a vascular cushion in the rectum with no evidence of blood coming from further proximal in the rectum. Even if the bleeding site is visualized, however, the clinician should consider a second source of bleeding, particularly if it is significant in quantity or dark in color. Stable, otherwise healthy patients with scanty bleeding may be referred for outpatient management within a few days. The nonoperative techniques used to treat prolapse are also used to control bleeding, with rubber band ligation currently the most commonly used technique in the United States. Bulk laxatives and avoidance of straining help to minimize bleeding until the procedure can be performed.

ANORECTAL ABSCESS

Anorectal abscess originates with infection in the anal crypts located in the dentate line. Inspissated secretions and fecal material lead to localized infection, which spreads deep to the anal sphincter and can then track in several directions (Fig. 49-31).

Diagnosis of anorectal abscess is often missed in the ED, with serious consequences. A high index of suspicion must be maintained, especially in patients com-

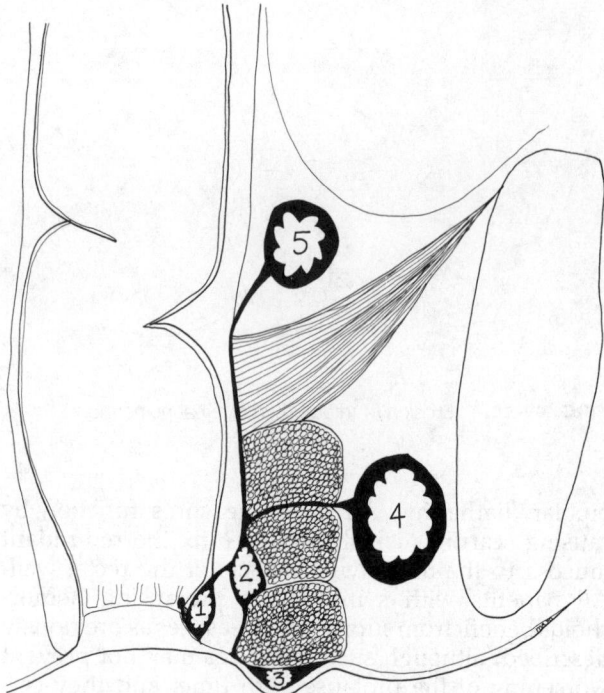

FIG. 49-31. Sites of spread of anorectal abscess (coronal cross section). 1 = submucosal, 2 = intersphincteric, 3 = subcutaneous (perianal), 4 = ischiorectal, 5 = supralevator.

plaining of continuous deep-seated rectal discomfort exacerbated by walking or sitting down. Fever and leukocytosis may or may not be present, especially in elderly or immunocompromised patients. The location and full extent of the infection are often impossible to determine without adequate sphincter relaxation and regional or general anesthesia. Subcutaneous perianal abscesses present as tender erythematous masses at the anal verge that are frequently mistaken for inflamed external hemorrhoids. Anorectal abscesses, particularly involving the deeper spaces, do not become fluctuant. *There is no place for expectant, nonsurgical management of this condition.*

The rate of recurrence of anorectal abscess after primary incision and drainage under local anesthesia has been found to be as high as 75%.[6] Many recurrent abscesses are associated with unrecognized fistulous tracts leading inside the anal canal. In a prospective study of 1023 consecutive patients with anorectal abscess managed with immediate examination under anesthesia and drainage in the operating room,[7] 34.5% of abscesses were found to be associated with primary fistulous tracts. Although this rate varies with location of the abscess, one third of patients with subcutaneous perianal abscess were found to have fistulas. Recurrence rates with 36 months of follow-up were as low as 1.8% in this study, suggesting that examination under anesthesia and formal operative drainage substantially reduce the risk of recurrence.

Many surgeons,[8] moreover, still feel that an initial trial of outpatient incision and drainage is warranted in patients with small subcutaneous abscesses. Patients with deep abscesses and those who are severely toxic, diabetic, or immunocompromised should be admitted and placed on broad-spectrum antibiotics effective against anaerobes and gram-negative enteric pathogens. Outpatient antibiotic use in the normal host is not necessary,[7] although some authors recommend perioperative antibiotics at the time of drainage. Adequacy of tetanus immunization should be checked in all patients with anorectal abscess.

If the emergency physician is to perform incision and drainage of a subcutaneous perianal abscess, the patient should be placed in a prone position and the buttocks spread and secured with tape to the examination table (see Fig. 49-30). A local field block should be induced. These blocks tend to be painful, and ample time for anesthetic potency should be allowed. The abscess can be drained with a generous radial incision to minimize disruption of the internal sphincter. After evacuation of pus and ensuring of adequate drainage of any loculated areas, the incision is packed loosely with iodoform gauze. Packing the cavity too tightly produces pain and inhibits drainage. A wad of gauze pads held in position by the intergluteal cleft and the patient's undergarments suffices as a dressing. Patients should be instructed to begin sitz baths two to four times daily after the initial 12 hours, and should be referred for follow-up and packing removal in 48 to 72 hours. It is prudent to inform patients that because of the high rate of recurrence, the ED treatment does not constitute definitive management.

PILONIDAL DISEASE

Pilonidal disease is an acquired suppurative process caused by ingrowth of hairs and folliculitis in the intergluteal cleft. Patients may complain of pain in the "tailbone" or may relate the pain to trauma, misleading the emergency physician. Physical examination reveals erythema, induration, and tenderness in the posterior midline. Fluctuance and sinus tracts may not be evident. In contrast to posterior perianal abscess, in pilonidal disease rectal examination demonstrates no induration or tenderness.

Treatment of pilonidal disease in the ED consists of incision and drainage. Definitive surgical management can be complex and may require wide excision down to the sacrum and full-thickness skin grafting. All patients with pilonidal disease should be followed closely for recurrence.

FISTULA IN ANO

Anal fistulas are openings in the perianal skin that lead to fibrotic tracts lined with infected granulation tissue. Most fistulas are caused by infection in the anal crypts and are associated with primary openings at the dentate line. Definitive management of a perianal fistula involves identification of the primary opening and debridement or excision of the granulomatous tract. Fistulous tracts can be multiple and convoluted, and identification of the primary opening can be difficult.

Patients with fistula in ano may present to the emergency department with complaints of purulent discharge and pruritus. Pain with fistula is usually caused by blockage of the secondary external opening, and can be greatly relieved by unroofing this area under local anesthesia. Fistulas can be readily identified on physical examination as small circles of red granulation tissue which, if patent, exude pus when compressed. The indurated tract is sometimes palpable on bidigital rectal examination. The epidermis surrounding the fistulous opening is normal, a helpful point in distinguishing fistula in ano from hidradenitis suppurativa. In the latter, the multiplicity of openings and widespread dermal scarring suggests the more superficial locus of infection. Fistula in ano may be seen in Crohn's disease and with infections caused by Actinomycetes or Chlamydia (LGV). Such fistulae do not heal without treatment of the underlying process. Carcinomas infrequently can present inside a fistulous tract. Except in the case of obstructed drainage or abscess formation, however, fistula in ano rarely requires emergency treatment.

ANAL FISSURE

Anal fissure may bring patients of any age to the ED or ambulatory care center. Patients with acute fissure complain of burning pain on defecation accompanied by the passage of a small amount of bright red blood, typically on the toilet paper. Chronic anal fissure may present with persistent discomfort, pruritus, and mucoid discharge.

Acute anal fissure is a linear disruption of the anoderm produced by stretching during defecation or trauma.[9] Caused by biomechanical vectors, over 90% of anal fissures are located in the posterior midline, with most others in the anterior or midline. Acute fissures are erythematous and bleed easily. They are commonly so tender that palpation requires the application of a topical anesthetic. Many fissures, however, are visible externally when the patient bears down.

Most acute anal fissures heal with supportive care. The most important adjunct to healing is the maintenance of a soft stool by use of a bulk laxative. Patients with acute fissure are frequently reluctant to defecate, and promoting a softer stool minimizes discomfort and reinjury. Frequent sitz baths also help reduce inflammation and aid hygiene. Use of topical anesthetics and steroid-containing salves, although initially soothing, may promote infection or lead to contact dermatitis.

Chronic anal fissure occurs when an acute fissure fails to heal. This is related to increased tone or spasticity of the internal sphincter, leading to repeated trauma with defecation. Chronic fissures deepen to the level of the internal sphincter, whose whitish fibers can be seen in the base of the lesion. Ongoing inflammation can lead to severe pruritus and the production of a "sentinel pile" or flap of redundant anoderm distal to the fissure. Chronic anal fissure frequently requires operative treatment. The most commonly recommended current procedure is lateral internal sphincterotomy. All operative treatments involve stretching or cutting the internal sphincter. The incidence of postoperative fecal incontinence can be as high as 15%.[10]

Many diseases can cause perianal fissuring and ulceration. Location off the midline, marked induration, multiplicity, or history of anal intercourse should prompt the emergency physician to consider further evaluation.

PRURITUS ANI

Pruritus ani, or perianal itching, is an extremely uncomfortable symptom with a multitude of possible causes (Table 49-36). A careful history should be obtained from the patient, including bowel habits, sexual practices, medications, diet, and usual clothing and hygiene. Many patients have attempted treatment with topical salves that may have exacerbated the original symptoms by producing contact dermatitis. Thorough general physical examination may suggest generalized dermatologic conditions or infestations. Anoscopy should be performed in all cases, and appropriate cultures and stains performed. Stool should be examined for parasites.

Specific therapy should be undertaken when the cause is identified. Unfortunately, even with thorough investigation, many causes of pruritus ani remain elusive. Patients should be instructed to keep the perianal skin clean and dry with frequent sitz baths in plain water without soap, and should avoid tight or synthetic underclothes. All topical ointments should be

TABLE 49-36. CAUSES OF PRURITIS ANI			
Dermatologic	**Anorectal**	**Infectious**	**Allergic**
Contact dermatitis	Fistula in ano	Candidiasis	Citrus
Lichen planus	Chronic anal fissure	Gonorrhea	Chocolate
Psoriasis	Prolapsed internal hemorrhoids	Trichomoniasis	Tomatoes
Atopic eczema		Chlamydia	Alcohol
Poor hygiene		Pediculosis pubis	Coffee
Psychogenic dermatitis		Pinworms	Tea
Alkaline soaps; benzocaine		Scabies	

stopped. Bulk laxatives should be used to treat loose or overly firm stool. Suspected food allergens should be avoided. In severe cases, antihistamines or sparing use of steroid creams may be helpful, although the latter can itself cause irritation.

FOREIGN BODIES AND ANORECTAL TRAUMA

Patients with retained rectal foreign objects or anorectal injuries due to anal intercourse, sexual assault, or anal instrumentation may present with varying complaints. The history of anal penetration is frequently not volunteered and sometimes denied; proper diagnosis requires a high index of suspicion in cases of unexplained rectal pain and hemorrhage.

Most foreign objects are palpable on rectal examination, but many are difficult to extract because of sphincter spasm or intraluminal suction proximal to the object. Plain radiographs should be taken in patients with retained large foreign bodies, both to document position and size of the object and to look for peritoneal free air. Many foreign objects can be removed under direct vision in the emergency department using an anoscope or a proctoscope and biopsy forceps. Local anesthesia using a circumanal sphincter block may simplify this process. Foreign objects held in position by intraluminal suction may be extracted by passing a Foley catheter proximal to the object and gently instilling air.

Patients with rectal foreign bodies that cannot be easily removed should be hospitalized for extraction under anesthesia. Because of the high likelihood of breakage, light bulbs and similar fragile objects should not be removed in the ED. Patients whose foreign bodies have been successfully removed and survivors of anorectal trauma should have careful examination by proctoscopy in the ED and should be admitted if there is any sign of mucosal perforation or bleeding. Obviously, patients with free air or signs of peritoneal irritation after rectal penetration require immediate laparotomy.

SEXUALLY TRANSMITTED ANORECTAL DISEASES

Many infections can be transmitted by anal intercourse, anilingus, and foreign object insertion (Table 49-37). These infections occur in both heterosexual and homosexual patients; history-taking should thus focus on specific sexual practices rather than sexual orientation.

Patients with acute proctitis may complain of pruritis, pain, tenesmus, bleeding, or rectal discharge. Physical examination and anoscopy can help narrow the diagnosis. Mucopurulent proctitis may be caused by gonorrhea or by non-LGV strains of chlamydia. Ulcerated lesions may represent syphilis, herpes, LGV, chancroid, or granuloma inguinale. Wartlike lesions may be condyloma acuminata or the condyloma lata of secondary syphilis.

It may be difficult to distinguish among the causes of acute proctitis on the initial visit. If available, slide testing with monoclonal antibodies, rapid RPR, and darkfield microscopy can be invaluable. Patients with anorectal herpes often have associated paresthesias in the sacral dermatomes and acute urinary retention, uncommon symptoms with any other infection. Giemsa staining may reveal the classic multinucleated giant cells. Patients with this distinct syndrome should be treated with acyclovir given orally or intravenously; acyclovir ointment is ineffective in anorectal herpes.

If immediate diagnosis is inconclusive in a patient with acute mucopurulent proctitis following anal sex, it is reasonable to treat empirically[11] with a combination of drugs effective against gonorrhea and chlamydia; e.g., ceftriaxone 250 mg. IM followed by doxycycline 100 mg bid for 7 days. Cultures should be obtained before treatment, and the patient should be referred for follow-up care.

Although this regimen is effective against incubating syphilis, chancroid, LGV, and granuloma inguinale, patients with syphilitic chancres or condyloma lata should be treated with benzathine penicillin, 2.4 million units IM.[12] Patients with anorectal syphilis who are coinfected with HIV may have persistently

TABLE 49-37. SEXUALLY TRANSMITTED PROCTITIS

Cause	Differential Diagnosis	Treatment[12]
Neisseria gonorrhoeae (Gonorrhea)	Diffuse inflammation with purulent discharge; gram stain or culture; IFA slide test	Ceftriaxone 250 mg IM or spectinomycin 2 g IM (not useful against incubating syphilis) PLUS treat for chlamydia
Chlamydia trachomatis (LGV and non-LGV chlamydial infections)	Culture, serology or IFA slide test; may be difficult to distinguish from GC clinically. LGV = ulcerated lesions; non-LGV strains = diffuse proctitis	(Consider empiric treatment for GC) PLUS doxycycline 100 mg bid for 7 days or erythromycin 500 mg qid for 7 days
Treponema pallidum (Syphilis)	RPR; ulcerated lesions with + IFA and + darkfield exam Condyloma lata are flat, moist verrucous lesions	Benzathine penicillin G 2.4 million units IM or doxycycline 100 mg IM for 7 days
Herpes simplex type II (Genital herpes)	Ulcerated lesions; + IFA exam, culture; + Giemsa stain	Acyclovir 400 mg 5 times daily for 10 days orally or 5 mg/kg intravenously tid for 5–7 days
Hemophilus ducreyi (chancroid)	Ulcerated lesions; culture; IFA	Ceftriaxone 250 mg IM or erythromycin 500 mg orally qid for 7 days
Human Papilloma virus (Condyloma acuminata genital warts)	Generally raised, dry verrucous lesions. Biopsy for dx	Cryotherapy with liquid nitrogen or surgical removal

TABLE 49-38. CAUSES OF SEXUALLY TRANSMITTED PROCTOCOLONIC INFECTIONS

Enteritis	Colitis/Proctitis	Proctitis
Giardia lamblia Cryptosporidium	Entamoeba histolytica Campylobacter	Neisseria gonorrhoeae Chlamydia trachomatis (non-LGV)
Isospora belli Mycobacterium-avium-intracellulare Cytomegalovirus	Salmonella Shigella	Treponema pallidum Hemophilus ducreyi
	Chlamydia trachomatis (LGV)	Herpes simplex
		Condyloma accuminata

negative serologic tests. Darkfield microscopy or biopsy may reveal spirochetes, but it can be difficult to distinguish treponemes from saprophytic spirochetes, which often colonize perianal skin. Immunofluorescence studies must be obtained in this situation. These patients should be treated empirically for syphilis. Consideration should be given to performing lumbar puncture to check for neurosyphilis in patients with coexistent HIV and syphilis.[12]

Patients with infections of the intestine proximal to the rectum usually complain of abdominal pain, bloating, and diarrhea. A multitude of pathogens are capable of causing sexually transmitted enteritis, colitis, or proctocolitis (Table 49-38). Because the treatment for different pathogens varies widely, therapy for

these infections should be specifically designed after obtaining the results of cultures and stool examination for ova and parasites. Patients requiring intravenous hydration and those with severe toxicity should be hospitalized, but most patients with sexually transmitted intestinal infections can be treated as outpatients.

Patients who are practicing anal intercourse, anilingus, or shared use of foreign objects are at higher risk for contracting HIV. There is an increasing trend toward early interventional therapy in the treatment of asymptomatic HIV infection. Thus the emergency physician is in a unique position to inform such patients of the usefulness of voluntary, confidential testing for HIV, and to advise them in safe sex practices.

Also, patients with AIS may develop severe anorectal infections and require surgery, although healing is often delayed and may be complicated by other infections (e.g., cytomegalic proctitis).[13]

REFERENCES

1. Hosking, S.W., Johnson, A.G., Smart, H.L., and Triger, D.R.: Anorectal varices, hemorrhoids, and portal hypertension. Lancet 1:349, 1989.
2. Bernstein, W.C.: What are hemorrhoids and what is their relationship to the portal venous system? Dis. Colon Rectum 26:829, 1983.
3. Goligher, J.: Surgery of the Anus, Rectum, and Colon. London, Baliere/Tindall, 1984.
4. Dennison, A.R., Whiston, R.J., Rooney, S., and Morris, D.L.: The management of hemorrhoids. Am. J. Gastroenterol. 84:5, 1989.
5. Dennison, A.R., Wheery, D.C., and Morris, D.L.: Hemorrhoids. Surg. Clin. North Am. 68:6, 1988.
6. Hughes, E.S.R.: Inflammation and Infection of the Anus. In Diseases of the Colon and Anorectum. 2nd ed. Edited by Turrell, R. Philadelphia, W.B. Saunders, 1969.
7. Ramanujan, P.S., Prasad, L., Abcarian, H., and Tan, A.: Perianal abscesses and fistulas. Dis. Colon Rectum 27:593, 1984.
8. Scoma, J.A., Salvati, E.P., and Rubin, R.J.: Incidence of fistulas subsequent to anal abscesses. Dis. Colon Rectum 17:3, 1974.
9. Notaras, M.J.: Anal fissure and stenosis. Surg. Clin. North Am. 68:6, 1988.
10. Walker, W.A., Rothenberger, D.A., and Goldberg, S.M.: Morbidity of internal sphincterotomy for anal fissure and stenosis. Dis. Colon Rectum 28:11, 1985.
11. Rompalo, A.M., Roberts, P., Johnson, K., and Stamm, W.E.: Empirical therapy for the management of acute proctitis in homosexual men. JAMA 260:3, 1988.
12. U.S. Centers for Disease Control: 1989 STD Treatment Guidelines. MMWR 38(S-8), 1989.
13. Holmes, J.W.C., and Nichols, R.L.: Anorectal infections. In Infectious Diseases. Edited by Gorbach, S.L., et al. Philadelphia, W.B. Saunders Co., 1992.

CHAPTER 50

INFECTIOUS DISEASES IN THE EMERGENCY DEPARTMENT

SEPTIC SHOCK

Charles B. Cairns and James T. Niemann

CAPSULE

Shock caused by infectious agents is an increasingly common, complex state that carries a high mortality rate. Early recognition and treatment of the hemodynamic abnormalities present a challenge to the emergency physician. The mainstay of therapy in the emergency department (ED) is volume replacement. Initial antibiotic therapy should be broad spectrum. Intensive care unit (ICU) admission and management are mandatory for all cases of septic shock.

INTRODUCTION

Sepsis is defined as the presence of pathogenic organisms or their toxins in the blood or tissues. Septic shock is the reduction of blood flow to multiple tissues and is clinically defined as systolic BP < 90 mm Hg or mean arterial pressure (MAP) < 60 mm Hg unresponsive to volume replacement.[1]

There are no reliable data on the incidence of sepsis and septic shock in patients presenting to the ED. Estimates of gram-negative rod bacteremia alone approach 300,000 per year (U.S.). The incidence of bacteremia is increasing and may be as high as 12 cases per 1000 admissions in large urban hospitals.

Sepsis may result from various pathogens, but is usually associated with gram-negative bacteremia. Septic shock occurs in 25 to 50% of the patients with culture-proven gram-negative bacteremia and 10% of those with gram-positive bacteremia. Other major organisms include fungi (e.g., Candida albicans) and perhaps viruses (e.g., cytomegalovirus).

The mortality rate of septic shock is approximately 50% and has been unchanged over the past 15 years.[2] All types of infecting organisms have approximately similar mortality rates. Pre-existing disease has been shown to have an adverse effect on survival.

The incidence of gram-negative and gram-positive bacteremia and fungal sepsis has steadily increased. Factors for this rise include increased use of intravascular catheters and invasive instrumentation, increasing numbers of patients with depressed immune function, including the elderly and patients with AIDS, and susceptible patients are living longer.

PATHOPHYSIOLOGY

Septic shock is a complex disease state that remains incompletely understood despite extensive study. Clearly this pathophysiologic state is caused by a wide variety of organisms and involves many endogenous biochemical intermediates.

Death from septic shock results from multiple organ failure in approximately 50% of patients, hypotension caused by persistent decrease in systemic vascular resistance (SVR) in 40%, and severe cardiac dysfunction in 10%. Figure 50-1 summarizes current understanding of the cascade that links a nidus of infection with the hemodynamic consequences characteristic of septic shock.[3]

The cascade is triggered by either invasion of the bloodstream by microorganisms or release of endotoxins. The most common sites for invasion include the urinary, respiratory, and gastrointestinal tracts. In approximately 30% of patients (and 50% of immunocompromised patients), however, the portal of entry is unknown. Approximately 50% of cases have negative blood cultures, thought to be caused by either

PATHOGENESIS OF HUMAN SEPTIC SHOCK

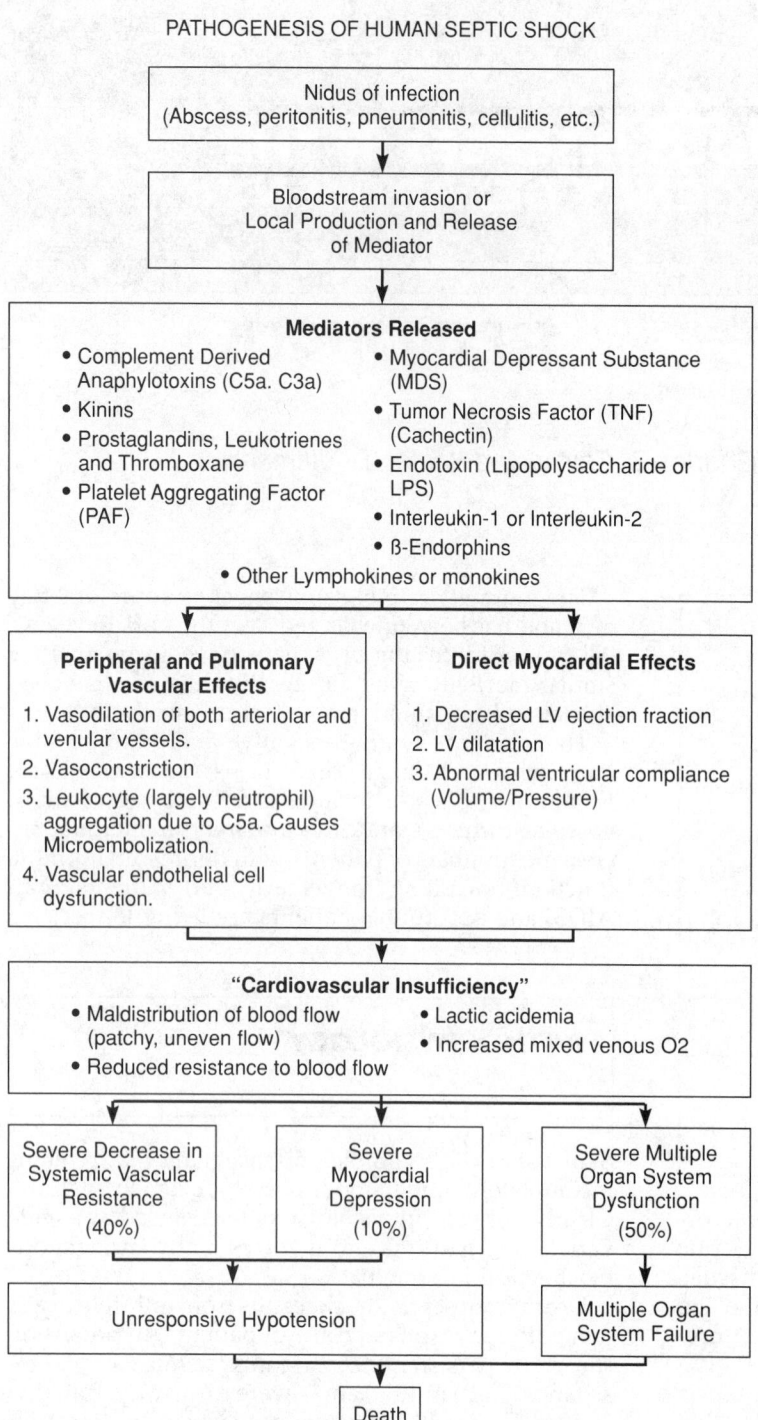

FIG. 50-1. A schematic flow diagram of the probable sequence of steps in a nonsurvivor of human septic shock. The diagram places emphasis on the cardiovascular effects of a wide variety of probable mediators. (With permission from Parrillo, J.E.: Biochemical mechanisms of critical illness. In Critical Decisions: Key Issues in the Recovery of the Critically Ill. Edited by Parrillo, J.E. Toronto, Decker, 1988, p. 28.)

intermittent bloodstream seeding or endotoxin release from a sequestered focus of infection.

Bloodstream invasion activates the metabolic cascade and allows dissemination to other secondary sites. Endogenous intermediates affect the peripheral vasculature, causing both generalized vasodilation and selective regions of marked vasoconstriction. This vasoconstriction, combined with microemboli of aggregated neutrophils, leads to ischemic tissue necrosis and organ dysfunction. Thus, clinical and laboratory signs of organ failure may occur without frank systemic hypotension. The end organs most commonly effected in septic shock are the kidneys, lungs, liver, brain, and heart. In addition, disseminated intravascular coagulation (DIC) of varying degrees of severity is commonly encountered.

The cardiac dysfunction associated with septic shock in humans has been well studied by Parrillo and colleagues.[4] Most patients develop a dilated left ventricle, decreased left ventricular ejection fraction, and normal to high cardiac outputs. The mechanism for myocardial contractile dysfunction is unclear, but a specific myocardial depressant substance has been implicated.[5] There is no evidence of decreased coronary blood flow or ischemia to account for the observed findings.

Several mediators are known to play key roles in the development of the septic shock syndrome. Complement activation by endotoxin leads to the release of C5a and other anaphylatoxins. These anaphylatoxins cause neutrophil aggregation and other mediator release. In addition to a direct effect of endotoxin,[6] mediators such as histamine, kinins, ecosinoids, and beta-endorphins probably contribute to the coagulopathy and cardiovascular dysfunction of severe sepsis.

Although histamine can cause vasodilation and could account for the decreases in SVR, levels of histamine are not elevated in septic shock.[1] The levels of kinins are elevated in septic shock and may account for the vasodilation and coagulation abnormalities seen.[2,7] Prostaglandins and analogues are implicated in regional vasocontriction. Beta-endorphins may have an important role in the hypotension of septic shock.[8]

CLINICAL PRESENTATION

Early recognition of severe sepsis may improve outcomes of patients with septic shock.[1] Important *symptoms* to recognize in sepsis include fever, chills, prostration, nausea, vomiting, and confusion. Additionally, sepsis should be suspected when immunocompromised patients exhibit a change in clinical status. The physiologic response to septicemia may be blunted in elderly patients. This phenomenon has been called "afebrile bacteremia."[9] Altered mental status or subtle changes in pulse, respiratory rate, or blood pressure may be the only clue to life-threatening infection.

Important *signs* to recognize include fever, hypotension, tachypnea, cyanosis, jaundice, and altered mental status. These signs reflect a maldistribution of organ blood flow and metabolic derangements.

Certain signs and laboratory findings predict septic shock and are listed in Table 50-1.[10] In particular, the presence of fever > 40.6 C or hypothermia (T < 35 C) in patients with sepsis frequently precedes hypo-

---

TABLE 50-1. PHYSICAL SIGNS AND LABORATORY DATA LIKELY TO PREDICT SEPTIC SHOCK*

1. Extremes of body temperature (T>40.6°C or T<35.0°C)
2. Altered mental status
3. Orthostasis
4. Decreased urine output
5. Unexplained edema
6. Tachypnea (with hypoxemia and/or metabolic acidosis)
7. Elevated serum lactate
8. Leukopenia
9. Thrombocytopenia (with or without rash)

*Adapted with permission from Sheagren, J.N.: Shock syndromes related to sepsis. *In* Cecil Textbook of Medicine. 18th Ed. Edited by Wyngaarden, J.B., and Smith, L.H. Philadelphia, W. B. Saunders, 1988.

---

tension. Altered mental status may indicate central nervous system involvement. Orthostatic hypotension may be caused by dehydration from vomiting or diarrhea or decreased SVR from early septic shock. Simple dehydration should respond rapidly to fluid replacement. Decreased urine output may reflect renal dysfunction or hypoperfusion. Unexplained edema, particularly associated with decreasing serum albumin, suggests hepatic dysfunction. Tachypnea, with or without cyanosis, can be associated with ARDS. Elevated lactate levels reflect peripheral hypoperfusion and thrombocytopenia reflects early DIC.[7]

Immunocompromised patients present a special challenge because over 50% do not manifest the clinical signs of sepsis. Additionally, half of these patients do not have an identifiable source of infection.[1]

DIFFERENTIAL DIAGNOSIS

Other disease processes (Table 50-2) can cause fever with or without hemodynamic instability and may mimic septic shock. Specifically, many hypersensitivity reactions present with hypotension, fever, and edema. Environmental hyperthermia, the neuroleptic malignant syndrome, drug withdrawal states, and

---

TABLE 50-2. DIFFERENTIAL DIAGNOSIS OF SEVERE SEPSIS

1. Hypersensitivity reactions
2. Neuroleptic malignant syndrome
3. Hyperthermia associated with cocaine or PCP use
4. Environmental hyperthermia (e.g., heat stroke)
5. Withdrawal (abstinence) syndromes (e.g., alcohol)
6. Systemic vasculitis
7. Pulmonary thromboembolism
8. Myocardial infarction (with fever)
9. Viral infections

systemic vasculitis can present with high fever, hemodynamic instability, and altered mental status. Pulmonary embolus and, infrequently, acute myocardial infarction may present with low-grade fevers and unstable vital signs.

The differential diagnosis of shock is addressed in another chapter. Septic shock is a form of distributive shock and must be distinguished from other forms such as hypovolemic shock. Briefly, hypovolemic shock, as opposed to septic shock, should rapidly respond to fluid infusion. Additionally, in septic shock, invasive hemodynamic monitoring usually shows the characteristic profile of high cardiac output (CO), low SVR, and low initial pulmonary capillary wedge pressure (PCWP).

INITIAL STABILIZATION

The priorities in initial management are to maintain adequate blood pressure and organ blood flow.

Initial stabilization requires intravascular access and fluid administration. The initial resuscitation fluid should be normal saline (0.9%). If the initial hematocrit is < 30%, packed RBCs can be given concomitantly.[1] If the patient does not respond to initial fluid replacement (up to a total of 15 to 20 cc per kg) and the systolic BP remains < 90 mm Hg or MAP < 60 mm Hg, immediate vasopressor therapy should be initiated with dopamine (begin with 2 to 5 μg per kg per minute and increase up to 20 μg per kg per minute).

Patients unresponsive to fluid replacement, especially those requiring vasopressors, are optimally managed with invasive hemodynamic monitoring.

LABORATORY AND OTHER PROCEDURES

After intravascular access has been achieved and either hemodynamic stability or monitoring has been established, appropriate cultures should be obtained and antimicrobial therapy initiated.

Aerobic and anaerobic blood cultures should always be obtained. All other potential nidi of infection identified by physical examination or history (such as genito-urinary tract, wound, respiratory tract, CNS) should be cultured and gram-stained. Additional ancillary laboratory studies should be obtained as shown in Table 50-3.

Laboratory data usually suggest bacteremia. The complete blood count (CBC) usually includes an elevated white blood cell (WBC) count (15,000 to 30,000), but occasionally neutropenia and even normal WBC

TABLE 50-3. LABORATORY STUDIES USEFUL IN SEVERE SEPSIS

1. Serum electrolytes, glucose, BUN, and creatinine
2. Complete blood count
3. Coagulation studies (PT, PTT)
4. Arterial blood gas
5. Serum lactate
6. Serum albumin
7. Radiologic studies (chest x ray; CT scan if needed)
8. Bacterial cultures (blood, urine, wounds, etc.)

---

counts occur.[11] The platelet count is usually low and the prothrombin time (PT), partial thromboplastin time (PTT), and fibrin split products may be elevated, reflecting DIC. Electrolyte values may vary considerably; however, the blood urea nitrogen (BUN) and creatinine are usually elevated. These elevations can reflect either prerenal azotemia or acute tubular necrosis (ATN). Prerenal azotemia caused by renal hypoperfusion is suggested by a fractional excretion of sodium of < 3%.

The arterial blood gas early in septic shock reveals a respiratory alkalosis. There may be rapid development of a metabolic acidosis as peripheral perfusion decreases, causing serum lactate to rise. Decreased tissue perfusion may lead to hepatic dysfunction ranging from mild elevations of liver enzymes to marked synthetic dysfunction with decreased serum albumin levels.

MANAGEMENT AND INDICATIONS FOR ADMISSION

All patients with suspected sepsis should be admitted for intravenous antibiotics and observation. All those with suspected septic shock should be admitted to intensive care units (ICU). Antibiotic therapy should be initiated in the ED.

ANTIBIOTICS

Although particular foci of infection may influence antibiotic choices, broad spectrum antibiotic therapy is mandatory in the emergent management of severe sepsis. The antibiotic regimen can be revised once culture results are available, 24 to 72 hours later. Table 50-4 lists possible initial antibiotic regimens for patients at risk for septic shock.

An aminoglycoside in combination with a cephalosporin (i.e., gentamicin and cefoxitin) provides broad initial coverage.[13] Alternatively, third-generation cephalosporins (such as ceftriaxone) have been touted as initial monotherapy.[12] In immunocompromised pa-

TABLE 50-4. SUGGESTED INITIAL ANTIBIOTIC REGIMENS FOR SEVERE SEPSIS*

Age/Condition	Organisms Covered	Suggested Regimen	Alternate Regimen†
Infant	Group B Streptococci, Escherichia coli, enterococci, listeria, staphylococcus aureus, hemophilus influenzae	Ampicillin (50 mg/kg IV q6h) and ceftriaxone (75 mg/kg) (initial dose)	
Child	H. influenzae, pneumococci, meningococci, S. aureus	Ceftriaxone (75 mg/kg) (initial dose)	Chloramphenicol (25 mg/kg IV q8h) and/or vancomycin (15 mg/kg IV q8h)
Adult	S. aureus, Group A and D streptococci, pneumococci, bacteroides species	Ampicillin/sublactam (3.0 g IV q6h) and antipseudomonal aminoglycoside (gentamicin 1.5 mg/kg IV initial)	Cefoxitin (2.0 g IV q4h) and gentamicin
IV drug abuser	S. aureus	Penicillinase resistant synthetic penicillin (oxacillin 2.0 g IV q4h) and gentamicin	Vancomycin 1 g q12h and gentamicin
Immunocompromised neutropenic (Adult doses)	Preceding organisms and pseudomonas sp.	Vancomycin and antipseudomonal penicillin (mezlocillin 3 g IV q4h) and gentamicin	Substitute ceftazidime (2 g IV q8h) for mezlocillin.

* Adapted with permission from Sanford, J.P.: Guide to Antimicrobial Therapy. West Bethesda, Antimicrobial Therapy, 1989. These are suggested regimens; other antibiotic combinations may be effective.
† Alternative regimens are for penicillin-allergic patients; if patient's penicillin allergy is anaphylactoid, the use of cephalosporins is not recommended.

tients (the elderly, diabetics, alcoholics, IV drug users, etc.), it is necessary to provide additional antipseudomonal coverage (i.e., mezlocillin, ceftazidime, or ciprofloxacin).[12]

ICU MONITORING

Invasive hemodynamic monitoring in an ICU is necessary for optimal management of the patient in septic shock. Monitoring includes the use of a balloon-tipped, flow-directed pulmonary artery catheter (for PCWP, SVR, CO measurements), an intra-arterial catheter (for BP, MAP measurements), and a Foley urinary catheter (for urine output measurements).

The PCWP should be maintained between 12 and 18 mm Hg with infusion of normal saline, blood products if the hematocrit is < 30%, and salt-poor albumin if serum albumin level is low.

VASOPRESSOR THERAPY

If the patient remains hypotensive, with the PCWP > 12 mm Hg, vasopressor therapy should be instituted. The current vasopressor of choice is dopamine. At low doses (2 to 5 μg per kg per minute), dopamine functions as an inotrope and increases renal blood flow. As the dose is increased to maintain the MAP > 60 mm Hg, dopamine becomes a powerful vasoconstrictor. For persistent hypotension refractory to dopamine, norepinephrine therapy (started at 2 μg per minute) is required. The dopamine dose should then be reduced to low (2 to 5 μg per kg per minute) doses to maximize renal blood flow.[14]

The prognosis is extremely poor for patients unresponsive to the combination of norepinephrine and low dose dopamine; however, some patients may respond to phenylephrine and epinephrine.[1] For patients with normal or elevated SVR, elevated PCWP, and cardiac dysfunction, dobutamine may be useful as an inotropic agent.[15]

For a select group of patients with continued evidence of poor organ blood flow despite a normal MAP and cardiac output, vasodilators, such as nitroprusside and nitroglycerin, may produce a beneficial redistribution of blood flow.[1] Nitroprusside (50 mg/250cc D_5W) is given by continuous intravenous infusion beginning at 0.5 μg per kg per minute with continous BP monitoring. The infusion rate is increased until evidence of improved organ function is obtained or until systolic BP < 90 mm Hg. Nitroglycerin (50 mg/250 cc D_5W) beginning at 10 to 20 μg per minute is given in a similar manner.

OTHER THERAPIES

The use of corticosteroids is discouraged in septic shock. Initial studies showing efficacy of steroids have been upstaged by recent clinical trials showing no benefit in septic shock.[16,17] In fact, steroid use may even be detrimental.[17]

Naloxone, which blocks endorphin receptors, has also been proposed as treatment for hypotension in sepsis. No large prospective controlled trial has been conducted to demonstrate the efficacy of naloxone treatment. In one study, there was a high incidence of adverse reactions and no therapeutic response.[18]

Surgical drainage is indicated for localized nidi of infection, particularly those with gas-forming organisms. Hyperbaric oxygen may prove useful in the treatment of infections with anaerobic organisms.

PROGNOSIS

The goal of therapeutic maneuvers is to recover normal arterial blood pressures, organ perfusion, and function, and eradicate the infection. Table 50-5 lists criteria developed by Parrillo to indicate therapeutic success in septic shock.[1] The major target organs include the liver, kidney, CNS, and lungs. The return of serum lactate to normal levels reflects adequate peripheral circulation.

Other factors are associated with unfavorable outcomes. Patients with serious underlying diseases (such as leukemia, lymphoma, diabetes, or heart disease) have a poor prognosis.[11] The development of ARDS or refractory hypotension during the course of sepsis also carries high mortality rates.

PITFALLS

The failure to recognize septic shock early and institute appropriate therapy is the major pitfall to therapeutic success. Particularly difficult are patients with atypical presentations, such as the elderly or debilitated or infants, who may be hypothermic or normothermic.

Another pitfall is inappropriate antibiotic therapy. The prognosis of a septic shock patient is significantly improved if the infecting organism is sensitive to the antibiotics administered.[19] The use of broad-spectrum antibiotics pending culture results and the clinical response is recommended.

The need for adequate initial fluid resuscitation and early vasopressor therapy for hemodynamic support cannot be overemphasized. Early, aggressive intervention has been shown to improve outcome in patients with hemodynamic compromise and severe sepsis.[1]

TABLE 50-5. CRITERIA INDICATING THERAPEUTIC SUCCESS IN HUMAN SEPTIC SHOCK*

1. Systolic blood pressure increases to 90 mm Hg or mean arterial pressure (MAP) increases to > 60 mm Hg and is maintained
2. Major organ blood flow is adequate (normal function in liver, CNS, lungs, kidneys: e.g., urine output remains > 20 cc/hr)
3. Arterial serum lactate returns to normal
4. Eradication of infection (through surgery and/or antibiotics)

* Adapted with permission from Parrillo, J.E.: Septic shock in humans. In Textbook of Critical Care. Edited by Shoemaker, W.C., et al. Philadelphia, W. B. Saunders, 1989.

HORIZONS

Antiserum directed against core lipopolysaccharide of a gram-negative organism to patients with septic shock was shown to reduce mortality in one series from 39% to 22%.[20]

Other monoclonal antibodies have been proposed to counteract other mediators of septic shock, including tumor necrosis factor, genetically engineered protease inhibitors, or the contact activation system inhibitors. Protein chemistry and molecular biology may soon generate agents to combat the pathophysiologic consequences of sepsis.[2]

A randomized double-blind, placebo-controlled trial of a human monoclonal antibody against antitoxin has been completed. In 543 septic patients, improved survival was found for those with gram-negative bacteremia. This agent should soon be available for clinical use from Centocor, Inc.[21]

REFERENCES

1. Parrillo, J.E.: Septic shock in humans: Clinical evaluation, pathogenesis, and therapeutic approach. In Textbook of Critical Care. Edited by Shoemaker, W.C., et al. Philadelphia, W.B. Saunders, 1989.
2. Colman, R.W.: The role of plasma proteases in septic shock. N. Engl. J. Med. 320:1207, 1989.
3. Cunnion, R.E., and Parrillo, J.E.: Myocardial dysfunction in sepsis: recent insights. Chest 5:941, 1989.
4. Parrillo, J.E., et al.: A circulating myocardial depressant substance in humans in septic shock. J. Clin. Invest. 76:1539, 1985.
5. Reilly, J.M., et al.: A circulating myocardial depressant is associated with cardiac dysfunction and peripheral hypoperfusion (lactic acidemia) in patients with septic shock. Chest 95:1072, 1989.
6. Suffredini, A.F., Harpel, P.C., and Parrillo, J.E.: Promotion and subsequent inhibition of plasminogen activation after administration of intravenous endotoxin to normal subjects. N. Engl. J. Med. 320:1165, 1989.
7. Mason, J.W., Kleesberg, U., Dolan, P., and Colman, R.W.: Plasma kallikrein and Hageman factor in Gram-negative sepsis. Ann. Intern. Med. 73:545, 1970.
8. Bernton, E.W., Long, J.B., and Holaday, J.W.: Opioids and neuropeptides: Mechanisms in circulatory shock. Fed. Proc. 44:290, 1985.
9. Gleckman, R.A., and Hilbert, D.: Afebrile bacteremia: A phenomenon in geriatric patients. JAMA 248:1478, 1982.
10. Sheagren, J.N.: Shock syndromes related to sepsis. In Cecil Textbook of Medicine, 18th Ed. Edited by Wyngaarden, J.B., and Smith, L.H. Philadelphia, W.B. Saunders, 1988.
11. Dale, D.C., and Petersdorf, R.G.: Septic shock. In Harrison's Principles of Internal Medicine. 11th Ed. Edited by Braunwald, E. New York, McGraw-Hill, 1987.
12. EORTC International Antimicrobial Therapy Cooperative Group: Ceftazidime combined with a short or long course of amikacin for empirical therapy of gram-negative bacteremia in cancer patients with granulocytopenia. N. Engl. J. Med. 317:1692, 1987.
13. Sanford, J.P.: Guide to Antimicrobial Therapy. West Bethesda, Antimicrobial Therapy, 1989, p. 34.
14. Schaer, G.L., Fink, M.P., and Parrillo, J.E.: Norepinephrine alone versus norepinephrine plus low-dose dopamine: En-

hanced renal blood flow with combination pressor therapy. Crit. Care Med. *13*:6:492, 1985.

15. Jardin, R., et al.: Dobutamine: A hemodynamic evaluation in human septic shock. Crit. Care Med. *9*:329, 1981.
16. Bone, R.G., et al.: A controlled clinical trial of high-dose methylprednisolone in the treatment of severe sepsis and septic shock. N. Engl. J. Med. *317*:11:653, 1987.
17. Veterans Administration Systemic Sepsis Cooperative Study Group: Effects of high-dose glucocorticosteroid therapy on mortality in patients with clinical signs of systemic sepsis. N. Engl. J. Med. *317*:659, 1987.
18. Rock, P., et al.: Efficacy and safety of naloxone in septic shock. Crit. Care Med. *13*:28, 1985.
19. Young, L.S., et al.: Gram-negative rod bacteremia: Microbiologic, immunologic, and therapeutic considerations. Ann. Intern. Med. *86*:456, 1977.
20. Zeigler, E.J., et al.: Treatment of Gram-negative bacteremia and shock with human antiserum to a mutant Escherichia coli. N. Engl. J. Med. *307*:1225, 1982.
21. Ziegler, E.J., Fisher, C.J., Sprung, C.L., et al.: Treatment of gram-negative bacteria and septic shock with HA-IA human monoclonal antibody against antitoxin. N. Engl. J. Med. *324*:429, 1991.

BIBLIOGRAPHY

Bone, R.C.: Sepsis syndrome, the diagnostic challenge. J. Critical Illness *6*:525, June 1991.

Parker, M.M., and Parrillo, J.E.: Septic shock and other forms of distributive shock. *In* Current Therapy in Critical Care Medicine. Edited by Parrillo, J.E. Toronto, Decker, 1987.

Parrillo, J.E.: Septic shock in humans: Clinical evaluation, pathogenesis, and therapeutic approach. *In* Textbook of Critical Care. Edited by Shoemaker, W.C., et al.: Philadelphia, W.B. Saunders, 1989.

Root, R.K., and Sande, M.M.: Septic Shock. New York, Churchill Livingstone, 1985.

ACQUIRED IMMUNODEFICIENCY SYNDROME (AIDS)

Richard E. Chaisson and Constance B. Wofsy

CAPSULE

AIDS is a uniformly fatal disease, and patients require extensive medical evaluation and treatment. Although the advent of antiviral therapy may extend the lives of many patients, their need for medical care remains substantial. Thus, given the projected scope of the AIDS epidemic, the geographical distribution of cases, and the severity of illnesses, it is essential that all primary care and emergency medicine practitioners be prepared to provide care to this patient population. This chapter reviews the epidemiology and pathogenesis of HIV infection and discusses the evaluation and management of HIV-related disease.

INTRODUCTION

The acquired immunodeficiency syndrome (AIDS) was first recognized in 1981, when an outbreak of Pneumocystis carinii pneumonia and Kaposi's sarcoma was reported in previously healthy homosexual men who were found to have severe defects in cellular immunity.

AIDS was defined in 1981 as the presence of diseases at least moderately indicative of underlying immunodeficiency in a patient without known cases of immunosuppression. In addition to Pneumocystis pneumonia and Kaposi's sarcoma, diseases reflecting immunodeficiency and diagnostic of AIDS include cerebral toxoplasmosis, cryptococcal meningitis, disseminated infection with Mycobacterium avium-intracellulare, cytomegalovirus disease, chronic herpes infection, and chronic cryptosporidiosis (Table 50-6). The agent that causes the syndrome, human immunodeficiency virus (HIV), was first identified in 1983 and cultured in 1984. Diagnostic tests for antibodies to HIV were first commercially available in March 1985, and widespread serologic studies of high-risk groups have helped define the scope of the epidemic.

AIDS is a reportable disease in the United States, although HIV infection and minor manifestations are not. Although tens of thousands of cases of AIDS have been reported in the United States, it is apparent that as many as one million Americans are infected with HIV and are at risk for subsequent disease. The United States Public Health Service predicts that, by 1991, a cumulative total of 271,000 cases of AIDS will have been diagnosed in the United States, 74,000 new cases

TABLE 50-6. CENTERS FOR DISEASE CONTROL SURVEILLANCE DEFINITION OF AIDS

The presence of reliably diagnosed disease at least moderately indicative of underlying cellular immunodeficiency in a person without a known cause of immunodeficiency other than HIV infection.

Diseases Diagnostic of AIDS

PROTOZOA
Pneumocystis carinii pneumonia
Toxoplasma gondii cerebritis
Chronic (> 1 month) cryptosporidiosis
BACTERIAL
Disseminated Mycobacterium avium-intracellulare infection
Mycobacterium tuberculosis infection (extrapulmonary)*
Salmonella infection*
VIRAL
Cytomegalovirus infection
Chronic mucocutaneous herpes simplex
Progressive multifocal leukencephalopathy (papovavirus)
FUNGAL
Candida esophagitis
Cryptococcus neoformans meningitis
Disseminated histoplasmosis
Disseminated coccidioidomycosis
MALIGNANT
Kaposi's sarcoma
Primary lymphoma of the brain
Non-Hodgkin's lymphoma*

* With positive HIV serology.

alone in 1991. Moreover, although more than 50% of AIDS cases through 1987 occurred in five cities (New York, San Francisco, Los Angeles, Newark, and Miami), in 1991, 75% of new cases will be diagnosed outside of the cities that have thus far borne the brunt of the epidemic.

EPIDEMIOLOGY

Since the beginning of the AIDS epidemic in the United States, the disease has been relatively confined to high-risk groups. Homosexual men (73%), intravenous drug users (17%), hemophiliacs, and transfusion recipients (4%), and heterosexual partners of any of the above (4%) constitute the majority of AIDS cases in this country. The concentration of AIDS in discrete geographic areas and among the high-risk groups was an early indication that a transmissible agent was the cause of the syndrome. The trend is changing to include more heterosexually contracted cases. Discovery of HIV and its isolation from patients with or at risk for AIDS established the viral cause of the syndrome. Seroepidemiologic surveys of at-risk group members have helped elucidate the mechanisms of HIV transmission and the natural history of the infection.

HIV is concentrated in blood and semen and has been found in lower concentration in cervical/vaginal secretions. It can be found in low titers in saliva, tears, amniotic fluid, and breast milk. Transmission of HIV is accomplished primarily through three routes:

1. *Sexual transmission.* The virus is transmitted by way of sexual intercourse by exposure to semen, female genital secretions, or blood. Coexistent genital ulcer disease is thought to facilitate transmission of the virus and may play an important role in the heterosexual transmission of HIV in developing countries. Receptive rectal intercourse is the predominant mode of transmission in homosexual men, although its role in heterosexual transmission is uncertain. Orogenital transmission has not been proved; however, it is likely that the virus could be transmitted in this fashion.

2. *Blood transmission.* Exposure to blood from infected individuals is a highly effective means of transmission. Intravenous drug users become infected by inoculation of infected blood where hypodermic needles are shared for drug injection. Both the frequency of drug injection and the amount of needle sharing by drug users have been linked to the prevalence of HIV infection. It appears that the amount of blood injected is an important determinant of subsequent infection; small inocula are unlikely to result in viral transmission. Recipients of a unit of infected blood, for example, have a greater than 90% likelihood of becoming infected, whereas health care workers accidentally injured by needle sticks from infected patients have a less than 0.1% likelihood of infection. The virus is transmitted by both whole blood and blood products. Contamination of Factor VIII and cryoprecipitate has led to widespread infection in hemophiliacs, and transmission has been documented from infected units of packed red cells, platelets, and transplanted organs.

3. *In utero transmission.* HIV-infected women may give birth to infected infants. Although transmission can occur during and after delivery, it clearly can occur in utero; the virus has been isolated from the tissues of aborted fetuses from HIV-infected women.

Although HIV transmission may occur by other routes (e.g., infected breast milk), the overwhelming majority of individuals infected with the virus were exposed by sexual contact, intravenous needle punctures, receipt of infected blood or blood products, or in utero transmission.

Populations at risk for AIDS vary geographically both within and between countries. In the United States, intravenous drug users now account for approximately 40% of AIDS cases in the metropolitan New York area, whereas homosexual and bisexual men account for 95% of cases in California. In developing countries, particularly Haiti and central African nations, heterosexual transmission is the primary mode of infection, and an almost 1:1 ratio of male to female AIDS cases has been observed. Heterosexual transmission is of increasing importance in developed countries, although homosexual and bisexual men will continue to account for the majority of AIDS cases in the next 5 years. Casual transmission of HIV is not thought to occur. There is no empiric or experimental evidence to suggest that transmission by means other than those outlined above occurs. This has important implications in the provision of health care, as will be discussed subsequently.

PATHOGENESIS OF HIV INFECTION

HIV is a previously unknown human retrovirus. Its ribonucleic acid (RNA) genome is carried inside highly conserved core proteins, which are in turn surrounded by a glycoprotein envelope. A unique characteristic of all retroviruses is the presence of the enzyme reverse transcriptase (RT), which uses host nucleotides to incorporate the viral genome into host deoxyribonucleic acid (DNA), whereby a latent infection is established. HIV preferentially infects human T lymphocytes of the helper/inducer subset (CD4$^+$). Helper T lymphocytes are central in controlling cellular immunity, and infection with HIV results in both qualitative and quantitative defects in helper-cell function. Latently infected helper T cells have defects in clonal proliferation, response to soluble antigen, and lymphokine production. Integration of cellular immune responses is also impaired, as evidenced by functional defects in suppressor T lymphocytes and killer lymphocytes. HIV-infected individuals show derangement in humoral immunity as well. A nonspecific polyclonal B-cell proliferation is seen concomitantly with an impaired ability for an antibody response to new antigens. Loss of helper T lymphocytes is associated with development of opportunistic disease, particularly infections, and of AIDS-defining conditions. Although uninfected individuals have on average more than 800 helper cells per μl of blood, patients with opportunistic infections frequently have less than 100 per μl.

The pathogenesis of HIV infection is chronic. Although unusual cases of individuals who developed AIDS 1 to 2 years after infection have been reported, the median time from HIV infection to development of AIDS may be 5 years or more. It is not clear whether all persons infected with HIV eventually develop AIDS. Long-term studies of infected persons, however, show that more than 25% do develop AIDS 7 to 8 years after infection, and more than 50% show signs and symptoms of disease. Virtually 100% of long-term infected individuals have laboratory evidence of cellular immunopathology.

The development of opportunistic disease is a marker of severe immunodeficiency, and the prog-

nosis after this point is extremely poor. Median survival beyond AIDS diagnosis is less than 1 year. Recently, survival of selected AIDS patients has been prolonged by administration of antiviral chemotherapy, although the overall impact of treatment on survival remains unclear. Treatment of infected individuals before the development of opportunistic disease may alter the natural history of HIV infection, and clinical trials of this strategy are under way. At present, however, HIV infection remains incurable, and AIDS remains fatal.

CLINICAL PRESENTATION

Infection with HIV can be manifested by signs ranging from inapparent seropositivity to fulminant opportunistic infection. Early descriptions of patients with AIDS focused on the terminal stages of HIV infection, particularly opportunistic pulmonary and central nervous system disease and disseminated Kaposi's sarcoma. When it became apparent that members of AIDS risk groups could suffer from a multitude of lesser ailments than the full syndrome, the terms AIDS-related complex (ARC) was coined to describe less life-threatening illnesses that were felt to be prodromal to AIDS. As the epidemic has progressed, an increasing number of clinical syndromes have been associated with HIV infection, and the incidence of infections not usually associated with immunodeficiency has been observed to be higher in HIV-infected patients. For example, both pulmonary and extrapulmonary tuberculosis, *Salmonella* infections, and infections caused by encapsulated bacteria have been found frequently in patients with AIDS or HIV infection.

Several classification systems of HIV infection have been proposed. The Walter Reed system has seven stages and relies on clinical findings, helper T lymphocyte counts, and response to cutaneous antigen testing. A practical classification system for both epidemiologic surveillance and clinical evaluation has been proposed by a panel convened by the Centers for Disease Control (CDC). The CDC system contains four categories of HIV infection and multiple subcategories for more advanced disease (Table 50-7). Group I refers to the mononucleosis-like syndrome associated with acute HIV infection. This syndrome has been described in homosexual men and in health care workers who have been documented to seroconvert for HIV antibody. Symptoms of acute infection include fever, headache, malaise, arthralgias, and myalgias. Photophobia and meningismus have also been reported. Lymphadenopathy is usually absent. A diffuse truncal exanthem is reported in up to 50% of patients. Laboratory findings are usually nonspecific but should include a negative Monospot test. The ill-

TABLE 50-7. CENTERS FOR DISEASE CONTROL SYSTEM FOR CLASSIFYING HIV INFECTIONS

Group I:	Acute infection
Group II:	Asymptomatic infection, with or without associated laboratory abnormalities
Group III:	Persistent generalized lymphadenopathy
Group IV:	Symptomatic disease
Subgroup A:	Constitutional disease, e.g., weight loss, prolonged fever, unexplained diarrhea
Subgroup B:	Neurological disease, e.g., dementia, aseptic meningitis, peripheral neuropathy
Subgroup C:	Secondary infectious diseases
Category C1:	Infections diagnostic of AIDS, e.g., *Pneumocystis* pneumonia, toxoplasmosis, cryptococcosis
Category C2:	Infectious complications not diagnostic of AIDS, e.g., oral hairy leukoplakia, disseminated herpes zoster, *Salmonella* bacteremia, tuberculosis
Subgroup D:	Malignancies: Kaposi's sarcoma, non-Hodgkin's lymphomas
Subgroup E:	Other diseases

(*From* Classification system for human T-lymphocyte virus type III/lymphadenopathy-associated virus infections. MMWR *35*:334, 1986.)

ness usually lasts for 1 to 2 weeks, after which the patient returns to normal health. Seroconversion for HIV antibody can be seen within several weeks of the acute illness and should be present by 3 months. The incubation period of acute infection is not well established but appears to be 2 to 6 weeks after exposure.

Group II of the CDC system refers to asymptomatic seropositive individuals without clinical signs or symptoms of disease. Laboratory evaluation of seropositive individuals, however, may reveal a variety of abnormalities including lymphopenia, reversal of the helper/suppressor ratio, elevation of the sedimentation rate and β_2-microglobulin, or mild anemia. Thrombocytopenia has been reported in a small proportion of seropositive patients and may be associated with purpura or mucosal bleeding. Hemodynamically significant bleeding, however, is rare.

Group III of the CDC system includes asymptomatic individuals who have persistent generalized lymphadenopathy (PGL). This condition is the result of HIV infection, and may develop in more than one half of HIV-seropositive persons. PGL is not a sign of more advanced HIV infection because individuals with this finding have no greater degree of immunologic impairment and do not progress to opportunistic disease at a rate greater than those seropositives without lymphadenopathy.

The proportion of asymptomatic seropositive persons, with or without lymphadenopathy, who go on to develop HIV-related diseases has been the subject of intense investigation. Studies of cohorts of seropositives followed prospectively reveal an ominous trend toward development of immunodeficiency and illness in a substantial proportion. Approximately 25% of seropositives observed for 3 to 6 years develop the full syndrome. An additional 25% to 30% of subjects

observed for up to 8 years develop HIV-related opportunistic disease. Further observation of such cohorts will determine the ultimate proportion who will progress to clinical illness after infection with HIV.

CDC group IV refers to individuals manifesting clinical disease associated with HIV or immunosuppression caused by HIV. Subgroup A includes constitutional disease such as persistent unexplained fever, weight loss greater than 10% of body weight, or persistent unexplained diarrhea. Subgroup B consists of neurologic disease caused by HIV, including encephalopathy, aseptic meningitis, and peripheral neuropathy. Subgroup C, secondary infectious diseases, refers both to infections diagnostic of AIDS (category C1), such as Pneumocystis pneumonia, toxoplasmosis, cryptococcosis, and to infectious complications of HIV that do not fulfill the CDC case definition for AIDS (category C2), including oral hairy leukoplakia, disseminated herpes zoster, Salmonella bacteremia, or tuberculosis. Patients who present with HIV-associated opportunistic infections generally have severe defects in cellular immunity, manifested by low $CD4^+$ lymphocyte counts. In the absence of therapy to restore immunocompetence, patients in this category can be expected to have frequent opportunistic infections and a high mortality rate.

Patients in subgroup D, secondary cancers, are those with malignant tumors associated with HIV infection. The most common cancer in AIDS patients is Kaposi's sarcoma, an endothelial tumor or that can involve the skin, mucosal membranes, lung, gastrointestinal tract, and other visceral organs (Fig. 50-2). Highly aggressive non-Hodgkin's lymphomas and primary lymphoma of the brain have also been reported with increased incidence in HIV-infected individuals. These malignancies carry a poor prognosis,

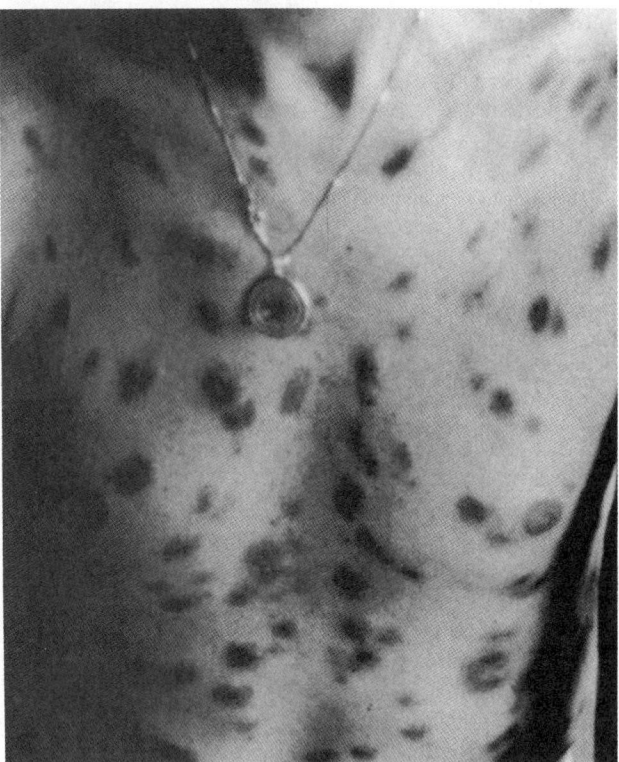

FIG. 50-2. *Skin lesions of Kaposi's sarcoma in an AIDS patient. (Courtesy of P. Volberding, MD.)*

TABLE 50-8. PULMONARY COMPLICATIONS OF AIDS

Pathogens Causing Infections
  PROTOZOA
    Pneumocystis carinii
  FUNGI
    Cryptococcus neoformans
    Coccidioides immitis
    Histoplasma capsulatum
  VIRUSES
    Cytomegalovirus
    Human immunodeficiency virus (?)
  BACTERIA
    Mycobacterium tuberculosis
    Mycobacterium avium-intracellulare
    Mycobacterium kansasii
    Streptococcus pneumoniae
    Haemophilus influenzae
Malignancies
  Kaposi's sarcoma
  Non-Hodgkin's lymphoma

because antitumor therapy is unlikely to result in a complete remission, and opportunistic complications are frequent.

Subgroup E in the CDC classification system refers to clinical manifestations of HIV infection not classified in the other categories, including chronic lymphoid interstitial Pneumocystis infection. As the clinical manifestations of HIV become better elucidated, it is likely that additional diseases or findings will be listed in this category.

CLINICAL PRESENTATION AND DIAGNOSIS OF HIV-RELATED DISEASE

RESPIRATORY DISEASE

The lungs are the organs most frequently involved in AIDS-related opportunistic disease. Various pathogens and disease processes cause respiratory signs and symptoms in patients with HIV infection (Table 50-8). Sixty-three percent of AIDS diagnoses are made on the basis of Pneumocystis pneumonia, and an additional 20% of AIDS patients are estimated to have Pneumocystis infection at some time during the course of their illness. Despite the frequency of Pneumocystis

infection in AIDS patients, the differential diagnosis of pulmonary disease is extensive, and a thorough evaluation, including the use of appropriate diagnostic tests, is essential in the work-up of patients known or suspected to be HIV seropositive.

Symptoms of AIDS-related pulmonary disease include fever, night sweats, weight loss, dyspnea, and cough (with or without sputum). Pleuritic chest pain is uncommon in Pneumocystis pneumonia but can be associated with bacterial (e.g., pneumococcus) pneumonias. The duration of symptoms is frequently 1 to 3 weeks, and constitutional symptoms may precede respiratory abnormalities by months. A history of HIV seropositivity, generalized lymphadenopathy, thrush, or hairy leukoplakia is often elicited. Physical examination may reveal fever, tachycardia, and elevated respiratory rate. Auscultation of the chest is often normal, although fine rales or occasionally wheezing may be present in some patients. Patients with a history of AIDS or known to be risk for AIDS who present with respiratory symptoms should undergo laboratory evaluation for opportunistic lung disease (Fig. 50-3).

Initial laboratory evaluation of respiratory symptoms begins with a chest radiograph. Diffuse, bilateral interstitial pulmonary infiltrates are commonly found in patients with Pneumocystis pneumonia (Fig. 50-4). Some patients may have local infiltrates or no radiographic abnormality (5% to 10%). Hilar or mediastinal adenopathy suggests Kaposi's sarcoma, lymphoma, or tuberculosis. Pleural effusions are a frequent consequence of pulmonary Kaposi's sarcoma but may also be seen with mycobacterial infections. Nodular infiltrates can be seen with fungal infections, lymphoma, and Kaposi's sarcoma. Patients suspected of having Pneumocystis pneumonia who have an abnormal radiograph should have a specific test for Pneumocystis performed. Patients with a normal ra-

Suggested Approach to Screening for Pneumocystis carinii

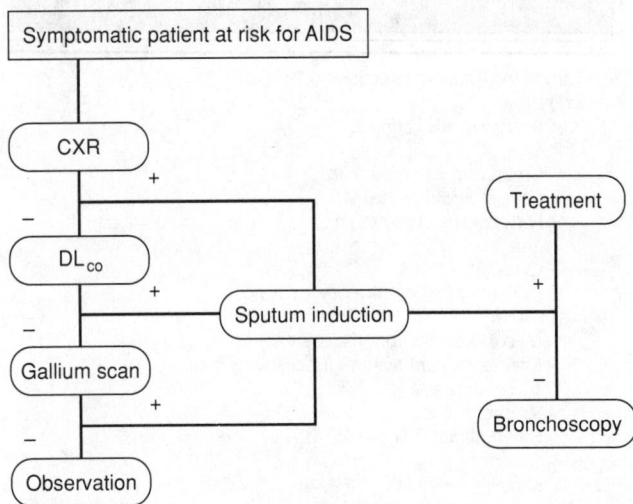

FIG. 50-3. Algorithm for evaluating respiratory disease in HIV-infected patients. CXR = chest x-ray, DL$_{co}$ = diffusing capacity of the lungs for carbon monoxide. (*Courtesy of* J. Curtis, MD.)

diograph but who have signs and symptoms of respiratory disease can be further evaluated with noninvasive screening tests, including arterial blood gas determination, pulmonary function tests, or gallium lung scanning. An increased alveolar-arterial (A–a) difference either at rest or with exercise is a highly

sensitive test for Pneumocystis pneumonia. Pulmonary function testing is a rapid and sensitive screening method for assessing the likelihood or Pneumocystis infection: a restrictive pattern and decreased diffusing capacity for carbon monoxide are both consistent with Pneumocystis pneumonia. Uptake of gallium citrate in the lungs suggests pulmonary infection and is sensitive for Pneumocystis. Patients with a normal chest radiograph and normal noninvasive tests can be observed for worsening of symptoms. Frequently, empiric antibiotic therapy for bronchitis is prescribed, particularly if sputum production is prominent. Individuals with a normal chest radiograph but with an abnormally large A—a difference, decreased diffusing capacity, or positive gallium scan should undergo testing for the presence of Pneumocystis.

Examination of Giemsa-stained sputum (induced by inhalation of nebulized saline) for Pneumocystis trophozoites and cysts is an efficient and noninvasive technique for diagnosing Pneumocystis pneumonia (Fig. 50-5). In selected patients, this method has a sensitivity of approximately 80%, although its negative predictive value is low. Patients who have organisms identified on induced sputum specimens should be treated in the manner subsequently outlined. A negative induced sputum result does not rule out pneumocystis, and patients with negative results should undergo fiberoptic bronchoscopy. Bronchoalveolar lavage and transbronchial biopsy are both highly specific and sensitive for diagnosing Pneumocystis infection. Lavage alone initially decreases the complication rate of bronchoscopy and has a high yield in establishing the diagnosis of Pneumocystis pneumonia. Patients with a negative lavage result may be restudied, and transbronchial biopsy performed. Open lung biopsy is rarely indicated in patients with AIDS-related pulmonary disease and does not appear to aid in the search for Pneumocystis. Treatment of AIDS-related pulmonary infections should be aimed at the causative organism, although empiric therapy is often initiated pending definitive evaluation.

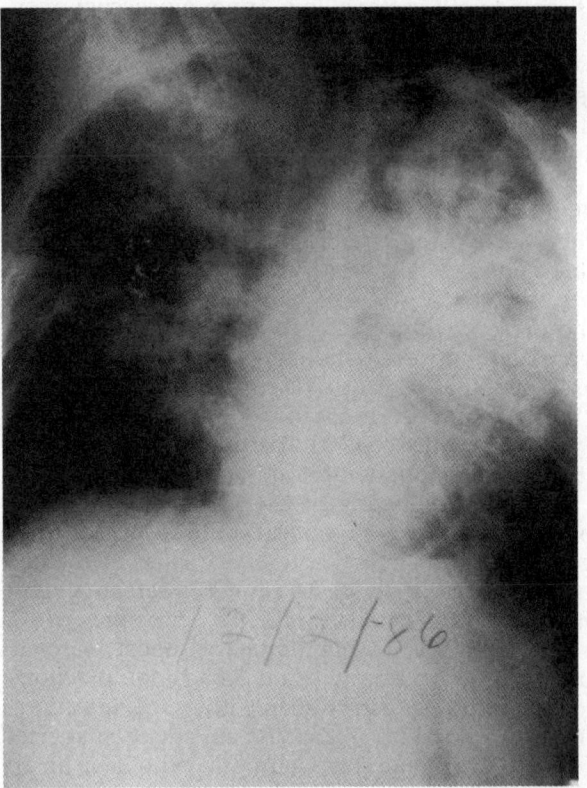

FIG. 50-4. Chest radiograph showing diffuse bilateral infiltrates in a patient with Pneumocystis carinii pneumonia (PCP).

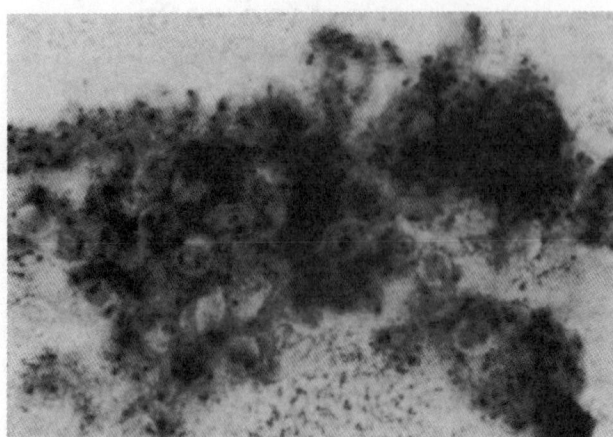

FIG. 50-5. Pneumocystis cysts and trophozoites in Giemsa-stained induced sputum. (*Courtesy of* WK Hadley, MD, PhD.)

Pneumocystis pneumonia can be treated with several regimens. Trimethoprim-sulfamethoxazole can be administered intravenously or orally at a dosage of 15 to 20 mg/kg body weight trimethoprim per day in divided doses and is considered the first-line choice by many clinicians. Toxic reactions are common, occurring in more than 50% of patients maintained on therapy for at least 2 weeks. Frequent severe toxic manifestations include a generalized maculopapular rash, neutropenia, hepatitis, hyponatremia, and nausea. Pentamidine is another effective agent and is administered intravenously in a single dose of 4 mg/kg body weight per day. Like trimethoprim-sulfamethoxazole, pentamidine can cause serious toxicity, including neutropenia, azotemia, hypoglycemia, and, rarely, ventricular dysrhythmias. With either therapy, the onset of symptoms of toxicity usually occurs between day 7 and 14 of therapy. Recently, aerosolized pentamidine in 600 mg doses by nebulizer has been used successfully to treat Pneumocystis pneumonia, with minimal toxicity. The combination of dapsone and trimethoprim has also been proved effective in the treatment of this condition. The regimen is given orally as 100 mg of dapsone daily and 15 to 20 mg/kg body weight trimethoprim daily in divided doses. Toxic reactions with this combination are significantly less than with trimethoprim-sulfamethoxazole, but are nevertheless frequent and include rash, hepatitis, nausea, and methemoglobinemia.

Other treatments are also being studied. The use of trimetrexate (an antifolate agent) can inhibit the folate metabolism enzyme dihydrofolate reductase 1500 times more than trimethoprim. This drug has undergone initial study and shows some promise, particularly for patients for whom conventional therapy has failed. Leucovorin (folinic acid) "rescue" must, however, be used to protect the host tissues from the antifolate activity. The use of a sulfonamide in addition to trimetrexate may enhance therapeutic efficacy.

Response to therapy for Pneumocystis can be slow, and patients should not be considered to have failed treatment before 5 to 7 days of therapy have elapsed. Seventy to eighty percent of patients with first episodes of Pneumocystis pneumonia recover, and higher mortality rates are associated with severe hypoxemia, elevated lactate dehydrogenase levels, and the severity of pathology seen on lung biopsy. Patients who fail an initial drug regimen usually do not respond when therapy is changed. Respiratory failure requiring mechanical ventilation is an ominous development, usually resulting in a mortality rate higher than 90%. Patients who require a change of therapy because of drug toxicity usually have a favorable outcome. The use of corticosteroids in the treatment of Pneumocystis pneumonia is unproved, but clinical trials are under way.

Recurrences of Pneumocystis pneumonia are extremely common after successful therapy. One half of patients surviving 1 year from an initial episode relapse without preventive therapy. Consequently, prophylactic antibiotics are recommended for all patients after a first episode of Pneumocystis pneumonia. Careful clinical trials of prophylactic therapy for AIDS patients have not been conducted, but extensive clinical data have been collected for a variety of regimens. Trimethoprim-sulfamethoxazole, two double-strength tablets daily, is effective for preventing Pneumocystis pneumonia in immunocompromised patients without AIDS. Use of these agents in AIDS patients is limited by frequent toxic reactions. The combination of pyrimethamine and sulfadoxine (Fansidar) given weekly appears effective for prophylaxis but is also associated with symptoms of toxicity. Other agents that are being examined for preventive therapy include oral dapsone and parenteral or aerosolized pentamidine. The use of prophylactic therapy in patients who have not had a primary episode of Pneumocystis pneumonia is not established.

NEUROLOGIC DISEASE

More than 10% of patients with AIDS present with a neurologic diagnosis, and at autopsy more than two thirds are found to have neurologic involvement (Table 50-9). Central nervous system involvement may manifest as dementia, meningitis, or focal neurologic disease with or without delirium. A painful neuropathy is a common finding in peripheral nervous system disease.

AIDS-related encephalopathy is a progressive dementia seen in HIV-infected individuals. Memory loss, inattention, confusion, and decreased cognitive function are characteristic. Magnetic resonance imaging (MRI) scans of the head may show severe cortical atrophy (Fig. 50-6). Therapy is supportive.

Aseptic meningitis is common in patients with HIV infection and usually is associated with headache, malaise, fever, and occasionally meningismus. Lumbar puncture usually reveals a slightly elevated protein level, mild pleocytosis (predominantly lymphocytes),

TABLE 50-9. NEUROLOGIC COMPLICATIONS OF AIDS

Syndrome	Agent(s)
Encephalopathy	HIV
	Cytomegalovirus (?)
Aseptic meningitis	HIV (?)
Meningitis	Cryptococcus neoformans
	Listeria monocytogenes
Cerebritis/abscess	Toxoplasma gondii
	Mycobacterium tuberculosis
	Cryptococcus neoformans
Progressive multifocal leukencephalopathy	Papovavirus
Peripheral neuropathy	?
Tumor	Kaposi's sarcoma
	NonHodgkin's lymphoma

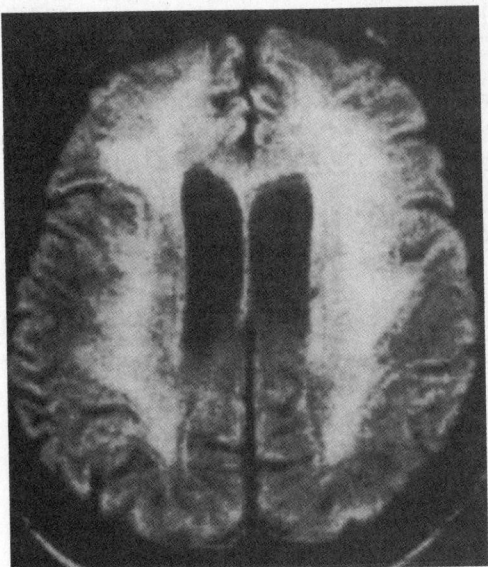

FIG. 50-6. Magnetic resonance scan of a patient with human immunodeficiency virus (HIV) encephalopathy. In addition to cortical atrophy and enlargement of the ventricles, diffuse white matter abnormalities are present. (*Courtesy of* S. McArthur, MD.)

and a normal glucose level. Routine cultures of the cerebrospinal fluid are generally negative. HIV may be cultured from the cerebrospinal fluid of patients with this presentation, although a causative role is not clear. Supportive care and anti-inflammatory analgesics are indicated.

Meningitis from Cryptococcus neoformans is a common infectious complication of AIDS and frequently manifests as a nonfulminant process. Headache with fever is the most common complaint and may be accompanied by other constitutional symptoms, such as nausea, vomiting, and sometimes meningismus. Serum cryptococcal antigen is usually present, and meningitis is confirmed by detecting cryptococcal antigen or culturing Cryptococcus from the cerebrospinal fluid. Prolonged therapy with amphotericin B is usually required, and relapses occur frequently in patients not on oral maintenance therapy with ketoconazole and fluconazole. Administration of 5-fluorocytosine is associated with frequent toxicity and is not considered necessary by many clinicians.

Focal neurologic disease is most frequently caused by Toxoplasma gondii, although primary or metastatic malignancies, brain abscesses, or tuberculosis may cause a similar presentation. Patients may have seizures associated with focal weakness, although delirium and weakness may be the presenting symptoms. Fever is present in only 50% of patients with toxoplasmosis. The diagnosis is suggested by the finding of ring-enhancing lesions on computed tomography or magnetic resonance imaging scans. Definitive diagnosis is made with brain biopsy, although lesions are often inaccessible. Empiric therapy with pyrimethamine and sulfadiazine often leads to dramatic improvement. A favorable response to a course

of empiric therapy is diagnostic if brain biopsy cannot be performed. Relapses are common when therapy is withheld; thus lifelong suppressive therapy is indicated. Drug toxicity, particularly with sulfa agents, is common. Treatment with diphenhydramine may be of benefit when drug rash occurs. Clindamycin may be substituted for sulfadiazine in the face of unacceptable toxic reactions. The role of corticosteroids in treating toxoplasmosis is not established.

GASTROINTESTINAL DISEASE

The gastrointestinal tract is frequently affected in patients with AIDS or HIV infection. Impairment of mucosal host defenses may result in infectious complications, and AIDS-related malignancies may involve all portions of the alimentary system.

Esophagitis can be suspected when dysphagia, odynophagia, or retrosternal burning and pain occur. Asymptomatic candidal esophagitis may be seen in patients with oropharyngeal thrush. Etiologic agents, in addition to Candida, are herpes simplex and cytomegalovirus. Gastric involvement in AIDS may be due to cytomegalovirus, Kaposi's sarcoma, or lymphoma.

Patients with suspected upper gastrointestinal lesions can be evaluated with barium radiographs or endoscopy. Candida, herpes virus, and cytomegalovirus can be diagnosed by biopsy and cultures. Lymphomatous involvement is seen in biopsy specimens. Kaposi's sarcoma is usually evident on visual inspection by endoscopy; biopsy may confirm the diagnosis, although the sensitivity is low because of the submucosal location of Kaposi's lesions.

Candida esophagitis is generally treated with oral ketoconazole, 200 to 400 mg per day; however, amphotericin B may be required for severe cases. Herpes esophagitis may be treated with acyclovir, whereas cytomegalovirus frequently responds to the experimental agent gancyclovir.

Diarrhea is a common complaint in AIDS patients and may be caused by a number of organisms (Table 50-10). Colitis is frequently associated with cramping,

TABLE 50-10. CAUSES OF DIARRHEA IN AIDS

Enterocolitis
   Entamoeba histolytica
   Giardia lamblia
   Cryptosporidium
   Shigella flexneri
   Campylobacter jejuni

   Salmonella
   Cytomegalovirus
Proctitis
   Neisseria gonorrhoeae
   Chlamydia trachomatis
   Herpes simplex

flatulence, and watery stools. Proctitis is suggested by tenesmus and painful defecation. Patients with diarrhea should be evaluated with routine stool cultures and an examination for ova and parasites, including Cryptosporidium, which may require special staining techniques. Blood cultures are helpful if fever is present, as infections with Salmonella and, to a lesser extent, Shigella may be bacteremic. If a diagnosis cannot be established with a noninvasive evaluation, patients should undergo proctosigmoidoscopy or colonoscopy with biopsy and appropriate cultures.

CUTANEOUS MANIFESTATIONS

Several diseases of the skin have been reported in patients with HIV infection and AIDS. Kaposi's sarcoma, a vascular endothelial tumor with a predilection for the skin, was among the first AIDS diagnoses reported in the United States. Kaposi's sarcoma occurs more frequently in homosexual men than in other risk groups in developed countries and is also common in Haitians with AIDS. For unclear reasons, the proportion of AIDS patients with Kaposi's sarcoma has declined dramatically in the past several years. Clinically, Kaposi's sarcoma presents as painless raised violaceous papules and nodules that do not blanch. Frequent sites of Kaposi's sarcoma are the face, extremities, and oral cavity (Figs. 50-2 and 50-7); however, it involves many internal organs, particularly the lungs and gastrointestinal tract.

Diagnosis of Kaposi's sarcoma is based on biopsy of suspicious lesions. Histologically, Kaposi's sarcoma appears as a vascular proliferation with erythrocyte extravasation, hemosiderin deposition, and numerous nonendothelialized channels. Diagnosis of pulmonary or gastrointestinal Kaposi's sarcoma can be made by observation of characteristic lesions during bronchoscopy or endoscopy, or by biopsy. Treatment is with vinca alkaloids or radiation therapy, although

many patients do not need or are unlikely to benefit from treatment. Severe visceral Kaposi's sarcoma is often progressive even in the face of therapy with vincas, doxorubicin, and bleomycin and can disseminate widely, often contributing to death.

Mucocutaneous herpes simplex virus infections are another syndrome seen frequently in AIDS patients. Genital infection with herpes simplex virus type 2 is a sexually transmitted disease commonly encountered in patients from AIDS risk groups, and recurrence may occur in a small proportion. In the presence of cellular immunodeficiency from HIV infection, however, herpes simplex virus type 2 can reactivate chronically and is diagnostic of AIDS when lesions are present for longer than a month. Recurrence of herpes simplex virus type 2 typically involves the genitals, rectum, and sacral region. Typically, painful small vesicles, usually unilateral, with an erythematous base are noted. Systemic complaints are unusual. Diagnosis is confirmed by viral culture. Syphilitic chancres and chancroids are other possible causes. Treatment is with acyclovir, 200 to 400 mg orally 5 times daily for 1 or 2 weeks. Because of the chronicity of some recurrences, patients may benefit from suppressive therapy with 400 to 600 mg of acyclovir daily.

The incidence of reactivation of varicella-zoster virus is increased in patients with HIV infection and AIDS. Presumably, defects in cellular immune function result in reactivation of latent varicella-zoster virus in nerve root ganglia. Most cases occur before an AIDS diagnosis, and the occurrence of varicella-zoster virus in an HIV-infected patient is often prodromal to AIDS. Most patients note a painful eruption of vesicles in one or two dermatomes, although dissemination occurs in a minority of patients. Case reports of meningitis concurrent with varicella-zoster infection have appeared. The diagnosis is made clinically and can be confirmed with viral culture. Treatment of disseminated disease requires intravenous acyclovir at 1500 mg/M^2 daily. For dermatomal outbreaks, many cli-

FIG. 50-7. Kaposi's sarcoma of the hard palate in a patient with AIDS. (*Courtesy of J.S. Greenspan, PhD.*)

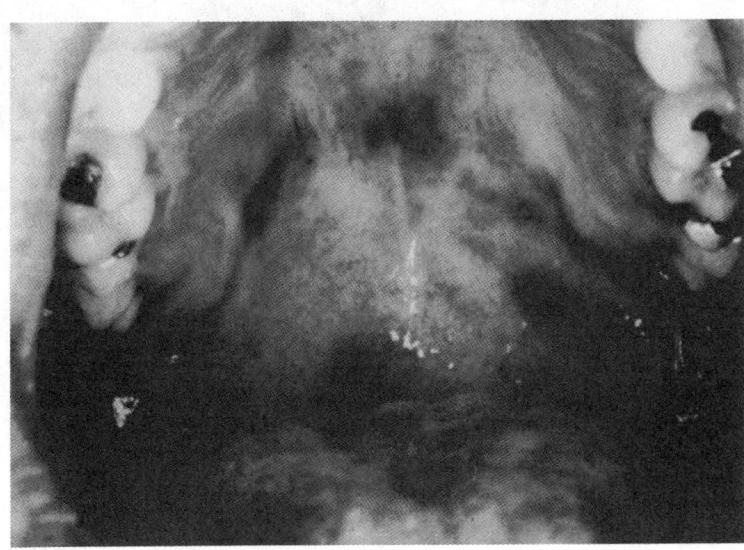

nicians use acyclovir, 400 to 800 mg 5 times daily, although this regimen has not been studied in AIDS patients. The course of varicella-zoster infection in AIDS patients is usually less than 2 weeks, and recovery is often complete. Cases of second and third episodes of varicella-zoster infection in AIDS patients have been observed.

ORAL MANIFESTATIONS

Oral lesions in HIV-infected subjects are a common clinical problem and may herald the onset of symptomatic immunodeficiency. Examination of the oral cavity by primary care physicians and dentists often provides the initial diagnosis of an AIDS-related condition.

Oral candidiasis is seen in most AIDS patients. In HIV-seropositive patients, thrush is a strong predictor of progression to AIDS. Thrush may appear as an exudative lesion—with typical "cottage cheese" material on the buccal mucosa, palate, and tongue—or as an erythematous lesion without exudate involving the palate. Diagnosis is confirmed by potassium hydroxide smears, although exudative thrush rarely requires this. Treatment is with topical agents, such as nystatin or clotrimazole. Oral ketoconazole is a highly effective agent for refractory thrush but may be associated with systemic toxicity. Thrush frequently recurs when therapy is withheld because of the patient's underlying immunodeficiency.

Viral hairy leukoplakia is a thrush-like lesion that is associated exclusively with HIV infection (Fig. 50-8). Hairy leukoplakia characteristically involves the lateral border of the tongue and appears as an exudative white lesion. Other parts of the tongue and buccal mucosa may also be involved. The cause of

hairy leukoplakia is thought to involve both HIV and Epstein-Barr virus. Hairy leukoplakia is rarely symptomatic, and specific therapy is generally not required.

Kaposi's sarcoma not uncommonly appears in the oral cavity of AIDS patients. Flat or nodular lesions are found on the hard and soft palates, gingiva, and tonsillar fossa (see Fig. 50-6). Large lesions may be painful or cause mechanical distortion of dentition, thereby impairing oral intake. Oral Kaposi's sarcoma can be treated with laser therapy or radiation in addition to systemic chemotherapy.

TREATMENT OF HIV INFECTION

Antiviral chemotherapy is an important strategy for retarding the progression of HIV infections. Various agents have shown activity against HIV in vitro, but currently only zidovudine (azidothymidine) is licensed for use in selected patients with HIV-related disease. Zidovudine has proved effective in reducing mortality and disease progression in patients with severe ARC or recent Pneumocystis carinii pneumonia. The drug is approved by the Food and Drug Administration for all HIV-infected patients who have had P. carinii pneumonia or who have symptomatic HIV infection and less than 200/CD4$^+$ lymphocytes μl. Therapy is extremely expensive, about $8000 per year. Although zidovudine has been shown to reduce circulating HIV antigen, it does not eradicate the infection and is not curative. Children have been treated with 180 mg/m^2 q6h, reduced to 120 mg/m^2 if severe anemia developed.

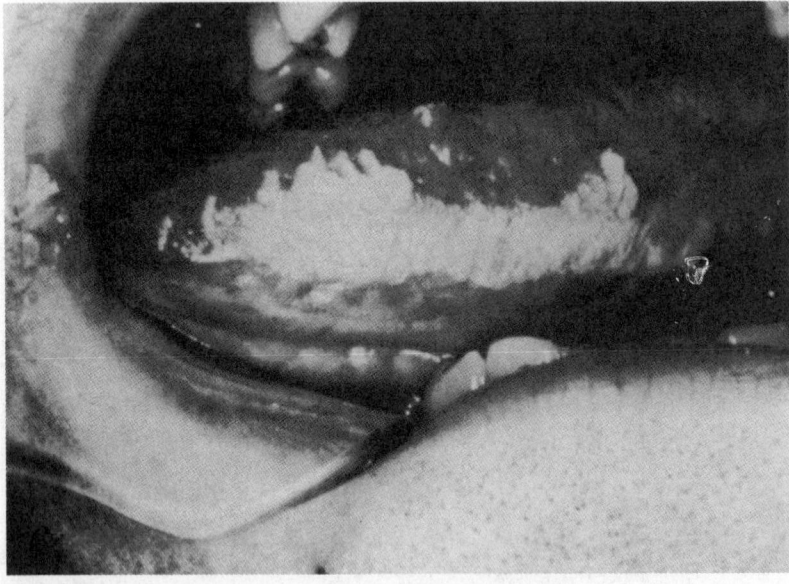

FIG. 50-8. Viral "hairy" leukoplakia on the margin of the tongue in an AIDS patient. (*Courtesy of J.S. Greenspan, PhD.*)

Zidovudine therapy is associated with bone marrow toxicity, and careful monitoring of patients is essential. Macrocytic anemia, granulocytopenia, and lymphopenia occur frequently and are more likely to appear in patients with low white blood cell counts and anemia at the onset of therapy. Zidovudine-related anemia is more severe in patients receiving high doses of acetaminophen, presumably because of acetaminophen's interference with glucuronidation of zidovudine. Children have been given IV immune globulin for prophylaxis.

RISK OF TRANSMISSION OF HIV TO AND FROM HEALTH CARE WORKERS

Since the identification of HIV as the cause of AIDS, the possibility of transmission of the agent to health care workers has been appreciated. Case reports of several health care workers shown to seroconvert to anti-HIV antibodies after exposure to HIV-infected patients has increased concern among individuals with potential occupational exposure to HIV. Occupational transmission of HIV has been documented in injuries involving needle stick punctures with transfer of blood and is strongly suspected in several instances of transmission by blood exposure to nonintact skin and mucous membranes. Several thousand health care workers, however, have been similarly exposed without seroconversion. Prospective studies of health care workers with known HIV needle stick exposure demonstrate that the risk of infection is substantially less than 0.5% per year.

Both the University of California, San Francisco, Task Force on AIDS and the CDC have issued recommendations for the prevention of occupational transmission of HIV. *Central to preventive measures are the use of latex gloves to prevent exposure to blood, secretions, saliva, and wounds; the use of protective eyewear and masks to prevent mucous membrane exposure; and careful attention to the disposal of needles and other instruments that may carry infectious material. Recapping of needles should be strictly avoided, as this practice is the most common cause of needle stick injuries.* All patients should be considered potentially infectious; asymptomatic individuals may be HIV-infected. A recent study of trauma patients in an urban emergency room showed a 3% seroprevalence of anti-HIV antibodies in individuals not known to be HIV-positive. *Routine screening of patients for anti-HIV antibodies is an impractical and inefficient preventive measure and should not be substituted for the broader policy of treating all patients and patient-derived specimens as capable of transmitting HIV.*

Transmission of HIV from physicians to patients has been reported. Careful use of protective equipment is essential.

EMERGENCY HEALTH CARE WORKERS AND PREVENTION OF AIDS

The Emergency Department (ED) may well be the place of first contact for unsuspected HIV-infected people and those at higher risk for infection (e.g., intravenous drug users, people with other sexually transmitted diseases). Because of the pivotal function of the emergency facility, opportunities for educating patients about modes of HIV transmission and "safer sex" should not be lost. Through posters, pamphlets, and direct counseling, there is great opportunity to reduce the epidemic spread of AIDS. Also, when a positive serologic result is returned, the patient may be referred to the local health department for contact tracing and notification, and should be directed to an appropriate source of medical care for evaluation and management—even if there are no obvious symptoms.

Some physicians, to protect the confidentiality of patients and families, resist recording AIDS as the cause of death. This practice is dangerous and rarely, if ever, suitable.

BIBLIOGRAPHY

GENERAL

Classification system for human T-lymphotropic virus type a III/lymphadenopathy-associated virus infections. M.M.W.R. 35:334, 1986.

Morgan, W.M., and Curran, J.: Acquired immunodeficiency syndrome: Current and future trends. Public Health Rep. 101:459, 1986.

Nzilambi N., DeCock, K.M., Forthal, D.N., et al.: The prevalence of infection with human immunodeficiency virus over a 10 year period in rural Zaire. N. Engl. J. Med. 318:276, 1988.

Revision of the CDC surveillance case definition for acquired immodeficiency syndrome. M.M.W.R. 36:Suppl, 1987, 1.

Update: AIDS—United States. M.M.W.R. 36:522, 1987.

PATHOGENESIS

Bowen, D.L., Lane, H.C., and Fauci, A.S.: Immunopathogenesis of the acquired immunodeficiency syndrome. Ann. Intern. Med. 103:704, 1985.

Ho, D.D., Pomerantz, R.J., and Kaplan, J.C.: Pathogenesis of infection with human immunodeficiency virus. N. Engl. J. Med. 317:278, 1987.

CLINICAL MANIFESTATIONS/DIAGNOSIS AND TREATMENT

Bigby, T.D., Margolskee, D., Curtis, J.L., et al.: The usefulness of induced sputum in the diagnosis of *Pneumocystis carinii* pneumonia in patients with the acquired immunodeficiency syndrome. Am. Rev. Respir. Dis. *138:*515, 1986.

Broaddus, C., Dake, M.D., Sulbarg, M.S., et al.: Bronchoalveolar lavage and transbronchial biopsy for the diagnosis of pulmonary infections in the acquired immunodeficiency syndrome. Ann. Intern. Med. *102:*747, 1985.

Chaisson, R.E., Schecter, G.F., Theuer, C.P. et al.: Tuberculosis in patients with acquired immunodeficiency syndrome: Clinical features, response to therapy and survival. Am. Rev. Respir. Dis. *136:*570, 1987.

Current trends: Classification system for human T lymphotropic virus type III/lymphadenopathy associated virus infections. M.M.W.R. *35:*334, 1988.

Ho, D.D., Rota, T.R., Schooley, R.T., et al.: Isolation of HTLV-III from cerebrospinal fluid and neural tissues of patients with neurologic syndromes related to the acquired immunodeficiency syndrome. N. Engl. J. Med. *313:*1493, 1985.

Hopewell, P.C. and Luce, J.M.: Pulmonary involvement in the acquired immunodeficiency syndrome. Chest *87:*104, 1985.

Leoung, G., Mill, J., Hopewell, P., et al: Dapsone-trimethoprim for *Pneumocystis carinii* pneumonia in the acquired immunodeficiency syndrome. Ann. Intern. Med. *105:*45, 1986.

Levy, R.M., Bredesen, D.E., and Rosenblum, M.L.: Neurological manifestations of the acquired immunodeficiency syndrome (AIDS): Experience at UCSF and review of the literature. J. Neurosurg. *62:*75, 1985.

Montgomery, A.B., Rebs, R.J., Luce, J.M., et al.: Aerosolized pentamidine as sole therapy for *Pneumocystis carinii* pneumonia in patients with acquired immunodeficiency syndrome. Lancet *2:*480, 1987.

Murray, J.F., Felton, C.P., Garay, S.M., et al.: Pulmonary complications of the acquired immunodeficiency syndrome: Report of a National Heart, Lung and Blood Institute workshop. N. Engl. J. Med. *310:*1682, 1984.

Redfield, R.R., Wright, D.C., and Tramont, E.C.: The Walter Reed staging classification of HTLV-III/LAV infection. N. Engl. J. Med. *314:*131, 1986.

Wharton, J.M., Coleman, D.L., Wofsy, C.B., et al.: Trimethoprim-sulfamethoxazole or pentamidine for *Pneumocystis carinii* pneumonia in the acquired immunodeficiency syndrome. Ann. Intern. Med. *105:*37, 1986.

HIV THERAPY

Fischl, M.A., Richman, D.D., Grieco, M.H., et al.: The efficacy of azidothymidine (AZT) in the treatment of patients with AIDS and AIDS related complex. N. Engl. J. Med. *317:*185, 1987.

INFECTION CONTROL

Baker, J.L., Kelen, G.D., Sivertson, K.T., and Quinn, T.C.: Unsuspected human immunodeficiency virus in critically ill emergency patients. JAMA *257:*2609, 1987.

Gerberding, J.L., and the University of California, San Francisco Task Force on AIDS: Recommended infection-control policies for patients with human immunodeficiency virus infection: An update. N. Engl. J. Med. *315:*1562, 1986.

Gerberding, J.L., Bryant-LeBlanc, C.E., Nelson, K., et al.: Risk of transmitting the human immunodeficiency virus, cytomegalovirus, and hepatitis B virus to health care workers exposed to patients with AIDS and AIDS-related conditions. J. Infect. Dis. *156:*1, 1987.

Henderson, D.K., Saah, A.J., Zak, B.J., et al.: Risk of nosocomial infection with human T-cell lymphotropic virus type III/lymphadenopathy-associated virus in a large cohort of intensively exposed health care workers. Ann. Intern. Med. *104:*644, 1986.

Recommendations for prevention of HIV transmission in health-care settings. M.M.W.R. *36*(Suppl):2S, 1987.

PULMONARY INFECTION IN THE HIV-INFECTED PATIENT

Sanjiv Sharma and Aaron E. Glatt

CAPSULE

Human immunodeficiency virus (HIV) infection causes a progressive and irreversible depletion of the T-helper lymphocytes. T-helper cells (T4 cells), besides being central to the integrity of the host's cellular immune defense system, also seem to significantly influence the function of the humoral and the phagocytic limbs of the immune system. Table 50-11 shows how derangements in the different parts of the defense system lead to an increased predilection to infection by certain specific pathogens. As can be expected, infections, especially those against which the cellular immune defenses play an important role, occur with increased frequency in HIV-infected patients. Therapy directed against the HIV is still in the early stages of development. Therefore, the major diagnostic and therapeutic energies of the clinician are currently directed toward the management of these opportunistic infections.

Pulmonary infections are by far the most frequent and life-threatening, and are of major importance in the differential diagnosis of the febrile HIV-infected patient. Table 50-12 lists the different infectious as well as noninfectious causes of lung disease in HIV infected patients.

This review focuses primarily on pulmonary Pneumocystis carinii and Mycobacterium tuberculosis and briefly discusses other pulmonary diseases encountered in HIV-infected patients.

TABLE 50-11. PREDILECTION TO INFECTION BY PATHOGENS

Host Defense Defect	Pathogens
Granulocytopenia	Gram-negative bacilli
	Escherichia coli
	Pseudomonas aeruginosa
	Klebsiella pneumoniae
	Gram-positive bacilli
	Staphylococcus aureus
	Staphylococcus epidermidis species
	Fungi
	Candida
	Aspergillus
T Cell Defect	Viruses
	Varicella zoster virus
	Herpes simplex virus
	Cytcomegalovirus
	JC virus
	? Adenovirus
	Bacteria
	Listeria monocytogenes
	Salmonella
	Mycobacteria
	Nocardia asteroides
	Legionella
	Mycobacteria
	Fungi
	Candida albicans
	Pneumocystis carinii*
	Cryptococcus neoformans
	Histoplasma capsulatum
	Coccidioides immitis
	Protozoa
	Toxoplasma gondii
	Isospora belli
	Cryptosporidium
	Helminth
	Strongyloides stercoralis
B cell defect	Streptococcus penumoniae
	Hemophilus influenzae

* Previously considered a protozoan

TABLE 50-12. PULMONARY COMPLICATIONS IN HIV INFECTED PATIENTS

I. Infectious Complications	
Protozoal:	Toxoplasma gondii
	Strongyloides stercoralis
Fungal:	Pneumocystis carinii*
	Cryptococcus neoformans*
	Candida albicans
	Coccidioides†
	Histoplasma capsulatum†
Mycobacterial:	Mycobacterium tuberculosis*
	Mycobacterium avium intracellulare complex
Bacterial:	Streptococcus pneumoniae*
	Hemophilus influenzae*
	Staphylococcus aureus
	Nocardia asteroides
Virus	Cytomegalovirus*
	Herpes simplex
II. Noninfectious Complications	
Neoplastic:	Kaposi's sarcoma
	Lymphoma
Non-neoplastic:	Lymphoid interstitial pneumonitis‡
	Nonspecific interstitial pneumonitis*

* Common in HIV infected patients.
† Common in endemic areas.
‡ Mostly in children.

GENERAL FEATURES OF PULMONARY INVOLVEMENT IN HIV-INFECTED PATIENTS

EPIDEMIOLOGY AND PATHOGENESIS

Pulmonary involvement occurs at some point in almost all HIV-infected patients. In two-thirds of these patients, Pneumocystis carinii pneumonia (PCP) occurs as the first opportunistic infection. Pneumocystis carinii infection in an HIV-infected patient is one of the Center for Disease Control's *AIDS case-defining* infection.[1] (See Chapter 50 for more details). Mycobacterium tuberculosis infection often precedes the diagnosis of AIDS and has been labeled a sentinel infection of AIDS. Extrapulmonary tuberculosis in an HIV-infected patient is now included in the Center for Disease Control's AIDS case-defining infection list; pulmonary tuberculosis *may* be added at a future date.

An increasing incidence of Mycobacterium tuberculosis infection and pyogenic pneumonia has been noted, and similarly childhood lymphoid pneumonia has been increasing in frequency. Legionella pneumonia appears to be decreasing.[2]

Most of the organisms that take advantage of the T-cell defect share common pathogenic characteristics. After initial infection, these organisms are capable of persisting intracellularly for years (latent phase) and can reactivate when cellular immunity wanes (as in worsening HIV-induced immunosuppression). This latent infection can sometimes be recognized, e.g., a significantly reactive tuberculin test indicating previous infection with Mycobacterium tuberculosis. Such individuals are candidates for preventive treatment, e.g., INH 300 mg per day to prevent reactivation of tuberculosis.

Knowledge of the place of origin and history of travel for an individual patient and the geographic distribution of different organisms helps in the diagnosis of HIV-associated pulmonary infections. For example, coccidioidomycosis is a major HIV-associated pulmonary pathogen in the Southwest United States (San Joaquin Valley Area); histoplasmosis is of great concern in the Ohio River Valley.

Multiple pulmonary pathogens may occur simultaneously, e.g., Pneumocystis carinii and concurrent Cytomegalovirus pneumonia; Pneumocystis and tuberculosis; and tuberculosis and bacterial pneumonias.

Pulmonary and other infections tend to be more severe and disseminated in an HIV-infected host than the same infection occurring in a non-HIV infected host.

Tuberculosis is the only common pulmonary pathogen that is contagious to the health care personnel taking care of the HIV-infected patient.

DIAGNOSTIC APPROACH

HISTORY AND PHYSICAL EXAMINATION

The history and physical examination form the base for building a differential diagnosis of HIV infection-associated pulmonary disease. By carefully assessing the duration of symptoms, their progression, severity, and associated findings, one may be able to form a clinical impression of the likely pathogen. In general, Pneumocystis carinii pneumonia has an indolent presentation with a history of progressive fatigue, exertional dyspnea, low-grade fevers and cough (usually only mildly productive if productive at all) stretching over the previous few weeks, or even months. Bacterial pneumonias tend to have a more acute course marked with higher fever, cough, expectoration of purulent phlegm, and marked dyspnea. When violaceous skin lesions are seen on a patient presenting with pulmonary symptoms and chest x-ray abnormalities, Kaposi's sarcoma involvement of the lung is a possibility. Likewise, exposure to tuberculosis, past PPD positivity, careful travel history, and geographic background may clue one into specific causes. Frequently, however, the presentation of many of these pulmonary pathogens is similar and the physical examination is equally nonspecific; further diagnostic work-up is required to allow more specific treatment.

CHEST X RAY

The chest x ray is abnormal in the vast majority of HIV-infected patients with pulmonary disease. Pneumocystis classically presents with diffuse bilateral infiltrates, as can cytomegalovirus pneumonia and Mycobacterium avium-intercellulare infections. Bacterial processes present more frequently as focal areas of consolidation. Tuberculosis in HIV patients is often associated with middle and lower lung zone infiltrates and hilar lymphadenopathy as opposed to the classic upper lobe/apical abnormalities previously seen. One must always keep in mind, however, that any process presents in many different ways in an HIV-infected patient, and exceptions are the rule.

COMPUTED TOMOGRAPHIC SCAN AND MAGNETIC RESONANCE IMAGING

Computed tomographic (CT) scan and magnetic resonance imaging (MRI) are of limited value in evaluating pulmonary problems in HIV-infected patients, and should be reserved for specific indications such as aiding thoracentesis or guiding the bronchoscopist or the mediastinoscopist to areas of high yield for biopsy. Newer techniques currently under investigation, however, may allow the earlier diagnosis and detection of pulmonary disease in patients with normal/nondiagnostic noninvasive workup.

GALLIUM SCAN

Gallium lung scanning may be useful in febrile HIV-infected individuals with minimal pulmonary symptoms, who have a normal or equivocal chest x ray. In such patients, a "negative" gallium scan usually indicates that the infection is probably extrapulmonary, and more invasive pulmonary procedures may be obviated. In the presence of objective respiratory abnormalities, however, further work-up may still be indicated. Abnormal gallium scans are usually nonspecific and require further diagnostic testing.

ARTERIAL BLOOD GAS STUDY

Arterial blood gas study is a most useful test in evaluating pulmonary disease in HIV-infected patients. Hypoxemia is common but *not* invariably present. Hypoxemia, with or without an elevated alveolar-to-arterial oxygen gradient, indicates significant disease and requires further investigation. A normal arterial blood gas study does not exclude pulmonary pathology, and if clinical suspicion is still present, further work-up is mandated.

SPUTUM EXAMINATION

Sputum induction and analysis is one of the most important, relatively noninvasive, tests, and can obviate the need for more dangerous diagnostic procedures. Pneumocystis carinii and Mycobacterium tuberculosis are the most important organisms that should be searched for with specific sputum staining techniques. Bacterial culture (other than mycobacterial) is unfortunately of little value in these patients, and currently no technology exists to culture Pneumocystis. Nonbronchoscopic lavage (usually in intubated patients) is also valuable in obtaining good specimens for staining.

BRONCHOSCOPY

Bronchoscopic bronchoalveolar lavage (with or without transbronchial lung biopsies) is the definitive procedure for most HIV-positive patients with pulmonary symptomatology. A combination of bronchoalveolar lavage and transbronchial biopsy carries a high diagnostic yield (especially for evaluating Pneumocystis carinii pneumonia and tuberculosis.)[2,3]

OPEN-LUNG BIOPSY

Open-lung biopsy is occasionally required to establish a diagnosis, especially in patients unable to tolerate fiberoptic bronchoscopy or when certain causes are especially considered (i.e., Kaposi's sarcoma, lymphoma). Otherwise, open-lung biopsy is an invasive and potentially dangerous procedure reserved for patients who have had full nondiagnostic evaluations, yet remain with significant disease and symptoms that are potentially treatable.

SPECIFIC PATHOGENS

PNEUMOCYSTIS CARINII

Pneumocystis carinii is the commonest cause of opportunistic infection in HIV-infected patients. Approximately 60 to 65% of AIDS patients have Pneumocystis carinii pneumonia, either alone or in combination with Kaposi's sarcoma as their index diagnosis.[2,4,5] Eventually, over 80% of AIDS patients develop P. carinii pneumonia, and it is projected that, by 1991, over 100,000 cases of P. carinii pneumonia will have been reported in the United States alone. Prophylaxis and earlier intervention and diagnosis are essential to combat this preventable and usually treatable disease.

Microbiology and Pathogenesis. Pneumocystis carinii was initially classified as a protozoan but has more recently been described as a fungus. Two different forms may be present in the pulmonary alveolar matrix: cysts (largest form, 6 to 7 microns in diameter) and trophozoites (1 to 5 microns). A complicated intra- and extracellular life cycle has also been described. Cysts stain brown-black with Grocott-Gomori methanamine silver nitrate and numerous other stains and

techniques can be used to show either the cysts, trophozoites, or both. Pneumocystis is ubiquitous in distribution. Asymptomatic "infection" is common at a young age in the immunocompetent host. HIV infection, Hodgkin's disease, acute lymphocytic leukemia, steroids, malnutrition, and immunosuppressive agents increase susceptibility to P. carinii pneumonia. Available evidence suggests that pneumonia results from reactivation of latent foci. Infection is usually confined to the lungs, although this changes with the advent of aerosolized pentamidine prophylaxis and therapy. Even before the advent of such therapy, over 25 reports documenting disseminated or localized extrapulmonary infection have been described.

Clinical Features and Screening Tests. The history and physical examination may be dominated by nonspecific features of HIV infection itself (fever, fatigue, weight loss) or concurrent pulmonary as well as nonpulmonary infections. Patients can occasionally present with an acute illness characterized by high fevers, cough, dyspnea, dry rales and respiratory failure; more often, however, there is a mild subtle prolonged (weeks to months) prehospitalization history of slowly progressive dyspnea on exertion, low-grade fevers, with a nonproductive (or minimally productive, white phlegm) cough. Aggressive investigation of new "minor" symptoms often leads to early diagnosis and presumbly better prognosis with earlier intervention.

The most common pattern seen on chest x ray is diffuse bilateral interstitial infiltrates,[2,5,6] however, a completely normal chest x ray is seen in 5 to 10% of cases. Atypical patterns are seen in about a third of x rays; these include unilateral infiltrates, localized infiltrates, lobar or segmental consolidation, solitary pulmonary nodules, cysts, honeycomb pattern, and rarely, pneumothorax. Isolated apical disease may be seen in patients on aerosolized pentamidine prophylaxis.

Pulmonary function tests lack specificity when applied to the diagnosis of P. carinii pneumonia and are not routinely indicated. Diffusion capacity of the lungs is decreased in P. carinii pneumonia and in patients with IV drug abuse history or any chronic diffuse pulmonary disease, and these tests fail to differentiate among them. Arterial blood gas study, however, is a relatively simple, readily available test that is useful in evaluating the significance of even minor complaints. In the setting of minimal symptoms and a normal chest x ray, a normal blood gas analysis may allow postponement (or a more leisurely work-up) of further tests. Significant hypoxemia or an elevated alveolar-to-arterial oxygen gradient (P (A-a)02 gradient) in a relatively healthy patient with mild pulmonary symptoms, however, suggests the need for a more definitive diagnostic work-up.

Measurement of P(A-a)02 after exercise is more sensitive than resting P(A-a)02 in the evaluation of the HIV-infected patient for Pneumocystis pneumonia. After 1½ minutes of exercise, a significant increase in the alveolar-to-arterial oxygen gradient is a sensitive indicator of P. carinii pneumonia in patients with normal chest x rays and mild pulmonary symptoms.[7]

Gallium scan of the lung is a sensitive test that lacks specificity. Specificity is improved if only a diffusely intense pulmonary uptake of gallium is considered to be "positive," but this may compromise sensitivity in patients on whom the test is most frequently used, i.e., those with minimal disease and minimal objective abnormalities. Thus, although both pulmonary function tests and gallium scan may have some clinically useful role in the evaluation of the HIV-infected patient with mild pulmonary symptoms and a normal or equivocal chest x rays, patients with more significant illness and/or objective abnormalities need a specific diagnostic test (or empiric trial of therapy).

P. Carinii Pneumonia.   *Diagnostic Studies.* Although patients with P. carinii pneumonia often have non-productive cough, adequate sputum specimens can be obtained by having the patient inhale an aerosol of hypertonic saline, produced by ultrasonic nebulization. With appropriate analysis, the reported yield for P. carinii by this technique is greater than 50% and in some hands approaches 90%. False positives are rare and are usually attributed to artifact or misreading. Unfortunately, not enough time is usually spent on obtaining a proper specimen, and an experienced observer (using the best stains or preparations) is essential to duplicate the successful yields of sputum induction technology. Bronchoscopic bronchoalveolar lavage alone has a high (more than 90%) sensitivity for the diagnosis of P. carinii pneumonia. Unless there is a focal abnormality of the chest x ray and/or transbronchial biopsy is indicated, the procedure is done without fluroscopic guidance. Transbronchial biopsy through the fiberoptic bronchoscope can be complicated by hemorrhage and pneumothorax, and is usually not necessary for diagnosing pneumocystis. In an HIV-infected patient presenting with a rapidly progressive clinical deterioration without pulmonary symptoms and abnormal chest x ray, fiberoptic bronchoscopy is the procedure of choice to rapidly establish the diagnosis of P. carinii pneumonia and document institution of appropriate treatment. Treatment can be begun before the procedure and does not appreciably decrease the sensitivity in HIV-infected patients. Open lung biopsy is rarely necessary and is reserved for the uncommon situations in which induced sputum and fiberoptic bronchoscopy (with bronchoalveolar lavage and biopsy) (possibly even repeated) have not yielded the diagnosis or cannot be technically done. Patients at a higher risk of developing complications from transbronchial biopsy (i.e., patients with an incorrigible coagulopathy) may also benefit from open-lung biopsy, if the bronchoalveolar lavage is negative for P. carinii.

Treatment. Treatment of pneumocystis is initiated with trimethoprim (15 to 20 mg per kg per day) and sulfamethoxazole (75 to 100 mg per kg per day, available as the combination Bactrim, Septra, Cotrimoxazole, etc.) Alternatively, pentamidine isethionate (4 mg. per kilogram of body weight per day) may be used.[2,4,5] Both regimens appear equally efficacious. Trimethoprim/sulfamethoxazole has the advantage of providing coverage against a concurrent bacterial pathogen (i.e, Hemophilus or pneumococcal pneumonia). Furthermore, in the mildly to moderately ill patient, it can be given orally if there is no question of compliance, gastrointestinal absorption, and tolerance, and thus may obviate the need for admission. Pentamidine should be considered in patients with a previous history of significant allergic reaction to sulfa-containing drugs. Patients who require stringent fluid restriction may also benefit from pentamidine because IV administration of trimethoprim/sulfamethoxazole often requires the administration of more than a liter of fluid daily.

The response rate to an initial infection with P. Carinii in the HIV-infected patient approaches 80 to 90%, with response somewhat poorer for subsequent episodes. Response to therapy, however, may be slow. Patients who truly fail on one regimen rarely respond to the other agent, but it is appropriate to try switching regimens after 5 to 7 days of treatment if there is no clinical response or the patient's condition worsens. Chest x ray may take weeks to months (if ever) to clear, and cystic forms of P. carinii may persist in the alveoli for weeks to months after initiation of effective treatment. Optimum duration of treatment is unclear; 3 weeks is commonly recommended, but shorter or longer courses may be necessary, and should be individualized by severity, rapidity of response, route of therapy, and toxicity.

In mild to moderate disease, outcome of therapy is unrelated to the route of administration. Trimethoprim/sulfamethoxazole should be given orally if compliance and absorption are not problems. This allows tremendous cost savings (in both hospitalization and drug costs), is highly beneficial to the patient, and mitigates somewhat the toxicity of treatment. Intramuscular pentamidine is associated with painful sterile abscesses and slow intravenous administration (over 1 to 2 hours) is the preferred method of administration. Preliminary data suggest that daily inhaled pentamidine may be equally effective and less toxic in mild to moderate cases, but requires further investigation for treatment of acute pneumocystis pneumonia.

The major problem with currently available therapy is the high incidence of adverse consequences. Of special concern are the irreversible and dose-limiting side effects.

An adverse reaction to either trimethoprim/sulfamethoxazole or pentamidine occurs in 20 to 85% of HIV-infected patients. Rash, fever, leukopenia, hyponatremia, and elevated levels of transaminases are frequently observed during therapy with trimethoprim/sulfamethoxazole. Leukopenia, azotemia, dysglycemias, hypotension, pancreatitis, and abnormal liver function tests are common with pentamidine. Irreversible diabetes mellitus is of particular concern because it is not predictable and may require life-long institution of insulin. Many cases of "drug toxicity"/allergy do *not* necessarily require discontinuation of therapy; reduction of dose or symptomatic treatment may be sufficient in many cases, and the patient will eventually be able to tolerate the drug.

Alternative regimens are under investigation. Dapsone (100 mg per day), plus trimethoprim, trimetrexate, eflornithine (DFMO), and others are being evaluated, but the research for a less toxic, more efficacious agent is still ongoing. Steroids remain controversial, but may benefit selected patients; they should not be routinely used in mild to moderate disease. They may be considered in rapidly worsening patients with respiratory distress, in whom it is felt that a steroid-responsive acute inflammatory process may be causing the sudden downward progression. Prospective double-blind studies, however, are lacking, and management must remain individualized.

Concurrent Infections. Concomitant pulmonary infections as well as noninfectious processes are frequently present in AIDS patients infected with Pneumocystis carinii. Kales and coworkers noted concurrent Mycobacterium tuberculosis, Mycobacterium avium intercellulare, Cytomegalovirus, Cryptococcus, or Toxoplasma pneumonitis in 10% of their HIV-infected patients with P. carinii pneumonia.[8] When patients do not respond to what appears to be appropriate treatment, a diligent search should be made for additional pathogens before the patient is labeled a treatment failure.

AIDS versus Non-AIDS Immunocompromised Patients. As discussed, HIV-related P. carinii pneumonia presents with a subacute insidious course, as opposed to the more rapidly progressive pulmonary decompensation seen in other immunocompromised hosts with P. carinii pneumonia. AIDS patients also seem to have a slower clinical and radiologic response to treatment than non-AIDS patients with P. carinii infections.[9]

Recurrence and Prophylaxis. After successful treatment, recurrence of Pneumocystis remains a major problem; relapse rates of 18% at 6 months, 46% at 9 months, and 65% at 18 months have been reported. Therefore, suppressive therapy (secondary prophylaxis) is necessary after treatment. Trimethroprim/sulfamethazole is an effective agent, but side effects may limit its use. If tolerated, Trimethoprim/Sulfamethoxazole appears to be essentially 100% effective (although most of the data are from non-HIV infected patients at high risk for PCP) and prevents systemic and upper lobe disease as well. It is relatively inexpensive, may provide prophylaxis and treatment against other HIV-associated infections, and is probably the preferred treatment at the present time.

Optimum dosage is unknown; a single daily or twice-daily double-strength tablet (160 to 800 mg) is frequently given.[4]

Preliminary information suggests that once monthly (300 mg) aerosolized pentamidine (using the Respirgard II4A system) is also effective in preventing recurrences. Problems, however, have arisen with aerosolization treatment. Efficacy is not 100%; atypical recurrences, especially upper lobe and disseminated Pneumocystis infections have occurred with alarming frequency. In addition, tuberculosis must be ruled out to prevent spread of tuberculosis throughout the staff and hospital, as has already been reported. Finally, this treatment is expensive ($2000 to 3000 per year), although toxicity and compliance problems are minimal.

Primary prophylaxis for high-risk patients is under intense investigation. HIV-infected patients with less than 200 T4 cells/cu mm are clearly at a righ risk of developing Pneumocystis carinii pneumonia, and should be placed on preventive therapy. Fischel et al. reported excellent efficacy with TMP/SMX (160 mg of trimethoprium and 800 mg of sulfamethoxazole) twice a day.[10] Preliminary work by Metroka and colleagues showed similar results with the use of dapsone (100 mg per day) in preventing P. Carinii pneumonia.[11] Among 250 patients with fewer than 200 T4 cells per cubic millimeter, only 1 patient acquired P. Carinii pneumonia, even though 55 other opportunistic infections were observed. Inhaled pentamidine is also effective (with the reservations outlined previously under secondary prophylaxis) and should be considered in patients unable to take the other regimens.

MYCOBACTERIUM TUBERCULOSIS

Of the mycobacteria, Mycobacterium avium-intracellulare complex is most frequently isolated in patients infected with HIV. Recent reports, however, verify an increasing incidence of Mycobacterium tuberculosis among patients with HIV infection. Tuberculosis is one of the few AIDS-related infections that is contagious. Furthermore, it shows a good response to therapeutic as well as preventive measures, even in this population. Therefore, it is important to expeditiously recognize and treat this infection in patients with HIV.

Epidemiology. Since national tuberculosis recording was started in 1953, there was a consistent decline in the number of new tuberculosis cases occurring in the United States until 1986, when an actual increase in the number of new reported cases was noted.[12,13] This increase is predominantly caused by the increasing incidence of tuberculosis in patients with HIV infection. Epidemiologic studies have shown that the association between tuberculosis and HIV infection is especially striking among groups in which there is a high prevalence of tuberculosis infection, e.g. Haitians, prisoners, IV drug abusers, and inner-city residents. Petchenik and colleagues reported a 79 to 91%

incidence of prior exposure (as shown by a significantly reacting tuberculin test) in Haitian immigrants in Florida.[14] They also showed that 60% of Haitian AIDS patients had tuberculosis. Although striking, these statistics should not be surprising. Tuberculosis is the prototypic infectious disease associated with a defective cellular immunity. The degree of immunosuppression required to reactivate *M. tuberculosis* appears to be lower than that required to reactivate other opportunistic pathogens; consequently, its occurrence in HIV-infected patients often predates the diagnosis of AIDS. Extrapulmonary tuberculosis occurs more commonly in HIV-infected patients, comprising 42 to 76% of all reported tuberculosis cases in this group, compared to 12.7% of national tuberculosis cases considered as a whole. Extrapulmonary tuberculosis and the presence of a positive HIV serology are now among the CDC criteria for defining AIDS.

Clinical Features. Tuberculosis usually precedes other opportunistic infections by 1 month to 2 or more years, but may occur concomitantly with or even after these other opportunistic infections strike the patient with HIV infection. Most tuberculous infections in this population occur as a result of reactivating of a latent tuberculous focus; however, HIV-infected individuals occasionally present with a progressive primary disease. Lymphatic and disseminated (i.e., miliary tuberculosis or the involvement of two or more noncontiguous sites) occurs frequently in HIV-infected patients, and brain abscesses, gastrointestinal tract fistulae, skin, rectal, testicular and soft tissue abscesses, abdominal masses, mediastinal and retroperitoneal lymphadenopathy are frequently seen. Tuberculosis may present still with the classical symptoms, i.e., an indolent course lasting weeks to months characterized by low-grade fevers, night sweats, malaise, anorexia, and weight loss, with or without pulmonary and/or extrapulmonary organ system symptomatology such as productive cough, hemoptysis, diarrhea, focal neurologic signs, frank meningitic features, and local masses.

Diagnosis The radiographic picture is often atypical. Although epidemiologic evidence indicates that most of the tuberculosis occurs as a result of reactivation, the chest x rays tend to follow the patterns seen in primary tuberculosis. This is understandable in view of the severe immune defect in the host. Thus, hilar or mediastinal lymphadenopathy with or without noncavitating pulmonary infiltrates is common. The infiltrates are located with approximately equal frequency in the upper and lower lung fields. Miliary infiltrates are common; cavity formation is uncommon.[2,6,14]

A high index of suspicion is recommended in all HIV-infected patients, especially in those at higher risk for tuberculosis; i.e., Haitians, IV drug abusers, prisoners, homeless, "shelter" dwellers, lower socioeconomic groups, inner-city residents, and patients with a history of a significant reaction to tuberculin test. Conversely, in patients with proven tuberculosis, the physician should have a high index of suspicion for concomitant HIV infection, especially if there is an atypical presentation or extrapulmonary disease. A detailed "risk" history is essential to help determine the likelihood of HIV infection, but HIV testing is suggested often, even with a noncontributory history.

HIV-infected persons with pulmonary tuberculosis are less likely to have positive acid fast sputum smears than are persons with pulmonary tuberculosis who are not infected with HIV. Sputum smears still show acid-fast bacilli in up to 45% of cases and should be carefully examined routinely in HIV patients presenting with pulmonary symptoms.

If the sputum smear is nondiagnostic and clinical evidence suggests intrathoracic pulmonary parenchymal disease (e.g., abnormal chest x ray, arterial blood gas, diffusion capacity), a fiberoptic bronchoscopy with bronchoalveolar lavage and transbronchial biopsy should be performed. Granuloma formation is less common in HIV-infected patients who develop tuberculosis, reflecting their poor helper T-cell function. M. tuberculosis can also be cultured from urine, blood, stools, and pleural fluid; culture as well as histopathologic examination may also be performed on biopsy specimens obtained from marrow, lymph nodes, brain, liver, and pleura.

The tuberculin test remains positive in many HIV-infected patients who develop tuberculosis, especially in those with less immunosuppression. A negative tuberculin test does *not* exclude previous exposure or currently active disease.

Treatment. Antituberculosis chemotherapy should be started whenever acid-fast bacilli are identified from a specimen obtained from a patient with proven or suspected HIV infection. There is a dearth of prospective data on the treatment of HIV-related tuberculosis, although the limited information available indicates that the initial response to therapy in HIV-infected patients is not substantially worse than in patients without HIV infection. Petchenik et al. demonstrated that the acid-fast bacilli were cleared from the sputum in 1 to 4 months.[14] The joint position paper of ATS/CDC (1986) recommends treatment with isoniazid (INH), rifampin, and pyrazinamide for the first 2 months (ethambutol or streptomycin may be added during these 2 months, especially if drug resistance is suspected or if disseminated disease or central nervous system disease is present). After that, INH and rifampin alone (if the patient is sensitive) should be continued for a minimum total of 9 months and for at least 6 months after documented culture conversion.[12]

Prophylaxis. Whether prolonged "maintenance" therapy with INH is necessary and of any benefit in preventing relapse is unknown and is not routinely advocated after completion of an antituberculous regimen. Any HIV-infected individual who shows a greater than 5 mm reaction to tuberculin skin test should be given a course of Isoniazid, 300 mg per day for prophylaxis (6 months to 1 year, or longer), regardless of age, provided that active tuberculosis infection has been excluded.

CYTOMEGALOVIRUS (CMV)

The pathogenic importance of CMV as a cause of pneumonitis is controversial. Epidemiologic studies do not show a relationship between "infection" and disease. Disseminated CMV is found in most AIDS patients at autopsy. Nearly 100% of homosexual HIV-positive men were found to be seropositive for CMV in one study, and more than half were shedding CMV in urine.[15]

Microbiology and Pathogenesis. CMV belongs to the herpesvirus group. Herpesviruses cause primary, latent, or recurrent infections. Primary infection refers to CMV infecting a previously uninfected host. In immunocompetent hosts, primary CMV infection is often a benign subclinical event, but in pregnant women it carries a risk of transplacental transfer to the fetus and resultant congenital CMV disease. After primary infection, the viral genome incorporates itself in the human DNA and persists silently for years. During periods of suppression of cellular immunity, the latent viral genome can lead to active recurrent infection with viral shedding.

Active CMV infection is common in HIV-positive patients, and pathologic findings of CMV infection may be seen in lungs, liver, GI tract, eyes, adrenals, and even the brain. (For detailed discussion of nonpulmonary CMV infection, see previous subchapter.)

Diagnosis of Cytomegalovirus Pneumonia. To clearly diagnose CMV as a cause of pneumonia in an AIDS patient, the following criteria must be met: (1) a clinical constellation of fever, hypoxemia and diffuse pulmonary infiltrates; (2) histopathologic evidence of CMV cytopathic effect (typical intranuclear and intracytoplasmic inclusion bodies) in lung tissue, usually with a positive cell culture, and (3) absence of evidence of other infectious or neoplastic pulmonary process. There is a dearth of cases in literature that meet these criteria, and the benefits of treatment remain controversial. Current review of the literature does not suggest a significant benefit using ganciclovir (formerly DHPG) routinely. Intense investigation is under way to determine the necessity and efficacy of therapy with other agents.

BACTERIAL PNEUMONIAS

Bacterial pneumonias occur with increased frequency in the HIV-infected population and appear to be associated with a higher morbidity, mortality, and recurrence risk. As expected, *Legionella pneumophila* and *Nocardia asteroides*, known to cause infections in patients with impaired T-cell function, have been reported in HIV-infected patients. However, as HIV affects other limbs of the immune system, i.e., B cells as well as neutrophils, pneumococcal and Hemophilus influenzae pneumonia and/or bacteremia are frequently encountered. Patients with HIV infection who require prolonged hospitalizations are at risk for nosocomial bacterial pneumonias; chemotherapy-induced neutropenia predisposes to bacterial infections, and alterations in mental status and multiple factors predispose to aspiration pneumonitis.

Diagnosis and Treatment. Most of the community-acquired pneumonias seen in HIV-infected patients are caused by either Streptococcus pneumoniae or Hemophilus influenzae. The clinical presentation is one of an acute onset of fever, productive cough, shortness of breath, and chest pain with infiltrates on the chest x ray. The clinical course is usually more severe, with a longer period before defervescence, slower response to antibiotics, and an increased incidence of complications (i.e., empyema). It is noteworthy that H. influenzae can cause diffuse bilateral infiltrates indistinguishable from those of Pneumocystis carinii pneumonia. HIV-infected patients presenting with more acute pulmonary symptoms and diffuse bilateral infiltrates should receive antibiotic(s) with H. influenzae, as well as Pneumocystis coverage. Pneumococcal pneumonia usually presents with focal infiltrates. Empiric therapy should be started according to the clinical presentation without waiting for the culture results.

FUNGAL PNEUMONIA: CRYPTOCOCCUS NEOFORMANS

Cryptococcal disease, usually meningitis, is a common opportunistic infection in HIV-infected patients and has been discussed elsewhere. Concomitant cryptococcal pneumonia occurs frequently, whereas isolated pulmonary involvement is seen in only 4 to 7% of cases. Patients present with fever, weight loss, productive cough, and occasionally chest pain. Chest radiographs can show localized or diffuse infiltrates, mass lesions, and hilar-mediastinal lymphadenopathy. If cryptococcal pneumonia is suspected, serum cryptococcal antigen should be obtained. Sputum examination is occasionally helpful. Bronchoscopic lavage, especially if combined with a transbronchial biopsy, is sensitive in isolating cryptococci. Once cryptococcal pneumonia is documented, it is important to carefully rule out central nervous system or disseminated cryptococcal disease. Treatment is the same as outlined subsequently for meningitis.

HISTOPLASMA CAPSULATUM

Epidemiologic evidence suggests that most histoplasmosis in HIV-infected patients occurs because of the reactivation of latent infections. Patients, either presently or at some time in the past, resided in endemic areas. In almost all cases, histoplasmosis presents as a disseminated disease with pulmonary and constitutional symptoms (weight loss, malaise, fever, and chills) similar to tuberculosis.

Chest x rays can show diffuse infiltrates, a miliary pattern, nodular or cavity lesions, or adenopathy. Diagnosis is based on the presentation, serologic tests, sputum and bronchoscopic specimen examination. The initial response to amphotericin B is usually good; frequent relapses mandate maintenance treatment. Here, too, fluconazole may play an important role in both treatment and prophylaxis.

COCCIDIODES IMMITIS

Like histoplasmosis, coccidiodes immitis is reported primarily among HIV-infected patients living in endemic areas. Respiratory symptoms are more prominent in this disease than in histoplasmosis and include dry or productive cough, shortness of breath, and pleuritic chest pain. The most common pattern on chest x rays is diffuse bilateral infiltrates, which may be interstitial or nodular. Recommended therapy is a course of amphotericin B followed by maintenance treatment indefinitely. Fluconazole may also play a major role here.

CANDIDA AND ASPERGILLUS

Although candidiasis is the most common fungal infection seen in HIV-infected patients, pulmonary involvement is infrequent. Usually the diagnosis of pulmonary candidiasis is made only at autopsy, and it is usually part of disseminated candidiasis. The recommended treatment in the few cases diagnosed antemortem is amphotericin B; the role of fluconazole is under intense investigation.

Aspergillosis only rarely causes pulmonary infections in HIV-infected patients. This may be because of the relatively well-preserved neutrophil function in these patients.

KAPOSI'S SARCOMA (KS)

Kaposi's sarcoma involves the lungs in approximately 20% of HIV-infected patients with cutaneous Kaposi's.[16] The latter presents with violaceous lesions. Associated visceral involvement of the gastrointestinal tract, lymph nodes, and other organ systems is frequently present, but isolated pulmonary KS does occur. Pulmonary KS must be considered in the differential diagnosis of the HIV-infected patient presenting with pulmonary symptoms and an abnormal chest x ray. Clinical presentation of pulmonary KS frequently simulates that of opportunistic infections discussed above, i.e., infiltrates, with a reticulonodular or nodular pattern. Most patients have varying degrees of hypoxemia and a widened alveolar-to-arterial oxygen gradient.

Localized lesions may cause hoarseness (because of laryngeal involvement), stridor with upper airway obstruction symptomatology, wheezes, and even hemoptysis. Hilar and mediastinal adenopathy and pleural effusions are common.

Diagnosis and Treatment. Diagnostic yield of bronchoscopic specimens (i.e., lavage, endobronchial biopsy, and transbronchial biopsy) is less than 10%.,[3,16] This is because of the small sample size of the biopsied lung tissue. Crush artifacts, granulation tissue, and hemorrhage can mimic pulmonary KS lesions, and the distribution of KS in the lung is patchy and may be missed when small biopsy samples are taken. Open-lung biopsy increases the diagnostic yield to about 50%. HIV-infected patients with documented pulmonary KS have a dismal prognosis, with median survival duration between 2 and 4 months. Whole lung field irradiation, interferon, and combination chemotherapy have been tried, but the results are poor. It is important to exclude treatable opportunistic pulmonary infections with certainty before proceeding to the palliative treatment of pulmonary KS.

ACKNOWLEDGMENT

The authors wish to thank Graceann Puccio for her secretarial skills in helping prepare this manuscript.

REFERENCES

1. Centers for Disease Control: Revision of the CDC Surveillance case definition for acquired immunodeficiency syndrome. MMWR 36:1s, 1988.
2. Murray, J.F., Garay, S.M., Hopewell, P.C., et al.: NHLBI workshop summary. Pulmonary complications of the acquired immunodeficiency syndrome: An update. Report of the Second National Heart, Lung and Blood Institute Workshop. Am. Rev. Respir. Dis. 135:504, 1987.
3. Broaddus, C., Dake, M.D., Stulbarg, M.S., et al.: Bronchoalveolar lavage and transbronchial biopsy for the diagnosis of pulmonary infections in the acquired immune deficiency syndrome. Ann. Intern. Med. 102:747, 1985.
4. Glatt, A.E., Chirgwin, K., and Landesman, S.H.: Current concepts: Treatment of infections associated with human immunodeficiency virus. N. Engl. J. Med. 318:1439, 1988.
5. Hughes, W.T.: Pneumocystis carinii pneumonitis. Chest 85:810, 1984.
6. DeLorenzo, L.J., Huang, C.T., Maguire, G.P., et al.: Roentgenographic patterns of Pneumocystis carinii pneumonia in 104 patients with AIDS. Chest 91:323, 1987.
7. Stover, D.E., White, D.A., Romano, P.A., et al.: Spectrum of pulmonary disease associated with the acquired immune deficiency syndrome. Am. J. Med. 78:429, 1985.
8. Kales, C.P., Murren, J.R., Torres, R.A., et al.: Early prediction of in-hospital mortality for Pneumocystis carinii pneumonia in

the acquired immunodeficiency syndrome. Arch. Intern. Med. *147*:1413, 1987.

9. Kovacs, J.A., Hiemenz, J.W., and Macher, A.M.: Pneumocystis carinii pneumonia: A comparison between patients with the acquired immune deficiency syndrome and patients with other immunodeficiencies. Ann. Intern. Med. *100*:663, 1984.

10. Fischel, M.A., Richman, D.D., Grieco, M.H., et al.: The efficacy of azidothymidine (AZT) in the treatment of patients with AIDS and AIDS-related complex: A double-blind, placebo-controlled trial. N. Engl. J. Med. *317*:185, 1987.

11. Metroka, C.E., Lange, M., Braun, N., et al.: Successful chemoprophylaxis for Pneumocystis carinii pneumonia with dapsone in patients with AIDS and ARC. Presented at the Third International Conference on AIDS. Washington, DC, June 1–5, 1987 (abstract).

12. Joint position paper of the American Thoracic Society and the Centers for Disease Control: Mycobacterioses and the acquired immunodeficiency syndrome. Am. Rev. Respir. Dis. *136*:492, 1987.

13. Centers for disease control: Tuberculosis, Final data—United States 1986. MMWR *36*:817, 1988.

14. Petchenik, A.E., Cole, C., Russell, B.W., et al.: Tuberculosis, Atypical mycobacteriosis and the acquired immunodeficiency syndrome among Haitian and non-Haitian patients in south Florida. Ann. Intern. Med. *101*:641, 1984.

15. Mintz, L., Drew, W.L., Miner, R.C., and Braff, E.H.: Cytomegalovirus infections in homosexual men: An epidemiologic study. Ann. Intern. Med. *98*:326, 1983.

16. Garay, S.M., Belenko, M., Fazzini, E., et al.: Pulmonary manifestations of Kaposi's sarcoma. Chest *91*:39, 1987.

SEXUALLY TRANSMITTED DISEASES OTHER THAN AIDS

GENERAL PRESENTATION

Ralph K. della Ratta and Aaron E. Glatt

CAPSULE

Sexually transmitted diseases (STDs) are among the most common infectious diseases. Despite the availability of effective treatment, there has been a resurgence of STDs in industrialized nations since the early 1960s. Classic STDs, in addition to previously unrecognized ones (acquired immunodeficiency syndrome, for example) have had a great impact on society, in terms of both economic costs and human suffering.

Patients with STD often present for medical evaluation to the Emergency Department (ED). Indeed, the majority of patients with STDs are cared for by primary care physicians, especially emergency physicians.[1] Emergency physicians must recognize these diseases and initiate an appropriate diagnostic evaluation (Table 50-13). Empiric treatment must be provided in the ED when the diagnosis is not clear or when results of diagnostic modalities are not available initially. Arrangement of follow-up care is imperative. Concurrent infection with multiple organisms is not uncommon, and there are potential serious sequelae for both male and female patients and their sexual contacts if correct treatment is not given.

This chapter section explores the clinical presentation, diagnostic evaluation, and treatment of the four STD syndromes dealt with most commonly in the emergency department: (1) male urethritis, (2) mucopurulent cervicitis, (3) pelvic inflammatory disease (PID), and (4) genital ulceration. The acquired immunodeficiency syndrome (AIDS, previous subchapters), the urethral syndrome and vaginitis (Chap. 57) are not discussed in this section.

EPIDEMIOLOGY

All of the etiologic agents of STD are epidemiologically intimate, with the exception of genital herpes. They are characterized by a higher incidence in sexually active adolescents and young adults in large urban areas, and are often associated with the economically disadvantaged. The clinician must be aware of regional differences in prevalence of each agent.

It is suspected that a core group of highly effective transmitters of these infections contribute dispropor-

TABLE 50-13. COMMON SEXUALLY TRANSMITTED PATHOGENS

Organism	Disease
Bacteria	
Neisseria gonorrhoeae	Urethritis, cervicitis, PID, pharyngitis, proctitis, epididymitis, conjunctivitis, arthritis-dermatitis syndrome.
Treponema pallidum	Syphilis (primary, secondary, tertiary stages)
Hemophilus ducreyi	Chancroid
Calymmatobacterium granulomatis	Granuloma inguinale
Chlamydiae	
Chlamydia trachomatis	Urethritis, cervicitis, PID, proctitis, lymphogranuloma venereum, conjunctivitis, epididymitis
Mycoplasmas	
Mycoplasma hominis	PID, urethritis
Mycoplasma genitalis	PID, urethritis
Ureaplasma urealyticum	PID, urethritis
Viruses	
Herpes simplex virus (HSV)	Genital ulceration, proctitis
Human papillomavirus	Condyloma acuminatum, cervical carcinoma
Molluscum contagiosum virus	Molluscum contagiosum
Human immunodeficiency virus (HIV)	Acquired immunodeficiency syndrome
Protozoa	
Trichomonas vaginalis	Occasionally urethritis, vaginitis
Fungi	
Candida species	Balanitis, vaginitis

tionately to endemic levels of disease. This group includes a community reservoir of asymptomatic infection with gonococcus and Chlamydiae. Increasing incidence rates for many STDs may reflect improved case detection and reporting rates. The sexual revolution of the 1960s, however, with subsequent changes in sexual practices including premarital intercourse at increasingly younger ages, has certainly heightened the risk of disease.[2] Also, changes in contraceptive use from barrier methods (condom, diaphragm) to nonbarrier methods (oral contraceptives, intrauterine device) has increased risk.

PATHOPHYSIOLOGY

The pathophysiology of STDs depends not only on characteristics of the individual microorganism, but also on the immunocompetence of the host. Examples of STDs with differing pathogenetic mechanisms of disease are gonorrhea, syphilis, and genital herpes.

Gonorrhea is a paradigm for many infectious diseases. The initial pathogenetic event in gonorrhea is mucosal colonization. There are cell surface structures of the gonococcus that contribute to its pathogenesis and virulence. These include pili, outermembrane

proteins, lipopolysaccharide (endotoxin activity), and the release of IgA proteases.

In contrast, Treponema pallidum (the causative agent of syphilis) may penetrate normal mucosal membranes. The organism then causes a focal endarteritis with rapid dissemination by way of the lymphatic and blood systems. In genital herpes, after mucosal surface exposure to the herpes simplex virus, the virus replicates in epidermal or dermal cells. Replication of the virus is followed by spread to contiguous cells, resulting eventually in infection of sensory and/or autonomic neurons. Progressive cell destruction leads to vesicle formation within the epithelial cell layer.

MALE URETHRITIS

Male urethritis is a common problem in patients seen by primary care and emergency physicians. It is invariably sexually transmitted, with most cases caused by Neisseria gonorrhoeae (gonococcal urethritis) and Chlamydia trachomatis (the major cause of non-gonococcal urethritis-NGU), although the differential diagnosis also includes Trichomonas vaginalis, Herpes simplex virus, and genital mycoplasmas. Concurrent infections are not uncommon. The symptoms of urethritis in the male include urethral discharge, dysuria, and occasionally meatal pruritus. Physical examination findings include urethral discharge (with leukocytes on Gram stain of that discharge) occasionally associated with arthritis, conjunctivitis, dermatitis, and epididymitis. Flank and abdominal pain, fever, and hematuria are usually not found, and their presence suggests an infection other than urethritis. Clinical signs and symptoms are not reliable enough to distinguish gonococcal and nongonococcal urethritis.

Since 1984, gonorrhea is increasing in the United States, after a steady decline from 1976 to 1984. In 1987, there were 750,000 reported cases of gonococcal male urethritis. The incubation period for gonococcal urethritis is approximately 2 to 5 days. Presentation is hallmarked by the abrupt onset of both dysuria and a urethral discharge which is frequently copious and purulent. In men, gonorrhea may be asymptomatic or cause mild symptoms; only 10% of cases of male urethritis truly present in an asymptomatic fashion. In follow-up studies of male sexual contacts of women with newly diagnosed gonorrhea, however, up to 50% of the men may have mild symptoms, asymptomatic urethritis, or urethral colonization with gonococcus without a true urethritis. Asymptomatic cases serve as a reservoir for spread of gonorrhea in the community, and if untreated usually persist for several months until natural host defenses eradicate it. Coinfection of the gonococcus and Chlamydia trachomatis occurs in 20 to 30% of cases of male urethritis.

Laboratory confirmation of suspected cases of gonorrhea requires both microscopic examination of the urethral discharge and culture. If the urethral discharge is not readily apparent on physical examination, urethral "milking" from the base of the penis forward may elicit the discharge. If no discharge is forthcoming, a swab may be inserted with a rotational motion, 2 to 3 cm into the urethra to obtain a specimen for analysis and culture. Microscopic examination of the centrifuged sediment of the first 5 cc of a urine specimen may also reveal the leukocytes. An inflammatory urethral exudate is defined as $\geq$ 5 polymorphonuclear leukocytes (PMNs) per high-powered field of a Gram-stained urethral smear, or $\geq$ 15 PMNs per high-powered field of the centrifuged urine sediment.[3] The inflammatory urethral exudate may be more easily found on early morning examination before urination; early morning re-evaluation may be warranted when the diagnosis is unclear.

If an inflammatory urethral exudate is found, the Gram stain must be reviewed for the presence of gram-negative gonococci ("kidney bean"-shaped diplococci) within the PMNs. For symptomatic urethritis, the sensitivity of the Gram stain urethral smear for gonorrhea is 90 to 95%; the specificity approaches 100%. If the gram-negative organisms are not present within PMNs or their shape is not of the classical description, the smear is equivocal and the possibility of nongonococcal urethritis (NGU) must be enter-

tained. Culture for gonococcus, on selective media such as Thayer-Martin or chocolate agar, has a sensitivity of 95% regardless of the status of symptoms. Cultures should be obtained routinely in the evaluation of urethritis. Antibiotic-resistant Neisseria gonorrhoeae is a growing problem in the United States. Resistant strains have been isolated in all 50 states, but are much more common in certain areas such as New York and Florida.

NGU is approximately twice as common as gonoccocal urethritis in the United States. Exact figures are difficult to come by, however, because it is not a reportable disease. Chlamydia trachomatis is the major cause of NGU, with Ureaplasma urealyticum ("T-strain" mycoplasmas) making up the bulk of remaining cases. Other genital mycoplasmas, Trichomonas vaginalis, and Herpes simplex account for a small percentage of cases of urethritis. Mycoplasma genitalium, a fastidious and recently described organism, and anaerobic organisms are postulated as a cause of urethritis in homosexual men with NGU. Interestingly, homosexual men with NGU are almost never found to be infected with either Chlamydia trachomatis or Ureaplasma urealyticum.[3] In up to 20% of cases of NGU, no cause can be found even after a thorough workup. NGU, for the most part, has a longer incubation period (7 to 21 days) and milder symptoms than gonococcal urethritis. The longer incubation period explains the "postgonococcal urethritis" syndrome originally seen when concomitant gonococcal and chlamydial infection was treated with antigonococcal therapy only. The urethral discharge in NGU is often thinner, mucoid or watery, less purulent, and smaller in quantity than in gonococcal urethritis. Asymptomatic NGU may approach 20% of cases; these cases serve as a reservoir of spread of NGU in the community.

Diagnosis of NGU is usually established by showing an inflammatory urethral exudate in the absence of gonococci. Specific laboratory diagnosis of Chlamydia can be accomplished by cell culture. Cell culture, the "Gold Standard" with an 80 to 90% sensitivity for the organism, is an expensive and time-consuming technique often unavailable to the practicing clinician. Fluorescent antibody testing, a rapid test for chlamydial antigens using monoclonal antibodies, is more widely used, but is less sensitive and specific than cell culture. Ureaplasma urealyticum is difficult to culture, and even when cultured is not conclusive proof of cause because of the high prevalence of this organism in the urethras of normal people, especially promiscuous men and women. Although evidence certainly exists to suggest that the organism is etiologically linked to male urethritis, it is not recommended to routinely culture for the organism because of its high prevalence in the normal population. Cases of *persistent* or *recurrent* nongonococcal urethritis should be evaluated for infection with genital mycoplasms (Ureaplasma urealyticum, etc.), Trichomonas vaginalis, and Herpes simplex virus, with the appropriate laboratory techniques.

Asymptomatic gonococcal and chlamydial urethritis serve as a reservoir that perpetuates spread of these infections in the community; therefore contact tracing and treatment of sexual partners of the infected individuals are imperative. For the emergency physician, this implies appropriate referral to follow-up agencies such as the State Health Department, etc. Contact tracing in cases of gonococcal urethritis depends on the presence of symptoms. For symptomatic cases, sexual partners over only the previous 2 weeks require contact tracing; however, if the urethritis was asymptomatic, partners over the previous month need evaluation. In the same vein, each case of gonococcal urethritis should be recultured to test for persistence of the organism within 1 week of completing antibiotic therapy, even if symptoms resolve. With Chlamydia urethritis, all sexual contacts in the previous month need appropriate evaluation.

MUCOPURULENT CERVICITIS

Mucopurulent cervicitis (MC) is the counterpart in women of urethritis in men. Whereas urethritis in men is readily recognized and treated, cervicitis is frequently missed. Even when it is recognized, the woman and her male sex partner are often not treated because MC is frequently asymptomatic despite its potential severe complications, such as PID.

Despite the long list of bacteria, viruses, and protozoa that are suspected causes of cervicitis, only three organisms, chlamydia trachomatis, Neisseria gonorrhoeae, and Herpes simplex virus, are consistently identified. C. trachomatis is responsible for the majority of cases, and this organism is more prevalent in cervicitis than it is in male urethritis. Herpes simplex virus, although frequently a cause of cervicitis, particularly the primary episode, usually does not cause a mucopurulent discharge, but rather there are cervical vesicles and ulcers with a mucoid discharge.

True mucopurulent cervicitis must be distinguished from cervical ectropion. The latter is simply endocervical columnar epithelium on exposed visible exocervix, which appears red in color and is a benign condition. True cervicitis must also be differentiated from cystitis, urethritis, and vaginitis (Chapter 57); they may share similar presentations, including increased vaginal discharge, dyspareunia, dysuria, and vulvar pruritus. Visualization of the cervical os for purulent discharge and microscopic Gram stain analysis and culture of that discharge are essential for the proper diagnosis of MC. After cleansing of the exocervix, identification of ≥10 PMNs per oil immersion field (1,000x) on a Gram-stained specimen of endocervical mucous (obtained by inserting a swab into the os) correlates highly with chlamydial or gonococcal

MC. These criteria (visualization of purulent endocervical discharge and the microscopic identification of the inflammatory component) hold true only for nonmenstruating women.[4] The finding of typical intracellular gram-negative diplococci is specific for the diagnosis of gonorrhea, but is at best only 60% sensitive. A negative Gram stain never excludes gonorrhea in a woman. Additional swabs of the mucopus must be obtained and placed on appropriate media for gonococcal culture. Cell culture or direct antigen tests for Chlamydia, as discussed previously in the section on male urethritis, are 75 to 95% sensitive in making this diagnosis in women. Rarely, the diagnosis of chlamydial MC is established by culposcopy or cervical cytology (Pap smear). Simultaneous gonococcal and chlamydial infection is frequent (30 to 60%) and must always be sought and treated.

Therapy for MC should include a regimen active against both C. trachomatis and N. gonorrheae. Antibiotics with good antichlamydial activity include doxycycline, 100 mg twice daily, or tetracycline hydrochloride, 500 mg four times daily, for 7 days. During pregnancy or if the patient is allergic to tetracycline, erythromycin, 500 mg four times daily for 7 days, can be used. For gonorrhea, single-dose ceftriaxone, 250 mg intramuscularly, is given whenever penicillin resistance is suspected, as it is in many places in the United States. All male sexual contacts of patients with documented cervicitis should be evaluated, cultured, and treated similarly.

PELVIC INFLAMMATORY DISEASE

Pelvic inflammatory disease (PID) is a clinical syndrome caused by ascending infection from the lower genital tract, usually the cervix, which results in inflammation in the fallopian tubes and adjacent structures. Endometritis, salpingitis, and peritonitis may all be part of the clinical presentation. PID is the sexually transmitted disease that most commonly requires hospitalization; approximately one million cases are diagnosed annually in the United States, with up to one quarter of the patients hospitalized. Additionally, surgical intervention is often necessary for acute or chronic complications of the disease.

Sequelae of PID are numerous and include (1) recurrent pelvic infections, (2) chronic pelvic pain, (3) ectopic pregnancy, (4) infertility (approximately 20%), (5) tubo-ovarian abscess, and (6) dyspareunia. Given the serious potential sequelae and the high incidence in sexually active teenagers, the cost of PID is especially high when measured in terms of economics and human suffering.[5] Because most cases first present in the emergency setting, the emergency physician must maintain a high index of suspicion for this entity.

Risk factors for the development of PID include (1) the occurrence of other STD, (2) previous episodes of PID, (3) multiple sexual partners, and (4) the use of an intrauterine device (IUD). Menstruation may be an additional risk factor, however, apparently only for gonococcal PID because most (66%) of these patients develop symptoms during or immediately (7 days) after the menses. In contrast, nongonococcal forms of PID show an even distribution throughout the menstrual cycle. Oral contraceptives and barrier methods of contraception decrease the risk of developing PID.

Pathogenesis of PID is believed to be by direct spread of the infection from the endocervix up to the endometrial surface, and subsequently to the fallopian tubal mucosa (endosalpingitis). Pus from the inflammatory process in the fallopian tube can spill over into the peritoneal cavity. Organisms capable of producing PID are numerous; most cases are believed to be combinations of sexually transmitted organisms and mixed endogenous genital tract flora. Causative microorganisms fit into four major categories: (1) Neisseria gonorrhoeae; (2) Chlamydia trachomatis, (3) mixed anaerobic and facultative bacteria (Bacteroides fragilis, Peptostreptococci, Peptococci, and Escherichia coli); and (4) genital mycoplasmas (Mycoplasma hominis, Ureaplasma urealyticum, and Mycoplasma genitalis).[6] While many of the anaerobic and facultative bacteria are part of the normal vaginal flora, after an episode of PID these organisms can gain access to tubal tissue and cause persistent or acute inflammation. Actinomyces israelii may occasionally be cultured from the upper genital tract in a case of PID, invariably related to extended use of an IUD.

Even in the hands of experienced personnel, the clinical diagnosis of PID may be difficult, and is correct only approximately 65% of the time. Mild cases are easily overlooked. It is preferable to overtreat, given the serious potential sequelae of PID. Symptoms frequently noted in proven cases of PID include fever, chills, malaise, anorexia, nausea, occasionally vomiting, dyspareunia, increased vaginal discharge, and abdominal pain that may be unilateral or bilateral (most commonly bilateral). Lower abdominal pain may be mild and misinterpreted as menstrual cramps, or severely incapacitating. Physical examination must be comprehensive, searching not only for signs of PID but also for other abdominal or pelvic conditions that may present in a similar fashion, such as appendicitis, ectopic pregnancy, septic abortion, ruptured ovarian cyst, and pyelonephritis. Physical examination findings of PID include fever ≥ 38°C, tachycardia, bilateral lower quadrant abdominal tenderness, yellowish endocervical discharge, unilateral or bilateral adnexal tenderness and/or mass, and cervical motion tenderness (the so-called "chandelier sign"). Gonococcal PID often presents with more pronounced and acute signs and symptoms in addition to a more purulent cervical discharge. When present, the constellation of abdominal tenderness, adnexal tenderness, and cervical mo-

tion tenderness, in addition to any one of the following criteria: (1) fever, (2) leukocytosis, (3) pelvic abscess on physical exam or ultrasound, (4) purulent material on culdocentesis, (5) elevated ESR, (6) gram-negative intracellular diplococci on Gram stain of purulent endocervical material, can identify most cases of severe PID.

Laboratory investigation often reveals a leukocytosis (greater than 10,000 WBCs/mm^2), with a leftward PMN shift, and an elevated erythrocyte sedimentation rate, although these are nonspecific indicators. Evaluation of purulent endocervical material for gonococci and Chlamydia with Gram stain, rapid ELISA tests, and culture is essential. Serum or urine tests for the beta subunit of human chorionic gonadotropin should be performed (ectopic pregnancy must be considered); of note, PID is uncommon during pregnancy. Most cases of gonococcal PID that occur during the first trimester of pregnancy end in septic abortion.

Culdocentesis, endometrial biopsy, and laparoscopy are additional diagnostic tests that may be useful in the evaluation of PID; the availability of these procedures varies widely among clinical centers. Laparoscopy can confirm the diagnosis in questionable cases, and remains the "Gold Standard" diagnostic test. Both aerobic and anaerobic cultures should be performed on any specimens obtained.

Most patients with PID are managed as outpatients. Close follow-up is essential, however, with reassessment within 48 hours of the initiation of treatment to evaluate response. For the emergency physician, the decision for outpatient therapy may present a dilemma, especially if there is no assurance that outpatient follow-up with either a gynecologist or primary care physician will occur. The patient should usually be hospitalized if any of the following criteria are present initially: (1) adnexal mass (rule out abscess), (2) peritoneal signs, (3) pregnancy, (4) temperature greater than 38°C, (5) uncertain initial diagnosis (admit to rule out potential surgical emergencies), (6) severe nausea and vomiting limiting the ability to tolerate oral medications, (7) the presence of an IUD (which should be removed only after intravenous antibiotics have been initiated), (8) if there has been no response to outpatient therapy, (9) adolescent age group (frequent noncompliance in addition to the risk of infertility in this younger age group), and (10) if outpatient follow-up cannot be arranged with certainty. Male contacts must be examined, and urethral cultures should be performed for N. gonorrhoeae and C. trachomatis. Presumptive treatment should be instituted for the exposed man, using any of the regimens for uncomplicated male urethritis. Treatment, whether inpatient or outpatient, must use antimicrobial agents broad enough to cover each of the four groups of common causative agents of PID. No single drug can accomplish this; multiple drug regimens are used. Please refer to the treatment section of this chapter for specific guidelines.

GENITAL ULCERATION

Genital ulcers may result from infection, carcinoma, gross trauma, or excoriation. Of the classic sexually transmitted diseases, i.e. gonorrhea, syphilis, herpes genitalis, lymphogranuloma venereum, chancroid, and granuloma inguinale, all but gonorrhea may present with genital ulcers and regional adenopathy.[7] Although clinical appearance of a genital ulcer may suggest a cause, clinical impression may be wrong in up to 50% of cases.[8] Diagnosis must, therefore, involve laboratory testing and incorporate epidemiologic information. The Centers for Disease Control (CDC) estimates that 500,000 new cases of genital herpes occur in the United States each year. In contrast, in 1984, 29,000 cases of early syphilis (chancres), 665 cases of chancroid, 170 of lymphogranuloma venereum (LGV), and 30 cases of granuloma inguinale were reported. The actual incidence figures are probably higher because of underreporting, and it is important to keep in mind that none of these lesions are mutually exclusive; multiple causes and/or concurrent disease are not uncommon.

Important points to determine from the history of a patient who presents with a genital ulcer include duration and time course of development of the ulcer, associated pain, and a thorough review of recent sexual contacts. Physical examination of the ulcer may aid in differential diagnosis and should include a description of the location, number, depth, size, presence of induration or purulence, and type of borders (sharp or irregular) of the ulcers. Associated regional adenopathy should be described in terms of time of onset compared to the ulcer, distribution, and presence of tenderness and fluctuance (Table 50-14). Inguinal adenopathy, when present, may be unilateral or bilateral. Significant unilateral inguinal adenopathy is more characteristic of lymphogranuloma venereum, chancroid, or pyogenic superinfection of a genital ulcer, in contrast to bilateral inguinal adenopathy, which is usually seen with syphilis and herpes genitalis. Exceptions abound, however. Inguinal adenopathy associated with sexually transmitted diseases that may present without genital ulceration, or after the ulcer has cleared, include LGV, occasionally chancroid, and lymphadenitis after bacterial superinfection. Large fluctuant inguinal lymph nodes may require aspiration (through uninflamed skin), both for culture and to provide drainage and relief of pain; aspiration may also prevent rupture through the skin and subsequent fistulization.

Classically, the lesion of primary syphilis (the chancre) begins as a single, round, indurated, painless papule that erodes to form an ulcer. The lesion is slow to develop, with a 2- to 6-week incubation period (average 3 weeks). The ulcer is indurated, nontender, and nonpurulent, with sharply defined borders. Atypical ulcers can occur, especially in the era of HIV infection, and every genital ulcer should be evaluated for syphilis. Inguinal adenopathy, characteristically

TABLE 50-14. DIFFERENTIAL DIAGNOSIS OF COMMON CAUSES OF GENITAL ULCERATION

	Ulcer Characteristics	Number of Ulcers	Inguinal Lymph Node Distribution	Systemic Symptoms*	Incubation Period	Diagnostic Methods†
Primary syphilis	Painless, indurated, sharp borders, no purulence	Single	Bilateral, non-tender	Absent	2–6 weeks	Darkfield examination, (successive days if first negative) Nonspecific serologic tests (VDRL, RPR) Specific serologic tests (FTA)
Herpes simplex virus	Painful, multiple, shallow, no exudate	Multiple vesiculo-ulcerative lesions in close proximity	Bilateral, mildly tender	Present (primary episode)	Often < 1 week	Viral culture Tzanck prep Rapid fluorescent antibody
Chancroid	Painful, deep, purulent base irregular borders	Usually single but can be multiple	Unilateral, fluctuant, tender	Absent	< 1 week	Selective culture media Gram stain of smear of lesion
Lymphogranuloma venereum	Small, superficial, painless, transient	Single	Unilateral, fluctuant, multiple sinus tracts, tender	Present	Variable, few days to several weeks	Cell culture (lymph node aspirate) Serologic tests

* Fever, myalgia, malaise, headache, meningismus
† Often presents only with inguinal adenopathy. Ulcer is transient and overlooked by patient
See text for discussion of diagnostic tests.

bilateral, nontender, mobile and firm, is present in 70 to 80% of cases of primary syphilis. Chancres may be multiple, and when secondarily infected can be painful and tender. Primary lesions of syphilis in women usually occur on the vulva and external genitalia, less frequently on the cervix (but not the vagina), and may also occur in the mouth or anus. Definitive diagnosis of primary syphilis requires darkfield examination of material from the ulcer to identify motile treponemes. Darkfield examination is difficult and largely observer-dependent; it should therefore be performed by experienced personnel only. Material obtained from ulcers in the mouth may contain nonpathogenic treponemes that are part of the normal flora of that area. Thus, the darkfield technique should be reserved for material obtained from genital ulcers only. Ideally, if the initial darkfield examination is negative, it should be repeated. Previous antibiotic therapy may cause a false negative darkfield examination.

Diagnosis may also be established by serologic testing using "nonspecific" (i.e., not antitreponemal) tests like the VDRL or the rapid plasma reagin (RPR). Early in the course of the chancre, these may be negative; the serologic test should be repeated weekly to confirm the diagnosis. Early antibiotic treatment, however, may never allow the test to become positive. Specific treponemal tests like the free treponemal antibody (FTA-Abs) will be positive sooner in the course of disease and can be obtained to establish the diagnosis. The FTA-Abs usually remains positive for life.

Herpes genitalis is the most common cause of genital ulcers in industrialized countries. Primary infection is characterized by groups of painful small vesicles on an erythematous base. When the vesicles rupture, painful ulcers occur. These are not usually exudative unless they are secondarily infected. Bilateral, painful, shotty inguinal lymphadenopathy is common. Lesions may occur in the anal and oral areas depending on sexual practices. Primary infection is often associated with constitutional symptoms, including fever, myalgia, headache, meningismus, paresthesias, and hyperesthesias.[9] Recurrent episodes are frequent but often less severe, with fewer lesions and little or no adenopathy or systemic symptoms. Exceptions abound, especially in immunocompromised hosts (i.e., HIV-infected patients). Herpes virus infection is usually diagnosed on clinical grounds, although many cases may be missed if diagnostic tests are not performed. The most reliable diagnostic technique is viral culture. A Tzanck smear, which is a Wright stain of vesicular fluid, may reveal multinucleated giant cells characteristic of herpes infection. Rapid fluorescent specific antibody tests are sensitive and readily available. Serologic testing, in particular the detection of HSV antibody, is not helpful in the diagnosis of HSV infection, but is an epidemiologic tool.

Chancroid is an extremely common cause of genital ulceration in developing countries and is now much more frequently seen in the United States, especially in large urban areas. After a short incubation period, patients present with a papule or pustule that will erode into a deep painful ulcer with a purulent base and irregular, undermined borders. They may be singular or multiple. More than half of the cases have concomitant tender inguinal lymph nodes, which often rupture to form inguinal ulcers or buboes. Hemophilus ducreyi, the etiologic agent of chancroid, is fastidious and difficult to culture, requiring selective media. Gram stain of a smear of the lesion may reveal gram-negative coccobacillary organisms in a "train-track" pattern. Frequently, these organisms are not seen and the diagnosis is established on clinical grounds. Herpes may mimic chancroid, and therefore evaluation for herpesvirus infection should also be performed with viral culture and/or Tzanck preparation of the material from the lesion.

Lymphogranuloma venereum, caused by LGV serovars of Chlamydia trachomatis, is rare in the United States. The genital ulcer is usually small, superficial, and painless, and heals quickly; it is so transient that it is usually not noticed by the patient and it is often not present at the time of medical evaluation. Approximately 2 to 6 weeks later, inguinal adenopathy dominates the clinical picture; the lymph nodes are matted and adherent to the overlying skin, which is characteristically of a violaceous hue. The lymph nodes, usually unilateral, are often fluctuant and large in size, and may form sinus tracts. Rarely, this may progress to chronic lymphatic disease with elephantiasis of the genital tissues. Nonspecific systemic symptoms (malaise, fatigue, fever, myalgias) are frequently also present. Diagnosis is by standard cell culture methodology (using McCoy cells usually); material may be obtained from lymph node aspirate, or the urethra, rectum or cervix if they are involved. Serologic tests such as the LGV complement fixation test, although insensitive and nonspecific, may be helpful. A fourfold increase or an isolated titer greater than 1:64 is pathognomonic.

Granuloma inguinale (donovanosis) is rare in the United States. It involves indolent painless granulation of infected superficial tissues; inguinal lymph nodes are not enlarged unless there is bacterial superinfection. Calymmatobacterium granulomatis, a fastidious gram-negative bacillus, is the causative organism. Diagnosis is established by identifying the organism in macrophages (Donovan bodies) in a biopsy specimen.

Evaluation and work-up of genital ulcers must therefore use historical and epidemiologic information in addition to the clinical examination and appearance of the lesions, plus associated laboratory tests. Of importance to the emergency physician, many patients with genital ulcers are often available for follow-up, which is necessary for proper diagnosis and treatment. Definitive virologic and bacteriologic results are often not available initially, and the diagnosis is frequently unconfirmed. Additionally, multiple causes can be present simultaneously. Empiric therapy is usually necessary, with additional care given to the possibility of incubating syphilis, given the preventable potential complications of this disease.

TREATMENT

Despite important advances in the treatment of STD, including improved understanding of the mechanisms and genetics of antimicrobial resistance for several pathogens, many of the recommended therapeutic regimens remain intuitive or based on limited data.[10]

Of particular concern is the treatment of gonorrhea, which is now complicated by the spread of strains that are resistant to various antimicrobial agents. Although these strains have been identified in all 50 states, they are more commonly encountered in large urban areas. Resistant strains comprise 1% of all isolates, but this number is rapidly increasing. Resistance occurs by two genetic mechanisms: (1) chromosomally mediated,

and (2) plasmid-mediated. Chromosomal mutations cause changes in the permeability of the organism's outer membrane (penicillin, tetracycline, erythromycin resistance) or ribosomal structure (aminoglycoside resistance). Homosexual men with gonorrhea demonstrate an especially high prevalance of chromosomally mediated resistance. After acquisition of plasmids for beta-lactamase production, the gonococci develop absolute resistance to the penicillins and some cephalosporins. There is a high prevalence of concurrent chlamydial infection in patients with gonorrhea (in men, up to 25%; in women, up to 50%). Therefore treatment regimens for gonorrhea must include antimicrobials with antichlamydial activity. The emergency physician, after providing initial treatment, must refer the patient for contact tracing and post-treatment (3 to 7 days) cultures to ensure eradication. Post-treatment cultures are not needed in pure chlamydial infection. Most treatment regimens for gonorrhea cure incubating syphilis (seronegative, no clinical signs of syphilis).

Table 50-15 lists the current recommendations for treatment of sexually transmitted diseases.[11,12]

TABLE 50-15. ANTIMICROBIAL THERAPY FOR SEXUALLY TRANSMITTED DISEASES

Organism/Syndrome	Regimen	Alternatives	In Pregnancy*
Neisseria gonorrhoeae† Urethritis, cervicitis, proctitis, pharyngitis	Ceftriaxone 250 mg IM one dose	Spectinomycin 2 g IM once or Ciprofloxacin 500 mg orally, one dose or Norfloxacin 800 mg orally one dose, or Cefuroxime 1 g with Probenecid 1 g orally one dose For penicillin-sensitive strains: Amoxicillin 3.0 g orally or Ampicillin 3.5 g orally or Procaine penicillin G 4.8 million units IM, each with probenecid, 1.0 g orally	Ceftriaxone or spectinomycin
Chlamydia trachomatis Urethritis, cervicitis§	Doxycycline 100 mg po bid for 7 days or Tetracycline HCL 500 mg po qid for 7 days	Erythromycin base, 500 mg po qid for 7 days Erythromycin ethylsuccinate 800 mg po qid for 7 days	Erythromycin
Treponema pallidum/ Syphilis# Early (primary, secondary, or late < 1 year)	Benzathine penicillin G 2.4 million units IM	Doxycycline 100 mg po bid for 14 days or Tetracycline HCL 500 mg po qid for 14 days	Penicillin (desensitize if penicillin allergic)
Late (> 1 year or cardio-vascular involvement)	Benzathine penicillin G 2.4 million units IM weekly for 3 weeks	Same as for early syphilis except duration is 30 days	Penicillin
Neurosyphilis	Aqueous penicillin G 2.4 million units IV q4h for 10–14 days	No data available (? ceftriaxone)	Penicillin

TABLE 50-15. CONTINUED

Organism/Syndrome	Regimen	Alternatives	In Pregnancy*
Herpes Simplex Virus Primary episode of genital herpes	Acyclovir 200 mg orally five times daily for 7–10 days (400 mg dosing for proctitis)	No data available	No data available
Pelvic inflammatory disease Outpatient Therapy	Cefoxitin 2 g IM with probenecid 1.0 g orally or Ceftriaxone 250 mg IM *plus* Doxycycline 100 mg orally bid for 10–14 days or Tetracycline HCL 500 mg po qid for 10–14 days	Not well studied	Cefoxitin or ceftriaxone plus erythromycin Cefoxitin or ceftriaxone plus erythromycin
Inpatient therapy**	Cefoxitin 2.0 g IV qid or Cefotetan 2.0 g IV q 12 hr *plus* Doxycycline 100 mg IV bid	Clindamycin 600–900 mg IV q8h plus Gentamicin 1.5 mg/kg IV q8h (adjust for renal clearance)	Clindamycin/gentamicin or Cefoxitin/erythromycin
Hemophilus ducreyi/ Chancroid	Ceftriaxone 250 mg IM or Erythromycin 500 mg orally qid for 7 days	Trimethoprim/sulfamethoxazole DS 1 tablet twice daily for 7 days or Ciprofloxacin 500 mg po bid for 3 days	Ceftriaxone
Genital mycoplasmas/Ureaplasma urealyticum			Erythromycin
Urethritis	Doxycycline 100 mg orally bid for 7 days	Tetracyline HCL or Erythromycin or Clindamycin or ? Quinolones	

* Also consider for children under 16 years old.
† Must always treat for presumed coincident chlamydial infection at the same time.
§ Treatment regimens for LGV are the same except that duration of treatment is 21 days.
# It is unclear if these treatment regimens are effective for HIV infected patients as well.
** Continue intravenous regimen for at least 48 hours after clinical response before switching to oral regimen. Total therapy should continue for 10 to 14 days.

MEDICOLEGAL PEARLS

- Use the local/state health departments as a resource for contact tracing.
- Gonorrhea in children presumed to be from sexual abuse (age 0–1 may be from inadvertent contact with an infected adult at birth).
- Patients with an STD (especially syphilis) should be referred for HIV counseling and HIV antibody testing.

NATIONAL CONTACTS

Sexually Transmitted Diseases National Hotline (American Social Health Association): 800-227-8922

REFERENCES

1. Larson, R.E., and Shapiro, M.A.: Sexually transmitted urogenital diseases. Emerg. Med. Clin. North Am. 6:487, 1988.
2. Medical News & Perspectives: Sexually transmitted diseases may reverse the revolution. JAMA 255:1665, 1986.
3. Hooton, T.M., and Barnes, R.C.: Urethritis in men. Infect. Dis. Clin. North Am. 1:165, 1987.
4. Brunham, R.C., Paavonen, J., Stevens, C.E., et al.: Mucopurulent cervicitis: The ignored counterpart in women of urethritis in men. N. Engl. J. Med. 311:1, 1984.
5. Landers, D.V., and Sweet, R.L.: Acute pelvic inflammatory disease. In New Surgical and Medical Approaches in Infectious Diseases. Edited by Root, R.K., Trunkey, D.D., and Sande, M.A. New York, Churchill Livingstone, 1987, pp. 189–200.
6. Westrom, L., and Mardth, P.A.: Salpingitis. In Sexually Transmitted Diseases. Edited by Holmes, K.K., Mardth, P.A., Sparling, P.F., et al. New York, McGraw-Hill, 1984, pp. 615–632.
7. Krockta, W.P., and Barnes, R.C.: Genital ulceration with re-

gional adenopathy. Infect. Dis. Clin. North Am. *1*:217–233, 1987.

8. Chapel, T.A., Brown, W.J., Jeffries, C., et al.: How reliable is the morphological diagnosis of penile ulcerations. Sex. Trans. Dis. *4*:150, 1977.

9. Corey, L., and Spear, P.G.: Infections with herpes simplex viruses (second of two parts). N. Engl. J. Med. *314*:749, 1986.

10. Handsfield, H.H.: Problems in the treatment of bacterial sexually transmitted diseases. Sex. Trans. Dis. *13*:179, 1986.

11. Centers for Disease Control: Sexually transmitted diseases treatment guidelines, 1989. M.M.W.R. *38*:1, 1989.

12. The Medical Letter: Treatment of sexually transmitted diseases. The Medical Letter *32*:5, 1990.

SPECIFIC DISEASES

Sumner E. Thompson

CAPSULE

This chapter section covers specific sexually transmitted diseases, and describes their clinical presentation, diagnosis, and treatment in men, women, and children. Also covered are sexually transmitted lower gastrointestinal infections in homosexual men.

GONOCOCCAL INFECTIONS

The gonococcus (Neisseria gonorrheae) may infect any mucosal surface. The most common site of infection in men is the anterior urethra; in women it is the uterine cervix. Other commonly infected sites are the female urethra and the rectal mucosa and posterior pharynx of both sexes. The gonococcus may enter the bloodstream from any of these sites, producing a syndrome of arthralgias and skin lesions ranging from petechiae to pustules, or of septic arthritis. The gonococcus is also a common cause of acute epididymitis and acute salpingitis. Spread of this organism from the fallopian tubes to the liver, probably through lymphatic vessels, is associated with a perihepatitis (Fitz-Hugh-Curtis syndrome), which is easily confused with viral hepatitis or acute gallbladder disease. All of the syndromes produced by the gonococcus, except disseminated syndromes, are mimicked by another common sexually transmitted pathogen, Chlamydia trachomatis. Because the antibiotic therapies for these agents differ, the clinician should attempt to distinguish between the two (see *Treatment*).

SYMPTOMS

Men. Symptoms of *acute urethritis* usually occur within a few days after sexual intercourse with an infected individual. Usually the patient has increasingly severe dysuria during all phases of micturition and a scant white to yellow urethral discharge, which becomes copious and purulent. *Rectal infections* may occur in homosexual men, with itching, burning, or tenesmus with or without discharge, but may also be asymptomatic. Men with *acute epididymitis* usually have unilateral testicular pain and swelling; a urethral discharge is not always present.

Women. *Gonococcal cervicitis* is often asymptomatic or associated with the relatively nonspecific symptoms of increased vaginal discharge, severe cramping during menses, and intermenstrual spotting. Women with *urethritis* complain of dysuria but rarely notice a urethral discharge. *Rectal infections* in women are almost always asymptomatic. Upper genital tract infections, i.e., salpingitis or pelvic inflammatory disease, are discussed elsewhere.

Both Sexes. *Pharyngeal infections* occur after orogenital contact with an infected individual of either sex. There is no correlation between symptoms of pharyngitis and colonization of the tonsils with N. gonorrhoeae. Patients with *hematogenous infections* (disseminated gonococcal infections) usually present in one of two ways: (1) with a few tender raised lesions on the extremities and aching of several joints in the hands, feet, wrists, or ankles, or (2) with complaints of swelling and pain on motion of a single joint, usually the knee, wrist, or ankle. On rare occasions, patients may develop *endocarditis* or *meningitis* with symptoms indistinguishable from those caused by other bacteria.

Children. Prepubescent girls may present with a *vulvovaginitis* and complain of vaginal itching or burning with or without dysuria. Boys usually present with *urethritis*. Gonorrhea in a child should be considered evidence of *sexual abuse* until proved otherwise. Any child with a sexually transmitted infection and any child or teenager who reports sexual abuse should be reported to the appropriate authorities for investigation of possible abuse. Sexually abused children are best managed by a team of professionals experienced in addressing their physical and psychologic needs. Children with genital gonococcal infections should also have pharyngeal and rectal cultures taken.

PHYSICAL FINDINGS

Men. The *urethral discharge* is usually copious and yellowish or greenish, but may be scant, requiring urethral stripping for demonstration. Inguinal adenopathy is not a feature. A Gram stain of the urethral exudate reveals large numbers of polymorphonuclear leukocytes and intracellular gram-negative diplococci. In gonococcal *proctitis*, there may be purulent discharge and severe pain on insertion of the examining finger into the rectum. Occasionally, a *prostatitis* is also present, along with urethritis. A Gram stain of the discharge often reveals a picture similar to that seen in urethritis. Anoscopy usually shows purulent cryptitis.

Women. The cervix may be difficult to visualize because of cervicovaginal discharge, usually yellowish and purulent. Occasionally, a small amount of discharge may be seen exuding from the endocervical canal. The cervix may appear normal or inflamed and swollen. In women with urethritis, discharge is best demonstrated by gently milking the urethra. A Gram stain of endocervical discharge may show the same features as urethritis in men but is often difficult to interpret because of the normal presence of other microorganisms. There are usually no objective findings in rectal infections. *Perihepatitis* presents as percussion tenderness over the liver, occasionally with a friction rub. Jaundice is rare. Signs of upper genital tract infection, e.g., salpingitis, may be present (see *Genital Chlamydial Infections*).

Both Sexes. There are no pathognomonic findings in *pharyngeal infections*. There is no correlation with exudative pharyngitis or cervical adenopathy. The skin lesions of *disseminated infections* are often distinctive. There are usually fewer than a dozen lesions, almost always limited to the extremities and often sensitive to touch. They may have various forms, often in the same patient: petechial, maculopapular, or pustular, sometimes with a greyish necrotic center. Small joints of the hands or feet are often red and tender, but careful examination reveals that tenderness is of the periarticular structures, not the joint itself (tenosynovitis). A true septic arthritis may be present, with pain on motion of the joint, redness, swelling, and the presence of intra-articular fluid. The cause of the septic arthritis cannot be suspected unless tenosynovitis is present as well, a combination occurring in fewer than 10% of cases. The objective findings of *meningitis* or *endocarditis* are the same as for other bacterial causes of those syndromes. A major confusion could be between meningococcemia with or without meningitis and disseminated gonococcal infection.

Infants and Children. The most common infection in infancy is *gonococcal ophthalmia*. The presence of unilateral or bilateral eyelid edema, chemosis, and a white or yellow purulent exudate is the hallmark. Prepubescent girls develop *vulvovaginitis* rather than cervicitis. There are redness and edema of the vaginal walls and labia, with a scant or copious vaginal discharge. The signs of urethritis in boys are the same as those in the adult male.

DIAGNOSIS AND TREATMENT

For urethral infections in men, a Gram-stained smear of the urethral exudate is sufficient to establish the diagnosis. In interpretation of the smear, care must be taken to count only intracellular gram-negative diplococci. Extracellular organisms are often not gonococci. Note that Chlamydia cannot be seen with Gram stain; thus Gram stain is not helpful in ruling out simultaneous chlamydial infection. In cervical infections, the results of the Gram stain are reliable if read by an experienced microscopist, but are much less sensitive than results in men. An endocervical culture is necessary to confirm the clinical impression. Cultures are best taken at the bedside and transferred directly to a selective medium. Transport media such as a "culturette" are much less satisfactory. For infections of other sites (throat, rectum, bloodstream, or joint), a culture is required; smears are seldom reliable. A Gram stain of pustular skin lesions may be helpful but cannot distinguish the meningococcus from the gonococcus.

Two special difficulties in treating gonococcal problems deserve comment. Up to one third of individuals with genital gonorrhea also have a simultaneous genital infection with Chlamydia trachomatis. Treatment with penicillin alone cures the gonorrhea but not the chlamydial infection. This persistent infection is responsible, in large part, for the postgonococcal urethritis syndrome commonly seen in men. Gonococci that produce penicillinase, which renders them highly resistant to penicillin, have been seen with increasing frequency in the United States since 1980 and are now endemic. Infection with one of these resistant organisms should be suspected in individuals who fail to respond to treatment. Two clues that should alert the clinician to the possibility of infection with a penicillinase-producing gonococcus are acquisition of gonorrhea from a prostitute or a person living overseas, particularly in Asia or Africa. Within the past 2 years, reports of gonococci resistant to tetracycline have appeared and may be a widespread problem in the United States.

Uncomplicated gonococcal infections in adults may be treated with any of four regimens:

1. 3.5 g ampicillin (or 3.0 g amoxicillin) orally with 1.0 g probenecid orally and 500 mg tetracycline orally, four times a day for 7 days (the tetracycline cotreats chlamydial infection).
2. 250 mg ceftriaxone (Rocephin) intramuscularly with 500 mg tetracycline orally, four times a day for 7 days.
3. 4.8 million U aqueous procaine penicillin G intramuscularly with 1.0 g probenecid and 500 mg tetracycline orally, four times a day for 7 days (penicillin-sensitive strains only).
4. For the penicillin-allergic patient, 2.0 g spectinomycin intramuscularly with 500 mg tetracycline orally, four times a day for 7 days (alternatives for tetracycline are 100 mg doxycline orally, twice a day for 7 days, or 500 mg erythromycin orally, four times a day for 7 days).
5. Ciprofloxicin, 500 mg orally; norfloxacin, 800 mg orally; or cephiroxine, 1 gram with 1.0 gram proterenol and 500 mg tetracycline orally, 4 times a day for 7 days.

The ampicillin or amoxicillin regimen may be less useful for treatment of gonorrhea in homosexual men because they tend to be infected with more resistant strains; additionally, this regimen is not always effective for pharyngeal infections. Because homosexual men are infrequently coinfected with *Chlamydia*, ceftriaxone is probably the drug of choice.

Penicillin-allergic patients and patients failing therapy on penicillin should be retreated with 2.0 g spectinomycin, intramuscularly. There have been reports of spectinomycin-resistant gonococci, but this is presently a rare phenomenon in the United States.

Patients with gonorrhea who also have syphilis or are contacts of syphilis patients should be given additional therapy appropriate to the stage of syphilis.

Examination and treatment of sexual partners should be considered a part of total patient care.

Follow-up cultures should be obtained from infected sites within a few days after completing initial therapy.

Patients with disseminated gonococcal infections should be initially hospitalized for observation and treatment. Therapy should not be initiated until blood and joint fluid cultures have been obtained.

Infants with gonococcal ophthalmia should be hospitalized for therapy.

GENITAL CHLAMYDIAL INFECTIONS

Chlamydia trachomatis, an obligately intracellular bacterium, is one of the most ubiquitous disease-pro-

ducing agents in humans. It is found in virtually all populations worldwide. It causes trachoma, a chronic eye infection that produces blindness, and is probably the most common sexually transmissible agent in the United States. The epidemiology of this agent in the genital tract is similar to that of the gonococcus, and indeed, the two are often transmitted together. Approximately half of all cases of nongonococcal urethritis in men are caused by this agent; it is also an important cause of epididymitis in men under age 35 and is a cause of Reiter's syndrome. Up to 25% of women attending sexually transmitted disease clinics are infected with this agent; many of these women are asymptomatic but are at risk for salpingitis, subsequent infertility, and perihepatitis by direct extension of the organism to the capsule of the liver. *Chlamydia* is also a major cause of cervicitis and lower urinary tract infections. Pregnant women with genital chlamydial infections can transmit the agent to their babies during delivery; the attack rate in exposed infants is 30% to 50% for inclusion conjunctivitis and approximately 10% for chlamydial pneumonitis.

SYMPTOMS

Men. The most common infection is acute urethritis. Symptoms usually occur within 7 to 14 days after sexual contact with an infected partner. The onset of dysuria is gradual and often mild; discharge is scanty and clear or white if present at all. Another common presentation is postgonococcal urethritis: the patient is infected simultaneously with the gonococcus and Chlamydia trachomatis (this occurs in up to 30% of all cases of gonorrhea). The incubation period of gonococcal urethritis is short, and the patient develops typical acute anterior urethritis diagnosed as gonorrhea. He is then treated with a penicillin, a short course of tetracycline or spectinomycin, or a cephalosporin, none of which can eradicate the chlamydial component of the infection. Seven to ten or more days later, he experiences onset of a new bout of mild urethritis, which is actually a chlamydial infection. Men with chlamydial urethritis are also at risk for developing acute epididymitis, which is not clinically distinguishable from gonococcal or other types of bacterial epididymitis. Homosexual men may develop proctitis caused by C. trachomatis. This can vary from a severe inflammatory response with rectal discharge, bloody stools, and tenesmus to a mild or asymptomatic condition.

Women. Chlamydial cervicitis is not associated with any specific symptoms. Occasionally, patients may complain of some increase in vaginal discharge and mild cramping during menstruation. Women with chlamydial urethritis complain of dysuria. Rectal and pharyngeal infections with this organism apparently do occur, but are asymptomatic. Upper genital tract infection (salpingitis) is common. The symptoms are similar to those of salpingitis caused by any other micoorganisms, but often fever is absent and women are not acutely ill.

PHYSICAL FINDINGS

Men. Urethral discharge is usually scant and clear or whitish. Urethral stripping is usually required to demonstrate it. A Gram stain of the discharge reveals many polymorphonuclear leukocytes (PMNs) and no intracellular organisms. The chlamydial inclusions are found in epithelial cells, not PMNs, but do not stain with Gram stain. Chlamydial proctitis may be indistinguishable from gonococcal proctitis (see the previous discussion) clinically. Both infections may coexist. Sigmoidoscopy may reveal lesions that can be confused with ulcerative colitis. Chlamydial epididymitis can be suspected only by finding the discharge typical of nongonococcal urethritis.

Women. The cervix may appear grossly normal despite infection with Chlamydia trachomatis. Endocervical discharge is the hallmark, however. It is usually scant and yellowish-white. There may be a follicular, hypertrophic appearance to the cervix, which is best appreciated with the colposcope. Gentle stripping of the urethra in women complaining of dysuria (up to 40% of women with cervicitis) may reveal a discharge similar to that seen in the male. A Gram stain of cervical or urethral material reveals PMNs without intracellular organisms. Examination of the first-void urine may also reveal PMNs and no free-swimming bacteria. The findings of salpingitis do not permit distinction from other causes, except that mild fundal tenderness (endometritis) is common. There are no findings associated with pharyngeal infection or rectal infection in women.

DIAGNOSIS AND TREATMENT

For urethral infections in men and women, or for endocervical infections, a carefully prepared and interpreted Gram stain that shows PMNs without gram-negative intracellular diplococci is presumptive evidence for a chlamydial infection. A culture for Neisseria gonorrhoeae, however, should always be done in this situation. Chlamydia are not visible on the Gram stain. A culture using a slender calcium alginate swab, which can be inserted 1 to 2 cm into the urethra, is the definitive means of making the diagnosis. The specimens require a special transport medium and proper temperature to be useful, and results are usually not available for at least 3 days. Recently, a smear technique using direct staining with a fluorescent monoclonal antibody has become commercially available. Although this technique is both sensitive and specific, it requires meticulous attention to specimen collection and interpretation of the slide. Results can be available within 30 minutes with this method.

The diagnosis of chlamydial salpingitis is difficult. The finding of nongonococcal cervicitis or a positive endocervical chlamydial culture in a patient with salpingitis is of some help. The demonstration of Chlamydia in an endometrial specimen collected with a shielded biopsy needle is stronger evidence. Best, but most difficult, is the demonstration of Chlamydia from a specimen obtained from the fallopian tubes with laparoscopy. A fourfold or greater titer change using either the complement-fixation test or microimmunofluorescence test is also strong evidence, but these tests are often unavailable.

Tetracycline hydrochloride is the treatment of choice for chlamydial infections. For uncomplicated urethritis or cervicitis, the regimen is 500 mg tetracycline hydrochloride four times a day for 7 days; 100 mg doxycycline twice a day may be substituted. Erythromycin in the same schedule may be substituted in those who cannot tolerate tetracycline, but may be slightly less efficacious. The sexual partners of patients should receive the same therapy. For the treatment of salpingitis and epididymitis, a tetracycline regimen of 10 to 14 days may be adequate, but this has not been well studied.

LYMPHOGRANULOMA VENEREUM

Certain strains of *Chlamydia trachomatis* are capable of causing a chronic infection of the lymphatic system, lymphogranuloma venereum (LGV). The symptoms are different in the two sexes because different chains of lymphatics are affected. The primary infection is a genital papule that ulcerates and heals rapidly. Patients rarely seek medical attention at this time because the process is asymptomatic. In the secondary stage of disease, at which the patient most commonly seeks out the physician, it is usually the man who is symptomatic. Unilateral or bilateral tender inguinal swellings appear, and may be associated with draining sinuses later in the disease's course. Constitutional symptoms of fever, malaise, and headache may also be present. Because it is usually the pelvic lymphatics that are involved in women, specific symptoms are lacking.

In men, unilateral tender inguinal adenopathy without lesions of the external genitalia is the most common finding. The adenopathy is usually firm, with matting of node groups. The finding of a large area of fluctuance that suggests an abscess cavity goes against the diagnosis because the abscesses within nodes are usually microabscesses. One or more sinuses draining purulent material may be seen. Both inguinal and femoral nodes may be involved, producing masses above and below Poupart's ligament, the groove sign. In homosexual men, the site of primary involvement may be the rectum, with signs of proctitis, or later, with involvement of node chains in that area, the finding of rectal stricture. In women, there may be no early secondary signs. With fibrosis of lymphatics, vulvar edema and ulceration may occur. Inguinal adenopathy is uncommon. Rectal stricture may also occur late in women because of fibrosis of deep pelvic perirectal lymphatics.

LGV is most easily diagnosed by serologic testing. A single complement fixation titer of 1:64 or greater is considered strong evidence of recent infection. Titers in established disease are often extremely high. Chlamydia may occasionally be cultured from a needle aspirate of a bubo. Frei's test, a measure of delayed hypersensitivity, is no longer commercially available. The test is not specific for LGV. Most often, the diagnosis is made on clinical grounds alone.

Treatment of LGV is similar to that of chlamydial urethritis or cervicitis (500 mg tetracycline four times a day or 100 mg doxycycline twice a day), but the treatment should continue for a minimum of 2 weeks. In later stages of the disease, treatment may have to be extended for several weeks to a month or more. Erythromycin is the second drug of choice. The patient's sexual partners should be treated.

CHLAMYDIAL DISEASE IN INFANTS

Inclusion conjunctivitis is usually a mild disease characterized by conjunctival and palpebral edema with a scant discharge causing the eyelids to be stuck together (sticky eye syndrome). Occasionally, the discharge may be purulent and rarely copious, causing confusion with other bacterial conjunctival infections—neisserial, staphylococcal, or hemophiliac. There is usually a follicular component, best demonstrated by everting the upper lid. Chlamydial pneumonia usually occurs several weeks to a month after birth. It is characterized by a dry cough, tachypnea, and an interstitial, bilaterally symmetrical infiltrate on radiographs of the chest.

Chlamydial inclusion conjunctivitis can be diagnosed with a Giemsa or Pap smear of the upper palpebral conjunctiva. The direct fluorescent smear appears to be useful in this situation. At the least, a Gram stain to detect other bacterial pathogens and a bacterial culture are necessary. Chlamydial pneumonia can be diagnosed by culture of endotracheal aspirate or by direct lung puncture; a rising antibody titer on serologic testing is also helpful.

Inclusion conjunctivitis can be prevented by the instillation of tetracycline ointment into the eyes of the newborn at delivery. This maneuver does not prevent pneumonia. Treatment of established conjunctivitis should include systemic, not just topical, therapy. Optimal therapy is erythromycin syrup, 50 mg/kg of body weight in four divided doses for 2 weeks. The treatment of chlamydial pneumonia is the same regimen for at least 3 weeks.

SYPHILIS

Syphilis is a chronic systemic infection caused by Treponema pallidum with protean manifestations. This organism can penetrate intact mucous membranes and apparently normal skin as well. It rapidly enters local lymphatics, gains access to the bloodstream, and disseminates from there to all tissues. The incubation period is 10 to 90 days, with a mean of 3 weeks. The first clinical manifestation is the *syphilitic chancre* (primary syphilis), usually located on the external genitalia, but in women, it may occur in the vagina or on the cervix. It may also be found in extragenital sites such as the rectum, mouth, or finger. The chancre heals spontaneously and is usually followed in several weeks by the *secondary stage* of disease. When hematogenous dissemination of spirochetes occurs, constitutional symptoms, malaise and fever, are often accompanied by generalized nontender lymphadenopathy and a generalized "measly" rash. This phase also subsides spontaneously, and the patient enters *latency*. During this phase of the disease, by definition, there are no signs or symptoms. This stage may last for the life of the patient, but spirochetes probably persist in the untreated individual for life. The disease may be reactivated at any time. The mechanisms or causes of this reactivation are not known. *Late*, or *tertiary syphilis*, may take a variety of forms. The basic pathologic lesions are an endarteritis and periarteritis. Occurrence in the central nervous system leads to meningovascular syphilis, general paresis, or tabes dorsalis; occurrence in the heart, to syphilitic aortitis with aneurysm formation and aortic insufficiency or to stenosis of the coronary arteries. Destructive mass lesions, syphilitic gumma, may occur in any tissue.

SYMPTOMS

Most patients are asymptomatic throughout the course of the disease, which is detected because of a reactive serologic test. The chancre is almost always painless. Patients with secondary syphilis occasionally present because of a nonpruritic skin rash and a flu-like syndrome. There are rarely any complaints during tertiary syphilis to bring a patient to the physician.

PHYSICAL FINDINGS

The chancre is usually a solitary, painless sore located on the genitals or rectum. It is characterized by a clean surface with rolled edges and an indurated, nonerythematous base. There is usually accompanying unilateral or bilateral nontender inguinal adenopathy. Occasionally, there may be two ulcers, and rarely, three. Nongenital lesions are accompanied by regional adenopathy as well. A sparse, generalized symmetric non-pruritic rash, which may range from macular to pustular (rarely vesicular), and generalized, shotty nontender adenopathy are characteristic of secondary syphilis. Whitish patches resembling leukoplakia (mucous patches) may sometimes be seen on the tongue and buccal mucosa, and broad-based warty excrescences (condylomata latum) can sometimes be found in moist perigenital locations. There is no clinical evidence of infection during the latent stage of the disease.

DIAGNOSIS AND TREATMENT

Serous material obtained by lightly abrading the chancre should be examined immediately by darkfield microscopy for the characteristic motile treponemes. A positive test result establishes the diagnosis of syphilis. If this test cannot be done on the spot, the patient should be referred to a clinical facility, such as a public clinic, where the test can be carried out. If none of these options are available or suitable lesions are not present, the clinician must rely on serologic testing. The RPR or other rapid tests that can be obtained while the patient is still in the clinic do not always yield positive results in early syphilis. These tests, however, are virtually always reactive during secondary syphilis and, in this stage of the disease, allow a presumptive diagnosis to be made and therapy to be initiated. In patients with neurologic manifestations in which syphilis is part of the differential diagnosis, a lumbar puncture, cell count, and Venereal Disease Research Laboratory (VDRL) test on cerebrospinal fluid are mandatory.

Patients with primary, secondary, or latent syphilis of a year or less in duration should receive benzathine penicillin G, 2.4 million U by intramuscular injection once, or aqueous procaine penicillin G, 600,000 U by intramuscular injection daily for 8 days (a total of 4.8 million U). Note: a single injection of 4.8 million U of procaine penicillin G is *not* adequate therapy. For penicillin-allergic patients, the treatment of choice is tetracycline, 500 mg orally four times a day for 15 days. Patients with syphilis of more than one year's duration or of unknown duration or with cardiovascular or gummatous syphilis should be treated with benzathine penicillin G, 2.4 million U by intramuscular injection weekly for 3 *consecutive* weeks (7.2 million U total). There is controversy over the therapy of central nervous system syphilis. My recommendation is for hospitalization for treatment with high-dose intravenous penicillin.

If therapy for other stages of syphilis is to be initiated on an outpatient basis, patients should be warned about the possibility of having a Herxheimer's reaction, a febrile reaction often accompanied by headache and occasionally worsening of the rash, which may occur within 1 to 4 hours of antibiotic therapy. Rest and antipyretic therapy are indicated for this limited reaction.

All patients should be referred to a public health facility for follow-up serologic testing to determine the adequacy of treatment and for interviewing for testing and treatment of sex partners. This most important part of the therapeutic plan is often overlooked in the Emergency Department (ED).

GENITAL HERPES VIRUS INFECTIONS

Herpes simplex of the genitalia may be caused by either type 1 virus (oral) or type 2 virus (genital). The lesions produced by these two types of virus cannot be distinguished clinically. There are three categories of infection:

1. *Primary infection:* the result of an individual's first contact with a herpes virus (i.e., there is no pre-existing antibody against herpes virus). These infections tend to be severe, associated with constitutional symptoms, and prolonged.
2. *Initial infection:* the first apparent clinical episode noted by the patient. Serologic testing shows antibody to be present, indicating previous inapparent infection (usually an early childhood type 1 virus infection). Because of partial immunity, the initial infection tends to be less severe than the primary episode.
3. *Recurrent infection:* the form most often seen clinically. These episodes are usually the least severe, recur in the same anatomic location, and tend to heal within a week.

SYMPTOMS

In primary infections, the patient notices the sudden onset of crops of blisters somewhere on the external genitalia, sometimes on the thighs and sometimes in the anal area. Itching is common initially, but eventually burning and severe pain, both at the site of the ulcer and in the nerve root distribution, occur. The lesions eventually ulcerate. New crops of lesions often continue to appear while old ones are ulcerating and crusting. Headache, malaise, and fever are common; dysuria is a common complaint in both sexes, but women in particular may have acute urinary retention. Rectal infections are characterized by severe rectal and perianal pain, which is worse during defecation; intense itching occurs at times and, occasionally, rectal discharge. Neuritic pain radiating down the legs is common, sometimes associated with motor weakness.

A prodrome consisting of tingling, burning, or itching sensations, occurring minutes to hours before lesions appear at the site of eruption, is the hallmark of recurrent infections; it occurs in about 85% of individuals. The prodrome tends to be exactly the same before each outbreak. Local pain at the site of the lesions tends to be most severe during the first few days of the episode, when new lesions are forming; systemic complaints are rare. Other symptoms depend on the location of the recurrent lesions, for example, dysuria in a urethral or periurethral infection.

PHYSICAL FINDINGS

The finding of multiple painful vesicular lesions on an erythematous base in association with tender inguinal adenopathy is almost pathognomonic of genital herpes, but, particularly in recurrent infections, the lesions are often ulcerated or crusted by the time the patient presents. In primary infections, there may be large numbers of lesions. The finding of lesions in several different stages is characteristic. Exceptionally tender inguinal adenopathy is almost universally present. Up to 10% of patients with primary genital herpes may have meningeal signs. In recurrent disease, there may be only one or two ulcers, and pain and adenopathy may be minimal. This wide spectrum of clinical presentations makes it imperative that herpes simplex be included in the differential diagnosis of all genital ulcers.

DIAGNOSIS AND TREATMENT

A Giemsa-stained smear (Tzanck preparation) or a Pap smear is at least 90% sensitive if prepared by scraping the base of a freshly unroofed vesicle. The sensitivity, however, drops to less than 50% if the smear is taken from an ulcer and is even less if taken from a crusted lesion. The ability to isolate virus by culture follows the same pattern for the three types of lesions. The chances for viral isolation are best during the first week to 10 days of a primary infection and during the first 2 or 3 days of recurrent infections. Serologic testing is not helpful (and usually not available) in the initial evaluation of patients suspected of having herpes. The finding of characteristic vesicles or a history of recurrent lesions at the same site is the most reliable guide to clinical diagnosis. Women with lesions of the external genitalia may also have silent lesions of the uterine cervix, which may sometimes be diagnosed by direct visualization. A Pap smear is said to be about 80% sensitive. Viral cultures are expensive and usually not necessary. In general, their use should be limited to patients with suspected primary infections, patients with atypical presentations, and pregnant women.

The cycloguanosine acyclovir (Zovirax), available orally, greatly decreases pain and viral shedding and speeds healing in patients with primary infections. It has a less dramatic effect on recurrent infections. Acyclovir does not eradicate virus from ganglia, where it resides during latency; hence, it is not curative. The recommended oral dosage is 200 mg in five divided doses daily for 5 to 7 days.

Daily doses of acyclovir have proved to prevent recurrences of herpes successfully in many individuals who have frequent, debilitating outbreaks. The drug has been studied in individuals for up to one year. Discontinuing use of the drug, however, has been associated with severe recurrent "rebound" infections. An intravenous form is also available, which is useful in severe primary infections, in infections in immunocompromised individuals, and for meningoencephalitis.

Nonspecific support consisting of bed rest, sedation, and pain medication are helpful in primary infections. Antibiotics rarely have a place in management because true superinfection of herpetic lesions is rare. Occasionally, patients require hospitalization for management, usually related to acute urinary retention, meningitis, or other neurologic manifestations. Dysuria, which can be severe, particularly in women, can often be managed by having the patient urinate by squatting in a partially-filled bathtub. Nonspecific topical creams and ointments should be avoided because they may interfere with healing. Intercourse should be avoided when lesions are present. The efficacy of the condom in providing protection for men from a woman with herpetic lesions is not known.

CHANCROID

Chancroid is an ulcerative infection of the genitalia caused by Hemophilus ducreyi, an organism that is difficult to grow in culture. It has been increasingly reported in the United States, usually in focal epidemics in relation to prostitution.

SYMPTOMS

Chancroid is most commonly seen in men, probably because the painful lesion is more easily seen on the penis. Women occasionally present with an ulceration on the labia or the fourchette. The patient complains of a foul-smelling, painful ulcer, and pain and swelling in the groin ipsilateral to the lesion. A history of self-medication with inexorable worsening of the ulceration, pain, and swelling is common.

PHYSICAL FINDINGS

The ulcer is most often single and is usually located in the coronal sulcus or first third of the shaft of the penis. Ulceration of the cervix may occasionally be seen on speculum examination of women. In both sexes, the ulcer may be shallow or deep, is always painful to touch, and appears "superinfected." Tender, fluctuant erythematous adenopathy, usually unilateral and ipsilateral to the lesion, is a hallmark of the disease. These buboes are abscesses of both nodal and perinodal tissue. They tend to point and rupture relatively early in the course of the disease.

DIAGNOSIS AND TREATMENT

Multiple small, shallow penile or vulvar ulcerations suggest herpes, whereas a single clean, painless ulcer is more suggestive of syphilis. Both may be accompanied by inguinal adenopathy, but fluctuance and rupture are uncommon in syphilis. Syphilis should be ruled out by direct darkfield microscopic examination of material scraped from the base of the ulcer. If this cannot be done, a rapid serologic test for syphilis [rapid plasma reagin (RPR)] should be performed, but a negative test result does not rule it out.

The only reliable method of diagnosing herpetic infection when lesions are in the ulcerative stage is a culture. Within several days after progression from vesicles to ulcers, however, the amount of virus in the lesion is usually low, and cultures are often negative. Serologic tests are not useful in diagnosing acute herpetic outbreaks, and a Tzanck or Pap smear of the ulcer is usually nondiagnostic. A few laboratories now have media available for the isolation of Hemophilus ducreyi, and swabs of the lesions can be submitted in transport medium, which must be sent immediately to the laboratory, plated immediately, and incubated in 5% carbon dioxide. Most often, however, the diagnosis must still be made on clinical grounds alone. In all cases of genital ulcers, a follow-up syphilis serologic examination is important because all three organisms can coexist in the same lesion.

In the United States, most H. ducreyi produce a β-lactamase, making them highly resistant to penicillin. Suggested antibiotic regimens are ceftriaxone, 250 mg intramuscularly in a single dose; erythromycin, 500 mg orally four times a day; trimethoprim-sulfamethoxazole, one double-strength tablet orally twice a day for a week, or ciprofloxacin, 500 mg b.i.d. for 3 days. Large fluctuant nodes should be aspirated to prevent rupture, but incision and drainage can result in a prolonged healing time. The aspirated material may occasionally grow H. ducreyi. Longer therapy may be necessary for deep, infected ulcers or large buboes. Sexual partners of infected persons should also be treated with the same regimens. Note that none of these regimens is adequate therapy for syphilis.

SEXUALLY TRANSMITTED LOWER GASTROINTESTINAL INFECTIONS IN HOMOSEXUAL MEN

Because of sexual practices that involve contact with fecal material, enteric infections are common in sexually active homosexual men. Many of the organisms that cause traditional sexually transmitted diseases are associated with gastrointestinal tract infection: Neisseria gonorrhoeae, Chlamydia trachomatis, Treponema pallidum, herpes simplex virus, and papillomavirus. Enteric bacteria, including Salmonella, Shigella, and Campylobacter, are a common cause of infection, as are the protozoans Entamoeba histolytica and Giardia lamblia. Although they are not diseases involving the gastrointestinal tract, hepatitis A and B are clearly transmitted through fecal contact and rectal intercourse. More recently, with the AIDS epidemic have come infections with two other protozoans, Cryptosporidium and Isospora belli, and other agents, such as Cytomegalovirus, Candida albicans, and Mycobacterium. With the educational efforts directed toward "safer sex" in the homosexual community, rectal gonorrhea and syphilis have declined in the past few years.

The clinical syndromes produced by these agents involve overlapping regions of the intestine and anorectum; therefore, the clinical picture alone is not usually distinct enough to help distinguish between the various entities. The availability of diagnostic microbiology laboratory testing is essential.

SYMPTOMS

The pattern of symptoms depends heavily on the portion of the gastrointestinal tract involved. *Proctitis*, inflammation of the anorectum, produces anal pain, or pain on defecation, sometimes a rectal discharge, and often constipation. *Enteritis*, infection of the small intestine, most commonly produces diarrhea associated with cramps, gas, and bloating. *Proctocolitis*, inflammation of the lower colon, may produce combined symptoms of proctitis and enteritis. Certain organisms are associated with a predilection for certain areas of the intestine.

Anorectum: gonococcus, Chlamydia, T. pallidum, herpes simplex virus, cytomegalovirus

Colonic: E. histolytica, some strains of Chlamydia, cytomegalovirus, Campylobacter, Shigella, Mycobacterium (M. avium-intracellulare)

Enteric: Giardia, Cryptosporidium, Isospora, Mycobacterium, cytomegalovirus

Most of these pathogens can cause asymptomatic infection. This is typical of gonococcus, Chlamydia, enteric bacteria, T. pallidum, and E. histolytica.

Rectal gonorrhea and chlamydial infections produce similar symptoms, often mild rectal pain, itching, and discharge. Occasionally, chlamydial infections may produce widespread colonic disease that mimics inflammatory bowel disease.

Enteric pathogens typically produce a syndrome of abdominal pain, diarrhea, and fever.

Cryptosporidial and isosporal infections are characterized by watery, chronic diarrhea and weight loss, almost exclusively in human immunodeficiency virus (HIV)-infected patients.

Mycobacterial infection, occurring in HIV-infected patients, is often asymptomatic until gut wall invasion becomes massive; then, diarrhea characterized by steatorrhea and malabsorption may occur.

PHYSICAL FINDINGS

N. Gonorrhoeae. A mucopurulent rectal discharge may be present. Anoscopy may show normal mucosa or some erythema and small ulcerations. The mucopurulent discharge consists predominantly of PMNs.

C. Trachomatis. The presentation is often identical to that of a gonococcal infection. Occasionally, severe infections involving large areas of the colonic mucosa may be seen and are easily confused with inflammatory bowel disease on sigmoidoscopy. Apparently, only certain strains of *Chlamydia*, those associated with lymphogranuloma venereum, produce this severe inflammatory reaction.

Herpes Simplex Virus. This is the most common cause of nongonococcal rectal infections in homosexual men. It is common in HIV-infected patients. The lesions are usually extremely painful, making anoscopy and sometimes even digital rectal examination difficult. The lesions rarely extend into colonic tissue. If vesicles are present, they are virtually pathognomonic of herpetic proctitis; however, the lesions are most often ulcerative and multiple, and extend out onto perirectal skin.

Cytomegalovirus. This herpes virus may be isolated from asymptomatic individuals. In HIV-infected patients, it may produce a severe ulcerative disease of the colon and small intestine, associated with bloody diarrhea and, occasionally, bowel perforation.

Syphilis. The rectal chancre of primary syphilis is usually a solitary lesion that is painless, but sometimes it is atypical and painful, resembling an anal fissure or trauma. Occasionally, it may be polypoid, resembling a hemorrhoid. Condyloma latum, a form of secondary syphilis, may be confused with common venereal warts.

Enteric Bacteria. Shigella, Salmonella, and Campylobacter species may be isolated from asymptomatic individuals. They should be specifically sought in patients developing diarrhea, cramps, and fever. Gross blood may occasionally be seen in the stool of patients with Shigella and Campylobacter infections.

E. histolytica. Most infections are asymptomatic. A syndrome of mild diarrhea to full-blown dysentery may be seen. Diffuse inflammation and ulceration of the distal colon may be seen on sigmoidoscopy.

Cryptosporidium and Isospora. Both organisms may produce a severe watery diarrhea that contains neither white nor red blood cells and may be associated with profound weight loss and dehydration.

Giardia. This organism is usually confined to the small intestine, producing frequent small, loose, foul-smelling stools, chronic diarrhea, and weight loss. Rectal and sigmoidoscopic examinations are normal.

DIAGNOSIS AND TREATMENT

N. Gonorrhoeae and Chlamydia. PMNs predominate in the rectal discharge. A Gram stain of this material may show typical gram-negative diplococci within PMNs. The sensitivity of a Gram stain from a blindly taken rectal swab is only about 50%. It is much higher if an anoscopically directed swab is taken from an ulceration or purulent material. A culture should always be taken for confirmation even when the results of a Gram stain are positive. Routine screening of homosexual men should always include rectal, urethral, and throat cultures for N. gonorrhoeae. Chlamydia cannot be seen on a Gram-stained smear. The diagnosis can be established only through culture or a direct immunofluorescent stain. The chlamydial enzyme-linked immunosorbent assay (ELISA) may yield falsely positive results in rectal specimens and is not reliable.

The recommended treatment for rectal gonorrhea is ceftriaxone, 250 mg intramuscularly, or spectinomycin, 2.0 intramuscularly. Penicillin or ampicillin in various combinations should not be used. Cotreatment with tetracycline, 500 mg orally four times a day, or doxycycline, 100 mg orally twice a day for 7 days, to cover Chlamydia is also recommended. For treating chlamydial infections alone, tetracycline or doxycycline is sufficient. For severe infections, continuation for 2 or 3 weeks may be necessary. Contact tracing and treatment should be a routine part of the treatment plan.

Herpes Simplex Virus. If vesicles are present, no further diagnostic tests need be used. For ulcerated lesions, a Tzanck's smear (Giemsa-stained smear of the ulcer) or a direct immunofluorescent smear can help confirm the diagnosis, but a culture is the most sensitive method for confirmation.

For symptomatic infections, acyclovir, 200 mg four or five days a day for a week to 10 days, appears to be efficacious. The value of continuous prophylactic therapy to prevent recurrences of rectal herpes has not been established.

Cytomegalovirus. Cultures are not usually helpful because they require weeks to yield positive results. Biopsy of ulcerated lesions may show cells with typical inclusions. Diagnostic findings on serologic testing are a high titer (more than 1:1028) or a fourfold rise in cytomegalovirus antibodies. Acyclovir is not useful. An experimental drug, DHPG (ganciclovir), has shown some activity against cytomegalovirus in AIDS patients with extensive bowel disease or cytomegalovirus retinitis.

Syphilis. A darkfield microscopic examination should be made of all suspicious lesions. This is the simplest and fastest method of establishing a diagnosis. The RPR or VDRL may occasionally yield negative results during the early stages of the chancre but yields strongly positive results in virtually all cases of secondary syphilis.

Benzathine penicillin G, 2.4 million U intramuscularly (two 1.2 million U injections) at a single session, is the treatment of choice for primary and secondary syphilis. Tetracycline, 500 mg orally four times a day for 15 days, may be used for seriously penicillin-sensitive subjects. Recently, serologic failures have been demonstrated in HIV-infected patients with syphilis. Individuals who do not respond to these regimens with an adequate serologic decrease should be retreated. Contact identification and treatment are important parts of the therapeutic plan.

Enteric Bacteria. When infection with these organisms is suspected, it is important to bring stool or swabs to the laboratory immediately after they are taken and to request isolation of these particular pathogens, because many laboratories do not always routinely use the special media and conditions required. A Gram-stained smear of the stool may be helpful if it shows fecal leukocytes, often seen in Shigella and Campylobacter infections.

Shigellosis usually responds to supportive treatment. In severe cases, trimethoprim-sulfamethoxazole (Septra, Bactrim), one double-strength tablet orally twice a day for 7 days, is sufficient. Multiple antibiotic resistance in Shigella is common, however, and antibiotic sensitivity patterns of isolates should be routinely requested. Campylobacter infections, asymptomatic or symptomatic, should be treated with erythromycin, 500 mg orally four times a day for 7 days. Salmonella infections should be treated for the most part with supportive measures alone. Antibiotics are said to prolong the excretion of the organism.

E. Histolytica and Giardia. The diagnosis of these pathogens is usually made through stool examination. A liquid stool is much more likely to yield the pathogens than a formed stool. Stools should be submitted to the laboratory while they are still warm unless preservatives are used. *E. histolytica* may be identified in lesion biopsy specimens obtained through the anoscope or sigmoidoscope. Occasionally, *Giardia* are difficult to find in stool, and duodenal aspirates or Crosby's capsule biopsy specimens may be required.

The most common regimen for eradication of amebae is metronidazole, 750 mg orally three times a day for 10 days, with iodoquinol, 650 mg three times a day for 20 days. For treating giardiasis, one may use either quinacrine hydrochloride, 100 mg orally three times a day for 1 week; or metronidazole, 250 mg orally three times a day for 1 week. Retreatment may be required in up to 20% of cases.

Cryptosporidium and Isospora. An acid-fast stain of stool that has been concentrated by one of several methods is the simplest method of making the diagnosis. No effective therapy for either agent has been reported. Spiramycin, a macrolide antibiotic not available in the United States, has been shown to have some activity against Cryptosporidium, but its use is controversial.

Mycobacterium. Occasionally, the stool is positive on acid-fast staining for Mycobacterium. More often, staining of biopsy specimens of bowel wall are required. Because the most common pathogen, M. avium-intracellulare, is usually resistant to the standard mycobacterial regimens, treatment attempts, usually unsuccessful, have used six or seven drug regimens.

MENINGITIS AND MENINGOENCEPHALITIS

Mary Anne Mangelsen

CAPSULE

In spite of an impressive armamentarium of drugs to combat organisms responsible for central nervous system (CNS) infections, these diseases still cause characteristically significant morbidity and mortality. Diagnostic acumen, early recognition of the likely etiologic agent, and institution of therapy are requirements in the effective management of meningitis and meningoencephalitis. Immediate treatment includes administering appropriate antimicrobial and antiviral agents, controlling intracranial hypertension, and correcting metabolic imbalances and possible sequelae, such as disseminated intravascular coagulopathy and inappropriate secretion of vasopressin. Any microorganism, whether it be bacterial, viral, fungal, or protozoan, can cause a meningitis that can be insidious or fulminant but is always a medical emergency until proved otherwise. Nonbacterial meningoencephalitis frequently defies clinical and diagnostic definition by immediate, routine procedures, but confirmation must nonetheless be pursued aggressively because effective early treatment may be available, as with herpetic meningoencephalitis.[1]

PATHOPHYSIOLOGY

Most cases of meningitis or meningoencephalitis are the result of the hematogenous spread of infection, such as pneumonia, to the meninges. Some organisms that cause otitis media, sinusitis, or retro-orbital abscesses can invade the meninges through adjacent bone, whereas trauma or surgery can allow a more direct inoculation of microbes into the CNS. Herpes simplex and varicella-zoster viruses infect the meninges by retrograde spread to the CNS by way of peripheral nerves. Once in the subarachnoid space, the organisms multiply easily because both complement and immunoglobulin levels are low, preventing adequate opsonization and phagocytosis. Organisms in high concentrations disrupt the blood-brain barrier and open capillaries, allowing the entrance of white blood cells.

CLINICAL PRESENTATION

Meningitis must be considered in the differential diagnosis of anyone presenting with one or some of the following: an unexplained fever, severe headache; vomiting; some degree of altered mental status ranging from irritability to lethargy; neck pain or stiffness, focal neurologic deficits; seizures; and an erythematous, macular, or petechial rash.

Although these signs and symptoms do not help to define the specific etiologic agents, an alteration of consciousness, seizures, neurologic deficit, and a high fever most frequently indicate infection by a bacterium rather than by a virus or fungus. Moreover, children, the immunocompromised, and the elderly may present with insidious, subtle symptoms that are poorly defined and confusing: lack of appetite, weight loss, nausea, abrupt deafness or blindness, irritability, lethargy, and changes in behavior.

INITIAL PHYSICAL EVALUATION AND STABILIZATION

A quick, thorough examination includes a search for conjunctival and cutaneous petechiae, nuchal rigidity, bulging fontanelles in an infant, Brudzinski's sign (passive neck flexion producing flexion of the hips and knees), and Kernig's sign (back or neck pain on passive extension of the knee past 120 degrees with the hips flexed). If papilledema or a focal neurologic deficit (such as a third or sixth nerve palsy) is present, empiric antibacterial therapy is started, and an immediate computed tomographic (CT) scan is indicated. Lumbar puncture should be delayed because it may be associated with tentorial herniation. If increased intracranial pressure is not present, a lumbar puncture should be performed immediately. Table 50-16 provides a

TABLE 50-16. SUPPORTIVE THERAPY FOR MENINGITIS AND ENCEPHALITIS

Intravenous Fluids
    5% dextrose in half normal saline if patient is older than 6 months.
    10% dextrose in half normal saline if patient is younger than 6 months and if
       serum glucose is less than 90 mg/dL.
    Maintenance water calculations for children: 100 mL/kg/24 hr for first 10 kg
       of weight, then 50 mL/kg/24 hr for next 30 kg.
    NaCl requirements: 3 mEq/kg/24 hr to a maximum of 45 mEq/day.
Dexamethasone Therapy for Bacterial Meningitis
    Dexamethasone (Decadron) 0.15 mg/kg IV every 6 hours for 4 days*
Increased Intracranial Pressure
    20% mannitol solution: 1–3 g/kg IV over 30 min.
    Dexamethasone (Decadron): 0.15 mg/kg IV q 6hr.
Seizure Activity
    Diazepam (Valium): 0.1–0.2 mg/kg IV, titrated slowly to point of control.
    Phenobarbital: 10–20 mg/kg IV, titrated slowly to point of control. An alter-
      nate to diazepam.
    Phenytoin (Dilantin): 1–3 mg/kg (neonate), 5 mg/kg (pediatric), 10–15 mg/kg
      (adult) IV; titrated slowly to point of control. An alternate to diazepam.
Sedation for Lumbar Puncture or Computed Tomography
    Midazolam (Versed): 0.15–0.35 mg/kg IV, titrated slowly to point of control.
      To be used only when necessary.
      Advantage: short half-life.
    Diazepam (Valium): 0.1–0.2 mg/kg IV, titrated slowly to point of control. To
      be used only when necessary. An alternate to midazolam.
    Morphine sulfate: 0.1–0.2 mg/kg IV, titrated slowly to point of control. An
      alternate to midazolam
      Advantage: can be reversed with naloxone (Narcan) at 0.01 mg/kg IV,
      titrated to patient response.

* Lebel, M.H., Freij, B.J., Syrogiannopoulos, G.A., et al.: Dexamethasone therapy for bacterial meningitis. N. Engl. J. Med. *319:*964, 1988.

guide for possible sedation needed during a lumbar puncture. If the puncture cannot be completed, however, an empiric antimicrobial program should be initiated without it, after consideration of the probable infectious organism and the age and condition of the host. A thorough examination (ears, pharynx, sinuses, chest, and genitourinary tract) may reveal a logical source of infection.

Seizures occur in 30% of patients with bacterial meningoencephalitis and in approximately 5% of patients with viral meningoencephalitis. Terminating a seizure requires establishing an adequate airway and immediately administering intravenous diazepam in a dose of 0.1 to 0.2 mg per kg; phenobarbital (10 to 20 mg per kg slowly intravenously) and phenytoin (10 to 15 mg per kg slowly intravenously for the adult) are alternates. Irritability, mottling of the skin, pallor, or confusion may indicate poor perfusion and demand immediate intervention before other diagnostic procedures are undertaken. Even in the presence of a normal blood pressure, initial treatment should involve an infusion of 5% dextrose in half normal saline if the patient is older than 6 months or 10% dextrose in half normal saline if the patient is younger than 6 months and if the serum glucose level is less than 90 mg per dL. In the elderly, an altered cardiac or renal status should be kept in mind when administering fluids. Signs of increased cranial pressure call for im-

mediate use of mannitol and dexamethasone (see Table 50-16). Other measures include restricting fluids, administering osmotic diuretics, and inducing hyperventilation. In one recent study, infants and children who received dexamethasone early in their meningitis became afebrile sooner and were less likely to have residual hearing loss.

Because the interval from the appearance of obvious symptoms to death may be only 4 to 10 hours, it is imperative that antimicrobial therapy start within 30 to 60 minutes for the fulminant presentation, although optimal timing is rarely achieved except during epidemics. If there is a confusing presentation or a delay in CT scanning or lumbar puncture, immediate intravenous antibiotic therapy is warranted until a specific diagnosis can be made. The age of the patient is the best guide for initial antimicrobial treatment (Table 50-17).

DIFFERENTIAL DIAGNOSIS

Although Rocky Mountain spotted fever rarely develops into an encephalitis, the possibility of confusing this disease with meningococcemia is real. Patients

TABLE 50-17. INITIAL ANTIMICROBIAL THERAPY FOR MENINGITIS AND ENCEPHALITIS*

Age/Condition	Most Common Organism	Antibiotics	Dosage	Alternate	Dosage
1–3 months	Gram-negative rods; Escherichia coli (50–60%)	Ampicillin and Gentamicin	50–100 mg/kg q 6 hr IV 2.5 mg/kg q 8 hr IV	Cefuroxime or ceftriaxone†	10 mg/kg q 12 hr IV 75 mg/kg × 1 dose, then 50 mg/kg q 12 hr IV (2 g q 12 hr for adults)
	Group B streptococci (20–40%)	Penicillin G‡	62,500 U/kg q 6 hr	Chloramphenicol	25 mg/kg q 12 hr IV
	Listeria monocytogenes (2–10%)	Ampicillin	As above		
3 months–10 years	Haemophilus influenzae (40–60%) Neisseria meningitidis (25–40%) Streptococcus pneumoniae (10–20%)	Ampicillin and Chloramphenicol	50 mg/kg q 4 hr IV 25 mg/kg q 12 hr IV (infant) 25 mg/kg q 6 hr IV (child)	Ceftriaxone†	75 mg/kg × 1 dose, then 50 mg/kg q 12 hr IV (2 g q 12 h for adults)
10 years–adult	Streptococcus pneumoniae (30–50%) Neisseria meningitidis (10–35%) Group A streptococcus (< 10%)	Penicillin G‡	50,000 U/kg q 4 hr IV (24,000 million U q day for adults)	Chloramphenicol	1 g q 6 hr IV (adult)
	Haemophilus influenzae (< 10%)	Ampicillin and Chloramphenicol	50 mg/kg q 4 hr IV (12 g q day for adult) 25 mg/kg q 6 hr IV (child)	Cefuroxime† or ceftriaxone†	60 mg/kg q 6 hr IV 75 mg/kg × 1 dose, then 50 mg/kg q 12 hr IV (2 g q 12 hr for adults)
Alcoholic	Streptococcus pneumoniae Listeria monocytogenes	Ampicillin	50 mg/kg q 4 hr IV (12 g q day for adult)	Chloramphenicol	1 g q 6 hr IV
CNS abscess, acute	Staphylococcus aureus Streptococci Streptococcus pneumoniae	Nafcillin and Chloramphenicol	25 mg/kg q 4 hr IV (child) 0.5–1 g q 4–6 hr IV (up to 10 g/day for adults) 25 mg/kg q 6 hr IV (child adult)		
CNS shunt	Staphylococcus aureus	Penicillinase-resistant penicillin, e.g., Nafcillin	As above (adult) As above (child)	Vancomycin	15 mg/kg q 8 hr IV (child) 500 mg q 6 hr IV (adult)
Asplenic	Streptococcus pneumoniae Haemophilus influenzae	Ampicillin and Chloramphenicol	50 mg/kg q 4 hr IV (child, adult) (12 g q day for adult) 25 mg/kg q 6 hr IV (child, adult)		
Trauma, recent craniotomy	Staphylococcus aureus Streptococcus pneumoniae Gram-negative rods	Penicillinase-resistant penicillin, e.g., Nafcillin or methicillin Antipseudomonal aminoglycoside, e.g., Amikacin or Gentamicin and Ceftriaxone†	As above 5 mg/kg q 8 hr IV (child, adult) 1.5 mg/kg q 8 hr IV (child, adult) 75 mg/kg × 1 dose, then 50 mg/kg q 12 hr IV (child) or 2 g q 12 hr (adult)	Vancomycin	15 mg/kg q 8 hr IV (child) 500 mg q 6 hr IV (adult)
Immunosuppressed	Listeria monocytogenes Gram-negative rods except:	Ampicillin and Ceftriaxone†	50 mg/kg q 4 hr (12 g q day for adults) As above	Trimethoprim-sulfamethoxazole	20 mg TMP/100 mg SMX/kg q day IV, divided into q 6 hr doses
	Pseudomonas Acinetobacter calcoaceticus	IV & intrathecal aminoglycoside, e.g., Gentamicin and Antipseudomonal cephalosporin, e.g., Ceftazidime†	1.5 mg/kg q 8 hr IV 4 mg intrathecally q 12–24 hr (adult) 2 g q 8 hr IV (adult) 50 mg/kg q 8 hr (child)		

TABLE 50-17. CONTINUED*

Age/Condition	Most Common Organism	Antibiotics	Dosage	Alternate	Dosage
All ages	Cryptococcus neoformans Aspergillus Mucor	Amphotericin B and	25 mg IV, moving gradually up to 50 mg q day after 42 days		
		5-Fluorocytosine	37.5 mg/kg IV q 6 hr for 6 wk		
		Intrathecal amphotericin B	0.1 mg q 2 days	Ketoconazole	400 mg q day po (adult)
	Herpes simplex	Acyclovir	5 mg/kg q 8 hr IV		
	Varicella-zoster	Acyclovir	As above		
	Rabies	No treatment			
	Rickettsial Rocky Mountain spotted fever	Tetracycline or	5 mg/kg q 6 hr IV (avoid in children less than 9 yr)		
		Chloramphenicol	25 mg/kg q 6 hr IV (child, adult)		
	Toxoplasma gondii	Pyrimethamine§ and	2 mg/kg q day orally in 2 doses for 1–3 days, then 1 mg/kg q day in two doses for 4 wk with a maximal dose of 25 mg q day		
		Sulfadiazine	Oral loading dose of 75 mg/kg, then 100 mg q day up to 8 g q day in 2 doses		
	Spirochete: Leptospira	Doxycycline	0.1 g q 12 hr 1st day, then 0.1–0.2 g q day IV (adult)	Penicillin G	≥ 10 million U q day
	Ameba: Naegleria fowleri	IV and intrathecal amphotericin B	1 mg test dose IV, then 25 mg IV, moving gradually up to 50 mg q day 0.1 mg intrathecally q 2 days		
	Mycobacterium tuberculosis	Rifampin and	600 mg q day po		
		Isoniazid and	8–12 mg/kg q day po (adult)‖ 15–20 mg/kg q day po (child)‖		
		Ethambutol and	15 mg/kg q day po	Streptomycin	0.75 g q day IM
		Pyrazinamide	25 mg/kg q day po		

* The doses are for patients with normal renal function and need to be adjusted for those with renal impairment.

† These agents alone are not adequate for eliminating *Pseudomonas* or *Acinetobacter* species unless minimal inhibitory concentrations (MIC) are available and cerebrospinal fluid antibiotic levels are known and are therapeutic. Third-generation cephalosporins provide incomplete coverage for group B streptococci and pneumococci and none at all for *L. monocytogenes*. First-generation cephalosporins should not be used in therapy for bacterial meningitis.

‡ 0.5% to 2% of pneumococcal strains are resistant to penicillin. All isolates should be screened for penicillin susceptibility.

§ Folinic acid may reduce toxicity: give 5–10 mg q day po or parenterally q 2 days.

‖ To be taken with pyridoxine: 100 mg q day.

with either disease may present with severe headache, lethargy, fever, and a petechial rash. The singular difference may be that in the rickettsial syndrome, the petechial rash is concentrated peripherally, generally over the hands and wrists, ankles, and feet, and specifically on the palms and soles; whereas the distribution in meningococcemia is symmetric and tends to involve sclerae and conjunctivae. The macular rash that becomes petechial or hemorrhagic is difficult to distinguish from underlying gonorrhea, syphilis, systemic lupus erythematosus, drug reactions, enterovirus infections (especially the echovirus type 9 infection), Kawasaki syndrome, leptospirosis, Lyme disease, or toxic shock syndrome. Petechiae may also be seen with pneumococcal and Staphylococcus aureus meningitis but rarely with Haemophilus influenzae. Disseminated intravascular coagulopathy frequently accompanies meningococcemia, which in its most dreaded form can progress to shock, characteristic of the Waterhouse-Friderichsen syndrome.

In meningitis caused by Neisseria meningitidis, a relatively nonspecific erythematous or macular rash can explode into a petechial-hemorrhagic rash within a few minutes to a few hours as opposed to a few days, which is more characteristic of Rocky Mountain spotted fever. Herpes simplex should be strongly suspected in a patient with acute hepatic necrosis, preceding risk factors (high-dose steroids, a compromised immune system, pregnancy), or skin or mucosal vesicles on the lips, mouth, vagina, penis, or perineum.

Bacterial meningitis and measles encephalitis most frequently occur in spring or winter, whereas the enterovirus, togavirus, and Listeria meningitises peak in late spring, summer, and early autumn (Table 50-18). H. influenzae, Streptococcus pneumoniae, and N. meningitidis remain the most common bacterial causes of meningitis, accounting for 80% of the reported cases. Pneumococcal meningitis tends to occur most frequently in young adults, alcoholics, and the immunosuppressed, particularly those with splenic abnormalities, hemoglobinopathies, Wiskott-Aldrich syndrome, nephrotic syndrome in children, Hodgkin's disease, leukemia, or multiple myeloma. It also tends to recur in patients with congenital or traumatic communications between the environment and the subarachnoid space. When the pneumococcus is the etiologic agent, coma is more frequent, as are ear infections, sinusitis, or pneumonia. Likewise, H. in-

fluenzae meningitis in adults is associated with otitis media and pharyngitis in over 50% of cases. The presence of another site of active infection is rare in patients with meningitis.

H. influenzae meningitis occurs most frequently in persons between 6 months and 3 years, who may present with deafness occurring within 24 to 36 hours of the onset of illness. H. influenzae type b has been noted in all age groups, however, and should be considered in initial antibiotic coverage. Listeria is the fourth most common bacterial cause of meningitis in all age groups and is most often associated with neonates, the elderly, or immunocompromised adults. Seizures with meningeal signs, especially in summer and early fall, increase the likelihood of Listeria as the causative agent. The cerebrospinal fluid (CSF) of persons with Listeria meningitis most frequently demonstrates mononuclear pleocytosis, as it does with infections by other, less common organisms (Table 50-19).

Meningitis caused by gram-negative rods occurs most frequently in neonates (as a nosocomial infection), in immunocompromised hosts and as the result of head trauma or neurosurgical procedures. Because

TABLE 50-18. IDENTIFYING CHARACTERISTICS OF VIRUSES CAUSING MENINGITIS AND MENINGOENCEPHALITIS

Virus	Peak Season	Comments
Enteroviruses (polio, echo, coxsackie)	Late summer–early autumn	Accounts for 50% of viral meningitis; encephalitis rare; associated with paralytic myelitis, myocarditis, pleurodynia
Mumps	April–July	Associated parotitis; 10% of viral meningitis
Measles	Winter–spring	Characteristic rash, conjunctivitis, Koplik's spots; encephalitis syndrome occurs during convalescent stage
Arenaviridae (lymphocytic choriomeningitis)	Winter, sporadic	Contact with rodents
Herpesviridae (Epstein-Barr virus, cytomegalovirus)	Sporadic	Associated with a mononucleosis syndrome; may be seen more often in immunoimpaired hosts
(varicella-zoster)	Sporadic	Vesicular rash precedes CNS symptoms; cerebellar ataxia; transverse myelitis (rare)
(herpes simplex)	Sporadic	Hemorrhagic encephalitis; focal neurological deficits with temporal localization
Togaviridae (St Louis encephalitis; western equine encephalitis, eastern equine encephalitis, dengue)	Late spring, early autumn	Mosquito-borne; primarily encephalitis syndrome
Bunyaviridae (California encephalitis)	Late spring, early autumn	Mosquito-borne; primarily encephalitis syndrome
Reoviridae (Colorado tick fever)	April–August	Tick transmission; "saddle bar" fever, myalgias
Rhabdoviridae (rabies)	Sporadic	Encephalomyelitis syndrome, may mimic Guillain-Barré syndrome; animal/bite exposure, hydrophobia, aerophobia
Human immunodeficiency retrovirus (HIV)	Sporadic	Immunocompromised host; frequently subacute presentation; polyneuropathy; vacuolar myelopathy

(Modified with permission from Benson CA, Harris, A.A.: Acute neurologic infections 70:993, 1986.)

TABLE 50-19. SELECTED LESS COMMON ORGANISMS IN CNS SYNDROMES

Organism	Comments
Borrelia burgdorferi Tick-borne spirochete	Lyme disease; cranial neuritis, especially of the 7th nerve; begins weeks to months after Lyme disease diagnosis
Brucella species Gram-negative coccobacillus	Brucellosis (undulant fever); contact with livestock or dogs; ingestion of contaminated milk or airborne spread; calcifications of old lesions in liver or spleen
Clostridium botulinum Spore-bearing bacillus	Botulism; muscle paralysis caused by toxin in food or wound; gastrointestinal symptoms; frequent drug abuse history
Clostridium tetani Spore-bearing bacillus	Lockjaw; syndrome produced by exotoxin causing intense activity of motor neurons resulting in severe muscle spasms
Coccidioides immitis Fungus	Coccidiodomycosis; endemic in southwestern US; frequently associated with pulmonary cavitation
Corynebacterium diphtheriae Gram-positive bacillus	Diphtheria; grayish adherent membrane on pharynx; paralysis of palate; similar to Guillain-Barré syndrome
Francisella tularensis Gram-negative bacillus	Important animal host: rabbit; also transmitted by insect vectors (such as deer flies), handling infected animals, inhaling infected aerosols; frequent primary ulcer; hepatomegaly; splenomegaly
Leptospira interrogans Spirochete	Leptospirosis; occurs frequently during hot weather; wide spectrum of animal hosts; found in animal urine for months to years; swimming in contaminated water accounts for outbreaks
Listeria monocytogenes Gram-positive bacillus	Inhalation, ingestion, or direct contact with contaminated food or animal products; disseminated granulomas and focal necrosis; clinically similar to infectious mononucleosis
Mima polymorpha Gram-negative bacillus	Easily confused on Gram's stain with members of the *Neisseria* group and *H. influenzae*; difficult to distinguish on clinical grounds also, but responds to tetracycline
Mycobacterium tuberculosis Acid-fast bacillus	May develop cranial nerve palsy; a complication of untreated miliary tuberculosis; long tract signs; frequent inappropriate secretion of antidiuretic hormone
Naegleria fowleri Ameba	Contact with brackish waters in southern states; abnormal olfactory sensation
Nocardia asteroides Bacterium with branching hyphae	Usually a pre-existing debilitating condition; frequent bronchopneumonia; presents as a brain abscess or purulent meningitis
Plasmodium falciparum Protozoan	Malaria; synchronous periodicity of fever; hepatomegaly; splenomegaly; thrombocytopenia
Taenia solium Cestode	Cerebral cysticercosis from ingesting inadequately cooked pork, even years before; asymptomatic subcutaneous cysts or skeletal muscle calcifications
Toxoplasma gondii Protozoan	Toxoplasmosis; contracted usually from uncooked meats and close association with cats; similar to mononucleosis syndrome; possible retinochoroiditis
Trypanosoma brucei Protozoan	Trypanosomiasis; bite of African tsetse fly; wasting; maculopapular rash; facial edema; hemorrhages into lung, bone marrow
Unknown	Reye's syndrome; antecedent viral illness; elevated ammonia and liver function tests[3]

humans have a natural immunity to Staphylococcus aureus, most cases of meningitis due to this organism are the result of invasive procedures: craniotomy or CNS shunt.

Viral meningitis and meningoencephalitis are often difficult to diagnose on clinical grounds alone. The identifying characteristics of the more prominent viruses are listed in Table 50-18. Rabies may manifest itself as a nonspecific encephalitis[4] or as a fulminant encephalomyelitis syndrome that characteristically includes hypersalivation, generalized convulsions, or a laryngeal/pharyngeal spasm provoked by the sight of water (hydrophobia) or by air blown in the face (aerophobia). Twenty percent of patients exhibit a paralysis that mimics the Guillain-Barré syndrome.

Although most viral infections of the CNS have a benign self-limited course, early specific diagnosis of a herpes simplex or varicella-zoster encephalitis is essential for initiating antiviral therapy, such as the use of acyclovir. The patient's level of consciousness at the time of treatment is a good prognostic sign. Nearly 90% of persons with meningitis caused by either of these two organisms present with severe headache or focal neurologic signs. On the other hand, infections

---

TABLE 50-20. INFECTIOUS AND NONINFECTIOUS CAUSES OF ASEPTIC MENINGITIS OR MENINGOENCEPHALITIS*

Infectious Agents and Diseases
  Bacteria: Partially treated meningitis, *Mycobacterium tuberculosis,* paramenin-
    geal focus (brain abscess, epidural abscess), acute or subacute bacterial
    endocarditis
  Viruses: Enteroviruses, mumps, lymphocytic choriomeningitis, Epstein-Barr,
    arboviruses (eastern equine, western equine, St Louis), cytomegalovirus,
    varicella-zoster, herpes simplex, retrovirus (HIV)
  Rickettsiae: Rocky Mountain spotted fever
  Spirochetes: Syphilis, leptospirosis, Lyme disease
  Mycoplasma: M. pneumoniae, M. hominis (in neonates)
  Fungi: *Candida albicans, Coccidioides immitis, Cryptococcus neoformans*
  Protozoa: *Toxoplasma gondii,* malaria, *Naegleria fowleri* (ameba)
  Nematodes: Rat lungworm larvae (eosinophilic meningitis)
  Cestodes: Cysticercosis (tapeworm larvae of *Taenia solium*)
Noninfectious Diseases
  Malignancy: Primary medulloblastoma, metastatic leukemia, Hodgkin's disease
  Collagen-vascular disease: Lupus erythematosus
  Trauma: Subarachnoid bleeding, traumatic lumbar puncture, neurosurgery
  Granulomatous disease: Sarcoidosis
  Direct toxin: Intrathecal injections of contrast media, spinal anesthesia
  Poison: Lead, mercury
  Autoimmune disease: Guillain-Barré syndrome
  Postviral disease: Reye's syndrome
  Unknown: Multiple sclerosis, Mollaret's meningitis, Behçet's syndrome, Vogt-
    Koyanagi syndrome, Harada's syndrome, Kawasaki disease

---

* Aseptic meningitis or meningoencephalitis is defined as meningitis or meningoencephalitis in the absence of evidence of a bacterial pathogen detectable in CSF by usual
laboratory techniques.
  (With permission from Klein, J.O., Feigin, R.D., and McCracken, G.H.: American Academy
of Pediatrics: Report of the task force on diagnosis and management of meningitis. Pediatrics
78:970, 1986.)

---

with the human immunodeficiency retrovirus (HIV) can be present in the CNS and cause headache alone, altered mental state, or no neurologic symptoms or signs at all. Furthermore, HIV can be isolated from the CSF of persons without clinically apparent immunosuppression.[5] The only reliable diagnostic test for severe encephalitis is culture of the virus from the infected tissue. A computed tomographic scan, a radionuclide scan, and possibly magnetic resonance imaging (MRI) of the head may be necessary before an open biopsy is performed.

Because several less common organisms sometimes cause the signs and symptoms of a meningoencephalitis, Table 50-19 outlines characteristics that may aid in their diagnosis. Furthermore, Table 50-20 lists many causative agents of aseptic meningitis, which so often presents a diagnostic dilemma.

PROCEDURES

If there is no evidence of increased intracranial pressure, a lumbar puncture should be performed after the patient's emergent need for fluids is met. The normal opening pressure is 150 ± 30 mm H_2O, with a 5 to 10 mm variation with respiration. If manometry is performed, the patient should be positioned on the side during normal respiration to avoid inaccurately elevated measurements. If the opening pressure is greater than 350 mm H_2O, the physician should take a small amount of fluid and withdraw the needle. If, during the lumbar puncture, the patient exhibits evidence of tentorial herniation (fixed, dilated pupils; decerebrate or decorticate posturing; Cheyne-Stokes respiration; or focal neurologic deficits), immediate measures must be taken to lower intracranial pressure. These measures include intubation, induction of hyperventilation, and administration of mannitol. A subsequent decompressive craniectomy may have to be performed.

LABORATORY PROCEDURES

CEREBROSPINAL FLUID

Laboratory tests performed on the CSF to diagnose meningitis include CSF pressure, Gram stain, culture for a bacterium and any other microbe that may be suspected, red blood cell and white blood cell counts,

TABLE 50-21. INITIAL INTERVENTION

Source for Immediate Testing	Possible Additional Tests
BLOOD	Toxic screen
Serum glucose	Urea nitrogen
Complete blood count	Osmolality
Blood cultures	Prothrombin time
Electrolytes	Thromboplastin time
Countercurrent immuno-electrophoresis*	Fibrin split products
	Fibrinogen
SPINAL FLUID	Platelet count
Cell count and differential	Type and cross-match for blood and plasma
Protein	Ammonia
Glucose	Acute serology for viral etiology
Culture for all microbes	Latex particle agglutination†
Gram's stain	Enzyme-linked immunosorbent assay (ELISA)
India ink preparation	Serology for toxoplasmosis, histoplasmosis, coccidioidomycosis, blastomycosis, Q fever
Countercurrent immuno-electrophoresis*	Cryptococcal antigen assay
URINE	Antinuclear antibody titer
Urine analysis	Fluorescent treponemal antibody absorption test
Urine culture	Fungal cultures
Countercurrent immuno-electrophoresis*	Mycobacterial cultures
	Acid-fast smear
	Viral cultures
	Cytology for malignant cells
	Total complement
	Anti-double-stranded DNA
	T- and B-cell subsets
	Cryoglobulins
	Rheumatoid factor
	Rapid plasma reagin
	Venereal Disease Research Laboratory serological test for syphilis
	Computed tomography
	Magnetic resonance imaging
	Cultures of nose, throat, stool
	Gram's stain of skin lesions and sputum
	Sputum cultures
	Needle aspiration of middle ear fluid
	Chest radiograph
	Appropriate cultures for family members

* Test for group B Streptococcus; K¹ strains of Escherichia coli; Haemophilus influenzae type B; Neisseria meningitidis groups A, B, C, Y, and W-135; Streptococcus pneumoniae; Listeria monocytogenes; Klebsiella pneumoniae; and Pseudomonas aeruginosa. A negative test result does not exclude a diagnosis of bacterial meningitis.

† Test for group B meningococci, H. influenzae type B, S. pneumoniae, N. meningitidis, and group B streptococci. Tests may yield positive results for up to 10 days after children have received H. influenzae polysaccharide vaccine.

cell type, and glucose and protein levels (Table 50-21). In a traumatic tap, one white blood cell per 700 red blood cells is considered normal. A 1 mg/dL rise in protein per 1000 red blood cells approximates the amount of contaminating serum protein. The CSF contains a preponderance of polymorphonuclear leukocytes in bacterial meningitis in contrast to viral meningoencephalitis (10 to 1000 white blood cells in which mononuclear cells predominate). These figures are by no means definitive, for a viral meningitis can be associated with neutrophils, whereas lymphocytes can predominate in 10% of bacterial CNS infections.

Counterimmune electrophoresis (CIE) and latex particle agglutination can detect the antigens of many microbes in the CSF, sputum, serum, and urine, and the testing can be completed within the hour. CIE can detect nonogram quantities of the antigens of group B streptococci, six strains of Escherichia coli, H. influenzae type b, N. meningitidis groups A, B, C, Y, and W-135, S. pneumoniae, L. monocytogenes, Klebsiella pneumoniae, and Pseudomonas aeruginosa. If one desires to increase a test's sensitivity, urine has the obvious advantage over CSF in quantity, and can be concentrated 10- to 100-fold. The diagnosis of bacterial meningitis by CIE may be enhanced by evaluation of urine in addition to CSF and serum, particularly in partially-treated patents. A negative CIE test, however, is inconclusive because there is a minimum threshold of antigen detection and crossreactivity occurs with certain organisms, reducing specificity.[7] The latex particle agglutination method has been found useful in detecting antigen in CSF infected with H. influenzae type b, N. meningitidis groups B and C, and S. pneumoniae. Indeed, it may be more sensitive than CIE for detection of the capsular antigen of H. influenzae.

An India ink slide preparation stains positive in approximately 50% of cryptococcal infections, and testing for the cryptococcal antigen can prove 90% successful for that disease. If tuberculosis meningitis is suspected, an acid-fast smear should be obtained. In addition, an enzyme-linked immunosorbent assay (ELISA) can detect the mycobacterial antigen and antibody, but because of limited sensitivity, a negative test result does not exclude the diagnosis of tuberculous meningitis.[8] Measurement of the CSF lactate level, once proposed as a confirmation of bacterial meningitis, is not routinely recommended now because of the rate of false-positive results. ELISA appears to be more specific than the CIE or latex particle agglutination method, but is cumbersome and takes 3 to 6 hours to complete. Although clinical data are limited, a more rapid ELISA method has been used to detect types 2 and 3 group B Streptococcus antigens in the CSF.[9] The Limulus lysate assay detects the presence of endotoxin. It identifies 90% of gram-negative meningitis but cannot distinguish between H. influenzae and N. meningitidis, and occasionally crossreacts with gram-positive organisms.

BLOOD

The most immediate blood studies needed are a complete blood count; a serum glucose test for metabolic status and comparison with the CSF glucose level (the normal CSF/serum glucose ratio is approximately 0.6; infants less than 6 months of age have a mean ratio of 0.81); a coagulation survey to detect possible disseminated intravascular coagulopathy; and blood cultures. Fifty percent of blood cultures are positive in cases of suppurative meningitis in the newborn, whereas the yield for older children is variable: 33% for N. meningitidis, 50% for S. pneumoniae, and 80% for H. influenzae.

INFECTIOUS AGENTS

When appropriate, sputum Gram stain and culture, urinalysis and culture, petechial scrapings for a Gram's stain, culture of fluid from an infected joint, and appropriate radiographs may help to confirm the causative agent, but their results should not be considered definitive.

AN INITIAL THERAPEUTIC APPROACH

The physician is sometimes faced with pleocytosis in the CSF fluid and a negative Gram stain. Possible causes are vast and outlined in Tables 50-18 through 50-20. Initial therapy should be based on the condition of the CSF (Table 50-22), the Gram stain, and the age and health of the individual. In an otherwise healthy individual over 3 months, chloramphenicol in combination with either penicillin or ampicillin, or chloramphenicol alone in penicillin-allergic patients covers N. meningitidis, H. influenzae, and S. pneumoniae,

TABLE 50-22. CSF FINDINGS

Diagnosis	RBC	Mono	PMN	CSF Pressure (mmHg)	Glucose (mg/dl)	Protein (mg/dl)
Normal CSF	0	< 5	0	< 200	40–75	15–55
Bacterial	N	+	+ + +	+	< 40	> 55
Aseptic meningitis	N	+ +	+	+	N	+
Amebic, protozoan, fungal, tubercular	N	+ + +	+	+	< 40	+
Spirochete, viral	N, +	+ +*	+	+	N	+
Subarachnoid hemorrhage	+ + +	+	+	+ +	N	+ +
CNS neoplasm	N	N	N	+ +	N	+ +

RBC = red blood cells, Mono = mononuclear leukocytes; PMN = polymorphonuclear leukocytes; N = normal; +, + +, + + + = increased.
*A PMN reaction can be seen in this early CNS infection. This usually converts within a short time to a mononuclear majority.

the most common causes of community-acquired meningitis. If the patient has hepatic or renal function abnormalities, hypotension, or persistent shock, it is preferable to avoid the use of chloramphenicol and the aminoglycosides, if possible, because of the patient's diminished ability to excrete them by the hepatic and renal routes. β-Lactam antibiotics are preferred in these cases unless the serum concentrations of chloramphenicol or aminoglycosides can be promptly determined.

Table 50-17 summarizes more specific antimicrobial therapy. Moxalactam has been successful in treating neonates, children, and adults with enteric gram-negative meningitis.[10] It has, however, poor activity against pneumococcal meningitis and has common significant side effects, hypoprothrombinemia and platelet dysfunction. The use of moxalactam is now avoided if possible. The spectrum of activity of ceftriaxone is similar to that of cefotaxime, except that ceftriaxone has a long half-life and can be administered once or twice a day. Ceftriaxone compares favorably with ampicillin-chloramphenicol therapy in the treatment of meningitis in children.[11] Ceftizoxime, a newer third-generation cephalosporin, may be effective in the management of meningitis caused by H. influenzae, S. pneumoniae, and N. meningitidis and possibly enteric gram-negative bacillary meningitis, but clinical data are limited.[12] Ceftazidime is a new cephalosporin with enhanced antipseudomonal activity. The placement of an Ommaya reservoir should be considered in situations requiring intrathecal administration of antibiotics.

WITHHOLDING THERAPY

If aseptic meningitis is diagnosed because of the inability of the usual laboratory techniques to clearly define the pathogen, some investigators advocate withholding antibiotic therapy and repeating the lumbar puncture after 6 to 8 hours of closely observing the patient in the hospital. This course of action *is not recommended* if the patient has been treated recently with antibiotics, is younger than 1 year, is clinically unstable, or begins to deteriorate during the observation period. Others advocate presumptive therapy after culturing appropriate body fluids if the physician assesses the meningitis or meningoencephalitis to be treatable. For example, if a definitive diagnosis of herpes simplex or varicella-zoster meningoencephalitis is not possible but the classic signs of behavioral changes and CSF with lymphocytosis and a normal glucose level are present, it is appropriate to administer intravenous acyclovir immediately and to continue for 5 days until a more specific diagnosis can be made.[13]

USE OF STEROIDS

The benefit of corticosteroids has not been conclusively shown. Three studies in children, however, support use of dexamethasone, 0.15 mg/kg, q6h for 4 days. Cefuroxime (80 mg q8h) or ceftriaxone (80 mg/kg) was also given IV immediately, then q12h for 2 days and once daily thereafter. The antibiotics were given for 10 days in Hemophilus influenzae type b or Streptococcus pneumoniae meningitis infections, and 7 days in Neisseria meningitidis infections. Benefit was seen in infants and children, particularly in preventing deafness.[16] Another study with cefotaxime and dexamethasone confirmed this result.[17]

FAMILY HISTORY AND PARTICIPATION

Obtaining a history from the family is a valuable adjunct to diagnosis. Helpful information includes the patient's and family's recent infections, travel history, contacts, and the presence of animals, especially cats and farm animals. Depending on the most likely diagnosis of the patient, prophylaxis for the family and contacts must be considered. (Table 50-23); if meningococcemia is suspected, it is appropriate to obtain nasopharyngeal cultures.

MEDICOLEGAL PEARLS

- No group of symptoms is absolute for meningitis or meningoencephalitis. Headache, fever, vomiting, meningeal irritation, lethargy, rash—any combination of these should heighten a physician's suspicion of a CNS infection.
- Timing is critical. The proper antimicrobial therapy should be initiated within the shortest time possible.
- Aggressive history-taking and prophylaxis for the family are keys to adequate management.
- The CSF may be normal, but the patient may still have meningitis according to clinical signs. Close observation with a repeat lumbar puncture in 6 to 8 hours usually demonstrates the infection. Thorough laboratory testing is necessary for defining occult sources of infection.
- Remember the new antiviral antibiotic (e.g., acyclovir), particularly for herpes simplex and cytomegalovirus.

TABLE 50-23. PROPHYLAXIS FOR CLOSE CONTACTS OF PERSONS WITH MENINGITIS OR MENINGOENCEPHALITIS

Organism	Drug	Dose
Hemophilus influenzae	Rifampin	20 mg/kg/day for 4 days, not to exceed 600 mg/day If < 1 yr, 5 mg/kg bid for 2 days Child: 10–20 mg/kg/day for 4 days, not to exceed 600 mg/day

Comment: In a day-care classroom in which a case of systemic H. influenzae b disease has occurred and in which one or more children under 2 years old have been exposed, strong consideration should be given to administering rifampin prophylaxis. Rifampin eradicates ampicillin-sensitive strains from the nasopharynx but does not eliminate the carrier state or ampicillin-resistant strains.[14]

Neisseria meningitidis types A and C	Polysaccharide vaccine	50 μg each of the respective capsular polysaccharides SQ

Comment: The vaccine is used in outbreaks and for immunization of military recruits. Group A vaccine is effective in children 3 months old and older; for children less than 18 months old, two doses 3 months apart have been given to control an epidemic. Group C vaccine is effective in children 2 years old and older. The vaccine is administered subcutaneously as a single 0.5 ml dose. Routine vaccination is not recommended.[15]

Neisseria meningitidis	Rifampin	Same as for H. influenzae

Comment: Members of the same household and intimate contacts are at risk for meningococcal spread, which typically occurs within 3 days of the initial case.

Streptococcus pneumoniae	23-valent serotype pneumococcal vaccine	0.5 mL dose SC orIM

Comment: High-risk individuals above 2 years of age should receive the vaccine because in spite of effective antibiotics, the mortality rate remains high at 20–30%.

Rabies virus	Human rabies immune globulin (RIG)	20 IU/kg in a single IM dose
	Human diploid cell vaccine (HDCV) globulin	5 1 mL IM doses on days 0, 3, 7, 14, 28

EMERGENCY CONTACTS

Centers for Disease Control, Atlanta, Georgia: 1-404-639-3311 (days, 8:00 AM to 4:30 PM), 1-404-639-2888 (evenings and weekends).

REFERENCES

1. Whitley, R.J., Soong, S., Linneman, C., et al.: Herpes simplex encephalitis. JAMA 247:317, 1982.
2. Benson, C.A., and Harris, A.A.: Acute neurologic infections. Med. Clin. North Am. 70:987, 1986.
3. Trauner, D.A.: Treatment of Reye syndrome. Ann. Neurol. 7:2, 1980.
4. Anderson, L.J., Nicholson, K.G., Tauxe, R.V., et al.: Human rabies in the United States, 1960 to 1979: Epidemiology, diagnosis, and prevention. Ann. Intern. Med. 100:728, 1984.
5. Hollander, H., Levy, J.A.: Neurologic abnormalities and recovery of human immunodeficiency virus from cerebrospinal fluid. Ann. Intern. Med. 106:692, 1987.
6. Klein, J.O., Feigin, R.D., and McCracken, G.H.: American Academy of Pediatrics: Report of the task force on diagnosis and management of meningitis. Pediatrics 78:959, 1986.
7. Martin, W.J.: Rapid and reliable techniques for the laboratory detection of bacterial meningitis. Am. J. Med. 75:119, 1983.
8. Watt, G., et al.: Rapid diagnosis of tuberculous meningitis by using an enzyme-linked immunosorbent assay to detect mycobacterial antigen. J. Infect. Dis. 158:681, 1988.
9. Polin, R.A., and Kennett, R.: Use of monoclonal antibodies in an enzyme immunoassay for rapid identification of a group B streptococcus, types II, and III. J. Clin. Microbiol. 1:332, 1980.
10. Landesman, S.H., Carrado, M.L., Shar, A.M., et al.: Past and current roles for cephalosporin antibiotics in treatment of meningitis: Emphasis on use in gram-negative bacillary meningitis. Am. J. Med. 71:693, 1981.
11. Reinis, C.M., and Sande, M.A.: Bacterial meningitis: Still a medical emergency. J. Crit. Illness. 2:62, 1987.
12. Overturf, G.D., Cable, D.C., Forthal, D.N., and Shikuma, C.: Treatment of bacterial meningitis with ceftizoxime. Antimicrob. Agents Chemother. 25:258, 1984.
13. Fekety, R.: Personal communication, 1987.
14. Broome, C.V., Mortimer, E.A., Katz, S.L., et al.: Use of chemoprophylaxis to prevent the spread of Hemophilus influenzae B in day-care facilities. N. Engl. J. Med. 316:1126, 1987.
15. American Academy of Pediatrics: Report of the Committee on Infectious Diseases, 20th Ed. Elk Grove Village, Illinois, American Academy of Pediatrics, 1986, p. 246.
16. Dexamethasone therapy for bacterial meningitis. Results of two double-blind placebo-controlled trials. N. Engl. J. Med. 319:964, 1991.

17. Odio, C.M., Faingezicht, I., Paris, M., et al.: The beneficial effects of early dexamethasone administration in infants and children with bacterial meningitis. N. Engl. J. Med. *324*:1525, 1991.

BIBLIOGRAPHY

Bolan, G., and Barza, M.: Acute bacterial meningitis in children and adults. Med. Clin. North Am. *69*:231, 1985.

Henry, K., and Crossley, K.: Meningitis: Principles of diagnosis, advances in treatment. Postgrad. Med. *80*:59, 1986.

Kaplan, S.C., and Feigin, R.D.: Clinical presentations, prognostic factors and diagnosis of bacterial meningitis. *In* Sande, M.A., Smith, A.L., and Root, R.K. (eds): Contemporary Issues in Infectious Diseases. New York, Churchill Livingstone, 1985, p. 83.

Lebel, M.H., Freij, B.H., Syrogiannopoulos, G.A., et al.: Dexamethasone therapy for bacterial meningitis. N. Engl. J. Med. *319*:964, 1988.

Lembo, R., and Merchant, C.: Acute phase reactants and risk of bacterial meningitis among febrile infants and children. Ann. Emerg. Med. *20*:36, 1991.

McCracken, G.H.: New developments in the management of neonatal meningitis. *In* Sande, M.A., Smith, A.L., and Root, R.K. (eds.): Contemporary Issues in Infectious Diseases. New York, Churchill Livingstone, 1985, p. 159.

McGee, Z.A., and Kaiser, A.B.: Acute meningitis. *In* Mandell, G.L., Douglas, R.G., Jr., and Bennet, J.E. (eds.): Principles and Practice of Infectious Diseases. New York, John Wiley & Sons, 1985, p. 560.

Tauber, M.G., and Sande, M.A.: Principles in the treatment of bacterial meningitis. Am. J. Med. *76*:224, 1984.

HERPES SIMPLEX MENINGOENCEPHALITIS

George R. Schwartz

CAPSULE

Herpes simplex meningoencephalitis, although relatively uncommon, is probably the most serious of all viral encephalitides seen in the United States. In its earliest manifestations, the condition has a predilection for the temporal lobes, probably because the virus enters the central nervous system through the olfactory nerves and pathways. The clinical symptoms of this condition were assessed by Whitley and associates,[1] who prepared tables of demographics and clinical findings in a large sample (Tables 50-24 and 50-25). The most common clinical symptoms were alteration of consciousness (97%) and fever (92%).

Early recognition of this condition is vital because early treatment with acyclovir and other antiviral agents markedly reduces the mortality rate and improves the overall neurologic outcome. Treatment must usually be instituted before definitive diagnosis by brain biopsy because of the disease's often rapid course and the clinical observation that the condition at the time of initiation of antiviral therapy is prognostic of eventual outcome.

INTRODUCTION

Herpes simplex meningoencephalitis, usually caused by herpesvirus Type I (HSV-I) is a severe condition with mortality approaching 90 to 100% in untreated cases. The herpesvirus Type II is more commonly involved in neonatal herpetic infections. Immunosuppressed patients (such as those with AIDS) appear to be at higher risk. The epidemiology does not show a strong seasonal variation, but does suggest some increased frequency in the late childhood and teenage years. Although HSV-I infection may be primary, the prevailing theory is that it usually results from reactivation of a pre-existing viral infection. The major advance has occurred over the last decade with development of effective antiviral therapies.

PATHOPHYSIOLOGY

Herpes simplex viruses usually infect the meninges and brain through retrograde spread to the CNS by

TABLE 50-24. COMPARISON OF DEMOGRAPHIC FEATURES IN "BRAIN-NEGATIVE" AND "BRAIN-POSITIVE" PATIENTS* WITH HERPES SIMPLEX ENCEPHALITIS

	Number (%) of Patients	
	Brain Positive (N = 113)	Brain Negative (N = 85)
Race		
White	97(86)	69(81)
Latin	3(3)	5(6)
Black	7(6)	6(7)
Asian	3(3)	2(2)
Other	3(3)	3(4)
Sex		
Male	61(54)	58(68)
Female	52(46)	27(32)
Age (years)		
0.5–10	13(12)	15(18)
10–20	22(19)	21(25)
20–30	16(14)	20(24)
30–40	7(6)	4(5)
40–50	13(12)	9(11)
50–60	22(19)	9(9)
≥ 60	20(18)	8(9)
Month of Diagnosis		
January–March	26(23)	18(21)
April–June	24(21)	15(18)
July–September	38(34)	24(28)
October–December	25(22)	28(33)

* "Brain negative" and "brain positive" refer to positive or negative brain tissue culture findings.
With permission from Whitley, R.J., Soong, S.J., Linneman, C., Jr., et al.: Herpes simplex encephalitis: Clinical assessment. JAMA 247:317, 1982. Copyright 1982, American Medical Association.

way of peripheral nerves. The disease is generally bilateral, and tends initially to affect, in addition to the meninges, the grey matter of the temporal and inferior frontal lobes as well as the hippocampus, amygdaloid nuclei, olfactory cortex, and cingulate gyrus. The viral infection within the neurons and glia is characteristically destructive with hemorrhagic necrosis (the reason for its old name of "acute necrotizing encephalitis"). Microscopically, one sees a mononuclear and polymorphonuclear inflammation with hemorrhagic necrosis. Intranuclear inclusions (so-called "cowdry" bodies) are seen. Rapid inflammation leads to the finding of cerebrospinal fluid pleocytosis in 97% of cases.

PREHOSPITAL ASSESSMENT AND STABILIZATION

The presenting symptoms may require emergency treatment with attention to the airway (e.g., seizures). Otherwise, the clinical symptoms might point to acute CNS infection. Fever with confusion or change in con-

sciousness can heighten suspicion. Initial management should include initiating an IV infusion of 5% dextrose in half normal saline. Seizures can be treated with small amounts of intravenous diazepam titrated slowly until the point of control is reached. Continuous attention to the airway is essential. Emergency medical technicians (EMTs) must be aware of the capabilities of the hospitals to which they transport such patients, particularly for diagnostic procedures if life-threatening delays are to be avoided. The three most important diagnostic tests are cerebrospinal fluid examination, CT scan, and brain biopsy (although treatment may have to be initiated before definitive diagnosis). Routine stabilization and supportive measures are needed with particular attention to avoiding vomiting with aspiration.

The possibility of acquired immunodeficiency syndrome (AIDS) should be kept in mind and suitable precautions taken.

CLINICAL PRESENTATION AND EXAMINATION

Tables 50-24 and 50-25 demonstrate the likely clinical signs from compilation of large series. Herpes simplex meningoencephalitis usually (in more than 95% of cases) begins with fever and signs of CNS dysfunction (e.g., confusion, alteration in consciousness). The onset is often rapid and progressive over hours, although occasionally insidious presentations with symptom development over several days have been reported. Seizures may occur (in 67%) and headache is relatively common (in 81%). So-called "personality changes" with combativeness have led to occasional initial errors in assessment, with resulting psychiatric referral or an impression of a drug- or alcohol-induced state.

DIFFERENTIAL DIAGNOSIS

Differential diagnosis must include other forms of meningoencephalitis (e.g., viral, bacterial, or fungal meningitis). Toxic effects of drugs or alcohol confuse the clinical picture. In AIDS patients, differentiation must be made between herpesvirus-caused CNS changes verus central nervous system AIDS.

DIAGNOSTIC TESTING

Computed tomography (CT) and magnetic resonance imaging (MRI) detect lesions in areas of central ner-

TABLE 50-25. COMPARISON OF FINDINGS IN "BRAIN-POSITIVE" AND "BRAIN-NEGATIVE" PATIENTS* WITH HERPES SIMPLEX ENCEPHALITIS†

	Number (%) of Patients	
	Brain Positive	Brain Negative
Historical findings		
Alteration of consciousness	109/112(97)	82/84(98)
CSF pleocytosis	107/110(97)	71/82(87)
Fever	101/112(90)	68/85(78)
Headache	89/110(81)	56/73(77)
Personality change	62/87 (71)	44/65(68)
Seizures	73/109(67)	48/81(59)
Vomiting	51/111(46)	38/82(48)
Hemiparesis	33/100(33)	19/72(26)
Memory loss	14/59 (24)	9/47(19)
Clinical findings at presentation		
Fever	101/110(92)	64/79(81)
Personality change	69/81 (85)	43/58(74)
Dysphasia	58/76 (76)	36/54(67)
Autonomic dysfunction	53/88 (60)	40/71(56)
Ataxia	22/55 (40)	18/45(40)
Hemoparesis	41/107(38)	24/81(30)
Seizures	43/112(38)	40/85(47)
Focal	28	13
Generalized	10	14
Both	5	13
Cranial nerve defects	34/105(32)	27/81(33)
Visual field loss	8/58 (14)	4/33(12)
Papilledema	16/111(14)	9/84(11)

* "Brain positive" and "brain negative" refer to positive or negative brain tissue culture findings.
† None of the differences were significant at the 5% level by X^2 tests.
With permission from Whitley, R.J., Soong, S.J., Linneman, C., Jr., et al.: Herpes simplex encephalitis: Clinical assessment. JAMA 247:317, 1982. Copyright 1982, American Medical Association.

vous system destruction; however, such lesions are found only in the later stages of the disease because viral destruction leads to necrosis.

Lumbar puncture usually shows a nonspecific pleocytosis and an elevation of the protein, with normal glucose levels.

Brain biopsy is a specific diagnostic test with a complication rate of 1 to 2%. The biopsy may be inaccurate in almost 4% of cases. Most centers do not have immediate capability for this biopsy. As a result, treatment should be initiated rapidly and modified later if necessary.

TREATMENT CONSIDERATIONS

Acyclovir, synthesized by Schaffer in the late 1960s as an inhibitor of the enzyme adenine deaminase, is a major improvement in the treatment of herpes simplex encephalitis. Although brain biopsy provides a definitive diagnosis, therapy should begin as soon as the diagnosis is suspected because of the often fulminant destructive course of untreated herpetic encephalitis. The dosage is 30 mg/kg/day, given at 8-hour intervals for at least 10 days. Patients with AIDS have markedly increased susceptibility to herpesvirus infections and are at increased risk for meningoencephalitis. The clinical picture may be confusing, owing to the CNS effects of AIDS.[2] Moreover, some strains of herpesvirus in AIDS patients have developed resistance to acyclovir.[3,4]

Vidarabine, although not as effective as acyclovir, still has a treatment role in this disease.[5] One study found a mortality rate of 54% in the vidarabine-treated group as compared with a 28% mortality rate in the acyclovirabine-treated group. The study also showed that at a 6-month follow-up of the survivors, 14% of the vidarabine-treated group versus 38% of the acyclovir-treated group were functioning normally.[1] These findings are in accord with studies by a Swedish group[5] who discovered a mortality rate of 19% in the acyclovir-treated group versus 50% in the vidarabine-treated group.

Herpetic encephalitis is difficult to diagnose early, but clinical suspicion must be raised if the physician sees any combination of symptoms and signs of personality change (combativeness, irritability), fever, headache, stiff neck, vomiting, seizures, disorientation, or confusion. In later stages of the disease, obtundation and coma occur. *The critical role of the acute care physician, however, is to suspect the diagnosis early and begin treatment immediately.* The most important prognostic factors are age and level of consciousness on admission.[1] One study[6] demonstrated a survival rate of 91% in lethargic patients under age 30, but only 21% of comatose patients over that age survived, and these people were all left with permanent neurologic sequelae.

The use of corticosteroids (e.g., dexamethasone, 0.1 to 0.2 mg/kg) in acute bacterial meningitis has gained support in the past several years. There is, however, no clear evidence supporting their use in herpetic meningoencephalitis. Some authorities consider them contraindicated.

PITFALLS

Early diagnosis of herpes simplex meningoencephalitis requires a high index of suspicion and continuing close assessment. Beware of ascribing "personality change" to psychiatric causes if other CNS signs are present. Alcohol use or intoxication can markedly confuse the clinical picture. Beware of herpesvirus infections in AIDS patients.

MEDICOLEGAL PEARLS

Few cases involving herpetic meningoencephalitis appear in the legal literature. The principal case (1987, Louisiana) focused on elements of transfer. This 18-year-old patient was transferred from a large, multispecialty facility to a small (less than 100 beds) community hospital where his condition worsened and he was not treated with antiviral substances. Despite clear and classic clinical signs, his condition went unrecognized and untreated for many hours and ended in his death. This case was eventually decided for the defense, based primarily on the rarity of the condition.

HORIZONS

If the trend of acyclovir-resistant herpes infection continues, new antiviral antibiotics will partially replace acyclovir. A viral vaccine is a possibility but has not yet had clinical trials.[4]

NATIONAL CONTACTS

Questions regarding treatments and new methods of diagnosis can be directed to the Centers for Disease Control (CDC) (404-639-3311). CDC also advises as to methods of sample collection for viral analysis.

REFERENCES

1. Whitley, R.J., Soong, S.J., Linneman, C., Jr., et al.: Herpes simplex encephalitis: Clinical assessment. JAMA 247:317, 1982.
2. Glatt, A.E., Chirgwin, K., and Landesman, S.H.: Treatment of infections associated with human immunodeficiency virus. N. Engl. J. Med. 318:22, 1988.
3. Drew, W.L., and Ehrlich, K.: Herpes virus in AIDS patients. J. Crit. Illn. 4:92, 1989.
4. Saral, R.: Management of mucocutaneous herpes simplex virus infections in immunocompromised patients. Am. J. Med. 85:57, 1988.
5. Skoldenberg, B., and Forsgren, M.: Acyclovir versus vidarabine in herpes simplex encephalitis. Scand. J. Infect. Dis. (Suppl) 47:89, 1985.
6. Rand, K.H.: Herpes simplex virus: Clinical syndromes and current therapy. Compr. Ther. 8:44, 1982.
7. Weman, W.M., Brunton, J.L., Lank, B.A., and Ronald, A.R.: Herpes simplex encephalitis: Poor outcome despite adenine arabinoside therapy. Can. Med. Assoc. J. 126:819, 1982.
8. Whitley, R.J., and Alford, A.A., Jr.: Toward therapy and prevention of herpetic infections. Semin. Perinatol. 7:64, 1983.

BIBLIOGRAPHY

Abramson, J.S., Roach, E.S., and Levy, H.B.: Postinfectious encephalopathy after treatment of herpes simplex encephalitis with acyclovir. Pediatr. Infect. Dis. 3:146, 1984.

Dayes, L.A., Cushman, A., Bache, R., et al.: Herpes simplex encephalitis and its neurological implications: Report of five cases. Int. Surg. 66:255, 1981.

Dix, R.D., Baringer, J.R., Panitch, H.S., et al.: Recurrent herpes simplex encephalitis: Recovery of virus after Ara-A treatment. Ann. Neurol. 13:196, 1983.

Koskiniemi, M.L., Vaheri, A., Valtonen, S., et al.: Trial with human leucocyte interferon and vidarabine in herpes simplex virus encephalitis: Diagnostic and therapeutic problems. Acta Med. Scand. (Suppl) 668:150, 1982.

Lunsford, L.D., Martinez, A.J., Latchow, R.E., and Pazin, G.J.: Rapid and accurate diagnosis of herpes simplex encephalitis with computed tomography stereotaxic biopsy. Surg. Neurol. 21:249, 1984.

Ommen, K.J., and Salazar-Calderon, V.H.: Herpes simplex virus (type 1) encephalitis: Report of a case treated with acyclovir. Ariz. Med. 42:313, 1985.

Whitley, R.J., Alford, C.A., Hirsch, M.S., et al.: Vidarabine versus acyclovir therapy in herpes simplex encephalitis. N. Engl. J. Med. *314*:144, 1986.

Whitley, R.J.: Herpes simplex virus infections of the central nervous system. Am. J. Med. *85*:61, 1988.

VIRAL INFECTIONS IN THE EMERGENCY DEPARTMENT

Michael R. Sayre and Emily Jean Lucid

CAPSULE

Emergency physicians see patients with viral illnesses every day. Many therapies and vaccinations are available for viral illnesses, and there are complications with which the physician should be familiar.

This chapter section covers many infections, including viral exanthems, viral gastroenteritis, herpesviruses, mumps, and rabies. Use of antiviral agents such as acyclovir is covered in depth. The emergency physician must know the use of these newer antiviral antibiotics, which can be life-saving in some cases.

GENERAL VIROLOGIC PRINCIPLES

Table 50-26 defines viral terms. A virus particle (virion) is covered with a protein shell that has a specific geometric shape. The inside of the virus is nucleic acid, which can be either RNA or DNA. Some viruses are covered with an envelope derived from the host cell membrane as the virion is made.

Viruses follow a simple life cycle. First they are taken up by a cell, and the viral capsid is removed. The free

TABLE 50-26. VIRAL TERMS

Capsid	Protein shell around nucleic acid
Capsomeres	Protein building blocks of capsid
Envelope	Proteins, lipids, and carbohydrates from host cell membrane
Hemagglutins	Glycoproteins that agglutinate red blood cells
Nucleic acid	Either RNA or DNA, single or double stranded
Virion	Virus particle

nucleic acid then begins its takeover of the cell protein building machinery. New nucleic acid is produced along with proteins for the capsid. These elements are assembled and released when the cell either dies or the viruses bud out through the membrane. These new virions infect adjacent cells or are expelled outside of the organism and lie dormant until they either are destroyed or come into contact with another organism that they can infect.

MACULOPAPULAR EXANTHEM AGENTS

MEASLES (RUBEOLA)

Measles is an acute epidemic disease caused by an RNA virus and characterized by cough, coryza, conjunctivitis (especially palpebral), a confluent erythematous maculopapular rash, and a pathognomonic exanthem in the mouth called Koplik spots. It is a highly contagious disease transmitted by infectious droplets or less commonly by airborne spread.[1] Measles is responsible for 2,000,000 deaths worldwide yearly.[2]

The incubation period lasts 8 to 12 days from exposure to onset of symptoms. The patient typically has 2 to 3 days of nonproductive cough, rhinorrhea, sore throat, and significant fever. The rash usually starts on the back of the neck and then spreads to involve all the body surfaces. The palpebral conjunctival injection is most marked in the lower lids. Koplik spots are bright red inflamed spots on the buccal and lingual mucosa. The patient may have right lower quadrant abdominal pain; and the diagnosis of measles is sometimes made by a pathologist who finds multinucleated giant cells in the appendix, confirming the diagnosis before the rash is present.

Complications of measles most commonly include otitis media and pneumonia. Encephalitis occurs in 1 of every 2000 cases reported in the U.S., and survivors of this complication frequently have permanent brain damage. Death, predominantly from repiratory and neurologic complications, occurs in 1 of every 3000 cases reported in the U.S.

The differential diagnosis before onset of the rash includes other viral causes of upper respiratory symptoms, streptococcal pharyngitis, Mycoplasma infection, TWAR-agent chlamydia, and infectious mononucleosis.

The treatment is supportive because no specific antiviral therapy is available. The introduction of a vaccine in the 1960s, with further improvement occurring in the 1970s, led to a dramatic reduction in the number of cases of measles. In 1978, the Department of Health, Education, and Welfare initiated a Measles Elimination Program, with a goal to eliminate indigenous measles from the United States by October 1, 1982. One of the hallmarks of this program was aggressive outbreak control. As a result of this program, the number of cases reported annually dropped from 26,871 in 1978 to an all-time low of 1497 in 1983. An increase occurred in 1986 (6282), with a decrease again in 1987 and 1988, but the number of cases rose again in 1989, when more than 14,000 cases were reported.[3]

The goal of eliminating measles in the United States has not been reached because of failure to implement the current vaccination recommendations, resulting in large numbers of unvaccinated preschool-age children in some areas and vaccine failure.[2]

In 1989, new recommendations were developed to achieve the goal of measles elimination (Tables 50-27 and 50-28). A routine regimen of two doses of vaccine is now recommended. Immunosuppressed patients such as those with leukemia, lymphoma, or generalized malignancy or those undergoing therapy with immunosuppressive drugs or radiation should not be given live measles virus vaccine. Patients with HIV infection, including the acquired immunodeficiency syndrome, (AIDS), should be vaccinated because measles in these patients can be severe.

RUBELLA

Rubella in the postnatal period is usually a mild disease characterized by a few days of malaise and low-grade fever, followed by a pink maculopapular rash lasting 2 to 3 days and associated with postauricular and suboccipital lymphadenopathy. The disease is commonly accompanied by transient polyarthralgia and polyarthritis in older individuals. Rare complications include encephalitis and thrombocytopenia. Transmission is through direct or droplet contact with nasopharyngeal secretions. The peak incidence of infection is late winter and early spring.

Before widespread use of the rubella vaccine, rubella was an epidemic disease with 6- to 9-year cycles. Because the vaccine is effective, the incidence of rubella has declined by more than 99% when compared to the prevaccine era. Outbreaks do still occur, usually in young adults. Recent serologic surveys have indicated that 10 to 20% of young adults are susceptible to rubella, predominantly because of underutilization

---

TABLE 50-27. 1989 RECOMMENDATIONS FOR MEASLES VACCINATION

Routine childhood schedule, United States	Two doses*†
Most areas	—first dose at 15 months
	—second dose at 4–6 years (entry to kindergarten or first grade)§
High-risk areas¶	Two doses*†
	—first dose at 12 months
	—second dose at 4–6 years (entry to kindergarten or first grade)§
Colleges and other institutions post-high school	Documentation of receipt of two doses of measles vaccine after the first birthday† or other evidence of measles immunity‡
Medical personnel employment	Documentation of receipt of two doses of measles vaccine after the first birthday† or other evidence of measles immunity‡

* Both doses should preferably be given as combined measles, mumps, rubella vaccine (MMR).

† No less than 1 month apart. If there is no documentation of any dose of vaccine, vaccine should be given at the time of school entry or employment and no less than 1 month later.

§ Some areas may elect to administer the second dose at an older age or to multiple age groups.

¶ A county with more than five cases among preschool-aged children during each of the last 5 years, a county with a recent outbreak among unvaccinated preschool-aged children, or a county with a large inner-city urban population. These recommendations may be applied to an entire county or to identified risk areas within a county.

‡ Prior physician-diagnosed measles disease, laboratory evidence of measles immunity, or birth before 1957.

TABLE 50-28. RECOMMENDATIONS FOR MEASLES OUTBREAK CONTROL*

Outbreaks in preschool-age children	Lower age for vaccination to as low as 6 months of age in outbreak area if cases are occurring in children < 1 year of age†
Outbreaks in institutions: day-care centers, K-12 grades, colleges, and other institutions	Revaccination of all students and their siblings and of school personnel born in or after 1957 who do not have documentation of immunity to measles§
Outbreaks in medical facilities	Revaccination of all medical workers born in or after 1957 who have direct patient contact and who do not have proof of immunity to measles§
	Vaccination may also be considered for workers born before 1957
	Susceptible personnel who have been exposed should be relieved from direct patient contact from the 5th to the 21st day after exposure (regardless of whether they received measles vaccine or IG) or, if they become ill, for 7 days after they develop rash.

* Mass revaccination of entire populations is not necessary. Revaccination should be limited to populations at risk, such as students attending institutions where cases occur.
† Children initially vaccinated before the first birthday should be revaccinated at 15 months of age. A second dose should be administered at the time of school entry or according to local policy.
§ Documentation of physician-diagnosed measles disease, serologic evidence of immunity to measles, or documentation of receipt of two doses of measles vaccine on or after the first birthday.

of the vaccine and not because of waning immunity in immunized persons.[1]

The most severe complication of rubella is transmission to unborn children (congenital rubella). It is acquired by transplacental infection of the fetus and is a devastating disease. A discussion of this syndrome is beyond the scope of this text, but the important point is that patients with rubella should be advised to stay away from any woman who may be pregnant. Contact isolation is required for 7 days after onset of the rash.

When a pregnant woman is exposed to rubella, a blood specimen should be obtained as soon as possible and tested for rubella antibody. The presence of antibody indicates that the individual is immune and not at risk. Those previously determined to be immune can also be reassured. If antibody is not detectable, further testing must be done 3 and 6 weeks after exposure to determine accurately whether or not infection has occurred. The routine use of immunoglobulin (IG) for postexposure prophylaxis in early pregnancy is not recommended because studies have shown that infants with congenital rubella have been born to mothers who were given IG shortly after exposure.

Congenital rubella can only be prevented by adequate immunization of the general population with live rubella virus vaccine (Table 50-29). Available data indicate that one dose confers long-term immunity.

Special efforts must continue to immunize postpubertal adolescents and adults, including college students and military recruits who have not been previously immunized or have not been proven serologically to be immune. For a detailed discussion of the recommended immunization guidlines for rubella, see the Report of the Committee on Infectious Diseases published by the American Academy of Pediatrics, affectionately known as "The Red Book."[1]

ERYTHEMA INFECTIOSUM (FIFTH DISEASE)

Erythema infectiosum is characterized by 1- to 4-day history of mild systemic symptoms followed by a characteristic rash, which may erupt in three stages. The typical first phase consists of intensely red cheeks with circumoral pallor, giving use to the descriptive term "slapped cheek." This is followed by a maculopapular lace-like rash on the arms. The rash then moves to the trunk, buttocks, and thighs. Reappearance of the rash may occur for several weeks after nonspecific stimuli such as a change in temperature, sunlight, or emotional stress.

Arthralgia and arthritis are commonly reported. Joints in the hands are most frequently involved, followed by joints in the knees and wrists. Joint symptoms are reported to be more common in adults and may occur as the sole manifestation of the infection.

In 1975, erythema infectiosum was found to be caused by human parvovirus B19. This virus has also been shown to be the primary cause of transient aplas-

TABLE 50-29. INDICATIONS AND CONTRAINDICATIONS FOR RUBELLA IMMUNIZATION

Indications	Contraindications
Children ≥ 15 months (with measles and mumps vaccines [as MMR])	Pregnancy
Susceptible individuals in the following groups:	Immunodeficiency or immuno-compromised state*†
• Pubertal girls	IG or blood in past 3 months§
• Postpubertal adults, especially women:	
—premarital	
—postpartum	
• College students	
• Day care personnel	
• Military personnel	
• Health care personnel	

* With permission from Peter, G., Hall, C.B., Lepaw, M.L., and Phillips, C.F. (eds): Report of the Committee on Infectious Diseases 21st edition, American Academy of Pediatrics, 1988.
† Exception is AIDS.
§ Rubella vaccine may be given postpartum concurrently or after the administration of anti-Rho (D) IG or blood products.

tic crisis in patients with chronic hemolytic anemias and chronic anemia with immunodeficiency, and it has been associated with fetal death. In addition to patients with chronic hemolytic anemias (e.g. sickle cell disease, hemoglobin SC disease, hereditary spherocytosis, β-thalassemia, and autoimmune hemolytic anemia), this virus can also cause transient aplastic crises in other conditions in which increased red cell production is necessary to maintain stable red cell indices, as may occur in anemia from blood loss. Chronic B19 infection can cause a severe anemia asociated with red cell aplasia in patients with immune deficiency diseases, including human immunodeficiency virus (HIV)-related immune deficiency as well as leukemias and congenital immune deficiencies.[4]

Erythema infectiosum outbreaks often occur from late winter to early spring and may persist until school recesses for summer. The incubation period is usually 4 to 14 days. Transmission is probably by respiratory secretions from viremic patients.

There is no vaccine to prevent B19 virus infection, and the role of IG in patients with immunodeficiency syndromes needs further study.

EXANTHEM SUBITUM (ROSEOLA)

Human herpesvirus-6 (HHV-6), also called the human B-lymphotropic virus (HBLV), was first isolated in 1986.[5] It was not clear what illness this agent caused until 1988, when HHV-6 was shown to be the cause of a common childhood illness formally called exanthem subitum and informally roseola. [6]Because HHV-6 is a herpesvirus, one might expect that it can reactivate under certain conditions, and indeed some patients with AIDS do have high levels of the virus

in their serum.[7] HHV-6 may also cause clinical illness in the form of lymphadenopathy syndromes.[8] At least 25% of the population has detectable antibody to HHV-6.[8]

Exanthem subitum is a disease of children between 6 months and 3 years. It is the most common exanthem in children under 2 years old.[9] The clinical course begins with the abrupt onset of a high fever, often to 40°C. The child usually does not appear particularly ill despite the high temperature. Febrile seizures are not uncommon, however. After 3 days, the fever ends, and a fine macular erythematous rash appears over the face, trunk, and extremities. This characteristic exanthem consists of small, pale pink, discrete macules or maculopapules. Periorbital edema is a common finding. The rash fades over the next 12 to 24 hours. HHV-6 can cause a similar febrile illness but without the characteristic rash.[9] There are no known sequelae of HHV-6 infection, but research into the life cycle of this virus has just begun.

The diagnosis of HHV-6 infection is based on the characteristic clinical course of the illness. There is an IgG antibody test available for research purposes (Cappel Laboratories, Cochranville, PA) to document seroconversion after a clinical illness.[9] No data exists to estimate the infectivity of HHV-6, but given the fact that cases are sporadic, it seems that it is low. A roseola-like illness has been associated with several other viral agents including enterovirus, echovirus, and several adenoviruses.

Exanthem subitum is a benign illness that requires no therapy other than comfort measures and reassurance. The principal challenge is differentiation from other more serious causes of high fever in infants. Frequently, therefore, it is a diagnosis of exclusion, used when pneumonia and occult bacteremia have

TABLE 50-30. COMMON MACULOPAPULAR EXANTHEMS

	Measles (Rubeola)	Rubella (German, 3-day measles)	Roseola (Exanthema Subitum)	Fifth Disease (Erythema Infectiosum)	Enterovirus	Scarlet Fever
Incubation Prodome	10–14 days 3 days high fever, cough, conjunctivitis, and coryza; child appears toxic, lethargic	14–21 days May be none; lymphadenopathy (especially postauricular, suboccipital), malaise, variable low-grade fever	10–14 days 3–4 days high fever in otherwise well child, preceding rash	7–14 days None	Variable (short) Variable; fever, malaise, vomiting, sore throat, rhinorrhea	2–4 days 1–2 days fever, vomiting, sore throat; often toxic
Exanthem	Reddish-brown; begins on face and progresses downward; generalized by second day; discrete; lasts 2–3 days, fades in order of appearance	Pink; begins on face and progresses rapidly downward; generalized by second day; discrete; lasts 2–3 days, fades in order of appearance	Appears after defervescence; rose, discrete; initially on chest, spreads to involve face and extremities; fades quickly	Erupts in 3 stages: (1) red-flushed cheeks with circumoral pallor (slapped cheek), (2) maculopapular eruption on extremities (lacelike), (3) may recur secondary to heat, sunlight, trauma	Maculopapular, discrete, nonpruritic, generalized; rubella-like; hand, foot, and mouth distribution	Erythematous, punctate, sandpaper texture; appears 1st in flexor areas, then generalized; most intense on neck, axilla, inguinal, popliteal skin fold; circumoral pallor; lasts 7 days, then desquamates

been ruled out. A clue to the correct diagnosis is the relatively well appearance of the child despite the elevation in temperature.

Table 50-30 compares the common maculopapular exanthems discussed in this section.

VESICULAR EXANTHEM AGENTS

Many of the agents that cause vesicular exanthems are members of the herpes-viridiae family. Herpesviruses are relatively complicated. They have a double-stranded, linear DNA with a regular icosahedral protein shell surrounded by a lipid, carbohydrate, and protein envelope. Generally, herpesviruses produce a pronounced primary infection and then a period of latency. At some point there can be reactivation with variability between infected individuals as well as species of herpesviruses.

CHICKENPOX

Varicella-zoster virus (VZV) causes chickenpox. The same virus has been shown by restriction endonuclease mapping to cause herpes zoster. There are about 2.8 million cases of chickenpox in the U.S. each year.[10]

Most cases occur from November through May. Half of all cases happen in 5- to 9-year-olds (Fig. 50-9). Therefore, by age 15, less than 10% of Americans remain susceptible.

Once the virus is introduced into a household, the attack rate for susceptible contacts is 87%.[11] Transmission of chickenpox is by respiratory droplet spread, but transmission by direct contact with infected vesicles or rarely on the hands of hospital personnel has also been reported.[12] VZV cannot be recovered from vesicular crusts or room dust.[13]

After a person inhales the respiratory droplets, primary replication begins in the nasopharynx. In a few days, a primary viremia seeds the reticuloendothelial system. The virus replicates there until the secondary viremia, beginning about 14 days after initial viral acquisition, infects the skin. As the secondary viremia begins, the patient often has mild fever, myalgias, and malaise. Within a day, the rash begins with small red macules, followed by development over 12 to 24 hours of the vesicle filled with clear fluid containing infectious virus, lymphocytes, and cellular debris. Initially, the rash appears on the trunk and spreads to the extremities. Then the vesicle becomes cloudy, ruptures, and forms a crust within 12 to 24 hours. Crusts can last up to 1 to 3 weeks. The secondary viremia continues about 5 days, and the patient with chickenpox remains contagious until all the vesicles have crusts. Itching is a prominent symptom.

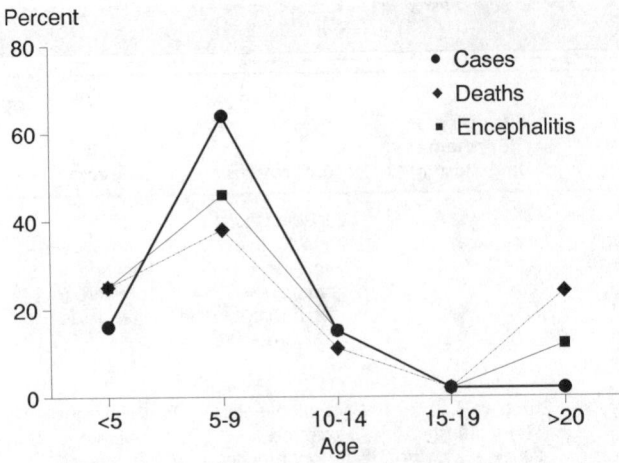

FIG. 50-9. *Age distribution of chickenpox and its complications. Adapted from Preblud S.R., D'Angelo L.J. Chickenpox in the United States, 1972–1977.* **J. Infect. Dis.** *140.257–260, 1979.*

Complications from chickenpox are unusual in the immune competent host. They include bacterial superinfection of the skin, acute cerebellar ataxia, Reye's syndrome, and death. Up to 33% of adults with chickenpox have radiographic evidence of pneumonitis.[14] If the pneumonia is to become clinically evident, it will do so about 3 to 5 days after the onset of the rash.

Many mothers of patients with chickenpox say, "I am pregnant. Will chickenpox hurt my baby?" Because most adult Americans are immune to chickenpox, it is unlikely that the expectant mother wil become infected. If she does, however, chickenpox in pregnant women is usually *no* more severe than in other adults although it was once thought to be so. Chickenpox with pneumonia in pregnant women, however, has led to reported deaths.[15]

There is a congenital varicella syndrome characterized by hypoplastic limbs and severe fetal scarring, but this is rare, even when the mother gets chickenpox late in first trimester. On the other hand, if virus is acquired transplacentally just before birth, i.e., if the mother's rash appears 5 days before through 2 days after delivery, the resulting perinatal disease is severe. In these cases, the baby has up to a 30% chance of death.[16]

In nearly all cases, the diagnosis of chickenpox can be made by the characteristic appearance of the rash. A Tzanck smear can be performed to demonstrate multinucleated giant cells. In addition, antibody tests can establish whether past infection was present. This is important for the management of nosocomial outbreaks.[17]

Acetaminophen generally has been recommended; however, this treatment was recently shown to be of no benefit and may prolong the illness.[18]

Aspirin should not be used because of the risk of Reye's syndrome. Simple measures such as trimming the fingernails and oatmeal baths in lukewarm water often help. If the patient is not an infant, antihistamines such as diphenhydramine (Benadryl) may be prescribed to help control itching.

There has been a great deal of interest in the use of acyclovir for the treatment of chickenpox. It is useful in immunocompromised children in preventing dissemination of the infection throughout the body,[19] and has a role in fulminating varicella. Acyclovir has been tested in normal children, and studies have shown that it shortens the clinical course and reduces morbidity.[19a] Its ability to reduce the rare serious complications is not proven. Because of the possibility that varicella pneumonia in pregnant women is more severe than in their nonpregnant counterparts, one paper did recommend that maternal varicella pneumonia be treated with intravenous acyclovir.[20,21] Until better antiviral agents are developed, there is little specific therapy for the ordinary varicella sufferer.

Prevention of chickenpox is difficult. Unfortunately, most people are exposed before a rash is present on the source, because viral shedding begins up to 24 hours before the rash. Partial temporary immunity is available in the form of varicella-zoster immune globulin for patients at high risk for disseminated disease.[22] Live varicella vaccine will probably be licensed soon, and it may eliminate most wild virus disease.[23] One study demonstrated a lower incidence of zoster in children with leukemia who received the live attenuated varicella vaccine.[23a]

SHINGLES (HERPES ZOSTER)

Herpes zoster represents reactivation of the varicella-zoster virus. The virus travels from the dorsal root ganglion along the peripheral nerves to the skin. Zoster is mainly a disease of the elderly, with about 5 to 10 cases per 1000 persons per year.[24] Between 2 and 10% of patients with one attack will have another some time in their lives.[24]

Shingles begins with a burning pain, usually in the T3 to L3 dermatome, 48 to 72 hours before the onset of the rash. New lesions form for about 3 to 5 days, and the illness generally runs its course in a little over a week. If the sensory branch of the facial nerve is involved, zoster may produce Bell's palsy (Ramsay-Hunt syndrome).

The diagnosis of zoster is usually made clinically. But it can be confused with herpes simplex (herpes gladiatorum) and coxsackievirus, which also cause dermatomally distributed vesicular rashes. In addition, zoster may be confused with many other causes of acute pain before the onset of the rash. Frequently, the correct diagnosis is made only in retrospect after the rash appears.

Unless generalized disease is present, patients with herpes zoster do not spread disease by respiratory droplets. The skin lesions that have not crusted are infectious, and good hand washing should prevent most spread. Elderly immunodeficient patients can probably acquire new varicella infections. These patients are susceptible to widely disseminated infection arising either endogenously from an outbreak of shingles or exogenously from a second case of chickenpox.[25,26]

Herpes zoster is feared mainly because of the complication of postherpetic neuralgia. This condition is defined as the persistence of pain after herpes zoster. It is uncommon in young people, but 50% of patients over age 50 have persistent pain in the involved dermatome after the resolution of the rash. This incidence is also increased in those with cancer.[27] In older patients or those with compromised cellular immunity, dissemination of varicella-zoster virus can happen with an outbreak of herpes zoster and have potentially fatal consequences. The VZV may infect the central nervous system, skin, and other systems or organs.

Management of zoster depends on the age of the patient as well as the presence of underlying disease. If the distribution of the rash involves the first branch of the trigeminal nerve, the patient should be referred to an ophthalmologist to be assessed for eye involvement. If the patient is immunocompromised, intravenous vidarabine or acyclovir can be given.

Oral acyclovir has been studied extensively to determine its effectiveness in treating zoster. It does have a beneficial effect when given in an adequate dose, which research studies have defined as 800 mg 5 times daily for 10 days.[28,29] Unfortunately, this treatment is rather expensive. Some patients respond to lower doses, but there is no way to identify them. An informal survey of pharmacies revealed that the cost of 200 acyclovir capsules ranged from $127.58 to $167.80. One author's strategy is to treat all patients over 60 years of age whose pain and rash have been present for less than 96 hours.[30] Pain relief in the form of a nonsteroidal antiinflammatory medication or narcotic is helpful as well.

Another area of concern is the prevention and control of postherpetic neuralgia. Acyclovir in the dose given above does decrease the incidence of postherpetic neuralgia, at least in the first 3 months.[29] Three small studies looked at the use of corticosteroids for the prevention of postherpetic neuralgia. Steroids were somewhat effective, but there were design problems in the studies that make generalizing the results hazardous.[31] Further studies show little effect of steroids when acyclovir is used.[32] A multicenter NIH now under way will try to answer the question of steroid effectiveness.

HERPES SIMPLEX

Herpes simplex virus (HSV) is the cause of several clinical illnesses characterized by localized ulcerations, typically on the oral or genital mucosa. Herpes simplex is divided into two antigenic types: Herpes simplex virus-1 and virus-2. Infection begins with invasion of cells not resulting in cell death. A typical herpesvirus latency period ensues, much shorter than that of other herpesviruses. Later reactivation happens.

Herpes simplex infection is common. About 40% of Americans between ages 25 and 29 have antibodies to HSV-1.[33] The age-specific prevalence rates for HSV-1 are decreasing, however, whereas visits to private practitioners for genital herpes increased ninefold in the U.S. between 1966 and 1981.[34] Herpes simplex-2 antibodies do not appear until puberty, and their prevalence correlates with the past sexual activity of the individual. Up to 80% of female prostitutes have antibodies against HSV-2. Interestingly, only about a third of individuals with antibodies against HSV-2 have a history of genital ulcerations.

Herpes simplex is usually acquired after direct contact with virus from another person's mucosa. About 5% of adults have asymptomatic salivary excretion of HSV-1. HSV, however is likely to be transmitted when the source has lesions.

Herpes infections have been found nearly everywhere on the body. After initial acquisition of the infection, there is an incubation period of about 1 week (range 1 to 26 days). Frequently, first episodes of the infection are accompanied by systemic symptoms. Both strains of the virus can infect the genital and oral regions. Each virus, however is more severe in its perferred site.

Oral-facial HSV infection is commonly referred to as a "cold sore." Usually these infections are caused by the HSV-1 serotype. First episodes of the infection are manifested by gingivostomatitis and pharyngitis. Systemic symptoms include fever, malaise, myalgias, irritability, and cervical adenopathy; and these may last between three and 14 days. The differential diagnosis includes bacterial pharyngitis, Stevens-Johnson syndrome, and other viral stomatitis (coxsackievirus, etc.)

The patient may never have a recurrence or may experience reactivation with a range from asymptomatic viral excretion to severe buccal ulcerations. The complications of oral-facial herpes simplex infections include generalization of infection in the immunocompromised host, superinfection, and erythema multiforme.

Genital herpes simplex infections were the most dreaded result of promiscuous sexual behavior, at least until AIDS made its appearance known in the early 1980s. Despite lack of recent publicity, HSV infection of the genital tract continues to occur. Between 20 and 50% of genital HSV infections are with HSV-1.[35]

A genital infection with HSV is characterized by fever, headache, malaise, myalgias, vaginal or urethral discharge, and tender inguinal adenopathy. The skin lesions range in appearance from vesicles to pustules to painful ulcers. When a woman is seen with a small vaginal tear, some clinicians have noted an association with HSV infection. Up to 80% of women with first-time episodes have uterine cervical involvement.

About 80% of genital HSV-2 infected individuals have their first recurrence within 1 year, compared with 55% of those with genital HSV-1 infections. In addition, superinfection with the other strain of HSV can occur, although it is frequently a milder disease.[35]

The complications of genital HSV infection are similar to those of oral-facial infections. In addition, genital herpes simplex infection is associated with increased risk of cervical and vulvar carcinoma.

Herpes simplex can infect the rest of the body as well. Of particular interest to health care workers is HSV infection of the finger which is called herpetic whitlow. It is most common in medical professionals who do not wear gloves when in contact with mucosa. Usually HSV-1 is cultured from medical personnel and HSV-2 from the general public.

Herpetic whitlow is characterized by the abrupt onset of edema, erythema, and localized tenderness around the base of the fingernail. These vescular and pustular lesions may appear like a bacterial paronychia. Fever and systemic symptoms are common. Surgical treatment of lesions mistaken for bacterial paronychia is thought to lead to delayed healing.

Herpes simplex infections of the first branch of the trigeminal nerve can lead to herpetic keratoconjunctivitis, which is the most common cause of corneal blindness in the U.S. Steroid treatment of such lesions allows spread of the disease. Proper treatment includes prompt ophthalmologic referral and antiherpetic therapy.

Herpes simplex virus can also infect the central nervous system, either as a complication of oral-facial or genital disease or spontaneously. Herpes simplex encephalitis is the most common cause of acute, sporadic viral encephalitis in the U.S. with two cases per 1,000,000 population each year. Nearly all are HSV-1. It generally spreads from exogenously acquired virus by way of the olfactory bulb. This disorder is characterized by fever and focal temporal lobe signs. A brain biopsy may be required for the diagnosis.

When herpes simplex virus is acquired during delivery, it can be devastating. Neonatal herpes simplex affects about 17 in 100,000 live births.[36] About 70% of infants with untreated neonatal herpes have CNS involvement, and if the CNS is involved, the mortality rate approaches 65%.[37] Between 55 and 70% of neonatal herpes simplex is caused by HSV-2,[36] but the risk of acquiring infection at time of vaginal delivery is less than 89.[38] The newborn can also acquire HSV-1 spread from family members or medical personnel. Antiviral chemotherapy has reduced the mortality to a still high 14%.[39]

The clinical diagnosis of HSV infection is accurate when classic findings are present. The best laboratory test is the tissue culture. It is usually positive 2 to 4 days after inoculation. Serologic testing for antibodies against HSV is not clinically useful.

ACYCLOVIR TREATMENT OF HERPETIC INFECTIONS

In the 1980s, a major advance was made in treating HSV infections. This treatment revolution has come about because of the introduction of acyclovir. Acyclovir effectively shortens the symptoms and duration of lesions in first-time infections of immunocompetent persons. The dose for initial infections is 200 mg 5 times daily for 10 to 14 days. Acyclovir's effect on recurrent lesions is less dramatic. The duration of symptoms and of viral shedding is shortened by one day. The dose is 200 mg five times daily for 5 days as long as it is begun within 2 days of the onset of the symptoms.[40] Oral acyclovir has also been shown to be effective in treating herpetic whitlow in a small retrospective study.[41]

The benefits of acyclovir for oral herpes simplex infections are much less pronounced. It has some benefit when administered orally for initial infections. Little benefit has been shown for recurrent infections.

Acyclovir can be given intravenously for severe infections. This therapy is needed in cases of disseminated infection or when the patient's cellular immunity is impaired. Intravenous acyclovir is also used for CNS infections. Resistance to acyclovir is becoming a problem.[41] When resistance occurs, another antiviral agents, foscarnet, appears to be effective.[43] Vidarabine is also effective for treating HSV encephalitis, but acyclovir appears to be superior. Chlorhexidine oral gel may offer some topical treatment for HSV.[44] There is also interest in the use of lidocaine cream to abort recurrences.[45]

Prevention of initial HSV infection is desirable because it will reduce the risks that a mother will be shedding virus or that someone will acquire HSV encephalitis. Currently, there is extensive research on a herpes simplex vaccine. Avoidance of sexual intercourse when lesions are present is a self-evident way of lessening the risk of HSV transmission, and good hand washing lessens the risks of herpetic whitlow. The use of condoms may decrease transmission during periods of asymptomatic viral secretion.

Acyclovir at a dose of 400 mg twice daily is efficacious in decreasing the risk of recurrent genital herpes reactivation.[46] Its long-term safety is unknown, and therefore it may make sense to use it only when recurrences are frequent (more than twice a year or so).

SYSTEMIC VIRAL INFECTIONS WITHOUT RASH

CYTOMEGALOVIRUS

Cytomegalovirus (CMV) is another herpesvirus that can cause either a lytic (active) or latent infection. Microscopically, CMV-infected cells appear as giant cells, and so the virus was named. Cytomegalovirus is found worldwide. Approximately 1% of newborns in U.S. are infected with CMV. The virus is transmitted because it is shed in milk, saliva, feces, and urine. It is not as easily transmitted as varicella, however.

Cytomegalovirus infection is common in some groups. For example, viral shedding is noted in 50 to 100% of 2-year-olds in day care centers.[47] Antibody titers approach 100% in female prostitutes and homosexual men. Sixty-three percent of the tested employees of the Children's Hospital of Alabama had antibody to CMV.[48] Once acquired, CMV persists for life but normally remains latent. Reactivation, however can occur in the presence of impaired T-lymphocyte immunity.

When CMV infects certain types of patients, it can have severe consequences. One feared complication of CMV is fetal deformity. The clinical features of congenital CMV include petechiae, hepatosplenomegaly, jaundice, microcephaly, intrauterine growth retardation, prematurity, inguinal hernias, and chorioretinitis. If an infant is severely affected it has about 20 to 30% mortality risk.

On the other hand, perinatal CMV is not as severe as congenitally acquired disease. About half of newborns breast-fed from seropositive mothers are infected within one month of birth. Usually the infection is asymptomatic, but some infants develop interstitial pneumonitis.

After the newborn period, CMV mononucleosis is the most common presentation. The typical patient is a sexually active young adult. Illness begins 20 to 60 days after acquisition of the virus, and it lasts from 2 to 6 weeks. The illness is characterized by myalgias, headaches, and splenomegaly. Unlike mononucleosis caused by Epstein-Barr virus, exudative pharyngitis is unusual. On diagnostic testing, there are frequently more than 10 atypical lymphocytes on the differential white cell count, but the heterophil-antibody test is negative. After primary infection, low-grade viral shedding may last for years.

Complications of CMV infection include reactivation and dissemination during periods of impaired-cellular immunity, as well as possible atherosclerosis.[49] CMV is the most important viral pathogen complicating organ transplants. CMV infection in AIDS patients is nearly universal and may worsen T-lymphocyte deficiency.

Each of the several diagnostic techniques for CMV has a pitfall. A positive culture of urine, blood, or genital secretions confirms infection, but does not prove that CMV is the cause of the patient's symptoms. Seroconversion of IgG antibody from negative to positive is diagnostic of primary infection, but it is not a rapid diagnostic technique. IgM antibody is usually indicative of primary infection in the immune competent patient but is highly unreliable in the immunocompromised. Finding CMV inclusion bodies on microscopic examination is diagnostic of infection, but the study is not sensitive.[50] There is another test under development called the granulocyte-associated immunoglobulin test that will reportedly rapidly diagnose CMV infection.[51] Because its specificity is only 82%, however, its clinical utility has been questioned.[52]

There is no treatment available or required for the majority of patients with CMV. These patients have intact immune systems and handle the virus well. If the patient has depressed cellular immunity, ganciclovir has shown some promise,[53] and can be used for treatment or prophylaxis (5 mg/kg IV twice daily for 2 weeks).[53a]

A live virus vaccine against CMV is undergoing clinical evaluation. It does not prevent disease, at least in renal transplant recipients, but it does seem to attenuate its severity.[54]

INFECTIOUS MONONUCLEOSIS

Infectious mononucleosis, a common illness among American teenagers, is caused by the Epstein-Barr virus (EBV). Epstein-Barr virus is transmitted primarily by saliva (kissing). In poor populations, primary infection frequently occurs at an earlier age. These early infections are mild and appear like most other upper respiratory viral illnesses. The peak incidence in the United States is between 14 and 18 for boys. The virus is shed continuously in the oropharynx for up to 18 months after primary infection. Then it is shed periodically without clinical illness.

When it is transmitted by saliva, the initial site of replication of the EBV is in the oropharynx. Epstein-Barr virus infects B lymphocytes. In addition, oropharyngeal epithelial cells contain virus in infectious mononucleosis. Within 24 hours after entry into B lymphocytes, Epstein-Barr nuclear antigens (EBNA) become detectable. Then Epstein-Barr virus stimulates these B lymphocytes to produce immunoglobulins, which react with sheep red blood cells (heterophil antibodies). Eventually some cells lyse and release virus, which infects other B lymphocytes.

The immune system produces antibody to viral capsid antigen and the nuclear antigen. In addition, there is a cellular immune response with T suppressor-cytotoxic lymphocytes (CD8). The EBV remains in a small number of B lymphocytes for life, and it can reactivate during periods of depressed cellular immunity such as organ transplantation, iatrogenic immunosuppression, or AIDS.

After an incubation period of about 4 to 8 weeks, the patient develops nonspecific symptoms including malaise, anorexia, and chills. Fatigue is often a prominent complaint. Physical findings include pharyngitis that can be exudative, fever, and lymphadenopathy. Ninety percent of patients have fever up to 39° or 40°C, and 50% have splenomegaly. Sometimes the diagnosis is made when the patient is given ampicillin to treat presumed streptococcal pharyngitis. Administration of ampicillin to a patient with infectious mononucleosis frequently results in a pruritic, maculopapular eruption. The pharyngitis generally lasts about 5 to 7 days, the fever 7 to 14 days, and the lymphadenopathy 3 weeks. The malaise is persistent. Most patients restart work or school in about 3 to 4 weeks.

Antibodies to sheep erythrocytes that can be removed by prior absorption with beef red cells, but not with guinea pig kidney cells, are termed heterophil antibodies. Heterophil antibodies are present in 50% of young children and 90 to 95% of adolescents and adults with infectious mononucleosis. Up to 15% of patients with infectious mononucleosis are heterophil-negative during the first 5 days of the illness. The Monospot test is a rapidly performed and accurate substitute for the standard heterophil differential antibody test. The heterophil antibody test remains positive for 9 to 12 months after the illness.

In addition to the antibody tests, the differential white cell count may show a relative and absolute lymphocytosis in 75% of cases. Frequently, a large number (10% or more) are atypical in appearance. Also, specific antibody tests can be performed, but are of limited utility in the emergency department (ED). IgM antibodies to viral capsid antigen are diagnostic of primary EBV infection. IgG antibodies appear early in the course of the illness and are present for life.

There are few complications to a primary infection with the EBV. About half of patients with infectious mononucleosis have mild thrombocytopenia. Spontaneous splenic rupture does occur rarely, usually in the second or third week of the illness.[55] Other complications include autoimmune hemolytic anemia, severe granulocytopenia, cranial nerve palsies, encephalitis, persistent headaches,[56] hepatitis, pericarditis, myocarditis, interstitial pneumonitis,[57] Burkitt's lymphoma, and B-cell lymphoma.

The diagnosis of infectious mononucleosis is usually made clinically with laboratory confirmation by way of a positive differential heterophil antibody test or positive Monospot. Severe pharyngitis may be caused by another virus (herpes simplex) or β-hemolytic streptococci. Streptococci may be found in up to 30% of patients with infectious mononucleosis. In addition, atypical lymphocytosis is sometimes found in rubella, hepatitis, toxoplasmosis, mumps, and drug reactions. The management of infectious mononucleosis is chiefly supportive. There is no evidence that bed rest hastens recovery, and the patient should be allowed to return to usual activities as tolerated. The patient should be advised to avoid contact sports for 6 to 8 weeks to decrease the risk of splenic rupture. No medications have yet been shown to influence the course of the illness.

CHRONIC FATIGUE SYNDROME

The "chronic fatigue syndrome" has evoked a great amount of interest in the popular press in recent years. This disorder has also been called chronic mononucleosis or chronic Epstein-Barr virus syndrome because it was thought to be related to the Epstein-Barr virus.[58] More recent work has shown that Epstein-Barr antibody titers, although elevated in patients with chronic fatigue syndrome, are no more statistically related to illness than antibodies to cytomegalovirus, herpes simplex virus, and measles virus.[59] There is a great similarity between the chronic fatigue syndrome and fibromyalgia; in fact, both disorders may be the same.[60]

A group of patients with nonspecific symptoms of malaise, fatigue, pharyngitis, fever, lymphadenopathy, and problems with higher cognitive function are heterophil-antibody-negative. The true cause or causes of their illnesses remain unknown. To improve the diagnostic accuracy of physicians and to provide a research tool, a case definition for chronic fatigue syndrome was put forward by the Centers for Disease Control (CDC), which provides major and minor criteria for a diagnosis of chronic fatigue syndrome (Table 50-31).[61] A case must have both major criteria, and the following minor criteria: at least 6 of the 11 symptom criteria and 2 or 3 of the physical criteria, or 8 or more of the 11 symptom criteria. The differential diagnosis is extensive (see Table 50-32). The laboratory evaluation of this illness is complex.

Unfortunately, although patients with chronic fatigue syndrome are sometimes severely ill, there is no effective treatment. One option is to offer supportive counseling and sometimes psychotherapy rather than specific antiviral treatment.[62] In fact, in the treatment strategies thus far tried, there is a strong placebo effect.[63] It seems appropriate for the emergency physician to leave specific therapy to the physician who will be following the patient in the long term.

MUMPS

Mumps is caused by a paramyxovirus. Since live virus mumps vaccine was released in 1967, the incidence of mumps in the United States has fallen dramatically. Almost 13,000 cases occurred in the U.S. in 1987, however, among those who were not vaccinated and those in whom the vaccine failed. The vaccine has an efficacy about 80%.[64]

TABLE 50-31. DIAGNOSTIC CRITERIA FOR CHRONIC FATIGUE SYNDROME*

Major Criteria
1. New onset of persistent or relapsing, debilitating fatigue severe enough to reduce activity by 50% for at least 6 months
2. Other clinical conditions have been excluded (see differential diagnosis box)

Minor Criteria
Symptom Criteria
1. Mild fever (37.5°C to 38.6°C) or chills
2. Sore throat
3. Painful cervical or axillary nodes
4. Generalized muscle weakness
5. Myalgia

6. Prolonged (≥ 24 hours) fatigue following exercise that was previously well tolerated
7. Generalized headaches
8. Migratory arthralgias
9. Neuropsychologic complaints (e.g. photophobia, forgetfulness, confusion, difficulty thinking)
10. Sleep disturbance
11. Development of the symptom complex over a few hours to days

Physical criteria (documented by a physician at least twice, at least one month apart)
1. Oral temperature 37.6°C to 38.6°C
2. Nonexudative pharyngitis
3. Palpable or tender cevical or axillary nodes

* (With permission from Holmes, G.P., et al.: Chronic fatigue syndrome: A working case definition. Ann. Intern Med. *108:*388, 1988.)

TABLE 50-32. DIFFERENTIAL DIAGNOSIS FOR CHRONIC FATIGUE*

Malignancy	Endogenous depression
Autoimmune disease	Hysterical personality disorder
Localized infection	Anxiety neurosis
Chronic or subacute bacterial disease	Schizophrenia
Lyme disease	Sarcoidosis
Tuberculosis	Wegener granulomatosis
Histoplasmosis	Chronic hepatitis
Blastomycosis	Multiple sclerosis
Coccidioidomycosis	Myasthenia gravis
Toxoplasmosis	Hypothyroidism
Amebiasis	Addison's disease
Giardiasis	Cushing's syndrome
Helminthic infection	Diabetes mellitus
Human immunodeficiency virus infection	Drug dependency or abuse
	Adverse reaction to medication or toxin

* (With permission from Holmes, G.P., et al.: Chronic fatigue syndrome: A working case definition. Ann Intern Med *108:*388. 1988.)

Mumps is characterized by painful swelling of the parotid gland lasting at least two days. Many cases are subclinical. Frequently the swelling is unilateral, and is usually followed by a moderate temperature. Other salivary glands may be involved. The illness usually lasts less than a week. Mumps virus has been transmitted up to 24 hours before the onset of the swelling, and the patient remains capable of transmitting virus as long as 3 days after symptomatic improvement. The incubation period is about 18 days.

Complications of mumps include meningoencephalitis, deafness, and orchitis.[65] The orchitis is usually unilateral and occurs in 20 to 30% of postpubertal males, but sterility is rare.[65] Death is also rare, but half of the deaths have been in adults.[65]

If the patient with mumps has any contact with someone who has not been vaccinated or is unsure of immune status and the contact was born after 1956, mumps vaccine should be administered to that contact.[65] No other treatment is available.

COLORADO TICK FEVER

Colorado tick fever is a febrile, benign, systemic illness caused by a virus transmitted by the bite of the tick Dermacentor andersoni.[66] The incubation period last about 4 days and the illness about 10 days. The central nervous system is involved in about a quarter of cases. This illness probably accounts for many apparent cases of Rocky Mountain spotted fever.[67] Treatment is supportive.

VIRAL GASTROENTERITIS

ROTAVIRUS

Rotavirus, the most common cause of diarrhea in infants and children, causes up to half of the cases of diarrhea in the winter months[68] and is responsible for most hospitalizations for diarrhea among American children.[69] Rotavirus tends to cause illness between October and April. Because the peak incidence of illness begins each year in the Southwestern U.S. and travels Northeast, transmission may be by means other than fecal contamination of food or water.[69]

Rotavirus infection is characterized by frequent diarrheal stools in children between 6 months and 3 years of age. Illness typically begins after an incubation period of 2 days. The patient usually has vomiting and a low-grade fever. About a fifth of children have red tympanic membranes with loss of landmarks.[70] The illness lasts from 1 to 5 days and usually resolves spontaneously. The diarrhea can be quite severe, and the patient may become significantly volume depleted. Dehydration and subsequent circulatory collapse is the mechanism of death in patients with severe untreated diarrhea.

The diagnosis of rotavirus infection depends on laboratory isolation of the virus from stool samples. Several rapid tests for rotavirus detection in the stool are now available.[71] In adults, in whom rotavirus infection is unusual, the presence of fecal white blood cells or fecal occult blood is helpful, but it is a poor screen in children for a bacterial cause of the diarrheal illness because about a third of rotavirus infections have fecal white blood cells or occult blood.[72] Serum electrolytes may reveal reduced plasma bicarbonate concentration, signifying the development of acidosis.

The treatment of rotavirus infection involves preventing or treating dehydration. Most children can be treated with oral rehydration. A few require intravenous fluids, either because of associated vomiting or because of the degree of volume depletion. The risk of death from diarrheal illness is closely related to an admission weight less than the third percentile for age.[73] For children who are less than 5% dehydrated, oral rehydration therapy with a glucose-electrolyte solution is nearly always as effective as intravenous therapy.[74] The oral rehydration solution is a balanced glucose and Na^+ mixture with a Na^+ concentration between 40 and 90 mEq/L. These solutions serve only to maintain fluid balance and have no effect on stool volume or the patient's nutritional status. Early feeding may help to resolve the illness. Drug therapy with either antibiotics or antidiarrheals is *not* recommended. As with many of the other viral illnesses discussed in this chapter, a rotavirus vaccine is in development.[75]

SMALL ROUND STRUCTURED VIRUS

The Norwalk agent is one of a group of viruses termed small round structured viruses, which can cause gastroenteritis. Many of these infectious agents have been found because of their link to food-borne outbreaks.[76] Norwalk agent in particular has been associated with shellfish contamination. Snow Mountain agent is another small round structured virus which causes disease apparently spread by contaminated food.[77] Airborne transmission of Norwalk virus in an emergency department has also been implicated.[78]

There is no treatment for these infections which are self-limited (i.e., "the 24-hour bug"). However, the public health implications include regarding food handlers and health care workers as potentially secreting virus until 48 hours after clinical recovery.[78,79]

ADENOVIRUS

Adenovirus group F has been shown to be a cause of diarrhea in all age groups. Adenovirus may be as common as rotavirus among hospitalized children in the 1- to 6-month age group.[80] Watery and nonbloody diarrhea begins after an 8- to 10-day incubation period and lasts up to 1 week. Most patients have some vomiting and a fever. No special treatment other than maintenance of hydration is required.[81]

CENTRAL NERVOUS SYSTEM AGENTS

POLIOVIRUS

Poliovirus infection is increasingly uncommon. In 1988, only 335 confirmed cases of poliovirus infection were reported in the Americas, and there appears to be a reasonable chance that wild poliovirus can be eliminated from the hemisphere by the end of 1990.[82] Poliomyelitis is characterized by the development of fever, headache, and myalgias followed by acute paralysis. The paralysis may be severe and cause respiratory insufficiency. Treatment is supportive, and many patients recover some or all of their motor function. A syndrome of delayed weakness is sometimes found years after the initial poliomyelitis.

The disease is vaccine-preventable, but whether killed or live virus is preferable remains controversial.[83] In some areas, both vaccines are given in combination.[84] Live polio vaccine can apparently be given to pregnant women without an increase in fetal malformation.[85] Poliovirus infection can occur in immunocompromised contacts of normal children immunized with live oral poliovirus vaccine.[86]

TABLE 50-33. STEPS IN POST-EXPOSURE PROPHYLAXIS FOR RABIES

Local wound care
- Wash with soap and water
- Debride devitalized tissue
- Avoid suturing

Update tetanus immunization

Passive immunization
- Rabies immune globulin 20 IU/kg
  ½ intramuscularly and ½ locally at wound site at time of active immunization, but can be given up to 7 days later
- Not required in patients with pre-exposure immunization

Active immunization
- Human diploid cell virus
  1 mL intramuscularly on days 0, 3, 7, 14 and 28
  1 mL intramuscularly on days 0 and 3 only in patients with pre-exposure immunization

RABIES

Rabies is an acute viral encephalitis caused by a rhabdovirus that is capable of producing infection in animals as well as humans. The virus cannot penetrate intact skin, and except for rare cases of infection by means of inhalation or corneal transplant, the virus requires a break in the skin or mucous membrane to establish local infection. Only 40 to 50% of victims of bites from rabid animals develop rabies, but the disease is almost uniformly fatal.

The average interval between exposure and clinical disease in man is 1 to 2 months, but may vary from 10 days to well over a year. Variables affecting the length of the incubation period include the age of the patient (shorter in children than adults), the size of the inoculum, the severity of the bite, and the location of the bite (shorter for wounds of the face and neck than for the extremities).

"Classic" rabies usually presents with a prodromal phase. Symptoms include fever, chills, malaise, and myalgias, and may also include nonspecific gastrointestinal and upper respiratory symptoms. This prodrome may begin with proximal radiation of pain, paresthesias, and pruritus from the site of the bite. This is followed by the symptoms of encephalitis, which include excessive motor activity and altered mental status followed shortly thereafter by spasm of the laryngeal and pharyngeal muscles. It is this last sign that led to the disease being called "hydrophobia." Facial grimacing, opisthotonos, and seizures also occur. During the latter stages of the illness, autonomic overactivity is common, along with cardiac dysrhythmias, cranial nerve palsies, syndrome of inappropriate antidiuretic hormone, and hallucinations. Cortical function is maintained until late in the disease, but ultimately the patient becomes comatose and soon dies.

The differential diagnosis of "classic" rabies includes tetanus, delirium tremens, other viral encephalitis and hysteria. The diagnosis of rabies is not made without a high index of suspicion. The CDC in Atlanta should be consulted concerning any patient suspected of having rabies.

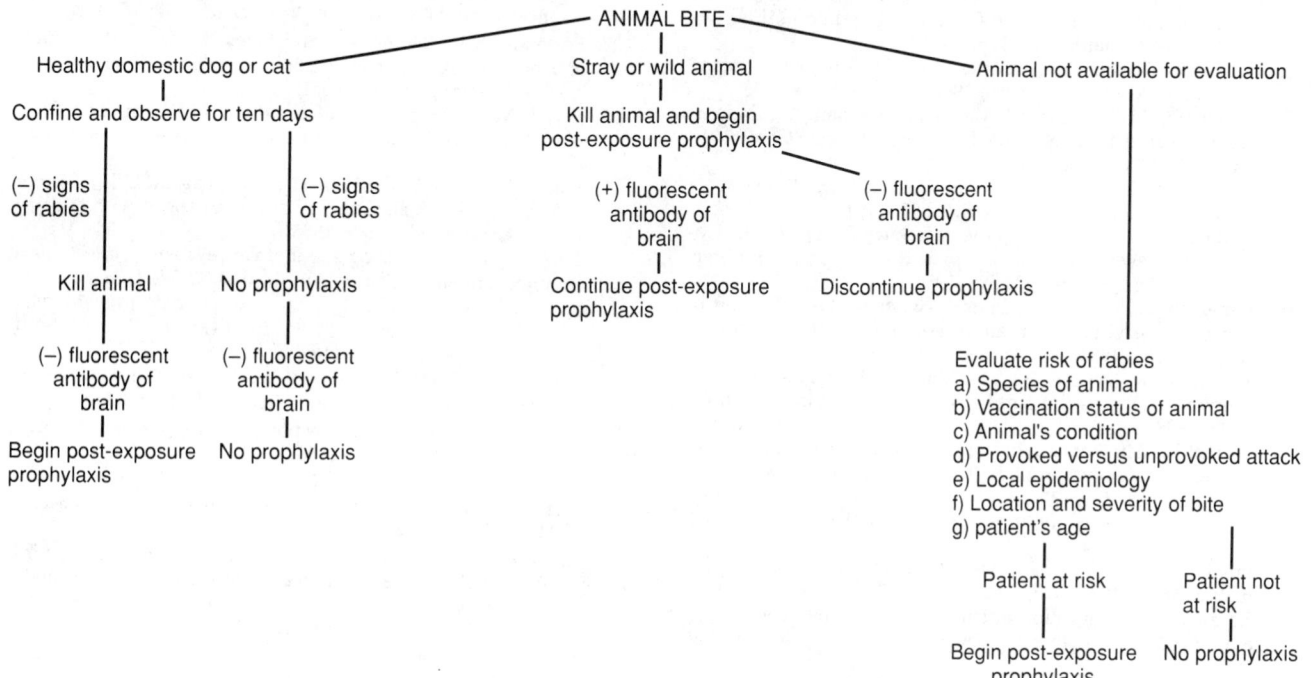

FIG. 50-10. Indication for rabies prophylaxis in animal bites. (+) = positive result; (−) = negative result. With permission from Kauffman, F.H., and Goldman, B.: Rabies. In Am. J. Emerg. Med. 4:529. Philadelphia, W.B. Saunders Co., 1986.

The most important issue for emergency physicians is the appropriate use of vaccines for the prevention of the disease. The method of administration of the vaccine is simple (Table 50-33). The difficult task, however, is determining whether or not the vaccine is needed (Fig. 50-10). The emergency physician must determine the patient's risk of developing rabies. Several points should be considered in making this decision: (1) the species of the animal, (2) its vaccination status, (3) its condition at the time of the bite, (4) whether the attack was provoked or unprovoked, and (5) the local rabies epidemiology.

Good local wound care cannot be overemphasized as the beginning of postexposure prophylaxis. The wound should be washed with copious amounts of soap and water and debrided of devitalized tissue. Consideration should be given to *not* closing the wound primarily. Tetanus immunization should be administered, based on the patient's immunization history.

After local wound care, simultaneous passive and active immunization should be instituted. The human diploid cell vaccine (HDCV) now available is much safer than older vaccines. Immunization is most effective when performed immediately after exposure to rabies. Table 50-33 outlines the regimen for this prophylaxis.[87]

REFERENCES

1. Peter, G., Hall, C.B., Lepaw, M.L., Phillips, C.F. (eds). Report of the Committee on Infectious Diseases, 21st edition. American Academy of Pediatrics, 1988, p.277-289.
2. Centers for Disease Control. International task force for disease eradication. M.M.W.R. 39:209, 1990.
3. Centers for Disease Control. Measles prevention: Recommendations of the Immunization Practices Advisory Committee (ACIP). M.M.W.R. 38:1, 1989.
4. Centers for Disease Control. Risks associated with human parvovirus infection B19. M.M.W.R. 38:81, 1989.
5. Salahuddin, S.Z., Ablashi, D.V., Markham, P.D., et al.: Isolation of a new virus, HBLV, in patients with lymphoproliferative disorders. Science 234:596, 1986.
6. Yamanishi,K., Okuno, T., Shiraki, K., et al.: Identification of human herpesvirus-6 as a causal agent for exanthem subitum. Lancet 1:1065, 1988.
7. Ablashi, D.V., Josephs, S.F., Buchbinder, A., et al.: Human B-lymphotropic virus (human herpesvirus-6). J. Virol. Methods 21:29, 1988.
8. Eizuru, Y., Minematsu, T., Minamishima, Y., et al.: Human herpesvirus 6 in lymph node (letter). Lancet 1:40, 1989.
9. Suga, S., Yoshikawa, T., Asano, Y., et al.: Human herpesvirus-6 infection (exanthem subitum) without rash. Pediatrics 83:1003, 1989.
10. Preblud, S.R.: Age-specific risks of varicella complications. Pediatrics 68:14, 1981.
11. Ross, A.H.: Modification of chickenpox in family contacts by administration of gamma globulin. N. Engl. J. Med. 67:369, 1962.
12. Leclair, J.M., Zaia, J.A. Levin, M.J., et al.: Airborne transmission of chickenpox in a hospital. N. Engl. J. Med. 302:450, 1980.
13. Weller, T.H.: Varicella-herpes zoster virus, in Evans, AS (ed): Viral Infections of Humans: Epidemiology and Control, 2nd ed. New York, Plenum Publishers, 1982, p. 569-595.
14. Preblud, S.R.: Age-specific risks of varicella complications. Pediatrics 68:14, 1981.
15. Fox, G.N., and Strangarity, J.W.: Varicella-zoster virus infections in pregnancy. Am. Fam. Phys. 39:89, 1989.
16. Preblud, S.R., Orenstein, W.A., and Bart, K.J.: Varicella: Clinical manifestations, epidemiology and health impact in children. Pediatr. Infect. Dis. 3:505, 1984.
17. Sayre, M.R., Lucid, E.J.: Management of varicella-zoster virus-exposed hospital employees. Ann. Emerg. Med. 16:421, 1987.
18. Doran, T.F., De Angelis, C., Baumgardner, R.A., and Mellits, E.D.: Acetaminophen: More harm than good for chickenpox? J. Pediatr. 114:1045, 1989.
19. Novelli, V.M., Marshall, W.C., Yeo, J., et al.: High dose oral acyclovir for children at risk of disseminated herpes virus infections. J. Infect. Dis. 151:372, 1985.
19a. Dunkle, L.M., Arvin, A.A., Whitley, R.S., et al.: A controlled trial of acyclovir for chickenpox in normal children. N. Engl. J. Med. 325:1539, 1991.
20. Davidson, R.N., Lynn, W., Savage, P., and Wanabrough-Jones, M.H.: Chickenpox pneumonia: experience with antiviral treatment. Thorax 43:827, 1988.
21. Brown, Z.A., Baker, D.A.,: Acyclovir therapy during pregnancy. Obstet. Gynecol. 73:526, 1989.
22. Immunization Practices Advisory Committee (ACIP), Varicella-zoster immune globulin for the prevention of chickenpox. M.M.W.R. 33:84, 1984.
23. Weibel, R.E., Neff, B.J., Kuter, B.J., et al.: Live attenuated varicella virus vaccine: Efficacy trial in healthy children. N. Engl. J. Med. 310:1409, 1984.
23a. Hardy, I., Gershon, A.A., Steinberg, S.P., et al.: The incidence of zoster after immunization with live attenuated varicella vaccine. N. Engl. J. Med. 325:1545, 1991.
24. Weller, T.H.: Varicella and herpes zoster: changing concepts of the natural history, control, and importance of a not-so-benign virus. N. Engl. J. Med. 309:1362, 1983.
25. Morens, D.M., Bregman, D.J., West, C.M., et al.: An outbreak of varicella-zoster virus infection among cancer patients. Ann. Intern. Med. 93:414, 1980.
26. Eckstein, R., Loy, A., and Jehn, U.: A spell of chickenpox on a cancer patients' ward. Klin. Wochenschr. 62:387, 1984.
27. Portenoy, R.K., Duma, C., and Foley, K.M.: Acute herpetic and postherpetic neuralgia: Clinical review and current management. Ann. Neurol. 20:651, 1986.
28. Wood, M.J., Ogan, P.H., McKendrick, M.W., et al.: Efficacy of oral acyclovir treatment of acute herpes zoster. Am. J. Med. 85:79, 1988.
29. Huff, J.C., Bean, B., Balfour, H.H., Jr., Laskin, O.L., Connor, J.D., Corey, L., et al.: Therapy of herpes zoster with oral acyclovir. Am. J. Med. 85:89, 1988.
30. Peterslund, N.A.: Management of varicella zoster infections in immunocompetent adults. Am. J. Med. 85:74, 1988.
31. Post, B.T., Philbrick, J.T.,: Do corticosteroids prevent postherpetic neuralgia? A review of the evidence. J. Am. Acad. Dermatol. 18:605. 1988.
32. Esmann, V., Geil, J.P., Kroon, S., et al.: Prednisolone does not prevent post-herpetic neuralgia. Lancet 2:126, 1987.
33. Corey, L., and Spear, P., Infections with herpes simplex virus. N. Engl. J. Med. 314:686, 1986.
34. Becker, T.M., Blount, J.H., Guinan, M.E.,: Genital herpes infections in private practice in the United States. 1966-1981. JAMA 253:1601, 1985.
35. Landry, M.L., and Zibello, T.A.: Ability of herpes simplex virus (HSV) types 1 and 2 to induce clinical disease and establish latency following previous genital infection with heterologous HSV type. J. Infect. Dis. 158:1220. 1988.
36. Selin, L.K., Hammond, G.W., and Aoki, F.Y.: Neonatal herpes simplex virus infection in Manitoba, 1980 to 1986, and implications for preventive strategies. Pediatr. Infect. Dis. J. 7:733, 1988.

37. Stagno, H., and Whitley, R.J.: Herpesvirus infections of pregnancy. N. Engl. J. Med. *313*:1327, 1985.
38. Prober, C.G., Sullender, W.M., Yasukawa, L.L., et al.: Low risk of herpes simplex virus infections in neonates exposed to the virus at the time of vaginal delivery to mothers with recurrent genital herpes simplex virus infections. N. Engl. J. Med. *316*:240, 1987.
39. Koskiniemi, M., Happonen, J.-M., Järvenpää, A.-L., et al.: Neonatal herpes simplex virus infection: A report of 43 patients. Pediatr. Infect. Dis. J. *8*:30, 1989.
40. Guinan, M.E.: Oral acyclovir for the treatment and suppression of genital herpes simplex virus infection. JAMA *255*:1747, 1986.
41. Davis, E.A., and Sayre, M.R.: The use of oral acyclovir in the treatment of herpetic whitlow (abstract). Ann. Emerg. Med. *18*:471, 1989.
42. Erlich, K.S., Mills, J., Chatis, P., et al.: Acyclovir-resistant herpes simplex virus infections in patients with the acquired immunodeficiency syndrome. N. Engl. J. Med. *20*:293, 1989.
43. Chatis, P.A., Miller, L.E., Schrager, L.E., and Crumpacker, C.S.: Successful treatment with foscarnet of an acyclovir-resistant mucocutaneous infection with herpes simplex virus in a patient with acquired immunodeficiency syndrome. N. Engl. J. Med. *320*:297, 1989.
44. Park, J.B., and Park, N.-H.: Effect of chlorhexidine on the in vitro and in vivo herpes simplex virus infection. Oral Surg. Oral Med. Oral Pathol. *67*:149, 1989.
45. Cassuto, J.: Topical local anesthetics and herpes simplex. Lancet *1*:100, 1989.
46. Baker, D.A., Blythe, J.G., Kaufman, R., et al.: One-year suppression of frequent recurrences of genital herpes with oral acyclovir. Obstet. Gynecol. *73*:84, 1989.
47. Pass, R.F., and Hutto, C.: Group day care and cytomegalovirus infections of mothers and children. Rev. Infect. Dis. *8*:599, 1986.
48. Balcarek, K.B., Bagley, R., Cloud, G.A., and Pass, R.F.: Cytomegalovirus infection among employees of a children's hospital: No evidence for increased risk associated with patient care. JAMA *263*:840, 1990.
49. Melnick, J.L., Adam, E., DeBakey, M.E.: Possible role of cytomegalovirus in atherogenesis. JAMA *263*:2204, 1990.
50. Drew, W.L.: Diagnosis of cytomegalovirus infection. Rev. Infect. Dis. *10*:S468, 1988.
51. Debure, A., Celton, J.L., Cartron, J., et al.: Granulocyte-associated immunoglobulins in renal transplant recipients with cytomegalovirus infection. Lancet *2*:1338, 1988.
52. Morris, D.J.: Rapid diagnosis of cytomegalovirus infection in renal transplant recipients. Lancet *1*:332, 1989.
53. Buhles, W.C., Jr., Mastre, B.J., Tinker, A.J., et al.: Syntex Collaborative Ganciclovir Treatment Study group. Ganciclovir treatment of life- or sight-threatening infection: Experience in 314 immunocompromised patients. Rev. Infect. Dis. *10*:S495, 1988.
53a. Schmidt, G.M., Norak, D.A., Niland, J.C., et al.: A randomized controlled trial of prophylactic gancyclovir for CMV infection (pulmonary) in recipients of allogenic bone marrow transplants. N. Engl. J. Med. *324*:1005, 1991.
54. Brayman, K.L., Dafoe, D.C., Smythe, W.R., et al.: Prophylaxis of serious cytomegalovirus infection in renal transplant candidates using live human cytomegalovirus vaccine: Interim results of a randomized controlled trial. Arch. Surg. *123*:1502, 1988.
55. Konvolinka, C.W., and Wyatt, D.B.: Splenic rupture and infectious mononucleosis. J. Emerg. Med. *7*:471, 1989.
56. Diaz-Mitoma, F., Vanast, W.J., and Tyrrell, D.L.J.: Increased frequency of Epstein-Barr virus excretion in patients with new daily persistent headaches. Lancet *1*:411, 1987.
57. Schooley, R.T., Carey, R.W., Miller, G., et al.: Chronic Epstein-Barr virus infection associated with fever and interstitial pneumonitis. Ann. Intern. Med. *104*:636, 1986.
58. Jones, J.F., Ray, C.G., Minnich, L.L., et al.: Evidence for active Epstein-Barr virus infection in patients with persistent, unexplained illnesses: Elevated anti-early antigen antibodies. Ann. Intern. Med. *102*:1, 1985.
59. Holmes, G.P., Kaplan, J.E., Stewart, J.A., et al.: A cluster of

60. patients with a chronic mononucleosis-like syndrome: Is Epstein-Barr virus the cause? JAMA *257*:2297, 1987.
60. Goldenberg, D.L.: Fibromyalgia and its relation to chronic fatigue syndrome, viral illness and immune abnormalities. J. Rheumatol. Suppl. *19*:91, 1989.
61. Holmes, G.P., Kaplan, J.E., Gantz, N.M., Komaroff, A.L., et al.: Chronic fatigue syndrome: A working case definition. Ann. Intern. Med. *108*:387, 1988.
62. Katz, B.Z., and Andiman, W.A.: Chronic fatigue syndrome. J. Pediatr. *113*:944, 1988.
63. Kaslow, J.E., Rucker, L., and Onishi, R.: Liver extract-folic acid-cyanocobalamin vs placebo for chronic fatigue syndrome. Arch. Intern. Med. *149*:2501, 1989.
64. Wharton, M., Cochi, S.L., Hutcheson, R.H., et al.: A large outbreak of mumps in the postvaccine era. J. Infect. Dis. *158*:1253, 1988.
65. Centers for Disease Control. Mumps prevention. M.M.W.R. *38*:388,397, 1989.
66. Cimolai, N., Anand, C.M., Gish, G.J., et al.: Human Colorado tick fever in southern Alberta. Can. Med. Assoc. J. *139*:45, 1988.
67. Wright, S.W., and Trott, A.T.: North American tick-borne diseases. Ann. Emerg. Med. *17*:964, 1988.
68. Bartlett, A.V., 3d, Reves, R.R., and Pickering, L.K.: Rotavirus in infant-toddler day care centers: epidemiology relevant to disease control strategies. J. Pediatr. *113*:435, 1988.
69. Ho, M.S., Glass, R.I., Pinsky, P.F., and Anderson, L.J.: Rotavirus as a cause of diarrheal morbidity and mortality in the United States. J. Infect. Dis. *158*:1112, 1988.
70. Rodriguez, W.J.: Viral enteritis in the 1980s: Perspective, diagnosis and outlook for prevention. Pediatr. Infect. Dis. J. *8*:570, 1989.
71. Prey, M.U., Lorelle, C.A., Taff, T.A., et al.: Evaluation of three commercially available rotavirus detection methods for neonatal specimens. Am. J. Clin Pathol. *89*:675, 1988.
72. Paccagnini, S., Fontana, M., Ceriani, R., Zuin, G., Galli, L., Quaranta, S., et al.: Occult blood and faecal leukocyte tests in acute infectious diarrhoea in children. Lancet *1*:442, 1987.
73. Hay, I.T.: Age and admission weight as predictors of mortality in gastro-enteritis. S. Afr. Med. J. *76*:483, 1989.
74. Santosham, M., Daum, R.S., Dillman, L., et al.: Oral rehydration therapy in infantile diarrhea: A controlled study of well nourished children hospitalized in the United States and Panama. N. Engl. J. Med. *306*:1070, 1982.
75. Lanata, C.F., Black, R.E., del Aguila, R., et al.: Protection of Peruvian children against rotavirus diarrhea of specific serotypes by one, two, or three doses of the RIT 4237 attenuated bovine rotavirus vaccine. J. Infect. Dis. *159*:452, 1989.
76. Iversen, A.M., Gill, M., Bartlett, C.L. et al.: Two outbreaks of foodborne gastroenteritis caused by a small round structured virus: evidence of prolonged infectivity in a food handler. Lancet *2*:556, 1987.
77. Guest, C., Spitalny, K.C., Madore, H.P., et al.: Foodborne Snow Mountain agent gastroenteritis in a school cafeteria. Pediatrics *79*:559, 1987.
78. Sawyer, L.A., Murphy, J.J., Kaplan, J.E., et al.: 25- to 30-nm virus particle associated with a hospital outbreak of acute gastroenteritis with evidence for airborne transmission. Am. J. Epidemiol. *127*:1261, 1988.
79. Reid, J.A., Caul, E.O., White, D.G., and Palmer, S.R.: Role of infected food handler in hotel outbreak of Norwalk-like viral gastroenteritis: implications for control. Lancet *2*:321, 1988.
80. Wood, D.J., Longhurst, D., Killough, R.I., and David, T.J.: One-year prospective cross-sectional study to assess the importance of group F adenovirus infections in children under 2 years admitted to hospital. J. Med. Virol. *26*:429, 1988.
81. Wood, D.J.: Adenovirus gastroenteritis. Br. Med. J. [Clin. Res.] *296*:229, 1988.
82. Centers for Disease Control. Progress toward eradicating poliomyelitis from the Americas. M.M.W.R. *262*:1443, 1989.
83. Moulia-Palat, J.P., Garanna, M., Schlumbergar, M., and Diouf, B.: Is inactivated polio vaccine more expensive? (letter) Lancet *2*:1424, 1988.
84. Tulchinsky, T., Abed, Y., Shaheen, S., et al.: A ten-year ex-

perience in control of poliomyelitis through a combination of live and killed vaccines in two developing areas. Am. J. Public Health 79:1648, 1989.
85. Harjulehto, T., Aro, T., Hovi, T., and Saxen, L.: Congenital malformations and oral poliovirus vaccination during pregnancy. Lancet 1:771, 1989.

86. Nkowane, B.M., Wassilak, S.G., Orenstein, W.A., et al.: Vaccine-associated paralytic poliomyelitis. United States: 1973 through 1984. JAMA 257:1335, 1987.
87. Kauffman, F.J., and Goldmann, B.J.: Rabies. Am. J. Emerg. Med. 4:525, 1986.

ANTIBIOTIC USE IN THE EMERGENCY DEPARTMENT

GENERAL PRINCIPLES AND DECISION MAKING

Robert D. Libke

CAPSULE

Many antibiotics have been introduced for use in clinical practice over the last few years. Some agents have replaced drugs frequently used in everyday practice, whereas others are only rarely used. In the Emergency Department (ED), initiation of antibiotic therapy is usually done empirically, on the basis of a clinical diagnosis, and treatment based on the results of culture and sensitivity tests is unusual. Because of this practice, the exact role of a newly introduced antibiotic is difficult to assess, especially when the previous therapy in a given clinical situation was clearly defined and effective, with minimal toxicity. This chapter reviews the antibiotic activity, doses, and advantages, if present, of the newer broad-spectrum penicillins, cephalosporins, carbapenems, monobactams, and quinolones.

Newer antibiotics may have several characteristics that give them a place in practice. Advantages to look for in any new drug include:

1. Expansion of antibiotic spectrum
2. Improved pharmacokinetics
3. Lessened toxicity
4. Lower cost

Expansion of the antibiotic spectrum over the older drugs in a chemical group has resulted in the largest number of newer agents. The best example of this has been the "third-generation"

cephalosporins that have become available. Organisms (such as Enterobacter, Pseudomonas, and Serratia) resistant to the earlier cephalosporins are often found to be sensitive to the newer agents in this group. Changes in pharmacokinetics considered advantageous include higher blood levels, longer half-lives, better penetration into body fluids or compartments, and better absorption after oral administration. Lessened toxicity within a class of antibiotics is often difficult to prove in small studies. Frequently, claims of better tolerance of one drug compared with another in the same class have not been verified by further experience. The broader spectrum of activity of many new agents makes possible the treatment of infections that required antibiotics with more potential toxicity, such as the aminoglycosides. In these cases, the replacement of one class of antibiotics with a less toxic group offers a major benefit.

Unfortunately, the unit cost of each newly introduced antibiotic is seldom lower than that of the drugs that are replaced. Often, however, because of the less frequent administration allowed by improved pharmacology, the actual cost may be competitive with that of older drugs. The cost of a therapeutic regimen may be reduced if the expanded spectrum of an antibiotic makes monotherapy possible in situations in which a combination of agents was previously used to provide adequate coverage. In addition, if lowered toxicity allows fewer tests to monitor for organ system dysfunction and negates the need for drug level determinations, the increased unit cost may be offset.

The potential advantages of the newer antibiotics do not come without potential disadvantages. The expanded spectrum of the newer antibiotics is often accompanied by greater disturbance of the normal flora of patients. This may result in such complications as antibiotic-induced colitis or suppression of vitamin K-producing bacteria leading to disturbances in coagulation. In addition, development of more resistant organisms in patients and within the hospital environment is a potential problem if widespread use of the newer drugs occurs. For these reasons, use of the newer antibiotics should be confined to situations in which the potential benefits outweigh the risks and increased costs involved. Certainly, substitution of the newer, broad-spectrum agents is not indicated for treatment of infections in well-defined clinical situations in which less toxic, narrower-spectrum agents can be used.

BROAD-SPECTRUM PENICILLINS

Carbenicillin and ticarcillin are the agents in the broad-spectrum penicillin group that have been in use for some time. They are active against organisms sensitive to ampicillin (including B-lactamase—negative Haemophilus influenzae, Escherichia coli, Proteus mirabilis, and some strains of Enterobacter) and most bacteria susceptible to penicillin. Carbenicillin and ticarcillin were the first B-lactam antibiotics to reliably cover Pseudomonas aeruginosa and a larger number of *Enterobacter* species. Several indole-positive Proteus species fall within the spectrum of these antibiotics. Ticarcillin is about twice as active as carbenicillin against P. aeruginosa and may be preferred for the treatment of infections caused by this organism. Of note is the fact that none of the broad-spectrum penicillins, with the exception of ticarcillin-clavulanate potassium (Timentin) and ampicillin-sulbactam (Unasyn), have activity against penicillin-resistant Staphylococcus aureus.

Although the organisms mentioned are considered susceptible to ticarcillin or carbenicillin, this is only with the high blood levels attained when high doses of 18 to 30 g per day are given to patients with normal renal function.

NEWER BROAD-SPECTRUM PENICILLINS

MEZLOCILLIN (MEZLIN)

Mezlocillin is a broad-spectrum penicillin that is active against the same organisms as carbenicillin and ticarcillin. Although it is slightly better in vitro against many of the gram-negative aerobic organisms, the main feature of mezlocillin is its enhanced activity against Klebsiella and Providencia. Mezlocillin's activity against Pseudomonas is comparable with that of carbenicillin and ticarcillin.

The pharmacology of mezlocillin is similar to that of carbenicillin and ticarcillin. Mezlocillin is a monosodium compound (compared with ticarcillin and carbenicillin, which are disodium), resulting in a lower sodium load, a feature that may be beneficial in patients with hemodynamic or renal dysfunction.

In the ED, the use of mezlocillin depends on the previous use of carbenicillin or ticarcillin. In light of its slightly expanded spectrum, mezlocillin may be a preferred agent if competitive pricing results in similar cost.

PIPERACILLIN (PIPRACIL)

Piperacillin is a uriedo-penicillin with a spectrum similar to that of mezlocillin, including good activity against Klebsiella species. In addition, piperacillin has considerably enhanced action against Pseudomonas aeruginosa when compared with other agents in this group. Like mezlocillin, it is a monosodium compound and has pharmacokinetic activity similar to the other broad-spectrum penicillins.

In the ED, piperacillin should be considered for use in patients who are likely to have Pseudomonas infections. Such patients may include those who have recently been on antibiotic therapy, those recently hospitalized or in a nursing home, or those who have been on chemotherapy. In general, however, piperacillin should be reserved for hospitalized patients with infection proved by culture and sensitivity reported to be susceptible to piperacillin but resistant to the older, narrower-spectrum, less expensive agents.

AZLOCILLIN (AZLIN)

Azlocillin has antipseudomonal activity comparable to that of piperacillin, but is less active than piperacillin or mezlocillin against other gram-negative bacteria. Its pharmacology is similar to that of the other expanded-spectrum penicillins. Azlocillin is used principally for treatment of pseudomonal infections and probably should not be used in the ED for empiric therapy unless it is combined with other agents to provide broad coverage.

TICARCILLIN-CLAVULANATE POTASSIUM (TIMENTIN)

When the potassium salt of clavulanic acid is combined with ticarcillin, the activity of ticarcillin is enhanced by inhibition of B-lactamases that inactivate ticarcillin. These enzymes are produced by various gram-negative and a few gram-positive organisms. As a result of enzyme inactivation, the spectrum of ticarcillin is expanded to include Staphylococcus aureus, B-lactamase-producing Hemophilus influenzae, and many Klebsiella species. In one study, combining ticarcillin with clavulate increased the susceptibility of Enterobacteriaceae strains from about 70% to about 90%. In addition, the activity against Bacteroides fragilis is increased. The combination does not improve the activity of ticarcillin against Serratia or Pseudomonas species.

The dosage of ticarcillin-clavulanate potassium for systemic infections is 3.1 g (3 g ticarcillin with 100 mg clavulanic acid) given every 4 to 6 hours. For urinary infections, 3.2 g (3 g of ticarcillin and 200 mg of clavulanic acid) is given intravenously every 8 hours. These doses should be adjusted in patients with renal dysfunction when the creatinine clearance falls below 60 ml per minute.

For patients with infection acquired outside the hospital setting, ticarcillin-clavulanate potassium may be used as monotherapy when the primary site of infection appears to be in the respiratory, urinary, or abdominal area. Some studies have suggested that the use of this combination antibiotic-β-lactamase inhibitor may replace the use of combinations containing aminoglycosides for broad-spectrum coverage, thereby avoiding the renal and eighth-nerve toxicity inherent in those drugs.

AMPICILLIN-SULBACTAM (UNASYN)

As with ticarcillin, combining ampicillin with a β-lactamase inhibitor, sulbactam, has extended its spectrum. Organisms such as β-lactamase-producing Staphylococcus aureus, Hemophilus influenzae, and many of the Enterobacteriaceae previously resistant to ampicillin now fall within the treatment range of this combination. Many resistant Bacteroides fragilis are found to be sensitive to ampicillin-sulbactam. The activity of ampicillin against Pseudomonas aeruginosa, however, is not particularly enhanced by combination with sulbactam.

The dosage used for systemic infection is 2 g of ampicillin with 1 g sulbactam given intramuscularly or intravenously every 6 hours.

The exact role of ampicillin-sulbactam in initial therapy has not yet been well established. The similarity of its spectrum of activity to that of ticarcillin-clavulanate potassium suggests that it may be used in a similar fashion.

The pencillins share similar side effects and cross-react with one another. Hypersensitivity reactions presenting as delayed onset skin rashes are seen in 5% and 10% of patients. Drug fever, diarrhea, and phlebitis may occur in some patients. Serum sickness, eosinophilia, leukopenia, and a positive reaction to Coombs' test have been reported but are infrequent clinical problems. Because of high-dose regimens used with the broad-spectrum agents, elevated transaminase levels, hypokalemia, and platelet dysfunction may occur, and rarely, hemolytic anemia is seen. Patients with renal failure can develop central nervous system toxicity (excitability, agitation, convulsions) if dose adjustments are not made.

CEPHALOSPORINS

A wide array of cephalosporin antibiotics have become available over the past few years. They have arbitrarily been divided into "generations" on the basis of the range of activity against gram-negative organisms: those with a moderately expanded spectrum are classified as second generation, whereas those with broad activity become third-generation agents. In reality, with the number of agents now available, precise categorization of a given drug may be difficult.

Although this is not universal, the increased action of the newer cephalosporins against gram-negative organisms is often accompanied by a loss of potency against gram-positive cocci, especially S. aureus. Enterococci and methicillin-resistant S. aureus are resistant and none of the cephalosporins should be used for treatment of infections with these organisms (even if standard in vitro tests indicate susceptibility).

FIRST-GENERATION CEPHALOSPORINS

CEPHALOTHIN, CEPHAPIRIN, CEPHRADINE, AND CEFAZOLIN

The first of the cephalosporins were introduced when there were a limited number of antibiotics active against gram-negative infections. Ampicillin, chloramphenicol, kanamycin, tetracycline, and the polymyxins were in use at the time cephalothin (Keflin, Seffin) was released. Like ampicillin, the principal β-lactam antibiotic with gram-negative activity then in use, cephalothin had activity against Escherichia coli and Proteus mirabilis but was also active against Klebsiella and Staphylococcus aureus. It was not as active as ampicillin against Hemophilus influenzae or anaerobes but was, nevertheless, a welcome addition to the antibiotic armamentarium because of the activity against organisms commonly encountered in clinical practice.

The other first-generation cephalosporins have spectrums like that of cephalothin. Unlike cephapirin

(Cefadyl), cephradine (Velosef, Anspor), and cephalothin, which have similar pharmacokinetics, cefazolin (Ancef, Kefzol) has pharmacologic advantages over the other older cephalosporins. It produces higher, more prolonged blood levels and is better tolerated locally when given intravenously or intramuscularly. With these pharmacologic advantages, cefazolin is the preferred first-generation cephalosporin in most clinical situations.

SECOND-GENERATION CEPHALOSPORINS

CEFAMANDOLE (MANDOL)

Cefamandole is one of the first expanded-spectrum cephalosporins. The main expansion of the spectrum was the addition of activity against Enterobacter species, against which the older cephalosporins had little activity. Cefamandole is also active against β-lactamase-producing H. influenzae and Neisseria gonorrhoeae. Its activity against S. aureus is somewhat less than that of the older cephalosporins.

Cefamandole has a longer half-life than cephalothin, but its pharmacokinetics do not compare favorably with those of cefazolin. The dosage in adults with normal renal function should be 1 to 2 g every 6 hours.

CEFONICID (MONOCID)

Cefonicid is a second-generation cephalosporin, with activity similar to that of cefamandole. Its major feature is a half-life of 4 hours. Cefonicid has been used predominantly in surgical prophylaxis for single-dose preoperative therapy (1 g). If used in therapy other than prophylaxis, doses of 1 to 2 g are given intravenously or intramuscularly every 12 hours.

CEFOXITIN (MEFOXIN)

Cefoxitin has slightly more activity against many of the Enterobacteriaceae than do the first-generation cephalosporins. It has unreliable action against Enterobacter species, however. The main advantage of cefoxitin is enhanced antianaerobic action, especially with respect to Bacteroides fragilis, which the older cephalosporins do not cover well. As with cefamandole, the susceptibility of Staphylococcus aureus to cefoxitin is diminished compared with the older agents.

Because of its slightly shorter half-life and lower levels in the blood, cefoxitin should be given in doses of 1 to 2 g at least every 6 hours.

CEFOTETAN (CEFOTAN)

Cefotetan is considered roughly equivalent to cefoxitin in its spectrum but with slightly better activity against some gram-negative organisms. Although cefotetan is active against B. fragilis, however, some of the other bacteroides species are less sensitive.

The principal advantage of cefotetan lies in its pharmacology. While cefoxitin has a half-life of approximately 0.8 hours, cefotetan's serum half-life is about 4 hours. Because of this, cefotetan can be given at a dose of 1 to 2 g every 12 hours.

CEFUROXIME (ZINACEF, KEFUROX)

Cefuroxime has a spectrum of activity similar to that of cefamandole. It has good activity against Hemophilus influenzae, including β-lactamase-producers. It is not as active as cefoxitin or cefotetan against anaerobic organisms. Good activity is seen against most gram-positive organisms; however, as with the other second-generation cephalosporins, S. aureus is less susceptible to cefuroxime.

Although the antibacterial spectrum of cefuroxime is similar to that of the other second-generation cephalosporins, improved pharmacokinetics give cefuroxime its main value. Not only are its levels in the blood somewhat higher than those achieved with cefamandole and cefoxitin, it also has a longer half-life (about 1.3 hours). An additional feature is increased penetration into the cerebrospinal fluid. All previously mentioned cephalosporins have inadequate penetration into the cerebrospinal fluid to allow their use in proven or suspected central nervous system infections. Clinical studies have shown cefuroxime effective in therapy for meningitis caused by most central nervous system pathogens in nonimmunocompromised patients, and it can be used in place of more traditional therapies, such as ampicillin and/or chloramphenicol.

The usual dosage of cefuroxime for adults with nonmeningeal infection is 750 mg to 1.5 g parenterally every 8 hours. For children, the dosage is 100 mg/kg of body weight per day in divided doses. In children with meningitis, doses up to 200 mg/kg per day are used. The dose and/or frequency of administration of cefuroxime should be altered for patients with severe renal dysfunction when the creatinine clearance is 20 mL per minute or less.

These parenteral second-generation cephalosporins may occasionally be used empirically for patients requiring hospitalization. Cefamandole, although at one time of some use, has largely been replaced by the newer second- and third-generation cephalosporins and broad-spectrum penicillins. Cefoxitin is often indicated for treatment of patients suspected of having anaerobes as part of their infecting flora. In anaerobic pulmonary disease, cefoxitin may be used as primary monotherapy, especially in penicillin-allergic patients. For patients with suspected abdominal or pelvic infections, it may be used as monotherapy or combined with an aminoglycoside in severely ill patients. Cefotetan has indications similar to those of cefoxitin, and in light of its pharmacokinetics, may be used preferentially for the advantage of dosing every 12 hours. Cefuroxime, as noted previously, may be used as initial therapy in the treatment of patients with meningitis. In adults with nonanaphylactoid penicillin allergy, cefuroxime is a reasonable therapeutic alternative to chloramphenicol for the treatment of meningitis.

THIRD-GENERATION CEPHALOSPORINS

CEFOTAXIME (CLAFORAN)

Cefotaxime is active against the gram-negative organisms covered by first- and second-generation cephalosporins and, in addition, reliably covers Citrobacter and Serratia. Milligram for milligram, cefotaxime is more potent against many gram-negative organisms than are the aminoglycosides. Cefotaxime has limited action against Pseudomonas and Acinetobacter. In vitro, the susceptibility of Bacteroides fragilis is variable; however, an in vivo metabolic breakdown product called desacetylcefotaxime has considerable antibacterial activity and enhances the usefulness of cefotaxime in patients with mixed infections. The sensitivity of Staphylococcus aureus to cefotaxime is less than its sensitivity to the older agents in the cephalosporin group, but cefotaxime has more antistaphylococcal potency than other third-generation cephalosporins. Like the older cephalosporins, cefoxtaxime and the other third-generation agents cannot be used for treatment of enterococcal infections.

Cefotaxime has the shortest half-life (1.5 hours) of the third-generation cephalosporins and should be given frequently to maintain adequate levels in the blood for marginally sensitive organisms. The dosage of cefotaxime for patients with systemic infection is 1 to 2 g every 8 hours and, when life-threatening disease is present, up to 12 g per day, with dosing every 6 hours, may be given. Cefotaxime and other third-generation cephalosporins penetrate into the cerebrospinal fluid adequately for treatment of infections caused by sensitive organisms.

CEFTRIAXONE (ROCEPHIN)

Ceftriaxone has a spectrum of activity much like that of cefotaxime. Like the other third-generation drugs, it is β-lactamase-stable and active against both gram-positive (except enterococci) and gram-negative organisms.

Ceftriaxone has a long half-life of 6 to 8 hours, which allows dosing once or twice daily. Single daily dosing has made this an appealing agent for home intravenous therapy regimens. It has good cerebrospinal fluid penetration and has been used successfully in the treatment of meningitis.

CEFTIZOXIME (CEFIZOX)

The spectrum of ceftizoxime is similar to that of cefotaxime. It has a slightly longer half-life and is recommended for dosing every 8 hours.

MOXALACTAM (MOXAM)

Moxalactam was one of the first broader-spectrum cephalosporins to become available. It is active against a wide variety of organisms, including anaerobes. It has considerably less activity than cefotaxime against Staphylococcus aureus and has limited antipseudomonal activity.

The serum half-life of moxalactam is about 2 hours and levels in the blood with similar doses are higher than those of cefotaxime. Moxalactam has been used successfully for the treatment of meningitis, including infections caused by gram-negative bacilli.

Bleeding caused by both platelet dysfunction and hypoprothrombinemia, induced by moxalactam, has limited its usefulness.

CEFOPERAZONE (CEFOBID)

Cefoperazone also has broad gram-negative coverage and was the first expanded-spectrum cephalosporin to have reasonably good activity against Pseudomonas aeruginosa. Coverage of *Acinetobacter* is marginal, and activity against Bacteroides fragilis is less than with the drugs previously mentioned.

Cefoperazone has a 2-hour half-life and can be used in dosing regimens of 1 to 2 g every 12 hours. For more severe infections, 6 to 12 g per day are recommended. Because cefoperazone is eliminated by both hepatic and renal routes, minimal adjustment of dosing is necessary for patients with renal dysfunction unless hepatobiliary disease is also present.

CEFTAZIDIME (FORTAZ, TAZIDIME, TAZICEF)

Ceftazidime is active against Enterobacteriaceae, like other third-generation cephalosporins. It is the most active of these agents against P. aeruginosa. It is less active than cefotaxime or ceftriaxone against gram-positive organisms and has unreliable activity against B. fragilis.

The half-life of ceftazidime is approximately 1.8 hours. It has been used in doses of 1 to 2 g every 8 to 12 hours. For treatment of meningitis caused by gram-negative bacteria, up to 6 g per day are recommended. In children, 30 to 50 mg/kg of body weight are given intravenously every 8 hours.

USE OF THIRD-GENERATION CEPHALOSPORINS IN THE ED

The use of third-generation cephalosporins in the ED is currently in a state of flux. Clearly, the expanded spectrum of activity has made them inviting drugs to be used in monotherapy in patients with moderate to severe infections. The inherent toxic and renal toxicity of the aminoglycosides, which were previously relied on to cover the more resistant gram-negative organisms, makes replacement with less toxic drugs a desirable goal. Broad-spectrum β-lactam antibiotics may serve that purpose in many clinical situations, but in severely ill patients infected by undefined organisms, further experience may be needed before the aminoglycosides are comfortably replaced. The combination of a β-lactam antibiotic (a cephalosporin or penicillin) with an aminoglycoside has been found in vitro to be synergistically active against many gram-positive and gram-negative organisms. Some of the reluctance to abandon aminoglycosides in more severely ill patients is founded partly on these in vitro observations and on studies in immunocompromised patients, who have been shown to do better when a synergistic combination is used. In studies of nonimmunocompromised hosts, a beneficial effect of such synergistic combinations is difficult to show.

For most patients who acquired infections outside a medical care facility or nursing home and who were not exposed to antibiotic treatment before presentation, the third-generation cephalosporins may be used for initial therapy, pending the results of appropriate cultures. Cefotaxime, ceftriaxone, or cefizoxime could be used in this situation as long as there is no suspicion of infection with methicillin-resistant S. aureus, enterococci, or Pseudomonas. If these agents are used in abdominal or pelvis infections, additional antianaerobic coverage is often needed. Cefoperazone or ceftazidime may be useful if the presence of *Pseudomonas* is highly suspected. In such situations, however, other hospital-acquired organisms may be present, and if the patient is severely ill, these drugs are often combined with an aminoglycoside, such as amikacin, for initial therapy. For patients with meningitis, initiation of treatment with a third-generation cephalosporin can be reasonable, with the addition of an antistaphylococcal penicillin if there is associated trauma or neurosurgery.

The continuation of any of these broad-spectrum agents depends on sensitivity reports of the organisms involved. Generally, after such information becomes available, it is prudent to select the narrowest-spectrum, least toxic, effective antibiotic with the lowest cost.

Like the penicillins, cephalosporins are relatively safe agents. Hypersensitivity reactions, most commonly in the form of maculopapular skin eruptions, occur in up to 8% of patients. Eosinophilia and dose-related neutropenia are seen occasionally. Although positive reactions to a Coombs' test are common in patients receiving cephalosporin therapy, hemolytic anemia is unusual. Bleeding caused by hypoprothrombinemia, thrombocytopenia, or platelet dysfunction has most often been described with the use

of moxalactam; some of these effects on coagulation have been associated with cefoperazone. Weekly vitamin K administration effectively prevents the hypoprothrombinemia caused by these drugs. Rarely, nephrotoxicity (often interstitial nephritis with eosinophiluria) has been attributed to the cephalosporin antibiotics. Diarrhea and pseudomembranous colitis occur with all of the broad-spectrum β-lactam antibiotics, including the cephalosporins.

Cross-hypersensitivity is seen in 5% to 10% of patients with a history of the delayed-onset type of penicillin allergy. With careful monitoring, such patients could be treated with a cephalosporin if other, safer alternatives cannot be found. Those with acute hypersensitivity (hives, bronchospasm, or anaphylaxis) to penicillins should rarely, if at all, receive therapy with a cephalosporin.

CARBAPENEMS

IMIPENEM-CILASTATIN (PRIMAXIN)

Imipenem is the first member of the carbapenem class of antibiotics. Derived from the patent compound, thienamycin, imipenem has the broadest spectrum of activity of the β-lactam antibiotics currently available. It has good activity against gram-positive bacteria, including enterococci and penicillinase-producing strains of Staphylococcus aureus. Imipenem has limited activity against methicillin-resistant staphylococci and some corynebacteria. The susceptibility of most gram-negative organisms, including Pseudomonas aeruginosa, Acinetobacter, Neisseria, and Haemophilus, to imipenem has been demonstrated, whereas Pseudomonas cepacia and Pseudomonas maltophilia have shown resistance. Imipenem also has broad antianaerobic action, including good potency against *Bacteroides* species; however, its action against Clostridium difficile is limited.

Imipenem undergoes extensive metabolic breakdown in the kidney by a brush-border dipeptidase. An inhibitor of this enzyme, cilastatin, increases the urinary concentration of imipenem and decreases the renal toxicity seen when imipenem was administered alone in early animal experiments. The dosage of imipenem-cilastatin given intravenously is 0.5 to 1.0 g every 6 hours. Moderate dose adjustments for patients with impaired renal function are required.

In spite of the broad spectrum of imipenem-cilastatin, it should not be regarded as a panacea for all clinical infections. Indeed, because many alternative broad-spectrum agents are currently available, imipenem should rarely be used for initial, empiric therapy. Rather, it should be reserved for patients who acquire infection in a hospital setting and who are proved, by culture and sensitivity report, to have organisms sensitive to imipenem and resistant to other narrower-spectrum agents.

MONOBACTAMS

AZTREONAM (AZACTAM)

Aztreonam is a monocylic β-lactam (monobactam) antibiotic that, like its novel monocylic structure, has a novel antibacterial spectrum. It has broad activity against aerobic gram-negative bacteria but little action against gram-positive bacteria or anaerobes. The spectrum of gram-negative activity includes organisms commonly encountered in nosocomial infections. Not only is aztreonam effective against most of the Enterobacteriaceae, but it also shows good activity against Neisseria, Haemophilus, and Serratia. It has moderate activity against P. aeruginosa and variable action against Enterobacter species. Acinetobacter, P. Maltophilia, and P. cepacia tend to be resistant.

Peak serum levels after administration of 2 g aztreonam intravenously are over 200 μg/mL immediately after the infusion and about 90 μg/mL one hour after infusion. The antibiotic is widely distributed throughout the body and diffuses well into the cerebrospinal fluid, especially in the presence of inflamed meninges. Aztreonam has an elimination half-life of about 1.7 hours in patients with normal renal function and about 8 hours in patients who are anephric. The dosage in patients with systemic infection is 1 to 2 g every 8 or 12 hours; dose adjustment is required in patients with renal dysfunction.

The exact use of aztreonam therapy in the ED is not well established. Aztreonam could be used as an alternative to aminoglycosides in the treatment of urinary tract infections shown by Gram stain to be caused by gram-negative rods. It should not be used as the single agent in empiric therapy if mixed infections with gram-positive or anaerobic species are suspected. Because aztreonam does not seem to show cross-sensitivity with other β-lactams, it may be useful in treating patients who are allergic to penicillin or cephalosporin—perhaps along with a non-β-lactam agent such as clindamycin or vancomycin for coverage of gram-positive bacteria.

QUINOLONES

Nalidixic acid has been used for many years in the treatment of urinary tract infections. This drug, along with oxolinic acid and cinoxacin, is an antimicrobial agent with a 4-quinolone nucleus. These quinolone group antibiotics have been joined by two new agents, norfloxacin and ciprofloxacin, and will probably be joined by a host of others. These compounds act by inhibiting bacterial deoxyribonucleic acid (CNA) gyrase, an enzyme required for formation of negative superhelical twists in bacterial DNA. Although this lethal action is common to all the members of this group, some of the newer, more potent agents may have additional mechanisms of action that are not well defined.

Stepwise resistance to the earlier quinolone antibiotics has been noted, and development of resistance during therapy with nalidixic acid has been seen. The frequency of occurrence of stepwise resistance with the newer quinolones is less than that seen with the older agents, but could potentially be a serious problem if there is uninhibited use in hospitals.

NORFLOXACIN (NOROXIN)

Norfloxacin is a fluoroquinolone that has enhanced antibacterial activity that includes Pseudomonas aeruginosa and most of the enteric and urinary pathogens (including enterococci). It is active against Neisseria gonorrhoeae, even those that produce penicillinase. Norfloxacin has activity against most gram-positive organisms, including methicillin-resistant strains of Staphylococcus aureus. Its action against streptococci is less than that against staphylococci.

At present, norfloxacin is indicated only for the treatment of urinary tract infections caused by susceptible organisms. It is available only for oral administration and is given in a dose of 400 mg twice daily. For uncomplicated infections, treatment is continued for 7 to 10 days, whereas in complicated infections, therapy may extend up to 3 weeks. In patients with impaired renal function and creatinine clearance less than 30 mL per minute, 400 mg once daily is used.

Because studies of the use of high doses in animals showed damage to the joints while growth was occurring, norfloxacin should not be used in children or pregnant women. This drug is contraindicated in patients with a history of hypersensitivity to any of the quinolone group of antibiotics.

In the ED, norfloxacin's use should generally be limited to patients who have infections proved resistant to the antimicrobials commonly used for treatment of urinary tract infection. Its broad spectrum and ability to be administered orally often negate the need for hospitalization of patients for parenteral therapy with more toxic drugs. Because most of these patients are seen in the ED, without the benefit of bacterial culture information, deciding on the appropriate antibiotic therapy is difficult.

CIPROFLOXACIN (CIPRO)

Ciprofloxacin is active against a wide variety of bacterial pathogens. It is active against most gram-positive organisms, including methicillin-resistant Staphylococcus aureus and enterococci. The minimal inhibitory concentrations for Streptococcus pneumoniae and Streptocccus viridans are slightly higher than for the other gram-positive bacteria. Ciprofloxacin is highly active in vitro against Neisseria meningitidis, N. gonorrhoeae, and Haemophilus species. Its in vitro activity against gram-negative bacilli is quite broad and includes Enterobacteriaceae, Pseudomonas aeruginosa, Serratia, and Citrobacter. Other organisms against which ciprofloxacin is active include Legionella and some mycobacterial strains.

After oral administration of ciprofloxacin, serum levels are adequate for treatment of systemic infection. This drug has been used in the treatment of bone, respiratory, skin and soft tissue, urinary, and gastrointestinal infections. It has also been used successfully in the therapy of gonorrhea and chancroid.

Ciprofloxacin should seldom be used empirically, except possibly for the treatment of bacterial gastroenteritis, because it has shown good activity against Salmonella, Shigella, and Campylobacter. Further clinical studies are needed before it can be certain that ciprofloxacin should be used in the treatment of patients presenting with diarrheal disease of undefined cause.

The possibility of oral therapy for infections for which only parenteral treatment was previously available, including those outside of the urinary tract, makes ciprofloxacin (and similar future agents) a welcome addition to our armamentarium. At present, however, its empirical use in the ED is poorly defined, and recommendations await the outcome of further clinical studies.

BIBLIOGRAPHY

Holmes, B., Richards, D.M., Brogden, R.N., and Heel, R.C.: Piperacillin. A review of its antibacterial activity, pharmacokinetic properties and therapeutic use. Drugs 28:375, 1984.

Lode, H., and Kass, E.H.: Enzyme-mediated resistance to β-lactam antibiotics: A symposium on sulbactam/ampicillin. Rev. Infect. Dis. 8:55, 1986.

Neu, H.C.: Aztreonam: A monocyclic beta-lactam antibiotic (proceedings of a symposium). Am J. Med. 78:2A, 1985.

Neu, H.C.: Beta-lactamase inhibition: Therapeutic advances (proceedings of a symposium). Am. J. Med. 79:513, 1985.

Neu, H.C.: New antibiotics: Areas of appropriate use. J. Infect. Dis. 155:403, 1987.

Remington, J.S.: Carbapenems: A new class of antibotics (proceedings of a symposium). Am. J. Med. 78:6A, 1985.

Rubinstein, E., Adam, E., Moellering, R., Jr., and Waldvogel, F.: International Symposium on New Quinolones. Rev. Infect. Dis. 10:S1, 1988.

SPECIFIC ANTIBIOTIC CHOICES

Mary Anne Mangelsen and Kenneth A. Murphy, Jr.

CAPSULE

This section of the chapter contains notes on antibiotic choices that may be helpful in clinical decision making. The antibiotics discussed are penicillins (including the penicillinase-resistant and broad-spectrum penicllins), cephalosporins, aminoglycosides, clindamycin, chloramphenicol, sulfonamides and trimethoprimsulfamethoxazole, erythromycin, tetracyclines, vancomycin, metronidazole, quinolones, spectinomycin, and rifampin.

Tables 50-34 and 50-35 at the end of this section give pediatric and neonatal dosages for many of these agents. Table 50-36 outlines initial antimicrobial therapy based on clinical indications, giving antibiotic dosages and their alternatives.

PENICILLIN

Penicillin is bactericidal. Its penetration into the cerebrospinal fluid is limited to approximately 5 to 10%

TABLE 50-34. PEDIATRIC ANTIBIOTIC DOSAGES*

Antibiotic	PO	IV
Amoxicillin or Amoxicillin/ clavulanic acid	20–40 mg Q8H	
Ampicillin	50–100 mg Q6H	200–400 mg Q4–6H
Cefaclor	40 mg Q8H	
Cefazolin		25–100 mg Q6–8H
Cefotaxime		50–200 mg Q4–6H
Cefoxitin		80–160 mg Q4–6H
Ceftazidime		90–150 mg Q8H
Ceftriaxone		50–100 mg Q12–24H
Cefuroxime		50–240 mg Q6–8H
Chloramphenicol	50–100 mg Q6H	50–100 mg Q6H
Clindamycin	10–25 mg Q6–8H	15–40 mg Q6–8H
Cloxacillin	50–100 mg Q6H	
Dicloxacillin	12½–100 mg Q6H	
Erythromycin	30–50 mg Q6–8H	20–50 mg Q6H
Furazolidone	8 mg Q6H max = 400 mg	
Gentamicin		6–7½ mg Q8H
Metronidazole	Depends on disease state	
Nafcillin	Not recommended	100–200 mg Q6H
Neomycin	50–100 mg Q6H	
Penicillin	40,000–80,000U Q6H	100,000–300,000U Q6H
Piperacillin		200–300 mg Q4–6H
Quinacrine	6 mg Q8H Max = 300 mg	
Ticarcillin		200–300 mg Q4–6H
Tobramycin		6–7½ mg Q8H
Vancomycin		30–45 Q8H

* Meningitis doses are not given. Neonatal doses are given in Table 50-35. Doses are in mg/kg/*day*.

TABLE 50-35. NEONATAL DOSAGES*

Antibiotic	Route	< One Week Old BW < 2000 grams (mg/kg/day)	< One Week Old BW > 2000 grams (mg/kg/day)	> One Week Old BW < 2000 grams (mg/kg/day)	> One Week Old BW > 2000 grams
Ampicillin	IV	50 Q12H	75 Q8H	75 Q8H	100 Q6H
Cefotaxime	IV	100 Q12H	100 Q12H	150 Q8H	150 Q8H
Chloramphenicol	IV/PO	25 Q24H	25 Q24H	25 Q24H	50 Q12H
Erythromycin	PO	20 Q12H	20 Q12H	30 Q8H	45 Q8H
Gentamicin	IV	5 Q12H	5 Q12H	7.5 Q8H	7.5 Q8H
Nafcillin	IV	50 Q12H	75 Q8H	75 Q8H	100 Q6H
Neomycin	PO	100 Q6H	100 Q6H	100 Q6H	100 Q6H
Penicillin G	IV	50,000 U Q12H	75,000 U Q8H	75,000 U Q8H	100,000 U Q6H
Ticarcillin	IV	150 Q12H	225 Q8H	225 Q8H	300 Q6H
Tobramycin	IV	5 Q12H	5 Q8H	7.5 Q8H	7.5 Q8H
Vancomycin	IV	20 Q12H	20 Q12H	30 Q8H	30 Q8H

* Given in mg/kg/day except for penicillin G (no meningitis doses) BW = birth weight

of serum levels. A "penicillin" is the term for a broad group of agents: penicillin G, penicillin V, methicillin, oxacillin, cloxacillin, dicloxacillin nafcillin, ampicillin, amoxicillin, carbenicillin, ticarcillin, mezlocillin, azlocillin, piperacillin, etc. Organisms affected are gram-positive aerobic cocci (Streptococcus), gram-negative aerobes (Neisseria, Pasteurella), anaerobes (Clostridium but not Bacteroides fragilis, Actinomyces israeli), and Treponema pallidum.

PENICILLINASE-RESISTANT PENICILLINS

With modification of the side chain of penicillin, penicillinase-resistant penicillins were developed to treat penicillinase-producing staphylococci. These agents include oxacillin, nafcillin, methicillin, cloxacillin and dicloxacillin. They are not effective against Escherichia coli, Klebsiella, Enterobacter, or Pseudomonas, and are not recommended in the treatment of gonorrhea.

TABLE 50-36. INITIAL ANTIMICROBIAL THERAPY*

Site	Clinical Diagnosis		Selected Empiric	Alternative	Second Alternate/ Comments
Abdomen	Appendicitis, perforation Bacterial gastroenteritis	Enterobacteriaceae Bacteroides Enterococci	Clindamycin 600 mg Q6H and Gentamicin 1–1.6 mg/kg Q8H and Ampicillin 2g Q4–6H	Cefoxitin 2 g Q4–6H or Cefotetan 2g Q8–12H and Gentamicin 1–1.6 mg/kg Q8H	Ampicillin/Sulbactam 3 g Q6H and Gentamicin 1–1.6 mg/kg Q8H
		Shigella	TMP/SMX ONE DS Q12H × 5d	Ampicillin 500 mg po Q6H × 5d or Tetracycline 500 mg po Q6H × 5d	Ciprofloxacin 500 mg Q12H × 5d
		Salmonella	Chloramphenicol 500 mg po Q6H × 7d	Amoxicillin 500 mg po Q8H × 7d or TMP/SMX 1 DS po Q12H × 7d	Ciprofloxacin 500 mg Q12H × 7d Antibiotics may prolong carrier state and select resistant strains
		Vibrio parahemolyticus	Tetracycline 500 mg Q6H (Antibiotic Tx may not be Indicated)	Ciprofloxacin 500 mg Q12H	Found in shellfish
		Campylobacter Invasive E. coli	Erythromycin 250 mg Q6H × 14d	Ciprofloxacin 500 mg Q12H	
	Cholera	Vibrio Cholerae	Tetracycline 250 mg Q6H × 2d	TMP/SMX 1 DS Q12H × 2d	
	Diarrhea/dysentery, no travel history, no neutrophils in stool	Rotovirus Norwalk agents Escherichia coli	None	Ampicillin 500 mg po Q6H × 5d	Mild: fluids, moderate (305) uni- formed stools/d; no fever, no bleeding: Doperamide: 4 mg followed by 2 mg after each stool: do not exceed 16 mg/d; or bismuth subsalicylate 262 mg po qid. Severe: less than 6 uniform stools with fever, blood. Rx: antimicrobial Tx (see subsequent table section)
	Infant Diarrhea Febrile; gross blood; neutrophils in stool; history of travel	E. coli Varies; Campylobacter jejuni, E. coli (enterotoxigenic, enteroinvasive, Enterohemorrhagic 157: H7); Shigella, Salmonella, Aero- monas, Vibrio Cryp- tosporidium	Neomycin po 25 mg Q6H Ciprofloxacin 500 mg Q12H or Norfloxacin 400 mg Q12H or TMP/SMX 1 DS Q12H	Doxycycline 100 mg Q12H	
	Premature infant enterocolitis	Echerichia Coli; staph- ylococcus epidermi- dis, Pseudomonas aeruginosa, Clos- tridium perfringens	Ampicillin and tobramycin (if staph and vancomy- cin) (see Pediatric dos- age)	Ticarcillin and cefotaxime or Ceftriaxone	
	Antibiotic associ- ated colitis	Clostridium difficile toxin	Metronidazole 250 mg po Q6H × 10d	Vancomycin 125 mg po Q6H × 10d	
	Food contamination	Yersinia enterocolitica, Y. Pseudotubercu- losis	Tobramycin 1–1.6 mg/kg Q8H	TMP/SMX 1 DS Q12H	Cefriaxone 2 mg IV Q24H
	Diverticulitis, no perforation	Enterobacteriaceae Bacteroides Enterococci	TMP/SMX 1 DS Q12H and Metronidazole 500 mg po Q6H	Cefoxitin 2 g Q4–6H or Gentamicin 1–1.6 mg/kg Q8H and Clindamycin 600 mg Q6H	
	Giardiasis	Giardia lamblia	Quinacrine 100 mg po tid × 5d Children under 9 yrs Furazolidone	Metronidazole 250 mg tid	
	Peritonitis, nephrotic or cirrhotic	Pneumococci Group A streptococci Enterobacteriaceae Staphylococcus aureus	Clindamycin 600 mg Q6H and Gentamicin 1–1.6 mg/kg Q8H and Ampicillin 2 g Q4–6H	Cefoxitin 2 g Q4–6H or Cefotetan 2 g Q8–12H and Gentamicin 1–1.6 mg/kg Q8H	Ampicillin/sulbactam 3 g Q6H or Ticarcillin/clavulanate 3.1 g Q4– 6H and Gentamicin 1–1.6 mg/kg Q8H or Imipenem/cilastatin 500 mg Q6H
	Bowel perforation	Enterobactericeae Enterococci Bacteroides	Same as previous		

TABLE 50-36. CONTINUED

Site	Clinical Diagnosis		Selected Empiric Therapy	Alternative	Second Alternate/ Comments
	CAPD catheter	Candida (~ 2%) Staphylococcus epidermides S. aureus Streptococcus Enterobacteriacea	Tobramycin 8 mg/1 + vancomycin 25 mg/1 in dialysate		
	Typhoid fever	Salmonella typhi S. paratyphi	Chloramphenicol 500 mg Q6H	TMP/SMX 1 DS Q12H	Ciprofloxacin 500 mg Q12H or Ceftriaxone 2 mg Q24H
Anus/ rectum	Anorectal abscess	Enterobacteriaceae Bacteriodes Enterococci	Cefoxitin 2 g Q4–6H or Cefotetan 2 g Q8–12H or Ampicillin/sulbactam 3 g Q6H or Ticarcillin/clavulanale 3.1 g Q4–6H	Clindamycin 600 mg Q6H and Gentamicin 1–1.6 mg/kg Q8H and Ampicillin 2 g Q4–6H	
Bone	Osteomyelitis, newborn	S. aureus Enterobacterioceae Group A, B streptococci	Gentamicin and nafcillin (see Pediatric dosage)	Nafcillin and cefotaxime	
	Children under 3 yrs	Hemophilus Influenzae Streptococcus	Cefuroxime or Ceftriaxone or Cefotaxime (see Pediatric dosage)	Cloxacillin 125 mg/kg/day Q6H Dicloxacillin 100 mg/kg/day Q6H	
	Children under 3 yrs	S. aureus	Appropriate pediatric dose or in Adults: Nafcillin (1–2 g) Q4–6H	Vancomycin 1 g Q12H	
Breast	Mastitis, postpartum	S. aureus	Nafcillin IV 1–2 g Q4–6H or Cloxacillin po 250 mg Q6H or Dicloxacillin po 250 mg Q6H	Vancomycin IV 1 g Q12H	
	Nonpuerperal	S. aureus Bacteriodes Peptococcus	Clindamycin IV 600 mg Q6H or Nafcillin IV 1–2 g Q4–6H and Metronidazole IV 7.5 mg/kg Q6H	Cefazolin 1 g Q8H or Vancomycin IV 1 g Q12H and Metronidazole IV 7.5 mg/kg Q6H	
Central nervous system	Brain abscess Complications of otitis media, mastoiditis, lung abscess, congenital heart disease	Streptococcus viridans anaerobic strep bacteriodes Enterobacteriaceae	Penicillin G IV 4 million units Q4H and Cefotaxime 2 g Q4H or Ceftriaxone 2 g Q12H and Metronidazole 7.5 mg/kg Q6H If Staph, Nafcillin 2 gm Q4H or Vancomycin 1 g Q12H	Penicillin G IV 4 mu Q4H and Chloramphenicol 500 mg–1 g Q6H	
Ear	External otitis, swimmer's ear	Pseudomonas Enterobacteriaceae Proteus species Fungus (rare)	Polymyxin B + Neomycin and Hydrocortisone drops 1–2 drops Q6H		
	Acute malignant otitis externa	Pseudomonas species	Piperacillin 3 g Q4H and Tobramycin 1–1.6 mg/kg Q8H or Ceftazidime 2 g Q8H and Tobramycin 1–1.6 mg/kg Q8H	Ciprofloxacin 750 mg Q12H	May be life-threatening
	Furuncle with cellulitis	S. aureus	Cloxacillin 250 mg Q6H or Dicloxacillin 250 mg Q6H	Cephalexin 250 mg Q6H or Clindamycin po 150 Q6H or Amoxicillin/clavulanate 250 mgQ8H	I&D

TABLE 50-36. CONTINUED

Site	Clinical Diagnosis		Selected Empiric Therapy	Alternative	Second Alternate/ Comments
	Acute otitis media, children under 4 yrs	Pneumococci H. influenzae B. catarrhalis S. aureus Group A streptococci Idiopathic	Amoxicillin or Erythromycin/sulfamethox-izole or TMP/SMX (see Pediatric Dosage)	Cefaclor or Amoxicillin/clavulanate	
	Children over 4 yrs (4–14 yrs)	Same as previous	Amoxicillin 500 mg Q8H Amoxicillin/clavulanate 250–500 mg Q8H Cefuroxime 250–500 mg Q12H or Cefaclor 250–500 mg Q8H	Erythromycin 500 mg Q6H	
	Mastoiditis, acute	Pneumococci H. influenzae B. Catarrhalis	Cefuroxime 500 mg Q12H or Cefaclor 500 mg Q8H or Amoxicillin/clavulanate 500 mg Q8H or Ceftriaxone 1 g IV Q24H	TMP/SMX 1 DS Q12H	
Eye	Blepharitis	S. aureus	Erythromycin ointment or Chloramphenizol Oint-ment to lid margins qid		
	Orbital cellulitis, adults	S. aureus Enterobacteriaceae	Naficillin 1–2 g Q4–6H and Tobramycin 1–1.6 mg/kg Q8H	Cefoxitin 2 g Q4–6H and Vancomycin 1 g Q12H or Ticarcillin/clavulanate 3.1 g Q4–6H	
	Children	H. Influenzae	Cefuroxime and Nafcillin (see Pediatric Dosage)	TMP/SMX or Ceftriaxone	
	Conjunctivitis a. Acute hemor-rhagic	Enterovirus Coxsackie Adenovirus H. influenzae Pneumococci Group A streptococci	None Neomycin and Polymxin B drops qid	Sulfacetamide 10% drops qid	
	b. Inclusion	Chlamydia trachoma-tis	Tetracycline 250 mg Q6H × 21d (minimum) and Topical tetracycline Q6H	Erythromycin 250 mg Q6H × 21d and Topical erythromycin Q6H	
	c. Trachoma	Chlamydia trachoma-tis	Topical erythromycin Q6H × 21d (minimum)	Topical tetracycline Q6H	
	Dacrocystitis	Pneumococci Streptococci S. aureus Pseudomonas	Penicillin G 3 mu Q6H or Nafcillin 1 g Q6H or Tobramycin 1–1.6 mg/kg Q8H		
	Stye with cellulitis	S. aureus	Cloxacillin 250 mg Q6H or Dicloxacillin 250 mg Q6H	Cephalexin 250 mg Q6H or Clindamycin po 150 Q6H or Amoxicillin/clavulanate 250 mg Q8H	
Foot	Diabetic foot cellulitis	Multiple	Ampicillin/sulbactam 3 g Q6H or Ticarcillin/clavulanate 3.1 g Q4–6H or Imipenem 500 mg Q6H	Clindamycin 600 mg Q6H and Aztreonam 2 g Q8H or Ciprofloxacin 750 mg Q12H and Metronidazole 500 mg Q6H	
Genital tract	Septic abortion	Bacteriodes Group B streptococci Enterobacteriaceae	Cefoxitin 2 g Q4–6H or Piperacillin 3 g Q4–6H or Ticarcillin/Clavulanate 3.1 g Q4–6H	Clindamycin 600 mg Q6H and Gentamicin 1–1.6 mg/kg Q6H	

TABLE 50-36. CONTINUED

Site	Clinical Diagnosis	Selected Empiric Therapy	Alternative	Second Alternate/ Comments
	Endomyometritis postpartum (2d–6 wk)	Same as for septic abortion		
	Endomyometritis (late)	Chlamydia trachomatis	Tetracycline 500 mg Q6H × 10d or Doxycycline 100 mg Q12H × 10d	Erythromycin 500 mg Q6H × 10d	
	Epididymo-orchitis < 35	Gonococcus Chlamydia trachomatis	Tx gonorrhea/nongonococcal Urethritis		
	Orchitis > 35	Enterobacteriaceae	TMP/SMX 1 DS Q12H	Ampicillin 500 mg Q6H or Tetracycline 500 mg Q6H	
	Cervicitis		Tx for gonorrhea or nongonoccal urethritis		
	Gonorrhea	Gonococcus	Ceftriaxone IM × 1 250 mg and Doxycycline 100 mg po Q12H × 7d	Newer quinolones or Spectinomycin 2 g IM × 1 and Doxycycline 100 mg po Q12H × 7d or Ampicillin 3.5 g po and Probenicid 1 g po × 1	Erythromycin 500 mg Q6H × 7d when Tetracycline contraindicated
	Postgonococcal or nongonococcal urethritis	Chlamydia Ureaplasma	Doxycycline 100 mg Q12H × 7d	Erythromycin 500 mg Q6H × 7d or Ciprofloxacin 750 mg Q12H × 7d	
	Acute prostatitis	Enterobacteriaceae	TMP/SMX 1 DS Q12H × 14d	Ampicillin 500 mg Q6H × 14d or Doxycycline 100 mg Q12H × 14d or Ciprofloxacin 500 mg Q12H × 14d	
	Chronic prostatitis	Pseudomonas	Ciprofloxacin 750 mg Q12H × 90d or TMP/SMX 1 DS Q12H × 90d		
	Salpingitis, outpatient	Gonococcus Chlamydia Bacteroides Enterobacteriaceae	Ceftriaxone 250 mg IM × 1 and Doxycycline 100 mg Q12H × 14d	Cefoxitin 2 g IM × 1 and Doxycycline 100 mg Q12H × 14d	Erythromycin 500 mg Q6H × 14d if doxycycline contraindicated
	Salpingitis, inpatient	Gonococcus Chlamydia Bacteroides Enterobacteriaceae	Cefoxitin 2 g Q6H and Doxycycline 100 mg IV Q12H	Gentamicin 1–1.6 mg/kg Q8H and Clindamycin 600 mg Q6H	At least 4 days or (without fever) 48 hours, then change to oral therapy to complete 14 days
	Syphilis, primary (< 1 year)	Treponema pallidum	Benzathine PCN G 2.5 mill. units IM × 1	Tetracycline 500 mg Q6H × 15d or Erythromycin 500 mg Q6H × 15d	
	> 1 year		Benzathine PCN G 2.4 mu Q week × 3	Tetracycline 500 mg Q6H × 30d or Erythromycin 500 mg Q6H × 30d	
	Neurosyphilis	Treponema pallidum	Penicillin G 2 mill. units IV Q4H × 10d and Benzathine PCN G 214 Mill. units IM Q week × 3 after the 10d IV therapy	Chloramphenicol 500 mgQ6H 15–30d	
	Chancroid	H. ducreyi	Ceftriaxone 250 mg IM × 1 or Erythromycin 500 mg Q6H × 7d	TMP/SMX 1 DS Q12H × 7d or Ciprofloxacin 500 mg Q12H × 7d	
	Lymphogranuloma venereum	Chlamydia trachomatis	Doxycycline 100 mg Q12H × 21d	Erythromycin 500 mg Q6H × 21d	

TABLE 50-36. CONTINUED

Site	Clinical Diagnosis		Selected Empiric Therapy	Alternative	Second Alternate/ Comments
	Granuloma inguinale	Calymmatobacterium granulomatis (Donovan bodies)	Tetracycline 500 mg Q6H or Chloramphenicol 500 mg Q8H po and Gentamicin 1 mg/kg Q12H	TMP/SMX 1 DS Q12H	
	Vaginitis	Candida	Miconazole topical × 7d or Clotrimazole topical × 7d	Nystatin 100,000 units bid × 14d	
		Trichomonas vaginalis	Metronidazole 2 mg po × 1		
	Malodorous	Gardnerella vaginalis Bacteroides nonfragilis Peptococci	Metronidazole 500 mg Q12H × 7d	Ampicillin 500 mg Q6H × 7d	
Joints	Septic arthritis, < 3 months	H. influenza Pneumococci	Nafcillin and Gentamicin (see Pediatric Dosage)	Clindamycin and Gentamicin	
	3 months–2 yrs	S. aureus Group A streptococci H. influenzae	Nafcillin and Cefuroxime (see Pediatric Dosage)	Vancomycin and Cefuroxime	
	Children under 2 yrs	Same as previous	Same as above		
	Adults	Gonococci S. aureus Group A streptococci Enterobacteriaceae	Nafcillin 1–2 g Q4–6H and Tobramycin 1–1.6 mg/kg Q8H	Vancomycin 1 g Q12H and Tobramycin 1–1.6 mg/kg Q8H	Imipenem 500 mg Q6H (Not in penicillin-allergic patients)
Mouth	Vincent's angina	Fusospirochetae species	Penicillin VK 500 mg Q6H	Erythromycin 500 mg Q6H or Tetracycline 500 mg Q6H	
	Orofacial infection, odontogenic origin	Oral microflora	Penicillin VK 500 mg Q6H	Erythromycin 500 mg Q6H or Clindamycin 150 mg Q6H or Amoxicillin/clavulanate 250 mg Q8H	
	Buccal cellulitis, children under 4 yrs	H. influenzae	Cefuroxime (see Pediatric Dosage)	Amoxicillin/clavulanate or Ceftriaxone	
Muscle	Gas gangrene, contaminated wound	Clostridium perfringens and other species	Penicillin G IV 4 mill. units Q4H	Gentamicin 1–1.6 mg/kg Q8H and Clindamycin 600 mg Q6H or Cefoxitin 2 mg Q4H and Gentamicin 1–1.6 mg/kg Q8H or Chloramphenicol 1 g Q6H and Gentamicin 1–1.6 mg/kg Q8H	
Skin	Acne, inflammatory Boils, to prevent recurrence	S. aureus	Tetracycline 250 mg Qd Mupirocin intranasally × 5 d	Erythromycin 250 mg Qd Rifampin 600 mg Qd × 14d and Cloxacillin 250 mg × 14d or Dicloxacillin 250 mg × 14d	
	Burns, infected	S. aureus Enterobacteriaceae Pseudomonas species Serratia species Providencia specie	Piperacillin 4 g Q4H and Tobramycin 1–1.6 mg/kg Q8H and Silver sulfadiazine, topical	Imipenem 1 g Q6H and Tobramycin 1–1.6 mg/kg Q8H and Silver sulfadiazine, topical	May need larger doses of aminoglycosides Ceftazidime 2 g Q6–8H (for penicillin allegic patient) and Tobramycin 1–1.6 mg/kg Q8H
	Cellulitis extremities (not with catheter)	Group A streptococci	Penicillin VK 500 mg Q6H × 7d or Penicillin G 1 mill. unit IV Q4H	Erythromycin 500 mg × 7d	
	Facial, adults	Group A streptococci S. aureus	Nafcillin 1 g Q4–6H or Cloxacillin 500 mg Q6H or Dicloxacillin 500 mg Q6H	Cephalexin 500 mg Q6H or Cefazolin 1 g Q8H or Vancomycin 1 g Q12H	
	Facial, children	H. influenzae	Cefuroxime IV (see Pediatric Dosage)	Amoxicillin/clavulanate p.o.	

TABLE 50-36. CONTINUED

Site	Clinical Diagnosis	Selected Empiric Therapy	Alternative	Second Alternate/ Comments
	Bullous lesions associated with raw fish	Vibrio vulnificus	Tetracycline 500 mg po Q6H and Tobramycin 1–1.6 mg/kg Q8H	Chloramphenicol 500 mg Q6H	Ciprofloxacin 500 mg Q12H or Ceftriaxone 1 g Q24H
	Diabetes	Group A streptococci S. aureus Occ. enterobacteriaceae	Nafcillin 1–2 g Q4–6H and Tobramycin 1–1.6 mg/kg Q8H or Nafcillin 1–2 g Q4–6H and Aztreonam 2 g Q8H	Cefazolin 1 g Q8H and Tobramycin 1–1.6 mg/kg Q8H or Ampicillin/sulbactam 3 mg Q6H or Ticarcillin/clavulanate 3.1 mg Q4–6H or Imipenem/cilastatin 500 mg Q6H	
	Decubitus ulcer with sepsis	S. aureus Group A streptococci Enterobacteriaceae Pseudomonas species	Clindamycin 600 mg Q6H and Tobramycin 1–1.6 mg/kg Q8H or Ticarcillin/clavulanate 3.1 g Q4–6H	Cefoxitin 2 mg Q4–6H and Tobramycin 1–1.6 mg/kg Q8H	
	Erythrasma	Corynebacterium minutissimum	Erythromycin 500 mg Q6H		
	Furunculosis with cellulitis and/or sepsis	S. aureus	Nafcillin 1–2 g Q4–6H or Cloxacillin 250 mg Q6H or Dicloxacillin 250 mg Q6H	Cefazolin 1 g Q8H or Cephalexin 500 mg Q6H or Vancomycin 1 g IV Q12H	
	Impetigo, nonbullous	Group A streptococci S. aureus	Penicillin VK 500 mg Q6H	Erythromycin 500 mg Q6H	
	Bullous	S. aureus	Cloxacillin 500 mg Q6H or Dicloxacillin 500 mg Q6H or Erythromycin 500 mg Q6H	Cephalexin 500 mg Q6H or Clindamycin 150 mg Q6H	
	Pediculus species (lice, crabs, mites)	Phthirus pubis	Pyrethrine	Lindane or permethrin	
	Scabies (mites)	Sarcoptes scabiei	Lindane		
	Wound traumatic (includes necrotizing fasciitis)	Without sepsis: S. aureus Group A streptococci Enterobacteriaceae Clostridium perfringens C. tetani	Cloxicillin 500 mg Q6H or Dicloxicillin 250 mg Q6H	Erythromycin po 500 mg Q6H or Clindamycin po 300 mg Q6H	
		With sepsis: C. tetani	Tobramycin 1.5 mg/kg Q8H + Cefoxitin 2 g Q4H or Tobramycin 1.5 mg/kg + Clindamycin 600 mg Q6H or Ampicillin/sulbactam 3.0 g Q6H + Tobramycin 1.5 mg/kg Q8H	Vancomycin 1 g Q12H + Tobramycin 1.5 mg/kg/Q8H	

* Based on clinical indication.

This group of penicillins is less active against penicillin-susceptible anaerobes than older penicillins.

BROAD-SPECTRUM PENICILLINS

This group, possessing variable activity against gram-negative bacilli, is divided into second-, third-, and fourth-generation penicillins.

SECOND-GENERATION PENICILLINS (Ampicillin, Amoxicillin, etc.)

These penicillins are more active than ordinary penicillin against enterococcus, Listeria monocytogenes, Hemophilus influenzae, some strains of Escherichia coli and Proteus, Salmonella, and Shigella.

Ampicillin/sulbactam (Unasyn) is a combination of ampicillin with a β-lactamase inhibitor (sulbactam) similar to the combination of amoxicillin/clavulanate. Ampicillin/sulbactam is effective as parenteral therapy for intra-abdominal, gynecologic, and other infections caused by susceptible organisms. Sulbactam inactivates many bacterial β-lactamases, thereby extending the activity of ampicillin. The combination is active against β-lactamase-producing strains of Hemophilus influenzae, B. catarrhalis, Neisseria, many anaerobes (including B. fragilis), Escherichia coli, Proteus, Klebsiella, Enterobacter aerogenes, Acinetobacter calcoaceticus, Staphylococcus aureus, and S. epidermidis.

Ampicillin/sulbactam is not active against Pseudomonas aeruginosa, E. cloacae, Serratia sp., and some Enterobacteriaceae. (Ticarcillin/clavulanate is more active against P. aeruginosa.)

THIRD-GENERATION PENICILLINS CARBENICILLIN AND TICARCILLIN

Both agents have increased activity against gram-negative bacteria. Ticarcillin has a lower sodium load, is less likely to cause hypokalemia alkalosis, has improved activity against Pseudomonas aeruginosa lung infections, and possibly has fewer bleeding diatheses. It is replacing carbenicillin in many institutions, and is seldom used as a single agent because of concern that resistance will develop rapidly. It is frequently used in combination with gentamicin or another aminoglycoside to provide synergism against gram-negative organisms, particularly pseudomonas. Ticarcillin is a second-line drug against Bacteroides fragilis. The combination of ticarcillin and clavulanic acid (Timentin) is active against β-lactamase-producing strains of Staphylococcus aureus, E. coli, Klebsiella species, Proteus, Hemophilus influenzae, Shigella, and some strains of Pseudomonas aeruginosa.

FOURTH-GENERATION PENICILLINS (AZLOCILLIN, MEZLOCILLIN, AND PIPERACILLIN)

These drugs have spectrums of activity similar to those of the third-generation penicillins, and the differences are probably not clinically important.

CEPHALOSPORINS

The β-lactam antibiotics (penicillins and cephalosporins) interfere with cell wall synthesis by acting on penicillin-sensitive enzymes. Bacterial resistance to β-lactam antibiotics other than production of β-lactamases (penicillinases, cephalosporinases) are under study.

As bactericidal agents, they are relatively resistant to the β-lactamases produced by Staphylococcus aureus. The first generation agents remain the most active against S. aureus. As a group, they are not active against the enterococci or Pseudomonas species, except for some third-generation agents. They have fewer allergic reactions than the penicillins and because of their high therapeutic-toxic ratio, they may be preferable to aminoglycosides when a choice is allowed. The newer β-lactam antibiotics (e.g., aztreonam and imipenem/cilastatin) and the quinolones have potential competing roles with the cephalosporins.

FIRST-GENERATION CEPHALOSPORINS

Parenteral drugs include cephalothin (Keflin), cefazolin (Ancef, Kefzol), cephapirin (Cefadyl), cephradine (Velosef); oral drugs include cephalexin (Keflex), cephradine (Velosef, Anspor), and cefadroxil (Duricef). These agents are active against gram-positive bacteria including penicillin-susceptible and penicillin-resistant Staphylococcus aureus, and streptococci. They are not active against enterococci. Some strains of Escherichia coli, as well as Klebsiella and Enterobacter species, are susceptible. Many Proteus and Enterobacter species, as well as Bacteroides fragilis, are resistant. Hemophilus influenzae is moderately susceptible at present; cefazolin is most frequently used in institutions.

SECOND-GENERATION CEPHALOSPORINS

Parenteral drugs include cefamandole (Mandol), cefoxitin (Mefoxin), cefuroxime (Zinacef), ceforanide (Precef), cefonicid (Monocid), and cefotentan (Cefotan); oral drugs include cefaclor (Ceclor) and cefuroxime axetil (Ceftin).

As an example of one of the more frequently used agents, cefuroxime is active against streptococci, but not as active against methicillin-susceptible S. aureus as the first-generation cephalosporins; still, it has good activity. Methicillin-resistant S. aureus, enterococci, and L. monocytogenes are resistant to this agent. Cefuroxime, however, is excellent for H. influenzae, Neisseria meningitidis, N. gonorrhae, and Pasteurella multocida.

The third-generation cephalosporins are more active against a wide range of gram-negative bacilli.

THIRD-GENERATION CEPHALOSPORINS

Parenteral agents include cefotaxime (Claforan), moxalactam (Moxam), cefoperazone (Cefobid), ceftizoxime (Cefizox), ceftriaxone (Rocephin), ceftazidime (Fortaz, Tazidime, or Tazicef). Investigational agents include cefsulodin and cefmenoxime.

Cefotaxime combined with ampicillin is a combination of choice as initial therapy for neonatal and infant meningitis. Ceftriaxone, considered a major milestone in antimicrobial milestone therapy, has the longest half-life of the currently available third-generation cephalosporins, making once or twice daily dosing possible. It is active against S. pneumoniae and groups A and B streptococci. Moderately useful against methicillin-susceptible S. aureus, it is not active against enterococci, L. monocytogenes, or co-agulase-negative or methicillin-resistant staphylococci, and does poorly against P. aeruginosa. Ceftriaxone is very active against H. influenzae and N. gonorrheae (including β-lactamase producers), N. meningitidis, and most Enterobacteriaceae (E. coli, Klebsiella, Serratia and Proteus species, etc.) When it is combined with an aminoglycoside, synergy is often demonstrated.

Cefoxitin or cefotetan is more active against anaerobes (e.g., Bacteroides fragilis) than ceftriaxone. The latter, however, is an important adjunct in meningitis, Lyme disease, and uncomplicated gonorrhea.

Third-generation cephalosporins are *not* indicated for single-agent therapy in suspected Pseudomonas aeruginosa infections. For enhanced P. aeruginosa activity in the patient in whom ticarcillin or piperacillin cannot be used because of a penicillin allergy, ceftazidime can be combined with an aminoglycoside for synergy.

AMINOGLYCOSIDES

These bactericidal agents include streptomycin, kanamycin, and more recently the popular four: gentamicin, tobramycin, netilmicin, and amikacin (a semisynthetic kanamycin). Many studies prefer ampicillin or a cephalosporin if susceptibility studies allow because aminoglycosides have more toxic side effects. Also, they provide poor oral absorption and penetrate the blood-brain barrier poorly.

Aminoglycosides are particularly useful in nosocomial infections because of the likelihood of resistant strains.

They have some activity against gram-positive aerobes, primarily Staphylococcus aureus, but even here they are not recommended as single agents. They are most often combined with a penicillin for synergy against enterococci and streptococci. They are not effective against pneumococci, but are particularly active against the gram-negative aerobes: Escherichia coli, Klebsiella, Proteus, Pseudomonas, Acinetobacter, and Providencia. Anaerobes or nonenterococcal streptococci are not affected by aminoglycosides.

Gentamicin, tobramycin, netilmicin, and amikacin have almost equal bactericidal levels. Nonetheless, when choosing an agent against a specific organism such as Pseudomonas aeruginosa, tobramycin has a 2 to 4 times greater bactericidal ratio than the ratios of gentamicin and amikacin. Gentamicin is preferred for Serratia, and with a penicillin has the greatest activity against enterococci. If one is treating a resistant organism, amikacin is the drug of choice. Streptomycin is the drug of choice for tularemia and brucellosis (with tetracycline).

CLINDAMYCIN

This antibiotic class can be used in penicillin-allergic patients and is the drug of choice for Bacteroides fragilis. Although effective against Staphylococcus aureus and group A streptococci, it is not useful against enterococci and gram-negative aerobes. Clindamycin is active against gram-positive and gram-negative anaerobes, including Clostridium perfringens. Diarrhea or inflammatory bowel disease is a relative contraindication to the use of this agent because of the potential complication of pseudomembranous colitis.

CHLORAMPHENICOL

This agent should be avoided when possible because of its rare but irreversible side effect of fatal aplastic anemia. It is a broad-spectrum antibiotic active against many gram-positive and gram-negative organisms, rickettsiae, Chlamydia, and mycoplasmas. Its potential use includes life-threatening Hemophilus influenzae infections or severe anaerobic infections.

SULFONAMIDES AND TRIMETHOPRIM-SULFAMETHOXAZOLE

When oral preparations are used in routine doses, bacteriostatic blood levels are usually achieved. These agents are still useful in uncomplicated urinary tract infections, against Nocardia asteroides, rheumatic fever prophylaxis, and an alternate for Chlamydia pneumonia.

Trimethoprim-sulfamethoxazole (TMP-SMZ) is a unique combination that sequentially blocks two steps in the synthesis of folic acid by bacteria. This agent is active against most staphylococci and streptococci, but not usually against enterococci. Salmonella, Shigella, H. influenzae, and Pneumocystis carinii are susceptible. It is not useful against gonococci, Pseudomonas, or anaerobes. Because of the risk of kernicterus, it is not recommended for infants under 2 months; because of its teratogenetic potential, it is contraindicated in pregnant or lactating women.

ERYTHROMYCIN

A macrolide, this bacteriostatic agent is thought to be one of the safest antibiotics today. It has a broad-spectrum and is active against gram-positive and gram-negative bacteria, mycoplasmas, chlamydiae, treponemas, and rickettsiae.

Erythromycin is the drug of choice for mycoplasma pneumonia, Legionella pneumophila, Chlamydia trachomatis pneumonia, Bordetella pertussis, Campylobacter, and Corynebacterium species. This agent is also an alternate for penicillin-allergic patients. The esolate base of erythromycin is no longer recommended by the authors because of its potential for hepatitis and because of other available, effective bases, including the erythromycin base, the stearate salt, and the ethylsuccinate esters. Parenteral forms are available for more serious infections.

TETRACYCLINES

These bacteriostatic agents (tetracycline hydrochloride, oxytetracycline, methacycline, doxycycline hydrate, and minocycline) act against many gram-positive and gram-negative bacteria, rickettsiae mycoplasmas, chlamydiae, spirochetes, and Actinomyces species. They are not the drugs of choice for staphylococci, streptococci, some pneumococci, and Bacteroides species. Many Enterobacteriaceae and pseudomonas species are resistant. Urinary concentrations are adequate for most community-acquired Escherichia coli, so that tetracycline can still be used for urinary tract infections.

Although IV preparations are available, the oral route is the usual mode of administration. Tetracyclines should be avoided or used with caution in patients with liver dysfunction. Doxycycline is considered the tetracycline of choice for extrarenal infections when the patient has underlying renal failure.

Tetracycline is the drug of choice for nonspecific

urethritis; other uses include brucellosis, bronchitis, pelvic inflammatory disease, traveler's diarrhea, acne, prostatitis, and as an alternate agent in the penicillin-allergic patient with syphilis or gonorrhea.

VANCOMYCIN

A bactericidal agent, vancomycin is structurally unrelated to other antibiotics and is therefore particularly useful in the penicillin- or cephalosporin-allergic patient. This agent is active against gram-positive aerobes, especially methicillin-resistant staphylococci. In an endocarditis regimen, vancomycin is joined with an aminoglycoside like gentamycin because vancomycin is bacteriostatic only against some enterococci.

Because high stool concentrations are achieved by oral administration, this agent is useful in antibiotic-induced colitis and staphylococcal enterocolitis.

Treatment failures in some meningitis cases are known.

METRONIDAZOLE

This agent is effective against Trichomonas vaginalis, Giardia lamblia, Gardnerella vaginalis, Entamoeba histolytica, and anaerobic bacteria inlcuding Bacteroides species, Clostridium, Peptococcus, and Peptostreptococcus species. Less active against anaerobic gram-positive cocci, it is not at all active against common aerobes.

Oral and intravenous preparations provide excellent serum levels. Metronidazole has a carcinogenic potential.

QUINOLONES

This newer group of bactericidal broad spectrum antibiotics includes norfloxacin, ciprofloxacin, pefloxacin, enoxacin, ofloxacin, and amifloxacin. They are active against gram-positive cocci (staphylococci, streptococci (Group B), Streptococcus pneumoniae, and enterococci); gram-negative susceptible organisms include Neisseria species, Hemophilus influenzae, Escherichia coli, Klebsiella, Enterobacter, Salmonella, Shigella, Campylobacter, Serratia, Acinetobacter, and Pseudomonas species. Other agents are preferred for anaerobes.

Ciprofloxacin, a frequently used quinolone, is well

absorbed and in the elderly, the dosing should not be more frequent than every 12 hours. This drug is most useful in urinary tract infections, sexually transmitted diseases, recurrent bacterial bronchitis, traveler's diarrhea, skin and soft tissue infections, and especially decubitus ulcers.

Because the quinolones have only limited activity against group A streptococci, these agents are not useful in pharyngitis. Nor are they the drugs of choice in otitis media or sinusitis. Other agents are preferred for community-acquired penumonia commonly caused by Streptococcus pneumoniae.

Additional study is needed to elucidate the precise role of the quinolones in respiratory infections as compared to other classes of antibiotics.

SPECTINOMYCIN

Spectinomycin is a bacteriostatic agent similar to the aminoglycosides but not identical. It is used primarily as an alternate for uncomplicated anogenital gonococcal infections. Ceftriaxone is now the drug of choice. Spectinomycin may even prolong the incubation period of syphilis.

RIFAMPIN

Rifampin is a broad-spectrum agent, active against bacteria, mycobacteria, and chlamydia.

Rifampin is officially approved only for use in the treatment of Mycobacterium tuberculosis infections and nasopharyngeal carriers of Neisseria meningitidis. Its use in the treatment of other infections is under active investigation.

CUTANEOUS ABSCESSES AND GAS GANGRENE

Patrick Connell and John I. Ellis

CAPSULE

Subcutaneous abscesses and other infections of skin and soft tissue are commonly seen and treated in emergency and acute care departments. Although most cases are fairly straightforward, these infections can cause a spectrum of disease ranging from the near-trivial to life and limb threatening. In addition, the complications arising from pre-existing disease, or improper or inadequate treatment may cause disfigurement or death. It is imperative that the emergency physician be familiar with both the outpatient treatment of simple abscesses and soft tissue infections, and with the indications for consultation, admission, and emergency surgical treatment.

INTRODUCTION

An abscess is "a localized collection of pus caused by suppuration buried in a tissue, organ, or confined space."[1] In its early stage, it appears as an area of tender inflammation, which later becomes fluctuant as a liquid or semiliquid exudate of leukocytes, necrotic material, and cellular debris accumulates in the closed space. A surrounding area of hyperemia and inflammation is present as the "abscess wall"; this can become fibrotic and tough in longstanding abscesses. Abscesses may be caused by bacterial seeding, by foreign bodies, or rarely by viral (the "herpetic whitlow") or autoimmune mechanisms.[1-3]

CAUSES AND TYPES OF ABSCESSES

The most common cause of abscess formation in the normal host is the plugging of the ducts of one of the superficial exocrine glands, such as the apocrine and sebaceous glands, especially those associated with hair follicles.[4] Any other gland, such as Bartholins' glands, the mucus glands in the rectum, or breast duct tissue may also become involved. When plugging of the duct occurs, the impacted secretions of the gland become infected, often with one of the organisms in the flora of the anatomic area of the gland.[4]

Perirectal abscesses are formed by inspissation of the perirectal mucous glands. They often extend much deeper and farther than readily apparent on physical examination. The periurethral abscess, which points into the perineum or scrotum, is often a sequela of urethritis. If not adequately treated, these lead to numerous complications such as urethral stricture and chronic urinary fistulae.

Additionally, congenital cysts and sinuses may become plugged and infected, leading to abscess formation. Commonly involved are branchial cleft cysts on the head and neck and pilonidal cysts or sinuses located near the midline of the superior part of the gluteal cleft.

Abscesses can also result from trauma resulting in a skin break. Foreign bodies are associated with slowly healing or recurrent abscesses. Both of these factors are often found in parenteral drug users.

Although unusual exceptions exist, abscesses are usually caused by bacterial infection. The primary determinant of the organism or organisms isolated from an abscess is the body area on which the abscess is found.[2,4-6] Meislin et al. reviewed 135 cutaneous abscesses in all age and gender groups; the results of this study are summarized in Tables 50-37 and 50-38. Contrary to popular assumption, Staphylococcus aureus is not universally present in dermal abscesses; isolation rates for S. aureus vary between 45 and 60%.[3,4,7,8.] Anaerobes are found in all body areas, with increased incidence in the perineum. The organisms in perineal abscesses parallel the flora of the lower GI tract. Neisseria gonorrheae is also commonly isolated from abscesses in the perineum, especially from Bartholin's cyst abscesses and periurethral abscesses. Four percent of all abscesses in this study yielded no growth or were "sterile abscesses."

The pilonidal cyst abscess, in contradistinction to the perirectal abscess, is a true dermal abscess, caused by the plugging of a congenital sinus by hair and debris. The flora of these is usually that of trunk or extremity abscesses.[9,10] The head and neck are affected most often by Staphylococcus species and by aerobic and anerobic mouth flora.

The anatomic location and bacteriology of abscesses among parenteral drug users differs from that of the general population. They occur most often as the result of subcutaneous drug injection ("skin popping") or from missed attempts at IV injection. Drug users' abscesses most commonly occur on the extremities, breasts, and lateral buttocks.[11] Abscesses found in these locations in the absence of other trauma should raise the physician's suspicion of parenteral drug abuse, with its other attendant risks, such as hepatitis and HIV infection. Drug users also often harbor for-

TABLE 50-37. INCIDENCE OF ABSCESS BY ANATOMIC LOCATION

Head and neck	19%
Trunk	8%
Axilla	16%
Extremity	12%
Hand	6%
Inguinal	5%
Vulvovaginal	10%
Buttock	9%
Perirectal	16%

* Adapted with permission from Meislin, H.W., et al.: Cutaneous abscesses: Anaerobic and aerobic bacteriology and outpatient management. Ann. Intern. Med. *87:*145, 1977.

TABLE 50-38. PERCENTAGE OF ORGANISMS CAUSING ABSCESS BY BODY SITE

	Staphylococcus aureus	Staphylococcus Epidermidis	Streptococci	Diphtheroids	Enterobacteriacea
Head and neck	16	24	12	8	24
Trunk	18	18	9	0	36
Axilla	50	9	9	5	40
Extremity	38	6	12	13	19
Hand	25	38	38	0	26
Inguinal	29	0	14	0	14
Vulvovaginal	8	0	29	0	8
Buttock	33	0	25	25	0
Perirectal	0	5	53	10	10

* Adapted with permission from Meislin, H.W., et al.: Cutaneous abscesses: Anaerobic and aerobic bacteriology and outpatient management. Ann. Intern. Med. *87:*145, 1977.

eign bodies, either microscopic adulterants of the drugs or broken needles.

Studies in drug users from different geographic areas report differing prevalences of organisms. In Los Angeles, 63% of abscesses were polymicrobial in origin, including 67% growing anaerobes. Only 19% contained S. aureus. In New York, most commonly isolated were gram negative aerobes and oropharyngeal flora.[11] The most common gram positives were beta hemolytic Streptococcus species. In Ireland, 90% of the abscesses in users were found to contain S. aureus.[12]

Although abscesses occur frequently in normal hosts, patients with diabetes mellitus, other chronic metabolic disorders, hematologic disorders such as sickle cell disease, and those immunosuppressed for any reason are susceptible to much more severe and progressive infection. What begins as a simple abscess may often cause generalized sepsis or involves deeper structures, giving rise to severe cellulitis, necrotizing fasciitis, or myonecrosis. These patients are also predisposed to infection with unusual organisms, such as fungi, Nocardia, parasites, or uncommon bacteria.[13–18] Patients with any of the above risk factors should be seriously considered as candidates for admission for surgical consultation and IV antibiotic therapy.

CLINICAL PRESENTATION

The classic abscess is a tender, fluctuant mass located in the dermal or subdermal tissue, demonstrating the classic inflammatory responses of rubor, tumor, dolor, and calor. Although the abscess itself may be exquisitely tender, the underlying muscle or other tissue should not be. Motion of the affected part should not cause extreme discomfort. In simple abscess, although the mass itself is erythematous, the surrounding area of erythema should be relatively small.

In most instances, the diagnosis of abscess is fairly obvious to the clinician. A few cases, however, warrant special mention. Early presentation may be somewhat confusing if fluctuance is not fully developed. Aspiration, although occasionally falsely negative, may be helpful. Even a drop of pus obtained is indication for incision and drainage.[2] If aspiration is negative, the patient should be seen again in 24 to 48 hours to check for development of more classic signs.

Conversely, some patients, especially those with underlying disease, may present with signs of spreading cellulitis, lymphangitis (red streaks radiating proximally from the lesion), endocarditis, or sepsis. For this reason, complete vital signs and a general physical examination should be done on all patients with abscesses. Obviously, any patient with the above findings should not be treated as an outpatient. Approx-

imately 5% of all patients with abscesses have bacteremia at the time of presentation.[2]

DIFFERENTIAL DIAGNOSIS

Early abscesses may be confused with cellulitis, especially if no fluctuance is found. This is an important differentiation because the primary treatment of abscess is drainage, whereas that of cellulitis is antibiotics, elevation, and immobilization. Again, aspiration can help.

Granulomatous diseases such as lymphogranuloma venereum, scrofula, and others may also mimic abscess. Usually in these cases, however, the inflammatory response is more subdued, indicating a chronic process. If doubt exists, consultation should be obtained before proceeding because aspiration or incision may exacerbate these processes.

Noninfectious masses, such as branchial cleft cysts, sebaceous cysts, and lipomata or other neoplasms should be differentiated by history and their absence of inflammation. Appropriate consultation should be arranged in these cases.

A rare but potentially disastrous misdiagnosis is the femoral or other aneurysm diagnosed as an abscess. Abscesses may lie over or near vital vascular or nervous structures. In all cases, the underlying and nearby anatomy should be kept in mind; any mass that is pulsatile or near vascular or nervous structures should be seen by an appropriate consultant before attempts at aspiration or incision are made.

Soft tissue infections accompanied by either disproportionately severe pain or lack of any pain should alert the examiner to the possibility of deeper infection, such as necrotizing fasciitis or myonecrosis. Both of these entities are true surgical emergencies because they may rapidly progress to limb loss and death.

Necrotizing fasciitis is an aggressive infection of the superficial fascia and subcutaneous tissue. The underlying muscle and superficial integument are usually spared early in the course of the infection. It may be difficult to distinguish from cellulitis because erythema, edema, leukocytosis, and fever are seen in both entities. Most cases are polymicrobial, although group A streptococci are often the predominant organisms.[19] Later in the course, the presentation is similar to that of gas gangrene.

Gas gangrene or clostridial myonecrosis should always be considered in the differential diagnosis of soft tissue infection because of its mortality rate of 80 to 90% in untreated cases.[20] Historically associated with wartime injury, it is seen in civilian practice as well. It is estimated that 900 to 1000 cases occur anually in the U.S.[21] In its classic, Clostridium-caused form, the process is one of rapid necrosis and liquefaction of fascia, muscle, and tendon. Clostridium perfringens,

Clostridia	Bacteroides Fragilis	Other Anaerobes	Average No. Species per Abscess	
			Aerobes	Anaerobes
0	4	88	1	2
0	9	99	1	2
0	5	50	1	1
19	0	37	1	1
0	0	13	2	0
0	0	157†	0	3
8	23	223	1	3
8	17	142	1	3
10	47	262	1	5

† Percentages greater than 100% represent isolation of more than one organism per abscess.

the causative organism in 50 to 98% of causes, liberates a number of exotoxins.[20,21] The primary or alpha toxin, a C-lecithinase, destroys cell walls, leading to necrosis and hemolysis; systemic secondary effects are anemia, hemoglobinuria, jaundice, and renal failure. Even with maximal therapy, the mortality rate from clostridial myonecrosis is 10 to 25%.[20–26]

Although classically associated with trauma, the insult may be as trivial as venipuncture. So-called "spontaneous" cases occur, most commonly in the patient with diabetes mellitus, colon cancer, burns, atherosclerotic vascular disease, or abdominal surgery.[21,22] There are 150 species of the genus Clostridium, all large gram-positive rods. They are ubiquitous soil and environmental saprophytes. As anaerobes, they require low tissue O_2 concentrations to reproduce and to elucidate their exotoxins; this explains the occurrence of gas gangrene only in individuals with some degree of vascular compromise or necrotic tissue.

Gas gangrene presents clinically as a markedly edematous "bronze" to purplish discolored area, often with flaccid bullae containing a watery, brownish, nonpurulent liquid. A foul odor is often prominent. The patient may complain of severe pain out of proportion to the superficial appearance of the infection; conversely, if necrosis of nerve endings has occurred, the patient may complain only of "heaviness" in the affected limb. Fever is usually moderate, but exam reveals tachycardia out of proportion to the temperature elevation. Crepitance or gross gas bubbles may be discovered in the affected part, and should always be sought. White blood cell (WBC) count is often normal or only modestly elevated. Later, in the fulminant stage, apathy or coma may present.

Other organisms may also cause infections that have similar clinical presentations, especially the production of foul gas in the tissues and rapid spread. This "nonclostridial gas gangrene" is usually caused by mixed gram-negative rods and enterococci.[21,27] Nonclostridial gas gangrene occurs almost exclusively in diabetics, and has a much more variable course than classic gas gangrene, resulting in a mortality of approximately 4% when appropriately treated.[27] While

penicillin is the drug of choice in the antibiotic therapy of clostridial gas gangrene, broad spectrum coverage should be obtained in nonclostridial cases. For this reason, it is imperative that aspiration and Gram stain be done in the emergency department (ED) on all suspected cases of gas gangrene.

PREHOSPITAL OR ED STABILIZATION

Although most patients presenting with soft tissue infections are stable, they may run the gamut to frank septic shock. Therefore, as with all patients in the ED, prompt vital signs and attention to the ABC's (airway, breathing, and circulation) must be given. Resuscitation of patients with abnormal vitals or ABC's is covered in depth elsewhere. A careful history concentrating on possible trauma including IV drug abuse, high fevers, and concomitant or antecedent illness, especially diabetes, atherosclerosis, valvular heart disease, or other chronic illness should be taken. A history consistent with Crohn's disease should be sought if a perineal abscess is present. Medications taken and drug allergy history should not be forgotten. Finally, a general physical examination, seeking signs of neurovascular compromise, heart murmurs, and the general condition of the patient is a must. Adequate tetanus immunization should be ensured.

Pretreatment with parenteral antibiotics to minimize the adverse effects of the bacteremia caused by the incision and drainage is advisable if there is any history of rheumatic or other valvular disease, immunocompromise, or sepsis. A first-generation cephalosporin should adequately prophylax the majority of abscess procedures. The decision to pretreat healthy individuals is less clear. Although there is no evidence that antibiotics given before drainage affect healing rates, there is some evidence that, when given one hour prior to the procedure, they do somewhat shorten healing times.[2,3,5,7,28] Contrary to some teaching, inhibitory or bactericidal levels of some antibiotics are achieved in the abscess cavity when given before drainage.[5]

An often overlooked part of the initial treatment and stabilization of the patient with an acute abscess is analgesia. In the otherwise stable patient, an appropriate parenteral narcotic can be helpful, alleviating pain and decreasing the anxiety surrounding the potentially painful procedure in the patient's near future.

PROCEDURES

LABORATORY

In the otherwise healthy individual, routine laboratory studies are not indicated. Unless the history is distinctly unusual, cultures of the abscess are likewise valueless because antibiotic therapy has not been shown to affect the course when given after incision and drainage (I&D).[4,28]

Patients with signs of toxicity or with chronic diseases or immunocompromise are a different matter because of the often devastating sequelae of their soft tissue infections. A complete blood count should be performed to check for leukopenia or toxic granulations. Electrolytes, BUN, creatinine, and glucose are necessary in diabetic patients or those suspected of harboring deep infection. Electrolyte abnormalities, most importantly, markedly increased potassium, may be seen in myonecrosis. Urinalysis should be performed to rule out hemo- or myoglobinuria. A positive chemical test for heme in the absence of cells on microscopic examination confirms this.

Patients with marked edema, erythema, abnormally severe pain, blebs, gas on examination, or toxic appearance should have microbiologic evaluation. Any material obtained from the site of infection should be immediately Gram-stained and examined for typical organisms—the typical large gram-positive rods of Clostridia, the mixed flora of so-called "synergistic" or nonclostridial gangrene, or the gram-positive cocci often seen in the more common abscess and cellulitis. If the patient is admitted for IV antibiotics, this can often give a good starting point for empiric therapy. Material should also be cultured both aerobically and anaerobically.

X RAY

Radiographs of the affected area should be included in the evaluation if there is a history of trauma, drug abuse, or evidence of deep infection. Foreign bodies and fractures are sometimes easily missed in the edema and tenderness caused by the infection. A broken needle encountered while digitally probing a cavity is not only a nasty surprise for the physician, but any retained foreign body may cause delayed healing or recurrence of the infection. While nonspecific and nonsensitive, when deep infection is suspected, gas seen on a radiograph is an ominous sign of gas gangrene.

INDICATIONS FOR ADMISSION OR NOT PROCEEDING WITH I&D

Although I&D of abscesses is a relatively simple and commonly performed procedure, it is advisable to first consider the patients for whom I&D in the ED is not appropriate (Table 50-39).

A deep foreign body, or proximity of infection to vascular or nervous structures necessitates considerable expertise and the controlled circumstances of the operating room to safely treat. Any involvement of the hands when associated with severe edema, passive stretch tenderness or tenderness along the course of a tendon, or involvement of any joint requires hospitalization and possible surgery.

Perirectal and periurethral abscesses are often fraught with problems when I&D in the ED is attempted. These abscesses often extend far deeper than they appear, and are associated with fistulous tracts to numerous areas. It must be emphasized that these should rarely, if ever, be drained in the ED.

The "danger triangle" of the face, the area defined by the corners of the mouth inferiorly and the glabella superiorly, undergoes venous drainage into the cavernous sinus. The infection itself or manipulation of an abscess may lead to cavernous sinus thrombosis. Any significant infection in this area should be dealt with by an otolaryngologist or ophthalmologist. Likewise, incision into the orbits should be left to the ophthalmologist.

Indications for admission include all the above factors. Additionally, any patient with signs of significant systemic toxicity needs IV antibiotic therapy and monitoring. Almost without exception, diabetics and immunosuppressed individuals should be admitted. Infection arising from human bite wounds should

---

TABLE 50-39. CONTRAINDICATIONS TO EMERGENCY DEPARTMENT I&D

- Inability to achieve adequate anaesthesia
- Deep foreign body
- Proximity to important vascular, nervous, or tendinous structures
- Hand or joint involvement
- Perirectal/periurethral
- "Danger triangle" of the face
- Orbits

usually be admitted because of the progressive, destructive nature of these infections. Abscesses associated with significant cellulitis or lymphangitis should be managed in an inpatient setting.

Again, with deeper involvement or gas in the tissues, admission is mandatory. The only hope to improve the dismal prognosis in gas gangrene is with full-scale surgical therapy. This includes IV penicillin G at 12 to 24 million units a day, and rapid surgical debridement of all necrotic tissue. Other procedures such as fasciotomy may be indicated. Penicillin allergic patients may be treated with tetracycline, 2 to 4 gs IV per day, or clindamycin, 600 mg IV q 6 hours.[21]

The role of hyperbaric oxygen therapy is somewhat controversial. Although there has never been a controlled study of its use in human gas gangrene, numerous studies report that the mortality and loss of tissue is significantly decreased.[20–26] This holds true especially when it is administered within 24 hours of presentation.[20] The best results were obtained by administering one hyperbaric treatment of 2.7 atmospheres of 100% oxygen before surgical treatment. Conservative debridement of only clearly necrotic tissue and other procedures such as fasciotomy were then performed. Two further hyperbaric treatments were then given the first day.[25] Unfortunately, although the benefits of early hyperbaric treatment seem clear, one study[23] showed that patients transferred to a hyperbaric facility before adequate surgical and/or antibiotic therapy had a higher mortality, proportional to the distance transported. It seems reasonable to suggest that, if hyperbaric oxygen is immediately available, it should be taken full advantage of; transport if necessary to a hyperbaric facility does not obviate the need, nor should it delay surgical and antibiotic treatment.

PREPARATION AND ANESTHESIA

The keys to successful, safe, and smooth incision and drainage, as in any other procedure, are collection of the proper equipment, good positioning of the patient, and a clear, uncluttered field.

Achieving good anesthesia is sometimes difficult. Incision and drainage are often and needlessly an excruciating procedure. IV analgesia with morphine, meperidine, or fentanyl does much to "dull the edge" of the pain. Small amounts of a benzodiazapine may be used to allay anxiety. Local anesthetic infiltration is often less than effective because the tissue pH in the infected tissue is often too low to allow ready diffusion of the agent into nerves. Although it is usual to have enough anesthesia to allow incision, any further manipulation of the abscess frequently is impossible because of pain. Alternative techniques, when location, size of abscess, and innervation allow, are regional, Bier, or field blocks which, being relatively distant from the infection, allow normal anesthetic pharmacodynamics.

Nitrous oxide/oxygen inhalation is safe and effective analgesia for incision and drainage.[29] At 50/50 concentrations, its onset and duration of action are sufficiently short to preclude the necessity of intensive patient monitoring during its use. Devices are available that deliver a fixed 50/50 ratio of the gases, self-administered by the patient from a demand-valve mask. The patient should begin inhaling the mixture during the preparations for the procedure, and continue throughout. As long as the mask remains handheld by the patient, the likelihood of overdosage and loss of consciousness are slight. Effects dissipate within 5 to 10 minutes of cessation of inhalation.

Again, if adequate anesthesia is impossible to obtain, the abscess should be drained under general anesthesia.

The administration of parenteral antibiotics, if used, should be done approximately 1 hour before the planned procedure.

It is usual practice to prepare the skin with providone-iodine and to drape the patient and the field, although this mainly serves to protect the operator and the room from the abscess contents.

The basic equipment needed for I&D are first, a scalpel. A No. 11 blade is most useful for small, localized abscesses. Larger abscesses are easier to adequately treat using a No. 15 or 10 blade. One or two pairs of Mayo or similar forceps are necessary for probing the cavity and breaking loculations. A pair of scissors is needed for trimming necrotic skin and cutting packing and dressings. Suction is helpful when draining larger abscesses to maintain a clear field and a clean room. One or more liters of normal saline for irrigation should be on the stand. Finally, a generous supply of gauze sponges and packing should be at hand.

INCISION AND DRAINAGE

The treatment of acute abscess is drainage. Without significant cellulitis, the administration of antibiotics after I&D is of no benefit, only adding to the cost of treatment and exposing the patient to the real risks of antibiotic therapy.[2,28,30] Many procedures have been proposed and studied for the drainage of abscess, but all have proven to be either more difficult and of equal effectiveness to standard I&D, or inferior to it.[2,30–32]

After achieving adequate anesthesia, an incision is made, following the superficial skin creases, across the entire area of fluctuance. This is important to achieve adequate drainage. A simple stab wound is inadequate. The most common cause of abscess recurrence is inadequate incision.[2] For large abscesses, an ellipse may be excised from the abscess roof to allow better access to the cavity. If the ellipse follows skin creases, the resulting scar will be identical to that resulting from linear incision.[2] Any necrotic or clearly devascularized skin should be removed. The cavity is then carefully probed, breaking up any encountered loculations. For small and moderate-sized cavities, this is efficiently done with a forceps or clamp by gently probing and spreading the clamp. For larger abscesses, a gauze covered finger does well.

The cavity should then be irrigated with a bulb syringe and saline to flush away all loosened purulent and necrotic material, then be loosely packed with an appropriately sized material. It is neither necessary nor desirable to tightly fill every cubic millimeter of potential space, as overtight packing will interfere with the inflammatory hyperemia necessary for healing. Special packing devices, such as the Word catheter for Bartholin's cyst abscesses, are convenient to use if available. Finally, an absorbent dressing is applied. Some creativity is often required here; a sanitary napkin, for example, is useful for wounds in the perineum.

The patient should be instructed to apply warm compresses to the area to facilitate drainage. Again, antibiotics are not indicated for outpatient therapy. The patient should be seen again in 24 to 48 hours to remove the packing and assess the response to therapy. If a large amount of drainage persists, the cavity may be repacked. Otherwise, the patient may be instructed to begin soaking the area with warm water 3 to 4 times a day to aid with hygiene and promote further drainage and healing. A clean, absorbent dressing should cover the wound at all other times. Healing occurs in 5 to 9 days in most cases.[2,30,32]

PITFALLS

- Always consider the possibility of deeper involvement or more serious infection than appears. Remember the vitals and ABC's! Gas gangrene and fasciitis require aggressive surgical therapy.
- Always inquire about or, if in doubt, investigate the possibility of diabetes mellitus or immunosuppression. These patients need admission for infections considered trivial in others.
- Perirectal and periurethral abscesses are often more severe than immediately apparent, and lead to numerous long-term complications. Often, the only sign of a perirectal abscess is a fever and a dull ache in the rectum. Perirectal abscesses may point anywhere from the anus to the lateral buttocks.
- All infected human bites should be considered for hospitalization.
- Keep the anatomy of the affected body part in mind. Nearby joints, nerves, vessels, and tendons will complicate the course of the disease or the therapy.
- The enlarged, tender, sometimes fluctuant inguinal nodes of lymphogranuloma venereum are often confused with acute subctuaneous abscesses. I&D of LGV lesions can lead to chronic draining sinuses.

MEDICOLEGAL PEARLS

1. Any patient with signs of systemic involvement warrants admission.
2. If there is any question as to the presence of an abscess, aspiration should be done. Even a drop of pus is indication for I&D. Realize that false negatives occur frequently.
3. Essentially all IV drug abusers with a fever should be admitted because the possibility of coexistent endocarditis cannot be ruled out in the ED.
4. When making the incision, follow skin creases for the best cosmetic result.
5. In infected sebaceous cysts, remember to inform the patient that I&D is not the definitive procedure and that removal of the entire cyst will be required once the acute process is resolved.
6. Ensure adequate tetanus prophylaxis.
7. Nearly all patients with abscesses of the hand, perirectal and periurethral abscesses, and human bites should be admitted.
8. The most important factors in avoiding medicolegal complications are to ensure that the patient fully understands the treatment plan and to arrange close, adequate followup.

REFERENCES

1. Robbins, S.L., and Cotran, R.S.: Inflammation and repair. *In* Pathologic Basis of Disease. 2nd Ed. Philadelphia, W.B. Saunders Company, 1979.
2. Burney, R.E.: Incision and drainage procedures: Soft tissue abscesses in the emergency service. Emerg. Med. Clin. North Am. *4*:527, 1986.
3. Halvorson, G.D., Halvorson, J.E., and Iserson, K.V.: Abscess incision and drainage in the emergency department. J. Emerg. Med. *3*:227, 1985.
4. Meislin, H.W., et al.: Cutaneous abscesses: Anaerobic and aerobic bacteriology and outpatient management. Ann. Interr. Med. *87*:145, 1977.
5. Blick, P.W.H., et al.: Antibiotics in the surgical treatment of acute abscesses. Br. Med. J. *281*:111, 1980.
6. Llera, J.L., Levy, R.C., and Staneck, J.L.: Cutaneous abscesses: Natural history and management in an outpatient facility. J. Emerg. Med. *1*:489, 1984.
7. Fine, B.C., Sheckman, P.R., and Bartlett, J.C.: Incision and drainage of soft-tissue abscesses and bacteremia. Ann. Intern. Med. *103*:645, 1985.
8. Brooks, I., and Finegold, S.M.: Aerobic and anaerobic bacteriology of cutaneous abscesses in children., Pediatrics *67*:891, 1981.
9. Raffman, R.A.: A re-evaluation of the pathogenesis of the pilonidal sinus. Ann. Surg. *150*:895, 1959.
10. Hanley, P.H.: Acute pilonidal abscesses. Surg. Gynecol. Obstet. *150*:9, 1980.
11. Orangio, G.R., et al.: Soft tissue infections in parenteral drug abusers. Ann. Surg. *199*:97, 1984.
12. O'Sullivan, M., Beattie, T., and Keane, C.T.: A review of drug addict abscesses. Ir. Med. J. *77*:68, 1984.
13. Kalb, R.E., Kaplan, M.H., and Grossman, M.E.: Cutaneous

nocardiasis: Case reports and review. J. Am. Acad. Derm. *13*:125, 1985.

14. Gleich, S.: Primary subcutaneous abscess due to *Streptococcus pneumoniae*. South. Med. J. *77*:1602, 1984.

15. Tsukamura, M., Hilosaki, K., Nishimura, K., and Hara, S.: Severe progressive abscesses and necrotizing tenosynovitis caused by *Rhodococcus auranticus*. J. Clin. Microbiol., *26*:201, 1988.

16. Boudreau, S., Hines, H.C., and Hood, A.F.: Dermal abscesses with *Staphylococcus aureus*, cytomegalovirus, and acid-fast bacilli in a patient with acquired immunodeficiency syndrome (AIDS)., J. Cutan. Pathol. *15*:53, 1988.

17. Podzamczer, D., Ribera, M., and Gudiol, F.: Skin abscesses caused by *Candida albicans* in heroin abusers (letter). J. Am. Acad. Derm. *16*:386, 1987.

18. Rimsza, M.E., and Berg, R.A.: Cutaneous amebiasis., Pediatrics *71*:595, 1983.

19. Sabacinski, K.A., et al.: Necrotizing fasciitis. J. Foot Surg. *28*:106, 1989.

20. Shupak, A., Halpern, P., Ziser, A., and Melamed, Y.: Hyperbaric oxygen therapy for gas gangrene casualties in the Lebanon War, 1982. Isr. J. Med. Sci. *20*:323, 1984.

21. Hart, G.B., Lamb, R.C., and Strauss, M.B.: Gas gangrene. J. Trauma *23*:991, 1983.

22. Gibson, A., and Davis, F.M.: Hyperbaric oxygen therapy in the management of Clostridium perfringens infections. N.Z. Med. J. *99*:617, 1986.

23. Hitchcock, C.R., Demello, F.J., and Haglin, J.J.: Gangrene infections: New approaches to an old disease. Surg. Clin. North Am. *55*:1403, 1975.

24. Holland, J.A., et al.: Experimental and clinical experience with hyperbaric oxygen in the treatment of clostridial myonecrosis. Surgery *77*:74, 1975.

25. Hirn, M., and Niinikoski, J.: Hyperbaric oxygen in the treatment of clostridial gas gangrene. Ann. Chir. Gynaecol. (Finland), *77*:37, 1988.

26. Turnbull, T.L., and Kline, K.S.: Spontaneous clostridial myonecrosis. J. Emerg. Med. *3*:353, 1985.

27. Bessman, A.N., and Wagner, W.: Nonclostridal gas gangrene. JAMA *233*:958, 1975.

28. Llera, J.L., and Levy, R.C. Treatment of cutaneous abscesses: A double-blind clinical study. Ann Emerg. Med. *14*:15, 1985.

29. Flomenbaum, N., et al.: Self administered nitrous oxide: an adjunct analgesic. JACEP *8*:95, 1979.

30. MacFie, J., and Harvey, J.: Treatment of acute superficial abscesses: A prospective clinical trial. Brit. J. Surg. *64*:264, 1977.

31. Sorensen, C., Hjortruop, A., Moesgaard, F., and Lykkegaard-Nielsen, M.: Linear incision and curettage vs. deroofing and drainage in subcutaneous abscesses: A randomized clinical trial. Acta. Chir. Scand. *153*:659, 1987.

32. Simms, M.H. et al.: Treatment of acute abscesses in the casualty department. Br. Med. J. *284*:1827, 1982.

Chapter 51

IMMUNOLOGY IN THE EMERGENCY DEPARTMENT

FAILURE OF HOST-DEFENSE MECHANISMS IN ACUTE EMERGENCIES

George R. Schwartz with contributions by
Alan Winkelstein and Edward J. Wing

CAPSULE

Major medical or surgical illnesses, including severe trauma and burns, are known to simultaneously cause prominent defects in several host-defense mechanisms. These abnormalities have important clinical manifestations; in total, the most important adverse effect is to greatly increase the risk of serious infections. This section reviews the normal host-defense systems and describes major abnormalities associated with several emergency disorders and therapeutic implications. In particular, immune deficiency conditions, immunosuppressive drugs, splenectomy, and malnutrition are important factors in emergency department (ED) practice. Early detection and treatment are necessary because of the higher morbidity and mortality from injection.

INTRODUCTION

The prototype of systemic failure in host defenses is extensive burn injury.[1] Factors related to the initial injury, plus secondary manifestations such as increased secretion of corticosteroids and malnutrition associated with excessive protein catabolism, all combine to produce measurable abnormalities in most host defenses. For example, these patients show transient decreases in the concentrations of serum immunoglobulins and complement components. Of potentially greater significance, there are prominent defects in the functions of fixed and mobilizable phagocytic cells. These abnormalities contribute to a limitation of the host's abilities to ingest and destroy invading bacteria and eliminate toxic materials. Concurrently, there are prominent abnormalities in cell-mediated immune defenses; these may result from the presence of serum inhibitory factors and overactive suppressor cells. In total, these abnormalities combine to greatly increase the susceptibility of burn patients to overwhelming infections and systemic organ failure.

To appreciate the pathophysiologic processes occurring in severely ill patients, it is necessary to consider the functions of each major host-defense mechanism. Classically, protective systems are divided into two general groups, those that are classified as specific (cell-mediated and humoral immune defenses) and a second group of nonspecific functions. The latter includes the several types of phagocytic cells as well as serum opsonizing factors such as complement. This division, however, is somewhat arbitrary, as the various systems function in a coordinated and interdependent manner; therefore, failure of one component frequently leads to dysfunction involving several others. This discussion does not cover in detail the acquired immunodeficiency syndrome (AIDS), which is covered in Chapter 50. AIDS has caused a resurgence of many diseases of immunodeficiency and has also increased understanding of the pivotal role of lymphocytes.

IMMUNE DEFENSES

The immune system is an essential host-defense mechanism specifically adapted to recognize self from foreign and to selectively react against the latter.[2,3] These reactions provide a highly efficient mechanism for eliminating foreign substances (antigens), thus protecting the host from environmental pathogens. Abnormalities in immune mechanisms can be categorized in two general groups: a failure to respond appropriately to pathogens (*immune deficiency syndromes*) and a loss of ability to distinguish self from foreign (*autoimmunity*).

There are two general types of immune responses, designated *cell-mediated* and *humoral* immunity. Cell-mediated immunity requires direct contact between the effector cells and the target antigen. In general, cell-mediated reactions are limited to the site of antigen deposition; manifestations of these responses develop slowly, and serum factors are not involved. Humoral immune responses are effected by circulating antibodies, proteins specifically modified to combine with the inciting antigen. The term "immunoglobulins" is used to designate the total pool of humoral antibodies. These reactions occur at sites distal to the antibody-producing cell; manifestations usually develop rapidly, and serum factors such as complement often participate, both by accelerating clearance of antigen-antibody complexes and by enhancing the associated inflammatory reactions.

Immune responses can also be differentiated on the basis of the history of antigen exposure. The initial contact with an immunogen elicits a *primary immune response*. By contrast, re-exposure to the same antigen produces a more accelerated reaction that is also of greater magnitude; this is termed the *secondary* or *anamnestic immune response*. The differences in reaction rates in an unsensitized and sensitized individual apply to both humoral and cell-mediated immunity. Furthermore, these differences form the basis for the concept of "immunologic protection." An individual sensitized to an antigen is capable of rapidly responding to a second challenge, thereby mounting protective immune responses before the onset of pathologic changes.

Although most antigens elicit both cell-mediated and humoral immune responses, the activity of one often predominates in maintaining homeostasis (Table 51-1). Humoral immunity is primarily required for the elimination of the encapsulated pyogenic bacteria. These include Streptococcus pneumoniae, Hemophilus influenzae, Neisseria meningitidis, and, to a lesser extent, other streptococci. Patients with immunoglobulin deficiencies are highly susceptible to infections by this limited spectrum of organisms. Humoral immunity, however, has other protective functions; it serves to neutralize soluble toxins (e.g., tetanus toxin) and can provide resistance during the incubation phase of several viral infections. Nevertheless, most hypogammaglobulinemic patients are not unduly susceptible to most viral illnesses. Humoral immunity has variable roles in transplantation rejection reactions and may act to protect tumors against cell-mediated immune destruction (immune enhance-

---

TABLE 51-1. ROLES OF CELL-MEDIATED AND HUMORAL IMMUNITY

I. *Cell-Mediated Immunity:*
   A. Resistance to intracellular organisms (many bacteria, most viruses, protozoa, and fungi)
   B. Transplantation rejection reactions
   C. Tumor immunity
   D. ? Autoimmune diseases
II. *Humoral Immunity*
   A. Resistance to encapsulated pyogenic bacteria (S. pneumoniae, H. influenzae, N. meningitidis)
   B. Neutralization of soluble toxins
   C. Protection against viral infections during incubation phase
   D. ? Transplantation and tumor immunity
   E. Autoimmune and allergic disease

---

ment). This mechanism is also the major pathogenic mechanism in many autoimmune and allergic diseases.

Cell-mediated reactions provide the major defense against intracellular pathogens. This mechanism is required for protection against many bacteria and most viruses, fungi, and protozoa. Individuals with severe defects in cellular immunity are susceptible to a wide range of microorganisms, including several usually not considered highly pathogenic. These immunocompromised hosts frequently succumb to overwhelming infections from such organisms as Mycobacterium tuberculosis, Cytomegalovirus, Cryptococcus neoformans, or Toxoplasma gondii. Patients with AIDS have particularly changed the spectrum of disease.

Recent studies suggest several other important functions for the cell-mediated immune system. These reactions provide the major mechanism involved in allogeneic organ transplant rejection. In fact, the major barrier to transplant therapy is the need to suppress the recipient's cell-mediated responses directed against the donor organ without severely compromising his ability to protect himself against microbial pathogens. A variant of the transplant rejection reaction is the graft versus host disease which is frequently observed in bone marrow transplant recipients. In this situation, the recipient is unable to reject foreign, immunologically competent cells. By contrast, the donor's cells can recognize the recipient's antigens as foreign and react against them.

Cell-mediated reactions appear to provide immune protection against neoplasms. Several different cellular immune mechanisms cause lysis of tumor cells. All involve direct cell contact between the tumor and effector cell. At present, it appears that these cytolytic reactions may be important in eliminating small numbers of tumor cells but are incapable of significantly influencing large tumors. A role for cell-mediated responses in autoimmune disease has been postulated but not yet defined.

LYMPHOCYTES

The principal cellular components of a functioning immune system are lymphocytes.[3] These mononuclear cells are capable of interacting with antigens, a process that initiates a coordinated sequence of events leading to a specific immune response directed at the inciting antigen. In parallel with the two types of immunologic reactions described above, there are two major populations of lymphocytes. These are designated *T* (*thymic-dependent*) and *B* (*bone marrow-derived*) cells. *T cells* are responsible for effecting cell-mediated reactions; *B cells* and their progeny, plasma cells, synthesize and secrete specific humoral antibodies. In addition, there is a third population of lymphocytes that lack characteristics of either T or B cells, i.e., *null cells*. Recent studies indicate that several different types of lymphoid cells are contained within this group. Some are precursors for the lymphoid and hematopoietic systems. Others are effectors for newly described mechanisms of target cell lysis, natural killing (NK) and antibody-dependent cellular cytotoxicity (ADCC) (see subsequent text).

Although these cellular divisions suggest that T and B cells act independently, there is increasing awareness of multiple cellular interactions between the two.[4] The best defined interdependence is the involvement of T cells in the B cell responses to most antigens. The initiating event in many humoral responses depends on a T cell-antigen interaction. These stimulated T cells, in cooperation with macrophages, act to instruct B cells to respond; it is the latter that then develop into antibody producing plasma cells. The T cell activity, termed "helper" function, is essential to stimulate the B cell response; if absent, antibodies will not

be elaborated. Antigens dependent on this T-B cell interaction are termed *thymic dependent*; there is also a smaller group of immunogens that can directly stimulate B cells (*thymic independent antigens*).

A second and important type of interaction is the ability of T cells to regulate the magnitude of B cell responses. Certain types of T cells, termed suppressor lymphocytes, can limit reactivity. Abnormally heightened suppressor cell activities are thought to be one of the mechanisms responsible for the acute depression of immune reactivity seen following severe trauma and burns. Suppression has proved to be an important homeostatic mechanism; it provides a means for maintaining *tolerance* (specific unresponsiveness to an antigen). Thus, the presence of suppressor cells serves to prevent the individual from mounting immune responses against antigens on his own tissues. Defective T suppressor function has been implicated in the pathogenesis of many autoimmune diseases.[5–7]

LYMPHOCYTE RESPONSES TO ANTIGENS

The cellular events involved in generating a B or T cell response to antigens constitute a complex sequence of events (Fig. 51-1).[3,8] The stimulus for lymphocyte activation is usually provided by macrophage-antigen complex. The phagocytic cells initially process and present antigens in an immunogenic form on their cell membranes. Lymphocytes, in turn, recognize the immunologic stimuli because of the presence of antigen specific receptors on their cell membranes; the cellular responses are initiated by the interaction between the receptors and the antigens. Stimulated lymphocytes are transformed from a resting to an actively

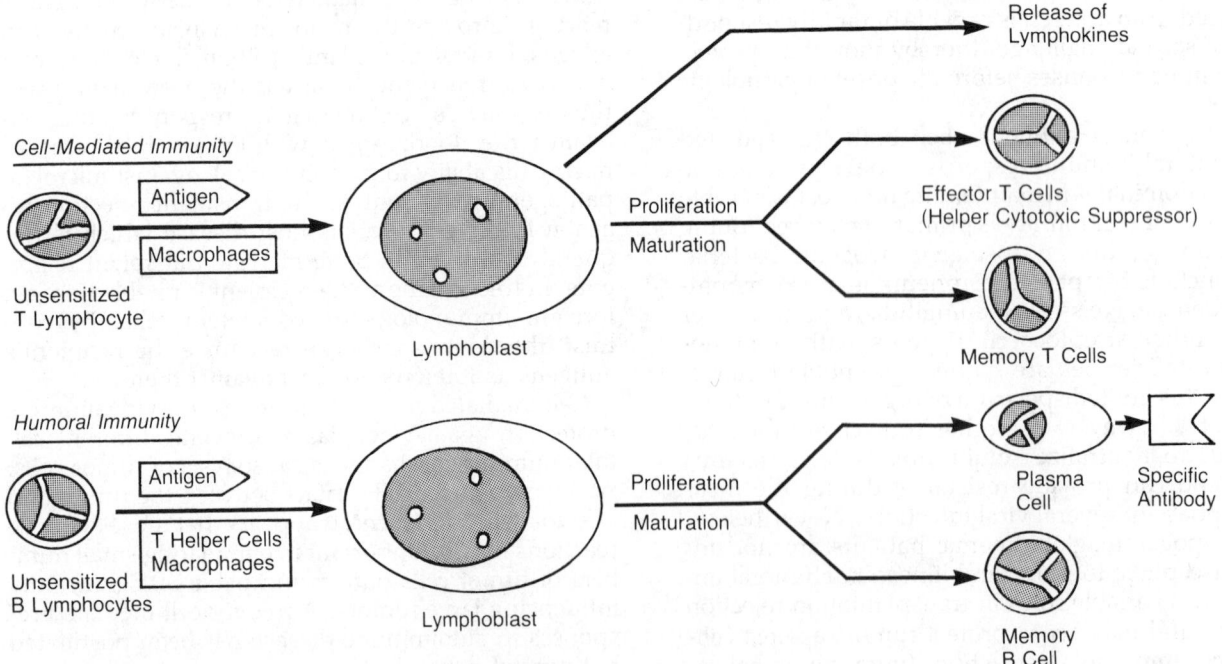

FIG. 51-1.   Interaction between lymphocyte antigens. For both T and B cells, macrophages are generally required to initiate the responses.

metabolic state; protein, RNA, and DNA synthesis is markedly increased. Morphologically, these cells de-differentiate into immature-appearing lymphoblasts (often designated as "atypical lymphocytes") that undergo a series of mitotic divisions. This proliferative expansion phase is then followed by maturation into immunologic effectors.

The initial sequence is similar in both the T and B cell systems, except that many B cell responses require the instructive functions of T helper cells. The immunologic effectors in the two systems are different, however. In the T cell system, these appear as small lymphocytes that are programmed to perform specific immunologic functions. These include the capacity to help B cell responses, to release biologically active substances, termed lymphokines, which mediate inflammation, to kill antigen-expressing target cells (cytolysis), and to regulate the magnitude of immune responses acting as suppressor cells. As discussed below, these activities may be mediated by different T cell subsets.

By contrast, effectors in the B cell system are plasma cells that are coded to synthesize and secrete antigen-specific humoral antibodies. All plasma cells derived from a single B lymphocyte elaborate only one type of antibody, which is specific for only a single antigen (monoclonality). In both the T and B cell systems, some daughter cells revert to small lymphocytes and function as memory cells. These are "programmed" lymphocytes, which upon rechallenge with the inciting antigen are capable of mounting the accelerated, secondary-type immune responses.

LYMPHOKINES (Table 51-2)

These are soluble products of T cells which are released in vivo or in vitro following antigen stimulation and help to mediate inflammation.[9,10] One of the principal effects of these mediators is to attract and stimulate a principal effector of cellular immunity, macrophages. One type of lymphokine induces macrophage migration to the site of inflammation (chemotactic factor), a second inhibits the random migration away from the involved area (migration inhibition factor, MIF), and a third activates intracellular killing mechanisms (macrophage activating factor, MAF).

The importance of T lymphocyte-macrophage interactions is shown in experiments investigating in vitro murine resistance to *Listeria monocytogenes*. These microorganisms can readily infect normal (nonactivated) macrophages and survive well in this intracellular environment. Once the macrophages are activated, however, they rapidly destroy these organisms. The activation process can be initiated by exposing normal macrophages to a soluble product generated by incubating Listeria antigens with sensitized T lymphocytes.[10a] Macrophage killing is nonspecific. The soluble product elicited by contact between Listeria antigens and Listeria-sensitized T cells is capable of activating macrophages to kill other intracellular pathogens, such as mycobacteria and toxoplasma. These activated macrophages also possess potent tumoricidal properties. This in vitro model closely correlates with the in vivo mechanisms mediating resistance to intracellular pathogens.[11-13]

In addition to macrophages, soluble factors derived from T lymphocytes affect the functions of numerous other cells. For example, mediators are released that are chemotactic for neutrophils, eosinophils, basophils, and lymphocytes. Other lymphokines induce proliferation of neutrophil, monocyte, and eosinophil precursors (colony-stimulating factors), other lymphocytes (mitogenic factor, T cell growth factor), and fibroblasts. Soluble factors can also lyse target cells

TABLE 51-2. REPRESENTATIVE LYMPHOKINE ACTIVITIES*

Cellular Function	Mediator	Activity
Mobility	Chemotaxis—macrophages, neutrophils, eosinophils, and basophils	Attraction of cells to site of antigen deposition
	Migration inhibition—macrophages (MIF), neutrophils (LIF)	Localizing inflammatory cells
Injury	Lymphotoxin	Killing of target cells
Activation	Helper and suppressor factors	Regulate activities of T and B cells
	Macrophage activation factor (MAF)	Activate intraenzymes in macrophages
	Augmentation of T cell cytotoxicity	Promotes target cell killing by T cells
	Interferon	Antiviral agent; increases NK activity
	Stimulation of collagen synthesis by fibroblasts	Induces secretion of this extracellular matrix protein
Growth	Mitogenic factor	T cell proliferation
	T cell growth factor (IL-2)	Perpetuates T cell growth
	Colony stimulating factor (CSF)	Induces growth of neutrophils and macrophages

(lymphotoxin) and induce collagen synthesis by fi-broblasts. Interleukins, interferons, and "tumor ne-crosis factor" are examples of cytokines produced by lymphocytes. Other functional properties of soluble products include augmentation of the activities of T cytotoxic and suppressor cells. Interferon, a potent antiviral compound, is also able to enhance the cy-tolytic activities of a specific type of lymphocyte,[13a] natural killer cells (see subsequent text). Certain lym-phokines may also be secreted by cells other than T lymphocytes. The multiple functions of lymphokines suggest that these soluble factors have a central role in regulating immunity, effecting cell-mediated re-actions, and promoting inflammatory responses.[13b]

CELL-MEDIATED CYTOTOXICITY (Table 51-3)

Another important activity of T cells is the ability to directly kill certain target cells (cytolysis).[14] This ac-tivity results from direct contact between an antigen-expressing target and the cytolytic T cell effector. In the killing reaction, the lymphocyte transiently binds to the target cell membrane; this cell-to-cell contact initiates a lytic injury to the membrane of the target cell.[15] Each effector lymphocyte is capable of killing multiple target cells. These targets may be histoin-compatible, tumor, or virus-infected cells; in fact, con-siderable data suggest that T cell cytotoxicity is a prime protective mechanism against many of these micro-organisms.

Cellular cytotoxicity is not a property restricted to T lymphocytes. Two types of killing reactions effected by null lymphocytes have been described. These are termed *natural killer (NK) cell activity*[16,17] and *antibody-dependent cellular cytotoxicity (ADCC)*.[14,18,19] Natural killing is a phenomenon that may be of major im-portance in the innate resistance to neoplasms. Ef-fectors in this reaction differ from cytotoxic T cells because they can lyse target cells in the absence of

prior antigen exposure. Thus, NK cytolytic activity can be expressed in naive animals, those that have never been exposed to target cell antigens. By contrast, T cell cytolysis depends upon presensitization of the effectors by target cell antigens.

Antibody-dependent cellular cytotoxicity is another form of target cell lysis, expressed by a subpopulation of null lymphocytes termed killer (K) cells. Monocytes can also act as ADCC effectors. In this reaction, an-tibodies of the IgG class react with surface antigens on the target cell. Once fixed, the antibodies react with specific (Fc) receptors on the K cells, enabling the latter to initiate a lytic reaction. In parallel with the NK phenomenon, ADCC effectors do not require prior sensitization. ADCC responses appear to be important in eliminating histoincompatible cells, tumor cells, and virally infected cells. They may also function as im-portant mechanisms in certain autoimmune diseases; in these, the host's own cells are coated by IgG au-toantibodies and subsequently lysed by K cells.

RECOGNITION OF LYMPHOID SUBSETS

On peripheral blood smears, lymphocytes appear as a relatively homogeneous cell population. Most are small cells lacking unique cytologic features. An oc-casional lymphocyte appears larger, with more abun-dant cytoplasm and a less condensed nuclear chro-matin. These cells are probably lymphocytes in the process of reacting to antigens. Morphologic criteria are inadequate to distinguish different subsets of lym-phocytes. Subpopulations of lymphocytes can be rec-ognized by characteristics of the cell membrane (Table 51-3).[8,21] T cells possess membrane receptors for sheep red blood cells and will bind these erythrocytes, pro-ducing a characteristic rosette. By contrast, other types of lymphocytes do not bind sheep cells. The most widely used technique for identifying B lymphocytes depends on the unique property of these cells to ex-

TABLE 51-3. RECOGNITION OF HUMAN MONONUCLEAR CELL SUBPOPULATIONS

	T Cells	B Cells	Null Cells	Macrophages
Sheep red blood cell rosettes	+	0	0	0
Reactivity with pan T cell reagents (OKT 3)	+	0	0	0
Surface immunoglobulins (endogenously produced)	0	+	0	0
Fc receptors	+*	+	±†	+
C receptors	0	+	±†	+
Expression of Dr antigens	0**	+	+	+

* These receptors are present on certain T cells but are demonstrable only by using specialized techniques.
** Dr antigens are also present on activated T cells.
† Expressed on a portion of null cells.

press immunoglobulins on their surface membrane.[22] These antibodies are formed intracellularly and rapidly incorporated into the cell membrane, where they function as antigen receptors. Surface-bound immunoglobulins can be recognized by reacting the cell suspension with a heterologous antibody to human immunoglobulins that has been labeled with a readily detectable dye, such as fluorescein.

The technique for producing a single homogeneous antibody (*monoclonal* antibodies) has been used to further identify lymphocyte subsets.[7,23] Antibody-producing cells are generated by immunizing mice with specific antigens. Spleen cells from these animals manifest a spectrum of antibody-producing lymphocytes, each cell producing a single antibody that reacts with only one antigen determinant. The splenic lymphocytes are fused with murine tumor cells, which permits exchange of genetic information between the two cells. A portion of the fused cells retain the property of the tumor cell of self-replication and the property of the antibody-producing cell to synthesize a specific antibody. Those producing the desired antibody are selected and allowed to grow in culture. The resultant clone, a homogeneous population of cells, will elaborate large amounts of monoclonal antibody with specificity for a single determinant of the inciting antigen.

Using this technique, it is possible to produce antibodies that recognize several subsets of T cells (Table 51-4). The three most widely used monoclonal antibodies are designated T3, T4, and T8.[7,23,24]

The T3 antiserum reacts with all peripheral blood T cells; thus it is a pan-T cell reagent. Lymphocytes capable of reacting with the T4 antiserum have been designated *T inducer/helper* cells. The T8 antiserum reacts with a second, non-overlapping subpopulation of T cells that mediates cellular suppression and cytolysis (*T suppressor/cytotoxic cells*).

Using these techniques, it is possible to define characteristics of the peripheral blood lymphocyte pool. In normal individuals, the total number of circulating lymphocytes averages 2500 cells/μL with a range of 1500 to 4000 cells/μL. A decrease in total number of circulating cells is termed *lymphopenia*, an increase,

lymphocytosis.[25] In a normal individual, the vast majority (60 to 70%) are identified as T cells. Only 5 to 10% of the circulating lymphoid pool are B cells. The remaining 20 to 30% are considered null cells. Monoclonal antibody studies indicate that approximately 65% of the circulating T cells belong to the inducer/helper class and 35% to the suppressor/cytotoxic subset.

Certain other receptors are also found on lymphocytes; these have provided alternate methods for cell identification.[26] Many B cells and some null cells have receptors for the Fc portion of IgG and for the C3b and C4b components of complement.[27] In addition, it appears that some T inducer/helper cells have receptors for the μ heavy chain of IgM immunoglobulins (Tμ cells), while certain T suppressor cells bear receptors for the gamma heavy chain of IgG (Tγ cells).[6,28]

FUNCTIONAL MEASURES OF LYMPHOCYTE ACTIVITIES

In addition to morphologic criteria, human lymphocytes can be examined in vitro for several functional activities. These include lymphoproliferation, ability to elaborate lymphokines, immunoglobulin synthesis, target cell cytolysis, and capacities to express helper or suppressor cell activities. Functional assays provide information that is distinct from that provided by morphologic subset identification. For example, many patients with hypogammaglobulinemia have normal numbers of circulating B lymphocytes; however, in culture, these cells will not synthesize normal amounts of immunoglobulins. Individual function assays are reviewed elsewhere.[8,29]

One specific reaction with clinical applications is the ability to stimulate lymphoproliferative responses in vitro. Lymphocytes proliferate only when exposed to a stimulating agent. The most widely used agents are nonspecific mitogens. Lymphocyte responses to these substances are independent of prior antigen sensitization. Examples of these nonspecific agents are phytohemagglutinin (PHA), concanavalin A (Con-A), and pokeweed mitogen. Each mitogen appears to react with a distinct population of cells. In addition to nonspecific mitogens, histoincompatible cells can also induce proliferation. Mononuclear cells from two unrelated individuals stimulate each other; this test, the mixed leukocyte culture (MLC), is widely used to type donors and recipients in preparation for organ transplantation. A third type of stimulus is specific antigens. These induce a proliferative response in an individual who is sensitized to the antigen. For example, tuberculin protein (PPD) induces a proliferative response in a normal individual who has been sensitized to this antigen, but not in a person who has not been exposed. In addition, serum factors that can inhibit immune response are frequently assessed by measuring reductions in the in vitro proliferation of lym-

TABLE 51-4. SUBSETS OF T LYMPHOCYTES

	Helper Cells	Suppressor/ Cytotoxic Cells
Sheep red blood cell rosettes	+	+
Reactivity with T3 sera	+	+
Reactivity with T4 sera	+	0
Reactivity with T8 sera	0	+
Tμ receptors	+	0
Tγ receptors	0	+

phocytes following the inclusion of small amounts of test serum.

DELAYED HYPERSENSITIVITY SKIN TESTS

The most common means of assessing cell-mediated immunity in man is the delayed hypersensitivity skin test, which measures cutaneous responses to antigens to which the individual has previously been sensitized. On intradermal injection of minute amounts of a specific antigen, a slowly developing reaction occurs at the local site; this consists of erythema and induration. Generally, the reaction is maximal after 48 to 72 hours. The PPD response is the prototype of a delayed hypersensitivity reaction. As the incidence of tuberculosis declines, however, most normal individuals are not sensitized to tuberculin antigens and thus do not react. To circumvent this, several common antigens that elicit delayed hypersensitivity responses in most normal individuals are used to test reactivity. Such antigens include Candida, mumps, and streptokinase-streptodornase. The inability to respond to a battery of these antigens is termed *anergy*; this phenomenon implies a temporary or permanent defect in cellular immunity. It should be recognized that skin test reactions are the expression of one form of cellular immunity; several other types of responses are not measured by delayed hypersensitivity testing. Furthermore, in many circumstances, the ability to mount cutaneous responses does not correlate closely with resistance to infection.

PHAGOCYTES

MACROPHAGES

Macrophages, which are one of the two principal types of phagocytes, are critical in defenses against microbial pathogens (Tables 51-5 and 51-6). Macrophages also play an essential role in a variety of other processes, including antigen presentation to lymphocytes, destruction of tumor cells, regulation of the immune response, and synthesis and secretion of soluble products responsible for acute and chronic inflammation.[30] The central role of the macrophage in host defenses is illustrated by the fact that no syndrome exists in which there is an absence or serious defect in macrophages—such a syndrome is presumably incompatible with life.

Macrophages are derived from mesodermal stem cells in the bone marrow; they mature and differentiate under the regulation of a glycoprotein, colony-stimulating factor, and enter the circulation as monocytes. The normal number of circulating monocytes is 150 to 800 cells/μL (3 to 8% of the total white cell count). Once released from the marrow, monocytes circulate for several days. These cells then migrate into extravascular sites, where a proportion mature into tissue macrophages and may persist for months.

Macrophages are large cells, ranging from 10 to 30

TABLE 51-5. PROPERTIES OF ACTIVATED MACROPHAGES COMPARED WITH UNSTIMULATED MACROPHAGES

Increased size and spreading
Increased glucose utilization through the hexose monophosphate shunt
Increased membrane enzyme adenylate cyclase and increased cytoplasmic enzyme lactate dehydrogenase
Increased production of plasminogen activator and prostaglandins
Increased Ca^{2+} influx
Increased cGMP
Increase in the number of cytoplasmic granules
Phagocytosis of C3b-coated particles
Increased pinocytosis
Increased bacterial killing
Tumor inhibition and killing

TABLE 51-6. REPRESENTATIVE LIST OF MACROPHAGE SECRETORY PRODUCTS

Enzymes
  Lysozme
  Neutral proteases (e.g., plasminogen activator)
  Acid hydrolases
Complement components
Fibronectin
Prostaglandins
Interleukin I
Interferon
Colony-stimulating factor
Factors inhibiting cell replication (cytolytic factor)
Endogenous pyrogens
Oxygen metabolites

μm in diameter. They have oval, indented nuclei, undulating cell membranes, numerous lysosomes—vacuoles containing hydrolytic enzymes—and phagocytic vacuoles. Their cell membrane contains receptors for the Fc portion of immunoglobulin and the complement product C3b. The functional activities, metabolism, and structure of macrophages are closely related to their anatomic location. For example, alveolar macrophages appear to function better in aerobic environments, whereas the metabolism of peritoneal macrophages is primarily anaerobic. In contrast, the overall bactericidal activities of peritoneal macrophages appear to be greater than those of alveolar macrophages.

Macrophage Activation. A central concept in macrophage physiology is the principle of activation.[31–33] Macrophages can become "activated" on exposure to secretory products of T lymphocytes (lymphokines), such as macrophage activating factor (MAF), interferon, and colony stimulating factor. The presence of endotoxin may be necessary in the activation process as a second signal. Metabolic and functional changes occur with activation (Table 51-5). Compared with resting macrophages, activated cells are larger, secrete increased amounts of mediators such as plasminogen activator, have increased metabolism by the hexose monophosphate shunt, and have increased pinocytic and phagocytic rates. The most important functional feature of activated macrophages is that they can readily kill intracellular pathogens such as *Toxoplasma gondii* and can destroy tumor cells, whereas unstimulated, resting macrophages cannot.

Monocytes and macrophages are amebalike cells with the capacity to migrate through tissues.[34] This migration may be random or highly directional toward a chemotactic stimulus. Principal chemotactic stimuli include activated components of complement (C5a, C3a, and the C567 complex), certain tripeptides that may be derived from bacteria, and chemotactic factors elaborated by T lymphocytes (lymphokines). Chemotaxis serves to attract macrophages to sites of inflammation, antigen deposition, infection, or tumor. This phenomenon is illustrated by Listeria infection in experimental animals. Within 24 hours of bacterial inoculation, large numbers of monocytes and macrophages migrate to areas of microbial multiplication. This accumulation of phagocytes is predominantly responsible for initially limiting bacterial proliferation.

The major function of macrophages is to phagocytize and kill microbial pathogens.[2] In normal individuals, these cells are primarily responsible for destroying or inhibiting the growth of intracellular organisms. These include many relatively resistant pathogens such as mycobacteria, protozoa, fungi, viruses, and certain helminths. Phagocytosis of these microbes begins with attachment or binding of a particle to a receptor on the cell membrane of the macrophage (Fig. 51-2).[34] This binding is greatly aided if the particle is coated with antibody and/or complement, a process termed opsonization. This process increases phagocytic rates up to 100 times. Binding itself appears to stimulate contractile proteins within microfilaments in the cytoplasm of macrophages; this, in turn, causes the macrophage to begin to surround the particle. With increasing engulfment, more receptors are brought into contact with the particle, leading to increased binding and subsequent activation of additional microfilaments.[35] Eventually, the particle is completely surrounded by the macrophage cell membrane, thus forming a vacuole (phagosome), which is interiorized into the cytoplasm of the macrophage. The particle, however, never directly enters the cell's cytoplasm; it is contained within the vacuole, whose limiting membrane is derived from the macrophage's membrane.

The process of phagocytosis simultaneously stim-

FIG. 51-2. *Phagocytosis of particulate material by macrophages. The coating of the particle by antibody and complement greatly accelerates ingestion. The initial attachment of ligand to cell receptors stimulates cytoplasmic movement, enabling more ligands to bind to receptors. Ultimately, the macrophage membrane completely surrounds the particles, leading to the formation of a phagosome. Destruction results from the release of lysosomal enzymes and H_2O_2 into the phagosome.*

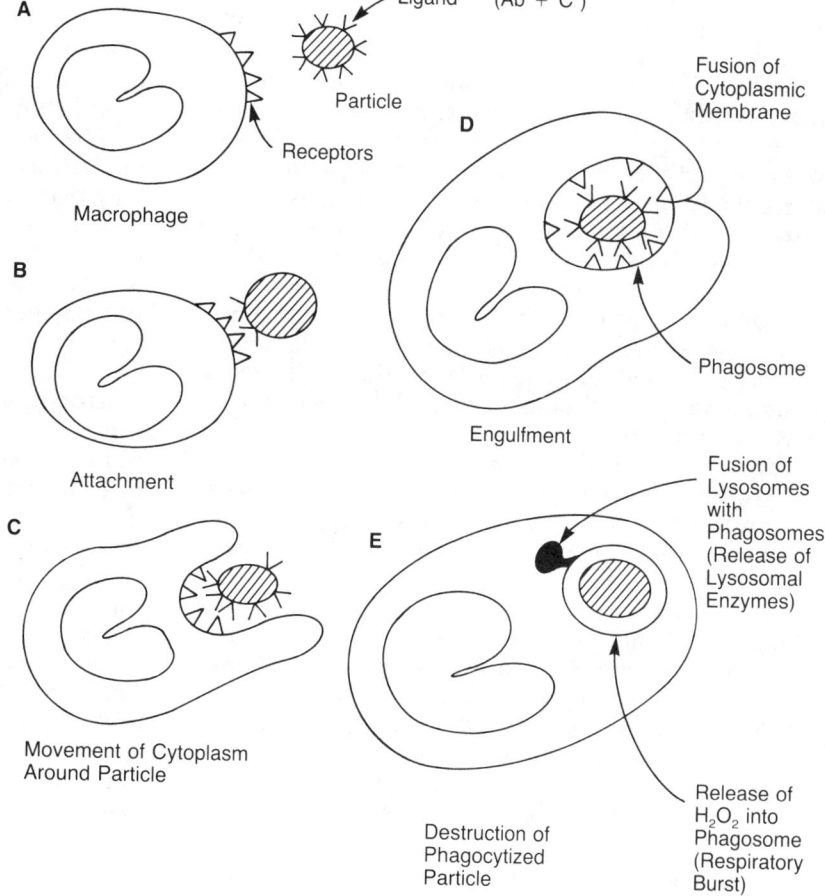

A
Ligand (Ab + C')
Particle
Receptors
Macrophage

B
Attachment

C
Movement of Cytoplasm
Around Particle

D
Fusion of Cytoplasmic Membrane
Phagosome
Engulfment

E
Fusion of Lysosomes with Phagosomes (Release of Lysosomal Enzymes)
Release of H_2O_2 into Phagosome (Respiratory Burst)
Destruction of Phagocytized Particle

ulates two sets of intracellular reactions.[36] The first, the "respiratory burst," involves the sequential reduction of oxygen to superoxide and then to hydrogen peroxide.[37] These oxygen products, possibly in concert with halide ions, result in the killing of phagocytized microorganisms. The second set of reactions, which occurs simultaneously, involves the fusion of intracellular lysosomes (cytoplasmic granules) with the membrane of the phagosome. This results in the discharge of hydrolytic enzymes into the vacuole; these are also capable of microbial killing.

Macrophages have important antitumor functions.[38] In vitro, activated macrophages can selectively kill certain malignant cells by non-phagocytic processes without damaging normal cells. Furthermore, there is circumstantial evidence suggesting that the tumoricidal functions of macrophages are important in vivo. For example, many neoplasms are extensively infiltrated by these phagocytic cells—histologic data suggesting an antitumor activity. This is also supported by studies showing an inverse correlation between tumor regression and macrophage infiltration. The presence of activated macrophages in experimental animals, as in those with chronic infections, confers increased resistance to transplanted tumors. The mechanisms responsible for macrophage tumoricidal effects are not known but may involve release of hydrogen peroxide and other oxygen radicals. Furthermore, macrophages can kill tumor cells by releasing a neutral serine protease, termed cytolytic factor. Macrophages can also lyse tumor cells coated with IgG antibodies by an ADCC mechanism.

Besides their antimicrobial and antitumor activities, macrophages have been shown to be essential in regulating the magnitude of immune responses.[39] These cells can both promote and suppress immune reactions; the balance between these two activities is dictated by the numbers of macrophages present and their state of activation. These cells are required as initiators of primary immune responses for both thymic dependent and thymic independent antigens. Macrophages process (degrade and chemically modify) antigens and present them on their cell membranes to responsive lymphocytes. This activity markedly increases the antigenicity of foreign material; immunogens presented to lymphocytes in this form are several thousand times more potent than those presented in a soluble form. Thus, macrophages are essential in initiating both humoral and cell-mediated responses. In general, only small numbers of macrophages are required for these initiating interactions. The process of antigen presentation is, in many models, genetically restricted—the macrophage and lymphocyte must have the same histocompatibility genes. These phagocytic cells also act through other mechanisms to enhance immune responses. Macrophages release a soluble product, a monokine, which enhances lymphocyte proliferation (interleukin 1 or IL-1).

By contrast, macrophages can also act to inhibit immune reactivity. Suppression is directly correlated with both the relative numbers of macrophages in an infiltrate and their state of activation. Large numbers of these cells, particularly if activated, exert an inhibitory effect on lymphocyte responses. A variety of inhibitory mechanisms have been described; these include the release of inhibitory prostaglandins, excessive thymidine, and other low molecular weight compounds. In some models, suppression requires direct cell-to-cell contact.

These observations suggest a model for macrophage regulation (Fig. 51-3). Initial antigen exposure serves to recruit small numbers of macrophages; these cells initiate lymphocytic responses. Once lymphoid cells are stimulated, they release lymphokines, which attract other macrophages to the local site (chemotactic factors) and activate these phagocytic cells (MAF). The subsequent accumulation of large numbers of activated macrophages not only promotes the destruction of the inciting antigen or microorganisms but also acts back on the stimulated lymphocytes to "shut off" the immune response.

Macrophages secrete a variety of biologically active compounds (see Table 51-6),[40] many of which are released in appreciable concentrations only by activated macrophages and are important in regulating inflammatory reactions. For example, lysozymes are enzymes that can produce extracellular lysis of certain bacteria. Plasminogen activator is a neutral protease that not only activates plasmin to lyse fibrin but also initiates the complement cascade and activates the bradykinin system. Acid hydrolases, including proteases and lipases, are active in the acid environment of inflammatory lesions. Additional secretory products include prostaglandins, interferon, colony stimulating factors, and endogenous pyrogen, all of which may play important roles in host defenses.

A recent factor termed cachetin or tumor necrosis factor (TNF) is involved with promotion of inflammation and tissue destruction. Modulation of this factor has therapeutic implications, which are in initial stages of application.[40a]

Macrophage Function Impairment. Macrophage function may be compromised by a number of conditions.[41] Any process that interferes with T lymphocyte function can affect macrophage function. Thus, if T cells do not respond normally to antigen, their production of lymphokines is reduced, and macrophage activation is impaired. Congenital defects in macrophage function include chronic granulomatous disease, in which a defect in the oxygen burst mechanism prevents normal killing of microbial pathogens, and chronic mucocutaneous candidiasis and Wiskott-Aldrich syndrome, in which chemotaxis is abnormal. Patients with these conditions show an increased susceptibility to infections. In addition, certain drugs, particularly corticosteroids, cause defects in monocyte function.

Monocyte function in patients with lymphoma, cancer, or infection may be abnormal. In one study, monocytes of untreated patients with lymphoma had normal phagocytic capacity but absent bactericidal activity. Furthermore, chemotaxis may also be abnormal in patients with malignancy and those with certain chronic infections.

Finally, several substances directly depress macrophage function and may be lethal for macrophages; these include silica particles, carrageenan, cigarette smoke, and antimacrophage serum. Patients exposed to silica, for example, are more susceptible to infection with intracellular pathogens, such as Mycobacterium tuberculosis, and tumors.

POLYMORPHONUCLEAR LEUKOCYTES

Polymorphonuclear leukocytes (or neutrophils), the second major type of phagocyte, operate primarily against bacteria that cause acute infection, particularly staphylococci and aerobic gram-negative rods.[42]

As with macrophages, neutrophils are derived from bone marrow stem cells under the control of colony stimulating factors.[43] The daily production of neutrophils is approximately 10^{11} cells. Neutrophils in the blood exist in two roughly equal and exchangeable pools, a circulating population and a marginated one adhering to vascular endothelium. The distribution between the two pools can be influenced by several factors; epinephrine, acute stress, and corticosteroids cause demargination, whereas certain acute infections increase neutrophil adherence. Neutrophils persist in the circulation for approximately 6 to 12 hours. The cells then move into extravascular tissues, where they survive for several hours to several days.

Neutrophils have polylobed nuclei, primary and secondary cytoplasmic granules, and microfilaments. By contrast, these cells contain few ribosomes and mitochondria. Receptors for the Fc portion of IgG and,

possibly, C3b complement can be found on the cell membrane. Primary or azurophilic granules, which form early in the maturation process, degranulate into phagosomes and are involved in killing phagocytosed microorganisms; secondary granules, formed later in the maturation process, are released outside of the cell and involved in extracellular inflammation.

The attraction of neutrophils to areas of bacterial multiplication or inflammation is a critical step in the response to inflammatory or infectious stimuli.[44] Granulocyte adherence to the vascular endothelium facilitates movement of these cells into extravascular tissues. Increased adherence or "stickiness" depends on plasma factors such as integrin and other cell adhesion molecules.[44a] Like macrophages, neutrophils respond chemotactically to concentration gradients of certain soluble attractants such as bacterial products (certain tripeptides), lymphocyte chemotactic factors, and complement components, particularly C3a, C5a, and the trimolecular complex C567.

Once a neutrophil is in an area of inflammation or near a foreign particle, phagocytosis begins by attachment of the particle to membrane receptors; this process is mediated by opsonins such as antibody and complement. Engulfment then occurs in a sequential fashion, similar to that described for macrophages.

As with macrophage phagocytosis, neutrophil phagocytosis stimulates two processes, the generation of hydrogen peroxide in the respiratory burst and the discharge of primary granules into the phagocytic vacuole.[45] The interaction of hydrogen peroxide, myeloperoxidase, and halide ions combines to effect halogenation of bacteria, a microbicidal event. In addition, other metabolites of oxygen such as superoxide (O_2-), singlet oxygen $(^1O_2)$, and oxygen radicals $(OH\bullet)$ may participate in killing events. Oxygen-independent bactericidal mechanisms, which are more important under anaerobic conditions, include

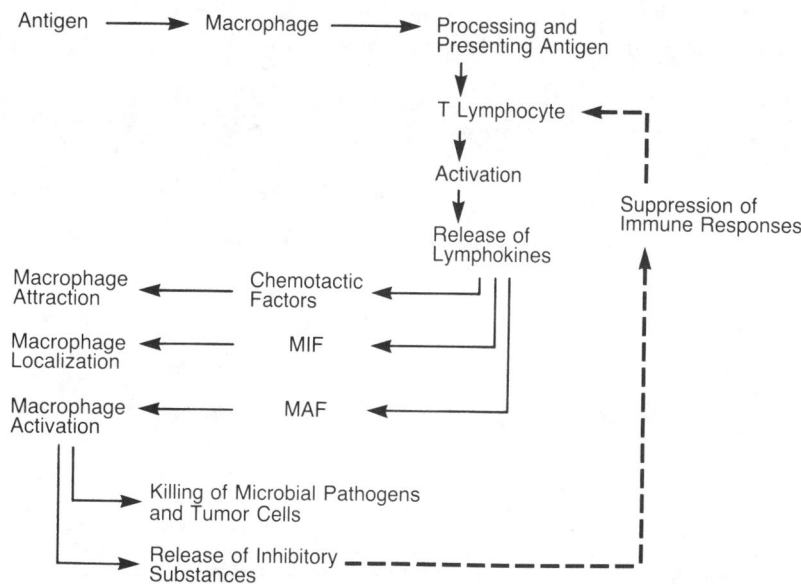

FIG. 51-3. *Schematic diagram of the interaction between macrophages and T lymphocytes. The macrophages have a dual function; they have the capacity to both facilitate and suppress T cell immune responses.*

acidification of the phagocytic vacuole and release of lactoferrin, lysozyme, and cationic proteins into the phagosome.

Granulocytopenia (Neutropenia). This is by far the most common cause of overall neutrophil dysfunction. An absolute neutrophil count (less than 1000 neutrophil cells/μL) is a life-threatening condition; patients with this abnormality are highly susceptible to overwhelming bacterial or fungal infections.[46,46a] This risk increases dramatically when the count is below 500 cells/μL. The most frequent cause of severe neutropenia is use of cytotoxic drugs for the treatment of underlying malignancies. Autoimmune diseases, bone marrow infiltration processes, aplastic anemia, or idiosyncratic reactions to drugs are other causes of severe neutropenia. Hallmarks are the rapidity and overwhelming nature of the associated infection. Patients may initially manifest a low grade fever without localizing signs, yet be dead 24 hours later of overwhelming sepsis. Thus, it is imperative to initiate treatment with antibiotics at the first sign of infection.

Neutropenic patients usually develop infections at epidermal and mucous membrane surfaces. The most common sites of infection are the oral cavity and pharynx, esophagus, lungs, perirectal area, urinary tract, and skin. On examination, it is important to evaluate these sites carefully for evidence of infection. Many of the usual symptoms and signs of a localized infection may be lacking. Inflammation is suppressed because of the lack of a neutrophilic response. Local pain is one of the consistent findings.

Almost 70% of infections in neutropenic hosts are caused by the following microorganisms: Escherichia coli, Klebsiella pneumoniae, Pseudomonas aeruginosa, Staphylococcus aureus, and Candida albicans.[22] The remaining pathogens include other aerobic gram-negative rods and other gram-positive cocci such as streptococci. These patients do not have an increased tendency to develop infections caused by pneumococci, anaerobic pathogens, Pneumocystis carinii, or other opportunistic intracellular pathogens.

Trials have shown that a combination of an aminoglycoside such as tobramycin and an anti-pseudomonas penicillin such as ticarcillin affords optimal initial antibiotic coverage in these patients.[46] Other equivalent combinations are an aminoglycoside plus a cephalosporin such as cefazolin, or trimethoprim-sulfamethoxazole plus ticarcillin. Addition of a third drug does not appear to add benefit. The third generation cephalosporins such as moxalactam or cefotaxime do not have adequate antipseudomonas coverage and should not be used alone, although one study in neutropenic patients compared ceftazidime alone with combination therapy, and concluded that there was little difference.[46a] If systemic fungal infection is suspected or proved, amphotericin B should be added. The value of granulocyte transfusions is highly debatable; at present, it is unclear if they offer advantages over antibiotics alone.[47] It has been shown that they should not be used prophylactically, and there is increasing evidence indicating that, in infected patients, they do not improve survival over that in patients treated only with antibiotics. Furthermore, they are expensive and can induce such complications as pulmonary dysfunction and cytomegalovirus infections. The granulocyte/macrophage-stimulating substances, however, will have a role in the future, and are more suitable because they stimulate the individual's own granulocyte production and release.[47a] Future promise is also shown for subcutaneous recombinant interferon in prophylaxis and probably treatment.[47b]

IMMUNOGLOBULINS

Immunoglobulins—a term used collectively to describe serum antibodies—are a heterogeneous group of proteins, each specifically modified to react with a particular antigen (Table 51-7).[48-50] Antibodies are primarily synthesized by plasma cells; however, small amounts are also produced by B lymphocytes. All antibodies of the same type, which are specific for a single

TABLE 51-7. PROPERTIES OF IMMUNOGLOBULINS

	IgG	IgA	IgM	IgD	IgE
Serum concentration (mg./ml.)	12.4	2.5	1.2	0.03	0.0003
Molecular weight	160,000	170,000 385,000*	900,000	180,000	200,000
Sedimentation coefficient	7S	7S (9S, 11S, 13S)	19S	7S	8S
Biological half-life (days)	23**	6	5	2.8	2.4
Synthetic rate mg./kg./day	34	24	3.3	0.4	0.0023
% Intravascular	45	42	80	75	51
Biological function	principal serum antibody	secretory antibody	initial response to antigen	unknown	anaphylactic reaction

* The molecular weight of serum IgA is 170,000. Secretory IgA consists of two units of IgA combined with "secretory piece" (m.w. 385,000).
** Biologic half life of IgG is a function of serum concentration. T 1/2 is prolonged with low levels, shortened with high concentrations. Half-lives of other immunoglobulins are independent of serum concentrations.

antigen, are believed to be derived from a single clone of cells. Thus, a *clone* represents a population of cells all originating from a single common precursor; each cell in the clone is programmed to respond by elaborating the same antibody.

Immunoglobulins (Ig) are subdivided into five classes in order of decreasing concentrations: IgG, IgA, IgM, IgD, and IgE (Table 51-7). Most antibodies belong to the IgG class. Further separation of IgG proteins indicates that four distinct subclasses are present: IgG_1, IgG_2, IgG_3, and IgG_4. Each subclass has slightly different biological properties. For example, IgG_1 and IgG_3 are effective in activating complement by the classic pathway. By contrast, IgG_2 is only minimally active in this reaction, and IgG_4 does not activate the classic complement pathway.

Although IgA is the immunoglobulin in the second highest concentration in the serum, its chief function is in external secretions.[51] This immunoglobulin predominates in lacrimal, nasopharyngeal, salivary, respiratory, and gastrointestinal fluids. Plasma cells located submucosally in these organs synthesize and secrete this immunoglobulin, which is then linked to a small protein produced by the epithelial cells, called secretory piece, and the complex is secreted externally. Secretory IgA provides an important barrier against tissue invasion by many pathogens.

The largest immunoglobulin is IgM (macroglobulin), with a molecular weight of approximately 900,000 daltons. IgM constitutes the first detectable antibody synthesized following antigenic challenge. A sensitive relationship exists between the circulating levels of IgG and IgM antibodies. Specific IgM antibodies may facilitate the production of IgG antibodies; in turn, the latter inhibit the further production of IgM. The levels of IgG antibodies generally rise to high concentrations and persist for appreciably longer times than do those of the IgM class. There is little information about the function of IgD; it is present in only minute quantities in normal blood. IgE is responsible for allergic reac-

tions. This immunoglobulin binds to and remains fixed to mast cells for prolonged periods. Reactions between these antibodies and appropriate antigens (allergens) serve to induce the mast cell to release histamine and other mediators of the allergic response.

The structure of the immunoglobulin molecule has been well defined (Figure 51-4). Each unit consists of four polypeptide chains—two identical light chains (L chains) and two identical heavy chains (H chains), held together by disulfide bonds. Light chains may be of two types, designated kappa (κ) or lambda (λ), and are common. For IgG, IgA, IgM, IgD, and IgE, the heavy chains are respectively designated gamma (γ), alpha (α), mu (μ), delta (δ), and epsilon (ε).

Portions of the molecule are frequently defined by fragments generated after digestion with the enzyme papain. The Fab fragments, composed of the light chain and portions of the heavy chain, contain the antigen combining sites. The remaining portion of the heavy chain is designated the Fc fragment.

Each unit contains two antigen-combining sites. Antigen specificity is determined by the amino acid sequence of the Fab portion of both the light and the heavy chains. The portion of each chain that specifically reacts with the antigen is designated the "variable region"; the remainder is called the "constant" region. The antigen-specific portion of the immunoglobulin molecule is unique for antibodies derived from each clone of B cells; this portion has been termed the *idiotype*. The Fc fragment has important biologic functions; it determines properties such as complement fixation attachment to phagocytes and lymphocytes, skin fixation, and placental transfer.

The same basic structure is common to all immunoglobulin classes. IgG, IgD, and IgE are monomers of this unit.

The serum concentration of each class of immunoglobulin is determined by several factors: the rate of synthesis, the rate of elimination, and the distri-

FIG. 51-4. Basic structure of immunoglobulins. This monomer contains four polypeptide chains, two identical light chains and two identical heavy chains. The antibody combining site is made up of portions of both heavy and light chains.

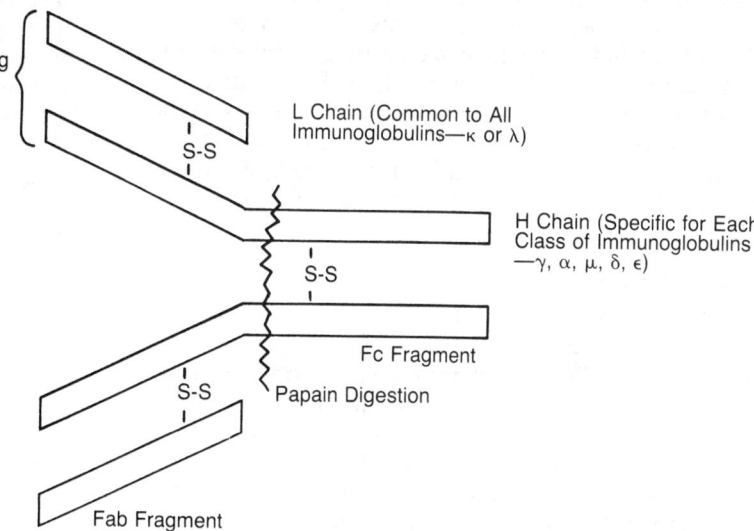

bution of immunoglobulin between the extra- and intravascular fluids. IgG, which is present in the highest concentration, has the longest half-life, 23 days, while both IgD and IgE are rapidly eliminated with half-lives of less than 3 days. IgM, because of its large molecular size, does not escape the vascular system in any significant amounts; therefore, more than 80% is intravascular. Except in the nephrotic syndrome, significant concentrations of immunoglobulins are not found in the urine.

FUNCTION OF IMMUNOGLOBULINS

In the maintenance of normal host defenses, immunoglobulins serve multiple functions. Of prime importance, they are essential in defense against polysaccharide-encapsulated pyogenic bacteria, particularly Streptococcus pneumoniae, Hemophilus influenzae, and Neisseria meningitidis. Antibody attachment to capsular antigens permits the fixation of activated complement components and phagocytosis. In addition, immunoglobulins neutralize soluble toxins (e.g., tetanus toxin); by similar processes, humoral antibodies can reduce the infectivity of viruses. Virus neutralization offers protection during the incubation phase; by contrast, these antibodies do not significantly alter the course of an established infection. IgA in external secretions may be particularly important in protection against respiratory and gastrointestinal pathogens. A recently described function for IgG is as a mediator for antibody dependent cellular cytotoxicity (ADCC). In these reactions, target cells coated with these antibodies are directly lysed by K cells (lymphocytes and/or monocytes). This form of cytolysis is independent of complement.

In an immunoglobulin-synthesizing plasma cell, the light and heavy chains are separately produced on different cytoplasmic polyribosomes. The rate-limiting factor in the production of antibody is the synthesis of the heavy chains. Light chains rapidly combine with heavy chains as the latter are formed, yielding a complete immunoglobulin molecule. In normal individuals, a balance exists between the production of light and heavy chains, so that there is virtually no excess of the former. In malignant diseases involving plasma cells, however, light chains may be synthesized in marked excess or, in some cases, exclusive of heavy chain production. Free light chains are rapidly and completely excreted in the urine.

COMPLEMENT

The complement system provides an important mechanism for amplifying inflammatory responses, particularly those involving humoral immune responses (Table 51-8).[52-55] There are at least 15 different complement components plus several known inhibitors; most, if not all, are synthesized by either macrophages or hepatic cells. The individual components normally circulate in an inactive form; activation results from

TABLE 51-8. BIOLOGICAL ACTIVITIES OF ACTIVATED COMPLEMENT COMPONENT

Activity	Complement Components
Chemotaxis	C3a, C5a, C567
Immune adherence	C3b
Anaphylatoxin (smooth muscle constriction, vasodilation, localized edema)	C3a, C5a
Viral neutralization	C1, C4, C2
Increased vascular permeability	C2
Cell lysis	C9, C8

limited proteolysis. In the activation of complement, one activated component often serves as the catalyst for the next factor; thus, activation proceeds as a cascade mechanism, much like that involved in blood clotting. During the process, activated factors not only serve as enzymes for subsequent reactions but also possess important biologic properties.

The biochemical reactions involved in activation can be conveniently subdivided into three groups—the *classic pathway*, the *alternate pathway*, and the *terminal pathway*. The first two serve to generate enzymes, termed C3 convertases, which activate the C3 component. Once activated C3 is generated, it triggers the terminal sequence of activation (C5 through C9) (Fig. 51-5).

CLASSIC PATHWAY

Antigen-antibody reactions involving IgM or IgG, particularly IgG_1 and IgG_3, serve to initiate complement activation through the classic pathway. In these, one molecule of IgM is capable of initiating the complement cascade, whereas two molecules of IgG are required. Furthermore, the IgG molecules must be spatially arranged such that they can combine with the first complement component. The first component in the classic system is a trimolecular complex termed C1. The binding of C1 to the Fc portion of IgG or Igm serves to generate an active enzyme, C1 esterase. In normal serum, there is a naturally occurring inhibitor, C1 esterase inhibitor; this factor is absent in patients with hereditary angioneurotic edema. Once formed, the C1 esterase catalyzes the proteolysis of two other components, C4 and C2, to their active forms. These components form a C42 complex, which is a potent C3 convertase. The next stage involves the activation of C3, the central component of the complement system, by C3 convertase. Proteolytic cleavage of C3 yields two fragments—C3b, which is primarily active when bound to cells or immune complexes, and C3a, which is present in the fluid phase.

ALTERNATE PATHWAY

It appears that two different C3 convertases are generated,[56] C3B and C3bBb. Alternate pathway activation can be effected by bacterial products (endotoxin), components of these cell walls (e.g., zymosam), or aggregated IgG₄, IgA, or IgE. It appears that, in normal individuals, there is an interaction between three components of the alternate pathway (factor B, factor D, and properdin) and C3 that leads to the formation of the slowly acting C3 convertase, C3B. This convertase serves to generate small amounts of C3b. The C3b then interacts with factors B and D, forming the complex C3bBb convertase; this is capable of rapidly converting large amounts of C3 into its active form. The complex is stabilized by the action of properdin. The formation of this convertase is regulated by two inhibitors, β1H and C3b inactivator. Normally, the inhibitory activity predominates; this limits the generation of this enzyme and the subsequent activation of the complement system. In the presence of one of the activating substances, however, the reaction is shifted to favor the formation of the C3 convertase. It is noteworthy that this system contains a positive feedback loop; the formation of C3b not only acts to initiate the terminal sequence of complement activation, but it also autocatalyzes the generation of additional convertase.

TERMINAL PATHWAY

This set of reactions initially serves to activate C5 by C3b. C5b, the bound component, fixes the last four components, C6 to 9, thereby completing the entire complement sequence. Thus, the terminal reactions depend on an activated C3; this can be achieved by either activation of the classic or alternate pathways.

BIOLOGICAL ACTIVITIES OF COMPLEMENT COMPONENTS

The complete sequence of complement activation results in target cell lysis (Table 51-8). The lytic activity is mediated predominantly by the C9 component; C8 also has weak lytic properties. Of greater importance, many of the intermediate components have significant biologic activities.[53,57,58] Of these, the cell or complex bound C3b is important in opsonization and subsequent phagocytosis. Several cells, including monocytes, neutrophils, erythrocytes, platelets, and B lymphocytes have receptors for C3b. Adherence results from the binding of a C3b coated particle to its receptor on phagocytes; this leads to particle ingestion and destruction. The function of C3b receptors on other cells is not known; it has been postulated that these receptors on B lymphocytes may serve an immunoregulatory function.

The C1, C4 and C2 components have viral neutralizing properties. Furthermore, a peptide derived from C2 has vasoactive properties; this component increases vascular permeability. The C3a and C5a components, along with the trimolecular complex C567, have chemotactic activities for neutrophils, eosinophils, and mononuclear cells. Thus, the presence of these factors serves to increase cellular exudation into

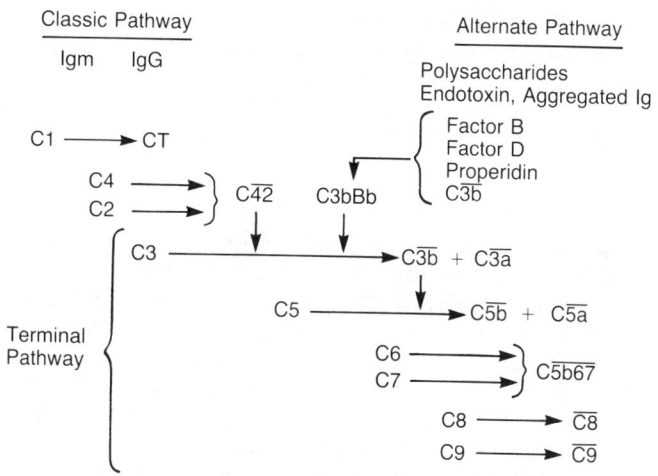

FIG. 51-5. *Schematic diagram of complement activation. A line over a complement component number indicates that component has been activated.*

areas of inflammation. Furthermore, both C3a and C5a have anaphylatoxic properties. These components induce histamine release from mast cells, which, in turn, causes increased vascular permeability, reduces arterial blood pressure, and causes smooth muscle contraction.

In addition, there are several links between activated complement components and blood coagulation. Products of coagulation are known to be a major component of inflammatory responses. Activation of C5, leading to the generation of C5a, causes the generation of tissue factors in neutrophils, which may initiate the clotting cascade through the extrinsic system. In addition, plasmin, the activating enzyme in the fibronolytic system, is capable of activating the complement sequence through both the classic and alternate pathways. The immediate activator of plasmin is Hageman factor (Factor XII), which also initiates the intrinsic clotting system.

The importance of complement in bacterial infections is illustrated by studies examining its role in the clearance of intravenous pneumococci in guinea pigs.[59] Immune guinea pigs clear these microorganisms at a greatly accelerated rate when compared with normal animals. Both IgM and IgG antipneumococcal antibodies can effect this phenomenon. If the classic pathway is inoperable, however, as in guinea pigs congenitally deficient in C4, IgM is unable to promote accelerated clearance. IgG-coated bacteria activate both the classic and alternate pathways; in animals deficient in C4, these organisms are removed from the circulation at a rate slightly greater than that measured in nonimmune animals. Neither antibody, however, is effective in guinea pigs in the absence of complement component C3. Additional studies suggest that activated C3b is primarily responsible for mediating this clearing phenomenon. Of the two antibodies, IgM is at least 10 times more potent than IgG, a finding that correlates with the observations that only one IgM molecule is required to activate complement, whereas two IgG molecules, spatially arranged to bind the first component, are required to recruit this host defense system.

COMPLEMENT-INDUCED GRANULOCYTE AGGREGATION

Jacobs et al. recently found that cellophane membranes, such as those used for hemodialysis, were capable of activating complement by the alternate pathway.[60] The C5a component generated in these reactions resulted in increased granulocyte adhesiveness. This caused the formation of circulating neutrophil aggregates, which can be trapped in the pulmonary microcirculation, leading to pulmonary dysfunction and arterial hypoxemia.

Preliminary studies suggest that a similar mechanism may be operative in the adult respiratory distress syndrome (ARDS, "shock-lung"). This syndrome occurs frequently in three groups of patients: those with gram-negative sepsis, those with severe trauma, and those with acute pancreatitis. In all three disorders, activated products of complement can be identified in the circulation. Correlative animal studies indicate that these components can induce neutrophil aggregation similar to that seen following exposure of blood to cellophane membranes. These leukoemboli deposit in the pulmonary vessels and help to initiate the pulmonary injury. It appears that neutrophils present in these emboli are activated, releasing toxic oxygen radicals, which mediate endothelial damage.[61] The end result is fluid exudation. It is of potential clinical importance that it may be possible to interrupt this sequence by massive doses of corticosteroids.

FIBRONECTIN

In the maintenance of internal homeostasis, the reticuloendothelial system has an essential function. This system, consisting of both fixed and mobilizable mononuclear phagocytes, acts as a highly discriminating clearing mechanism, removing endogenous cellular debris, denatured proteins, effete cells, and numerous particulates. A major component of the reticuloendothelial system consists of fixed or sessile phagocytic cells lining vascular channels. The chief elements of this system are localized to the liver (Kupffer cells), spleen, and bone marrow. These cells monitor the circulation for blood-borne toxins and particulate matter and effect their removal. The activity of the fixed reticuloendothelial system is compromised in many medical and surgical illnesses; furthermore, defective function has been postulated as a factor contributing to the syndrome of multiple organ failure, a sequela of many severe illnesses.[62–65]

The function of the reticuloendothelial system is, in part, governed by a circulating protein, *plasma fibronectin*, also termed cold insoluble globulin or opsonic α_2SB glycoprotein.[63,65,66] This factor can coat particulate substances such as cellular debris, denatured collagen, fibrin monomers, and certain bacteria. As a result, the coated particles adhere to reticuloendothelial cells, a process that appears to initiate phagocytosis and subsequent destruction. The major site of particulate clearance is the liver. The action of fibronectin is independent of immune reactants, including complement.

The concentration of plasma fibronectin correlates with the activity of the reticuloendothelial system as measured by the clearance of test particles. Particulate clearance and fibronectin concentrations are depressed in patients with severe bacterial infections, advanced malignancies, diseases of aberrant immunity, disseminated intravascular coagulation, severe trauma, and extensive burns and in those undergoing major surgery.[63,67] Reduced plasma fibronectin concentrations may result in depressed reticuloendothelial clearance of toxic materials. The concentration of these harmful substances would then build up in the circulation and, through processes that are not well understood, promote formation of microthrombi in such organs as the lungs and kidneys. These initiate reactions that can contribute to damage to vascular integrity and the accumulation of extravascular fluid. The end result is multiple organ dysfunction including pulmonary and renal failure and disturbances in peripheral microvascular circulation.[68]

Fibronectin is an α_2 globulin with a total molecular weight of approximately 450,000 daltons. Binding sites on the molecule have been identified for denatured collagen, Staphylococcus aureus fibrin, and actin. There is also a portion of the molecule that is capable of reacting with receptors on macrophages and probably also on neutrophils.[65]

The potential clinical importance of fibronectin is suggested by uncontrolled studies in which cryoprecipitates of fresh plasma are infused into patients with trauma and burns and into surgical patients with sepsis.[63] This therapy is associated with prompt correction in plasma opsonizing activity. Several beneficial systemic changes are detected, including improvement in pulmonary function and increased limb perfusion. An infusion of cryoprecipitates restores levels of fibronectin to normal for 1 to 2 days. It has not yet been established that this form of therapy will increase survival or if the observed effects are entirely due to fibronectin.

HOST DEFENSE DEFECTS ASSOCIATED WITH SURGERY, TRAUMA AND BURNS

Numerous studies indicate that a generalized impairment in host defense mechanisms occurs in traumatized patients, those with extensive burns, and those undergoing major operative procedures. Furthermore, the magnitude of the defects closely correlates with the risks of infection and may be related to the overall death rates. It should be recognized, however, that the precise relationship between measurable abnormalities and infectious complications is not well defined. In some circumstances, the defects appear to be epiphenomena rather than a true pathogenic factor.

One correlation that has been noted is that the preoperative status of cellular immunity, as defined by delayed hypersensitivity skin tests, has been found to relate to both the risk of sepsis and mortality in surgical patients.[69] Patients who are anergic preoperatively or who lose reactivity during the postoperative period show a greatly increased incidence of severe infection and a higher mortality than reactive individuals. Similar findings have been reported in burn patients; again, anergy is closely related to both morbidity and mortality. In these two patient groups, it is difficult to define a cause-and-effect relationship because infections are generally not due to intracellular organisms. More likely, both anergy and susceptibility to infections are manifestations of an underlying and, at present, undefined abnormality.

In traumatized, burned, and postoperative patients, several other specific host defense abnormalities have been identified. Immunoglobulin levels appear to be transiently reduced,[70,71] however, antibody responses are usually not depressed.[72,73] Furthermore, the immunologlobulin levels rapidly return to normal. Similarly, the complement components are reduced for only brief periods except in patients with sepsis.[71,74] More significant abnormalities in various parameters of cellular immunity, reticuloendothelial clearance functions,[63,75] and neutrophil activities[76–81] have been identified. With respect to the cell-mediated responses, most studies suggest reduced levels of circulating T cells,[82–84] decreased in vitro lymphoproliferative responses,[85,86] and abnormalities of effector cell functions such as cell-mediated cytotoxicity. There is a general correlation between the extent of the injury and the cellular abnormalities; similarly, defects in one or more parameters tend to correlate with increased rates of sepsis and mortality.

SERUM INHIBITOR EFFECTORS

Increasing evidence suggests that a spectrum of cellular responses is regulated by circulating serum factors.[87,87a] Furthermore, it appears that in severely ill patients the concentrations of these inhibitory factors are often increased, and these may be of major importance in the generalized suppression of host defense mechanisms. Several circulating inhibitors, such as alphafetoprotein, C reactive protein, and inhibitory lipoproteins, have been identified; the specific role of each is unclear at present. In most circumstances, it appears that inhibitors are normally circulating substances that increase markedly during stressful events.

IMMUNOREGULATORY ALPHA GLOBULIN (IRA)

Of the serum inhibitory factors, one of the best characterized is immunoregulatory alpha globulin. This polypeptide has been found to be present in trace amounts in normal sera; its concentrations are strikingly elevated in several groups of severely ill patients and correlate closely with the anergic state. It is characterized as a low molecular weight protein ($< 10,000$ daltons) that exists in the circulation bound to an α_2 globulin.[88]

Immunologic studies indicate that IRA will suppress many T cell functions in experimental animals. Administration prolongs skin allograft survival,[89] inhibits antibody production to sheep erythrocytes (a thymic-dependent antigen),[90] reduces elaboration of migration inhibition factor, and suppresses lymphocyte mediated cytotoxicity.[91] It does not appear to affect responses to T independent antigens. IRA is maximally immunosuppressive in experimental models if given prior to or simultaneously with the antigen. By contrast, it has comparatively little activity if administered in the interval following antigen stimulation.

In clinical studies, IRA is usually assessed by its ability to inhibit lymphoproliferative responses to PHA. It also impairs reactivity to other nonspecific mitogens, allogeneic cells (MLC reactions), and specific antigens. Studies have shown that IRA will bind weakly to T lymphocytes. It is not, however, cytotoxic for these cells. IRA levels are markedly elevated in severely traumatized patients, regardless of the cause of the injury.[92] Furthermore, increased concentrations can be closely related to the anergic state. Similar data have been reported in patients with burns;[93] again, the extent of the burn is correlated with the development of abnormally high levels of IRA. It is also increased in anergic patients with cancer.[94]

SUPPRESSOR CELLS

Another potential mediator of the impaired immune responsiveness seen in traumatized patients is suppressor cells. These elements negatively regulate immune responses, and, in many clinical states, excessive inhibitory activity has been noted. There appear to be several types of cells capable of mediating suppression; these include both T lymphocytes[95,96] and macrophages.[97] Both types have been shown to be activated in the suppression seen in injured patients. In addition, B lymphocytes may also be involved in mediating inhibitory activities; these cells have been found to provide an activating stimulus for suppressor T cells.[98,99] To date, the relative importance of each of the various types of inhibitory cells has not been defined, and whether there is a subpopulation of cells with a suppressor function exclusively is not established.

A study in burn patients interrelated serum suppressor factors, reduction in the PHA responses of patient's lymphocytes, and the presence of suppressor cells with both sepsis and mortality.[100] Several notable findings were apparent. Most (15 of 18 patients) developed serum inhibitory activity. This usually appeared during the first week after the burn and reached a peak between the second and third week. It appeared before systemic infection. The presence of inhibitory serum, however, did not prove highly discriminatory in distinguishing patients who were to develop infections, nor did it define the group likely to succumb to the injury. In contrast, reduced response of autologous lymphocytes to PHA was a sensitive predictor of both sepsis and mortality. Furthermore, this decrease in mitogenic reactivity correlated with the presence of nonadherent suppressor cells, presumably T cells.

HOST DEFENSE FAILURES IN MEDICAL ILLNESSES

Systemic failure of host defense mechanisms may occur physiologically in association with the aging process, pathologically as a complication of many acute and chronic illnesses, and iatrogenically as a result of the administration of drugs capable of altering resistance. In most circumstances, multiple protective mechanisms are simultaneously compromised. Thus, it is common to find concomitant defects in both phagocytic and immune mechanisms. As in surgical patients, the immediate consequence of compromised defense systems is an increased risk of serious infection.

In diseases that affect primarily one host defense mechanism, there is an excellent correlation between the defect and the susceptibility to specific infection (Table 51-9). For example, patients with primary hypogammaglobulinemia are at great risk to develop overwhelming respiratory infections from Streptococcus pneumoniae and Hemophilus influenzae. These organisms are also the principal causes of infections in patients with untreated malignancies involving B lymphocytes (chronic lymphocytic leukemia, multiple myeloma, macroglobulinemia); this group of neoplasms is characterized by a failure to synthesize polyclonal humoral antibodies. By contrast, patients with Hodgkin's disease show a primary failure of cell-mediated immune responses and often develop infections from a variety of intracellular pathogens. These patients frequently develop fatal illnesses due to listeria, salmonella, cytomegalovirus, cryptococcus, nocardia and mycobacteria. As noted, granulocytopenic patients are highly susceptible to gram-negative bacteremia.

A major factor causing defective host defenses is drugs, particularly corticosteroids and cancer chemotherapeutic agents. Steroids have a wide range of

TABLE 51-9. PRINCIPAL MICROBIAL PATHOGENS IN IMMUNOCOMPROMISED HOSTS

Granulo-cytopenia	Hypogamma-globulinemia	Suppressed Cell-mediated Immunity
Escherichia coli	Streptococcus pneumoniae	Mycobacterium tuberculosis
Klebsiella pneumoniae	Hemophilus influenzae	Listeria monocytogenes
Pseudomonas aeruginosa	Neisseria meningitidis	Salmonella sp.
Staphylococcus aureus		Nocardia sp.
Candida albicans		Herpes simplex
Aspergillus sp.		Herpes zoster
		Cytomegalovirus
		Cryptococcus neoformans
		Candida albicans
		Toxoplasma gondii
		Pneumocystis carinii
		Strongyloides stercoralis

effects on host defense systems;[101,102] in essence, virtually all protective components are impaired (Table 51-10). With respect to the blood leukocytes, these agents cause neutrophilia, lymphopenia, monocytopenia, and eosinopenia. The increase in blood neutrophils results from release of cells from marrow storage pools, from demargination, and from a decreased rate of egression of cells from the blood into tissue sites. It is not the result of accelerated production. The inability of circulating cells to escape from the vascular compartment limits their ability to gain access to inflammatory sites, a detrimental effect.

Changes in normal blood lymphocytes appear to result from altered circulation, not from after lympholysis. Studies indicate that after a single large dose of steroids, blood lymphocytes decrease to a nadir, which is reached after 4 to 6 hours. This reduction is caused by sequestration of these cells in the marrow and other lymphoid tissues. The decrease in circulating lymphocytes is transient; by 24 hours, the lymphocyte count has returned to normal. T cells, primarily T helper cells, show the most pronounced decreases. The changes in blood monocytes and eosinophils also appear to result from sequestration.

Anergy is frequently associated with steroid therapy. The factors leading to the inability to respond to cutaneous antigens are not fully known. It appears that therapy with high doses of steroids for 10 to 14 days is usually required to cause this immune failure. Of importance, the inability to mount a delayed hypersensitivity response is often associated with widespread infections by intracellular pathogens; for example, steroid therapy can lead to reactivation of tuberculosis.

Another important effect of steroids is to block reticuloendothelial functions. This activity is used therapeutically in the treatment of autoimmune blood dyscrasias, in which the steroids act primarily to reduce the phagocytosis of antibody-coated particles (e.g., red cells coated with IgG antibodies). This effect, how-

TABLE 51-10. EFFECTS OF CORTICOSTEROIDS

1. Cellular changes
   A. Transient increase in neutrophils
      (1) Demargination
      (2) Release from bone marrow
      (3) Decreased egress into inflammatory sites
   B. Lymphocytes
      (1) Not lympholytic
      (2) Decrease in blood lymphocytes due to seques-
          tration
      (3) Recovery within 24 hrs
      (4) T helper cells maximally affected
   C. Monocytopenia
   D. Eosinopenia
2. Immune responses
   A. Cellular
      (1) Decreased reactivity to skin tests
      (2) Increased risk of disseminating intracellular infec-
          tions
   B. Humoral
      (1) Slow decrease in immunoglobulin production
      (2) No acute changes in antibody titers
3. Phagocytic functions
   A. Decreased reticuloendothelial function
   B. Decreased microbial killing
   C. Decreased responses to lymphokines
   D. Stabilizing of lysosomal membranes (anti-inflamma-
      tory)

ever, may be detrimental to the host, as these drugs simultaneously decrease the clearance of bacteria and can reduce the killing of intracellular pathogens. The anti-inflammatory activities of steroids on cellular immune responses are multifactorial; migration of T cells and monocytes into inflammatory sites, decreased release of lymphokines and blocking of the activities of these mediators on monocytes all appear to occur. It is obvious that these effects in vivo compromise this host defense mechanism, thereby increasing susceptibility to overwhelming infections.

Cytotoxic drugs, such as those used in the treatment of neoplasms, also alter host defense mechanisms.[103] These drugs have the potential for killing any replicating cell line. They affect, to varying degrees, hematopoietic and lymphoid cells, gastrointestinal epithelial cells, and gonadal cells. The most common cause of infection in patients receiving cytotoxic therapy is a decrease in granulocytes. Typically, the nadir of the granulocyte count is seen 10 to 14 days after a single large therapeutic dose. Long-term therapy with cytotoxic drugs can also predispose to a wide variety of infections, including those caused by intracellular organisms. This effect has been attributed to the chronic suppression of immune defense mechanisms. Patients on long-term cytotoxic drugs also appear to be predisposed to development of malignancies.

AIDS

Although the acquired immunodeficiency syndrome (AIDS) and human immunodeficiency virus (HIV)

type 1 infection are covered in depth in Chapter 50, the cytopathic effects should be mentioned here. The ability of the HIV-1 virus to injure the CD4+ subset of human T lymphocytes is an important contribution to the state of profound immunodeficiency resulting from the infection. The total count becomes progressively reduced because of multiple pathologic processes. The protection from the usual immune mechanisms of viral destruction causes inability to contain or reverse active disease, and results in myriad destructive infections.

TRANSPLANT PATIENTS

Recipients of organ transplants have chronically impaired immune defense mechanisms. These patients require long-term therapy with immunosuppressive drugs to inhibit graft rejection mechanisms. The agents currently used, however, do not selectively inhibit those responses directed at the transplant organ. Rather, they act nonspecifically to suppress a wide range of immune response and also alter other protective mechanisms such as phagocytosis. In transplanted patients, two major complications of therapy have been recognized—the susceptibility to infection and the increased risk of malignancies.

Studies in renal transplant patients suggest a typical time table that characterizes the infectious complications.[104] In the first post-transplant month, the major causes of infection are bacterial. The period between 1 and 6 months is most critical in terms of life-threatening infections. This time interval coincides with the maximum use of immunosuppressive drugs. During this period, transplant patients are particularly prone to develop infections from a wide range of opportunistic organisms. One common infecting organism is cytomegalovirus (CMV); clinical or laboratory evidence of CMV infections can be found in 60 to 96% of transplant patients. A lower risk is seen in the late transplant period (after 6 months); this is probably related to the lesser amounts of immunosuppression required for graft survival. These individuals, however, are still prone to viral infections, particularly hepatitis and CMV, and opportunistic organisms such as Cryptococcus neoformans.

There is a greatly increased risk of malignancy in transplant patients receiving immunosuppressive drugs. The incidence of de novo neoplasms is approximately 100 times that in age-matched controls. Two types of malignancies predominate: skin cancers and lymphomas. Lymphoid tumors are most commonly of the histiocytic or immunoblastic cell types. Not infrequently, these tumors involve the central nervous system, a site not commonly affected by the usual types of lymphomas.

SPLENECTOMY

Splenectomized patients are at risk for severe sepsis, a syndrome termed overwhelming post-splenectomy syndrome (OPSI).[105] The vast majority of episodes of OPSI occur within 3 years of splenectomy, but cases can occur many years afterward. The overall risk of OPSI ranges from 1 to 25%, depending on the underlying condition for which the splenectomy was performed. The risk is greatest in patients splenectomized for diffuse disease of the reticuloendothelial system, such as thalassemia and lymphoreticular malignancy. It also occurs, however, in patients without underlying illnesses, such as those splenectomized for trauma.[106] The most common infecting organism is Streptococcus pneumoniae (approximately 50%); this is followed by Hemophilus influenzae, Neisseria meningitidis, Escherichia coli, other streptococci, and staphylococci.

Patients with this syndrome may present with nonspecific symptoms and low-grade fever. There may be no evidence of localized infection. Of great clinical significance, the syndrome has a fulminant course; within hours, the patient may develop shock and die. The overal mortality of OPSI is greater than 50%. Two factors appear to be responsible for the rapidity of this syndrome—the loss of the splenic reticuloendothelial function and a decrease in immunoglobulin synthesis, particularly IgM. As a result, the concentration of bacteria in the peripheral blood is dramatically increased; it may reach levels as high as 10^6 organisms/μL. Furthermore, the huge numbers of circulating organisms can initiate the syndrome of disseminated intravascular coagulation (DIC); this may be the immediate cause of the multiple organ failure complicating OPSI.

Because of the potential for overwhelming sepsis, splenectomized patients who present with fever should be treated empirically with intravenous antibiotics even before culture results are available. Ampicillin plus tobramycin covers the major pathogens responsible for OPSI.

Patients should be vaccinated with pneumococcal and meningococcal vaccine at least 2 weeks before splenectomy if possible. No convincing evidence exists that prophylactic antibiotics are effective in preventing OPSI. Hospitals that keep records of splenectomized patients have been advised by the CDC to alert such patients to possible complications.

MALNUTRITION

Nutritional status has a profound effect on immune function.[107,108] Numerous studies have demonstrated that chronic protein-calorie malnutrition (PCM) exerts a suppressive effect on the functions of T lymphocytes.

TABLE 51-11. SELECTED IMMUNOMODULATORS
Bacille Calmette-Guerin (BCG)
Killed Corynebacterium parvum
Brucella abortus extract (Bru-Pel)
Muramyl dipeptide (MDP)
Transfer factor
Interferon

Delayed hypersensitivity reactions, lymphocyte proliferative responses to mitogens and antigens, and T cell-dependent antibody responses are all decreased by PCM. B lymphocyte and macrophage function tend to be less severely affected. Antibody levels in malnourished individuals may be normal, or if infection is present, increased. However, neutrophil bactericidal activity has been shown to be decreased in PCM. Geriatric patients are particularly susceptible to immune impairment from nutritional deficiency or impaired intake or absorption (see Chap. 60).

Immune suppression has also been documented in deficiencies of trace elements such as zinc and copper, and certain vitamins such as thiamine and folate. As with PCM, T lymphocyte function is affected most. In all of these conditions, replacement of the deficient nutritional component results in restoration of immune function.

By contrast, certain nutritional abnormalities may result in enhanced immune function. Short-term starvation has been shown, in both laboratory and clinical situations, to increase resistance to infection. Similarly, protein and calorie deprivation may prevent the onset of autoimmune phenomena and inhibit tumor growth in laboratory animals. The clinical importance of these findings remains to be determined.

IMMUNOMODULATION

Attempts to modify the immune system began as early as Koch's work with extracts of *Mycobacterium tuberculosis*. Although his protocols aimed at treating clinical tuberculosis with mycobacterial extracts failed, his work stimulated a large number of trials aimed at enhancing beneficial immune responses (Table 51-11).[109,110] Intravenous immune globulin has been used extensively, but its exact role is still not clear. Definite indications, apart from immunodeficiency states, are acute autoimmune thrombocytopenia and Kawasaki's syndrome. There is a basis for use in some cases of myasthenia gravis, chronic demyelinating polyneuropathy (Guillain-Barré syndrome), HIV infection in children, asthma in some children, juvenile rheumatoid arthritis, and possibly recurrent abortion.[113]

It is important to realize that immunomodulators can enhance immune functions in different ways. For example, many agents, such as Corynebacterium parvum and muramyl dipeptide (MDP), act as adjuvants, enhancing antibody responses to antigens.

Macrophage function can be enhanced either directly or indirectly by agents such as extracts of brucella and MDP. Administration of these components to experimental animals affords protection against tumors and a variety of microbial pathogens. Similarly, interferon stimulates both macrophage and NK cell tumoricidal activity. Purified interferon is currently undergoing trials as an antitumor and antiviral agent.

Although immunomodulators hold promise, none is currently licensed for clinical use. Problems with their administration include their toxic side effects, their inability to alter the courses of established tumors or infections, and their lack of specificity.

More research and interest in these possibilities have come about through work done on AIDS and various approaches to treatment, most still largely unsuccessful.[111] In terms of wounds, however, the epidermal growth factor is an immunomodulator that has shown promise in enhancing wound healing.[112]

MEDICOLEGAL PEARLS

- A relevant case involved a granulocytopenic 45-year-old woman after cytotoxic medication for breast cancer. Treatment was delayed and she was erroneously considered "terminal." This led to her death and a large court settlement.

- In another case, not detecting prior splenectomy resulted in failure to diagnose fulminant pneumococcal sepsis in a 40-year-old man. He died, and the resulting lawsuit was settled for a large amount.

- Delay in diagnosis and treatment of meningococcemia has resulted in numerous lawsuits, particularly in immunosuppressed individuals.

- Inability to correlate an enormous increase in "band" cells (30%) led to false security in a septic patient with peritonitis. The white blood count was only slightly elevated, most likely from a "consumption" phenomenon.

- Neutropenia may mute signs of inflammation, and extremely severe pneumonia may not be clearly indicated on chest x rays. One case involved failure to recognize such results of decreased immunologic response.

REFERENCES

1. Meakins, J.L.: Clinical importance of host resistance to infection in surgical patients. Adv. Surg. 15:225, 1981.
2. Wing, E.J., and Remington, J.S.: Lymphocytes and macrophages. In Mandell, G.L., Douglas, R.G., Jr., and Bennett, J.E. (eds.): Principles and Practices of Infectious Diseases. New York, John Wiley and Sons, 1979, pp. 83–103.
3. Winkelstein, A., and Rabin, B.S.: Lymphocyte biology. Bull. Rheum. Dis. 25:816, 1975.
4. Cantor, H., and Boyse, E.A.: Regulation of immune response by T-cell subclasses. Contemp. Top. Immunol. 7:47, 1977.
5. Chess, L., and Schlossman, S.F.: Human lymphocyte subpopulations. Adv. Immunol. 25:213, 1977.
6. Moretta, L., Mingari, M.C., and Moretta, A.: Human T-cell subpopulations in normal and pathologic conditions. Immunol. Rev. 45:163, 1979.
7. Reinherz, E.L., and Schlossman, S.F.: Regulation of immune response—inducer and suppressor T-lymphocyte subsets in human beings. N. Engl. J. Med. 303:370, 1980.
8. Winkelstein, A.: The anatomy and physiology of lymphocytes. In Lichtman, M.A. (ed.): The Science and Practice of Clinical Medicine, Vol. 6: Hematology and Oncology. New York, Grune and Stratton, 1980, pp. 165–168.
9. Cohen, S., Mayer, M., Pick, E., et al.: Current state of studies of mediators of cellular immunity: A progress report. Cell Immunol. 33:233, 1977.
10. Rocklin, R.E., Bendtzen, K., and Greineder, D.: Mediators of immunoty: Lymphokines and monokines. Adv. Immunol. 29:56, 1980.
10a. Kaufmann, S.H.: Which + cells are relevant to resistance against Listeria monocytogenes infection? Adv. Exp. Med. Biol. 239:135, 1988.
11. Mackaness, G.B.: Cellular resistance to infection. J. Exp. Med. 116:381, 1962.
12. Mackaness, G.B.: The monocyte in cellular immunity. Semin. Hematol. 7:172, 1970.
13. Rosenstreich, D.L.: The macrophage. In Oppenheim, J.J., Rosenstreich, D.L., and Potter, M. (eds.): Cellular Functions in Immunity and Inflammation. New York, Elsevier/North Holland, 1981, pp. 127–159.
13a. Siegel, J.P.: Effects of interferon on the activation of human "+" lymphocytes. Cell Immuno. 111:461, 1988.
13b. Horohov, D.W., and Siegal, J.B.: Lymphokines—Progress and promise. Drugs 33:289, 1987.
14. Cerottini, J.C., and Brunner, K.T.: Cell-mediated cytotoxicity, allograft rejection and tumor immunity. Adv. Immunol. 18:67, 1974.
15. Allison, A.C., and Ferluga, J.: How lymphocytes kill tumor cells. N. Engl. J. Med. 295:165, 1976.
16. Herberman, R.B., Djeu, J.Y., Kay, H.D., et al.: Natural killer cells: Characteristics and regulation of activity. Immunol. Rev. 44:43, 1979.
17. Herberman, R.B., and Ortaldo, J.R.: Natural killer cells: Their role in defenses against disease. Science 214:24, 1981.
18. Lovchik, J.C., and Hong, R.: Antibody dependent cell-mediated cytolysis (ADCC): Analysis and projections. Prog. Allergy 22:1, 1977.
19. Nelson, D.L.: Cell-mediated cytotoxicity. In Oppenheim, J.J., Rosenstreich, D.L., and Potter, M. (eds.): Cellular Functions in Immunity and Inflammation. New York, Elsevier/North Holland, 1981, pp. 187–205.
20. The International Chronic Granulomatous Disease Study Group: A controlled trial of Interferon gamma to prevent infection in chronic granulomatous disease. N. Engl. J. Med. 324:8, 1991.
21. Robbins, D.L., and Gershwin, M.E.: Identification and characterization of lymphocyte subpopulations. Semin. Arthritis Rheum. 7:245–277, 1978.
22. Kunkel, H.G.: Surface markers of human lymphocytes. Johns Hopkins Med. J. 137:216, 1975.
23. Reinhenz, E.L., Kung, P.C., Goldstein, G., et al.: Separation of functional subsets of human T cells by a monoclonal antibody. Proc. Natl. Acad. Sci. U.S.A. 76:4061, 1979.
24. Bach, M.A., and Bach, J.F.: The use of monoclonal anti-T cell antibodies to study T-cell imbalances in human diseases. Clin. Exp. Immunol. 45:449, 1981.
25. Winkelstein, A.: Lymphocytosis and lymphopenia. In Lichtman, M.A., (ed.): The Science and Practice of Clinical Medicine. Vol. 6: Hematology and Oncology. New York, Grune and Stratton, 1980, pp. 168–171.
26. Rowlands, D.T., Jr., and Daniele, R.P.: Surface receptors in the immune response. N. Engl. J. Med. 293:26, 1975.

27. Nussenzweig, V.: Receptors for immune complexes on lymphocytes. Adv. Immunol. *19*:217, 1974.
28. Moretta, L., Ferrarini, M., and Cooper, M.D.: Characterization of human T-cell subpopulations as defined by specific receptors for immunoglobulin. Contemp. Top. Immunobiol. *8*:19, 1978.
29. Rose, N.R., and Friedman, H. (eds.): Manual of Clinical Immunology. Washington, D.C., American Society of Microbiology, 1980.
30. Wing, E.J., and Remington, J.S.: Delayed hypersensitivity and macrophage functions. *In* Fudenberg, H.H., Stites, D.P., Caldwell, J.L., et al. (eds.): Basic and Clinical Immunology. 3rd ed. Los Altos, CA, Lange Medical Publications, 1980, pp. 129–143.
31. Cohn, Z.A.: The activation of mononuclear phagocytes: Fact, fancy, and future. J. Immunola. *121*:813, 1978.
32. Karnovsky, M.L., and Lazdins, J.K.: Biochemical criteria for activated macrophages. J. Immunol. *121*:809, 1978.
33. North, R.J.: The concept of the activated macrophage. J. Immunol. *121*:806, 1978.
34. Snyderman, R., and Mergenhagen, S.E.: Chemotaxis of macrophages. *In* Nelson, D.S. (ed.): Immunobiology of the Macrophage. New York, Academic Press, 1976, pp. 323–349.
35. Griffin, F.M., Jr., Griffin, J.A., and Silverstein, S.C.: Studies on the mechanism of phagocytosis. II. The interaction of macrophages with anti-immunoglobulin IgG-coated bone marrow-derived lymphocytes. J. Exp. Med. *144*:788, 1976.
36. Densen, P., and Mandell, G.L.: Phagocyte strategy vs. microbial tactics. Rev. Infect. Dis. *2*:817, 1980.
37. Babior, B.M.: Oxygen-dependent microbial killing by phagocytes. N. Engl. J. Med. *298*:659, 721, 1978.
38. Adams, D.O., Meitzer, M.S., and Nathan, C.F.: Macrophage activation and secretion: A mini symposium. Fed. Proc. *41*:2193, 1982.
39. Unanue, E.R., and Rosenthal, A.S. (eds.): Macrophage Regulation of Immunity. New York, Academic Press, 1980.
40. Nathan, C.F., Murray, H.W., and Cohn, Z.A.: The macrophage as an effector cell. N. Engl. J. Med. *303*:622, 1980.
40a. Beutler, B. and Carami A.: The biology of cachetin (TNF)— A primary mediator of the host response. Ann. Rev. Immun. *7*:625, 1989.
41. Cline, M.J., Lehrer, R.I., Territo, M.C., et al.: Monocytes and macrophages: Functions and diseases. Ann. Intern. Med. *88*:78, 1978.
42. Densen, P.: Granulocytic phagocytes. *In* Mandell, G.L., Douglas, R.G., Jr., and Bennett, J.E., (eds.): Principles and Practice of Infectious Diseases. New York, John Wiley and Sons, 1979, pp. 63–82.
43. Walker, R.I., and Willenze, R.: Neutrophil kinetics and the regulation of granulopoiesis. Rev. Infect. Dis. *2*:282, 1980.
44. Gallin, J.I.: Abnormal phagocytic chemotaxis: Pathophysiology, clinical manifestations and management of patients. Rev. Infect. Dis. *3*:1196, 1981.
44a. Albelda, S.M., and Buck, C.A.: Integrins and other cell adhesion molecules. F.A.S.E.B. J. *4*:2868, 1990.
45. Root, R.K., and Cohen, M.S.: The microbicidal mechanisms of human neutrophils and eosinophils. Rev. Infect. Dis. *3*:565, 1981.
46. Schimpff, S.C.: Therapy of infection in patients with granulocytopenia. Med. Clin. North Am. *61*:1101, 1977.
46a. Pizzo, P.A., Hathorn, J.W., Hieninz, J. et al.: A randomized trial comparing ceftazidime alone with combination antibiotics in cancer patients with fever and neutropenia. N. Engl. J. Med. *315*:552, 1986.
47. Young, L.S.: Prophylactic granulocytes in the neutropenic host. Ann. Intern. Med. *96*:240, 1982.
47a. Mitsuyasu, R.T., and Golde, D.W.: Clinical role of granulocyte-macrophage colony stimulating factor. Hematol. Oncol. Clin. North Am. *3*:411, 1989.
47b. The International Granulomatous Disease Study Group: A Phase III study establishing efficacy of human recombinant interferon for infection prophylaxis in chronic granulomatous disease. N. Engl. J. Med. *324*:509, 1991.

48. Natvig, J.B., and Kunkel, H.G.: Human immunoglobulins. Classes, subclasses, genetic variants, and idiotypes. Adv. Immunol. *16*:1, 1973.
49. Solomon, A., and McLaughlin, C.L.: Immunoglobulin structure determined from products of plasma cell neoplasms. Semin. Hematol. *10*:3, 1973.
50. Spiegelberg, H.L.: Biological activities of immunoglobulins of different classes and subclasses. Adv. Immunol. *19*:259, 1974.
51. Waldman, R.H., and Ganguly, R.: Role of immune mechanisms on secretory surfaces in prevention of infection. *In* Allen, J.C. (ed.): Infection and the Compromised Host. Baltimore, Williams & Wilkins Co., 1976, pp. 29–48.
52. Cooper, N.R.: The complement system. *In* Fudenberg, H.H., Stites, D.P., Caldwell, J.L., et al. (eds.): Basic and Clinical Immunology. 3rd ed. Los Altos, CA, Lange Medical Publications. 1980, pp. 83–95.
53. Ruddy, S., Gigli, I., and Austen, K.F.: The complement system of man. N. Engl. J. Med. *287*:489, 545, 592, 642, *1972*.
54. Sandberg, A.L.: Complement. *In* Oppenheim, J.J., Rosenstreich, D.L., and Potter, M. (eds.): Cellular Functions in Immunity and Inflammation. New York, Elsevier/North Holland Publishers, pp. 397–410, 1981.
55. Spitzer, R.E.: The complement system. Pediatr. Clin. North Am. *24*:341, 1977.
56. Fearon, D.T., and Austin, K.F.: Current concepts in immunology: The alternative pathway of complement—a system for host resistance to microbial infections. N. Engl. J. Med. *303*:259, 1980.
57. Agnello, V.: Complement deficiency states. Medicine *57*:1, 1978.
58. Schur, P.H.: Complement testing in the diagnosis of immune and autoimmune diseases. Am. J. Clin. Pathol. *68*:647, 1977.
59. Brown, E.J., Hosea, S.W., Hammer, C.H., et al.: A quantitative analysis of the interactions of antipneumococcal antibody and complement in experimental pneumococcal bacteremia. J. Clin. Invest. *69*:85, 1982.
60. Jacob, H.S., Craddock, P.R., Hammerschmidt, D.E., et al.: Complement-induced granulocyte aggregation. N. Engl. J. Med. *302*:789, 1980.
61. Hammerschmidt, D.E., Harris, P.D., Wayland, J.H., et al.: Complement-induced granulocyte aggregation in vivo. Am. J. Pathol. *102*:146, 1981.
62. Kaplan, J.E., and Saba, T.M.: Humoral deficiency and reticuloendothelial depression after traumatic shock. Am. J. Physiol. *230*:7, 1976.
63. Saba, T.M., and Jaffe, E.: Plasma fibronectin (opsonic glycoprotein): Its synthesis by vascular endothelial cells and role in cardiopulmonary integrity after trauma as related to reticuloendothelial function. Am. J. Med. *68*:577, 1980.
64. Scovill, W.A., Saba, T.M., Kaplan, J.E., et al.: Deficits in reticuloendothelial humoral control mechanisms in patients after trauma. J. Trauma *16*:898, 1976.
65. Mosher, D.F.: Fibronectin. Progr. Hemos. Thromb. *5*:111, 1980.
66. Pearlstein, E., Gold, L.I., and Garcia-Pardo, A.: Fibronectin: A review of its structure and biological activity. Mol. Cell. Biochem. *29*:103, 1980.
67. Lanser, M.E., and Saba, T.M.: Opsonic fibronectin deficiency and sepsis. Ann. Surg. *195*:340, 1982.
68. Sata, T.M.: Disturbances in plasma and cell surface fibronectin: Relationship to altered vascular permeability and host defense. J. Trauma *21*:679, 1981.
69. Christou, N.V., Meakins, J.L., and MacLean, L.D.: The predictive role of delayed hypersensitivity in preoperative patients. Surg. Gynecol. Obstet. *152*:297, 1981.
70. Arturson, G., Hogman, C.F., Johnsson, S.G.O., et al.: Changes in immunoglobulin levels in severely burned patients. Lancet *1*:546, 1969.
71. Parker, D.J., Cantrell, J.W., Karp, R.B., et al.: Changes in serum complement and immunoglobulins following cardiopulmonary bypass. Surgery *71*:824, 1972.
72. Kinnaert, P., Mahieu, A., and Van Geertruyden, N.: Stimulation of antibody synthesis induced by surgical trauma in rats. Clin. Exp. Immunol. *32*:243, 1978.

73. Markley, K., Smallman, E., and Evans, G.: Antibody production in mice after thermal and tourniquet trauma. Surgery *61*:896, 1967.
74. Farrell, M.F., Day, N.K., Tsakraklides, V., et al.: Study of lymphocyte depletion and serum complement perturbations following acute burn trauma. Surgery *73*:697, 1973.
75. Berghem, L., Lahnborg, G., and Jarstrand, C.: Role of phagocytic cells in host defense in relation to trauma—a brief review. Acta Chir. Scand. Suppl. *489*:231, 1979.
76. Christou, N.V., and Meakins, J.L.: Neutrophil function in anergic surgical patients. Ann. Surg. *190*:557, 1979.
77. Christou, N.V., McLean, A.P.H., and Meakins, J.L.: Host defense in blunt trauma: Interrelationships of kinetics of anergy and depressed neutrophil function, nutritional status and sepsis. J. Trauma *20*:833, 1980.
78. Davis, J.M., Dineen, P., and Gallin, J.I.: Neutrophil degranulation and abnormal chemotaxis after thermal injury. J. Immunol. *124*:1467, 1980.
79. Heck, E., Edgar, M.A., Hunt, J.L., et al.: A comparison of leukocyte function and burn mortality. J. Trauma *20*:75, 1980.
80. Loose, L.D., and Turinsky, J.: Macrophage dysfunction after burn injury. Infect. Immun. *26*:157, 1979.
81. Meakins, J.L., McLean, A.P.H., Kelly, R., et al.: Delayed hypersensitivity and neutrophil chemotaxis: Effect of trauma. J. Trauma *18*:240, 1978.
82. Neilan, B.A., Taddeini, L., and Strate, R.G.: T lymphocyte rosette formation after major burns. JAMA *3348*:493, 1977.
83. Slade, M.S., Simmons, R.L., Yunis, E., et al.: Immunodepression after major surgery in normal patients. Surgery *78*:363, 1975.
84. Wood, G.W., Volenec, F.J., Mani, M.M., et al.: Dynamics of T-lymphocyte subpopulations and T-lymphocyte function following thermal injury. Clin. Exp. Immunol. *31*:291, 1978.
85. Miller, C.L., and Baker, C.C.: Changes in lymphocyte activity after thermal injury. J. Clin Invest. *63*:202, 1979.
86. Salo, M., Merikanto, J., Eskola, J., et al.: Impaired lymphocyte transformation after accidental trauma. Acta Chir. Scand. *145*:367, 1979.
87. Cooperband, S.R., Nimberg, R., Schmid, K., et al.: Humoral immunosuppressive factors. Transpl. Proc. *8*:225, 1976.
87a. Hirohata, S., Davis, L.S., and Lipsley P.: Role of Interleukin in generation of CD4+ Suppressor of Human B-cell responsiveness. J. Immunol. *142*:3104, 1989.
88. Constantian, M.B., Menzoian, J.O., Nimberg, R.B., et al.: Association of a circulating immunosuppressive polypeptide with operative and accidental trauma. Ann. Surg. *185*:73, 1977.
89. Manzoian, J.O., Glasgow, A.H., Nimberg, R.B., et al.: The prolongation of renal allograft survival by an immunosuppressive peptide isolated from human plasma. Transplantation *18*:391, 1974.
90. Badger, A.M., Merluzzi, V.J., Mannick, J.A., et al.: Immunosuppressive activity of IRA on the plaque-forming response to SRBC in vitro: Reversal with educated T cells. J. Immunol. *118*:1228, 1977.
91. Cooperband, S.R., Badter, A.M., Davis, R.C., et al.: The effect of immunoregulatory α globulin (IRA) upon lymphocytes in vitro. J. Immunol. *109*:154, 1972.
92. McLoughlin, G.A., Wu, A.V., Saporoschetz, I., et al.: Correlation between anergy and a circulating immunosuppressive factor following major surgical trauma. Ann. Surg. *190*:297, 1979.
93. Constantian, M.B.: Association of sepsis with an immunosuppressive polypeptide in the serum of burn patients. Ann. Surg. *88*:209, 1978.
94. Glasgow, A.H., Nimberg, R.B., Menzoian, J.O., et al.: Association of anergy with an immunosuppressive peptide fraction in the serum of patients with cancer. N. Engl. J. Med. *291*:1263, 1974.
95. Miller, C.L., and Claudy, B.J.: Suppressor T-cell activity induced as a result of thermal injury. Cell Immunol. *44*:201, 1979.
96. Winchurch, R.A., and Munster, A.M.: Post-traumatic activation of suppressor cells. J. Reticul. Soc. *27*:83, 1980.
97. Wang, B.S., Heacock, E.H., Wu, A.V.O., et al.: Generation of suppressor cells in mice after surgical trauma. J. Clin. Invest. *66*:200, 1980.
98. Ninnemann, J.L., and Stein, M.D.: Bacterial endotoxin and the generation of suppressor T cells following thermal injury. J. Trauma *20*:959, 1980.
99. Ninnemann, J.L.: Immunosuppression following thermal injury through B cell activation of suppressor T cells. J. Trauma *20*:206, 1980.
100. Wolfe, J.H.N., Saporoschetz, I., Young, A.E., et al.: Suppressive serum, suppressor lymphocytes and death from burns. Ann. Surg. *193*:513, 1981.
101. Fauci, A.S., Dale, D.C., and Balow, J.E.: Glucocorticosteroid therapy: Mechanisms of action and clinical considerations. Ann. Intern. Med. *84*:304, 1976.
102. Haynes, B.F., and Fauci, A.S.: The differential effect of in vivo hydrocortisone on the kinetics of subpopulations of human peripheral blood thymus-derived lymphocytes. J. Clin. Invest. *61*:703, 1978.
103. Webb, D.R., Jr., and Winkelstein, A.: Immunosuppression and immunopotentiation. *In* Fudenberg, H.H., Stites, D.P., Caldwell, J.L., et al. (eds.): Basic and Clinical Immunology. 3rd ed. Los Altos, CA, Lange Medical Publications, 1980, pp. 313–326.
104. Rubin, R.H., Wolfson, J.S., Cosimi, A.B., et al.: Infection in the renal transplant recipient. Am. J. Med. *70*:405, 1981.
105. Francke, E.L., and Neu, H.C.: Post-splenectomy infection. Surg. Clin. North Am. *61*:135, 1981.
106. Gopal, V., and Bisno, A.L.: Fulminant pneumococcal infections in "normal" asplenic hosts. Arch. Intern. Med. *137*:1526, 1977.
107. Gross, R.L., and Newberne, P.N.: Role of nutrition in immunologic function. Physiol. Rev. *60*:188, 1980.
108. Suskind, R.M. (ed.): Malnutrition in the Immune Response. New York, Raven Press, 1977.
109. Chedid, L., Miescher, P.A., and Muller-Eberhard, H.J. (eds.): Immunostimulation. Berlin, Springer Verlag, 1980.
110. Mackowiak, P.A.: Clinical uses of microorganisms and their products. Amer. J. Med. *67*:293, 1979.
111. Greene, W.C.: The molecular biology of human immunodeficiency virus type I infection. N. Engl. J. Med. *324*:308, 1991.
112. Brown, G.L., Nanney, L.B., Griffen, J., et al.: Enhancement of wound healing by topical treatment with epidermal growth factor. N. Engl. J. Med. *321*:76, 1989.
113. Dwyer, J.M.: Manipulating the immune system with immune globulin. N. Engl. J. Med. *326*:107, 1992.

BIBLIOGRAPHY

Allen, P.M.: Antigen processing at the molecular level. Immunol. Today *8*:270, 1987.

Baker, C.C., Miller, C.L., Trunkey, D.D., et al.: Identity of mononuclear cells which compromise the resistance of trauma patients. J. Surg. Res. *26*:478, 1979.

Bauer, A.R., McNeil, C., Trentelman, E., et al.: The depression of T lymphocytes after trauma. Am. J. Surg. *136*:674, 1978.

Bjornson, A.B., Altemeier, W.A., and Bjornson, H.S.: Complement, opsonins and immune response to bacterial infection in burned patients. Ann. Surg. *191*:323, 1980.

The EORTC International Antimicrobial Therapy Project Group: Three antibiotic regimens in the treatment of infection in febrile granulocytopenic patients with cancer. J. Infect. Dis. *137*:14, 1978.

Gallin, J.I., Goldstein, I.M., and Snyderman, R. (Eds.): Inflammation: Basic Principles and Clinical Correlates. New York, Raven Press, 1988.

Glenn, J., Funkhouse, W.K., and Schneider P.S.: Acute illnesses necessitating urgent abdominal surgery in neutropenic cancer patients. Surgery 105:778, 1989.

Goldstein, S.A., and Elwyn, D.H.: The effects of injury and sepsis on fuel utilization. Ann. Rev. Nutrition 9:445, 1989.

Horwitz, M.A.: Phagocytosis of microorganisms. Rev. Infect. Dis. 4:104, 1982.

Malech, H.L., and Gallin, J.I.: Neutrophils in human disease. N. Engl. J. Med. 317:687, 1987.

Neilsen, H.E., Kochy, C., Magnussen, P., and Lind, I.: Complement deficiencies in selected groups of people with meningococcal disease. Scand. J. Infect. Dis. 21:389, 1989.

Roth, J.A. (ed.): Virulence Mechanisms of Bacterial Pathogens. American Society of Microbiology, Washington, D.C., 1988.

Stites, D.P.: Clinical laboratory methods of detecting cellular immune functions. In Fudenberg, H.H., Stites, D.P., Caldwell, J.L., et al. (eds.): Basic and Clinical Immunology. 3rd ed. Los Altos, CA, Lange Medical Publications, 1980, pp. 382–397.

Winkelstein, J.A., Gorbach, S.L., Bartlett, J.G., and Blacklow, N.R. (Eds.): The Complement System in Infectious Diseases. Philadelphia, W.B. Saunders Co., 1992.

ANAPHYLAXIS

David N. Zull

CAPSULE

Early recognition and treatment of the initial manifestations of anaphylaxis are crucial in preventing mortality as well as in limiting the severity of such reactions. Upper airway obstruction is the most common cause of death in anaphylaxis, so that any sign (uvular, tongue, or lip edema) or symptom (hoarseness, lump in throat, dysphagia) of oropharyngeal and laryngeal edema must be treated with great urgency.

Epinephrine by the subcutaneous or intramuscular route is the mainstay of therapy; however, intravenous epinephrine may be life-saving in progressive airway obstruction or shock refractory to fluid resuscitation and intramuscular epinephrine. Paradoxically, intravenous administration of epinephrine is the most common cause of iatrogenic death in anaphylaxis, resulting from cardiac arrhythmias and myocardial ischemia. Glucocorticoids should be administered early in all but the mildest or most transient allergic reactions, with the intent of preventing a biphasic or protracted clinical course.

The physician must be an undaunted detective in determining the cause of anaphylaxis. Although penicillin, hymenoptera sings, and radiopaque contrast media are the most common causes of fatal anaphylaxis, foods, nonsteroidal anti-inflammatory drugs, and exercise are increasingly recognized causes of life-threatening reactions.

INTRODUCTION

Anaphylaxis (Fig. 51-6) is an acute life-threatening systemic reaction manifested by urticaria, angioedema, upper airway obstruction, bronchospasm, hypotension, and gastrointestinal disturbances. All features of the anaphylactic syndrome may be present; however, it is more common to see a single manifestation or some combination of organ involvement. In fact, it is the often limited expression of anaphylaxis that results in delays in diagnosis and treatment. Acute isolated lip swelling and sudden development of urticaria without other symptoms are frequently categorized as minor nuisance symptoms; however, this clinical presentation may be a harbinger of a severe, multisystem reaction in progress and should be treated urgently.[1-6]

The clinical manifestations of anaphylaxis result from the massive release of chemical mediators (e.g., histamine, kinins, leukotrienes) from mast cells and basophils throughout the body. This mast cell degranulation classically results from antigen-IgE interaction; however, complement activation, changes in prostaglandin metabolism, and direct chemical effects on mast cells may cause an identical clinical picture. Effective therapy of anaphylaxis, which includes epinephrine, corticosteroids, and antihistamines, focuses on preventing mast cell degranulation and/or inhibiting mediator and organ effects.[1-6]

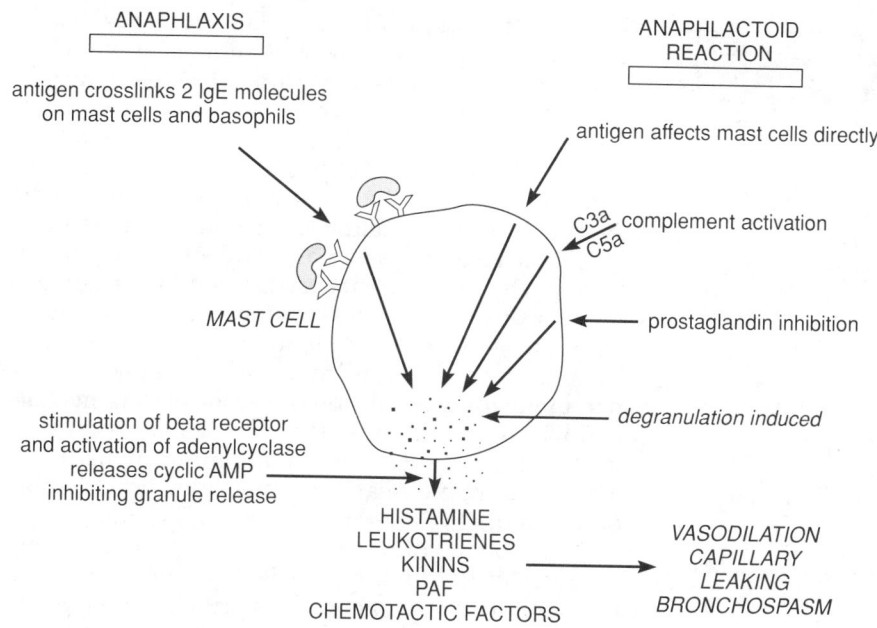

ANAPHLAXIS

antigen crosslinks 2 IgE molecules
on mast cells and basophils

ANAPHLACTOID
REACTION

antigen affects mast cells directly

$C3a$
$C5a$ complement activation

MAST CELL

prostaglandin inhibition

stimulation of beta receptor
and activation of adenylcyclase
releases cyclic AMP
inhibiting granule release

degranulation induced

HISTAMINE
LEUKOTRIENES
KININS
PAF
CHEMOTACTIC FACTORS

*VASODILATION
CAPILLARY
LEAKING
BRONCHOSPASM*

FIG. 51-6.   Macrophages regulate magnitude of immune responses through release of a variety of biologically active substances.

PATHOPHYSIOLOGY

In classic anaphylaxis from antigen-IgE interaction, previous sensitization to a foreign antigen is requisite. On exposure to a foreign substance, B lymphocytes are stimulated to transform into plasma cells, which produce a variety of immunoglobulins specific to the antigen. After repeated exposure, antibody production is increased, and after a long absence, subsequent antigen contact stimulates an amnestic antibody response.[7]

For allergic sensitization to occur, an adequate concentration of antigen-specific IgE must be produced, which then binds to the cell membranes of mast cells and basophils. IgE binds to these cells with its Fc portion, leaving its Fab arms free to interact with antigen, which on re-exposure crosslinks the Fab arms of two adjacent IgE molecules. This cell membrane reaction results in release of cytoplasmic granules, which contain preformed mediators like histamine, kallikreins, eosinophil chemotactic factor, and neutrophil chemotactic factor. In addition, other mediators are released that are formed with cell stimulation, including leukotrienes, prostaglandins, and platelet-activating factor.[7,8]

These chemical mediators result in increased vascular permeability and vasodilation, which account for many of the clinical manifestations of anaphylaxis. The resultant tissue swelling and edema may cause upper airway obstruction if localized to the larynx or oropharynx. Urticaria and/or angioedema of the skin result, depending on whether the swelling is in the up-

per dermis (urticaria) or deep dermis (angioedema). Even edema of the intestinal mucosa may occur, causing cramping, vomiting, and diarrhea. Vasodilation and third-spacing are also responsible for the hypotension in anaphylaxis. In addition, bronchospasm may be partly attributed to respiratory mucosal edema, although leukotriene-mediated bronchial smooth muscle constriction is primarily responsible.[8]

The release of chemical mediators from mast cells and basophils may be provoked by mechanisms separate from the IgE-antigen interaction. Certain compounds like opiates, curare, radiopaque contrast media, and dextran have a direct degranulating effect on mast cells. Provocation of the complement cascade by immune complexes or a direct effect results in release of $C3_a$ and $C5_a$, so-called anaphylotoxins, which cause mast cells to degranulate. Blood products like plasma, immunoglobulins, and whole blood are the classic examples of complement-mediated anaphylaxis. Physical factors such as exercise and cold exposure may provoke mediator release from mast cells by a direct effect also. Lastly, modulators of prostaglandin metabolism, the prototypes being aspirin and the nonsteroidal anti-inflammatory drugs, cause mast cell degranulation by a mechanism separate from IgE-antigen interaction. In addition, it should be noted that NSAIDs inhibit the cyclo-oxygenase enzyme, thereby shunting prostaglandin metabolism to leukotriene production and further aggravating anaphylaxis as well as bronchial asthma.[9]

An important modulator of mast cell mediator release is the level of intracellular cyclic AMP, which inhibits degranulation. Stimulation of the beta-adrenergic receptor activates adenylcyclase, resulting in increased production of cyclic AMP. As a result, the

TABLE 51-12. SYMPTOMS AND SIGNS OF ANAPHYLAXIS

Reaction	Symptom	Sign
Urticaria	Itching, flushing	Raised wheals, diffusely wandering, evanescent
Angioedema	Nonpruritic tingling	Swelling of lips, eyes, hands, no heat or erythema
Laryngeal edema	Hoarseness, dysphagia, lump in throat, airway obstruction sudden death, drooling	Inspiratory stridor, intercostal and clavicular retractions, cyanosis, uvular, tongue, and lip edema, supraglottic edema
Bronchospasm	Cough, dyspnea, chest tightness	Wheezing, high respiratory rate, retractions
Hypotension	Dizziness, syncope, confusion, sense of doom	Hypotension (mild to severe), tachycardia, oliguria
Rhinitis	Nasal congestion, itching, sneezing	Mucosal edema, rhinorrhea
Conjunctivitis	Tearing, itching	Lid edema and injection
Gastroenteritis	Cramping, diarrhea, vomiting, hematochezia	Normal examination

beta-agonist agent epinephrine is critical in the management of allergic reactions because it inhibits ongoing mediator release in addition to its additional benefits of bronchodilation (beta effect) and vasoconstriction (alpha effect).[6]

Theophylline increases cyclic AMP levels by inhibiting the phosphodiesterase enzyme. which degrades cyclic AMP. The benefit, however, is greatest in asthma prophylaxis. Antihistamines have no effect on mediator release, but rather competitively inhibit histamine at its vascular and smooth muscle receptors. Steroids' mechanism of action in anaphylaxis is probably multifactorial, including inhibition of leukotriene production, stabilization of the mast cell membrane, and anti-inflammatory and antichemotactic effects, which may prevent a biphasic or protracted anaphylactic reaction.[3,6]

CLINICAL PRESENTATION

Anaphylaxis is an acute allergic reaction, usually beginning within 30 minutes of antigen exposure, but often immediately. In fact, the more immediate the reaction, the more severe it will be. Delays from 2 to 3 hours may be seen in antigens by the oral route, which may confuse identification of the etiologic factors.

Symptoms of anaphylaxis (Table 51-12) usually reach their peak within several minutes of onset, but may persist for hours afterward. Mild reactions may resolve in less than 30 minutes, but more severe cases may persist beyond 24 hours. A small percentage of patients demonstrate a biphasic course in which there is recrudescence of the anaphylactic syndrome within 24 hours of initial complete resolution.[10] Rarely, restrictions have been described days after a bee sting.[11]

Frequent, intermittent exposure to a foreign antigen increases the risk of sensitization, but in many cases no prior exposure can be identified. Antigen exposure by any route may lead to a reaction; however, the parenteral route usually produces the most immediate and life-threatening reactions. Routes of exposure in descending order of severity are intravenous, intraarterial, intramuscular, subcutaneous, intradermal, oral, conjunctival, vaginal, rectal, and dermal.[1]

At the outset of anaphylaxis, before development of any physical findings, patients often note certain premonitory symptoms such as pruritus of the palms and soles, tingling of the lips and tongue, generalized warmth, lump in the throat, tightness in the chest, or a feeling of impending doom.

Some patients may present with syncope or sudden death secondary to anaphylactic shock, yet lack other manifestations of the anaphylactic syndrome. Although there is great variability in hypotension in anaphylaxis, a 20 to 30 mm Hg drop in blood pressure is typical. Hypotension, however, is a leading cause of death from anaphylaxis, second only to upper airway obstruction.[12–14]

Laryngeal edema is the principal cause of death in anaphylaxis, often presenting as sudden death or "café coronary." Like shock, laryngeal edema may be the only manifestation of anaphylaxis; however, angioedema of adjacent tissues of the pharynx often de-

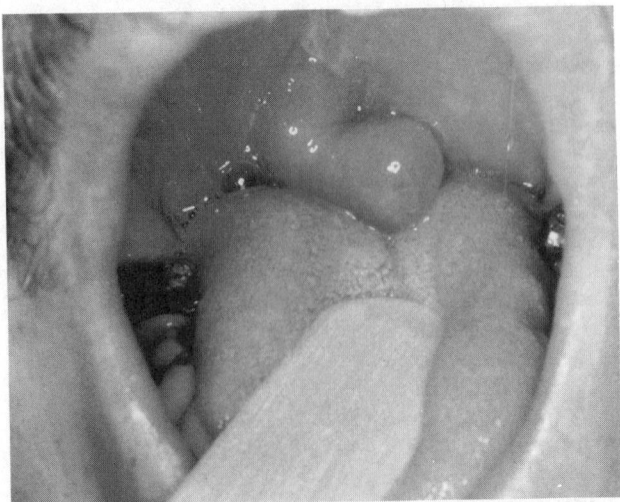

FIG. 51-7. Marked angioedema of the uvula and soft palate as the primary manifestation of acute anaphylaxis in a patient sensitive to peanuts. Onset after ingestion was less than 15 minutes, but complete resolution took 48 hours. Uvular swelling is a common physical finding in acute anaphylaxis, sometimes heralding concomitant laryngeal edema.

velops concomitantly and thereby acts as a helpful marker of potential laryngeal involvement. Uvular edema (Fig. 51-7) in particular, as well as angioedema of the lips, tongue, and oropharynx, should be treated aggressively, not so much for the fear of oropharyngeal obstruction, but rather for incipient laryngeal obstruction. Patients often complain of "hoarseness" or "a lump in my throat" but the physician finds the oropharyngeal examination normal. Although indirect laryngoscopy is appropriate at this point, administration of epinephrine should not be delayed in a patient with these complaints.[3,12]

Wheezing secondary to bronchospasm and lower airway edema is commonly seen in anaphylaxis, but is generally mild. If the patient has a pre-existing history of asthma, however, severe status asthmaticus may be provoked. Noncardiogenic pulmonary edema is also described in anaphylaxis, but is a rare phenomenon associated with drugs in anesthesia[4] or as a terminal event.[15]

The most common and clinically obvious feature of anaphylaxis is skin involvement, with over 90% of patients developing urticaria, angioedema, or both. Urticaria appears as raised, erythematous wheals covering most of the body in evanescent, pruritic patches. Angioedema, on the other hand, is characterized by nonpruritic, nonerythematous, puffy areas of skin that do not pit. Patients with angioedema complain of tingling and a swollen sensation that is painless, found most prominently about the face, lips, and hands. In some instances, patients may present with a diffuse body flush without typical hives or angioedema.[2,3]

Gastrointestinal involvement is common in anaphylaxis, and is manifested by nausea, vomiting, diarrhea, and rarely hematochezia. These symptoms are usually mild and overshadowed by the other manifestations of anaphylaxis. Similarly, rhinitis and conjunctivitis are common, nonlife-threatening feature of anaphylaxis.

Cardiac anaphylaxis has been described, featuring nonspecific ST-T wave changes, ventricular arrhythmias, and even myocardial infarction. These abnormalities, however, are felt to be secondary to hypoxia, hypotension, and overzealous epinephrine therapy, and not from stimulation of H_2 receptors in the heart as is often hypothesized.[16–18]

It should be noted that fever is not a characteristic of allergic reactions, with the exception of serum sickness and drug fever, which are delayed phenomena.[11]

DIFFERENTIAL DIAGNOSIS

The physician must maintain a high index of suspicion for anaphylaxis in shock of unknown cause, especially if blood loss, volume depletion, sepsis, or cardiac causes are not evident.

Upper airway obstruction from infectious causes such as croup, epiglottitis, and retropharyngeal abscess may have a presentation similar to that of angioedema of the larynx and supraglottic region, but the appearance of the pharynx usually distinguishes these entities. Foreign body aspiration is another important consideration in acute airway obstruction.

Hereditary angioedema may present with acute upper airway obstruction, gastrointestinal symptoms, and angioedema of the skin that mimics anaphylaxis. This is an autosomal dominant disorder, caused by a C_1 esterase inhibitor deficiency. Attacks usually begin in adolescence and can recur intermittently throughout life, often precipitated by stress or trauma. Gastrointestinal symptoms may be prominent, with abdominal pain mimicking an acute abdomen. Urticaria is absent in this disorder. Fresh frozen plasma is effective in abolishing attacks, whereas epinephrine is often ineffective.[19]

Scombroid fish poisoning may present with acute urticaria, headache, nausea, vomiting, and dysphagia. This syndrome occurs from the ingestion of fish with a high histidine content (mahi, tuna). When these fish spoil, the histidine is broken down to histamine.[20]

Acute flushing, chest discomfort, and nausea as seen in the "Chinese restaurant syndrome," better termed the MSG syndrome, may resemble anaphylaxis, but the frequent prominence of headache and the usual lack of hives or angioedema are distinguishing features. Monosodium glutamate (MSG) is responsible for this syndrome.[21]

Carcinoid syndrome and systemic mastocytosis may present with episodes of flushing and hypotension, but are rare neoplastic disorders.

Status asthmaticus and acute urticaria are localized forms of anaphylaxis, treated with similar urgency.

Occasionally, patients feign stridor and respiratory distress, known as globus hystericus or Munchausen's anaphylaxis. They should be treated in a standard manner unless indirect laryngoscopy demonstrates a completely normal examination.[22]

Serum sickness is a delayed allergic reaction characterized by urticaria, but differentiated by the presence of fever, joint pains, and lymphadenopathy.

CAUSES (Table 51-13)

PENICILLIN AND CEPHALOSPORINS

Penicillin and its derivatives (ampicillin, dicloxacillin, etc.) are the most common causes of life-threatening anaphylaxis, with over 100 deaths per year reported in the United States. Of these deaths, the great majority are by the parenteral route. In fact, only 6 cases have been cited in the literature of fatal anaphylaxis from oral penicillin. It is estimated that 1% of the population is sensitive to penicillin, most manifesting urticaria alone. Anaphylaxis, however, occurs in 15

TABLE 51-13. CAUSES OF ANAPHYLAXIS

I. Proteins
   A. Venoms
      1. Insect: Hymenoptera (yellowjacket, honeybee, hornet, wasp, fire ant). Other insects (kissing bugs, bedbugs)
      2. Animal: Rattlesnake, gila monster, jellyfish
   B. Foods
      1. Plant: nuts, legumes, seeds
      2. Animal: shellfish, fish, eggs
      3. Additives: sulfites, tartrazine
   C. Allergy extracts
      (pollens of ragweed, trees, grass; animal danders)
   D. Foreign sera
      1. Human: immune globulin, blood, plasma
      2. Equine: antitoxin (botulism), antivenom (snake)
   E. Hormones
      (animal and human insulin, corticosteroids)
   F. Enzymes
      (streptokinase, chymopapaine, protamine)
   G. Vaccines
      (tetanus toxoid, egg-based like MMR and Influenza)
   H. Seminal fluid
II. Haptens:
   A. Penicillins, cephalosporins, and imipenem
   B. Other antibiotics (tetracycline, nitrofurantoin, streptomycin, sulfonamides)
III. Prostaglandin inhibition
   A. Aspirin (not sodium salicylate or Disalcid)
   B. Nonsteroidal anti-inflammatory drugs (indomethacin, tolmetin, ibuprofen, naproxen, etc)
IV. Physical factors
   A. Exercise-induced anaphylaxis
   B. Food or NSALD-dependent exercise-induced anaphylaxis
   C. Cold-induced urticaria and anaphylaxis
V. Multifactorial or unknown (complement activation, direct mast cell degranulation, IgE, effects on kinins or clotting)
   A. Radiopaque contrast media (IVP dye, etc.)
   B. Polysaccharides
   C. Thiamine, vitamin K, morphine, protamine
   D. Local anesthetics (procaine, methylparaben)
   E. Drugs in general anesthesia (muscle relaxants, etc.)

to 40 per 100,000, and fatal anaphylaxis in 1 to 2 per 100,000.[23]

Cephalosporins crossreact in 5 to 16% of penicillin-allergic patients; however, the likelihood is much greater if a life-threatning reaction has occurred. As a result, cephalosporins should be used with caution in patients with a history of penicillin allergy. In regard to other penicillin analogues, imipenem crossreacts with penicillin, whereas azotreonam does not.[24] Other classes of antibiotics are much less commonly implicated in anaphylaxis, but urticaria and serum sickness are not unusual, especially with sulfonamides.

BITES AND STINGS

Hymenoptera envenomation includes stings of yellowjackets, honeybee, hornets, wasps, bumblebees, and fire ants, and constitutes the second most com-mon cause of life-threatening anaphylaxis in the USA. Such stings cause over 50 deaths per year, mostly in late summer. The incidence of bee sting allergy is about 1% in the general population, and although large local reactions are not predictive of anaphylactic sensitivity, any systemic reaction is, especially in adults. Interestingly, over 90% of stings occur in patients under 20 years, whereas 93% of the deaths are in patients over 20 years.[12,25] Anaphylaxis to other bites and stings is much less common, but includes reactions to kissing bugs, bedbugs, snakes, jellyfish, and gila monsters.[26]

IODINATED CONTRAST MEDIA

This is the third most common cause of anaphylactic death in the United States, with 40 to 50 deaths reported per year. One to two percent of patients studied experience an anaphylactoid reaction. Most of these reactions are mild and self-limited; however, fatal reactions have been reported at a rate of 1 to 10 per 100,000. Factors that place a patient at high risk of radiocontrast reactions include a previous severe reaction, advanced age, atopy, asthma, dehydration, cardiac disease, and renal or hepatic dysfunction. Nonionic contrast media may provide partial protection from systemic reaction; however, pretreatment with prednisone (50 mg by mouth 13 hours, 7 hours, and 1 hour before administration) and diphenhydramine (50 mg intramuscularly 1 hour before) is the most reliable method of reducing the frequency and severity of radiocontrast media reactions.[27]

FOODS

Foods are among the most common causes of mild anaphylaxis in the outpatient setting; however, there is an increasing awareness of fatalities secondary to food-induced anaphylaxis. Shellfish, legumes, nuts, eggs, and seeds are commonly implicated. Exercise may be a permissive factor in the precipitation of some reactions. Food additives, such as tartrazine and sulfites, may occasionally be responsible.[28–30]

ASPIRIN AND NONSTEROIDAL ANTI-INFLAMMATORY DRUGS

These drugs are also common causes of anaphylaxis in the ambulatory setting. Their use is so prevalent that they are often overlooked as a potential cause. Aspirin and the NSAIDs all crossreact as does the food dye tartrazine; however, nonacetylated salicylates like sodium salicylate and acetaminophen are well tolerated.[31,32]

EXERCISE

Exercise, by itself or in conjunction with food or NSAID ingestion, is another underdiagnosed cause of anaphylaxis. Exercise-induced anaphylaxis is not predictable or reproducible in most patients, but is more common in those with a personal or family history of atopy and during hot, humid weather. Prevention involves avoidance of food or medications 4 hours before exercise, stopping exercise at the first hint of pruritus, and exercising with a partner carrying an epinephrine emergency kit.[30,33] Cold exposure is another physical factor that can induce urticaria and rarely anaphylaxis.[3]

OTHER CAUSES

Any complete protein antigen may provoke anaphylactic sensitivity in a susceptible person. Such agents include streptokinase, chymopapaine, insulin, vaccines (egg products), toxoids, allergy extracts, blood products (including antisera), and seminal fluid.[3,9]

Numerous drugs by the intravenous route have been associated with anaphylaxis, including anesthetic induction agents, paralyzing drugs, morphine, thiamine, vitamin K, protamine, and hydrocortisone.[3,4,6]

True allergic reactions to local anesthetics are rare, and are generally attributed to the preservative methylparaben. The ester group of anesthetics (tetracaine, procaine, benzocaine) do not crossreact with the amide group (lidocaine, mepivacaine, bupivacaine); in addition, agents within the amide group do not crossreact with each other. If allergy is suspected and the agent is unknown, skin testing with pure lidocaine without preservatives (cardiac lidocaine) is suggested if use of a local anesthetic is absolutely necessary.[6]

Enalapril and other ACE inhibitors have been associated with facial and upper airway angioedema that is gradual in onset and resistant to therapy.[34] Beta blockers, although not a precipitant of anaphylaxis, may make allergic reactions refractory to epinephrine and other treatment.[35]

UNKNOWN CAUSES

Even after thorough evaluation by an allergist, about 25% of cases of anaphylaxis have no identifiable cause. The course of idiopathic anaphylaxis is variable, but deaths have not been reported. Prophylactic therapy with steroids and antihistamines is effective, and epinephrine kits are indispensable.[36]

PREHOSPITAL ASSESSMENT AND STABILIZATION

The diagnosis of anaphylaxis by prehospital personnel is usually straightforward, especially when all components of the syndrome are present. If only one clinical feature predominates, however, such as upper airway obstruction or shock, the proper diagnosis and

---

TABLE 51-14. TREATMENT OF ANAPHYLAXIS

1. Remove antigen, delay absorption.
2. Maintain an adequate airway.
3. Epinephrine
   If a mild episode:
     —0.3 cc subcutaneously (0.01 cc/kg in a child) 1/1000
     —Repeat at 10 to 20 minute intervals.
   If more severe episode:
     —0.3–0.5 mL intramuscularly 1/1000
     —Repeat at 5- to 10-minute intervals.
   If in shock or incipient airway obstruction:
     —1/100,000 dilution intravenously, 1–2 cc per minute up to a total of 10 cc (0.1 mg)
     —If persistent shock, may repeat dose or start a drip: 1 mg in 250 cc D5W, 1–4 μ per minute.
   If patient is elderly (over 50) or has a cardiac history, and life-threatening symptoms exist:
     ——Test dose of 0.1–0.15 cc subcutaneously or IM.
     —If shock is resistant to other measures or there is imminent airway closure, consider a drip as noted previously.
4. Volume expansion with saline or lactated ringer's
   Shock:
     Adult: 1 L over 15 minutes, then reassess
     Child: 20 cc/kg bolus
5. Methylprednisolone
   125 mg IV push, may repeat every 4 hours if persistent symptoms. (or hydrocortisone 500 mg)
   If discharging home, prednisone 40 mg per day, for 2 to 3 days.
6. Diphenhydramine
   25–50 mg IV push, IM, or by mouth depending on severity, repeat every 2–4 hours as needed.
   If patient is being discharged, 50 mg q6hr prn for 3 days
7. If resistant hypotension
   A. MAST suit, Trendelenburg position[37]
   B. Dopamine infusion
   C. Naloxone, 0.4–0.8 mg IV[6]
   D. Cimetidine 300 mg IV[38]
8. If beta blocker accentuated anaphylaxis (epinephrine-resistant)
   A. Glucagon, 1–2 mg IV over 2 minutes, then drip
   B. Terbutiline 0.25 mg subcutaneously
   C. Isoproterenol drip

---

treatment (Table 51-14) may be delayed unless a high index of suspicion exists.

The first priority in prehospital management is establishing and maintaining an airway. Oxygen should be administered, and bag mask ventilation started if necessary. Upper airway angioedema with partial obstruction may benefit from an upright posture; however, this position may aggravate hypotension. If significant angioedema is present, tracheal intubation by both the oral and nasal routes should be attempted; however, prompt administration of epinephrine may avert obstruction and make intubation unnecessary. In fact, early administration of epinephrine in anaphylaxis treatment is as critical as the basic ABCs of resuscitation.[3,6]

If hypotension is present, the patient should be placed in a Trendelenberg position (if airway patency allows), and a large-bore intravenous line started. Normal saline or lactated Ringer's solution should be infused wide open initially after the blood pressure response, but watch for the development of rales. Application and inflation of a military antishock trousers (MAST) suit should also be considered by the rescue squad if hypotension persists.[37] Concomitantly, prompt administration of epinephrine (0.3 mL of 1:1000 dilution in an adult or 0.01 mL per kg in a child) by the subcutaneous or intramuscular route is critical. If hypotension is profound or refractory to treatment, intravenous epinephrine may be necessary (see Emergency Department management, subsequently).[18]

In the case of a bee sting, local measures include application of a loose tourniquet above the site (if it is on an extremity), cold application, dependency of the extremity, and careful removal of the stinger if present.

In addition to the above measures, antihistamines and corticosteroids may be administered in the field if available (see subsequent text). After initial stabilization, prompt transport to the nearest emergency department (ED) should be facilitated.

Regarding self-treatment in the prehospital setting, most patients with idiopathic anaphylaxis, as well as those with bee sting and food-related anaphylaxis, should carry an Epi-Pen, a spring-loaded automatic injector that delivers 0.3 cc of 1:1000 epinephrine. An epinephrine inhaler (Primatene) is another option, delivering 0.2 mg of epinephrine per puff.

EMERGENCY DEPARTMENT MANAGEMENT

All patients with anaphylaxis, even those with a single manifestation (acute urticaria), should be treated with similar urgency, remembering that the severity of a reaction is proportional to its rapidity of onset. Standard initial measures include supplemental oxygen, a large-bore intravenous line (infusing normal saline or lactated Ringer's solution), and placement on a cardiac monitor.

Prompt administration of epinephrine is critical in the management of anaphylaxis. Its beta-agonist effect on mast cell increases production of intracellular cyclic AMP, thereby inhibiting further release of mediators. In addition, the beta-adrenergic effects product bronchodilation, as well as positive inotropic and chronotropic effects on the heart. The alpha-adrenergic action of epinephrine causes vasoconstriction, resulting in a rise in systemic blood pressure and a decrease in angioedema of skin and mucous membranes.

The usual dose of epinephrine in mild to moderate anaphylaxis is 0.3 mL of 1:1000 dilution, administered subcutaneously, repeated at 10- to 20-minute intervals for three doses. In moderate to severe anaphylaxis (hypotension, upper airway angioedema), epineph-

rine should be given IM and the dose may be increased to 0.5 mL per 1:1000, repeated at the same intervals.[6,18]

If hypotension is unresponsive to fluid resuscitation and intramuscular epinephrine or if upper airway obstruction appears imminent despite repeated doses of epinephrine (IM or SQ), the intravenous route of administration must be considered. Great caution, however, must be taken in the use of intravenous epinephrine because it may lead to malignant ventricular arrhythmias, myocardial infarction, and sudden death. The recommended dose is 1.0 cc of 1:10,000 epinephrine further diluted in 10 cc of normal saline given by slow IV push over 5 to 10 minutes. If shock or airway obstruction is not improving, this IV dose may be repeated several times, limited, of course, by the development of chest pain or ventricular arrhythmias. An alternative strategy is preparation of an epinephrine drip composed of 1.0 mg of epinephrine in 250 cc of D5W, infused at 1 to 4 µg per minute. Once a clinical response is demonstrated, switching back to the IM or SQ route is indicated.[6,18]

The emergency physician must focus constant attention on the patency of the upper airway, as well as the patient's hemodynamic status, because laryngeal edema and shock are the principal causes of death in anaphylaxis. Any degree of angioedema of the uvula, tongue, soft palate, or lips should alert the physician to possible concomitant laryngeal edema. Any complaints of hoarseness, dysphagia, or lump in the throat should be approached aggressively, rather than waiting for audible stridor and drooling to develop. If complete obstruction occurs or the patient's airway remains tenuous despite IV epinephrine, endotracheal intubation should be attempted. The oral route is preferred to directly visualize the anatomy, but supraglottic angioedema may make this technically difficult. Nasotracheal intubation may be attempted as a last resort before proceeding with a surgical airway. Nebulized racemic epinephrine may have some benefit in decreasing airway edema, but it is a temporizing measure and not definitive therapy. If the patient remains in extremis despite the above measures, cricothyrotomy or needle cricothyrotomy (in patients under 6 years) should be performed.[6]

Hypotension in anaphylaxis generally respond to fluid resuscitation and epinephrine administration. Crystalloids started in the field should be continued in the ED, anticipating that most patients will require 1 or 2 L over the first hour. Insertion of a Foley catheter and a CVP catheter may aid in monitoring volume status. Keeping the patient in Trendelenberg position and applying a MAST suit are other adjuncts often started in the field. Epinephrine or dopamine infusion is a last-resort measure in refractory shock.[13,14,35,37]

Antihistamines are an integral component in the therapy of anaphylaxis. Diphenhydramine (Benadryl), an H_1 antagonist in a dose of 25 to 50 mg, can be administered by the oral, IM, or IV route depending on the severity of the reaction. Concomitant use of H_2 antagonists such as cimetidine, 300 mg or ranitidine,

50 mg IV, may offer significant benefits, but the literature is anecdotal.[6,38]

Corticosteroids should be routinely admnistered in all but the most mild and transient anaphylactic reactions. Although steroids have never been documented to have any immediate benefit in anaphylaxis, the benefit of early steroid treatment in status asthmaticus suggests probable usefulness in other allergic emergencies.[39] More importantly, however, steroids appear to have their greatest benrfit in preventing reexacerbation of anaphylaxis and reducing swelling from angioedema. Common dosage recommendations include methylprednisolone, 125 mg, or hydrocortisone, 500 mg IV push STAT, repeating the same or a smaller dose at 4-hour intervals according to symptoms and signs.[3]

Bronchospasm in anaphylaxis is treated in a standard manner, with therapy including aerosolized beta-2 agonists and aminophylline infusion (see Chap. 46).

An individualized approach should be taken in patients over 50 and those with cardiac disease. Fluid administration should be done cautiously, monitoring the patient for development of rales. Epinephrine may be more toxic in these patients, but should not be withheld in patients with signs of upper airway obstruction or those with hypotension unresponsive to crystalloid administration.[40] Epinephrine, 0.1 to 0.15 cc at 1:1000 dilution, may be administered IM or SQ as a test dose, repeating it if no arrhythmias or chest pain are provoked. Intravenous epinephrine should be avoided in this patient group unless death appears imminent without its use.[18]

Anaphylaxis in patients on beta blockers presents another special treatment situation. Epinephrine therapy has limited efficacy in these patients; in fact, its effect is alpha-adrenergic stimulation only. In this situation, glucagon, 1 to 2 mg intravenously over 5 minutes, may have great benefit. In theory, glucagon works by stimulating adenylcyclase by a receptor separate from the beta receptor. Pure beta agonists such as isoproterenol by infusion or terbutaline subcutaneously, as well as an anticholinergic like atropine, are indicated if bradyarrhythmias develop.[35]

Measures to prevent absorption of an antigen should not be overlooked. A honeybee stinger should be flicked off and a loose tourniquet applied proximal to the injection site. Gastric emptying and charcoal administration should be considered for ingested antigens.

LABORATORY TESTS

The laboratory is of little help in the initial assessment and treatment of a patient with anaphylaxis. Peak expiratory flow measurements may be useful in following patients with prominent bronchospasm, and ar-

terial blood gases should be considered in anyone with persistent respiratory distress. An ECG should be performed in patients with moderate to severe anaphylaxis because myocardial ischemia and infarction have been reported in anaphylaxis; however, nonspecific ST-T wave changes and sinus tachycardia are commonly observed.[16] Patients should be on a cardiac monitor. If a strong suspicion of hereditary angioedema exists, low serum complement levels may be diagnostic.

DISPOSITION AND INDICATIONS FOR ADMISSION

Patients with mild anaphylaxis who have a rapid clinical response to treatment and never develop angioedema of the upper airway or persistent hypotension may be discharged home after observation in the ED for at least 3 hours, with close follow-up. Patients are generally discharged on a 2- to 3-day course of prednisone, 40 mg once daily and diphenhydramine, 25 to 50 mg at 6-hour intervals.

Any patients who has had life-threatening manifestations including shock or upper airway compromise should be admitted to the hospital for observation, even if symptoms and signs completely resolve in the ED. The reason is that up to 20% of these patients may have a recurrence of symptoms in the next 8 hours. A slow or incomplete response to therapy or any worsening of symptoms during therapy in the ED mandates admission. Finally, elderly, debilitated, or cardiac patients should be admitted for observation.

PITFALLS AND MEDICOLEGAL PEARLS

1. Take a careful history of all events in the 3 to 4 hours before the reaction. Common but underrecognized causes of anaphylaxis should be sought, including antibiotics, nonsteroidal anti-inflammatory drugs (especially over-the-counter aspirin and ibuprofen), foods (shellfish, nuts), exercise, and antihypertensives (beta blockers, ACE inhibitors).
2. Remember that uvular and pharyngeal edema is a warning sign of laryngeal involvement.
3. Do not ignore symptoms of hoarseness, dysphagia, or foreign body sensation because they may be harbingers or upper airway obstruction.
4. Remember that IV epinephrine is extremely toxic, and recommended dosage regimens should not be exceeded (1 cc of epinephrine 1:10,000, further diluted in 10 cc of saline

given over 5 to 10 minutes). IV use should be reserved for refractory shock and incipient airway obstruction only.

5. Do not withhold epinephrine in the elderly or cardiac patient if life-threatening manifestations develop.

6. Remember that recurrence of the anaphylactic syndrome may occur in 4 to 8 hours after complete resolution of initial symptoms and signs.

7. Do not prescribe cephalosporins in patients with severe systemic reactions to penicillin. The same is true of all penicillin derivatives including the monobactam, Imepenum.

8. Remember that prompt therapy may be life-saving, and keep a high index of suspicion of anaphylaxis, even if only one component of the syndrome is present (e.g., urticaria).

REFERENCES

1. Kelly, J.F., and Patterson, R.: Anaphylaxis: Course, mechanisms, and treatment. JAMA 227:1431, 1974.
2. Lucke, W.C., and Thomas, T.H.: Anaphylaxis: Pathophysiology, clinical presentations, and treatment. J. Emerg. Med. 1:83, 1983.
3. Weiszer, I.: Allergic emergencies. In Allergic Diseases: Diagnosis and Management (3rd Ed.) Edited by Patterson, R. Philadelphia, J.B. Lippincott Co., pp. 418–439, 1985.
4. Fisher, M.: Anaphylaxis. DM 33:433, 1987.
5. Terr, A.I.: Anaphylaxis. Clin. Rev. Allergy 3:3, 1985.
6. Lindzon, R.D., and Silvers, W.S.: Anaphylaxis. In Emergency Medicine, Concepts, and Clinical Practice (2nd Ed.) Edited by Rosen, P., Baker, F.J., Barkin, R.M., et al. St. Louis, The C.V. Mosby Co., pp. 203–231, 1988.
7. Ishizaka, K., and Ishizaka, T.: Immunology of IgE-mediated hypersensitivity. In Allergy: Principles and Practice (2nd Ed.). Edited by Middleton, E., Reed, C.E., and Ellis, E.J.: St. Louis, C.V. Mosby & Co., 1983.
8. Wasserman, S.I.: Mediators of Immediate Hypersensitivity. J. Allergy Clin. Immunol. 72:101, 1983.
9. Sheffer, A.L.: Anaphylaxis. J. Allergy Clin. Immunol. 75:227, 233, 1985.
10. Stark, B.J., and Sullivan, T.J.: Biphasic and protracted anaphylaxis. J. Allergy Clin. Immunol. 78:76, 1986.
11. Reisman, R.E., and Livingston, A.: Late-onset allergic reactions, including serum sickness after insect stings. J. Allergy Clin. Immunol. 84:331, 1989.
12. Patterson, R., and Valentine, M.: Anaphylaxis and related allergic emergencies including reactions due to insect stings. JAMA 248:2632, 1982.
13. Smith, P.L., Kagey-Sobotka, A., Bleecker, E.R., et al.: Physiologic manifestaions of human anaphylaxis. J. Clin. Invest. 66:1072, 1980.
14. Silverman, H.J., Van Hook, C., and Haponik, E.F.: Hemodynamic changes in human anaphylaxis. Am. J. Med. 77:341, 1984.
15. Carlson, R.W., Schaeffer, R.C., Puri, V.K., et al.: Hypovolemia and permeability pulmonary edema associated with anaphylaxis. Crit. Care. Med. 9:883, 1981.
16. Booth, B.H., Patterson, R.: Electrocardiographic changes during human anaphylaxis. JAMA 211:627, 1970.
17. Levine, H.D.: Acute myocardial infarction following wasp sting. Am. Heart J. 91:365, 1976.
18. Barach, E.M., and Nowack, R.M.: Epinephrine for treatment of anaphylactic shock. JAMA 25:2118, 1984.
19. Moore, G.P., Hurley, W.T., Pace, S.A.: Hereditary angioedema. Ann. Emerg. Med. 17:1082, 1988.
20. Russell, F.E., and Maretic, Z.: Scombroid poisoning: Mini-review with case histories. Toxicon 24:967, 1986.
21. Zautcke, J.L., Schwartz, J.A., and Mueller, E.J.: Chinese restaurant syndrome: A review. Ann. Emerg. Med. 15:1210, 1986.
22. Snyder, H.S., Weiss, E.: Hysterical stridor: A benign cause of upper airway obstruction. Ann. Emerg. Med. 18:991, 1989.
23. O'Leary, M.R., and Smith, M.S.: Penicillin anaphylaxis. Am. J. Emerg. Med. 4:241, 1986.
24. Saxon, A., Beall-Gelden, N., Rohr, A.S., et al: UCLA conference: immediate hypersensitivity reactions to beta-lactam antibiotics. Ann. Intern. Med. 107:204, 1987.
25. Settipane, G.A., and Boyd, G.K.: Anaphylaxis from insect stings: Myth, controversy, and reality. Postgrad. Med. 86:273, 1989.
26. Piacentine, J., Curry, S.C., and Ryan, P.J.: Life-threatening anaphylaxis following a Gila monster bite. Ann. Emerg. Med. 15:959, 1986.
27. Greenberger, P.A.: Contrast media reactions. J. Allergy Clin. Immunol. 74:600, 1984.
28. Yunginger, J.W., Sweeney, K.G., Sturner, W.Q., et al.: Fatal food-induced anaphylaxis. JAMA 260:1450, 1988.
29. Amlot, P.L., Kemeny, D.M., Zachary, C., et al.: Oral allergy syndrome (OAS): Symptoms of IgE-mediated hypersensitivity to foods. Clin. Allergy 17:33, 1987.
30. Novey, H.S., Fairshter, R.D., Salness, K., et al.: Postprandial exercise-induced anaphylaxis. J. Allergy Clin. Immunol. 71:498, 1983.
31. Stevenson, D.D.: Diagnosis, prevention, and treatment of adverse reactions to aspirin and nonsteroidal anti-inflammatory drugs. J. Allergy Clin. Immunol. 74:617, 1984.
32. Sandler, R.H.: Anaphylactic reactions to zomepirac. Ann. Emerg. Med. 14:171, 1985.
33. Sheffer, A.L., and Austen, K.F.: Exercise-induced anaphylaxis. J. Allergy Clin. Immunol. 73:699, 1984.
34. Slater, E.E., Merrill, D.D., Guess, H.A., et al.: Clinical profile of angioedema associated with angiotensin converting-enzyme inhibition. JAMA 260:967, 1988.
35. Perkin, R.M., and Anas, N.G.: Mechanisms and management of anaphylactic shock, not responding to traditional therapy. Ann. Allergy 54:202, 1985.
36. Wiggins, C.A., Dykewicz, M.S., and Patterson, R.: Idiopathic anaphylaxis: A review. Ann. Allergy 62:1, 1989.
37. Oertel, T., and Loehr, M.M.: Bee-sting anaphylaxis: The use of the military antishock trousers. Ann. Emerg. Med. 13:459, 1984.
38. Mayumi, H., Kimura, S., Asana, M., et al.: Intravenous cimetidine as an effective treatment for systemic anaphylaxis and acute allergic skin reactions. Ann. Allergy 58:447, 1987.
39. Littenberg, B., Gluck, E.H.: A controlled trial of methylprednisolone in the emergency treatment of acute asthma. N. Engl. J. Med. 314:150, 1986.
40. Cydulka, R., Davison, R., and Grammer, L.: The use of epinephrine in the treatment of older adult asthmatics. Ann. Emerg. Med. 17:322, 1988.

VACCINES AND IMMUNOPROPHYLAXIS

David N. Zull and Nancy Clark

CAPSULE

Every year, both children and adults develop vaccine-preventable diseases because they have not received the recommended pediatric immunizations and adult boosters. For example, in epidemics of measles and mumps reported in the United States, over 10% of cases occurred in adults.[1,2] In addition, more than 50% of Americans over 60 lack protective antibodies against tetanus and diphtheria.[2]

The emergency physician is in a position to recognize deficiencies in standard immunizations and provide such immunizations or referrals when appropriate. For many patients, Emergency Department (ED) care is the only form of medical care available. More commonly, the emergency physician is asked to provide postexposure prophylaxis, as in rabies, tetanus, hepatitis A, hepatitis B, and erythroblastosis fetalis. Last, the emergency physician should be aware of the side effects and contraindications of vaccinations, both for his or her medicolegal protection and recognition of hypersensitivity and infectious complications in vaccine recipients. The second part of this chapter reviews immunization controversies, including pertussis, polio, Hemophilus influenzae type b, influenza, and pneumococcal vaccines.

INTRODUCTION

Immunization is a process in which protective antibodies are actively induced or passively provided to a person who is susceptible because he or she has not acquired the natural disease in the past. Active immunization mimics acute infection by introducing the patient to a foreign antigen that is alive or killed or some antigenic component of the organism that induces protective antibodies. If there has been no prior exposure to the antibody, response usually takes 7 to 21 days. If there has been prior exposure to vaccine or natural infection, secondary antibody production after repeat immunization occurs within 4 days.[3] A vaccine may be a live attenuated virus (measles, mumps, rubella, polio, and yellow fever) or a killed microorganism (rabies, influenza, pertussis, cholera, and typhoid). A vaccine may also contain highly defined antigens (the polysaccharide of Hemophilus influenzae type B and the pneumococcus, or the surface antigen of hepatitis B). Active immunity may also be achieved with a toxoid, which is a modified bacterial toxin that has been rendered nontoxic (tetanus, diphtheria). Vaccines made from live organisms or polysaccharide components generally provide lifelong immunity, whereas killed vaccines and toxoids require repeated primary vaccinations and periodic boosters to maintain antibody titers.[3,4]

Passive immunization refers to the provision of temporary immunity by administering preformed antibodies. Immune globulin is a sterile solution for intramuscular use, fractionated from large pools of human plasma and used in the prophylaxis of hepatitis A and measles. Intravenous immune globulin is especially prepared for IV use, but is limited to therapy of immunodeficiency states and immune disorders like idiopathic thrombocytopenic purpura (ITP). Specific immune globulin preparations pooled from previously infected or hyperimmunized donors is available against hepatitis B, rabies, tetanus, and varicella zoster. None of these human immune globulin preparations has been shown to transmit human immunodeficiency virus or other infectious diseases.[4] Antitoxin refers to a solution of antibodies derived from horses immunized against specific poisons; such solutions include diphtheria antitoxin, botulinum antitoxin, and snake antivenoms.

PRE-EXPOSURE IMMUNIZATIONS

Emergency physicians should be familiar with the recommended immunizations for children (Table 51-15) and adults (Table 51-16) so as to identify patients at risk for infection. Immigrants, the elderly, and lower socioeconomic groups are the most likely patients who have not been adequately vaccinated. Tetanus and diphtheria immunizations are initiated in the ED as part of a postexposure prophylaxis (see Post-exposure Immunizations), whereas the need for other pre-

TABLE 51-15. RECOMMENDED IMMUNIZATION SCHEDULE FOR INFANTS AND CHILDREN*

Age	Vaccines	Comments
2 months	DPT #1†, OPV #1‡, Hib #1‖	
4 months	DPT #2, OPV #2, Hib #2‖	
6 months	DPT #3, Hib #3‖	OPV #3 in high risk areas
15 months	MMR§, DPT #4, OPV #3, Hib #4‖	
4–6 years	DPT #5, OPV #4, MMR #2‖	At or before school entry
11 years	MMR§	Booster given here if not given earlier, i.e., 4–6 years
14–16 years	Td + +#	Repeat every 10 years

* With permission from Advisory Committee on Immunization Practices: General recommendations on Immunization. M.M.W.R. *38*:205, 1989.
† Diphtheria and tetanus toxoids and pertussis, adsorbed
‡ Oral poliovirus vaccine, live oral, trivalent
§ Measles-mumps-rubella virus vaccine, live. Not to be given (15 months)
‖ Hemophilus influenza b polysaccharide antigen conjugated to a protein carrier, H to C
Tetanus and diphtheria toxoids, adsorbed

exposure vaccinations should be identified and appropriately referred.

MEASLES

Measles is a highly contagious illness traditionally seen in preschool children. Although there has been a 75% reduction in measles cases since the 1970s, the early 1980's showed a progressive rise in measles with most of the outbreaks in children from 10 to 19 years of age and in young adults (especially on college campuses).[5] In the measles epidemic of 1989, however, there was a resurgence of cases in inner-city children under 5 years old. These children had not received their routine primary immunizations or were too young for routine immunization (under 15 months old).[5–8]

Measles vaccine is a live attenuated virus vaccine that should provide lifelong immunity with a single dose; however, in recent inner-city outbreaks, over half of the reported cases had been previously vaccinated. As a result, the Centers for Disease Control (CDC) now recommends a two-dose immunization schedule. The initial dose should be given at age 15 months, except in areas at high risk for preschool transmission, where it should be given at 12 months. The second dose should be given at school entry (5 years), although older children and young adults should be vaccinated during urban epidemics. Vaccination as early as 6 to 9 months may be considered during inner-city outbreaks, followed by two additional shots at 15 months and 5 years.[9,10] Regarding adults, individuals born before 1956 are likely to have been infected naturally and are thereby considered immune. Adults born after 1956 should be immunized during outbreaks or if they are in a high-risk profession (e.g., health care); this need is obviated only by documentation of rubeola antibody titers.[5–7,9,10]

As was demonstrated in a Chicago measles epi-

demic, EDs may be called on to vaccinate susceptible children with uncertain follow-up plans.[8] In addition, modifying the severity of the illness by postexposure vaccination makes ED administration appropriate. Immune serum globulin may modify the infection in doses of 0.25 mL per kg if given within 6 days of exposure in infants under 1 year old, in immunosuppressed hosts (dose 0.5 cc per kg), or in children over 1 year after 72 hours of exposure. Infants as young as 6 months may receive preexposure prophylaxis in measles-prevalent areas, but it should not be given within 3 months of giving immune serum globulin.

Measles vaccine is available alone or combined with mumps and rubella vaccines (MMR). Both forms are equally effective against measles, and while MMR may be preferred in children, it often results in transient arthritis and arthralgia in adults and thereby should be used selectively in older patients. Other untoward reactions include fever up to 39.4°C in 5 to 15% of recipients, transient rashes in 5%, and encephalitis in less than one per 1 million vaccinations.[3,6,8]

MUMPS

From 1985 to 1987, the number of reported cases of mumps increased fourfold, and the reported peak incidence rate shifted from 5- to 9-year-olds to individuals 10 to 19 years old, with outbreaks in adults as well. It is complicated by meningitis in 15% of cases and by orchitis in 20% of postpubertal men.

A large cohort of young adults currently entering the work force are susceptible to mumps infection. This susceptibility has occurred because it was not until 1977 that a live attenuated mumps vaccine was required for routine childhood immunizations to produce prolonged immunity in over 90% of recipients. Before this time, there had been only partial use of mumps vaccinations including both live attenuated

TABLE 51-16. RECOMMENDED ADULT IMMUNIZATIONS AND PROTOCOLS FOR MISSED PRIMARY IMMUNIZATIONS

Vaccine	Age	Primary Immunization	Immunization Recommendation
Tetanus-diphtheria	Any	Yes	Td at 10-year intervals
	>6 years	No	Td at initial visit, 1 month, and 6–12 months
	<6 years	No	DPT at initial visit, 1 month, 6–12 months
Measles	Born before 1956	Yes or no	No vaccine
	Born after 1956	Yes	Immunize if given before 12 months of age
			Immunize if vaccinated 1963–1967
			Immunize if school outbreak and vaccinated before 1980
	Born before 1956	No	Vaccinate with measles vaccine or MMR
Mumps	Born before 1956	Yes or no	Do not vaccinate
	Born after 1956	Yes	Do not vaccinate
	Born after 1956	No	Immunize with mumps vaccine or MMR unless physician-documented illness
Rubella	Any	Yes	Do not vaccinate
	Any	No	Vaccinate all women of childbearing years and health care workers who are susceptible by serologic testing
Pneumovax	>65 years		One-time vaccination (booster in 5–10 years if immunocompromised)
Influenza	<65 years		If chronically ill (see text)
	>65 years		Yearly vaccinations
	<65 years		Yearly vaccinations if chronically ill (see text)

and killed virus preparations (the latter which was ineffective). Partial vaccine use kept the disease at a low incidence so that a large number of unvaccinated children never acquired natural immunity.[11,12] As with measles, persons born before 1956 are presumed immune by natural infection, whereas those born after 1956 should be vaccinated if there is any uncertainty of their mumps disease history or vaccination status. It is available either in monovalent form or as part of the MMR, and should be given to children at 15 months of age and also to susceptible adults. There is no contraindication to vaccination of persons previously infected or immunized, and side effects are minimal (one case of meningitis is described). Postexposure mumps immunization does not appear to be protective, yet taking this opportunity to immunize high-risk patients is reasonable.[11–14]

RUBELLA

Rubella is a self-limited viral syndrome with exanthem that is sometimes complicated by transient arthritis. If infection occurs in the first trimester of pregnancy, congenital rubella syndrome may result in up to 80% of fetuses. As a result, the objective of rubella im-

munization in children at 15 months of age and susceptible adults is the prevention of infection in women of childbearing age. An estimated 10 to 15% of young adults are susceptible. Unless there is documentation of vaccination after the first birthday or a positive serologic test, susceptible adults should be vaccinated, especially if they are in the health care profession. Women who are pregnant or planning pregnancy in the next 3 months should not be vaccinated, although no case of the congenital rubella syndrome has been documented in women inadvertently immunized.[15] Adverse effects associated with rubella vaccine include low-grade fever and rash in 5 to 10% of recipients, and arthralgias with or without arthritis. The rheumatologic symptoms are age-dependent, with less than 3% in children and as many as 40% in adult women. This fact may temper the use of MMR in adults, although rubella vaccine is available in the monovalent form.[3,10,15,16]

DIPHTHERIA

Diphtheria classically involves the respiratory tract. Symptoms include serosanguinous nasal discharge, acute pharyngitis with membrane formation on the tonsils and soft palate, and laryngotracheitis. Diphtheria may also infect the skin, and is characterized by chronic nonhealing ulcers with a dirty grey membrane. Respiratory diphtheria is often associated with toxin production, resulting in myocarditis and polyneuropathy. Cutaneous infection is more indolent, and signs of intoxication are unusual.

Widespread immunization has almost eliminated diphtheria from the United States, with only two to three cases per year reported. Nevertheless, 50 to 70% of Americans over 60 lack adequate antibodies against diphtheria and tetanus because of inadequate immunization, accounting for the predominance of disease in older adults.[2] In addition, large outbreaks of predominantly cutaneous diphtheria have been reported in the urban, indigent alcoholic population and Native Americans.[17] Current recommendations are that diphtheria toxoid be given routinely in conjunction with tetanus toxoid, as outlined in Table 51-17. Minimal to no increase in adverse reactions is seen with the combination of tetanus and diphtheria toxoids over tetanus toxoid alone.[18]

Diphtheria antitoxin produced in horses is a cornerstone of therapy for acute respiratory diphtheria in conjunction with penicillin or erythromycin therapy.

HEALTH CARE WORKER PRE-EXPOSURE IMMUNIZATION

Universal immunization to measles, mumps, and rubella is recommended unless a health care worker has documented immunity. Occasional cases of poliomyelitis occur in the United States, and it is recommended that all health care personnel be immune. For

those without proof of completed primary series, completion with inactivated poliomyelitis vaccine is recommended. Intravenous poliovirus vaccine (IPV) is preferred over oral poliovirus vaccine (OPV) in susceptible adults because of the slightly increased risk of vaccine-associated paralysis after administration of OPV.[19]

Annual immunization of health care workers with influenza vaccine is recommended to reduce morbidity and the likelihood of transmission of influenza to debilitated patients who are at risk of complications from this disease. Hepatitis B vaccination is recommended for all health care workers who have contact with blood and blood products.

TRAVELERS' PRE-EXPOSURE IMMUNIZATIONS

An awareness of immunization requirements for international travelers is worthwhile to help emergency physicians to better recognize vaccine side effects and the potential infectious diseases that may be acquired during travel.

First of all, routine immunizations should be updated before travel, including tetanus-diphtheria boosters and measles vaccination. Regarding tetanus-diphtheria, the problem is not increased risk of infection subsequent to injuries occurring overseas, but rather the issue of availability and safety of this vaccine outside the U.S. The risk of measles may be substantially greater overseas, and all who are at risk should be immunized.[20]

Yellow fever and cholera immunizations are compulsory for entry into certain countries. Yellow fever, which occurs in parts of tropical Africa and South America, is a fulminant febrile illness characterized by hepatitis, hemorrhagic diathesis, and nephropathy. It is a mosquito-borne viral illness with a 50% fatality rate. The vaccine is a live virus preparation given 10 days before travel and is available only in designated vaccination centers. Up to 10% of vaccinees develop headache, fever, and myalgias 5 to 10 days after vaccination.[20,21]

The risk of cholera among travelers is low, but cholera immunization is still required for travel to Southeast Asia, the Indian subcontinent, and the Middle East. The vaccine is of limited efficacy and is commonly associated with local reactions and occasional fever and malaise. In fact, this severe diarrheal illness is best prevented by careful food and water hygiene.[20,22]

Other diseases encountered by travelers to specific endemic areas in which immunizations are sometimes recommended include typhoid, hepatitis A, polio, meningococcal disease, plague, rabies, and hepatitis B. Side effects of the vaccines for these diseases consist primarily of local reactions, with occasional mild systemic symptoms.[20] One follow-up study from an immunization center revealed that travelers returned

TABLE 51-17. TETANUS PROPHYLAXIS IN WOUND MANAGEMENT*

Immunization History	Clean, Minor Wounds		All Other Wounds†	
	Td+	TIG	Td+	TIG
Unknown or <3 doses	Yes	No	Yes	Yes
>3 doses				
<5 yrs since last dose	No	No	Yes	No
>5 yrs since last dose	No	No	Yes	No
>10 yrs since last dose	Yes	No	Yes	No

* With permission from Advisory Committee on Immunization Practices: Diphtheria, tetanus, and pertussis: Guidelines for vaccine prophylaxis and other preventative measures. M.M.W.R. *34*:405, 1985.
† Examples are wounds contaminated with dirt, feces, soil, saliva, etc.; puncture wounds; avulsions; wounds resulting from missiles, crushing, burns, and frostbite; wounds > 24 hours old
§ For children <7 years of age, DPT preferred; for persons ≥ 7 years old, Td preferred.

with diarrhea (25%), upper respiratory infections (5%), rashes (1%), and malaria ($\frac{1}{2}$%). Of these travelers, 27% were noncompliant with chloroquine prophylaxis[23] (see Chapter 76).

POSTEXPOSURE IMMUNIZATIONS

It is in the prevention or modification of disease after exposure that the proper administration of immunizations by the emergency physician is so critical. Preventable diseases after exposure include tetanus, diphtheria, rabies, hepatitis A, measles, and erythroblastosis fetalis.

TETANUS

Tetanus, with its characteristic clinical manifestations of trismus, paroxysmal muscle spasms, and generalized muscle hypertonia, is caused by a potent exotoxin elaborated by Clostridium tetani, which is ubiquitous in the environment and causes 300,000 to 500,000 cases of tetanus worldwide each year. In the U.S., 60 to 100 cases are reported each year, and more than 70% of these occur in persons over 50 with unknown or incomplete immunization status.[24,25]

An analysis of 147 cases of tetanus in the U.S. during 1985 to 1986 showed that 70% of cases occurred after an acute injury, 20% were associated with chronic wounds, 1% were related to intravenous drug use, and 9% had no known cause.[24]

Because of the high fatality rate of tetanus (30 to 50%), appropriate wound care and administration of tetanus toxoid (preferably in combination with diphtheria toxoid) and human globulin are important.

To reduce the likelihood of Clostridium tetani proliferation, the wound site should be thoroughly cleansed, pus drained, foreign bodies removed, necrotic tissue meticulously debrided, and antibiotic prophylaxis considered.

Table 51-17 summarizes the current recommendations for tetanus prophylaxis in wound care in an adult or a child 7 years or older. In children under 7 years, DPT should be given unless there is a history of hypersensitivity to pertussis, in which case DT is recommended. Adults and children 7 years and older should receive lower-dose diphtheria immunization (Td) at a dose of 0.5 mL IM. Patients who have received the full immunization series or a booster dose within 10 years and have a clean, minor wound require no additional immunoprophylaxis; whereas if the last dose was more than 5 years previously and the wound is tetanus-prone, Td should be given without tetanus immunoglobulin (TIG). Tetanus-prone wounds include those contaminated with dirt, feces, or saliva; puncture wounds; avulsions, wounds neglected for more than 24 hours; crush injuries; burns; wounds from missiles; and frostbite.[18,25]

If the patient has not received the full tetanus series or the immunization status is unknown, Td and TIG should be given for tetanus-prone wounds, whereas Td alone is recommended for clean, minor wounds. Studies of tetanus prophylaxis in EDs have shown significant numbers of patients that had been both overtreated (12 to 17%) and undertreated (2 to 6%).[26,27] Undertreatment places the patient at risk for tetanus, and overimmunization increases the risk of adverse reactions and unnecessarily increases health care costs.

The most common adverse reaction is local erythema, with induration and tenderness at the injection site. Fever and systemic reactions are uncommon unless the patient has been hyperimmunized. This Arthus-type hypersensitivity reaction occurs 2 to 8 hours after the injection. It is self-limiting and rarely serious. Anaphylaxis, urticaria, angioedema, and neurologic complications have been reported rarely.[18,28]

The only contraindication to administering tetanus-diphtheria toxoids is a history of severe hypersensitivity reaction or neurologic reaction after a previous dose. If a patient relates a history of an extensive local reaction or systemic anaphylaxis to tetanus toxoid, he or she probably has a high titer of protective antibodies to tetanus. If the physician is confronted with a tetanus-prone wound in a tetanus-allergic patient whose last dose was more than 5 years ago, TIG alone may be the safest alternative. Concomitant administration of penicillin or metronidazole seems prudent, but has never been proven effective. In a clean, minor wound, determination of serum antitoxin levels may be helpful. A high antitoxin titer precludes the need for Td or TIG, whereas a low titer indicates that the administration of Td is safe as well as necessary.

Human TIG is given IM at a dose of 250 IU. TIG does not need to be given in the wound site, and care should be taken to use separate sites with separate needles and syringes when Td is given concomitantly. The TIG dose may be increased to 500 IU in highly tetanus-prone wounds. In clinical tetanus, TIG in a dose of 500 to 1000 IU IM is a critical part of management in conjunction with intensive care unit (ICU) supportive measures and muscle relaxants.[18,25]

RABIES

Rabies is a viral encephalitis with virtually 100% mortality that progresses inexorably once symptoms have developed. With timely administration of rabies vaccine and rabies immune globulin in the ED, this tragedy can be avoided. Although over 20,000 deaths per year secondary to rabies are reported to the World Health Organization (WHO), these cases are confined primarily to tropical regions such as India, Thailand, Brazil, and the Philippines. In the U.S., there were only 51 cases of rabies from 1960 to 1989, and only 12 of these since 1980.[29,30]

Because rabies is acquired from the bite or mucous membrane exposure of mammalian carnivores, the risk of human cases is determined by the local incidence of rabies in wild and domestic animals. Before the nationwide animal vaccination programs of the 40s and 50s, domestic dogs and cats were the major source of rabies in the U.S. Since 1960, the prevalence of animal rabies has shifted to wildlife, principally skunks, bats, raccoons, and foxes; however, one third of cases of human rabies in this period resulted from exposure to rabid dogs outside the U.S. (especially Mexico). Interestingly, over 20% of human rabies cases in the last 30 years had no known animal exposure.[29,30] Nonbite exposures like scratches, licking, mucous membrane exposure, and inhalation must be kept in mind. Human-to-human spread of rabies has never been documented except in corneal transplantation.[31]

In assessing the risk of rabies from an animal bite seen in the ED, the physician must consider the species involved, the local epidemiology of rabies, and the animal's behavior and domestication. Ninety percent of animal rabies in the U.S. is reported in skunks, bats, raccoons, and foxes; therefore, animals and humans exposed to these and related wild species should be considered rabid. In contrast, rodents, rabbits, and all nonmammals are considered virtually free of rabies risk. As a result, bites of dogs, cats, and domesticated wild animals pose the most difficult decision regarding rabies prophylaxis for the emergency physician.[32]

Regarding dog and cat bites, if the animal is captured and appears healthy, it should be confined and observed for 10 days after biting a person. If it appears ill or vicious (unprovoked attack) on capture or during quarantine, it should be sacrificed and the brain analyzed with rabies fluorescent antibody. At this point, the patient should have prophylaxis initiated pending the results. Quarantine is generally not recommended for wild animals because incubation periods may be variable or prolonged. Exceptions to immediate sacrifice are domesticated wild animals (e.g., ferrets) or rare or valuable animals. In either circumstance, rabies prophylaxis should be initiated. The epidemiology of animal rabies in your locale may influence your decision regarding prophylaxis, but this information is useful only when an area has been consistently rabies-free (e.g., Hawaii and New York City).[32,33]

If there is definite bite or nonbite (saliva into a wound or mucous membrane) exposure to a species in which there is risk of rabies, in a locale where animal rabies has been reported, the physician should initiate prophylaxis and appropriate wound care. It has been shown in experimental animals that thorough cleansing and irrigation of the wound with a 20% soap solution may reduce the risk of rabies by as much as 90%, especially if the wound is superficial. Other irrigants such as benzalkonium chloride and 70% ethanol are also rabicidal, but are irritating to tissues. Wounds to the face and those with extensive tissue destruction are of particularly high risk and should be treated aggressively. During irrigation, vigorous swabbing is recommended. Thorough removal of foreign bodies and debridement of devitalized tissue should be performed, and wounds should not be sutured. If the size of the wound allows, infiltration with human rabies immune globulin (up to one half the dose) should be performed.[34,35]

Rabies immune globulin (RIG) is a plasma concentrate, obtained from hyperimmunized adults, which provides immediate and short-term immunity while awaiting the antibody response from vaccination. RIG and human diploid cell vaccine (HDCV) should be administered concomitantly (different sites) within 24 hours of exposure. Further delays may significantly decrease its protective benefit, but it is never too late to try. If RIG is not given concomitantly with HDCV, it can be given up to the eighth day after vaccination, after which time endogenous antibody production has begun.[36] See Table 51-18 for further recommendations.

Several cases of clinical rabies have resulted when vaccination alone was administered as prophylaxis, emphasizing the critical importance of RIG. Twenty IU per kg is the recommended dose, with up to half that amount infiltrated at the wound site and the remainder IM. If aerosol or mucous membrane exposure occurs, the entire RIG dose should be given IM. The only exception to RIG use is the patient who has received pre-exposure prophylaxis so that a prompt amnestic response to vaccination would be expected.[32,34,36]

Side effects from RIG are minimal, with occasional local pain and low-grade fever. Hepatitis or systemic allergic reactions have never been reported.

Human diploid cell vaccine is a killed-virus vaccine, grown on human tissue culture, which replaced the duck embryo vaccine (DEV) in 1980. The DEV was immunogenically weak, requiring 23 serial injections, and had a high incidence of side effects.

HDCV in conjunction with RIG should be given as soon as possible after possible rabies exposure (preferably within 24 hours). Additional doses of HDCV alone are administered on days 3, 7, 14, and 28. HDCV, 1.0 mL for both adults and children, should be given IM in the deltoid in an adult or in the thigh in a child. The gluteal area should be avoided because antibody response to HDCV vaccination may be submaximal in this area compared to the deltoid. A reduced antibody response to gluteal injection has been clearly demonstrated for hepatitis B vaccine, and two recent failures of rabies prophylaxis have been partially attributed to gluteal injection.[37,38]

Selected high-risk individuals such as veterinarians, animal handlers, spelunkers (cave explorers), and travelers to areas of endemic canine rabies should receive pre-exposure rabies prophylaxis, consisting of

	TABLE 51-18. RABIES POSTEXPOSURE PROPHYLAXIS*	

The following recommendations are only a guide. In applying them, take into account the animal species involved, the circumstances of the bite or other exposure, the vaccination status of the animal, and presence of rabies in the region. Local or state public health officials should be consulted if questions arise about the need for rabies prophylaxis.

Animal Species	Condition of Animal at Time of Attack	Treatment of Exposed Person†
Domestic: Dog and cat	Healthy and available for 10 days of observation	None, unless animal develops rabies§
	Rabid or suspected rabid	RIG‖ and HDCV
	Unknown (escaped)	Consult public health officials. If treatment is indicated, give RIG‖ and HDCV
Wild: Skunk, bat, fox, coyote, raccoon, bobcat, and other carnivores	Regard as rabid unless proven negative by laboratory tests#	RIG‖ and HDCV
Other: Livestock, rodents, and lagomorphs (rabbits and hares)	Consider individually. Local and state public health officials should be consulted on questions about the need for rabies prophylaxis. Bites of squirrels, hamsters, guinea pigs, gerbils, chipmunks, rats, mice, other rodents, rabbits, and hares almost never call for antirabies prophylaxis.	

* With permission from Advisory Committee on Immunization Practices: Rabies prevention—United States, 1984. M.M.W.R. *33*:393, 1984.

† *All bites and wounds should immediately be thoroughly cleansed with soap and water.* If antirabies treatment is indicated, both rabies immune globulin (RIG) and human diploid cell rabies vaccine (HDCV) should be given as soon as possible, *regardless* of the interval from exposure. Local reactions to vaccines are common and do not contraindicate continuing treatment. Discontinue vaccine if fluorescent-antibody tests of the animal are negative.

§ During the usual holding period of 10 days, begin treatment with RIG and HDCV at first sign of rabies in a dog or cat that has bitten someone. The symptomatic animal should be killed immediately and tested.

‖ If RIG is not available, use antirabies serum, equine (ARS). Do not use more than the recommended dosage.

The animal should be killed and tested as soon as possible. Holding for observation is not recommended, unless there is a special circumstance.

three doses of HDCV on days 0, 7, and 28. This prophylaxis does not preclude the need for repeated vaccination if the patient is subsequently bitten by a potentially rabid animal. Such patients should receive HDCV 1.0 mL on days 0 and 3; concomitant RIG is not necessary. See Table 51-19 for further details.

Adverse reactions to HDCV consist of local pain, erythema, swelling, and pruritus in 25% of cases; mild systemic symptoms including myalgias, headache, nausea, abdominal pain and dizziness occur in about 20%. Immune complex reactions manifested by urticaria, arthralgias, arthritis, and fever are seen in up to 6% of patients receiving booster shots after preexposure prophylaxis; however, such reactions are rare during primary immunizations. Three neuroparalytic illnesses have been reported in association with HDCV: two cases resembling Guillain-Barré syndrome and one characterized by a subacute focal CNS disorder.[32,36]

Because of the virtual 100% mortality rate of human rabies (only three reported survivors in the literature), there are no absolute contraindications to rabies prophylaxis. Although data in pregnancy is limited, fetal abnormalities have not been reported, and rabies pro-

phylaxis should not be withheld. Even allergy to HDCV does not preclude its use in high-risk exposures; pretreating with antihistamines and keeping epinephrine on hand is suggested.

HEPATITIS

Hepatitis A (HAV) accounts for over one third of cases of acute hepatitis reported in the U.S. It is spread by person-to-person contact through fecal contamination, which is facilitated by poor personal hygiene, poor sanitation, and intimate (household or sexual) contact. The incubation period is 15 to 50 days (average 30 days), and the period of greatest infectivity is the 2-week interval before the onset of jaundice.

Before treatment of contacts is considered, serologic diagnosis of the index case must be confirmed by the finding of IgM-class anti-HAV serum antibodies. Serologic screening of contacts for anti-HAV antibodies is not recommended because it would delay therapy and incur greater cost.[39]

Immune globulin is effective in preventing hepatitis A when administered within 14 days of exposure; be-

TABLE 51-19. TREATMENT APPROACH FOR HIGH-RISK RABIES EXPOSURE

Local Wound Care
 Vigorous scrub with soap and water
 Irrigate with 20% soap solution
 Follow-up irrigation with high-pressure saline
 Debride devitalized tissue
 Do not suture
 Tetanus toxoid and antibiotic prophylaxis
Rabies Immune Globulin (Human)
 Dose: 20 IU/kg (150 IU/mL) intramuscularly
 One half of dose infiltrated into the wound
 If the site permits, the remainder IM
 Entire dose IM if mucus membrane or aerosol exposure
 Administer the same time as the vaccine, but different site
 If not given with vaccine initially, there still may be benefit up to 7 days later
 Should be given within 24 hours of exposure but is never too late
 No absolute contraindications
 Not required in patients who have received pre-exposure vaccinations (e.g., veterinarians)
 Virtually free of side effects
 If not available, equine antisera (ARS) 40 IU/kg IM
Human Diploid Cell Vaccine
 Dosage: 1.0 mL intramuscularly
 Site: Deltoid in adults, thigh in children
 If no previous immunizations, give vaccine on days 0, 3, 7, 14, and 28
 If pre-exposure prophylaxis, give vaccine alone, days 0 and 3
 No absolute contraindications except severe allergy
 Side effects: 20% local RXN, 25% mild systemic symptoms

yond that point, it is not indicated. The nature of exposure determines the need for ISG. The following are clear-cut indications for prophylaxis: all household and sexual contacts, residents and staff of custodial care institutions, and children and staff of day care centers. Routine administration of ISG in schools or hospital exposures is not indicated unless there is an outbreak or exposure to feces of infected individuals. Office and factory contacts should not be treated. Common source food-borne or water-borne exposure is usually not treated because, once cases have begun to appear, the 2-week period after exposure will have been exceeded. If a food handler is diagnosed as having acute hepatitis, fellow food handlers should receive ISG, but patrons are not treated unless the following criteria are satisfied: the patron can be identified within 2 weeks of exposure, the food handler's hygienic practices are shown to be deficient, and the food was not cooked after handling.[39]

For postexposure prophylaxis, a single IM dose of 0.02 mL per kg of ISG is recommended. Pre-exposure prophylaxis in a dose of 0.02 to 0.06 mL per kg has been proven effective in international travelers to endemic areas. Adverse reactions to ISG include local tenderness and, rarely, immune complex or anaphy-

lactic reactions, the more severe reactions often seen in IgA deficient individuals who have antibody to IgA.

POSTEXPOSURE PROPHYLAXIS IN MISCELLANEOUS DISEASES

MEASLES

ISG or measles vaccine administered within a few days of exposure may modify disease or perhaps prevent it.[3]

ERYTHROBLASTOSIS FETALIS

Rh Immune globulin, prepared from donors with high Rh antibody titer, is recommended for Rh-negative women who give birth to Rh-positive infants or who undergo abortion. It must be given within 72 hours.

BOTULISM

Trivalent equine antitoxin (1 to 3 vials IM) may modify the course of the disease.

HEPATITIS B

See next chapter section.

CONTRAINDICATIONS (Table 51-20)

PREGNANCY

It has generally become common practice to avoid all unnecessary drugs or procedures that may interfere with fetal development, including immunizations. Most data concerning adverse effects to vaccines in pregnancy are accumulated from cases in which vaccines were unknowingly given during pregnancy; as a result, the data is scanty. When vaccination is advisable in a pregnant patient, waiting until the first trimester is over is a reasonable precaution against teratogenicity. Exceptions to this rule include high-risk exposures to rabies or hepatitis B.[40]

Live-virus vaccines (measles, mumps, rubella, polio, and yellow fever) are contraindicated in pregnant women or those who are likely to become pregnant within 3 months of receiving the vaccine. The fetal risk, however, appears to be small as evidenced by data collected by the CDC on 988 women receiving

TABLE 51-20. IMMUNIZATIONS: CONTRAINDICATIONS AND TOXICITY

Vaccine	Type	Contraindications	Toxicity
Cholera	Killed bacteria	Previous severe local or systemic reaction	Local pain and induration for 1–2 days, occasional fever and malaise
Hemophilus influenza B	Polysaccharide	Vaccine hypersensitivity	Mild local reactions <10%
Hepatitis A	Gamma globulin	IgA deficiency or allergy	Local discomfort, anaphylaxis (rare)
Influenza	Killed virus	Egg allergy, first trimester of pregnancy	Mild local reaction <33%, malaise and myalgia 6–12 hours post vaccination, rare, allergic reaction
Measles	Live virus	Pregnancy, egg allergy, immunocompromised host, neomycin sensitivity	5–15% fever >39.4, 5–21 days post-vaccination, 5% transient rash, local reactions (rare), encephalitis (<1 in a million)
Mumps	Live virus	Pregnancy, immunocompromised host, egg or neomycin allergy	Mild allergic reaction (rare), parotitis (rare), meningitis (reported)
Pertussis	Killed bacteria	Serious febrile illness, active pertussis, neurologic illness	Fever and local reaction >60%, encephalopathy (reported), seizures or hypotonia 1 in 1750
Pneumovax	Polysaccharide	First trimester of pregnancy	Local reaction 50%
Polio	Live virus	Immunocompromised host, pregnancy	Paralysis (rare)
Rabies	Killed virus	Severe allergy	Local reaction 25%, headache, myalgia, nausea and dizziness 20%, guillain-barre (rare)
Rubella	Killed virus	Immunocompromised host, pregnancy	Arthralgias (1–3 weeks later) <40%, arthritis <2%
Tetanus-diphtheria	Toxoids	First trimester of pregnancy (unless high-risk wound), severe local or systemic reaction	Local reactions, systemic allergy, or arthus reaction (rare), mild fever, malaise
Typhoid	Killed bacteria	Previous reaction	Local reaction, mild systemic symptoms
Yellow fever	Live virus	Immunocompromised host, pregnancy, egg allergy	Fever and mild systemic symptoms <5% delayed allergic reaction

rubella vaccinations within 3 months before or after conception. No cases of congenital rubella syndrome were identified among the children borne by these women.[41]

There are no data to suggest risk to the fetus from immunizing pregnant women with inactivated viral or bacterial vaccines or toxoids. Tetanus and diphtheria toxoids should be given to pregnant women when the clinical circumstances indicate a risk of disease, but waiting until the second trimester is preferred.

ALLERGY TO VACCINE COMPONENTS

Allergic reactions to vaccines may range from mild local reactions to systemic anaphylaxis. Various vaccine components may cause hypersensitivity, including animal proteins, antibiotics, preservatives, and stabilizers. The most common allergen identified is egg protein, found in measles, mumps, influenza, and yellow fever vaccines. Patients with anaphylactic sensitivity to egg products should not be vaccinated, but those able to eat eggs can be treated safely.

Certain vaccines contain trace amounts of antibiotics, such as neomycin, which is found in measles, mumps, and rubella vaccines. Although rare, anaphylactic sensitivity to this component precludes its use. No currently available vaccines contain penicillin or its derivatives. Most local reactions and fever to vaccines are thought to be toxic rather than allergic reactions; however, sensitivity may occur to the vaccine itself, as in the case of tetanus toxoid.[28,40]

IMMUNOCOMPROMISED STATES

Administration of live, attenuated virus vaccines in an immunocompromised host may cause rapid virus replication and severe systemic illness. As a result, patients with leukemia, lymphoma, generalized malignancy, chemotherapy induced immunosuppression, and symptomatic HIV infection should not be given live vaccines. Immunization recommendations for children with HIV infection are given in Table 51-21. Toxoids, polysaccharides, and killed-virus vaccines may be given, but may have decreased effectiveness.[40]

TABLE 51-21. RECOMMENDATIONS FOR ROUTINE IMMUNIZATION OF HIV-INFECTED CHILDREN, UNITED STATES

Vaccine	Known HIV Infection	
	Asymptomatic	Symptomatic
DTP*	Yes	Yes
OPV†	No	No
IPV§*	Yes	Yes
MMR‖	Yes	Yes#
HbCV**	Yes	Yes
Pneumococcal	Yes	Yes
Influenza	No††	Yes

* DTP = Diphtheria and tetanus toxoids and pertussis vaccine, adsorbed. DTP may be used up to the seventh birthday.
† OPV = Poliovirus vaccine live, oral, trivalent.
§ IPV = Poliovirus vaccine Inactived.
‖ MMR = Measles, Mumps, and Rubella Virus Vaccine, Live.
Should be considered.
** HbCV = Vaccine composed of Hemophilus influenzae b polysaccharide antigen conjugated to a protein carrier.
†† Not contraindicated.

FEBRILE ILLNESS

Febrile illness is not a contraindication per se to vaccination, but if the illness is severe, postponement is appropriate to avoid superimposing vaccine side effects on the underlying illness or mistakenly attributing symptoms to the vaccination.[4]

REFERENCES

1. Centers for Disease Control (CDC): Progress toward achieving the national 1990 objectives for immunizations. M.M.W.R. 37:613, 1988.
2. CDC: National Adult Immunization Awareness Week. M.M.W.R. 38:708, 1989.
3. Hinman, A.R., Orenstein, W.A., Bart, K.J., et al.: Immunization. In Principles and Practice of Infectious Diseases. 3rd Ed. Edited by Mandell, G.L., Douglas, R.G., and Bennett, J.E. New York, Churchill Livingstone, 1990, pp. 2320–2334.
4. Advisory Committee on Immunization Practices (ACIP): General recommendations on immunization. M.M.W.R. 38:205, 1989.
5. Medical Letter: Measles revaccination. Med. Lett. 31:69, 1989.
6. CDC: Measles—United States, 1988. M.M.W.R. 38:601, 1989.
7. Markowitz, L.E., Preblud, S.R., Orenstein, W.A., et al.: Patterns of transmission of measles outbreaks in the United States, 1986–1987. N. Engl. J. Med. 320:75, 1989.
8. CDC: Update: Measles Outbreak—Chicago, 1989. M.M.W.R. 39:317, 1990.
9. ACIP. Measles prevention: Supplemental statement. M.M.W.R. 38:11, 1989.
10. ACIP: Measles prevention. M.M.W.R. 38:1, 1989.
11. ACIP: Mumps prevention. M.M.W.R. 38:388, 1989.
12. Kaplan, K.M., Marder, D.C., Cochi, S.L., et al.: Mumps in the workplace. JAMA 260:1434, 1988.
13. Murray, M.W., and Lewis, M.J.: Mumps meningitis after measles, mumps, and rubella vaccination. Lancet :677, 1989.
14. ACIP. Mumps Prevention. M.M.W.R. 33:301–318, 1984.
15. CDC. Rubella vaccination during pregnancy—United States, 1971–1988. M.M.W.R. 38:289, 1989.
16. Polis, M.A., Davey, V.J., Collins, E.D., et al.: The emergency department as part of a successful strategy for increasing adult immunization. Ann. Emerg. Med. 17:1016, 1988.
17. Harnisch, J.P., Tronca, E., Nolan, C.M., Turch, M., and Holmes, K.K.: Diphtheria among alcoholic urban adults—a decade of experience in Seattle. Ann. Intern. Med. 111:71, 1989.
18. ACIP: Diphtheria, tetanus, and pertussis: Guidelines for vaccine prophylaxis and other preventative measures. M.M.W.R. 34:405, 1985.
19. ACIP: Poliomyelitis prevention. M.M.W.R. 31:22, 1982.
20. Hill, D.R., and Pearson, R.D.: Health advice for international travel. Ann. Intern. Med. 108:839, 1988.
21. World Health Organization (WHO): Yellow Fever in 1987. Bull. W.H.O. 67:451, 1989.
22. Wolfe, M.S.: Protection of travelers. In Principles and Practice of Infectious Diseases. 3rd Ed. Edited by Mandell, G.L., Douglas, R.G., and Bennett, J.E. New York, Churchill Livingstone, 1990, pp. 2334–2342.
23. Hilton, E., Edwards, B., and Singer, B.: Reported illness and compliance in U. S. travelers attending an immunization Facility. Arch. Intern. Med. 149:178, 1989.
24. CDC: Tetanus—United States, 1985–1986. M.M.W.R. 36:477, 1987.
25. Cate, T.R.: Clostridium Tetani (Tetanus). In Principles and Practice of Infectious Diseases. 3rd Ed. Edited by Mandell, G.L., Douglas, R.G., and Bennett, J.E. New York, Churchill Livingstone, 1990, pp. 1842–1846.
26. Giangrasso, J., and Smith, R.K.: Misuse of tetanus immunoprophylaxis in wound care. Ann. Emerg. Med. 14:573, 1985.
27. Brand, D.A., Acampora, D., Gottlieb, L.D., Glancy, K.E., and Frazier, W.H.: Adequacy of antitetanus prophylaxis in six hospital emergency rooms. N. Engl. J. Med 309:636, 1983.
28. Jacobs, R.L., Lowe, R.S., and Lanier, B.Q.: Adverse reactions to tetanus toxoid. JAMA 247:40, 1982.
29. Bernard, K.W. and Fishbein, D.B.: Rabies virus. In Principles and Practice of Infectious Disease. 3rd Ed. Edited by Mandell, G.L., Douglas, R.G., and Bennett, J.E. New York, Churchill Livingstone, 1990, pp. 1291–1303.
30. Anderson, L.J., Nicholson, R.G., Tauxe, R.V., et al.: Human rabies in the United States, 1960 to 1979: Epidemiology, diagnosis and prevention. Ann Intern. Med. 100:728, 1989.
31. Houff, S.A., Burton, R.C., Wilson, R.W., et al.: Human to human transmission of rabies virus by corneal transplant. N. Engl. J. Med. 300:603, 1979.
32. Fishbein, D.B., Dobbins, J.G., Bryson, J.H., et al.: Rabies surveillance, United States, 1987. M.M.W.R. 37:1, 1988.
33. NASPHV: Compendium of Animal Rabies Control, 1988. M.M.W.R. 37:19, 1988.
34. Zull, D.N.: Rabies: Disease epidemiology and prophylaxis, Part 2. Crit. Decis. Emerg. Med. 3:1, 1988.
35. Morrison, A.J., and Wenzel, R.P.: Rabies: A review and current approach for the clinician. South. Med. J. 78:1211, 1985.
36. ACIP: Rabies prevention—United States, 1984. M.M.W.R. 33:393, 1984.
37. Shill, M., Baynes, R.D., and Miller, S.D.: Fatal rabies encephalitis despite appropriate post-exposure prophylaxis. N. Engl. J. Med. 316:1257, 1987.
38. Lumbiganon, P., Bunyahotra, V., and Pairojkul, C.: Human rabies despite treatment with rabies immune globulin and human diploid cell vaccine—Thailand. M.M.W.R. 36:759, 1987.
39. AICP. Protection against viral hepatitis. M.M.W.R. 39:1, 1990.
40. ACIP: General Recommendations on Immunization. Ann. Intern. Med. 111:133, 1989.
41. CDC: Rubella vaccination during pregnancy—United States, 1971–1988. M.M.W.R. 38:289, 1989.

IMMUNIZATION CONTROVERSIES

James McCarty

PERTUSSIS VACCINE

Pertussis remains a major cause of morbidity and mortality. It begins with mild upper respiratory tract symptoms and progresses to a severe paroxysmal cough accompanied by an inspiratory whoop. Pertussis may lead to apnea, seizures, encephalopathy, pneumonia, and death. It is most severe in children under 1 year and leads to hospitalization in 75% of them. In this age group, it causes pneumonia in 20%, seizures in 2%, and encephalopathy in 0.4%. Atypical forms of pertussis occur in partially immune or non-immune older children and adults.

Current pertussis vaccines are prepared from either an inactivated whole-cell suspension or partially purified cell products. Pertussis vaccine is effective and provides protection in 90 to 95% of those vaccinated. Protection has been demonstrated in young infants, who are most at risk for severe complications.

Adverse reactions associated with pertussis vaccine are common and include mild to moderate fever, erythema and tenderness at the injection site, irritability, drowsiness, vomiting, and occasional persistent crying. The frequency of these reactions increases with subsequent doses. Rare but more severe adverse reactions associated with pertussis immunization include high fever with temperatures of 40.5°C or greater (1 in 330 doses), seizures (1 in 1750 doses), collapse with a shock-like hyporesponsive state (1 in 1750 doses), and encephalopathy (1 in 110,000 doses). Permanent neurologic deficits occur in one in 310,000 doses; however, the exact association of pertussis vaccination with encephalopathic reactions remains controversial because temporal association does not prove causality. For instance, sudden infant death syndrome (SIDS) and infantile spasms have been temporally associated with pertussis immunizations. Studies have shown that pertussis vaccinations are unlikely to cause either. Unfortunately, these temporal associations have led to decreased acceptance of pertussis immunization. Decreased immunizations in Great Britain between 1977 and 1979 led to a large epidemic with 102,500 cases of pertussis resulting in 5000 hospitalizations and 36 deaths. Pertussis is an ever-present and dangerous disease.

Contraindications to further doses of pertussis vaccine include encephalopathy within 7 days of administration, seizures occurring within 3 days of administration, persistent uncontrollable screaming or crying for 3 or more hours or an unusual high-pitched cry within 48 hours, collapse or a shock-like hyporesponsive state within 48 hours, unexplained temperature of 40.5°C or higher within 48 hours, or an allergic reaction to the vaccine, such as anaphylaxis. Pertussis vaccine should not be given to children with a progressive neurologic disorder or a history of seizures unless, perhaps, they are exposed to an outbreak of pertussis. Pertussis vaccine should not be given to children 7 years and older. A family history of seizures is not a contraindication for pertussis vaccine.

Whole-cell pertussis vaccine will probably be replaced by an acellular pertussis vaccine (APV) in the United States within several years. APV has been used in Japan since 1981. The vaccine has not been studied well in younger infants, however, and these data are pending the outcome of ongoing trials in the United States. Some experts have argued that the introduction of APV will have little impact on the rate of encephalopathy and SIDS temporally associated with pertussis because these events occur frequently during the first 6 months of life, and there are no good data showing that whole-cell pertussis vaccine causes either.

POLIO VACCINES

Polio is now rare in the United States since the introduction of the vaccine. Most adults are already immune and do not need vaccination unless they may be exposed because of travel or a health-care occupation.

Two trivalent polio vaccines are available: live oral polio vaccine and inactivated polio vaccine. A primary vaccination series induces immunity in over 95% of recipients. Adults have a higher risk than children of associated paralysis with oral vaccine. Therefore, inactivated vaccine is preferred for adults who require vaccination. Unimmunized adults who are about to travel to a high-risk area within 4 weeks, however, should receive a single dose of oral polio vaccine.

Polio vaccine is given to children at 2, 4, and 15 months and at 4 years. The vaccine is given orally to induce intestinal immunity. Immunization is also indicated for susceptible persons at risk of exposure to wild virus: those traveling through areas where the virus is endemic and health-care workers who may handle patients shedding, or lab specimens containing, wild poliovirus.

Oral polio vaccine has been rarely associated with paralysis in healthy recipients or their close personal contacts (1 in 7 to 9 million doses). Persons with anaphylactic reactions to neomycin should not receive the live vaccine.

Antibody-containing blood products do not interfere with immunity to oral polio vaccine. This vaccine should not be given to immunocompromised persons *or* to their household contacts. Inactivated vaccine should be used in these situations. Pregnant women should not be vaccinated.

HEMOPHILUS INFLUENZAE TYPE B CONJUGATE VACCINE

Hemophilus influenzae type b (Hib) is the leading cause of meningitis in the United States and also a common cause of pneumonia, bacteremia, septic arthritis, and epiglottitis in children under 5 years. The first Hib vaccine licensed in the United States consisted of purified Hib polysaccharide, which was primarily effective in children over 24 months. H. influenzae type b conjugate vaccine (HBCV), composed of Hib polysaccharide conjugated to a carrier protein, is immunogenic and effective in children under 24 months. The ACIP now recommends giving one of two available conjugated vaccines licensed for use in 2-month doses: at 2, 4, and 6 months of age with a booster and final dose given at 15 months for HbOC vaccine* and at 2 and 4 months with a booster at 12 months for PRP-OMP vaccine.† Children under 5 who were vaccinated with H. influenzae polysaccharide vaccine should be revaccinated with one dose of a conjugate vaccine. Vaccination may be indicated in children 5 years and older with conditions found to be associated with an increased risk for H. influenzae type b disease, such as asplenia and Hodgkin's disease. Adverse reactions are uncommon and include fever and local tenderness.

INFLUENZA VACCINE

Influenza is characterized by the sudden onset of fever, chills, malaise, headache, myalgia, and cough. It

---

* Lederle-Praxis.

† Merck Sharp & Dohme.

leads to increased mortality worldwide each year, and only 20 to 30% of high-risk patients are immunized. New vaccines must be developed annually because of the tendency for the virus to undergo frequent antigenic changes. Vaccines contain several viral subtypes in anticipation of the expected prevalent strains, and are available as whole-virus split-virus preparations. Because of increased febrile reaction in children, whole-virus preparations should be given only to persons over 12 years of age.

Those at high risk of developing serious or complicated influenza should be vaccinated annually. These include anyone 65 years of age and older and persons of any age with congenital or acquired heart disease, pulmonary dysfunction, diabetes mellitus or other metabolic diseases, chronic/severe anemia (including sickle-cell disease), and immunodeficiency. In addition, health-care workers, family members, or close contacts of high-risk persons and nursing home residents should be vaccinated annually. Influenza vaccine should be given during September, October, and November, anticipating outbreaks in January and February.

Adverse reactions are uncommon and include tenderness and induration at the injection site and occasional fever and myalgias. Hypersensitivity reactions are rarely seen in persons allergic to eggs. An increased frequency of Guillain-Barré syndrome was seen in association with the 1976 swine influenza vaccine but not with subsequent vaccines. Amantadine may be effective in protecting against influenza A in those who cannot be vaccinated.

PNEUMOCOCCAL VACCINE

Streptococcus pneumoniae is responsible for thousands of deaths annually in the United States. Pneumococcal pneumonia is the most widespread serious community-acquired respiratory infection. The mortality rate is higher in the elderly and immunocompromised; however, many of the population for whom the vaccine is indicated have not been immunized. Patients who have undergone splenectomy are at a higher risk of developing pneumococcal sepsis and should be immunized.

Pneumococcal vaccine contains purified capsular polysaccharide from the 23 strains of S. pneumoniae that cause approximately 90% of serious infections. It is given as a single injection and should not be repeated. It is indicated for all persons 65 years of age and older as well as for those with congenital or acquired heart disease, pulmonary dysfunction, anatomic or functional asplenia, renal failure, diabetes mellitus, alcoholism, multiple myeloma, lymphoma, and drug-induced immunosuppression. Local adverse reactions are seen in approximately 50% of recipients and include erythema and mild pain. Systemic reactions are less frequent and include fever, rash, and arthralgia in 1 to 5% of adult recipients. Revaccination is usually not indicated because it leads to increased incidence of both local and systemic reactions.

FUTURE VACCINES

New vaccines are being developed, and it is likely that we will soon see routine vaccinations to protect against organisms such as rotavirus and varicella. More immunogenic H. influenzae type B vaccines are being developed by conjugating the capsular polysaccharide with proteins. These should be effective in children less than 2 years of age. Work is continuing on a number of vaccines, including those to protect against infection with herpes simplex virus, rotavirus, cytomegalovirus, respiratory syncytial virus, and human immunodeficiency virus. It is possible that, in the future, many common infectious diseases will become relics of the past.

NATIONAL CONTACTS

In addition to the references listed subsequently, the Division of Immunization of the Centers for Disease Control in Atlanta, Georgia offers technical advice on vaccines (telephone 404-639-3311).

BIBLIOGRAPHY

American Academy of Pediatrics: Report of the Committee on Infectious Disease, 21st Ed. Evanston, Illinois, American Academy of Pediatrics, 1988.

American College of Physicians: Guide for Adult Immunization, 2nd Ed. Philadelphia, American College of Physicians, 1990.

Change in administration schedule for Haemophilus b conjugate vaccines. M.M.W.R. 39:232, 1990.

Fulginiti, V.A.: The current state of pertussis and pertussis vaccines. Am. J. Dis. Child. 143:532, 1989.

General Recommendations on Immunization. M.M.W.R. 38:205, 1989.

Measles Prevention: Recommendations of the Immunization Practices Advisory Committee (ACIP). M.M.W.R. 38:69, 1989.

Polis, M.A., Davey, V.J., Collins, E.D., et al.: The Emergency Department as part of a successful strategy for increasing adult immunization. Ann. Emerg. Med. 17:1016, 1988.

Rubella Vaccination during Pregnancy—United States, 1971–1988. M.M.W.R. 38:289, 1989.

NEEDLE-STICK PROTOCOL

Michael R. Sayre and Emily Jean Lucid

CAPSULE

Exposure to blood and body fluids is a well-known occupational hazard of the health care professions. Management of exposure requires ascertaining clinical information about the source, if known, the type of exposure, and the immune status of the victim. Appropriate postexposure prophylaxis for tetanus, hepatitis B, and possibly human immunodeficiency virus should be initiated in the Emergency Department (ED) when indicated. Emergency physicians can be leaders in their departments and hospitals in preventing exposure by implementing universal precautions as well as safe needle-handling techniques.

INTRODUCTION

In most EDs, the emergency physician is frequently confronted with hospital employees who have been stuck by needles. The purpose of this chapter is to outline a rational approach to management of these patients. We describe the magnitude of the problem, methods for determining significant blood or body fluid exposure, techniques for prevention of needle-stick injuries, and management of those injuries that do occur.

Interest in the problem of needle-stick injury has grown dramatically since the human immunodeficiency virus made its presence known in the early 1980s. In 1988, 5.2% of all patients presenting to the Johns Hopkins ED were seropositive for HIV,[1] and 7.8% of the critically ill or injured patients were seropositive.[2] At the time of this writing (winter 1990), 61 health care workers had HIV seroconversion documented and thought to be occupationally acquired.[3] Of those cases, two have developed AIDS. After needle-stick exposure, the risk of seroconversion with development of antibodies against HIV is thought to be about 0.4%.[4]

Nonetheless, concern remains high because many health care professionals have or will be exposed to HIV-infected serum. For example, in New York City, 17% of pediatric house officers had sustained a needle-stick injury with HIV-infected blood at some time during their residencies.[5] Unfortunately, the studies have only addressed exposures to patients with known disease. Because the large majority of HIV-infected individuals are unaware of their antibody status, no studies have addressed the issue of risk of seroconversion after exposure to the blood of these individuals.[6] The highest-risk infectious agent that health care workers face, however, is hepatitis B.

Hepatitis B virus kills at least 250 health care workers each year from occupationally acquired disease, and about 1000 workers become chronic carriers. Thousands more become ill and lose time from work.[7] This means that the emergency provider is more likely to die from hepatitis B than occupationally acquired HIV disease or even than being struck by lightning (115 deaths per year, U.S.). People who want to live do not stand under trees at the golf course in a thunderstorm, nor should health care providers fail to take steps to protect themselves from hepatitis B.

Many different infectious agents have been transmitted by needle stick. These include the previously mentioned human immunodeficiency and hepatitis B viruses. In addition syphilis, non-A, non-B hepatitis (hepatis C), malaria, diphtheria, Rocky Mountain spotted fever, tuberculosis, and many other agents have all been communicated by parenteral exposure.[8]

Prehospital care providers are also at risk. They suffer from the added disadvantage of not having the same degree of access to patient's health status, and may not be notified when they have been exposed to infectious agents.[7]

PATHOPHYSIOLOGY

MECHANISM OF EXPOSURE

The primary method of parenteral exposure to infectious material is through an accidental needle-stick. Nearly 35% of needle-stick injuries occur during recapping.[8] The risk of injury depends on the type of device (Fig. 51-8). The disposable syringe is the lowest-risk device, and the highest is the IV tubing and needle combination (piggyback).[8] This study did not address the risk of disease transmission with the different devices. Intuitively, an IV piggyback setup, especially when attached to an IV mainline some distance from the IV catheter, seems a low-risk device for transmitting disease, even if it has the highest rate of injury. Exposure can also occur through splashes of blood or other body fluid into the eye or other mucous membranes such as the mouth.

RISK OF ACQUIRING DISEASE

Hepatitis B virus infection is common in hospital workers. Of 5697 persons studied, 807 (14%) were seropositive for either past or present HBV infection.[9] Among those with frequent blood contact, the rate of new HBV infections was 1.05 per 100 people per year.[9] Emergency workers had the highest initial prevalence of HBV infection markers (20%), but unlike adult ICU

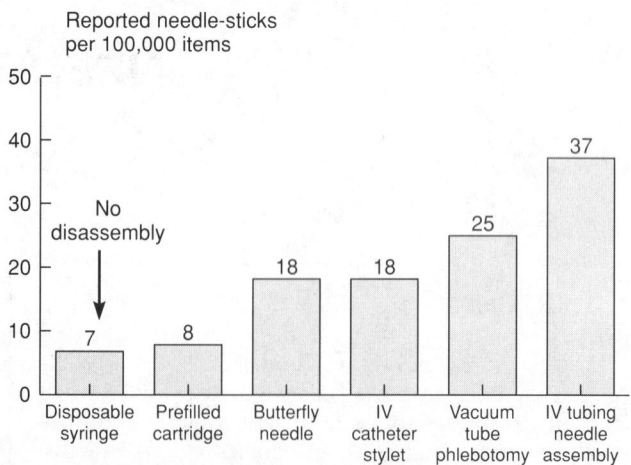

FIG. 51-8. Needle-stick injury rates per 100,000 items purchased. With permission from N. Engl. J. Med. *319:785,* 1988.

workers, they did not show an increase in these markers with longer time on the job.[9]

As mentioned earlier, the risk of acquiring HIV infection from a needle-stick injury with infected blood is about 0.4%.[4] So far, epidemiologic evidence implicates only blood, semen, vaginal secretions, and possibly breast milk in HIV transmission.[10,11]

Acquisition of infectious agents other than hepatitis B or HIV by needle-stick injury is possible but unlikely. If syphilis were acquired, a chancre should appear at the site of the injection. Hepatitis C virus can presumably be transmitted by needle-stick injury, but this risk is not quantified.

PREVENTION OF EXPOSURE

BARRIER TECHNIQUES

Universal precautions were implemented at the suggestion of the CDC in 1985.[12] These guidelines recommend assuming that every patient and blood sample is potentially contaminated with an infectious agent. Unfortunately, there is little experimental evidence that universal precautions work in reducing acquisition of disease. In fact, the use of gloves and other barrier devices was shown not to be highly protective against infection with hepatitis B virus in oral surgeons.[13] A moderate protective effect could not be excluded because of the limitations of the sample size.[13] Considering the amount of blood exposure in EDs and the fact that HIV and hepatitis testing require days to complete, it is prudent to practice universal precautions in the ED.

The universal precaution recommendations specifically address the handling of "sharps." Needles should not be recapped, bent or broken, removed from disposable syringes, or otherwise manipulated by hand. Needles and other sharp items should be disposed of in puncture-resistant containers placed as close as possible to the area of use. These recommendations apply to *all* patients.[11]

HANDLING "SHARPS"

Because needle-stick injuries are the most important means of transmitting infectious agents to health care workers, researchers are making special efforts to reduce them.[10] Several new methods of handling sharp instruments and needles have been introduced in the past few years to limit the number of injuries with these devices. One such method is the "point of use" disposal system. In this system, puncture-resistant containers are placed in the immediate vicinity of the area in which sharps are used, preferably within an

arm's reach of the bedside. When this is not practical, the containers are at least in the same room. The goal is to eliminate a walk down the hall by a worker carrying a fistful of needles waiting to stick a passerby. Traditionally, nurses recognized that risk, and recapped the needles before their walk down the hall. This led to many recapping injuries. The point-of-use disposal system reduces the temptation to recap needles by providing a handy box in which to place uncapped needles.[14] Indeed, such a system appears to reduce the number of needle-stick injuries.[15]

Other techniques focus on reducing the number of needles a worker handles. For example, it is unnecessary to change needles after drawing blood for culture before injecting the sample into the culture bottles.[16] "Heparin locks" do not need to be flushed with heparin to prevent clotting. Regular saline flushes work just as well and eliminate the need for a saline flush of the heparin before drug administration.

Some writers advocate teaching the safe use of sharp instruments as a part of instruction in surgical technique. One suggestion is that no two people handle the same sharp instrument at the same time. In the operating room, a magnetic pad can be used between the Mayo stand and the operative field whereon sharp instruments are placed as they are passed back and forth between surgeon and scrub nurse.[17] An operative technique easily adapted to emergency medicine is the use of double gloves. A British study demonstrated that 11% of outer gloves but only 2% of inner gloves had punctures at the end of general surgical operations. Interestingly, the wearers were aware of only half the punctures. The use of double gloves may be tempered by reduced dexterity and sensation.[18]

Outside the operating theatre, the person using a needle must be responsible for its safe disposal. It is not acceptable to leave loose needles on a suture tray for a nurse to try to find later. Too often, loose, unaccounted-for needles become the source of an injury. The physician performing the procedure must personally be sure that the needles and other "sharps" are disposed of in a puncture-resistant container as soon as feasible after use.

Recently, new designs for needles have been developed to offer more protection for the worker. One design, based on the premise that a recapped needle is safer than an uncapped needle, is a needle recapping device that has reduced needle-stick injuries fourfold.[19] Another technique uses a protective blunting member that protrudes past the needle tip after the needle is withdrawn from the skin. A third technique uses a valve in the bore of the needle that allows only fluids to be injected into the body and prevents blood from being aspirated back into the syringe. A new design in use in many hospitals now is the "hands-off" Tubex injector. This design keeps the operator's hands away from the tip of the needle. It is hoped that these and other new needle designs will reduce the chances of a needle-stick injury.[20]

POSTEXPOSURE MANAGEMENT

Management of parenteral exposure to potentially infectious material requires a hospital-wide program administered by a knowledgeable nurse or physician. Responsibilities of such a program include identification and tracking of victims of needle-stick injuries, follow-up on laboratory tests on the source, administration of hepatitis B vaccine, and identification of risk-reduction techniques in the workplace.

The CDC has defined an exposure as a percutaneous injury (needle-stick or cut), contact of mucous membranes, or contact of skin (when abraded or chapped) with blood, tissues, or other body fluids to which universal precautions apply.[21]

Following exposure to blood or body fluids, the following laboratory tests might be obtained on the *source:* hepatitis B surface antigen (HBsAg, active infection), hepatitis B surface antibody (anti-HBs, past infection), aspartate aminotransferase (if elevated, may suggest non-A, non-B hepatitis or hepatitis C), and RPR or VDRL (syphilis). In addition, the Centers for Disease Control recommend testing the source patient for HIV as long as consent is obtained.[21] Hospitals should develop a policy for HIV testing when consent cannot be obtained (e.g., cardiopulmonary arrest and death).[11] Some states have enacted legislation allowing testing for HIV infection even when the source refuses to be tested.[10] In addition, some high-risk source patients may be retested for HIV at 12 weeks after the incident if they are initially seronegative and thought likely to be infected with HIV.[7] The tetanus status of the victim should be ascertained and appropriate immunization administered as needed.

HEPATITIS PROPHYLAXIS

The main risk to the potential needle-stick victim is that of acquiring hepatitis B.[22,23] The management of hepatitis B exposure is dealt with in depth in the previous chapter section.

HIV PROPHYLAXIS

If the source is found to be positive for HIV or if the source refuses to be tested, the victim should be counseled about the risks of HIV infection. The victim should be tested for HIV at the time of exposure. Seronegative victims should be retested at 6, 12, and 26 weeks after exposure. In addition, the exposed worker should be enrolled in the CDC surveillance program (telephone 404–639–1644). The worker should be advised to report any acute febrile illness in the first 3 months after exposure, and to follow the recommendations for prevention of transmission of HIV. In addition, exposed workers should follow the Public Health Service recommendations for the prevention of HIV transmission for at least 6 to 12 weeks after exposure.[21] Of course, confidentiality must be maintained by the health care provider.[7]

There has been some interest in the post-exposure prophylaxis of HIV infections with zidovudine (AZT), which has been shown to prolong life for patients with AIDS[24] and patients with low CD4 lymphocyte counts.[25] This aggressive use of AZT has been extended by some to postexposure prophylaxis of HIV infection.[21] There is at least one trial under way that is trying to answer the question of whether zidovudine begun within hours or days of exposure and continued for a period of 4 to 6 weeks will prevent development of seroconversion and subsequent HIV disease. Another similar trial was stopped because of the difficulty in finding subjects.

Some hospitals that treat large numbers of AIDS patients and therefore have a high number of exposed employees have begun to provide zidovudine in the absence of scientific data regarding its efficacy or the lack thereof. If it is to be given, it seems logical that the drug be administered as soon as possible after the exposure. Zidovudine, however, is not without adverse reactions. Nausea and headaches are common. Acetaminophen and probenecid should be avoided. Complete blood counts should be taken every other week for eight weeks to identify those who will become anemic or leukopenic.[26] Considering the low risk of seroconversion from a single needle-stick, the known high mortality rate from HIV infection, and the potential toxicity of zidovudine, the decision to initiate postexposure prophylaxis is difficult. If exposure comes from a known HIV-positive source and therapy is to be given, it makes sense to begin therapy when the victim is first seen for the exposure—usually in the ED. One option is to begin the therapy in the ED, and let the victim consider the risks and benefits of continuing the treatment while taking the drug because treatment can always be stopped. The CDC recommends obtaining written informed consent.[21] The usual dose is 200 mg every 4 hours around the clock for 6 weeks. This therapy currently costs about $1000. Lower doses may be just as effective in patients with AIDS.[25] Perhaps the same lower dose will work for postexposure prophylaxis.

REFERENCES

1. Kelen, G.D., Fritz, S., Qaquish, B., et al.: Unrecognized human immunodeficiency virus infection in emergency department patients. N. Engl. J. Med. *319*:1645, 1988.
2. Kelen, G.B., Fritz, S., Qaquish, B., et al.: Substantial increase in human immunodeficiency virus (HIV-1) infection in critically ill emergency patients: 1986 and 1987 compared. Ann. Emerg. Med. *18*:378, 1989.
3. Barnes, D.M.: Health workers and AIDS: Questions persist. Science 241:161, 1988.

4. Marcus, R., and CDC Cooperative Needlestick Surveillance Group. Surveillance of health care workers exposed to blood from patients infected with the human immunodeficiency virus. N. Engl. J. Med. 319:1118, 1988.
5. Melzer, S.M., Vermund, S.H., and Shelov, S.P.: Needle injuries among pediatric housestaff physicians in New York City. Pediatrics 84:211, 1989.
6. Kelen, G.D.: Reanalysis of surveillance data regarding health care worker risk of nosocomial acquisition of HIV (editorial). Ann. Emerg. Med. 17:1101, 1988.
7. Centers for Disease Control (CDC): Guidelines for prevention of transmission of human immunodeficiency virus and hepatitis B virus to health-care and public-safety workers. M.M.W.R. 38:3, 1989.
8. Jagger, J., Hunt, E.H., Brand-Elnaggar, J., and Pearson, R.D.: Rates of needle-stick injury caused by various devices in a university hospital. N.Engl. J. Med. 319:284, 1988.
9. Hadlers, S.C., Doto, I.L., Maynard, J.E., et al.: Occupational risk of hepatitis B infection in hospital workers. Infect. Control Hosp. Epidemiol. 6:24, 1985.
10. Becker, C.E., Cone, J.E., and Gerberding, J.: Occupational infection with human immunodeficiency virus (HIV): Risks and risk reduction. Ann. Intern. Med. 110:653, 1989.
11. CDC: Recommendations for prevention of HIV transmission in health-care settings. M.M.W.R. 36:3S, 1987.
12. CDC: Recommendations for preventing transmission of infection with human T-lymphotropic virus type III/lymphadenopathy-associated virus in the workplace. M.M.W.R. 34:681, 691, 1985.
13. Reingold, A.L., Kane, M.A., and Hightower, A.W.: Failure of gloves and other protective devices to prevent transmission of hepatitis B virus to oral surgeons. JAMA 259:2558, 1988.
14. Ribner, B.S., Landry, M.N., Gholson, G.L., and Linden, L.A.: Impact of a rigid, puncture resistant container upon needlestick injuries. Infect. Control Hosp. Epidemiol. 8:63, 1987.
15. Sanborn, C., Luttrell, N., and Hoffmann, K.: Creating a safer environment for health care workers: Implementing a point-of-use sharps disposal system. Nurs. Admin. Q 12:24, 1988.
16. Isaacman, D.J., and Karasic, R.B.: Lack of effect of changing needles on contamination of blood cultures. Pediatr. Infect. Dis. J. 9:274, 1990.
17. Bessinger, C.D. Jr.: Preventing transmission of human immunodeficiency virus during operations. Surg. Gynecol. Obstet. 167:287, 1988.
18. Matta, H., Thompson, A.M., and Rainey, J.B.: Does wearing two pairs of gloves protect operating theatre staff from skin contamination? Br. Med. J. 297:597, 1988.
19. Goldwater, P.N., Law, R., Officer, J.A., and Cleland, J.F.: Impact of a recapping device on venepuncture-related needlestick injury. Infect. Control Hosp. Epidemiol. 10:21, 1989.
20. Zimmerman, D.: Health workers' fears spur changes in needle design. Med World News 9:57, 1988.
21. CDC: Public Health Service statement on management of occupational exposure to human immunodeficiency virus, including considerations regarding zidovudine postexposure use. M.M.W.R. 39:1, 1990.
22. Grady, G.F., Lee, V.A., Prince, A.M., et al.: Hepatitis B immune globulin for accidental exposures among medical personnel: final report of a multicenter controlled trial. J. Infect. Dis. 138:625, 1978.
23. CDC: Protection against viral hepatitis: Recommendations of the Immunization Practices Advisory Committee (ACIP). M.M.W.R. 39:1, 1990.
24. Fischl, M.A., Richman, D.D., Grieco, M.H., et al.: The efficacy of azidothymidine (AZT) in the treatment of patients with AIDS and AIDS-related complex. N. Engl. J. Med. 317:185, 1987.
25. Drugs for HIV infection. Med. Lett. Drug. Ther. 31:11, 1990.
26. Bartlett, J.A.: HIV therapeutics: An emerging science (editorial). JAMA 260:3051, 1988.

HEPATITIS B VACCINATION

Donald A. Romig

CAPSULE

The main risk to needlestick victims is that of acquiring hepatitis B. This chapter focuses on the management of possible hepatitis B virus exposure with its preventive interventions, including a review of the available hepatitis B vaccines. AIDS precautions and recommendations are covered in previous chapter sections.

RISK OF HBV EXPOSURE

Hepatitis B infection can have serious consequences including massive hepatic necrosis, chronic active hepatitis and cirrhosis of the liver. Sixty to 80% of patients and 6 to 10% of adults who are infected in the United States become carriers. It has been estimated that more than 170 million people in the world today are persistently infected with the hepatitis B virus (HBV). These patients who become chronic carriers can infect others and are at increased risk of developing hepatocellular carcinoma. Considering the serious consequences of infection, immunization should be considered for all persons at potential risk of exposure to the hepatitis B virus.

Many epidemiologic studies have demonstrated which groups of individuals have a higher incidence of hepatitis B serum markers.[1-5] The overall risk of the general population, according to the prevalence of all hepatitis B serologic markers in healthy adults, is 3% to 5%. The relative risk of the health care workers varies: emergency nurses, 30%; surgeons, 28%; emergency medical technicians, 18% to 25%; laboratory technicians, 19% to 25%; internists, 18%; and emergency physicians, 12%.[6] The following groups are at high risk of developing hepatitis B and should be immunized: health care professionals, renal dialysis patients, institutionalized patients, patients requiring repeated transfusions, male homosexuals, sexual partners of Hepatitis B surface antigen (HB_sAg)-positive persons, and neonates of HB_sAg-positive mothers.[7] In addition, although with a lower priority, vaccination has been recommended for household contacts of HB_sAg-carriers, children and susceptible adults in areas of high HBV endemicity, and military and foreign service personnel assigned to HBV-endemic areas.

The above recommendations apply to United States population groups. The greatest potential use of the vaccine, however, is in the third-world countries with high HBV endemicity. These recommendations have stood the test of time since the introduction of Heptavax-B in 1981.

VACCINES

Three vaccines are currently available for protection against hepatitis B, Heptavax-B,* licensed in 1981, Recombivax HB,* licensed in 1986, and Engerix-B,** licensed in 1989.

Heptavax-B is produced from the serum of blood donors with high titers of hepatitis B surface antigen (HB_sAg). Each lot of plasma is processed with multiple steps to remove or inactivate infectious HBV particles or other known viruses that may appear in the bloodstream, including slow viruses, retroviruses, herpes virus, and many others. The final product is alum-absorbed and tested in animals before release for human use.

Recombivax HB is a noninfectious viral vaccine produced in yeast cells cloned to produce HB_sAg with the yeast's own protein. The yeast cells are disrupted and the purified protein is harvested. This protein is treated with formalin and adsorbed by aluminum hydroxide as an adjuvant. Engerix-B is genetically engineered by this same process.

Although the two types of vaccines differ slightly with regard to physical and chemical properties, the quality of the antibodies produced by both types of vaccines is identical.[8]

There has been no evidence that human immunodeficiency virus (HIV) has been acquired from the use of Heptavax-B. Because Recombivax HB and Engerix-B are harvested from yeast cells, they cannot contain HIV.

The risks of using either type of vaccine are minimal because the vaccines are purified protein (albeit de-

rived from different sources) that, when given to humans intramuscularly, provides an immune response and the production of antibodies to HB_sAg. The most common side effect with either vaccine is local swelling with slight discomfort at the site of the injection. Generally, both types of vaccines are well tolerated; hypersensitivity reactions and severe central nervous system disorders have been reported but are rare.

Both vaccines, if properly administered intramuscularly in the arm, not the buttock, are immunogenic. Hepatitis B surface antibodies (HB_sAb) can be detected in 85% to 92% of recipients of Heptavax-B, in 92% to 97% of recipients of Recombivax HB and in approximately 96% of recipients of Engerix-B. These numbers are comparable, and as experience with Recombivax HB increases, these figures may become identical.

The vaccines' efficacy in preventing disease has been documented by several well-controlled studies that have demonstrated the presence of HB_sAb in the serum of vaccinated individuals.[1,2,9] These studies were performed with the Heptavax-B vaccine but demonstrate that with an adequate response (defined as $\geq$ 10 SRV by radioimmunoassay, or positive by enzyme immunoassay), the production of HB_sAb is protective against acquisition of infection. In addition, Recombivax HB and Engerix-B have been shown to prevent hepatitis B in neonates who received one dose of hepatitis B immune globulin (HBIG) at birth and three subsequent doses of vaccine.[10] Pregnancy is not a contraindication to hepatitis B vaccine because hepatitis during pregnancy may have long-term deleterious effects for the fetus.

The recommended schedule of injection of the vaccines is at months 0, 1, and 6, but an alternate schedule (injections at months 0, 1, and 2) has been designed for certain populations (i.e., neonates born of hepatitis B-infected mothers, individuals who have or may have been recently exposed to the virus, and certain travelers to high-risk areas. See package inserts for more details). In addition, patients on hemodialysis may need booster injections, depending on their antibody levels, because of lower seroconversion rates and lower titers. Drug abusers may have suboptimal response.

PRETESTING

Some controversy surrounds the concept of testing candidates for vaccination before administration of the vaccine. Several methods have been proposed: (1) no serum testing, (2) testing for Hb_sAb and HB_sAg, or (3) testing for hepatitis B core antibody (HB_cAb).

Not testing serum before the administration of vaccine eliminates the testing cost but immunizes many people who already have hepatitis markers in their serum. At a vaccine cost of over $100 per person, a significant saving can be realized with pretesting of

---

*Merck & Co, Inc.
**SmithKline Biologicals

vaccine candidates for HB$_c$Ab, HB$_s$Ag, or HB$_s$Ab. If any of these tests are positive, the candidate can be excused from receiving the vaccine. HB$_s$Ab-positive or HB$_c$Ab-positive individuals do not need the vaccine; they are immune. No reliable information is available about the immune status of individuals with low HB$_s$Ab titers; laboratories generally report the test results as simply positive or negative. HB$_s$Ag-positive individuals will not convert to HB$_s$Ab-positive, but there are no contraindications for them to receive the vaccine.[11] In general, the development of a consistent policy with regard to pretesting is advisable within each vaccine program. Most programs advocate pretesting on the basis of cost and individual information. A false sense of security may arise if immunization proceeds without prior knowledge of immune or carrier status.

TREATMENT

Hepatitis B immune globulin (HBIG) has been shown to reduce the incidence of hepatitis, but is expensive,

with an average patient cost of $400 to $600 per dose. Administration is recommended for a susceptible person who has had contact with blood or body fluids of a known carrier of HB$_s$Ag.[12] The main weapon in the prevention of hepatitis B is hepatitis B vaccine. It is well-accepted that the combined use of HBIG and vaccine immediately after exposure to a known HB$_s$Ag carrier provides improved protection from hepatitis B, or at least a moderation of the disease if it occurs.[13] The efficacy of HBIG in neonates of HB$_s$Ag-positive mothers is also well documented.[10] Because presence of HB$_c$Ab may be a clearer marker of immunity in unimmunized individuals, testing for HB$_c$Ab should proceed after exposure to hepatitis B. Current treatment recommendations include testing for HB$_c$Ab immediately after exposure, administering HBIG, preferably within 24 hours at a dose of 0.06 mL per kg and administering the first dose of hepatitis B vaccine within one week after exposure.[13] If the person tests positive for HB$_c$Ab, HB$_g$Ag, or HB$_s$Ab, further doses of vaccine are unnecessary. Vaccination proceeds in HB$_c$Ab-negative (susceptible) persons, with the second and third doses per prescribed schedule at 1 month and 6 months (see alternate schedule in package insert). A person who has had a needle stick from a person in a low-risk group (when a sample is not

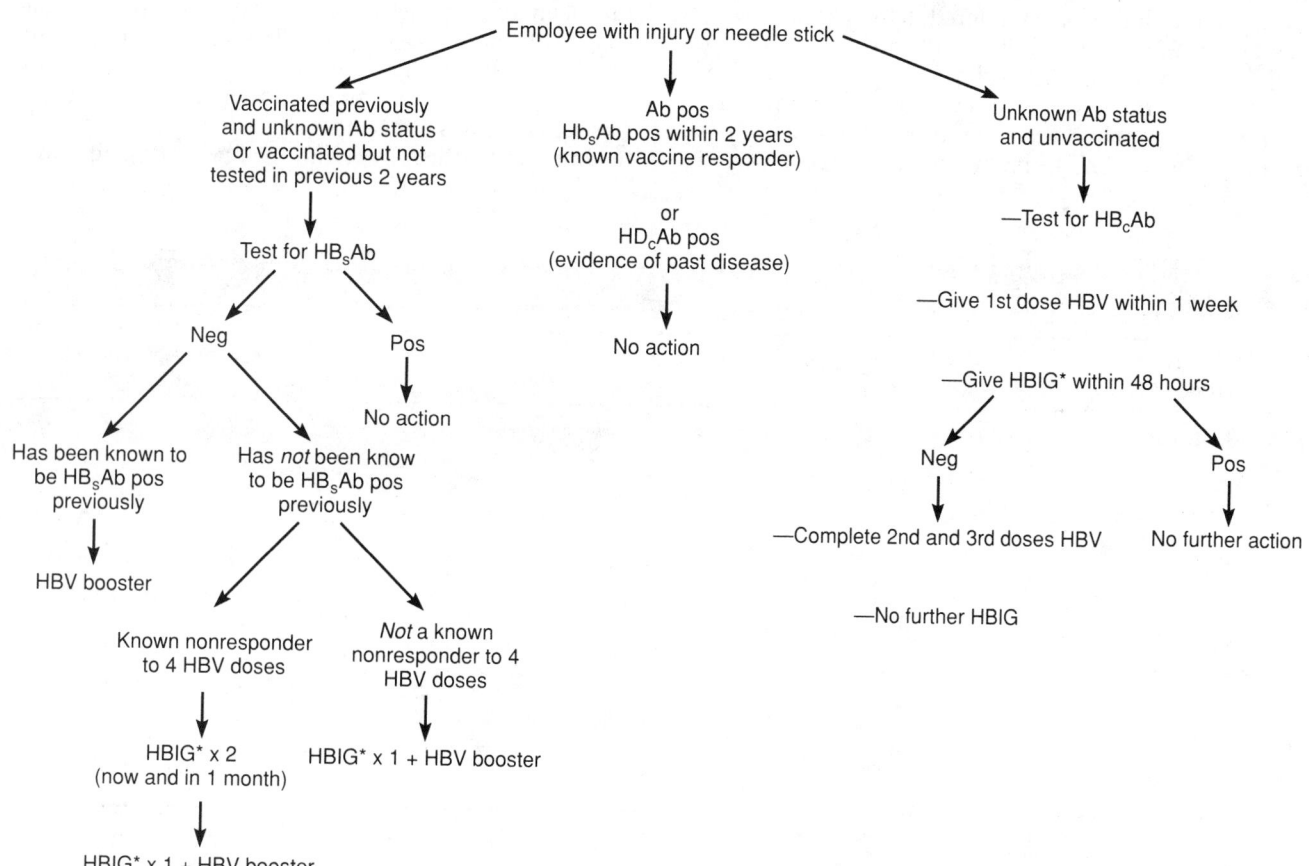

FIG. 51-9. *Algorithm for treating "sharp" injury or needle stick contaminated with blood from a donor of unknown hepatitis status. Ab = antibody; pos = positive; Hb$_s$Ab = hepatitis B surface antibody; Hb$_c$Ab = hepatitis B core antibody; HBIG = hepatitis B immune globulin; neg = negative; Hb$_s$Ag = hepatitis B surface antigen; HBV = hepatitis B vaccine.*

available), or an unknown needle stick, rarely needs hepatitis immune globulin. In these fearful times, however, it is often administered to catch the rare circumstance of transmission. The algorithm for the management of an accidental needle-stick is presented in Figure 51-9.

Screening after vaccination is usually not recommended. Individuals who received vaccine in the buttock or persons employed in specific high-risk areas are candidates for postvaccination screening. The single screening test for HB$_s$Ab is done, as this is the only antibody produced by the vaccine.[13]

Accidental percutaneous exposure in the previously immunized individual necessitates testing for HB$_s$Ab in that individual unless the previous antibody status is known. The exposed person needs no further care if HB$_s$Ab is present. The management of a previously vaccinated needlestick victim is reviewed in Table 51-22 and Figure 51-9.

Although the algorithm generally addresses a needle stick from an unknown source, if the source is known to be HB$_s$Ag-positive and the victim has inadequate antibodies, HBIG is given. Any person who has been previously vaccinated and who has not been tested for HB$_s$AB within the previous 2 years should be tested at the time of evaluation. If that result shows adequate antibody, nothing further needs to be done. Otherwise, further treatment depends on whether the vaccine series has been completed. If the vaccine series has not been completed, it should proceed, possibly with the addition of HBIG depending on the risk of the donor. If the vaccine series is completed and the victim is a known vaccine nonresponder, HBIG is given. If the victim is known to have seroconverted

in the past but is now negative, he or she is probably immune, but should still receive a booster dose of the vaccine. There is no evidence that Recombivax HB or Heptavax-B has any ability to prevent hepatitis A. Serum immune globulin is no longer recommended in any schemata involving hepatitis B.

Vaccination of family contacts or day care contacts of HB$_s$Ag-positive individuals is generally not recommended, unless they fall in the high-risk groups discussed previously.

Hepatitis C virus has been described, but no vaccine currently exists to prevent its transmission.

CASE ILLUSTRATION: WHEN IS VACCINATION INDICATED?

During the late evening shift at the hospital, a nursing employee reports to the nursing supervisor that she has sustained a needle stick, which occurred during a cardiorespiratory arrest in the intensive care unit. The patient died. The hepatitis B status of the patient is unknown, and no blood is available for testing. The steps in decision making are outlined in Figure 51-9.

Depending on the status of the injured employee (vaccinated, antibody-positive, or unknown) and the risk of the donor patient for HBV exposure, a decision can be made quickly by the nursing supervisor or employee health personnel. This schema eliminates the need for repeated testing, does not require the testing of donor blood if none is available, and can be applied to any individual receiving the needle stick or "sharp" injury from an unknown donor. Of course, this schema does not address decision making for HIV testing, preventing syphilis, or preventing tetanus.

TABLE 51-22. TREATMENT ACCORDING TO SOURCE*

Exposed Person	Source HB$_s$Ag-Positive	Source HB$_s$Ag-Negative	Source Not Tested or Unknown
Unvaccinated	HBIG × 1* and initiate HB vaccine†	Initiate HB vaccine†	Initiate HB vaccine†
Previously vaccinated Known responder	Test exposed for HB$_s$AB 1. If adequate,‡ no treatment 2. If inadequate, HB vaccine booster	No treatment	No treatment
Known nonresponder	HBIG × 2 or HBIG × 1 plus 1 dose HB vaccine	No treatment	If known high-risk source, *may treat as if source were HBsAg-positive*
Response unknown	Test exposed for anti-HB$_s$ 1. If inadequate,‡ HBIG × 1 plus HB vaccine booster dose 2. If adequate, no treatment	No treatment	Test exposed for HB$_s$Ab 1. If inadequate, HB vaccine booster dose 2. If adequate, no treatment

* With permission from Centers for Disease Control: Protection against viral hepatitis: Recommendations of the Immunization Practice Advisory Committee. M.M.W.R. 39:1, 1990.
* HBIG dose 0.06 ml/kg IM.
† HB vaccine dose depends on manufacturer. See package literature.
‡ Adequate anti-HBs is ≥ 10 SRU by RIA or positive by EIA.

Attention should be directed to reducing needlestick injury by new designs to reduce needle recapping and device assembly.[14]

REFERENCES

1. Szmuness, W., Stevens, C.E., Harley, E.H., et al.: Hepatitis B vaccine. N. Engl. J. Med. *303*:833, 1980.
2. Francis, D.P., Hadler, S.C., Thompson, S.E., et al.: The prevention of hepatitis B with vaccine Ann. Intern. Med. *97*:362, 1982.
3. Lewis, T.L., Alter, H.J., Chalmers, T.C., et al.: A comparison of the frequency of hepatitis B antigen and antibody in hospital and nonhospital personnel. N. Engl. J. Med. *289*:648, 1973.
4. Breuer, B., Friedman, S.M., Millner, E.S., et al.: Transmission of hepatitis B virus to classroom contacts of mentally retarded carriers. JAMA *254*:3190, 1985.
5. Mosley, J.W., Edwards, V.M., Casey, G., et al.: Hepatitis B virus infections in dentists. N. Engl. J. Med. *293*:729, 1975.
6. Trott, A.: Hepatitis B exposure and the emergency physician. Am. J. Emerg. Med. *5*:54, 1987.
7. Editorial: The evolution, implications, and applications of the hepatitis B vaccine. JAMA *247*:2272, 1982.
8. Emini, E.A., Ellis, R.W., Miller, W.J., et al: Production and immunological analysis of recombinant hepatitis B vaccine. J. Infect. *13*(Suppl A):3, 1986.
9. Dienstag, J.L., Werner, B.G., Polk, B.F., et al.: Hepatitis B vaccine in health care personnel: Safety, immunogenicity, and indicators of efficacy. Ann. Intern. Med. *101*:34, 1984.
10. Beasley, R.P., Hwang, L., Stevens, C.E., et al.: Efficacy of hepatitis B immune globulin for prevention of perinatal transmission of the hepatitis B carrier state: Final report of a randomized double-blind, placebo-controlled trial. Hepatology *3*:135, 1983.
11. Dienstag, J.L., Stevens, C.E., Bhan, A.K., et al.: Hepatitis B vaccine administered to chronic carriers of hepatitis B surface antigen. Ann. Intern. Med. *96*:575, 1982.
12. Seeff, L.B., Wright, E.C., Zimmerman, H.J., et al.: Type B hepatitis after needle-stick exposure. Prevention with hepatitis B immune globulin. Ann. Intern. Med. *88*:235, 1978.
13. Valenti, W.: Hepatitis B prevention part 1: A review of ACIP's newest guidelines. Infect Control *7*:74, 1986.
14. Jagger, J., Hunt, E.H., Brand-Elnaggar, J., and Pearson, R.D.: Rates of needle-stick injury caused by various devices in a university hospital. N. Engl. J. Med. *319*:284, 1988.
15. Centers for Disease Control: Protection against viral hepatitis: Recommendations of the Immunization Practice Advisory Committee (ACIP). MMWR *39*:No. RR-2:1, 1990.

Chapter 52

EMERGENCY RHEUMATOLOGY

SYSTEMIC RHEUMATIC DISEASES

Rita K. Cydulka and Steven B. Sorin

CAPSULE

The key to differentiating between the systemic rheumatic diseases depends on obtaining a clear history and through physical examination, with attention to evidence of progressive joint damage and evidence of systemic involvement. Emergency Department (ED) laboratory examination is rarely helpful, although radiography may help distinguish between diseases.

Both rheumatoid arthritis (RA) and systemic lupus erythematosus (SLE) may present with polyarticular joint involvement, as well as multi-system and generalized somatic complaints. In patients with RA, aspiration of synovial fluid is helpful only when one joint is inflamed out of proportion to disease activity elsewhere. Venography may be indicated to differentiate a Baker's cyst from thrombophlebitis. Patients with SLE who suffer from cardiac, pulmonary, renal, or central nervous system (CNS) disease should be started on high-dose corticosteroids and admitted to the hospital. Patients with renal involvement in scleroderma and accelerated hypertension require aggressive treatment with angiotensin-converting enzyme inhibitors.

Polymyositis and dermatomyositis both present with progressive proximal muscle weakness. They can be differentiated from each other on the basis of the violaceous skin rash. The level of CPK reflects the extent and activity of muscle breakdown. Myoglobinuria indicates severe disease. Polymyalgia rheumatica (PMR) presents with proximal pain and stiffness, rather than weakness. Physical examination reveals normal strength. A markedly elevated Westergren erythrocyte sedimentation rate (ESR) may be noted. Response to moderate dose steroids is dramatic.

The diagnosis of giant cell arteritis should be considered in all patients over 50 who present with a headache. Laboratory findings are similar to those found in patients with polymyalgia rheumatica (PMR). Treatment with high-dose corticosteroids should never be delayed pending biopsy confirmation of the diagnosis to avoid potentially disastrous sequelae.

INTRODUCTION

Over the years, the systemic rheumatic diseases have had various misnomers, such as connective tissue diseases or collagen diseases. One of the major recent advances in rheumatology has been the recognition of the diversity of rheumatic disease and the importance of accurate diagnosis for prognosis and specific treatment.

RHEUMATOID ARTHRITIS

Rheumatoid arthritis (RA) is the most common cause of chronic joint inflammation. The disease most commonly begins between ages 40 and 60, although it may have its onset as early as 6 months of age or as late as 80 years.[1] Its cause remains unknown. A genetic predisposition has been noted in population studies. Current theory suggests that some unknown environmental factor, such as a long-standing viral infection, may initiate the disease process in predisposed hosts.[1,2] Once it is established, autoimmune factors perpetuate the inflammatory process. Rheumatoid factors, antibodies to immunoglobulin G, are made,

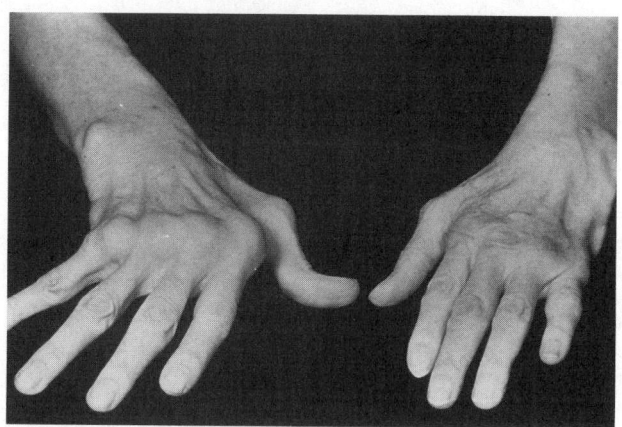

FIG. 52-1. Ulnar deviation, subluxation of the metacarpophalangeal joints, joint swelling, and muscular atrophy seen in the hands of patients with rheumatoid arthritis. With permission from Clinical Slide Collection on the Rheumatic Diseases, The Arthritis Foundation, Atlanta, Georgia, 1972.

and immune complexes of rheumatoid factor and normal IgG activate the complement cascade, increase local prostaglandin synthesis, and attract inflammatory cells to affected joints.[2] Cellular immunity may also be important in disease pathogenesis because involved synovium becomes heavily infiltrated with T cells and lymphocytes. Early events include microvascular injury and edema of the subsynovial tissues leading to mild synovial lining cell proliferation.[3] With continued disease activity, the synovium begins to hypertrophy into pannus. Pannus is composed of proliferating fibrous tissue and capillaries, which grow from the synovial margin into and over the articular cartilage and subchondral bone. The formation of pannus ultimately leads to cartilage and bone damage and produces the characteristic radiographic findings and clinical deformities of RA (Fig. 52-1). Pannus formation is unique to RA.[3]

RA is a systemic disease, although the synovium is the primary site of inflammation. Patients often complain of malaise, fatigue, low-grade fever, and a pe-

culiar morning stiffness. The duration of morning stiffness is actually the single best subjective indicator of disease activity.[1] Joint inflammation and swelling are usually present, although they may be subtle and episodic early in the course of the disease. The pattern of joint involvement is typically symmetric. The metacarpophalangeal joints and wrists are frequently involved, whereas the DIP joints are relatively spared.[1] The knees, feet, and ankles may also be affected. Some of the more unusual joints involved include the sternoclavicular, temporal mandibular, and cricoarytenoid joints.[4] Involvement of the laryngeal joints may cause hoarseness and sore throat. Involvement of the axial skeleton is limited to the upper cervical spine, especially at the level of C1-C2.[1] Periarticular disease and carpal tunnel syndrome may be presenting manifestations of RA.[5] Tendonitis and ruptured tendons, involving the hand flexor tendons and wrist extensor tendons as well as the rotator cuff, are common in later stages of disease, leading to severe functional impairment and deformities.[5]

The differential diagnosis of rheumatoid arthritis is extensive and includes systemic lupus erythematosus, mixed connective tissue disease, progressive systemic sclerosis, sarcoidosis, inflammatory bowel disease, Whipple's disease, amyloidosis, chronic infection and malignancies, gout or pseudogout, polymyalgia rheumatica, and Lyme disease.[1] These conditions share some similarities with RA, but can generally be recognized on the basis of extra-articular manifestations, absence of progressive joint damage, and characteristic laboratory findings. Perhaps the most common diagnostic dilemma is between rheumatoid arthritis and osteoarthritis. Features that may help to distinguish between RA and OA are listed in Table 52-1.

Laboratory findings are not a reliable guide to the diagnosis of rheumatoid arthritis.[4] A modest normocytic normochromic or hypochromic anemia is common, but a hematocrit of less than 30 should prompt a search for other associated factors, such as gastrointestinal bleeding. Elevated acute phase reactants are also common, but again nonspecific. A pos-

TABLE 52-1. DIAGNOSTIC FEATURES OF RHEUMATOID ARTHRITIS AND OSTEOARTHRITIS

	Rheumatoid Arthritis	Osteoarthritis
Joints affected	PIP, MCP, wrist, elbow, shoulder, hip, knee, ankle, MTP	DIP, PIP, hip, knee, cervical and lumbar spine
Symptoms	Morning stiffness, systemic	Pain with use, crepitus
Findings	"Boggy" swelling	Bony enlargement
Laboratory findings	Anemia, Rheumatoid factor	None
X ray findings	Osteoporosis, erosions, symmetric joint space narrowing	Osteophytes, cysts, asymmetric narrowing

itive rheumatoid latex fixation test, which measures the presence of immunoglobulin M rheumatoid factors (RF), is found in almost 80% of patients at some time, but less than 50% during the first year of illness.[4] Higher titers of RF are generally more significant, but may be found in other systemic rheumatic diseases, particularly in Sjögren's syndrome, chronic liver disease, and sarcoidosis. Up to 25% of normal elderly women also have a low-titer rheumatoid factor.[4] A positive antinuclear factor may also be found in 10 to 15% of patients with RA. This finding alone does not alter the diagnosis.[6]

Radiographic findings progress from early soft tissue swelling to juxta-articular demineralization, to erosions and joint space narrowing in advanced disease.[7] These findings imply pannus growth and a poor functional outcome.

EMERGENCY CONDITIONS ASSOCIATED WITH RHEUMATOID ARTHRITIS

Several crisis situations are likely to bring the patient to the ED: acute septic arthritis, Baker's cyst, and atlantoaxial subluxation. Patients with RA are at higher-than-normal risk for all infections, especially superimposed joint sepsis.[5,8,9] It is often difficult to differentiate between infection and a monoarticular flare-up of disease. Any joint that is inflamed out of proportion to disease activity elsewhere mandates synovial fluid aspiration and culture. Increasing intra-articular pressure in the knee joint may lead to formation of a popliteal or Baker's cyst. Fluid from the knee is forced into the cyst during motion, and cannot be returned to the joint space because of a one-way valve mechanism. Eventually the cyst ruptures into the calf and/or occludes the popliteal vein, creating a clinical picture indistinguishable from deep vein thrombosis, so called "pseudophlebitis." The correct diagnosis can be established by means of arthrography or ultrasound.[7] Finally, rheumatoid involvement at C1-C2 may cause subluxation with potential for cervical cord compression.[10] Patients present with poor balance and a spastic gait, and may also manifest quadriplegia. Additional findings include hyperreflexia and Babinski signs. Radiographs with the neck in gentle flexion demonstrate the subluxation (Fig. 52-2). Critical cervical narrowing warrants urgent admission and neurosurgical evaluation.

SYSTEMIC LUPUS ERYTHEMATOSUS

Systemic lupus erythematosus (SLE) is another systemic rheumatic disease of unknown cause that may lead to emergency presentation. As in rheumatoid arthritis, SLE is autoimmune in nature, and there is clearly a

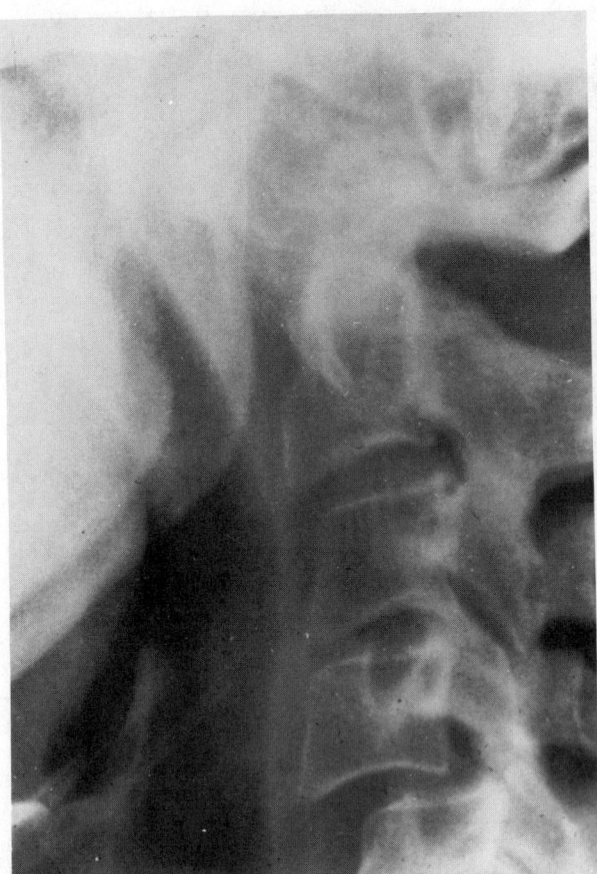

FIG. 52-2.   Atlantoaxial subluxation in a patient with rheumatoid arthritis. The preodontoid space is markedly widened. Note also anterior displacement of vertebral body 4 on 5. With permission from Clinical Slide Collection on the Rheumatic Diseases. The Arthritis Foundation, Atlanta, Georgia, 1972.

hereditary predisposition.[11] Virtually all patients with SLE demonstrate autoantibodies, so-called antinuclear factors. The laboratory hallmark of SLE is the finding of antibodies to native, double-stranded DNA.[4] Such antibodies are found in only about 60% of patients with SLE, however.[4] There is convincing experimental and clinical evidence that these antibodies play a pathogenetic role in the clinical manifestations of SLE. The cause of immune regulatory breakdown is still unknown, although lack of adequate suppressor T-cell function can be demonstrated.[11] In many respects, SLE resembles chronic immune complex mediated serum sickness. Immune complexes of antigen and antibody are deposited in target organs, i.e., renal glomeruli, small blood vessels, basement membrane of the skin, and the choroid plexus of the brain. These immune complexes can then activate the complement system producing local inflammation and tissue damage.[11]

Of patients with SLE, 90% are women, mostly of childbearing age. SLE is not a rare disease; it affects up to one in 250 black women between the ages of 15 and 64.

Joint disease is the most common manifestation of SLE, and may lead to diagnostic confusion with rheumatoid arthritis. Actual synovitis is present in 70 to 80% of patients at diagnosis, and ultimately 95% of patients develop arthritis or arthralgias during their illness. Joints involved are similar to those in rheumatoid arthritis, but without pannus formation or radiographic evidence of bone or cartilage damage.[12] Cutaneous lesions are also common and often lead to the correct diagnosis. The classic facial butterfly erythema is present in nearly 50% of patients at diagnosis.[13] Other nonspecific erythematosus maculopapular eruptions, as well as sun sensitivity, are also common. Overt cutaneous vasculitis may also be noted. Raynaud's phenomenon occurs in about 20% of patients, although it is more common and severe in overlap syndrome and scleroderma.[14] Serositis, with involvement of the pleura or pericardium, is another common manifestation of SLE and may be a presenting manifestation. Clinical evidence of renal disease is present in about 50% of patients with SLE.[15] Early manifestations include proteinuria, nephrotic syndrome, and active urinary sediment with cellular elements and casts. Hypertension and renal insufficiency may ensue.[14] Involvement of the central nervous system may present as organic brain syndrome, seizures, and pure psychosis. Focal lesions, presumably on the basis of infarcts, also occur.[12] Myocardial infarction may occur even without significant coronary artery disease.

The most typical patient is a young woman, often black, with multiple organ involvement. At the time of diagnosis, symptoms of fatigue, weight loss, and fever may dominate. Although almost 40% of patients have a temperature above 102° F at time of diagnosis, fever in a patient with SLE should prompt a search for a site of infection.

EVALUATION IN THE EMERGENCY SETTING

Evaluation of the patient with SLE in the ED must have three objectives: (1) to confirm the proper diagnosis; (2) to establish an index of disease severity, and (3) to search for evidence of multiorgan disease involvement and complications. Serum should be sent for antinuclear factor and other auto-antibodies. A negative antinuclear antibody (ANA) virtually excludes the diagnosis of SLE. Anemia of chronic disease and elevated acute phase reactants are nonspecific findings. Levels of specific complement components may be a general guide to disease activity because complement proteins are consumed during active immune complex disease. Echocardiography may detect pericardial or myocardial disease if chest x-ray and ECG are inconclusive. A serum creatinine determi-

nation and a urinalysis, including microscopic examination of the sediment, should also be performed.[4]

Admission to the hospital and aggressive treatment with corticosteroids and possibly immunosuppressive agents should be considered for patients with serious systemic manifestations, as well as those with serious cardiac, pulmonary, renal, CNS, or psychiatric disease. Other patients may be sent home on nonsteroidal anti-inflammatory drugs (NSAIDS), such as ibuprofen or naproxen, or even low-dose steroids if careful follow-up is ensured.[15]

SCLERODERMA

Scleroderma or systemic sclerosis is another, presumably autoimmune, multisystem disorder characterized by microvascular damage and fibrosis of the skin and target organs. Almost all patients with scleroderma have severe Raynaud's phenomenon.[16] In early stages, Raynaud's phenomenon is often the most prominent manifestation. Over time, the puffy skin of the hand noted early in the course of the disease gives way to the typical hidebound cutaneous changes of scleroderma.[16] Even in early stages of the disease, microscopic evaluation of the nailfold capillary bed reveals areas of ischemia alternating with large, dilated capillary loops.[16] As vascular disease progresses, clearly visible telangiectasia develops, often on the face, anterior chest, and hands.

Although the skin changes and Raynaud's phenomenon may be of most concern to the patient, involvement of internal organs has a much more serious effect on long-term prognosis. Involvement of the lower esophagus occurs in almost 90% of patients with classic scleroderma, although only 50 or 60% of patients complain of dysphagia or serious reflux.[17]

Diffuse interstitial lung disease is often insidious. It is the third leading cause of death in scleroderma, from either pulmonary insufficiency or secondary pulmonary hypertension. Cardiac disease caused by microvascular insufficiency and subsequent myocardial infarction are also common. Patients may present with arrhythmias or congestive heart failure in late-stage disease. The scleroderma patient with angina may have normal coronary arteriograms because ischemia is secondary to microvascular disease.[18]

Fortunately, renal involvement in scleroderma is rather uncommon, occurring in less than 10% of patients.[19] Damage to the capillaries and mesangium causes renal ischemia and stimulates increased renin production, manifest as abrupt accelerated hypertension and rapidly progressive renal failure.[19] Aggressive treatment with angiotensin-converting enzyme (ACE) inhibitors can ameliorate or even reverse the disease.[20]

POLYMYOSITIS AND DERMATOMYOSITIS

Polymyositis/dermatomyositis is a systemic autoimmune disease whose primary target organ is muscle. Polymyositis is uncommon, with an incidence one third to one fifth that of systemic lupus erythematosus. Women are affected twice as often as men.[21] The mean age of onset is around 50. While the cause remains obscure, cell-mediated autoimmune factors appear to play some role in muscle damage.[21] Biopsy of involved muscle often reveals inflammatory lymphocytic infiltrates with occasional plasma cells and polymorphs. Variation in muscle fiber size and shape attests to the damage.[21]

The typical patient with polymyositis presents with insidious onset of painless weakness of the proximal muscles, which usually progresses over several months before the diagnosis is established.[22] Patients most commonly complain of inability to rise from the floor or a low chair, climb stairs, raise their arms overhead, or lift heavy objects. Weakness in the upper extremities is somewhat less common. Upper esophageal dysphagia, caused by involvement of striated pharyngeal muscles, and dyspnea, caused by involvement of the diaphragm and muscles of respiration, are uncommon on presentation, but are generally ominous signs.[23] Occasionally, patients with polymyositis present with acute, severe weakness associated with massive muscle breakdown and myoglobinuria. This condition must be differentiated from other causes of acute rhabdomyolysis, particularly crush injury and acute alcoholic myopathy. Fewer than 50% of patients experience significant muscle pain. Thus, complaints of severe myalgias are more suggestive of polymyalgia rheumatica or hypothyroidism.

The typical erythematous or violaceous skin rash differentiates dermatomyositis from polymyositis. Most typically, the eyelids, nose, cheeks, and the extensor services of the extremities are involved. Erythema overlying the knuckles, called Gottron's patches, are highly suggestive of dermatomyositis. There is poor correlation between the severity of the skin involvement and muscle involvement.[23]

An elevated CPK is found in a vast majority of patients at time of presentation. The level of CPK reflects the extent and activity of muscle breakdown. Urine myoglobin is generally found only in the most severe cases. Once the diagnosis of polymyositis/dermatomyositis is suspected, patients should be referred for further evaluation and treatment.[4]

POLYMYALGIA RHEUMATICA

The patient with polymyalgia rheumatica (PMR), as opposed to the one with polymyositis, presents with proximal pain and stiffness, rather than weakness.[24]

As in polymyositis, symptoms are generally localized to the shoulder and hip girdles, with aching extending down the proximal extremities. Peripheral joints may also be involved, especially the knees and wrists, making it virtually impossible to distinguish between PMR and seronegative rheumatoid diseases. A hallmark of PMR is severe and prolonged morning stiffness: patients often complain that they can barely roll out of bed or need assistance in getting up in the morning.[25] This stiffness may last for several hours, unlike the brief morning stiffness of osteoarthritis. About half of patients with PMR also complain of systemic symptoms such as low-grade fever, fatigue, and weight loss.

Polymyalgia rarely occurs before age 50, and its incidence rises rapidly with age. By age 80, PMR is almost as common as RA. Women are affected twice as often as men. The cause remains obscure.[26]

Physical examination is generally most helpful for negative findings. Despite complaints of weakness, muscle testing reveals normal strength. Minimal joint swelling may be present but significant synovitis, especially of the small joints of the hands and feet, should lead toward a diagnosis of rheumatoid arthritis. Laboratory studies are also either negative or nonspecific.[4] A modest anemia of chronic disease may be present, but serologies are negative. Acute phase reactants, however, are markedly elevated in almost all patients. The Westergren ESR is greater than 35 mm per hour in most patients, and values exceeding 100 mm per hour are common. Elevated fibrinogen and C reactive protein levels also reflect the inflammatory state. All acute phase reactant levels return to normal with adequate treatment.[5]

Symptoms of PMR invariably respond to low- or moderate-dose corticosteroid therapy. Response is usually so rapid and complete that it can be used as a criterion for diagnosis. Divided doses of 15 to 20 mg of prednisone per day may lead to complete resolution of symptoms within 48 to 72 hours. Lack of response generally means that the diagnosis is in error.[25]

GIANT CELL ARTERITIS

A condition closely associated with polymyalgia rheumatica is temporal or giant cell arteritis (GCA). Temporal arteritis also affects predominantly elderly patients, especially women. There is a clear-cut association between giant cell arteritis and PMR. Symptoms of PMR have been noted in 40 to 60% of patients with GCA, and is the initial symptom in 20 to 40%.[25] Conversely, from 8 to 80% of patients presenting with PMR are found to have giant cell arteritis on biopsy of an asymptomatic temporal artery.[26]

Although the onset of giant cell arteritis may be acute or insidious, most patients are symptomatic for several weeks or months before the diagnosis is established. About 60% of patients complain of headache at the time of diagnosis.[26] The pain, described as boring or lancirating, is usually localized to the occiput or temple, with associated scalp pain and tenderness. Examination may reveal tenderness or loss of pulse in the affected arteries. Involvement of other arteries of the head and neck produces other typical symptoms. Involvement of the facial artery causes intermittent claudication of the jaw and/or tongue. Involvement of the central retinal or ciliary arteries may lead to optic nerve infarct and irreversible blindness. Although a patient may have warning signs such as amaurosis fugax or diplopia, blindness most often occurs abruptly and may be bilateral. Involvement of other large elastic arteries, the aortic arch and its branches, may also occur, leading to a syndrome similar to Takayasu's disease. Finally, the diagnosis of giant cell arteritis should be considered in the differential diagnosis of elderly patients presenting with fever, weight loss, and anemia of chronic disease because constitutional symptoms may predominate. Laboratory findings are similar to those found in patients with PMR; almost all patients have markedly elevated acute phase reactants. Westergreen ESR is rarely less than 50 and often greater than 100.[4]

Treatment with corticosteroid should be initiated as soon as the diagnosis is strongly considered. Treatment with steroids for up to 5 or 7 days will not affect biopsy results; thus treatment should never be withheld for this reason. Patients with visual symptoms are best admitted to the hospital for intravenous corticosteroids, whereas patients with somewhat less urgent symptoms may be started on 60 to 80 mg of prednisone in divided daily doses pending biopsy. Corticosteroids provide prompt symptomatic relief, and prevent the potentially disastrous sequelae.[25]

REFERENCES

1. Bennett, J.C.: Rheumatoid arthritis. Edited by Wingaarden, J.B. and Smith, L.H. Cecil Textbook of Medicine. In Philadelphia, W.B. Saunders Co., 1985, p. 1911.
2. Ziff, M.: Systemic rheumatoid disease: Immunological aspects. Adv. Inflam. Res. 3:123, 1982.
3. Schumacher, H.R.: Synovial membrane and fluid morphologic alterations in early rheumatoid arthritis. Microvascular injury and virus-like particles. Ann. N. Y. Acad. Sci. 256:39, 1975.
4. Cohen, A.S. (ed): Laboratory Diagnostic Procedures in the Rheumatic Diseases. 2nd edition. Boston, Little, Brown and Co. 1975.
5. Hollingsworth, J.W.: Local and systemic complications of rheumatoid arthritis. Philadelphia, W.B. Saunders Co., 1968.
6. Tan E.: Autoantibodies to nuclear antigens (ANA): The immunobiology and medicine. Adv. Immunol. 33:167, 1982.
7. Short, C.L., Bauer, W. and Reynolds, W.S.: Rheumatoid Arthritis. Cambridge, Harvard Press, 1957.
8. Morley, P.K., Hull, R.G., and Hall, M.A.: Pneumococcal septic arthritis in rheumatoid arthritis. Ann. of Rheum. Dis. 46:482, 1987.
9. Rowe, I.S., Deans, A.C., and Keat A.C.S.: Pyogenic infection and rheumatoid arthritis. Postgrad. Med. J., 63:19, 1987.
10. Sorin, S., Askari, A., and Moskowitz, R.W.: Atlantaxial subluxation as a complication of early ankylosing spondylitis. Arthritis Rheum. 22:1, 1979.
11. Smith, H.R., and Steinberg, A.D.: Autoimmunity—A prospective. In Annual Review of Immunology, Volume I. Edited by Paul, W.E., Fatham, E.G., Metzgar, H. Palo Alto, Annual Reviews Inc., 1983, p. 175.
12. Rothfield, M.F.: Systemic Lupus Erythematosus. Clin. Rheum. Dis. Volume I, Dec. 1975.
13. Steinberg, A.D.: Systemic lupus erythematosus. In Cecil Textbook of Medicine. Edited by Wingaarden, J.B., and Smith, L.H. Philadelphia, W.B. Saunders Co., 1985, p. 1924.
14. Ropes, M.W.: Systemic Lupus Erythematosus. Cambridge, Harvard University Press. 1976.
15. American Journal of Kidney Disease, 11(suppl 1), July 1982.
16. Rodnan, G.P., Myerowitz, R. L., and Justh, G.O.: Morphologic changes in the digital arteries in patients with progressive systemic sclerosis (scleroderma) and Raynaud's phenomenon. Medicine 59:393, 1980.
17. Ninelstein, S.H., Brody, S., McShane, D., and Holman, H.R.: Mixed connective tissue disease: A subsequent evaluation of the original 25 patients. Medicine 59:239, 1980.
18. Follansbee, W.P., Curtiss, E.I., Medsger, T.A., et al.: Physiologic abnormalities of cardiac function in progressive systemic sclerosis with diffused scleroderma. N. Engl. J. Med. 310:142, 1984.
19. Traub, Y.M., Shapiro, A.P., Rodnan, G.P., et al.: Hypertension and renal failure (scleroderma renal crisis) in progressive systemic sclerosis. Review of a 25 year experience with 68 cases. Medicine 62:335, 1983.
20. Witman, A.J., Case, O.B., Larugh, J.H., et al.: Variable response to oral angiotensin-converting enzyme blockage in hypertensive scleroderma patients. Arthritis Rheum. 25:241, 1982.
21. Messner, R.P.: Dermatomyositis and polymyositis. In Cecil Textbook of Medicine. Edited by Wingaarden, J.B., Smith, L.H. Philadelphia, W.B. Saunders Co., 1985, p. 1947.
22. Kagen, L.J.: Approach to patient with myopathy. Bull. Rheum. Dis. 33:2, 1983.
23. Bohan, A., Peter, J.B., Bowman, R.L., and Parson, C.N.: A computer-assisted analysis of 153 patients with polymyositis dermatomyositis. Medicine 56:255, 1977.
24. Healey, L.A.: Polymyalgia rheumatica. In Cecil Textbook of Medicine. Edited by Wingaarden, J.B. and Smith, L.H. Philadelphia, W.B. Saunders Co., 1985, p. 1946.
25. Healey, L.A., Wilske, K.R.: The systemic manifestations of temporal arteritis. New York, Grune and Stratton, 1978.
26. Chuang, T.-Y., Hunder, G.G., Islterup, D.M., and Kurland, L.T.: Polymyalgia rheumatica. A 10 year epidemiologic and clinical study. Ann. Intern. Med. 97:672, 1982.

NONSTEROIDAL ANTI-INFLAMMATORY DRUGS (NSAIDS)

Rita K. Cydulka and Steven B. Sorin

CAPSULE

The widely used nonsteroidal anti-inflammatory drugs (NSAIDS) are a heterogeneous group of compounds that share certain therapeutic actions and can have significant side effects. The prototype is aspirin. NSAIDs are used primarily to treat pain of low to moderate intensity, such as chronic postoperative pain and that secondary to inflammation and musculoskeletal disorders such as rheumatoid arthritis, osteoarthritis, and ankylosing spondylitis. Pain associated with hollow viscera is usually not relieved. While the NSAIDs provide symptomatic relief from pain and inflammation, they do not arrest the progression of pathologic injury to tissue. Side effects associated with NSAIDs include gastrointestinal upset, sodium and water retention, renal dysfunction, and central nervous system (CNS) problems. Patients with known hypersensitivity to aspirin may experience hypersensitivity reactions to NSAIDs. The use of NSAIDs in patients with renal or hepatic insufficiency should be avoided. Continuous combination therapy with more than one NSAID is best avoided because little extra benefit is achieved and the incidence of side effects is increased. The NSAIDs do not cause dependence or change perception of sensory modalities other than pain.

INTRODUCTION

The nonsteroidal anti-inflammatory drugs are often chemically unrelated, but share certain therapeutic actions and side effects. The prototype anti-inflammatory drug, aspirin, and most other NSAIDs have antipyretic and analgesic effects in addition to their anti-inflammatory actions. The chief indication for anti-inflammatory agents is to treat low- to moderate-intensity pain associated with musculoskeletal disorders and musculoskeletal injuries. They are rarely effective against pain associated with hollow viscera, except for the injectable ketorolac (Toradol). The NSAIDs provide symptomatic relief from pain and inflammation, but do not arrest the progression of pathologic injury to tissue.

The NSAIDs inhibit the biochemical pathway responsible for biosynthesis of the prostaglandins and related lipoxygenase, which cause inflammatory changes and sensitize pain receptors to mechanical and chemical stimulation.[1] Most NSAIDs irreversibly inhibit cyclo-oxygenase. Drugs that inhibit both cyclo-oxygenase and lipoxygenase have better anti-inflammatory actions than those that only inhibit cyclo-oxygenase.[2] Individual agents have different modes of inhibitory activity on cyclo-oxygenase. Inhibition of other enzymes probably contributes to the toxic effects of the NSAID.

Most NSAIDs are tightly bound to plasma proteins and may displace other drugs from binding sites. Therefore, concurrent administration of NSAIDs with other plasma protein-bound drugs should be avoided. If two plasma protein-bound drugs must be administered together, drug dosages must be adjusted and drug levels monitored.[1] Such drugs include warfarin, sulfonylurea hypoglycemic agents, and methotrexate. Tolmetin is an exception because it does not interfere with other protein-bound drugs and may be freely used with other drugs that bind plasma proteins.

Side effects generally appear in the first few weeks of therapy.[3] The most common side effects involve the gastrointestinal (GI) tract. Complaints range from mild dyspepsia to ulceration of the stomach or small intestine, with secondary edema and blood loss. The drugs vary considerably in their tendency to cause such erosions. Gastric damage is induced by at least two mechanisms: local irritation that allows retrograde diffusion of acid into the stomach mucosa and thus induces tissue damage; and inhibition of biosynthesis of gastric prostaglandins PGI_2 and PGE_2 which inhibit gastric acid secretion and promote secretion of cytoprotective mucus in the intestine.[4]

The renal effects of the NSAID are manifold. NSAIDs decrease renal blood flow and glomerular filtration rate in patients with diminished circulatory volumes, in addition to inhibiting renal prostaglandins.[5,6] Therefore, extreme caution should be exercised when prescribing NSAIDs for patients with conditions causing decreased effective plasma volume, renal disease, renal vascular hypertension, hydronephrosis, ureteral obstruction, and Bartter's syndrome.[5] NSAIDs promote salt and water retention, resulting in concentrated urine, hypervolemia, and peripheral edema. Patients who use NSAIDs should be carefully monitored for fluid and electrolyte disturbances. The NSAID should be discontinued at the first sign of hypervolemia, congestive heart failure, or hyponatremia.

Renal dysfunction induced by NSAIDs is characterized by a rapid rise in blood urea nitrogen and serum creatinine following the initiation of therapy. In addition, one may note a precipitous decrease in urine output, significant fluid weight gain, and sodium retention. The serum potassium may rise out of proportion to the degree of renal insufficiency. The urinalysis is without active sediment.

Persons at risk for developing NSAID-induced renal dysfunction are generally over 60, are concomitantly using diuretics, and have renovascular disease, diabetes mellitus, or coronary artery disease.[7] The drug most commonly implicated in causing renal disease is indomethacin. Sulindac is reported to spare the kidneys.[5] Rapid recovery of renal function on cessation of NSAID is the rule.

Persons who use NSAIDs for prolonged periods or in high doses may develop analgesic nephropathy. Within the United States, persons who live in the southeast have the highest prevalence of NSAID-induced analgesic nephropathy because of the warm climates, which lead to dehydration.[5] Worldwide, an increased prevalence of analgesic nephropathy is reported in Australia and Switzerland. Additionally, there is a 4:1 ratio of women to men suffering from this complication. Tubular concentration is defective early in the course of analgesic nephropathy. Acidosis is noted out of proportion to the increase in blood urea nitrogen and creatinine because of the presence of concomitant renal tubular acidosis. Proposed mechanisms for development of analgesic nephropathy include direct toxicity of compounds or metabolites on the kidney, metabolic alterations that decrease available ATP, immunologic mechanisms, and ischemia secondary to prostaglandin inhibition.[5] This condition is reversible if it is detected early and further consumption of NSAID is avoided.

The NSAIDs affect several other organ systems, including the hematopoietic system, the central nervous system, and the endocrine system. Disturbances include abnormal platelet function, prolonged bleeding time, aseptic meningitis, prolonged gestation, spontaneous labor, and cognitive dysfunction.[1]

Twenty to twenty-five percent of middle-aged patients with asthma, nasal polyps, or chronic urticaria are intolerant of aspirin and most aspirin-like drugs. This response is believed to be related to the inhibition of cyclo-oxygenase.[3] The use of aspirin or any NSAID must be avoided in any patient who reports an aspirin hypersensitivity reaction.

NSAID therapy should be initiated in low doses. Marked variation in an individual's response to different but closely related drugs may be noted. Continuous combination therapy with more than one NSAID is best avoided because little extra therapeutic benefit is achieved and the incidence of side effects is increased.

The dramatic relief of pain and inflammation that the NSAIDs afford patients should not prevent the emergency physician from searching for treatable causes of musculoskeletal pain, such as gout. Failure to do so may lead to neglect of an underlying metabolic problem and allow multisystem progression of the joint disease.[8]

ACETYLSALICYLIC ACID (ASPIRIN)

The medicinal effect of willow bark has been known to several cultures for centuries. The active ingredient, salicin, was finally isolated in its pure form in 1829 and introduced as aspirin in 1899.[1] Aspirin, or acetylsalicylic acid, relieves pain from myalgias, arthralgias, and skin structures. It does not lead to tolerance or addiction. Its usefulness as an anti-inflammatory, antipyretic, and analgesic agent is often underrated by laymen because it is so easily available. It does, however, have a potential for serious toxicity if used improperly.

After oral ingestion, aspirin is absorbed rapidly from both the stomach and upper small intestine. It is found in the plasma within 30 minutes after oral ingestion, and peak plasma concentrations are noted within 2 hours. The rate of absorption is determined by the disintegration and dissolution rate of tablets, mucosal pH, and gastric emptying time. The presence of food in the stomach delays the absorption of orally administered aspirin. Rectal absorption of aspirin is slower, less complete, and less reliable, and is therefore not the preferred route of administration. Acetylsalicylic acid is readily absorbed through the skin.[1]

Aspirin is distributed throughout most body tissues and most transcellular fluids by pH-dependent passive processes.[9] It readily crosses the placental barrier.[10] Aspirin competes with thyroxine, triiodothyronine, penicillin, thiopental, phenytoin, sulfinpyrazone, bilirubin, tryptophan, uric acid, naproxen, and possibly steroids for plasma-binding sites. Aspirin is metabolized in many tissues, particularly the hepatic endoplasmic reticulum and mitochondria, and is excreted mainly by the kidneys. Excretion rates depend on urinary pH.[9] The plasma half-life of aspirin is 15 minutes. At low doses, the plasma half-life of salicylate is 2 to 3 hours. At anti-inflammatory doses, the plasma half-life of salicylate increases to 12 hours and, at high or toxic doses, it increases to 15 to 30 hours.[9]

The most common side effects of aspirin involve the GI tract. These include epigastric distress, nausea, vomiting, gastric ulceration, and gastric hemorrhage.[11] A single dose of aspirin alters bleeding time for up to 4 to 7 days. Other side effects include mild hemolysis in patients with glucose-6-phosphate dehydrogenase deficiency and hypersensitivity reactions on persons with asthma and nasal polyps.[12] The use of aspirin should be avoided in patients with severe hepatic disease, hypoprothrombinemia, vitamin K deficiency, hemophilia, and renal insufficiency.

Table 52-2 gives formulations and route of administration of aspirin and other salicylates.

DIFLUNISAL

Diflunisal is a difluorophenyl derivative of salicylic acid that is not converted to salicylic acid in vivo. Although it is a more potent anti-inflammatory than aspirin, it is devoid of antipyretic effects and is primarily used as an analgesic agent in the treatment of osteoarthritis and other musculoskeletal disorders.[1] Diflunisal produces fewer and less severe GI side effects than does aspirin.

This drug is almost completely absorbed after oral administration. Peak plasma concentrations appear within 2 to 3 hours after oral administration. It is 99% bound to plasma protein. Diflunisal readily appears in the milk of lactating women. Diflunisal is metabolized in the liver and excreted in the urine. As with salicylic acid, concentration-dependent pharmacokinetics prevail.[13]

PYRAZOLONE DERIVATIVES

The pyrazolone derivatives include phenylbutazone, oxyphenbutazone, antipyrine, aminopyrine, dipyrone, and apazone (not yet available in the United States).

PHENYLBUTAZONE

Phenylbutazone was introduced in the United States in 1949 for the treatment of rheumatoid arthritis and other arthritides. It is an effective anti-inflammatory agent but a poor analgesic-agent for nonrheumatoid pain.[1] Phenylbutazone's toxic side effects preclude its routine use as an analgesic or antipyretic agent.

Phenylbutazone is rapidly and completely absorbed from both the upper GI tract and the rectum. It achieves peak plasma concentrations within 2 hours and is 96% protein-bound, thus displacing other protein-bound drugs such as the NSAID agents, oral anticoagulants, oral hypoglycemic agents, and sulfonamides. In addition, phenylbutazone induces hepatic

microsomal enzymes, increases the effects of insulin, and complicates the interpretation of thyroid function tests.[1] The plasma half-life of phenylbutazone is 50 to 65 hours, but high concentrations persist in the synovial spaces for up to three weeks after discontinuing the medication. Phenylbutazone is metabolized in the liver and excreted in the urine.[14]

Phenylbutazone is poorly tolerated by 10 to 45% of patients who initiate therapy and must be discontinued in 10 to 15% of these patients. The most common side effects are nausea, vomiting, epigastric pain, and skin rashes. Additional side effects include diarrhea, vertigo, insomnia, euphoria, nervousness, hematuria, and blurred vision. Water and electrolyte retention may lead to significant edema, congestive heart failure, and pulmonary edema. Phenylbutazone reduces the uptake of iodine by the thyroid gland and may cause a goiter or myxedema. More serious side effects caused by phenylbutazone include peptic ulcer disease with hemorrhage or perforation, hypersensitivity reactions, serum sickness, ulcerative stomatitis, hepatitis, nephritis, leukopenia, thrombocytopenia, aplastic anemia, and agranulocytosis. The use of phenylbutazone is best avoided in the elderly, in whom toxic side effects are more severe.[3]

See Table 52-2 for information on administration and dosage.

OXYPHENBUTAZONE

Oxyphenbutazone is an active metabolite of phenylbutazone and has the same spectrum of activity, drug interactions, toxicity, and contraindications as its parent drug, but causes less gastric irritation.[14]

ANTIPYRINE AND AMINOPYRINE

These two drugs are no longer available in the United States because of drug-induced agranulocytosis. Antipyrine is still used in analgesic mixtures in some countries.[1]

APAZONE (AZAPROPRAZONE)

Apazone is the newest pyrazolone derivative. It has a similar spectrum to that of anti-inflammatory, analgesic, antipyretic, and uricosuric activity as phenylbutazone but causes much less toxicity. Apazone is particularly useful in the treatment of acute gouty arthritis but is not currently available in the United States.[15]

Apazone is rapidly and completely absorbed from the GI tract. Peak plasma concentrations are noted within 4 hours of oral ingestion, whereas peak synovial fluid concentrations are not noted for many more hours. Apazone is over 95% protein-bound and therefore displaces other protein-bound drugs. Apazone has significant enterohepatic cycling. The plasma

TABLE 52-2. SUMMARY OF POPULAR NONSTEROIDAL ANTI-INFLAMMATORY DRUGS

Drug	Formulation	Route of Administration	Dosage	Uses	Comments
Salicylate Derivatives Acetylsalicylic acid	65–975 mg capsules, tablets, also time release capsules, suppositories	Oral Per rectum	Adults: 325–650 mg q4h Children: should not be used as antipyretic in children. Rheumatoid arthritis: 4–6 g daily in divided doses	Anti-inflammatory Acute muscular disorders Rheumatoid arthritis, ankylosing spondylitis, osteoarthritis	Take with full glass of water to minimize gastric irritation Absorption from enteric-coated tablets is sometimes incomplete Preparation containing alkali or buffer may have a shorter plasma half-life, secondary to urine alkalization Contraindications: persons with hypersensitivity, asthma, and nasal polyps
Sodium salicylate	325 mg, 650 mg tablets, injection solution	Oral, parenteral	325–650 mg q4h		
Diflunisal (Dolobid)	250–500 mg tablets	Oral	Initial dose: 500–1000 mg Followed by: 250–500 mg q8–12h	Analgesic, osteoarthritis	
Pyrazolon Derivatives Phenylbutazone (Azolid, Butazolidin)	100 mg coated tablets, capsule	Oral	Initial dose: 800 mg in one dose Followed by 100–400 mg per day in divided doses	Acute gouty arthritis May be considered in acute exacerbations of rheumatoid arthritis, ankylosing spondylitis, osteoarthritis	Take with meals to lessen gastric irritation Take for 1 week maximal Discontinue drug and report to physician if the following occurs: fever, sore throat, oral lesions, rash, pruritis, jaundice, weight gain, or melena Complete blood count and weight checks must be done frequently Contraindications: hypertension, cardiac renal hepatic dysfunction history of peptic ulcer disease, history of aspirin sensitivity
Oxyphenbutazone (Oxalid, Tandearil)	100 mg tablets	Oral	100 mg tid to qid	same as phenylbutazone	Same as phenylbutazone
Apazone (Rheumox)	300 mg capsules 600 mg tablets	Oral	Initial dose: 600 mg qid × 1 day 600 mg 1200 mg per day in divided doses	Gout, rheumatoid arthritis, osteoarthritis	Not available in the United States Ulcerogenic Contraindications: aspirin-induced bronchospasm
Indoles Indomethacin (Indocin)	25 mg/50 mg Capsules Sustained release capsules 50 mg suppositories	Oral Per rectum	Initial dose: 25 mg bid-tid May increase up to 100–200 mg per day	Acute gouty arthritis, ankylosing spondylitis, osteoarthritis	Take with food or immediately after meals to lessen gastric distress Contraindications: aspirin hypersensitivity, pregnancy or nursing, persons operating machinery, psychiatric disease, seizure disorder, Parkinsonism, renal disease, stomach or intestinal disease
Sulindac (Clinoril)	100 mg/200 mg tablets	Oral	100–200 mg bid, up to 400 mg per 24 hours	Acute gouty arthritis, rheumatoid arthritis, osteoarthritis, ankylosing spondylitis	Take with food if gastric discomfort If taken with food, absorption may be delayed and concentrations may be reduced in the plasma Kidney sparing Contraindications: aspirin hypersensitivity, bleeding dyscrasias

TABLE 52-2. CONTINUED

Drug	Formulation	Route of Administration	Dosage	Uses	Comments
Fenamates Mefamic acid (Ponstel)	250 mg capsules	Oral	Initial dose 500 mg, followed by 250 mg q 6 hours	Analgesia	Take with food Not recommended for children under 14 years or pregnant females Discontinue if diarrhea or skin rash results The maximal clinical trial is 7 days Contraindications: gastrointestinal disease, aspirin hypersensitivity
Meclofenamate sodium (Meclomen)	500/100 mg capsules	Oral	200–400 mg per 24 hours divided tid to qid	Rheumatoid arthritis, osteoarthritis (however, not as initial treatment)	Not recommended for children Discontinue if diarrhea or skin rash develops Contraindications: gastrointestinal disease, aspirin hypersensitivity
Tolmetin (Tolectin)	200 mg/400 mg capsules	Oral	400 mg tid, up to 2 g/day, 20 mg/kg/day in children over 2 years old	Osteoarthritis, rheumatoid arthritis, juvenile rheumatoid arthritis, ankylosing spondylitis	May be given with meals, milk, or antacid to decrease abdominal discomfort Contraindications: aspirin hypersensitivity Reports of anaphylactoid reactions in non-aspirin sensitivity patients have been reported
Propionic Acid Derivatives Ibuprofen (Motrin, Rufen, Advil, Nuprin)	200 mg/300 mg/400 mg/600–800 mg tablets Available only as 200 mg tablets without prescription	Oral	Up to 2400 mg/day in divided doses	Acute muscular conditions, rheumatoid arthritis, osteoarthritis, ankylosing spondylitis, acute gouty arthritis	May be given with food to decrease gastrointestinal side effects Recently approved for use in children over 6 months of age Caution in patients with peptic ulcer disease Discontinue use if ocular side effects are noted Contraindications: pregnancy, breast feeding
Naproxen (Naprosyn)	250/375 mg/500 mg tablets	Oral	250–375 mg bid Initial: 750 mg Followed by 250 mg q8h until attacks subside Initial: 500 mg Followed by 250 mg q8h	Rheumatoid arthritis, osteoarthritis, ankylosing spondylitis Acute gout Bursitis, acute tendonitis	May be given with meals to decrease gastric comfort Advantage: bid dosing is easier for patient compliance
Naproxen sodium (Anaprox)	275 mg	Oral	275 mg bid	Same as Naprosyn	Same as Naprosyn
Fenoprofen calcium (Nalfon)	200–600 mg capsules and tablets	Oral	300–600 mg bid–qid Up to 3.2 g/day 200 mg q4–6h	Rheumatoid arthritis, osteoarthritis, gouty arthritis Moderate pain	May be given with meals to decrease gastrointestinal upset Not recommended for children Exercise caution when prescribing this drug for patients with a history of gastrointestinal pathology
Flurbiprofen (Ansaid)		Oral	Initial: 400 mg in first 24 hours Followed by: 200 mg/day in divided doses for 5 days	Acute gouty arthritis	Same as ibuprofen
Piroxicam (Feldene)	10 mg/20 mg capsules	Oral	10 mg bid	Rheumatoid arthritis, osteoarthritis, ankylosing spondylitis, acute muscular skeletal disorders, acute gouty arthritis	Neither food nor antacids alter the rate or extent of absorption Contraindications: aspirin hypersensitivity

TABLE 52-2. CONTINUED

Drug	Formulation	Route of Administration	Dosage	Uses	Comments
Diclofenac sodium (Voltaren)		Oral	150–200 mg per day in divided doses 100 mg divided bid-pid 25 mg qid plus 25 mg qhs	Rheumatoid arthritis Osteoarthritis Ankylosing spondylitis	Monitor liver function tests within 8 weeks of beginning treatment and frequently thereafter Discontinue drug if any abnormality persists Monitor blood counts frequently
Colchicine	0.5 mg/0.6 mg tablets 0.5 mg/mL sterile solution	Oral IV	Oral: initially 1–1.2 mg Followed by 0.5–1.2 mg q 1–2 h up to 4–10 mg Discontinue when pain disappears or GI symptoms appear Intravenous: 2 mg diluted in 10–20 mL of water or 0.9% normal saline, up to 4 mg		Discontinue as soon as GI symptoms occur Oral medications must be stored in a tight, light-resistant container Do not repeat acute course dosage within 3 days Tissue necrosis may occur if intravenous solution is extravasated Caution must be exercised when prescribing this medication for the aged, patients with cardiac disease, renal disease, or gastrointestinal disease Patients should be advised to take the first dose of colchicine at the first twinge of pain

half-life of apazone is 20 to 24 hours, and 65% of it is excreted in the urine unchanged.[3]

Apazone is generally well tolerated and rarely needs to be discontinued because of side effects.[3] Only 3% of patients complain of GI side effects, such as nausea, epigastric pain, dyspepsia, and heartburn; 3% also complain of skin rashes. Less common complaints include headache and vertigo. Apazone does not cause agranulocytosis.[1]

For more information regarding dosage and administration, see Table 52-2.

INDOLES

INDOMETHACIN

Indomethacin, a methylated indole derivative, was introduced in 1963 to treat rheumatoid arthritis and related disorders. It is a potent inhibitor of cyclooxygenase that exhibits prominent anti-inflammatory, analgesic, and antipyretic properties. In fact, it is 10 to 40 times more potent than acetylsalicylic acid. Unfortunately, its use is limited by its toxicity.

Indomethacin is rapidly absorbed from the GI tract after oral ingestion. In fasting subjects, peak plasma concentrations are noted within 2 hours. Peak synovial fluid concentrations are reached within 5 hours. Absorption is delayed when indomethacin is taken after meals. The plasma concentration of indomethacin and its metabolites may be increased with concurrent administration of probenecid. After absorption, indomethacin is 90% bound to plasma proteins and extensively bound to tissue. The plasma half-life of indomethacin varies from 2 to 11 hours, primarily because of extensive enterohepatic circulation. Indomethacin is converted to inactive metabolites in the liver and is excreted in the urine, bile, and feces.[1] Indomethacin antagonizes the natriuretic and antihypertensive effects of furosemide and the thiazide diuretics, as well as the antihypertensive effects of beta-adrenergic blocking agents. Acute renal failure has been reported with concomitant administration of indomethacin and triamterene.[6] The concurrent administration of indomethacin with oral anticoagulants does not affect either agent.[16]

Of patients taking indomethacin, 30 to 50% experience side effects that cause 20% to discontinue the drug. Most adverse reactions are dose-related. The most common side effect noted by patients who use indomethacin on a chronic basis is a severe frontal headache.[1] Other side effects noted involve the GI system, the central nervous system, and the hematopoietic system. GI side effects include anorexia, nausea, abdominal pain, upper GI tract ulcers with perforation and hemorrhage, occult GI blood loss, ulceration, acute pancreatitis, diarrhea, and (rarely) hepatitis. Central nervous system (CNS) side effects include dizziness, vertigo, lightheadedness, mental confusion, severe depression, psychosis, and hallucinations. Hematopoietic side effects include thrombocytopenia, neutropenia, and aplastic anemia. Hypersensitivity reactions including rash, pruritis, urticaria, and bronchospasm have been noted. Contraindications to the use of indomethacin include aspirin hypersensitivity, pregnancy, nursing mothers, psychiatric disease, seizure disorders, Parkinson's disease, renal disease, and stomach or intestinal ulcerative disease.[14] Persons whose jobs require the operation of dangerous or heavy machinery should also avoid the use of indomethacin. For further information on dosage and administration, see Table 52-2.

SULINDAC

Sulindac is a pro-drug with weak anti-inflammatory properties. Its sulfide metabolite, however, is 500 times more potent an inhibitor of cyclo-oxygenase than the parent substance. Fewer GI side effects are noted with the use of sulindac because the gastric and intestinal mucosa is exposed to the pro-drug rather than the active drug after oral administration.[3] In addition, sulindac is said to spare the kidneys if taken in recommended dosages.[5]

Sulindac is 90% absorbed after oral administration and reaches peak plasma concentrations within 1 hour. Its sulfide metabolite reaches peak concentrations within 2 hours. Sulindac is transformed in the liver and has extensive enterohepatic circulation. After absorption, it is 93% bound to plasma proteins. The plasma half-life of sulindac is 7 hours, whereas the plasma half-life of the active sulfide is 18 hours. It is largely excreted in the feces, with a small amount excreted in the urine.[1] Side effects are seen in 25% of patients who take sulindac. The most common side effects reported are abdominal pain, nausea, and constipation. GI bleeding is uncommon. CNS side effects, including headache, drowsiness, dizziness and nervousness, are seen in 10% of patients, and 5% complain of rash or pruritis. Fewer than 5% of patients experience transient elevations in hepatic enzymes.[3,14]

Like other NSAIDs, sulindac impairs platelet function and increases bleeding time.[3]

FENAMATES

The fenamates are a family of aspirin-like drugs derived from N-phenylanthranilic acid with anti-inflammatory, antipyretic, and analgesic properties. The fenamates include mefanamic acid, meclofenamic acid, flufenamic acid, tolfenamic acid, and etofenamic acid. Although they were discovered in the 1950s, the fenamates have not gained widespread popularity because they frequently cause severe diarrhea and have no clear advantage over several other aspirin-like drugs. The fenamates inhibit cyclo-oxygenase and antagonize the inflammatory effects of prostaglandins. Only mefanamic acid and meclofenamate are available in the United States.[14]

After oral ingestion, meclofenamate is more rapidly absorbed than meclofenamic acid. Meclofenamate reaches peak plasma concentrations within 30 minutes to 2 hours after oral ingestion, whereas meclofenamic acid does not reach peak plasma concentrations for 2 to 4 hours. Both drugs are conjugated within the liver and have a plasma half-life of 2 to 4 hours. Both drugs are bound to plasma proteins and thus displace other drugs that are also bound to plasma proteins. They are both excreted in the urine (50%) and in the feces (20%).[1]

Of patients using the fenamates, 25% experience gastrointestinal side effects such as dyspepsia, epigastric pain, inflammatory bowel changes, severe diarrhea, constipation, bleeding ulcers, and steatorrhea. Less common side effects include transient abnormalities of hepatic and renal function, CNS effects, rashes, and hemolytic anemia. The fenamates also inhibit platelet function. The use of fenamates is contraindicated in persons with gastrointestinal disease or aspirin hypersensitivity and must be discontinued immediately if diarrhea or a skin rash appears.[14] For further information on use of the fenamates and their derivatives and dosage, see Table 52-2.

TOLMETIN

Tolmetin is an anti-inflammatory, analgesic and antipyretic agent introduced in the United States in 1976. It is equivalent in efficacy to moderate doses of aspirin, but better tolerated.

Tolmetin is rapidly and completely absorbed in the GI tract after oral administration and reaches peak plasma concentrations within 20 to 60 minutes. Concomitant administration of antacids does not affect absorption of tolmetin. Although tolmetin is 90% protein-bound, it does not displace other protein-bound medications. Its plasma half-life is 1 to 2 hours. Tolmetin is conjugated in the liver and excreted in the urine.[17]

In 25 to 40% of patients taking tolmetin, side effects cause 5 to 10% to discontinue treatment. The most common problems noted are mild GI side effects including epigastric pain, dyspepsia, nausea, and vomiting. Gastric and duodenal ulcers are reported less frequently. CNS side effects, which include nervousness, anxiety, insomnia, and visual disturbances, are infrequently noted. Occasional skin rashes and urticaria are reported.[17] Persons who experience hypersensitivity reactions to aspirin also experience hypersensitivity reactions to tolmetin. Several reports of severe anaphylactoid reactions in patients without aspirin hypersensitivity have been documented.[18]

For further information on dosage and administration, see Table 52-2.

PROPIONIC ACID DERIVATIVES

Propionic acid derivatives include ibuprofen, naproxen, fenoprofen, fenbufen, plurbiprofen, indoprofen, ketoprofen, and suprofen. As a group, propionic acid derivatives are effective anti-inflammatory, analgesic and antipyretic agents and are better tolerated than other NSAIDs. Ibuprofen was the first propionic acid derivative available for general use and is now available for sale without a prescription in the United States.

All are effective inhibitors of cyclo-oxygenase, although naproxen is 20 times more potent an inhibitor of cyclo-oxygenase than aspirin, ibuprofen and fenoprofen.[1] All propionic acid derivatives alter platelet function and therefore prolong bleeding time. GI side effects, as well as renal side effects, are frequently noted. Several propionic acid derivatives have prominent inhibitory effects on leukocyte migration.[19] Persons who have experienced aspirin hypersensitivity reactions should avoid using propionic acid derivatives. Although all propionic acid derivatives are highly protein-bound, most do not alter the effects of oral hypoglycemic agents or warfarin. Nevertheless, caution should be exercised when using warfarin and propionic acid derivatives simultaneously. The propionic acid derivatives reduce the antihypertensive effects of the thiadize diuretics, beta-adrenergic antagonists, prazosin, and captopril, and reduce the diuretic and natriuretic effect of furosemide.[3,6]

IBUPROFEN

Ibuprofen is rapidly absorbed after oral administration and reaches peak plasma concentrations within 1 to 2 hours. Absorption from the rectum takes slightly longer. After absorption, ibuprofen is 99% bound to plasma protein, but occupies only a fraction of the total available drug binding sites.[1] Ibuprofen slowly diffuses and then remains in the synovial spaces. High synovial fluid concentrations of the drug are noted even as the plasma concentration drops. Its plasma half-life is 2 hours. Ibuprofen is metabolized in the liver and excreted in the urine.[20]

In 5 to 15% of patients using ibuprofen, GI side effects including epigastric pain, nausea, heartburn, abdominal discomfort, and sensations of fullness are seen, and 10 to 15% discontinue the drug because of these side effects. Less frequent side effects include thrombocytopenia, skin rashes, headache, dizziness, blurred vision, toxic amblyopia, fluid retention, and edema.[20] Ibuprofen readily crosses the placenta, and its use should be avoided by pregnant or lactating women.[1] For further information on dosage and administration, see Table 52-2.

NAPROXEN

Naproxen is fully absorbed when administered either rectally or orally. After oral administration, the rapidity but not the extent of absorption is influenced by the presence of food in the stomach. Peak plasma concentrations are achieved within 2 to 4 hours and are noted even sooner after ingestion of naproxen sodium. The absorption of naproxen is accelerated by concurrent administration of sodium bicarbonate, but is reduced by concomitant administration of magnesium oxide or aluminum hydroxide. After absorption, naproxen is 99% bound to plasma protein and readily crosses the placenta. Its plasma half-life is 14 hours. Naproxen is conjugated in the liver and excreted in the urine.[21]

Patients using naproxen complain of GI and CNS side effects with equal frequency. Side effects include mild dyspepsia, epigastric discomfort, heartburn, nausea, vomiting, gastrointestinal bleeding, drowsiness, headache, dizziness, sweating, fatigue, depression, and ototoxicity. Less common reactions include pruritus, rashes, jaundice, renal impairment, angioneurotic edema, thrombocytopenia, and agranulocytosis.[21]

For further information on dosage and administration, see Table 52-2.

FENOPROFEN

Fenoprofen is incompletely absorbed after oral administration. When it is taken on an empty stomach, peak plasma concentrations of the drug are achieved within 2 hours. Although the presence of food in the stomach retards absorption and diminishes the peak plasma concentrations achievable, concomitant administration of antacids does not alter the peak plasma concentrations achieved. Fenoprofen is 99% plasma bound, with a plasma half-life of 3 hours. Over 90% of the drug is metabolized in the liver and 100% is excreted in the urine.[1,22]

Side effects are noted less frequently with fenoprofen than with equipotent doses of aspirin. Fifteen percent of patients complain of gastrointestinal problems including abdominal discomfort, dyspepsia, constipation, and nausea. Additional side effects include rash, tinnitus, dizziness, lassitude, confusion, and anorexia. Caution must be used when prescribing this drug to patients with gastrointestinal pathology. See Table 52-2 for information concerning dosage and administration.

FLURBIPROFEN

Clinical trials have demonstrated that flurbiprofen is as effective as indomethacin and phenylbutazone in the treatment of acute gouty arthritis.[23,24] Absorption and metabolism of flurbiprofen are similar to those of fenoprofen.[1,22] Side effects of flurbiprofen include GI side effects and fluid retention.[1] For further information concerning dosage and administration, see Table 52-2.

PIROXICAM

Piroxicam is anti-inflammatory, antipyretic, and analgesic. It is equivalent to aspirin, indomethacin, or naproxen for long-term treatment of rheumatoid arthritis or osteoarthritis, but is better tolerated than either aspirin or indomethacin and needs less frequent dosage because of its long plasma half-life.[25]

Piroxicam is completely absorbed after oral administration. Neither food nor antacids alter the rate or extent of absorption. Piroxicam reaches peak plasma concentrations within 2 to 4 hours, and after absorption is 99% bound to plasma proteins and exhibits extensive enterohepatic circulation.[25] High synovial fluid concentrations are not reached for 7 to 10 days after ingestion. Thus maximum therapeutic responses are not achieved for 2 weeks. The plasma half-life is estimated at 45 hours. Piroxicam is largely excreted in the urine and feces.[1,25]

In 11 to 46% of patients using piroxicam, side effects necessitate discontinuing the drug. The most common side effects observed are mild GI problems. Peptic ulcers or gastric erosions are observed in fewer than 1% of patients. Like all anti-inflammatory agents, piroxicam alters platelet function and increases bleeding time. Patients who experience hypersensitivity reactions to aspirin should avoid using piroxicam.[25] For further information on dosage and administration, see Table 52-2.

DICLOFENAC SODIUM

Diclofenac sodium is a potent anti-inflammatory, analgesic, and antipyretic agent that was recently introduced in the United States. It has been available in other countries since 1974 and has been promoted as "the number one prescribed antiarthritic in the world." Diclofenac sodium is a chlorophenyl amino derivative of benzine acidic acid whose mechanism of action is unknown, but it is presumed to inhibit prostaglandin synthesis.[3,14,26]

Diclofenac sodium is well absorbed when administered orally. Peak plasma concentrations are reached within 2 hours if the drug is taken on an empty stomach. Concomitant food, drink, or use of antacids delays but does not decrease absorption. Synovial fluid concentrations exceed those achieved in the plasma.

The plasma half-life of diclofenac sodium is 1 to 2 hours. Diclofenac sodium is metabolized in the liver and excreted in the feces and urine.[3,14,26]

Side effects of diclofenac sodium are similar to those of ibuprofen. Most commonly noted are GI side effects, including nausea, dyspepsia, and diarrhea. Gastric ulceration and GI bleeding are uncommon. Renal toxicity, fluid retention, and hypersensitivity reactions have been noted. Elevation in liver enzymes and clinical hepatitis, autoimmune hemolytic anemia, and renal failure have been described.[27] The risk of aplastic anemia when using this drug is similar to the risk associated with the use of phenylbutazone.[27] Diclofenac sodium decreases the effectiveness of diuretic and antihypertensive agents, such as furosemide and thiazides. It decreases the renal clearance of lithium and increases the toxicity of methotrexate.[14,26] For further information on dosage and administration, see Table 52-2.

COLCHICINE

Colchicine is an alcohol derivative of colchicinum autumnale, which has been used to relieve articular pain since the 6th century AD and more specifically for the treatment of acute gouty arthritis since 1763.[1]

Colchicine is not an analgesic agent. Its anti-inflammatory effect is specific for acute gouty arthritis and several other limited conditions. It is an antimyotic agent that inhibits the migration of granulocytes into an inflamed area, breaking the inflammatory response cycle. It is thought to prevent production and release of glycoprotein from leukocytes, thereby decreasing joint pain and inflammation.[28]

Colchicine is rapidly absorbed after oral administration and reaches peak plasma concentrations within 30 minutes to 2 hours. The onset of therapeutic effect is more rapid when colchicine is administered intravenously, but the drug is equally effective by mouth. It is metabolized in the liver and excreted 90% in the feces and 10% in the urine.[1]

Colchicine enjoys the smallest benefit-to-toxicity ratio of all drugs that are effective for acute gouty arthritis. In the past, relief of joint pain after the administration of colchicine was considered a diagnostic test for acute gouty arthritis. At present, microscopic examination of synovial fluid for crystals is the gold standard for diagnosis of acute gouty arthritis.[29] Nausea, vomiting, diarrhea, and abdominal pain are noted within several hours of oral ingestion of the drug because of its action on the rapidly proliferating gastrointestinal tract epithelial cells.[30] Colchicine must be discontinued at the onset of these symptoms to avoid further toxicity. Ahern and colleagues reported that patients undergoing treatment with colchicine for acute gouty arthritis experienced diarrhea before pain relief.[30] Although most authors suggest that colchicine is more effective in treating acute gouty arthritis if begun within 6 hours of the onset of symptoms, Ahern et al. and Rodran did not find that the duration of symptoms before initiating colchicine therapy had any effect on the outcome at 48 hours.[30,31] In addition, they recommend that oral colchicine be used only in patients in whom less toxic NSAIDs are contraindicated.

Side effects noted with chronic administration of colchicine include agranulocytosis, aplastic anemia, myopathy, alopecia, azospermia, volume depletion, hyponatremia, hypocalcemia, cytopenias, renal failure, sepsis, and disseminated intravascular coagulation. Tissue necrosis can result from local extravasation of colchicine.[1,32] Acute overdose of colchicine can cause hemorrhagic gastroenteritis, vascular disease, nephrotoxicity, muscular compression, and ascending paralysis.[1]

Hepatic or renal disease is a relative contraindication to the use of colchicine. For further information on dosage and administration, see Table 52-2.

REFERENCES

1. Flower, R.J., Moncada, S., and Vane, J.R.: Analgesic anti-pyretic and anti-inflammatory agents; drugs employed in the treatment of gout. Chapter 29. Goodman and Gillman's The Pharmacological Basis of Therapeutics, 7th Ed. New York, MacMillan Publishing Co., 1985, pp. 674–715.
2. Higgs, G.A., and Flower, R.J.; Anti-inflammatory drug and the inhibition of Arachidonate Lipoxygenase in SRS-A and Leukotrienes. Edited by Piper, P.J. London, John Wiley and Son, Limited, 1981, pp. 197–207.
3. A Symposium: Anti-Rheumatic Drugs, Edited by Huskisson, E.C. New York, Praeger Publishers, 1983.
4. Bjarnason, I., Zanelli, G., Smith, T., et al.: The pathogenesis and consequence of non-steroidal anti-inflammatory drug induced small intestinal inflammation in man. Scand. J. Rheumatol. 64:55, 1987.
5. D'Angio, R.G.: Non-steroidal anti-inflammatory drug-induced renal dysfunction related to inhibition of renal prostaglandins. Drug Intell. Clin. Pharm. 21:954, 1987.
6. Clive, D.M., and Stoff, J.S.: Renal syndromes associated with non-steroidal anti-inflammatory drugs. N. Engl. J. Med. 310:563, 1984.
7. Blackshear, J.L., Davidman, M., and Stillman, M.T.: Identification of risks for renal insufficiency from non-steroidal anti-inflammatory drugs. Arch. Intern. Med. 143:1130, 1983.
8. Scopelitis, E., and McGrath, H.: NSAID-masked gout. South. Med. J. 80:1464, 1987.
9. Furst, D.L., Tozer, T.N., and Melmon, K.L.: Salicylate clearance, the resultant of protein binding and metabolism. Clin. Pharmacol. Ther. 26:380, 1979.
10. Collins, E.: Maternal and fetal effects of acetaminophen and salicylates in pregnancy. Obstet. Gynecol. 58:575, 1981.
11. Leonards, J.R., and Levy, G.: Gastrointestinal blood loss during prolonged aspirin administration. N. Engl. J. Med. 289:1020, 1983.
12. Mathison, D.A., Stevenson, D.D., and Simon, R.A.: Precipitating factors in Asthma: Aspirin, sulfites, and other drugs and chemicals. Chest. 87:505, 1985.
13. Brogden, R.N., Heel, R.C., Pates, G.E., et al.: Diflunisal: A review of its pharmacological properties and therapeutic use in pain in muscular skeletal strains and sprains and pain in osteoarthritis. Drugs 19:84, 1980.
14. Hart, F.D., and Huskisson, E.L.: Non-steroidal anti-inflammatory drugs. Current status and rational therapeutic use. Drugs 27:232, 1984.
15. Yu, T.F.: Milestones in the treatment of gout. Am. J. Med. 56:676, 1974.
16. Pullar, T., and Capell, H.A.: Interaction between oral anticoagulant drugs and non-steroidal anti-inflammatory agents: A review. Scott. Med. J. 28:42, 1983.
17. Brogden, R.N., Heel, R.C., Speight, T.M., and Avery, G.S.: Tolmetin: A review of pharmacological properties and therapeutic efficacy in rheumatic diseases. Drugs 15:429, 1978.
18. Rake, G.W., Jr., and Jacobs, R.L.: Anaphylactoid reactions to tolmetin and zomepirac. Ann. Allergy 50:323, 1983.
19. Ham, E.A., Cirrillo, V.J., Zanetti, M., Shen, T.Y., and Kuehi, F.A., Jr.: Studies on the mode of action of non-steroidal anti-inflammatory agents. In Prostaglandins in Cellular Biology. Edited by Ramwell, P.W., and Pharris, B.B., New York, Plenum Press, 1972, pp. 345–352.
20. Cantor, T.G.: Ibuprofen. Ann. Intern. Med. 91:877, 1979.
21. Brogden, R.N., Heel, R.C., Speight, T.M., and Avery, G.S.: Naproxen: A review of its pharmacologic properties and therapeutic efficacy in rheumatic diseases. Drugs. 13:241, 1977.
22. Brogden, R.N., Pinder, R.M., Speight, T.M., and Avery, G.S.: Fenoprofen: A review of its pharmacological properties and therapeutic efficacy in rheumatic diseases. Drugs 13:241, 1977.
23. Butler, R.C., Goddard, D.H., Higgens, C.S., et al.: Double-blinded trial flurbiprofen and phenylbutazone in acute gouty arthritis. Br. J. Clin. Pharmacol. 20:511, 1985.
24. Lomen, P.L., Turner, L.F., Lamborne, K.R., et al.: Flurbiprofen in the treatment of acute gout: A comparison with indomethacin. Am. J. Med. 80:134, 1986.
25. Symposium: Pharmacology, efficacy and safety of a new class of anti-inflammatory agents: A review of piroxicam. Am. J. Med. 72:1, 1982.
26. Diclofenac. In The Medical Letter 30:109, 1988.
27. International Agranulocytosis and Aplastic Anemia Study. JAMA 256:1749, 1986.
28. Malawista, S.E.: The action of colchicine in acute gouty arthritis. Arthritis Rheum. 18:835, 1975.
29. Roberts, W.N., Liang, M.H., and Stern, S.H.: Colchicine in acute gout: Re-assessment of risks and benefits. JAMA 257:1920, 1987.
30. Ahern, M.J., Reid, C., Gordon, T.P., et al.: Does colchicine work? The results of the first controlled study in acute gout. Aust. J. Med. 17:301, 1987.
31. Rodran, G.P.: Treatment of the gout and other forms of crystal-induced arthritis. Bull. Rheum. Dis. 32:43, 1982.
32. Ferrannini, E., and Pentimone, F.: Marrow aplasia following colchicine treatment for gouty arthritis. Clin. Exp. Rheumatol. 2:173, 1984.

CHAPTER 53

HEMATOLOGIC DISORDERS IN THE EMERGENCY DEPARTMENT

ANEMIA

Ronald L. Rhule

CAPSULE

Anemia is a common and distracting emergent finding. Discovery of unsuspected anemia can often misorient the physician, creating diversions in management and initial therapy. The accidental discovery of anemia can yield clues to the diagnosis and management of the disease process that is causing it, and with proper guidelines may direct the physician to the proper diagnostic pathway and subsequent laboratory "work-up."

INTRODUCTION

DEFINITION OF ANEMIA

Anemia is usually defined as a reduction in hematocrit or hemoglobin level. This reduction of the O_2-carrying capacity of the blood is a reflection of the actual reduction in the red blood cell (RBC) count. Normal range varies with age and sex. For practical purposes, 12 g/dL of hemoglobin may be accepted as the dividing line for adult women and 13.5 g/dL for adult men. Values below these indicate varying levels of anemia.

The loss of hemoglobin with consequent reduction in the oxygen-carrying capacity of the blood is the most conspicuous feature of anemia and the pathologic basis for most of the associated signs and symptoms such as dyspnea, tachycardia, weakness, and so on. Anemia is not a stand-alone diagnosis or a valid basis for treatment. In most instances, anemia occurs as a sign or complication of other processes which must be defined.

Anemia may be caused by many disease states, and thereby has varied and complex presentations. It is important to remember that *anemia itself is not a disease* but a manifestation of an underlying illness, and therefore its presence should lead to further search for the cause. The most important aspect of the early definition of anemia is to determine if it is acute or chronic.

With the myriad signs or symptoms of the various diseases associated with the anemias, there is no clinical means of establishing a firm diagnosis other than the measurement of the hemoglobin and hematocrit. For example, the presenting signs of dehydration and subsequent volume depletion complicated by anemia are similar to, and confused with, acute blood loss symptoms, and must be ruled out. The patient with acute dehydration and accidentally discovered low hemoglobin is a difficult and challenging combination. The signs of volume depletion can be differentiated from those of acute blood loss in the appearance of the hemogram. The mean red cell volume (MCV) and mean corpuscular hemoglobin concentration (MCHC) must be determined, as well as whether signs of dehydration exist. Early signs of dehydration reveal that the hemoglobin remains stable but the hematocrit suggests concentration.

The various signs and symptoms associated with acute blood loss are discussed subsequently in this chapter, but remember that no matter how stringent your personal rules are in screening patients for clinical signs of anemia, it is difficult to establish this diagnosis in the well compensated patient. Various adaptations in fluid displacement and relative intervascular volume levels, developed through a millennium of evolution in the mammalian species, have allowed us to survive in the face of great extremes in hemoglobin values.

A physical examination coupled with an ever-present high degree of suspicion will serve well in establishing this diagnosis in the otherwise asymptomatic patient. The cause of an anemia cannot be finalized until specific laboratory tests are performed. Anemia

TABLE 53-1. TESTS FOR DIFFERENTIAL DIAGNOSIS OF ANEMIA

1. CBC with differential (hand-performed)
2. Electrolytes with BUN and creatinine
3. Coagulation profile (PT, PTT, platelets, reticulocyte count)
4. Glucose level
5. Blood for type and screen
6. Clot to "hold" for subsequent studies. This is important in that immediate treatments may alter the basic studies, making exact diagnosis unclear
7. Urinalysis, including strip testing for urobilinogen

can be suspected on clinical grounds, but must be confirmed by a hemoglobin level, RBI count, or hematocrit. A battery of tests can help the physician to sift through the rough differential (Table 53-1).[1,2]

The hematocrit measures the volume of RBCs as a fraction (percentage) of the total blood volume (Table 53-2). The hemoglobin is expressed as a concentration in g per 100 mL of whole blood. These tests do not measure the volume of blood in the body or the total body mass of red blood cells. This simple concept is important in understanding the lack of early reduction in hemoglobin and hematocrit in the face of acute blood loss. Acute blood loss does not affect the measured levels of hemoglobin and hematocrit until certain compensatory mechanisms come into play.

In the acute situation, decreases in blood volume caused by bleeding (or other fluid loss) may be detected by orthostatic changes in pulse and blood pressure. This produces symptoms of volume depletion, including postural dizziness. Occasionally, orthostatic syncope weakness, cardiogenic strain, and shock ensue if the process of inadequate circulating volume is not interrupted.

Because of the potential for end-organ compromise, early and accurate assessment of the level of loss and anemia is essential. The evaluation of the anemic patient should be based on a firm understanding of pathophysiologic principles incorporating the three basic mechanisms of anemia: blood loss, underproduction, and hemolysis (Table 53-3).

The changes seen in chronic anemia are associated with the hypoxic side effects and also the fatigue that accompany tissue demand for oxygen. So fatigue, irritability, difficulty in breathing, palpitations, and cardiac hypoxia including angina are commonly seen, and in fact may represent the most classic presentation of chronic anemia, that of unusual and unexplained fatigue. Cardiac strain occurs if the symptoms are left unabated.

Often chronic anemia is discovered during evaluation of the patient's other problems, and if not suspected may be missed completely. Our best defense in this issue is the persistent pursuit of the common problems that plague mankind. "Common problems occur commonly" is good advice that serves us well in the chronic anemias.[3,4]

PATHOPHYSIOLOGY

RBC PRODUCTION

RBCs (erythrocytes) are derived from the bone marrow as a multipotential cell called the pluripotent stem cell, which is capable of both self-renewal and differentiation. It is implicit, therefore, that this primordial cell

TABLE 53-2. HEMOGRAM NORMAL VALUES

Age	Hemoglobin (g/dL)	Hematocrit (md/dL)	Red Blood Cell (count)
3 months	10.4 to 12.2	30 to 36	3.4 to 4.0
3–7	11.7 to 13.5	34 to 40	4.4 to 5.0
Adult (men)	14.0 to 18.0	40 to 52	4.4 to 5.9
Adult (women)	12.0 to 16.0	35 to 47	3.8 to 5.2

TABLE 53-3. BASIC MECHANISMS OF ANEMIA

Blood Loss	Underproduction	Hemolysis
Test stool for occult blood	Reticulocyte count RBI indexes and bone marrow are informative	Reticulocyte count
List obvious sites of bleeding		Bilirubin haptoglobin
Orthostatic changes		Abnormal RBI

is capable of evolving granulocytes, monocytes, and platelets. The actual drive for specific differentiation is poorly understood. The erythroid burst-forming unit (BFU) is responsive to the hormone erythropoietin. Monocytes and lymphocytes act synergistically with erythropoietin. The more mature form in this cascade is the erythroid colony-forming unit (CFU). This produces a smaller clone of the erythroid cell that resembles a mature lymphocyte and is sensitive to erythropoietin levels.

Biochemically erythropoietin has a molecular weight of about 36,000. Erythropoietin is produced primarily by the kidneys in response to hypoxic stimuli. When anemia develops, the resultant tissue hypoxia leads to elevated levels of erythropoietin in the plasma. Erythropoietin is a glycoprotein enhanced in the kidney and activated in the liver. Resultant normoblastic hyperplasia produces more erythrocytes for delivery to the circulation. This hormone can be readily assayed by radioimmunoassay, and interacts with the erythroid stem cells resulting in the production of recognizable blastic erythroid series, type cells.[5-7]

In addition to this function, erythropoietin stimulates hemoglobin synthesis. RBC maturation in the bone marrow requires approximately 7 days before cells are released as reticulocytes. At the completion of this differentiating cellular series, at the last division, the pyknotic nucleus is removed from the normoblast, forming the reticulocyte that rests in the formative focus in the bone marrow.

The reticulocyte is released to a 24-hour circulation time, losing its mitochondria and ribosomes and then resembling the mature RBC. Because the RNA of the reticulocyte disappears about a day after its entry into the blood, enumeration of *reticulocytes measures the number of cells being delivered by the marrow to the blood.*

This is a measure of effective erythropoiesis. The normal absolute reticulocyte count is approximately 50,000 per microliter, or 1% of the circulating erythrocytes.

If the erythrocyte count is determined, one can calculate the absolute reticulocyte count by multiplying the reticulocyte percentage by the erythrocyte count.[8,9]

HEMOGLOBIN BIOSYNTHESIS

Studies have demonstrated that 98% of the protein in the cytoplasm of circulating red cells is hemoglobin. In normal adults, 97% of the total hemoglobin is composed of hemoglobin A. The remaining 3% is in the form of hemoglobin A_2. This minor component is increased in patients with thalassemia. An additional component in adult blood is fetal hemoglobin or HbF, accounting for less than 1%. This hemoglobin is persistently high in certain disease processes. Other than in specific disease processes, the alpha and beta chains are evenly balanced. The biochemical characteristic of the thalassemias, on the other hand, is hallmarked by asymmetric chain construction.

Oxygen transportation is the single most important task of the RBC, along with movement of carbon dioxide from the capillary beds. Reviewing the anatomy and physiology of circulation, we note that the RBC becomes fully saturated with oxygen as it passes through the pulmonary bed. During the capillary phase of circulation the oxygen saturation is depleted. This dissociation can be plotted and also predicted using standard dissociation curves. The bases for the curves are the variables pH, temperature, and 2, 3, DPG (Fig. 53-1).

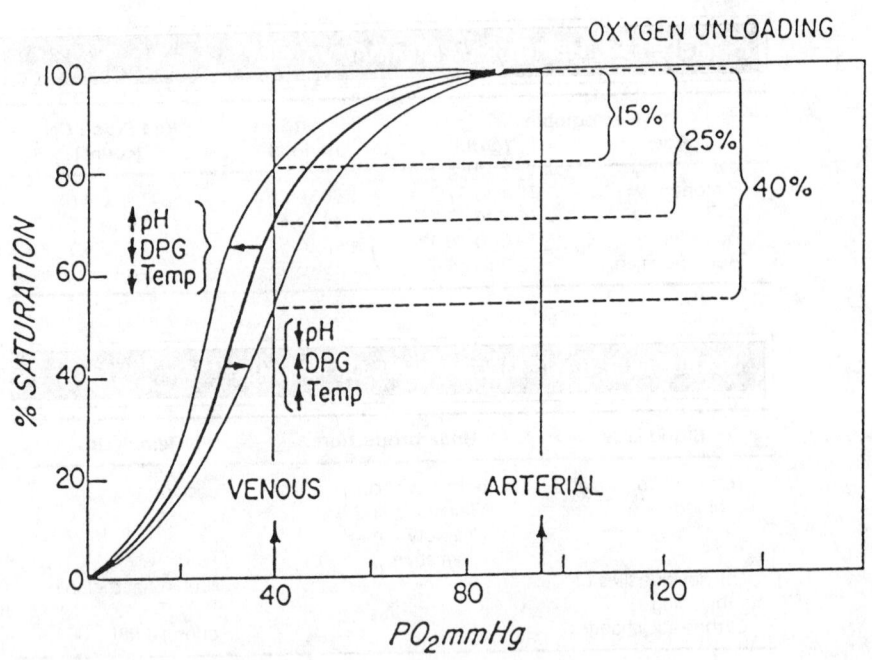

OXYGEN UNLOADING

FIG. 53-1. The oxyhemoglobin dissociation curve of normal blood. The major factors influencing the position of the curve are pH, temperature, and the intracellular concentration of 2,3-DPG. An increase in plasma pH or a decrease in temperature and 2,3-DPG causes an increase in oxygen affinity (shift to the left) and a relative decrease in oxygen unloading when going from an arterial Po_2 of 95 mmHg to a venous Po_2 of 40 mmHg. Conversely, a decrease in pH or an increase in temperature and 2,3-DPG causes a decrease in oxygen affinity (shift to the right) and a relative increase in oxygen unloading.

The RBC obtains all of its energy from the anaerobic glycolytic pathways (Embden-Meyerhof and hexose monophosphate shunt). Deficiencies involving any of the enzymes required in this cascade lead to depleted energy production and a hemolytic anemia. Glucose-6-phosphate dehydrogenase deficiency is the most common clinical problem encountered. The production of 2, 3, DPG is a biochemical result of the Embden-Meyherhof pathway, which then binds with hemoglobin and pushes the dissociation curve to the left. (High levels of 2, 3, DPG mean that hemoglobin easily unloads oxygen; low levels of 2, 3, DPG mean that hemoglobin does not unload). This shifts the curve to the left, allowing hemoglobin to hold more tightly to oxygen (higher saturation at lower partial pressure of O_2, Fig. 53-1).[10–12]

APPROACH TO ANEMIA

In reviewing the diseases that face primary care physicians, it becomes apparent that anemia is one of the leading causes of concern, and also one of the most commonly seen disorders. Anemia may be clinically difficult to diagnose, and a well-defined approach at the bedside is required to establish the diagnosis with efficiency. The symptoms depend greatly on the specific defect causing the anemia and also the duration from onset.

The hemoglobin and hematocrit are both good measurements of anemia. The accuracy of the reflection of anemia depends on the method of determining the actual laboratory value. Because anemia is not a disease but rather a signal or reflection of a disease, it should be a marker to look further for an active disease process. Anemia may be best classified according to the pathophysiologic mechanism, appearance of the RBC's, or gross cause.

Anemia of rapid onset may first be detected by the symptoms of rapid fluid depletion, high pulse rate, low blood pressure, and orthostatic changes, leading to shock. Other physical complaints may accompany these symptoms, including thirst and mild disorientation with low level confusion, depending on the aggression and length of time of the bleeding. The age of the patient may play an important role in our assessment; the elderly are generally more labile and infants and children relatively resistant to early changes associated with rapid blood loss. Additionally, other processes affect each subgroup that may confuse the subjective picture (underlying medical problems, current medications, distracting injuries, language skill deficits [no history]). Common sites of occult bleeding in the acutely ill patient with trauma include the liver, spleen, pleural cavity, pelvis, and kidneys including the retroperitoneal space. Adolescents are particularly prone to traumatic disease and

TABLE 53-4. HISTORY AND PHYSICAL EXAMINATION FOR EMERGENT ANEMIA

History
General
    Prehospital status, therapy, and response to therapy
    Bleeding diathesis
    Previous blood transfusion
    Underlying diseases, including allergies
    Current medications, platelet inhibition?
Trauma
    Nature and time of injury
    Blood loss at scene
    Tetanus immunization
    Time of last meal
Nontrauma
    Skin: Petechiae, ecchymoses
    Gastrointestinal: Hematemesis, hematochezia, peptic ulcer
    Genitourinary: Menorrhagia, metrorrhagia, last menstruation, hematuria
Physical Examination
Vital Signs Measured Serially
    Blood pressure, pulse, respiratory rate
    Three-positioned orthostatic blood pressure and pulse
    Level and content of consciousness
Skin
    Pallor
    Diaphoresis
    Jaundice
    Diagnosis
    Purpura, ecchymoses, petechiae
    Examine completely for penetrating wounds
Cardiovascular
    Murmurs, S3, S4
    Quality of femoral and carotid pulse
Abdomen
    Hepatosplenomegaly
    Pain, guarding, rebound on palpation
Rectal and pelvic examination
    Masses
    Pain, guarding, rebound on palpation
    Stool hemoglobin testing

should be highly suspect for these sites of injury. Patients with well compensated chronic anemia may have obviously "normal" vital signs, and perhaps complain of fatigue or reduced exercise tolerance, but have a markedly reduced residual capacity for changes in blood volume. Chronically anemic patients can be likened to an alkaline battery, with the declining slope of energy vertical and not angular (Table 53-4).

The hallmark of chronic and slower anemias is the revelation that the patient can sustain "normal" function at significantly reduced levels of hemoglobin. The primary symptoms of chronic anemia are derived from the tissue hypoxia that occurs: fatigue, headache, angina, and orthopnea. Chronic anemia is a symptom of gastrointestinal bleeding until proven otherwise, and gastrointestinal (GI) bleeding is a symptom of carcinoma until defined otherwise. It is therefore imperative that the actual cause of low-level anemia be accurately defined and catalogued for the patient.

The origin of the anemia is critical in understanding the patient's symptoms. Each particular category of anemia is host to signs and symptoms that are classic in medical literature (vitamin B12 deficiency meaning glossitis and oral changes, iron deficiency meaning inflammation of the oral mucosa, classic pica food cravings, and "spooning" of the nailbeds). One must remember that the vast bulk of anemias produce no symptoms whatsoever until the levels achieve depressions that are disruptive to the blood pressure and pulse.

The definition and categorization of anemia cannot be finalized, however, until appropriate laboratory studies are performed. Even with this symptomology, the actual definition requires a hemogram. The standard "Coulter counter" electronic analyzer is accurate and simple to obtain. The services of a trained hematologist are not necessary to establish the criteria for diagnosis. Important, however, is the establishment of a solid set of guidelines to feel your way through the maze.

CLINICAL PRESENTATION AND EXAMINATION

PHYSICAL SIGNS

Pallor is the physical finding most commonly associated with anemia. The usefulness of this sign, however, is limited by other factors that affect the color of the skin. Furthermore, the blood flow to the skin can undergo wide fluctuations. Normal individuals appear sallow when blood is shunted away from the skin, whereas anemic patients may appear flushed when overheated or during periods of excitement. One cannot ignore the melanin concentration as another important determinant of skin color, and therefore a distracting element in assessing pallor.

The underlying disease process (the real reason why the patient is in your department) may confuse the picture, diseases such as Addison's disease, hemochromatosis, hyperbilirubinemic states, and other "discoloring" disorders affect our initial approach. As mentioned previously, a patient with a sudden onset of anemia is acutely ill, with high pulse rate and low blood pressure, and quick to comment on fatigue and lightheadedness. Usually, in this abrupt state, there are other blatant symptoms of blood loss.

GI bleeding is common in many patients, but most cannot accurately decipher what GI blood loss looks like. Establishing the apparent from the covert is your goal. Demonstration of bleeding from the GI tract may require the insertion of a nasogastric tube. Remember that frank blood is what we are looking for; if the lavage is clear, occult testing is distracting and inappropriate

and the nasal passage irritation from the tube alone may cause the test to become positive.

Our first task is to assess the patient's ability to cope with gravity. The following questions should be answered: Can the blood pressure be maintained in various angular positions? Can the pulse rate be held to reasonable levels while the patient persists with the ability to perform routine tasks?

Another question is whether skin changes bespeak coagulation defects or reveal unusual purpuric discoloration. Are there large bruises or hemorrhagic lesions? These changes are often seen in the elderly, revealing senile skin changes, and rarely associated with underlying anemia, other than the anemia of old age. Therefore other considerations must be incorporated into our assessment.

The "discovery" of anemia is usually a fortuitous event following the results of a routine CBC, the patient being basically asymptomatic for the anemic process and really presenting with the overt signs and symptoms of some other problem instead. Anemia rarely causes symptoms until the hematocrit drops below 30%, at which time the oxygen delivery is decreased unless the anemia is of rapid onset. Increased O_2 delivery can be facilitated by several mechanisms. Exercise intolerance with heavy exertion is experienced with even minor drops in hematocrit, but at levels below 30%, daily activities cause increasing problems in performance. Predictably, most patients experience exertional dyspnea and weakness, tiredness, and occasionally dizziness at low levels of performance. This is inconsistent if the anemia is of long duration.

All bets are off when trying to establish physical criteria for the detection of anemia in the "chronic" patient, in that the nail beds are usually pink and the conjunctiva are not pale. Two factors contribute to the development of pallor in patients with anemia. There is, of course, a decrease in the hemoglobin concentration of blood perfusing the skin and mucous membranes. Also, blood is shunted away from the skin and other peripheral tissues, permitting enhanced blood flow to vital organs. Redistribution of blood flow is an important mode of compensation in anemia.[13–20]

DIFFERENTIAL DIAGNOSIS

Anemias can be subdivided into distinct groups that aid us in approaching the cause and origin.[21] Three specific categories are analyzed in these groupings: (1) acute blood loss, (2) increased RBC destruction, and (3) decreased RBC production (Table 53-5).

TABLE 53-5. CLASSIFICATION OF ANEMIAS

Anemias caused by decreased production (blood loss)
  Anemias resulting from deficiencies of nutrients
    Iron deficiency
    Vitamin B12 and folate deficiency
  Anemias resulting from hypoproliferative disorders
    Anemia of chronic disease
    Anemia of renal disease
    Anemia of liver disease
    Anemia of endocrine disease
  Anemias resulting from stem cell defect
    Aplastic anemia
    Pure RBC aplasia
    Sideroblastic anemia
Anemias caused by increased destruction of RBCs
  Anemias from extrinsic defects (immune)
    Drug-induced
    Autoimmune
    Paroxysmal cold hemoglobinuria
    Isoimmune
    Hemolytic disease of the newborn
  Anemia resulting from extrinsic RBC defects
    Microangiopathic
  Anemias resulting from intrinsic (membrane) defect
    Heredity spherocytosis and elliptocytosis
    Paroxysmal nocturnal hemoglobinuria
  Anemias resulting from intrinsic RBC defects (hemoglobino-
    pathies)
    Sickle cell syndromes
    Unstable hemoglobins
    Hemoglobins with altered oxygen affinity
    Thalassemias
  Anemias: intrinsic (enzymopathies)
    Glucose-6-phosphate dehydrogenase deficiency
    Pyruvate kinase deficiency
  Anemias due to dilution of mature RBCs
    Anemia of pregnancy
    Iatrogenic volume overexpansion[21]

TABLE 53-6. DISEASES CAUSING AUTOIMMUNE HEMOLYTIC DISORDERS

Drug immune reactions
  Hapten type with antibodies to the drug
    Complement-fixing antibody: Quinidine, quinine, phenac-
    etin, ethacrynic acid, sulfa drugs
    Noncomplement fixing: Penicillin in doses > 20 million units
    per day
  Autoimmune type with antibodies to RBC membrane:
    Methyldopa, 1-dopa, mefenamic acid, chlordiazepoxide
  Cephalosporins at large (>4 g/day) doses may cause hemolysis
    by direct membrane injury
Collagen vascular disease
  Systemic lupus erythematosus
  Periarteritis nodosa
  Rheumatoid arthritis
Neoplastic
  Malignant: Chronic lymphocytic leukemia, lymphoma, my-
    eloma, thymoma, chronic myeloid leukemia
  Benign: Ovarian teratoma, dermoid cyst
Infections
  Mycoplasma
  Syphilis
  Malaria
  Bartonella
  Viral infections: Mononucleosis, hepatitis, influenza coxac-
    kievirus, cytomegalovirus
Miscellaneous
  AIDS, thyroid disorders, ulcerative colitis

ACUTE BLOOD LOSS

Of these categories, acute blood loss with hemodynamic alteration causes the usual and most dramatic initial emergency presentation.

INCREASED DESTRUCTION

The normal RBC survival is 100 to 120 days. The pathology of the hemolytic anemias is a shortening of this life span. The cell membrane is the "target" during hemolysis; thus any disorder that affects the membrane may shorten RBC survival. Both intrinsic and extrinsic mechanisms are categorized, depending on whether the defect is within the cell or affecting the cell from without. The intrinsic defects are congenital, and the extrinsic ones are acquired.

The basic response of the bone marrow to the hemolytic event is erythropoiesis. The bone marrow has the capacity to increase basal rate from 5 to 8 times normal production. Depending on the parallel marrow production in the face of hemolysis, the patient either demonstrates anemia or is classified as having "compensated" hemolytic anemia. The bone marrow production can be monitored by the reticulocyte count and, classically, the presence of increased reticulocytosis and the absence of blood loss conclude a probable hemolysis. The classification of hemolytic anemias is based on RBC survival studies, and the anemias are subcategorized as corpuscular or extracorpuscular (Table 53-6).

Corpuscular defects are classified as hereditary (membrane, metabolic, and hemoglobin abnormalities) and acquired (paroxysmal nocturnal hemoglobinuria). Extracorpuscular (acquired) defects have multiple causes: chemical (e.g., from drugs or metals), hemolytic to G-6-PD-deficient cells (also chemically induced), physical agents (e.g., heat and severe thermal burns), and poisons (e.g., fava beans, Castor beans, etc.). Further hemolysis can be caused by snake venoms, infectious agents, and immune reactions.

Laboratory findings differ according to the site of the hemolysis, the amount of destroyed blood, and the rate of destruction. If the destruction is intravascular and the quantity of destroyed blood is large, free hemoglobin and methemalbumin are present in the plasma (hemoglobinemia and methemalbuminemia). Free hemoglobin is distributed bound to haptoglobin, and the hemoglobin-haptoglobin complex is catabolized by the reticuloendothelial system. This process normally prevents hemoglobin from being excreted unchanged in the urine. When sufficient amounts of hemoglobin are absorbed by the proximal tubules, the

TABLE 53-7. RBC INDICES: CLASSIFICATION OF DECREASED RBC PRODUCTION DISEASE

Macrocytic:
  B12 deficiency
  Folate deficiency
  Infectious
  Malignancy
  Dialysis
Microcytic: (three subtypes, iron, porphyrin, and globin)
  Iron deficiency
  Blood loss (1 mg iron/2 mL blood loss)
  Hemoglobinemias (thalassemia)
  Heavy metal poisoning (porphyrin)
  Sideroblastic (porphyrin)
Normocytic
  Primary (bone marrow suppression; aplastic, metaplasia with myelofibrosis, myelophthisic anemia)
  Secondary: Cirrhosis, uremia, endocrinopathies

hemoglobin iron is converted to hemosiderin. When these tubular cells are later shed into the urine, hemosiderinuria results. If the amount of hemoglobin present in the tubule exceeds the absorption rate, measurable hemoglobinuria is the byproduct. This mechanism is the reason for the hemoglobinuria present in acute hemolytic transfusion reactions.

Normal plasma hemoglobin level is 2 to 3 mg per dL. A rise of 5 to 10 imparts a yellow or orange color to the plasma, and yields the icteric discoloration typical of these conditions. Levels up to 20 or greater are often seen in hemolytic anemia. Increased haptoglobin levels may be present in any inflammatory disease or intense steroid therapy. During the metabolism of the free hemoglobin and the binding limitations of hemoglobin-haptoglobin, urobilinogen is produced. The normal urobilinogen in a 24-hour specimen is up to 3.5 mg in the urine and up to 280 mg in the stool. Hemolysis may produce up to 180 to 200 mg. in the urine and 300 to 400 mg. in the stool.[22–33]

DECREASED RBC PRODUCTION

Anemias from decreased RBC production are hallmarked by slow onset and low reticulocyte count. RBC indices coupled with an accurate smear are essential. The emergency physician can often isolate but not define the actual cause of the anemia (Table 53-7).

Hypoproduction anemias are hallmarked by close scrutiny of the RBC indices, although typically not "picked up" at a casual contact in the ED. Attention to the mean corpuscular hemoglobin (MCH) and the MCHC are the critical measurements. As noted in Table 53-7, the hypoproduction anemias can be classified as iron deficiency, porphyrin deficiency, and globin alteration. In terms of frequency, iron deficiency is the most common, and in our ED is seen with some regularity. Exploring the actual cause for this process is generally limited to a brief examination

of the patient's skin (bruising), oral cavity (ulceration, ecchymosis), and rectum (occult blood). This brief examination, coupled with a more elaborate history, often leads in the correct direction in a fascinating number of cases. The actual laboratory workup is, in most cases, inappropriate in the ED setting.

The thalassemias are represented by decreased globin production and therefore reduced hemoglobin construction and resultant altered erythropoiesis. There are three major thalassemias. *Homozygous beta-chain thalassemia* (thalassemia major, mediterranean anemia) is often associated with severe anemia, and in many patients leads to accelerated premature death. In *heterozygous beta-chain thalassemia* (thalassemia minor), the indices appear similar to those of patients with iron deficiency anemia, but more exaggerated. *Alpha-thalassemia* is the least symptomatic, and is most commonly seen in Orientals and blacks.

The impaired hemoglobin production in sideroblastic anemia results in mitochondrial deposition of iron. This alteration results in elevated levels of transferrin, ferritin, and serum iron. This particular type of anemia is seen more frequently because it is linked to the elderly population and is therefore becoming more and more common. Unfortunately, the most obvious signs, pallor and fatigue, are often confused in the elderly population, making this particular definition difficult at best. One reversible, and potentially catastrophic cause of this anemia is lead poisoning. The suspicion of this, coupled with an elevated serum lead level, establishes the diagnosis.

MEGALOBLASTIC AND MACROCYTIC ANEMIAS

It is fair to say that the hemogram results of vitamin B$_{12}$ deficiency and folate deficiency are vitually identical. Only through elaborate and expensive testing can the two be ideally differentiated. Poor erythropoiesis and pancytopenia result from general body alteration in DNA synthesis, whether it is due to vitamin B$_{12}$ or folate deficiency and therefore the initial presentation is similar. The clinical picture involves tissues with rapid cell turnover, the GI tract being the most common. Folic acid is obtained usually from green vegetables, cereals, fruit, and multivitamins. The minimum daily requirement (MDR) is about 100 mg. Careful preparation of food is required because folate is heat-labile. The causes of folate deficiency are overcooked food, malabsorption syndromes, alcoholism, and enzymatic deficiency. Increased requirements caused by pregnancy, malignancy, hemolytic anemia, and chronic blood loss also cause relative deficiency.

Vitamin B$_{12}$ is a heat-stable, easily absorbed vitamin, found only in animal sources. This vitamin is absorbed in the ileum after binding with the "intrinsic factor." The daily requirement is 1.5 mg, the body being able to store 5 mg. It may therefore, take up to 4 years to develop overt anemia. The obvious causes of B_{12} anemia are vegetarianism, intrinsic factor deficits, abnormalities in the absorption surface (ileum), and rapid transit bowel disease.[34–37]

PROCEDURES AND LABORATORY CONSIDERATIONS

Laboratory analysis reveals the level of the anemia in terms of hematocrit, hemoglobin, and actual measure of the number of RBCs present, but when considering which laboratory tests to perform, one must first consider the underlying causes of anemia as categorized in the three subgroups mentioned previously: defective RBC production, increased RBC destruction (hemolysis), and gross blood loss.

The possibility of blood loss as either the sole cause or a contributing factor must always be considered. The occult blood test on stool is requisite in *all* patients with discovered anemia. The reticulocyte count is the most useful laboratory test for answering this question. Reticulocytosis is a reflection of the release of an increased number of young cells from the bone marrow. The degree of erythropoiesis can then be assessed more quantitatively by determining the reticulocyte index, which uses the hematocrit or packed cell volume (PCV). The patient's PCV is divided by a normal PCV and then multiplied by the reticulocyte percentage. This yields the reticulocyte index. This measure fails to consider the distribution of reticulocytes between the bone marrow and the peripheral blood. When the marrow is greatly stimulated, marrow reticulocytes enter the circulation prematurely.

A failure to produce red cells is reflected in an inappropriately low reticulocyte count. In contrast, a significant elevation of reticulocytes suggests hemolysis. Patients with rapid blood loss or recently treated vitamin B_{12} anemia also produce brief elevations in the reticulocyte count and must be considered (see previous discussion of reticulocyte count).

The measurement of unconjugated bilirubin in the serum is a particularly useful guide to the presence of accelerated red blood cell breakdown. After collection of this data, the essential cause of the anemia can be determined. Three additional baseline studies are of critical importance in the initial work up of the patient with anemia: measurement of red cell indexes, examination of the peripheral blood smear, and in many patients, bone marrow examination.

RBC INDEXES

Red cell indexes can be calculated from determinants of hematocrit, hemoglobin concentration, and RBC count. Measuring the hematocrit or PCV is the simplest and one of the most precise ways to ascertain the concentration of red cells in the blood. The PCV is the ratio of the volume of packed red cells to the total volume. The mean red cell volume (MCV) is determined by dividing the PCV by the calculated RBC volume. The mean corpuscular hemoglobin concentration (MCHC) is determined by dividing the hemoglobin by the PCV and is expressed in g per dL. A third RBC index, the mean corpuscular hemoglobin (MCH) is determined by dividing the hemoglobin by the RBCs. When calculated by an electronic counter, the MCHC is unreliable and of little use to the clinician. Generally an automated system provides a printout which includes hemoglobin concentration, RBC count, PCV, and the three RBC cell indexes, MCV, MCHC, and MCH.

EXAMINATION OF THE BLOOD SMEAR

The technologist may miss certain elements in the smear if not targeted to search for abnormalities. The clinician can approach the specimen with a prepared mind and can scrutinize it for specific abnormalities. The examination can confirm the size and color of RBCs as estimated by RBC indexes. Furthermore, although these indexes provide mean statistical values, the microscopic examination can reveal variation in RBC size (anisocytosis) or shape (poikilocytosis), changes that are helpful in the diagnosis of specific anemias. Examination of the blood smear is particularly important in evaluating the patient with a hemolytic anemia. The finding of rouleaux suggests the presence of dysproteinemia as occurs in multiple myeloma. The examination may provide the initial clue that the patient has significant thrombocytopenia.

ANEMIA FROM BLOOD LOSS

The presentation of acute blood loss depends greatly on the rapidity of loss, and also to underlying contributing factors (other medical problems, medicines, drugs, etc.). But generally, the clinical presentation depends on the site, severity, and speed of loss. The typical trauma patient with moderate to severe loss exhibits symptoms secondary to hypoxia and hypovolemia. The patient has weakness, fatigue, lightheadedness, stupor, or coma, and often appears pale, diaphoretic, and irritable. The increased sympathetic tone creates a stabilized and "compensated" patient, with symptoms of anxiety, hyperventilation, mild tachycardia, and often diaphoresis.

The nonspecific signs of compensated shock from rapid blood loss are often confusing and highly dependent on the general health status of the patient. A narrow pulse pressure is generated by the relatively low cardiac output coupled with a catecholamine-driven increase in peripheral resistance.

ACUTE BLOOD LOSS

In acute blood loss, as in other categories of potential disasters, the emergency physician must practice as a preventive medicine specialist and attempt to prevent the patient from imminent threat. This is best accomplished by carefully assessing the orthostatic blood pressure curves and noting measures. Careful evaluation and anticipation reward the physician by avoiding the unnecessary resuscitation required for the shock patient. The simple exercise of caution with appropriate clinical evaluation provides sufficient data to salvage the great majority of patients.

Impaired delivery of oxygen and removal of metabolic waste products, both products of severe hypovolemia, may lead to widespread cellular dysfunction and organ damage.[38]

Examination of all patients with acute blood loss anemia or shock reveals trauma as the expected cause in the majority of cases. Motor vehicle accidents, various person-to-person assaults, and acute GI bleeding give us sufficient direction for the clinical orientation. Physiologic responses to acute hypovolemia that favor maintenance of sufficient blood pressure to perfuse the coronary and carotid arteries, such as tachycardia and increased peripheral vascular resistance, and movement of extravascular water, salt, and protein into the plasma allow a healthy individual to tolerate an acute blood loss of as much as 25% of the total blood volume.

Autopsy confirmation of massive exsanguination is still a logged cause of death in this country, and should push us to seek this diagnosis with vigor. The sensation of weakness that the patient expresses is a result of the early cerebral hypoxia seen in even "compensated" patients. Many organ systems are affected by the volume contraction in the patient with acute blood loss, including shifting of elemental ions and loss of electrolyte stability. This alteration results in decreased capacity to manage redirected blood flow. Mitochondrial damage from decreased oxygen distribution and altered circulating blood volume result in lysosomal autolysis and subsequent damage at a cellular level. Target organs for basic cellular shock states can be demonstrated to be affected, based upon the needed blood flow and underlying organ compromise.

Metabolic acidosis is a result of the anaerobic metabolism and production of CO_2. Lactate levels are increased and shock is found to be a significant cause of metabolic acidosis. The rise and fall of the serum lactate levels are good general indicators of outcome, with persistent lactic acidosis being an ominous predictor. The initial respiratory compensation for shock induced acidosis is often displayed as an alkalotic overcompensation for the initial insult. As the shock continues, the patient undergoes decompensated mixed metabolic and respiratory acidosis.[39]

Initial stabilization and transfer of patients from the field with suspected trauma induced shock can be treated with two large bore IVs of lactated ringer's solution, oxygen, and, if needed, MAST trousers (see Hypovolemic Shock, Chap. 7). When the shock is not accompanied by an obvious source of bleeding several entities can be identified. Of the problems that we can include are dissecting aneurysm, transection of the spinal cord, and tension pneumothorax, not forgetting restrictive pericarditis.[40]

RESUSCITATION AND FLUID THERAPY

Blood component therapeutic intervention is both lifesaving and life-threatening. The value of whole blood in the acutely bleeding, decompensating patient is in the prompt restoration of blood volume through replacement of fluids so that tissue perfusion and delivery of oxygen are maintained. Nonblood-component fluids given promptly and in adequate volume are usually satisfactory for correcting the blood volume deficit of mild to moderate shock. Blood component replacement is generally unsuitable as the initial fluid of choice in the primary resuscitative effort; its use is associated with potential risks of transmitted infectious diseases, and component reactions. Physiologic responses to acute hypovolemia that favor maintenance of sufficient blood pressure to perfuse the coronary and carotid arteries, such as tachycardia, increased peripheral vascular resistance, and movement of extravascular water, salt, and protein into the plasma, allow one to tolerate as much as 25% reduction in volume.

The choice of crystalloid solutions for volume replacement in hemorrhagic shock is recommended. Crystalloid solutions move quickly into interstitial tissues, providing a necessary vehicle for continued metabolism. The relationship of this interstitial "deficit" to the pathophysiology of shock is not well studied or understood. In light of the fact that 75% of the infused crystalloid becomes interstitial fluid, the volume of crystalloid replacement to measured blood loss is skewed, requiring a 3:1, to 4:1 replacement ratio (crystalloid to blood loss).[41,42]

BLOOD COMPONENT USAGE

Circulating blood volume has a critical mass effect in terms of vital organs, but beyond the sheer volume involved, consideration must be given the oxygen-carrying capacity of that fluid. At some juncture, the tissue hypoxia must be addressed. So what is the threshold for transfusion? The classic directive was a hematocrit of 30%, or hemoglobin and hematocrit are "unadjusted" in early massive hemorrhage. In the saline-loaded versus the "dry" patient, the actual measurements are obviously distorted, and this distortion is true of the acutely bleeding patient as well.

The decision to transfuse red cells must include not only the hemoglobin and hematocrit, but also the patient's general medical "gestalt" (cardiac, cerebrovascular, and chemical considerations). Is the patient orthostatic; can the patient tolerate exercise (movement); what are the limits of physiological endurance for *this* patient? Compiling all of the data and subtracting from this formula the potential for AIDS, hepatitis, coagulation disorders, and anaphylaxis, we can make the major decision to transfuse, which used to be so simple.

RBCs may be transfused as whole blood or as a modified component. Packed cells (PRBCs) are prepared by removing approximately two thirds of the plasma from a unit of whole blood, resulting in a residual hematocrit of 65 to 70%. The advantage of PRBCs is that a substantial volume of RBCs can be given in relationship to the number of "units" of blood transfused. Care must be exercised when considering the loss of coagulation factors, and other essential factors that may be lost in the storage of fresh blood. Many formulas exist for the calculation of replacement, but the importance to adequate therapy is that you consider the use of cryoprecipitate, fresh frozen plasma, and platelets.

Vital signs are a reflection of cardiovascular compensation for the acute blood loss. The patient has hypotension and tachycardia in proportion to the degree of hemorrhage. Orthostatic changes are useful in the initial evaluation of patients with acute blood loss. If the pulse rises 25% or more, or the systolic blood pressure falls 20 mm Hg or more on going from a supine to a standing position, the patient is likely to have significant hypovolemia (blood loss >1000 mL) and requires prompt replacement.

Acute blood loss in excess of 1500 mL usually leads to cardiovascular collapse. If the blood loss is acute, the CBC may not reveal a significant decrease in packed cell volume or hemoglobin because the red blood cell mass and plasma volume are contracted in parallel. There are often moderate leukocytosis and a "shift to the left" in the whole cell differential count. An increased platelet count and a shortened coagulation time are the earliest manifestations and may be demonstrable in less than an hour. The next development is a moderate leukocytosis from 10,000 to 35,000 and a shift to the left reaching the peak in 2 to 5 hours. Twenty-four to 48 hours later, an outpouring of reticulocytes begins and becomes maximal 4 to 7 days after the hemorrhage.

There is a progressive decrease in serum iron. Thrombocytosis may be encountered in both acute and chronic blood loss, particularly if the patient is iron-deficient. The immediate posthemorrhage period shows the patient to have a spurious macrocytic red cell index (MCV = 95 to 105) and also shows peripheral reticulocytosis. Sustained reticulocytosis is evident if bleeding continues.[43–49]

MANAGEMENT AND INDICATIONS FOR ADMISSION

The criteria for blood replacement have been modified in recent years, mainly because of the intrinsic hazards of human blood usage.

The patient's tolerance to the current anemia, coupled with any extenuating history, aid us in the decision to admit. The vast bulk of patients with new-onset anemia are managed in an outpatient setting, but some stricter guidelines should be followed. Hemodynamically unstable patients and those with significant concomitant disease and newly discovered hematocrit values less than 30% should be admitted for full evaluation. Also, concern for the patient's cardiovascular status is of paramount importance, and should be the hallmark of the initial therapeutic intervention.

Therapy in acute bleeding requires immediate and vigorous intervention. A large-bore intravenous line should be placed. While blood is being typed and crossmatched, saline, Ringer's lactate, and, if warranted, 5% albumin should be infused to correct hypovolemia. Whole blood is then administered as soon as it is available. Monitoring of vital signs and central venous pressure is useful in determining the appropriate amount of volume replacement.

During the immediate evaluation period and concurrently with the "workup" on arrival at the ED, diagnostic studies may reveal the site or sites of occult bleeding. If the bleeding is unexplained, coagulation studies should be obtained and a nasogastric tube inserted. If any rigidity or unusual pain is observed, evaluation of the peritoneal space should be performed.

HORIZONS

A new, third-generation automated hematology system (Technicon Instruments H-1) can furnish a full range of values including erythrocyte parameters and a leukocyte differential count. Particular attention is focused on erythrocyte morphometric parameters, including measurement of cell size and hemoglobin content on a cell-by-cell basis.

New parameters derived from these measurements, such as mean corpuscular volume and red blood cell distribution width (which characterize cell size), mean corpuscular hemoglobin concentration and hemoglobin distribution width (which characterize cell size), and mean corpuscular hemoglobin concentration and hemoglobin distribution width (which characterize cell hemoglobinization) give the practicing physician more useful information concerning the oxygen-carrying capacity of the blood being analyzed.

An expert system is being developed to aid in the classification of anemias. Input for this system consists of limited demographic information on each patient and the results of the CBC, with the incorporation of the results of further chemical testing (serum iron, total iron-binding capacity/ferritin and serum B_{12}/serum folate/red blood cell folate). Performance of this system resulted in accurately classifying 74 of 84 (88%) of cases according to previously established criteria.[50,51]

REFERENCES

1. Daly, M.P.: Anemia in the elderly. Am. Fam. Phys. 39:129, 1989.
2. Mannix, F.: Hemorrhagic shock. In Emergency medicine: Concepts and clinical practice. Edited by Rosen, P., et al. St. Louis, The C.V.Mosby Co.
3. Gretz, N., Unger, R., Grittman, S., and Strauch, M.: Renal function, anemia and blood pressure in patients with chronic renal failure. Scand J. Urol. Nephrol. 108:57, 1988.
4. Walker, R.E., Parker, R.I., Kovacs, J.A., et al.: Anemia and erythropoiesis in patients with the acquired immunodeficiency syndrome (AIDS) and Kaposi sarcoma treated with zidovudine. Ann. Intern. Med. 108:372, 1988.
5. Howard, A.P., Moore, J., Jr., Welch, P.G., and Gouge, S.F.: Analysis of the quantitative relationship between anemia and chronic renal failure. Am. J. Med. Sci. 297:309, 1989.
6. Kellermeyer, R.W.: General principles of the evaluation and therapy of anemia. Med. Clin. North Am. 68:633, 1984.
7. Fukamachi, J., Urabe, A., Saito, T., Takaku, F., and Kubota, M.: Burst-promoting activity in anemia and polycythemia. Inter. J. Cell Cloning 4:74, 1986.
8. Paganini, E.F., Garcia, J., Abdulhadi, M., et al.: The anemia of chronic renal failure. Overview and early erythropoietin experience. Cleve. Clin. J. Med. 56:79, 1989.
9. Najean, Y., Deschryver, F., and Dresch, C.: Radio-ion kinetic studies in anemia and the measurement of dyserythropoiesis. Nouv. Rev. Fr. Hematol. 30:167, 1988.
10. Wallerstein, R.O.: Role of the laboratory in the diagnosis of anemia. JAMA 236:490, 1976.
11. Segal, G.M., Eschbach, J.W., Egrie, J.C., et al.: The anemia of end-stage renal disease: Hematopoietic progenitor cell response. Kidney Int. 33:983, 1988.
12. Nonnast-Daniel, B., Creutzig, A., Kuhn, K., et al.: Effect of treatment with recombinant human erythropoietin on peripheral hemodynamics and oxygenation. Nephrology 66:185, 1988.
13. Cundall, D.B., Whitehead, S.M., and Hechtel, F.O.: Severe anemia and death due to the pharyngeal leech Myxobdella africana. Trans. R. Soc. Trop. Med. Hyg. 80:940, 1986.
14. Reich, P.R.: Hypochronic anemia. In Hematology: Pathophysiologic Basis for Clinical Practice. Edited by Reich, P.R. Boston, Little, Brown & Co., 1978.
15. Wilson, R.F., et al.: Shock in the emergency department. JACEP 5:678, 1976.
16. Wintrobe, M.M. (Ed.): Blood, Pure and Eloquent. New York, McGraw-Hill, 1980.
17. Sapira, J.D.: Contemporary use of the disease concept: II. The question of anemia. Aourh Mws J. 80:55, 1987.
18. Fitzpatrick, S., Johnson, J., Shragg, P., and Felice, M.E.: Health care needs of Indochinese refugee teenagers. Pediatrics. 79:118, 1987.
19. Wurapa, F.K., Bulsara, M.K., and Boatin, B.A.: Evaluation of conjunctival pallor in the diagnosis of anemia. J. Trop. Med. Hyg. 89:33, 1986.
20. Bugge, P.M., Hendriksen, C., Jensen, A.M.: A critical evaluation of the clinical diagnosis of anemia. Am. J. Epidemiol. 124:657, 1986.
21. Jacobs, H.S.: A pathogenic classification of the anemias. Med. Clin. North Am. 50:1679, 1966.
22. Maslow, W.C., et al.: Disorders associated with accelerated erythrocyte turnover Hematologic disease: Practical diagnosis. Boston, Houghton Mifflin Co., 1980.
23. Huguley, C.M., Lea, J.W., and Butts, J.A.: Adverse hematologic reactions to certain drugs. Progr. Hematol. 5:105, 1966.
24. Castle, W.B.: From man to molecule and back to mankind. Semin. Hematol. 13:159, 1976.
25. Alter, B.P.: Advances in the prenatal diagnosis of hematologic diseases. Blood 64:329, 1984.
26. Jaffe, E.F.: Methemoglobinemia. Clin. Hematol. 10:99, 1981.
27. Bunn, H.F., and Forget, B.G.: Hemoglobin: Molecular genetic and clinical aspects. Philadelphia, W.B. Saunders Co., 1986.
28. Hershko, C.: The fate of circulating hemoglobin. Br. J. Haematol. 29:199, 1975.
29. Beutler, E.: Glucose-6-phosphate dehydrogenase deficiency. In Hematology. Edited by Williams, W.F., et al. New York, McGraw-Hill Book Co., 1983.
30. Beutler, E.: Red cell enzyme defects as nondiseases and as disease. Blood 54:1, 1979.
31. Soff, G.A., and Kadin, M.C.: Tocainide-induced reversible agranulocytosis and anemia. Arch. Intern. Med. 147:598, 1987.
32. Miescher, P.A.: Blood dyscrasias secondary to non-steroidal anti-inflammatory drugs. Med. Toxicol. 1:57, 1986.
33. Stenke, L., Hast, R., Osby, E., et al.: Dilution and hemolysis causing anemia after artificial heart implantation. Blut. 54:127, 1987.
34. Herbert, V.: Megaloblastic anemias. In Cecil Textbook of Medicine. Edited by Beeson, P.B., Mcdermott, W., and Wyngaarden, J.F. Philadelphia, W.B. Saunders Co., 1979.
35. Hamilton, G.C., and Jurisic, M.A.: Hematologic manifestations of alcoholism. Top. Emerg. Med. 6:74, 1984.
36. Howard, A.D., Moore, J., Jr., Welch, P.G., and Gouge, S.F.: Analysis of the quantitative relationship between anemia and chronic renal failure. Am. J. Med. Sci. 297:309, 1989.
37. Pagnotta, I.: Transient vitamin B12 malabsorption in a patient with mixed nutritional anemia. J. Am. Board. Fam. Pract. 2:130, 1989.
38. Moss, G.S., et al.: Traumatic shock in a man. N. Engl. J. Med. 290:724, 1974.
39. Vincent, J.L., Dufaye, P., Berre, J., et al.: Serial lactate determinations during circulatory shock. Crit. Care Med. 2:449, 1983.
40. Kaplan, B.C., Civetta, J.M., Nagel, E.L., et al.: The military anti-shock trouser in civilian pre-hospital emergency care. J. Trauma. 13:843, 1973.
41. Takaori, J., and Safar, P.: Treatment of massive hemorrhage with colloid and crystalloid solutions: Studies in dogs. JAMA 199:297, 1976.
42. Crystal, R.G., and Baue, A.E.: Influence of hemorrhagic hypotension on measurements of the extracellular fluid volume. Surg. Gynecol. Obstet. 129:576, 1969.
43. Nicolaides, K.H., Thilaganathan, B., Rodeck, C.H., and Mibashan, R.S.: Erythroblastosis and reticulocytosis in anemic fetuses. Am. J. Obstet. Gynecol. 159:1063, 1988.
44. Bower, R.J., Bell, M.J., Ternberg, J.L.: Diagnostic value of white blood count and neutrophil percentage in the evaluation of abdominal pain in children. Surg. Gynecol. Obstet. 152:424, 1981.
45. Roberts, W.H., and Speicher, C.E.: The medical laboratory and the emergency department. In Emergency Medicine Annual: 1984. Norwalk, CT. Appleton-Century-Crofts, 1984.

46. Carson, J.L., Poses, R.M., Spence, R.K., and Bonavita, G.: Severity of anemia and operative mortality and morbidity. Lancet 1:727, 1988.
47. Beutler, E.: The common anemias. JAMA 259:2433, 1988.
48. Johnson, C.A., and Chester, M.I.: Pathophysiology and treatment of the anemia of renal failure. Clin. Pharm. 7:117, 1988.
49. Crosby, W.H.: Acute anemia in the severely wounded battle casualty. Military Medicine 153:25, 1988.
50. Blomberg, D.J., Ladley, J.L., Fattu, J.M., and Patrick, E.A.: The use of an expert system in the clinical laboratory as an aid in the diagnosis of anemia. Am. J. Clin. Pathol. 87:608, 1987.
51. Fossat, C., David, M., Harle, Jr., et al.: New parameters in erythrocyte counting. Value of histograms. Arch. Pathol. Lab. Med. 111:1150, 1988.

ACQUIRED HEMOLYTIC DISORDERS

Rajalaxmi McKenna

CAPSULE

The onset of a bleeding disorder in a person with previously normal hemostasis may involve derangements of plasma coagulation, the primary hemostatic mechanism that consists of the platelet-fibrinogen-von Willebrand factor-vessel wall axis, or both. Rapid availability of the results of specific coagulation tests allows identification of the precise abnormalities in hemostasis and permits one to tailor the therapy to individual circumstances.

CONSUMPTIVE THROMBOHEMORRHAGIC SYNDROMES (DISSEMINATED INTRAVASCULAR COAGULATION)

PATHOPHYSIOLOGY

The major abnormality in consumptive thrombohemorrhagic syndromes is excessive production of thrombin because of activation of the coagulation mechanism by one or more pathways.[1-6] The normal vascular endothelium has special properties that allow it to maintain blood in a fluid state: a negatively charged surface, presence of thrombomodulin and glycosoaminoglycans, and ability to release plasminogen activator. Illnesses that injure the endothelial cell/vessel wall disrupt this physiologic antithrombotic mechanism by altering the endothelial cell and/or exposing the subendothelial structures to flowing blood and activating the contact system (factors XII, high molecular weight kininogen, prekallikrein, and XI).

The several consequences of this process are shown in Figure 53-2. Tissue injury can activate another pathway of coagulation through tissue factor, a plasma membrane glycoprotein that can combine with factor VII or VII$_a$ and finally cause thrombin generation (Fig. 53-3). Platelets can be activated by several factors, including ADP, thrombin, and damaged endothelium; the procoagulant phospholipids that appear on the platelet surface after activation along with factor V can accelerate the coagulation process. Platelets may also contribute to the activation of factors XII, XI, and IX. A simplified schema of the coagulation cascade is shown in Figure 53-3. Because of activation of these pathways, thrombin is generated, and its effects on several hemostatic parameters are listed in Table 53-8. The sudden generation of thrombin in large amounts can cause bleeding from severe reductions in hemostatic factors and thrombotic manifestations caused by fibrin deposition in the smaller vessels; both of these processes can occur simultaneously. When thrombin is generated slowly and in smaller amounts, the changes in the coagulation factors are less pronounced, and there may be no clinical manifestations related to the coagulopathy, or the patient may present with thrombotic complications or minor bleeding. The fibrinolytic system is activated by plasminogen activator released by injured endothelial cells at sites of thrombus formation and also by contact phase factors, resulting in the generation of plasmin. This increased plasmin, usually secondary to activation of the coagulation mechanism or rarely a primary disorder, can reduce the levels of several coagulation factors (Fig. 53-4). Fibrin degradation products (FDP) are produced by the actions of plasmin on native fibrin, which has been crosslinked by factor XIII or by the degradation of fibrinogen; these interfere with fibrin monomer polymerization and platelet function. Degradation products resulting from the action of plasmin on crosslinked fibrin distinguish disseminated intravascular coagulation (DIC) from the rare syndrome of primary fibrinolysis.[7] The FDPs are cleared by the liver and

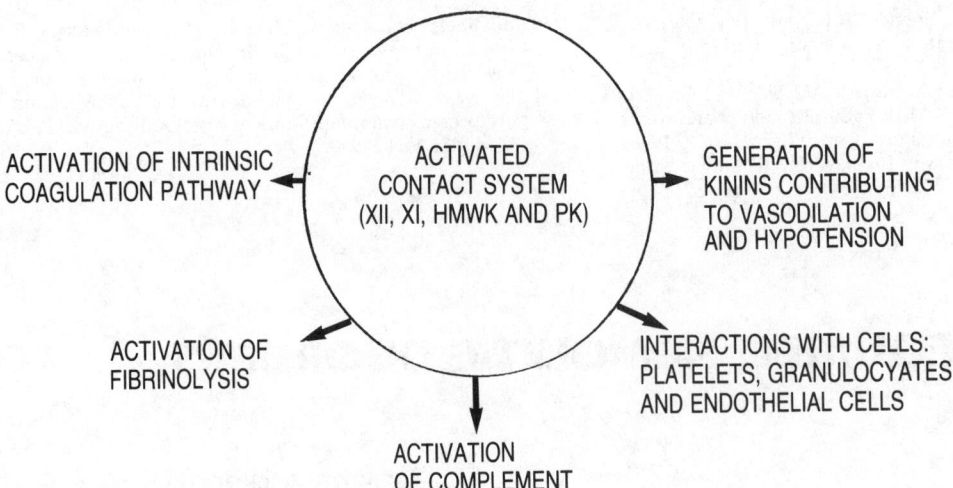

FIG. 53-2. Consequences of activation of the contact system.

act as positive feedback, causing the liver to increase fibrinogen production rapidly and raise the level of fibrinogen in the circulation. The thrombocytopenia that develops during DIC is caused by the presence of thrombin and other inducers of platelet aggregation; the platelet aggregates are then cleared from the circulation and cause a drop in the platelet count. Unlike the liver, which responds to DIC by rapidly increasing the synthesis of fibrinogen, normal bone marrow responds slowly to an increased need for platelets, so that thrombocytopenia may persist for several days after DIC is controlled. The physiologic inhibitors in plasma temper DIC through a broad spectrum of effects and are an important determinant of the extent of activation of hemostasis (Table 53-9). The reticuloendothelial system, in particular the liver, also has an important modulating influence on the outcome of DIC by participating in the production of procoagulants and inhibitors and clearing activated coagulation factors and fibrin from the circulation. Thus, the circulating level of any coagulation factor depends on the balance between its rate of production and its rate of consumption. Liver dysfunction can adversely influence this process; the details are discussed in this chapter under liver disease. Finally, the underlying disease state influences the final outcome of activation of the coagulation system. For example, in pregnancy the hemostatic thermostat is tilted in favor of thrombosis. Therefore, activation of the coagulation system during pregnancy is manifested primarily by thrombotic rather than bleeding complications in the mother. Interestingly, thrombotic complications can also develop in the neonate because of transplacental passage of the stimuli.[8] In acute pancreatitis, the disordered coagulation mechanism results from a nonspecific degradation of the coagulation proteins by the proteases released into the circulation. After snakebites, there may be unusual modes of activation of the coagulation system.

Because of activation of the coagulation mechanism, fibrin and platelet thrombi develop in the microcirculation, causing ischemia, infarction, and bleeding into the affected tissues, with subsequent development of organ dysfunction. Although this process can occur in any organ, there is a predilection for the following organ systems: the skin, with hemorrhagic-necrotic lesions with a dark center and erythematous periphery (Fig. 53-5); the kidneys, with renal dysfunction caused by thrombi in the glomerular capillaries and afferent arterioles (Fig. 53-6); the gastrointestinal system, with bleeding from multiple submucosal ulcerations; the central nervous system with CNS dysfunction; the lungs, with variable degrees of pulmonary dysfunction; and, less often, the cardiovascular system, with persistent hypotension from hemorrhagic necrosis destroying both adrenals (Waterhouse-Friderichsen syndrome).

CLINICAL PRESENTATION AND LABORATORY FINDINGS

The clinical manifestations of this syndrome are extremely variable and depend on the rapidity with which the precipitating illnesses appear; they can be sudden in onset (acute) or appear slowly (chronic). When the extent of "consumption" of the hemostatic factors is severe and sudden in onset, acute DIC can present with generalized bleeding from numerous sites: venipunctures or other recently operated or invaded sites, gastrointestinal bleeding from superficial ulcerations; hematuria, and bleeding into the skin, CNS, and lungs. Varying degrees of acute renal failure reflect the underlying thrombotic process. In chronic DIC, on the other hand, patients may have no clinical symptoms or only minor bleeding or thrombotic manifestations. The skin lesions seen in patients with the

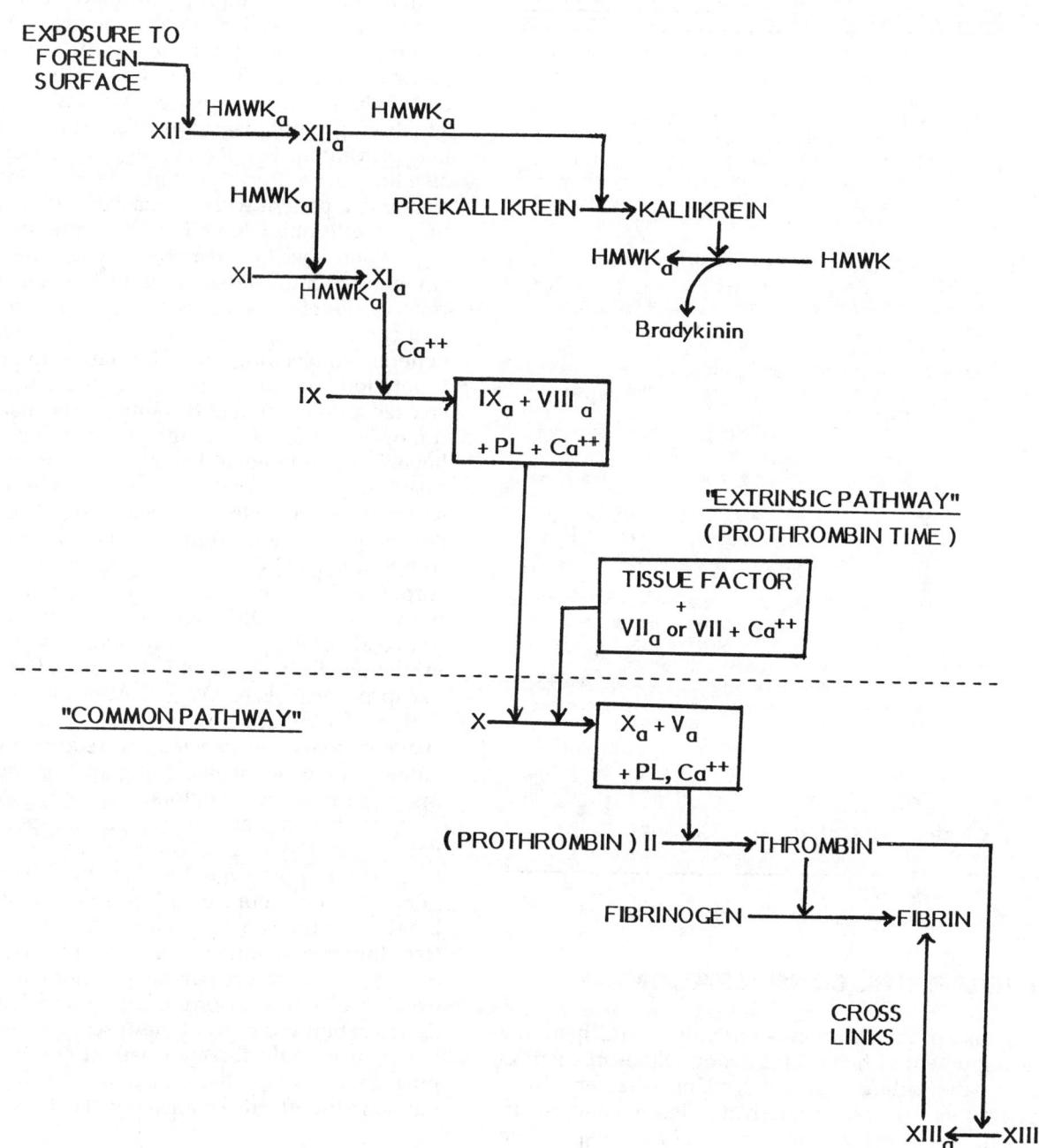

FIG. 53-3. *Simplified schema of the coagulation cascade.*

Kassabach-Merritt syndrome are diagnostic (Fig. 53-7). Various disease states associated with DIC are listed in Table 53-10. Laboratory test results can also be extremely variable; Tables 53-11 and 53-12 list abnormalities in clotting tests that may occur in patients with acute and chronic DIC. The fibrinogen level can help to classify DIC as decompensated, compensated, or overcompensated, and is a useful parameter in conjunction with the clinical findings to determine the need for therapy. In acute decompensated DIC, severe reductions in fibrinogen and factors V and VIII-C should be expected, whereas in chronic overcompensated DIC, present in patients with metastatic carcinoma, one finds an increased level of fibrinogen.[9–12] The specific finding of increased levels of D-dimer, a specific type of FDP, is useful in the diagnosis of DIC.[7] A microangiopathic hemolytic anemia is uncommon in patients with DIC.

TABLE 53-8. HEMOSTATIC FACTORS AFFECTED BY THROMBIN

1. **FIBRINOGEN (FACTOR I):** Thrombin releases fibrinopeptides A and B from fibrinogen, causing the generation of fibrin, which polymerizes to form a fibrin clot. Fibrinogen, the target protein, is thereby reduced with variable reductions in the level of prothrombin (factor II). The plasma level of fibrinogen is determined by the balance between the rate of production by liver and the rate of use by conversion to fibrin by thrombin.
2. **FACTORS V AND VIII:** Thrombin alters factors V and VIII, resulting in a temporary increase of their coagulant activity (V$_a$, VIII$_a$).
3. **PROTEINS C AND S:** Thrombin bound to thrombomodulin on the endothelial cell surface converts protein C to activated protein C; the latter rapidly degrades V$_a$ and VIII$_a$, causing reduced levels and hypocoagulability. Both proteins C and S (the latter a cofactor for protein C) can be reduced, causing a thrombotic tendency. In some animals, activated protein C has been shown to increase fibrinolysis by inhibiting the inhibitors of plasminogen activator.
4. **PLATELETS:** Thrombin is a potent, physiologic platelet-aggregating agent causing shape change, availability of procoagulant platelet phospholipids (PF 3), release of granule contents, and aggregation, with subsequent thrombocytopenia and a bleeding tendency. A functional deficiency can also occur because of the circulation of "storage pool deficient" platelets (platelets circulating after release of granule contents).
5. **FACTOR XIII:** Thrombin activates Factor XIII (an enzyme that crosslinks fibrin), resulting in a "stable" fibrin clot, which is less susceptible to plasmin degradation. Factor XIII$_a$ also crosslinks fibrin to platelet proteins and fibronectin.
6. **PLASMINOGEN ACTIVATOR:** Thrombin releases plasminogen activator and plasminogen activator inhibitor from the endothelial cells, thereby influencing the fibrinolytic process.
7. **ANTITHROMBIN III:** This is an important physiologic serine protease inhibitor that binds to thrombin, thereby inhibiting it and being reduced in the process. A 50% level of AT III can predispose to thrombosis.
8. **OTHER EFFECTS:** Chemotactic activity, initiation of cell division, and cleavage of complement components C$_3$, C$_5$.

THERAPEUTIC CONSIDERATIONS

The task of the clinician is not only to anticipate the development of hemostatic abnormalities in a particular patient, but to also determine whether appropriate therapy of the underlying disease alone is sufficient to correct the hemostatic abnormalities. The need to use blood products and/or pharmacologic agents to improve the coagulopathy should be based on a careful evaluation of the patient's overall status and serial laboratory test results. In all instances of DIC, it is essential to identify the precipitating factor(s) because correction or removal of those factors is likely to halt the process of DIC and prevent further deterioration of the hemostatic parameters. In patients with self-limited clinical disorders, the DIC is also self-limited, and appropriate therapy of the precipitating factor(s) alone may correct the coagulopathy. Such spontaneous correction may occur after delivery of the baby and removal of the placenta in a patient with abruptio placentae, after treatment of hypotension

and acidosis in a patient in shock, or appropriate antibiotic treatment of a septic patient. The routine performance of coagulation profiles (APTT, PT, fibrinogen level, fibrin split products, factors II, V, VII and X and platelet count) in patients with major illnesses known to trigger DIC could detect the coagulopathy even when patients are clinically stable. In such a situation, prompt institution of appropriate measures may prevent further deterioration and onset of clinical bleeding, even if precipitating factor(s) continue. For example, a patient with a metastatic adenocarcinoma may have chronic DIC without clinically evident bleeding. When specific chemotherapy for the adenocarcinoma is administered, lysis of tumor may release procoagulants, which cause further consumption and reduction of coagulation factors. This may precipitate generalized bleeding. In this instance, to prevent deterioration, one may counteract the anticipated increased autoinfusion of thromboplastic material from tumor lysis after chemotherapy by starting low-dose heparin before chemotherapy. An approach to the treatment of patients with acute or chronic DIC is summarized in Tables 53-11 and 53-12. There is much debate about the usefulness of heparin in acute decompensated DIC, with a suggestion that antithrombin III concentrates may be useful in patients with shock and DIC, but a clear warning has been issued about the possible thrombotic consequences of inhibiting fibrinolysis with the use of epsilon-aminocaproic acid (EACA).[8,13–15] Atypical modes of initiation of coagulopathy, such as those induced by snake venoms and pancreatitis, require atypical modalities of treatment, including antivenoms, antitoxins, or proteolytic inhibitors.

In conclusion, determination of the specific precipitating factor(s) in DIC provides the most effective therapeutic approach to treating DIC. The hemostatic derangement should be addressed by using a combination of the clinical context, the ability to rapidly treat the precipitating factor(s), and the degree of aberration of laboratory parameters, not only to treat an existing bleeding disorder but to anticipate further deterioration and prevent the onset of excessive bleeding, which could threaten patient survival. General measures to keep vital organs functioning are mandatory in the effective management of these disorders.

THROMBOTIC THROMBOCYTOPENIC PURPURA (TTP)

The traditional concept of this syndrome required the presence of the following five components to diagnose this disorder: microangiopathic hemolytic anemia, thrombocytopenia, renal failure, neurologic dysfunction, and fever.[16] Patients may present with only some of these manifestations, but a sine que non for this

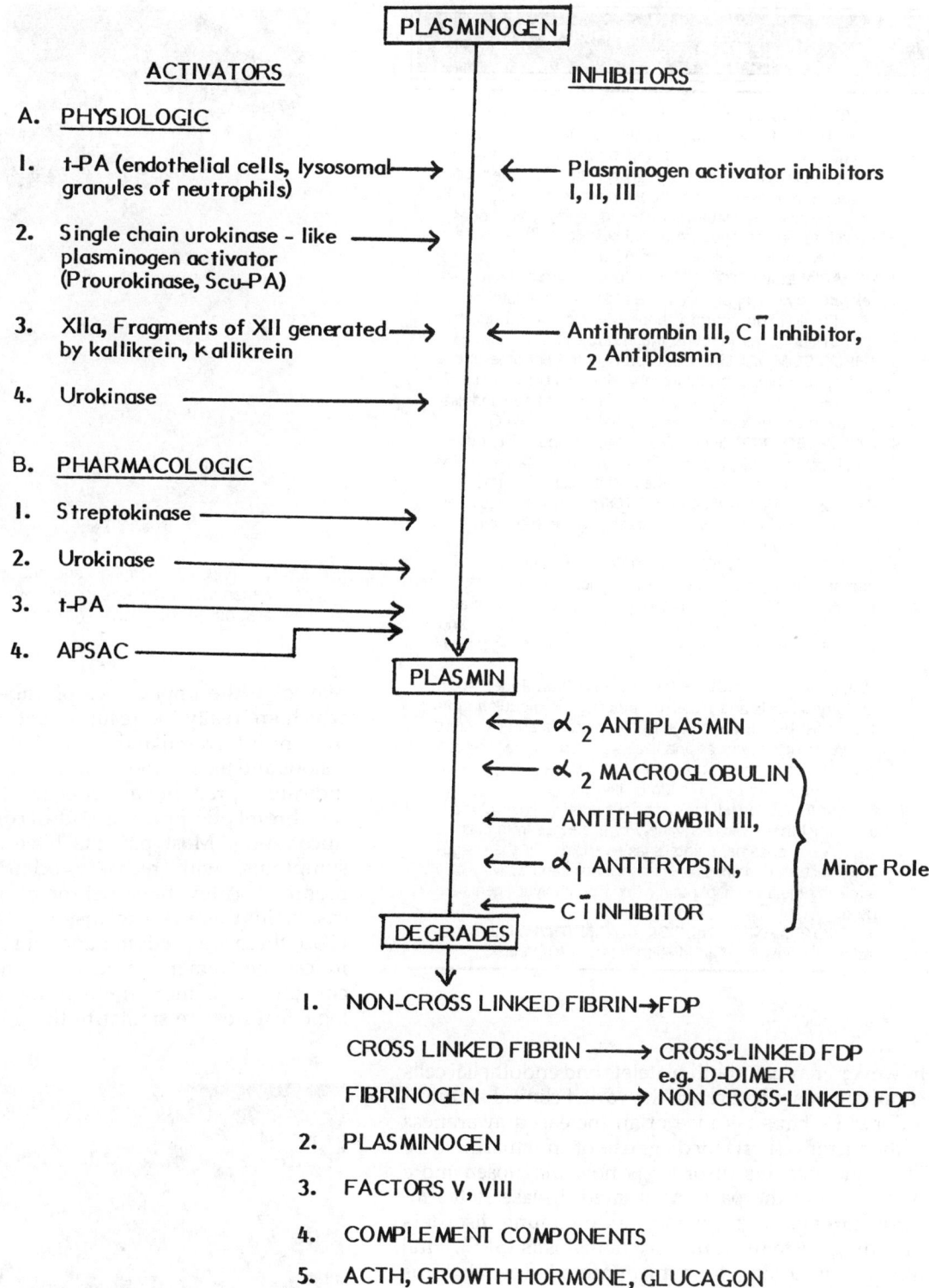

PLASMINOGEN

ACTIVATORS   INHIBITORS

A. PHYSIOLOGIC

I. t-PA (endothelial cells, lysosomal⟶   ⟵ Plasminogen activator inhibitors
    granules of neutrophils)   I, II, III

2. Single chain urokinase - like ⟶
    plasminogen activator
    (Prourokinase, Scu-PA)

3. XIIa, Fragments of XII generated⟶   ⟵ Antithrombin III, C̄I Inhibitor,
    by kallikrein, kallikrein   ₂ Antiplasmin

4. Urokinase ⟶

B. PHARMACOLOGIC

I. Streptokinase ⟶

2. Urokinase ⟶

3. t-PA ⟶

4. APSAC ⟶

PLASMIN

                        ⟵ α₂ ANTIPLASMIN

                        ⟵ α₂ MACROGLOBULIN

                        ⟵ ANTITHROMBIN III,   } Minor Role

                        ⟵ α₁ ANTITRYPSIN,

                        ⟵ C̄I INHIBITOR

DEGRADES

I. NON-CROSS LINKED FIBRIN⟶FDP

    CROSS LINKED FIBRIN ⟶ CROSS-LINKED FDP
                                  e.g. D-DIMER
    FIBRINOGEN ⟶ NON CROSS-LINKED FDP

2. PLASMINOGEN

3. FACTORS V, VIII

4. COMPLEMENT COMPONENTS

5. ACTH, GROWTH HORMONE, GLUCAGON

FIG. 53-4.   *Activation of the fibrinolytic system with conversion of plasminogen to plasmin. The several substrates of plasmin are also shown.*

disorder is the presence of a microangiopathic hemolytic anemia with schistocytes in the peripheral smear, in association with thrombocytopenia. Over the years, several causes have been postulated for this syndrome. The presence of a platelet-aggregating activity in the patient's plasma has been consistently demonstrated by several investigators. Whether this is caused by a platelet-aggregating protein in the plasma, large molecular vWF multimers, absence of a protective immunoglobulin in the patient's plasma, endothelial cell damage, or alterations in prostacyclin remains a matter of debate. The precipitating factor(s),

TABLE 53-9. PROTEINS WITH INHIBITORY EFFECTS ON HEMOSTASIS

1. **ANTITHROMBIN III:** Inhibits several serine proteases: Thrombin, X_a, IX_a, XII_a, XI_a, and plasmin. The inhibitory effect of AT III is markedly potentiated by heparin. Isolated inherited deficiency of this protein can be associated with recurrent venous thromboembolic disease. Its major role is as an intravascular antithrombotic agent in the fluid phase, as well as on the endothelial cell surface. Heparin sulfate on the endothelial cell activates AT III.
2. **HEPARIN COFACTOR II:** Neutralizes thrombin slowly. Accelerated by mucopolysaccharides (dermatan sulfate) of the vessel wall. Main antithrombotic role may be outside the endothelium, after injury to the endothelium.
3. **THROMBOMODULIN:** A receptor on the endothelial cell surface that binds thrombin, inhibiting its ability to clot fibrinogen and aggregate platelets. This thrombomodulin-thrombin complex, however, can activate protein C.
4. **ACTIVATED PROTEIN C:** Causes hypocoagulability by degrading V_a and VIII_a. Protein S is an important cofactor. Major antithrombotic action is on the endothelial cell surface.
5. **ACTIVATED PROTEIN C INHIBITOR:** Inactivates activated protein C, is also capable of inhibiting X_a and thrombin, and is potentiated by heparin.
6. **EXTRINSIC PATHWAY INHIBITOR:** Newly discovered inhibitor of tissue factor–factor VIII complexes.
7. **α_2-ANTIPLASMIN:** The primary inhibitor of plasmin. It also interferes with the binding of plasminogen to fibrin, and inhibits Hageman factor fragments, kallikrein, XI_a, X_a, thrombin, and t-PA.
8. **PLASMINOGEN ACTIVATOR INHIBITORS:** Type I from endothelial cells and platelets, important in modulating fibrinolysis. Type II is secreted by the placenta and increases as pregnancy advances and is also present in monocytes.
9. **PROSTACYCLIN:** A potent inhibitor of platelet aggregation, synthesized by the endothelial cells.
10. **α_2-MACROGLOBULIN:** An ancient protein (in evolutionary terms) that inhibits a variety of proteases from plasma, white cells, bacteria, plants, snake venoms. Of the coagulation factors, it inhibits plasmin, thrombin, and X_a. May play a role in regulation of plasmin when thrombolytic agents are used.
11. **α_2-PROTEINASE INHIBITOR (α_1-ANTITRYPSIN):** Minor role in hemostasis. Can inhibit thrombin, XI_a, and X_a.

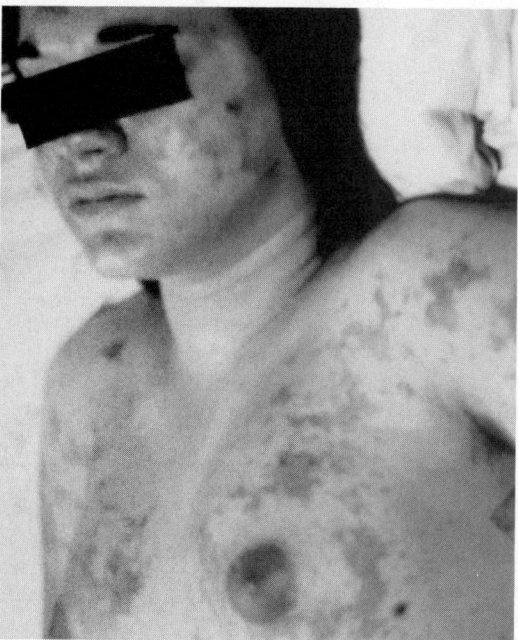

FIG. 53-5. Typical hemorrhagic and necrotic skin lesions of DIC in a young woman with meningococcemia, acute decompensated DIC, and the Waterhouse-Friderichsen syndrome.

may give the appearance of subendothelial lesions which are really the result of endothelial cell growth over the intravascular thrombi. Both the microvascular lesions and tests of the plasma coagulation mechanism indicate a predominant consumption of platelets in the thrombotic process, and decompensated DIC is uncommon. Most patients have an acute onset of symptoms, with recovery occurring in weeks to months.[17] A few have a chronic, slow onset, and occasionally there is a relapsing or a familial form. In HUS, there is a predominance of renal failure without much involvement of other organs; it may occur in clusters and is more frequent in children. The histologic features are similar to those of TTP.

however, may alter both platelets and endothelial cells simultaneously and cause the varied clinical manifestations. Perhaps because of an increased awareness of the current criteria for diagnosis or an actual increase in frequency, this disorder is now diagnosed more often than in the past. Associated disease states include toxemia of pregnancy; autoimmune disorders including systemic lupus erythematosus (SLE), viral illnesses including human immunodeficiency virus (HIV); and bacterial infections after use of chemotherapeutic agents such as mitomycin, cisplatin, vinca alkaloids, and other drugs. Histologic confirmation is obtained by the finding of intracapillary and intra-arteriolar hyaline thrombi in virtually all organs; these consist of platelet and fibrin thrombi in varying stages of development (Fig. 53-8). The vessel wall in the vicinity of the thrombus does not have a cellular infiltrate, and an accompanying endothelial hyperplasia

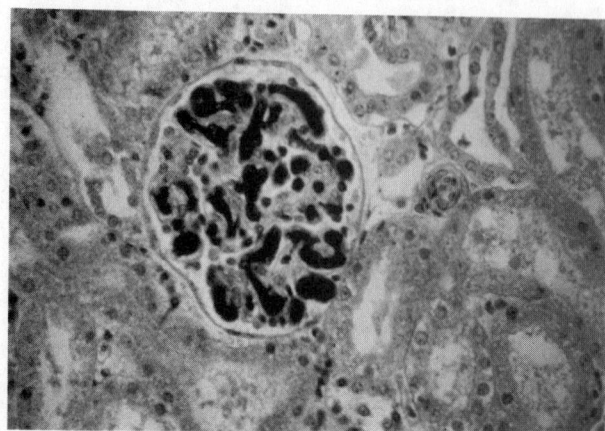

FIG. 53-6. Thrombi in the glomerular capillaries of a woman with abruptio placentae and an acute decompensated DIC.

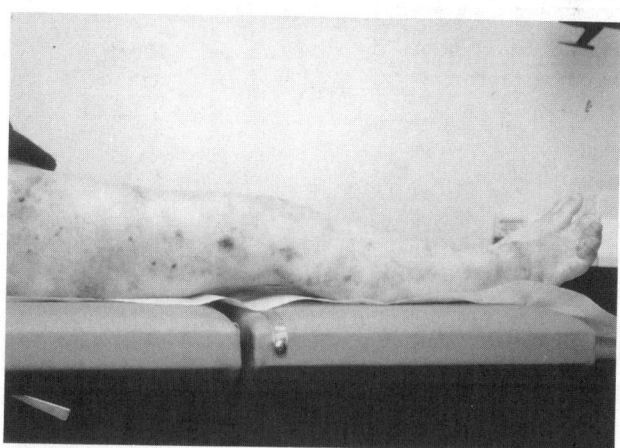

FIG. 53-7. *Characteristic extensive skin lesions with dilated tortuous veins involving the entire right lower extremity, in a patient with the Kasabach-Merritt syndrome and a chronic decompensated DIC.*

Untreated patients with TTP have a high mortality rate. Survival has improved dramatically in these patients with recently used therapeutic approaches.[18] Based on currently available data, it is appropriate to start these patients on a combination of prednisone in a dose of at least 60 mg per day and infusions of fresh frozen plasma. The latter should be replaced by 2 to 3 L plasma exchanges as soon as feasible because this procedure requires good venous access and technical expertise. The highest remission rates have been reported with plasma exchanges using fresh frozen plasma as a replacement fluid, and this has become the treatment of choice in seriously ill patients. If a critically ill patient arrives at the Emergency Department (ED) of an institution that does not have the capability of performing plasma exchanges, whole blood exchanges may be performed while arrangements are being made to transfer the patient to a tertiary care center. Despite the assumption that platelet aggregation is of fundamental importance in the pathogenesis of this disease, there is a reluctance to administer antiplatelet drugs during the severely thrombocytopenic phase, particularly when it is accompanied by neurologic dysfunction. This is driven by the concern about precipitating bleeding at sites of thrombosis and infarction when platelet dysfunction is superimposed on severe thrombocytopenia. This concept is further strengthened by recent reports documenting clinical deterioration after use of antiplatelet drugs. These findings explain the wide variability in the frequency with which antiplatelet drugs are used in the acute phase. Platelet transfusions may be associated with acutely worsening thrombotic symptoms in patients with severe thrombocytopenia caused by TTP, indicating the necessity for a cautious evaluation of the need for such therapy in these patients.[19] Because of the suggested association between recovery thrombocytosis and thrombotic complications, it seems logical to administer acetylsalicylic acid in a dose of 325 mg per day when the platelet counts start to rise above 40,000 per mm.[3] The frequency and duration of plasma exchanges are predicated by the overall clinical status of the patient with platelet and reticulocyte counts and LDH levels serving as useful laboratory parameters. A gradual tapering of steroids should be instituted when clinical and laboratory parameters indicate a remission. Splenectomy is not used as frequently as in the past, perhaps because of the risks of surgery in these patients.

LIVER DISEASE

PATHOPHYSIOLOGY

The hepatocyte is a critical determinant of hemostasis because it is involved in the synthesis of (1) all the coagulation factors except factor VIII, (2) some components of the fibrinolytic system, and (3) many of the physiologic inhibitors of hemostasis and fibrinolysis. The gamma-carboxyglutamic acid cycle is involved in the vitamin K-dependent carboxylation of glutamic acid residues in the precursors of the vitamin K-dependent factors; this is another important function of the liver.[20–21] Liver disease damages this carboxylation cycle and disrupts the synthesis of both vitamin K-dependent and vitamin K-independent coagulation factors. Alterations in other physiologic functions of the liver contribute to the coagulopathy of liver disease. Impairment of the clearance of activated coagulation factors from the circulation can increase the consumptive process (DIC). Another consequence of impaired clearance is accelerated catabolism of coagulation factors such as fibrinogen, caused by the prolonged presence of plasmin and other proteases. A combination of abnormalities in the synthesis of coagulation factors and persistence of serine proteases, which result in increased thrombin generation and catabolism of factors, occurs in patients with liver disease. Two other interesting facets of liver disease play a minor role in its coagulopathy. Abnormal molecular forms of the vitamin K-dependent factors are produced because of hypocarboxylation of the precursor proteins (PIVKA); these can interfere with the prothrombin time test. A variable degree of dysfibrinogenemia can occur, because of the synthesis of fibrinogen molecules containing an excess of sialic acid, which impairs fibrin monomer polymerization and slightly prolongs the thrombin time.[22] Hepatomas may synthesize a totally abnormal fibrinogen.

Derangements of primary hemostasis frequently accompany the coagulopathy of liver disease. In cirrhotics, mild to moderate thrombocytopenia is mainly caused by splenic sequestration with up to 60% to 90% of the circulating platelet mass being present in the

TABLE 53-10. DISEASE STATES PRECIPITATING DIC

A. VESSEL WALL/ENDOTHELIAL INJURY (CONTACT PHASE ACTIVATION)
1. **SEPSIS:** Gram-negative (endotoxinemia), gram-positive (Staphylocoagulase from Staphylococcus aureus forms a catalytically active complex with human prothrombin), fungal, viral (hemorrhagic fevers), rickettsial (Rocky Mountain spotted fever), parasitic (malaria).
2. **EXTRACORPOREAL CIRCULATION:** Exposure to foreign surfaces.
3. **VASCULAR MALFORMATIONS:** Kasabach-Merritt Syndrome, giant hemangiomas, or lymphangiomas (may be localized to one organ) or malignant vascular disorders (hemangioendotheliomas).
4. **ANTIGEN-ANTIBODY COMPLEXES:** Syndrome of purpura fulminans.
5. Large **AORTIC ANEURYSM** with or without a false channel.
6. **TRANSPLANT REJECTION,** e.g., hyperacute kidney rejection.
7. **HEAT STROKE** with endothelial injury and factor XII activation.
8. **HYPOTENSION, ACIDOSIS and SHOCK,** e.g., cardiogenic shock.
9. **TTP–HUS:** Primarily platelet consumption with red cell destruction; a coagulopathy is uncommon.

B. TISSUE INJURY (EXTRINSIC SYSTEM ACTIVATION)
1. **MALIGNANCIES:** Tissue factor or tissue thromboplastin, (solid tumors, acute promyelocytic leukemia). Mucinous extract of adenocarcinomas can directly activate FX. Increased thromboplastic activity of circulating monocytes can also be found in patients with malignancies.
2. **SEPSIS, ENDOTOXIN, SURGICAL PROCEDURES** can induce increased thromboplastic activity on the surface of circulating monocytes. Tissue thromboplastin from tissue injury may escape into the circulation in extensive burns or orthopedic procedures. In Rocky Mountain Spotted fever, extrinsic pathway is also activated.
3. **OBSTETRIC CAUSES:** Abruptio placentae, amniotic fluid embolism, intrauterine fetal death, pre-eclampsia-eclampsia syndrome, abortions including septic abortion, extensive dilation and curettage, chorioamnionitis, and endomyometritis during delivery.
4. **HEAD INJURY** or other **EXTENSIVE TRAUMA.**
5. **LIGHTNING** and **BURNS.**
6. **TUMOR NECROSIS FACTOR:** A cytokine that causes a marked increase in cell-associated tissue factor (tissue thromboplastin) activity.

C. MISCELLANEOUS MECHANISMS THAT ALTER HEMOSTATIC FACTORS
1. **MASSIVE HEMOLYSIS:** Caused by immune mechanisms such as mismatched blood transfusions. Nonimmune mechanisms of hemolysis, e.g., paroxysmal nocturnal hemoglobinuria, G6PD deficiency, hypotonic hemolysis (river water drowning) may be associated with a coagulopathy.
2. **ADULT RESPIRATORY DISTRESS SYNDROME (ARDS)** is primarily associated with thrombosis and dysfunction of the lungs, but other organs may be involved.
3. **LEVEEN SHUNTING,** massive acute **HEPATIC NECROSIS, RAPID RATE OF INFUSION** of concentrates of coagulation factors containing activated products such as **KONYNE, PROPLEX** in patients with **LIVER DISEASE, LIVER TRANSPLANT.**
4. **SNAKEBITES** can cause a bleeding diathesis. These venoms have many actions, including, thrombin-like, activating factors II, V, IX or X; thromboplastic activity; increase fibrinolysis; activate/aggregate platelets; have generalized proteolytic effects, or cause hemolysis. Many venoms have multiple actions. Snakebites by vipers (Malayan pit viper, Russell's viper, boomslang, sawscaled viper), rattlesnakes, mambas, tiger snakes, cobras (a few) have been known to induce variable degrees of hemostatic abnormalities.
5. Release of proteolytic enzymes: **ACUTE PANCREATITIS.**
6. Extravascular proteolytic degradation of fibrinogen: **LEUKOCYTE ELASTASES.**
7. Platelet activating/aggregating activity: **TUMORS.**
8. **INCREASE IN FIBRINOLYSIS.** Release of activator(s) of plasminogen by certain lung tumors.
9. **DRUGS: L-ASPARAGINASE** and **ADRIAMYCIN.**

spleen, in contrast with the normal individual in whom only one third of the circulating platelet mass is in the spleen. Varying degrees of mild to moderate platelet dysfunction have been described and presumed to be caused by alterations in platelet membrane lipid composition and fibrin split products. Thus several different abnormalities contribute to abnormal hemostasis in liver disease.

CLINICAL PRESENTATION AND LABORATORY FINDINGS

Patients with chronic liver disease can present with easy bruisability, nosebleeds, bleeding from the gastrointestinal tract from underlying lesions such as varices, or bleeding from the urinary tract. Unless the thrombocytopenia and coagulopathy are severe, gen-

TABLE 53-11. CLINICAL MANIFESTATIONS, DIAGNOSTIC PARAMETERS, AND TREATMENT OF ACUTE DECOMPENSATED DIC

Clinical Manifestations	Test Results	Treatment
Severe generalized bleeding from GI tract caused by superficial ulcers, GU tract, upper airway, vagina, particularly in obstetric cases, venipuncture, and arterial puncture sites. Varying reductions in renal function. May have prominent necrotic-hemorrhagic skin lesions. Hypotension and shock may accompany activation of contact factors.	Severely reduced levels of fibrinogen, factors V, VIII-C, platelets. Variable reductions in levels of vitamin K-dependent factors, depending on concomitant liver dysfunction Increased level of fibrin degradation products as measured by serial D-dimer levels and staphylococcal clumping test; the latter measures large molecular fibrin degradation products Shortened euglobulin lysis time (fibrinogen level in sample should be corrected before inference that this test reflects increased fibrinolysis) Reduced levels of proteins C and S, plasminogen, factor XIII Reductions in inhibitors such as antithrombin III and α_2 antiplasmin	Determine precipitating factor(s) by history Correct precipitating factor(s): hypotension, hypovolemia, acidosis, shock, poor cardiac output Treat sepsis with broad spectrum antibiotics If patient is bleeding actively, improve level of hemostatic factors by judicious use of FFP and platelets. Use cryoprecipitate only when fibrinogen levels are severely reduced, i.e., 80 mg%, and patient has active bleeding Monitor patient and coagulation tests serially to assess results of treatment and to ensure minimal use of blood products Rarely, when the precipitating factor is not readily correctable, heparin may be necessary in addition to blood products. Dosage recommendations vary widely; I recommend starting with low-dose IV infusions of heparin with q 4° monitoring of coagulation parameters (APTT, prothrombin time, fibrinogen level and quantitation of fibrin split products) to determine the need for further increases. A large dose of heparin could cause bleeding into infarcted tissues The use of inhibitors of fibrinolysis such as EACA (AMICAR) is not indicated in the vast majority of patients and should be instituted only after special coagulation tests are performed in a careful, sequential manner to establish a dominant and deleterious role of excessive fibrinolysis Avoid unnecessary invasive procedures and perform only those essential for stabilization.

TABLE 53-12. CLINICAL MANIFESTATIONS, DIAGNOSTIC PARAMETERS, AND TREATMENT OF CHRONIC DIC

Clinical Manifestations	Test Results	Treatment
Localized or migratory venous thrombosis including deep vein thrombosis CNS and renal dysfunction caused by small vessel thrombosis Localized bleeding at sites of invasive procedures, rarely systemic bleeding In patients with adenocarcinomas, arterial occlusions can occur because of nonbacterial thrombotic endocarditis (Libman-Sacks) Occasionally a major hemolytic process with thrombocytopenia (HUS-TTP) can develop in patients with ovarian carcinomas, hemagioendotheliomas and toxemia of pregnancy Consumptive process may be localized to an organ such as a large aortic aneurysm or hemangiomas	Fibrinogen level may be increased, normal, or reduced Routine tests such as APTT, PT may be normal or only minimally abnormal. Abnormal test results depend on the extent of reduction of fibrinogen and other factors Severe reduction in fibrinogen without concomitant severe reduction in factor V and VIII-C can occur Levels of other coagulation factors dependent on liver dysfunction Variable degree of thrombocytopenia Increased level of fibrin split products by the D-dimer and staphylococcal clumping tests	Ultra low-dose heparin (1–5 u/kg/hr) by IV infusion without a bolus at the start Monitor coagulation parameters, particularly levels of fibrinogen and fibrin split products serially to document efficacy and to determine the need for further increase in dosage Heparin should be started and DIC controlled before an anticipated increase in the stimulus for coagulation, e.g., before the start of effective chemotherapy in patients with malignancies

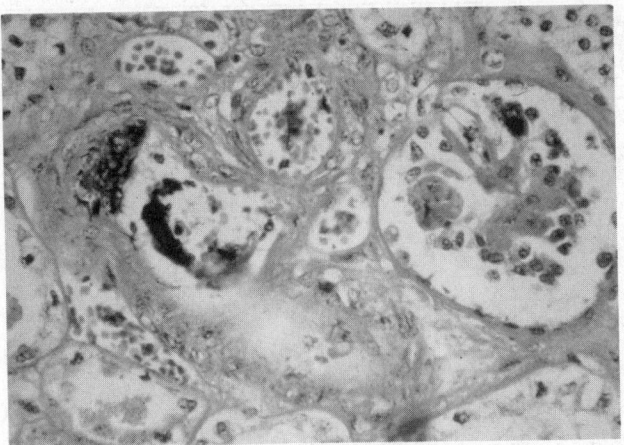

FIG. 53-8. Intra-arteriolar crescentic subendothelial lesions with fibrin deposition in the kidney of a patient with TTP.

eralized manifestations of bleeding are uncommon. In general, there is concordance between the biochemical and coagulation findings in patients with chronic liver disease, but there can be a discrepancy between the two. For instance, patients who have relatively good preservation of hepatocyte function, as in severe biliary cirrhosis, may have reasonable coagulation factor synthesis despite having advanced liver disease by biochemical parameters. The laboratory findings in chronic, slowly progressive liver disease may be arbitrarily divided into stages (Table 53-13). The first manifestation may be a mild reduction in the levels of the vitamin K-dependent factors, caused by gamma-carboxyglutamic acid cycle being most sensitive to injury.[23] In moderately advanced liver disease, there is a further reduction in the levels of the vitamin K-dependent factors, accompanied by mild reductions in factor V and fibrinogen. In advanced liver disease, all factor levels may be severely reduced and the profile may be indistinguishable from that of acute decompensated DIC, except for a normal or increased level of factor VIII-C. There is a concomitant reduction in

some factors participating in the fibrinolytic system as well as the levels of the physiologic inhibitors such as antithrombin III and α_2 antiplasmin. The development of additional complications in a patient with severe liver disease, e.g., sepsis, hypotension, LeVeen shunting, etc., can precipitate DIC; rarely, excessive fibrinolysis may predominate. In stable patients with severe liver disease, the major cause of the hemostatic abnormalities resides in poor synthetic liver function (Table 53-13); DIC and/or excessive fibrinolysis play only an accessory role. Each patient must be evaluated by special hemostatic tests, however, to determine whether decreased production of factors or DIC/fibrinolysis is the current major determinant of the coagulopathy. In these patients, defects in primary hemostasis are present with severe thrombocytopenia or a prolonged bleeding time when the platelet counts are $\geq 60,000$ per mm^3.

Acute massive hepatic necrosis, which occurs secondary to acute viral hepatitis, shock liver, and partial hepatectomy can cause a rapid drop in the level of the coagulation factors, including the vitamin K-dependent factors, fibrinogen, and factor V.[24] In this instance, a reduction in the level of factor VIII-C is the primary clue to the extent of thrombin generation and DIC because VIII-C levels are usually increased in liver disease because of its production by the reticuloendothelial cells of the liver; there is a simultaneous increased production of VIII-vFW. The level of the coagulation factors varies according to the extent and duration of the acute hepatic injury. Rapid spontaneous recovery from the coagulopathy may occur in patients with shock liver when the blood pressure normalizes, but severe persistent coagulopathy, causing bleeding, may develop if hepatocyte function does not recover.

Patients with advanced liver disease and massive ascites are candidates for the LeVeen type of peritoneovenous shunting. Preoperatively, they present with the severe coagulopathy of advanced liver disease. After shunting, they have a further reduction in coagulation factors from at least two causes; (1) DIC

TABLE 53-13. EXAMPLES OF TYPICAL CHANGES IN LIVER DISEASE

| Tests | Slowly Progressive Liver Disease | | | Acute Massive Hepatic Necrosis |
	Mild	Moderate	Severe	
APTT (21–31 sec)	25	32	50	50
PT ($\geq$70%)	60	40	20	20
TT (12–14 sec)	13	15	20	30
Fibrinogen (200–400 mg%)	300	200	100	80
FDP < 10 (latex)	<10	10–40	10–40	>40
ELT (180–360 mins)	320	180	80	50
F II	60	40	15	20
F V	100	55	35	10
F VII	55	35	15	20
F X	65	45	20	30
F VIII-C	150	200	350	40

caused by activation of hemostasis by both soluble and cellular elements in the ascitic fluid, and (2) a dilutional component caused by the massive autoinfusion of ascitic fluid. Immunoglobulin levels before and after the procedure can help to quantify the latter. Thrombosis of the shunt is another hemostatic problem that can occur in these patients, and shunt patency can be easily monitored with a hand-held Doppler device to document alterations in flow.[25,26]

THERAPEUTIC CONSIDERATIONS

A simple rule in treating patients with liver disease and hemostatic abnormalities is parenteral vitamin K_1 to correct a possible deficiency; lack of response of the prothrombin time to vitamin K indicates hepatocellular dysfunction. In patients with bleeding and advanced liver disease, replacement of coagulation factors is best achieved by the slow infusion of fresh frozen plasma (FFP), which contains all the coagulation factors and physiologic inhibitors. Serious fluid overload may be caused by the large volumes of FFP needed to elevate factors II, V, and X to an ~40% level, thus improving the prothrombin time to within $2\frac{1}{2}$ seconds longer than the control. If diuretics are contraindicated because of a hepatorenal syndrome, an exchange transfusion may be necessary at first, followed by a continuous infusion of FFP to maintain factors at an ~30 to a 40% level. Although prothrombin complex concentrates (Proplex and Konyne) contain

high concentrations of the vitamin K-dependent factors, they (1) may precipitate DIC because of the presence of activated coagulation factors, particularly if the infusion is rapid; (2) can cause venous thrombotic complications; (3) do not correct levels of the nonvitamin K-dependent factors and physiologic inhibitors, and (4) carry a high risk of transmission of viral illnesses. The minimum level of the various coagulation factors needed for adequate hemostasis and the dose and type of blood product to be used is indicated in Table 53-14. Patients with liver disease are exquisitely sensitive to heparin because the liver is involved in degrading heparin; even small amounts of heparin may cause a large anticoagulant effect in these patients. Therefore, the presence and continuing deleterious role of a DIC should be clearly established by sequential monitoring of coagulation profiles including VIII-C and D-dimer levels, before using heparin in patients with acute or chronic liver disease. We have used low-dose continuous infusion of heparin (2.5 to 5.0 u per kg per hour) starting immediately after LeVeen shunting to prevent shunt thrombosis.[26] When thrombocytopenia and platelet dysfunction are associated with prolonged bleeding time and excessive bleeding, platelet transfusions may be necessary to improve hemostasis; 1-deamino-8-D-arginine vasopressin (DDAVP) can be used to correct defects in primary hemostasis.[27,28] The use of inhibitors of fibrinolysis, such as epsilon-aminocaproic acid (AMICAR), is rarely indicated.

TABLE 53-14. MINIMUM COAGULATION FACTOR LEVELS NEEDED FOR ADEQUATE HEMOSTASIS AND INITIAL DOSE OF REPLACEMENT PRODUCT

Factor	Minimum Level for Adequate Hemostasis	Replacement Product and Initial Suggested Dose
Fibrinogen	50%–100 mg%	a. Cryoprecipitate: 1 bag/5 kg
II, V, X	20%–30%	FFP: 10–20 ml/kg
V	~30%	FFP: 20 ml/kg
VIII-C		a. Cryoprecipitate 1–3 bags/5 kg
Minor bleed, postoperative	~25%	
Major bleed, intraoperative	~80%	b. Factor VIII concentrate 15–40 u/kg
XI	~25%	FFP: 15 ml/kg
VIII-vW	a. Improve bleeding time	a. DDAVP 0.3–0.4 ug/kg IV infusion in type I and some type II patients.
	b. Normalize VIII-C	b. Cryoprecipitate: 1 bag/10 kg.
XIII	>1% but <5%	a. FFP: 500 mL or cryoprecipitate: 5 bags every 3 weeks.
Platelets	≥20,000/mm³ in patients with bone marrow disorders	1 unit platelet concentrate will raise platelet count by 5,000–10,000/mm³ in 70 kg adult
	≥60,000/mm³ or a bleeding time ≤12 mins. in surgical bleeding	1 unit single donor concentrate obtained by apheresis will increase platelet count by 30,000–60,000/mm³ in a 70 kg adult

VITAMIN K DEFICIENCY

Vitamin K, a series of homologous fat-soluble compounds, is necessary for adequate synthesis of procoagulant factors II, V, VII and X by the liver.[20,29] These procoagulants are synthesized by the vitamin K-dependent addition of γ carboxy groups to the glutamic acid residues in the precursor proteins (PIVKA). Other important vitamin K-dependent proteins include proteins C, S, M, and Z. Normally, the diet, particularly green leafy vegetables, and normal gut flora are the major sources of vitamin K. Bleeding disorders from critical reductions in the levels of the vitamin K-dependent factors because of vitamin K deficiency can occur in newborns, elderly patients with poor diets, or patients receiving total parenteral nutrition and antibiotics simultaneously. They can also occur in patients with malabsorption syndromes including biliary obstruction or with chronic renal failure, particularly those undergoing hemodialysis; and in patients taking oral anticoagulants or (intentionally or accidentally) rat poison.[30-32] It has been suggested that large doses of vitamins A and E, and salicylates antagonize vitamin K. As much as 50% of parenterally administered vitamin K_1 appears in the liver within the first hour, indicating its rapid availability for the synthetic processes in the liver.

The prothrombin time can be used as a simple measure of adequacy of vitamin K in all patients. The parenteral administration of ~150 μg of vitamin K_1 per day provides adequate replacement therapy to patients who are on broad spectrum antibiotics and are not receiving oral feeding. All patients with bleeding disorders and a prolonged prothrombin time should receive 1 mg of vitamin K_1 parenterally. Patients with a marked prolongation of the prothrombin time caused by accidental ingestion of rat poison or overdosage with oral anticoagulants, require larger, repeated doses of vitamin K_1 intravenously to improve hemostasis. Thus, in most instances of a reduction in vitamin K-dependent factors, intravenous vitamin K_1 rapidly corrects the abnormality if liver function is normal. If severe active bleeding or bleeding into vital organs is present, there may be a need to perform a plasma exchange using fresh frozen plasma, or rarely, to use concentrates of the vitamin K-dependent factors. The latter is infrequently used now because of problems associated with its use, which have been discussed previously under liver disease. Table 53-15 summarizes the laboratory features of severe vitamin K deficiency, advanced liver disease, and acute decompensated DIC.

ACQUIRED HEMOSTATIC DISORDERS IN SURGICAL PATIENTS

EXTRACORPOREAL CIRCULATION

Exposure of blood to artificial surfaces in the cardiopulmonary bypass system or other artificial organs results in activation of the contact system.[6] This leads to thrombin generation with resultant release of fibrinopeptides and fibrin formation, despite the massive heparinization routinely used in these patients.[33] Varying degrees of red cell hemolysis caused by shear stress, turbulence, osmotic changes, and alteration in temperature also contribute to activation of the coagulation system. These changes are minimized by hemodilution, which occurs from priming of the bypass system with crystalloids and colloids. The use of autotransfusion techniques, which recycle the bloody fluid aspirated from the surgical field by the suction device, allow tissue factor to enter into the circulation. Thus this artificial extracorporeal circulation system is heavily geared toward clot formation. A persistent decompensated DIC is, however, uncommon because of the adequacy of heparinization, even though a drop

TABLE 53-15. DIFFERENCES IN THE COAGULOPATHY OF SEVERE VITAMIN K DEFICIENCY, ADVANCED LIVER DISEASE, AND ACUTE DECOMPENSATED DIC

Parameter	Severe Vitamin K Deficiency	Advanced Chronic Liver Disease	Acute Decompensated DIC
APTT	Prolonged	Prolonged	Prolonged
PT	Prolonged	Prolonged	Prolonged
Thrombin time	Normal	Prolonged	Prolonged
Fibrinogen	Normal	Reduced	Reduced
Factors VII/X/II	Reduced	Reduced	Variably reduced
Factor V	Normal	Reduced	Reduced
Factor VIII-C	Normal	Normal or increased	Reduced
Platelets	Normal	Usually reduced	Reduced
Proteins C, S	Reduced	Reduced	Reduced
Euglobulin lysis time	Normal	Normal or short	Usually short
D-dimer	Normal	Normal	Increased

in the basal fibrinogen level with an increase in FDP is present postoperatively.[34] The presence of additional nonsurgical factors such as heart failure, liver disease, prolonged hypotension, and sepsis could perpetuate a decompensated DIC in these patients. After bypass, the prothrombin time and APTT are a few seconds longer than the preoperative value in most patients. But the factors participating in these tests are usually ≥ 50% of normal, and therefore without an effect on hemostasis.[34] Another consequence of the bypass is occurrence of microemboli caused by fibrin, cellular aggregates/debris, fat, foreign materials from the perfusion system, and air from the suction devices and oxygenators. Varying degrees of thrombocytopenia and platelet dysfunction develop during extracorporeal circulation because of exposure of this highly reactive cell to artificial surfaces; this interaction is further increased by the presence of fibrinogen on those surfaces. Both thrombin and ADP (from tissue injury and hemolysis) activate platelets, which aggregate and release their contents. These changes in the platelets cause a prolongation of the bleeding time in most patients, although the extent of this abnormality varies.[33,35]

Clinically, the hemostatic problems encountered after bypass procedures include CNS damage caused by microemboli and excessive bleeding, generally from the operated site because of the presence of a surgical bleeder, thrombocytopenia, and platelet dysfunction. Infrequently, excessive bleeding is attributable to decreased plasma coagulation factor levels from dilution, DIC, heparin excess from inadequate neutralization with protamine, or a heparin rebound phenomenon from the re-entry of extravascular heparin after initial adequate neutralization with protamine, or excess protamine. The emergency physician is the first person to encounter the rare patient who returns within 7 to 10 days after exposure to homologous blood products, with the acute onset of a severe bleeding disorder caused by the occurrence of a severe thrombocytopenia. This is the potentially lethal syndrome of post-transfusion purpura, which is caused by the the development of alloantibodies to the Pl^{A1} or other antigens.[36,37] The development of severe thrombocytopenia within a few hours of the transfusion of blood products could be caused by the passive transfer of such antibodies.[37]

Patients with pre-existing bleeding disorders from abnormalities in primary hemostasis benefit from the intraoperative use of DDAVP to reduce blood loss. The benefit of administering DDAVP routinely to a patient with normal hemostasis who is undergoing bypass surgery is, however, still being debated. Postoperative management after bypass surgery requires careful monitoring of the chest tube output of blood, along with an assessment of the platelet count and coagulation profile (APTT, PT, thrombin time, fibrinogen level, fibrin split products, and factors II, V, VII, and X).[34] If excessive bleeding occurs within 48 to 72 hours of surgery, platelet transfusions should be given

to patients with significant thrombocytopenia (≤ 60,000/mm³) or prolonged bleeding time.[35] DDAVP can also be used to improve defects in primary hemostasis. Patients who have received heparin before bypass are more likely to develop a heparin rebound phenomenon after bypass, thus aggravating postoperative bleeding. The coagulation profile should be used to confirm the presence of excess heparin or DIC because excessive bleeding caused by these disorders would necessitate the use of protamine sulfate or blood products.

MASSIVE TRANSFUSION

Massive hemorrhage requiring rapid transfusions of large volumes of banked whole blood within a few hours can cause hemostatic abnormalities related to alterations in platelet numbers and function and decreases in coagulation factors in stored blood, as well as accompanying DIC from concomitant acidosis, tissue injury, hypotension, and sepsis in the patient. The major hemostatic defect ascribable to massive transfusions is a decrease in platelet count and function. Storage of blood at 4°C for 2 days causes morphologic and metabolic changes in platelets.[38] Transfusion of this platelet-poor blood causes a dilutional thrombocytopenia, which is not rapidly compensated because of the slow response rate of the bone marrow. Additionally, ADP released from hemolyzing red cells and tissue injury may not only reduce circulating platelet numbers by aggregating them but cause the remaining platelets to become refractory to aggregating agents, thereby contributing to platelet dysfunction. Filters used to avoid particulate emboli because of the debris and cellular aggregates in stored blood may also trap functional platelets. Generation of serine proteases such as thrombin, caused by DIC, can cause a further reduction in platelets. The extent of thrombocytopenia and platelet dysfunction varies from patient to patient, but may be anticipated in patients receiving large volumes of banked blood in a few hours.[39,40]

Coagulation factors VIII-C and V are severely depleted in stored blood. Factor VIII-C activity falls to ~30% within 5 days, whereas factor V activity falls to that level within 3 weeks of storage.[41] Levels of other coagulation factors are not significantly affected. Various transfusion reactions and metabolic abnormalities can cause changes that potentiate coagulation abnormalities. Finally, the presence of major organ dysfunction such as shock liver and adult respiratory distress syndrome (ARDS) can perpetuate the coagulopathy.

In a patient with massive bleeding, platelet transfusions should be used empirically to prevent the anticipated decline in platelet number and function when more than 5 units of banked blood have been transfused within a few hours. Whenever feasible, such therapy should be guided by the use of serial platelet counts and bleeding times. The APTT, PT, and fibrinogen level can be used as screening tools to detect significant reductions in plasma coagulation factor levels. When these screening tests are abnormal, the rapid availability of assays of factors II, V, VII, and X, and thrombin time facilitates not only an understanding of the abnormalities but also assists in the decision to use fresh frozen plasma to maintain the coagulation factors at the minimal levels needed for adequate hemostasis (see Table 53-7). The use of cell savers during extensive surgical procedures allows recycling of the patient's own shed blood and minimizes volume loss. The frequency with which blood products are needed can be best judged by serial testing of hemostatic parameters because recovery, consumption, and endogenous rate of factor synthesis and cardiovascular tolerance vary from patient to patient.

OTHER CAUSES OF BLEEDING

THROMBOCYTOPENIA AND/OR PLATELET DYSFUNCTION

Thrombocytopenia can contribute to a hemorrhagic diathesis, manifested by petechiae and ecchymoses (Fig. 53-9). A few of the causes are briefly considered here. Significant reductions in the platelet count can occur in patients with septicemia caused by bacteria (gram-negative or gram-positive), viruses, rickettsiae, and parasites. This may be on an immunologic basis or from platelet aggregation caused by the organisms or DIC. The possibility of drug-induced thrombocytopenia should be considered in all patients.[36,37] All

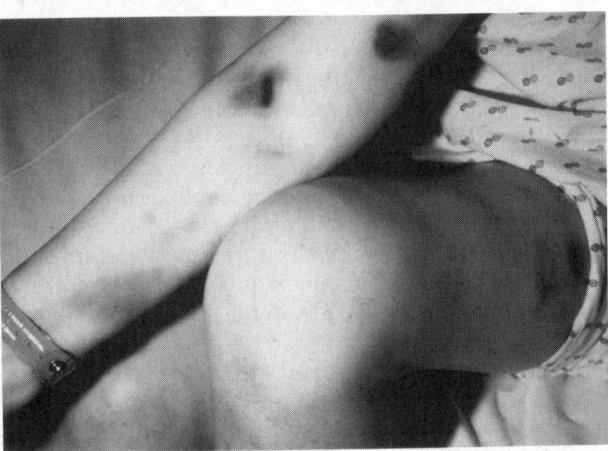

FIG. 53-9.   Bruises and petechiae in a patient who was overanticoagulated with warfarin sodium and developed an acute ITP at the same time.

drugs suspected of causing thrombocytopenia should be stopped; this does not usually pose a problem because alternative agents are available. In vitro tests to detect a drug-platelet antibody should be performed, but may not be helpful. Heparin-induced thrombocytopenia, although infrequent, requires prompt cessation of the heparin when arterial embolic complications or severe thrombocytopenia develops in the patient. In vitro testing with patient's serum, ABO-compatible platelet-rich plasma, and porcine/bovine heparin for platelet aggregation/lysis is a rapid but relatively insensitive test for heparin platelet antibodies.

Numerous drugs have been implicated as a cause of a drug-induced platelet dysfunction.[42] The combination of alcohol and aspirin can cause marked prolongation of the bleeding time; the frequency with which these drugs are used should alert the emergency physician to look for this drug combination as a cause of bleeding.[43] Some antimicrobials such as ticarcillin, carbenicillin, and moxalactams have significant effects on the bleeding time, particularly in patients with renal dysfunction.

Other systemic disorders associated with platelet dysfunction and not discussed thus far include acute and chronic renal failure and a variety of bone marrow disorders. **Uremia** has been associated with defects in platelet activation, adhesion to the subendothelium, aggregation/secretion, and platelet factor 3 availability in response to a variety of agonists. Qualitative defects in the von Willebrand factor have also been described. Guanidinosuccinic and phenolic acids, along with poorly characterized "middle" molecular weight substances, and an increased production of prostacyclin by endothelial cells and anemia have all been implicated as causative factors for platelet dysfunction in renal failure. Despite the above findings and the fact that uremia is an important cause of prolonged bleeding time, not all patients with renal failure have prolonged bleeding time. The template bleeding time must be performed to evaluate this facet. Another hemostatic complication is the exaggerated response to standard drugs such as heparin, acetylsalicylic acid, and antibiotics; their concomitant administration may markedly potentiate bleeding in uremic patients. Improvement of the bleeding disorder can be achieved by adequate dialysis, maintaining a hematocrit of at least 30% and avoiding excess heparin or the concomitant use of antiplatelet drugs. Sometimes other modalities of treatment such as DDAVP (0.3 μg per kg IV over 15 minutes), conjugated estrogens (0.6 mg per kg per day IV for 5 days), or the use of cryoprecipitate may be required to improve the markedly prolonged bleeding time.[27,28,44-46]

Primary bone marrow disorders such as essential thrombocythemia, polycythemia vera, chronic granulocytic leukemia, agnogenic myeloid metaplasia, myelodysplastic syndromes, and acute leukemias have been associated with a wide variety of platelet functional defects. The platelet dysfunction has been ascribed to defects in the arachidonate and lipoxygenase pathways, alteration of receptors, abnormal metabolic activity, and altered platelet membrane constituents including membrane glycoproteins. Generally, correlation has not been good between in vitro platelet functional abnormalities and bleeding or thrombotic manifestations. Thrombocytopenia and platelet dysfunction have traditionally been corrected by the use of platelet transfusions when they cause bleeding.

ANTICOAGULANT AND FIBRINOLYTIC AGENTS

The most important complication to be anticipated with the use of these agents is bleeding. A generally applicable rule is that excessive anticoagulant effect with either heparin or warfarin sodium is likely to be associated with a risk of bleeding. The presence of underlying lesions (such as a colonic polyp), the performance of invasive procedures (such as arterial blood gases) and the simultaneous administration of antiplatelet drugs, which impair primary hemostasis, can precipitate bleeding even in patients who are not excessively anticoagulated (Fig. 53-10).

HEPARIN

There is clearly a relationship between the use of large doses of heparin, a markedly prolonged clotting test (usually the APTT), and an increased frequency of bleeding complications.[47] There is also a strongly held clinical opinion that an excessive anticoagulant effect of heparin, as judged by an APTT beyond the desired therapeutic limit of 2 times the control value, is associated with an increased risk of bleeding. Patients receiving a continuous infusion of heparin have a lower frequency of bleeding than those receiving intermittent injections of heparin. The kinetics of heparin are altered in patients with liver disease and renal failure, causing them to be more sensitive to a given dose of heparin. Elderly women appear to be at a higher risk for bleeding complications. Therefore these patients should be monitored more carefully. The development of life-threatening bleeding in a patient receiving heparin warrants the slow intravenous infusion of protamine sulfate (1 mg neutralizes 100 units of heparin). But the dosage of protamine sulfate to be given depends on the time elapsed since heparin was last administered because of the short biologic half-life of heparin in the plasma (~60 minutes). Therefore, only 50% of the calculated dosage of protamine sulfate should be given if an hour has elapsed since heparin was last administered. I make an additional 25% reduction in the calculated dose of protamine sulfate because of the substantial amount of heparin that equilibrates with the extravascular space. Thus large doses of protamine sulfate in the 50 mg to 100 mg range are seldom necessary. It is essential to monitor

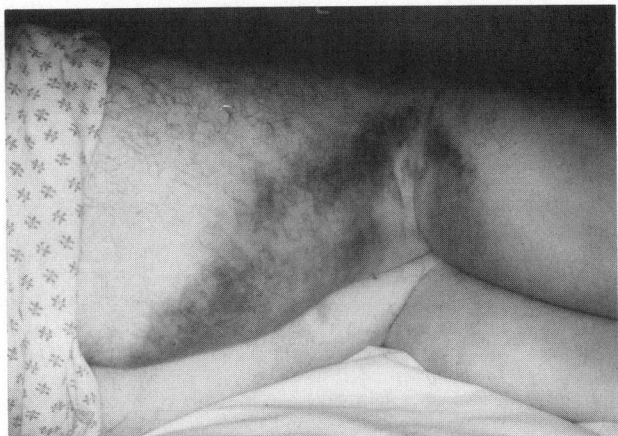

FIG. 53-10. A patient with a ruptured Baker's cyst developed progressive, massive bleeding into the thigh and calf after receiving therapeutic doses of intravenous heparin for calf and popliteal pain, which had mistakenly been diagnosed as a DVT.

the APTT immediately after protamine sulfate is given to ascertain that shortening of the APTT has been achieved. The patient may develop hypotension or anaphylaxis during the administration of protamine sulfate. Simultaneous administration of intravenous nitroglycerin to patients receiving heparin reduces the anticoagulant effect of a given dose of heparin.[48]

WARFARIN SODIUM

Careful monitoring of the prothrombin time and awareness of drug interactions play a critical role in the use of warfarin sodium.[49] The frequency of bleeding complications increases along with prothrombin time in patients receiving this drug.[50] A common cause of oral anticoagulant-related bleeding is the inadvertent administration of drugs that potentiate warfarin sodium effect (Table 53-16). To minimize bleeding complications, all ED personnel should not only ascertain that the patient's prothrombin time is in the desired therapeutic range (ratio of patient to control prothrombin time of 1.4 to 1.5 for venous thromboembolic disease and higher ratios of ~1.8 for patients with other special indications)[51] but also educate the patient about drug interactions. Emphasis on maintenance of written records by the patient, with entries of doses of warfarin and all other drugs taken along with all prothrombin time test results (including the control value) not only facilitates the physician's ability to quickly correct excesses but educates the patient. Such measures may help to minimize the higher risk of bleeding in patients who are not only receiving oral anticoagulants over a prolonged period of time but also have other underlying diseases. If the prothrombin time is slightly longer than desired, simple measures such as reduction in dosage, removal of the potentiating drug, or withholding warfarin for a few days may be sufficient to correct the problem. If

---

TABLE 53-16. DRUG INTERACTIONS BETWEEN WARFARIN SODIUM AND COMMONLY USED DRUGS

A. Drugs That Potentiate Warfarin Effect

1. **Anti-inflammatory drugs**
   Acetylsalicylic acid
   Phenylbutazone
   Indomethacin
   Naproxen (Naprosyn)
   Ibuprofen (Motrin, Advil)
   Others
2. **Antibiotics**
   Trimethoprim sulfamethoxazole
      (Bactrim, Septra)
   Metronidazole (Flagyl)
   Third-generation cephalosporins

3. **Others**
   Allopurinol
   Androgenic steroids
   Antabuse
   Cimetidine, ranitidine
   Dilantin sodium
   Liver disease/large doses of alcohol
   Poor diet
      Sulfinpyrazone (Anturane)
   Vitamin E

B. Drugs That Reduce Warfarin Effect
   Barbiturates
   Carbamazepine
   Cholestyramine
   Diet rich in vitamin K, i.e., greens
   Glutethimide
   Griseofulvin
   Hereditary resistance
   Oral contraceptives
   Rifampin
   Spironolactone

---

moderately severe bleeding complications are also present or the prothrombin time is markedly prolonged in the absence of active bleeding, repeated small intravenous infusions of vitamin K_1 (1 mg IV over 10 minutes) could rapidly improve the vitamin K-dependent factors to the 30 to 40% range or higher and reduce bleeding. If gastrointestinal absorption is not a problem and the clinical circumstances could tolerate a slower rate of correction of the prothrombin time, oral doses of vitamin K may suffice. If bleeding is potentially life-threatening, despite their disadvantages, concentrates of the vitamin K-dependent factors or a plasma exchange may be necessary in addition to intravenous vitamin K_1. Patients who have taken large doses of warfarin sodium, accidentally or intentionally, require repeated large doses of vitamin K_1 (10 mg IV as a slow infusion over 10 minutes) because of the expected high plasma levels and known long half-life of warfarin sodium. The phenomenon of coumarin necrosis is discussed elsewhere in this chapter.

THROMBOLYTIC AGENTS

Two fibrinolytic agents, streptokinase and t-PA, are currently being used with increased frequency in patients with acute myocardial infarction. With the trend toward early administration of these agents for an acute MI, it is possible that patients may arrive in the ED after having received these agents in the ambulance en route to the hospital. Patients who come to the ED with recent onset of a popliteal or more proximal deep vein thrombosis should receive thrombolytic therapy starting in the ED before admission. The beneficial effect of thrombolytic therapy in patients with massive or submassive acute pulmonary embolism has been well established. All these patients should obviously have an objectively diagnosed proximal deep vein thrombosis or pulmonary embolism and not have major contraindications to thrombolytic therapy. The risk of bleeding complications in these patients is related to the presence of a systemic fibrinolytic state. Bleeding complications develop because plasmin lyses fibrin at all sites regardless of whether the fibrin has been deposited in response to a physiologic or a pathologic stimulus, and does not depend particularly on the extent of drop in the fibrinogen level.[52] The performance of invasive procedures, including repeated venipunctures, is a major cause of bleeding and can be easily avoided by placing an intracatheter with a three-way stopcock before the start of thrombolytic therapy to be used for drug infusions and blood sampling. The potential for CNS bleeding in older patients must be kept in mind. Because of the short half-life of plasmin, rapid correction of the hemostatic defect can be achieved by stopping the thrombolytic agent; epsilon-aminocaproic acid and fresh frozen plasma may also be used when required.

INHIBITORS: SPECIFIC AND NONSPECIFIC

Acquired inhibitors of hemostasis or circulating anticoagulants are generally immunoglobulins, which may be directed against specific coagulation proteins or may be nonspecific and interfere with in vitro coagulation reactions.

SPECIFIC INHIBITORS

The commonest of these are **factor VIII-C inhibitors,** which can develop in hemophiliacs, patients with autoimmune disorders, in the postpartum period, after drug reactions, in association with malignancies, after surgery, or spontaneously. A smaller number of patients with an acquired von Willebrand syndrome from either specific **antibodies to the von Willebrand factor** or binding of the von Willebrand protein to malignant cells have also been described. Less frequently, inhibitors to other coagulation proteins such as factors IX, V, XIII, and fibrinogen have been described. Treatment of specific coagulation factor inhibitors is complex and usually prompted by the presence of significant bleeding. **Monoclonal gammopathies** have been associated with prolongation of the thrombin time and abnormalities of fibrin monomer polymerization with abnormal fibrin clots; various platelet functional defects have also been described. In most instances, clinically significant bleeding is uncommon; if it is a problem, plasmapheresis is used to remove the abnormal protein along with therapy of the underlying disorder. Increased bruising and the development of periorbital hemorrhages after procedures requiring the head to be in a dependent position have been described in **amyloidosis** (Fig. 53-11). Rarely, patients with amyloidosis have an acquired isolated factor X deficiency, associated with severe bleeding. The reduction in factor X is because of its selective clearance from the circulation as a result of binding to the amyloid fibrils; infusions of factor X are ineffective in this disorder. Splenectomy may be beneficial.

NONSPECIFIC INHIBITORS

The lupus-type anticoagulants are a nonspecific type of coagulation inhibitor, and are not directed against specific coagulation factors or associated with a bleeding disorder.[53] An association between these and venous thrombosis, strokes, and recurrent spontaneous abortions has been suggested, but a prospective cause-and-effect relationship has not yet been shown. Their importance lies in the fact that they are directed against phospholipids, thereby interfering with phospholipid-dependent in vitro coagulation tests such as the APTT, PT (more so in the dilute thromboplastin PT test), dilute Russell's viper venom test, and others. The VDRL and anticardiolipin antibody tests may also be positive. The in vitro coagulation test abnormalities can cause confusion in management; for example, FFP may be used in patients with this inhibitor to correct the prolonged APTT/PT before a surgical procedure. It is important to recognize that patients with prolonged in vitro coagulation tests caused by the lupus-type anticoagulants do not experience a bleeding disorder even when invasive procedures are performed. This is contrary to the usual rule, in which the presence of a prolonged APTT/PT dictates the avoidance of sur-

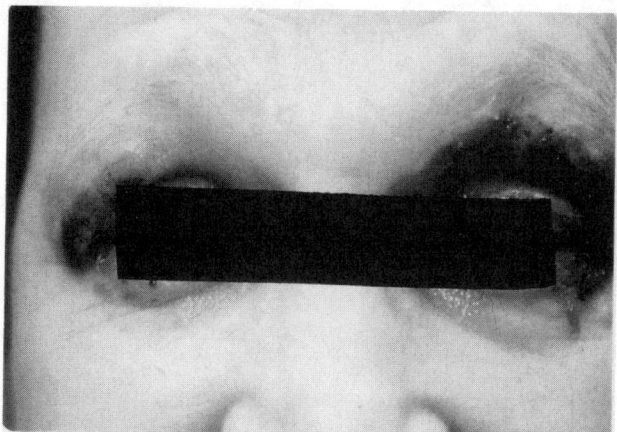

FIG. 53-11.   *Periorbital hemorrhages following proctoscopy in a patient with amyloidosis.*

gical procedures because of the potential risk for bleeding.

ACQUIRED VASCULAR DISORDERS

HENOCH-SCHÖNLEIN PURPURA

Henoch-Schönlein purpura or allergic purpura is a group of disorders that may be caused by the deposition of IgA-containing immune complexes in the vessels, causing leukocytoclastic vasculitis.[54] There is a predominant neutrophilic perivascular infiltrate with fibrinoid necrosis, platelet thrombi, IgA, and components of complement in the lesions. It has been suggested that this disease may represent a collagen vascular disorder. Comparisons have also been made between the renal lesions in Henoch-Schönlein and primary IgA nephropathy, with the suggestion that the latter represents the chronic progressive renal phase of a disease which, in the acute form, consists of findings seen in the Henoch-Schönlein syndrome.

This form of purpura primarily affects young children and is characterized by the sudden onset of crops of a copper-colored itchy skin rash, which may recur over 4 weeks (Fig. 53-12). The rash is symmetric in distribution and generally involves the lower extremities; it is often preceded by an upper respiratory infection. The purpuric lesions are accompanied by malaise, fever, colicky abdominal pain, polyarthralgias, and edema of the extremities. The abdominal pain is associated with gastrointestinal bleeding, usually in the form of guaiac positive stools or melena, and may proceed to an intussusception or bowel perforation. Kidney involvement develops in the second to third week of the illness; hypertension and renal failure are less common. Although swelling and pain are seen around the joints, the latter are not hot and swollen. Edema of the hands, feet, scalp, and scrotum, sometimes painful, occurs in young children; hemorrhage into and torsion of the testes has also been reported.

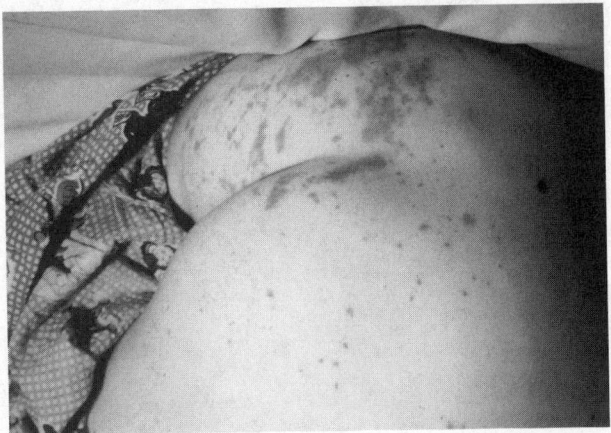

FIG. 53-12. Characteristic location and appearance of copper-colored purpuric skin lesions in a child with Henoch-Schönlein purpura.

The vasculitis may involve the central nervous system and cause focal paresis, convulsions, or cranial nerve palsies. Focal changes in the heart and lungs have also been described. Occasionally, recurrences characterized by the reappearance of skin rashes and abdominal pain are seen.[55]

Despite the widespread vasculitis with bleeding manifestations, routine coagulation tests are normal and the platelet count is either normal or increased. The white blood cell (WBC) count may be increased and the presence of anemia depends on the extent of bleeding. Urinalysis may show varying degrees of hematuria, proteinuria, red cells, and granular casts. Skin and kidney biopsies confirm the presence of vasculitis. Symptomatic treatment of the acute syndrome usually suffices because the overall prognosis is good and most young patients recover completely. Corticosteroids have been successfully used to reduce the edema and prevent complications in patients with serious abdominal and joint involvement; the skin rash and renal disease do not seem to be positively influenced by steroids.

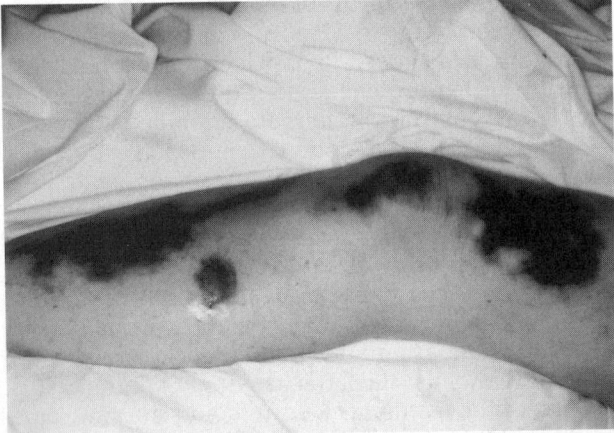

FIG. 53-13. Extensive necrotic skin lesions of purpura fulminans in a critically ill patient.

OTHER CAUSES OF VASCULAR PURPURA

Other causes of vascular purpura include **simple purpura,** usually benign and found over the extremities in young women, and **senile purpura,** occurring in older people and typically present on the dorsum of the hands. Degenerative changes in the supportive connective tissue are responsible for the latter disorder. **Steroid purpura** has a similar pathogenesis and is seen in patients receiving glucocorticoids over a prolonged period. **Factitial** and **psychogenic purpura** occur in patients with psychologic aberrations and may be difficult to diagnose; the atypical location of the bleeding site, such as recurrent bleeding from an old healed scar or the presence of fixed shape purpuras, should raise suspicion about the cause of such abnormalities. **Infectious purpura** is caused by various bacterial, viral, rickettsial, and protozoan infections, which damage the vessel wall. In certain **dysproteinemias** such as **macroglobulinemia** and **cryoglobulinemia,** vascular injury can cause small purpuric skin lesions; removal of the abnormal protein along with treatment of the underlying disorder is necessary in these instances. **Autoimmune diseases** with **vasculitis** can present with a similar purpura. Perifollicular hemorrhages are associated with **vitamin C deficiency,** although petechiae may be the first manifestation. Other serious bleeding caused by scurvy, such as intramuscular hematomas and subperiosteal bleeding, may occur in patients who have been maintained on hyperalimentation for months, alcoholics with a poor diet, and infants who have been solely breast-fed for prolonged periods.

PURPURA FULMINANS

Purpura fulminans is a rare disease in which painful unusual purpuric lesions develop over the extremities, buttocks, face, and back in critically ill patients. In children, streptococcal infections or varicella may be followed by the development of this syndrome; in adults, it may be more difficult to identify a specific cause. The lesions have a dark, firm, blackish center with an erythematous border; some may develop a central area of necrosis (Fig. 53-13). An acute decompensated DIC is simultaneously detected in these patients. A biopsy of the involved area shows widespread thrombosis of the capillaries and venules with a perivascular inflammatory infiltrate. Recognition of this abnormality and prompt institution of intravenous heparin are necessary to control and reverse this process.

COUMARIN NECROSIS

The sudden onset of painful purpuric skin lesions, which can progress to skin and muscle necrosis, was originally described in patients receiving warfarin sodium and has been referred to as "Coumarin necrosis" (Fig. 53-14). This phenomenon has been reported in patients who have pre-existing moderate reductions in protein C or protein S (due to a congenital or acquired cause) before the start of warfarin therapy.[56] Because of the short half-life of protein C of ~ 6 hours, an additional rapid drop in the level of protein C occurs in these patients after starting warfarin therapy. This causes a severe reduction in the level of protein C before an adequate reduction of the other vitamin K-dependent factors (II,IX,X) can inhibit hemostasis and result in a therapeutic anticoagulant effect. Thus patients whose protein C levels are initially only moderately reduced and in the range of a heterozygous deficiency (~40% -60%) before the start of warfarin therapy have a further drop in these levels toward those seen in the homozygote with protein C deficiency (<10%). This appears to trigger the development of the thrombotic-hemorrhagic-necrotic skin lesions. Infants with a severe reduction in protein C levels from an inherited homozygous state for protein C deficiency develop the syndrome of purpura fulminans. Thus the phenomenon of coumarin necrosis appears to develop in patients who have an acquired severe reduction in protein C level. Clinically and histologically, the lesions are identical to those described for purpura fulminans. The immediate administration of therapeutic doses of intravenous heparin and intravenous vitamin K_1, with discontinuation of warfarin sodium, not only aborts the further progression of these lesions but causes regression of the changes and healing. Successful reintroduction of warfarin sodium while patients are being adequately heparinized is feasible.[57] Heparin should be stopped when the factor II level (the vitamin K-dependent factor with the longest half-life) is less than 30%.[58]

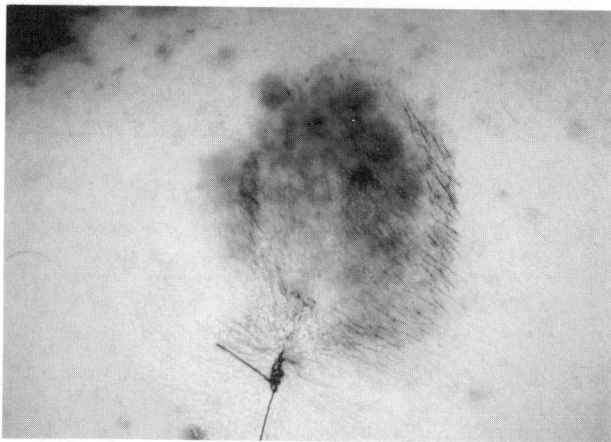

FIG. 53-14.   Skin lesions that developed within 36 hours of starting warfarin sodium in a patient who was receiving inadequate doses of intravenous heparin and had an advanced metastatic adenocarcinoma of the lung.

DIAGNOSTIC APPROACH TO BLEEDING DISORDERS (TABLE 53-17)

The history determines whether a person has an inherited or acquired bleeding disorder; a negative family history for a bleeding diathesis should be obtained in most patients with acquired bleeding disorders. The relationship of the onset of bleeding to any preceding or known underlying disease process, worsening by the ingestion of antiplatelet drugs, a poor dietary intake in a debilitated individual on antibiotics are all clues to the type of defects to anticipate. The development of spontaneous bleeding is a sign of a serious hemostatic defect, although mild trauma may precede the problem. Excessive bleeding only after recent surgical procedures could date the onset of the bleeding disorder. Defects in primary hemostasis can manifest as petechiae, bruises, nosebleeds, and other mucosal-type bleeding and may occur spontaneously or follow mild trauma. Mild plasma coagulation defects manifest themselves by bruises and bleeding from invaded sites or underlying lesions. When these defects are

severe, they may present with large deep hematomas, bleeding from multiple sites, or even retroperitoneal hemorrhages. Other physical findings such as the presence of diffuse angiomas or lesions of purpura fulminans, although rare, may be diagnostic. Excessive bleeding from a specific surgical site could be related either to a surgical bleeder or defects in hemostasis induced by the type of procedure, i.e. massive blood transfusions or open heart surgery.

Initial screening laboratory tests in all patients who are seriously ill with or without a hemostatic disorder should consist of an APTT, PT, fibrinogen, FDP, and a platelet count. If these preliminary tests are abnormal, further evaluation is necessary to understand the types of defects. If the APTT is prolonged and all other tests are normal, the next step should involve mixing experiments with normal plasma and patient's plasma to determine whether a deficiency or an inhibitor is the cause of the prolonged APTT. This has to be accompanied by specific assays of the early coagulation factors, with VIII-C, IX, and XI of importance as a cause of the bleeding disorder. Based on these results, further specialized tests may be necessary to determine the presence of specific or nonspecific inhibitors. Such tests include a Bethesda titer of a specific inhibitor, or tests such as the dilute Russell's viper venom time and dilute thromboplastin PT test, to detect a phospholipid type of inhibitor. Abnormalities of the PT should be pursued by assays of factors II, V, VII, and X, which are easily performed and in conjunction with the APTT, PT, fibrinogen level and screening FDP levels determine the presence of DIC, liver disease, vitamin K deficiency, or other coagulopathy. A factor VIII-C and D-dimer levels are useful in differentiating a DIC from other causes of a coagulation disorder. Concurrently, there is a need to evaluate primary hemostasis. If the platelet count is >60,000 per mm^3, there is a need to perform a bleeding time test. If that is prolonged, the abnormalities may reside in platelet

TABLE 53-17. ESSENTIAL COMPONENTS OF A DIAGNOSTIC APPROACH TO A BLEEDING PATIENT

1. *HISTORY:* Inherited or acquired bleeding disorder, drugs currently being taken, recent hospitalization, surgery, or infusion of blood products, events precipitating visit to ED.
2. *ASSOCIATED DISEASE STATE:* Liver disease, chronic renal failure, massive trauma, massive bleeding, sepsis, shock, malignancies, pregnancy, administration of anticoagulant/thrombolytic or other pharmacologic agents.
3. *BLEEDING SITE:*
   LOCALIZED: From nose, site of surgery or trauma, vagina, gastrointestinal tract, genitourinary tract, skin, into specific organs.
   GENERALIZED: Gingiva, skin, epistaxis, gastrointestinal, genitourinary, vagina, venipuncture, recent sites of surgery, into other organs.
   OTHERS: Petechiae, ecchymoses, vascular malformations, necrotic-hemorrhagic skin lesions, lesions localized to fingertips, toes, earlobes, tip of nose.
4. *LABORATORY TESTS:*
   INITIAL: APTT, PT, thrombin time, fibrinogen, FDP, platelet count.
   ADDITIONAL: Factors II, V, VII, X if PT prolonged; if APTT is prolonged, APTT inhibitor test (mixing experiments with normal plasma to confirm deficiency or inhibitor), template bleeding time, D-dimer, VIII-C, IX, XI, euglobulin lysis time.
   SPECIALIZED TESTS: Heparin neutralization test, specific inhibitor assays, VIII vW, VIII-vW multimer analysis, thromboplastin dilution test, dilute Russell's viper venom time, platelet function studies, urea solubility test (Note: a normal APTT and PT canot exclude dFXIII deficiency), and other tests.

dysfunction, abnormal F VIII-vW, or other less common disorders. Other specialized testing includes a heparin neutralization test, the euglobulin lysis time, platelet function studies, factor VIII-vW multimer analysis, and tests for factor XIII deficiency. It is important to understand that a normal APTT and PT cannot exclude the presence of mild reductions of coagulation factors or of factor XIII or α_2 antiplasmin deficiencies or vascular disorders. Active bleeding indicates a defect in hemostasis, but the absence of active bleeding in a seriously ill patient does not preclude the presence of a coagulopathy, which may manifest itself after even minor invasive procedures.

MEDICOLEGAL PEARLS AND PITFALLS

- Detailed history always yields a clue to the diagnosis.
- Types of skin lesions and sites of bleeding are a clue to the type of hemostatic defect (plasma coagulation defect versus a defect in primary hemostasis).
- Do not perform invasive procedures, other than venipunctures, in patients with an uncorrected hemostatic disorder except as a life-saving measure.
- Apply pressure and ice packs to active bleeding sites whenever feasible. Do not apply heat.
- Do not mistake the skin lesions of DIC, coumarin necrosis, and purpura fulminans for bruises.

- Check history for recent blood product transfusion in patients with an acute onset of thrombocytopenia because post-transfusion purpura requires urgent plasmapheresis.
- Do not allow patients with suspected or confirmed proximal DVT to ambulate, whether or not they are on thrombolytic therapy.
- Onset of bleeding, generally superficial but occasionally serious in a patient who is otherwise healthy, should raise suspicion about the surreptitious use of anticoagulants or self-induced trauma.
- Poor choice of venipuncture sites such as small dorsal hand veins, use of small-gauge needles with poor blood flow, use of excessive suction force to collect the blood, or femoral "stick" blood samples can cause in vitro activation and consumption of coagulation factors and ex vivo coagulation test abnormalities.
- Errors in specimen acquisition such as inadequate filling of tubes with blood, use of the wrong anticoagulant for coagulation tests (i.e., use of EDTA tubes for APTT, PT) result in abnormal test results.
- The proportion of anticoagulant to blood, usually 1 volume of 3.8% sodium citrate to 9 volumes of whole blood, should be changed to 0.5 volume citrate to 9 volumes of whole blood in patients with an increased hematocrit of >60% to avoid excess citrate causing ex vivo coagulation test abnormalities.
- Screening tests of hemostasis should be sent as a STAT and must include an APTT, PT, fibrinogen, FDP, and platelet count in all patients who have serious systemic illnesses, are critically ill, or are bleeding.
- Additional coagulation tests as indicated in Table 53-17 must be pursued if preliminary test results are abnormal.
- If screening coagulation tests are severely abnormal in an otherwise normal-appearing patient or normal in a critically ill patient, question the results and repeat the tests. Errors in specimen labeling and laboratory testing can occur.
- In patients receiving heparin, avoid drawing a blood sample for an APTT from an area proximal to the site of heparin infusion.
- Monitor the PT in all patients on warfarin sodium to check adequacy, and educate the patient about drug interactions.
- Correct hypovolemia, acidosis, and shock promptly and start treatment for sepsis if there is no obvious cause for a DIC.
- Intravenous streptokinase may be associated with allergic reactions; symptoms generally develop within a few minutes of starting the drug. Protamine sulfate, when given intravenously to neutralize excess heparin, may cause an anaphylactic reaction.
- If DDAVP is used to improve hemostasis, IV fluids must be reduced for about 12 to 18 hours after the last dose of DDAVP and the patient monitored for hyponatremia.

NATIONAL CONTACTS

Refer to the American Society of Hematology or the International Society of Thrombosis and Hemostasis directory for experts in your local area.

ACKNOWLEDGMENTS

I am grateful to my colleagues, Drs. E.R. Cole and W.F. Fried, for their incisive comments; and to Mrs. C.M. Lambert for her patience and typing skills.

REFERENCES

1. McKay, D.G.: Disseminated intravascular coagulation: An intermediary mechanism of disease. New York, Harper and Row, 1965, p. 1–493.
2. Hardaway, R.M.: Syndromes of disseminated intravascular coagulation with special reference to shock and hemorrhage. Springfield, Il., Charles C Thomas, 1966, p. 1–466.
3. Bachmann, F.: Disseminated intravascular coagulation. Dis. Mon. Chicago, Il., Year Book Medical Publishers Inc., Dec. 1969, p. 3–44.
4. Colman, R.W., Robboy, S.J., Minna, J.D.: Disseminated intravascular coagulation. A reappraisal. Annu. Rev. Med. 30:359, 1979.
5. Marder, V.J., Martin, S.E., Francis, C.W., et al.: Consumptive thrombo-hemorrhagic disorders. In Hemostasis and Thrombosis. Basic Principles and Clinical Practice, 2nd ed. Edited by Colman, R.W., et al. Philadelphia, J.B. Lippincott Co., 1987, p. 975.
6. Colman, R.W.: Surface mediated defense reactions: The plasma contact activation system. J. Clin. Invest. 73:1249, 1984.
7. Rylatt, D.B., Blake, A.S., Cottis, L.E., et al.: An immunoassay for human D dimer using monoclonal antibodies. Thromb. Res. 31:767, 1983.
8. Dairaku, M., Sueishi, K., Tanaka, K.: Disseminated intravascular coagulation in newborns: Prevalence in autopsies and significance as a cause of death. Pathol. Res. Pract. 174:106, 1982.
9. Corrigan, J.J., Jr., Ray, W.L., and May, N.: Changes in the blood coagulation system associated with septicemia. N. Engl. J. Med. 279:851, 1968.
10. Spero, J.A., Lewis, J.H., and Hasiba, U.: Disseminated intravascular coagulation: Findings in 346 patients. Thromb. Haemost. 43:28, 1980.
11. Pineo, G.F., Regoeczi, E., and Hatton, M.W.C.: The activation of coagulation by an extract of mucus: A possible pathway of intravascular coagulation accompanying adenocarcinomas. J. Lab. Clin. Med. 82:225, 1973.
12. Owen, C.A., Jr., and Bowie, E.J.W.: Chronic intravascular coagulation syndromes. A summary. Mayo Clinic Proc. 49:673, 1974.
13. Feinstein, D.I.: Diagnosis and management of disseminated intravascular coagulation: The role of heparin therapy. Blood 62:288, 1982.
14. Blauhut, B., Kramar, H., Vinazzer, H., et al.: Substitution of antithrombin III in shock and DIC: A randomized study. Thromb. Res. 39:81, 1985.
15. Ratnoff, O.D.: Epsilon aminocaproic acid—A dangerous weapon. N. Engl. J. Med. 180:1124, 1969.
16. Amorosi, E.L., and Ultmann, J.E.: Thrombotic thrombocytopenic purpura: Report of 16 cases and review of the literature. Medicine 45:139, 1966.
17. Bukowski, R.M.: Thrombotic thrombocytopenic purpura: A review. Prog. Hemost. Thromb. 6:287, 1982.
18. Shepard, K.V., and Bukowski, R.M.: The treatment of thrombotic thrombocytopenic purpura with exchange transfusions, plasma infusions and plasma exchange. Sem. Hematol. 24:178, 1987.
19. Gordon, L.I., Kwaan, H.C., and Rossi, E.G.: Deleterious effects of platelet transfusions and recovery thrombocytosis in patients with thrombotic microangiopathy. Semin. Hematol. 24:194, 1987.
20. Stenflo, J., Fernlund, P., Egan, W., et al: Vitamin K dependent modifications of glutamic acid residues in prothrombin. Proc. Natl. Acad. Sci. U.S.A. 7:2730, 1974.
21. Suttie, J.W.: Metabolism, and properties of a liver precursor to prothrombin. Vitam. Horm., 32:463, 1974.
22. Martinez, J., Palascak, J.E.: Hemostatic alterations in liver disease. In Zakim, D., et al (eds); Hepatology. A Textbook of Liver Disease. Philadelphia, W.B. Saunders, 1982, p. 546.
23. Blanchard, R.A., Furie, B.C., Jorgensen, M., et al.: Acquired vitamin K-dependent carboxylation deficiency in liver disease. N. Engl. J. Med. 305:242, 1981.
24. Rake, M.O., Flute, P.T., Panell, G., et al.: Intravascular coagulation in acute hepatic necrosis. Lancet 1:1533, 1970.
25. Stein, S.F., and Harker, L.A.: Kinetic and functional studies of platelets, fibrinogen and plasminogen in patients with hepatic cirrhosis. J. Lab. Clin. Med. 99:217, 1982.
26. McKenna, R., and Jensen, D.: Unpublished observations from a randomized prospective trial of saline versus low dose heparin in prevention of thrombosis in LeVeen shunts.
27. Kobrinsky, N.L., Israels, E.D., Gerrard, J.M., et al.: Shortening of bleeding time by 1-deamino-8-arginine vasopressin in various bleeding disorders. Lancet 1:1145, 1984.
28. Manucci, P.M., Vicente, V., Vianello, L., et al.: Controlled trial of desmopressin in liver cirrhosis and other condition with a prolonged bleeding time. Blood 67:1148, 1986.
29. Suttie, J.W.: Mechanism of action of vitamin K: Synthesis of γ-carboxyglutamic acid. Crit. Rev. Biochem. 8:191, 1980.
30. Olson, R.E.: Vitamin K. In Hemostasis and Thrombosis. Basic Principles and Clinical Practice, 2nd ed. Edited by Colman, R.W., et al. Philadelphia, J.B. Lippincott Co., 1982, p. 846.
31. Ansell, J.E., Kumar, R., and Deykin, D.: The spectrum of vitamin K deficiency. JAMA 238:40, 1977.
32. Lipsky, J.J.: N-Methyl-thio-tetrazole inhibition of the gamma carboxylation of glutamic acid: Possible mechanism for antibiotic-associated hypoprothrombinemia. Lancet 2:192, 1983.
33. Edmunds, L.H., Jr., and Addonzio V.P., Jr.: Extracorporeal circulation. In Hemostasis and Thrombosis. Basic Principles and Clinical Practice, 2nd ed. Edited by Colman, R.W., et al. Philadelphia, J.B., Lippincott Co., 1982, p. 901.
34. Bachmann, F., McKenna, R., Cole, E.R., et al.: The hemostatic mechanism after open heart surgery. J. Thorac. Cardiovasc. Surg. 70:76, 1975.
35. McKenna, R., Bachmann, F., Whittaker, B., et al.: The hemostatic mechanism after open heart surgery. J. Thorac. Cardiovas. Surg. 70:298, 1975.
36. Shulman, N.R., and Jordan J.V., Jr.: Platelet immunology. In Hemostasis and Thrombosis. Basic Principles and Clinical Practice, 2nd ed. Edited by Colman, R.W., et al. Philadelphia, J.B. Lippincott Co., 1982, p. 452.
37. Aster, R.H., and George, J.N.: Thrombocytopenia due to enhanced platelet destruction by immunologic mechanisms. In Hematology, 4th ed. Edited by Williams, W.J., et al. New York, McGraw-Hill, 1990, p. 1370.
38. Murphy, S., and Gardner, F.H.: Platelet preservation: Effect of storage temperature on maintenance of platelet viability-del-

eterious effect of refrigerated storage. N. Engl. J. Med. *280*:1094, 1969.

39. Krevans, J.R., and Jackson, D.P.: Hemorrhagic disorder following whole blood transfusions. JAMA *159*:171, 1955.
40. Counts, R.B., Haisch, C., Siuron, T.L., et al.: Hemostasis in massively transfused trauma patients. Ann. Surg. *190*:91, 1979.
41. Miller, R.D., Robbins, T.O., Tong, M.J., et al.: Coagulation defects associated with massive blood transfusions. Ann. Surg. *174*:794, 1971.
42. Shattil, S.J., and Bennett, J.S.: Acquired qualitative platelet disorders. *In* Hematology, 4th ed. Edited by Williams, W.J., et al. New York: McGraw Hill, 1990, p. 1420.
43. Deykin, D., Janson, P., and McMahon, L.: Ethanol potentiation of aspirin-induced prolongation of the bleeding time. N. Engl. J. Med. *306*:852, 1982.
44. Fernandez, F., Goudable, C., Sie, P., et al.: Low hematocrit and prolonged bleeding time in uraemic patients: Effect of red cell transfusions. Br. J. Haematol. *59*:139, 1985.
45. Janson, P.A., Jubeliner, S.J., Weinstein, M.S., et al.: Treatment of bleeding tendency in uremia with cryoprecipitate. N. Engl. J. Med. *303*:1318, 1980.
46. Livio, M., Manucci, P.M., Vigano, G., et al.: Conjugated estrogens for the management of bleeding associated with renal failure. N. Engl. J. Med. *315*:731, 1986.
47. Norman, C.S., and Provan, J.L.: Control and complications of intermittent heparin therapy. Surg. Gynecol. Obstet. *145*:338, 1977.
48. Habbab, M.A., and Haft, J.I.: Heparin resistance induced by intravenous nitroglycerin. A word of caution when both drugs are used concomitantly. Arch. Intern. Med. *147*:857, 1987.
49. O'Reilly, R.A., and Aggeler, P.M.: Determinants of the responses to oral anticoagulant drugs in man. Pharmacol. Rev. *22*:35, 1970.
50. Hull, R., Hirsh, J., Jay, R., et al.: Different intensities of oral anticoagulant therapy in the treatment of proximal vein thrombosis. N. Engl. J. Med. *307*:1676, 1982.
51. Hirsh, J., Poller, L., and Deykin, D.: Therapeutic range for the control of oral anticoagulant therapy. Chest *89*:11, 1986.
52. Marder, V.J., and Bell, W.R.: Fibrinolytic therapy. *In* Hemostasis and Thrombosis. Basic Principles and Clinical Practice, 2nd Ed. Edited by Colman, R.W. et al. Philadelphia, J.B. Lippincott Co., 1982, p. 1393.
53. Triplett, D.A.: Laboratory diagnosis of lupus anticoagulants. Semin. Thromb. Hemost. *16*:182, 1990.
54. Giangiacomo, J., and Tsai, C.C.: Dermal and glomerular deposition of IgA in anaphylactoid purpura. Am. J. Dis. Child. *131*:981, 1977.
55. Gottlieb, A.J.: Allergic purpura. *In* Hematology, 4th ed. Edited by Williams, W.J., et al. New York, McGraw Hill, 1990, p. 1443.
56. Comp, P.C.: Clinical implications of the protein C/protein S system. Ann. N.Y. Acad. Sci. *509*:149, 1987.
57. Green, D.: Protein C and protein S. *In* Clinical Thrombosis. Edited by Kwaan, H.C., et al. Florida, CRC Press, 1989, p. 243.
58. McKenna, R.: Personal observations.

HEMOPHILIA AND ALLIED DISORDERS

Wadie F. Bahou, Paula L. Bockenstedt, and David Ginsburg

CAPSULE

The hemophilias and von Willebrand's disease (vWD) are the most common congenital bleeding disorders in man.[1-3] Because of the potentially serious acute and long-term consequences of hemorrhagic episodes, rapid diagnosis and institution of appropriate measures are necessary to minimize patient morbidity and mortality. Over the past two decades, tremendous progress has been achieved in the purification and preparation of human plasma products, supplying physicians with a broad armamentarium of readily available therapeutic options. Partially offsetting these advances in therapy is the high prevalence of human immunodeficiency virus (HIV) infections in frequently transfused patients. Although this complicating factor rarely influences the emergency treatment of bleeding episodes, the physician should be alert to potential manifestations of the acquired immunodeficiency syndrome (AIDS), and appropriate precautions must be maintained to minimize exposure to allied health personnel. The mainstays of therapy in bleeding patients involve precise diagnosis of the congenital disorder, assessment of complicating factors (i.e., presence of inhibitor antibodies), and initiation of the appropriate form of replacement therapy.

INTRODUCTION

Congenital disorders of hemostasis characteristically involve a deficiency or functional abnormality of a single coagulation protein with familial transmission of the defect. Hemophilia A accounts for approximately 80 to 90% of the hemophilias, and is caused by an inherited deficiency of the procoagulant Factor VIII (FVIII), also known as the antihemophilic factor. This disorder is X-linked recessive, so that female carriers (heterozygotes) transmit the disorder to half of their sons and the defective allele to half of their daughters. Female carriers may manifest mild hemorrhagic tendencies, not infrequently seen in the postpartum state. In *approximately 25 to 30% of cases,* hemophilia A is caused by spontaneous mutations, and *no family history is obtainable.* Factor IX deficiency (hemophilia B) is clinically indistinguishable from FVIII deficiency, and is also an X-linked recessive disorder. Management of bleeding episodes involves a different concentrate than that used for hemophilia A. Factor XI deficiency is a rare and generally mild autosomal recessive bleeding disorder that occurs primarily in Jews of European descent (Ashkenazi). Not infrequently, it may present later in life as persistent postsurgical or post-traumatic hemorrhage. Congenital deficiency of factors V, VII, X and prothrombin is extremely rare. Congenital factor XII deficiency should not be confused with hemophilia, is usually asymptomatic, and paradoxically may predispose to thrombotic tendencies.

Von Willebrand's disease is an autosomal dominant disorder that may affect up to 1% of the general population. It is generally a mild hemostatic defect, although rare severely affected individuals have hemorrhagic patterns similar to those of patients with severe hemophilia.

PATHOPHYSIOLOGY

Normal hemostatic responses to injury include vasoconstriction and platelet plug formation as an immediate response, with subsequent activation of the

coagulation cascade and fibrin clot formation. Von Willebrand factor (vWF) is a large multimeric adhesive glycoprotein that is produced in endothelial cells and megakaryocytes, and acts as a primary mediator of platelet adhesion to the subendothelium in areas of vessel wall injury. It circulates in plasma as a noncovalently linked complex with FVIII, thereby playing a critical role in maintaining stability of the latter protein. Patients with quantitative (Type I) or qualitative (Type II) disorders of vWF exhibit a bleeding tendency that is clinically similar to that seen in patients with primary platelet disorders (primary hemostatic defect). FVIII serves as a cofactor in the activation of Factor X by Factor IXa in the intrinsic pathway of coagulation. Deficiencies of this protein serve as the prototype for hemostatic defects associated with procoagulant deficiency. Unlike vWD or primary platelet defects, which are associated with skin and mucosal bleeding, disorders of the coagulation cascade frequently involve visceral, intra-articular, and intramuscular hemorrhages. Fibrin clot formation is delayed, and the absence of this firm meshwork results in a more prolonged and potentially serious hemorrhagic state. The pattern of bleeding correlates relatively well with the baseline procoagulant activity (Table 53-18).

ASSESSMENT AND STABILIZATION

The introduction of factor concentrates and the advent of home self-therapy programs have revolutionized

TABLE 53-18. CLINICAL CHARACTERISTICS OF HEMOPHILIA AND VON WILLEBRAND'S DISEASE

	Hemophilia	vWD
Family history	Positive in approximately 75% of individuals	Usually positive
Inheritance	X-linked recessive	Autosomal dominant
Type of bleeding	Intra-articular, visceral and intramuscular deep hematomas; frequently after trauma	Mucosal surfaces (frequently epistaxis), skin (petechiae and ecchymoses), menorrhagia in females
Duration	Delayed after trauma and persistent	Immediate after trauma, short-lived
Local pressure	Not effective, except with minor lacerations	May stop bleeding
Severity of bleeding associated with FVIII coagulant activity		N/A
25–50%	May occur after major trauma.	
5–24% (Mild)	Severe bleeding after surgical procedures and some bleeding after trauma, no spontaneous bleeding.	
1–4% (Moderate)	Severe bleeding after injury, occasional spontaneous hemorrhage.	
<1% (Severe)	Severe hemophilia with spontaneous bleeding into muscles and joints.	

health-care management of patients with hemophilia. Early outpatient therapy of bleeding disorders has remarkably altered the quality of life, and secondarily led to a high level of patient sophistication. Because of patients' familiarity with their disease, the physician *should not hesitate to discuss the proposed treatment plan* and alternative options. Not infrequently, admission to an Emergency Department (ED) is prompted by continual bleeding not responsive to standard outpatient regimens, the need for evaluation of unusual bleeding sites, or for a life-threatening hemorrhage. In patients with a well-established diagnosis of hemophilia, *prompt evaluation and replacement therapy* are indicated.

INITIAL ASSESSMENT AND DIFFERENTIAL DIAGNOSIS

Hemophilia should be suspected if there is an X-linked inheritance pattern in the patient, a positive family history, a lifelong disorder, and a characteristic pattern of bleeding (Table 53-18). Laboratory testing should confirm the diagnosis. In patients with hemophilia, the bleeding time, platelet count, thrombin time, and prothrombin time are usually normal. The characteristic abnormality is an isolated prolongation of the activated partial thromboplastin time (aPTT), the hemostatic test designed to evaluate the integrity of the intrinsic pathway of coagulation. Specific factor assays establish the diagnosis, and should correlate with the level of severity. Concomitant prolongation of the bleeding time may suggest outpatient ingestion of platelet-inhibiting agents (aspirin, nonsteroidal anti-inflammatory agents, etc.), or an alternative diagnosis (von Willebrand's disease). Isolated prolongation of the aPTT is also characteristic of deficiencies of Factors IX, XI and XII, which may be confirmed by specific factor assays. Isolated prolongation of the aPTT with no prior bleeding history suggests either a previously unrecognized mild form of hemophilia or an acquired inhibitor to a coagulation protein. The failure of the aPTT to normalize when incubated at 37°C in a 1:1 mix with normal plasma ("mixing study") is presumptive evidence for the presence of an inhibitor. Such inhibitors are usually directed against FVIII, and may be associated with the postpartum state, lymphoma, or medication (diphenylhydantoin), or may be idiopathic in nature. The lupus anticoagulant may also present with an isolated aPTT abnormality, but is infrequently associated with a hemorrhagic diathesis.

The diagnosis of vWD rests on a high index of suspicion in the appropriate clinical setting because standard testing fails to confirm the diagnosis in up to 30% of patients. In most patients, the bleeding time and aPTT are prolonged, and the diagnosis is established by documenting approximately 50% or greater reductions in vWF antigen, FVIII coagulant activity, and ristocetin cofactor activity. Precise classification

may be established by multimer gel analysis, usually performed by specialty reference laboratories.

SITES OF HEMORRHAGE

HEMARTHROSES

Spontaneous bleeding into joints occurs in severe hemophiliacs, but those with hemophilia of any severity may develop bleeding with trauma. The joints most frequently involved (in order of descending frequency) are the knees, elbows, ankles, shoulders, hips, and wrists. An "aura" lasting up to several hours may precede the onset of bleeding, and usually consists of a vague warmth or tingling sensation. If treatment is not instituted promptly, the joint becomes progressively painful, range of motion becomes limited, and joint swelling and cutaneous warmth become evident. Early intervention before the development of severe joint impairment delays the onset of chronic synovitis, a process that predisposes the joint to recurrent hemorrhage.[4] Ice and elastic bandages are often helpful to such patients, and additional support to the ankles may be given with firm, high-laced boots. Short-term splinting may relieve pain, but long-term splinting is unnecessary and may delay recovery of normal range of motion. If a bleeding episode progresses to cause tense distention of the joint, orthopedic consultation followed by aspiration may be indicated after replacement therapy is given, and should be followed by a firm elastic bandage. Although aspiration is generally unnecessary with prompt and adequate replacement therapy, it should be seriously considered with a distended hip hemarthrosis to prevent the development of avascular necrosis of the femoral head. Osteomyelitis should be suspected in a chronically painful joint, and the diagnosis established by plain films and radionuclide scanning (Fig. 53-15). Acute septic arthritis may be difficult to differentiate from hemorrhage, and diagnostic aspiration may be performed after factor replacement and orthopedic consultation.

HEMATOMAS

Hematomas are either subcutaneous or intramuscular, and may follow even trivial episodes of trauma. Bleeding into the deep muscles may cause fever, leukocytosis, severe pain, and hyperbilirubinemia, and not infrequently leads to delayed skin discoloration. With sufficient blood loss, anemia or rarely shock may complicate untreated bleeding episodes. Muscle and subcutaneous hemorrhage in the extremities is especially dangerous if it occurs within a closed compartment. Optimal management of such hemorrhages should include appropriate factor replacement with careful neurovascular checks to obviate the development of a *compartment syndrome*. Upper extremity bleeding should be complemented with elevation and splinting

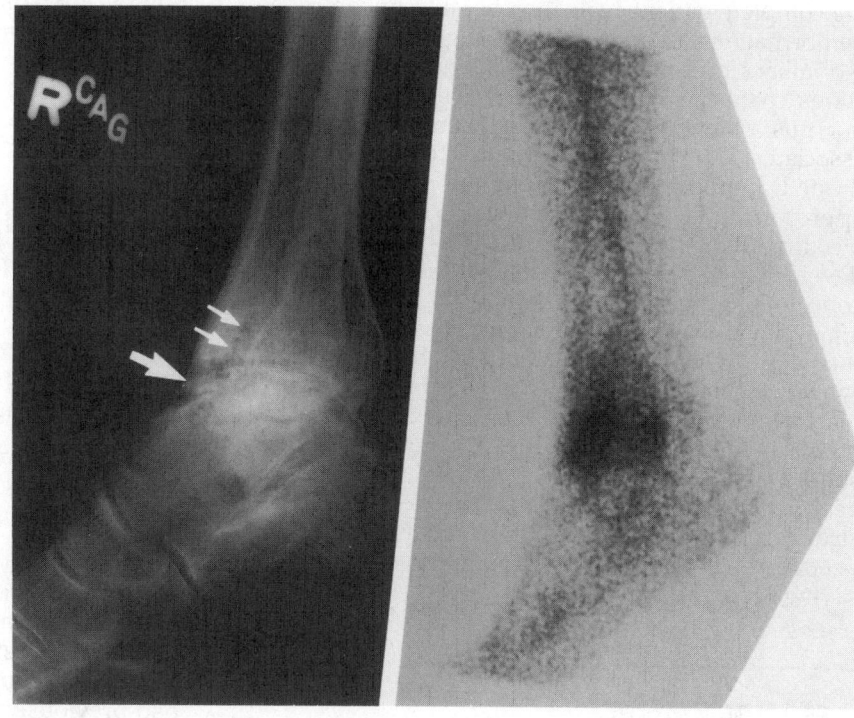

FIG. 53-15. A patient with severe hemophilia A complained of progressive pain and swelling of his right ankle that did not respond to factor infusion. A. X ray of the ankle reveals narrowing of the articular surface of the ankle joint (large arrow) and subchondral cystic changes (small arrows) typical of hemophilic arthropathy. B. ⁹⁹ᵐtechnetium radionuclide scanning reveals tracer uptake in the tibia that extends more superiorly than is usually seen with hemophilic arthropathy. Although not pathognomonic, the history and diagnostic studies are more consistent with acute osteomyelitis superimposed on chronic hemophilic arthropathy.

A   **B**

of the involved arm. Surgical intervention with fasciotomy may be required if a compartment syndrome complicates management. *Psoas muscle* or *retroperitoneal hematomas* may cause pain in the abdominal lower quadrant (which may mimic appendicitis if it occurs on the right) or pain referred to the groin (which may be mistaken for hemarthrosis of the hip). Iliopsoas muscle hemorrhage is associated with loss of hip extension, whereas an intra-articular hip hemarthrosis is associated with a greater loss of internal rotation. Referred pain to the anterior surface of the thigh from femoral nerve compression, with resultant loss of deep tendon reflexes, may also be observed. A flat plate of the abdomen may reveal loss of the involved psoas shadow, and the diagnosis confirmed by pelvic ultrasound or CT scan. Rarely, repeated hemorrhage into the soft tissue or bones results in the development of a *pseudotumor*, which may require surgical extirpation.

HEMATURIA

More than half of hemophiliacs experience at least one episode of hematuria, which is usually painless, renal in origin, and occasionally associated with colic from a ureteral or renal pelvis clot. Intravenous pyelography is generally safe, although not necessarily indicated unless hematuria is chronic or recurrent. Use of the antifibrinolytic agents epsilon-aminocaproic acid (EACA, Amicar) or tranxemic acid is contraindiated in such situations because of the risk of preventing the lysis of clots, which may then obstruct the collecting system.

OTHER SITES OF HEMORRHAGE

Gastrointestinal hemorrhage is unusual and should prompt the physician to search for an associated underlying disease. Rarely, *submucosal intestinal hemorrhage* may present as acute abdominal pain. A high index of suspicion, along with confirmation by plain film, ultrasound, or CT scan should confirm the diagnosis.

Prolonged *gingival hemorrhage* is common with eruption of new teeth or following instrumentation. EACA is usually sufficient to control the hemorrhage, and infusion of factor concentrates is required only occasionally. Epistaxis in a severe hemophiliac is not unusual, although an associated nasal lesion should be suspected in mild hemophilia.

HAZARDOUS BLEEDING AREAS

Intracranial hemorrhage and *retropharyngeal hemorrhage* represent potentially life-threatening situations that require immediate attention. Retroperitoneal bleeding may also be lethal because of persistent hemorrhage into a surreptitious site (see previous text). A history of head trauma may be obtained in approximately 50% of patients with intracranial bleeding; subarachnoid hemorrhage carries a better prognosis than intracerebral hemorrhage. Patients who sustain even minimal head trauma should be admitted for observation and, in most cases, treated prophylactically with factor replacement for at least 24 hours if the CT scan reveals no evidence of intracranial hemorrhage. *Appropriate factor replacement should not be delayed* pending complete patient evaluation because uncontrolled hemorrhage is associated with a high mortality. Hemophiliacs presenting to the ED with acute mental status changes should be fully evaluated for central nervous system (CNS) bleeding, meningitis, or HIV-associated CNS opportunistic infections. When indicated, lumbar puncture should be performed after appropriate factor replacement. Retropharyngeal bleeding frequently accompanies pharyngitis, or may develop after suturing of gingival margins without concomitant replacement therapy. In the latter situation, blood may dissect down into the soft tissues of the neck, giving rise to a potentially obstructing pharyngeal hematoma. Patients may subjectively complain of discomfort, swelling, or inability to swallow their saliva. A soft-tissue lateral x ray of the neck should help confirm the diagnosis of a retropharyngeal hematoma, and delineate the extent of the obstruction. With appropriate replacement therapy, the need for a tracheostomy—although potentially life-saving—may be obviated.

MANAGEMENT

Therapy of coagulation factor deficiencies is based on replacement of the missing factor with plasma, purified plasma fractions, or concentrates (see Type of Replacement Therapy in subsequent text). Because concentrates are prepared from pooled plasma derived from thousands of donors, various methods have been instituted to minimize the risks associated with viral contamination (hepatitis and HIV). Such methods include dry heat, pasteurization (heating in aqueous solution), treatment with organic solvent/detergent solutions, and most recently immunoaffinity chromatography.[5] Preliminary studies suggest that these methods may eliminate some or all of the viral risks, although identification of a clearly superior product must await more exhaustive clinical testing.[6] The choice of products available to the practitioner is generally restricted by the policies of individual hospital formularies.

The optimal dose is determined by certain general principles, such as the location and extent of the bleeding, the potential danger to the patient, and the half-life of the factor. The duration of therapy also varies with different clinical situations. The dose of replacement factor is calculated in units. One unit is defined as the amount of factor found in 1.0 mL of pooled, normal plasma, and is equivalent to 100% clotting factor activity. Both FVIII and vWF have half-lives of approximately 8 to 12 hours, whereas Factor IX has a larger volume of distribution and a longer half-life of 18 to 24 hours. When prolonged treatment is required, the appropriate dose is generally repeated at these intervals or may alternatively be administered by continuous infusion with monitoring of the specific factor coagulant activity to maintain the desired replacement level.

DOSAGE CALCULATION

The dose of factor replacement may be readily calculated by applying the following calculation:

1. One unit of FVIII per kg of body weight raises the patient's plasma level by 2%,

   OR

2. One unit of FIX per kg of body weight raises the patient's plasma level by 1%.

Because of the cost of these products (up to one dollar per unit), the actual amount infused should be rounded off to the nearest reconstituted vial.

Example: A 36-year-old, otherwise healthy man with hemophilia A is admitted to the ED complaining of progressive pain and swelling of his left knee. The bleeding had started 24 hours previously, at which time the patient self-infused 1400 units of FVIII. He had previously undergone a right prosthetic knee replacement for hemophilic arthropathy. His physical examination is remarkable primarily for deformities of both elbows and right ankle, consistent with his chronic hemophilic synovitis. The left knee is slightly warm and erythematous, with readily palpable soft tissue swelling of the joint, and limited range of motion. Because of his debilitating arthropathy, you assume that he has severe disease with less than 1% coagulant activity. You order a FVIII assay and inhibitor screen, wrap and ice the joint, and initiate a treatment plan that would result in a level of 50%, with a calculation as follows:

> 25 units per kg × 70 kg = 1750 units. The vials each contain 300 units, and the patient is infused with 1800 units (6 vials).

TYPE OF REPLACEMENT THERAPY

The form of replacement depends on the degree of severity (mild, moderate, severe) and the clinical situation. Other considerations should include prior hepatitis exposure, hepatitis B vaccination status, and human immunodeficiency status. In general, patients with mild or moderate hemophilia should be managed with donor-designated cryoprecipitate or DDAVP (described subsequently) whenever possible. As previously mentioned, however, the newer viral attenuation methods seem to be highly effective in eradicating contaminating organisms, and these products may become the standard form of replacement if their safety record is confirmed with further clinical experience. Consultation with a blood bank or a hematologist familiar with these products and with treatment of such patients should be obtained whenever possible.

The resultant search for pharmacologic compounds to replace blood products for the management of hemophilia A and vWD has led to the clinical application of a vasopressin analog as an effective alternative in certain clinical situations. Desmopressin (DDAVP, 1-deamino-8-D-arginine vasopressin) has been shown to reduce bleeding during dental extractions or surgical procedures in patients with mild or moderate hemophilia A or vWD. At a dose of 0.3 mg/kg IV, FVIII and vWF increase on the average two to four times above basal levels. Because of considerable patient variability, prior response to DDAVP should be documented before its use. In known responders, DDAVP should be considered the initial agent of choice in select clinical situations in mild or moderate hemophiliacs and in patients with Type I vWD.[7] It is generally ineffective in hemophiliacs or vWD patients with severe disease, and may be contraindicated in patients with certain qualitative forms of vWD. Table 53-19 highlights the features of the various preparations and their clinical indications.

THERAPEUTIC RECOMMENDATIONS

Although a certain dogma exists about therapeutic regimens for hemophilia, variability in the disease and in the bleeding episodes mitigate against a clear consensus. For example, adequate therapy for many bleeding episodes may be two thirds to one half the conventional dose if given within 4 hours of bleeding.

A proposed treatment schedule with general guidelines is outlined in Table 53-20.

ADJUVANT DRUG THERAPY

Symptomatic control of painful bleeding episodes may necessitate the use of analgesics as adjuvant measures. Because aspirin inhibits platelet aggregation and prolongs the bleeding time, it should not be used in patients with vWD or hemophilia. Acetaminophen, codeine, or other more potent narcotics may be safely used for pain control. In general, the nonsteroidal anti-inflammatory drugs (NSAIDs) may also interfere with platelet function in vivo. For this reason, these agents should be used primarily for control of chronic arthritis, and not for pain control during acute bleeding episodes. Of the NSAIDs, ibuprofen and naproxen are generally well tolerated, and associated with few hemorrhagic episodes. Concomitant use of alcohol should be strongly discouraged. Steroids have been used safely at doses of 1 to 2 mg/kg/day, and may be used for their anti-inflammatory effect.

MANAGEMENT OF PATIENTS WITH INHIBITORS

Approximately 10 to 15% of patients with severe hemophilia A develop inhibitor alloantibodies that neutralize exogenously transfused FVIII. This development is far less common in patients with hemophilia

TABLE 53-19. PLASMA REPLACEMENT PRODUCTS AND THEIR INDICATIONS

	Enriched in	Approximate Concentrations	Indications	Limitations/Toxicity
Fresh frozen plasma	All factors	0.7–1 IU/mL of each factor	Any congenital bleeding disorder Factor XI deficiency	Replacement limited by volume in patients w/severe disease
Cryoprecipitate	I, VIII, vWF, XIII	80–100 U FVIII/10 cc bag	von Willebrand's disease Hemophilia A	Viral hepatitis unless from donor-designated pool Rare allergic reactions
Factor VIII concentrates	VIII	Specified by manufacturer	Hemophilia A	Viral hepatitis; large doses of intermediate purity may cause hemolytic anemia in recipients with Type A or B blood from contaminating isohemagglutinins
Factor IX concentrate (Prothrombin complex concentrate)	II, VII, IX, X	25 IU/mL	Hemophilia B Hemophilia A patients with inhibitors	Viral hepatitis Potentially thrombogenic Should be used with caution in patients with pre-existing liver disease or vascular disease
Porcine factor VIII	VIII	Specified by manufacturer	Hemophilia A patients with inhibitors	Allergic reactions
DDAVP	—	—	Type I vWD* Mild/moderate Hemophilia A*	Tachyphlaxis with recurrent use. Possible hyponatremia/fluid overload

* Patients should have trial infusion of 0.3 micrograms per kg to establish efficacy.

TABLE 53-20. GENERAL GUIDELINES FOR TREATMENT OF BLEEDING EPISODES

Clinical Situation	Hemophilia A Desired Level	Hemophilia B Desired Level	Additional Recommendations	Moderate to Mild vWD*
Mild hemorrhage (Early hemarthrosis or hematoma; epistaxis, hematuria, or dental bleeding unresponsive to EACA)	30–40%	20–30%	1. Ice, elastic bandage 2. Repeat infusion following day if joint still painful 3. Consult orthopedist for aspiration if hemorrhage is extensive, if hip is involved, or if problem persists longer than 1 week.	DDAVP†§
Mucosal hemorrhage (Mouth, deciduous teeth)	30–40%#	20–30% Treatment as per hemophilia A, although if Factor IX concentrate is used, wait 6–8 hrs prior to EACA initiation	1. EACA§‖ × 6D 2. May use DDAVP simultaneously 3. If tooth is loose, extract and give factor replacement	DDAVP†§ with EACA‖
Epistaxis	30–40%#	20–30% See hemophilia A	1. Bilateral pressure for 30 minutes 2. If unsuccessful, pack with thrombin-soaked gauze 3. EACA as above 4. Replacement if above fail	DDAVP†§
Hematuria	30–40%#	20–30% Treatment as in hemophilia A	1. Bed rest, force fluids 2. Prednisone 2 mg/kg (maximum 60 mg) × 2 days 3. If no response after 1–2 days, initiate factor replacement 4. EACA contraindicated	DDAVP†§
Major hemorrhage (hemarthrosis with pain and swelling, gastrointestinal)	50%	40% As per hemophilia A	Consult hematologist for long-term recommendations	Cryoprecipitate 20 u/kg
Life-threatening hemorrhage (CNS, retropharyngeal or retroperitoneal bleed; major trauma, "compartment syndromes")	80–100%	60–80% As per hemophilia A	Consult hematologist for long-term recommendations	Cryoprecipitate 20 u/kg

* Use cryoprecipitate 20 u/kg for severe disease or in patients with Type IIB vWD.
† DDAVP 0.3 mg/kg in 25–50 cc NS IVPB over 15 minutes. May be repeated at 12 hour intervals prn. Usage limited to patients with previously demonstrated response.
§ If unresponsive to more conservative measures.
# Epsilon-aminocaproic acid (EACA) 200 mg/kg po loading dose, then 100 mg/kg po Q6H (Adults: 8–12 g loading followed by 4–6 g Q6H. If ineffective, use cryoprecipitate 20 u/kg. May be repeated at 8–12 hour intervals.

Special Situations
Guidelines for managing hemophilia patients who require surgery.

Recommendations

1. Invasive procedures (L P, paracentesis, joint aspiration, etc.)	Give one dose calculated to raise patient's plasma level to 100% 1 hour before
2. Minor surgical procedures	Dose to 50–100% level 1 hour before surgery, then maintain 30–50% level for 4–5 days post-operatively.**
3. Major surgical procedures	Dose to 100% level 1 hour before surgery, then maintain 40–60% level for 5–7 days, followed by 20–30% level for 5–7 days.**
4. Dental procedures	Give EACA 200 mg/kg 4 hours before surgery and 100 mg/kg Q6H for 7 days. Give factor to 40–60% 1 hour before surgery if block anesthesia is required. May repeat factor replacement in 1–2 days if procedure is extensive.

** May use continuous infusion drip. Follow FVIII levels 1–2 times daily.

B or severe vWD. Although these antibodies may be transient, reappearance may occur with repeated exposure. Their presence should be suspected in any bleeding episode that does not respond to factor replacement, or in a patient whose aPTT or FVIII coagulant assays do not respond to appropriate replacement therapy. Most clinical laboratories quantify the level of these inhibitors by the Bethesda assay, with results reported in Bethesda units (BU). Patients with low-titer (< 10 BU per mL) antibodies are less likely to develop an anamnestic response to factor replacement than are high-titer inhibitor patients (> 10 BU

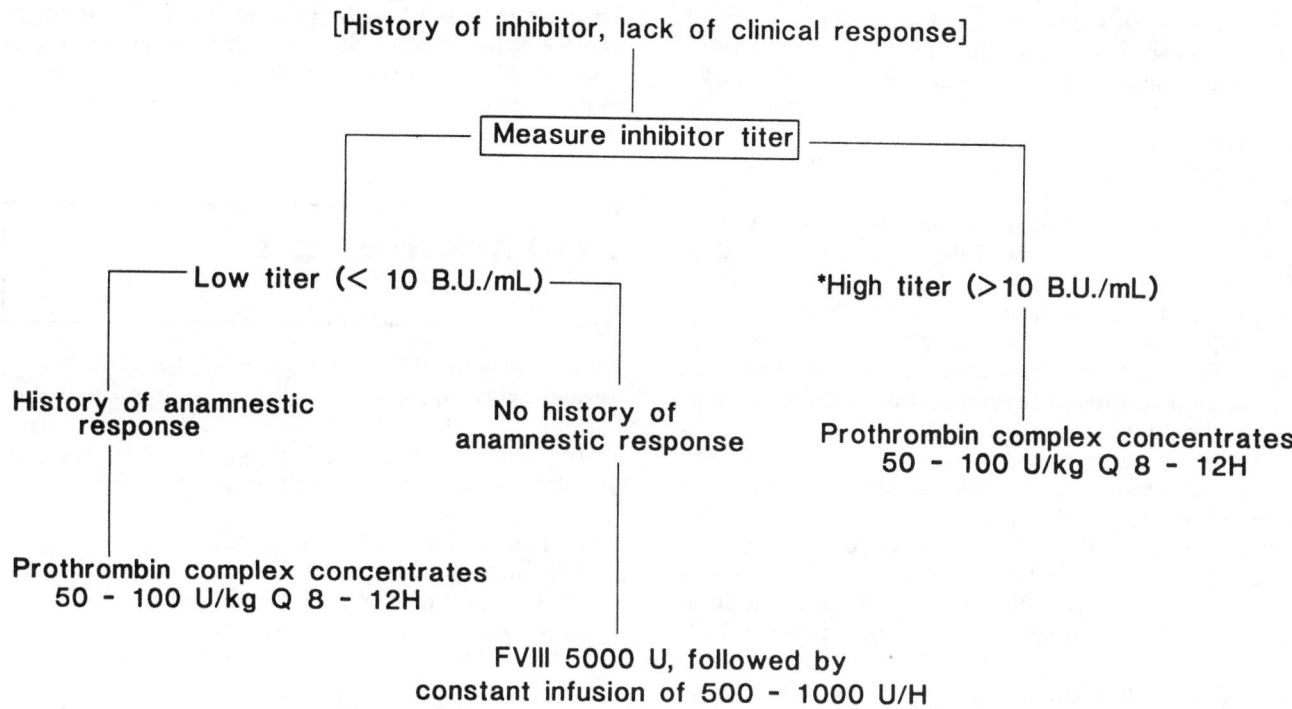

[History of inhibitor, lack of clinical response]

Measure inhibitor titer

Low titer (< 10 B.U./mL)

*High titer (>10 B.U./mL)

History of anamnestic response

No history of anamnestic response

Prothrombin complex concentrates 50 - 100 U/kg Q 8 - 12H

Prothrombin complex concentrates 50 - 100 U/kg Q 8 - 12H

FVIII 5000 U, followed by constant infusion of 500 - 1000 U/H

*Consider porcine FVIII, high dose FVIII in life-threatening situations

FIG. 53-16.   *Management of FVIII inhibitor patients.*

per mL). Low-titer inhibitor patients may generally be treated with conventional therapy (at higher doses), whereas those with high-titer inhibitors may be treated with prothrombin complex concentrates (PCC) (which are thought to "bypass" the inhibitor), pharmacologic doses of FVIII or porcine factor VIII.[8] The general management of these patients is outlined in Figure 53-16. Because the care of these patients is complex, the assistance of a hemophilia center is highly recommended.

COMPLICATIONS

Occasionally patients develop allergic reactions to cryoprecipitate or fresh frozen plasma, rarely associated with bronchospasm or anaphylaxis. Such side effects are uncommon in patients receiving concentrates, and prior reactions to plasma products do not preclude use of these concentrates. Rarely, patients who are IgA-deficient may develop anaphylaxis when infused with plasma products, although this adverse toxicity is not limited to hemophiliacs. Headache and abdominal pain may be seen with concentrate usage and are related to the rate of infusion. Large doses of FVIII concentrates, as typically used in patients undergoing surgery or involved in major trauma, may

cause a Coombs-positive hemolytic anemia because of the simultaneous transfer of high-titer anti-A or anti-B antibodies in the concentrate. If severe red blood cell (RBC) destruction is observed, steroids and infusion of Type O blood may control the hemolysis. Commercial concentrates prepared by immunoaffinity chromatography have no significant titer of isohemagglutinins.

As previously mentioned, prothrombin complex concentrates (PCCs) and activated prothrombin complexes (aPCCs) may be indicated in patients with inhibitors to factor VIII and with hemophilia B. Both these products are associated with thrombotic risks, sometimes complicated by disseminated intravascular coagulation (DIC). This risk is increased in patients at prolonged bed rest or those with underlying hepatocellular dysfunction. In addition, concurrent administration of PCCs with antifibrinolytic agents (EACA or tranxemic acid) is generally contraindicated for similar reasons. High-risk patients should be periodically monitored for incipient DIC, mobilized if at all possible, and the efficacy of the products confirmed before repeated infusions.

Viral infections are a frequent cause of morbidity for patients receiving pooled plasma products. The great majority of hemophiliacs have detectable levels of hepatitis B surface antibody, documenting prior exposure to this virus. Only a minority (approximately 5%) are chronic carriers, however. Newly diagnosed hemophiliacs should receive the hepatitis B vaccine to minimize this risk. Persistent mild elevation of transaminases is observed in most treated hemophiliacs. Histopathologic examination of small cohorts reveals a pattern of chronic persistent hepatitis most consistent with non-A, non-B hepatitis. Prevalence estimates for chronic active hepatitis are as high as 20 to 30% in some studies.

Human immunodeficiency virus (HIV) syndromes represent the most serious long-term health threat to the hemophiliac population. Three separate studies using the enzyme-linked immunosorbent assay (ELISA) for presence of HIV antibody confirmed that 50 to 90% of hemophiliacs intensively treated with factor concentrates were seropositive by 1984, and that approximately half converted during 1981 and 1982. Duration of seropositivity and age are probably the most important determinants of the actuarial incidence of acquired immunodeficiency syndrome (AIDS), which is 18% at 6 years in one reported study.[9] The clinical manifestations of AIDS are discussed in more detail in Chapter 50. Because of state and federal regulations concerning patient rights of privacy, HIV status may not be readily available to health care personnel providing medical care to hemophiliacs. The emergency physician should take all appropriate measures to minimize possible exposure to other members of the ED staff. Caution in handling factor concentrates should also be emphasized to all involved medical personnel. Fortunately, the risk of HIV infection to seronegative patients has been reduced markedly—if not eliminated—by newly implemented donor screening practices and by the refinement of methods to inactivate the thermolabile virus.

HORIZONS

Blood banking technology has had a tremendous impact on quality-of-life issues for most hemophiliacs. These advances in treatment modalities have been clouded by the morbidity associated with transfusion-associated hepatitis, and more recently by the devastating impact of HIV-related illnesses. Improved donor screening, viral detection, and viral attenuation methods have recently been successfully implemented, although the absolute efficacy of these methods is still being investigated. Greater sensitivity in the detection of non-A, non-B-infected blood products should be achieved with the recent molecular identification of the causative agent.

The isolation and cloning of the genes for factors VIII and IX allow application of DNA technology to mass-produce recombinant factor in unlimited supply that should theoretically be free from contaminating human viruses. Successful infusion of one such product (FVIII) in hemophiliacs has been reported and appears to be functionally comparable to its human plasma counterpart.[10] Although liver transplantation

has been used as a curative modality in highly selected patients with hemophilia, this approach has minimal general applicability. Gene replacement therapy is currently in its infancy, but may eventually offer a feasible method for definitive therapy.

NATIONAL CONTACTS

Over 100 centers in the United States specialize in providing comprehensive care to patients with hemophilia. A Directory of Hemophilia Treatment Facilities may be obtained through the National Hemophilia Foundation at the following address:

The National Hemophilia Foundation
The SoHo Building
110 Greene Street, Room 406
New York, New York 10012
212–219–8180

REFERENCES

1. Coller, B.S.: Von Willebrand's disease. *In* Hemostasis and Thrombosis. Basic Principles and Clinical Practice. Edited by Colman, R., Hirch, J., Marder, V., and Salzman, E. Philadelphia, J.B. Lippincott Company, 1987.
2. Levine, P.: Clinical manifestations and therapy of hemophilias A and B. *In* Hemostasis and Thrombosis. Basic Principles and Clinical Practice. Edited by Colman, R., Hirch, J., Marder, V., and Salzman, E. Philadelphia, J.B. Lippincott Company, 1987.
3. Ruggeri, Z., and Zimmerman, T.: Von Willebrand factor and von Willebrand disease. Blood *70*:895, 1987.
4. Brettler, D., Forsberg, A., O'Connell, F., et al.: A longterm study of hemophilic arthropathy of the knee joint by a program of factor VIII replacement given at time of each hemarthrosis. Am J. Haematol. *18*:13, 1985.
5. Brettler, D., and Levine, P.: Factor concentrates for treatment of hemophilia: Which one to choose? Blood 73:2067, 1989.
6. Schimpf, K., Mannucci, P., Kreutz, W., et al.: Absence of hepatitis after treatment with a pasteurized factor VIII concentrate in patients with hemophilia and no previous transfusions. N. Engl. J. Med. *316*:918, 1987.
7. De la Fuente, B., Kasper, C., Rickles, F., and Hoyer, L.: Response of patients with mild and moderate Hemophilia A and von Willebrand's disease to treatment with desmopressin. Ann. Intern. Med. *103*:6, 1985.
8. Sjamsoedin, J., Heijnen, L., Mauser-Bunschoten, E, et al.: The effect of activated prothrombin-complex concentrate FEIBA on joint and muscle bleeding in patients with hemophilia A and antibodies to factor VIII: A double-blind clinical trial. N. Engl. J. Med. *305*:717, 1981.
9. Goedert, J., Kessler, C., Aledort, L., Biggar, R., et al.: A prospective study of human immunodeficiency virus Type I infection and the development of AIDS in subjects with hemophilia. N Engl. J. Med. *321*:1141, 1989.
10. White, G., McMillan, C., Kingdon, H., and Shoemaker, C.: Use of recombinant and antihemophilic factor in the treatment of two patients with classic hemophilia. N. Engl. J. Med. *320*:166, 1989.

THROMBOCYTOPENIC DISORDERS

Steve Hulsey and Joseph C. Howton

CAPSULE

Platelets are integral to hemostasis. A low platelet count may lead to life-threatening hemorrhage. The thrombocytopenic patient may present to the Emergency Department (ED) with obvious external bleeding or subtle hemorrhage in the eye, central nervous system (CNS) or gastrointestinal (GI) tract. A thorough history is essential to narrow the differential, which is divided into defects in platelet production, disorders of peripheral destruction, sequestration, and platelet loss. Stabilization of the platelet-deficient patient involves quick attention to the ABCs, a careful search for occult bleeding, and possible transfusion of platelets and other blood products. ED evaluation should include routine laboratory tests, review of the peripheral smear, and a search for infection and DIC. Management beyond initial stabilization is usually carried out by the specialist.

PATHOPHYSIOLOGY

Platelets are anucleate 1 to 2 μg blue bodies with red and purple Giemsa-stained granules. They are fragments of megakaryocyte cytoplasm produced in bone marrow which mature from a multipotential stem cell. Platelet production can be augmented up to eightfold in times of thrombocytopenia. The normal platelet count is 150,000 to 400,000 per mm^3. That of thrombocytopenia is a count below 100,000. There is an approximate relation between the number of platelets and the severity of bleeding. Patients with >40,000 platelets may bleed after injury or surgery, but spontaneous hemorrhage is unlikely. Levels of 20,000 to 30,000 lead to common spontaneous bleeding, whereas with levels below 10,000, bleeding is usual and often severe. Platelet number remains stable throughout life. The exact regulatory mechanism, however, is not fully understood. Thrombopoetin, synthesized in the kidney, can directly stimulate platelet production, but is clearly not the only factor. Platelets normally live for 8 to 12 days, and clearing of senescent platelets occurs primarily in the marrow, but also in the liver and spleen. The exact mechanism

of platelet aging and death is unknown. One third of the total platelet pool is normally sequestered in the spleen and exchanges freely with the general circulation.

Immediate hemostasis depends on vasoconstriction of the vessel wall and plug formation by aggregated platelets. Maintenance of the clot consists of fibrin made from the coagulation cascade. In response to vascular damage, platelets adhere to the subendothelium, using the von Willebrand factor as a bridge. Platelet activation occurs through ADP or thrombin and ultimately forms a receptor for fibrinogen. This produces aggregation. The clustered platelets then release their granular contents, which aid in hemostasis, and actinomycin retracts the clot. Platelets also play a key role in coagulation by providing surface features for the cascade system.

CLINICAL PRESENTATION

HISTORY

In narrowing the differential of a thrombocytopenic patient, one needs to take a careful history of exposure to drugs and environmental toxins. Patients may neglect to mention over-the-counter medications unless they are specifically asked. Some drugs may be part of nonmedical products, including quinine in gin and tonic and antibiotics in food. Patients should be asked about recent transfusions. In the review of systems, attention should be paid to symptoms of headache in regard to CNS hemorrhage, visual changes for retinal bleeding, epistaxis (frequent and prolonged), melena or hematemesis, bleeding from gums, hematuria, and menorrhagia. Most importantly, patients must be asked about petechiae and ecchymoses.

Thrombocytopenic bleeding occurs most often in the skin and mucosal surfaces and is spontaneous. If bleeding occurs after mild trauma, it is immediate and relatively short-lived, with local pressure usually successful in hemostasis. The family history of similar events is usually negative. On the other hand, bleeding from coagulation cascade defects after trauma is delayed and usually occurs in the form of deep hematomas in the viscera, joints, and muscle. Local pressure is often ineffective.

PHYSICAL EXAMINATION

Petechiae are painless, 1 to 3 mm, round red or brown lesions secondary to hemorrhage into the skin. They occur primarily in areas of high venous pressure such as the lower legs and those where clothing constricts. They do not blanch, which may be discerned by compressing with a microscope slide. Ecchymoses are red, purple, blue, or yellow; of various sizes; tender; and possibly elevated. A careful fundoscopic exam is important to rule out retinal hemorrhage. The oral mucosa should be checked for hemorrhagic bullae (classic for thrombocytopenic bleeding). A palpable spleen is almost always a significant finding but easy to miss, whereas the normal liver may be palpable up to 5 cm below the lower costal margin.

DIFFERENTIAL DIAGNOSIS

PRODUCTION DEFECTS (Insufficient Megakaryocyte Number or Poor Platelet Production)

In *aplastic anemia*, numbers of all cell lines are decreased. Cause of the acquired form stems from exposure to drugs, toxins, and ionizing radiation. The hereditary *Fanconi syndrome* usually presents at age 6 to 8 years. *Thrombocytopenia with absent radius, and Wiskott-Aldrich and May-Hegglin anomaly* are examples of hereditary stem cell defects that affect only the platelet line and may be associated with other bodily malformations. Pancytopenia secondary to *infiltration* by tumor or fibrosis may also occur. *Drugs, alcohol, and infection* can produce a marrow with inadequate megakaryocytes but sufficient in other cells. *Thiazides* can cause thrombocytopenia in some patients by their toxicity to megakaryocytes. *Ethanol* decreases platelet lifespan, but also impairs the marrow's ability to increase production.[1] Alcoholic thrombocytopenia reverses within 1 to 3 weeks after abstinence. A reversible thrombocytopenia may also be associated with *estrogen* use. *Cyclic thrombocytopenia*, a disorder found in otherwise normal women, has in some studies been associated with the 2 weeks before menstruation. The thrombocytopenia may rarely become severe, but abnormal bleeding is unusual. *Vitamin B12, folate, and iron deficiency, paroxysmal nocturnal hemoglobinuria, renal failure, and hyperbaric oxygen* may cause ineffective platelet production from initially normal megakaryocytes.[2] In hyperbaric exposure, there is a progressive decrease in platelet levels to about 75% of normal over 3 days.

PLATELET DESTRUCTION (Abundant Normal Megakaryocytes, Short Platelet Life)

IMMUNE FORM

Immune thrombocytopenic purpura (ITP) is a common disorder in which an IgG produced in the spleen and marrow binds to platelets. Antibody-covered platelets are trapped in the monocyte-macrophage system and destroyed. ITP may have a genetic predisposition. The acute form (permanent remission <3 months) is seen in children (peak age 2 to 9 years) and young adults and is common after a viral illness. It usually presents with sudden bleeding from the gingiva and the genitourinary (GU) or GI tract, and florid purpura and petechiae of a few days duration. The chronic form, most common in adults, has also recently been found prevalent in HIV risk groups.[3] With rapid platelet destruction, minor changes in production (drugs, infection) can cause dangerously low platelet levels. *Drug-induced platelet destruction* is clinically indistinguishable from ITP, and therefore a thorough drug history must be taken. Numerous drugs have been reported to cause immunologic thrombocytopenia. Many of these reports may be coincidental. The most common offending agents are quinine, quinidine, heparin, and gold salts. Other possible drugs include sulfonamides, rifampin, and indomethacin. The mechanism is not firmly understood but probably involves coating of platelets by the drug or drug/antibody complex. Except for the possible HLA association with gold salts, there is no way to predict who will develop the reaction.[4,5] There are two types of *heparin thrombocytopenia.*[6] The mild form occurs within 5 days of exposure and usually requires no treatment. The severe form begins a few days later and may be associated with arterial thrombosis. The thrombosis is probably caused by aggregation of antibody-coated platelets. A thrombocytopenic purpura has recently been noticed in *chronic narcotic abusers*, many who had not injected for months. Average platelet count was 53,000 and associated with elevated levels of antiplatelet IgG.[7] Low platelets have also been found in homosexual men, with a large percentage positive for *HIV*.[8] *Post-transfusion purpura* occurs 2 to 10 days after transfusion of a product containing platelets. It occurs mainly in women over 40 and leads to severe thrombocytopenia (often <10,000). The pathophysiology is obscure, but may be secondary to a genetically determined antigen which is lacking in affected patients.

NON-IMMUNE FORM

Distinction between the immune and nonimmune forms is somewhat arbitrary because of the poorly understood mechanisms of many thrombocytopenic disorders. Much overlap exists. Possible nonimmune mechanisms include vessel wall abnormalities causing platelet activation, blood agglutinating agents and hyperthrombinemia causing DIC.

Erythroblastosis fetalis, prematurity, pre-eclampsia, and large hemangiomas are disorders causing congenital nonimmune platelet destruction.[9] *Thrombotic thrombocytopenic purpura (TTP) and hemolytic uremic syndrome (HUS)* may be a spectrum of one disease. TTP is a life-threatening illness occurring in adults (peak incidence at age 25) with five major manifestations:

1. Severe hemolytic anemia with marked fragmentation of RBCs and high LDH
2. Thrombocytopenia with increased megakaryocytes and short platelet survival
3. Fever
4. Fluctuating CNS symptoms from headache to coma
5. Renal disease. HUS has many similarities to TTP, but occurs in infancy and early childhood.

In HUS, the renal involvement is severe, whereas the CNS manifestations are mild. Many pathophysiologic mechanisms are postulated for TTP/HUS, but none are proven. An abnormality of small vessels is the primary lesion. There may also be a deficiency of platelet aggregation inhibition. A rarer adult form of HUS occurs, predominantly in postpartum patients and those using birth control pills.[10] *Disseminated intravascular coagulation (DIC)* causes thrombocytopenia. Activation of the coagulation cascade from various stimuli produces high levels of thrombin. Thrombin activates platelets, aiding intravascular coagulation and decreasing platelet numbers. *Infection* can cause thrombocytopenia through DIC, but also through a separate, poorly understood mechanism. Examples of infections associated with thrombocytopenia are listed in Table 53-21. Approximately 15% of *pre-eclampsia* patients experience moderate thrombocytopenia. The bite of certain species of *snakes* can produce a severe form. This is sometimes caused by DIC, but may also be secondary to platelet-activating proteins in venom. The *hypoxic state* as seen in cyanotic heart disease, adult respiratory distress syndrome (ARDS), chronic obstructive pulmonary disease (COPD), and burns over more than 10% of the body surface area, and *renal transplant rejection* can lead to a nonimmune thrombocytopenia. The mechanism in these cases is probably trapping of platelets in damaged tissue.

PLATELET SEQUESTRATION

Hypersplenism from various causes usually produces moderate thrombocytopenia without significant bleeding problems unless there is an associated coagulopathy. Sequestration of up to 90% of circulating platelets is secondary to an increase in the splenic vascular bed with resulting slow passage through sinus channels. The spleen must be easily palpable to

TABLE 53-21. INFECTIONS ASSOCIATED WITH THROMBOCYTOPENIA	
Varicella	Dengue
Mononucleosis	Malaria
Mumps	Typhus
Herpes	Tuberculosis
CMV	Histoplasmosis
Gram-negative sepsis	Rocky Mountain spotted fever
Bacterial endocarditis	
Toxic shock	

cause significant thrombocytopenia. Platelet production is increased only up to twofold because the body's total number of platelets is not decreased.[11] *Hypothermia* has been noted to produce platelet levels as low as 30,000. The suspected mechanism is sequestration in the liver and spleen and platelet clumping. A body temperature below 35° C is required. Platelet levels are rarely severe enough to cause bleeding, and rise to normal within 1 to 2 weeks after rewarming.[12]

PLATELET LOSS

Bleeding with subsequent *transfusion* causes a washout of functioning platelets. The degree of thrombocytopenia is directly related to the number of transfusions, and may become clinically significant after 10 units of stored blood. If it is untreated, the low platelet levels persist for 3 to 5 days.

INITIAL STABILIZATION

Always remember to attend to the airway first. Obtain vital signs and completely undress the patient. Search for and tamponade any external bleeding sites with hand pressure over clean gauze. Do not use arterial or venous tourniquets unless absolutely necessary. Look carefully for occult bleeding from posterior epistaxis, oral hemorrhage, or rectal or vaginal bleeding. If you are unable to stop hemorrhage and unsure as to the patient's hemostatic defect, crystalloid should be infused rapidly to maintain circulatory balance. Blood should be ordered for type and cross match and requests placed for both platelets and fresh frozen plasma. If an immunologic mechanism is known or suspected, high-dose steroids (e.g., prednisone) may be given. If severe uterine bleeding is present, 25 mg conjugated estrogen IV may be helpful. These therapies are based on a widely held belief in steroid protection of platelets.

LABORATORY

An estimate of platelet number may be made on viewing the stained peripheral smear. In an oil immersion field, each platelet seen equals approximately 20,000/mm^3. Three to 10 platelets per oil field is an adequate count for hemostasis. Pseudothrombocytopenia, the agglutination of platelets in the transport tube, may falsely lower a normal platelet count, but is recognized on review of the smear. The integrity of the platelet plug is measured by the bleeding time. This is performed by inflating a blood pressure cuff to 40 mmHg around the arm, making three 1 cm incisions (with a standard device) on an avascular area of the forearm, and blotting until clotted. Normal time is less than 9.5 minutes. Most commonly, the platelet count is used to determine the risk of hemorrhage, but not all patients with severe thrombocytopenia bleed. Platelet size is also important because large platelets are hemostatically more active. New Coulter counters are capable of providing mean platelet volume, which may help in predicting the risk of hemorrhage in thrombocytopenic patients.

In patients with a history of exposure to a drug definitely known to cause thrombocytopenia, with a marrow rich in megakaryocytes, the clinician usually does not make any further attempt to prove the relationship. Other causes of thrombocytopenia must be ruled out, however. Diagnosis of ITP is one of exclusion. There is no readily available test for increased platelet destruction, although a rough estimate may be made by transfusion of six units of platelets. If the platelet count returns to baseline or below in less than 24 hours, increased removal is involved. The amount of platelet bound IgG is usually not increased in the nonimmunologic causes of platelet destruction. Blood cultures are important to exclude bacterial infection as a cause, through either direct effects or DIC. Urinalysis is used to evaluate for infection, pre-eclampsia, or renal disease.

Thrombocytopenia may be an early manifestation of the disorders listed in Table 53-22. Efforts should be made to exclude these diseases if the clinical picture is appropriate.

TABLE 53-22. DISEASES IN WHICH THROMBOCYTOPENIA MAY BE AN EARLY MANIFESTATION

Lymphoma/leukemia	Systemic lupus erythematosus
Thyrotoxicosis	Hashimoto's disease
Cancer	Scleroderma
Evans syndrome	Myasthenia gravis

MANAGEMENT

Management of the thrombocytopenic patient in the ED involves the following procedures:

1. Stop any current bleeding, stabilize, and transfuse if necessary.
2. Recognize the severity of thrombocytopenia and risk of hemorrhage.
3. Attempt to discern the cause of thrombocytopenia and ensure appropriate follow-up care.
4. Stop any possible offending agents.
5. Begin nutritional supplementation if implicated.

The approach to every disorder depends on the degree of thrombocytopenia and severity of hemorrhagic manifestations.

IDIOPATHIC THROMBOCYTOPENIC PURPURA

ITP is a relatively benign disorder with mortality of 1 to 5% (usually from intracranial hemorrhage). Risk of hemorrhage is greatest during the first 2 weeks. Steroids are used in mild cases, and interfere with macrophage phagocytosis of platelets and decrease synthesis of antiplatelet antibody. Long-term remission is reported in up to 20% of cases with steroids alone. Splenectomy, which eliminates the major site of platelet removal and antiplatelet antibody production, is indicated when steroids fail. Other interventions, for severe cases, include intravenous gamma globulin, plasmapheresis, and immunosuppressive agents.

THROMBOTIC THROMBOCYTOPENIC PURPURA

TTP mortality has been much reduced with the onset of newer therapeutic modalities. Remission rates of 60 to 80% have been achieved in recent years. Steroids are used early; aspirin and dipyrimadole may be given to block platelet aggregation. Severe TTP is treated with plasmapheresis. Splenectomy is controversial. Management of HUS is similar to that of TTP except that treatment of renal failure and hypertension may be required.

Post-transfusion purpura may last up to 6 weeks untreated. Steroids may be used and plasmapheresis is suggested in severe cases. For thrombocytopenia secondary to infection, pre-eclampsia, and sequestration, it is best to treat the primary disease. Drug-induced immune platelet destruction is primarily treated by removal of the offending agent, but if bleeding is severe or the course expected to be prolonged, steroids and/or chelation (as in gold salts) may be used. In combating heparin-induced thrombocytopenia, the best measure is to begin oral anticoagulants along with heparin. If heparin becomes a problem, it may then be discontinued without untoward effects. A level below 50,000/m³ is a basis for consultation if there is a known or potential bleeding site (e.g., GI, GU).

INDICATIONS FOR ADMISSION

Any patient with severe thrombocytopenia (levels below 10,000 to 20,000) or bleeding manifestations should be hospitalized. If the diagnosis is unsure, hospitalization and consultation are necessary.

PLATELET TRANSFUSIONS

Random donor platelets are those isolated from one unit of donor blood. It is not necessary to worry about ABO or Rh incompatibility, although HLA matching may be necessary in patients with a transfusion history because repeated transfusions can result in destructive antibody formation. They can be stored for 3 to 5 days at room temperature; chilling decreases their half-life. Fresh whole blood loses its platelet activity within several hours because of the chilling. Each unit of platelets raises the platelet count approximately 10,000 mm³ per m² of body surface area. For the average adult with 1.73 m² of body surface area, 10 units of platelets raise the count by approximately 50,000. Disorders of platelet destruction blunt this rise.

Indications for platelet transfusion:

1. Thrombocytopenia or prolonged bleeding time with life-threatening bleeding.
2. Massive stored blood transfusion (usually >10 units).
3. Acute leukemia with severe thrombocytopenia (possible benefit).

Transfusion of platelets in patients with ITP and hypersplenism is not effective because of consumption and pooling, but may be temporarily effective in controlling life-threatening bleeding. Transfusing platelets in patients with DIC, TTP, or heparin thrombocytopenia with thrombosis may actually be harmful because of the induction of further microvascular clotting. In life-threatening bleeding with thrombocytopenia, however, platelets are generally used. Be sure that any underlying condition (e.g., infection) is treated immediately.

Use standard macroaggregate filters in blood tubing for transfusion. In the bleeding patient, transfuse 6 to 8 units and repeat every 8 hours as needed. Fever and chill reactions are common and may be secondary to immunization by previous transfusions. It is not necessary to stop transfusion; nonaspirin antipyretics may be given.

DISCHARGE INSTRUCTIONS

If a thrombocytopenic patient is to be discharged, the patient should be instructed to:

1. Refrain from any activity that may produce bodily trauma.
2. Remain at bed rest, avoid Valsalva maneuvers, and keep stools loose if the platelet count is low.
3. Discontinue any possible offending agent.
4. Take no medications with antiplatelet activity.
5. Wear a medical-alert tag if thrombocytopenia is known to be secondary to a drug.
6. Return immediately if headache or new or worsening bleeding manifestations develop.

Careful follow-up should always be ensured.

PITFALLS AND MEDICOLEGAL PEARLS

- Never make the diagnosis of thrombocytopenia without review of the peripheral smear.
- It is not the absolute number of platelets which is most important clinically, but the bleeding manifestations.
- Take a thorough drug history in every thrombocytopenic patient.
- Always rule out sepsis and DIC in the platelet-deficient patient.
- You probably will not make the definitive diagnosis in the ED. Your job is to recognize the patient with low platelets, stabilize, rule out occult bleeding, hospitalize when necessary, and ensure careful follow-up care.

REFERENCES

1. Cowan, D.H.: Thrombokinetic studies in alcohol-related thrombocytopenia. J. Lab. Clin. Med. *81*:23, 1973.
2. Valeri, C.R., et al: Effects of hyperbaric exposure on human platelets. Aerospace Med. *45*:610, 1974.
3. DiFino, S., Lachant, N., Kirshner, J., and Gottlieb, A.: Adult idiopathic thrombocytopenic purpura. Am. J. Med. *69*:430, 1980.
4. Miescher, P.: Drug-induced thrombocytopenia. Semin. Haematol. *10*:311, 1973.
5. Miescher, P., and Graf, J.: Drug-induced thrombocytopenia. Clin. Haematol. *9*:505, 1980.
6. King, D., and Kelton, J.: Heparin-associated thrombocytopenia. Ann. Intern. Med. *100*:535, 1984.
7. Savona, S., et al.: Thrombocytopenic purpura in narcotics addicts. Ann. Intern. Med. *102*:737, 1985.
8. Walsh, C., Krigel, R., Lennette, E., and Karpatkin, S.: Thrombocytopenia in homosexual patients. Ann. Intern. Med. *103*:542, 1985.
9. Shim, W.: Hemangiomas of infancy complicated by thrombocytopenia. Am. J. Surg. *116*:896, 1968.
10. Ponticelli, C., et al.: Hemolytic uremic syndrome in adults. Arch. Intern. Med. *140*:353, 1980.
11. Cooney, D., and Smith, B.: The pathophysiology of hypersplenic thrombocytopenia. Arch. Intern. Med. *121*:332, 1968.
12. Gower, P.: Thrombocytopenia in hypothermia. Br. Med. J. *291*:23, 1985.

BIBLIOGRAPHY

Cuttner, J.: Thrombotic thrombocytopenic purpura: A ten-year experience. Blood 56:302, 1980.

Corrigan, J.J.: Thrombocytopenia: A laboratory sign of septicemia in infants and children. J. Pediatr. 85:219, 1974.

Ridolfi, R., and Bell, W.: Thrombotic thrombocytopenic purpura. Med. (Balt.) 60:413, 1981.

Counts, R.B., et al.: Hemostasis in massively transfused trauma patients. Ann. Surg. 190:91, 1979.

Eldor, A., et al.: Prediction of haemorrhagic diathesis in thrombocytopenia by mean platelet volume. Br. Med. J. 285:397, 1982.

Rubenstein and Federman (eds.): Scientific American Medicine. New York, Scientific American, Inc. 1989.

Oberman, H., et al. (eds.): General principles of blood transfusion. American Medical Association, 1985.

Isselbacher, et al. (eds.): Harrison's Principles of Internal Medicine (ninth edition). McGraw-Hill, 1980.

Williams, W., Beutler, E., Erslev, A., and Lichtman, M.: Hematology (third edition). New York, McGraw-Hill, 1983.

LEUKOCYTE DYSFUNCTION AND NEUTROPENIA

Martin R. Klemperer and Joseph C. Howton

CAPSULE

Of all the leukocyte disorders, neutrophil dysfunction is the most devastating. Alterations in the capacities of neutrophils to contain bacterial infections can occur by way of several mechanisms. There may be a decrease in the absolute number of neutrophils, a decreased capacity of the neutrophils to migrate to the site of infection, and a diminished ability to ingest bacteria or to kill ingested bacteria. Because neutrophils provide an important initial defense against bacterial infection, adequate neutrophil function is necessary to prevent disseminated bacterial disease. The fate of the septic patient with functional neutropenia may be determined by the rapidity with which they are given antibiotics. After an expeditious history and physical and the drawing of appropriate cultures, broad spectrum antibiotics should be administered emergently, particularly covering for gram-negative organisms. Further emergency department (ED) evaluation and preparation for admission may then proceed at a less hurried pace.

INTRODUCTION

Five types of circulating leukocytes are identified by their morphology on blood smears: neutrophils, eosinophils, basophils, lymphocytes, and monocytes. Inferences are often made regarding the severity of an illness based on the total leukocyte count and the differential expressed as a percentage. It is more precise to determine the absolute count of cells per milliliter of blood by multiplying the total leukocyte count by the percent value. The normal individual has an average of 3650 neutrophils per mL of blood. Neutropenia, an absolute neutrophil count of less than 2500 per mL, is the most common defect in adequate neutrophil function. Occasionally neutropenia occurs in healthy adults with no apparent cause, most often in black individuals.[1] Patients may be neutropenic, yet have elevated white blood cell counts (WBCs). In such cases, neutrophils constitute a minor percentage of the white blood cells.

The normal functions of neutrophils are phagocytosis, microbicidal action, digestion of foreign material, and chemotaxis. Various illnesses, including diabetes mellitus, uremia, and the collagen vascular diseases, may cause defects in neutrophil function. Tissue neutrophil response may be impaired by drugs such as glucocorticoids and alcohol, which inhibit neutrophil adherence to the vascular endothelium.

PATHOPHYSIOLOGY

Neutropenia is the most common pathogenic cause of decreased neutrophil function. Neutropenia is usually part of generalized marrow failure, resulting in decreased granulocyte pools. Therefore, most individuals who present with symptoms referable to neutropenia, such as infection, have evidence of a panmyelopathy.[2] The diseases in which widespread marrow dysfunction is present are characterized by decreased production. An example is aplastic anemia, in which a decrease in both the precursors and all mature formed elements of the blood is present.[3] In rarer causes, the committed neutrophil stem cell is absent or has variable proliferative capacity. These diseases are seen in children and result in chronic severe neutropenia, Kostman's agranulocytosis, or cyclic neutropenia.

The acute leukemias are the most common group of panmyelopathies. Neutropenia is common in acute lymphoblastic and in the acute nonlymphocytic leukemias. Although the bone marrow is usually hypercellular, production of normal blood elements is decreased.[4] Simplistically, the acute leukemias result in functional aplastic anemia.

Solid tumors may metastasize to the bone marrow and replace normal cellular elements. This displacement rarely causes significant peripheral neutropenia, but this may be present in children with neuroblastoma and rarely in adults with carcinoma of the breast or lungs. Metastatic tumors disrupt the marrow architecture and may be associated with the release of immature white blood cells as well as red blood cells. This is termed a "leukoerythroblastic reaction."

Adults and children with neoplastic disease commonly have episodes of transient neutropenia as a direct result of bone marrow toxicity caused by the administration of chemotherapy and radiation therapy. The nadir in granulocyte count usually occurs 10 to 21 days after the therapy, and then the count gradually returns to normal. Patients infected with HIV may develop significant neutropenia associated with the administration of AZT or trimethoprim-sulfamethoxazole. Individuals who have drug-induced neutropenia frequently have counts of less than 2000 per mL. Among the drugs most commonly implicated are sulfonamides, salicylates, phenylbutazone, antithyroid agents, and phenothiazines.[5,6]

Certain infections may be accompanied by neutropenia. Viral hepatitis, mononucleosis, measles, HIV, and many other viral illnesses may cause neutropenia. Typhoid, paratyphoid, tularemia, yellow fever, and rickettsial diseases have also been associated. These neutropenias are mostly mild and may be caused by redistribution of cells into an enlarged marginal pool. In overwhelming infections such as gram-negative bacteremia or miliary tuberculosis, neutropenia correlates with a poor prognosis.

Neutropenia may result from immune destruction of neutrophils through antineutrophil antibodies. Such antibodies are usually of IgG class and directed against specific neutrophil antigens. Destruction of the antibody-coated neutrophils occurs primarily in the fixed macrophages of the spleen and liver. In neonatal alloimmune neutropenia, the antibody of IgG class is of maternal origin. It is directed against paternal antigens present on the infant's neutrophils and transferred across the placenta. An autoimmune cause may bring about prolonged neutropenia because the antibody is produced by the patient. This condition is most frequently associated with connective tissue diseases such as systemic lupus erythematosus.

Severe neutropenia may be seen in patients with splenic sequestration as seen in Banti's syndrome, Gaucher's disease, Hodgkin's disease, and other lymphoreticular malignancies. Generally, the degree of neutropenia in patients with splenic sequestration is not below 1000 neutrophils per mL.

Chronic neutropenia without splenomegaly has been described in numerous conditions. Cyclic neutropenia is characterized by the periodic absence of neutrophils from the blood and bone marrow associated with fever, malaise, mouth ulcers, and cervical adenopathy. Patients are well between episodes, which usually occur in 21-day cycles. Symptoms usually begin in early childhood, although adult onset is occasionally seen. Chronic idiopathic neutropenia may have onset at any age; frequently the syndrome is recognized on a routine blood count. There is usually a family predisposition for the abnormality, and the patient may be asymptomatic despite neutrophil counts as low as 200 per mL.[7]

True disorders characterized by neutrophil dysfunction are exceedingly rare and are the result of several distinct pathophysiologic mechanisms. Disorders of chemotaxis, the accumulation of neutrophils in response to inflammation, are present in inherited disorders such as deficiencies of the membrane glycoproteins. In the *lazy leukocyte syndrome*, patients have gingivitis, stomatitis, and otitis with relatively few severe infections. Deficiencies in cellular enzymes or in the degranulation of neutrophil lysosomes are inherited disorders characterized by increased infections beginning in childhood. Among these rare disorders are chronic granulomatous disease, myeloperoxidase deficiency, severe glucose-6-phosphate-dehydrogenase deficiency, and Chediak-Higashi syndrome. In all of these diseases, the neutrophil count may be normal or elevated at the time of infection.

CLINICAL PRESENTATION AND EXAMINATION

The patient with dysfunctional neutrophils has no absolute physical findings to confirm the diagnosis. The condition may be suspected in any patient with recurrent infections such as stomatitis, or with a family history of frequent bacterial infections and early childhood deaths. Underlying illnesses such as malignancy and collagen vascular disease should be considered in directing the history and physical examination, and the patient should be questioned as to all medications he or she has taken. Timing of chemotherapy is relevant. Most chemotherapeutic agents have their lowest neutrophil count 10 to 21 days after administration except for the nitrosureas, which have their nadir at 4 to 6 weeks.

Patients with neutropenia caused by a lack of stem cells or myeloid progenitor cells have no positive findings attributable to their basic disease. Therefore, the findings of splenomegaly and generalized lymphadenopathy are more consistent with a diagnosis of malignant disease such as leukemia or lymphoma. This is particularly true of the patient who has purpura, either petechial or ecchymotic, and pallor. Patients with aplastic anemia of the Fanconi type may have skeletal anomalies such as short thumbs, abnormalities of the radii, microphthalmia, and abnormal pigmentation such as café-au-lait spots.

Most infected neutropenic patients are febrile except for the neonates and young infants who may present with hypothermia. Findings of localized infection should be sought, such as sinusitis, pneumonia, skin or perirectal abscesses, and meningitis. Tachycardia, hypotension, poor capillary filling of the nail beds, cool extremities, decreased urine output, and changes in consciousness are indications of septic shock.

INITIAL STABILIZATION

An ill-appearing patient with suspected neutropenia represents a medical emergency. The greatest im-

mediate threat to life is sepsis and resulting shock caused by the release of endotoxins and exotoxins. While a directed history and physical examination are performed, crystalloid infusion and pressors should be administered as needed to maintain adequate perfusion. Supplemental oxygen should be provided and the patient placed on a cardiac monitor. Appropriate cultures should be rapidly obtained, and the patient should be given broad spectrum antibiotics as quickly as possible. The choice of initial antibiotics is guided by patient characteristics (Table 53-23).

LABORATORY AND OTHER PROCEDURES

Any patient in whom a defect in neutrophil function is postulated should have a CBC with differential and platelet count obtained immediately. If the patient appears septic, blood cultures should be drawn from at least two different sites. If the patient has an indwelling, long-term central venous line such as a Hickman catheter, blood cultures should be obtained from the line as well. Additional blood should be sent to the laboratory for a chemistry panel, PT/PTT, fibrinogen and fibrin split products, type and crossmatch for packed RBCs. Cultures from additional sites such as sputum, pleural or joint effusions, open wounds, superficial abscesses, urine, and CSF should be planted for aerobic and anaerobic organisms as well as fungal cultures. Gram stain should be performed

TABLE 53-23. ANTIBIOTIC SELECTION IN THE FEBRILE NEUTROPENIC PATIENT*

Patient Characteristics	Antibiotics	Adult Dosage	Pediatric Dosage
No localizing findings	Ticarcillin plus Tobramycin	3 g q 4 hr given over ½ to 2 hr IV 3–5 mg/kg/d IV, divided q 8 hr	200–300 mg/kg/d IV divided q 4–6 h 6–8 mg/kg/d IV divided q 8 hr
Known high percentage gram-negative rod resistance (>80%) to first-choice therapy	Piperacillin or Mezlocillin or Ticarcillin-Clavulanate plus Amikacin	3 g q 4 hr given over ½ hr IV 3.1 g q 4–8 hr IV 15 mg/kg/day divided q 8 or q 12 hr IV	Not approved 200–300 mg/kg/d IV divided q 4–6 h 15–30 mg/kg/d IV divided q 8 h
Known Staphylococcus aureus carrier, previous staphylococcal infections, or central venous catheter.	Add Vancomycin	1 g q 12 hr IV	40–60 mg/kg/d IV divided q 6 h
Penicillin allergy immediate in type (good history) Delayed in type (or doubtful history)	Aztreonam plus aminoglycoside Ceftazidime plus aminoglycoside	2 g q 6 hr IV as above 1–2 g q 8–12 hr IV as above	Not approved, as above 100–150 mg/kg/d IV divided q 8 h as above
Renal failure	Piperacillin or mezlocillin plus single dose of aminoglycoside followed by double B-lactam (e.g., continue piperacillin, add ceftazidime); dose both according to renal function dosing nomograms		As above, but do not use piperacillin
Congestive heart failure	Piperacillin or mezlocillin or ceftazidime plus aminoglycoside	See above	As above

* Adapted with permission from Lauter, C.B.: Antibiotic therapy of life-threatening infectious diseases in the emergency department. Ann. Emerg. Med. *18*:1341, 1989.

on all suitable samples. Appropriate radiologic studies should be obtained.

In most cases of neutrophil dysfunction, the CBC is diagnostic. The presence of white cell blasts indicates a leukemic process. A decrease in the WBC count, platelet count and RBC parameters is highly suggestive of marrow failure. If neutropenia is associated with a decreased platelet count in which the platelets are large, an immunologic cause can be suspected. This is also true if spherocytes and polychromasia of the red cells is noted.

Functional neutrophil defects need metabolic studies such as nitroblue tetrazolium (NBT) reduction, chemiluminescence or specific enzyme assays performed to define the defect precisely. Defects in chemotaxis can be defined by in vitro tests of chemotaxis or by the Rebuck skin window technique. All of these require expert consultive support.

MANAGEMENT AND INDICATIONS FOR ADMISSION

A healthy-appearing individual who has the incidental finding of neutropenia on a CBC does not necessarily need admission. Similarly, a cancer patient in remission found to be neutropenic during the expected period following chemotherapy, who is afebrile and has no signs of infection, can usually be managed as an outpatient. It is generally advisable to consult with a hematologist or oncologist in either setting.

For the febrile, neutropenic patient, antibiotic treatment should be started with as little delay as possible. Coverage should be broad enough to include in the spectrum relatively resistant organisms such as Pseudomonas aeruginosa, Serratia marcescens, and Enterobacter species in addition to the more usual Escherichia coli and Klebsiella species. Most authorities recommend broad spectrum coverage consisting of an aminoglycoside in combination with an antipseudomonal penicillin (such as ticarcillin) or third-generation cephalosporin (cefoperazone or ceftazidime).[8–11] Gram-positive coverage with vancomycin is usually held in the absence of specific indications, such as the finding of an exudate around the exit site of a permanent indwelling venous catheter. The majority of catheter-related bacteremias in neutropenic patients can be successfully treated with appropriate antibiotics alone. Patients with infection extending along the subcutaneous tunnel tract of the catheter, however, should have the device removed expeditiously, because antibacterial therapy alone is generally inadequate in this circumstance.[8]

The concept of granulocyte transfusion for the infected neutropenic patient has been all but abandoned. Current transfusion technology does not allow the transfer of functional granulocytes in sufficient quantities to adequately replenish the neutropenic pa-

tient. Also, leukocyte transfusion carries inherent risks, such as transmission of CMV and toxoplasmosis and untoward interactions with drugs such as amphotericin B.

PITFALLS

Use of the WBC count for decision making in emergency medicine is problematic. One should never be lulled into a false sense of security by a "normal" leukocyte count in a patient suspected of bacterial infection. Factors such as overwhelming sepsis, nutritional deficiencies, or underlying malignancy may impair the expected neutrophil response.

MEDICOLEGAL PEARLS

The prevalence of automated Coulter counters has been a boon, enabling EDs to obtain CBC results rapidly. Many laboratories, however, do not perform a differential count in a timely manner on patients with a WBC in the normal range. In a patient with suspected neutrophil dysfunction, it is up to the emergency physician to insist that a manual differential be performed, even in the presence of a normal WBC count, and especially when the count is low.

HORIZONS

New antibiotics are continually being developed and refined, resulting in greater survival and fewer side effects. The recent introduction of imipenem-cilastin (a penem) and aztreonam (a monobactam) has increased the clinical choices available for managing patients with special needs. Patients with penicillin allergy, and hepatic or renal disease may now be treated optimally with minimum adverse effects.

Improvements in granulocyte transfusion technology may eventually rekindle interest in its use. In addition, a substance known as "granulocyte/macrophage colony stimulating factor" has been demonstrated in clinical trials to cure cyclic neutropenia and shorten the period of neutropenia in patients receiving chemotherapy.

REFERENCES

1. Karalycin, G., Rosner, F., and Switsky, A.: Pseudo-neutropenia in American Negroes. Lancet 2:387, 1972.

2. Athens, J.W., et al.: Leukokinetic studies IV. The total blood, circulating and marginal granulocyte pools, and granulocyte turnover rate in normal subjects. J. Clin. Invest. *40*:989, 1961.

3. Bottiger, L.E., and Bottiger, B.: Incidence and cause of aplastic anemia, hemolytic anemia, agranulocytosis and thrombocytopenia. Acta Med. Scand. *210*:475, 1981.

4. Boggs, D.R., Wintrobe, M.M., and Cartwright, G.E.: The acute leukemias: analysis of 322 cases and a review of the literature. Medicine *41*:163, 1962.

5. Young, G.A., and Vincent, P.C.: Drug-induced agranulocytosis. Clin. Haematol. *9*:438, 1980.

6. Miller, D.R., and Baehner, R.L. (eds.): Disorders of granulopoiesis. *In* Blood diseases of infancy and childhood., 6th Ed. St. Louis, C.V. Mosby Company, 1989.

7. Dale, D.C.: Abnormalities of Leukocytes. *In* Harrison's Principles of Internal Medicine, 11th Ed. Edited by Isselbacher, et al. New York, McGraw Hill.

8. Rubin, M., Hathorn, J.W., Pizzo, P.A.: Controversies in the management of febrile neutropenic cancer patients. Canc. Invest. *6*:767, 1988.

9. Van den Broek, P.J.: Infection control during neutropenia. J. Hosp. Infect. *11*:7, 1988.

10. Mitchell, C.D.: Management of infections in the neutropenic child with cancer. Pediat. Ann. *17*:680, 1988.

11. Lauter, C.B.: Antibiotic therapy of life-threatening infectious diseases in the emergency department. Ann. Emer. Med. *18*:1339, 1989.

POLYCYTHEMIAS

Eric Stirling

CAPSULE

The polycythemias are a broad group of disorders manifested clinically by symptoms of vascular congestion or compromise and chemically by an increased hemoglobin concentration and hematocrit. Emergency phlebotomy may be necessary in severe cases, and rapid differentiation of primary and secondary causes is critical to initiate management.

INTRODUCTION

The polycythemias are a relatively common group of disorders that cause increased hemoglobin concentration and hematocrit. The increased hematocrit reflects a state of increased viscosity, which causes many of the symptoms. Further investigation of an elevated hematocrit is necessary because the primary and secondary causes have markedly different management algorithms. In general, the severity of the symptoms determines the urgency of treatment. Absolute levels of the hematocrit demand treatment regardless of the presence or absence of symptoms to prevent serious morbidity.

PATHOPHYSIOLOGY

There are many causes of a decreased plasma volume with a normal absolute red cell mass (Table 53-24). Patients with major burns, acute severe dehydration (plasma volume decreases with red blood cells (RBCs) maintaining near normal volume), and pheochromocytoma have normal RBC mass and rarely manifest hyperviscosity syndromes or a hematocrit over 55%. Stress polycythemia (Gaisbock's syndrome) is found in stocky middle-aged men who usually develop hypertension and cardiac disease. The RBC mass is at the top of normal, and the plasma volume low. Smoker's polycythemia involves a high normal RBC volume and a decreased plasma volume. When polycythemia is chronic or with the onset of COPD (chronic obstructive pulmonary disease), the worsening hypoxia stimulates erythropoietin and RBC mass increases beyond the normal range.

A number of diseases have a common denominator of hypoxia. The renal sensors monitor tissue hypoxia, and erythropoietin is released. This appropriate release (Table 53-25) causes secondary erythrocytosis and an absolute increase in RBC mass. All the feedback loops are intact and resolution of the hypoxic state shuts off erythropoietin release. Cardiac patients presenting with high hematocrits must be separated into those who have an underlying primary erythrocytosis and those in whom tissue hypoxia drives erythropoietin. Symptoms are usually severe, with dyspnea at rest, cyanosis, clubbing, and class IV functional levels. A room air pO_2 of less than 65 mm Hg or a saturation of less than 90% is necessary to produce a high hematocrit. If the pO_2 or saturation is higher than these levels in patients with cardiac disease, and the hematocrit is over 60%, polycythemia vera is likely. The same values can be used to help differentiate the patient with recurrent pulmonary embolism who is suspected of having polycythemia vera as the underlying disease. High altitude causes increases in RBC mass and hematocrit. Levels start to rise in patients who live over 6000 feet (1830 meters). At 10,000 feet, an appropriate hematocrit for a man is 55%.

There are hundreds of hemoglobinopathies, which must be distinguished from polycythemia rubra vera (PRV). The platelet count, leukocyte count, and pO_2 are normal in these hemoglobinopathies. Measuring the p_{50} confirms the presence of an abnormal hemoglobin if it is low. Methemoglobinemia, if chronic, causes increased RBC mass. The chocolate appearance of whole blood in this condition is nearly diagnostic.

Heavy smokers not only have the relative polycythemia already described, but because of the chronic carbon monoxide poisoning, have increased RBC mass. Carboxyhemoglobin levels of 5 to 8% help to confirm the suspicion of smoker's polycythemia. The leukocyte and platelet counts should be normal and there should be no splenomegaly on physical examination before confirming smoking as the cause of the high hematocrit.

In some rare syndromes, erythropoietin is produced inappropriately (Table 53-26). In patients with a normal spleen, leukocyte and platelet counts, and normal pO_2s, a workup for renal disease or malignant syndromes should be undertaken.

PRV is a myeloproliferative disorder involving the pleuripotential stem cell and thus all cell lines. There is some epidemiologic suggestion that exposure to ionizing radiation plays a part in the origin of this disease. It is most often seen in patients 60 to 80 years old. The hyperviscosity syndrome and added underlying frequent atherosclerotic disease combine to produce transient ischemic attacks and deep lacunar infarcts. Thrombocytosis contributes to the high incidence of vascular thromboses, and a congestive hepatosplenomegaly is common. Without treatment, 50% of patients die within 18 months, usually from vascular disease. Myelofibrosis or leukemic degeneration follows if the vascular disease is not fatal.

PREHOSPITAL CARE

There is no current capability for diagnosing primary or secondary polycythemia in the field. Care is limited

TABLE 53-24. RELATIVE POLYCYTHEMIA/ DECREASED PLASMA VOLUME

Dehydration	Requires severe volume depletion
Stress polycythemia	Male, smoker, hypertension, coronary disease
Pheochromocytoma	Variable, mechanism unknown

TABLE 53-25. APPROPRIATELY INCREASED RED CELL MASS

COPD	pO_2 less than 65 mmHg, hypoxia Stimulated erythropoietin
CHF/AV shunt	Same mechanism as COPD
High altitude	Requires residence over 6000 feet
Hemoglobinopathies	SaO_2 normal, P_{50} and O_2 dissociation Curves abnormal

TABLE 53-26. INCREASED RED CELL MASS WITH INAPPROPRIATE ERYTHROPOIETIN

Renal disorders	Hydronephrosis, renal transplant, polycystic kidneys
Malignancies	Renal, ovarian, cerebellar, adrenal, leiomyomas

to support of the patient's cardiac and neurologic status. If the patient has altered mental status, the standard 25 g of 50% dextrose in H_2O and naloxone 2 mg IV are administered. Cardiac monitoring, supplemental oxygen, airway support, and vital signs are uniformly indicated. Phlebotomy is not indicated in the field, even in symptomatic patients with known PRV.

CLINICAL PRESENTATION

Patients complain of malaise, pruritus (without rash), burning feet, ulcer symptoms, and fullness in the head. Lesser symptoms include tinnitus, vertigo, increased sweating, and weight loss. During a crisis, neurologic syndromes from lacunar infarcts or hemorrhagic problems may occur. The physical examination usually shows plethora, engorged retinal veins, hypertension, scattered ecchymoses, and hepatosplenomegaly. Tender ribs and sternal areas are occasionally seen. Positive stool heme testing may occur in the presence of gastrointestinal hemorrhage.

DIFFERENTIAL DIAGNOSIS

The major problem in differential diagnosis is in separating primary from secondary causes of erythrocytosis. Once a significantly elevated hematocrit is discovered, the question of the relationship of the presenting symptoms to the elevation must be answered, and then the cause of the elevation. Because the hematocrit is universally available, the suspicion of elevation or the fortuitous discovery of the elevation is soon known.

INITIAL STABILIZATION

The patient presenting with cardiac, neurologic or hemorrhagic symptoms and findings needs ABCs, cardiac monitoring, and IV access. Secondary causes should have the underlying cause addressed as promptly and completely as possible. Phlebotomy is rarely needed unless the hematocrit is over 60%, and then only small amounts (250 cc) should be withdrawn. PRV patients should be phlebotomized 500 cc over 30 to 60 minutes with replacement of plasma volume by saline, and then worked up more thoroughly for the presenting problem (CT head scan, etc.). Symptomatic patients with PRV should be admitted, generally to a medical ward. ICU admission is necessary only if cardiac or neurologic instability warrants. The hematocrit needs reducing to 40 to 42% over a period of days. In the long term, phlebotomy alone results in a much higher rate of thrombotic complications than if radioactive phosphorus or chlorambucil is added to the program. Prophylactic aspirin or dipiridamole increases the hemorrhagic risk without reducing the thrombotic rate. With close management, median survival now exceeds 10 years.

LABORATORY AND OTHER PROCEDURES

In the Emergency Department (ED), the essential tests include the hematocrit, leukocyte count, platelet count, pO_2, and SaO_2. A hematocrit above 60% is 100% associated with an increase in the RBC mass. Between 50 and 60%, there is much overlap between the primary and secondary syndromes. In PRV, the platelet count is over 400,000 and the leukocyte count over 12,000 with a normal SaO_2 (Table 53-27). Renal and liver function tests are important adjuncts. Definitive

TABLE 53-27. DIAGNOSTIC CRITERIA FOR PRV	
Hematocrit	Over 50%, usually over 60%
RBC mass	Over 32 mL/kg in women, 35 mL/kg in men
Platelet count	Over 400,000
Leukocyte count	Over 12,000
SaO$_2$	Normal
Leukocyte alkaline phosphatase	Over 100 units
Serum B12	Over 900 pg/mL

tests include the RBC mass, neutrophil alkaline phosphatase, and serum B12 levels. Admission chest x ray and electrocardiogram, CT head scan if indicated, and appropriate tests for secondary causes complete testing. If emergency phlebotomy is needed, 500 cc should be withdrawn over 30 to 60 minutes, either in a standard blood bank donor setup or with sterile technique in 50 cc aliquots at the bedside. Close monitoring of vital signs is necessary.

PITFALLS

The patient who presents with pruritus is often relegated to a quick diphenhydramine prescription and referral. If no rash is present, the hematocrit is a simple and quick screen.

The patient with PRV who has been phlebotomized repeatedly becomes iron-deficient, with a reasonable hematocrit. The leukocyte and platelet counts may still be high, and thrombotic complications occur. History regarding the diagnosis of PRV must be sought.

Polycythemic patients undergoing emergency surgery may need more aggressive management of the hematocrit. Levels over 55% predispose to increased complications in the perioperative period. Consultation is often needed regarding phlebotomy under these circumstances.

The known PRV patient who nonspecifically feels "worse" must be assessed carefully for leukemic degeneration, which often has a subtle presentation.

MEDICOLEGAL PEARLS

The labeling of a PRV patient as a secondary erythrocytosis (for example, mistaking PRV for smoker's polycythemia) delays the diagnosis, and irreversible complications may occur.

The risk of moderately severe polycythemia (hematocrit 55 to 60%) is significant. If no urgent treatment is done, good documentation of phone consultation or a documented reason for nontreatment is essential.

BIBLIOGRAPHY

Adamson, J.W.: The polycythemias: Diagnosis and treatment. Hosp. Pract. *18:*49, 1983.

Berlin, N.I.: Diagnosis and classification of the polycythemias. Semin. Hematol. *12:*339, 1975.

Pearce, J.M.S., Chandrasekera, C.P., and Ladusand, E.J.: Lacunar infarcts in polycythemia with raised packed cell volumes. Br. Med. J. *287:*935, 1983.

Schrier, S.J.: Polycythemias. *In* Scientific American Medicine. Edited by Rubenstein, E. New York, Scientific American, 1989.

SICKLE CELL DISEASE

Elliott P. Vichinsky

CAPSULE

Sickle cell disease is a common medical problem that is characterized by sudden and life-threatening complications in a previously stable patient. Early and aggressive treatment of these acute events can dramatically improve patient survival. Many of these treatments do not require tertiary care centers. Rehydration, oxygen, antibiotics, and attention to respiratory status can be critical interventions. Transfusions may become necessary with precipitous hemoglobin drops.

PATHOPHYSIOLOGY

Sickle cell anemia refers to the doubly heterozygote inheritance of the sickle cell gene. The pathophysiology and treatment guidelines described in this article also apply to other forms of sickle cell disease such as sickle hemoglobin C (SC disease) and sickle thalassemia (S thal). In sickle cell disease, the abnormal hemoglobin polymerizes under deoxygenation, converting the normally biconcave red blood cell (RBC) into a sickle-shaped cell.

Sickle cells are less deformable than normal cells and fragment in the circulation, resulting in shortened RBC survival. This accounts for the chronic hemolytic anemia observed in patients. Alterations in the erythrocyte membrane, caused partly by the hemoglobin polymerization, cause the sickle cells to adhere to vascular endothelium. The combination of these physical properties gives rise to the vaso-occlusive phenomena

associated with this disease. Occlusion of capillaries and small vessels results in chronic and often clinically asymptomatic organ damage.

In the infant, functional asplenia develops, and with age, progressive renal, pulmonary, liver, and cardiac damage occurs. Acute occlusion of larger vessels results in sudden symptoms such as pain, cerebrovascular accidents, acute splenic sequestration crisis, pulmonary infarction, and others. Diagnosis and management of these acute events are reviewed subsequently.

INFECTION

Patients with sickle cell anemia are immunocompromised hosts. The absence of splenic function, defects in the alternate complement pathway, and other factors make sickle cell disease patients susceptible to bacterial infections. *In younger patients, sudden infection is the most common cause of death and remains a factor as the patient ages.* The organisms to which patients are susceptible include Streptococcus pneumoniae, Hemophilus influenzae, Escherichia coli, Salmonella, and Mycoplasma.

CLINICAL PRESENTATION

Bacterial sepsis must be considered in all sickle cell disease patients who present with an unexplained fever of 101° or higher (Table 53-28). A 3- or 4-hour delay in an asplenic patient with pneumococcal sepsis can make a significant difference in survival. Therefore, quick but thorough examination searching for the source of infection should be performed. Because pneumonia commonly occurs, increased respiratory rate and abnormal auscultory findings should be carefully evaluated. In childhood, acute sequestration crises are commonly associated with fever.

1. During the physical examination, the physician should look for evidence of:
   Respiratory distress
   Meningitis
   Sepsis
   Splenomegaly
   Degree of jaundice
   Localized bone pain
   CVA tenderness
   The physical findings detected during this examination should be compared to those of the patient's steady-state examination.
2. After the examination is completed, the following laboratory evaluation should be undertaken:
   CBC and reticulocyte count
   Blood culture
   Chest x ray
   Urinalysis, culture and sensitivity
   Mycoplasma titer (optional)
   Stool culture (if diarrhea is present)
   Lumbar puncture: performed in all patients under 1 year or with even minimal signs suggesting meningitis
   Evaluation for osteomyelitis: if a patient has severe localized bone pain and high fever, an orthopedic consultation should be obtained, and bone scan, skeletal films, and culture of the involved bone by direct aspiration of the inflamed site are indicated.
3. All patients under age 5 with a documented oral temperature above 101°F are admitted to the hospital.
4. If meningitis is not suspected or has been ruled out, the patient is placed on cefuroxime sodium or other antibiotic to cover Streptococcus pneumoniae and H. influenzae at a dose of 150 mg/kg/day. If the evaluation for the fever reveals no cause, the antibiotics are continued until the blood cultures are negative for 72 hours.
5. The patient may be discharged after 72 hours on oral Ceclor or Augmentin if he or she is afebrile and nontoxic, and has a safe hemoglobin level. During the hospitalization, the CBC and reticulocyte counts should be ordered at least every other day.
6. All patients must be re-evaluated within a week of discharge.

Patients should undergo a rapid laboratory evaluation, which should include a CBC and reticulocyte count to exclude a concomitant acute anemic event. Sepsis should be evaluated by a blood culture, urine culture, and chest x ray. Infants under 1 year should have a lumbar puncture for the slightest indication. Once the diagnostic testing is completed, parenteral antibiotics should be started. Particularly in children under 5 years, administration of antibiotics should not be delayed.

A child in whom bacterial infection is suspected should be promptly treated with parenteral antibiotics, for example, cefuroxime (150 mg per kg every 24 hours in three divided doses). In healthy-appearing older children and adults, a parenteral dose of ceftriaxone (100 mg per kg every 24 hours in two doses to a maximum of 4 g in 24 hours) can be given, followed by oral antibiotics.

In the febrile patient with severe localized bone pain, osteomyelitis must be rapidly differentiated from bone infarct. Direct aspiration of the involved area for culture, and blood and stool cultures should be obtained with special emphasis on the identification of salmonella species. Orthopedic consultation and nuclear imaging can be helpful. After laboratory evaluation, antibiotics that cover salmonella and staphlococcus should be started.

PULMONARY COMPLICATIONS

Acute pulmonary disease characterized by pulmonary infiltrates, fever, and chest pains often represents a medical emergency. These episodes account for greater than 15% of deaths in patients with sickle cell disease and cause significant morbidity in all age groups. In adults, most acute pulmonary disease results from in situ pulmonary vascular thrombosis. The clinical picture is similar to that of infectious pneumonia, except that chest pain is the chief complaint. Occasionally, the chest symptoms may be secondary to bone marrow emboli. In children, acute pulmonary disease is usually caused by infection. Pneumonia in patients with sickle cell disease can be severe and rapidly progressive despite adequate antibiotic therapy. Pulmonary infarction-induced focal pulmonary hypoxemia may cause sudden pulmonary failure in a patient who was previously adequately oxygenated. In older patients, recurrent episodes of pulmonary infarction and pneumonia cause progressive decreased pulmonary function and may lead to pulmonary hypertension, right ventricular hypertrophy, and cor pulmonale.

CLINICAL DIAGNOSIS

Fever, coughs and tachypnea are usually found in young children. In adults, pleuritic chest pain is often the major symptom. Occasionally the chest pain is secondary to sternal or rib infarction. Chest pain can mimic angina or myocardial infarction; however, coronary artery disease is extremely rare in young adult sickle cell patients.

LABORATORY DIAGNOSIS

Often the chest x ray shows an infiltrate in one or more lobes, but it may be normal for the first 2 to 3 days. Measurement of arterial blood gas is necessary in the initial assessment of the disease. Knowledge of the steady-state arterial blood gas is helpful because many adult patients have mild to moderate chronic hypoxemia. Severe hypoxemia (Pa 0_2 <60 mmHg in adults, <70 mmHg in children), however, indicates a life-threatening disease. CBC, reticulocyte, and blood culture should be obtained on all patients because a falling hemoglobin contributes to hypoxemia. The protocol we follow for patients is indicated in Table 53-29. All patients with acute chest syndrome must be admitted to the hospital. Those with mild respiratory symptoms may deteriorate rapidly within a short time. Therefore, observation for 24 hours is usually necessary. Analgesics should be administered, but narcotic induced hypoventilation must be avoided. Oxygen therapy is indicated for hypoxemia and should be monitored by frequent arterial blood gases. Intravenous hydration should be given, but fluid overload must be avoided. Antibiotics to treat streptococcal pneumonia and Hemophilus influenzae should be started. Oral erythromycin should be added if mycoplasma pneumonia is suspected. Exchange transfusions should be done if rapidly progressive disease or signs of respiratory insufficiency are present.

TABLE 53-29. PROTOCOL FOR ACUTE CHEST SYNDROME

1. All patients with chest or lung symptoms must be examined immediately. Review medical record to determine patient's previous steady-state respiratory rate, arterial blood gas, chest x ray, and VQ scan.
2. Patients should undergo the following investigations:
    Chest x ray
    CBC, reticulocyte count
    Blood culture, sputum culture (if possible)
    Arterial blood gas in room air
    Mycoplasma titer (acute and follow up)
    VQ scan (this scan is indicated when chest signs exist with a negative chest x ray)
    ECG (optional)
    Viral studies (optional)
    Type and hold blood (optional)
3. All patients with evidence of acute pulmonary pathology should be admitted to the hospital. IV hydration should be given. IV + PO should equal a minimum of 1.0 times maintenance fluids.
4. Oxygen should be administered if the patient has hypoxia (PO$_2$ < 70 mmHg) demonstrated by arterial blood gas measurements.
5. IV cefuroxime sodium (100 to 150 mg/kg/day) should be started immediately. Optional erythromycin can be added if mycoplasma is suspected.
6. If pleural fluid is present on a chest x ray and contributing to respiratory distress, thoracentesis is indicated.
7. Arterial blood gas should be closely monitored.
8. A partial exchange transfusion should be initiated for any of the following criteria:
    PaO$_2$ < 70 mm Hg
    25% drop in the patient's baseline PaO$_2$
    Acute congestive heart failure or acute right heart strain
    Rapidly progressive pneumonia
    Marked dyspnea with tachypnea
9. After recovery from an acute pulmonary event, patients should undergo baseline pulmonary function tests, arterial blood gas measurement, and a steady-state VQ scan. This will facilitate future evaluation for acute pulmonary disease.

ACUTE ANEMIC COMPLICATIONS

Sickle cell anemia patients usually have a steady-state hemoglobin, generally in the range of 6 to 9 g per dL. At times, the hemoglobin falls acutely or chronically. Sudden drops in the hemoglobin are called anemic episodes and are produced by either splenic sequestration of red blood cells or episodes of transient erythroid hypoplasia. It is important to be knowledgeable of each patient's steady state hemoglobin and reticulocyte count to evaluate his or her hemoglobin during an Emergency Department (ED) visit.

Acute splenic sequestration crisis is the second most frequent cause of death in patients under 5 years with sickle cell disease. Viral infections often appear to precede most episodes. Splenic sequestration can develop rapidly, with sudden enlargement of the spleen, pooling of peripheral blood, and hypovolemic shock. During severe sequestration crises, hemoglobin level can precipitously drop to less than 2 g/dL, resulting in death. Two clinical forms of acute sequestration crises are noted: a major sequestration crisis in which the anemia is life-threatening, and a minor sequestration crisis in which the anemia is less severe. Because many young patients have mild splenomegaly, it is important to determine splenic size during steady-state periods.

The usual clinical findings of this complication are sudden weakness, pallor, increased respiratory rate, and abdominal enlargement.

The protocol that we follow for children with acute splenic sequestration is indicated in Table 53-30. Im-

---

TABLE 53-30. SPLENIC SEQUESTRATION CRISIS

Major Acute Sequestration Crisis
Rapid enlargement of spleen compared with baseline size
Fall in hemoglobin low enough to require transfusion:
    Absolute hemoglobin value < 6 g/dL
    Drop in hemoglobin value > 3 g/dL compared with baseline value
    Elevated reticulocyte count
Minor Acute Sequestration Crisis
Enlargement of spleen compared with baseline value
Fall in hemoglobin, but absolute value > 6 g/dL
Indications for Surgery
One major or two minor acute splenic sequestration episodes
Treatment of Acute Splenic Sequestration Crisis
Transfuse to hemoglobin of 9 to 10 g/dL
Use exchange transfusion if any signs of cardiorespiratory distress
    Remove ¾ blood volume and replace with packed RBC/normal saline (50/50)
If there are no signs of cardiorespiratory distress, give two separate transfusions using Lasix to prevent fluid overload
Splenectomy if patient age > 2 years or patient age < 2 years and no evidence of splenic function
Chronic transfusion program until age 2, maintain hemoglobin S < 30 per cent if patient is < 2 years and splenic function is intact

mediate transfusion therapy is given to patients with severe sequestration crisis. After the patient's clinical course is stabilized, he or she should be considered for splenectomy.

Aplastic episodes often present with increased fatigue and shortness of breath. Laboratory evaluation shows a low hemoglobin and absent reticulocytes. Recent studies suggest that many aplastic episodes are secondary to infections by B19 parvovirus. These aplastic episodes spontaneously resolve in 1 to 2 weeks. Treatment is symptomatic. Transfusions with packed RBCs should be given if the degree of anemia is severe (less than 5 g per dL) or cardiorespiratory compromise is noted.

CENTRAL NERVOUS SYSTEM COMPLICATIONS

Complications involving the CNS occur in over 15% of patients with sickle cell disease. Strokes, seizures, and meningitis are most common. Neurologic manifestations can be focal (e.g., hemiparesis) or more generalized (e.g., coma and seizures).

Strokes usually first occur in childhood and are secondary to cerebral infarction. Subarachnoid and intracerebral hemorrhages are increasingly more common in older patients.

Patients suspected of having a cerebrovascular accident should be immediately evaluated and treated. Nonfocal abnormalities such as dizziness and headaches are relatively common in sickle cell disease, and may or may not be caused by cerebral infarction. Transient ischemic attacks causing focal neurologic deficits may occur and require immediate evaluation and intervention. The use of nuclear magnetic resonance (MRI) has improved the evaluation of patients with CNS complications. Its use eliminates the potential hazards of contrast material in patients with sickle cell disease. Lumbar puncture should be considered if meningitis is suspected or the MRI shows no evidence of increased intracranial pressure. Arteriography may be used in follow-up studies to evaluate more fully the cerebral infarction. For the patient who has experienced an acute cerebrovascular accident, rapid treatment is necessary. This patient should be admitted to the intensive care unit (ICU). Parenteral hydration is immediately started to maintain fluid balance. Exchange transfusion, with the goal to lower the hemoglobin S level to 30%, is performed. This can be accomplished by a one-volume exchange transfusion. Simple transfusion is not recommended because of the problem of hyperviscosity. Pharmacologic agents to decrease cerebral edema and assist in controlling seizures are often necessary. Neurosurgical

and neurologic consultation may be helpful. After stabilization of the patient, rehabilitation therapy should be started. Long-term, chronic transfusions maintaining a hemoglobin S level below 30% are necessary.

VASO-OCCLUSIVE CRISIS

One of the most frequent and debilitating problems in sickle cell disease patients is vaso-occlusive crisis from ischemic tissue injury caused by obstruction of blood flow. The reduced blood flow causes further tissue hypoxia, which increases the sickling process. Hypoxia, infection, acidosis, dehydration, and extreme cold may precipitate painful events. In most cases, however, no precipitating event can be identified. The frequency of vaso-occlusive crises is extremely varied. One third of patients experience pain only rarely, but 5% of patients have more than 30 events a year. Such patients are frequently at EDs seeking pain relief, and may become addicted to analgesics.

No clinical or laboratory finding is diagnostic of a painful event. The possibility of the pain being precipitated by a concurrent medical problem always exists. The physician should rule out a precipitating illness in every instance. Musculoskeletal pain is common. At times, sickle cell crisis may be difficult to distinguish from osteomyelitis, septic arthritis, or even gout. Sickle cell disease is also an important cause of osteonecrosis of the femoral head (almost 10% of cases followed over 6 years). Acute abdominal pain is the second most common type of pain and may be confused with acute surgical abdomen, such as in cholecystitis or pelvic inflammatory disease. The low back area is also a common site for pain in adults.

It is recommended that patients seek immediate care by a physician if they are febrile and experiencing severe abdominal or pulmonary symptoms, or if any neurologic symptoms occur. Many patients can manage painful events at home with conservative measures such as aspirin, fluid, and bed rest. Acute care should be sought when these measures have failed.

The laboratory evaluation of the patient in pain should include a CBC and reticulocyte count. Normally, the patient's hemoglobin level is unchanged during a vaso-occlusive event; however, occasionally aplastic or sequestration crisis can occur. If a fever over 101° F is present, an aggressive evaluation for its source should be made. Similarly, if acute chest symptoms are present, a chest x ray and arterial blood gas should be performed. If osteomyelitis is suspected, aspiration of the bone and cultures are often required. In a dehydrated patient, serum electrolytes and blood pH are necessary because of the high frequency of renal salt wasting.

MANAGEMENT

Dehydration, which promotes sickling, frequently occurs in sickle cell patients because of hyposthenuria. Intravenous hydration is recommended for patients in severe pain. Oral hydration is adequate for mild to moderate pain. The goal is to hydrate the patient at a rate of one and one-half to twice the daily maintenance once deficiencies are corrected. D5W and one third normal saline are usually adequate. Parenteral hydration should be monitored closely to avoid iatrogenic congestive heart failure and pulmonary edema.

Analgesic therapy is the mainstay of treatment of vaso-occlusive crisis. The goal of analgesic therapy is to provide prompt pain relief. The choice of therapy is based on the severity of pain (Table 53-31). The effect of the route of administration and drug absorption must be considered. Continuous intravenous infusion of narcotic and PCA devices provides excellent pain control, but should be performed only by institutions

familiar with its use. The oral route is less than one half as effective as the parenteral route. Oral administration of narcotics, however, avoids the complications of parenteral pain medication infusion.

If potent narcotics are used, one should keep in mind the side effects, which include respiratory depression, pruritis, hypotension, and changes in seizure threshold. Synthetic narcotics such as pentazocine and butorphanol should be avoided in patients receiving narcotics because of their induction of withdrawal symptoms. Non-narcotic analgesics are used alone to treat mild pain. In patients with severe pain, adding these analgesics to narcotic therapy increases analgesia. Diazepam and other antianxiety sedative medications do not potentiate the analgesic effects and should be avoided.

Oxygen therapy does not benefit vaso-occlusive episodes unless hypoxemia is present. Similarly, sodium bicarbonate and vasodilators have not proven efficacious in the management of painful episodes.

After the administration of analgesic medication and fluids, a decision about hospitalization or discharge should be made. If the patient remains comfortable after 3 hours, administering an oral narcotic

TABLE 53-31. RECOMMENDED INITIAL DOSE AND INTERVAL OF ANALGESICS NECESSARY TO OBTAIN ADEQUATE PAIN CONTROL IN SICKLE CELL DISEASE

	Maximum Dose (mg)	Route*	Interval	Comments
Severe Pain				
Morphine	0.15 mg/kg/dose (max. 10 mg)	SC, IM	Q3h	Drug of choice
Meperidine	1.5 mg/kg/dose (max. 100 mg)	IM	Q3h	Increased incidence of seizures; avoid in patients with renal or neurologic disease
Moderate Pain				
Oxycodone (Percocet or Percodan)	1 to 2 tablets/dose (1 tablet = 5 mg)	PO	Q4h	Patients over age 5
Methadone	0.15 mg/kg/dose	PO	Q6h	Effective in patients usually requiring parenteral narcotics. NOT FOR ROUTINE USE.
Meperidine	1.5 mg/kg/dose (max. 100 mg/dose)	PO	Q3½h	
Mild Pain				
Codeine	0.75 mg/kg/dose	PO	Q4h	May be effective up to 6 hours
Aspirin	1.5 g/m²/24 h divided into six doses	PO	Q4h	May be given with a narcotic for added analgesia
Acetaminophen	1.5 g/m²/24 h divided into six doses	PO	Q4h	May be given with a narcotic for added analgesia
Motrin (Ibuprofen)	300 to 600 mg/dose	PO	Q6h	

and observing for 1 hour are often helpful. If significant pain persists, the patient should be considered for hospitalization. If a holding unit is available, a repeat parenteral narcotic dose followed by observation is indicated. Patients who require continuing treatment with parenteral analgesics and intravenous fluids should be admitted to the hospital.

A few patients are almost always in pain. These patients often appear in the Emergency Department (ED) several times a week. Regardless of the cause of the pain, chronic depression and anxiety often amplify these patients' symptoms. Adequate treatment plans developed by a multidisciplinary team program should be used. *Drug addiction should not be the primary concern of the physician treating a sickle cell patient in the ED.* If a patient is addicted, he or she should be referred to a pain center equipped to manage this problem.

PRIAPISM (see also Chap. 48)

Priapism is a persistent, painful erection caused by obstruction of venous flow in the corpus cavenosa. Most attacks are spontaneous, but they can be precipitated by hypoxemia, alcohol ingestion, and sexual intercourse. Two common patterns of priapism have been described: short, transient episodes lasting less than 3 hours and severe, prolonged attacks lasting longer than 24 hours. Severe attacks often cause impotence.

Initial evaluation should include detailed history concerning prior episodes, duration of the present episode, and possible causes. Initial examination should include prostatic massage and examination of prostatic fluid for infection. Immediate treatment with intravenous hydration and parenteral narcotics to relieve pain is helpful. Insertion of a Foley catheter may be necessary to alleviate bladder obstruction. If detumescence does not occur within hours, RBC exchange transfusion should be done.

There is a controversy as to the correct surgical treatment of severe priapism in sickle cell disease. In cases that do not respond rapidly to fluid and transfusion, a urologist should be consulted. Sometimes penile aspiration or a "Winter" procedure is necessary in these resistant cases. Without early, aggressive interventions, severe priapism is likely to cause impotence.

TRANSFUSIONS

Transfusion therapy is one of the most commonly used treatments for sickle cell complications and has been mentioned throughout this review. The common use of transfusion in sickle cell disease is based upon its ability to increase oxygen carrier capacity and improve blood flow. Routine transfusions in sickle cell disease are not indicated. Under certain circumstances, however, transfusions are necessary.

Symptoms such as respiratory and cardiac or CNS dysfunction caused by a falling hemoglobin less than 5 mg/dL can sometimes be corrected by transfusion therapy. A rapidly falling hemoglobin associated with sequestration crisis requires earlier intervention. Life-threatening complications of sickle cell disease such as stroke, respiratory distress, priapism, and acute chest syndrome may be improved by lowering the hemoglobin S-containing cells by exchange transfusion.

The choice of blood product varies according to the patient's transfusion history. Sickle cell disease patients have a high frequency of alloimmunization and iron overload. Before transfusion, history of transfusion reactions and alloantibodies should be sought. In general, sickle-negative packed RBCs should be used. Washed cells eliminate febrile reactions seen in recurrently transfused patients.

HORIZONS

There is presently no cure for sickle cell disease. Multiple clinical trials have been started with experimental agents. Antisickling agents that alter hemoglobin polymerization are under investigation, and pharmacologic agents that increase hemoglobin F in RBCs are in clinical trial. Preliminary data suggest that an increase in total hemoglobin and a decrease in vaso-occlusive crises may result from the use of these agents, but long-term effects of these cytotoxic agents are yet unknown. Hydroxyurea is the safest and most widely used experimental drug available to increase sickle cell patients' fetal hemoglobin level. Adult patients seeking information concerning clinical research trials should contact a Sickle Cell Center listed in the National Institute of Health's manual, Management and Therapy of Sickle Cell Disease.

BIBLIOGRAPHY

Charache, S., Lubin, B., and Reid, C. (Eds.): Management and Therapy of Sickle Cell Disease. U. S. Department of Health and Human Services, NIH Publication No. 89–2117, September, 1989.

Edmond, A.M., Holman, R., Hayes, R.J., and Serjeant, G.R.: Priapism and impotence in homozygous sickle cell disease. Arch. Intern. Med. 140:1434, 1980.

Russell, M.O., Goldberg, H.I., Hodson, A., et al.: Effect of transfusion therapy on arteriographic abnormalities and on the recurrence of stroke in sickle cell disease. Blood 63:162, 1984.

Sprinkle, R.H., Cole, T., Smith, S., and Buchanan, G.R.: Acute chest syndrome in children with sickle cell disease. A retrospective analysis of 100 hospitalized cases. Am. J. Pediatr. Hematol. Oncol. 8:105,110, 1986.

Vichinsky, E., and Lubin, B.: Suggested guidelines for the treatment of children with sickle cell anemia. Clin. Hematol. 1:483, 1987.

Vichinsky, E., Johnson, R., and Lubin, B.: Multidisciplinary approach to pain management in sickle cell disease. Am. J. Pediatr. Hematol. Oncol. 4:328, 1982.

SPLENOMEGALY

Lawrence Dall and Wendy Moffatt

CAPSULE

Determination of the cause of splenomegaly can present a diagnostic challenge to the emergency physician. It is often difficult to determine the exact cause of splenomegaly by noninvasive procedures, but diagnostic guidelines do exist. Splenic enlargement can be difficult to detect by physical examination and may require enlargement of 2 to 4 times normal before it can be palpated.[1] The spleen is normally slightly enlarged in 30% of newborns, 15% of young children, and 3% of college freshmen.[2] Although an enlarged spleen can occasionally be normal, the finding of a definitely enlarged spleen should incite an evaluation for the more likely benign or malignant causes (Tables 53-32 and 53-33).

PATHOPHYSIOLOGY

The pathophysiology of splenomegaly is related to its functions in the immune, circulatory, and hematologic systems. Infectious causes produce splenomegaly by inducing hyperplasia of germinal centers in response to blood-borne antigens. This form of splenic enlargement may also occur in immunologically mediated illness such as rheumatoid arthritis and systemic lupus erythematosus (SLE).

Splenomegaly may also be congestive, related to portal hypertension and stasis of blood in the red pulp. Frequently this form is overshadowed by associated signs of esophageal varices, ascites, or hepatic failure. Histologically, accumulation of erythrocytes in the red pulp and proliferation of cells lining the pulp sinuses and cords is found. A similar histologic picture occurs in diseases associated with abnormal morphology of erythrocytes.

The spleen is a primary site of hematopoiesis until the fifth gestational month. It can resume a significant role in hematopoietic function under any circumstances in which the bone marrow is unable to meet the demand for blood components, producing enlarged and dilated pulp sinuses.

Many inherited disorders are characterized by abnormal accumulation of materials in phagocytic cells, with resultant enlargement of the spleen and other reticuloendothelial organs. Most often, this defect is caused by the absence of a critical enzyme (Gaucher's disease and Niemann-Pick disease).

PHYSICAL DIAGNOSIS

The normal adult spleen lies under the left diaphragm, with its convex surface separated from the thoracic

TABLE 53-32. DIFFERENTIAL DIAGNOSIS OF INFECTIOUS CAUSES OF SPLENOMEGALY

1. Bacteremia (Typhoid fever—Salmonella, bacterial endocarditis)
2. Viral infections (infectious mononucleosis, hepatitis, measles, cytomegalovirus)
3. Rocky Mountain spotted fever
4. Psittacosis
5. Malaria
6. Disseminated tuberculosis
7. Disseminated histoplasmosis
8. Toxoplasmosis
9. Secondary syphilis
10. Relapsing fever
11. Splenic abscess
12. Brucellosis
13. Congenital syphilis
14. Chronic meningococcemia
15. Kala-azar
16. Schistosomiasis
17. Echinococcosis
18. Trypanosomiasis

TABLE 53-33. DIFFERENTIAL DIAGNOSIS OF NONINFECTIOUS CAUSES OF SPLENOMEGALY

A. *Inflammatory*
   1. Felty's syndrome
   2. Sarcoidosis
   3. Berylliosis
B. *Circulatory*
   1. Cirrhosis
   2. Portal vein obstruction
   3. Splenic vein obstruction
   4. Congestive heart failure
C. *Hyperplastic*
   1. Hemolytic anemia
   2. Hemoglobinopathies
   3. Myeloplastic anemia
   4. Systemic lupus erythematosus
   5. Thrombotic thrombocytopenic purpura
   6. Graves' disease
   7. Polycythemia vera
D. *Infiltrative*
   1. Storage diseases
   2. Amyloidosis
   3. Diabetes mellitus
E. *Cysts and neoplasms*
   1. Cysts
   2. Hamartomas
   3. Leukemia/lymphoma
   4. Histiocytosis
   5. Metastatic neoplasm

cage by the pleura. The normal-sized spleen is not palpated on physical examination. Rarely, the presence of emphysema or a low left hemidiaphragm may make a normal-sized spleen palpable. The long axis of the spleen (12 cm) lies behind the parallel to the oblique tenth rib in the midaxillary line. The width (7 cm) that determines the area of splenic dullness is between the ninth and eleventh ribs. Percussion of this area allows the examiner to determine if a large spleen is present. Other causes for dullness to percussion in this area include fluid in the stomach and feces in the colon.

Normally, the spleen weighs about 150 g, but in disease the weight may increase to 6000 g or more.[3] Because the superior aspect of the spleen is bounded by fixed structures, enlargement pushes the spleen downward and toward the right iliac fossa. Acute infections produce enlarged soft spleens, whereas chronic disorders produce hard spleens with sharp edges. The spleen, even when enlarged, should not be tender. If tenderness is elicited, peritonitis or infarction should be suspected.

DIAGNOSTIC APPROACH

The causes of splenomegaly are many and varied. Without an orderly systemic approach, many needless laboratory tests are performed, and unfortunately needless abdominal surgical explorations may occur.

The evaluation of splenomegaly should always begin with a careful history and physical examination. This usually leads to performing laboratory tests to confirm the diagnosis. In a child or a young adult, the cause of splenomegaly is usually viral; *infectious mononucleosis* caused by the Epstein-Barr virus is the major etiologic agent. The history of pharyngitis, muscle aches, fever, and the finding of lymphadenopathy, particularly in the posterior cervical region, splenomegaly or palatal petechiae make this diagnosis likely. The finding of atypical lymphocytes in the blood, along with a positive monospot test or heterophil titer, confirms the diagnosis. At week 1 of the disease, approximately 80 to 85% of patients have more than 10% atypical lymphocytes and a positive rapid slide monospot test. At the peak of the illness, both tests have sensitivities of greater than 90%.[4] Other agents may be responsible for a mononucleosis-like clinical picture such as that of cytomegalovirus (CMV) or toxoplasmosis. Patients with the cytomegalovirus mononucleosis syndrome tend to be older than the Epstein-Barr group (age 20 to 40 as opposed to 16 to 25).[5] Severe pharyngitis and lymphadenopathy are less common. In these cases, it is acceptable to follow the patient carefully without resorting to other testing. If a definitive diagnosis is desired, IgM antibody titers against CMV and toxoplasma can be obtained.

Other infectious causes of splenomegaly include bacterial endocarditis, malaria, and typhoid fever. History is helpful, especially in judging whether patients were in endemic areas of disease. Blood cultures and smears are helpful in these cases, although blood cultures may be sterile in typhoid fever. In some of the other esoteric infectious diseases responsible for splenomegaly, more invasive procedures are required. Liver biopsy and bone marrow aspiration with culture are valuable in diagnosing many of the systemic granulomatous diseases (tuberculosis, histoplasmosis, and sarcoidosis).

Splenomegaly has both malignant and nonmalignant hematologic causes. The differentiation requires examination of the peripheral blood, bone marrow, and lymph nodes. The differential diagnosis of the leukemias can be accomplished by examination of the blood and bone marrow with appropriate cytochemical, immunologic, and chromosomal analysis. When malignant lymphoma is expected, the diagnosis can usually be made by the biopsy of a peripheral lymph node. When intra-abdominal lymphoma is expected in the absence of peripheral lymphadenopathy, the diagnosis can often be made in the bone marrow. If this is unsuccessful, this is one of the few justifications for surgical exploration in the patient with splenomegaly.

The nonmalignant hematologic causes of splenomegaly are usually hemolytic anemias. The cause of splenomegaly in this situation is overwork or hypertrophy of the spleen. Hemolysis can be suspected if there is an elevated reticulocyte count. Careful examination of the peripheral blood smear may show spherocytes, target cells, elliptocytes, or stomatocytes, which indicate hemolysis. These hemolytic anemias can be either hereditary or acquired. If acquired hemolytic anemia is possible, a history including that of medications is important and a Coombs test should be ordered. Rarely, splenomegaly has been associated with chronic iron deficiency anemia, and megaloblastic anemia.

The patient with erythrocytosis and splenomegaly is likely to have polycythemia vera. The combination of an elevated red blood cell (RBC) volume, an arterial oxygen saturation of greater than 92%, and splenomegaly satisfies the diagnosis.[6]

Connective tissue diseases such as rheumatoid arthritis and SLE are associated with splenomegaly. Felty's syndrome consists of rheumatoid arthritis, splenomegaly, and neutropenia. Serologic testing is helpful in diagnosing these diseases.

Congestive causes of splenomegaly are common and sometimes difficult to diagnose. The two most common are intrinsic liver disease (portal hypertension) and chronic congestive heart failure. In most cases, physical examination along with liver function tests, particularly the prothrombin time, allows the differentiation.

An enlarged spleen may lead to hypersplenism, defined as hyperfunctioning of the spleen associated with reduction in RBCs, white blood cells, and platelets with compensatory bone marrow hyperplasia. The granulocytopenia and thrombocytopenia rarely lead to clinical problems, but the anemia can be profound. But when qualitative platelet disorders also exist (drugs, Banti's syndrome), bleeding can be profound.

Splenic infarction may occur in any large spleen. Although the patient is often asymptomatic, he or she may also present with acute left upper quadrant pain and an audible rub. This is more common in sickle cell disease or thalassemia. Only supportive and preventive treatments are available.

DIAGNOSTIC IMAGING

Physical examination is insensitive to mild splenomegaly. Nearly one half of radionucleotide proven splenomegaly may be missed by physical examination, and up to 28% are missed by abdominal radiography.[7] When the cause of splenomegaly is unknown, CT scanning is the preferred technique because it is more likely to demonstrate conditions that may be responsible for the splenic enlargement (abdominal lymph node enlargement in lymphoma, changes in size and shape of the liver, and prominence of venous structures in the splenic hilum suggesting cirrhosis and portal hypertension).

Infrequent sequelae of splenomegaly are rupture and infarction. CT scan is the procedure of choice, showing a low-density region in the spleen in infarct, and crescent-shaped collections of fluid that flatten or indent the lateral margin of the spleen in subcapsular hematomas.

MANAGEMENT

The most important aspect of the management of splenomegaly is to determine the cause and treat the underlying disease. In the unlikely case of splenic rupture, emergency surgery is indicated. When the sequelae of hypersplenism are progressive and severe, and cannot be improved by the treatment of the underlying disease, splenectomy or splenic irradiation may be indicated.

REFERENCES

1. Eichner, E.R.: Splenic function: Normal, too much, and too little. Am. J. Med. 66:311, 1979.
2. Westin, J., Lanner, L., and Larsson, A.: Spleen size in polycythemia. Acta Med. Scand. 191:263, 1972.
3. Degowin, E.L., and Degowin, R.L.: Splenomegaly. In Bedside Diagnostic Examination. London, The Macmillan Company, 1965, p. 485.
4. Griner, P.F.: Infectious mononucleosis. In Clinical Diagnosis and the Laboratory: Logical Strategies for Common Medical Problems. Edited by Griner, P.F., Panzer, R.J., and Greenland, P. Chicago, Year Book Publishers, Inc., 1986, p. 57.
5. Klemola, E.: Infectious mononucleosis-like disease with negative heterophil agglutination test: Clinical features in relation to Epstein-Barr virus and cytomegalovirus antibodies. J. Infect. Dis. 121:608, 1970.
6. Berlin, N.I.: Diagnosis and classification of the polycythemias. Semin. Hematol. 12:339, 1975.
7. Koehler, R.E.: Spleen. In Computed Tomography. Edited by Lee, J.K.T., Sagel, S.S., Stanley, R.J. New York, Raven Press, 1983, p. 115.

TRANSFUSION THERAPY IN EMERGENCY MEDICINE

Steven J. Davidson

CAPSULE

Transfusion of blood and blood products is relatively infrequent for emergency physicians, but is always fraught with tension and a sense of urgency. Preplanning and advance arrangements with hospital and local/regional blood banks can reduce the chaos and the stress. Newer technologies can shorten the time required for typing recipient blood, thus speeding the availability of blood for transfusion. Widespread use in trauma centers of "universal donor" and "type-specific" blood has given sanction in the civilian sector to long-standing practices in military medicine.

Clinical studies over the last decade have suggested that "dilutional coagulopathy" is a misnomer, and thus prophylactic administration of fresh frozen plasma is not required to maintain adequate clotting in most patients, even those massively transfused. On the other hand, the data have supported the use of platelet transfusion in bleeding, massively transfused patients with low platelet counts. Limiting the transfusion of single donor products makes sense, given the risk of disease transmission.

Disease transmission by blood transfusion remains an overriding concern. The newest donor prescreening questionnaires, combined with recent developments in serologic testing, have reduced the transfusion recipient's risk immensely in the United States from 1 in 40,000 (worst case) to 1 in 1 million. Elsewhere, especially in the Third World and Eastern Europe, the risk of acquiring hepatitis, HIV, or other viruses is variously estimated at 1 in 40 to 1 in 1000 units transfused.

STANDARDS AND ORGANIZATIONS

Blood for transfusion is commonly supplied through regional blood banking agencies that belong to consortia organized through the American Association of Blood Banks (AABB) or the American Red Cross (ARC). Emergency physicians (among others) confront limited availability of blood products and other problems in blood utilization so the American College of Emergency Physicians (ACEP) and these two organizations, together with the National Institutes of Health (NIH), consumers, donors, insurers and other professionals, formed the American Blood Commission (ABC) to evaluate problems facing blood banking and attempt to solve them.

The Department of Health and Human Services, through the Food and Drug Administration, enforce federal regulations regarding blood transfusion services that require proper storage, record keeping, typing and cross-matching, and other requirements to maintain a safe blood supply. In addition, the AABB and ARC maintain voluntary standards for their member blood services. These standards contribute to the overall consistency, safety and affordability through which voluntarily donated blood is available throughout our country.

Naturally, we emergency physicians take these entities and their activities for granted, not even realizing the full range of their impact. Only when we demand instantaneous availability of blood for transfusion to a patient in extremis do the realities of these organizations' activities become real. The regulation and control of transfusion practice in modern emergency medicine are not capricious and arbitrary. Rather, they are designed to protect both the patient and practitioner in an environment where laboratory and clinician meet with no correlation of data whatsoever. Crossmatching of blood for transfusion is the only "routine" laboratory practice that allows for no clinical correlation.

DONATION (VOLUNTEER VERSUS PAID DONORS)

A large body of work over many years has clarified the relative safety of blood collected from volunteer donors compared to blood collected from paid donors. This conclusion, originally based on data regarding the transmission of hepatitis B and later non-A, non-B hepatitis, resulted in the implementation of a totally volunteer donor system for the collection of whole blood and untreated fractions resulting therefrom. *All* whole blood, cellular fractions, and fresh frozen plasma transfused in the United States today come from volunteer donors.

Plasmapheresis of hyperimmunized donors is the major source of hyperimmune gamma globulins for serotherapy of tetanus (HyperTet), rabies (HypeRab) and others. The donors who participate in these plasmapheresis programs are paid. The process used to purify the plasma and make hyperimmune gamma globulins, however, is believed to result in a noninfectious product. No infectious complications have been traced to immunoglobulins prepared using currently available technologies.

BLOOD BANKING

Modern surgical practice and trauma care are indebted to blood banking. Without the ready availability of functioning red blood cells (RBCs) for transfusion, many patients cared for by emergency physicians would perish. The community blood center is the source of this invaluable resource, and whether it functions through the AABB consortium or under the aegis of the ARC, it adheres to certain consistent and inviolable standard practices. Emergency physicians may sometimes find some of these burdensome.

Insistence by a blood bank technician that a specimen be redrawn, rather than a current specimen relabeled, although a distraction, is a standard required practice that ensures patient safety. Because no clinical correlation exists for an individual patient's blood type, and this determination is entirely laboratory-based, absolute identification of patient, specimen, and blood components for transfusion is essential. The overwhelming majority of complications and bad results traced to the transfusion of blood components is subsequently traced to misidentification. Thus, the use of specimens drawn by prehospital care providers (paramedics) is highly variable and not widely sanctioned. Individual hospitals in some rural locales may permit such an arrangement with a regional blood center.

In the emergency department (ED) setting, blood bank directors often cooperate and permit the use of a unique, code-numbered wristband for the patient which provides tear-off stickers for the specimen tube and blood unit. This practice may obviate the requirement of full patient identification at times of greatest need and stress when all that is available is "John Doe, a man in his 20s or 30s."

The following criteria are useful for identifying patients who require type and cross match for donor units:[1]

1. Shock
2. Observed 100 mL or greater blood loss
3. Gross gastrointestinal bleeding
4. Hemoglobin less than 10 mg/dL or hematocrit less than 30
5. Probability of a blood-losing operation (e.g., laparotomy for trauma, ectopic pregnancy, etc.).

There are no guidelines for determining the appropriate number of units to prepare for any given patient. The number of units requested is a clinical judgment, based on an estimate of ongoing and future losses. For patients who do not meet any of these criteria, a type and screen for atypical antibodies suffice as long as the antibody screen is negative. If it is not, the clinician should be notified by the blood bank so that the ordering of blood for crossmatch may be considered. This is the standard policy in blood banks operating under AABB or ARC standards.

CROSSMATCHING PROCESS

The properly labeled "clot tube" is centrifuged on arrival in the laboratory. Slide-typing techniques, using modern potent reagents, can be completed in 60 seconds. The immediate spin phase of the crossmatch can be completed in another 3 to 5 minutes. Within 5 minutes of arrival, incompletely crossmatched blood can be available in most cases. These techniques are not necessarily those routinely used for more leisurely or elective crossmatches, but are considered reliable, and when prearranged protocols are agreed on by both emergency center and blood bank, they are helpful in shortening the interval until blood for transfusion is available.

Full crossmatching requires antibody screening in albumin and Coombs serum, both of which require time-consuming incubations at 37°C. These techniques, requiring up to an additional 30 minutes, can be completed after blood is released for transfusion in cases of extreme urgency. In all cases, these steps are completed so that the clinician can be apprised of any incompatibility potentially resulting in a delayed transfusion reaction.

EMERGENCY RELEASE OF BLOOD

The administration of type-specific but incompletely crossmatched blood or type O blood carries a risk of transfusion reaction, yet may be life-saving. When possible, the additional 5 minutes necessary to secure type-specific rather than universal donor blood for emergency transfusion is preferred. The clinical decision to use incompletely cross-matched or universal donor blood, however, is justifiable in the following circumstances:

1. Exsanguinating hemorrhage with no or insufficient initial response to the rapid infusion of crystalloid volume expanders,
2. Profound shock resulting from exsanguination in patients with cardiopulmonary, cerebral or vascular disease,
3. Profound shock from blood loss in infants and small children because of their smaller blood volume,

4. Any situation in which the typical additional delay of 20 to 30 minutes from crossmatched blood would further endanger the patient.

The civilian use of type O universal donor blood is generally limited to the early resuscitative phase of trauma management.[2] Military experience in the use of group O packed red blood cells (PRBCs) documents the safety of their use in a young male population. Nearly $\frac{1}{4}$ million units were transfused in a 20-month period during the Vietnam conflict. Only one of the 24 hemolytic transfusion reactions resulting was caused by something other than misidentification of donor blood.[3,4] Smaller-scale civilian population studies have shown a small risk of transfusion reactions in previously transfused individuals and in parous women.[5]

All the military studies used Rh-positive blood because only men were transfused and large quantities of Rh-negative blood are unavailable. The civilian studies and most civilian practice call for the use of Rh-negative blood because demand is far more episodic and local stores can more easily be replenished. In any case, whether one used Rh-positive type O in men, Rh-negative for women, or Rh-negative for all patients requiring critically urgent transfusions, only PRBCs should be transfused so as to limit the volume of antibody-containing plasma transfused. Type-specifc crossmatched PRBCs should be given as soon as available unless more than four units of universal donor blood has already been transfused.

Neither fluorocarbons nor pyridoxinated hemoglobin polymer have yet been shown to be effective substitutes for red blood cells.

AUTOTRANSFUSION

As practiced in the ED, autotransfusion is the collection of exsanguinated blood from the thorax or (rarely) the peritoneal cavity, and reinfusion into the same patient. Intraperitoneal blood reinfusion, when used, is usually accomplished with cell washing and antibiotic administration because the extent of intraperitoneal contamination is unknown.

The patient with traumatic hemothorax is the most suitable candidate for autotransfusion because only known intrathoracic infection, malignancies, and enteric contamination are contraindications to performing the procedure. Hemothorax blood is drained through a chest tube and then screen-filtered to remove gross clots and debris. Citrate-phosphate-dextrose (CPD) solution may be added, either by premeasurement or simultaneously with the collection of blood, to inhibit coagulation in the system. The blood may be reinfused through a micropore filter.

Autotranfusion provides a rapidly available, warm, type-specific source of blood for the patient in urgent need. Blood collected from the chest has functioning white blood cells (WBCs) and near-normal levels of all noncellular coagulation factors except fibrinogen. Platelets are apparently altered in the collection process, and the few that pass through the micropore filter do not function normally.

Complications of autotransfusion are rare and mostly dose-related. Reinfusion of less than 4000 mL of autotransfused blood is rarely associated with clinical complications. Hemoglobinemia and hemoglobinuria occur in varying degrees after autotransfusions. In most reported series, they have not been associated with renal failure. Disseminated intravascular coagulation (DIC) has been a reported complication.

BLOOD COMPONENTS: DESCRIPTIONS AND INDICATIONS

Whole blood consists of cellular and noncellular components. Cellular components include red blood cells (RBCs), platelets, and granulocytes. Noncellular components include albumin, plasma protein fraction (PPF), fresh frozen plasma (FFP), cryoprecipitate, and other soluble coagulation factors. Component transfusion, rather than whole blood transfusion, is preferred to correct a specific physiologic deficiency and to make the most efficient use of a limited resource.

The emergency physician most frequently uses red blood cell concentrates and has secondary needs for fresh frozen plasma, coagulation factor concentrates, platelets, albumin, and PPF. Whole blood transfusions are currently rarely used, generally only for infant transfusion.

Transfusion of all but the chemically and heat-treated components (albumin, PPF), carries with it the risk of hepatitis. Other infectious illnesses, including AIDS, can also be transmitted by blood transfusion. Incompatibility, isoimmunization, and allergic and toxic reactions are all potential complications.

WHOLE BLOOD

Even whole blood is no longer "whole" at the time of administration. Within 24 hours of initiating storage in citrate-phosphate-dextrose-adenine (CPDA-1) solutions, blood stored at 4°C has no functioning granulocytes, and only 50% of the functional activity of platelets and coagulation factor VIII remains. Both platelet function and factor VIII activity are negligible by 72 hours.

Continued refrigerated storage of whole blood causes 50% reductions in factor V at 3 to 5 days and increased affinity of hemoglobin for oxygen at 4 to 6 days with decreasing RBC viability and deformability beginning at about the same time. About the fifth day, hydrogen ion, ammonia, and potassium concentrations begin to rise and microaggregates of platelets, fibrin, and leukocytes collect rapidly. Viability of at least 70% of the administered RBCs at 24 hours is the standard by which all storage of blood products is judged. CPDA-1 permits 35-day storage to meet this standard. Decreased RBC deformability limits the ability of RBCs to travel through capillaries in tissues, and increased RBC oxygen affinity reduces tissue oxygenation. These latter effects are reversed 24 to 48 hours after the RBCs are returned to the more "natural" environment of the vascular tree. Detriments to the use of whole blood include limited concentrations of labile clotting factors, excessive accumulations of metabolic by-products, volume overload, contamination with viruses or bacteria, and exposure to antigens. Usually, RBC concentrations and crystalloid infusions suffice when volume and RBC mass repletion are necessary. Fresh whole blood, when available, however, is appropriate in massive transfusion. Autotransfusion may be a helpful adjunct in these circumstances.

CELLULAR CONCENTRATES

PACKED RED BLOOD CELLS (PRBCs)

PRBCs are transfused when RBC mass repletion is the primary aim. They are prepared in closed systems to a hematocrit no greater than 80 and have a 35-day refrigerated shelf-life. PRBCs and crystalloid solutions are ideal volume and RBC repletion fluids in the overwhelming majority of emergency transfusions. The infusion rate is maximized by using wide tubing and a large-bore infusion catheter, and by diluting the blood with warmed normal saline solution. Infusing warm rather than cold blood also reduces the patient's metabolic workload and reduces the risk of hypothermia.

PRBCs do not provide volume or noncellular coagulation factors. Approximately 10% of the original donor plasma remains in each unit of PRBCs, but, except in exchange or massive transfusions, hepatic synthesis of coagulation proteins rapidly replenishes intravascular stores.

The advantages of PRBCs include: (1) decreased burden of citrate, ammonia and organic acids; (2) reduced risk of alloimmunization because fewer antigens are infused; and (3) reduced risk of volume overload when multiple units are infused.

WASHED RED BLOOD CELLS

Washed RBCs provide a pure PRBC unit with a 24-hour shelf-life. They are most often used for patients with known allergic reactions to platelet, granulocyte, or plasma antigens, and are rarely used in the ED.

PLATELETS

Platelets are administered for bleeding resulting from thrombocytopenia or inadequate platelet function. A platelet pack increases platelet count by 4000 to 8000 in a 70 kg patient, and 10 packs are generally given at a time. ABO matching is not necessary, although human lymphocyte antigen (HLA) matching may be performed in special circumstances. In surgical or trauma patients with normal platelet function, platelet counts of 40,000 to 100,000 per cubic millimeter (cmm) may rarely cause bleeding correctable by platelet administration. More than 20,000 platelets per mm^3 spontaneous bleeding is uncommon, but is frequent and severe at platelet counts below 10,000 per mm^3.

NONCELLULAR COMPONENTS

FRESH FROZEN PLASMA (FFP)

FFP contains all noncellular coagulation factors in near-normal levels. Units come from a single donor, are approximately 250 mL in volume, thawed to order, and ABO-matched before transfusion. Because hepatitis and other disease transmission risks are identical to those of whole blood and PRBCs, FFP should not be used for simple colloid volume replacement or expansion.

An NIH consensus conference concluded that FFP is the most overused blood product. FFP's only unequivocal indication is for the correction of clinically significant deficiencies of clotting factors. For example, FFP might be transfused to a patient who is taking coumadin and who has significant bleeding or needs immediate surgery. Even in this case, it is inefficient because coagulation factors are not concentrated in FFP. Cryoprecipitate (see subsequent text) is a more rational choice to correct a deficiency in the factors it contains. For the patient with an acute, undiagnosed bleeding disorder, FFP is the only source of all noncellular coagulation factors. At the risk of volume overload, FFP in adequate volume corrects any deficiency. Once a diagnosis is made, however, the specific factor that is deficient should be given.

Prophylactic administration of FFP should be eschewed. Historically, many practitioners administered 1 unit of FFP for every 5 to 6 units of PRBCs. Apparently, a concern regarding "dilutional coagulopathy" drives this practice. The mathematics of exchange transfusion, however, demonstrate the irrationality of this practice. Furthermore, evaluation in individual patients seldom demonstrates consistent findings—a situation typical of the clinical environment. Some patients bleed abnormally; others do not. Those who do have abnormalities in coagulation beyond those that can be explained by dilution alone. Fibrin-split products found in the blood of these patients and limited transient response to coagulation factor repletion suggest consumption of clotting factors as found in disseminated intravascular coagulopathy.

SPECIFIC FACTOR THERAPY

Classic hemophilia (a factor VIII deficiency, also known as hemophilia A) accounts for approximately 85% of patients with congenital abnormalities of coagulation factors. Most patients are aware of the diagnosis and their usual therapeutic requirements. Treatment of this disorder is replacement of the specific factor deficiency through the use of cryoprecipitate, usually obtained through standard blood bank resources. Recently, a commercially available factor VIII product produced through the use of recombinant DNA technology has become available. Because it is highly standardized in factor VIII content, there is an apparent advantage to its use, especially because there is no hepatitis risk or risk of transmission of HIV. Its cost, however, is substantially greater than that of cryoprecipitate, and this marketplace concern currently limits its use. At the time of this writing, a bill has been introduced in Congress to fund the use of this product for hemophiliacs in the future.

Cryoprecipitate is prepared by first freezing individual units of plasma and then thawing at 4°C. The small amount of protein precipitated in the process is rich in factor VIII and fibrinogen. When packaged separately and provided as individual units, it is commonly known as cryoprecipitate. Cryoprecipitate does not require crossmatching before administration. Factor VIII potency may vary significantly between units of cryoprecipitate. Thus, cryoprecipitate is commonly administered in multiple packs based on the patient's usual requirements for the extent of the injury being treated. The usual error made by the treating physician is not related to the estimate of total dose but rather to the failure of early initiation of treatment and adequate continuation through the course. The goal of treatment is to raise factor VIII levels sufficiently to ensure adequate function dependent on a clinical situation. For example, early superficial hematomas may be treated by raising factor VIII levels to 25%, whereas deep muscle hematomas or dental bleeding may require levels of 50%. Treatment of a hemophiliac patient with intracranial bleeding or serious trauma requires levels of up to 80%.

Fibrinogen is also present in large quantities in cryoprecipitate. The rare individual with congenital hypofibrinogenemia may be treated with cryoprecipitate.

Factor-IX deficiency (Christmas disease, hemophilia B) is a far less common congenital coagulopathy. Formerly available commercial products to treat episodes contained all the Vitamin K-dependent coagulation factors, including factors II, VII, IX and X. These products, prepared from pooled plasma collected from paid donors, carried the risk of disease transmission, and

so are no longer available. FFP is generally substituted. A recombinant DNA-produced product may become available in the future.

ALBUMIN AND PLASMA PROTEIN FRACTION (PPF)

Colloid administration for maintenance or restoration of oncotic pressure remains controversial. Both albumin and PPF are chemically and heat treated to eliminate the risk of hepatitis and HIV transmission. Albumin is available as a 25% "salt-poor" preparation (which in reality contains 160 mEq/L of sodium) hyperoncotic to plasma, and a 5% buffered solution iso-oncotic to plasma. The typical 25 mL ampule (12.5 g) has an oncotic effect approximately equal to one unit of FFP.

PPF contains 88% albumin and 12% globulins. It is iso-osmotic with plasma containing 130 to 160 mEq/L of sodium. Current methods of preparation have eliminated the risk of hypotension caused by the presence of pre-kallikrein activator.

IMMUNE GLOBULINS

Immune globulins such as tetanus (Hypertet), hepatitis B (H-BIG), and rabies (HypeRab) are prepared by hyperimmunizing donors who undergo plasmapheresis. Immune serum globulin is prepared by routine fractionating of plasma separated from whole blood. Hyperimmunized donors are not used. It is often used in an attempt to modify or prevent viral illnesses such as rubella, poliomyelitis, or rubeola, and to treat acquired or congenital hypoglobulinemias or agammaglobulinemias. Although it is sometimes suggested for prophylaxis after inadvertent needlestick exposure, there is no evidence of any efficacy or reduction in risk of acquiring transmitted diseases in such situations. The nature of the separation and processing of immune serum globulin precludes any risk of hepatitis or AIDS transmission.

BLOOD TRANSFUSION PRACTICES

BLOOD ADMINISTRATION HARDWARE

Patients who receive blood in the ED are likely to have multiple units transfused. The use of micropore fibers, blood-warming systems, pressure infusion pumps, and special tubing can contribute positively to outcome.

Blood can be administered with large-bore IV extension tubing, or with Y-type administration sets that have one inlet for the blood and another for the IV solution. Warmed saline solution can be run through the one arm of the Y, and when blood is infused, it is warmed and diluted to flow faster. Calcium- or glucose-containing solutions should not be used. Normal saline rather than hypotonic saline solutions should be used to prevent RBC lysis.

Micropore ("millipore") filters, available in 20- to 40-μm pore sizes, may be used to filter microaggregates of platelets, fibrin, and leukocyte fragments, thereby relieving the lung of the burden of doing so. They slow the rate of transfusion.

The energy and oxygen demand placed on a patient to warm a blood volume from 4° to 37°C is significant, and potentially life-threatening hypothermia can occur with massive transfusion. All too often, the patient is unclothed during resuscitation, massively transfused, and subsequently subjected to a surgical procedure in an air-conditioned operating room. Warming of the blood and other fluids tends to be overlooked.

Most warming systems in current use operate by maintaining a thermostatically controlled water bath or heating plate through which blood in a closed tubing system, designed to expose a maximum surface area, is circulated. The major deficiency with these systems is the reduction in rate of flow through the system and thus, reduced rate of infusion. Pressurized infusions systems may help to maintain adequate flow and, to some extent, offset this liability of warming systems. Pressure infusion devices operate by applying pneumatic pressure of no more than 300 torr (mm of mercury) to the blood bag. Systems should be closed to use such pressure infusion devices, and any puncture of a port in the system is likely to cause leakage upon pressurization.

Recently, warming devices with high-flow, large-bore manifolds and heat exchangers, using high volume counter-current flow of thermostatically regulated warmed water, have become available. These systems are expensive, but effective at warming large quantities of blood while maintaining high rates of flow. The most widely available comes from Level-1 Technologies and is called the Level 1 Fluid Warmer.

An alternative, readily available approach in most EDs, however, is to warm the sterile normal saline solution to approximately 110°F through the use of a thermostatically controlled oven or standard microwave oven. The warmed saline solution may then be used to dilute cold packed RBCs, warming the entire infusion toward a more physiologic temperature.

MASSIVE TRANSFUSION

Massive transfusion is transfusion of one-half of the patient's blood volume at one time, or transfusion of one blood volume within a 12-hour period. Massively transfused patients suffer complications of the underlying disease or trauma as well as potential complications of transfusion such as impaired hemostasis,

hypothermia, hyperkalemia, citrate toxicity, and adult respiratory distress syndrome (ARDS). Coagulopathies may result from platelet deficiency/destruction and DIC in the presence of dilution of labile clotting factors. The mathematics of exchange transfusion, however, demonstrate that 37% of the circulating volume originally present is still present after a 10-unit transfusion of packed red blood cells and supplemental crystalloid.[6]

The deficiencies of factors VIII and V present in all refrigerated blood are rapidly made up by liver-maintained stores. Even when huge quantities of blood are transfused, the liver rapidly corrects for dilution by rapid synthesis. Indeed, factors V and VIII are particularly well maintained, regardless of their depletion in refrigerated blood. Massively transfused patients with clinically significant bleeding and impaired hemostasis invariably have deficits much greater than can be explained by the dilution. Thus routine "prophylactic" administration of FFP is unwarranted. A massively transfused and bleeding patient, however, may well require supplementation with FFP. Thus, although prophylaxis is no longer appropriate, treatment certainly is.

Dilutional thrombocytopenia should be anticipated after transfusion of more than one blood volume in less than 6 hours. Ten platelet packs should be given if continued transfusion is anticipated.

Cold blood can cause hypothermia, which increases the metabolic workload and depresses cardiac function. Hypothermia is also a major and frequently overlooked cause of impaired hemostasis. In massive transfusion, blood must be warmed as it is infused.

Microaggregates contained in refrigerated blood, once implicated in post-traumatic and post-transfusion ARDS, are no longer thought to be relevant to the pathogenesis of the syndrome. Micropore filtration relieves the lung of the burden of removing microaggregates from the circulation, but the use of micropore filters does not appear to affect the incidence of ARDS.

Citrated blood infusion at rates greater than one mL/kg/min is rarely associated with perioral tingling and carpopedal spasm. At greatest potential risk are infants and those with hepatic dysfunction. Citrate chelates ionized calcium, and this effect continues until the citrate is metabolized. Myocardial depression has been demonstrated at ionized calcium levels one third of normal. Total calcium levels are variable, and in hemorrhagic shock are unreliable predictors of the need for calcium supplementation.

Calcium supplementation is not routinely necessary for massively transfused patients, but could be considered for the patient who is not responding to adequate volume replacement or who has acute heart failure. Prolongation of the corrected QT interval is a good, albeit late, indicator of decreased calcium ion concentration.[7] When used, 5 to 10 cc of calcium gluconate should be given slowly intravenously at a site distant from the blood transfusion.

Hyperkalemia, hyperphosphatemia, hyperammonemia, and acid-base disturbances are theoretic considerations that are rarely of clinical significance.

COMPLICATIONS OF TRANSFUSION

IMMEDIATE TRANSFUSION REACTIONS

Immediate transfusion reactions are classified as febrile, allergic, and hemolytic. Febrile reactions, the most common transfusion reactions, are characterized by the development of fever, chills and malaise. They rarely progress to hypotension or respiratory distress. Febrile reactions are thought to be the result of the infusion of platelets and leukocytes to which the recipient has antibodies. The use of leukocyte-poor blood or washed PRBCs for this type of reaction prevents its occurrence.

Once a febrile reaction is recognized, the transfusion should be terminated because it is impossible to differentiate on clinical grounds between a simple febrile reaction and the more serious immediate intravascular hemolytic transfusion reaction. A search for RBC destruction (described subsequently) should immediately ensue. Once the reaction is determined to be nonhemolytic in nature, transfusion may be resumed. The use of acetaminophen as an antipyretic may add to patient comfort. Anesthetized patients, infants incapable of shivering, and unconscious patients do not demonstrate, and obviously do not report, the symptoms of a febrile reaction.[8]

ALLERGIC REACTIONS

True anaphylactic reactions to blood transfusion are rare, occurring approximately once in 20,000 transfusions. The genetically IgA-deficient recipient is most at risk. Individuals with a history of multiple allergies should be carefully observed during transfusion. Those with a history of previous allergic reaction to transfusion should be premedicated with antihistamines. Ideally, these individuals should be given washed PRBCs or blood from IgA-deficient donors.

The treatment of immediate hypersensitivity reaction to blood is the same as the treatment of any anaphylactic reaction: epinephrine, fluids, and antihistamines. The transfusion should be stopped immediately.

HEMOLYTIC REACTIONS

Intravascular hemolysis, the most serious immediate reaction, is most often the result of misidentification of patient, specimen or blood unit. This antibody-mediated reaction results in the rapid destruction of transfused red cells within minutes of administration. The resulting release of free hemoglobin produces hemoglobinemia, hemoglobinuria, depletion of haptoglobin and subsequent bilirubin elevation. Clinical manifestations include fever, chills, low back pain and other myalgias, and a burning sensation at the site of infusion and along the vein centrally. Later manifestations include a feeling of breathlessness or chest tightness, hypotension, and bleeding. Anesthetized and unconscious patients may manifest only hypotension, bleeding, and hemoglobinuria. The damaged red cells activate complement leading to DIC, renal, or respiratory failure.

Laboratory evaluation includes determination of haptoglobin and free hemoglobin in blood serum and hemoglobin in urine, direct and indirect Coombs test, and coagulation and renal function profiles. A quick, simple screen can be performed by saving a complete-blood-count tube and centrifuging it. A pale pink color suggests a free hemoglobin level of 50 to 100 mg/dL. A pale brown color may be evident at levels as low as 20 mg/dL. This "naked eye" screen does not supplant the need for full laboratory evaluation.

Treatment begins with discontinuing the current transfusion and instituting crystalloid infusion. Furosemide in 80 to 100 mg doses intravenously increases renal cortical blood flow and helps protect renal function. Mannitol, which increases urine flow by decreasing tubular absorption, does not improve renal blood flow and therefore should not be used. Large amounts of fluids must be administered to maintain intravascular volume. Urinary output should be maintained at 0.5 to 1.0 mL per kg per hour. Monitoring central venous pressures or pulmonary capillary wedge pressures ensures that volume depletion is not mistaken for renal failure subsequent to the hemolytic transfusion reaction.

DELAYED REACTIONS

Extravascular hemolysis is the most common type of delayed transfusion reaction. An unexplained decrease in hemoglobin days after transfusion is the most common clinical manifestation of delayed extravascular hemolytic transfusion reactions. Transfused red blood cells become coated by nonagglutinating antibodies and are removed by tissue-bound macrophages, primarily in the spleen.

Treatment includes fluid administration and redetermination of the compatibility for transfusion of all blood units destined for transfusion to the patient. Blood specimens for the determination of hemoglobin, bilirubin, and haptoglobin help to differentiate between extravascular and intravascular hemolysis. Repeat searches for atypical antibodies may now reveal the presence of a previously undetected antibody as a result of the anamnestic immunologic response.

INFECTIONS

Infections resulting from blood transfusion include hepatitis, HIV (AIDS), HIV-II, HTLV-I, HTLV-II, cytomegalovirus, Epstein-Barr virus, syphilis, and malaria. Viral hepatitis is the most common and most severe infectious complication, occurring at a rate of 30,000 cases per year and causing perhaps 1500 to 3000 deaths annually.

Antibody to the hepatitis B and hepatitis C viruses can be tested for directly. The use of indirect screening tests for blood units to determine the presence of chronically elevated liver enzymes, in particular alanine amino transferase (ALT), once widely debated, has been implemented because of the growing concern about the safety of the blood supply. The loss of 6% of the currently available units for transfusion has still further strained the already stressed blood supply system.

No therapeutic or prophylactic modality has been shown effective in avoiding post-transfusion hepatitis. Prophylactic administration of immune serum globulin may reduce the risk in patients receiving multiple transfusions, but extensive washing of RBCs has not been useful.

Human immunodeficiency virus (HIV) and related retroviruses (HIV-II, HTLV-I, HTLV-II) have become a concern only in the last decade. The rapid development and implementation of serologic testing for HIV has been a major stride in control of disease transmission. All single-donor blood products transfused since 1985 have been screened by such tests. Because viremia is present before the development of antibody, not all infected units are excluded by testing. The continuing use of guidelines excluding donors at high risk, in conjunction with serologic testing, have reduced the risk of transmission of HIV to between one in 100,000 and one in 1,000,000. The next generation of assays, which identifies specific viral antigens of HIV in blood, reduces the risk even further. Testing for antibody to HTLV-I, a leukemia virus, has been recently implemented and concern about transmission of a second AIDS virus (HIV-II) may lead to testing for its antibodies.[8]

Cytomegalovirus (CMV) and the Epstein-Barr virus can also be transmitted by transfusion. A serologic test for antibody to cytomegalovirus has been approved and is being implemented for screening. Because most normal adults have antibody to CMV, however, units are not automatically screened and excluded from the blood supply. Rather, CMV seronegative units are sought and reserved for immunocompromised patients such as seronegative organ-transplant recipients, premature neonates, and seronegative pregnant women.[9]

Syphilis may be transmitted by fresh, untested blood units, but this is rare.because all banked blood is treated for its presence and Treponema pallidum do not survive in citrated blood for more than 2 or 3 days. Malaria is rarely transmitted because blood is not accepted from donors who have traveled in endemic areas 6 months before the donation, or who have ever contracted the disease.[10]

REFERENCES

1. Clarke, J.R., Davidson, S.J., Bergman, G.E., et al: Blood ordering for emergency department patients. Ann. Emerg. Med 9:2, 1980.
2. Sohmer, P.R., and Dawson, R.B.: Transfusion therapy in trauma: A review of the principles and techniques used in the M.I.E.M.S. program. Am. Surg. 45:109, 1979.
3. Barnes, A.: Status of the use of universal donor blood transfusion. CRC Critical Reviews in Clin. Lab. Sci. 4:147–160, 1973.
4. Barnes, A.: Transfusion of universal donor and uncrossmatched blood: Surgical hemotherapy. Bibl. Haematol., 46:132, 1980.
5. Schwab, C.W., Shayne, J.P., and Turner, J.: Immediate trauma resuscitation with Type O uncrossmatched blood: A two-year prospective experience. J. Trauma 26:897, 1986.
6. Marsaglia, G., and Thomas, E.D.: Mathematical consideration of cross circulation and exchange transfusion. Transfusion 11:216, 1971.
7. Rutledge, R., Sheldon, G.F., and Collins, M.L.: Massive transfusion in critical care management of the trauma patient. Crit. Care Clin. 2:791, 1986.
8. Shulman, I.A.: Adverse reactions to blood transfusion. Tex. Med. 85:35, 1989.
9. Bove, J.R.: Transfusion-transmitted diseases: Current problems and challenges. In Progress in Hematology, Volume XIV. New York, Grune and Stratton, pp. 123, 1986.
10. Berkman, S.A.: Infectious complications of blood transfusion. Blood Rev. 2:206, 1988.

BIBLIOGRAPHY

American Association of Blood Banks: Standards for Blood Banks and Transfusion Services (12th ed.). Washington, D.C., AABB, 1987.

Collins, J.A.: Current status of blood therapy in surgery. Adv. Surg. 22:75, Chicago, Yearbook Medical Publishers, 1989.

Mollison, P.L., Engelfriet, C.P., and Contreras, M: Blood Transfusion in Clinical Medicine (8th ed.). Oxford, Boston, Blackwell Scientific Publications, 1987.

Oberman, H., Chaplin, H., Poleshy, H.F., et al. (eds.): General Principles of Blood Transfusion. Chicago, AMA, 1985.

Chapter 54

ENDOCRINE AND METABOLIC EMERGENCIES

ACID-BASE BALANCE

Jamie Dananberg

CAPSULE

Maintenance of acid-base equilibrium is accomplished by various blood buffering systems and through dynamic changes in renal and pulmonary function. A variety of processes can shift this balance by altering acid or base loads and clearance or by affecting the two organ systems' homeostatic mechanisms. These processes are categorized by the type of shift that occurs and by the system affected. This chapter describes physiologic concepts of acid-base homeostasis and discusses the alterations in metabolic or respiratory function that lead to abnormalities in arterial hydrogen ion concentration.

PHYSIOLOGIC CONCEPTS

The hydrogen ion (H^+) concentration in arterial blood is closely regulated. Under normal circumstances, the negative logarithm concentration of H^+ (pH) is maintained between 7.35 and 7.45. Although there are several acid-base systems in the body, the primary determinant of arterial pH is the bicarbonate system. The bicarbonate equilibrium is shown in Equation 1. As predicted by the Henderson-Hasselbach equation (Equation 2), the final pH is determined by the ratio of pCO_2 and HCO_3^- and not by the absolute amounts of either individually. Because the pCO_2 concentration is regulated by the lung excretion and HCO_3^- concentration by the kidney, the maintenance of steady state pH is accomplished by an interaction between respiratory and renal processes. This interplay is outlined subsequently.

Under basal conditions, the body tends toward acidosis because of the continuous production of volatile acids from metabolic processes in the form of H_2CO_3 and the metabolism of dietary foodstuffs producing the fixed acids in the form of sulfates, phosphates, ketoacids, and lactic acid. Volatile acid is excreted as CO_2 by the lungs. Fixed acids consume HCO_3^-, which is regenerated by the kidney during the tubular excretion of H^+. Changes that occur in the metabolic production or ingestion of acids or bases must be quickly and efficiently dealt with to maintain pH homeostasis. The systems responsible for maintaining acid-base equilibria are chemical buffers and physiologic compensation.

The buffering capacity of blood is achieved through four systems: bicarbonate, as mentioned, and phosphate, protein, and hemoglobin buffers. These equilibria are shown in Equations 2 through 5.

The most rapid systems for controlling sudden changes in acid-base status are the bicarbonate system and the proteins present in serum. The other systems equilibrate over a period of hours.

When these buffers fail to maintain pH adequately within physiologic parameters, compensatory changes in respiratory or metabolic function occur in an attempt to restore acid-base homestasis by shifting the bicarbonate system in one direction or the other. The changes that occur in organ function are such that pCO_2/HCO_3^- ratio remains constant. For example, a decrease in HCO_3^- elicits a response to decrease pCO_2 by increasing alveolar ventilation. This compensatory secondary change occurs for each possible primary change in pCO_2 or HCO_3^-.

There are a number of important considerations regarding compensation. First, respiratory changes occur rapidly, often within minutes after a primary metabolic change in acid-base status. The maximal response, however, may require 12 to 24 hours. Renal changes in HCO_3^- production and H^+ excretion typically require 2 to 5 days to compensate fully for pri-

[Equation 1]:

$$\text{Bicarbonate: } HCO_3^- + H^+ \Leftrightarrow H_2CO_3 \Leftrightarrow H_2O + CO_2$$

[Equation 2]:

$$\text{Henderson-Hasselbach Equation: } pH = pK + \log \frac{HCO_3^-}{H_2CO_3}$$

$$pH = 6.1 + \log \frac{HCO_3^-}{0.03 \times pCO_2}$$

[Equation 3]:

$$\text{Serum/intracellular Protein: } Protein^- + H^+ \Leftrightarrow HProtein$$

[Equation 4]:

$$\text{Phosphate: } HPO_4^{2-} + H^+ \Leftrightarrow H_2PO_4^-$$

[Equation 5]:

$$\text{Hemoglobin: } Hgb^- + H^+ \Leftrightarrow HHgb$$

mary respiratory disorders. Second, the compensatory mechanisms counterbalance the primary effect; however, the degree of compensation is not perfect. Compensation only rarely returns acid-base status to normal ranges. For this reason, a normal pH in the face of alterations of both pCO_2 and HCO_3^- represents at least two primary acid-base disorders (mixed disorder). Third, the actual degree of compensation is held within relatively narrow ranges. These ranges are shown in Table 54-1. When there appears to be compensation outside the values predicted by these rules, one must suspect a mixed disorder. In that metabolic compensation for respiratory disorders takes time, as mentioned previously, these values vary by the amount of time a primary respiratory disorder has been present. Expected compensation may fall outside the rules when estimates of time are wrong.

The mechanisms by which the kidney maintains blood bicarbonate concentration are complex, involving a series of steps in the bicarbonate-buffer system and occurring at most points along the tubule. Because bicarbonate is freely filtered at the glomerulus, the nephron must either reabsorb or regenerate an equal amount. This system is graphically illustrated in Figure 54-1. The HCO_3^- ion is impermeable to the tubular membrane. The strategy is to combine the ion with a proton (H^+), thereby forming carbonic acid (H_2CO_3), which is then readily translocated from luminal to intracellular sites. The hydrogen ion is derived from the cleavage of H_2CO_3, which occurs in the tubular cell. In addition to providing H^+ for excretion into the tubular lumen, this reaction also generates HCO_3^-, which is reabsorbed from the cell into the blood stream. Finally, H_2CO_3 is formed in the tubule and reabsorbed into the cell, where it can serve as a template for the generation of additional HCO_3^- and H^+ ions. This perpetuates the system of H^+ excretion and HCO_3^- generation and uptake. The overall effect of the cycle is the generation of a HCO_3^- ion for each HCO_3^- filtered at the glomerulus and the process is termed bicarbonate reclamation.

In addition to bicarbonate reclamation, the kidney serves as the primary site for elimination of nonvolatile acids produced by metabolism and ingested in the diet. The precise mechanisms by which H^+ ion excretion occurs vary along the length of the tubule.[1] Many of the known processes are shown in Figure 54-1. In the proximal tubule, the primary vehicle by which urinary acidification occurs is Na^+-H^+ exchange.[2] This exchange is fueled by the Na^+ concentration gradient established by Na^+-K^+ pump ATPase activity. In addition to the activity of Na^+-H^+ exchange, evidence suggests a role for direct ATPase activated H^+ transport.[3] Another possible transport

TABLE 54-1. RANGES OF COMPENSATORY CHANGE

Primary Defect	Expected pCO_2	Expected $[HCO_3^-]$	Compensatory Change
Metabolic acidosis	<35	<18	$\Delta pCO_2 = [1 - 1.5] \times (\Delta HCO_3^-)$
Metabolic alkalosis	>35	>28	$\Delta pCO_2 = \{0.5 - 1.0\} \times (\Delta HCO_3^-)$
Acute respiratory acidosis	>45	>20	$\Delta HCO_3^- = 0.1 \times (\Delta pCO_2) \pm 3$
Chronic respiratory acidosis	>45	>28	$\Delta HCO_3^- = 0.4 \times (\Delta pCO_2) \pm 4$
Acute respiratory alkalosis	<35	>18 and <24	$\Delta HCO_3^- = \{0.1 - 0.3\} \times (\Delta pCO_2)$
Chronic respiratory alkalosis	<35	>14 and <20	$\Delta HCO_3^- = \{0.2 - 0.5\} \times (\Delta pCO_2)$

Bold numbers indicate the primary change. Change in pCO_2 is calculated from 40 mm Hg. Change in HCO_3^- is calculated from 24 mEq/L.

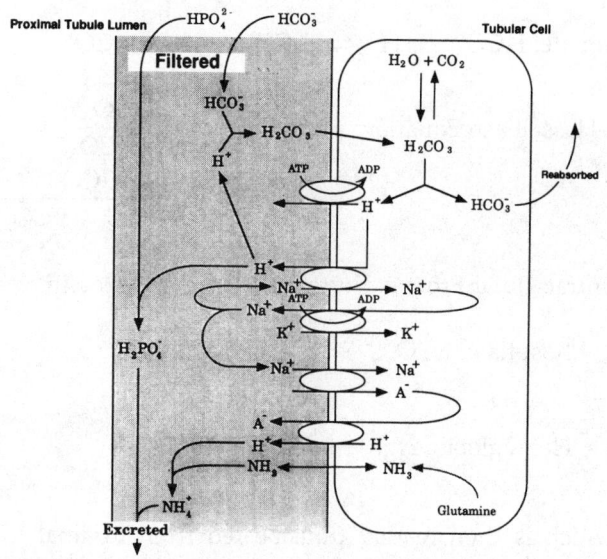

FIG. 54-1. *Representation of the various mechanisms of tubular bicarbonate reclamation and acid excretion.*

system involves sodium-anion coupling.[4] The Na^+-anion species crosses into the cell and dissociates. The free anion species is then co-transported with H^+ back into the lumen. The role of this system in H^+ excretion has yet to be fully determined. Many of these mechanisms exist in other parts of the tubule. In addition, H^+-K^+-coupled transport may also exist in collecting duct segments.

Once in the tubular lumen, H^+ ions must be excreted. Two mechanisms by which this occurs are titratable acid and ammonia excretion. Phosphate, uric acid, and creatinine can all serve as weak acids which are filtered by the glomerulus. The dibasic phosphate species HPO_4^{2-} combines with luminal H^+ to form the monobasic $H_2PO_4^-$, which is excreted. This process is depicted in Equation 4. The other entities play a much smaller role in H^+ ion excretion. Ammonia is produced in the tubular lumen cell during glutamine metabolism. This species diffuses into the lumen, combines with H^+, forming ammonium, and is excreted.

Generally, the proximal tubule reabsorbs about 80% of the total filtered load of bicarbonate through the mechanisms stated above. The remaining segments each reabsorb additional bicarbonate. Although their contribution is small, each system must work effectively to avoid bicarbonate losses. Acid secretion is primarily active in the proximal tubule and the thick ascending limb.

The respiratory control of acid-base status resides in the medullary and pontine brain stem regions, although there is higher cortical input to this region so that some element of conscious override can occur. There are three main areas of control. The medullary respiratory center is located in the reticular formation of the medulla and controls the rhythmic aspects of inspiration and expiration. The lower pons has some control over respiration as well because transection of

the brain stem above this location leads to apneustic breathing. The pneumotaxic center, located in the upper pons, is responsible for controlling the upper set point of respiration.

At the ventral surface of the medulla are chemoreceptors that, if stimulated by H^+ or CO_2, rapidly stimulate breathing. Because these receptors are bathed in cerebrospinal fluid (CSF), changes in CSF pH are immediately reflected by changes in respiratory patterns. Carbon dioxide crosses the blood-brain barrier easily so that changes in arterial pCO_2 are reflected in alterations in respirations.[5] In addition to central receptors, the carotid body appears to be sensitive to pH as well.

PRIMARY ACID-BASE DISORDERS

Before describing the physiologic mechanisms involved, it is important to consider certain terms. Acidosis refers to a disease process that, if unopposed, leads to accumulation of hydrogen ions, resulting in acidemia and a lowered arterial pH. Similarly, alkalosis refers to a disease process that, if unopposed, leads to an excess of bicarbonate ions, resulting in alkalemia and a raised arterial pH. Respiratory disturbances of acid-base equilibria are the result of the abnormal excretion of carbon dioxide (CO_2) leading to a deficit or excess of carbonic acid (H_2CO_3). This relationship is described by the Henderson-Hasselbach equation, discussed previously and shown as Equation 1. Alternatively, metabolic disturbances are those in which there is an excess intake or production of bicarbonate (HCO_3^-) or a decreased excretion of acids (other than carbonic acid). A simple acid-base disorder is one in which a single, primary acidosis or alkalosis occurs from respiratory or metabolic causes, followed by a compensatory change in the uninvolved system. A mixed acid-base disorder results when two or more primary processes occur in a single patient. See Tables 54-2 and 54-3 for illustrations of some specific cases.

METABOLIC ACIDOSIS

PATHOPHYSIOLOGY

Normal Anion Gap. These disorders encompass processes that cause a primary decrease in the concentration of extracellular HCO_3^- with a subsequent decrease in arterial pH. The lowering of bicarbonate may be from direct losses through gastrointestinal or renal sources or titration by acid. One of the clues used to distinguish among the causes of metabolic acidosis is the measurement of the difference between measured extracellular cations (namely, Na^+) and extracellular anions (HCO_3^- plus Cl^-). This difference, known as

TABLE 54-2. DISTURBANCES OF ACID-BASE BALANCE

Conditions	pHa	Paco$_2$	Standard HCO$_3^-$	BD	Compensatory Mechanisms	Treatment	Causes
Metabolic acidemia						Buffers	Shock-cardiac arrest Diabetic ketoacidosis
Uncompensated	↓ ↓	Normal	↓ ↓	↑ ↑			Diarrhea
Compensated	↓	↓	↓ ↓	↑ ↑	Respiratory Spontaneous hyperventilation	(Hyperventilation?) Increase minute ventilation	Renal failure Hypoventilation ↓ ↓
Respiratory acidemia							
Uncompensated	↓ ↓	↑ ↑	normal	none			
Compensated	↓	↑ ↑	↑	↓	Renal		
Metabolic alkalemia						Administration of acids Prevention of Cl loss Modest hypoventilation	Vomiting Bicarbonate administration
Uncompensated	↑ ↑	Normal	↑ ↑	↓ ↓			
Compensated	↑	Slightly ↑	↑ ↑	↓ ↓	Minimal respiratory		
Respiratory alkalemia						Normoventilation	Hyperventilation
Uncompensated	↑ ↑	↓ ↓	normal	none	Renal		
Compensated	↑	↓ ↓	↓	↑		Paco$_2$ normalization by controlled ventilation, addition of deadspace, or FICO$_2$	

Note: Box indicates site of lesion.
Abbreviations: pHa = Arterial pH; Paco$_2$ = arterial carbon dioxide pressure; HCO$_3^-$ = bicarbonate; BD = base deficit, FICO$_2$ = inspired carbon dioxide concentration.

the anion gap, represents an unmeasured amount of anions that must be present to maintain electroneutrality. Therefore, as bicarbonate is depleted, another anion must increase. If the other anion is chloride, a measured electrolyte, the anion gap remains unchanged. Alternatively, if bicarbonate is replaced by an anion that is not measured, the anion gap increases. In most situations, a normal gap is 8 to 14 mEq/L. Several circumstances can falsely alter the anion gap. Most proteins in plasma carry a negative charge, accounting for some of the unmeasured anions. In hypoproteinemia, the anion gap may therefore become elevated. Similarly, in patients with excess proteins, an example being multiple myeloma, the anion gap can approach zero. If cation concentrations are abnormal, the anion gap may also be affected. Changes in calcium, magnesium, or potassium are usually not of a magnitude to cause significant changes in the measured anion gap; however, in severe cases, this may occur.

Generally, normal anion gap metabolic acidoses are caused by gastrointestinal or renal losses of bicarbonate with concomitant increases in chloride transport. For this reason, normal anion gap metabolic acidosis is also termed hyperchloremic acidosis.

The various causes of a normal anion gap metabolic acidosis are listed in Table 54-4. *The most common cause of hyperchloremic acidosis is diarrhea.* These gastrointestinal fluids are rich in bicarbonate, sodium, and potassium, but are poor in chloride. Individuals with severe diarrhea develop hypobicarbonatemia as well as hypokalemia and hyperchloremia. Additionally, these individuals are usually volume-depleted. Biliary and pancreatic fluids are also high in bicarbonate and low in chloride, so that substantial losses of either can also cause hyperchloremic acidosis.

Renal tubular acidosis (RTA) is another cause of hyperchloremic acidosis. Because this disorder specifically affects the kidney's ability to acidify the urine, because of either excess HCO$_3^-$ loss or diminished H$^+$ ion excretion, any patient with a normal anion gap acidosis and a urinary pH of greater than 5.5 should be suspected of having RTA. This is in contrast to gastrointestinal losses, in which the urine is normally acidified. RTA is classified according to the site and source of the defect.

Type I RTA consists of a defect in the distal tubular excretion of H$^+$. In its classic form, there is an abnormality in ATP-dependent proton movement into the tubular lumen.[6] The urine is therefore not normally acidified. Because mineralocorticoid-dependent sodium reabsorption proceeds normally, the exchange cation for H$^+$ is potassium, causing hypokalemia, a characteristic finding in type I RTA.[6] Type II RTA involves a defect in proximal tubular HCO$_3$ reabsorption.[6] The exact abnormality is not clear; however, the derangement appears to be related to sodium-hydrogen exchange. Although direct evidence for this hypothesis is not available, it is supported by the fact that type II RTA is associated with other, more generalized defects in proximal tubular transport such as Fanconi's syndrome, in which there are problems with

TABLE 54.3. TYPES OF METABOLIC ACIDEMIA

Type of Acidemia	History	Clinical	Laboratory	Therapy
Diabetic ketoacidosis	• Often insulin-dependent • Antecedent stress, illness, missed insulin	Nausea, vomiting Dehydration Kussmaul breathing Coma Polyuria	Hyperglycemia Ketonemia/ketonuria Hyperkalemia ↑ Anion gap	• Hydration, vigorous • Titrated insulin • Rarely, bicarbonate
Alcoholic ketoacidosis	• Young chronic alcoholics • Drinking binge • Anorexia, hyperemesis • Usually seen about 48 hr. after cessation of drinking	Vomiting Semicoma	Near-normal blood sugar Marked ketosis ↑ Anion gap	• Glucose • Vigorous hydration • Insulin not necessary • Occasionally bicarbonate
Lactic acidosis	• r/o phenformin • r/o underlying malignancy	Toxic	Elevated serum lactate and lactate/pyruvate ↑ Anion gap	• Massive doses of bicarbonate • Hydration with diuresis • May need dialysis
Salicylate intoxication	• 80% pediatric • Suicide attempt	Early hyperventilation Hyperthermia Dehydration Delirium, seizures	Salicylate level over 50 mg./100 ml. ↑ Anion gap	• Hydration with forced diuresis • Cautious bicarbonate • External cooling • Gastric lavage/emesis
Methanol poisoning	• Usually chronic alcoholic	Asymptomatic latent period 8–36 hr. Headache, vertigo Vomiting Abdominal, back pain Dyspnea, apnea Peripheral vasoconstriction Coma Blindness	Methanol/formate in blood and urine Milk ketonemia Albuminuria ↑ Anion gap	• Hydration • Ethanol • Dialysis
Ethylene glycol poisoning	• Chronic alcoholic • Pediatric	Euphoria followed by deepening coma Tachycardia Paralysis Respiratory distress Renal failure	↑ Anion gap	• Emesis/lavage • Oxygen • Titrated bicarbonate

TABLE 54-4. CAUSES OF NORMAL ANION GAP METABOLIC ACIDOSIS AND SOURCE OF REDUCED BICARBONATE

A. Gastrointestinal disease ....GI HCO_3^- loss
  1. Diarrhea
  2. Fistula
B. Renal disorders
  1. RTA type I ....Reduced renal H^+ excretion
  2. RTA type II ....Renal HCO_3^- loss
  3. Early renal failure ....Reduced renal H^+ excretion
  4. Nephritis ....Reduced renal H^+ excretion
C. Hyporeninemic hypoaldosteronism ....Reduced renal H^+ excretion
D. Ureterosigmoidostomy/ileostomy ....GI Cl^- absorption/HCO_3^- loss
E. Hyperalimentation ....HCl administered with amino acids
F. Drugs
  1. Acetazolamide (Diamox) ....Renal HCO_3^- loss
  2. Chloride-containing compounds
    Calcium, magnesium chloride salts ....GI Cl^- absorption/HCO_3^- loss
    HCl, arginine HCl ....HCl administration

amino acid, glucose, and phosphate exchange mechanisms with sodium.

In early renal failure, there is often a modest defect in distal urinary hydrogen ion excretion resulting in a normal anion gap metabolic acidosis. This occurs before the accumulation of uremic byproducts which would increase the anion gap. Other specific renal disorders can lead to abnormalities in H^+ ion excretion. Interstitial nephritis, lupus nephritis, sickle cell nephropathy, and amyloid renal disease are included in this group.

Various drugs can cause hyperchloremic acidosis. Diamox, a carbonic anhydrase inhibitor, essentially causes a type II RTA by limiting normal bicarbonate reabsorption in the proximal tubule. Several chloride-containing compounds also lead to a normal anion gap acidosis. When large amounts of calcium or magnesium chloride are ingested, the chloride is readily absorbed by the intestine but the cations are not. A certain amount of these cations complex with HCO_3^-, leading to a net exchange of HCO_3^- for Cl^-. Similarly, direct infusion of HCl or HCl-containing materials (NH_4Cl, arginine HCl) increases to the chloride pool while depleting stores of HCO_3^-. Occasionally, hyperalimentation solutions may contain excess amino acids-HCl salts, thereby causing hyperchloremic acidosis. Current commercially available formulas for hyperalimentation do not present this problem.

Ureteral diversion procedures can lead to normal anion gap acidosis; however, current surgical protocols lessen the likelihood of this complication considerably. Previously, when the ureter was diverted to the sigmoid colon, the urine remained in contact with intestinal mucosa for prolonged periods. This leads to a reabsorption of chloride in urine with subsequent exchange for HCO_3^-. Most surgical procedures today have smaller amounts of intestine used in the loop, and the drainage through a stomal site is immediate. If there is an obstruction to urine flow, particularly at the stoma, hyperchloremic acidosis is possible.

Hyporeninemic hypoaldosteronism is a disorder seen primarily in older individuals with underlying renal disease and frequently coexisting diabetes mellitus. Aldosterone secretion is low, related to the low renin levels. The actual cause of abnormal renin secretion is unknown. Although these patients can develop hyperchloremic acidosis, the major ramification is hyperkalemia. Because the acidosis appears to be renally mediated, and is distinguishable from types I and II RTA, this disorder has also been termed type IV RTA.

Elevated Anion Gap. When acidosis is present and the anion gap is found to be elevated, the decrease in HCO_3^- is made up for by an anion that is otherwise unmeasured. The causes of high anion-gap metabolic acidosis and the unmeasured anion in each case are given in Table 54-5.

Renal failure may result in metabolic acidosis for several reasons. In cases of significant failure, the reduced nephron mass and the tubular abnormalities lower the kidney's ability to secrete an acid load or generate additional bicarbonate.[7] In mild insufficiency, there may be an enhanced proximal uptake of chloride leading to electrical potential inhibition of hydrogen ion excretion.[7] In patients with prerenal azotemia, there may be peripheral hypoxia, caused by poor cardiac output, which may lead to lactic acidosis (see subsequent text) in addition to the decrease in renal perfusion causing a decrease in acid excretion.

Ketoacidosis is a life-threatening abnormality that occurs primarily in type I diabetes mellitus but can be seen in severe alcoholism and starvation. The cause of diabetic ketoacidosis (DKA) can be specifically traced to insulinopenia, which can be absolute (patient not taking insulin) or relative (usual dose in face of infectious process). The reduced insulin levels cause hepatic production of ketoacids, namely β-hydroxybuterate (β-HB) and acetoacetate (AcOAc), the reduction in tissue uptake and metabolism of these compounds, and an increase in free fatty acid production by adipose tissue with a net effect of increases in serum concentrations of β-HB, AcOAc, and acetone. It is primarily acetone, because of its low vapor pressure, that can be detected on the breath of patients with DKA. The acidosis in this illness is often exacerbated by coexisting dehydration and excess lactate production. Alcoholic ketoacidosis is seen in patients with

---

TABLE 54-5. CAUSES OF HIGH ANION GAP METABOLIC ACIDOSIS AND ASSOCIATED UNMEASURED ANION

A. Renal failure/uremia . . . . .Phosphates, sulfates, organic anions
B. Ketoacidosis . . . . .β-hydroxybutyrate, acetoacetate
    1. Diabetes mellitus
    2. Alcoholism
    3. Starvation
C. Lactic acidosis . . . . Lactate
D. Toxins
    1. Aspirin . . . . Salicylate, organic anions
    2. Methanol . . . . Formate
    3. Ethylene glycol . . . . Glycolate
    4. Paraldehyde . . . . Unknown

chronic alcoholism who have co-existing malnutrition and repeated emesis. These individuals become dehydrated and develop an increase in serum ketones, primarily β-HB, so that tests for presence of ketones may be lower than expected.

Lactic acidosis occurs in accumulation of lactate because of either an increase in production or a decrease in utilization. Lactate is a metabolic end product of glycolysis, the anaerobic metabolism of glucose. It is produced from pyruvate by lactate dehydrogenase (LDH) in a reaction that is NADH-dependent. The reaction is reversible and given by the following equation:

[Equation 6]:

$$\text{Pyruvate-H} \underset{\text{NADH}}{\overset{\text{NAD}}{\rightleftharpoons}} \text{Lactate-H}$$

Under normal circumstances, pyruvate enters the Krebs cycle to yield additional energy during oxidative metabolism. Under conditions of tissue hypoxia, pyruvate accumulates and the reaction is shifted to the right. The accumulation of lactic acid depletes bicarbonate thereby causing a high anion gap acidosis.

A series of toxins and compounds also cause metabolic acidosis. *Salicylates* can cause complicated changes in acid-base status by virtue of its effect on respiratory drive and as a cause of metabolic acidosis. Given the concomitant respiratory alkalosis that may be present, patients may present with high, low, or normal pH. In terms of metabolic effects, the salicylate anion replaces bicarbonate, thereby causing a high anion gap; however, lactic acid and ketoacids may also be responsible for metabolic acidosis in severe abuse or overdose cases. Because salicylates are considerably more common than the other agents listed in Table 54-3, any patient with an unexplained high anion gap metabolic acidosis should be suspected of aspirin intoxication. This is especially true if a respiratory alkalosis is also present.

The ingestion of methanol may cause a severe metabolic acidosis. Methanol is metabolized by the enzyme alcohol dehydrogenase in the same fashion as ethanol. The end products of formaldehyde and formic acid deplete bicarbonate and increase the anion gap. In addition to the acid-base disturbance, formic acid may cause severe neurologic sequelae.

Ethylene glycol, a frequent ingredient in automotive antifreeze and organic solvents, can cause marked metabolic acidosis. Like methanol, it is metabolized by hepatic alcohol dehydrogenase to glycolate, hippurate, and oxalate, but glycolic acid appears to be the primary source of toxicity and acidosis.[8] (See Chap. 84 for treatment of poisoning.) Aside from the acid-base disturbance, glycolic acid also has serious neurologic manifestations. Because ethylene glycol also has significant osmolar characteristics, the osmolarity

of blood may be elevated. The presence of an "osmolar gap" should heighten suspicion for this diagnosis. The osmolar gap is that measured in the laboratory minus that calculated by Equation 7. The existence of such a gap indicates that another osmolar substance is present in the serum. It is important to bear in mind that only the presence of ethylene glycol increases the osmolarity. Glycolate replaces bicarbonate one for one so that osmolarity does not change because of the associated anion.

[Equation 7]:

$$Posm = 2([Na] + [K]) + ([Glucose]/18) + (BUN/2.8)$$

[Na] and [K] are given as mEq/L
[Glucose] and BUN are given as mg/dl

Administration or ingestion of *paraldehyde* also yields a metabolic acidosis because of its metabolism to acetaldehyde and acetic acid. Paraldehyde has been primarily used as an anticonvulsant in the past, particularly for status epilepticus. Its difficulty in administration and potential toxicity, however, and the availability of other effective alternatives have significantly limited its use. The actual anion responsible for increasing the anion gap has not been well established.

CLINICAL PRESENTATION

The clinical presentation of patients with metabolic acidosis depends on several factors, including the rate of development of acidemia and the chronicity of its presence. In general, the clinical signs and symptoms of acidemia are multisystem. The effects of acidemia on the cardiovascular system represent the most serious expression of lowered arterial pH. The overall effects on any part of the cardiovascular system rely on the balance of positive and negative factors. Positively, at mild levels of acidemia, catecholamines are released, and this enhances most measures of cardiovascular performance, including cardiac inotropy and chronotropy, cardiac output, and peripheral vascular resistance. At more significant levels of acidemia, usually at arterial pH less than 7.20, the direct effect of H^+ ions predominate. These latter effects include negative inotropy and bradycardia, reduced cardiac output, and peripheral vasodilation. Prolonged severe acidemia can therefore cause life-threatening hypotension.

The pulmonary manifestations of acidemia include respiratory compensation (i.e., hyperventilation) and increased pulmonary vascular resistance. Oxygen delivery can be affected in divergent ways. Acidemia shifts the oxygen-hemoglobin dissociation curve to facilitate tissue release of oxygen. Continued acidemia, however, lowers red blood cell levels of 2,3-DPG, which hampers peripheral oxygen dissociation. The net effect is frequently an unchanged delivery of oxygen.

Although changes in mental status are often seen in patients with a significant metabolic acidosis, it is

[Equation 8]:

$$HCO_3^- \text{ deficit} = 0.5 \times \text{body weight (kg)} \times (24 - [HCO_3^-])$$
$$\text{where } [HCO_3^-] \text{ is the electrolyte total } CO_2 \text{ in mEq/L.}$$

felt that this is primarily from the effects of decreased perfusion associated with hypotension and changes in osmolality that may occur in associated diseases.

Most cases of normal anion gap metabolic acidosis do not have a substantially severe enough acidemia to cause more than a primary hyperventilatory response. For this reason, most individuals who are otherwise healthy are able to maintain arterial pH near normal levels and frequently not less than 7.30.

In contrast, individuals with an anion gap acidosis may have a large source of continued acid production, which overwhelms the normal buffering capacity and drives arterial pH to values less than 7.20. In general, the rate of change of arterial pH seems to be the most predictive indicator for the presence of symptoms. Patients with chronic renal failure may have few, if any, symptoms of acidemia, and no pertinent signs may be present. Alternatively, patients with acute renal failure may be markedly symptomatic and require bicarbonate infusion and/or acute hemodialysis.

Patients with ketoacidosis may display a variety of symptoms. The clinical presentation and treatment of such patients are specifically discussed in Chapter 00. Other useful indicators of DKA are the presence of urinary or serum ketones, ketone breath, and hyponatremia.

Patients with acidosis on the basis of toxins may develop various symptoms, depending on the specific agent used. Individuals with salicylate intoxication may develop hyperventilation because of the direct effect of the agent on respiratory centers. A frequent coexisting symptom in significant overdose is tinnitus. In large doses, hyperthermia may also occur. Cardiovascular pathology is reported but uncommon. Obtundation and coma can be seen in severe toxicity. Gastrointestinal effects such as nausea and vomiting are common, with bleeding and perforation occuring less frequently. The direct effect of salicylates on the hematologic system causes a prolonged bleeding time.

DIAGNOSIS AND TREATMENT

The treatment of individuals with metabolic acidosis depends on the causative factors. Although the identified abnormality is a decrease in the serum HCO_3^- concentration, treatment with sodium bicarbonate to increase its concentration may sometimes prove harmful. Although this is seemingly counterintuitive, the administration of sodium bicarbonate carries with it the attendant risks of hypervolemia, hyperosmolality, and iatrogenic hypokalemia. Rapid administration of sodium bicarbonate can also adversely affect tissue oxygen delivery by altering the oxygen-hemoglobin dissociation curve. It is not considered prudent to treat metabolic acidosis aggressively with bicarbonate ther-

apy, particularly in patients with mild acidosis (pH > 7.20). In those with immediately life-threatening acidosis (pH < 7.00), however, more directed use of sodium bicarbonate is advisable, along with other supportive measures aimed at correcting abnormalities in hemodynamic and respiratory function. In any event, the primary goal of therapy should always be aimed at improving the underlying disorder.

When repletive therapy is determined to be in order, it is helpful to calculate the bicarbonate deficit. This serves as a useful starting point for determining appropriate amounts of bicarbonate to avoid both over- and undertreatment. The deficit may be determined by Equation 8. The rate and route of administration are discussed subsequently.

NON-ANION GAP ACIDOSIS

Gastrointestinal losses of bicarbonate can usually be treated by slowing diarrheal losses. Once the patient is rehydrated, the renal capacity to regenerate lost bicarbonate makes up the deficit in a timely fashion. In the case of severe losses, oral repletion can be used. Both type I and type II RTA are treated with oral bicarbonate therapy on a chronic basis. Because proximal type II RTA is a disease of bicarbonate wasting, these individuals' requirements are frequently greater than in distal RTA. Type II RTA should be treated with 5 to 15 mEq per kg per day, whereas type I RTA can usually be effectively treated with 1 to 3 mEq per kg per day.[9] The renal failure-related causes of non-anion gap acidosis generally require either no treatment or low- to moderate-dose chronic oral replacement of bicarbonate. These cases usually involve early and mild renal impairment, and repletive therapy is unusual.

Patients with hyporeninemic hypoaldosteronism rarely require bicarbonate replacement. The level of acidosis is typically mild, with serum bicarbonate concentrations almost always greater than 15 mEq/L. The more significant impairment is that of potassium excretion, and individuals may have serum potassium concentrations of 5.0 to 6.2 mEq/L. Many of these patients have diabetes mellitus with underlying renal impairment. The degree of acidosis appears to correlate with the level of renal dysfunction. The thrust of therapy in these patients is glycemic control. Improvements in this parameter invariably improve acidosis and hyperkalemia.

Patients who have undergone ureteral diversion procedures and subsequently develop acidosis secondary to this can be treated in several ways. Most importantly, acceptable function of the diversion must be verified. Any strictures or other obstructions to flow cause or worsen the hyperchloremic acidosis. Oral bicarbonate therapy, in lieu of surgical reconstruction, can be helpful.

The remaining causes relate to drugs or hyperalimentation. It is clear that the mainstay of therapy is to withdraw the offending agent. The chloride-containing salts may be switched to carbonate preparations.

ANION-GAP ACIDOSIS

The treatment of anion gap metabolic acidosis is removal of the offending acid by reversing its metabolic production or by removal. The causes of this form of acidosis are relatively limited to the four main categories listed in Table 54-3. Patients with severe acidosis caused by uremia can generally be managed most rapidly and efficiently by hemodialysis. These individuals, however, frequently have chronic acidosis in which the degree of acidosis can fluctuate widely. Acidosis is often tolerated well in this case, and emergent therapy is often not required.

In contrast, diabetic ketoacidosis (DKA) is an acute alteration in acid-base homeostasis requiring prompt attention. The level of acidosis has been used as a guide to the severity of the illness; however, the possibility of rapid deterioration is always present, and frequent clinical re-evaluation is critical. Patients require multiple therapeutic modalities. In general, the mainstays of therapy are fluid repletion and insulin therapy. Immediate infusion of fluids is the initial therapy in all cases of DKA. Volume expansion diminishes any contributing lactic acidosis and hypotension. Furthermore, renal clearance of acid and glucose is enhanced with the increase in renal blood flow. Finally, some patients with severe volume depletion can maintain sufficient intravascular volume and blood pressure because of the osmotic forces attributed to glucose. Reduction of glucose concentrations in these individuals with insulin without prior fluid repletion can precipitate life-threatening hypotension and shock.

There has been considerable discussion regarding the use of bicarbonate in the treatment of DKA. Physiologically, there are substantial reasons not to administer bicarbonate. The oxidation of AcOAc and β-HB results in HCO_3^- production and insulin administration prevents the reaccumulation of these acids. Therefore, pH returns toward normal without exogenous alkali. Similarly, administration of bicarbonate during insulin and fluid therapy of DKA can easily lead to a metabolic alkalosis. Additionally, rapid increases in arterial pH may adversely affect the hemoglobin oxygen dissociation curve as well as causing paradoxic decreases in cerebrospinal fluid pH. It can also be argued that when arterial pH falls to less than 7.0 cardiovascular and central nervous function may be significantly depressed. A pragmatic approach calls for administration of small to moderate doses of bicarbonate (1 to 2 mEq/kg) added to one liter of 0.45%

saline to patients with arterial pH less than 7.00 or in those in whom the plasma bicarbonate concentrations are less then 5 mEq/L. Additional therapy should be dictated only by repeat measurement of arterial pH 1 to 2 hours after all modalities of therapy have been instituted.

Alcoholic ketoacidosis is treated by administration of dextrose and fluids. These maneuvers clear the high levels of ketoacids in these individuals. The primary acid is β-HB, which does not react with the urine nitroprusside test to indicate the presence of ketones. Early on, therefore, these patients may have weakly positive tests. With treatment, however, the β-HB is converted to AcOAc during oxidation, and urinary ketones may become markedly positive despite appropriate therapy. As always, other treatment protocols must be followed in treating patients with alcoholic ketoacidosis because of the high prevalence of other deficiency syndromes, particularly thiamine, B_{12}, magnesium, and phosphorus.

The diagnosis of *lactic acidosis* may be made by direct measurement of blood lactate. It is advised that this assessment be made in any individual with an elevated anion gap acidosis in whom other causes have been ruled out or felt to be highly unlikely. Other helpful laboratory determinations include the presence of hyperphosphatemia and hyperuricemia. In the therapy of lactic acidosis, it is essential to treat the underlying cause of lactate production as well as the resultant acidemia. In terms of correction of the acid-base disturbance, the use and amount of sodium bicarbonate depend on the level of acidemia and the degree to which further lactate production can be reduced. Individuals with arterial pH below 7.2 should be treated with sodium bicarbonate. The amount given can be calculated by the base deficit as given by Equation 8. The overall goal is to bring the pH to values between 7.2 and 7.3 and the serum bicarbonate concentration to greater than 12 mEq/L. Half of the calculated deficit should be given immediately, and the remaining sodium bicarbonate can be given by adding it to 5% dextrose and infusing over 8 to 12 hours.[10] Any ongoing lactate production alters the actual amount of bicarbonate required to reverse the acidemia. Although there is continued discussion regarding the appropriateness of bicarbonate use, substantial evidence exists regarding the above protocol.[11]

PHYSIOLOGIC GUIDE TO TREATMENT OF TOXIN-INDUCED METABOLIC ACIDOSIS

The initial treatment of toxin-induced metabolic acidosis is identical for all poisonings, i.e., to reduce absorption and increase elimination. Salicylate overdosage is the most common cause of toxin-induced acid-base disturbances. The initial treatment is to reduce elimination by gastric lavage, emesis with syrup of ipecac (30 mL in adult or child greater than 90 pounds; 15 mL in children aged 1 to 12; 5 mL in infants 6 to 12 months), or with single or repeated doses of activated charcoal (given as a slurry: 30 to 100 mg in adults, 15 to 30 mg in children, or 1 to 2 mg/kg, mixed in 240 mL of diluent per 30 g of charcoal; repeated doses are usually half initial dose). The initial dose of charcoal is followed by a cathartic, usually sorbitol or magnesium sulfate. Charcoal is probably as effective as emesis in reducing elimination and should be the primary treatment if ingestion was more than 2 to 3 hours before presentation.

As discussed previously, the metabolic effects of salicylates are complex. Acidosis should be treated with intravenous sodium bicarbonate, 1 to 2 mEq per kg added to hypotonic fluid. In addition to correcting the acid-base disturbance, delivering bicarbonate alkalinizes the urine, which enhances the renal excretion of the acid. Adequate alkalinization requires 44 to 132 mEq of sodium bicarbonate per liter of D5W given at a rate of 2 to 3 mL/kg per hour and producing a similar urine flow. Because potassium deficits are common and alkalinization is not effective without potassium repletion, 20 to 30 mEq of KCl should also be added to each liter. Urine pH should be maintained at 7 to 8. All patients should be closely monitored for mental and respiratory status. Frequent measurement of serum potassium and pH and urine output is essential.

In patients with salicylate levels greater than 130 mg per dL at 6 hours after ingestion or those with persistent acidemia or further clinical worsening, hemodialysis is recommended.

Ingestions of methanol are serious and must be treated rapidly. Gastrointestinal absorption of methanol is rapid, so that lavage or emesis may be effective for only 30 minutes after ingestion. Activated charcoal can absorb small to moderate amounts of methanol but does not inhibit ethanol absorption. The acid-base disturbances in methanol ingestion can be severe. Because the acid-base derangements are caused by the products of methanol metabolism, acidosis may be delayed for 18 to 48 hours. If ethanol has been simultaneously ingested, methanol metabolism may be slowed further and acidemia may occur days later. The acidosis is managed by infusion of sodium bicarbonate, 1 to 2 mEq per kg with careful monitoring of arterial pH. Ethanol infusion is the primary modality of therapy in this condition and substantially prevents the metabolism of methanol. If significant metabolism of methanol has already occurred, or in large ingestions, hemodialysis is a highly effective means of therapy.

Ethylene glycol is also metabolized by alcohol dehydrogenase to substances that are responsible for toxicity. As with methanol, treatment of the acidosis is with sodium bicarbonate, 1 to 2 mEq per kg given every 2 to 3 hours as dictated by arterial pH measurements. Ethanol infusions are also effective in this ingestion. Hemodialysis is also highly useful in large ingestions. Paraldehyde may cause significant acidosis. Treatment of acidosis is primarily bicarbonate

infusion, as described. (See Chaps. 83 and 84 for further treatment of these toxicities.)

METABOLIC ALKALOSIS

PATHOPHYSIOLOGY

Metabolic alkalosis leads to an excess of serum bicarbonate concentrations. This process is best understood by examining its production, maintenance, and clearance. The processes that initiate metabolic alkalosis can be different from the factors that promote its maintenance. Furthermore, certain pathophysiologic conditions must exist for metabolic alkalosis to persist. Normally, the kidney can completely excrete any excess bicarbonate presented to it. Factors must exist to limit this ability for hyperbicarbonatemia to persist. Once these factors are overcome, recovery from alkalosis occurs.

The initial mechanisms that can produce metabolic alkalosis take one of three forms. First, there may be a loss of H^+ ions from the extracellular space. These losses may be from gastrointestinal or renal sources or from shifts of H^+ ions into the intracellular compartment. Second, HCO_3^- or substances that can generate it are added to the extracellular fluid in excess of daily acid production and consumption. Third, loss of chloride-rich and bicarbonate-poor fluids causes bicarbonate to rise so that electrochemical neutrality is preserved.

In contrast to initiating mechanisms, maintenance factors have their primary effect by impeding renal excretion of alkali. On occurrence of metabolic alkalosis, buffer systems in the blood, respiratory hypoventilation, and renal bicarbonate excretion all work together to return arterial pH to normal. Several conditions can hinder the kidney's ability to excrete the alkali load.

Volume depletion and activation of mineralocorticoid excess states are two of the major maintenance causes of alkalosis. In hypovolemia, sodium and chloride are lost and proximal tubular sodium reabsorption is maximized. Because of the chloride deficit, sodium transport linked to this anion is hampered (Na^+-A^- transport, depicted in Figure 54-1). Sodium uptake associated with Na^+-H^+ ion exchange is enhanced. The H^+ excretion causes a reciprocal and obligate increase in the production of HCO_3^-, thereby reducing the net excretion of alkali. Furthermore, during volume depletion, aldosterone concentration is increased. This steroid has been shown to have several effects on renal acid production. It enhances tubular hydrogen excretion independent of its effects on sodium and potassium handling.[12] Additionally, increases in distal sodium reabsorption are linked, in part, to hydrogen excretion. Finally, mineralocorticoid-induced hypokalemia can lead to increased losses of hydrogen ions by exchange with the intracellular compartment.[13] In mineralocorticoid excess, these effects can occur in the absence of volume depletion.

TABLE 54-6. CAUSES OF METABOLIC ALKALOSIS

A. Chloride-responsive (low urine chloride [<10 mEq/L])
  1. Diuretics
  2. NG suction/vomiting
  3. Colonic villous adenoma
  4. Recovery from respiratory acidosis
  5. Cystic fibrosis
B. Chloride-unresponsive (high urine chloride [>20 mEq/L])
  1. Aldosteronism (primary, secondary, congenital)
  2. Cushing's syndrome/disease
  3. Bartter's syndrome
  4. Licorice ingestion
  5. Severe potassium deficiency
C. Other
  1. Excess alkali intake/administration
  2. Milk-alkali syndrome
  3. Refeeding after starvation
  4. Large doses of poorly reabsorbable anion (e.g. carbenicillin, penicillin)
  5. Massive transfusions of citrate-containing blood products

---

Chloride depletion alone may also play a role in the maintenance of metabolic alkalosis. Renal bicarbonate excretion must be balanced electrically by another ion. Under conditions of chloride deficits, no other anions in adequate concentrations are available to provide this balance.[14] Cation co-excretion is theoretically possible, but excretion of large amounts of sodium leads to volume depletion. The effects of volume depletion and subsequent sodium reabsorption take precedence over the need for bicarbonate excretion.

In light of this discussion, *the causes of metabolic alkalosis can be divided into conditions related to sodium, chloride, and volume depletion* (chloride-responsive), *and those unrelated to these circumstances* (Table 54-6). The former group includes gastrointestinal fluid losses. Gastric fluid secretions are in acid and can amount to 2 liters daily. The fluid H^+ ion normally combines with pancreatic HCO_3^- to allow excretion of acid and alkali. With large acid losses from NG suctioning or prolonged vomiting, the bicarbonate is not excreted, and hyperbicarbonatemia develops. This condition is maintained if gastric losses are sufficient to cause sodium and chloride depletion and dehydration.

The renal cause of chloride-responsive alkalosis is diuretics. Because patients using diuretics are also placed on salt-restricted diets, these individuals may become mildly alkalemic. The diuretic induces mild to moderate dehydration with subsequent increases in sodium avidity along with chloride deficits. Sodium is reabsorbed preferentially to maintain volume status and acid secretion is increased to handle the sodium uptake. Acid generation is coupled to bicarbonate production, and a metabolic alkalosis results.

When individuals have chronic respiratory acidosis, the appropriate compensatory correction is a rise in bicarbonate. When the acidosis is corrected, the renal compensatory response takes days to recover, so that alkalemia may result. If dehydration and chloride de-ficiency are also present, the alkalosis is maintained. Rarely, children with cystic fibrosis have been reported to develop a metabolic alkalosis based on large losses of chloride in excess of HCO_3^- ion.

The chloride-unresponsive group of conditions are primarily a state of excess mineralocorticoid activity. Primary, secondary, or congenital aldosteronism may all cause metabolic alkalosis. The sources of primary hyperaldosteronism include bilateral adrenal hyperplasia, unilateral adrenal autonomous nodule aldosterone secretion, adrenal carcinoma, and increased endogenous or exogenous glucocorticoid administration with crossover mineralocorticoid activity. Secondary aldosteronism can occur in renal artery stenosis or renin-secreting juxtaglomerular cell tumors. Glucocorticoid excess causes some element of mineralocorticoid excess unless the source of glucocorticoid is exogenous and is devoid of mineralocorticoid activity. Congenital adrenal hyperplasia caused by 11-β or 17-α hydroxylase deficiency leads to mineralocorticoid excess states. In all these cases, mineralocorticoid increases distal tubular sodium reabsorption in exchange for potassium and hydrogen ions as well as directly stimulated distal hydrogen ion excretion. Administration of mineralocorticoid in humans does not lead to alkalosis or persistent positive sodium balance (mineralocorticoid escape), suggesting that other mechanisms are also coming in to play in the development of metabolic alkalosis. Bartter's syndrome is a rare condition of hyperreninemic hyperaldosteronism with marked hypokalemia and metabolic alkalosis and is seen most commonly in children. Black licorice contains glycyrrhizic acid, which has mineralocorticoid activity, and large intakes of this substance can simulate hyperaldosteronism.

The final cause of metabolic alkalosis is potassium deficiency. Although no data suggest the mechanism by which potassium deficiency causes alkalosis, several cases have been reported in which serum potassium concentrations of less than 2 mEq/L were associated with persistence in an established alkalosis and treatment with sodium chloride was effective only after the potassium deficit was itself corrected.[15]

Several causes of metabolic alkalosis that do not fit clearly into the above classification scheme are also listed in Table 54-6. Although the kidney is capable of secreting large amounts of bicarbonate, continuous administration of excess alkali overwhelms the kidney and causes metabolic alkalosis. This is more pronounced in renal insufficiency because decreased renal function also diminishes intrinsic bicarbonate excretion ability.

Milk-alkali syndrome is an interesting disease in which there is oral intake of large amounts of calcium and alkali such as calcium carbonate or milk and sodium bicarbonate. Currently, this syndrome is rare because absorbable alkali has been replaced by nonabsorbable alkali in the treatment of peptic ulcer disease and development of the syndrome requires more than 4 g of elemental calcium daily.

Individuals who are refed with carbohydrate meals after prolonged fasting develop a metabolic alkalosis, although the mechanisms by which this occurs are unknown. Patients who receive large doses of poorly reabsorbable anion in antibiotics can be found to have a metabolic alkalosis. It is presumed that the large amount of nonreabsorbed anion delivered to the distal tubule stimulates acid and potassium excretion, thereby increasing bicarbonate generation and reabsorption. Massive transfusions of citrate-containing blood products cause a metabolic alkalosis because citrate is metabolized to bicarbonate.

CLINICAL PRESENTATION

Many systems can be adversely affected by the presence of systemic alkalemia. The respiratory system may be altered in several ways. Increases in plasma bicarbonate concentration decrease central respiratory drive, causing a rise in arterial pCO_2 (as predicted by the equations in Table 54-1). Other associated metabolic changes, particularly hypokalemia, may reduce respiratory muscle function. These conditions may cause hypoxia and its attendant symptoms and signs.

Neuromuscular effects include neurologic irritability as evidenced by the presence of Chvostek and Trousseau signs, generalized weakness, muscle spasm or tetany, or frank seizures. Depression in mental status may also result. These changes occur partly because of decreases in ionized calcium induced by the alkalemia, coexisting hypokalemia, and changes in cerebral blood flow.

Cardiovascular changes are also seen. The heart is particularly prone to excitability, with an increased incidence of tachyarrhythmias. These arrhythmias are poorly treated by classic antiarrhythmics unless acid-base status is returned closer to normal.[16]

DIAGNOSIS AND TREATMENT

The approach to the patient with metabolic alkalosis includes a full assessment of possible causative factors in both the generation and maintenance of the disorder. Concurrent disease or processes are of the utmost importance and include diarrhea, vomiting, heart failure, and medication use. In general, the degree of alkalemia is related to the level of volume, chloride, and potassium depletion as well as the degree of renal insufficiency, if present. In the assessment of patients with metabolic alkalosis, a measurement of urinary chloride aids in the differentiation of various etiologic processes and guides management.

Urinary chloride concentrations less than 10 mEq/L point to processes that are chloride-responsive. Alternatively, concentrations greater than 20 mEq/L point to mineralocorticoid excess states and other causes primarily related to renal pathophysiology.

The treatment of metabolic alkalosis requires restoration of the kidney's ability to excrete the excess bicarbonate and correction of any of the possible causes that generated the alkalosis initially. In chloride-responsive alkalosis, the former goal is accomplished by infusion of 0.9% saline solutions to provide sufficient volume and chloride. Potassium concentrations must be monitored and repleted as necessary. A discussion regarding appropriate routes and rates of potassium administration can be found in the subchapter Fluids and Electrolytes. In general, unless potassium concentrations are less than 2.0 mEq/L or life-threatening conditions referable to hypokalemia exist, oral administration of potassium chloride is preferred over intravenous repletion.

In cases in which volume expansion is difficult or impossible because of cardiovascular or renal pathology, infusion of isotonic hydrochloric acid (HCl) can be helpful in restoring arterial pH toward normal. Calculation of the appropriate dose requires estimation of bicarbonate excess. To avoid possible overtreatment with this agent, an assumption of bicarbonate distribution can be made conservatively. If bicarbonate is presumed to distribute to a space confined to 20% of body weight, bicarbonate excess is given by Equation 9.

One-half of the alkali excess can be corrected with infusion of equal milliequivalents of 0.1 N (100 mEq/L) HCL solution at a maximal rate of 0.3 mEq per kg per hour. Careful observation of changes in arterial pH and serum electrolytes must be made so that the infusion rate can be appropriately adjusted. HCL infusion should always be through a central venous catheter. There are many reports of its safety when the above guidelines are followed,[17,18] but there are also reports of mediastinitis, chest wall necrosis, and catheter deterioration when infusion is at higher concentrations.[19-21]

Correction of the initiating cause of alkalosis requires a determination of the possible causes. Diuretics should be curtailed or discontinued if necessary, antibiotic administration altered, NG suction reduced or removed, emesis or diarrhea controlled as much as possible, and supplemental alkali administration discontinued.

Patients with chloride-unresponsive metabolic alkalosis are approached similarly in that both initiating and maintaining factors must be treated to arrive at

[Equation 9]:

$$HCO_3^- \text{ excess} = 0.2 \times \text{body weight (kg)} \times ([HCO_3^-] - 30 \text{ mEq/L})$$

where $[HCO_3^-]$ is the electrolyte total CO_2 given as mEq/L a satisfactory outcome. Patients with mineralocorticoid excess states should be placed on sodium restriction and given potassium chloride supplementation. The addition of a mineralocorticoid antagonist, spironolactone (Aldactone) can be beneficial. Often, the dose of spironolactone required is 200 mg daily in divided doses to have a substantial effect. Because spironolactone also has androgen-blocking effects, this dose is also associated with untoward effects in men. Removal of the source of mineralocorticoid excess (e.g., by tumor excision) is the ideal treatment, but is often not possible. The treatment of Bartter's syndrome is difficult. Large supplements of oral or intravenous potassium chloride, along with potassium sparing diuretics (spironolactone, triamterene, or amiloride), are the primary therapy. Serum potassium concentrations may be kept above 3.0 mEq/L but occasionally may require massive supplements. Prostaglandin synthesis inhibitors have been shown to provide short-term improvement,[22,23] but long-term studies of efficacy are unavailable.

TABLE 54-7. CAUSES OF RESPIRATORY ACIDOSIS

A. Mechanical abnormalities of the thorax
  1. Airway obstruction
    croup
    epiglottitis
    foreign body
    laryngeal edema
    aspiration
  2. Pleural effusion
  3. Pneumothorax
  4. Trauma
    flail chest
    ruptured airway
  5. Scoliosis
B. Pulmonary diseases
  1. Chronic obstructive pulmonary disease
  2. Bronchospasm
  3. Pneumonia
  4. Pulmonary edema
  5. Interstitial pulmonary disease
  6. Smoke inhalation
C. CNS depression decreasing respiratory drive
  1. Drug overdose/effect
  2. Primary-secondary CNS lesions
  3. CNS infection
D. Neuromuscular diseases affecting the thoracic muscular compartment
  1. Guillain-Barré syndrome
  2. Poliomyelitis
  3. Myasthenia gravis
  4. Muscular dystrophy
  5. Paralyzing toxins/drugs
    succinyl choline, pancuronium
    botulinum toxin
E. Inadequate respiratory settings
  1. Low tidal volume and/or frequency
  2. Large dead space
F. Myxedema

RESPIRATORY ACIDOSIS

PATHOPHYSIOLOGY

Respiratory acidosis is defined as a process that causes primary elevation in arterial pCO_2. Because the lungs are so efficient at expiring CO_2, any abnormal increase in carbon dioxide content can be directly attributed to an abnormality affecting this organ system. Carbon dioxide readily diffuses across the alveolar membrane, so that increases in pCO_2 are always caused by ventilation-perfusion mismatches or to alveolar hypoventilation. *Factors that cause these basic abnormalities can be divided into several categories, including mechanical abnormalities of the thorax, pulmonary diseases, CNS depression, neuromuscular disease, inadequate respirator settings, and myxedema.* Pathophysiologically, pulmonary disease causes ventilation-perfusion mismatches and the other causes of respiratory acidosis lead to alveolar hypoventilation. This schema is given in Table 54-7.

Mechanical Abnormalities or Obstructions. Inadequate ventilation can occur at any point in the respiratory hierarchy. Patients with airway obstruction have inadequate minute ventilation which, under most conditions, leads to alveolar hypoventilation. These obstructions can be from any cause including, but certainly not limited to, croup, epiglottitis, lodged foreign body, laryngeal edema from any cause, or aspiration of fluid, gastric contents, etc. Large pleural effusions of greater than 2 L prevent maximal lung expansion. Pneumothorax may drastically diminish ventilatory capacity. Traumatic injury to the chest wall may significantly impair respiration because of pain or to a flail segment. Marked scoliosis can also interfere with the normal costovertebral and costochondral articulation so that lung volume cannot be increased sufficiently.

Pulmonary Disease. Various pulmonary diseases may adversely affect the ability of the lungs to excrete CO_2 by causing areas of perfusion which are not ventilated. Most commonly, this type of picture is seen in chronic obstructive pulmonary disease (COPD; bronchitis, bronchiectasis, emphysema, and asthma). Although CO_2 retention is less typical in interstitial pulmonary disease, it may occur. More acute illnesses such as pneumonitis, acute pulmonary edema, or smoke inhalation may cause effective decreases in alveolar ventilation, thereby causing an increase in arterial pCO_2.

Central Nervous System. The CNS is essential in the control of respiration. This function resides primarily in groups of neurons located in the medulla and pons. Chemoreceptors responding to changes in acid-base status are located at the base of the medulla. Changes in pH at these receptors can alter respiratory status in seconds. Given the highly sensitive nature of these respiratory centers, it is not surprising that a variety of agents can decrease pontine and medullary respiratory drive. These agents are typically those that alter level of consciousness. Drugs that fall into this category include narcotics, hypnotics, amnesics, barbiturates, and alcohol. Lesions in the CNS such as stroke, hemorrhage, or tumor may also alter respiratory patterns, causing respiratory acidosis. These lesions either involve the brainstem or, by virtue of their size, increase intracranial pressure and compress the brainstem. Infectious processes may also alter respiratory patterns by changing cerebrospinal fluid pH, increasing intracranial pressure, or by altering cerebral blood flow characteristics.

Neuromuscular Disease. Diseases or drugs that affect the muscles of respiration may compromise normal patterns of breathing. Guillain-Barré syndrome causes a nonpermanent ascending paralysis that can extend cephalad to affect breathing musculature. Other neuromuscular diseases such as poliomyelitis, myasthenia gravis, amyotrophic lateral sclerosis, and muscular dystrophy may all diminish respiratory capacity. Drugs and toxins that are primarily neuromuscular blocking agents can cause paralysis and death. Succinylcholine and pancuronium, a synthetic relative of curare, are in this class. The clinical effects of botulism are mediated by a neurotoxin that can cause respiratory paralysis.

An important cause of respiratory acidosis that occurs uniquely during acute care settings is *improper settings on a mechanical ventilator*. Large amounts of dead space that are not accounted for in tidal volume calculations, or inadequate minute ventilation for a given patient, cause increases in pCO_2 and subsequent decreases in pH.

Severe hypothyroidism presenting as myxedema coma is associated with multi-system hypofunction. Respiratory depression is a frequent finding in these individuals so that respiratory acidosis is common.

CLINICAL PRESENTATION

The clinical findings in cases of respiratory acidosis depend on the rate of development of the acid-base disturbance. Patients with acute hypercapnia differ from those with chronic respiratory acidosis and those with an acute decompensation of chronic acidosis.

Patients with acute respiratory acidosis uniformly develop hypoxia, the sequelae of which are the predominant clinical finding. If obtundation has not developed, patients may complain of increasing shortness of breath and restlessness. The remaining signs and symptoms frequently depend on the degree of acidosis. When pH falls to less than 7.20, hemodynamic function is compromised and signs of cardiovascular dysfunction such as hypoperfusion and hypotension can become evident.

In contrast to those with acute acidosis, patients who have a primary respiratory acidosis lasting more than several days have had a greater degree of metabolic compensation. These individuals have few if any overt symptoms or signs. Arterial pH in these patients approaches normal and, if pO_2 is maintained, the physical findings present may relate only to chronic obstructive lung disease or cor pulmonale. Patients with pre-existing chronic respiratory acidosis who develop a superimposed illness that increases pCO_2 further may present much like those individuals with an acute acidosis. These patients, however, have a smaller increment in pH for a given rise in pCO_2 than those previously discussed, partly because of the already high levels of buffering capacity in the blood and the kidney's enhanced ability to excrete acid.

DIAGNOSIS AND TREATMENT

Patients with primary respiratory acidosis are found to have an elevated pCO_2, an elevated HCO_3^-, and lowered pH. The degree of elevation of bicarbonate depends on the length of time the acidosis has persisted. The parameters for changes in bicarbonate as a function of changes in pCO_2 are given in Table 54-1. As seen in the table, in acute respiratory acidosis, HCO_3^- changes little for changes in pCO_2. Bicarbonate concentrations do not generally exceed 30 mEq/L.

During chronic respiratory acidosis, the kidney has had the necessary time to increase and maximize H^+ ion excretion. Under these circumstances, pCO_2 is elevated but now HCO_3^- has risen to a greater extent so that pH is less severely affected. Patients with acute acidosis superimposed on chronic hypercapnia develop further increases in pCO_2, decreases in pH, and a modest further increase in bicarbonate.

In most cases, the determination of causality of a respiratory acidosis is easily determined by clinical examination. The historical events suggesting airway obstruction can usually be obtained immediately on a patient's arrival to the ED. Gross congenital or traumatic deformities are also self-evident. The presence of a pleural effusion or pneumothorax significant enough to cause hypercapnia should be discernible on physical examination.

Similarly, patients with underlying pulmonary disease can be assessed clinically. Historical evidence of COPD is almost always obtained from the patient unless obtundation is present. Bronchospasm, pneumonitis, and pulmonary edema are associated with specific and clear physical findings.

CNS sources of respiratory acidosis usually present primarily with an altered level of consciousness. A complete discussion of neurogenic causes of respiratory failure is given in Chapter 47. The development of respiratory acidosis from neuromuscular disease is usually of subacute onset. Other symptoms referable to a neuromuscular cause such as weakness or muscle pain can often be elicited.

As previously discussed, patients with myxedema coma can present with multiple system dysfunctions. Therefore, in any patient presenting with hypoventilation, hypothermia, hyponatremia, and/or hypoglycemia, the diagnosis of hypothyroidism should be entertained.

GENERAL TREATMENT

With respect to the treatment of respiratory acidosis, the primary mode of therapy is the support of oxygenation and ventilation. Because acute increases in pCO_2 are buffered poorly and rapid development of acidemia is likely, mechanical ventilation is mandatory in any individual showing signs of impending respiratory failure. Although assessment of acid-base status in these patients is important, the determination to intubate a patient should be a clinical decision. Waiting for the results of arterial blood gases is inadvisable, and any individual in acute respiratory distress in whom the work of breathing is overwhelming should be placed on ventilatory support.

Once respiratory support has been established, all attention is directed at reversing the underlying cause of the respiratory depression. The direction in which treatment proceeds depends on the level at which the cause is acting. The use of intravenous sodium bicarbonate therapy is recommended only in severe acidosis, in which correction of respiratory depression with mechanical ventilation is not rapidly achievable. Use of sodium bicarbonate therapy may actually worsen the CNS consequences of acidosis. Sodium bicarbonate increases peripheral pH, but equilibration of HCO_3^- across the blood–brain barrier is much slower than that of CO_2. CSF levels of CO_2 rise out

of proportion to changes in HCO_3^-, and CNS acidosis may increase.

RESPIRATORY ALKALOSIS

PATHOPHYSIOLOGY

Respiratory alkalosis is a condition in which an increase in minute ventilation is accompanied by a decrease in arterial pCO_2 with a secondary increase in pH and a modest decrease in HCO_3^-. Because CO_2 is excreted only by the lungs, the only cause of respiratory alkalosis is hyperventilation. This syndrome is felt to be the most common acid-base disturbance among seriously ill patients.[24] The causes of hyperventilation and respiratory alkalosis are given in Table 54-8.

The changes that occur during respiratory alkalosis are similar in magnitude but opposite in direction to those in respiratory acidosis. During acute alkalosis, there is little renal compensation. To reduce blood HCO_3^-, intracellular buffers release H^+ ions. As Table 54-1 indicates, the change in HCO_3^- is small compared to the change in pCO_2, so that the change in pH may be great. After 1 to 2 days, renal compensatory mechanisms are complete and bicarbonate excretion is increased or bicarbonate generation reduced.

Cortical override of respiration is possible and hyperventilation arising from upper level input is one of the more common causes of respiratory alkalosis. Anxiety reactions from any stimulus may cause hyperventilation. The degree of hypocapnia or alkalemia does not help in establishing one diagnosis over another, and in anxiety disorders, severe alkalosis with the concomitant clinical features is possible.

Hypoxia from any cause can markedly stimulate respiration. Common causes of hypoxia also cause respiratory alkalosis as long as another process has not intervened. Bronchospasm, congestive heart failure, and pneumonitis are among the most likely causes. Pulmonary emboli may present with tachycardia and tachypnea. In early interstitial lung disease, the presence of hypoxia caused by a diffusion defect in the lung stimulates respiratory centers to increase minute ventilation. Individuals who travel but are not acclimated to high altitude may increase their minute ventilation to make up for the reduction in oxygen tension.

CNS pathology is another cause of hyperventilation. This includes CNS tumors as well as primary infectious diseases, cerebrovascular accidents, and head trauma. Several drugs that probably act directly on the respiratory centers include acetylsalicylic acid (ASA, aspirin), catecholamines, progestins, and stimulants (e.g., caffeine). Pregnancy has been associated with mild respiratory alkalosis and is felt to be related to the high levels of circulating progesterone.

Hyperthyroidism is associated with overactivity of

TABLE 54-8. CAUSES OF RESPIRATORY ALKALOSIS

A. Anxiety/hyperventilation syndromes
B. CNS pathology
  1. Tumors, infection, trauma, stroke
C. Hypoxia
  1. Bronchospasm
  2. Congestive heart failure
  3. Change in altitude
  4. Pneumonia
  5. Pulmonary emboli
  6. Early interstitial pulmonary disease
D. Drugs
  1. Catecholamines
  2. Progestins
  3. Stimulant overdose (e.g. caffeine)
  4. Salicylates
E. Pregnancy
F. Pain
G. Hyperthyroidism
H. Hepatic dysfunction
I. Fever/sepsis
J. Inappropriate ventilator settings

many organ systems. Among the pulmonary findings of hyperthyroidism is an increase in minute ventilation.[25] Hepatic dysfunction and the early phases of sepsis can cause hyperventilation; however, the exact nature of this response is unknown.

As discussed in the section on respiratory acidosis, patients with inappropriate ventilator settings may be prone to acid-base disturbances. Those in whom the minute ventilation is set too high have a lowered arterial pCO_2. Prolonged ventilation in this fashion causes an expected compensatory decrease in HCO_3^-. When a patient is weaned from the ventilator, the minute ventilation must be high to prevent acidosis from occurring, given the lowered serum bicarbonate.

CLINICAL PRESENTATION

The symptoms of mild to moderate alkalosis are generally related to neuromuscular irritability. As pH is altered, calcium-protein binding is affected so that, during alkalosis, ionized free calcium levels fall. For this reason, many of the severe symptoms of acute respiratory alkalosis mimic those of hypocalcemia.

The most common early finding is circumoral and peripheral paresthesias. These are followed by muscle cramping and even tetany. Carpopedal spasm is a possible sign of severe acute alkalosis. Seizures have been reported. It is often possible to elicit Chvostek's and Trousseau's signs in patients with hyperventilation and hypocapnia. When alkalosis is particularly severe, cardiac arryhythmias may intercede and prove impossible to treat effectively. In addition to these conditions, alkalosis can cause a reduction in cerebral blood flow. This may explain the presence of headache or of an altered level of consciousness, including syncope.

DIAGNOSIS AND TREATMENT

Laboratory findings in respiratory alkalosis include a diminished pCO_2 and HCO_3^- and an increased pH. The level to which the HCO_3^- concentration is lowered depends on the length of time the alkalosis has been present. As previously discussed, renal compensatory mechanisms take approximately 24 to 48 hours to activate fully.

As in all cases of acid-base disturbance, the main modality of therapy is the correction of the underlying disorder. In most serious cases, improving oxygenation is the most important step in improving acid-base homeostasis. In general, oxygen therapy provides more benefits than does correction of alkalosis alone. In patients with anxiety-based hyperventilation, paper bag breathing increases arterial pCO_2 and may break the cycle. It is vitally important to ensure that the patient is adequately oxygenated before using such treatments. The availability of portable oxymeters in many EDs makes this assessment rapid.

MIXED ACID-BASE DISORDERS

RATIONAL APPROACH TO ARTERIAL BLOOD GASES

The proper interpretation of arterial blood gases is essential in appropriate diagnosis of acid-base abnormalities. Incorporating a knowledge of the patient's clinical condition and medication profile vastly aids in this interpretation. The approach to arterial blood gases and a discussion of mixed acid-base disorders requires an understanding of the normal compensatory mechanisms that occur after a change in acid-base status. When the actual and theoretic changes diverge, as determined by the blood gases, the clinician must suspect a mixed acid-base disorder. A mixed acid-base disorder may, however, develop in which the "numbers" fall within expected limits. Aside from the history, the anion gap may be the only clue that multiple disorders are simultaneously present. For this reason, a patient's clinical state must be considered when interpreting measurements of acid-base status. Also, some medications can cause confusing alterations of hypoglycemia.

There are several combinations of mixed acid-base disorders. The severity of any mixed disorder depends on whether the two primary conditions change the pH in the same or opposite directions. For example, a patient with COPD and a chronic respiratory acidosis is placed on diuretics and develops a mild metabolic alkalosis. This individual does not develop severe symptoms referable to his acid-base disturbance. Alternatively, another individual with diabetic ketoacidosis has a severe metabolic acidosis. If this patient develops respiratory failure related to aspiration or mental status changes, the ensuing respiratory acidosis could push the arterial pH to critical levels.

Another circumstance that might, at first glance, appear unusual is the concurrent existence of a metabolic acidosis and alkalosis. This occurs when two separate processes develop in which changes in bicarbonate concentration move in opposite directions. The clue to the presence of such a set of conditions is the anion gap. A classic example serves to illustrate this well. Consider an individual with a metabolic alkalosis caused by persistent vomiting. The arterial blood gases in such an individual might be pH of 7.50, pCO_2 of 48, and HCO_3^- of 36; and the calculated anion gap is 12. If the vomiting continues and dehydration and lactic acidosis develops, the following blood gases may be obtained: pH of 7.32, pCO_2 of 28, and HCO_3^- of 14 with an anion gap of 34. The clue to the presence of more than one process is the anion gap. If the second set of blood gases were caused only by a primary metabolic acidosis, we would expect the drop in bicarbonate to be balanced by a rise in the unmeasured anion, in this case lactate. The anion gap should be

22 (normal bicarbonate of 24 mEq/L less the measured of 14 mEq/L plus the normal level of anion gap of 12). The anion gap is 34 and not 22 because the bicarbonate fell from a level of 36 mEq/L and not 24 mEq/L. The significantly increased anion gap tells us that bicarbonate fell from an abnormally high level, indicating the pre-existing metabolic alkalosis.

To make matters slightly more complicated, it is further possible that the patient becomes anxious and begins to hyperventilate. The pCO_2 falls and the patient develops a third primary acid-base disturbance in addition to the first two, namely a respiratory alkalosis. The new blood gases could be: pH of 7.48, pCO_2 of 18, and HCO_3^- of 13 with an anion gap of 36. Again, the anion gap is the key to deciphering the acid-base disorder.

The overall interpretation of arterial blood gases therefore requires information about the clinical setting in which the disorder occurred, a measurement of arterial blood gases, and the calculation of anion gap from the measured electrolytes. Once the pH of arterial blood is assessed as alkaline or acid, the pCO_2 helps to differentiate between primary respiratory or metabolic disturbances. A comparison of the pCO_2 and the HCO_3^- determines, for a given pH, whether the compensatory change was appropriate. If outside the expected range of correction, a second primary disorder should be suspected. In all cases, the anion gap should be calculated because an elevation in the gap may be the only clue as to the presence of a metabolic process.

REFERENCES

1. Breyer, M.D., and Jacobson, H.R.: Mechanisms and regulation of renal H⁺ and HCO₃⁻ transport. Am. J. Nephrol. 7:150, 1987.
2. McKinney, T.D., and Burg, M.B.: Bicarbonate and fluid absorption by renal proximal straight tubules. Kidney Int. 12:1, 1977.
3. Kinne-Saffran, E., Beauwens, R., and Kinne, R.: An ATP-driven proton pump in broush-border membranes from rat renal cortex. J. Membrane Biol. 357:209, 1982.
4. Malnic, G.: Role of the kidney in controlling acid-base balance. Child. Nephrol. Urol. 9:241, 1989.
5. West, J.B.: Respiratory physiology—The essentials. 2nd ed. Baltimore, Waverly Press, 1979.
6. Maher, E.R.: Renal tubular acidosis. Br. J. Hosp. Med. 42:116, 1989.
7. Schwartz, W.B., and Cohen, J.J.: The nature of the renal response to chronic disorders of acid-base equilibrium. Am. J. Med. 64:417, 1978.
8. Riley, L.J., Jr., Ilson, B.E., and Narins, R.G.: Acute metabolic acid-base disorders. Crit. Care Clin. 5:699, 1987.
9. Riley, L.J., Jr., Ilson, B.E., and Narins, R.G.: Acute metabolic acid-base disorders. Crit. Care Clin. 5:699, 1987.
10. Hazard, P.B., and Griffin, J.P.: Sodium bicarbonate in the management of systemic acidosis. South. Med. J. 73:1339, 1980.
11. Narins, R.G., and Cohen, J.J.: Bicarbonate therapy for organic acidosis: The case for its continued use. Ann. Intern. Med. 106:615, 1987.
12. Seldin, D.W.: Metabolic acidosis. In Brenner, B.M., and Rector, F.C. (Eds): The Kidney. Philadelphia, W.B. Saunders, 1976, p. 615.
13. Sebastian, A., Sutton, J.M., Julter, H.M., et al.: Effect of mineralocorticoid replacement therapy on renal acid-base homeostasis in adrenalectomized patients. Kidney Int. Dec. 18:762, 1980.
14. Galla, J.H., and Luke, R.G.: Chloride transport and disorders of acid-base balance. Ann. Rev. Physiol. 50:141, 1988.
15. Garella, S., Chazan, J.A., and Cohen, J.J.: Saline-resistant metabolic alkalosis or "chloride-wasting nephropathy". Report of four patients with severe potassium depletion. Ann. Intern. Med. 73:31, 1970.
16. Slivinski, M., Hoffman, M., Biederman, A., et al.: Association between hypokalemic alkalosis and development of arrhythmia in early postoperative period. Anesth. Resusc. Intens. Care 2:193, 1974.
17. Brimioulle, S., Vincent, J.L., Dufaye, P., et al.: Hydrochloric acid infusion for treatment of metabolic alkalosis: Effects on acid-base balance and oxygenation. Crit. Care Med. 13:738, 1985.
18. Worthley, L.I.: The rational use of i.v. hydrochloric acid in the treatment of metabolic alkalosis. Br. J. Anaesth. 49:811, 1977.
19. Narins, R.G., Rudnick, M.R., Townsend, R., et al.: Metabolic acid-base disorders: Pathophysiology, classification, and treatment. In Arieff, A.I., and DeFronzo, R.A. (Eds.): Fluid, Electrolyte, and Acid-Base Disorders. New York, Churchill Livingstone, 1985, pp. 335–67.
20. Jankauskas, S.J., Gursel, E., and Antonenko, D.A.: Chest wall necrosis secondary to hydrochloric acid use in the treatment of metabolic alkalosis. Crit. Care Med. 17:963, 1989.
21. Kopel, R.F., and Durbin, C.G., Jr.: Pulmonary artery catheter deterioration during hydrochloric acid infusion for the treatment of metabolic alkalosis. Crit. Care Med. 17:688, 1989.
22. Norby, L., Flamenbaum, W., Lents, R., and Ramwell, P.: Prostaglandins and aspirin therapy in Bartter's syndrome. Lancet 2:604, 1976.
23. Verberckmoes, R., von Damme, B., Clement, J., Amery, A., and Michielsen, P.: Bartter's syndrome with hyperplasia of renomedullary cells: Successful treatment with indomethacin. Kidney Int. 9:302, 1976.
24. Kaehny, W.D.: Pathogenesis and management of respiratory and mixed acid-base disorders. In Schrier, R.W. (Ed.): Renal and Electrolyte Disorders, 3rd ed. Boston, Little, Brown, 1986, pp. 187–206.
25. Stein, M., Kimbel, P., and Johnson, R.L., Jr.: Pulmonary function in hyperthyroidism. J. Clin. Invest. 40:348, 1961.

BIBLIOGRAPHY

Atkinson, D.E., and Bourke, E.: Metabolic aspects of the regulation of systemic pH. Am. J. Physiol. 252:F947, 1987.

Brewer, E.D.: Disorders of acid-base balance. Pediatr. Clin. North Am. 37:429, 1990.

Galla, J.H., and Luke, R.G.: Chloride transport and disorders of acid-base balance. Ann. Rev. Physiol. 50:141, 1988.

Hyneck, M.L.: Simple acid-base disorders. Am. J. Hosp. Pharm. 42:1992, 1985.

Kaehny, W.D., and Gabow, P.A.: Pathogenesis and management of metabolic acidosis and alkalosis. In Schrier, R.W. (Ed.): Renal and Electrolyte Disorders, 3rd ed. Boston, Little, Brown, 1986, pp. 141–86.

Kearns, T., Wolfson, A.B.: Metabolic acidosis. Emerg. Med. Clin. North Am. 7:823, 1989.

Sagy, M., Barzilay, Z., and Boichis, H.: The diagnosis and management of acid-base imbalance. Pediatr. Emerg. Care 4:259, 1988.

Shaprio, B.A. Arterial blood gas monitoring. Crit. Care Clin. 4:479, 1988.

FLUIDS AND ELECTROLYTES

Jamie Dananberg

CAPSULE

The patient presenting with, or found to have, disturbances in electrolyte and/or water metabolism represents an especially difficult problem in diagnosis and management. Cause and effect are hard to dissociate, yet this distinction is critically important if appropriate interventions are to be undertaken. Furthermore, the clinical problems discussed here are unique in that they are often brought to light by reports of blood chemistries and not by history or physical examination. Despite this reliance on laboratory results, the important determinations of causality require a careful physical assessment of the patient rather than a dependence on data accrual. In that volume status stands as a central focus for many of the diagnostic algorithms, the basic observations inherent in a complete physical examination are indispensable in the appraisal of these individuals.

This section of the chapter deals with a group of abnormalities with an exceptionally diverse group of causes. Although they are interrelated, each electrolyte and water disturbance is discussed individually for clarity.

DISORDERS OF SODIUM METABOLISM

PHYSIOLOGIC CONCEPTS

The understanding of sodium metabolism requires a discussion of water balance because the two are inextricably linked. The serum sodium concentration depends on water balance and, in turn, serum osmolality depends on the sodium concentration. To best illustrate the movement of sodium and water, it is helpful to divide the body into intracellular and extracellular compartments. This differentiation is used throughout the remainder of this chapter.

Total body water represents approximately 60% of body weight. Of this, two thirds are intracellular, with the remaining one third extracellular. With the exception of specialized brain cells, cells lining the collecting ducts, and transitional epithelium, water moves freely across cell membranes so that the tonicity of the two compartments is equal. On the other hand, cell membranes are not freely permeable to electrolytes. The movement of ions is closely regulated by ATPase-dependent pumps and ion channels whose conductance can be varied by resting membrane potential, acid-base status, hormonal controls, and drugs. The extracellular space can be further subdivided into intravascular and interstitial spaces. For the purposes of this discussion, we will assert that there is no gradient between the two spaces, so that ion concentrations are equivalent between them.

In the extracellular space, sodium is the most abundant cation. Except on rare occasions that will be discussed subsequently in the Pathophysiology section, sodium concentration establishes the tonicity of serum. Unless other agents which have a high osmotic potential are present in serum, plasma osmolality can be defined by Formula 1:

$$Posm = 2([Na] + [K]) + ([Glucose]/18) + (BUN/2.8)$$

[Na] and [K] are given as mEq/L
[Glucose] and BUN are given as mg/dL

Sodium concentration is not directly regulated. The two vital physiologic parameters that are regulated and that secondarily affect sodium metabolism are osmolality and blood pressure. Sodium probably stimulates "osmoreceptors" better than glucose, and certainly better than urea. Plasma osmolality is tightly controlled by hormonal and neural mechanisms originating in the hypothalamus and affecting the renal handling of water and the thirst drive to water intake, respectively. In fact, given the usually close relationship between serum sodium and plasma osmolality, sodium concentration is held within a narrow range.

The primary hormonal regulation of osmolality is by antidiuretic hormone (vasopressin, ADH). Stimulation and inhibition of ADH secretion is closely tied to the plasma osmolality. ADH secretion is also affected by hemodynamic, emetic, glycemic, environmental, and drug factors. Changes in both blood pressure and blood volume are negatively and exponentially correlated with changes in plasma ADH. The interaction between hemodynamic and osmolal factors is seemingly contradictory. As blood pressure falls and ADH secretion increases, one would expect to see a fall in plasma osmolality. This fall should diminish ADH secretion. The compromise is a resetting of the osmostat to a lower level so that osmolal regulation can still occur, but at a new set-point. Nausea is a potent stimulus for ADH release. Although hypoglycemia also induces ADH release, it is not as robust as that induced by nausea. Although the mechanisms by which they act have not been worked out, it is believed that the renin-angiotensin axis interacts with ADH secretion also. Furthermore, physical and environmental factors such as pain, exertion, temperature, stress, oxygenation, and acid-base status have been reported to affect ADH release. A large assortment of pharmacologic agents can affect ADH secretion.

In the presence of ADH, the distal and collecting tubules become permeable to solute-free water, allowing water to diffuse down the osmotic gradient from tubular fluid to renal cortex or medulla. The net effect is to increase the overall osmolality of the urine up to a maximum of 1200 to 1400 mOsm/kg. In the absence of vasopressin, the distal and collecting tubules are impermeable to diffusion of water. Urine flow increases up to 20 mL per minute, and urine becomes hypotonic, as low as 60 mOsm/kg. It must be noted that the urinary responses to vasopressin can vary with other circumstances. In glucose diuresis, for example, a much larger volume of fluid with solutes is delivered to the distal tubule because the osmotic agent has overcome the capacity of the proximal tubule to actively reabsorb the solutes. In this case, even with maximally high vasopressin levels, the ability of the distal tubule to reabsorb the large volume of water is overwhelmed; hence the urine is not maximally concentrated and urine flow is high.

The efficaciousness of the renal response to the disappearance of antidiuretic hormone (vasopressin; ADH) ensures that osmolality will not decrease below 280 mOsm/kg. In contrast, the upper limit of serum osmolality is controlled by central thirst mechanisms. The intensity of the thirst mechanism ensures that the upper limit of plasma osmolality will not increase to levels beyond 296 mOsm/kg. Thirst ensures adequate water intake in virtually all circumstances. The slopes of the magnitude of these homeostatic mechanisms are such that osmolality, in the vast majority of circumstances, is maintained within 285 and 290 mOsm/kg.

Mineralocorticoids represent the other class of hormonal agents that regulate sodium. Aldosterone secretion is regulated by the renin-angiotensin axis as well as by serum potassium, adrenocorticotrophic hormone (ACTH), and several other factors. Several other adrenal steroids, including cortisol and deoxycorticosterone (DOC), have mineralocorticoid activity; however, the importance of these compounds in causing abnormalities in sodium metabolism is usually limited to excess or deficiency states. Angiotensin II (AII) is the primary regulator of aldosterone secretion. It is at the midpoint in a cascade that is initiated by the enzyme renin. Renin activity is stimulated by baroreceptors activated by decreases in blood pressure from volume loss or posture changes. Renin activity is also stimulated by adrenergic stimulation and so-

dium depletion. Plasma potassium has been clearly shown to exert a positive effect on aldosterone secretion. ACTH has a limited but positive effect on aldosterone secretion.

Other systems interact with the kidney to alter sodium homeostasis. Because sodium reabsorption depends on the filtered load of sodium, changes in GFR could potentially lead to large changes in sodium excretion. By mechanisms that are not fully known, sodium reabsorption can vary, based on GFR maintaining a relatively constant sodium excretion rate. For many years, evidence has accumulated suggesting that changes in hematocrit and plasma protein concentration can modulate tubular sodium reabsorption. Renal hemodynamics, including renal arterial pressure, renal vascular resistance, and renal blood flow, can exert a substantial influence on sodium homeostasis. Atrial natriuretic factor, a small peptide secreted by cardiac atria in response to stretch and volume expansion, can markedly increase fractional sodium excretion. The adrenergic nervous system has also been shown to regulate sodium excretion as well.

The effect of aldosterone on renal sodium handling is to increase tubular sodium reabsorption. Although only a small portion of filtered sodium reabsorption is altered by mineralocorticoids, changes in sodium balance can be affected. In mineralocorticoid excess, sodium retention occurs initially; however, an escape phenomenon occurs within 1 to 3 days and sodium balance is restored.

Under clinical conditions, we generally determine not osmolality but serum sodium concentration. As discussed, this gives a reasonable reflection of osmolality. It does not, however, reflect total body sodium stores. Because body sodium does reflect overall volume status of the individual, we can use the assessment of hydration to help direct therapy of the many causes of abnormalities in sodium and water metabolism.

HYPERNATREMIA

PATHOPHYSIOLOGY

In virtually all circumstances, hypernatremia is associated with elevations in plasma osmolality. Elevations in sodium concentration can occur under conditions of increased, decreased or normal total body sodium. Extracellular fluid (ECF) status parallels body sodium, so that patients may show evidence of hyper-, hypo-, or isovolemia. This differentiation helps to classify, for purposes of treatment, the various causes of hypernatremia. This categorization of groups by volume status is listed in Table 54-9.

The hypovolemic causes of increased serum sodium concentration are conditions in which total body sodium and water stores are insufficient to maintain postural blood pressure or tissue turgor adequately. These conditions are caused by water losses associated with, but in excess of, sodium losses. They are caused by drugs, hormones, or intrinsic renal disease, or by fluid losses from gastrointestinal, pulmonary, or dermatologic pathology. These fluids are all hypotonic compared to serum, so that excess losses from these systems always results in a greater water than sodium deficit. It must be kept in mind that, under normal circumstances, a rise in serum sodium by even marginal amounts (>145 mEq), with concomitant increases in serum osmolality of as little as 5 to 8 mOsm/kg above normal levels, triggers a potent thirst drive. Furthermore, the intensity of thirst rises steeply from this point. At a serum osmolality above 300 mOsm/kg, the thirst drive is intense. When individuals have adequate access to water and this drive is intact, there is a prompt correction of hypernatremia. Therefore, in addition to the causes listed in Table 54-9, a superimposed defect in water consumption must be present. Bedridden patients and those with mental status changes, physical impairments, inaccessibility to water, oral or esophageal pathology or swallowing dysfunction are among the individuals susceptible to hypernatremia.

The renal causes of excessive water and sodium loss often depend on external drug or hormonal influences. Diuretics are the most common pharmacologic agents in this category. They cause sodium and water losses; however, urinary sodium concentrations are always lower than serum concentrations during diuresis. In most patients, the free water is replaced normally with dietary intake. In cases when free water is not accessible or when a patient is overtreated, hypovolemic hypernatremia can occur. Other compounds causing a hypotonic diuresis act similarly, such as glycosuria in uncontrolled diabetes mellitus or mannitol administration. Intrinsic renal dysfunction can also lead to chronic loss of hypotonic urine, with concomitant development of hypernatremia. Despite the relative hypotonicity of gastrointestinal, pulmonary, and dermatologic fluids, they contain significant amounts of electrolytes, and persistent losses can cause hypovolemia. Generally, these losses are severe and not clinically subtle. Gastrointestinal losses from sustained emesis can lead to these changes relatively quickly, even in otherwise healthy individuals, because of the inability to replace free water.

The hypervolemic causes of hypernatremia are straightforward. In virtually all cases, either hypertonic saline or tube feedings in patients without access to water have been administered, or there is a mineralocorticoid excess state. Primary aldosteronism is the classic example of this latter condition. The renal effect of aldosterone is to increase reabsorption of sodium and water and enhance potassium excretion. These patients are typically hypertensive and have mild hypernatremia and mild to moderate hypokalemia. Because cortisol has both glucocorticoid and mineralocorticoid effects, in Cushing's syndrome (endogenous or exogenous), hypervolemic hypernatremia can also result.

In patients with isolated water losses, water shifts

TABLE 54-9. CAUSES OF HYPERNATREMIA

A. Hypovolemic: water loss in excess of sodium loss
  1. Renal causes
    —Diuretics/drugs
    —Glucose, urea diuresis
    —Renal failure
    —Partial urinary tract obstruction
  2. GI, pulmonary, skin losses
B. Isovolemic: water loss alone
  1. Central diabetes insipidus
  2. Nephrogenic diabetes insipidus
  3. Reset osmostat
  4. Skin losses
  5. Iatrogenic causes
C. Hypervolemic: sodium gain in excess of water gain
  1. Iatrogenic
  2. Mineralocorticoid excess syndromes

TABLE 54-10. CAUSES OF DIABETES INSIPIDUS

A. Central diabetes insipidus (ADH deficiency)
  1. Familial/idiopathic
  2. Trauma
  3. Neoplasms
  4. Granulomatous disease
  5. Infectious
  6. Drugs
  7. Vascular lesions
  8. Rheumatic diseases
B. Nephrogenic diabetes insipidus (diminished ADH action)
  1. Renal causes
  2. Electrolyte abnormalities
  3. SS or SC disease
  4. Congenital
  5. Miscellaneous
  6. Drugs
C. Excess water intake
  1. Psychogenic polydipsia
  2. Reset osmostat

from the intracellular to the extracelluar compartments, thereby buffering the losses. Therefore, unless losses have been extreme, intravascular volume is usually well preserved. This group of hypernatremias can therefore be termed isovolemic. There is, however, an increase in the concentration of electrolytes. Additionally, the loss of water without sodium quickly increases serum osmolality, which rapidly and potently stimulates thirst centers. Therefore, only individuals in whom access to water is restricted become dehydrated. Because exclusive water loss with maximal sodium retention rarely occurs outside the renal tubule, the cause in most patients with this disturbance is diabetes insipidus (DI), or the loss of ADH secretion or action in the face of increased serum osmolality. The causes of DI are found in Table 54-10.

The cause of central diabetes insipidus generally is related to destruction of the neurosecretory neurons whose axons terminate in the posterior pituitary and originate in the supraoptic nucleus in the hypothalamus. Studies have corroborated the fact that about 80% loss of these neurons is required before the clinical syndrome becomes evident. Tumors located exclusively in the pituitary sella are unlikely to cause this degree of neuronal loss and therefore rarely cause DI. In the emergency department (ED), the diagnosis must be kept in mind in victims of head trauma. Patients with tumors, primarily craniopharyngiomas, superiorly expanding pituitary macroadenomas, and metastatic disease from lung or breast cancer or lymphoma, are all susceptible to DI. Granulomatous diseases such as sarcoid, histiocytosis X, or tuberculosis have been known to cause DI when the diseases involve hypothalamic sites. Central nervous system (CNS) infections (meningitis, encephalitis) have been shown to be associated with DI, possibly from compromise of the hypothalamic vasculature. Familial causes of DI have also been established.[1]

Central DI is caused by an absolute deficiency in the secretion of vasopressin; nephrogenic DI is caused by renal tubular resistance to the effects of the hormone. There is a relative insensitivity to ADH. Nevertheless, a problem does not exist until the kidney is unable to appropriately concentrate urine at vasopressin levels normally achievable at rising serum osmolality at the level that stimulates thirst. It has been shown that the renal tubular response to ADH must be diminished approximately tenfold for this condition to occur.

The causes of nephrogenic DI are listed in Table 54-10. Intrinsic renal diseases can cause DI, as well as acute tubular necrosis and partial or postobstructive syndromes. Patients with recent renal transplants are also known to display DI. Pyelonephritis, particularly when chronic, can be responsible for DI as well. Patients with polycystic kidney disease can also demonstrate insensitivity to ADH. Other electrolyte abnormalities, such as hypokalemia and hypercalcemia, have also been linked to diabetes insipidus. Sickle cell anemia probably induces ADH resistance because of ischemia or infarction in the renal medulla secondary to sickling in and occlusion of the vasa recta.

In addition to the diseases mentioned, several conditions, otherwise unclassified, should be discussed. Infiltrative and rheumatologic diseases can be responsible for the induction of insensitivity to ADH. These include multiple myeloma, sarcoidosis, Sjögren's syndrome, and amyloidosis. Patients with severe malnutrition have also been found to have syndromes consistent with nephrogenic DI. An inherited, congenital form of nephrogenic diabetes insipidus has been described. The pharmacologic causes of DI are numerous and are listed in Table 54-11. Many of these agents cause DI by different mechanisms at the cellular level.

The final category of diseases that cause DI are excessive water-drinking states. Although psychogenic causes of water engorging can cause excessive urine volumes which are of low osmolality, and therefore mimic DI, the patients always have serum sodiums that are normal or slightly low in contrast to the other causes of DI. This condition is dealt with further in the discussion of hyponatremia.

CLINICAL PRESENTATION

Although alterations in serum sodium concentration can manifest as many symptoms, most frequently the symptoms are related to the underlying pathophysiologic status. As sodium concentration increases, however, neurologic and neuromuscular symptoms predominate. This is presumed to occur because of the hypertonicity and CNS dehydration caused by hypernatremia.

The predominant neurologic symptom of hypernatremia is profound thirst if the patient is awake and has intact thirst centers. As hypernatremia worsens, mental status is depressed from lethargy to obtundation and coma. Seizures have been documented also. Neuromuscular symptomalogy is consistent with hyperactivity, with cramps, hyperreflexia, and spasticity.

DIAGNOSIS AND TREATMENT

The initial assessment of hypernatremia depends on the clinical determination of volume status. Unlike hyponatremia, conditions causing an elevation in serum sodium are always associated with hyperosmolality so that the measurement of serum osmolality does not help differentiate among the causes of this syndrome. Volume status, on the other hand, is helpful in determining causality. The hypernatremias can be divided into those associated with salt and water loss (hypovolemia), water loss alone (isovolemia), and sodium gain (hypervolemia). Although the extremes are easier to categorize, most patients have more modest fluid shifts making the assessment of volume status difficult. Adjuncts to the physical examination to help

TABLE 54-11. DRUG CAUSES OF DIABETES INSIPIDUS

A. Barbiturates
B. Lithium
C. Tetratcyclines (demeclocycline)
D. Glyburide
E. Vinca alkaloids
F. Platinum
G. Methoxyflurane
H. Ethyl alcohol
I. Diphenylhydantoin (Dilantin)
J. Acetohexamide
K. Tolazamide
L. Amphotericin B
M. Propoxyphene
N. Colchicine

establish volume status include the measurement of hemoglobin and hematocrit, blood urea nitrogen (BUN), and creatinine.

The causes of hypovolemic hypernatremia are best classified as renal and extrarenal losses of salt and water. In hypernatremia of renal origin, the loss can be measured in the urine by assessing urinary sodium concentration. There are losses of both sodium and water, with water in excess, and there are generally sufficient amounts of salt, so that urinary sodium concentration will be greater than 20 mEq/L. In extrarenal losses, primarily from GI, pulmonary, and skin sources, the ensuing hypovolemia causes the kidney to maximally reabsorb water and sodium. The findings in this case demonstrate urinary sodium concentrations of less than 10 mEq/L. Treatment of these patients depends on the severity of the salt and water loss and the degree of symptoms. In mild hypernatremia (serium sodium between 145 and 155 mEq/L) without hemodynamic compromise, infusion of hypotonic solutions, typically 0.45% saline, lowers serum osmolality and restores total body salt levels simultaneously. Patients with more marked volume depletion should have it replaced with 0.9% saline to allow more rapid restoration of ECF volume. Because 0.9% saline contains 154 mEq/L of sodium and has an osmolality of 290 mOsm/kg, this solution is hypotonic relative to the patient's serum.

Isovolemic hypernatremia encompasses diabetes insipidus (central and nephrogenic), osmoreceptor dysfunction, skin losses, and iatrogenic causes. Historical information can usually establish diagnoses other than DI. The lack of thirst in patients with hypernatremia and serum osmolality > 295 mOsm/kg is diagnostic for this disorder. In the ED, all instances of isovolemic hypernatremia should be treated with free water, preferably by the oral route, but intravenous 5% dextrose or 5% dextrose with 0.25% saline is also adequate. The rate of fluid replacement is described subsequently. Patients with a known history of central DI can also be treated with desamino-8-D-arginine vasopressin (DDAVP), a synthetic analogue of vasopressin with greater antidiuretic effect and longer duration of action. Ten to 25 μg intranasally or 1 μg intravenously should quickly reverse the free water loss.

Hypervolemic hypernatremia, most commonly from exogenous administration of excess sodium, is treated with potent diuretics to reduce the total body sodium load along with free water administration, usually with 5% dextrose. Although it is uncommon in an emergency setting, patients with mineralocorticoid excess states may rarely present with hypernatremia, often in conjunction with hypertension. Emergent treatment of these patients is not necessary. These individuals are more likely to have a threatening problem with hypokalemia. Spironolactone, at least 200 mg daily in divided doses, is required to treat primary hyperaldosteronism. In cases associated with secondary hyperaldosteronism, the factors that stim-

ulate aldosterone secretion invariably lead to water retention as well, so that hypernatremia rarely, if ever, occurs.

In all cases, hypernatremia should not be corrected faster than over 48 hours. Rapid changes in serum sodium may cause marked volume shifts in the CNS, precipitating seizures and/or coma. A standard rule is to correct no more than half of the sodium abnormality over the first 24 hours.

HYPONATREMIA

PATHOPHYSIOLOGY

The investigation for causes of hyponatremia depends on the determination of serum osmolality and body sodium and volume status. Unlike hypernatremia, disorders of decreased serum sodium can be associated with increased, decreased, or normal osmolality in addition to these same changes in volume status. This classification aids in the diagnostic differentiation of the causes of hyponatremia and clarify therapeutic options. The causes of hyponatremia are listed in Table 54-12.

When serum osmolality is normal (280 to 285 mOsm/kg) and serum sodium concentration is low (< 130 mEq/L), the patient may not have true hyponatremia. The pseudohyponatremic syndromes are caused by changes in the proportion of lipid or protein in a given volume of serum. Sodium is confined to the water fraction of a given volume of plasma. If this fraction is diminished because of a concomitant increase in lipid or protein, the proportion of sodium relative to the entire sample diminishes. The concentration of sodium in the water fraction, however, remains normal.

TABLE 54-12. CAUSES OF HYPONATREMIA

A. Isotonic syndromes
 1. Hyperlipidemia
 2. Hyperproteinemia
 3. Moderate hyperglycemia
 4. Infusion of hypertonic solution (Mannitol)
B. Hypertonic syndromes
 1. Severe hyperglycemia
 2. Excessive infusion of hypertonic solution
C. Hypotonic syndromes
 1. Hypovolemia
  —Diuretic use/abuse
  —Prolonged fluid losses (GI, skin, renal, pulmonary) with replacement by solute free water
  —Addison's disease
 2. Hypervolemia
  —Congestive heart failure
  —Chronic hepatic failure
  —Renal failure
  —Nephrotic syndrome
 3. Euvolemia
  —Inappropriate secretion of ADH (SIADH)
  —Psychogenic polydipsia

Another circumstance may arise in which a patient may have isotonic hyponatremia. This group of patients will have a true hyponatremia; however, the serum tonicity may be increased by infusions of hypertonic solutions. The coincident finding of true hyponatremia and marked hyperglycemia may result in a normal serum osmolality. These two circumstances can also lead to the hypertonic causes of hyponatremia if the substance adding tonicity to the serum is elevated substantially. Large mannitol infusions or profound hyperglycemia are such cases.

The hypotonic causes of hyponatremia are the most common. These can be conveniently divided into those associated with hypo-, hyper-, and isovolemia. Among the hypovolemic sources of hyponatremia are many of the diseases also causing hypernatremia in patients who are unable to increase fluid intake. The most common cause of this condition is diuretic use or abuse. As stated previously in the discussion of hypernatremia, any prolonged fluid loss from gastrointestinal, skin, renal, or pulmonary derivation causes sodium and water loss, water in excess of sodium. Patients with these syndromes, in contrast to those with hypernatremic syndromes, replace these losses with free water so that there is a net decrease in the water deficit. Sodium continues to be lost, however, and the combined result is hyponatremia. The same

set of conditions can be applied to many of the other causes of hyponatremia listed in Table 54-12. The renal loss of salt and water is also hypotonic compared to that of serum, and tends to cause hypernatremia. Nevertheless, patients who restore water balance with solute-free oral intake become hyponatremic. Addison's disease is a more specialized situation. The disorder stems from deficiency of both glucocorticoids and mineralocorticoids. The kidney appears unable to normally excrete water in the face of cortisol deficiency, although the mechanism by which this occurs is not clear. In some cases, ADH appears elevated; however, water excretion defects have been detected in patients with glucocorticoid deficiency and normal ADH levels. It has been suggested that changes in renal hemodynamics occur in cortisol deficiency states. Loss of mineralocorticoid causes sodium wasting in the urine with excess reabsorption of potassium. The net hypovolemia reduces GFR and increases ADH with a net increase in water reabsorption all of which leads to hyponatremia.

Patients with hyponatremia and volume overload are commonplace because of the prevalence of the diseases leading to this condition. Among the causes of hypervolemic hyponatremia, congestive heart failure is most common, with chronic liver failure, nephrotic syndrome, and renal disease also seen. In all cases, the volume expansion is noted as the presence of peripheral edema. Except in renal disease, the defect is primarily related to a decrease in effective intravascular volume which stimulates baroreceptors leading to increased ADH secretion. This leads to an increase in proximal tubular reabsorption of water and solutes which, in turn, diminishes the amount of filtrate delivered to the distal tubule and collecting duct. The net result is a decrease in water excretion. Furthermore, baroreceptor stimulation also activates thirst centers so that these patients have an increase in water intake. The combined result is hyponatremia and effective hypovolemia in the face of increased total body sodium and water.

Syndromes of euvolemia and hyponatremia encompass the diverse group of diseases grouped under the heading of syndrome of inappropriate secretion of ADH (SIADH) (Table 54-13). The hallmarks of this entity are a lowered serum sodium and a defect in water excretion in conjunction with normal blood volume and normal total body water stores. The syndrome has been noted to occur across a wide spectrum of diseases and pharmacologic agents. The most common systems involved are the pulmonary and central nervous systems. SIADH is a frequent paraneoplastic syndrome stemming from an assortment of tissue types. With respect to the pathophysiology of ADH-induced hyponatremia, the defect specifically affects urinary dilution and not concentration so that, under conditions of low water intake, hyponatremia generally does not occur. This highlights the primary therapy of water restriction in the treatment of this syndrome as discussed subsequently.

TABLE 54-13. CAUSES OF SIADH

A. Neoplasm
   1. Pulmonary malignancies
   2. Carcinoma of duodenum, pancreas, prostate, bladder, ureter
   3. Lymphoma
   4. Mesothelioma
   5. Thymoma
   6. Ewing's sarcoma
B. Trauma
C. Pulmonary disease
D. Hypothyroidism
E. Central nervous system disease
   1. Meningitis, abscess, encephalitis
   2. Guillain-Barré syndrome
   3. Subarachnoid hemorrhage
   4. Acute intermittant porphyria
   5. Cerebrovascular disease
   6. Delirium tremens
   7. Multiple sclerosis
   8. Psychosis
F. Drugs
   1. Chlorpropamide
   2. Thiazides
   3. Carbamazepine
   4. Nicotine
   5. Clofibrate
   6. Vincristine
   7. Cyclophosphamide
   8. Phenothiazines
   9. Tricyclic antidepressants
   10. MAO inhibitors
G. Idiopathic

Psychogenic polydipsia or water intoxication is cited as a cause of isovolemic hyponatremia. In the face of normal renal function and normal vasopressin physiology, water intake is highly unlikely to cause a significant depression in serum sodium. This is because of the kidney's ability to excrete up to 15 to 20 liters of water daily.

CLINICAL PRESENTATION

Most symptoms and signs referable directly to hyponatremia are unusual if serum sodium concentrations are above 125 mEq/L. Furthermore, concentrations below this point vary markedly in clinical presentation, presumably in relation to the rate at which sodium abnormalities have occurred.

The principal effects of hyponatremia are manifested by alterations of neurologic, neuromuscular, and gastrointestinal function. Neurologic effects are seen as changes in mental status and can range from disorientation and confusion to stupor and coma. Neuromuscular symptomatology often consists of the nonspecific complaints of weakness and muscular cramping. Gastrointestinal complaints may be present even when hyponatremia is mild, and are predominantly anorexia and nausea.

As in hypernatremia, the severity of symptoms is related to the rate at which sodium disturbances develop. Individuals with chronic hyponatremia may have surprisingly normal cognitive function, whereas acute lowering of serum sodium may precipitate seizures and significant alterations in mental status.

DIAGNOSIS AND TREATMENT

The diagnosis of hyponatremia relies on the determination of serum osmolality and assessment of volume status. The measurement of urinary sodium concentration can frequently add information toward diagnostic and therapeutic decision-making. Because sodium is the single most influential solute determining serum osmolality, we expect osmolality to be low in all cases of hyponatremia. If osmolality is found to be normal or elevated, the focus turns to pseudohyponatremia or the presence of other solutes present in the serum. In cases of normal serum osmolality, the diagnosis of pseudohyponatremia is established and serum protein and lipids should be measured. If serum osmolality is increased, serum glucose must be measured and the possibility of hypertonic infusion investigated. Patients in these groups often do not need specific therapy directed at hyponatremia because the sodium abnormality corrects itself once the underlying cause is satisfactorily treated. Patients with marked hyperglycemia from diabetic ketoacidosis often present with hyponatremia; however, these patients are often significantly volume-depleted. In these cases, a rapid reduction of glucose should not be undertaken. In many conditions, the tonicity provided by the hyperglycemia maintains intravascular volume. Because these patients are often grossly dehydrated and sodium-depleted, a rapid reduction in the serum glucose without first repleting salt and water losses may lead to vascular collapse.

In patients with depressed serum osmolality, the next step requires an estimation of ECF state. Patients at either end of the spectrum of extracellular volume are easily categorized. Individuals with milder alterations in fluid status present difficult clinical problems. Patients found to have edema have expansion of both total body water and sodium with a proportionally greater increase in water volume thus depressing sodium concentration. This group of patients with hypervolemic hyponatremia can be further subgrouped into those with adequate intravascular volume and those with an effective decrease in circulating blood volume. In both cases, the primary defect is the inability of the kidney to excrete the excess water load. Urinary sodium concentration can differentiate between the two subgroups. Sodium concentrations greater than 20 mEq/L suggest intrinsic renal disease, whereas the sodium retention states of congestive heart failure, liver failure, and nephrotic syndrome are associated with maximal sodium reabsorption and urinary sodium concentration of less than 10 mEq/L. Given the large water surplus in these patients, therapy consists of sodium and water restriction. In patients with chronic congestive heart failure who do not have evidence of cardiovascular or pulmonary compromise and in the remaining group of patients, the use of diuretics, particularly in the ED, is discouraged. These patients rarely have profound depression of serum sodium, and additional aggressive intervention is rarely necessary.

Patients found to have signs of dehydration fall into the group of hypovolemic hyponatremia. These patients all have significant losses of total body water with greater losses of total body sodium. These patients can be divided into subgroups of those with renal losses and those with extrarenal losses. This differentiation can be made with the measurement of urinary sodium. Extrarenal losses classically stimulate mechanisms that maximize sodium reabsorption, thereby reducing urinary sodium concentration to less than 10 mEq/L. Renal losses, on the other hand, develop partly because of circumstances that tend to preserve water conservation in preference to sodium so that sodium concentration in urine frequently rise to greater than 20 mEq/L. With the total body losses, these individuals need replacement sodium and water in amounts relative to their dehydration and hyponatremia. These patients should be treated with 0.9% saline at 100 to 150 mL per hour to replace volume losses. The treatment of severe hyponatremia is covered subsequently.

In some individuals, a history of fluid loss cannot be obtained. These patients appear to have a slight increase in total body water, but edema is not present. This group comprises those with isovolemic hyponatremia. It is useful to measure urinary osmolality and sodium concentration to help differentiate the possible causes of this condition. In the ED, these patients should be treated with water restriction as their evaluation proceeds.

Despite the straightforward management of most cases of hyponatremia, the treatment of severe depression in serum sodium (less than 120 mEq/L) still generates debate. It is generally accepted that sodium concentrations of this level are associated with significant morbidity and mortality, particularly from neurologic causes. Marked CNS depression has been clearly demonstrated. Rapid correction of hyponatremia to normal or elevated levels can lead to more problems than the treatment was meant to solve. A link between rapid changes in serum sodium and central pontine myelinosis, a syndrome of myelin loss in the pons, leading to severe neurologic sequelae, has been implied in several studies.[2] In light of these circumstances, guidelines in the management of severe hyponatremia can be established. Firstly, hypertonic saline (3 or 5% solution) is indicated only in cases of serum sodium below 120 mEq/L associated with clear symptoms requiring prompt intervention. Serum sodium below 110 mEq/L with only minimal symptoms is a relative indication for the use of hypertonic saline. The rate of administration should be adjusted so that serum sodium changes no more than 0.5 to 0.75 mEq/hour over the first 24 hours. The maximum serum sodium concentration achieved within this time frame should be kept below 125 mEq/L. Because of the risks associated with rapid changes in serum sodium, these infusions must be done under close observation, specifically in intensive care unit settings. The use of hypertonic saline in the ED should be restricted to the sickest individuals. Volumetric pumps for the infusion, frequent verification of the amounts actually infused, careful input and output values for the patient, and hourly measurements of serum sodium are essential features of the treatment of severe hyponatremia. The amount of hypertonic saline to be infused is given in Formula 2.

only a fraction of total body potassium is extracellular, even small changes in potassium balance can potentially alter serum potassium concentration drastically. The daily intake of potassium, up to 100 mEq, is itself more than the potassium found in the entirety of extracellular stores. Similarly, the amount of filtered potassium in the kidney is in vast excess of this extracellular quantity. It becomes clear, therefore, that small perturbations in the systems which control potassium balance can lead to clinically evident hyper- or hypokalemia. Gastrointestinal and insensible losses of potassium are negligible, and potassium elimination is primarily through urine. The renal handling of potassium is varied by a number of factors. The vast majority of filtered potassium is reabsorbed in the proximal tubule, and therefore potassium elimination depends on distal secretion. The kidney is able to maintain potassium balance by altering potassium secretion over a wide range. Under conditions of large potassium turnover (increased diet, increased tissue release), urinary potassium can reach up to 100 mEq/L. During potassium depletion, urinary potassium concentration diminishes greatly, although there is a small obligatory loss. Potassium secretion is mineralocorticoid-dependent. Aldosterone raises tubular potassium secretory rates with accompanying reabsorption of sodium. Aldosterone secretion is, in turn, stimulated by hyperkalemia. Additionally, aldosterone is controlled by the renin-angiotensin axis and in conditions associated with decreases in effective intravascular volume, aldosterone secretion is increased. Potassium excretion also varies directly with tubular fluid flow rates. Also, the actual amounts of sodium delivered in glomerular filtrate also affect potassium secretion. When large volumes of sodium are delivered to the distal tubule, sodium reabsorption may outpace the uptake of diffusable anion. In this case, to maintain electroneutrality, potassium excretion increases. The converse is also true, and in states of sodium restriction, potassium excretion is inhibited even in the face of increased mineralocorticoid.

Shifts of potassium between the intra- and extra-

Formula 2

$$\text{Rate of infusion (ml/hr)} = \frac{\text{Sodium to be infused (mEq/hr)}}{\text{[Na]Infusate (mEq/100 ml)}}$$

where:

$$\text{Sodium to be infused (mEq/hr)} = \text{TBW} \times \text{rate of change [Na]serum (mEq/hr)}$$
$$= 0.6 \times \text{weight (kg)} \times \text{rate of change [Na]serum (mEq/hr)}$$

DISORDERS OF POTASSIUM METABOLISM

PHYSIOLOGIC CONCEPTS

Potassium homeostasis represents a balance between daily input and output and cellular shifts. Because

cellular compartments also affect the serum potassium concentration. Hormonal milieu, acid-base status, plasma osmolality, and drugs will all affect the movement of potassium to and from the large intracellular pool to the small extracellular compartment. Insulin, β-agonists, and aldosterone all increase cellular potassium uptake thereby diminishing serum potassium. The hydrogen ion also affects cellular potassium shifts. During systemic acidosis, hydrogen ions shifts from extracellular fluid into cells because of a concentration gradient. This is accompanied by an ionic shift of potassium to maintain electroneutrality, tending to increase serum potassium. The opposite occurs during alkalosis.

HYPERKALEMIA

PATHOPHYSIOLOGY

The causes of hyperkalemia are listed in Table 54-14. Generally, the appearance of hyperkalemia requires the presence of a combination of defects. In patients with preserved homeostatic control, large amounts of oral or intravenous potassium are required to increase serum potassium above normal levels. This explains the observation that many causes of hyperkalemia are associated with the use of oral potassium supplements or specific medications which affect renal handling of potassium.

The various causes of hyperkalemia can be divided into subgroups. These include an increase in intake, an increase in cellular loss or transcompartmental shift, a decrease in renal clearance, and finally, laboratory error. An increase in potassium intake may be derived from several sources. Most obvious is the oral supplementation many individuals take with diuretic therapy. Although thiazide and loop diuretics cause kaliuresis, these patients may be prone to hypovolemia, which tends to increase potassium reabsorption. Furthermore, the combination of potassium-sparing diuretics and oral potassium supplementation

---

TABLE 54-14. CAUSES OF HYPERKALEMIA

A. Exogenous administration
  1. Cellular loss/transcompartmental shift
    —Acidosis
    —Diabetic ketoacidosis (hypoinsulinemia)
    —Drugs
      Succinylcholine cardiac glycosides
    —Periodic paralysis
    —Massive cellular lysis
      Tissue crush injury, rhabdomyolysis
      Massive hemolysis (GI bleeding, intravascular hemolysis)
  2. Decreased renal excretion
    —Intrinsic renal disease
      Relative insufficiency (e.g., CFH, hypovolemia)
      Acute tubular necrosis
      Obstructive uropathy
      Chronic renal insufficiency
    —Drugs
      NSAIDS
      Angiotensin-converting enzyme inhibitors
      Potassium sparing diuretics
    —Mineralocorticoid deficiency
      Addison's disease
      Congenital adrenal hyperplasia syndromes
      Hyporeninemic hypoaldosteronism
  3. Pseudohyperkalemia
    —Hemolysis during phlebotomy
    —Thrombocytosis ($>1 \times 10^6$)
    —Marked leukocytosis

---

may be dangerous. Intravenous potassium can rapidly lead to hyperkalemia. As a general rule, in nonemergent therapy, the rate of potassium replacement should not exceed 10 to 20 mEq/hour, and the concentration of potassium should be no more than 40 mEq/L. Other less obvious sources of exogenous potassium are transfused blood and antibiotics. Banked blood contains a large supply of potassium based on intracorpuscular supply. Any hemolysis that occurs before or during transfusion can alter serum potassium. The soluble salt of many antibiotics has potassium as the accompanying cation.

Movement of potassium from intra- to extracellular locations can cause hyperkalemia. This movement can be from hormonal, acid-base, or drug effect or may be caused by cell death with subsequent efflux of potassium. Acidosis, particularly of the metabolic type, can lead to significant increases in serum potassium. Hypoinsulinemia, as occurs in diabetes, diminishes cellular uptake of potassium. In conjunction with acidosis, as occurs in diabetic ketoacidosis, the rise in serum potassium can be life-threatening. Several drugs act specifically on cellular mechanisms that control potassium transport. Cardiac glycosides and the paralytic agent succinylcholine decrease cellular uptake of potassium. Succinylcholine should be avoided in several conditions because of a likelihood of exaggerated hyperkalemic reponse. These include spinal cord injury, tetanus, muscle injury, stroke, encephalitis, and thermal injury.[3] Several other agents that have been reported to cause hyperkalemia include fluoride, nifedipine, lithium, and arginine HCl.[4] Cellular injury is an important cause of hyperkalemia. Any patient presenting with crush injury, severe motor vehicle accident, hypotension, or large thermal burn should be evaluated for the presence of hyperkalemia. The release of large stores of intracellular potassium can be immediately life-threatening. In muscle injury, myoglobin release may also cause acute tubular necrosis, which itself may increase the likelihood of hyperkalemia. Massive cell death can also occur during the chemotherapeutic treatment of leukemia. Hemolysis is another potentially large source of cellular potassium. During gastrointestinal bleeding, large amounts of hemolyzed blood lead to large quantities of intraluminal potassium, which can be absorbed, causing hyperkalemia. Other intravascular hemolytic diseases such as sickle crisis or G6PD deficiency can also lead to the same.

The causes of diminished renal excretion of potassium can be intrinsic renal disease itself or drugs or hormones that affect the kidney's ability to normally handle potassium. When renal function decreases to the point where glomerular filtration rate is below 5 mL per minute, the kidney is no longer able to excrete a typical daily intake of potassium. As patients approach this level of renal function, they should be placed on potassium-restricted diets. Acute tubular necrosis or a complete obstructive uropathy also severely restricts the kidney's ability to handle a potassium load. Nephritis caused by drugs or chronic infection or the renal dysfunction seen in sickle cell disease may adversely affect potassium handling by the kidney.[5] Among the drugs that can interfere with renal potassium excretory function are nonsteroidal anti-inflammatory drugs, angiotensin-converting enzyme inhibitors, and potassium-sparing diuretics. Any cause of mineralocorticoid deficiency, including Addison's disease, hyporeninemic hypoaldosteronism, or postsurgical removal of an aldosterone secreting tumor can cause hyperkalemia.

Factitious hyperkalemia is an important cause of laboratory-determined elevations of serum potassium. This occurs under several circumstances. Poor blood drawing technique increases the likelihood of iatrogenic hemolysis leading to a laboratory determination of hyperkalemia. A serum sample taken from patients with significant thrombocytosis (greater than $1 \times 10^6/mm3$) or leukocytosis (greater than 5×10^5) can yield a falsely high concentration because of release of potassium during clotting. In patients with these findings, a measurement of *plasma* potassium (as compared to the serum determination) clarifies this potential problem.

CLINICAL PRESENTATION

Severe hyperkalemia is a life-threatening condition. The primary action that causes mortality and morbidity is the effect on cardiac rhythm. The effect of hyperkalemia on the heart is discussed in greater detail in Chapter 45. The risk of sudden death from ventricular standstill or fibrillation increases with increasing potassium concentrations. Many patients complain of weakness, fatigue, muscle cramping, and nausea. Other neurologic complaints are rare and, unlike disorders of sodium metabolism, hyperkalemia does not induce encephalopathic symptoms. As noted, the most common cardiac effects are found on the electrocardiogram. Specifically, with increasing potassium concentrations, one can find progressive peaking of the T wave, QT interval shortening, and PR interval lengthening. Eventually, there is QRS prolongation, initially appearing similar to an intraventricular conduction delay and finally assuming the classic sine-wave pattern. The likelihood of an unstable arrhythmia occurring at this point is high; however, arrhythmias can occur at any time, particularly at potassium concentrations above 6.0 mEq/L. Heart block is a rare finding.[6] Clearly, coexisting electrolyte disturbances, myocardial injury, or drugs can alter these electrocardiographic findings.

DIAGNOSIS AND TREATMENT

The simple and rapid determination of serum electrolytes obtained for a wide variety of clinical circumstances has made the determination of hyperkalemia straightforward. In most laboratories, potassium concentration above 5.0 mEq/L is considered abnormal.

In general, patients with hyperkalemia in the range below 6.0 mEq/L are not at high risk for an untoward event. Serum potassium above this level, however, should be aggressively evaluated and treated. Even in suspected cases of pseudohyperkalemia, the patient should be assumed to have elevation of serum potassium and assessed more fully while repeat blood determinations are carried out. The underlying cause of the disorder can usually be quickly divided into two broad groups. The first group resulting from an increased potassium load includes patients with exogenous sources of potassium ingestion or infusion, patients with illnesses causing transcellular shifts, and patients with crush injuries or burns are diagnosed by history and physical examination. Additionally, patients with other cellular sources, such as leukemia or marked intravascular hemolysis, are diagnosed by physical findings and adjunct laboratory examination. The second group is caused by inadequate potassium excretion and includes causes of renal origin. These include cases caused by intrinsic renal disease, mineralocorticoid deficiency syndromes, and drug-induced hyperkalemia.

Before discussing general treatment guidelines, several of the causes of hyperkalemia deserve special attention because of their especially high mortality and morbidity. Patients with severe crush injuries and hyperkalemia must also be strongly considered to have rhabdomyolysis. A positive urine dipstick for heme with few or no observable red blood cells should raise suspicions. Urinary myoglobin can be directly measured; however, these results are not universally available on an emergent basis. These patients should have treatment for hyperkalemia instituted immediately; however, dialysis should also be strongly considered to prevent the possibility of acute renal failure. Another circumstance involves the patient with hyperkalemia associated with hypotension or shock, fever, nausea, diffuse muscle aching and weakness, and possibly hyperpigmentation. These individuals must be presumed to have adrenalcortical insufficiency until proven otherwise. Blood should be drawn for ACTH and cortisol and patients should then be treated immediately with a water-soluble preparation of cortisol, specifically hydrocortisone sodium succinate (Solu-Cortef), 100 mg intravenously. This treats the life-threatening glucocorticoid deficiency and also provides sufficient mineralocorticoid activity. When fluids are instituted simultaneously, hyperkalemia often responds fairly quickly. Any degree of hyperkalemia that causes ECG changes should be treated as outlined subsequently.

Because the greatest risk of death from hyperkalemia is from cardiac arrhythmias, the order of treatment of hyperkalemia is first to reverse the toxic effects of potassium on the heart, followed by actions that shift potassium out of the extracellular and into the intracellular compartment. Finally, treatments that lower the total body potassium are administered. All patients should first have a 12-lead electrocardiogram performed, and all treatment should be done with continuous cardiac monitoring.

Infusion of intravenous calcium is the most rapid modulator of adverse effects of potassium. The effect of calcium is to increase cardiac transmembrane potential toward normal levels so that the heart becomes less refactory to depolarization. Calcium for intravenous administration is available in several preparations. The recommended solution is calcium gluconate, which comes in 10 mL ampules as a 10% solution and contains 0.45 mEq calcium per mL. Up to 50 mL of this solution can be administered safely if given slowly. The first 10 mL may be given over 1 to 2 minutes, with subsequent ampules given over 5 to 10 minutes each. Under emergency conditions, the drug may be given intramuscularly if necessary. Calcium chloride, which may be more readily available, may be a more effective drug because free ionized calcium concentrations are usually higher and sustained longer after its administration. This preparation, however, available as a 10% solution containing 1.36 mEq calcium per mL, is acidifying and can cause phlebitis. If injected into tissue directly or through a catheter that has infiltrated subcutaneously, it can cause necrosis and ulceration. For this reason, the drug is a second-line agent. The ability of calcium to antagonize the effects of hyperkalemia should be noted within minutes of infusion; however, the duration of action is less than 1 hour.

Phase 2 of treatment is to drive extracellular potassium into cells. The most rapid way to induce this effect is by alkalinization, particularly if the patient is acidotic initially. An ampule of 50 mEq of sodium bicarbonate can be injected intravenously over 5 minutes. This agent is effective within minutes and lasts for up to 2 hours. Repeated infusions should be diluted and given more slowly to avoid hypertonicity and sodium overload, particularly in patients with congestive heart disease. In conjunction with bicarbonate, the effect of glucose on insulin secretion and potassium uptake can be used. Theoretically, 50% dextrose infusion can increase serum tonicity and exacerbate hyperkalemia. To avoid this potential problem, 500 mL of a 10% dextrose infusion can be given over 1 hour. This adequately stimulates insulin secretion in normal individuals to achieve the desired effect. Alternatively, 10 to 15 units of insulin can be added to the solution to ensure adequate insulin levels. The effect of this treatment is seen within 30 minutes and lasts for several hours. An additional therapeutic modality has recently been described. The use of a nebulized mist treatment (NMT) with the β-agonist albuterol has been shown to effectively shift potassium into the intracellular compartment.[7] Albuterol, 10 to 20 mg, given as an NMT is effective within 30 minutes and acts for up to 2 hours. It has the advantage of easy administration and few side effects.

The final phase in the treatment of hyperkalemia is the removal of potassium from the body. The most effective mechanism of potassium extraction is with the use of a binding resin given orally or rectally. Sodium polystyrene sulfonate (Kayexalate) is such a resin, which exchanges sodium for potassium in the GI tract without the drug itself being absorbed. When given orally, it must be given with an osmotic agent to keep fluid in the gut so that the resin is eventually passed. Typically, 20 g is mixed with 70% sorbitol solution. The oral preparation is more effective in that the resin is in contact with a larger area of bowel and for longer periods of time. For the same reason, however, its onset of action is not for 1 to 2 hours after administration. This dose may be repeated every 2 hours; however, care must be taken that patients do not develop sodium overload because of the cation exchange or constipation from retained resin. When 50 g of resin is given rectally by retention enema, the onset of action is within 20 to 30 minutes. The enema may be repeated once an hour as necessary. These treatments are successful in most patients, with even severe hyperkalemia, in a relatively short time. Nevertheless, hemodialysis is also available for patients who are resistant to these treatments or have other complications that render some of these modalities impossible to use.

HYPOKALEMIA

PATHOPHYSIOLOGY

The causes of hypokalemia are given in Table 54-15. These can be conveniently grouped to aid in diagnosis and treatment. The groupings include renal losses, gastrointestinal losses, redistribution from extra to intracellular compartments, and miscellaneous causes.

The most common cause of renal potassium wasting is that induced by diuretics. There are several additive mechanisms by which this occurs. The drug causes an increase in the delivery of sodium and filtrate to the distal tubule and collecting duct. This stimulates the mechanism that attempts to reabsorb the excess sodium in exchange for potassium, thereby inducing a kaliuresis. Furthermore, the diuretic often establishes some degree of hypovolemia, which stimulates the renin-angiotensin-aldosterone axis, further enhancing potassium secretion. Other factors such as the induction of magnesium depletion and the development of mild alkalosis from stimulated hydrogen ion excretion may also contribute to hypokalemia. Osmotic diuresis may also lead to hypokalemia. High amounts of filtrate formed from glycosuria or mannitol prevent most potassium from being absorbed proximally. Because little potassium is reabsorbed more distally, this leads to potassium wasting and possible hypokalemia.

Excess mineralocorticoid alters normal sodium-potassium exchange in the distal tubule, thereby causing kaliuresis. The most abundant endogenous mineralocorticoid, aldosterone, is secreted by the adrenal cortex under control of the renin-angiotensin axis. Serum potassium, acid-base status, and adrenocorticotrophic

---

TABLE 54-15. CAUSES OF HYPOKALEMIA

A. Renal losses
  1. Drugs
     —Diuretic use/abuse
  2. Osmotic diuresis
  3. Excess mineralocorticoid
     —Primary aldosteronism
     —Secondary aldosteronism
        Bartter's syndrome
        Renin secreting J-G cell tumor
     —Cushing's syndrome/disease
     —Glycyrrhizic acid (licorice)
  4. Renal tubular acidosis (Types I and II)
  5. Magnesium depletion
B. Gastrointestinal losses
  1. Profound nausea, vomiting, diarrhea
  2. Villous adenoma
  3. Laxative abuse
  4. Nasogastric suction
  5. Kayexelate
C. Compartment redistribution
  1. Aklalosis
  2. Insulin
  3. β-agonists
  4. Periodic paralysis
  5. Vitamin B_{12} therapy
  6. Barium poisoning
D. Miscellaneous
  1. Pseudohypokalemia
  2. Excess sweating
  3. Ureterosigmoidostomy

---

hormone (ACTH) can also regulate aldosterone secretion independently. Primary hyperaldosteronism can be caused by a unilateral adenoma of the adrenal gland (Conn's syndrome), or less commonly to bilateral hyperplasia. These patients often present with hypertension that is difficult to control and a history of borderline or moderate hypokalemia resistant to most therapy. In several other disease states, there is a physiologic increase in aldosterone secretion, usually related to a decrease in intravascular volume. These states include congestive heart failure and liver disease. It is infrequent, however, for these conditions to cause hypokalemia without other factors intervening. Rarely, renin-secreting tumors arising from juxtaglomerular cells have been reported. Cortisol has weak mineralocorticoid effect and when circulating levels are substantially elevated from endogenous or exogenous sources, this effect may become clinically evident. Among the other causes of hypokalemia is Bartter's syndrome, a disease that usually presents in childhood with hypokalemia and polyuria. Although these patients are found to have elevated plasma renin activity and aldosterone levels, the hypokalemia is not fully mineralocorticoid-dependent. In adults with Bartter's syndrome, it is exceedingly difficult to increase serum potassium through any modality.

Renal tubular acidosis (RTA) is another cause of hypokalemia. In RTA type I, there is an abnormality in hydrogen ion excretion by the distal tubule, caused by either back diffusion of hydrogen ion or an inability to secrete hydrogen ions against a steep gradient. It has been proposed that potassium excretion makes up partly for the decrease in hydrogen ion excretion. RTA type II is a disorder of bicarbonate wasting in the proximal tubule in the face of normal serum bicarbonate. Because the increase in bicarbonate delivery increases distal fluid delivery and the excess bicarbonate is excreted partly as a potassium salt, there is potassium wasting and hypokalemia. For this reason, the hypokalemia of RTA type II is exacerbated by oral administration of bicarbonate.

Gastrointestinal fluids can be relatively high in potassium. Unreplaced losses may therefore lead to hypokalemia. Normal colonic concentration of potassium can be upward of 25 mEq/L. The potassium concentration of diarrheal stool can range from 20 to 80 mEq/L and is particularly high in villous adenoma. Gastric potassium concentrations are significantly less than this, and therefore loss of gastric fluid from prolonged emesis usually does not lead to significant potassium losses. It does, however, lead to volume contraction, which can cause potassium wasting in the kidney because sodium is preferentially retained by the distal tubule. Laxative abuse also causes excess potassium to be lost from colonic sources. Nasogastric suctioning may also induce hypokalemia for the same reasons discussed for emesis. Excess loss of gastric fluid may also cause a metabolic alkalosis, which tends to shift potassium into intracellular compartments as well. Patients who have been given excess potassium binding resin such as Kayexalate may develop hypokalemia. This is especially true in patients who have been given repeated oral doses.

The shift of potassium into the intracellular compartment may also lead to hypokalemia. Individuals with alkalosis are prone to hypokalemia. Unlike shifts of potassium out of cells caused by acid-base changes, potassium shifts inward in exchange for hydrogen ions occur in both respiratory and metabolic alkaloses. During treatment of diabetic ketoacidosis, administration of fluids and insulin, as well as the correction of acidosis, causes potassium to shift to the intracellular compartment. Because these patients are frequently depleted of potassium, significant hypokalemia may occur. One form of familial periodic paralysis, an inherited disorder associated with periods of hypokalemia, has also been described and can be provoked by high carbohydrate meals or exercise. Patients with pernicious anemia who are treated with B_{12} have been reported to develop hypokalemia as potassium is taken up by the burst growth activity in the bone marrow.

Several miscellaneous causes of hypokalemia should be discussed. Laboratory error should be considered as a potential factor when the report of a low potassium does not fit with the clinical history. In cases of significant leukocytosis, the cellular elements continue to actively take up potassium. Under normal circumstances, this has little effect on the potassium determination. If the sample is not assayed for a lengthened period, however, falsely low potassium concentrations may be reported. Sweat has enough potassium in it to make the possibility of hypokalemia a reality in cases of profound skin losses.

CLINICAL PRESENTATION

The prominent symptoms and signs of hypokalemia are related to the effect of potassium on muscle of all types. The specific cellular effects were discussed previously. Potentially the most important effect of hypokalemia is on cardiac muscle. Symptoms related to cardiac electrical instability are palpitations and "skipped beats." Underlying rhythms found in hypokalemia include premature ventricular depolarizations, ventricular tachyarrhythmias including fibrillation, intraventricular conduction abnormalities, and heart block.[18] Patients with a history of ischemic heart disease using potassium-wasting diuretics are particularly at risk for hypokalemia induced arrhythmia.[19] Electrocardiographic findings in patients with hypokalemia include the presence of U waves greater than 1 mm and larger than the corresponding T wave in the same lead. The ECG changes, the arrhythmia potential, and the clinical symptoms have been found to be closely correlated with the degree of potassium depletion. It is rare to have cardiac muscle effects until serum potassium concentrations fall below 3.0 mEq/L. It is of particular importance to note that many of the electrocardiographic changes and many of the arrhythmias described are more likely to occur in patients taking cardiac glycosides. It is for this reason that patients taking both a digitalis preparation and a diuretic must be carefully monitored for hypokalemia. It has been suggested that these patients be maintained with serum potassium greater than 4.0 mEq/L to decrease the chances of hypokalemia in the future.

The effect of hypokalemia on cardiac tissue is paralleled in striated muscle. Many patients complain of weakness, especially as potassium levels fall below 2.5 mEq/L. The degree of weakness is correlated with the degree of potassium depression and may become profound at severely low levels. Patients have been described with paralysis, which may include chest wall muscles, leading to respiratory failure. In more moderate cases, patients frequently complain of muscle cramps and twitching unrelated to lower extremity position unlike those with nocturnal gastrocnemius cramps. Severe, prolonged hypokalemia has also been reported to cause rhabdomyolysis. When this occurs, muscle destruction and subsequent potassium shifts in the extracellular compartment may transiently reverse hypokalemia making the diagnosis difficult.

The effects on smooth muscle are primarily manifested as abnormal gastrointestinal function. It is not uncommon for patients with significant hypokalemia to develop a paralytic ileus. Other, more nonspecific symptoms include nausea and vomiting, bloating, and abdominal cramping.

DIAGNOSIS AND TREATMENT

Important areas of interest in the assessment of the patient with hypokalemia include a history of diuretic use, hypertension, diabetes, recent drug treatments, diarrhea, and emesis. The exclusion of redistributive causes of hypokalemia is accomplished by historical features. Patients on insulin, β-agonists, or other hypokalemic drugs should first have their management altered. After this, it is most convenient to separate renal from nonrenal causes. This characterization can most easily be carried out with the measurement of 24-hour urinary potassium excretion. The only caveat to this procedure is related to sodium balance. It is essential to provide adequate sodium when measuring urinary potassium excretion. Under conditions of sodium deficiency, aldosterone is stimulated, thereby causing urinary potassium excretion despite hypokalemia. Therefore, a simultaneous urinary measurement of 24-hour sodium excretion greater than 100 mEq/day verifies adequate sodium stores. In this circumstance, urinary potassium losses less than 20 mEq/day lead to the diagnosis of extrarenal potassium loss or redistribution.

The renal causes of hypokalemia are varied. Several clues help lead to a definitive diagnosis. Patients with concomitant acidosis should be considered to have RTA until proven otherwise. Because ketoacidosis and gastrointestinal losses are the only other causes of simultaneous hypokalemia and acidosis, this is an important clue in the diagnostic evaluation. The inability to maintain serum potassium greater than 3.0 mEq/L despite large supplemental doses can be ascribed to four conditions. Patients with significant sodium depletion are not able to conserve potassium, as noted previously. Individuals with Bartter's syndrome usually have serum potassum concentrations less than 3.0 mEq/L despite therapeutic measures. Patients with this syndrome can be differentiated from those with aldosteronism by virtue of an elevated plasma renin activity (PRA), which is suppressed in the latter condition. Patients with profound hypomagnesemia do not correct the potassium defect until magnesium has been repleted (see subsequent text). Finally, patients abusing diuretics often have "untreatable" hypokalemia. This is due to continued abuse of the agent or to non-compliance with supplementation regime. In this case, a urine screen for diuretics is essential. One must be careful about diagnostic manipulations in these patients. These individuals are often admitted to the hospital, where supplements may be continued but diuretics are unknowingly stopped. The kidney quickly becomes potassium-avid and hyperkalemia may ensue. In all patients with suspected renal hypokalemia, a plasma aldosterone and PRA should be measured before treatment.

The method of treatment of hypokalemia depends

on the actual level of serum potassium, the mechanism by which hypokalemia has occurred, and the presence of neuromuscular or cardiac effects. Potassium levels greater than 2.5 mEq/L in asymptomatic individuals can usually be corrected with oral supplementation. Patients with any evidence of arrhythmia, ECG changes, digitalis use, angina pectoris, objective muscle weakness and/or respiratory insufficiency, or ileus should be treated by intravenous infusion of potassium. In virtually all circumstances, repletion should be accomplished with potassium chloride.

The rate of administration is restricted by two factors. The administration of potassium too quickly increases serum potassium to dangerously high concentrations before a new equilibrium between extra- and intracellular spaces can take place. Furthermore, high concentration potassium is a strong irritant and may cause significant phlebitis. Under most circumstances, 10 to 20 mEq of potassium may be added to 100 mL of solution in a piggyback infusion device. This solution can then be infused over 1 hour. The primary line must be well established, however, and infusing must be at a substantial rate. Mild to moderate hypokalemia can usually be substantially corrected by repeating this therapy for several hours. A repeat serum potassium measurement determines the need for additional therapy. No more than a 1-hour supply should be set up at any given time to avoid the risk of iatrogenic hyperkalemia. In more severe forms of hypokalemia, the rate of infusion can be increased to 40 mEq/hour; however, this should be done only with extreme caution. Infusion rates of up to 60 mEq/hour have been used under conditions of life-threatening arrhythmias; however, this must be given by central venous route and is not otherwise recommended. As a guideline, 40 mEq of infused potassium will raise serum concentration by 1 mEq/L. All patients who are being so treated should be placed on a cardiac monitor. Any electrocardiographic evidence of hyperkalemia should halt the infusion immediately. Serum potassium levels must be frequently checked and, as concentrations approach 3.5 mEq/L, the supplements should be discontinued. At that time, 20 to 40 mEq of potassium may be placed in each liter of solution and infused at normal maintenance rates. Furthermore, oral repletion can begin at this time also. Although potassium is well absorbed from the GI tract, there is a substantial reduction in the likelihood of ensuing hyperkalemia from this route of administration.

Patients with diabetic ketoacidosis present a special circumstance. Total body potassium stores are almost always depleted in these individuals, but they often present with hyperkalemia for reasons discussed under Pathophysiology of Hyperkalemia. Generally, the first liter of replacement fluids should be normal saline without added potassium until results of serum electrolytes are obtained. Once the potassium concentration is below 4.0 mEq/L, potassium can be safely administered.

DISORDERS OF CALCIUM METABOLISM

PHYSIOLOGIC CONCEPTS

Calcium is the most abundant divalent cation found in the body. In a 70 kg individual, there is approximately 1 kg of elemental calcium, the vast majority of which exists in bone. Of this large source pool, about 5 to 10 gm of calcium can be freely mobilized. Dietary intake of calcium is on the order of 1 g daily. Despite these relatively large amounts, the serum concentration of ionized calcium is held in the narrow range of 4 to 4.5 mg/dL (1.0 to 1.15 mOsm/L). This task is accomplished by complex interactions among several hormones acting on absorption and excretion of calcium at the level of the gastrointestinal, renal, and skeletal systems. For this section, the following brief discussion highlights important aspects of calcium metabolism.

The important hormones responsible for calcium homeostasis include parathyroid hormone (PTH), 1,25-dihydroxy Vitamin D (calcitrol), and calcitonin. Each hormone has specific effects on the target tissues. PTH secretion by the parathyroid glands is controlled primarily by serum ionized calcium concentration. Although magnesium in its normal physiologic concentrations does not seem to regulate PTH secretion, deficiency of this cation severely impedes the normal PTH secretory response to hypocalcemia. Hypermagnesemia may also inhibit PTH secretion as well. Multiple other agents have been tested for their effect on PTH secretion. In each case, either no effect is noted or conflicting data have been reported. These agents include catecholamines, serotonin, histamine, vitamin D and its metabolites, phosphorus, calcitonin, and glucagon. PTH is important in the control of calcium metabolism by virtue of its effect on calcium transport and vitamin D metabolism in the kidney and mobilization of calcium from bone. The effects of PTH on bone are several. An initial fast response causes the mobilization of calcium from bone by osteocytes. A later phase, occurring within 12 hours of exposure, stimulates osteoclast-mediated resorption of bone to further increase transfer of calcium, causes differentiation of precursor elements into osteoclast cell types, and inhibits osteoblast function. The direct effect of PTH on calcium handling by the kidney is to increase distal reabsorption. Although most calcium is reabsorbed proximally, this system is not PTH-dependent. Proximal calcium handling is tightly linked to sodium, so that conditions that alter sodium delivery or reabsorption cause parallel changes in calcium absorption. Only 10% of the filtered calcium reaches the distal tubule, representing approximately 1 g of calcium. This allows for the short-term regulation of serum calcium concentration by PTH. Furthermore, PTH can act to increase 1-hydroxylase activity in the kidney used in the synthesis of the active 1,25-(OH)$_2$D moiety.

Vitamin D, in turn, affects calcium homeostasis by activity directed at the intestine, kidney, and bone. Vitamin D (cholecalciferol) stores are supplied from two sources. Vitamin D is synthesized in skin, where the vitamin D precursor, 7-dihydrocholesterol, is converted to previtamin D by exposure to ultraviolet irradiation from sun exposure. There are relatively small amounts of naturally occurring vitamin D in foodstuffs. Most dietary vitamin D$_2$ and D$_3$ are from additives to milk, cereals, and breads. Absorption of vitamin D occurs in the duodenum and jejunum and is substantially reduced in fat malabsorption syndromes. Circulating vitamin D, bound to a specific binding globulin, is converted to 25-(OH)D efficiently by the liver. There does not appear to be any significant physiologic control over the 25-hydroxylation step. The 25-(OH)D is converted to 1,25-(OH)$_2$D or 24,25-(OH)$_2$D by the kidney by two separate enzyme systems. Of the two forms, 1,25-(OH)$_2$D is the primary active form responsible for end-organ control of mineral homeostasis. The major control over vitamin D action is, therefore, the activity of the 1-hydroxylase enzyme. Under normal circumstances, 24,25-(OH)$_2$D is the major circulating dihydroxy form of vitamin D. Although the systems are separate, they are inversely regulated by PTH, phosphorus, 1,25-(OH)$_2$D, and possibly calcium. As mentioned previously, PTH directly stimulates 1-hydroxylase activity and inhibits 24-hydroxylase. Phosphorus has the opposite effect on enzymatic conversion to the dihydroxy vitamin D forms. This is discussed in the next section on disorders of phosphorus metabolism. 1,25-(OH)$_2$D acts in a parallel manner to phosphorus, so that increased levels of this form feed back and inhibit its own biosynthesis.

The primary effect of vitamin D on the intestine is to significantly increase the active uptake of calcium from luminal contents. Although calcium is also absorbed by passive diffusion as well, this appears to be physiologically less important. It is believed that the regulator of intestinal calcium transport is 1,25-(OH)$_2$D and not PTH or calcium. The direct bone effect of 1,25-(OH)$_2$D is an increase in bone resorption. This seems to be additive to the PTH effect. Osteoid mineralization is thought to occur passively, given the appropriate mineral milieu. Renal responses to vitamin D and its metabolites have not been fully worked out; however, there seems to be an increase in calcium reabsorption.

Calcitonin, a 32 amino acid peptide secreted by the thyroid C-cells, has clearly demonstrable effects on bone and kidney. Acute infusion of calcitonin in animals causes a rapid decrease in serum calcium. Nevertheless, no clear physiologic role in mineral metabolism has been assigned to this peptide. No changes in calcium or phosphorus homeostasis have been found in patients with calcitonin deficiency after total thyroidectomy or in those with the drastically elevated calcitonin levels seen in medullary thyroid carcinoma. Because clinical syndromes of calcitonin deficiency or excess have not been identified, a further discussion of end-organ responses will not be undertaken. The primary use of calcitonin is presently in the treatment of Paget's disease of bone and potentially in osteoporosis.

The integrated control of calcium homeostasis occurs as follows. A decrease in serum ionized calcium stimulates PTH secretion. The increase in PTH raises renal calcium reabsorption and 1,25-(OH)$_2$D levels. The elevation of 1,25-(OH)$_2$D stimulates an increase in calcium uptake from the intestines. Both PTH and 1,25-(OH)$_2$D operate in concert to mobilize bone sources of calcium. The controls against hypercalcemia are essentially the opposite of the previous scenario.

HYPERCALCEMIA

PATHOPHYSIOLOGY

Hypercalcemia is a condition in which calcium delivery to the extracellular compartment overwhelms the ability of the kidney to excrete the excess load. Because the normal kidney can excrete up to 1000 mg of calcium daily, hypercalcemia occurs only when calcium influx is massive and/or renal calcium handling is altered hormonally or by intrinsic renal disease. The causes of hypercalcemia are listed in Table 54-16.

The most common cause of hypercalcemia is hyperparathyroidism. Population studies have suggested an incidence on the order of 50,000 new cases annually in the United States. The disease is rarely found in individuals under 30 years, and is twice as common in women as in men. In most of these cases, a single functional parathyroid adenoma is present.

TABLE 54-16. CAUSES OF HYPERCALCEMIA

A. Primary hyperparathyroidism
B. Hypercalemia of malignancy
    1. Locally destructive metastases
    2. Hypercalcemia associated with squamous carcinomas
    3. Hypercalcemia associated with lymphoma
C. Thyrotoxicosis
D. Addison's disease
E. Neuroendocrine tumors (VIPoma, pheochromocytoma)
F. Drugs
    1. Thiazide diuretics
    2. Hypervitaminosis A or D
    3. Lithium
    4. Estrogens
G. Milk-alkali syndrome
H. Granulomatous disease
    1. Sarcodosis, eosinophilic granulomatosis
    2. Tuberculosis, coccidioidomycosis, histoplasmosis, candiasis
    3. Berylliosis, silicosis
I. Immobilization
J. Familial hypocalcuric hypercalcemia

As many as 10 to 15% of patients may have parathyroid hyperplasia in which part or all of the 4 parathyroid glands are pathologically involved. Patients with multiple endocrine neoplasia syndromes display this form of hyperparathyroidism. Parathyroid carcinoma is rare; however, most of these are functional and therefore present with hypercalcemia.

The hypercalcemia associated with malignancy can be divided into two large groups on the basis of causality. The first group consists of tumors that metastasize to bone and by direct mechanisms cause bone resorption and mobilization of calcium. Prostaglandin E_2 and a set of proteins collectively grouped under the heading osteoclast activating factor have been implicated in the mechanisms by which these tumors induce hypercalcemia. The second class encompasses malignancies that may or may not metastasize to bone but are believed to secrete a humoral substance called PTH-like protein, which causes osteocytic mediated calcium mobilization or activates osteoclastic bone resorption. As listed in Table 54-16, hypercalcemia associated with lymphoma has been listed separately. Although these cancers most frequently cause hypercalcemia by the direct mechanisms described previously, it has been shown that, in certain cases, these tumors may secrete $1,25-(OH)_2D$.

Several endocrinopathies have been shown to be causative factors in hypercalcemia. Hyperthyroidism causes an increase in bone resorption and formation, the former to a greater extent, hence the elevation in serum calcium. The severity of hypercalcemia is mild and rarely, if ever, symptomatic itself. Serum calcium greater than 11.5 mg/dL should arouse suspicion of other hypercalcemic factors operating. Addison's disease has been reported to cause hypercalcemia; however, the mechanisms by which this occurs have not been established. Concentration of the extravascular space with concomitant elevations in calcium levels has been proposed as a likely cause, although this is probably not the only causal component. Tumors of neuro-endocrine origin such as pheochromocytoma and VIPoma have also been associated with hypercalcemia. These tumors include those that are seen outside the scope of multiple endocrine neoplasia syndromes and may act through a humorally mediated substance.

Drugs are an important group of causes of hypercalcemia particularly because of the ease in treatment they usually represent. The most common agent among the pharmacologic agents is thiazide diuretics. The actual effect at the level of the nephron is still debated, although the fact that these agents cause hypocalcuria after several days of treatment is well established. Vitamin D preparations, when used in excess, can cause hypercalcemia. This effect is not expected to be noticed until doses of vitamin D are greater than 100,000 U. Patients with liver or renal disease who are maintained on the hydroxy or dihydroxy vitamin D agents are considerably more likely to develop this toxicity. Hypervitaminosis A is rare but clearly implicated among the causes of hypercalcemia. Lithium, acting by increasing PTH secretion or by diminishing renal calcium excretion, has also been linked to hypercalcemia. Estrogens and anti-estrogens are reported to cause hypercalcemia, although those reports are from patients with metastatic breast carcinoma.

Milk-alkali syndrome is among the rare causes of hypercalcemia. This disease is infrequently noted, partly because of the especially large amounts of elemental calcium required in the development of the syndrome.

Granulomatous diseases represent an interesting collection of illnesses that have been shown to cause hypercalcemia. Sarcoidosis, the most carefully studied, causes elevated serum calcium by virtue of granulomata participation in the conversion of $25-(OH)D$ to $1,25-(OH)_2D$. Other granulomatous diseases also cause hypercalcemia, possibly by similar mechanisms.

Immobilization is a known cause of hypercalcemia, although the populations at risk tend to be adolescents and patients with Paget's disease. In this disorder, patients are more or less completely disabled by orthopedic or neurologic disorders. The hypercalcemia is felt to be caused by an increase in bone turnover, with a particular emphasis on resorption. The pathogenesis of this is unknown. It is important to note that immobilization hypercalcemia has not been reported in elderly individuals who are similarly immobilized without other etiologic factors present.

Familial hypocalciuric hypercalcemia is a disorder that elevates plasma calcium levels by unclear mechanisms. Several important features of the syndrome are the virtual lack of complications related to hypercalcemia, the uniform decrease in the fractional excretion of both calcium and magnesium, and the high prevalence among family members with an autosomal dominant inheritance pattern and almost complete penetrance.

CLINICAL PRESENTATION

The disorders causing hypercalcemia listed in Table 54-16 have substantial clinical symptoms themselves, in addition to any caused by elevations in serum calcium. Furthermore, hypercalcemic symptoms, like those of most electrolyte disturbances, tend to be nonspecific. As such, suspicion and diagnosis of hypercalcemia are difficult. Manifestations of changes in calcium homeostasis are displayed as alterations in mental status or cardiovascular, renal, or gastrointestinal function.

The CNS is probably the most severely affected by hypercalcemia. Patients can display the full range of changes in mental status from lethargy and confusion to obtundation and coma. Renal manifestations vary somewhat, depending on the acuity of calcium elevations. Under acute conditions, there are diuresis and natriuresis, causing extracellular volume contraction with its attendant symptoms. If hypercalcemia has been present chronically, there is a distinct abnormality in the urine-concentrating ability, leading to chronic dehydration, polyuria, and polydipsia. There may also be renal stones and nephrocalcinosis. The cardiovascular system is often not directly affected significantly by hypercalcemia, although orthostatic hypotension may ensue. The ECG often shows a shortened Q-T interval. The gastrointestinal findings are all centered around hypofunction. Nausea is common and is related to a calcium-induced ileus. Calcium-stimulated gastrin secretion may lead to the development of peptic ulcer disease.

DIAGNOSIS AND TREATMENT

In the ED, calcium determinations are often obtained as part of a consolidated biochemical profile of patients. It is in this light that hypercalcemia comes to attention. There are several circumstances in which determinations of calcium must be deliberately ordered prospectively. Patients with a known history of malignancy, particularly of breast or squamous cell origin, who present with mental status changes, dehydration with or without polyuria/polydipsia, or anorexia, nausea, and bloating should stimulate suspicion of hypercalcemia. Other groups of patients at higher risk are those with a known history of hyperparathyroidism, Paget's disease, familial hypercalcemic syndromes, or those on specific medications including lithium, thiazide diuretics or prescription vitamin supplements. Individuals with these risk factors who develop any of the hallmark symptoms of hypercalcemia should be investigated further.

When an elevated serum calcium is reported in a patient in whom clinical suspicion was not initially present, additional investigation is warranted. Patients should be asked specifically about the diseases known to be associated with hypercalcemia. A careful and thorough medication profile must be obtained, including specific queries concerning over-the-counter preparations.

Most hypercalcemia is caused by malignancy, hyperparathyroidism, or drug therapy. In the ED, the diagnostic evaluation is limited to the history, which frequently yields the essential information. If no historical cause is known, blood should be obtained for simultaneous measurement of total and ionized calcium and PTH. At present, various PTH assays are commercially available, based on the portion of the molecule to which specific antibodies are directed. Currently, the intact PTH assay is felt to be the best measurement for most circumstances. The measurement of PTH with antibody specific for the c-terminal fragment of the peptide is acceptable except in patients with renal dysfunction, in whom these levels are significantly elevated. The only other adjuncts to these assessments are related to clinical suspicion. Patients

suspected of having malignant disease should have at least a chest radiograph and careful breast examination. Individuals with other signs or symptoms of the respective endocrinopathies may need blood determinations for thyroid or adrenocortical function.

There are several treatment modalities for hypercalcemia, each depending on the severity of the calcium elevation and the presence and degree of symptoms. Generally, the most important emergency decision is determination of the need for hospitalization. Any patient with significant symptoms referable to hypercalcemia should be admitted. Patients with serum calcium concentrations greater than 14 mg/dl should be admitted as well.

Volume expansion and saline diuresis are the foundations of treatment for all causes of hypercalcemia. These significantly increase glomerular filtration rate (GFR) and decrease proximal tubular calcium reabsorption, thereby markedly increasing fractional calcium excretion. Most patients with significant hypercalcemia are modestly volume-depleted. Rapid administration of 1 to 2 liters 0.9% saline corrects this defect. Continued infusion of 200 to 300 mL per hour of 0.9% saline induces a natriuresis which further diminishes proximal tubular calcium reabsorption. The addition of furosemide (Lasix) 80 to 120 mg intravenously every 2 to 4 hours to this regime once volume is repleted further enhances urinary calcium loss and helps prevent undue volume overload and the development of congestive heart failure. Monitoring for the latter conditions is particularly important in elderly patients, those with renal dysfunction, or those with other cardiovascular pathology. These patients must be assessed frequently during treatment, and the use of invasive hemodynamic monitoring to follow volume status should be considered in difficult cases. In addition to following the reduction in calcium with treatment, concentrations of serum magnesium and potassium must be measured at intervals during saline diuresis because urinary excretion of these cations will substantially increase. The direct measurement of urinary magnesium and potassium at 1 to 2 hourly intervals allows replacement of these cations in administered fluids.

Several other emergent therapies may be used in specialized circumstances. Patients with renal failure cannot be treated with large volumes of saline and instead can undergo hemodialysis or peritoneal dialysis using calcium-free dialysate. This temporarily but effectively lowers serum calcium.

The emergency physician should be aware of several newer pharmacologic therapies for the treatment of hypercalcemia. Patients will present to the department taking these drugs for chronic hypercalcemia. Mithramycin, a cytotoxic antibiotic, inhibits osteoclast activity in resorbing bone and is effective in reducing serum calcium levels. It is given once every 1 to 2 weeks. It has been used primarily in cancer patients. It can cause hepato- and nephrotoxicity as well as significant thrombocytopenia. Phosphates have been used to lower serum calcium, although their use is limited by the potential of raising serum phosphorus levels too high and causing tissue calcification. Calcitonin has been used as well, particularly in patients with Paget's disease; however, it appears to lose effectiveness after some time. Diphosphonates are a group of medications that are highly effective, especially in malignancy-induced hypercalcemia, and are available for intravenous administration.

HYPOCALCEMIA

PATHOPHYSIOLOGY

The pathogenetic classification of hypocalcemia is given in Table 54-17. Hypocalcemia in general is an uncommon disorder. Because calcium is approximately 50% protein-bound, depression of total calcium concentration as determined by routine laboratory examination is most frequently related to a decrease in binding associated with hypoalbuminemia. These patients are not symptomatic because ionized calcium is normal. The remaining causes of hypocalcemia can be conveniently divided among those conditions associated with parathyroid hormone dysfunction and those associated with other mechanisms.

Hypoparathyroidism is an infrequent disorder, but the most common clinical disorder causing hypocalcemia. These conditions can be separated into those related to surgery and those from other causes. Patients who have undergone parathyroid exploration may develop mild hypocalcemia (~ 8.0 mg/dL), the nadir occurring 3 to 6 days postoperatively. In the

---

TABLE 54-17. CAUSES OF HYPOCALCEMIA

A. Pseudohypocalcemia: hypoalbuminemia
B. Hypoparathyroidism
  1. Postoperative
  2. Hypomagnesemia
  3. Idiopathic
  4. Parathyroid injury/infiltration
C. Pseudohypoparathyroidism syndromes
D. Renal insufficiency
E. Disorders of vitamin D absorption/synthesis
F. Acute pancreatitis
G. Acute bone mineralization
H. Hyperphosphatemia
  1. Iatrogenic intake
  2. Laxative abuse
  3. Rhabdomyolysis
  4. Tumor lysis
I. Drugs
  1. Calcitonin
  2. Mithramycin
  3. Heparin
  4. Anticonvulsants
  5. Glutethimide
  6. Citrated blood
  7. Fluoride
  8. Propylthiouracil
  9. Colchicine
J. Transient ionized hypocalcemia from alkalosis

---

hands of experienced endocrine or neck surgeons, most of these are partial and transient, although a certain number are more profound and permanent. Hypoparathyroidism may also develop after thyroid exploration and resection and is related to injury of the parathyroid vascular supply. The number of patients who experience transient or permanent impairment of parathyroid function following this type of neck exploration is related to the amount of thyroid tissue resected and the skill of the surgeon. Parathyroid dysfunction must be differentiated from hypocalcemia, which can occur after thyroid resection for thyrotoxicosis. As discussed in the previous section, hyperthyroidism can lead to bone demineralization and resorption with hypercalcemia. This condition physiologically suppresses parathyroid function. The rapid removal of thyroid hormone by surgical intervention can therefore rarely lead to mild, transient hypocalcemia, which readily reverses when remineralization is established.

The nonsurgical causes of hypoparathyroidism are uncommon. Most importantly, any patient with hypocalcemia must also have a determination of serum magnesium concentration. Magnesium is essential for normal PTH synthesis and secretion. Individuals with hypomagnesemic hypocalcemia will not correct this calcium abnormality until the magnesium has been repleted. Other unusual forms of hypoparathyroidism include an idiopathic variety which is probably autoimmune in nature and is often associated with autoimmune endocrinopathies, particularly Addison's disease. Malignant replacement of parathyroid tissue has been noted in a substantial number of reports; however, functional impairment of the parathyroid glands is rare. Evidence of infiltrative diseases such as amyloidosis or hemochromatosis affecting the parathyroid glands has also been reported, but clinically evident hypoparathyroidism is exceptional.

An interesting group of diseases causing hypocalcemia are those known as pseudohypoparathyroidism (PHP). Most of these patients display a typical phenotype known as Albright's hereditary osteodystrophy (AHO), which includes short stature, round facies, short fourth and fifth metacarpals and metatarsals, poor dentition, and subnormal intellect. The basic defect in these patients is end-organ insensitivity to PTH. A somewhat complicated categorization of these patients has been made based on the presence or absence of an underlying defect at the cellular level that appears to be a dysfunctional G-protein subunit of the adenylate cyclase system. Patients with pseudohypoparathyroidism are those with the phenotype AHO but with normal serum calcium.

The remaining disorders in Table 54-17 are extrinsic to the parathyroid gland and, in fact, frequently cause secondary hyperparathyroidism. In renal insufficiency, abnormalities in the synthesis of 1,25-$(OH)_2$D may lead to hypocalcemia. Renal failure is also associated with hyperphosphatemia, and can cause hypocalcemia (see subsequent text). Other diseases associated with alterations in vitamin D absorption or synthesis include dietary deficiency and fat malabsorption. These disorders usually become evident as skeletal abnormalities but may also present as hypocalcemia. Anticonvulsants and glutethimide can reduce 25-hydroxylation of vitamin D by the liver. Patients with acute pancreatitis can develop severe hypocalcemia with extreme sequelae. Acute bone mineralization occurs after surgical treatment of hyperparathyroidism (hungry bone syndrome) and after vitamin repletion in patients with severe vitamin D-deficient rickets. Hyperphosphatemia from various causes has been classically thought to lead to hypocalcemia by causing precipitation of calcium phosphate in tissues. It may also lower serum calcium by decreasing distal tubular calcium reabsorption partly because of calcium-phosphate complexing in tubular filtrate and by inhibition of $1,25\text{-}(OH)_2D$ formation.

Many drugs can induce hypocalcemia. Calcitonin, as noted in a previous section, can lower serum calcium concentrations. In patients with rapid bone turnover (e.g., in Paget's disease), hypocalcemia may occur when large doses are administered. Mithramycin can also cause hypocalcemia. Heparin has been associated with decreases in total serum calcium in patients on hemodialysis. It is proposed that intravenously administered heparin activates lipoprotein lipase, which can increase amounts of free fatty acids that, in turn, bind calcium. Ionized calcium remains normal. Citrated blood products chelate calcium, and patients receiving more than 3 units of blood or those requiring rapid transfusions should have serum calcium concentrations followed closely and should probably have them replaced prophylactically. Use of large doses of fluoride causes hypocalcemia by forming complexes with calcium. Acute overdose with sodium fluoride can be a medical emergency. The induced profound hypocalcemia can cause cardiac asystole. Colchicine and propylthiouracil have been reported to cause hypocalcemia, presumably by inhibiting PTH secretion.

One final group of patients with hypocalcemia have neuromuscular impairment from a sudden decrease in ionized calcium. In these disorders, alkalosis, particularly acute respiratory alkalosis because of the rapidity of its onset, causes an increase in the binding of ionized calcium to albumin. Patients with marked primary central hyperventilation will develop a marked, uncompensated alkalosis with a significant and profound drop in ionized calcium. Many of these individuals develop the most impressive symptoms of hypocalcemia despite their rapid reversibility.

CLINICAL PRESENTATION

Neurologic, neuromuscular, and cardiovascular signs and symptoms dominate the clinical presentation of hypocalcemia. The most common symptoms of hypocalcemia is muscle cramping and peripheral and circumoral paresthesias caused by neuromuscular irritability. In severe cases, carpopedal spasm may intervene. Carpopedal spasm is also induced by hyperventilation because this disorder causes a rapid reduction in ionized calcium due to the sudden respiratory alkalosis with subsequent shift in calcium-albumin binding. Whereas extremity muscles are primarily affected, respiratory and truncal muscles may be rarely involved. This neuromuscular hyperexcitability can be demonstrated on physical examination with a positive Chvostek's and/or Trousseau's sign. The former is performed by tapping on the facial nerve 2 to 3 cm anterior to the ear, eliciting a contraction of the facial muscles and a drawing up of the lip. A percentage of normal individuals show traces of this sign; however, an individual with hypocalcemia can demonstrate clear lip and facial retraction. The Trousseau's sign is the induction of distal arm and hand spasm from the placement of a sphygmomanometer cuff on the upper arm and inflating it 20 mm beyond systolic blood pressure. The spasms are caused by localized irritation and ischemia under the cuff rather than distal ischemia from a reduction in arterial flow.

The CNS effects of hypocalcemia include seizures, mental status changes, and extrapyramidal symptoms. Generalized, focal, petit mal, and syncopal type seizures have all been described with hypocalcemia. It is not clear whether the lowered calcium itself can initiate seizures or if there is a lowering of epileptic threshold stimulating activity in seizure-prone areas. The alterations in mental status can range from psychosis and irritability to lethargy. Extrapyramidal effects appear to be limited to patients with chronic hypocalcemia from hypoparathyroidism who have developed basal ganglia calcifications.

The cardiovascular manifestations of lowered serum calcium is primarily reported as decreased cardiac function. Cases of congestive heart failure resolving when serum calcium has been restored to normal have been reported.[11,12] Electrocardiographic abnormalities are common and include shortened QTc, prominent U waves, T wave abnormalities, and right axis deviation.[13]

DIAGNOSIS AND TREATMENT

The emergency evaluation of hypocalcemia is relatively limited. The most useful laboratory evaluations include serum albumin, pH, magnesium, and phosphate. If true hypocalcemia exists, without magnesium deficiency, the serum phosphate helps to differentiate some of the causative factors.

The vast majority of cases of hypocalcemia are caused by hypoalbuminemia. The simplest calculation of ionized calcium in this setting is to increase the serum calcium by 0.8 mg/dL for each 1 g/dL depression in albumin below 4.5 g/dL. Many clinical laboratories are capable of measuring ionized calcium, and this is the preferable assessment if symptoms referable to hypocalcemia are suspected. Patients presenting with carpopedal spasm should have an arterial blood gas obtained to document the presence of hyperventilation and a determination of serum calcium concentration. Finally, any patient with hypocalcemia must have a concomitant measure of magnesium. To the extent that magnesium is deficient, the calcium cannot be restored until the magnesium is repleted.

The treatment of acute, symptomatic hypocalcemia is the administration of intravenous calcium. Several intravenous calcium preparations are available. Calcium chloride, 10%, in 10 mL ampules have been widely available, primarily because of their earlier use in cardiac arrest protocols. Despite much evidence against its use under arrest conditions and its removal from all but rare arrest protocols, calcium chloride continues to be widely available. There are 272 mg in a 10 mL ampule, amounting to 13.6 mEq of calcium. This form, however, is acidic and caustic, and other agents should be used. Calcium gluceptate, 23% containing 180 mg (0.9 mEq) of calcium, and calcium gluconate 10% containing 90 mg (0.45 mEq) calcium each in 10 mL ampules, are the preferred forms for intravenous administration. The initial therapy is 200 mg of elemental calcium, diluted in 50 to 100 mL of 5% dextrose and administered over 5 to 10 minutes. This can be repeated at 6- to 8-hour intervals if necessary. Calcium infusions can be given in the most severe cases at a rate of 1 to 2 mg/kg/hour but with caution and only with electrocardiographic and physiologic monitoring. Because intravenous calcium potentiates cardiac glycoside toxicity, patients using digoxin should be treated with special caution. Intravenous infusion of calcium should be discontinued when serum calcium approaches 8.0 mg/dL and symptoms resolve.

The treatment of chronic hypocalcemia is with oral calcium supplementation and moderate doses of vitamin D analogues to increase the intestinal absorption of the calcium. Several vitamin D preparations are available, including cholcalciferol (vitamin D_3), ergocalciferol (vitamin D_2), dihydrotachysterol (DHT, reduction product of vitamin D_2), and calcitriol (1,25-dihydroxycholecalciferol). The two latter analogues do not require renal 1-hydroxylation for activity.

Hypocalcemia in Pregnancy. The discovery that pregnant patients who receive supplemental calcium (2 g/day) have reduced risk of hypertensive disorders has resulted in re-evaluation of calcium metabolism in such patients.[15] Serum levels of calcium were "normal," but there is a significant question of metabolic differences in handling calcium.

DISORDERS OF PHOSPHATE METABOLISM

PHYSIOLOGIC CONCEPTS

The control of phosphate homeostasis is closely associated with calcium regulation. The major hormones, PTH and vitamin D, and organ systems involved (kidney, intestines, and bones) are the same. Calcitonin does increase urinary excretion of phosphorus when administered in pharmacologic doses; however, the importance of calcitonin-regulated proximal tubular phosphorus reabsorption under physiologic conditions is unclear. For a substantive overview of the regulation of these hormones, the reader is referred to the section on calcium metabolism. Despite similar agents and sites of action, phosphorus is less tightly regulated than is calcium. The primary site of phosphorus control is the renal tubule.

Phosphorus is primarily found in the intracellular compartment and in the skeleton. Of an average daily intake of about 1000 to 1400 mg of elemental phosphorus, 75 to 85% is absorbed. The extracellar pool of orthophosphate is only 10 to 15% protein bound, in several different binding states, and expressed as a concentration of total elemental phosphorus. This pool is in equilibrium with the phosphorus stored in bone and the intracellular compartment. The kidney excretes an amount equal to the absorbed phosphorus each day. Under normal conditions, the filtered load of phosphorus is 5000 to 7000 mg daily. The proximal tubule reabsorbs phosphorus in a cotransport with sodium. The distal tubule probably plays no role in phosphorus handling, and any anion not reabsorbed proximally is excreted in the urine. In spite of the lack of excretory phosphate activity in the nephron, the system is designed to accommodate excess states as well. The reabsorption system is saturable and varies with the GFR. There is, in effect, a tubular threshold for phosphate reabsorption beyond which filtered phosphate is excreted. Several regulatory conditions alter the phosphate threshold, providing a mechanism for maintaining serum phosphate concentrations.

The effects of PTH on phosphorus homeostasis reflect its activity on bone, vitamin D metabolism, and the kidney. The ability of PTH to increase calcium mobilization from bone is also reflected in a simultaneous increase in phosphorus reabsorption from the same source. Despite the large potential source of phosphorus, this represents only a minor control over serum phosphate. The effect on renal phosphate handling is more important. PTH decreases proximal tubular phosphate reabsorption, lowering the tubular threshold for phosphate, thereby enhancing urinary thereby enhancing urinary excretion.

Vitamin D interacts with phosphate metabolism at several levels. Renal 1-hydroxylase activity is inversely regulated by serum phosphorus concentration. Under conditions of phosphorus deprivation, 1,25-$(OH)_2D$ levels are maximally stimulated within 3 days. Although PTH-regulated 1-hydroxylase activity appears more important in the control of vitamin D metabolism, phosphorus does play a role, which can become clinically evident. Intestinal absorption of phosphorus can be regulated partly by 1,25-$(OH)_2D$, which acts to increase orthophosphate transport. Unlike calcium, however, phosphorus absorption is less tightly regulated and its active carrier transporter system is of exceptionally high capacity. The effect of vitamin D on bone, as stated previously in the calcium metabolism discussion, is to increase bone resorption in conjunction with PTH. By mechanisms that are not clear, 1,25-$(OH)_2$D increases the tubular phosphate threshold, thereby increasing phosphorus reclamation.

HYPERPHOSPHATEMIA

PATHOPHYSIOLOGY

The causes of hyperphosphatemia are generally restricted to renal dysfunction, phosphate loading from exogenous or endogenous sources, and increased phosphorus reabsorption. A comprehensive list of causes is found in Table 54-18. In addition, there appears to be a trend toward increases in the tubular phosphate threshold in adolescents and younger children, which is considered normal. This leads to a tendency toward slight elevations in serum phosphate above the upper limits of normal for adults.

Chronic renal insufficiency is the most common disease in which hyperphosphatemia is seen. As GFR falls to less than 30 mL/min, there is a progressive increase in the fractional proximal phosphate reabsorption so that serum phosphate will rise. Hyperphosphatemia is seen in acute forms of renal failure as well. In these circumstances, oliguric renal failure is much more likely to develop elevations in serum phosphate concentration. Marked elevations in phosphate can be seen in acute tubular necrosis caused by rhabdomyolysis-induced myoglobinuria.

Although hyperphosphatemia is unlikely in the face of normal renal function, large quantities of phosphate, from exogenous or endogenous sources, can overcome homeostatic mechanisms and lead to elevations of this electrolyte. Some sources of exogenous phosphorus that could lead to hyperphosphatemia include sodium phosphate laxatives and enemas, and overzealous addition of phosphate-containing salts to intravenous solutions. Hyperphosphatemia from endogenous sources is caused by the rapid nonphysiologic transit of phosphorus from the intracellular to the extracellular compartment. This circumstance occurs in rhabdomyolysis and in massive cell death and lysis, which may occur in the chemotherapeutic treatment of some malignancies. Malignant hyperthermia has also been associated with hyperphosphatemia. Because lactic acidosis is associated with cell death, it is also associated with elevations in serum phosphate.

Under hormonal stimulation, the tubular phosphate threshold can be increased so that a new higher steady state in serum phosphate will be reached. This situation is clear in hypoparathyroidism. In many patients with hyperthyroidism, serum phosphate is elevated. The change is modest and without consequences and believed to occur because of alterations in renal phosphate reabsorption.

CLINICAL PRESENTATION

Hyperphosphatemia is a nondescript entity with a relative lack of clear-cut signs and symptoms related to its excess. Symptoms related to the underlying cause of hyperphosphatemia are much more likely to be manifested. In that renal failure causes the vast majority of these cases, uremic signs and symptoms are the most common at presentation. If calcium is also elevated, soft tissue calcifications may occur.

DIAGNOSIS AND TREATMENT

The cause of hyperphosphatemia is almost always evident historically. As noted previously, the most common cause is chronic renal insufficiency. These patients typically have a concomitant decrease in serum calcium. Difficulty arises in cases in which calcium concentration is relatively normal and phosphate concentration rises. The calcium-phosphate product may predispose these individuals to complications of soft tissue calcifications, including nephrocalcinosis which may worsen the renal function, further hastening the possibility of dialysis. These patients are well managed with phosphate binding antacids which contain aluminum salts. This antacid may affect bioavailability of several other oral medications, including digoxin and oral anticoagulants. Aluminum-containing antacids may also cause significant constipation.

In hypoparathyroidism, patients rarely develop severe hyperphosphatemia or present on an emergent basis. In respect to phosphate metabolism, these patients are well managed on oral vitamin D and calcium supplementation. The hyperphosphatemia found in hyperthyroidism is transient and mild, and it is unnecessary to treat it.

HYPOPHOSPHATEMIA

PATHOPHYSIOLOGY

Much like the changes in potassium homeostasis, disorders leading to substantial depression in serum phosphate concentration (Table 54-19) can be cate-

---

TABLE 54-18. CAUSES OF HYPERPHOSPHATEMIA

A. Acute/chronic renal failure
B. Physiologic: childhood and adolescence
C. Phosphate loading
  1. Exogenous
    —Phosphate containing laxatives or enemas
    —Iatrogenic intravenous phosphate administration
  2. Endogenous
    —Rapid tumor lysis
    —Rhabdomyolysis
    —Malignant hyperthermia
    —Associated with lactic acidosis
D. Increased phosphate reabsorption
  1. Hypoparathyroidism
  2. Hyperthyroidism
  3. Postmenopausal

TABLE 54-19. CAUSES OF HYPOPHOSPHATEMIA

A. Disorders of phosphate intake or absorption
  1. Poor dietary intake
    —Malnutrition
    —Vomiting, nasogastric suction
  2. Malabsorption syndromes
  3. Aluminum-containing antacids
B. Renal phosphate losses
  1. Hyperparathyroidism
  2. Hypercalcemia
  3. Diuretic use
  4. Associated with malignancy (elaboration of phosphar-
    turic substance)
  5. Fanconi's syndrome
  6. Vitamin D-resistant rickets (familial X-linked hypophos-
    phatemic rickets)
  7. Recovery from acute tubular necrosis
  8. Post-transplantation
C. Redistribution
  1. Glucose/insulin administration
  2. Therapy of diabetic ketoacidosis
  3. Respiratory (± metabolic) alkalosis
  4. Acute bone mineralization (hungry bone syndrome)

gorized as deficiency in intake or reduced absorption, excess renal losses, or redistributive changes from the extracellular to the intracellular compartment.

Disorders of dietary phosphorus deficiency are rare, considering the ubiquitous nature of phosphates in most foods. Furthermore, intestinal absorption of orthophosphate is efficient, particularly if phosphorus levels are low. In most cases of dietary insufficiency, there will be concomitant evidence of protein-calorie malnutrition as well. Alcoholic beverages contain little or no phosphate and individuals who consume these as their primary caloric staple are at high risk of developing hypophosphatemia. This is particularly true at the time when these individuals are hospitalized and given regular meals as increased insulin drives phosphorus into cells. Prolonged nasogastric suction has been reported to cause hypophosphatemia, although this is likely to be a consequence of prolonged food deprivation. Individuals given parenteral nutrition with adequate phosphorus additives do not become hypophosphatemic. Malabsorption and diarrhea can result in a relative decreased intake of phosphates. The cause of hypophosphatemia in these cases is more likely to be vitamin D deficiency causing hypocalcemia and secondary hyperparathyroidism. Overzealous use of aluminum-containing antacids, which bind the phosphate anion in the intestinal lumen, preventing its absorption, can subsequently lower serum phosphorus. This is, however, uncommon for individuals on regular diets.

Because the kidney represents the most important regulator of serum phosphorus, it stands to reason that many disorders that affect the renal tubule directly or through endocrine intermediates result in abnormalities in phosphorus homeostasis. Hyperparathyroidism of any cause can lead to hypophosphatemia

unless other conditions supervene. Any form of induced diuresis can enhance urinary phosphorus excretion if extracellular volume is not contracted. Malignant conditions have been reported to be associated with hypophosphatemia. These include all those associated with hypercalcemia of malignancy (see previous Pathophysiology section under Hypercalcemia), in addition to prostatic cancer, mesenchymal tumors, fibrous dysplasia, and epidermal nevus syndrome.[14] It has been considered possible that these latter tumors may express a humoral factor with phosphaturic properties. A proximal renal tubular transport defect known as Fanconi's syndrome is described, in which phosphate wasting occurs in conjunction with amino acid, glucose, uric acid, and bicarbonate wasting. Various conditions can give rise to this syndrome, including cystinosis, hereditary amyloidosis, Wilson's disease, tyrosinemia, fructose intolerance, type I glycogen storage disease, and acute lead toxicity. The condition known as vitamin D resistant rickets, an X-linked inherited genetic disorder, also results in hypophosphatemia associated with osteomalacia and the characteristic skeletal deformities of the rickets syndrome. Pharmacologic doses of vitamin D are unable to restore phosphate levels to normal. Patients recovering from acute tubular necrosis or those shortly following renal transplantation can demonstrate marked phosphaturia and subsequent hypophosphatemia.

Shifts of phosphate from the extracellular compartment into cells or bone represents another mechanism by which hypophosphatemia can occur. Glucose administration, with or without exogenous insulin, can facilitate this shift of phosphorus. This is particularly true in malnourished individuals who are started on a refeeding program. Similarly, patients with diabetic ketoacidosis can develop severe hypophosphatemia within 12 to 24 hours after the institution of therapy. As previously discussed for calcium, removal of a parathyroid adenoma or vitamin repletion of vitamin D deficiency rickets results in rapid bone mineralization and can cause a rapid decline in serum phosphate. Excessive hyperventilation with ensuing respiratory alkalosis can also cause hypophosphatemia.

CLINICAL PRESENTATION

Phosphorus is essential in such a wide variety of biochemical pathways that attributing symptoms and signs to any cellular event is impossible. Nevertheless, because it is so important, severe hypophosphatemia is life-threatening and must be treated as a medical emergency. The normal range for phosphorus is generally 2.5 to 4.5 mg/dL. Patients can be considered to have mild hypophosphatemia when serum concentrations are between 1.5 and 2.5, moderate between 1.0 and 1.5, and severe less than 1.0 mg/dL. The primary symptoms are neurologic and neuromuscular.

CNS effects are especially diverse. Alterations in mental status can take the form of irritability and lethargy to frank obtundation and coma. Many of these symptoms have been ascribed to alcohol intoxication, alcohol withdrawal, or delirium tremens in the alcoholic patient, highlighting the need to consider hypophosphatemia in any patient with evidence of metabolic encephalopathy. Seizures, paresis, paralysis, and paresthesias have all been reported. A neuromuscular syndrome of ascending paralysis similar to Guillain-Barré has been described. Frank hemolysis, myopathy, and rhabdomyolysis can occur, and may temporarily raise serum phosphate levels, obscuring the underlying basis of the disorder.

DIAGNOSIS AND TREATMENT

The cause of hypophosphatemia is often determined by history. If careful questioning is unable to clarify a cause, the measurement of urinary phosphate concentration can be useful. Renal wasting can be excluded if serum phosphate is below 2 mg/dL and urinary phosphate is less than 4 mg/dL. Any other values of phosphate excretion are nondiagnostic; urinary phosphate concentration can vary much, even if renal wasting syndromes are not the underlying cause.

The nonrenal causes of hypophosphatemia of decreased intake, decreased absorption, and redistribution are usually easily differentiated historically. Of these, redistribution syndromes are the most common. Renal causes of phosphate wasting can often be sorted out with the determination of total calcium, PTH, vitamin D levels, and the measurement of urinary glucose and amino acids.

All patients who are at risk to develop hypophosphatemia must be closely observed. These patients, many of whom present to the ED, include diabetic ketoacidosis, alcoholic or malnourished individuals being refed, and patients receiving parenteral nutrition. There is some controversy over the routine addition of phosphate to intravenous solutions in patients with DKA because phosphate-induced hypocalcemia with subsequent tetany has been reported following treatment. It would be prudent, therefore, to measure phosphate concentration early on and during the course of therapy and replace phosphate as necessary. Hyperalimentation solutions should routinely have 1000 mg of elemental phosphorus added to the daily supply. Oral phosphorus agents (e.g., Neutra-Phos) can be given to undernourished patients; however, diarrhea may become problematic.

In patients who are severely hypophosphatemic (less than 1.0 mg/dL) or with significant symptoms referable to phosphate deficiency, intravenous phosphorus supplementation should be given. The dose is 2.5 to 5 mg/kg of elemental phosphorus administered over 6 hours. For an individual weighing 70 kg, the addition of 2 to 4 mL of potassium phosphate to 1 liter of solution is adequate. This supplies 6 to 12 mOsm (175 to 350 mg) of phosphate and 8.8 to 17.6 mEq of potassium. Phosphorus supplementation should not be continued once serum concentrations are 2.0 mg/dL or greater.

DISORDERS OF MAGNESIUM METABOLISM

PHYSIOLOGIC CONCEPTS

Magnesium, a divalent cation, is plentiful in the body, stored as part of the mineral content of bone and in the intracellular compartment. Only a small fraction of the total body magnesium is in the extracellular space. Of the extracellular fraction, approximately 45% is protein bound or complexed. The protein-bound and ionized fraction are in equilibrium, which, like calcium, is affected by changes in acid-base status.

The homeostatic control of magnesium, unlike any of the previously discussed electrolytes, is not regulated by any known hormone or humorally acting substance. It is relatively well absorbed from the gastrointestinal tract, varying the percentage uptake inversely to the amount ingested. Renal excretion is the primary regulator of serum magnesium concentration. Magnesium is reabsorbed along the entire length of the tubule, with the greatest uptake occurring at the thick ascending loop of Henle. Neither PTH, calcitonin, nor vitamin D affects the tubular reabsorption of magnesium.

The mechanisms by which magnesium shifts between the extracellular and intracellular compartments are poorly understood. Because the serum magnesium is poorly correlated with total body magnesium stores, some regulation over the movement of magnesium must occur. In an analogous situation, movement of magnesium to and from bone mineralization stores must occur, although the factors that regulate this movement have not been identified.

HYPERMAGNESEMIA

PATHOPHYSIOLOGY

The disorders causing hypermagnesemia are listed in Table 54-20. This syndrome is rare, owing to the remarkable efficiency of the kidney at eliminating excess magnesium. Overwhelming the renal mechanisms of magnesium clearance requires a massive ingestion or intravenous administration. Even in these cases, clinically significant elevations in serum magnesium are unlikely to occur, but can be dangerous (as in magnesium sulfate administration in eclampsia).

Renal insufficiency, on the other hand, is the single condition in which hypermagnesemia is more likely to occur. In fact, patients with chronic renal failure should specifically avoid excess magnesium, particularly that found in antacids and laxatives.

TABLE 54-20. CAUSES OF HYPERMAGNESEMIA

A. Massive exogenous intake
   1. Laxative, antacids
   2. Intravenous administration
B. Renal insufficiency/failure
C. Drugs
   1. Milk-alkali syndrome
   2. Lithium therapy

Magnesium is being increasingly thought of as a therapeutic agent. Clinical applications include its use in eclampia and premature labor, epilepsy, malignant ventricular arrhythmias including torsades de pointes and cardiac glycoside toxicity, and in acute asthma. Despite these uses, hypermagnesemia rarely occurs except with coexisting renal failure. There are reports of hypermagnesemia occurring with the milk-alkali syndrome and associated with lithium therapy.

CLINICAL PRESENTATION

Magnesium in high concentrations acts as a nonspecific calcium-channel blocker. This activity may be responsible for the known cardiovascular, neurologic, and neuromuscular effects of hypermagnesemia.

The cardiovascular effects of magnesium will be discussed in more detail in Chapter 45. At toxic levels, magnesium can cause hypotension and intraventricular conduction delays and at very high levels, heart block and asystole. Electrocardiographic findings include a prolonged PR and QRS interval and bradycardia.

The CNS effects referable to hypermagnesemia are confusion, obtundation, and coma, but a direct causality is controversial. The mechanisms and rate by which magnesium crosses the blood-brain barrier are poorly understood. Magnesium, in its role as a calcium-channel blocker, has well defined neuromuscular effects. The reduction of the slow phase of the action potential (calcium influx) at the presynaptic myoneural junction diminishes neurotransmitter release and muscle contractile responses. These effects have been well established by electromyography. If neuromuscular depression deepens, respiratory failure may ensue. Prior to this degree of depression, the clinical sign of a decrease or loss of deep tendon reflexes will occur. This has become a standard obstetric evaluation procedure in the assessment of eclamptic patients receiving magnesium therapy.

Endocrinologic effects of magnesium are also well established. Hypermagnesemia, probably working through mechanisms similar to hypercalcemia, inhibits PTH release and can result in hypocalcemia. As noted subsequently, a certain amount of magnesium is necessary for normal PTH responsiveness, and hypermagnesemia can also lead to hypoparathyroidism.

DIAGNOSIS AND TREATMENT

Based on the limited etiologic spectrum of hypermagnesemia, the cause of such a finding should generally be readily apparent. If no serious adverse effects of hypermagnesemia are present, most patients can be observed, providing that the source of magnesium has been removed. Saline diuresis with moderate doses of furosemide is the treatment of choice as described in the treatment of hypercalcemia. Similarly, patients with renal dysfunction may require larger doses of diuretic for a substantive effect, and individuals with more marked renal failure may be considered for dialysis.

Treatment of the severe consequences of hypermagnesemia is aimed at supporting cardiorespiratory function and reversing the relative calcium-channel blockade. Marked respiratory depression must be treated, including intubation and mechanical assistance if necessary. Conduction disturbances, hypotension, and heart block can be treated with intravenous infusion of calcium until the ECG normalizes. These patients should receive 200 mg of elemental calcium. This can be conveniently administered as 20 mL of 10% calcium gluconate diluted into 50 mL of 5% dextrose and given over 5 minutes. This dose can be repeated every 5 to 10 minutes until cardiovascular and neurologic status has stabilized. Patients may require calcium infusions to maintain the reversal of the hypermagnesemic effect until magnesium levels fall substantially. Patients with pre-existing renal disease or those resistant to diuresis and calcium infusions frequently require hemodialysis, which is highly effective at reducing serum magnesium to nontoxic levels.

HYPOMAGNESEMIA

PATHOPHYSIOLOGY

The causes of magnesium depletion are listed in Table 54-21. These are divided among the basic causes of decreased oral intake or gastrointestinal absorption of magnesium, increased renal and nonrenal losses, redistribution of magnesium from the extracellular to the intracellular compartment, and several miscellaneous causes.

Any discussion of magnesium depletion must discuss the relationship of magnesium stores and serum concentration. Magnesium is the primary intracellular divalent cation, and its overall availability is poorly correlated with serum measurements. Significant depletion of magnesium as measured in leukocytes or skeletal muscle may occur with essentially normal serum concentrations. The discussion that follows concerns magnesium depletion per se. Because intracellular magnesium measurements are not available on a clinical basis, suspicion of magnesium deficiency must occur in any patient at risk. The concomitant find-

TABLE 54-21. CAUSES OF MAGNESIUM DEPLETION

A. Decreased intake
  1. Dietary deficiency
  2. Kwashiorkor
  3. Malabsorption syndromes, steatorrhea
  4. Primary hypomagnesemia
B. Increased losses—nonrenal
  1. Prolonged diarrhea
  2. Prolonged nasogastric suctioning
C. Increased losses—renal
  1. Diuresis
     —Osmotic, saline, drugs
     —Post-obstructive, recovery of ATN, post-transplant
  2. Intrinsic renal tubular disorders
  3. Hereditary magnesium wasting
  4. Drugs
     —Loop diuretics
     —Aminoglycosides
     —Amphotericin
     —Digoxin
     —Cisplatin
  5. Hyperaldosteronism, Bartter's syndrome
  6. Other disorders
     —Alcohol ingestion
     —Hypercalciuria
     —Thyrotoxicosis
     —SIADH
     —Phosphate depletion
     —Hypokalemia
D. Redistribution
  1. Glucose, amino acid, insulin administration
  2. Treatment of diabetic ketoacidosis
  3. Hungry bone syndrome (primary hyperparathyroidism)
  4. Acute pancreatitis
E. Miscellaneous
  1. Multiple blood transfusions
  2. Hypoparathyroidism
  3. Hypoalbuminemia

ing of low or low-normal serum magnesium in such a patient should initiate the treatment modalities.

Decreases in magnesium intake over time lead to magnesium deficiency. Children with kwashiorkor have been well studied and have clear evidence of magnesium depletion and hypomagnesemia. There is a wide variety of malabsorption syndromes, including pancreatic insufficiency, short bowel syndrome, ileal diversions or resections, and intrinsic bowel disease, which cause hypomagnesemia and magnesium depletion. There may also be primary hypomagnesemia in which there is selective magnesium malabsorption. This is a congenital, inherited disorder.

Increased loss of magnesium can be divided between renal and nonrenal causes. The nonrenal sources are essentially gastrointestinal. Although upper gastrointestinal fluids are relatively low in magnesium, prolonged removal caused by emesis or nasogastric suction can lead to magnesium depletion, particularly in patients whose fluids are replaced intravenously with magnesium-free solutions. The lower gastrointestinal tract, however, has five to ten

times higher magnesium content; therefore losses from diarrhea of any cause can lead to magnesium depletion.

The renal losses of magnesium are varied. Diuresis decreases the reabsorption of magnesium, leading to negative balance. The diuresis that is known to occur after successful renal transplantation, relief of a renal outflow obstruction, or recovery from acute tubular necrosis tends to deplete magnesium stores. Disorders of the renal tubule can lead to abnormalities in magnesium reabsorption. Interstitial nephritis, pyelonephritis, hydronephrosis, congenital magnesium wasting, renal tubular acidosis, and Bartter's syndrome may all affect renal magnesium handling. A series of drugs can induce magnesium wasting directly or through toxic renal affects. Loop diuretics increase delivery of magnesium into more distal tubular sections leading to greater excretion. Cardiac glycosides also seem to increase renal magnesium wasting. Cisplatin, aminoglycosides, and amphotericin B are nephrotoxic and can lead to magnesium depletion. Both primary and secondary hyperaldosteronism have been associated with magnesium depletion. A series of diseases that are apparently otherwise unrelated increase urinary magnesium losses. Ethanol is known to decrease tubular magnesium reabsorption. This fact, along with other factors related to chronic alcoholism, namely poor diet, malabsorption, and secondary aldosteronism can lead to significant magnesium depletion states. Because magnesium and calcium reabsorption are linked, disorders causing hypercalciuria lead to magnesium losses as well. Thyrotoxicosis is associated with excess magnesium losses and mild hypomagnesemia. The syndrome of inappropriate secretion of ADH has been reported to occur with hypomagnesemia; however, magnesium depletion probably does not occur to any great degree. Hypophosphatemia and hypokalemia are reported to be associated with magnesium depletion, although this appears to be caused by coexisting diseases that are likely to cause multiple fluid and electrolyte abnormalities.

The redistributive causes of hypomagnesemia relate to various conditions that cause a relatively rapid shift of magnesium from the extracellular to the intracellular compartment. Magnesium influx into cells seems to be coupled with the movement of glucose and amino acids, which in turn can be stimulated to occur with insulin. Administration of any of these agents, therefore, can precipitate hypomagnesemia. Similarly, patients with diabetes mellitus are at a particularly high risk for magnesium depletion. Poorly controlled diabetes mellitus with concomitant glycosuria diuresis can predispose individuals to excess magnesium losses. Insulin therapy tends to drive magnesium into cells, as occurs with potassium and phosphorus. Therefore, poorly controlled diabetics who develop ketoacidosis and are subsequently treated are at high risk to develop magnesium depletion and hypomagnesemia. As discussed with calcium and phosphorus, patients who have had significant hyperparathyroidism and then undergo surgical removal of the adenoma can develop a syndrome of extreme bone avidity for mineralization ions. A significant hypomagnesemia, known as hungry bone syndrome, can occur along with depression of serum calcium and phosphate. Acute pancreatitis may be associated with alcoholism and diabetes mellitus, both of which predispose individuals to magnesium loss. Furthermore, saponification may lead to deposition of magnesium salts in addition to the usual calcium salts.

Several miscellaneous disorders have been linked to hypomagnesemia. As in the case of calcium, magnesium is a divalent cation that is chelated to the added citrate in stored blood products. Many facilities have policies regarding the administration of calcium following multiple transfusions; however, the same may not be true for magnesium supplementation. Patients with chronic hypoparathyroidism treated with calcium supplements and vitamin D can rarely develop hypomagenesemia, possibly related to the induced excess urinary calcium secretion. Finally, total magnesium may be lowered somewhat in the face of normal ionized levels if hypoalbuminemia leads to a decrease in the protein-bound fraction.

CLINICAL PRESENTATION

The precise nature of the clinical manifestations of magnesium deficiency are difficult to underscore. In large part, this is because of the simultaneous disturbances in potassium, phosphate, and calcium homeostasis that accompany significant hypomagnesemia. These accompanying disturbances may be caused by the underlying disorder which also affects the handling of these electrolytes, but may also be related to direct effects of magnesium deficiency. Magnesium's role as a cofactor in normal cellular ion pump ATPase activity leads to many symptoms that are identical to those noted for other electrolyte abnormalities, most notably hypocalcemia. Broadly, these effects can be divided into those affecting cardiovascular, neurologic, and neuromuscular function and electrolyte balance.

Potassium, phosphate, and calcium regulation depend on magnesium at various levels. As mentioned, magnesium plays a crucial role in trans-membrane ion movement. Additionally, magnesium is necessary for normal PTH secretion as well. Many of the patients found to have significant magnesium depletion are also found to have hypokalemia, often associated with substantial total body potassium losses. Hypocalcemia is also a prominent feature of hypomagnesemia for several reasons. In addition to alterations in PTH secretion, bone responses to PTH may be decreased. Furthermore, depressed serum magnesium stimulates release of magnesium from bone with resultant uptake of calcium. For reasons that are not clear, hypomagnesemia lowers the tubular phosphate threshold, leading to phosphaturia and hypophosphatemia. The fact that magnesium is a vital part of the regulatory mechanisms which control these electrolytes is verified by the fact that these secondary disturbances are often resistant to standard therapy until magnesium has been repleted.

The main effect of magnesium depletion on cardiovascular function is the increased potential for cardiac arrhythmias. Magnesium is important in membrane electrophysiology and dysrrhythmias related to disturbances of this cation include ventricular tachyarrhythmias, torsade de pointes, ventricular fibrillation, atrial fibrillation, and supraventricular tachycardia. Additionally, because magnesium is critical to normal sodium-potassium pump ATPase activity, an ion channel affected by cardiac glycosides, magnesium deficiency potentiates digitalis toxicity and predisposes individuals taking this class of drug to arrhythmia. As is the case for electrolytes, these digitalis-induced arrhythmias may not respond to conventional therapy until magnesium depletion is at least partially corrected. The CNS is also affected by magnesium deficiency. Cognitive and personality changes have been described. Frank confusion, agitation, and delirium may occur. Rarely, seizures have been reported also. It has been suggested that alcohol withdrawal seizures may be exacerbated by magnesium deficiency. Cerebellar ataxia is another finding associated with hypomagnesemia.

The overt neuromuscular symptoms of magnesium depletion can be indistinguishable from hypocalcemia. In both, patients may have Chvostek's and Trousseau's signs, carpopedal spasm, muscle cramping, and tetany. The mechanisms by which these signs and symptoms develop are unknown. It is likely, however, that they represent the net effect of membrane potential changes caused by magnesium-induced alterations in intracellular ion concentration, changes in axonal release of acetylcholine, and abnormalities in magnesium-dependent actinomyosin interaction.

DIAGNOSIS AND TREATMENT

As discussed previously, the diagnosis of magnesium deficiency may be difficult to make because plasma concentration may not reflect intracellular pool size. Any patient at risk of developing magnesium depletion with associated symptoms should be further evaluated and probably treated. Additionally, as stated, a low-normal value of magnesium concentration should be considered significant in a target population. The most important groups at risk include patients with diabetes mellitus (particularly after treatment for ketoacidosis), alcoholism, pancreatitis, chronic diuretic use, nutritional deficiency, and chronic malabsorption or diarrhea.

In the ED, low magnesium in plasma under the proper circumstances suggests magnesium deficiency, and treatment should be instituted. The division of causes of magnesium deficiency can be made on the basis of 24 hour urinary magnesium excretion. In the face of hypomagnesemia, loss of greater than 40 mg (2 mOsm) per day indicates excess renal losses of magnesium. Patients with normal plasma magnesium, in whom the diagnosis is suspected, may be investigated with a loading test. These individuals are given 600 mg (30 mOsm) of magnesium sulfate ($MgSO_4$) in 500 mL of 5% dextrose over 12 hours. A 24-hour urine collection is obtained, beginning at the start of the infusion. Magnesium deficiency is diagnosed if less than 15 mOsm is excreted in the urine over the 24 hour period.

The treatment of this disorder is administration of magnesium. Magnesium sulfate is the most commonly used agent. Although intramuscular administration is effective, it is painful, and therefore the intravenous route is preferred. Several preparations are available in 10, 20, and 50% solutions, but the latter should be reserved for intramuscular use unless diluted. Patients with renal insufficiency should be treated with extreme caution, and parenteral therapy should be avoided if possible.

Patients with symptoms referable to magnesium deficiency should receive 8 g $MgSO_4$ (600 mg [30 mOsm] of elemental magnesium) in 500 mL of 5% dextrose over 4 hours. An additional 10 g of $MgSO_4$ should then be given in 1000 mL of 5% dextrose over the next 18 to 20 hours. In individuals without intravenous access, 2 gm of 50% $MgSO_4$ can be given intramuscularly, usually in 2 sites, every 4 hours for 1 day. In emergent conditions, 2 g of $MgSO_4$ (160 mg [8 mOsm] elemental magnesium) can be diluted in 10 mL and given over 10 minutes. Other electrolyte deficiencies should be corrected simultaneously. Patients should be treated with ECG monitoring during infusions.

Several authors have recommended prophylactic use of magnesium in patients at risk. Patients being treated for diabetic ketoacidosis, acute pancreatitis, or acute alcohol withdrawal may have 600 mg of $MgSO_4$ added to each 1000 mL of replacement fluids.

Interest has focused on magnesium use in refractory ventricular fibrillation.[16] Whether this represents hypomagnesemia is not known, but ACLS conferences are increasingly concerned with magnesium's role in resuscitation.

REFERENCES

1. Cannon, J.F.: Diabetes insipidus: Clinical and experimental studies with consideration of genetic relationships. Arch. Intern. Med. 96:215, 1955.
2. Sterns, R.H.J., Riggs, J.E.R., and Schochet, S.S.: Osmotic demyelination syndrome following correction of hyponatremia. N. Engl. J. Med. 314:1535, 1986.
3. Zull, D.N.: Disorders of Potassium Metabolism. Emerg. Med. Clin. North Am. 7:771, 1989.
4. Williams, M.E., Rosa, R.M., and Epstein, F.H.: Hyperkalemia. Adv. Intern. Med. 31:265, 1986.
5. Gabow, P.A., and Pertson, L.N.: Disorders of potassium metabolism. In Renal and Electrolyte Disorders, 3rd edition. Edited by Schrier, R.W. Boston, Little, Brown, & Co., 1986, pp. 207–49.
6. Przybojewski, J.Z., and Knott-Craig, C.J.: Hyperkalaemic complete heart block. A report of 2 unique cases and a review of the literature. S. Afr. Med. J. 63:413, 1983.
7. Allon, M., Dunlay, R., and Copkney, C.: Nebulized albuterol for acute hyperkalemia in patients on hemodialysis. Ann. Intern. Med. 110:426, 1989.
8. Ohmae, M., and Rabkin, S.W.: Hyperkalemia-induced bundle branch block and complete heart block. Clin. Cardiol. 4:43, 1981.
9. Stewart, D.E., Ikram, H., Espiner, E.A., and Nicholls, M.G.: Arrhythmogenic potential of diuretic induced hypokalemia in patients with mild hypertension and ischaemic heart disease. Br. Heart J. 54:290, 1985.
10. Godolphin, W., Cameron, E.C., Frohlich, J., and Price, J.D.: Spurious hypocalcemia in hemodialysis after heparinization. In-vitro formation of calcium soaps. Am. J. Clin. Pathol. 71:215, 1979.
11. Connor, T.B., Rosen, B.L., Blaustein, M.P., Applefeld, M.M., and Doyle, L.A.: Hypocalcemia precipitating congestive heart failure. N. Engl. J. Med. 307:869, 1982.
12. Levine, S.N., and Rheams, C.N.: Hypocalcemic heart failure. Am. J. Med. 68:1033, 1985.
13. Vered, I., Vered, Z., Perez, J.E., Jaffe, A.S., and Whyte, M.P.: Normal left ventricular performance documented by Doppler echocardiography in patients with long-standing hypocalcemia. Am. J. Med. 86:413, 1989.
14. Singer, F.R.: Metabolic bone disease. In Endocrinology and Metabolism. Edited by Felig, P., Baxter, J.D., Broadus, A.E., and Frohman, L.A. New York, McGraw-Hill Book Company, 1987, pp. 1454–1499.
15. Belizan, J.M., Villar, J., Gonzalez, L., et al.: Calcium supplementation to prevent hypertensive disorders of pregnancy. N. Engl. J. Med. 325:1399, 1991.
16. Tobey, R.C., Birnbaum, G.A., Allegra, J.R., et al.: Successful resuscitation and neurologic recovery from refractory ventricular fibrillation after magnesium sulfate administration. Ann. Emerg. Med. 21:92, 1992.

BIBLIOGRAPHY

Felig, A.F., Baxter, J.D., Broadus, A.E., and Frohman, L.A. (Eds.): Endocrinology and Metabolism, 2nd ed. New York, McGraw-Hill Book Co., 1987.

Glorieux, F.H.: Rickets: The continuing challenge. N. Engl. J. Med. 325:1875, 1991.

Narins, R.G., Jones, E.R., Stom, M.C., Rudnick, M.R., and Bastl, C.P.: Diagnostic strategies in disorders in fluid, electrolyte and acid-base homeostasis. Am. J. Med. 1982; 7:496, 1982.

Schrier, R.W. (Ed.): Renal and Electrolyte Disorders, 3rd ed. Boston: Little, Brown & Co, 1986.

Stoff, J.S.: Phosphate homeostasis and hypophosphatemia. Am. J. Med. 7:489, 1982.

Endocrine and metabolic emergencies. Emerg. Med. Clin. North Am. Nov. 7:1989.

DIABETIC KETOACIDOSIS

Joseph C. Howton and David K. English

CAPSULE

Diabetic ketoacidosis (DKA) is a life-threatening metabolic disruption characterized by hyperglycemia, ketonemia, and acidosis. It is the end result of a relative or absolute lack of insulin and is therefore exclusively a disease of diabetics. It may be triggered by severe physiologic stress, including infection, myocardial infarction, or pregnancy, or by the omission of the diabetic's usual insulin. Lack of insulin and excess of counter-regulatory hormones leads to profound acidosis and marked fluid and electrolyte losses. Successful resuscitation requires aggressive therapy with crystalloid solutions, insulin, and careful monitoring with frequent re-evaluation. The underlying cause must be sought and corrected if the patient is to recover.

PATHOPHYSIOLOGY

Most of the cells in the body are absolutely dependent on the presence of insulin to take up glucose. In the liver, insulin promotes the storage of glycogen and inhibits gluconeogenesis. It promotes fat storage and inhibits the breakdown of triglycerides to fatty acids. In muscle cells, insulin promotes the uptake of amino acids and the synthesis of protein. Without insulin, these cells must reverse the metabolic pathways to produce energy. The breakdown of fat releases free fatty acids, which are converted in the liver to the organic acids beta-hydroxybutyric acid and acetoacetic acid. The normal 3:1 ratio of these acids is increased because of the reductive metabolism seen in DKA (Fig. 54-2). The breakdown of proteins releases amino acids, causing azotemia and muscle wasting. Glycogen is broken down to release glucose, and hepatic gluconeogenesis increases, resulting in hyperglycemia.

At the same time, stress hormones are produced in excess. Corticosteroids, catecholamines, growth hormone, and most importantly glucagon, all have effects opposite to insulin. Actions of the stress hormones are essential to the development of ketoacidosis. An excess can produce ketoacidosis, even in the face of normal insulin levels.

High levels of glucose and ketone bodies lead rapidly to an osmotic diuresis, with profound losses of water, sodium, chloride, and potassium. Other solutes such as calcium, magnesium, and phosphorus are lost in varying but usually large amounts (Table 54-22). The increasing acidosis and osmolality, combined with insulin lack, cause a shift of intracellular potassium to the extracellular compartment. Serum levels of potassium remain relatively elevated even as massive total body deficits develop. The patient may actually have cardiac arrhythmias associated with hyperkalemia despite the total body deficit of potassium. Similar factors promote the loss of phosphorus.

As the extracellular osmolality rises, water is drawn from the cells, diluting the remaining sodium. For every 100 mg per dL, the glucose level rises and measured sodium concentration drops by 1.6 mEq/L.[1] This is a true, albeit transient, hyponatremia that causes the expected clinical effects of lowered serum sodium. In addition, the lipemic serum often seen in DKA causes a falsely lower sodium reading than is actually present. Some patients have a true dilutional hyponatremia and a pseudohyponatremia simultaneously.

With the loss of fluid and electrolytes (Table 54-22), the patient becomes profoundly dehydrated and may present in shock. Lactic acidosis may be superimposed from poor tissue perfusion and poor oxygen delivery. Nausea and vomiting are common, and greatly exacerbate the fluid and solute losses. By increasing the respiratory rate and creating a compensatory respiratory alkalosis, the profound metabolic acidosis is partially corrected. Occasional patients may actually present with a near-normal pH despite severe ketoacidosis when there have been massive losses of hydrochloric acid during protracted vomiting. Hyperglycemia, hyperosmolality, hypovolemia, electrolyte disturbances, and the precipitating illness can all contribute to alteration of consciousness, although only the increase in osmolality correlates well with the mental status.

There is a significant precipitating illness in most patients who present with DKA (Table 54-23). Up to 50% are eventually found to have an infection. Approximately 20% of patients are found to have omitted their insulin for various reasons; some will do so repeatedly. Other important conditions that can trigger DKA include myocardial ischemia and infarction, cerebrovascular accident, trauma, pregnancy, hyperthyroidism, pancreatitis, steroid usage, and emotional upset. Pregnant diabetics can develop ketosis with much less stress than nonpregnant ones; this may

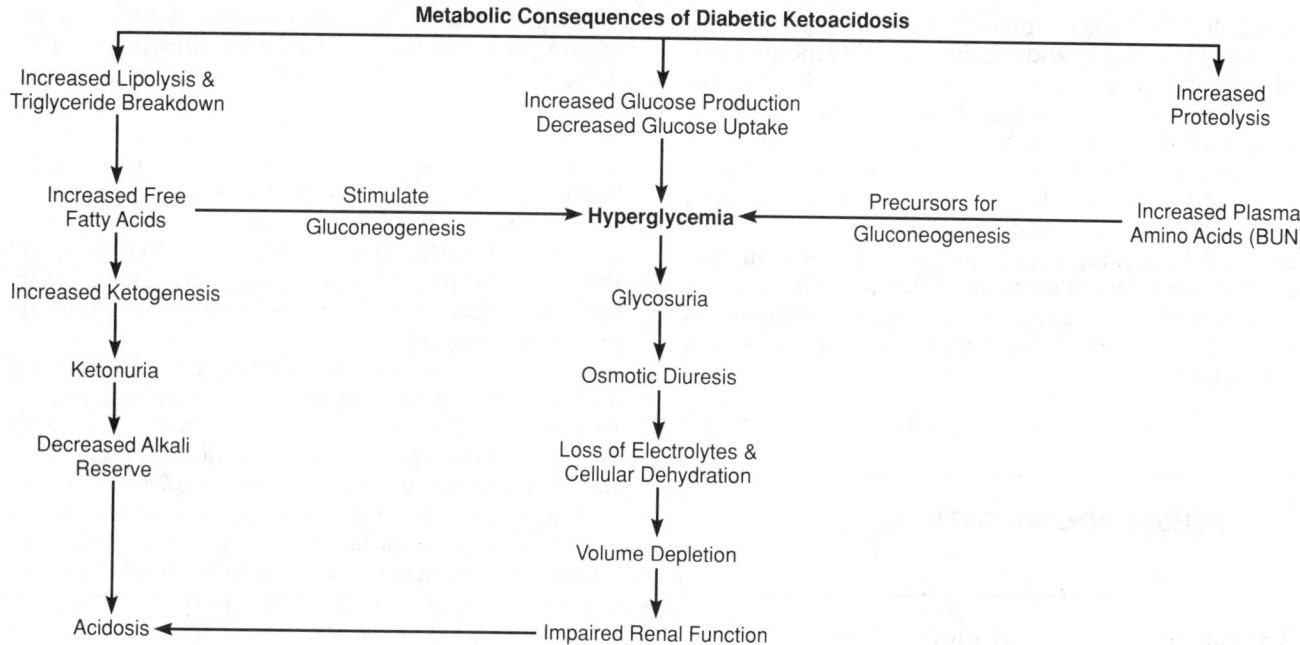

FIG. 54-2.   *Altered carbohydrate, lipid, and protein metabolism in diabetic ketoacidosis with resultant water and electrolyte imbalances, impaired renal function, and acidosis. (Modified with permission from Kitabchi, A. E., and Murphy, M. B.: Diabetic ketoacidosis and hyperosmolar hyperglycemic nonketotic coma. Med. Clin. North Am. 72:1549, 1988.)*

TABLE 54-22. TYPICAL WATER AND ELECTROLYTE LOSSES IN DKA

Water	5–10 liters
Sodium	400–700 mOsm
Potassium	300–500 mOsm
Phosphate	60–80 mOsm
Magnesium	30–50 mOsm

TABLE 54-23. COMMON PRECIPITATING FACTORS IN DKA

Infection
Myocardial ischemia or infarction
Cerebrovascular accident
Trauma
Pregnancy
Steroid usage
Hyperthyroidism
Pancreatitis
Noncompliance, insulin lack
Surgery
Delayed diagnosis of diabetes

carry a poor prognosis for the fetus. Also, the pregnant diabetic may not develop the usual degree of hyperglycemia as the fetus and placenta continue to metabolize glucose.

PREHOSPITAL ASSESSMENT AND STABILIZATION

Maintenance of adequate airway and breathing, followed by circulation, are the most important immediate considerations. With altered consciousness and greatly increased minute ventilation, the patient is at risk for respiratory failure. If intubation and mechanical ventilation are necessary, the clinician must remember the likelihood of severe metabolic acidosis with respiratory compensation and hyperventilate the patient accordingly. Failure to do so could result in a sudden and profound drop in the pH as the patient's physiologic hyperventilation is impaired.

After adequate airway and oxygenation, the patient needs immediate and vigorous fluid resuscitation. In the short term, shock is deleterious to the patient. Adequate hydration alone partially reduces many of the pathologic processes. Resuscitation should start with large-bore intravenous lines containing isotonic crystalloid solutions. Patients in severe DKA may have fluid deficits of 5 to 10 L, and it is therefore essential to restore the intravascular volume. For a typical adult patient, a 1 or 2 L initial fluid bolus is not excessive. Pediatric patients can usually tolerate a 20 mL/kg initial bolus. Although insulin replacement is necessary for the ultimate resolution of the process, it can wait until the diagnosis is better established at the hospital.

Patients suspected of DKA should be treated as critically ill. They need immediate and frequent monitoring of vital signs and continuous ECG monitoring. Myocardial infarction is a common precipitant of ketoacidosis in the long-term diabetic, and the combination carries a 50% mortality in some series. Hyperkalemia or hypokalemia may cause dysrhythmias and sudden death. The prehospital provider should deliver the patient rapidly to the emergency department (ED), making every attempt to prevent further deterioration. In systems with Advanced Life Support (ALS) capability, supplemental oxygen, intravenous (IV) fluid and cardiac monitoring may greatly benefit the patient.

CLINICAL PRESENTATION

The patient who presents early in diabetic ketoacidosis may complain only of malaise, polyuria, and polydipsia. The classic late presentation includes nausea and vomiting, abdominal pain, hyperventilation progressing to Kussmaul respirations, weight loss, dehydration, hypotension, tachycardia, and the fruity smell of acetone on the breath. There are even case reports of DKA presenting as sudden death. The progression may occur over a period of hours or days, depending on the patient's underlying condition and intake of food, fluids, and insulin.

History may be unobtainable at times, especially from the most desperately ill patients. The patient who is fairly alert may relate malaise, polyuria, and polydipsia of varying duration. Nausea, vomiting, and abdominal pain are seen in 50 to 75% of cases. The pain may mimic almost any intra-abdominal catastrophe and has occasionally led to unnecessary laparotomy. It should resolve with hydration and insulin. The patient who is suspected of true surgical pathology needs frequent reassessment. If there is convincing evidence of acute abdomen or failure to improve, lifesaving surgery should not be delayed because of the ketoacidosis. Women of childbearing age must always be questioned about the possibility of pregnancy.

Patients often present with complaints of dyspnea. Commonly, it is caused by the acidosis, but it may represent cardiac disease or pulmonary infection. The patient should be questioned closely about chest pain or other symptoms of cardiac disease. Unfortunately, painless myocardial infarction is all too common in diabetics, and a negative history may not exclude heart disease. Symptoms of infection must be sought, but the patient in ketoacidosis is often inappropriately normothermic or even hypothermic because of a lack of substrate at the cellular level to generate heat. Hypothermia with DKA may also indicate overwhelming infection.

The patient must be questioned about diet and medication. Some patients mistakenly stop their insulin when they become ill on the the premise that they do not need insulin if they are not eating. Others intentionally, sometimes surreptitiously, stop their insulin as a way of seeking attention or other secondary gain. Such patients can be difficult management problems.

Sometimes acute ketoacidosis is the initial presentation of diabetes. This is particularly common with the pediatric patient. Lack of a previous history of diabetes should not dissuade the clinician from appropriate treatment.

Physical examination usually reveals tachypnea and a varying degree of dehydration. The patient may appear only mildly ill or may seem moribund. The classic "fruity" breath odor of acetone is helpful but not entirely reliable because some individuals are much more sensitive to it than others. Examination of the tongue is helpful in ascertaining the degree of dehydration. Diffuse, sometimes severe abdominal tenderness is a common finding. Occult infections are a common precipitant to DKA, and the patient must be carefully checked for a hidden abscess in areas such as the perineum. Patients with severe DKA may have a depressed level of consciousness that correlates with the degree of serum hyperosmolality. In one series of 123 patients, there were no patients with an osmolality of greater than 330 mOsm/kg who were fully alert.[2] Patients with hyperglycemic hyperosmolar nonketotic coma (HHNC) tend to have a much higher serum osmolality than that seen in DKA. It is not surprising, therefore, that deep coma is unusual in DKA, whereas it is common in HHNC. An altered level of consciousness may also be caused by a serious underlying condition such as meningitis, and cannot be safely attributed to DKA alone.

DIFFERENTIAL DIAGNOSIS

Many other illnesses can mimic some of the initial clinical manifestations of DKA, but there should be little doubt of the diagnosis if the triad of hyperglycemia, ketosis, and acidosis (Fig. 54-3) is recognized. Hyperosmolar nonketotic coma, discussed in the next subchapter, is the other significant diabetic emergency that must be distinguished. By definition, it does not include significant ketone production, although there may be a small component of acidosis from dehydration or starvation. Alcoholic ketoacidosis may present with ketonuria and acidosis, but the glucose is usually normal to mildly decreased. The history, if available, includes poor food intake and the sudden cessation of heavy alcohol intake. Lactic acidosis and uremia may produce altered consciousness and acidosis, but the glucose is not elevated.

Other toxic and metabolic causes of altered consciousness should always be considered. Hypogly-

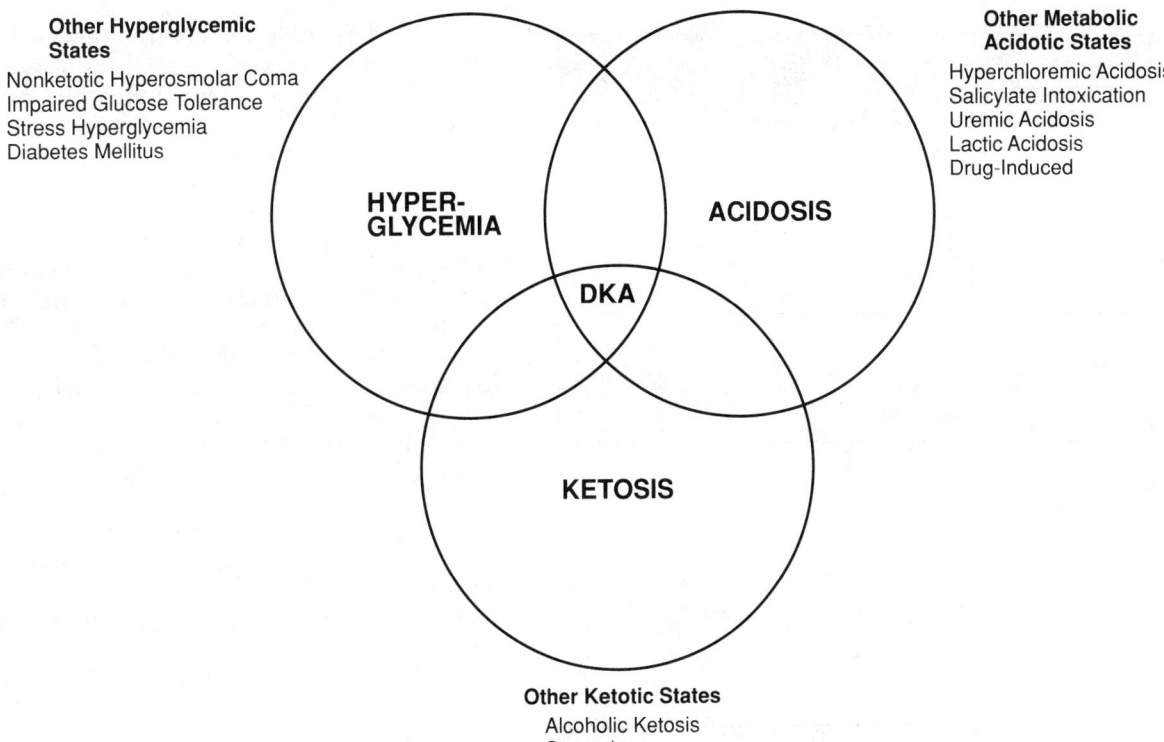

Other Hyperglycemic States
Nonketotic Hyperosmolar Coma
Impaired Glucose Tolerance
Stress Hyperglycemia
Diabetes Mellitus

Other Metabolic Acidotic States
Hyperchloremic Acidosis
Salicylate Intoxication
Uremic Acidosis
Lactic Acidosis
Drug-Induced

HYPER-GLYCEMIA

ACIDOSIS

DKA

KETOSIS

Other Ketotic States
Alcoholic Ketosis
Starvation

FIG. 54-3.   *Symptom complex in diabetic ketoacidosis. (With permission from Kitabchi, A. E., and Fisher, J. N.: Diabetes mellitus. In Clinical Studies in Medical Biochemistry. Edited by Glew, R. H., and Peters, S. P. New York, Oxford University Press, 1987, p. 105.*

cemia is a common cause of coma and should not be missed. Intoxications that can produce an altered level of consciousness and acidosis include those from aspirin, ethylene glycol, methanol, isopropyl alcohol, isoniazid, and paraldehyde. Ethylene glycol and industrial acetylene may cause an acetone odor on the breath. Iron may cause coma and acidosis, but the serum glucose is low.

Diabetic patients are always at increased risk of infection, and sepsis may mimic DKA as well as precipitate it. In fact, patients in shock from any cause may present with tachycardia and "air hunger" similar to those of a patient in DKA.

LABORATORY AND OTHER PROCEDURES

The initial rapid laboratory evaluation (Tables 54-24 to 54-27) should include blood glucose, urinalysis, and arterial blood gas. The blood glucose can be estimated within minutes at the bedside with a commercial reagent glucose oxidase strip. Urine should be immediately obtained and tested for glucose and ketones. Therapy can be started immediately with just these few tests; it should not wait for the more time-con-

TABLE 54-24. RECOMMENDED PROCEDURES IN DKA

Stat:	Dextrose stick, urine dipstick, arterial blood gas, ECG
	Electrolytes, BUN/Cr, glucose, Ca^{++}, Mg^{++}, Phos
	CBC with differential
	Chest radiograph
Optional procedures:	
	Lactate level
	Blood cultures
	Wound and other bodily fluid cultures
	CSF analysis
	KUB, extremity radiographs when evidence of infection
	Serum ketones (probably not particularly useful)

suming studies. Because the renal threshold for ketone bodies is so low, the absence of ketones in the urine effectively excludes the possibility of ketonemia. The arterial blood gas shows whether the patient is adequately oxygenated, the severity of the acidosis, and whether the patient has reached the limits of respiratory compensation. As a general rule of thumb, the pCO_2 should drop by 10 mmHg for every 0.08 unit decrease in the pH. A patient who is not maximally hyperventilating in the face of a severe acidosis is in danger of imminent arrest. For example, a patient with

TABLE 54-25. KCL REPLACEMENT IN DKA (AFTER FIRST LITER OF PLAIN NSS OR 1/2 NSS)

Initial serum K⁺ value

	Recommendation
Marked hyperkalemia (>6.0)	Hold K⁺
Mild hyperkalemia (5.0–6.0)	10 mEq/hr
Normokalemia (3.5–5.0)	20–40 mEq/hr
Hypokalemia (<3.5)	40–60mEq/hr (with MD at bedside)

TABLE 54-26. LABORATORY FINDINGS IN DKA

Anion Gap: $Na^+ - (Cl^- + HCO3^-)$
Normal range: 10–15

Osmolarity: $2(Na^+) + (Glu/18) + (BUN/2.8)$
Normal range: 285–295

K Elevation/pH fall: As pH falls by 0.1, K^+ rises by 0.6

Na Fall/Glucose rise: As glucose increases by 100 mg/dL, Na falls by 1.6 mEq/L

TABLE 54-27. TYPICAL DKA LABORATORY VALUES

	Mild to Moderate	Severe
Glucose	500–700	900–1000
Sodium	130	125
Potassium	5–6	6–7
HCO₃	6–10	0–6
BUN	25–30	30 +
pH	7.1	Below 7.0
pCO₂	15–20	Above 20

a pH of 7.0 and a pCO_2 of 28 may have reached the limits of respiratory compensation and is now fatigued. One may then see a steadily rising pCO_2 and a falling pH, which cause death without timely intervention.

Other appropriate laboratory tests include electrolytes, BUN, creatinine, magnesium, calcium, and phosphorus (Table 54-24). Serum ketones are frequently measured but are not particularly helpful. Most laboratories provide only a semiquantitative measurement of acetoacetate. As the patient improves, more beta-hydroxybutyrate may be converted to acetoacetate and the patient's measured ketones rise despite the improvement. An elevated serum amylase might suggest pancreatitis, but it is often falsely elevated in DKA because of interference with the assay by ketones. Serum creatinine may be falsely elevated as well as secondary to ketone bodies interfering with the serum assay. Lipase more accurately reflects pancreatic inflammation in DKA, and often does not correlate with the amylase. Lactate levels may be indi-

cated to determine the contribution of lactic acid to the metabolic acidosis.

A CBC should be obtained, but the white blood cell count is usually elevated. A recent study reported that an increase in the percentage of band forms was highly sensitive and fairly specific for infection.[4] A pregnancy test is advisable for women. If there is any possibility of infection, appropriate cultures should be obtained. A microscopic urinalysis is important in the search for infection. Appropriate x-ray films should be obtained in the search for an underlying cause, including at least a chest film. Extremities with evidence of soft tissue infection may be radiographed to rule out gas gangrene. A KUB should be considered when urosepsis is present to rule out emphysematous pyelonephritis.[5] Both of these conditions are indications for emergent surgery.

An ECG is essential early in the ED course. It may reveal changes of hyperkalemia or hypokalemia, as well as myocardial infarction or ischemia. Because hyperkalemia and DKA can produce electrocardiographic changes that mimic acute infarction, the ECG should be repeated after appropriate treatment has begun.[6]

MANAGEMENT

After initial stabilization of breathing and circulation, fluid and electrolyte replacement should continue. The physician must frequently reassess the vital signs and clinical appearance of the patient. The initial goal is to restore the intravascular volume. Intake and output should be closely monitored, and a urinary catheter is desirable. In the elderly or debilitated, central venous pressure monitoring or even pulmonary artery catheter measurements allows more precise management of fluids. The choice of fluid is controversial, but most authors would start with isotonic saline for the first liter. Some advocate starting with half normal saline in the normotensive patient on the premise that the patient's losses are approximately equal to half normal saline and giving normal saline may prolong the hyperosmolar state.[7] Others claim that hypotonic fluid promotes cellular swelling and cerebral edema, a rare but often fatal complication. Still other authors favor colloid solutions.[8] The only consistent finding is that patients do poorly with inadequate volume replacement.[9]

As soon as the diagnosis is established, the patient should receive short-acting, regular insulin. Various dosing schedules have been proposed by IV, IM, and subcutaneous routes. Intramuscular and especially subcutaneous routes can have unpredictable and delayed effects, especially in the hypovolemic patient. Intravenous insulin is preferred initially because absorption is certain. All hypotensive patients should receive their insulin intravenously. There is no role for long-acting insulin preparations in the initial management of DKA. Insulin drips provide a more consistent and physiologic level of insulin, but require more intensive monitoring and titration and are not always practical in a busy ED. Intravenous boluses of insulin given hourly work nearly as well. Although insulin's half-life in the serum is only 4 to 5 minutes, its functional half-life at the cellular level is 20 to 30 minutes.

A reasonable starting dose of regular insulin is 0.15 units per kg by IV push, followed by 0.1 units per kg per hour on an infusion pump or as hourly boluses (Table 54-28). The glucose should be measured every hour at first, the goal being a fall in blood sugar of 80 to 120 mg/dL per hour. More rapid reduction carries the unacceptable risks of cerebral edema and hypoglycemia. If the blood sugar has not fallen by 10% after the first hour, the initial loading dose may be repeated.

The primary goal of insulin therapy is to stop the production of ketones and acids. Much less insulin is needed to inhibit gluconeogenesis than to inhibit ketogenesis. Therefore it is important not to stop or decrease the insulin just because the glucose has normalized. Instead, supplemental glucose should be given and the insulin continued until the acidosis and ketonemia have resolved. When the serum glucose has fallen to between 200 and 300 mg/dL, glucose should be added to the intravenous fluids to prevent hypoglycemia. One unit of insulin is required to metabolize 4 g of dextrose. A liter of D5 solution contains 50 g of dextrose. Therefore, one approach would be to place 10 to 12 units of insulin in a liter of D51/2 NS (with potassium added if necessary) to run at a rate of 250 cc per hour. In insulin resistance, patients may need 100 to 200 u of insulin daily.[10]

Patients with DKA are often profoundly acidotic. The clinician is often tempted to administer bicarbonate, but there is little reason to do so even with a pH as low as 7.0. The acidosis improves rapidly with proper fluid and insulin therapy. Ketone bodies are metabolized to produce alkali, and excess hydrogen can be excreted by the kidneys as soon as adequate volume is restored. Bicarbonate may result in a metabolic alkalosis as the DKA resolves, and it may cause a paradoxical CSF acidosis. It may produce severe and even dangerous hypokalemia. Alkalinization also shifts the oxyhemoglobin dissociation curve to the left, impeding oxygen delivery at the tissue level. Most studies have been unable to show any improvement in outcome with bicarbonate, even when the pH was as low as 6.9.[11] Bicarbonate should probably be given only under special circumstances, such as with a pH below 6.9 or with dysrhythmias secondary to hyperkalemia. It should be given slowly by intravenous drip (e.g., two amps in a liter of fluid) unless the patient is pulseless because of dysrhythmias, in which case it may be pushed.

The initial serum potassium may be normal or even high, but as the acidosis resolves and glucose is taken up by cells, the true potassium deficit rapidly becomes apparent. Soon after the initial treatment with insulin and fluids, almost every patient is hypokalemic. The only exception is the anuric patient. After the first or second liter of IV fluids, 20 to 40 mEq/liter of potassium should be added to the infusions and the serum potassium monitored frequently, perhaps hourly at first (see Table 54-25). Severe hypokalemia during treatment has resulted in unexpected respiratory arrest. Some authors add a small quantity of potassium to the initial fluid, but the possibility that the patient is already hyperkalemic makes this hazardous.

Magnesium and phosphorus are also depleted, but the need for supplementation is less clear. Hypophosphatemia causes a fall in erythrocyte 2,3-diphosphoglycerate, resulting in a shift of the hemoglobin-oxygen dissociation curve to the left and decreased delivery of oxygen. In addition, low phosphorous levels (less than 1.5 mg/dL) are associated with respiratory muscle weakness, hemolysis, congestive heart failure, and altered mental status. Despite these ill effects, studies using routine phosphate replacement in DKA have not shown any improved outcome.[12,13] Phosphate replacement does have risks, such as hypocalcemia, hypomagnesemia, renal failure, and hyperphosphatemia. It is important to remember that most DKA patients are initially hyperphosphatemic even though total body stores are depleted. Hypophosphatemia may develop during treatment, as correction of the acidosis and administration of insulin and fluids causes phosphate to move into cells. In severe hypophosphatemia, potassium phosphate may be used at a dose of 1/4 of the potassium requirement given as K_2PO_4. Each mL of K_2PO_4 contains 4.4 mEq KCL and 3 mOsm of PO_4.

Most patients with DKA require admission to the hospital. Only a few compliant patients with mild early illness can be managed as outpatients. Those who are moderately or severely ill require admission to the intensive care unit. Most patients with DKA have a serious underlying illness which precipitated the ketoacidosis. If there is any suspicion of infection, the patient should receive broad spectrum antibiotics for the most likely sources immediately in the ED.

Table 54-28 summarizes the treatment of DKA.

HORIZONS

Better understanding of the acid-base and electrolyte derangements of DKA and the use of low-dose insulin infusions has helped reduce mortality significantly over the past 10 years. The next decade may bring advances in our understanding of the pathogenesis and prevention of cerebral edema in DKA, especially in regard to the choice of fluid used for resuscitation.

TABLE 54-28. SUMMARY OF TREATMENT OF DKA

Large-bore IV, start with NSS wide open
Oxygen, cardiac monitor
Load with 20 u regular insulin, IV push
Alternate NSS and 1/2 NS at 1000 mL/hr for first 3–4 hours
Consider LR for hyperchloremic patients or cardiac and elderly patients with severe acidosis
Add KCL to bottles
Maintain insulin infusion at 10 u/hr or give 5–10 u IM/IV qhr
Follow hourly glucose, K⁺, bicarbonate
When blood glucose is 200–300, switch infusion to D51/2NS with 10 u insulin per bottle, add KCl if indicated
Follow glucose
Feed patient

PITFALLS AND MEDICOLEGAL PEARLS

- DKA is always an emergency. Failure to recognize the condition or its severity is the leading cause of death.
- Fluid deficits are large, and replacement must be vigorous.
- Electrolyte shifts are massive during both the illness and treatment. Failure to anticipate the drop in potassium can be deadly.
- Patients in DKA frequently have an underlying serious illness.
- Pregnant diabetics are especially prone to DKA with minimal physiologic stress. DKA is particularly harmful to the fetus and must be treated vigorously.
- Patients in severe DKA are often at the limits of their respiratory compensation. Anything which hinders their ventilation can cause a fatal downward spiral.
- Always look out for infection and sepsis in patients with DKA.

ACKNOWLEDGMENT

The authors would like to thank Dr. Corey Slovis for his invaluable assistance in designing the summarized tables used in this chapter.

REFERENCES

1. Katz, M.A.: Hyperglycemia-induced hyponatremia calculation of expected serum sodium depression. N. Engl. J. Med. 289:843, 1973.
2. Fisher, J.N., et al.: Diabetic ketoacidosis: Low dose insulin therapy by various routes. N. Engl. J. Med. 297:238, 1977.
3. Vinicor, F., et al.: Hyperamylasemia in diabetic ketoacidosis: Sources and significance. Ann. Intern. Med. 91:200, 1979.
4. Slovis, C.M., et al.: Diabetic ketoacidosis and infection: Leukocyte count and differential as early predictors of serious infection. Am. J. Emerg. Med. 5:1, 1987.
5. Oullet, L.M., and Brook, M.P.: Emphysematous pyelonephritis: An emergency indication for the plain abdominal radiograph. Ann. Emerg. Med. 17:22, 1988.
6. Simon, B.S.: Pseudomyocardial infarction and hyperkalemia: A case report and subject review. J. Emerg. Med. 6:511, 1988.
7. Kitabchi, A.E., and Murphy, M.B.: Diabetic ketoacidosis and hyperosmolar hyperglycemic nonketotic coma. Med. Clin. North Am. 72:1545, 1988.
8. Hillman, K.: Fluid resuscitation in diabetic emergencies—A reappraisal. Intensive Care Med. 13:4, 1987.
9. Axelrod, L.: Diabetic emergencies and the Loch Ness monster (editorial). Intensive Care Med. 13:1, 1987.
10. Moller, D.E., and Flier, J.S.: Mechanisms of disease: Insulin resistance—mechanisms, syndromes, and implications. N. Engl. J. Med. 325:938, 1991.
11. Morris, L.R., et al.: Bicarbonate therapy in severe diabetic ketoacidosis. Ann. Intern. Med. 105:836, 1986.
12. Wilson, H.K., et al.: Phosphate therapy in diabetic ketoacidosis. Arch. Intern. Med. 142:517, 1982.
13. Fisher, J.N., et al.: A randomized study of phosphate therapy in the treatment of diabetic ketoacidosis. Clin. Endocr. Metabl. 57:177, 1983.

HYPOGLYCEMIA

R. Carter Clements

CAPSULE

Hypoglycemia occurs when a mismatch of endogenous glucose need with exogenous and endogenous glucose availability derails the metabolic engine of normal glucose homeostasis. There are many causes, and it is the duty of the emergency physician both to establish the cause of the episode and to treat the resultant sympathetic and cerebral dysfunction. In practice, the sequence of these events may be reversed. The diabetic population is at greatest risk for the development of hypoglycemia. The occurrence of this disorder without obvious cause should be of grave concern to the emergency physician. Several treatment modalities are available to prehospital and definitive care providers; intravenous D50W, 25 to 50 g, is the most commonly used in the acute setting.

As the care of diabetic patients in the future becomes more sophisticated, we should see a decrease in the incidence of hypoglycemia. Current emphasis on aggressive, tight control of diabetes, however, may result in an increase in the number of hypoglycemia related visits in the short term.[1] For the present, it is a common, severe, and potentially lethal pathologic state about which we must have intimate knowledge and understanding.

In the regulation of serum glucose, insulin is the major endocrine agent in the induction of hypoglycemia. Glucagon and epinephrine are its major antagonists. Excess of insulin is the most common cause of hypoglycemia. Its most likely source is exogenous and its most frequent causes are iatrogenic and therapeutic complications. Symptoms are classic or nonclassic. Classic hypoglycemia shows adrenergic symptoms and signs followed by the progressive neurologic dysfunction ending in coma and death if untreated. Nonclassic presentations, especially focal neurologic lesions, are myriad. Diagnosis must be swift to minimize the chances of complications, permanent neurologic damage, and death. Focus is placed on identifying the cause of the episode, which is mandatory before discharge. Therapy should be rapid, with glucose stat intravenously and thereafter by maintenance infusion. Difficult-to-control cases may require high-percentage dextrose solution infusion or adjunctive glucagon, cortisol, or diazoxide. Inability to control hypoglycemia with therapy or inability to state the cause with accuracy and assurance are the indications for admission. Because of the complex nature of this diagnosis, the potential to err is high. It is incumbent on the emergency physician to make a measured, organized, conservative approach to diagnosis and management of hypoglycemia in all its forms if therapeutic and medicolegal misadventures are to be avoided.

INTRODUCTION

Hypoglycemia is a common problem in the Emergency Department (ED). Potter et al. have reported their ED experience with adult hypoglycemia in a large urban population. They found that excessive insulin administration was the most likely cause (98%) in their population and a minimum of 9% of their diabetic patients have hypoglycemic episodes requiring emergency treatment, with 64% of these severe cases requiring admission.[2] Another study looked at the cases of severe hypoglycemia presenting to an inner-city urban ED over a 1-year period and found that 73% of cases were secondary to either a missed meal (52%) in diabetics or alcohol (21%) consumption.[3] Fischer et al. reported episodes of hypoglycemia in hospitalized patients and found that 45% of patients were diabetic, with 90% of their episodes secondary to excessive insulin. In addition, renal disease alone was found to be the single predisposing factor in 28% of admitted patients. Hypoglycemia as a complication of the treatment of hyperkalemia was seen in 9% of their patients. They reported an in-hospital mortality of 27%, although none of the patient deaths were directly the result of hypoglycemia.[4] Malouf and Brust reported a year of experience with symptomatic hypoglycemia in the Harlem Hospital ED. Diabetes, sepsis, or alcoholism caused 90% of 125 cases. For all episodes, stupor or coma was seen in 52%, affective derangement or confusion in 30%, seizures in 7%, anxiety in 8%, and hemiparesis in 2%. Fourteen patients died but only one from hypoglycemia.[5]

A universal standard definition is elusive but a serum glucose level of ≤ 50 mg per deciliter (≤ 2.75 mOsm per liter) with appropriate symptoms that resolve on return of serum glucose to normal is powerfully suggestive.[6] It should be kept in mind that some individuals may have normal serum glucose levels of less than 50 mg/DL, without hypoglycemic symptoms. Such a finding is more common in the pediatric and female populations.[7] Hypoglycemia's array of symptoms arises from excessive adrenergic activity and progressive central nervous system (CNS) dysfunction in the presence of depressed serum glucose level. Depending on the rapidity of onset of hypoglycemia, the expression of these symptoms may be variable, but ultimately, if no treatment is forthcoming, the patient develops an altered level of consciousness.[8] It is no surprise that the care of these patients frequently falls to the emergency practitioner.

The symptoms of hypoglycemia have frequently resolved before the evaluation of the patient by a physician because the characteristically rapid response to treatment with $D_{50}W$ either in the field by prehospital care providers or in the ED by nursing staff. This may cause the physician to underestimate the severity of the event.

This entity has a complex pathophysiology with numerous causes. The emergency physician must not only treat the metabolic derangement but also avidly seek and correct the underlying cause. The diagnosis should read "Hypoglycemia secondary to _____ ." If the preceding "blank" is not known with certainty, the patient should be admitted to definitively establish the cause. The most frequent culprits are exogenous insulin, sufonylureas, and ethyl alcohol, with insulin by far the leader. Hypoglycemia is frequently the complication of a previous treatment, but because of the acuity and severity of the symptoms, the patient is most likely to be treated in the ED when it occurs.

Many patients with hypoglycemia can be rapidly evaluated and released after counseling and education on changes in therapy or lifestyle. This assumes that they are at their baseline level of function, and the cause is clear. It is incumbent on the emergency physician to convey information about the hypoglycemic episode to the patient's primary care provider to prevent recurrence and limit the potential for morbidity and possible mortality to the patient.

PATHOPHYSIOLOGY AND ANATOMY

Euglycemia is the ultimate goal of the complex system of neurohormonal and organ interactions involved in glucose homeostasis in the human body. This homeostasis is absolutely necessary to preserve normal brain metabolism and function. The metabolism of the CNS is essentially totally driven by the oxidation of about 150 g per day of glucose that must be immediately available from the circulation. Mild to moderate hypoglycemia can cause abnormal cognitive function even in the absence of other symptoms in normal men.[9] Cryer and Gerich reported that brain glucose uptake is directly proportional to the arterial glucose concentration.[1] The brain's reserves of glucose are minimal, at best sufficient for only a few minutes of continued normal activity. Auer has suggested that hypoglycemic brain damage may begin rapidly after hypoglycemic coma has become clinically manifest.[10] Hypoglycemia is therefore a pathologic condition that presents an immediate threat to life.

In the euglycemic state, the body's demand for glucose is balanced by ingestion of glucose or endogenous production of glucose. The time since the last meal will determine which of these mechanisms is dominant. The latter mechanism achieves primacy in the postabsorptive state which is at least 5 to 6 hours after the last meal. An overnight fast of 8 to 14 hours definitely places the patient in the postabsorptive group. The internal mechanisms of glucose production are hepatic glycogen breakdown (glycogenolysis) and de novo glucose synthesis (gluconeogenesis) using lactate, pyruvate, glycerol, and alanine. The immediate clinically important site of these activities is the liver, although in starvation (2 to 3 day fast), the kidney is capable of gluconeogenesis and muscle regularly produces glucose for its own consumption by glycogenolysis; releasing lactate in the process of anaerobic catabolism. Glycogen stores are sufficient only for the first day of starvation in the average individual. After that, gluconeogenesis provides the lion's share of endogenous glucose supply.[8]

The coordination of these activities is endocrine and neurohormonal. Insulin is the major hormone in the control of serum glucose. It has a hypoglycemic effect and inhibits glycogenolysis and gluconeogenesis. The hyperglycemia-inducing arm of this euglycemia feedback loop is populated by several humeral factors including glucagon, epinephrine, growth hormone, and cortisol. These factors considered as a group are referred to as the "counterregulatory hormones" of glucose metabolism.[11] That is, they act to return serum blood glucose levels toward normal levels from hypoglycemic levels. Glucagon is the most powerful, followed closely by epinephrine with the rest of minor importance for the normal subject. Insulin is produced in the pancreatic beta islet cells, glucagon in the pancreatic Å islet cells, growth hormone in the pancreatic β islet cells, epinephrine in the adrenal medulla, and cortisol from the hypophyseal pituitary axis.

Hypoglycemia results when excessive use or inadequate production of glucose causes a fall in the serum level, resulting in end organ deprivation of this primary energy metabolism precursor. The terminal event in the natural history of this process is neuroglycopenia, as initially described by Marks et al.[12] with progressive failure of central neural metabolism and function causing coma, neuronal death, and ultimately the death of the patient if treatment is not available.

PREHOSPITAL ASSESSMENT AND STABILIZATION

In patients who have had prior episodes of hypoglycemia and have home care providers who have received diabetic instruction, hypoglycemic episodes are frequently subject to early recognition and treatment. If that fails, 911 EMS calls are necessary. Severe episodes of hypoglycemia are defined as those that require a hospital visit or the intervention of another person.

Prehospital care providers are skilled in the diagnosis and symptomatic treatment of hypoglycemia because this diagnosis is universally addressed in the EMS treatment protocols of altered level of consciousness. Once diagnosed, mild cases are treated with oral sugar-containing fluids and intravenous fluids as needed. The hypoglycemic patient, however, may present with nonclassic symptoms that may be beyond the diagnostic ability of prehospital personnel.

The administration of intravenous glucose or intramuscular glucagon will increase serum glucose levels in patients who are otherwise systemically intact. The effect of glucose is rapid unless the patient has sustained prolonged neurologic insult. The effect of glucagon is much less dramatic, taking 10 to 20 minutes to be clinically apparent. The previously hypoglycemic patient may be postictal because of hypoglycemic seizures, may have suffered significant trauma during the episode, or may show persistent neurologic or cardiovascular signs and symptoms caused by the episode. All these factors can limit efforts at field stabilization.

CLINICAL PRESENTATION AND EXAMINATION

Hypoglycemia may exhibit classic or nonclassic constellations of symptoms. The classic presentation includes sympathomimetic symptoms followed by those of neuroglycopenia. The adrenergic or sympathomimetic symptoms include (but are not limited to) pallor, palpitations, tachycardia with or without hypertension, tremor, diaphoresis, anxiety, and affective hyperactivity. The intensity of the counterregulatory response and adrenergic symptoms is proportional to the depth of the patient's fall in serum glucose level more than the rate of fall or the absolute decrease in serum glucose.[1] Counterregulation begins at higher

glucose levels than do symptoms. Cardiac ischemia[13] and arrhythmias from hypoglycemia have been reported. In rapidly evolving hypoglycemia, the adrenergic phase may be transient as symptoms of cerebral dysfunction quickly become dominant.

If neuroglycopenia evolves, the patient may have any of the myriad signs or symptoms. The patient may complain of weakness, headache, or decreased visual acuity or blindness. Confusion or coma with muscle laxity is common but the patient may exhibit altered cognitive function while awake,[9] visual hallucinations,[14] hemiplegia (strangely, the right side is affected more often than left),[15,16] aphasia, tetany, seizures, or flaccid coma. Cardiac or respiratory arrest is not unknown. If the patient has had a seizure from hypoglycemia, he or she may have shoulder dislocation(s) or other orthopedic trauma.[17,18] Such dislocations, when present, are often posterior. Their occurrence should be a clue to grand mal seizures from any cause. These findings are summarized in Table 54-29.

The physical examination usually shows a decreased level of consciousness with or without excessive adrenergic outflow. Signs of the long-term complications of diabetes may be present and should be sought. Evidence of liver failure, renal disease, endocrinopathies, neoplastic disease, or psychiatric disease may be present. Examination of the fundus to

TABLE 54-29. SYMPTOMS AND SIGNS OF HYPOGLYCEMIA

Sympathomimetic Symptoms
  Pallor
  Palpitations
  Tachycardia
  Hypertension
  Tremor
  Diaphoresis
  Anxiety
  Affective hyperactivity
  Cardiac ischemia
  Arrythmias
Neuroglycopenia
  Weakness
  Headache
  Decreased visual acuity
  Visual hallucinations
  Blindness
  Confusion or altered cognitive function while awake
  Hemiplegia
  Aphasia
  Tetany
  Seizures
  Flaccid coma
Nonclassical Signs and Symptoms
  Any of above as isolated finding or
  Any of above in conjunction with major systemic disease
  Shoulder dislocation(s), especially posterior
  Other orthopedic trauma
  Facial flushing
  Urticaria

look for retinopathy and papilledema is mandatory. Tachycardia should be seen but may be abolished by severe neuroglycopenia or beta blockade. Hypertension is variably present. Diaphoresis is common and may be the only adrenergic symptom in the hypoglycemic patient on a nonselective beta blocking agent. Facial flushing and urticaria have been reported. Evidence of liver failure is ominous because more than 80% loss of hepatic function must be present to cause hypoglycemia.

DIFFERENTIAL DIAGNOSIS

The initial differential diagnosis for the hypoglycemic patient is most often that of altered level of consciousness. The diagnosis should be confirmed by demonstration of decreased serum glucose, with adrenergic excess or neurologic dysfunction, and resolution of normal function after restoration of physiologic serum glucose levels after a suitable interval (Whipple's triad).[19]

Once the diagnosis of hypoglycemia has been firmly established, the emergency physician must determine if the episode was reactive (postprandial) or fasting (postabsorptive). The differential diagnosis of hypoglycemia is summarized in Table 54-30.

Postprandial or reactive hypoglycemia may be alimentary in cause. That is, it is seen in patients who have undergone surgery that alters the normal anatomy of the upper gastrointestinal system, such as pyloroplasty, partial or complete gastrectomy, and gastrojejunostomy, among others. In this condition, there is rapid absorption of ingested glucose causing increased release of insulin, followed in 2 to 3 hours by hypoglycemia. Patients with prediabetic syndromes may show glucose intolerance with initial hyperglycemia and subsequent postprandial hypoglycemia. Other causes of postprandial hypoglycemia are rare, they include galactosemia, hereditary fructose intolerance, and inborn enzymatic deficiencies. These all become apparent when the patient is a child.[20]

Despite the love of the lay public for the diagnosis of functional postprandial/reactive hypoglycemia, this diagnosis is uncommon in the adult population. Most often, signs and symptoms cannot be consistently demonstrated to coincide with depressed glucose levels after mixed meals, and the diagnosis is psychiatric for the vast majority of patients in this group.[7]

Hypoglycemia after fasting is designated as postabsorptive and is potentially more ominous because it implies relative or absolute failure of counterregulatory mechanisms. In the fasting state, the patient's glucose homeostasis is under primary control by counterregulatory hormones, which should be protective against the development of hypoglycemia. Fasting hy-

TABLE 54-30. DIFFERENTIAL DIAGNOSIS OF HYPOGLYCEMIA

Postprandial or Reactive Hypoglycemia
  Alimentary—abnormal anatomy
  Prediabetic glucose intolerance
  Galactosemia
  Hereditary fructose intolerance
  Inborn enzymatic deficiencies
  Functional or idiopathic hypoglycemia
Fasting (Postabsorptive) Hypoglycemia
  Exogenous insulin excess
    Therapeutic
      Diabetes
      Acute management of hyperkalemia
    Iatrogenic complications
    Factitious
      Munchausen's syndrome
      Suicide attempt
      Homicide attempt
      Child abuse
  Endogenous Insulin Excess
    Beta cell islet tumors (insulinoma) and hyperplasia
  Extrapancreatic Tumors
    Insulin-like factors
  Organ Failure
    Hepatic failure
    Renal failure
    Congestive heart failure
    Cardiogenic shock
    Adrenal failure
    Hypothyroidism
    Hypopituitarism
  Drug-Induced (see Table 54-31)
    Excessive insulin secretion—sulfonylureas
    Failure of counterregulation—alcohol, tylenol, others
  Counterregulatory Hormone Deficiencies
    Congenital
      Glucagon
      Epinephrine
      Cortisol
      Growth hormone
    Acquired
      Glucagon
      Epinephrine
      Cortisol
      Growth hormone
  Systemic Disease
    Malnourished state
    Sepsis
    Shock
    Agonist insulin or insulin receptor antibodies
      Autoimmune diseases
        Systemic lupus erythematosus
        Grave's disease
        Scleroderma
      Lymphoreticular neoplasms
        Hodgkin's disease
Differential Diagnosis of Pediatric Hypoglycemia
  Neonatal hypoglycemia
  Hypoglycemic ketosis
  Prolonged starvation
  Child abuse
    Starvation
    Factitious
  Multiple inborn enzyme defects

poglycemia is caused by an excess of circulating insulin relative to available serum glucose.

Exogenous, therapeutic insulin excess is the most common cause of fasting hypoglycemia. Other causes of fasting hypoglycemia include excessive pancreatic beta cell insulin production, extrapancreatic tumors, organ failure, drugs that cause excessive insulin secretion or failure of counterregulation, counterregulatory hormone deficiencies, and several systemic diseases.

Excessive pancreatic beta cell insulin production may be seen in beta cell islet tumors and hyperplasia as well as with drugs that cause increased secretion of endogenous insulin such as the sulfonylurea oral hypoglycemic drugs. Extrapancreatic tumors can produce insulin-like factors that may produce hypoglycemia despite normal serum insulin levels.

Hepatic and renal failure have been associated with decreased serum glucose with or without frank hypoglycemia. In liver disease, this may be caused by glycogen depletion or deficient gluconeogenesis either alone or in conjunction. The kidney and liver are the primary sites of elimination of insulin. Thus, for the renal failure patient with diabetes, insulin requirements decrease as the disease progresses. Also, the kidney is gluconeogenic during prolonged fasting. These factors, in combination with the chronically malnourished state of most renal failure patients, contribute to the hypoglycemia that may be seen. It should be noted that both diabetic and nondiabetic renal failure patients are at increased risk of profound hypoglycemia versus normal controls during the acute management of hyperkalemia.[21]

Patients with congestive heart failure or cardiogenic shock may have hypoglycemia, thought to be caused by liver dysfunction induced by passive congestion or hypoperfusion. Infarction or ablation of the adrenals or pituitary may result in hypoglycemia secondary to counterregulatory hormone deficit. Hypothyroidism may also cause hypoglycemia.

Multiple drugs are known to cause hypoglycemia by either increasing serum insulin or inhibiting counterregulation. Insulin and the sulfonylureas produce hypoglycemia in overdosage and may even do so in therapeutic doses. Both agents may be taken in overdosage when the patient is attempting suicide or seeking admission because of covertly induced (factitious) hypoglycemia.[22] Ethanol is a well known cause of hypoglycemia from inhibition of gluconeogenesis in glycogen-deficient individuals. Salicylate-induced hypoglycemia has been repeatedly reported to be associated with overdosage, especially in the pediatric population.[7] Tylenol-induced hypoglycemia is caused by liver necrosis, seen in overdosage. Numerous other drugs implicated in hypoglycemia[23–26] are listed in Table 54-31.

Seltzer reviewed 1418 cases of hypoglycemia secondary to drugs. Sulfonylureas caused 63% of cases, with alcohol, propranolol, and aspirin causing another

TABLE 54-31. HYPOGLYCEMIA-INDUCING DRUGS	
Insulin	Sulfa antibiotics
Sulfonylureas	Chloramphenicol
Ethanol	Co-trimazole
Salicylate	Sublactam/ampicillin
Tylenol	Tetracyclines
Disopyramide	Mebendozole
Beta-adrenergic antagorists	Amphetamine
Phenothiazines	Cocaine
Butyrophenones	Non-steroidal anti-inflammatory
Lithium	drugs
Calcium	Pyridoxine
Manganese	Bromocriptine
Ethylenediaminetetra-acetate	Clofibrate
Monoamine oxidase inhibitors	ACE inhibitors
Dextropropoxyphene	Orphenadrine
Coumadin	Cibenzoline
Pentamidine	Theophylline
	Quinine

19%. Pentamidine, disopyramide, ritodrine, and quinine yielded 7% more.[23] Recently hypoglycemia has been reported from inadvertent dispensing of sulfonylurea agents to nondiabetic patients. This pharmacy error was caused by the similarity of proprietary names and drug appearance.[27]

Deficiencies of glucagon, epinephrine, cortisol, and growth hormone can cause failure of counterregulation with subsequent hypoglycemia episodes. These deficits may be congenital or acquired. Congenital deficiencies become obvious early in life. Acquired disease is associated with disease or trauma of the liver, pancreas, adrenals, and pituitary. Of particular note to the emergency physician are long-standing insulin-dependent diabetics and patients on long-term steroid treatment. The long-term diabetics have acquired deficiency in secretion of glucagon and epinephrine.[8] These patients are prone to hypoglycemia, which is likely to be severe if nonselective beta adrenergic blockers are prescribed. If long-term steroid patients suddenly discontinue their medication, they may present with hypoglycemia as a symptom of Addisonian crisis. For them, parenteral steroids with glucocorticoid and mineralocorticoid activity constitute mandatory, life-saving emergency therapy.

Systemic disorders such as sepsis and shock can cause hypoglycemia, primarily from liver failure. This is especially true for patients wth pre-existing liver disease. Autoimmune diseases, such as systemic lupus erythematosus and Grave's disease, and lymphoreticular neoplasms, such as Hodgkin's disease, can cause generation of autoantibodies to insulin or insulin receptors that may have agonist rather than antagonist activity.[28,29]

The differential diagnosis of pediatric hypoglycemia deserves special mention. In addition to the causes discussed already, the emergency physician must add the following to his differential when confronted with the hypoglycemic child: neonatal hypoglycemia, hypoglycemic ketosis, prolonged starvation, child abuse, and multiple inborn errors or metabolism.[30] Essentially, all children born out of asepsis or in the ED should be considered at risk for neonatal hypoglycemia and rapidly screened. Blood glucose less than 40 mg per dL should be treated as indicated with intravenous D50W in a dose of 1 to 2 mL per Kg, repeated as needed. Response to therapy should be documented by heel stick. Oral glucose supplementation is also administered.

Pediatric starvation or drug-induced hypoglycemia should raise a high suspicion of child abuse or pediatric psychiatric disease in the previously healthy child or adolescent.[31] I refer the reader to other chapters in this text and pediatric texts for further study of this matter.

INITIAL STABILIZATION

On arrival in the ED, the adult patient should undergo rapid history and physical assessment, with the usual emphasis on airway, breathing, and circulation (the ABCs). History attained from prehospital care providers or family can be diagnostic and valuable. The history should focus on precipitating, predictive, or exacerbating factors in the genesis of hypoglycemia. The time since the last meal, the presence of diabetes, prior episodes of hypoglycemia, and drug therapy (especially with insulin and sulfonylureas) must be documented. Potential clues to the etiology of hypoglycemia include concurrent liver, renal, endocrine, or neoplastic disease, recent prescriptions, signs of depression, alcohol or stimulant abuse, and other diseases that cause the patient to be chronically malnourished (see Table 54-30).

An intravenous line should be rapidly established and blood specimens obtained for initial serum glucose evaluation as well as other studies that may be indicated if the cause of the hypoglycemic episode is not immediately obvious. Blood should be tested with a reagent strip at the bedside to speed diagnosis. The older "dextro-sticks" are less accurate and read lower. If the patient is conscious, history can be taken at this time and the patient treated with oral glucose solution. If not, 25 to 50 g of 50% glucose in water solution is given by intravenous push and the patient should be placed on supplemental oxygen and a cardiac monitor. Thiamine, 100 mg IM, should be given concomitantly. If immediate intravenous access is not possible, the patient should be treated with 1 to 2 mg of intramuscular glucagon. This may be repeated once in 10 to 20 minutes, although the utility of higher doses is suspect. Intravenous administration of 5 or 10% dextrose in water in volumes of at least 2 to 3 mL per minute should be administered after bolus therapy

has been given. The patient should be given oral glucose supplementation in addition, preferably a mixed snack or meal to ensure against recurrence if mental status permits. Patients who do not respond to this therapy must be evaluated for other causes of the altered level of consciousness.

The patient should undergo a repeat examination to document any response to initial therapy and to be evaluated for nonpharmacologic causes of the episode as previously discussed if the cause is unknown. Blood sampling for post-treatment serum glucose analysis should done. Other laboratory and diagnostic studies as indicated by the clinical situation should be ordered.

LABORATORY FINDINGS

The patient should have a serum blood glucose that is 50 mg per dL or below on the initial specimen and should show a serum glucose rise of at least 100 to 200 mg per dL on post-treatment analysis if therapy is successful. Blood should not be allowed to stand for a protracted period before separation because elevated leukocyte counts from hematologic malignancy or reactive leukocytosis may accelerate glucolysis in vitro causing artifactual hypoglycemia.[22] Hypoglycemia has been reported in a leukemic patient (AML) who did not have leukocytosis.[32] Further glucose testing should be done in severe reactions to document failure of recurrence of hypoglycemia. The patient should have serum electrolyte analysis. In the hyperinsulinemic state, the administration of high doses of intravenous glucose may cause electrolyte abnormalities, in particular, hypokalemia.

Serum obtained at the time of initial examination may be analyzed for levels of insulin, proinsulin, C-peptide, and antibodies to insulin or its receptor as indicated by the clinical presentation and course. Insulin levels are elevated in exogenous insulin excess or endogenous insulin excess from sulfonylureas or pancreatic beta cell islet tumors. Proinsulin levels are elevated only when endogenous insulin secretion is elevated. Alternately, C-peptide levels indirectly measure proinsulin levels because C-peptide is liberated during the proteolytic conversion of proinsulin to insulin. Antibodies to insulin occur in autoimmune diseases and when heterologous insulins such as those derived from pork or beef or (to a much lesser extent) homologous insulins have been administered. Insulin receptor antibodies are seen only in autoimmune diseases. The levels of these various compounds should be measured in patients in whom the cause of hypoglycemia is not evident. Specific patterns of measured levels may be diagnostic or suggestive. Such testing is beyond the scope of ED care.

Qualitative blood and urine toxicologic testing can be done to seek drug-induced hypoglycemia. Cerebrospinal fluid glucose concentration is depressed after an episode of hypoglycemia and may take several hours to recover. This can be an important diagnostic modality in the patient who does not respond well to therapy and in whom no other cause of CNS dysfunction is found.[33] An ECG should be done.

MANAGEMENT AND INDICATIONS FOR ADMISSION

After initial stabilization has been achieved, the patient should be monitored for a time for recurring hypoglycemia. The duration of the period of observation is somewhat arbitrary, but should be at least 3 to 6 hours while receiving treatment. An intravenous glucose solution of 5 or 10% should be administered during this observation and the trend of serum glucose followed at regular intervals by either fingerstick or laboratory measurement. Patients requiring 10% dextrose infusion during emergency therapy should be admitted for further treatment and observation.

Patients whose hypoglycemia is due to "regular" insulin excess, nutritional deficit, or alcohol can be amenable to ED stabilization and subsequent discharge. On the other hand, episodes of hypoglycemia caused by "intermediate" or "long-acting" insulins and first-generation (tolbutamide, chlorpropamide, tolazamide, and acetohexamide) or to second-generation (glyburide, glipizide, and gliclazide) sulfonylurea oral hypoglycemic agents are at risk of prolonged hypoglycemic secondary to the extended half-life of these agents. It is improvident to discharge them. Seltzer recommends that all patients with severe drug-induced hypoglycemia be treated with intravenous 10% glucose for at least a day until sustained hyperglycemia can be documented.[23]

Further episodes of hypoglycemia should be treated with increased concentrations of intravenous glucose (up to 20% dextrose) and consideration given to addition of glucagon, cortisol, or diazoxide to the treatment regimen. The drug treatments for hypoglycemia are given in Table 54-32.

Failure to stabilize the serum glucose by initial emergency bolus and maintenance therapy, hypoglycemia requiring escalating intensity of treatment, or an episode of unexplained hypoglycemia warrants medical admission for observation, treatment, and further diagnostic workup, as indicated. If the planned disposition is discharge, the patient should be watched for a minimum of 1 to 2 hours after discontinuing supplemental glucose, and continuation of euglycemia quantitatively documented.

PITFALLS

Failure to determine the cause of a hypoglycemic episode is cause for serious concern to the emergency physician. These patients must be admitted because no guarantee can be given that hypoglycemia will not recur. This situation is fraught with potential morbidity and mortality for the patient and extreme medicolegal risk for the physician. Inadequate treatment or an insufficient period of observation can cause recurrence of hypoglycemia and have the same attendant risks.

Somogyi reaction is defined as morning hyperglycemia caused by nocturnal hypoglycemia, related to excessive doses of intermediate or long-acting insulin. This effect is controlled through counterregulatory mechanisms. The treatment of this complication of diabetes is reduction not increase, of the insulin dose. Thus good communication between the emergency practitioner and the primary care provider is imperative. The ED often sees and treats the hypoglycemic event, but the primary care provider may be aware only of elevated fasting glucose levels if the patient is a poor historian and the emergency physician is not assiduous in reporting.

The increasing use of human recombinant insulin has several potential negative effects. Human-source insulin as compared to animal-source insulin is less likely to cause the patient to recognize impending hypoglycemia since it causes fewer adrenergic symptoms.[34] The potential for more frequent severe reactions is obvious, especially in patients on tight glycemic control protocols. Additionally, human-source insulin is much less immunogenic than animal-source insulin, and this may make the diagnosis of factitious hypoglycemia more difficult.

One should not rely on historical evidence of abnormal

TABLE 54-32. DRUGS USED IN THE TREATMENT OF HYPOGLYCEMIA

Drug	Dose	Interval	Route
50% Glucose solution	25–50 g	As needed	IV
Glucagon	1–2 mg	10–20 minutes × 2*	IM/IV
Hydrocortisone†	25–50 mg	Daily	IV/IM
Dyazoxide	3–8 mg/kg	8–12 hours	PO

* Higher doses in hypoglycemia from beta blocker overdose
† Normal daily endogenous production is approximately 20 mg

glucose levels on a 5-hour oral glucose tolerance test to diagnose hypoglycemia.[7] The test has poor specificity and may show up to 50% of patients to be hypoglycemic, although hypoglycemia is seldom demonstrated after physiologic mixed nutrient meal testing of serum glucose.

Patients with hypoglycemia from hyperinsulinism caused by pancreatic or other tumors frequently respond well to ED treatment and may have stable blood glucose levels on short-term observation. They may need up to 72 hours of enforced in-hospital fasting to manifest another bout of hypoglycemia.[35] Despite the patient's apparent stability, he or she must be admitted if there is no known diagnosis making the cause of the hypoglycemic episode clear. At the least, these patients must receive extremely urgent follow-up.

Administration of 50% glucose solution by peripheral vein is frequently done, but has the risk of subcutaneous infiltration with tissue necrosis because of the osmotic load of the solution. The potential for local venous thrombosis and vein sclerosis is high.

MEDICOLEGAL PEARLS

Hypoglycemia at the extremes of age may result from child abuse or elder abuse, and this should always be kept in mind while considering the differential diagnosis in the pediatric and geriatric populations. Notification of child or adult protective services is mandatory and legally protective to the patient and physician if the suspicion arises.

The hypoglycemic patient is often the victim of chronic disease. He may become depressed and the hypoglycemic episode may be the result of a suicide attempt by drug overdose. The physician should be sensitive to the subtle signs of depression, especially if the hypoglycemic patient is not diabetic or has a history of psychiatric disease, and have no fear to act to prevent the possibility of another attempt. Failure to diagnose suicidal intent may incur physician liability. This is also true for the patient with factitious hypoglycemia.

Any patient involved in a motor vehicle accident with an altered sensorium should have serum glucose determination.[36,37] Many states require reporting of episodes of loss of consciousness to public health agencies, who route the information to the Department of Motor Vehicles. Failure to diagnose hypoglycemia in this event is a medical and legal disservice to the patient. Failure to report the episode undermines the public health and safety and places the emergency physician liable in the event of further traffic mishaps involving the patient. This liability may include wrongful death of the patient or his victim.

All of the points considered in the section entitled "Pitfalls" are potential medicolegal jungles. It is especially important to document instructions given to the patient as to changes in therapeutic regimen and lifestyle and the required follow-up. If possible, contact the patient's physician and document that contact.

HORIZONS

It is hoped that our generation may come to see the cure of diabetes, or at least vast improvements in the therapy and technology aimed at what has been the therapeutic "Grail" of diabetic euglycemia. When this comes to pass, the community of emergency care providers will see far less of the scourge of iatrogenic hypoglycemia. This rosy prognostication is dimmed somewhat by the prospect of the increasing demographic reality of the geriatric population explosion. It will bring increased prevalence of many of the disease states that admit patients to the cohort of those at great risk of hypoglycemia. The ultimate balance of these factors can only be guessed at.

Pontiroli et al. have reported the use of an intranasal glucagon preparation that may have great utility in the treatment of impending hypoglycemia in outpatient and prehospital care.[38]

REFERENCES

1. Cryer, P.E., and Gerich, J.E.: Glucose counterregulation, hypoglycemia, and intensive insulin therapy in diabetes mellitus. N. Engl. J. Med. *313*:232, 1985.
2. Potter, J., Clarke, P., Gale, E.A., et al.: Insulin-induced hypoglycaemia in an accident and emergency department: The tip of an iceberg? Br. Med. J. *285*:1180, 1982.
3. Feher, M.D., Grout, P., Kennedy, A., et al.: Hypoglycaemia in an inner-city accident and emergency department: A 12-month survey. Arch. Emerg. Med. *6*:183, 1989.
4. Fischer, K.F., Lees, J.A., and Newman, J.H.: Hypoglycemia in hospitalized patients. Causes and outcomes. N. Engl. J. Med. *315*:1245, 1986.
5. Malouf, R. and Brust, J.C.: Hypoglycemia: Causes, neurological manifestations, and outcome. Ann. Neurol. *17*:1985.
6. Field, J.B.: Hypoglycemia. Definition, clinical presentations, classification, and laboratory tests. Endocrinol. Metab. Clin. North Am. *18*:27, 1989.
7. Nelson, R.L.: Hypoglycemia: Fact or fiction? Mayo. Clin. Proc. *60*:844, 1985.
8. Campbell, P.J., and Gerich, J.E.: Mechanisms for prevention, development, and reversal of hypoglycemia. Adv. Intern. Med. *33*:205, 1988.
9. Stevens, A.B., McKane, W.R., Bell, P.M., et al.: Psychomotor performance and counterregulatory responses during mild hypoglycemia in healthy volunteers. Diabetes Care *12*:12, 1989.
10. Auer, R.N.: Progress review: Hypoglycemic brain damage. Stroke *17*:699, 1986.
11. Gerich, J.E., and Campbell, P.J.: Overview of counterregulation and its abnormalities in diabetes mellitus and other conditions. Diabetes Metab. Rev. *4*:93, 1988.
12. Marks, V., Marrack, D., and Rose, F.C.: Hyperinsulinism in the pathogenesis of neuroglycopenic syndromes. Proc. R. Soc. Med. *54*:747, 1961.
13. Pladziewicz, D.S., and Nesto, R.W.: Hypoglycemia-induced silent myocardial ischemia. Am. J. Cardiol. *63*:1531, 1989.
14. Nakanishi, T.: Visual hallucination without the disturbance of consciousness in hypoglycaemic attack: Report of an unusual case—Consideration on psychic symptoms related to hypoglycaemia. Igaku Kenkyu *58*:421, 1988.

15. Foster, J.W., and Hart, R.G.: Hypoglycemic hemiplegia: Two cases and a clinical review. Stroke *18*:944, 1987.
16. Lala, V.R., Vedanarayana, V.V., Ganesh, S., et al.: Hypoglycemic hemiplegia in an adolescent with insulin-dependent diabetes mellitus: A case report and a review of the literature. J. Emerg. Med. *7*:233, 1989.
17. Hepburn, D.A., Steel, J.M., and Frier, B.M.: Hypoglycemic convulsions cause serious musculoskeletal injuries in patients with IDDM. Diabetes Care *12*:32, 1989.
18. Litchfield, J.C., Subhedar, V.Y., Beevers, D.G., and Patel, H.T.: Bilateral dislocation of the shoulders due to nocturnal hypoglycaemia. Postgrad. Med. J. *64*:450, 1988.
19. Whipple, A.O.: The surgical therapy of hyperinsulinism. J. Int. Chir. *3*:237, 1938.
20. Betteridge, D.J.: Reactive hypoglycaemia. Br. Med. J. *295*:286, 1987.
21. Williams, P.S., Davenport, A., and Bone, J.M.: Hypoglycaemia following treatment of hyperkalaemia with insulin and dextrose. Postgrad. Med. J. *64*:30, 1988.
22. Horwitz, D.L.: Factitious and artifactual hypoglycemia. Endocrinol. Metab. Clin. North Am. *18*:203, 1989.
23. Seltzer, H.S.: Drug-induced hypoglycemia. A review of 1418 cases. Endocrinol. Metab. Clin. North Am. *18*:163, 1989.
24. Bailey, C.J., Flatt, P.R., and Marks, V.: Drugs inducing hypoglycemia. Pharmacol. Ther. *42*:361, 1989.
25. Schattner, A., Rimon, E., Green, L., et al.: Hypoglycemia induced by co-trimoxazole in AIDS. Br. Med. J. *297*:742, 1988.
26. Aron, D.C.: Endocrine complications of the acquired immunodeficiency syndrome. Arch. Intern. Med. *149*:330, 1989.
27. Huminer, D., Dux, S., Rosenfeld, J.B., and Pitlik, S.D.: Inadvertent sulfonylurea-induced hypoglycemia. A dangerous, but preventable condition. Arch. Intern. Med. *149*:1890, 1989.
28. Moller, D.E., Ratner, R.E., Borenstein, D.G., and Taylor, S.I.: Autoantibodies to the insulin receptor as a cause of autoimmune hypoglycemia in systemic lupus erythematosus. Am. J. Med. *84*:334, 1988.
29. Walters, E.G., Tavare, J.M., Denton, R.M., and Walters, G.: Hypoglycaemia due to an insulin-receptor antibody in Hodgkin's disease. Lancet *1*:241, 1987.
30. Haymond, M.W.: Hypoglycemia in infants and children. Endocrinol. Metab. Clin. North Am. *18*:211, 1989.
31. Dershewitz, R., Vestal, B., Maclaren, N.K., and Cornblath, M.: Transient hepatomegaly and hypoglycemia. A consequence of malicious insulin administration. Am. J. Dis. Child. *130*:998, 1976.
32. Al Hilali, M.M., Majer, R.V., and Penney, O.: Hypoglycaemia in acute myelomonoblastic leukaemia: Report of two cases and review of published work. Br. Med. J. *289*:1443, 1984.
33. Kaplinsky, N., and Frankl, O.: The significance of the cerebrospinal fluid examination in the management of chlorpropamide-induced hypoglycemia. Diabetes Care *3*:248, 1980.
34. Heine, R.J., van der Heyden, E.A., and van der Veen, E.A.: Responses to human and porcine insulin in healthy subjects. Lancet *2*:946, 1989.
35. Service, F.J., Dale, A.J., Elveback, L.R., and Jiang, N.S.: Insulinoma: Clinical and diagnostic features of 60 consecutive cases. Mayo Clin. Proc. *51*:417, 1976.
36. Ratner, R.E., and Whitehouse, F.W.: Motor vehicles, hypoglycemia, and diabetic drivers. Diabetes Care *12*:217, 1989.
37. Stevens, A.B., Roberts, M., McKane, R., et al.: Motor vehicle driving among diabetics taking insulin and nondiabetics. Br. Med. J. *299*:591, 1989.
38. Pontiroli, A.E., Calderara, A., Pajetta, E., et al.: Intranasal glucagon as remedy for hypoglycemia. Studies in healthy subjects and type I diabetic patients. Diabetes Care *12*:604, 1989.

NONKETOTIC HYPEROSMOLAR COMA

Eric Stirling and Kristi Koenig

CAPSULE

Nonketotic hyperosmolar coma (NHC) is a syndrome of severe hyperglycemia, alteration of consciousness, hyperosmolality, and cellular dehydration without severe ketoacidosis, usually occurring in elderly noninsulin-dependent diabetics. Although uncommon, NHC has a high mortality rate. Rapid emergency department (ED) recognition, aggressive but closely monitored fluid and insulin therapy, and a thorough search for precipitating causes substantially decrease morbidity and mortality. Of special note is new evidence correlating the serum sodium concentration to the level of coma.[1]

PATHOPHYSIOLOGY

A thorough comprehension of the underlying pathophysiology in NHC is crucial to guide therapy. Under normal circumstances, there is an increase in insulin release by the beta cells in the pancreas after a meal so that glucose can be utilized by the tissues. When there is severe beta cell deficiency, the resulting insulin release is inadequate to maintain normal glucose levels. The beta cells are presumably working maximally, even in the fasting state, and thus there is no increase in insulin release after a meal or glucose load, and hyperglycemia results.

Along with the relative insulin deficiency, elevated

levels of the counter-regulatory hormones glucagon, cortisol, and catecholamines are present. This allows decreased peripheral glucose utilization and increased hepatic glucose production. Hyperglycemia, resulting in an osmotic diuresis, ensues. Dehydration eventually leads to a decrease in glomerular filtration rate and an increase in stress, which causes an increase in counter-regulatory hormone production. A spiraling hyperglycemia and worsening dehydration results.

The exact mechanism by which serum glucose levels are allowed to continue to rise without production of ketones is poorly understood, and multiple theories have been proposed.[2-4] Some experiments suggest that dehydration and hyperosmolarity limit lipolysis and ketogenesis.[5,6] It may be that sufficient insulin is present from endogenous or exogenous sources to prevent excessive lipolysis and the resultant production of ketoacids, but not to prevent hyperglycemia. The patient thus does not develop ketoacidosis. If dehydration leading to extracellular fluid depletion occurs, however, NHC may develop. The key concept is that severe dehydration at the cellular level results from these metabolic abnormalities, and this dehydration is responsible for the clinical presentation.

PREHOSPITAL CARE

Prehospital care workers should realize that, although most patients with NHC are elderly, patients of any age, including infants, have been reported. About one third of patients are known noninsulin-dependent diabetics on oral hypoglycemic agents. A history of recent prior illness is common. Precipitating causes include infection, myocardial infarction, cerebrovascular accident, and hypothermia. Prominent symptoms include alteration of consciousness, weakness, polyuria, vomiting, and abdominal pain.

Prehospital protocols should treat the altered level of consciousness with 25 g of 50% dextrose in water; thiamine, 100 mg intramuscularly or intravenously; and naloxone, 2 mg IV. Supportive care, including cardiac monitoring, frequent assessment of vital signs, and appropriate fluids for the dehydration should be instituted. Rapid transport is essential.

There is controversy over the use of intravenous (IV) dextrose in patients with altered levels of consciousness who may have increased intracranial pressure, or in those whose glucose levels are already markedly elevated. The current accepted viewpoint is that the glucose load given has a minor effect on brain edema compared to the major effect created by uncorrected hypoglycemia. The glucose load given to an already markedly hyperglycemic patient does not cause further deterioration because the percentage amount added is small.

CLINICAL PRESENTATION

The usual patient with NHC is an elderly, noninsulin-dependent diabetic over 60 with a history of progressive illness over a few days or weeks. It must be remembered that NHC may be the first manifestation of diabetes, or a complication of insulin-dependent diabetes when the patient has taken enough insulin to prevent ketosis but not hyperglycemia.[7] Younger patients, especially obese borderline diabetics with severe intercurrent illness, may develop NHC.

The most common precipitating factors are gram-negative pneumonias, uremia with vomiting, and acute viral syndromes.[8] Other bacterial infections, pancreatitis, discontinuation of oral hypoglycemic agents, silent myocardial infarction, cerebrovascular accidents, or trauma may also trigger NHC. In the hospital, causes include vigorous diuretic use, steroids, hyperalimentation, and propranolol use. The mechanism of action of diuretics is thought to be volume depletion, hypokalemia, and insulin suppression. Propranolol blocks insulin release and masks the autonomic responses to hypoglycemia.

Patients clinically present with dehydration, fever, obtundation, and either polyuria or oliguria. One third are hypotensive. Various neurologic presentations, including seizures, focal deficits, full stroke syndromes which resolve with therapy, and global dysfunction occur. In one study, 12 of 33 patients later shown to have NHC were given the admitting diagnosis of "probable acute stroke."[8] Toxidromes secondary to poisoning or overdose may predominate. Cardiac or respiratory failure may be either a cause or an effect.

DIFFERENTIAL DIAGNOSIS

Several metabolic disorders can mimic NHC. The most common is diabetic ketoacidosis. Hypoglycemic coma presents with a more rapid onset and without dehydration. Uremia may have a similar onset and alteration of consciousness, but dehydration is not present. Sepsis with lactic acidosis may also yield hyperglycemia, and it may be difficult to identify the primary cause. Alcoholic ketoacidosis rarely produces the degree of obtundation and dehydration seen with NHC. Structural coma may also present with hyperglycemia and dehydration but to a much lesser degree than NHC. Myxedema coma has a similar onset, but physical signs and the absence of significant hyperglycemia serve to differentiate. Severe hypernatremia

TABLE 54-33. DIFFERENTIAL DIAGNOSIS OF NONKETOTIC HYPEROSMOLAR COMA

Syndrome	Onset	Clinical Presentation	Glucose Level	pH	BUN	Hyperventilation
NHC	Days	Sick, obtunded	Extremely high	Normal	Increased	No
Diabetic ketoacidosis (DKA)	Days	Sick	High	Decreased	Increased	Yes (marked)
Alcoholic ketoacidosis	Days	Variable	Variable	Decreased	Normal	Yes
Hypoglycemia	Hours	Healthy, altered mental status	Low	Normal	Normal	No
Hypernatremia (severe)	Days	Sick, obtunded	Normal	Normal	Increased	No
Lactic acidosis	Hours	Sick	Variable	Decreased	Normal	Yes
Uremic acidosis	Weeks	Sick	Normal, increased	Decreased	Decreased	Yes

may mimic all the findings of NHC, with only the serum glucose to differentiate (Table 54-33).

INITIAL STABILIZATION

Therapy must be started immediately, even as the diagnosis is being considered. Once the patient is stabilized, therapy can proceed more slowly. This prevents the patient with little reserve from worsening, while allowing a gradual correction of the metabolic abnormalities. It is helpful to keep a time flow sheet to record vital signs, laboratory data, all therapy, and changes in physical and mental status. If the patient is hypotensive, isotonic saline should be infused to restore extracellular volume. One to two L are required in the first 2 hours. The IV should then be switched to 0.45% NS to prevent excessive extracellular volume repletion. This may be used initially if hypotension is absent. Total water deficits average 100 cc per kg of body weight, and one-half should be given over the next 24 hours, with the fluid type either 5% Dextrose in water or 5% Dextrose in 0.45% saline depending on volume status and serum sodium.

Ventilatory status and airway are the first priority and should be managed by clinical assessment and arterial blood gases. Oxygen and cardiac monitoring should be instituted, and dysrhythmias should be managed according to standard advanced cardiac life support (ACLS) protocols. Much of the irritability seen in NHC resolves with fluid and insulin therapy.

Insulin therapy is of less importance than fluids. Many NHC patients are sensitive to small doses, and no more than 10 units IV should be given initially. After this, a continuous infusion of 0.1 units per kg per hour, or hourly IV or intramuscular (IM) 5 to 10

unit boluses can be administered. Hourly measurement of serum glucose should be performed until levels of 300 mg% are reached, at which point a 5% dextrose-in-salt solution should be started.

LAB PROCEDURES

Initial laboratory measurements should include serum glucose, electrolytes, BUN, creatinine, magnesium, and phosphorus. Serum ketones, arterial blood gases, CBC, and urinalysis complete the basic workup. If deemed clinically necessary, creatine phosphokinase, thyroid studies, toxicology screens, serum amylase, liver function studies, blood cultures, and specific blood levels of medications should be drawn. Osmolality can be calculated using the formula (Na + K) (2) + (serum glucose)/18 + BUN/2.8. In NHC, the osmolality is usually more than 350 (normal 280 to 300). Measured serum osmolality is not necessary unless an osmolar gap is suspected (e.g., in methanol poisoning).

The serum glucose is often over 1000 mg% and may reach 2000 mg%. Potassium is variable but total body potassium is decreased. Bicarbonate levels are normal unless the patient has a concomitant metabolic acidosis or chronic hyperventilation. The anion gap is normal in uncomplicated NHC. Leukocyte counts may be elevated without demonstrable infection, and a normal leukocyte count may be present in sepsis with NHC. The serum sodium is now thought to be a useful index of cerebral cellular hydration and in identifying patients at risk for coma or neurologic abnormalities. It must first be corrected for the serum glucose with the formula that states that serum sodium will fall 1.6 meq/liter for each 100 mg% increment above normal of the serum glucose.[9] For example, the expected serum sodium for a serum glucose of 1100 mg% would be 140 (normal serum Na) − (1100 − (100 × 1.6)) = 124 meq per liter. If the corrected serum sodium is more than 140 meq per liter, more free water depletion than predicted is present. More aggressive replacement of water is then indicated.

The patient with focal neurologic syndromes should undergo CAT scanning even though resolution may occur with NHC treatment. Foley catheter, nasogastric intubation, and central venous pressure (CVP) monitoring are usually required in NHC. Oxygen administration and cardiac monitoring have already been discussed.

MANAGEMENT AND ADMISSION CRITERIA

Although mortality has dropped from about 40%, which it was 20 years ago, it remains at approximately 10%. Because of the high mortality rate and need for continuous monitoring, an intensive care unit (ICU) setting is preferred for the management of NHC. Although patients may be severely hypertonic, rapid fluid replacement is essential to restore blood pressure and urine output and to prevent cardiovascular collapse and death. Careful intake and output records are mandatory. CVP monitoring is recommended in elderly or hemodynamically unstable patients and those with underlying cardiac disease.

Fluid replacement should result in a maximum of 2 meq/liter/hour drop in the serum sodium. Rebound cerebral edema and seizures may result if this is exceeded. Glucose should be added to the IV solution when the serum level drops below 300 mg%. Potassium should be added when the level drops below 5 meq/liter and urine output is ensured. If potassium phosphate is used, it must be remembered that the formula is K_2PO_4, and the potassium twice that in KCl. Insulin in the amount of 0.1 unit per kg body weight per hour, or hourly 5 to 10 unit boluses IM or IV, provides smooth decrease in the serum glucose.

Seizures are especially problematic in the NHC patient. The differentiation between overvigorous therapy and underlying causes must be made rapidly. Hypoxia, meningitis, or structural lesions, drugs causing seizures, or an underlying seizure disorder must be distinguished. Phenytoin (Dilantin) is relatively contraindicated because of its inhibition of insulin secretion and its predilection to worsen existing metabolic abnormalities. Diazepam and phenobarbital are preferred for seizure control.

It is tempting to just "correct the numbers" in NHC. The underlying pathophysiology and precipitating factors are the determinants of survival, and must be addressed.

Communication with the family is critical, both to obtain history and to convey the severity of the patient's condition.

PITFALLS

- Look for unsuspected sepsis, meningitis, myocardial infarction, or overdose in the NHC patient who remains obtunded or refractory to timely fluid and insulin therapy.
- There is a fine line between the necessarily aggressive volume replacement and fluid overload in the elderly patient. Invasive monitoring is frequently needed. Persistent oliguria mandates a workup for acute tubular necrosis.
- Hypokalemia, hypophosphatemia, or hypomagnesemia may delay recovery as well as increase respiratory failure and cardiac dysrhythmias. Appropriate supplementation avoids these pitfalls.
- The serum glucose may fall rapidly with therapy. If the level is not checked hourly, hypoglycemia may occur, with seizures or continued coma.

MEDICOLEGAL PEARLS

Beware of iatrogenic precipitants of NHC—hyperalimentation, steroids, diuretics, and beta blockers.

Beware of nursing home or family neglect—deprivation of fluids, noncompliance with oral hypoglycemic agents, bedsores with sepsis, etc.

Beware of poisonings in the elderly diabetic precipitating NHC or obscuring the diagnosis.

HORIZONS

The population of America is growing older, and survival with chronic disease is increasing. With an increase in the population of diabetics, nursing home residents, and patients on complex medications, there will be an increase in NHC. There is no long-term prevention. ED workers must maintain vigilance to ensure early therapy of this often fatal condition.

REFERENCES

1. Daugirdas, J.T., et al.: Hyperosmolar coma: Cellular dehydration and the serum sodium concentration. Ann. Intern. Med. *110*:855, 1989.

2. Kitabchi, A.E., and Murphy, M.B.: Diabetic ketoacidosis and hyperosmolar hyperglycemic nonketotic coma. Med. Clin. North Am. 72:1545, 1988.
3. Malone, J.K., et al.: The hyperglycemic hyperosmolar syndrome. Indiana Med. 81:766, 1988.
4. Butts, D.E.: Fluid and electrolyte disorders associated with diabetic ketoacidosis and hyperglycemic hyperosmolar nonketotic coma. Nurs. Clin. North Am. 22:827, 1987.
5. Gerich, J., et al.: Effect of dehydration and hyperosmolarity on glucose, free fatty acid and ketone body metabolism in rats. Diabetes 22:264, 1973.
6. Gerich, J., et al.: Clinical and metabolic characteristics of hyperosmolar nonketotic coma. Diabetes 20:228, 1971.
7. Geheb, M.A.: Clinical approach to the hyperosmolar patient. Crit. Care Clin. 3:797, 1987.
8. Arieff, A.I., and Carroll, H.J.: Nonketotic hyperosmolar coma with hyperglycemia: Clinical features, pathophysiology, renal function, acid-base balance, plasma-cerebrospinal fluid equilibria and the effects of therapy in 37 cases. Medicine 51:73, 1972.
9. Katz, M.A.: Hyperglycemia-induced hyponatremia—calculation of expected serum sodium depression. N. Engl. J. Med. 289:843, 1973.

LACTIC ACIDOSIS

Douglas M. Salyards

CAPSULE

Lactic acidosis is the most common form of metabolic acidosis and the form most commonly encountered by the emergency physician. Two broad categories of lactic acidosis exist: type A, associated with tissue hypoxia; and type B, associated with other disease conditions.

LACTATE METABOLISM

Lactate is a metabolic byproduct of glycolysis and is in equilibrium with pyruvate in the following reaction:

$$\text{Pyruvate} + \text{NADH} + \text{H} \xrightarrow{\text{LDH}} \text{Lactate} + \text{NAD}$$

This reaction is catalyzed by lactate dehydrogenase (LDH) and requires nicotinamide adenine dinucleotide (NADH) and hydrogen ion (H).

Three main factors determine the level of lactate. First, lactate cannot be used in any other intracellular reaction, and is therefore dependent on the ultimate fate of pyruvate.[1] Pyruvate is used as a substrate for glucose in gluconeogenesis and is oxidized in mitochondria to CO_2 and H_2O. Secondly, NADH is reoxidized to NAD along the electron transport chain. This process is halted during anoxia, hence the effect on the redox state and resultant buildup of lactate and acidosis during shock and tissue hypoxia. Finally, the lactate concentration is affected by intracellular pH and its effects on lactate transport, enzymatic reactions, and the lactate/pyruvate ratio. A decrease in pH causes a resultant decrease in uptake of lactate by the liver, and when pH falls below 7.0, the liver may begin to produce lactate.[2] A lowering of pH, however, generally causes decreased lactate production, whereas raising the pH causes elevated lactate production.

Lactate is used primarily by the liver and kidneys, although under some circumstances skeletal and even cardiac muscle is capable of extracting some lactate from the circulation.[3]

The liver normally clears up to 50% of the lactate produced through the process of gluconeogenesis.[3] The kidney normally clears about 30% of lactate, also through gluconeogenesis rather than by clearance. The ability of the liver to clear lactate during certain pathologic states such as seizures and shock, however, is not clearly defined. Studies of hemorrhagic shock induced in dogs with low flow states to the liver have shown variable rates of clearance of lactate by the liver, from markedly reduced to normal.[3] Also, it has been shown that, in low flow states, the liver may actually produce lactate, contributing to the acidosis.[3] It is felt that lactic acidosis can be caused by increased production from tissues other than the liver, by decreased uptake in the liver, and when blood flow and oxygenation to the liver are reduced, by increased production by the liver. All these contributions are variable depending on the underlying cause.[3]

The kidney reabsorbs lactate up to concentrations of 6 to 10 mM to provide the necessary substrate for production of bicarbonate and reversal of the acidosis.[4] This is why rebound alkalosis can occur with administration of bicarbonate after underlying factors are corrected.

DEFINITION OF LACTIC ACIDOSIS

Lactic acidosis is an ion gap metabolic acidosis associated with an elevated blood lactate concentration. The lactate concentration is normally 0.5 to 5 mEq/L. The general consensus is that a lactate concentration of 4 mEq/L or greater with a significant lowering of pH is evidence of a lactic acidosis.[1] No firm criteria for pH has been agreed upon. The pH may even be normal if an underlying alkalosis is present.

DIAGNOSIS OF LACTIC ACIDOSIS

The diagnosis of lactic acidosis is usually not difficult, and can initially be suspected on the basis of clinical conditions. The presence of an anion gap metabolic acidosis associated with a clinical disorder in which lactic acidosis is known to occur, most often in a patient with compromised cardiovascular function, provides a high degree of certainty for the diagnosis of lactic acidosis.[5] Other causes of anion gap metabolic acidosis must, of course, be excluded, and this is usually possible with a rapid determination of the blood lactate level (Fig. 54-4).

CLASSIFICATION AND CLINICAL PRESENTATION OF LACTIC ACIDOSIS

Lactic acidosis is classified into two broad categories. Type A lactic acidosis is associated with tissue hy-

Signs and symptoms consistent with lactic acidosis, especially when shock and/or tissue hypoxia occur

↓

Laboratory values consistent with an elevated anion-gap metabolic acidosis (pH may be elevated or normal with a coexisting alkalosis)

↓

Check lactate level. Greater than 4.0 mEq/L is strongly suggestive of lactic acidosis

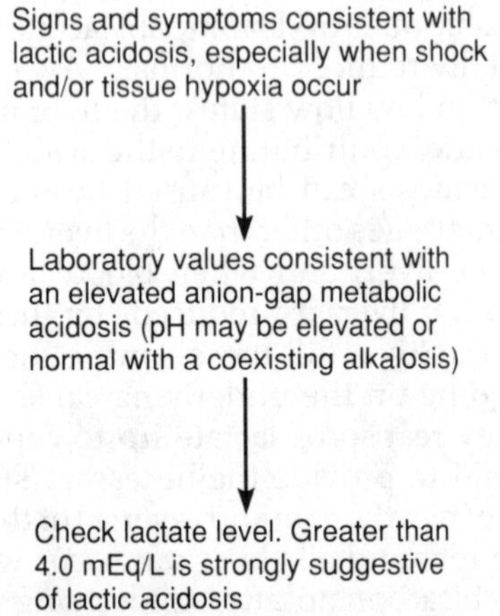

FIG. 54-4.   Initial workup of lactic acidosis

TABLE 54-34. CLASSIFICATION OF LACTIC ACIDOSIS

TYPE A: Associated with tissue hypoxia
1. Shock (e.g., hemorrhagic, septic, cardiogenic)
2. Severe hypoxia (e.g., status asthmaticus, pulmonary embolism, acute exacerbation of chronic obstructive pulmonary disease)

TYPE B: Not associated with tissue hypoxia
1. Underlying clinical disorders
   a. Diabetes mellitus
   b. Grand mal seizures
   c. Primary hepatic disease
   d. Malignancies, particularly acute lymphocytic leukemia
   e. Thiamine deficiency
   f. Metabolic acidosis
   g. Acute and chronic renal failure
   h. Reye's syndrome
2. Drugs, toxins
   a. Ethanol
   b. Biguanides (phenformin)
   c. Salicylates
   d. Catecholamines
   e. Fructose
   f. Sorbitol
   g. Sodium nitroprusside
   h. Methanol
3. Enzyme defects
   a. Pyruvate dehydrogenase
   b. Fructose 1,6 diphosphatase
   c. Type I glycogen storage disease
   d. Pyruvate carboxylase
   e. Subacute necrotizing encephalomyelopathy
   f. Others

poxia, and type B is associated with all other disease states (Table 54-34).[6]

TYPE A LACTIC ACIDOSIS

Type A lactic acidosis, associated with tissue hypoxia, is the most common type seen in the emergency department (ED). Any condition causing shock can lead to this condition. These conditions include hemorrhage, sepsis, myocardial infarction with cardiogenic shock, poisoning, and pulmonary embolism. It is important to remember that decreased tissue perfusion may be present without an initial measurable drop in blood pressure and that hypoxemia may not be present. Lactate is accumulated as tissue hypoxia causes increased production of lactic acid and hydrogen ion, and this may be exacerbated by decreased blood flow to the liver causing reduced clearance or even production of lactate by the liver.

Clinically, the patient may initially develop nausea, vomiting, and agitation, which may develop into stupor and frank coma if the shock is severe. The acidosis causes compensatory hyperventilation in a patient who is not obtunded, and this may be the most common feature.

Hypoxia without shock, as seen in pulmonary edema, status asthmaticus, severe exacerbation of chronic obstructive pulmonary disease, and asphyxiation may also cause type A lactic acidosis. The hypoxia is usually severe and acute and is most often associated with an inability to compensate for the respiratory insult.

TYPE B LACTIC ACIDOSIS

Type B lactic acidosis occurs with an elevated blood lactate level and no evidence of tissue hypoxia or shock. Many of these disorders are uncommon and therefore may go undiagnosed initially. This type may appear slowly or abruptly with no apparent cause. The pH may be lowered, normal, or even elevated.

Type B lactic acidosis is further divided into types associated with systemic disorders, types associated with drugs, toxins, and hormones, and types associated with enzyme defects.

Diabetes mellitus is the clinical disorder most often associated with lactic acidosis.[7] Despite various theories and findings under experimental conditions, the occurrence of lactic acidosis in diabetes mellitus since the withdrawal of phenformin from the market has become virtually nonexistent. The association of lactic acidosis and diabetes remains unclear.[3]

Lactic acidosis is common in grand mal seizures, probably because of an overproduction of lactate. This condition is self-limited and requires no treatment. When the seizure ends, lactate serves as a substrate for the production of bicarbonate, and the acidosis is corrected.

Although lactic acid levels are often increased in primary hepatic disease, frank lactic acidosis is rare, probably because of large functional reserves for hepatic uptake of lactate by the liver. Lactic acidosis can occur when additional stresses are placed on the liver, particularly by ethanol consumption or hypoglycemia.[3]

Lactic acidosis has occasionally been associated with malignancies, particularly acute lymphocytic leukemia and solid tumors.[3]

Other disease states in which lactic acidosis has been reported include thiamine deficiency, metabolic acidosis, acute and chronic renal insufficiency, and Reye's syndrome. No clear causal relationships have been defined.

In type B lactic acidosis caused by drugs, hormones, and toxins, alcohol is the most common cause. The increase in lactate levels associated with ethanol is caused by decreased clearance by the liver rather than by increased production.[8] This is seldom severe, and the lactate level rarely exceeds 3 mM.[8] Lactic acidosis can occur with consumption of ethanol when other factors such as liver disease, seizures, hypoglycemia, or diabetes mellitus are present. Lactic acidosis in the alcoholic is easily reversible by the administration of glucose.[9]

Other drugs associated with lactic acidosis include the oral hypoglycemic phenformin (which has been withdrawn from the market), salicylates, fructose, sorbitol, catecholamines, and methanol.

Type B lactic acidosis associated with enzyme defects are included in Table 54-34. Lactic acidosis has been associated with hypoglycemia, but this is usually in association with enzyme defects in gluconeogenesis or glyconeogenesis, primarily in children, or in adults with underlying hepatic or renal disease or alcoholism.[1,3] When hypoglycemia and lactic acidosis occur together, the acidosis may not be reversible until the hypoglycemia is corrected, and often glucose may be all that is needed.[3]

TREATMENT OF LACTIC ACIDOSIS (Fig. 54-5)

The existence of lactic acidosis implies a serious underlying pathologic disease state. There is uniform agreement that the primary aspect of treatment in lactic acidosis consists of identification and treatment of the underlying cause. In the most common form, type A, associated with shock, this implies restoration of blood pressure, cardiac output, and tissue perfusion. Volume replacement is obtained with fluids, plasma, or whole blood as necessary. Ventilation and oxygenation must be ensured. In this scenario, vasopressors are to be avoided because they may increase tissue hypoxia. In type B, underlying causes must also be addressed but are usually much more difficult to determine.

Controversy surrounds the use of sodium bicarbonate in the treatment of lactic acidosis, although it has long been a mainstay of therapy. Severe lactic acidosis has numerous adverse effects, including de-

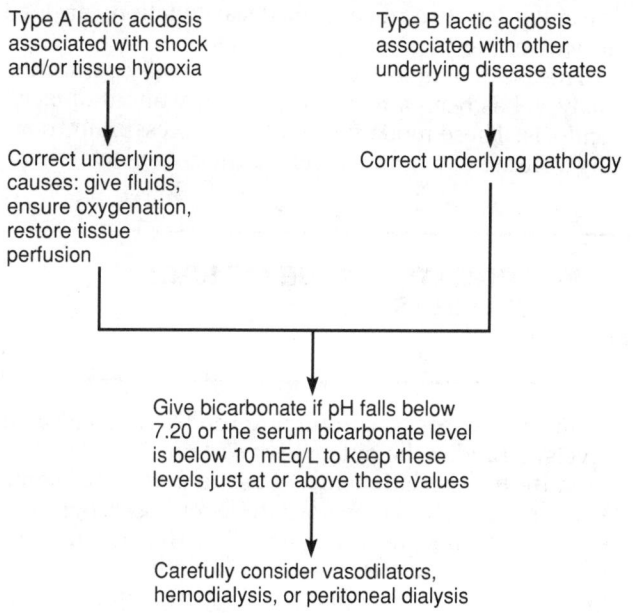

FIG. 54-5. Treatment of lactic acidosis.

pression of myocardial contractility and cardiac output, increased occurrence of ventricular arrhythmias, and impairment of response to catecholamines. Theoretically, treatment with sodium bicarbonate should have beneficial effects by lessening the adverse hemodynamic effects of the acidosis and restoring the myocardial responsiveness to catecholamines. The early aggressive use of bicarbonate may produce adverse effects such as volume overload and congestive failure from the high sodium load, a left shift of the oxyhemoglobin dissociation curve and reduced tissue oxygenation, rebound alkalosis secondary to conversion of lactate to bicarbonate, and electrolyte disturbances. Use of bicarbonate in initial CPR treatment has been curtailed.

Studies on dogs with phenformin-induced lactic acidosis have shown the use of bicarbonate to be associated with worsening acidosis and 100% mortality.[3] Their clinical relevance to the treatment of lactic acidosis in humans is unknown. Considering the clinical conditions associated with lactic acidosis, it is not surprising that treatment with bicarbonate has not been shown effective in the absence of correction of underlying pathology. Because of the seriousness of this condition and the grave prognosis without bicarbonate, however, a recommendation against its use is not justifiable. Bicarbonate is generally indicated whenever the pH falls below 7.20 or the serum bicarbonate level is below 10 mEq/L.[3] Bicarbonate should be used sparingly to raise the pH and bicarbonate above these values to minimize adverse effects. This is particularly true in patients with malignancies to avoid accelerated production of lactate by the tumor.

Vasodilating drugs such as nitroprusside have occasionally been used successfully in the treatment of lactic acidosis.[3] Theoretically, the reduction in afterload might increase cardiac output, tissue perfusion, and tissue oxygenation. These agents must be used carefully because uncontrolled vasodilation can lead to worsening hypoxia and acidosis.

The use of hemodialysis and occasionally peritoneal dialysis has been attempted in the treatment of lactic acidosis. These modalities may be successful in treating volume overload as well as the hyperlactatemia.

PROGNOSTIC VALUE OF LACTIC ACID LEVELS

Controversy exists surrounding the use of lactic acid levels to predict the outcome of certain clinical states. Because of its relationship to tissue perfusion, some studies have shown the lactate level has prognostic significance for the outcome.[3,10,11] This occurs primarily in disease states associated with a low tissue perfusion, such as septic, cardiogenic, and hemorrhagic shock and pulmonary embolism. Other studies

have both supported and refuted these findings. A variety of underlying clinical states could account for these differences, including liver disease and nutritional state. Perez et al.[10] noted that mortality increased from 18% to 73% in patients with a lactate level above 4.4 mEq/L. Weil and Afifi[11] found that only 11% of patients with a lactate greater than 4 mEq/L survived circulatory shock.

Others have noted that a more rapid clearance of lactate during therapy has more prognostic significance than the peak lactate concentration.[12,13] During rewarming of hypothermic patients, a washout may occur, causing increased lactate levels even though the patient is actually improving.[14]

MEDICOLEGAL PEARLS

- In lactic acidosis, the pH may be normal or even elevated if underlying alkalosis is present.
- The most common early sign of lactic acidosis may be a compensatory hyperventilation.
- Severe hypoxia causing tissue hypoxia may produce lactic acidosis without shock.
- Bicarbonate should be used sparingly in malignancies because its use may stimulate neoplasms to increase production of lactate.
- During rewarming of a hypothermic patient, washout may occur, causing the lactate level to increase even though the patient is improving clinically.

REFERENCES

1. Relman, A.S.: Lactic Acidosis. Acid-base and Potassium Homeostasis. New York, Churchill Livingston, 1978, pp. 65–100.
2. Lloyd, M.H., Iles, R.A., Simpson, B.R., et al.: The effect of stimulated metabolic acidosis on intracellular pH and lactate metabolism in the isolated perfused rat liver. Clin. Sci. Mol. Med. 45:543, 1973.
3. Kreisberg, R.A.: Lactate homeostasis and lactic acidosis. Ann. Intern. Med. 92:227, 1980.
4. Yudkin, J., Cohen, R.D., and Slack, B.: The haemodynamic effects of metabolic acidosis in the rat. Clin. Sci. Mol. Med. 50:177, 1976.
5. Waters, W.C., Hall, J., and Swartz, W.B.: Spontaneous lactic acidosis. Am. J. Med. 35:781, 1963.
6. Cohen, R.D., and Woods, H.F.: Clinical and biochemical aspects of lactic acidosis. Boston, Blackwell Scientific Publications, Inc., 1976.
7. Oliva, P.B.: Lactic acidosis. Am. J. Med. 48:209, 1970.
8. Kreisberg, R.A., Owen, W.C., and Soegal, A.M.: Ethanol-induced hyperlactatemia; inhibition of lactate utilization. J. Clin. Invest. 50:166, 1971.
9. Miller, P.D., Heinig, R.E., and Waterhouse, C.: Treatment of alcoholic acidosis. Arch. Intern. Med. 138:67, 1978.
10. Perez, D.I., Scott, H.M., Duff, J., et al.: The significance of lactic acidemia in the shock syndrome. Ann. N.Y. Acad. Sci. 119:1133, 1965.
11. Weil, M.H., and Afifi, A.A.: Experimental and clinical studies of lactate and pyruvate as indicators of the severity of acute circulatory failure (shock). Circulation 41:989, 1970.

12. Vincent, J.L., Dufaye, P., Berre, J., et al.: Serial lactate determination during circulatory shock. Crit. Care Med. *11*:449, 1983.
13. Falk, J.L., Rackow, E.C., Leavy, J., et al.: Delayed lactate clearance in patients surviving circulatory shock. Acute Care *11*:212, 1985.
14. Reuler, J.B.: Hypothermia: Pathophysiology, clinical settings, and clinical management. Ann. Intern. Med. *89*:519, 1978.

BIBLIOGRAPHY

Harrison: Principles of Internal Medicine. 1983, pp. 679–682.

Jay, S.: Internal Medicine 1987, pp. 827–828.
Kreisberg, R.A.: Lactate homeostasis and lactic acidosis. Ann. Intern. Med. 92:227, 1980.
Mizock, J.: Controversies in lactic acidosis. JAMA *258*:497, 1987.
Ragland, G.: Lactic Acidosis. *In* Emergency Medicine: A Comprehensive Study Guide. Edited by Tintinalli, J.E., Rothsytein, R.J., and Krome, R.L., 1985, pp. 628–633.

ADRENAL INSUFFICIENCY AND ADRENAL CRISIS

David Baldwin, Jr.

CAPSULE

Although relatively uncommon, decompensated adrenal insufficiency in an important diagnostic consideration in a wide variety of acute medical presentations. Decompensation is typically provoked by another superimposed acute medical or surgical process that may overshadow underlying cortisol deficiency. Clues for this diagnosis are often nonspecific, yet prompt institution of parenteral corticosteroid therapy is essential to successfully stabilize these patients. Acute adrenal insufficiency may occur from a wide range of causes and in patients of any age, from neonates to the elderly.[1]

PATHOPHYSIOLOGY

The adrenals are highly vascular glands that secrete the glucocorticoid cortisol and the mineralocorticoid aldosterone. Cortisol is critical for the maintenance of arterial vascular tone and blood pressure and helpful in the maintenance of a variety of metabolic functions. Cortisol secretion is strictly regulated by the pulsatile secretion of hypothalamic corticotrophin releasing factor (CRF), which triggers the release of pituitary ACTH. The latter directly stimulates the cortisol-producing cells of the adrenal. The operational integrity of these cells is critically dependent on the presence of ACTH. In its absence, these cells atrophy and lie dormant. During periods of stress, CRF, ACTH, and cortisol secretion are increased many times their basal rates.

Aldosterone has two important roles in the regulation of renal tubular function. The first is its stimulation of the retention of salt and water. The second is its stimulation of the secretion of potassium by the distal nephron. Aldosterone secretion is not regulated by the pituitary but directly by potassium ion concentration and by the renin-angiotensin system. A fall in renal blood flow triggers release of the enzyme renin which catalyzes the conversion of hepatic angiotensinogen to angiotensin I. Angiotensin-converting enzyme (ACE) converts this to the potent vasoconstrictor angiotensin II, which raises systemic blood pressure and directly stimulates the release of aldosterone from the adrenals. Thus, salt and water are retained, blood pressure is raised, and renin release decreases as renal perfusion is improved.

PREHOSPITAL ASSESSMENT

Most patients with adrenal crisis have a history of chronic adrenal insufficiency or exogenous steroid treatment. All such patients should ideally wear an emergency bracelet that identifies their need for exogenous steroids in times of stress. Such bracelets should be sought during the initial prehospital assessment. Ideally, these patients and their families should have available, and be taught to give, 100 mg of cortisone acetate IM or 4 mg dexamethasone IM at the first sign of severe stress such as infection or an accident.

CLINICAL PRESENTATION

Patients may present with adrenal crisis at any age. The typical infant with severe salt wasting congenital adrenal hyperplasia exhibits vomiting, weight loss, and dehydration between 2 and 4 weeks of life. Hyponatremia, hyperkalemia, hypoglycemia, and acidosis are usually present and should immediately suggest this diagnosis. Ambiguous genitalia or precocious virilization are important clues on physical examination.[2]

The clues to diagnosis in adults may be more subtle. Patients with chronic adrenal insufficiency complain of weight loss, weakness, anorexia, orthostasis, and abdominal pain. Acute stress may provoke adrenal crisis with vomiting, fever, shock, confusion, or coma. The most common stress factor is acute infection, which must be sought diligently in all such patients. Trauma, the acute surgical abdomen, and myocardial infarction are other common examples.

Alternatively, an acute medical illness may cause acute adrenal destruction and add adrenal crisis to the patient's underlying condition. The classic example of this is the Friderichsen-Waterhouse syndrome of overwhelming sepsis, often caused by the meningococcus. Another example being recognized with greater frequency is acute adrenal hemorrhage associated with anticoagulants or seen in hypotensive postoperative patients.[3] Hyperpigmentation, especially of knuckles and palmar creases, is an important clinical clue to chronic primary adrenal insufficiency, but is missing in patients with the other variety of adrenal insufficiency, that related to pituitary failure with ACTH deficiency. The most common example of ACTH deficiency or secondary adrenal insufficiency is in a patient who has been chronically treated with exogenous corticosteroids such as prednisone. Recovery of the pituitary-adrenal response to stress may take up to 1 year after prior high dose chronic steroid therapy.

LABORATORY ABNORMALITIES

In primary adrenal insufficiency, the following laboratory abnormalities are seen:

1. Hyponatremia (80%)
2. Hyperkalemia (60%)
3. Hypoglycemia (25%)
4. Azotemia
5. Metabolic acidosis
6. Hypercalcemia (6%)
7. Eosinophilia
8. Anemia

Secondary adrenal insufficiency (pituitary failure) produces the following laboratory abnormalities:

1. Hypoglycemia (50%)
2. Hyponatremia (15%)
3. Eosinophilia (20%)
4. Anemia

DIFFERENTIAL DIAGNOSIS

Acute adrenal insufficiency is seen in:

1. Congenital adrenal hyperplasia or hypoplasia in infants
2. Adrenal hemorrhage (often secondary to anticoagulants or hypotension)
3. Adrenal infarction secondary to overwhelming sepsis (Friderichsen-Waterhouse syndrome)

Chronic adrenal insufficiency ± crisis is seen in:

1. Autoimmune adrenal destruction (accounts for 70% of all primary adrenal insufficiency). This is associated with hypoparathyroidism, Hashimoto's hypothyroidism, Type I diabetes, pernicious anemia, hypogonadism, and vitiligo
2. Tuberculosis (still accounts for 10 to 15% of primary adrenal insufficiency)
3. Primary or metastatic malignancy
4. Fungal infection such as histoplasmosis
5. Surgical resection
6. Drugs:
   —Mitotane, aminoglutethemide
   —Ketoconazole (inhibits cortisol synthesis)
   —Rifampin (accelerates cortisol degradation and clearance)
7. Cytomegalovirus adrenalitis (common in patients with the acquired immunodeficiency syndrome (AIDS). Acute adrenal insufficiency may occur especially in patients receiving ketoconizole or rifampin[4]

Acute pituitary insufficiency is seen in:

1. Postpartum Sheehan's syndrome
2. Trauma
3. Meningitis
4. Rupture of an internal carotid aneurysm
5. Post-operative
6. Apoplexy (hemorrhage of a pituitary tumor)

Chronic pituitary insufficiency is seen in:

1. Tuberculosis, fungal infections, syphilis
2. X-irradiation
3. Primary or metastatic tumors
4. Sarcoidosis or hemochromatosis
5. Hand-Schüller-Christian syndrome
6. Autoimmune hypophysitis

INITIAL MANAGEMENT

Once the diagnosis of adrenal crisis is suspected, the following should be done:

1. Establish reliable intravenous access. Consider a central line.
2. Perform rapid physical examination assessing volume status, neurologic status, cardiopulmonary status, possible sites of infection such as CNS, lungs, abdomen, urinary tract, extremities, and possible sites of traumatic injury.
3. Obtain fingerstick blood glucose measurement and give 50 cc of 50% dextrose IVP if blood glucose is less than 80. Send blood for STAT chemistries, CBC and arterial blood analysis, and catheterized urine for analysis.
4. In patients who are obviously volume-depleted and hypotensive, begin to administer D5/.9% NaCl 500 to 2000 cc/hour. Care must be taken to avoid volume overload in older patients.
5. Give 40 mg of methylprednisolone (Solu-Medrol) immediately IVP.
6. Obtain ECG and chest x ray.
7. In severe symptomatic hyponatremia, carefully administer 3% NaCl 100 cc/hour after serum sodium every 2 hours. Severe hyperkalemia associated with ECG changes (peaked T waves) should be treated with regular insulin 10 units IVP and 10 units IM and 50 cc of 50% dextrose IVP and 50 cc of sodium bicarbonate IVP. Repeat 50% dextrose in 60 minutes if fingerstick glucose is less than 100. If idioventricular complexes are present, 10 cc of 10% calcium chloride should be given slowly IVP (3 to 5 min). Kayexalate (sodium polystyrene sulfonate), 100 g, be administered as an enema.
8. After appropriate cultures are obtained, administer empiric antibiotics to any patients with obvious infection or clues of possible infection such as a history of sickle disease or splenectomy, significant leukocytosis, respiratory alkalosis not explained by hypoxia, and significant hypothermia or hyperthermia.
9. In infants with vomiting, dehydration, and hypotension associated with hyponatremia, hypoglycemia, and hyperkalemia, take a rapid therapeutic approach. The diagnoses of pyloric stenosis, congenital adrenal hyperplasia and congenital adrenal hypoplasia must be considered. Infants

should be treated with D5/.9NS 20 cc/kg. in 1 hour and then 2000 to 3000 cc/m^2 per 24 hours. Additionally, they should receive hydrocortisone, 3 mg/kg. IVP and then 25 mg/m^2 IV each 6 hours.

FOLLOW-UP MANAGEMENT

Once the patient has been stabilized in the first 1 to 4 hours, then testing of the pituitary-adrenal axis should be performed. This is most rapidly and reliably accomplished by administering 0.25 mg of synthetic ACTH (cosyntrophin) IVP and obtaining red-top tube 60 minutes later for measurements of serum cortisol. Stimulated values greater than 20 are normal and rule out significant chronic pituitary failure and acute or chronic adrenal failure.[5] Patients with acute hypopituitarism may, of course, have a normal adrenal response to ACTH despite clinical adrenal insufficiency. The rapid ACTH test cannot differentiate between adrenal and pituitary disease; a 3-day continuous ACTH stimulation test is required for this purpose. Once this stimulated cortisol level has been obtained, all patients should receive hydrocortisone, 50 to 75 mg IV every 6 hours or 10 mg per hour by continuous IV infusion. Solu-Medrol is given as the initial dose of steroid so that there is no interference with the subsequent measurement of endogenous cortisol secretion. Patients should continue to receive 200 to 300 mg of hydrocortisone IV every 24 hours for several days until the results of the rapid ACTH stimulation test are available. Patients with an abnormal test may be slowly tapered to a maintenance dose of 30 mg per day of hydrocortisone over 4 to 8 days as clinical stability and underlying medical problems permit. Most patients with primary adrenal insufficiency (Addison's disease) should also receive fludrocortisone (Florinef), usually 0.1 mg per day, for mineralocorticoid replacement. All patients with newly diagnosed Addison's disease should have computed tomogram (CT) or magnetic resonance imaging (MRI) of their adrenal galnds to look for hemorrhage, malignancy, tuberculosis, or fungal infection.[6] All patients with newly diagnosed pituitary failure should have CT or MRI imaging of the sella as well as a full battery of pituitary function tests (T$_4$, TSH, PRL, etc.).[7]

PITFALLS AND MEDICOLEGAL PEARLS

Whenever the diagnosis of acute adrenal insufficiency is suspected, empiric stress dose IV steroids must be given until the results of a rapid ACTH stimulation test are known. Steroids should never be withheld from an unstable or symptomatic patient while awaiting such results. The sole clue to the underlying presence of adrenal insufficiency may be hypotension, especially hypotension refractory to vasoconstrictive pressors. The differential diagnosis for "pressor-resistant" hypotension includes:

1. Adrenal insufficiency
2. Myxedema
3. Severe hypocalcemia
4. Sepsis
5. Severe left ventricular failure
6. Severe right ventricular failure, e.g., massive pulmonary emboli
7. Pericardial constriction/tamponade
8. Severe acidosis

An emergency bracelet stating that the patient has adrenal insufficiency and takes steroids should be ordered for all newly diagnosed patients before their hospital discharge.

REFERENCES

1. Burke, C.W.: Adrenocortical insufficiency. Clin. Endocrinol. Metab. *14*:947, 1985.
2. Kannan, C.R.: The Adrenal Gland. Plenum, New York and London, 1988.
3. Rao, R.H., Vagnucci, A.H., and Amico, J.A.: Bilateral massive adrenal hemorrhage: Early recognition and treatment. Ann. Intern. Med. *110*:227, 1989.
4. Biglieri, E.G.: Adrenocortical function in the acquired immunodeficiency syndrome [AIDS] [Medical Staff Conference]. West. J. Med. *148*:70, 1988.
5. May, M.E., and Carey, R.M.: Rapid adrenocorticotropic hormone test in practice. Am. J. Med. *79*:679, 1985.
6. Vita, J.A., Silverberg, S.J., Goland, R.S., et al.: Clinical clues to the cause of Addison's disease. Am. J. Med. *78*:461, 1985.
7. Abboud, C.F.: Laboratory diagnosis of hypopituitarism. Mayo Clin. Proc. *671*:35, 1986.

INAPPROPRIATE SECRETION OF ANTIDIURETIC HORMONE

David L. Vesely

CAPSULE

The syndrome of inappropriate secretion of antidiuretic hormone (SIADH) is a common cause of hyponatremia, with 34% of all cases of hyponatremia secondary to SIADH.[1] This syndrome, originally described by Schwartz et al.[2] in 1957, is characterized by: (1) Hyponatremia accompanied by a decreased serum osmolality (< 270 mOsm/L); (2) urine osmolality, usually 50 mOsm/L greater than the serum osmolality, and (3) urine sodium greater than 20 meq/L. Other laboratory features of SIADH are low serum concentrations of blood urea nitrogen (BUN), creatinine, uric acid, and albumin. Increased concentrations of antidiuretic hormone (ADH) result in retention of free water, increased excretion of sodium, and hyponatremia. Symptoms generally occur only when the hyponatremia is below 125 meq/L, and early ones may include anorexia, nausea, vomiting, and lethargy. With further decrease in the serum sodium (usually below 115 meq/L), these symptoms may progress to confusion, irritability, muscle weakness, and seizures. If treatment is not instituted, stupor, coma, and death may occur when the serum sodium decreases below 110 meq/L.

SIADH results from malignancy (two thirds of cases), but pulmonary disease, central nervous system (CNS) disease, and drugs such as chlorpropamide, vincristine, and cyclophosphamide are also important causes. Treatment of mild or moderate water intoxication (SIADH) is water restriction to 800 mg per day and treatment of the underlying cause. Patients with severe water intoxication associated with mental confusion, convulsions, or coma should receive intravenous administration of 200 to 500 mL of 3% saline solution over 6 hours, the goal being to raise the serum sodium to 125 meq/L to cause the symptoms to improve. To prevent cardiac overload, 1 mg per kg of furosemide should be given simultaneously intravenously. Once the serum sodium reaches 120 to 125 meq/L, the intravenous sodium infusion and furosemide should be stopped because trying to correct the serum sodium to "normal" may result in central nervous system (CNS) damage.

PATHOPHYSIOLOGY

The serum osmolality is normally maintained between 285 and 290 mOsm/kg H_2O. Maintenance of osmolality within this narrow range is accomplished largely by regulation of salt intake and output of free water with small changes in plasma osmolality being detected by sensitive osmoreceptors in the hypothalamus. The information obtained by these osmoreceptors is then transmitted by way of the nervous system to modify the thirst response and the secretion of antidiuretic hormone (ADH, vasopressin). Under normal conditions in a healthy individual, ADH is secreted only by the neurohypophysis in response to an increase in plasma osmolality. A decrease in plasma osmolality, on the other hand, normally inhibits ADH secretion.

The syndrome of inappropriate ADH secretion (SIADH) is a disorder in which there is a continual release of ADH unrelated to plasma osmolality. With the continual reabsorption of free water secondary to ADH, patients are unable to excrete a dilute urine, and ingested fluids are retained. This retention results in expansion of extracellular fluid volume and the development of a dilutional hyponatremia. Recently it has been found that this increased plasma volume also stretches the volume receptors in the atrium of the heart, releasing atrial natriuretic peptides, which, in turn, increase the fractional excretion of sodium[3,4] which further decreases the serum sodium concentration.

SIADH occurs in association with a large number of clinical disorders, but two thirds of the episodes are associated with malignancy[5] (Table 54-35). Of the various causes of ectopic production of ADH by malignancies, the major cause (80%) is oat cell (small cell) carcinoma of the lung.[5] Nonmalignant pulmonary tissues also possess the capability of synthesizing ADH. The most frequent nonmalignant pulmonary diseases causing SIADH are tuberculosis, lung abscesses, and pneumonia, particularly when caused by staphylococcus.[6] In recent years, it has become apparent that several drugs used in medical practice cause SIADH. These drugs are listed in Table 54-35. A few of them deserve special mention. In diabetics, many cases of chlorpropamide (Diabinase)-induced water intoxication have been reported.[7] Chlorpropamide stimulates ADH release and enhances the antidiuretic action of submaximal concentrations of ADH.[7] The antineoplastic drugs vincristine and cyclophosphamide (Cytoxan) cause SIADH by eliciting an increased release of ADH from the neurohypophysis.[8,9] The tendency to water retention in patients treated with anticancer agents is further aggravated by the common practice of recommending a large fluid intake to prevent formation of uric acid calculi and the occurrence of chemical cystitis in these patients.

TABLE 54-35. CAUSES OF THE SYNDROME OF INAPPROPRIATE SECRETION OF ANTIDIURETIC HORMONE (SIADH)

I. MALIGNANCY (2/3)
  A. Bronchogenic carcinoma (80% oat cell)
  B. Carcinoma of duodenum
  C. Carcinoma of pancreas
  D. Thymoma
  E. Carcinoma of ureter
  F. Lymphoma
  G. Ewing's sarcoma, Hodgkin's disease
  H. Carcinoma of the prostate

II. DRUGS
  A. Vasopressin and desmopressin
  B. Oxytocin
  C. Vincristine
  D. Chlorpropamide
  E. Chlorothiazide, hydrochlorothiazide, hydrofluomethiazide, and cyclothiazide (thiazide diuretics)
  F. Clofibrate (Atromid-S)
  G. Tegretal
  H. Nicotine
  I. Phenothiazines
  J. Cyclophosphamide
  K. Narcotics and haloperidol
  L. Barbituates
  M. Monoamine oxidase inhibitors
  N. Tricyclic antidepressants

III. NON-NEOPLASTIC DISEASES
  A. Trauma
  B. Pulmonary disease
    1. Pneumonia (bacterial, especially staphylococcus), viral
    2. Cavitation (aspergillosis) or abscess (staphylococcus)
    3. Tuberculosis
    4. Positive-pressure breathing or pneumothorax
  C. Central nervous system disorders
    1. Meningitis, bacterial or viral
    2. Head injury with skull fracture
    3. Brain abscess
    4. Encephalitis
    5. Guillain-Barré syndrome
    6. Subarachnoid or subdural hemorrhage
    7. Acute intermittent porphyria
    8. Peripheral neuropathy
    9. Psychosis (physical or emotional stress)
    10. Delirium tremens
    11. CSF leak
    12. Lupus erythematosis
  D. SIADH In endocrine disease
    1. Addison's disease
    2. Myxedema
    3. Hypopituitarism
  E. "Idiopathic" SIADH

TABLE 54-36. SYMPTOMS ASSOCIATED WITH THE SYNDROME OF INAPPROPRIATE SECRETION OF ANTIDIURETIC HORMONE RELATED TO THE SERUM SODIUM CONCENTRATION

Serum Sodium meq/L	Symptoms
>125	No symptoms
115–125	Anorexia, nausea, malaise, lethargy, headache
<115	Confusion, irritability, muscle weakness, seizures
<110	Coma, death

CLINICAL PRESENTATION

The clinical presentation of persons with the syndrome of inappropriate secretion of antidiuretic hormone (SIADH) depends on the amount of free water retained and the resulting degree of hyponatremia as outlined in Table 54-36. Persons with serum sodiums above 125 meq/L may have no clinical symptoms. These patients may have experienced weight gain, but clinically evident edema is rare. With a serum sodium below 125 meq/L, brain swelling ensues, producing the first clinical symptoms of anorexia, nausea, vomiting, and lethargy.[10] With further decrease in the serum sodium (usually below 115 meq/L), the symptoms may progress to confusion, irritability, muscle weakness and seizures. At this time the person often has a delayed relaxation to deep tendon reflexes. If treatment is not instituted, stupor, coma, and death may result when the serum sodium decreases below 110 meq/L. Untreated acute water intoxication is nearly uniformly fatal, and represents a true medical emergency. The above symptoms also depend on how rapidly the sodium is reduced; the quicker the fall in the concentration of the serum sodium, the lower the threshold for symptoms.[10]

PREHOSPITAL ASSESSMENT AND STABILIZATION

A quick, thorough physical examination should be made to rule out bacterial meningoencephalitis, which may present with a similar clinical picture of confusion and seizures, searching for conjunctional and cutaneous petechiae, nuchal rigidity, Kernig's sign (back and neck pain on passive extension of the knee past 120 degrees with the hips flexed) and Brudzinki's sign (passive neck flexion producing flexion of hips and knees). In children with bacterial meningitis, up to 50% have associated SIADH. Thus, meningitis is especially important in the differential diagnosis in children with these symptoms (see Chaps. 50, 59). Lack of the above meningitis signs with no fever or papilledema suggests a possible metabolic cause of the confusion rather than an infectious cause. With a metabolic cause of the confusion such as hypoglycemia or hyponatremia, the physical examination is essentially normal, with no edema or hypertension.

Thus, with an essentially normal general physical and neurologic examination, the routine laboratory evaluation, including plasma glucose (to rule out hypoglycemia), electrolytes, BUN, and urine sodium becomes important in determining the cause of the confusion. SIADH should be suspected in any patient with hyponatremia who excretes urine that is hypertonic relative to plasma. The finding that the urinary sodium concentration is greater than 20 meq/L provides further support for the diagnosis of SIADH. The serum sodium concentration is generally lower than 130 meq/L with SIADH and below 125 meq/L when symptoms are present. The plasma osmolality is below 270 mOsm in SIADH. Although a plasma osmolality may not be initially ordered in the initial evaluation of a patient with confusion, it can be easily calculated from the following formula, using the results of routine laboratory evaluation.

$$\text{Osmolality: } 2 \times Na^+(meq/l) + \frac{\text{glucose (mg/dl)}}{18} + \frac{\text{BUN(mg/dl)}}{2.8}.$$

BUN is included in this equation so that the calculated osmolality will agree with the measured osmolality obtained from the laboratory; however, BUN does not affect osmolality in vivo. Other laboratory

Serum Na+ > 120 meq/L and mild, moderate, or no symptoms

↓

Fluid restriction (800 mL/day) as only treatment

Serum Na+ < 120 meq/L/day and mild to moderate symptoms

↓

Fluid restriction (800 mL or less per day) as initial treatment only

Serum Na+ < 120 meq/L and coma, convulsions, or severe mental confusion

↓

200 to 500 mL of 3% saline intravenously over 6 hours to raise serum sodium concentration to 125 meq/L

FIG. 54-6. Treatment of SIADH based on initial serum sodium and symptoms.

TABLE 54-37. DIFFERENTIAL DIAGNOSIS OF HYPONATREMIA

Condition	Plasma Osmolality	Urine Osmolality	Urine Sodium Concentration	Edema	Dehydration
SIADH	↓	↑	↑	−	−
Adrenal insufficiency	↓	↑	↑	−	+
Diuretic use, diarrhea	↓	↑ or NC	↑	−	+
Congestive heart failure	↓	↑	↓	+	−
Liver cirrhosis	↓	↑	↓	+	−
Nephrosis	↓	↑	↓	+	−
Pseudohyponatremia	NC or ↑	NC or ↑	NC	−	−
Primary polydipsia	↓	↓	↓	−	−

NC = no change, ↑ = increased, ↓ = decreased, + = present, − = absent

features in SIADH are low serum concentrations of BUN, creatinine, uric acid, and albumin.

Initial treatment with mild or moderate symptoms of water intoxication should be treated only by restricting fluid intake to 800 mL or less daily. Occasionally, patients with severe water intoxication associated with mental confusion, convulsions, or coma must be treated more vigorously. Intravenous administration of 200 to 500 mL of 3% saline solution over 6 hours is usually sufficient to raise the serum sodium to 125 meq/L to cause the symptoms to improve. A greater or more rapid correction in the serum sodium may carry a risk of central neurological system damage (central pontine myelinolysis). The simultaneous administration of 1 mg per kg of furosemide intravenously usually causes a diuresis sufficient to reduce cardiac overload.[12] Figure 54-6 provides a guide based on serum sodium and symptoms for treatment of SIADH in the emergency department (ED).

DIFFERENTIAL DIAGNOSIS

The syndrome of inappropriate secretion of antidiuretic hormone (SIADH) must be differentiated from other causes of hyponatremia. Factitious hyponatremia or pseudohyponatremia due to hyperglycemia, hyperlipedemia, or hyperglobulinemia can be excluded by appropriate blood tests of glucose, etc., or by demonstrating that the plasma osmolality is decreased in proportion to plasma sodium. In hyperglycemia, the serum sodium level decreases 1.6 mEq/L for each increase in glucose of 100 mg/dL.[13] Nonosmotic stimuli of ADH secretion, such as hypovolemia, hypotension, nausea, or adrenal insufficiency, can usually be excluded by the clinical history, physical examination, and laboratory evaluation as observed in Table 54-37 (see previous subchapter for adrenal insufficiency). Patients with depletional hyponatremia usually have physical findings of dehydration, including decreased skin turgor, tachycardia,

and orthostatic hypotension, which are not present in patients with SIADH. Other characteristics of depletional hyponatremia include hemoconcentration, increased blood urea nitrogen (BUN), and renal conservation of sodium, whereas patients with SIADH usually have a low BUN and renal wasting of sodium. Congestive heart failure, cirrhosis, and nephrosis should also be excluded because they can cause both vasopressin-dependent and vasopressin-independent defects in free water metabolism (Table 54-37). These diseases, in contrast to SIADH, usually result in clinically evident edema and renal sodium conservation (Table 54-37). Psychogenic polydipsia should also be excluded because extreme water intake can cause dilutional hyponatremia if the intake exceeds the capability of the kidney to dilute urine adequately. This condition is usually easily distinguished from SIADH because the urine excreted is maximally dilute. Unfortunately, measurement of plasma vasopressin has little or no value in the differential diagnosis because neither the absolute level nor the dynamic response to osmotic stimuli is uniquely characteristic of SIADH or any of the other forms of hyponatremia.

LABORATORY PROCEDURES

The diagnosis of inappropriate secretion of antidiuretic hormone, is a diagnosis of exclusion after the conditions in the differential diagnosis of hyponatremia have been ruled out. The diagnosis of SIADH in a person with normal renal and adrenal function is strongly suggested by the following triad:

1. Hyponatremia accompanied by a decreased serum osmolality (<270 mOsm per L).
2. Urine osmolality usually greater than 50 mOsm/L higher than the serum osmolality.
3. Urine sodium greater than 20 meq per liter.

The response to water loading is useful means of establishing the diagnosis of SIADH.[14] Before water loading is carried out, the serum sodium must be brought to a safe level, generally above 125 meq per liter, by appropriate fluid restriction and sodium administration if necessary as described previously. The patients must be free of the symptoms of hyponatremia. Because all patients with symptomatic hyponatremia should be admitted to the hospital to evaluate the correct long-term treatment and cause of SIADH, this water load test is usually performed after the patient is admitted to the hospital. The water loading test is performed as follows:[14] (1) An oral water load of 20 mL per kg of body weight is given over 15 to 20 minutes; (2) Urine is collected hourly for the next 5 hours while the patient is recumbent.

In normal individuals, more than 80% of the water load is excreted by the 5th hour, and urinary osmolality falls to less than 100 mOsm/kg (specific gravity = 1.005). Patients with hyponatremia who excrete the water load normally are usually said to have a "low-set" osmoreceptor. In marked contrast, patients with SIADH excrete less than 40% of the water load in the fifth hour, and fail to dilute urine to hypotonic levels. When a water load has been given to a patient with SIADH, no further water intake should be permitted over the next 24 hours to prevent symptomatic water intoxication.

This water load test cannot distinguish people with adrenal insufficiency from those with SIADH. Usually hyperkalemia and/or hypoglycemia with or without increased skin pigmentation in a patient with a picture of SIADH suggests the correct diagnosis of adrenal insufficiency.[15]

INDICATIONS FOR ADMISSION

All persons with the described picture of SIADH should be admitted to the hospital to determine the cause. With the large number of possibilities (Table 54-35), it is imperative to do an immediate workup as to the source and begin corrective treatment.

TREATMENT

Restriction of water intake is the key to all therapy for SIADH after the initial treatment in the emergency department. Without adherence to strict fluid restriction, the patient usually presents again to the ED with water intoxication after only a short period at home. Treatment should be directed to the underlying problem. The withdrawal of drugs that might have been causing water retention usually results in prompt resolution. Likewise, SIADH occurring with CNS dis-

orders is usually transient and clears with improvement of the underlying disease. The resolution of SIADH associated with tuberculosis and bacterial lung abscesses is usually slower and correlates with resolution of the abscess or tuberculosis. Combination antineoplastic therapy for oat cell carcinoma has been reported to cause resolution of SIADH with associated regression of tumor in 16 of 17 patients studied.[16] In all of these diseases, persistence or recurrence of SIADH can serve as a means of monitoring disease activity.

With respect to water restriction, a normal diet contains almost 1500 mL of water, and thus, often no additional fluids of any kind are recommended. Because such a regime is difficult for many patients to follow, it is often necessary to use an additional form of therapy. Of the proposed drugs for treating SIADH, at present demeclocycline (Declomycin) is probably the best.[17] Administration in doses of 900 to 1200 mg of demeclocycline causes a reversible form of nephrogenic diabetes insipidus in almost all patients with SIADH.[17] At this writing, there are no drugs that consistently inhibit ADH release from the neurohypophysis or from a tumor. Diphenylhydantoin inhibits ADH release but is clinically ineffective in most patients with SIADH.

PITFALLS

The major pitfall in treating a patient with SIADH in the ED is in correcting the serum sodium too rapidly or trying to correct the sodium completely to "normal." Once the serum sodium reaches 120 to 125 meq/L, the symptoms (coma, seizure, or confusion) usually disappear. Thus, once the serum sodium reaches 120 to 125 meq/L, the intravenous sodium infusion should be stopped and the serum sodium allowed to increase gradually secondary to fluid restriction to prevent CNS toxicity (central pontine myelinolysis).

MEDICOLEGAL PEARLS

No group of symptoms is absolute for SIADH. Confusion, convulsion, or coma should make one think of SIADH in addition to meningitis or metabolic disturbance as a cause of this picture.

Remember that adrenal insufficiency and hypothyroidism may give an identical laboratory picture to that of a person with SIADH, and that the former two diseases need to be ruled out.

With a serum sodium of 125 meq/L or above and no symptoms, do not give intravenous saline. Water restriction alone is better (and less hazardous) treatment.

HORIZONS

Extensive research on the treatment of SIADH is being aimed at developing specific vasopressin antagonists that specifically antagonize V_2 receptors[18] so that diuresis can occur without causing a possible cardiovascular risk by negating the vasoconstrictive effects of vasopressin (V_1 receptors).

REFERENCES

1. Anderson, R.J., Chung, H.M., Kluge, R., and Schrier, R.W.: Hyponatremia: A prospective analysis of its epidemiology and the pathogenic role of vasopressin. Ann. Intern. Med. *102:*164, 1985.
2. Schwartz, W.B., Bennett, W., Curelop, S., and Bartter, F.C.: A syndrome of renal sodium loss and hyponatremia probably resulting from inappropriate secretion of antidiuretic hormone. Am. J. Med. *23:*529, 1957.
3. Epstein, M., Loutzenhiser, R., Norsk, P. et al.: Responsiveness of prohormone atrial natriuretic peptides during immersion-induced central hypervolemia in normal humans. Am. J. Hypertension *1:*128, 1988.
4. Cogan, E., Debieve, M.F., Pepersack, T., and Abramow, M.: Natriuresis and atrial natriuretic factor secretion during inappropriate antidiuresis. Am. J. Med. *84:*409, 1988.
5. Bartter, F.C., and Schwartz, W.B.: The syndrome of inappropriate secretion of antidiuretic hormone. Am. J. Med. *42:*790, 1967.
6. Rosenow, E.C., Segar, W.E., and Zehr, J.E.: Inappropriate antidiuretic hormone secretion in pneumonia. Mayo Clin. Proc. *47:*169, 1972.
7. Moses, A.M., Numann, P., and Miller, M.: Mechanism of chlorpropamide-induced anti-diuresis in man: Evidence for release of ADH and enhancement of peripheral action. Metabolism *22:*59, 1973.
8. Robertson, G.L., Bhoopalam, N., and Zelkowitz, L.J.: Vincristine neurotoxocity and abnormal secretion of antidiuretic hormone. Arch. Intern. Med. *132:*717, 1973.
9. DeFronzo, R.A., Braine, H., Colvin, M., et al.: Water intoxication in man after cyclophosphamide therapy. Ann. Intern. Med. *78:*861, 1973.
10. Arieff, A., Llach, F., and Massry, S.: Neurological manifestations and morbidity of hyponatremia. Correlation with brain water and electrolytes. Medicine *55:*121, 1976.
11. Beal, T., Anderson, R.J., McDonald, K.M., et al.: Clinical disorders of water metabolism. Kidney Int. *10:*117, 1976.
12. Hantman, D., Rossier, B., Zohlman, R., et al.: Rapid correction of hyponatremia in the syndrome of inappropriate secretion of antidiuretic hormone: An alternative treatment to hypertonic saline. Ann. Intern. Med. *78:*870, 1973.
13. Katz, M.A.: Hyperglycemia-induced hyponatremia—Calculation of expected serum sodium depression. N. Engl. J. Med. *289:*843, 1973.
14. Moses, A.M., Miller, M., and Streeten, D.H.P.: Pathophysiologic and pharmacologic alterations in the release and action of ADH. Metabolism *25:*697, 1976.
15. Vesely, D.L.: Hypoglycemic coma: Don't overlook acute adrenal crisis. Geriatrics *37:*71, 1982.
16. Hainsworth, J.D., Workman, R., and Greco, F.A.: Management of the syndrome of inappropriate antidiuretic hormone secretion in small cell lung cancer. Cancer *51:*16, 1983.
17. DeTroyer, A.: Demeclocycline: Treatment for syndrome of inappropriate antidiuretic hormone secretion. JAMA *237:*2723, 1977.
18. Manning, M., and Sawyer, W.H.: Development of selective agonists and antagonists of vasopressin and oxytocin. *In* Vasopressin. Edited by Schrier, R.W. New York, Raven Press, 1985, pp. 131–144.

BIBLIOGRAPHY

Abbott, R.: Hyponatremia due to antidepressant medications. Ann. Emerg. Med. *12:*708, 1983.

Buerkert, J.: The pathophysiological basis for alterations in water balance. *In* The kidney and body fluids in health and disease. Edited by Klahr, S. New York, Plenum Publishing Company, 1983, pp. 149–198.

Narins, R.G., Jones, E.R., Stom, M.C., et al.: Diagnostic strategies in disorders of fluid, electrolyte, and acid-base homeostasis. Am. J. Med. *72:*496, 1982.

Schrier, R.W.: Treatment of hyponatremia. N. Engl. J. Med. *312:*1121, 1985.

Weise, K., and Zaritsky, A.: Endocrine manifestations of critical illness in the child. Pediat. Clin. North Am. *34:*119, 1987.

HYPOTHYROIDISM AND MYXEDEMA COMA

Joseph C. Howton

"You know the thyroid gland in your throat—the one that stokes the engine and keeps the old brain working. In some people the thing doesn't work properly, and they turn out cretinous imbeciles . . . But feed'em the stuff, and they come out absolutely all right. . ."

LORD PETER WIMSEY IN DOROTHY SAYERS' Hangman's Holiday, 1933

CAPSULE

Hypothyroidism is a common clinical problem with presentations that may be quite subtle. As a result, the diagnosis is frequently delayed. Once diagnosed, however, patients usually respond quite well to current therapy. Table 54-38 demonstrates the range of symptoms. Frequently, this condition is not diagnosed in the elderly.

Myxedema coma is the life-threatening end point of untreated hypothyroidism. Until the twentieth century, this was a uniformly fatal illness; nevertheless, mortality is still high at 30 to 40%, even with optimal therapy. Frequently, the diagnosis must be made clinically and treatment undertaken before obtaining the results of confirmatory tests. A solid understanding of the pathophysiology of myxedema coma is essential to effectively manage the critical patient with this disorder.

PATHOPHYSIOLOGY

Primary hypothyroidism, that caused by thyroid gland dysfunction, accounts for over 90% of cases of hypothyroidism.[1] Autoimmune (Hashimoto's) thyroiditis is the most common cause of gland destruction, followed by iatrogenic damage as a result of radioiodine or surgical ablation of the gland in the course of treating hypothyroidism (Table 54-39). Regardless of the cause, hypothyroid patients eventually manifest multisystem pathology caused by deceleration of cellular metabolic processes and the accumulation of hygroscopic mucoplysaccharides in connective tissues. Effusions, which often have a high protein content, occur in various serous cavities.

Myxedema coma occurs as a result of decompensated hypothyroidism. Thermoregulation is defective and mental status altered because of hypothalamic dysfunction.[2] The most common precipitating events for this life-threatening condition include hypothermia, infection, and drug effect (Table 54-40). Drugs and hormones are metabolized at a much slower rate than normal in hypothyroidism. If dosages are not adjusted in a timely manner, predictable adverse consequences occur.

CLINICAL PRESENTATION AND EXAMINATION

The signs and symptoms of hypothyroidism reflect the systemic nature of the disease; virtually every organ system may be affected. Presentation tends to be most subtle at the extremes of age. Classic signs and symptoms include fatigue, cold intolerance, constipation, hoarseness, dry skin with hyperkeratosis, delayed relaxation time of deep tendon reflexes, brittle hair, periorbital puffiness, and nonpitting pretibial edema. Central nervous system (CNS) dysfunction may be manifest by diminished activity, flattened affect, and confusion ("myxedema madness"). Often patients cannot give subjective impressions because of mental obtundation, and the family may be the only available provider of an accurate history. Neurologic symptoms may mimic other illnesses such as multiple sclerosis (MS), myasthenia gravis, and CNS tumor. Cerebellar findings such as ataxia may be present. Peripheral neuropathies, including carpal tunnel syndrome and Bell's palsy, have been well described. Finally, seizures may occur in up to 25% of patients with long-standing hypothyroidism. In some cases, this may be caused by hyponatremia or hypoglycemia.[3–5]

Patient complaints are frequently referable to the musculoskeletal system. Muscle cramping may correspond to objective findings of weakness with paradoxic hypertrophy. Arthralgias and joint effusions may occur, often with typical findings of gout or pseudogout on joint fluid analysis.

Exertional dyspnea may be a prominent symptom, possibly secondary to chest muscle weakness, myxedematous changes in the oropharynx and upper airway, or pleural effusions. In addition, there is a blunted response to hypoxemia and hypercapnea in hypothyroid patients. Such patients are at increased risk for atelectasis and pneumonia.

Unopposed alpha-adrenergic stimulation may cause diastolic hypertension and bradycardia. With increased peripheral vasoconstriction there are cool, pale, dry extremities, cold intolerance, and a reduction of total blood volume of up to one liter. Pericardial effusions may develop, although tamponade is rare. ECG findings, in addition to bradycardia and low voltage, include prolonged Q-T intervals occasionally leading to torsade de pointes and other ventricular arrhythmias. Although the lowered basal metabolic rate seen in hypothyroidism diminishes demands on the heart, increased atherogenesis is seen from abnormal lipid metabolism. In fact, an elevated cholesterol is a reasonable marker for checking thyroid function.

Myxedema coma presents as a maximal deterioration of the processes described above. Unrecognized impending respiratory failure is a common cause of death, and expeditious intubation is frequently necessary. Unlike many illnesses, this disease lives up to its name in that coma is a common finding. Hypothermia, usually profound, is a sine qua non of this disorder.

DIFFERENTIAL DIAGNOSIS

Not all comatose patients presenting with an old surgical scar on the neck are in myxedema coma. Other possibilities that must be considered include drug or

TABLE 54-38. SYMPTOMATOLOGY OF MYXEDEMA* (77 Cases: 64 Women, 13 Men)

Symptom	Percent of Cases	Symptom	Percent of Cases
Weakness	99	Constipation	61
Dry skin	97	Gain in weight	59
Coarse skin	97	Loss of hair	57
Lethargy	91	Pallor of lips	57
Slow speech	91	Dyspnea	55
Edema of eyelids	90	Peripheral edema	55
Sensation of cold	89	Hoarseness or	
Decreased sweating	89	aphonia	52
Cold skin	83	Anorexia	45
Thick tongue	82	Nervousness	35
Edema of face	79	Menorrhagia	32
Coarseness of hair	76	Palpitation	31
Pallor of skin	67	Deafness	30
Memory impairment	66	Precordial pain	25

* With permission from Ingbar, S. H., and Woeber, K. A.: The thyroid gland. In Textbook of Endocrinology, 6th ed. Edited by Williams, R. H. Philadelphia, W. B. Saunders Company, 1981, p. 213.

TABLE 54-39. CAUSES OF HYPOTHYROIDISM

A. Primary Hypothyroidism
  1. Acquired
    a. Destructive lesions
      Hashimoto's thyroiditis
      Subtotal thyroidectomy
      Radioiodine therapy for hyperthyroidism
      Radiation therapy to the neck
      Cystinosis
    b. Impaired function of near-normal gland
      Endemic goiter
      Drug-induced: lithium, phenylbutazone, sulfonamides, others
      Iodine excess (>6 mg/day)
  2. Congenital
B. Secondary Hypothyroidism
  1. Pituitary dysfunction
    a. Sheehan's syndrome
    b. Neoplasms, trauma, idiopathic
    c. Dopamine infusion, severe illness
C. Tertiary Hypothyroidism
  1. Hypothalamic dysfunction
    a. Neoplasms, eosinophilic granuloma, irradiation
D. Tissue Resistance to Thyroid Hormone

TABLE 54-40. COMMON PRECIPITATING FACTORS FOR MYXEDEMA COMA

Infection
Exposure to cold
Drug effect—alcohol, sedatives, diuretics, digitalis
Hypoglycemia
Stroke
Trauma, surgery
CO_2 narcosis

alcohol overdose, hypoglycemia, nonketotic hyperosmolar coma, head trauma, cerebrovascular accident, and sepsis. Several of these entities may coexist or precipitate myxedema coma.

INITIAL STABILIZATION

The patient who is stuporous or comatose from myxedema coma is at a high risk of respiratory failure. Aggressive airway management with early intubation and oxygen supplementation may be lifesaving. A large-bore intravenous line of normal saline should be started, but fluids should be given cautiously because of impaired water excretion and the danger of fluid overload. Although profound hypothermia is usually present, only passive external warming with blankets should be used initially. Active rewarming with heated blankets or heated inhaled mist may cause peripheral vasodilation and a precipitous drop in blood pressure. Cardiac monitoring and pulse oximetry are useful as laboratory tests are drawn and definitive management planned.

TABLE 54-41. RECOMMENDED DIAGNOSTIC STUDIES IN MYXEDEMA COMA

Stat glucose estimation by glucose oxidase strip
Arterial blood gas
Rectal temperature
CBC, lytes, BUN, CR, GLU, Mg, Ca, Phos
T4, T3RU, TSH (frequently not available on a stat basis)
Cortisol level
ECG
Chest radiograph
Urinalysis
Optional studies: Cardiac enzymes (may be falsely elevated),
    liver function tests, CT of brain, CSF analysis, cultures of
    blood and other sites

TABLE 54-42. MANAGEMENT OF MYXEDEMA COMA

Oxygen administration, early intubation when indicated
Passive rewarming with blankets
Large bore IV, cautious hydration with normal saline
Cardiac monitor, pulse oximetry
Thyroxine, 6 ug/kg slow IV push; watch for cardiac ischemia
Hydrocortisone, 100 mg IV
Consider hypertonic saline for seizures caused by hypo-
    natremia
Look for precipitating causes

LABORATORY AND OTHER PROCEDURES (Table 54-41)

For the patient in myxedema coma, an arterial blood gas should be one of the initial tests obtained for evaluation of pulmonary status. A baseline hemoglobin and hematocrit should be checked because many hypothyroid patients are anemic. Values may change as a patient becomes euvolemic. The white blood cell (WBC) count is often low or normal even in the face of infection; however, an elevated band count is a useful marker for bacteremia. Hyponatremia is common and, because of SIADH, may lead to intractable seizures if untreated. Hypoglycemia is rare in myxedema coma alone, but may occur in diabetics with hypothyroidism who develop diminishing insulin requirements as the basal metabolic rate declines. Thyroid function tests should be limited to T4, T3RU, and TSH. Some laboratory order forms list the option "free thyroxine index" or FTI, which is the product of T4 and T3RU. A low FTI is indicative of hypothyroidism. When the TSH is elevated, primary hypothyroidism occurs because of thyroid gland failure. A low TSH in conjuction with a low FTI implies pituitary or hypothalamic dysfunction. A cortisol level is useful initially because adrenal insufficiency sometimes coexists with hypothyroidism.

Work-up of the patient should be guided by history and physical examination. If there is any hint of infection, cultures of blood, urine, and any other appropriate sites should be obtained, and antibiotics begun without delay. CT scan of the head may be indicated if there is any possibility of head trauma or a cerebrovascular accident. An ECG should be performed to look for signs of ischemia or infarction as well as toxic drug effect such as from digitalis. Serum CPK, SGOT, and LDH values are frequently elevated, possibly because of altered membrane permeabilities. There are several reports in the literature of the erroneous treatment of myocardial infarction because of elevated CKMB fractions in myxedema coma.[6,7]

MANAGEMENT (Table 54-42)

An otherwise healthy patient who complains of cold intolerance, muscle aches, lethargy, and constipation may be followed as an outpatient after initial studies such as T4, T3RU, and TSH. A patient with suspected hypothyroidism with any degree of altered mental status or defective thermoregulation manifest by below normal temperature should be admitted and started on synthetic thyroid hormone. The moribund patient in myxedema coma should have the aggressive work-up and management as described previously. The critical interventions in such a patient are:

1. Airway management (oxygen followed by blood gases). Ventilator treatment may be needed in severe cases.
2. Prompt administration of synthroid, 6 μg per kg, slow IV push while constant cardiac surveillance is maintained to watch for signs of ischemia.
3. Significant signs of increased metabolism are evident by 6 hours. Subsequent doses should be 50 μg per day IV until the oral form is tolerated. Hydrocortisone, 100 mg IV, should be given as well to prevent adrenal crisis, which may occur if the patient has any underlying adrenal suppression. Alternatively, the first steroid dose can be given as dexamethasone, 2 mg IV, so that a 1-hour cosyntropin stimulation test can be started concomitantly. This measure will help assess more thoroughly the possibility of adrenal insufficiency. To perform this test, cosyntropin, 0.25 mg, is given IV; cortisol levels are checked before giving the drug and at 1 hour after drug administration.
4. Administration of normal saline for sodium replacement requires the utmost caution. Patients are usually hyponatremic because of impaired glomerular filtration, and fluid restriction is sometimes necessary to restore a normal sodium balance. Some patients have hyponatremia severe enough to cause seizures, especially when the serum sodium drops below 110 mEq/L. Hypertonic saline is indicated in such patients, but extreme caution is necessary to prevent congestive heart failure.

5. Any possible underlying conditions such as infections or drug overdose must be aggressively sought and treated. Septicemia may be present with myxedema coma.

PITFALLS

Active rewarming is a tempting procedure in hypothermic, myxedamatous patients. It should be avoided, however, because it may lead to cardiovascular collapse from vasodilation in these volume-depleted patients. By the same token, diuretics are generally not indicated despite the appearance of pedal edema. Another common pitfall is a delay in intubating a patient with signs of respiratory insufficiency. Pressors should not be given because profound vasoconstriction is already present, and they may contribute to the development of tachyarrhythmias.[8] Finally, failure to consider all possible precipitating factors may lead to delays in administration of antibiotics to a septic patient or glucose to a patient with hypoglycemia.

HORIZONS

Although we have come a long way in our understanding of thyroid gland function, myxedema coma still carries a remarkably high mortality rate. Alternative forms of thyroid hormone administration, such as nasogastric or parenteral triiodothyronine (T_3) continue to be studied.[9] Most authorities, however, continue to recommend IV thyroxine in the management of myxedema coma. As in many areas of medicine, the most room for improvement lies in prevention and early diagnosis. Routine, widespread screening for thyroid disease

is gaining acceptance, and should eventually help to reduce morbidity from this disorder.

REFERENCES

1. Mazzaferri, E.L.: Adult hypothyroidism—Manifestations and clinical presentation. Postgrad. Med. 79:7, 1986.
2. Nicoloff, J.T.: Thyroid storm and myxedema coma. Med. Clin. North Am. 69:1005, 1985.
3. Tachman, M.L., and Guthrie, G.P.: Hypothyroidism: Diversity of presentation. Endocr. Rev. 5:456, 1984.
4. Klein, I., and Levy, G.S.: Unusual manifestations of hypothyroidism. Arch. Intern. Med. 144:123, 1984.
5. Bastenie, P.A., Bonnyns, M., and Vanhaelst, L.: Natural history of primary myxedema. Am. J. Med. 79:91, 1985.
6. Hickman, P.E., et al.: Cardiac enzyme changes in myxedema coma. Clin. Chem. 33:622, 1987.
7. Nee, P.A., et al.: Hypothermic myxedema coma erroneously diagnosed as myocardial infarction because of increased CKMB. Clin. Chem. 33:1083, 1987.
8. Bagdade, J.D.: Endocrine emergencies. Med. Clin. North Am. 70:1111, 1986.
9. Pereira, V.G., et al.: Management of myxedema coma: Report on three successfully treated cases with nasogastric or intravenous administration of triiodothyronine. J. Endocr. Invest. 5:331, 1982.

BIBLIOGRAPHY

Goldstein, B.J., and Mushlin, A.I.: Use of a single thyroxine test to evaluate ambulatory medical patients for suspected hypothyroidism. J. Gen. Intern. Med. 2:20, 1987.

Jordan, R.M.: Endocrine emergencies. Med. Clin. North Am. 67:1193, 1983.

Mitchell, J.M.: Thyroid disease in the emergency department. Emerg. Med. Clin. North Am. 7:885, 1989.

Sawin, C.T.: Hypothyroidism. Med. Clin. North Am. 69:989, 1985.

HYPERTHYROIDISM AND THYROID STORM

Joseph C. Howton

CAPSULE

Hyperthyroidism is a common endocrinologic derangement that may present with vague constitutional complaints. After obtaining initial laboratory tests, most patients may be worked up as outpatients. Initiating treatment with beta-blockers should be considered in the absence of contraindications.

Thyroid storm is a life-threatening metabolic event characterized by hyperthermia, unremitting tachycardia, and altered mental status. The diagnosis must often be made clinically. Rapid intervention with cooling measures, beta-blockade when appropriate, and inhibition of thyroid hormone production and secretion are essential to prevent an adverse outcome. Any underlying causes must be sought and treated.

PATHOPHYSIOLOGY

The thyroid hormones thyroxine (T_4) and triiodothyronine (T_3) are formed in the thyroid gland by the iodination of tyrosine and the coupling of iodoamino acid residues. The thyroid gland is the only source of endogenous T_4; T_3, on the other hand, is primarily formed in the periphery by deiodination of the outer ring of T_4. The thyroid hormones exert their effects through a variety of mechanisms, including stimulation of mitochondrial oxidative metabolism, potentiation of catecholamine-induced lipolysis, and modulation of the linkage between the catecholamine receptors and adenylate cyclase. Thyroid hormones in the bloodstream are tightly but reversibly bound to several plasma proteins, the most important being thyroid hormone-binding globulin (TBG). It is the unbound ("free") T_4 and T_3 that are the active moieties. The small quantities of T_4 (0.03%) and T_3 (0.3%) that are not protein-bound are in rapid equilibrium with the protein-bound fraction. Variations of TBG levels are common. Most of the changes of measured T_4 concentration (which measures both bound and unbound fractions) that occur in clinically euthyroid patients are caused by predictable fluctuations in the TBG level. For example, pregnant patients or those on oral contraceptives have elevated levels of TBG and have an elevated T_4 on assay. They are, however, usually clinically euthyroid because the amount of free hormone is unchanged. In some pathologic states, the affinity of T_4 to TBG is affected, resulting in more free hormone without affecting the T_4 level seen on assay.

TABLE 54-43. COMMON PRECIPITATING FACTORS IN THYROID STORM

Trauma
Sepsis
Pulmonary embolism
Adrenocortical insufficiency
DKA
Childbirth
Iodinated dyes
Bowel infarction
Congestive heart failure
Psychiatric dis-

Measurement of actual free T_4 is a cumbersome procedure. Instead, the resin uptake test is used: the serum is enriched with labeled hormone and incubated with a resin that binds hormone. The percent of labeled hormone taken up by the resin varies inversely with the concentration of unoccupied binding sites on TBG. T_3 is usually chosen for labeling because it is less tightly bound than T_4, yielding higher and more accurate uptake values. Normal values for resin-T_3 uptake (RT_3U) range from 25 to 35%. The product of the serum T_4 concentration and the RT_3U is the "free T_4 index" (FTI) and varies directly with changes in the free T_4. The FTI therefore corrects for fluctuations in TBG levels and gives a close approximation of the amount of active thyroid hormone in the extra-thyroidal tissues.

Hyperthyroidism or thyrotoxicosis is a clinical state resulting from an excess of free thyroid hormone. In most cases, both T_4 and T_3 are elevated. Thyrotoxicosis with only elevation of T_3 and a normal T_4 has been described, however. Among the many causes of hyperthyroidism, in descending order of frequency, are Graves' disease, toxic nodular goiter, thyroiditis, exogenous iodide, TSH excess (pituitary tumor, choriocarcinoma), thyroid carcinoma, and hyperthyroidism factitia from exogenous thyroid. Although there are findings of excessive adrenergic stimulation, levels of circulating catecholamines are usually normal in hyperthyroidism. It is postulated that thyroid hormone causes heightened responsiveness of tissues to catecholamines in addition to direct effects that the hormones may have by binding to cellular receptors.

The pathophysiology of thyroid storm is that of decompensated hyperthyroidism. In the past, this dreaded complication was most often seen in hyperthyroid patients inadequately treated before surgery. Currently, major stresses such as sepsis, DKA, or adrenocortical insufficiency are the most common precipitating factors (Table 54-43). Interestingly, thyroid hormone levels are not much different when comparing patients with simple thyrotoxicosis to those in thyroid storm. The precise mechanism by which patients are "tipped over the edge" into the maelstrom of fulminant storm remains to be elucidated. Factors regulating thyroid hormone binding to globulins and cellular receptors as well as tissue sensitivity to catecholamines are paramount.

CLINICAL PRESENTATION

A patient with hyperthyroidism may present with numerous vague complaints. Insomnia, palpitations, hyperdefecation, neck swelling, weakness, weight loss, and heat intolerance are common symptoms (Table 54-44). The classic physical findings of Graves' dis-

TABLE 54-44. INCIDENCE OF SYMPTOMS AND SIGNS OBSERVED IN 247 PATIENTS WITH THYROTOXICOSIS*

Symptom	Percent	Symptom	Percent
Nervousness	99	Increased appetite	65
Increased sweating	91	Eye complaints	54
Hypersensitivity to heat	89	Swelling of legs	35
Palpitation	89	Hyperdefecation (without diarrhea)	33
Fatigue	88	Diarrhea	23
Weight loss	85	Anorexia	9
Tachycardia	82	Constipation	4
Dyspnea	75	Weight gain	2
Weakness	70		

Sign	Percent	Sign	Percent
Tachycardia†	100	Eye signs	71
Goiter‡	100	Atrial fibrillation	10
Skin changes	97	Splenomegaly	10
Tremor	97	Gynecomastia	10
Bruit over thyroid	77	Liver palms	8

* With permission from Ingbar, S. H., and Woeber, K. A.: The thyroid gland. *In* Textbook of Endocrinology, 6th ed. Edited by Williams, R. H. Philadelphia, W. B. Saunders Company, 1981, p. 187.
† In other studies, thyrotoxic patients with normal pulse rate have been observed.
‡ The data shown in this table are taken from Williams, R. H.: J. Clin. Endocr. 6:1, 1946.

ease are diffuse goiter, ophthalmopathy, and dermopathy. The thyroid is palpably enlarged in 95% of cases, and bruits are common. Exophthalmos occurs from orbital deposition of mucopolysaccharides and is often asymmetric. Increased sympathetic tone leads to lid retraction with increased scleral visibility. The dermopathy of Graves' disease is manifest as raised plaques with an orange peel appearance that may be intensely pruritic. They occur most commonly on the shins (hence the misnomer "pretibial myxedema").

Elderly patients are especially susceptible to deleterious cardiac effects, and may present with congestive heart failure or atrial fibrillation. In addition, in older patients the clinical picture may be one of apathy rather than hyperactivity. The only complaints may be of weakness and weight loss without obvious signs of a hypermetabolic state. Therefore, it is important to consider hyperthyroidism in all patients with unexplained cardiac failure or arrhythmias, especially those of atrial origin.

THYROID STORM

Thyroid storm typically presents with manifestations of decompensated hyperthyroidism. The patient appears toxic, with fever up to 106°F or more, unremitting tachycardia, and delirium. Hypotension, vomiting, and diarrhea are common. Essential for the diagnosis is altered mental status manifested by anything from mild confusion to deep coma.[2,3] A precipitating event or illness is usually uncovered after careful evaluation.

DIFFERENTIAL DIAGNOSIS

Signs and symptoms of certain nonthyroid disorders may overlap those of hyperthyroidism. Anxiety and tremulousness, prominent features of hyperthyroidism, may also occur from a purely emotional basis. Hyperthyroid patients, however, usually have warm and moist extremities as opposed to the cold and clammy hands of the patient with an anxiety syndrome. Patients experiencing alcohol or drug withdrawal may appear diaphoretic, tremulous, and tachycardic. A careful history is invaluable in this circumstance. Pheochromocytoma shares some of the symptoms of a hypermetabolic state. Such patients, however, are typically hypertensive and have a remitting course. Thyrotoxicosis factitia may be suspected when hyperthyroidism is present in the absence of a palpably enlarged thyroid. It occurs most frequently in medical personnel with easy access to thyroid hormone preparations.

Although exophthalmos may occur in patients with Graves' disease in the absence of thyrotoxicosis, other possibilities should be considered. Cavernous sinus thrombosis, retrobulbar tumors, accelerated hypertension, COPD, chronic alcoholism, and uremia are among the many causes of exophthalmos.

Thyroid storm should be considered in hyperthyroid patients with fever, tachycardia, and any degree of altered mental status. A patient not known to be hyperthyroid may be thought to have malignant hyperthermia. Patients in thyroid storm, however, do not have the muscle rigidity and rhabdomyolysis usually seen in this disorder. Overwhelming sepsis from toxic shock or meningitis may present with pyrexia, tachycardia, and altered mental status, but the extremities are usually cold and clammy because of peripheral vasoconstriction.

INITIAL STABILIZATION AND MANAGEMENT

A patient suspected of being in thyroid storm needs prompt, aggressive therapy if he or she is to survive. It is often necessary to begin therapy without waiting for confirmatory test results. Even if an occasional patient is found to have an illness other than thyroid storm, initial antithyroid therapy rarely proves to have been harmful.

Successful treatment of thyroid storm involves a multifaceted approach. The danger of imminent cardiovascular collapse is reduced by cooling measures, diminishing peripheral vascular shunting, and lowering cardiac work load. Cooling may be initiated with ice packs in the groin and axillae, fanning, and a cooling mattress. Prevention of the shivering response is essential, and may be accomplished by pharmacologic blockade of central nervous system (CNS) thermoregulatory centers with 25 to 50 mg of chlorpromazine and 25 to 50 mg meperidine intravenously every 4 to 6 hours.

Aggressive use of beta-blockers may be life-saving when excessive adrenergic stimulation is present. Contraindications to beta-blockade, such as bronchoconstrictive disease or congestive heart failure, must be considered. Beta-blockade may be initiated with 1 mg propranolol given slowly IV every 5 minutes until a substantial drop in pulse occurs. Then a propranolol infusion is given at the rate of 5 to 10 mg per hour to sustain the effect. The goal is to achieve a heart rate between 90 and 110 in the afebrile thyrotoxic patient. In febrile patients, the heart rate may not fall below 140 until a normal body temperature is restored.

General supportive measures to replace fluids, glucose, and electrolytes are essential in light of the hypermetabolic state. Glucocorticoids are generally advocated for the hypothetic benefits of correcting relative adrenal insufficiency and inhibiting peripheral conversion of T_4 to T_3. A full replacement dose (i.e., 300 mg cortisol every 24 hours or its equivalent) is generally given in divided doses.

Production and secretion of thyroid hormones may be inhibited by administering antithyroid drugs in high doses. Propylthiouracil (PTU) and methimazole can prevent organic binding of iodide within an hour. Nicoloff suggests a regimen of 200 mg of PTU, 2 mg of dexamethasone, and 5 drops of saturated solution of iodine (SSKI) given orally or through a nasogastric tube every 6 hours.[4]

Ideally, the PTU should be given 1 hour before the SSKI. Patients unable to receive antithyroid drugs orally may be given sodium iodide, 1 g IV every 8 hours. No thioamide preparations are available for IV use; however, methimazole, 40 mg in tablet form, may be crushed and placed in aqueous solution for rectal administration every 6 hours.

Metabolic effects of thyroid hormones may be combated by catecholamine-depleting agents in addition to beta-adrenergic blockers. Reserpine, 5 mg IM as an initial dose with repeated doses of 2.5 mg every 4 to 6 hours may be life-saving in patients with propanolol-resistant hyperthyroid crisis or those with contraindications to propanolol.[5] Guanethidine, 50 to 150 mg orally, is effective in 24 hours, but maximal effect may not be reached for several days.[6]

Patients who fail to improve with conventional therapy may be candidates for aggressive measures to remove circulating hormone. Thyroxine may be readily removed by plasma exchange or peritoneal dialysis; these therapeutic modalities should always be considered when pharmacologic intervention alone is unsuccessful.[7] One such treatment involves removing 500 cc of blood every 3 hours and returning only the red blood cells to the patient. This can be repeated several times.

LABORATORY AND OTHER PROCEDURES

Although thyroid storm is primarily a clinical diagnosis, many tests are useful in managing the patient. A serum T_4 and RT_3U should be obtained for a baseline to calculate the free thyroxine index. Unfortunately, these results are usually not available on an emergency basis. As part of an investigation for a triggering event for a patient's thyroid storm, a chemistry panel should be sent to rule out DKA or look for clues of adrenal insufficiency. A leftward shift on CBC may point to the presence of an occult infection, and blood cultures should be considered. CPKs should be followed for the possibility of rhabdomyolysis and myocardial infarction. Because pulmonary emboli may trigger thyroid storm, arterial blood gases should be obtained. ECG and cardiac monitoring are important in any patient with a profound tachycardia. Chest radiograph and urinalysis should be checked as possible sources of infection. A technique has been described by Goldfarb et al. that may help diagnose thyroid storm on an emergency basis.[8] Technetium 99-m pertechnetate is injected with a flow study concentrated over the anterior neck. This is followed 15 minutes later by static images of the thyroid gland. In a hyperthyroid state there is markedly increased trapping of Tc-99m.

When there is no available history of hyperthyroidism, this technique may be especially useful.

INDICATIONS FOR ADMISSION

A patient in fulminant thyroid storm needs aggressive intervention that may be started in the ED and continued in the intensive care unit. A hyperthyroid patient with a febrile illness who is alert and appears well may usually be managed as an outpatient. It is important to note that an infectious process may precipitate thyroid storm, and close follow-up is mandatory.

A patient presenting with signs and symptoms of new-onset hyperthyroidism or exacerbation after running out of medications may usually be managed as an outpatient in consultation with an endocrinologist. Patients who are unreliable or who appear unable to care for themselves adequately, however, should be admitted for initial management.

PITFALLS

Failure to recognize and treat an underlying cause, such as infection or pulmonary embolism, is the most common pitfall in the management of thyroid storm. Other errors include allowing shivering induced by cooling and undertreatment of a patient because of rapid drug metabolism. Neglecting consideration of alternative modes of therapy such as plasma exchange when pharmacologic therapy is unsuccessful could be a deadly pitfall. Look out for deliberate thyroid hormone overdose, which can provoke marked hyperthyroidism. Symptoms may include fever, tachycardia, and seizures. If the overdose is a suicide attempt, accurate history may not be attainable.

HORIZONS

With advances in our understanding of thyroid hormone production and utilization, mortality from fulminant storm has declined over the past few decades. Further elucidation of the complex relationship between thyroid hormones and catecholamines should bring forth new methods for managing this rare but catastrophic disease.

REFERENCES

1. Shalet, S.M., Beardwell, C.G., Lamb, A.M., and Gowland, E.: Value of routine serum-triiodothyronine estimation in diagnosis of thyrotoxicosis. Lancet *2*:1008, Nov. 1975.
2. Wartofsky, L.: Thyroid Storm. *In* Werner's The Thyroid: A Fundamental and Clinical Text. Edited by Ingbar, S.H., and Braverman, L.E. Philadelphia, J.B. Lipincott, 1986, pp. 974.
3. Howton, J.C.: Thyroid storm presenting as coma. Ann. Emerg. Med. *17*:343, 1988.
4. Nicoloff, J.T.: Thyroid storm and myxedema coma. Med. Clin. North Am. *69*:1005, 1985.
5. Anaissie, E., and Tohme, J.F.: Reserpine in propranolol-resistant thyroid storm. Arch. Intern. Med. *145*:2248, 1985.
6. Mackin, J.F., Canary, J.J., and Pittman, C.S.: Thyroid storm and its management. N. Engl. J. Med. *291*:1396, 1974.
7. Tajiri, J., Katsuya, H., Kiyokawa, T. et al.: Successful treatment of thyrotoxic crisis with plasma exchange. Crit. Care Med. *12*:536, 1984.
8. Goldfarb, C.R., Varma, C., and Roginsky, M.: Diagnosis in delirium: Prompt confirmation of thyroid storm. Clin. Nucl. Med. *5*:66, 1980.

BIBLIOGRAPHY

Cooper, D.S., and Ridgway, E.C.: Clinical management of patients with hyperthyroidism. Med. Clin. North Am. *69*:953, 1985.

Ingbar, S.H.: Thyrotoxic Storm. N. Engl. J. Med. *274*:1252, 1966.

Roth, R.N., and McAuliffe, M.J.: Hyperthyroidism and thyroid storm. Emerg. Med. Clin. North Am. *7*:4, 1989, pp. 873–883.

Tennenbein, M.: Thyroid hormone poisoning. *In* Clinical Emergency Medicine. Edited by Harwood-Nuss, A., Linden, C., Luten, R., et al. Philadelphia, J.B. Lippincott Co., 1991.

PHEOCHROMOCYTOMA

Sushma Reddy and James R. Sowers

CAPSULE

Pheochromocytomas are catecholamine-secreting tumors that arise from the chromaffin cells of the sympathoadrenal system. Patients commonly present with paroxysms of headache, sweating, palpitations, and hypertension. The diagnosis of pheochromocytoma requires a high index of suspicion. Twenty-four hour urine for metanephrines is the most reliable screening test, but for more definitive diagnosis, elevated plasma or urinary catecholamine levels should be demonstrated. Phentolamine, an alpha receptor blocker, and sodium nitroprusside are the drugs of choice in the acute management of pheochromocytoma. Beta-blockers are used to control arrhythmias only after adequate alpha-blockade is achieved. Preoperative preparation for resection of pheochromocytoma involves adequate alpha-blockade, volume re-expansion, and control of arrhythmias.

INTRODUCTION

Pheochromocytomas are relatively rare catecholamine-producing tumors that arise from the chromaffin cells of the sympathoadrenal system. The majority of pheochromocytomas arise from the adrenal medulla (90%), more commonly the right adrenal. These tumors may also arise from the paraganglia cells of the sympathetic nervous system and the organ of Zuckerkandl (8%). Rarely, they may occur extra-abdominally in the neck or thorax (2%). Pheochromocytomas occur at any age with a peak incidence in the fourth and fifth decades of life. In adults, 50 to 60% of these tumors occur in women. Approximately 10% of pheochromocytomas are bilateral or arise from multiple sites. In children, approximately two thirds occur in boys and 30 to 35% of these arise from multiple sites. Pheochromocytomas are an uncommon cause of hypertension, accounting for approximately 0.1% of patients with persistent diastolic hypertension.[1] The early diagnosis of pheochromocytoma, however, is important not only as a surgically correctable cause of hypertension, but also because these patients are at risk for potentially lethal hypertensive emergencies. Malignancy occurs in approximately 10% of pheochromocytomas (more often extra-adrenal). Familial pheochromocytomas usually arise in the adrenal medulla and may be associated with other endocrine or nonendocrine disorders. Up to 70% of these tumors are bilateral.

PATHOPHYSIOLOGY

Pheochromocytomas are usually vascular, encapsulated tumors, averaging 5 cm in diameter, although there is considerable variation in size and weight. Most of these tumors secrete both norepinephrine and epinephrine, with norepinephrine being the predominant catecholamine. Rarely, these tumors may predominantly secrete dopamine. Anatomically, extra-adrenal tumors mainly secrete norepinephrine, whereas adrenal tumors secrete epinephrine, norepinephrine, and occasionally dopamine. The clinical manifestations of pheochromocytoma are determined by the release of the various catecholamines from the tumor tissue. There is, however, poor correlation between the size of the tumor or its catecholamine content and clinical and laboratory manifestations.[1] Nonetheless, smaller tumors often have a rapid turnover of catecholamines, causing the release of large amounts of norepinephrine and epinephrine into the circulation. Rarely, various other peptides (vasoactive intestinal peptide, opioids, vasopressin, somatostatin) may be secreted by these tumors.

CLINICAL PRESENTATION

Patients with pheochromocytoma usually present with paroxysmal symptoms associated with elevations in blood pressure. A severe, throbbing bilateral headache, often located in the occipital or frontal region and accompanied by nausea and vomiting, is typically seen. Sweating is seen in 60 to 70% of patients and is more pronounced in the upper portion of the body. Palpitations, usually accompanied by tachycardia, occur in patients with sustained (51%) or paroxysmal hypertension (73%). The absence of this symptomatic triad of headache, generalized sweating, and palpitations in a hypertensive patient makes the diagnosis of pheochromocytoma less likely. Anxiety occurs in 28 to 60% of patients during the attacks. Other associated features are nausea, vomiting, constipation, epigastric or chest discomfort. There is an unexplained increased incidence of cholelithiasis in pheochromocytoma. Megacolon, ischemic enterocolitis, and intestinal obstruction have been observed. Transient vasoconstriction may present as pallor of the face, paresthesias, arm pain, and even Raynaud's phenomenon. These symptoms are more common in patients with paroxysmal hypertension. Episodic loss of vision or blurred vision may be experienced during an attack.

The symptoms experienced by patients with pheochromocytoma vary in intensity and tend to occur episodically. Symptomatic episodes vary in frequency from once every few months to as often as 24 to 30 per day. Approximately 75% of patients experience one or more attacks per week. Symptomatic episodes also vary in duration from less than a minute to as long as 1 week. About 80% of patients experience attacks lasting less than 1 hour. The symptoms experienced and the order of occurrence remain relatively constant during each episode. As time passes, the attacks usually increase in frequency, but not in severity. Symptoms may also occur dramatically because of the sudden explosive discharge of catecholamines into the circulation. Postural changes, anxiety, pressure in the vicinity of the tumor, smoking, micturition, hyperventilation, ingestion of alcoholic beverages, and various drugs may elicit an attack. Factors precipitating an attack are listed in Table 54-45. Patients with pheochromocytoma may present with a hypertensive crisis or unexplained shock precipitated by general anesthesia, intubation, operative procedures, angioplasty, or parturition.

Sustained hypertension is seen in up to 50% of patients with pheochromocytoma, whereas paroxysmal hypertension occurs in 40 to 50%. Most patients with sustained hypertension also have superimposed paroxysms. Patients with pheochromocytoma characteristically have wide fluctuations in blood pressure, with the severity of symptoms correlating with the level of blood pressure. The hypertension is typically difficult to control, with a paradoxic response to various drugs such as beta-blockers, hydralazine, guanethidine, and ganglionic blockers. The presence of orthostatic hypotension in an untreated hypertensive patient suggests the possibility of underlying pheochromocytoma. Transient electrocardiographic changes suggestive of myocardial ischemia and tachyarrhythmias resistant to treatment may occur in patients with pheochromocytoma. Patients may be hypermetabolic, with characteristics similar to those of hyperthyroidism. Marked weight loss, fatigue, and exhaustion have been observed. Fine tremor and slight elevation of temperature may occur. Glycosuria and hyperglyce-

TABLE 54-45. FACTORS PRECIPITATING AN ATTACK IN PHEOCHROMOCYTOMA
Pressure in the vicinity of the tumor
Anxiety, trauma, pain, hyperventilation
Exercise, postural changes
Micturition, bladder distention, sexual intercourse
Increased abdominal pressure, straining at stool
Valsalva maneuver, pressure on the carotid sinuses
Sneezing, laughing, shaving, gargling, smoking
Changes in body temperature, certain odors
Foods containing tyramine (cheese, beer, wine) or synephrine (citrus fruit)
Intubation, general anesthesia, parturition
Angiography, operative procedures
Drugs
Antihypertensives: beta-blockers, hydralazine, guanethidine, ganglionic blockers
Tricyclic antidepressants: imipramine, desipramine
Morphine, meperidine, nalozone
Cholinergic agents: succinylcholine, methacholine
Phenothiazines, metoclopramide, droperidol
Cytotoxic drug therapy
Saralasin, angiotensin II analogues
Sympathomimetics: epinephrine
Histamine, nicotine, tyramine
Glucagon, adrenocorticotrophic hormone (ACTH), thyrotropin-releasing hormone (TRH)

mia are commonly seen. The combination of diabetes mellitus, hypermetabolism, and hypertension is suggestive of pheochromocytoma.

The clinical symptoms and signs encountered in the Mayo Clinic series of 76 patients with pheochromocytoma are shown in Tables 54-46 and 54-47, respectively.[2] The clinical features may suggest the predominant catecholamine secreted by the tumor. Epinephrine-secreting tumors present with tachycardia, disproportionate systolic hypertension, sweating, flushing, and rarely hypotension and syncope. The rare patient with a predominantly dopamine-secreting tumor typically presents with normotensive paroxysmal attacks. Although unusual, both epinephrine- and dopamine-secreting tumors are more common as part of familial syndromes. Norepinephrine-secreting tumors are commonly associated with hypermetabolism and diastolic hypertension.

PHYSICAL EXAMINATION

Patients with actively secreting pheochromocytomas are often thin, feel warm, perspire, and have cool and moist extremities. Pallor of the face and chest may be present. Patients are anxious, tachycardic, and hypertensive. Orthostatic hypotension may be present. Grade II to III retinopathy, similar to that seen in essential hypertension, may be seen in 55% of patients

TABLE 54-46. SYMPTOMS OF PHEOCHROMOCYTOMA*

Symptom	Occurrence (%)
COMMON	
Headache	72–92
Sweating	60–70
Palpitations with or without tachycardia	51–73
Nervousness	35–40
Weight loss	40–70
Chest or abdominal pain	22–48
Nausea with or without vomiting	26–43
Weakness or fatigue	15–38
LESS COMMON	
Visual disturbance	3–21
Constipation	0–13
Paresthesias or pains in arms	0–11
Polydipsia, polyuria	0–2
Flushing	~18
Dyspnea	11–19
Dizziness	3–11
Convulsions (grand mal)	3–5
Bradycardia (noted by patients)	3–8
Warmth with or without heat intolerance	13–15
Tightness in throat	~8
Tinnitus, dysarthria, gagging	3

* With permission from Sowers, J. R.: Pheochromocytoma. *In* Manual of Endocrinology and Metabolism. Edited by Lavin, N. Boston, Little, Brown and Company, 1986, p. 131.

with persistent hypertension. These retinal changes improve after removal of the pheochromocytoma and normalization of blood pressure. A palpable abdominal mass may be present only in 10 to 20% of patients with pheochromocytoma. Abdominal palpation in such patients may precipitate severe hypertension and other clinical manifestations.

ATYPICAL MANIFESTATIONS

Most children with pheochromocytoma have sustained hypertension (90%). Polydipsia, polyuria, and seizures occur in approximately 25% of these patients. Impaired growth is a typical feature. Nausea, vomiting, weight loss, sweating, and visual symptoms are more common in children than in adults. Acrocyanosis may be seen.

Pheochromocytomas complicating pregnancy may be confused with preeclampsia, eclampsia, or a ruptured uterus if the patient develops shock following labor. All pregnant patients with unexplained sustained or paroxysmal hypertension must be evaluated for the presence of pheochromocytoma. This tumor, if untreated, is associated with increased maternal and fetal mortality.[1] In postmenopausal women, paroxysmal attacks of pheochromocytoma may be confused with hot flashes. The diagnosis of pheochromocytoma

TABLE 54-47. CLINICAL SIGNS OF PHEOCHROMOCYTOMA*

Blood Pressure Changes (seen in 98% of patients):
  Sustained hypertension in 50 to 60% with superimposed paroxysms in 50%
  Hypertension is intermittent in up to 50%; rarely, there is paroxysmal hypotension or hypertension alternating with hypotension
  Hypertension induced by a physical maneuver such as exercise, postural change, or palpation and massage of flank or mass elsewhere
  Orthostatic hypotension with or without postural tachycardia
  Paradoxic blood pressure response to some antihypertensive drugs and marked pressor response with induction of anesthesia
Other Signs of Catecholamine Excess
  Hyperhydrosis
  Tachycardia or reflex bradycardia, forceful heartbeat, arrhythmia
  Pallor of face and upper part of body (seen in 28 to 60%)
  Anxious, frightened, troubled appearance
  Hypertensive retinopathy (seen in 50 to 70%)
  Dilated pupils; rarely, exophthalmus, larcrimation, scleral pallor or injection; pupil may not react to light
  Leanness or underweight
  Tremor
  Raynaud's phenomenon or livedo reticularis; occasionally, puffy, red cyanotic hands in children; skin of extremities wet, cold, clammy, and pale; gooseflesh; cyanotic nailbeds (occasionally)
  Fever
Mass Lesion
  Palpable tumor in abdomen (rare)
  Neck pheochromocytoma or chemodectoma
  Thyroid carcinoma (in MEN-II)
  Thyroid swelling (very rare and seen only during hypertensive paroxysms)
Signs Caused by Encroachment on Adjacent Structures or by Invasion and Pressure Effects of Metastases
Manifestations Related to Complications or Coexisting Diseases or Syndromes
  Sudden death after minor trauma
  Arrhythmias, tachycardia, unexplained hypotension, or cardiac arrest after induction of general anesthesia
  Congestive heart failure with or without cardiomyopathy
  Fever, leukocytosis, and sustained hypotension simulating gram-negative shock
  Myocardial infarction
  Cerebrovascular accident
  Azotemia
  Ischemic enterocolitis with or without megacolon
  Dissecting aneurysm
  Hypertensive encephalopathy
  Severe pre-eclampsia during pregnancy; fever, shock, or sudden death pre- or postpartum
  Cholelithiasis

Key: MEN-II = multiple endocrine neoplasia, type II.
* With permission from Sowers, J. R. Pheochromocytoma. *In* Manual of Endocrinology and Metabolism. Edited by Lavin, N. Boston, Little, Brown and Company, 1986, p. 131.

must be entertained when hormonal therapy fails to alleviate the postmenopausal symptoms.

Pheochromocytomas of the urinary bladder occur more frequently in the second decade of life. These tumors account for 10% of extra-adrenal pheochromocytomas. Bladder pheochromocytomas must be suspected in patients presenting with painless hematuria and micturitional attacks, i.e., palpitations, headache, sweating and nausea during or immediately after voiding. The diagnosis may be further suggested by the presence of elevated blood pressure during micturition or massage of the bladder.[1]

FAMILIAL SYNDROMES

Pheochromocytomas can occur as an inherited disorder and may be associated with other endocrine or nonendocrine disorders, as follows:

1. Multiple endocrine neoplasia type II-a: This syndrome comprises medullary carcinoma of the thyroid, parathyroid adenoma or hyperplasia, and rarely bilateral adrenocortical hyperplasia in patients with pheochromocytoma.
2. Multiple endocrine neoplasia type II-b: Pheochromocytoma in association with medullary thyroid carcinoma, mucosal neuromas, thickened corneal nerves, alimentary tract ganglioneuromatosis, and occasionally marfanoid habitus are seen in this familial syndrome.
3. Neurofibromatosis: This occurs in 5% of patients with pheochromocytomas. Café-au-lait spots may be present.

DIAGNOSIS

All patients with suspected pheochromocytoma presenting with hypertensive crisis must be admitted to the hospital. Indications for workup are listed in Table 54-48. Conditions that must be considered in the differential diagnosis of pheochromocytoma are given in Table 54-49.

The diagnosis of pheochromocytoma is established by the demonstration of elevated urinary or plasma catecholamine levels. Measurement of total metanephrines, 3-methoxy metabolites of norepinephrine and epinephrine, in a 24-hour urine collection is the most reliable screening test. A single voided spot urine metanephrine correlates closely with the results of the 24-hour urine collection.[3] Measurement of urinary vanillylmandelic acid, although readily available, is associated with a higher incidence of false negatives and false positives. False elevation in urinary metanephrines may occur from administration of chlorpromazine, benzodiazepines, or sympathomimetics. Determination of urinary free catecholamines may be used to confirm an elevated urinary metanephrine or

TABLE 54-48. INDICATIONS FOR SCREENING PATIENTS FOR PHEOCHROMOCYTOMA*

1. Severe sustained or paroxysmal hypertension associated with
   Diabetes mellitus
   Hypermetabolism
   Grade 3 or 4 retinopathy
2. Recurrent symptomatic episodes suggestive of pheochromocytoma
3. Hypertension in children
4. Family history of pheochromocytoma or MEN-II-a or II-b syndromes
5. Paradoxic increase in blood pressure with beta-blockers, hydralazine, guanethidine, or ganglionic blockers
6. Unexplained or paroxysmal hypertension during pregnancy
7. Hypertensive episodes during anesthesia, surgery, labor, or radiologic procedures
8. Unexplained circulatory shock following parturition, anesthesia or surgery
9. Radiographic evidence of a suprarenal mass
10. Unexplained pyrexia

* Adapted with permission from Manger, W. M., Gifford, R. W., Jr., and Hoffman, B. B.: Pheochromocytoma: A clinical and experimental overview. Curr. Probl. Cancer 9:1, 1985.

TABLE 54-49. DIFFERENTIAL DIAGNOSIS OF SUSPECTED PHEOCHROMOCYTOMA*

All forms of hypertension (sustained and paroxysmal)
Anxiety, tension states, psychoneurosis, psychosis
Diabetes mellitus
Paroxysmal tachycardia
Hyperdynamic circulatory state
Menopause (flushing, sweating)
Vasodilating headache (migraine and cluster headaches)
Coronary insufficiency syndrome
Acute hypertensive encephalopathy
Hyperthyroidism
Renal parenchymal or renal arterial disease with hypertension
Focal cerebral arterial insufficiency
Intracranial lesions, with or without increased intracranial pressure
Autonomic hyperreflexia
Diencephalic seizure and syndrome
Toxemia of pregnancy
Hypertensive crises associated with monoamine oxidase inhibitors
Carcinoid syndrome
Hypoglycemia
Mastocytosis
Familial dysautonomia
Acrodynia
Neuroblastoma, ganglioneuroblastoma, ganglioneuroma
Acute infectious disease
Amphetamines, cocaine
Rare causes of paroxysmal hypertension (acute porphyria, lead poisoning, tabetic crisis, encephalitis, clonidine withdrawal, hypovolemia with inappropriate vasoconstriction, pulmonary artery fibrosarcoma, pork hypersensitivity, dysregulation of hypothalamus, tetanus, Guillain-Barré syndrome, factitious)
Fortuitous circumstances simulating pheochromocytoma

* Adapted from Sowers, J.R.: Pheochromocytoma: In Manual of Endocrinology and Metabolism. Edited by Lavin, N. Boston, Little, Brown and Company, 1986, p. 131.

vanillylmandelic acid. This assay is also useful in patients with only epinephrine or dopamine-secreting tumors, as is seen in familial tumors and multiple endocrine neoplasia type II syndromes. Measurement of plasma catecholamines is useful in diagnosing a tumor that secretes episodically. Bravo et al. have found fasting basal supine plasma catecholamine levels more reliable than urinary metanephrines or vanillylmandelic acid.[4] Spurious plasma catecholamine results, however, may be obtained from elevation of catecholamines as a result of various conditions such as anxiety, smoking, volume depletion, anoxia, exercise, marked obesity, renal failure, acidosis, increased intracranial pressure, and drugs such as methyldopa or L-dopa.

Various suppressive and provocative tests are used to diagnose pheochromocytoma in patients in whom the above-mentioned hormonal studies are inconclusive. The clonidine suppression test is used to differentiate pheochromocytoma from essential hypertension. Patients with essential hypertension demonstrate suppression of their plasma norepinephrine levels into the normal range within 3 hours after oral administration of 0.3 mg of clonidine, whereas patients with pheochromocytoma show no such suppression.[5] Changes in plasma catecholamine levels after intravenous administration of pentolinium may be useful in the diagnosis of pheochromocytoma. Rarely, in patients with infrequent episodes, glucagon or histamine may be used to provoke an attack. These provocative tests may be potentially dangerous, and phentolamine should be available when these provocative tests are performed.

After biochemical evidence of elevated catecholamine levels is demonstrated, anatomic localization of the tumor is indicated. Computed tomography (CT) of the adrenals with contrast is the initial procedure of choice and visualizes over 90% of pheochromocytomas. Recently, radioisotope scanning with metaiodine-131-iodobenzylguanidine has been found sensitive and specific in detecting adrenal and extraadrenal tumors; in certain centers this may be the initial procedure of choice.[6] Magnetic resonance imaging (MRI, T-2 weighted image) is also useful in localizing pheochromocytoma.[7] Arteriography and adrenal venography have been largely supplanted by CT and metaiodine-131-iodobenzylguanidine scanning, except in unusual circumstances.

ACUTE MEDICAL MANAGEMENT

Patients with suspected pheochromocytoma must have complete bed rest with the head of the bed elevated at 45 degrees. Phentolamine, an alpha receptor blocker, is administered at 2 to 5 mg intravenously every 5 minutes until blood pressure is stabilized. Sodium nitroprusside, 100 mg in 500 mL of 5% dextrose as an intravenous infusion, can also be used for acute blood pressure control. Propranolol, 1 to 2 mg intravenously every 5 to 10 minutes, is used to control arrhythmias. Esmolol, a short-acting beta blocker, 0.5 mg/kg intravenously over 1 minute followed by an intravenous infusion of 0.1 to 0.3 mg/kg/minute may be a useful alternative.[8] Beta-blockers, however, should be used only after adequate alpha blockade is achieved because severe hypertension may result from unopposed alpha receptor stimulation. Patients can be switched to an oral alpha receptor blocker after blood pressure is stabilized.

MAINTENANCE AND PREPARATION OF PATIENT FOR SURGERY

Preoperative preparation of patients with pheochromocytoma involves achievement of adequate alpha blockade, blood volume re-expansion, and control of arrhythmias. Although most patients require only a few days for preoperative preparation, prolonged medical therapy is often necessary in patients who have evidence of catecholamine cardiomyopathy or recent myocardial infarction, or who are in the last trimester of pregnancy.

Phenoxybenzamine, an oral alpha receptor blocker, is the drug of choice in preoperative management of patients with pheochromocytoma. The initial dose of 10 mg twice daily is gradually increased by 10 to 20 mg per day, as needed to achieve optimal blood pressure control, to a maintenance dose of 40 to 200 mg per day. After alpha-adrenergic blockade is achieved, propranolol can be used to treat arrhythmias at a dose of 20 to 40 mg every 6 hours. Prazosin, an exclusive alpha$_1$ receptor blocker, and labetalol, a combined alpha and beta receptor blocker, have been used with varying success.[9,10] Isolated case reports of success with nifedipine and captopril in the setting of hypertrophic cardiomyopathy and congestive heart failure respectively have been reported.[11,12]

Alpha-methyl-p-tyrosine, an inhibitor of tyrosine hydroxylase, is used primarily in patients who are inoperable or who have metastatic malignant pheochromocytoma.[13] Recent reports suggest that combination therapy with cyclophosphamide, vincristine, and dacarbazine is effective in advanced malignant pheochromocytoma.[14]

In pregnancy, adequate alpha blockade before surgical removal of the tumor has been shown to decrease fetal mortality. When the diagnosis of pheochromocytoma is made in the third trimester of pregnancy, maintenance of adequate alpha blockade, followed by combined cesarean section and tumor removal, is recommended.[15]

OPERATIVE MANAGEMENT

Alpha receptor blockers are continued until surgery. Intraoperative hemodynamic and electrocardiographic monitoring is necessary to assess intravascular volume status. Sodium nitroprusside is used to control hypertensive episodes during surgery. Lidocaine and beta-blockers are used to treat arrhythmias.[16]

REFERENCES

1. Manger, W.M., and Gifford, R.W., Jr.: Pheochromocytoma. New York, Springer-Verlag, 1977.
2. Gifford, R.W., Jr., Kvale, W.F., Mater, F.T., et al.: Clinical features, diagnosis and treatment of pheochromocytoma: A review of 76 cases. Mayo Clin. Proc. 39:281, 1964.
3. Oishi, S., Sasaki, M., Ohno, M., and Sato, T.: Urinary normetanephrine and metanephrine measured by radioimmunoassay for the diagnosis of pheochromocytoma: Utility of 24-hour and random 1-hour urine determinations. J. Clin. Endocrinol. Metab. 67:614, 1988.
4. Bravo, E.L., Tarazi, R.C., Gifford, R.W., and Stewart, B.H.: Circulating and urinary catecholamines in pheochromocytoma. Diagnostic and pathophysiologic implications. N. Engl. J. Med. 301:682, 1979.
5. Bravo, E.L., et al.: Clonidine suppression test: A useful aid in the diagnosis of pheochromocytoma. N. Engl. J. Med. 305:623, 1981.
6. Shapiro, B., et al.: Iodine-131-metaiodobenzylguanidine for the locating of suspected pheochromocytoma: Experience in 400 cases. J. Nucl. Med. 26:576, 1985.
7. Quint, L.E., et al.: Pheochromocytoma and paraganglioma: Comparison of MR imaging with CT and I-131 MIBG scintigraphy. Radiology 165:89, 1987.
8. Nicholas, E., Deutschman, C.S., Allo, M., and Roch, P.: Use of esmolol in the intraoperative management of pheochromocytoma. Anesth. Analg. 67:1114, 1988.
9. Nicholson, J.P., et al.: Pheochromocytoma and prazosin. Ann. Intern. Med. 99:477, 1983.
10. Rosca, E.A., et al.: Treatment of pheochromocytoma and clonidine withdrawal hypertension with labetalol. Br. J. Clin. Pharmacol. 3:809, 1976.
11. Serfas, D., Shoback, D.M., and Lereu, B.H.: Pheochromocytoma and hypertrophic cardiomyopathy: Apparent suppression of symptoms by calcium channel blockade. Lancet 2:711, 1983.
12. Israeli, A., Gottehrer, N., Gavish, D., and Melmed, R.N.: Captopril and pheochromocytoma. Lancet 2:278, 1985.
13. Gittow, S.E., Pertsemlidis, D., and Bertani, L.M.: Management of patients with pheochromocytoma. Am. Heart J., 82:557, 1971.
14. Auerbuch, S.D., et al.: Malignant pheochromocytoma: Effective treatment with a combination of cyclophosphamide, vincristine and dacarbazine. Ann. Intern. Med. 109:267, 1988.
15. Burgess, G.E., III: Alpha blockade and surgical intervention of pheochromocytoma in pregnancy. Obstet. Gynecol. 53:266, 1979.
16. Pullerits, J.: Continuing medical education article. Anesthesia for pheochromocytoma. Can. J. Anesth. 35:526, 1988.

BIBLIOGRAPHY

Bravo, E.L., and Gifford, R.W., Jr.: Pheochromocytoma: Diagnosis, localization and management. N. Engl. J. Med. 311:1298, 1984.

Cryer, P.E.: Pheochromocytoma. Clin. Endocrinol. Metab. 14:203, 1985.

Dequattro, V., Myers, M., and Campese, V.M.: Pheochromocytoma: Diagnosis and therapy. In Endocrinology. Edited by DeGroot, L.J. et al. Philadelphia, W.B. Saunders Company, 1989, p. 1780.

Manger, W.M., Gifford, R.W., Jr., and Hoffman, B.B.: Pheochromocytoma: A clinical and experimental overview. Curr. Probl. Cancer 9:1, 1985.

Ross, N.S., and Aron, D.C.: Hormonal evaluation of the patient with an incidentally discovered adrenal mass. N. Engl. J. Med. 323:1401, 1990.

Sheps, S.G., Jiang, N.S., and Kleps, G.G.: Diagnostic evaluation of pheochromocytoma. Endocrinol. Metab. Clin. N.A. 17:397, 1988.

Sowers, J.R.: Pheochromocytoma: In Manual of Endocrinology and Metabolism. Edited by Lavin, N. Boston, Little Brown and Company, 1986, p. 131.

THE PORPHYRIAS

Barbara H. Greene

CAPSULE

The porphyrias are a group of disorders that result from partial deficiencies in the activity of specific enzymes along the pathway of heme biosynthesis. In each disorder, accumulation and corresponding excretion of porphyrins and their precursors occur. Clinically, the porphyrias are expressed by the presence of photosensitivity of the skin and/or acute attacks of abdominal pain with or without neurologic dysfunction or both. The diagnosis is established by demonstrating the excessive excretion of the characteristic porphyrin or its porphyrin precursors or the decreased activity of a specific enzyme. Management and supportive therapy of acute attacks is similar regardless of the specific enzyme defect. High carbohydrate intake and parenteral hematin administration may modify an attack clinically and biochemically. The use of luteinizing hormone-releasing hormone (LHRH) agonists to prevent recurrent attacks in selected women is under investigation.

INTRODUCTION

The biosynthesis of heme, an essential component of hemoglobin, myoglobin, the cytochromes, catalases and other oxidative enzymes involved in drug metabolism, requires production of porphyrins and porphyrinogens. The porphyrias are a family of disorders that result from enzymatic abnormalities in this metabolic pathway. All but one of the porphyrias have a dominant autosomal pattern of inheritance. The exception is congenital erythropoietic porphyria (CEP), which is transmitted in an autosomal recessive fashion. The porphyrias are distinguished one from another biochemically by the type of porphyrin or precursor excreted. The major sites of heme production are the bone marrow (erythrocytes) and liver. The porphyrias may be classified into three groups: (1) erythropoietic, (2) hepatic, and (3) erythrohepatic, depending on which production site is primarily responsible for the abnormal accumulation of metabolites as a result of substrate-enzyme mismatch.

PATHOPHYSIOLOGY

The porphyrias are best understood by examining the basic scheme of heme synthesis (Figure 54-7). For a more detailed account of this biosynthetic pathway, the reader is referred to Kappas, 1989.[1] Rate of synthesis is controlled by the initial enzyme, delta-aminolevulinic acid (ALA) synthase in the mitochondrion. Porphyrins and porphyrinogens are cyclic tetrapyrroles. The tetrapyrrole rings in cytoplasm remain in the reduced state, but the number of carboxyl residues per ring is progressively decreased from eight to two. The loss of these carboxyl groups makes each successive compound less water-soluble. The immediate product at each step is a porphyrinogen, which in turn is the substrate for the next step. The only exception is the final step in which a porphyrin, protoporphyrin, is the substrate for ferrochelatase in the production of heme. This final enzymatic reaction takes place in mitochondrion and results in heme, the volume of which, in turn, exerts a repressive action on the activity of the initial enzyme, ALA synthase.

The intermediate porphrinogens in this pathway readily oxidize under air to porphyrins. The more water-soluble of these intermediates are excreted in the urine, and the less soluble ones are excreted in the bile and thus present in the stool.

In each of the hepatic porphyrias, the basic defect is a partial deficiency in the activity of a nonrate-limiting enzyme (see Fig. 54-7). Although this specific genetic and enzymatic defect is present throughout life, clinical expression usually occurs after puberty. The course of these disorders is characterized by long latent periods interrupted by acute attacks. During latency, with normal levels of heme production in the liver, the defect may be well tolerated, and urinary excretion of porphyrins and their precursors ranges from minimal to moderate. When ALA synthase production in the liver is induced by environmental factors, such as sunlight, fasting, infection, hormonal changes, alcohol and drugs, increased precursor production overwhelms the defective step in the pathway and biochemical tests for these products become positive. Intermediates proximal to the partial block accumulate and spill out of the liver into the circulation. Depending on the enzyme involved and the extent to which ALA synthase has been induced, this surplus may consist of the porphyrin precursors, ALA and

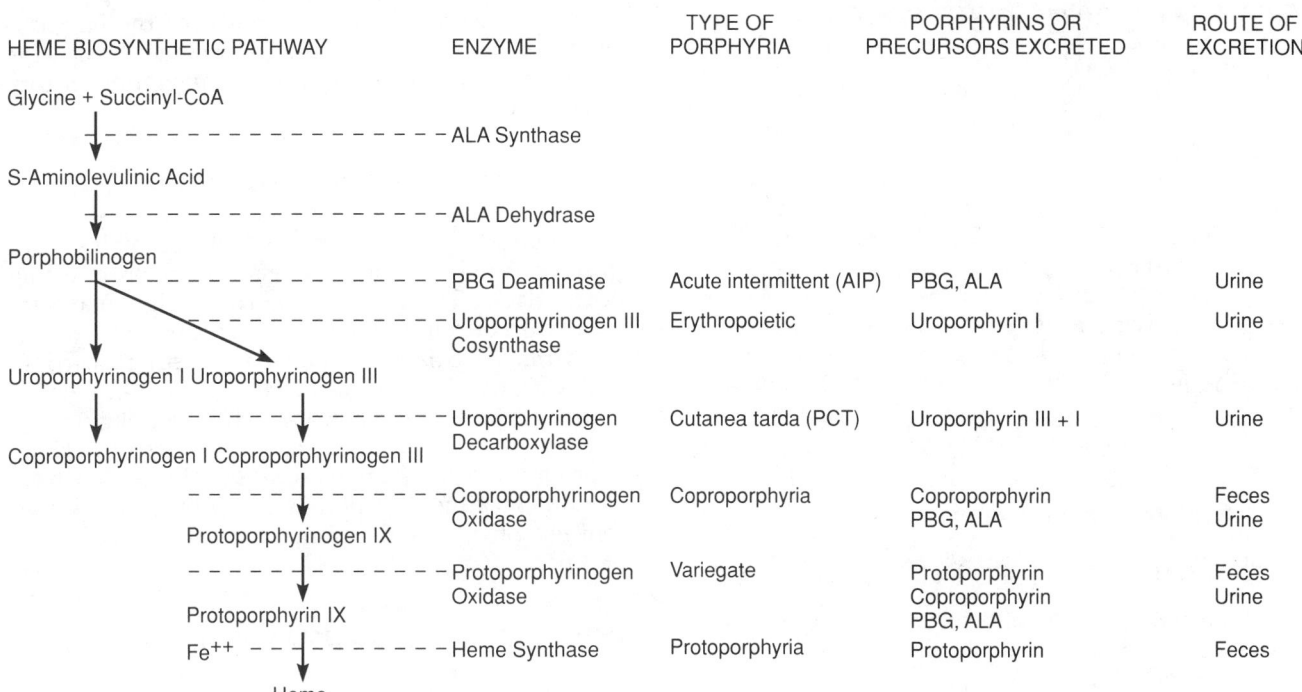

HEME BIOSYNTHETIC PATHWAY	ENZYME	TYPE OF PORPHYRIA	PORPHYRINS OR PRECURSORS EXCRETED	ROUTE OF EXCRETION
Glycine + Succinyl-CoA	ALA Synthase			
S-Aminolevulinic Acid	ALA Dehydrase			
Porphobilinogen	PBG Deaminase	Acute intermittent (AIP)	PBG, ALA	Urine
	Uroporphyrinogen III Cosynthase	Erythropoietic	Uroporphyrin I	Urine
Uroporphyrinogen I Uroporphyrinogen III	Uroporphyrinogen Decarboxylase	Cutanea tarda (PCT)	Uroporphyrin III + I	Urine
Coproporphyrinogen I Coproporphyrinogen III	Coproporphyrinogen Oxidase	Coproporphyria	Coproporphyrin PBG, ALA	Feces Urine
Protoporphyrinogen IX	Protoporphyrinogen Oxidase	Variegate	Protoporphyrin Coproporphyrin PBG, ALA	Feces Urine
Protoporphyrin IX				
Fe++ Heme Synthase	Heme Synthase	Protoporphyria	Protoporphyrin	Feces
Heme				

FIG. 54-7.   *Basic scheme of home synthesis. Modified with permission from Kushner, J. P.: The Porphyrias. In Criteria for Diagnosis. Edited by Hurst, J. W. Stoneham, MA, Butterworth Publishers, 1989, p. 267.*

porphobilinogen (PBG), either alone or in combination with various amounts of uroporphyrinogen, copro-porphyrinogen, and protoporphyrinogen. Porphyrinogens oxidize to their respective fluorescent porphyrins. The excretion of ALA, PBG, and porphyrins is usually measured in urine and stool. This induction of ALA synthase, by direct stimulation of the enzyme or by inadequate repression of ALA synthase because of a paucity of available heme, appears to explain the apparent contradiction between a fixed genetic defect and a relapsing clinical pattern.

The mechanism by which certain drugs precipitate the induction of ALA synthase is uncertain, but possibilities include (1) the induction of cytochrome P450, (2) direct inhibition of hepatic PBG deaminase, as may be the case with sulfonamide antibiotics, or (3) increased heme catabolism, as has been implicated with progesterone. The mechanism by which glucose suppresses the production of ALA and PBG is not clearly defined.

Therapy of acute attacks is designed to reduce the stimulation of ALA synthase by the administration of glucose and/or the administration of hematin to reduce the demand for heme.

Although the genetic and biochemical basis for these disorders is established, the pathogenesis of the clinical manifestations remains speculative. Photosensitivity is directly related to increased tetrapyrroles deposited in the skin or within dermal vessels. Neurologic dysfunction coincides with the excess production of ALA and PBG, but the precise cause of the neurologic dysfunction is not known. Possibilities include a direct neurotoxic effect by excess production of delta ALA, a deficiency of heme, or both.[2]

CLASSIFICATION AND SPECIFIC PORPHYRIAS

A more extensive review of each disorder can be found in Kappas et al.[1]

ERYTHROPOIETIC PORPHYRIAS

CONGENITAL ERYTHROPOIETIC PORPHYRIA (CEP)

This rare disorder is the only purely erythropoietic and the only autosomal recessive porphyria. It is caused by a severe deficiency of uroporphyrinogen III cosynthase activity. Massive amounts of uroporphyrin I are excreted into the urine and impart a reddish-brown color. Erythrodontia (red teeth), hemolysis, anemia, hirsutism, splenomegaly and severe photomutilation characterize the disorder. The stool contains increased amounts of uroporphyrin I and coproporphyrin I (see Fig. 54-7). The erythroid precursors in bone marrow contain uroprophyrin I, which fluoresces intensely under ultraviolet light. Management includes avoidance of sunlight and treatment of secondary skin infections.

ERYTHROHEPATIC PORPHYRIAS

PROTOPORPHYRIA

This autosomal dominant disorder is characterized by mild to marked nonbullous photosensitivity of the skin, leading to scarring, altered pigmentation, lichenification, and premature aging of the skin. Onset is usually by age 4 years. This disorder may be associated with cholelithiasis and chronic liver disease. Preliminary data indicate a 50% deficiency of ferrochelatase activity in hepatic cells as well as erythrocytes. Increased amounts of protoporphyrins are excreted in feces and excess protoporphyrin is present in both circulating erythrocytes and plasma. There is no uroporphyrin in the urine (see Fig. 54-7).

HEPATIC PORPHYRIAS

ACUTE INTERMITTENT PORPHYRIA (AIP)

This autosomal dominant disorder, caused by a 50% deficiency of porphobilinogen deaminase activity, is characterized clinically by acute attacks of abdominal pain and other neurologic dysfunctions. There is no associated photosensitivity. Induction of ALA synthase leads to the accumulation of precursors ALA and PBG, which are excreted in increased amounts in the urine. The diagnosis requires the demonstration of increased urinary excretion delta-aminolevulinic acid and prophobilinogen with normal fecal porphyrin excretion (see Fig. 54-7). The direct measurement of erythrocytic PBG deaminase activity is the procedure of choice for acute attacks and screening, but is not universally available. There is some overlap between the values of PBG deaminase activity in normal patients and patients with AIP, and the measurement of ALA synthase in peripheral blood cells can be helpful in borderline cases.[3] Treatment is outlined under Initial Stabilization and Management.

VARIEGATE PORPHYRIA (VP)

The primary defect of this autosomal dominant disorder lies in a 50% deficiency of protophyrinogen oxidase activity. Photosensitivity, resembling that seen in PCT, or acute attacks, identical to those seen in AIP, occur alone or together. During acute attacks, urinary excretion of ALA and PBG is increased and fecal coproporphyrin is increased, but the fecal excretion of protoporphyrin is elevated at all times (see Fig. 54-7). Photosensitivity is managed by protective clothing and by shielding the patient from sunlight by sunscreen barriers that exclude light within the wave length of 390 to 420 nm. Unfortunately, these preparations usually contain zinc or titanium oxides, which are not cosmetically pleasing because of their heavy consistency. Oral beta-carotene may be useful. The yellow discoloration of the skin caused by the β-carotene can be converted to a more cosmetically pleasing tan by the simultaneous oral administration of canthaxanthin.[4]

HEREDITARY COPROPORPHYRIA (HCP)

Hereditary coproporphyria (HCP) resembles AIP. Photosensitivity, if present, may occur only during acute attacks. The skin's reaction to sunlight may vary from mild burning or itching to urticaria and edema and from vesiculation or bullae to crusting, scarring, and atrophy. The defect in HCP is a deficiency of coproporphyrinogen oxidase. HCP can be distinguished from VP by fecal porphyrin analysis. In HCP, coproporphyrin excretion exceeds protoporphyrin excretion. Treatment of photosensitivity is identical to that used for VP and treatment of acute attacks is as in AIP.

PORPHYRIA CUTANEA TARDA (PCT)

Photosensitivity and skin lesions are the predominant clinical manifestations. From age 40 to 50, there is an insidious onset of hypertrichosis of the forehead and increased fragility of light-exposed parts of the skin. Varying degrees of hepatic injury occur, most often associated with ethanol abuse. The exact nature of the metabolic defect is uncertain, although a deficiency in the activity of uroporphyrinogen decarboxylase has been proposed. Urinary uroporphyrin is increased. The diagnosis may be suspected by observing pink- or brown-colored urine (Table 54-50). Biopsy of the liver may show hepatic hemosiderosis, hepatocellular necrosis, and fluorescence from porphyrin overload. Biopsy of the skin may establish the diagnosis by characteristic porphyrin fluorescence.

CLINICAL PRESENTATION AND EXAMINATION

The two features characteristic of the porphyrias are skin lesions of photosensitivity and acute attacks of abdominal pain with or without other neurologic dysfunction. One or the other is always present.

Mild manifestations of photosensitivity include erythema, skin fragility, and bullous lesions restricted to hands and face; those of a more severe nature include automutilation and hirsutism. For management of photosensitivity, see specific disorders under Classification and specific porphyrias.

Acute attacks occur in acute intermittent porphyria, variegate porphyria, and hereditary coproporphyria. Recurrent attacks begin after puberty and are inducible

TABLE 54-50. SOME CONDITIONS PRODUCING SECONDARY PORPHYRINURIA*

Anemias	Miscellaneous disorders
Aplastic	Bronze baby syndrome
Hemolytic	Diabetes mellitus
Pernicious	Infections
Hodgkin's disease	Myocardial Infarction
Leukemias	Pregnancy
Liver disease	Starvation
Acute hepatitis	Toxins
Alcoholic liver disease	Alcohol
Chronic hepatitis	Benzene and benzene congeners
Cirrhosis (alcoholic and non-alcoholic)	Haloalkanes (carbon tetrachloride and congeners)
Hereditary conjugated hyperbilirubinemias (Dubin-Johnson syndrome, Rotor's syndrome)	Haloaromatic hydrocarbons
	Heavy metals (arsenic, gold, iron, lead)

* With permission from Bonkovsky, H. L.: Porphyria: Practical advice for the clinical gastroenterologist and hepatologist. Dig. Dis. 5:179, 1987.

by (1) low carbohydrate intake or fasting, (2) medicines or hormonal changes (notable causes include barbiturates, anticonvulsants, estrogens, contraceptives, and alcohol (Table 54-51) or (3) intercurrent illnesses. Abdominal pain, often the initial and most prominent symptom, results from autonomic neuropathy. The abdominal pain ranges from mild to severe and is often colicky, diffuse, and frequently associated with nausea and vomiting. It may be accompanied by anorexia and constipation. Diarrhea has been reported. The abdomen is usually soft with only mild tenderness. Rectal examination is negative. Fever, leukocytosis, and tachycardia may accompany the abdominal pain and lead to the mistaken diagnosis of an acute surgical abdomen.

Other autonomic neuropathic signs may include sinus tachycardia, labile hypertension with postural hypotension, urinary retention, and excessive sweating. Cerebral manifestations include behavioral changes, irritability, anxiety, hallucinations, confusion, depression, and seizures. Overt psychiatric disturbances such as mania, psychosis, delirium, and depression may occur. Cranial neuropathy may lead to optic nerve atrophy, ophthalmoplegia and dysphagia. Peripheral neuropathy is predominantly motor, with varying degrees of weakness, paresis and paralysis to the point of paraplegia or flaccid quadriplegia. If intercostal nerves are involved, severe ventilatory insufficiency may lead to death from respiratory failure. A sensory component may be present with hyperesthesia and paresthesia. Deep tendon reflexes may be diminished or absent. Typically, attacks may last for several days to weeks.

The urine may be dark brown or reddish-brown. If it is of normal color when first passed, it will darken rapidly on standing while exposed to light because of the spontaneous production of porphyrins from the excreted precursors.

DIFFERENTIAL DIAGNOSIS

The hepatic porphyrias must be included in the differential diagnosis of otherwise unexplained abdominal pain, acute psychiatric disturbances, and acute polyneuropathies. A positive family history, background of skin photosensitivity, the presence of pain in the back and extremities as well as in the abdomen, or the onset of hypertension with an acute attack may help in establishing the correct diagnosis. Suspicion should be heightened if symptoms occur with menses or after fasting or exposure to certain drugs (see Table 54-51).

The clinician should be aware that several different diseases, especially hepatobiliary disorders, may be associated with a mild to moderate increase in urinary porphyrins, especially coproporphyrin. These "secondary porphyrias" can be distinguished by normal urinary levels of ALA and PBG (see Table 54-50).

INITIAL STABILIZATION AND MANAGEMENT

MONITORING

Provision should be made for the detection of (1) progressive polyneuropathies by serial neurologic examinations; (2) ventilatory insufficiency including, as indicated, serial assessment of vital capacity and arterial blood gases; (3) dehydration and electrolyte ab-

TABLE 54-51. REPORTED DRUG EXPERIENCE IN ACUTE PORPHYRIAS*

1. Unsafe	2. Potentially Unsafe	3. Probably Safe	4. Safe
Antipyrine	Alfadolone acetate	Adrenaline	Acetaminophen
Amidopyrine	Alfaxolone	Chloramphenicol	Amitryptyline
Aminoglutethimide	Alkylating agents	Chlordiazepoxide	Aspirin
Barbiturates	2-Allyloxy-3-methylbenzamide	Colchicine	Atropine
Carbamazepine	Bemegride	Diazepam	Bromides
Carbromal	Clonidine	Dicumarol	Chloral hydrate
Chlorpropramide	Chloroform	Digoxin	EDTA
Danazol	Choroquine	Diphenhydramine	Ether
Dapsone	Colistin	Guanethidine	Glucocorticoids
Diclophenac	Etomidate	Hyoscine	Insulin
Diphenylhydantoin	Erythromycin	Ibuprofen	Narcotic analgesics
Ergot preparations	Fluroxene	Imipramine	Penicillin and derivatives
Ethclorvynol	Food additives	Indocin	Phenothiazines
Ethinamate	Heavy metals	Labetalol	Propranolol
Glutethimide	Hydralazine	Lithium	Streptomycin
Griseofulvin	Ketamine	Mandelamine	Succinylcholine
Isopropylmeprobamate	Methyldopa	Mefanamic acid	Tetracycline
Mephenytoin	Metoclopramide	Methylphenidate	
Meprobamate	Metyrapone	Naproxen	
Methylprylon	Nalidixic acid	Neostigmine	
N-butylscopolammonium bromide	Nikethamide	Nitrofurantoin	
Novobiocin	Nitrazepam	Nitrous oxide	
Phenylbutazone	Nortryptyline	Paracetamol	
Primadone	o,p'-DDD	Penicillamine	
Pyrazolone preparations	Pargyline	Procaine	
Succinimides	Pentazocine	Propanid	
Sulfonamide antibiotics	Pentylenetetrazole	Propoxyphene	
Sulfonethylmethane	Phenoxybenzamine	Prostigmin	
Sulfonmethane	Pyrazinamide	Rauwolfia alkaloids	
Synthetic estrogens, progestins	Rifampicin	Thiouracil	
Tolazamide	Spironolactone	Thyroxine	
Tolbutamide	Theophylline	Tubocurarine	
Trimethadione	Tolazamide	Vitamin B	
Valproic acid	Tranylcypromine	Vitamin C	

* Modified with permission from Kappas, A., et al.; The Porphyrias. *In* The Metabolic Basic of Inherited Disease, 6th Ed., Edited by Scriver, C. R., Beaudet, A. L., Sly, W. S., and Valle, D., New York, McGraw-Hill Book Company, 1989, p. 1327.

normalities including, as indicated, serum and urinary electrolytes and osmolality; and (4) hypertension and tachycardia by serial vital signs. Precautions should be taken to prevent aspiration and protect the patient if seizures occur.

Facilities should be available to provide suctioning, tracheal intubation, and respiratory assistance.

SUPPORTIVE CARE

Dehydration and/or hyponatremia should be corrected with appropriate IV fluids. These derangements may be caused by (1) excessive losses from the gastrointestinal tract, (2) presence of antidiuretic hormone secretion, or (3) a primary defect of the renal tubule.

Pain may be relieved by the administration of simple analgesics such as acetaminophen, aspirin, or dihydrocodeine, but meperidine, other narcotics, and phenothiazines often are required. Chloral hydrate

and/or diazepam is suitable to induce sleep or sedation.

Tachycardia and hypertension may be controlled with beta-adrenergic blockade, usually with propranolol. When possible, a low oral starting dose of 10 mg every 6 hours is recommended. Undue sensitivity, manifested by marked hypotension and bradycardia, has been reported.[5] Doses of up to 480 mg per day intravenously may, however, be necessary to control the hypertension and tachycardia.[6]

Seizures may be present in up to 10% of acute attacks. Specific therapy is frequently not required. All commonly used anticonvulsants are potentially capable of inducing an acute attack. **Phenytoin and phenobarbital are contraindicated.** If, however, seizures are prolonged or recurrent, the establishment of an adequate airway and immediate administration of intravenous diazepam in a dose of 0.1 to 0.2 mg/kg have been used successfully. Other causes of seizures such as hyponatremia must be excluded.

Depression, insomnia, and emotional lability often do not require specific therapy. If psychiatric presentations, such as hypomania or hallucinations, require intervention then the use of psychotropic agents such as chlorpromazine may be advisable.

SPECIFIC THERAPY

The first step is to identify a precipitating cause and remove the inciting agent. Questioning should be directed at obtaining a history of an intercurrent illness, fasting, or use of oral steroid contraceptives, barbiturates, or any medication known to induce an acute attack (see Table 54-51).

Suppress induction of ALA synthase by administering a high-carbohydrate diet. Polycose may be administered orally or through a fine-bore nasogastric tube. If the patient is unresponsive or parenteral administration is desirable, intravenous infusion of glucose at a rate approaching 20 g per hour (400 to 500 g per day) is recommended. If hyperglycemia or glycosuria occurs, small doses of insulin may be given.

Promote autosuppression of ALA synthase by providing heme. Hematin administration is indicated if rapid symptomatic improvement does not occur or if motor neuropathy is present. The role of hematin is to promote autosuppression of ALA synthase by providing heme. The dosage is 3 to 4 mg per kg, dissolved in normal saline and given intravenously **over 20 to 30 minutes** every 12 or 24 hours. Duration of therapy is usually 4 to 7 days. A lyophilized hematin preparation (Panhematin) is available from Abbott Laboratories (see Pitfalls subsequently in this chapter). Administration through a large peripheral vein or preferably a central venous line is advisable because of the potential for thrombophlebitis. Plasma and urine levels of ALA and PBG usually return to normal within 1 to 2 days, with accompanying resolution of pain and discomfort. Peripheral neuropathies are not immediately reversed, but their progression ceases. The effectiveness of hematin must be weighed against the risk of transfusion of a blood product and the seriousness of the acute attack.

LABORATORY PROCEDURES

See section entitled Classification and Specific Porphyrias for more details of specific testing.

Each of the porphyrias is associated with a unique pattern of porphyrin precursors or porphyrins in hepatic or erythropoietic tissues, urine, and feces. In an emergency setting, a Watson-Schwartz test or Hoesch test may be used to screen urine for the presence of porphobilinogen. Nevertheless, obtain qualitative analysis of urine for ALA, PBG, coproporphyrin, and

uroporphyrin; and stools for fecal coproporphyrin and protoporphyrin. If levels are abnormal, quantitative determinations of precursors or porphyrins in feces and urine should be performed (see Fig. 54-7). Demonstration of reduced PBG deaminase activity in erythrocytes is definitive in establishing the diagnosis of AIP.

Request serum and urinary electrolytes and osmolality. Hyponatremia, hypokalemia, hypochloremia, hypercholesterolemia, and hyperamylasemia are seen.

ADMISSION

Admission is recommended if rapid symptomatic improvement does not occur or if motor neuropathy is present.

REHABILITATION

Prevent contractures and overstretching of tendons if muscle weakness or limb paralysis exists by physiotherapy and splinting. Passive exercises should be started early. A program of active movements must continue until full recovery occurs.

EDUCATION AND PREVENTION

Prevention remains the primary goal of management of patients with porphyria. Counsel all patients with genetic defects as to the nature of the disorders and how to avoid known precipitating factors. In particular, patients should be encouraged to provide adequate nutritional intake and to avoid fasting. Prompt treatment of intercurrent illnesses or other diseases is important. In such settings, adequate intake may be compromised and oral supplementation with Polycose (Abbott Laboratories) may be advisable to maintain a high carbohydrate intake. Patients should avoid drugs known to exacerbate the acute porphyrias and abstain from alcohol. The patient and family members should be provided with a list of drugs considered safe and unsafe. Patients should wear "medical alert" bracelets.

Women with cyclic exacerbation of acute porphyria in relation to their menses may benefit from exogenous steroids, which suppress ovulation. Nasal or subcutaneous administration of a long-acting agonist of

LHRH, D-His, has been shown to inhibit ovulation and greatly reduce the incidence of perimenstrual attacks. The safety of the long term treatment with these agents, however, needs to be established.

SCREENING

Screening of relatives is important; 90% of individuals with acute intermittent porphyria remain asymptomatic. Those with the genetic trait should be informed about the nature of the inherited disorder and advised to take necessary precautions.

In screening relatives of patients with hereditary coproporphyria and variegate porphyria, fecal measurements of porphyrins must be performed in addition to urinary assays. The most sensitive way of identifying the latent case is by the demonstration of reduced activity of appropriate heme enzymes in their peripheral erythrocytes.

Variegate porphyria and hepatic coproporphyria may manifest episodic increased excretion of ALA and porphobilinogen as well as excess tetrapyrroles. In variegate porphyria, in the absence of an easily available assay for protoporphyrinogen oxidase, quantitative tests for porphyrins in the urine and feces of family members must be performed to permit genetic counseling and diagnosis. Negative tests should not be considered definitive unless family members have reached puberty.

PITFALLS

In the hepatic porphyrias (AIP, VP, HCP), the absence of photosensitivity, rarity of the disorder, and latency until puberty, when induction of acute attacks occurs, make this diagnosis particularly challenging to a clinician. Failure to recognize the disorder may lead to (1) an unnecessary laparotomy, (2) administration of medications likely to exacerbate the disorder, or (3) failure to monitor for progressive neuropathies leading to respiratory death.

Therapeutic effectiveness of hematin depends critically on its method of preparation and storage because of its instability.[8] Moreover, the decayed hematin, unlike the fresh material, has anticoagulant properties.[9] There is some evidence that some of the side effects of hematin infusions, phlebitis in particular, may be caused by the breakdown products of hematin. The use of lyophyilized hematin, as a panhematin, provides a stable product and should prevent this complication if administered **promptly.**

HORIZONS

Whether genetic engineering will lead to the elimination of this disease is still speculative.

REFERENCES

1. Kappas, A., et al.: The porphyrias. *In* The Metabolic Basis of Inherited Disease. 6th ed. Edited by Scriver, C.R., Beaudet, A.L., Sly, W.S., and Valle, D. New York, McGraw-Hill Book Company, 1989, p. 1305.
2. Bloomer, J.R., and Bonkovsky, H.L.: The porphyrias. Dis. Mon. *35*:13, January, 1989.
3. McColl, K.E.L., Moore, M.R., Thompson, G.G., and Goldberg, A.: Screening for latent acute intermittent porphyria: The value of measuring both delta-aminolaevulinic acid synthase and erythrocyte uroporphyrinogen-1-synthase activities. J. Med. Genet. *19*:271, 1982.
4. Eales, L: The effects of canthaxanthin—a beta-carotene analogue—on the photocutaneous manifestations of EHP, VP and SP. S. Afr. Med. J. *54*:25, 1978.
5. Bonkovsky, H.L., and Tschudy, D.P.: Hazard of propranolol in treatment of acute porphyria. Br. Med. J. *4*:47, 1974.
6. Brezis, M., Ghanem, J., Weiler-Ravell, D., et al.: Hematin and propranolol in acute intermittent porphyria: Full recovery from quadriplegic coma and respiratory failure. Eur. Neurol. *18*:289, 1979.
7. Anderson, K.E.: LHRH Analogues for hormonal manipulation in acute intermittent porphyria. Semin. Hematol. Jan; *26*:10, 1989.
8. Goetsch, C.A., and Bissell, D.M.: Instability of hematin used in the treatment of acute hepatic porphyria. N. Engl. J. Med. *24*:315, 1986.
9. Jones, R.L., Sorette, M., and Sassa, S.: Hematin-derived anticoagulant activity: Generation *in vitro* and *in vivo* (abstract). Blood *62*:275, 1983.

BIBLIOGRAPHY

Kappas, A., et al.: The porphyrias. *In* The Metabolic Basis of Inherited Disease, 6th ed. Edited by Scriver, C.R., Beaudet, A.L., Sly, W.S., and Valle, D. New York, McGraw-Hill Book Company, 1989, p. 1305.

Laiwah, A.C., and McColl, K.E.: Management of attacks of acute porphyria. Drugs *34*:604, 1987.

Chapter 55

EMERGENCIES OF THE EYES, EARS, NOSE, AND THROAT

SECTION ONE: OPHTHALMOLOGY IN THE EMERGENCY DEPARTMENT

ACUTE VISUAL LOSS

Douglas D. Brunette and Steven R. Bennett

CAPSULE

Acute visual loss, as discussed here, is the loss of vision, usually in only one eye, that occurs over a period ranging from a few seconds to a day or two. The vision is reduced to a low level, usually 20/200 or worse. The causes of sudden, severe visual loss are diverse. As a general rule, an acute, sudden, and significant visual loss is an ophthalmologic emergency until proven otherwise. Patients must be quickly evaluated to determine whether a treatable lesion exists. The differential diagnosis of acute visual loss not related to trauma includes optic neuritis, optic neuropathy, vascular occlusion, retinal detachment, vitreous hemorrhage, macular disorders, and hysteria. Table 55-1 lists the common causes of acute visual loss. Most of these patients need ophthalmic or neurologic referral for a complete work-up. Patients with acute visual loss who present within an hour or two of visual loss should be seen immediately and quickly evaluated for the possibility of central retinal artery occlusion.

CLINICAL PRESENTATION AND EXAMINATION

Patients often present complaining of acute visual loss when in fact they may have neither an acute process nor a visual loss caused by the eye. For example, a patient with a visual field cut secondary to a neuro-ophthalmologic lesion may present with acute visual loss when the patient discovers the field cut. A patient with hemianopia usually has normal visual acuity even though both eyes are affected. An accurate history as to how the patient discovered the visual loss, as well as the timing of the loss, is vitally important. For example, a patient may notice the visual loss in one eye only when something requires monocular viewing, such as sighting a rifle.

OPTIC NEURITIS AND OPTIC NEUROPATHY

These can both cause sudden visual loss. Optic neuritis is a subacute monocular loss of vision caused by focal demyelination of the optic nerve. The causes of optic neuropathy include ischemic, toxic, and metabolic disorders and conditions such as multiple sclerosis. Optic neuritis and optic neuropathy are discussed in further detail in the next chapter section, Neuro-ophthalmologic Emergencies.

VASCULAR OCCLUSION

Acute visual loss can occur as a result of vascular occlusion of the central retinal artery or vein. Central retinal artery and central retinal vein occlusion cause painless monocular visual loss.

Central retinal artery occlusion results in an ischemic stroke of the retina. The most common cause is embolization into the central retinal artery. Patients who are susceptible to central retinal artery occlusion

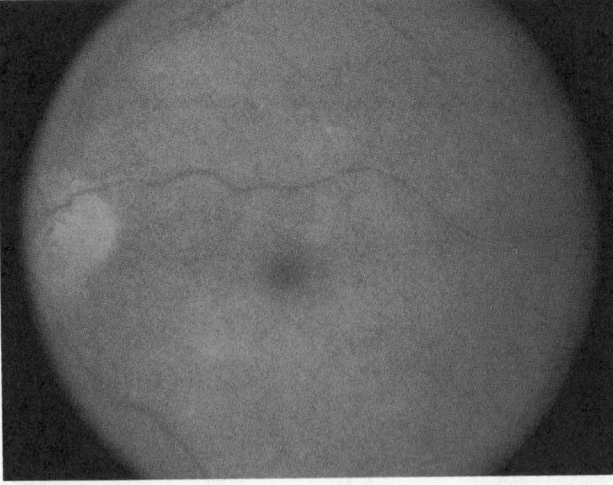

FIG. 55-1. Central retinal artery occlusion.

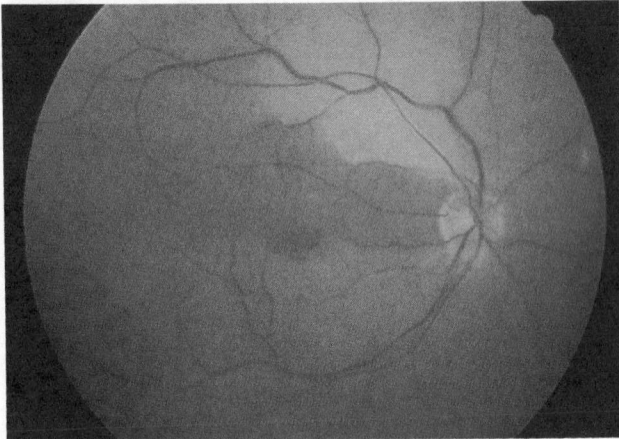

FIG. 55-2. Central retinal artery occlusion with partial sparing of the retina due to a cilioretinal artery.

are those with hypertension, cardiac disease, diabetes, collagen vascular disease, vasculitis, and sickle cell disease. Patients with increased orbital pressure are also at risk, including those with acute glaucoma, retrobulbar hemorrhage, and endocrine exophthalmos. Examination reveals markedly reduced visual acuity with an afferent pupillary defect. On ophthalmoscopic examination, the posterior pole of the retina is edematous, with a pale gray-white appearance, and the fovea appears as a cherry-red spot (Fig. 55-1). Approximately 15 to 20% of the population have retinas that receive some of their blood supply from a cilioretinal artery. The presence of a cilioretinal arteriole from the optic nerve head leads to partial sparing of the retina during a central retinal artery occlusion (Fig. 55-2). Therapy for this condition should be instituted immediately after diagnosis. The mainstays of therapy are directed at dislodging or dissolving the embolus, dilating the artery to promote forward blood flow, and reducing intraocular pressure to allow an increase in perfusion gradient. Specifically, digital global massage and inhalation of a 95% oxygen 5% carbon dioxide mixture or rebreathing into a brown paper bag should be immediately begun in the Emergency Department (ED) even while awaiting ophthalmologic consultation. Global massage is performed by applying direct digital pressure through closed eyelids. This pressure can be applied for 5 to 10 seconds, then released for 5 to 10 seconds. Significant increases in pCO_2 can be obtained by rebreathing into a paper bag for 10 minutes. Intraocular pressure may be reduced by instilling timolol maleate 0.5% topically into the affected eye, and administering acetazolamide 500 mg IV. Prompt ophthalmologic consultation should be obtained because additional therapeutic modalities, including anterior chamber paracentesis, heparin anticoagulation,

low molecular weight dextran, and thrombolytic therapy may be tried. Central retinal artery occlusion may be seen as one component of the visual loss from temporal arteritis. Because central retinal artery occlusion is usually an embolic phenomenon, a complete neurologic and cardiovascular evaluation is necessary to diagnose treatable lesions that might otherwise lead to a larger central nervous system (CNS) event.

Vasospasm may cause transient monocular blindness, characterized by brief periods of visual loss that may recur throughout the day.

CENTRAL RETINAL VEIN OCCLUSION

Central retinal vein occlusion also presents as a painless loss of vision. Central retinal vein occlusion leads to edema, hemorrhage, and vascular leakage. The disease process has a wide spectrum of clinical appearances that depend on the degree of venous obstruction present. Loss of vision can range from minimal to recognition of hand motion only. Central retinal vein occlusion can be further divided into ischemic and nonischemic types. The nonischemic type shows macular edema with dilated, leaking capillaries. These patients tend to have less severe visual loss, and macular vision often improves over time. Ischemic central retinal vein occlusion is associated with capillary closure, eventually leading to neovascular glaucoma. The ophthalmoscopic appearance can vary, but classically includes dilated and tortuous veins, retinal hemorrhages, and disc edema (Fig. 55-3). Branch retinal vein occlusions occur just distal to an arterial/venous crossing, and hemorrhages occur distal to the site of occlusion. The differential diagnosis of central retinal vein occlusion includes hypertension, diabetes mellitus, hyperviscosity syndromes, and papilledema. All four of these diagnoses tend to be bilateral processes, whereas central retinal vein occlusion is generally a unilateral process. The treatment of central retinal vein occlusion is not effective. Patients should receive a complete medical evaluation aimed at the diagnosis of hypertension, blood dyscrasias, diabetes mellitus, vascular disease, and glaucoma. Various therapeutic modalities have been tried to alleviate the venous obstruction and improve outcome, with little success. The prognosis varies according to the degree of obstruction and resultant complications.

RETINAL DETACHMENT

The retina has two layers, the inner neuronal retinal layer and the outer retinal pigment epithelial layer. The retinal pigment epithelium meets the pigmented ciliary body epithelium at the ora serrata anteriorly. Retinal detachment is a separation of the two layers of the retina caused by fluid accumulation. Retinal detachment can occur by three mechanisms, namely rhegmatogenous, exudative, and tractional. Rhegmatogenous retinal detachment occurs as a result of a tear or hole in the neuronal layer, causing fluid from the vitreous cavity to leak between and separate the two retinal layers. A common cause of rhegmatogenous retinal detachment is protein vitreous separation. As a consequence of aging, the vitreous gel develops changes that lead to its pulling away from the posterior retina. This often happens acutely, and is called a posterior vitreous separation. In some patients this is accompanied by symptoms of flashing lights and new floaters. Sometimes in the process of separating from the retina, the vitreous tears the retina, allowing fluid to seep through and the retina to detach. Rhegmatogenous retinal detachment generally occurs in patients over 45 years of age, is more common in men than women, and is associated with degenerative myopia. Trauma may be associated with rhegmatogenous detachment by causing tears in the retina or a disinsertion of the retina from its attachment at the ora serrata anteriorly. Traumatic retinal detachment can occur at any age. Exudative retinal detachment occurs as a result of fluid or blood leakage from vessels

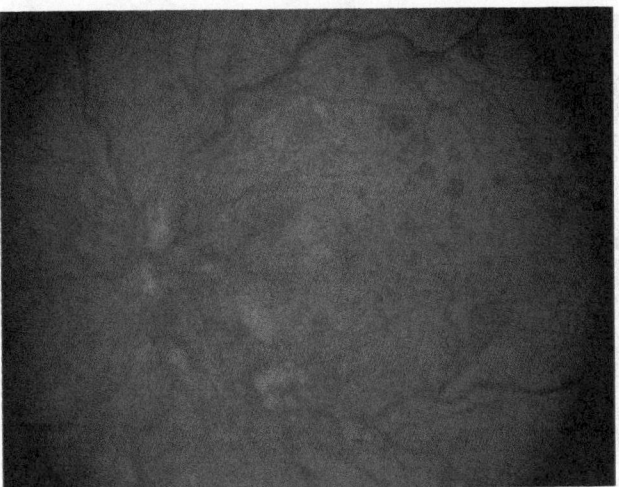

FIG. 55-3.   Central retinal vein occlusion.

within the retina. Conditions leading to secondary retinal detachment include hypertension, toxemia of pregnancy, central retinal venous occlusion, glomerulonephritis, papilledema, vasculitis, and choroidal tumor. Traction retinal detachment is a consequence of fibrous band formation in the vitreous and contraction of these bands. These fibrous bands result from the organization of inflammatory exudates or blood from prior vitreous hemorrhage.

The signs and symptoms of retinal detachment vary according to the location, size, and acuteness of the detachment. Typically, patients complain of flashes of light related to the traction on the retina, floaters related to vitreal blood or pigmented debris, and visual loss. The visual loss is frequently described as a filmy, cloudy, or curtain-like appearance. Pain is absent. On physical examination, visual acuity is preserved unless the macula is involved, in which case severe visual loss will have developed. There are visual field cuts related to the location of the retinal detachment, and an afferent pupillary defect if the detachment is large enough. When the detachment is visualized by means of ophthalmoscopy, the retina appears out of focus at the site of the detachment. In large retinal detachments when much fluid accumulation has occurred, the bullous detachment, with retinal folds, can be easily seen (Fig. 55-4). Direct ophthalmoscopic examination through a dilated pupil only examines the posterior pole of the retina. Therefore retinal detachment cannot be completely ruled out by this method of examination. Indirect ophthalmoscopy by an ophthalmologist is needed to visualize more anterior portions of the retina. Treatment of retinal detachment depends on its type. Rhegmatogenous and tractional detachment are amenable to surgical repair, whereas treatment of exudative detachment is often aimed at treating the underlying cause or use of laser photocoagulation. Retinal detachments that are diagnosed or suspected in the ED need immediate ophthalmologic consultation.

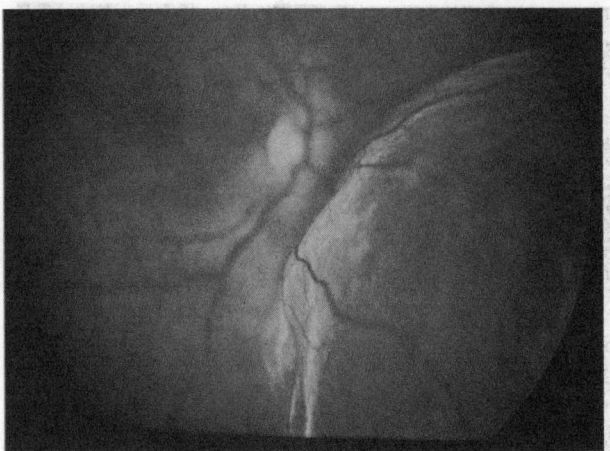

FIG. 55-4. Large retinal detachment.

FIG. 55-5. Early stages of senile macular degeneration, with scattered drusen appearing in the fundus.

VITREOUS HEMORRHAGE

Vitreous hemorrhage results from bleeding into the preretinal space or the vitreous cavity itself. The most common causes are neovascularization from diabetic retinopathy and retinal tears. Additional causes include neovascularization associated with branch vein occlusion, sickle cell disease, retinal artery microaneurysms, trauma, and aging macular degeneration. The symptoms of vitreous hemorrhage often begin with floaters or "cobwebs" in the vision, and may progress over a few hours to severe visual loss. Direct ophthalmoscopy reveals a reddish haze in mild cases to a black reflex in severe cases. Details of the fundus are usually difficult to visualize because of the hemorrhage. Vitreous hemorrhage alone does not cause an afferent pupillary defect, and if present indicates a retinal detachment behind the vitreous hemorrhage. The hemorrhage itself can take on varying appearances, depending on the size of the hemorrhage and

the time that has passed since the event. The hemorrhage may be evenly distributed throughout the vitreous, or focally located. Long-standing preretinal hemorrhage can become a white mass that may be misdiagnosed as a tumor, exudate, or infection. The treatment of vitreous hemorrhage depends on the cause. Most cases of vitreous hemorrhage are caused by diabetic retinopathy. In these instances, initial therapy consists of bed rest with elevation of the head of the bed. Panretinal photocoagulation to cause regression of the neovascularization can be performed once the hemorrhage clears, which can take days or never occur. If the hemorrhage fails to clear or the retina is detached, the blood can be removed with vitrectomy surgery. Ultrasonography can be used to determine if a retinal detachment is present, and may also be helpful in determining the cause.

MACULAR DISORDERS

Many disease processes can cause acute changes in the macula leading to acute visual loss. The role of the emergency physician is to recognize the existence of a maculopathy, and initiate ophthalmologic consultation. Keys to the diagnosis of macular dysfunction include loss of central vision with preservation of peripheral vision, complaints of central visual distortion, and anatomic changes in the retina on ophthalmoscopic examination.

Degenerative maculopathies occur as the result of trauma, radiation exposure, inflammation, vascular disease, toxins, or hereditary disease; or may be idiopathic in nature. The most common form is related to aging macular degeneration. This maculopathy is most common after age 65, but has an unknown cause. It is the leading reason for legal blindness in the United States. In the early stages, ophthalmoscopic examination reveals scattered drusen (Figure 55-5). Drusen are small, sharply defined yellow-white masses. Some patients with drusen develop blood vessel membranes that arise from the choroid and grow in an abnormal place under the retina. If left untreated, the neovascularization leads to hemorrhage, transudation, and scar formation (Fig. 55-6). The process causes an exudative detachment of the retina with resultant blurring of vision. If a large hemorrhage occurs from the neovascular membrane, it can cause severe central visual loss, and may break through the retina into the vitreous, causing peripheral visual loss. The choroidal neovascular membrane can be best visualized by fluorescein angiography, and treatment is photocoagulation. However, only 10 to 15% of those with this disease process are candidates for therapy.

INFLAMMATORY DISEASE OF THE RETINA

Inflammatory processes involving the retina may also cause visual loss, especially if the macula is involved.

Bacterial, viral, and protozoal agents have been shown to cause maculopathy. The presenting symptoms and signs vary according to the disease process and severity. Inflammatory debris from exudative processes may fill the vitreous, leading to a cloudy appearance. Changes in the retina may be seen with the ophthalmoscope. Infections within the eye are often associated with severe pain, redness, and periocular edema. If the retina and choroid are obliterated, the lesions appear white. Patients suspected of having an inflammatory maculopathy need immediate ophthalmologic consultation, along with a complete medical evaluation.

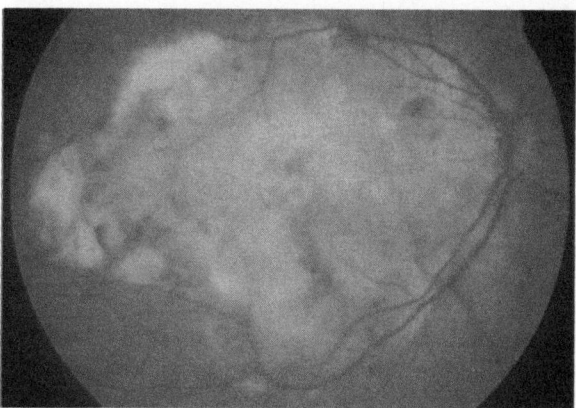

FIG. 55-6.   *Advanced senile macular degeneration.*

FUNCTIONAL VISUAL LOSS

Patients who present with functional visual loss fall into two categories, hysterical conversion reactions and malingering. Patients with hysterical conversion reactions, usually caused by underlying psychopathology, present with a nondeliberate but nonetheless imagined visual loss. Typically, the patient has a flatter affect than one would expect under the circumstances of acute visual loss. Indeed, the patient might appear completely unaffected emotionally by the acute visual loss. The malingerer, on the other hand, is a patient who is well aware that no visual loss exists, yet deliberately feigns visual loss for some secondary gain. This patient is typically overemotional about the visual loss.

Frequently, cortical blindness is mistaken for functional blindness because patients with both lesions have normal fundoscopic examinations and intact pupillary reflexes. Anton's syndrome is characterized by bilateral blindness, normal pupillary reflexes, bilateral occipital lesions, and denial of blindness. It is this denial of blindness that may lead the physician to incorrectly diagnose a functional cause.

In beginning the history and physical examination, it should be determined if the blindness is bilateral or unilateral. Patients with real bilateral equal visual loss do not have an afferent pupil defect, and patients with real cortical blindness will have normal pupils. The cause of unilateral visual loss can be difficult to diagnose, and is more often real. If a patient claims to have no light perception, there is always an afferent pupil defect present. In milder forms of unilateral visual loss, ophthalmic consultation is usually necessary, but may not be urgent.

Examination of a patient with a suspected functional visual loss should be conducted in exactly the same manner as every other ophthalmologic examination, with particular attention paid to possible neuro-ophthalmologic deficits. Normal pupillary reflexes and the absence of an afferent pupillary defect, together with a normal fundoscopic examination, point toward functional visual loss. There are multiple other tests that the examiner can perform to ascertain whether a visual loss is organic or functional. Patients with feigned visual loss are hesitant about trying to appose the index fingers of each hand, and often write their names in a disorderly fashion, whereas even acutely and genuinely blind patients can sign their names without difficulty. One effective test involves placing a large mirror directly in front of the patient's face and asking him or her to look straight ahead. The mirror is then tilted slightly back and forth. Most patients follow the reflection of their eyes in the mirror as it changes position, proving feigned visual loss. In some difficult cases, more sophisticated tests must be performed, including optokinetic nystagmus tests, stereopsis prism shift tests, and red/green glasses. If the diagnosis of feigned visual loss cannot be definitively made, ophthalmologic consultation is required to rule out neuro-ophthalmologic visual loss.

MEDICOLEGAL PEARLS

As a general rule of thumb, the more acute the onset and the more severe the visual loss, the more urgent the problem. Sudden and severe visual loss is an emergency demanding immediate evaluation. No patient who presents with a chief complaint of sudden and profound visual loss should be allowed to wait for medical examination.

BIBLIOGRAPHY

Burde, R.M., Savino, P.J., and Trobe, J.D.: Clinical Decisions in Neuro-ophthalmology. St. Louis, C.V. Mosby Company, 1985.

Ellenberger, C., and Epstein, A.D.: Ocular complications of atherosclerosis: What do they mean? Semin. Neurol. 6, 1986.

Folk, J.C.: Aging macular degeneration. Ophthalmology: 92, 1985.

Gombos, G.M.: Handbook of Ophthalmologic Emergencies. 2nd Edition. New Hyde Park, New York, Medical Examination Publishing Co., Inc., 1977.

Hayreh, S.S.: Classification of central retinal vein occlusion. Ophthalmology 90:458, 1983.

Kini, M.M.: Retina and vitreous. *In* Manual of Ocular Diagnosis and Therapy. Edited by Pavan-Langston, D. Boston, Little, Brown, & Co., 1981.

Marcus, D.F., and Bovino, J.A.: Retinal detachment. JAMA: 247, 1982.

Newell, F.W.: Ophthalmology Principles and Concepts. 6th ed. St. Louis, The C.V. Mosby Company, 1986.

Paton, D., Hyman, B.N., and Justice, J.: Introduction to Ophthalmoscopy. Kalamazoo, Upjohn Company, 1981.

SanBorn, G.E., Magargal, L.E., and Jaeger, E.A.: Venous occlusive disease of the retina. *In* Clinical Ophthalmology. Edited by Duane, T.D., and Jaeger, E.A. Philadelphia, Harper & Row, 1986.

Stern, W.H., and Archer, D.B.: Retinal occlusion. Ann. Rev. Med. 32:101, 1981.

Vaughan, D., and Asbury, T.: Retina. *In* General Ophthalmology. Edited by Vaughan, D., and Asbury, T. Los Altos, Lange Medical Publications, 1986, pp. 163–183.

Walsh, F.B., and Hoyt, W.F.: Clinical neuro-ophthalmology. 4th Edition. Baltimore, Williams and Wilkins, 1983.

Winslow, R.L., and Taylor, B.C.: Spontaneous vitreous hemorrhage: Etiology and management. South. Med. J.: 1450, 1980.

Zun, L.S.: Acute visual loss. *In* Ophthalmologic Emergencies and Ocular Trauma. Edited by Mathews, J., and Zun, L.S. Emerg. Med. Clin. North Am. 6:1, 1988.

NEURO-OPHTHALMOLOGIC EMERGENCIES

Douglas D. Brunette and Steven R. Bennett

CAPSULE

Neuro-ophthalmologic emergencies constitute a small, diverse, and important group of ophthalmologic problems seen in the emergency department (ED). Table 55-2 lists common causes of neuro-ophthalmologic conditions. Neuro-ophthalmologic visual loss can be defined as visual loss not explained by obvious abnormalities of the eye. Anisocoria, nystagmus, extraocular movement disorders, and an abnormal optic disc can all be classified as neuro-ophthalmologic conditions. Patients who present to the ED with a history and physical examination compatible with optic neuropathy, chiasmal or postchiasmal compression, papilledema, third-nerve compression, cavernous sinus disease, and new-onset nystagmus that is not vestibular or benign in orgin need immediate ophthalmologic and neurologic consultation. Those diagnosed as having optic neuritis should receive ophthalmologic follow-up within 24 hours.

PATHOPHYSIOLOGY AND ANATOMY

Neuro-ophthalmologic emergencies represent a myriad of clinical entities. The anatomic relationships are generally constant, however, and a thorough understanding of the anatomy of the neuro-optic system is mandatory for comprehension of the individual disease processes. Figure 55-7 demonstrates the pathway of neuronal transmission of the optic system. Note that prechiasmal disease affects monocular vision, and disease processes affecting the optic chiasm or optic tracts generally result in binocular visual loss. The nasal retinal optic nerve fibers decussate at the optic chiasm and receive light stimulation from the temporal visual field.

TABLE 55-2. COMMON CAUSES OF NEURO-OPHTHALMOLOGIC DISEASE

I. Neuro-ophthalmologic Visual Loss
  A. Prechiasmal disease
    1. Optic neuritis
    2. Ischemic optic neuropathy
      a. Temporal arteritis
      b. Idiopathic
    3. Compressive optic neuropathy
    4. Toxic/metabolic optic neuropathy
  B. Chiasmal disease
    1. Compression by tumor
  C. Postchiasmal disease
    1. Infarction
    2. Tumor
    3. Arteriovenous malformation
    4. Migraine disorders
    5. Hemorrhage
II. Anisocoria
  A. Adie's tonic pupil
  B. Pharmacologic blockade
  C. Third nerve palsy
  D. Horner's syndrome
  E. Benign anisocoria
III. Abnormal optic disc
  A. Papilledema
  B. Hyaline bodies
  C. Anterior ischemic optic neuropathy
  D. Severe hypertension
  E. Central retinal vein occlusion
  F. Congenital anomalous disc
  G. Optic neuritis
IV. Nystagmus
  A. Congenital
  B. Acquired
    1. Toxic exposure
    2. Defective retinal impulses
    3. Labyrinth/vestibular disease
    4. Central lesions
V. Disorders of Extraocular Movement
  A. Monocular diplopia
    1. Refractive errors
    2. Feigned disease
  B. Binocular diplopia
    1. Local mechanical defects
    2. Cranial nerve palsy
    3. Thyroid disease
    4. Multiple sclerosis
    5. Myasthenia gravis
    6. Progressive ophthalmoplegia

CLINICAL PRESENTATION AND EXAMINATION

NEURO-OPHTHALMOLOGIC VISUAL LOSS

Visual loss not readily explained by an obvious abnormality on physical examination of the eye can be called neuro-ophthalmologic visual loss.[1] Patients can be divided into those who complain of decreased vi-sion and have a reduced visual acuity and those patients who complain of visual loss, but have a normal visual acuity. It is imperative to conduct careful visual field testing in this latter group.

Neuro-ophthalmologic visual loss can be further divided into processes involving the prechiasmal, chiasmal, or postchiasmal anatomic areas.

PRECHIASMAL DISEASE

Patients with prechiasmal disease present with decreased visual acuity or visual field loss in the eye on the affected side. Prechiasmal disease may be a unilateral or bilateral process, depending on the cause. The swinging flashlight test reveals an afferent pupillary defect on the side involved, unless the process is bilateral. In such cases, the relative degree of afferent defect determines the results. Visual field testing demonstrates a field defect that does not respect the vertical meridian, and is often localized to the center of the visual field. Causes of prechiasmal visual loss include optic neuritis, ischemic optic neuropathy, compressive optic neuritis, and toxic and metabolic optic neuritis.

Optic Neuritis. Optic neuritis is an acute monocular loss of vision caused by focal demyelination of the optic nerve. The patient's age ranges from 15 to 45 years. The classic presenting symptoms are a progressive loss of vision over several hours or days and ocular pain with eye movement.[2] This is described as an ache behind the eye made worse by moving the eyes. Physical examination reveals a decreased visual acuity that can range from minimal loss to no light perception. An afferent pupillary defect (Marcus Gunn pupil) is always present, and direct ophthalmoscopic examination is generally normal.[3] The natural history of optic neuritis is for visual acuity to reach its poorest within 1 week, and then slowly improve over the next several weeks. Visual acuity recovers to 20/40 or better in 85% of patients.[4] Approximately one third of patients experience Uhthoff's syndrome, an episodic blurring of vision after recovery precipated by exercise or a hot shower. Steroids have been the standard therapy. Whether the use of steroids improves the prognosis for visual acuity or merely shortens the symptomatic period is not known.[3,5] Approximately 35% of patients with optic neuritis subsequently develop multiple sclerosis, most within 4 years of the initial episode. The diagnosis of optic neuritis is initially made on clinical grounds. Formal visual field testing and visually evoked potentials, however, are often needed to make the definitive diagnosis. All patients presenting with a clinical picture compatible with optic neuritis should have ophthalmologic and neurologic follow-up as soon as possible. Treatable lesions, such as tumors causing optic nerve compression, can mimic optic neuritis. In cases where the etiology of a prechiasmal visual field loss is not clear, neuroradiologic testing is indicated.

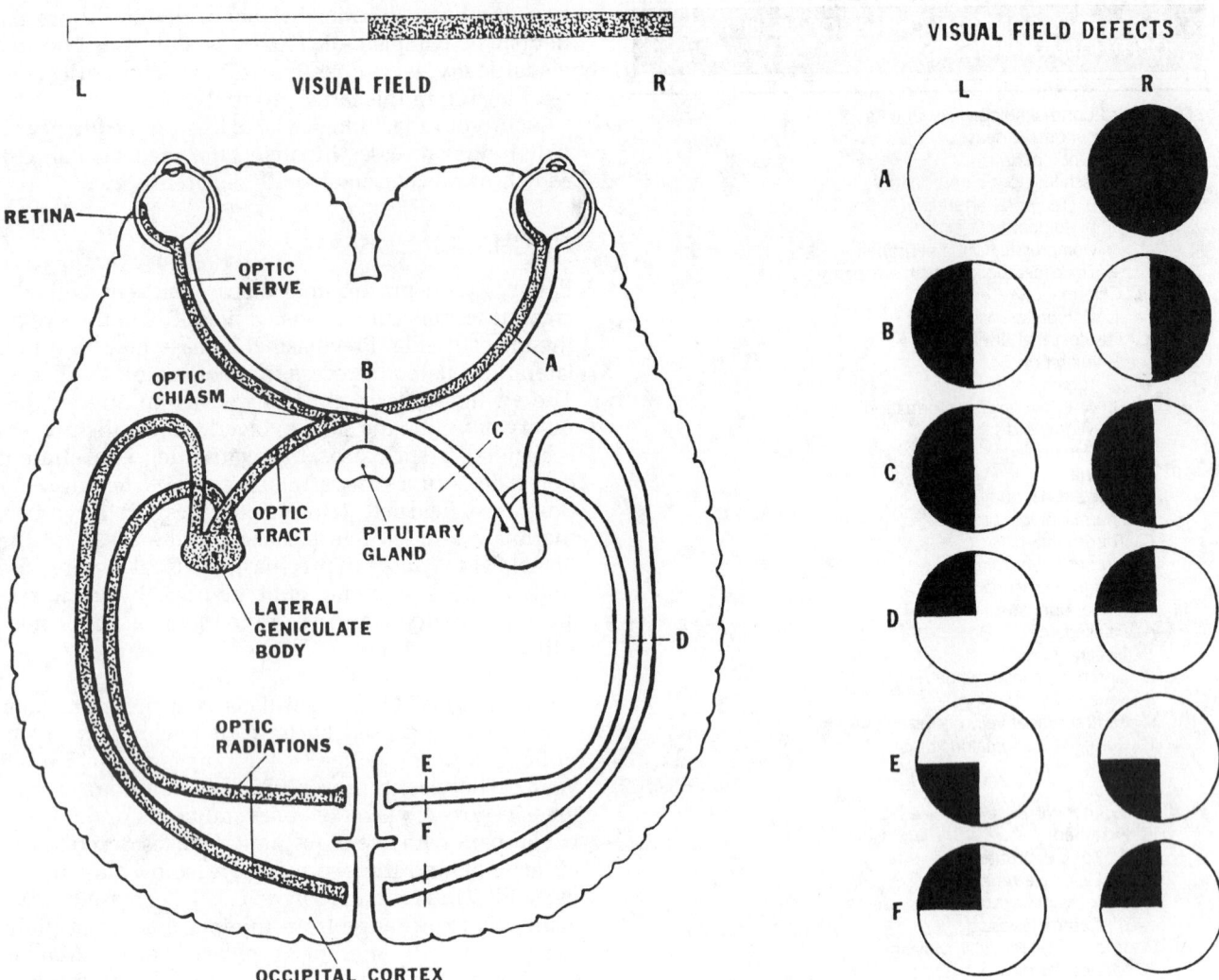

FIG. 55-7. Anatomy of the neuronal transmission of the optic system. Note the visual field defects caused by lesions located at different points along the pathway.

Ischemic Optic Neuropathy (ION). ION is the most common cause of optic neuropathy and one of the most common causes of visual loss after middle age.[6] ION can be divided into giant cell arteritis and idiopathic categories. Giant cell arteritis (temporal arteritis) is characterized by weight loss, malaise, jaw pain, headache, scalp tenderness, polymyalgia rheumatica, and low-grade fever. It is extremely rare under age 50, and the incidence rises with each subsequent decade. One third of patients with temporal arteritis develop severe visual loss if the condition is untreated, and visual loss is often abrupt.[7] Occasionally, visual loss is preceded by episodes of amaurosis fugax. Generally, one eye is affected first, with the second eye becoming involved in a high percentage of patients within hours to days. Physical examination reveals a large afferent pupillary defect, visual loss, and a visual field defect that may respect the horizontal meridian. The optic disc shows pallor and swelling. The diagnosis can be clinically con-firmed by demonstration of an elevated erythrocyte sedimentation rate (ESR). The ESR is above 50 mm per hour (Westergren) in 90% of patients with temporal arteritis, and frequently is higher.[8] C-reactive protein is also usually elevated, and should be drawn before steroid therapy. The diagnosis is made definitively by temporal artery biopsy. Temporal arteritis (TA) is an emergency that can cause a significant visual loss in the absence of effective therapy. The standard treatment is high-dose corticosteroids, which should be started as soon as the diagnosis is suspected, before biopsy. Steroids do not bring about recovery of lost vision, but often prevent progression of the disease and involvement in the second eye.[1] Patients should generally be admitted to the hospital for intravenous steroid therapy, and medical consultation obtained.

Idiopathic ischemic optic neuropathy is much more common than temporal arteritis. Patients lack the classic symptoms of temporal arteritis and do not have an elevated ESR. Most have systemic vascular disease, diabetes, or hypertension, and tend to be younger than temporal arteritis patients. They present, however, with painless visual loss, afferent pupillary defects, disc swelling, and visual field defects that respect the horizontal meridian. The visual loss is less severe than that seen with TA, and improvement does occur in one third of patients.[9] Steroids have been advocated, but the results are less than convincing. If there is any doubt as to whether a particular patient has TA versus an idiopathic form of ischemic optic neuropathy, treatment with high-dose steroids should be started until a temporal artery biopsy is performed.

Compressive Optic Neuritis. This has numerous causes, including tumor, aneurysm, sphenoid sinusitis or mucocele, blunt trauma, and dysthyroid disorders. Therefore optic nerve compression can occur at any age. Although this neuropathy is defined as a prechiasmal disorder, compression can occasionally occur far enough posteriorly to affect the optic chiasm. Patients with compressive optic neuropathy have visual loss that continues to progress beyond 7 days. Compressive optic neuropathies are ophthalmologic emergencies requiring neuroradiographic evaluation and rapid medical and surgical intervention. Optic neuritis, a self-limited and generally benign process, can be difficult to distinguish from a compressive optic neuropathy. Compressive syndromes tend to involve other cranial nerves, and patients frequently have a history of cancer, thyroid disease, neurofibromatosis, or other endocrine disorders. As a general rule of thumb, if the signs and symptoms do not closely fit optic neuritis or ischemic optic neuropathy, a compressive lesion exists until proven otherwise.

Toxic and Metabolic Neuropathies. There are a large number of toxic and metabolic neuropathies. Common toxic causes include barbiturates, chloramphenicol, emetine, ethambutol, ethylene glycol, isoniazid, and methanol.[3] Causes of metabolic optic neuropathies include thiamine deficiency, pernicious anemia, and heavy metal poisoning. These processes are bilateral, progressive, and symmetric. Visual loss can be severe, and visual field testing reveals central defects. Treatment is aimed at the underlying toxin or metabolite involved.

CHIASMAL DISEASE

Chiasmal disease represents the second category of neuro-ophthalmologic visual loss. Chiasmal compression by tumor is the most common cause of chiasmal visual loss. Pituitary tumors (50%), craniopharyngiomas (25%), and meningiomas (10%) are the most common tumors affecting the optic chiasm.[1] Visual loss is generally gradual and progressive, and may be present for a prolonged time before it is discovered by the patient. The diagnosis is made by visual field testing. Although formal visual field testing by an ophthalmologist is necessary to stage the patient preoperatively or pretherapy, and to follow improvement and monitor for recurrence, the diagnosis can usually be made by confrontation visual field testing. The classic defect is a bitemporal hemianopsia. Tumors, however, frequently compress the optic chiasm and optic nerves asymmetrically, resulting in combined central and temporal defects. Any time a visual field defect respects the vertical meridian from a neuro-ophthalmologic visual loss, the lesion is out of the globe, and must be either chiasmal or postchiasmal. Chiasmal visual loss demands an immediate ophthalmologic, neurosurgical, and endocrinologic consultation.

POSTCHIASMAL DISEASE

Postchiasmal disease represents the third category of neuro-ophthalmologic visual loss. The most common causes are infarction, tumor, arteriovenous malformation, and migraine disorders. The patient often presents with vague complaints related to difficulty in performing a certain task, such as reading. Lesions can be located from the immediate postchiasmal optic tract to the occipital cortex. The classic visual field defect is the homonymous hemianopsia. Patients that present with such lesions have a focal neurologic deficit, and need immediate neurologic consultation to rule out cerebral infarction, hemorrhage, and tumor. Cortical blindness is a special cause of neuro-ophthalmologic visual loss that is most commonly caused by bilateral occipital cortical lesions secondary to infarction. Frequently, cortical blindness is mistaken for functional blindness because patients with both lesions have normal fundoscopic examinations and intact pupillary reflexes. Anton's syndrome is characterized by bilateral blindness, normal pupillary reflexes, bilateral occipital lesions, and denial of blindness, which may be incorrectly assumed to be evidence of a psychiatric process.

ANISOCORIA

This is a commonly encountered clinical problem in the ED. Pupillary size is determined by the interaction of two groups of smooth muscles within the iris. The sphincter muscle receives its innervation from the parasympathetic nerve supply; the dilator is innervated by way of the sympathetic system. Anisocoria results from defects in the nerves or muscles that control the iris musculature, and is not related to retinal or optic nerve function.

The clinical setting in which anisocoria occurs is important. Anisocoria in a patient with head trauma or a decreased level of consciousness demands immediate and aggressive therapeutic intervention because the aniscoria may be third-nerve compression from uncal herniation. In a patient who is awake and alert, without signs of trauma, and presents with anisocoria of unknown cause, the first question to ask is "which is the abnormal pupil?" If one pupil constricts to a light stimulus poorly, it is likely the abnormal one.[10] If anisocoria exists in a patient with a normal afferent visual system, either an innervational or structural defect in the iris sphincter exists.[1] Most structural defects in the iris can be diagnosed by slit lamp examination, and many of these patients relate a history of previous eye surgery or trauma. If both pupils react well to light, and no iris abnormalities are seen with slit lamp examination, the next step is to determine whether the anisocoria increases in light or darkness. In Adie's tonic pupil, pharmacologic blockade, and third-nerve palsy, anisocoria increases in light.[10] In benign anisocoria and Horner's syndrome, anisocoria increases in darkness.[10] Comparing pupillary size in a brightly and dimly lit room is the easiest way to evaluate the effect of lighting on anisocoria.

ADIE'S TONIC PUPIL

This is a disorder in which patients present complaining of blurred near vision but normal distant vision. Adie's syndrome is seen in young women 70% of the time, and has associated symmetrically reduced deep tendon reflexes. Physical examination reveals poor accommodation, with a slow constriction to near testing. The pupil redilates slowly when the vision is again made distant. Examination with the slit lamp often reveals sector palsies of the iris. The diagnosis is confirmed when a weak cholinergic agent (pilocarpine, 0.1%) causes an intense pupillary constriction as a result of cholinergic supersensitivity. Patients need to be referred to an ophthalmologist non-emergently for cholinergic agent therapy and bifocal corrections. Approximately 50% of patients with Adie's tonic pupil recover full accommodation within 2 years.[11]

PHARMACOLOGIC MYDRIASIS

A wide variety of agents can cause a pharmacologic mydriasis. Pharmacologic mydriasis can be caused by the deliberate or inadvertent local administration of both sympathomimetic and parasympatholytic agents. Phenylephrine and cocaine are two sympathomimetic substances that can be responsible for iatrogenic anisocoria. These substances are frequently used as nasal premedicants for nasotracheal intubation, and careless administration may lead to anisocoria as a result of ocular contamination. Many parasympatholytic agents, such as atropine and scopolamine, have been implicated in the development of anisocoria. The transdermal patches placed for the prevention of motion sickness frequently have a parasympatholytic agent, and have been known to cause anisocoria. Pilocarpine, 1.0%, can be used in special circumstances to help differentiate a third-nerve palsy from pharmacologically mediated mydriasis. The administration of pilocarpine, 1.0% rapidly constricts the pupil that is dilated secondary to a third-nerve palsy. Pilocarpine, 1.0%, however, does not produce miosis in pupils that are dilated secondary to parasympatholytic agents.[12] It is important to note that pilocarpine, 1.0% rapidly constricts pupils that are dilated secondary to the administration of sympathomimetic agents.[12]

THIRD-NERVE PALSY

Patients who present with anisocoria that increases in light, without evidence of Adie's tonic pupil or pharmacologic mediation, should be suspected of having third-nerve palsy. Patients with anisocoria secondary to third-nerve palsy almost always have other signs of third-nerve involvement, including ptosis and extraocular muscle dysfunction. Typically, the patient complains of diplopia, and the involved eye is turned down and out. Patients may present with ptosis and extraocular dysfunction with or without pupil dilation. Any patient who presents with a new-onset third-nerve lesion involving the pupil should be urgently admitted to the hospital and undergo neuroradiographic studies to rule out aneurysm.

HORNER'S SYNDROME

This syndrome consists of ptosis, miosis, and facial anhydrosis resulting from an interruption of sympathetic innervation. Dilation lag is a classic finding in Horner's syndrome. The anisocoria caused by Horner's syndrome is increased in darkness, and the dilation lag results from the Horner's pupil requiring up to 15 seconds to dilate fully.[13] Thus, the anisocoria is greater at 3 to 5 seconds of darkness than at 15 seconds of darkness, although the anisocoria is still more pronounced than in light. The diagnosis of Horner's syndrome and the localization of the point of sympathetic interruption can be accomplished by pharmacologic testing performed by an ophthalmologist. Preganglionic interruptions cause major concern because they may be from intrathoracic or intraspinal malignant neoplasms. Patients with preganglionic Horner's syndrome require a full medical evaluation. Postganglionic Horner's syndromes are usually benign.[14]

SIMPLE ANISOCORIA

As much as 20% of the general population may have simple anisocoria,[15] which may be transient or prolonged and may alternate pupils. The difference in pupillary size is generally under 1 mm, and although the anisocoria increases in darkness, there is no dilation lag as seen with Horner's syndrome.

ABNORMAL OPTIC DISC

The optic nerve contains approximately one million nerve fibers, and is generally yellowish in color. The physiologic cup is an area of lighter-colored central excavation through which the central retinal artery and vein traverse. One important acquired cause for an abnormal optic disc is papilledema. This term refers to the changes in the optic disc as a result of increased intracranial pressure. One of the earliest signs of increased intracranial pressure is the absence of venous pulsations. Half of the general population do not have venous pulsations, however, and therefore their absence in any particular patient is generally not helpful. The presence of venous pulsations makes increased intracranial pressure unlikely. As the papilledema progresses, there is blurring of the disc margins, hyperemia, and loss of physiologic cupping. Flame-shaped hemorrhages and yellow exudates appear near the disc margins as the edema progresses. Patients may present with a history of significant headaches or be completely asymptomatic. Visual acuity is generally not affected until the papilledema is long-standing.[16] Brief obscurations of vision, enlargement of the physiologic blind spot, and nasal inferior visual field loss are common. Papilledema is a bilateral process, but may be asymmetric. The causes of increased intracranial pressure are numerous, including tumor, brain abscess, hemorrhage, hydrocephalus, meningitis, and pseudotumor cerebri. Any patient with newly diagnosed papilledema should be admitted to the hospital for neuroradiographic evaluation.

Many disorders can cause a papilledema-like appearance in the optic disc. Hyaline bodies, anterior ischemic optic neuropathy, severe hypertension, central retinal vein occlusion, congenital anomalous disc, and optic neuritis can all be mistaken for papilledema. Hyaline bodies are present from birth, and have characteristic multiple elevations at the nerve head. Although the disc margins may be blurred, there is no engorgement of the veins, and no other changes associated with papilledema. Ischemic optic neuropathy, caused by vascular insufficiency or temporal arteritis, causes a pale papilledema, which is almost never seen with increased intracranial pressure. Central retinal vein occlusion and optic neuritis are unilateral processes, and associated with acute visual loss. Should the diagnosis of papilledema be in question on physical examination, immediate consultation with an ophthalmologist is warranted.

NYSTAGMUS

Clinically significant nystagmus is an oscillation of the eyes that occurs within 30 degrees of the midline.[17] Nystagmus can be classified according to many different characteristics. Pendular nystagmus is a nystagmus in which the oscillations are of equal velocity in both directions. Jerk nystagmus is an oscillation in which the velocity of movement is obviously faster in one direction. In jerk nystagmus, the pathologic component is the slow movement, but the nystagmus is named according to the direction of the fast component. For example, right nystagmus is an oscillation

in which the slow, abnormal drift is to the left, and the fast correctional component is to the right. Nystagmus can also be divided into monocular versus binocular, conjugate (both eyes moving in the same direction) versus disconjugate (eyes moving in opposite directions), and primary gaze position versus gaze position nystagmus. A careful history is important in the initial evaluation of nystagmus. Important questions include the presence of tinnitus, nausea, vomiting, oscillopsia, and vertigo.

CONGENITAL NYSTAGMUS

This is noted at birth or within the perinatal period. This nystagmus is usually horizontal, conjugate, bilateral, symmetric, and pendular. On lateral gaze, however, this nystagmus may become jerky in nature. The nystagmus remains horizontal despite upward or downward gaze. Congenital nystagmus is damped by convergence, increased with fixation, accentuated by covering one eye, and abolished with sleep. Patients do not have oscillopsia or other neurologic complaints. Some carry their heads in a position that minimizes their nystagmus. Almost all have recognized their nystagmus previously, and the diagnosis is generally straightforward. Infants with decreased vision or blindness from birth develop nystagmus from failure to develop fixation reflexes. Any infant that presents with nystagmus should have a thorough examination by an ophthalmologist to look for a treatable lesion or reduced vision as a cause of the nystagmus.

There are many causes of acquired nystagmus. General categories of disease that result in nystagmus include toxic exposure, defective retinal impulses, diseases of the labyrinths or of the vestibular nuclei, and lesions of the central pathways controlling ocular posture.

VESTIBULAR NYSTAGMUS

This is caused by an acute loss in vestibular function. The most common causes of this nystagmus are vascular disease, viral infection, traumatic injury, and Ménière's disease. This nystagmus is almost always unidirectional, and the fast component is away from the affected side. Vertical or pure rotary movement is never present in vestibular nystagmus, and visual fixation inhibits the nystagmus. Patients may present with nausea, vomiting, and diaphoresis. Vertigo is almost universally present.[4] Additionally, both hearing loss and tinnitus are often present.

CENTRAL NYSTAGMUS

This is caused by lesions involving the brain stem, cerebellum, or their pathways. The nystagmus can be unidirectional or bidirectional, and may be horizontal, rotary, or vertical. Any nystagmus that is vertical and/or multidirectional must be assumed to be central in origin. The causes are diverse, but commonly are toxic, metabolic, or structural. Included in these categories are phenytoin toxicity, multiple sclerosis, tumor, and vertebrobasilar insufficiency. The most common cause is toxic drug exposure. Anticonvulsants, barbiturates, lithium, tranquilizers, and phenothiazines can all cause a central nystagmus. Vertigo, if present, is mild, tinnitus and decreased hearing are not present, and visual fixation does not inhibit the nystagmus.

POSITIONAL NYSTAGMUS

The lesion in positional nystagmus may be either peripherally or centrally located. The key to diagnosis lies in determining that the nystagmus is produced by altering the position of the body or head. The chief complaint is generally vertigo, and the patient is distressed when the vertigo is elicited. To determine whether the nystagmus is positional in origin, the patient is asked to sit up for a few minutes, and then is rapidly laid supine, head just over the edge of the bed, and turned to one side. Positional nystagmus caused by a peripheral lesion has a latent period of 3 to 15 seconds after the head has been turned, decreases measurably within 1 minute, and is difficult to reproduce in the next several minutes. Usually, peripherally caused positional nystagmus is invoked in only one head position, and is associated with severe nausea and vertigo. This condition is almost always benign. Centrally caused positional nystagmus does not have a period of latency, but rather develops immediately on head turning. This nystagmus does not fatigue, and can be elicited repeatedly. The patient's symptoms tend to be milder, and vertigo is less than that seen with peripherally located lesions. It is important to diagnose a centrally generated positional nystagmus because these are often produced by posterior fossa lesions. In trying to discriminate between a peripheral and central positional nystagmus, the examiner should always look carefully for associated focal neurologic signs.

Many other types of nystagmus exist. Rebound, seesaw, periodic alternating, upbeat and downbeat, and horizontal pursuit defect nystagmus have all been characterized.[18] Nystagmoid-like disturbances, such as opsoclonus, superior oblique myokymia, ocular bobbing, and voluntary nystagmus can all be confused with nystagmus. As a general rule of thumb, any patient with nystagmus who does not easily fit into one of the more common and benign varieties, such as congenital, vestibular, or benign positional vertigo, should have a thorough neurologic examination.

DISORDERS OF EXTRAOCULAR MOVEMENT

Patients typically present with the chief complaint of diplopia, produced or exacerbated by certain eye movements. The first step in the diagnosis is to determine whether the diplopia is monocular or bin-

ocular. Binocular diplopia disappears with either eye covered. Monocular diplopia is less concerning because it is caused most commonly by refractive errors and feigned disease.

Binocular diplopia from misalignment of the eyes can be caused by a multitude of disease processes. Local mechanical defects such as hematoma, orbital floor fractures, and abscess formation can limit ocular motility. Cranial nerve palsy of the third, fourth, or sixth cranial nerve can lead to motility problems. Many miscellaneous processes, such as thyroid disease, progressive ophthalmoplegia, extraocular muscle fibrosis syndrome, multiple sclerosis, and myasthenia gravis can lead to newly acquired extraocular movement dysfunction.

Hematoma and orbital floor fractures are readily suspected with the history of recent trauma. Patients with dysfunction of the extraocular movement secondary to infectious processes are easy to recognize from other manifestations of their disease, such as local erythema and warmth, and systemic signs of toxicity such as fever and tachycardia. Thyroid ophthalmoplegia is secondary to hypertrophy of the extraocular muscles. Upward gaze is generally the most affected. Myasthenia gravis usually produces ptosis, and weakness of convergence and upgaze is manifested. A classic sign of multiple sclerosis is intranuclear ophthalmoplegia (INO). This represents dysfunction of the medial longitudinal fasciculus located in the brainstem. The description of an INO is a lag of the agonist medial rectus muscle in a conjugate gaze movement, i.e., the adduction lag.[1] Patients under 40 who present with an INO are usually afflicted with multiple sclerosis; those over 50 generally have vertebrobasilar vascular disease.

The most common cause of newly acquired extraocular movement dysfunction is cranial nerve palsy. To appropriately diagnose a cranial nerve disorder affecting the extraocular muscles, the examiner must understand the innervation of the extraocular muscles and their normal function.

Patients who have brainstem disease as a cause for their cranial nerve palsy frequently have involvement of other cranial nerves, disturbances in level of consciousness, and sensorimotor loss. Isolated third nerve lesions produce a palsy in which the patient develops ptosis, an inability to turn the eye inward or upward, and pupillary mydriasis. The causes of third-nerve palsy are varied and foreboding. Newly acquired third-nerve palsy demands prompt neurologic and radiographic evaluation.

Isolated fourth-nerve palsy is an easily missed disorder. Patients present complaining of double vision, which is made worse in downgaze, or gaze away from the paretic side. On physical examination, these patients typically present with a head tilt to the opposite shoulder to compensate for the vertical extorsion, and have weakness in downward gaze. Trauma and vascular disease account for most cases of isolated fourth-nerve palsy, but aneurysm, intracranial tumor, and myasthenia gravis have been implicated. Prompt neurologic and radiographic evaluation is appropriate in these patients.

Sixth-cranial-nerve palsies are the most frequently reported ocular motor palsies. Patients have an esotropia that is worsened by lateral gaze, and often turn the head laterally toward the paretic side to compensate. Because sixth-nerve palsy is caused by various diseases, detection is of no localizing value. Aneurysm, vascular disease, trauma, neoplasm, multiple sclerosis, and meningitis may all cause dysfunction.[19] The initial management and workup of patients with isolated sixth-nerve palsy depend on the patient's age, clinical presentation, and associated signs. It is best to obtain immediate neurologic and ophthalmologic consultation for these patients.

PITFALLS

A careful visual field examination should be performed on all patients complaining of a visual loss who have normal visual acuity.

MEDICOLEGAL PEARLS

The signs and symptoms of neuro-ophthalmologic disease can be subtle. Do not diagnose a psychiatric condition until you have fully evaluated other possible causes. Many significant neuro-ophthalmologic disease processes need to be diagnosed as early as possible. Consultants should be involved early. These patients have probably a higher than average medicolegal risk of liability. Only through careful history taking and thorough physical examination can neuro-ophthalmologic disorders be reliably diagnosed and managed.

REFERENCES

1. Burde, R.M., and Savino, P.J., and Trobe, J.D.: Clinical Decisions in Neuro-ophthalmology. St. Louis, C.V. Mosby, 1985.
2. Perkin, G.D., and Rose, F.C.: Optic neuritis and its differential diagnosis. Oxford, Oxford Medical Publications, 1979.
3. Miller, N.R.: Walsh and Hoyt's Clinical Neuro-ophthalmology. 4th Edition. Baltimore, Williams and Wilkins, 1983.
4. Savino, P.J.: Neuro-ophthalmology. San Francisco, American Academy of Ophthalomology, 1985.
5. Bird, A.C.: Controversy in ophthalmology. Philadelphia, W.B. Saunders Co., 1977.
6. Hayreh, S.S.: Anterior ischemic optic neuropathy. Arch. Neurol. 38:367, 1981.
7. Keltner, J.L.: Giant cell arteritis. Ophthalmology 89:1101, 1982.
8. Goodman, B.W.: Temporal Arteritis. Am. J. Med. 67:839, 1979.
9. Wray, S.H.: Neuro-ophthalmology: Visual fields, optic nerve, and pupil. In Manual of Ocular Diagnosis and Therapy. Edited by Pavan-Langston, D. Boston, Little, Brown, and Co., 1981.
10. Thompson, H.S., and Pilley, S.F.: Unequal pupils. A flow chart for sorting out the anisocorias. Surv. Opthalmol. 21:45, 1976.
11. Weinstein, J.M., Zweifel, T.J., and Thompson, H.S.: The clinical diagnosis of pupil disorders. J. Clin. Exp. Ophthalmol. 41:15, 1979.
12. Anatasi, L.M., Ogle, K.N., and Kearns, T.P.: Effect of pilocarpine in counteracting mydriasis. Arch. Ophthalmol. 79:710, 1968.
13. Pilley, S.F., and Thompson, H.S.: "Dilation lag" in Horner's syndrome. Br. J. Ophthalmol. 59:731, 1975.
14. Zweifel, T.J., and Thompson, H.S.: The pupil in clinical diagnosis. Neurol. Neurosurg. (weekly update) 1:1978.
15. Loewenfeld, I.E.: "Simple central" anisocoria: A common condition seldom recognized. Trans. Am. Acad. Ophthalmol. Otolaryngol. 83:832, 1977.
16. Victor, M., and Adams, R.D.: Common disturbances of vision, ocular movement, and hearing. In Harrison's Principles of Internal Medicine. 9th Edition. Edited by Isselbacher, K.J., et al. New York, McGraw-Hill, 1980.
17. Harrison, M.J.G.: Contemporary neurology. London, Butterworth & Co., 1984.
18. Walton, J.: Brain's Diseases of the Nervous System. Oxford, Oxford University Press, 1985.
19. Rush, J.A., and Younge, B.R.: Paralysis of cranial nerves III, IV, and VI. Cause and prognosis in 1,000 cases. Arch. Ophthalmol. 99:76, 1981.

THE ACUTE PAINFUL EYE

Michael E. Whiting

CAPSULE

Virtually all eye complaints include pain, redness, or change in vision; most include two and many all three of these cardinal symptoms. Optic disorders are commonly caused by infections or trauma, or are manifestations of systemic disease. Ophthalmic disease may present as a change in vision or as a neurologic problem. This chapter, however, focuses on the painful eye, which is not readily explained by trauma, infection, or systemic disease. Most commonly, the differential includes glaucoma, allergic reaction, toxic reaction, and iritis/uveitis. Infectious causes and chlamydia must be considered, however. Table 55-3 illustrates the differential diagnosis.

ACUTE ANGLE CLOSURE GLAUCOMA

Glaucoma is characterized by elevated intraocular pressure, progressive loss of vision, and optic nerve head cupping. Chronic open angle glaucoma is usually insidious in onset and diagnosed by screening examination or in evaluation of severe gradual vision loss. In contrast, acute angle closure (narrow angle) glaucoma results from a sudden rise in intraocular pressure, followed by a red, painful eye and a decrease in vision.

In the normal eye, aqueous is produced by the ciliary body and flows anteriorly around the iris to the anterior chamber, exiting the eye by way of the trabecular meshwork. Aqueous then collects in the canal of Schlemm, which communicates with the episcleral veins. Patients who are at risk for angle closure are often short-eyed (far-sighted) with shallow anterior chambers, or have large lenses, particularly the elderly. In either case, the angle through which the aqueous flows narrows abnormally, causing the iris to block the trabecular meshwork. Attacks often begin in low light conditions when the pupil is mid-dilated, maximizing the impingement of the iris upon the trabecular meshwork. The intraocular pressure rises, causing pain and ocular ischemia.

Patients usually present with acute onset of severe pain, blurry vision, and a red eye. The pain may be a generalized headache and nausea and vomiting may be present. The examination reveals a red eye, usually with a mid-dilated pupil and an edematous (steamy) cornea. The affected eye is quite hard (marble-like) when compared with the unaffected eye. A narrow angle may be visible on penlight or slit lamp examination. The intraocular pressure should be measured using the Shiotz or pneumotonometer. Pressures up to 20 are considered normal; in an acute attack, pressures are usually high (40 to 70) and require immediate treatment. Angle closure glaucoma may also be subacute or intermittent. The finding of a shallow chamber and a red, painful eye should alert the examiner to obtain a history of previous episodes of pain and to document intraocular pressures.

Mainstays of treatment in the Emergency Department (ED) include acetazolamide 500 mg PO or IV, timolol 0.5% drops, and pilocarpine 1% drops every 15 minutes as needed. Mannitol 1 to 1.5 mg/kg IV may be given as an osmotic load to promote diuresis. Because of ocular ischemia, the topical drops have little effect until the attack is broken by the systemic agents.

Once the acute attack is broken, laser iridotomy or surgical peripheral iridectomy can remove the risk of recurrent attacks. A prophylactic peripheral iridotomy is usually performed on the contralateral eye as well so that the possibility of angle closure bilaterally is eliminated. Prognosis is good if the patient is treated in the early stages of the attack, but blindness can result from delay in recognition or treatment.[1,2,3]

ED physicians must be especially aware of glaucoma in blacks, which is often undertreated.[3a]

TABLE 55-3. THE ACUTE PAINFUL EYE: DIFFERENTIAL DIAGNOSIS

Allergy
  Rhinoconjunctivitis
  Atopic conjunctivitis
  Giant papillary conjunctivitis
  Vernal conjunctivitis
Glaucoma
  Acute angle closure
Trauma
  Abrasion
  Laceration
  Iritis
Infectious
  Viral conjunctivitis
  Bacterial conjunctivitis
  Herpes simplex
  Herpes zoster
  Orbital cellulitis
  Keratoconjunctivitis
Systemic Disease
  Temporal arteritis
  Uveitis
    Sarcoid
    Tuberculosis
    Syphilis
    Behçet's disease
    Reiter's syndrome
    Toxoplasmosis
    Traumatic
    Idiopathic
  Headache syndromes
  Scleritis/episcleritis

ALLERGY

Red, painful, itchy eyes are a common chief complaint in the ED, and allergy accounts for a large fraction. The most common type of ocular allergy is rhinoconjunctivitis. The history usually reveals a seasonal allergen exposure, with resulting bilateral red, itchy eyes and accompanying coryza. The examination shows edematous conjunctiva, giving the eye a watery or glassy appearance. There may be a pink or milky discharge. Papillae are typically present in allergic conjunctivitis; they are heaped-up collections of inflammatory cells surrounding a vascular core. A smear taken from the conjunctiva reveals eosinophils or eosinophilic granules, which are virtually pathognomonic of allergy. Treatment includes cool compresses, topical antihistamines and decongestants, and cromolyn drops for severe cases.[4,5] (See the section of this chapter entitled Ophthalmologic Pharmacotherapy in Emergencies.)

Patients with atopic dermatitis are also at risk for atopic keratoconjunctivitis, an allergic conjunctivitis. In addition to the signs and symptoms described previously, the lids may demonstrate atopic lesions or staphylococcal blepharitis. Atopic keratoconjunctivitis may require topical steroids as well as decongestants, antihistamines, and cromolyn. Because the use of steroids incurs the risk of glaucoma, cataracts, and corneal thinning, all patients who may need steroids should be referred to an ophthalmologist.[6]

Vernal keratoconjunctivitis occurs in children or teenagers and is frequently associated with other allergic problems. Vernal keratoconjunctivitis is similar in presentation to atopic or rhinoconjunctivitis, but is notable for the presence of giant papillae on the upper lid conjunctiva. Complications include corneal ulcers or pseudomembranes. Treatment includes topical and systemic steroids under the direction of an ophthalmologist, and cromolyn. Vernal keratoconjunctivitis is usually self-limited, resolving after 5 to 10 years.[5,6]

CONJUNCTIVITIS

Contact conjunctivitis may result from ocular exposure to cosmetics, drugs, soaps or detergents, or other noxious stimulus. A notorious and common cause of contact conjunctivitis is the thimerosal preservative in many eyedrops and contact lens solutions. Usually withdrawal of the offending substance is sufficient treatment, but this may require persistence by the physician when the suspect agent is a drug of long-standing use, such as over-the-counter eyedrops.[6]

In allergic conjunctivitis, more often than in viral or bacterial conjunctivitis, itching is the chief complaint.[5] Usually the vision is unaffected after the mucus and discharge are wiped away. Unlike the bright red conjunctiva and purulent discharge of bacterial conjunctivitis, allergic conjunctivitis is marked by a milky or glassy eye and a stringy clear or milky discharge.[6]

Viral conjunctivitis may be similar to allergic con-

junctivitis in presentation; however, viral conjunctivitis is often associated with upper respiratory infections at the onset, begins unilaterally, and may be persistent. Viral conjunctivitis is marked by clear, watery discharge and conjunctival follicles. Follicles are small, white tufts of lymphoid tissue that are avascular, but may be surrounded by vessels; follicles are usually on the lower conjunctival surface and are visible with the slit lamp.[6,7]

Follicles are also found in chlamydial (inclusion) conjunctivitis, along with a mucopurulent discharge and bright red bulbar conjunctiva. It is usually bilateral, associated with local lymph node enlargement, and may be associated with nonocular chlamydial or other sexually transmitted diseases. Patients with inclusion conjunctivitis are generally young and sexually active.[8] In any patient whose conjunctivitis lasts longer than 3 weeks and particularly in patients who are at risk for sexually transmitted disease, chlamydial cultures and/or a trial of tetracycline 250 mg PO for 2 weeks is indicated before concluding that the conjunctivitis is of allergic cause.

IRITIS/UVEITIS

Iritis and anterior uveitis are nearly synonymous terms for inflammation of any cause occurring in the anterior chamber, iris, and ciliary body. Trauma and local infection are the most obvious causes; however, systemic diseases (see Table 55-3) may be an occult cause, and in many cases no specific cause is ever identified.[2] Although the association of acute anterior uveitis with HLA-B27 is well known (50% of white patients with acute anterior uveitis are HLA-B27 positive[2]), recent studies have shown that uveitis is highly correlated with numerous other autoimmune syndromes with HLA associations.

Patients with anterior uveitis present with pain, redness, and photophobia. Examination reveals a small, often irregular, and poorly reactive pupil. Slit lamp examination shows cell and flare in the anterior chamber and the acuity is often decreased because of this haze. Other findings may include collections of white cells, keratic precipitates, on the iris, lens, or posterior cornea. Fibrous adhesions (synechiae) may form between the iris and the lens, causing the pupil to be irregular.

Treatment includes intermittent dilation and paralysis of the pupil with homatropine to relieve the ciliary spasm and to prevent the formation of synechiae, along with topical steroids and occasionally systemic anti-inflammatories. Referral to an ophthalmologist is essential because the sequelae can include cataracts, glaucoma, neovascularization, and macular edema.

EPISCLERITIS/SCLERITIS

Episcleritis is a localized inflammation and dilation of the episcleral vessels, usually in one quadrant of the eye. The reaction may be to external irritants or viral disease, or may be idiopathic. The episcleral edema and inflammation may be nodular, are often salmon-pink, and are mobile over the underlying sclera. Episcleritis is usually self-limited, but may persist for weeks.[2,7,9]

Scleritis is a more serious inflammation of the sclera proper, usually caused by underlying collagen vascular disease or infection. The eye may appear bluish in the areas of inflammation and is deeply painful, particularly with ocular motion. Referral to an ophthalmologist is essential because an extensive workup is often required to elucidate the cause. Scleritis is usually treated with topical steroids and systemic anti-inflammatory medications.[2]

CONTACT LENSES

Contact lenses have become nearly ubiquitous in the last decade, resulting in increasing numbers of complications and ED visits. The most serious complication is infectious keratitis (see next chapter section, Common Eye Infections), but noninfectious complications are probably more common. Most frequent is the overuse syndrome—corneal abrasions or ulcers secondary to prolonged wear or minor trauma on insertion or removal.[10] After removal of the lens, the abrasion or ulcer is easily seen on slit lamp examination with the use of fluorescein. Unlike simple abrasions, these should not be patched but treated with antibiotic drops or ointment and left open because some data suggest that patching these abrasions increases the risk of infection.[11] If infection is suspected, the patient should be immediately referred to an ophthalmologist.

Giant papillary conjunctivitis (GPC) is an allergic conjunctivitis often associated with contact lens wear. The hallmarks of GPC are pruritus, watery discharge, and large papillae on the upper lid. Symptoms usually resolve when lenses are discontinued; for those unwilling to sacrifice their lenses, meticulous hygiene, new lenses, and often a switch to gas-permeable, hard, or disposable lenses will cure the problem.[6,7,10]

MEDICOLEGAL PEARLS

- Visual acuity is the vital sign of the eyes, and must be recorded for every patient with ocular complaints.
- A complete examination, including acuity, fundoscopy, slit lamp, and tonometry is essential if the diagnosis is at all in doubt.
- Prescribe ophthalmic steroids *only* after consultation with an ophthalmologist who will follow the patient, or based on prior agreements.
- Never prescribe topical anesthetics for continued outpatient use.
- Angle closure glaucoma is a vision-threatening medical emergency that requires aggressive treatment and immediate consultation.
- Exclude chlamydial conjunctivitis before making the diagnosis of chronic allergic conjunctivitis or epidemic keratoconjunctivitis.

REFERENCES

1. Elkington, A.R., and Khaw, P.T.: The glaucomas. Br. Med. J. 297:677,1988.
2. Yanofsky, N.N.: The acute painful eye. Emerg. Med. Clin. North Am. 6:21, 1988.
3. Greenidge, K.C.: Angle-closure glaucoma. Int. Ophthalmol. Clin. 30:177, 1990.
3a. Javitt, J.C., McBean, A.M., Nicholson, G.A., et al.: Undertreatment of glaucoma among black Americans. N. Engl. J. Med. 325:1419, 1991.
4. Friedlaender, M.H., Okumoto, M., and Kelley, J.: Diagnosis of allergic conjunctivitis. Arch. Ophthalmol. 102:1198, 1984.
5. Friedlaender, M.H.: Ocular allergy. Postgrad. Med. 79:261, 1986.
6. Friedlaender, M.H.: Ocular allergy. J. Allergy Clin. Immunol. 76:645, 1985.
7. Elkington, A.R., and Khaw, P.T.: The red eye. Br. Med. J. 296:1720, 1988.
8. Bienfang, D.C., Kelly, L.D., Nicholson, D.H., and Nussenblatt, R.B.: Ophthalmology. N. Engl. J. Med. 323:956, 1990.
9. Watson, P.G., and Hayreh, S.S.: Scleritis and episcleritis. Br. J. Ophthalmol. 60:163, 1976.
10. Cohen, E.J., Laibson, P.R., Arentsen, J.J., et al.: Corneal ulcers associated with cosmetic extended wear soft contact lenses. Ophthalmology 94:109, 1987.
11. Grutzmacher, R.D.: Ocular disease from wearing contact lenses. Postgrad. Med. 86:90, 1989.

COMMON EYE INFECTIONS

Theodore Rabinovitch, Scott S. Weissman, and Robert A. Nozik

CAPSULE

Most ocular infections that confront the emergency physician affect the external ocular structures. Most of the common infections of the lids and conjunctiva are not immediately vision-threatening and may be treated with local antibiotics and or compresses. A red eye, in addition to being caused by acute glaucoma, scleritis and iritis, may be the result of ulcerative keratitis, acute endophthalmitis, or orbital cellulitis, all of which may cause blindness. It is the task of the emergency physician to recognize the source, nature, and severity of the infection so that proper treatment can be instituted. Awareness of the more serious eye infections will lead to prompt referral to an ophthalmologist and may save the patient's sight.

PATHOPHYSIOLOGY AND ANATOMY

The eyelids are complex structures whose main function is to protect the globe from dessication through their barrier effect and by means of secretion of mucus, oil, and aqueous elements to add to the tear film. The meibomian glands' normal function is to secrete oil to the external tear film layer. They are sandwiched between the inner conjunctival surface and the outer muscle and skin within the dense tarsal plates of the eyelids. Obstruction of the meibomian gland orifices causes extrusion of lipid within the eyelid, with subsequent granulomatous inflammation called chalazia. Hordeola (styes) are acute staphylococcal inflammations of the superficial sweat and sebaceous glands and hair follicles of the eyelids.

The inner surface of the eyelid is lined with the conjunctiva, a secretory squamous epithelial surface rich in goblet cells which provide the mucus component to the tear film that lubricates the globe and lids. Bacteria and viruses can infect the conjunctiva as a result of contact with infected secretions or direct inoculation from trauma or foreign bodies.

The corneal epithelium is an excellent barrier to organisms. Direct trauma to the epithelium through contact lenses, corneal abrasions, or chronic neurotrophic epithelial defects may cause contamination of the corneal stroma and lead to corneal ulcers. Koch-Weeks bacillus, Corynebacterium diphtheriae, and Neisseria

gonorrhea can penetrate the intact epithelium without antecedent injury. Pseudomonas infections are particularly dangerous because of the quick spread to surrounding ocular structures. In all instances, however, compromise of local immune factors from topical steroid treatment may lead to devastating infection of the cornea and globe.

The lacrimal sac lies in a bony depression along the inferomedial aspect of the bony orbit. It receives tears from the eye by way of the puncta, two tiny openings located at medial aspect of the upper and lower eyelid margins. The lacrimal sac empties its contents by means of a tubular duct that enters the nose beneath the middle turbinate. Chronic obstruction of the nasolacrimal duct may lead to acute or chronic dacryocystitis by organisms commensal to the conjunctiva. In infants, the obstruction is normally caused by congenital blockage of the lower end of the lacrimal duct as it empties into the nose. In adults, the cause is often idiopathic, presumably from underlying anatomic predispositions, or from trauma.

The globe is enclosed within the bony orbit. This space is surrounded by the frontal, maxillary, and ethmoid sinuses. Acute sinusitis or direct orbital trauma may cause orbital cellulitis. Abscess formation may cause compression to the optic nerve and may lead to loss of vision. Retrograde transmission of organisms to the cavernous sinus causes cavernous sinus thrombosis.

INITIAL EYE EVALUATION

HISTORY

In all eye infections, the history can guide the physician to correct diagnosis in many cases. For example, the presence of pain versus itching can help differentiate between a keratitis and an allergic conjunctivitis. In a contact lens wearer who presents with pain, redness, and blurred vision, a corneal abrasion should be suspected. A red eye that develops shortly after an upper respiratory infection is often caused by viral conjunctivitis. In a patient with a history of tearing and the development of a red, painful lump near the nose, dacryocystitis should be suspected.

PHYSICAL EXAMINATION

The recording of visual acuity is essential. Most external eye infections do not affect the cornea and there-

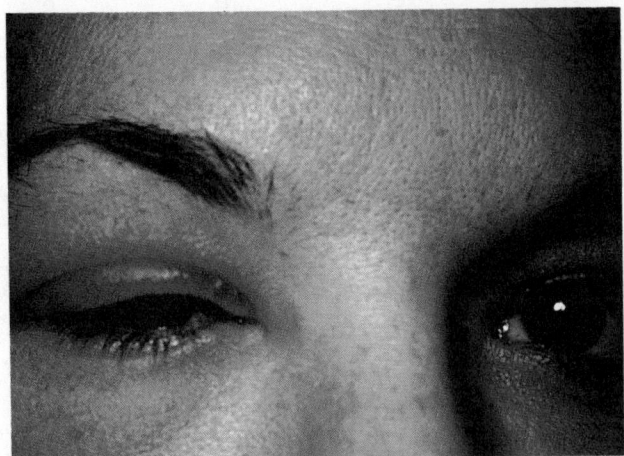

FIG. 55-8. Inflamed lid secondary to hordeolum.

fore do not severely diminish vision. Pus from a purulent conjunctivitis, however, may temporarily blur the vision. Similarly, a viral keratitis associated with conjunctivitis may significantly reduce visual acuity.

Visual inspection of the periorbita, lids, conjunctiva, and cornea often reveals the primary site of the infection. Slit-lamp examination aids in the detection of conjunctival follicles or papillae, keratitis, or iritis. Ophthalmoscopic evaluation of the fundus may reveal vitritis, retinitis, choroiditis, or optic nerve disease.

LABORATORY INVESTIGATIONS

The eye is subject to infection by a host of different organisms, including bacteria, viruses, and fungi. In some instances, i.e., viral conjunctivitis and herpetic keratitis, clinical evaluation may be sufficient to sort out the cause, thereby avoiding the need for bacterial cultures. In other instances, the microbiology laboratory can be helpful in isolating the offending organisms. In stubborn conjunctivitis and corneal ulcers, scrapings of the infected tissue are taken for Gram and Giemsa staining. Swabs from infected tissue should be cultured on blood agar because it supports growth of most organisms that infect the eye. Often

only a small number of organisms may be responsible for certain ocular infections. Therefore a liquid nutrient broth provides an excellent medium for growth and detection. Chocolate agar is an excellent medium for detection of Hemophilus and Neisseria; Sabouraud's dextrose agar permits growth of most fungi and yeasts.[1]

CLINICAL PRESENTATION, PHYSICAL EVALUATION, AND STABILIZATION

INFECTIONS OF THE EYELIDS

EXTERNAL HORDEOLUM (STYE) (FIG. 55-8)

Clinically, this presents as a painful, red, localized pustule on the eyelids. Treatment consists of hot compresses. Topical antibiotics are usually helpful. Rarely, incision and drainage are required.

CHALAZION

This presents as an uninflamed, nontender mass in the upper or lower lid. Hot compresses and topical antibiotics result in disappearance or shrinkage, but incision and curettage are often necessary in persistent cases.

INFECTIONS OF THE CONJUNCTIVA

The differential diagnosis to consider in conjunctivitis includes bacterial, viral, chlamydial, fungal, parasitic, chemical, and allergic causes. By and large, all cause red eyes, but specific differences in symptoms and signs allow a reasonable diagnosis, indicating appropriate management (Table 55-4).

GIANT PAPILLARY CONJUNCTIVITIS (GPC)

GPC presents with grossly enlarged papillae on the upper palpebral conjunctiva (described as "cobble-

TABLE 55-4. SIGNS AND SYMPTOMS OF CONJUNCTIVITIS

	Viral	Bacterial	Allergic

Symptoms	Burning
	Irritation
	Lids and lashes
	  slightly sticky
	  in AM
		Burning
		Irritation
		Lids and lashes stuck
		  together
		  in AM
			Itching
			Tearing

Laterality	Bilateral	Unilateral > Bilateral	Bilateral
Discharge	Watery	Purulent	Watery
Conjunctiva	Follicles	Papillae	Pale edema
Preauricular nodes	Present	Usually not	None

stone" in appearance). This condition is most often related to contact lens wear, particularly with extended-wear contact lenses. Various preservatives in the contact lens solutions have been most often implicated. This condition may also be observed in relation to exposed suture material or a prosthetic eye.

Symptoms consist most often of severe itching, excessive mucus production, and excessive contact lens movement with blinking.

Treatment consists of removing the sensitizing factor, for example, eliminating contact lens wear for 1 to 4 months. When resumption of contact lens wear is recommended, the patient should consider only daily-wear contact lenses, use of nonpreserved contact lens solutions, and even frequent replacement of the lenses (such as every 4 to 6 months). Elimination of an irritating suture or polishing or complete replacement of a prosthesis are therapeutic considerations. The medication most commonly used is cromolyn sodium (Opticrom 4%) four to six times daily.

BACTERIAL CONJUNCTIVITIS

Acute bacterial conjunctivitis (pink eye) is most often caused by Staphylococcus aureus, Streptococcus pneumoniae, and Hemophilus influenzae; more chronic forms may be caused by Pseudomonas, coliform bacteria, and Moraxella. Hyperacute purulent conjunctivitis (Fig. 55-9) may be caused by Neisseria gonorrheae. At-risk populations include sexually active adults, especially homosexuals, and neonates.

The contagious nature of most bacterial and viral conjunctivitis should be emphasized. The examiner should wear gloves for the examination, and hand washing on the part of the patient should be thorough. The patient should be warned about contagion and given appropriate instructions in hygiene.

Bacterial conjunctivitis usually presents with mucopurulent discharge and a red eye. The patient complains of sticking and matting of the lids and lashes, mostly in the morning. Vision is blurred when copious amounts of discharge are present. The disease may be bilateral, but usually begins with one eye. Dilation

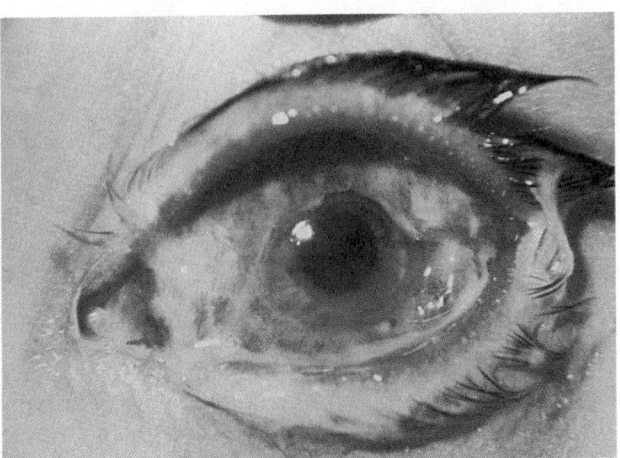

FIG. 55-9. Hyperacute bacterial conjunctivitis.

of conjunctival vessels, mucopurulent discharge, and papillae on the tarsal conjunctiva are present. Disease may affect one or both eyes and is usually self-limited.

Use of topical antibiotics such as polymyxin, bacitracin, and erythromycin is adequate in most cases. If there is no drug allergy history, a 10% solution of sulfacetamide q.i.d. is an appropriate consideration. In most cases, a broad-spectrum antibiotic such as sulfacetamide 10% or an antibiotic combination drug such as polytrim (trimethoprim sulfate and polymyxin B sulfate) four times daily up to 7 to 10 days is effective. Polytrim is preferable to neosporin (neomycin-bacitracin-polymyxin B) because of the significant incidence of hypersensitivity to neomycin.

Other ophthalmic preparations such as gentamicin or tobramycin are effective for gram-negative organisms, including pseudomonas, but because they are toxic and may cause emergence of resistant organisms, they should not be the drugs of first choice. With appropriate antibiotic therapy, the infection begins to improve within 2 to 4 days. If no improvement occurs, one should consider resistant organisms or improper diagnosis. These patients should be referred to an ophthalmologist. Cultures are important to isolate the specific bacteria and determine drug sensitivities.

Topical antibiotics are usually sufficient for treatment of most bacterial conjunctivitis (Tables 55-5 and 55-6). Systemic antibiotics do not provide any additional benefit unless Neisseria sp. is isolated. This conjunctivitis is not self-limited. It presents with hyperpurulent discharge, severe chemosis, redness of the conjunctiva, and swelling of the lids. Corneal ulcers may develop because the organism can penetrate the intact corneal epithelium. These patients should be considered acute emergencies and should have an immediate referral to an ophthalmologist.

VIRAL CONJUNCTIVITIS (FIG. 55-10)

Viral conjunctivitis presents with an acute red eye with watery discharge. The lashes are usually not matted in the morning. There is often a history of recent URI or exposure to other infected individuals. The second eye often becomes affected within days. Tender preauricular adenopathy is often present. The eye is injected, and follicles are seen on the conjunctiva. In epidemic keratoconjunctivitis (EKC) caused by an adenovirus, the mild keratitis may cause photophobia and blurred vision.[2]

In viral conjunctivitis, supportive therapy such as cool compresses, artificial tears, and cleansing of the lids and lashes is sufficient. Use of topical antibiotics is optional if a viral cause is suspected. The patient should be made aware of the natural history of the disease: that the infection will completely clear without sequelae within 2 to 4 weeks. These infections are highly contagious, and patients should be instructed to wash their hands often and avoid direct contact of their ocular secretions with other people through use of separate towels, pillows, etc.

TABLE 55-5. PARTIAL LIST OF COMMERCIALLY AVAILABLE ANTIBIOTIC EYEDROPS*

Antibiotic	Trade Name	Concentration
Gentamicin	Garamycin, Gentacidin	0.3%
Tobramycin	Tobrex	0.3%
Sulfacetamide	Bleph 10 & 30	10%, 30%
	Sodium Sulamyd 10%, 30%	10%, 30%
	Sulfacel-15	15%
Sulfisoxasole	Gantrisin	4%
Tetracycline	Achromycin	1%
Ciprofloxacin	Ciloxan	0.3%
Polymyxin B-Neomycin	Neosporin, AK Spore	Polymyxin B 5000 U–10,000 U/mL
Gramicidin		Neomycin sulfate 1.75 U–2.5 U/mL
		Gramicidin 0.025 mg/mL
Trimethoprim-Polymyxin B	Polytrim	Trimethoprim sulfate 0.1%
		Polymyxin B sulfate 10,000 U/mg

* With permission from Baum, J.L.: Antibiotic use in ophthalmology. *In* Duane's Clinical Ophthalmology, volume 4, chapter 26. Edited by Tasman, W., and Jaeger, E. A. Philadelphia, J.B. Lippincott Company, 1988.

TABLE 55-6. PARTIAL LIST OF COMMERCIALLY AVAILABLE ANTIBIOTIC OINTMENTS*

Antibiotic	Trade Name	Concentration
Tetracycline	Achromycin	1%
Gentamicin	Garamycin, Gentacidin	3 mg/g
Erythromycin	Ilotycin	0.5%
Tobramycin	Tobrex	0.3%
Sulfacetamide	Cetamide	10%
	Sodium Sulamyd	10%
	Sulten-10	10%
	Ak-Sulf	10%, 15%, 30%
Sulfisoxasole	Gantrisin	4%
Bacitracin	Baciquent	Baciguent 500 U/g
Polymyxin B-Neomycin	Neosporin, Ak-Spore	Polymyxin B sulfate 5000–10,000 U/g
		Neomycin sulfate 3.5 mg–5.0 mg/g
Polymyxin B-Bacitracin	Polysporin	Polymyxin B sulfate 10,000 U/g
		Zinc Bacitracin 400–500 U/g
Polymyxin B-Neomycin	Statrol	Polymyxin B sulfate 6,000 U/g
		Neomycin sulfate 3.5 mg/g

* With permission from Baum, J.L.: Antibiotic Use in Ophthalmology. *In* Duane's Clinical Ophthalmology, volume 4, chapter 26. Edited by Tasman, W. and Jaeger, E. A. Philadelphia, J.B. Lippincott Company, 1988.

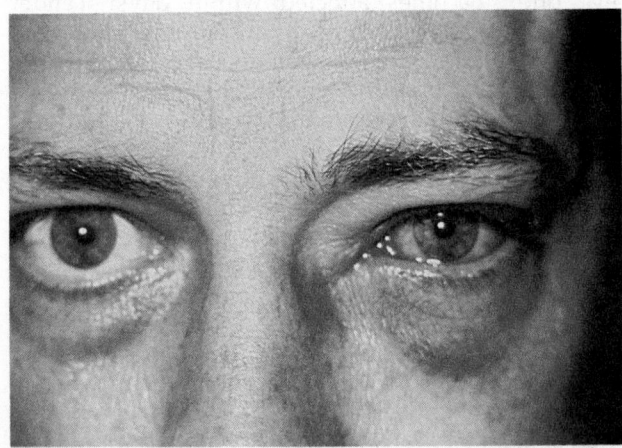

FIG. 55-10. Viral conjunctivitis with watery discharge.

CHLAMYDIAL CONJUNCTIVITIS

Chlamydial conjunctivitis is seen in sexually active adults, who often have an associated vaginitis or urethritis, and newborn infants of infected mothers. A chronic unilateral conjunctivitis of more than 4 weeks' duration) associated with follicular reaction (Fig. 55-11) and mild mucopurulent discharge are seen. Treatment is given by systemic tetracycline or erythromycin for 3 weeks. Systemic treatment of sexual partners is essential to break the cycle of recurrent infection. In neonates, the diagnosis may be made by identifying inclusion bodies on Giemsa stain of conjunctival scrapings. A monoclonal antibody test is available and highly specific.[2a]

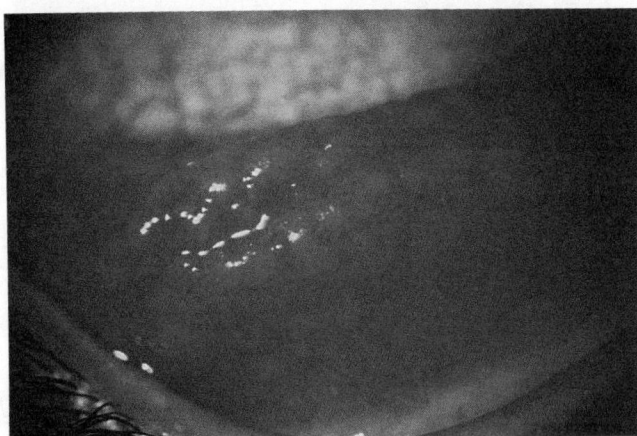

FIG. 55-11. Follicular reaction on superior tarsal conjunctiva in Chlamydial conjunctivitis. Follicular changes also occur with viral conjunctivitis.

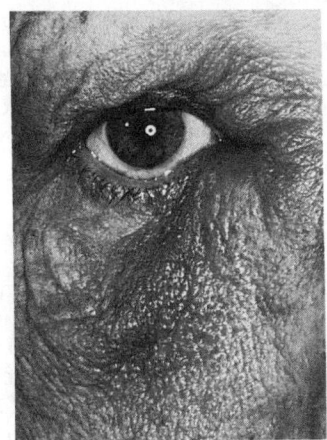

FIG. 55-12. Dacryocystitis.

ALLERGIC CONJUNCTIVITIS

Prominent itching is the main symptom of allergic conjunctivitis. Mild to severe redness is accompanied by lacrimation, often associated with a stringy discharge. Swelling of the conjunctivae and papillae is often present. There may be a history of contact with common allergens. Avoidance of the offending agent plus treatment with cool compresses is often sufficient in mild disease. More severe cases may be treated with topical antihistamine-decongestant drops three to four times daily. Topical cromolyn is useful as prophylactic treatment; topical steroids may be helpful in severe cases but should be prescribed only by an opthalmologist. Steroids may cause increased intraocular pressure, provoke rampant spread of herpes simplex infection of the cornea, delay corneal healing, allow overgrowth of bacteria and fungi, and mask underlying inflammatory conditions.

INFECTIONS OF THE LACRIMAL SAC

DACRYOCYSTITIS (FIG. 55-12)

In acute dacryocystitis, the lacrimal sac is red and tender and may display fluctuance. Chronic dacryocystitis demonstrates smoldering infection without severe distention of the sac. Tearing is a common complaint of both, as well as chronic unilateral conjunctivitis.

Common bacterial causes of dacryocystitis include pneumococci, streptococci, and staphylococci. Other causative organisms, including gram-negative bacteria and actinomyces, may infect the lacrimal sac.

Treatment of acute dacryocystitis consists of warm compresses and antibiotics. Topical agents are occasionally sufficient, but usually systemic treatment is necessary. Penicillins or cephalosporins are the agents of choice. Incision and drainage are often necessary but may lead to chronic draining fistulas.

INFECTIONS OF THE CORNEA

ULCERATIVE KERATITIS (CORNEAL ULCERS)

Ulcerative lesions of the cornea are an emergency. A Pseudomonas infection can devastate the eye within 24 hours. Corneal ulcers present with a red, often painful eye and blurred vision. Purulent discharge may be present. A white infiltrate can often be seen with the unaided eye, and with the slit lamp the ulcer appears as an epithelial defect with a central crater filled with purulent debris (Fig. 55-13). An infiltrate may be present in the corneal stroma. There may be a hypopyon, a layering of white blood cells and inflammatory debris that has settled to the bottom of the anterior chamber. Initial recognition of this as an ocular emergency with immediate referral to an ophthalmologist is vital. If the patient is to be seen by the ophthalmologist, treatment should not be initiated until cultures with scrapings are performed. Patients are often hospitalized for around-the-clock hourly instillation of prepared fortified topical antibiotics. Systemic

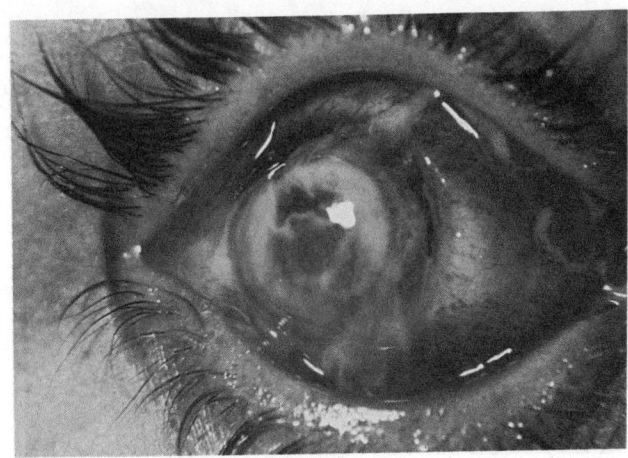

FIG. 55-13. Bacterial corneal ulcer.

antibiotics are usually not necessary because the local application penetrates the cornea better than systemic circulation. Fortified antibiotics are instilled topically in the eye every half hour around the clock. No patching is ever incorporated in the therapy. Systemic antibiotics are appropriate in severe cases.

HERPES SIMPLEX KERATITIS (FIG. 55-14)

The common cold sore virus (herpes simplex I) can cause secondary infection of the cornea. The virus may lie dormant in the trigeminal ganglion and the cornea, and under conditions of stress, ultraviolet light, menstruation, and fever, can be activated and reinfect the cornea. The eye is diffusely reddened and the patient has photophobia, pain, foreign body sensation, and tearing. A typical dendritic figure that stains with fluorescein dye is best seen by slit-lamp examination. The cornea is hypesthetic at the margin of the dendrite. Effective treatment includes the use of topical antiviral agents (trifluoridine or idoxuridine drops) for 7 to 10 days. Alternatively, one can debride the infected corneal epithelium with a cotton swab and patch the eye. These corneas are at risk of developing permanent corneal scarring and should be managed only by the ophthalmologist. Acyclovir is unproven in this condition; its use depends on the consultant and the severity of infection.[2b]

HERPES ZOSTER OPHTHALMICUS

When herpes zoster affects the ophthalmic division of the fifth cranial nerve, ocular lesions may occur. This is especially true if the nasociliary branch innervating the tip of the nose is affected. Typical skin lesions appear on the forehead, eyelids, and nose. Conjunctivitis is common; the cornea is involved less often. When the cornea is involved, there are fine dendritic figures and a superficial punctate keratitis seen at the slit lamp. Severe iritis may occur with elevation of intraocular pressure. Specific therapy can be effective and includes the use of systemic acyclovir

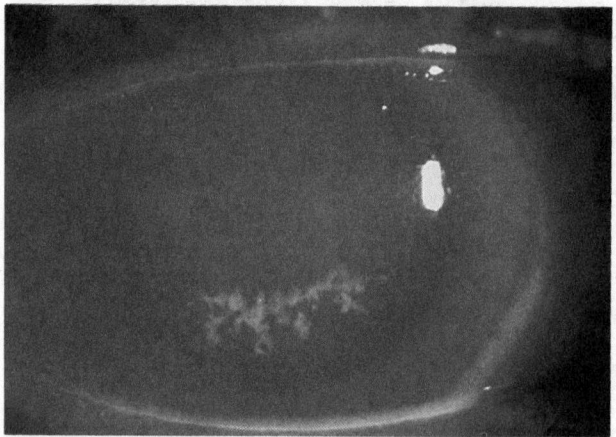

FIG. 55-14.   Herpes simplex dendrite of the corneal epithelium.

(800 mg five times a day) if the disease is recognized in the first 10 days after infection.[3] This may limit the duration of the skin lesions and may aid in decreasing ocular complications. Topical antibiotics may prevent secondary bacterial conjunctivitis. If iritis is present, the patient should be referred to the ophthalmologist without delay. Dilation of the pupil with 5% homatropine twice daily alleviates some discomfort by putting the eye at rest. The use of topical and systemic corticosteroids is controversial.

OPHTHALMIA NEONATORUM

Many opportunistic organisms found in the female genital tract are capable of producing disease. Although silver nitrate 1% prophylaxis has dramatically reduced the incidence of gonococcal disease of the newborn eye, it is not always effective. Gonococcus causes a hyperacute bilateral conjunctivitis (see Fig. 55-9) and is serious because it can rapidly penetrate intact epithelial cells and cause corneal ulceration. The incubation period is 2 to 3 days. Traditionally, infected infants are treated with systemic penicillin G, 50,000 units per kg IM or IV every 12 hours for 7 days, as well as topical penicillin G, 10,000 to 20,000 units every hour around the clock until the disease subsides. Newer protocols suggest the use of ceftriaxone 50 mg per kg IM (one dose) for simple conjunctivitis. If the cornea is also involved, ceftriaxone, 25 to 40 mg per kg IV every 12 hours for 3 days, is recommended.[4]

Chlamydia infection is the most common cause of neonatal conjunctivitis. The incubation period is 5 to 12 days. Babies with chlamydial conjunctivitis may contract chlamydial pneumonia if the conjunctivitis is untreated.[5] Treatment is with 10% sulfacetamide ointment four times daily plus systemic erythromycin, 40 mg per kg per day in divided doses for 3 weeks.

Herpes simplex type 2 infections are less common but serious because they may be associated with chorioretinitis or encephalitis. Blepharoconjunctivitis and typical herpetic vesicles on the lid margins are the normal presenting signs. Treatment is with topical trifluorithymidine 1% drops every 2 hours while the patient is awake. For systemic disease, intravenous acyclovir should be considered.

Other bacteria such as Pneumococcus and Hemophilus can infect the infant's eyes. Therefore, in the neonate, it is essential to perform appropriate bacterial cultures on blood agar as well as on chocolate and Thayer Martin media for Neisseria. Viral and chlamydial cultures should be performed, as well as scrapings for Giemsa staining of inclusion bodies seen in chlamydial disease.

INFECTIONS OF THE ORBIT

PRESEPTAL CELLULITIS

Preseptal cellulitis usually presents as an acute, tender swelling of the lids. A slight fever may accompany this condition, but there is no proptosis or limitation of ocular movement.

An acute chalazion may present as a preseptal cellulitis; it can be differentiated from diffuse inflammation because there is usually no fever and the tenderness can usually be localized by the physician with an applicator stick lightly applied to the lid over the region of the acute glandular (meibomian gland) swelling.

Treatment of chalazion usually consists of warm compresses and massage. Occasionally, surgical excision may be necessary. Depending on the systemic symptoms, oral antibiotics may be indicated.

ORBITAL CELLULITIS (FIG. 55-15)

Acute sinus infection, periorbital deep skin infection, or trauma may lead to orbital cellulitis. Extension into the cavernous sinus or epidural space may be life-threatening. Patients present with periorbital swelling and edema associated with fever and a high white blood cell count. The eye is red and chemotic, and in advanced cases may be proptotic. Patients usually have pain and limitation of eye movement, and may have blurred vision if the optic nerve is compressed by an orbital abscess. The patient may appear toxic or febrile. Skull films detect sinus involvement, but CT scan and MRI demonstrate involvement of the orbit and surrounding sinuses with greater sensitivity.[6] Orbital cellulitis is a serious infection that may lead to loss of vision, intracranial infection, sepsis, and death. Therefore, admission to hospital for intravenous antibiotic therapy is essential. Use of second- and third-generation cephalosporins such as cefoxitin and ceftriaxone, respectively, offers broad-spectrum antibacterial coverage to treat the common organisms that cause sinusitis (pneumococcus, strepto-

coccus, and staphylococcus). Localized abscesses within the orbit often do not respond to antibiotics, and surgical drainage may be necessary. These patients should have cultures of the nasopharynx and blood and should be hospitalized for intravenous antibiotic therapy and close observation.

HORIZONS

Research into advanced drug delivery systems is beginning to pave the way to contemporary ophthalmic drug therapy. Controlled-release dosage forms using polymers, liposomes, mucoadhesives, bioadhesives, colloidal carriers, gel-forming devices, and collagen shields are making great advances. Newer antibiotics such as the fluoroquinolones[7] have been shown effective in treating some common eye infections.

MEDICOLEGAL PEARLS

- Always obtain a culture, Gram stain, and Giemsa stain on all newborns with conjunctivitis.
- Use great caution in prescribing steroids from the ED.
- Refer all patients who are not responding to initial therapy to ophthalmology.
- Culture if the patient returns within 24 hours with worsening symptoms.

REFERENCES

1. Smolin, G., and Thoft, R.A. (Eds.): The Cornea—Scientific Foundations and Clinical Practice, 2nd Ed. Boston, Little, Brown & Company, 1987.
2. Dawson, C.R., et al.: Adenovirus type 8 keratoconjunctivitis in the United States. Am. J. Ophthalmol. 69:473, 1970.
2a. Sheppard, J.D., Kowalski, R.P., Meyer, M.P., et al.: Immunodiagnosis of adult chlamydial conjunctivitis. Ophthalmology 15:434, 1988.
2b. Schwab, J.R.: Oral acyclovir in the management of Herpes simplex ocular infections. Ophthalmology 94:423, 1988.
3. Cobo, L.M., et al.: Oral acyclovir in the therapy of acute herpes zoster ophthalmicus. Ophthalmology 93:763, 1986.
4. Ullman, S., Roussel, T.J., and Forster, R.K.: Gonococcal keratoconjunctivitis. Surv. Ophthalmol. 32:199, 1987.
5. Harrison, J.R., et al.: Chlamydia trachomatis infant pneumonitis. N. Engl. J. Med. 298:702, 1978.
6. Weiss, A., et al.: Bacterial periorbital and orbital cellulitis in childhood. Ophthalmology 90:195, 1983.
7. Kestelyn, P., et al.: Treatment of adult gonococcal keratoconjunctivitis with oral Norfloxacin. Am. J. Ophthalmol. 108:516, 1989.

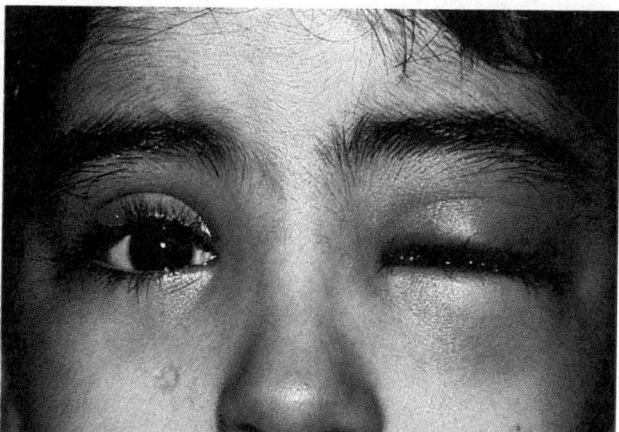

FIG. 55-15.   Orbital cellulitis.

THE EYE AND SYSTEMIC DISEASE

Scott S. Weissman, Theodore Rabinovitch, and Robert A. Nozik

CAPSULE

Ophthalmologic symptoms or signs may be a harbinger of systemic disease, and may be the presenting feature in many cases. The prompt recognition of the underlying systemic disease may be facilitated by an awareness of these oculosystemic associations. The first part covers ophthalmologic emergencies that are commonly associated with systemic disease; the second covers systemic emergencies that may have characteristic eye findings; and the third lists the more important ocular side effects of systemic drugs.

OPHTHALMIC EMERGENCIES ASSOCIATED WITH SYSTEMIC DISEASE[1,2]

CENTRAL RETINAL ARTERY OCCLUSION (SEE ALSO CHAPTER SECTION ENTITLED ACUTE VISUAL LOSS)

Commonly associated conditions include arteriosclerosis and embolization. The latter usually results from cardiac vegetations or carotid atheromas, but is also seen with mitral valve prolapse, after cardiac or carotid surgery, or after cardiac catheterization. Hyperviscosity syndromes and the antiphospholipid antibody syndrome (see subsequent text) also increase the risk of developing central retinal artery occlusion.

CENTRAL RETINAL VEIN OCCLUSION (SEE ALSO CHAPTER SECTION ENTITLED ACUTE VISUAL LOSS)

Common systemic disease associations include cardiovascular disease (74%), hypertension (57%), diabetes (34%), hyperviscosity syndromes, anti-phospholipid antibody syndrome, and other systemic diseases producing ocular vasculitis (e.g., syphilis, sarcoidosis, lupus).

UVEITIS (SEE ALSO CHAPTER SECTION ENTITLED THE ACUTE PAINFUL EYE)

This may be defined strictly as an inflammation of the iris (iritis), ciliary body (cyclitis), choroid (choroiditis), or combinations of these (e.g., iridocyclitis), but retinal inflammation (retinitis) is also included under this heading. Pain, redness, and photophobia typify an acute iridocyclitis, whereas insidious loss of vision with many floaters suggests a retinitis or vitritis. Protein (flare) and circulating white blood cells are typically observed by slit lamp examination in the anterior chamber in an active anterior uveitis, and a perilimbal injection may also be seen (ciliary flush). To ascertain whether causative systemic disease is present and identify it, it is crucial to determine by symptoms and ophthalmoscopic examination: (1) the primary site of inflammation, because different systemic diseases have a predilection for different ocular structures (e.g., toxoplasmosis and cytomegalovirus produce a retinitis, whereas histoplasmosis is thought to cause a choroiditis), and (2) whether the inflammation is granulomatous or nongranulomatous (Table 55-7). Only granulomatous uveitis exhibits any or all of the following signs: greasy or "mutton-fat" deposits on the corneal endothelium by slit lamp examination; iris nodules; and iris, retinal or choroidal granulomas.

TEMPORAL (CRANIAL) ARTERITIS (SEE ALSO CHAPTER SECTION ENTITLED NEURO-OPHTHALMOLOGIC EMERGENCIES)

The inflammation may involve any medium or large artery, usually in patients over 60. It is slightly more common in women, and is rarer in blacks and Asians than in whites. The most dreaded manifestation of temporal arteritis is blindness, which is generally sudden and irreversible. Involvement of the short posterior ciliary arteries may lead to optic nerve ischemia and infarction, manifested by a pale, swollen optic disc, often with peripapillary hemorrhages and an afferent pupillary defect. Amaurosis fugax, extraocular muscle palsies, and central or branch retinal artery occlusion occurs in a few patients. The contralateral eye often becomes involved within 1 to 10 days, underscoring the need for rapid diagnosis and institution of high-dose oral corticosteroids (80 to 100 mg of prednisone per day).

Although the ocular manifestations of temporal arteritis usually follow the systemic ones, they may be the presenting or only symptoms of the disease. Sys-

TABLE 55-7. SYSTEMIC DISEASES ASSOCIATED WITH UVEITIS

PREDOMINANTLY ANTERIOR UVEITIS*

Systemic Disease	Comments
1. Reiter's syndrome (NG)†	*1–4:* Acute, recurrent iridocyclitis. Severe pain, redness and photophobia. Both eyes not involved simultaneously, anterior chamber fibrin or hypopyon, HLA B27+ (especially 1 and 2). Uveitis related to activity of colitis (3). Uveitis unrelated to activity of arthritis (1, 2, and 4)
2. Ankylosing spondylitis (NG)	
3. Inflammatory bowel disease (NG)	
4. Psoriatic arthritis (NG)	
5. Juvenile rheumatoid arthritis (NG)	Minimal symptoms, no red eye. Uveitis more common in periarticular form and in those who are ANA+
6. Kawasaki disease (NG)	Optic disc edema, dilated retinal veins
7. Anterior segment ischemia (NG)	Ocular pain, poorly reactive pupil
8. Acute interstitial nephritis (NG) (rare)	

PREDOMINANTLY POSTERIOR UVEITIS‡

Multiple sclerosis (NG)	Mild vitritis, retinal periphlebitis. Characteristic vitreous opacities, retinal vasculitis
Whipple's disease (NG)	
Cytomegalovirus (G§)	Retinitis, often hemorrhagic, may simulate retinal branch vein occlusion, seen in immunocompromised host, minimal vitreous inflammation
Presumed ocular histoplasmosis syndrome (G)	Peripheral and peripapillary choroidal maculopathy, no vitreal inflammation, thought to occur many years after systemic histoplasmosis infection
Other fungal infections (i.e., Candida, Cryptococcus) (G)	Vitreous fluff balls with Candida in immunosuppressed host
Tuberculosis (G/NG)#	Often no obvious systemic manifestations
Pneumocystis carinii (NG)	Multifocal choroiditis, minimal vitreous inflammation, seen after aerosolized pentamidine for *P. carinii* pneumonia

ANTERIOR AND/OR POSTERIOR UVEITIS

Sarcoidosis (G/NG)#	Serum ACE may be normal if total body granulomatous load is low
Endogenous (metastatic) bacterial endophthalmitis	May be fulminant onset, nonocular foci present in most cases (meningitis, wound or urinary tract infection, endocarditis)
Vogt-Koyanagi-Harada syndrome (NG/G)	Prodrome of meningismus; tinnitus, dysacousia, alopecia, poliosis, and vitiligo occur later. Exudative retinal detachment may occur. American Indians, Japanese, Blacks predisposed
Syphilis (G/NG)#	Uveitis usually occurs in secondary or tertiary disease, interstitial keratitis, pigmentary retinopathy, Argyle-Robertson pupils, optic atrophy occur in some cases
Behçet's syndrome (NG/G)	Blinding uveitis, often with hypopyon and retinal vasculitis; most patients of Japanese or Mediterranean descent
Lymphoma (intraocular) (masquerade syndrome) (NG)	Suspect in elderly with neurologic symptoms. Must rule out CNS lesion, although uveitis may precede CNS disease
Lyme disease (G/NG)	Uveitis usually occurs in stage II. Optic nerve involvement

* Anterior = iritis/iridocyclitis
† NG = Nongranulomatous
‡ Posterior = retinitis/choroiditis
§ G = Granulomatous
# (Nongranulomatous form is rarer)

temic manifestations such as polymyalgia rheumatica, temporal headaches, jaw claudication, weight loss, malaise, and anemia are supportive, and the erythrocyte sedimentation rate is elevated in over 90% of the cases, often to a marked degree.

Temporal artery biopsies should include at least a 3 cm segment, as skip areas have been demonstrated; some authors advocate bilateral biopsies. In the face of progressive visual loss despite high-dose oral prednisone, administration of intravenous methyprednisone (1000 mg every 12 hours for 5 days) may prevent further visual loss. Steroids may be tapered gradually, with vigilant monitoring for signs and symptoms of recurrent disease. *Any elderly patient with the typical ocular manifestations of temporal arteritis with an elevated ESR or associated systemic features must be treated im-*

mediately with high-dose oral corticosteroids even before performing a temporal artery biopsy. Fragmentation of the internal elastic lamina is not affected by as much as a week of corticosteroid therapy, thus permitting pathologic confirmation of the clinical diagnosis.

SUBLUXATION/DISLOCATION OF THE LENS

In the absence of significant ocular trauma, one should search for the following predisposing conditions: Marfan's syndrome (bilateral, often symmetric, superotemporal lens subluxation eventually seen in 50 to 80% of patients); homocystinuria (usually an inferonasal subluxation); and Weill-Marchesani syndrome (the small round lens may dislocate into the anterior chamber, producing acute angle-closure glaucoma by blocking aqueous flow through the pupil). Less common causes of subluxated lenses include syphilis, hyperlysinemia, sulfite oxidase deficiency, and Ehlers-Danlos syndrome. Most cases of lens malposition can be managed with nonsurgical treatment.

SCLERITIS (SEE ALSO CHAPTER SECTION ENTITLED THE ACUTE PAINFUL EYE)

This inflammation produces deep, boring pain and tenderness of the globe that is commonly referred to the jaw, forehead, or temple. More than 50% of cases are bilateral, and in 50% of cases an associated systemic disease may be present, usually rheumatoid arthritis (Table 55-8). Examination of the sclera in natural light reveals a bluish or violaceous-reddish hue in the area of scleritis, caused by deep vascular engorgement.

Scleritis can be divided into anterior and posterior forms. Anterior scleritis is further divided into diffuse, nodular, and necrotizing forms, the latter subdivided into forms with and without inflammation. The necrotizing forms of scleritis are generally associated with severe, long-standing systemic disease, with a significant improvement in 5-year survival when systemic immunosuppression is used (Fig. 55-16).

Findings associated with scleritis include peripheral ulcerative keratitis (also an indicator of severe underlying systemic disease), uveitis, glaucoma, and scleral thinning and perforation. Topical corticosteroids are only minimally effective and do not address the underlying disease, and often oral nonsteroidal anti-inflammatory agents are used in non-necrotizing

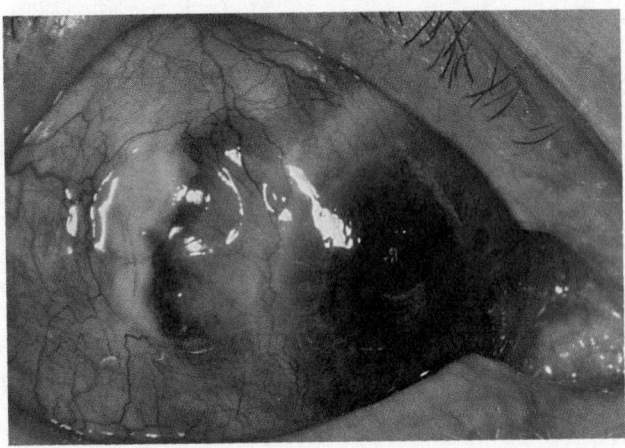

FIG. 55-16. Necrotizing scleritis, with underlying uveal tissue visible.

TABLE 55-8. SYSTEMIC DISEASES ASSOCIATED WITH SCLERITIS

Systemic Disease	Associated Features
Rheumatoid arthritis*	Painless peripheral corneal thinning; keratoconjunctivitis sicca frequent
Polyarteritis nodosa, Wegener's granulomatosis, relapsing polychondritis, psoriatic arthritis, Crohn's disease	Peripheral corneal thinning and/or infiltration
Systemic lupus erythematosis	Retinal vasculitis, with frank occlusion if lupus anticoagulant is present
Temporal arteritis	Central retinal artery occlusion, cranial nerve palsies, ischemic optic neuropathy
Gout	Brown band keratopathy, corneal crystals
Herpes zoster	Unilateral, history of zosteriform eruption in V_1 distribution, corneal pseudodendrite decreased corneal sensation, sector iris atrophy uveitis, glaucoma
Herpes simplex	Unilateral, corneal dendrite, corneal stromal scar, decreased corneal sensation, mild iris atrophy, uveitis, glaucoma
Cogan's disease	Interstitial keratitis
Tuberculosis, syphilis	Interstitial keratitis, uveitis
Lyme disease	Conjunctivitis, keratitis, uveitis

* Most frequent systemic disease associated with scleritis

cases, with oral prednisone and/or immunosuppressive agents such as cyclophosphamide often used in unresponsive or progressive cases. Intravenous pulse corticosteroids (1 g of methylprednisone), often in combination with cytotoxic agents such as cyclophosphamide, may be required in rare cases.

External ocular redness, which is sectorial and associated with deep ocular pain or nodule formation, but not with purulent discharge, is not due to conjunctivitis, but represents a deeper, more serious scleral inflammation; such signs and symptoms may be associated with a life-threatening systemic disease, and require aggressively systemic therapy.

OPTIC NEURITIS (SEE CHAPTER SECTION ENTITLED NEURO-OPHTHALMOLOGIC EMERGENCIES)

SYSTEMIC EMERGENCIES WITH CHARACTERISTIC OCULAR FINDINGS

ENDOCRINE (TABLES 55-9 AND 55-10)

GRAVES' DISEASE

Hyperthyroidism often presents with ocular findings before systemic manifestations, and there may be little correlation between the course of eye disease and the level of circulating thyroid hormones. The principal ocular signs include lid retraction (Dalrymple's sign); lid lag on downgaze (von Graefe's sign), both of which are effects of increased adrenergic innervation to Müller's muscle, which helps to elevate the upper lid; periorbital and conjunctival edema; conjunctival injection over the medial and lateral rectus muscle insertions; restrictive extraocular myopathy often with vertical diplopia (inferior rectus muscle most frequently involved); proptosis with resultant corneal exposure;

TABLE 55-9. GRAVES' DISEASE: OCULAR FINDINGS (NO SPECIFICATIONS) (Modified Werner's Classification)

N: No signs or symptoms
O: Only signs, no symptoms: upper lid retraction, stare, +/− lid lag, +/− mild proptosis
S: Soft tissue involvement: conjunctival edema and injection (especially over horizontal rectus muscle insertions)
P: Proptosis
E: Extraocular muscle involvement; inferior rectus most frequently involved may produce vertical diplopia)
C: Corneal involvement: exposure keratitis
S: Sight loss (compressive optic nerve involvement)
Some cases may not progress through these stages in a predictable fashion; e.g., optic neuropathy may occur without proptosis.

TABLE 55-10. OCULAR MANIFESTATIONS OF ENDOCRINOLOGIC EMERGENCIES

Disease	Ocular Manifestations
Hyperthyroidism	NO specifications
Hypothyroidism	Temporal eyebrow or eyelash loss, conjunctival and periorbital edema, night blindness, optic neuritis or atrophy
Cystic fibrosis	Retinal vascular dilation and hemorrhages, optic neuritis, papilledema
Hypoparathyroidism	Lens opacities* in 50 to 60% (may be polychromatic); keratoconjunctivitis and papilledema
Addison's disease	Hyperpigmentation of the lids, conjunctiva, and uveal tract in a minority of patients
Hypercalcemia (Hyperparathyroidism, hypophosphatasia, hypervitaminosis D)	Scleral, conjunctival, and corneal calcifications, the latter usually within the palpebral fissure and separated from the limbus by a clear interval (band keratopathy)
Diabetes mellitus	Background retinopathy: Microaneurysms, dot and blot hemorrhages, hard exudates (edema residue), cotton wool spots; Preproliferative retinopathy: Extensive retinal hemorrhages, many cotton wool spots intra-retinal microvascular abnormalities (IRMA), venous beading; Proliferative diabetic retinopathy: neovascularization of the optic nerve and/or the retina; fibrovascular proliferation along vitreous surface; vitreous hemorrhage and retinal detachment, rubeosis iridis, neovascular glaucoma

* Lens opacities may also be seen in many other systemic diseases, including pseudohypoparathyroidism, pseudo-pseudohypoparathyroidism, Lowe's syndrome, hypocalcemia, hypo- or hypermagnesemia, galactosemia, Wilson's disease, phenylketonuria, diabetes mellitus, homocystinuria, Alport's syndrome, myotonic dystrophy, and the congenital rubella syndrome.

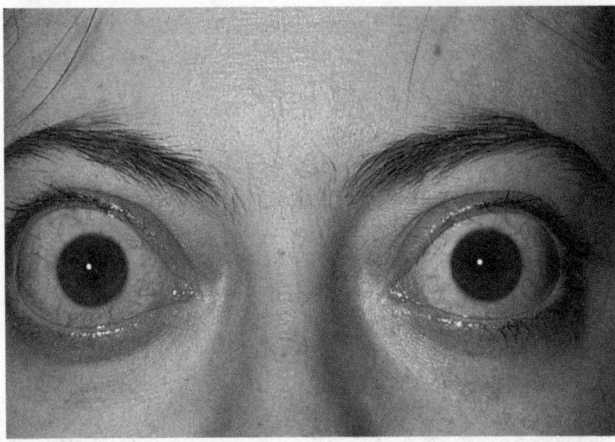

FIG. 55-17. *Graves' disease demonstrating bilateral exophthalmos and lid retraction.*

and optic neuropathy from nerve compression at the orbital apex by markedly swollen extraocular muscles (Fig. 55-17, Table 55-9).

Treatment of the primary disease may exacerbate the ocular disease. Specific ocular therapy includes vigorous ocular lubrication with tear substitutes; pharmacologic (guanethidine drops) and surgical correction of severe lid retraction; and surgical correction of extraocular muscle imbalances if disabling diplopia is present. Nonemergent surgical procedures should be deferred until ocular signs have remained stable for several months.

Thyroid optic neuropathy represents an ophthalmologic emergency and treatment includes high-dose systemic corticosteroids, possibly combined with cyclosporin A, radiation directed at the posterior orbit (1500 to 3000 rads), or orbital decompression.

DIABETIC RETINOPATHY

This generally appears 10 to 15 years after the diagnosis of diabetes is made; the retinal microangiopathy correlates with that in other organs, e.g., the kidney. The retinopathy can be divided into background, preproliferative, and proliferative phases (see Table 55-10). Panretinal photocoagulation, for proliferative and advanced preproliferative diabetic retinopathy, significantly reduces the risk of severe visual loss. The beneficial effect of laser treatment may be from an increase in retinal oxygenation or a decrease in formation of vasoproliferative factors by ischemic retina.

CARDIOVASCULAR

HYPERTENSION[3]

Hypertensive changes in retinal arterioles mirror the changes in vessels elsewhere in the body. Because retinal vessels are directly observable, fundus exam-

ination provides a noninvasive guide to the severity of systemic hypertensive vasculopathy.

In mild to moderate hypertension, retinal arterioles may demonstrate arteriolar narrowing, generalized sclerosis with "copper" or "silver wiring" appearance, focal constrictions, and arteriovenous crossing changes. In more severe hypertensive retinopathy, "flame" hemorrhages, located in the retinal nerve fiber layer, and deeper intraretinal "blot" hemorrhages are seen. "Cotton wool spots" (areas of retinal infarction) appear as fluffy, greyish white areas with feathery, blurred edges. (Cotton wool spots may also be seen in diabetic retinopathy, collagen vascular disease, infective endocarditis, and acquired acute immunodeficiency syndrome). Yellow, lipid exudates may accumulate in the posterior pole, taking on the appearance of a macular star.

In malignant hypertension, as seen with advanced renal disease, pheochromocytoma, and toxemia of pregnancy, a severe hypertensive retinopathy and vasculopathy are seen, and papilledema is an essential finding (Fig. 55-18). Spontaneous venous pulsations may be present because this swelling of the optic nerve is not necessarily from increased intracranial pressure, but may be from local ischemia from arteriolar occlusion. Serous retinal detachments and choroidal detachments and choroidal ischemia also occur; the latter two are well seen with fluorescein angiography.

Prompt antihypertensive treatment is usually successful in resolving cotton wool spots, hemorrhages, and papilledema.

CAROTID ARTERY INSUFFICIENCY (COARCTATION OF THE AORTA, PULSELESS DISEASE)

Carotid insufficiency may present with ocular symptoms or signs including transient monocular blindness lasting anywhere from seconds to minutes (amaurosis

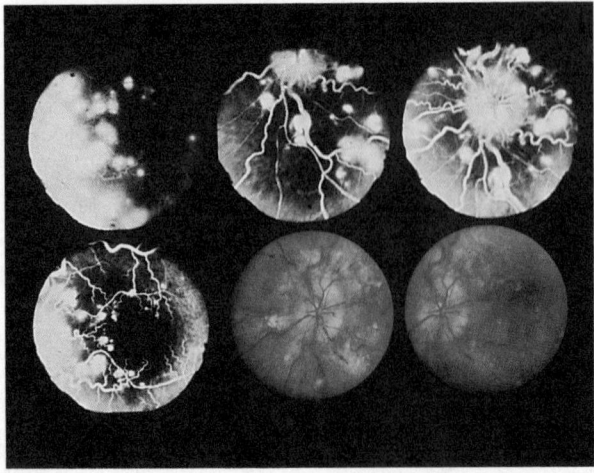

FIG. 55-18. *Papilledema and cottom wool spots in malignant hypertension (b.p. 280/150).*

fugax) or chronic anterior segment ischemia, which is manifested by dull ocular pain, corneal folds, rubeosis iridis, or uveitis. Central or branch retinal artery occlusion and anterior ischemic optic neuropathy may also occur. A search for retinal emboli is important if carotid disease is suspected; cholesterol emboli (Hollenhorst plaque) comprise about 85% of all retinal emboli and appear refractile; platelet-fibrin emboli are dull grey-white; and calcific emboli are chalky white and may appear larger than the vessel lumen.

Ipsilateral central retinal artery pressure is low, as measured by ophthalmodynamometry, and there may be an ipsilateral venous stasis retinopathy characterized by retinal hemorrhages, retinal capillary microaneurysms, and engorged retinal veins. Sometimes there is less hypertensive and/or diabetic retinopathy in the eye ipsilateral to the carotid occlusion, compared to the contralateral eye.

SUBARACHNOID HEMORRHAGE

One third of patients with subarachnoid hemorrhage have associated intraocular hemorrhage, and about 6% have vitreous hemorrhage (Terson's syndrome). The source of the vitreous hemorrhage is unknown but is thought to be a retinal vessel rupture caused by a sudden increase in venous pressure after a sudden increase in intracranial pressure.

INFECTIVE ENDOCARDITIS

Characteristic findings include conjunctival petechiae; retinal cotton wool spots; flame-shaped, often white-centered retinal hemorrhages (Roth spots may also be seen in anemia, leukemia, etc.); retinal arterial occlusions; metastatic endophthalmitis; and papillitis.

DERMATOLOGIC

ERYTHEMA MULTIFORME MAJOR

Ocular complications occur in 50% of cases and include purulent, pseudomembranous or cicatricial conjunctivitis with goblet cell loss and tear mucous deficiency; conjunctival squamous metaplasia with keratinization; lid scarring with misdirected lashes (trichiasis); and corneal epithelial defects with subsequent corneal ulceration and vascularization. Less severe conjunctivitis may be seen in toxic epidermal necrolysis (Lyell's disease).

HEMATOLOGIC

SICKLE CELL DISEASE

Characteristic retinal manifestations include peripheral retinal artery occlusions and arteriovenous anastomoses (seen only with indirect ophthalmoscopy); angioid streaks; salmon patch hemorrhages; black sunbursts; peripheral retinal neovascularization, typically in a sea fan configuration; vitreous hemorrhage; and retinal detachment. Retinal complications are more common in SC and S-thal disease than in SS disease because of the higher hematocrit generally found in the former conditions. Laser photocoagulation of retinal neovascularization is effective in reducing the incidence of visual loss. Comma-shaped conjunctival vessels may also be seen with sickle hemoglobinopathies.

SYSTEMIC VASCULITIDES

Keratoconjunctivitis sicca, episcleritis, scleritis (see Table 55-7), peripheral ulcerative keratitis, and retinal cotton wool spots may be associated with these diseases.

DISSEMINATED INTRAVASCULAR COAGULATION

Occlusion of choroidal vessels by platelet and fibrin thrombi and hemorrhage is the most striking ocular abnormality, producing a discolored and often hemorrhagic choroid, often with serous retinal detachments. Less frequently, conjunctival, iris, anterior chamber, or vitreous hemorrhages may occur.

ANTIPHOSPHOLIPID ANTIBODY SYNDROME (LUPUS ANTICOAGULANT)

Retinal arterial occlusions (rarely venous also), ischemic optic neuropathy, transient visual field loss, or diplopia have been associated with this syndrome.

GASTROINTESTINAL

WILSON'S DISEASE

A gold or gray-brown Kayser-Fleisher ring represents a deposition of copper in a deep layer of the cornea (Descemet's membrane). It is seen in the vast majority of Wilson's patients with neurologic abnormalities, and may precede neurologic or hepatic disease. A sunflower cataract may also be present.

ONCOLOGIC (SEE ALSO TABLE 55-11)

METASTATIC TUMORS

The vast majority of tumors metastatic to the eye and adnexa are carcinomas, with lung carcinoma in men and breast carcinoma in women being the most frequent primary sites. Carcinoma of the gastrointestinal tract, renal cell carcinoma, thyroid carcinoma, carcinoid tumor, and cutaneous malignant melanoma occasionally metastasize to the eye.

TABLE 55-11. OCULAR MANIFESTATIONS OF ONCOLOGIC DISEASES

Disease	Ocular Manifestations
Lymphoma (intraocular)	Masquerade syndrome with first onset of "uveitis" with neurologic findings in the elderly
Lymphoma (orbital)	Proptosis or painless lacrimal gland swelling
Multiple endocrine neoplasia type IIb	Markedly enlarged corneal nerves, neuromas of the conjunctiva, keratoconjunctivitis sicca
Leukemia	Retina most often involved clinically: retinal hemorrhages, cotton wool spots, Roth's spots, hard exudates (edema residue), retinal vascular dilation papilledema (leukemic optic nerve infiltration)
Pediatric oncologic diseases	
Wilm's tumor	Aniridia (in sporadic form only) associated with severe photophobia; glaucoma and corneal scarring may also occur with aniridia
Metastatic neuroblastoma	Eyelid ecchymosis in 50% of the cases (may be bilateral); proptosis
Intestinal polyposis (Gardner's syndrome)	Congenital retinal pigment epithelial hypertrophy
Peutz-Jegher's syndrome	Hyperpigmentation of eyelid skin, conjunctiva, sclera, cornea, and iris

Most metastases in children involve the orbit and often produce exophthalmos, most notably from Ewing's sarcoma or neuroblastoma, the latter of which is often heralded by bilateral eyelid ecchymoses.

Metastatic scirrhous ductal breast carcinoma characteristically produces enophthalmos because of contraction of the fibrotic orbital tumor.

Cancer of the prostate may metastasize to orbital bones, but rarely to ocular structures.

Most intraocular metastases in adults are to the posterior choroid and may result in retinal detachment. The iris and ciliary body are less frequent sites for metastases to the eye. Ophthalmoscopy, ultrasonography, CT, and MRI are often useful in the diagnostic work-up; management may include chemotherapy or radiotherapy.

METABOLIC

CYSTINOSIS

Refractile cystine crystals appear in the cornea by 1 year of age, and photophobia is a prominent symptom. Crystals may also appear in the conjunctiva and iris, along with peripheral retinal pigmentary abnormalities. Conjunctival biopsy may be diagnostic by revealing crystals.

FABRY'S DISEASE

Corneal epithelial whorls (Table 55-12), aneurysmal dilation and tortuosity of conjunctival and retinal vessels, and upper eyelid edema may be present. Conjunctival or corneal epithelial biopsy may show birefringent inclusions.

GALACTOSEMIA

Oil droplet cataract (dulcitol generated from galactose by aldose reductase accumulates within the lens) is often a sign of galactosemia.

REFSUM'S DISEASE AND BASSEN-KORNZWEIG DISEASE

Both can produce pseudoretinitis pigmentosa with progressive night blindness, constriction of peripheral visual fields, posterior subcapsular cataracts, retinal vessel attenuation, macular degeneration, ophthalmoplegia, ptosis, and late optic atrophy. Both diseases are treatable, in contrast to true retinitis pigmentosa.

RETINOPATHY OF PREMATURITY (ROP) (FORMERLY CALLED RETROLENTAL FIBROPLASIA)

This is a proliferative retinopathy of premature and low birth weight infants. The American Academy of Pediatrics recommends examination of all high-risk infants (less than 36 weeks gestation or birth weight less than 2000 g who have received oxygen therapy) at 7 to 9 weeks of age, and again at 3 to 6 months. Because the temporal retinal vasculature is the last to develop, oxygen therapy may cause toxicity to the endothelium of the vascular precursors in this area. On indirect ophthalmoscopy, the temporal periphery of both eyes is avascular and gray. In severe disease, dilation of retinal vessels in the posterior pole may also occur; new blood vessels may proliferate above the retinal surface in response to the peripheral

TABLE 55-12. DRUG-INDUCED OCULAR SIDE EFFECTS

Drug	Ocular Side Effects
Digoxin	Cone dysfunction with decreased vision, xanthopsia (yellow vision)
Vitamin A	Papilledema, pseudotumor cerebri (also seen with tetracycline, nalidixic acid, phenytoin), strabismus and diplopia, eyelash or eyebrow loss
Ethambutol (> 25 mg/day)	Dyschromatopsia, optic neuritis, optic atrophy, toxic amblyopia, retinal vascular dilation, retinal hemorrhage
Isoniazid	Optic neuritis, dyschromatopsia, optic atrophy, papilledema, toxic amblyopia, photophobia
Phenobarbital, phenytoin	Nystagmus, disturbed smooth pursuit, visual hallucinations, paralysis of extraocular muscles, ptosis
Chloroquine, Hydrochloroquine	Corneal epithelial whorls (also seen with indomethacin, amiodarone, and chlorpromazine, corneal and lenticular deposits, toxic amblyopia, pigmentary retinopathy, bull'seye maculopathy (most of these effects are dose-related; early changes may be reversible)
Phenothiazines (thoridazine, chlorpromazine)	Hyperpigmentation of lid skin, conjunctiva and cornea. Also conjunctival, corneal, lenticular deposits; oculogyric crises, paralysis of accommodation, myopia, pigmentary retinopathy (most effects are dose-related)
Chloramphenicol	Toxic amblyopia, dyschromatopsia, optic neuritis, optic atrophy
Oral contraceptives	Myopia, optic neuritis, retinal vascular occlusions, papilledema, keratoconjunctivitis sicca
Oral corticosteroids	Glaucoma, posterior subcapsular cataracts, pseudotumor cerebri (also seen with tetracycline, nalidixic acid), glaucoma, papilledema in children, exophthalmos
Sulfonamides	Transient myopia
Niacin	Reversible cystoid maculopathy (seen with high doses)

ischemia, sometimes causing vitreous hemorrhage, retinal detachment, and fibrous tissue proliferation.

Milder cases usually vascularize normally without treatment. In progressive disease, cryopexy significantly reduces the rate of severe visual loss, and vitrectomy and retinal detachment repair may be indicated in selected cases. The use of systemic Vitamin E remains controversial.

INFECTIOUS

ACQUIRED IMMUNODEFICIENCY SYNDROME (AIDS)[4]

The eye is frequently affected in AIDS. A noninfectious microangiopathy consisting of cotton wool spots with or without retinal hemorrhages is seen in over 50% of AIDS patients (Fig. 55-19). Kaposi's sarcoma can involve the eyelids and conjunctiva. Neuro-ophthalmic lesions such as optic neuropathy, papilledema, and cranial nerve palsies may occur, sometimes as a result of cryptococcal meningitis, herpes zoster ophthalmicus, viral encephalitis, or central nervous system toxoplasmosis or lymphoma. Pneumocystis choroiditis may occur after the use of aerosolized pentamidine for treatment of Pneumocystis carinii pneumonia.

By far, cytomegalovirus (CMV) retinitis is the most common ocular opportunistic infection seen in AIDS patients, occurring in approximately 25% of them. In fact, 10% of patients with AIDS have CMV retinitis as the presenting sign. CMV causes a necrotizing retinitis with retinal opacification and often intraretinal hemorrhage and vasculitis (Fig. 55-20). Early peripheral lesions usually do not cause symptoms other than

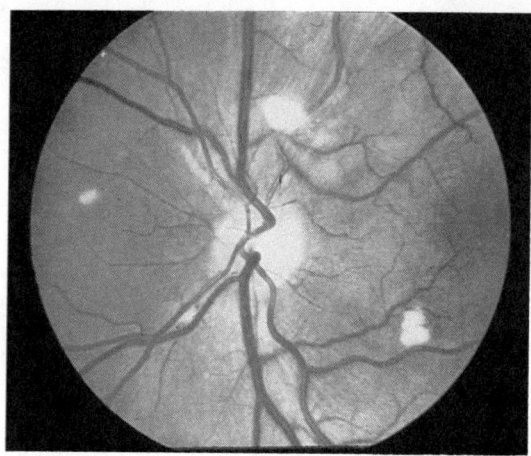

FIG. 55-19.   Retinal cotton wool spots in AIDS.

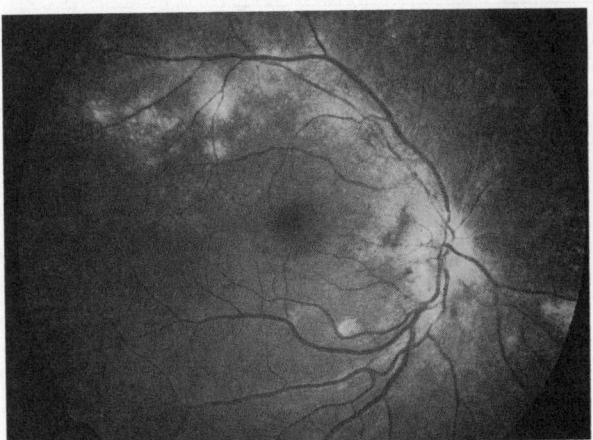

FIG. 55-20. CMV retinitis.

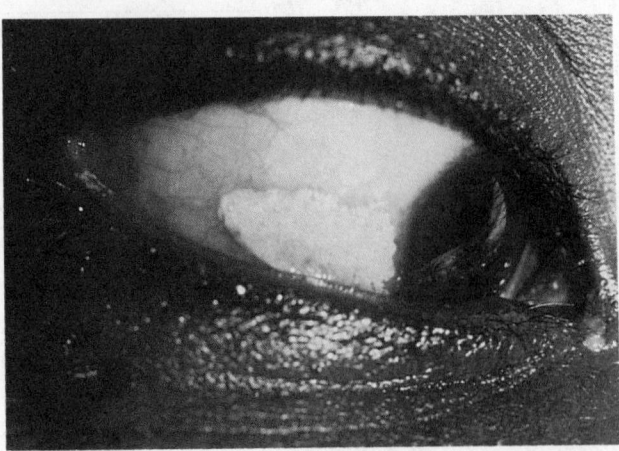

FIG. 55-21. Bitot's spot seen in vitamin A deficiency.

floaters and visual field changes. Without treatment, however, CMV causes a relentless, progressive retinitis resulting in blindness from macular or optic nerve involvement, or retinal detachment associated with retinal necrosis.

Ganciclovir (9-[1,3-dihydroxy-2-propoxymethyl]-gaunine) is a virostatic agent that arrests the progression of CMV retinitis after intravenous induction (10 mg per kg daily for 10 to 14 days). Because breakthrough retinitis often occurs, maintenance therapy (5 mg per kg daily, 5 days per week) is required. Even on this maintenance therapy, recurrence develops in 30 to 50% of patients. In 13 to 38% of patients, bone marrow toxicity results in profound leukopenia, and discontinuation of the drug is required. Zidovudine (AZT) also induces neutropenia, which may force a choice to be made between vision-preserving therapy with ganciclovir and life-prolonging treatment with AZT. Alternative treatment modalities that allow for both anti-CMV and anti-HIV (human immunodeficiency virus) drugs to be used together include intravitreal ganciclovir injections, and the use of Foscarnet (trisodium phosphonoformate hexahydrate), an alternative nonmyelosuppressive agent with both anti-HIV and anti-CMV properties.

MENINGOCOCCEMIA

Conjunctival petechiae, panophthalmitis, and sixth cranial nerve paresis may be associated with this infection.

NUTRITIONAL

Vitamin A deficiency (may be seen in this country in patients with cystic fibrosis, in those who have had gastrointestinal surgery, and in malnourished patients): night blindness, white retinal opacities, conjunctival and corneal xerosis, Bitot's spot (pathognomonic paralimbal, triangular, white collection of

keratin and diphtheroids, Fig. 55-21), and keratomalacia with corneal perforation, are the characteristic findings in vitamin A deficiency.

1. Gold, D.H., and Weingest, T.A.: The Eye in Systemic Disease. Philadelphia, J.B. Lippincott Co., 1990.
2. Roy, F.H.: Ocular Syndromes and Systemic Diseases, Second Edition. Philadelphia, W.B. Saunders Company, 1989.

3. Breshin, D.J., Gifford, R.W., Fairbairn, J.F., and Kearns, T.P.: Prognostic importance of ophthalmoscopic findings in essential hypertension. JAMA *91*:195, 1966.
4. Holland, G.N., et al.: Acquired immune deficiency syndrome:

ocular manifestations. Ophthalmology *90*:859, 1983.
5. Fraunfelder, F.T., and Meyer, S.M.: Drug-Induced Ocular Side Effects and Drug Interactions. Third Edition. Philadelphia, Lea & Febiger, 1989.

OPHTHALMOLOGIC PHARMACOTHERAPY IN EMERGENCIES

Scott S. Weissman, Theodore Rabinovitch, and Robert A. Nozik

CAPSULE

By virtue of high local drug concentrations achievable, topical therapy is preferable in most ophthalmologic emergencies. Rather than providing an encyclopedic listing of currently available pharmacologic agents, we provide the emergency physician with the indications, dosage schedules, and side effects of prototypic drugs from each class of agents.

DIAGNOSTIC AGENTS

DYES

FLUORESCEIN

Fluorescein sodium is a yellow water-soluble dye used to check for corneal epithelial defects. The intact corneal epithelium resists penetration of water-soluble fluorescein. Any breach in integrity of the epithelial barrier, whether it results from trauma or viral or bacterial infection, permits fluorescein to diffuse among the intercellular spaces and stain the underlying anterior corneal stroma. Hence, after fluorescein administration, an area of abraded corneal epithelium appears bright green with ordinary light or bright yellow if a cobalt blue filter is used.

For topical ocular use, fluorescein may be administered as a 2% solution (which often contains both a preservative and a topical anesthetic), or by fluorescein-impregnated filter paper strips.

ROSE BENGAL

Rose bengal, an iodine derivative of fluorescein, stains devitalized corneal or conjunctival epithelial cells. In contrast to fluorescein staining, an epithelial defect is not required for rose bengal staining, and the devitalized areas appear red after rose bengal administration. It is commonly used to demonstrate drying of the interpalpebral conjunctival and corneal epithelium in keratoconjunctivitis sicca, to identify virally infected corneal epithelial cells at the edges of a herpes simplex dendrite, and to demonstrate keratinization in various ocular surface disorders.

For topical ocular use, application of a solution is preferable to the use of moistened filter paper strips. A topical anesthetic must be used in conjunction with rose bengal, which produces significant ocular irritation. It can stain the eyelids and clothing, and excess dye should be irrigated to prevent these complications.

AGENTS FOR EVALUATION OF MYASTHENIA GRAVIS

EDROPHONIUM CHLORIDE (TENSILON)

When myasthenia gravis is suspected as a cause of a ptosis or extraocular muscle palsy, 2 mg of edrophonium chloride (10 mg per mL) may be injected intravenously as a test dose, while monitoring the ptosis and extraocular motility disturbances. This may be followed 45 seconds later by an additional 8 mg intravenously if no response was noted with the test dose. A positive test, in which ptosis and/or motility disturbances improve, is highly suggestive of myasthenia gravis. False positive and false negative Tensilon tests may occur, however. Atropine sulfate, 0.6 mg., should immediately be given intravenously to treat serious parasympathetic toxic effects, such as bradycardia or hypotension.

AGENTS FOR EVALUATION OF ANISOCORIA (INEQUALITY OF PUPILLARY SIZE) (TABLE 55-13)

ABNORMAL PUPIL IS MIOTIC: SUSPECTED HORNER'S SYNDROME

Significant anisocoria (> 1 to 2 mm of difference in pupillary diameters), exaggerated in dim illumination, often with a lag in dilation of the miotic pupil, suggests an interruption of sympathetic tone to the iris dilator muscle, resulting in a miotic pupil. This may occur in combination with ptosis, anhidrosis, and apparent enophthalmos on the side of the miotic pupil. Pharmacologic testing can be used to confirm the presence of a Horner's syndrome and localize the lesion to a postganglionic, or more proximal (preganglionic or central) location.

ABNORMAL PUPIL IS DILATED: SUSPECTED ADIE'S PUPIL

An Adie's pupil, characterized by a dilated pupil, with slow constriction to light, and a slow or tonic redilation, is postulated to result from damage to the ciliary ganglion, a structure located in the orbit. Methacholine, 2.5% or pilocarpine, $\frac{1}{8}$% causes an Adie's pupil to constrict because of denervation hypersensitivity. In contrast, a normal pupil or a dilated pupil on the basis of 3rd cranial nerve compression by tumor or aneurysm does *not* constrict in response to these weak parasympathomimetic agents.

AGENTS FOR DIFFERENTIATION OF PARASYMPATHETIC INTERRUPTION VERSUS PHARMACOLOGIC CAUSE OF A DILATED PUPIL

PILOCARPINE, 1%

Following topical administration of Pilocarpine 1%, the dilated pupil resulting from instillation of an at-ropine-like drug *fails* to constrict after topical pilocarpine 1%, whereas the dilated pupil caused by interruption of parasympathetic innervation (i.e., tumor, aneurysm) *will* constrict.

AGENTS FOR PUPILLARY DILATION (RED-TOPPED BOTTLES) (TABLE 55-14)

Pupillary dilation may be optimally achieved with the use of both a topical sympathomimetic (pure mydriatic) and a topical parasympatholytic (mydriatic-cycloplegic) agent. Sympathomimetic agents produce mydriasis by stimulating the iris dilator muscle. Parasympatholytics block the effect of acetylcholine released from cholinergic neurons at the iris sphincter and ciliary muscles. The former effect produces pupillary dilation, and it also prevents constriction of the pupil during ophthalmoscopy.

The latter effect prevents accommodation, precluding performance of near tasks, and thus only shorter-acting parasympatholytic agents should be used for routine pupillary dilation.

PHENYLEPHRINE HYDROCHLORIDE

Phenylephrine 2.5% (Neosynephrine, Mydfrin) is the synthetic alpha-receptor agonist most commonly used for pupillary dilation.

TROPICAMIDE (MYDRIACIL, TROPICACYL)

Because of its relatively fast onset, short duration and intensity of mydriatic effect, tropicamide 0.5% or 1%, is the parasympatholytic of choice for pupillary dilation.

TABLE 55-13. TESTING FOR ABNORMAL PUPILS*

Clinical Problem	Drug	Abnormal Pupil	Normal Pupil
Horner's syndrome	Cocaine, 10%	Fails to dilate†	Dilates
Preganglionic or central	Hydroxyamphetamine, 1% (Paredrine)	Dilates†	Dilates
Postganglionic	Hydroxyamphetamine, 1% (Paredrine)	Fails to dilate†	Dilates
Adie's (Tonic) pupil	Pilocarpine, 1/8% Methacholine, 2.5%	Constricts‡	No reaction
Pharmacologically dilated pupil	Pilocarpine, $\frac{1}{2}$–1%	Fails to constrict‡	Constricts

*Adapted with permission from Basic and Clinical Science Course, San Francisco, American Academy of Ophthalmology, 1989, Section 5, page 126.
† Abnormal pupil is miotic
‡ Abnormal pupil is dilated

TABLE 55-14. MYDRIATICS AND CYLOPLEGICS (RED-TOPPED BOTTLES)			
Mydriatic only			
Phenylephrine hydrochloride (Neosynephrine, Mydfrin)	2.5%, 10% drops	15–60 minutes	3 hours
*Mydriatic-Cycloplegic**			
Tropicamide (Mydriacil, Tropicacyl)	0.5%, 1% drops	20–30 minutes	4–6 hours
Cyclopentolate hydrochloride (Cyclogyl, Pentolair, Ak-Pentolate)	0.5%, 1%, 2% drops	15–30 minutes	24 hours
Homatropine hydrobromide (Isopto Homatropine)	2%, 5% drops	10–30 minutes	1–3 days
Scopolamine hydrobromide (Isopto Hyoscine)	0.25% drops	15–30 minutes	3–7 days
Atropine sulfate	0.5%, 1%, 2%, 3% drops 1% ointment	30–40 minutes	7–12 days

* The duration of mydriasis differs from that of cycloplegia with these agents.

For performing dilated ophthalmoscopy in the ED, the following regimen is recommended: one drop of tropicamide 0.5% or 1% every 5 minutes × 3, and one drop of phenylephrine 2.5%. These agents tend to be less effective in dark-eyed individuals, and may necessitate allowing additional time, or administering more drops, to achieve adequate dilation.

Longer-acting parasympatholytics are available primarily to produce ciliary muscle paralysis to relieve pain and photophobia and prevent intraocular scarring (synechiae) associated with uveitis, or to aid in refraction of infants and children by preventing inappropriate accommodation.

CONTRAINDICATIONS

Relative contraindications to pupillary dilation include pupillary involvement from neurologic disease and a history of, or anatomic predisposition toward, angle-closure glaucoma (which may be noted with tangential penlight illumination).

Phenylephrine *10%* should *not* be used in an ED setting, but instead reserved for ophthalmologic use only when other dilating agents have not been successful. It is especially dangerous in infants and small children, patients taking monoamine oxidase inhibitors or tricyclic antidepressants, and patients with hypertension or coronary artery disease because systemic toxicity including marked elevation of blood pressure, cardiac arrhythmias, and subarachnoid hemorrhage have been associated with topical phenylephrine, 10%.

PRECAUTIONS

Infants and young children may develop central nervous system and respiratory compromise resulting from systemic absorption of topical cycloplegics, especially after atropine, scopolamine, and cyclogyl.

ANESTHETIC AGENTS

LOCAL

These permit the emergency physician to remove conjunctival or corneal foreign bodies and measure the intraocular pressure by either applanation or Schiotz tonometry.

Proparacaine hydrochloride, 0.5% (Ak-taine, Alcaine, Ophthaine, Ophthetic), and tetracaine hydrochloride, 0.5% (Anacel, Pontocaine), are the most commonly used agents. One drop of either agent has an onset of action of less than one minute, with a duration of action between 10 and 20 minutes. On instillation, these agents may sting and produce punctate areas of corneal epithelial fluorescein staining. Topical lidocaine 4% (xylocaine) provides a deeper anesthesia than proparacaine or tetracaine, and may be used instead of regional anesthetic injections when suturing conjunctival lacerations or performing conjunctival biopsies. Cocaine (1 to 4%) is rarely used as an anesthetic agent because it dilates the pupil and damages the corneal epithelium. Under *no circumstances* should topical anesthetics be prescribed for continued use because this may ultimately result in ocular infection and even perforation.

REGIONAL

These are used to allow repair of lid lacerations. Local infiltration of lidocaine 2% (Xylocaine) is adequate for shorter procedures, whereas bupivacaine 0.25% to 0.75% (Marcaine) may be combined with an equal amount of lidocaine for longer procedures. The addition of epinephrine to promote hemostasis is recommended by some ophthalmic plastic surgeons. The anesthetic injections should be given in a manner that minimizes distortion of the eyelid anatomy. When blepharospasm interferes with the surgical repair, the facial nerve that supplies the orbicularis oculi muscles responsible for lid closure should also be anesthetized. Various techniques for blocking the facial nerve at or distal to its emergence from the stylomastoid foramen have been described (Nadbath, O'Brien, Atkinson, Van Lindt).

AGENTS FOR TREATMENT OF ANGLE-CLOSURE GLAUCOMA (TABLE 55-15)

Angle-closure or narrow-angle glaucoma is an opthalmologic emergency. Prompt lowering of the intraocular pressure is imperative to prevent or minimize optic nerve damage. Medical treatment is used as a first step before performing definitive laser or surgical re-establishment of normal aqueous outflow.

TOPICAL PARASYMPATHOMIMETICS (GREEN-TOPPED BOTTLES)

In treating narrow-angle glaucoma, these miotic agents stimulate muscarinic receptors in the iris sphincter muscle. This pulls the peripheral iris out of the anterior chamber drainage angle, improving aqueous outflow.

PILOCARPINE

Pilocarpine, 1% or 2%, is generally used in this setting because higher concentrations may increase iris vascular congestion.

The iris sphincter muscle is often ischemic in the face of markedly elevated intraocular pressure, and pilocarpine may have no effect (as evidenced by the lack of miosis) until other agents applied concomitantly begin to reduce the pressure by other mechanisms.

TOPICAL ADRENERGIC ANTAGONISTS

Blockade of the beta-adrenergic receptors in the ciliary body lowers intraocular pressure, mainly by decreasing aqueous humor secretion. Timolol (Timoptic), 0.25 to 0.50%, and levobunolol (Betagan) 0.25 to 0.50%, are nonselective beta-blockers, whereas betaxolol (Be-

---

TABLE 55-15. DRUGS FOR TREATMENT OF ANGLE-CLOSURE GLAUCOMA*

| | | Topical Medications | |
Generic Name	Trade Name	Drop Concentration	Dosage During Acute Attack
Miotic Agents (Green-topped)			
Pilocarpine hydrochloride	Pilocar, Isoptocarpine Pilocel, Pilomiotin Almocarpine, Akarpine Adsorbocarpine	1–2%**	q15 min × 1st hr, q½ × 1 hr thereafter‡
Beta-Blockers (Blue- or Yellow-topped)			
Timolol maleate	Timoptic	0.25%, 0.5%	Hourly
Betaxolol hydrochloride	Betoptic	0.25%, 0.5%	Hourly
Levobunolol hydrochloride	Betagan	0.5%	Hourly
		Parenteral Medications	
Generic Name	Trade Name	Preparation	Dosage
Carbonic Anhydrase Inhibitors			
Acetazolamide	Diamox Ak-Zol Cetazol	250 mg tablet§	2 tablets stat, then 2 tablets q12h
Acetazolamide sodium	Diamox (parenteral)	500 mg	1 dose IV or IM stat, then q12h
Hyperosmotic Agents			
Glycerin	Glyrol Osmoglyn	50%, 75% solution	1–1.5 g/kg PO stat, repeat q6–8h
Isosorbide	Ismotic	45% solution	1.5 g/kg PO stat, repeat q6–12h
Mannitol	Osmitrol	20% solution	1.5–2 g/kg IV over 30–60 mins., repeat dose with caution

* Only the most effective, rapidly acting agents in each class are listed.
† Higher concentrations of pilocarpine should not be used in this setting because they increase iris vascular congestion.
‡ Pilocarpine is ineffective until the intraocular pressure has been decreased by other agents to a level that relieves iris ischemia.
§ More rapid onset than 500 mg timed-release preparation.

toptic), 0.25 to 0.50%, is a cardioselective beta-blocker, and may be preferable in patients with pulmonary disease or advanced heart block.

CARBONIC ANHYDRASE INHIBITORS

Carbonic anhydrase is required for ion transport across the ciliary epithelium during aqueous humor secretion. Carbonic anhydrase inhibitors noncompetitively inhibit this enzyme and reduce aqueous humor secretion and hence the intraocular pressure. These agents are given by the oral, intramuscular or intravenous route, depending on the magnitude of the intraocular pressure elevation.

RELATIVE CONTRAINDICATIONS

Contraindications include acid-base disturbances, especially in the setting of adrenal insufficiency or chronic obstructive pulmonary disease; severe renal or hepatic disease; sulfonamide hypersensitivity, pregnancy.

ADVERSE EFFECTS

Reactions common to sulfonamides including bone marrow depression, renal stones (especially after acetazolamide), metabolic acidosis, generalized side effects: malaise, fever, weight loss, loss of libido, paresthesias, and rarely flaccid paralysis or convulsions.

HYPEROSMOTIC AGENTS

These agents are generally administered orally or intravenously to acutely decrease a markedly elevated intraocular pressure. These agents lower intraocular pressure by creating an osmotic gradient between the ocular fluids and the now hyperosmotic plasma of ocular blood vessels. A significant drop in intraocular pressure may result within 15 to 60 minutes. This effect can last up to 6 hours. Chronic administration is contraindicated.

Mannitol (Osmitrol) is the hyperosmotic often used and is the most effective agent to lower intraocular pressure acutely. It is not absorbed from the GI tract, and therefore is unsuitable for oral use. Because it is not metabolized and is excreted in the urine, it can be used in diabetic patients, but should be used with caution in patients with renal disease. Glycerin (Glyrol) and isosorbide (Ismotic) are both readily absorbed from the GI tract, and hence useful oral agents. Glycerin undergoes the metabolism typical of other carbohydrates, and must be given cautiously to diabetics. Isosorbide is not metabolized and can be given safely to diabetic patients. Urea (Ureaphil) is the least effective hyperosmotic, and is rarely used in the setting of angle-closure glaucoma.

RELATIVE CONTRAINDICATIONS

Anuria, severe dehydration, pulmonary edema, and cardiac decompensation are contraindications to hyperosmotic agents.

ADVERSE EFFECTS

Nausea, vomiting, headache, confusion, disorientation, subarachnoid hemorrhage, severe dehydration, and hyperosmotic coma have been seen.

TOPICAL CORTICOSTEROIDS

These agents are used to treat the anterior segment inflammation that accompanies an attack of acute angle-closure glaucoma. The recommended initial dosage is one drop hourly (see Topical Ophthalmic Corticosteroids, subsequently in this chapter).

Many of the agents described previously, with the exception of hyperosmotic agents, are also used to treat chronic open-angle glaucoma, a non-emergent condition in the vast majority of cases. Another class of topical agents used to treat chronic open-angle glaucoma, epinephrine derivatives (epinephrine bitartarate, epinephrine borate, epinephrine hydrochloride, and dipivalyl epinephrine), are not used to treat angle-closure glaucoma, as they increase both iris vascular congestion and intraocular inflammation.

PUPILLARY BLOCK TYPE OF ANGLE-CLOSURE GLAUCOMA

Angle-closure glaucoma may be produced in some cases by an inability of aqueous to flow freely from the posterior chamber to the anterior chamber, known as a pupillary block mechanism. This generally occurs in the setting of a small pupil or a large intraocular lens. Treatment of this situation includes both sympathomimetics and cycloplegics (see previous text) as pupillary dilation will help to re-establish the normal flow of aqueous. This is in contrast to recommended treatment of angle-closure glaucoma without a pupillary block component (see previous text), in which miotics are employed.

TOPICAL OCULAR DECONGESTANTS (TABLE 55-16)

Because much of the symptomatic picture of conjunctival Type I hypersensitivity reactions (redness, swelling, and itching) is caused by mast cell release of histamine, antihistamines are usually effective in relieving annoying symptoms. These agents are often

TABLE 55-16. TOPICAL OCULAR DECONGESTANTS*

Drug	Vasoconstrictors Trade Names
Naphazoline hydrochloride	Prefrin, Neo-synephrine, Isoptofrin, Degest
Phenylephrine hydrochloride	Albalon, Naphcon, Vasocon Regular, Vasoclear, Degest 2, Ak-Con, Op-con, Clear Eyes
Tetrahydrozoline hydrochloride	Visine, Murine Plus, Soothe, Tetracon

Generic Name of Antihistamine	Antihistamine/Vasoconstrictor Combinations Trade Name of Combination	Preparation
Antazoline	Vasocon-A Albalon-A	0.5% antazoline phosphate plus 0.05% naphazoline
Pheniramine	Naphcon-A Opcon-A Ak-Con-A	0.3% pheniramine maleate plus 0.025% naphazoline
Pyrilamine	Preferin-A	0.1% pyrilamine maleate plus 0.12% phenylephrine plus 0.1% antipyrine†

* The usual dosage of ocular decongestants is 1 drop to the affected eye 3 to 4 times a day p.r.n.
† A weak local anesthetic.

given with decongestants and are usually administered topically.

The vasoconstrictor effect of the adrenergic agonists (i.e., phenylephrine and the imidazole derivatives) makes them useful as topical ocular decongestants. After instillation, conjunctival vessels constrict within minutes, causing the eye to whiten. Minor ocular irritation can be relieved.

Because of the relatively low concentrations required for ocular decongestion, phenylephrine and the imidazole derivatives generally do not cause systemic side effects. These products should be used on a short-term basis because they mask signs and symptoms of more serious ocular disease, and a rebound hyperemia may follow cessation after chronic use.

SYMPATHOMIMETICS

Phenylephrine hydrochloride, naphazoline hydrochloride, and tetrahydrozoline hydrochloride are useful to decrease ocular irritation and injection from allergic conjunctivitis. Astringents such as zinc sulfate may be combined with these sympathomimetics.

CONTRAINDICATIONS

See previous section entitled Pupillary Dilation above.

ANTIHISTAMINES/SYMPATHOMIMETIC COMBINATIONS

Antazoline, pheniramine maleate, and pyrilamine maleate are H1-blockers, and are indicated when ocular itching is present. An A following the trade name of the sympathomimetic indicates the presence of an antihistamine (i.e., Vasocon-A).

Warning: Topical antihistiminics may produce a local sensitivity reaction. They should be used with caution in persons with a narrow angle or past history of angle-closure glaucoma.

MAST CELL STABILIZER

Cromolyn sodium (Optichrom 4%) is a mast cell stabilizer that is effective in vernal and atopic keratoconjunctivitis, and somewhat effective in other forms of allergic conjunctivitis, including contact lens-related conjunctivitis. Two to four weeks of treatment are usually required before symptomatic improvement is noted. It is therefore more useful as a prophylactic than as acute treatment of these conditions. Cromolyn sodium has no intrinsic vasoconstrictor, antihistaminic, or anti-inflammatory activity. Rare hypersensitivity reactions after topical cromolyn sodium have been reported, but no other ocular side effects have been noted.

For severe allergic eye diseases, or when rapid relief of symptoms is mandatory, topical corticosteroids may be justified only on a *short-term* basis. Refills for topical corticosteroids should *never* be dispensed for allergic ocular diseases because of the propensity of these agents to cause serious ocular morbidity (see subsequent text). Antihistaminic/sympathomimetic agents and mast cell stabilizers are considerably safer than topical corticosteroids for treatment of the vast majority of allergic ocular disease.

ANTIBIOTICS

The clinical presentation and laboratory data should guide the choice of initial antimicrobial therapy. By virtue of the high local antibiotic concentrations achievable with topical therapy, the preferred antibiotic for a particular ocular infection may be different from the antibiotic recommended for treatment of systemic infections with these organisms, i.e., topical aminoglycosides may be used to treat corneal ulcers caused by gram-positive organisms.

Alternate routes of antibiotic administration are required when infections are located in the deeper ocular or periocular structures, i.e., vitritis, endophthalmitis, preseptal or orbital cellulitis. These routes include periocular (subconjunctival or subTenon's) and intravitreal injections and oral and intravenous administration.

TOPICAL ANTIVIRALS (TABLE 55-17)

Topical antivirals are used to treat herpes simplex infections of the corneal epithelium. Triflurthymidine (Viroptic) produces the most rapid epithelial healing, but idoxuridine (IDU, Stoxil, Herplex) and vidarabine (Vira-A, ARA-A) are alternatives for cases resistant to Viroptic.

Acyclovir is indicated in the acute treatment of herpes zoster ophthalmicus (800 mg PO 5 times a day). Its efficacy in the treatment of herpes simplex stromal keratitis and iridocyclitis is also being investigated in a prospective randomized trial.

TOPICAL OPHTHALMIC CORTICOSTEROIDS (TABLE 55-18)

These agents are effective for inflammations of the lids, conjunctiva, cornea, iris, and ciliary body. In posterior uveitis, topical therapy may require supplementation with periocular injection or systemic corticosteroids. Weaker steroids (HMS) are recommended for minor lid and conjunctival inflammations. The type and location of inflammation determines which route of administration is appropriate. **The minimal effective dose should be used for the shortest time possible.** The incidence of adverse effects appears to rise significantly as dosages are increased. Many are also available as ointments for night-time administration, and as corticosteroid/antibiotic combinations (Table 55-19). Caution must be exercised in prescribing cortisone preparations from the ED.

CONTRAINDICATIONS

The contraindications to these corticosteroids are herpes simplex epithelial keratitis, ocular viral or fungal infections, and documented elevations of intraocular pressure after steroid use (steroid responders). Warning: **Prolonged use may result in glaucoma, cataract formation, and secondary ocular bacterial, viral, or fungal infections.**

Periocular corticosteroids may be needed to achieve higher levels in the posterior portions of the eye than are possible with topical therapy, such as when treating vitritis or cystoid macular edema. The two depot preparations most commonly used are triamcinolone acetonide (Kenalog, 40 mg per mL), and Solumedrol

TABLE 55-17. TOPICAL OPHTHALMIC ANTIVIRALS*

Generic Name	Trade Name	Preparation	Dosage
Idoxuridine (IDU)	Dendrid, Herplex	0.1% drops	q1h daytime q2h nighttime
	Stoxil	0.1% drops or 0.5% ointment	5× daily 5× daily (last dose at hs)
Trifluridine	Viroptic	1% solution	5×/day–q2h while awake (maximum 9×/day)
Vidarabine	Vira-A, ARA-A Adenine arabinoside	3% ointment	5×/day
Acyclovir ophthalmic (not available in U.S.A.)	Zoovirax	3% ointment	5×/day and hs

* Adapted with permission from Walsh, J.B., Gold, A., and Charles, C. (eds.): Physician's Desk Reference for Ophthalmology. 18th Ed. Oradell, Medical Economics Company Inc., 1990, Section 2, Table 6.

TABLE 55-18. TOPICAL OPHTHALMIC CORTICOSTEROIDS

Generic Name	Trade Name	Concentration
I. Prednisolone		
Acetate suspension*	Pred Mild/Pred Forte	0.12%/1.0%
Acetate suspension	Econopred/Econopred Plus	0.125%/1.0%
Acetate suspension	Ak-Tate, I-Pred	1.0%
	Predulose	0.25%
Sodium phosphate solution	Inflamase/Inflamase Forte	0.12%/1.0%
Sodium phosphate solution	Ak-Pred	0.125%/1.0%
Sodium phosphate solution	Metretron, Hydeltrasol	0.5%
Sodium phosphate ointment	Hydeltrasol	0.25%
II. Dexamethasone		
Phosphate suspension	Maxidex	0.1%
Phosphate solution	Decadron, Ak-Dex	0.1%
Phosphate ointment	Decadron, Ak-Dex	0.05%
III. Hydrocortisone		
Acetate suspension	Hydrocortone acetate	2.5%
Acetate solution	Optef drops	0.2%
Acetate ointment	Hydrocortone acetate	1.5%
IV. Progesterone-like Compounds		
Medrysone	HMS	1.0%
Fluorometholone susp.	FML/FML Forte	0.1%/0.25%
Fluorometholone susp.	Fluor-Op	0.1%
Fluorometholone ung.	FML	0.1%

* Adapted with permission from Walsh, J.B., Gold, A., and Charles, C. (eds.): Physician's Desk Reference for Ophthalmology. 18th Ed. Oradell, Medical Economics Company Inc., 1990, Section 2, Table 12.

† Acetate preparations of topical corticosteroids penetrate the intact corneal epithelium better than the phosphate preparations, and are thus preferable for most corneal and intraocular inflammations. The acetate preparations are suspensions, and therefore must be well shaken before each use.

TABLE 55-19. TOPICAL CORTICOSTEROID-ANTIBIOTIC COMBINATIONS

Trade Name	Steroid	Antibiotic
Drops		
Poly-Pred suspension	Prednisolone acetate 0.5%	Neomycin 0.35% plus 10,000 u polymyxin-B-sulfate/ml
Pred-G suspension	Prednisolone acetate 1%	Gentamicin 0.3%
Dexacidin*	Dexamethasone 0.1%	Neomycin 0.35% plus 10,000 u polymyxin-B-sulfate/ml
Dexasporin*		
AK-Trol*		
Maxitrol*		
TobraDex suspension	Dexamethasone 0.1%	Tobramycin 0.3%
Neo-Decadron solution†	Dexamethasone phosphate 0.1%	Neomycin 0.35%
Chloromycetin hydrocortisone	Hydrocortisone acetate 0.5%	Chloramphenicol 0.25%
Neo-Cortef suspension	Hydrocortisone acetate 0.5%	Neomycin 0.35%
Ointments		
Ophthocort	Hydrocortisone acetate ·0.5%	Chloramphenicol 1% plus 10,000 u polymyxin-B-sulfate/gm
Cortisporin	Hydrocortisone 1%	Neomycin 0.35% plus 400 u bacitracin zinc plus 10,000 u polymyxin-B-sulfate/gm

* Also available as ophthalmic ointment
† Also available as ophthalmic ointment (dexamethasone 0.05% plus neomycin 0.35% plus 10,000 u polymyxin-B-sulfate/g)

(Depo-Medrol, 40 mg per mL and 80 mg per mL). One cc of either medication may be injected into the posterior subTenon's space by an ophthalmologist, with less frequent scarring and hypersensitivity reactions following Kenalog, by virtue of the relative inertness of its vehicle.

Oral corticosteroids are generally indicated in severe ocular inflammatory disease such as cicatricial ocular pemphigoid, peripheral corneal melting disorders, Grave's ophthalmopathy, vitritis, and scleritis. Oral nonsteroid anti-inflammatory drugs (NSAIDs) are sometimes useful alone or as steroid-sparing agents, in these conditions. NSAIDs are seldom of use topically. Oral corticosteroids may prevent permanent, severe visual loss in temporal arteritis. The efficacy of oral corticosteroids in the treatment of optic neuritis has not been clearly demonstrated.

ARTIFICIAL TEARS

A multitude of over-the-counter tear substitutes are available. These agents are used to treat patients with dry eye disorders and to prevent a recurrence of epithelial breakdown in recently healed corneal abrasions. They are composed of various inorganic electrolytes to maintain ocular tonicity, preservatives to maintain sterility, and buffers to adjust pH and water-soluble polymeric systems. Refresh, containing polyvinyl alcohol and povidone, is preservative-free, and is available in single-use dispensers.

Formulations to treat dry eyes should replace the deficient component(s) of the tear film, including lipid, aqueous and mucin.

Methylcellulose and its derivatives (i.e., gum cellulose, celluvisc) and polyvinyl alcohol enhance viscosity and are more mucomimetic than other tear substitutes. These agents are therefore preferred in settings of conjunctival goblet cell deficiency with resultant mucin deficiency, i.e., cicatrizing conjunctivitis after chemical injuries. The frequency of tear solution administration depends on the severity of ocular signs and symptoms, and may vary from every half hour to 3 times daily.

Many artificial tear preparations exist, and trade names include: Tears Naturale I and II, Liquifilm Tears, Tears Plus, Akwa-Tears, Duolube*, Duratears*, Hypotears*, and Lacri-lube S.O.P.* (* = ointment).

OINTMENTS

These include petrolatum, lanolin, and mineral oil ointments. They have the advantage of longer retention in the conjunctival cul-de-sac, but blur vision for some hours after instillation. Lubricants are frequently administered at bedtime only to supplement daytime drops.

OPHTHALMIC IRRIGATING SOLUTIONS

For irrigation of chemical injuries, in which irrigation with large volumes of fluid are mandatory, standard intravenous solutions of normal saline are recommended. When smaller volumes are required, a variety of sterile, over-the-counter isotonic solutions are available, and include: AK/Rinse, Aqua-Flow, Blinx, Collyrium Eye Lotion, Dacriose, Eye Stream, Irigate, M/Rinse, I Rinse, Eye Wash, I-Sol, Lauro, Lavoptik Eye Wash, Murine Regular Formula, Ocu-Bath Eye Lotion, Ocu-Drop, Surgisol, Neo-Flow, and Trisol.

MEDICOLEGAL PEARLS

A significant fraction of an ophthalmic eyedrop is systemically absorbed, and may produce life-threatening toxic effects in susceptible individuals.

HORIZONS

The following agents are under development:

Topical prostaglandin inhibitors and topical NSAIDs to control ocular inflammatory disease.

Topical carbonic anhydrase inhibitors to treat glaucoma.

Topical retinoids to treat keratinizing ocular surface disorders.

Corneal collagen shields as an ophthalmic drug delivery system.

BIBLIOGRAPHY

Bartlett, J.D., Ghormley, N.R., Jaanus, S.D., Rowsey, J.J., and Zimmerman, T.J. (eds.): Ophthalmic Drug Facts. Philadelphia J.B. Lippincott Company, 1989.

Fraunfelder, F.T., and Roy, F.H. (eds.): Current Ocular Therapy. 3rd Ed. Philadelphia, W.B. Saunders Company, 1990.

Walsh, J.B., Gold, A., and Charles, C. (eds.): Physician's Desk Reference for Ophthalmology. 18th Ed. Oradell, Medical Economics Company Inc., 1990.

SECTION TWO: EAR, NOSE, AND THROAT EMERGENCIES

SUDDEN HEARING LOSS

Wallace Rubin

CAPSULE

Sudden hearing loss is an emergency. No audiologic test can differentiate patients whose hearing will return spontaneously from those whose hearing loss will be permanent. It is therefore imperative that all patients be seen as soon after the hearing insult occurs as possible. If the decision not to treat the hearing loss is made, the patient must be informed that the optimum time for treatment may have been lost.[1]

INTRODUCTION

Sudden deafness is practically always a unilateral, abrupt loss of hearing, sensorineural in type. It is important to differentiate known causes from the idiopathic varieties.[2] The known causes are generally excluded by history. These causes include mumps, measles, meningitis, encephalitis, skull fracture, concussive trauma, and ototoxicity. Other causative mechanisms such as Ménière's disease, perilymph fistula, and acoustic neuroma must be differentiated by further audiologic and vestibular function testing.

Patients with Ménière's disease usually give a history of dizziness, tinnitus, and/or fullness in the ear. Perilymph fistula patients frequently describe an insult such as sneezing, coughing, or lifting a heavy object before the onset, and neuroma patients may describe a combination of the above.

Vascular incidents, vasospasm, and autonomic imbalance have all been suggested and occasionally incriminated as etiologic mechanisms. Therefore a complete medical history and a general physical examination is indicated at the outset. Table 55-20 illustrates aspects of evaluation.

CLINICAL EVALUATION

Sudden hearing loss can occur at any age, and the history related by the patient establishes the sudden concept. It it usually unilateral and abrupt, occurs within hours, and may or may not be accompanied by dizziness and/or buzzing in the affected ear. The patient may awaken from sleep with the hearing loss and notice a stuffy, full feeling with the loss. It may also occur suddenly with the feeling of a pop or crack in the affected ear. The hearing loss may be mild or moderate, or the hearing may be completely absent. As stated in the capsule, there may or may not be a significant medical history of a viral, vascular, or other clinically significant problems.

The emergency physician must first recognize the urgency of the problem based on the history. The physician should follow the following protocol:

1. Take an extensive history, especially in regard to:
   a. Prior hearing or balance problems
   b. Trauma
   c. Cardiovascular status
   d. Drugs
   e. Infection, especially viral
2. Physical examination, especially directed to:
   a. Ear examination
   b. Cardiovascular status
   c. Tuning fork testing, especially Weber and Rinne tests
3. If there is any question at all after the history and physical examination, request an immediate otologic consultation (see Table 55-20)

The otolaryngologist who sees the patient should be knowledgeable in regard to hearing and balance evaluation procedures.

The complaint of sudden unilateral hearing loss should trigger a hearing evaluation which is part of a neurotologic workup. This should be performed only after a complete ear, nose and throat physical examination. The purpose of the hearing evaluation is to document the hearing loss and differentiate coch-

TABLE 55-20. SUDDEN HEARING LOSS

Cause	Evaluation	Action
Viral infection (e.g. mumps, herpes, cytomegalic)	History* Audiogram* ENG* Physical examination usually shows no specific abnormalities although viral vesicles may be present	Referral
Bacterial infection	History Physical examination shows inflammation and bulging of tympanic membrane	Treat with antibiotics
Head trauma	X-ray skull CT scan, MRI	If other test results are negative, labyrinthine disruption is likely diagnosis
Rupture of round or oval window	History of blast, pressure changes Audiogram, ENG	Refer for possible exploratory surgery
Tumor (e.g., acoustic neuroma)	History of slowly developing loss CT scan	Referral for full work-up
Postoperative	Document with audiogram ENG	Immediate referral to operating surgeon
Endolymphatic hydrops and Ménière's disease	History shows "dizziness," nausea, vomiting, vertigo Audiogram, ENG	Refer for treatment; immediate treatment includes diuretic and an anti-nauseant, anti-vertigo agent
Metabolic causes	History of ototoxic drugs, (aminoglycoside antibiotics, streptomycin, ethacrynic acid, salicylates) Audiogram, ENG	Stop medication; referral
Disturbance of lipid metabolism	Check for elevated triglycerides and other forms of hyperlipidemia Check for diabetes as well	Refer for long-term treatment
Vascular causes (e.g., hypertension, ischemia)	Check for other causes, history of vascular problems Audiogram, ENG	Treat with bed rest, stool softener, daily audiograms; possible use of heparin, ACTH, papaverine, low MW dextran, carbon dioxide, prednisone; these agents have been reported to have some success—although benefits are not clearcut and risks are involved that must be weighed

* Emergency Departments can easily be equipped with a small audiometer to assess hearing as well as electronystagmography to aid recognition of vestibular problems. History should include the presence of tinnitus, vertigo, "imbalance," ataxia, nausea, vomiting.
Source: From Frederick Fiber, M.D., Ear and Vertigo Association, Albuquerque, N.M.
Abbreviations: ENG = Electronystagmography; CT = computed tomography; ACTH = adrenocorticotropic hormone.

TABLE 55-21. DIFFERENTIAL DIAGNOSIS[3,8]

	Normal	Middle Ear	Inner Ear
History	Not hearing as well as before	Upper respiratory infection Allergy Tinnitus Fullness	Viral Infection Tinnitus Fullness Dizziness
Physical	Normal	Normal or signs of serous otitis media	Normal
Auditory	Normal	Conductive	Sensorineural
Tuning fork evaluation			
Weber	Normal	Lateralizes to involved ear	Lateralizes to noninvolved ear
Rinne	Normal	Bone conduction louder than air	Bone and air conduction equal

lear from retrocochlear neural hearing losses (Table 55-21).

The hearing evaluation should include at least air and bone conduction threshold levels regardless of the air conduction results; impedance audiometry, both typanometry and the stapedial reflexes; the acoustic stapedial reflex; and auditorily evoked potentials.[3]

If the patient has any symptoms of dysequilibrium, evaluation of the balance system is necessary.[4]

This can best be accomplished with the use of electronystagmography. The significance of documenting vestibular abnormality in patients with sudden hearing loss is that the prognosis for recovery of hearing is much worse when there is vestibular abnormality.

RELATIONSHIP TO OTHER BIOCHEMICAL SYSTEMS

Mechanical energy signals that are processed and interpreted as sound originate in the environment. Other mechanical energy signals occur as a result of body movements. These mechanical energy signals must be converted to electrical energy to be transmitted to the appropriate areas of the brain by way of the eighth cranial nerve. This conversion or transduction takes place in the inner ear. The transduction process is accomplished by the chemicals within the inner ear fluids.

Once this role is appreciated, the pathway and mechanisms necessary to transport the chemicals ingested in our food to the inner ear become significant. It is this transport through the circulatory system to the cerebrospinal fluid system and then to the inner ear by way of the endolymphatic duct and sac that is of significance in our thinking and testing for inner ear etiologic mechanisms. It is also important to recognize that the adrenal gland, the pituitary gland, the immune system, the hormonal system, and the hypothalamus also influence the chemical constituents of the inner ear fluids as a result of their interrelated homeostatic mechanisms. These simple concepts but complicated mechanisms are important in deciding which testing procedures are applicable for use in determining the causes of inner ear abnormalities such as sudden hearing loss.

The biochemical, metabolic, hormonal, and neurotransmitter influences as they relate to hearing and balance problems have just begun to be explored. The inner ear is, in fact, an internal body organ. The diagnostic and therapeutic direction for the evaluation of the neurotologic patient should be oriented to confirm the cause. This can be accomplished only if our testing modalities are used in a way that is topographically diagnostic. This approach would then logically culminate in a systematic etiologic investigation.

After confirming the hearing loss, further testing should be done to treat the hearing loss etiologically.[5–7] The biochemical and imaging evaluation should include the following:

1. Cholesterol
2. Triglyceride
3. Thyroid
4. Glucose tolerance response—ENG monitored
5. Blood urea nitrogen
6. Serum glutamic-oxaloacetic transaminase (SGOT)
7. Complete blood count (CBC)
8. Sedimentation rate
9. Fluorescent treponemal antibody absorption (FTA-ABS)
10. Prolactin level in females
11. Uric acid
12. Radioallergosorbent test (RAST) immunologic studies
13. Fasting blood sugar (FBS)
14. MRI of brain and IAC

The bottom line is that sudden hearing loss is an emergency, and patients need a complete hearing and balance evaluation as soon as possible. If this topographic evaluation is not performed, the etiologic investigation that will direct treatment cannot be accomplished in a timely fashion.

REFERENCES

1. Wilson, W. Sudden sensorineural hearing loss. Otolaryngology. Edited by Gerald M. English 1:1, 1988.
2. Simmons, F.B.: Sudden idiopathic sensori-neural hearing loss: Some observations. Laryngoscope 83:1221, 1973.
3. Brookler, K.H., Berko, D.R., and Feder, T.: Contemporary office audiology. Am. J. Otol. 5:438, 1984.
4. Rubin, W.: Harmonic acceleration tests as a measure of vestibular compensation. Ann. Otol. Rhinol. Laryngol. 91:489, 1982.
5. Seigel, L.G.: The treatment of idiopathic sudden sensorineural hearing loss. Otolaryngol. Clin. North Am. 8:467, 1975.
6. Jaffe, B.F.: Sudden deafness—a local manifestation of systemic disorders: Fat emboli, hypercoagulation and infections. Laryngoscope 80:788, 1970.
7. Rubin, W.: Biochemical Evaluation of the Patient with Dizziness. Semin. Hearing 10:151, 1989.
8. DeWeese, D., and Saunders, W.H.: Textbook of Otolaryngology. St. Louis, The C.V. Mosby Company, 1960, pp. 296–298.

BIBLIOGRAPHY

Bordley, J.E., Brookhouser, P.E., and Worthington, E.L.: Viral infections and hearing: A critical review of the literature, 1969–1970. Laryngoscope: 82:557, 1972.

Byl, Jr., F. Sudden hearing loss: Eight years' experience and suggested prognostic table. Laryngoscope 94:647, 1984.

Byl, F.M.: Seventy-six cases of presumed sudden hearing loss occuring in 1973: Prognosis and incidence. Laryngoscope 87:817, 1977.

Currier, W.D.: Metabolic errors and sudden deafness. Otolaryngol. Clin. North Am. 8:501, 1975.

Jaffe, B.F.: Hypercoagulation and other causes of sudden hearing loss. Otolaryngol. Clin. North Am. 8:395, 1975.

Matsuki, K., Harada, T., Juji, T., et al.: Human leukocyte antigen in childhood unilateral deafness. Arch. Otolaryngol. Head Neck Surg. 115:46, 1989.

Mattox, D.E., and Simmons, F.B.: Natural history of sudden sensorineural hearing loss. Ann. Otol. 86:463, 1977.

Nakashima, T., Kuno, K., and Yanagita, N. Evaluation of prostaglandin E1 therapy for sudden deafness. Laryngoscope 99:542, 1989.

Saunders, W.H.: Symposium on ear diseases. Sudden deafness and its several treatments. Laryngoscope 82:1206, 1972.

EAR INFECTIONS

Donald R. Paugh and Steven A. Telian

CAPSULE

The initial or emergency evaluation of the patient with localized ear pain, edema, drainage, or erythema must differentiate infection of the external ear (auricle, external auditory canal, or lateral surface of the tympanic membrane) from otitis media. Uncomplicated otitis externa is treated with topical agents. Systemic antibiotics are reserved for patients with cellulitis, folliculitis or perichondritis. Acute otitis media requires systemic antibiotic therapy, whereas active chronic otitis media (perforated tympanic membrane and purulent drainage) may require topical and systemic antibiotics. Prompt diagnosis and appropriate therapy should prevent suppurative complications in the temporal bone, surrounding soft tissues, and intracranial cavity.

ANATOMY AND PHYSIOLOGY

EXTERNAL EAR

The external ear includes the auricle, external auditory canal, and lateral tympanic membrane. The auricle is composed of convoluted elastic cartilage bound by perichondrium and skin. The avascular cartilage derives its blood supply from the adjacent perichondrium. The lobule, or ear lobe, is formed of skin and soft tissue. Thus the lobule may be involved in cellulitis but not perichondritis. The tragus is that portion of the auricle just anterior to the external auditory canal. It may become tender to pressure if external otitis (a skin infection) advances to frank cellulitis of the periauricular soft tissues. The structures of the auricle are illustrated in Figure 55-22. The skin of the auricle is tightly bound to perichondrium laterally. Medially (behind the ear) and around the lobule, the skin is more loosely draped. In these areas, sebaceous cysts and furuncles are more common. The conchal bowl

or concha cavum is the anterior-central portion of the auricle, which funnels into the external auditory canal (EAC). The lateral third of the EAC is lined by thick skin abundant with hair follicles, sebaceous and apocrine glands. These glands produce a waxy secretion, which combines with sloughed skin to form cerumen. Cerumen is a water-repellent, acidic coating which forms a protective barrier to infection of the EAC skin. The fissures of Santorini are tiny dehiscences in the cartilage of the EAC. These areas are potential routes for spread of infection from the EAC to the soft tissues anterior and inferior to the ear, including the temporomandibular joint and parotid gland.

The medial two thirds of the EAC is surrounded by bone, with a thin layer of stratified squamous epithelium directly applied to the periosteum. There are no skin appendages medial to the bony-cartilaginous junction. Figure 55-23 shows a coronal section of the external ear. The EAC is about 2.5 cm long in the adult. The lateral, cartilaginous portion proceeds medially in a rostral and slightly posterior course. At the bony-cartilaginous junction, the EAC swerves anteriorly and inferiorly. To examine the tympanic membrane effectively, the auricle must be pulled superiorly and

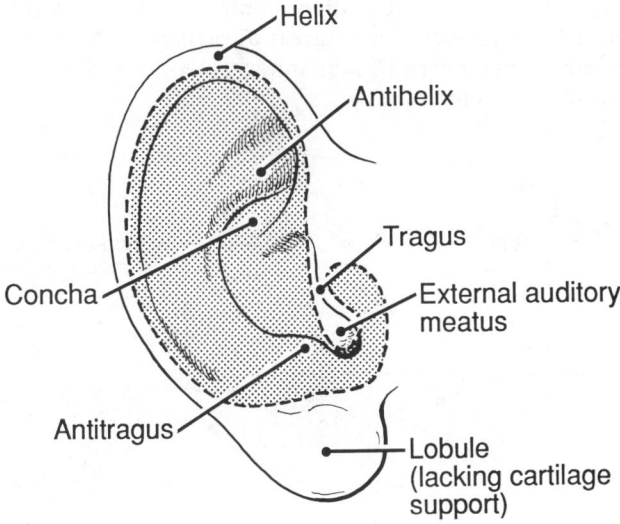

FIG. 55-22.   *Anatomy of the auricle. The shaded area denotes the extent of the cartilage framework.*

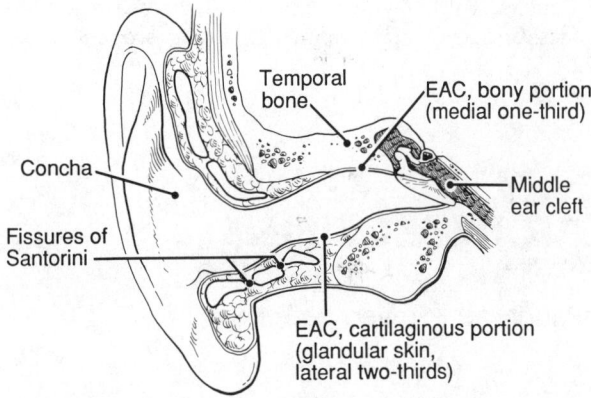

FIG. 55-23. Coronal section of the middle ear, external auditory canal, and auricle. The fissures of Santorini are dehiscences in the cartilage, which may allow infection to spread into adjacent soft tissues.

posteriorly, aligning the cartilaginous lateral EAC with the bony medial EAC. In infants, pulling the auricle laterally displays the tympanic membrane for examination. For best results, the largest speculum possible is used for examination. The speculum should be inserted to the bony-cartilaginous junction, which is approximately at the point where hair follicles are no longer seen. Advancing the speculum tip more medially causes undue discomfort because the periosteum is sensitive, and does not improve visualization.

The blood supply to the external ear is from the external carotid artery by way of the superficial temporal and posterior auricular arteries. Venous drainage occurs in a parallel fashion, with superficial temporal and posterior auricular veins joining the posterior facial vein, ultimately flowing into the deep jugular system. Preauricular and postauricular lymph nodes drain into the superior cervical lymph node chain, between the mandible and the sternocleidomastoid muscle. Sensory innervation to the auricle and EAC is mediated by the fifth, seventh, and tenth cranial nerves, and the anterior branches of the second and third cervical roots (great auricular nerve). The ninth cranial nerve IX may innervate a portion of the tympanic membrane.

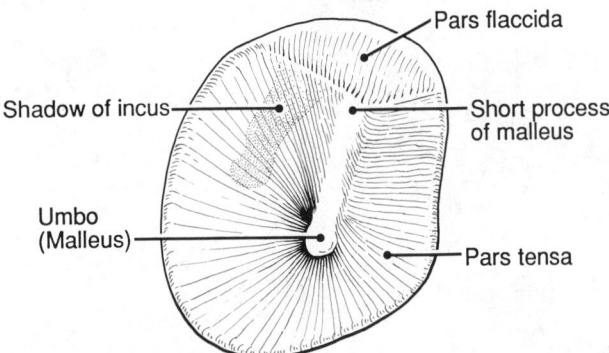

FIG. 55-24. Right tympanic membrane viewed through the external auditory canal. Note the superior posterior orientation of the Incus. Please see text for further description.

The tympanic membrane (TM), or ear drum, is depicted in Figure 55-24. The TM is formed of three layers: outer (lateral) skin, a middle fibrous layer, and a medial mucosal layer continuous with the mucosa of the middle ear. The fibrous layer is a barrier to encroaching inflammation from the EAC. The primary bony landmark of the TM is the long process of the malleus. The inferior tip of the malleus is the umbo. The TM is conical, with the tip projecting medially. The apex of the cone is the umbo. Superiorly, above the short process of the malleus, is the pars flaccida of the TM. This area is prone to retraction of skin and subsequent chronic infection. The major part of the TM has a taut appearance and is called the pars tensa.

MIDDLE EAR

The pneumatized portion of the temporal bone includes the bony eustachian tube, the middle ear cleft with the ossicular chain, and the mastoid air cell system. The eustachian tube (ET) connects the nasopharynx with the middle ear cleft and is approximately 3 cm long. It travels anteriorly, inferiorly, and medially as it descends to the nasopharynx. The ET is lined by a simple cuboidal respiratory epithelium with occasional ciliated cells. It functions to aerate the middle ear on yawning and swallowing. ET dysfunction may result in negative middle ear pressure, retracted TM, and a fluid-filled middle ear.

The middle ear cleft lies medial and superior to the TM. Its contents include the malleus, incus, stapes, and tympanic portion of the facial nerve. The footplate of the stapes lies in the oval window in the posterosuperior portion of the middle ear. The round window membrane is tucked under a cornice of bone just inferior to the oval window. All of these structures may be affected by suppurative processes.

The mastoid cavity lies posterior to the middle ear cleft and EAC in the mastoid portion of the temporal bone. The mastoid cavity is not well developed in the newborn. By age 2 years, the mastoid air cells show signs of inferior, posterior, and medial expansion. In the adult, the mastoid cavity is bordered anteriorly by the EAC and the vertical portion of the facial nerve, posteriorly by the sigmoid sinus and posterior fossa, superiorly by the middle foss dura, and anteromedially by the middle ear cleft and the bony labyrinth of the inner ear.

CLINICAL PRESENTATION

OTITIS EXTERNA

Otitis externa may present as an acute or chronic process. Acute diffuse otitis externa (swimmer's ear) is a common infection and is associated with hot, humid climates or chronic exposure to water. Patients usually experience moderate to severe pain and "blockage of the ear." Senturia[1] describes three clinical stages of acute diffuse otitis externa: preinflammatory, acute inflammatory, and chronic inflammatory.

The pre-inflammatory stage begins when hot, humid conditions or multiple exposures to water decrease the protective lipid layer on the EAC skin. The aqueous content of the stratum corneum increases and the resulting edema blocks the drainage of the apopilosebaceous unit. The skin of the lateral EAC appears slightly edematous and erythematous. The patient may complain of intense pruritis, usually with minimal or no other discomfort.

The acute inflammatory stage is manifested by increasing edema, pruritis, and often severe pain. A clear drainage mixed with epithelial debris is usually observed. As the infection progresses, green drainage may develop and edema may increase to completely occlude the EAC. Because the skin overlying the medial bony EAC does not contain glandular structures, the edema and obstruction primarily involve the lateral, cartilaginous EAC. As the infection progresses, exudate and squamous epithelial debris collect medially, causing inflammation of the TM. Pseudomonas is the organism most commonly cultured in acute diffuse otitis externa. Staphylococcus aureus and other gram-negative organisms may also play a significant role.

The chronic inflammatory stage results from multiple recurrences or incompletely resolved episodes of acute diffuse otitis externa. Chronic manipulation of the external auditory canal leads to lichenification of the skin and varying degrees of EAC stenosis. The entire length of the EAC may become involved, and the tympanic membrane often appears pale and dull to otoscopic examination. The TM is usually mobile. Pain is not usually a prominent symptom, although pruritis may be intense. Underlying gram-negative infection or chronic dermatitis contribute to ongoing symptoms. Otomycosis (mycotic external otitis) occurs more frequently in hot and humid climates. Patients with a history of chronic topical antibiotic use are highly susceptible. Otomycosis is generally associated with intense pruritis. Physical examination may be unimpressive, demonstrating only mild erythema of the EAC. When hyphae are abundant, grossly evident white, grey, or black fungal debris may be visible. The tympanic membrane may be involved. In patients with otomycosis that is recurrent or unremitting despite appropriate treatment, evidence of immune deficiency should be sought. Among the more common fungi seen are Aspergillus, yeasts, dermatophytes, and Mucormycosis.

OTITIS MEDIA

Otitis media implies inflammation of the mucosal surfaces of the middle ear cleft and the mastoid cavity.

The spectrum of otitis media includes acute otitis media, otitis media with effusion, and chronic otitis media. Acute otitis media is synonymous with acute suppurative, purulent, or bacterial otitis media. Typically, otalgia and fever are hallmarks of this infection. Infants may constantly pull on the affected ear. Otoscopy classically demonstrates a bulging, erythematous TM with limited or no mobility to pneumatic otoscopy. The EAC appears normal. The moderate to severe pain of acute otitis media may subside with spontaneous perforation of the tympanic membrane and the appearance of purulent drainage in the EAC. Acute otitis media may also occur in patients with patent tympanostomy tubes, as evidenced by acute onset of purulent drainage, usually without fever. Early in the course of acute otitis media, otoscopy may demonstrate an erythematous or dull TM with normal mobility to pneumotoscopy. This signifies inflammation of the tympanic membrane mucosa without exudate. This condition is called myringitis, and because it usually progresses to acute otitis media, it should be treated as such.

OTITIS MEDIA WITH EFFUSION

This implies the presence of a subacute or chronic middle ear effusion that is usually asymptomatic except for a mild conductive hearing loss. The effusion may be serous, mucoid, or mucopurulent in nature. The TM has markedly decreased or absent mobility. If the TM has an amber or bluish appearance, a diagnosis of otitis media with serous effusion is made. Often the TM is opaque and retracted; therefore no conclusion can be drawn as to the nature of the fluid. The most important distinction between this type of disease and acute (suppurative) otitis media is that the signs and symptoms (otalgia, fever) are lacking in otitis media with effusion. Hearing loss is often present in both conditions.[2]

CHRONIC OTITIS MEDIA

By definition this implies a permanent perforation of the tympanic membrane, with or without active drainage. Inactive chronic otitis media implies a nonhealing perforation without active mucosal disease or drainage. Healthy middle ear mucosa appears glistening white, laced with fine, pink blood vessels. Diseased middle ear mucosa appears thickened, erythematous, and sometimes polypoid. A permanent perforation of the TM may result from trauma or previous infection.

ACTIVE (SUPPURATIVE) CHRONIC OTITIS MEDIA

This condition is defined by the presence of purulent drainage through a permanent perforation of the tympanic membrane. The drainage may be described as mucoid or purulent. The presence of profuse clear, watery drainage should alert the clinician to the rare possibility of cerebrospinal fluid (CSF) leak. Before examining an ear filled with purulence or debris, the contralateral (normal) ear should be examined to observe depth of the TM and normal landmarks. The EAC should then be gently aspirated with a 5 French (Fr) diameter suction tip. Care should be taken not to traumatize the bony EAC or TM. Often erythematous and polypoid granulation tissue may be seen extruding from the TM perforation. The use of a binocular microscope is helpful in cleaning and examining a draining ear. If the primary care physician is uncomfortable cleaning a draining ear, early otolaryngologic consultation is appropriate. Intermittent suppurative otorrhea implies reversible mucosal disease. Chronic unremitting otorrhea, possibly associated with a foul odor, indicates chronic mastoiditis, a mastoid abscess, or cholesteatoma.

A *cholesteatoma* is a focus of proliferating stratified squamous epithelium within the pneumatized spaces of the temporal bone. Its origins are usually associated with retraction of the posterior and superior TM into the middle ear. Skin may also migrate into the middle ear through a perforation in the TM. Perforations near the posterior rim and the superior TM (pars flaccida) are most prone to this complication. All patients with retraction pockets or perforations in the tympanic membrane must be followed by an otologist. These patients are at higher risk for recurrent infection and other temporal bone complications, including hearing loss, vestibular dysfunction, and facial nerve injury.

DIFFERENTIAL DIAGNOSIS AND CLINICAL MANAGEMENT

OTITIS EXTERNA

The differential diagnosis of otitis externa is listed in Table 55-22. The diagnosis is made by history and physical examination. A history of previous ear infections or underlying medical illness, such as diabetes, may be valuable clues to the type of infection present. The onset, duration, and severity of symptoms such as erythema, pain, and drainage must be

determined. Complications such as hearing loss, vertigo, and facial nerve weakness must be sought.

Physical examination begins with inspection of the normal ear, and includes careful cleaning of the EAC, otoscopy, and pneumotoscopy to assess mobility of the TM. Figure 55-25 shows equipment useful for examining the EAC and TM. The auricle, lobule, and tragus of the diseased ear are carefully inspected for erythema or skin lesions and palpated for pain. Dry cerumen or skin debris may be carefully cleaned from the EAC by gentle teasing with a cerumen spoon. Mucoid or purulent drainage is suctioned from the lateral EAC with a Fraser tipped suction as previously described. The diagnosis of diffuse external otitis is confirmed by observing an intact, mobile TM and diffuse inflammation of the EAC. Uncomplicated acute otitis media is a common diagnosis confirmed by a bulging, erythematous TM with decreased mobility. The EAC appears normal. In a chronically draining ear, the EAC may be secondarily inflamed from exposure to purulence, although the primary pathology lies in the middle ear or mastoid.

Uncomplicated acute otitis externa is treated with topical agents effective against pseudomonas and staphylococci. Hydrocortisone, 1%, neomycin sulfate, and polymyxin B (Cortisporin Otic Suspension) three drops t.i.d. is usually effective. For patients with neomycin hypersensitivity, gentamicin (Garamycin Ophthalmic Solution) may be equally effective. Narcotic analgesic combinations containing codeine or oxycodone with aspirin or acetaminophen are prescribed to control pain. If the lateral EAC is totally occluded by edema, a wick must be placed in the EAC to allow distribution of topical antibiotics into the medial canal. The wick is best inserted to a depth of one

TABLE 55-22. DIFFERENTIAL DIAGNOSES OF EXTERNAL OTITIS
Otitis Media (acute or chronic)
Perichondritis
Furunculosis
Bullous myringitis or bullous external otitis
Herpetic otitis externa
Necrotizing otitis externa
Malignant neoplasm

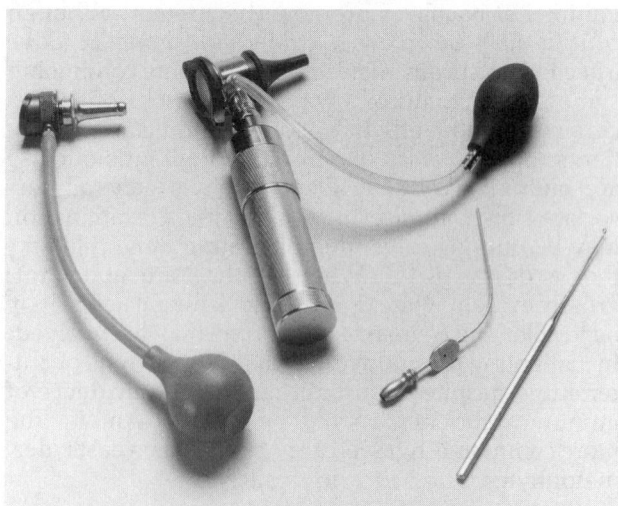

FIG. 55-25. Equipment useful for examining the external auditory canal and tympanic membrane. The Siegel pneumatic otoscope (left) and the hand held otoscope (center) are used to visualize the TM and assess its mobility. A small Fraser tipped suction and blunt curet are used to gently clean the ear of debris.

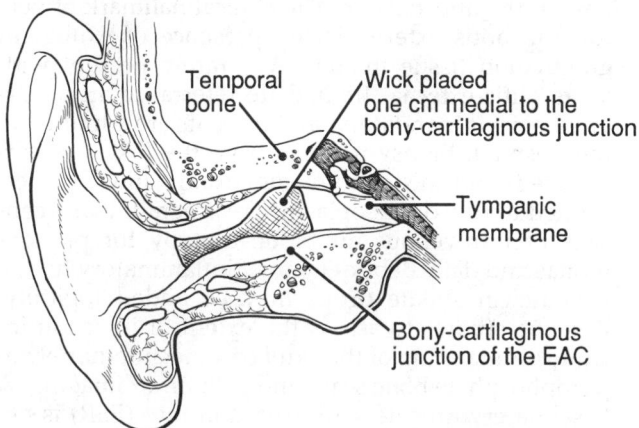

FIG. 55-26. Inflammation associated with acute external otitis occurs laterally in the external auditory canal. A cotton or gauze wick transmits topical antibiotics medial to occlusive edema.

cm medial to the point of restriction, usually just lateral to the bony-cartilaginous junction (Fig. 55-26). Commercial products such as the Pope otowick are ideal for this purpose. Alternatively, a folded piece of $\frac{1}{4}$ inch strip gauze may be inserted. Insertion of a wick is a painful procedure in the best of hands, and should be performed in a firm but compassionate manner. Gentle dilation of the stenosis with progressively larger speculae may be required. In milder forms of external otitis, the EAC skin may be moist and slightly edematous or dry and eczematous. The moist ear should be treated with acidifying and anti-inflammatory agents. Acetic acid preparations (VoSol, Domeboro) are effective antibacterial agents and function to restore the physiologic pH of the EAC. Alternatively, half-strength white vinegar (diluted with water) irrigation of the EAC may be equally effective and is significantly less expensive. A simple device for irri-

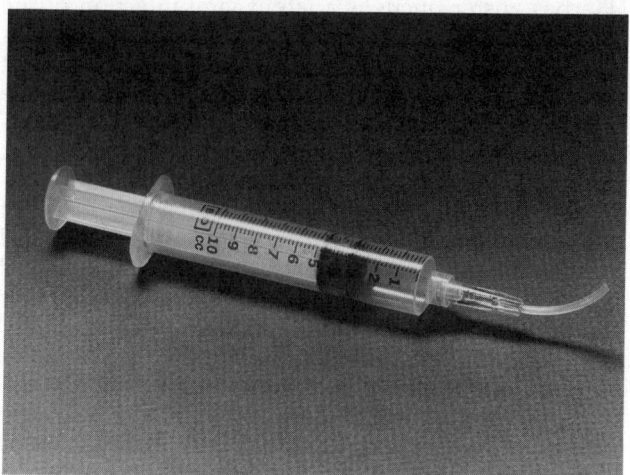

FIG. 55-27. A 10 cc syringe fitted with 3 cm of butterfly catheter tubing is useful for irrigating the external auditory canal in chronic infection.

gating the EAC is shown in Fig. 55-27. The pruritic, eczematous EAC is treated with acetic acid and steroid combinations (VoSol HC) or 0.025% triamcinolone cream applied sparingly with a cotton-tipped applicator.

Systemic antibiotics are reserved for severe acute otitis externa with cellulitis of surrounding soft tissues. Antistaphylococcal penicillins (Dicloxacillin) or first-generation cephalosporins (Velosef, Keflex) are usually effective. Ciprofloxacin (a fluoroquinolone derivative) has excellent activity against pseudomonas and other gram-negative organisms, and may be useful in refractory cases.

In refractory cases in which fungal external otitis is suspected, the EAC should be cleaned, and scrapings should be added to 10% aqueous potassium hydroxide and examined microscopically for hyphae and spores. Treatment is similar to that of mild inflammatory external otitis. Acetic acid solutions (such as Cresylate) are fungistatic. If the EAC is dry, topical antifungal creams such as tolnaftate (Tinactin) or clotrimazole (Lotrimin) may be applied with a cotton-tipped applicator.

Follow-up for uncomplicated cases of acute external otitis is usually directed towards the primary care physician. In cases in which examination is incomplete because of severe edema or purulence, or if symptoms progress despite initial therapy, otolaryngologic follow-up is mandatory.

FURUNCULOSIS

Furunculosis is an infection of the hair follicles in the external auditory canal, usually caused by staphylococci. Typically, a well-circumscribed raised, erythematous pustule is seen in the lateral portion of the EAC. The lesion is usually moderately painful. Treatment consists of antistaphylococcal antibiotics (dicloxacillin, clindamycin, first- or second-generation cephalosporins) and mild narcotic analgesia. Warm saline soaks applied locally may induce spontaneous drainage of the furuncle. If drainage has not occurred in 2 days, aspiration of purulence under local anesthesia may hasten resolution.

PERICHONDRITIS

Infection of the perichondrium or cartilage of the auricle is uncommon, and may result from surgical or accidental trauma to the external ear. Rarely perichondritis may result from extension of acute otitis externa. We have recently seen two cases associated with piercing of the auricle for earrings. The initial clinical feature is diffuse erythema of the cartilage skeleton with sparing of the lobule. As the infection advances, auricular swelling and pain develops, with or without fever. Treatment of early, spontaneous perichondritis with oral antibiotics active against staphylococcus and other gram positive organisms is usually effective. Perichondritis associated with trauma and extension of external otitis is usually caused by pseudomonas, and should be treated with intravenous antipseudomonal penicillins and aminoglycosides. Alternatively, ciprofloxacin may be prescribed for oral therapy. It has a wide spectrum of activity against gram-positive and gram-negative organisms including pseudomonas; thus it has developed a secure role in the treatment of external ear infections. (It is contraindicated in children because of the risk of abnormal cartilage maturation and failure of normal long bone development.) If a subperichondrial abscess is evident by local fluctuance, it must be drained and cultured promptly and treated with a pressure dressing to minimize cartilage necrosis leading to collapse of the cartilaginous auricular skeleton. If the patient is not admitted for IV antibiotics, daily follow-up by the managing otolaryngologist is indicated.

Polychondritis, sometimes mistaken for auricular cellulitis, may be differentiated by history, elevated ESR, and other cartilage involvement.[2a]

BULLOUS MYRINGITIS AND BULLOUS EXTERNAL OTITIS

Bullous myringitis is usually associated with an upper respiratory infection, and presents with severe otalgia. Physical examination reveals hemorrhagic bullae exclusively on the tympanic membrane. The causative agent is usually viral, but the infection may be associated with acute otitis media, often caused by Mycoplasma pneumoniae. Management includes an attempt to rupture all bullae, resulting in a dramatic reduction in pain. The ear canal should be allowed to dry spontaneously after decompression.[3] Erythromycin, 500 mg qid, is recommended.

Bullous external otitis is also a viral illness presenting with acute otalgia. Examination reveals multiple hemorrhagic bullae of the bony external canal. Spontaneous rupture and hemorrhage may occur. The TM appears normal. No effort should be made to decompress these bullae as in bullous myringitis. Treatment consists of oral codeine or oxycodone analgesics with topical antibiotics (Cortisporin Otic Suspension) and topical benzocaine (Auralgan Otic). Systemic antibiotics are not routinely administered.

NECROTIZING OTITIS EXTERNA

Necrotizing otitis externa (malignant otitis externa) is a potentially life-threatening infection that begins in the EAC. This infection classically occurs in elderly diabetics, although it may occur in younger (usually immunocompromised) patients. If it is not aggressively treated, a fulminating soft tissue infection and osteitis of the skull base ensue, with substantial risk for multiple cranial neuropathies, vascular sequelae, intracranial abscess, and sepsis. Pseudomonas aeruginosa is almost always the infecting organism. Patients present with symptoms of diffuse acute otitis externa: otalgia, purulent drainage, and sense of full-

ness in the affected ear. The clinical hallmark of necrotizing otitis externa is the presence of exuberant granulation tissue in the EAC, rarely present with acute otitis externa. Immediate referral to an otolaryngologist is mandatory, and patients are admitted to the hospital. Biopsy material from the EAC tissue is cultured and histopathologic examination is performed to rule out neoplasm. Treatment initially consists of intravenous antibiotic therapy for pseudomonas and daily debridement of inflammatory tissue. Gentamicin sulfate drops may be added topically. Baseline studies to assess the extent of infection include CT scanning of the skull base, technetium-99m-pyrophosphate bone scan, and gallium-67 imaging. A baseline erythrocyte sedimentation rate (ESR) is obtained to begin monitoring the course of disease. Traditionally, patients with radiographic evidence of bone destruction are treated with an IV antipseudomonal penicillin and aminoglycoside for 4 to 8 weeks. Adjunctive hyperbaric oxygen therapy has been reported to hasten resolution of infection.[4] Successful treatment of necrotizing otitis media with oral ciprofloxacin and rifampin[5] has been reported, significantly decreasing the cost of treating this serious infection. Aggressive local management of the ear canal disease is mandatory until epithelialization is complete.

MALIGNANT NEOPLASM OF THE EXTERNAL EAR

An adequate description of the external ear malignancies is beyond the scope of this chapter. Malignancy is relatively rare, and most often involves squamous cell or basal cell carcinoma. Any patient with a nonhealing ulcer, mass, or polyp should be referred to the specialist for biopsy.

HERPES ZOSTER OTICUS

Herpes zoster oticus is a latent viral infection of the geniculate ganglion (seventh cranial nerve). It is included in this discussion of ear infections because it presents with a painful, burning vesicular rash of the pinna, posterior EAC, and postauricular skin. Secretomotor neurons and taste-mediating neurons that pass through the geniculate ganglion may also be affected, causing a serpiginous vesicular enanthem of the lateral nasal wall, soft palate and anterolateral tongue. When herpes zoster oticus presents with facial paralysis or involvement of the cochlear-vestibular nerve (i.e., vertigo and sensorineural hearing loss), the infection is called Ramsey-Hunt syndrome. The vesicles may rupture, coalesce, and form honey-colored crusts. Treatment is generally supportive. Warm, moist compresses and narcotic analgesic combinations should be evident. Topical or systemic antibiotics active against gram-positive flora are prescribed only if a secondary bacterial infection is evident. Acyclovir cream, 5% has been shown to decrease duration of rash and otalgia in immunocompromised patients. This same benefit, however, has not been demonstrated in immunocompetent patients.[6] These patients must be followed closely for bacterial superinfection, facial paralysis, and cochlear-vestibular nerve involvement. Neurologic complications are best treated with intravenous acyclovir. Oral acyclovir (800 mg five times daily) can accelerate healing in severe cases.

OTITIS MEDIA

Otitis media is a common infection in children and is less frequently diagnosed in adults. In children, acute otitis media often occurs after an upper respiratory infection. Recurrent otitis media is associated with eustachian tube dysfunction, serous otitis media, allergy, and adenoid hypertrophy. The diagnosis of acute otitis media is made when the patient presents with fever, otalgia, and a bulging erythematous TM. The most common organisms cultured are Streptococcus pneumoniae, Hemophilus influenzae and Branhamella catarrhalis. Staphylococcus aureus, Streptococcus pyogenes, and other organisms play a minor role. Amoxicillin and ampicillin are preferred initial antibiotics of choice, unless oral administration cannot be accomplished. If that is the case, parenteral ampicillin can be given initially. In penicillin-allergic patients, erythromycin or erythromycin-sulfamethoxazole is effective. Recently, the incidence of beta-lactamase-producing strains of H. influenzae and B. catarrhalis has been estimated as 40% in all ears cultured.[7] Therefore, beta-lactamase resistant antibiotics such as amoxicillin-potassium clavulanate (Augmentin), cefaclor (Ceclor), or trimethoprim-sulfamethoxazole (Bactrim, Septra) are prescribed if initial antibiotic therapy fails. Decongestants have not been demonstrated to shorten the course of illness. Initially, mild narcotic analgesics may be prescribed. These patients should be re-examined after a 10- to 14-day course of antibiotic therapy. Otolaryngologic referral and consideration for myringotomy and culture are indicated for immunocompromised patients, seriously ill or toxic patients, those suppurative complications, neonates, and patients with recurrence despite multiple courses of appropriate antibiotics.

Initial treatment of active chronic otitis media consists of gentle suctioning of the EAC and initiating antibiotic drops. The microbiology of the draining ear may be similar to that of acute otitis media, but there is an increased incidence of S. aureus, anaerobes, and gram-negative organisms. Neomycin-polymyxin B-hydrocortisone (Cortisporin Otic Suspension), sulfamethoxazole-hydrocortisone (Vasocidin), or chloramphenicol (Chloromycetin Otic) three drops qid are prescribed. Alternatively, one-half strength white vinegar with tap water irrigation is effective treatment of chronic middle ear infection and drainage. Irrigations are started twice daily. All patients with chronic otitis media should be followed to resolution of otorrhea. If a permanent perforation or cholesteatoma is sus-

pected, patients should be referred to an otolaryngologist.

Systemic antibiotics are effective in selected cases of chronic otitis media. Patients with a previously dry TM perforation who develop otorrhea associated with an upper respiratory infection should be treated with oral antibiotics active against the usual pathogens of acute otitis media.[8] Patients with a chronically draining ear, with or without infected cholesteatoma, are prone to infection by S. aureus and gram-negative organisms including Pseudomonas and Proteus. Most oral antibiotics are ineffective against these organisms. Oral ciprofloxacin (500 mg PO bid) may be effective antibiotic therapy, however. If chronic otitis media is associated with cellulitis of the EAC or surrounding soft tissues, beta-lactamase resistant antibiotics (Ceclor, Ceftin, Augmentin, Bactrim) should be initiated with topical care.

COMPLICATIONS OF EAR INFECTIONS

Complications of ear infections may involve the soft tissues and cartilage of the external ear or the deeper structures of the temporal bone and intracranial cavity. Prompt recognition and appropriate management of these infectious complications can prevent unacceptable morbidity. Generally, complications are associated with chronic purulent otitis media. Intratemporal complications, however, particularly serous or suppurative labyrinthitis and facial nerve paralysis, may occur with an intact TM (acute otitis media.)[9]

OTITIS EXTERNA

Complications of external otitis include cellulitis, perichondritis, and stenosis of the external auditory canal. Moderate cellulitis of the EAC and periauricular soft tissues may be treated with oral antibiotics and warm compresses. If extensive cellulitis, perichondritis, lymphadenopathy, or sepsis is present, IV antibiotics are required. Stenosis of the EAC results from hypertrophic scarring following repeated inflammation. Treatment is excision of EAC skin, enlarging the bony canal with a drill, and split thickness skin grafting.

OTITIS MEDIA

The litany of complications of otitis media includes osteitis, subperiosteal abscess, Bezold's abscess, serous or suppurative labyrinthitis, facial nerve weakness, epidural abscess, brain abscess, meningitis, and sigmoid sinus thrombosis (Table 55-23). The complications of otitis media can occur with or without an

TABLE 55-23. COMPLICATIONS OF EAR INFECTIONS

Otitis Externa
  Cellulitis
  Perichondritis
  Osteomyelitis
  Stenosis of the EAC
Otitis Media (temporal bone and intracranial complications)
  Serous labyrinthitis
  Facial nerve paralysis or paresis
  Meningitis
  Subperiosteal abcess (including Bezhold's abcess)
  Brain abcess
  Epidural abcess
  Subdural empyema
  Sigmoid sinus thrombosis

intact TM, and usually require aggressive medical therapy and often surgical drainage.

Acute coalescent mastoiditis involves destruction of the mastoid air cell septations in the temporal bone by necrotizing osteitis. It may occur as a complication of acute otitis media that fails to respond to treatment or relapses within the first 10 days. Destruction of the bony septae of the mastoid air cell system is usually evident on CT scan. This complication is relatively uncommon, and requires intravenous antibiotic therapy and a simple mastoidectomy. If infection progresses through the bony cortex, subperiosteal abscess may occur. In these cases, fluctuance in the superior postauricular crease causes anterior and inferior displacement of the auricle. Bezold's abscess occurs when subperiosteal purulence extends medially and inferiorly from the mastoid tip, deep to the origin of the sternocleido-mastoid muscle. Treatment is surgical drainage and IV antibiotics guided by culture and sensitivity.

Serous labyrinthitis may occur with acute or chronic infection, and the patient may complain of vertigo, nausea, or hearing loss. Toxic products irritative to the labyrinthine structures may diffuse across the round window membrane, causing vestibular symptoms or transient sensorineural hearing loss. Patients usually respond to systemic antibiotics and symptomatic treatment. When these symptoms are associated with high fever and toxemia, suppurative labyrinthitis and/or an intracranial complication is implied.

Acute facial paralysis occurring with acute or chronic otitis media requires prompt surgical drainage, usually by mastoidectomy and wide myringotomy. IV antibiotics are initiated empirically and guided by culture.

Meningitis is the most common intracranial complication of otitis media.[10] Lethargy, headache, papilledema and nuchal rigidity are the most common presenting signs and symptoms. In children, otitic hydrocephalus can occur. If an intracranial infection is suspected, CT scanning with contrast should be performed before lumbar puncture to rule out brain abscess. Other intracranial suppurative complications are far less common. In order of decreasing frequency, brain abscess, subdural empyema, sigmoid sinus thrombosis, and epidural abscess may occur.

When the diagnosis of temporal bone or intracranial complication of acute or chronic ear infection is suspected, immediate consultation with the otolaryngologist is indicated. Prompt surgical and medical treatment of the complication and initial focus of infection must be initiated to prevent fulminant infection, permanent loss of cranial nerve function, or other neurologic sequelae.

INDICATIONS FOR ADMISSION

Acute otitis media is by far the most common ear infection treated by the emergency physician. Acute otitis externa (swimmer's ear) and chronic otitis media are also common infections. The remaining infections of the ear described in this chapter are relatively uncommon, but the initial diagnosis is important because specific therapy may be required. Although temporal bone and intracranial complications of acute and chronic otitis media are distinctly uncommon in a primary care practice, early diagnosis is paramount to prevent potentially catastrophic sequelae.

Most acute ear infections are treated on an outpatient basis. Severe cases of acute diffuse otitis externa with widespread erysipelas or cellulitis, or severe otitis media require admission for IV antibiotics. Diabetics or other immunocompromised patients must be considered for admission if the infection does not improve in 24 to 48 hours.

Patients with acute otitis media are hospitalized under the following conditions: systemic toxicity, age under 2 months (high risk for meningitis), temporal bone or intracranial complications, or a significantly compromised immune system. Patients with chronic suppurative otitis media require admission only under the following circumstances: persistent drainage with fever or deep, boring pain (suggestive of necrotizing abscess, osteitis or neoplasm) despite adequate topical and oral antibiotic therapy; and the presence of temporal bone or intracranial complication.

FOLLOW-UP CARE

All chronically draining ears must be followed by an otologist because permanent TM perforations are associated with recurrent infection and cholesteatoma. Many of these patients have surgically correctable conductive hearing losses after resolution of chronic infection. Acute otitis media is routinely followed up by the primary care physician after a 10- to 14-day course of antibiotics. Patients who fail to resolve following a second course of beta-lactamase resistant antibiotics, or patients with complaints of hearing loss and middle ear effusion should be referred to the otolaryngologist for a thorough head and neck evaluation and consideration for placement of ventilation tubes. Unilateral serous otitis media requires examination of the nasopharynx to rule out a lesion obstructing the eustachian tube.

Acute otitis externa demands follow-up for subsequent ear cleaning and to assess improvement in edema and pain. Chronic otitis externa is best managed by a physician experienced in treating dermatitis and inflammation of the EAC. Patients with unusual anatomy or sufficient inflammation to distort normal landmarks should be referred to the otolaryngologist for definitive diagnoses. The specialist often has the advantage of binocular microscopy and specialized instruments to satisfactorily identify pathology in difficult cases.

REFERENCES

1. Senturia, B.H., Marcus, M.D., and Lucente, F. E.: Diseases of the External Ear. 2nd ed. Orlando, Grune and Stratton, 1980.

2. Bluestone, C.D.: Management and therapy of otitis media. *In* Otologic Medicine and Surgery, Vol. 2. Edited by Alberti, P.W., and Ruben, R.J. New York, Churchill Livingstone, 1988.

2a. Coppola, M., and Yealy, D.M.: Relapsing polychondritis: An unusual cause of painful auricular swelling. Ann. Emerg. Med. 21:81, 1992.

3. Smith, P.G., and Lucente, F.E.: Infections of the external ear. *In* Otolaryngology/Head and Neck Surgery, Vol. 4. Edited by Cummings, C.W., Fredrickson, J.M., Harker, L.A., Krause, C.J., and Schuller, D.E. St. Louis, C.V. Mosby Co., 1986.

4. Moder, J.T., and Love, J.T.: Malignant external otitis: Cure with adjunctive hyperbaric oxygen therapy. Arch. Otolaryngol. 108:38, 1982.

5. Rubin, J., et al.: Efficacy of oral ciprofloxacin plus rifampin for treatment of malignant external otitis. Arch. Otolaryngol. 115:1063, 1989.

6. Mandal, B.K., et al.: A double-masked placebo controlled trial of acyclovir cream in immunocompetent patients with herpes zoster. J. Infec. 17:57, 1988.

7. Bluestone, C.D.: Unpublished data from the Pittsburgh Otitis Media Research Center. Presented at the Lamberson Lectureship, May, 1989.

8. Kemink, J.L., Telian, S.A., and Niparko, J.K.: Evaluation and treatment of the Draining Ear. Modern Med. 56:76, 1988.

9. Samuel, J., and Fernandes, C.M.C.: Otogenic complications with an intact tympanic membrane. Laryngoscope 95:1387, 1985.

10. Gower, D.J., McGuirt, W.F., and Kelly, D.L.: Intracranial complications of ear disease in a pediatric population with special emphasis on subdural effusion and empyema. South. Med. J. 78:429, 1985.

INFECTIONS OF THE UPPER AIRWAY

Suzanne M. Shepherd and Gerard R. Cox

CAPSULE

Few emergencies produce more fear in patients or their family members than sudden difficulty in breathing. Few emergencies demand more rapid evaluation by prehospital care providers and physicians than entities causing acute airway obstruction. Failure to address the airway expeditiously and definitively places the patient at risk for unnecessary morbidity and mortality. The emergency care provider must rapidly assess the level of airway involvement, the probable nature of the problem, and the degree of distress and decide on appropriate intervention, while maintaining a calm and reassuring manner.

Causes of obstruction may be divided into three major groups: (1) those causing sudden unexpected obstruction, i.e., foreign bodies; (2) those producing fixed airway obstruction, i.e., congenital abnormalities; and (3) those of infectious origin. This chapter focuses on the infectious causes of airway compromise. These have been reported with increasing frequency in the last two decades. Practitioners in large hospitals in the United States can expect to see several pediatric and adult cases each year.

Infections of the airway have been reported more frequently in the last 20 years, at least partly because of increased sensitivity to the diagnosis of these illnesses by practicing physicians. These illnesses present a significant threat of rapid airway compromise. The emergency physician should be facile with recognition, and aggressively but appropriately use airway management techniques. Expeditious mobilization of an "airway team" is best accomplished using well-publicized and practiced protocols. The patient care team, functioning in a well-coordinated and effective fashion, can do much to reassure a frightened patient and family and thus ensure better cooperation.

HISTORICAL PERSPECTIVE

Holmes first described what today is known as croup in 1765. In 1797, George Washington died of quinsy, after his personal physician ignored the opinion of two other physicians that he needed an emergency tracheostomy. In 1900, Theison reported three cases of infectious membranous croup in children. In 1936, LeMierre published the first case report of epiglottitis and cervical abscess in a 49-year-old woman who presented with fever, dyspnea, and pharyngeal obstruction.[1] Sinclair identified Hemophilus influenzae as the major cause of epiglottitis in 1941. In 1948, Rabe proved epiglottitis and croup to be two separate entities. Bouchan, in 1974, showed Parainfluenzae types I and III to be the major causative agents of croup.[1,2,3]

Current controversies in the treatment of airway infections center around aggressiveness of initial airway management in adults and length of time of intubation, sedation, and paralysis in children. Newer reports focus on more unusual causative agents of supraglottitis in the immunocompromised host.

ANATOMIC AND MECHANICAL CONSIDERATIONS

The upper airway can be divided into three sections: supraglottic, intraglottic, and infraglottic. Alignment of the hyperextended head and neck in the "sniffing position" allows maximum air flow between these axes [4] (Fig. 55-28).

During inspiration pressure on the extrathoracic airway increases, narrowing the lumen, while pressure on the intrathoracic airway decreases, enlarging the lumen. Expiration reverses the pressures and thus the lumen sizes. Lesions causing a fixed wall narrowing would limit flow during inspiration and expiration equally because airway caliber cannot change with changes in airway pressure. An extrathoracic lesion that compressed the airway but allowed it to be mobile at the site of obstruction would affect inspiratory flow to a significantly greater degree than expiratory flow.

Poiseuille's law further delineates the significant impact of airway narrowing on flow: the pressure to produce a given air flow varies directly with the length of the tube and indirectly with the fourth power of the radius. A person must therefore work exponentially to maintain normal air flow, even in the presence of a small degree of obstruction. At a critical level of narrowing, minimal further swelling, or the presence of secretions, may suddenly prevent adequate flow. It has been estimated that 1 mm of mucosal edema in

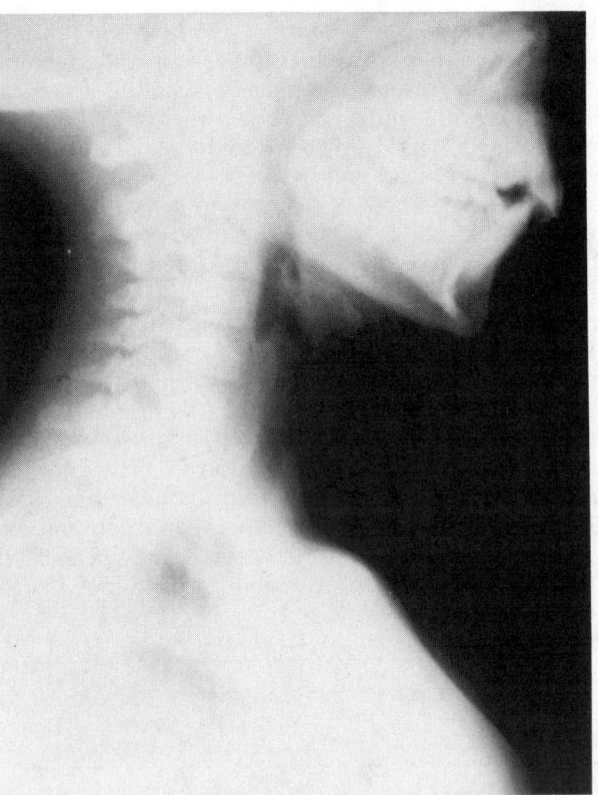

FIG. 55-28.   Normal lateral soft tissue neck radiograph in an adult. Courtesy of Dr. Margaret Stull, Department of Radiology, Georgetown University Hospital.

a newborn reduces airway flow by 30%. Secretions further limit air flow by producing turbulence.

The degree of laxity of the submucosal tissues in the upper airway tends to localize infections, and provides the careful examiner with further clues to determine the level of airway involvement. Swelling caused by inflammation in the supraglottic airway progresses anteriorly along the lingual surface because tissues are more loosely adherent here. The epiglottis, with its relatively lax submucosal adherence, is particularly vulnerable.

As the epiglottis swells, it is transformed from its usual thin curved sheet of tissue to a large, posteriorly facing C-shaped structure. This causes symptoms of odynophagia and severe sore throat. The patient may begin to drool in an attempt to avoid swallowing his secretions. As swelling extends beyond the pharyngoepiglottic fold into the arytenoepiglottic fold, worsening respiratory distress and inspiratory stridor develop. The voice quality becomes muffled rather than hoarse because the relatively firm adherence of the submucosal tissues in the true glottic structures prevents the development of massive edema and prevents the spread of edema into the subglottic region.[5,6] The patient may assume an upright "sniffing" position, often with the tongue extended, in an attempt to maximize airway diameter.

Subglottic tissues have relatively loosely adherent submucosa, allowing the development of significantly greater edema. Individuals with subglottic inflammation have a hoarse voice and often a brassy or barking cough. Assumption of the "sniffing" position is unusual in patients with subglottic swelling because it does not alter the subglottic diameter. Stridor may be present during both inspiration and expiration.

Although supraglottitis was first described in an adult, it has been primarily discussed in the pediatric population. Increased reporting in the adult literature in the last two decades probably reflects an increase in sensitivity to the diagnosis rather than an actual increase in the incidence of adult cases. The adult airway is relatively protected from serious compromise from inflammatory causes by its larger diameter, its more rigid cartilaginous structure, the change in anatomic configuration of the epiglottitis with age, and the relative lack of reactive lymphoid tissue. These several factors may cause the adult presentation of epiglottitis to be only subtly different from that of pharyngitis.[7–10] When an adult's symptoms appear out of proportion to the clinical examination of the pharynx, it is prudent to consider this potentially lethal entity.

GENERAL MANAGEMENT

Because of the high risk of sudden significant airway compromise in the patient with infections of the upper airway, particularly those of bacterial origin, history taking and physical evaluation must be brief and well directed. The examiner should initially note the patient's general appearance, color, level of consciousness, vital signs, presence of audible (stridor) or visible (retractions, use of accessory muscles or nasal flaring) signs of respiratory distress, presence or absence of drooling, and findings on direct examination of the external neck and chest. Any portion of the examination that seems to be significantly distressing to the child should be abbreviated or abandoned because strap muscle tightening or laryngospasm may convert subcritical to critical airway compromise. Examination of the mouth is traditionally avoided in children because it may cause laryngospasm. Children may remain less agitated if examined in the arms of a parent. Numerous reports in the adult literature describe mirror evaluation in the stable patient without difficulty.[2,3,9]

Humidified high-flow oxygen by mask should be provided. Children may not tolerate the mask on the face, but may tolerate a mask held close to the face by a parent. A bag-valve mask and intubation and surgical airway trays must be readily available because sudden airway loss may occur without warning. If the patient decompensates in transit to the hospital, laryngospasm can usually be overcome by bag-valve mask ventilation if a good seal is ensured.[2]

Ideally, definitive airway evaluation and management are done under controlled conditions in the operating room by appropriate surgical and anesthesia personnel. Many institutions have developed "airway" or "epiglottitis" protocols, which help to ensure the most rapid, safe and methodic care of the pediatric patient by expeditious notification of the pediatrician, the otolaryngologist, the anesthesiologist, the radiologist, and the operating room on the patient's arrival. The emergency physician coordinates initial care, maintains constant contact with the patient, and must be ready to provide an airway if needed while the team is assembling. Under no circumstances should a patient be left unattended by medical personnel able to provide immediate definitive airway management.

WHICH PATIENTS REQUIRE IMMEDIATE AIRWAY MANAGEMENT?

Certainly, individuals in obvious distress with stridor, drooling, and lethargy require immediate management. Cyanosis is an obvious but late sign of critical airway compromise. Other accepted indications for airway intervention include significant tachycardia, tachypnea, hypoxemia, fatigue, presence of pneumonia, congestive heart failure, or significant secretions.[2,3,7–9,11] Children who present with stridor and drooling associated with fever and toxicity routinely receive prophylactic definitive airway management. Prophylactic airway management in this population has reduced mortality from an unacceptable 6% percent to under 1%.[9,10]

The preferred method of providing an airway in both the adult and pediatric patient is nasotracheal intubation. Nasotracheal intubation is easy and rapidly performed, and avoids the complications of tracheostomy, including hemorrhage, pneumothorax, fistula formation and tracheal stenosis. It is relatively well tolerated in an awake patient, shortens the duration of intubation and hospitalization, and leaves no scar.[3,9,10,12,13] A suggestion by Heeneman and Ward[14] that intubation might promote abscess formation has not been substantiated in the literature.[3,10,13] Tube size is chosen to produce a slight air leak so that postextubation edema is minimized. Tracheostomy may be preferable, however, if continuous intensive monitoring is not available.[10,15] Induction of anesthesia is usually accomplished using halothane. Sedation with diazepam (Valium) or midazolam (Versed) may be useful adjuncts. Positive pressure ventilation by means of CPAP or PEEP is used to minimize pulmonary edema, increase functional residual capacity, decrease shunt, and prevent small airway closure.[2,12,16] Routine use of prolonged sedation, paralysis, and mechanical ventilation remains controversial.[2,15,17]

Intravenous access, diagnostic testing and further evaluation of the child are of second priority and may prove agitating. They should be delayed until the airway is satisfactorily secured.

DIFFERENTIAL DIAGNOSIS

In the patient who appears nontoxic and has no obvious signs of respiratory compromise, a more thorough history and physical examination and diagnostic tests may be performed to better define the illness. The infectious entities to be considered in the differential diagnosis are several: supraglottitis (epiglottitis); viral laryngotracheobronchitis (croup); bacterial tracheitis; lingual tonsillitis; retropharyngeal abscess or cellulitis; prevertebral abscess; and diphtheria. One must also always consider aspirated foreign material. Optimal management varies according to the diagnosis, the age of the patient, and the degree of illness.

The two diagnostic modalities most widely used to aid in differentiating these entities are laryngoscopy and soft tissue radiography (Fig. 55–29) The emergency physician must be facile with both.

Laryngoscopy may be done with a mirror or a flexible fiberoptic laryngoscope or bronchoscope. Laryngoscopy is more reliable than soft tissue radiography, but requires some technical expertise.[9,11,17,18] Its use has not been favored in the acute evaluation of the pediatric population for the reasons noted, but it has been used safely and effectively in adults.

Lateral and anteroposterior soft tissue radiography is fairly sensitive and does not carry the risk of producing laryngospasm, but carries the risk of time. Ei-

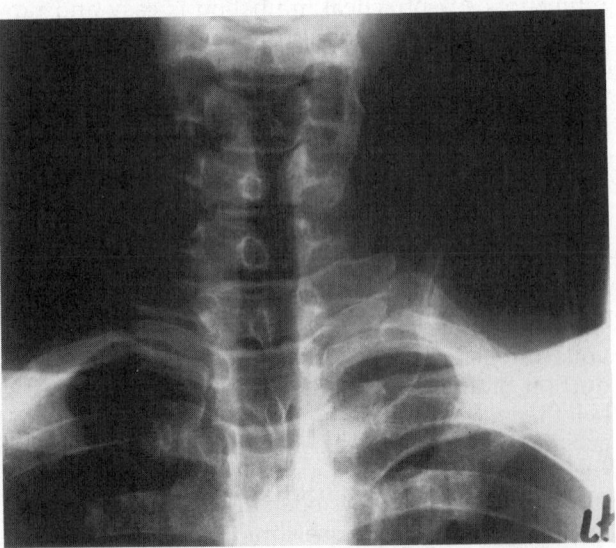

FIG. 55-29.   Normal anteroposterior soft tissue radiograph of the neck in a child. Courtesy of Dr. Clifton Leftridge, Department of Radiology, Georgetown University Hospital.

ther the patient should remain in the Emergency Department (ED) and have portable films obtained, or appropriate personnel should accompany the patient to the radiology suite for expeditious films. Radiographic evaluation of the supraglottic structures has been suggested to be up to 90% sensitive in demonstrating supraglottitis.[9] Interpretation of films can be adversely affected by patient flexion, rotation, age, and the presence of an omega-shaped epiglottis (normal variant in the population).[13,19–22] Jones reported a 30% false positive rate in their series because of noninflammatory thickening of the epiglottis, hypopharyngeal ballooning, and subglottic stenosis.[19] Lindquist suggested that xeroradiographs might provide clearer detail[5] as may CT scan and MRI, but the latter may not be available or cause dangerous delays.

History and physical examination, supported by radiographic or laryngoscopic findings, help the practitioner to differentiate these illnesses. The specific management of each is discussed.

SUPRAGLOTTITIS (EPIGLOTTITIS)

Supraglottitis, classically, is most commonly caused by Hemophilus influenzae in both pediatric (70 to 90%) and adult patients. Hemophilus parainfluenzae has also been isolated. In the immunocompetent adult population, Streptococcus viridans and Staphylococcus aureus have also been implicated. Streptococcus pneumoniae is more frequently isolated in the immunocompromised host.[23–25] Other causative organisms identified in immunocompromised patients include Klebsiella[22] and Candida albicans.[26–28] Viruses such as Influenza B[29] and Parainfluenza type III,[30] have been cultured from patients with epiglottitis. Definitive viral causality has not been demonstrated[23] except in one reported case of necrotizing epiglottitis and pneumonia in a patient with mononucleosis.[31] Either these viruses represent colonization, or a preceding viral infection may predispose to bacterial superinfection by damaging the mucosal barrier.[9,25] In fact, pharyngeal isolates in the patient with supraglottitis, such as Neisseria meningitidis, may represent normal respiratory flora or colonization.[3,7,23]

Blood cultures often do not correlate with pharyngeal isolates. In adults, up to 70% of blood cultures have been reported to be sterile.[9] Twenty-three to 35% of adults infected with Hemophilus influenzae are bacteremic, as compared to 60 to 90% of children.[7,32,33] One retrospective study found that bacteremia appears to correlate with more severe disease, occurring more often in patients who died or required early airway intervention.[9]

An early peak in incidence of supraglottitis occurs in children 2 to 6 years old. A second peak occurs in adults 20 to 40 years old. Supraglottitis at the extremes of age often occurs with unusual presentations.[11,26,34] The incidence is slightly higher during the summer months. Men predominate slightly over women.[11]

Because of the bacterial nature of this illness, patients tend to present abruptly, often within 12 to 16 hours of symptom occurrence. Although symptoms of respiratory distress do not appear to be sensitive or specific predictors of airway obstruction,[35] the risk of obstruction is highest in patients who present early.[9,13] Supraglottitis may present as a localized cellulitis with variable degrees of drooling, dysphonia, dysphagia, and respiratory distress. Abscess formation or ulceration may occur. Supraglottitis may also present as a systemic infection with toxicity including high fever (> 39 C), leukocytosis and associated otitis media, cervical adenitis, pneumonia, or rarely meningitis.[6,11,36]

Adults, because of the previously discussed differences in anatomy and physiology of their airway, often have a longer prodrome and less serious course.[2,3,11] This benign presentation may mislead the examiner. The disease may, however, have a particularly fulminant course in immunocompromised adults.[39] In a prospective evaluation of 155 children, Mauro et al. attempted to delineate symptoms that might reliably differentiate epiglottitis from croup. *The three clinical findings associated with epiglottitis were drooling, agitation, and absence of spontaneous cough, but their absence could not exclude the diagnosis.*[35]

Seven percent of children develop pulmonary edema as a complication of epiglottitis. Three proposed mechanisms have been suggested: increase in venous return secondary to highly negative intrathoracic pressure and shunting of blood from the peripheral to the central circulation; decreased interstitial hydrostatic pressure accompanying high negative intrathoracic pressure; and disruption of the anatomic integrity of capillary walls secondary to hypoxia and

transmission of abnormally high negative intrathoracic pressure to the peribronchial spaces.[2,16,37,38]

Soft tissue radiographs in these patients classically reveal swelling of the epiglottis and surrounding structures to form the "thumb sign" on the lateral view (Fig. 55-30). In adults, epiglottic width greater than 8 mm, aryepiglottic folds larger than 7 mm, a decrease in the angle of the valleculae, and an increase in the ratio of hypopharyngeal to tracheal air column strongly and more reliably suggest the diagnosis.[19,20,36,40,40a]

Laryngoscopy in children with Hemophilus influenzae supraglottitis usually reveals a large, swollen, cherry-red epiglottis with surrounding erythema and edema. In adults, often only a mild erythema or pale, watery edema is present.[9,11]

THERAPY OF EPIGLOTTITIS

The therapy of choice in children with epiglottitis is intubation, administration of humidified oxygen, sedation with or without paralysis, and mechanical ventilation[2,15,17] in the intensive care unit setting. As previously noted, 4 to 5 cm of CPAP or PEEP is often used.[2,6,12,16]

Appropriate airway management in adults with supraglottitis remains a matter of debate in the literature. Most adults do well with less aggressive airway management, avoiding prolonged intensive care unit stays and the potential complications of nasotracheal intubation or tracheostomy.[3,7,15,41] Mayo-Smith et al. retrospectively reviewed 56 cases of adult epiglottitis in Rhode Island. Four patients died, two of them without warning while being carefully observed.[9] They feel that the currently reported mortality rate of 4.6% in

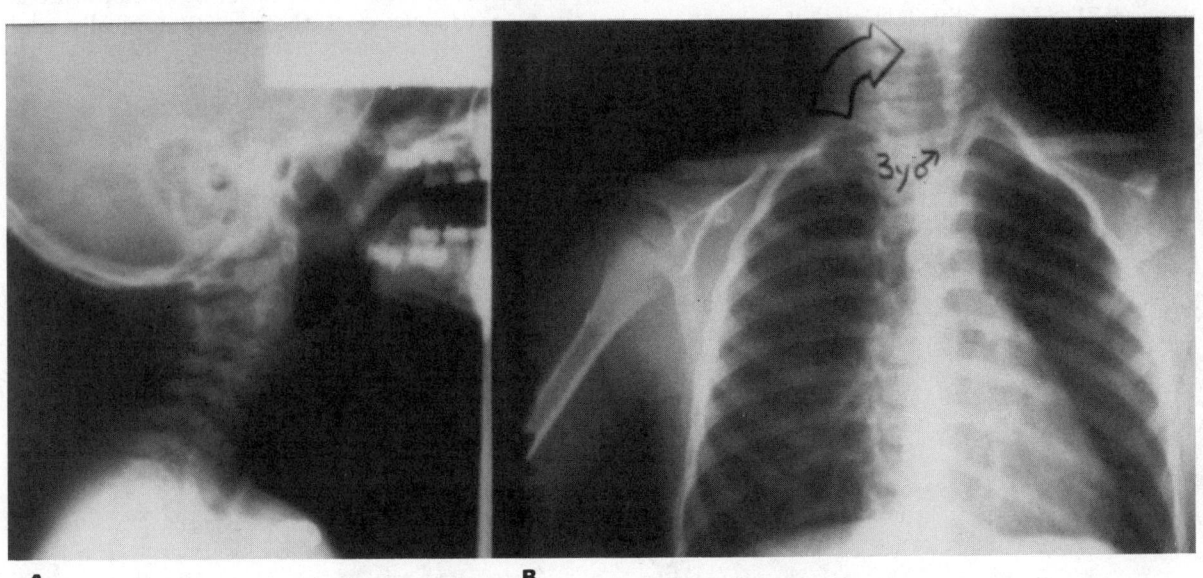

FIG. 55-30.   A. Lateral and B. anteroposterior soft tissue radiographs of a 3½-year-old child with supraglottitis. Note the classic thumb-shaped swelling of the epiglottitis and surrounding structures on the lateral radiograph. Courtesy of Dr. Clifton Leftridge, Department of Radiology, Georgetown University Hospital.

adults with epiglottitis is excessive, and support earlier recommendations of routine intubation.[9,42]

Choice of intravenous antibiotics is predicated on a 25% incidence of plasmid-mediated beta-lactamase production in strains of Hemophilus influenzae. Ampicillin (200 mg per kg per day) and chloramphenicol (100 mg per kg per day) or a third-generation cephalosporin such as ceftriaxone (50 to 75 mg per Kg per day) or cefuroxime (100 mg per kg per day) are recommended. In adults, cefazolin (1 g IV every 6 hours) is often added. Intravenous antibiotics are continued for 48 to 72 hours, followed by a 10-day course of oral medication such as trimethoprim-sulfamethoxazole or cefaclor.[3,11]

Racemic epinephrine is not effective in supraglottitis.[3] The use of parenteral steroids remains controversial in regard to benefit as opposed to risk.[23,43,44]

Most patients are extubated within 24 to 72 hours, based on clinical improvement and repeat laryngoscopy. Postextubation edema may respond to nebulized racemic epinephrine or require reintubation with an endotracheal tube one size smaller than the original and treatment with parenteral steroids (dexamethasone, 0.5 to 1 mg per kg every 6 hours for 24 hours).[2,6,12,16]

LARYNGOTRACHEOBRONCHITIS (CROUP)

Croup is usually caused by Parainfluenzae virus type I (74%). Respiratory syncytial virus, Influenzae A and B viruses, rhinovirus, echovirus, adenovirus, coxsackie virus, and measles virus have also been isolated.[2,45] Viral replication in the epithelial mucous glands causes cell degeneration and inflammation.

Croup is usually seen in children under 3, with a peak incidence at 21 to 24 months. It is felt that children at this age are more susceptible developmentally to significant illness because of their relatively small airway diameter, relatively loose and vascular mucosa and the small rigidly confined space in their subglottic airway.[2,45] The illness is predominant in boys and tends to occur in early fall and winter, with a peak incidence in November. Fifteen percent of children with croup have a positive family history.[2]

Because of the viral nature of the illness, croup is often gradual in onset. Mild upper respiratory symptoms, such as mucoid nasal drainage and mild cough, progress to a harsh barking cough, hoarseness, and a variable degree of stridor and respiratory distress. The child's symptoms may wax and wane, often becoming worse at night. The temperature is usually less than 39°C (38.1 to 38.5°C). Many medical centers use scoring systems based on degree of stridor, retractions, air entry, color, and level of consciousness to initially evaluate and follow a child's course.[2,45,46]

Anteroposterior soft tissue radiographic evaluation of the neck classically shows subglottic narrowing to form the "steeple," "wine bottle," or "Washington monument" sign (Fig. 55-31). Laryngoscopy reveals swelling below the cords, often with visible exudate and secretions.[2,45]

Many children respond to humidification provided by a shower or vaporizer at home or exposure to colder air outside the home. Cool mist is safer to use than steam because burns are avoided.

The child who does not respond to mist at home should be brought to the hospital for further evaluation and management. Antipyretics may be given as indicated. Mist therapy is continued and the child is hydrated. Children unresponsive to mist and hydration are given racemic epinephrine (0.5 cc of 2.25% racemic epinephrine diluted in 3 cc NS) over 15 minutes by nebulization or IPPB. Racemic epinephrine is believed to vasoconstrict the airway topically and

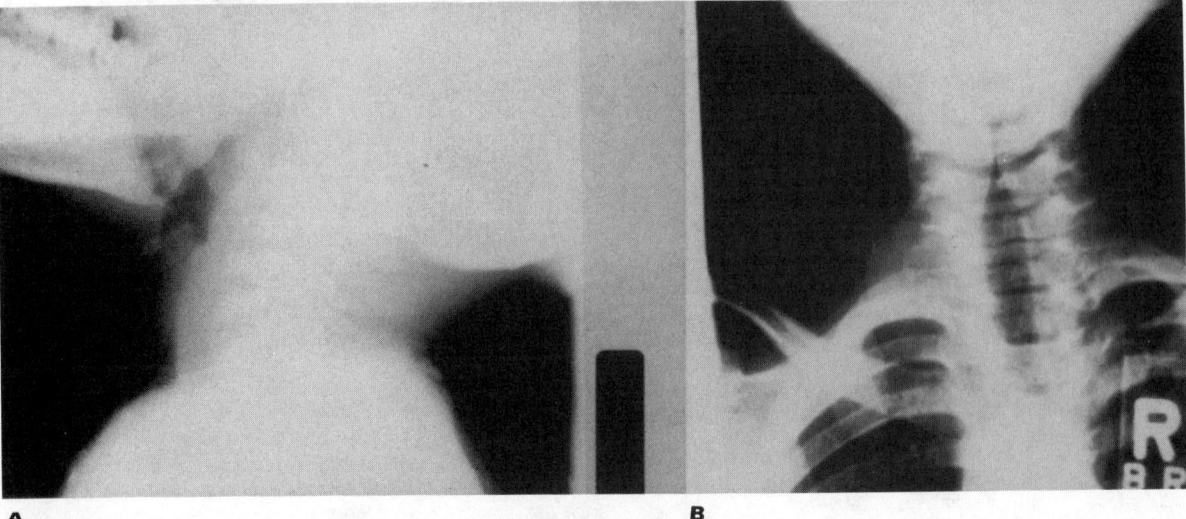

A **B**

FIG. 55-31.   A. Lateral and B. anteroposterior soft tissue radiographs of a child with croup. Note the characteristic steepling on the anteroposterior radiograph. Courtesy of Dr. Clifton Leftridge, Department of Radiology, Georgetown University Hospital.

thereby decrease edema. Controlled trials have demonstrated the efficacy of racemic epinephrine compared to normal saline.[46,47] Children usually respond promptly, but may develop rebound edema in 1 to 2 hours. Once the decision to give racemic epinephrine is made, the child is admitted for observation.

Studies suggest that 5 to 10% of children with croup require hospitalization. One to two percent of these hospitalized children require airway intervention, based on clinical and arterial blood gas parameters (hypoxia, hypercarbia and acidosis).[2] Antibiotics have not been shown to be beneficial.[2,45] Sedation should be avoided because it decreases respiratory drive. Clinical trials of parenteral steroids have shown widely varying results, partly because of significant differences in methodology. The most promising results have been seen with the use of a single high dose of dexamethasone (1.0 to 1.5 mg per kg, maximum 30 mg).[2,45,48]

BACTERIAL TRACHEITIS

Although Influenza A can produce severe croup with purulent secretions, clinicians in the late 1970s and early 1980s saw the reemergence of "membranous croup," an illness common in the 1920s through the 1940s. Staphylococcus aureus is cultured in 65% of these cases. Streptococcal species, Escherichia coli, Neisseria species, Hemophilus influenzae, Klebsiella, Pseudomonas, Chlamydia trachomatis and Branhamella catarrhalis have also been isolated.[49–52] These organisms are felt to represent true infection rather than colonization. Gram stains of the secretions have been found to be an accurate predictor of culture results.[52] Blood cultures are usually sterile.

Bacterial tracheitis should be considered in children resistant to the usual therapy for croup. It should also be considered in the child with croupy symptoms who has a significant leukocytosis and high band count[49,53] or in a toxic-appearing child with a barking cough who does not have the drooling or voice-muffling suggestive of supraglottitis.[50,52,54]

Soft tissue radiography of the neck may demonstrate shadows in the airway that represent secretions. A shaggy outline of the mucosa is noted in addition to the steeple sign.[45,49,52,55] Endoscopy reveals reddened, swollen mucosa with thick purulent exudate.[49,52,55]

Children often require intubation or tracheostomy. Airway obstruction may occur despite intubation because of the thick, purulent, tenacious exudate produced. Frequent suctioning is necessary. These secretions may also contribute to the lack of efficacy of nebulized racemic epinephrine in membranous croup because the drug may not reach the heavily coated mucous membranes.[49] Antibiotic choice should include antistaphylococcal coverage, i.e., cefuroxime (100 mg per kg per day) or a combination of oxacillin (150 mg per kg per day) and chloramphenicol (100 mg per kg per day). The mortality rate of bacterial tracheitis is relatively high. The mean duration of hospitalization is 12 days, roughly 4 times that of the patient with croup.[49]

RETROPHYARYNGEAL ABSCESS OR CELLULITIS

Retropharyngeal abscess or cellulitis is usually a complication of nasopharyngitis that has extended into the lymphoid tissue located in the space formed by the deep layers of the cervical fascia. This space extends from the base of the occiput to T_2. It is bounded anteriorly by the posterior wall of the pharynx and posteriorly by the prevertebral deep fascia. It is divided in half by the pharyngeal constrictor muscles. This retropharyngeal lymphoid tissue drains the sinuses, posterior nose, and nasopharynx. This lymphoid tissue atrophies with age, and therefore these infections are seen most commonly in children under six years of age.

Retropharyngeal abscess or cellulitis is less common today than in the preantibiotic era. The most common causative organisms are Staphylococcus aureus, Group A beta-hemolytic streptococci and oral flora. Other predisposing factors include trauma, intubation, otitis media, parotitis, and cervical osteomyelitis or discitis. A recent history of pharyngitis may be elicited.

The patient usually presents with severe sore throat, dysphagia, drooling, stridor, and neck pain, and often holds the neck stiffly in extension. Gentle palpation of the neck in the adult may demonstrate a unilateral mass, but a mass may not be apparent in young children.[2,4,22,45] The abscess may cause meningismus.

Soft tissue lateral radiography may demonstrate the abscess as soft tissue swelling in the retropharyngeal space, with anterior displacement of the airway and a loss of the normal lordotic curve of the spine.[22] (Fig. 55-32). Films must be obtained during inspiration with the neck extended. The retropharyngeal soft tissues of young children balloon during expiration, which may lead to a false positive diagnosis of abscess. Generally, the prevertebral soft tissues should be less than one half of the width of the adjacent vertebral body.[22,56] Lack of soft tissue swelling may indicate cellulitis without abscess. Computerized tomography (CT) of the neck is a helpful adjunct to delineate the extent of abscess spread (Fig. 55-33).

Treatment involves placement of an endotracheal tube to protect and maintain the airway, followed by surgical drainage of the abscess. Antibiotic choices include intravenous aqueous penicillin (100,000 units per kg per day) plus a semisynthetic penicillin such as oxacillin (150 mg per kg per day), or a third-generation cephalosporin such as cefuroxime (100 mg per kg per day).[4,22,45] Potential complications of retropharyngeal abscess include hemorrhage, mediastinitis, and rupture into the esophagus.

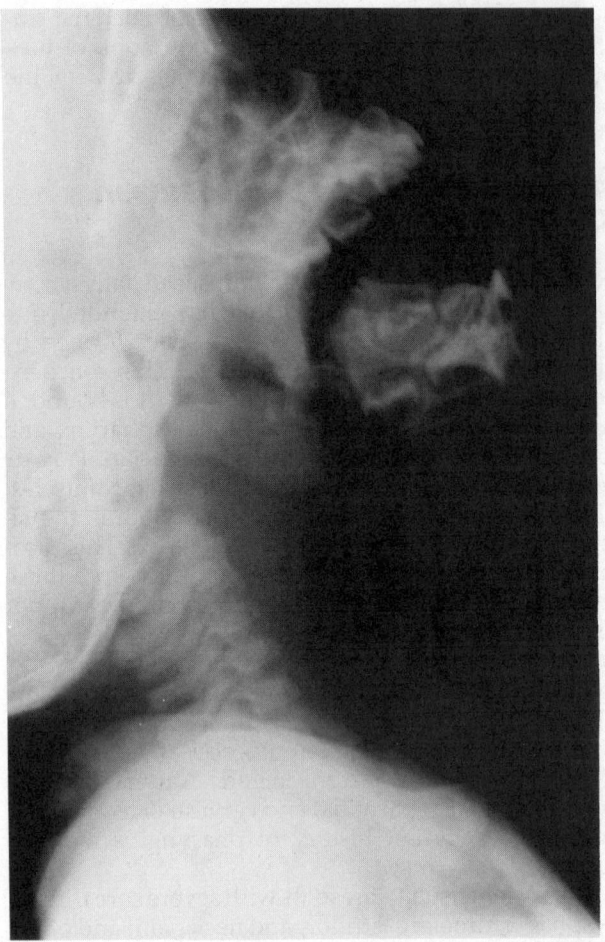

FIG. 55-32. Lateral soft tissue radiograph of a child with a retropharyngeal abscess. Note the neck and head position, marked widening of the retropharyngeal soft tissue, and anterior displacement of the air column. Courtesy of Dr. Margaret Stull, Department of Radiology, Georgetown University Hospital.

Other abscesses of the head and neck are covered subsequently.

DIPHTHERIA

This process, caused by toxigenic Corynebacterium diphtheriae, is rarely seen in the United States (5 to 10 cases per year). Infection usually localizes in the pharynx, middle ear, nose, larynx, and occasionally the skin. The primary route of transmission is by contact with respiratory secretions in the form of aerosolized droplet or on fomites. Conditions of poor hygiene, overcrowding, and poor medical care promote spread.

Diphtheria toxin is produced as an inactive polypeptide (MW 61,000), which is then cleaved and reduced to two subunits. The B subunit attaches to a specific glycoprotein receptor on the host cell. The internalized A subunit then interrupts cellular protein synthesis, ultimately leading to cell death.

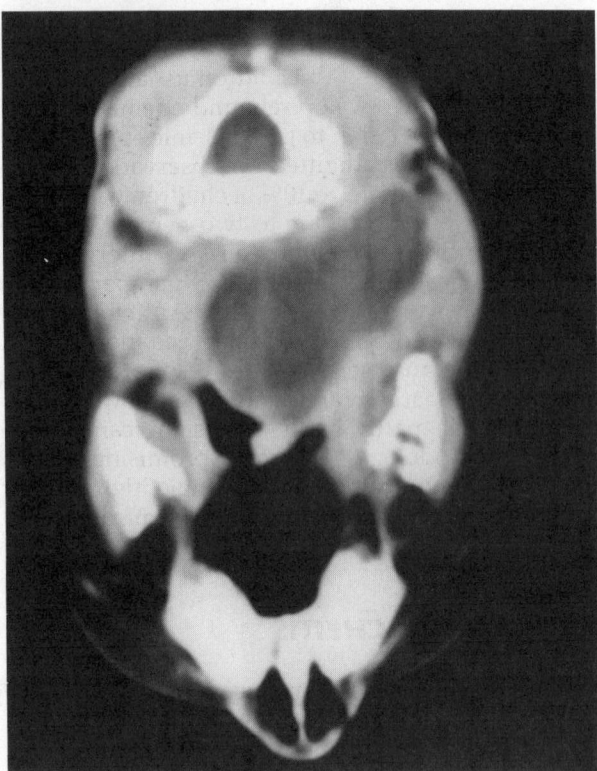

FIG. 55-33. Computerized tomograph of a retropharyngeal abscess. Courtesy of Dr. Margaret Stull, Department of Radiology, Georgetown University Hospital.

The incubation period is approximately 1 week. Patients with nasal or otic diphtheria may be relatively asymptomatic. Patients with pharyngeal diphtheria may note low-grade fever, sore throat, fatigue, or headache or may be extremely ill on presentation. The classic diphtheritic membrane is comprised of inflammatory exudate and has a foul odor. It is gray-green, necrotic, and adherent and bleeds easily if disturbed. Soft tissue edema may result in a "bull neck." Toxic myocarditis is seen in 50% of cases, and 10 to 20% of patients demonstrate neural toxicity such as cranial nerve palsies, neuropathy, or paralysis.[57-59] Airway obstruction is caused by a combination of toxin-mediated palatal and laryngeal paralysis, and mechanical occlusion by the false membrane.

The diagnosis of diphtheria is confirmed bacteriologically. Swabs from affected areas are planted on Loeffler slants and blood and tellurite agar. Toxigenicity is tested by the Elek test.[60]

Treatment is directed at several issues: control of infection, prevention of further toxin elaboration, neutralization of produced toxin, support of vital functions, and prevention of transmission. Critically ill patients need intensive monitoring. Intubation and secretion control may be required for airway maintenance. Management of myocarditis may require antiarrhythmic drugs, temporary pacing, or treatment of congestive heart failure. The only antitoxin currently available in the United States is derived from equine serum. Twenty to 40 thousand units of antitoxin are administered intravenously to patients with 2 days or less of mild pharyngeal disease. Individuals with more significant involvement may require 80,000 to 100,000 units intravenously. Hypersensitivity testing and desensitization should precede antitoxin administration.[57,59] Penicillin (600,000 U benzathine IM) and erythromycin (250 mg four times a day for 7 days) are both appropriate antibiotic choices.[57]

Contacts should be cultured. A diphtheria booster immunization should be given to contacts who have not been immunized during the preceding 5 years. Contacts without prior immunization should be treated with penicillin or erythromycin. Because of the re-emergence of this illness in the United States, immunization with combined tetanus and reduced dose diphtheria toxoids (Td) is recommended at 10-year intervals.

REFERENCES

1. LeMierre, A., Meyer, A., and LePlane, R.: Les septicèmes à bacille de Pfeiffer. Ann. Med. 39:97, 1936.
2. Davis, H.W., Gartner, J.C., Galvis, A.G., Michaels, R.H., et al.: Acute upper airway obstruction: Croup and epiglottitis. Ped. Clin. North Am. 28:859, 1981.
3. Stair, T.O., and Hirsch, B.E.: Adult Supraglottitis. Am. J. Emerg. Med. 3:512, 1985.
4. Dailey, R.H.: Acute upper airway obstruction. Emerg. Med. Clin. North Am. 1:261, 1983.
5. Lindquist, J.R., Franzen, R.E., and Ossoff, R.H.: Acute infectious supraglottitis in adults. Ann. Emerg. Med. 9:256, 1980.
6. Hirschmann, J.V., and Everett, E.D.: Hemophilus influenzae infections in adults: Report of nine cases and a review of the literature. Medicine 58:80, 1979.
7. Chaisson, R.E., Ross, J., Geberding, J.L., and Sande, M.A.: Clinical aspects of adult epiglottitis. West. J. Med. 144:700, 1986.
8. Morgenstein, A.L., and Abrahamson, A.L.: Acute epiglottitis in adults. Laryngoscope 81:1066, 1971.
9. Mayo Smith, M.F., Hirsch, P.J., Wordzinski, S.F., and Schiffman, F.J.: Acute epiglottitis in adults. N. Engl. J. Med. 314:1133, 1986.
10. Cantrell, R.W., Bell, R.A., and Morioka, W.T.: Acute epiglottitis: Intubation versus tracheostomy. Laryngoscope 58:994, 1978.
11. Mace, S.E.: Acute epiglottitis in adults. Am. J. Emerg. Med. 3:543, 1985.
12. Gerber, A.C., and Pfenniger, J.: Acute epiglottitis: Management by short duration of intubation and hospitalization. Int. Care Med. 12:407, 1986.
13. Deeb, Z.E., Yenson, A.C., and DeFries, H.O.: Acute epiglottitis in the adult. Laryngoscope 95:289, 1985.
14. Heeneman, H., and Ward, K.M.: Epiglottic abscess: Its occurrence and management. J. Otolaryngol. 6:31, 1977.
15. Brett, W., Shann, F., Walker, C., et al.: Acute epiglottitis: A different approach to management." Crit. Care Med. 16:43, 1988.
16. Lee, S.C., Meislin, H., and Iserson, K.V.: Epiglottitis presenting as pulmonary edema. Ann. Emerg. Med. 14:60, 1985.
17. Gershan, W.M., Gillman, K., Baxter, M., et al.: Acute Airway Obstruction in a 7 month old infant with epiglottitis. Pediatr. Emerg. Care 4:197, 1988.
18. Cox, G.J., Bates, G.J., Drake-Lee, A.B., and Watson, D.J.: The use of flexible nasoendoscopy in adults with acute epiglottitis. Ann. Roy. Coll. Surg. Eng. 70:361, 1988.
19. Jones, J.L.: False positives in lateral neck radiographs used to diagnose epiglottitis. Ann. Emerg. Med. 12:797, 1983.
20. Schumaker, H.M., Doris, P.E., and Birnbaum, G.: Radiographic parameters in adult epiglottitis. Ann. Emerg. Med. 13:588, 1984.
21. Kirchner, S.G.: Nontraumatic emergencies. In Radiology in Emergency Medicine. Edited by Dalinka, M.K., and Kaye, J.J. New York, Churchill Livingstone, 1984, p. 183.
22. Berthiaume, J., and Pieu, F.: Acute Klebsiella epiglottitis: considerations for initial antibiotic coverage. Laryngoscope 92:799, 1982.
23. Guss, D.A., and Jackson, J.E.: Recurring epiglottitis in an adult. Ann. Emerg. Med. 16:441, 1987.
24. Cohen, E.L.: Epiglottitis in Adults. Ann. Emerg. Med. 13:588, 1984.
25. Westerman, E.L., and Hutton, J.P.: Acute uvulitis associated with epiglottitis. Arch. Otolaryngol. Head Neck Surg. 112:784, 1986.
26. Haberman, R., Becker, M., and Ford, C.: Candida epiglottitis. Arch. Otolaryngol. Head Neck Surg. 109:770, 1983.
27. Cole, S., Zawin, M., Lundberg, B., et al.: Candida epiglottitis in an adult with acute nonlymphocytic leukemia. Am. J. Med. 82:662, 1987.
28. Walsh, T.J., and Gray, W.C.: Candida epiglottitis in immunocompromised patients. Chest 91:482, 1987.
29. Grattan-Smith, T., Forer, M., Kilham, H., et al.: Viral supraglottitis. J. Ped. 110:434, 1987.
30. Schwartz, R., Knerr, R., and Hermansen, K.: Acute epiglottitis caused by B hemolytic Group G streptococci. Am. J. Dis. Child. 136:558, 1982.
31. Biem, J., Roy, L., Halik, J., and Hoffstein, V.: Infectious mononucleosis complicated by necrotizing epiglottitis, dysphagia and pneumonia. Chest 96:204, 1989.
32. Goldhagen, J.L.: Supraglottitis in Three Young Infants. Pediatr. Emerg. Care 5:175, 1989.
33. LaScolea, L., Roseales, S., Welliver, R., et al.: Mechanisms underlying the development of meningitis or epiglottitis in children after hemophilus influenzae type B bacteremia. J. Infect. Dis. 151:1162, 1985.
34. Singer, J.I., and McCabe, J.B. Epiglottitis at the extremes of age. Am. J. Emerg. Med. 6:228, 1988.
35. Mauro, R.D., Poole, S.R., and Lockhart, C.H.: Differentiation of epiglottitis from laryngotracheitis in the child with stridor. Am. J. Dis. Child. 142:679, 1988.
36. Schuh, S., Huang, A., and Fallis, J.C.: Atypical epiglottitis. Ann. Emerg. Med. 17:168, 1988.
37. Travis, K.W., Toddes, D., and Shannon, D.C.: Pulmonary edema associated with croup and epiglottitis. Pediatrics 59:695, 1977.
38. Galvis, A.G., Stool, S.E., and Bluestone, C.D.: Pulmonary edema following relief of acute upper airway obstruction. Ann. Otol. Rhinol. Laryngol. 89:124, 1980.
39. Rothstein, S.G., Persky, M.S., Edelman, B.A., et al.: Epiglottitis in AIDS patients. Laryngoscope 99:389, 1989.
40. Schabel, S.I., Katzberg, R.W., and Burgener, F.A.: Acute inflammation of the epiglottitis and supraglottic structures in adults. Diag. Radiol. 122:601, 1977.
40a. Rothrock, S.G., Pignatello, G.A., and Howard, R.M.: Radiologic criteria for epiglottitis. Ann. Emerg. Med. 19:978, 1990.
41. Black, M.J., Harbour, J., Remsen, K.A., and Baxter, J.D.: Acute epiglottitis in adults. J. Otolaryngol. 10:237, 1981.
42. Bishop, M.J.: Epiglottitis in adults. Anesthesiol. 55:701, 1981.
43. Diaz, J.H.: Controversies in the diagnosis and management of common upper airway infections. E. R. Reports 4:25, 1983.
44. Strome, M., and Jaffe, B.: Epiglottitis: Individualized management with steroids. Laryngoscope 84:921, 1974.
45. Mendelsohn, J.: Pediatric respiratory emergencies. Topics Emerg. Med. 2:25, 1980.
46. Gardner, H.G., Powell, K.R., Rodes, V., et al.: The evaluation of racemic epinephrine in the treatment of infectious croup. Pediatrics 52:52, 1973.

47. Westley, C.R., Cotton, E.K., and Brooks, J.G.: Nebulized racemic epinephrine by IPPB for the treatment of croup. Am. J. Dis. Child. *132*:484, 1978.
48. Tunnesen, W.W., and Feinstein, A.R.: The steroid croup controversy: An analytic review of methodologic problems. J. Ped *96*:751, 1980.
49. Jones, R., Santos, J.I., and Overall, J.C.: Bacterial tracheitis. JAMA *242*:721, 1979.
50. Nelson, W.E.: Bacterial croup: A historical perspective. J. Pediatric. *105*:52, 1984.
51. Bass, J.L., Axel, S.M., Mehta, K.A., and Bennett, L.I.: Bacterial tracheitis caused by Branhamella catarrhalis. Pediatr. Emerg. Care *5*:171, 1989.
52. Sofer, S., Duncan, P., and Chernick, V.: Bacterial tracheitis: An old disease rediscovered. Clin. Pediatr. *22*:407, 1983.
53. Campbell, T.P., Paris, P.M., and Stewart, R.D.: Tracheitis: The "other" cause of upper airway obstruction. Ann. Emerg. Med. *17*:66, 1988.
54. McNamera, R.M., Altreuter, R.W., and Malone, D.R.: Bacterial tracheitis: A resurfacing airway emergency. Am. J. Emerg. Med. *5*:224, 1987.
55. Goldhagen, J.L.: Cricoarytenoiditis as a cause of acute airway obstruction in children. Ann. Emerg. Med. *17*:532, 1988.
56. Schuit, K., and Johnson, J.: Infections of the head and neck. Pediatr. Clin. North Am. *28*:965, 1981.
57. Chen, R.T., Broome, C.V., Weinstein, R.A., et al.: Diphtheria in the United States 1971-1981. Am. J. Public Health *75*:1393, 1985.
58. Barksdale, L.: Diphtheria bacilli and other corynebacteria. *In* Microbiology. Edited by Braude, A.I. Philadelphia, W.B. Saunders, 1982, p. 295.
59. McClosky, R.V., Ellner, J.J., Green, M., et al.: The 1970 Epidemic of Diphtheria in San Antonio. Ann. Intern. Med. *75*:495, 1971.
60. Sack, R.B., and Barker, L.R.: Immunization to prevent infectious disease. *In* Principles of Ambulatory Medicine. Edited by Barker, L.R., Burton, J.R., and Zieve, P.D. Baltimore, Williams and Wilkins. 1986, p. 397.

ACUTE PHARYNGITIS

Jean T. Martin

CAPSULE

Although acute pharyngitis is one of the most commonly diagnosed problems in the ambulatory population, its management remains controversial. Evidence now suggests that multiple organisms may be responsible for causing pharyngitis, but group A beta-hemolytic streptococcus (GABHS) remains the pathogen of greatest concern for the clinician. The goals of treating GABHS pharyngitis are to shorten the clinical course, decrease the transmission rate, prevent suppurative complications, and decrease the incidence of rheumatic fever.[1] The throat culture has been the "gold standard" in the diagnosis of GABHS infection, but now several rapid tests are available that may affect management decisions. The issues of when and how to treat pharyngitis, how to distinguish potentially life-threatening or treatable causes in the differential diagnosis, which diagnostic tests to use, and patient compliance and follow-up are of particular concern to the emergency or primary care physician dealing with a transient patient population. Airway obstruction from deep neck infections is a rare but potentially lethal complication.

INTRODUCTION

Sore throat is the third most common complaint among patients seeking medical care, accounting for 3% of all office visits.[2] The treatment of GABHS infection has been the primary focus in pharyngitis because of the risks of rheumatic fever and suppurative complications. Recent outbreaks of acute rheumatic fever have led to renewed interest in this area.[3,4] In current practice, patients with a positive throat culture for GABHS are treated with antibiotics, and those with a negative culture receive symptomatic therapy only. There are several problems with this approach.

Recent studies have implicated a variety of organisms, such as Chlamydia trachomatis, Mycoplasma pneumonia, and Corynebacterium haemolyticum, as causative agents in pharyngitis in addition to viruses and GABHS. These potentially treatable infections cannot be diagnosed if a throat culture for GABHS alone is used, and penicillin may be ineffective in treating copathogenic organisms.[5] The technique used in obtaining a throat culture may result in false negative cultures.[6] A positive throat culture can represent a carrier state of GABHS as well as an acute infection. Depending on the practice population, it may be difficult to achieve adequate follow-up for all patients with positive throat cultures, particularly if the results take several days to return. Even if GABHS is correctly diagnosed by culture, treatment with penicillin is often inadequate. Noncompliance with the prescribed ten day course of oral antibiotics is well-documented.[3,7] Recent studies show a 20 to 30% treatment failure rate even when penicillin is dosed appropriately.[5] Recognition of these problems as well as new information regarding causative pathogens and rapid diagnostic tests have resulted in alternative approaches to the management of acute pharyngitis.

PATHOPHYSIOLOGY

In most cases of acute pharyngitis, the cause is unknown. It is felt that most of these are caused by viral infections, which are difficult to detect using standard laboratory techniques.[8] Viruses are generally felt to be transmitted by inhalation of contaminated secretions and aerosol spread of infection is enhanced by crowding in closed areas. Young children are common carriers of these infections because of their limited previous exposure.[9]

Of the bacterial causes of pharyngitis, GABHS is the most well-studied. Group A streptococci are transmitted primarily by means of droplets from respiratory secretions. Many strains have a predilection for the upper respiratory tract. Nasopharyngeal carriage is increased during the winter months.[9] Group C streptococci can be isolated in healthy individuals as well as those with pharyngitis. Except for one reported epidemic in which Group C pharyngitis was followed by glomerulonephritis, poststreptococcal sequelae do not occur. Group D streptococci are common among the normal flora of the upper respiratory tract. Pharyngitis is apparently caused by invasion of these normal flora rather than person-to-person transmission.[9] Groups C and G can produce epidemic infections. Some data have shown a greater recovery rate of the non-group A streptococci from children, with GABHS being more commonly isolated from adults with clinical pharyngitis.[10]

Mycoplasma pneumoniae infection is usually endemic, with an increased incidence during the winter months. Epidemics are unusual except in physically confined populations. The organism is transmitted in aerosolized droplets produced during coughing or sneezing.[9] Corynebacterium diphtheriae is also transmitted by aerosolized droplets. Because of childhood immunization it is seen most frequently in adults of lower socioeconomic status. Pharyngeal infections may also be contracted from organisms shed from other sites, such as skin ulcers.[2]

Several sexually transmitted diseases are associated with pharyngeal infection. Neisseria gonorrhoeae is generally felt to produce asymptomatic colonization of the pharynx, but local suppurative complications as well as dissemination from the pharynx can occur. Gonococci can be cultured from the saliva of infected individuals, and it is likely that transmission occurs through oral-oral, oral-anal, and oral-genital contact.[11] Chlamydia trachomatis is capable of oro-genital transmission, but the importance of this mechanism as a cause of adult pharyngitis is unknown.[8] Treponema pallidum, the causative agent of syphilis, may produce pharyngeal symptoms in both the primary and secondary stages. The primary mode of transmission is by sexual or direct oral contact.[9]

The Candida yeast species are part of the normal flora, but can cause candidiasis of the mucous membranes in the immunocompromised patient.[9]

CLINICAL PRESENTATION

The overlap in signs and symptoms associated with the various viral and bacterial pharyngitides generally prevents their differentiation on a clinical basis alone. Certain clinical features along with appropriate diagnostic studies, however, are useful in diagnosing some causes of pharyngitis. These are outlined in Table 55-24.

Infectious mononucleosis, caused by the Epstein-Barr virus, is most commonly diagnosed in older children and young adults, particularly those in higher socioeconomic groups. Young children in lower socioeconomic groups may be exposed to the virus earlier and have a more clinically inapparent infection. Prominent generalized lymphadenopathy and splenic enlargement, when present, help to distinguish infectious mononucleosis from other causes of pharyngitis. Hepatitis, thrombocytopenia, pneumonitis, and central nervous system involvement can occur.[9]

Group A beta-hemolytic streptococcus pharyngitis occurs most commonly in children between the ages of 5 and 10 and decreases in frequency with age. In the United States, the seasonal peak occurs in winter and early spring.[12] The patient presents primarily with fever, a sore throat, and lymphadenopathy but headache, malaise, vomiting, and abdominal pain can also occur.[13] Cough is uncommon. Children under 3 often have a more non-specific presentation with coryza and anorexia.[8] The presence of a scarlatinal rash, caused by an erythrogenic toxin elaborated by certain strains of streptococci, is virtually diagnostic of a GABHS infection. This appears as a fine, erythematous, "sandpaper" textured rash that blanches on pressure. It

TABLE 55-24. CLINICAL FEATURES AND MANAGEMENT OF PHARYNGITIS*

Syndrome	Causative Agent(s)	Clinical Features	Diagnostic Studies	Management
Viral	Rhinovirus, coronavirus, adenovirus, respiratory syncytial virus, parainfluenza, influenza	Compared with GABHS, more gradual onset and more often associated with rhinorrhea, hoarseness, and cough	(Rarely used) Late and convalescent sera antibody titers, viral cultures, indirect immunofluorescence techniques	Symptomatic
	Coxsackie A, herpesvirus	Ulcerative lesions of the oropharynx	Tzanck smear-multinucleated giant cells	Antiviral agents for symptomatic relief
Infectious mononucleosis	Epstein-Barr virus	Young adults, associated headache, fever, fatigue, lymphadenopathy, splenic enlargement, membranous exudate, hepatitis, pneumonitis	Heterophil antibody test	Symptomatic, systemic corticosteroids in severe cases
Streptococcus	Group A beta-hemolytic streptococcus (GABHS)	Fever, tonsillar exudates, cervical lymphadenopathy, "strawberry" tongue, erythrogenic toxin causes scarlatinal rash with certain strains, nonsuppurative complications: rheumatic fever, glomerulonephritis	Throat culture, rapid diagnostic tests (see text)	Penicillin, erythromycin, penicillin with rifampin for carriers
	Groups C D G	Similar to GABHS, but nonsuppurative complications extremely rare		
Diphtheria	*Corynebacterium diphtheria*	Malaise, fever, chills, tachycardia, anterior cervical lymphadenopathy, gray, pharyngeal membrane, exotoxin effects on cardiac and central nervous systems	Culture on Loeffler's medium	Diphtheria antitoxin, penicillin or erythromycin to prevent secondary infections and treat chronic carriers
Mycoplasma	*Mycoplasma pneumoniae*	Clinically indistinguishable from other causes of pharyngitis	Culture with special medium, serologic tests-cold agglutinins	Tetracycline, erythromycin
Chlamydia	*Chlamydia trachomatis*	Clinically indistinguishable from other causes of pharyngitis	Tissue culture, serologic techniques, direct immunofluorescent staining for elementary bodies	Erythromycin, tetracycline
Gonorrhea	*Neisseria gonorrhoeae*	Usually asymptomatic colonization of the pharynx, but may have suppurative complications and dissemination from the pharynx	Culture with rayon swab on Thayer-Martin medium under low oxygen tension	Ceftriaxone, procaine penicillin plus probenecid, tetracycline
Syphilis	*Treponema pallidum*	Primary—painless, erythematous ulcer of the oropharynx Secondary—white, patchy lesions of the mucous membranes, lymphadenopathy, rash involving palms and soles	Direct visualization of motile spirochetes by dark-field microscopy or fluorescent antibody techniques, serologic tests	Penicillin, tetracycline, erythromycin
Vincent's angina	*Fusobacterium* and *Bacteroides* species	Underlying gingivitis, foul-smelling pseudomembranous ulceration of the oropharynx	Direct visualization of spirochetes with phase contrast or dark-field microscopy, anaerobic culture	Treat underlying periodontal disease, penicillin, erythromycin
Tularemia	*Francisella tularensis*	Insect or animal vector, may present as severe exudative pharyngitis	Serum agglutination test	Streptomycin
Yeast	*Candida* species	Immunocompromised patients, consider HIV infection, patchy, white "thrush" lesions	Hyphae or pseudohyphae on microscopic exam	Antifungal agents in an oral suspension
Toxoplasmosis	*Toxoplasma gondii*	Rarely presents with pharyngitis, lymphadenopathy, fever, malaise and a rash	Serologic tests	Synergistic therapy with pyrimethamine and a sulfonamide

* Adapted with permission from Mandel, J.H.: Pharyngeal infections: Causes, findings, and management. Postgrad. Med. *77*:187, 1985.

occurs initially on the neck and upper trunk, then spreads to the extremities, sparing the palms and soles. Areas of hyperpigmentation called Pastia's lines can occur in the skin folds. The face may appear flushed, but characteristically has a circumoral pallor. During the recovery phase of scarlet fever, generalized desquamation of the rash occurs.[13]

The clinical manifestations of Corynebacterium diphtheriae infection vary with the virulence of the organism and the host sensitivity. On examination, the patient may be tachycardic out of proportion to the fever. Anterior cervical lymphadenopathy is present, and swelling can produce a bullneck appearance. Classically, a grayish membrane covers the pharynx that may extend to the larynx, causing obstruction.[7,9] The most serious late complications are caused by the exotoxin produced and involve the cardiac and nervous systems. Myocardial degeneration can cause cardiac dysfunction and eventual circulatory collapse if it is not reversed. The most common late neurologic findings are paralysis of the soft palate, affecting the ability to swallow, and polyneuritis of the lower extremities.[9] Corynebacterium hemolyticum can cause fever, pharyngitis, and occasionally a pharyngeal membrane, but does not produce the systemic symptoms seen with diphtheria.

Mycoplasma pneumoniae is well recognized as a cause of pneumonia, but its importance as a pathogen in pharyngitis is unclear. The incidence of Mycoplasma pneumoniae cultured in patients with pharyngitis is approximately 5 to 15%.[5,14–16] A similar rate of recovery has been found in asymptomatic patients, however, suggesting that a carrier state can occur.[15,16] In clinical studies, the presentation of patients with pharyngitis in whom M. pneumonia was isolated was similar to that seen when viruses or other bacterial organisms were found.[14,15]

Various studies have shown conflicting results as to the significance of Chlamydia trachomatis in pharyngitis. Chlamydia species have been identified in fewer than 1 to 21% of patients presenting with sore throat. Elevated levels of antibody to C. trachomatis may actually indicate cross reactivity with other chlamydial organisms.[15–18] A recent study indicated a relatively high recovery rate (8%) of the Chlamydia species strain TWAR in patients with pharyngitis. This organism has been shown to be associated with respiratory tract infections, including pharyngitis.[14,19]

DIFFERENTIAL DIAGNOSIS

The initial evaluation of any patient with the complaint of sore throat must include a consideration of potential life-threatening conditions. The airway can be compromised as a result of infection, trauma, bleeding, neoplasm, or local inflammation. Acute supraglottitis (epiglottitis) caused by Haemophilus influenzae usually presents as sore throat, odynophagia, and drooling in a young child, and may rapidly progress to stridor and complete airway obstruction.[20] Adults have a less acute presentation, but they are also at risk for airway compromise. A Corynebacterium diphtheriae infection can also cause acute airway obstruction. This is discussed further in the "Clinical Presentation" section of this chapter.

Patients with retropharyngeal or prevertebral abscesses can prevent similarly, with odynophagia, drooling, and a muffled voice. On examination, the head is characteristically held in extension and a bulging posterior pharyngeal wall may be apparent. Any patient with a deep neck abscess is at risk of airway compromise from obstruction or rupture of the abscess into the upper airway.[21]

Ludwig's angina is an infection of the submandibular space usually arising from the mandibular dentition. Patients classically present with dysphagia, drooling, a muffled voice, and an inability to move the tongue. The submandibular abscess may grow rapidly and force the tongue upward, resulting in airway occlusion.[21]

A peritonsilar abscess is a complication of bacterial pharyngitis that can be differentiated from simple pharyngitis by examination of the pharynx. Characteristically, the involved tonsillar pillar is erythematous, indurated, and full, causing the uvula to deviate to the opposite side. An area of fluctuance may be palpable in the posterior pharynx. In advanced cases the patient presents with dysphagia, drooling, a "hot potato" voice, and trismus. If the infection is allowed to spread untreated, airway obstruction is possible.[7]

Retropharyngeal bleeding should be considered in any patient with a history of a bleeding diathesis or on anticoagulant therapy with the complaint of sore throat. Local trauma to the pharynx can cause airway obstruction from accompanying bleeding, inflammation, and edema. Certain head and neck tumors may cause sore throat and have the potential to rapidly or gradually compromise the airway. Inhalation of gaseous or chemical irritants can cause pharyngitis from local irritation, laryngeal edema, bronchospasm, or toxic effects from the substance itself. Unless the victim is a child or mentally impaired adult, the history is generally sufficient to make the diagnosis in these cases.[7]

Once the potential life-threatening conditions have been considered, attention can be given to differentiating the more common infectious causes of pharyngitis. Of these, Group A beta-hemolytic streptococcus (GABHS) remains the greatest concern. Scoring systems have been devised to identify patients with a high probability for GABHS infection who are candidates for empiric antibiotic therapy.[5,7] In one study using a pediatric scoring system, the diagnosis of GABHS was positively correlated with fever greater than 100.5°F, sore throat, headache, abnormal pharynx, cervical adenopathy, a white cell count greater than 20,400/mm³, age between 5 and 10 years, occurrence in late winter/early spring, and the absence of cough.[22] In a similar scoring system study for adults, the findings most strongly correlated with the diagnosis of GABHS were fever, recent streptococcal exposure, exudative pharyngitis, cervical adenopathy, and the absence of cough.[23] In most cases, however, the symptom complex is too indistinct to clinically differentiate GABHS from the other common types of bacterial or viral pharyngitis.[14]

Certain historical or clinical features are useful in determining the cause of infectious pharyngitis. Known exposure to contagious infections, such as GABHS or infectious mononucleosis, may suggest the diagnosis. Organisms such as herpesvirus, Chlamydia species, Neisseria gonorrhoeae, and Treponema pallidum are capable of orogenital transmission, and should be considered in patients with both pharyngitis and a genital infection.[8] An opportunistic mycosis may be seen in the immunocompromised patient. AIDS complications often include pharyngitis from various organisms. Toxic shock syndrome, originally described with tampon use in menstruating women, has been discovered as possibly arising from upper respiratory infection (URI). The syndrome described includes fever, hypotension, and erythroderma (followed by desquamation), caused by toxins elaborated by staphylococcal or streptococcal organisms with URI.[8a]

PROCEDURES AND LABORATORY STUDIES

Despite the availability of several rapid diagnostic tests for streptococcal pharyngitis, the throat culture remains the standard for diagnosis. A recent study found that recovery was greatest from specimens obtained from the tonsil. Specimens obtained from saliva or other areas of the oropharynx gave unreliable results.[6] Once obtained, the swab can be transported dry or using transport media. Plating on sheep's blood agar can be delayed for more than 24 hours without affecting recovery of GABHS.[7] If a zone of beta hemolysis surrounds the colony, it can be further grouped using a bacitracin-impregnated disk. Over 95% of Group A streptococci are bacitracin-sensitive; most other hemolytic streptococci are resistant.[24]

Because 24 to 48 hours are required to obtain throat culture results, several rapid diagnostic tests for GABHS have been developed.[25] The basis of most of these tests is a reaction, such as agglutination or a color change, between an antibody and the group-specific polysaccharide extracted from the cell wall. The specificities of most of these tests range from 90% to greater than 95%, a positive result indicating a high likelihood that a throat culture will also be positive. The sensitivities, however, range from 60% to 95%, and the chance of false negatives with these tests is higher.[24,26]

MANAGEMENT

When the clinical presentation suggests a condition with the potential for airway compromise, this must be addressed first. If acute supraglottitis is suspected, time spent in the emergency department (ED) should be minimized. A lateral radiograph of the soft tissue of the neck in the young child or indirect laryngoscopy in cooperative older children or adults can confirm the diagnosis. The airway should be secured in the operating room under direct visualization, preferably with an experienced anesthesiologist and otolaryngologist in attendance.[20]

Patients with deep neck infections, such as retropharyngeal or prevertebral abscesses, lateral pharyngeal space infections, or submandibular abscesses (Ludwig's angina) are at risk for airway obstruction or rupture of the abscess into the upper airway. Emergency airway equipment, including a set-up for tracheostomy, should be readily available at all times. A lateral soft-tissue film can confirm the diagnosis of a retropharyngeal abscess if widening or an air-fluid level is seen in the retropharyngeal space. A chest film may show evidence of mediastinal infection, and a CT scan may be needed to differentiate an abscess from cellulitis. All of these patients require hospitalization for intravenous fluid hydration and antibiotics. Admission laboratory studies including serum electrolytes, glucose, blood urea nitrogen, creatinine, and blood cultures should be obtained. Penicillin or clindamycin can be used initially pending culture results. A localized cellulitis may respond to antibiotics alone, but once an abscess develops, surgical drainage is usually necessary.[21]

An untreated peritonsilar abscess may cause a deep space infection of the neck and threaten airway patency. Spontaneous rupture of the abscess during sleep can lead to aspiration of pus. These patients require incision and drainage of the abscess followed by a course of antibiotics and analgesia as indicated. Antibiotic therapy, penicillin or a cephalosporin, should be initiated pending culture results of the abscess fluid. Unreliable patients or those unable to tolerate oral intake should be admitted for intravenous hydration and antibiotics.[27]

Membranous pharyngitis may be present with a Corynebacterium species infection, infectious mononucleosis, or Vincent's angina (Table 55-24). Because of the risk of airway compromise and the serious late sequelae in untreated diphtheria, this disease should be the primary concern in managing membranous pharyngitis. Treatment should be initiated on the basis of the clinical diagnosis, rather than waiting for laboratory confirmation. Diphtheria antitoxin is the only specific treatment and is given as a single intramuscular or intravenous dose.

If a sexually transmitted disease is suspected by either the history or clinical presentation, appropriate cultures should be taken. If the patient has a known genital infection, or has had sexual contact with a person with known infection, treatment should be initiated before obtaining culture results.[7] The clinical features and management of gonorrhea, syphilis, chlamydia, and herpesvirus infection are outlined in Table 55-24.

When considering the diagnosis of GABHS, management depends on the patient population and available resources as well as the individual patient's clinical presentation. Decisions as to whether or not to use rapid diagnostic tests for GABHS, perform throat cultures, treat with antibiotics empirically, or use oral or parenteral therapy are influenced by such factors as patient compliance, ability to achieve follow-up, laboratory and medication costs, the clinical presentation, and the patient's risk factors.

Certain patients with the clinical possibility of GABHS should be treated empirically. These include immunocompromised patients, patients with a history of rheumatic fever who are at risk for recurrence, children (except infants) with an associated scarlatinal rash, and those who have already taken antibiotics, which render any diagnostic tests invalid.[7,13,28]

The duration of symptoms associated with GABHS is shortened if antibiotic therapy is initiated within the first 24 to 48 hours of the onset of illness.[3,7,29,30] As previously discussed, several scoring methods have been devised to assist the physician in identifying clinically the patients with a high probability of having GABHS who would benefit from early antibiotic therapy. When such scoring systems are used, the probability of a positive throat culture, given a certain clinical score, varies with the prevalence of GABHS in the practice population.[29] This can change with the season of the year or make-up of the patient population, for instance, during a large influx of college students or military recruits.

To minimize the risks of untreated GABHS infection, all patients with pharyngitis should be treated either empirically or on the basis of a throat culture. To decrease the costs associated with testing, patients with a high clinical probability of GABHS infection should receive empiric antibiotic therapy and all others should be cultured.[31] This strategy does not take into account the delay for throat culture results, which may

increase the number of patients lost to follow-up and prevent some patients with GABHS infection from receiving the benefits of early treatment. These problems can be reduced with the use of rapid diagnostic tests for GABHS. Studies have shown that when these tests are used and the results are readily available to the clinician, the initial and overall treatment rates improve.[25,26,32]

Because the rapid diagnostic tests for GABHS have high specificities, patients with a positive result should receive antibiotic therapy, and a confirmatory throat culture is not indicated. Because of the lower sensitivities with these tests, a negative result is less significant and if the diagnosis is in question, a throat culture should be performed.[10]

Penicillin remains the drug of choice for the treatment of GABHS pharyngitis and the prevention of rheumatic fever.[33] In areas where rheumatic fever is prevalent and compliance or follow-up cannot be ensured, intramuscular benzathine penicillin G should be given in a dose of 600,000 units for children weighing less than 27 kg and 1,200,000 units in patients weighing more than 27 kg. A less painful alternative is a combination of 900,000 units of benzathine penicillin G and 300,000 units of procaine penicillin G given intramuscularly.[34] An oral regimen of 250 mg of penicillin V given three to four times daily for 10 days is equally effective for properly educated patients with good compliance.[33] An alternative for adults is erythromycin in a dose of 250 mg four times daily for 10 days. In children, erythromycin estolate is the preferred form in a dosage of 20 mg per kg per day in two divided doses for 10 days. Oral first-generation cephalosporins are equally effective, but significantly more expensive.[33] Post-treatment cultures are not indicated in asymptomatic patients.[28,35]

Patients who remain symptomatic with positive throat cultures after appropriate treatment for GABHS may represent tolerance of the organism to penicillin, the presence of beta-lactamase-producing bacteria in the pharynx, or carriers with a viral or other infection.[10] Evidence showing improved eradication of GABHS when beta-lactamase-resistant antibiotics are used supports the theory that beta-lactamase plays a role in treatment failures.[4,10] There is no consensus on the definition of the GABHS carrier state or the need to eradicate the organism in these patients. One definition of a carrier is the patient with a positive throat culture, no host response as measured by a rise in antistreptococcal antibody titers, and persistent positive cultures despite treatment.[29] These patients appear to be at less risk for the development of rheumatic fever, and are less likely to transmit the organism to close contacts.[33] Attempts should be made to eradicate the organism in carriers when there is a history of rheumatic fever or recurrent GABHS infections in the family, or if there is an outbreak of rheumatic fever in the community.[28,33] The concurrent use of oral penicillin for 10 days or a one-time intramuscular dose of penicillin with rifampin for 4 days (20 mg per kg per day up to 600 mg per day divided once or twice daily) has proven effective in eradicating GABHS from carriers.[28]

Except for infectious mononucleosis, the etiologic agent for viral pharyngitis is rarely sought. Lymphocytosis with increased numbers of atypical lymphocytes supports the diagnosis of infectious mononucleosis, but the inexpensive heterophil antibody spot test is more specific. Treatment of viral pharyngitis is directed toward symptomatic relief. In severe cases of infectious mononucleosis with significant splenomegaly or serious hematologic or neurologic complications, hospitalization and administration of systemic corticosteroids may be indicated.[8]

PITFALLS

In current practice, when a patient with uncomplicated pharyngitis has a negative throat culture for GABHS, he or she is assumed to have a viral infection requiring symptomatic treatment only. This is significant when the results of inadequate throat cultures are used to make management decisions. False negative results occur when a proper specimen cannot be obtained from an uncooperative patient or if the patient has recently taken an antibiotic. Error can also be introduced during the culturing process.[24]

Other treatable causes of pharyngitis may be missed if GABHS is the only organism considered. Potential life-threatening conditions, such as the membranous pharyngitis of diphtheria or infectious mononucleosis, may resemble common viral pharyngitis in the early stages.

The patient population must be considered when making management decisions. Although throat cultures are considered the "gold standard" in diagnosing GABHS, they may be useless in a setting where most patients are lost to follow-up.

HORIZONS

The significance of other potentially treatable causes of pharyngitis, such as Chlamydia trachomatis or Mycoplasma pneumoniae, has yet to be determined. In one controlled study, when erythromycin was given empirically to patients with non-streptococcal pharyngitis, there were significantly fewer new illnesses among household members. This lends support to the theory that bacteria other than GABHS may cause a large percentage of adult pharyngitis.[36]

There is some evidence to suggest that the initiation of

antibiotics within the first 24 to 48 hours of GABHS infection may increase the risk of subsequent infection, possibly because of suppressed antibody production. This must be weighed against the benefits of early treatment including earlier symptom relief and a decreased rate of infection among household contacts.[30]

Although the incidence of rheumatic fever has declined markedly since the widespread availability of antibiotics, there have been recent isolated outbreaks of the disease. Bacterial surveys performed at the time of two of these outbreaks revealed the presence of mucoidal Group A streptococcal strains of M-types 3 and 18. Such mucoid strains have been associated with rheumatic fever outbreaks in the past suggesting that certain strains have increased rheumatogenic potential. Rheumatic fever has always been more common among those living in poor, crowded conditions, but recent outbreaks have occurred primarily among middle-class children. This points out the need for continued vigilance in the management of GABHS infection to prevent this devastating disease. If the trend continues, previous mainstays of therapy, including administering intramuscular antibiotics to ensure compliance, culturing household contacts, and performing post-treatment cultures to ensure eradication of GABHS, may need to be reconsidered.[37,38]

REFERENCES

1. Wald, E.R.: Management of pharyngitis revisited. J. Fam. Pract. 26:367, 1988.
2. Cypress, B.K.: Patient's Reasons for Visiting Physicians: Vital and Health Statistics, Series 13, Data from the National Health Survey, No. 56, U.S. Department of Health and Human Services publication No. (PHS) 82-1717, p. 26, 1982.
3. Randolph, M.F., Gerber, M.A., DeMeo, K.K., and Wright, L.: Effect of antibiotic therapy on the clinical course of streptococcal pharyngitis. J. Pediatr. 106:870, 1985.
4. Smith, T.D., Huskins, W.C., Kim, K.S., and Kaplan, E.L.: Efficacy of beta-lactamase-resistant penicillin and influence of penicillin tolerance in eradicating streptococci from the pharynx after failure of penicillin therapy for group A streptococcal pharyngitis. Pediatr. Pharmacol. Ther. 110:777, 1987.
5. Sinkinson, C.A., Pichichero, M.E., and Centor, R.M.: The compromises of managing acute pharyngitis. Emerg. Med. Reports 9:162, 1988.
6. Brien, J.H., and Bass, J.W.: Streptococcal pharyngitis: Optimal site for throat culture. J. Pediatr. 106:781, 1985.
7. Hedges, J.R., and Lowe, R.A.: Approach to acute pharyngitis. Emerg. Med. Clin. North Am. 5:335, 1987.
8. Mandel, J.H.: Pharyngeal infections: Causes, findings, and management. Postgrad. Med. 77:187, 1985.
8a. Gallo, U.O., Fontanarosa, P.B.: Toxic streptococcal syndrome. Ann. Emerg. Med. 19:1332, 1990.
9. Joklik, W.K., Willett, H.P., and Amos, D.B. (eds.): Zinsser Microbiology. New York, Appleton-Century-Crofts, 1980.
10. Denny, F.W.: Current problems in managing streptococcal pharyngitis. J. Pediatr. 111:797, 1987.
11. Hutt, D.M., and Judson, F.N.: Epidemiology and treatment of oropharyngeal gonorrhea. Ann. Intern. Med. 104:655, 1986.
12. Markowitz, M.: A clinical approach to the diagnosis of group A beta-hemolytic streptococcal pharyngitis in children. Clin. Ther. 10:17, 1988.

13. Tanz, R.R., and Shulman, S.T.: Streptococcal pharyngitis: What's new. Postgrad. Med. *84*:203, 1988.
14. Huovinen, P., et al.: Pharyngitis in adults: The presence and coexistance of viruses and bacterial organisms. Ann. Intern. Med. *110*:612, 1989.
15. Reed, B.D., Huck, W., Lutz, L.J., and Zazove, P.: Prevalance of *Chlamydia trachomatis* and *Mycoplasma pneumoniae* in children with and without pharyngitis. J. Fam. Pract. *26*:387, 1988.
16. McMillan, J.A., et al.: Viral and bacterial organisms associated with acute pharyngitis in a school-aged population. J. Pediatr. *109*:747, 1986.
17. Huss, H., Jungkind, D., Amadio, P. and Rubenfeld, I.: Frequency of *Chlamydia trachomatis* as the cause of pharyngitis. J. Clin. Microbiol. *22*:858.
18. Komaroff, A.L., et al.: Serologic evidence of chlamydial and mycoplasmal pharyngitis in adults. Science *222*:927, 1986.
19. Kuo, C.C., and Grayston, J.T.: *Chlamydia* spp. strain TWAR: A newly recognized organism associated with atypical pneumonia and other respiratory tract infections. Clin. Microbiol. Newslett. *10*:137, 1988.
20. Deeb, Z.E.: Approach to supraglottitis. Emerg. Med. Clin. North Am. *5*:353, 1987.
21. Ortiz, J.A., Hudkins, C., and Kornblut, A.: Adenitis, adenopathy, and abscesses of the head and neck. Emerg. Med. Clin. North Am. *5*:359, 1987.
22. Breese, B.B.: A simple scorecard for the tentative diagnosis of streptococcal pharyngitis. Am. J. Dis. Child. *131*:514, 1977.
23. Walsh, B.T., Bookheim, W.W., Johnson, R.C., and Tompkins, R.K.: Recognition of streptococcal pharyngitis in adults. Arch. Intern. Med. *135*:1493, 1975.
24. Kaplan, E.L.: Laboratory diagnosis of group A streptococcal pharyngitis. Clin. Ther. *10*:22, 1988.
25. Redd, S.C., Facklam, R.R., Collin, S., and Cohen, M.L.: Rapid group A streptococcal antigen detection kit: effect on antimicrobial therapy for acute pharyngitis. Pediatrics *82*:576, 1988.
26. Lieu, T.A., Fleisher, G.R., and Schwartz, J.S.: Clinical evaluation of a latex agglutination test for streptococcal pharyngitis: performance and impact on treatment rates. Pediatr. Infect. Dis. J. *7*:847, 1988.
27. Abelson, T.I., and Witt, W.J.: Otolaryngologic procedures. *In* Clinical Procedures in Emergency Medicine. Edited by Roberts, J.R., and Hedges, J.R. Philadelphia, W.B. Saunders Company, 1985.
28. McCracken, G.H.: Diagnosis and management of children with streptococcal pharyngitis. Pediatr. Infect. Dis. *5*:754, 1986.
29. Centor, R.M., Meier, F.A., and Dalton, H.P.: Throat culture and rapid tests for diagnosis of group A streptococcal pharyngitis. Ann. Intern. Med. *105*:892, 1986.
30. Pichichero, M.E., et al.: Adverse and beneficial effects of immediate treatment of group A beta hemolytic streptococcal pharyngitis with penicillin. Pediatr. Infect. Dis. J. *6*:635, 1987.
31. DeNeef, P.: Selective testing for streptococcal pharyngitis in adults. J. Fam. Pract. *25*:347, 1987.
32. Lieu, T.A., Fleisher, G.R., and Schwartz, J.S.: Clinical performance and effect on treatment of latex agglutination testing for streptococcal pharyngitis in an emergency department. Pediatr. Infect. Dis. *5*:655, 1986.
33. Kaplan, E.L.: How, and how not, to treat group A streptococcal pharyngitis. Clin. Ther. *10*:28, 1988.
34. Bass, J.W.: Treatment of streptococcal pharyngitis revisited. JAMA *256*:740, 1986.
35. Dillon, H.C.: Streptococcal pharyngitis in the 1980's. Pediatr. Infect. Dis. J. *6*:123, 1987.
36. McDonald, C.J., et al.: A controlled trial of erythromycin in adults with nonstreptococcal pharyngitis. J. Infect. Dis. *5*:1093, 1985.
37. Bisno, A.L., Shulman, S.T., and Dajani, A.S.: The rise and fall (and rise?) of rheumatic fever. JAMA *259*:728, 1988.
38. Massell, B.F., Chute, C.G., Walker, A.M., and Kurland, G.S.: Penicillin and the marked decrease in the morbidity and mortality from rheumatic fever in the United States. N. Engl. J. Med. *318*:280, 1988.

ABSCESSES OF THE HEAD AND NECK

John R. Jacobs and Arthur W. Weaver

CAPSULE

The ability to distinguish between adenopathy, inflammatory mass, and abscess remains critical to the successful emergency management of the patient presenting with a tender mass of the neck. History and physical examination are assisted greatly by selected radiographic tests and fine needle aspiration. Although antibiotic therapy has benefitted these patients, prompt surgical drainage of neck abscesses is necessary to minimize development of complications.

PATHOPHYSIOLOGY AND ANATOMY

Before the development of antibiotics, most neck abscesses were caused by infections of the pharynx and tonsil; only 20% were thought to be secondary to dental infections. With the introduction of antibiotics, these numbers have changed; and now only 30% are thought to be secondary to infection of the pharynx and tonsil and 30 to 40% are of dental origin. The remaining 40% are from cervical adenitis, otitis, intravenous drug abuse, mastoiditis, sialoadenitis, infected cysts, and thyroiditis.[1]

FASCIAL PLANES OF THE HEAD AND NECK

Connective tissue envelops the visceral structures of the neck, forming fascial planes and defining potential spaces for the spread of infection in the neck and occasionally into the thorax. Immediately surrounding the vertebral column and the paraspinal muscles is the prevertebral fascia. This plane extends from the base of the skull to the diaphragm. Infection of the vertebral bodies can extend into this potential space.

Anterior to the prevertebral space and immediately beneath the pharyngeal wall is the retropharyngeal space. This space extends from the skull base to approximately the level of the tracheal bifurcation. This potential space is the location of the retropharyngeal abscess, seen primarily in children. This age preference reflects the atrophy with advancing age of the lymph node bearing tissue contained within the space. These nodes drain the nasopharynx, sinus, and posterior nasal spaces.

The pharyngeal space is adjacent to the retropharyngeal space. It forms a cone starting with the base at the skull and extending inferiorly to the point at the level approximately of the hyoid bone. Contained within this space are the carotid artery, jugular vein, the sympathetic chain, and the ninth through twelfth cranial nerves. Infection contained within this poten-

tial space tends to cause a bulge in the pharyngeal wall. This problem must be differentiated from a bulge resulting from a peritonsillar abscess.

The submandibular space is divided by the mylohyoid muscle into the sublingual superiorly and the submental inferiorly. Involvement of the sublingual space can cause a condition known as Ludwig's angina, with retrusion of the tongue and potential airway compromise. Involvement of the submental space usually presents as a mass in the neck.

MICROBIOLOGY

The microbiology of deep-space neck infections reflects the indigenous flora of the oral cavity. This flora is effected by age, diet, nutritional status, dentition, periodontal disease, and prior antibiotic exposure. It is important to remember the importance of anaerobic flora in these infections when deciding on the choice of antibiotic.

CLINICAL PRESENTATION AND PHYSICAL EXAMINATION

Patients with deep-space neck infections present with local and systemic signs of infection, usually with pain and tenderness associated with fever and leukocytosis. One must remain cognizant of the possibility of airway compromise in this patient population. This is especially true for patients with Ludwig's angina. The patient with Ludwig's angina has a swollen, tender neck, especially in the submandibular submental area. Later in the course of the disease, the tongue becomes elevated, with a resulting threat to the airway.

Retropharyngeal abscess is usually identified in younger patients and presents with a swollen posterior pharyngeal wall associated with drooling. Parapharyngeal space abscess also results in a mass effect in the region of the posterior pharynx. The majority of the swelling, however, is lateral, and the patient experiences trismus, making the examination difficult. Differentiation of a parapharyngeal space abscess from a peritonsillar abscess may be difficult. The diagnostic key is usually associated torticollis from the pharyngeal abscess. Other more indolent processes may present at the Emergency Department (ED) as masses of the neck. Within the list of possibilities must be included metastatic tumor, congenital cyst, benign tumors, and granulomatous infections. Often the location of the mass helps to limit the diagnostic possibilities and direct the evaluation process. Figure

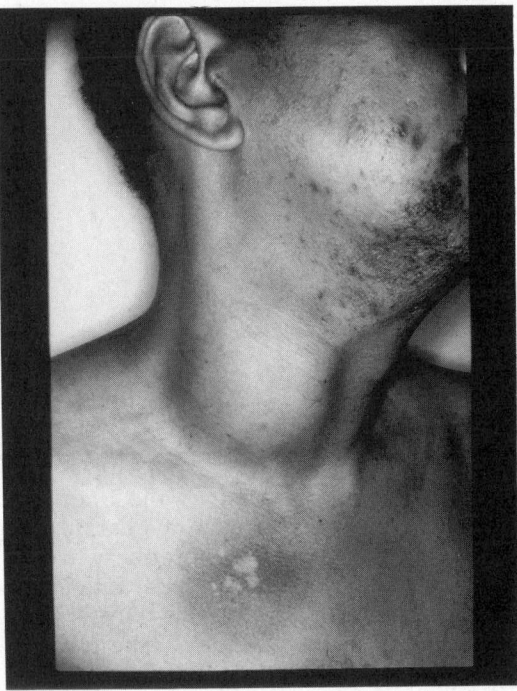

FIG. 55-34. Patient with a large left cervical mass. Differential diagnosis includes infection, thyroid, tumor, or congenital cyst.

55-34 displays by location a common neck mass. These masses are usually nontender, nonfluctuant, and not associated with signs of system illness such as fever and leukocytosis.

LABORATORY PROCEDURES

The use of fine-needle aspiration often yields important information on which to base treatment plans. It can potentially differentiate between abscess and cellulitis. The aspirate can be useful for Gram stain and cytology. It is important to culture for both anaerobic and aerobic organisms when dealing with infections of the head and neck.

RADIOGRAPHIC PROCEDURES AND ANTIBIOTIC SELECTION

A lateral neck film can often confirm the diagnosis of retropharyngeal abscess. Similarly, a panorex film or a mandible series can potentially render the diagnosis of a periapical root abscess on its way to becoming a Ludwig's angina. Computed tomography (CT) and ultrasound can help to differentiate abscess from cellulitis. One should not rely solely on a single test in determining the treatment plan and antibiotic selection. Antibiotic selection varies according to Gram stain, culture results, and identification of newer and hopefully more effective agents. Until culture results are received or Gram stain clearly defines the probable organism, for deep space neck infections in adults, cefoxitin (1 g q8h to 2 g q4h) plus Gentamicin (3 to 5 mg/kg/day) is recommended, with alternatives of clindamycin (300 to 900 mg q8h) plus gentamicin or cefoperazone (1 to 2 g q4 to 6h) or ceftazidime (1 to 2 g q8 to 12h).[2] Surgical drainage is still mandatory.

AIRWAY MAINTENANCE

The potential for airway compromise exists and has a distressing capability of changing rapidly with spread of the infection in the neck. Intubation may rapidly become impossible when tissue distortion or trismus prevents satisfactory visualization of the glottis. If concern arises as to the safety of the airway, one should proceed on the side of caution and secure it under controlled circumstances. Emergency tracheostomy through the grossly distorted neck tissues is fraught with hazard and associated with significant risk even when performed by skilled surgeons.

Once the diagnosis of abscess is established, incision and drainage should be performed expeditiously to minimize spread and assist in resolution of the infectious process. Antibiotics are not a substitute for adequate drainage. The details of the operative approaches are beyond the scope of this chapter but the usual approach involves opening the potential infected spaces and placement of drains. At the time of surgery, an assessment should be made as to the possibility of vascular compromise and steps initiated to avoid vascular obstruction. If the patient fails to improve after drainage, a search must be made for the presence of a nonrecognized abscess or additional abscess formation. Consideration should also be given to reculturing and possibly changing the antibiotic coverage.

MEDICOLEGAL PEARLS AND DIAGNOSTIC TIPS

1. If the history even suggests the possibility of a foreign body, a well documented search for it must be made. Beware of swallowed items such as fishbones.
2. Ultimate antibiotic selection must reflect culture results.
3. Be aware of the possibility of a fungal cause in the susceptible patient (diabetic or immunosuppressed).
4. Consider the possibility of a pseudoaneurysm communicating with the abscess cavity in the intravenous drug abuser. If the mass pulsates, an arteriogram is necessary.
5. Dental abscesses from mandibular teeth present in the mouth if the abscessed root tips above the mylohyoid insertion, and in the neck if the bone abscess is below the mylohyoid insertion.
6. Alcoholics frequently have enlarged salivary glands.
7. A submaxillary salivary gland that fluctuates in size may have a stone in the duct. This may be confirmed by bimanual palpation of the floor of the mouth. Submental-vertex films made with a film plate in the mouth may show the stone.
8. Thyroglossal duct cysts and branchial cleft cysts may become infected and present as an abscess.
9. Metastatic cancer in neck nodes may be cystic and tender. Biopsy should be done at the time of drainage if there is any question.
10. Submental and submaxillary enlarged nodes in black men are frequently caused by infected hair root follicles of the face.

REFERENCES

1. Fairbanks, D.: Anti-microbial therapy in otolaryngology. *In* Head and Neck Surgery. American Academy of Otolaryngology, Head and Neck Surgery Foundation Inc., Washington, D.C., 1987, p. 57.
2. Adkins, W.: Deep neck infection. *In* Current Therapy in Otolaryngology Head and Neck Surgery. Edited by Gates, G., Decker, B.C., Toronto 1987, pp. 216–217.

DYSPHONIA

Andrew Blitzer

CAPSULE

Dysphonia is an impairment of the voice, more precisely of phonation. It must be distinguished from dysarthria, in which a dysfunction with articulation interferes with the formation of sound into fluent speech. Patients may have a breathy, soft, or whispering voice quality because of a mechanical disability or weakness of the muscles of the larynx. Some disorders present with a low or harsh voice; others may be squeaky with loss of pitch variation. Still other disorders might produce a strained voice quality, with breaks in speech, or a tremulous quality. Some of these abnormalities of sound production may be accompanied by noisy breathing or stridor.

EVALUATION

HISTORY

The history of the dysphonia is important in making a diagnosis for the abnormality.[1] It is important to know about the onset; other associated symptoms; association with pain, swallowing disability, dyspnea, or hemoptysis; previous trauma, surgery, or anesthesia; occupation and avocation with possible voice abuse; and other illnesses or medications.

PHYSICAL EXAMINATION

A complete head and neck examination should be performed to evaluate the patient for cranial nerve deficits, stridor, neck masses, tremor, facial spasms, or scars. It is highly important to listen to the voice and observe for dyspnea or stridor, which often indicate the location of the lesion. In the supraglottis, there may be inspiratory without expiratory stridor, a muffled voice, and a normal sound generator. At the level of the glottis, sound may be abnormal inspiratory and expiratory stridor may be present. At the level of the subglottis, the sound generator may be normal with inspiratory and expiratory stridor.[2]

LARYNGOSCOPIC EXAMINATION

A thorough laryngoscopic examination is obviously crucial to evaluate for degree of airway obstruction; vocal cord integrity and shape; vocal cord motion or paralysis; vocal cord nodules, laryngeal tumors or cysts; red, white, or ulcerative areas in the larynx; and areas of infection.[3–5] A voice analysis by a speech pathologist should be performed on many of these patients. This should include evaluation of the production of a sustained vowel, loudness analysis, pitch analysis, endurance, reading of standard passages, and analysis of spontaneous speech. An evaluation of the articulatory mechanism is also important. The therapist also notes how the patient uses breath control during speaking. This is important for therapy in patients who abuse their voices.[6]

Patients with vocal cord paralysis should also have an examination of the thyroid to look for an occult carcinoma, which may have destroyed the recurrent laryngeal nerve. Chest x rays evaluate the possibility of thoracic tumor. Skull base x rays should also be taken to look for a lesion affecting the vagus nerve at its exit from the cranium.[7]

X-RAY STUDIES

Radiologic imaging of the larynx allows morphologic and functional assessment of the airway as well as a method of viewing structures that are not easily seen on endoscopy (e.g., the laryngeal ventricle or subglottis). The laryngeal framework and surrounding soft tissues can also be evaluated. Patients with potential airway compromise should not be sent for radiographs: they may obstruct during the procedure. Radiographs should not supersede the need for a thorough direct inspection of the glottis and airway.[8,9]

Patients with a motion disorder of the larynx (spasms, tremor, jerks, etc) should have a full neurologic examination for other subtle motion disorders. A videostroboscopy allows slowing of the laryngeal motion for greater understanding of the basis of the abnormal motion. Laryngeal electromyography can evaluate the regularity and rate of a tremor, document the rate of myoclonic jerks, and evaluate for signs of myopathy or denervation.[10,11]

DIFFERENTIAL DIAGNOSIS

Dysphonia or abnormal voice production is a symptom of a disorder of the sound generator. Insufficient air delivered to the sound generator (vocal apparatus) can cause dysphonia. Other causes are related to abnormalities of the vocal apparatus. Paralysis, paresis, or mechanical limitation of motion of the vocal cords causes weakness of the resonator. In patients with paralysis, as the subglottic pressure is increased, the weakened vocal cord is pushed laterally, leaving an open chink and a breathy quality of the voice. The pitch variance is also hampered. With the limitation of abduction, the patient may also experience dyspnea on vigorous exertion. In patients with a mechanically fixed vocal cord, the voice may be relatively normal if the cord is fixed in the midline, but may have dyspnea on exertion. If the vocal cord is fixed in a more lateral position, the patient has a breathy, weak voice with little or no dyspnea. In bilateral vocal cord paralysis, the patient may have a good voice but an imperiled airway with some stridor, or if the cords are in the paramedian position, the voice may be weak or just a whisper, with dyspnea on exertion. A similar picture is seen with bilateral vocal cord fixation.

The resonator is also impaired if the vibratory surface is irregular from webs, nodules, cysts, tumors, or trauma. Atrophy of the vocal cords produces poor vibration and sound generation and a resultant breathy voice. There is usually no associated dyspnea.

The vocal cords can be swollen, causing poor vibration and sound generation. In the acute situation, edema of the vocal cords causes a muffled sound, as in voice abuse or viral laryngitis. In subacute or chronic swelling, infection or endocrine or autoimmune conditions may be responsible.

The sound generator may also produce abnormal sound when affected by a tremor disorder. There may be an audible tremor or some harshness in speech pattern, depending on the frequency of the tremor. Essential tremor, myoclonus, Parkinson's disease, and dystonia are some of the more common examples. Occasionally, the dysphonia is related to spasms of the vocal cords, as seen in laryngospasm. Voice production and respiration are severely impaired during spasms. Dystonia may also cause brief spasms during phonation, producing a choppy sound termed by some "laryngeal stuttering" or "spastic dysphonia."

The resonator of the voice is the chamber above the sound generator (vocal cords). This chamber includes the pharynx, nasal cavity, and oral cavity. Cysts and tumors of the epiglottis or supraglottic structures or pharynx, or infectious swelling as in epiglottitis, may produce a muffled or a "hot potato" voice. The airway is likely to be compromised in these situations.

MANAGEMENT

The most important decision to be made emergently is whether there is an indication of already present or impending airway compromise. Patients who have vocal cord paralysis and stridor should be admitted and observed and possibly intubated and/or tracheotomized. Other patients with an increasingly obstructive disorder may have minimal symptoms when first examined, but later deteriorate rapidly. This group includes patients with infectious processes such as epiglottitis; cysts or tumors of the larynx or pharynx; cysts, tumors, or hemorrhage of the thyroid; foreign bodies; trauma of the airway with hemorrhage; or neuromuscular diseases such as myasthenia gravis. Any evidence of airway compromise or stridor should be taken seriously, and an immediate examination of the larynx and airway must be performed. Once the status of the airway is established, a therapeutic plan can be established.[12]

If the patient with dysphonia is found to have no dyspnea, stridor, aspiration, or dysphagia, a laryngeal examination is planned. If a cyst, tumor, or ulcerative lesion is found, the patient should have a laryngoscopy and biopsy. This is often a diagnostic and curative. If the patient is found to have nodules from voice abuse, voice therapy should be used to stop the abuse. If the lesion does not disappear while the patient is receiving voice therapy, a laryngoscopy and vocal cord stripping should be used to remove the nodules or polyps. The patient should then be put back into voice therapy to prevent recurrence.[13]

If the patient is found to have unilateral vocal cord paralysis but no dyspnea, stridor, aspiration, or dysphagia, usually observation is sufficient. Evaluation for a chest, thyroid or skull base lesion should be instituted. If no lesion is found, time usually allows the paralyzed vocal cord to medialize slowly, along with compensation by the contralateral vocal cord. The vocal cord function may recover with time: 6 months to a year on the right side and 9 months to 1 ½ years on the left. A laryngeal electromyogram is useful after 2 to 3 months to assess potential regeneration.[11] This test can be repeated every 3 months to evaluate progression of electrical improvement and for direct visualization of the vocal cords. Speech therapy concentrating on breath control is helpful to many patients. If the voice remains weak and/or the patient has some aspiration, a direct laryngoscopy with gelfoam injection can be performed to medialize the vocal cord, giving better glottic closure on phonation and swallowing. The gelfoam is usually resorbed by 3 to 4 months, when the normal function may return. In patients with chronic loss, either Teflon injection or a laryngoplasty with cartilage or alloplastic implant can be used to medialize the vocal cord for better glottic closure on phonation and swallowing.[14–24]

If no stridor or airway distress is present but the voice is nonexistent or weak, one should consider the possibility of an open glottis. It is important to ask questions related to cough or aspiration, particularly when the patient is drinking. Patients with a history of laryngeal trauma, rheumatoid arthritis with cricoarytenoid fixation, or neuromuscular diseases may have an open glottic chink with no airway distress, but no voice and poor laryngeal closure on swallowing, allowing the possibility of aspiration. If the symptoms are severe, the patient should be admitted and observed. If the chest radiograph shows evidence of pneumonitis, the patient should have oral intake restricted and be fed intravenously or by nasogastric tube. If the situation is chronic, a gastrostomy may be needed. If the patient still has problems, even with oral secretions, parasympatholytic drugs, tracheostomy, or laryngeal closure procedures may be necessary to prevent chronic pneumonia and pulmonary insufficiency.[25–33]

In patients who have poor voice because of an ulcerative lesion with erythema, viral causes are common. These are usually self-limiting diseases with quick recoveries. The treatment is usually symptomatic. If the lesions persist, or more generalized signs of ulcerative diseases are seen, the spectrum of collagen-vascular diseases or tuberculosis should be made. Biopsy with prompt treatment can prevent progression of disease and more disastrous complications.[12]

PITFALLS AND MEDICOLEGAL PEARLS

The most important way of preventing trouble is to follow the standard rules. If the patient has airway compromise, it must be dealt with quickly, and then more thorough investigation can be made. If there is no acute distress, a thorough history

should be taken, with particular attention to airway, swallowing, aspiration or cough, recurrent pneumonia, neurologic deficits, medications, trauma, fever, etc. A thorough examination should be performed. No treatment should be given for dysphonia without a direct inspection of the larynx and pharynx. Often practitioners decide that the patient has an infection and put him or her on a course of antibiotics, only to find out several weeks later that the patient has a large tumor. The evaluation should proceed according to the examination. If there is any question about a possible impending airway compromise or aspiration, the patient should be admitted to the hospital for careful monitoring or treated acutely in the Emergency Department (ED). The treatment options are based on the severity of the symptoms and the diagnosis.

REFERENCES

1. Spofford, B.: History and physical examination. In Otolaryngology—Head and Neck Surgery. Edited by Cummings, C., et al. St. Louis, C.V. Mosby Co., 1986, pp. 1789–98.
2. Sasaki, C.T., and Isaacson, G.: Functional anatomy of the larynx. Otolaryngol. Clin. North Am. 21:595, 1988.
3. Fujimura, O.: Fiberoptic observation and measurement of vocal fold movement. In. Proceedings of the conference on the Assessment of Vocal Pathology—ASHA Reports II, Rockville MD, 1981.
4. Kelly, J.H.: Methods of diagnosis and documentation. Otolaryngol. Clin. North Am. 17:29, 1984.
5. Silberman, L.E.: Advances in the optical examination of the upper airway. Otolaryngol. Clin. North Am. 11:355, 1978.
6. Painter, C.: Neurophysiologic testing. In Otolaryngology—Head and Neck Surgery. Edited by Cummings, C., et al. St. Louis, C.V. Mosby Co., 1986, pp. 1799–1845.
7. Tucker, H.M.: Laryngoscopy, endoscopic surgery, and special techniques. In The Larynx. Edited by Tucker, H.M. New York, Thieme Medical Publishing Co., 1987, pp. 163–179.
8. Glazer, H.S., and Siegel, M.J.: Radiology of the larynx. In Otolaryngology—Head and Neck Surgery. Edited by Cummings, C., et al. St. Louis, C.V. Mosby Co., 1986, pp. 1847–1865.
9. Noyek, A.M., and Shulman, H.S.: Diagnostic imaging. In The Larynx. Edited by Tucker, H.M. New York, Thieme Medical Publishing Co., 1987, pp. 79–134.
10. Brin, M.F., and Younger, D.: Neurologic Disorders and Aspiration. Otolaryngol. Clin. North Am. 21:691, 1988.
11. Blitzer, A., Lovelace, R.E., Brin, M.F., et al.: Electromyographic findings in focal laryngeal dystonia (spastic dysphonia). Ann. Otol. Rhinol. Laryngol. 94:591, 1985.
12. Biller, H.F., and Lawson, W.: Management of Acute Laryngeal Trauma. In Surgery of the Larynx. Edited by Bailey, B.J., and Biller, H.F. Philadelphia, W.B. Saunders Co., 1985, pp. 149–154.
13. McNeill, R.: Non-surgical conditions of the Larynx. In Surgery of the Larynx. Edited by Bailey, B.J., and Biller, H.F. Philadelphia, W.B. Saunders Co., 1985, pp. 207–228.
14. Arnold, G.E.: Vocal Rehabilitation of Paralytic Dysphonia. Arch. Otolaryng. 76:358, 1962.
15. Lewy, R.B.: Glottic rehabilitation with Teflon injection—The return of voice, cough, and laughter. Acta Otolaryngol. 58:214, 1964.
16. Rontal, E., Rontal, M., Morse, G., and Brown, E.M.: Vocal cord injection in the treatment of acute and chronic aspiration. Laryngoscope 86:625, 1976.
17. Schramm, V.L., May, M., and Lavorato, A.S.: Gelfoam paste injection for vocal cord paralysis: temporary rehabilitation of glottic competence. Laryngoscope 88:1268, 1978.

18. Ward, P.H., Hanson, D.G., and Abemayor, E.: Transcutaneous Teflon injection of the paralyzed vocal cord: A new technique. Laryngoscope 95:644, 1985.
19. Dedo, H.H., et al.: Intracordal injection of Teflon in the treatment of 135 patients with dysphonia. Ann. Otol. Rhinol. Laryngol. 82:661, 1973.
20. Rubin, H.J.: Misadventures with injectable polytef (Teflon). Arch. Otolaryngol. 101:114, 1975.
21. Opheim, O.: Unilateral paralysis of the vocal cord, Acta Otolaryngol. 45:226, 1955.
22. Levine, H.L., and Tucker, H.M.: Surgical management of the paralyzed. In Larynx. Surgery of the Larynx. Edited by Bailey, B., and Biller, H.F. Philadelphia, W.B. Saunders Co., 1985, pp. 117–47.
23. Smith, G.W.: Aphonia due to vocal cord paralysis corrected by medial positioning of the affected vocal cord with a cartilage autograft. Can. J. Otolaryng. 1:295, 1972.
24. Isshiki, N.: Recent Advances in Phonosurgery. Folia Phoniatr. 32:119, 1980.
25. Nahum, A.M., Harris, J.P. and Davidson, T.M.: The patient who aspirates—diagnosis and management. J. Otolaryngol. 10:10, 1981.
26. Logemann, J.: Evaluation and Treatment of Swallowing Disorders. San Diego, College Hill Press, 1983.
27. Blonsky, E.R., Logemann, J.A., Boshes, B., and Fisher, H.B.: Comparison of speech and swallowing function in patients with tremor disorders and in normal geriatric patients: A cineflourographic study. J. Gerontol. 30:299, 1975.
28. Buchin, P.J.: Swallowing Disorders: Diagnosis and medical treatment. Otolaryng. Clin. North Am. 21:663, 1981.
29. Montgomery, W.W.: Surgical laryngeal closure to eliminate chronic aspiration. N. Engl. J. Med. 292:1390, 1975.
30. Habel, M.B., and Murray, J.E.: Surgical treatment of life endangering chronic aspiration pneumonia. Plast. Reconstr Surg. 49:305, 1972.
31. Strome, M., and Fried, M.P.: Rehabilitative surgery for aspiration. Arch. Otolaryngol. 109:809, 1983.
32. Lindeman, R.A.: Diverting the paralyzed larynx: A reversible procedure for intractable aspiration. Laryngoscope 85:157, 1975.
33. Blitzer, A.: Evaluation and management of chronic aspiration. N.Y. State J. Med. 87:154, 1987.

BIBLIOGRAPHY

Bailey, B.J., and Biller, H.F. (eds.): Surgery of the Larynx. Philadelphia, W.B. Saunders Co., 1985.

Blitzer, A., Brin, M.F., Sasaki, C.T., et al.: Neurological Disorders of the Larynx. New York, Thieme Medical Publishing Co., 1990. In Press.

Krespi, Y.P., and Blitzer, A.: Aspiration and Swallowing Disorders. Otolaryngol. Clin. North Am. 28:1988.

Tucker, H.M.: The Larynx. New York, Thieme Medical Publishing Co., 1987.

SINUSITIS

Arnold M. Cohn and John R. Jacobs

CAPSULE

The complaint "Doctor, I've got sinus trouble" is often heard in the Emergency Department (ED). With persistent frequency, patients continue to attribute various modalities of facial pain, headaches, nasal obstruction, and nasal drainage to sinus disease. The number of decongestants, antihistamines, and sprays on the commercial market reflect the earnings that these patients provide to a host of corporations. Only some of these patients, however, truly have purulent sinusitis.

Purulent sinusitis is a result of viral or bacterial infection of the sinuses, and is frequently associated with specific predisposing factors such as anatomic nasal deformity and nasal allergy. Although time alone does not distinguish between an acute infection and a chronic infection in an otherwise healthy host, some concept of duration is usually incorporated into this distinction in an arbitrary manner.

Acute suppurative sinusitis may be defined as an infectious process lasting up to 3 weeks. Subacute suppurative sinusitis may last as long as 3 months, but observable disease and pathologic changes in the sinus mucosa are reversible. Chronic sinusitis exists in patients whose sinus symptoms persist more than 3 months, with evidence of some elements of irreversible change by biopsy or x ray. Chronic sinusitis is a result of inadequate or untreated acute and subacute sinusitis, or occurs when these conditions are incompletely treated or fail to respond to conventional management.

ANATOMY AND PATHOPHYSIOLOGY

The perinasal sinuses are air-containing cavities that surround the nose but also lie adjacent to the orbit and the anterior cranial fossa. They originate from the nasal cavity and share the characteristics of the nasal lining and its diseases. The mucosal lining contains glands and cilia, not as numerous as those in the nose; the surface of the mucosa is covered by a mucous blanket mobilized toward the ostia by the surface cilia.

The ethmoid and maxillary sinuses are present at birth and reach full development by the teens, when the permanent teeth fully descend. The ethmoid sinuses are frequently clinically involved in children, but it is unusual for the maxillary sinus to be clinically involved before age 10. The frontal sinus begins to develop at 1 year and becomes clinically important after age 6. The sphenoid sinus first shows itself at age 3, reaching full development at age 12.

The neurovascular supply to the nasal mucosa is by the preganglionic parasympathetic fibers arising from the superior salivatory nucleus, which joins the facial nerve as the nervus intermedius, then joins the greater superficial petrosal nerve, which in turn joins with postganglionic fibers from the sympathetic plexus to form the vidian nerve. The vidian nerve enters the sphenopalatine ganglion, where the preganglionic parasympathetic fibers synapse and the resulting full postsynaptic vidian nerve is distributed to the upper respiratory tract mucosa.

Stimulation of these parasympathetic fibers causes an increase in minor salivary gland secretion, vasodilation, and nasal obstruction. Stimulation of the sympathetic plexus component causes vasoconstriction and decreased glandular secretion.

The function of the sinuses is uncertain. Some speculate that the sinuses lighten the skull, act as resonators for the voice, further produce mucus to moisten the nose, and are really rudimentary in humans, with little if any function. The nasal mucosa, and to some degree that of the sinus, produces a fluid high in protein, containing glycoprotein, muramidase, and immunoglobulin A. Approximately 75% of the mucus, however, is water and has a pH of 7.0.

The nasal mucosa reacts to various stimuli, usually with an increase in secretion, vasodilation, and obstruction. Any disturbance of the mucosa around the ostia may disturb ciliary function and propelling of the mucous blanket. Postural change alone may influence function; when an individual is in the recumbent position with the head turned towards one side, the downward nasal chamber becomes "stuffy" and the upper chamber clear. This reverses as the head is turned in the opposite direction, as frequently occurs during normal sleep and is aggravated by concurring stimuli. The nasal mucosa cycle may also react to such stimuli as physical injury; changes in temperature; drugs; infection; antibody-antigen reactions, in which serotonin and ahistamine are also secreted; and hormonal changes such as may occur during menses, sexual intercourse, and pregnancy.

Anatomic causes of obstruction may include unilateral choanal atresia, septal deviation, neoplasm in the nose or nasopharynx, adenoid hypertrophy, and foreign body in the nose.

The nasal mucosa as a target receptor in allergic rhinitis reacts with increased secretion and nasal obstruction as a specific inflammatory response to an inhaled or ingested antigen, with the resulting secretion tending to be thin and watery.

Vasomotor rhinitis results from neural imbalance of the autonomic nervous system with excessive parasympathetic nervous system activity, such as may occur on stepping into an air-conditioned building from an intensely hot outdoor environment, or when going outdoors in the winter from a heated facility. Certain migraine equivalent disorders may behave in a similar way. Again, the mucosa tends to be swollen and pale and the secretion modest and thin.

The normal flora of the nose usually contains Staphylococcus epidermis, Neisseria catarrhalis and the diphtheroids. The more common pathogens include Hemophilus influenzae, particularly in children, Streptococcus pyogenes, Streptococcus pneumonia, and Staphylococcus aureus. Rarely, primary Pseudomonas aeruginosa sinusitis is seen. Usually there is only one pathogen and frequently nasal cultures may be negative in the presence of obvious sinusitis on x ray. Nasal cultures do not necessarily correspond to the sinus pathogen.

The distinction between acute and chronic sinus infection is not clear or necessarily related to time alone. The implication is, nonetheless, that the acute infection was not successfully or incompletely treated and predisposing factors not successfully managed.

Predisposing factors of sinus infection include such local factors as nasal septal pathology; rhinitis causing edema obstructing the ostia, yet allowing micro-organisms to gain access to the sinuses; use of drugs such as reserpine derivatives, topical vasoconstrictors, or narcotics; allergic diathesis; repeated barotrauma; nasal polyps; and foreign bodies. Regional factors affecting nasal function include poor dentition, especially caries in the premolars whose roots may penetrate the maxillary sinuses, and any mechanical basis for nasopharyngeal obstruction. Systemic factors include metabolic malnutrition and depletion, diabetes, systemic steroid use, and immunosuppression.

SIGNS AND SYMPTOMS

The symptoms and signs of acute sinusitis include pain and tenderness over the involved sinus or sinuses, nasal obstruction, nasal discharge, erythema and edema of the nasal turbinates, and systemic symptoms including nonpulsating headaches, malaise, and a low-grade fever. Inquiries should be made as to the onset and periodicity of the nasal obstruction and secretion; exposure to environmental irritants such as various chemicals, weather changes, prescribed and other drugs such as narcotics and tobacco, and associated facial pain and headache. Exudate occurs when bacteria interact with polymorphonuclear leukocytes. The nasal discharge in acute sinusitis is mucopurulent green or yellow, and is unilateral or bilateral depending on the sinus or sinuses involved.

Sensory nerve fibers transmitting head and neck pain and headache include cranial nerves V, VII, IX, X, C_2, and C_4. They are stimulated by mechanical toxic irritants and diagnosis requires skill and patience. In *acute maxillary sinusitis,* pain and tenderness are experienced over the cheek, in the canine and bicuspid teeth (whose roots may extend to the maxillary sinus) and sometimes the eye. The pain is more intense on stooping and in the afternoon. In *frontal sinusitis,* the pain and tenderness are over the forehead and anterior wall of the sinus, and a localized frontal swelling is possible. In *ethmoid sinusitis,* there may be a constant dull pain behind the eyes, pain on eye movement, occasional sore throat, tenderness over the medial canthal ligament, and periorbital edema. In *sphenoid sinusitis,* there is a generalized headache that radiates to the occiput. A superior orbital fissure syndrome may develop because of irritation of the second, third, fourth, and sixth cranial nerves, which surround the sinus. There may be periorbital edema, upper eyelid ptosis, ophthalmoplegia, diplopia, and proptosis. Chronic sinusitis is associated with less defined pain but a sense of "headache" and some posterior nasal obstruction and discharge. Few if any systemic symptoms are experienced, although recurrent headache and chronic cough are reported. In recurring acute and chronic sinusitis, cultures should include aerobic and anaerobic bacteria, acid-fast bacteria, and fungi.

The physical examination is done after shrinking the nasal mucosa with 2% ephedrine or ½% neosynephrine solution or other commercial decongestant. This is accomplished with a fixed-sized speculum attached to an otoscope or an adjustable nasal speculum. It has been said that a pale-body mucosa suggests allergy or vasomotor rhinitis, and an engorged red mucosa suggests infection or rhinitis medicamentosa. These distinctions, however, frequently fail to corroborate diagnosis. The mucosa may be thin and crusted, and have ulcerations from atrophic rhinitis; the septum may be perforated as a result of disease such as syphilis or after surgery. Mucopus may be seen coming from the middle meatus; a confusing pitfall is cerebrospinal fluid from mere rhinitis.

DIAGNOSTIC PROBLEMS

Patients may insist that they have "sinus" even when advised that sinus infections share the symptoms and signs of other disorders in the same region. More common disorders to consider, but not listed in decreasing frequency, include:

1. Viral rhinitis
2. Allergic rhinitis
3. Vasomotor rhinitis
4. Rhinitis medicamentosa
5. Tumor, benign or malignant, in the nose, nasopharynx or orbit
6. Dental abscess
7. Antihypertensive medications
8. Endocrine-related effects such as menstrual period, pregnancy, and "honeymoon rhinitis" during intercourse
9. Environmental contaminants
10. Unilateral choanal atresia in children
11. Nasal foreign body, especially in children or mentally retarded patients
12. Cerebrospinal fluid rhinorrhea secondary to tumor or trauma

DIAGNOSTIC AIDS

IMAGING

X rays are not necessary in every case. Patients with classic symptoms of maxillary sinusitis may be started on treatment without confirmatory x-ray films. It may be argued that x rays may be withheld if treatment is not affected by accurate distinction between purulent sinusitis and purulent rhinitis. Furthermore, sinus x rays from many normal patients with no symptoms may show variable mucosal thickening. On the other hand, sinus x rays can indicate significant mucosal disease, demonstrate an air-fluid level or show complete opacification. Computed tomographic (CT) scans can further detail the extent of pathology.

CULTURES

Cultures of sinus material usually require an invasive procedure and thus are infrequently performed. Cultures of the nose do not always reflect the pathogen in the sinus.

TREATMENT

MEDICAL MANAGEMENT

Successful primary medical management is directed toward three principal end results: relief of pain, control of infection, and restoring mucosal ciliary activity.

To relieve pain, simple analgesics such as acetaminophen, with or without codeine, and ibuprofen suffice for most acute sinus infections. The pain associated with acute frontal and sphenoid sinusitis may, however, demand a stronger narcotic. Applying local heat may also increase patient comfort as well, as will providing adequate humidification and ensuring sufficient hydration.

Topical decongestants such as 2% ephedrine solution as ½% phenylephrine solution or other commercial products, are available to help open the sinus nasal ostium as well as help nasal breathing, but their use beyond 5 days should be discouraged to avoid rhinitis medicamentosa. Systemic decongestants such as phenylpropanolamanine and pseudoephedrine are less dramatic in their effects but better tolerated; they are found in many commercial products. Topical steroids may assist in reducing the inflammatory response but are best used in noninfectious rhinitis. Antibiotics of choice are penicillin or amoxicillin, because most pathogens are gram-positive, with Hemophilus influenzae excepted. The duration of treatment is 7 to 10 days, and can be on an outpatient basis unless a complication is also present. For patients who are allergic to penicillin, or with organisms resistant to amoxicillin, trimethoprim and sulfamethoxazole are the alternatives.

Successful medical management of acute sinusitis includes addressing not only the problem at hand, but also the predisposing factors influencing the natural course of the disorder. Thus, if allergy is involved, testing, desensitization, and avoidance are appropriate. If a labile autonomic vasomotor reaction is implicated, appropriate avoidance supports systemic treatment. If an anatomic abnormality is present, such as a deviated septum, engorged mucosa, or nasal polyps, a secondary surgical procedure may be required.

SURGICAL TREATMENT

Surgery may be needed for relief of severe pain, impending complications, or when the patient is not responding as expected. Surgery can facilitate sinus drainage and sinus ventilation. Nasal surgery including septoplasty, turbinate reduction procedures, nasal polypectomy, and the like, may be required to relieve some of the disposing factors. Primary surgical procedures on the sinus include irrigation, trephination, drainage procedures, and, of course, excision.

TREATMENT FAILURES

Treatment failure may be the result of several factors. One of the principal reasons for patients not responding to conventional management is failure to recognize the underlying causes or predisposing factors such as:

1. Systemic allergy
2. Anatomic deformity such as deviated nasal septum
3. A unilateral choanal atresia
4. Nasal polyps
5. Irreversible mucosal changes
6. Exposure to environmental irritants either in the home or at the place of employment
7. Patient use of nasal medications and topical nasal constrictors
8. Patient social habits (use of intranasal narcotics)
9. Nasal foreign body, particularly in children and the emotionally disturbed patients

COMPLICATIONS

Complications with sinusitis are usually the result of delayed consultation, but may occur if a particularly virulent organism i.e., pseudomonas aeruginosa, is the offender, or if host defenses are compromised by concurrent systemic illness, i.e. diabetes mellitus; immuno-deficiency syndromes of one sort or another. Complications are usually local and related to the sinus involved, though the orbit is particularly at risk.

With *maxillary sinusitis*, it is common to note concurrent otitic or pulmonary infection; should a tooth be extracted when there is co-existent sinusitis an oral-antral fistula may develop. When there is *frontal sinusitis* the infection may spread into the diploic bone to develop an osteomyelitis of the frontal bone, or a sub-periosteal abscess. Pain is exquisite and may require urgent trephination to relieve the pressure, concurrent with parenteral antibiotics, as definitive treatment is planned. When the mucosa around the ostia of the nasal-frontal duct obstructs the frontal sinus, a mucocoele may develop that may cause pressure necrosis of surrounding bone and invade surrounding structures which include the orbit and the anterior frontal fossa. Involvement of the *sphenoid sinus* may progress and cause a superior orbital fissure syndrome which would include paralysis of the third to sixth cranial nerves as they envelop the cavernous sinus and sphenoid. Certainly an infection of any of the sinuses can extend into the central nervous system (CNS) and produce *meningitis*.

The *orbit* is particularly at risk. A *subperiosteal abscess* can occur as a result of maxillary, ethmoid or frontal sinusitis. Upper and lower eyelids are edematous and some proptosis is evident, but extraocular muscle mobility and vision remain intact. Medical treatment is vigorous in this stage, with the patient hospitalized on parenteral antibiotics. As the orbital contents become involved, *cellulitis* develops in the enveloping fat and muscle, proptosis increases and extraocular muscle mobility is reduced. The orbit should be surgically explored at this juncture to prevent development of an expanding abscess. When visual acuity begins to deteriorate, suggesting abscess formation, surgical drainage is urgent if vision is to be preserved.

The *cavernous sinus* may be infected by direct spread from the sphenoid sinus and by the venous circulation from any sinus by way of the pterygoid vessels. Spiking fever, mental change, and ophthalmoplegia appear along with the signs and symptoms of the infection in the offending sinus.

Danger signals of impending complications discussed above therefore include:

1. Headache as a new finding, or increasing in severity
2. Nausea or vomiting
3. Chills and fever
4. Stiff neck
5. Forehead or eyelid swelling and proptosis
6. Visual change
7. Personality change
8. Convulsions
9. Eye ground changes
10. White blood cell counts greater than 20,000.

SINUSITIS IN CHILDREN

The ethmoid and maxillary sinuses are the most frequently involved, but nonetheless are rarely a significant problem in young children. The maxillary sinus, although present at birth, lies high in the maxilla above the permanent teeth. As the teeth erupt, the floor of the sinus descends. Because of the distance between the floor of the sinus and the erupted teeth in young children, dental problems as a cause of sinusitis is less frequent than in adults. On the other hand, in unilateral choanal atresia, nasal foreign body and a nasopharyngeal mass, either benign as with adenoids, or malignant, are the more frequent causes of sinusitis in children as compared to older patients.

A small child has difficulty in articulating his symptoms, and thus, these patients' difficulties with rhinorrhea, otitis media, cough, and fever are frequently attributed to chronic upper respiratory tract infection or allergy. Because of a reluctance to take x rays, diagnosis is frequently delayed.

Treatment of sinusitis in children is similar to that in adults except for the difficulty in arriving at a diagnosis. Hemophilus influenzae is more common as the causative organism in this age group, making amoxicillin the drug of choice, with trimethoprim and sulfamethoxazole, or cloromycetin as alternatives for amoxicillin-resistant organisms or the penicillin-allergic patients. The displacement procedure of Proetz is frequently useful in infants and children for evacuating the mucopurulent material as well as obtaining material for culture. Surgery is infrequent because of the permanent teeth being in the anterior maxillary wall. Occasionally, a sinus may be irrigated, but this is uncommon until the child is older. The frontal sinus is seldom clinically involved until approximately age 10, and then may rarely require trephination. Complications affect the lower respiratory tree more frequently in children than in adults, but are otherwise similar to those in older patients.

ALLERGIC RHINITIS

Rajesh Shah

CAPSULE

Allergic rhinitis is a common condition affecting 20 to 30 million people in the United States and associated with a high incidence of morbidity and considerable cost. Frequently it is a symptom accompanying other conditions in the Emergency Department (ED). The prevalence of this disease among adolescents is estimated at 25 to 30%.

Allergic rhinitis is an antibody-mediated inflammatory disease of nasal mucous membranes. It is classified as seasonal or perennial depending on the timing and duration of symptoms. The characteristic symptoms are paroxysms of sneezing, nasal pruritus and obstruction of nasal passages (nasal polyps), mucus secretion resulting in post nasal drainage, conjunctival and pharyngeal itching, and lacrimation.

The most common type of allergic rhinitis is seasonal, related to airborne pollens and most common in young people.

PATHOPHYSIOLOGY AND CAUSES

Allergic rhinitis represents exaggerated responses to environmental allergens mediated through the immune system, primarily IgE producing reversible tissue changes.

The nasal mucosa is rich in mast cells. With exposure and re-exposure to allergens, it activates biologic processes in mast cells and leads to degranulation and immediate release of preformed mediators that are responsible for clinical symptoms of allergic rhinitis.

Etiologic factors include an array of substances inhaled, ingested, or injected into the body that trigger an allergic reaction, for example:

Pollens
Animal dander
House dust
Certain foods or drugs
Physical stimuli such as heat, cold, sunlight, tobacco smoke, exercise
Exposure to certain chemicals

Weeds and certain grass and tree pollens elicit seasonal rhinitis. Molds and decaying organic matter may be contributing causes.

Perennial rhinitis occurs in response to allergens that are present throughout the year, such as animal dander, dust accumulating at home and work, processed materials and chemicals used in industrial settings, and fibers such as feathers from pillows.

These conditions may be seen in the emergency medicine setting, and must be differentiated from upper respiratory infections.

MANIFESTIONS

Symptoms of allergic rhinitis include episodic rhinorrhea, often watery and profuse; paroxysmal sneezing; nasal obstruction; lacrimation (itching, tearing, and redness of eyes); conjunctival pruritus; and irritation of the nasal mucosa and throat (palate and pharynx). The nasal mucosa is pale and boggy. Swelling of the turbinates and mucous membranes, with obstruction of sinus ostia and eustachian tubes, precipitates secondary infection of the sinuses and middle ear, common in perennial rhinitis but rare in seasonal rhinitis. Nasal polyps often arise with edema and/or infection.

Patients with allergic rhinitis especially children, have a distinctive appearance. They have dark circles under their eyes and a nasal crease from rubbing the nose upward to open the nasal airway, known as the "allergic salute." Mouth breathing is also typical, but the appearance of these symptoms does not prove that a person has an allergy.

Table 55-25 outlines the diagnosis of seasonal and perennial allergic rhinitis.

TREATMENT

Treatment can be divided in three parts:

1. Avoidance of offending allergens
2. Immunotherapy administered by an allergist for allergens that cannot be avoided
3. Drug therapy for symptomatic relief

AVOIDANCE

The most desirable therapeutic option is avoidance of the offending allergens. This is difficult and impractical, but a great deal can be done to eliminate exposure, for example:

Removal of pets from home to avoid animal dander
Use of air filtration devices and dehumidifers
Use of 1:750 solution of zephiran chloride, an effective agent in controlling mold growth
Travel to nonpollinating areas during the critical periods to minimize airborne pollens

DRUG THERAPY

For symptomatic relief during the allergy season, antihistamines are extremely useful and are the only specific end-organ antagonists available to control mast-cell-derived reactions. Antihistamines neutralize the effect of histamine by blocking receptor sites. Other agents in use are cromolyn sodium and corticosteroids.

TABLE 55-25. DIAGNOSIS OF ALLERGIC RHINITIS

Seasonal Allergic Rhinitis	Perennial Allergic Rhinitis
A. Depends on accurate history	A. Also needs accurate history
B. Occurrence with pollination	B. Symptomatic all year. Intermittent or continuous symptoms
C. Offending allergen, windborne pollens of weeds, grass, and trees	C. Indoor inhalants: allergen-house dust, feathers, danders of household pets, mold spores; high-humidity climate
D. Prevalence is age-related. Common in children; ragweed and hay fever rare before 4 to 5 years of age	D. Problems in adult women more than men
E. Characteristic pale, almost bluish nasal turbinates coated with clear watery secretion	E. Manifest as nasal polyps; clear, glistening white grape-like masses.
F. Predominance of eosinophils in nasal secretion	F. Increase eosinophils in nasal secretion and peripheral eosinophilia
G. Total serum IgE is elevated.	G. Total serum IgE is elevated
	H. Thickening of sinus membranes on x ray

Note: Specificity of elevated serum IgE is critical to an etiologic diagnosis.

MANDIBULAR DYSFUNCTION

Cherie A. Hargis

CAPSULE

Temporomandibular disorders (TMDs) can be subdivided into masticatory muscle and intrinsic temporomandibular joint (TMJ) problems.[1] Major factors common to both groups include trauma, repetitive loading, arthritis, and stress-induced muscle tension.[2] Key signs of TMD are pain, joint noises, and limited jaw movement.[3]

The most common muscular disorders are myofascial pain dysfunction (MPD), muscle spasm, muscle splinting, myositis, contracture, and hypertrophy. The most common joint problems are disc displacements, arthritis, dislocations, and ankylosis.[2]

Always rule out life-threatening causes of craniofacial pain before diagnosing TMD. Emergency Department (ED) treatment of most TMDs is supportive except for acute anterior dislocations which require immediate manual reduction. Refer patients to dental clinicians who specialize in TMDs.

ED physician understanding of mandibular function is not merely academic. Adequate jaw mobility is a crucial factor for successful oral intubation.

INTRODUCTION

Temporomandibular disorders (TMDs) comprise a subset of the cluster of extracranial causes of craniofacial pain or headache.[1] The two main TMD subdivisions are masticatory muscle disorders and intrinsic joint problems.[2]

Four to 28% of the general population may experience TMD;[3] and 5 to 15% may require treatment.[4] Women are affected three times more often than men, but the reason is unknown.[3]

FUNCTIONAL ANATOMY

The temporomandibular joint (TMJ) is a complex hinge-gliding "joint with a movable socket."[5] The con-

vex mandibular condyle articulates with the glenoid fossa and the convex articular eminence of the temporal bone. The articular surfaces are covered by fibrocartilage. A uniquely shaped fibrocartilaginous disc rests between the condyle and the temporal bone (Fig. 55-35A). The firm but pliable biconcave disc acts as a movable socket that accommodates the mismatched shapes of the condyle and the articular eminence. The disc also creates an upper and lower joint space (Fig. 55-35B).

The jaw opens by hinge and gliding movements called rotation and translation. First, the condyle rotates on the disc within the glenoid fossa, in the lower joint space. Then, within the upper joint space, the disc-condyle translates down the posterior slope of the articular eminence to rock on its apex (Fig. 55-36). The mechanism that governs disc movement with the condyle is unknown.[6] During jaw closure, the actions occur in reverse. Because the TMJs are connected by the mandible, all motions occur in tandem. A problem on one side eventually affects the other.

The disc attaches by means of collateral ligaments to the medial and lateral poles of the condyle and appears ridged in the sagittal plane. The posterior ridge or band is thicker than the anterior band or the thin intermediate zone (Fig. 55-37). The bulk of the disc is noninnervated and avascular except peripherally. The bilaminar retrodiscal (posterior attachment) tissue however, is highly vascular and well innervated.

Anteriorly, the disc (Fig. 55-38) blends with the capsule (Fig. 55-39) and fascia of the upper head of the lateral pterygoid muscle. Although most of this muscle inserts on the condylar neck, some fibers may directly insert on the anteromedial disc.

The retrodiscal surfaces and joint spaces have a synovial lining. The loose, thin capsule enclosing the outer edges of the disc also has a synovial lining and a rich neurovascular supply.

Branches of the mandibular division of the trigeminal nerve innervate the temporomandibular region. The auriculotemporal nerve innervates the TMJ, retrodiscal tissue, posterior capsule, and lateral ligament. The masseteric and posterior deep temporal nerves innervate the anterior capsule. The vascular supply is provided by the superficial temporal artery and masseteric branches of the maxillary artery.[7]

The TMJ is reinforced laterally by the strong temporomandibular ligament and medially by the weaker sphenomandibular and stylomandibular ligaments.

The three principal mandibular movements are: opening-closing, protrusion-retrusion, and lateral ex-

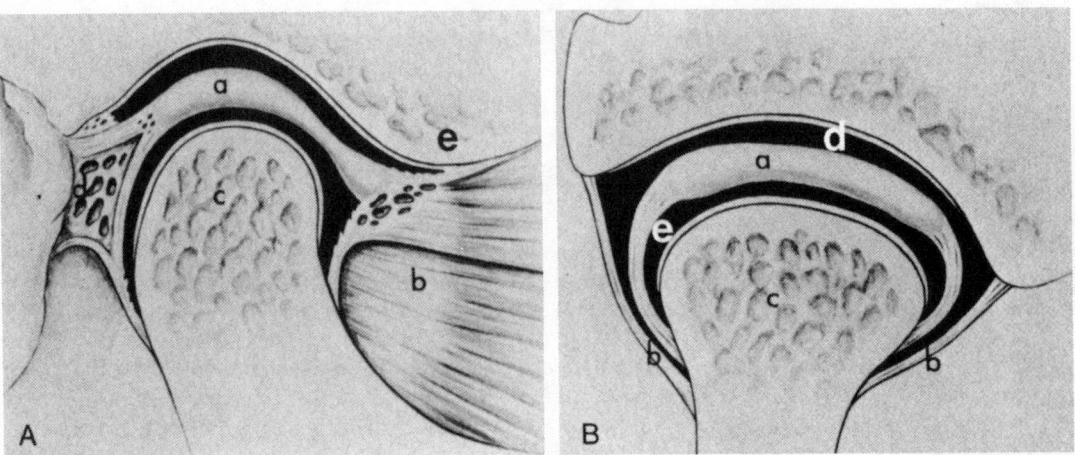

FIG. 55-35. A. Sagittal section of the temporomandibular joint demonstrating the disc (meniscus) (a), lateral pterygoid muscle with insertion into disc and condylar head (b), condylar head (c), bilaminar zone in posterior attachment (retrodiscal tissue) of the disc, allowing translatory motion (d), and articular eminence of the temporal bone (e). B. Coronal section of the temporomandibular joint. The disc (a) separates the joint into two separate compartments (d and e). The capsule of the joint (b) is shown in relation to the condylar head (c). With permission from Greenberg, S.A., Jacobs, J.S., and Bessette, R.W.: Temporomandibular joint dysfunction: Evaluation and treatment. Clin. Plast. Surg. 16:707, 1989.

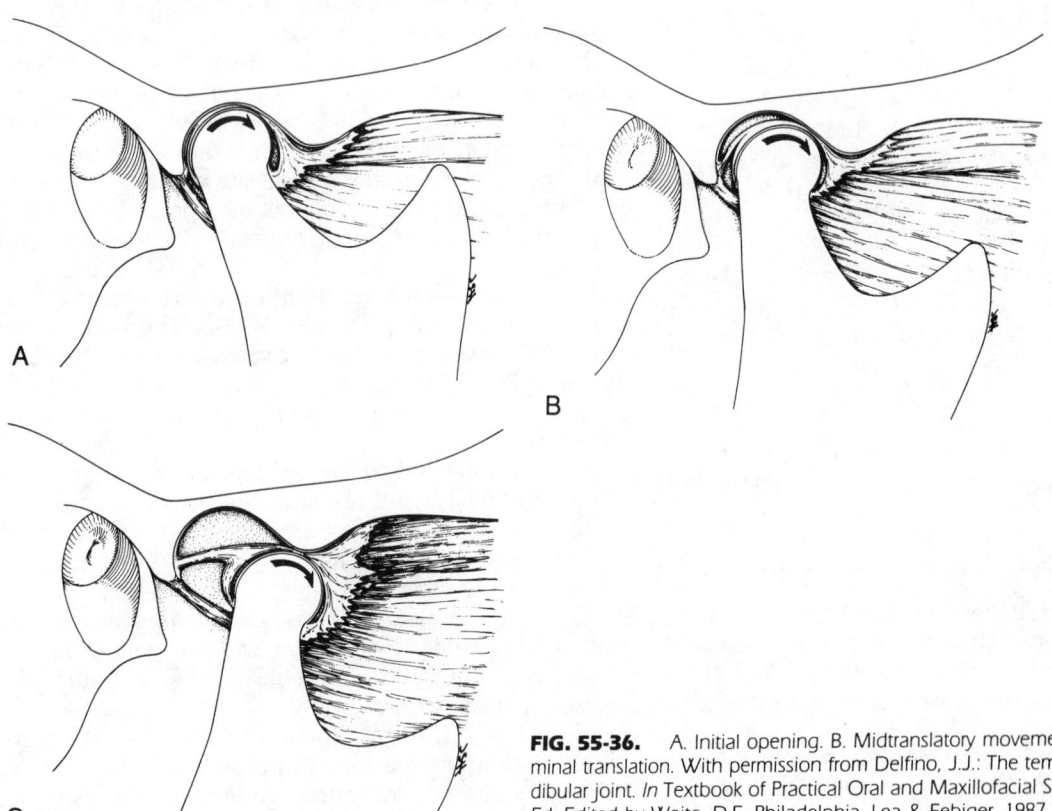

FIG. 55-36. A. Initial opening. B. Midtranslatory movement. C. Terminal translation. With permission from Delfino, J.J.: The temporomandibular joint. In Textbook of Practical Oral and Maxillofacial Surgery, 3rd Ed. Edited by Waite, D.E. Philadelphia, Lea & Febiger, 1987.

cursion. The inferior heads of the lateral pterygoids, anterior digastrics, and mylohyoids open or depress the mandible. The superior heads of the lateral pterygoids are inactive during opening.

The masseters, medial pterygoids, and temporalis muscles close or elevate the mandible. Bilateral contractions of the inferior heads of the lateral pterygoids

cause protrusion. Retrusion involves the posterior temporalis, masseters, mylohyoids, and digastrics. Lateral excursion enlists the lateral and medial pterygoids on one side and on the opposite, the temporalis.[8] For example, the right-sided pterygoids pull the chin to the left of midline.

The TMJ is a phylogenetically recent addition to the

mammalian jaw and is the last joint to develop in the human embryo.[5,9] The TMJ and mandible develop from the first branchial arch, as do the malleolus and the incus. The joint of the primitive reptilian jaw forms the malleolar-incus joint in mammals.[5] Hence, the middle ear and the TMJ are intimately related, and TMJ pain may refer to the ear or elicit otologic symptoms. In 1934, Costen reported one of the first "TMJ syndromes"—severe ear and sinus pain, tinnitus, vertigo, and occipital headache, purportedly from malocclusion.[2,3]

Normal TMJ function depends on the harmonious balance between the muscles, which close the jaw, and the teeth, which signal a fixed endpoint to closure. The TMJ capsule and the periodontal ligament receptors of the teeth provide afferent input to guide mandible positioning.[3] Changes in dental occlusion can cause mandibular deviation during closure or masticatory muscle spasm.

Various jaw positions reflect the balance between muscle forces and the teeth. In the rest position, the lips touch but there is a 1.3 to 3.0 mm "freeway space" between the upper and lower teeth.[10] The rest position is dynamic, however, and changes with head position, body posture, activity, fatigue, and emotional tension. The rest position allows the muscles time to repair. A loss or decrease of the freeway space places the teeth in constant contact and leads to muscle fatigue and stress on the TMJ structures and eventual soft-tissue remodeling.

Yawning triggers an inverse stretch reflex, which inhibits contraction and enhances full relaxation of the elevator muscles. Clenching triggers an inverse stretch reflex in the depressor muscles. Excessive clenching,

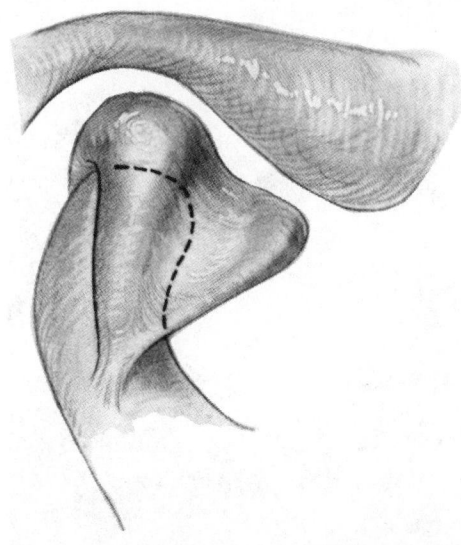

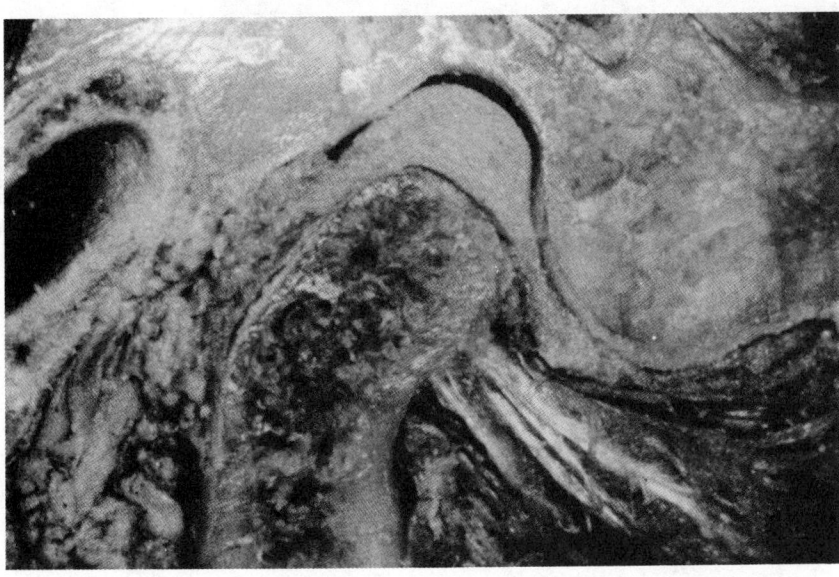

A

FIG. 55-37.   A. In the closed-mouth position, the thick posterior band of the disc envelops the superior portion of the condyle. The intermediate zone and anterior band lie between the condyle and posterior slope of the articular eminence.

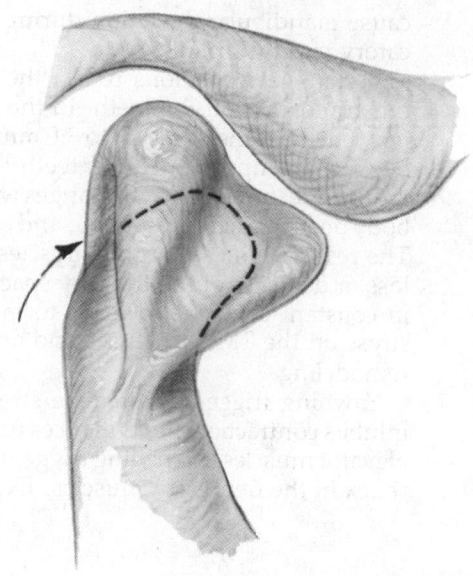

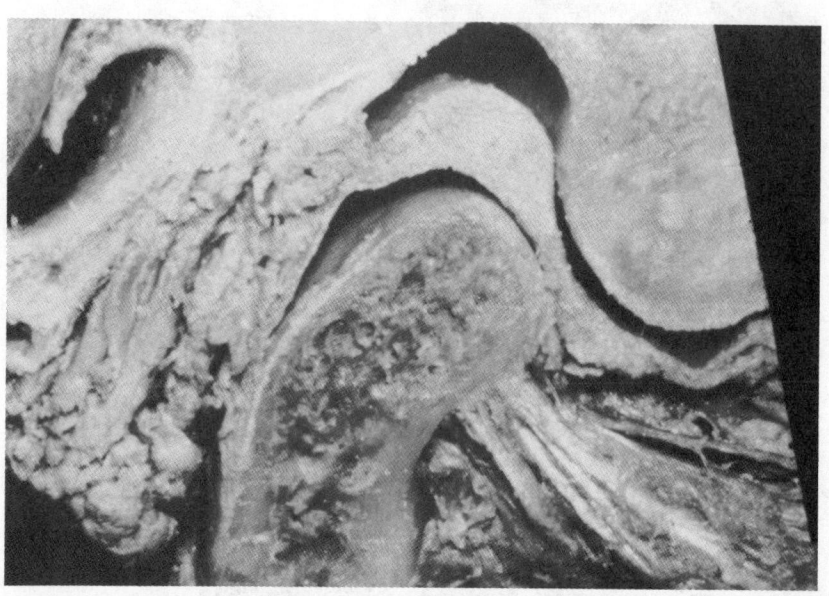

B

FIG. 55-37 Continued. B. During opening, the posterior band assumes a more posterior relationship to the condyle as condylar rotation occurs. The intermediate zone becomes the articulating surface between the condyle and articular eminence. This condyle-disc relationship is maintained during most jaw movements.

bruxism and other parafunctional oral habits, however, repetitively load and stress the joint and cause muscle imbalances. Bruxism is a rhythmic or spasmodic grinding of the teeth unrelated to chewing. It occurs especially during REM sleep and may reflect a stress-induced state of partial arousal which manifests as increased muscle activity. Clenched jaws can generate pressures of 55 to 280 lbs psi, but patients who habitually brux can generate six times of the bite force of nonbruxers. Dentures can reduce biting forces to 15% of normal.[10]

PATHOPHYSIOLOGY

In the past, malocclusion and psychologic stress were considered primary causes of TMDs. Current theories cite four major factors: trauma, repetitive loading, arthritic disease, and stress-induced muscle tension.[2] Trauma can occur from direct impact, overstretching,

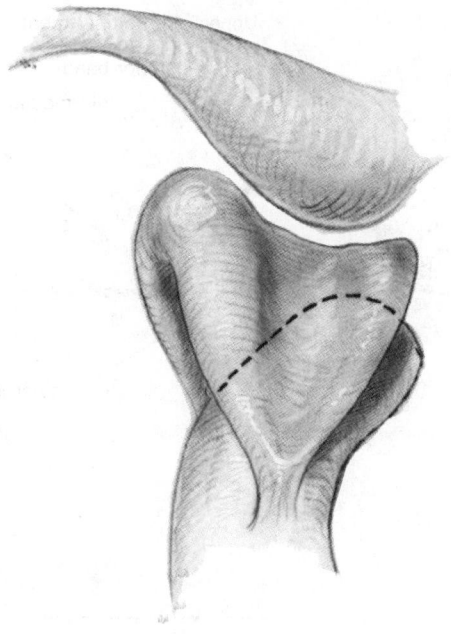

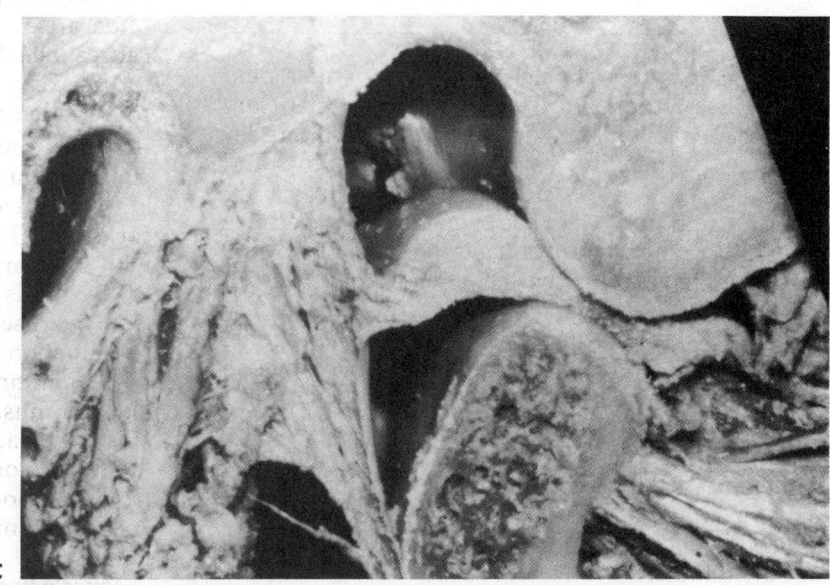

FIG. 55-37 Continued.   C. During maximum opening of the mandible, the condyle may rotate under the anterior band of the disc. The vascular posterior attachment tissues fill with blood to occupy the space created as the condyles move anteriorly from the mandibular fossa. During closure or retrusion, the blood-filled posterior attachment tissues empty as the condyles return to the fossa. With permission from Dolwick, M.F., and Sanders, B.: TMJ Internal Derangement and Arthrosis. St. Louis, C.V. Mosby, 1985.

or dental procedures. Some clinicians cite cervical whiplash as a cause of TMD and have coined the controversial term "mandibular whiplash."[11,12]

Repetitive loading such as bruxism and clenching stress the TMJ and fatigue the muscles. Hard and soft-tissue adaptations in the joint may develop over time. Both degenerative and rheumatoid arthritis produce joint pain and dysfunction. Stress-induced muscle tension can play a substantial role in some TMDs.

Psychologic profiles have shown that some TMD patients are "more likely to have emotional problems and difficulties dealing with life events."[2]

TMDs can be divided into masticatory muscle disorders and joint disorders. There is considerable overlap of signs and symptoms in both major groups. Muscle disorders are the most common cause of TMDs, followed by TMJ internal derangements and osteoarthritis.

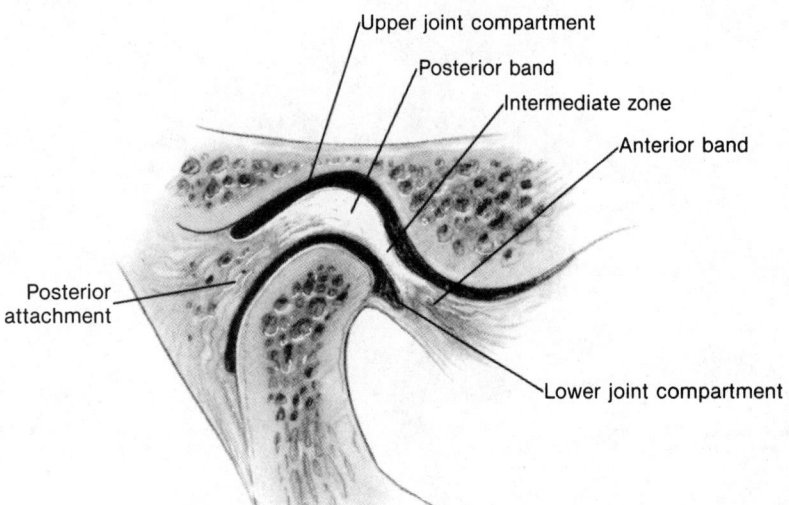

Upper joint compartment
Posterior band
Intermediate zone
Anterior band
Posterior attachment
Lower joint compartment

FIG. 55-38. View of disc. Note thin anterior band, very thin intermediate zone and thick posterior band. With permission from Dolwick, M.F., and Sanders, B.: TMJ Internal Derangement and Arthrosis. St. Louis, C.V. Mosby, 1985.

MASTICATORY MUSCLE DISORDERS

Common disorders characterized by muscular pain and stiffness leading to limited jaw movement are myofascial pain dysfunction (MPD), spasm, reflex splinting, contracture, myositis, hypertrophy, and neoplasms.

Past definition of MPD has been confusing because of variable nomenclature and symptomatology. MPD has been called mandibular stress syndrome, TMJ syndrome, and "tension headache of the masticatory muscles." Its cause is unclear, but bruxism, emotional stress, and malocclusion are thought to play roles in MPD. For most clinicians, MPD signs and symptoms include masticatory muscle tenderness; lack of joint tenderness with endaural palpation; pre-auricular pain, joint clicking or crepitus; limited mandibular function; and lack of positive radiographic findings.[13] Both MPD and internal derangement share the latter four symptoms.

Other clinicians consider that key diagnostic criteria for MPD include: discrete trigger points and diffuse masticatory muscle tenderness; associated symptoms and contributing factors.[14] Trigger points are hard, tender bands in musculoskeletal tissue. Stimulated trigger points produce consistent patterns of referred pain.[14] Various associated symptoms include bitemporal headache, visual and otologic disturbances, paresthesias, dermal flushing, heat or cold hypersensitivity, and GI distress. Contributing factors include stress, parafunctional oral habits, and sleep disturbances. The lateral pterygoid is commonly involved and refers pain to the ear and zygoma. The similarities between MPD and fibromyalgia are striking; MPD may be a localized form of fibromyalgia.[14]

Muscle spasm is an acute involuntary tonic contraction that continues even at rest. The muscle is shortened and painful, and has a limited range of motion. A self-perpetuating cycle of pain-spasm-pain often arises.[15] Isolated jaw spasm is rare.[2] Possible causes include local injury or central nervous system (CNS) excitation (consider tetanus). Untreated spastic muscles become painless but contracted over time.

Muscle splinting (trismus) causes painful restricted jaw movement on attempted use. The hypertonicity is a protective response to local injury, pain or other coexistent TMDs. Jaw tremor and incoordination occur with movement but not at rest.[2]

Myositis is an inflammatory response to local injury from overuse, trauma, or infection. The muscle is sore to palpation, even at rest. Movement worsens the pain. Splinting occurs and jaw motion is limited. The elevator muscles are chiefly affected. Prolonged myositis may lead to contracture.

Muscle contracture produces painless shortening from scars or adhesions in the muscle or its fascia. Associated muscle hypertrophy or ankylosis may occur.

Muscle hypertrophy can be idiopathic or can reflect severe bruxism. It is usually painless and associated with contracture. Enlargement may occur unilaterally or bilaterally.

Neoplasms that affect the TMJ structures are rare. Tumors may arise from intrinsic joint tissues, from metastasis to the joint, or from direct extension of nearby tissues. Clinical signs include swelling over the affected area, motor paresis, sensory paresthesia, and altered mandibular function such as trismus or occlusal changes. Eighth cranial nerve involvement is common too, including auditory changes, tinnitus, and vertigo. Note that pain is not considered a specific symptom of neoplasm. Early malignancy may present as a painless restriction of joint movement.[16]

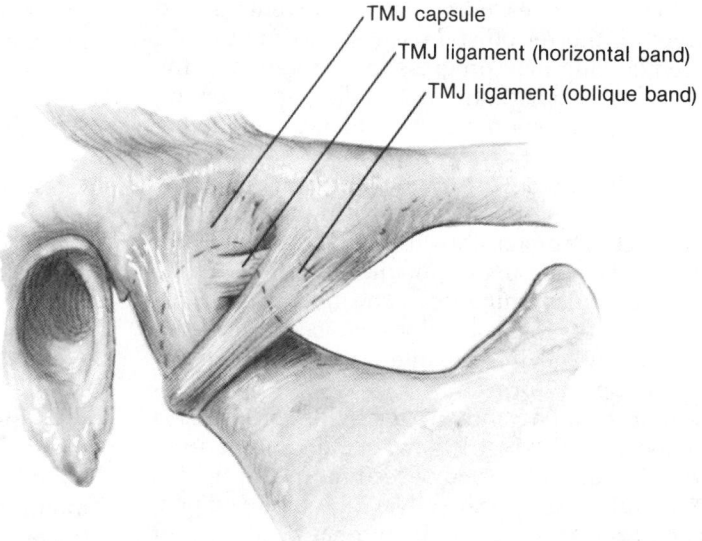

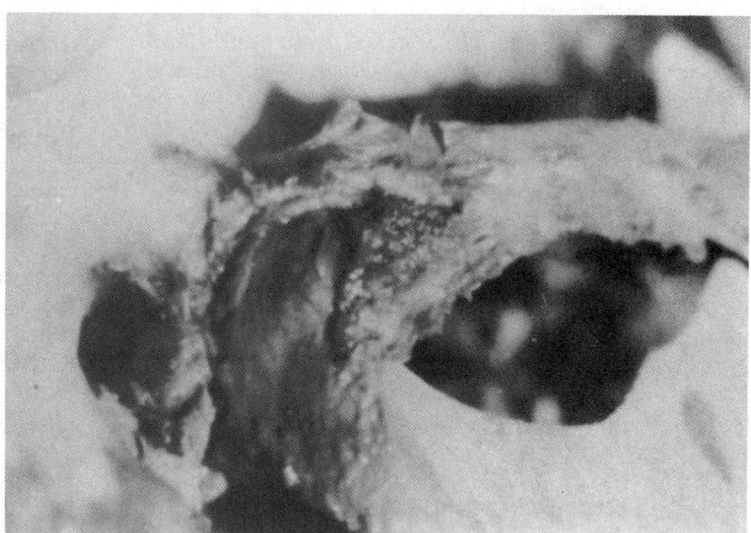

FIG. 55-39.   The articular capsule is strongly reinforced laterally by the temporomandibular ligament, which has a superficial oblique band and a deeper horizontal band. The temporomandibular ligament "checks" or limits retrusion and anterior movement of the condyle. With permission from Dolwick, M.F., and Sanders, B.: TMJ Internal Derangement and Arthrosis. St. Louis, C.V. Mosby, 1985.

TEMPOROMANDIBULAR JOINT DISORDERS

TMDs caused by intrinsic joint pathology include internal derangement (ID), arthritis, dislocations, and ankylosis. ID and arthritis are the most prevalent problems, but only dislocations require definitive ED treatment.

INTERNAL DERANGEMENT (DISC DISPLACEMENT)

The term internal derangement (ID) generally pertains to any abnormal relationship between the TMJ articular components. More often, the term denotes aberrant disc-condyle relationships such as disc displacement. Three major stages of progressive ID are: disc displacement with reduction; without reduction; and with perforation.[17] The continuum starts when the disc's thick posterior band subluxes anterior to the condyle and impedes normal joint movement and overstretches the retrodiscal tissues. Over time, soft tissue remodeling may progress to perforation of the disc or of the retrodiscal tissues. Radiographs remain normal until perforation occurs and bony remodeling ensues.

Disc displacement with reduction is heralded by reciprocal clicks on opening and closing the jaw. The opening click occurs as the anteriorly subluxed disc reduces to its normal position just as the condyle strikes the articular eminence.[17] The more subtle closing click occurs as the disc dislocates again just before the teeth nearly touch in the intercuspal position. Radiographs appear normal.

Disc displacement without reduction produces a "closed lock," which restricts jaw opening. Joint noise is absent, but a prior period of reciprocal clicking has existed and then disappeared. Now the subluxed posterior band never returns to its normal position as it obstructs the condyle's path and overstretches the retrodiscal tissues. Radiographs remain normal.

Disc displacement with perforation is the most advanced stage of ID and is marked by crepitus and osteoarthritis. Perforation of the disc or the retrodiscal tissues exposes the rough articular surfaces to one another.[17,18] Radiographs may show degenerative changes.

OSTEOARTHRITIS

Osteoarthritis (osteoarthrosis) is the second most common joint TMD. Its hallmarks are crepitus, joint tenderness to palpation, joint pain worsening with movement, and radiographic changes. The primary form is an age-related degeneration of the articular surfaces.[3] It affects up to 20% of the general population over 40.[19] Patients with the primary form have relatively mild symptoms but significant radiographic findings.[3] The second degenerative form affects younger people and is often post-traumatic, but can be idiopathic.[2,3] Their symptoms are more severe, but the radiographs are less striking.[3] Degenerative arthritis often occurs from internal derangement.[20]

POLYARTHRITIS

Systemic, polyarthritic conditions also affect the TMJ. Fifty to 60% of patients with rheumatoid arthritis have TMJ involvement.[18,21] On rare occasions, the TMJ may be the first or only affected joint.[22,23] Rheumatoid arthritis is usually more severe than TMJ osteoarthritis. Clinically there is tenderness, restricted motion, crepitus and an anterior open bite caused by condylar destruction. Radiographic findings include osteopenia, joint space narrowing, bony erosion or proliferation, and flattening of the posterior slope of the condyle.[18,20] Other polyarthritic conditions that may affect the TMJ include ankylosing spondylitis, gout, systemic lupus erythematosis, Sjögren's syndrome, systemic sclerosis, and psoriatic arthritis.[3,21,23]

AVASCULAR NECROSIS

Avascular necrosis of the TMJ is rare. It is usually a post-traumatic, postsurgical, or postradiation complication, but it can also result from systemic disease such as sickle cell anemia.[3,24]

ANKYLOSIS

Ankylosis caused by fibrous adhesions or bony fusion results in complete or partial restriction of jaw movement. Translation is lost but rotation is preserved for mouth opening to 25 mm.[25] Ankylosis is usually unilateral, but can be bilateral; it results from trauma, infection or rheumatoid arthritis. Ankylosis affects appearance, speech, chewing, and oral hygiene and may preclude oral intubation.[3] A depressed zygomatic arch fracture can cause pseudoankylosis.[25]

INFLAMMATORY CONDITIONS

The synovial linings of the TMJ and capsule are vulnerable to inflammatory processes. Inflammation can be caused by trauma, overuse, metabolic imbalances, arthritis, infection, or foreign body reactions to surgical implants. Synovitis and capsulitis are clinically indistinguishable. Both conditions produce a fluctulent effusion, synovial fluid changes, palpable joint tenderness, and pain with jaw movement. An acute effusion may produce a posterior open bite. Infectious processes may arise secondary to trauma, surgical or invasive imaging procedures, local spread from otitis media, malignant otitis externa; mastoiditis, parotitis, oral infection, or from hematogenous seeding.[3,20,23] TMJ septic arthritis is most commonly caused by staphylococci.[26] Reports exist of TMJ infections from Hemophilus influenzae, Neisseria meningitidis, Neisseria gonorrhoeae, viruses, mycobacteria, and spirochetes.[22,26,27] Antibiotics and drainage may prevent joint destruction and ankylosis.

DISLOCATION

The mandibular condyle can dislocate in an anterior, posterior, lateral, or superior direction. Anterior dislocation is most common. The condyle translates anterior to the articular eminence. Muscular spasm and the bony eminence itself prevent spontaneous reduction. Anterior dislocation frequently occurs without a concomitant mandibular fracture. Anterior dislocations are classified as acute, chronic recurrent, and chronic prolonged, depending on the duration and frequency of displacement.[28]

Posterior condylar displacement is usually associated with a fracture of the anterior bony auditory canal or a basilar skull fracture. The patient presents with restricted jaw opening, TMJ pain, and an external auditory canal laceration. Treatment requires manual reduction and otologic care.

Lateral subluxation (Type 1) and dislocation (Type 2) involve a coexistent mandibular body fracture. In a lateral subluxation, the condyle is a palpable protuberance in the preauricular area. In a Type 2 dislocation, the condyle is driven laterally and then superiorly into the temporal area, where it is palpable. The patient exhibits a crossbite. Treatment involves reduction of the condyle and the fracture.[28]

Superior dislocations drive the condyle up through the thin articular fossa roof into the middle cranial fossa. Cerebral contusion, facial nerve paralysis, and deafness can occur. The patient displays restricted jaw opening and ipsilateral deviation, preauricular tenderness, hemotympanum and external auditory canal bleeding. Superior dislocations rarely occur without a fracture. Treatments include condylotomy, condylectomy, elastic traction, manual reduction, or conservative management.[28]

ANTERIOR DISLOCATION

Factors that predispose the mandible to anterior dislocation include an overstretched capsule, a shallow eminence, and muscle fatigue from overuse. Up to 70% of the general population can sublux the mandible but then spontaneously reduce it.[28]

Acute anterior dislocations are painful and tend to be bilateral, but can be unilateral. Dislocation occurs from wide opening during yawning, laughing, eating, dental treatment, convulsions, or trauma. The ensuing muscle spasms of the lateral pterygoid and temporalis preclude spontaneous reduction.

The patient presents with an inability to close the mouth (open lock), preauricular pain, and a preauricular depression from displacement of the condyle from the glenoid fossa. The lower jaw protrudes and enunciation is poor. If the dislocation is unilateral, the chin deviates to the contralateral side.

The differential diagnosis includes mandibular fracture-dislocation, hemarthrosis, disc displacement without reduction, MPD and dystonic reaction. An oral panoramic radiograph demonstrates the dislocation and any mandibular fracture. The condyle appears anterior and superior to the articular eminence.[28]

TREATMENT

Because the anteriorly dislocated condyle is on the "wrong side" of the articular eminence, the goal of reduction is to push the condyle down and back around the eminence into the glenoid fossa. Most commonly, the patient is seated with the head against the wall or a headrest. The operator stands facing the patient. The patient's mandible should be at or below the operator's elbows to allow sufficient leverage.

Latex gloves are highly recommended. The thumbs can be placed posteriorly along the oblique mandibular ridge lateral to the molars while the other digits curl under the angle and body of the mandible. Lateral oblique ridge placement obviates the risk of crushed thumbs when the reduced jaw snaps closed. The thumbs should be wrapped in gauze if they are placed directly on the molars.[28]

The operator first applies downward, then backward pressure to achieve reduction. Some clinicians recommend lifting the chin anteriorly before applying the backward pressure.[18] Bilateral dislocations should be reduced sequentially.[28]

In a second method, the patient is supine and the operator stands at the head of the gurney. The operator pushes the mandible down toward the patient's feet and then back toward the ears.[28]

In a third and unusual method, the operator stimulates the pharynx to induce a gag reflex. The jaw depresses during the efferent loop of the reflex.[29]

Sedation may be necessary for the patient who displays marked apprehension. Some clinicians use intravenous diazepam (5 to 10 mg) or midazolam (2.5 to 3.0 mg). Maintain extreme vigilance for respiratory depression.

Other clinicians advocate the use of local anesthesia into the joint or into the lateral pterygoid muscle. Injection into the TMJ is fraught with the risks of infection and disc or capsular trauma, and should not be performed by inexperienced operators. Intraoral injection into the lateral pterygoid muscle is an alternative. Two to three mL of 2% lidocaine with 1:100,000 epinephrine are injected posterior to the maxillary tuberosity, using a 25-gauge needle.[28]

If reduction is successful, the patient is advised to avoid wide mouth opening for 3 to 4 weeks, place a hand under the chin when yawning to support the jaw, maintain a soft diet, and use a nonsteroidal anti-inflammatory drug for several days. The patient is referred to a dental professional for follow-up. If reduction is unsuccessful, the patient must be admitted for general anesthesia with muscle relaxation. Intermaxillary fixation is not required for an initial anterior dislocation. Patients with chronic recurrent dislocations may require surgical intervention such as capsular plication, augmentation of the eminence, or removal of the eminence.[28]

PREHOSPITAL ASSESSMENT AND STABILIZATION

Most patients with nontraumatic TMD who present to the ED are ambulatory. The only exception might be a patient with an acute jaw dislocation. Allow the patient to sit upright and lean forward to protect the airway from pooled secretions. If a dystonic reaction from phenothiazines is suspected administer diphenhydramine, 50 mg IM or IV.

CLINICAL PRESENTATION AND EXAMINATION

The key signs of a TMD are preauricular pain, joint noise, and limited jaw movement. Other signs and symptoms include jaw deviation to the affected side, shoulder and neck tenderness, headache, and ear stuffiness. Acute pain symptoms are more likely to respond to simple therapies; resolution of chronic symptoms is more challenging. The patient may relate the onset of symptoms to a specific event such as acute trauma or a dental procedure. More often, the triggering event is unknown. A screening history and physical examination delineate patients who require referral for further TMJ imaging and evaluation (Tables 55-26 and Table 55-27).

PAIN

Patients with disc displacement tend to localize the pain directly over the TMJ just anterior to the ear. Patients with muscle disorders describe a more diffuse pattern. Patients with both joint and muscle disorders describe the chief component as most severe. Joint pain is described as a constant, dull pain of variable intensity. The pain is worsened by jaw movement and

---

TABLE 55-26. RECOMMENDED SCREENING QUESTIONNAIRE FOR TMD.*

1. Do you have difficulty or pain, or both, when opening your mouth, as for instance, when yawning?
2. Does your jaw get "stuck," "locked," or "go out"?
3. Do you have difficulty or pain, or both, when chewing, talking, or using your jaws?

---

4. Are you aware of noises in the jaw joints?
5. Do you have pain in or about the ears, temples, or cheeks?
6. Does your bite feel uncomfortable or unusual?
7. Do you have frequent headaches?
8. Have you had a recent injury to your head, neck, or jaw?

---

9. Have you previously been treated for a jaw joint problem? If so, when?

---

* With permission from McNeill, C., Mohl, N.D., Rugh, J.D., and Tanaka, T.T.: Temporomandibular disorders: Diagnosis, management, education, and research. J. Am. Dent. Assoc. *120*:253, 1990.
Note: If any one of the first three questions is answered affirmatively, the clinician should complete a comprehensive history and examination; for questions 4 through 8, two should be answered affirmatively, and for question 9, a positive answer to two other questions (4–8) is required to warrant further evaluation.

TABLE 55-27. RECOMMENDED SCREENING EXAMINATION PROCEDURES FOR TMD*

1. Measure range of motion of the mandible an opening and right and left laterotrusion.
2. Palpate for preauricular TMJ tenderness.
3. Palpate for TMJ crepitus.

---

4. Palpate for TMJ clicking.
5. Palpate for tenderness in the masseter and temporalis muscles.
6. Note excessive occlusal wear, excessive tooth mobility, fremitus, or migration in the absence of periodontal disease, and soft tissue alterations, for example, buccal mucosal ridging, lateral tongue scalloping.

---

7. Inspect symmetry and alignment of the face, jaws, and dental arches.

---

* With permission from McNeill, C., Mohl, N.D., Rugh, J.D., and Tanaka, T.T.: Temporomandibular disorders: Diagnosis, management, education, and research. J. Am. Dent. Assoc. *120*:253, 1990.
Note: Any positive finding for procedures 1 through 3 warrants consideration for a comprehensive history and examination, whereas any two positive findings for procedures 4 through 6 suggest the same consideration; procedure 7 requires two other positive findings (4–6) to suggest the same consideration.

---

diminished by rest. Joint pain is minimal on awakening. Muscle pain is cyclic, intermittent, and of variable intensity. It is often worse on awakening because of nocturnal bruxism. At other times, the patient can be pain-free.[29]

JOINT NOISE

Joint noise presents as clicking, crepitus, or both. Joint noise that is changing may herald a progressive dysfunction. Clicks or pops may be constant or related to activities such as bruxism or eating. Clicks from nocturnal bruxism occur only on awakening, whereas clicks caused by eating may signal an occlusal imbalance. Clicks associated with pain often occur with disc displacement; pain may be worse before the click and better afterward. Crepitus is considered a sign of advanced TMJ disease; it signals a perforation of the disc or its attachment.[30]

JAW MOBILITY

Jaw mobility can be limited on opening, protrusion, or lateral excursion. Average vertical (interincisal) excursion is 40 to 50 mm; rotation occurs in the first 20 to 25 mm and translation in the last 15 to 20 mm.[3,30] No deviation should occur on opening. Normal protrusion is 10 mm and lateral excursion is 10 mm.[30]

Limited opening caused by a closed lock occurs in disc displacement without reduction. The closed lock can be intermittent, progressive, or permanent. Some patients can unlock their jaws by specific jaw movements. Muscular disorders usually produce a sensation of jaw tightness rather than immobility.[30]

ASSOCIATED SYMPTOMS

Bruxism may produce tooth pain or soreness, but odontogenic factors should be eliminated first. Headaches precipitated or worsened by jaw usage suggest an extracranial cause such as TMD. Headaches secondary to disc displacement are often described as vascular, unlike the bandlike pain of muscle disorders.

An intimate anatomic relationship exists between the TMJ and the middle ear. Hence, earaches, ear stuffiness, tinnitus, and occasionally dizziness may be caused by TMJ pathology. First rule out obvious otologic sources. Myofascial trigger points in the lateral pterygoid and sternocleidomastoid can also refer pain to the ear.[31] Patients with TMD commonly have musculoskeletal symptoms in the cervical and upper back too.[2]

PSYCHOSOCIAL FACTORS

Carefully evaluate the effect of TMD symptoms on the patient's daily activities. The patient may have altered his or her diet or jaw movement, but rarely do the symptoms cause complete disruption of lifestyle without coexistent psychologic factors. Make tactful inquiries about significant life stresses, depression, narcotic or sedative use, and prior treatments for TMD.[30]

PHYSICAL EXAMINATION

Carefully evaluate the TMJ, muscles of mastication, dentition, and cervical region. The TMJ is palpated laterally in front of the ear and posteriorly through the external auditory canal (endaural palpation). Check for joint tenderness, clicks, crepitus, and range of motion. One can also auscultate the TMJ using the bell of the stethoscope as the patient slowly moves the jaw.

Check for a reciprocal click caused by disc displacement with reduction.

The TMJ is tender and the jaw deviates to the affected side before the click and returns to midline afterwards.

Check for a closed lock caused by disc displacement without reduction. Opening is limited to 35 mm or less.[32] The TMJ may be tender, and the jaw deviates to the affected side without a click. Lateral movement to the opposite side is also limited to 7 mm or less.[32] One may be able to reduce an acutely locked disc by applying downward pressure over the mandibular molars, then forward and medial traction.[33] Remember, "The joint that clicks is not locked and joint that is locked does not click."[33]

Crepitus occurs in disc displacement with perforation. The TMJ is tender and jaw opening limited.

Palpate the masticatory muscles for tenderness, spasm, and trigger points. The masseters and medial pterygoids are palpable at the lateral and medial angle of the jaw, respectively. Hook a finger under the jaw to feel the medial pterygoid or palpate it intraorally on the lingual side of the mandible. The lateral pterygoid is palpable in the vestibule posterior and superior to the maxillary tuberosity behind the third molar.[30] Almost all patients, however, report tenderness by this method.[15] A more objective, functional palpation of the lateral pterygoid is done by providing resistance as the patient opens, protrudes, or moves the jaw laterally.[15,34] Palpate the temporalis internally where it inserts on the coronoid process. Externally palpate its anterior, middle, and posterior fibers.

Evaluate the dentition for abnormal wear, mobility, tenderness, caries, malocclusion and missing teeth. Evaluate the cervical region for asymmetry, muscle hypertrophy, range of motion, crepitus, muscle spasm and tenderness. Palpate the sternocleidomastoid because it can refer pain to the TMJ and ear.[31]

DIFFERENTIAL DIAGNOSIS OF TMDS

First rule out serious or life-threatening causes of craniofacial pain. Intracranial disorders include bleeding, trauma, neoplasm, and infection. Then consider vascular disorders such as migraine, cluster headache, temporal arteritis, and toxic-metabolic or substance withdrawal headache. The neuralgic disorders include trigeminal neuralgia, glossopharyngeal neuralgia, atypical facial neuralgia, post-herpetic neuralgia and Eagle's syndrome. Also consider causalgia and reflex sympathetic dystrophy.[35] See Chapter 16 on headache.

Next consider extracranial causes of headache and facial pain. Rule out odontogenic and periodontogenic infections, inner ear disorders, sinusitis, intranasal disease, parotitis, and cervical disease.[35] Referred jaw pain from myocardial infarction must be considered too.

Disorders that affect the ability to open or close the mouth include tetanus, dystonic reactions, tumors, mandible fractures, depressed zygomatic arch fractures, scleroderma, myasthenia gravis, and Bell's palsy.[7]

Psychiatric disorders such as conversion reaction and malingering are diagnoses of exclusion.[35]

LABORATORY PROCEDURES AND IMAGING

The only emergent TMD procedure is reduction of a dislocated mandible as described earlier. Patients who present with craniofacial trauma require cervical spine radiographs and a "facial series"—submental vertex,

Townes, and Water's view. An oral surgical consultant may also require a panoramic view.

Refer patients with TMDs for further radiographic evaluation such as transcranial lateral views and tomographs.[3,20] Patients who demonstrate pathology by means of such conventional imaging techniques may require further imaging. Current advanced modalities include computed tomography (CT), magnetic resonance (MRI), arthography, and arthroscopy.[3,20,36] Videoarthrography of both upper and lower joint spaces is considered the "gold standard" of TMJ evaluation. It can evaluate the structure and function of the disc as well as joint capsule perforation and disc perforation. MRI generally produces excellent soft-tissue resolution of the TMJ and is considered by many the imaging of choice.[3] Meniscal perforations are difficult to diagnose with MRI, and a high percentage of false-positive diagnoses occurs.[3] MRI is superior to arthrography for detecting certain internal derangements and condylar avascular necrosis.[3]

Laboratory tests are limited to patients with trauma, inflammatory disorders or polyarthritic conditions.

MANAGEMENT

Initial ED treatment modalities for both muscular and joint disorders include a soft diet, ice, or moist heat applications and non-narcotic analgesics with anti-inflammatory properties. Instruct the patient to rest the jaw muscles for 3 to 4 days. The patient should try to avoid hard foods, taking large bites, clenching, bruxing, gum-chewing, and other parafunctional habits. Remind the patient to keep the teeth slightly apart in the rest position. Jaw relaxation is enhanced when the tip of the tongue gently touches the palate just behind the central incisors.[36,37] After several days, the jaw can be gently stretched by placing a finger across the mouth so that the PIP joint is between the central incisors; gradually one more finger is added.[36]

Refer the patient to an oral surgeon or general dentist with TMD expertise. Centers or clinics that specialize in TMDs use a multidisciplinary team involving dentists, oral surgeons, physicians, physical therapists and psychologists or behavioral therapists.

Further treatment may involve use of an occlusal splint, physical therapy (jaw exercises, TENS, ultrasound, myofascial release, postural training), and stress management (biofeedback, relaxation techniques, counseling).[36,37] Some patients may benefit from restorative work or orthodontics.

Surgery is a treatment option of last resort and is restricted to TMDs involving joint and not muscular disorders. TMJ arthroscopy, disc repositioning and plication, or discectomy may be surgically indicated for ID.[3,18] After a discectomy, the articular surfaces are recontoured and a temporary implant or autogenous graft can be inserted to replace the disc.[18]

Patients with severe craniofacial trauma or irreducible dislocations that require general anesthesia will require admission.

MEDICOLEGAL PEARLS

"Mandibular whiplash" is a term used by some practitioners to describe a TMJ injury from rapid acceleration-deceleration forces. During deceleration, the mandible flies open and overstretches the retrodiscal tissues and ligaments. Patients may present with neck pain and TMJ pain. With the current medicolegal climate, perhaps the evaluation of a cervical hyperextension injury should include TMJ function.

PITFALLS

Always consider more serious causes of craniofacial pain when assessing TMDs: intracranial bleeding, neoplasms, and infections as well as migraines, temporal arteritis, sinusitis, parotitis, odontogenic infections, inner ear disorders, and dystonic reactions. One should also consider myocardial infarction because the pain may be referred to the jaw.

HORIZONS

Reconstructive arthroplasty using vascularized autogenous materials to create a new disc or condylar head is considered the future trend of TMJ surgery.[18]

TMJ arthroscopy is a relatively recent imaging procedure. It can also be used to lavage and lyse joint adhesions. Complications include hematoma, infection, facial nerve injury, disc damage, and middle cranial fossa perforation.[38]

NATIONAL CONTACTS

American Dental Association
312-440-2500

American Academy of Craniomandibular Disorders
415-947-0237

American Association of Oral and Maxillofacial Surgeons
1-800-822-6637

Craniomandibular Institute
415-284-5014

REFERENCES

1. McNeill, C., Mohl, N.D., Rugh, J.D., and Tanaka, T.T.: Temporomandibular disorders: Diagnosis, management, education and research. J. Am. Dent. Assoc. 120:253, 1990.
2. Clark, G.T., Solberg, W.K., and Monteiro, A.A.: Temporomandibular disorders: New challenges in clinical management, research and teaching. In Perspectives in Temporomandibular Disorders. 1st Ed. Edited by Clark, G.T., and Solberg, W.K. Chicago, Quintessence Publishing Co., Inc., 1987.
3. Greenberg, S.A., Jacobs, J.S., and Bessette, R.W.: Temporomandibular joint dysfunction: Evaluation and treatment. Clin. Plast. Surg. 16:707, 1989.
4. Schiffman, E., and Fricton, J.R.: Epidemiology of TMJ and craniofacial pain: An unrecognized societal problem. In TMJ and Craniofacial Pain: Diagnosis and Management. 1st Ed. Edited by Fricton, J.R., Kroening, R.J., and Hathaway, K.M. St. Louis, Ishiyaku EuroAmerica Inc., 1988.
5. Bell, W.E.,: Chapter 2. Normal craniomandibular structure. In Temporomandibular Disorders: Classification, Diagnosis and Management. 3rd Ed. Chicago, Year Book Medical Publishers, Inc., 1990.
6. Dolwick, M.F., and Sanders, B.: Chapter 1. Anatomy. In TMJ Internal Derangement and Arthrosis. Anatomy. St. Louis, C.V. Mosby Co., 1985.
7. Delfino, J.J.: The temporomandibular joint. In Textbook of Practical Oral and Maxillofacial Surgery. 3rd Ed. Edited by Waite, D.E. Philadelphia, Lea & Febiger, 1987.
8. Friedman, M.H., Weisberg, J., and Nathan, H.: Anatomy and function of the temporomandibular joint (TMJ). In Temporomandibular Joint Disorders. Diagnosis and Treatment. 1st Ed. Edited by Friedman, M.H., Weisberg, J., Nathan, H., and Agus, B. Chicago, Quintessence Publishing Co. Inc., 1985.
9. Ogus, H.D., and Toller, P.A.: Common Disorders of the Temporomandibular Joint. 2nd Ed. Bristol, J. Wright & Sons, Ltd., 1986.
10. Bell, W.E.: Chapter 3. Normal craniomandibular function. In Temporomandibular Disorders: Classification, Diagnosis, and Management. 3rd Ed. Chicago, Year Book Medical Publishers, Inc., 1990.
11. Ramer, E.: Controversies in temporomandibular joint disorders: Dent. Clin. North Am. 34:125, 1990.
12. Schellhas, K.P.: Temporomandibular joint injuries. Radiology 173:211, 1990.
13. Ware, W.H.: Clinical presentation. In Internal Derangements of the Temporomandibular Joint. 1st Ed. Edited by Helms, C.A., Katzberg, R.W., and Dolwick, M.F. San Francisco, Radiology Research and Education Foundation, 1983.
14. Fricton, J.R., Kroening, R.J., and Haley, D.: Muscular disorders: The most common diagnosis. In TMJ and Craniofacial Pain: Diagnosis, and Management. 1st Ed. Edited by Fricton, J.R., Kroening, R.J., and Hathaway, K.M. St. Louis, Ishiyaku EuroAmerica, Inc., 1988.
15. Bell, W.E.: Chapter 9. Masticatory muscle disorders. In Temporomandibular Disorders: Classification, Diagnosis, and Management. 3rd Ed. Chicago, Year Book Medical Publishers, Inc., 1990.
16. Bavitz, J.B., and Chewning, L.C.: Malignant disease as temporomandibular joint dysfunction: Review of the literature and report of case. J. Am. Dent. Assoc. 120:163, 1990.
17. Dolwick, M.F., and Sanders, B.: Chapter 2. Pathology. In TMJ Internal Derangement and Arthrosis. St. Louis, C.V. Mosby, Co., 1985.
18. Dolwick, M.F.: Management of temporomandibular disorders. In Contemporary Oral and Maxillofacial Surgery. 1st Ed. Edited by Peterson, L.J., Ellis, E., Hupp, J.R., and Tucker, M.R. St. Louis, C.V. Mosby Co., 1988.
19. Hansson, T.L.: Temporomandibular joint anatomical findings relevant to the clinician. In Perspectives in Temporomandibular Disorders. 1st Ed. Edited by Clark, G.T., and Solberg, W.K. Chicago, Quintessence Publishing Co., Inc., 1987.
20. Murphy, W.A.: Temporomandibular joint. In Bone and Joint Imaging. 1st Ed. Edited by Resnick, D. Philadelphia, W.B. Saunders Co., 1989.
21. Norman, J.E. de B., and Bramley, P.: Chapter 4. Medical diseases. In Textbook and Color Atlas of the Temporomandibular Joint. Diseases, Disorders, Surgery. Chicago, Year Book Medical Publishers, Inc., 1990.
22. Vamvas, S.J.: Differential diagnosis of TMJ disease. In Diseases of the Temporomandibular Apparatus. A Multi-Disciplinary Approach. 2nd Ed. Edited by Morgan, D.H., House, L.R., Hall, W.P., and Vamvas, S.J. St. Louis, C.V. Mosby Co., 1982.
23. Bell, W.E.: Chapter 11. Inflammatory disorders. In Temporomandibular Disorders. Classification, Diagnosis, Management. 3rd Ed. Chicago, Year Book Publishers, Inc., 1990.
24. El-Sabbagh, A.M., and Kamel, M.: Avascular necrosis of temporomandibular joint in sickle cell disease. Clin. Rheumatol. 8:393, 1989.
25. Bell, W.E.: Chapter 12. Chronic hypomobility and growth disorders. In Temporomandibular Disorders. Classification, Diagnosis, Management. 3rd Ed. Chicago, Year Book Medical Publishers, Inc., 1990.
26. Norman, J.E. de B., Bramley, P.: Chapter 12. Unusual Surgical Disease and Disorders. In Textbook and Color Atlas of the Temporomandibular Joint. Diseases, Disorders, Surgery. Chicago, Year Book Medical Publishers, Inc., 1990.
27. Lader, E.: Lyme disease misdiagnosed as a temporomandibular joint disorder. J. Prosthet. Dent. 63:82, 1990.
28. Luyk, N.H., and Larsen, P.E.: The diagnosis and treatment of the dislocated mandible. Am. J. Emerg. Med. 7:329, 1989.
29. Awang, M.N.: A new approach to the reduction of acute dislocation of the temporomandibular joint: a report of three cases. Br. J. Oral Maxillofac. Surg. 25:244, 1987.
30. Dolwick, M.F., and Sanders, B.: Chapter 3. Diagnosis. In TMJ Internal Derangement and Arthrosis. St. Louis, C.V. Mosby Co., 1985.
31. Kroening, R.: Neural blockade in the differential diagnosis of craniofacial pain. In Perspectives in Temporomandibular Disorders. 1st Ed. Edited by Clark, G.T., and Solberg, W.K. Chicago, Quintessence Publishing Co., Inc., 1987.
32. Schiffman, E.L., Fricton, J.R., Haley, D.P., and Shapiro, B.L.: The prevalence and treatment needs of subjects with temporomandibular disorders. J. Am. Dent. Assoc. 120:295, 1990.
33. McCarty, W.: Diagnosis and treatment of internal derangements of the articular disc and mandibular condyle. In Temporomandibular Joint Problems. Biologic Diagnosis and Treatment. Chicago, Quintessence Publishing Co., Inc., 1980.
34. Fricton, J.R., Bromaghim, C., and Kroening, R.J.: Physician evaluation: The need of a standardized examination. In TMJ and Craniofacial Pain: Diagnosis and Management. 1st Ed. Edited by Fricton, J.R., Kroening, R.J., and Hathaway, K.M. St. Louis, Ishiyaku EuroAmerica, Inc., 1988.
35. Fricton, J.R., Kroening, R.J., and Schellhas, K.P.: Differential diagnosis: The physical disorders. In TMJ and Craniofacial Pain: Diagnosis and 1st Ed. Edited by Fricton, J.R., Kroening, R.J., and Hathaway, K.M. St. Louis, Ishiyaku EuroAmerica, Inc., 1988.
36. Fricton, J.R., Kroening, R.J., Braun, B.L., et al.: Joint disorders: Derangements and degeneration. In TMJ and Craniofacial Pain: Diagnosis and Management. 1st Ed. Edited by Fricton, J.R., Kroening, R.J., and Hathaway, K.M. St. Louis, Ishiyaku EuroAmerica, Inc., 1988.
37. Hertling, D.: The temporomandibular joint. In Management of Common Musculoskeletal Disorders. 2nd Ed. Edited by Hertling, D., and Kessler, R.M. Philadelphia, J.B. Lippincott, 1990.
38. Forman, D.: Success with temporomandibular joint arthroscopic surgery. Dent. Clin. North Am. 34:135. 1990.

SECTION THREE: DENTAL AND PERIODONTAL EMERGENCIES

ODONTOGENIC PAIN

Bruce R. Rothwell

"For there was never yet philosopher that could bear the toothache patiently"

William Shakespeare
Much Ado About Nothing

CAPSULE

Pain of dental origin is one of the more common predicaments confronting patients and emergency care providers alike. Despite significant advances in preventive and restorative dental care, toothaches and more advanced dental problems continue to be an urgent treatment need for many people. Although most individuals seek attention from dentists when pain originates in the oral region, many obtain care through emergency medical care facilities. In addition to the relatively straightforward diagnosis and short-term management of the uncomplicated toothache, orofacial pain may indicate more serious underlying maladies. A differential diagnosis of other varieties of orofacial pain syndromes must be considered in the workup of odontogenic pain.

Most simple toothaches without infection or involvement of other oral structures can be managed by elementary measures to alleviate pain until more definitive dental care can be obtained. Hospitals or other emergency care facilities with dental support can arrange to provide timely dental diagnosis and treatment even for relatively complex situations. Individuals performing triage operations in the emergency room may need to separate patients requiring immediate care from those in whom a delay in extensive treatment does not pose a problem. Odontogenic pain may be referred to regions distant from the site of the affliction and may mimic a number of other conditions including sinusitis, neuralgias, and arthritis. In addition, in many cases, pain appearing to emanate from the sinuses, the temporomandibular point, or other facial structures may in fact be of dental origin. Thus appropriate history, examination, and diagnosis are essential for proper management.

INTRODUCTION

Despite significant reductions in the prevalence of dental diseases in the U.S., pain of dental origin continues to be a presenting complaint of many patients contacting emergency treatment facilities. With the changing frequency of dental disease, there has been a shift in the demographics of those most likely affected.[1] Dental problems are now more common in lower socioeconomic groups and those less likely to receive regular dental care. These people are also more likely to seek only episodic medical care and go to emergency facilities for acute dental problems.

Although most oral diseases are chronic, with little associated discomfort, some situations produce acute, severe pain. This pain may follow carious destruction of dental tissues, involvement of pulpal tissue resulting in periapical abscesses, or periodontal infections. Most of these conditions are lumped into the "toothache" category. Other, less dentally-oriented ailments can result in orofacial pain. These include dentoalveolar trauma, bacterial and viral infections of soft tissues, neuralgias of facial nerves, sinusitis, and temporomandibular disorders. Sometimes dental pain can result directly or indirectly from dental treatment. Recently placed dental restorations can cause mild to severe discomfort, and older fillings can deteriorate to a state in which teeth become painful. Teeth with large fillings can lose structural integrity after repeated masticatory stress and become cracked, with or without displacement of the broken fragment, and often with pain on biting.

Toothaches are often baffling in behavior. Teeth are visceral structures with sensory capabilities similar to those of other visceral organs. Dental pulps are individual, separate organs with discrete connections to the neural system. Pain of dental origin can occur acutely with little or no forewarning, or can be a chronic condition with either increasing severity or diminishing tolerance on the part of the sufferer. Truly acute problems are less common and can result from fractured teeth, pulp exposures, or infectious processes that impact vital structures. More commonly, there is some portent of an affliction with mild or intermittent discomfort that, when ignored, later develops into more intense distress. Although the result may seem similar, there is often considerable difference in the extent and progress of the underlying disease process.

For many reasons, some people do not seek timely and regular dental care. Although monetary considerations may prevent some individuals from receiving regular dental treatment, it is more likely that anxiety and fear are the underlying obstacle. Because apprehension keeps some people from developing a care relationship with a dentist, developing problems may propel them to seek care from a hospital emergency department (ED). In addition, the underlying anxieties often dissuade some people from seeing a dentist during regular office hours, and they then present to an ED at night or in the early morning.

Management of odontogenic pain can vary from definitive treatment to simple pain relief. Depending on the nature of the presenting situation and the availability of dental services, a treatment decision can be formulated as to the extent of management. In most cases of uncomplicated toothaches, relief of pain with analgesics or local anesthetics allows a patient to seek more definitive dental therapy later. When infections are present, particularly those involving vital structures of fascial spaces, more definitive treatment is necessary, along with appropriate antibiotics.

PATHOPHYSIOLOGY AND ANATOMY

ORAL ANATOMY AND TERMINOLOGY

Teeth and the immediately adjacent supporting soft tissues and bone are most likely to be the affected structures in painful processes. Teeth are comprised of enamel, dentin, and cementum, and contain neural and vascular elements in the pulpal tissue. Teeth are embedded in the alveolar bone, attached and supported by periodontal soft tissues. Connection between root surfaces and bone is effected through periodontal ligament fibers. The five exposed surfaces of the teeth are referred to as buccal or facial (lateral), mesial (anterior), distal, lingual, or palatal (medial), and occlusal (the top biting surface) (Fig. 55-40).

There are generally 20 teeth in the deciduous dentition and up to 32 adult teeth, although third molars (wisdom teeth) are often missing because of previous extraction or lack of eruption. The deciduous teeth erupt between the ages of 6 months and 2½ years,

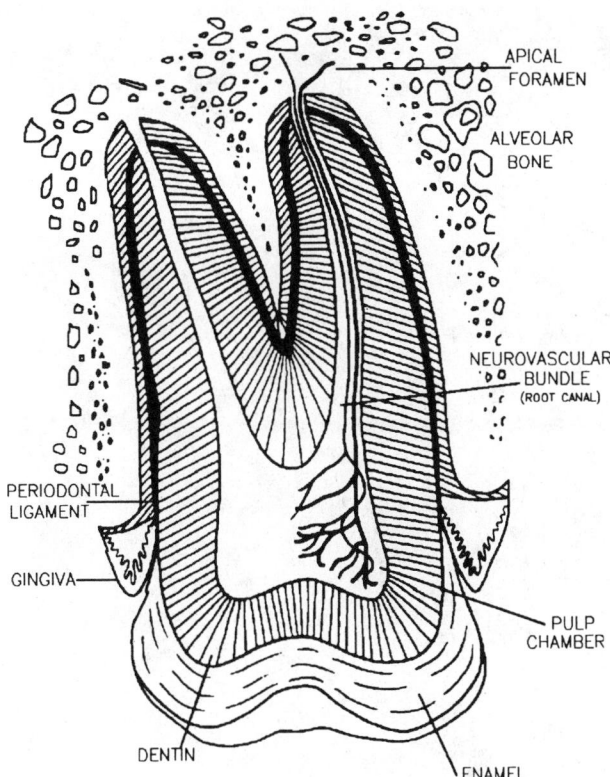

FIG. 55-40.   Tooth anatomy, sagittal section.

and the permanent teeth begin to erupt around age 6. The oral cavity can be divided into four parts and referred to by quadrant designations such as upper right (UR) or lower left (LL). The permanent dentition is commonly designated by a 1 to 32 numbering system, beginning with number 1 in the maxillary right posterior (third molar) and moving sequentially in a clockwise direction to the maxillary left (No. 16), mandibular left (No. 17), and back to mandibular left posterior (No. 32) (Fig. 55-41).

DENTAL CARIES

Although reduced considerably in prevalence, caries continues to be one of the most common afflictions of the oral cavity. Dental caries is caused by bacteria, which produce substances that destroy mineralized tooth structures and can ultimately result in infections of pulpal tissues. It is often an asymptomatic process because enamel is not innervated, and involvement of the dentin may be only mildly and intermittently painful. The development of dental caries is a lengthy course, commonly extending over months or years. This chronic process can become acutely painful when the decay involves extensive amounts of dentin or invades the pulpal tissue.

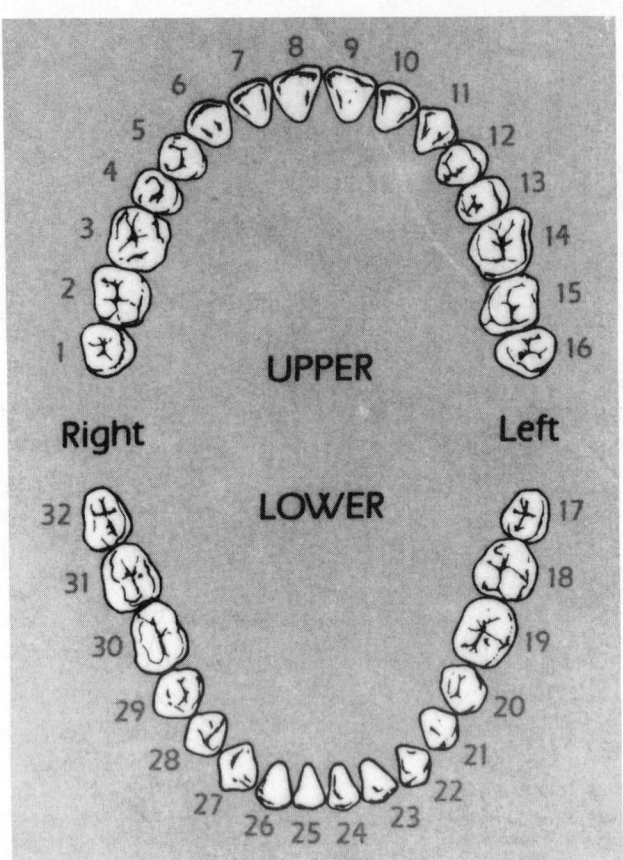

FIG. 55-41. Normal adult dentition with full complement of 32 teeth.

Although caries can occur insidiously, it is more likely to be a result of long-term dental neglect. Most cases of dental pain involve extensive carious destruction of several teeth. Caries often undermines existing dental restorations, with resultant fracture of the teeth or displacement of the filling material. Carious exposure of dental pulp can lead to intense toothaches and eventually to bacterial infection of pulp and periapical tissues.

INFLAMMATORY CONDITIONS

Many conditions that can result in orofacial pain may appear to originate in the dental structures. Most are infectious or inflammatory conditions involving the periodontal structures. Gingivitis is inflammation of the gingival tissues immediately adjacent to the teeth, and periodontitis is the extension of that inflammation to the periodontium and alveolar supporting bone. These are often painless processes and thus will not often be confused with odontogenic pain, but some acute varieties (e.g., necrotizing ulcerative gingivitis) produce symptoms not unlike simple tooth pain. In patients with dental neglect, caries, periodontal disease, and other conditions exist concurrently, and it may be difficult to sort out the primary cause of the acute complaints.

Extension of the process of caries or exposure of pulpal tissues by other means produces inflammation of the neurovascular tissues of the dental pulp. Pulpitis can be confined to the tooth or extend to affect the periapical tissues at the end of the root. Most of what is commonly referred to as "dental abscess" is a result of pulpitis or other periapical pathology.

These conditions are covered in more detail in other chapters.

THE UNCOMPLICATED TOOTHACHE

One of the early decisions that must be made in managing a patient with pain of apparent dental origin is the assessment of the level of involvement and extent of the process. Clearly, most "toothaches" are not serious problems, but extension of infections to fascial spaces of the head and neck or dentoalveolar trauma are situations that require expeditious management.[2] Pain originating from the teeth, usually as a result of caries, without involvement of other structures or systemic reaction, may be classed as an uncomplicated toothache and managed accordingly.

These uncomplicated situations are not accompanied by fever, swelling, lymphadenopathy, or other signs of infection. In addition, traumatic avulsion of teeth and fractures are not present in the history. The cause is usually readily apparent and limited to the dental structures. Caries is the usual underlying process, with production of varying degrees of pulpal inflammation (pulpitis). Reversible pulpitis produces dental pain of short duration on specific stimuli such as cold, heat, or percussion. Irreversible pulpitis produces pain produced by specific provocation or no exact cause, and the painful episode often extends well beyond the inciting event. Irreversible pulpitis often awakens people from sleep or may keep them from sleeping. It is not uncommon for an individual suffering from a toothache to present to an ED in the early morning hours after unsuccessful attempts to sleep.

Dental pain may also result from previously placed dental restorations that have become defective. This process usually involves a course of slowly developing, slowly increasing pain on chewing hot, cold, or sweet foods. It may be something as overt as a large filling that has fallen out or a crown or bridge that has become dislodged. Defective restorations that are not dealt with expeditiously often develop caries around the leaking or open margins of the restorations. Longstanding fillings that are reported as having "fallen out" are frequently associated with grossly carious teeth.

Recently placed dental restorations may also become acutely painful. Most restorative materials are dental pulp irritants, good thermal conductors, or both. It is relatively common for people to have increased hot/cold sensitivity following the placement of amalgams or gold alloy crowns, and many dentists advise patients of this possibility. Generally, this tenderness is relatively minor and usually resolves over a few weeks. More prolonged or intense pain could indicate irreversible pulpal distress.

Trauma often causes dental pain, either immediately after the injury or as a delayed phenomena. Generally, the history of an injury is clear, but it may not be readily apparent to the practitioner, particularly if time has elapsed. Even patients with no clear history of trauma to the dentition can present with dental pain from injuries to the teeth. Posterior teeth with pre-existing restorations are particularly prone to the "cracked tooth syndrome," in which repeated occlusal forces have caused a cusp to become incompletely fractured from the body of the tooth. Continuing occlusal forces produce pain in the tooth on chewing or percussion. This condition is particularly difficult to diagnose because there is often no clinical or radiographic evidence of the incomplete fracture. Patients may experience several weeks of discomfort before the fragment is finally dislodged from the remainder of the tooth. Somewhat paradoxically, the associated pain is often diminished at that point.

CLINICAL PRESENTATION AND EXAMINATION

HISTORY

A pertinent medical history should be obtained from patients with dental complaints, particularly regarding allergies, current medications, medical problems, and difficulties with dental treatment. The history of the chief complaint should include a description of the nature, severity, and character of the pain. The location of the painful area and factors (hot, cold, percussion) that elicit the distress should be obtained along with the duration after removal of the stimulus. A history of any recent dental care, particularly in the same region as the current complaints, should be ascertained.

PHYSICAL EXAMINATION

For even apparently routine toothaches, standard vital signs of pulse, blood pressure, and temperature should be obtained. Although most dental complaints are localized phenomena, infectious processes may produce fever, and patients with more complicated oral abnormalities may have diminished water intake and resultant fluid imbalances.

Before the intraoral examination, particular extraoral and facial structures should be examined and palpated. Because most oral structures are drained by lymph node chains in the neck, the sublingual, submental, anterior cervical, and preauricular lymphatics

should be palpated to distinguish inflammatory enlargement or soreness. In addition, facial structures should be inspected for localized swelling, comparing both sides for alterations in symmetry. Percussion and palpation can be carried out over the maxillary and frontal sinuses to help rule out involvement of these structures. As pain related to tooth pain is often referred to the preauricular region, the temporomandibular joint (TMJ) and surrounding structures should be palpated for associated manifestations to aid in the differentiation of the source. Even toothaches with pain radiating to the TMJ should not generally produce pain on palpation directly over the joint region.

After the extraoral examination, intraoral structures can be examined by visual inspection, palpation, and percussion methods. Soft tissues are generally examined before the periodontium and teeth, with particular regard for swellings, erythema, and alterations in normal anatomy. The oral mucosa consists of three general types: the masticatory mucosa covering the hard palate and gingiva, the lining mucosa of the lips and cheeks, and the specialized mucosa covering the dorsum of the tongue.[3] All tissues are normally various shades of pink, from the coral pink of the gingiva to the more vermilion hue of the lining mucosa. Intense erythema of the mucosa generally indicates local or underlying inflammation. Inflammation of the periodontium, particularly the gingiva immediately adjacent to the teeth, is usually readily apparent with moderate to intense erythema. If available, periodontal probes can be used to scrutinize the gingival sulcus.

After the mucosal and periodontal examination, the dentition can be examined visually along with percussion, palpation, and other tests. Individual teeth should be examined for obvious carious lesions, fractures, defective restorations, or cracks. If the pain can be localized to a specific quadrant, closer attention can be paid to those teeth, with percussion of each tooth to elicit the offending site. The blunt end of a small instrument, such as a dental mirror, can be used to tap on the occlusal (biting) surface of each tooth. About 80% of the teeth with painful pulpitis will react positively to percussion.[4] If an intraoral, high-intensity fiber optic light source is available, teeth can be transilluminated to check for cracks, and interproximal carious lesions. In many cases, application of heat or cold to teeth can elicit temperature-dependent symptoms. Cold applied to individual teeth is a relatively simple diagnostic aid for many forms of pulpitis. Cold testing can be done by using small chips of ice or cotton rolls sprayed with ethyl chloride. Although some toothaches are relieved by cold, most are aggravated by direct application of ice, allowing localization of the problem. Dentists often use an electric pulp tester to determine the vitality of individual teeth, but this instrument may not be available to the physician in the ED. Teeth with inflamed periapical regions are often tender on biting. It is also possible for traumatic occlusion to be the underlying cause for odontogenic pain when a tooth in premature contact produces acute or chronic damage to the adjacent periapical tissues and resultant pain. Thus, an examination of the occlusion often elicits at least the region of involvement.

Radiographs are valuable diagnostic tools to determine the cause of odontogenic pain. Although it is possible to have pain emanating from a tooth without demonstrable changes on radiography, more commonly the underlying cause is readily apparent. Intraoral periapical films are the best method of imaging individual teeth and surrounding periodontium. If these are not available in the ED, extraoral films can be used instead. Panoramic radiographs depict a broad overview of the jaws, dentition, and TMJs, and are a good screening tool. If no "dental" radiographs are accessible, traditional plane films of the jaws such as right and left lateral jaw surveys can be used to evaluate for gross problems. The resolution and detail of extraoral films, particularly lateral jaw radiographs, is not sufficient to determine subtle periapical or dental changes.

Although many cases of odontogenic pain have obvious causes, in some situations the origin is difficult to discern. Pain of high intensity may result even when the changes on diagnostic tests are subtle and inconclusive. The final diagnosis may be elusive when the patient first presents, and palliative measures should be used until more definitive conclusions can be reached later.

DIFFERENTIAL DIAGNOSIS

When pain is suspected to be originating from the dentition, other sources must be considered in the differential diagnosis (Table 55-28), for structures both in and out of the oral cavity. The enigmatic behavior and variable nature of dental pain makes the precise diagnosis troublesome. As Bell characterizes the analysis of dental pain, "The extreme variability of toothache is such that a good rule for any examiner is to consider all pains about the mouth and face to be of dental origin until proved otherwise."[5]

TABLE 55-28. DIFFERENTIAL DIAGNOSIS— DENTAL DISORDERS

- Pulpitis (reversible or irreversible)
- Periapical inflammation or pathosis (abscess)
- Cracked tooth syndrome
- Traumatic occlusion
- Post-treatment situations (iatrogenic causes)
- Acute gingivitis e.g. ANUG
- Periodontal abscess
- Fractured tooth (acute traumatic episode)

There are, however, some common characteristics of all dental pain. The discomfort is described most frequently as a dull aching, often throbbing sensation with paroxysms of lancinating pain. Because pain arising from the dental pulp is poorly localized, it is frequently difficult to discern which arch is involved, let alone which particular tooth. There is considerable variation in the relationship between the stimulus and the severity of the pain, both between groups and in the same individual. As indicated previously, percussion, biting, and thermal factors often provoke responses, but the initiation can also be spontaneous.

Involvement of the periodontal structures is more likely to manifest pain that is more readily localized. Thus pulpal conditions that have extended to the periapical tissues are more easily delineated, which often makes the diagnosis of early pulpal inflammation difficult.

In formulating a differential diagnosis for suspected odontogenic pain, an inventory of dental conditions is reasonably prudent as a first step. Pulpitis, either reversible or irreversible, is by far the most common underlying cause of pain emanating from the dentition, and pulpal involvement that has spread to the surrounding periapical tissues is next in probability. Cracked teeth or defective restorations are less common and generally less intensely painful, and may be the result of recurrent caries. Teeth that are in premature contact may become tender, and recent dental care that has caused either pulpitis or occlusal trauma often causes localized tooth pain. Other, less common conditions such as acute necrotizing ulcerative gingivitis (ANUG), periodontal abscess, or acute trauma are unlikely to be confused with other dental conditions.

Other nondental situations (Table 55-29) can produce pain that may appear to be of dental origin. Although they are far less common than odontogenic ailments in causing facial and perioral pain, they must be considered in situations in which the cause is not apparent. Teeth can become tender from pharyngeal or nasal inflammations, and maxillary sinusitis often causes teeth in an entire quandrant to be tender on percussion or biting.

Temporomandibular disorders (TMD) and myofascial pain dysfunction syndromes (MPD) will often mimic tooth pain, particularly when the masseter or temporalis muscles are involved. Additionally, toothache pain is often referred to the ear or preauricular region on the same side. There are several reports of cardiac pain referred to the jaws, particularly the mandible, that may mimic dental pain.[6,7] Conditions such as trigeminal neuralgia and other neuritis states often produce facial pain that closely mimics tooth pain. Less common antecedents for toothache-like pain include local malignancies, Herpes zoster exacerbations, elongated styloid process (Eagle syndrome)[8] and distant malignancies such as leukemias and lymphomas.[9] Several other unrelated ailments can cause pain of this sort.

PROCEDURES

Simple diagnostic maneuvers can be used to define the diagnosis of pain arising in the dentition. As previously indicated, the dental examination (Table 55-30) begins with the history, vital signs, and evaluation of extraoral structures. After assessment of any facial swelling, lymphadenopathy, or TMJ involvement, the attention can move to the intraoral structures, including soft tissues and teeth. Any swelling, erythema, purulent exudate, or altered form in the mucosa or gingiva should be noted, and the gingival sulcus area can be investigated with periodontal probes for pocketing. Gross caries or fractured teeth are generally immediately apparent on visual examination, but other conditions may be more subtle. If the patient can localize the pain to a particular area, percussion of the teeth in that quandrant will help to clarify the specific site. If available, transillumination can be used to scrutinize teeth for caries or cracks. The application of ice or ethyl chloride helps to determine teeth with pulpitis. Occlusal prematurities may be distinguished by palpation of individual teeth during biting.

Radiographs are extremely helpful in the analysis of dental problems, in the investigation of both coronal caries and periapical involvement. Carious destruction is visualized as a radiolucency in the relatively opaque enamel and dentin. Periapical involvement may not produce any apparent changes in surrounding bone in early stages, but later exhibits discrete or diffuse radiolucencies of alveolar bone. Intraoral dental films (periapical, bite-wing) render the greatest detail of dental structures, but may not be available to hospital EDs. Extraoral films such as panoramic or lateral jaw films are more readily available, but do not provide the fine detail often necessary for accurate diagnosis of subtle problems.

INITIAL STABILIZATION AND MANAGEMENT

TOOTHACHE

In providing treatment for dental pain, it is important to determine the extent of involvement and whether or not other orofacial structures are involved. For the purposes of this section, it is assumed that the main goal will be the relief of pain in the uncomplicated toothache (Table 55-31). Because other situations produce pain that may simulate tooth pain, it is important to establish that the problem in question is indeed a simple toothache (Table 55-32). Odontogenic pain is

TABLE 55-29. NONDENTAL ORIGINS FOR FACIAL PAIN

- Temporomandibular disorders (TMD)
- Myofascial pain dysfunction (MPD)
- Neuralgia/neuritis
- Sinus, pharyngeal, nasal inflammation
- Herpetic infections
- Headaches, migraines
- Salivary gland disorders
- Malignancies

TABLE 55-30. DENTAL EXAMINATION

- History, vital signs
- Extraoral examination
- Exam of mucosa, gingiva
- Visual inspection of teeth
- Percussion
- Transillumination
- Thermal tests, occlusion
- Radiographs

usually sharp or dull, with throbbing intensity localized to the jaws. There is often an obvious dental problem (caries, lost restoration, etc.), but usually no facial swelling, lymphadenopathy, or fever. Likewise, the intraoral inspection does not reveal any soft tissue masses or purulent exudates. Involved teeth are likely to be sensitive to percussion and thermal (particularly cold) tests. Radiographs, if available, do not demonstrate any large radiolucent periapical lesions.

PAIN RELIEF

Although it really has no effect on the underlying dental causes, the immediate management goal in these situations is relief of pain. It is not reasonable to expect a patient presenting to an emergency medical facility to receive definitive treatment of dental problems, even if a dentist is available. Attention is therefore directed to short-term pain management.

Probably the safest and most effective way to provide pain relief for an isolated dental problem is the provision of local anesthetic nerve blocks. With longer-duration anesthetics, patients can receive 4 to 12 hours of pain relief in a segment of the dentoalveolar process. Local anesthetics generally allow effective pain relief without the side effects and abuse potential of narcotic analgesics. The newer extended-duration local anesthetics such as bupivacaine and etidocaine are particularly useful to afford overnight pain relief for patients until they can seek care from a dentist the next day.

TABLE 55-31. DIAGNOSIS AND MANAGEMENT OF SIMPLE TOOTHACHE

	Reversible Pulpitis	Irreversible Pulpitis	Apical Abscess
Cause	Mild trauma, e.g., small blow to tooth Exposed dentin, recent dental treatment Smaller areas of caries	Moderate to severe trauma Deep caries—near pulp Recent dental treatment	Deep caries/pulp exposure Necrotic pulp
History/Complaint	Sharp, sometimes throbbing pain Short duration, always with stimulus Thermal incitement common	Sharp or dull throbbing pain Longer duration (seconds to minutes) Induced by stimulus or spontaneous	Dull, possibly throbbing pain Spontaneous/intermittent pain Pain on chewing, percussion
Typical examination findings	Dental caries Chipped tooth Cold air sensitive—short duration	Deep dental caries Deep restorations Sensitive to cold—beyond stimulus	Caries, recent dental treatment, trauma Percussion sensitive Localized swelling/adenopathy
Immediate treatment	Mild to moderate analgesics Local anesthetics Refer to dentist Sedative/temporary fillings	Dental consultation Moderate to strong analgesia Long-acting local anesthetics Definitive dental treatment	Dental consultation Moderate analgesics Antibiotics e.g., penicillin Immediate treatment if T > 39, facial swelling Incision/drainage, fluids, IV Ab

TABLE 55-32. SIMPLE TOOTHACHES

- Dull, throbbing pain
- Afebrile
- No lymphadenopathy
- No swellings
- Percussion sensitive
- Thermal sensitive
- Negative radiographs

Oral analgesics are a mainstay for pain relief in dental patients either in place of, or as a complement to, local anesthesia. Tooth-related pain can be categorized as mild, moderate, or severe, and distinct analgesics or combinations prescribed for pain relief. Orofacial pain appears to respond differently to oral analgesics, based upon the underlying cause. Acute pain of surgical or traumatic origin responds well to nonsteroidal anti-inflammatory drugs (NSAIDs), particularly when a loading dose is available. Toothaches of longer duration, however, appear not to be well relieved by NSAIDs and often require more potent narcotic analgesics. Tooth pain originates either in the dentin or from inflammation of pulpal tissues.[10] Typically, dental pain can be managed at the peripheral inflammatory source, the site of pain perception in the CNS, or both. Combinations of narcotics that act centrally to obtund the perception of pain and prostaglandin-inhibiting analgesics to manage the peripheral inflammatory pain are generally quite effective.

For mild pain, simple oral analgesics such as aspirin, 600 mg or one of the NSAIDs such as ibuprofen, 200 to 400 mg are effective for adults. For those in whom a NSAID or aspirin is inappropriate, acetaminophen 600 to 1000 mg is a reasonable alternative.

Management of moderate dental pain generally requires combination drugs for effective analgesia. For surgical pain, NSAIDs such as ibuprofen 600 to 800 mg are effective, particularly with a loading dose and regular administration. Combinations of codeine and either aspirin or acetaminophen have a long-term track record of effectiveness in the management of dental pain. These combinations allow pain to be attacked both centrally and peripherally with smaller doses of each component, but encompass some of the undesirable narcotic side effects. In addition to codeine, oxycodone provides equally effective pain relief in combination with either aspirin or acetaminophen. For both types of pain, extremely effective pain relief can be obtained with local anesthetic blocks using longer-duration drugs such as bupivacaine or etidocaine.

Most dental pain is not of the severe variety, and more potent narcotic analgesics are rarely necessary. Local anesthetics are also effective in this category, and allow time to acquire appropriate dental care. Higher doses or more frequent doses of the codeine or oxycodone combinations may be effective to manage pain of the severe type. Because of the side effects and abuse potential, stronger opioid narcotics should be used with care.[11] Oral drugs such as methadone 10 mg or hydromorphone 2 mg are effective for the short-term management of severe pain. In a small

TABLE 55-33. ANALGESIC CHOICES FOR DENTAL PAIN

	Mild Pain	Moderate Pain	Severe Pain
Toothache pain	ASA 600 mg q6h Acetaminophen 600–1000 mg q4h Ibuprofen 200–400 mg q6h	ASA 300 mg/codeine 30 mg q4h Acetominophen 300 mg/codeine 30 mg q4h Oxycodone 5 mg/ASA or Acetaminophen	ASA 600 mg/codeine 60–90 mg Acetaminophen 600–1000/codeine Hydromorphone HCl 2 mg q4h Local anesthesia (bupivacaine or etidocoine)
Surgical pain	Ibuprofen 200–600 mg q6h ASA 600 mg q6h Acetaminophen 600–1000 mg q4h	Local anesthesia (bupivacaine or etidocoine) Ibuprofen 600–800 mg q4h ASA/codeine or Acetaminophen/codeine ASA/oxycodone or acetaminophen/codeine	ASA or acetominophen/codeine 60–90 mg Ibuprofen 600–800 mg +/− codeine Hydromorphone HCl 2 mg q4h Local anesthesia (bupivacaine or etidocoine)

number of situations, truly severe pain and anxiety unrelieved by oral medications may require administration of parenteral narcotics such as meperidine or morphine (Table 55-33).

The use of antibiotics should be limited to specific situations when there is a clear ongoing infectious process. The presence of swelling, lymphadenopathy, fever, or other similar signs often indicates an infectious process that has spread beyond the confines of the tooth. If a culture is not available, penicillin remains the first-choice antibiotic in minimum adult doses of 500 mg four times a day for 7 to 10 days. Erythromycin is the typical alternative for penicillin-allergic patients, and first-generation cephalosporins may be another alternative in selected patients. Antibiotics directed specifically at coagulase-positive *staphylococcus* are not useful in most dental infections and are definitely not the antibiotic of choice in these situations. Somewhat contrary to the clear indications for antibiotics listed, clinical experience has shown that penicillin or similar antibiotics seem to be helpful in relieving the pain associated with early periapical pathosis without other signs of infection.

Aside from the pharmacologic methods to deal with simple dental problems, there are productive local temporary treatment measures for the relief of pain. Eugenol in one form or another has been used for centuries to relieve toothaches. Eugenol is the essential ingredient in oil of cloves, and many over-the-counter toothache remedies have similar constituents that can be applied topically. Patients should be cautioned never to apply aspirin to oral tissues because it is extremely caustic to mucosa and gingiva.[12] Local anesthetics such as benzocaine, 20% or lidocaine, 2 to 5% are available as gels that can be applied topically to oral tissues. They are not particularly effective in tooth-related pain, but may provide temporary amelioration of mucosal irritations.

Carious lesions or defective or missing fillings can be temporarily restored and/or exposed dentin cov-

ered with a variety of sedative filling materials. Zinc oxide/eugenol preparations provide antiseptic qualities along with adequate sealing and thermal insulation.[13] Loose debris can be removed with gentle irrigation or cotton swabs and the opening dried. The filling material is then mixed and condensed into the cavity with a small instrument[14] (Fig. 55-42). In many cases, fractured cusps or large missing fillings cannot be restored simply because of a lack of retention for the temporary filling material.

Depending on the extent of involvement of dental services with the emergency medical facility, it may be more prudent to consult a dentist early in the diagnosis and treatment phases. If dentists are less directly available to the ED, a triage mechanism should be developed regarding situations in which dental consultation is absolutely necessary. A dentist or oral and maxillofacial surgeon should be involved in dentoalveolar trauma and avulsed teeth, orofacial or through-and-through lacerations, facial swellings from odontogenic infections, and other moderate to severe oral infections. Many simple dental problems and uncomplicated toothaches can be adequately managed in the short term by emergency medical personnel until the patient can be seen by a dentist for definitive care.

PITFALLS

DIAGNOSIS

The main determinant of ultimate management of apparent odontogenic pain in the emergency medical setting is the origin of the pain and extent of involvement. For uncomplicated toothache, relatively short-term pain relief is the goal of treatment. One should take care to ensure that the pain is ema-

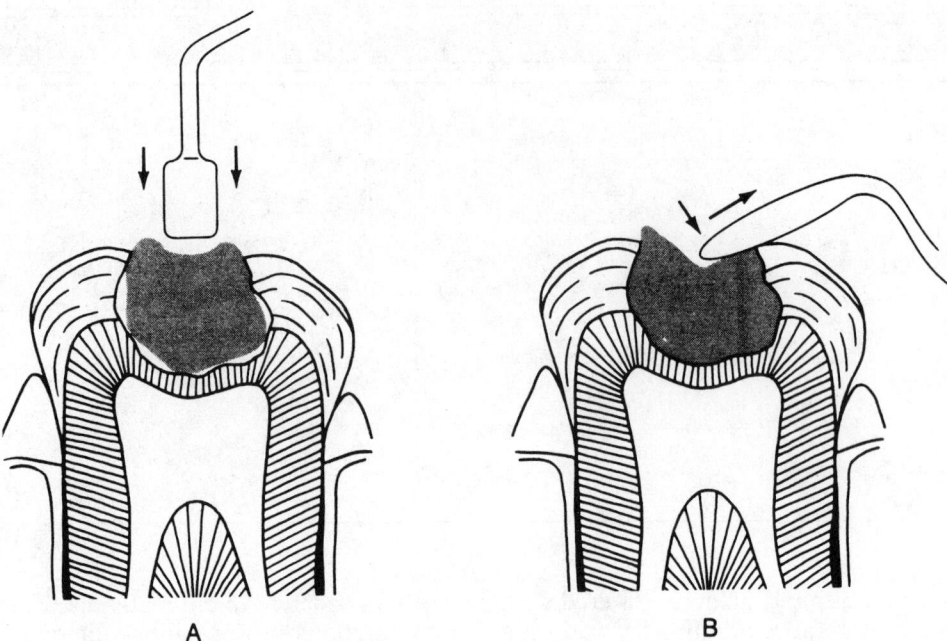

FIG. 55-42. Placement of temporary filling material with condenser (A) and carver (B). With permission from Klokkevold, P.: Common Dental Emergencies, Emerg. Med. Clin. North Am., 7:29-63, 1989.

nating from the dentition and that no other structures are involved.

As mentioned previously, most orofacial pain is of odontogenic origin, and it is generally reasonable to assume that the dentition is the cause. There are, however, exceptional circumstances in which disorders in other structures produce similar pain. The characteristic of pain from maxillary sinusitis, TMD, MPD, neuralgias, migraine headaches, and viral infections should be kept in mind when investigating facial pain of apparent dental origins. It is also useful to recognize that dental pain is often poorly localized and commonly referred to structures somewhat distant from the source.

TREATMENT

In most uncomplicated toothaches, antibiotics are of little value. Their use should be reserved for overt infections extending to involve other elements in the face. In the absence of a culture and sensitivity analysis, penicillin, erythromycin, or first-generation cephalosporins are the drugs of choice for odontogenic infections.

When pain relief becomes the primary goal of immediate therapy, analgesics are the primary modality of management. The prescription of narcotic analgesics entails the potential for drug abuse. Although most patients with dental pain have a sincere need for pain relief and a low potential for abuse, some with known dental problems seek care for the sole purpose of obtaining narcotic analgesics. It is probably wise to avoid prescriptions for drugs with known higher-abuse potentials and use other formulations. Alternatives to narcotic prescriptions are local anesthetics that can relieve dental pain for 4 to 12 hours, and these should be considered.

NATIONAL CONTACTS

If the emergency medical facility does not have a dental department or regular dental consultants, there are a number of local and national sources for information and referral. On a regional level, the state or local dental society will be able to supply information regarding emergency dental care programs, referral mechanisms, and dentists trained in hospital dentistry or oral and maxillofacial surgery.

Some national sources for dental care information are:

American Association of Hospital Dentists
211 East Chicago Avenue
Chicago, IL 60611
312-440-2661

American Dental Association
211 East Chicago Avenue
Chicago, IL 60611
800-621-8099

American Association of Oral and Maxillofacial
  Surgeons

9700 West Bryn Mawr Avenue
Rosemount, IL 60018

REFERENCES

1. Miller, A.J., Brunelle, J.A., Carlos, J.P., et al.: Oral Health of United States Adults, U.S. Dept. Of Health and Human Services, August 1987.
2. Rothwell, B.R.: Odontogenic infections. Emerg. Med. Clin. *3*:161, 1985.
3. Sicher, H., and DuBrul, E.L.: Oral anatomy. Fifth Ed. Saint Louis, C.V. Mosby, 1970.
4. Dickey, D.M.: Evaluation of pain of dento-alveolar origin. Dent. Clin. North Am. *17*:391, 1973.
5. Bell, W.D.: Orofacial pains. 4th Ed. Chicago, Year Book Publishers, 1989.
6. Graham, L.L., and Schinbeckler, G.A.: Orofacial pain of cardiac origin. J. Am. Dent. Assoc. *104*:47, 1982.
7. Batchelder, B.J., Krutchkoff, D.J., and Amara, J.: Mandibular pain as the initial and sole clinical manifestation of coronary insufficiency, J. Am. Dent. Assoc. *115*:710, 1987.
8. Eagle, W.W.: Symptomatic elongated styloid process. Arch. Otolaryngol. *49*:490, 1949.
9. Kant, K.S.: Pain referred to teeth as sole discomfort in undiagnosed mediastinal lymphoma: Report of case. J. Am. Dent. Assoc. *118*:587, 1989.
10. Hargreaves, K.M., Troullos, E.S., and Dionne, R.A.: Pharmacologic rationale for the treatment of acute pain. Dent. Clin. North Am. *31*:675, 1987.
11. Terezhalmy, G.T., Bowen, L.L., and Rye, L.A.: Pharmacotherapeutics in urgent dental care. Dent. Clin. North Am. *30*:399, 1986.
12. Maron, F.S.: Mucosal burn resulting from chewable aspirin: Report of a case. J. Am. Dent. Assoc. *119*:279, 1989.
13. Accepted Dental Therapeutics, 40th Ed. Chicago, American Dental Association, 1984.
14. Klokkevold, P.: Common dental emergencies. Dent. Clin. North Am. *7*:29, 1989.

GINGIVAL AND PERIODONTAL ABSCESSES

James T. Amsterdam

CAPSULE

Periodontal and gingival problems are usually chronic and insidious. Many patients are unaware that they have gum inflammation (gingivitis). Minor problems such as bleeding during toothbrushing, however, may cause alarm and motivate the patient to seek care in the emergency department (ED). Other conditions such as an acute periodontal abscess are painful and may be a more likely cause for seeking immediate attention. Management of these conditions in the ED is conservative, and referral back to the general dentist or periodontist is important.

PATHOPHYSIOLOGY

NORMAL PERIODONTIUM

The normal periodontium can be divided into two major components, the *gingival unit* and the *attachment apparatus*.[1]

GINGIVAL UNIT

The gingival unit is composed of the soft tissues investing the teeth and the alveolar bone. The *gingiva* is covered by stratified squamous keratinized epithelium. It extends from the free gingival margin to the mucogingival junction. Apical to the mucogingival junction is the *alveolar mucosa,* which is covered by nonkeratinized, stratified squamous epithelium and is continuous with the mucosa of the lip and cheek.

In healthy individuals, the gingiva is attached tightly to the tooth and has a stippled appearance similar to that of an orange peel.[2] From a level that is coronal to the margin of the alveolar bone to the level of the cementoenamel junction, connective tissue fibers from the gingiva insert into the cementum covering the root of the tooth.

Coronal to the epithelial attachment is a space bounded on one side by enamel and on the other by a continuation of the gingival epithelium. This space, called the *gingival sulcus,* is the cuff that is formed around the necks of the teeth by the gingival tissues. The gingiva lining this space is not attached to the tooth and is therefore called *free gingiva.* The gingiva apical to the base of the gingival sulcus is called *attached gingiva.* In the healthy periodontium, the gingival sulcus is rarely more than 2 to 3 mm deep.

ATTACHMENT APPARATUS

The attachment apparatus is the group of structures that attach the teeth to the jaws. It consists of the cementum covering the root, the alveolar bone surrounding the root, and the periodontal ligament. The periodontal ligament is composed of collagen fibers that insert on one end in the alveolar bone and on the other end in the cementum thus serving as a double

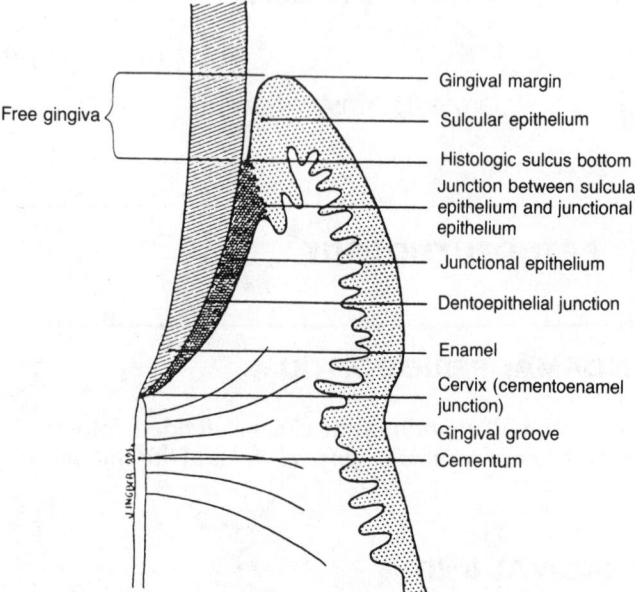

FIG. 55-43. *Histologic relationships of marginal gingiva. (With permission from Loe, H., and Listgarten, M.: Periodontium. In Periodontal Therapy. 5th Ed. Edited by Goldman, H., and Cohen, D. St. Louis, C.V. Mosby, 1973).*

Labels in figure:
Free gingiva
Gingival margin
Sulcular epithelium
Histologic sulcus bottom
Junction between sulcular epithelium and junctional epithelium
Junctional epithelium
Dentoepithelial junction
Enamel
Cervix (cementoenamel junction)
Gingival groove
Cementum

periosteum. The union of the tooth to the alveolar bone is not a calcific union but a fibrous attachment. The anatomy of the attachment apparatus is illustrated in Figure 55-43.

Periodontal abscesses can be a direct result of periodontal disease or mechanical problems. Gingivitis is an inflammation of the gingiva in response to an irritant such as dental bacterial plaque or other factors (e.g., hormonal changes from puberty or menopause, diabetes, other immune deficiencies).[3] Once the alveolar bone is involved (periodontitis), there is a breakdown of the attachment apparatus. Alveolar bone is destroyed, and the gingival sulcus develops into a *periodontal pocket* of several millimeters in depth as compared to the 2 to 3 mm. of depth of a healthy sulcus. This pocket then becomes a reservoir for plaque and other debris. If it becomes obstructed, a true abscess develops. Stretching of these tissues causes pain. A similar mechanical obstruction can occur in a relatively healthy gingival sulcus from something as simple as a popcorn kernel and also result in an abscess.

Because these abscesses result from entrapped dental bacterial plaque, numerous dental microorganisms are involved.[3] In addition, many anaerobic organisms are present. These organisms appear to be susceptible to penicillin, cephalosporins, and erythromycin. Moreover, the anaerobic organisms seem susceptible to the tetracyclines.

CLINICAL PRESENTATION

Patients with gingival abscess present with a localized swelling of the gingiva adjacent to the area involved. There may or may not be some spontaneous drainage in the area of the gingival margin or an area of pointing and maximum fluctance. On palpation with the gloved finger or tongue blade, the area is usually very tender. There should be no spontaneous pulsations or thrills over the swelling. The patient may be febrile. The gingival abscess may be the focus of more extensive infection of the head and neck, but this should be obvious on initial examination.

DIFFERENTIAL DIAGNOSIS

PERIODONTAL ABSCESS

As described previously, the periodontal abscess is a swelling of the gingiva secondary to the entrapment of plaque and debris in a pocket. Abscesses of this nature usually respond to local curettage, warm saline irrigation, and antibiotics (phenoxymethyl penicillin, 250 mg qid; tetracycline, 250 mg qid; doxycycline, 100 mg bid, or erythromycin, 250 mg qid). Because local curettage in the ED may be difficult, sometimes conservative incision and drainage are indicated (See Procedures). The periodontal abscess may also be secondary to a mechanical obstruction such as a popcorn kernel or piece of food. This problem will ultimately have to be treated with local curettage to remove the offending agent.[3]

PARULIS

Occasionally a periodontal abscess is the direct result of infection at the apex of a tooth from a necrotic pulp. A periapical abscess may erode through the cortical plate of the alveolar bone, extend subperiosteally, and give the impression of a periodontal abscess ("parulis"). Although the treatment is the same as that for the periodontal abscess, ultimately the tooth itself will have to be treated with endodontics (root canal work) or extracted.[3]

COMBINED PERIODONTAL/ENDODONTIC LESION

A complicated type of periodontal abscess, somewhat similar to the parulis, has a focus of infection from both the mechanical properties of a periodontal pocket and periapical infection associated with a necrotic pulp. Until both conditions are managed, recurrent bone destruction and periodontal involvement continue. Referral to a dentist is important to manage this complex entity.[4]

ACUTE NECROTIZING ULCERATIVE GINGIVITIS (ANUG)

An acute destructive disease of the periodontium, ANUG is found most often in adolescents and young adults, especially those under stress.[5] It is the only periodontal lesion in which bacteria invade non-necrotic tissue. Other signs and symptoms include fever, malaise, and localized lymphadenopathy.

ANUG begins most often as painful, edematous interdental papillae (tissue between the teeth). The affected areas ulcerate and a grayish pseudomembrane forms, leaving a tender bleeding surface when removed (Fig. 55-44). Necrosis of the interdental papillae follows, and the interdental tissue appears "punched out." The patient complains of foul breath and a metallic taste in the mouth.

The oral bacteria involved in this process consist of large numbers of fusobacteria and spirochetes. Other fusospirochetal disease (such as Vincent's angina, extension of ANUG to the fauces and tonsils, cancorum oris, and pulmonary abscesses) are also characterized as necrotizing ulcerative processes. In addition to bacteria, immunologic factors have been reported to contribute to the pathogenesis of ANUG. Other factors that contribute to the development of ANUG include fatigue, emotional stress, and smoking.[2]

ANUG commonly occurs in large numbers of people living together in close quarters, such as in the

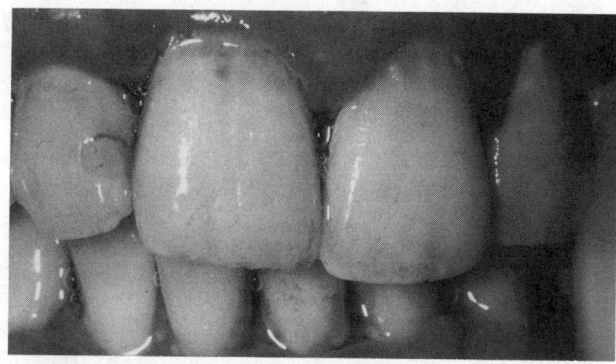

A

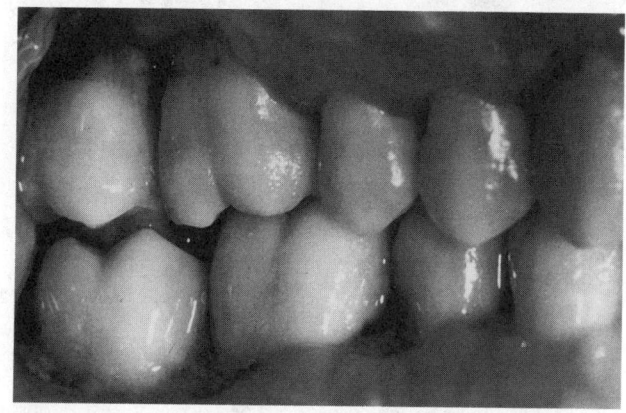

B

FIG. 55-44.   Acute necrotizing ulcerative gingivitis involving A. maxillary and B. mandibular anterior gingiva. (With permission from Amsterdam, J., Hendler, B., and Rose, L.: Dental emergencies. *In* Principles and Practice of Emergency Medicine. 2nd Ed. Edited by Schwartz, G., et al. Philadelphia, W.B. Saunders, 1986.)

trenches during World War I (hence the name "trench mouth)," college dormitories, and military barracks. This has fostered the belief that ANUG is a communicable disease; however, to date no evidence exists to support this belief.[6]

Patients present to the ED complaining of painful gums, bad breath, and a metallic taste in the mouth. Frequently, periodontal abscesses may be associated with the condition because underlying periodontal disease is a predisposing factor and recurrent ANUG distorts gingival morphology, making the periodontium more susceptible to pocket formation.

Patients achieve dramatic relief with the application of saline rinses and the administration of either penicillin or tetracycline. Follow-up with a general dentist or periodontist is important, however. ANUG leaves behind bony destruction that makes the patient more susceptible to periodontal infection. Minor to major periodontal therapy may be required to restore a healthy architecture to the periodontium so that the patient can perform adequate home care to remove plaque and prevent further disease. The need for referral should be well documented in the chart.

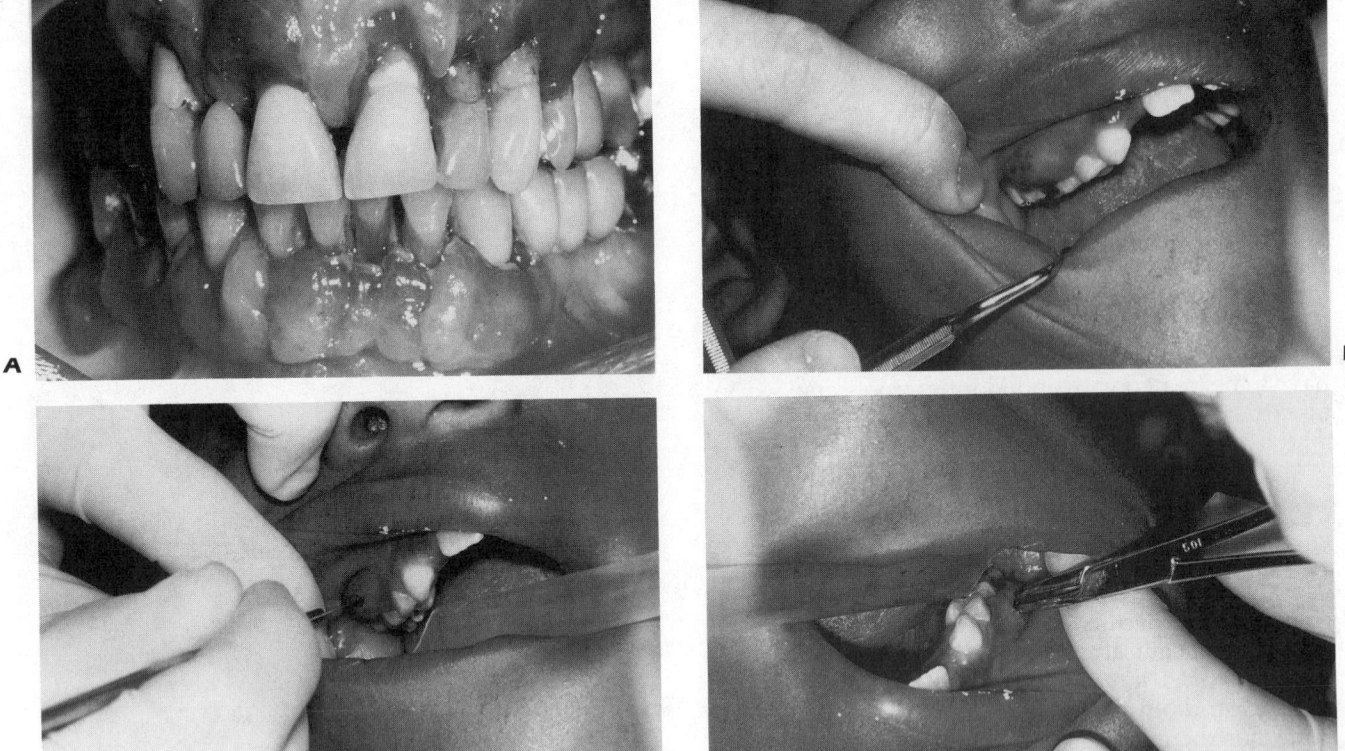

FIG. 55-45. Incision and drainage of a periodontal abscess. A. Abscess. B. Incision. C and D. Blunt dissection and drainage. (With permission from Amsterdam, J., Hendler, B., and Rose, L.: Emergency dental procedures. *In* Clinical Procedures in Emergency Medicine. 1st Ed. Edited by Roberts, J., and Hedges, J. Philadelphia, W.B. Saunders, 1985.)

PROCEDURES

Incision and drainage may be required in the treatment of a periodontal abscess. Contrary to the classic teaching of opening the abscess to its full extent as opposed to a stab incision, a stab incision is all that is required to drain a periodontal abscess.[7] A small amount of spreading can be performed with a mosquito hemostat, and there may or may not be room for a drain (Penrose or iodoform), depending upon the size of the abscess (Fig. 55-45). The patient performs intraoral warm saline rinses, which continue drainage. Follow-up with a dentist should occur in 1 to 2 days.

MANAGEMENT

The management of the periodontal abscess has been outlined previously. Strictly speaking, management is conservative. Admission is warranted for a periodontal abscess if the lesion is the focus of a more serious infection of the head and neck. Occasionally, a patient with ANUG may be dehydrated and require admission for intravenous fluids. Before draining a periodontal abscess, care should be taken to determine whether the patient requires systemic bacterial endocarditis (SBE) prophylaxis because significant bacteremia occurs during the incision and drainage procedure.[8]

PITFALLS

Before performing an incision and drainage or a periodontal abscess, care should be taken to ensure that one is indeed dealing with a abscess. The area should be fluctuant and nonpulsatile (e.g., an AVM). All stab incisions should be made directly toward alveolar bone to avoid any aberrant vessels.

MEDICOLEGAL PEARLS

SBE prophylaxis should be carefully undertaken in patients who require it. Especially in ANUG, referral to a general dentist or periodontist is important for further treatment. The patient should understand the importance of this, and it should be documented in the chart. The patient should also be aware of the signs and symptoms of spread of infection to the head and neck, and return if he or she feels worse.

REFERENCES

1. Linde, J.: Textbook of Clinical Periodontology. Copenhagen, Munksgaard, 1983, Chapter 1.

2. Loe, H., and Listgarten, M.: Anatomy and histology, Part I. *In* Periodontal Therapy, 6th ed. Edited by Goldman, H.M., and Cohen, D.W. St. Louis, C.V. Mosby, 1980.
3. Weisgold, A., et al.: Dental medicine. *In* Fundamentals of Internal Medicine, 1st Ed. Edited by Kaye, D., and Rose, L.F. St. Louis, C.V. Mosby, 1983.
4. Amsterdam, M.: Periodontal prosthesis: Twenty-five years in retrospect. Alpha Omegan, December, 1974.
5. Barnes, G.P., Bowles, W.F., and Carter, H.G.: Acute necrotizing ulcerative gingivitis: A survey of 218 cases. J. Periodontol. *44*:35, 1973.
6. Schluger, S.: Necrotizing ulcerative gingivitis in the army: Incidence, communicability, and treatment. J. Am. Dent. Assoc. *38*:174, 1949.
7. Amsterdam, J., Hendler, B., and Rose, L.: Emergency dental procedures. *In* Clinical Procedures in Emergency Medicine. Edited by Roberts, J., and Hedges, J. Philadelphia, W.B. Saunders, 1985.
8. Klokkevold, P.: Common dental emergencies. Dent. Clin. North Am. 7:29, 1989.

GINGIVAL HEMORRHAGE

James T. Amsterdam

CAPSULE

Oral hemorrhage may be spontaneous from the gingiva or, more commonly, a result of dental treatment, especially the surgical extraction of teeth. A systematic approach to oral hemorrhage identifies the cause in most cases and aids in overall management.

PATHOPHYSIOLOGY

Gingival bleeding originates from capillaries within the gingiva. Postextraction bleeding usually results from oozing of blood from the alveolar bone, but also might originate from capillary bleeding from the traumatized gingiva around the socket or from an arteriole.[1] Major vessel bleeding is not a problem. Therefore, such bleeding usually responds to local measures such as direct pressure, suture ligation, or hemostatic agents. Dental trauma, periodontal surgery (even scaling or curettage), and especially tooth extraction may reveal the first manifestation of an unrecognized coagulopathy (e.g., factor IX deficiency, platelet dysfunction).[2]

PREHOSPITAL ASSESSMENT AND STABILIZATION

Patients requiring prehospital care for gingival hemorrhage are likely to have significant bleeding. Attention should first be directed toward the airway. If the patient is unable to control the airway because of massive bleeding, intubation is required. The prehospital care provider should exercise extreme infection control precautions (gloves, goggles, mask) because much blood is likely to splatter. Once adequate ventilation has been established, the circulatory status should be evaluated. If the patient has inadequate perfusion, a large bore line should be established and volume replacement initiated with crystalloid. At the same time, local measures should be initiated to control bleeding, i.e., direct pressure to the bleeding site. Fortunately, most patients with gingival hemorrhage are not in extremis. Transport in a position of comfort with the patient biting down on gauze is all that is usually required.

CLINICAL PRESENTATION

The history from a patient presenting with bleeding gingiva should include any recent dental scaling, curettage, or prophylaxis; dental extraction; and trauma. Like the prehospital care provider, the emergency physician should examine the patient with a minimum of gloves and mask; eye protection is strongly recommended. Patients with gingival bleeding are prone to coughing and gagging. There should be adequate lighting, good suction, and a large supply of gauze. Begin the examination by having the patient rinse with saline and expectorate any clots and debris. Dry the mouth with suction and gauze and evaluate the bleeding, which may be localized to an extraction or surgical site, or diffusely involving all of the gingiva.

DIFFERENTIAL DIAGNOSIS AND PROCEDURES

POSTEXTRACTION BLEEDING

Patients commonly present with bleeding secondary to dental extraction.[3] This bleeding may be secondary to local trauma or excessive intraoral negative pressure (spitting, smoking, use of straws). A medication history is also useful. Patients may have been taking a lot of aspirin, alone or in combination with a narcotic, for pain before or immediately after the extraction. The effects of as much as one aspirin may linger for a week or more.[2]

If clots are present in the oral cavity, they should be removed with suction and gauze. The patient should be encouraged to do no further spitting and to bite down on gauze for 20 minutes. If the bleeding has not stopped, the area of the socket should be infiltrated with 1% to 2% lidocaine combined with 1:100,000 epinephrine.[4] The resulting anesthesia allows the patient to bite harder, and the local vasoconstrictor also helps to stop bleeding. Gauze pressure is then reapplied for 20 minutes. Continued bleeding

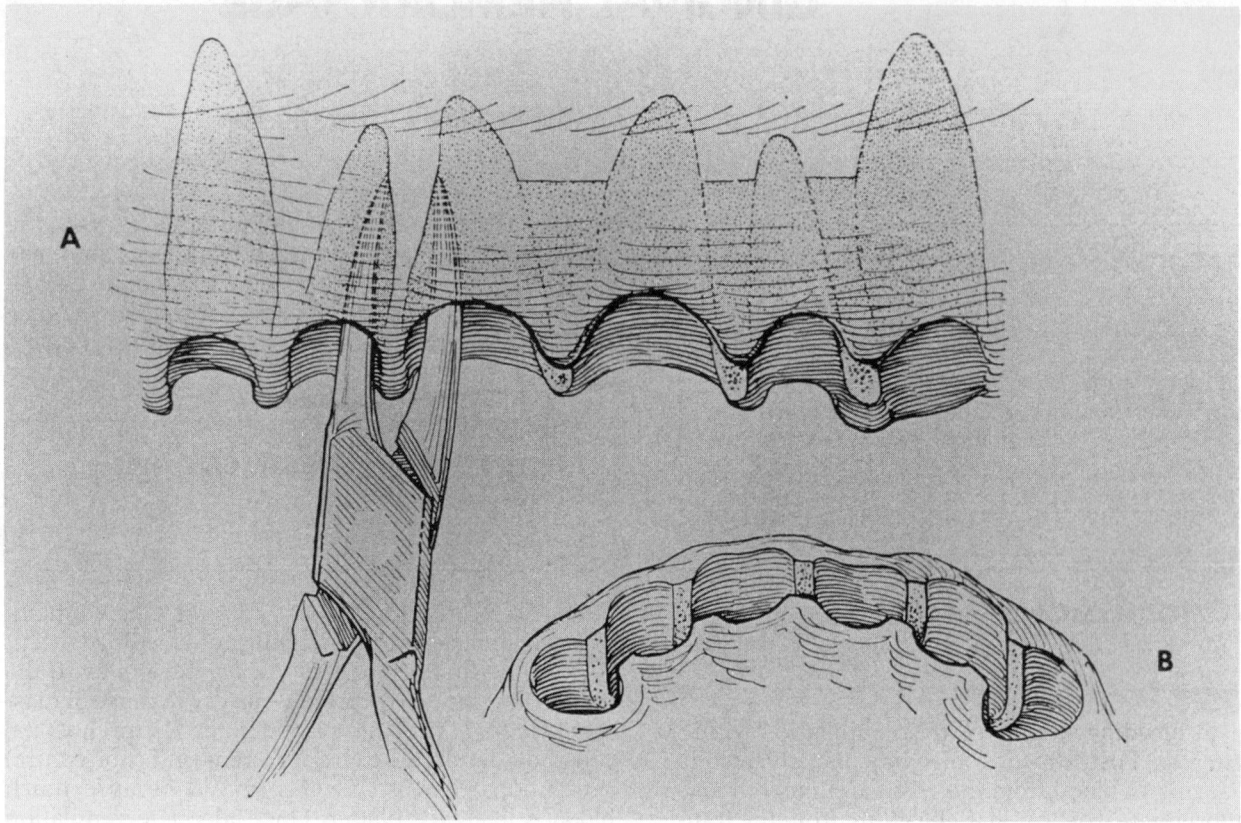

FIG. 55-46. Interradicular alveoloplasty. A. Narrow-beaked rongeur removes septa without raising a flap or destroying the labial plate. B. Weakened labial plate is collapsed to palatal plate by thumb pressure. The gingiva is then sutured. (With permission from Kruger, G.O.: Complicated exodontics. *In* Textbook of Oral and Maxillofacial Surgery. 6th Ed. Edited by Kruger, G.O. St. Louis, C.V. Mosby, 1984, p. 68.)

after the 20 minutes may respond to the placement of small piece of absorbable knitted fabric (Surgicel) or gelatin foam (Gelfoam) in the socket, secured with a 3–0 or 4–0 black silk suture. Continued oozing despite these procedures warrants a coagulation profile (CBC, platelet count, PT/PTT) because many coagulapathies first present after dental extraction.

Postextraction bleeding may also be the result of poor surgical technique. Multiple extractions without a surgical flap or bony recontouring may be prone to bleeding. Such areas may need additional sutures or a complete alveoloplasty by the oral and maxillofacial surgeon[5] (Figures 55-46 and 55-47).

BLEEDING AFTER PERIODONTAL SURGERY

Bleeding is frequently seen after periodontal surgery. Periodontal therapy may involve deep scaling and curettage of the tissues or surgery involving gingival flaps and grafts. The tissue at the surgical site is usually covered with a dressing called a periodontal pack (e.g., Coe-Pak). This surgical dressing is extremely critical to the healing of the wound.[6] Therefore, if it is dislodged, the periodontist should be notified at once. If there is bleeding around the pack, care should be taken not to disturb or remove the pack. This type of hemorrhage usually responds to peroxide rinses and local pressure. Sustained vigorous hemorrhage should be evaluated in a manner similar to that used for postextraction bleeding.

BLOOD DYSCRASIAS

Periodontal disorders have been described in association with blood dyscrasias such as leukemia, cyclic neutropenia, thrombocytopenia, pancytopenia, and other coagulopathies including all the factor deficiencies, which might not be apparent until the system is stressed, e.g., from postextraction or periodontal surgery.[7]

Acute leukemia, particularly the acute granulocytic form, causes massive infiltration of leukemic cells into the gingival tissues. The hyperplastic gingivitis thus produced may be so marked as to almost cover the teeth. The gingiva is edematous and bluish-red in color. Varying degrees of gingival inflammation have been described, and the tissue is subject to bleeding either spontaneously or from trauma (Fig. 55-48).

Thrombocytopeniac purpura may initially present with gingival bleeding, intramucosal hemorrhages, and prolonged bleeding from trauma. Thrombocytopenia from various causes including alcoholism and quinidine sensitivity may present with gingival bleeding.

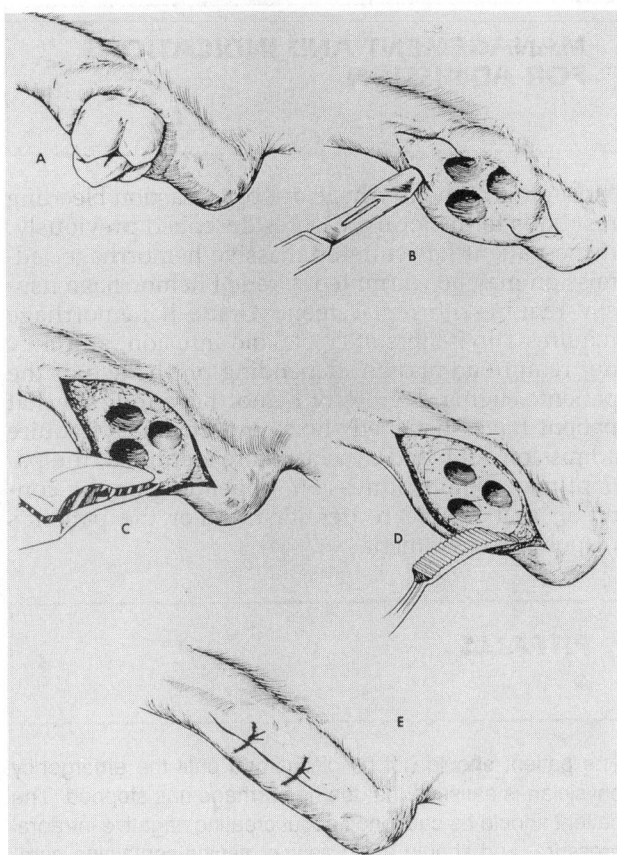

FIG. 55-47.   Single tooth alveoloplasty. A. Isolated tooth with high alveolar bone (pre-extraction). B. After tooth removal, wedge-shaped portions of gingiva are removed from the socket. C. Bony reduction with rongeur. D. Smoothing with bone file. E. Final suturing. (With permission from Guernsey, L.H.: Preprosthetic surgery. In Textbook of Oral and Maxillofacial Surgery. 6th Ed. Edited by G.O. Kruger. St. Louis, C.V. Mosby, 1984, p. 115.)

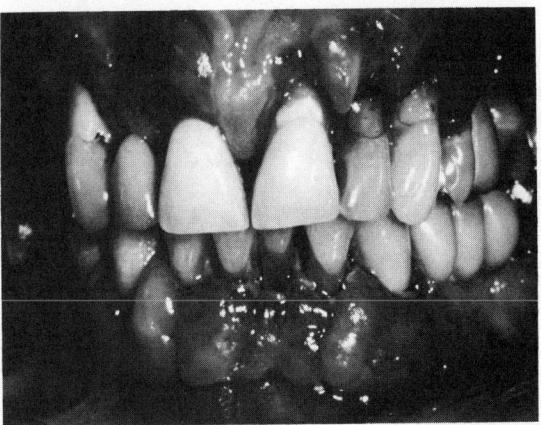

FIG. 55-48.   Periodontal manifestations of acute leukemia. (With permission from Amsterdam, J., Hendler, B., and Rose, L.: Dental emergencies. In Principles and Practice of Emergency Medicine. 2nd Ed. Edited by Schwartz, G., et al. Philadelphia, W.B. Saunders Co., 1986, p. 1583.)

MANAGEMENT AND INDICATIONS FOR ADMISSION

Most gingival hemorrhage or postextraction bleeding responds to the local measures described previously. If the patient has suffered massive hemorrhage, admission may be warranted. Grade I hemorrhage usually requires no replacement; Grade II hemorrhage requires 1 to 2 liters of crystalloid infusion, and may not require admission, depending on the age of the patient. Higher degrees of hemorrhage indicate that patient have sustained shock and obviously require admission.[8] If blood dyscrasias are identified, the patient may require admission, depending on the condition that has been identified and/or the patient's response to treatment.

PITFALLS

The patient should not be discharged until the emergency physician is satisfied that the hemorrhage has stopped. The patient should be cautioned about creating negative intraoral pressure, and should avoid aspirin, aspirin-containing compounds, and similar agents.

MEDICOLEGAL PEARLS

All patients with gingival or postextraction bleeding do not need a coagulation profile. Patients who do not respond to local measures, however, may have an underlying blood dyscrasia, and this should be pursued. Patients who have required a hemostatic pack, especially Surgicel, should be cautioned that they are likely to develop an acute alveolar osteitis (dry socket). These patients should be warned that, if they experience extreme pain and a bad taste in 2 to 3 days, a dry socket is the likely diagnosis. The patient should either contact the dentist immediately, or return to the ED for treatment.

REFERENCES

1. Alling, D., and Alling, R.: Hemorrhage and shock. *In* Textbook of Oral and Maxillofacial Surgery. 6th Ed. Edited by Kruger, G.O. St. Louis, C.V. Mosby, 1984.
2. Lynch, M.A.: Bleeding and clotting disorders. *In* Burket's Oral Medicine. 8th ed. Edited by Lynch, M.A., Brightman, V., and Greenberg, M. Philadelphia, J.B. Lippincott Co., 1984.
3. Reynolds, D.C.: Special considerations in exodontics. *In* Textbook of Oral and Maxillofacial Surgery. 6th Ed. Edited by Kruger, G.O. St. Louis, C.V. Mosby, 1984.
4. Amsterdam, J., Hendler, B., and Rose, L.: Emergency dental procedures. *In* Clinical Procedures in Emergency Medicine. Edited by Roberts, J., and Hedges, J. Philadelphia, W.B. Saunders, 1985.
5. Kruger, G.O.: Complicated exodontics. *In* Textbook of Oral and Maxillofacial Surgery. 6th Ed. Edited by Kruger, G.O. St. Louis, C.V. Mosby, 1984.
6. Corn, H.: Mucogingival surgery and associated problems. *In* Periodontal Therapy. 5th ed. Edited by Goldman, H., and Cohen, D.W. St. Louis, C.V. Mosby, 1973.
7. Greenberg, M.S.: Hematologic disease. *In* Burket's Oral Medicine. 8th ed. Edited by Lynch, M.A., Brightman, V., and Greenberg, M. Philadelphia, J.B. Lippincott Co., 1984.
8. Textbook of Advanced Trauma Life Support. Chicago, American College of Surgeons, Committee on Trauma, 1988.

TOOTH AVULSIONS AND FRACTURES

Jeffrey B. Dembo

CAPSULE

It is important to understand the treatment of dentoalveolar injuries because of the frequency with which they occur and the complications that may result. If not promptly recognized and treated, these injuries in children may interfere with tooth eruption, facial development, and occlusion. In adults, they can result in loss of esthetics, loss of function, collapse of the dental arch through tooth migration, and potential chronic infection. Emergency physicians may find themselves needing to evaluate and treat these conditions, particularly in remote areas where dental care may not be immediately accessible.

INTRODUCTION

Tooth fractures and avulsions are examples of dentoalveolar trauma, i.e., trauma involving the dentition and supporting hard and soft tissue structures. Dentoalveolar trauma occurs frequently and may be isolated or associated with other injuries. The injury may affect teeth alone, but is more likely to involve soft tissue as well. Children represent the population most likely to suffer dentoalveolar trauma. By age 14, it is possible that 30% of children will have sustained injuries to the primary dentition and 22% to the permanent dentition.[1] Boys appear to be twice as prone to dentoalveolar trauma as girls. The highest incidence of trauma occurs at ages 8 through 10.

PREDISPOSING FACTORS

The many predisposing factors to dentoalveolar trauma are described in the following paragraphs.

AGE

Dentoalveolar trauma is rare in children under 1 year old, but injuries can occur (e.g., a fall from a table). A significant cause of injury in the infant can be child abuse (see Medicolegal Pearls, subsequently in this chapter). At 1 to 3 years, once the child begins walking and running, the incidence of injury increases because of adventuresome activity combined with lack of coordination. At school age, playground and bicycle injuries are most common. During the teen years, sports injuries are frequent causes. In adulthood, sports injuries, motor vehicle accidents, industrial and farming accidents, altercations, and spouse abuse are potential causes of trauma.

SPORTS ACTIVITIES

Hockey, football, soccer, and basketball are frequent causes, most often involving contact with a fist or elbow. Horseback riding may also be a significant source of dentoalveolar injury.

MEDICAL HISTORY

A higher frequency of dental injuries has been noted among patients with mental retardation and cerebral palsy.[2] Substance abuse may also increase the likelihood of dentoalveolar injury.

DENTAL ANATOMY

Protruding maxillary incisors or inability to close the lips at rest may increase the chance for injury.

PATHOPHYSIOLOGY AND ANATOMY

Trauma to dentoalveolar structures can be *direct* (tooth-object contact) or *indirect* (force transmitted by blow to soft tissue of lip, gingiva, etc.). The nature of the trauma influences the type of injury. Injuries may

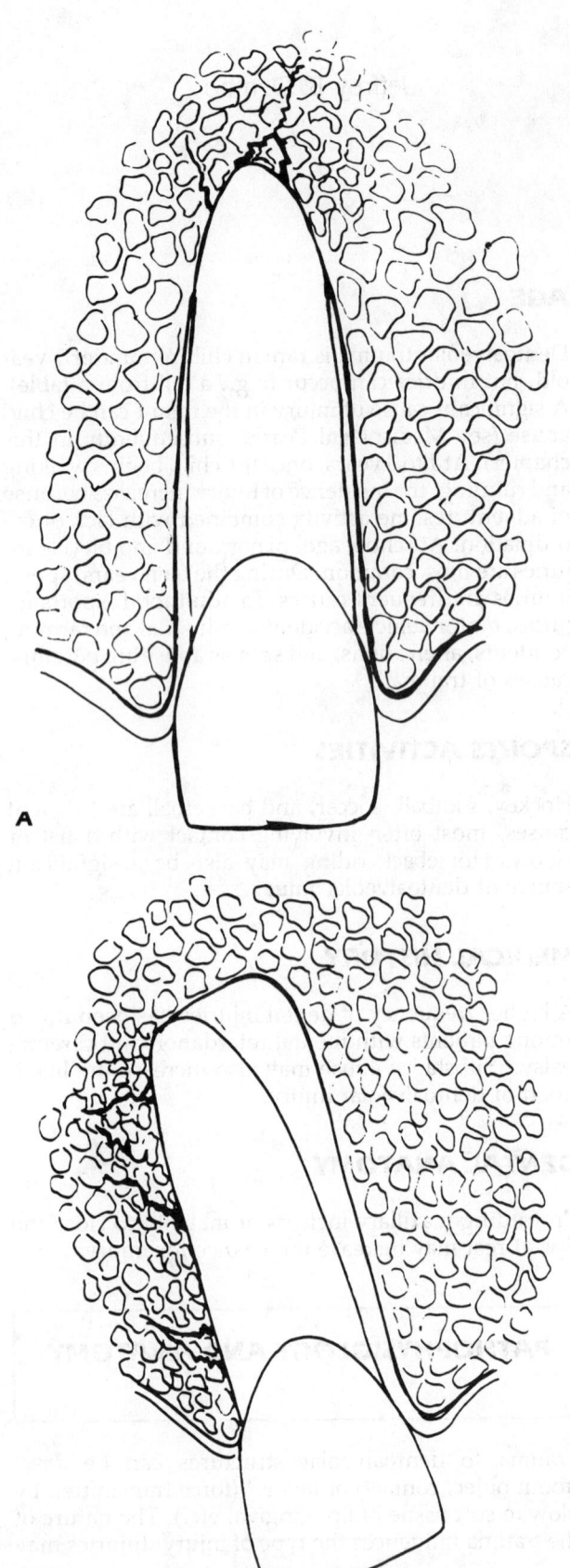

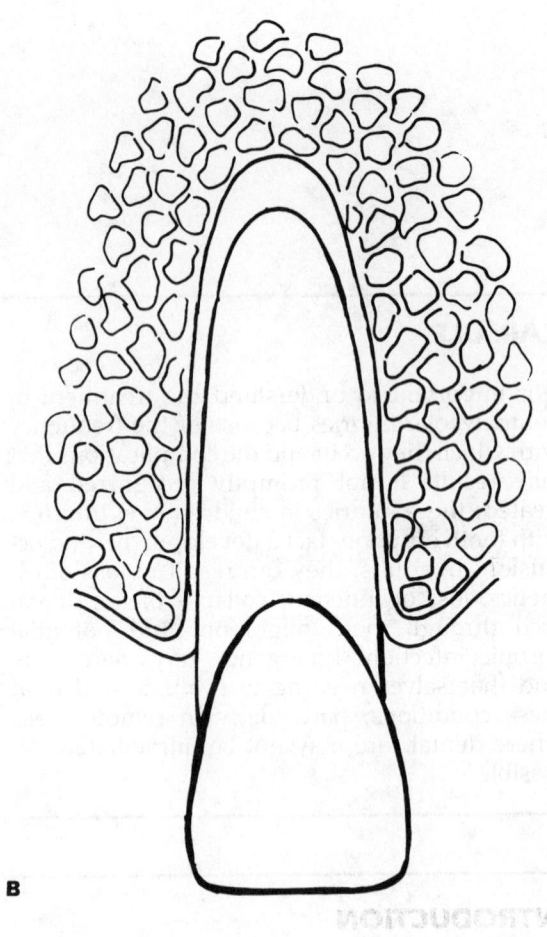

FIG. 55-49. A. Partial displacement with intrusion. B. Partial displacement with extrusion. C. Partial displacement laterally.

be classified as subluxation, displacement (partial or total), or fracture.

Subluxation refers to abnormal loosening of the tooth without evidence of displacement from the socket.

Displacement may be partial or total. In partial displacement the tooth position has been traumatically altered, resulting in intrusion, extrusion, and anteroposterior or lateral movement (Fig. 55-49). In total displacement (avulsion), the tooth has been totally dislodged from the bony socket.

Fracture may involve only tooth substance or both tooth and alveolar bone. In tooth fracture, tooth substance has been injured, resulting in fracture of enamel, dentin, cementum, and/or pulp in the crown or root (Fig. 55-50). In dentoalveolar fracture, single or multiple teeth and supporting alveolar bone are injured and are mobile as a unit.

Displacement is the most common type of injury in children. The teeth have short crowns and are vertical, and the alveolar bone is elastic with a thin cortex. Thus, tooth integrity is usually spared because the supporting structures absorb much of the impact. In contrast, the adult dentition is characterized by large tooth crowns and dense supporting bone, making tooth fractures more likely.

CLINICAL PRESENTATION AND EXAMINATION

A careful history is important for accurate diagnosis of dentoalveolar injuries and for ensuring the best prognosis of treatment. The following questions need to be addressed:

1. How did the injury occur?
   The traumatic event can offer clues as to the nature and types of injuries sustained. For example, one should consider the energy of impact, direction of force, and resiliency and shape of the object.
2. When did the injury occur?
   The time elapsed between injury and treatment can be one of the most significant factors in the prognosis of the injured area, especially in the case of avulsed teeth.
3. Where did the injury occur?
   Antibiotic or tetanus prophylaxis may be indicated if a dirty wound is suspected.
4. What treatment has already been provided?
   Previous treatment records or a verbal report from witnesses can be helpful in treatment planning. For example, how was the tooth stored in the case of an avulsion?
5. What is the past dental history, including dental injuries?
   Is the fractured incisor a new injury or an old one? Was the tooth previously root canal treated?

6. What are the patient's subjective symptoms?
   Has there been spontaneous pain from any teeth? Is there any sensitivity to touch or extremes of temperature?

The clinical examination must be systematic, and specific attention should be paid to the following areas:

1. The ability to open the mouth fully, assessing for damage to the jaws or temporomandibular joint. Does the mouth open fully without deviation? A temporomandibular joint injury causes deviation toward the affected side.
2. Dental occlusion.
   Can the teeth be brought together in the usual manner, or does the patient state that the "bite is off?" Do all teeth appear to occlude evenly, or does one area occlude prematurely?
3. Presence of fractured, displaced, or loosened teeth.
4. Change in tooth coloration.
   Pulpal congestion or necrosis from injury can cause color changes (e.g., pink or grey-blue hue visible through the dentin and enamel).
5. General dental condition of the patient.
   Is a tooth loosened from trauma or from pre-existing periodontal disease?
6. Presence of soft tissue trauma.
   Lacerations or ecchymosis of the gingiva or mucosa can often provide clues to presence and location of dentoalveolar injuries. Hemorrhage in the gingival crevice of the tooth may indicate subluxation (Fig. 55-51). Care should be taken to examine soft tissues thoroughly (e.g:, in lip laceration) because foreign bodies and tooth fragments may be embedded and remain undetected.
7. Missing teeth or prostheses.
   If a partial denture or avulsed tooth cannot be located, be suspicious that the object may have been swallowed or aspirated.

Radiographs useful for an accurate diagnosis include a panoramic film ("panorex"), periapical radiographs of the dentition, and soft tissue films to rule out foreign bodies. Unless the beam of radiation passes directly through a line of cleavage, a tooth fracture may remain undetected; hence, radiographs taken from several directions are useful (Fig. 55-52). A tooth fracture typically appears as a radiolucent line extending to the edge of the tooth but not beyond. Subluxation or displacement presents as a widening or irregularity of the periodontal ligament space around the root.

A digital examination is a vital part of the evaluation. A finger or instrument (e.g., tongue blade) can be used to place pressure on a tooth to determine if mobility is present. Only a gentle motion should be used to prevent iatrogenic displacement of a loosened tooth. If mobility is present, note if a single tooth or a group of teeth exhibits movement. Mobility of several teeth may indicate the presence of an alveolar fracture. Remember that deciduous teeth near the time of exfo-

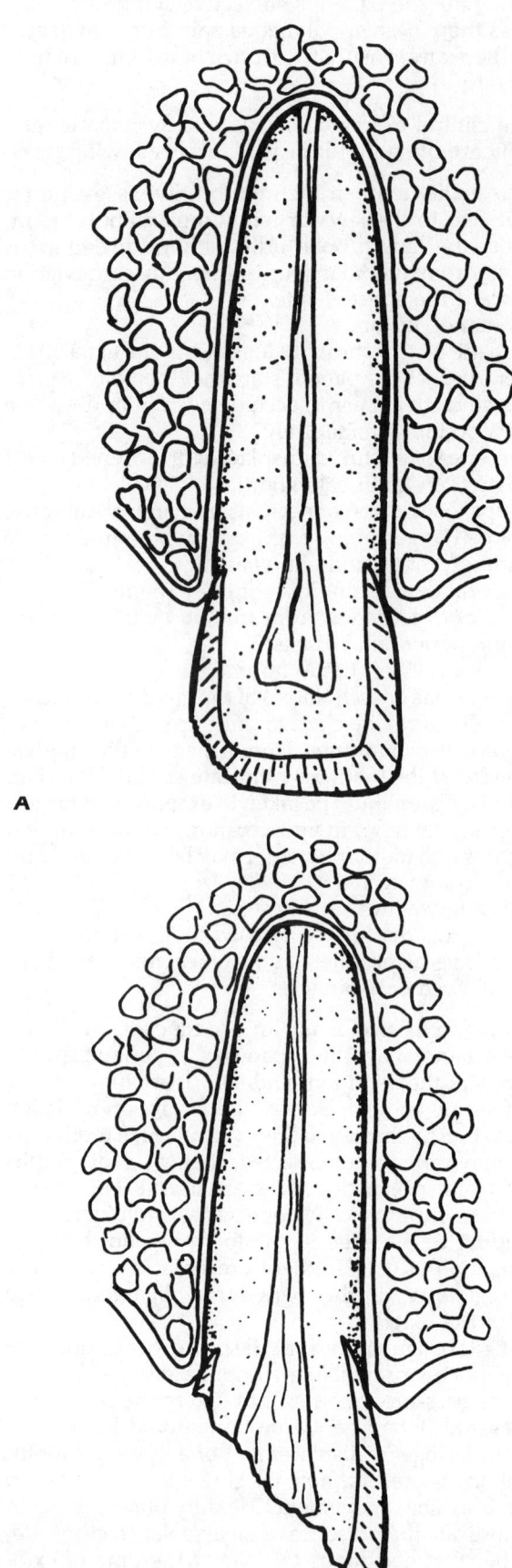

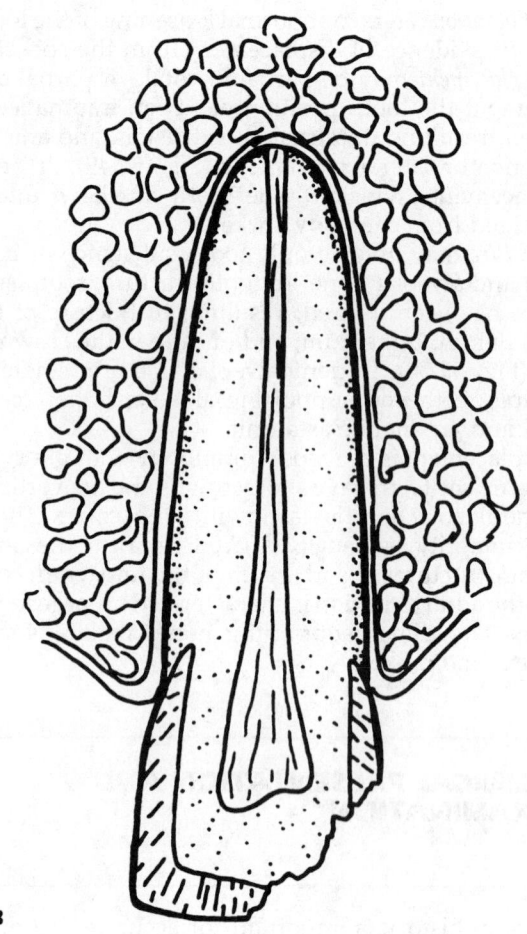

FIG. 55-50. A. Crown fracture through enamel only. B. Crown fracture through enamel and dentin. C. Crown fracture through enamel and dentin with pulp exposure.

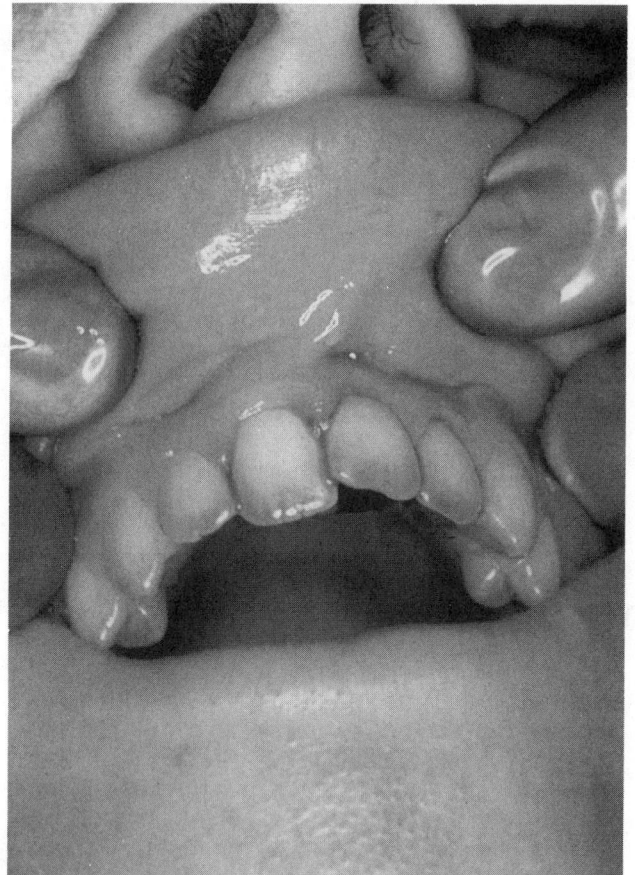

FIG. 55-51.   Hemorrhage in the gingival crevice is a common finding with subluxated and displaced teeth.

liation normally exhibit mobility because of root resorption. A finger or instrument should also be used to gently tap on the occlusal edge of the teeth. Sensitivity to percussion indicates damage to the periodontal ligament, supporting a diagnosis of subluxation.

On the basis of the clinical and radiographic findings, the injury can be assigned to one of three categories: subluxation, displacement, or fracture. Perhaps the most common emergency handled by Emergency Department (ED) personnel is the avulsed tooth. This is a true emergency because the success of reimplantation of traumatically avulsed teeth is directly related to the *length of time* the tooth remains out of the socket before replacement and *how it is handled* during that time. When reimplanted teeth have been outside the alveolus more than 2 hours, 95% ultimately show signs of root resorption; only 10% show resorption if reimplanted within 30 minutes.[3] Dessication of the periodontal membrane is thought to be the major explanation for this time-dependent phenomenon, although continued exposure of the root to mechanical trauma and foreign substances plays a role.[4]

Storage of the tooth during the extraoral period is also crucial. Teeth can be successfully stored in saliva for about 2 hours. Keeping a tooth under the tongue or in the buccal vestibule is one method for storage before replantation. The length of storage time is somewhat limited by the hypotonicity and high bacterial count of saliva. Recent studies indicate that milk taken directly from the refrigerator can be an excellent medium for storage.[5,6] A high percentage of viable cells in the periodontal membrane are seen even after 6 hours of storage in milk. A third choice of storage medium is isotonic saline. Tap water should be used only as a last resort because it is not isotonic.

This emergency may be handled by phone, usually by a parent or teacher calling to ask about treatment. Important recommendations are described below. In the case of all tooth and tooth-related injuries, prompt referral to a general dentist, pediatric dentist, or oral and maxillofacial surgeon means that the patient will receive early definitive care, improving the prognosis for success.

INITIAL STABILIZATION AND DEFINITIVE TREATMENT (TABLE 55-34)

SUBLUXATED TEETH

Subluxated teeth usually need no immediate stabilization, but further trauma to the tooth must be prevented. This includes avoidance of additional forceful facial contact. Diet should be limited to liquids or extremely soft solids. Referral to a dentist is recommended for more definitive care and follow-up. The dentist may grind the occlusal surface of the opposing tooth to prevent contact and performs periodic pulp vitality tests over the next 8 to 12 weeks to determine if root canal therapy is indicated for pulpal necrosis.

DISPLACED TEETH

PARTIAL DISPLACEMENT

Primary Tooth. If the tooth has been intruded or posteriorly displaced, or appears radiographically to be in close proximity to an unerupted permanent tooth, the displaced tooth should be carefully extracted. Fewer abnormalities develop in the permanent teeth when this treatment is provided. An extruded tooth should also be extracted, as well as a tooth that is expected to exfoliate within the next 6 months. A tooth that is about to exfoliate generally has less than half its root structure remaining because of resorption.

If the deciduous tooth is not in proximity to the

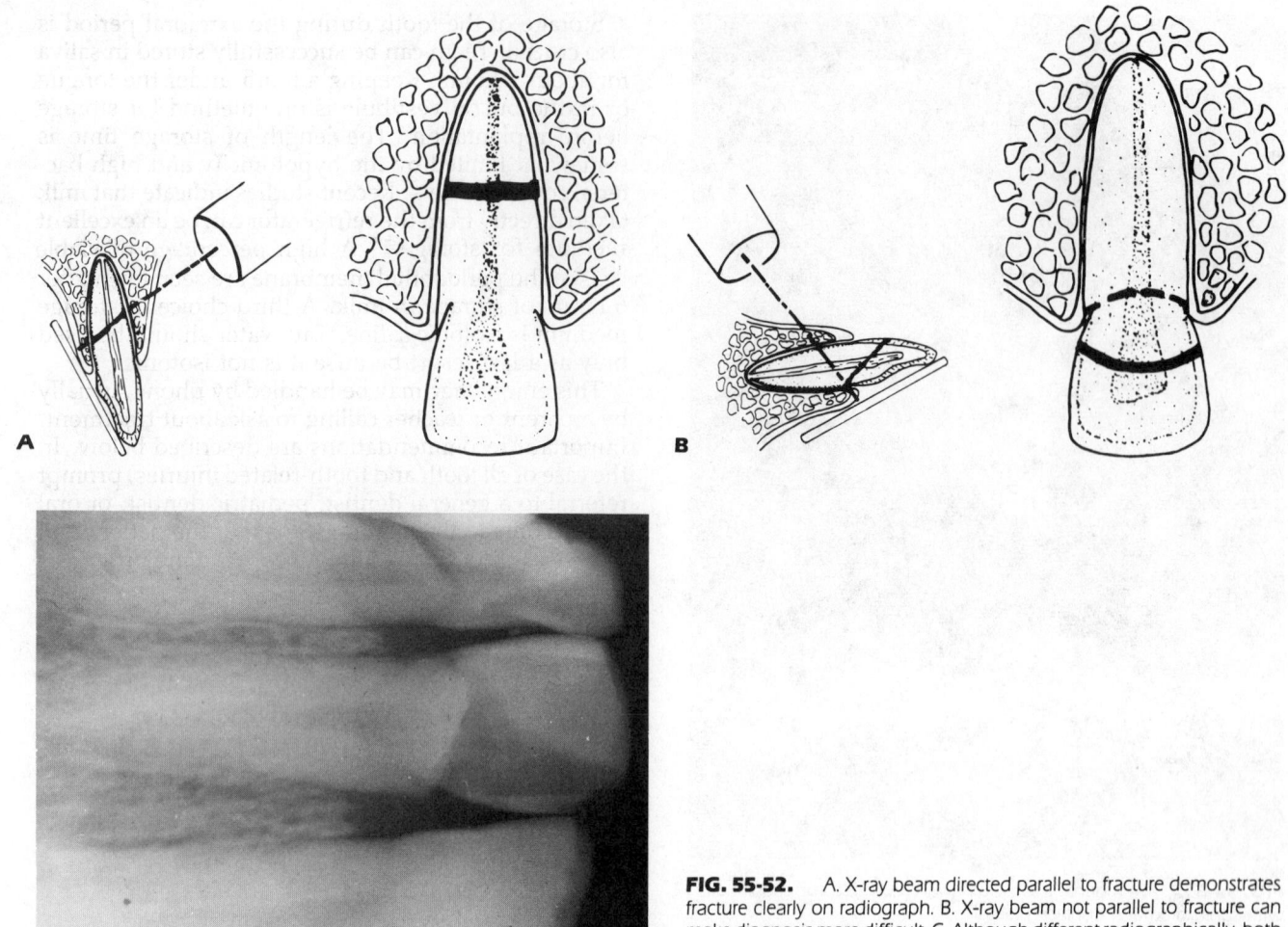

FIG. 55-52. A. X-ray beam directed parallel to fracture demonstrates fracture clearly on radiograph. B. X-ray beam not parallel to fracture can make diagnosis more difficult. C. Although different radiographically, both incisors have sustained similar fractures.

underlying permanent tooth (e.g., anterior or lateral displacement, or minimal intrusion), it can be allowed to re-erupt. Good oral hygiene should be stressed, and a soft diet maintained for 1 to 2 weeks. Usually, spontaneous repositioning occurs within 6 months.[7] In some cases, orthodontic appliances may be needed to move the tooth into correct position.

Permanent Tooth. All permanent teeth that have been displaced should receive definitive treatment from a dentist. If there is no gross mobility of the displaced tooth, no immediate stabilization is needed. This existing stability may be from consolidation of a blood clot in the alveolus or wedging of the tooth against the alveolar wall, locking it in position. If mobility is evident, temporary stabilization may be achieved by digitally repositioning the tooth. The purpose of splinting is to stabilize the injured tooth and prevent further damage to the pulp and periodontal ligament. Further methods of temporary stabilization include moist gauze or cotton rolls placed in the labial vestibule against the teeth or tying a figure-of-eight suture around the occlusal aspect of the affected tooth

and adjacent tooth (Fig. 55-53). Ensure that this suture is placed as close to the occlusal edge as possible; placing it too close to the gingiva causes extrusion of the tooth. Aluminum foil or foil from a dental film packet can be crimped around the tooth surfaces to provide temporary stabilization. A periodontal dressing, if available, is an excellent means of stabilizing teeth and is easy to apply (e.g., COE-pak, Coe laboratories, Chicago, IL). Equal lengths of two pastes are mixed on a paper pad, and the material is adapted around the teeth and tissues, which have been cleaned and dried. The paste hardens in a short time, and provides the temporary stability needed. In most cases of permanent tooth displacement, the dentist more definitively splints the affected tooth. It is frequently accomplished with a tooth-colored composite resin applied to the enamel surface of the affected and adjacent tooth (Fig. 55-54). The enamel is prepared to accept this resin by application of an acid to "etch" the surface, aiding in retention of the resin. Splinting may also be accomplished with orthodontic appliances and wire, or by application of a metal arch bar with circumdental wiring of the bar (see Fig. 55-57B).

TABLE 55-34. TREATMENT SUMMARY		
	Primary Tooth	**Permanent Tooth**
Subluxation	No stabilization needed Soft or liquid diet Refer to dentist	No stabilization needed Soft or liquid diet Refer to dentist
Displacement	Extract if: 1. Intruded and close to permanent tooth OR expected to exfoliate within 6 months 2. Extruded Otherwise, allow to re-erupt	Nonmobile: No active treatment needed Refer to dentist for stabilization Mobile: Digital repositioning Temporary stabilization
Avulsion	Reimplantation not indicated	Cleanse the tooth—no scrubbing Examine and cleanse socket Reimplant tooth within 30 minutes If unable to reimplant immediately, store tooth in saliva or milk
Fractures		
Crown	Achieve hemostasis, pain control Protect/stabilize area Remove tooth fragment if aspiration risk Refer to dentist for restoration and/or endodontics	Same as primary teeth
Root	Apical or middle third: Reposition tooth and stabilize Refer to dentist for immobilization	Same as primary teeth
	Coronal third: Remove crown Protect and stabilize remaining root	Same as primary teeth
Dentoalveolar	Reposition and stabilize segments Remove loose bone fragments not attached to periosteum Refer to dentist or oral surgeon for definitive immobilization	Same as primary teeth

TOTAL DISPLACEMENT (AVULSION)

Primary Tooth. Reimplantation is not indicated because an avulsed deciduous tooth has a poor chance of survival if reimplanted.[8] Referral to a dentist is necessary to determine if some form of space maintainer is required to prevent the dental arch from collapsing before the permanent tooth erupts. If space is lost, permanent teeth could erupt ectopically or show a delayed eruption pattern.

Permanent Tooth. Immediate action is required whether the patient is seen in the dental office or ED or consulting over the telephone. A few simple steps can ensure the best chance for long-term retention of the tooth. If the case is discussed over the telephone, the practitioner can give the instructions to the patient or person accompanying him or her so that prompt reimplantation can be accomplished. The practitoner should:

1. Ascertain the history of the trauma and the time elapsed since the avulsive injury.
2. Determine the extent of associated injuries; if there has been contact with soil or other contaminants, consider tetanus prophylaxis.
3. Inspect the tooth for fractures and to evaluate the stage of root development. (Handle the tooth only by the crown if possible.) An incompletely formed root (open apex) may yield a better prognosis even if the tooth has been avulsed for a longer than ideal time.[9] The alveolus should be examined for signs of fractures or damage to adjacent teeth.
4. Cleanse the tooth. Care should be taken to avoid mechanical trauma to the root surface during handling. Do not rub or scrape the root surface because this denudes the remaining periodontal membrane. Simple rinsing with water (without drying) usually removes any foreign debris.
5. Advise on tooth storage. If the tooth is to be stored, storage in one of the following will suffice until reimplantation can be performed:
   —tongue or buccal vestibule of patient
   —tongue or buccal vestibule of parent, etc.
   —container of milk
   —container of normal saline
6. Reimplantation of the tooth should be accomplished as quickly (within 30 minutes) and atraumatically as possible. If there is a blood clot in the socket preventing the tooth from seating, suction, or curettage will dislodge the clot to allow for reim-

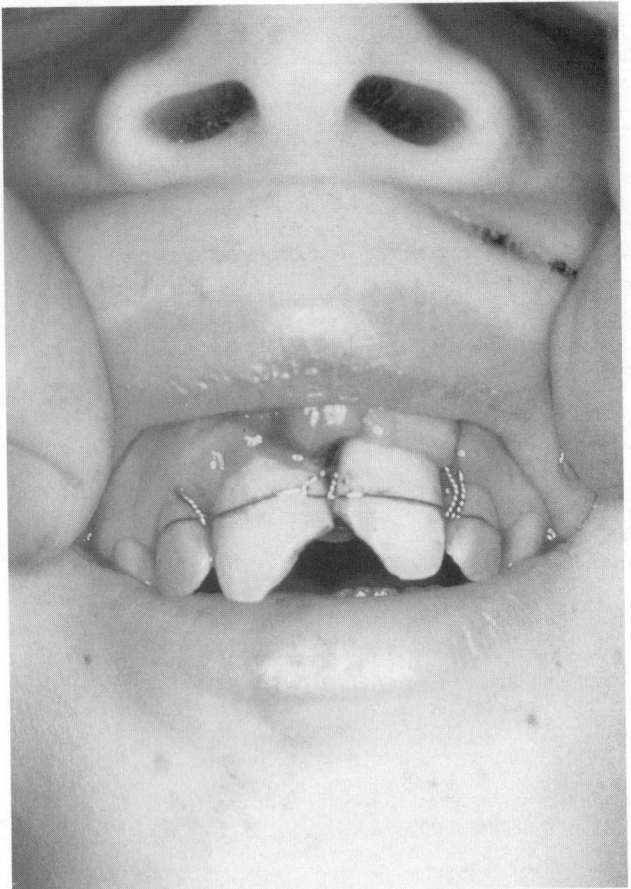 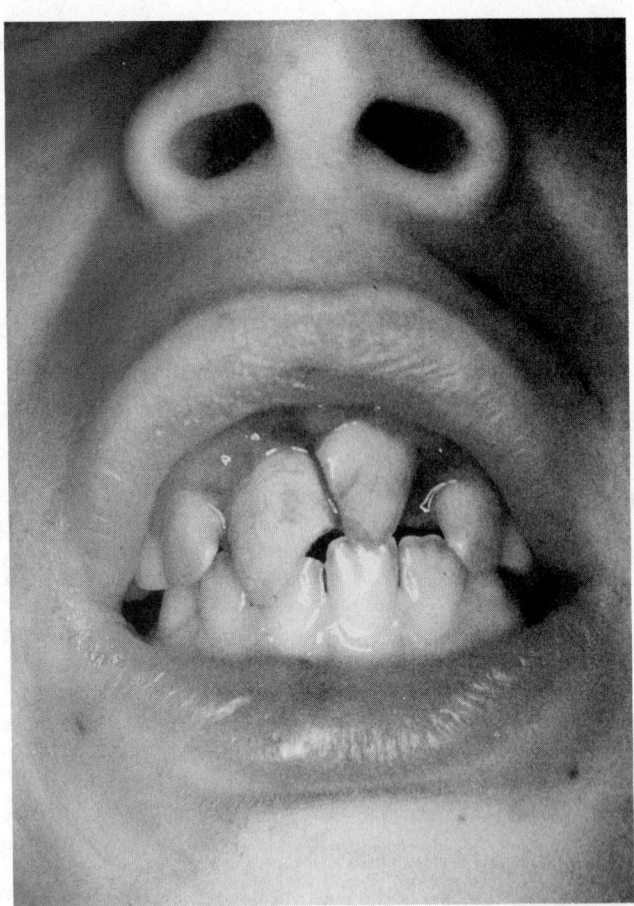

FIG. 55-53. A and B. This anteriorly displaced central incisor was manually repositioned and stabilized with a figure-of-eight stainless steel wire.

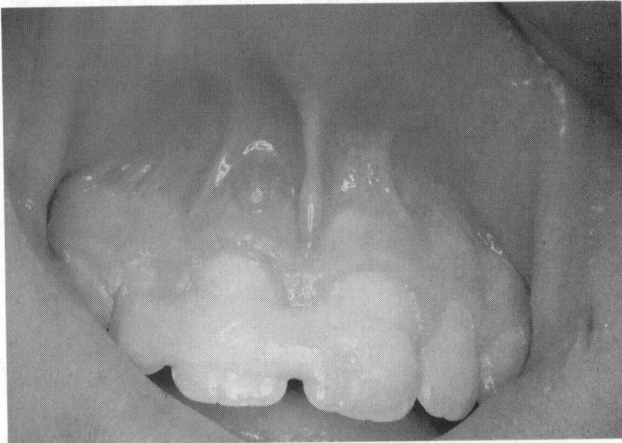

FIG. 55-54. A typical resin splint used by the dentist for stabilization.

plantation. The tooth should be reimplanted by digital pressure alone. Local anesthesia can be administered as necessary.

7. Treat soft tissue injuries.
8. Antibiotics should be prescribed (preferably penicillin) and achieve temporary stabilization until referral to a dentist for definitive splinting and endodontic (root canal) treatment if required.

Several factors may contraindicate reimplantation of an avulsed tooth. A nonfunctional tooth or one contained within an overcrowded dental arch should probably not be reimplanted. The presence of frank periodontal disease or severe caries contraindicates reimplantation. It is undesirable to reimplant a tooth with a fracture of the middle or cervical third of the crown, or when a fractured alveolar socket cannot support the tooth.[10]

After reimplantation, referral to a dentist is necessary for stabilization of the tooth. Acid-etch resin bonding is used most frequently and is kept in place for a period of 1 week. This short stabilization allows resumption of normal physiologic movement of the periodontal ligament, which has been shown to minimize the chance of root resorption. Root canal therapy is most often instituted several days to 1 week after reimplantation. Once the splint is removed, some tooth mobility still persists, and a soft diet is maintained for several weeks. Despite adequate stabilization and follow-up, a tooth that was not promptly reimplanted has a 75 to 96% chance of undergoing external root resorption (Fig. 55-55).

FRACTURED TEETH

In general, fractured teeth may require as urgent treatment as avulsed teeth. Prompt referral to a dentist ensures that definitive therapy will be instituted with as little delay as possible. The most frequent forms of dental therapy involve endodontics or repair with acid-etch resin techniques. Fractured deciduous teeth are treated in the same manner as permanent teeth. Several distinct types of injuries may occur, and are described below.

CORONAL (CROWN) FRACTURES

The fracture line may extend through enamel alone or enamel and dentin. Hemorrhage from the tooth or a small pink/red dot or line within the fractured area indicates that a pulp exposure has occurred. Hemorrhage can be easily controlled by using gentle pressure on the site with sterile cotton soaked in local anesthetic combined with a vascoconstrictor. Pain may be controlled by infiltration or appropriate nerve blocks. Avoid injecting anesthetic directly into the pulp tissue. If a small (several millimeters) pulp exposure is noted, the vitality of the tooth may be preserved if a dentist can apply a pulp "cap" of calcium hydroxide within several hours. If a large exposure is seen, endodontic therapy should be performed as soon as possible, with removal of all or part of the pulp contents. While a brief delay does not adversely affect the final treatment, remember that the patient is likely to have persistent pain and sensitivity until the exposure is treated. If it is left untreated for more than 24 to 48 hours, there is a significant chance for infection to develop. Infection can also develop without pulp exposure because dentin contains microtubules that can channel bacteria into the pulp chamber.

A fractured tooth fragment that is mobile but retained within the socket may have residual gingival attachment onto the tooth surface. If there is danger of aspiration of a loose fragment, the fragment should be gently removed with a hemostat, taking care to sever the remaining attachment without tearing tissue. Otherwise, temporary stabilization of the fragment without removal is desirable. Definitive dental treatment for the tooth structure may involve merely smoothing rough edges, or may require full restoration with a tooth-colored composite material or a crown.

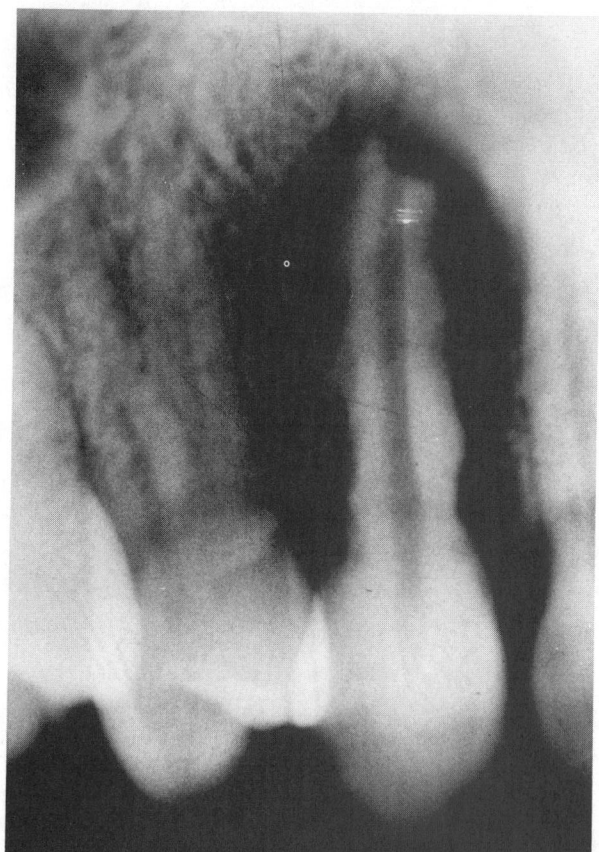

FIG. 55-55.   External root resorption after replantation of an avulsed tooth.

ROOT FRACTURES

Generally, the closer the root fracture is to the apex of the tooth, the better the prognosis for healing through repair or bony union. The location of the fracture can be assessed through radiographs and by clinically observing the mobility characteristics of the tooth. If the root fracture is within the middle third or apical third (nearest the root tip), the tooth should be immediately repositioned using finger pressure and firm stabilization. The dentist places a splint to immobilize the affected tooth for 1 to 3 months, with a good chance for healing to occur (Fig. 55-56). If the fracture is within the coronal third (near the junction of the crown and root), the crown portion should be removed if definitive endodontic therapy will not begin within a short time. A small, tightly folded gauze square can be placed over the retained root for protection and hemostasis. The dentist determines the final treatment (i.e., restoration or extraction) based on the location of the fracture and the restorability of the tooth.

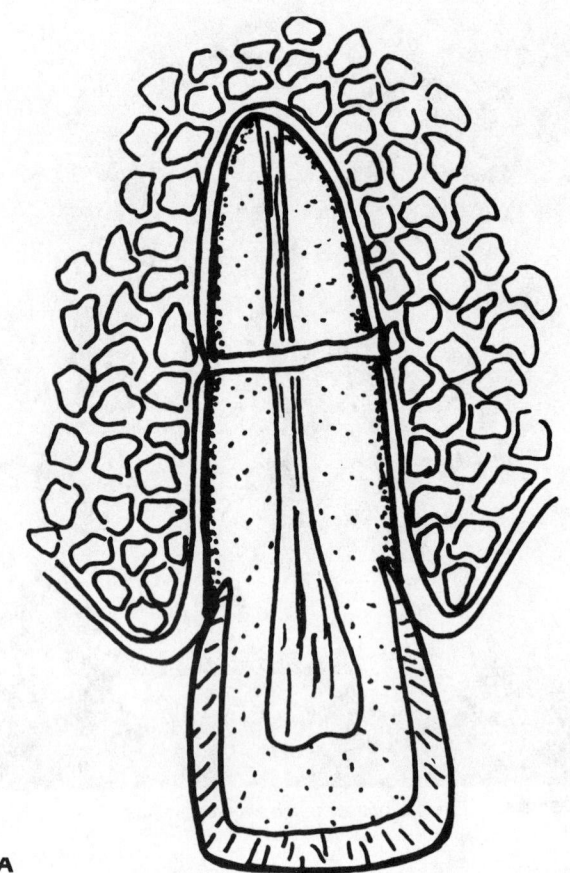
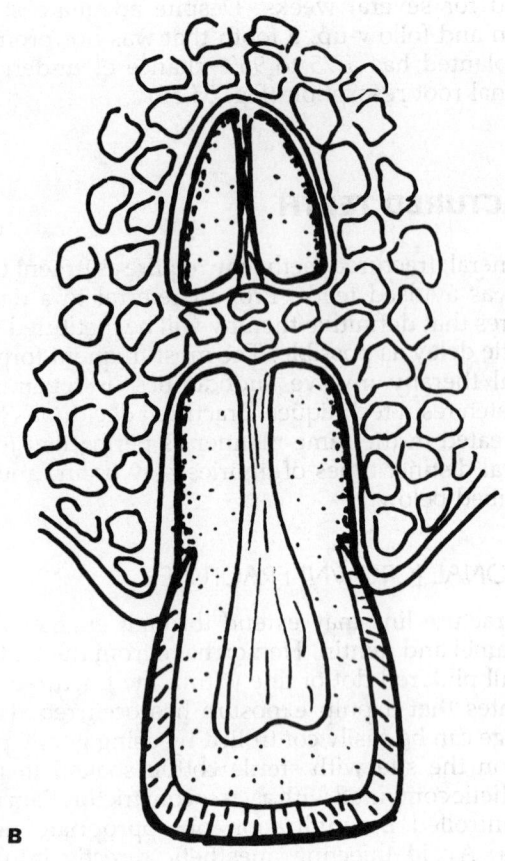

FIG. 55-56. A and B. A fracture of the apical third of the root has a good prognosis for healing if properly immobilized.

DENTOALVEOLAR FRACTURES

If a tooth and its alveolar segment are mobile, gentle repositioning of the segment is indicated. Loose bony pieces not attached to periosteum should be removed. If any attachment still remains, the bone should be conserved and not disturbed. Indiscriminate removal of bone can make future restoration of function and cosmetic appearance in the area difficult. The fractured segment can be stabilized by any of the methods described previously, or immobilized by placement of a metal arch bar of the type used in treatment of jaw fractures (Fig. 55-57).

SEQUELAE

Adverse sequelae of dentoalveolar trauma can compromise esthetics, function, and development of the dentofacial structures. These may include loss of tooth vitality, ankylosis (tooth fusing to bone), external or internal root resorption, infection, discoloration, loss of space in the dental arch with tooth migration, malformation of permanent teeth, premature loss of teeth, and compromised mastication and speech. Emotional distress can be common, especially when the injury involves the anterior teeth and is readily apparent during smiling or talking.

MEDICOLEGAL PEARLS

It is estimated that half of the children involved in child abuse sustain facial or oral injuries.[11] The dentoalveolar injuries described previously can be manifestations of child abuse. Suspicion should be aroused when a child under 3 years presents with dentoalveolar injuries that are poorly explained by par-

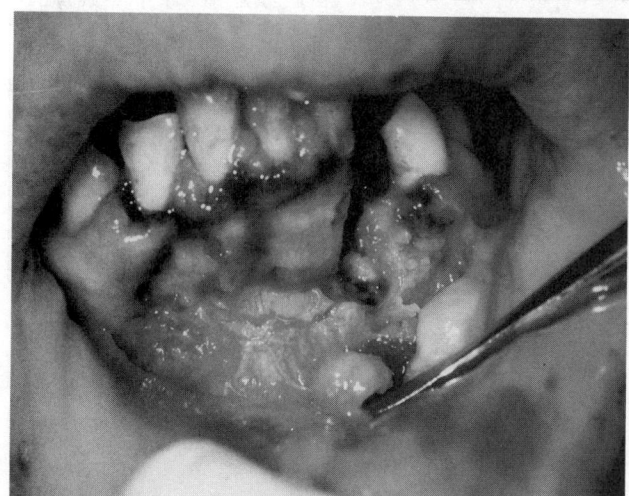

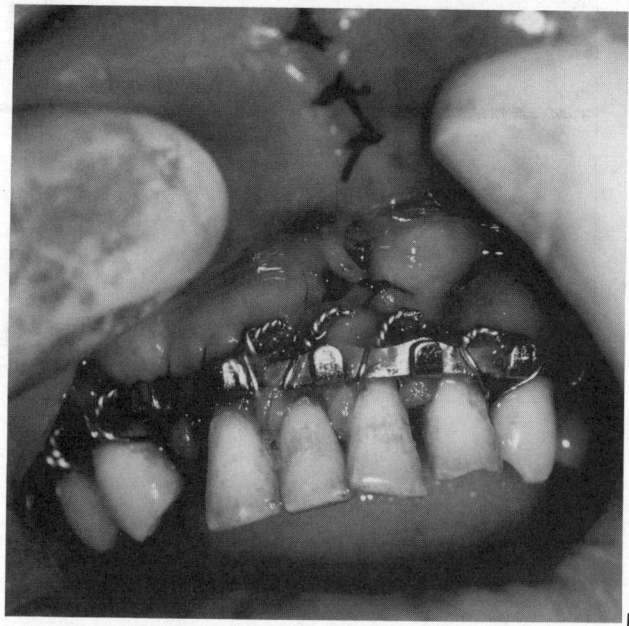

FIG. 55-57.   A. Dentoalveolar fracture with accompanying soft tissue injuries. B. Repositioned alveolar segment with arch bar stabilization.

ents, or when there is a delay of hours or days in seeking treatment. Further examination may be needed, and may disclose generalized bruising, broken bones, and other evidence of abuse.

NATIONAL CONTACTS

State and local dental societies are the best resources for information and referrals.

REFERENCES

1. Andreasen, J.O., and Ravn, J.J.: Epidemiology of traumatic dental injuries to primary and permanent teeth in a Danish population sample. Int. J. Oral Surg. *1*:235, 1972.
2. Andreasen, J.O.: Traumatic Injuries of the Teeth. Philadelphia, W.B. Saunders Co., 1981, p. 30.
3. Andreasen, J.O., and Hjorting-Hansen, E.: Replantation of teeth I: radiographic and clinical study of 110 human teeth reimplanted after accidental loss. Acta Odontol. Scand. *24*:263, 1966.
4. Soder, P.O., Otteskog, P., Andreasen, J.O., et al.: Effect of drying on viability of periodontal membrane. Scand. J. Dent. Res. *85*:164, 1977.
5. Blomlof, L., Andersson, L., Lindskog, S., et al.: Storage of experimentally avulsed teeth in milk prior to replantation. J. Dent. Res. *62*:912, 1983.
6. Courts, F.J., Mueller, W.A., and Tabeling, H.J.: Milk as an interim storage medium for avulsed teeth. Pediatr. Dent. *5*:183, 1983.
7. Schreiber, C.K.: The effect of trauma on the anterior deciduous teeth. Brit. Dent. J. *106*:340, 1959.
8. Needleman, H.L.: Total tooth displacement and reimplantation. *In* The Management of Traumatized Anterior Teeth of Children. Edited by Hargreaves, J.A., Craig, J.W., and Needleman, H.L. New York, Churchill Livingstone, 1981, p. 98.
9. Ibid., p. 103.
10. Olson, R.A.J.: Dentition and Alveolar Process Injuries. *In* Maxillofacial Trauma. Edited by Alling, C.C., and Osbon, D.B. Philadelphia. Lea & Febiger, 1988, p. 390.
11. Becker, D.B., Needleman, H.L., and Kotelchuck, M.: Child abuse and dentistry: orofacial trauma and its recognition by dentists. J. Am. Dent. Assoc. *97*:24, 1978.

BIBLIOGRAPHY

Andreasen, J.O.: Traumatic Injuries of the Teeth. Philadelphia, W.B. Saunders Co., 1981.

Chapter 56

DERMATOLOGY IN THE EMERGENCY DEPARTMENT

THE DERMATOLOGIC EXAMINATION

Philip D. Shenefelt and Neil A. Fenske

CAPSULE

Dermatologic examination and diagnosis require visual pattern recognition combined with information obtained from the history, and if necessary, special procedures, laboratory tests, and skin biopsies. It is important for the examiner to establish a personal methodic routine or habit pattern to follow when performing the examination, taking the history, considering a differential diagnosis, and arriving at the diagnosis. A recommended routine for dermatologic examination is outlined.

INTRODUCTION

Dermatologic diagnosis requires a mental process of rapid pattern recognition based primarily on visual perception. Recent studies show that chance favors the prepared mind. For example, accuracy of diagnosis was 21% for second-year medical students using 100 slides of common skin conditions as a test. For fourth-year medical students, accuracy was 31% and for second year family practice residents, it was 55%. General practitioners scored 66%, and dermatologists attained 87% accuracy. Correct diagnoses were associated with quick response times, whereas errors were associated with much longer response times. This finding suggests that errors result from confusion in pattern recognition rather than carelessness or haste. Hence, der-

matologic diagnosis is based more on visual pattern than on mastery of complex rules.[1]

EVALUATION PATTERN FOR SKIN LESIONS

Because visual pattern recognition is the key to dermatologic diagnosis, the dermatologic physical examination is usually performed before rather than after extensive history-taking. First you, as the examiner, elicit the chief complaint and a brief history of the timing of onset and development of the lesions and associated events. Then proceed directly to the physical examination. Based on the types and pattern of skin lesions seen, mentally place the findings in one or more categories of differential diagnoses, such as papulosquamous or eczematous. At this point, obtain a more detailed history, focusing on questions that will help to include or exclude the various diagnostic possibilities within the differential diagnosis categories under consideration. Re-examination of the types and patterns of skin lesions may then be indicated, based on new information from the history. When needed, special office examinations, laboratory tests, or skin biopsies are performed to assist in arriving at a working diagnosis. For some diagnoses, one glance at the skin lesions is all that is necessary. Common examples are typical acne, typical psoriasis, typical pityriasis rosea, and typical herpes zoster. For other diagnoses, considerably more time and effort may be required. Once you have established the working diagnosis or limited set of differential diagnoses, it is sometimes necessary to follow the patient through several visits to confirm the diagnosis or determine the cause. This is frequently the case with contact dermatitis when the history does not reveal the cause.

2254

CHIEF COMPLAINT AND BRIEF HISTORY

The history should begin with statements of the patient's race, sex, age, and chief complaint. Do not assume that an obvious, visible skin condition such as acne or psoriasis is what brought the patient to see you. The patient's chief complaint may be another unrelated skin condition. Asking the patient what problem he or she has come to see you about will save you and the patient from embarrassment or hostility.

The patient comes to see you motivated by concerns reflected in the chief complaint. At one extreme, a condition that may be psychologically distressing to the patient may seem medically trivial to you. At the other extreme, a skin condition that may not bother the patient may appear to you to warrant medical treatment. It is important to recognize the psychologic impact of the skin disease on the patient. You may anger or embarrass the patient if you dismiss the chief complaint as medically trivial. It is important to treat the patient's concerns with respect and address the concerns rather than brushing them aside. Patient education and reassurance may be all that are necessary.

Occasionally you see a patient who is too embarrassed to tell you the true chief complaint initially. Such a patient may have you examine some nevi or other apparently trivial condition while working up the courage to ask you about a genital lesion. Rushing the patient may inhibit him or her from communicating the true chief complaint to you.

After eliciting the chief complaint, you should obtain a brief history of the present illness: duration of the problem with time sequence, symptoms, environmental exposure including occupation and hobbies, oral and topical medications, family history, and sexual history if appropriate.

PHYSICAL EXAMINATION OF THE SKIN

The patient should be undressed and draped. You should perform a full body skin examination in all instances when it is not refused by the patient. Refusal of full skin examination should be noted in the medical record. Not performing a full body skin examination can result in missed diagnoses. The physician must nonetheless use discretion and be sensitive to the modesty of the patient so as not to alienate the patient and lose cooperation.

Adequate lighting is essential for proper examination of the skin. A portable light and a magnifying lens can greatly assist you when close scrutiny of the skin is required. Inadequate illumination can cause you to miss the diagnosis.

When examining the skin, you should inspect and palpate in a systematic, thorough, and organized manner. If you suspect infection or the eruption is moist or oozing, you should wear examination gloves when palpating the lesions. Start with the global examination and work to the specific. Note the locations of the lesions, their arrangement in terms of symmetry and configuration, types of primary and secondary lesions present, size, shape, color, and any induration, tenderness, or mobility (Table 56-1). Also note any

TABLE 56-1. PHYSICAL EXAMINATION OF THE SKIN

LOCATION OF LESIONS
  SITES
  EXTENT
  ARRANGEMENT
    SYMMETRY
    CONFIGURATION
CHARACTERISTIC LESIONS
  PRIMARY AND SECONDARY
    FLAT
      MACULE
        NONSCALY
        SCALY
      PETECHIAE
      ECCHYMOSIS
    FLAT OR DEPRESSED
      ATROPHY
      SCLEROSIS
      INFARCT
      GANGRENE
    FLAT OR ELEVATED
      TELANGIECTASIA
      PURPURA
    FLAT, ELEVATED, OR DEPRESSED
      ABSCESS
      CYST
      NODULE
      SCAR
    ELEVATED
      WHEAL
      VESICLE
      BULLA
      PUSTULE
      PAPULE
        NONSCALY
        SCALY
      PLAQUE
        NONSCALY
        SCALY
      VEGETATION
      KERATOSIS
      LICHENIFICATION
    ELEVATED OR DEPRESSED
      EXUDATE (CRUSTS)
    DEPRESSED
      EROSION
      EXCORIATION
      FISSURE
      ULCER
  SIZE
  SHAPE
  COLOR
    HYPER- OR HYPOPIGMENTATION
    SHADE
    INTENSITY
    SURROUNDINGS
  INDURATION
  TENDERNESS
  MOBILITY
NONCUTANEOUS FINDINGS
  ORAL
  SATELLITE ADENOPATHY
  INTERNAL

associated noncutaneous findings such as adenopathy, oral lesions, or internal findings.[2]

LOCATION OF LESIONS

Determining the sites of the lesions helps to narrow the diagnostic possibilities. Each type of skin disease has predilections for certain body areas. The skin areas usually considered as separate units are the scalp, face, eyelids, mouth, trunk, axillae, anogenital area, arms and forearms, thighs and legs, hands and feet, nails, and hair. Be alert to recognize certain regional distributions such as photoexposed, intertriginous, flexural, extensor, hair-bearing, acne-prone, apocrine, and palmar-plantar areas.

Also note the extent of the lesions in terms of skin areas affected and the amount of involvement within each area. To estimate the percentage of total skin involved, you can use the burn formula rule of nines for body surface. Estimate the percentage of involvement in each area of skin, multiply that by the percentage of total body area represented by that region, and add up the results for each area to get total body involvement. For example, if about 70% of each leg is involved, and each leg is about 18% of the total body area, 70% times 18% times 2 legs is about 25% of the total body area.

ARRANGEMENT OF LESIONS

The overall arrangement of the lesions in terms of symmetry and configuration or grouping also helps to narrow the diagnostic possibilities. Bilateral symmetry of the lesions implies generalized internal factors or symmetric external exposure. Asymmetry implies localized internal factors or localized external exposure. Configuration is the pattern produced by the spatial relationships of the various lesions or parts of the lesion. Common terms used to describe configurations or groupings are as follows:

ANNULAR: ring-like; only the outer edge of the circle (Fig. 56-1).
ARCUATE: curved; only the border of the curve (Fig. 56-2).
CIRCINATE: circular, involving the whole area of the circle (Fig. 56-3).
CONFLUENT: running together (Fig. 56-4).
DISCOID: disk-like; solid, round, and slightly raised.
DISCRETE: separate (Fig. 56-4).
GROUPED: clustered (Fig. 56-5).
GUTTATE: scattered like drops (Fig. 56-6).
GYRATE: coiled or winding around.
HERPETIFORM: creeping (Fig. 56-7).
IRIS OR TARGET: concentric circles (Fig. 56-8).
LINEAR: line-like (Fig. 56-9).
NUMMULAR: coin-like.
POLYCYCLIC: borders of irregular curves (Fig. 56-10).

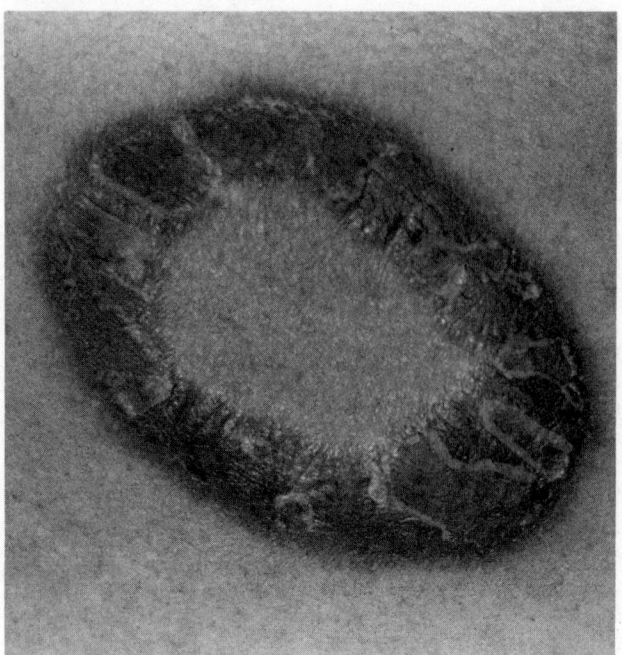

FIG. 56-1.   Annular lesion of psoriasis with central clearing.

RETIFORM: net-like (Fig. 56-11).
SERPIGINOUS: crawling like a snake (Fig. 56-12).
ZOSTERIFORM or DERMATOMAL: belt-like on one side of the body (Fig. 56-13).

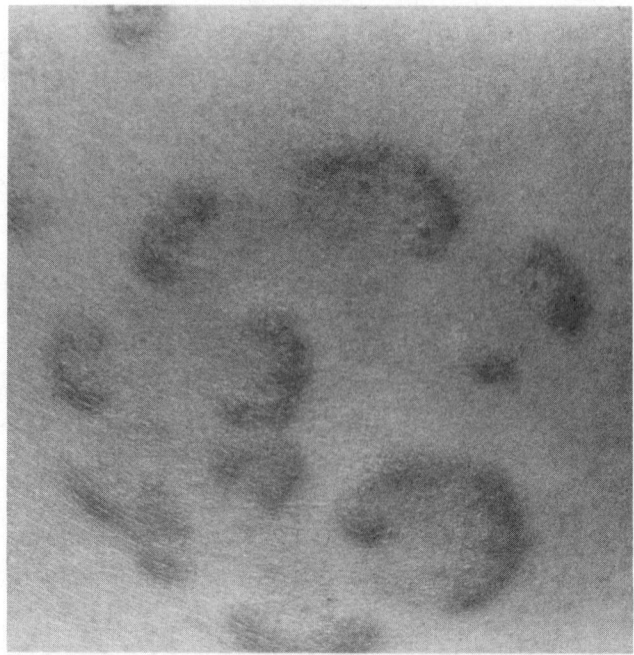

FIG. 56-2.   Arcuate lesions of granuloma annulare.

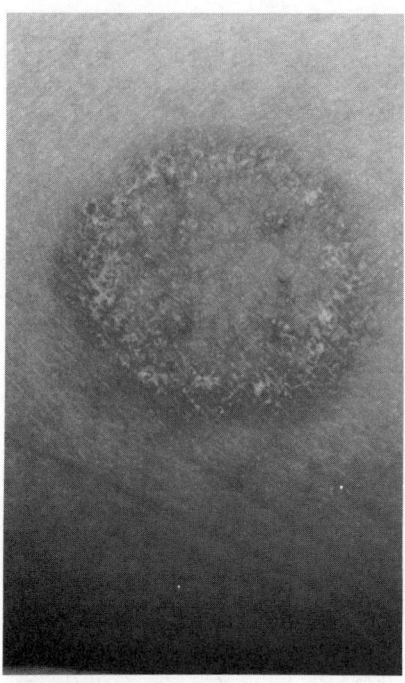

FIG. 56-3. Circinate macular lesion of tinea corporis.

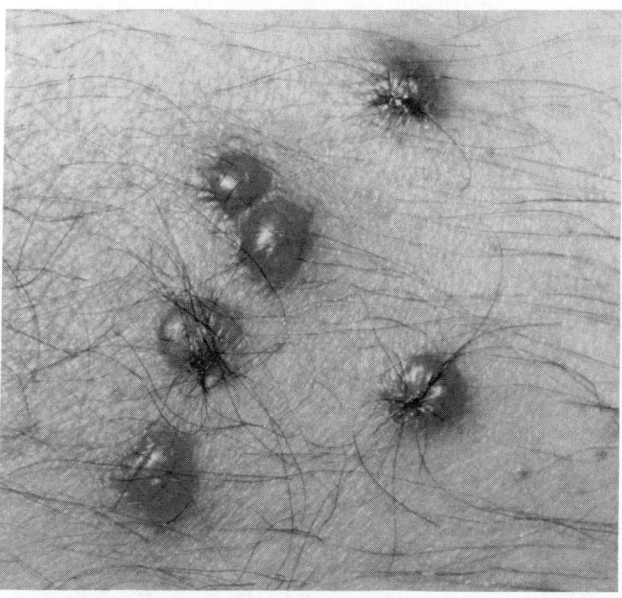

FIG. 56-5. Grouped vesicular insect bite reactions.

CHARACTERISTIC LESIONS OR MORPHOLOGY

Primary lesions are those not altered by secondary factors such as infection, eczematization, healing, or therapy. Accurate recognition of the primary lesion is the key to diagnosis. Details of small lesions can be better appreciated with an illuminated magnifying glass. Examples of primary lesions are macules, papules, nodules, tumors, cysts, plaques, wheals, vesicles, bullae, pustules, and burrows. Secondary lesions appear after the primary lesions are altered by healing or exogenous factors. Examples of secondary lesions are crusts, scales, fissures, erosions, ulcerations, excoriations, lichenification, atrophy, and scarring. Following are definitions of common primary and secondary lesions. They are grouped according to flatness, elevation, or depression with respect to the skin surface.

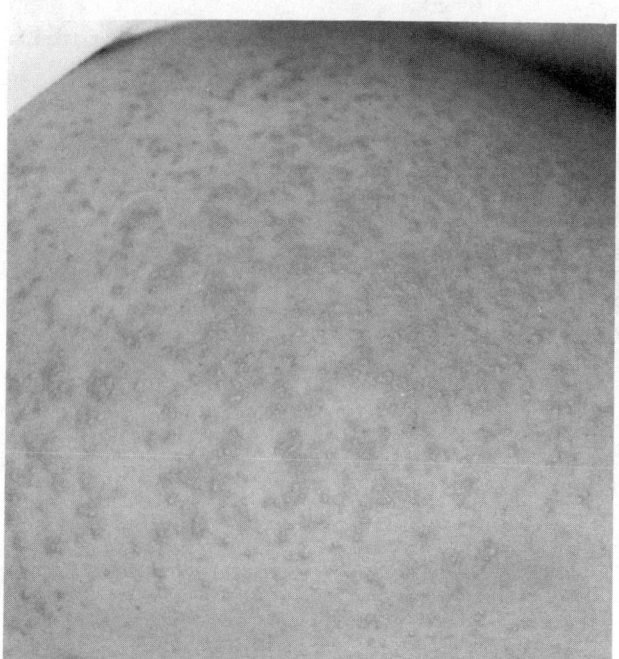

FIG. 56-4. Discrete peripheral and confluent central lesions of contact dermatitis on thigh.

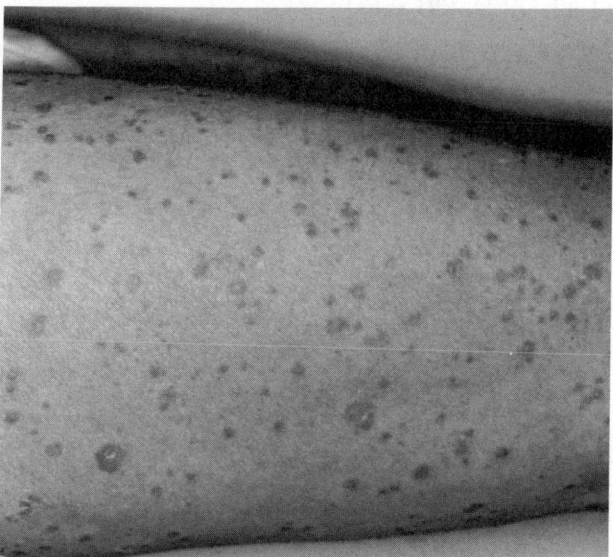

FIG. 56-6. Guttate lesions of guttate psoriasis on thigh.

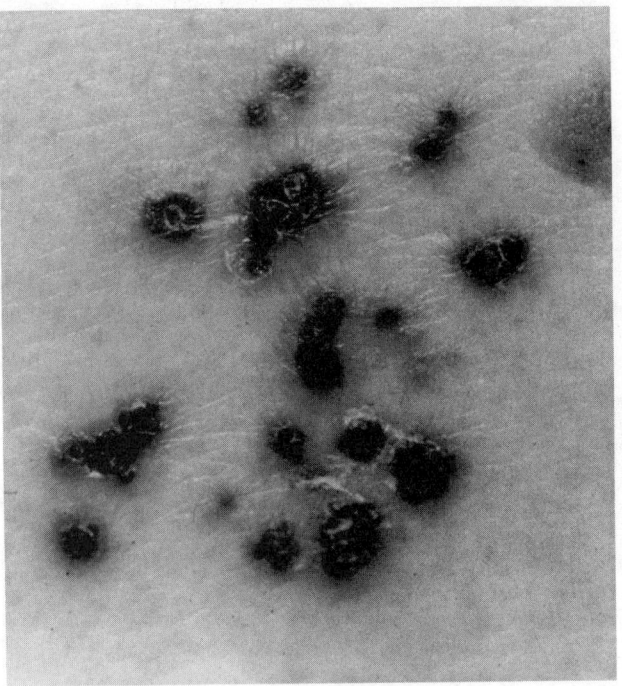

FIG. 56-7. Herpetiform crusts of herpes simplex lesions several days old.

PRIMARY AND SECONDARY SKIN LESIONS

FLAT

MACULE: a flat, circumscribed change in skin color 1 cm or less in diameter, smooth or scaly, with whitish fine to coarse flakes (Fig. 56-3).

PETECHIAE: tiny nonblanching purple spots, 1 to 2 mm in diameter.

FLAT OR DEPRESSED

ATROPHY: thinning of one or more skin components, with fine "cigarette paper" wrin-

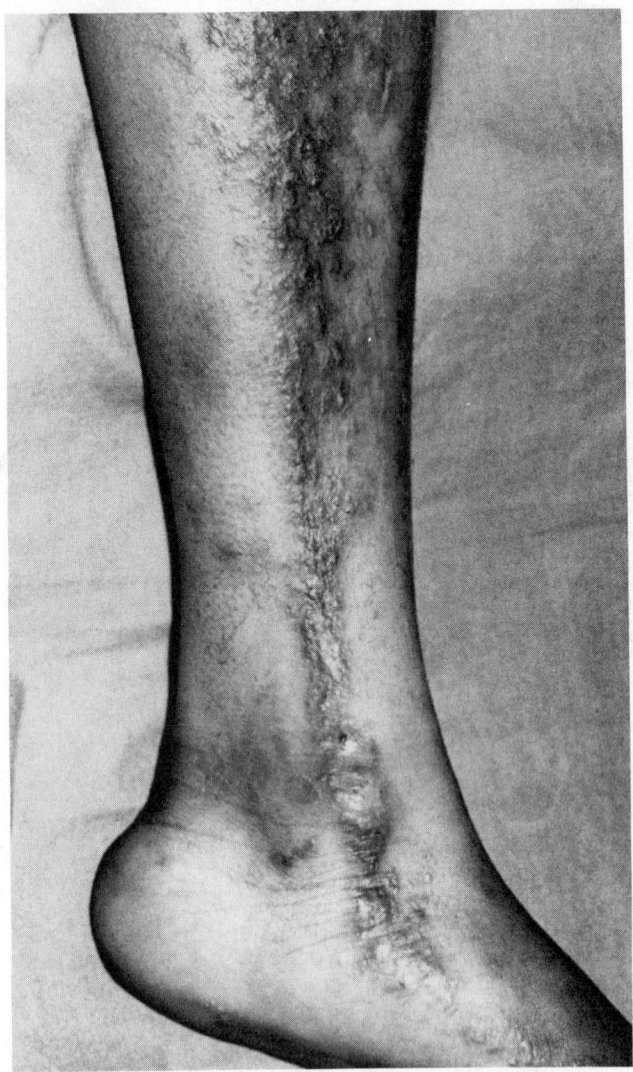

FIG. 56-9. Linear band of lichen striatus on lower leg.

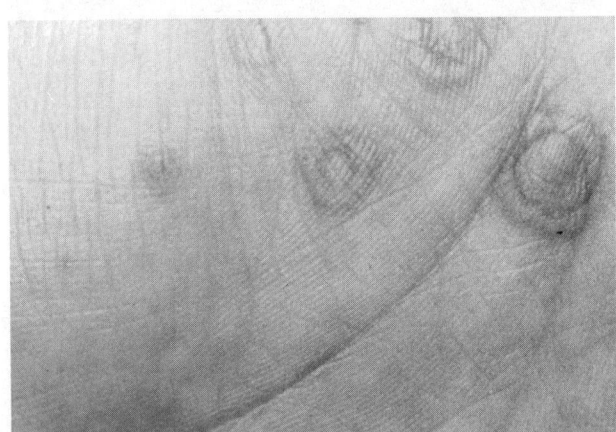

FIG. 56-8. Target lesions of erythema multiforme on palm.

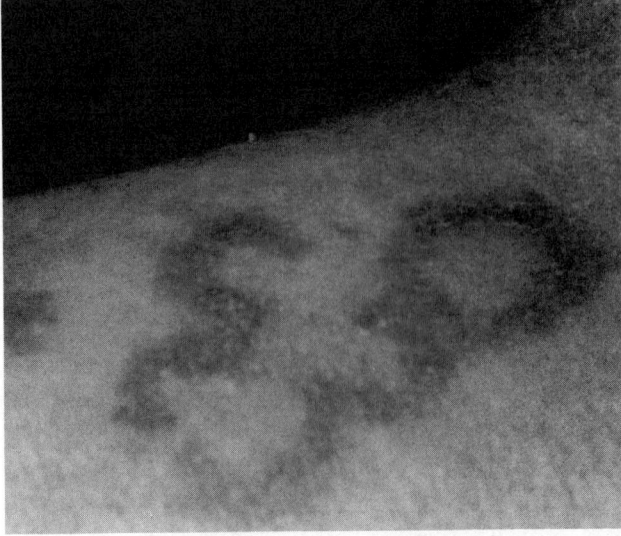

FIG. 56-10. Polycyclic lesions of subacute cutaneous lupus erythematosus on upper back.

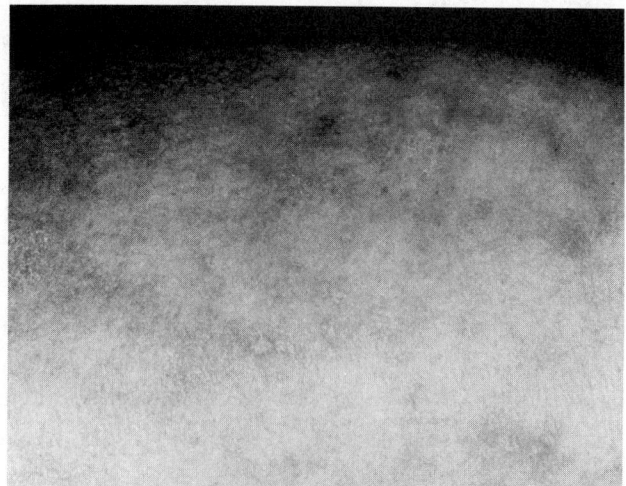

FIG. 56-11.   Retiform pattern of livedo reticularis on leg.

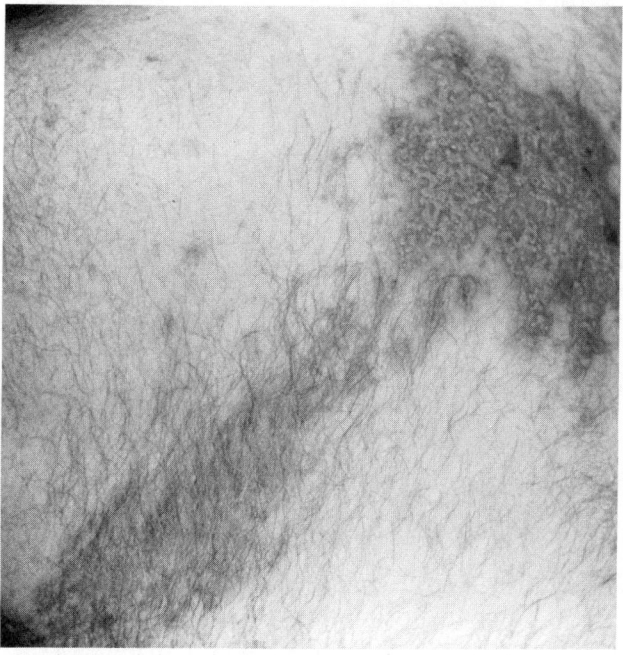

FIG. 56-13.   Zosteriform band of herpes zoster on back.

kling if epidermal, and depression if dermal (Fig. 56-14).

SCLEROSIS: firm, indurated skin.

INFARCT: cutaneous necrosis, usually reddish gray.

GANGRENE: tissue necrosis, usually bluish-black in color, then sloughing, often malodorous.

FLAT OR ELEVATED

TELANGIECTASIA: blanchable small superficial dilated capillaries.

PURPURA: a nonblanching purple discoloration from extravasation of blood in the skin.

FLAT, ELEVATED, OR DEPRESSED

ABSCESS: a tender red fluctuant nodule, sometimes with a draining sinus.

CYST: a spheric sac containing fluid or semisolid material (Fig. 56-15).

NODULE: a palpable solid lesion, deeper than a papule in the dermis or subcutaneous tissue, 1 cm or less in diameter.

TUMOR: a nodule more than 1 cm in diameter (Fig. 56-16).

SCAR: a fibrotic area following dermal damage, usually with loss of normal skin lines.

ELEVATED

WHEAL: an evanescent, edematous papule or plaque, usually lasting only a few hours, with peripheral redness (Fig. 56-17).

VESICLE: a circumscribed, thin-walled, elevated skin lesion containing fluid and 5 mm or less in diameter (Fig. 56-5).

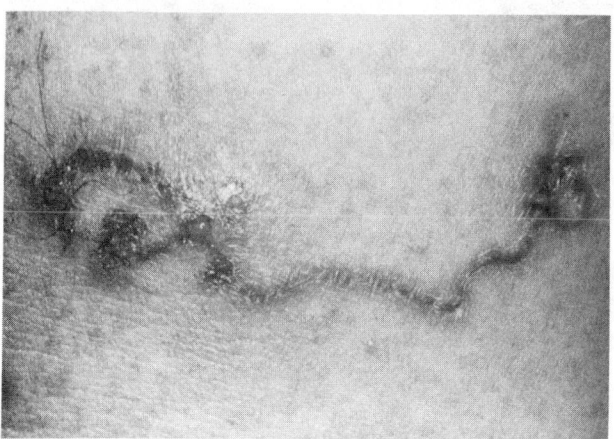

FIG. 56-12.   Serpiginous track of cutaneous larval migrans.

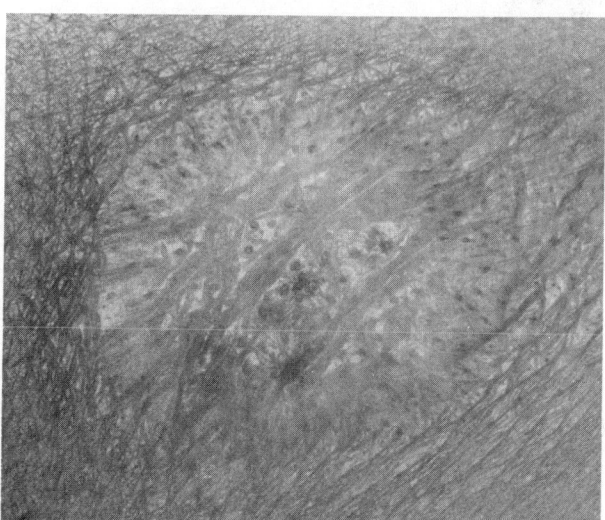

FIG. 56-14.   Atrophic "cigarette paper" wrinkling of lichen sclerosis et atrophicus.

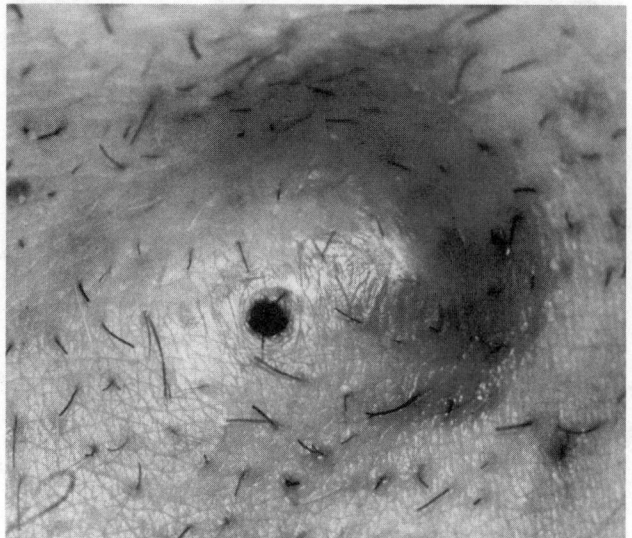

FIG. 56-15.   Cyst with comedo.

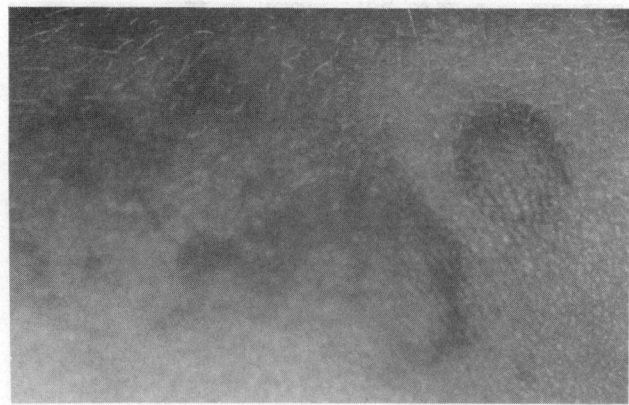

FIG. 56-17.   Wheals of urticaria.

BULLA: a vesicle more than 5 mm in diameter (Fig. 56-18).

PUSTULE: a vesicle containing purulent material.

PAPULE: a solid, palpable, elevated skin lesion 1 cm or less in diameter, smooth or scaly (Fig. 56-19).

PLAQUE: a flat-topped elevation, often formed by a confluence of papules, with a smooth or scaly surface (Fig. 56-20).

VEGETATION: multiple small closely packed projections on a papule or plaque.

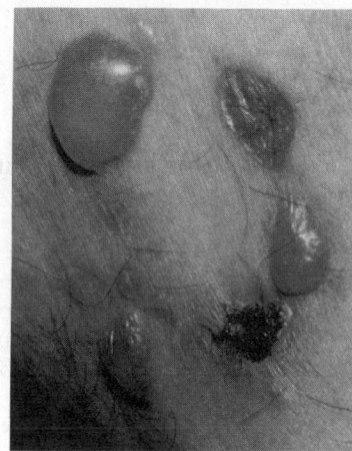

FIG. 56-18.   Bullae of bullous pemphigoid.

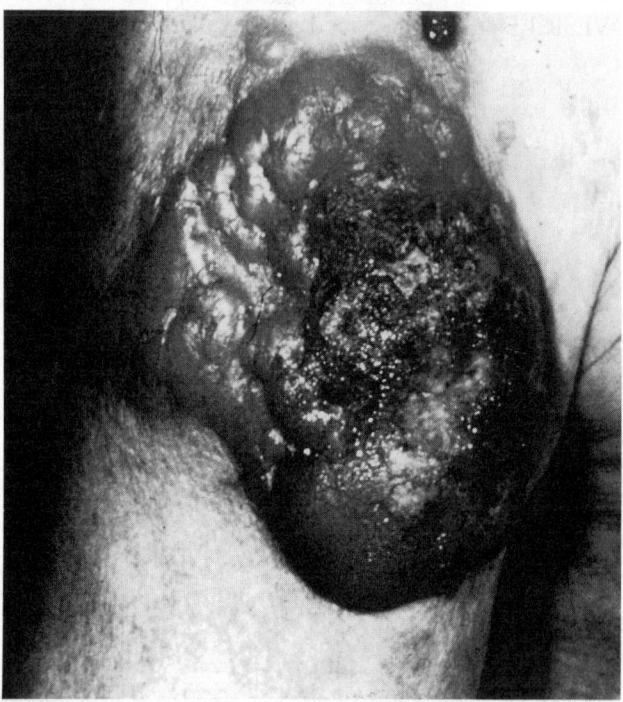

FIG. 56-16.   Tumor of mycosis fungoides on arm.

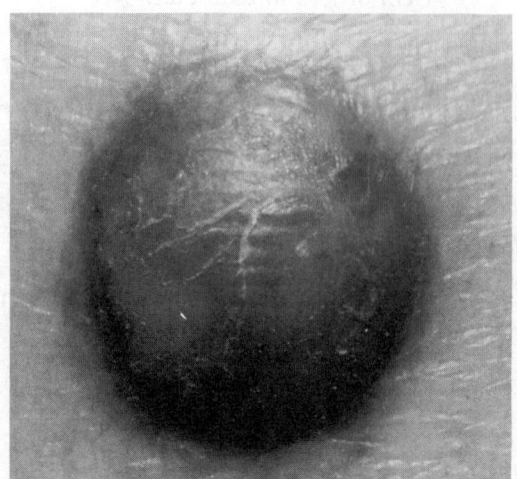

FIG. 56-19.   Papule of fibroxanthoma.

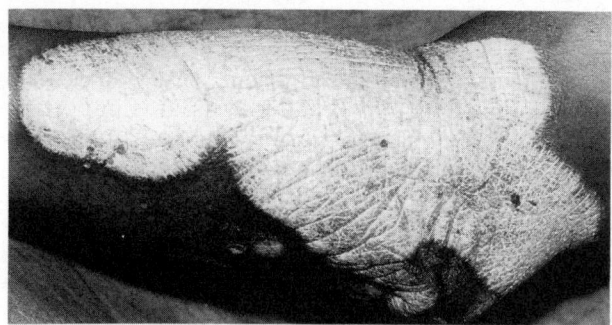

FIG. 56-20.   Plaque of psoriasis on forearm.

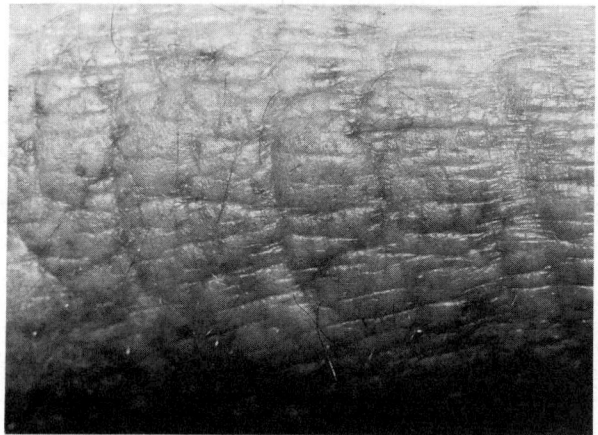

FIG. 56-21.   Lichenification in lichen simplex chronicus.

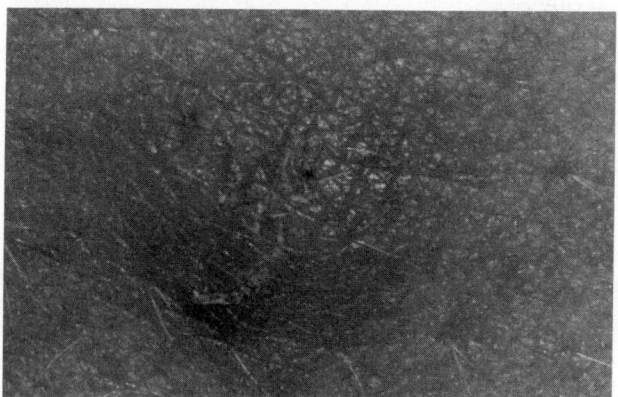

FIG. 56-22.   Scabies burrow.

KERATOSIS: a papule with excessive cornification.
LICHENIFICATION: thickened skin with accentuated skin marking lines (Fig. 56-
21).
COMEDO: a papule centering on an impacted pilo-
sebaceous unit (Fig. 56-15).
BURROW: a small linear papule usually associated
with scabies (Fig. 56-22).

ELEVATED OR DEPRESSED

EXUDATE (CRUSTS): oozing or dried concretions,
yellow to brown to black (Fig.
56-7).

DEPRESSED

EROSION: ruptured vesiculobullous lesion denuding
the epidermis but not involving dermis
(Fig. 56-23).
EXCORIATION: linear erosions produced by scratch-
ing.
FISSURE: linear cracks in skin surface.
ULCER: loss of epidermis and part or all of dermis
(Fig. 56-24).

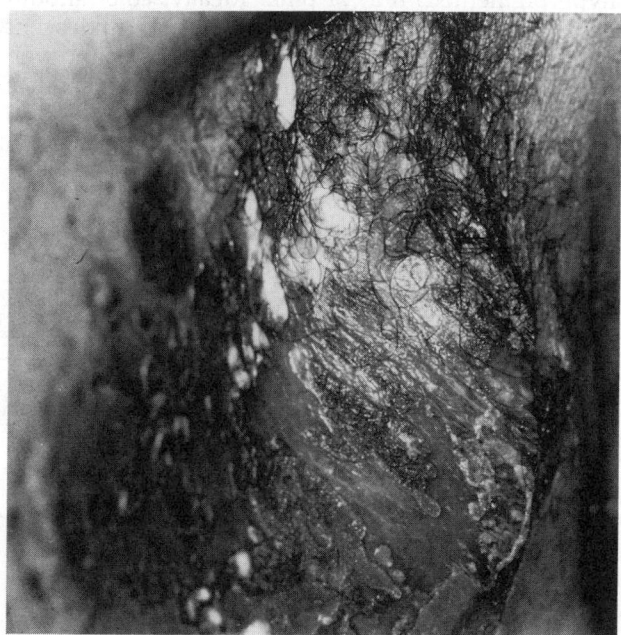

FIG. 56-23.   Erosions of pemphigus vulgaris on inner thigh.

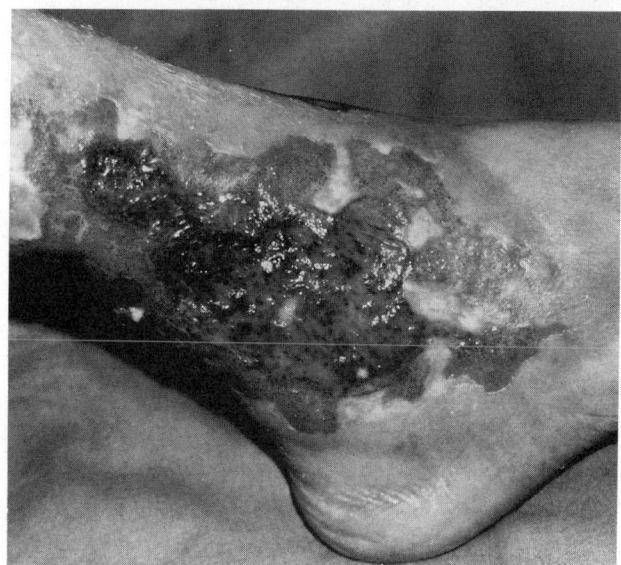

FIG. 56-24.   Ulcer as complication of stasis dermatitis.

The size of the average lesions should be estimated or measured in millimeters or centimeters. If the shape is not round, the dimensions of its long axis and short axis should be given. A flexible clear plastic ruler is useful for making the measurements.

The shape of the individual lesions should be described. The lesions may be circular, annular, oval, polygonal, or linear. Lesions may be monomorphous or polymorphous.

The color of the lesions should be described. There may be hyperpigmentation or hypopigmentation. The color may be red, pink, salmon, orange, yellow, green, blue, violaceous, purple, brown, black, white, or gray. Intensity of color may be described as dull or bright. The surroundings may be normal skin color, pale, hyperpigmented, red, or pink. Ideally, color should be evaluated under natural sunlight. Incandescent lighting shifts the appearance toward reds and yellows; most fluorescent lighting shifts the appearance toward blues.

Induration or woodiness is detected by palpation of the lesions. At the same time, the patient can report any tenderness. You can also check nodules for mobility over underlying structures and for fluctuance.

NONCUTANEOUS FINDINGS

Certain skin diseases may present with oral, ocular, or genital mucous membrane lesions. It is important to check these areas as part of the general cutaneous examination and also to check for regional satellite adenopathy and generalized adenopathy. If indicated by diagnostic considerations or patient complaints, check internal organ systems by physical examination.

HISTORY OF THE SKIN LESIONS

ONE LESION OR SEVERAL DISCRETE LESIONS

When an eruption consists of one or several discrete lesions, elicit from the history its development, course, and treatment (Table 56-2). Determine the duration of the eruption, its character at onset, its course of development, and any secondary changes that have occured. Elicit the symptoms. In the case of an inflamed lesion, does it itch or hurt? For a tumor, has it grown or changed in shape or color? Has it bled or drained? If the lesion is systemic, has there been associated fever, malaise, or weight loss? Do any family mem-

---

TABLE 56-2. HISTORY OF THE SKIN LESIONS

IF THERE IS AN ERUPTION OF ONE OR SEVERAL DISCRETE
  LESIONS
  DURATION
  CHARACTER AT ONSET
  COURSE OF DEVELOPMENT
  SECONDARY CHANGES
  SYMPTOMS
  THERAPY
    DATES
    NATURE
    BY WHOM
    RESULTS
      IMMEDIATE
      SUBSEQUENT
  BIOPSY (?)—RESULTS
IF THERE IS AN ERUPTION OF MULTIPLE LESIONS OR OF A
  DIFFUSE NATURE
  ONSET
    SITE
    NATURE AT START
  TIME (DATE OR SEASON)
  ASSOCIATED EVENTS
    ILLNESS
    MEDICATIONS
    VOCATION
    HOBBIES
    EMOTIONAL STATUS
    CONTAGION
    GEOGRAPHIC LOCALE
  COURSE
    SEQUENCE
      CONTINUOUS
      INTERMITTENT
      CYCLIC
      IRREGULAR
      RELATED ASSOCIATIONS
    PROGRESSION
      ADDITIONAL LESIONS

      SEQUENCE OF SITES
      COALESCENCE
      REGRESSION
      CURRENT TREND
  SYMPTOMS
    CUTANEOUS
      ITCHING
      PAIN
    SYSTEMIC
      PRECEDING
      CONCURRENT
      SUBSEQUENT
  TREATMENT
    PROFESSIONAL (BY WHOM?) OR NONPROFESSIONAL
    DATES AND DURATION
    NATURE (EXTERNAL, INTERNAL)
    RESULTS
      INFLUENCE ON ERUPTION
      ALLERGY OR TOXICITY
  GENERAL CUTANEOUS HISTORY
    PREVIOUS ERUPTIONS (SIMILAR OR APPARENTLY UN-
      RELATED)
      DATES
      DURATION
      COURSE
      RESPONSE TO TREATMENT
  FAMILIAL CUTANEOUS HISTORY
GENERAL NONCUTANEOUS HISTORY (AS A RULE, BRIEF)
  PREVIOUS SYSTEMIC OR SERIOUS ILLNESS
  ANY IMMEDIATELY PRECEDING ILLNESS
  CONCURRENT OR SUBSEQUENT ILLNESS
  SEXUAL
  ATOPY OR OTHER ALLERGY (PERSONAL OR FAMILIAL)
  ALLERGY TO ANY MEDICATIONS
  MEDICATIONS (PRECEDING, CONCURRENT, OR SUBSE-
    QUENT)
  SPECIAL FOR SPECIFIC DERMATOSES (LIPIDS, DIABETES,
    ETC.)

bers, friends, or coworkers have similar lesions? Has the patient been exposed to anything different lately at work or through hobbies or travels? Has the patient had any previous laboratory tests, skin scrapings, or biopsies?

Regarding previous treatment, what prescription and nonprescription agents, home remedies, etc., has the patient used? What were the dates of treatment, who performed the treatments, and what were the results, both immediate and subsequent? Sometimes, when asked in a general way about treatments, a patient denies using any treatment, but when asked about specific treatments, is prompted to remember using one or several treatments. What kind of skin care does the patient practice? What soaps, clothing, laundry detergents, fabric softeners, perfumes, lotions, or cosmetics does the patient use?

MULTIPLE LESIONS OR LESIONS OF A DIFFUSE NATURE

When the lesions are multiple or of a diffuse nature, elicit from the history the onset, development, spread, associated events, course, and treatment (see Table 56-2). Determine the date and site of onset, nature at the beginning, season of the year, and any associated events such as illness, medications, vocation, hobbies, emotional status, contagion, and geographic locale. Ask about the course of the lesions in terms of sequence and progression. Has it been continuous, intermittent, cyclic, or irregular? Were there any associated illnesses, activities, or events? Have there been any additional lesions? What has been the sequence of lesion sites? Have they coalesced? Have any regressed? What is the current trend? What kind of cutaneous symptoms has the patient had in terms of itching, pain, burning sensation, etc.? Has the patient had any systemic symptoms preceding, concurrent with, or subsequent to the eruptions? Regarding previous treatment, has it been professional or nonprofessional and by whom? What were the dates and duration of treatment? What was the nature of the treatment, and was it external or internal? What were the results of treatment in terms of influence on the eruption and any allergy or toxicity from the treatment?

GENERAL CUTANEOUS HISTORY

Elicit whether the patient has had any previous eruptions, either similar or apparently unrelated. Obtain the dates, duration, course, and response to treatment. Also inquire about the cutaneous history of other family members who are blood relatives.

GENERAL NONCUTANEOUS HISTORY

As a rule, the noncutaneous history should be brief. Ask about any previous systemic or serious illness, any immediately preceding illness, or any concurrent or subsequent illness. Note any previous hospitalizations, surgery, or injuries. Ask about any allergies to medications and, when appropriate, take a sexual history. Inquire about a personal or family history of atopy or other allergy. Take a history of all medications, whether preceding, concurrent, or subsequent to the present skin problem. Inquire about abnormal laboratory tests, especially if there may be an associated condition such as a lipid abnormality, diabetes, etc.

DIFFERENTIAL DIAGNOSIS

The next step is to formulate a differential diagnosis by combining the information from the chief complaint, the physical examination, and the history. If you are unsure about any of the information, you can recheck it at this point. Based on your clinical findings, choose one or more of the cutaneous reaction patterns that fit reasonably with the information obtained.[3,4]

CUTANEOUS REACTION PATTERNS

Cutaneous reaction patterns, superficial and deeper, are outlined as follows (see also Table 56-3).

SUPERFICIAL

URTICARIA: wheals or hives lasting less than 24 hours.

TABLE 56-3. DIFFERENTIAL DIAGNOSIS

CUTANEOUS REACTION PATTERNS
  SUPERFICIAL
    URTICARIA
    TOXIC ERYTHEMA/MORBILLIFORM/SCARLATINIFORM
    ERYTHEMA MULTIFORME
    PAPULES
    PAPULOSQUAMOUS
    LICHENIFIED/HYPERKERATOTIC
    ECZEMATOUS/DERMATITIS
    EXUDATIVE/IMPETIGINIZED
    VESICLES/BULLAE
    PUSTULES/PAPULOPUSTULAR
    ERYTHRODERMA/EXFOLIATIVE DERMATITIS
    PURPURA
    HYPERPIGMENTED/HYPOPIGMENTED
    POIKILODERMA/ATROPHIC
    ICHTHYOSIFORM
  DEEPER
    ACNEIFORM
    NODULES
    INDURATION/SCLEROSIS
    ULCERS
    CUTANEOUS INFARCTION

TOXIC ERYTHEMA/MORBILLIFORM/
SCARLATINIFORM: pink to red symmetric eruption, macular or papular.

ERYTHEMA MULTIFORME: target or iris lesions.

PAPULES: small, nonscaly, elevated, discrete lesions.

PAPULOSQUAMOUS: papules or plaques covered with scales.

LICHENIFIED/HYPERKERATOTIC: thickened skin surface with or without accentuated skin lines.

ECZEMATOUS/DERMATITIS: pink to red roughened areas of skin with or without vesicles, oozing, crusts, or excoriations.

EXUDATIVE/IMPETIGINIZED: oozing, or yellowish to brownish crusts on a circumscribed area of skin.

VESICLES/BULLAE: blisters.

PUSTULES/PAPULOPUSTULAR: purulent blisters, either by themselves or surmounted on papules.

ERYTHRODERMA/EXFOLIATIVE
DERMATITIS: generalized dermatitis or redness with scaling.

PURPURA: petechiae or ecchymoses.

HYPERPIGMENTED/
HYPOPIGMENTED: altered amount of pigment compared with normal skin.

POIKILODERMA/ATROPHIC: thinned or depressed areas of skin with or without hyperpigmentation, hypopigmentation, and telangiectasias.

ICHTHYOSIFORM: dry skin with fish scale appearance.

DEEPER

ACNEIFORM: acne-like appearance with comedones or papules or pustules in a typical distribution on the face, chest, or upper back.

NODULES: palpable lesions more deep-seated (deep dermis, subcutis) than papule (superficial dermis).

INDURATION/SCLEROSIS: thickened or woody hardness, deep in the skin.

ULCERS: loss of epidermis and part or all of dermis locally.

CUTANEOUS INFARCTION: necrosis of skin.

SPECIAL OFFICE EXAMINATIONS

Further procedures may be necessary to help establish the diagnosis. Some, such as blood tests, bacterial cultures, etc., are sent to the laboratory. Other procedures discussed subsequently can be performed in the office (Table 56-4). It is important to learn how to do these properly.[5]

DIASCOPY

Diascopy means applying downward pressure on a lesion with a clear glass or plastic slide while observing the lesion. This procedure is useful to ascertain that a purpuric-looking lesion does not blanch on diascopy, confirming that it is truly purpuric. With diascopy, you can also compress blue-black, vascular-looking lesions to be sure that they do not blanch and are not a melanoma or other pigmented lesion. You can also use diascopy to check granulomatous-appearing lesions for the appearance of apply-jelly nodules, seen in diseases such as sarcoidosis and cutaneous tuberculosis.

SCRAPINGS AND SMEARS

KOH PREP or potassium hydroxide preparation is done on scaling lesions to detect dermatophyte hyphae or candidal pseudohyphae. To obtain a specimen, scrape the lesion with a No. 15 scalpel blade or the edge of a glass slide and put the scrapings on a glass slide. Then apply a 10% potassium hydroxide solution and add a cover slip. Heat the slide gently

---

TABLE 56-4. SPECIAL EXAMINATIONS

SPECIAL OFFICE EXAMINATIONS
  DIASCOPY
  SCRAPINGS/SMEARS
    KOH PREP
    MINERAL OIL OR SALINE PREP FOR SCABIES
    TZANCK SMEAR
    GRAM STAIN
  WOODS LIGHT EXAM
LABORATORY
    HEMATOLOGIC—CBC, DIFFERENTIAL, PLATELETS, PT, PTT
  BLOOD CHEMISTRIES
  URINALYSIS
  SEROLOGIC—VDRL, ANA, ASO, ETC.
SKIN BIOPSY
  H & E
  SPECIAL STAINS
  DIRECT IMMUNOFLUORESCENCE

over a flame and examine it under a microscope.

MINERAL OIL OR SALINE PREP FOR SCABIES is done on burrows or small papules to look for scabies. Wet the No. 15 scalpel blade with the mineral oil (if available) or saline, scrape the lesion until it almost bleeds, and put the scraping on a clean glass slide. Add a drop of the mineral oil or saline to the slide, cover with a cover slip, and examine under the microscope for mites, mite eggs, or mite scybellae (droppings).

TZANCK SMEAR is used most commonly to look for multinucleated giant cells to confirm herpes simplex or herpes varicella/zoster infections. Remove the top of a vesicle with a No. 15 scalpel blade, scrape the base of the blister, and smear the material on a clean glass slide. Allow it to air-dry. If you have Giemsa or Wright's stain, you may stain the slide yourself. Otherwise, you can send the slide to the laboratory to be stained in the blood smear stainer. Examine the slide under a microscope with or without a cover slip and a drop of mineral oil.

GRAM STAIN is done to look for bacteria from a lesion. After using a Q-tip cotton applicator to obtain a specimen and smear it on a slide, you can either perform the Gram stain yourself or send it to the laboratory for staining. Examine the slide under the microscope using oil immersion to look for bacteria.

WOODS LIGHT EXAMINATION is done with a blacklight, long wavelength ultraviolet light 340 to 450 nanometers with a peak at 365 nanometers. With a Woods lamp, you can detect pigmentary disorders more clearly. Areas with complete loss of pigment appear bluish-white. You can also detect erythrasma with its coral-red fluorescence or pseudomonas with its yellow-green fluorescence. A few tinea infections also fluoresce, but the majority do not. You can also check a urine specimen acidified with a few drops of 10% hydrochloric acid for coral-red fluorescence if you suspect porphyria cutanea tarda.

LABORATORY TEST

Depending on the differential diagnosis, laboratory tests may be required to help determine the diagnosis. The following is a list of common laboratory tests used in dermatology.

HEMATOLOGIC: CBC, differential, platelets, PT, PTT

BLOOD CHEMISTRIES: enzymes, lipids, glucose, etc.

URINALYSIS

SEROLOGIC: VDRL, ANA, ASO, etc.

SKIN BIOPSY

Sometimes a skin biopsy is required for diagnosis. If you are sure the process is superficial, a shave biopsy may suffice. For deeper processes, a punch biopsy of epidermis and dermis and upper subcutis is indicated. If the process is deep or if you need to know the depth of invasion of a tumor, do an excisional biopsy. For ordinary staining with hematoxylin and eosin, you can submit the specimen preserved in formalin. If you need special stains, consult with the pathologist before taking the specimen. Biopsy specimens for direct immunofluorescence may be sent fresh on saline-soaked gauze if the laboratory is immediately available. Otherwise they should be sent in Michelle's medium.

TABLE 56-5. TWENTY ETIOLOGIC FACTORS TO CONSIDER

ITCH MAP MNEMONIC
   6 EYES (i's)
   4 TOES (t's)
   2 OF EVERYTHING ELSE
I T C H
6 i's
   IMMUNE ABNORMALITIES
   INFECTIONS
      BACTERIAL
      VIRAL/CHLAMYDIAL
      AFB/ACTINO/NOCARDIA
      FUNGAL
      RICKETTSIAL
      PROTOZOAL
   INFESTATIONS
   INFLAMMATORY OF UNKNOWN CAUSE
   INSECT BITES/STINGS
   IRRITANT
4 t's
   TOXIC
   TRAUMATIC
   TREATMENT-INDUCED (IATROGENIC)
   TUMORS (NEOPLASIA)
2 c's
   COLLAGEN-VASCULAR (CONNECTIVE TISSUE DISEASE)
   CONGENITAL
2 h's
   HEREDITARY
   HORMONAL
M A P
2 m's
   METABOLIC/NUTRITIONAL
   METASTATIC
2 a's
   ALLERGY
      IMMEDIATE
      DELAYED CONTACT
   ATOPIC
2 p's
   PHYSICAL
      COLD
      HEAT
      LIGHT
      PRESSURE
   PSYCHOGENIC

DIAGNOSIS

Arriving at a diagnosis may be as simple as glancing at the skin lesions or as complex as requiring a complete history and physical, laboratory and office tests, a biopsy, and several follow-up visits to follow the progression of the skin lesions. Once you have reached one or more differential diagnosis categories, you can use the "itch map" mnemonic in Table 56-5 to jog your memory for etiologic categories of possible diagnoses. Then it is a matter of further evaluation and testing to narrow the diagnostic possibilities until you reach the one most likely diagnosis.

REFERENCES

1. Norman, G.R., et al.: The development of expertise in dermatology. Arch. Dermatol. *125*:1063, 1989.
2. Fitzpatrick, T.B., Eisen, A.Z., Wolff, K., et al.: Dermatology in General Medicine. 3rd. Ed. New York, McGraw-Hill, 1987.
3. Fitzpatrick, T.B., and Walker, S.A.: Dermatologic Differential Diagnosis. Chicago, Year Book Medical Publishers, 1962.
4. Korting, G.W., and Denk, R.: Differential Diagnosis in Dermatology. Philadelphia, W. B. Saunders, 1976.
5. Fenske, N.A., and Cohen, L.E.: The dermatologic exam. Emerg. Med. Clin. North Am. 3:643, 1985.

CUTANEOUS SIGNS OF SYSTEMIC DISEASE

Eric Stirling

CAPSULE

Many systemic diseases give clues to their presence in the skin. Prediction of hemorrhage, malignancy, or systemic infection may be made by the astute physical examiner. A potentially fatal outcome may be prevented by a thorough skin examination, as illustrated by the petechiae of meningococcemia or the hyperpigmentation of adrenal insufficiency. The emergency practitioner must first learn to describe basic skin lesions accurately to be able to use this and other dermatologic references.

INTRODUCTION

This text progresses by functional systems. Specific lesions or signs are grouped in the tables and shown in Figures 56-25 through 56-58. The reader should review other chapters in this or other standard texts for more complete descriptions of diseases identified. Exceedingly rare diseases are not covered unless the Emergency Department (ED) presentation mandates immediate and life-saving treatment.

PREHOSPITAL CARE

Dermatologic diagnosis is difficult in the field. The patient is not undressed, lighting is insufficient, and the disease spectrum vast. Rashes must be presumed contagious, and universal precautions taken. A strong emphasis on recognizing purpuric lesions should be taught, and extra precautions should be taken after intravenous (IV) attempts as well as monitoring for blood loss.

CLINICAL PRESENTATIONS

HEMORRHAGIC AND HEMATOPOIETIC DISORDERS

The cardinal sign of these disorders is purpura. Petechiae are purpura of 3 mm or less. Ecchymoses are larger. Lever has categorized these lesions into inflammatory (bacterial, drug allergy, allergic vasculitis, periarteritis nodosa, Wegener's granulomatosis) and noninflammatory (stasis purpura, thrombocytopenic purpura, coagulation disorder-related, senile purpura, scurvy, cryoglobulinemic purpura, purpura fulminans).

Only a few causes of purpura *do not* need a work-up. The syndrome of purpura on the extensor surfaces of arms and hands in the elderly from solar elastosis is called senile purpura. These lesions are benign. Some patients may say that they have always "bruised easily." If no systemic symptoms are present, and the ecchymoses are minor without a change in pattern, no work-up is necessary. "Appropriate" ecchymoses for a traumatic event do not need further work-up. Virtually all other patients with petechiae or ecchymoses need investigation. Complete blood count (CBC), platelet count, partial thromboplastin time (PTT), urinalysis (UA), stool heme testing, serum creatinine, and chest x ray complete the basic testing. A good organ system history must be taken. *A high degree of suspicion must be maintained for the life-threatening syndromes of meningococcemia, disseminated intravascular coagulation, sepsis, thrombocytopenic and thrombotic purpura, hemophilia, and von Willebrand's disease.* A patient with altered level of consciousness (ALOC) may not be able to give the history of a bleeding disorder. On the physical examination, petechiae present in pressure point areas first. Ecchymoses must be evaluated for uniformity. A greenish hue indicates lesions that are days old and a yellowish hue those a week or more old. Purpura that are palpable signify an epidermal component and a significant cutaneous necrotizing venulitis (Table 56-6).

The most common infections that precipitate palpable purpura are hepatitis B and group A hemolytic streptococci. Medications most commonly incriminated are sulfonamides, thiazides, penicillins, and serum products. Palpable purpura must be worked up and explained because inadvertent rechallenge may be life-threatening.

SKIN MANIFESTATIONS IN HEMATOPOIETIC DISEASES

Skin manifestations in hematopoietic diseases are varied. Pernicious anemia presents with vitiligo (Fig. 56-25, Table 56-7 for differential diagnosis), glossitis, and stomatitis. Sickle cell anemia causes leg ulcers that are sharply marginated with little undermining. These ulcers heal slowly and are prone to recur in the same area. Hand-foot syndrome presents in children as a distal extremity cellulitis with fever. It is often misdiagnosed as a bacterial infection, but resolves spontaneously over a period of weeks. Iron deficiency anemia presents with angular cheilitis, glossitis, and atrophy of the tongue papillae. Hair loss, koilonychia, and oral candidiasis may be present.

Multiple myeloma may have xanthomas, dermal plasmacytomas, and pyoderma gangrenosum in addition to the constitutional symptoms (see Table 56-8 for differential diagnosis of pyoderm gangrenosum). Pyoderma gangrenosum begins as pustules or nodules that evolve into ulcers with an undermined violaceous border. It may occur anywhere on the body. Mycosis fungoides is a malignancy primarily located in the skin. It is often misdiagnosed as eczema, and consists of annular erythematous plaques found in the "bathing trunks" area; these plaques may ulcerate. The plaques themselves are not pruritic, but generalized

TABLE 56-6. PURPURA	
Thrombocytopenic	Idiopathic thrombocytopenic purpura
	Thrombotic thrombocytopenic purpura
	Drugs
	Post-transfusion
	Disseminated intravascular coagulation
	Wiskott-Aldrich syndrome
Nonthrombocytopenic	Coagulation defects
	Platelet function disorders
	Severe thrombocytosis
	Gardner-Diamond syndrome
Connective tissue support defects	Corticosteroid administration
	Solar elastosis, trauma, scurvy, amyloidosis
	Pseudoxanthoma elasticum
	Ehlers-Danlos
Palpable purpura	Infections—hepatitis B, hemolytic streptococci, leprosy
	Drugs—sulfonamides, thiazides, penicillin, serum products
	Chronic disease—SLE, rheumatoid arthritis, lymphoproliferative disorders, Sjögren's syndrome, cryoglobulinemia, hyper-gammaglobulinemia
	Unknown cause—angioedema, Henoch–Schönlein purpura

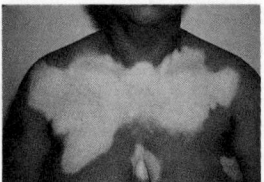

FIG. 56-25. Vitiligo.

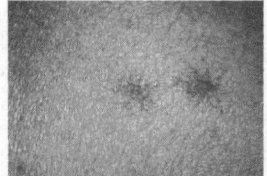

FIG. 56-26. Spider angioma in liver disease.

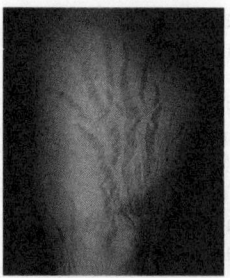

FIG. 56-27. Striae in patient on long-term steroids.

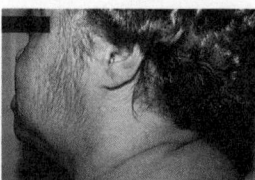

FIG. 56-28. Buffalo hump and hirsutism secondary to systemic steroids.

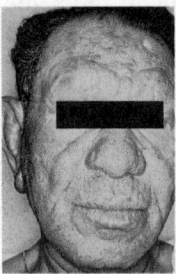

FIG. 56-29. Leprosy showing lepromatous "leonine facies." Note absence of eyebrows.

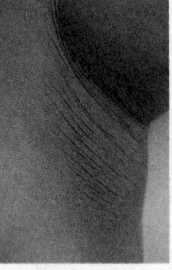

FIG. 56-30. Acanthosis nigricans.

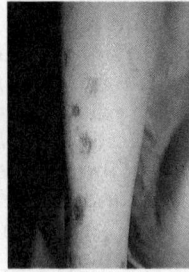

FIG. 56-31. Diabetic dermopathy.

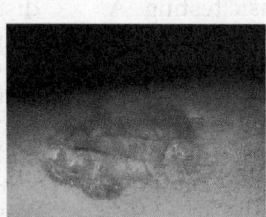

FIG. 56-32. Necrobiosis lipoidica diabeticorum.

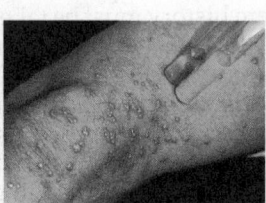

FIG. 56-33. Eruptive xanthomatosis. Note patient's turbid serum as compared to normal control serum.

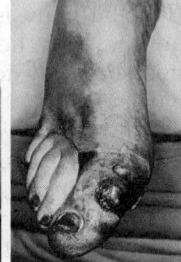

FIG. 56-34. Diabetic gangrene.

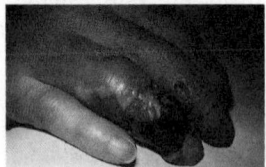

FIG. 56-35. Diabetic peripheral neuropathy and gangrene.

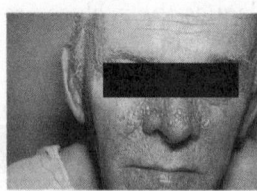

FIG. 56-36. Tuberous sclerosis. Classic angiofibromas of nose and cheeks.

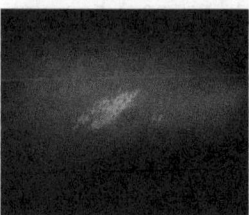

FIG. 56-37. Tuberous sclerosis "ash leaf" spot.

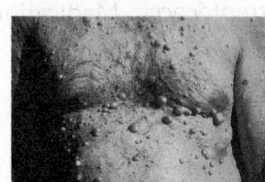

FIG. 56-38. Von Recklinghausen's neurofibromatosis.

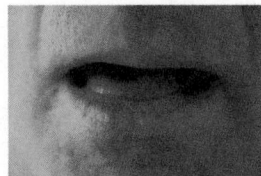

FIG. 56-39. Osler-Weber-Rendu disease. Patient also had epistaxis.

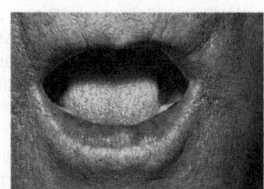

FIG. 56-40. Peutz-Jeghers syndrome. Patient has intestinal polyposis.

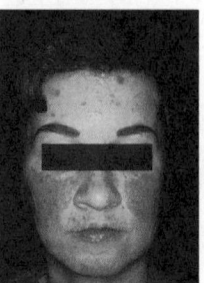

FIG. 56-41. Systemic lupus erythematosus.

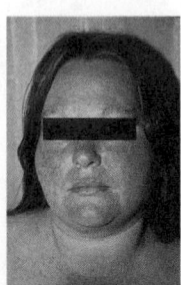

FIG. 56-42. Phototoxic eruption caused by a diuretic (sulfonamide). Original diagnosis was SLE.

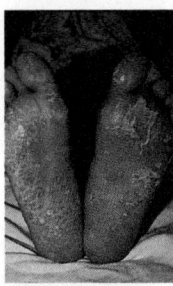

FIG. 56-43. Reiter's syndrome showing keratotic soles. Original diagnosis was secondary lues or psoriasis.

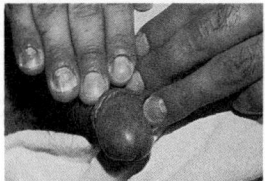

FIG. 56-44. Reiter's syndrome with erosive balanitis and nail lesions. Original diagnosis was psoriasis.

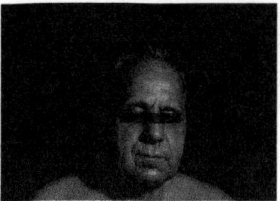

FIG. 56-45. Dermatomyositis (heliotrope). Violaceous areas over eyelids.

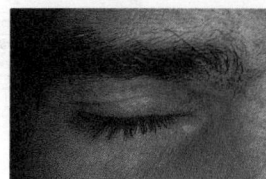

FIG. 56-46. Dermatomyositis showing erythema of eyelids (heliotrope).

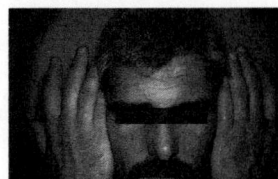

FIG. 56-47. Dermatomyositis showing photosensitivity and Gottron's papules.

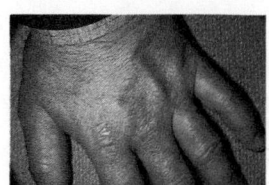

FIG. 56-48. Dermatomyositis. Gottron's papules over knuckles.

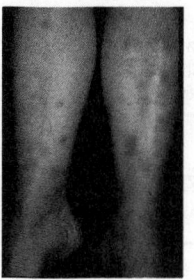

FIG. 56-49. Erythema nodosum (sarcoid).

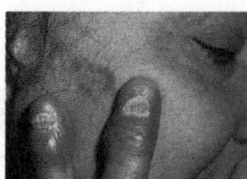

FIG. 56-50. Sarcoidosis. Lupus pernio of fingers and annular sarcoid.

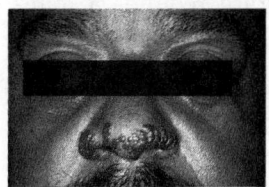

FIG. 56-51. Sarcoid. Classic location of firm papules and nodules.

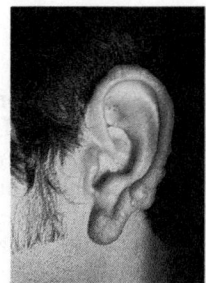

FIG. 56-52. Leprosy. Lepromatous classic nodules on cooler skin areas.

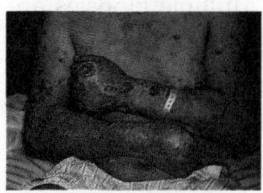

FIG. 56-53. Leprosy. Lepromatous lucio phenomenon.

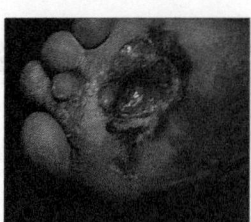

FIG. 56-54. Malam perforans in leprosy.

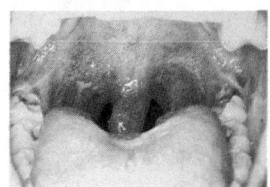

FIG. 56-55. Tuberculosis of pharnyx secondary to severe pulmonary tuberculosis.

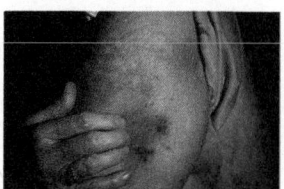

FIG. 56-56. Neurotic excoriations. Patient's husband is an alcoholic. Note easy access areas.

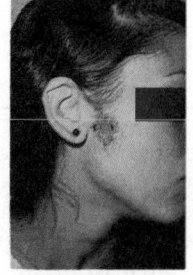

FIG. 56-57. Factitious excoriations.

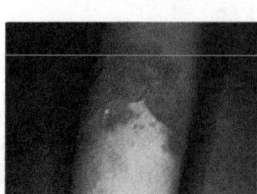

FIG. 56-58. Factitious lesions. Note scalloped appearance. Patient denied producing these lesions.

TABLE 56-7. VITILIGO	
Systemic disorders	Grave's disease
	Thyroiditis
	?Myxedema, thyroid cancer
	Adrenal insufficiency
	Pernicious anemia
Idiopathic	Familial autosomal dominant with incomplete penetrance
Post-traumatic	Koebner phenomenon, probably an expression of idiopathic form
Miscellaneous	?Psoriasis

TABLE 56-8. PYODERMA GANGRENOSUM	
Mimicking lesions	Pyogenic abscess, tuberculosis, syphilis
Diseases found in	Ulcerative colitis, regional enteritis, gastric ulcer, gastrointestinal polyposis, dysproteinemias, rheumatoid arthritis

TABLE 56-9. SKIN FINDINGS IN LIVER DISEASE	
Jaundice	Carotene, lycopene, quinacrine can mimic
Vascular	Spider angiomata, purpura, telangiectasias rosaceae, collateral veins, rhagades, striae
Hormonal	Gonadal atrophy, secondary hair loss, gynecomastia, xanthelasma, acne vulgaris
Other	Palmar erythema, Terry's nails (white nails), Mee's lines (transverse lines), clubbing, watchglass nails, Dupuytren's contractures, edema

itching may sometimes occur. Multiple biopsies are needed to establish the diagnosis. Leukemias may present as randomly distributed flesh-colored erythematous to plum-colored papules or nodules that are rubbery and less than 2 cm in size. Nonspecific findings in hematologic malignancies include pallor, exfoliative dermatitis, urticaria, or severe pruritis with neurodermatitis. A good history is necessary to correlate subtle constitutional symptoms with these non-specific findings.

LIVER DISEASE

It is no surprise that, with the central role the liver plays in body homeostasis, the list of skin manifestations is long and varied. This section concentrates on findings that are clearly related to the underlying liver disease and also clearly related to ED practice. (Table 56-9).

Jaundice may vary from a light golden color to a bright yellow or even a dark green (from increased biliverdin). Perception of jaundice requires a minimum of 2.5 mg per dL. The deeper the constitutional pigment, the higher the level required for recognition. In neonates, clinical jaundice is not evident until levels reach 6.0 mg/dL.[2] Jaundice lags behind hyperbilirubinemia in both appearance and resolution. Bilirubin is not intrinsically harmful to the skin. It must be remembered that all yellow skin discoloration is not jaundice. Carotene (carrots, squash, spinach), lycopene (tomatoes, rose hips, bittersweet berries), and administration of quinacrine may all induce pigmentation. Only jaundice, however, causes yellowish discoloration of the sclerae as well.

Pruritus is prominent in both obstructive jaundice and primary biliary cirrhosis (PBC). PBC is poorly understood, involves refractory pruritus, and has no effective treatment. The serum alkaline phosphatase is high, and jaundice is a late finding.

Hyperpigmentation in liver disease occurs with hemochromatosis. It is a metallic grey coloration, most prominent on sun-exposed surfaces. The differential diagnosis includes porphyria, adrenal insufficiency, pituitary tumors, lymphoma, tuberculosis, malabsorption syndromes, and, rarely, cirrhosis.

Nail changes in liver disease are common but inconstant and nonspecific. Terry's nails are completely whitish, and may involve from one to several nails at a time. Transverse white lines (Mee's lines) rarely occur in cirrhosis but should always raise the question of arsenic or heavy metal poisoning. Spoon-shaped nails (koilonychia), clubbing, or watch-glass nails (mild clubbing) without hypertrophic osteoarthropathy are found rarely in chronic liver disease, but are much more common in iron deficiency anemia.

Hormone-related changes include gynecomastia, loss of secondary hair growth, acne, striae, and pseudo-Cushing's syndrome. Dupuytren's contractures are frequent but nonspecific. Xanthomas are often prominent but do not necessarily correlate with an underlying lipid disorder.

Vascular changes are nonspecific but common in chronic liver disease. The classic spider angiomas (Fig. 56-26) consist of a central punctum and branching vessels with a background erythematous blush. They are rarely seen below the diaphragm level. They may also be seen in pregnant patients, those with rheumatoid arthritis, hormone recipients (estrogens), patients with thyrotoxicosis, and occasionally normal patients. Palmar erythema may be seen as increased mottling or a blanchable hypothenar patch. Telangiectasias, increased collateral vessels, corkscrew scleral vessels, and purpuric lesions are common.

ENDOCRINE DISEASE

Many endocrine diseases present unique skin features, and a positive diagnosis can be made by appearance only. The examiner must beware of the multiple endocrine syndromes or partially treated syndromes in which the skin findings remain and may mislead. Iatrogenic causes may mimic endocrine syndromes, as in steroid therapy.

Excess glucocorticoids produce thin, atrophic, shiny skin. The dermis becomes loose and the skin friable, with ecchymoses at pressure points. Wound healing is poor, with frequent infection resulting. Purplish mottling of dependent parts (cutis marmorata) and stasis ulcers may be presenting complaints. Broad purple striae (Fig. 56-27) occur on the trunk secondary to loss of integrity of the dermal connective tissue. Plethora and telangiectasia of the face, hypertrichosis, hirsutism, and acne are alone highly suggestive. Late findings include central obesity with limb fat atrophy (moon facies, buffalo hump) (see Fig. 56-28). Exogenous steroids tend to cause less androgenic effects (acne, hirsutism, hypertrichosis).

A decrease in glucocorticoids is much less striking. Hyperpigmentation, the most common skin finding, occurs most intensely in areas of recent trauma and at pressure points (elbows, knees, skin folds, palmar creases). Skin in sexual areas (nipples, areolas, peri-

neum) is also disproportionately affected. Paradoxically, vitiligo occurs in 15% of patients. Some hair loss is usually present.

Excess androgens present with virilizing syndromes. There is excessive oiliness of the skin, with enlarged pores, acne, and coarse body hair. The skin is thickened and coarse, and the genitalia are masculinized.

Decreased androgen levels create the opposite picture. Fine, nonoily skin, sparse body hair with no beard or axillary or pubic growth, and marked skin pallor are present. Features vary with the age of onset. Androgens reverse all of the skin changes.

Much of skin function depends on thyroid hormone. Turnover of dermal collagen, sebum production, cutaneous blood flow, thickness of the epidermis, and maintenance of hair growth all depend on the amount of thyroid hormone present.

Excessive thyroid hormone causes warm, moist, smooth skin with persistent flushing of the face and palms. Nails show onycholysis with achropachy of the fingers. Patchy hyperpigmentation and vitiligo may coexist: alopecia is a common concomitant. Pretibial myxedema starts as raised pink to brown nodules that become verrucous and sometimes elephantine. They do not resolve with treatment.

Decreased thyroid hormone produces cold, dry, pale skin that is coarse with an ivory-yellow hue. The hair is coarse and brittle. Loss of the lateral third of the eyebrow hair (also found in leprosy, as shown in Fig. 56-29, and syphilis), decreased sebum production, and generalized nonpitting puffiness is typical. There is a classic facies with a broad nose, thickened lips, a large smooth tongue, droopy eyelids, and expressionless features. This appearance resolves with appropriate hormone replacement.

Excess parathyroid hormone does not cause cutaneous changes. Decreased levels, however, cause dry, scaly, puffy skin. Eczematous dermatitis results. Mucocutaneous candidiasis that is refractory to treatment is well documented, and should cause a serum calcium level to be drawn in the ED.

Growth hormone excess causes many skin changes besides the obvious acromegaly. The skin is thickened, with prominent pores. There is excessive sweating resulting in frequent axillary and gluteal abscesses. Hyperpigmentation is common. Acanthosis nigricans (Fig. 56-30) has been reported in 10% of patients.[3]

Panhypopituitarism produces a prominent pallor with a yellowish tinge to the skin. The skin is dry but smooth, with puffiness of the face, which seems expressionless. There is marked loss of body hair; sweating and sebaceous secretions are diminished.

The skin manifestations of diabetes mellitus (Figs. 56-31 through 56-35) are protean, but correlate poorly with metabolic changes or control of the glucose levels. Diabetic dermopathy (Fig. 56-31) consists of atrophic, well circumscribed brownish lesions up to a few centimeters in size on the lower extremities. It presents in crops and resolves over a period of years. Redness of the face (rubeosis facii) and extremities occurs in long-standing diabetes and does not correlate with metabolic control. Necrobiosis lipoidica diabeticorum (Fig. 56-32) starts as a small, dusky red nodule that enlarges and becomes irregular. Coalescence then occurs; vessels are seen on the surface, and ulcerations follow. The lesions remain well circumscribed and rarely become infected. There is no effective treatment. Cutaneous manifestations of insulin therapy include lipodystrophy and lipoatrophy. These lesions seem related to the purity of the insulin preparation, and are seen much less frequently with recombinant human insulin. They last for years once they are developed, and there is no specific treatment.

NEUROCUTANEOUS DISEASE

This category encompasses a vast number of mostly obscure and unpronounceable syndromes. Therefore, only a few representative examples are described.

Somatic motor denervation leads to a characteristic set of skin signs. Aside from the flaccid paralysis and severe atrophy, the skin is cool, pale, and moist from preserved autonomic function. There is no alteration in piloerection or sebaceous activity. In sensory denervation, the skin is prone to trauma and damage. If the denervation is partial, paresthesias and hypersensitivity may be so severe that basic skin care is neglected. Sebum, debris, and sweat accumulate, the nails grow long and ridged, and yellowish crusts form. Ulceration from minor trauma may progress to abscess. Autonomic function depends on the lesion.

Tuberous sclerosis (Fig. 56-36) is a congenital disease with protean manifestations. The triad of adenoma sebaceum, epilepsy, and mental retardation is often sufficient to make the diagnosis. The seizures and retardation are manifest by age 5, and the adenoma sebaceum by age 10. Fifty percent of patients also have yellow retinal plaques (phakoma). Eighty-five percent have "ash leaf" spots (Fig. 56-37) on the trunk and limbs consisting of hypomelanotic areas up to 2.0 cm seen best with a Wood's light. Adenoma sebacea are actually angiofibromas with a red to pink nodular appearance localized to the face and scalp. There is no treatment for this disease, and 50% of patients die before adulthood.

Neurofibromatosis (von Rechlinghausen's disease) involves many organ systems, but is characterized by its skin lesions (Fig. 56-38). Cranial nerve syndromes, seizures, and mental retardation may be presenting features but are uncommon. Café-au-lait spots are patches of cutaneous pigmentation ranging from a few millimeters to many centimeters with a light brown color. Any patient with more than six spots exceeding 1.5 cm is presumed to have the disease. Axillary freckling is nearly pathognomonic for this disease.[4] The

cutaneous tumors are soft or firm papules of varied shapes, flesh-colored, and are able to be invaginated by means of a small opening in the dermis. These can vary in number in the individual patient from a few to thousands. These tumors can be found in internal organs, and present problems varying from hydrocephalus to cardiac abnormalities.

Several syndromes involve skin telangiectasias or hemangiomas. Most involve the face and scalp, along with underlying cerebral structures. The clinician must always assume that large surface hemangiomas have underlying life-threatening cerebral lesions and proceed accordingly.

GASTROINTESTINAL DISEASE

There are many well described examples of gastrointestinal (GI) abnormalities with skin lesions or markers. Many are associated with GI hemorrhage, some with polypoid changes, and some with connective tissue or endocrine disease. It is incumbent on the clinician to examine the skin of any patient with GI bleeding, both for the classically associated syndromes as well as signs that signify some other systemic bleeding disorder (purpura, etc.). Similarly, patients with positive occult blood in the stool may be well on the way to a specific diagnosis if the skin marker is present for intestinal polyposis or malignancy.

Osler-Weber-Rendu disease (hemorrhagic hereditary telangiectasia) is an autosomal dominant disease with multiple vascular lesions in the skin and internal organs. In the skin, 1 to 3 mm macular telangiectasias are present, especially on the face (Fig. 56-39). Epistaxis occurs in 50% and GI hemorrhage in 25%. Pulmonary AV fistulas occur, and bleeding may occur in any organ system.

Connective tissue disorders include pseudoxanthoma elasticum and Ehlers-Danlos syndromes. Both have hyperextensible skin and joints. The former also has characteristic yellow papules, giving a pebbled appearance to the skin. Ehlers-Danlos syndrome has fragile, translucent skin. Both are associated with GI hemorrhage.

Several papers have associated achrocordons (skin tags) with GI polyps and malignancy. The major flaw in methodology revolves around the statistic that more than 50% of patients over age 50 have skin tags. No study has been large enough to clearly associate the two. Current recommendations do not advise GI workup in the patient with skin tags.[5]

Many GI polyposis syndromes have skin manifestations, all uncommon, but malignant change is likely and preventive colectomy often indicated. Gardner's syndrome involves colonic polyps, bone osteomas, and multiple epidermal cysts and dermoid tumors (benign fibrous tumors in musculoaponeurotic soft tissues). Malignant changes in the colon have occured as early as age 9. Peutz-Jeghers syndrome (Fig. 56-40) involves hamartomatous polyps, and mucocutaneous melanin pigmentation. Pigmented areas are most commonly on the lips and buccal mucosa, but may occur on the palms and soles.

Crohn's disease is well known for its inflammatory bowel syndromes and other internal problems. The skin may show aphthous ulcers in the mouth, ulcerated nodules in the skin, pyoderma gangrenosum, and erythema nodosum. Ulcerative colitis does not have ulcerated nodules, but may present with erythema multiforme or primary pustular lesions.

Neurofibromatosis (von Recklinghausen's disease) is usually diagnosed by its skin manifestations, but may present with bleeding GI polyps.

AUTOIMMUNE DISEASE

Systemic lupus erythematosus (SLE) is a multisystem disease of great variability found in young women. The clinical presentation of fever, rash, and arthritis is accompanied by a wide variety of skin manifestations (Fig. 56-41). It behooves the ED clinician to know these well because life-threatening crises may occur as the initial presentation of the disease. Discoid lupus, with its follicular plugging, atrophy, telangiectasias, and scarring, may accompany SLE or exist with no systemic problem. Erythematous patches around the fingertips with telangiectasias are common but not specific to SLE. Alopecia may be either diffuse thinning on a normal scalp, or accompanied by erythema, scaling, and atrophy. Mouth ulcerations are common and painful. Purpura may be from vasculitis with normal platelet counts, or from thrombocytopenia. Raynaud's phenomenon and photosensitivity are less common. There are suggestive laboratory tests (ANA, LE cells, proteinuria, leukopenia), but the diagnosis is clinical, and the skin signs essential. Differential diagnosis may include phototoxic eruptions seen as a reaction to drugs (Fig. 56-42). Because patients may present with bleeding, pleuritic chest pain, pericarditis pain, arrythmias, congestive heart failure (CHF), renal failure or nephrotic syndrome, seizures, psychosis, or confusion, the clinical suspicion and skin examination are both of paramount importance.

The rheumatic diseases may have specific skin lesions that help considerably in the diagnosis. Rheumatic fever may have multiple 2 to 5 mm subcutaneous nodules over the bony prominences, and a ringed erythematous, rapidly spreading rash (erythema marginatum) on the trunk and lower limbs. Still's disease (juvenile rheumatoid arthritis) presents with an erythematous macular scattered rash that usually accompanies fever and joint symptoms. The rash may last for years. The similar-appearing rash of Coxsackie and Echovirus infection tends to be fleeting and more diffuse. Reiter's syndrome, with its triad of arthritis, urethritis, and conjunctivitis, also has discrete hyperkeratotic scaling lesions resembling those of psoriasis on the palms and soles (Fig. 56-43). These start as vesicles that become purulent and thickened and end as the classic keratoderma blenorrhagicum. Papular scaling lesions of the penis (circinate balanitis) complete the picture (Fig. 56-44).

Dermatomyositis is a rare disease with muscular weakness and soreness, most often in the shoulder and pelvic girdle areas. Skin lesions may precede active disease. The heliotrope rash is diagnostic, and consists of edema and a purplish red periorbital discoloration, especially over the upper lids (Figs. 56-45, 56-46). A butterfly rash commonly accompanies the heliotrope component. Gottron's sign is a scaly maculopapular rash over extensor joint surfaces, usually the fingers (Figs. 56-47, 56-48). Older patients have a high rate of underlying malignancy. Severe myopathy may present with aspiration pneumonia. Creatine phosphokinase (CPK) is uniformly elevated.

Scleroderma is a systemic disease with diagnostic skin signs. Tissue edema gives a masklike facies, constriction of mouth opening, and sausage-like fingers. Other features include telangiectasias of the face and neck, loss of hair, hyperpigmentation, ulcerations of the fingertips, and a curious calcification of the fingertips.

Morphea is a form of localized cutaneous scleroderma without systemic complications, characterized by sclerotic placques with a pale or ivory-colored center and a violaceous halo. Patients with systemic variants of scleroderma present with calcinosis cutis, Raynaud's phenomenon, sclerodactyly, and telangiectasias (CRST syndrome). Both CRST and primary scleroderma may present with severe dyspnea, esophageal malfunction, aspiration pneumonia, CHF, or pericarditis.

Scleredema consists of a sudden onset of a nonpitting symmetric induration of the skin, especially in the posterior cervical area. The edema then spreads to the face, chest, arms, and shoulders. Normal skin markings are lost, and the skin feels woody with a waxy appearance. It follows some infectious process (usually streptococcal)and is a self-limited problem without major systemic manifestations. Other diseases presenting with facial edema (scleroderma, dermatomyositis, myxedema, amyloidosis, and hypoalbuminemic edema from a cardiac or renal source) must be ruled out before scleredema is diagnosed.

MISCELLANEOUS CONDITIONS (Figs. 56-49 through 56-58)

Sarcoidosis is a disease of unknown cause usually found in young black women. Many cases are diagnosed after a routine chest radiograph shows hilar adenopathy. Other presentations include restrictive airway disease with pulmonary infiltrates, fever of unknown origin, cardiac dysrhythmias or heart block, uveitis, nephrocalcinosis, and cranial nerve palsies. Skin lesions may be the only clue to the underlying systemic disease. Erythema nodosum (Fig. 56-49) is often the presenting complaint, and is characterized by shiny, red, rounded intradermal lesions on the shins that are elevated and quite painful. The redness becomes purplish after a week and then gradually fades. Other diseases must be excluded before erythema nodosum is attributed to sarcoidosis.

Lupus pernio (Fig. 56-50) presents as persistent violaceous placques, classically on the ear lobes and less frequently on the nasal and cheek areas, signifying upper respiratory involvement. Nasal ulceration (Fig. 56-51) and septal perforation occur rarely. Other scars previously present may become purplish and inflamed, probably because of a hypersensitivity reaction from sarcoidosis. Violaceous plaques on the limbs and buttocks tend to correlate with lymphadenopathy and splenomegaly. Maculopapular rashes are often the presenting feature in the ED and correlate with uveitis and intrathoracic involvement.

No quick diagnostic test is available. Tissue biopsy, angiotensin-converting enzyme and the Kveim test have been used with varying accuracy. Steriods are still the mainstay of treatment in symptomatic disease.

Malignant acanthosis nigricans is a dermatosis strongly associated with internal adenocarcinomas, 80% involving the GI tract. The skin lesions may precede the malignancy by months or years. Early lesions are in body folds, especially the axillae, umbilicus, nipples, and knuckles. The lesions are composed of confluent hyperkeratotic hyperpigmented verrucosities. Diffuse keratoderma of the palms and soles may be seen late in the course of the disease.

A benign form of acanthosis nigricans, not associated with malignancy, is commonly seen in dark-skinned overweight people and cannot be distinguished clinically or histologically from the malignant type. Sudden onset of acanthosis nigricans in an adult warrants careful evaluation to rule out GI or pulmonary malignancy.

HORIZONS

The history and physical examination are still the most cost-effective areas in the practice of medicine. For emergency medicine practitioners, the correlation of skin findings with systemic disease is of much greater importance than the management of other more indolent skin conditions. It is especially important in advancing one's expertise in skin diagnosis to follow up patients admitted or referred for consultation to learn the manifold variants of presentation.

REFERENCES

1. Domonkos, A.N., Arnold, H.L., and Odom, R.B. (eds): Andrew's Diseases of the Skin. Philadelphia, W. B. Saunders, 1989.
2. Arris, I.M.: Hepatic aspects of bilirubin metabolism. Ann. Rev. Med. 17:257, 1966.
3. Fitzpatrick, T.B., et al. (eds): Dermatology in General Medicine. New York, McGraw-Hill, 1988.
4. Weber, F.P.: Cutaneous pigmentation in von Recklinghausen's disease. Br. J. Dermatol. 21:49, 1909.
5. Callen, J.P. and Jorizzo, J.L. (eds): Dermatology Clinics. Philadelphia, W. B. Saunders, July 1989.

DERMATITIS

Joseph F. Fowler, Jr.

CAPSULE

The term dermatitis or eczema denotes a group of inflammatory skin disorders that may be acute or chronic and may result from endogenous or exogenous factors or both. Acute and chronic dermatitis frequently occur simultaneously in the same patient. The diagnosis of dermatitis is essentially made on clinical grounds, although skin biopsy may be used to confirm the clinical impression. Eczema is a term essentially synonymous with dermatitis, although many dermatologists use the term to imply an acute, vesicular, weeping process and the term dermatitis to imply a more chronic, lower-grade disease.

SUBSETS OF DERMATITIS

Dermatitis may be subdivided into a group of related conditions that show distinct clinical morphology and/or distinct causative factors. Although other classifications and categories may exist, the following are the commonly seen types of dermatitis.

ATOPIC DERMATITIS

The term atopy indicates a specific type of immunologic hyperreactivity that may manifest as dermatitis, hay fever, asthma, or any combination of these. Atopic dermatitis almost always appears first during childhood or adolescence. For unexplained reasons, atopic individuals develop itching much more readily than other individuals. Stimuli that may not cause an itching response in most people may lead to severe itching in the atopic. It is felt that much of the clinical appearance of the atopic individual is from rubbing and scratching as a result of this intense itch response. In more severe cases, the skin may thicken, become hypertrophic or even nodular, and develop fissures. In other words, the itching precipitates scratching, which in turn precipitates clinical findings, rather than the other way around. In infants, sites of dermatitis are usually localized over extensor areas where they are able to rub against the bed. The scalp, upper back, and dorsal lateral arms and legs are therefore affected. The more typical pattern is seen when the child can direct his scratching and progresses to the classic atopic picture of dermatitis in the antecubital and popliteal spaces and on the face. The periorbital areas may show dermatitis and edema as a result of the atopic dermatitis as well as allergic rhinitis and conjunctivitis. The basic cause of atopic dermatitis remains unclear, although some investigators have found elevated levels of antistaphylococcal IgE in these patients. Treatment with antibiotics to decrease cutaneous colonization with Staphylococcus may be of benefit in some atopics. Food hypersensitivity has been shown to occur in only about 10% of atopic dermatitis.

TREATMENT

The thrust of treatment in these individuals is to decrease inflammation and reduce itching. Systemic antihistamines such as diphenhydramine or hydroxyzine should therefore be used liberally. Initial topical therapy consists of emollients to lubricate the skin, providing an environment for the skin to heal itself and also reducing the itching stimulus. Because large areas of the body may be involved, mildly to moderately potent topical steroid ointments may be used, but high-potency topical steroids generally should be avoided because of the risk of cutaneous atrophy and systemic absorption. Systemic steroids may occasionally be of benefit, but should be used cautiously because the disease process is chronic. Occasionally systemic antibiotics such as erythromycin or dicloxacillin may benefit by reducing cutaneous Staphylococcus colonization.

Although many atopic children "grow out of it" by puberty, some continue to have sensitive skin throughout their lives. Accordingly, much of the treatment must be directed toward assisting the patient in coping with the condition and developing awareness of his or her need for continuing skin care.

CONTACT DERMATITIS

Contact dermatitis is a cutaneous reaction pattern caused by interaction with exogenous environmental factors. Contact dermatitis may be further split into irritant and allergic contact dermatitis.

Irritant contact dermatitis is caused by the direct toxic effect of an environmental agent on the skin. The immune system is not involved. Detergents, solvents, acids, and alkalis are all capable of causing an irritant contact dermatitis. The amount of exposure determines whether dermatitis may occur, as does the variable sensitivity of an individual's skin. For instance, a dilute solvent or detergent may not cause skin irritation, whereas a more concentrated agent or prolonged exposure may break down the skin's natural barriers and cause irritant dermatitis, which most often affects the hands. Other areas of the body exposed to the environment or irritation from clothing may also develop it (Fig. 56-59).

In contrast, *allergic contact dermatitis* is caused by an immunologic hypersensitivity to an allergen in contact with the skin (Fig. 56-60). Therefore the immune system, specifically cell-mediated immunity, must be intact for allergic contact dermatitis to develop. Poison ivy or oak (Rhus) is by far the most common cause of allergic contact dermatitis in North America. Some attempt should be made to differentiate irritant versus allergic contact dermatitis because the treatments for each are somewhat different. History is of great benefit because there is often a known precipitating source of irritant contact dermatitis such as acid or solvent exposure, excessive hand washing, etc. In allergic contact dermatitis, history may also be helpful, especially in cases of possible exposure to poison ivy or related plants. Skin changes may not appear until 10 to 12 days after exposure to the plant. The initial lesions are usually on the hands, arms, or fingers, but frequently spread to the eyes, genitalia, or elsewhere. Poison ivy may be carried to the patient indirectly by long-haired dogs or even by droplets on a windy day. Pruritus is prominent.

Skin involvement may be mild or severe, depending on the amount of exposure and degree of sensitivity of the individual. The eruption is usually asymmetric, often shows vesicles in a linear arrangement, and may

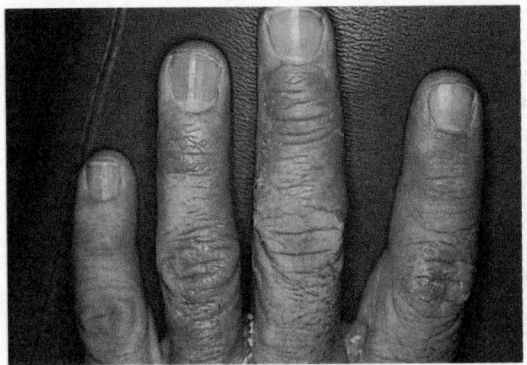

FIG. 56-59. Typical appearance of chronic irritant dermatitis with scaling, erythematous lesions on hands.

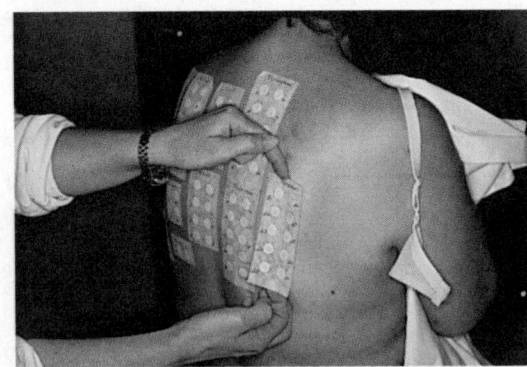

FIG. 56-61. Applications of patch tests to a patient's back.

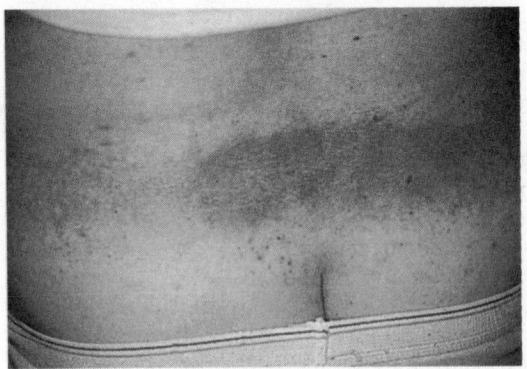

FIG. 56-60. Allergic contact dermatitis caused by elastic in underwear.

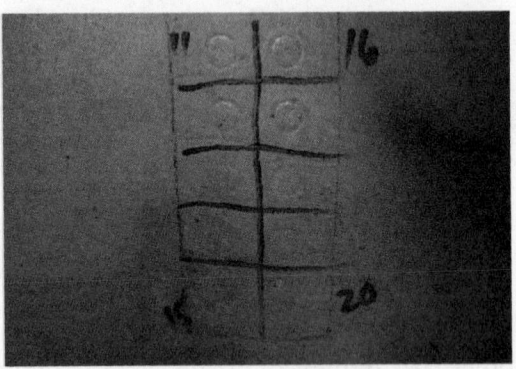

FIG. 56-62. Patch test reading showing two positive reactions.

show considerable edema, especially of the eyelids or face. A characteristic clinical finding is the presence of groups of fluid-filled lesions of varying sizes.

TREATMENT

Acute contact dermatitis with vesiculation and weeping should be treated by topical drying agents such as tap water or Burrow's solution soaks. Contact dermatitis and the various forms of atopic dermatitis may be difficult to tell apart, and occasionally the two conditions may occur together, as when a patient develops a contact dermatitis in response to a medication that has been applied to an area of atopic dermatitis. Patients with other primary skin conditions such as seborrheic dermatitis, lichen planus, and psoriasis may develop superimposed contact dermatitis or secondary eczematization, and the physician can identify the primary process only by finding undisturbed lesions at other locations. Although it is helpful for the physician to be able to explain the process to the patient, most cases of eczematous dermatitis can be treated satisfactorily until subsequent re-evaluation gives more precise definition of the underlying problem. Cool or cold compresses are applied three or four times daily for 30 minutes, and although water is ef-

fective, Burrow's solution offers enough advantage to merit its routine use. This solution is a 1:40 mixture consisting of a powder packet (provided by several pharmaceutical companies) dissolved into 1 pint of cold water. Between applications, the Burrow's solution is refrigerated so that the proper temperature of the compresses is ensured. This coldness reduces pruritus, removes heat from the inflamed surfaces, and provides topical anesthesia. These values should be explained to the patient. A corticosteroid cream or lotion may be applied to reduce inflammation. In poison ivy dermatitis, systemic steroids are extremely helpful. They should not be used in mild cases or situations in which they are contraindicated by other illnesses. A course starting at 40 to 60 mg of prednisone tapering over a 2-week period usually provides prompt and prolonged relief from the allergic contact response if the patient is seen early in the course of the illness. Because the average case of poison ivy reaches peak severity after about 3 to 5 days, the required dose may be minimal if a patient with poison ivy is started on systemic corticosteroids on day 6. Thorough questioning may reveal whether the patient is already improving and the course and severity of previous episodes of poison ivy, all of which may provide some predictive information. A common mistake is to treat the patient for too short a time, allowing recurrence of the eruption. Irritant contact dermatitis, in contrast, is not benefitted by systemic steroids because an immune hypersensitivity response is not occurring. Systemic antihistamines may be helpful for sedation and control of pruritus, although in allergic contact dermatitis the pruritus is much better controlled by systemic steroids. The patient should avoid hot water and overheating, both of which exacerbate pruritis. Chronic contact dermatitis is best managed by the use of topical steroids and emollients and by making an effort to avoid the source of the problem. Patch testing is the only method that can determine the causative agent in allergic contact dermatitis (Figs. 56-61 and 56-62).

LICHEN SIMPLEX CHRONICUS

This term is used to denote a localized area of dermatitis in which rubbing and scratching by the patient is a prominent feature. This results in lichenification, a thickening of the skin markings and production of a small amount of scale. Lichenification directly results from chronic trauma such as repeatedly rubbing a particular area of the skin. Another term for lichen simplex chronicus (LSC) is neurodermatitis. This term, however, may imply a neurotic basis for the condition, which is not always the case. In LSC, no underlying reason for the pruritus and dermatitis can be found. LSC is most often seen in older individuals. Common sites of involvement are areas that can be easily rubbed by the patient, such as the posterior neck, hands and forearms, and the lower legs. It does not occur in areas that the patient cannot rub, such as the middle of the back.

TREATMENT

The mainstay of treatment for this condition consists of local application of topical steroids, along with application of strong lubricating agents to soften the skin and relieve itching. Systemic antihistamines are also valuable for this purpose. High-dose systemic steroids are usually not indicated in this condition, although a low-dose, long-acting preparation, such as triamcinolone acetonide 40 mg intramuscularly, may be helpful. Behavior alteration to try to get the patient to avoid continuous rubbing and scratching is also of great importance.

SEBORRHEIC DERMATITIS

This is one of the most common forms of dermatitis. Although usually affecting adults, it may be seen in the neonate for the first several months of life as a result of an influence of maternal hormones. Simple dandruff is a mild manifestation of seborrheic dermatitis. More severe manifestations include scaling and crusting in the scalp with erythema and pruritus, but other areas of the skin that contain sebaceous glands may also be affected, such as the face, especially the eyebrows and nasolabial folds, and the axillae, chest, and pubic area. Seborrheic dermatitis should not be confused with psoriasis, although the conditions are similar. Seborrheic dermatitis may sometimes be accompanied by seborrhea, an increased amount of sebaceous gland secretions, but the underlying cause of seborrheic dermatitis is uncertain. It appears that colonization with the yeast organism *Pityrosporum folliculAris* or the Demodex mite, both of which are common inhabitants of the normal skin flora, may be related to seborrehic dermatitis in some individuals.

TREATMENT

As in other forms of dermatitis, topical steroids are particularly useful. Liquid forms of these agents are especially helpful in hair-bearing areas. Tar-containing shampoos are also commonly used. Generally, seborrheic dermatitis has a chronic course and may require intermittent treatment throughout life.

STASIS DERMATITIS

Stasis dermatitis may occur on the legs of individuals with poor venous circulation. Generally, the anterior lower legs are affected in a diffuse erythematous eruption with minimal scale. Often the skin feels somewhat thickened and is shiny in appearance and, in many of these individuals, lower leg edema may also be present. Chronic stasis dermatitis may lead to ulceration.

TREATMENT

Palliation of the conditions leading to pooling of blood in the lower extremities is of paramount importance in the treatment of stasis dermatitis. Elevation of the legs and wearing support stockings is crucial. Without improvement in the underlying circulatory conditions, other treatments may fail. Medium- to lower-strength topical steroids are helpful, but high-strength topical steroids are generally not needed unless the skin is severely thickened. Occasional use of triamcinolone acetonide intramuscularly may be beneficial, allowing a temporary resolution of the condition. This, however, cannot take the place of management of the underlying venous problem.

XEROTIC DERMATITIS

Xerosis simply means dry skin. In some individuals, especially the elderly or those with hereditary abnormalities of the stratum corneum, excessive drying of the skin may cause an actual dermatitis manifested by low grade chronic inflammation with redness, scal-

TABLE 56-10. TREATMENT OF DERMATITIS

Dermatitis Type	Topical	Systemic
Allergic contact (e.g., poison ivy)	Cool, wet dressings with Burrow's solution Strong steroid creams, e.g., betamethasone or fluocinonide b.i.d. Calamine lotion	Prednisone, 40–60 mg/day in divided doses Taper over 10–14 day period Antihistamine, e.g., hydroxyzine, 10 mg qid, prn, or diphenhydramine 25–50 mg qid prn
Irritant contact	Emollient lotions Low-strength steroid ointments, e.g., desonide, hydrocortisone valerate	Rarely needed
Atopic	Emollient lotions Low- to medium-strength steroid creams, e.g., desonide, hydrocortisone valerate, or triamcinolone	Antihistamines as for allergic contact Occasionally antibiotics, e.g., erythromycin, 250 mg tid for 7 days Rarely, systemic steroids
Lichen simplex chronicus	Keratolytic agent, e.g., glycolic acid, lactic acid, or urea lotion Strong steroid cream, e.g., betamethasone or fluocinonide	Antihistamine as for allergic contact
Seborrheic dermatitis	Tar shampoo Steroid lotion, e.g., fluocinonide or hydrocortisone	Rarely needed
Stasis dermatitis	Elevation of leg Support hosiery Low- to medium-strength steroid creams as for atopic dermatitis	Antihistamines as above Triamcinolone Acetonide, I.M.
Xerotic dermatitis	Same as for irritant contact dermatitis Avoidance of harsh soaps and excessive bathing	

NOTE: This table should serve as a guideline only. The large number of corticosteroid creams and systemic antihistamines available preclude listing all, although their therapeutic efficacy may be equal to those listed above.

ing, and mild to moderate pruritus. Although this may occur anywhere on the body, the head and neck are almost never affected, whereas the lower extremity and trunk are most commonly involved.

TREATMENT

Emollients are needed to replace the natural skin moisture that is lacking in individuals with xerotic dermatitis. Simple over-the-counter skin lotions and bath oils are effective. The addition of low-strength topical steroids may help decrease secondary inflammation and itching.

Autosensitization (id reaction) is an acute eczematous dermatitis that appears, often suddenly, in a patient who has a more localized eczematous condition elsewhere on the body. In the typical case, a patient's stasis dermatitis or tinea pedis exacerbates, and an acute eczematous dermatitis appears symmetrically on the arms, hands, upper trunk, or face.

Autosensitization is not uncommon in infants who develop candidiasis of the diaper area. In most cases, adequate therapy of the localized process produces rapid involution of the secondary skin lesions. Autosensitization is frequently misdiagnosed as a drug eruption, and only awareness of this condition can prevent discontinuance of valuable drugs.

SUMMARY

Many of the described types of dermatitis are seen incidentally in the ED, but are not the primary focus of the patient's complaints. Allergic contact dermatitis, however, is frequently seen in the ED. Poison ivy, oak, and sumac (Rhus) dermatitis is by far the leading cause of contact dermatitis in North America and may result in significant morbidity. In some areas of the country, and in some occupations such as forestry workers, Rhus dermatitis is a major cause of loss of time from work. Several products have been promoted as being able to block the penetration of the Rhus allergens through the outer layer of the skin, thereby blocking the development of allergic contact dermatitis. One is a P-P-6-3 diamine dilinoleate preparation, Stokogard. Its effectiveness is improved when it is washed off within 8 to 12 hours.

It is usually helpful to determine which subtypes of dermatitis are present. Exploration of the cause and appropriate treatment can then be carried out. A summary of treatment is given in Table 56-10.

BIBLIOGRAPHY

Adams, R.A.: Occupational Skin Disease. New York, Grune & Stratton, 1983.

Domonkos, A.N., Arnold, H.L., Jr., and Odom, R.B.: Andrew's Diseases of the Skin, 7th ed. Philadelphia, W.B. Saunders, 1982.

Fisher, A.A.: Contact Dermatitis, 3rd ed. Philadelphia, Lea & Febiger, 1986.

Maiback, H.I.: Occupational and Industrial Dermatology, 2nd ed. Chicago, Yearbook Medical Publishers, 1987.

PURPURA

Howard M. Simons

CAPSULE

Purpura is an indication of several possible diseases, including anaphylactoid purpura, systemic vasculitis, systemic infections, and purpura fulminans. The recognition, differential diagnosis, and management are reviewed.

INTRODUCTION

Purpura is a change in color of the skin, mucous membranes, or both that results from extravasation of red blood cells. Although usually pink or red in color, various shades from orangish-brown to bluish-black are seen as the red cells break down to form various pigments. Smaller lesions, 3 mm or less, are called *petechiae*; larger ones are known as *ecchymoses*. *Hematoma* refers to a palpable ecchymotic mass, often the result of trauma. In contrast, small purpuric lesions are almost always macular unless an associated inflammatory infiltrate makes them palpable.

Purpura is recognized by failure of a suspected lesion to blanch under application of firm pressure. Although finger pressure is most often used, diascopy, in which the pressure is applied with a glass slide provides better visualization of the lesion. Differentiating purpura from macular inflammatory lesions or telangiectasia may be especially difficult on the lower legs, and in such cases diascopy should always be used. In some cases, purpura can be identified only with the help of a skin biopsy, but the latter is usually not considered an emergency department (ED) procedure.

Like pruritus or anemia, purpura is an indication of disease, not a disease per se. Although the diseases that cause purpura are numerous, only the small number that may present as an emergency condition are discussed here. This number is further reduced by the omission of thrombocytopenic purpuras and coagulation defects, which are discussed in Chapter 53.

ANAPHYLACTOID PURPURA (HENOCH-SCHÖNLEIN PURPURA)

This syndrome (Fig. 56–63) results from acute or subacute inflammation of small blood vessels in the skin and, less commonly, in the gastrointestinal tract, joints, and kidneys. When purpura and gastrointestinal changes occur together, the term *Henoch's purpura* is often applied; *Schönlein's purpura* is used when joint changes are prominent. Physicians, however, now avoid this unnecessary splitting of the syndrome by using the term *Henoch-Schönlein purpura* synonymously with *anaphylactoid purpura*.

This is primarily a condition of children and young adults, with peak incidence in the 4- to 7-year-old

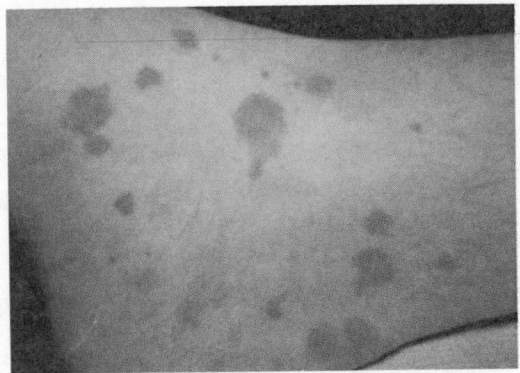

FIG. 56-63. Anaphylactoid (Henoch-Schönlein) purpura.

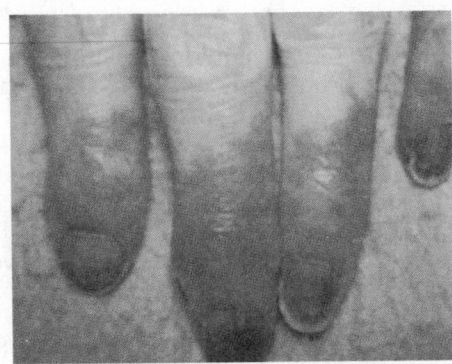

FIG. 56-66. Purpura fulminans.

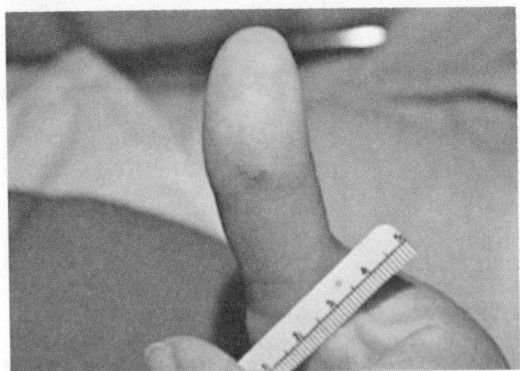

FIG. 56-64. Gonococcemia.

infections. Although numerous drugs have been incriminated as causative agents, there is no drug history in the vast majority of cases. The possibility that the syndrome results from hypersensitivity to an occult virus has been considered but never proved, although some experimental work suggests that an antigen-antibody reaction occurs in or near the small blood vessels.

Indeed, any mechanism that produces dilation and altered permeability of the small vessels could account for the cutaneous hallmarks of anaphylactoid purpura, exudation and hemorrhage. On dilation of the small vessels, the initial lesions are pink and macular, but within hours they become edematous or even urticarial. As hemorrhage occurs, their color darkens to red, then purple; the subsequent variable hues of resolving purpura are seen during the next several days.

Most cases of anaphylactoid purpura resolve spontaneously in 3 to 5 weeks, although recurrences are seen in a small minority of patients.

RECOGNITION

The skin of patients with anaphylactoid purpura shows more than purpura, although few skin lesions resolve without displaying at least some petechial

group. Twice as many boys as girls are affected. The syndrome is most common in early spring and follows upper respiratory infections in many patients. Despite the reported high incidence of preceding infections, no relationship between infection and this syndrome has been clearly established. Antistreptolysin O titers are not found to be elevated, and the renal involvement of anaphylactoid purpura differs qualitatively from the glomerulonephritis that follows streptococcal

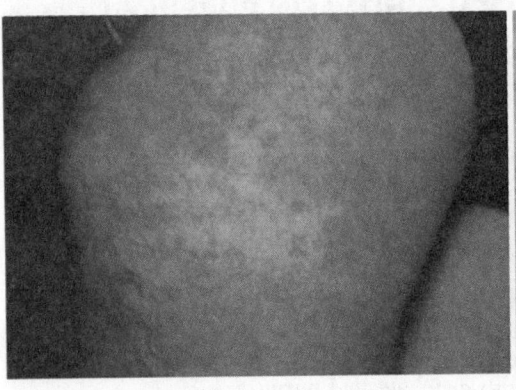

A   B

FIG. 56-65. Progressive pigmentary purpura.

component. The skin changes are polymorphous. Macules, papules, urticarial edematous lesions, palpable purpura and, if the exudation is severe in the upper dermis, hemorrhagic bullae may be seen. Erosions, ulcers, and crusts are not common. Lesions are seen most commonly on the lower legs and ankles, but the buttocks, elbows, and forearms are also frequently involved. Localized edema of the face, hands, and feet often occurs in younger children and is apparently unrelated to any underlying renal involvement.

Gastrointestinal involvement usually produces colicky pain that is difficult to localize on abdominal examination. Vomiting, hematemesis, and melena are also frequently seen. The abdominal pain may be severe enough to cause confusion with an "acute abdomen," and this is especially likely if skin changes are minimal. In some cases, intussusception does occur, requiring surgical correction.

The typical joint pain of anaphylactoid purpura is acute at onset, involves the knees and ankles most often, and occurs in the absence of joint swelling and redness. The pain may be transient and variable during the attack.

Recognition of anaphylactoid purpura is easy if the triad of palpable purpura, abdominal colic, and joint pain is present. Recognition may also be easy if purpuric lesions are present with involvement of only *one* of the other systems, provided that the examining physician has an appreciation of the distribution and polymorphous appearance of the cutaneous changes. Because the syndrome recurs in some patients, a history of prior involvement may be obtained.

Laboratory tests are not especially helpful, although a normal platelet count rules out a thrombocytopenic cause for the purpura. The sedimentation rate is frequently elevated to a moderate degree. Although urinary abnormalities reflecting renal vascular involvement are found in most patients, these are almost always absent in the early stages. Eventually, most of the patients show microscopic hematuria, and approximately 40% have gross hematuria, proteinuria, or both. A small number of patients develop severe renal involvement that may lead to permanent kidney damage. As with gastrointestinal involvement, the severity of the renal changes does not correlate with the severity of the cutaneous lesions.

Because noninflammatory diseases and coagulation defects usually cause purpura that is monomorphous and macular, confusion with anaphylactoid purpura is unlikely. In contrast, separation from conditions that produce inflammatory purpura or elevated lesions may be difficult, and one or more of the conditions described subsequently may have to be considered in the differential diagnosis.

SYSTEMIC VASCULITIS

This entity, also known as leukocytoclastic angiitis because of its characteristic histologic features, may

show skin lesions similar to those of anaphylactoid purpura, but is a more chronic process and more variable in its clinical presentation. Although anaphylactoid purpura and systemic vasculitis appear to be related by their occasionally identical cutaneous changes and similar vascular pathologic processes, anaphylactoid purpura should be viewed as a well-defined, more acute clinical syndrome. In contrast, systemic vasculitis is seen more commonly in adults, has large vessel involvement resulting in cardiopulmonary and central nervous system changes, and causes fever in 75% of cases. Skeletal involvement produces myalgia, stiffness, and weakness, in contrast to the transient joint pain of anaphylactoid purpura.

GONOCOCCEMIA

In a small percentage of gonococcal infections, the infecting organism invades the blood stream and produces the triad of fever, arthritis, and skin lesions. The skin changes are typically either hemorrhagic or vesiculopustular on an erythematous base and usually accompanied by an intermittent fever, chills, and mild to moderate prostration. The arthritis is mild and polyarticular at first, later becoming localized in one or two joints, and, unlike anaphylactoid purpura, may produce heat, tenderness, and swelling. The gonococcemic lesions are palpable and most often involve the hand and fingers (Fig. 56–64), unusual sites for the skin lesions of anaphylactoid purpura. The latter condition is seen most commonly in children, whereas gonococcemia is limited to persons, usually women, who are sexually active. Unfortunately, the gonococcus is difficult to demonstrate in the skin lesions by either culture or direct smear, although fluorescent antibody techniques have shown the organism to be present.

MENINGOCOCCEMIA

Although most patients with meningococcemia are prostrate, febrile, and either obtunded or comatose, milder cases in which an alert patient complains of muscle aches, nausea, or cough may be difficult to separate from anaphylactoid purpura. As in the latter condition, the cutaneous changes of acute meningococcal diseases show purpura on a background of polymorphous lesions. The purpura is typically palpable, decidedly grayish in color, varies in size from a few millimeters to several centimeters, and is irregular in outline—much like the coast of Maine. It has a more generalized distribution, but the buttocks and legs are predominantly involved. Except for epidemics in the military, meningococcemia attacks the same age group as that subject to anaphylactoid purpura.

Any problems in differentiating anaphylactoid purpura from mild forms of acute meningococcemia are usually solved by laboratory tests. Leukocytosis is almost always present in acute meningococcemia, and spinal fluid examination may show a polymorphonuclear pleocytosis and gram-negative diplococci on culture or smear. Direct examination of material from a skin lesion is much less likely to demonstrate the organism.

Recurrent episodes of anaphylactoid purpura could be confused with chronic meningococcemia, a condition in which a transient bacteremia occurs every 1 to 4 days, resulting in distinct episodes of fever, chills, myalgias, anorexia, and skin lesions. The cutaneous changes appear in showers after the onset of the fever and evolve and fade as the fever and other signs of the bacteremia resolve, only to reappear with the next episode. The morphology of the skin lesions is much less regular. Poorly demarcated erythematous macules and papules are more common, but hemorrhagic lesions are also described, as well as a variety of vague intermediate lesions. Culturing the organism from the blood confirms the diagnosis.

RHEUMATIC FEVER

Erythema marginatum occurs in 10 to 15% of patients with acute rheumatic fever and may be confused with the skin changes of anaphylactoid purpura because of the associated joint involvement and its occurrence in a similar age group. Erythema marginatum begins as an erythematous macule or papule that enlarges peripherally, leaving a paler inactive center and producing an annular or polycyclic pattern. The advancing borders may be macular or elevated; their color may be pink, red, or dusky, but the papules are *always* blanchable. Erythema marginatum typically enlarges rapidly, rarely lasts more than a few days, and leaves no residual marks. Recurrent crops, however, may prolong the skin changes for several weeks or longer. It is usually asymptomatic and is more common on the trunk and extremities than on the acra.

The evanescence, the rapid peripheral spread, and the immunologic relationship to streptococcal organisms suggest that erythema marginatum is probably a variant of urticaria. Occasionally, when the pale central part of the lesion is edematous, the similarity to a hive is striking. The lesion may be viewed as an inferior form of hive, a hive with scanty exudation and little or no pruritus.

The lesions of anaphylactoid purpura may be differentiated from erythema marginatum by the absence of peripheral spread and by the presence of purpura. Recognition of the former requires that one take an adequate history; identification of the latter requires a microscopic slide for diascopic examination.

PROGRESSIVE PIGMENTARY PURPURA

Although this chronic condition is seen almost exclusively in adults, it merits brief inclusion here, more because of its importance to the diagnosis of purpura in general than because of its only superficial resemblance to anaphylactoid purpura. The use of the term *progressive pigmentary purpura* permits elimination of at least seven cumbersome eponymic designations, of which *Schamberg's disease* is probably the best known. Researchers have not yet determined its cause or causes.

Irregular orangish-brown or yellowish-brown patches typically begin on the lower legs or feet and spread proximally. The most characteristic clinical finding is the delicate pinpoint petechiae (cayenne pepper spots) seen within and at the periphery of older lesions (Fig. 56–65). Although pruritus is usually minimal or absent, some variants are pruritic and show a more generalized distribution. The process seems unrelated to other medical problems and may resolve spontaneously over many months or years.

Progressive pigmentary purpura is clinically differentiated from anaphylactoid purpura by the absence of ecchymoses, elevated lesions, and other epidermal changes; by its chronic course without other system involvement; and by its frequency in middle-aged persons, especially men. Progressive pigmentary purpura could be confused more easily with a drug eruption, venous insufficiency, and Waldenström's hyperglobulinemic purpura.

ROCKY MOUNTAIN SPOTTED FEVER

Six or 7 days after a tick bite, the infected patient usually develops grippelike symptoms (headache, myalgia, and malaise) and subsequently fever, chills, and joint symptoms. On the third or fourth day of fever, a blanchable erythema begins on the wrists and ankles and spreads to the palms and soles as well as centrally to the arms, legs, trunk, and face. In time, the erythema becomes dusky or bluish and, finally, petechial.

Although the typical case of Rocky Mountain spotted fever is not easily confused with anaphylactoid purpura, a patient with a milder prodrome might be puzzling. In a more severely ill patient, meningococcemia may be difficult to rule out. Because routine laboratory tests are within or close to normal limits in Rocky Mountain spotted fever, its diagnosis must be clinical. The patient should be questioned carefully about recent tick bites, possible exposure to ticks, and the progression of the eruption and its relationship to early symptoms. The treatment of choice is tetracycline, 1 g every 8 hours in adults, taken on an empty stomach.

MANAGEMENT

Although anaphylactoid purpura is an acute self-limited process, most patients are best treated in the hospital. Management generally centers around reassurance of the patient and his family, relief of the acute symptoms, and bed rest. Only in the mildest cases should this be attempted on an outpatient basis. Another reason for hospitalization is the uncertainty of the diagnosis (i.e., the possible confusion with rheumatic fever or sepsis).

Despite the large number of cases that appear to follow upper respiratory infections, antibiotics should not be given unless a specific infection is present or suspected. Joint pain is best treated by bed rest, as it allows the patient to assume the position that provides the most comfort. Since aspirin and phenacetin have gastrointestinal and renal side effects, respectively, they should be strictly avoided. Acetaminophen or propoxyphene hydrochloride is appropriate if analgesics are needed. The skin changes do not appear to be helped by topical corticosteroids.

Systemic corticosteroids are most valuable in treating painful arthritis, abdominal pain, and gastrointestinal hemorrhage. This last condition is the most dangerous acute problem in anaphylactoid purpura and should be treated with systemic corticosteroids as soon as the possibility of intussusception has been ruled out. Prednisone should be given in daily doses of 40 to 60 mg. (in adults), depending on the age of the patient and the severity of the hemorrhage or pain. Localized soft tissue edema also responds rapidly to systemic corticosteroids, although other cutaneous changes do not.

Intussusception occurs in about 3% of affected children, and surgical consultation should be obtained if abdominal symptoms are severe. Renal changes in anaphylactoid purpura are slower to appear and are, therefore, usually not the concern of the emergency physician. The value of treating these changes with systemic corticosteroids or immunosuppressive agents has not yet been established.

PURPURA FULMINANS

This rare entity is characterized by the sudden appearance of large ecchymotic areas that often become necrotic or gangrenous (Fig. 56–66). These fulminating ecchymoses usually are on the extremities, although acral parts of the face may be involved. The skin changes are accompanied or soon followed by fever, chills, and vascular collapse, which may lead to death within 1 or 2 days. In patients who survive, gangrenous digits often either self-amputate or require surgical amputation.

The cause of purpura fulminans is better understood by its relationship to the syndrome of disseminated intravascular coagulation. Although purpura fulminans is most often described as occurring in children recovering from mild viral or bacterial infections, it is also seen in certain obstetric disorders, following pulmonary surgery, in prostatic carcinoma, and following certain snake bites. All of these conditions have been reported to show altered intravascular coagulation and increased fibrinolytic activity.

Apparently, clots form continuously in blood vessels as a normal occurrence, and this process may increase in various conditons, even without clinical thrombotic disease. In purpura fulminans and the diseases mentioned in the preceding paragraph, intravascular clotting is more extreme and more generalized, and results in the consumption of circulating fibrinogen. Thus, coagulation in distal vessels and generalized defibrination explain the acral gangrene and large ecchymotic areas, respectively, that occur in purpura fulminans.

RECOGNITION

The combination of rapidly progressing hemorrhagic skin lesions with signs of prostration, fever, and shock is suggestive of purpura fulminans. The ecchymoses are palpable and usually limited to the extremities initially, although they often spread centripetally, show some blistering necrosis, and may be joined by gangrene of the digits or of hemorrhagic areas. The typical patient is an otherwise healthy youngster who is convalescing from a minor infection.

Less severe forms of purpura fulminans merge with the syndrome of disseminated intravascular clotting, and it may be better to use the latter term in such cases, reserving "purpura fulminans" for the more explosive condition just described. The diagnosis of disseminated intravascular clotting is most often made on patients hospitalized with various ailments such as septicemias, leukemias, obstetric problems, and various carcinomas. As more sophisticated hematologic testing becomes available, it seems likely that all or most patients with these ailments will be shown to have increased clotting tendencies, even in the absence of clinical bleeding.

It is important to note that patients with the intravascular coagulation syndrome come to the ED with signs of hemorrhage (purpura, hemoptysis, hematuria, etc.) or because of their underlying disease (septicemia, carcinoma, etc.), but without both present together, the correct diagnosis is difficult to make clinically. Any patient with *palpable* purpura should be questioned thoroughly about underlying cardiopulmonary conditions that could produce hypoxia; the presence of cancers, especially of the prostate; recent treatment with chemotherapeutic agents; and infections of any kind. Areas of acral and facial cyanosis are seen occasionally and are usually gun-metal or purplish and sharply outlined, and do not blanch with pressure.

The diagnosis of purpura fulminans or disseminated intravascular coagulation can almost always be confirmed by laboratory tests, which show a prolonged prothombin time and decreased fibrinogen and platelets. In patients with liver disease or in milder cases in which tests may be equivocal, a skin biopsy is helpful.

MANAGEMENT

Although the intravascular coagulation syndrome is usually managed by treatment of the underlying disease, purpura fulminans produces such severe hemorrhage that it should be treated immediately with anticoagulation. Although the dose of intravenous heparin has not been clearly established for this condition, somewhere in the range of 80 to 100 units per kg every 4 hours seems reasonable. The hemorrhage will continue for at least 18 to 24 hours before responding to heparin; treatment is usually continued for 3 or 4 days longer. Monitoring of the hemostatic factors usually shows a more rapid return to normal of fibrinogen than of platelets.

Supportive measures are essential, and acidosis and hypotension in particular should be treated vigorously to increase the already decompensated tissue perfusion. Blood transfusion may be indicated. Local skin care is aimed at preventing and treating infections that are expected to occur as the large ecchymotic areas become necrotic or gangrenous. Gentle compression with an antibacterial soap and applications of gentamicin ointment will be helpful.

Milder forms of disseminated intravascular coagulation rarely require heparin, because therapy for the primary process is usually available. The one exception is in acute leukemias, in which heparin may halt a hemorrhagic episode until the malignancy can be brought under effective long-term control by chemotherapy.

DRUG ERUPTIONS

Jeffrey P. Callen and Carol L. Kulp-Shorten

CAPSULE

Cutaneous eruptions are commonly seen in the emergency department (ED). Rashes or pruritus can be rapid in their onset, and may cause a great deal of alarm for the patient. Often the cutaneous problem is the primary reason for the visit to the ED. New rashes are commonly caused by drugs; in other circumstances, a drug eruption is considered within the differential diagnosis. In this chapter we focus on the form in which a drug eruption may occur, the differentiation of an eruption caused by a drug from other causes, the identification of the causative agent, and the therapy of the drug eruption.

INTRODUCTION

No currently available laboratory test can identify a drug as a cause of an eruption or which drug has caused the eruption. Despite the lack of a diagnostic test, knowledge of the reaction rates for a drug, the history of drug ingestion, the morphology of the rash, and specific drugs as causing a "specific" type of eruption, allow the physician to establish a diagnosis of a drug eruption. Almost any drug must also be considered. As a general rule, drugs that have been recently administered should be considered first, even though the onset of a drug rash can occur after the offending drug has been stopped.

INCIDENCE

Drug reactions are common,[1] accounting for 1 in 20 courses of drug administration. The rates of various drugs causing an eruption, however, are usually estimated from data derived from hospitalized patients. Thus the rate may be quite different when considering patients in the outpatient setting. Bigby et al. reported that 2.2% of hospitalized patients develop a drug eruption.[2] Thus, drug eruptions occurring in hospitalized patients may represent 60,000 to 90,000 reactions per year. In addition, some drugs are known to be rare causes of drug eruptions (Table 56-11), whereas others are common causes (Table 56-12).

FINDING THE GUILTY DRUG

Most often, the adverse reaction is caused by a drug that has been recently ingested (within the last 7 days).[3] It is not, however, impossible for drugs used continuously for a long time to cause a drug reaction. Although cutaneous reactions are listed in the PDR as a possible side effect for most drugs, the frequency of drugs causing reactions per use varies greatly from penicillin, which causes a reaction in up to 52 patients

TABLE 56-11. DRUGS THAT RARELY CAUSE CUTANEOUS DRUG REACTIONS

Digitalis
Antacids
Acetaminophen
Nitroglycerin
Spironolactone
Methyldopa
Aminophylline
Propranolol
Prednisone
Diazepams
Insulin
Antihistamines
Codeine
Iron
Milk of magnesia

TABLE 56-12. DRUGS ACCOUNTING FOR MOST FREQUENT ERUPTIONS

Antibiotics (penicillins and sulfonamides)
Allopurinol
Barbiturates
Nonsteroidal anti-inflammatory agents
Furosemide
Thiazide diuretics

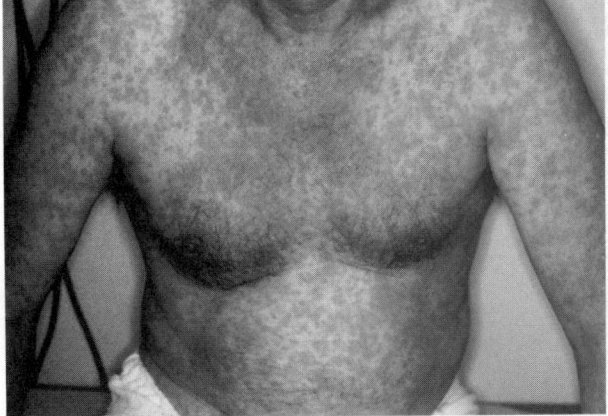

FIG. 56-67. Generalized, confluent erythematous macules, the result of an ampicillin reaction.

per 100 uses to digitalis, which has rarely, if ever, been implicated in causation of a drug reaction.

When considering the agents that the patient has been taking, the physician can use certain guidelines to identify a potential causative agent. First, which drugs are new? Second, which drugs are more likely to cause a reaction? Third, what is the morphology of the reaction? Finally, are there possible causes for the eruption other than a drug? In the following discussion, the morphologic reactions are presented in their order of frequency. The most common cutaneous patterns observed are urticarial and morbilliform reactions. Although drug reactions, when recognized, usually have a benign outcome, some cutaneous reactions such as toxic epodermal necrolysis (TEN) can end in death.

MORBILLIFORM ERYTHEMATOUS ERUPTION

Probably the most common cutaneous pattern is the morbilliform erythematous macular and/or papular exanthem (Fig. 56-67). Antibiotics, particularly the penicillins and sulfonamides, nonsteroidal anti-in-

flammatory drugs (NSAIDS), and diuretics are among the most common causative agents.

This eruption does not portend a life-threatening process. It is more worrisome to the patient because of pruritus, which may also be present, and because of its existence. Therapy is aimed at control of symptoms and removal of the potential offending agents. Oral antihistamines (diphenhydramine HCl and hydroxyzine) and topical antipruritics (menthol-based creams or lotions such as Sarna, Pramagel, etc.) are the primary therapy. Corticosteroids administered topically are often used, but probably do not have any demonstrable benefit. Systemic corticosteroids are generally unnecessary. Repeat administration of the offending agent should not occur, but when it does, the reaction continues to be non–life-threatening.

URTICARIA

Acute urticaria (hives) (Fig. 56-68) is frequently related to drug ingestion, whereas chronic urticaria (>2 months duration) is rarely caused by drugs. Some patients also manifest angioedema in addition to the urticaria. Last, there are patients who have angioedema without hives, but drugs are an unusual cause.[4] Most urticarial reactions from drugs are not life-threatening, but with severe angioedema, airway problems can occur. Also, some patients develop such severe vascular leakage that irreversible hypotension may occur. Thus, re-exposure to the offending drugs should be avoided because the reaction may become progressively more severe. The reaction often persists up to 2 weeks after drug removal, but may resolve quickly in some cases. Also, the reaction may have its onset shortly after completion of therapy.

Most often, this reaction appears to be IgE-mediated

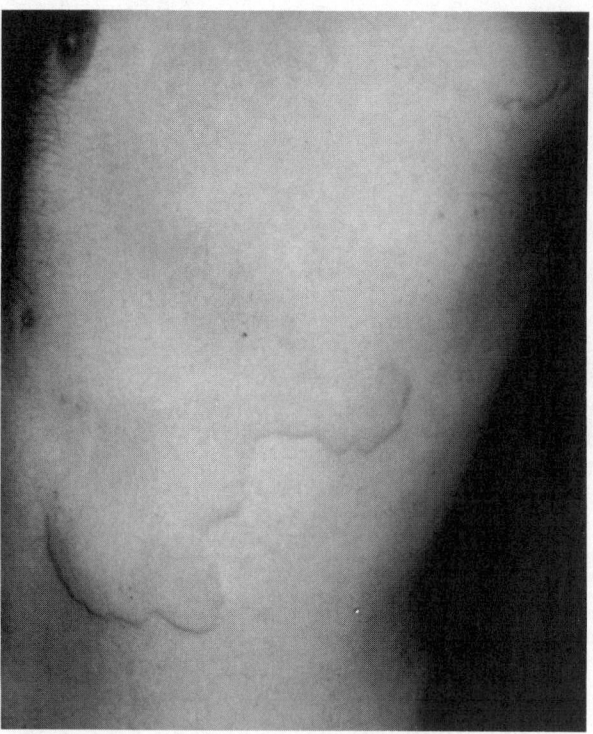

FIG. 56-68.   *Giant urticaria caused by penicillin therapy.*

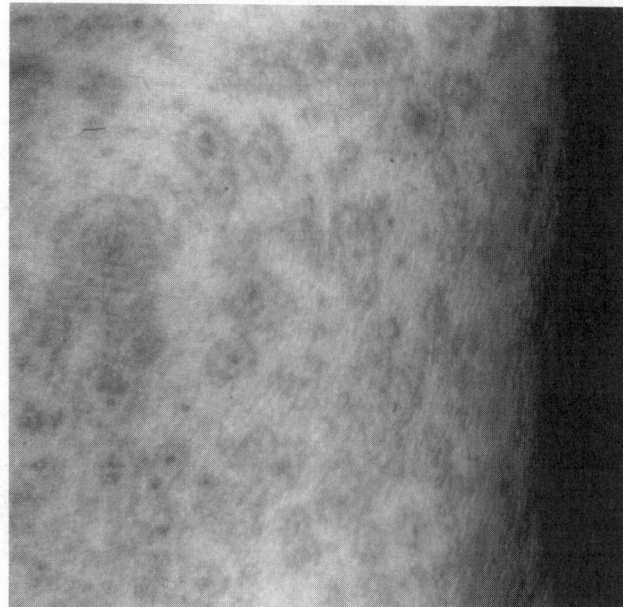

FIG. 56-69.   *Drug-induced erythema multiforme. Multiple typical "targetoid" lesions are present.*

(type I hypersensitivity) with mast cell degranulation occurring, but occasionally the reaction is caused by immune complex disease (type III hypersensitivity). Serum sickness usually begins 7 to 14 days after antigenic exposure, and its usual symptoms of urticaria, arthralgia, fever, and lymphadenopathy begin immediately. The most common causes of drug-induced urticaria are antibiotics (penicillins or sulfonamides), NSAIDs and salicylates, barbiturates, foreign antisera, radiocontrast materials, and opiates. The latter two cause urticaria by nonimmunological means, by direct mast cell degranulation.

As with exanthems, most urticarial reactions are more bothersome than life-threatening. Control can usually be achieved with oral antihistamines. Topical agents are rarely necessary. Severe reactions and anaphylaxis require aggressive management with airway support, enhanced oxygenation, intravenous fluids, and subcutaneous or intramuscular epinephrine. Intravenous epinephrine is reserved for the rare individual with cardiac arrest.[5] Corticosteroids given in high doses intravenously or orally are useful over a short time frame (1 to 2 days), although their onset of action is often delayed.

ERYTHEMA MULTIFORME AND ITS VARIANTS

Erythema multiforme (EM) is characterized by macules, urticarial papules, and vesiculobullous lesions, which typically form a target-like appearance (Fig. 56-69). The lesions are most common on acral surfaces, but can be generalized, with symmetric involvement being usual. Mucous membranes may be involved (Fig. 56-70), with the lesions manifesting most often as painful erosions. A severe variant of erythema multiforme, known as Stevens-Johnson syndrome, or erythema multiforme major, is characterized by vesiculobullous lesions, involvement of two or more mucosal surfaces, and systemic findings such as fever, lethargy, hypotension, etc. This reaction can be life-threatening if left untreated. Another process, known as toxic epidermal necrolysis (TEN), may be another variant of severe EM. This presents as the sudden denudation of large areas of epidermis, usually ac-

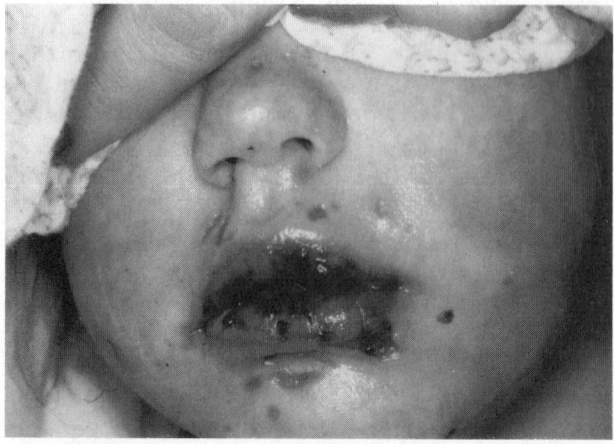

FIG. 56-70.   *Sulfonamide-induced Stevens-Johnson syndrome. Severe mucosal involvement is present.*

companied by mucosal lesions and systemic findings.

The drugs that cause EM are similar to those that cause urticaria. The most common offenders are antibiotics such as penicillins and sulfonamides, NSAIDs, hydantoins, and barbiturates.[6] TEN has been commonly linked to allopurinol administration, as well as the above mentioned drugs. Although the categories mentioned are the most common, the list of drugs presumed to have caused EM reactions is extensive. Furthermore, EM may be caused by drugs administered topically, such as eyedrops. In addition, one must keep in mind that EM is not always drug-related. EM is often secondary to an infectious agent, the most common of which is recurrent herpes simplex virus. It is not rare for the patient to present with an EM reaction and be on an antibiotic for a presumed upper respiratory tract infection. In this case, it may be difficult to sort out the cause.

EM minor is usually a self-limited process, and if the causative agent is removed or treated, the reaction clears. Severe EM can be life-threatening; thus, hospitalization, fluid and electrolyte therapy and prevention and/or treatment of infections are necessary. The use of systemically administered corticosteroids is controversial. They may shorten the course of EM, but with TEN or Stevens-Johnson syndrome, they may prolong the hospitalization and lead to an increased risk of infection. In patients with involvement of the eyes, an experienced ophthalmologist should be actively involved in management to prevent blindness.

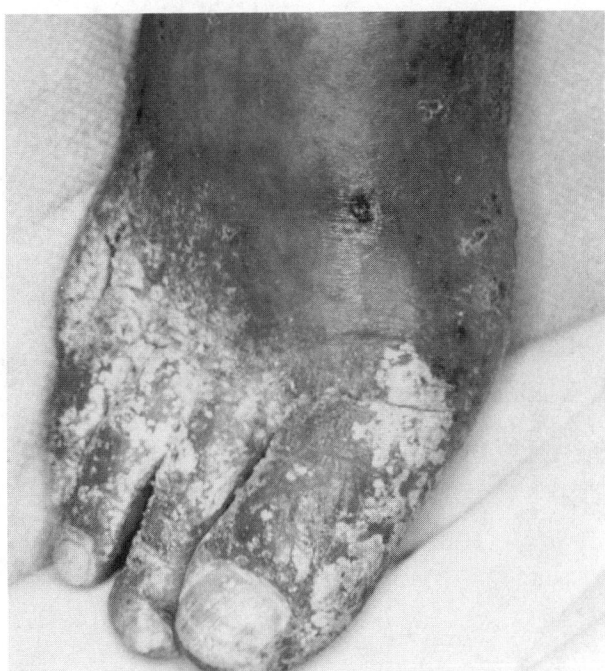

FIG. 56-71. Neomycin-induced contact dermatitis on the lower extremities.

ECZEMATOUS ERUPTIONS

Eczema or dermatitis is a general term used to describe a variety of processes that manifest as a pruritic eruption. In acute phases, vesicles are often present, but in chronic forms the manifestations are lichenification, excoriations, and slight scaling. This pattern may be present in a variety of disorders including seborrheic dermatitis, atopic dermatitis, photodermatitis, and contact dermatitis. Drugs can cause both photodermatitis and contact dermatitis.

Contact dermatitis caused by a medicament is often subtle, and the patient often continues to apply the offending agent. This eruption is a manifestation of classical delayed hypersensitivity (type IV cell-mediated immune response). Thus, the eruption requires sensitization first, and then a sensitive patient can develop the eruption upon rechallenge. Interestingly, the risk of sensitization seems greater for patients with pre-existing dermatitis, particularly of the lower legs, e.g., stasis dermatitis (Fig. 56-71). The most common causes of allergic contact dermatitis include neomycin, topical anesthetics such as benzocaine, topical anti-

histamines, and agents used in creams and lotions as stabilizers. Treatment consists of removal of the offending agents, compresses, and topical or systemic corticosteroids. After resolution of the eruption, patch testing can confirm the suspected sensitivity.

Photodermatitis occurs through two types of mechanisms: photoallergic dermatitis and phototoxic dermatitis. The difference is that in allergic dermatitis there must be sensitization, and only a few patients given the drug are sensitized, whereas in phototoxicity, the reaction is possible in most of the people receiving enough drug and enough light. Furthermore, the skin rash is of a different character, with an eczematous eruption in the photoallergic reaction and an exaggerated sunburn in the phototoxic reaction (Fig. 56-72). The most common causes of phototoxicity are tetracyclines, sulfonamides, sulfonylureas, thiazides, quinidine, psoralens, griseofulvin NSAIDs, and phenothiazines. Photoallergic dermatitis occurs more frequently with topically applied medicaments. Therapy for photodermatitis includes recognition of the offending agent(s) and cessation of therapy, if possible. If the agent cannot be stopped, the patient can alter his or her exposure to light by altering habits and perhaps applying an appropriate sunscreen. The decision as to what is an appropriate sunscreen is difficult because the agent chosen must be effective against the wavelength involved in the reaction. Most phototoxic drug reactions involve activation by ultraviolet A radiation. Therefore, one of the broad spectrum sunscreens such as Photoplex should be recommended.

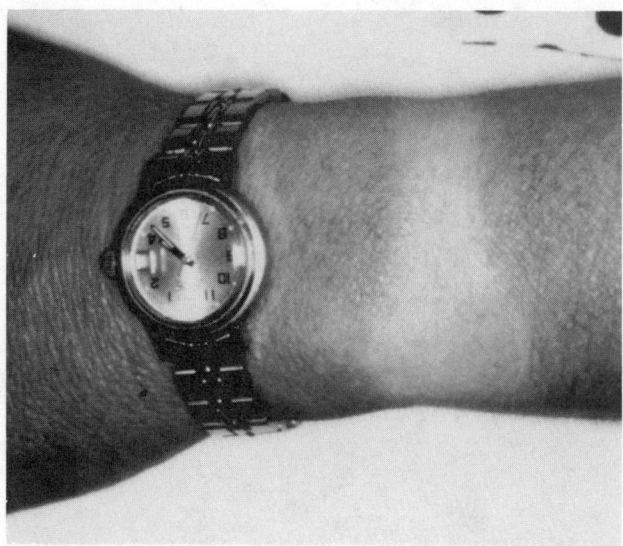

FIG. 56-72. Phototoxic reaction caused by Thorazine therapy.

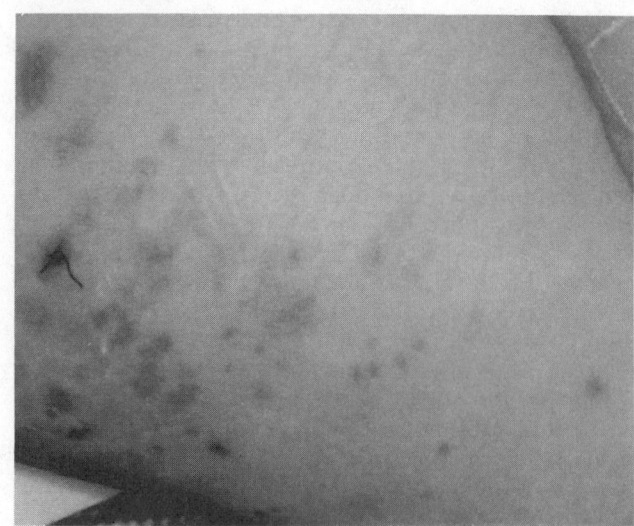

FIG. 56-73. Gold-induced lichenoid drug eruption.

ERYTHEMA NODOSUM

Erythema nodosum (EN) is characterized by tender, erythematous, subcutaneous nodules, most often on the anterior shins. Drugs can induce EN but probably account for less that 5% of cases. The mechanism by which a drug causes EN is not known. The most common drugs involved are oral contraceptives, although occasionally an antibiotic has been implicated. In a patient with acute EN, the differential diagnosis includes infections such as beta-streptococcal, fungal or mycobacterial sarcoidosis, inflammatory bowel disease, pregnancy, or an oral contraceptive or other drug. Treatment is nonspecific and includes rest, elevation, and antiinflammatory agents. If an underlying cause is found, treatment of the process may improve the EN.

LICHENOID DRUG ERUPTION

Certain drugs can cause an unusual eruption, similar in appearance to lichen planus. Patients often present with pruritic, violaceous to hyperpigmented plaques (Fig. 56-73) on their extremities, but occasionally the plaques become generalized. Reticulated, lacy patches on the buccal mucosa occur in idiopathic lichen planus, but may also be present in patients with lichenoid drug eruptions. The most common cause is gold, but antimalarials, penicillamine, thiazides, and sulfonamides may also cause this reaction. Therapy involves removal of the offending agent and topical corticosteroids. On rare occasions, systemic corticosteroids are necessary.

FIXED DRUG ERUPTION

This unusual reaction is manifest as a violaceous and/or vesicular plaque (Fig. 56-74), which repeatedly appears in the same areas of the body on ingestion of the offending agent. The lesions are frequently on the genitalia, hands, and face. The most common cause is phenolphthalein, used in over-the-counter laxatives. In addition, tetracyclines, sulfa drugs and some nonsteroidal anti-inflammatory agents may cause the eruption. The process, when recognized, needs only to be treated by removal of the offending agent.

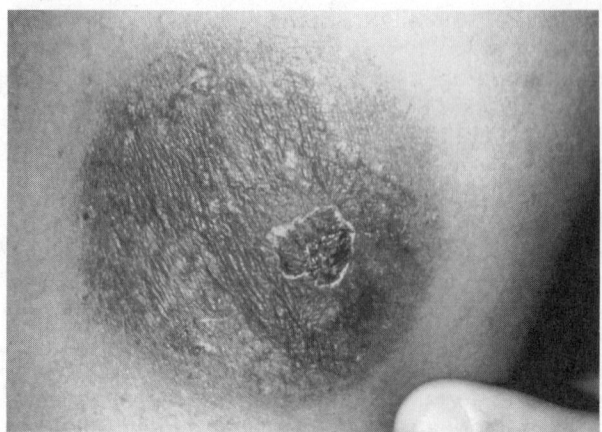

FIG. 56-74. Thorazine-caused recurrent violaceous fixed drug eruption.

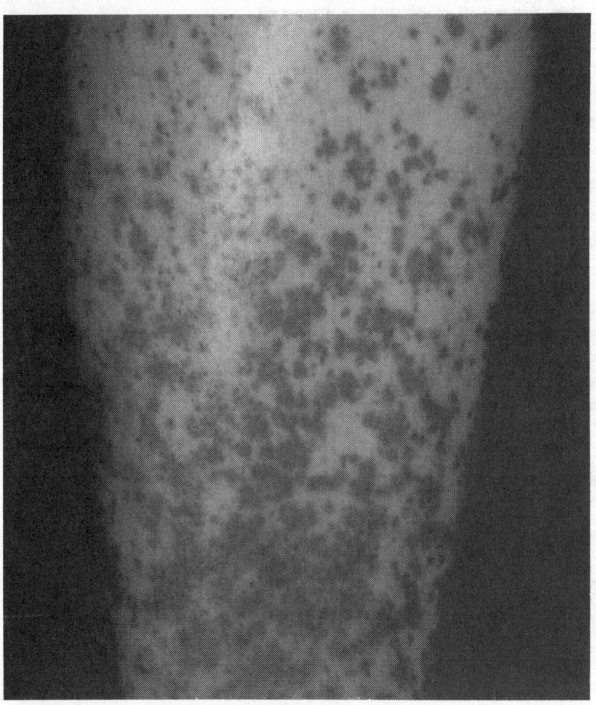

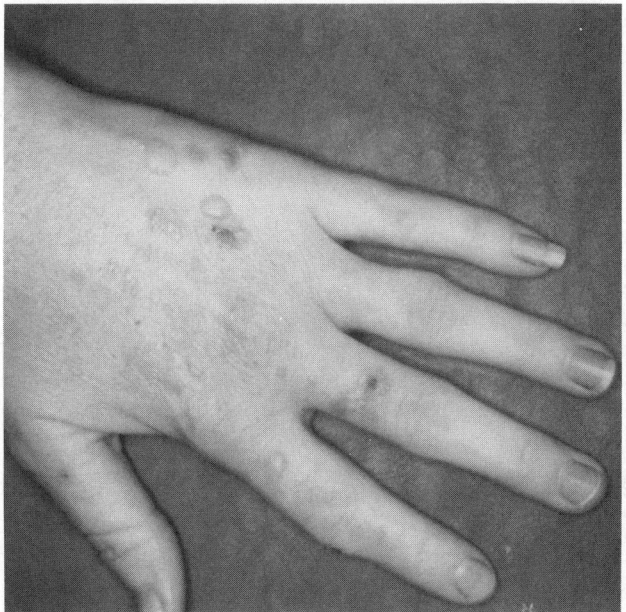

FIG. 56-76. Naproxen-induced photoeruption with blisters and milia on the hands (pseudoporphyria).

FIG. 56-75. Cutaneous leukocytoclastic vasculitis caused by a cephalothin.

CUTANEOUS VASCULITIS

Cutaneous vasculitis, or hypersensitivity angiitis, is manifested most commonly by palpable purpura on the lower extremities (Fig. 56-75). In some patients, the reaction is urticarial, bullous, or ulcerative. Vasculitis is caused by the formation of immune complexes with deposition in the small vessels (postcapillary venules). Although the reaction may occur only in the skin, it is caused by circulating immune complexes; thus the kidney, joints, or gastrointestinal tract can also be involved. In studies of large groups of patients with vasculitis, drugs are found as the cause in only 5 to 10%, and the most frequent agents are those found with urticaria or erythema multiforme. Treatment of drug-induced LV in selected patients involves removal of the offending agent, oral antihistamines, oral colchicine, and/or systemic corticosteroids.

MISCELLANEOUS

Several reactions are worthy of brief mention. Naproxen may cause a blistering eruption on the dorsum of the hands, clinically like porphyria cutanea tarda and known as pseudoporphyria (Fig. 56-76). Penicillamine can induce a blistering epidermal process known as pemphigus, which can be life-threatening. Thiazide diuretics and griseofulvin have been reported to cause nonscarring cutaneous lupus erythematosus in susceptible individuals. Coumarin may cause infarcted lesions that manifest as deep, bizarre, asymmetric ulcers. These appear 3 to 10 days after the anticoagulant has been started, and the initial lesions are tender red areas that progress to purpuric swellings and ulceration with hemorrhagic eschars.

REFERENCES

1. Swinyer, L.J.: Drug eruptions in an emergency department setting. Emerg. Med. Clin. N.A. 3:717, 1985.
2. Bigby, M., Jick, S., Jick, H., and Arndt, F.: Drug-induced cutaneous reactions. JAMA 256:3358, 1986.
3. Wintroub, B.U., and Stern, R.: Cutaneous drug reactions: Pathogenesis and clinical classifications. J. Am. Acad. Dermatol. 13:167, 1985.
4. Kaplan, A.P.: Drug-induced skin disease. J. Allergy Clin. Immunol. 74:573, 1984.
5. Sussman, G.L., and Dolovich, J.: Prevention of anaphylaxis. Semin. Dermatol. 8:158,1989.
6. Genvert, G.I., Cohen, E.J., Donnenfeld, E.D., and Belcher, M.H.: Erythema multiforme after use of topical sulfacetamide. Am. J. Ophthalmol. 99:465, 1985.

LIFE-THREATENING DERMATOSES

Jeffrey P. Callen and Carol L. Kulp-Shorten

CAPSULE

The saying goes that dermatologic disease neither kills nor is curable. Although this is generally true, there exists a group of disorders in which the skin is either an early sign of severe disease or one of the major organs involved in the process. Most of the disorders discussed in this chapter can result in death if not recognized and promptly treated (Table 56-13). In some cases, however, even with the best current therapy and early recognition, a fatal outcome is inevitable. Death can be caused by a loss of the epidermal barrier function, as in toxic epidermal necrolysis or pemphigus; dissemination of infection, as in gonorrhea; or systemic manifestations of the disease, as in Kawasaki's disease.

Death can occur from a number of diseases in an insidious fashion such as metastases from a cutaneous melanoma or death that occurs secondary to AIDS. These disorders, although part of the "life-threatening" diseases, are only tabulated rather than discussed (Table 56-14). This chapter concentrates on the disorders in which imminent death can occur. This group is the more likely to be seen in an Emergency Department (ED) setting, whereas the recognition of pigmented lesions is more likely to occur in an ambulatory care clinic.[1]

TABLE 56-13. DERMATOSES THAT CAN BE RAPIDLY FATAL

Infections
- Erysipelas
- Toxic shock syndrome
- Necrotizing fasciitis
- Staphylococcal scalded skin syndrome
- Meningococcemia
- Disseminated gonococcemia
- Rocky Mountain spotted fever
- Disseminated herpes simplex
- Disseminated herpes zoster

Bullous Diseases
- Pemphigus vulgaris
- Stevens-Johnson syndrome (toxic epidermal necrolysis)

Purpuric or Hemorrhagic Diseases
- Disseminated intravascular coagulation
- Purpura fulminans
- Antiphospholipid syndrome
- Vasculitis
- Brown recluse spider bites
- Thrombocytopenia
- Child abuse

Miscellaneous
- Pustular psoriasis
- Exfoliative dermatitis (erythroderma)
- Anaphylaxis

TABLE 56-14. SKIN DISEASES THAT CAN LEAD TO OR BE ASSOCIATED WITH A FATAL OUTCOME OVER A MORE PROLONGED PERIOD

- Melanoma
- Cutaneous T-cell lymphoma (mycosis fungoides)
- Cutaneous lupus erythematosus
- Behcet's syndrome
- Skin lesions in the AIDS patient
  —Infections
  —Kaposi's sarcoma
- Bullous pemphigoid
- Skin lesions in the organ transplant patient
  —Bone marrow (graft-versus-host disease)
  —Kidney (squamous cell carcinoma)
  —Miscellaneous (heart, lung, liver, pancreas, etc)

INFECTIONS

ERYSIPELAS

Erysipelas is a specific type of cellulitis most often caused by group A beta hemolytic streptococcal infection. The lesions are tender, warm, sharply marginated, expanding erythema. The patient is usually systemically ill, with high fever, chills, leukocytosis, and malaise. Erysipelas must be treated promptly with systemic antibiotics given intravenously.

KAWASAKI'S DISEASE (MUCOCUTANEOUS LYMPH NODE SYNDROME)

Kawasaki's disease (KD) is an acute febrile illness that occurs primarily in children. The major clinical features include prolonged fever (>5 days) that is nonresponsive to antibiotics, conjunctivitis, lymphadenopathy, mucosal changes, polymorphous skin eruptions, and acral erythema and desquamation. The exact cause of KD is not known, but it may represent a reaction to an infectious agent or environmental toxin. In addition to the above common problems, which are used as major criteria for diagnosis, 15 to 25% of these patients develop coronary artery aneurysms. This manifestation can result in sudden death and requires appropriate recognition and treatment. In KD there appears to be a marked immune activation; and therefore, treatment has consisted of aspirin therapy and intravenous immune globulin (IVIG).[2] Recent studies of IVIG suggest that this therapeutic maneuver effectively produces immunomodulation and prevents or allows reversal of endothelial cell injury, which is the presumed mechanism of the coronary artery aneurysm.

TOXIC SHOCK SYNDROME (TSS)

Toxic shock syndrome (TSS) is an acute multisystem illness with prominent dermatologic features.[3] The illness is caused by toxin-producing strains of Staphylococcus aureus, phage type I. This syndrome was initially recognized in menstruating women and linked to super-absorbent tampon usage. Since the initial reports, however, both nonmenstruating women and men have been reported with toxic shock syndrome. The Center for Disease Control (CDC) has issued a set of criteria for TSS which include: fever >102°F, rash with desquamation, hypotension, clinical or laboratory abnormalities in 3 or more organ systems, and exclusion of other causes. The cutaneous manifestations include both early and late changes. Early in the course, the patient has a sudden onset of a generalized erythroderma or nonpitting edema. Later the rash may become urticarial or papular. Desquamation occurs between 10 days and 3 weeks. Two to six months afterward, diffuse hair loss (telogen effluvium) may occur, and Beau's lines may be seen on examination of the fingernails.

The therapy of TSS involves removal of potentially infected foreign bodies or drainage of infected sites. Appropriate cultures should be taken, then intravenous antistaphylococcal beta-lactamase-resistant antibiotics should be given in maximal doses. Fluid and electrolyte imbalance should be corrected and carefully managed, and organ involvement should be aggressively managed with appropriate consultation with subspecialists. The role for corticosteroids or intravenous immunoglobulin is controversial. TSS may recur, with recurrence rates as high as 30% reported.

NECROTIZING FASCIITIS

Necrotizing fasciitis is a rapidly progressive process that occurs in the superficial fascia undermining the skin. It often follows minor trauma, surgery, or injury to the skin. Immunocompromised patients are predisposed to this rare infectious process, as are patients with a history of drug abuse, diabetes, obesity, atherosclerotic vascular disease, alcoholism, and malnutrition.[4] Necrotizing fasciitis may be caused by a wide variety of organisms, but beta-hemolytic streptococcus is the most common offender.[5] Erythema and edema are almost universal cutaneous findings, with ulceration, necrosis or bullae developing in later stages. The lesions are painful, and the patient is toxic. Appropriate care is directed at the causative organism, combined with surgical debridement of involved tissue. Death is a common outcome of undiagnosed cases.

STAPHYLOCOCCAL SCALDED SKIN SYNDROME (SSSS)

The staphylococcal scalded skin syndrome (SSSS) usually occurs in children. The disorder is produced in an individual infected with Staphylococcus aureus group 2 phage type 71, which produces an exotoxin. The toxin causes a split within the granular layer of the epidermis. The skin is initially red and tender, and then develops vesicles, bullae, erosions and crusts (Fig. 56-77). In general, patients also appear toxic. This disorder must be differentiated from erythema multiforme and toxic epidermal necrolysis, in which the epidermal split occurs in the basal layer. Antibiotics and supportive care are usually effective, with complete recovery in >98% of cases.

DISSEMINATED GONORRHEA

Gonococcal septicemia occurs within 3 to 21 days after local infection. It often occurs during menstruation or pregnancy, or in conjunction with gynecologic surgery or delivery. The patient presents with fever, arthritis, and skin lesions. The skin lesions appear in crops, are few in number, and tend to be acral in their distribution, often overlying joints. The individual lesion is typically an umbilicated pustule with surrounding erythema or hemorrhage with necrosis (Fig. 56-78). The arthritis usually involves only a few joints, and is asymmetric. Cultures of appropriate orifices (rectum, pharynx, urethra, and/or cervix) effectively identify the responsible organism, whereas cultures from the skin and/or joints rarely identify the gonococcus. Treatment with systemically administered antibiotics is effective and may, under the appropriate circumstances, be administered on an outpatient basis.

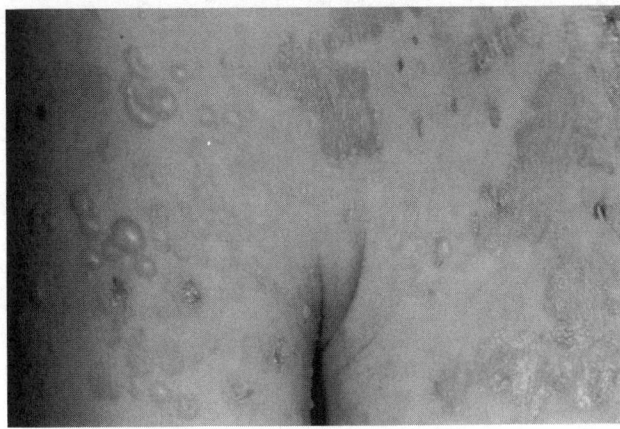

FIG. 56-77. *Staphylococcal scalded skin syndrome. This patient has crusts and small bullae on a noninflammatory base.*

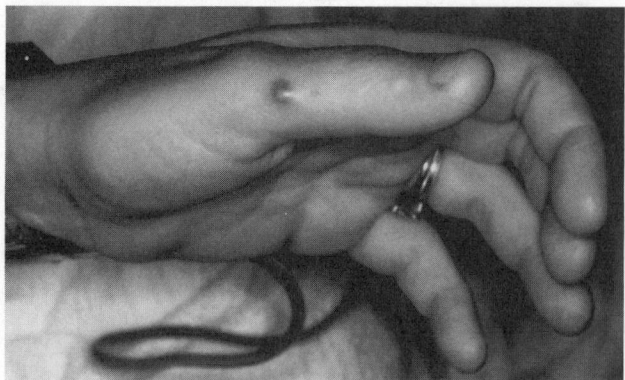

FIG. 56-78. Disseminated gonococcemia. A pustule is present in this young woman who presented with fever and arthritis.

DISSEMINATED HERPES SIMPLEX

Herpex simplex virus (HVS) infection is a common problem that can occur on any surface of the body but is most common on the lips and genitalia. Two varieties of the virus exist—HSV-1 and HSV-2. In immunocompetent individuals, an infection with either virus is a benign self-limited process, but the virus remains in a latent phase within a nerve ganglion after the initial infection. Recurrence rates vary from 16% to 45% for oral HSV infection,[6] and are similar for genital HSV. In addition to clinically recognizable reactivation, asymptomatic viral shedding may occur in 0.75% to 10% of infected individuals. Thus, primary infection can occur in an individual exposed to asymptomatic shedding. In neonates (immunologically immature) and patients with atopic dermatitis, malignancies, iatrogenic immunosuppression, or AIDS, the herpes virus infection can be atypical, or can disseminate. Disseminated HSV may not have the classical grouped lesions, but appear as widespread vesicles and occasionally pustules (Fig. 56-79). The patient may be febrile, and internal involvement is sometimes present and can be life-threatening. Diagnosis of herpetic infection can be confirmed by performing a Tzanck smear and demonstrating the typical multinucleated giant cells. Culture can later differentiate herpes simplex from herpes zoster. Therapy includes careful in-hospital monitoring and parenterally administered acyclovir.

DISSEMINATED HERPES ZOSTER

Herpes zoster is a self-limited recurrence of a varicella (chickenpox) infection caused by the varicella zoster (VZ) virus. In the noncompromised patient, herpes zoster usually involves only one dermatome. Its initial manifestations include pain, burning, and itching, accompanied or followed shortly by a grouped vesicular rash. The process is self-resolving within 2 to 3 weeks, but residual neuralgia (postherpetic neuralgia) occurs

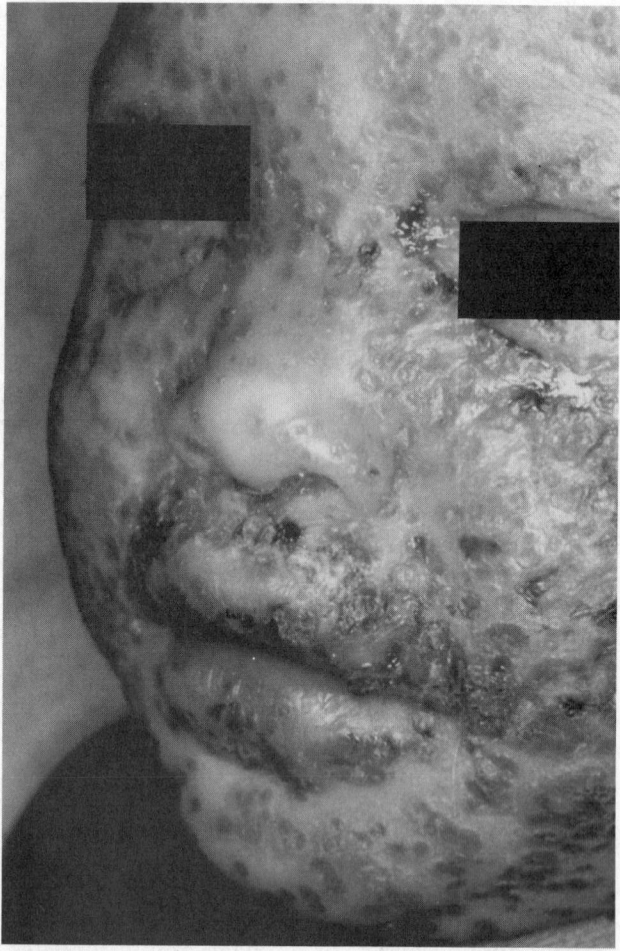

FIG. 56-79. Eczema herpeticum. This child with mild atopic dermatitis developed disseminated herpes simplex after being kissed by a relative with a "cold sore" on his lip.

commonly in elderly patients. Prevention of postherpetic neuralgia is possible with pharmacologic doses of prednisone for 2 weeks when given within the first few days of the eruption. The immunosuppressed host may have a dermatomal presentation or may develop widespread vesicles with or without evidence of a dermatomal distribution (Fig. 56-80). Treatment with an antiviral agent is helpful, and acyclovir and vidarabine have been most commonly used.

BULLOUS DISEASES

PEMPHIGUS

Pemphigus is a rare group of disorders characterized by intraepidermal blister formation. Pemphigus vulgaris is the most common form of the disease. If un-

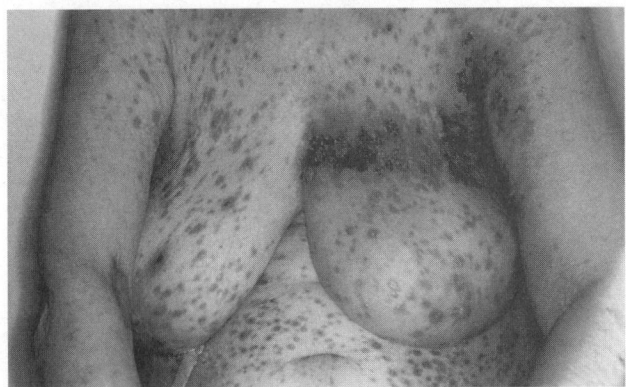

FIG. 56-80. Disseminated herpes zoster with a residual dermatomal eruption.

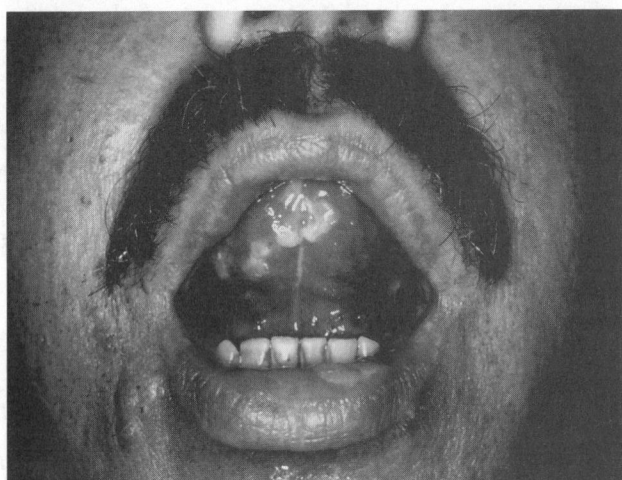

FIG. 56-81. These painful oral erosions were the initial manifestation of pemphigus vulgaris.

treated, it is associated with a high frequency of death. These disorders are characterized by deposition of antibody in the epidermal intercellular cement, but the exact mechanism of blister formation is not completely understood. The pemphigus antibody may be found

in the serum and the titer can be used with clinical information to adjust therapy. Pemphigus often presents with painful oral erosions (Fig. 56-81) followed by the development of widespread cutaneous flaccid bullae or erosions and crusts. Biopsy and immunofluorescence studies can help confirm the diagnosis. Treatment should be begun promptly after diagnostic confirmation. The mainstay of initial therapy is systemic corticosteroids given in moderate or high doses (80 to 120 mg/day of prednisone or an equivalent). The dose can be raised if the patient fails to respond properly. In advanced disease, hospitalization may be necessary for fluid and electrolyte management as well as treatment of secondary infections. For patients who do not respond to corticosteroids, immunosuppressive agents, apheresis, or gold may be used.

STEVENS-JOHNSON SYNDROME AND TOXIC EPIDERMAL NECROLYSIS

Stevens-Johnson syndrome (SJS) is severe, often bullous erythema multiforme with systemic symptoms and involvement of multiple mucosal surfaces. Toxic epidermal necrolysis (TEN) is almost identical to SJS except that the typical lesion of erythema multiforme is not seen and the skin is lost in sheets (Fig. 56-82). TEN is also almost always drug-induced, whereas SJS may be drug-induced or secondary to a variety of infectious agents. It is possible that TEN and drug-induced SJS are identical processes. Nevertheless, both processes often begin with a prodrome, fever, and malaise, followed by either a generalized morbilliform erythema (TEN) or erythematous targetoid lesions (SJS). Skin tenderness is marked. Conjunctivitis and oral mucosal erosions are common. The Nikolsky sign involves further desquamation by gentle pressure on normal-appearing skin. In each case, the process must be aggressively managed with an approach similar to that for a burn patient, and the mortality rate is high. The use of corticosteroids is controversial, and has been linked to prolonged hospitalization and more

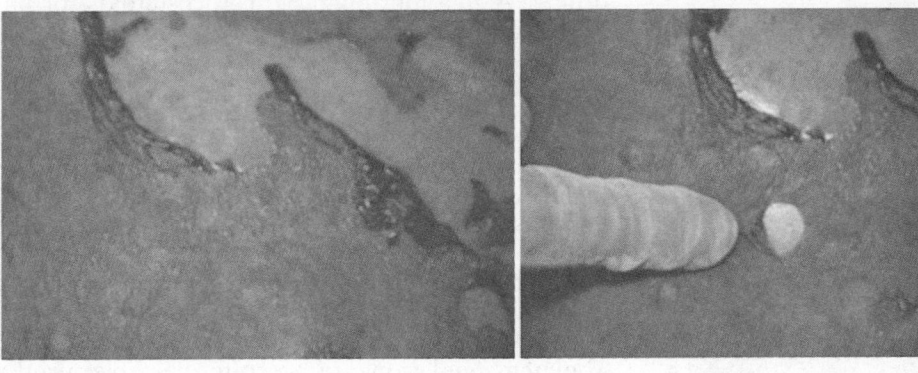

A   B

FIG. 56-82. A. Toxic epidermal necrolysis. B. The Nikolsky sign of toxic epidermal necrolysis. Courtesy of Howard Simons, M.D.

frequent bacterial infections. Skin care, fluid and electrolyte balance, ophthalmologic care and infection surveillance are of primary importance. Thus a team approach to these life-threatening processes is necessary.

PURPURIC OR HEMORRHAGIC DISEASES

DISSEMINATED INTRAVASCULAR COAGULOPATHY (DIC)

Disseminated intravascular coagulopathy (DIC) is a term synonymous with consumptive coagulopathy and represents a condition in which systemic bleeding occurs because of the consumption of platelets and coagulation factors. The process can be initiated within a local area, such as an aneurysm or hemangioma, or can begin systemically following an infection, massive trauma, complicated pregnancy, or in the presence of a tumor. Bleeding from and within the skin and widespread purpura or ecchymoses are signs of DIC (Fig. 53-83). The diagnosis is confirmed by a reduced platelet count, prolonged prothrombin time, decreased fibrinogen level, and the presence of fibrin split products. Appropriate hematologic consultation and hospitalization should follow immediately on recognition of this process.

PURPURA FULMINANS

Purpura fulminans is probably a variant of DIC that is most common in children after an infection, but may occur in neonates secondary to homozygous protein C deficiency, or in adults heterozygous for protein C deficiency who are given coumadin (coumadin necrosis).[7] The disease is manifested by large areas of ecchymotic plaques, which eventually become ne-

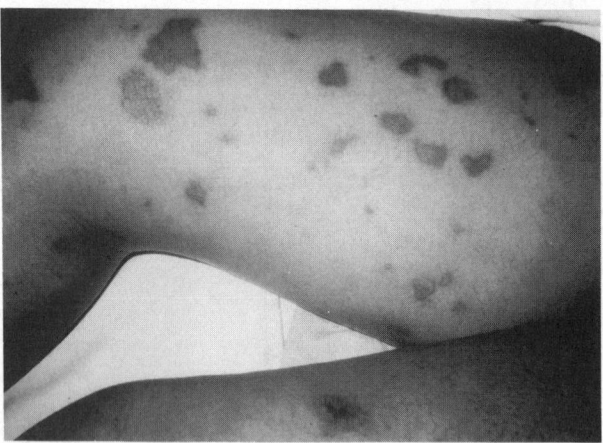

FIG. 56-83.   DIC due to meningococcemia.

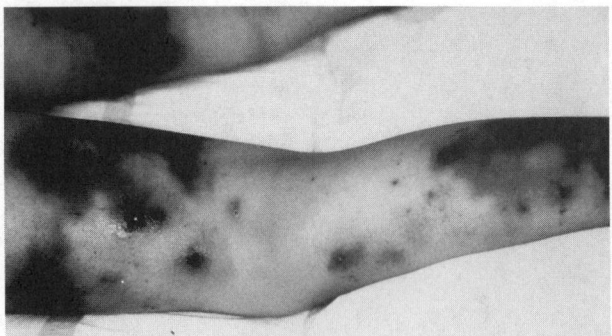

FIG. 56-84.   Purpura fulminans following varicella infection.

crotic and may result in bullae, ulceration, or both (Fig. 56-84). Purpura fulminans is a noninflammatory process that can be differentiated from leukocytoclastic vascultis on biopsy. Treatment is similar to that for DIC.

ANTIPHOSPHOLIPID SYNDROME

Patients with antibodies to neutral or negatively charged phospholipids may have life-threatening disease. These antibodies are also known as anticardiolipin antibodies or the lupus anticoagulant. This latter term is a misnomer because patients may or may not have lupus erythematosus, and the presence of these antibodies has been associated with thromboembolic phenomenon, manifest as recurrent fetal loss, arterial and venous thromboses, and progressive CNS disease. Many of these patients have no skin lesions; others have livedo reticularis, a netlike purpuric condition of the skin, ulceration or hemorrhage, or necrosis of the skin. Patients with noninflammatory purpura, unexplained ulcers, livedo reticularis, or recurrent thrombophlebitis should perhaps be tested for antiphospholipid antibodies. The best therapy for this process has not yet been determined, but anticoagulants such as heparin or coumadin and platelet inhibitors such as aspirin or persantine have been recommended as treatment of various aspects of the syndrome. A role for apheresis, corticosteroids, or immunosuppressives has not yet been established.

VASCULITIS

Leukocytoclastic vasculitis (LCV) is a common inflammatory cause of cutaneous purpura. Often the clinical term "palpable purpura" is used as a synonym. LCV is an immune complex disease that may be manifest only in the skin, or may have accompanying systemic involvement. The common systemically involved areas are the joints, kidneys, and gastrointestinal tract. The cutaneous lesions are most often palpable purpura on the lower extremities or other dependent areas of the body, although some patients manifest urticaria-like lesions that may have a residual ecchymosis upon resolution. This disorder has been commonly related to drugs, infections, collagen-vascular diseases, and dysproteinemias or may be idiopathic. Diagnosis is confirmed by skin biopsy. The evaluation should rule out embolic phenomena and infections such as subacute bacterial endocarditis, and should assess the cause and extent of the process. A variant known as Henoch-Schönlein purpura (HSP) is caused by IgA immune complexes and is more frequently seen in children. Treatment is first directed at removal of a causative factor (drug) or treatment of an associated condition. In the absence of an identifiable factor, treatment is based on severity of and presence of organ involvement. Severe necrotizing vasculitis requires aggressive management with corticosteroids and/or immunosuppressives.

BROWN RECLUSE SPIDER BITES

The bite of Loxosceles reclusa or the brown recluse spider (fiddler spider) causes a hemorrhagic necrotic area in the skin. The spider is reclusive and nocturnal and lives in warm, dry areas. Bites are probably most common through exposure in attics or crawlspaces of houses that have been undisturbed for long times. Not all bites are dangerous, but those in which venom is injected can cause a life-threatening systemic disease process.[9] Local reaction involves pain and erythema at the site of the bite, followed by necrosis of the skin (Fig. 56-85). The systemic symptoms are more common in children and include fever, chills, nausea, vomiting, arthralgias, convulsions, and hemolysis. Severe hemolysis can trigger DIC or result in hemoglobinuria and acute renal failure. Diagnosis of the brown spider bite is difficult unless the spider is brought by the patient. This is not likely because the bite is often not recognized until hours after it took place. Treatment is directed at local measures. Excision of the necrotic tissue is controversial, but once the borders have been established this may be helpful. Early therapy with oral dapsone has been suggested, but only anecdotal information exists.

THROMBOCYTOPENIA

Thrombocytopenia, regardless of its cause, can result in a petechial rash or small areas of nonpalpable purpura (Fig. 56-86). The rash, often accompanied by bleeding such as epistaxis, may be the presenting manifestation of the thrombocytopenia. Thrombocytopenia can be caused by decreased production (drugs, infection, radiation, tumors), sequestration (hemangioma or spleen), or increased destruction (immunologic or consumptive). Recognition and appropriate treatment of the cause can prevent fatal hemorrhage.

CHILD ABUSE

Purpura and ecchymoses in various stages of resolution are the most frequent cutaneous signs of child abuse, one of the most frequent causes of death in young children (1 to 4 years of age). It should be suspected by examining physicians in the ED. Suspicion of child abuse is reportable to the child protective services in all states, and failure to report it is punishable.

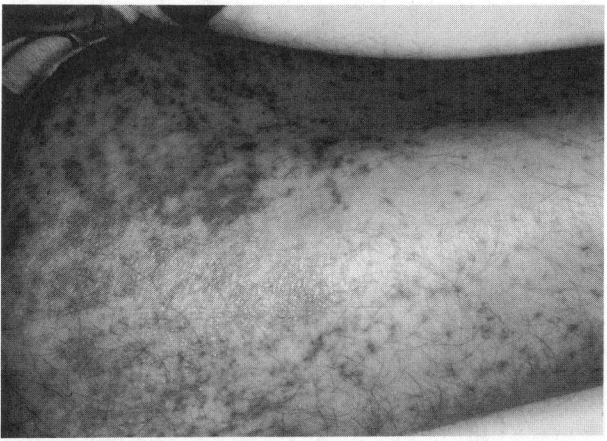

A

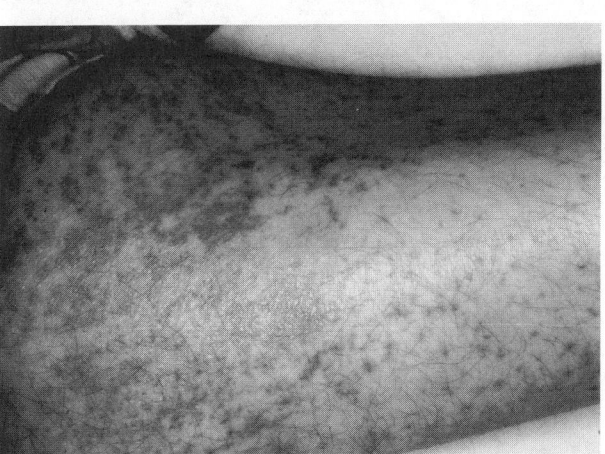

B

FIG. 56-86.   Nonpalpable purpura from thrombocytopenia.

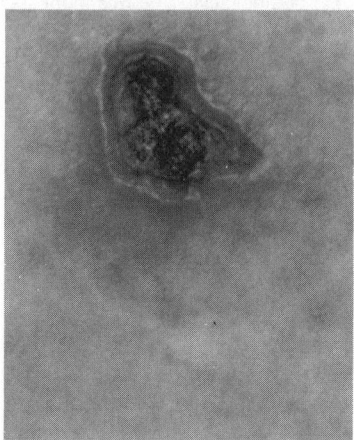

FIG. 56-85.   Brown recluse spider bite.

In addition to strangely configured and distributed purpura, burns, bite marks, hemorrhage in the shape of a hand, or abrasions may be manifestations. More severe abuse can cause broken bones or internal hemorrhage. Only with recognition can the child be protected and removed from the abusive environment. Because children who are abused frequently become abusive parents, treatment and behavior modification are needed to prevent the continued spread of this disorder.

MISCELLANEOUS CONDITION

PUSTULAR PSORIASIS

Most patients with psoriasis have a chronic non-life-threatening disease. In a rare individual, however, a generalized pustular process with systemic symptoms can occur. The patient may or may not have a personal or family history of psoriasis. The eruption spreads rapidly, and is characterized by small pustules on an erythematous base or polycyclic areas of erythema with pustules. The patient is frequently toxic, with a high fever, and may become hypotensive. Various drugs have been implicated in the cause of this reaction, including lithium, beta blockers, nonsteroidal anti-inflammatory agents, and withdrawal from systemic corticosteroids. In addition, infections and pregnancy have sometimes provoked this reaction pattern. Pustular psoriasis is a serious condition. The patient should be hospitalized, any provocative factor removed or treated, and fluid and electrolyte balance maintained. Topical emollients and soaks are helpful and useful systemic agents include methotrexate and corticosteroids. Recently, with the availability of oral retinoids (isotretinoin or etretinate) the condition can be quickly brought under control in most patients.

EXFOLIATIVE DERMATITIS (ERYTHRODERMA)

A generalized exfoliative erythroderma is a diffuse erythematous rash with desquamation. The patient is often uncomfortable and severely pruritic and skin pain may also be a symptom. Because of a defective epidermal barrier, heat control may be problematic, with some patients experiencing constant chills. Also, fluid and electrolyte imbalance may occur. Frequently a high output cardiac failure is evident, particularly in the elderly. Exfoliative dermatitis develops in preexisting dermatoses in about 40 to 50% of cases, and has occurred with psoriasis, any type of dermatitis, lichen planus, or scabetic infestation. A specific contactant is responsible for some cases. Severe drug eruptions account for 10 to 20% of cases, and a lymphoreticular malignancy accounts for another 10 to 15%. Only about 20% are idiopathic. The patient with exfoliative erythroderma is best managed in the hospital, but can be occasionally treated in an outpatient setting. A careful evaluation to locate a treatable cause or associated condition is necessary. Treatment with soaks, topical emollients, and topical corticosteroids may be sufficient. Occasionally small doses of ultraviolet light are helpful. Systemic corticosteroids are reserved for recalcitrant cases.

This chapter has briefly dealt with a potpourri of conditions that may be seen in an ED or urgent care center. Recognition, appropriate evaluation, hospitalization, and aggressive therapy can often be lifesaving.

REFERENCES

1. Krusinski, P.A., and Flowers, F.P.: Life-threatening dermatoses. In Dermatology in Ambulatory and Emergency Medicine. Edited by Flowers, F.P., and Krusinski, P.A.: Chicago, Year Book Medical Publishers, 1984, pp. 412–433.
2. Leung, D.Y.M.: Immunomodulation by intravenous immune globin in Kawasaki's disease. J. Allergy Clin. Immunol. 84:588, 1989.
3. Chesney, P.J.: Clinical aspects and spectrum of illness of toxic shock syndrome: Overview. Rev. Infect. Dis. 2:A1, 1989.
4. Wojno, K., and Spitz, W.U.: Necrotizing fasciitis: A fatal outcome following minor trauma. Am. J. Med. Pathol. 10:239, 1989.
5. Umbert, I.J, Winkelmann, R.K., Oliver, G.F., and Peters, M.S.: Necrotizing fasciitis. A clinical, microbiologic, and histopathologic study of 14 patients. J. Am. Acad. Dermatol. 20:774, 1989.
6. Scully, C.: Orofacial herpes simplex virus infections: Current concepts in the epidemiology, pathogenesis, and treatment and disorders in which the virus may be implicated. Oral Surg. Oral Med. Oral Pathol. 68:701, 1989.
7. Rick, M.E.: Protein C and Protein S. JAMA 263:701, 1990.
8. Callen, J.P.: Cutaneous vasculitis and its relationship to internal disease. Dis. Mon. 28:1, 1981.
9. Gendron, B.P.: Loxosceles reclusa envenomation. Am. J. Emerg. Med. 8:51, 1990.

URTICARIA

Marc D. Brown

DEFINITION AND CLASSIFICATION

Urticaria, commonly referred to as hives, is a frequently encountered skin condition affecting as much as 10 to 20% of the population. The cutaneous reaction of urticaria consists of raised, erythematous pruritic papules and plaques (wheals), which represent localized areas of edema in the superficial dermis. These wheals of urticaria are usually well circumscribed but can enlarge and become confluent. Fortunately, urticaria is usually a transient condition, and individual lesions resolve within several hours, rarely persisting more than 24 hours. As individual lesions resolve, however, new lesions may continue to arise. When individual lesions persist for more than 24 hours, the term "urticarial reaction" is used and an underlying vasculitis must be considered.[1] Urticaria may represent an early phase of anaphylaxis, and attention must be given to vital signs to note any tachycardia or hypotension.

The inflammatory dermatosis of urticaria results from vasodilation, increased vascular permeability, and subsequent extravasation of protein and fluids into the dermis. When the edema is localized in the superficial dermis, it is referred to as urticaria, and may give the skin an "orange peel" appearance. When the edema is in the deep dermis or subcutaneous tissue, the dermatosis is classified as angioedema. Angioedema can be either acquired or inherited.

The various classification systems for urticaria have been multiple and complex and, at times, confusing. The classification of acute versus chronic urticaria, however, is well accepted and helps to determine the appropriate evaluation and treatment plan. Acute urticaria is defined as that lasting less than 6 weeks.

Most episodes of urticaria are acute and self-limited, and symptoms generally resolve whether or not definitive causes have been determined. Recurrent urticarial lesions that come and go for longer than 6 weeks are termed chronic urticaria.

PATHOGENESIS

The pathogenesis of urticaria is multifactorial and cannot easily be ascribed to one specific mechanism. Mast cells and mast cell-dependent mediators appear to play the major role, which leads ultimately to an increase in vascular permeability and leakage of plasma fluids.[2] Histamine is the primary mediator of this event and the major cause of the associated itching. Other related pathogenic mechanisms include alterations in arachidonic acid pathways, complement-mediated responses, and an IgE-dependent hypersensitivity response.[3] More prolonged or delayed responses may be caused by chemotactic factors and leukocyte infiltration.

The histopathology of urticaria is characterized by edema in the papillary and reticular dermis. Vessels are dilated, but there is no evidence of endothelial destruction. Neutrophils are always present, usually mixed with eosinophils, lymphocytes and monocytes. Mast cells are prominent.

CLINICAL PRESENTATION

URTICARIA

Urticaria is usually not difficult to diagnose. The lesions evolve rapidly as an area of localized swelling. The typical lesion appears red and raised (Fig. 56-87). The patient usually complains of itching and, at times, burning or stinging. The individual wheals vary in size from a few millimeters to several centimeters. Urticaria may be localized to one small area or extended over the entire body. It is not necessarily limited to the skin, but also can involve the mucosal surfaces. Urticarial plaques are usually well circumscribed, but may enlarge and become confluent by peripheral extension. Lesions enlarge and result in

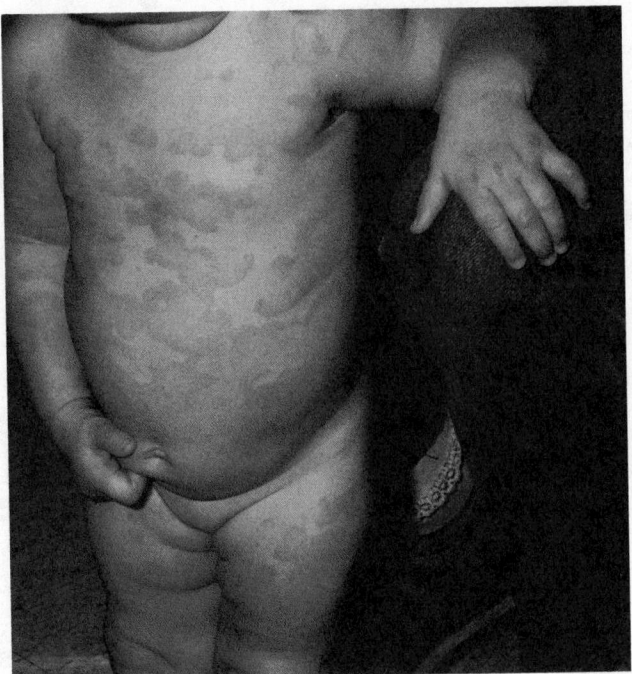

FIG. 56-87. Red, raised lesions in a child with urticaria.

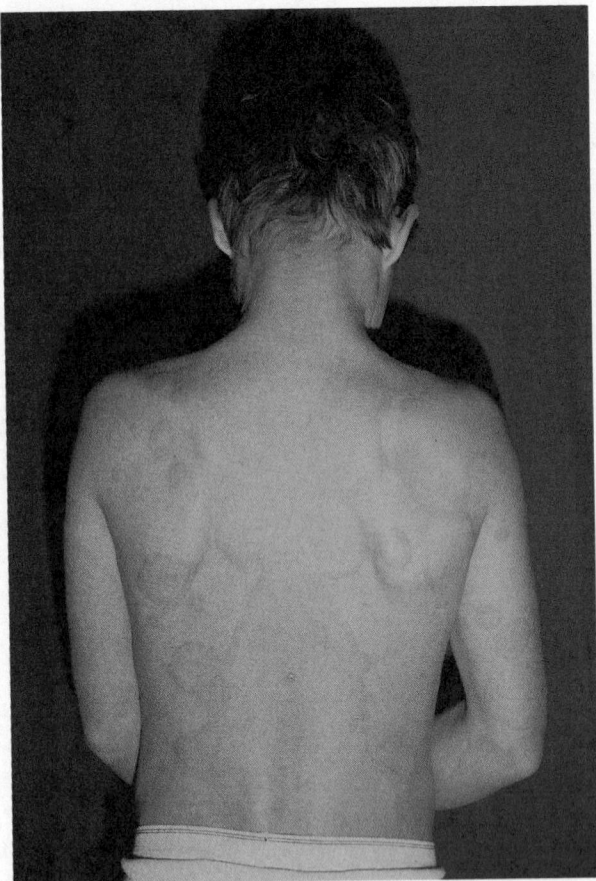

FIG. 56-88. Bizarrely shaped lesions in a patient with urticaria.

bizarre geographic configurations (Fig. 56-88). The individual urticarial plaques can be surrounded by a ring of erythema or pallor. Men and women are equally affected with acute episodes of urticaria, but with chronic urticaria it appears that women in the 30 to 40 age range are more commonly affected. Lesions usually disappear without the subsequent skin changes often seen with other types of dermatitis. There are usually no scales or pigmentary changes. Although individual lesions involute within several hours, there may be multiple stages, making urticaria appear to be a more or less consistent eruption.

ANGIOEDEMA

Angioedema can be considered a more severe form of urticaria with exudation of plasma into deeper perivascular spaces. Any area of the body can be involved, but it occurs most commonly around the mouth, lips, eyes, tongue, earlobes, palms, soles, and genital area.[4] When swelling occurs in these soft tissue and mucous membrane areas, it can appear grotesque in proportion and alarm the patient. Angioedema, unlike urticaria, can be nonpruritic. The edema is nonpitting and often asymmetric. Angioedema can be acquired or hereditary. The hereditary form is caused by a deficiency of C-1-esterase inhibitor, which inhibits the activated first component of the complement system.[5] It is inherited in an autosomal dominant pattern with two genetic types. In type I, there is an absolute decrease in the serum level of the C-1 inhibitor and in type II a dysfunctional mutant form of the C-1 in-

hibitor. Hereditary angioedema is usually not associated with urticaria elsewhere on the body. In addition to swelling, gastrointestinal symptoms are common, including nausea, vomiting, and colicky abdominal pain caused by localized gastrointestinal wall edema and swelling. Laryngeal edema can occur, causing difficulty with breathing, and at times becomes a medical emergency.

Acquired angioedema (the more common form of the disease) often occurs simultaneously with urticarial plaques elsewhere.[6] Many patients with chronic urticaria have episodic bouts of acquired angioedema, which occurs equally in both sexes and in all age groups. Acute episodes are more frequent in young adults, whereas chronic angioedema is more common in middle-aged women.

If an individual urticarial plaque or wheal persists for more than 24 hours, there must be a strong suspicion that the cutaneous reaction is not simply hives but may be caused by an underlying vasculitis. At the mild end of the spectrum, these patients may have only skin lesions that may be indistinguishable from true urticaria. When lesions are more severe, there may be evidence of multisystem disease.[7] An important diagnostic feature distinguishing between true urticaria and urticarial vasculitis (aside from the historical data that these lesions are not transient) is the association with systemic symptoms of fever, malaise, polyarthralgia, and abdominal pain. With time, these urticarial-appearing lesions may become petechial or purpuric in appearance. They may be painful and burn or sting, and pruritis is less common than with true urticaria. Associated angioedema can be seen with urticarial vasculitis. When these urticarial vasculitic plaques resolve, they can leave a persistent postinflammatory hyperpigmentation, not seen with true urticaria. Careful inspection of the skin may also reveal livedoid changes, small blisters, or targetoid lesions, which all suggest a diagnosis of vasculitis. When the history shows that individual urticarial lesions have persisted for more than 24 hours, vasculitis needs to be ruled out with a skin biopsy. A 4 mm punch biopsy is usually adequate. As a general rule, urticaria rarely needs to be biopsied except when there is a suspicion of a vasculitis. Histology reveals a leukocytoclastic vasculitis with fibrinoid necrosis of the vessel wall. Urticarial vasculitis has been associated with hepatitis B, mononucleosis, serum sickness, systemic lupus erythematosis, and Sjögren's syndrome.[8]

CAUSES

Although the clinical diagnosis of urticaria is usually straightforward, determining the cause is not. Table 56-15 lists the general causes of urticaria. Its cause in many patients with acute episodes and most with chronic episodes cannot be determined even with extensive and expensive diagnostic workups. With chronic urticaria, only 10% of cases are usually attributed to a specific cause.[9] Thus, many patients are simply labeled as having "idiopathic urticaria," although this is equally frustrating to both patient and physician. When a cause can be determined for acute urticaria, it is usually a drug or infection. Common *medications* that can cause urticaria include aspirin and salicylate products, penicillin and related antibiotics, sulfa drugs, nonsteroidal anti-inflammatory drugs (NSAIDs), insulin, codeine or other narcotic drugs, and hormones (Table 56-16). Acute *infectious causes* that can be related to urticaria include mononucleosis, serum hepatitis, varicella, and certain respiratory viruses. Chronic urticaria can be related to underlying occult infections, including sinusitis, dental abscess, cholecystitis, prostatitis, urinary tract infections, parasitic infections (e.g., Girardia), Epstein-Barr virus infections, and gastrointestinal candidiasis (Table 56-17).

Certain *foods and other ingested items* can cause urticaria (Table 56-18). The most common foods that cause repeated attacks of urticaria are shellfish, nuts, eggs, beans, chocolate, fresh fruits (especially strawberries), cheese, tomatoes, mushrooms, corn, and

---

TABLE 56-15. CAUSES OF URTICARIA

1. Drugs
2. Ingestants
   a. Foods
   b. Additives
   c. Dyes
   d. Diagnostic agents
3. Inhalants
   a. Molds
   b. Dust
   c. Pollen
   d. Volatile chemicals
   e. Aerosols
   f. Smoke
4. Contactants
   a. Foods
   b. Cosmetics
   c. Animals
   d. Plant materials
   e. Plastics
   f. Textiles and fabrics
   g. Chemicals
5. Physical and Environmental Stimuli
   a. Cold
   b. Heat
   c. Exercise
   d. Sun
   e. Pressure and vibration
   f. Aquagenic
   g. Dermographism
6. Infections
   a. Acute
   b. Occult

TABLE 56-16. COMMON DRUG CAUSES OF URTICARIA

Aspirin and salicylates
Codeine and narcotic pain medications
Penicillin and related antibiotics
Sulfa drugs
Nonsteroidal anti-inflammatory drugs
Insulin
Hormones

TABLE 56-17. INFECTIOUS CAUSES OF URTICARIA

1. Acute
   a. Mononucleosis
   b. Viral hepatitis
   c. Varicella
   d. Respiratory viruses
2. Occult
   a. Sinusitis
   b. Dental abscess
   c. Prostatitis
   d. Urinary tract infection
   e. Cholecystitis
   f. Parasitic (Giardia)
   g. Epstein-Barr virus
   h. Intestinal candidiasis
   i. Vaginitis

TABLE 56-18. COMMON FOODS THAT CAUSE URTICARIA

Fresh fruits
Nuts
Chocolate
Tomatoes
Shellfish
Eggs
Cheese
Beans
Corn
Mushrooms
Pork
Seasonings

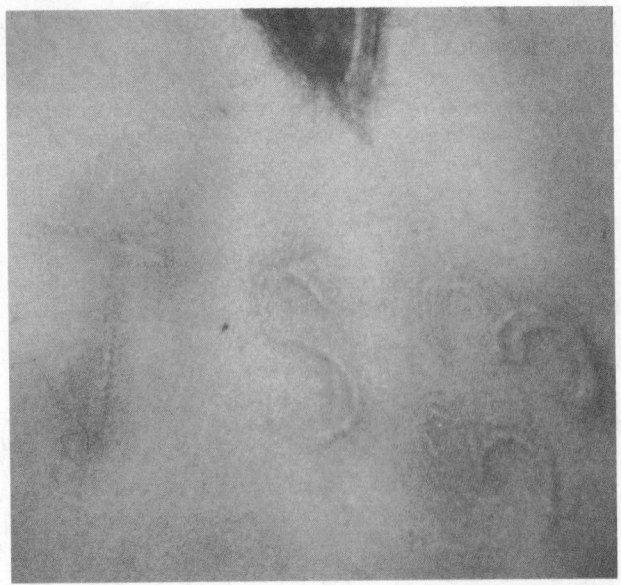

FIG. 56-89. Dermographism. Mild trauma produces "writing" on skin.

pork. Fresh foods appear to cause more frequent episodes of urticaria than do cooked foods. Foods derived from yeast fermentation can also cause urticaria in selected individuals.[10] Food additives, preservatives, and dyes (especially yellow dye #5) may be responsible for both acute and chronic episodes of urticaria.[11] Dairy products (especially those containing penicillin) can cause urticaria in sensitized individuals. Even fluoride in drinking water and toothpaste has been implicated as a cause of chronic urticaria.

Inhalants including molds, dust, and pollen can trigger urticaria, particularly in patients with an atopic history (asthma, allergic rhinitis and eczema). Aerosols, volatile chemicals, and smoke are other common inhalants that cause urticaria.

Contact urticaria is a relatively common condition in which urticaria is induced by simple contact of a substance with the skin or mucous membrane. The contact urticarial reaction occurs quickly, usually within 30 to 60 minutes, and resolves within 24 hours. The reaction can be mild, appearing only as localized erythema; patients often view this only as an irritation and do not seek medical attention. Reactions, however, can be severe, generalized, and symptomatic. The list of substances that cause both immunologic and nonimmunologic contact urticaria is extensive and beyond the scope of this chapter.[12] The more common contact urticants, however, include foods (food handlers are at an increased risk), cosmetics, animals, plant materials, certain textiles and fabrics, plastics, insects, topical medications, and chemicals. The bites of certain insects (mosquitoes, fleas, chigger mites, bedbugs) cause crops of small, pruritic wheals commonly referred to as *papular urticaria*.

Another major etiologic classification for urticaria is the *physical urticarias*. This group is characterized by urticaria and/or angioedema induced by various physical or environmental stimuli including cold, heat, water, exercise, pressure and vibration, and sun exposure.[13] The physical urticarias are the most common identifiable cause in patients with chronic urticaria. Although usually not a lifelong disorder, these physical urticarias can persist from months to years.

Dermographism, the most common physical urticaria, presents as a wheal and flare response caused by mild trauma to the skin such as stroking or scratching (Fig. 56-89).[14] This phenomenon is seen in about 5% of the population but is common in as many as 15% of patients with chronic urticaria. Some patients have symptomatic itching with the onset of dermographism. Testing for dermographism is easily performed by applying moderate pressure from a tongue depressor over a linear area of about 10 cm on the upper back. A linear wheal of erythema develops in 3 to 5 minutes and usually lasts for 20 to 30 minutes. Occasionally, this response can be delayed for 30 minutes up to several hours (delayed dermographism). *Delayed pressure urticaria* can also result from prolonged stimulation or trauma such as walking a long distance. The most commonly affected sites are the palms and soles, and the lesions are sometimes painful.

Cholinergic urticaria is produced by exercise or heat and often associated with an elevation in body temperature. Severe emotional stress exacerbates the condition and sometimes precipitates it, as does ingestion of spicy foods. It is most common in young adults between 15 and 25. The primary symptom is a warm or hot feeling of the skin followed by the development of pruritic, erythematous plaques and wheals. Common sites of involvement are the upper chest, back, and face. The urticarial lesions are distinctive, being only 1 to 2 cm in size and surrounded by a large red flare. The lesions appear relatively quickly after the triggering event and resolve in 30 to 60 minutes. Urticaria usually develops when patients begin to sweat. A small percentage of patients with cholinergic urticaria develop coexisting angioedema, sometimes associated with hyperactive airway disease.[15] This associated angioedema is frequently localized to the eyelids and perioral areas. Having the patient take a hot shower or bath or exercise until sweating begins usually reproduces the urticarial lesions.

Cold urticaria can be inherited or acquired.[16] Urticaria is produced at sites where the skin has been cooled and then rewarmed. Hands, face, and extremities are the common sites of involvement. As in cholinergic urticaria, most patients are young, usually under 30. Familial cold urticaria is inherited as an autosomal dominant trait and is rare. Patients are more likely to have associated systemic symptoms such as fever, arthralgias, myalgias, swelling of hands and feet, and abdominal pain.[17] Laboratory examination is significant for leukocytosis. This condition usually starts early in childhood with worsening of symptoms between the first and second decade and gradual improvement in the young adult years. Eating cold food or drinks can produce angioedema of the lips or tongue. Acquired (essential) cold urticaria is the more common form. Five to ten minutes of cold exposure trigger the onset of pruritic wheals at the exposed site after it has been rewarmed. This condition is more common in young adults than in children (as opposed to familial cold urticaria). If the cold exposure is prolonged, or if the patient is extremely sensitive to cold, large amounts of histamine can be released and the patient may develop generalized urticaria with associated symptoms of asthma, flushing, syncope, tachycardia, or headache. Patients with cold urticaria must be extremely careful about swimming in cold water because a generalized reaction may cause unconsciousness. It is estimated that as many as 70% of patients with acquired cold urticaria are at risk of drowning if the water temperature is less than 80°F. Secondary acquired cold urticaria can be associated with underlying diseases such as cryoglobulinemia, cryofibringenemia, cold hemolysins, and hematopoietic malignancies.[18]

Rare causes of the physical urticarias include solar and aquagenic urticaria. *Solar urticaria* is caused by sun exposure. Urtication appears in sun-exposed areas after short exposure times.[19] The wheals usually disappear within 60 minutes, but at times can be more persistent. The major differential diagnosis is polymorphic light eruption, a much more common cutaneous reaction to sun exposure. Polymorphic light eruption is usually not urticarial and usually takes hours to days to develop after exposure to ultraviolet light and persists for longer periods of time. *Aquagenic urticaria* is from contact with water regardless of the temperature of the water. Lesions can be elicited by the application of a wet towel placed on the back for approximately 30 minutes.

Many aggravating factors exist in addition to these causes of urticaria. These commonly include emotional stress, dry or irritated skin, alcohol, caffeine, heat, and prolonged pressure. Hormonal changes associated with pregnancy and menopause can trigger episodes of urticaria, as can thyroid function abnormalities.

EMERGENCY EVALUATION (Table 56-19)

In an emergency setting, it is impractical and usually nonproductive to embark on an overzealous workup. The primary task at hand is to establish the diagnosis, determine whether the condition is acute or chronic, rule out the more obvious causes by means of an accurate and thorough history, and ascertain whether there may be any associated systemic symptoms. Follow-up with a dermatologist or allergist is often necessary if it is a chronic condition that will require long-term extensive testing. On the other hand, if urticaria is an early sign of a severe systemic reaction (e.g., anaphylaxis), emergency treatment may be life-saving.

In evaluating patients with urticaria, there is absolutely no substitute for a complete history. Various history and questionnaire forms have been developed as evaluation aids, and sometimes serve as a guide to help uncover any obvious or more subtle causes of urticaria when the patient presents in the emergency department.[10] The historical checklist should include the following:

1. History of the urticaria: is this an acute or chronic episode of urticaria? How frequently does the pa-

---

TABLE 56-19. EVALUATION OF URTICARIA

1. Acute urticaria
   a. Thorough history and physical examination only
2. Chronic urticaria
   a. Hematologic
      —CBC with differential
      —Chemistry profile
      —Sedimentation rate
      —U/A with micro
      —ANA
      —Serum complement
      —Thyroid function profile
      —Hepatitis profile
      —Cryoglobulin and cryofibrinogen
      —EB virus titer
   b. Micro
      —Stool for O & P, Candida
      —Urine for C & S
      —Vaginal smear for Candida
      —Sputum culture
      —KOH of skin (dermatophyte or scabies)
   c. X ray
      —Teeth
      —Sinus
      —Chest
   d. Provocative tests for physical urticaria
3. Urticarial vasculitis
   a. Skin biopsy
4. Angioedema
   a. C1 inhibitor
   b. C4

tient develop urticaria? How long does an individual urticarial lesion last? It is useful at times to draw a circle around several typical urticarial lesions with a marking pen. During the course of an Emergency Department (ED) visit, the lesions may disappear, ruling against a diagnosis of urticarial vasculitis. If the patient requires follow-up by a dermatologist or allergist, these skin markings are a helpful aid. Do urticarial lesions come and go in a continuous fashion or are there periods when the patient is free of lesions? Is there any associated pruritis, pain, burning or stinging? How large are the lesions and how extensive do they become? Is there any swelling of the hands, feet, eyes, mouth, ears or face (angioedema)?

2. Are there any associated systemic symptoms? Does the patient have fever, chills, myalgias, arthralgias, headaches, wheezing, or tachycardia? Is there an atopic history (asthma, hay fever, eczema)? Are there any symptoms suggesting an intercurrent illness and/or infection? Ask specifically about symptoms of vaginitis, sinusitis, dental abscess, acute or chronic upper respiratory infections, cholecystitis, prostatitis, urinary tract infections, diarrhea or rectal itching (parasitic). Is the patient pregnant or menopausal? Could the patient be hyperthyroid?

3. Are there any trigger factors? What makes the urticaria worse? Is it associated with exercise, heat, cold, sweating, swimming, bathing, sun exposure, pressure or rubbing, emotional upset, prolonged trauma, clothing fabrics, tight-fitting clothing, or contact with any specific chemicals or materials? Have there been any recent insect bites (mosquitoes, chigger mites, fleas, spiders, etc.)? Does the ingestion of any substance cause the urticaria? Ask about the common foods that can cause urticaria and ask about ingestants that may contain dyes or preservatives.

4. What have been the environmental exposures, including hobbies, occupations, pets, or recent travel?

5. What medications does the patient take? An accurate medication history, including over-the-counter preparations, is critical. Ask about vitamin supplements, laxatives, pain medications, antibiotics, hormones, insulin, diet pills, sleeping pills, cough syrups, and topical medicaments. Ask about any recent injections of blood products, immunoglobulins, or contrast dyes.

The physical examination is equally important. What do the urticarial lesions look like? Are they small, large or confluent? Are they painful on palpation, or is there purpura or a hemorrhagic component to the lesions to suggest an underlying vasculitis? Where are the lesions located? Are they primarily exposed or nonexposed areas (is the sun a precipitating factor)? Is there associated angioedema or respiratory compromise? Does the physical examination suggest an underlying infection or systemic illness?

Some relatively simple provocative physical tests can be performed, but not all are necessarily practical in an ED setting. Cold urticaria can be induced by the application of an icebag to the skin for 5 minutes and then rewarming the area. Dermographism is produced by stroking the skin on the back with a blunt instrument. Cholinergic urticaria can be precipitated by exercising until sweating is induced. Cholinergic urticaria can also be reproduced by the intradermal injection of methacholine (0.05 mL of a 0.02% solution).[18] A typical wheal rejection occurs in 20 to 30 minutes. Aquagenic urticaria follows the application of a wet towel to the skin.

The extent of laboratory testing should usually be of a limited nature in an ED setting. If the urticaria is acute and without associated angioedema or systemic symptoms, generally no laboratory examinations are indicated. Remember that an acute episode of urticaria is likely to be transient and self-limited and the cause elicited most often by a careful history. If the urticaria is chronic, general laboratory screening is indicated and initially includes a CBC with differential, chemistry profile, urinalysis, antinuclear antibody, and serum complement level. Controversy exists, however, as to the value of laboratory screening.[20] If an underlying occult infection is suspected, a chest x ray, sinus films, dental x ray, stool examination for ova and parasites, or vaginal smear for Trichomonas or Candida may be indicated. If any coexisting cutaneous lesions suggest a dermatophyte or yeast infection (e.g., tinea pedis or tinea corporis) or a scabetic infestation, a KOH scraping is easily performed. If angioedema is present, the condition is considered more serious and levels of C1 inhibitor and complement (especially C4) should be drawn. Complete laboratory testing also includes hepatitis antigen and antibody, Epstein-Barr virus antibody, thyroid function tests, and cryoglobulin levels. Patch testing for suspected contact urticaria and phototesting for solar urticaria should be done, when indicated, on an outpatient basis. If individual urticarial lesions are present for more than 24 hours, a skin biopsy is required to rule out an underlying vasculitis. The patient should understand that it is unusual for these extensive laboratory tests to define the exact cause of the urticaria, and that most of the time with chronic urticaria, the patient is labeled as idiopathic. Although potentially nonproductive and expensive, however, a complete evaluation can reassure patient and physician that no systemic causes are being overlooked.

TREATMENT

The best treatment for chronic urticaria is not necessarily the simplest: to determine the cause and then eliminate it. It is possible to determine the causative agent or stimulus for urticaria in only a minority of patients. Therefore, most patients must be treated empirically and symptomatically. First, it is helpful to avoid aggravating factors such as alcohol, aspirin, coffee, exertion, heat or emotional stress. For the physical urticarias, avoidance of the specific triggering factor is imperative. For example, patients with symptomatic dermographism should try to avoid scratching, rubbing, or wearing tight clothing. In cholinergic urticaria, patients should avoid exercise or heat to the point of sweating. Cold avoidance is common sense for patients with cold urticaria, but this may mean not swimming in colder water for fear of drowning. Patients should avoid any rapid decrease in skin surface temperature or prolonged cold exposure to the arms, legs or face. At times, induction of tolerance to cold can be considered, but this is time-consuming and uncomfortable for the patient.[18] For solar urticaria, episodes can be minimized by the use of sunscreens with a sun protection factor of 15 or greater; blocking both ultraviolet A and ultraviolet B rays is important. When urticaria is severe, a buddy system for exercise (cholinergic) or swimming (cold) should be encouraged and the patient instructed in the proper use of a self-injection epinephrine kit.

When an urticarial reaction to food is suspected, an elimination diet may be helpful. The patient is placed on a strict diet, sometimes initially consisting only of rice and water. If no new urticarial lesions develop, normal foods are gradually reintroduced to detect the possible offending food sources. Food diaries are also helpful to determine patterns of particular food ingestion with the development of new urticarial lesions.

ACUTE URTICARIA

MILD CASES

Most cases of acute urticaria are self-limited and usually persist for only a few days. Any possible offending drug or ingested item should be discontinued. Underlying infections should be treated appropriately. Oral antihistamines are the mainstay of symptomatic treatment. Hydroxyzine hydrochloride (Atarax, Vistaril) and diphenhydramine (Benadryl) are the most popular choices and work equally well in most patients. Diphenhydramine has the advantage of being over-the-counter, but must be taken at an adequate dose (50 mg) to be beneficial. Hydroxyzine comes as 10 mg tablets, but usually a minimum dose of 25 mg. qid is required for symptomatic relief. The side effect profiles are similar and include drowsiness and anticholinergic symptoms. Antipruritic lotions (Sarna, Pramasone) and cool compresses also give symptomatic relief.

SEVERE CASES

For severe forms of acute urticaria (angioedema), subcutaneous injection of epinephrine (0.3 ml of 1:1000

solution) is needed. With angioedema associated with bronchospasm, airway maintenance is imperative. A long-acting epinephrine (Susphrine) may be needed to control rapid recurrence of bronchospasm. Subcutaneous epinephrine is usually successful and can be followed by oral Benadryl or Atarax. Twenty-four-hour observation is recommended. With hereditary angioedema from C1 inhibitor deficiency, anabolic steroids are prescribed (Danazol 200 mg).[21] Analgesics and intravenous fluids are sometimes necessary for angioedema associated with abdominal symptoms. Danazol, 200 mg once a day, can help to prevent recurrent attacks of angioedema. For cold urticaria, cyproheptadine (Periactin) 2 to 4 mg tid is the treatment of choice and highly effective.[22] Patients should be warned that weight gain with cyproheptadine is common.

Patients who present in the ED with *chronic* urticaria and/or angioedema are more challenging. These patients have often been on different antihistamines with variable success. Keep in mind, however, that there are 6 chemical classes of H_1 antihistamines, and different antihistamines from the various classes should be implemented. A 12 week trial of a new antihistamine is usually necessary to determine its efficacy. Newer nonsedating antihistamines have gained in recent popularity.[23] Terfenadine (Seldane) 60 mg bid and astemizole (Hismanal) 10 mg qd are currently approved for use. Astemizole requires 2 days for onset of action and 2 to 3 weeks to reach a steady state and therefore has little use as an acute treatment and is best used prophylactically on a long-term basis. Sometimes combining H_1 antihistamines from different classes is helpful. To avoid a cumulative sedating effect, combining terfenadine or astemizole with an around-the-clock antihistamine such as hydroxyzine is beneficial. Various studies have examined the combination of H_1 and H_2 blockers such as cimetidine and ranitidine, with mixed results to date. It should be considered, however, as a therapeutic option for refractory cases. The tricyclic antidepressant doxepin (Adapin, Sinequan) has been shown to be a potent inhibitor of histamine-induced urticarial reactions and may also exert H_2 antihistamine properties. A dose of 50 to 75 mg at bedtime or 10 to 25 mg tid is recommended.[24] Beta-adrenergic agents have been tried in an attempt to block the release of histamine and related mediators from the mast cell.[25] Terbutaline (Brethine) 2.5 mg has had mixed results in clinical studies. Ephedrine sulfate (25 mg) has also been used. Cardiac disease mitigates against the use of this class of drugs.

Finally, systemic steroids have been used. Because the risks of chronic steroid use outweigh its potential benefits in the treatment of chronic urticaria, one should at all times avoid the use of steroids. All attempts should be made to find a safer management strategy. Unfortunately, many patients with chronic urticaria end up with chronic steroid use primarily because it works so well. At times, a short course (1 to 2 weeks with rapid tapering) of prednisone may be

TABLE 56-20. TREATMENT OF URTICARIA

1. Antihistamines (H₁ Blockers)

	Dose
Sedating	
—Diphenhydramine	25–50 mg qid
—Hydroxyzine	25 mg qid
—Cyproheptadine	2–4 mg tid
Nonsedating	
—Terfenadine	60 mg bid
—Astemizole	10 mg qid

2. Combination of H₁ Blockers
3. Combination of H₁ Blocker + H₂ Blocker
4. Tricyclic Antidepressant

a. Doxepin	50–75 mg qhs or 10–25 mg tid

5. Beta-Adrenergic

a. Terbutaline	2.5 mg tid
b. Ephedrine sulfate	25 mg tid

6. Anabolic steroid (angio-edema)

a. Danazol	200 mg tid

7. Systemic steroids

a. Prednisone	60 mg qd with rapid tapering over 1–2 wks

used to help break a cycle of acute urticaria, but repeated treatments with steroids should be avoided. The only true indication for long-term steroid use is life-threatening refractory angioedema. Table 56-20 outlines treatment approaches.

REFERENCES

1. Jorizzo, J.L.: Classification of urticaria and the reactive inflammatory vascular dermatoses. Dermatol. Clin. 3:3, 1985.
2. Kaplan, A.P.: The pathogenic basis of urticaria and angioedema. Am. J. Med. 70:755, 1981.
3. Keahey, T.M.: The pathogenesis of urticaria. Dermatol. Clin. 3:13, 1985.
4. Champion, R.H., Roberts, S.O.B., Carpenter, R.G., and Roger, J.H.: Urticaria and angioedema: A review of 554 patients. Br. J. Dermatol. 81:588, 1969.
5. Frank, M.M.: Hereditary angioedema: The clinical syndrome and its management. Ann. Intern. Med. 84:580, 1976.
6. Farnam, J., and Grant, A.: Angioedema. Dermatol. Clin. 3:85, 1985.
7. Monroe, E.W.: Urticarial vasculitis: an updated review. J. Am. Acad. Dermatol. 5:88, 1981.
8. Gammon, W.R.: Urticarial vasculitis. Dermatol. Clin. 3:97–105, 1985.
9. Green, G.R., Koelsche, G.L., Kierland, R.R.: Etiology and pathogenesis of chronic urticaria. Ann. Allergy 23:30–36, 1965.
10. Guin, J.: The evaluation of patients with urticaria. Dermatol. Clin. 3:29, 1985.
11. Michaelson, G., and Juhlin, L.: Urticaria induced by preservatives and dye additives in food and drugs. Br. J. Dermatol. 88:525, 1973.
12. Burdick, A.E., and Mathias, C.G.: The contact urticaria syndrome. Dermatol. Clin. 3:71, 1985.
13. Jorizzo, J.L., and Smith, E.B.: The physical urticarias: An update and review. Arch. Dermatol. 18:194, 1982.
14. Wong, A.: Dermographism: A review. J. Amer. Acad. Dermatol., 11:643–652, 1984.
15. Lawrence, C.M., Jorizzo, J.L., and Kobrablack, A.: Cholinergic urticaria with associated angioedema. Br. J. Dermatol. 105:543, 1981.
16. Neittaanmaki, H.: Cold urticaria. J. Amer. Acad. Dermatol. 13:636, 1985.
17. Doeglas, H.M.G., and Bleumink, E.: Familial cold urticaria: Clinical findings. Arch. Dermatol. 110:382, 1974.
18. Sibbald, R.G.: Physical urticaria. Dermatol. Clin. 3:57, 1985.
19. Ramsay, C.A.: Solar urticaria. Int. J. Dermatol. 19:233, 1980.
20. Jacobson, K.W., Branch, L.B., and Nelson, H.S.: Laboratory tests in chronic urticaria. JAMA 243:1644, 1980.
21. Gelfard, J.A., Sherins, R.J., Alling, D.W., and Frank, M.M.: Treatment of hereditary angioedema with danazol: Reversal of clinical and biochemical abnormalities. N. Engl. J. Med. 295:1444, 1976.
22. Wanderer, A.A., and Ellis, E.F.: Treatment of cold urticaria with cyroheptadine. J. Allergy Clin. Immunol. 48:366, 1971.
23. Monroe, E.W.: Chronic urticaria: Review of nonsedating H₁ antihistamines in treatment. 19:842, 1988.
24. Green, S.L., Reed, C.E., and Schroeter, A.L.: Double-blind crossover study comparing doxepin with diphenhydramine for treatment of chronic urticaria. J. Amer. Acad. Dermatol. 12:669, 1985.
25. Kennes, B., DeMaubeuge, J., and Delespesse, S.: Treatment of chronic urticaria with beta-adrenergic stimulant. Clin. Allergy 7:35, 1977.

SKIN INFECTIONS

Howard M. Simons

CAPSULE

Considering the large area of the skin surface, it is surprising that cutaneous life-threatening emergencies are relatively infrequent. Even in urticaria and erythema multiforme, both of which occur fairly often, only a small percentage of cases require emergency treatment.

Although each emergency dermatologic condition is uncommon in its full-blown form, less severe variants occur often enough. More important, perhaps, only through a working knowledge of these entities can one prevent misdiagnoses, thus avoiding unnecessary laboratory studies and undue alarm to the patient and his or her family.

This section reviews the presentation, identification, and treatment of skin infections.

Aside from cultures and microscopic examination for organisms, specific laboratory tests are rarely available, and clinical impression remains the basis of diagnosis. A careful history and precise description of the skin lesion therefore assume the greatest importance.

Although few dermatologic conditions are life-threatening, patients with acute skin conditions frequently present at Emergency Departments (EDs). This probably reflects the suddenness of onset, the high visibility of the lesions, and the frequent severe pruritis. Reassurance of the patient and family are an important component of treatment.

INFECTIONS

BACTERIAL INFECTIONS

IMPETIGO CONTAGIOSA

This common superficial pyoderma is caused by either group A streptococci or Staphylococcus aureus, and frequently both bacteria are found together in skin lesions. Although investigators continue the debate over which organism causes the primary lesion and which is the secondary invader, there is little doubt that at least two clinical forms exist. Impetigo is much more common in children, but may occur in any age group.

Recognition. The characteristic lesion in the streptococcal form is an irregularly rounded cluster of tiny vesiculopustules that quickly rupture and become covered by heavy yellowish crusts. As these crusts enlarge on addition of new layers of dried seropurulent discharge, the underlying erythema is often obscured. Smaller lesions in an earlier phase of development may be found in adjacent skin areas. The face, hands, and arms are most commonly involved.

Although rheumatic fever does not follow group A streptococcal infection of the skin, many cases of acute glomerulonephritis have been preceded by streptococcal pyodermas. Lymphadenopathy may occur.

The staphylococcal form of impetigo typically shows flaccid bullous lesions, thin scalelike crusts, and circinate lesions with central healing. The lesions spread to other parts of the body, apparently by autoinoculation. Although these lesions bear a superficial resemblance to fungal infection, the latter is much more delicate and never so exudative. Satellite lesions are frequently present in staphylococcal impetigo.

Leukocytosis is present occasionally in streptococcal impetigo but rarely in the staphylococcal form. Smear from moist lesions shows characteristic gram-positive cocci. Although cultures demonstrate the presence of one or both causative organisms, such procedures are economically impractical and rarely necessary. Nephritic changes seldom occur earlier than at least 1 week after streptococcal impetigo, but a baseline urinalysis is helpful.

Usually, the two forms of impetigo are distinct enough clinically to permit differentiation, but milder forms may cause confusion. Because treatment is similar in both, however, culturing and other efforts to tell them apart are not indicated.

Management. Although topical measures alone are adequate in early uncomplicated cases, there is an increasing tendency to use systemic antibiotics in all cases of impetigo. Perhaps systemic antibiotics are most valuable when the patient is unreliable in carrying out local care. Oral penicillin is effective in all streptococcal and most staphylococcal cases, but dicloxacillin should be used when the presence of penicillinase-producing staphylococci is suspected. Dosage is 250 mg of either medication taken four times daily. More severe cases need parenteral methicillin.

Topical measures should include warm water compresses or soaks two or three times daily to remove crusts, followed by application of gentamicin or another antibiotic ointment.

Although suppurative complications are rare in healthy patients with impetigo, persons with atopic dermatitis, diabetes, or other debilitating conditions are at greater risk. All patients should be evaluated at least superficially for upper respiratory infections, lymphangitis, and bacteremia and re-evaluated in 3 to 5 days so that the physician can ascertain that the pyoderma has responded to therapy. Because treatment with penicillin *does not* always prevent nephritis, urinalysis 4 weeks after skin infection is indicated.

ECTHYMA AND ERYSIPELAS

These two skin infections are discussed together because both are caused by group A streptococci. Ecthyma can be considered a deeper form of impetigo, whereas erysipelas is a superficial cellulitis characteristically seen on the face, scalp, or lower legs.

Recognition. Ecthyma appears as superficial rounded erosions, often a centimeter or more in diameter, surrounded by indurated erythema. Multiple lesions are often present on the involved area, which is usually on the lower legs. Children are commonly affected, and trauma appears to precede the infection.

In erysipelas, group A streptococci (and group G rarely) enter through a break in the skin and produce a not uncommon superficial cellulitis that is always hot, erythematous, and sharply demarcated from normal skin. Patients are usually febrile and at least mildly toxic. The fiery red lesion typically spreads peripherally but shows no central clearing. Erysipelas involves the lower legs in debilitated patients, apparently secondary to stasis dermatitis, chronic tinea pedis, or excoriations. In these patients, repeated episodes may occur, resulting in chronic edema as lymph channels and nodes are replaced by fibrotic scar.

A moderate leukocytosis should be expected, and antistreptolysin O titer eventually rises. Like most streptococcal diseases elsewhere in the body, the lesion is nonexudative, making culture or smear of the organism difficult.

Erysipelas could be confused clinically with angioedema or acute contact dermatitis, and unilateral facial involvement might mimic herpes zoster. Angioedema does not show the deep erythema or heat of erysipelas, and contact dermatitis usually has more eczematous changes. The fever and leukocytosis of erysipelas are further differentiating features.

Streptococcal cellulitis may occur as a complication of erysipelas, or more commonly, as a rapidly spreading erythema around a wound or other injury to the skin. Because subcutaneous tissues as well as skin may be involved, lymphangitis and septicemia are more likely complications. The process is tender, hot, and edematous, and is associated with fever and systemic symptoms, as may occur in erysipelas. Many cases *cannot* be distinguished from the latter, although the advancing border of cellulitis is usually less distinct than the more superficial and less serious erysipelas. In cases that are clinically confusing, it seems prudent to diagnose and treat the more dangerous condition.

Management. The usual treatment for ecthyma and erysipelas is oral penicillin, although erythromycin is substituted if there is history of penicillin allergy. Antibiotic therapy should begin at once. Although ecthyma is treated on an outpatient basis, hospitalization for erysipelas may be indicated by the severity of the process, possibility of associated cellulitis, or presence in the patient of other conditions that reduce defenses against infection. Parenteral medication may be needed in severe cases with lymphatic spread.

Ecthyma usually benefits from application of warm water compresses two or three times daily to remove crusts, followed by topical gentamicin. The localizing effect of heat on infection, however, is of little value in erysipelas and cellulitis when compared with the marked symptomatic relief afforded by cool compresses. Here, bed rest, elevation of the infected area, and protection of the lesion from trauma are helpful. Because of their tendency to retain heat, ointments should be avoided; hydrating creams are beneficial in the scaly healing stages.

Systemic signs and symptoms usually improve within 48 hours of penicillin treatment, but the inflammatory changes of the skin resolve rather slowly. Both erysipelas and cellulitis recur frequently in patients with chronic lymphedema of the lower legs. In such cases, prophylactic penicillin therapy over long periods may be indicated.

FOLLICULAR INFECTIONS

Coagulase-positive staphylococci are the most common cause of infections that begin in the hair follicle. Young, active adults are involved typically. Irritation or inflammation of the skin may underlie folliculitis, as in dry skin, chemical exposures, scabies, or atopic dermatitis. Friction and maceration account for this condition after close shaving and in wrestlers or other athletes. A rather mysterious recurrent folliculitis occurs in children on the buttocks and thighs in the absence of predisposing causes such as malnutrition or hematologic disease.

Recognition. *Folliculitis* is the term applied to a mild form of follicular infection that appears as erythema, slight tenderness and swelling, and perhaps pus formation at the follicular opening. Folliculitis is common but usually trivial when only one or several lesions occur, and it is frequently left untreated.

A recurrent variant called *sycosis barbae* occurs in males in the beard area as perifollicular papules and pustules in association with scaling and erythema. This process slowly spreads to involve larger areas of skin and may affect the eyebrows and eyelashes, even producing blepharoconjunctivitis. *Tinea barbae,* fungal infection in the same general area, may be difficult to distinguish clinically from sycosis barbae, although scrapings from tinea barbae usually show fungal hyphae on potassium hydroxide examination.

Furuncles and *carbuncles* are deeper, more severe forms of follicular infection. The former is essentially a boil, a deep-seated perifollicular inflammation that usually follows folliculitis. It is indurated, always tender, and usually uncomfortable or frankly painful, especially when on the nose and ears, where it is bound down against cartilage by overlying skin. The favored sites are hairy areas exposed to friction such as the neck, face, buttocks, and waistline.

Furuncles look like acne, but the latter appears in limited distribution and is usually accompanied by comedones and a variety of inflammatory lesions. In hidradenitis suppurativa, painful nodular lesions are sharply localized to the inguinal and axillary areas.

A carbuncle, infection of numerous contiguous hair follicles, begins as a painful, firm, erythematous lump. As suppuration occurs within it, pus appears from the numerous follicular orifices. The nape is the most common site. The patient is often febrile and appears ill. Although carbuncles are usually solitary, furuncles and folliculitis may be present in adjacent skin.

Management. The purpose of therapy in most follicular infections is to promote drainage of pus and necrotic material through the follicle itself. *Early lesions* must *never* be opened, picked, incised, or otherwise traumatized, as such procedures increase local inflammation and may lead to cellulitis or bacteremia. Therapy centers around warm (or hot) water compresses for 30 minutes three or four times daily to encourage "pointing" and subsequent drainage through follicular orifices. Thin applications of gentamicin ointment prolong effectiveness of the heat and may also reduce bacteria in adjacent skin areas. As pointing occurs, a gentle incision through the follicular orifice with a No. 11 blade guarantees continuation of drainage.

Systemic antibiotics are used for deeper furuncles, carbuncles, and milder follicular infections in patients with diabetes, immunoglobulin deficiency states, and malnutrition. Although penicillin is surprisingly effective, in view of the large number of coagulase-positive staphylococci resistant to this medication it seems more prudent to use erythromycin or one of the synthetic penicillins effective against penicillinase-producing bacteria. Furuncles around the nares and upper lip carry the additional risk of cavernous sinus thrombosis and meningitis and should be treated with maximum antibiotic doses. Bed rest is helpful in severe cases.

Painful carbuncles of the nape are less responsive to therapy. The physician is best advised to avoid immediate incision, however, preferably relying upon local applications of heat, analgesics, and high doses of systemic antibiotics.

In recurrent furunculosis, occasionally a most baffling problem, local treatment must be thorough and persistent. Gentamicin ointment should be applied to the nares, fingernails, and perineum as well as to the sites of infection. Frequent use of antibacterial soaps is indicated, even at the risk of overdrying the skin, and dressings should be avoided except on actively discharging lesions. Because furuncles recur after cessation of systemic antibiotics, the latter are best avoided unless their prolonged use is acceptable.

VIRAL INFECTIONS

HERPES SIMPLEX

This worldwide viral infection, one of the most common infections of humans, has various primary and secondary (or recurrent) forms. Although almost the entire population is infected with the virus, more than 98% of all primary infections are either subclinical or so mild as to be unrecognized. Symptomatic primary infections are characterized by mild to moderate systemic reactions and localized lesions at the portal of entry of the virus.

Recognition. The most common form of primary herpes simplex infection is *gingivostomatitis,* usually occurring in young children as painful widespread oral vesicles in association with fever and malaise. The gums are characteristically swollen, bloody, and erythematous, and eating and drinking produce severe discomfort. Tender submandibular lymphadenopathy commonly occurs. Other viral and bacterial infections usually involve only the posterior pharynx, and erythema multiforme is much more exudative. The triad of fetid breath, severe gingivitis, and anterior buccal involvement suggests the diagnosis of herpetic gingivostomatitis.

Herpetic *vulvovaginitis* produces similar constitutional symptoms, rapidly eroding vesicles on the vaginal mucosa and adjacent skin areas, pain, and inguinal lymphadenopathy. Dysuria and dyspareunia usually are present, and pruritus is a common complaint. In men, multiple vesicles often center around the urethral meatus and, in the absence of fever, are difficult to differentiate from recurrent herpes simplex.

Herpetic *keratoconjunctivitis* is usually unilateral, may appear alarmingly severe and destructive, and occasionally displays swelling, exudation, and superficial ulceration of the cornea. *Kaposi's varicelliform eruption* may be either a primary or recurrent infection in a person with an underlying dermatitis.

Inoculation herpes simplex is a primary infection that

occurs in abraded or injured skin and is an occupational hazard of physicians and nurses. It occurs most commonly on fingertips as clusters of tense papulovesicles that are usually painful. The patient is often febrile and more or less ill and has regional lymphadenopathy. Careful clinical evaluation is required to differentiate this condition from bacterial infections, monilial paronychia, and recurrent herpes simplex infections.

Recurrent herpes simplex infections are many times more common than all of the primary forms taken together. They differ strikingly from the latter by their localized distribution and absence of fever and systemic symptoms. Recurrent infections frequently recur in the same general areas but usually not at the exact sites. The most commonly involved areas are the lips and around the mouth, the face generally, and the genitalia, although the palms and buttocks are not uncommon sites.

Following a brief prodrome of burning or itching discomfort, one or several rounded clusters of tiny discrete vesicles appear on an erythematous base. The lesions become crusted in a day or two, almost always in the absence of a preceding oozing phase. With the one exception of palmar involvement, recurrent herpes infections are rarely complicated by secondary pyoderma or lymphangitis.

Whereas recurrent infections are usually recognized easily by their typical appearance and history, primary infections show less consistent changes and, being less common, are often misdiagnosed. The absence of a history of prior herpes lesions, however, supports the diagnosis of primary infection, especially in older children and adults. Of the four clinical features of primary herpes infections (fever, lymphadenopathy, constitutional symptoms, and vesicular lesions), it is the cutaneous changes that most aid recognition. Oral and vulvar vesicles often slough rapidly, producing whitish plaques or superficial erosions that are easily seen against the edematous and erythematous background mucosal surfaces. The fever of primary infections is almost always low-grade and often precedes by several days the onset of mucosal or cutaneous lesions.

The most helpful laboratory aid in the recognition of herpes infections is the Tzanck smear, in which contents from an intact vesicle are examined microscopically. After removal of the roof of the vesicle with a fine iris scissors, the fluid is blotted with gauze carefully so as not to disturb the cells below. Cloudy material from the floor of the lesion is then gently scraped with a dull No. 15 scalpel onto a glass slide as thinly as possible. After fixation in methyl alcohol, the slide is treated with Giemsa stain according to the technique used for blood smears and then examined under the microscope. Finding multinucleate giant epithelial cells confirms the diagnosis of herpes simplex, although similar bizarre viral cells also are characteristic of herpes zoster and varicella. In most primary herpes infections, the patient's hemogram shows a low normal or decreased number of white blood cells and an increase in lymphocytes or monocytes.

Management. The antiviral agent acyclovir has been approved for primary herpes infections and recurrent infections in immunosuppressed patients. Its cost is also a limiting factor and will probably restrict its use to more severe infections and to patients at risk. It is hoped that related compounds that are both more effective and less expensive will be developed for topical use. Acyclovir (Zovirax) capsules are now available (200 mg capsules for oral use) to reduce the duration of acute infection and speed lesion healing in some cases. Acyclovir capsules reduce frequency and/or severity of recurrence in more than 90% of cases. Recommended dose is 400 to 800 mg q.i.d.

Few cases of primary herpes simplex infection produce enough discomfort and functional impairment to require hospitalization. Patients with severe gingivostomatitis, almost always infants or young children, may require parenteral alimentation or fluid balance that should be initiated in the ED.

Although vidarabine has proved valuable in the management of herpes simplex keratitis, it has been much less effective on skin lesions. Assuming that this chemical is absorbed more readily on mucous membranes, the physician should prescribe this agent for the buccal and vaginal mucosae, with directions to apply it hourly during the waking hours and every 3 hours during the night. Keratoconjunctivitis should be managed by an ophthalmologic consultant.

Nonspecific symptomatic measures for primary infections include analgesics, which must often be administered parenterally, and intraoral lidocaine for patients old enough to hold this anesthetic in their mouths for several minutes before swallowing it. Use of lidocaine before meals may allow oral intake of food and liquid that would be otherwise intolerable. Cool or cold water compresses to the vulvar region are comforting, but, to avoid maceration, applications should not exceed 15 minutes four times daily. Spread-eagle positioning of the legs is also helpful.

The patient or family or both should be reassured that the pain and discomfort of primary infections subside in 5 to 8 days, although complete healing may require several weeks. They must also be warned, however, that herpes simplex lesions contain millions of viral particles that may infect susceptible persons, especially infants and children without prior exposure. Family members with eczematized or injured skin are especially at risk.

The physician facilitates management of *recurrent* herpetic infections by dividing the course of infection into two phases: an early phase, the first 36 to 48 hours, in which the viruses are replicating and spreading; and a second phase, in which viral activity is dormant and injured tissues are healing. Treatment during the early phase can markedly shorten the course of the recurrent infection, whereas second-phase therapy is much less spectacular, consisting of symptomatic measures. The emergency physician appears to have the unique opportunity to initiate early-phase treatment in many cases.

Early-phase treatment with frequent applications of vidarabine or acyclovir and orally administered acyclovir (800 mg q.i.d.) reduces the lesions and shortens the clinical course.

HERPES ZOSTER

Both varicella and zoster are caused by the same virus, *Herpesvirus varicellae.* Whereas varicella occurs as a primary infection in patients without immunity to the virus, zoster represents activation of the virus in a person with partial immunity. Varicella-zoster infection may be compared superficially with herpes simplex infection in which distinctive primary infections may be followed by activation of the virus to produce localized herpes simplex lesions. Unlike herpes simplex, however, zoster almost never recurs.

The factors that cause activation of the varicella-zoster virus are basically unknown, although greater frequency of zoster in patients with Hodgkin's disease, lymphomas, leukemias, and other cancers is well established. In patients who have received antimetabolites or radiation therapy, it is difficult to know whether subsequent zoster is the result of therapy or of the disease under treatment.

Recognition. The typical clusters of papulovesicles occurring in the skin of one or two contiguous dermatomes produce one of the most characteristic clinical pictures seen in dermatology. New lesions may appear over a period of several days' duration in a centripetal fashion such that the first cluster of lesions is often on the back, somewhat lateral to the midline. The clusters are initially discrete and separated by normal skin, but may become confluent in severe cases. Unilateral involvement with sharp cut-off at the midline is occasionally helpful in ruling out an acute eczematous dermatitis (like contact dermatitis) when the dermatomal distribution is not apparent.

When the ophthalmic branch of the trigeminal nerve is involved, ocular changes are likely. These may vary from a mild keratoconjunctivitis to a deeper keratitis with ulceration or scarring. Because ocular changes may lag behind the skin lesions by several days, it is prudent to obtain early ophthalmologic consultation. Ocular involvement is supposedly more likely when the side of the nose shows vesicular lesions, indicating involvement of the nasociliary nerve. Involvement of the maxillary or mandibular divisions of the trigeminal nerve, although much less common, produces unilateral vesicles in the mouth.

Although motor system involvement in zoster is not common, partial paresis of an extremity is occasionally

noted. Even though motor function returns, early recognition of the paralysis is crucial so that prompt physiotherapy can be used to prevent disuse atrophy of large muscle masses. A more characteristic example of motor involvement is the Ramsay-Hunt syndrome, in which the geniculate ganglion is affected. This produces vesicles of the external auditory canal and ear lobe along with persistent earache and facial nerve paralysis that is occasionally permanent. Zoster in the sacral dermatomes (S2 to S4) may be accompanied by bladder dysfunction, manifested by either acute urinary retention or urinary frequency.

Pain is a prominent symptom in most older patients with zoster and may be a diagnostic challenge when it precedes the skin lesions. Involvement of thoracic or lumbar dorsal roots may mimic myocardial infarction, peritonitis, or other painful syndromes, although careful clinical evaluation usually reveal the pain's superficial location. The finding of itching, paresthesias, hypesthesia, or hyperesthesia in a dermatomal distribution is suggestive of zoster. Pain is almost always minimal or absent in young adults.

Zoster is frequently accompanied by regional lymphadenopathy and occasionally by mild constitutional symptoms. Although milder cases may heal uneventfully in 2 to 4 weeks, severe reactions with necrosis or hemorrhage may require several months to heal with scar formation. Elderly patients and those with reticuloendothelial diseases usually show more devastating skin changes, and the latter also may show disseminated or bilateral lesions.

Recognition of zoster rests almost totally on clinical findings, and rarely is recourse to laboratory aids indicated or helpful. The hemogram and sedimentation are normal unless secondary bacterial infection has occurred. The Tzanck smear distinguishes zoster from erythema multiforme and dermatitis herpetiformis but not from herpes simplex occurring in a zosteriform distribution. The latter's history of recurrence, however, rules out zoster.

Management. Milder cases are managed by supportive outpatient treatment that centers around reassurance about anticipated duration and course of the viral illness and symptomatic measures. Aspirin or propoxyphene hydrochloride should be tried first, although codeine compounds or stronger narcotics may be needed. Pruritus can be reduced by cool water compresses and oral antihistamines, along with calamine lotion, which can be applied as often as needed to relieve itching. Topical steroids are of little value in either reducing pruritus or accelerating resolution of skin lesions. If compresses are prescribed, maceration is reduced by use of compresses for no longer than 15 minutes four times daily. Similarly, immersion of affected skin in bath water must be avoided in favor of short, coolish showers. It is doubtful that bed rest or other restrictions are necessary in these milder cases, although the patient should be warned of his contagion for children who have not had varicella.

Pain by itself is not necessarily an indication for hospitalization, although for a patient with other illnesses or debilitation, management may be aided by the hospital setting. Severe, hemorrhagic, or gangrenous skin changes require inpatient treatment and dermatologic consultation.

Acyclovir (800 mg q.i.d.) reduces the duration of the clinical course and improves symptoms. The incidence of postherpetic neuralgia may be reduced. Systemic corticosteroids may also reduce postherpetic neuralgia, but must be used with care. It is best for the emergency physician to begin the antiviral (acyclovir) treatment and refer the patient to a dermatologist for long-term treatment. Be aware of the possibility of AIDS in this patient group.

FUNGAL INFECTIONS

Tinea, dermatophytosis, and "ringworm" refer to fungal infections caused by a related group of fungi that includes the three genera *Microsporum, Trichophyton,* and *Epidermophyton.* The term "ringworm," despite the clinical picture it evokes, has been a source of confusion for the nondermatologist, and preference should be given to the other two terms. By stressing the ringed morphology, this term has been misapplied all too often to erythema annulare, various eczematous lesions, and the herald patch of pityriasis rosea, and it has slowed appreciation of the nonringed appearance of dermatophytosis of the hands, feet, and beard areas.

Dermatophytes, like bacteria, exist only as saprophytes or parasites and, being essentially necrophilic, are found only in such dead tissue as hair, nails, and the stratum corneum. Although all dermatophytes invade the skin, some species appear to be excluded from hair and nails. Anthropophilic species of dermatophytes tend to produce milder and more chronic cutaneous lesions, whereas zoophilic fungi, which usually infect people from an animal source, evoke a more inflammatory skin lesion.

Enumeration of species and the clinical conditions they produce would be lengthy and inconsistent with the aims of this chapter. The following discussion by regions of the body should facilitate recognition of common dermatophyte infections while avoiding details and terms more valuable to mycologists or dermatologists. Additional information is available in mycology textbooks.

Recognition of fungal infections is aided immensely by *direct microscopic examination* of material from suspected lesions. The scales, nail scrapings, or hairs are placed on a glass slide. Add one or two drops of 15% potassium hydroxide and a coverslip, and heat the preparation gently for several seconds with a Bunsen burner. Although boiling should be avoided, any bubbles that appear can be removed by tapping the coverslip. Let the preparation stand, preferably on the microscope light, for 20 minutes to enhance clearing. Using reduced light, examine the slide under low power initially; switch to high power for details. The microscopic elements to look for are discussed below.

TINEA INFECTIONS: TINEA UNGUIUM

More common on the toenails than the fingernails, this infection typically begins at the distal edge of the nail as a whitish or yellow patch that slowly spreads proximally in irregular fashion. The nail plate thickens, becomes deformed, and is eventually lifted off the nail bed by the accumulation of subungual material, although many variations of the above changes are seen. The process is almost always asymptomatic.

Psoriasis is easily confused with tinea unguium, and it is usually necessary to examine all areas of skin in search of other lesions of psoriasis. The characteristic superficial pits of the nail plate in psoriasis are not found in fungal infection. Psoriasis is more symmetric, whereas tinea unguium frequently involves only one hand.

To identify fungal elements on direct microscopy (see above), use a sterile scalpel blade to obtain scrapings from the whitish areas on the surfaces of the diseased nails. A caveat here is to avoid the temptation to collect the luxurious subungual dermis of these dystrophic nails; fungal elements are notably absent in such scrapings. The finding of translucent, branching linear filaments (hyphae), often segmented into arthrospores, confirms the diagnosis of dermatophyte infection. Hyphae must be carefully differentiated from the so-called "mosaic artifact," which is less translucent and follows the outlines of the keratinized cells.

TINEA CAPITIS

The most common form of dermatophytosis of the scalp is caused by *Microsorum audouini* and typically occurs as epidemics in prepubertal school children. These noninflammatory lesions are oval to round, are covered by a grayish scale, and contain hair that is uniformly broken off about 2 mm from the scalp surface. The more inflammatory form of tinea capitis is contracted from young pets, is usually caused by *Microsporum canis,* and often shows slight edema, vesiculation, and peripheral spread. In both forms, the lesions are asymmetric and variable in size. Kerion is an even more inflammatory reaction in the scalp that begins with follicular pustules that coalesce to produce a solitary boggy swelling resembling an abscess.

The finding of several irregularly rounded areas of partial alopecia with broken-off hairs (with or without scaling) suggests tinea capitis. History of similar changes in siblings or schoolmates all but confirms the diagnosis. Sporadic cases and infections in adults are more easily mistaken for alopecia areata, although the latter is never scaly.

Examination of scalp lesions with Wood's light* reveals bright green or yellowish-green fluorescence of hairs in *Microsporum* infections but not in the much less common *Trichophyton* infections. In early infections in which hyphae are still below the skin surface, no fluorescence is seen. In such cases, the physician should epilate several hairs with a forceps and examine their roots under Wood's light. If this examination is still negative or equivocal, a potassium hydroxide mount should be prepared for microscopic examination. Broken or lusterless hairs or hairs from the edges of suspected lesions should be selected. In *Microsporum* infections, small arthrospores form sheaths around hairs, and under low power these hairs appear to have a granular coating. With higher magnification, individual spores can be identified along the outside of the hairs in a so-called "mosaic pattern." In *Trichophyton* infections, the arthrospores are larger and appear in parallel chains, either outside the hair shafts or within the hairs.

TINEA CORPORIS

Dermatophytosis of the glabrous skin is more common in tropical areas and is a summertime disease in temperate climates. Its more common occurrence on exposed parts such as the face, hands, and arms supports the thesis that the disease is usually contracted from an animal or another human, even though some lesions appear to result from self-inoculation. All known dermatophytes can produce tinea corporis, and the causative organisms appear to reflect prevailing fungi of the particular area.

The most common form begins as a mildly pruritic inflammatory papule that enlarges peripherally to produce a papulosquamous lesion with an elevated, vesicular, scaling border. With central clearing, an annular lesion is seen, although occasionally secondary areas of activity appear within the circle. Other lesions show a variable morphology, ranging from severely scaling eczematous patches to granulomatous nodules.

Most lesions of tinea corporis are solitary or few in number, totally asymmetric, round or oval, and discrete. These features aid differentiation from the other

papulosquamous eruptions that usually are more widespread in their distribution. Tinea corporis, however, can be confused with the "herald patch" of pityriasis rosea, impetigo, contact dermatitis, and even psoriasis on occasion. With few exceptions, all solitary papulosquamous lesions should be examined for presence or absence of fungal elements.

TINEA CRURIS

Dermatophytosis of the crural or perineal folds is relatively common in men but rare in women. It displays the same peripheral spread as tinea corporis but has a more irregular, often scalloped border and variable central clearing. Extension to the perianal skin or down the medial thighs occurs commonly. The process is usually bilateral.

Examination of scales treated with potassium hydroxide verifies the diagnosis. Erythrasma produces a brownish-pink discoloration of intertriginous skin that fluoresces coral red with Wood's light. It never shows an active border or significant inflammation. In contrast to tinea cruris, candidiasis involves the vulvar and scrotal skin. It is fairly common in females. Intertrigo of the crural folds often shows striking similarities to tinea cruris, and the potassium hydroxide scraping may be the only way to make the correct diagnosis in such cases.

TINEA PEDIS

Only the acute form, consisting of vesiculation between the toes or on the plantar surfaces or both is likely to challenge the emergency physician. It usually is caused by *Trichophyton mentagrophytes*. The process begins between or under the toes as a slight maceration and scaling that is invariably pruritic and is usually followed by fissuring and accumulation of hyperkeratotic debris. Acute episodes are marked by increased erythema, vesiculation, and extension of the vesiculobullous lesions to the plantar surfaces. Secondary bacterial infection may occur in the fissures or deepseated button-like vesicles. If the patient tries to treat himself, the infected acute tinea pedis is likely to be further irritated by various antifungal medications (which are more or less irritating to start with). The clinical picture of tinea pedis thus varies from slight scaling of the fourth interspace (the most common site of initial involvement) to a crusted, oozing, edematous mess.

This acute process and its complications are more common in men and in persons who wear occlusive footwear and work on their feet. Plantar hyperhidrosis, warm weather, and poor bathing habits are contributing factors. Tinea pedis is exceedingly rare in prepubertal children.

---

*Wood's light is an ultraviolet light fitted with a nickel oxide filter. It emits maximum radiation with wavelengths of about 3650 angstrom units and is useful in the diagnosis of erythrasma and tinea versicolor as well as tinea capitis. Always use Wood's light in a darkened room.

Recognition of tinea pedis is aided by a history of recurrence in warm weather and improvement with antifungal preparations. The scaling hyperkeratotic and fissured phase displays a characteristic clinical picture, and its interdigital location is somewhat unique. In the vesiculobullous phase, microscopic examination of keratinous material is essential to recognition, and vesicle roofs are the best source of fungal elements. The roof should be removed with a fine scissors, thinned extensively before and after heating, and placed on the microscope light for 20 minutes for additional clearing.

Shoe contact dermatitis and dyshidrotic eczema rarely involve the intertoe spaces, typically involve the dorsal surfaces of the toes and feet, and usually produce more eczematous changes rather than discrete vesiculobullous lesions. Because pustular psoriasis is extremely difficult to differentiate from some cases of tinea pedis, the emergency physician should examine for the nail changes of psoriasis and psoriatic lesions elsewhere on the patient's body. Wood's light should be used to detect the coral red fluorescence of erythrasma, a superficial bacterial infection found commonly in interdigital or other intertriginous areas.

In the acute form of tinea pedis with superimposed pyoderma or contact dermatitis, it is more essential to recognize and treat these complications than the underlying, often unrecognizable, fungus infection.

In marked contrast to this acute form is the chronic variety of tinea pedis most frequently caused by *Trichophyton rubrum*. This condition is recognized by its extreme chronicity, faint or absent erythema, and diffuse fine scaling that often involves the entire plantar surface and extends around the sides of the foot in the so-called "moccasin distribution." It is usually bilateral and, unlike its acute counterpart, occasionally produces a unilateral tinea manuum of similar appearance. Its increased incidence in patients with Cushing's disease or lymphomas suggests that reduced cell-mediated immunity may be an important underlying factor. Although patients rarely request therapy for it, *T. rubrum* infection is extremely common in men, should not go unrecognized, and at least provides the emergency physician with an opportunity to practice and perfect his potassium hydroxide scraping technique.

Management of Tinea Infections. Orally administered griseofulvin is effective in the treatment of dermatophytosis, although its value in the treatment of the different tineas is variable. It is most valuable in the treatment of *Tinea capitis,* for which the curative dose in children is 1 g four times daily for a total dose of 4 g. Higher blood levels are obtained if griseofulvin is taken with a fatty meal. The young patient and his parents should be warned of the contagiousness of this condition, and the patient should be advised not to share his hat, comb, brush, and towel with others.

Mild shampooing two or three times weekly may help eliminate infectious scales and hairs. Siblings and other household children should be examined with Wood's light and re-examined along with the patient 3 weeks after treatment.

Griseofulvin is not without side effects, but appears to be especially well tolerated by children. Headache, gastrointestinal distress, and diarrhea are the most common complaints, but the physician can eliminate these problems by lowering the dosage or stopping and then starting the medication again. Although preliminary toxicologic studies had indicated that griseofulvin produced serious adverse hepatic and bone marrow reactions, no such side effects have been experienced during almost 15 years of clinical use. Occasionally, there is a reduction in leukocyte counts, and even though this is transient and reversible, some caution is warranted in patients already receiving other bone marrow–depressing drugs. Because of its action on the liver enzyme system, griseofulvin reduces the effectiveness of coumarin anticoagulants; for the same reason, barbiturates reduce the antifungal activity of griseofulvin.

It the emergency physician feels inexperienced in the use of griseofulvin, a prudent alternative is referral of the patient to a dermatologist for initiation of this therapy, especially because some follow-up evaluation of the patient and his family is usually necessary. Ketoconazole, a newer and more potent oral antifungal agent, has hepatotoxicity and should not be prescribed in the ED for dermatophyte infections.

In tinea corporis and tinea cruris, topical antifungal therapy is effective, usually making griseofulvin unnecessary. Tolnaftate, haloprogin, and miconazole nitrate are valuable in these conditions, and the latter two agents appear to be effective in candidiasis as well. The cream form should be applied three times daily to lesions of the glabrous skin, whereas lotion is preferable in intertriginous infections in order to reduce maceration. Crural lesions are additionally benefited by cool water compresses to remove sweat and debris and by avoidance of tight-fitting or occlusive underclothing. The patient should be seen for follow-up 2 weeks after treatment is begun.

In the vesicular type of tinea pedis, emergency treatment centers around warm water soaks three times daily to soften the skin and remove debris, followed by applications of either tolnaftate, haloprogin, or miconazole nitrate cream. The cream should be spread thinly over the entire plantar surface and usually between and under the toes as well. If excessive hyperkeratosis or deep-seated vesiculobullae are present, a thin layer of Whitfield's ointment should be applied over the antifungal cream. Whitfield's ointment, a keratolytic containing 3% salicylic acid and 6% benzoic acid, should not be used in ambulatory patients because it may increase maceration. It should also be avoided if secondary contact dermatitis or bacterial infection is present.

CANDIDIASIS

This fungal infection principally involves skin and mucous membranes and only rarely produces systemic disease. The causative organism is almost always Candida albicans, although other Candida species are implicated occasionally. Because C. albicans (as well as other Candida species) is a harmless resident of normal skin, mucous membranes, and the gastrointestinal tract, its isolation from pathologic conditions in these areas is difficult to evalute.

The virulence of all Candida species seems low, and it is generally assumed that in all cases of candidiasis local or systemic factors predispose the patient to this fungal disease. Diabetes mellitus, antibiotic or corticosteroid therapy, use of oral contraceptives, obesity, and lymphoreticular disease are some of the better known processes associated with candidal infection. Infancy, pregnancy, and old age produce certain physiologic changes that also allow the yeast to assume a pathogenic role.

Recognition. Oral candidiasis (thrush) shows well-defined, creamy white patches on any portion of the oral mucous membranes. This creamy material, often compared with curds of milk, appears crumbly when disturbed, and its removal reveals an erythematous base. Its incidence in infants has decreased greatly, and it is now more a problem of premature infants and of adults with debilitating disease or AIDS, or following antibiotic therapy.

A similar reaction occurs in Candidal vaginitis, but here the process is exudative and more inflammatory. A yellowish-white milky discharge that may contain curd-like material dominates the clinical picture. The vaginal mucosa and usually the vulvar skin are erythematous, swollen, and extremely pruritic. Scratching may cause excoriations, erosions, and additional inflammation, often with extension of the process over the perineum and into the crural areas.

Candidal intertrigo is the most common *skin* infection, usually seen in inguinal, axillary, and inframammary folds. The intergluteal cleft and the spaces between the fingers and toes show occasional involvement. Candidiasis in these areas is almost always superimposed on intertrigo or seborrheic dermatitis and frequently is difficult to separate clinically from these two underlying conditions. Clues to its presence are (1) an *intense erythema* that is surprisingly nontender and nonedematous; (2) sharply demarcated, peripherally spreading *scalloped* borders; and (3) *satellite vesiculopustules*. Interdigital candidiasis shows a moist red macerative lesion surrounded by scaling overhanging borders, and because of this eroded appearance has been termed "erosio interdigitalis blastomycetica."

Candidal paronychia produces erythema, fusiform swelling, and tenderness in the paronychial tissues. Although slight pus formation usually occurs, it is not clear whether this is caused by the yeast infection or an associated bacterial overgrowth. Widening and/or deepening of the nail groove is almost pathognomonic of candidal infection in this area. These paronychial changes are chronic, interrupted by more acute intermittent episodes, and usually produce secondary dystrophic changes in the nail plate.

Paronychial infection *always* precedes the nail changes of candidiasis, and a diagnosis of the latter is untenable without at least some history of paronychial inflammation. These nail changes are directly proportional to the amount of nail matrix injury resulting from paronychial activity and can be differentiated from tinea unguium by their proximal location and absence of subungual debris. One or several fingers may be involved. Candidal paronychia is almost totally confined to persons whose hands are frequently wet, such as bartenders, housewives, and waitresses.

In the presence of clinical changes suggestive of candidiasis, the diagnosis should be confirmed by demonstration of large numbers of fungal elements in material from mucosal or skin lesions. Scrapings may be examined microscopically with the potassium hydroxide technique, but use of either Gram or Giemsa stain facilitates identification of the small (2 to 4 μ), oval, thin-walled cells. Pseudohyphae* and budding yeast cells are usually also present. It should be stressed that, because C. albicans may be found normally in the vagina and gastrointestinal tract and may colonize intertriginous areas under special circumstances, demonstration of this organism in clinical lesions is significant *only* if these lesions are consistent with clinical changes generally accepted as being produced by the organism.

Recognition of candidiasis is further aided by the presence of one or more underlying conditions known to predispose the patient to this infection. The physician should inquire about immunosuppressive drugs, systemic corticosteroids, and antibiotics. History and physical examination may reveal a tendency toward excessive sweating, obesity, or intertrigo. Candidiasis could be the first sign of pregnancy, diabetes, or immune deficiency. Although it seems unreasonable to expect the emergency physician to investigate all these possibilities, a blood glucose determination usually is indicated.

Management. Specific anticandidal *topical* agents have generally replaced Castellani's paint and gentian violet in the mangement of this fungal infection. Although ketoconazole was initially felt to be a safe and effective *systemic* agent, questions about its safety have been raised; its use should be restricted to special situations and only after consultation with a dermatol-

---

*Pseudohyphae are filaments composed of elongated budding cells that have failed to detach. Unlike true hyphae, they have unequal diameters along their length.

ogist or infectious disease specialist. Griseofulvin is ineffective in yeast infections.

For oral lesions, the patient should be directed to suck on one nystatin oral tablet (three times daily) until it completely dissolves in the mouth. In infants and children, 1 cc of nystatin oral suspension is placed in the mouth four times daily. For candidal vaginitis, nystatin vaginal tablets are prescribed twice daily for 2 weeks inserted into the vagina with an applicator that comes with this product.

Amphotericin B or haloprogin should be prescribed in lotion form for candidal intertrigo or other skin lesions. Sweating and maceration can be reduced by avoidance of hot water, tight-fitting clothing, and excessive physical activity. Cool water compresses provide cleanliness, remove debris and perspiration, reduce pruritus, and soothe inflamed skin at the same time, but they should be used only two or three times daily for no longer than 10 minutes. Candidal paronychia requires scrupulous avoidance of moisture, and a simple way to achieve this is by application of clear nail lacquer on top of the antifungal lotion. Finger cots should be suggested for unavoidable wet work.

BIBLIOGRAPHY

Ackerman, A.B., Miller, R.C., and Shapiro, L.: Gonococcemia and its cutaneous manifestations. Arch. Derm. 91:227, 1965.

Allen, D.M., Diamond, L.K., and Howell, D.A.: Anaphylactoid purpura in children (Schönlein-Henoch syndrome). Am. J. Dis. Child. 99:833, 1960.

Ansell, B.M.: Henoch-Schönlein purpura with particular reference to the prognosis of the renal lesion. Br. J. Dermatol. 82:211, 1970.

Ashton, H., Frenk, E., and Stevenson, C.J.: The management of Henoch-Schönlein purpura. Br. J. Dermatol. 85:199, 1971.

Baker, H., and Levene, G.M.: Cutaneous reactions to anticoagulants. Br. J. Dermatol. 81:236, 1969.

Benoit, F.L.: Chronic meningococcemia. Am. J. Med. 35:103, 1963.

Berger, R.S.: A critical look at therapy for the brown recluse spider bite. Arch. Dermatol. 107:298, 1973.

Callaway, J.L., and Tate, W.E.: Toxic epidermal necrolysis caused by "gin and tonic." Arch. Dermatol. 109:909, 1974.

Champion, R.H., et al.: Urticaria and angio-edema. Br. J. Dermatol. 81:588, 1969.

Cullen, S.I.: Understanding and treating seborrheic dermatitis. Hosp. Med. January 1985, p. 226.

Daughters, D., Zackheim, H., and Maibach, H.: Urticaria and anaphylactoid reactions after topical application of mechlorethamine. Arch. Dermatol. 107:429, 1973.

Deykin, D.: The clinical challenge of disseminated intravascular coagulation. N. Engl. J. Med. 283:636, 1970.

Dillaha, C.J., et al: North American loxoscelism. JAMA 188:33, 1964.

Everett, E.D., and Overholt, E.L.: Hemorrhagic skin infarction secondary to oral anticoagulants. Arch. Dermatol. 100:588, 1969.

Fardon, D.W., et al.: The treatment of brown spider bite. Plast. Reconstr. Surg. 40:482, 1967.

Gardner, L.W., and Acker, D.W.: Triamcinolone and pyoderma gangrenosum. Arch. Dermatol. 106:599, 1972.

Higgins, P.G., and Crow, K.D.: Recurrent Kaposi's varicelliform eruption in Darier's disease. Br. J. Dermatol. 88:391, 1973.

Juel-Jensen, B.E.: Severe generalized primary herpes treated with cytarabine. Br. Med. J. 2:154, 1970.

Kahn, G., and Danielsson, D.: Septic gonococcal dermatitis. Arch. Dermatol. 99:421, 1969.

Kahn, S., Stern, H.D., and Rhodes, G.A.: Cutaneous and subcutaneous necrosis as a complication of coumarin-congener therapy. Plast. Reconstr. Surg. 48:160, 1971.

Kazmier, F.J., et al.: Treatment of intravascular coagulation and fibrinolysis (ICF) syndromes. Mayo Clin. Proc. 49:665, 1974.

Kelly, J.F., and Patterson, R.: Anaphylaxis. Course, mechanisms and treatment. JAMA 227:1431, 1974.

Koch-Weser, J.: Coumarin necrosis (Editorial). Ann. Intern. Med. 68:1365, 1968.

Lowney, E.D., et al.: The scalded skin syndrome in small children. Arch. Dermatol. 95:359, 1967.

Lyell, A.: A review of toxic epidermal necrolysis in Britain. Br. J. Dermatol. 79:662, 1967.

Moschella, S.L.: Pyoderma gangrenosum. Arch. Dermatol. 95:121, 1967.

Nalbandian, R.M., et al.: Petechiae, ecchymosis and necrosis of skin induced by coumarin congeners. JAMA 192:603, 1965.

Nalbandian, R.M., et al.: Coumarin necrosis of skin treated successfully with heparin. Obstet. Gynecol. 38:395, 1971.

Nielsen, L.T.: Chronic meningococcemia. Arch. Dermatol. 102:97, 1970.

Perry, H.O.: Pyoderma gangrenosum. South. Med. J. 62:899, 1969.

Raab, B.: Acyclovir: The drug and its uses. Resident and Staff Physician 30:90, 1984.

Radimer, G.F., Davis, J.H., and Ackerman, A.B.: Fumigant-induced toxic epidermal necrolysis. Arch. Dermatol. 110:103, 1974.

Robboy, S.J., et al.: The skin in disseminated intravascular coagulation. Br. J. Dermatol. 88:221, 1973.

Ross, C.M.: The acute defibrination syndrome. Arch. Dermatol. 87:213, 1963.

Sahn, D.J., and Schwartz, A.D.: Schönlein-Henoch syndrome. Pediatrics 49:614, 1972.

Shelley, W.B.: Consultations in Dermatology I. Philadelphia, W. B. Saunders Co., 1972, pp. 166–170.

Shelley, W.B.: Consultations in Dermatology II. Philadelphia, W. B. Saunders Co., 1974, pp. 250–255.

Strauss, S.E., et al.: Acyclovir. N. Engl. J. Med. 310:1545, 1984.

Wheeler, C.E., and Abele, D.C.: Eczema herpeticum, primary and recurrent. Arch. Dermatol. 93:162, 1966.

VESICULOBULLOUS ERUPTIONS

Howard M. Simons

CAPSULE

Some dermatologic diseases present as vesiculobullous eruptions. These include life-threatening conditions such as toxic epidermal necrolysis, and relatively benign ones such as erythema multiforme. Pemphigus, Behçet's disease, bullous pemphigoid, and Kaposi's varicelliform eruption are all reviewed in terms of presentation, differential diagnosis, and treatment.

INTRODUCTION

Considering the large area of the skin surface, it is surprising that cutaneous life-threatening emergencies are relatively infrequent. Even in urticaria and erythema multiforme, both of which occur fairly often, only a small percentage of cases require emergency treatment.

Although each emergency dermatologic condition is uncommon in its full-blown form, less severe variants occur often enough. More important, perhaps, is that only through a working knowledge of these entities can one prevent misdiagnoses, thus avoiding unnecessary laboratory studies and undue alarm to the patient and his or her family.

Much of the discussion in dermatologic diseases is organized from the standpoint of major symptoms and signs. Classification by etiologic agent or agents is theoretically more desirable, but in most instances, the cause is obscure. Similarly, aside from cultures and microscopic examination for organisms, specific laboratory tests are rarely available, and clinical impression remains the basis of diagnosis. A careful history and precise description of the skin lesion therefore assume the greatest importance.

Although few dermatologic conditions are life-threatening, patients with acute skin conditions frequently present at emergency departments (EDs) because of the suddenness of onset, the high visibility of the lesions, and the frequent severe pruritus. Reassurance of patient and family is an important component of treatment.

TOXIC EPIDERMAL NECROLYSIS

Toxic epidermal necrolysis is a cutaneous syndrome heralded by erythema, fever, bullae, and widespread exfoliation of the skin. This desquamation is probably its most characteristic feature and is similar in appearance to wet paper peeling off a wall (see Fig. 56-82A). The Nikolsky sign, in which gentle pressure on normal skin causes bullae or further desquamation, is invariably present (see Fig. 56-82B). As the exfoliation progresses, the denuded surface appears moist, erythematous, and glistening, similar in appearance to a severe thermal burn—hence the alternative term for this condition, *scalded skin syndrome*. The process begins suddenly, and initial lesions usually appear around the eyes, oronasal area, and genitalia, with subsequent mucous membrane involvement.

The most common symptom, skin tenderness, is often severe. Even before clinical changes are seen in the skin, infants and younger children remain still because of the discomfort produced by movement. Other symptoms include anorexia, lethargy, diarrhea, and vomiting.

CAUSES

The causes of toxic epidermal necrolysis fall into two main groups. In infants and children up to 7 years, most cases are caused by epidermolytic toxin elaborated by staphylococci. In almost all cases of this milder form of the disease, the toxin is produced by group 2 staphylococci, usually phage type 71 or 55/71, but more recent reports have implicated group 1 as well. The mortality rate for infants is high, but drops to around 5% in the 1- to 6-year-old group.

In adults, various drugs and chemicals cause a more severe form of toxic epidermal necrolysis characterized by more extensive mucous membrane involvement and a mortality rate of 30 to 40%. The drugs most often cited are sulfonamides, phenylbutazone, salicylates, penicillins, and barbiturates, although a complete list of all drugs mentioned in the literature would exceed 100 preparations. One patient who developed the syndrome after the ingestion of gin and tonic was exquisitely sensitive to small quantities of quinine. Carbon monoxide and a fumigant containing acrylonitrile have been reported to produce toxic epidermal necrolysis after inhalation.

Although toxic epidermal necrolysis is reported in adult patients with a variety of diseases, it is not clear if the skin changes are caused by these diseases or one of the many medications that the patients receive.

RECOGNITION

In more severe forms of toxic epidermal necrolysis, the combination of widespread painful erythema and sheetlike exfoliation with flaccid bullae usually permits a rapid clinical diagnosis. In erythema multiforme, there is also periorificial involvement (Fig. 56-90), but typical iris or target lesions (Fig. 56-91), a negative Nikolsky sign, and discrete lesions rather than widespread exfoliation are often present. Erythema multiforme and toxic epidermal necrolysis are both reaction patterns to a variety of agents, and, in cases that cannot be separated clinically, both entities may be present at the same time.

Milder toxic epidermal necrolysis in children may be less easy to recognize clinically, and a high index of suspicion is essential. About 90% of children are febrile and 50% show leukocytosis, suggestive of an infectious process but otherwise nonspecific. Although erythema may be absent, skin tenderness is an almost constant finding, resulting in an irritable, febrile child who appears afraid to move. There is usually a history of sore throat, earache, or rhinorrhea.

Division of toxic epidermal necrolysis into two major types should aid recognition. The milder staphylococcal type is seen mainly in children, whereas the more severe "drug" type shows more mucous membrane involvement and may be confused clinically with erythema multiforme. It should be remembered, however, that the "drug" type may be seen in children as well as adults and that a few staphylococcal cases have been reported in adults.

Although the histology of the two types differs, frozen section techniques are usually unavailable, making this an impractical means of differentiating between the two.

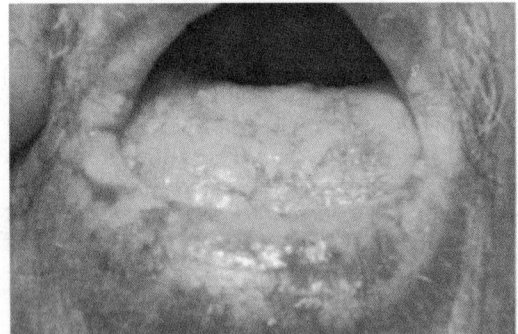

FIG. 56-90. Erythema multiforme.

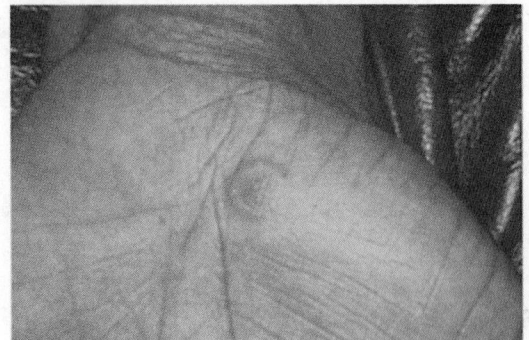

FIG. 56-91. Erythema multiforme, indicating the iris lesion.

MANAGEMENT

As soon as the presumptive diagnosis of toxic epidermal necrolysis is made, cultures should be obtained from the nasopharynx, blood, urine, unruptured bullae, skin, eyes, and ears. One should immediately begin an intravenous drip to facilitate therapy and maintenance of fluid balance and nutrition. Although almost all patients require hospitalization, patients 10 years old and under (and most older patients as well) should be started on treatment for penicillinase-producing Staphylococcus aureus infection while still in the ED. Sodium nafcillin or sodium methicillin is the drug of choice, although the former has been used more widely in treating this condition. It is given intravenously in dosages of 50 mg per kg daily in divided doses every 4 hours for children and 0.5 to 1 g every 4 hours for adults. Cultures and sensitivity tests may detect methicillin-resistant Staphylococcus aureus. Erythromycin is also effective and should be used if the patient is allergic to penicillin. If parenteral medication is necessary, however, a cephalosporin antibiotic can be used cautiously.

In drug-induced cases, systemic steroids are clearly indicated, and moderate to high doses should be given, depending on the presence of relative contraindications to their use. The intravenous route should be used initially. One of the most challenging problems confronting the emergency physician is the severely ill child whose history and clinical appearance do not permit differentiation between toxic epidermal necrolysis and erythema multiforme, even though one or the other seems more likely. The child may be toxic, febrile, and dehydrated and may have already received small doses of numerous medications. In such a patient, high-dose steroids should be combined with appropriate antibiotics, with the possibility of a drug-induced syndrome kept in mind. Systemic steroids do not appear to affect Staphylococcus aureus–induced toxic epidermal necrolysis adversely, provided that an effective antibiotic is given simultaneously.

Local care of the skin may be life-saving in the seriously ill patient with the drug-induced variety and should be started in the ED if admission to the hospital will be delayed more than a few hours. Warmed silver nitrate, 0.5% aqueous, should be applied as a compress to denuded areas to reduce the number of gram-negative organisms in these areas. Use of a rotating frame aids compressing and also reduces trauma to the intact skin. Placing the patient in a warm, humidified room can help reduce loss of heat, and strict isolation procedures reduce the chances of a life-threatening secondary infection. Fluids, electrolytes, and nutrition must be monitored and maintained, especially in infants.

ERYTHEMA MULTIFORME

Erythema multiforme (Figs. 56-90 and 56-91), an acute disorder primarily affecting the skin and mucous membranes, has distinctive clinical lesions and multiple causes. Unfortunately, dermatologists, because of their tendency to describe in detail and to give adjectival names to minor variations of this entity, have encouraged nondermatologists to lump together under this heading conditions that do not belong there. The lesions of erythema multiforme are well defined and characteristic. The multiforme appearance is related to the severity of the process and the tendency for new crops of lesions to continue to appear.

CAUSES

The causes of erythema multiforme are many, and each year several new "causes" are added to the list. Although little is known about the specific mechanisms of disease production, various investigations suggest that sensitivity to bacterial, viral, or chemical products is followed by deposition of circulating immune complexes in the small blood vessels in the skin. A large number of recurrent cases are caused by, or at least associated with, Mycoplasma pneumoniae and the virus of herpes simplex, and this may include the common "idiopathic" erythema multiforme that occurs in children and young adults during the winter and early spring. Other infections that may be related include histoplasmosis, trichomoniasis, influenza, ECHO and coxsackie viremias, and fungal infections. Vaccinations with the viruses of vaccinia, mumps, and poliomyelitis have also been implicated.

Although many drugs have been reported to produce erythema multiforme, those most often cited are the penicillins, sulfonamides, and barbiturates. Phenolphthalein, used as a laxative or as a dye in inexpensive red wines, produces a localized erythema multiforme reaction of the genitalia or lips. Radiographic therapy, internal malignancies, and collagen diseases are other causes.

RECOGNITION

Erythema multiforme occurs most commonly in a mild form, but for unknown reasons also may appear as a more severe toxic process often referred to as the Stevens-Johnson syndrome. Episodes of both forms resolve spontaneously in 2 to 4 weeks. Rarely, however, a fulminating course with secondary infection may lead to a fatal outcome.

The initial lesions of the mild form are bright red macules that typically appear suddenly on the hands and feet in symmetric distribution. Other common sites are the forearms, elbows, and lower legs, and all these sites may be involved together. The lesions may coalesce and become generalized, but rarely is the trunk involved before the extremities. Mucosal lesions, present in about 30% of cases, begin as vesicles or bullae that become eroded or crusted.

The red macules evolve to violaceous papular swellings or more frequently to the characteristic iris (or target) lesions. The latter are pathognomonic of erythema multiforme and show a thin peripheral red border, a middle pale zone, and a dusky center that may be vesicular. Iris lesions are edematous at first but later persist as macules until they fade, 8 to 12 days after their initial appearance. Resolution occurs without scarring, but hyperpigmentation may persist for weeks to months. Pruritus is variable.

The Stevens-Johnson syndrome is characterized by severe mucosal involvement, especially of the mouth and eyes, although the vagina and urethra often show changes as well. The palate and oral mucosa show raw, tender surfaces covered by a sticky gray exudate; the lips may be swollen, bloody, crusted, and exquisitely tender. The patient cannot eat, drink, or open the mouth to permit examination. The eyes are bilaterally involved, with a purulent conjunctivitis; the lids are edematous, and crusting causes them to stick together. Corneal involvement with ulceration may occur, probably owing to secondary bacterial infection. Genital lesions show a similar exudative clinical pattern, but the anal and nasal mucosae are rarely involved.

The skin may show the iris and maculoedematous lesions of the milder form or may display severe vesiculobullous lesions, frequently with hemorrhage. In other cases, severe mucosal involvement occurs without skin changes. Stevens-Johnson syndrome may be ushered in with fever, malaise, prostration, and a prodrome of flulike symptoms, but these changes, along with pneumonitis, may be caused by an underlying respiratory virus.

Recognition of erythema multiforme depends on the characteristic appearance of the eruption, and diagnosis is almost impossible during the prodromal period. If the patient is seen during the prodrome, an upper or lower respiratory infection may be suspected. Erythema multiforme, however, is often recurrent in children and young adults, and by taking a thorough history, the astute emergency physician may be able to predict the appearance of the eruption.

In sum, erythema multiforme is recognized by its characteristic symmetry, acral and mucosal distribution, and cutaneous iris or vesiculobullous lesions. By using rigorous clinical standards, one may avoid false-positive diagnosis. There are no specific laboratory tests for erythema multiforme, and any abnormal findings usually reflect an underlying process or secondary infection. Recognition of erythema multiforme occasionally requires consideration of the following mucocutaneous disorders:

PEMPHIGUS

In this more chronic and indolent process, the bullae are larger, break easily, and leave eroded lesions that tend to enlarge by detachment of the epidermis at the periphery. Involvement of the trunk is common, and erythema is rarely prominent. Mouth lesions are the first site of activity in more than one half of cases; however, they are typically erosive and show little tendency toward crust formation. Nikolsky sign is present and may account for the localization of skin lesions to areas of the trunk that are exposed to friction or pressure (Fig. 56-92). If pemphigus is suspected, a Tzanck test performed on material scraped from the floor of a bulla shows *acantholytic* cells, swollen epidermal cells whose cytoplasm has condensed peripherally at the cell walls.

BEHÇET'S DISEASE

This rare clinical entity, reported most often from eastern Mediterranean countries, is characterized by recurrent oral and external genital ulcerations in association with iritis and other destructive inflammatory changes of the eyes. The mouth lesions are similar to the erosions of recurrent aphthous stomatitis, and Behçet's disease is more easily confused with the latter than with erythema multiforme. Ocular involvement is usually progressive and severe, although it is initially unilateral in one half of cases, in contrast to erythema multiforme, in which eye lesions are symmetric. Behçet's disease may show varying multisystem involvement. Its other skin lesions are described as acneiform or pyodermatous when present.

BULLOUS PEMPHIGOID

In this skin disease of the elderly, large, tense bullae appear in association with erythema in a wide distribution, although the axillae, groin regions, and flexor

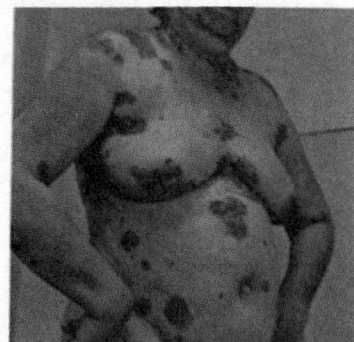

FIG. 56-92. Pemphigus.

arm areas are more commonly involved (Fig. 56-93). Oral mucosal lesions occur in one third of patients but are few in number, rarely painful, and never progress to severe stomatitis. Bullous pemphigoid may be further differentiated from erythema multiforme by (1) its gradual onset and more chronic course; (2) the absence of iris lesions, although gyriform erythematous lesions are seen; (3) the sparing of acral areas; and (4) its rarity in patients under 50 years of age, even though occasional childhood cases have been seen.

TOXIC EPIDERMAL NECROLYSIS

In most cases, the sheetlike exfoliation of this entity contrasts well with the more discrete vesiculobullous eruptions of erythema multiforme, and yet confusion between the two entities does occur. Favoring toxic epidermal necrolysis are a positive Nikolsky sign, exfoliation *around* the mouth rather than crusting of the lips, unilateral eye involvement, and the symptom of tender skin.

MANAGEMENT

The mild form of erythema multiforme usually requires little more than symptomatic treatment, reas-

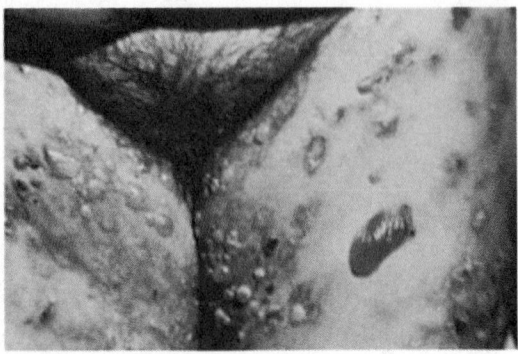

FIG. 56-93. Bullous pemphigoid.

surance about the benign prognosis, and an explanation to the patient about likely causes of this
mucocutaneous disorder. With regard to the last, a
thorough history and physical examination must aim
at uncovering latent infections and must record all
medications (including "over-the-counter" preparations) that the patient has taken. The patient should
be asked specifically about fever sores, herpes infections, and cold sores present now or in the past and
about any other cutaneous lesions he has noticed. A
chest radiograph is indicated for even the mildest of
respiratory symptoms associated with skin manifestations. Antibiotic treatment of Mycoplasma pneumoniae infection should be instituted if this underlying condition is found.

The discomfort of oral lesions may be reduced by
warm saline gargles, aspirin, and viscous lidocaine.
One tablespoon of lidocaine should be swished
around in the mouth, held there for 1 minute, and
then swallowed just before meals. Applications of petrolatum soften superficial crusting around the eyes
and lips.

In more severe cases of erythema multiforme, systemic steroids are indicated and should be started immediately as hydrocortisone 80 to 120 mg. every 8
hours intravenously, or 60 to 90 mg. of oral prednisone
daily in one stat dose if oral ingestion is tolerated.
Because hospitalization is indicated in severe cases,
antibiotics should be reserved for treatment of specific
infections that may be uncovered later. All suitable
cultures should be taken before institution of any antibiotic therapy.

KAPOSI'S VARICELLIFORM ERUPTION

This somewhat cumbersome term refers to an infection by the viruses of either herpes simplex or vaccinia
that occurs *only* in persons with a predisposing skin
disease. The terms "eczema herpeticum" and "eczema
vaccinatum" have the advantage of being more specific but have not completely displaced the older term
because (1) the two viral conditions are almost identical clinically, and (2) a third agent, coxsackievirus
A16, has also been shown to produce Kaposi's varicelliform eruption.

Although atopic dermatitis is by far the most common condition in which these infections occur, they
are also known to infect patients with Darier's disease,
seborrheic dermatitis, pemphigus, ichthyosis, contact
dermatitis, and AIDS.

RECOGNITION

The cutaneous eruption typically begins with the sudden appearance of massive crops of small vesicles that

enlarge rapidly, develop characteristic central umbilications, and become pustular and crusted. Although
abnormal skin usually shows the earliest involvement,
the process may later become generalized. Crops of
new lesions appear as the patient develops high fever,
constitutional symptoms, and marked regional lymphadenopathy. The face frequently shows the most severe involvement and may be markedly edematous
(Fig. 56-94).

Depending on the severity of the infection, the lesions may become confluent, severely erosive, or hemorrhagic. Secondary bacterial infection may obscure
the primary lesions and occasionally contribute to
mortality, although viremia and viral visceral involvement appear to be the main causes of death in this
condition.

The most severe cases occur in infants and other
patients who have no antibodies against the causative
viruses; therefore, recurrent attacks in the same individual are almost always milder. In eczema vaccinatum, a history of vaccination in the patient or a close
family member is usually obtained. The herpes simplex virus is more ubiquitous and thus more apt to
cause recurrent attacks. Usually, healing occurs in 2
to 3 weeks.

Because most patients (or their parents) assume that
the skin problem is merely an exacerbation of atopic
dermatitis, close examination of the clinical lesions and
a high index of suspicion are required to recognize
this occasionally fatal condition. The physician must
steer away from the crusted or hemorrhagic confluent
areas of the face and look for discrete lesions with
characteristic central umbilications. Fever and prostration also suggest that this is more than just an acute
dermatitis.

The diagnosis of eczema vaccinatum is confirmed
by a history of recent vaccination or exposure to a
vaccinated person. Although eczema herpeticum may
also have historical support, its diagnosis should be
confirmed in the emergency department by examination of a smear (Tzanck test) taken from one of the
lesions. The roof of an early vesicle or pustule is removed with a scalpel blade or fine iris scissors, and
the residual fluid is gently removed with a small gauze

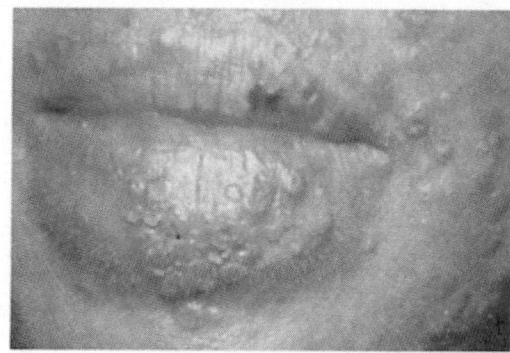

FIG. 56-94. *Kaposi's varicelliform eruption.*

sponge. The base of the vesicle or pustule is then scraped onto a glass slide with a scalpel blade and is stained with Giemsa or Wright stain. Finding multinucleated epithelial giant cells allows one to confirm the diagnosis of eczema herpeticum; these changes are absent in eczema vaccinatum and smallpox.

Differentiation of the latter two diseases may be difficult in geographic areas in which smallpox occurs; here, the emergency physician may have to base his working diagnosis on the absence of severe prodromal symptoms and consistently centrifugal distribution of the skin lesions of smallpox. Subsequent changes in antibody titers will make the distinction quite clear.

MANAGEMENT

Acyclovir, an antiviral agent effective against most herpesvirus infections, is the drug of choice if Kaposi's varicelliform eruption is caused by herpes simplex virus. Acyclovir has been found to be free of significant toxicity and appears to be rapidly effective whether given intravenously, intramuscularly, or orally. It is also active against varicella-zoster virus and Epstein-Barr virus; however, it is not effective against vaccinia virus, for which hyperimmune gamma globulin should be used. Until the use of acyclovir becomes more standardized, a dermatologist or other experienced physician should be consulted regarding proper dosage and method of administration. The range is 200 to 800 mg four times daily. The higher dose (800 mg q.i.d.) is gaining wide use for severe infections.

Patients who have moderate to severe involvement with Kaposi's varicelliform eruption require hospitalization. Bacterial cultures of the skin should be taken, and penicillin or cephalosporin antibiotics may be necessary for the streptococcal or staphylococcal bacterial overgrowth often present in this condition. Cool compresses of a 1 to 40 solution of aluminum subacetate (Burow's solution) should be applied four times daily for 30-minute periods to facilitate crust removal, although localized pyodermatous areas benefit more from warm aqueous compresses and gentamicin ointment.

Strict isolation technique should begin in the ED, and it is the responsibility of the emergency physician to ensure that it is continued during the patient's transferral to the hospital floor. The severely ill patient already has a viremia and overgrowth of resident bacteria on the skin; an additional pathogen may be more than he or she can handle. Also, isolation separates the patient from medical personnel and from other patients who may be susceptible to the viruses of Kaposi's varicelliform eruption.

PHARMACOTHERAPY FOR SKIN DISEASES

Ben Lerman

CAPSULE

To the busy emergency physician, skin diseases often seem to be a nuisance. They are rarely life-threatening, are frequently difficult to diagnose in the Emergency Department (ED), and only occasionally is specific, curative therapy available. No wonder that many of us are content to "dry what's wet, wet what's dry, and if that fails use steroids!" In fact, most skin diseases are not true emergencies, and could be referred from the ED without treatment. But the patient paying for your expertise is expecting treatment, not triage. And the indigent patient may never get to see the dermatologist to whom you would like to refer him or her. This chapter is intended to help the emergency physician initiate appropriate therapy for skin diseases in the ED, including the use of corticosteroids, antibiotics, antifungal agents, pediculocides, scabicides, and antipruritics.

INTRODUCTION

Skin is a distinctive organ in that drugs can be applied to it directly. This favors topical administration in many instances. On the other hand, systemic administration may lead the patient to be more compliant by avoiding the mess, the smell, the stained clothing, the frequent application and the expense of topicals. Also, some skin diseases (e.g., cellulitis, or fungal infections of the fingernails) are dramatically more responsive to systemic agents. When the topical route is chosen, factors influencing absorption must be considered. Absorption is enhanced by higher concentration of the drug, well-hydrated stratum corneum, damaged skin, and skin with a thinner stratum corneum (i.e., the skin of premature infants and elderly patients, and the skin of flexor surfaces and genitals).

The vehicle chosen for the drug is important for both its intrinsic properties and for its effect on drug absorption. The vehicle itself may be cooling, protective, emollient, occlusive, or astringent, depending on its composition. The classification of vehicles as lotions, creams, ointments, and so forth is confusing (Fig. 56-95) and variable. Creams and lotions are the most pleasant vehicles to the touch and consequently the most popular. Ointments have a greater emollient effect (useful for dry skin) and enhance drug absorption. They should not be used in hairy or sweaty areas, where creams are more appropriate. Lotions (e.g.,

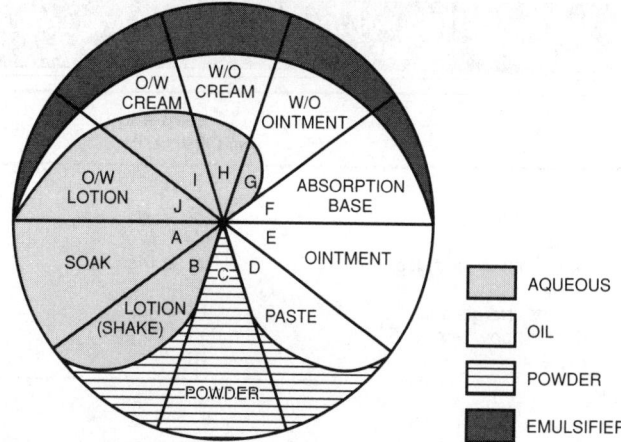

FIG. 56-96.   A universe of topical medication (*From* Katz, M.: The design of topical drug products: pharmaceutics. With permission from Arriens, E.J. (ed.): Drug Design, vol 4. New York, London, p. 108.

calamine lotion) have a cooling and drying effect, which is most valuable in acute erythematous and papular dermatoses that are not weeping. Soaks, such as dressings wet with Burow's solution or saline, are useful for acute weeping dermatoses. Dry powdered milk may also help to dry such lesions and is inexpensive.

Topical drugs (Fig. 56-96) are generally applied three to four times a day. Even when the drug itself has prolonged action (e.g., corticosteroids), the therapeutic properties of the vehicle often warrant more fre-

FIG. 56-95.   Interrelationship of the seven basic forms of topical application.

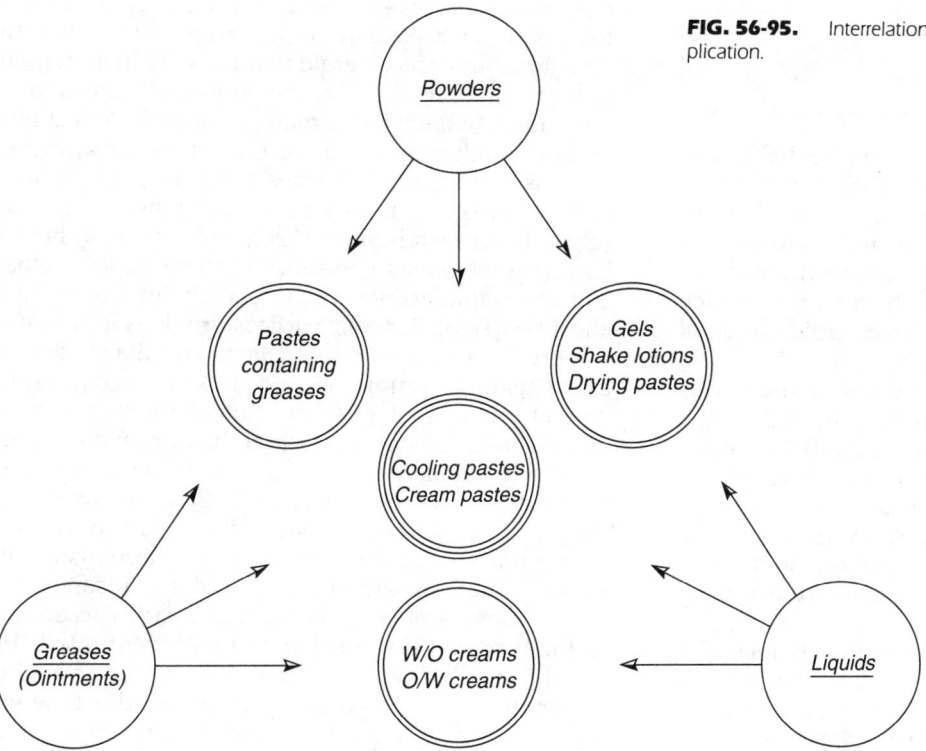

TABLE 56-21. QUANTITY OF OINTMENTS AND LOTIONS NEEDED FOR ONE WEEK'S APPLICATION

	Creams and Ointments	Lotions (mL)
Face	5–15 g	100
Both hands	25–50 g	200
Scalp	50–100 g	200
Both arms or both legs	100–200 g	200
Body	200 g	500
Groins and genitalia	15–25 g	100
Dusting powders	50–100 g	
Paints	10–25 ml	

quent application. This may be accomplished in such instances at less expense by alternating nonspecific and drug-containing preparations. Corticoid-containing preparations should not be used simply as lubricants. The patient needs instruction to apply a thin film to the entire affected area. Shlagel found that unsupervised patients, each asked to anoint his whole body, used anywhere from 8 to 114 g.[1] Patient education can help to standardize the dose received. Prescribing the proper total amount also helps to clue the patient as to how much should be used at each application. Table 56-21 may be used as a guide to the quantities required for 1 week of tid application of a preparation. One ounce (30 g) of a cream generally allows one application to the entire adult body.

CORTICOCORTICOIDS

The introduction of corticosteroids in the 1950s radically improved our ability to help patients with skin diseases. The initial excitement was eventually tempered by a recognition of the local and systemic toxicities of these drugs. Although an unfortunate correlation does exist between the therapeutic potency and toxicity of the different corticosteroids, careful prescribing minimizes side effects.

Hydrocortisone, originally called compound F, was introduced to dermatologists in 1952 by Sulzberger and Witten.[2] Currently more than 50 different compounds, alone and in combination with other drugs, are available, and most of these are available in a range of concentrations. The plethora of available corticosteroid preparations is at once a testimony to the usefulness of this class of drugs and a pitfall to the unwary physician.

Systemic hydrocortisone has multiple activities. The mineralocorticoid and glucocorticoid effects are best understood, but are essentially side effects in the treatment of skin diseases. The catabolic effect on muscle

and collagen is also undesired and manifests as atrophy of the dermis. The inhibition of DNA synthesis in many cells may be advantageous in proliferative disorders such as psoriasis and keloids, but also contributes to atrophy. The most useful properties, the anti-inflammatory and immunosuppressive effects, are also the least understood. Hydrocortisone is known to inhibit vasodilation, capillary permeability, and margination of leukocytes. Corticosteroids bind with receptors in the cytosol, which then interact with DNA in the nucleus to release mRNA which programs for a variety of anti-inflammatory proteins. The varying affinity for these receptors in the cytosol of the different corticosteroids accounts partly for their varying potency.

The list of possible indications for corticosteroids is *almost* as long as the list of skin diseases. (Possible exceptions include rosacea and pruritus without a cutaneous cause.[3] Even infectious conditions amenable to specific therapy may improve more rapidly with simultaneous corticosteroid treatment if inflammation is significant. In the ED, the common indication is dermatitis, whether eczematous, allergic, infectious or photo-induced. A special indication for systemic corticosteroids may be herpes zoster in patients over 60 years of age, to reduce the risk of subsequent neuralgia. If the rash is generalized and severe, systemic corticosteroids may be useful. In the absence of specific contraindications such as diabetes mellitus, a short course of systemic corticosteroids is fairly safe. Suppression of the hypothalamic pituitary-adrenal axis, Cushing's syndrome, and growth retardation are side effects of systemic (and potent topical) corticosteroids that are not seen when the duration of treatment is less than 3 weeks. Less serious but more common side effects include water retention and insomnia; the patient should be warned of these. The most common route of systemic corticosteroid administration in the outpatient setting is oral, and prednisone is by far the most popular choice. Dosage varies according to the disease being treated and its severity, but the usual range is 0.5 to 1.0 mg per kg of body weight. Other drugs may be used by adjusting the dose for their potency. A high initial dose should be tapered rapidly as the condition improves. Ideally, this is guided by a physician observing the patient's progress, which is often impractical. Generally, the emergency physician must try to forecast at the outset what sort of tapering is appropriate. One to two weeks is long enough for most acute dermatoses (e.g., contact dermatitis), although rhus dermatoses may require 3 to 4 weeks of systemic corticoids. A single daily dose in the morning minimizes the risks of adrenal suppression.[4] Alternatively, the patient may be given a single intramuscular injection of a long-acting corticosteroid in the ED. This avoids the potentially confusing instructions of how to taper the prednisone pills. Triamcinolone acetonide (Kenalog), 40 mg IM, gives 3 to 4 weeks of anti-inflammatory effect.[5,6] Betamethasone, dexamethasone, and methylprednisolone are all shorter-acting, with effects lasting 7 to 10 days.[4,6,7] Methylprednisolone sodium acetate (Depomedrol), in a dose of 80 mg IM, has been compared favorably with a 1-week oral tapering of the same drug in treating acute asthma. Controversy about long-term intermittent use of intramuscular corticosteroids and their effect on the hypothalamus, pituitary, and adrenal glands exists, but it is generally agreed that a one-time dose is as safe as prednisone tapering of similar duration.[5–7] A needle long enough to reach a large muscle should be used to avoid fat atrophy.

TOPICAL CORTICOSTEROIDS

For a more localized or less severe rash, topical corticosteroid preparations may be chosen. These are theoretically safer, especially in diabetic and hypertensive patients, and the benefits of the vehicle may be helpful as well. The selection and dosage of the preparation may be confusing, but in the emergency setting, a few guidelines will suffice. Topical corticosteroids are rated according to various potency tables devised by the AMA Drug Evaluation, the Medical Letter, the British National Formulary, and many individuals, using anywhere from three to six categories. Of course, no two of these lists are identical, and in rare instances a low-potency drug from one list is considered high potency elsewhere. The discrepancies may be attributed to different rating systems (e.g., clinical trials vs. laboratory tests) or different preparations of a drug (concentration or vehicle tested). See Table 56-22 for a useful rating of some drugs available in the U.S.

Hydrocortisone is the prototypical low-potency topical corticosteroid. It is available over the counter at 0.5% concentration and by prescription up to 2.5% in a variety of vehicles. It is almost free of side effects and is a safe choice for use on the face, genitals, and flexures, and in children. It is relatively ineffective on thickened skin and psoriasis. Hydrocortisone with urea and hydrocortisone butyrate and valerate are more potent and may have more side effects.

Moderately potent drugs include triamcinolone acetonide, 0.1% (e.g., Kenalog and Aristocort); fluoci-

nolone acetonide, 0.05% (e.g., Synalar); and many others. These are useful for a more severely inflamed rash or one occurring in an area of thicker skin (e.g., trunk, extensor surfaces, scalp). Side effects such as striae, atrophy, and ecchymoses should not be a problem during a short (less than 4-week) course of this class of drugs provided that they are not used on the face or genitals or in infants. Systemic side effects with these drugs when used for less than 2 months should

TABLE 56–22. RELATIVE EFFICACY OF SOME TOPICAL CORTICOSTEROIDS IN VARIOUS FORMULATIONS

Lowest efficacy
0.25–2.5%	Hydrocortisone
0.25%	Methylprednisolone acetate (Medrol)
0.04%	Dexamethasone* (Hexadrol)
0.1%	Dexamethasone* (Decaderm)
1.0%	Methylprednisolone acetate (Medrol)
0.5%	Prednisolone (Meti-Derm)
0.2%	Betamethasone* (Celestone)

Low efficacy
0.01%	Fluocinolone acetonide* (Fluonid, Synalar)
0.01%	Betamethasone valerate* (Valisone)
0.025%	Fluorometholone* (Oxylone)
0.05%	Aclometasone dipropionate (Aclovate)
0.025%	Triamcinolone acetonide* (Aristocort, Kenalog, Triacet)
0.1%	Clocortolone pivalate* (Cloderm)
0.03%	Flumethasone pivalate* (Locorten)

Intermediate efficacy
0.2%	Hydrocortisone valerate (Westcort)
0.1%	Mometasone furoate (Elocon)
0.1%	Hydrocortisone butyrate (Locoid)
0.025%	Betamethasone benzoate* (Benisone, Flurobate, Uticort)
0.025%	Flurandrenolide* (Cordran)
0.1%	Betamethasone valerate* (Valisone)
0.05%	Desonide (Tridesilon, Desowen)
0.025%	Halcinonide* (Halog)
0.05%	Desoximetasone* (Topicort L.P.)
0.05%	Flurandrenolide* (Cordran)
0.1%	Triamcinolone acetonide*
0.025%	Fluocinolone acetonide*

High efficacy
0.05%	Betamethasone dipropionate* (Diprosone)
0.1%	Amcinonide* (Cyclocort)
0.25%	Desoximetasone* (Topicort)
0.5%	Triamcinolone acetonide*
0.2%	Fluocinolone acetonide* (Synalar-HP)
0.05%	Diflorasone diacetate* (Florone, Maxiflor)
0.1%	Halcinonide* (Halog)
0.05%	Fluocinonide* (Lidex, Topsyn)

Highest efficacy
0.05%	Betamethasone dipropionate* in optimized vehicle (Diprolene)
0.05%	Diflorasone diacetate* in optimized vehicle (Psorcon)
0.05%	Clobetasol propionate* (Temovate)

* Fluorinated steroids.

TABLE 56-23. GUIDELINES FOR TOPICAL CORTICOIDS
Hydrocortisone for face, flexures, genitals, and in children Moderate potency for thick skin severe eruption High potency—small quantities, no refills

not be seen at doses of less than 100 g per week in adults.

There is no reason for the emergency physician to *initiate* therapy with the high potency drugs. The occasional patient requesting a refill of a high-potency drug should be given a limited quantity to encourage the close follow-up with a dermatologist mandated by these drugs.

The general guidelines about vehicles and dosage discussed at the start of this chapter apply to the topical corticosteroids. It should be noted, however, that once- or twice-daily applications achieve the full therapeutic effect of the drug in this instance, and may avoid tachyphylaxis (and increased expense) of more frequent applications.[3] A bland (nonmedicated) vehicle may be prescribed for interval application.

Many corticosteroid combination drugs are available. The most useful in the emergency setting are those combining a low- or moderate-strength corticosteroid with an antifungal for treatment of inflamed candidiasis or tinea infections. Examples include Lotrisone (clotrimazole and betamethasone) and Mycolog (nystatin and triamcinolone).

Obviously the physician must be aware of the components of the drug used and select appropriately for the infection being treated and the skin site involved. See Table 56-23.

ANTIBIOTICS

Skin infections are a common problem. Although acne is the most common, even teenagers rarely perceive it as an emergency and it will not be discussed further. Bacterial skin infections are generally caused by staphylococci and streptococci, and manifest clinically as impetigo, folliculitis, furuncles, carbuncles, erysipelas, and cellulitis. These diseases are referred to collectively as pyodermas. Although topical antibiotics have been used, systemic antibiotics are preferred for several reasons. Most important is their efficacy; topical antibiotics generally do not penetrate well. Other concerns are sensitizing the patient to a drug that might be needed later for a more serious infection and selecting resistant strains by indiscriminate use. A relatively new drug, mupirocin (Bactroban), is more effective than other topicals and has a low incidence of sensitization and no systemic applications. It seems

as effective as systemic antibiotics for impetigo,[8] but this remains to be well documented.[9]

In impetigo, the uncommon (less than 1%) sequela of poststreptococcal glomerulonephritis is another theoretic reason for systemic antibiotics, but their efficacy in preventing this has not been demonstrated.[9,10]

Because staphylococcus is such a common skin pathogen and culture results are rarely available in the ED, a penicillinase-resistant drug should be selected. Dicloxacillin (250 to 500 mg every 6 hours) or cloxacillin (500 to 1000 mg every 6 hours) are first choices for oral therapy.[11] Alternatives include Augmentin (250 to 500 mg every 8 hours) or a cephalosporin such as cephalexin. The manufacturer states that Keflex may be given in a 500 mg every 12 hours dose for soft tissue infections. Ceftriaxone may be used in select cases for once-a-day outpatient therapy. Erythromycin is a third-line agent, although, because of its low cost, some physicians have recommended it as a first choice for impetigo. Ciprofloxacin is a good alternative for patients unable to take penicillin or erythromycin. Finally, soft tissue infections resistant to the above agents might be treated with clindamycin, but diarrhea is a frequent problem with this drug, and pseudomembranous colitis may occur in 0.1 to 10% of those treated, limiting its use.[12]

TOPICAL ANTIBIOTICS

Topical antibiotics are used chiefly in the ED as part of wound dressings. Antibiotics with systemic uses are not used frequently to avoid selection of resistant organisms and avoid sensitization of the patient. Polymyxin B, bacitracin, and neomycin are often used in an ointment. Silver sulfadiazine (silvadene and povidone iodine) are also used. Benefits include less adherence of dressings, less coagulum formation, and possibly faster wound healing.[13] There is little information regarding their efficacy in preventing wound infection, but it is dubious.[14] The use of topical antibiotics at IV sites is of marginal benefit at best.[9]

Other uses of topical antibiotics in dermatology are for acne, rosacea, and hidradenitis, but these are rarely treated by the emergency physician. Two special uses deserve note. To treat aphthous stomatitis, tetracycline, 125 mg/5 cc is recommended as a 10 cc rinse tid.[15] Triamcinolone in orabase has also been recommended. Silvadene cream applied qid to herpes zoster lesions quickly relieves the skin pain and dries the lesions.[16]

ANTIFUNGALS

Various antifungal agents are available in both systemic and topical forms. Patients requiring systemic therapy (e.g., those with extensive diseases, tinea capitis, resistance to topical therapy) may best be referred to a dermatologist, and this discussion is limited to topical drugs. Candida and dermatophytes are the primary indications for antifungals in the ED. The imidazoles include clotrimazole (Lotrimin), econazole (Spectazol), miconazole (Micatin, Monistat), and Ketoconazole (Nizorol). These agents act by disrupting the cell membrane. All are effective against dermatophytes, yeasts, and gram-positive bacteria. Nystatin and amphotericin B are polyenes effective only for Candida.

Because Candida and dermatophyte infections are easily confused clinically and polyenes offer no advantage over the imidazoles, a case can be made for exclusive use of the latter agents.[17,18] Tinea versicolor is an exception in that it is susceptible to less expensive agents such as selenium sulfide shampoo, $2\frac{1}{2}\%$ (Exsel, Selsun) for 30 minutes a day for 1 to 2 weeks. Dermatophytes and yeast should be treated well beyond clinical resolution to prevent recurrence, generally for 2 to 4 weeks. Lotrimin 1% is available in a cream combined with 0.05% betamethasone dipropronate (Lotrisone), which may relieve symptoms more rapidly in patients with moderate inflammation.[19]

PEDICULICIDES AND SCABICIDES

Lindane 1% (Kwell), pyrethrins (RID), permethrin 1% (NIX), and other drugs not available in the U.S. are used against lice. They are all fairly effective against the lice, but less so against the unhatched eggs (nits). Consequently, a second application 1 week later is recommended to eradicate newly hatched larvae that survived the original treatment as eggs.[17,20,21] There is some evidence that NIX is more effective than Kwell for head lice.[21] Lindane toxicity has been reported in small infants but it is generally considered safe for children over 1 year.[21]

Scabies may be best treated with 5% permethrin. It is also susceptible to a single overnight application of Kwell lotion. It must be applied to every square inch of skin from the neck down. Because there is a large allergic, inflammatory component to scabies (and often to pediculosis), symptoms may persist for weeks after treatment. After treatment of the infestation, topical or systemic corticosteroids bring quicker relief.[21]

ANTIVIRALS

Herpes simplex (especially of the genitals), varicella, and herpes zoster are the usual viral skin diseases seen in the ED. The only oral agent widely available against the viruses responsible for these diseases is acyclovir (Zovirax). This is supplied in 200 mg tablets and as a 5% ointment. For the first episode of genital herpes, oral acyclovir, in a dose of 200 mg five times a day for ten days, substantially shortens the period of dysuria and pain, the time to healing of lesions, and the period of viral shedding. Its use during the primary episode does not alter the pattern of subsequent episodes. When used early during a recurrent outbreak, it is still effective but less dramatically so, reducing the duration of symptoms only by 1 to 2 days.[22,23] Consequently, most authorities recommend treatment for all primary episodes, but treatment for recurrences must be individualized. Some patients who suffer frequent or severe recurrences are maintained on a daily dose of 200 mg tid or 400 mg bid. Others may keep a supply at home, allowing them to initiate full doses at the earliest symptoms of a recurrence. Topical acyclovir is marginally effective at best, and because systemic therapy is safe, offers no advantages.[22,23]

The role of antiviral therapy for varicella zoster is evolving. For immunocompromised patients and those with complications (pneumonia, encephalitis), early treatment with parenteral acyclovir or vidarabine certainly seems helpful for both varicella and zoster.[24,25] For otherwise healthy patients, with uncomplicated varicella or zoster, most authorities limit antiviral treatment to particular high-risk categories, especially neonatal varicella, ophthalmic zoster, or zoster in patients over age 60 (with a higher risk for postherpetic neuralgia).[24–27] Some also consider adults with varicella a high-risk group warranting acyclovir. In zoster, acyclovir, intravenously or in high oral doses (600 to 800 mg five times per day), significantly decreases pain, time to healing and viral shedding, and the incidence of ocular complications.[25,28] High-dose oral acyclovir seems as effective in this setting as by the intravenous route, at least when given within the first 96 hours of pain.[29] Unfortunately, most studies fail to show marked effects of acyclovir in preventing postherpetic neuralgia.[24,25,30] Table 56-24 summarizes the above recommendations for management of varicella and zoster.

ANTIPRURITICS

Pruritus is, of course, a symptom, not a disease. Common medical sense dictates that therapy be directed primarily at the cause. Unfortunately, a cause is often not evident in the ED, and even when it is evident, it generally takes time to eliminate. Bear in mind that unexplained pruritus in the ED merits further evaluation because it may be a manifestation of various

TABLE 56-24. SUGGESTED TREATMENTS FOR ACUTE VARICELLA AND ZOSTER INFECTIONS

Infection	Host	Complication	Drug	Regimen	Comment
Varicella	Normal	None	None	—	—
		Frank pneumonia	Acyclovir	10 mg/kg i.v. q8h × 7d	Unproven
	Compromised	None, any	Acyclovir	10 mg/kg i.v. q8h × 10d	Early treatment
			or		
			Vidarabine	10 mg/kg i.v. QD × 10d	Early treatment
Zoster	Normal	None	None	—	—
		Ophthalmic	Acyclovir	600–800 mg p.o. q4h × 10d	
	Compromised	None	None	—	Mild immune deficiency
			or		
			Acyclovir	10 mg/kg i.v. q8h × 7–10d	Early treatment
			or		
			Vidarabine	10 mg/kg i.v. QD × 7–10d	Early treatment
		Dissemination	Acyclovir	10 mg/kg i.v. q8h × 10d	—
			or		
			Vidarabine	10 mg/kg i.v. QD × 10d	—

serious diseases (tumor, parasites, hepatic or renal disease, thyroid disorders, etc).

The mainstay of nonspecific treatment of pruritus are antihistamines and emollients. The mechanism of the former is unclear. Although a blunting of the effects of histamine as an itch mediator in the skin has been suggested,[17,31] the sedative side effect of antihistamines is probably most important. The nonsedating antihistamines have clarified this because they seem beneficial only for urticarial (i.e., histamine related) itching.[32-34] One study found them effective in nonurticarial itching, but was limited by its small sample size.[31]

Any systemic antihistamine may be tried; if the patient has failed to benefit from one antihistamine, an alternative or an increased dose may still be helpful. Topical antihistamines should not be used.

Emollients (e.g., Eucerin) are helpful because they cool and soothe. In addition, they may treat one of the specific causes of pruritus, namely dry skin. Patients should be advised to avoid overheating their homes and bathing too frequently.

The long list of other drugs used for itching proves the adage that many treatments mean that none works well. Cimetidine, charcoal, tranquilizers and sedatives, antidepressants, carbamazepine cholestyramine, iron, aspirin, intravenous lidocaine, and, of course, naloxone have all been used in the battle against the itch. Some of these are effective in specific circumstances, another reason to refer the patient with a recalcitrant itch to a dermatologist.

ACKNOWLEDGMENT

The author wishes to thank Howard Maibach, M.D. for reviewing this manuscript.

REFERENCES

1. Schlagel, C.A., and Sanborn, E.C.: The weight of topical preparations required for total and partial body inunction. J. Invest. Dermatol. 42:253, 1964.
2. Sulzberger, M.B., and Witten, V.H.: The effect of topically applied Compound F in selected dermatoses. J. Invest. Dermatol. 19:101, 1952.
3. Clement, M., and Yirier, A.D.: Topical Steroids for Skin Disorders. Oxford, Blackwell Scientific Publications, 1987.
4. Bickers, D.R., Hazen, P.G., and Lynch, W.S.: Clinical Pharmacology of Skin Disease. New York, Churchill Livingstone, 1984.
5. Storrs, F.J.: Intramuscular corticosteroids: A second point of view. J. Am. Acad. Dermatol. 5:600, 1984.
6. Arnold, H.L., Jr.: Comments on "A second point of view." J. Am. Acad. Dermatol. 5:604, 1981.
7. Hoffman, I.B., and Fiel, S.B.: Oral vs. repository corticosteroid therapy in acute asthma. Chest 93:11,
8. Dux, P.H., Fields, L., and Pollock, D.: 2% topical mupirocin versus systemic erythromycin and cloxacillin in primary and secondary skin infections. Curr. Ther. Res. 40:933, 1986.
9. Hischmann, J.V.: Topical antibiotics in dermatology. Arch. Dermatol. 124:1691, 1988.

10. Carruthers, R.: Prescribing antibiotics for impetigo. Drugs *36*:364, 1988.
11. Reboli, A.C., and DelBene, V.E.: Oral antibiotic therapy of dermatologic conditions. Dermatol. Clin. *4*:497, 1988.
12. Bartlett, J.G.: Antimicrobial agents implicated in clostridium difficile toxin associated diarrhea or colitis. Johns Hopkins Med. J. *149*:6, 1981.
13. Geronemus, R.G., Mertz, P.M., and Englstein, W.H.: Wound healing: The effects of topical antimicrobial agents. Arch. Dermatol. *115*:1311, 1979.
14. Heinrich, J.J., Brand, D.A., and Cuong, C.B.: The role of topical treatment as a determinant of infection in outpatient burns. J. Burn Care Rehabil. *9*:253, 1988.
15. Rook, A., Parish, L.C., and Bease, J.M.: Practical Management of the Dermatologic Patient. Philadelphia, J.B. Lippincott Company, 1986.
16. Montes, L.F., Muchinik, G., and Fox, C.H.: Response of varicellar zoster virus and herpes zoster to silver sulfadiazine. Cutis *38*:363, 1986.
17. Shelley, W.B., and Shelley, E.D. Advanced Dermatologic Therapy. Philadelphia, W.B. Saunders Company, 1987.
18. Landon, R.K.: Handbook of Dermatologic Treatment. Greenbrae, California, Jones Medical Publications, 1983.
19. Katz, H.L., Bard, J., Cole, G.W., et al.: Sch 370 (Clotrimazole-betamethasone dipropionate) cream in patients with tinea cruris or tinea corporis. Cutis *34*:183, 1984.
20. Kalter, D.C., Sperbe, J., Rosen, T., and Matarasso, S.: Treatment of peduculosis pubis—clinical comparison of efficacy and tolerance of 1% lidane shampoo vs. 1% permethrin creme rinses. Arch. Dermatol. *123*:1315, 1987.
21. Reeves, J.T.: Head lice and scabies in children. Pediatr. Infect. Dis. J. *6*:598, 1987.
22. Webb, D.H., and Fife, K.H.: Genital herpes simplex virus infections. Infect. Dis. Clin. North Am. *1*:97, 1987.
23. Mertz, G.J.: Diagnosis and treatment of genital herpes infections. Infect. Dis. Clin. North Am. *1*:341, 1987.
24. Nicholson, K.G.: Antiviral therapy: Varicella-zoster virus infections herpes labialis and mucocutaneous herpes, and cytomegalovirus infections. Lancet *2*:677, 1984.
25. Whitley, R.J., Soong, S.J., Dolin, R.M., et al.: Early vidarabine therapy to control the complications of herpes zoster in immunocompromised patients. N. Engl. J. Med. *307*:971, 1982.
26. Peterslund, N.A.: Management of varicella zoster infections in immunocompetent hosts. Am. J. Med. *85*:74, 1988.
27. Straus, S.E., Ostrove, J.M., Inchauspe, G., et al.: NIH conference. Varicella-zoster virus infections. Biology, natural history, treatment, and prevention. Ann. Intern. Med. *108*:221, 1988.
28. Esmann, V., Ipsen, J. Peterslund, N.A., et al.: Therapy of acute herpes zoster with acyclovir in the nonimmunocompromised host. Am. J. Med. *73*:320, 1982.
29. Peterslund, N.A., Esmann, V., Ipsen, J., et al.: Oral and intravenous acyclovir are equally effective in herpes zoster. J. Antimicrob. Chemother. *14*:185, 1984.
30. Straus, S.E.: The management of varicellar and zoster infections. Infect. Dis. Clin. North Am. *2*:367, 1987.
31. Doherty, V., Sylvester, D.G., Kennedy, C.T., et al.: Treatment of itching in atopic eczema with antihistamine with a low sedative profile. Br. Med. J. *298*:96, 1989.
32. Paul, E., and Bodeker, R.H.: Comparative study of astemizole and terfenadine in the treatment of chronic idiopathic urticaria. A randomized double blind study of 40 patients. Ann. Allergy *62*:318, 1989.
33. Rubenstein, R.: Pruritus: A new look at an old problem. J. Fam. Pract. *24*:625, 1987.
34. Krause, L., and Shuster, S.: Mechanism of action of antipruritic drugs. Br. Med. J. *287*:1199, 1983.

Part VI

Obstetric and Gynecologic Emergencies

Chapter 57

OBSTETRIC EMERGENCIES

EMERGENCY DELIVERY

Stephen D. Higgins

CAPSULE

A significant number of pregnant women presenting to the emergency department (ED) are at high risk, with a greater chance of death and disability for mother and baby. Proper triage, conduct of delivery, and recognition and treatment of life-threatening emergencies increase the likelihood of a good outcome. The emergency physician should also be prepared for the unusual possibility and need for perimortem cesarean section to save the fetus, and possibly also the mother, during cardiorespiratory arrest.

Table 57-1 presents a glossary of terms used in obstetrics.

INTRODUCTION

An inordinate number of patients presenting in the prehospital care arena or to the ED are high-risk pregnant patients. A high-risk pregnancy is defined as one in which the mother or the fetus has a significantly increased chance of death or disability. This is compared to a low-risk pregnancy in which optimal outcome is expected for both mother and baby. For high-risk pregnancies, the perinatal infant mortality rate is as great as 3.5 to 14.5%, whereas in low-risk pregnancies, the perinatal infant mortality rate is as little as 0.04%. In a study of 738 patients, Hobel has shown that, in the prenatal period, approximately 34% of pregnant patients can be categorized as high risk.[1] When labor begins, an additional 20% are added to this category. A recent study by Brunette confirms the increased mortality and morbidity of patients delivering in the prehospital care setting or the ED.[2] These authors, in a study of 80 patients delivering in the

field or the ED, showed an infant mortality rate of 9%. There was an increased incidence of shoulder dystocia, postpartum hemorrhage, prolapsed cord, and meconium staining. Because of the significant and yet unpredictable number of high-risk pregnancies in the field and the ED, as well as the predictable increased incidence of complications associated with these high-risk pregnancies, it is important for the emergency physician to strongly discourage prehospital deliveries whenever possible and to encourage transfer of pregnant patients to the appropriate facility as soon as feasible. The type of facility also has an effect on outcome. Paneth has shown that patients with high-risk pregnancies have a 24% higher risk of death if birth occurred outside of a level III perinatal center.[3] A high-risk pregnancy was easily determined in this study as either preterm (<37 weeks) or low birth weight (<2251 g). A level III perinatal center is one in which all types of perinatal care are provided, including obstetric and neonatal intensive care as well as a broad range of subspecialty consultative services.

PATHOPHYSIOLOGY OF LABOR

True labor is defined as pain and progress (Table 57-2). The pain occurs at regular intervals, which progressively shorten while the intensity of the pain gradually increases. The pain can occur in the back as well as in the abdomen, and can be interpreted also as mere discomfort. This is especially true in early or preterm labor. For a diagnosis of true labor, however, there must not only be pain, but also progress, i.e., documented progressive cervical dilatation and effacement. Two or more serial examinations may be necessary to properly document progress in early labor. In contrast to true labor, false labor is characterized by pain occurring at irregular intervals with the intervals remaining long and the intensity remaining

TABLE 57-1. GLOSSARY OF OBSTETRIC TERMS

ABORTION:	The termination of pregnancy by any means (natural or induced) before 20 weeks of gestation.
GRAVIDA:	A pregnant woman.
GRAVIDITY:	The number of pregnancies a woman has had, irrespective of outcome.
MULTIGRAVIDA:	A woman who has been pregnant more than once.
MULTIPARA:	A woman who has completed two or more pregnancies to the stage of viability.
NULLIGRAVIDA:	A woman who is not now and has never been pregnant.
PARITY:	The number of pregnancies carried to the stage of viability irrespective of outcome and number of fetuses in a single pregnancy.
PRIMIPARA:	A woman who has completed one pregnancy.
PRIMIGRAVIDA:	A woman pregnant for the first time.
TOCOLYSIS:	The process of stopping labor; tocolytic drugs are now available to stop preterm labor and allow fetal maturation.
VERNIX:	Thick, white, cheesy substance composed of sebum and desquamated epithelial cells which covers the skin of the fetus in late-term pregnancy.

TABLE 57-2. CHARACTERISTICS OF TRUE VERSUS FALSE LABOR

TRUE LABOR
  Pain at regular intervals
  Intervals gradually shorten
  Intensity gradually increases
  Progressive cervical dilation and effacement
FALSE LABOR
  Pain at irregular intervals
  Intervals remain long
  Intensity remains unchanged
  No cervical dilation or effacement

unchanged or diminishing. More importantly, on repeated examinations, there is no cervical dilatation or effacement.

There are three stages of labor (Fig. 57-1). The first stage of labor starts with pain and cervical dilation and effacement, and ends when the cervix is fully dilated. The second stage begins with full dilation and effacement of the cervix, and is completed with delivery of the infant. This is the stage during which the mother is actively pushing. The third stage begins with the delivery of the infant and ends with the delivery of the placenta and fetal membranes.

The first stage of labor has commonly been divided into two distinct phases, latent and active. The latent phase can be anywhere from a few hours to as long as 20 hours in nulliparas and 14 hours in multiparas.

This phase is characterized by uterine contractions of milder intensity and shorter duration. The cervical dilation and effacement occur at a slower rate. During the active phase, in contrast, the cervix dilates rapidly at 1 to 2 cm per hour. The active phase begins at about 4 cm dilation. During the active phase of labor, dilation occurs in nulliparas at a minimum of 1.2 cm per hour and in multiparas at a minimum of 1.5 cm per hour. Generally speaking, mothers with a higher gravidity and parity have a faster labor. It must be assumed, however, when trying to anticipate these patterns, that obstetrics is predictably unpredictable.

The rapid nature of the second phase of labor is probably one of the factors that results in the delivery of some mothers in the field or the ED. More importantly, a few of these mothers are likely to be the victims of precipitate labor. Precipitate labor and delivery are those that are extremely rapid. A rapid, uncontrolled delivery with the mother pushing vigorously can cause rupture of the uterus or extensive lacerations of the cervix, vagina, vulva, or perineum. In addition, the fetus is subjected to an increased mortality and morbidity, as a result of poor uterine blood flow and oxygenation of the fetal blood during the vigorous labor, as well as direct trauma to the intracranial contents of the fetus as it is expelled explosively through the introitus. It is vitally important, therefore, for the ED personnel or physician to be available to control the delivery and prevent injury to the mother and fetus as well as be available for any needed resuscitation after the delivery.

PHYSICAL EXAMINATION

The basic documentation of the initial physical examination should always include a reference to amniotic fluid, cervical dilation and effacement, presenting part, and station. If the membranes have ruptured, the character of the fluid should be noted. Presence of vernix indicates a mature fetus and presence of meconium suggests fetal distress and mandates the need to prevent meconium aspiration during delivery. The amount of cervical dilation is determined by estimating the diameter of the cervical opening with two fingers in the vagina. The cervix is said to be maximally dilated when the diameter is 10 cm across or it can no longer be palpated. Cervical effacement is the length of the cervix compared to that of an uneffaced cervix. On the basis of previous experience, the examiner has a general idea of the normal length of a cervix, which is approximately 2 cm. When this cervix is reduced by one half, it is said to be 50% effaced. A cervix is 100% effaced when it becomes almost paper-thin, i.e., has no thickness. Presenting part refers to either cephalic or breech presentation. It is important for later management to be absolutely sure of the presenting

FIG. 57-1.   Progress of labor.

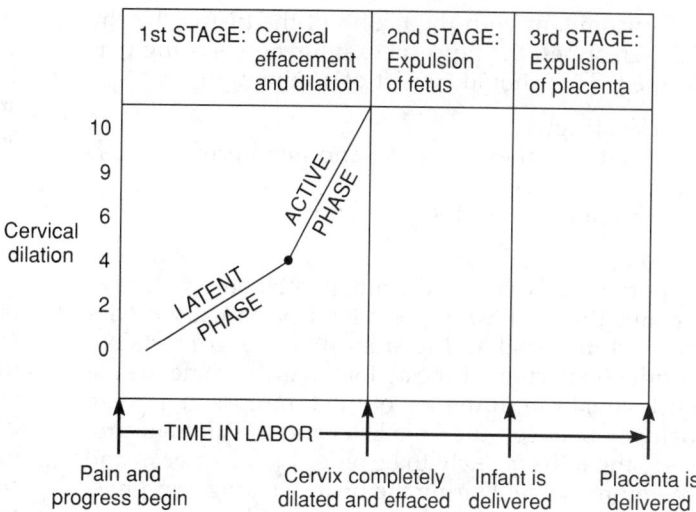

1st STAGE: Cervical effacement and dilation	2nd STAGE: Expulsion of fetus	3rd STAGE: Expulsion of placenta

Cervical dilation 10 9 6 4 2 0

ACTIVE PHASE
LATENT PHASE

— TIME IN LABOR —

Pain and progress begin Cervix completely dilated and effaced Infant is delivered Placenta is delivered

part as ascertained in the first examination. Station is the level of the presenting fetal part in the birth canal. The ischial spines felt as bony prominences in the vagina are about halfway between the pelvic inlet at the top of the birth canal and the pelvic outlet at the introitus. When the presenting part or top of the head is at the ischial spine, it is said to be at 0 station. When the presenting part is at the pelvic inlet, it is at a −3 station, and when it reaches the perineum, it is at a +3 station. When the presenting part is at 0 station and happens to be the vertex, engagement is said to have occurred. That is, the biggest part of the head must have passed through the pelvic inlet, and there is less likelihood for the umbilical cord to occupy the birth canal and therefore less chance of cord prolapse.

PREHOSPITAL ASSESSMENT AND STABILIZATION

The minimum amount of history to be obtained by the ED personnel includes:

Gravidity, parity, and abortion
Last normal menstrual period
Estimated date of confinement
Presence or absence of ruptured membranes
History of bleeding
Pregnancy or medical problems

The gravidity, parity, and abortion give some idea as to the rapidity with which delivery will occur. A primigravida (woman with her first pregnancy) has a slower labor than a multigravida (woman with several pregnancies).

The last normal menstrual period is important to know to estimate where the mother is in the course of this pregnancy. Be sure to note that the last normal

menstrual period is defined as the first day of the last menstrual period. A pregnancy wheel is most convenient for measuring the mother's gestational age. In general, fetuses with less than 26 weeks' gestation are considered pre-viable. In pregnancies of 26 to 37 weeks, fetuses are obviously premature and at higher risk. In pregnancies after 37 weeks and up to 42 weeks, fetuses are considered term. In pregnancies after 42 weeks, fetuses are post-term and again are at high risk.

It is also important to ask the mother her due date or estimated date of confinement. This might be different from what you calculate because her obstetrician might have changed it, based on his or her earlier examination or an ultrasound or other information.

Documentation of ruptured membranes is important because it may alert you to increased risk of infection if the membranes have been ruptured for a prolonged period of time (longer than 24 hours). Also, as noted earlier, the presence of vernix may indicate a term fetus and the presence of meconium may indicate a distressed fetus with the need for measures to prevent meconium aspiration at delivery.

The presence of bleeding may indicate serious complications such as placenta previa and placental abruption. A small amount of blood mixed with mucus indicates a bloody "show," and represents expulsion of the mucus plug from the cervix. If the mother states that a small amount of blood was mixed with mucus, it can be safely presumed that this is bloody show. If the mother states, however, that there has been bleeding without the presence of mucus and/or that the bleeding has been "more than a menstrual period," it must be presumed that there is a placenta previa until proven otherwise with ultrasound.

It is important also for ED personnel to ask the obvious question as to whether or not there have been any problems with the pregnancy. This may include not only problems with the pregnancy itself, but also any pre-existing medical problems.

Concomitant with the taking of the history by the ED personnel, the physical examination is being performed. This should consist of a minimum of:

Vital signs
Abdominal examination and monitoring of uterine contractions
Examination of the perineum

Among the vital signs, blood pressure is especially important because, by definition, a blood pressure of greater than 140/90 is pre-eclampsia, a cause of increased maternal and fetal morbidity and mortality. A brief inspection of the abdomen gives some idea of gestational age. If the top of the fundus is more than halfway between the umbilicus and the xiphoid process, the fetus is likely to be older than 26 weeks and therefore viable. During the history taking and physical examination, the examiner should have his or her hand on the patient's abdomen, monitoring for uterine contractions. The absence of frequent uterine contractions is somewhat reassuring in the prehospital setting because imminent delivery (delivery about to occur imminently or immediately) is not likely. Frequent and vigorous uterine contractions, however, may be predictive of imminent delivery, precipitate delivery, or placental abruption. If there is any possibility of imminent delivery, personnel should examine the perineum for perineal bulging, rectal bulging, and crowning of the fetal head.

PREHOSPITAL DELIVERY

Imminent delivery is characterized by uncontrollable pushing by the mother. At this time, the basic principle

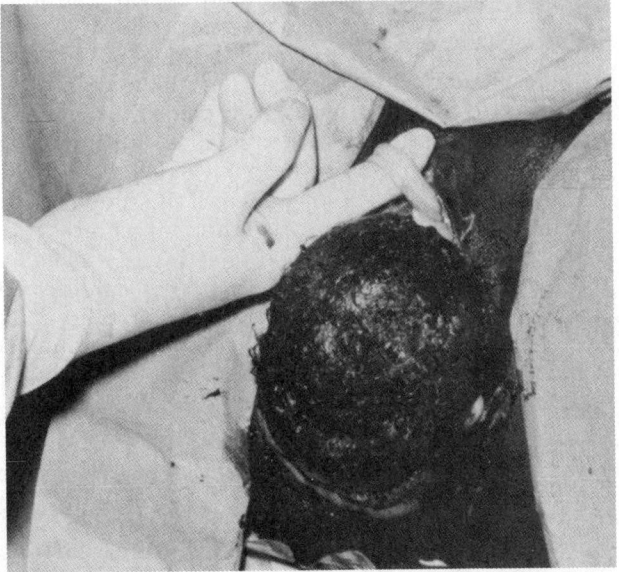

FIG. 57-2. Cord identified around the neck. It readily slipped over the head. With permission from Cunningham, F.G., MacDonald, P.C., and Gant, N.F.: Williams Obstetrics, 18th edition. Norwalk, CT, Appleton and Lange, 1989, p. 317.

must turn away from rapid transport of the mother to the hospital and instead change to immediate preparation for delivery in the field. Any attempt to restrain or delay delivery at this point by holding the baby's head back or crossing the mother's legs are absolutely contraindicated. Preparation should be made for a safe delivery with special emphasis on preventing trauma to the birth canal and fetus. In preparing for an imminent delivery, if time permits, a large-bore intravenous line is started to administer 5% dextrose and normal saline solution at approximately 100 cc per hour. A clean sheet is placed under the mother and the ED personnel should allow her to assume whatever position is most comfortable. This may be on her back with her knees flexed and her thighs separated, or perhaps on her side. When she is lying in the supine position, a pillow or firm pad can be placed under the buttocks to allow room for delivery of the fetal head and shoulders. The ED personnel, as time permits, should put on mask and eye protection, wash their hands, and put on sterile gloves. As noted earlier, whether or not these preparations are possible, the overriding principle is still delivery with minimal trauma to the mother and without injury to the child. The ED personnel should be instructed now to control the delivery of the presenting head. The palm of the hand is placed on the fetal head, and gentle pressure is exerted to provide a slow, controlled delivery. The mother is instructed to "pant" and not to push between contractions. Many times the uterine contractions alone deliver the head. If not, the mother can be asked to perform controlled pushing on command when the uterine contractions commence. After the uterine contraction is over, again the mother should be asked not to push.

As the head is delivered, it rotates to one side. At this time, wipe dry the face and suction the infant's nose and mouth with bulb suction. When meconium is present, special attention should be directed to removing the meconium to prevent its aspiration by the infant during or after delivery, which can cause significant and possibly fatal lung damage. When meconium is present, bulb suction can be used, but a 10 French (Fr) catheter or a DeLee suction catheter has been described to be more efficient for this purpose. The DeLee catheter or 10 Fr catheter should be hooked up to a suction unit and therefore avoid contact with the mouth of the operator. After suctioning of the fetus, the EMS personnel should palpate the top of the neck for loops of cord. If loops of cord are around the neck, gentle traction with the index finger will slip the cord down over the head (Fig. 57-2). After delivery of the fetal head and suctioning of the nose and mouth, gentle downward traction on the head and neck delivers the anterior shoulder first. Following delivery of the anterior shoulder, upward traction delivers the posterior shoulder, followed by the rest of the infant. A firm grip is maintained on the infant, holding it along the length of the operator's arm with the head slightly lower than the feet.

TABLE 57-3. APGAR SCORE			
	0	1	2
Heart rate	Absent	<100 min.	>100 min.
Respirations	Absent	Weak cry; hyperventilation	Good, strong cry
Muscle tone	Limp	Some flexion	Active
Reflex flexibility	No response	Grimace	Cough or sneeze
Color	Blue or pale	Body pink; blue extremities	Completely pink

After completion of the delivery, an Apgar score should be assigned to the infant at 1 minute and 5 minutes after birth (Table 57-3). The 1-minute Apgar score indicates need for immediate resuscitation, and the 5-minute Apgar score indicates increased risk of infant mortality and morbidity later on in the nursery. A score of less than 5 indicates severe neonatal depression at 1 minute, and a high-risk neonatal course at 5 minutes.

After delivery and suctioning, while the child is being vigorously dried, the umbilical cord should be cut by placing two clamps approximately 6 cm from the fetal abdomen. Cut between these two clamps, which have been placed approximately 2 cm apart. If the baby has a lusty cry, a heart rate greater than 100, and good muscle tone after wrapping, it should be presented to the mother. The placenta need not be delivered in the field but can be left in situ while the mother and baby are transported to the nearest ED.

It is important for ED personnel during a field delivery to document:

The precise time of birth (the time after the infant is completely delivered)
The Apgar score
The child's gender.

EMERGENCY DEPARTMENT MANAGEMENT

TRIAGE

All women who are pregnant and complaining of pain or bleeding are of highest priority and should be seen immediately. It is imperative to rule out in any pregnant woman the possibility of labor, abnormal presentation such as breech, or other complications such as a prolapsed cord. Any pregnant woman after rupture of her membranes should have a vaginal examination to rule out prolapsed cord. Vaginal bleeding may indicate placenta previa or placental abruption, and there is always a possibility of ongoing fetal distress, which may occur in a woman who is post-term or has pre-eclampsia, or a fetus with cord complications. The woman who is relatively comfortable in her second trimester, but is complaining of mild abdominal pain, may actually be in active labor with a premature fetus and is in need of immediate tocolysis to stop her labor and save her baby. Many pregnancy complications requiring emergency intervention might not be evident in the average pregnant patient waiting her turn for care. Therefore, because of the occult nature of these emergencies, these patients should be seen as a highest priority in the ED.

Once a diagnosis of active labor is made, it should be understood that the best place for delivery is in the labor and delivery suite. In most situations, the ED is a difficult place to keep a dedicated space available for deliveries with the capability of maintaining aseptic technique and all the equipment and personnel available to help in a delivery. More importantly, there is no capability in the emergency department to perform the most definitive therapy for most major complications, that is, cesarean section. Therefore, after the patient has been properly evaluated in the ED, there should be a policy and procedure to allow a patient who is about to deliver to be transported rapidly to the labor and delivery suite, where she may be monitored by trained obstetric nurses, who are more comfortable with this type of patient. Even if the obstetrician or gynecologist is not available at the time, it is still safer for the emergency physician to deliver the mother in the labor and delivery suite, where perinatal nurses and neonatologists who are experts in resuscitation are most comfortable with this task and, more importantly, have their necessary warmers, airway equipment, umbilical lines, and other equipment.

When the delivery is imminent, however, and the mother is about to deliver before she can be safely transported to the labor and delivery suite, preparations for delivery in the ED must be made and there should be policies and procedures and adequate equipment in place to facilitate the emergency delivery wherever the patient happens to be.

DELIVERY

Delivery of the patient in active labor in the ED department should proceed the same as in the labor and delivery suite. A brief history and physical examination are done while the patient is receiving a large-bore intravenous line to instill a crystalloid solution. In the history, special attention is, of course, aimed at gravidity, parity, estimated date of confinement, problems with this pregnancy, and whether or not the patient has had ruptured membranes, bloody show, or vaginal bleeding. If there is a history of ruptured membranes and delivery is not imminent, this should be confirmed using nitrazine paper. The method is to insert a sterile speculum into the vagina. A cotton-tipped applicator is used to retrieve secretions from the vaginal vault. The cotton-tipped applicator is then pressed against a strip of nitrazine paper, and if the nitrazine strip turns blue, indicating a basic pH, the membranes are likely to be ruptured. Normally, the vagina is acidic and the paper stays yellow or green. Amniotic fluid is more basic and therefore turns the nitrazine paper blue. Contamination with blood, however, is also basic and confuses the test by also turning the nitrazine paper blue.

If the patient states that she has had vaginal bleeding, the physician needs to determine whether this is simply bloody show or an actual episode of pathologic bleeding. The differentiation is critical. Bloody show occurs early in labor and is a result of expulsion of the mucus plug from the cervix along with a little blood. Bloody show is characterized by a small amount of bleeding mixed with mucus. This is common, and when there is a clear history of a bloody show, the physician can go ahead and perform a pelvic examination without worry. If there is a significant amount of blood with no mucus mixed with it, however, one must consider the possibility of third-trimester bleeding. An important cause of third-trimester bleeding is placenta previa, and if an examination is performed on a patient with placenta previa, trauma to the placenta by the physician's fingers causes disruption of the placental vessels and resultant immediate catastrophic exsanguination of the mother on the examining table. It is therefore vitally important to defer pelvic examination on any pregnant woman having third-trimester bleeding. Patients with third-trimester bleeding should be immediately taken to the labor and delivery suite where the routine procedure is to institute large-bore intravenous lines, external fetal monitoring, appropriate blood studies including type and cross, and emergency ultrasound to obtain a definitive diagnosis. Antibiotics may be needed and should be given *early* to avoid infectious complications in mother and child.

If the history confirms that there has been no significant vaginal bleeding, a vaginal examination can be done. The first vaginal examination should be done with a clean glove, using sterile lubricant if the membranes have not ruptured. After the membranes have ruptured, a betadine solution may be used as a lubricant. The reason why the betadine solution is not used initially is that it may discolor the vaginal secretions, and when the membranes do rupture, the dark color of the betadine solution will be confused for meconium. The vaginal examination should determine the effacement and dilation of the cervix, the presenting part, and its station. Early on, it is again vitally important to be definitely sure of the presenting part because it is dangerous to allow a breech or shoulder or cord presentation to labor benignly without appropriate preparations for delivery.

Recommendations for monitoring fetal heart tones have been outlined in *Guidelines for Perinatal Care* (Table 57-4). Low-risk patients are monitored by auscultation of the fetal heart every 30 minutes after a contraction in the active phase of the first stage of labor and at least every 15 minutes in the second stage of labor. High-risk patients are monitored by either continuous electronic fetal monitoring or by more diligent auscultation at intervals of 15 minutes during the active phase of the first stage of labor and 5 minutes during the second stage of labor. Auscultation should be done immediately after a uterine contraction. When electronic fetal monitoring is used, the tracing should be monitored and initialed at comparable times during the first and second stages of labor.

In preparation for the delivery, the mother is placed in a position that is comfortable for her as well as effective for the physician who will be involved in administering analgesia and controlling the delivery. In the United States, the lithotomy position is generally used for vaginal delivery; however, many physicians have experience with and prefer the lateral or partial sitting position. The vulva and perineum are cleansed and sterile drapes applied. The physician dons scrub suit, mask, headgear, and protective eyewear; scrubs hands and forearms; and puts on water-

	First Stage (Active Phase)	Second Stage
High risk	Auscultate every 15 minutes	Auscultate every 5 minutes
Low risk	Auscultate every 30 minutes	Auscultate every 15 minutes

TABLE 57-4. RECOMMENDED FETAL HEART RATE MONITORING

repellant gown and gloves. The major goal now is to prevent a precipitous delivery, which would cause maternal or fetal trauma.

An episiotomy is an incision of the perineum and vaginal mucosa made just before delivery of the fetal head to avoid tearing of this area and prevention of later pelvic relaxation to avoid cystocele, rectocele, and urinary incontinence (Fig. 57-3). The procedure is simply performed by taking a straight scissors and, just before the fetal head is delivered, cutting down the perineum as well as up into the vaginal mucosa. (This same incision can be actually extended into the rectum for emergency situations such as shoulder dystocia and breech delivery.) There has been much debate recently, however, regarding whether or not the attributes of episiotomy are merely theoretic. In general, the episiotomy can be avoided in multiparous patients with a controlled delivery of the fetal head. In primiparous patients, when a laceration is considered likely, a midline episiotomy should be performed. Episiotomy is contraindicated in only a few conditions. These include cases of inflammatory bowel disease, lymphogranuloma venereum, severe perianal scarring and malformation, and perhaps coagulation disorders such as idiopathic thrombocytopenic purpura. A method of repair for episiotomy is found in Figure 57-4. As delivery proceeds, the goal is to prevent a precipitous delivery that would cause maternal or fetal trauma. This can be done by gently applying guidance to the fetal head and slight pressure on the perineum of the mother, and asking her to control her pushing by intermittently panting or blowing (Fig. 57-5). The normal expulsive forces of the uterus, combined with the controlled pushing of the mother, result in a controlled delivery of the fetal head, slow and progressive and not quick and explosive. After the fetal head is delivered, external rotation of the head to the side occurs and the mouth and nose are suctioned with a bulb aspirator. The neck should be checked for loops of umbilical cord (see subsequent section of this chapter). Next, the anterior shoulder is delivered by gently pulling the head by the neck in a downward position, then the posterior shoulder, and finally the body.

The third stage of labor, or delivery of the placenta, takes place after placental separation. Signs of placental separation include the following:

1. The uterus becomes globular and more firm. This is the earliest sign to appear.
2. A sudden gush of blood.
3. The uterus rises into the abdomen as the placenta passes into the vagina, where its bulk pushes the uterus upward.
4. The umbilical cord protrudes 2 or 3 inches farther out of the vagina, an indication that the placenta is descending.

Placental separation usually occurs anywhere from 1 to 20 minutes after delivery of the baby. If the physician is not sure if there has been placental separation

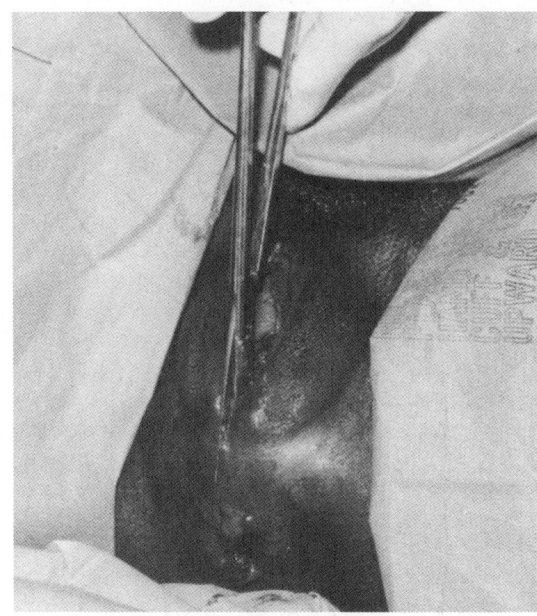

FIG. 57-3. Vulva partially distended by fetal head. Midline episiotomy being made. With permission from Cunningham, F.G., MacDonald, P.C., and Gant, N.F.: Williams Obstetrics, 18th edition. Norwalk, CT, Appleton and Lange, 1989, p. 316.

or not, the gloved examination hand can be placed up into the vagina to confirm that the placenta is actually sitting in the vagina, away and distinct from the cervix and uterus. Gentle traction on the cord then delivers the placenta, which should be checked for its integrity. If parts of the placenta are missing, retained products of conception should be considered and the obstetrician/gynecologist should be so informed.

Special mention should be made of proper airway management in the fetus with meconium staining. Meconium is the greenish-black contents of the fetal bowel; it consists of undigested debris from swallowed amniotic fluid as well as desquamated gastrointestinal cells and other products of secretion and excretion from the bowel. Its greenish-black color is produced by biliverdin. Normally, there is no evacuation of the bowel while the fetus is in utero. The presence of meconium staining has a strong correlation with fetal distress. Meconium staining of the amniotic fluid occurs in approximately 10% of all pregnant patients at delivery. It may occur in 44% of postdate pregnancies. If the meconium is aspirated by the fetus, meconium aspiration syndrome occurs. This syndrome has a mortality rate as high as 28%, and therefore, the ideal method of care is to prevent the aspiration. The infant should be suctioned immediately after delivery of the head, before the fetus has a chance to expand its lungs. The nose and then the mouth, oropharynx, and hypopharynx are suctioned using a DeLee suction catheter or 10 Fr suction catheter. To prevent injury to the fetus's airway, use suction pressures of less than 100 mm Hg. While the body is still in the birth canal, the chest is compressed and there is no chance of the fetus

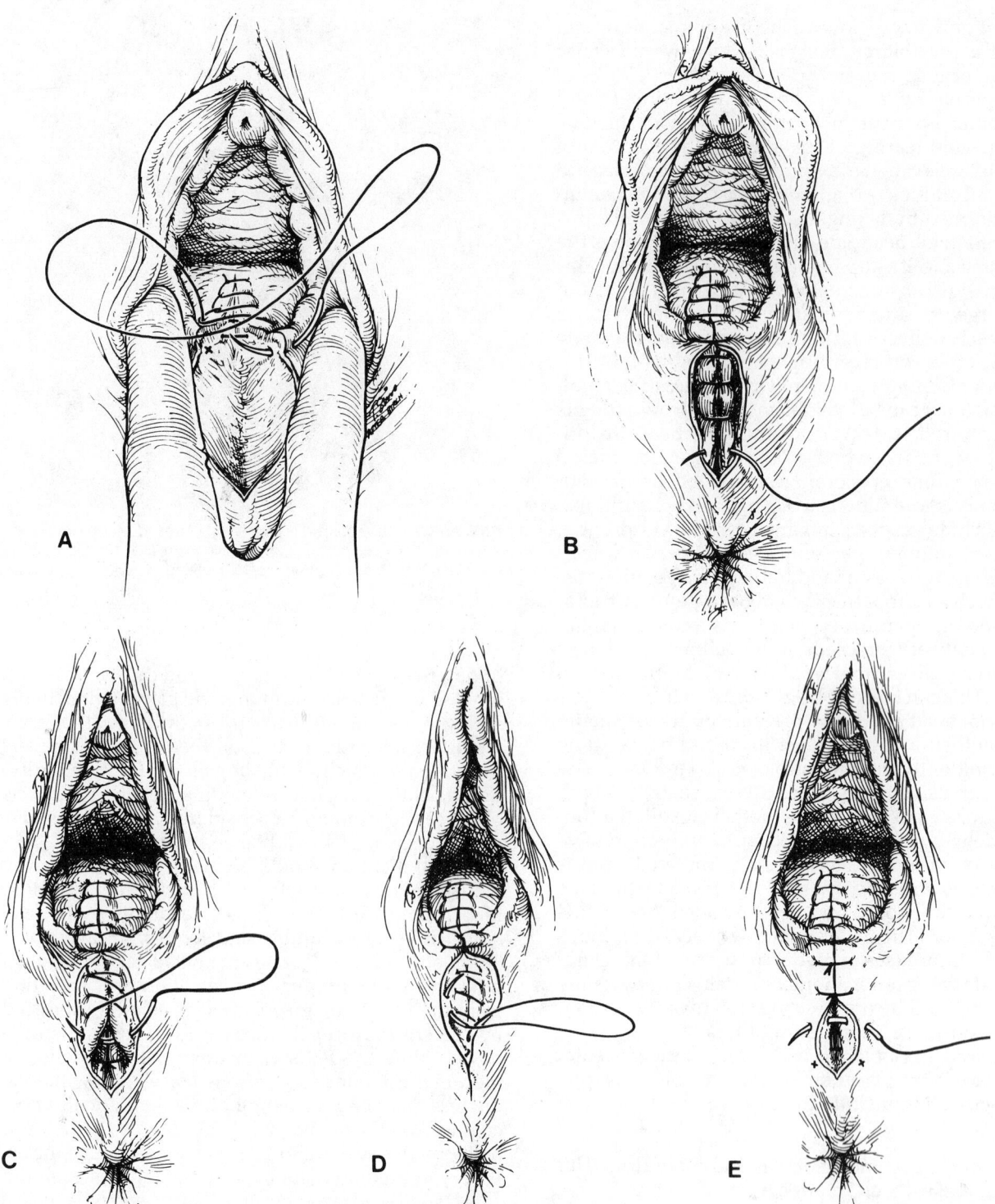

FIG. 57-4. Repair of median episiotomy. A. Chromic catgut 00, or preferably 000, is used as a continuous suture to close the vaginal mucosa and submucosa. B. After closing the vaginal incision and reapproximating the cut margins of the hymenal ring, the suture is tied and cut. Next, three or four interrupted sutures of 00 or 000 catgut are placed in the fascia and muscle of the incised perineum. C. A continuous suture is now carried downward to unite the superficial fascia. D. Completion of repair. The continuous suture is carried upward as a subcuticular stitch. (An alternative method of closure of skin and subcutaneous fascia is illustrated in E.) E. Completion of repair of median episiotomy. A few interrupted sutures of 000 chromic catgut are placed through the skin and subcutaneous fascia and loosely tied. This closure avoids burying two layers of catgut in the more superficial layers of the perineum. With permission from Cunningham, F.G., MacDonald, P.C., and Gant, N.F.: Williams Obstetrics, 18th edition. Norwalk, CT, Appleton and Lange, 1989, p. 324.

expanding its lungs to take a breath and aspirating the meconium. After thorough suctioning of the nose, mouth, oropharynx, and hypopharynx, the rest of the delivery proceeds. After delivery, the infant is placed on the examination table and laryngoscopy is used to visualize the cords. If meconium is present in the hypopharynx or on the cords, then endotracheal intubation is done and further suctioning below the cords is performed.

After the placenta is delivered, the primary mechanism by which hemostasis is achieved is the contraction of the myometrium, which compresses the uterine vessels and thus stops bleeding. Agents used to assist in this myometrial contraction include oxytocin, ergonovine, and methylergonovine. Because of the tendency for ergonovine and methylergonovine to cause a precipitous rise in blood pressure, oxytocin is the drug of choice because it is much easier and safer to use. The route of administration is 20 units of oxytocin in one liter of crystalloid solution to run in at approximately 100 cc per hour. Oxytocin can be given in 10 units intramuscularly, but should never be given as an intravenous bolus because this latter route can result in episodes of hypotension. Also, oxytocin should always be given in a crystalloid solution (lactated Ringer's or normal saline) because of its antidiuretic effect. If it is given in a dextrose and water solution, the antidiuretic effect may cause water intoxication and seizures in the mother.

The final, most important step in completing delivery is to check for genitourinary trauma. Immediately after delivery of the placenta, when the vagina has been stretched to its maximum, the best examination can be done with the least discomfort to the mother. The physician should be vigorous in putting four fingers of the left hand well into the vagina, thus pushing down the posterior floor of the vagina to reveal the cervix. Ring forceps are then used to grasp the anterior lip of the cervix and traction is applied in a downward and then upward motion to expose the entire cervical os. Only in this way can the physician be 100% assured that there are no actively bleeding tears on the cervix. When this has been ascertained, the ring forceps are disengaged, and several 4 × 4 gauze sponges are placed in the ring forceps. This bulky probe is then placed back into the vagina to push the cervix up and out of the way of the posterior vaginal wall. By continued pressure with the left hand pushing the floor of the vagina down and now pushing the cervix out of the way with the gauze bandages on the end of the forceps, the posterior wall of the vagina over the ischial spines can be visualized. It is not uncommon for a tear to occur over the ischial spines, i.e., the inferolateral wall of the vagina. These tears can be deep and not necessarily extend out into the introitus, and therefore can be missed if not checked for. This is the ideal time to diagnose this lesion, not several hours later when the mother is hemorrhaging. Next, the vulva should be examined, including the periurethral structures. Minor periurethral tears can be ignored, but

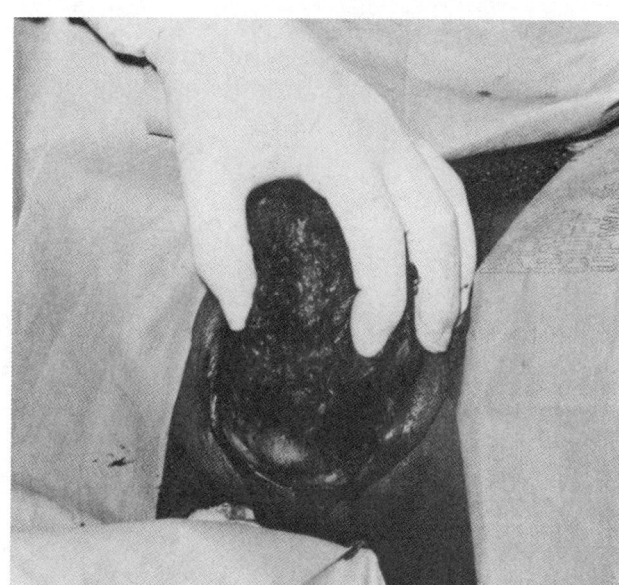

FIG. 57-5. Pressure is applied through the towel covering the hand on the underside of the chin of the infant as soon as the occiput is behind the symphysis. This extends the head. At the same time, the fingers of the other hand simultaneously elevate the scalp to help extend the head. With permission from Cunningham, F.G., MacDonald, P.C., and Gant, N.F.: Williams Obstetrics, 18th edition. Norwalk, CT, Appleton and Lange, 1989, p. 317.

any periurethral tears involving subcutaneous tissues or those with active bleeding should be reapproximated with absorbable suture. Whenever suturing around the urethra, a Foley catheter should always be in place to ensure proper localization of the urethra so that no sutures can be placed through this structure. The most common site of tears, however, are the lacerations that occur in the perineal areas. These are labeled first-, second-, third-, and fourth-degree lacerations (Table 57-5) and are repaired as illustrated (Fig. 57-6).

COMPLICATIONS OF DELIVERY

A detailed analysis and understanding of all obstetric emergencies is beyond the scope of practice of emergency physicians for several reasons. First of all, the management for many obstetric emergencies is ce-

TABLE 57-5. CLASSIFICATION OF LACERATIONS OF THE VAGINA AND PERINEUM

FIRST-DEGREE:	Laceration of the fourchet, perineal skin, and vaginal mucosa
SECOND-DEGREE:	First degree with extension into the fascia and muscle of the perineal body
THIRD-DEGREE:	Second degree with extension into the anal sphincter
FOURTH-DEGREE:	Third degree with extension into the rectal mucosa

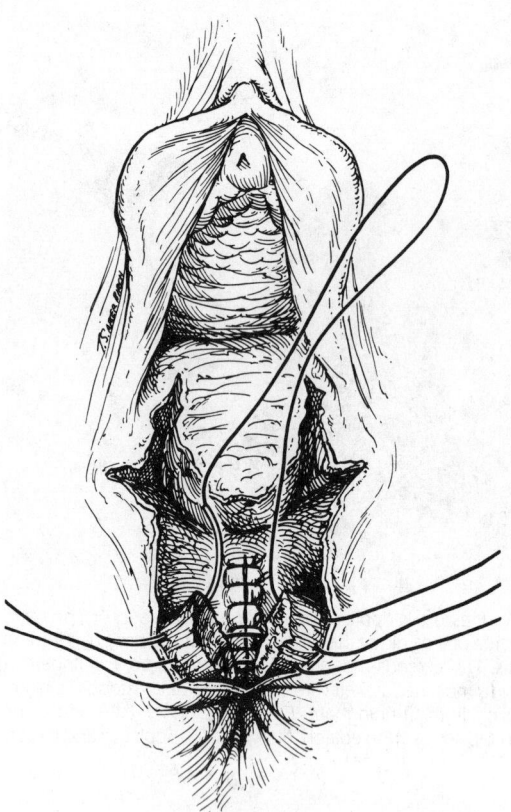

FIG. 57-6.   Repair of complete perineal tear. The rectal mucosa has been repaired with interrupted, fine chromic catgut sutures. The torn ends of the sphincter ani are next approximated with two or three interrupted chromic catgut sutures. The wound is then repaired, as in a second-degree laceration or an episiotomy. With permission from Cunningham, F.G., MacDonald, P.C., and Gant, N.F.: Williams Obstetrics, 18th edition. Norwalk, CT, Appleton and Lange, 1989, p. 325.

sarean section, which can be done neither in the field nor in the ED. In a study by Cavanaugh,[4] *almost 90% of the obstetric emergencies occurring in a prehospital setting are related to hemorrhage.* Therefore, most obstetric emergencies cannot be definitively cared for in the field or in the ED. Second, many obstetric complications are extremely rare. For example, acute uterine inversion occurs in 1 in 5,000 to 1 in 20,000 cases.

When the emergency physician does see such a complication, it is vitally important to know what to do to save the life of the mother or fetus. Certain complications should be recognized and immediately referred to the labor and delivery suite for definitive care. These include breech presentation, which is likely to need cesarean section or at least delivery by an experienced obstetrician/gynecologist. Patients with third-trimester bleeding should also be immediately referred to rule out the possibility of placenta previa or placental abruption. After placenta previa is diagnosed by emergency ultrasound, the patient must have a cesarean section. And finally, of course, fetal distress, when there is no chance of imminent delivery, must be referred to labor and delivery for immediate cesarean section.

PROLAPSED CORD

Other complications also need definitive care in the labor and delivery suite, but certain antecedent maneuvers can be undertaken to stabilize the situation. For example, prolapsed cord, when identified, is handled by placing the mother in the Trendelenburg or knee-chest position, and elevating the fetal part to prevent compression of the cord between the fetal presenting part and the pelvic bones of the mother. If compression of the cord can be prevented in this manner, the mother is rapidly transferred to the labor and delivery suite for emergency cesarean section.

UTERINE INVERSION

Another entity that can occur in the prehospital setting or the ED after delivery is acute uterine inversion. This occurs when the umbilical cord is tugged too vigorously in an attempt to deliver the placenta and the placenta and uterus, in an inside-out fashion, prolapse out of the vagina. This presents as a large, bleeding mass the exact size of a postpartum uterus but inverted on the outside of the vagina, often with the mother in shock. The treatment is to replace the uterus back in the vagina immediately by applying pressure to the inverted tip of the uterus and folding it back inside itself as if turning a sock inside out (Fig. 57-7). After the uterus is placed back into the vagina, the physician's hand, in the form of a fist, should be held up into the now normally placed uterus inside the mother until the uterus has a chance to clamp down around the fist and hemostasis is accomplished.

POSTPARTUM HEMORRHAGE

Another complication that can be stabilized in the ED before transfer to labor and delivery is early postpartum hemorrhage, defined as the loss of 500 mL or more of blood after delivery. As noted earlier, a thorough examination most often delineates the cause of a potential postpartum hemorrhage before it occurs. After the placenta is delivered, it is carefully examined for any missing cotyledons. If parts of the placenta are missing, retained products of conception are likely to be the cause of bleeding. A thorough examination of the vagina as described previously reveals whether or not the bleeding source is from laceration of the cervix, vagina, or vulva. If these have all been checked beforehand and postpartum hemorrhage does occur, the most likely cause is uterine atony or an inability of the uterus to contract down, compress its vessels, and therefore control its hemorrhage. The immediate therapy is to massage the uterus vigorously through the abdominal wall, encouraging uterine contractions and therefore, hemostasis. At the same time, the mother is receiving oxytocin in a crystalloid infusion, approximately 20 units per liter at 200 cc per hour. If

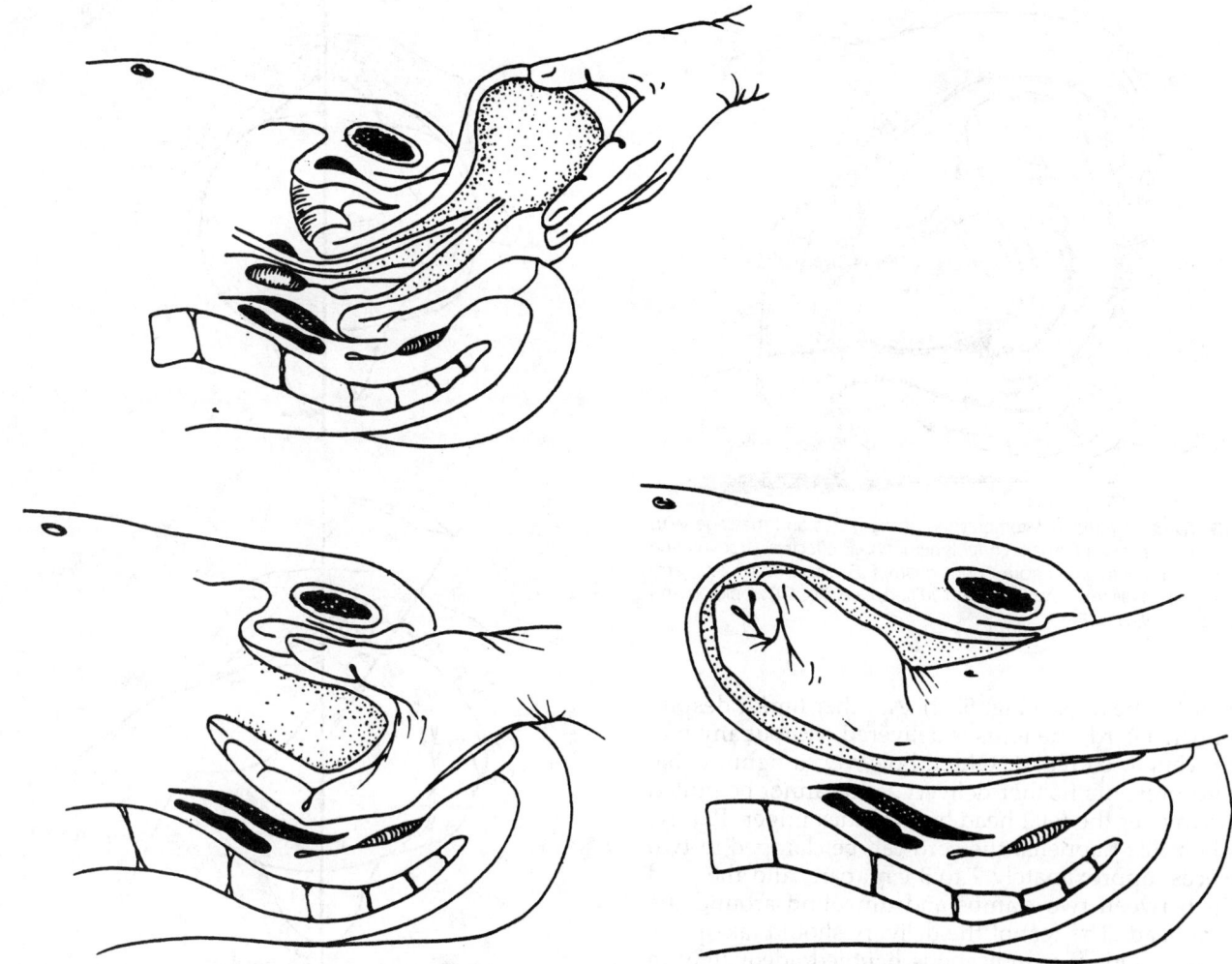

FIG. 57-7.   To reposition an inverted uterus, first push it gently toward the back of the vagina (left). Once the organ is inside, aim it with steady pressure upward toward the umbilicus (below, left). When the organ is back in place and the placenta has been detached, put your hand back inside the uterus to make sure that it is not reinverting (below).

this does not work, methylergonovine (Methergine), 0.2 mg, is administered intramuscularly or intravenously. Great care should be taken when giving methylergonovine because it may cause hypertension and exacerbate pre-eclampsia. Prostaglandin F-2 alpha (Prostin/15 M) has been approved by the Food and Drug Administration (FDA) for the treatment of postpartum hemorrhage from uterine atony. If this is available in the ED, it should be given as a 250 mcg (0.25 mg) dose intramuscularly. This is repeated if necessary at 15- and 90-minute intervals. Again, prostaglandin F-2 alpha should be monitored carefully because it may cause precipitous hypertension. If none of these rapid sequence measures seem to help, bimanual uterine compression can be used to control hemorrhage until help arrives (Fig. 57-8). Help consists of ensuring additional intravenous lines for fluid resuscitation, appropriate blood studies including clotting studies, type, and cross, and calling the obstetrician for possible surgical intervention including emergency cu-

rettage as well as exploratory laparotomy, which may entail uterine artery ligation, hypogastric artery ligation, and/or emergency hysterectomy.

Late postpartum hemorrhage occurs after the first 24 hours postpartum, in the puerperium. It is most often caused by retained products of conception, but can be caused by infection, subinvolution of the placental site, episiotomy breakdown, or dehiscence of a cesarean section incision.

NUCHAL CORD

Some obstetric emergencies can be handled adequately in the ED if they happen to occur there. The first of these is nuchal cord, or cord wrapped tightly around the neck noticed after delivery of the fetal head. Most times, an index finger can be placed over the top of the fetal neck and the cord pulled down

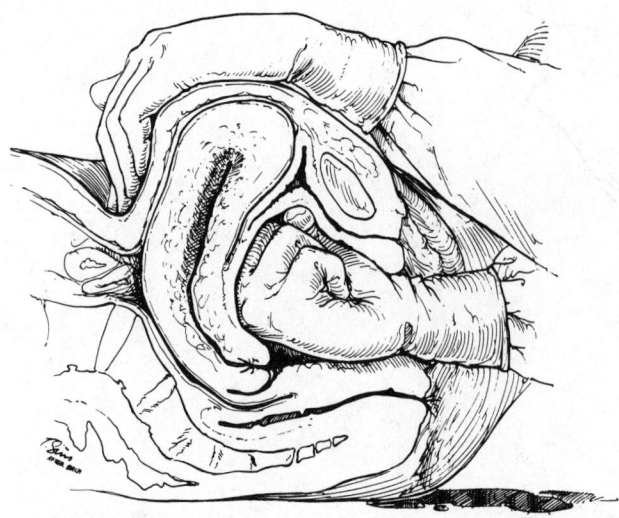

FIG. 57-8. Bimanual compression of the uterus and massage with the abdominal hand usually controls hemorrhage effectively from uterine atony. With permission from Cunningham, F.G., MacDonald, P.C., and Gant, N.F.: Williams Obstetrics, 18th edition. Norwalk, CT, Appleton and Lange, 1989, p. 418.

over the head (see Fig. 57-2). At other times, despite a nuchal cord, the fetus is delivered without any maneuvers to correct it. Often, however, a tight nuchal cord prevents further delivery, and cannot be pulled down over the fetal head by the index finger. Rarely, when this happens, the cord can be clamped in two places, approximately 2 to 3 cm apart, and the cord cut between two clamps and unwound around the fetal head. The rest of the delivery should take place rapidly. Other complications handled adequately in the ED have been discussed previously and include management of meconium staining and repair of vulvar and perineal lacerations.

SHOULDER DYSTOCIA

Finally, attention should be directed toward one of the most serious complications of delivery, which must be handled immediately regardless of where the delivery occurs. Shoulder dystocia occurs after the delivery of the fetal head and is a result of the shoulders being too large for the birth canal and the anterior shoulder impacting itself against the symphysis pubis. The fetus is essentially stuck in this position, with its cord already drawn into the pelvis and compressed between the fetus and the bony parts of the pelvis. Pressure above the symphysis may occasionally bring the shoulder into the pelvis. Immediate delivery must ensue or the fetus will die in a matter of minutes. If pressure does not work, the quickest, easiest method to relieve this situation is to make a proctoepisiotomy by cutting the episiotomy all the way into the rectum to achieve the greatest room possible. The physician should then try to rotate the shoulders one way or the other in a "corkscrew" maneuver (Fig. 57-9). By

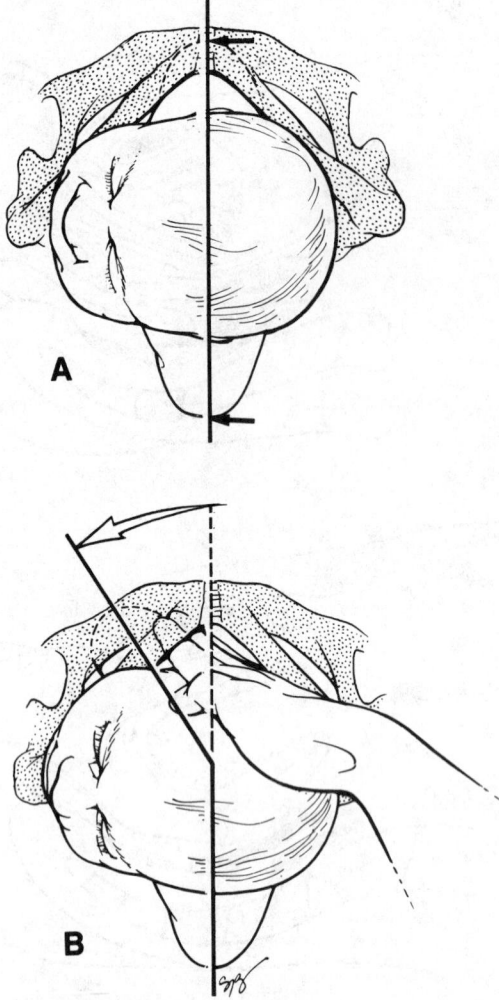

FIG. 57-9. Rubin's (second) maneuver. A. The shoulder-to-shoulder diameter is shown as the distance between the two small arrows. B. The most easily accessible fetal shoulder (the anterior is shown here) is pushed toward the anterior chest wall of the fetus. Most often, this results in abduction of both shoulders, reducing the shoulder-to-shoulder diameter and freeing the impacted anterior shoulder. With permission from Cunningham, F.G., MacDonald, P.C., and Gant, N.F.: Williams Obstetrics, 18th edition. Norwalk, CT, Appleton and Lange, 1989, p. 369.

taking two fingers of the examining hand, putting them into the vagina, and pushing the most easily accessible shoulder toward the chest, the physician reduces the shoulder-to-shoulder diameter, which may free the impacted anterior shoulder. If this does not work by pushing the shoulder away from the chest, rotation of the entire thorax can also result in dislodgement. If this is not successful, a final attempt is now made to grasp the posterior hand and deliver the posterior shoulder to relieve the obstruction. The physician should place the examining hand into the vagina along the fetus's posterior humerus. When this is identified, the humerus is then swept across the chest of the fetus; the hand is then grasped and the arm and shoulder are pulled out of the vagina. Delivering the posterior arm and therefore the shoulder

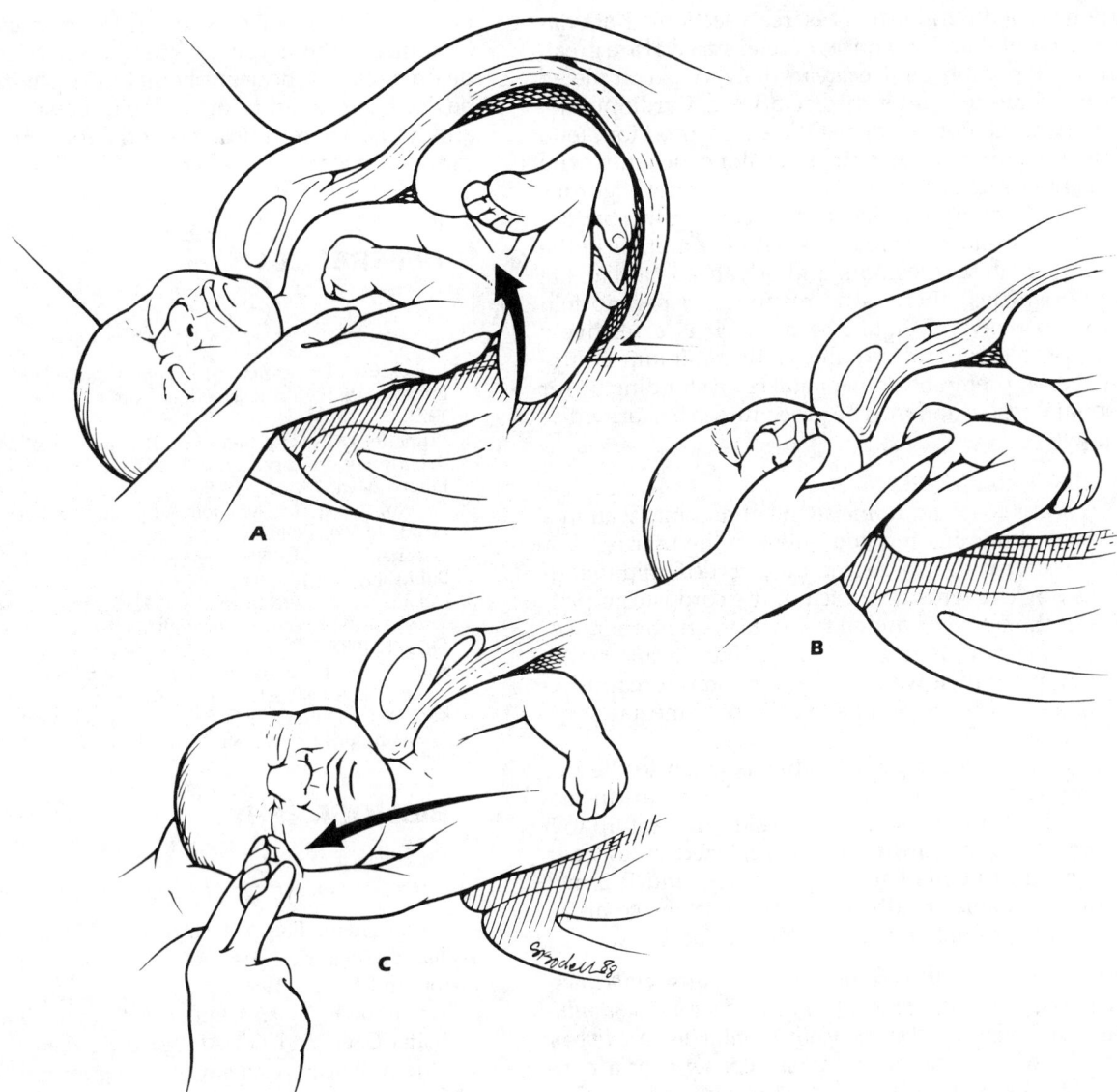

FIG. 57-10.   Shoulder dystocia with impacted anterior shoulder of the fetus. A. The operator's hand is introduced into the vagina along the fetal posterior humerus, which is splinted as the arm is swept across the chest, keeping the arm flexed at the elbow. B. The fetal hand is grasped and the arm extended along the side of the face. C. The posterior arm is delivered from the vagina. With permission from Cunningham, F.G., MacDonald, P.C., and Gant, N.F.: Williams Obstetrics, 18th edition. Norwalk, CT, Appleton and Lange, 1989.

disimpacts the anterior shoulder and delivery can ensue (Fig. 57-10).

PERIMORTEM SALVAGE

PERIMORTEM/POSTMORTEM CESAREAN SECTION

Postmortem cesarean sections have been performed since antiquity. There are many reports in the literature of the survival of the infant after a postmortem cesarean section done because of the sudden, unexpected death of the mother from trauma or other catastrophic medical complication. The fear has always been of performing a cesarean section too soon when the mother is actually not yet dead. *Several recent cases from the literature, however, have indicated that a postmortem cesarean section not only is an opportunity for saving the fetus, but also may result in greater likelihood for maternal survival.* Several cases have now been reported in which a postmortem cesarean section has resulted in survival of the mother, which might not have occurred if the postmortem cesarean section had not been immediately done.[5,6] Because these postmortem cesarean sections are done not only to save the fetus but also possibly to save the mother, they should properly be called perimortem cesarean sections. Katz has pointed out that the chances of fetal survival are greatest if the perimortem cesarean delivery is completed within 5 minutes after cardiac arrest.[7] Cardiopulmonary resuscitation is not an efficient method for blood flow dynamics for the mother, let alone the fetus, who quickly becomes anoxic. Therefore, if after vigorous cardiopulmonary resuscitation (including intubation, external cardiac compressions with the mother in the lateral decubitus position, and advanced cardiac life support drugs) there is no response, a perimortem cesarean delivery should be done. It is a relatively easy procedure and requires only minimum equipment and, preferably, a neonatal team standing by for neonatal resuscitation. The procedure is performed as follows:

1. CPR is continued.
2. A scalpel is used to incise the abdominal wall in a vertical midline incision down to the uterus.
3. The uterus is also incised by a vertical midline incision. The fetus is extracted, the cord is clamped, and the fetus is handed to the team in attendance.
4. The placenta is removed next. The uterine cavity and abdominal wall can be temporarily reapproximated with towel clips to control hemostasis.
5. Continue CPR.
6. If survival occurs, the mother is taken to the operating suite for definite repair of her cesarean section incision. Although survival is greatest up to 5 minutes after cardiac arrest, reported cases have been documented for longer times, and it is not unreasonable to attempt a perimortem cesarean section up to 25 minutes after cardiac arrest.

The perimortem cesarean section, in view of these guidelines, is truly an emergency procedure in which seconds and minutes may decide whether the mother and fetus will live or die. Therefore, whether to obtain consent for a perimortem cesarean section from the family is a moot point. It is well established in the medical and legal literature that emergency situations involving life and death circumstances imply that the right thing should be done at the right time in the interest of the mother and fetus. There is little potential for criminal offense in this strategy.

REFERENCES

1. Hobel, C.J., Hyvarinen, M.A., and Okada, D.M.: Prenatal and intrapartum high risk screening. Am. J. Obstet. Gynecol. *117*:1, 1973.
2. Brunette, D.D., and Sterner, S.P.: Prehospital and emergency department delivery: A review of eight years' experience. Ann. Emerg. Med. *18*:1116, 1989.
3. Paneth, N., et al.: The choice of place of delivery. Am. J. Dis. Child. *141*:60, 1986.
4. Cavanagh, D.: Obstetric emergencies. New York, Harper & Row Publishers, 1982.
5. DePace, N.L., Betesh, J.S., and Kotle, M.N.: Post-mortem cesarean section recovery of both mother and offspring. JAMA *248*:971, 1982.
6. Marx, G.F.: Cardiopulmonary resuscitation of late pregnant women. J. Anesthesiol. *56*:156, 1982.
7. Katz, V.L., Dotters, D.J., and Druegemueller, W.: Perimortem cesarean delivery. Obstet. Gynecol. *68*:571, 1986.

BIBLIOGRAPHY

Cunningham, F.G., MacDonald, P.C., and Gant, N.F.: Williams Obstetrics, 18th ed. Norwalk, Connecticut, Appleton and Lange, 1989.

Frigoletto, F.D., and Little, G.A. (eds.): Guideline for Perinatal Care, 2nd Ed. American Academy of Pediatrics and the American Academy of Obstetrics and Gynecology, 1988.

ECTOPIC PREGNANCY

Russell J. Carlisle

CAPSULE

Ectopic pregnancy remains a leading cause of maternal mortality. Despite a decrease in the overall mortality from this disorder, the incidence continues to rise because of epidemic increases in sexually transmitted diseases, pelvic surgery and instrumentation, and changing patterns of contraception, especially the use of IUDs. In the United States, it remains the leading cause of first-trimester death and the third leading cause of nontraumatic maternal death overall. Improved rates of diagnosis will certainly result from increased clinical suspicion and the prompt use of improved pregnancy tests in reproductive-age women who present with gynecologic, obstetric, and gastrointestinal complaints. Because serum hCG levels in ectopic pregnancy are often lower than in normal pregnancy, tests for the beta subunit or intact molecule of human chorionic gonadotrophin must be sensitive to <10 mIU/mL to detect at least 99% of ectopic pregnancies. Such tests are now widely available and rapidly performed. Ultrasonography, now of higher resolution and availability, can then be used in most instances to establish an intrauterine or extrauterine location of the pregnancy. Traditional diagnostic tests such as culdocentesis, laparoscopy, or laparotomy can supplement or replace sonography in more urgent or less optimal situations. Observation, stabilization, and consultation with the gynecologist remain essential. Women with possible ectopic pregnancy should not leave the Emergency Department (ED) until pregnancy has been excluded, intrauterine pregnancy has been confirmed, or gynecologic consultation and definite followup have been arranged.

GENERAL CONSIDERATIONS

Ectopic pregnancy is a potentially lethal disorder that is increasingly encountered in the ED. Diagnosis may be difficult, especially with early presentation. The incidence of ectopic pregnancy continues to increase dramatically, but despite improved diagnostic techniques and a decrease in the death rate, ectopic pregnancy remains the leading cause of maternal death in early pregnancy.[1] Many preventable deaths still occur, both among women with early presentation of the disorder and those seeking their first health care late in the course of the disorder when rapid intervention may still not be lifesaving. Prompt diagnosis at any stage of the disorder is essential to ensure maternal survival, decrease disability, and conserve reproductive ability.

DEFINITION

Pregnancy is defined as ectopic when the fertilized ovum implants elsewhere than the endometrial cavity of the uterus. Tubal pregnancies constitute more than 95% of all ectopic pregnancies. These occur primarily in the ampulla and isthmus and, much less commonly, in the infundibulum (or fimbria) and interstitium. Nontubal ectopic pregnancy may occur in the uterine cornua or cervix, or be attached to the ovary or elsewhere in the abdomen (attached to the broad ligament or peritoneal lining) (Fig. 57-11).

EPIDEMIOLOGY

The incidence of ectopic pregnancy has increased dramatically in the last two decades in both the United States and the rest of the world.[1-5] In the United States, from 1970 to 1987, the rate of ectopic pregnancy increased 3.7 times from 4.5 to 16.8 per 1000 reported pregnancies and the absolute annual number of ectopic pregnancies increased by almost 5 times from 17,800 to 88,000[2] (Fig. 57-12). The rate of ectopic pregnancy for the same time period was consistently higher for black and other nonwhite women than for white women. In either group, the rate is increased with maternal age.

The rising incidence of ectopic pregnancy has increased its importance as a cause of maternal death despite a fall in the mortality rate. Ectopic pregnancy

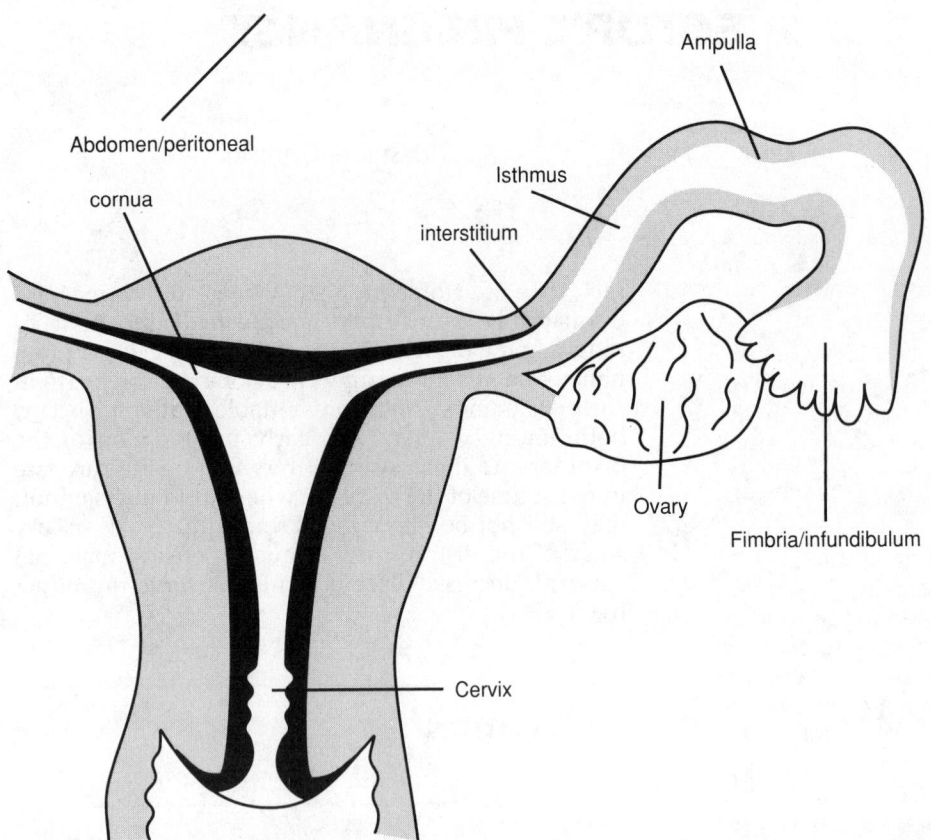

FIG. 57-11. Sites of ectopic implantation.

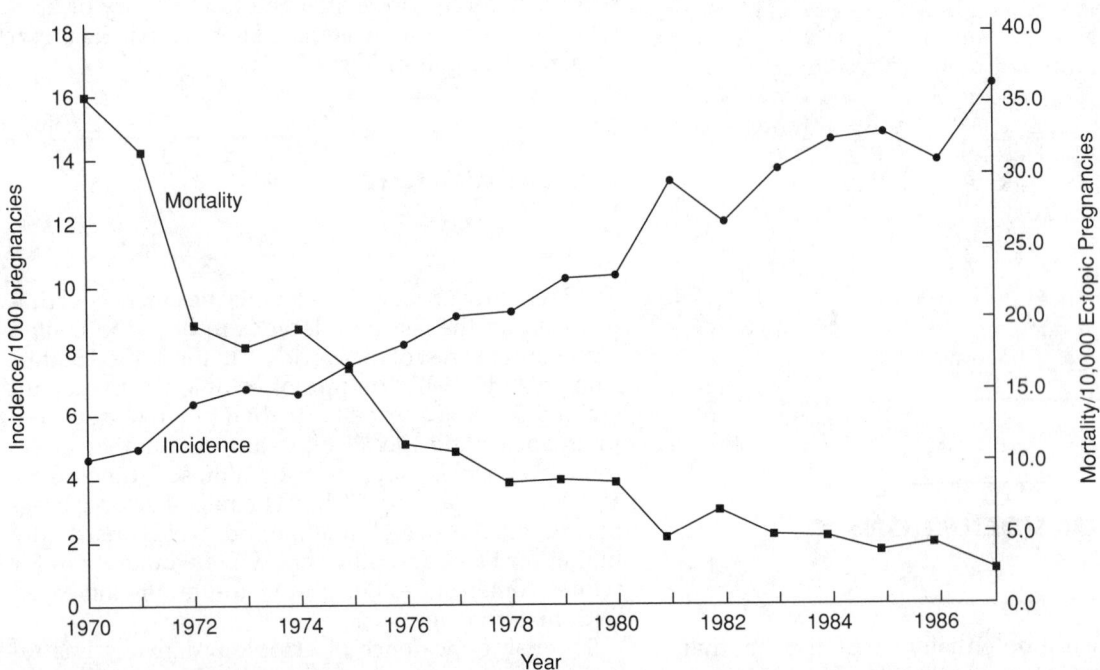

FIG. 57-12. Ectopic pregnancy incidence and mortality.

TABLE 57-6. MATERNAL DEATHS, MORTALITY RATIOS, AND RELATIVE RISKS*

Maternal Mortality Collaborative, 1980–1985, U.S., 19 areas

	601 Deaths	Age Group			Race Group		
Cause of Death	%	<30 Ratio	≥30 Ratio	RR	White Ratio	Other Ratio	RR
Embolism	17	2.0	5.5	2.7	1.4	4.4	2.6
Hypertensive disease	12	1.5	3.7	2.5	1.1	3.4	3.0
Ectopic pregnancy	10	1.1	3.3	3.0	0.7	3.5	5.3
Hemorrhage	09	0.8	3.2	3.8	1.1	1.5	1.3
Infections	09	0.7	0.4	0.6	0.4	0.8	1.8
Cerebrovascular accidents	08	1.1	2.7	2.4	1.3	1.8	1.4
Anesthesia complications	07	0.9	2.1	2.4	0.6	2.3	4.2
Abortions	05	0.7	1.5	2.1	0.4	1.8	4.1
Other/All causes	23	12.3	31.3	2.5	10.0	26.7	2.7
Total	100						

Ratio = crude cause-specific ratio per 100,000 live births for each age or race group
RR = relative risk
* Modified with permission from Rochat, R.W., Koonin, L.M., Atrash, H.K., Jewett, J.F., and the Maternal Mortality Collaborative: Maternal mortality in the United States: Report from the Maternal Mortality Collaborative. Obstet. Gynecol. 72:91, 1988.

is the major cause of maternal death in the first trimester of pregnancy and one of the three leading nontraumatic causes of maternal death overall[1,2,6] (Table 57-6). Blacks and other nonwhites have the highest mortality rates, with an overall 3.5 times increased risk of death. As a result, black women have a greater than 5 times risk of dying of ectopic pregnancy than white women when the net effect of the increased mortality rate and incidence rate for black women are considered together. Teenagers in any racial group have the highest age-dependent risk of death.

The increased incidence of ectopic pregnancy has been noted in association with certain predisposing factors, which include:

1. **Sexually transmitted diseases (STDs).** The increased incidence of ectopic pregnancy closely parallels the dramatic increase in STD in the recent past. Numerous studies have associated a history of previous STD with ectopic pregnancy or found evidence of previous tubal infection on pathology following surgery for ectopic pregnancy.[3,5,7–11] The association appears much stronger with upper tract disease, especially chlamydial and gonococcal salpingitis and pelvic inflammatory disease.
2. **Intrauterine device (IUD) use.** Despite the contraceptive effectiveness of the IUD, pregnancies occur with IUD use and have an increased incidence of ectopy. The greatest risk has been noted for current IUD users with a continued risk for at least 1 year after removal.[3,10,11]
3. **Pelvic surgery.** Ectopic pregnancy occurs more commonly after instrumentation of the upper pelvic tract, especially tubal surgery for treatment of infertility, prevention of fertility (tubal sterilization), and treatment of previous ectopic pregnancy.

Ectopic pregnancy occurs in 15 to 20% of the pregnancies that follow tubal sterilization.[5] Ectopic pregnancy recurs in approximately 25% of pregnancies after previous ectopic pregnancy and in higher numbers after multiple previous ectopic pregnancies.[5,12] One study of ectopic pregnancy following previous ectopic pregnancy or tubal infertility surgery found pre-existent salpingitis to be the predominant causative factor for ectopic implantation.[11] Previous nontubal abdominal surgery does not appear to increase the risk of ectopic pregnancy. Because tubal sterilization is the second most common ob/gyn procedure and the frequency of tubal reconstructive surgery has more than doubled in the United States, the increased incidence of ectopic pregnancy is expected to continue.[11]

4. **Changes in contraceptive use.** The decreased use of traditional oral contraceptives, which prevent ectopic pregnancy by depressing ovulation, may increase the incidence of ectopic pregnancy. Additionally, the use of tubal surgery, IUDs, and low-dose progestagen contraceptives in place of traditional estrogen/progestagen contraceptives may also have led to an increase in ectopic pregnancy incidence. Low-dose progestagens are felt to alter tubal motility, thereby leading to ectopic implantation.
5. **Other.** Use of ovulatory agents, fetal diethylstilbestrol (DES) exposure, induced abortion, and postponed timing of first pregnancy have also been noted to be associated with an increase in ectopic pregnancy incidence in some studies, although their independent contribution is less certain.

Additionally, it has been noted that an increased suspicion and rate of detection of ectopic pregnancy may have contributed to the observed increase in incidence. Earlier detection may now include some of the 10 to 50% of ectopic pregnancies that resorb spontaneously and previously went uncounted.

ANATOMY AND PHYSIOLOGY

In the normal sequence leading to pregnancy, a mature ovarian follicle ruptures, releasing the ovum into the abdominal cavity. The ovum is picked up by the fimbriated ends of the fallopian tube, fertilized by the spermatozoon in the ampulla, and transported for 3 days through the fallopian tube as the resultant zygote develops into the blastocyst. Roughly 6 days after ovulation, the blastocyst implants, first adhering and then eroding through the endometrial epithelium, and becomes buried in the endometrium. Human chorionic gonadotropin (hCG) production by the fetal trophoblast begins immediately with or just before implantation and is detectable in maternal blood within the first day of implantation. The maximum level of hCG is reached at 10 to 12 weeks of pregnancy, after which it declines. In response to stimulation from hCG, the corpus luteum produces the estrogens and progesterone to maintain the pregnancy for the first 6 weeks until placental production of estrogens, progesterone, and human placental lactogen (hPL) takes over.

In ectopic pregnancy, this sequence is altered drastically by the aberrant implantation. Ectopic implantation may result from anatomic or functional factors that delay or prevent passage of the fertilized ovum into the uterus or from embryonic abnormalities. These factors may include alterations of ciliary function, tubal morphology or patency as a consequence of salpingitis, tubal surgery, IUD use, or hormonal manipulation, as noted earlier. Ectopic implantation is tubal, most often in the ampulla, less often in the isthmus, and rarely in the interstitium or fimbria. Nontubal sites of ectopic pregnancy are felt to result from a primary tubal implantation and subsequent tubal rupture or abortion with secondary implantation in the nontubal site.

The blastocyst, once adherent to the tubal lumen, burrows through the epithelium and into the muscular wall. Trophoblastic invasion of maternal blood vessels follows, most often with intraluminal spread of trophoblast, intraluminal hemorrhage, and often subsequent leakage of blood out the abdominal end of the tube. Growth of the embryo is limited by the musculature and vasculature of the wall and does not always correspond with gestational age. Human chorionic gonadotropin is formed by the ectopic embryo and released into the maternal circulation at levels detectable with sensitive tests in nearly 100% of cases. Maternal serum hCG levels correlate best with tro-

phoblast mass, only roughly with degree of development of the embryo, and poorly with its age.[13] Corpus luteum production of estrogen and progestogens is usually sufficient to produce some degree of early uterine changes, including formation of decidua, softening of the cervix and isthmus, and an increase in uterine size. External bleeding associated with ectopic pregnancy is usually secondary to degeneration and sloughing of the uterine decidua.

COURSE OF TUBAL PREGNANCY

Tubal pregnancy may terminate in several ways, depending partly on the initial site of implantation: abortion, resorption, rupture, rupture and reimplantation, and surgical termination. Tubal abortion, most common with ampullary implantation, occurs when the products of conception separate from the tubal wall and are extruded through the fimbria and into the peritoneal cavity, where they are absorbed. Partial tubal abortion may result in hematosalpinx or placental polyp in the tube and cause pain for weeks. Tubal resorption occurs with in situ death of the products of conception. Tubal abortion and resorption are estimated to occur in from 10 to 50% of ectopic pregnancies. Tubal rupture usually occurs spontaneously but may result from trauma suffered accidentally or during sexual activity or pelvic examination. Isthmic pregnancies rupture earlier and more frequently, and although their rupture is less commonly preceded by bleeding or hemoperitoneum, they are usually accompanied by greater hemorrhage. Ampullary pregnancies are less prone to rupture, and their rupture is more often preceded by hemorrhage.[13,14] Profuse hemorrhage following tubal rupture results in circulatory collapse and maternal death in the absence of surgical intervention. Tubal rupture with limited hemorrhage results most commonly in resorption of conceptual products. In rare instances, an abdominal pregnancy occurs when the undamaged early zygote is delivered whole into the peritoneal cavity after tubal rupture and reimplants elsewhere. Alternatively, an intact gestational sac may be freed by tubal rupture with its placenta still attached to the ruptured tube. Interstitial pregnancy is less common (3 to 4%) and generally ruptures later (eighth to sixteenth menstrual week) than ampullary or isthmic pregnancies (fourth to twelfth menstrual week), is accompanied by more profuse bleeding because of its more advanced development and proximity to uterine and ovarian arteries, and is harder to diagnose clinically because of its easy confusion with a uterine pregnancy on examination. The incidence of simultaneous tubal and uterine pregnancies varies from 1 in 6000 to 30,000 pregnancies and is increased in patients undergoing ovulation induction. Bilateral tubal pregnancy occurs even less frequently, with an incidence of 1 in 200,000 pregnancies.

CLINICAL PRESENTATION

Ectopic pregnancy may present in a multitude of ways, some much more easily diagnosed than others. Classically, a young woman presents 6 to 10 weeks after her last menses with a history of amenorrhea, abnormal bleeding, and the relatively sudden onset of abdominal pain and symptoms of hypovolemia including dizziness or syncope. Examination is notable for postural or absolute hypotension, abdominal tenderness or rebound, cervical motion tenderness, and sometimes adnexal mass or cul-de-sac fullness. In such a classic presentation, diagnosis is relatively straightforward. Such presentations, however, are not uniform and are less common in women seeking medical attention earlier in the course of the disease. Additionally, the large number of women who have had several medical visits before the diagnosis was made or who were diagnosed at time of death or postmortem testifies to the varied and atypical presentations that may occur with ectopic pregnancy. In Dorfman's study of the 86 known fatal ectopic pregnancies in the U.S. in 1979, 77% of the women had been previously seen by clinicians (70% of whom were gynecologists), and physician misdiagnosis or deferral of the first visit contributed to the delay in diagnosis and death in over half of the cases.[9] In two larger studies of surgically diagnosed ectopic pregnancies 30 to 50% of the patients had been evaluated at least once before the correct diagnosis; 10% were evaluated three or more times.[8,15] A large study of ectopic pregnancy diagnosis in the ED revealed 55% were correctly diagnosed on the first visit.[16]

SYMPTOMS

Abdominal pain, amenorrhea, and abnormal vaginal bleeding are present in about two thirds of patients. See Table 57-7. Their absence does not mean there is no ectopic pregnancy.

PAIN

Abdominal or pelvic pain is the most often experienced symptom of ectopic pregnancy, occurring in over 90% of cases. Pain may be unilateral or bilateral, localized to the lower or upper abdomen or generalized throughout the abdomen. The pain may be sharp, stabbing, cramping, dull, or aching. Pain may be referred to the shoulders or back in 10 to 20% of cases indicating diaphragmatic irritation by intraperitoneal blood. Less severe or cramplike pain may indicate tubal distention or localized bleeding; more severe, sharp, and generalized pain generally indicates rupture. Pain is most often aggravated by motion. In

TABLE 57-7. SYMPTOMS AND SIGNS OF ECTOPIC PREGNANCY*

SYMPTOMS
  Abdominal pain
  Amenorrhea
  Vaginal bleeding/spotting
  Dizziness and syncope
  Symptoms of pregnancy
  Gastrointestinal symptoms
SIGNS
  Abdominal tenderness
  Adnexal tenderness
  Cervical motion tenderness
  Adnexal mass
  Hypotension
  Fever

* Listed in approximate order of decreasing frequency of occurrence; with increased diagnosis before rupture the occurrence of both symptoms and signs has decreased. Table based on references 5, 7, 8, 9, 14, 15, 16, 43, and 45.

roughly 50% of presentations, pain is of less than 24 hours' duration but in the remainder may be of longer duration or have occurred intermittently. The reported incidence of pain is less in ectopic pregnancies diagnosed from high-risk groups by screening and when increased percentages are diagnosed before rupture.[16]

AMENORRHEA

Roughly three quarters of women presenting with ectopic pregnancy have a history of a missed menses. The other quarter give no history of a missed period, although on detailed questioning some say that their last period was atypical in duration or amount or may have been off by a few days representing confusion of decidual bleeding with a normal menses. Time since the last period until presentation is most often 6 to 10 weeks. Later presentations are not infrequent, especially with cornual or interstitial implantation, present most often at 8 to 16 weeks.

VAGINAL SPOTTING OR BLEEDING

Roughly three quarters of women presenting with ectopic pregnancy have a history of abnormal vaginal bleeding. Most often, the bleeding is dark brown, scanty or spotting, and intermittent. Usually it represents uterine decidual reaction from inadequate hormonal support by the ectopic trophoblast. Less often, bleeding is moderate, and even less often it is profuse. Moderate and profuse bleeding are often confused respectively with menstrual bleeding and threatened or incomplete abortion. Profuse bleeding may be associated with cornual or interstitial pregnancies in up to 25% of cases.

SYMPTOMS OF PREGNANCY

Symptoms of pregnancy, including morning sickness, breast engorgement, and production of colostrum are not common and occur in one quarter or less of cases. Nausea may be more common but interpreted as a gastrointestinal symptom.

GASTROINTESTINAL SYMPTOMS

Gastrointestinal symptoms including nausea, vomiting, urge to defecate, and abdominal cramping have been noted with greatly varying incidence. In Dorfman's study of fatal ectopic pregnancies, 80% of the patients were noted to have gastrointestinal symptoms, and 25% were misdiagnosed as suffering from gastrointestinal disorders.[9]

DIZZINESS AND SYNCOPE

Dizziness, weakness, or less commonly syncope are found in roughly a third of cases.

HISTORICAL FACTORS

Inquiry should be made for a history of salpingitis, PID, tubal surgery, use of fertility agents, past or present IUD use or previous ectopic pregnancy.

PHYSICAL EXAMINATION (SIGNS)

Findings on physical examination may vary because of differences in location or chronologic stage of the ectopic gestation. Abdominal and adnexal tenderness are most consistent.

GENERAL EXAMINATION AND VITAL SIGNS

Most women with ectopic pregnancy have a normal appearance and normal vital signs. Signs of hypovolemia, including diaphoresis, pale skin, tachycardia, orthostatic changes, hypotension, and shock are found in 10 to 20% of cases. In contrast, in Breen's study of 654 ectopic pregnancies from 1947 to 1967, 80% were ruptured at the time of surgery and 48% presented in shock.[7] In Dorfman's study of fatal ectopic pregnancies, roughly 40% had a systolic blood pressure under 90 mm Hg and/or a pulse greater than 100 per minute.[9] Fever, usually low grade, is also present in perhaps 5 to 10% of patients, although Breen found temperatures of 99 to 103°F in 50%.[7]

ABDOMINAL AND PELVIC EXAMINATION

Abdominal tenderness is elicited in most cases. In unruptured cases, tenderness is usually less severe and better localized. It may sometimes be absent. Once rupture has occurred, examination is more likely to reveal generalized or rebound tenderness and rigidity, decreased or absent bowel sounds, and/or distention, all consistent with intraperitoneal bleeding.

Pelvic examination reveals adnexal tenderness or cervical motion tenderness in 75 to 90% of cases. An adnexal mass is found in about one half of cases, although in 20% of these the mass, usually the corpus luteum, is contralateral to the ectopic gestation. Cul-de-sac fullness is found in one to two thirds of cases. Uterine enlargement secondary to the effect of placental hormones is also commonly found, and uterine size frequently coincides with that of an intrauterine pregnancy, with a similar period of amenorrhea.

INITIAL STABILIZATION

An initial assessment of diagnosis and management should be made once the history and physical examination have been completed. Once the diagnosis of ectopic pregnancy is entertained, it can be categorized into three general diagnostic and management categories: obvious and critical, probable and urgent, and possible and stable. Obvious ectopic pregnancy with hypovolemia or shock demands immediate treatment of hypovolemia; preparation for surgery including administration of cross-matched, type-specific, or universal donor blood as indicated by the situation; and surgical exploration by the gynecologist or, in his or her absence, the general surgeon. Culdocentesis may be performed if time allows to confirm the diagnosis and guide laparotomy. In cases of probable ectopic pregnancy without obvious or marked hypovolemia, gynecologic consultation should be obtained and hypovolemia protocol instituted (IV access and fluid administration, orthostatic testing, blood for hemoglobin and hematocrit, and type and cross-match), coincident with blood work including serum pregnancy test and pelvic ultrasound or culdocentesis. In less probable cases, diagnostic testing may precede or obviate the need for institution of the hypovolemia protocol or gynecologic consultation.

DIAGNOSTIC TESTING: LABORATORY AND OTHER PROCEDURES

Diagnostic testing includes laboratory testing of blood or urine and procedures performed while the patient is in the ED, including pelvic ultrasound and culdocentesis as well as procedures performed by the consulting surgeon/gynecologist such as laparoscopy, curettage, or laparotomy.

The two principal goals of diagnostic testing in workup of suspected ectopic pregnancy are confirmation of pregnancy and, when it is confirmed, localization of the products of conception. Additional testing is performed to evaluate for anemia, infection, or other disorders coincident or confused with ectopic pregnancy. Initial blood work includes complete blood count with platelets, serum pregnancy test for hCG by a method sensitive to 5 to 10 mIU/ml such as radioimmunoassay (RIA), immunoradiometric assay (IRMA), or other or, in its absence, sensitive urine pregnancy test by enzyme-linked immunosorbent assay (ELISA), as well as blood typing, electrolytes, BUN, and creatinine. These are frequently followed by a diagnostic procedure of pelvic ultrasonography or culdocentesis or by direct visualization by the consultant gynecologist by means of laparoscopy or laparotomy. As noted, in the clinically unstable patient in whom diagnosis is most often apparent, laboratory testing may be limited to preparation for surgery and possibly culdocentesis.

COMPLETE BLOOD COUNT (CBC)

Complete blood count does not usually contribute substantially to diagnosis. Hemoglobin and hematocrit may not reflect acute blood loss because of the time required for restoration of blood volume and resultant hemodilution. A decrease in these values usually reflects severe or chronic blood loss, and in the presence of acute bleeding the degree of hemorrhage may be underestimated. Leukocyte count is usually normal, but in a substantial percentage of cases may be elevated secondary to catechol effect from hypovolemia and thus cannot reliably differentiate between pelvic infection and ectopic pregnancy.

PREGNANCY TESTS

Pregnancy testing is a pivotal point in diagnosis of ectopic pregnancy. The exclusion of pregnancy excludes ectopic pregnancy. Patient history can be remarkably inaccurate. In a study by Ramoska et al., only 47 (63%) of 68 women with positive pregnancy tests correctly thought that they were pregnant. Twenty-eight women who thought they were pregnant were not. In women whose last menstrual period was on time, who did not believe that they were pregnant, or who stated that there was no chance of pregnancy, more than 10% were found to be pregnant. Furthermore, 4% of women who used birth control and had experienced a normal previous period were pregnant.[17] In contrast, in a study of women with suspected ectopic pregnancy, only 20% had a positive pregnancy test, but of these almost half had an ectopic pregnancy.[18] Understanding the limitations of the currently available pregnancy tests as well as the endocrine physiology of normal and ectopic pregnancy may be critical in reaching the right diagnosis.

PHYSIOLOGY

Trophoblastic production of hCG begins at implantation and increases through the eighth week of conception, doubling every 1.4 to 2.1 days. Corpus luteum production of progesterone begins immediately after ovulation and, in response to hCG, continues until gradually replaced by placental production during the sixth through tenth menstrual weeks. Progesterone levels are significantly elevated by the third menstrual week, rise steadily through the fifth week, and rise gradually thereafter through the pregnancy. Because of limited space and vascular support, the production of hCG and consequent production of progesterone by the corpus luteum are significantly reduced in ectopic gestations, and the doubling time for hCG is prolonged. Serum hCG levels roughly correlate with trophoblastic mass and embryonic development but not with total ectopic size or gestational age.

In rare instances, ectopic pregnancy has been found with nondetectable hCG levels, but less than 1% of patients have an hCG level of less than 10 mIU per mL, and the great majority have levels of over 100 mIU per mL.[5,8,13,14,18–21] In a study of 184 ectopic pregnancies, Romero et al. found that 0.5% had a level of less than 10, 1% had a level of less than 20, 5% had a level less than 100, and 12% had a level less than 200 mIU per mL.[20] In a comparable study of 131 ectopic gestations (hCG values converted from 2nd IS to IRP using a factor of 1.67; see subsequent text), none had levels under 25 mIU/mL, and 20 (15%) cases had levels under 167. Mean hCG levels were 6924 and 16,418 mIU/mL for ampullary and isthmic locations respectively, and were higher when ruptured in either location.[13] About 10 to 20% of ectopic gestations have an hCG level greater than 10,000 mIU/mL. In summary, to detect at least 99% of ectopic pregnancies, one needs a test for hCG that can detect a serum level of 5 to 10 mIU/mL.

HUMAN CHORIONIC GONADOTROPIN

Discussion of hCG is complicated by the variety of reference standards and published discrepancies in their interconversion.[22–25] Measurements of hCG in serum or urine are generally expressed as units of activity using either the older Second International Standard (Second IS) established in 1964 or the highly purified CR 119 International Reference Preparation (IRP) established in 1974. The latter is also referred to as the Third International Standard for Chorionic Gonadotropin (WHO 3rd IS 75/537). All hCG values reported in this chapter are expressed in terms of the IRP standard. One nanogram of the IRP standard has a potency of 9.3 mIU (IRP) and about 5 mIU (2nd IS),[22,24] although a frequently cited study found it equal to 6.5 to 7.5 mIU (IRP) and 2.3 to 4.0 mIU of the 2nd IS.[25] Based on this, levels of serum measured with the IRP are roughly felt to be 100% higher than with the 2nd IS, although Fossum et al. found the IRP to be only 34% higher.[23]

Sensitive tests for hCG use antibodies directed against the beta subunit or the intact molecule (alpha and beta subunit) because the alpha subunit is shared in common with luteinizing hormone (LH), follicle-stimulating hormone (FSH), and thyroid-stimulating hormone (TSH). Assays sensitive to <5 mIU/mL are now available by various methodologies including radioimmunoassay (RIA), immunoenzymetric assay (IEA), immunoradiometric assay (IRMA), and others that can be performed in a matter of hours. Semi-quantitative tests for serum hCG levels less than 10, between 10 and 25 and greater than 25 mIU/mL can be performed by IEA or ELISA in less than 30 minutes. A qualitative urine hCG test with a sensitivity of 20 mIU/mL can be easily performed using the same methodology (Hybritech Tandem ICON II HCG) in the ED in 5 to 10 minutes. Dilute urine (specific gravity of <1.015) decreases the reliability of the test. Other urine tests that use hemagglutination and latex agglutination inhibition are rapidly performed but less sensitive (sensitivity of 150 to 200 and 500 to 800 mIU/mL, respectively).

When both sensitivity and rapidity of diagnosis are important, a two-assay protocol can be used, with a rapid urine assay for initial testing followed by a serum assay with a more sensitive method. Or if qualitative testing only appears indicated, a sensitive urine test alone can be used. The validity of either approach was confirmed by a study comparing paired urine and blood samples for 95 ectopic and 10 intrauterine gestations analyzed by 4 quantitative tests and two qualitative tests. All 105 women were correctly classified as pregnant by both the serum and urine qualitative assays (Hybritech Tandem ICON). Quantitative tests for intact hCG showed a roughly unitary relationship between concentrations in both fluids except in the presence of dilute urine.[19]

SERIAL HCG TESTING

A positive pregnancy test in a clinically stable woman, even with abdominal pain, uterine bleeding, and adnexal mass, still does not indicate ectopic pregnancy in most cases. Although the normal values for serum hCG at different conceptual ages are relatively well known for normal pregnancies, a single quantitative hCG determination cannot differentiate normal from abnormal pregnancies without the exact date of ovulation or the last period. Consequently, it has been advocated that the doubling time or slope of the increase in hCG be used to differentiate normal from abnormal pregnancies during the time when ultrasound cannot discriminate between the two. Kadar et al. proposed that abnormal pregnancies were associated with less than a 66% increase in hCG concentration over a 48-hour period (shorter periods were found to give too much variation). Using this criterion, they found that 15% of normal pregnancies would be

misclassified as abnormal and 13% of ectopic pregnancies misclassified as normal.[26] Using a 63% increase as a cutoff, Daus et al. found 13% of normal pregnancies to be misdiagnosed as abnormal and 6% of ectopics as normal.[27] In an evaluation of asymptomatic women at high risk for ectopy, however, Shepherd et al. found that 64% of ectopic gestations were misclassified as normal using the same criteria and early paired hCG measurements. With additional measurements, 85% of ectopic gestations were correctly identified.[28] In the ED setting, sequential sampling may be unsuitable because of the prolonged sampling period and the unavailability of rapid quantitative hCG testing. Patients with a diagnosis of "rule out ectopic," however, are likely to be seen more frequently because gynecologists use serial measurements to evaluate clinically stable patients with possible ectopic pregnancy.

PROGESTERONE

A single serum progesterone measurement has been suggested to aid in diagnosis of ectopic pregnancy.[16,29–31] Because progesterone levels remain relatively stable from the third through eighth weeks of pregnancy, neither serial determinations nor precise knowledge of gestational age are needed to differentiate normal from abnormal pregnancies. Additionally, the short half-life of progesterone (<10 minutes) versus that of hCG (>36 hours) may reflect changes in viability more rapidly. Initial studies found serum progesterone levels of <15 ng/mL in patients with ectopic pregnancies and levels of >15 ng/mL in patients with normal pregnancies.[29,30] Stovall et al. screened all urine hCG-positive women presenting to the ED of a large hospital with a high observed incidence of ectopic pregnancy with quantitative serum hCG and progesterone measurements. Patients with significant risk factors or significant symptoms received additional evaluation. All those with progesterone of <25 ng/mL and not initially diagnosed were called back for further evaluation and repeat quantitative hCG assay and endovaginal ultrasonography. Overall, of the 161 ectopic pregnancies found, 97% had progesterone values of <25, 55% were detected at first visit, and of the 45% detected on follow-up with aid of serum progesterone only one had a progesterone of >25. The apparent early diagnosis of ectopic pregnancy using this protocol resulted in a decrease in the rate of rupture from 79 to 39% compared with a retrospective control group.[16,30] Shortcomings of this approach are the lack of uniformity in normal progesterone values among hospitals and the lack of availability and rapidity of testing, all of which can be expected to improve with its increased use.

The urinary metabolite of progesterone, pregnanediol glucuronide (PG), is also correspondingly lower in abnormal pregnancies, and its use has also been proposed to aid in diagnosis of ectopic pregnancy.[21] Advantages ascribed to its use are that urine is more easily obtained than serum and a sensitive semi-quantitative enzyme immunoassay is available and can be performed in less than 10 minutes without special equipment or personnel, thus making it suitable for ED use. Sauer et al. found in a study of 60 ectopic and 34 intrauterine pregnancies that the urinary PG level was significantly depressed in ectopic gestations (4.8 µg/mL versus 24.5 µg/mL).[21] PG levels of <9 and <15 µg/mL were found in 75 and 90% of ectopic pregnancies, respectively, and levels of >9 and >15 µg/mL were found in 100% and 91% of intrauterine pregnancies, respectively. With further refinement and testing, this method may hold promise for emergency department use.

ULTRASONOGRAPHY

Once the existence of pregnancy has been established, pelvic ultrasonography is often used to further evaluate the clinically stable women suspected of having ectopic pregnancy. Its advantages are that it is non-invasive and relatively painless. Disadvantages are that it is often not available rapidly or on a 24-hour basis, it takes longer to perform, and it frequently has inadequate resolution. In fact, only 10 to 20% of ectopic pregnancies are visualized by ultrasonography, depending on ultrasonographic approach and the development and size of the ectopic gestation. Thus ultrasonography is most often used to establish the presence of an intrauterine pregnancy (IUP) and thereby exclude ectopic pregnancy statistically because of the extremely rare occurrence of simultaneous ectopic and intrauterine pregnancies.

The resolution of ultrasonography is limited even in establishing the presence of an IUP. The range of serum hCG concentration above which an IUP can be reliably diagnosed is referred to as the discriminatory zone, a concept first advanced by Kadar et al. in 1981.[32] Using transabdominal ultrasound (TAUS), they found that a normal IUP could be visualized 94% of the time with serum hCG levels above 6500 mIU/mL and that absence of visualization of a gestational sac above this level was diagnostic of an ectopic pregnancy in 86% of cases.[33] At levels below 6000 mIU/mL, they were unable to consistently identify the gestational location. The presence of a sac below these levels was more often associated with an abnormal pregnancy—either a missed abortion or an ectopic pregnancy. The concept of discriminatory zone has become commonly recognized and found to vary with ultrasonographic method, equipment, and operator.

Transabdominal ultrasonography has been more commonly available. It requires a full bladder for visualization of pelvic structures, which many women find uncomfortable. At most institutions, the discriminatory zone for TAUS is 5500 to 6500 mIU/mL (about 6 menstrual weeks). Above this level, about 90% of IUPs can be visualized as a gestational sac (a sonolucent area surrounded by a dense echogenic rim).

Absence of visualization of an IUP above this level is diagnostic of ectopic pregnancy in about 90% of cases.[32–34] Only about 25% to 40% of ectopic pregnancies have hCG levels above 6,000 mIU/mL.[32,33] Visualization of a sac below this level implies an abnormal pregnancy over half of cases, most often a spontaneous abortion, but occasionally an ectopic pregnancy in which event it represents the decidual reaction and is called a "pseudogestational" sac of ectopic pregnancy. Definitive evidence of gestational location, the presence of a fetal heartbeat, intrauterine or adnexal, is seen at even higher levels of hCG (about 17,000 mIU/mL) and later (7 to 8 menstrual weeks). Adnexal findings are thus infrequently definitive but may still be helpful. Adnexal masses are visualized in up to two thirds of ectopic pregnancies but are more often associated with spontaneous abortion (SAB) or IUP. Noncystic adnexal masses are found less often but are more often associated with ectopic pregnancy. The combined presence of noncystic adnexal mass and free peritoneal fluid occurs in roughly one quarter to one half of cases and is associated with ectopic pregnancy in over 90% of occurrences. Peritoneal fluid is visualized in up to one half of ectopics, but in the absence of a coincidental mass is more often associated with SAB or IUP.[35,36]

The more recently introduced endovaginal ultrasonography (EVUS) provides better resolution with less discomfort and increased rapidity because it does not require a full bladder and is less affected by obesity. Visualization of intrauterine pregnancy, embryonic structures, and abnormal pregnancy may be made about 1 week earlier than with TAUS.[23,37,38] EVUS allows visualization of the gestational sac at 1000 to 2000 mIU/mL (4 to 5 menstrual weeks), visualization of cardiac activity at 11,000 to 27,000 mIU/mL (the end of the 5th to 6th week); differentiation between head and body may be possible at 6 to 7 menstrual weeks. Additionally, EVUS allows better visualization of adnexal structures and peritoneal fluid. An ectopic sac is found in about two thirds of ectopic pregnancies.[37,39,40] Cardiac activity may be seen in 10 to 25% of ectopic pregnancies. Findings of a noncystic adnexal mass imply a risk for ectopic of 85%, and with pelvic fluid the risk increases to 90%.[40–42]

In review, the use of ultrasonography for diagnosis of ectopic pregnancy in the ED is limited by availability, resolution, and, in most cases, the absence of rapidly available quantitative hCG levels. Because most ectopic pregnancies present with hCG values below the discriminatory zone of TAUS and sizeable numbers with values below the discriminatory zone for EVUS, ultrasonic evidence for ectopic gestation is largely exclusionary (absence of an IUP) or based on probability or association (noncystic adnexal mass, peritoneal or cul-de-sac fluid). Definite visualization of ectopic gestation occurs in a few cases. When quantitative hCG values are available, diagnosis may be better guided. Nonvisualization of an IUP with values above the discriminatory zone of the ultrasonographic technique available makes the presence of ectopic pregnancy nearly certain. A normal ultrasonogram with hCG level below the discriminatory zone allows serial hCG monitoring or repeat ultrasonography at the time of predicted attainment of the discriminatory zone or both as long as the patient is clinically stable. In less stable patients, nonvisualization indicates the need for a more invasive procedure such as culdocentesis or laparoscopy.

CULDOCENTESIS

Culdocentesis is a simple procedure that may be rapidly performed by the emergency physician in the department with available equipment. Conflicting opinions have been reached by different investigators on the role and usefulness of culdocentesis despite similar findings in the probabilities and predictive values associated with the procedure. Its role has been questioned in both the evaluation of the stable patient, when sensitive pregnancy testing and ultrasonography are available, have similar predictive values and are less painful and invasive, and in the evaluation of the less stable or more probable patient when laparoscopy has a higher predictive value and may lead to less delay in ultimate operative treatment.[5,43,44] The continued value of culdocentesis has been argued by other investigators, especially when ultrasonography is either nondiagnostic or not rapidly available and in earlier presentations when culdocentesis has a relatively higher predictive value.[45,46]

Culdocentesis has a positive predictive value for both hemoperitoneum and ectopic pregnancy of about 85% in patients suspected of having ectopic pregnancy.[5,43-45] Surprisingly, hemoperitoneum occurs in most unruptured as well as ruptured ectopics.[44,45] As a consequence, culdocentesis does not accurately differentiate the two. The overall sensitivity of culdocentesis for ectopic pregnancy is about 70 to 90% and is slightly better for ruptured than for unruptured cases.[5,43-46] False negative rates of 1 to 15% (including aspiration of >10 cc of serous fluid) and nondiagnostic rates of 15 to 30% have been noted in association with surgically proven ectopic pregnancies. Additionally, false positive results have been noted in similar percentages in association with spontaneous abortion, intrauterine pregnancy, ruptured ovarian cyst, retrograde menstruation, and endometriosis. Negative or nondiagnostic culdocentesis does not exclude the diagnosis of ectopic pregnancy and may occur in up to 75% of clinically suspected cases with such results.

Culdocentesis is performed with the patient in the lithotomy position with the upper torso elevated. After insertion of a full-size vaginal speculum, cleansing of the vagina with antiseptic, and displacement of the cervix toward the symphysis with tenaculum, a long 16- or 18-gauge needle attached to a partially air-filled syringe is inserted through the posterior fornix. When air can be easily injected, an attempt is made to aspirate fluid. Anesthesia can be given either just before with parenteral fentanyl or coincident with needle insertion if several mL of 1% lidocaine is added to the syringe and injected on mucosal entry. Aspiration of >5 mL of nonclotting blood or bloody fluid with a hematocrit of >15% is considered positive, although in the presence of active bleeding larger amounts of clotting blood may be obtained. A small amount of clotting blood may indicate perforation of a local vessel by the needle at time of aspiration and is nondiagnostic. Aspiration of serous fluid is generally considered indicative of a ruptured ovarian cyst and a negative tap but has been reported in association with ectopic pregnancy. Failure to obtain fluid indicates failure to reach the cul-de-sac and is nondiagnostic.

OTHER PROCEDURES

Other procedures are available to aid in diagnosis of ectopic pregnancy but are more often performed by the consultant gynecologist. Laparoscopy allows excellent visualization of adnexal structures, except in the presence of adhesions or obesity. Additionally, it can be used for treatment immediately after confirmation of the diagnosis. False-positive and false-negative rates of less than 5% occur. Dilation and curettage may also be helpful when there is no objection to pregnancy termination. Finding of evidence of an intrauterine pregnancy grossly or on frozen section statistically excludes ectopic pregnancy, similarly to finding an IUP with ultrasonography. Laparotomy remains the definitive diagnostic as well as curative procedure, and when time is limited is the best diagnostic approach. A carefully performed early laparotomy has little morbidity if negative, and if positive may avoid a later emergent laparotomy with significant morbidity.

DIFFERENTIAL DIAGNOSIS

Misdiagnosis of ectopic pregnancy may result in fatality or, with later diagnosis, serious morbidity, including a decreased chance of future successful pregnancy. As noted, a substantial percentage of women have seen a physician at least once before correct diagnosis.[8,9,15] Perhaps half of the deaths from ectopic pregnancy might have been avoided if diagnosis had been made and treatment instituted more promptly.[9] Conditions most often confused with ectopic pregnancy include threatened or incomplete abortion, ruptured or torsed ovarian cyst, salpingitis, appendicitis, dysfunctional bleeding, and gastrointestinal disorder. Less commonly confused conditions include endometriosis, urinary tract infection, fibroid degeneration, ureterolithiasis, diverticulosis, and ulcer disease. Gastrointestinal disorder was the most common misdiagnosis in Dorfman's study of fatal ectopic pregnancies. A sensitive pregnancy test would help to differentiate most of these conditions, except abortions and some ovarian cysts, from ectopic pregnancy. See Tables 57-8 and 57-9.

Threatened or incomplete abortion may be confused with ectopic pregnancy in the presence of a positive pregnancy test. Bleeding is usually more profuse, pain is crampy, midline, and less severe, and onset is usually later after the last normal period. Shock, if present, is usually proportionate to visible blood loss. The finding of products of conception is usually diagnostic (except in the rare simultaneous uterine and ectopic pregnancy). Failure to send presumed products of conception for pathologic examination can be a serious or fatal error. Patients sent home with this diagnosis should receive prompt follow-up and serial hCG testing, sonography, or curettage to confirm the diagnosis.

Salpingitis may be easily differentiated from ectopic pregnancy with a sensitive pregnancy test in most cases. Treatment of salpingitis with a tetracycline antibiotic to treat possible chlamydial infection mandates such testing to avoid fetal exposure. Salpingitis is less often associated with bleeding or spotting and more often associated with fever and leukocytosis. Pain is more often bilateral. Unilateral salpingitis should prompt consideration of ectopic pregnancy.

A ruptured or torsed ovarian cyst may be especially difficult to differentiate from ectopic pregnancy in the presence of an intrauterine pregnancy. Abnormal vaginal bleeding and amenorrhea may be less common. Culdocentesis or ultrasonography may not be able to differentiate the two reliably. Ultimate diagnosis may be revealed at laparoscopy or laparotomy.

Pain of appendicitis may mimic a right-sided ectopic pregnancy. In appendicitis, the pain usually begins periumbilically and ultimately localizes higher. A pregnancy test is usually negative. Amenorrhea, vaginal bleeding, and adnexal mass are usually absent.

Gastrointestinal disorders may be mistaken for ectopic pregnancy. The absence of diarrhea should make the diagnosis of gastroenteritis less certain. Pregnancy testing should be considered, especially because gastrointestinal complaints, including nausea, vomiting, and abdominal pain, may occur in normal as well as ectopic pregnancies.

MANAGEMENT (Table 57-10)

A woman presenting to the ED with signs and symptoms consistent with ectopic pregnancy and hemodynamic instability needs immediate gynecologic

TABLE 57-8. CONDITIONS CONFUSED WITH ECTOPIC PREGNANCY
Spontaneous abortion
Ovarian cyst
Salpingitis/PID
Appendicitis
Dysfunctional bleeding
Gastrointestinal disorder
Endometriosis
Urinary tract infection
Ureterolithiasis
Diverticulosis
Ulcer Disease

consult and preparations for surgery. Volume resuscitation should be instituted immediately with crystalloid through two large-bore intravenous lines while blood is obtained for hemoglobin and hematocrit and type and crossmatch. Urine should be sent for stat pregnancy test. Crossmatched, type-specific, or universal donor blood should be given as indicated by availability and the patient's hemodynamic status. Culdocentesis may be performed at the discretion of the gynecologist or in less obvious cases. Laparotomy is diagnostic and life-saving, and should not be delayed while waiting for other confirmatory evidence because such delay may prove fatal.

The hemodynamically stable patient with probable or possible ectopic pregnancy can be more fully evaluated in the ED. If a question exists as to the patient's hemodynamic stability, intravenous access should be established with a large-bore intravenous line and postural blood pressures obtained. Instability revealed at this time indicates a need for a more urgent approach to diagnosis such as immediate ultrasonography, culdocentesis, or laparoscopy by the consultant gynecologist and immediate urine or serum hCG testing and blood for hematocrit and crossmatch. Approach to the still stable patient usually continues with sensitive urine or serum hCG testing and, if positive, endovaginal or transabdominal ultrasonography. If neither intrauterine nor ectopic pregnancy is found and quantitative hCG level is below the discriminatory zone for ultrasonography, arrangements should be made for prompt gynecologic consultation and follow-up. When gestational location is not found and quantitative hCG is not available or above the discriminatory zone, the patient should be admitted to the gynecologist for further evaluation, including possible laparoscopy. Culdocentesis can be used to further evaluate a patient in the ED, but should be used only to "rule in" ectopic pregnancy and not to give a false sense of security as to its nonexistence. Serum progesterone can also be used to help in evaluation, if available, with serum values <25 ng/mL indicating an abnormal pregnancy and increased risk of ectopic gestation and the need for prompt re-evaluation if the patient is discharged from the ED.

TABLE 57-9. DIFFERENTIAL DIAGNOSIS OF ECTOPIC PREGNANCY*

Diagnosis	Adnexal Mass	Amenor-rhea	Serum Pregnancy Test	Pain	Vaginal Bleeding	Other Comments
Tubal ectopic pregnancy	+ (50%)	+ (75%)	+ (99%)	+ (90%)	+ (75%)	May have GI symptoms or low-grade fever
Nontubal ectopic pregnancy	±	+	+	+	+	Rare
Threatened or incomplete abortion	± (if corpus luteum cyst)	+	+	Crampy, pelvic, midline	+ (may be profuse)	May be difficult to differentiate early from ectopic pregnancy
Intrauterine pregnancy with corpus luteum cyst	+	+	+	+	±	Vaginal probe ultrasound shows intrauterine sac at 1500 mIU/mL serum BH$_C$G
Ovarian cyst (follicular, corpus luteum, endmetriotic, benign or malignant)—torsed or ruptured	+	±	− (unless also pregnant)	Pelvic, usually sudden onset	±	Cervical motion tenderness/may require diagnostic laparoscopy
Salpingitis (PID)	± (if TOA)	−	−	Often bilateral	−	Fever, leukocytosis, vaginal discharge, cervical motion tenderness
Appendicitis	−	−	−	Pain migrates to RLQ	−	GI history usually precedes pain
Dysfunctional uterine bleeding	−	± (menses may be early or late)	−	Crampy, pelvic	+	Diagnosis of exclusion
Endometriosis	± (if ovarian cyst present)	−	−	Pelvic, bilateral	±	Maximal symptoms usually with menses
Fibroid—torsed or degenerating	−	−	−	+	±	Uterine nodules palpated
Urinary tract infection/ureterolithiasis	−	−	−	Back and abdomen	−	Abnormal U/A
Gastrointestinal, i.e., PUD, diverticulitis, gastroenteritis	−	−	−	+	−	

* Table prepared by Barbara Hanke, M.D.

Discharge of the pregnant patient from the ED without firm diagnosis of intrauterine pregnancy, normal or abnormal, should be considered only after consultation with the obstetrician/gynecologist and arrangement for definite follow-up has been made. Before discharge, quantitative serum hCG measurement should be ordered and the patient given clear instructions as to her responsibility to return immediately if any signs of hemodynamic instability (weakness, dizziness, or fainting) or increasing abdominal pain occur. Patients seen for re-evaluation, either scheduled or unscheduled, can be evaluated with repeat quantitative serum hCG measurement, looking for an appropriate increase in level of >66% per 48 hours and repeat ultrasonography, especially if hCG level is now in the discriminatory zone. Failure to find either an appropriate increase in hCG value or an IUP on ultrasonography mandates laparoscopy or other evaluation by the gynecologist.

Definitive treatment of ectopic pregnancy is the responsibility of the consultant gynecologist or surgeon, with the primary aim of preserving life and secondary

TABLE 57-10. MANAGEMENT OF POSSIBLE ECTOPIC PREGNANCY

Initial Clinical Assessment		Management	
Diagnostic	Hemodynamic	Diagnostic	Therapeutic

Obvious	Critical
	Hypovolemia
	Shock
		UCG/serum hCG
		CBC, type-cross
		  culdocentesis
			Fluid resuscitation
			Transfusion: 0-/type
			  specific/X matched
			Gynecologic consult

		Laparoscopy/laparotomy (definitive diagnosis and treatments not to be delayed by these)	
Probable	Urgent ± Hypovolemia ? Early perito- neal signs	UCG/qual hCG Orthostatic bp CBC, type/hold Ultrasound Culdocentesis	IV access Fluid resuscitation Gynecologic consultation Laparoscopy
Possible	Stable	Orthostatic bp—if + go to previous section	
		UCG/qual hCG Ultrasound Progesterone Culdocentesis Serial hCG Repeat UTZ	Gynecologic consultation Definitive follow-up Laparoscopy

aim of preserving tubal and reproductive function. Traditionally, treatment has been surgical, with salpingectomy in emergent situations and tube-conserving procedures when the situation allows, such as salpingostomy (tubal incision and evacuation), salpingotomy (tubal incision, evacuation, and closure), and segmental tubal resection and anastomosis. Laparoscopic surgery has gained increasing favor and use in stable patients. Expectant management has been advocated in patients with falling hCG levels and no evidence of bleeding or tube disruption as resorption will occur in the great majority of these cases. Systemic methotrexate and direct tubal instillation of methotrexate, KCl, and other agents have also been used to induce tubal abortion and resorption.

Persistent ectopic pregnancy has been reported after surgical tube-conserving procedures and should be suspected in symptomatic patients presenting after such procedures with persistent hCG elevation. In most patients, the hCG level is undetectable by the 12th postoperative day, although in some it has remained detectable for 3 weeks.[47,48]

Prognosis for further normal reproduction has improved with earlier diagnosis and increased use of tube-conserving surgical technique. Earlier studies of women treated with either salpingectomy or salpingostomy demonstrated a subsequent intrauterine pregnancy rate of roughly 40%. With increased use of conservative surgical technique, subsequent intrauterine pregnancy rates of 40 to 90% have been demonstrated. The rate for recurrent ectopic pregnancy has changed less and remains at about 15% depending on pre-existent tubal disease as well as time of diagnosis and surgical technique.[5,12,24]

Abdominal pregnancy, usually the result of a ruptured or aborted tubal pregnancy, represents a rare and special type of ectopic gestation. The mortality is higher than for tubal pregnancies, and diagnosis may be more difficult and occur much later in the course of the pregnancy. Management in the ED consists of prompt gynecologic consultation and admission, treatment of any hemodynamic instability, and, if any instability is present, preparation for possibly massive transfusion requirements. The reader is referred to several excellent reviews of the subject.[14,49,50]

PITFALLS AND MEDICOLEGAL PEARLS

A common pitfall is failure to consider possibility of pregnancy or ectopic pregnancy in women of childbearing age in the ED. Women of reproductive age with gynecologic, gastrointestinal, or other vague symptomology should be considered pregnant and ectopic until proven otherwise. Patient self-assessment of pregnancy is relatively unreliable.

Do not rely too heavily on insensitive urine or serum pregnancy tests. Urine pregnancy tests are less reliable with dilute urine (SG <1.015). Ectopic pregnancy can occur with serum hCG values as low as 5 to 10 mIU/mL. Know the sensitivities of your laboratory test.

Do not fail to consider ectopic or intrauterine pregnancy when diagnosing salpingitis. Salpingitis usually occurs in reproductive-age women, and its diagnosis should indicate the need for pregnancy testing, both to exclude ectopic pregnancy and to avoid fetal exposure to tetracycline antibiotics.

Avoid too much reliance on a "negative ultrasound." Ultrasonography is only definitive when intrauterine or extrauterine cardiac activity is seen. A "negative ultrasound" with an hCG value above the ultrasonographic discriminatory zone is "positive."

Do not fail to confirm intrauterine pregnancy pathologically when diagnosing missed, incomplete, or complete spontaneous abortion. Ectopic pregnancy should always be considered when diagnosing threatened abortion.

Do not delay definitive diagnosis and treatment (laparoscopy or laparotomy) of unstable patients while awaiting confirmatory evidence of pregnancy or gestational location.

REFERENCES

1. Lawson, H.W., Atrash, H.K., Saftlas, A.F., and Finch, E.L.: Ectopic pregnancy in the United States, 1970–1986. MMWR CDC Surveill. Summ. 38:1SS, 1989.
2. CDC: Current trends: Ectopic pregnancy—United States, 1987. MMWR 39:401, 1990.
3. Makinen, J.I., Erkkola, R.U., and Laippala, P.K.: Causes of the increase in the incidence of ectopic pregnancy, a study of 1017 patients from 1966 to 1985 in Turku, Finland. Am. J. Obstet. Gynecol. 160:642, 1989.
4. Stock, R.J.: The changing spectrum of ectopic pregnancy. Obstet. Gynecol. 71:885, 1988.
5. Weckstein, L.N.: Current perspective on ectopic pregnancy. Obstet. Gynecol. 40:259, 1985.
6. Rochat, R.W., et al.: Maternal mortality in the United States: Report from the maternal mortality collaborative. Obstet. Gynecol. 72:91, 1988.
7. Breen, J.L.: A 21 year survey of 654 ectopic pregnancies. Am. J. Obstet. Gynecol. 106:1004, 1970.
8. Brenner, P.F., Roy, S., Mishell, D.R.: Ectopic pregnancy: a study of 300 consecutive surgically treated cases. JAMA 243:673, 1976.
9. Dorfman, S.F., et al.: Ectopic pregnancy mortality, United States, 1979 to 1980: clinical aspects. Obstet. Gynecol. 64:386, 1984.
10. Marchbanks, P.A., et al.: Risk factors for ectopic pregnancy, a population based study. JAMA 259:1823, 1988.
11. Stock, R.J.: Histopathology of fallopian tubes with recurrent tubal pregnancy. Obstet. Gynecol. 75:9, 1990.
12. Mehta, L., and Young, I.D.: Recurrence risks for common complications of pregnancy—a review. Obstet. Gynecol. Surv. 42:218, 1987.
13. DiMarchi, J.M., Kosasa, T.S., and Hale, R.W.: What is the significance of the human chorionic gonadotropin value in ectopic pregnancy? Obstet. Gynecol. 74:851, 1989.
14. Cunningham, F.G., MacDonald, P.C., and Gant, N.F.: Williams Obstetrics. 18th Ed. East Norwalk, CT, Appleton & Lange, 1989.
15. Hughes, G.J.: The early diagnosis of ectopic pregnancy. Brit. J. Surg. 66:789, 1979.
16. Stovall, T.G., Kellerman, A.L., Ling, F.W., and Buster, J.E.: Emergency department diagnosis of ectopic pregnancy. Ann. Emerg. Med. 19:1089, 1990.
17. Ramoska, E.A., Sacchetti, A.D., and Nepp, M.: Reliability of patient history in determining the possibility of pregnancy. Ann. Emerg. Med. 18:48, 1989.
18. Schwartz, R.O., and DiPietro, D.L.: B-hcg as a diagnostic aid for suspected ectopic pregnancy. Obstet. Gynecol. 56:197, 1980.
19. Norman, R.J., Buck, R.H., Rom, L., and Joubert, S.M.: Blood or urine measurement of human chorionic gonadotropin for detection of ectopic pregnancy? A comparative study of quantitative and qualitative methods in both fluids. Obstet. Gynecol. 71:315, 1988.
20. Romero, R., et al.: The effect of different human chorionic gonadotropin assay sensitivity on screening for ectopic pregnancy. Am. J. Obstet. Gynecol. 153:724, 1985.
21. Sauer, M.V., et al.: Rapid measurement of urinary pregnanediol glucuronide to diagnose ectopic pregnancy. Am. J. Obstet. Gynecol. 159:1531, 1988.
22. Bangham, D.R., and Storring, P.L.: Standardization of human chorionic gonadotropin, HCG, subunits, and pregnancy tests (editorial). Lancet 1:390, 1982.
23. Fossum, G.T., Davajan, V., and Kletzky, O.A.: Early detection of pregnancy with transvaginal ultrasound. Fertil. Steril. 49:788, 1988.
24. Leach, R.E., and Ory, S.J.: Modern management of ectopic pregnancy. J. Repro. Med. 34:324, 1989.
25. Rasor, J.R., Farber, S., and Braunstein, G.D.: An evaluation of 10 kits for the determination of human chorionic gonadotropin in serum. Clin. Chem. 29:1828, 1983.
26. Kadar, N., Caldwell, B.V., and Romero, R.: A method of screening for ectopic pregnancy and its indications. Obstet. Gynecol. 58:162, 1981.
27. Daus, K., Mundy, D., Graves, W., and Slade, B.S.: Ectopic pregnancy: What to do during the 20-day window. J. Repro. Med. 34:162, 1989.
28. Shepherd, R.W., Patton, P.E., Novy, M.J., and Burry, K.A.: Serial B-hcg measurements in the early detection of ectopic pregnancy. Obstet. Gynecol. 75:417, 1990.
29. Matthews, C.P., Coulson, P.B., and Wild, R.: Serum progesterone levels as an aid in the diagnosis of ectopic pregnancy. Obstet. Gynecol. 68:390, 1986.
30. Stovall, T.G., Ling, F.W., Cope, B.J., and Buster, J.E.: Preventing ruptured ectopic pregnancy with a single serum progesterone. Am. J. Obstet. Gynecol. 160:1425, 1989.
31. Yeko, T.R., et al.: Timely diagnosis of early ectopic pregnancy using a single blood progesterone measurement. Fertil. Steril. 48:1048, 1987.
32. Kadar, N., DeVore, G., and Romero, R.: Discriminatory hcg zone: Its use in the sonographic evaluation for ectopic pregnancy. Obstet. Gynecol. 58:156, 1981.
33. Romero, R., et al.: Diagnosis of ectopic pregnancy: Value of the discriminatory human chorionic gonadotropin zone. Obstet. Gynecol. 66:357, 1985.
34. Batzer, F.R., et al.: Landmarks during the first forty-two days of gestation demonstrated by the B-subunit of human chorionic gonadotropin and ultrasound. Am. J. Obstet. Gynecol. 146:973, 1983.
35. Mahony, B.S., Filly, R.A., Nyberg, D.A., Callen, P.W.: Sonographic evaluation of ectopic pregnancy. J. Ultrasound Med. 4:221, 1985.
36. Romero, R., et al.: The value of adnexal sonographic findings in the diagnosis of ectopic pregnancy. Am. J. Obstet. Gynecol. 158:52, 1988.
37. Bree, R.L., et al.: Transvaginal sonography in the evaluation of normal early pregnancy: correlation with hcg level. Am. J. Roentgenol. 153:75, 1989.
38. Timor-Tritsch, I.E., et al.: The use of transvaginal ultrasonography in the diagnosis of ectopic pregnancy. Am. J. Obstet. Gynecol. 161:157, 1989.
39. Cacciatore, B., Stenman, U.H., and Ylostalo, P.: Comparison of abdominal and vaginal sonography in suspected ectopic pregnancy. Obstet. Gynecol. 73:770, 1989.
40. Nyberg, D.A., Mack, L.A., Laing, F.C., and Jeffrey, R.B.: Early pregnancy complications: endovaginal sonographic findings

correlated with human chorionic gonadotropin levels. Radiology *167*:619, 1988.
41. Shapiro, B.S., Cullen, M., Taylor, K.J.W., and DeCherney, A.H.: Transvaginal ultrasonography for the diagnosis of ectopic pregnancy. Fertil. Steril. *50*:425, 1988.
42. Bateman, B.G., et al.: Vaginal sonography findings and hcg dynamics of early intrauterine and tubal pregnancies. Obstet. Gynecol. *75*:421, 1990.
43. Kim, D.S., Chung, S.R., Park, M.I., and Kim, Y.P.: Comparative review of diagnostic accuracy in tubal pregnancy: A 14-year survey of 1040 cases. Obstet. Gynecol. 70:547, 1987.
44. Vermesh, M., Graczykowski, J.W., and Sauer, M.V.: Reevaluation of the role of culdocentesis in the management of ectopic pregnancy. Am. J. Obstet. Gynecol. *162*:411, 1990.
45. Romero, R., et al.: Value of culdocentesis in the diagnosis of ectopic pregnancy. Obstet. Gynecol. 65:519, 1985.
46. Schwab, R.A.: Ultrasound versus culdocentesis in the evaluation of early and late ectopic pregnancy. Ann. Emerg. Med. *17*:801, 1988.
47. Bell, O.R., Awadalla, S.G., and Mattox, J.H.: Persistent ectopic syndrome: a case report and literature review. Obstet. Gynecol. *69*:521, 1987.
48. DiMarchi, J.M., Kosasa, T.S., Kobara, T.Y., and Hale, R.W.: Persistent ectopic syndrome. Obstet. Gynecol. *70*:555, 1987.
49. Martin, J.N., et al.: Abdominal pregnancy: current concepts of management. Obstet. Gynecol. *71*:549, 1988.
50. Martin, J.N., and McCaul, J.F.: Emergent management of abdominal pregnancy. Clin. Obstet. Gynecol. *33*:438, 1990.

HYPERTENSIVE DISORDERS OF PREGNANCY

Russell J. Carlisle

CAPSULE

The role of the Emergency Department (ED) physician in the care of pregnant women with associated hypertension includes: (1) recognition and diagnosis, especially in those without prenatal care or previous diagnosis; (2) obstetric consultation and hospital admission for those with pre-eclampsia; and (3) initiation of stabilizing treatment in those with severe pre-eclampsia or eclampsia coincident with obstetric consultation and hospital admission.

Any pregnant woman with sustained systolic or diastolic elevation of >140/90 mm Hg should be questioned for history of previous hypertension, blood pressure values during previous prenatal visits, recent weight gain, edema, headache, epigastric pain, or visual disturbances. Physical examination and laboratory evaluation should be performed to ascertain the presence of edema, hyperreflexia, proteinuria, consumptive coagulopathy, or altered renal function.

Hypertensive women with less than 20 weeks of gestation and without other abnormality should be referred for prompt obstetric care. Physical or laboratory abnormality indicates a need for prompt obstetric consultation. Hypertensive women with longer than 20 weeks of gestation without previous hypertension or with proteinuria, edema, consumptive coagulopathy, or altered renal function should be considered pre-eclamptic and admitted for obstetric care. Women with severe pre-eclampsia (blood pressure of >160/110, marked proteinuria, headache, visual disturbance, oliguria, or upper abdominal pain) or eclampsia (seizures) need immediate treatment with intramuscular or parenteral magnesium sulfate and parenteral hydralazine and prompt admission for definitive treatment. The cure for pre-eclampsia and eclampsia is delivery. Therefore, patients should be stabilized when necessary and admitted immediately for obstetric care.

GENERAL CONSIDERATIONS

INCIDENCE, MORBIDITY, AND MORTALITY

Hypertensive disease is a common complication of pregnancy. It may be of new onset or be aggravated by pregnancy in previously hypertensive women. In the U.S., hypertensive disease in pregnancy has an average reported incidence of 6 to 7% with marked variations, with a higher incidence in nonwhites, especially blacks, and possibly in lower socioeconomic groups.[1] Hypertensive disorders continue to be a major cause of maternal mortality and were reported as the second most common cause of maternal death in two recent national maternal mortality surveys, accounting for 12 to 17% of maternal deaths[2-4] (Tables 57-11 and 57-12). The relative risk of maternal death from hypertensive disease is increased more than twofold in women over 30[5,6] and in black and other nonwhite women (Table 57-12). Maternal hypertension is also an important cause of perinatal morbidity and mortality. In the Collaborative Perinatal Project 13-year prospective study, the fetal death rate was noted to be three times higher in association with hypertension (diastolic >95 mmHg) alone and to increase with the severity of hypertension especially in the presence of proteinuria.[7] Frequency of occurrence and perinatal mortality rates for placental infarcts, placental growth retardation, and abruptio placentae increase with increasing maternal blood pressure.

DEFINITIONS AND CLASSIFICATION

Much confusion has arisen in the past over definitions and classification of hypertensive diseases of pregnancy. The recent classification by the American College of Obstetrics and Gynecology in 1986, with minor modifications by the authors of Williams Obstetrics, 18th edition, 1989,[1] is well accepted and simple (see Table 57-11). Hypertension is diagnosed when the blood pressure is 140/90 mmHg or when an increase of 30 mmHg systolic or 15 mmHg diastolic over previous values is noted on two or more occasions more than 6 hours apart. Women without a history of preexisting hypertension are considered to have pregnancy-induced hypertension (PIH). Women with pre-existing hypertension that has been exacerbated by pregnancy are considered to have pregnancy-aggravated hypertension (PAH). Women with pre-existent hypertension unaffected by pregnancy are considered to have coincidental or chronic hypertension. Others have advocated different blood pressure values for hypertension (greater than 125/75 mmHg with less than 32 weeks of gestation and greater than 175/85 with more than 32 weeks, or greater than 130/80 at any time during pregnancy) based on decreased fetal survival with increasing blood pressure elevation.[7,8] Thus it should be apparent that individual variations may preclude the use of any one value as an absolute indicator of hypertensive disease.

PRE-ECLAMPSIA

Pre-eclampsia is diagnosed when hypertension coexists with proteinuria and/or edema after 20 weeks of gestation, or earlier if there are extensive hydatiform changes in the chorionic villi (trophoblastic disease). Pre-eclampsia is considered severe when the blood pressure is >160/110 mmHg or in the presence of headache, epigastric pain, visual disturbances, severe proteinuria, or evidence of consumptive coagulopathy such as thrombocytopenia, hemoglobinuria, or hyperbilirubinemia. Eclampsia is diagnosed in a gravid woman having convulsions with no other cause and the clinical criteria for pre-eclampsia. Pre-eclampsia and eclampsia are considered to be superimposed when they develop in a woman with preexistent hypertension.

Proteinuria, defined as >300 mg per 24-hour period or >100 mg/dL in two random urine samples collected more than 6 hours apart is an important sign of pre-eclampsia, and some question the diagnosis in its absence. Proteinuria, however, may be late in occurrence or difficult to detect on a one-time visit with dilute urine. The presence of edema may indicate pre-eclampsia, but its occurrence is common in normotensive pregnant women. The edema should be path-

---

TABLE 57-11. HYPERTENSIVE DISORDERS OF PREGNANCY—CLASSIFICATION*

HYPERTENSION:
  Diastolic ≥ 90 mmHg or increase over previous ≥ 15 on ≥ 2 occasions at least 6 hours apart
  Systolic ≥ 140 mmHg or increase over previous ≥ 30 on ≥ 2 occasions at least 6 hours apart

PREGNANCY-INDUCED HYPERTENSION (PIH):
  Hypertension that develops as a consequence of pregnancy and regresses postpartum
  1. Hypertension without proteinuria or pathologic edema
  2. Preeclampsia—with proteinuria and/or pathologic edema
     a. Mild
     b. Severe (bp ≥ 160/110 mmHg)
  3. Eclampsia—proteinuria and/or pathologic edema with convulsions

PREGNANCY-AGGRAVATED HYPERTENSION (PAH):
  Pre-existent hypertension worsened by pregnancy
  1. Superimposed pre-eclampsia
  2. Superimposed eclampsia

CHRONIC OR COINCIDENT HYPERTENSION:
  Chronic hypertension that antedates pregnancy or persists postpartum

* Modified with permission from Cunningham, F.G., MacDonald, P.C., and Gant, N.F. In Williams Obstetrics 18th edition. Norwalk, CT, Appleton and Lange, 1989.

TABLE 57-12. SELECTED CAUSES OF MATERNAL DEATHS

Cause of Death	Kaunitz et al., 1974–1978, 50 States, 2475 States		Rochat et al., 1980–1985, 19 Selected Areas, 601 Deaths	
	No.	%	No.	%
Embolism	491	20	102	17
Hypertensive disease	421	17	74	12
Ectopic pregnancy	254	10	60	10
Hemorrhage	331	13	55	09
Infections	199	08	55	09
Cerebrovascular accidents	117	04	51	08
Anesthesia complications	98	40	42	07
Abortions	141	06	31	05
Cardiovascular (preexisting)			31	05
Cardiomyopathy			25	04
Other	423	17	75	12
Total	2475	100	601	100

* Modified with permission from Kaunitz, A.M., Hughes, J.M., Grimes, D.A., et al.: Causes of maternal mortality in the United States. Obstet. Gynecol. 65:605, 1985; and Rochat, R.W., Koonin, L.M., Atrash, H.K., et al.: Maternal mortality surveillance, United States, 1980–1985. MMWR 37:19–29, 1988.

ologic, not just dependent, involve the hands and face, and not resolve with activity or upright posture.

Emergent differentiation between pregnancy-induced hypertension, pregnancy-aggravated hypertension, and coincidental hypertension may be difficult. Patients may lack knowledge of previous blood pressure or hypertension or not have received prenatal care, or records may be unavailable. Additionally, it should also be kept in mind that, in both normotensive and previously hypertensive women, the blood pressure usually falls in the first two trimesters, reaching a nadir by the end of the second or early in the third trimester, and rises during the third trimester to a level above initial values. In the ED, distinction between types of hypertension may not be possible or relevant, and classification and diagnosis may be restricted to hypertension, pre-eclampsia, severe pre-eclampsia, or eclampsia.

The severity of pre-eclampsia roughly correlates with blood pressure and degree of proteinuria (Table 57-13). No one criterion, however, is entirely dependable. Convulsions may occur in the presence of mildly elevated blood pressure or with mild proteinuria, or rarely, even in its absence. Severe persistent proteinuria, however, is an indicator of severe preeclampsia, as is a markedly elevated blood pressure. Other ominous signs include severe headache or visual disturbances, right upper quadrant or epigastric pain (from stretching of the hepatic capsule secondary to edema or necrosis), and evidence of hemolysis (thrombocytopenia, hemoglobinemia or hemoglobinuria or hyperbilirubinuria). Many authors have noted an increased risk of multiple organ failure and poor maternal and fetal outcome associated with a condition known as the HELLP syndrome (Hemolysis, Elevated Liver enzymes, and Low Platelet count), which appears to involve progressive disseminated intra-

TABLE 57-13. INDICATORS OF SEVERE PRE-ECLAMPSIA

Blood pressure of ≥ 110 mmHg diastolic
　　　　　　　　 ≥ 160 mmHg systolic
Proteinuria of ≥ 2+
Headache or visual disturbances
Hyperreflexia or clonus
Epigastric or right upper quadrant pain
Oliguria
Pulmonary edema, cardiac failure, or hypoxia
Azotemia
Hemoconcentration
Hemolysis
Elevated liver enzymes or hyperbilirubinemia
Thrombocytopenia
Fetal growth retardation
HELLP (Hemolysis, elevated liver enzymes, low platelets)

vascular coagulation.[9,10] Seizures of eclampsia are generalized and may appear before, during, or up to 48 hours postpartum.

RISK FACTORS

The incidence of hypertensive disease of pregnancy can be related to several factors, including parity, age, race, genetics, and fetal number. Pre-eclampsia occurs most often in nulliparous women. In both nulliparous and multiparous women, the incidence of preeclampsia increases with age, with an overall two- to fourfold increase for older women, reflecting the increased incidence of hypertension with age. Primiparas aged 25, 35, and 40 have rates of pre-eclampsia of 6, 9, and 15% respectively, and multiparas of the same ages rates of 3, 5, and 7%. Thus nulliparity and increasing age are both independent risk factors for the development of pre-eclampsia[5,6] (see Table 57-14). Risk is also influenced by race, adjusting for parity, with lowest incidence in whites, increasing in Hispanics, and highest in blacks. This may reflect in part the increased incidence of hypertension in blacks. Pre-eclampsia also appears to be inherited, with an increased risk in offspring of mothers who had pre-eclampsia. Multiparas who had pre-eclampsia with their first pregnancy have a higher risk of recurrence than multiparas without such a history, and the severity of recurrence seems to parallel the severity of disease in the first pregnancy. The overall estimated risk of recurrence is about 7.5% in women who had severe pre-eclampsia in their first pregnancy.[11] Multiple gestational pregnancies are also associated with an increase in hypertensive disease.

PATHOGENESIS AND PATHOPHYSIOLOGY

Current understanding of the cause of pre-eclampsia and eclampsia seems to involve an aberrant immunologic response to the presence of fetal trophoblastic tissue or chorionic villi. This hypothesis is supported by observations that PIH is more likely to occur with first-time exposure to chorionic villi (nulliparas), later in pregnancy (beginning and increasing in incidence after the 20th week in normal pregnancies), in women with an overabundance of chorionic villi (multiple fetal and molar pregnancies), and in pregnancies with a new antigenic identity (multiparas impregnated by new consort or donor insemination). But the exact mechanisms involved are far from clear, and multiple other theories have been proposed.[12-15]

The basic pathophysiology of pre-eclampsia and eclampsia seems better elucidated. In perhaps the most commonly accepted theory, altered prostaglandin metabolism is felt to cause increased vascular reactivity, with resultant widespread maternal vasospasm, endothelial damage, platelet activation, and increased endothelial damage.[1,12,13] Vascular constriction causes increased vascular resistance and consequent arterial hypertension.[1] This theory is felt to be supported by the finding that the normal refractoriness of pregnant women to the pressors such as angiotension II is lost in women who develop pre-eclampsia even before it is clinically obvious. Friedman postulates that the altered prostaglandin metabolism is a result of uterine hypoperfusion, caused by the unexplained inability of the spiral arteries to dilate, with fetoplacental release of lipoxygenase products and the elevation of the maternal thromboxane A2/prostacyclin ratio.[12] Thromboxane A2 is a potent va-

soconstrictor and platelet aggregation activator that is manufactured primarily by platelets. Prostacyclin is a potent vasodilator and platelet aggregation inhibitor produced by the endothelium. Supportive of this is work that shows thromboxane A2 to be increased and prostacyclin decreased in pre-eclampsia.[1,12] Additionally, recent studies show a possibly decreased occurrence of pre-eclampsia in predisposed gravid women taking low-dose aspirin, which presumably alters the thromboxane/prostacyclin ratio.[12,16,17] A recent alternative theory for the pathophysiology of pre-eclampsia is the hyperdynamic model in which increased cardiac output and compensatory vasodilation mediate end-organ damage. Renal hyperperfusion causes hypertension and proteinuria. Systemic vasodilation causes diffuse endothelial damage with platelet activation, altered prostaglandin metabolism, and a feedback loop of increased endothelial damage, vasospasm, and development of clinical disease with a change to a hypodynamic state.[15]

Maternal vasospasm causes multiple changes in maternal physiology. Maternal blood volume, which normally increases in pregnancy by 1500 mL to a total of 5000 mL, remains at 3500 mL, presumably as a result of vasoconstriction. Systemic vascular resistance (SVR) is increased, as is blood pressure, and cardiac output is decreased, while cardiac contractility and left ventricular function are usually unchanged. The pre-eclamptic woman is left unduly sensitive to either vigorous fluid therapy or blood loss. Maternal hematologic abnormalities are common and are characterized by a consumptive coagulopathy with thrombocytopenia, and less often by microangiopathic hemolysis and decreased levels of plasma clotting factors and elevated levels of fibrin degradation products. Endocrine changes associated with preeclampsia include an absence of elevation of renin, angiotensin II, and aldosterone levels seen in normal pregnancies. Fluid distribution is altered, with an even greater extracellular fluid volume increase than seen in normal pregnancy. Renal perfusion and glomerular filtration fail to increase as in normal pregnancy, and in severe disease may even be lower than nonpregnant levels. Proteinuria is a part of the diagnostic definition of preeclampsia, but may not occur at significant levels until late in the disease. Hepatic abnormalities, including elevated serum liver enzymes, may result from periportal hemorrhagic necrosis and indicate serious disease, usually occurring in the presence of other organ involvement. Changes seen in the brain include edema, hyperemia, focal thrombosis, and hemorrhage, and may result in seizures or coma. Visual disturbances are associated with severe pre-eclampsia, although blindness is uncommon. Uteroplacental vasospasm causes decreased uteroplacental perfusion, and thus is probably the major cause of perinatal morbidity and mortality associated with preeclampsia. Microscopic study of uteroplacental arteries reveals endothelial damage, myointimal proliferation, and medial necrosis.

CLINICAL PRESENTATION

Most patients with hypertensive disease of pregnancy (PIH, PAH, or pre-eclampsia) who present to the ED are undiagnosed on their presentation. Diagnosed cases are generally already hospitalized or admitted directly to the obstetric ward. Therefore a high index of suspicion must be maintained when seeing pregnant women in their second and third trimesters. The two most reliable criteria for pre-eclampsia are abnormalities of which the patient is usually unaware, hypertension and proteinuria. Edema is a common finding and less discriminative. The patient may also be unaware of recent weight gain. By the time the patient is symptomatic, the disease is advanced, and its presence is indicated by headache, abdominal pain, visual disturbance, or even seizures. Lack of prenatal care denotes a high risk for the possible presence of undetected hypertensive disease because both quiescent and symptomatic abnormalities are routinely screened for during obstetric care. Other historical clues that may denote increased risk are, as noted previously, nulliparity, advanced maternal age, previous hypertension, diabetes, race, multiple fetal pregnancy, molar pregnancy, family history of pre-eclampsia, or previous pre-eclamptic pregnancy (Table 57-14).

HYPERTENSION

Blood pressure elevation is the only criterion for PIH or PAH, and is the most reliable indicator of pre-eclampsia. A confirmed elevation of blood pressure above 140/90 mmHg, the diastolic value being more reliable, or a confirmed elevation of 30 mmHg systolic or 15 mmHg diastolic from a known baseline denotes probable hypertensive disease.

PROTEINURIA

Significant proteinuria (≥1+ on the urine dipstick or >300 mg in 24 hours) is a later-occurring but more reliable sign of pre-eclampsia. In the ED, where timed collection is precluded, its reliability is decreased by normally varying urine concentration. Strongly positive urine should be regarded as indicating pre-eclampsia in the presence of hypertension.

EDEMA AND WEIGHT GAIN

Edema may occur commonly in pregnancy, but its occurrence may indicate pre-eclampsia, especially if it is nondependent, with swollen fingers or face. Onset

TABLE 57-14. RISK FACTORS FOR HYPERTENSIVE DISEASE OF PREGNANCY

Nulliparity
Age—increases with age in both nulliparas and multiparas
Race—increased in Hispanics, most increased in blacks
Previous hypertension
Diabetes
Family history of pre-eclampsia
Previous pregnancy with severe pre-eclampsia
Hydatiform mole
Multiple fetal pregnancy
Multipara with impregnation by new consort or donor insemination
Lower socioeconomic group—uncertain if independent influence

of edema may be preceded by sudden weight gain in excess of the normally expected 1 pound per week.

HEADACHE

Progressive severe headache, initially mild at onset and frontal to frontooccipital, may signify cerebral ischemia or inflammation. Headache usually precedes convulsions.

VISUAL DISTURBANCES

Visual disturbances associated with pre-eclampsia may include blurring of vision, scotomata, or rarely partial or complete blindness, and indicate ischemia or inflammation of the occipital cortex, retina, or ophthalmic vasculature.

EPIGASTRIC OR RIGHT UPPER QUADRANT PAIN

Epigastric or right upper quadrant pain may signify hepatic swelling or impending rupture from ischemia, edema, or hemorrhage.

CONVULSIONS

Convulsions are generally tonic-clonic and may occur antepartum, intrapartum, or postpartum. The tonic phase generally lasts less than 30 seconds, followed by a clonic phase of usually less than 1 minute, followed in turn by a postictal period. The convulsions may recur, and in untreated severe cases, recurrences may be multiple or the patient may develop status epilepticus. Pre-eclampsia nearly always precedes convulsions, as do severe headache and nervous system irritability. Coma may follow convulsions, but its occurrence alone is regarded as part of pre-eclampsia.

PHYSICAL EXAMINATION

In addition to checking of vital signs, the physical examination should specifically include:

1. Soft tissue examination looking for signs of non-dependent edema.
2. Chest auscultation, especially to ascertain presence of pulmonary edema, one of the most serious complications of pre-eclampsia.
3. Abdominal examination to elicit right upper quadrant tenderness, indicating hepatic edema or impending rupture, fundal height for estimation of gestational age, uterine tenderness to exclude abruptio placentae, and fetal heart tones to ascertain fetal viability.
4. Pelvic examination to check cervical dilation and effacement and fetal presentation and station.
5. Deep tendon reflexes to elicit hyperreflexia or clonus, indicators of central nervous system irritability or impending seizures.

LABORATORY TESTS

In the presence of suspected pre-eclampsia, laboratory tests should include:

1. Complete blood count (CBC), including platelets, to look for signs of hemoconcentration, hemolysis, or DIC.
2. Urinalysis to ascertain presence of proteinuria, renal disease, or oliguria.
3. Electrolytes, creatinine, and BUN to ascertain electrolyte status and renal function.
4. Coagulation studies, which may indicate coagulopathy or DIC, and possibly uric acid and liver function tests: bilirubin, LDH, and AST, all of which may be elevated in pre-eclampsia.

See Appendix 57A, at the end of this chapter.

SEVERITY

The severity of disease is generally but not reliably proportional to the degree of blood pressure elevation. Other criteria may also indicate increased severity of disease (see Table 57-13). These include the presence of proteinuria, especially if persistent and severe, symptoms of headache, disturbed vision, abdominal pain, oliguria, and convulsions; laboratory abnormalities of azotemia, liver dysfunction, or consump-

tive coagulopathy; or findings of fetal growth retardation or pulmonary edema. The more diffuse or severe the abnormalities, the more severe the disease and the greater the need for emergent stabilization and pregnancy termination.

MANAGEMENT

Once the diagnosis of hypertensive disease of pregnancy is made, whether it is PIH, PAH, pre-eclampsia or eclampsia, management includes hospitalization. Pregnancy-induced and pregnancy-aggravated hypertension are sometimes managed by the obstetrician on an outpatient basis after initial hospitalization, but for the emergency physician, diagnosis of hypertensive disease of pregnancy mandates hospitalization to the service of the obstetric specialist. In suspected pre-eclampsia, prompt hospitalization is absolutely indicated. In severe pre-eclampsia (see Table 57-13), stabilizing treatment should be instituted immediately in conjunction with hospitalization to the obstetric service.

Stabilizing treatment has two primary objectives: termination and/or prevention of convulsions and lowering of dangerously elevated blood pressure, both of which present a threat to the health of the mother and fetus. Pre-eclampsia persists until delivery of fetus and placenta, which is the only true cure.

Convulsions are controlled or prevented with magnesium sulfate (Table 57-15). An initial loading dose of 4 g of magnesium sulfate is diluted in 20 to 100 mL of D5W and given intravenously at a rate not to exceed 1 g per minute, usually over 10 to 30 minutes. This is then followed by the intravenous infusion of dilute magnesium sulfate at a rate of 1 to 3 g per hour by infusion pump with regular and continual monitoring of the patellar reflex for signs of toxicity (absent reflexes, or need for increased medication, hyperactivity, or clonus). Alternatively, after the initial intravenous loading dose of 4 g, deep intramuscular administration of 10 g of magnesium sulfate (50% solution divided in two equal doses of 10 mL with 1 mL of 1% or 2% lidocaine added to the syringe to minimize discomfort) is given in the upper outer quadrants of the buttocks. At 4-hour intervals, an additional 5 g of 50% magnesium sulfate is given in alternating buttocks as long as patellar reflex is present, respirations are not depressed, and urine output of at least 25 mL per hour is maintained. Although it is less comfortable, use of the intramuscular regimen may be advantageous in situations in which the patient may have to be transferred or transported or personnel or infusion pumps are limited. In either regimen, if seizures persist, additional magnesium sulfate is given intravenously in 1 to 2 g doses at rates no faster than 1 g per minute. Plasma magnesium levels may be helpful to assess efficacy or possible toxicity of therapy. The therapeutic range is 4 to 6 mEq/L, patellar reflexes disappear at 8 to 10 mEq/L, and respiratory depression and cardiac arrest generally occur at higher levels.

Some women may experience toxic symptoms at lower dosages, and caution must be used. Patients on magnesium sulfate *must* be under constant observation and nursing supervision. Calcium gluconate, 1 g given intravenously as 10 mL of 10% solution, usually reverses signs of serious toxicity. Otherwise prompt intubation and mechanical ventilation is necessary. If seizures persist despite therapeutic or elevated levels of magnesium, intravenous sodium amobarbital may be given in doses of up to 250 mg or diazepam in 5 to 10 mg doses.[1,14,18-20]

ANTIHYPERTENSIVE THERAPY

Antihypertensive therapy is indicated if the diastolic blood pressure is elevated above 110 Hg. Hydralazine is given intravenously as a 5 mg dose and blood pressure monitored at 5 minute intervals. Hydralazine is readministered at intervals no more frequent than 15 to 20 minutes in 5 to 10 mg doses until the desired diastolic level of 100 mmHg is reached. The initial dose should never exceed 5 mg (some advocate a 1 mg test dose). Subsequent doses should not exceed 5 to 10 mg. Increasing severity of hypertension does not predict the need for increasing dose of hydralazine. Some authors have observed that response to hydralazine correlates with severity of hypertension. An alternative is hydralazine by IV infusion (100 mg/250 cc NS) titrated by infusion pump to maintain a diastolic blood pressure of 100 mm Hg. Overzealous lowering of blood pressure or hypotension is to be avoided to prevent decreased placental perfusion and fetal jeopardization. In the rare circumstance that hydralazine does not effectively lower blood pressure, or in more precise temporal control of blood pressure (such as in an eclamptic undergoing caesarean section under general anesthesia), nitroglycerin infusion has been advocated because of its short half-life and lack of fetal toxicity.[21] In cases complicated by oliguria and/or pulmonary edema, invasive monitoring may also be needed to optimize pharmacologic and fluid management.[22] Use of beta-blockers to control hypertension has also been advocated.

Use of diuretics and hyperosmotic agents is to be avoided. This is because, although overall body fluid may be increased, the increase is in the extravascular component and the intravascular component is constricted. Excessive fluid therapy is also to be avoided because this would only exacerbate the existing maldistribution of fluid and increase the risk of pulmonary or cerebral edema.[1,14,18-20]

Complications seen with pre-eclampsia include pulmonary edema, intracranial bleeding, abruptio pla-

centae and fetal distress, growth retardation, and demise. Pulmonary edema is the most common cause of maternal death. Maternal mortality increases dramatically with maternal age.[23,24]

TABLE 57-15. MAGNESIUM SULFATE THERAPY*

Intravenous Regimen:
  Initial loading dose of 4 g magnesium sulfate (6 g in larger women) is diluted in 100 mL D5W and given over 30 minutes (more rapidly in presence of convulsions)
  Maintenance infusion by intravenous pump of 1 to 3 g magnesium sulfate per hour given as a 10% solution (20 g in 200 mL D5W—1 g per 10 mL) at a rate of 10 to 30 mL per hour
  Hourly assessment of deep tendon reflexes, urine output, and urine protein
  Magnesium level 2 hours after initial dose and repeated every 6 hours or every 4 hours for infusion rates > 2 g per hour
Intramuscular Regimen:
  Initial intravenous loading dose of 4 g of 20% magnesium sulfate solution (dilute 4 g to 20 mL with D5W) at a rate not to exceed 1 g per minute
  Follow promptly with 10 g of 50% solution, one half (5 g = 10 mL) injected deeply in the upper outer quadrant of both buttocks through a 3-inch, 20-gauge needle. Addition of 1 mL of 2% lidocaine to each syringe decreases discomfort. If convulsions persist after 15 minutes, give 2 g more intravenously as the 20% solution at a rate not greater than 1 g per minute.
  Every 4 hours thereafter, give 5 g of a 50% solution injected deeply in the upper outer quadrant of alternating buttocks, but only after ascertaining that:
    the patellar reflex is present
    respirations are not depressed
    urine output for the previous 4 hours exceeds 100 mL
Magnesium levels:
  Therapeutic 4 to 6 mEq/L
  Loss of patellar reflex 8 to 10 mEq/L
  Respiratory depression or arrest ≥ 12 mEq/L
Antidotal therapy for magnesium toxicity:
  Calcium gluconate 10 mL of 10% solution is given intramuscularly over 3 minutes
  Endotracheal intubation and mechanical ventilation if inadequate response to calcium gluconate

* Modified in part, with permission, from Cunningham, F.G., MacDonald, P.C., and Gant, N.F.: Williams Obstetrics, 18th Ed. East Norwalk, CT, Appleton and Lange, 1989, p. 680.

PITFALLS AND MEDICOLEGAL PEARLS

With severe pre-eclampsia, some maternal deaths have occurred from delays in delivery despite the fact that the infant was full-term. The emergency physician should treat this condition as possibly life-threatening.

Legal cases have been settled for substantial sums because of injury or maternal death associated with administration of magnesium sulfate in excess or without constant observation. In one illustrative case, the patient was in a private room and experienced respiratory and cardiac arrest that were detected only on routine nursing assessment.

REFERENCES

1. Cunningham, F.G., MacDonald, P.C., and Gant, N.F.: Williams Obstetrics, 18th Edition. Norwalk, Connecticut, Appleton and Lange, 1989.
2. Kaunitz, A.M., Hughes, J.M., Grimes, D.A., et al.: Causes of maternal mortality in the United States. Obstet. Gynecol. 65:605, 1985.
3. Koonin, L.M., Atrash, H.K., Rochat, R.W., and Smith, J.C.: Maternal mortality surveillance, United States, 1980–1985. MMWR 37:19, 1988.
4. Rochat, R.W., Koonin, L.M., Atrash, H.K., et al.: Maternal mortality in the United States: report from the maternal mortality collaborative. Obstet. Gynecol. 72:91, 1988.
5. Hanson, J.P.: Older maternal age and pregnancy outcome: A review of the literature. Obstet. Gynecol. Surv. 41:726, 1986.
6. Fonteyn, V.J., and Isada, N.B.: Nongenetic implications of childbearing after age thirty-five. Obstet. Gynecol. Surv. 43:709, 1988.
7. Friedman, E.A., and Neff, R.K.: Pregnancy outcome as related to hypertension, edema, and proteinuria. In Hypertension in Pregnancy. Edited by Lindheimer, M.D., Katz, A.I., and Zuspan, F.P. New York, Wiley, 1976, p. 13.
8. Ferris, T.F.: How should hypertension during pregnancy be managed? An internist's approach. Med. Clin. North Am. 68:491, 1984.
9. Weinstein, L.: Syndrome of hemolysis, elevated liver enzymes, and low platelet count: A severe consequence of hypertension in pregnancy. Am. J. Obstet. Gynecol. 62:751, 1982.
10. Van Dam, P.A., Renier, M., Baekelandt, M., et al.: Disseminated intravascular coagulation and the syndrome of hemolysis, elevated liver enzymes, and low platelets in severe pre-eclampsia. Obstet. Gynecol. 73:97, 1989.
11. Mehta, L., and Young, I.D.: Recurrence risks for common complications of pregnancy—A review. Obstet. Gynceol. Surv. 42:218, 1987.
12. Friedman, S.A.: Pre-eclampsia: A review of the role of prostaglandins. Obstet. Gynecol. 71:122, 1988.
13. Gant, N.F., and Gilstrap, L.C.: Pharmacologic approaches to prevent pregnancy-induced hypertension. In supplement no. 5 to Williams Obstetrics. 18th Ed. Norwalk, Appleton and Lange, 1990.
14. Doan-Wiggins, L.: Hypertensive disorders of pregnancy. Emerg. Med. Clin. North Am. 5:495, 1987.
15. Easterling, T.R., and Benedetti, T.J.: Pre-eclampsia: A hyperdynamic disease model. Am. J. Obstet. Gynecol. 160:1447, 1989.
16. Schiff, E., Peleg, E., Goldenberg, M., et al.: The use of aspirin to prevent pregnancy-induced hypertension and lower the ratio of thromboxane a2 to prostacylin in relatively high risk pregnancies. N. Engl. J. Med. 321:351, 1989.
17. Benigni, A., Gregerini, G., Frusca, T., et al.: Effect of low-dose aspirin on fetal and maternal generation of thromboxane by platelets in women at risk for pregnancy-induced hypertension. N. Engl. J. Med. 321:357, 1989.
18. Cunningham, F.G., and Pritchard, S.A.: How should hypertension be managed? Experience at Parkland Memorial Hospital. Med. Clin. North Am. 68:505, 1984.
19. Pritchard, J.A., Cunningham, F.G., and Pritchard, S.A.: The Parkland Memorial Hospital protocol for treatment of pre-eclampsia. Am. J. Obstet. Gynecol. 148:951, 1984.
20. Taber, B.: Manual of Gynecologic and Obstetric Emergencies, 2nd ed. Philadelphia, W.B. Saunders Co., 1989, pp. 212–229.
21. Cotton, D.B., Longmire, S., Jones, M.M., et al.: Cardiovascular alterations in severe pregnancy-induced hypertension: Effects of intravenous nitroglycerin coupled with blood volume expansion. Am. J. Obstet. Gynecol. 154:1053, 1986.
22. Clark, S.L., Greenspoon, J.S., Aldahl, D., and Phelan, J.P.: Severe pre-eclampsia with persistent oliguria: management of hemodynamic subsets. Am. J. Obstet. Gynecol. 154:490, 1986.
23. Lehmann, D.K., Mabie, W.C., Miller, J.M., and Pernoll, M.L.: The epidemiology and pathology of maternal mortality: Charity Hospital of Louisiana in New Orleans, 1965–1984. Obstet. Gynecol. 69:833, 1987.
24. Lopez-Llera, M., Linares, G.R., and Horta, J.L.H.: Maternal mortality rates in eclampsia. Am. J. Obstet. Gynecol. 124:149, 1976.

MEDICAL DISORDERS OF PREGNANCY

Van H. Miller

CAPSULE

Pregnant patients can be expected to present to the Emergency Department (ED) with routine concerns of normal pregnancy and complications of pregnancy induced by pre-existing medical disorders and acquired disorders. Diagnostic and therapeutic modalities used to evaluate life-threatening medical problems in pregnancy are, for the most part, the same as in nonpregnant patients; in general, maternal well-being ensures fetal well-being.

The emergency physician is required to have a thorough understanding of the normal physiology of pregnancy to properly evaluate and treat pregnancy complicated by medical disorders. Table 57-16 summarizes important physiologic changes of pregnancy. Table 57-18 lists medical disorders discussed in this chapter by organ system and separates disease into pre-existing and acquired disorders. These two tables may be used as an index to find specific medical problems that may complicate pregnancy. Expected changes in laboratory values secondary to normal pregnancy are enumerated in Table 57-17. Tables 57-19 through 57-23 summarize important management guidelines and clinical information.

PHYSIOLOGY OF PREGNANCY (TABLE 57-16)

CARDIOPULMONARY

CARDIOVASCULAR

Normal cardiovascular changes of pregnancy include an increase in cardiac output, which begins to rise during the first 10 weeks of pregnancy and peaks at the 20th week at 30 to 45% above resting cardiac output. Approximately 25% of maternal cardiac output goes to the uteroplacental unit, which functions as a large low-resistance arteriovenous shunt. Blood pressure is expected to fall or remain the same in relation to decreased systemic vascular resistance coupled with expanded blood volume and reduced arteriolar vasomotor tone. Dyspnea, edema, functional systolic heart murmurs, and the presence of a third heart sound are frequent occurrences in normal pregnancy. The enlarging uterus can interfere with venous and, to a lesser extent, arterial blood flow by compressing the inferior vena cava and aortofemoral vessels when the pregnant patient is in the supine position. Changing from the supine position to the left lateral decubitus position can increase cardiac output by as much as 22%.

PULMONARY

Two changes in the respiratory tree occur to increase breathing efficiency in pregnancy. There is a decrease in dead space in the lungs because of elevation of the diaphragm and increase in the chest diameter from thoracic wall intercostal muscle relaxation; also, the air bronchiolar resistance decreases from bronchiolar dilation.

Minute ventilation is increased up to 40% by increasing tidal volume without increasing respiratory rate. Respiratory rates above 20 indicate pathology. The developing fetus increases maternal oxygen consumption by approximately 20%, but the increase in ventilation is greater than the increase in oxygen consumption, and consequently maternal acid-base status is characterized by a mild respiratory alkalosis (Table

---

TABLE 57-16. PHYSIOLOGIC CHANGES IN PREGNANCY*

1. *Cardiopulmonary*
   Cardiovascular
   ↑ Blood volume, cardiac output
   ↓ Systemic vascular resistance, uterine circulation functions as A—V shunt
   Arteriovenous return of lower extremities subject to uterine compression
   Dyspnea, edema, and third heart sound frequently found
   Pulmonary
   ↑ O_2 consumption, ↑ minute ventilation by increasing tidal volume, subjective dyspnea

2. *Endocrine-Metabolic*
   Endocrine
   Hypermetabolic state, mimics hyperthroidism
   Principal hormones of pregnancy induce relative glucose intolerance, also produce benign clinical syndromes
   Metabolic
   Weight gain, first trimester average gain 2–3 lbs, second and third trimester gains of 11 lbs, total weight gain of 24 to 28 lbs.
   Retention of sodium and water, lower extremity edema common.
   Altered protein metabolism with ↓ albumin, ↑ thyroglobulin, and ↑ fibrinogen concentration, also in clotting cascade ↑ in procoagulants over circulating inhibiters of coagulation producing a so-called hypercoagulable state.

3. *Hematologic/Immunologic*
   Hematologic
   Expanded blood volume (45%), with ↑ in plasma volume greater than ↑ in circulating RBCs (33%), maximum effect in second trimester with resultant decrease in hematocrit (15%). Blood leukocyte count generally elevated, often markedly during labor and early puerperium.
   Immunologic
   Material immune hyporesponsiveness allows maternal-fetal coexistence. Proximity of fetal and maternal circulation presents risk of isoimmunization.

4. *Renal*
   30 to 50% ↑ glomerular filtration rate (GFR). Δs in tubular reabsorption coupled with ↑ GFR lead to glucosuria in 16%, proteinuria < 300 mg/24 hrs, ↑ renal plasma flow (RPF) result ↓ creatinine and urea concentration. Δs in drug clearance from ↑ in GFR and RPF. Physiologic hydronephrosis.

---

* Modified with permission from Barron, W.M.: The pregnant surgical patient: *Medical Evaluation and Management. Ann. Intern. Med. 101*:683, 1984.

57-17). Despite this increase in breathing efficiency, many pregnant women complain of breathlessness or feeling short of breath.

ENDOCRINE-METABOLIC

ENDOCRINE

Early normal pregnancy has a large increase in estrogen and progesterone levels; the former stimulates insulin secretion and enhances peripheral use of glucose. The first 20 weeks of pregnancy are characterized by a decrease in fasting plasma glucose and improved glucose tolerance. The latter 20 weeks of pregnancy

TABLE 57-17. LABORATORY VALUES IN PREGNANCY

Value	Nonpregnant Women	Pregnant Women
Electrolytes and Acid-Base Values		
Sodium (mEq/L)	135–145	132–140
Potassium (mEq/L)	3.5–5.0	3.5–4.5
Chloride (mEq/L)	100–106	90–105
Bicarbonate (mEq/L)	24–30	17–22
pCO_2 (mm Hg)	35–50	25–30
pO_2 (mm Hg)	98–100	101–104
Base excess (mEq/L)	0.7	3–4
Arterial pH	7.38–7.44	7.40–7.45
BUN (mg/dL)	10–18	4–12
Creatinine (mg/dL)	0.6–1.2	0.4–0.9
Creatinine clearance (mL/min)	3.5–5.0	2.0–3.7
Osmolality (mOsm/kg)	275–295	275–285
Fasting whole venous blood glucose (mg/dL)		<90†
Fasting venous plasma glucose (mg/dL)	75–115	<105†
Lipids and Liver Function Tests		
Total bilirubin (mg/dL)	1.0	1.0
Direct bilirubin (mg/dL)	0.4	0.4
Alkaline phosphatase (IU/mL)	13–35	25–80
SGOT (IU/mL)	10–40	10–40
Total protein (g/dL)	6.0–8.4	5.5–7.5
Albumin (g/dL)	3.5–5.0	3.0–4.5
Globulin (g/dL)	2.3–3.5	3.0–4.0
Total lipids (mg/dL)	460–1000	1040
Total cholesterol (mg/dL)	120–220	250
Triglycerides (mg/dL)	45–150	230
Free fatty acid (µg/L)	770	1226
Phospholipids (mg/dL)	256	350
Hematologic Laboratory Values		
Complete blood count		
Hematocrit (%)	37–48	32–42
Hemoglobin (g/dL)	12–16	10–14
Leukocyte (count/mm³)	4,300–10,800	5,000–15,000
Polymorphonuclear cells (%)	54–62	60–85
Lymphocytes (%)	38–46	15–40
Fibrinogen (mg/dL)	250–400	600
Platelets (count/mm³)	150,000–350,000	Normal or slightly decreased
Serum iron (µg)	75–150	65–120
Iron binding capacity (µg)	250–410	300–500
Iron saturation (%)	30–40	15–30
Ferritin (ng/mL)	35	10–12
Erythrocyte sedimentation (mm/hour)	<20	30–90

 * Adapted with permission from Carlson, J.A.: The role of the medical consultant in pregnancy. Med. Clin. North Am. Medical Problems in Pregnancy 73:54, 1989.
 † Greater than or equal to this value suggests glucose intolerance and indicates need for further testing

are characterized by a state of insulin resistance.[1] The reasons for this are not completely understood but probably related to increased levels of human placental lactogen (hPL), prolactin, cortisol, and progesterone. Thus normal pregnancy is characterized by fasting hypoglycemia with exaggerated postprandial insulin and glucose levels. The placenta is impermeable to insulin and glucagon. Fetal pancreatic insulin secretion begins between 9 and 11 weeks of gestation and may be stimulated by both glucose and amino acids. It is believed that fetal insulin is the major growth factor in the fetus.[1]

METABOLIC

Normal pregnancy is characterized by a 2- to 3-pound weight gain in the first trimester and approximately 11 pounds of weight gain in both the second and third trimesters, for an average total weight gain of 24 to 28 pounds. Extremity edema is present in up to 80% of normal pregnancies, partly as a result of decreased serum albumin and amino acids.

Because of the hormonal effects of pregnancy, the maternal response to feeding is characterized by elevated postprandial blood sugar, free fatty acids, ketones, and triglycerides. The maternal response to fasting is accelerated catabolism with a tendency for early ketosis and acidemia. The placenta regulates delivery of metabolic substrate to the fetus. Glucose is transported by facilitated diffusion, amino acids by active transport; ketones diffuse across freely, but fatty acids diffuse across in limited quantities by a gradient dependent on diffusion. The purpose is to ensure fatty fuels for maternal needs and promote carbohydrate transfer to the fetus. Maternal hyperglycemia results in fetal hyperinsulinemia.[1,2]

HEMATOLOGIC-IMMUNOLOGIC

HEMATOLOGIC

Normal pregnancy produces a 45% increase in blood volume at term. The increase in circulating red blood cells is relatively less than the increase in plasma volume, leading to an approximately 15% drop in hematocrit by the second trimester. Average-term hemoglobin concentration is 12.5 g %, and levels below 11 g % should be considered abnormal. Blood leukocyte counts are generally elevated during pregnancy, and often markedly so during labor and the early puerperium.

Pregnancy is frequently described as a hypercoagulable state, with a rise in most procoagulants.[3] It is also thought that the placenta modifies fibrinolytic activity, favoring clot formation over clot lysis.[3]

IMMUNOLOGIC

Maternal immune hyporesponsiveness allows maternal-fetal coexistence. The proximity of fetal and maternal circulation presents risk of isoimmunization.

RENAL

Values of serum creatinine and BUN are reduced in pregnancy. A serum creatinine and BUN greater than 0.9 mg/dL and 12 mg/dL should be suspect. Ideally, glomerular filtration rate (GFR), based on the clearance of serum creatinine, is used as a measure for renal function. Normal pregnancy produces a 30 to 50% increase in GFR and an increase in renal plasma flow. These increases produce the observed lowered concentrations of serum creatinine and blood urea nitrogen (BUN), and also increased drug clearance. As a result of increased GFR, drug dosages in pregnancy frequently have to be increased to remain therapeutic. Changes in tubular reabsorption coupled with increased glomerular filtration rate lead to glucosuria in 16% of normal pregnancies. Proteinuria is considered abnormal when urinary protein excretion exceeds 300 mg in 24 hours.[4] Hormones of pregnancy also produce a physiologic hydronephrosis.

GASTROINTESTINAL

The decreased peristalsis of smooth muscles of the gastrointestinal tract reduces the emptying time of the stomach, large intestines, and gallbladder, resulting in gastric reflux into the esophagus, constipation from increased water reabsorption of stool, and a propensity for gallstone formation.

MUSCULOSKELETAL

Low back pain and discomfort are common complaints of pregnant women. The increased incidence of nocturnal leg cramps during pregnancy remains unexplained.

MEDICAL COMPLICATIONS OF PREGNANCY (TABLE 57-18)

CARDIOVASCULAR PRE-EXISTING DISORDERS

CONGESTIVE HEART FAILURE AND CARDIOVASCULAR DISEASE

Since 1979, a clinical classification system provided by the New York Heart Association (NYHA), based on the functional status of the heart, has been widely used to determine the prognosis for successful pregnancy. In essence, this system divides all cardiac disease into four functional classes. Classes I and II are defined as having no functional limitation of activity and no cardiac symptoms with mild functional limitations and symptoms with physical activity. These patients do well during pregnancy. Class III patients have limited ability to perform most physical activities, but are asymptomatic at rest. Severe class III patients develop symptoms with minimal physical activity. Class IV patients have severe limitation of activity and some symptoms at rest with any physical activity producing cardiac symptoms. As might be expected, these patients do poorly and have a 30 to 50% chance of significant hemodynamic morbidity and a 25 to 50% chance of maternal mortality.

Management of congestive heart failure is similar in pregnant and nonpregnant patients. Functional class I and II patients may be allowed to labor and deliver with minimal intervention. Management involves close monitoring of input, output, pulse rate, respiratory rate, and dyspnea. Conventional delivery and relief of pain and apprehension without undue depression of the infant or the mother are all that are required.

TABLE 57-18. MEDICAL COMPLICATIONS OF PREGNANCY

Preexisting Disorders	Acquired Disorders
Cardiopulmonary	*Cardiopulmonary*
Cardiovascular	*Cardiovascular*
Congestive heart failure	Obstetrical shock/hemorrhage
Coronary heart disease/arrhythmias	Third trimester bleeding: Abruptio placentae
Organic heart disease/prosthetic heart	Placentae previa
valves	Eclampsia
Bacterial endocarditis prophylaxis	Peripartum heart failure
Hypertensive disorders	
Pulmonary	*Pulmonary*
Obstructive/restrictive pulmonary disease	Acute respiratory failure
	Carbon monoxide poisoning
	Thromboembolic disease: Pulmonary embolism
	Deep vein thrombosis
Endocrine/Metabolic	*Endocrine/Metabolic*
Overt diabetes mellitus	Gestational diabetes mellitus, hyperemesis
Hyperthyoidism	gravidarum, benign clinical syndromes
Hematologic/Immunologic	*Hematologic/Immunologic*
Anemias	Anemias
Nutritional	(see Cardiovascular/Obstetric Shock)
Sickle cell hemoglobinopathy	*Thrombocytopenia*
Thrombocytopenia	Without consumptive coagulopathy:
Idiopathic thrombocytopenia	Thrombotic thrombocytopenia
	Hemolytic uremia syndrome
	Postpartum renal failure
	With consumptive coagulopathy:
	Disseminated intravascular coagulation
Immunologic	*Immunologic*
Rheumatoid arthritis	Rh isoimmunization
Systemic lupus erythematosus	
Myasthenia gravis	
Renal	*Renal*
Impaired renal function (↓ GFR)	Acute Renal Failure
Renal transplant	UTI: Asymptomatic bacteriuria
	Cystitis/urethritis
	Pyelonephritis
Miscellaneous	*Miscellaneous*
Neurologic	*Gastrointestinal*
Seizures	Appendicitis
Infections	*Infections*
HIV	Viral: Rubella, rubeola, mumps, varicella-zoster, Epstein-Barr virus, erythema infectiosum, hepatitis A and B, herpes simplex, cytomegalovirus, enteroviruses.
	Bacterial: Group B streptococcus, Listeria monocytogenes, tuberculosis.
	Venereal/Bacterial: Syphilis, Chlamydia, gonorrhea.

Patients in the NYHA functional class III and IV categories have hemodynamically significant cardiac disease and often pulmonary hypertension and are at much higher risk during labor and delivery. Increases in pulse rate above 100, respiratory rate above 24, particularly when associated with dyspnea, suggest cardiac decompensation and require immediate medical intervention.[5]

Vaginal delivery is more desirable than cesarean section for patients with cardiac disease caused by attendant volume shifts, greater blood loss, and the effects of anesthesia on the cardiovascular system. Major surgical procedures are poorly tolerated by pa-

tients in heart failure, and the decision for cesarean section is reserved for the usual obstetric indications.

Coronary Artery Disease and Arrhythmias. Symptomatic coronary artery disease is rare in women of childbearing age. Most women with ischemic heart disease present for the first time during pregnancy. The rarity of this disease, with an estimated incidence of 1 in 10,000 pregnancies, makes low clinical suspicion a problem in making the diagnosis in the setting of pregnancy. The trimester in which infarction occurs has a major impact on survival. The mortality rate for third-trimester infarct is

45%, and 66% of infarctions occur during this trimester. An increased maternal mortality is seen when infarction occurs within 14 days of delivery.

Management goals are the same as for the nonpregnant patient. The unique stress of labor superimposed on the ischemic or recently infarcted heart calls for intense management.

In the emergency setting, the presentation and management of a tachyarrhythmia in a pregnant patient do not differ from those of the nonpregnant patient. Patients with arrhythmias resistant to medical therapy may undergo D/C cardioversion at low to moderate energy settings with little risk to the fetus, i.e., 25 to 50 joules.[6]

Organic Heart Disease and Prosthetic Heart Valves. Septal defects, patent ductus, ductus arteriosus (left-to-right shunts), and ductus arteriosus and tricuspid valve defects are low-risk organic cardiac lesions. These patients tolerate pregnancy well in the absence of pulmonary hypertension.

Pregnant patients with valvular regurgitation, i.e., mitral regurgitation and aortic regurgitation, tolerate pregnancy well. These patients are able to increase cardiac output in the face of the normal physiologic stresses of gestation and labor.

Stenotic lesions, i.e., aortic stenosis and mitral stenosis, are poorly tolerated in pregnant patients who have a fixed cardiac output and thus can poorly accommodate changes in blood volume and heart rate. They are particularly at risk for developing acute pulmonary edema during labor, when each uterine contraction transfuses 300 to 500 mL of blood into the systemic circulation.

Despite an overall decline in rheumatic heart disease, the occurrence of mitral stenosis is common enough to warrant familiarity with its course. Mitral stenosis remains one of the most dangerous cardiac complications of pregnancy. Life-threatening pulmonary edema, atrial flutter or fibrillation, and systemic embolization are often present in previously asymptomatic pregnant patients. Management does not differ from that of the nonpregnant patient, and is directed at decreasing heart rate, fluid restriction or diuretic therapy, and digitalis. Preferred delivery is vaginal, with epidural anesthesia for pain control.

Patients with organic heart disease producing pulmonary hypertension, cyanotic heart disease, coarctation of the aorta, and Marfan's syndrome do poorly during pregnancy. These patients must be identified early for appropriate counseling regarding interruption of a life-threatening pregnancy versus early intensive obstetric care. The emergency physician is frequently the first to identify such patients.

Women who have successfully undergone valve replacement and are pregnant are faced with the problems of anticoagulation. Although placement of bioprosthetic devices in women of childbearing age avoids these problems, these devices are of less durability than their mechanical counterparts, and re-

TABLE 57-19. AMERICAN HEART ASSOCIATION RECOMMENDATIONS FOR BACTERIAL ENDOCARDITIS PROPHYLAXIS AT THE TIME OF DELIVERY*

Drug	Dosage and Route
Ampicillin	2 g IV
Gentamicin	1.5 mg/kg IV/IM
In penicillin-allergic patients:	
Vancomycin	1 g IV
Gentamicin	1.5 mg/kg IV/IM to be administered in three doses every 8 hours

* Adapted with permission from Giannopoulos, J.G.: Cardiac disease in pregnancy. Med. Clin. North Am. *73*:3, 1989.

ports indicate that pregnancy may accelerate the degeneration of tissue valves.[7] Heparin is the anticoagulant of choice in pregnant patients with mechanical heart valves. Warfarin compounds are contraindicated during pregnancy because they readily cross the placenta and are teratogenic. Heparin is associated with no adverse fetal effects but may produce long-term maternal effects of reversible bone demineralization, thrombocytopenia, hyperkalemia, and dermatologic reactions. Fortunately, these complications are rare.

Although prophylaxis against bacterial endocarditis is not recommended by the American Heart Association for women undergoing vaginal delivery with organic heart disease, most cardiologists recommend prophylaxis for patients with structural heart disease undergoing vaginal delivery, as well as cesarean section and other surgical procedures. Administration should begin during labor and be continued for at least one dose after delivery. Table 57-19 gives the American Heart Association recommendations for bacterial endocarditis prophylaxis at delivery.

Hypertensive Disorders. Hypertension (HTN) is one of the most common medical complications encountered in pregnancy. The term pregnancy-induced hypertension (PIH) encompasses HTN alone and HTN from pre-eclampsia and eclampsia. Most women with HTN have uneventful pregnancies and actually show improvement of their blood pressure control during pregnancy; others experience dangerous worsening of their HTN accompanied by proteinuria, pathologic edema, and convulsions. These patients are indistinguishable from severe pre-eclampsia–eclampsia patients unless it is known that their HTN antedated the pregnancy. These patients are classified as having pregnancy-aggravated hypertension (PAH). The significance of differentiating severe chronic HTN presenting in preterm pregnancy from severe pre-eclampsia cannot be overstated.

Antihypertensive therapy in the management of severe HTN without PAH allows prolongation of pregnancy and lessening of perinatal mortality from 50%

untreated to the level of the general population. Also, antihypertensive therapy for mild pre-eclampsia is acceptable while awaiting maturation of the preterm fetus. But attempting to prolong pregnancy in the severe pre-eclamptic with aggressive antihypertensive therapy is not in the interest of the mother or fetus. The goal of treatment of chronic hypertension in pregnancy is to prevent the usual complications of HTN, i.e., intracranial hemorrhage, hypertensive congestive heart failure, and progressive renal failure. The prognosis for outcome during pregnancy is related to the severity of the disease before pregnancy. Although HTN in pregnancy has increased the risk of placental abruption, intrauterine fetal demise, and intrauterine fetal growth retardation, treatment of mild to moderate HTN does not appear to change the incidence of these complications. In fact, most pregnancies do well with mild to moderate HTN, whether or not antihypertensive therapy is given. Even with severe HTN, adverse outcomes are related to superimposed pre-eclampsia (PAH).

The decision to place the HTN patient on ongoing antihypertensive therapy requires consideration of the severity of HTN, the effects of treatment on the uteroplacental blood flow, and possible effects of the drugs themselves on the developing fetus. The usual standard of care is to treat with antihypertensive drugs if the BP is above 150/110 mmHg or the patient was receiving antihypertensive medication before the pregnancy and her HTN is well controlled. Methyldopa is probably still the drug of first choice, with labetalol and beta blockers reasonable but less well studied alternatives. Diuretics are usually not effective when used alone for the treatment of HTN in pregnancy.

ACQUIRED CARDIOVASCULAR DISORDERS

OBSTETRIC SHOCK AND HEMORRHAGE

The normal physiology of pregnancy delays the usual clinical signs of hemorrhagic shock. By the third trimester, a 40 to 50% increase in blood volume has occurred, allowing the approximate 600 mL blood loss seen in the average normal vaginal delivery to occur without physiologic compromise.[8,9] This physiologic increase in blood volume allows the pathologic loss of up to 35% of blood volume before tachycardia, hypotension, and other signs of hypovolemia are manifest. In the face of life-threatening exsanguination, mechanisms for self-preservation place maternal welfare over fetal welfare. Even in relatively well-compensated hypovolemia, the fetus may be in severe jeopardy before the usual clinical signs associated with significant hypovolemia in the nonpregnant patient are manifest.

In obstetric shock, the emphasis must be on early and aggressive volume replacement before the onset of the usual clinical signs of shock to avoid decreased uteroplacental blood flow. Use of vasopressors is discouraged because the uteroplacental arterioles appear to be maximally vasodilated under normal physiological conditions of pregnancy and the alpha-adrenergic activity seen in pharmacologic doses of most pressor agents can cause further reductions in uteroplacental blood flow from direct vascular constriction and effects on uterine muscle tone. If a vasopressor is needed, ephedrine has beta- as well as alpha-adrenergic activity and more favorable effects on uterine blood flow.

THIRD TRIMESTER BLEEDING

Abruptio Placentae. Premature separation of the normally implanted placenta, or abruptio placenta, has an incidence from 1 in 77 to 1 in 250 pregnancies.[3] Its cause is unknown, but its association with maternal HTN is well documented. Trauma is rarely a cause of abruption; for the most part abruption is equally associated with chronic maternal HTN and preeclampsia/eclampsia, and to a lesser extent with underlying renal insufficiency.[3,9] The most common cause of death is postpartum hemorrhage. The classical presentation is painful vaginal bleeding, often with shock out of proportion to the clinical evidence of bleeding. Most abruption affects less than 25% of the placenta area and is often not diagnosed until after delivery. Abruption of more than 50% of placental surface is severe and can lead to significant bleeding, disseminated intravascular coagulation (DIC), and intrauterine fetal demise (IUFD). Abruption severe enough to cause IUFD can be expected to cause a 2500 mL blood loss on presentation.[3]

Treatment is immediate delivery, with vaginal delivery the preferred route. Stabilization of maternal hypotension with blood and crystalloid and treatment of DIC before delivery is often necessary, particularly in patients with uterine inertia and failure to progress, who often face cesarean section (Table 57-20 and Chapter 44, Trauma in Pregnancy).

Placenta Previa. Placenta previa, low-lying placenta that encroaches on the internal cervical os, varies from partial to complete. Its cause is unknown but is associated with multiparity, advancing age, and prior uterine incisions. The incidence of placenta previa is approximately one in 260 pregnancies. Maternal mortality is approximately 0.1% and fetal mortality approximately 15 to 20%.[10]

The classical clinical presentation is painless uterine bleeding. Shock corresponds to clinical blood loss. Bleeding is generally not life-threatening unless the placenta is disrupted by digital examination. Suspected diagnosis in the stable patient can be confirmed by ultrasound. No pelvic examination should be attempted unless the patient is in an operating suite with full capabilities for emergency cesarean section.

Treatment is generally delivery by cesarean section. The stable patient who is not in labor, with minimal bleeding, can be admitted for observation.

Eclampsia. Eclampsia, a disease that has been called the great imitator, can also present as obstetric shock. Hepatic subcapsular hematomas can rupture, producing hypovolemic shock.

PERIPARTUM HEART FAILURE

Obstetric patients occasionally present in the third trimester or postpartum period with CHF of no apparent cause. These patients have been labeled as having peripartum cardiomyopathy (PPCM), defined on the basis of CHF in the last month of pregnancy or within 5 months of delivery and the absence of other discernible causes of heart failure. Studies of these patients have shown a low incidence of PPCM, one in 15,000 deliveries, with many of the patients actually having cardiomyopathies of discernible cause. Over 75% of patients initially thought to have PPCM are later found to have CHF secondary to chronic HTN, iatrogenic volume overload, previously unrecognized valvular heart disease, morbid obesity, or prior undiagnosed viral myocarditis.

The distinction between PPCM and peripartum heart failure of discernible cause is important. Recognition and treatment of the underlying condition in peripartum heart failure usually have a course consistent with the underlying lesion. The prognosis in PPCM corresponds to the degree of cardiomegaly persisting beyond delivery; patients with cardiomegaly beyond 6 months have a 5-year mortality greater than 75% from unrelenting CHF or complications of pulmonary or systemic emboli. Patients with PPCM not responding to medical management of CHF are candidates for transplantation.

PRE-EXISTING PULMONARY DISORDERS

OBSTRUCTIVE AND RESTRICTIVE PULMONARY DISEASE

Pulmonary diseases are commonly categorized into obstructive and restrictive disorders. Obstructive disorders include asthma, by far the most common pulmonary disease seen in pregnancy, with an incidence of 0.4 to 1.3%, chronic obstructive pulmonary disease (COPD), and emphysema. The latter two disorders are clinical amalgams of several disorders and are relatively uncommon during the childbearing years. Patients with a heavy smoking history, alpha 1 antitrypsin deficiency, or cystic fibrosis occasionally present with pregnancy complicating their management. The course of COPD is by nature variable and unpredictable, but the management does not generally differ between pregnant and nonpregnant patients. Most patients remain unchanged during pregnancy, but symptoms are more likely to get worse than to improve. Therapeutic modalities must not be harmful to mother or fetus. The symptomatic pregnant patient with COPD who does not respond to initial

---

TABLE 57-20. MANAGEMENT OF DIC IN PREGNANCY*

1. Identification and treatment of the underlying triggering mechanism must be sought and corrected aggressively.
2. Hemodynamic stabilization and vaginal delivery are the obstetric goals.
3. Blood component therapy guidelines are:
   a. Maintain fibrinogen more than or equal to 100 ng per mL. Most often this can be achieved with fresh frozen plasma (FFP); expect a rise of 10 mg per 100 mL per unit of FFP. Should the initial fibrinogen level be less than 50 mg per mL, infusion of cryoprecipitate is indicated. The expected rise of fibrinogen is 2 to 5 mg per 100 mL bag of cryoprecipitate.
   b. Maintain platelet count of greater than or equal to 50,000 per μL. Platelet packs should increase the platelet count approximately 5000 to 10,000 per μL per unit.
   c. Maintain hematocrit at 30% with transfusion of pRBCs. Each unit of pRBCs is expected to increase the hemoglobin by 1.5 g per mL and hematocrit by 3%.
   d. Correct factor deficiencies (evidenced by prolonged PT/PTT) with FFP. One unit of FFP for each 4 to 5 units of pRBCs or stored whole blood transfused is usually sufficient.

* Adapted with permission from Finley, B.E.: Acute coagulopathy in pregnancy. Med. Clin. North Am. Medical Problems in Pregnancy 73:723, 1989.

---

bronchodilator therapy should be considered for admission.

Restrictive pulmonary disease, with kyphoscoliosis the most common example, generally has a stable course, and these patients tend to tolerate pregnancy well. A vital capacity (VC) of less than 1 L, or 20% of predicted value represents a critical level of restrictive pulmonary disease, and these patients should be considered for therapeutic abortion or a planned cesarean section.[11]

Sarcoidosis is the most common interstitial lung disease to complicate pregnancy. Patients with sarcoid frequently do better during pregnancy, and the treatment is unchanged.

Myasthenia gravis, a rare autoimmune disorder involving the neuromuscular endplate, can present as subtle respiratory decompensation. A low threshold for obtaining arterial blood gases (ABGs), and a measure of the VC can prevent an obstetric catastrophe. It should be remembered that any drug with a curare-like effect must be used with extreme caution. Magnesium sulfate and aminoglycoside antibiotics are examples of such drugs.

Dyspnea and wheezing are the two most common respiratory complaints in pregnancy. The sensation of dyspnea is reported in 60 to 70% of normal pregnancies. Tachypnea, a respiratory rate greater than 18 to 20, is abnormal. Objective tachypnea should induce a search for a cause. Wheezing, the clinical hallmark of airway obstruction, does not indicate a cause and correlates poorly with the degree of obstruction and the response to therapy. Use of accessory muscles of respiration, pulsus paradoxus of 18 mmHg or more, and tachycardia greater than 120 beats per minute are reliable signs of respiratory distress.

Arterial blood gases (ABGs) give critical information and should be obtained early and often in pregnant patients with respiratory distress. Cyanosis, a late finding, should be anticipated through timely arterial blood gas measurements and avoided by appropriate interventions. In normal pregnancy, the pH is in the range of 7.40 to 7.45, the $paCO_2$ in the range of 27 to 32 mmHg, and the paO_2 in the range of 95 to 105 mmHg. This physiologic hyperventilation and mild respiratory alkalosis coupled with the fetus's poor tolerance to acidemia and hypoxemia changes the threshold for which intubation should be considered in the pregnant patient. The maternal arterial oxygen tension should be kept greater than 70 mmHg and the $paCO_2$ less than 50 mmHg. Deviations of 5 mmHg below and 50 mmHg above these values respectively is an ominous finding and should prompt immediate corrective measures, including intubation.[11]

The alveolar-arterial oxygen tension gradient, $(A-a)O_2$, is a useful indicator of gas exchange. An elevated $(A-a)O_2$ gradient along with tachypnea and hypercarbia are early signs of respiratory failure. The $(A-a)O_2$ gradient is normally increased in pregnancy, especially in the third trimester, but an $(A-a)O_2$ gradient greater than 20 mmHg should precipitate a search for wheezing, consolidation, or pulmonary edema.

Chest x rays should be obtained when there is a change in previous pulmonary disease or new pulmonary disease. Fetal radiation exposure is a theoretic risk. There is an estimated 1 to 3% incidence of congenital anomaly with exposure to 5000 mrad. A posterior-anterior chest x ray is 36 mrad, or the equivalent of the amount of radiation exposure in a cross-country plane flight.[11] When x rays are felt to be indicated, the abdomen should be shielded to avoid emotional issues.

There are no strict guidelines to determine the level of pulmonary function necessary for safe pregnancy. Despite tremendous pulmonary reserve, an FVC or FEV_1 of less than 1 liter can predict difficulties. Such patients breathe at more than 50% of their maximal breathing capacity at term and are dyspneic at rest.

The treatment goals are unchanged in the pregnant and nonpregnant patient with pulmonary disease. Medical regimens for patients with bronchospasm usually begin with inhaled beta 2 sympathomimetic agents. Albuterol is probably as safe as metaproterenol, but is a newer drug and its effects on pregnancy are less well known. Although the inhaled route of administration is becoming the most popular, subcutaneous administration of epinephrine or terbutaline is still considered the treatment of choice by some. Terbutaline, used as a tocolytic agent in preterm labor, should be avoided in active labor. Ephedrine is an over-the-counter adrenergic agent that has not been shown to be harmful to the fetus, but should be avoided because there are better agents with fewer side effects.

Although still controversial, corticosteroids are now frequently recommended over theophylline compounds for the patient with severe bronchospasm not responding to inhaled bronchodilators in the first 1 to 2 hours of treatment. Although some studies have shown slight increases in the incidence of congenital malformation (cleft palate), most studies of large groups of patients exposed to glucocorticoids at some time during pregnancy showed no significant increase in fetal morbidity and mortality. For the patient with severe bronchospasm who is unresponsive to inhaled bronchodilators, the risk of fetal hypoxia is significantly greater than the potential risk of exposing the fetus to corticosteroids.[12] The onset of action is 4 to 6 hours, and usage does not mandate chronic prednisone therapy. The dosage can be tapered over 10 to 14 days. Patients with steroid-dependent pulmonary disease must be covered with stress doses of hydrocortisone (100 mg parenterally every 8 hours).

Although controversial, theophylline will probably become a third-line drug for the treatment of bronchospasm. Although pregnancy is associated with increased clearance of theophylline in the first and second trimester, this clearance is significantly reduced in the third trimester, necessitating a reduction in dosage to avoid maternal and fetal toxicity.

Mucolytic agents and any agent that contains iodine are contraindicated in pregnancy because they are concentrated in the fetal thyroid and are teratogenic.

ACQUIRED PULMONARY DISORDERS

ACUTE RESPIRATORY FAILURE

Obstetric patients develop respiratory failure from the usual causes of decompensated restrictive and obstructive pulmonary disease. In addition, many obstetric complications lead to the so-called adult respiratory distress syndrome (ARDS). Any process that results in injury to the pulmonary vascular endothelium and increased fluid in the lungs, with progressive hypoxemia and pulmonary infiltrates, can be defined as ARDS. This high-mortality syndrome (60 to 70% mortality) is seen in conjunction with aspiration pneumonia, hemorrhagic shock, amniotic fluid embolism, sepsis, abruptio placenta, and pre-eclampsia. Although the triggering mechanisms are different, the management is remarkably similar. Intubation and mechanical ventilation with increased oxygen concentration and positive end expiratory pressure (PEEP) to keep the damaged alveoli open are usually necessary while attempts to correct the underlying disorder are undertaken.

In the pregnant patient with acute respiratory failure from any cause, the emergency physician must realize the significance of the 20% increase in maternal oxygen consumption and the demands of the uteroplacental unit. The fetal environment is relatively hypoxemic or hypercarbic relative to the mother with fetal umbilical vein pO_2 of 28.5 mmHg and pCO_2 10 mmHg higher than maternal pCO_2.[8] Fetal aerobic metabolism occurs because of greater affinity for oxygen by fetal hemoglobin, left-shifted oxygen dissociation curve, and other factors that allow increased oxygen extraction from the mother's blood by the fetus. Thirty seconds of apnea can produce a fall in maternal arterial pO_2 of 50 to 60 mmHg, placing the fetus at severe risk for hypoxemic insult. Maternal respiratory embarrassment or impending respiratory arrest must be anticipated to avoid significant fetal morbidity and mortality.

Management of respiratory failure in pregnancy requires an understanding of the rapidity of development of hypoxemia, the need for rapid intubation, and knowledge of the changes in the respiratory and gastrointestinal tracts. If intubation cannot be accomplished within 30 seconds, the pregnant patient needs preoxygenation with 100% O_2 for 3 to 4 minutes or, in extreme emergency, for at least four deep breaths.[11]

During pregnancy, the respiratory tract has increased vascularity resulting in some level of edema to the pharynx, larynx, and vocal cords. It is often wiser to use a smaller endotracheal tube to avoid trauma or significant bleeding from the friable tissues of the hypopharynx or vocal cords.

Chemical aspiration pneumonitis, or Mendelson's syndrome, was originally described in postanesthesia obstetric patients. It accounts for 30 to 50% of the maternal deaths associated with anesthesia. Delayed gastric emptying, decreased lower esophageal sphincter tone, increased gastric pressure from labor or uterine displacement, and the effects of magnesium sulfate or sedatives are some of the reasons for the high risk of aspiration in pregnant patients. Cricoid pressure, meaning manual application of pressure on the cricoid cartilage to compress the esophagus and prevent passage of stomach contents into the pharynx, is recommended during intubation of the pregnant patient. This pressure should be held until the proper position of the endotracheal tube is verified. Extubation of the pregnant patient should not occur until the patient is awake and competent enough to control gastric secretions.

CARBON MONOXIDE POISONING

Carbon monoxide (CO) is a relatively common toxic gas that produces functional tissue hypoxia by having a hemoglobin binding affinity 250 times greater than oxygen. Its consequences for the fetus in pregnancy are even graver than those for the mother.

Generally, maternal symptoms can be expected at a carboxyhemoglobin (COHgb) concentration of 20%. It appears that fetal COHgb levels may be 10 to 15% higher than those of the mother. COHgB concentrations that are asymptomatic for the mother may be fatal to the fetus. Furthermore, it appears that maternal COHgb levels at the time of clinical presentation do not correspond with the true risk of associated fetal morbidity and mortality, but that maternal COHgb levels at the site of exposure may predict more accurately the risk of fetal morbidity.

It takes five times longer to reduce an elevated fetal COHgb level using 100% normobaric oxygen to a safe level than to reduce a given elevated maternal COHgb level. Hyperbaric oxygen therapy should be strongly considered in the pregnant patient with even a low-level exposure to CO.[13]

THROMBOEMBOLIC DISEASE

Thromboembolic disease (TED) is felt to be a major cause of obstetric morbidity and mortality. TED is five times more likely in the pregnant patient than in the nonpregnant patient. Hypercoagulability, vascular damage, and stasis, events that occur regularly in pregnancy, increase the risk for TED. TED includes deep venous thrombosis (DVT) of the veins of the leg and pelvis, and associated pulmonary embolization (PE). About two thirds of TED occur in the puerperium, most often in the first 72 hours, and in women with other complications. Although DVT and PE do occur during pregnancy, their incidence is probably in the range of 4 and 1 per 10,000 pregnancies respectively.[14] Both are distinctly rare in early pregnancy. Because there are significant maternal and fetal complications from long term anticoagulation, it is as important to rule out, as well as rule in these potentially fatal disorders.

The clinical signs of DVT and PE are nonspecific. About half of patients with suspected deep venous disease have negative tests for thrombosis. A careful physical examination is necessary to exclude other disorders that may mimic DVT, such as ruptured Baker's cyst, muscle strain or hematoma, arterial insufficiency, neurogenic pain, and superficial thrombophlebitis. PE occurs in 50% of patients with documented DVT; of these only half are symptomatic for PE. Classical findings of dyspnea, pleuritic pain, and hemoptysis are seen in only 25% of patients with PE. The most common finding is a respiratory rate greater than 16. The frequency of this finding in PE is so common that a respiratory rate of less than 16 should rule against the diagnosis. The nonspecificity of clinical examination for TED makes objective tests essential for diagnosis.

The diagnosis of DVT in pregnancy is achieved through a combination of clinical suspicion, noninvasive, and (if necessary) invasive testing. Impedance plethysmography (IP), which measures volume changes within the leg, and Doppler ultrasound are the primary noninvasive tests used in pregnancy. Doppler ultrasound testing is highly subjective; correct interpretation of the results depends on the skill of the technician and patient positioning. Both have a higher degree of sensitivity for proximal thrombosis than for distal thrombosis. Both are affected by the physiologic alterations of pregnancy; most commonly, uterine occlusion of the venous system produces false positive results. After 20 weeks of gestation, a positive test should be confirmed by venogram before committing a patient to anticoagulation. For pregnant patients suspected of having DVT, start with noninvasive tests, either IP or Doppler ultrasound. A negative or normal noninvasive study all but precludes an occlusive proximal vein thrombus. Venography is indicated to confirm a positive IP or Doppler study or to evaluate suspected calf thrombosis.

Iodine[125] fibrinogen scanning is also a noninvasive study for diagnosis of DVT. It is particularly accurate for calf and lower thigh thrombosis with a sensitivity exceeding 90%. Sensitivity for proximal venous collecting system ranges between 60 and 80%. Radioactive iodine is contraindicated in pregnancy because it crosses the placenta and enters the fetal circulation, where it is concentrated in the fetal thyroid. Because it appears in breast milk, its use postpartum in the breast-feeding mother is also contraindicated.

Venography is the most definitive test available for the diagnosis of DVT, but is still subject to poor technique and errant interpretation. In addition, it is estimated to cause approximately a 3% incidence of chemical phlebitis. Unfortunately, venography and other studies miss pelvic thrombosis, the origin of many serious emboli. Venography is abnormal when evaluating a patient with suspected acute DVT superimposed on prior obstructive venous disease. In the nonpregnant patient the iodine[125] scan is used to differentiate acute from chronic disease because the study involves the incorporation of radioactively labeled fibrin into developing thrombus. In the pregnant patient, an indirect route can be used. Normal levels of fibrinopeptide A and antithrombin III are incompatible with an active ongoing thrombotic process.[15]

In the pregnant patient with the clinical scenario of PE, ventilation/perfusion lung scanning is indicated. Radiologists sometimes hesitate to perform this study, but the risks of not diagnosing PE or committing a pregnant patient and her fetus to long-term anticoagulation are greater than the theoretic risks of radiation exposure. Furthermore, proper interpretation of V/Q scans can eliminate the need for pulmonary angiography in 85% of patients with a high index of suspicion for PE.[14]

Intravenous administration of technetium[99] microspheres represents the perfusion scan. This is a sensitive but nonspecific test; any process that alters the lung architecture or blood flow alters the perfusion scan. A completely normal perfusion scan essentially eliminates the diagnosis of PE. The radiation from the injected material is excreted in the urine, the bladder contents contributing 85% of the dose to the fetus. Brisk diuresis and frequent voiding can minimize exposure.[14] The amount of radiation exposure has been estimated to be at 50 mrem, a level generally considered safe and not significantly different from the amount of radiation received from a CXR. An abnormal perfusion scan can be combined with the ventilation scan, and is performed by inhalation of an isotope of xenon. Perfusion/ventilation mismatches are consistent with PE.

V/Q scans are interpreted as low, average, or high risk for PE. Occasionally the radiologist commits to unequivocally positive for PE or normal V/Q scan, and further diagnostic studies can be stopped and appropriate treatment given. Low and indeterminate scans require pulmonary angiography to rule in or rule out the diagnosis of PE.

Pulmonary angiography is considered the "gold standard" for the diagnosis of PE. The procedure is not considered any more dangerous during pregnancy, and the fetus can be shielded to minimize radiation exposure. The morbidity and mortality are reported as less than 4% and 0.5% respectfully; deaths are principally from undiagnosed pulmonary HTN. The importance of accurately ruling out the diagnosis of PE and avoiding the risk of anticoagulation in pregnancy, with its attendant complications during labor and delivery, cannot be overstated. The decision to obtain pulmonary angiography is related to the individual and the locality. It depends on the skill of the institution in performing and reading the angiogram; there are reports of false-negative angiograms.[15] Table 57-21 lists indications for obtaining an angiogram in the pregnant patient.

The treatment of the antepartum patient with documented DVT or PE is heparin, which does not cross the placenta or is excreted in breast milk. Opinions differ regarding the duration of anticoagulation for patients with DVT or PE. The most widely practiced regimen involves subcutaneous heparin throughout pregnancy, up to labor and delivery, after an initial 7 to 10 days of intravenously administered heparin. A loading dose of 5000 to 10,000 units of heparin is usually given to start therapy. The dose frequency and magnitude are also controversial, but daily heparin doses in the range of 20,000 to 40,000 units appear to be appropriate. Mid-dosing partial thromboplastin times (PTT) should be 1.5 to 2.0 times the control value. After the hematocrit or PTT, urinanalysis can often detect the overanticoagulated patient. PTT has been found relatively insensitive for detecting bleeding. Complications of long-term heparin also include heparin-associated thrombocytopenia and osteoporosis.

Oral anticoagulants, or warfarin compounds, are currently avoided in pregnancy because of teratogenic effects in the first trimester and maternal-fetal hemorrhage at delivery. Some feel that the toxicity of warfarin during the second and third trimester has been overestimated, and furthermore that patients with artificial heart valves and recent thromboembolism are not adequately anticoagulated with subcutaneous heparin.[16] Under these circumstances, a risk-benefit analysis of the individual may favor use of oral anticoagulant therapy.

Pregnant patients with prior history of TED, anemia, planned operative delivery, or pre-eclampsia–eclampsia are at high risk for recurrent TED, and prophylactic subcutaneous heparin is indicated. The usual dosage is 5000 units subcutaneously two to three times a day throughout pregnancy. Heparin should be stopped at the time of labor and delivery, but prophylaxis must be reinstituted during the high-risk puerperal period. The administration of aspirin for TED in pregnancy is without foundation, can enhance the likelihood of hemorrhage, and should be avoided.

ENDOCRINE AND METABOLIC

PRE-EXISTING OR OVERT DIABETES MELLITUS AND ACQUIRED GESTATIONAL DIABETES MELLITUS

Diabetes mellitus can be broken down to two major classifications in regard to pregnancy, gestational diabetes mellitus (GDM) and pre-existing or overt diabetes mellitus. The prevalence of GDM, 0.15% to 12.3%, varies according to the blood glucose concentration used to define the disorder and the population screened. In the strictest definition, GDM is asymptomatic acquired glucose intolerance found in the latter half of pregnancy. More than half of the patients with GDM are ultimately found to have overt diabetes mellitus. Morbidity in GDM is primarily from complications of delivering a large infant that develops in an unchecked hyperglycemic environment.

The diagnosis of overt diabetes mellitus is based on the presence of fasting hyperglycemia found on two or more occasions. The difference between noninsulin-dependent diabetes mellitus (NIDDM) and insulin-dependent diabetes mellitus (IDDM) is based on the degree of fasting hyperglycemia/postprandial hyperglycemia and the ability to control these values with diet. Oral hypoglycemic agents have no place in the management of pregnant diabetics. It is estimated that 1% of women of childbearing age have overt diabetes mellitus, and one quarter of these women have IDDM.

The maternal morbidity of pregnancy complicated with IDDM has largely stabilized since the introduction of insulin, and is primarily related to underlying vascular disease. Pregnancies with IDDM are more likely to have complications of pre-eclampsia/eclampsia, infection, polyhydramnios, and postpartum hemorrhage.[17] Neonatal mortality can approach 1 to 2% of the general population, with meticulous control of diabetes starting preconceptually, intense multispecialty team care addressing obstetric, metabolic and neonatal management, and an involved, motivated mother. Even with optimal management, infants of mothers with IDDM have a 2 to 4 times greater incidence of congenital anomalies. Poor metabolic control before and during the period of organogenesis, 3 to 8 weeks of gestational age, may result in an incidence of congenital anomalies of 22%.[1]

TABLE 57-21. INDICATIONS FOR PULMONARY ANGIOGRAPHY IN THE PREGNANT PATIENT*

Clinical story overwhelming with a negative perfusion scan
Indeterminate or low-probability lung scan
Suspected pulmonary embolism in the presence of pulmonary parenchymal lung disease or congestive heart failure
Positive lung scan in a previously healthy young patient with an unlikely clinical history
High risk for anticoagulation, i.e. peptic ulcer disease, bleeding diathesis, recent aspirin
Diagnosis of pulmonary embolism infers high-risk follow-up treatment such as inferior vena cava interruption, surgical embolectomy, or use of thrombolytic agents

* Adapted with permission from Brunader, R.E.: Diagnosis and evaluation of thromboembolic disorders. J. Am. Board Fam. Pract. 2:106, 1989.

With poor management, pregnant diabetic women suffer intrauterine fetal demise (IUFD), increased perinatal death, dystocia with cesarean section rates as high as 80%, newborn respiratory distress syndrome, and metabolic disturbances of the newborn exposed to prolonged hyperglycemia. These latter disturbances of the newborn are characterized by hypoglycemia, hypocalcemia, polycythemia, and hyperbilirubinemia. A tenfold increase in maternal mortality and a 17% fetal mortality rate can be expected in the pregnancy of the IDDM patient complicated by maternal neglect, PIH, ketoacidosis, and infection.[17,18]

As discussed in the section on physiology of pregnancy, normal pregnancy is "diabetogenic." Increasing degrees of insulin deficiency result in greater postprandial glucose fluctuations and increasing fasting hyperglycemia. The natural facility for catabolism in pregnancy lowers the threshold for ketosis and acidemia. Diabetic ketoacidosis (DKA) occurs at much lower levels of hyperglycemia and carries grave consequences, with maternal and fetal death rates reported at 10 and 50%, respectfully.[1,19]

As in preoperative and operative surgical diabetic patients, stressed diabetic pregnant patients unable to take anything by mouth often require insulin and carbohydrate during an emergency or during labor and delivery. The diabetic pregnant woman exposed to further insulin antagonism, i.e., catecholamines, cortisol, and glucagon, can rapidly develop hyperglycemia, a resultant osmotic diuresis, and significant dehydration/tissue ischemia, if not incipient DKA. In the emergency setting, this scenario is far more common than hypoglycemia in the pregnant patient who has taken her insulin but is unable to take nutrition by mouth.[20] Under these circumstances, long- and intermediate-acting insulin should be discontinued and insulin requirements met by sliding scale regular (crystalline) insulin based on frequent bedside blood glucose measurements. Intravenous constant infusion insulin offers good control and is recommended.[1,2,20] The usual constant infusion rates are 0.02 to 0.04 units of regular insulin/kg/hr.[2] In DKA, with greater insulin antagonism from acidemia, infusion rates are 0.1 units of regular insulin per kg per hr.[20,21] Intravenous solutions should contain dextrose when blood glucose reaches 150 to 250 mg per dL.[21] Glucose requirements in the lean individual can be met by the equivalent of 5 to 10 gm per hour (50 to 100 cc per hr of D5W 0.45, or D5W 0.9% saline).[2,21]

The pregnant patient with IDDM has increased sensitivity to insulin during the first trimester. The evaluation of an unexplained hypoglycemic attack in an otherwise stable woman of childbearing age should prompt a pregnancy test. After delivery, the factors causing natural insulin resistance rapidly dissipate, and insulin dosages should be reduced accordingly. Many IDDM patients require no insulin on the day after delivery.

Diabetics with active retinopathy at conception can expect progression of their disease in 15 to 85% of pregnancies. Nephropathy shows temporary deterioration with increased proteinuria and increased incidence of PIH and IUGR and perinatal mortality goes from 2 to 10%. Although diabetic nephropathy tends to improve after delivery, its presence heralds the inevitable downward course of diabetic renal failure. Diabetic enteropathy and gastric paresis often result in hospital admissions for correction of dehydration and acidemia secondary to nausea and vomiting.[1]

Glucosuria is present in 16% of normal pregnancies. Its presence is an indication to check blood glucose. With the development of bedside glucometers, use of urinary glucose to direct insulin dosages is outmoded and too inaccurate to be useful. Urinalysis is more valuable for the early detection of ketosis, and its presence for longer than 8 hours warrants admission.

Note that finding a fasting plasma glucose greater than 105 mg/dL (fasting whole venous blood glucose greater than 90 mg/dL) suggests abnormal glucose tolerance and should prompt referral for a screening or formal glucose tolerance test (GTT). A screening GTT is recommended for all pregnancies between 24 and 28 weeks of gestational age. The desired "tight" metabolic control for pregnancies with IDDM is to maintain fasting serum glucose between 70 to 95 mg per dL and 2-hour postprandial glucose less than 140 mg per dL (see Table 57-17). Although this level of control is desirable, it should not be sought in the face of frequent hypoglycemic attacks.

Management of the acutely ill pregnant diabetic patient does not differ from that of her nonpregnant counterpart. Generally, well-managed pregnant diabetic patients should not present to the ED. Conversely, pregnancies complicated by diabetes showing clinical symptoms require immediate intervention and/or admission. The emergency physician has a unique opportunity to counsel and/or refer the nonpregnant diabetic patient contemplating pregnancy, and this should be kept in mind when caring for diabetic patients of childbearing years.

OTHER ENDOCRINE AND METABOLIC ACQUIRED DISORDERS

Hyperemesis Gravidarum. Nausea and vomiting are common complaints in pregnancy, usually seen beginning around 6 to 8 weeks of gestational age and dissipating around 14 weeks of gestational age, although they can persist throughout pregnancy. Nausea and vomiting are felt to be related to the principal hormones of pregnancy, particularly HCG, but the actual relationship is unknown. When nausea and vomiting become severe enough to cause weight loss, dehydration, and starvation, the condition is termed hyperemesis gravidarum (HG).

Presentation with clinical signs of dehydration, most notably evidence of ketosis/acidosis, is significant and demands immediate correction and/or admission. Other causes of nausea and vomiting in pregnancy must be considered and excluded, i.e., pyelonephritis, cholelithiasis, pancreatitis, hepatitis, and peptic ulcer disease.

Laboratory studies can demonstrate varying degrees of hyponatremia, azotemia, hypokalemia, alkalosis, and acidosis. Evidence of anaerobic metabolism with ketosis is the most significant finding. HG can have low-level elevations of liver transaminases and bilirubin. These values should return to normal when the dehydration is corrected. Differentiation of HG from hyperthyroidism can be problematic. Stabilization of HG usually allows differentiation from thyrotoxicosis but frequently requires hospital admission and consultation.

Beside the obvious correction of fluid and electrolyte disorders, management includes a regimen of frequent small feedings and the exploration of emotional factors often found in association with HG. Use of promethazine, prochlorperazine, and trimethobenzamide for control of nausea is acceptable.

Benign Clinical Syndromes. The normal physiologic changes of pregnancy produce a number of benign clinical syndromes likely to be encountered by the emergency physician. The hormonal changes that produce increased vascularity of the vagina also affect the nasal mucosa and, coupled with increased blood volume, lead to nasal stuffiness and a predisposition to epistaxis. Progesterone produces decreased peristalsis, delayed gastric emptying time, and lowered lower esophageal sphincter tone. An expanding uterus produces increased pressure on the stomach, and these two phenomena produce a 30 to 70% incidence of heartburn (the clinical term is esophagitis).[22] Decreased peristalsis also predisposes to constipation and hemorrhoids.

During the early middle trimester, as the uterus becomes an abdominal organ, tension is placed on the round ligaments of the uterus, causing episodic contractions that produce sharp pains in one or the other lower quadrants. Often referred to as round ligament syndrome, these pains typically last several minutes, are associated with movement, and tend to recur until the end of the second trimester. Backache is also frequently seen in normal pregnancy as the hormones of pregnancy produce relaxation of ligaments and the enlarging uterus produces a change in the center of gravity and increased lumbar sacral lordosis. Pubic symphysis separation can be seen with relatively minor trauma.

PRE-EXISTING HEMATOLOGIC AND IMMUNOLOGIC DISORDERS

ANEMIA

Nutritional Anemia. Anemia, the most common medical complication of pregnancy, is seen in about 50% of pregnancies in the U.S. Nutritional anemia from iron or folate deficiency represents 75 and 22% of the causes of anemia, and addressing these two conditions corrects over 90% of anemias seen during the reproductive years.[23] The developing fetus of the mother deficient in iron or folate does not suffer from these abnormalities because the placenta is able to absorb sufficient iron and folate from even severely depleted mothers. Because normal gestational requirements for iron and folate exceed available supply, blood loss from parturition from one pregnancy with inevitable iron and folate loss is often the cause of severe nutritional anemia in subsequent pregnancies. Vitamin B_{12} deficiency in pregnancy is rare; when present in patients of childbearing years, it is often accompanied by infertility.

Although the approach to the pregnant patient with anemia is the same as in the nonpregnant patient, the clinical and laboratory diagnosis of anemia is altered by pregnancy. Symptoms suggesting anemia in a nonpregnant patient, such as pallor, malaise and anorexia, may be present in pregnancy without actual anemia. A physiologic anemia (see section on normal physiology of pregnancy) is seen because of the relatively greater increase in plasma volume over red blood cell volume. The severely iron-deficient pregnant patient shows the usual morphologic changes in serum iron, total iron-binding capacity and serum ferritin; the moderately iron-deficient patient does not demonstrate classic laboratory findings (see Table 57-17).

Knowledge of the increased requirements for folate and iron in pregnancy make routine supplementation during normal pregnancy rational. Mild anemia, with Hgb less than 10 to 11 g % and Hct less than 30 volume %, has been associated with intrauterine growth retardation, polycythemia, and other fetal complications.[23] Delayed wound healing, higher incidence of infection, and prolonged hospitalization can be seen in moderately anemic patients, i.e., Hgb less than 8 g % and Hct less than 25 volume %. Maternal deterioration is not usually noted until Hgb concentration is less than 4 to 6 g % and Hct less than 12 to 18 volume %. The postpartum patient who is stable no longer faces the likelihood of further hemorrhage, can ambulate without symptoms, and is not febrile can generally tolerate a Hgb of 7 g % and be managed with iron supplementation rather than blood transfusion.[23]

Sickle Cell Hemoglobinopathy. Sickle cell disease (SSD) is the clinical manifestation of one of a number of biochemical hereditary defects in the alpha or beta hemoglobin chains that leads to decreased red blood cell life span through sickling and hemolysis. Pregnancy is a serious burden in SSD. The maternal death rate is 125 to 150 times greater and the perinatal mortality is 5 to 13 times greater for sickle cell SS disease and SC disease respectively than the same rate for non-white normal pregnancies.[24] Prenatal care and preventive treatment can reduce morbidity, mortality, and perinatal loss.

Pregnancies complicated by SSD are especially at risk for covert bacteremia and its complications. Rapid diagnosis and aggressive treatment of common infections such as pneumonia and pyelonephritis is essential. Pregnant patients with SSD are often misdiagnosed as having a vaso-occlusive crisis when they are suffering from an ectopic pregnancy, placental abruption, or pyelonephritis.

The stable pregnant SSD patient generally maintains and tolerates her hemoglobin concentration around 7%. These patients must be monitored closely for any factor that impairs their intense erythropoiesis, and supplemental folic acid is essential for the pregnant (and nonpregnant) patient with SSD. Critical changes in the hemoglobin/hematocrit can be seen secondary to sequestration of sickled red blood cells (RBCs) during a vaso-occlusive crisis or caused by increased hemolysis seen with infections.

Exchange transfusions have been recommended for hemoglobin levels below 6.0 g% or a drop in the hemoglobin level greater than 2 g per 24 hours. The issue of prophylactic RBC transfusions to maintain maternal Hgb concentration greater than 10 g % and to minimize the relative concentration of Hgb SS to normal Hgb A is controversial.[25] Although prophylactic transfusion definitely decreases maternal morbidity, recent studies have shown no change in perinatal outcome.[26] Transfusion morbidity from isoimmunization, hepatitis, and risk of HIV infection make repeated pregnancies and prophylactic transfusions especially troublesome.

Labor management for women with SSD is similar to that for women with cardiac disease. The woman should be kept comfortable and not oversedated, and oxygen therapy instituted. If cesarean section or complicated vaginal delivery is expected, the Hgb concentration should be elevated with consideration that these women are more prone to ventricular failure, circulatory overload, and pulmonary edema.

THROMBOCYTOPENIA

Idiopathic thrombocytopenia (ITP), also called auto-immune thrombocytopenia, is a syndrome that produces isolated but sometimes clinically significant thrombocytopenia by the presence of an IgG immunoglobulin that binds to platelets. It is seen commonly in women of childbearing years and seems to be exacerbated by pregnancy.[27] IgG antibodies cross the placenta and can cause thrombocytopenia in the fetus and neonate. Although steroids and splenectomy often produce a clinical remission, they may not produce an immunologic remission, and a mother may have a normal platelet count with continued fetal risk for bleeding, especially intracranial bleeding, during the trauma of labor and delivery.[27]

Women at term with active disease, generally with a platelet count less than 50,000 per mm^3 but perhaps better assessed by bleeding time, can be treated with corticosteroids or high-dose intravenous immune globulin. Steroid therapy appears to increase infant platelet count at birth, and it is postulated that steroid treatment can produce a safe platelet count for the infant and thus avoid routine cesarean section for women with ITP.[27] High-dose intravenous immune globulin appears to increase maternal platelet counts temporarily and benefit women with critical thrombocytopenia facing imminent surgery or vaginal delivery. The effect on neonatal platelet count cannot be determined.[27] Unfortunately there is no strong correlation between maternal and fetal platelet counts, nor does monitoring of platelet-associated antibody counts or levels of circulating platelet antibody correlate with the fetal level of thrombocytopenia. Intrapartum fetal scalp blood samples are used to detect significant fetal thrombocytopenia. When the fetal platelet count is less than 50,000 per mm^3, an immediate cesarean section is performed.[27] Thrombocytopenic patients with platelet counts between 20,000 and 50,000 per mm^3 rarely have spontaneous bleeding, but the patient with a platelet count under 50,000 per mm^3 facing surgery or vaginal delivery is at risk for excessive bleeding.[28] In the mother with active disease, the best route of delivery for the affected infant is unfortunately hazardous for the thrombocytopenic mother.

IMMUNOLOGIC DISORDERS

Rheumatoid Arthritis and Systemic Lupus Erythematosis. The most commonly encountered connective tissue disorders are rheumatoid arthritis (RA) and systemic lupus erythematosis (SLE). These diseases are of unknown cause but have in common the presence of autoimmune antibodies that induce inflammatory responses. They occur during childbearing years and, except in severe disease, do not affect fertility.

RA generally improves in pregnancy and has no adverse effects on the fetus. Remission in one pregnancy generally implies remission in subsequent pregnancies. Anti-inflammatory drugs, aspirin, indomethacin, and naproxen are felt to be relatively nontoxic in early pregnancy; later in pregnancy there are reports of prolonged gestation, increased antepartum and postpartum hemorrhage, and early closure of the ductus arteriosus. Steroids are used for active disease, but gold, penicillamine, azathioprine, and cyclophosphamide are to be avoided. Patients inadvertently using methotrexate during pregnancy have a 50% chance of producing an abnormal infant and should be advised to consider a therapeutic abortion.[29]

SLE patients with severe disease requiring high-dose corticosteroids, cyclophosphamid, or azothioprine regimens have a significant incidence of amenorrhea, anovulation, or premature ovarian failure, and successful pregnancy may not be possible.[30,31] In SLE patients who are able to conceive, an exacerbation of SLE is seen in approximately 50%. These flare-ups can be expected to be seen postpartum for one third of the patients, the rest equally divided throughout the antepartum. Disease at the onset of gestation is associated with subsequent disease, particularly in the third trimester and postpartum. Women in remission at the time of conception have a 35% chance of flare-up. A small but significant portion of SLE patients, varying from 7 to 9%, have permanent deterioration in renal function as a complication of pregnancy.[32,33] Thirty percent of SLE patients improve during pregnancy, but the course in one pregnancy does not predict the course in another.[29]

Overall fetal deaths have been reported as greater than 40%.[29] The fetal survival is 75% in women with established SLE before conception. If these women are in clinical remission before conception, the success rate is 88 to 100%. If pregnancy occurs in the presence of active disease, the survival is decreased between 50 and 75%. Finally, the onset of SLE during pregnancy or puerperium produces the highest death rate, with fetal survival reported at 50 to 64%.[29]

Asymptomatic patients, known SLE patients, or patients with nonspecific autoimmune disorders not meeting the diagnostic criteria for SLE sometimes present with arterial or venous thrombosis, habitual miscarriage, IUFD, or neonatal lupus syndrome (congenital complete heart block, neonatal dermatitis). These patients often have one of several autoantibodies that portend poor maternal or fetal outcome and can be serologic markers for eventual overt autoimmune disease in previously asymptomatic patients.[31]

The stable SLE patient should continue with corticosteroids without change in dosage when pregnancy is discovered. The guideline for use of steroids in pregnancy is similar to that in nonpregnant patients: the lowest dose that controls the disease should be used. Active disease at conception requires higher doses of steroids. The adverse effect of the uncontrolled flare-up on fetal growth and development far outweighs actual or theoretic risks attributable to maternal drug therapy. Therapeutic abortion does not reduce flare-ups or change the course of remissions. Delivery is vaginal, with steroid coverage.

Patients with HTN and renal disease from any cause have increased risk of developing eclampsia, and therefore SLE patients with nephropathy have a greater incidence of superimposed pre-eclampsia. The importance of differentiating maternal lupus with a flare-up from pre-eclampsia is underscored in the patient presenting in the third trimester with HTN, proteinuria, and edema. The treatment for eclampsia is timely delivery. The treatment for lupus nephritis is increased steroid dosage and immunosuppressive drugs if the flare-up is severe. Helpful laboratory studies are platelet counts (which tend to decrease in pre-eclampsia), rising titers of anti-DNA antibodies, and falling C3, C4 complement levels. Rising titers of anti-DNA antibodies and falling C3 levels can be indications of active SLE, even though the patient is clinically well. Evidence of uteroplacental compromise or decreased fetal well-being require preparation for timely delivery regardless of difficulties in separating active lupus nephritis from pre-eclampsia.[4,31]

ACQUIRED HEMATOLOGIC AND IMMUNOLOGIC DISORDERS

ANEMIA

Acute blood loss is discussed in the section on obstetric shock.

THROMBOCYTOPENIA

Thrombotic Thrombocytopenia, Adult Hemolytic Uremia Syndrome, and Postpartum Renal Failure. Thrombotic thrombocytopenia (TTP), the adult form of hemolytic uremia syndrome (HUS), and the syndrome of postpartum renal failure (PPRF) are relatively rare conditions that share an alteration in the hemostatic system. They produce microangiopathic hemolytic anemia and thrombocytopenia without consumption coagulopathy (normal PT and PTT), and lead to the formation of thrombi in the microvasculature, causing arteriolar fibrinoid necrosis. The clinical expression of this process is bleeding diathesis, neurologic complications, and renal failure. The cause is unknown, but pregnancy appears to predispose to these disorders. Differentiating pregnancy complicated by TTP/HUS/PPRF from other complications of pregnancy producing disseminated intravascular coagulation (DIC) is difficult. DIC is seen in association with obstetrically related acute renal failure, postpartum hemorrhage, puerperal sepsis, abruptio placentae, amniotic fluid embolism, IUFD, saline abortion, and pre-eclampsia/eclampsia (see subsequent section on DIC). Furthermore, early presentation of TTP/HUS/PPRF is often mild to moderate. Thrombocytopenia

with or without evidence of hemolytic anemia can be confused with ITP. SLE can present with some or all of the same clinical symptoms and findings.

Early recognition and management of these disorders is essential because the untreated or advanced state can have high mortality rates, and the mother and fetus undergoing premature anesthesia, induction of labor, or surgery can be placed at greater risk.[34] Still, a far more common clinical situation for progressive HTN, renal failure, and neurologic abnormalities is prompt delivery or termination of the pregnancy to prevent further maternal or fetal morbidity and mortality from pre-eclampsia/eclampsia.

Disseminated Intravascular Coagulation. The placenta contains the highest concentration of thromboplastin of any tissue in the body.[3] Clinical conditions producing exposure of the general circulation to placental material with tissue factor activity induces the phenomenon known as DIC. The fulminance or severity of DIC is based on the concentration and the rapidity with which the material with tissue factor activity is discharged into the maternal circulation. DIC-associated obstetric problems are listed in the section on TTP/HUS/PPRF.

Management of the pregnant patient with DIC is directed at aggressive identification and removal of the triggering insult while replacing circulatory volume and coagulation component deficits. Cardiopulmonary support is often needed in fulminant DIC. Therapeutic guidelines for blood component therapy for the patient with fulminant DIC is listed in Table 57-20.

IMMUNOLOGIC DISORDERS

Rh Iso-Immunization. In approximately 10% of pregnancies in Caucasian women, 5% in Black women, and 1% in Asian women, an Rh-negative woman gives birth to an Rh-positive infant. The Rh antigen is one of the most antigenic of the ABO and Rh systems and induces IgG isoantibodies in the mother if she is exposed or immunized to fetal blood with the Rh antigen. IgG immunoglobulin to Rh antigen is produced from this sensitization and can cross the placenta into the fetal circulation. Once sensitization occurs, the duration of fetal exposure and the titer of maternal anti Rh IgG antibodies determine the prognosis for the infant.

The timing of exposure is usually on delivery, miscarriage or abortion, or possibly ectopic pregnancy. Unusually large exposure to fetal blood cells occurs with abruptio placentae, cesarean section, and traumatic vaginal delivery.

When an Rh-negative mother is exposed to any of these conditions, an indirect Coombs test should be performed to alert the physician to prior isoimmunization. The previously unsensitized Rh-negative mother exposed to small amounts of fetal blood can be prevented from Rh isoimmunization by administration of a standard dose of 300 μg of anti-Rh immune globulin (RhoGAM) within 72 hours of exposure. This dose is felt to inactivate the Rh antigen in 15 mL of red blood cells or 30 mL of fetal blood. Unusually large exposue to Rh antigen requires more than the standard dose of RhoGAM. A quantitative estimate of the amount of RhoGAM to give can be estimated based on the information from a Kleihauer-Betke acid elution test on a maternal differential count, the maternal Hct, and an estimate of maternal blood volume.

PRE-EXISTING RENAL DISORDERS

IMPAIRED RENAL FUNCTION

Pregnancy in women with impaired renal function is accompanied by an increase in such complications as HTN, proteinuria, fetal prematurity, and fetal loss.[35] Maternal and fetal prognosis generally depend on the extent of renal compromise and the presence of HTN more than the specific underlying disease process.[4,30]

Pregnancy complicated by impaired renal function can be divided into mild, moderate, and severe disease on the basis of the prepregnancy serum creatinine. Mild renal dysfunction is considered to be present with a serum creatinine less than 1.4 mg per dL, with proteinuria and HTN absent before onset of pregnancy. These patients tolerate pregnancy well. Pregnancy does not appear to affect the course of their disease. Exceptions are seen in pregnancies complicated by active lupus nephritis with onset during pregnancy, polyarteritis nodosa, and scleroderma. Fortunately, the latter two are seldom seen in conjunction with pregnancy. In any event, pregnancy is poorly tolerated and can lead to significant deterioration in renal function and unacceptable maternal and fetal mortality.[4,29] The deterioration in renal function seen in some patients in the category of mild renal dysfunction is felt to represent the natural progression of the underlying disorder, and pregnancy is not felt to influence that progression.[4] Examples are amyloidosis, polycystic kidney disease, focal glomerulosclerosis, and some forms of glomerulonephritis.

Moderate to severe renal insufficiency is considered to be present with a prepregnancy serum creatinine greater than 1.4 mg per dL. These patients' chances for successful pregnancy are generally good, but fetal death rates of approximately 30% are reported.[4] Some patients with moderate renal insufficiency and pregnancy suffer irreversible damage to their renal function, but this again is felt to be part of the relentless course of the underlying disease process.[4]

Severe renal insufficiency is felt to be present with a prepregnancy serum creatinine level greater than 3 mg per dL, and normal pregnancy is uncommon at this level.

Management of the pregnant patient with impaired renal function is directed at control of HTN, maximization of existing renal function, and monitoring of fetal well-being.

When a pregnant patient with evidence of deterioration in renal function is seen, reversible causes of renal deterioration should be sought. Urinary tract infection, dehydration, and fluid and electrolyte disorders are correctable causes of deteriorating renal function. Control of HTN is also of great importance. Pregnancy is allowed to continue as long as there is no evidence of relentless renal deterioration or uncontrollable HTN compromising uteroplacental function or forewarning pre-eclampsia or eclampsia. Proteinuria without a decrease in GFR or the presence of HTN does not necessarily imply renal deterioration, and the pregnancy can be allowed to continue.[4] The exception to this is in SLE nephritis, in which increasing proteinuria is a sign of renal deterioration and calls for increasing steroid dosage.[31] If there is objective deterioration in renal function and no reversible causes, the pregnancy should be interrupted or the delivery induced.

Renal insufficiency, regardless of cause, has adverse effects on the fetus.[30] Patients with moderate renal disease develop PIH or PAH in slightly more than half of the cases, and early delivery is frequently forced. HTN is the accompanying problem that poses the greatest risk to the mother and fetus with impaired renal function.[35]

RENAL TRANSPLANT

Fertility problems are seen with serum creatinine levels in the range of 2.0 mg per dL.[30] Newer drug regimens introduced to limit the rate of lupus nephritis are also associated with impaired fertility.[31] Dialysis patients of child-bearing years seldom achieve pregnancy, and their rate for successful outcome is no more than 20 to 23%.[35] Renal transplant patients can achieve pregnancy, although such pregnancies are complicated and associated with increased maternal and fetal risk.

Complications include increased risk of graft deterioration and progressive HTN for the mother and increased fetal risk for prematurity, growth retardation, and infection. Continuation of immunosuppressive drugs is necessary because their withdrawal can precipitate acute rejection in a transplant patient who has otherwise been stable for years. The dosage of immunosuppressive drugs should be kept to a minimum.[36]

HTN is common and usually severe. Life-threatening HTN can occur suddenly. Its treatment does not differ from treatment of HTN in PIH and PAH. Decisions about terminating a pregnancy or premature delivery have to be made on the basis of the difficulty in controlling HTN.[36] Pre-eclampsia is seen in 30% of patients and signs of rejection in 9%. Differentiation of acute pyelonephritis, recurrent glomerulopathy, and/or pre-eclampsia is difficult.[36]

ACQUIRED RENAL DISORDERS

ACUTE RENAL FAILURE

Acute renal failure (ARF) can be caused by hypovolemia or thrombotic events in the renal vasculature. In pregnancy, the most common causes are abruptio placentae, pre-eclampsia or eclampsia, prolonged IUFD, hemorrhagic shock, and pyelonephritis complicated by endotoxemia. Most patients recover with supportive measures appropriate for ARF. Some patients, particularly those with ARF from placental abruption, pre-eclampsia or eclampsia, or endotoxin-induced shock develop renal cortical necrosis and are left with varying degrees of permanent renal failure.

URINARY TRACT INFECTION

Urinary tract infection (UTI) is the most common bacterial infection in pregnancy. It can be divided into three major types, asymptomatic bacteriuria, cystitis and urethritis, and pyelonephritis. Hormonal changes of pregnancy promote urinary stasis, diminished ureteral tone, and peristalsis. These same hormonal effects, coupled with ureteral compression by the enlarging uterus, produce hydronephrosis of pregnancy, and further predispose to UTI.[8]

Asymptomatic bacteriuria has an incidence of 2 to 12% and is typically present early in pregnancy. Twenty five percent of patients with untreated asymptomatic bacteriuria progress to develop acute symptomatic UTI. Symptoms of cystitis and urethritis are no different in pregnant women from those in nonpregnant women. Forty percent of pregnant women with acute pyelonephritis had preceding symptoms of cystitis. Pyelonephritis has an incidence of 1%. Fifty percent of cases are unilateral and right-sided, and 25% are bilateral. Symptoms must be differentiated from labor, appendicitis, and placental abruption. The usual infecting organism is Escherichia coli. The endotoxin produced can cause septic shock on first exposure in a pregnant woman rather than requiring an initial sensitizing inoculation as in nonpregnant persons. Also, gram-negative bacteria can produce phospholipase A_2 activity that can initiate the arachidonic acid cascade to produce prostaglandins in the pregnant uterus and induce premature labor. One can see the efficacy of bactericidal antibiotic treatment of asymptomatic bacteriuria in pregnant women.

Asymptomatic bacteriuria and cystitis can be treated with a 10- to 14-day course of antibiotics. There is a 30% recurrence rate in the eradication of asymptomatic bacteriuria, which is likely to be a relapse of the original infection. Antibiotic choices are typically nitrofurantoin, sulfisoxazole, ampicillin, or a cephalosporin. Single-dose treatment regimens have a 75% success rate. There is a 97% success rate for the 10- to 14-day treatment plan of cystitis. Return of a sterile urine culture in the symptomatic lower tract infection should prompt one to consider erythromycin treatment for possible Chlamydia urethritis. Pyelonephritis is treated with hospitalization and hydration. A 10-day drug course is begun empirically with ampicillin, a cephalosporin, extended-spectrum penicillin, or a combination of gentamicin or tobramycin plus ampicillin for suspected infections caused by resistant Escherichia coli bacteria. Serum creatinine levels and peak antibiotic serum levels should be followed for patients receiving gentamicin or tobramycin.[36]

Treatment of pyelonephritis leads to reversal of decreased GFR, dehydration, ketosis, and the risk of premature labor. Patients who fail to respond to treatment in 48 to 72 hours should be evaluated for urinary obstruction, usually by renal calculi that can be seen by abdominal flat plate x rays in 90% of cases, and for perinephric abscess, which can also cause prolonged fever. Recurrent infection rate is 30 to 40%, necessitating frequent urinalysis. Continued bacteriologic suppression with nitrofurantoin throughout the remainder of pregnancy can reduce relapse but can cause hemolysis for the fetus with glucose 6 phosphatase deficiency.[37]

MISCELLANEOUS

PREEXISTING NEUROLOGIC DISORDERS

Seizure Disorders. Seizures are the most common neurologic disorder seen in pregnancy. In general, 50% of pregnant patients with seizures show no change in seizure frequency, 25% a decrease, and 25% an increase in their seizure frequency. Seizures in one pregnancy do not imply similar seizures in subsequent pregnancies.[38] There is generally no increase in the frequency of spontaneous abortion, prematurity, and pre-eclampsia between epileptic pregnant women and controls. Major morbidity and mortality are caused by poorly controlled seizures, with resultant fetal hypoxia and acidemia. In the first trimester, these lead to malformations in organogenesis, and in the third trimester they lead to cerebral palsy and mental retardation. Status epilepticus does not occur more frequently during pregnancy but, when present, it can cause fetal death.[38,39]

A major controversy in management of seizures in pregnancy is the effects of anticonvulsants on the fetus or infant. All anticonvulsant drugs have been implicated with some overlap in the so-called "fetal hydantoin syndrome." This syndrome consists of varying degrees of craniofacial anomalies, usually cleft lip and palate, distal limb dysmorphosis, mental retardation, and congenital heart lesions. Of key significance in the decision to treat epileptic patients with anticonvulsant drugs is the roughly twofold greater incidence of congenital anomalies and mental retardation in treated and untreated epileptics over the general population.[38]

TABLE 57-22. MANAGEMENT GUIDELINES FOR SEIZURES IN PREGNANCY*

Patient Counseling

1. An attempt at drug withdrawal should be made for the patient who has remained seizure-free for some years and is seeking pregnancy.
2. For patients who experience regular seizures, the risk of seizures during pregnancy outweighs the risk of anticonvulsant teratogenesis.
3. For the well-controlled patient on phenytoin, there is no reason to switch to another drug of which less is known.
4. The epileptic woman should be informed that the risk of malformations and mental retardation in epilepsy is twice that of the general population. The chance of having a normal child is over 90%, however.

Anticonvulsant Agents

Medication	Daily Dosage Serum Level	Maternal Side Effects
Carbamazepine (Tegretol)	200–1200 mg/day 4–8 µg/mL	Drowsiness, blurred vision, GI upset
Phenobarbital	30–200 mg/day 10–35 µg/mL	Drowsiness, ataxia, rash
Phenytoin (Dilantin)	300–1200 mg/day 10–20 µg/mL	Drowsiness, ataxia, gum hyperplasia, hypertrichosis
Ethosuximide (Zarontin)	500–1500 mg/day 40–100 µg/mL	GI upset Headache

* Adapted from Naronha, A.: Neurologic disorders during pregnancy and the puerperium. Clin Perinatol. *12*:700, 1985, and Patterson, R.M.: Seizure disorders in pregnancy. Med. Clin. North Am. Medical Problems in Pregnancy, *73*:665, 1989.

An additional complication of anticonvulsant therapy is increased neonatal bleeding. Hemorrhagic disease of the newborn has an onset of bleeding in the first several days of life. With anticonvulsant-induced interference of the vitamin K-dependent clotting factors, bleeding develops in the first 24 hours. An estimated 10% prevalence is seen in pregnancies of patients treated with phenobarbital or phenytoin.[38]

Management guidelines are listed in Table 57-22. Differentiating recurrence of epileptic seizures in the third trimester from eclampsia is problematic. Eclampsia has persistent proteinuria and HTN, and evidence of clotting abnormalities and abnormal liver function tests also suggest eclampsia.[38] Magnesium sulfate controls the seizures of epilepsy as well as eclampsia. The treatment of status epilepticus is not altered by the presence of pregnancy.

Carbamazepine, a tricyclic anticonvulsant, is now being recommended for new-onset epilepsy in pregnancy. It has been in use since 1962, and clinical experience is of relatively short duration. Because there is currently no intravenous form of the drug, its use in the ED is limited. The lowest dose of phenytoin or carbamazepine to control active seizures is probably the "lesser of evils" to control active grand mal seizures in pregnancy.

Phenobarbital is also associated with "hydantoin-like" malformations. In addition, it can cause neonatal addiction and a withdrawal syndrome. It is not a benign drug.

Trimethadione and valproic acid, used for treatment of petit mal seizures, have unacceptable rates of birth defects and should be avoided in pregnancy. Etho-suximide is the drug of choice for petit mal seizures in pregnancy.

ACQUIRED GASTROINTESTINAL DISORDERS

APPENDICITIS

The incidence of appendicitis is about 1 in 2000 pregnancies. Pregnancy does not predispose to appendicitis but makes the diagnosis more difficult. Anorexia, nausea, and vomiting are fairly common symptoms of normal pregnancy. The physical examination is complicated by pain that is typically felt in the right middle to upper quadrant because of uterine enlargement displacing the appendix upward with advancing gestation. In addition, pregnancy is accompanied by leukocytosis.

Missed appendicitis increases the likelihood of abortion or preterm labor. The fetal loss rate is about 15%. Appendiceal rupture in the third trimester is more likely to cause generalized peritonitis. Regardless of the stage of gestation, if appendicitis is suspected, surgical exploration is indicated.

INFECTIONS

Table 57-23 summarizes important aspects of pregnancy and infection. Maternal effects, fetal/neonatal effects, diagnostic features, and management points are listed in regard to the most important viral and bacterial infections.

TABLE 57-23. INFECTIONS IN PREGNANCY

		Viral[40-42]		
Virus	**Maternal Effect**	**Fetal/Neonatal Effect**	**Diagnostic Features**	**Management**
Rubella	Mild viral illness, no change from non-pregnant course	Transplacental infection can produce congenital rubella syndrome	Maternal disease: fourfold rise in antirubella acute and convalescent antibody titers. Neonatal disease: Presence of IgM antibody, congenital rubella syndrome	Detection of infection up to 20 weeks of pregnancy requires referral for counseling. Vaccination of susceptible nonpregnant women
Rubeola	Possibly increases risk of pneumonia and heart failure	Transplacental infection may cause premature delivery. Perinatal measles has 33% mortality	Maternal disease: fourfold rise in antirubeola acute and convalescent antibody titers. Neonatal disease: Presence of IgM antirubeola antibody	Perinatal maternal infection requires passive immunization with immune serum globulin, the mother before birth and the infant immediately after birth
Mumps	No change in disease course	Twofold increase in spontaneous abortion rate when infection occurs in the first trimester, probably increased risk of preterm labor	Usually a clinical diagnosis; serologic tests are available	Symptomatic treatment, patient reassurance
Varicella-zoster	Significantly higher risk of morbidity and mortality from Varicella pneumonia	Maternal first trimester infection has low risk of producing congenital varicella syndrome. Maternal zoster infection poses no threat to fetus or neonate. Perinatal maternal infection within 4 days of birth can produce congenital Varicella infection	Diagnosis is by clinical presentation. Varicella antibody titers can be obtained but are not generally available.	Varicella-zoster immunoglobulin (VZIG): May be given to susceptible pregnant women within 5 days of exposure to modify disease but has not been shown to prevent birth defects. In primary maternal infection within 4 days of delivery; mother should receive VZIG before delivery and infant at birth or soon after
Epstein-Barr virus	No change in disease course	Infection in first trimester has increased risk of spontaneous abortion, prematurity, and intrauterine growth retardation. No evidence that mononucleosis produces congenital anomalies	Various serologic tests (heterophil antibodies, monospot test)	Reassurance and referral
Erythema infectiosum (fifth disease)[41] (Paravirus 319)	No change in disease course	Maternal parvovirus infection results in 30 to 40% fetal death. If fetus survives, no congenital abnormalities are seen. Intrauterine infection is not related to the stage of gestation or the severity of maternal infection	Parvovirus specific serum IgM antibodies	In suspected cases, draw serum specimen for acute phase serology and referral to obstetrician. There is no treatment as yet and patients are followed with maternal alpha-fetoprotein determinations and ultrasound
Enteroviruses Coxsackie A	No change in disease course, nonspecific febrile illness	Perinatal illness, rare event	Laboratory diagnosis for specific enteroviruses depends on various serologic and tissue culture techniques	Usually nonspecific viral illness, but possibility of transplacental or perinatal infection must be considered. Specific treatment does not exist, but referral and counseling for suspected infections is appropriate

TABLE 57-23. INFECTIONS IN PREGNANCY (CONTINUED)

		Viral[40-42]		
Virus	**Maternal Effect**	**Fetal/Neonatal Effect**	**Diagnostic Features**	**Management**
Coxsackie B	Nonspecific febrile illness	Transplacental infection produces congenital malformations. Neonatal infection can lead to myocarditis and CNS disease		
Echovirus	Nonspecific illness	Neonatal infection is life-threatening		
Poliovirus	Nonvaccinated women have increased susceptibility to infection	Low incidence of spontaneous abortion, low birth weight, stillbirth, and neonatal poliomyelitis		Susceptible individuals should be vaccinated with inactivated poliomyelitis vaccine (Salk) during pregnancy
Adenovirus	No change in disease course	No risk to fetus		
Respiratory syncytial virus	No change in disease course	No risk to fetus		
Hepatitis A	No change in disease course. Possible increase in preterm delivery	Perinatal infection associated with low incidence of chronic infection	Anti-HAV IgM is an indicator of acute infection or recent past infection	Immune serum globulin can be given to pregnant women and/or their infants for recent exposure
Hepatitis B[42]	No change in disease course. Possible increase in preterm delivery. Third-trimester infection carries a 60% chance of transmittal to neonate	Perinatal infection varies from asymptomatic to fulminant disease and 85 to 90% of infected infants become carriers, with 25% of the carriers eventually dying of complications of the infection	HBsAg is still the principal screening test for current infection and carrier state. HBsAg is marker of high infectivity and even higher rate of mother-to-infant transmission. Anti-HBsAg is a marker for recovery or immunity	Screening of all pregnant women for the presence of HBsAg. Neonates of chronic carriers or acutely infected mothers immunized with HBIG within 12 to 48 hours and Hepatitis B vaccine within 12 hours to 7 days with repeat doses at 1 month and 6 months. Strong consideration should be given for administering HBIG to infants of high-risk mothers with unknown HBsAg status.
Human immune deficiency virus (HIV)	Physiologic immune suppression of pregnancy would suggest accelerated disease course, but insufficient data to support this theory at present. Most women who deliver infants that subsequently develop AIDS are asymptomatic during pregnancy.	Perinatal transmission rates estimated from 20 to 75% of affected pregnancies. Prognosis is extremely poor for infected children	Congenital HIV infection: difficult to diagnose, tests based on presence of anti-HIV antibody of IgG class. In babies under 15 months of age, diagnosis depends on isolation of virus or persistent seropositivity associated with abnormal laboratory and physical findings	HIV-infected patients should be referred for counseling, with stress placed on the importance of the prevention of pregnancy. Opportunistic infections should be treated with standard regimens as the disease risks outweigh risks to fetus from therapy. Health care providers should observe universal precautions while caring for patients in labor and delivery
Herpes simplex virus (HSV) Type 1 Type 2	Increased frequency of recurrence, no change in disease course	Primary infection in first trimester has increased risk of abortion or fetal CNS malformation. Primary or recurrent infections near term associated with significant perinatal infection	Virus isolation in tissue culture in appropriate clinical setting. Cytology of lesions can give indirect evidence	Mothers with visible lesions at term should undergo cesarean section. Active HSV lesions with PROM and prematurity requires obstetric consultation
Cytomegalovirus (CMV)	Increased frequency of reoccurrence, usually a subclinical infection	In utero infection during first two trimesters has been associated with congenital infection and birth defects. The vast majority of infected newborns are asymptomatic	Common, usually benign maternal infection, rarely diagnosed, requires demonstration of seroconversion; problems in immunosuppressed	Mothers with documented CMV infection during first 20 weeks of pregnancy should be referred for counseling

TABLE 57-23. INFECTIONS IN PREGNANCY (CONTINUED)

Bacterial

Agent	Maternal Disease	Fetal/Neonatal Disease	Diagnostic Features	Management
Group B streptococcus	Asymptomatic colonization in 10–40% of pregnancies. A cause of chorioamnionitis in women with preterm labor and PROM	Early onset: Usually within 48 hrs of delivery, presents as basic. Rule out sepsis with neonatal work-up. Has a 30 to 90% mortality Late disease: Onset a week or more after birth, presents as meningitis but has lesser mortality rate than early onset disease	Usually associated with PROM or prematurity but more than half of infections are in term neonates	Transmission is intrapartum, prevention of maternal carrier state antenatally has proven ineffective. Immediate postpartum treatment with penicillin decreases incidence of disease but increases mortality of penicillin-resistant nonstreptococcal diseases. Intrapartum treatment of colonized mothers with penicillin can decrease the incidence of neonatal colonization and disease but requires universal screening for maternal carrier state. Passive neonatal immunity may be provided with maternal vaccination with capsular polysaccharide antigen
Listeria monocytogenes	From asymptomatic febrile illness confused with influenza or pyelonephritis to chorioamnionitis without ruptured membranes	Early onset: A cause of neonatal sepsis Late onset: A cause of meningitis after 3 to 4 weeks of age	Positive blood or stool culture is often the first clue to infection	Treatment of maternal listeriosis may be effective for fetal infection
Mycobacterium tuberculosis	Disease unchanged by pregnancy. With adequate treatment of active disease, pregnant women have the same excellent prognosis as their nonpregnant counterparts	Congenital tuberculosis is rare, even in the presence of active maternal disease. The newborn is susceptible to infection and therefore should be isolated from mother thought to have active disease	Maternal: Intradermal tuberculin skin tests (PPD) are valid during pregnancy. Chest radiographs have low yield unless the patient has positive skin test and evidence of active disease. Physiologic changes of pregnancy may conceal radiographic evidence of active disease. Neonatal: Can present as failure to thrive, tuberculin skin test is usually negative. Positive smear and culture results can be obtained from gastric washings, spinal fluid, or live biopsy specimens	Pregnant patients with positive skin test and no evidence of disease may have their isoniazid (INH) prophylaxis delayed until after delivery. If the patient is a recent converter with close contact to active disease, prophylaxis should be begun during pregnancy. Because mechanical effects of pregnancy tend to conceal active disease, treatment sometimes has to be undertaken with less objective evidence of active disease. Tuberculosis is always treated with at least two drugs. Combinations of INH, ethambutol, and rifampin have been well tolerated during pregnancy. Supplemental pyridoxine is recommended when pregnant patients are taking INH.

Venereal-Bacterial

Agent	Maternal Disease	Fetal/Neonatal Disease	Diagnostic Features	Management
Syphilis	No change in disease course. Because the disease is difficult to detect clinically, the first evidence of maternal disease can be stillbirth or birth of in-	Maternal syphilis at any time during pregnancy can result in fetal infection. Despite recommended treatment for maternal disease, approximately 20% of new-	Maternal syphilis: Serological tests (VDRL, RPR) are required as part of prenatal care. They can be expected to be positive by 4 to 6 weeks after contracting the disease. Rein-	Maternal syphilis: For nonpenicillin-allergic women the treatment is unchanged from treatment in nonpregnant women. Recommendations have been for penicillin-allergic pregnant women to be treated

TABLE 57-23. INFECTIONS IN PREGNANCY (CONTINUED)

Virus	Maternal Effect	Fetal/Neonatal Effect	Diagnostic Features	Management
	fant with severe congenital syphilis	borns have congenital syphilis	fection or inadequate treatment is determined by following monthly quantitative serologic tests. Women showing a fourfold or greater rise in titer should be retreated Congenital syphilis: Every neonate with suspected or proven disease should have a spinal tap before treatment. Their serology should be followed at monthly intervals until tests are negative or serofast	with erythromycin, but its effectiveness for treatment of fetal syphilis is not known. Likewise, cephalosporin effectiveness is not known. Tetracyclines are generally not recommended in pregnancy, but should be strongly considered for truly penicillin-allergic pregnant patients with syphilis. The risk is for staining of deciduous, not permanent teeth. Penicillin desensitization is also recommended. Congenital syphilis: Neonates born of mothers treated with erythromycin for syphilis during pregnancy should be retreated as though they have congenital syphilis
Chlamydia	Maternal cervical carriage rate of 3 to 26% Lower genital tract infections are generally minimally symptomatic Acute urethral syndrome is persistent dysuria, frequency, and pyuria with sterile urine cultures	Silent chorioamnionitis may cause preterm labor or PROM Conjunctivitis is one of the most common causes of preventable blindness in undeveloped countries. Inclusion conjunctivitis develops in approximately 33% of mothers with cervical infection. Approximately 10% of infants delivered through an infected cervix develop pneumonitis within 1 to 3 months.	Culturing requires special techniques. The organism does not show up in routine urine culture. A fluorescence-tagged chlamydia monoclonal antibody test is accurate to confirm the infection. Long latency periods and indolence characterize chlamydial infections, neonatal conjunctivitis appears later than the same disease caused by N. gonorrhoeae. Pneumonitis can present as chronic cough bilateral pulmonary infiltrates and failure to thrive.	Maternal disease: Confirmed maternal genital infection is treated with erythromycin. In absence of techniques to confirm infection but highly suspicious clinical settings, it is reasonable to treat empirically. Late third-trimester treatment of cervical infection substantially decreases the incidence of neonatal chlamydial infections. Male consort must be treated with tetracycline or erythromycin. Neonatal disease: Oral erythromycin is given for both conjunctivitis and pneumonitis.
Neisseria gonorrhoeae	Acute gonococcal salpingitis is not seen or rarely seen after 12 weeks of gestation. The pregnant patient may have asymptomatic local infection involving any combination of the lower genital tract, rectum, or pharynx	The newborn exposed to gonorrhea in the birth canal is at risk to develop gonorrheal ophthalmia. Routine prophylaxis at birth with silver nitrate, various topical ophthalmic ointments, or a single dose of parenteral penicillin is used to prevent gonococcal or chlamydial conjunctivitis	Gonococcal ophthalmia has traditionally required inpatient therapy with parenteral penicillin or more recently ceftriaxone, and therefore differentiation of symptomatic neonatal conjunctivitis by either culture or gram or Giemsa stain is important to differentiate between chlamydial and gonococcal infection. Ideally, all pregnant women should have an endocervical culture for gonorrhea at the time of their first prenatal visit	Maternal infection: Uncomplicated infection for nonpenicillin-allergic women in areas of low incidence of plasmid-mediated, penicillinase-producing organisms can be treated with usual regimen used for nonpregnant women. In areas of resistant gonococcal infection, spectinomycin or ceftriaxone is currently recommended. Incubating syphilis may not be treated by these drugs. Oral ampicillin, amoxicillin, or spectinomycin is not effective against pharyngeal infection. In pregnant patients, recommended coverage for possible coexistent chlamydial infection requires erythromycin, because tetracycline is not recommended during pregnancy Neonatal infection: Infants of mothers with gonorrhea are treated with a single injection of aqueous penicillin G

REFERENCES

1. Barss, V.A.: Diabetes and Pregnancy. Med. Clin. North Am. Medical Problems in Pregnancy 73:685, 1989.
2. Buchanan, T.A., Unterman, T.G., and Metzer, B.E.: The medical management of diabetes in pregnancy. Clin. Perinatol. Symposium on Medical Disorders During Pregnancy 12:625, 1985.
3. Finley, B.E.: Acute coagulopathy in pregnancy. Med. Clin. North Am. Medical Problems in Pregnancy 73:723, 1989.
4. Davison, J.M., Katz, A.I., and Lindheimer, M.D.: Kidney disease and pregnancy: Obstetric outcome and long-term renal prognosis. Clin. Perinatol. Symposium on Medical Disorders During Pregnancy 12:497, 1985.
5. Gianopoulos, J.G.: Cardiac disease in pregnancy. Med. Clin. North Am. Medical Problems in Pregnancy 73:639, 1989.
6. Carlson, J.A.: The role of the medical consultant in pregnancy. Med. Clin. North Am. Medical Problems in Pregnancy 73:541, 1989.
7. Sterling, W.M., et al.: Pregnant women with prosthetic heart valves. Clin. Obstet. Gynecol. 32:76, 1989.
8. Barron, W.M.: Medical evaluation of the pregnant patient requiring nonobstetric surgery. Clin. Perinatol. 12:481, 1985.
9. Higgins, S.D.: Caring for the injured pregnant patient. Contemp. OB/GYN Update on General Surgery. Med. Econom. Co. Inc., March, 1983.
10. Lockwood, C.J.: Placenta previa and related disorders. Contemp. Obstet. Gynecol. Jan. 1990, 47.
11. Noble, P.W., Lavee, A.E., and Jacobs, M.M.: Respiratory diseases in pregnancy. Obstet. Gynecol. Clin. North Am. 15:391, 1988.
12. Roberts, J.: Asthma during pregnancy. Emerg. Med. News, Dec. 1989, 6.
13. Caravati, E.M., et al.: Fetal toxicity associated with maternal carbon monoxide poisoning. Ann. Emerg. Med. 17:714, 1988.
14. Roberts, J.: Pulmonary embolism during pregnancy. Emerg. Med. News, Jan. 1990, 4.
15. Brunader, R.E.: Diagnosis and evaluation of thromboembolic disorders. J. Am. Board Fam. Pract. 2:106, 1989.
16. Stults, B.M., Dere, W.H., and Caine, T.H.: Long-term anticoagulation, indications and management. Clin. Rev. West. J. Med. 151:414, 1989.
17. Cousins, L.: Pregnancy complications among diabetic women: Review 1965–1985. Obstet. Gynecol. Surv. 42:140, 1987.
18. Diamond, M.P., et al.: Reassessment of White's classification and Pedersen's prognostically bad signs of diabetic pregnancies in insulin-dependent diabetic pregnancies. Am. J. Obstet. Gynecol. 156:599, 1987.
19. Brumfield, C.G., and Huddleston, J.F.: The management of diabetic ketoacidosis in pregnancy. Clin. Obstet. Gynecol. 27:50, 1984.
20. Gavin, L.A.: Management of diabetes mellitus during surgery: Clin. Rev. West. J. Med. 151:525, 1989.
21. Nolan, T.E., Hess, W.L., Hess, D.B., and Morrison, J.C.: Severe medical illness complicating cesarean section. Obstet. Gynecol. Clin. North Am. 15:697, 1988.
22. Bjorkman, D.J., Randall, B.W., and Tolman, K.G.: Primary care of women with gastrointestinal disorders. Clin. Obstet. Gynecol. 31:974, 1988.
23. Morrison, J.C.: Anemia associated with pregnancy. In Gynecology and Obstetrics. Edited by J.J. Sciarra. Hagerstown, MD: Harper & Row, Vol. 3, 1980.
24. Morrison, J.C.: Hemoglobinopathies and pregnancy. Clin. Obstet. Gynecol. 22:819, 1979.
25. Mclaughlin, B.N., Martin, R.W., and Morrison, J.C.: Clinical management of sickle cell hemoglobinopathies during pregnancy. Clin. Perinatol. 12:585, 1985.
26. Koshy, M., et al.: Prophylactic red-cell transfusions in pregnant patients with sickle cell disease, a randomized cooperative study. N. Engl. J. Med. 319:1447, 1988.
27. Hoffman, P.C.: Idiopathic thrombocytopenic purpura in pregnancy. Clin. Perinatol. 12:599, 1985.
28. Fellin, F., and Murphy, S.: Hematologic problems in the preoperative patient. Med. Clin. North Am. 71:477, 1987.
29. Nicholas, N.S.: Rheumatic diseases in pregnancy. Brit. J. Hosp. Med. pg 50, Jan. 1988.
30. Hayslett, J.P., and Reece, A.E.: Systemic lupus erythematosus in pregnancy. Clin. Perinatol. 12:539, 1985.
31. Dombroski, R.A.: Autoimmune disease in pregnancy. Med. Clin. North Am. 73:605, 1989.
32. Samuels, P., and Pfeifer, S.M.: Autoimmune diseases in pregnancy, the obstetrician's view. Rheum. Dis. Clin. North Am. 15:307, 1989.
33. Ransey-Goldman, R.: Pregnancy in systemic lupus erythematosus. Rheum. Dis. Clin. North Am. 14:169, 1988.
34. Kwaan, H.C.: Thrombotic thrombocytopenic purpura and hemolytic uremic syndrome in pregnancy. Clin. Obstet. Gynecol. 28:101, 1985.
35. Hou, S.: Pregnancy in women with chronic renal disease. Medical intelligence, N. Engl. J. Med. 312:836, 1985.
36. Hou, S.: Pregnancy in organ transplant recipients. Medical Problems in Pregnancy. Med. Clin. North Am. 73:667, 1989.
37. Sinkinson, C.S., Coustan, D.R., and Rayburn, W.F.: How to use drugs safely and effectively for pregnant patients. Emerg. Med. Rep. 10:115, 1989.
38. Patterson, R.M.: Seizure disorders in pregnancy. Medical Problems in Pregnancy. Med. Clin. North Am. 73:661, 1989.
39. Noronha, A.: Neurologic disorders during pregnancy and the puerperium. Symposium on Medical Disorders During Pregnancy. Clin. Perinatol. 12:695, 1985.
40. Ellis, G.L., Melton, J. and J., and Filkins, K.: Viral infections during pregnancy. A guide for the emergency physician. Ann. Emerg. Med. 19:802, 1990.
41. Jenista, J.A., McMillan, J., and MacDonald, N.: Erythema Infectiosum and Roseola: Avoiding the trap of misdiagnosis. Emerg. Med. Rep. 11:73, 1990.
42. Arevalo, J.: Hepatitis B in pregnancy. West. J. Med. 150:668, 1989.

BIBLIOGRAPHY

Pritchard, MacDonald, and Gant (eds.): Williams Obstetrics. Norwalk, CT, Appleton-Century-Crofts, 18th Ed., 1989.

Hayashi, R.H.: Emergency Care of the Pregnant Woman. In Schwartz, G.R., et al.: Emergency Medicine, The Essential Update. 1st Ed. Edited by Lamsback, W. Philadelphia, W. B. Saunders, 1989.

DRUG USE IN PREGNANCY

Robert R. Whipkey

CAPSULE

All practicing emergency physicians must be aware of the possible adverse effects of prescribed or over-the-counter medications in pregnant women and women of child-bearing age. Both mother and fetus may be affected. Potential teratogenic effects and altered physiology or metabolism of drugs must be taken into consideration in assessing the need for medication and the correct dosage. Prescribed and recreational drugs, along with the basic principles of prescribing, are covered in depth in this subchapter.

INTRODUCTION

The general public and medical professionals have become increasingly concerned with the potential teratogenic effects of drugs taken during pregnancy.[1] The altered metabolic effects and the possibility of drug-induced toxicity must be considered when treating pregnant patients and all women of childbearing age. Even with widespread physician and patient education regarding devastating teratogenic effects, misuse still occurs, as has been demonstrated with the effects of isotretinoin (Accutane), introduced to treat cystic acne in 1982. This medication carries a strong warning that it is contraindicated in women who are pregnant or unwilling to prevent pregnancy while under treatment. Despite this warning, 62 birth defects have been reported, and the FDA estimates between 900 and 1300 birth defects nationwide. In addition, 700 to 1000 spontaneous abortions and 5000 to 7000 induced abortions have been reported in women who became pregnant while taking isotretinoin.[2] As a result, Hoffman-LaRoche is re-emphasizing the warnings, clarifying the limited group of patients who actually need this drug, and recommending that only patients who can understand and carry out oral instructions and those given as written informed consent receive Accutane. The packaging is also being redesigned so that each time the patient takes a capsule, she sees the pregnancy warning.

Drugs cross the placenta by passive diffusion across a concentration gradient. A lipid-soluble, nonionized drug of low molecular weight crosses the placenta more rapidly than one that is less lipid-soluble, of higher molecular weight, or less lipid-soluble.

Teratogens are agents that increase the frequency of congenital malformations or fetal damage. Neither patient nor physician may be aware of pregnancy when the rapidly differentiating organs are most susceptible to teratogens, in the period spanning days 15 through 60 of gestation.[3] The teratogenic effects of agents are influenced by the genetic susceptibility of the fetus. Teratogenicity is generally considered to involve gross morphologic changes, but recently more subtle physiologic, biochemical, or behavioral effects have been noted. Early in pregnancy, in the first 8 to 10 weeks of fetal life, teratogenic agents may induce more severe alterations in development leading to gross malformations or spontaneous abortion. Drug exposure should be minimized during this period. As mentioned, however, many patients are unaware of being pregnant during this time. Later in pregnancy, adverse effects are more likely to be from unexpected influences on the immature and sensitive fetal metabolism or to maternal changes, such as hypotension or hypoxemia, secondarily harming the fetus.[4]

CATEGORIES OF MEDICATION

In 1979, the Federal Drug Administration (FDA) established five categories to be assigned to all drugs according to their potential for causing birth defects when given during the first trimester. The classification, as outlined by the FDA, includes the following:

Class A Medications—Controlled human studies have failed to demonstrate a risk to the fetus during the first trimester, and the possibility of fetal harm seems remote.

Class B Medications—Animal studies indicate no fetal risk, and there are no controlled human studies; or animal studies do show an adverse effect on the fetus, but well-controlled human studies do not.

Class C Medications—Teratogenic or embryocidal effects are shown in animals, but no controlled studies are available in either animals or human beings.

Class D Medications—Positive evidence of human fetal risks exists, but benefits may outweigh risks in certain situations.

Class X Medications—Studies or experience have shown fetal risk that clearly outweighs any possible benefits.

Of special note is the FDA's statement that even the medications deemed safest should be used only when clearly indicated.[5] The limitations of these classifications is further exemplified by the fact that animal studies failed to reveal any teratogenic effects of the drug Thalidomide before the appearance of its devastating effects on limb formation in human fetuses.

Relatively few drugs have been proven to directly harm the developing fetus. To reduce any unknown risks, a few general principles should be followed with all medications:[6]

1. Decrease exposure by giving the minimum effective dose for the shortest possible time to achieve the desired effect.
2. Prescribe oral or aerosolized forms when possible.
3. Choose well-known preparations rather than newer medications about which less is known.
4. Be aware of the potentially teratogenic components included in many combination formulations.

With some prescription drugs, the physiologic changes of pregnancy can lead to clinically important alteration of blood concentrations. Because of an increased volume of drug distribution, decreased albumin binding sites, and increased liver metabolism and renal flow, drugs metabolized by the liver or cleared by the kidney are excreted more rapidly. For example, phenytoin and theophylline are cleared at twice the rate found in nonpregnant women. Measurement of drug concentrations can be helpful in these circumstances.

Increased awareness of potential adverse effects of drug use in pregnancy among both physicians and the general public has had a positive effect, with a continuous decrease in analgesic and tranquilizer use since 1964, but not in the use of antiemetics, antibiotics, or vitamins.[7] The efficacy of alternative therapies available to treat various complaints in pregnancy is verified by the lower levels of labor pain perceived by mothers who use natural childbirth methods of delivery. Modalities such as heat therapy, cryotherapy, massage, transcutaneous electrical nerve stimulation, and hypnosis may be safe and effective for treatment of pregnant patients.[8] Situations continue to occur, however, in which alternative methods are impractical and a thorough knowledge of the teratogenic potentials of more commonly prescribed medications must be available to allow the physician to prescribe medications with full informed consent of pregnant patients. Physicians must also be aware of the risks associated with so-called recreational drugs to advise patients appropriately.

SPECIFIC MEDICATIONS

ANTIBIOTICS

A prospective study of 7765 nonpregnant hospitalized patients, conducted by Caldwell and Cluff,[9] showed the overall incidence of adverse side effects to be 4.4%. There have been no studies examining the incidence of pharmacologic side effects or changes in drug action in pregnant women. The hemodynamic changes of pregnancy influence the metabolism and distribution of antibiotics as they do those of other drugs because of increased intravascular volume, renal blood flow, and glomerular filtration rate. Pregnant patients have been shown to have lower antibiotic serum concentrations than those of nonpregnant patients receiving equivalent doses.[10–13]

The penicillins, including the semisynthetic forms, are considered safe in pregnant patients who do not exhibit an anaphylactic type of allergic reaction.[14] Based on widespread use and extensive experience, the penicillins cross the placental barrier readily without teratogenicity, decreased efficacy, or adverse effects on the mother. The newer synthetic compounds such as mezlocillin (Mezlin) and azlocillin (Azlin), all FDA Class B, generally should not be used because of lack of clinical experience unless they are relatively indicated by the potential outcome of an infection inadequately treated by other agents. For patients with immediate type sensitivity to penicillin, erythromycin base is the preferred alternative therapy.[15] For nonanaphylactic reactions, cephalosporins are the preferred alternative therapy.[16] It can safely be recommended that the cephalosporin ceftriaxone (Rocephin) replace spectinomycin as the alternative therapy to penicillin for gonorrhea infections during pregnancy.

Erythromycin base is safe and effective for use during pregnancy, particularly in the treatment of community-acquired pneumonias and in the management of syphilis in patients with penicillin sensitivity.

Erythromycin estolate should not be used because there is evidence of an increased risk of cholestatic hepatitis in the mother.[15] After 4 months of gestational age, intravenous erythromycin is needed to achieve therapeutic levels in fetal serum.[17]

Cephalosporins (FDA Class B) have no reported teratogenicity, decreased efficacy, or adverse metabolic effects in the fetus and no reported cases of problems in their history.[14]

Chloramphenicol appears to be safe without increased incidence of adverse side effects on the fetus or mother when used during pregnancy.[15,18] Of special interest is its association with a severe, rare idiosyncratic toxic reaction seen especially in premature infants. The "grey syndrome" was first observed in 1959 in neonates who exhibited cardiovascular collapse after chloramphenicol therapy.[19] Onset is usually 3 to 4 days into therapy, beginning with vomiting, irregular and rapid respirations, and abdominal distention. This progresses to flaccidity, ashen grey cyanosis, and decreased body temperature. Approximately 40% survive if chloramphenicol therapy is discontinued. The incidence of this reaction is extremely low and should not deter the use of chloramphenicol when indicated in pregnant women or neonates, provided that serum drug levels are followed.

The *aminoglycosides* cross the placenta poorly, but still expose the fetus to the risk of ototoxicity.[20] Their role in pregnancy is as backup therapy for organisms resistant to chloramphenicol. Overall, the use of aminoglycosides in pregnancy has been too infrequent to allow their unqualified recommendation, and we must rely on the proverbial risk-to-benefit ratio in clinical decision making.

The *sulfonamides* (FDA Class C), including those in combination preparations such as Bactrim and Septra, should be avoided in the third trimester, when their use is associated with an increased risk of kernicterus in the newborn.[21] There is also theoretic concern for adverse effects on fetal development during the first trimester as a result of the antifolate activity of sulfonamides. It may be prudent to use alternative antibiotics in this period if possible, but treatment should not be withheld on this basis alone when no effective options exist.

Tetracycline is contraindicated during pregnancy because of its effects on both fetus and mother. The normal risk of hepatotoxicity is increased in the mother during pregnancy.[22,23] This increased risk may be the result of altered renal clearance from the hemodynamic effects discussed earlier being accentuated in pyelonephritis, resulting in higher than therapeutic levels. The chelating property of tetracycline results in tetracycline-calcium orthophosphate complexes. This poses a risk of discoloration of the teeth in the offspring of pregnant women treated with tetracycline. The period of greatest damage seems to be after the fourth month of gestation.[24] This same chelating property can also cause deposition in bones with depression of bone growth.

Nitrofurantoin (Macrodantin) may be safely used during the first two trimesters of pregnancy. This drug should not be used in patients with known or potentially compromised renal function, such as those with toxemia, hypertension, or diabetes. There are no special considerations for the use of this drug beyond those in nonpregnant patients.[4]

The *quinolones,* norfloxacin (Noroxin) and ciprofloxacin (Cipro), FDA Class C, are nalidixic acid derivatives that can cause central nervous system reactions, intracranial hypertension, rare blood dyscrasias, and hemolytic anemia in young children.[25] This class of medications should be avoided in pregnancy.

During pregnancy, changes in the vaginal environment occasionally allow overgrowth of normal organisms. Candida is a normal component of vaginal flora and requires no treatment unless bothersome symptoms exist. Should these infections be transmitted during birth, they are easily treated in the normal newborn. Clotrimazole is safe for use during pregnancy in women presenting with symptomatic Candida vaginitis.[26] Trichomonas is found in 3 to 15% of asymptomatic women at gynecology clinics and in 20 to 50% of women at sexually transmitted disease clinics.[27] The growth of trichomonas is stimulated by the more alkaline environment of the vagina during pregnancy.[28] The infectious process associated with trichomonas vaginitis during pregnancy does not appear to harm the fetus. The initial therapy should be directed towards symptomatic relief, with tub baths twice daily and biweekly douches with a weak vinegar and water solution. Clotrimazole has been shown to be occasionally effective against trichomonas in cases when conservative therapy fails.[26] Metronidazole (Flagyl) use in pregnancy is controversial, with studies showing it to be carcinogenic in rodents and mutagenic in bacteria. As a result of these studies, metronidazole should be used in cases that remain symptomatic despite the therapies outlined, and then only during the second half of pregnancy.[28]

GASTROINTESTINAL MEDICATIONS

Heartburn is a frequent complaint during pregnancy because of either esophageal reflux of gastric contents or reflux of bile through the pyloric and lower esophageal sphincters. In general, antacid preparations are well tolerated and safe in the usual doses during pregnancy. Sodium bicarbonate should be avoided because it is absorbed in greater proportion than other antacids,[14] and if used excessively may alter both maternal and fetal pH with effects on enzyme function, oxygen-hemoglobin dissociation, and many other sensitive metabolic processes in the fetus.

Hemorrhoids are best treated with increased dietary fiber and/or one of the bulk-forming fiber preparations available to avoid constipation. Anal analgesia may also help, with either sitz baths or one of the non-steroidal soothing ointments or suppositories, such as Anusol.[29,30]

The standard initial treatment for nausea and vomiting associated with pregnancy is reassurance that it is a transient problem and advice to avoid instigating factors.[29] For vomiting associated with disease states, it is customary to rest the gastrointestinal tract for several hours and then slowly advance the diet, beginning with clear liquids. When these modalities fail, early aggressive treatment with intravenous fluids is encouraged to avoid maternal dehydration and altered fetal circulation. Many alternatives exist for the pharmacologic treatment of vomiting. There is great concern in the general public over the pharmacologic treatment of nausea in pregnancy, based primarily on the drug Bendectin. The Fertility and Maternal Health Advisory Committee of the FDA reviewed both published and unpublished data on Bendectin and was unable to demonstrate a direct increase in birth defects with its use.[31] The manufacturers, however, voluntarily removed the drug from the market because of the mounting costs of defending Bendectin's safety. Trimethobenzamide (Tigan) is an antinauseant that appears to be safe for use during pregnancy.[32] Prochlorperazine (Compazine), a phenothiazine, is also probably safe. The phenothiazines should be regarded as second-line therapy because of the small risk of maternal hypotension associated with phenothiazines and resultant placental insufficiency.[14]

Meclizine (Antivert), pregnancy category B, is an antihistamine used primarily to prevent motion sickness. Rodent studies show teratogenicity at high doses, but human studies do not indicate any risk in humans. It may be prudent to notify patients of this theoretic risk before prescribing.[30,33]

ANTICONVULSANTS

Seizure control during pregnancy requires diligent attention to serum concentrations of anticonvulsant medications to maintain therapeutic drug levels during the hemodynamic and metabolic changes of pregnancy. Phenytoin may be cleared at twice the rate seen in nonpregnant women. One study has shown that seizure frequency during pregnancy increases in 45% of patients, decreases in 5% and remains unchanged in 50% of women.[33] The level of control during pregnancy is best predicted from the level of control during the preceding two years.

No current evidence exists to contraindicate the rapid intravenous use of standard drugs to control status epilepticus, although the shorter-acting preparations may be preferred to shorten the exposure time.[34] Although the FDA has deemed benzodiazepines as Class D, their use is justified by research showing that levels and duration of hypoxia and acidosis, even with a short seizure, are significant and comparable to those seen with asphyxiated newborns.[35] Benzodiazepines are not advised in pregnancy except for short-term use in status epilepticus.

Major malformations occur at a slightly higher rate in the offspring of epileptic patients; these cannot always be related to a specific medication.[36,37] Maternal complications, including hyperemesis, vaginal bleeding, toxemia, delayed labor, and forceps delivery, are increased twofold in epileptic pregnancies.[38,39] The cause of all these changes is unclear, but they may be attributable to many factors including the disease itself, common genetic predisposition to epilepsy and other malformations, specific drugs, and deficiency states induced by drugs or seizures.

The known teratogenic potential of anticonvulsants has changed with recent evidence of associations between the use of some anticonvulsants and malformations. Trimethadione is strongly associated with fetal malformation and mental retardation in a high proportion of those exposed.[40] Sodium valproate appears to cause a greatly increased risk of spina bifida.[41] Prenatal testing for neural tube defects should be offered to patients exposed to this medication during pregnancy. Carbamazepine (Tegretol) has a significant risk of minor craniofacial and limb malformations and developmental delays.[42] The fetal hydantoin syndrome includes craniofacial anomalies, limb deformities, deficient growth, and mental retardation observed in the offspring of women on phenytoin therapy. The proven incidence of this syndrome is low and has never been shown prospectively.

The avoidance of seizures during pregnancy is of paramount importance to protect the developing fetus. When control of seizures is impossible without using medications that carry a teratogenic risk, patients should be counseled on these risks and informed consent should be obtained before use of potentially teratogenic medications.

ANTIASTHMATICS

Asthmatics have a slightly higher incidence of complications and adverse outcomes of pregnancies than nonasthmatics. Higher infant mortality rates are noted in patients with continually active asthma throughout their pregnancies. The offspring of asthmatics have a higher incidence of hypoxemia at birth when compared with controls, but no significant differences in the rates of malformation, disease, or birth injury.[43,44]

Minute ventilation and oxygen consumption both increase significantly during pregnancy. The major concern in pregnant asthmatics is maintaining fetal oxygenation. Probability is nearly equal that an asthmatic will deteriorate, improve, or remain unchanged throughout pregnancy.[45]

Beta-adrenergic drugs cause peripheral vasodilation and may shunt blood from the fetus as the uterine vessels constrict; however, the true significance of this effect is unknown. The Perinatal Collaborative Project[46] found a statistically significant increase in malformations in a group of mother-child pairs exposed to epinephrine in the first 4 months of pregnancy. It is unclear if the severity of asthma itself or the treatments required caused these malformations. When possible, epinephrine should be avoided during pregnancy if other modalities will suffice. Isoproterenol (FDA Class D) and ephedrine (FDA Class C) have not been well studied in pregnancy, but no increased risk of malformation has been shown clinically. These medications should not be used in pregnancy unless the clinical situation leaves no alternative but to expose the fetus to unknown risk.

Terbutaline (FDA Class B) and other beta-two stimulants are also given by continuous infusion to arrest premature labor through inhibition of uterine activity. Theoretically, beta-two stimulants near term could prolong labor, although this seems unlikely with the low dosages used to treat asthma. Although no controlled studies have been performed, no adverse effects from the use of terbutaline have been found in humans.[14,47] Terbutaline should be reserved for situations in which safer forms of therapy have failed.[46]

Metaproterenol (FDA Class C) is safe in both the aerosol and oral forms. No adverse effects in human fetuses or increased incidence of side effects in pregnant women has been noted in 20 years of clinical use. Although animal studies have shown high doses to be harmful,[44,48] the aerosol form requires only one tenth the oral dose and should be considered safe.

The Perinatal Collaborative Project failed to demonstrate any increased risk with the use of aminophylline or theophylline. The side effects of theophylline preparations remain the same in pregnant as in nonpregnant patients. Close attention must be paid to serum theophylline levels during pregnancy to avoid neonatal theophylline toxicity. Theophylline is also cleared at twice the rate found in nonpregnant women. Theophylline levels should be maintained in the lower therapeutic range, although cases have been reported in which neonatal toxicity was associated with maternal levels of 11 to 13 mg per milliliter.[49]

Cromolyn sodium has not been studied prospectively, but no fetal damage has been observed over its long clinical history of use.[50]

Many combination products used in asthmatics contain phenobarbital. There is no evidence to suggest that its use causes undue risk to the mother or fetus. The value of phenobarbital in asthma therapy, however, has not been shown.

Oral glucocorticoids are highly effective in the treatment of severe asthma. Three groups of mothers were studied retrospectively, including those using prednisone for short-course therapy, daily prednisone initiated during pregnancy, and continued daily prednisone initiated before pregnancy.[51] The study failed to reveal any adverse effects in the offspring during the first 2 years of life. Corticosteroids should not be withheld when indicated during pregnancy, but the lower doses required with aerosol forms may be preferred.[52]

Decongestants may be indicated for certain conditions during pregnancy. Many of these products are combination medications, and the clinician should be aware of any potential adverse effects of all components. Pseudoephedrine has not been studied and cannot be condoned for use during pregnancy. The cautious use of phenylephrine appears to be safe.[14,52]

Antihistamines may be needed to treat various conditions, including urticaria, angioedema, drug reactions, and allergic and vasomotor rhinitis. The well established antihistamines appear to be safe for use in pregnancy, with the exception of brompheniramine, which shows a statistically significant correlation with malformed offspring.[46] Diphenhydramine (Benadryl) appears to be safe, although an unconfirmed study suggests a correlation with cleft palate.[53] Current data suggest its safety.[52]

IMMUNIZATIONS

The commonly used tetanus/diptheria toxoid and tetanus immunoglobulin appear to be safe for use during pregnancy when indicated. Hepatitis B vaccine is a killed virus vaccine and appears to be safe for use during pregnancy, though not proven in a controlled study.[54] Live virus vaccines such as those for smallpox, measles, mumps, varicella, and rubella carry a small, theoretic risk of viremia with resultant fetal infection and thus are contraindicated in pregnancy according to the Centers for Disease Control (CDC) and others.[55–58]

ANALGESICS

The analgesic and antipyretic of choice in pregnancy is acetaminophen. It appears to have no teratogenic effects when taken in the usual doses, although renal changes may occur in offspring of heavy acetaminophen users.[59] The second-line analgesic antipyretics are the salicylates. In the past, aspirin was the most frequently used drug during pregnancy. Salicylates readily cross the placental barrier and are more slowly eliminated by the fetus because of the immaturity of the glucuronidation and renal excretory pathways. Numerous studies of the effect of salicylates on pregnancy outcome have failed to be definitive. The antiprostaglandin effect of these medications may inhibit uterine contraction and have been shown in animals and humans to increase the average length of gestation, the frequency of postmaturity, and the mean duration of spontaneous labor.[60] Of theoretic concern is premature closure of the ductus arteriosus as a result of prostaglandin inhibition.[61] Nonsteroidal anti-inflammatory drugs have similar effects and should also be avoided.

The FDA panel on "over-the-counter medications" concluded that aspirin was a potentially hazardous medication in pregnancy. The FDA recommended that all labels of aspirin-containing products include the warning, "Do not take this product during the last two months of pregnancy except under the advice and supervision of a physician."[62]

Local anesthetics are weak bases and, as with narcotics, are subject to ion trapping in the fetal circulation.[63,64] Weak bases can be converted to the nonionic form as a result of hyperventilation associated with pain. The nonionic form then crosses the placental blood barrier to the relatively acidotic fetal circulation and converts to its ionized form, and is trapped until cleared by fetal metabolism. Local anesthetics have been shown to be myocardial depressants with an even greater negative inotropic effect when combined with acidemia.[65] Therefore prolonged exposure to local anesthetics during labor, as with epidural blocks, should be avoided, especially when signs of fetal distress are present. The vascularity of the pelvic region causes a rapid rise in maternal plasma anesthetic levels during perivaginal and paracervical blocks. This direct diffusion can result in higher levels in the fetal serum than in the maternal serum.[66,67] In a study of 17 fetuses treated with 200 mg paracervical blocks, seven had episodes of significant bradycardia.[68] Those with bradycardia had a mean mepivacaine level of 4 μg per mL, whereas those with levels below 3 μg per mL showed no adverse effects. A similar 3 μg per mL threshold was found for lidocaine. Zador et al.[69] have developed a protocol for peridural anesthesia which successfully maintains umbilical vein lidocaine levels below 0.6 μg per mL. Other research has shown that the addition of epinephrine (1:400,000) to bupivicaine halved the maternal levels and decreased the fetal level by 30%.[70]

Local infiltration for various outpatient procedures appears to be safe during pregnancy. Using a 1% solution generally results in a total dosage of less than 5 mg of lidocaine. Nearly complete absorption from a subcutaneous site occurs over a 4-hour period and thus should not exceed the threshold established.[71] Interestingly, subcutaneous intercostal nerve blocks with 400 mg of lidocaine resulted in a mean peak level of only 2.0 μg per mL.[72]

Narcotic use (therapeutic as well as recreational) during pregnancy can affect the fetus and neonate in two ways. It may cause fetal hypoxia and acidosis secondary to maternal respiratory depression and by direct fetal or neonatal depression once the narcotic has crossed the placental barrier. Narcotics remain in the fetal circulation for prolonged periods because of underdeveloped degradation pathways and ion trapping. For example, meperidine has a half-life of 18 hours in the neonate compared with 3 hours in adults.[63] Retrospective studies of narcotic-addicted mothers indicate a higher incidence of meconium-stained amniotic fluid, anemia, low birth weight, and stillbirth.[73,74] To minimize the effects of narcotics on the fetus or neonate, guidelines should be followed:

1. Avoid prolonged use of narcotics during pregnancy.
2. Avoid acute detoxification, as with naloxone in suspected or known narcotic addicts because of possible deleterious effects on the fetus.[14]
3. Approach deliveries in narcotic-addicted mothers as high risk with potential for serious neonatal depression. Keep antidotes at hand.
4. Administer IV medications for pain control in labor only during uterine contractions. Placental blood flow from the maternal side ceases as the uterine intramural pressure rises during contractions, thus decreasing the bolus reaching the fetus.[75]

Both morphine sulfate and meperidine appear safe for cautious use during pregnancy. Careful titration to the desired effect must be followed to minimize the risk of respiratory depression in either the mother or the neonate.[76]

Nitrous oxide in a 50% oxygen and 50% nitrous oxide mixture is frequently used as an analgesic in the prehospital setting and during labor. No significant differences in mean Apgar scores at 1 and 5 minutes were observed in babies of mothers receiving continuous nasal nitrous oxide with supplemental nitrous oxide during contractions.[77] Nitrous oxide does not seem to impair adjustment to early life or have ill effects when used during labor. Exposure of health care personnel to low levels of nitrous oxide has been implicated in an increased incidence of spontaneous abortion and fetal malformations in these workers.[78] The FDA warns health professionals who may become pregnant that chronic occupational exposure to nitrous oxide may pose a risk to the fetus.[79] No evidence to date, however, implicates the short-term intermittent use of 50:50 nitrous oxide and oxygen mixture in causing adverse effects during pregnancy.

SUBSTANCES OF ABUSE

The effects of individual drugs of abuse or recreation are difficult to isolate because studies indicate that most abusers use multiple drugs. Use of alcohol, tobacco, caffeine, and cocaine has been related to retarded fetal growth and developmental delays.

Alcohol is associated with the group of manifestations known together as the *fetal alcohol syndrome*.[80] This syndrome includes growth retardation, tremulousness, hyperactivity, attention deficits, and at least two of the following facial anomalies: narrow eye width, ptosis, thin upper lip, and hypoplasia of the midfacial area. The critical period for alcohol teratogenicity appears to be around the time of conception.[81] The typical levels of alcohol intake have not been shown to be teratogenic,[82] yet abstinence should be encouraged because the more subtle behavioral findings of the alcohol syndrome may manifest themselves at lower levels of maternal use.

The deleterious effects and potential sudden death associated with cocaine use have been well documented elsewhere. The vasoconstriction, sudden hypertension, decreased uterine blood flow, cardiac arrhythmias, and anorexic effects of cocaine appear to result in growth retardation and an association with abruptio placenta.[83]

NATIONAL CONTACTS

In response to the need for information on medical, environmental, and occupational exposures during pregnancy, consultation services such as the Florida Teratogenic Information Service have been established. This service can be contacted at:

University of Florida, 904-392-4104
University of Miami, 305-547-6549
University of South Florida, 813-974-2262

REFERENCES

1. LaFauce, L., Williams, C., Osborne, W., and Moffett, M.: The Florida Teratogen Information Service. Florida Medical Association, December, 1988, Vol. 75, No. 12, pp. 814–816.
2. Marwick, C.: FDA ponders approaches to curbing adverse effects of drug used against cystic acne. JAMA 259:3225, 1988.
3. Moore, K.L. (Ed.): The Developing Human. Clinically Oriented Embryology, 2nd Ed. Philadelphia, W.B. Saunders Co., 1977, p. 133.
4. Lewis, B.V.: Drug Therapy in Pregnancy. Practitioner 221:566, 1978.
5. Pregnancy Categories for Prescription Drugs. FDA Drug Bulletin, September, 1979.
6. Whipkey, R.R., Paris, P.M., and Stewart, R.D.: Drug Use in Pregnancy. Ann. Emerg. Med. 13:346, 1984.
7. Harjulehto, T., Aro, T., and Saxen, L.: Long term changes in medication during pregnancy. Teratology 37:145, 1988.
8. Paris, P. (Ed.): Pain Management in Emergency Medicine. Norwalk, Connecticut, Appleton and Lange, 1988, p. 420.
9. Caldwell, J., and Cluff, L.: Adverse reactions to antimicrobial agents. JAMA 230:77, 1974.
10. Philipson, A.: Pharmacokinetics of ampicillin during pregnancy. J. Infect. Dis. 136:370, 1972.
11. Bernard, B., Barton, L., Abate, M., et al.: Maternal fetal transfer of cefazolin in the first twenty weeks of pregnancy. J. Infect. Dis. 136:377, 1977.
12. Weinstein, A.J., Gibbs, R.S., and Gallagher, M.: Placental transfer of clindamycin and gentamycin in term pregnancy. Am. J. Obstet. Gynecol. 124:688, 1976.
13. Good, R., and Johnson, G.: The placental transfer of kanamycin during late pregnancy. Obstet. Gynecol. 38:60, 1976.
14. Berkowitz, R.L., Coustan, D.R., and Michizuki, T.K. (Eds.): Handbook for Prescribing Medications During Pregnancy. Boston, Little, Brown and Company, 1986, pp. 221–224.
15. Weinstein, A.J.: Treatment of Bacterial Infections in Pregnancy. Drugs 17:56, 1979.
16. Weinstein, L.: Antimicrobial agents. Penicillin and cephalosporins. In The Pharmacologic Basis of Therapeutics, 7th Ed. Edited by Goodman, L., and Gillman, A. New York, MacMillan, 1985.
17. Fenton, L.J., and Light, I.J.: Congenital syphilis after maternal treatment with erythromycin. Obstet. Gynecol. 47:492, 1976.
18. Weinstein, L.: Antimicrobial agents. Tetracyclines and chloramphenicol. In The Pharmacologic Basis of Therapeutics, 7th Ed. Edited by Goodman, L., and Gillman, A. New York, MacMillan, 1985.
19. Burns, L.E., Hoggman, J.E., and Cass, A.B.: Fatal circulatory collapse in premature infants receiving chloramphenicol. N. Engl. J. Med. 261:13, 1959.
20. Conway, N., and Birt, B.D.: Streptomycin in pregnancy. Effect on the fetal ear. Br. Med. J. 2:260, 1965.
21. Brumfitt, T.W., and Purswell, R.: Trimethoprim—Sulfa Methoxazole in the Treatment of Bacteriuria in Women. J. Infect. Dis. 128:657, 1973.
22. Kunelis, C.T., Peters, R.L., and Edmondson, H.A.: Fatty liver of pregnancy and its relationship to tetracycline therapy. Am. J. Med. 38:359, 1965.
23. Davis, J.S., and Kaufman, R.H.: Tetracycline toxicity. A clinicopathologic study with special reference to liver damage and its relation to pregnancy. Am. J. Obstet. Gynecol. 95:523, 1966.
24. Weyman, J.: Tetracycline and teeth. Practitioner 195:661, 1965.
25. New, H.C.: Quinolones: A new class of antimicrobial agents with wide potential uses. Med. Clin. North Am. 72:623, 1988.
26. Haram, K., and Digraines, A.: Vulvovaginal candidiasis in pregnancy treated with chlotrimazole. Acta Obstet. Gynecol. Scand. 57:453, 1978.
27. Rein, M.F., and Chapel, T.A.: Trichomonas, candidiasis and the minor venereal diseases. Clin. Obstet. Gynecol. 18:73, 1975.
28. Fouts, A.C., and Krauss, J.: Trichomonas vaginalis: Reevaluation of its clinical presentation and laboratory diagnosis. J. Infect. Dis. 141:137, 1980.
29. Landers, D.V., Green, J.R., and Sweet, R.L.: Antibiotic use during pregnancy and the post partum period. Clin. Obstet. Gynecol. 26:401, 1983.
30. Biggs, J.S.G., and Vesey, E.J.: Treatment of gastrointestional disorders of pregnancy. Drugs 19:70, 1980.
31. Dworken, H.J. (Ed.): Gastroenterology. Pathophysiology and Clinical Applications. Boston, Butterworth Inc., 1982, pp. 512–513.
32. Indications for Bendectin Narrowed. FDA Drug Bulletin 2:5, 1981.
33. Millovich, L., and Van Den Berg, B.J.: An evaluation of teratogenicity of certain antinauseant drugs. Am. J. Obstet. Gynecol. 125:244, 1976.
34. Knight, A.H., and Rhind, E.G.: Epilepsy in Pregnancy—A study of 153 pregnancies in 59 patients. Epilepsia 16:99, 1976.
35. Montouris, G.D., Fenichel, G.M., and McLain, L.W.: The pregnant epileptic, a review and recommendations. Arch. Neurol. 36:601, 1979.
36. Orringer, C.E., Eustace, J.C., Wunsch, C.D., et al.: Natural history of lactic acidosis after grand mal seizures. N. Engl. J. Med. 297:796, 1977.
37. Shapiro, S., Sloane, D., Harty, S.C., et al.: Anticonvulsants and parental epilepsy in the development of birth defects. Lancet 1:272, 1976.
38. Shapiro, S., Sloane, D., Harty, S.C., et al.: Hydantoins (Phenytoins)—Human Teratogens? J. Pediatr. 90:673, 1977.
39. American Academy of Pediatrics Committee on Drugs: Anticonvulsants in pregnancy. Pediatrics 63:331, 1979.
40. Bjerkedal, T., and Bahna, S.L.: The course and outcome of pregnancy in women with epilepsy. Acta Obstet. Gynecol. Scand. 52:245, 1973.
41. Feldman, G.L., Weaver, D.D., and Lourien, E.W.: The fetal trimethadione syndrome report of an additional family and further delineation of this syndrome. Am. J. Dis. Child. 131:1389, 1977.
42. Munro, J. (Editorial): Valproate, spina bifida, and birth defects registries. Lancet 2:1404, 1988.
43. Jones, K.L., Lacro, R.V., Johnson, K.A., and Adams, J. (Eds.): Pattern of malformations in the children of women treated with carbamazepine during pregnancy. N. Engl. J. Med. 320:1661, 1989.
44. Bahna, S.L., and Bjerkedal, T.: The course and outcome of pregnancy in women with bronchial asthma. Acta Allergiol. (KBH) 27:397, 1972.
45. Turner, E.S., Greenberger, P.A., and Patterson, R.: Management of the pregnant asthmatic patient. Ann. Intern. Med. 6:905, 1980.
46. Sinaiko, R.J., and German, D.F.: Perceptive on asthma in pregnancy. West. J. Med. 131:315, 1979.
47. Heinonen, O.P., Slone, D., and Shapiro, S.: Birth Defects and Drugs in Pregnancy. Littleton, MA Publishing Sciences Group, Inc., 1977.
48. Bergman, B., and Hedner, T.: Antipartum administration of terbutaline and the incidence of hyaline membrane disease in pre-term infants. Acta Obstet. Gynecol. Scand. 58:217, 1978.
49. Arwood, L.L., Dasta, J.F., and Friedman, C.: Placental transfer of the theophyllin. Two case reports. Pediatrics 63:844–846, 1979.
50. Dykes, M.H.M.: Evaluation of an antiasthmatic agent chromolone sodium. JAMA 227:1061, 1974.
51. Synder, R.D., Synder, D.: Corticosteroids for asthma during pregnancy. Ann. Allergy 41:340, 1978.
52. Greenberger, P., and Patterson, R.: Safety of therapy for allergic symptoms during pregnancy. Am. Intern. Med. 89:234, 1976.
53. Saxen, I.: Cleft palate and maternal diphenhydramine intake. Lancet 1:407, 1974.

54. Barry, M., and Bia, F.: Pregnancy in Travel. JAMA *261*:728, 1989.
55. Epidemiology—Unnecessary small pox vaccination. Br. Med. J. *2*:1155, 1979.
56. Levine, M.M., Edsall, G., and Bruce-Chwatt, L.J.: Live virus vaccines in pregnancy: Risks and recommendations. Lancet 34, 1974.
57. Adverse reactions to small pox vaccination. MMWR *28*:265, 1978.
58. American Centers for Disease Control Rubella Vaccine Registry: Rubella vaccination during pregnancy—United States, 1971–1981. MMWR *31*:477, 1982.
59. Schenkel, B., and Vorherr, H.: Nonprescription drugs during pregnancy. Potential teratogenic and toxic effects upon embryo and fetus. J. Reprod. Med. *12*:27, 1974.
60. Lewis, R.B., and Schulman, J.D.: Influence of acetylsalicylic acid, an inhibitor of prostaglandin synthesis, on the duration of human gestation and labor. Lancet *2*:11, 1973.
61. Goodman, L., and Gillman, A. (Eds.): The Pharmacologic Basis of Therapeutics. New York, MacMillan, 1985, pp. 678–679.
62. Corby, D.J.: Aspirin and pregnancy. Maternal and fetal effects. Pediatric *62*:930, 1978.
63. Caldwell, J., and Notarianni, L.J.: Disposition of pethadine in childbirth. Br. J. Anaesth *50*:307, 1978.
64. Brown, W.U., Bell, G.C., Lorie, A.O., et al.: Newborn blood levels of lidocaine and mepivacaine in the first postnatal day following maternal epidural anesthesia. Anesthesiology 42:698, 1975.
65. Anderson, K.E., Gennser, G., and Nilson, E.: Influence of mepivacaine on isolated fetal hearts at normal and low Ph. Acta Physiol. Scand. *343*:34, 1970.
66. Petrie, R.H., Paul, W.L., Miller, F.C., et al.: Placental transfer of lidocaine following paracervical block. Am. J. Obstet. Gynecol. *120*:791, 1974.
67. Staffenson, J.L., Shnider, S.M., and DeLurimier, A.A.: Transarterial diffusion of lidocaine. Anesthesiology 32:459, 1970.
68. Asling, J.H., Shnider, S.M., Margolis, A.J., et al.: Paracervical block anesthesia in obstetrics. Am. J. Obstet. Gynecol. *107*:626, 1970.
69. Zador, G., Willdeck-Lund, G., and Nillson, B.A.: Low dose intermittent epidural anesthesia with lidocaine for vaginal delivery. Acta Obstet. Gynecol. Scand. *34*:3, 1974.
70. Beazly, J.M., Taylor, G., and Reynolds, F.: Placental transfer of bupivacaine after paracervical block. Obstet. Gynecol. *39*:2, 1972.
71. Ballard, B.E.: Lidocaine hydrochloride absorption from a subcutaneous site. J. Pharm. Sci. *64*:781, 1975.
72. Scott, D.B., Jebson, P.J.R., Braid, D.P., et al.: Factors affecting plasma levels of lignocaine and prilocaine. Br. J. Anaesth. *44*:140, 1972.
73. Ostrea, E.M., and Charez, C.J.: Perinatal problems in maternal drug addiction: A study of 830 cases. J. Pediatr. *94*:292, 1979.
74. Stone, M.L., Salerno, L.J., Green, M., and Zelson, C.: Narcotic addiction in pregnancy. Am. J. Obstet. Gynecol. *109*:716, 1971.
75. Albright, G.A.: Anesthesia in obstetrics. Menlo Park, CA, Addison-Wesley, 1978, pp. 140–148.
76. Morrison, J.C., Wiser, W.L., and Rosser, J.I.: Metabolites of meperidine related to fetal depression. Am. J. Obstet. Gynecol. *115*:1132, 1973.
77. McAneny, D.M., and Daughty, A.G.: Self-administered nitrous oxide/oxygen analgesia in obstetrics. Anesthesia *18*:488, 1963.
78. Cohen, E.N., Brown, B.W., Wu, M.L., et al.: Occupational disease in dentistry and chronic exposure to trace anesthestic gases. J. Am. Dent. Assoc. *101*:21, 1980.
79. Vessy, M.P.: Epidemiological studies of the occupational hazards of anesthestics—A review. Anesthesia *33*:430, 1978.
80. Rosett, H.: Clinical perspectives of the fetal alcohol syndrome. Alcoholism *4*:119, 1980.
81. Ernhart, C.B., Sokol, R.J., Martier, S., et al.: Alcohol teratogenicity in the humans; ADTL assessment and specificity, critical period, and threshold. Am. J. Obstet. Gynecol. *156*:33, 1987.
82. Plant, M., and Plant, M.: Family alcohol problems among pregnant women: Links with maternal substance use and birth abnormalities. Ireland, Elsevier Scientific Publishers, Ltd., pp. 213–219, 1987.
83. Acker, D., Sachs, B., Tracey, K., and Wise, W.: Abruptio Placentae Associated with Cocaine Use. Am. J. Obstet. Gynecol. *146*:220, 1983.

DRUGS AND BREAST MILK

Ronald K. Smith

CAPSULE

The evolution of pharmacologic management regarding maternal illness, in concert with possible effects in the breast-fed neonate and infant, presents a serious responsibility for all practicing physicians. Much of our knowledge concerning drugs in breast milk has been limited to case reports and research studies of limited size, making unequivocal guidelines impossible. The best general recommendations that can be made are to consider all medications transferable to the infant through breast milk, become familiar with the routes of metabolism and secretion of the drugs used, and select the least toxic agent after considering its half-life and pattern for maternal dosing. Breast-feeding should be initiated before maternal dosing and withheld for a reasonable period, usually 4 hours, to minimize the infant's exposure to medications. The risk benefit ratio and prudence should always be the guidelines in considering prescription to the lactating mother and her breast-fed infant.

INTRODUCTION

"Primum non nocere." Never has this adage been more appropriate than when considering the maternal/neonatal relationship and pharmacologic intervention. The warning that "all drugs cross into breast milk" is good advice to heed, but provides little assistance in deciding treatment regimens. Our goal is to review the pharmacokinetics involved in maternal and neonatal systems and establish reasonable guidelines for the emergency practitioner in prescribing medications for breast-feeding mothers.

The question of which drugs are safe during breast-feeding probably had its origin in antiquity. In 1908, C.B. Reed expressed such concerns and difficulties as:

"The transmission of medical substances through the milk of the mother to the baby is a subject of more than usual interest and more than usual obscurity. Many cases have been reported with the object of putting the phenomenon on a real scientific basis, but owing to the prevalence of tradition and the absence of thorough and accurate methods in correcting the data, the observations are for the most part quite valueless."[1,2]

Today the concerns persist and with the resurgence of interest in breast feeding, especially in the more industrialized countries, the treatment problems facing the prescribing physician are accentuated. Emergency physicians have faced a profound lack of information in this area and were often forced to rely on anecdotal reports citing adverse reactions in small numbers of patients, in some reports in only one patient.[3,4] In this chapter the known data of the 1980s are brought into view.

PHYSIOLOGY

Breast milk is a complex solution of water, protein, and fats in an emulsified state. Its ratio of the aforementioned products of fat and protein also varies from initiation of lactation with colostrum formation to that of mature human milk. Colostrum is high in protein content, with lesser amounts of fat and lactose, and in lesser volumes than mature milk.[5] The colostrum phase persists for approximately 1 week. This is followed by transitional milk, whose volume and fat content increase and protein content diminish. The final phase of mature milk shows its contents to be 95% water, with fat increasing and ranging from 8.7 to 120.5 mg per mL, and protein content decreasing but ranging from 7 to 20 mg per mL, with albumin relatively constant at 0.4 mg per mL.[6] The pH of breast milk ranges from 6.35 to 7.65, but generally is more acidic than that of human plasma.[2] Daily human milk production ranges from 600 to 1000 mL per day.[6]

The chemical characteristics of breast milk in association with the body's plasma content and mechanisms of passive diffusion, lipid solubility, molecular weight, pH, ionization, protein binding, distribution to maternal tissues, and maternal dosage determine the drug concentration found in human breast milk.[2,3,5,7] Of these physiochemical factors, fat solubility is the most important and pH/pKa are prime considerations.[3,5] Partitioning of drugs between maternal plasma and breast milk can occur readily if drugs remain ionized and poorly soluble. In the nonionized state, drugs become more lipid-soluble, less protein-bound, and more diffusible into breast milk. Medications and pollutants presenting as relatively weak bases pass into breast milk because of its more acidic state relative to plasma, whereas weak acids with low pKs remain trapped within the maternal plasma. A milk-to-plasma ratio concept of drugs has been developed and researched.[3–7] The significance of the M/P ratio is that drug presentation by breast milk shows variations in bioavailability because of time, constituent content, and dosage in the maternal system.

In presenting breast milk to the nursing infant, the mother has performed an initial semiselective screening for transmissible xenobiotics. The neonatal and infant gastrointestinal, hepatic, and renal systems and body water content influence total drug availability within the body.

Neonatal and infant extracellular fluid volume and total body fat content are age-dependent and are reviewed in Table 57-24.

A lower relative fat content in infants results in reduced sequestration of fat-soluble drugs in adipose tissue, and greater availability and potential toxicity in the brain despite low breast milk concentration of medications. The infant GI mucosa has a high permeability for macromolecules and delayed emptying time, with resultant absorption variation because of compartment trapping in the stomach and small intestine. After absorption from the gastrointestinal tract, limited protein binding occurs because of the low albumin content, and then biotransformation occurs in the liver. Two phases of drug metabolism have been described in the liver and are phase 1 reactions of the oxidative reductive and hydrolysis type and phase 2 reactions of the synthetic conjugation type. Primates and humans appear unique in their ability to perform phase 1 degradation using cytochrome p450 and its coenzyme complexes, but with limited activity and rate of these systems compared to those of adolescents and adults. Phase 2 reactions include glucuronidation, sulfation, and glutathione conjugation. The range of this activity is from almost nonexistent to 100% of adult activity.[8]

Renal metabolism demonstrates that neonatal glomerular function is first to mature and reaches peak activity in 3 weeks from the birth of a full-term baby, whereas tubular renal activity is delayed until 6

TABLE 57-24. BODY WATER AND TOTAL BODY FAT CONTENT[3]

Age	ECF Volume	Total Body Fat
Premature infant	50%	3%
Term infant	50%	12%
6/12-month-old infant	45%	30%
Adult	20–25%	18%

months of age.[3,9] These delayed elimination mechanisms account for increased drug accumulation in neonates despite low breast milk concentrations.

SPECIFIC MEDICATIONS

ANTIBIOTICS

Considering the medications used by emergency physicians, antibiotics represent the largest group prescribed to lactating mothers. The penicillin medications are readily used in treatment of common infections and represent a group of weak acids that are thought to cross poorly into breast milk. They are, however, found in low levels in early breast milk and can present a problem following absorption by the infant gastrointestinal system as macromolecules, because of increased GI permeability. Low concentrations of these medications in breast milk probably are not enough to cause therapeutic effects, except to decrease the suckling infant's oral or possibly gastrointestinal flora. They have also been postulated to cause sensitization, which could cause effects later in life with allergic-type reactions.[10–12] Cephalosporins of cephalexin, cephadroxil, cephalothin, cefazolin, cefotaxime, cephaprin, cefoxatin, ceftriaxone, and moxalactam have been investigated. This group of medications also represent weak acids with a relative degree of protein binding. Low levels of transmissibility to breast milk with some of these cephalosporins seem to increase with their long-term chronic use.[11,13–16] The risk to the suckling infant is that there may be a decrease in the oral and gastrointestinal flora, and then sensitization to these medications with allergic phenomenon. Of note, the third-generation cephalosporins like moxalactam have significant MICs against gram-negative organisms and may potentially allow gram-positive organisms to flourish and therefore resistant organisms to develop in the neonatal systems.[16] Generally, first- and second-generation cephalosporins appear to be safe in breast-feeding, but use of some third-generation cephalosporins may warrant cessation of breast-feeding.

The sulfonamides and nalidixic acid have been recognized for many years as dangerous because of induction of hemolytic anemia even when transferred by breast milk.[17–19] The administration and passage of sulfonamides also poses the potential problem of displacing bilirubin from albumin binding sites and resultant deposition of bilirubin in neonatal cerebral tissues, leading to kernicterus.

Tetracycline passage in milk has been questioned by some authors because of calcium and magnesium chelation. Yet some tetracycline forms, such as doxycycline and minocycline, have high lipid solubility and low affinity for calcium binding, and may have greater absorption.[20] The theoretic risk of mottled teeth in children bodes against tetracycline use in nursing mothers.[10] Two other low-occurrence risks have been reported with tetracycline: depression of bone growth, which appears to be dose-dependent and reversible, and pseudotumor cerebri, a condition of increased intracranial pressure, and these should be considered before use of tetracyclines.[19]

Clindamycin has been investigated and is found to be a basic drug of pKa 7.45 that accumulates in breast milk. Research findings demonstrated that clindamycin is widely concentrated in human serum, making prediction of secretion into breast milk difficult, but cessation of breast feeding during clindamycin administration is recommended.[21]

Metronidazole, often used for trichomonas vaginalis, has been assessed for breast milk passage. Present recommendations are for interruption of breast feeding for 12 to 24 hours because of metronidazole's half-life of 9 hours, and its primary elimination by the kidneys. The safety and effects in suckling infants are still unknown, but allowing a 24-hour hiatus of breast feeding ensures greatly reduced exposure in the neonates and infants.[22]

Chloromycetin is a potent antibiotic, often reserved for the most serious illnesses. Its reputation and theoretic risk for inducing the grey baby syndrome are well recognized but probably limited in nature from transmission in breast milk. The greater risk exists from the idiosyncratic reaction of bone marrow aplasia with even small doses of chloromycetin and is best avoided if breast feeding is not to be terminated.[10] The resurgence of tuberculosis in the United States and its pharmacologic management may some day face lactating women. Agents such as p-aminosalicylic acid and pyrazinamide have been found in single-agent treatment to be well below the therapeutic levels in breast milk, and can be considered safe in nursing mothers. The combination therapy of p-aminosalicylic acid with INH has been found to raise INH's serum and breast milk concentration and warrant limitation of breast feeding.[23]

Tropical illnesses such as malaria are rarely encountered in the United States, but remain large-scale problems in some areas. Agents such as *chloroquine, dapsone,* and *pyrimethamine* are all weak bases with plasma protein binding. They are all transmissible into breast milk, with concentrations ranging from 4.2% to 14.3% to 45% of maternal dose, respectively, and are unlikely to be harmful in infants. The reported problems associated with these agents are hemolytic anemia (with dapsone), insufficient coverage for plasmodium falciparum or plasmodium vivax, and possible induction of drug-resistant strains of these parasites.[24]

PULMONARY DRUGS

The methylxanthine agent theophylline has been investigated for transmission into breast milk. Two studies have found a milk/serum ratio of approximately 0.7, a half-life of 4 hours, and exposure of the nursing infant to about 1% of the total maternal dose. The full-term infant should not find this level a problem, but premature infants, who bind less theophylline to protein, may need serum monitoring of theophylline levels, especially if clinical signs of cardiac dysrhythmia, seizure, or pronounced irritability are witnessed.[25,26] Terbutaline has been found to have a pKa of 8.8 to 11.2, with resultant concentration in milk higher than in maternal plasma. Of the maternal dose of terbutaline, 0.2 to 0.7% has been observed to be ingested by the nursing infant without evidence of beta-adrenergic stimulation, and breast feeding need not be interrupted.[27,28]

Information in the literature on other beta-adrenergic agents such as metoproterenol and albuterol is limited, but on the basis of their low systemic absorption when administered by inhalation, they should be safe and not necessitate termination of breast feeding.

CARDIOVASCULAR DRUGS

Digitalis has long been known as a derivative of the foxglove plant. Until 1978, there appeared to be no literature on its transmission into breast milk despite its wide use for conditions such as paroxysmal atrial tachycardia, rheumatic heart disease, and congestive heart failure.

Digoxin is reported to be transmissible into breast milk, but at insignificant levels despite maternal doses as high as 0.75 mg per day. Breast feeding may continue safely in digitalized lactating mothers because the absorbed dose in the infant is approximately 1/100 of the daily recommended dosage therapeutically needed in children.[29,30] An explosion of beta-blocking agents has occurred since the 1960s because of their use as antihypertensive and anti-anginal interventions. The research on these medications in breast milk has extended to propranolol, atenolol, labetolol, oxyprenolol, timolol, nadolol, and some metabolites. Propranolol and its metabolites are weak bases, are lipophilic, and accumulate in the breast and breast milk. This accumulation, however, appears to be only 1/100 of the recommended dosage and these agents are probably safe for continued breast feeding. Observation for hypoglycemia and bradycardia in premature neonates and full-term newborns is warranted.[31,32] Agents such as oxyprenolol, timolol, nadolol, and metoprolol appear safe for breast feeding as well, despite the interesting kinetics of nadolol and metoprolol, with which breast milk preferentially shows a 3.5- to 5-fold increase without significant effect on the suckling child.[33–35]

Use of *calcium channel blockers* has increased in the 1970s and 1980s. Verapamil, norverapamil, and diltiazem have been investigated for transmissibility into breast milk, and all three agents sustain measurable levels. Verapamil appears to be safe, with levels of 0.01% to 0.5% of the maternal dose and from 0.0% to 0.4% of the therapeutic dose for the infant.[36–38] The information on diltiazem appears to be limited to case reports showing breast milk levels approaching maternal serum levels, but no sampling of infant levels has been completed. Pending further information, breast feeding should probably be withheld with use of this medication.[39] Antiarrhythmic therapy provides limited knowledge of transmission into breast milk. Lidocaine and mexilitine have been shown in case reports to appear in breast milk, but in significantly low levels that make continuous breast feeding safe.[40,41]

Antihypertensives are readily used worldwide for preeclampsia and toxemia of pregnancy, but information on many of these agents is limited. Clonidine has been recognized as crossing into breast milk readily and achieving twofold concentration levels compared to maternal serum. Evaluations of these breast-fed infants failed to show abnormalities of neurologic function or alteration in electrolyte or blood glucose levels, or any other typical side effects of sedation or xerostomia.[42] Captopril, an angiotensin II enzyme-converting antagonist, is excreted in breast milk at 1% blood levels. This should result in dosages of 0.03% of the child's maximum therapeutic dose as presented by breast milk, but could be higher because of reduction of renal function in neonates. In a study of 12 patients receiving Captopril, several subjects, despite proper warning, nursed their children without adverse effects.[43] Chlorthalidone, a potent, long-acting diuretic, should be terminated for 3 days after ingestion because of maternal milk concentrations approaching serum concentrations and an extended half-life, with resultant reduced excretion in the neonate.[44]

TABLE 57-25. RECOMMENDATIONS FOR NEUROPSYCHIATRIC AGENTS

Agent	Breast Feeding Recommendation	Reference/Comment
Antipsychotics		
Amitriptyline	Continue	Monitor neonatal and breast milk levels[53,54]
Amoxapine	Discontinue	Active metabolites, limited knowledge of effects[55]
Chlorpromazine	Continue	See Blacker et al.[56]
Doxepin	Continue	See Kemp et al.[57]
Haloperidol	No clear recommendation	See Stewart et al.[58]
Trazadone	Continue	Active metabolites[59]
Stimulants		
Amphetamine	Discontinue	High M/P concentration Alkaline pKa Possible psycho-behavioral or Dopamine receptor interference[60]
Sedatives		
Diazepam	Cautious use	Delay feeding at least 4 hours to avoid infant sedation, 8 hour delay best[3,61,62]
Lorazepam	Continue	Appears safe for single-dose pre-operative sedation.[63]
Miscellaneous		
Pyridostigmine	Continue	Handell et al.[84]
Baclofen	Continue	Eriksson et al.[5]

ANTINEOPLASTIC AGENTS

Doxorubicin, cisplatin, cyclophosphamide, and methotrexate have been investigated for passage into breast milk. All these agents have been shown to appear in breast milk, and because of their potential for adverse effects, even at low levels, necessitate cessation of breast-feeding.[45–47]

ANALGESIC DRUGS

Pain and its control often motivate patients to seek medical attention. The abuse liability of pain medication concerns every physician, and its potential has come to the forefront in the 20th century. Acetaminophen and aspirin represent a large group of over-the-counter, readily available pain medications that have been investigated for breast milk transmission. Acetaminophen and phenacetin are relatively weak acids, are hydrophilic, and can cross into maternal milk. The levels achieved by acetaminophen are significantly low and appear safe for continued breast feeding.[48,49] Salicylates are acidic and polar, and poorly cross lipid membranes, and although they appear in breast milk, do not necessitate cessation of nursing if taken at recommended dosages.[48] The recognition of the antiplatelet effect of salicylates should

be considered at higher doses when used by nursing mothers.[10] Nonsteroidal anti-inflammatory drugs such as tolmetin, naproxen, ibuprofen, piroxicam, and mefenamic acid have been noted to appear in breast milk. The piroxicam family achieves the highest maternal serum levels per presented maternal dose, but does not appear to be detectable in sampled infant plasma. The nonsteroid anti-inflammatory drugs, as a group, should be safe and allow continuance of nursing.[19,50–52] Narcotic agents such as codeine, morphine, and methadone have been shown to appear in breast milk, and although they appear safe at recommended therapeutic doses, their effects in neonates at excessive doses, in concert with low liver detoxification, raise many doubts of their safety.[10,48]

NEUROLEPTIC AND ANTICONVULSANT DRUGS

Postpartum depression and chronic psychiatric problems are increasingly recognized and the need for medication in these nursing mothers presents a difficult dilemma. The world's literature on anxiolytic and psychotropic agents is limited to case studies and a few trials of small numbers. The available recommendations for neuropsychiatric agents are summarized in Table 57-25.

Lithium carbonate, a well known agent used for bipolar affective disorders, is an absolute contraindication to breast feeding because of its reported breast milk accumulation and toxicities of lethargy, hypotonia, and cyanosis.[6]

Epilepsy in its various forms, from tonic-clonic to absence seizures, covers a broad spectrum of pharmacologic management options. Often the need for long-term management with multiple agents must be balanced against the desire of the mother to breast-feed. Carbamazepine, phenytoin, phenobarbital, and ethosuximide have been reviewed in the literature. Phenytoin and carbamazepine have been shown to produce maximum dosage levels of 0.4 mg per kg and 2.5 to 4 mg respectively, and therefore appears to be safe for continued breast-feeding.[66,67] Phenobarbital has been variably reported to cause sedation and induction of liver enzymes in infants, requiring avoidance in ingestion by way of breast milk.[68]

Ethosuximide is an agent with high bioavailability and lipid solubility, limited protein binding, and an extended half-life, resulting in moderate concentrations in breast milk. This increasing concentration compares to that of agents such as lithium, and has been shown to result in sedation of breast-fed infants. Termination of breast feeding is currently recommended during treatment of absence seizures with ethosuximide.[3]

MISCELLANEOUS DRUGS AND ENVIRONMENTAL POLLUTANTS

Warfarin is an orally active anticoagulant often used in cardiovascular disease and thrombophlebitis. It is now widely accepted that its transmission into breast milk is too low to pose a risk to nursing infants, but current recommendations still include giving vitamin K to the neonate whose mother requires high doses of anticoagulants. Other anticoagulants such as phenindione are contraindicated in continued breast-feeding.[19] Heparin, in contrast, appears to pose little risk to the breast-feeding infant because it does not appear in breast milk.[6]

Alcohol and its use in modern society have always posed multiple problems. Reports of fetal alcohol syndrome have stirred great concern worldwide. Research has demonstrated that ethanol can be found in breast milk with concentrations approaching that of blood and infant ingestions approaching 20% of the maternal dose.[19] A case report of pseudo-Cushing's syndrome was noted in an infant whose mother consumed at least 50 12 oz. cans of beer weekly in addition to other alcoholic beverages.[70] Current recommendations of occasional ethanol ingestion with avoidance of excess appears to be prudent.

Nicotine, as acquired by smoking, is transmissible to breast milk, although in low concentrations, and some authors have suggested possible clinical ramifications.[4,19] Reduction in cigarette consumption and subsequent nicotine ingestion appears to be wise, with avoidance the best general recommendation.

Corticosteroids like prednisolone and prednisone appear in breast milk in low levels and do not appear to pose a problem, but caution should be advised in nursing mothers.[71,72,78] Estradiol and oral contraceptives also appear in breast milk without harm to the suckling child despite reports of gynecomastia in breast-fed infants.[73]

Iodines appear to pass into breast milk in moderate levels, including absorption from vaginal sources such as povidone-iodine suppositories.[74] This could affect infant thyroid function and should be terminated during iodine use in nursing mothers. Propylthiouracil has been variably reported to concentrate in breast milk with dosages of 41 to 462 mg daily as presented by breast milk, but is unlikely to interfere with neonatal thyroid metabolism and nursing may continue.[75]

Atropine has long been recognized as crossing the plasma milk barrier, with recorded concentrations high enough to stimulate anticholinergic effects, necessitating termination of breast-feeding.[10] Ergotism, reported as a common problem from use of ergot alkaloids, also necessitates its cessation. Radiopharmaceuticals such as gallium citrate and iodine,[131] radioactive sodium, and technetium products are best avoided in lactating mothers.[19,68] Trace elements such as fluoride, magnesium, and calcium have been detected in breast milk from mothers who have required treatment with magnesium sulfate or live in regions where fluoride has been added to public water. These agents appear to pose little threat to the breast-fed child.[76,77] Over-the-counter medications represent an important class of readily available agents in modern society. In general, these multiple agents, when taken

TABLE 57-26. SUMMARY OF DRUG USE IN BREAST-FEEDING MOTHERS

Agents Contraindicated

Antineoplastics	Radiopharmaceutical
Lithium	Chloramphenicol
Atropine	Ergot alkaloids
Tetracyclines	Phenindione
Iodides	Metronidazole

Agents to be Used with Caution

Ethosuximide	Phenobarbital
Phenytoin	Diazepam
Carbamazepine	Lorazepam
Sulfonamides	Nalidizic acid
INH	Aspirin (high dose)
Tricyclic antidepressants	Haloperidol
Codeine	Morphine
Methadone	Alcohol
Oral contraceptives	Corticosteroids
Nonsteroidal anti-inflammatories	

Noncontroversial Agents

Acetaminophen	Aspirin (occasional use)
Most other antibiotics	Beta blockers
Warfarin	Most over-the-counter medications

as directed by the manufacturer, should be safe in lactating women because they represent the least toxic formulations of medications with the lowest effective dosage.[3] Environmental pollutants have increasingly presented themselves in the 20th century as toxins to consider in biologic change. PCB, PBB, DDT, and other multiple insecticides, as well as heavy metals and hydrocarbons, pose definite problems, but their final transmission and toxicity await further research.[4]

Table 57-26 is a summation of agents that are contraindicated, to be used with caution, and noncontroversial in breast-feeding mothers.

REFERENCES

1. Reed, C.B.: A study of the conditions that require the removal of the child from the breast. Surg. Gynecol. Obstet. 6:514, 1908.
2. Nation, R.L., and Hotham, N.: Drugs and breast feeding. Med. J. Aust. 146:308, 1987.
3. Rivera-Calimlim, L.: The significance of drugs in breast milk. Clin. Perinatol. 14:51, 1987.
4. Giacoia, G.P., and Catz, C.S.: Drugs and pollutants in breast milk. Clin. Perinatol. 6:181, 1979.
5. Syversen, G.B., and Ratkje, S.K.: Drugs distribution within human milk phases. J. Pharm. Sci. 74:1071, 1981.
6. Beeley, L.: Drugs and breast feeding. Clin. Obstet. Gynecol. 8:291, 1981.
7. Giacoia, G.P., and Catz, C.S.: Drug therapy in the lactating mother. Postgrad. Med. 83:211, 1988.
8. Mannering, G.J.: Drug metabolism in the newborn. Fed. Proc. 44:2302,
9. Morselli, P.L.: Clinical pharmacokinetics in neonates. Clin. Pharmacokinet. 1:81, 1976.
10. Medical Letter: Drugs in Breast Milk. 16:25, 1976.
11. Kafetzis, D.A., Siafas, C.A., Georgakopoulos, P.A., and Papadatos, C.J.: Passage of cephalosporins and amoxicillin into the breast milk. Acta Paediatr. Scand. 70:285, 1987.
12. Rasmussen, F.: Mammary excretion of benzylpenicillin, erythromycin and penethamate hydro iodide. Acta Pharmacol. Toxicol. 16:194, 1959.
13. Yoshioka, H., Cho, K., Takimoto, M., Maruyama, S., and Shimizu, T.: Transfer of cefazolin into human milk. J. Pediatr. 94:151, 1979.
14. Dresse, A., Lambotte, R., DuBois, M., et al.: Transmammary passage of cefoxitin: Additional results. J. Clin. Pharmacol. 23:438, 1983.
15. Kafetzis, D.A., Brater, D.C., Fanourgakis, J.E., et al.: Ceftriaxone distribution between maternal blood and fetal blood and tissues at parturition and between blood and milk postpartum. Antimicrob. Agents Chemother. 23:870, 1983.
16. Miller, R.D., Keegan, K.A., Thrupp, L.D., and Brann, J.: Human breast milk concentration of moxalactam. Am. J. Obstet. Gynecol. 148:348, 1984.
17. Rasmussen, F.: Mammary excretion of sulphonamides. Acta Pharmacol. Toxicol. 15:139, 1958.
18. Belton, E.M., and Jones, R.V.: Hemolytilanemia due to nalidixil acid. Lancet 691, 1965.
19. Atkinson, H.C., Begg, E.J., and Darlow, B.A.: Drugs in human milk. Clinical pharmacokinetic considerations. Clin. Pharmacokinet. 14:217, 1988.
20. Neavonen, P.J.: Interactions with the absorption of tetra-cyclines. Drugs 2:45, 1976.
21. Steen, Bengt, Rane, Anders: Clindamycin passage into human milk. Br. J. Clin. Pharmacol. 13:661, 1982.
22. Erickson, S.H., Oppenheim, G.L., and Smith, G.H.: Metronidazole in breast milk. Obstet. Gynecol. 57:48, 1981.
23. Holdiness, M.R.: Anti-tuberculosis drugs and breast feeding. Arch. Intern. Med. 144:888, 1984.
24. Edstein, M.D., Veenendaal, J.R., Newman, K., and Hyslop, R.: Excretion in chloroquine, dapsone and pyrimethamine in human milk. Br. J. Pharmacol. 22:733, 1986.
25. Berlin, J., and Cheston, M.: Excretion of the methylxanthines in human milk. Semin. Perinatol. 5:389, 1981.
26. Stec, G.P., Greenberger, P., Rao, T.I., et al.: Kenetics of theophylline transfer to breast milk. Clin. Pharmacol. Ther. 28:404, 1980.
27. Boreus, L.O., DeChateau, P., Lindberg, C., and Nyberg, C.: Terbutaline in breast milk. Br. J. Clin. Pharmacol. 13:731, 1982.
28. Lunnerholdm, G., and Lindstrom, B.: Terbutaline excretion into breast milk. Br. J. Clin. Pharmacol. 13:729, 1982.
29. Loughnan, P.M.: Digoxin excretion in human breast milk. J. Pediatr. 92:1019, 1977.
30. Finley, J.P., Waxman, M.B., Wong, P.Y., and Lickrish, G.M.: Digoxin excretion in human milk. J. Pediatr. 94:339, 1979.
31. Bauer, J.H., Pape, B., Zajicek, J., and Groshong, T. Propranolol in human plasma and breast milk. Am. J. Cardiol. 43:860, 1979.
32. Smith, M.T., Livingstone, I., Hooper, W.D., et al.: Propranolol, propranolol gluconide, and naphthoxylactic acid in breast milk and plasma. Ther. Drug Monit. 5:87, 1983.
33. Devlin, R.G., Duckin, K.L., and Fleiss, P.M.: Nadolol in human serum and breast milk. Br. J. Clin. Pharmacol. 12:393, 1981.
34. Fidler, J., Smith, V., and Deswiet, M.: Excretion of oxyprenolol and timolol in breast milk. Br. J. Obstet. Gynecol. 90:961, 1983.
35. Sandstrom, B.: Metoprolol excretion into breast milk. Br. J. Clin. Pharmacol. 9:518, 1980.
36. Andersen, H.J.: Excretion of verapamil in human milk. Eur. J. Clin. Pharmacol. 25:279, 1983.
37. Miller, M.R., Withers, R., Bhamra, R., and Holt, D.W.: Verapamil and breast feeding. Eur. J. Clin. Pharmacol. 30:125, 1986.
38. Anderson, P., Bondesson, U., Mattiason, I., and Johansson, B.W.: Verapamil and norverapamil in plasma and breast milk during breast feeding. Eur. J. Clin. Pharmacol. 31:625, 1987.
39. Okada, M., et al.: Excretion of diltiazem in human milk. N. Engl. J. Med. 312:992 (April 11, 1985).
40. Zeisler, J.A., Gaarder, T.D., and DeMesquita, S.A.: Lidocaine excretion in breast milk. Drug Intell. Clin. Pharm. 20:691, 1986.
41. Lewis, A.M., Johnston, A., Patel, L., and Turner, P.: Mexilitene in human blood and breast milk. Postgrad. Med. J. 57:546, 1981.
42. Hartikainen-Sorrt, A.L., Heikkinenk, J.E., and Koivisto, M.: Pharmacokinetics of clonidine during pregnancy and nursing. Obstet. Gynecol. 6:598, 1987.
43. Devlin, R.G., and Fleiss, P.M.: Captopril in human blood and breast milk. J. Clin. Pharmacol. 21:110, 1981.
44. Mulley, B.A., Parr, G.D., Pau, W.K., et al.: Placental transfer of chlorthalidone and its elimination in maternal milk. Eur. J. Clin. Pharmacol. 13:129, 1978.
45. Egan, P.C., Costanza, M.E., Dodion, P., et al.: Doxorubicin and cisplatinin excretion into human milk. Cancer Treat. Rep. 69:1387, 1985.
46. Wiernik, P.H., and Duncan, J.H.: Cyclophosphamide in human milk. Lancet 1:912, 1971.
47. Johns, D.G., Rutherford, L.D., Leighton, P.C., and Vogel, C.L.: Secretion of methotrexate into human milk. Am. J. Obstet. Gynecol. 112:978, 1972.
48. Findlay, J.W.A., DeAngelis, R.L., Kearney, M.F., et al.: Analgesic drugs in breast milk and plasma. Clin. Pharmacol. Ther. 29:625, 1981.
49. Bitzen, P.O., Gustafson, B., Jostell, K.G., et al.: Excretion of paracetomol in human breast milk. Eur. J. Clin. Pharmacol. 20:123, 1981.
50. Seagraves, R., Waller, E.S., and Goehrs, H.R.: Tolmetin in breast milk. Drug Intell. Clin. Pharm. 19:55, 1985.
51. Jamali, F., Stevens, D.R.S.: Naproxen Excretion in Milk and its Uptake by the Infant. Drug Intell. Clin. Pharm. 17:910, 1983.
52. Buchanan, R.A., Eaton, C.J., Koeff, S.T., and Kinkel, A.W.: The breast milk excretion of mifanamic acid. Curr. Ther. Res. 10:592, 1968.

53. Bader, T.F., and Newman, K.: Amitriptyline in human breast milk and the nursing infant's serum. Am. J. Psychiatry 137:855, 1980.
54. Brixen-Rasmussen, L., Halgrener, J., and Jorgensen, A. Amitriptyline and nortriptyline excretion in human breast milk. Psychopharmacology 76:94, 1982.
55. Gelenberg, A.J.: Amoxapine, a new antidepressant, appears in human milk. J. Nerv. Ment. Dis. 167:635, 1979.
56. Blacker, K.H., Weinstein, B.J., and Ellman, G.L.: Mother's milk and chlorpromazine. 178, 1962.
57. Kemp, J., Ilett, K.F., Booth, J., and Hackett, L.P.: Excretion of doxepin and N-desmethyldoxepin in human milk. Br. J. Clin. Pharmacol. 20:497, 1985.
58. Stewart, R.B., Karas, B., and Springer, P.K.: Haloperidol excretion in human milk. Am. J. Psychiatry 137:7, 849, 1980.
59. Verbeeck, R.K., Ross, S.G., and McKenna, E.A.: Excretion of trazodone in breast milk. Br. J. Clin. Pharmacol. 22:367, 1986.
60. Steiner, E., Villen, T., Hallberg, M., and Rane, A.: Amphetamine secretion in breast milk. J. Clin. Pharmacol. 27:123, 1984.
61. Erkkola, R., and Kanto, J.: Diazepam and breast feeding. Lancet 1:1235, 1972.
62. Brandt, R.: Passage of diazepam and desmethyldiazepam into breast milk. Arzneim-Forsch. (Drug Res.) 26:454, 1976.
63. Summerfeld, R.J., and Neilsen, M.S.: Excretion of lorazepam into breast milk. Br. J. Anesth. 1042, 1987.
64. Hardell, L.I., Lindstrom, B., Lonnerholm, G., and Osterman, P.O.: Pyridostigmine in human breast milk. Br. J. Clin. Pharmac. 14:565, 1982.
65. Eriksson, G., and Swahn, C.G.: Concentration of baclofen in serum and breast milk from lactating women. Scand. J. Clin. Lab. Invest. 41:185, 1981.
66. Steen, B., Rane, A., Lonnerholm, G., et al.: Phenytoin excretion in human breast milk and plasma levels in nursed infants. Ther. Drug Monit. 4:331, 1982.
67. Froescher, W., Eichelbaum, M., Niesen, M., et al.: Carbamazepine levels in breast milk therapeutic drug monitoring 6:266, 1984.
68. O'Brien, T.E.: Excretion of drugs in human milk. Amer. J. Hosp. Pharm. 31:844, 1974.
69. Baty, J.D., et al.: May mothers breast feeding their infants take warfarin? Proc. BPS. 969, 1976.
70. Binkiewicz, A., Robinson, M.J., and Senior, B.: Pseudo-Cushing syndrome caused by alcohol in breast milk. J. Pediat. 93:965, 1978.
71. McKenzie, S.A., Selley, J.A., and Agnew, J.E.: Secretion of prednisolone into breast milk. Arch. Dis. Child. 50:894, 1975.
72. Katz, F.H., and Duncan, B.R.: Entry of prednisone into human milk. N. Engl. J. Med. 293:11, 1975.
73. Nilsson, S., Nygren, K.-G., Johansson, E.D.B.: Transfer of estradiol to human milk. Am. J. Obstet. Gynecol. 132:653, 1978.
74. Postellon, D.C., and Aronow, R.: Iodine in mother's milk. JAMA 247:463, 1982.
75. Kampmann, J.P., Hansen, J.M., Johansen, K., Helweg, J.: Propylthiouracil in human milk. Lancet 1:736, 1980.
76. Ekstrand, J., Spak, C.J., Falch, J., Afseth, J., and Ulvestad, H.: Distribution of fluoride to human breast milk. Caries Res. 18:93, 1984.
77. Cruikshank, D.P., Varner, M.W., and Pitkin, R.M.: Breast milk magnesium and calcium concentrations following magnesium sulfate treatment. Am. J. Obstet. Gynecol. 143:685, 1982.
78. Lawrence, R.A.: Corticosteroid effect on lactation. JAMA 265:2409, 1991.

POSTPARTUM INFECTIONS

Mark D. Westfall and Leslie Zun

CAPSULE

The postpartum patient who presents to the emergency department (ED) with fever or other evidence of infection is of growing concern to the emergency physician. As obstetricians move for earlier discharge of their "uncomplicated patients" and home delivery grows in popularity, the potential for the emergency physician to see more patients with acute postpartum infections will increase. The emergency physician needs an increased awareness of these disorders as well as a high index of suspicion for the patient with a serious postpartum infection.

INTRODUCTION

PREHOSPITAL CARE

The major concern for the paramedical personnel and base station attendants regarding postpartum infections is for hypovolemia, sepsis, and shock. Initial management should include a brief but thorough physical examination with attention to the abdomen, frequent review of vital signs, and aggressive fluid administration with an isotonic solution. The patient should be placed on a cardiac monitor and low-flow oxygen.

DIFFERENTIAL DIAGNOSIS

The differential diagnosis of the febrile postpartum or postoperative patient who complains of fever or other evidence of infection is listed in Table 57-27.[1,2] After a thorough history and physical examination including breast, perineum, and pelvic examination, laboratory studies should include a complete blood count, urinalysis, and possibly a chest x ray and flat plate radiograph. Strong consideration should be given to obtaining an ultrasound to look for retained products of conception and a pelvic mass or abscess.[2,3] If the urine is positive for red blood cells, without significant white blood cells, an intravenous pyelogram is also indicated to look for renal lithiasis and hydronephrosis. Many of the diagnoses on the list of differentials are discussed in other sections of this text. The following discussion is limited to the diagnoses unique to the postpartum patient: mastitis, endometritis, septic pelvic thrombosis, cellulitis of the perineal and pelvic floor, and parametritis. Other causes of fever are dealt with in the appropriate chapters.

TABLE 57-27. DIFFERENTIAL DIAGNOSIS OF ACUTE POSTPARTUM FEVER OR OTHER EVIDENCE OF INFECTION
Endometritis
Mastitis (epidemic or endemic)
Pneumonia
Pyelonephritis
Perineal cellulitis
Pelvic abscess/cellulitis
Retained products of conception
Septic pelvic thrombosis
Thrombophlebitis
Other wound infections

MASTITIS

Mastitis is found in 1 to 2% of postpartum women.[1] It has been identified as occurring in two forms. The first is an epidemic or nosocomial form, acquired from an infant whose nasopharynx has become colonized with Staphylococcus aureus. Infection of the deep glandular tissues and abscess formation are not uncommon. The nonepidemic or endemic form of the disease, unusual today, develops after sporadic nursing or when the infant is being weaned. The bacteria responsible for the infection include a variety of both aerobic and anaerobic organisms. S. aureus is found in 50% of the cases.[1] In the nonepidemic form of mastitis, the periglandular tissues become inflamed and a superficial cellulitis is often noted. Abscesses of the breast are rare in this form as compared to the epidemic form of the disease.

The diagnosis is most often clinical, based on symptoms of pain, fever, edema, local erythema, and purulent discharge. Examination of the breast milk often shows numerous polymorphic nucleocytes and gram-positive cocci. Breast milk may be cultured to help identify the offending organism. The emergency physician's responsibility lies in making the diagnosis, sending laboratory specimens for culture, and initiating appropriate antibiotics. The antibiotic coverage must reflect the fact that S. aureus is a common and virulent etiologic organism for this infection. Dicloxacillin and nafcillin are often the drugs of choice because the staphylococcus strain may be penicillinase-producing.[1] Parenteral treatment may be necessary. Other common therapies include warm moist packs to the breast and breast pumping or feeding. For abscesses, incision and drainage are commonly performed under general anesthesia.

ENDOMETRITIS

Endometritis is well known as the most identifiable cause of infectious morbidity in the postpartum patient. Patients who undergo cesarean section have a twentyfold greater risk of endometritis over those having vaginal delivery.[1] Studies show that from 20 to 50% of patients undergoing abdominal delivery may develop endometritis.[2] Risk factors include a classical uterine incision during cesarean section, increased blood loss during surgery, premature labor, premature rupture of membranes, frequent vaginal examinations during labor, low socioeconomic status, and the presence of chorioamnionitis before delivery.[1] Intrapartum bacteriuria is also associated with a high risk of endometritis.

PATHOPHYSIOLOGY

The pathophysiology of endometritis is thought to involve ascending cervicovaginal flora as a cause of infection. The difficult aspect of this disease is identification of the bacteriologic cause. The bacteria of the noninfected woman and the incidence of occurrence are noted[4] (Table 57-28). Because the common pathogens for endometritis are found within the vagina as normal flora, the prediction of a potential group of pathogens is not difficult[1] (Table 57-29). This finding also necessitates the use of a broader spectrum of antibiotics because specific bacterial identification requires culture results. Some of the more common anaerobic pathogens include peptococcus, peptostreptococcus, clostridium, and bacteroides species. Common aerobic pathogens include Neisseria gonorrhea, Escherichia coli, Klebseilla, and Gardnerella vaginalis.[5,6]

TABLE 57-28. MICROORGANISMS FOUND IN THE GENITOURINARY TRACT

Microorganism	Range of Incidence (Percent)
Kidneys and urinary bladder normally sterile	
Female and male urethra usually sterile except for short anterior segment.	
Vagina and uterine cervix	
Lactobacillus	50–75
Bacteroides	60–80
Clostridium	15–30
Peptostreptococcus	30–40
Bifidobacterium	10
Eubacterium	5
Aerobic corynebacteria (diphtheroids)	45–75
Staphylococcus aureus	5–15
Staphylococcus epidermidis	35–80
Enterococci (group D streptococcus)	30–80
Streptococcus pyogenes (usually group B)	5–20
Enterobacteriaceae	18–40
Moraxella osloensis	5–15
Acinetobacter	5–15
Candida albicans	30–50
Trichomonas vaginalis	10–25

Reprinted with permission from Sommers, H.M.: The indigenous microbiota of the human host. In The Biologic and Clinical Basis of Infectious Diseases. 3rd Ed. Edited by Youmans, G.P. Philadelphia, W.B. Saunders, 1985, pp. 76–78.

TABLE 57-29. POSTPARTUM INFECTION PATHOGENS

Aerobes
Gram-positive cocci:
Group A streptococcus (Streptococcus pyogenes)
Group B streptococcus (S. agalactiar)
Group D streptococcus (S. faecalis, S. bovis)*
Staphylococcus aureus (rare)
Gram-negative cocci:
Neisseria gonorrhea*
Gram-negative bacilli:
Gardnerella vaginalis*
Enterobacteriaceae (escherichia, klebsiella, enterobacter, proteus, and citrobacter)*

Anaerobes
Gram-positive cocci:
Peptococcus*
Peptostreptococcus*
Streptococcus (Streptococcus mutans, S. mitis)*
Gram-positive bacilli:
Clostridia species (Clostridia perfringens)*
Listeria monocytogenes (rare)
Gram-negative bacilli:
Bacteroides (Bacteroides bivius, B. fragilis)*

Miscellaneous
Chlamydia, trachomatous

* Indicates common postpartum pathogen

CLINICAL PRESENTATION

The signs and symptoms of puerperal morbidity (endometritis) as outlined by the United States Joint Committee on Maternal Welfare are abdominal pain, fever, and an odorous discharge. The temperature must be 100.4° F or higher on 2 consecutive days within the first 10 postpartum, exclusive of the first 24 hours. A temperature of 100.4° F or greater within the first 24 hours may signify a more serious and virulent infection, possibly streptococcus.[6]

On physical examination, uterine tenderness in association with a foul-smelling lochia and fever may be the only presenting symptoms. Other symptoms that can be associated with endometritis include malaise, nausea, and vomiting. The laboratory evaluation of these patients must include cultures of blood, urine, and cervical secretions. The latter should include aerobic, anaerobic, gonococcal, and chlamydial studies.

TREATMENT

The current recommendations for treatment include intravenous fluids, antipyretics, and high-dose penicillin (10 to 20 million units per day) or ampicillin 8 to 12 g per day.[1,7] If a dramatic defervescence does not occur within 24 to 48 hours or the patient has a more toxic presentation, a regimen of clindamycin (900 mg per day) and an aminoglycoside or piperacillin (3 g every 6 hours) and an aminoglycoside (gentamicin 1.0 to 1.5 mg per kg every 8 hours) may be used.[5,7,8] If the patient fails to improve after an additional 48 hours, strong consideration should be given to the presence of a pelvic mass or septic pelvic thrombosis and a repeat examination and computed tomographic (CT) scan are in order.[1,9]

PROPHYLAXIS

Antibiotic therapy is prudent in all patients in labor who have a fever, particularly those who belong to the high-risk category for endometritis (premature labor, abdominal surgery during labor, premature rupture of membranes, and cesarean section). These patients should receive prophylactic parenteral antibiotics before or up to 1 hour after delivery.[1]

SEPTIC PELVIC THROMBOSIS

Another clinical syndrome that occurs in the febrile postpartum patient is septic pelvic thrombosis (SPT). This disease may be seen in the immediate postpartum period. It is an uncommon complication of pregnancy affecting 1 out of 2000 deliveries and 1 to 2% of patients with postpartum endometritis. Although it is rare, septic pelvic thrombosis is increasing in incidence as the cesarean section rate rises.[1,3]

PATHOPHYSIOLOGY

Numerous factors make pregnant and postpartum women at a greater risk for this disease. First, the pregnant woman is known to be hypercoagulable secondary to increased level of clotting factors. Second, the pelvic veins are sensitive to estrogen and demonstrate changes that increase their chances for injury. Lastly, the pregnant or postpartum woman is noted to have a relative venous stasis in the pelvic veins which causes increased venous capacity and decreased blood flow.[1]

CLINICAL PRESENTATION

The patient presents with a fever, tachycardia out of proportion to the fever, and possibly a palpable pelvic vein on pelvic examination. Occasionally the patient with septic pelvic thrombosis presents with respiratory complaints of dyspnea, tachypnea, and pleuritic chest discomfort from the occurrence of pulmonary embolus. In the patient with suspected postpartum endometritis, a persistent fever after treatment with appropriate antibiotics should suggest the presence of a septic pelvic thrombosis. The diagnosis is made by pelvic venography and abdominal/pelvic CT scan. If pulmonary involvement is a consideration, blood gas analysis, chest x ray, electrocardiogram, and ventilation perfusion lung scan are in order.[1]

TREATMENT

The therapy for septic pelvic thrombosis is heparin. In this disease, heparin is both diagnostic and therapeutic. The fever should decrease within 24 to 48 hours. Heparin is most often given concomitantly with antibiotics for a 7- to 10-day period. If the fever and abdominal symptoms do not improve after a 36- to 48-hour trial of heparin and antibiotic therapy, pelvic and abdominal CT scan should be performed to look for surgical pathology such as a pelvic abscess.[9]

CELLULITIS OF THE PERINEUM AND PELVIC FLOOR

Postpartum vaginal secretions can contain between 10^8 and 10^9 organisms per gram of fluid.[1] It is remarkable that only 1% of patients who have episiotomies, vaginal lacerations, and paracervical or pudendal blocks end up with an infection related to these procedures. In general, the etiologic organisms are staphylococcus, streptococcus, and gram-negative organisms such as the bacteroides species.[1] The diagnosis is made after the patient complains of persistent perineal discomfort, occasional worsening of her vaginal discharge, and fever. The patient is found to have erythema, edema, and occasionally a tender mass on physical examination. The treatment for local cellulitis wound consists of a penicillinase-resistant penicillin, or a first- or second-generation cephalosporin. If an abscess is identified, surgical drainage is the definitive treatment.

PARAMETRITIS

Parametritis, also termed pelvic cellulitis, is commonly suspected after the patient has failed to respond to adequate antibiotic therapy in 48 to 72 hours. This uncommon diagnosis is rarely made in the ED. Repeat examination may reveal continued tenderness in the lower abdominal and pelvic regions. The patient has a persistent fever of 100° F or higher in the absence of another source of infection.[6] Ultrasonography and computerized tomography are rarely useful, but occasionally they identify a localization of fluid that would require surgical drainage. The pathophysiology is an extension of a puerperal infection in which the bacteria enter the parametrial tissue by direct extension, by means of lymphatic spread, or across the wall of an infected vein of thrombophlebitis. The common pathogens are similar to those found in endometritis. The therapy for pelvic cellulitis includes prolonged intravenous antibiotics, repeated examinations to rule out surgical pathology, and repeated cultures to look for resistant organisms. Heparin therapy is a consideration for septic pelvic thrombosis.[9] Long-term complications of this disorder include extensive scarring throughout the affected tissues.

CONCLUSION

All sources of infection must be considered: water, wind, wounds, and walking. Often the source may be a superficial cellulitis such as endemic mastitis or cellulitis of the episiotomy, or even Candida. The emergency physician must realize that he or she may see deep tissue and more complex infections such as epidemic mastitis, endometritis, or pelvic cellulitis. Patients require hospitalization, intravenous antibiotics, and occasionally surgical exploration or drainage. The treatment regimens reflect the severity of the infection. If the patient does not respond to appropriate antibiotic therapy or presents with pulmonary symptoms in the absence of pneumonia, the diagnosis of septic thrombosis should be considered. Heparin in this case is both diagnostic and therapeutic. If the patient does not respond to antibiotics and heparin, a CT scan should be performed to rule out other pelvic pathology such as pelvic abscess.

REFERENCES

1. Isada, N.B., and Grossman, J.H.: Perinatal infections. *In* Obstetrics: Normal and Problem Pregnancies. New York, Churchill Livingstone, 1986, pp. 979–1047.
2. Sweet, R.L., et al.: Appropriate use of antibiotics in serious obstetric and gynecologic infections. Am. J. Obstet. Gynecol. *146*:719, 1983.
3. Lee, C.Y., Madrazo, B.L., Parks, S., and Sandler, M.: Ultrasonic evaluation in the management of postpartum infection. Henry Ford Hosp. Med. J. *35*:58, 1987.
4. Sommers, H.M.: The indigenous microbiota of the human host. *In* The Biologic and Clinical Basis of Infectious Diseases. 3rd Ed. Edited by Youmans, G.P., Philadelphia, W.B. Saunders Co., 1985, pp. 76–78.
5. Gunning, J.E.: A comparison of piperacillin and clindamycin plus gentamycin in women with pelvic infections. Surg. Gynecol. Obstet. *163*:1, 1986.
6. Pritchard, J.A., MacDonald, P.C., and Gant, N.F.: Williams Obstetrics. 17th Ed. Appleton Century Crofts, 1985, pp. 719–726.
7. Landers, D.V., Green, J.R., and Sweet, R.L.: Antibiotic use during pregnancy and the postpartum period. Clin. Obstet. Gynecol. *26*:391, 1983.
8. Yonekura, M.L.: The treatment of endomyometritis. J. Reprod. Med. *33*:579, 1988.
9. Gibbs, R.S.: Postpartum infection. *In* Current Therapy in Obstetrics. Edited by Charles, D. Philadelphia, B.C. Decker, Inc., 1988, pp. 184–189.

APPENDIX 57A.   DIFFERENTIAL DIAGNOSIS OF PRE-ECLAMPSIA

The differential diagnosis of pre-eclampsia includes:

1. Chronic hypertension
2. Gestational and dependent edema
3. Renal disease including the many types of glomerulonephritis, nephrotic syndrome, and chronic renal disease.

In addition, pre-eclampsia/eclampsia may mimic or be confused with other disorders, including:

1. Ocular disorders such as retinal detachment and hemorrhage
2. Abdominal conditions such as appendicitis, cholelithiasis, hepatitis, and pancreatitis
3. Central nervous system disorders such as stroke, TIA, cerebritis, and epilepsy
4. Multisystem, immunologic or hematologic disorders such as systemic lupus erythematosus (SLE), idiopathic thrombocytopenic purpura (ITP), thrombotic thrombocytopenic purpura (TTP), and disseminated intravascular coagulation (DIC).

In the acute setting, diagnosis may depend largely on history, and in the presence of elevated blood pressure, treatment of pre-eclampsia should be instituted along with hospitalization to the obstetric service with appropriate other consultations as indicated.

Chapter 58

GYNECOLOGIC EMERGENCIES

VAGINAL INFECTIONS

Christopher K. Wuerker and Joseph C. Howton

CAPSULE

Vaginitis is a common Emergency Department (ED) complaint in which 90% of cases are caused by Candida albicans, Gardnerella vaginalis (bacterial vaginosis), or Trichomonas vaginalis. Vaginal discharges with pH >4.5 can be treated with metronidazole. The thick white discharge of candidiasis, along with any vulvocutaneous involvement is treated with an imidazole cream. Recurrent infection is usually caused by reinfection by sexual partners or underlying disease. Wet preparation of vaginal secretions, revealing large amounts of white cells, requires investigation for cervicitis and pelvic inflammatory disease (PID). Vulvovaginal abscess is usually caused by polymicrobial infection and obstruction of Bartholin's gland. Treatment is incision and drainage with placement of a drain. See Table 58-1 for characteristics of common vaginitides.

INFECTIOUS CAUSES OF VAGINITIS

BACTERIAL

Bacterial vaginosis (also called Gardnerella vaginitis) is a shift in the normal vaginal flora from lactobacilli toward anaerobes, including Gardnerella, Bacteroides, and Mobiluncus. Gardnerella vaginalis is probably a normal occupant because it is found in up to 70% of healthy, asymptomatic women.[1] Although Gardnerella is found in all cases of bacterial vaginosis by definition, the clinical syndrome probably requires coinfection with other organisms, which disrupts the normal vaginal flora.[1]

Bacterial vaginosis presents with increased gray or yellow foul or fishy-smelling vaginal discharge. Itch and vulvar irritation are minimal. On examination, the characteristic discharge and odor are noted, although the cervix and vaginal mucosa appear normal. pH testing of the discharge reveals a relative alkaline environment caused by the lack of lactobacilli.

Diagnosis using the method of Amsel et al. requires three of the following four criteria: (1) characteristic discharge, (2) positive sniff test, (3) pH > 4.5, and (4) clue cells on wet mount.[2] Clue cells are stippled-appearing epithelial cells seen on wet-mount preparation of vaginal secretions. The granular bodies of clue cells are believed to be caused by adherent Gardnerella and other organisms attached to the external cell wall. Although they were once thought pathognomonic, clue cells may be seen in normal secretions. The sniff test (amine test) refers to release of a fishy odor when 10% or 20% KOH is added to vaginal secretions, although the odor is detected during the pelvic examination in most cases.

The treatment of choice is metronidazole in either a 2 g dose repeated once in 48 hours or 500 mg twice daily for 7 days.[3] In pregnant or metronidazole sensitive patients, clindamycin 300 mg three times a day or ampicillin 500 mg four times daily for 7 days is a less effective alternative.

In cases of relapse, evaluate for underlying disease, use of a broad spectrum antibiotic, coinfection with Candida albicans, and possible inoculation of Gardnerella by an asymptomatic male partner.

FUNGAL

Candida vulvovaginitis (monilia) is a fungal infection most commonly due to Candida albicans. Candida is

			Wet Slide					
	Pruritus	Discharge Quantity	Color	Viscosity	Odor	pH	NS	KOH
Bacterial vaginosis	Mild	Small	Gray or yellow	Thin	Fishy	>4.5	Clue cells	+ Sniff
Candidal vaginitis	Moderate	Small	White	Thick	None	<4.5		Hyphae
Trichomonal vaginitis	Severe	Large	Gray or yellow/green	Thin	None or fishy	> or <4.5	Trichomonads	
Normal vaginal discharge	None	Variable	Clear or white	Thick	None	<4.5		

a ubiquitous organism; vaginitis is caused by overgrowth of the yeast in an altered host environment from antibiotics, diabetes, or immunoincompetence (AIDS, cancer, chemotherapy, corticosteroids, and pregnancy).

Women complain of an itchy, thick, white vaginal discharge. Vulvar involvement causes burning irritation, external dysuria, and dyspareunia. On examination, the vaginal mucosa appears erythematous with adherent white fungal plaques and occasional fissures in addition to the characteristic discharge. Vulvar-cutaneous candidiasis appears as geographic erythema with satellite lesions. Although hyphae are classically seen on KOH wet preparation of vaginal secretion (one to two drops 10%/20% KOH), diagnosis should be made on the clinical picture because KOH preparations are falsely negative in up to 50% of cases.[4]

Treatment of choice is topical application of one of the imidazole creams (clotrimazole, miconazole, butoconazole, or terconazole). Current dosage options for clotrimazole are 100 mg vaginally for seven days, 200 mg for three days, and 500 mg once. Creams have the advantage of also being applied externally for vulvar involvement. Less effective alternatives include nystatin or boric acid capsules.

Recurrent infections are common and frequently frustrating, especially in patients with diabetes or impaired cell-mediated immunity. Treatment strategies include prolonged treatment for two to three weeks, treatment of sex partners (check for balanitis), and chronic suppressive treatment using an imidazole daily or for the 5 days before menses. Oral ketoconazole has been effective for suppressive treatment.[5] Attempts at eradicating Candida from the GI tract using oral nystatin have not proven effective.

PROTOZOAN

TRICHOMONAS VAGINALIS

Trichomonas vaginalis is a sexually transmitted protozoan that infects the vagina and lower urinary tract.

Women complain of a gray or yellow/green discharge (classically frothy but commonly not), and odor is minimal. Pruritus is usually severe and associated with vulvar irritation and dysuria. Trichomonas, however, may be asymptomatic in up to 50% of cases.[6]

On examination, the characteristic discharge is noted, along with mild vaginal erythema. A brightly erythematous "strawberry lesion" of the cervix is pathognomonic but rare. Ph of vaginal secretions may be normal (<4.5) or elevated. Sniff testing with KOH may be positive. Microscopic evaluations of normal saline wet preparations of vaginal secretions reveal trichomonads in 60% of cases when compared to culture and monoclonal antibody tests.[7] Detecting trichomonas on wet saline preparations can be optimized by promptly adding the saline and examining the slide before evaporation produces a hypertonic solution. Such a solution may kill the organisms, making their identification difficult. Although future testing by ELISA may become commonplace, current diagnosis is based on the clinical picture.

The treatment of choice is a 2 g dose of metronidazole for both the patient and sex partner(s).[8] Alternative dosage is 500 mg twice daily for 7 days. A less effective therapy for pregnancy is hypertonic 20% saline douches. Topical clotrimazole may offer some relief of symptoms, but is not therapeutic. Treatment failure is usually caused by reinfection by a sex partner or occasionally by resistant organisms requiring high dose and prolonged treatment with metronidazole.

PINWORM

Rare cases of vaginitis due to Enterobius vermicularis (pinworm) have been found in both adults and children with intestinal involvement. Patients complain of vaginal and perianal pruritus along with vaginal discharge. Diagnosis is by the "scotch tape" test treated with pyrantel or mebendazole.

VAGINITIS FROM NONINFECTIOUS CAUSES

ATROPHIC VAGINITIS

Atrophic vaginitis presents with burning irritation, mild itch, and dyspareunia in postmenopausal women. It is believed to be caused by loss of estrogen-dependent glycogen from the vaginal mucosal cells. On speculum examination, the mucosa appears dry and erythematous. Treatment is by restoration of estrogens, which is best achieved acutely by topical application of estrogen cream.

FOREIGN BODY VAGINITIS

Most commonly caused by lost tampons, foreign body vaginitis presents with foul-smelling yellow discharge and occasionally discomfort. Toilet paper is a common cause in children. The cause is obvious on speculum examination. In addition to removal of the offending body, douching with dilute vinegar and water or betadine may be beneficial in copious discharge.

CHEMICAL VAGINITIS

Chemical vaginitis is an uncommon cause of vaginal itching and discomfort, associated with mucosal irritation from disinfectants, deodorants, fragrances, and cosmetics. Women complain of vulvar tenderness, vaginal itch, and serous discharge. The diagnosis is made by history and resolution after discontinuation of the offending agent.

ALLERGIC VAGINITIS

Allergic vaginitis has been described, caused by sensitivity to topical medication, douches, and rarely spermatozoa.

VULVOVAGINAL CELLULITIS AND ABSCESS

Cellulitis is most commonly caused by infection of Bartholin's gland, located just lateral to the posterior vaginal fourchette. Infection is usually polymicrobial, including normal vaginal and gastrointestinal flora, but may be caused by Neisseria gonorrhoeae and Chlamydia trachomatis.[9] Cellulitis rapidly proceeds to abscess formation. Women complain of severe localized vulvar pain and tenderness that usually interfere with ambulation. On examination, unilateral vulvar edema and erythema are obvious, along with a palpable, tender, fluctuant mass adjacent to the posterior introitus. ED management is incision and drainage with placement of a drain. The abscess should be incised over the mucosal (medial) aspect lateral to the hymenal ring over the point of maximal fluctuance. A Ward catheter (5 cm, 10 French latex drain with 5 cc balloon tip) placed within the cavity and filled with water may be left in place for 2 to 3 weeks for fistualization. Appropriate antibiotic coverage is indicated for cellulitis or other concurrent pelvic infection. Patients should be instructed to take sitz baths until symptoms resolve. Specimens from either the abscess or the cervix should be cultured for gonorrhea and Chlamydia. Sequelae include recurrent abscess formation, cyst formation, and rarely necrotizing fascitis. Recurrent Bartholin's abscess requires referral for marsupialization.

Skene's periurethral glands may become infected and present with anterior vulvar cellulitis and abscess. Management should be referred to a gynecologist. Simple cutaneous abscesses are common in the perineal area and, if superficial, may be managed with incision, drainage, and packing. Abscesses posterior to Bartholin's glands are perianal, require a rectal examination and should be referred to a surgeon.

MEDICOLEGAL PEARLS

- Always investigate for pregnancy.
- Assess your responsibility for sequelae when writing a prescription for your patient's sex partner(s).
- Warn patents of metronidazole's interaction with alcohol.
- Patients with recurrence of symptoms need a complete re-evaluation; concurrent infections are common, and initial therapy may eradicate only one of the pathogens.
- Recurrent candidiasis requires an investigation for underlying disease.
- Consider empiric treatment when suspicious of gonorrhea or chlamydia infection in areas with high incidence of sexually transmitted diseases and poor patient follow-up, especially in the setting of trichomonas or Bartholin's abscess.

REFERENCES

1. Holmes, K.K.: Lower genital tract infections in women: Cystitis/urethritis, vulvovaginitis, and cervicitis. Sexually Transmitted Diseases. In Holmes, K.K., Mardh, P.A., Sparling, P.F., et al. New York, McGraw-Hill, 1984, pp. 557–575.
2. Amsel, R., et al.: Nonspecific vaginitis, diagnostic criteria and microbial and epidemiologic associations. Am. J. Med. 74:14, 1983.

3. Hovik, P.: Comparison of three dose regimens of metronidazole. Scand. J. Infect. Dis. *40:*107, 1983.
4. Rothenburg, R.B., et al.: Efficacy of selected diagnostic tests for sexually transmitted diseases. JAMA *253:*49, 1976.
5. Sobel, J.D.: Recurrent vulvovaginal candidiasis, a prospective study of the efficacy of maintenance ketoconazole therapy. N. Engl. J. Med. *315:*1455, 1986.
6. Rein, M.F., and Muller, M.: Trichomonas vaginalis. *In* Sexually Transmitted Diseases. Edited by Homes, K.K., Mardh, P.A., Sparling, P.F., et al. New York, McGraw-Hill, 1984, pp. 525–536.
7. Kreiger, J.N., et al.: Diagnosis of trichomoniasis, comparison of conventional wet-mount examination with cytologic studies, cultures, and monoclonal antibody staining of direct specimens. JAMA *259:*1223, 1988.
8. Hager, W.D., et al.: Metronidazole for vaginal trichomoniasis, seven-day vs single-dose regimens. JAMA *244:*1219, 1980.
9. Bleker, O.P., Smalbroak, D.S., and Schulte, M.F.: Bartholin's abscess, the role of Chlamydia trachomatis. Genitourin. Med. *66:*24, 1990.

MENSTRUAL DISORDERS

Arthur Shapiro

CAPSULE

Gynecologic complaints related to vaginal bleeding or menses are common in any Emergency Department. This chapter reviews menstrual disorders in the nonpregnant patient, including dysfunctional uterine bleeding, amenorrhea, dysmenorrhea, oligomenorrhea, and premenstrual syndrome.

INTRODUCTION

One of the most common reasons why a woman presents to the Emergency Department (ED) is vaginal bleeding. Obviously, it is most important to rule out intra- or extrauterine pregnancy. Because these latter problems are discussed elsewhere, we deal only with the nonpregnant patient in this chapter.

DYSFUNCTIONAL UTERINE BLEEDING

Abnormal bleeding that occurs in a nonpregnant woman is referred to as **dysfunctional uterine bleeding (DUB).** It can be defined as abnormal bleeding—irregular, excessive, scant or prolonged—in the absence of neoplasia, infection, pregnancy, trauma, blood dyscrasia, or exogenous hormone administration. Other terms that have been used such as **menorrhagia** (heavy menstrual flow) or **metrorrhagia** (ir-

regular flow other than at the time of the expected period) can be used to better describe the pattern of bleeding; the bleeding pattern itself also may suggest a cause and treatment for the problem.

The normal frequency of menstrual periods is generally between 26 and 35 days with a mean of about 28 days; the flow is present for 3 to 7 days. The amount of blood loss is 20 to 80 mL (mean, 40 mL).[1] Dysfunctional uterine bleeding can be classified into two types: ovulatory (10%) and anovulatory (90%) (Table 58-2).

One pattern of **ovulatory** DUB is characterized by midcycle staining and is caused by a greater-than-usual drop of estrogen levels at the time of ovulation. Another type of ovulatory DUB is polymenorrhea, defined as frequent, regular bleeding at intervals of 18 to 25 days; this may be caused by either a short proliferative or secretory phase of the cycle. Lastly, a bleeding pattern in ovulatory DUB may be characterized as oligomenorrhea (that is, infrequent, irregular bleeding at intervals longer than 36 to 45 days). In general, this pattern is caused by prolongation of the proliferative phase of the cycle.

Corpus luteum insufficiency, also known as inadequate luteal phase, is a progesterone deficiency

TABLE 58-2. CLASSIFICATION OF DYSFUNCTIONAL UTERINE BLEEDING

Ovulatory (10% incidence)
Mid-cycle bleeding
Short cycle
(shortened proliferative phase)
Oligo-ovulation
Corpus luteum insufficiency
Prolonged corpus luteum
(Halban's syndrome)
Anovulatory (90% incidence)

state. Corpus luteum insufficiency can be characterized by premenstrual spotting, menorrhagia (regular uterine bleeding with excessive amount of flow at the time of the period), or polymenorrhea, in which there is regular bleeding at intervals of less than 25 days associated with infertility and early abortions.

Prolonged corpus luteum, called Halban's syndrome, is characterized by intervals of oligomenorrhea with cycles longer than 36 to 45 days, caused by the persistence of a corpus luteum with irregular endometrial shedding. It is easily diagnosed by showing the presence of progesterone in the absence of beta-hCG levels. These patients can also present with heavy menstrual periods at regular intervals.

The most common type of dysfunctional uterine bleeding is anovulatory, caused by persistent "unopposed" estrogen levels (absence of progesterone) as opposed to the ovulatory type, which is associated with abnormal estrogen or progesterone secretion. **Anovulatory dysfunctional uterine bleeding** can present as either oligomenorrhea with an interval greater than 36 to 45 days in **menorrhagia** (heavy menstrual flow) or metrorrhagia (irregular but not excessive flow). A combination of these, which has been referred to as menometrorrhagia, refers to frequent, irregular, excessive, and prolonged periods of uterine bleeding. During the proliferative phases of the cycle, the endometrium grows in response to estrogen stimulation. This steroid also can cause increased intrauterine blood flow and vasodilation. If ovulation and corpus luteum formation fail, the ovary then continues to produce mostly estrogen, and the endometrium continues to grow and progress from a proliferative to a more hyperplastic pattern. The endometrium then either outgrows its blood supply, in which case the bleeding is classified as **breakthrough** of the endometrium. In addition, the unopposed estrogen may cause a negative feedback on the pituitary gland, decreasing the gonadotropin levels, which in turn lowers estrogen secretion. The resultant bleeding is caused by a withdrawal of the estrogen stimulation, with the surface of the endometrium sloughing irregularly and producing heavy, painless, **withdrawal** bleeding.

Although sporadic anovulatory bleeding is common in normal women, it tends to be rather frequent, if not physiologic, during the first few years after menarche and during the 2 to 3 years before menopause. Therefore, although a woman may present with a heavy menstrual flow at virtually any time during her reproductive life, the problem is more prominent and characteristic of the perimenarcheal and perimenopausal phases.

To diagnose and treat DUB, it is important to take a careful menstrual history of the patient and determine if her bleeding is acute or a chronic symptom of a long-standing problem. Obviously, the first responsibility should always be to rule out a pregnancy by using a rapid beta-hCG assay. Next, the physician must exclude organic disease, especially malignant neoplasm. The greater the patient's age, i.e., age 40

or over, the more likely is the possibility of the latter. Therefore, by the time a patient is menopausal, the presence of postmenopausal bleeding carries a 5% risk of a uterine cancer.

Other laboratory data that should be obtained are complete blood count, platelets, bleeding time, prothrombin time, and partial thromboplastin time to rule out a blood dyscrasia. If the patient is presenting with chronic menstrual irregularity, thyroid (thyroid stimulating hormone, T4, and T3 uptake) and prolactin studies should be done. The vagina and cervix should be carefully inspected to make sure that the source of the bleeding is in fact intrauterine, and a careful pelvic examination should be done to exclude any associated pathology such as fibroids or adnexal masses. Endometrial biopsy to diagnose the type of endometrium is especially important when considering which type of therapeutic modality will best suit the patient, and the patient should be referred for obstetric/gynecologic consultation.

TREATMENT

Usually, if a patient presents to the ED because of vaginal bleeding, the bleeding is likely to be of a profuse nature. The patient may actually be hemorrhaging and require emergency curettage. A simple guideline to determine if a patient requires a curettage is as follows: (1) profuse bleeding or associated severe anemia (hemoglobin of 8 g or less) is present; (2) the patient is over 35 to 40; and (3) the patient has not responded to previous hormonal therapy.

A nonemergent patient who requires dilation and curettage (D&C) may first undergo a simple office suction curettage under paracervical anesthesia. A suction-type curettage, such as vabra aspiration, compares favorably with the conventional D&C in accuracy of tissue diagnosis and has the advantage of being low-risk and cost-effective.[3] If the response to therapy is not as expected, tissue sampling by conventional D&C should be considered, with direct visualization of the endometrium by hysteroscopy so that lesions such as polyps, retained placenta, submucous myomas, or cancer can be localized and directly biopsied.

In patients under 35, particularly postmenarcheal teenage girls, an attempt can be made to stop the bleeding by use of intravenous conjugated estrogen in doses of 20 mg every 3 to 4 hours, repeated 2 to 3 times. If the bleeding abates, the patient can be discharged from the ED on oral estrogen, 2.5 to 10 mg of conjugated estrogens daily for 2 to 3 weeks, adding an oral progestin, Provera, for the last 12 days of the estrogen therapy. Progestagens have an antiestrogen effect, and the estrogen-stimulated endometrium requires a prolonged exposure of 10 to 13 days per month to effectively prevent the overgrowth of the endometrial tissue. Chronically anovulatory patients can be managed with cyclical progesterone therapy to prevent the endometrium from becoming hyperplastic. In fact, the cyclic use of progestagens can prevent patients from requiring repetitive D&Cs or hysterectomy. Therefore, if the patient is less than 35 to 40 and not hemorrhaging, consideration can be given to progestogen therapy alone (medroxy/progesterone acetate: Provera; norethenodrone acetate: Norlutate, or Aygestin). The medication should be given as 10 mg of Provera or 5 mg of Norlutate/Aygestin, 1 to 3 times daily each month for 10 to 12 days. Because of previous blood loss, iron therapy should also be instituted. An alternative to the oral estrogen/progesterone regimen is the progestin-dominant oral contraceptive (for example, Loestrin or LoOvral), using 2 to 4 pills per day for 7 to 21 days.[4] The patient who has a chronic problem of anovulatory dysfunctional uterine bleeding is discussed in the section on oligomenorrhea.

Patients should not be given oral contraceptives if they smoke and are over 30. These contraceptives are best avoided in any woman over 40. This is because of the increased risk of myocardial infarction and thrombovascular disease associated with oral contraceptive use in these patients. In addition, birth control pills can cause or exacerbate DUB, and patients frequently present with dysfunctional uterine bleeding secondary to use of these pills.

Lastly, a word should be said about endometrial ablation. As first reported by Goldrath,[5] the yttrium aluminum garnet (YAG) laser is used to agglutinate the endometrium and create an iatrogenic Asherman's syndrome (that is, intrauterine adhesions and amenorrhea). It is indicated only in patients who are no longer interested in fertility and who have dysfunctional uterine bleeding unresponsive to both hormonal therapy and curettage with no organic pathology. It is done by hysteroscopic visualization and, using a quartz fiber and the YAG laser, the endometrial tissue is agglutinated and heals as a fibrotic scar.

AMENORRHEA/OLIGOMENORRHEA

A woman may present to the ED complaining of the absence of menstruation, with or without associated infrequent vaginal bleeding. Once pregnancy is ruled out, the differential diagnosis of amenorrhea and oligomenorrhea is made as outlined in Figure 58-1. The baseline hormonal blood tests that should be obtained are: luteinizing hormone (LH) follicle-stimulating hormone (FSH), and thyroid-stimulating hormone (TSH); radioimmunoassay prolactin; T4 and T3 resin uptake; and a rapid beta-hCG assay. An intramuscular shot of progesterone in oil, 100 mg, can then be given to the patient, with instructions to see a gynecologist and to report whether or not withdrawal bleeding occurs. If it does occur, endogenous estrogen is present because progesterone has no effect on an unstimulated

endometrium. The work-up is done to rule out thyroid disease, pituitary adenoma, and polycystic ovarian syndrome. Patients who do not demonstrate withdrawal bleeding on intramuscular progesterone are given estrogen to induce a proliferative endometrium. If they still do not bleed, a diagnosis of endometrial failure is made. Asherman's syndrome (intrauterine adhesions) can be confirmed by hysterosalpingogram and/or hysteroscopy. This problem can occur after a D&C for an incomplete abortion or for retained placental tissue. Elevated FSH in the menopausal range confirms primary ovarian failure as in premature menopause. Patients with low to normal gonadotropins in association with elevated prolactin levels must have a pituitary computerized tomographic (CT) scan to rule out a prolactin-producing pituitary adenoma. Bromocriptine is effective in reducing prolactin levels and shrinking pituitary prolactinomas and in re-establishing normal ovulatory cycles. Cases of hyperprolactinemia secondary to primary hypothyroidism can be easily diagnosed by elevated TSH levels.

Most patients with chronic anovulatory bleeding patterns or amenorrhea can be classified as chronic anovulators and should be treated with replacement progestogen therapy on a cyclic basis (that is, Provera, 10 mg, 10 to 12 days per month). If the patient is interested in fertility, clomiphene citrate can be used to induce ovulation. In addition, pergonal, human menopausal gonadotropin, or purified FSH (Metrodin) can also be used to induce ovulation. The use of birth control pills is generally superfluous; in these anovulatory patients, birth control pills can cause such problems as postpill amenorrhea. These patients are best treated with barrier contraceptive methods along with concomitant cyclic progestagen therapy.

DYSMENORRHEA

A common reason for a woman presenting to the ED is pain associated with menstruation (dysmenorrhea), classified as primary or secondary. Primary dysmenorrhea is that occurring in patients with no identifiable pelvic pathology. Secondary dysmenorrhea occurs in patients with clearly associated pelvic pathology. More than 50% of menstruating women are affected by primary dysmenorrhea, and 10% have episodes severe enough to incapacitate them for 1 to 3 days each month.

PRIMARY

Primary dysmenorrhea is characterized by ovulatory cycles in which the pain begins hours before or after the onset of menstruation. It is located in the lower midabdomen and may spread across the lower abdomen

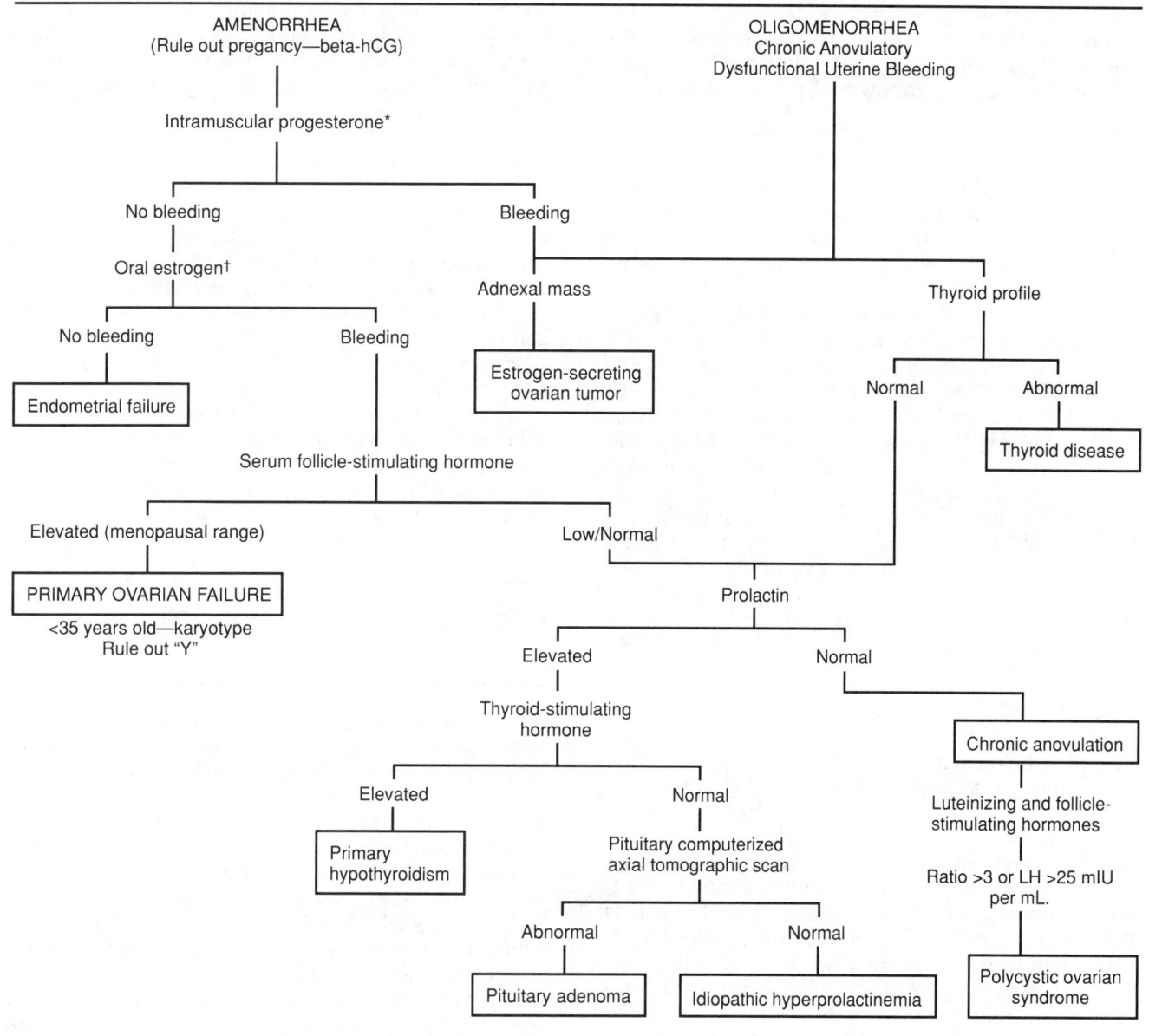

FIG. 58-1.   *Differential diagnosis of amenorrhea and oligomenorrhea. With permission from Emerg. Clin. North Am. 5:563, 1987.*

*100 mg progesterone in oil intramuscularly.
†2.5 mg conjugated estrogen daily for 7 to 14 days.

or radiate to the lower back and inner and/or anterior aspects of the thighs. It can be associated with gastrointestinal symptoms such as diarrhea, nausea, and vomiting as well as other associated symptoms such as headache, dizziness, and fainting spells. It may last for only a few hours to not more than 2 to 3 days during menstruation. The diagnosis of primary dysmenorrhea is made only after organic causes of pelvic pain are ruled out. It is usually associated with a history of dysmenorrhea dating back to menarche or shortly thereafter. Primary dysmenorrhea has been attributed to various factors. Recent evidence, however, has clearly shown that patients with severe dys-

menorrhea have an increased production and release of endometrial prostaglandins (PGs).[6] These higher levels of PG cause increased uterine activity and severe uterine cramping secondary to myometrial hypoxia and ischemia. The higher-than-normal levels of PGs also explain the associated gastrointestinal symptoms of nausea, vomiting, and diarrhea. Evidence that prostaglandins are involved in the pathogenesis of primary dysmenorrhea can be summarized as follows: (1) exogenous prostaglandins can reproduce the pain of dysmenorrhea; (2) late secretory endometrium has high concentrations of prostaglandins; (3) significantly higher levels of prostaglandins are noted in patients with primary dysmenorrhea; and (4) prostaglandin synthetase inhibitors (PGSIs) and nonsteroidal anti-inflammatory drugs (NSAIDs) have been shown effective in controlling the pain of primary dysmenorrhea.

Many PSGIs are available, and certainly, in many cases, one type may be more effective than another in an individual patient. If the patient does not respond to a change in the PGSI treatment, however, laparoscopy is definitely indicated to rule out pelvic pathology such as endometriosis or pelvic inflammatory disease (PID).

Another form of treatment for primary dysmenorrhea, especially if the patient desires effective contraception, is the use of birth control pills. In general, 65% of patients with primary dysmenorrhea may obtain relief with oral contraceptives, and in cases in which relief is only partial, PGSIs can be added at the time of menstruation. Other forms of therapy that have been advocated are cervical dilation or disruption of the nerve fibers to the uterus, such as is done with the presacral neurectomy. One technique, reported by Daniell and Feste, is the use of the CO_2 laser laparoscope to vaporize the uterosacral ligaments in the hope of disconnecting the nerve fibers that pass through these ligaments on the way to the uterus.[7]

SECONDARY

Patients who present to the ED with severe pelvic pain at the time of menstruation and state that this is a relatively new symptom are likely to have secondary dysmenorrhea. These patients should be evaluated for possible pelvic infection with gonococcal and chlamydia cultures of the cervix, complete blood count, and sedimentation rate. Because treatment of PID is discussed in another chapter, it is not reviewed here. PID without fever, elevated white blood cell count, and sedimentation rate, however, is difficult to differentiate from endometriosis. Both are associated with adnexal tenderness, cyclic pelvic pain, and adnexal masses. Ultrasound may be of some diagnostic help, but laparoscopic examination of the pelvis is more definitive and allows proper diagnosis and appropriate therapy.

ENDOMETRIOSIS

Pain associated with endometrioisis may be caused by the ectopic endometrial tissues of endometriosis producing higher amounts of prostaglandins than normal endometrium. This has not been substantiated, however, and the exact connection between endometriosis, dysmenorrhea, and pelvic pain is not clearly understood. The PGSIs are generally less effective in controlling the pain of endometriosis, and to establish clearly the diagnosis of endometriosis, a laparoscopy should be performed. With the use of laparoscopic laser techniques, endometriotic implants and associated adhesions can be vaporized and may not require an extensive laparotomy. In addition, Danazol has been shown effective in suppressing ovarian function and ovulation, usually producing an amenorrheic state. Along with its biologic property of being a weak androgen, Danazol has been successful in controlling the symptoms of endometriosis and for the regression of endometriotic implants. The new GnRH analogues[1] may be an alternative to Danazol therapy because they can virtually shut off all ovarian function, thereby relieving the patient of the cyclic pain associated with endometriosis. One such drug for treating prostatic cancer is leuprolid acetate (Lupron), an analogue of gonadotropin-releasing hormone with a more prolonged and potent action that suppresses pituitary gonadotropin secretion by "downregulation" of the gonadotropin cells.[8]

PREMENSTRUAL SYNDROME

The ED physician is often called on to deal with problems occurring in the postovulatory phase of the cycle, which may at times be diagnosed as "premenstrual syndrome" (PMS). Sutherland and Stewart define PMS as "any combination of emotional or physical features which occur cyclically in a female before menstruation and which regress or disappear during menstruation."[9] Many symptoms have been associated with PMS, such as irritability, anxiety, depression, mood and personality changes, abdominal bloating, weight gain, and breast tenderness. Patients complain of increased thirst and appetite, especially a craving for sweets and salty foods, as menses approach. Some women also note inability to concentrate, forgetfulness, and impaired judgment (to the point of being reluctant to drive a car or handle their interpersonal relationships both at work and at home). It usually occurs in patients in their mid to late 30s, although it can be seen as early as in the late teens.

The symptoms occur after ovulation and commonly start 1 week before menstruation and cease with the onset of menses. Because of the cyclic variation, PMS has been thought to be related to hormonal activity. No correlation with hormonal levels is seen in women complaining of PMS, however. One hypothesis is that endogenous opiates, peptides, and endorphins may be responsible for the symptoms of PMS. The blood levels of opiates, specifically **endorphins,** parallel those of estrogen; estrogen levels fall premenstrually along with the opiate blood levels. The theory has been advanced that these patients become autoaddicted to their own brain opiates, and that the sudden premenstrual deprivation of these compounds leads to anxiety and agitation.[10] Other neurotransmitters have been incriminated in the pathogenesis of PMS, i.e., melanocyte-stimulating hormone (MSH), a deficiency of which may cause inattention, depression, and lethargy.[11] Endogenous opiates can also inhibit dopamine secretion, which in turn can inhibit the pulsatile release of luteinizing hormone giving rise to progesterone deficiency and luteal phase defects. It has been theorized that the premenstrual syndrome is caused by progesterone deficiency, and in fact this syndrome has been treated with progesterone therapy. Careful evaluation of patients with complaints of premenstrual syndrome, however, has failed to show progesterone deficiency.[4]

Although PMS has been treated with diuretics, specifically aldosterone-inhibiting agents such as spironolactone,[12] symptomatic patients generally do not show enough weight gain consistent with fluid retention. Therefore, the abdominal bloating and breast tenderness sometimes associated at times with PMS may be from redistribution of fluid without significantly associated increase in weight.

It is important that the patient keep a record of her symptoms to determine whether they are confined to the 7- to 10-day period before menstruation. If a woman has symptoms that persist throughout the month and worsen only in the late luteal phase, she is unlikely to have premenstrual syndrome and may require psychotherapy and specific psychotropic medication.

TREATMENT OF PMS

Although no specific evidence shows that any of the therapeutic regimens used for PMS are based on proven clinical studies, many medications are used for these patients, such as:

1. Progesterone in the form of progesterone suppositories intravaginally (100 to 400 mg per day starting 2 to 3 days before the expected onset of symptoms)
2. Diuretics of the aldosterone-inhibiting type such as spironolactone, 25 mg 4 times a day
3. Bromocriptine (Parlodel), 1.25 to 2.5 mg with meals and at bedtime (particularly useful for breast engorgement problems)
4. Progesterone-only birth control pills such as Ovrettes, used daily. Standard cyclic birth control pills, per se, usually provoke a worsening of the symptoms because of an amplified decrease in hormone levels, which occurs every 3 weeks before menstruation. The progesterone-only birth control pills are given on a daily basis and therefore may dampen the variation of the endorphin MSH levels.

Other medications that can be used are medroxyprogesterone acetate (Provera), 10 to 30 mg orally every day, or Depo-Provera, 150 mg to 400 mg intramuscularly every 1 to 3 months.[13] Other treatments advocated have been Danazol (200 mg, 2 to 3 times daily) and vitamin B6 (100 to 500 mg daily). Bromocriptine and Danazol are particularly useful in controlling the painful breasts often associated with PMS. In any case, treatments should always start with a diet low in free sugar and salt, high in protein, including six small meals daily with no caffeine. In addition to diet, exercise is encouraged because it has been shown that regular exercise elevates the endorphins in the brain and may prevent the fluctuations and decreases that occur in the premenstrual phase of the cycle. Alcoholic beverages and smoking both may exacerbate the symptoms of PMS.

Lastly, severe mood changes, secondary to PMS or otherwise, may lead to aggressive (external or internal) behavior, and in extreme cases, patients may become suicidal or homicidal. Others may manifest their symptoms by child abuse or have severe anxiety produced by fear of abusing their children. In any case, these patients should be referred for appropriate psychiatric evaluation and treatment.

REFERENCES

1. Spellacy, W.N.: Dysfunctional uterine bleeding. Postgrad. Obstet. Gynec. 4:1, 1984.
2. Kempers, R.D.: Dysfunctional uterine bleeding. In Gynecology and Obstetrics. Volume 5, Chapter 20. Edited by Sciarra, J.J. Philadelphia, J.B. Lippincott, 1982.
3. Walters, D., Robinson, D., Park, R.C., et al.: Diagnostic outpatient aspiration curettage. Obstet. Gynecol. 46:160, 1975.
4. Speroff, L., Glass, R.H., and Kase, H.G.: Clinical Gynecology, Endocrinology, and Infertility. Baltimore, Williams & Wilkins, 1983, p. 236.
5. Goldrath, M.H., Fuller, T.A., and Segal, S.: Laser photovaporization of endometrium for the treatment of menorrhagia. Am. J. Obstet. Gynecol. 104:14, 1981.
6. Daywood, M.Y. (ed.): Dysmenorrhea. Baltimore, Williams & Wilkins, 1981.
7. Daniell, J.F., and Feste, J.R.: Laser laparoscopy. In Laser Surgery in Gynecology and Obstetrics. Edited by Key, W.R., Jr. Boston, G.I. Hall Medical Publishers, 1985, pp. 156–158.
8. Schriocke, E., Monroe, S.E., Henzel, M., et al.: Treatment of endometriosis with a potent agonist of gonadotropin releasing hormone. Fertil. Steril. 44:583, 1985.
9. Sutherland, H., and Stewart, I.: A critical analysis of the premenstrual syndrome. Lancet 1:1189, 1965.
10. Speroff, L.: PMS—Looking for new answers to an old problem. Contemp. Obstet. Gynec. 22:109, 1983.
11. Reid, R.L., and Yen, S.S.C.: Premenstrual syndrome. Am. J. Obstet. Gynecol. 139:185, 1981.
12. O'Brien, M.S., Cravend, D., Selby, C., et al.: Treatment of premenstrual syndrome by spironolactone. Br. J. Obstet. Gynaecol. 86:142, 1979.
13. Nader, S.: Premenstrual syndrome—Tailoring treatment to symptoms. Postgrad. Med. 90:173, 1991.

THE SEXUALLY ASSAULTED PATIENT

Stephen D. Higgins
With Contributions by George R. Schwartz

CAPSULE

Although management of the sexually assaulted patient may be facilitated by a checklist or protocol, it is nevertheless critical for the emergency physician to understand the emotional and medical pathophysiology of the victim. Treatment in the Emergency Department (ED) directly determines the patient's mental, medical, and legal recovery.

INTRODUCTION

The word "rape" comes from the Latin word "rapere," which means to take by force. It is a legal rather than a medical term. Definitions vary from state to state, but the most common generic definition is "the unlawful carnal knowledge of a woman by force and against her will."[1] Case law more specifically defines rape as "any sexual penetration, however slight." This means exactly that penile penetration of the labia majora or labia minora is "sufficient to complete the crime."[2] Essential elements in the definition include penetration, lack of consent, and force.

More important than the legal definition is the understanding that the real crime of rape is manifested in the outrage and horror of the victim. It must also be understood that rape perpetrated by fear and threats of violence is just as repugnant as rape perpetrated by physical force.

FBI statistics show a frightening trend in the incidence of rapes in this country. In 1960, there were 15,560 forcible rapes with an incidence of 17 per 100,000 women. In 1990, the projected number of rapes was 96,000, indicating an incidence of 85 per 100,000 women. These numbers are even more staggering when statisticians point out that they represent only between 10 and 50% of the actual rapes committed every year.

A random study of 3132 residents in Los Angeles County, done by Sorenson in 1984, revealed that the lifetime prevalence of sexual assault during adulthood (at or after age 16) was 10.5% of all women questioned in the sample. They defined sexual assault as "touching your sexual parts, you touching their sexual parts, or sexual intercourse."[3]

PATHOPHYSIOLOGY

The study of the behavior motivation of the rapist is in its infancy. Ground work in the understanding of the rapist began in 1977 with an article published by Abel, who studied two groups of men, rapists and nonrapists.[4] By measuring penile tumescence as a sign of sexual arousal, and exposing both groups of men to audiotapes representing alternately episodes of rape and mutually enjoyable intercourse, he was able to study the differing responses of the two groups. He found an almost perfect correlation between sexual arousal of the rapist and the audiotape depiction of aggression and rape.

Burgess goes on to further explain the rapist and states, "When life events impact on the offender in such a way as to activate . . . fears of helplessness and vulnerability, of worthlessness and emptiness, and/or of rejection and abandonment, sexual assault becomes his defense against the resulting pain."[5]

Burgess classifies rapists into three categories: The anger rapist, the power rapist, and the sadistic rapist.

The anger rapist uses physical brutality to express rage, contempt, and hatred for the victim. The attack is usually an unplanned assault and the rapist seldom feels sexually aroused when he initiates the attack. The rape is of relatively short duration. More force is characteristically used, however, than is necessary to overpower the victim, and the assault is one of physical violence to the whole body.

In contrast, the power rapist begins the attack to overcome feelings of inadequacy and insecurity and to accomplish sexual intercourse as evidence of conquest. The attack is usually premeditated, and although there is seldom physical injury beyond the act itself, the assault may be of extended duration. Power rapes outnumber anger rapes two to one. Therefore, the typical adult rape victim sustains relatively minor physical injuries.

In contrast, the sadistic rapist eroticizes physical force, and the rape itself may involve torture, be of extended duration, and involve mutilation or even murder. This may be the only way the sadistic rapist is able to achieve sexual satisfaction. Fortunately, this is the most uncommon type of rapist.

The sexually assaulted patient is most likely to be a woman under 40, nonHispanic white, with some college education. These characteristics vary greatly according to the population served by the ED. Most sexual assault victims know their assailant as an acquaintance, relative, intimate, or other person such as employer, teacher, or date. Only half experience harm or threat of harm.[3] It is thus evident that use of physical force and subsequent trauma are actually unusual. This is further substantiated by studies of rape victims who had objective evidence that penile penetration of the vagina had occurred, yet genital injury was found in only 28%.[6] The important point is that when you find physical evidence of rape, or trauma is found, it helps to confirm that the patient has actually been physically and sexually assaulted. Trauma is, however, a rare finding, and often rape victims have no evidence of physical, specifically genital, trauma.

RAPE TRAUMA SYNDROME

Burgress and Holmstrom, in their classic 1974 article, describe the rape trauma syndrome.[7] They analyzed 92 adult women rape victims and outlined a cluster of symptoms experienced by these women after being raped. This syndrome is divided into two parts (Table 58-3). The first part, called the acute phase, is characterized by disorganization. The second part, the long-term process, is characterized by reorganization.

In the acute phase, the clinician first sees one of two types of impact reactions (immediate reactions), which occur after the rape and may be exhibited in the ED. The first type of reaction is known as the expressed style, is characterized by fear, anger, and anxiety shown by crying, sobbing, restlessness, or tenseness. It is seen in about 50% of patients. In the other 50%, a controlled style is exhibited: the feelings are masked or hidden, and the patient appears calm and composed with subdued affect. This reaction goes against the myth of what a rape victim should look like. These patients are not beaten and brutalized, crying and sobbing. Often they have no physical findings and their demeanor can be that of calm composure. Also occurring during the acute phase are somatic reactions, which reveal themselves during the first several weeks after the rape. If there has been physical trauma, the woman often complains bitterly of bruising or soreness left from the attack. For example, if there has been oral intercourse, she complains of oral irritation. Tension headache and sleeplessness are common manifestations of somatic reactions. Gastrointestinal irritability such as stomach pains and nausea, as well as genitourinary disturbances such as dysuria and vaginal discharge, can occur. It is often difficult to tell somatic reactions from the side effects of postcoital contraception or the symp-

TABLE 58-3. RAPE TRAUMA SYNDROME

1. Acute Phase: Disorganization
   A. Impact reactions (immediate):
      —expressed style (50%): fear, anger, anxiety shown through crying, sobbing, smiling, restlessness, tenseness.
      —controlled style (50%): feelings masked or hidden; patient calm and composed with subdued affect.
   B. Somatic reactions (first several weeks):
      —physical trauma
      —skeletal muscle tension
      —GI irritability
      —GU disturbance
   C. Emotional reactions:
      Fear of physical violence and death
2. Long-Term Process: Reorganization (2 to 3 weeks after attack)
   A. Motor activity increased
   B. Nightmares increased
   C. Traumatophobia

Compounded Reaction: Past or current history of physical, psychiatric, or social difficulties along with rape trauma syndrome; this group has developed additional symptoms such as depression, psychotic behavior, acting-out behavior associated with ethanolism, drug use, sexual activity.

Silent Rape Reaction: Occurs in victim who has not told anyone of the rape, has not settled her feelings and reactions on the issue, is carrying a tremendous psychgologic burden. Symptoms include increased anxiety, avoidance of relationships with men, marked phobias, and loss of self-confidence and self-esteem.

Compounded reactions and silent rape reactions need psychotherapy referral.

toms of sexually transmitted diseases. The most common emotional reaction during this acute phase is fear of physical violence and death. A range of other emotions from humiliation and embarrassment to anger, revenge, and self-blame may be seen, however.

The long-term process begins approximately 2 to 3 weeks after the attack. It is characterized by increased motor activity such as the victim's need to get away, take a trip, or change her telephone number. Almost half of the victims change their residence, and many turn to their family members for support. Also, during the long-term process, there is an increased incidence of nightmares and traumatophobias. A traumatophobia can be manifested as fear of being indoors, especially if the victim was attacked while indoors. There can also be a fear of being alone, fear of people behind the victim, and sexual fear or difficulty in resuming sexual functioning with a loved one.

Two additional types of rape responses described by Burgress and Holmstrom are often seen in the ED. One is the compounded reaction, seen in patients who have been raped and have a past or current history of physical, psychiatric, or social difficulties. These patients develop additional symptoms such as severe depression, psychotic behavior, psychosomatic disorders, and suicidal behavior. Often they develop acting-out behavior associated with alcoholism, drug use, and sexual activity. The other type of rape response is the silent one, occurring in victims who have not told anyone of the rape, have not settled their feelings and reactions on the issue, and carry a tremendous psychologic burden. The symptoms are increased anxiety, avoidance of relationships with men, marked phobias, and loss of self-confidence and self-esteem. It is important to identify the rape trauma syndrome as distinct from the compounded reactions and silent rape reactions. Patients with rape trauma syndrome respond to crisis counseling and are issue-oriented, whereas those with compounded reactions and silent rape reactions need psychotherapy and should be appropriately referred. Most compounded reactions and silent rape reactions are manifested weeks, months, or years after the actual rape. It is important to identify the patient who has had repeated visits back to the ED because of drug use, alcoholism, and suicide ideation and intent, and to seek this type of history.

In 1980, the DSM-III described the post-traumatic stress disorder and included within its scope the rape-trauma syndrome. In later articles, Burgess also concluded that the rape-trauma syndrome was actually a variant of, if not the same as, the post-traumatic stress disorder described earlier in her article.

PREHOSPITAL ASSESSMENT AND STABILIZATION

Once the ED personnel have encountered a rape victim, someone should be assigned to stay with the patient at all times. She should never be left alone. Most textbooks state that it is preferable that a female health care giver be assigned this task of staying with the victim at all times. More important than male versus female, however, is the attitude of the health care giver. The ED personnel should introduce themselves to the victim and reassure her that she is safe. The care giver should exhibit sensitivity, allow the patient to set the pace in giving her history, keep her informed of her present physical condition in a supportive way, and explain to her what is going to happen during the transport and subsequent arrival at the ED.

Most importantly, from a forensic standpoint, the ED personnel should collect all evidence found at the scene. All the clothes are collected, as well as any other evidence such as towels, tissues, tampons, condoms, bedding, and foreign bodies. These are transported in a paper bag along with the patient to a nearby ED as soon as possible.

CLINICAL PRESENTATION AND EXAMINATION OF ADULT RAPE VICTIM

Most rape protocols require the examiner to describe the patient's initial response. It is important to do this without being judgmental. As noted previously, the patient's initial response can vary anywhere from sobbing and crying to a calm, quiet demeanor.

The examination should proceed as quickly as possible. Long delays not only lead to added stress but cause deterioration of physiologic enzymes that must be collected in hope of identifying the rapist. Privacy for patients is provided promptly on their arrival in the ED. A quiet, separate room is necessary for this privacy. As noted earlier, the patient is never left alone unless she specifically requests it. Throughout this time, continued attempts are made to allow the patient to regain control of her life. For example, the physician introduces himself or herself to the patient, and allows the patient to determine the rate of questioning. Permission for the examination is obtained from the patient, and the patient is informed of what is being done and what is going to be done in the process of the examination. When taking the history, ask only what is necessary to collect evidence and complete a thorough examination. By showing understanding and empathy, as well as informing the patient of the physical findings using terminology that is clearly understood, the examiner can build a rapport and continue to lead gradually to more sensitive questions. A compendium of important questions is presented in Figure 58-2.

Collection of evidence begins first with the material brought in with the patient, by the police, ED personnel, or the patient herself. This evidence, as well as the patient's clothes, is collected, labeled, and properly stored. Fingernail scrapings can be retrieved at this time as well, when indicated. Use a wooden instrument to scrape under the fingernails and try to avoid mixing any of the patient's blood resulting from trauma with the scrapings themselves. All evidence, including laboratory specimens, must be clearly marked with the following:

1. Full name of the patient
2. Name of hospital and patient identification number
3. Date and time of evidence collection
4. Description of evidence, including the location from whence it was collected
5. Name and signature of the person who collected the evidence and placed it in the container

Examination gloves should be worn by those collecting, labeling and storing this evidence to prevent cross contamination.

There should be no disruption in the chain of ev-

OBTAIN PATIENT HISTORY. RECORDER SHOULD ALLOW PATIENT OR OTHER PERSON PROVIDING HISTORY TO DESCRIBE INCIDENT(S) TO THE EXTENT POSSIBLE AND RECORD THE ACTS DESCRIBED BELOW. DETERMINE AND USE TERMS FAMILIAR TO THE PATIENT. FOLLOW-UP QUESTIONS MAY BE NECESSARY TO ENSURE THAT ALL ITEMS ARE COVERED.

1. Name of person providing history	Relationship to patient	Date/time of assault(s)

2. Location and physical surroundings of assault (bed, field, car, rug, floor, etc.)

3. Name(s), number and race of assailant(s)

4. Acts described by patient
(Any penetration, however slight, of the labia or rectum by the penis or any penetration of a genital or anal opening by a foreign object or body part constitutes the act. Oral copulation and masturbation only require contact.)

	Yes	No	Attempted	Unsure	If more than one assailant, identify person.
Penetration of vagina by					
Penis					
Finger					
Foreign object					
Describe the object					
Penetration of rectum by					
Penis					
Finger					
Foreign object					
Describe the object					
Oral copulation of genitals					
of victim by assailant					
of assailant by victim					
Oral copulation of anus					
of victim by assailant					
of assailant by victim					
Masturbation					
of victim by assailant					
of assailant by victim					
other					
Did ejaculation occur outside a body orifice?					
if yes, describe the location on the body.					
Foam, jelly, or condom used (circle)					
Lubricant used					
Fondling, licking or kissing (circle)					
If yes, describe the location on the body.					
Other acts					

5. Physical injuries and/or pain described by patient

_____
_____
_____
_____
_____
_____
_____
_____
_____

	Yes	No
Lapse of consciousness:		
Vomited:		
Pre-existing physical injuries:		

If yes, describe: _____
_____
_____

8. Pertinent medical history

Last menstrual period:
[   ]

Any recent (60 days) anal-genital injuries, surgeries, diagnostic procedures, or medical treatment which may affect physical findings? ( ) Yes ( ) No

If yes, record information in separate medical chart.

Consenting intercourse within past 72 hours? ( ) Yes ( ) No

Approximate date/time:
[   ]

DO NOT RECORD ANY OTHER INFORMATION REGARDING SEXUAL HISTORY ON THIS FORM.

6. Methods employed by perpetrator

	Yes	No	Area of body
Weapon inflicted injuries			
Type of weapon(s)			
Physical blows by hands or feet (circle)			
Grabbing/grasping/holding (circle)			
Physical restraints Type(s) used			
Bites			
Choking			
Burns (including chemical/toxic)			
Threat(s) of harm			
To whom:			
Type of threat(s)			
Other method(s) used			
Describe:			

_____

7. Post-assault hygiene/activity

( ) Not applicable if over 72 hours

	Yes	No
Urinated		
Defecated		
Genital wipe/wash		
Bath/shower		
Douche		
Removed/inserted tampon, sponge, diaphragm (circle)		
Brushed teeth		
Oral gargle/swish		
Changed clothing		

HOSPITAL IDENTIFICATION INFORMATION

FIG. 58-2. Protocol for questioning rape victim. With permission from the State of California Medical Report—Suspected Sexual Assault OCJP 923. Sacramento, Office of Criminal Justice.

CONDUCT A GENERAL PHYSICAL EXAM AND RECORD FINDINGS. COLLECT AND PRESERVE EVIDENCE FOR EVIDENTIAL EXAM

1. Blood pressure	Pulse	Temperature	Respiration	2. Height	Weight	Eye color	Hair color

3. Note condition of clothing upon arrival (rips, tears, presence of foreign materials)

4. Collect outer and underclothing worn during or immediately after assault.

5. Collect fingernail scrapings, if indicated.

6. Record general physical appearance:

- Record injuries and findings on diagrams: erythema, abrasions, bruises (detail shape), contusions, induration, lacerations, fractures, bites, burns and stains/foreign materials on the body.
- Record size and appearance of injuries. Note swelling and areas of tenderness.
- Collect dried and moist secretions, stains, and foreign materials from the body including the head, hair, and scalp. Identify location on diagrams
- Scan the entire body with a Wood's Lamp. Swab each suspicious substance or fluorescent area with a separate swab. Label Wood's Lamp findings "W.L."
- Collect the following reference samples at the time of the exam if required by crime lab: saliva, head, hair, and body/facial hair from males.
- Record specimens collected on Section 11.

7. Examine the oral cavity for injury and the area around the mouth for seminal fluid. Note frenulum trauma.
- If indicated by history: Swab the area around the mouth. Collect 2 swabs from the oral cavity up to 6 hours post-assault for seminal fluid Prepare two dry mount slides.
- If indicated by history, take a GC culture from the oropharynx and offer prophylaxis. Take other STD cultures as indicated.
- Record specimens collected on Section 11.

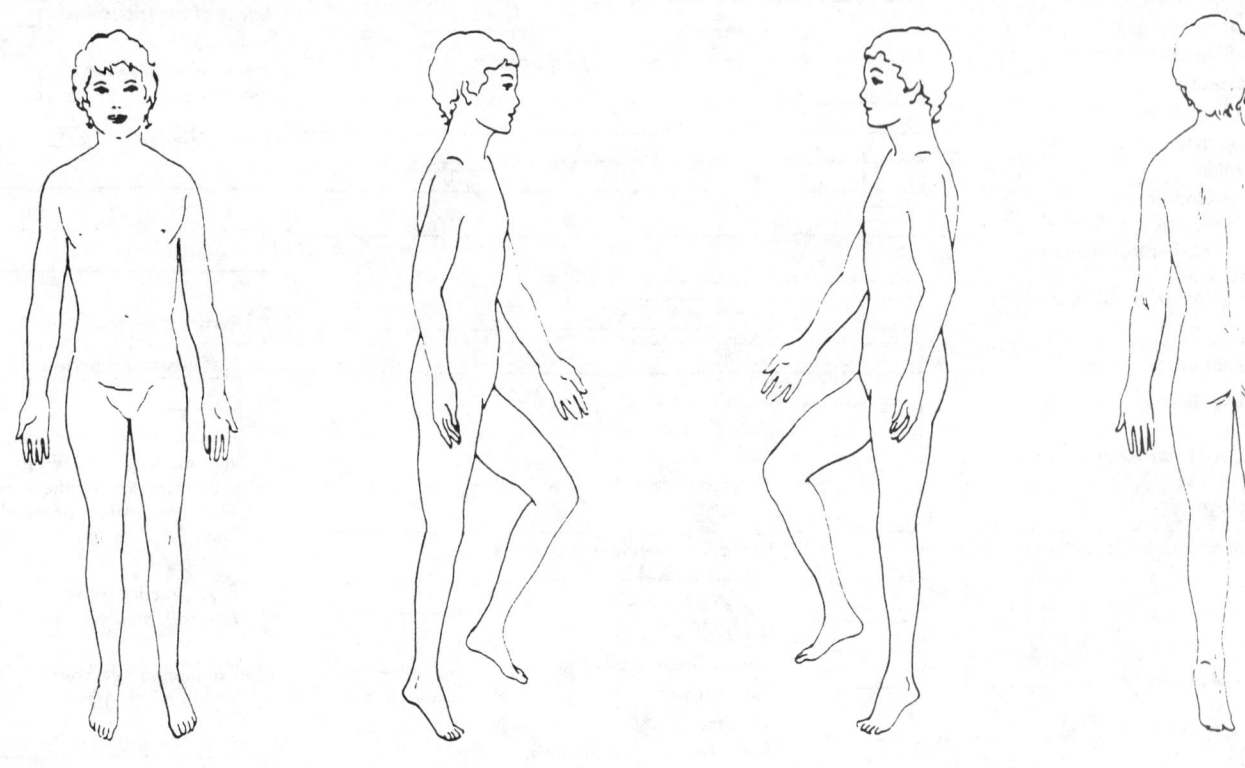

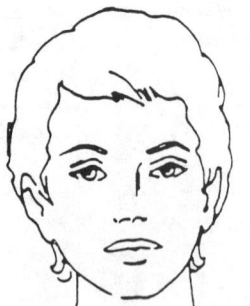

HOSPITAL IDENTIFICATION INFORMATION

FIG. 58-2. CONTINUED

8. External genitalia
- Examine the external genitalia and perianal area including the inner thighs for injury and foreign materials.
- Collect dried and moist secretions and foreign materials. Identify location on diagrams.
- Cut matted pubic hair. Comb pubic hair to collect foreign materials.
- Scan area with Wood's Lamp. Swab each suspicious substance or fluorescent area. Label Wood's Lamp findings "W.L."
- Collect pubic hair reference samples at time of exam if required by crime lab.
- For males, collect 2 penile swabs if indicated. Collect one swab from the urethral meatus and one swab from the glans and shaft. If indicated by history, take a GC culture from the urethra and offer prophylaxis. Take other STD cultures as indicated.
- Record specimens collected on Section 11.

9. Vagina and cervix
- Examine for injury and foreign materials.
- Collect 3 swabs from vaginal pool. Prepare 1 wet mount and 2 dry mount slides. Examine wet mount for sperm. Take a GC culture from the endocervix and offer prophylaxis. Take other STD cultures as indicated.
- If the assault occurred more than 24 hours prior to the exam, collection of cervical swabs may be indicated up to 2 weeks post-assault if no possibility exists of contaminating the specimen with semen from previous coitus. Label cervical swabs and slides to distinguish them from the vaginal swabs and slides.
- Aspirate/washings to detect sperm are optional.
- Record specimens collected on Section 11.
- Obtain pregnancy test (blood or urine).

10. Anus and rectum
- Examine the buttocks, perianal skin, and anal folds for injury.
- Collect dried and moist secretions and foreign materials. Foreign materials may include lubricants and fecal matter.
- If indicated by history and/or findings: Collect 2 rectal swabs and prepare 2 dry mount slides. Avoid contaminating rectal swabs by cleaning the perianal area and dilating the anus using an anal speculum.
- Conduct an anoscopic or proctoscopic exam if rectal injury is suspected.
- If indicated by history, take a GC culture from the rectum and offer prophylaxis. Take other STD cultures as indicated.
- Record specimens collected on Section 11.
- Take blood for syphilis serology. Offer prophylaxis.

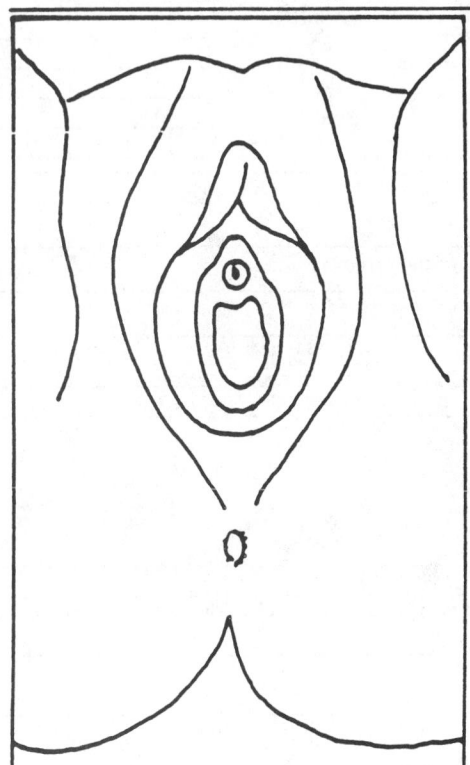
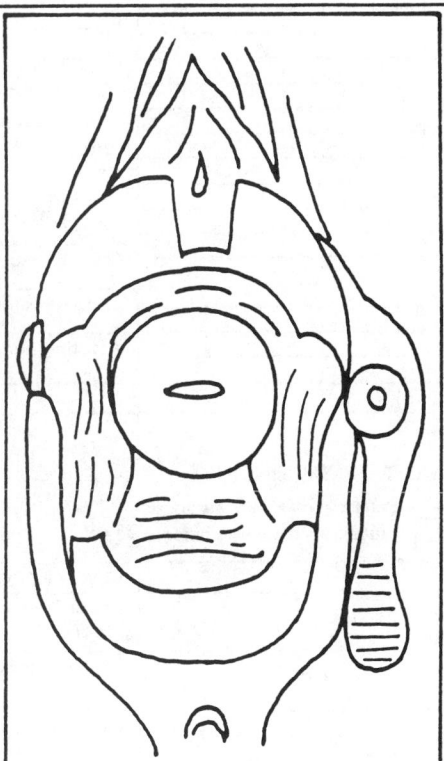
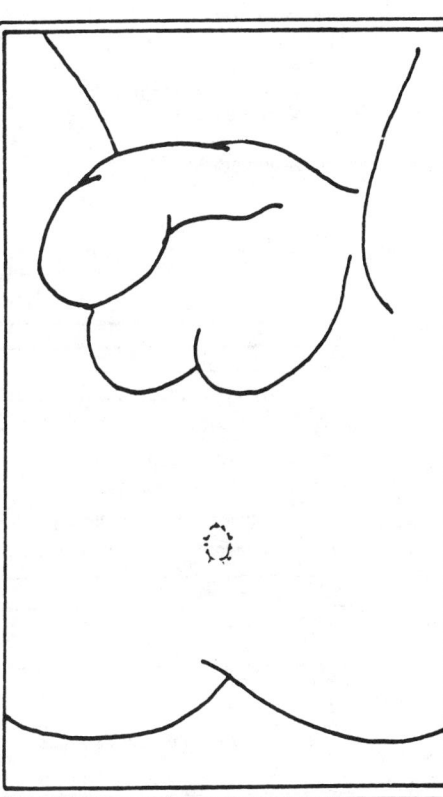

HOSPITAL IDENTIFICATION INFORMATION

FIG. 58-2. CONTINUED

11. Record evidence and specimens collected.

ALL SWABS AND SLIDES MUST BE AIR DRIED PRIOR TO PACKAGING (PENAL CODE § 13823.11). AIR DRY UNDER A STREAM OF COOL A
FOR 60 MINUTES. Swabs and slides must be individually labeled, coded to show which slides were prepared from which swabs, and time take
All containers (tubes, bindles, envelopes) for individual items must be labeled with the name of the patient, contents, location of the body whe
taken, and name of hospital. Package small containers in a large envelope and record chain of custody. See the State of California Medic
Protocol for Examination of Sexual Assault and Child Sexual Abuse Victims published by the state Office of Criminal Justice Planning, 1130
Street, Sacramento, CA 95814   (916) 324-9100 for additional information.

SPECIMENS FOR PRESENCE OF SEMEN, SPERM MOTILITY, AND TYPING TO CRIME LAB

	Swabs	Dry mount slides	Yes	No	N/A	Taken by	Time
Oral							
Vaginal							
Rectal							
Penile							
Aspirate/washings (optional)							

Vaginal wet mount slide examined
  for spermatozoa, dried, and submitted to crime lab
Motile sperm observed
Non-motile sperm observed

OTHER EVIDENCE TO CRIME LAB

	Yes	No	N/A	Taken by
Clothing				
Fingernail Scrapings				
Foreign materials on body				
Blood				
Dried secretions				
Fiber/loose hair				
Vegetation				
Dirt/gravel/glass				
Matted pubic hair cuttings				
Pubic hair combings				
Comb				
Swabs of bite marks				
Control swabs				
Photographs				

Area of the body _____
Type of camera _____
Other _____

_____
_____
_____

REFERENCE SAMPLES AND TOXICOLOGY SCREENS TO CRIME LAB

Reference samples and toxicology screens can only be collected with the consent of the patient. Reference samples can be collected at the time of the exam or at a later date according to crime lab policies. Toxicology screens should be collected at the time of the exam upon the recommendation of the physical examiner or law enforcement officer.

Reference samples

	Yes	No	N/A	Taken by
Blood typing (yellow top tube)				
Saliva				
Head hair				
Pubic hair				
Facial/body hair				

Toxicology screens

Blood/alcohol toxicology (grey top tube)				
Urine toxicology				

EXAM INFORMATION (print)

Anoscopic exam				
Proctoscopic exam				
Genital exam done with:				
Direct visualization				
Colposcope				
Hand held magnifier				

PERSONNEL INVOLVED (print) | PHONE

History taken by:

Physical examination performed by:

Specimens labeled and sealed by:

Assisting nurse:

FINDINGS

Report of sexual assault, exam reveals:

☐ PHYSICAL FINDINGS   ☐ NO PHYSICAL FINDINGS
  ☐ Exam consistent with history   ☐ Exam consistent with history
  ☐ Exam inconsistent with history   ☐ Exam inconsistent with history

SUMMARY OF FINDINGS

PHYSICAL EXAMINER

Print name of physical examiner

Signature of physical examiner

License number of physical examiner

LAW ENFORCEMENT OFFICER

I have received the indicated items as evidence and the original of this report.

Law enforcement officer

Law enforcement agency   ID number   Date

HOSPITAL IDENTIFICATION INFORMATION

ARRANGE FOLLOW-UP FOR STD, PREGNANCY, INJURIES, AND PROVIDE REFERRALS FOR PSYCHOLOGICAL CARE.

FIG. 58-2.   CONTINUED

idence. That is, the collected material must go from the physician to the nurse and the law enforcement officer without its ever having to be unattended. Transfers, when necessary, should be kept to a minimum, ideally to the three people just mentioned. A break in the chain of evidence may invalidate the evidence.

A complete physical examination and a mental status examination should be performed on all patients.

If the collection of evidence occurs within 72 hours of the rape, a complete evidential examination should be done. If more than 72 hours have elapsed, a modified evidential examination may be indicated as the prospect of recovering evidence diminishes rapidly after this period. A modified evidential examination consists of collecting of vaginal or, more important, cervical samples to look for the presence of sperm.

Bodily injury should be reported diagrammatically, on the chart, with special reference to areas of swelling and tenderness. The examiner is likely to be asked later in court to give an opinion as to the age of the injury. The presence of swelling and tenderness are criteria that place the injury as less than 2 days old. The evaluation of bruising and coloration is difficult at best, and can be extrapolated from guidelines in Table 58-4.

Special attention should be given to bite marks. A forensic dentist should be consulted immediately if these are present, usually through the law enforcement office. Proper photographs and/or casts of the injury can then be made and be used later to identify the perpetrator. Each bite mark should be swabbed with a swab moistened in distilled water to collect salivary residue. A swab should also be made of a nonbite mark area on the victim's body to be used by the laboratory for control purposes. Distilled water is used in this process because saline would interfere with the electrophoresis that must be done on the sample in the laboratory. These and all swabs collected subsequently should be labeled and air-dried before packaging.

Attention is turned now to the collection of bodily specimens. Look for and collect any dried and moist

TABLE 58-4. DATING OF BRUISES*

Age	Color
0–2 days	Swollen, tender
0–5 days	Red, blue, purple
5–7 days	Green
7–10 days	Yellow
10–14 days (or longer)	Brown
2–4 weeks	Cleared

*Adapted with permission from Helfer, R. E., and Kemp, R. S. (Eds.): The Battered Child. 4th Ed. Chicago, University of Chicago Press, 1987, p. 192.

secretions, stains, or foreign materials from any part of the body, from head to toe. This can be facilitated by scanning the patient with a Wood's lamp scan (long wave ultraviolet light). This is best done in a darkened room and more clearly shows up dried semen stains, rope marks, recent contusions, and other subtle injuries. Positive fluorescence of dry or moist material is not specific to seminal fluid, however, and confirmation of findings should be done in the laboratory. Examine the mouth and oral cavity for injury and evidence of seminal fluid. Swabs are taken of the oral cavity when indicated. Seminal fluid can be present up to 6 hours after the assault. Also, a gonorrhea culture is taken of the oropharynx when indicated.

Trauma to the oral cavity as a result of oral intercourse has been described as the fellatio syndrome. This is seen as erythema, petechiae, purpura, and/or ecchymosis of the soft palate, with or without separate hemorrhages.[8]

Attention is now turned toward the pelvic examination. Carefully examine the patient while she is in the lithotomy position and document any signs of injuries to the thighs, perineum, rectum, and vulva. Scan again with a Wood's lamp and collect dried or moist secretions and foreign materials from fluorescent areas. Dried specimens on the pubic hair are collected by cutting the matted hair. Also, the pubic area is combed to collect any loose hair or foreign materials and the combings sent, along with the comb, to the laboratory. Describe injuries on the vulva in reference to the face of a clock. For example, injuries in the posterior fourchette are at 6 o'clock, injuries toward the mons pubis at 12 o'clock, injuries on the right side of the vulva at 9 o'clock, etc. The most common location for sexual assault injuries is at 6 o'clock, specifically, in the area of the posterior fourchette.

Genital injuries have been reported in 5 to 30% of women who have been raped. They are mostly minor in nature and many are even asymptomatic. Investigators have identified methods of highlighting small tears and abrasions in the area of the posterior fourchette with toluidine blue.[9] By delineating these small abrasions or lacerations with the dye and then magnifying them with a colposcope, pictures can be taken for use in court at a later date. It must be noted, however, that these minor abrasions or lacerations are not proof of rape because studies have shown that they can occur with consensual intercourse.

A few rape victims suffer severe genital injuries that may require repair in the ED or operating room. Fortunately, the incidence of deep vaginal lacerations, dissecting hematomas, and similar injuries requiring fluid resuscitation is rare.

Next, the vaginal examination is done with a Graves speculum moistened in sterile water. No lubricant is used because this interferes with drying and specimen analysis. This is a good time to ask the patient if she wiped herself with any tissues at home or even in the ED. If so, this tissue is collected, labeled, dried, and submitted with other evidence. Place the speculum into the vagina and examine the vagina and cervix for injuries and foreign materials. Injury may occur anywhere but is most likely to be in the posterior vagina, characterized by lacerations, abrasions, ecchymoses, or hematomas. At this time, collect specimens from the vaginal pool. Sperm can be found in the vaginal pool up to 3 days after intercourse, but can be found in the cervix up to 2 weeks later. In an assault occurring less than 72 hours before, the vaginal pool is the most likely source for semen or sperm identification. If intercourse occurred more than 72 hours before, swabs can be taken of the cervix to look for sperm. One of the swabs can be used to prepare a wet mount slide, using saline as the medium. This is examined immediately under the microscope. The presence of motile sperm indicates recent intercourse. The absence of motile sperm on the slide does not, however, rule out the possibility of sperm being present. The wet mount is also searched for Trichomonas at this time. The wet mount and other slides are then labeled, dried, and presented as evidence. Next, a gonorrhea culture and a chlamydial culture or enzyme test (optional) are obtained from the cervix.

If there is no significant vaginal pool, a vaginal aspirate can be obtained by instilling 10 cc of saline into the vagina, aspirating it back into a syringe, and submitting it in a sealed test tube to the forensic laboratory.

Attention is next turned toward the rectal area. Again, note the presence of dried or moist secretions before and after scanning with the Wood's lamp. If indicated, rectal swabs for specimens as well as gonorrhea and chlamydial cultures or enzyme tests (optional) are taken using the following method: Cleanse the perianal area and dilate the anus using an anal speculum. Swabs are passed through the speculum for collection of specimens. If rectal injuries are suspected, the patient must have an anoscopic or proctoscopic examination.

The examination is completed after the bimanual examination is performed. The latter is useful for identifying hematomas as well as vaginal tears that may be missed by the speculum examination.

Collection of controls depends on the requirements of the local law enforcement jurisdiction and the state protocol. Some protocols request that blood, saliva, and hair be collected at the initial examination. Other protocols require that these be collected only after the alleged perpetrator has been apprehended.

Semen contains three genetic markers at high enough levels in the semen and low enough levels in the vagina to allow routine typing for evidence. These markers are ABO blood group antigens and the enzyme markers peptidase A (PepA) and phosphoglucomutase (PGM). ABO antigen testing is done by semiquantitative agglutination inhibition assay. The enzyme markers, PepA and PGM, and their phenotypes are analyzed using electrophoresis. It is important when collecting samples for genetic typing, therefore, that distilled water be used because saline, as

stated, interferes with the electrophoresis process. Because these genetic markers occur in variable proportions in different populations, their presence or absence in combination with each other can be used to arrive at a percentage likelihood that the suspect is the perpetrator or not.

PepA and PGM activities decrease rapidly in the vagina after intercourse. PepA is gone after 3 hours and PGM does not appear to survive longer than 6 hours. Therefore, for proper genetic typing, i.e., to provide the patient with the forensic evidence that will lead to her legal recovery, she must be examined promptly after being admitted to the ED, before these genetic markers have deteriorated. Specimens must be promptly collected on swabs and slides, labeled, dried, and packaged.

On arrival of the evidence in the forensic laboratory, the slides are first stained with an appropriate stain and sperm are looked for to substantiate the presence of ejaculate. If no sperm are found, prostatic antigen (P30) is looked for as evidence of ejaculation. There is a high incidence of sexual dysfunction among rapists, and 34% do not ejaculate in the vagina during the rape.[10] Also, the rapist may have had a vasectomy, making the absence of sperm understandable. If sperm or P30 is found, then genetic markers are sought. If the stained slide shows no sperm and the P30 is negative, the victim's clothes, tissues, towels, or other material are examined. Success in finding semen samples is more frequent with material brought in with the patient.

The following laboratory tests should be obtained on the rape victim:

1. Serology for syphilis
2. Pregnancy test
3. Gonorrhea culture of suspected sites
4. Chlamydia culture or enzyme test (optional)
5. HIV serology (optional)
6. Hepatitis B serology (optional).

Whether or not the patient receives antibiotics to combat potential sexually transmitted disease and whether or not she receives prophylaxis against pregnancy, she should nevertheless be followed up at 2 and again at 6 weeks for a repeat serology for syphilis, pregnancy test, and gonorrhea culture. Repeat chlamydial culture or enzyme test and/or HIV serology may be performed. Table 58-5 provides an overall checklist for evaluation.

MANAGEMENT AND INDICATIONS FOR ADMISSION

Psychologic as well as medical support is of paramount importance in the treatment of the rape victim from the time of the incident through recovery, which may

TABLE 58-5. CHECKLIST FOR EVALUATION OF ALLEGED RAPE*

Introductory Procedures
1. Obtain written consent for examination, photographs, tapes, laboratory tests, release of information, and laboratory samples
2. Contact local organization (if not already involved)
3. Retain typed copies for medical record
4. Save all clothing

History
1. Establish rapport
2. Find quiet environment
3. Use "high-touch" support team
4. Determine age, marital status, and parity
5. Obtain menstrual and contraceptive history
6. Determine time of last coitus prior to assault
7. Was there a change of clothes, bath, or douche?
8. Determine use of drugs or alcohol by patient or assailant
9. Obtain full description of incident—who, what, when, where, why (use patient's own words as much as possible) (See Fig. 58-2)
10. Specifically ask about penetration, ejaculation, condom, extragenital acts
11. Deal with fears and apprehensions of patient

General Physical Examination
1. Check vital signs and general appearance
2. Look for extragenital trauma—mouth, breasts, neck
3. Photograph cuts, bruises, or scratches
4. Evaluate emotional state and mental status

Pelvic Examination
1. Vulvar trauma, erythema, hymen, anal and rectal status
2. Matted hairs or free hairs
3. Vaginal exam—use unlubricated speculum; look for foreign body, discharge, blood, lacerations; examine hymenal area
4. Note uterine size or any sign of pregnancy
5. Check adnexa, especially hematomas

Laboratory Samples
1. Label samples carefully
2. Ensure "chain" of evidence
3. Vaginal swab: measure acid phosphatase, blood groups, male semen, forensic tests of sperm identity (PCR) DNA type
4. Take vaginal smears (Gram stain, Pap smear)
5. Take oral or rectal swabs and smears if indicated
6. Evaluate clotted blood, 3 tubes: serology, blood type, alcohol; pregnancy test, possible test for AIDS
7. Take cultures—cervix plus other areas, if indicated; check for Chlamydia, gonorrhea, syphilis
8. Evaluate urine—drugs; check for hematuria, routine urinalysis
9. Comb and clip hairs
10. Take fingernail scrapings as needed
11. Inspect wet mount for motile spermatoza

Treatment
1. Give care for injuries and emotional trauma
2. Give antibiotic prophylaxis for venereal disease; use CDC guidelines (see Chap. 50) and remainder of this section
3. First check for pregnancy. If none, protect against pregnancy unless patient wishes otherwise. Use the birth control pill, norgestrel and ethinyl estradiol (Ovral), 2 tablets orally immediately plus 2 tablets 12 hours later.
4. Protect legal rights; maintain confidentiality
5. Recommend continued follow-up and services of rape crisis center, psychiatrist, and emergency department as needed
6. Repeat gonorrhea culture and serology at 2 and 6 weeks
7. Test for AIDS initially and in 1 month and 6 months. There is no postexposure prophylaxis
8. Postexposure acyclovir (800 mg q.i.d.) may prevent herpes simplex, but there have been no conclusive studies

* Not all these procedures may be applicable for all cases. Circumstances and police and forensic laboratory capabilities determine other aspects. Table revised by George R. Schwartz.

be months to years later. From the time the victim is encountered in the field by the ED personnel, she is never left alone, and care and attention are always provided to her during the process of medical and forensic evaluation. The rape trauma syndrome responds to crisis counseling, and the patient can be specifically steered to agencies in the community. Any deviation from the rape trauma syndrome that would indicate a compounded reaction or a silent rape reaction is immediately referred to psychotherapy. These deviant symptoms and manifestations include severe depression, psychotic behavior, psychosomatic disorders, suicidal behavior, alcohol or drug use, aberrant sexual activity, marked increased anxiety, avoidance of relationships with men, marked phobias, and loss of self-confidence and self-esteem. Most often, these symptoms are noted on subsequent visits to the ED and can be discovered when old charts are sought and reviewed.

Prophylaxis to prevent sexually transmitted disease is offered to all rape victims. If they refuse prophylaxis, this is carefully documented on the chart. The prevalence of infection after sexual assault is difficult to study. Generally, the incidence of Neisseria gonorrheae after a sexual assault varies from 2 to 13% and the incidence of syphilis is probably less than 1%. Information on the other sexually transmitted diseases is not available because it cannot be adequately studied. Other sexually transmitted organisms include Chlamydia, Trichomonas, condyloma acuminatum virus, human immunodeficiency virus (HIV), hepatitis B virus, herpes simplex virus, and cytomegalovirus.

The minimum amount of searching for sexually transmitted disease includes culture for gonorrhea as well as serology for syphilis. Cultures or enzyme tests for Chlamydia can also be obtained; however, this may be unnecessary if the patient is going to receive prophylactic antibiotics anyway. It is debatable whether or not the patient needs serology testing for HIV and hepatitis B virus. At the initial examination, it is also advised to obtain a sample of serum to be frozen and saved for future testing. Any suspicious lesions suggesting herpes simplex virus are cultured.

Prophylaxis against the most common sexually transmitted disease, mainly gonorrhea and syphilis, consists of ceftriaxone, 250 mg IM, followed by oral tetracycline hydrochloride (500 mg four times a day) or doxycycline (100 mg twice daily) for 7 days. This regimen is effective in uncomplicated anogenital gonococcal infections as well as in Chlamydia trachomatis infection, and it also prevents the development of syphilis. Patients who are pregnant or allergic to tetracycline can receive ceftriaxone, 250 mg IM, followed by a regimen of erythromycin base or stearate, 500 mg four times a day for 7 days, or erythromycin ethylsuccinate, 800 mg four times a day for 7 days.[11]

The patient should also be offered the benefit of postcoital contraception. If she refuses, it is important to document this refusal on the chart. The patient must understand clearly that after sexual assault, the incidence of pregnancy is somewhere between 2 and 4% with a single unprotected sexual intercourse exposure at any time during the cycle. If the exposure occurs at midcycle, however, the chance of pregnancy goes up to 20%. That is, the closer the intercourse occurs to ovulation (about 2 weeks before the beginning of the next period), the greater the chance of pregnancy. If postcoital contraception is used within 72 hours after the unprotected intercourse, the chance of becoming pregnant is far less than 1%. The current recommended method of postcoital contraception is Ovral, commercially available as a birth control pill. It is a combination of an estrogen (ethinyl estradiol, 50 mcg) and a progesterone (norgestrel, 0.5 mg). The regimen is to administer two tablets within 72 hours after unprotected intercourse, then give an additional two tablets 12 hours later. Nausea and vomiting are common in patients after this regimen, and the dose must be repeated if vomiting occurs within 1 hour after administration. It is a good idea to give the patient an antiemetic suppository to combat the effects of nausea and vomiting. Because any estrogen and/or pro-

gesterone is teratogenic, it is important that the patient and physician know that she is not pregnant at the time when she takes the postcoital contraception pills. This can be further confirmed with a sensitive beta-HCG pregnancy test. Other contraindications include past or present tumors of the breast or reproductive organs and a history of thrombophlebitis. A relative contraindication is a strong family history of these disorders. After informing the patient of the availability of postcoital contraception, its effectiveness, and its side effects and contraindications, she should sign a consent stating that she understands and accepts the treatment. The patient should have available to her, when leaving the ED, a list of rape crisis centers. She should also be reassured that she may return to the ED at any time for problems that may ensue and need immediate attention. Importance of follow-up with her family doctor at 2-week and 6-week intervals is reinforced. At the 2-week medical follow-up, not only is there a repeat physical examination and psychologic evaluation but collection of gonorrhea cultures and Chlamydia cultures or enzyme tests (optional), as well as a search for other sexually transmitted disease such as Trichomonas, condylomata, or herpes. At the 6-week medical follow-up, repeat physical and psychologic evaluations are done, as well as repeat gonorrhea and chlamydial cultures or enzyme tests (optional). Evidence of Trichomonas, condylomata, or herpes is again sought. At this time also, serologic testing for syphilis is repeated. As indicated earlier, it is debatable whether or not hepatitis B and HIV serology should be done.

SPECIAL SITUATIONS

SEXUAL ABUSE OF MEN AND BOYS

When speaking of rape, we often think exclusively of women as victims. Men and boys, however, can be abused sexually by other men or by women. Rape does occur in jails and other institutions where men are confined. The psychologic trauma can be as great as or greater than for women, and subsequent counseling is essential. Such persons are victims of violence and characteristically go into states of shock and emotional withdrawal.

Sexual abuse of young boys, a form of a child abuse, is usually initiated by an older man. It is also being reported with increasing frequency. The pornographic film and videotape markets have expanded enormously, and increased sexual exploitation of children of both sexes is occurring.

The issues surrounding rape become more complex as society changes. Such problems as "spousal" rape and incest have come to the forefront of attention.

RAPE AND INCEST IN CHILDHOOD OR ADOLESCENCE*

Sexual intercourse with a child under the age of consent (usually 16 years) is considered statutory rape. The raped child or adolescent presents the physician with multiple problems and issues. He or she must first determine whether rape has occurred and, if so, determine the extent of any bodily damage and the possibility of pregnancy or infection. Rapport should be established with the victim and parents. If penetration has occurred, examination should proceed only after parental and patient consent has been obtained. Vaginal aspirate can be examined for sperm and used for bacterial culture. Treatment for gonorrhea may be necessary, and an anti-implantation pill may be used. A Venereal Disease Research Laboratories (VDRL) test is necessary several weeks after the rape. It is appropriate to obtain adequate records for use by police, if they are to be informed. In some areas, this is not an automatic procedure but depends on the parents' decision.

The parents may be as upset as the victim, who may feel frightened, angry, violated, and guilty. The physician should help the patient in a supportive way to ventilate feelings about this extremely traumatizing experience. Immediate psychiatric help may be indicated by the degree of upset experienced by the victim or parents or both. In some instances, more severe psychologic reactions may occur some time after the rape. Contact should be maintained for up to three months, and psychiatric help should be made available if and when necessary. Hospitalization may be needed for very young victims. Often the rapist is known to the family, who must be counseled against retribution other than legal prosecution.

Incest is probably more common than suspected. It may come to the attention of the physician on routine examination of a child with frequent vaginal infections or as part of a pattern of parental abuse or neglect. In most states, it must be reported and legally constitutes abuse. The most common pattern is father-daughter or stepfather-stepdaughter incest. Surprisingly often, the mother knows of the incestuous relationship. Its incidence is greatest in disturbed families in which the daughter has, in a sense, taken the mother's place or in which there is severe psychopathology in family members. Psychiatric consultation is imperative if the physician has proof of the existence of incest.

PITFALLS

The importance of expeditious collection of evidence cannot be overemphasized. The biochemical action of bacterial and vaginal enzymes continues to work at destroying evidence as long as any material is wet and not dry. If swabs or slides are left wet and are expected to dry with simple ventilation, this process will take 10 to 20 hours, and most evidence will be destroyed by the bacterial and vaginal enzymes. If a swab or slide is placed under a stream of air at room temperature for 1 hour, sufficient moisture is removed to arrest the degradation of genetic markers. It is therefore important that the physician obtain the samples from the patient as soon as possible, dry them properly, and, maintaining chain of evidence, pass them on to the law enforcement officer for laboratory storage and/or evaluation.

MEDICOLEGAL PEARLS

The importance of proper documentation also cannot be understated. A rape assault form destined for court with legible and understandable terms to describe injuries, as well as diagrams and even possibly photographs, often saves the physician an unnecessary trip to court to explain the chart. If it is necessary for the physician to go to court, written documentation of injury, especially presence or absence of tenderness and swelling, along with diagrams and photographs, will freshen the memory of the physician and allow better court testimony. The final test of proper collection, labeling, and storage often occurs in a courtroom when the prosecuting or defense lawyer opens in front of the physician on the witness stand the packaged specimens that he or she collected and which have been subsequently analyzed. This is certainly not the time for the physician to realize suddenly that he or she forgot to label properly all the slides and swabs. Nor is it the time to have to say under oath that he or she is unsure of the chain of evidence or the procedures in the ED for transfer of evidence.

Invariably, the emergency physician is called to court to testify in a rape case. Generally, the physician is required as either a "percipient" or an "expert" witness. A percipient witness is one who has examined, prescribed for, or cared for the patient, and is required to testify as to the patient's condition and the treatment rendered. An expert witness, in contrast, has not necessarily treated the patient but has been called as an "expert" to aid the court in evaluating the patient's physical condition and the prognosis of the case. As a percipient witness, the physician who cared for the patient is sometimes eligible for a minimum statutory fee (varying from state to state) for testifying. As an expert witness, the physician has special expertise in an area and will be qualified on the stand before testimony as to proof of this expertise. The expert witness is eligible for reasonable compensation for professional time, determined before the testimony. Whether you are a percipient or expert witness, certain guidelines should always be followed.

* See also Appendix 58A at the end of this chapter.

1. Always insist on preparation for your testimony and consultation with the attorney who called you as a witness. Never appear for your testimony without the benefit of this prior consultation. Take the role of medical witness seriously and prepare thoroughly and in depth for your testimony.
2. Listen to all questions carefully and answer only those that you understand. If you do not understand the question, say so. If you do not know the answer, say so. By answering all questions honestly and fairly, you will avoid any display of embarrassment or reluctance, which will discredit your testimony.
3. Do not allow yourself to be forced into a flat "yes" or "no" answer if a qualified answer is required. You have a right to explain or qualify your answer if it is necessary for a truthful answer.
4. Look at the jury when answering a question. Display in your demeanor your true interest and concern, and never look angry.
5. Be familiar with your notes and reports, but do not attempt to memorize them. You may refer to them whenever necessary for exact quotes, figures, or any other observation about which your memory is not crystal clear. Be alerted, however, that any notes that you bring into the courtroom can at any time be looked at by the opposing attorney. Do not bring anything with you that is not professional and germane to the case.
6. Present your information in an unbiased and unprejudiced manner. Look at this as an opportunity to educate the jurors, who want to understand what you have to say. Keep your voice up and always speak loudly enough for every juror to hear you.
7. It is, of course, understood that the physician will dress in a professional, conservative manner, sit erect in the witness stand, and leave the courtroom in a confident and professional manner.

are detected with x-ray film. This produces a picture of a strip of 30 to 40 dark bands that look something like the bar code used to identify items at the grocery store. This DNA fingerprint is highly individual and, with the exception of identical twins, varies from person to person, much as real fingerprints do. The chances of two people having the same "genetic fingerprint" ranges from 1 in 200,000 to 1 in 30 billion, depending on how many probes are used for the test. In contrast, the chances of two conventional fingerprints being identical are 1 in 64 billion. DNA fingerprinting can be seen to be exact because there are only 5 billion people on earth. One drawback of the test is that at least 1 μg of DNA is required for a single analysis. This limits the use of the test to blood stains larger than 50 μL, semen stains containing more than 10 μL, and bundles of at least 15 hairs. This sensitivity problem, however, can be overcome by enzymatically amplifying or growing more DNA from the original sample before analysis.

In the future, a sample of semen, blood, or hair taken from a sexual assault victim will be translated into DNA fingerprints and then fed into data banks holding genetic fingerprints of known criminals.

ANTI-HIV SUBSTANCES FOR RAPE VICTIMS

Nonoxynol 9 has been shown to inactivate sexually transmitted disease pathogens including HIV in vitro. Preliminary studies show that use of nonoxynol 9 has no effect on subsequent collection and analysis of acid phosphatase, the antigen P30, peptidase-A, phosphoglucomutase, or ABO antigens. Preliminary studies also show that DNA can be isolated from sperm cells after exposure to nonoxynol 9 in vivo. In the future, it is likely to be the standard of care to administer nonoxynol 9 or other topical anti-HIV agent as soon as possible after the assault, or at least immediately after arrival in the ED.

HORIZONS

NATIONAL CONTACTS

DNA FINGERPRINTING

In 1985, British geneticist Alec Jeffreys first reported the discovery of DNA fingerprinting, a method of identifying an individual's DNA and comparing this identification or "fingerprint" to those of other individuals. To obtain a DNA fingerprint, a small sample of cells is broken open to extract the DNA. An enzyme (restriction enzyme) is used to cut the DNA at specific sites into fragments, which are then separated according to size by gel electrophoresis. Jeffreys then produced probes, which are short pieces of radioactively labeled DNA that bind to specific combinations of nucleotide bases. The locations of the fragments that bind the radioactive probes

National Coalition Against Sexual Assault
2428 Ontario Road N.W.
Washington D.C. 20009
(202) 483-7165

REFERENCES

1. Schiff, A.F.: Rape in the United States. J. Forensic Sci. *23*:845, 1978.
2. Annotation: Rape—What Constitutes "Penetration"? American Law Review (3rd Ed.): *163*:178, 1977.

3. Sorenson, S.B., et al: The prevalence of adult sexual assault. Am. J. Epidemiol. *126*:1154, 1987.
4. Abel, G.G., et al.: The components of rapists' sexual arousal. Arch. Gen. Psychiatry *34*:895, 1977.
5. Burgess, A.W., and Baldwin, B.A. (Eds.): Crisis Intervention Theory and Practice. Englewood Cliffs, NJ, Prentice-Hall, Inc., 1981.
6. Cartwright, P.S., Moore, R.A., Anderson, J.R., and Brown, D.H.: Genital injury and implied consent to alleged rape. J. Reprod. Med. *31*:1043, 1986.
7. Burgess, A.W., and Holmstrom, L.L.: Rape trauma syndrome. Am. J. Psychiatry *131*:981, 1974.
8. Elam, A.L., and Ray, V.G.: Sexually related trauma: A review. Ann. Emerg. Med. *15*:576, 1986.
9. Lauber, A.A., and Souma, M.L.: Use of toluidine blue for documentation of traumatic intercourse. Obstet. Gynecol. *60*:644, 1982.
10. Groth, N.G., and Burgess, W.B.: Sexual dysfunction during rape. N. Engl. J. Med. *297*:764, 1977.
11. 1989 Sexually Transmitted Diseases Treatment Guidelines: U.S. Department of Health and Human Services. MMWR *38*:40, 1989.

BIBLIOGRAPHY

American Academy of Pediatrics: Rape and the adolescent. Pediatrics *72*:738, 1983.

Diamond, E.F.: Estrogen treatment for victims of rape. N. Engl. J. Med. *312*:988, 1985.

Graves, H.C.B., Sensabaugh, G.F., Blake, E.T.: Postcoital detection of male-specific semen protein. N. Engl. J. Med. *312*:338, 1985.

Halleck, S.: The physician's role in management of victims of sex offenders: JAMA *180*:273, 1962.

Polak, P.R., Reres, M., and Fish, L.: The management of family crises. *In* Resnik, H.L.P., and Ruben, H.L. (eds.): Emergency Psychiatric Care. Bowie, Md., Charles Press, 1975.

APPENDIX 58A.   ADDENDA TO RAPE AND INCEST IN CHILDHOOD AND ADOLESCENCE

George R. Schwartz

This complex topic is covered only briefly in this book. The emergency physician must recognize its many aspects and seek suitable consultation when available.

Examination of children should proceed as for adults, but speculum examination is not usually necessary. Findings should be documented carefully. Photographs may be helpful in court proceedings. Physicians in the ED must know the state laws regarding mandatory reporting as well as local custom.

The hymenal area may appear irregular or scarred, or have visible tears. Documentation of findings is critical for later courtroom testimony. Not all hymenal irregularities are caused by abuse. Masturbation, irritation from bubble baths, and urinary tract infections can cause abnormal appearance.

In cases of incest, the physician must know when and where to report suspected incest or family child abuse. (See also Chap. 59.)

ED directors should meet with appropriate law enforcement and social service officials to ensure adequate protocols and cooperation. Similarly, they should meet with groups such as "Rape Crisis Centers" and leaders of support groups for rape victims. A new pattern of care involves nurses specifically trained in evaluating patients of this type. In many rural or isolated emergency care facilities, however, the emergency physician has primary medical responsibility, and is often called upon for courtroom testimony. This frequent legal involvement has spawned a subspecialty in emergency medicine, with physicians becoming experts in rape evaluation and medical advisors to community groups.

Part VII

Pediatric Emergencies

Chapter 59

OVERVIEW OF PEDIATRIC EMERGENCY MEDICINE

PEDIATRIC CARE IN THE GENERAL EMERGENCY DEPARTMENT

Thom A. Mayer

CAPSULE

Most pediatric emergency care is delivered, not in children's hospitals or major academic centers, but in general Emergency Departments (EDs) spread throughout communities. Because of this, it is incumbent on all hospital EDs to ensure that they are able to offer the best possible standards of care to the children of their community.

The four essential components of a pediatric emergency medicine program, both in children's hospitals and university medical centers and in the community, are:

1. A clear and deep commitment to the unique needs of children in the ED
2. The development of a systems approach to the pediatric emergency patient
3. Adequate training of emergency personnel
4. Appropriate equipment for pediatric emergencies

INTRODUCTION

Of the nearly 90 million emergency department visits that are expected to occur each year, nearly 30% will be comprised of pediatric emergency patients. These 27 to 30 million patient encounters will, for the most part, occur in general community EDs throughout the country. For example, of the 100 member institutions of the National Association of Children's Hospitals and Related Institutions (comprising both children's hospitals and major academic medical centers throughout the country), only 59% have active EDs. These EDs account for only 7 to 10% of all pediatric emergency visits around the country. Thus, the vast majority of pediatric emergency care is delivered, not in children's hospitals or major academic centers, but in general emergency departments spread throughout the communities of this nation. Because of this, it is incumbent upon each hospital emergency department to ensure that they are able to offer the best possible standards of care to the children of their community. What are the best means of ensuring this goal?

To begin with, it is important to understand that the specialty of pediatric emergency medicine is, in many respects, younger and less well developed than emergency medicine itself. The first fellowship training programs in pediatric emergency medicine were begun in the early 1980s, although there are now over 30 such programs across the country. These programs originated as additional years of training for physicians who had completed pediatric residencies. As the specialty has evolved, however, the training programs have become staffed with nearly equal proportions of physicians who have completed emergency medicine residencies or pediatric residencies. In addition to expanding training programs, a large body of knowledge has evolved within pediatric emergency medicine, including literature on pediatric trauma, pediatric resuscitation, acute care of pediatric infectious diseases, etc. Perhaps the clearest benchmark of the development of the subspecialty of pediatric emergency medicine is the fact that the American Board of Emergency Medicine and the American Board of Pediatrics have cooperated in two important regards. Both boards have approved the concept of issuing certificates following a certification examination in the specialty of pediatric emergency medicine. In addition, joint training programs resulting in potential certification in both emergency medicine and pediatrics after 5 years of training have been developed. Thus the body of knowledge comprising pediatric emergency medicine, as well as potential pathways for educating physicians and ensuring that they are trained in this specialty, has developed rapidly.

Although the concept of ensuring that there is adequate *commitment* to the pediatric emergency medicine program may seem self-evident, it is important to ensure that each facility, including the medical staff, administration, hospital operating board, nursing staff, and emergency physicians, recognizes that an ongoing commitment to the care of the pediatric emergency patient requires significant expertise and dedication. Simply planning for the usual adult emergencies does not ensure that any given facility or the health care providers working therein have the ability to deliver the best possible pediatric emergency care.

Because a systems approach and appropriate training are required, it is extremely important to ensure that the level of commitment to a pediatric emergency medicine program is sufficient to allow it to meet its goals. This in no way implies that effective pediatric emergency care cannot be delivered in each ED across the country, but simply recognizes that such a goal requires a clear understanding of the level of commitment necessary.

Second, the care of the pediatric emergency patient is not confined to the walls of the ED, but is integrated within the community as a whole. To begin with, most pediatric patients have some association with their own private pediatrician or some form of pediatric clinic. As EDs seek to meet the needs of pediatric patients, it is essential to integrate their efforts with the child's existing health care system. Further, a systems approach to emergency medicine requires dedication to the needs of prehospital care providers, emergency department personnel, critical care units, pediatric floors, and staff pediatricians, as well as appropriate follow-up for the children and their families. Emergency physicians have increasingly realized the importance of prevention programs as a significant responsibility of the ED. Nowhere is this more apparent than in the care of the ill or injured pediatric patient, in which prevention is truly the best cure. In hospitals in which tertiary pediatric care will not be delivered, it is essential to ensure that the ED care is as carefully integrated as possible with the treatment protocols of the receiving pediatric tertiary care center. In addition to signed transfer agreements, it is important to ensure that the ED in the community setting cooperates carefully and *prospectively* with the pediatric critical center to ensure the best care available. In this respect, how long it takes a child to get to a pediatric critical care center is far less important than ensuring that the level of expertise available at the pediatric critical care center is present for the child at the earliest possible time. This is best delivered through a system in which this expertise is available in community EDs throughout the referral area.

The issue of training for pediatric emergency medicine is in some respects the least and in some the most controversial area of the care of ill and injured children. On one hand, the general consensus is that prehospital care providers, emergency department nurses, and ancillary emergency department personnel all need specific training in the needs of the pediatric emergency patient. Children presenting to the

ED have enough physiologic, pathophysiologic and anatomic differences that such training is generally considered essential for optimal care by EMTs, paramedics, nurses, and other health care providers in the ED. This should be provided during the initial training of these personnel, but continued on an ongoing basis through in-service educational programs.

In addition, it is important to ensure that the quality improvement program of the ED also addresses pediatric issues on an ongoing basis. Thus, the continuing in-service training should reflect these pediatric quality assurance activities. Nonetheless, some controversy still exists regarding the appropriate level of training for physicians providing pediatric emergency care. Emergency physicians are required, as part of their training, to gain significant expertise and experience in the evaluation and resuscitation of acutely ill pediatric patients. The Residency Review Committee (RRC) for Emergency Medicine lists such expertise as a firm requirement and, indeed, the RRC has aggressively enforced this concept in its site reviews. At the same time, the specialty of pediatric emergency medicine is developing so rapidly and includes so many areas of expertise that emergency medicine residency training alone is unlikely to keep a physician current with the evolving body of knowledge in pediatric emergency care. For that reason, and many others, pediatric emergency medicine fellowships have become popular with graduates of emergency medicine training programs.

In some cases, hospitals have chosen to segregate the pediatric emergency patient from the adult patients in the ED and essentially run a separate pediatric ED. In this setting, it may be possible to use physicians trained in pediatrics who have completed pediatric emergency medicine fellowships as the sole physicians staffing the facility. If such physicians see only pediatric patients, it is reasoned that training in pediatrics plus fellowship-level expertise in pediatric emergency medicine, is adequate. Although this arrangement has been successfully used in some institutions, it has drawbacks. First, many of these EDs are not open 24 hours a day for pediatric patients, which may create separate levels of care for such patients, depending on whether they are evaluated in the pediatric versus the "adult" section. In addition, it is difficult to integrate the practices of the pediatric and adult emergency physicians in this situation because it is virtually impossible for the pediatric emergency physicians to cross-cover the adult side if they do not have sufficient training and experience in adult emergency medicine. Finally, such an arrangement has a tendency to create an "exclusivist" approach to the practice of emergency medicine at a time when it is much more important to build bridges and ensure an inclusivist approach.

For that reason, one of the most successful models in creating a level of expertise in pediatric emergency medicine is the integrated model. In this situation, one or more physicians with fellowship level expertise in the care of the pediatric emergency patient can be recruited to an existing community ED group. These physicians are usually residency-trained or board-certified in emergency medicine, with additional training and/or expertise in pediatric emergency medicine. This allows them to comfortably practice in the adult acute care setting while developing the level of expertise of the hospital's ED regarding pediatric emergency care. The physician or physicians responsible for the section of pediatric emergency medicine develop protocols for the treatment of acute pediatric emergencies; educate their fellow physicians as to the evolving nature of the practice of pediatric emergency medicine; educate nursing, ancillary services, and prehospital personnel in regard to caring for ill and injured children; assist with appropriate pediatric quality improvement activities, develop outreach, educational, and prevention programs for children, etc. We have successfully used this model of staffing at our institution, which sees nearly 60 thousand ED visits per year. Thus, instead of creating a separate section of pediatric emergency medicine, we have recruited and maintained physicians with specific expertise in pediatric emergency care, who have assisted their colleagues in raising the standards of the entire department to that of the most sophisticated subspecialists in pediatric emergency medicine.

Regardless of the staffing model chosen or the specific training of the emergency physicians in pediatric emergency medicine, it is essential to ensure an ongoing commitment to continuing medical education in pediatric emergency care. Virtually all areas of pediatric emergency care are undergoing significant change as newer and newer treatment modalities are being developed in every area of the specialty.

Finally, the general emergency department must commit resources to *equipment*. Appropriate-sized, resuscitation equipment (possibly including the Broselow Length-Based System), infant scales, appropriate blood pressure cuffs, pediatric splints, etc. must all be present in the ED. The types of equipment that are necessary have been well described elsewhere, and the level of sophistication of such equipment varies according to the needs and budgets of individual EDs. Even the most sophisticated pediatric resuscitative and monitoring equipment, however, requires minimal capital outlay from the hospital. Some hospitals have also used separate pediatric waiting areas, which have been universally appreciated by pediatric emergency patients and their families.

Except in rare circumstances, every ED across the country is likely to see a fairly large proportion of pediatric patients. Generally, 25 to 33% of patients presenting to any community ED are children, most of whom do not require referral to a pediatric critical care center for definitive care because fewer than 10% of all pediatric emergencies require tertiary pediatric care. Each of these emergencies, however, deserves the best possible care available to the children of the community. As the specialty of pediatric emergency medicine continues to develop, it is likely that more and more resuscitative measures and treatment modalities will be developed that may improve the health and well-being of our children. Ensuring that the hospital has the appropriate level of commitment; dedication to a systems approach; training of emergency physicians, emergency nurses, and prehospital care personnel; and appropriate equipment, makes possible a true pediatric emergency medicine system within the community hospital setting. The best investment in the future is the health and well-being of our children, and emergency physicians in the community can have a substantial impact.

NEONATAL RESUSCITATION AND SELECTED NEONATAL EMERGENCIES

Kent F. Argubright and Kristi Watterberg

CAPSULE

The Emergency Department (ED) physician often approaches resuscitation of the newborn infant with great trepidation. The treatment of these tiny patients evokes discomfort even in the minds of physicians who are experienced with resuscitation procedures in adults. In this chapter, we provide the information necessary to allay those fears. The principles used in adults and children can be applied to the resuscitation of the newborn. An adequate understanding of the physiologic changes that occur at birth, however, is crucial to successful resuscitation. The latest treatment, intratracheal surfactant, can be used as prophylaxis and treatment of neonatal respiratory distress syndrome. Principles of pediatric ALS, important in the organized approach to neonatal resuscitation, include basic ABCs, venous access, warmth, dextrose, cultures and antibiotics, fluids, and naloxone if needed.

INTRODUCTION

The most common situation requiring neonatal resuscitation in the ED is a precipitous delivery before or after arrival. These neonates usually require simple resuscitative measures. Neonates who are the product of a planned home delivery are brought in because of failure to respond to simple resuscitative efforts. These infants often suffer severe respiratory and circulatory depression. Rapid and appropriate action on the part of the emergency physician is needed in such cases.

NEONATAL PROGNOSIS

Resuscitative efforts should not be withheld because of prolonged depressed states or prematurity.

ASPHYXIA

Clinicians often overestimate the long-term sequelae of neonatal depression and asphyxia. In a survey of 172 health professionals, more than 80% overestimated the incidence of handicap in surviving infants.[1] The outlook is surprisingly good for severe neonatal depression in term neonates. Studies of the neurologic and intellectual outcome of infants who have undergone perinatal asphyxial insults have demonstrated a remarkably low incidence of permanent sequelae.[2-12] Affected infants do have severe multiple handicaps, mostly neuromotor in nature.[13]

The United States Collaborative Perinatal Project prospectively followed 49,000 infants delivered in 12 medical centers. All infants were assigned Apgar scores by an independent observer at 1 and 5 minutes and additionally at 10, 15, and 20 minutes if the 5-minute Apgar score was less than 8. Eighty-five per cent of infants whose birth weights were over 2500 g and whose Apgar scores were 0 to 3 at 5 minutes after birth survived the first year of life. These infants had a 90 to 95% probability of having no significant neurologic sequelae. Reports with much smaller numbers from the United Kingdom support these results.[8,9] Increased use of surfactant therapy will improve statistics, even in this group.

PREMATURITY

Clinicians also underestimate the prognosis of preterm neonates.[14] In a survey, 10 to 37% of physicians, depending on specialty and years of practice, overestimated neonatal morbidity and mortality in premature infants. Improvement in survival of the premature infant has been dramatic, even in the recent past.[15] Increased weight-specific survival rates in the Newborn Intensive Care Unit at the University of New Mexico Hospital (Table 59-1) parallel those in other tertiary care referral centers nationwide. These results are caused partly by a more aggressive approach in the resuscitation of the very premature neonate at the time of delivery. In one prospective controlled study from Australia, survival rates in extremely low birth-weight infants (501 to 1500 g) improved from 51 to 77% with aggressive management of resuscitation.[16] The use of intratracheal surfactant as immediate prophylaxis to prevent or reduce the severity of respiratory distress syndrome has increased survival in even the most premature infants, and has an effect (somewhat lesser) on infants weighing more than 1250 g.[16a,16b] The introduction of surfactant allows emergency treatment.

CARDIOPULMONARY TRANSITION

Birth requires dramatic changes in cardiopulmonary function. Inflation of the lungs and rearrangement of the central circulatory pathways must take place to ensure successful oxygenation and an appropriate acid-base balance.[17,18]

The primary site of oxygenation in the fetus is the placenta. Approximately 40% of the fetal cardiac output flows out of the umbilical arteries from the fetal descending aorta to the placenta. This blood is oxygenated and returns to the fetus by way of the umbilical vein. Disruption of fetal respiratory gas exchange or oxygen transport can occur at several sites in this pathway. They include inadequate maternal uterine blood flow (e.g., maternal hypotension or uterine artery vasospasm), inadequate diffusion from the maternal to the fetal circulation (e.g., abruption, placental insufficiency), or inadequate fetal transport (e.g., fetal anemia, cord occlusion).

The fetal circulation (Fig. 59-1) depends on several "right-to-left" shunts.[19,20] Oxygenated blood return-

1978–1979		1991[16a,16b]	
Birthweight (g)	% Survival	Birthweight (g)	% Survival
		500–749	38
500–999	60	750–999	81–88
		1000–1249	92
1000–1499	84	1250–1499	96
		1500–1749	96
1500–1999	95	1750–1999	97
		2000–2249	98
2000–2499	90	2250–2499	95

TABLE 59-1. WEIGHT-SPECIFIC SURVIVAL RATES (%) IN THE UNIVERSITY OF NEW MEXICO HOSPITAL NEWBORN INTENSIVE CARE UNIT

* Discharged alive.

ing through the umbilical vein passes through the portal vein and into the inferior vena cava (IVC) by way of the ductus venosus. On entering the right atrium, this blood is directed through the foramen ovale to the left atrium. Deoxygenated blood returning by the superior vena cava (and a fraction by the IVC) passes from the right atrium to the right ventricle and out of the pulmonary artery. Only a small portion of this blood enters the pulmonary circulation, whereas the majority passes through the ductus arteriosus to the descending aorta. Pulmonary vascular resistance (PVR) in the fetus is high and secondary to pulmonary vasoconstriction. Because of the relatively low resistance of the placental vascular bed, systemic vascular resistance (SVR) in the fetus is low. This differential (PVR>>SVR) shunts blood away from the pulmonary circulation through the ductus arteriosus to the descending aorta and out to the placenta.

The fully developed fetal lung at term contains thousands of alveoli in close approximation to pulmonary capillaries.[18] These alveoli contain adequate amounts of surfactant to maintain alveolar patency once ventilation and respiration begin.[18a] The fetal lung at term contains approximately 100 to 120 mL of fluid. Birth initiates the cardiopulmonary changes necessary for neonatal survival (Fig. 59-2). Pulmonary fluid is expelled through the mouth and nose as the fetus passes down the birth canal. Residual fluid is forced down the airways with the infant's initial

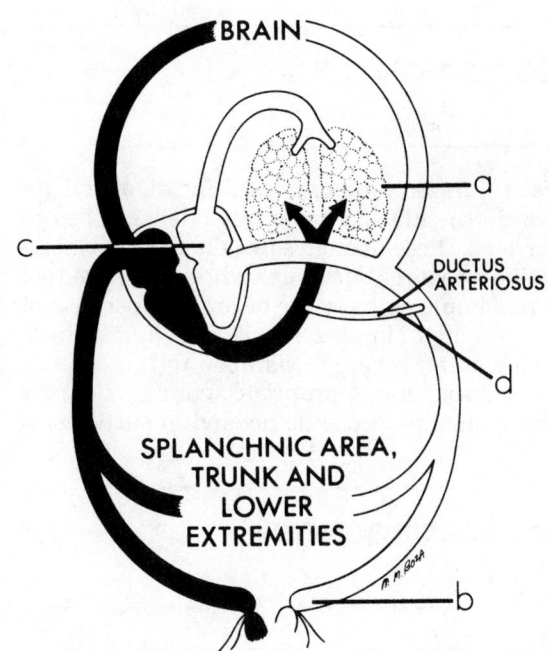

FIG. 59-2. Neonatal circulation. With expansion of the lungs (a), pulmonary vascular resistance (PVR) diminishes and pulmonary flow increases. Occlusion of the umbilical arteries (b) causes systemic vascular resistance (SVR) to increase. Right and left atrial pressures equilibrate, causing functional closure of the foramen ovale (c). Continued oxygenation maintains this flow pattern and causes the ductus arteriosus (d) to close. With permission from Schiarra, J. J., and Eschenbach, D. A. (eds.): Gynecology and Obstetrics, vol. 3: Maternal-Fetal Medicine, rev. ed. Philadelphia, Harper & Row, 1983, p. 2.

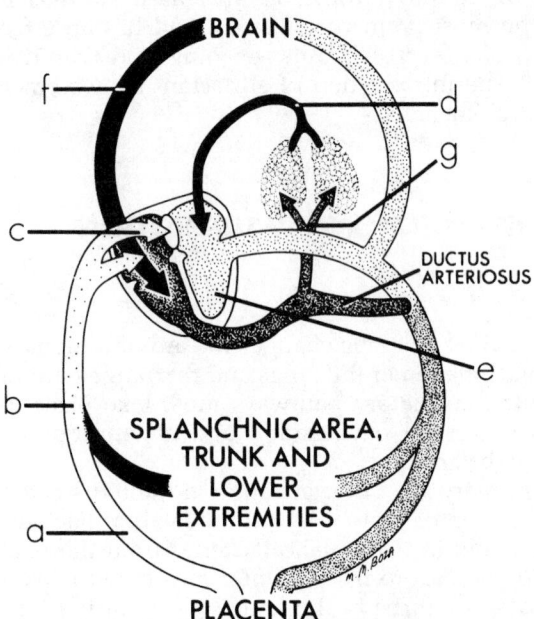

FIG. 59-1. Fetal circulation. Oxygenated blood from the placenta (a) enters the inferior vena cava (b) and preferentially passes through the foramen ovale (c). This mixes with a small amount of blood from the pulmonary veins (d) and passes to the left ventricle (e) and out the ascending aorta. Deoxygenated blood returning from the brain and upper body (f) enters the right atrium from the superior vena cava, passes through the right ventricle to the ductus arteriosus and the descending aorta. Only a small amount of this flow enters the pulmonary artery (g). With permission from Schiarra, J. J., and Eschenbach, D. A. (eds.): Gynecology and Obstetrics, vol. 3: Maternal-Fetal Medicine, rev. ed. Philadelphia, Harper & Row, 1983, p. 2.

breaths and is absorbed from the alveoli by the interstitial lymphatics.[21] With the onset of regular respirations, functional residual capacity is established and oxygen tension rises. Expansion of the lungs causes PVR to decrease. Increasing umbilical vessel occlusion (by either cord clamping or vasospasm) initiates conversion from fetal to neonatal circulatory patterns. Cutaneous vasoconstriction augments this increase in SVR. Over the following days, oxygenation results in closure of the ductus arteriosus. The left and right atrial pressures gradually equalize and the foramen ovale closes. The neonate converts to a circulatory pattern consistent with survival in its new air-breathing state.[22–24]

These patterns of circulatory change all depend on the establishment of adequate ventilation. If it is disrupted or prevented, fetal circulatory patterns persist or resume. Persistent fetal circulatory patterns may be seen in the neonate with birth asphyxia or meconium aspiration syndrome.

Asphyxia causes PVR to remain elevated; this results in diminished pulmonary flow, which causes further hypoxia and acidosis and maintains the patency of fetal shunts (i.e., foramen ovale and ductus arteriosus).[19,20] A vicious cycle is initiated. Fetal acidosis and hypoxia result in a pattern of persistent pulmonary hypertension and circulatory shunting, which prolongs and even worsens acidosis and hypoxia (Fig. 59-3).

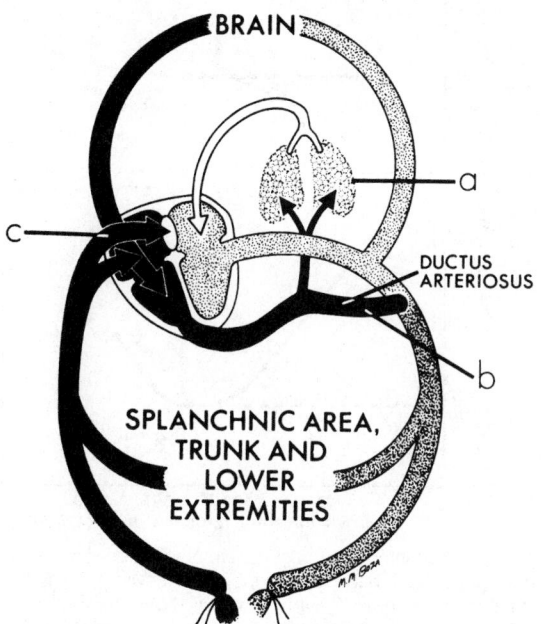

FIG. 59-3. Asphyxia-induced circulatory pattern. Poor lung expansion (a) leads to hypoxia, acidosis, and increased pulmonary vascular resistance (PVR), causing diminished pulmonary flow. Hypoxia causes maintenance of a patent ductus arteriosus with continued right to left shunting (b). The foramen ovale (c) also continues to shunt right to left because of low left atrial pressures from diminished pulmonary flow. With permission from Schiarra, J. J., and Eschenbach, D. A. (eds.): Gynecology and Obstetrics, vol. 3: Maternal-Fetal Medicine, rev. ed. Philadelphia, Harper & Row, 1983, p. 3.)

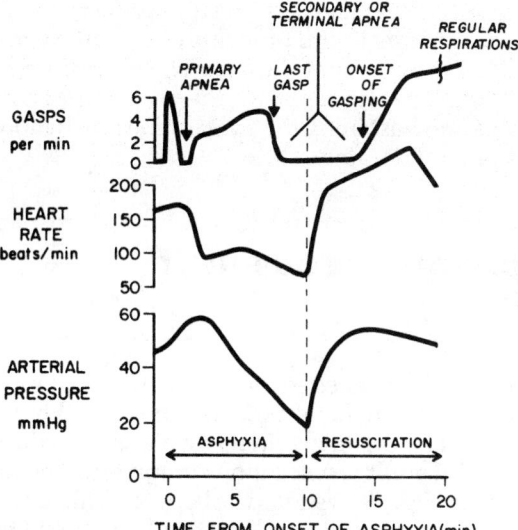

FIG. 59-4. Physiology of asphyxia and resuscitation. Physiologic variables in rhesus monkeys undergoing total asphyxia followed by resuscitation with positive pressure ventilation. With permission from Klaus, M. H., and Fanaroff, A. (eds): Care of the High-Risk Neonate, 2nd ed. Philadelphia, W. B. Saunders Company, 1979, p. 24

Aspiration of meconium causes ventilation-perfusion inequalities in the lung.[25] This may result in acidosis and hypoxemia, causing increased PVR and initiation of the cycle just described. Fetal hypotension may also cause persistence of the fetal pattern of right to left shunting.[20,23] Hypotension can result from direct fetal blood loss, which may be apparent (e.g., fetal laceration, hematoma, hemorrhage from the cord vessels), or from occult fetal blood loss (e.g., placenta previa, abruption, maternal-fetal hemorrhage, or fetal hemolysis).

PHYSIOLOGY OF RESUSCITATION

The neonatal response to resuscitation after an asphyxial stress may be delayed. The classic studies of Dawes and associates[26,27] have delineated the pathophysiology of asphyxia and the response to resuscitation. These investigators used the rhesus monkey as a model for total asphyxia. Before delivery, catheters were placed in the fetal vessels, and the fetal head was enclosed in a saline-filled bag. The fetus was then delivered by cesarean section. The umbilical cord was tied immediately at delivery. Various clinical parameters were monitored during the asphyxial stage and the subsequent resuscitative stage (Fig. 59-4).

After delivery and the onset of asphyxiation, the monkeys initially made rapid gasping efforts and wild thrashing movements. These efforts lasted for a little more than 60 seconds, at which time apnea ensued. During this state of *primary apnea*, the monkeys responded to external sensory stimuli with resumption of gasping efforts. After approximately 8 minutes of total asphyxia, gasping on stimulation ceased altogether. This was called the *last gasp*, and defined the onset of *secondary apnea*. During secondary apnea, no gasping efforts could be induced, in spite of sensory stimuli. During this period, heart rate and arterial pressure, which had initially dropped during primary apnea, continued to fall. Death occurred if resuscitation was not instituted within minutes after the onset of secondary apnea.

Resuscitation was limited to positive pressure ventilation. Dawes and associates[26,27] observed that the time to the *first gasp* following initiation of resuscitation was related to the duration of secondary apnea in a 2:1 manner (e.g., 1 minute of secondary apnea to 2 minutes of resuscitation before the first gasp was seen). The relationship of the resumption of rhythmic breathing to the duration of secondary apnea was more than 4:1.

Parallels to the clinical situation in the human neonate must be drawn with care. Clinical asphyxial episodes in humans are more commonly intermittent and not absolute. The severity of the asphyxia usually increases *slowly* during labor and delivery. This may alter the duration of primary apnea and delay the last gasp phenomenon. In addition, the human fetus is physically and neurologically less mature than the rhesus monkey fetus and therefore may tolerate hypoxia and acidosis for a longer period of time.[27]

Several direct parallels to the treatment of human neonates can be drawn:

1. If apnea is encountered, resuscitation should be instituted immediately, with the presumption of a severe asphyxial episode and secondary apnea. Only in retrospect will it be possible to decide whether asphyxia was present or if the apnea was secondary to other causes (e.g., maternal medications).
2. If secondary apnea is present, resuscitative efforts may have to be quite prolonged before spontaneous respirations are seen.
3. Gasping efforts during asphyxial episodes may cause in utero aspiration of amniotic fluid containing meconium or vernix. This may severely compromise initial ventilatory function and complicate resuscitation.

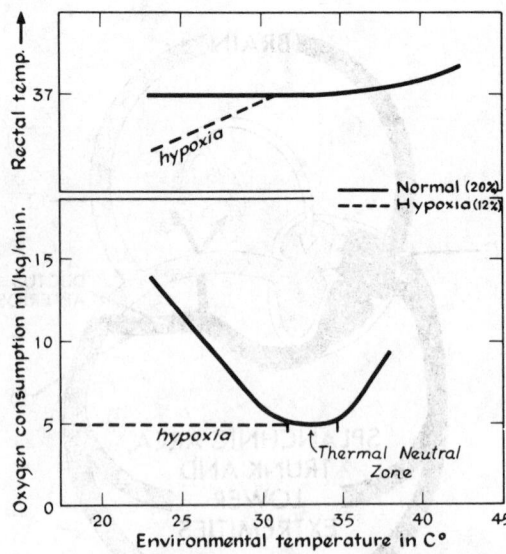

FIG. 59-5. Oxygen consumption and thermoregulation. Changes in oxygen consumption with decreasing or increasing environmental temperatures (breathing room air (20%) or a hypoxic (12%) mixture). With permission from Klaus, M., and Fanaroff, A. (eds.): Care of the High-Risk Neonate, 2nd ed. Philadelphia, W. B. Saunders Company, 1979, p. 95.

NEONATAL THERMOREGULATION

The maintenance of an appropriate thermal environment has profound effects on the survival of the low-birthweight or asphyxiated infant. As early as 1907, Pierre Budin, writing in *The Nursling*, noted that mortality increased from 33 to 90% when the rectal temperature was allowed to drop from 36 to 37°C to 32.5 to 33.5°C or 96.8 to 98.6°F to 90.5 to 92.3°F.[28]

Newborn infants lose heat by evaporation, convection, radiation, and conduction.[29] Evaporative heat losses can be substantial if the neonate is not dried immediately after delivery. Approximately 0.5 calorie of body heat is lost for every gram of water that evaporates. Conduction involves heat transfer from one solid object to another (i.e., neonate to blanket or mother). This can be reduced if contact is limited to *warmed surfaces*. Convection is heat transfer from a solid object (e.g., neonate) to the gaseous surroundings. Heat loss by convection can be limited by warming the ambient air and eliminating drafts. Radiant heat loss is direct infrared transfer from a warm object (e.g., neonate) to any surrounding cooler one (e.g., walls, carpet, chairs). This effect can be overcome with a radiant heater.

The neonate responds to the sudden environmental temperature change at birth in several ways. In the normal situation, this stimulus causes the initial breath.[23] In addition, cutaneous vasoconstriction adds to the increased SVR, aiding in normal neonatal cardiopulmonary transition.[23]

Although neonates are homothermic, their thermal regulatory capacity is limited.[11,30] The newborn depends primarily on chemical thermogenesis for maintenance of body temperature. This heat is generated from brown fat stores.[31] The ability to combat cold stress is limited further by prematurity, asphyxia, and low glucose.

The thermoregulatory range is narrow in the newborn. Thus, minimal cold stress can cause hypothermia. Because the primary mechanism of thermogenesis is consumption of brown fat, oxygen consumption increases dramatically with decreasing environmental temperature (Fig. 59-5). This increased oxygen demand may result in substrate depletion and acidosis in the premature or asphyxiated neonate.[32] Asphyxia may also *directly* compromise thermoregulation[33] by reducing the duration of primary apnea and hastening the onset of the much more ominous secondary apnea.[34]

RESUSCITATIVE EQUIPMENT

The basic equipment needed for neonatal resuscitation in the ED is listed in Table 59-2 and shown in Figure 59-6. It should be organized in its own area to reduce confusion with adult resuscitation equipment. The radiant warmer (Fig. 59-7) should be kept on at all times. This reduces conduction heat loss. Blankets should be placed in the warmer. A large, flat, stable area is most appropriate for neonatal resuscitation. Small cribs or bassinettes restrict access and may make procedures difficult or impossible.

TABLE 59-2. RECOMMENDED EQUIPMENT FOR NEONATAL RESUSCITATION

Flat, open, stable area under a radiant warmer
Warmed blankets
Apgar scoring system on wall
Wall clock with sweep second hand
Respiratory therapy equipment
  CPAP ventilation bags
  100% oxygen source, warmed and humidified if possible
  Neonatal ventilation masks
  Aneroid manometer
  Neonatal laryngoscope with Miller No. 1 and No. 0 blades
  Neonatal endotracheal tubes of various sizes (see Table 59-6) and stylets
Suction equipment
  Bulb syringes
  Suction catheters, if wall suction is available
  DeLee suction traps
Intravenous supplies
  3.5 and 5.0 Fr umbilical catheters
  Umbilical tape
  Volumetric pump
  Syringes and needles
  Intravenous solutions (D5W, D10W)
  Three-way stopcocks

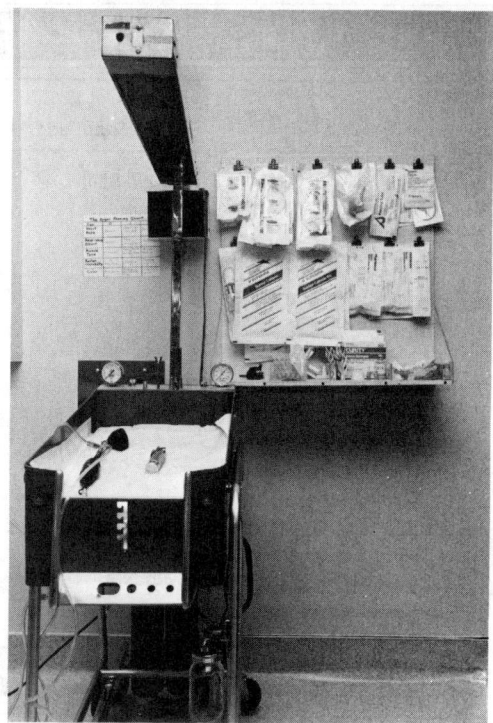

FIG. 59-7. Neonatal resuscitation area. Shown is a prewarmed radiant heater with oxygen and suction hookup. All equipment is organized on a wall board for immediate availability.

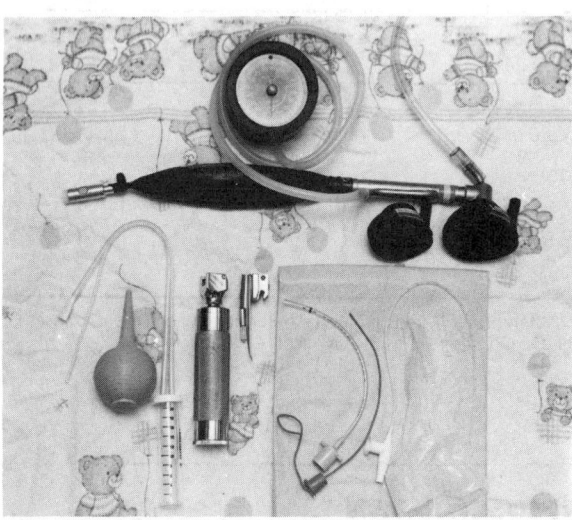

FIG. 59-6. Equipment for neonatal resuscitation. Illustrated are an aneroid manometer, continuous positive airway pressure (CPAP) ventilation bag, term and premature masks, bulb syringe, DeLee suction trap, laryngoscope with a Miller No. 0 blade, endotracheal tube with stylet, and suction catheter with glove.

MEDICATIONS

Only a limited number of medications are needed for neonatal resuscitation. They are listed, along with dosages and routes of administration, in Table 59-3 and include sodium bicarbonate, dextrose solutions, atropine, calcium gluconate, epinephrine, human serum albumin, and naloxone. Special comments regarding sodium bicarbonate and naloxone are appropriate.

SODIUM BICARBONATE

Because the normal-term neonate has a mixed respiratory and metabolic acidosis at birth (Table 59-4), care must be taken in the interpretation of blood gases.

Administration of alkali must be approached judiciously. Several studies have shown a correlation between hypernatremia secondary to alkali administration and intracranial hemorrhage,[32,35] whereas others have not.[24,36] Clearly, adequate ventilation must be established before administration of sodium bicarbonate or pCO_2 rises and acidosis worsens.

Use of alkali may be appropriate under the following conditions:

1. When the infant is intubated and adequate ventilation is documented.
2. When the infant is severely acidotic (arterial pH ≤ 7.10).
3. When the situation is life-threatening.
4. When blood gases are available to assess the effect of administration before a second dose of alkali is given.
5. When a central line (umbilical venous catheter) is in place through which the alkali can be infused.

TABLE 59-3. MEDICATIONS FOR NEONATAL RESUSCITATION

Agent	How Supplied*	Dosage	Dosage Dilution	Route of Administration
Sodium bicarbonate†	1 mEq/mL	1–3 mEq/kg (1–3 mL/kg)	1:3 with sterile water	IV slow push
Epinephrine	1:10,000	0.01 mg/kg (0.1 mL/kg)	None	IV push, endotracheal, intracardiac, sublingual
Calcium gluconate†	10% solution	100 mg/kg (1 mL/kg)	1:3 with sterile water	IV push
Naloxone	0.02 mg/mL	0.01 mg/kg (0.5 mL/kg)	None	IV push, or IM
Human serum albumin	25% solution	1 mL/kg (4 mL/kg)	1:4 with normal saline	IV infusion over 15–20 minutes
Atropine	0.4 mg/mL	0.01 mg/kg Give 0.1 mL to all neonates	None	IV push

* Neonatal solutions.
† Note: Calcium will precipitate with $NaHCO_3$. Intravenous lines must be well flushed between administration of these two medications.

TABLE 59-4. CHANGES IN BLOOD GASES BETWEEN FETUS AND NEONATE*

	Fetus		Neonate† (Arterial)		
	Umbilical Artery	Umbilical Vein	4 Minutes (± 1 SD)	16 Minutes (± 1 SD)	64 Minutes (± 1 SD)
pH	7.25	7.30	7.20 (±0.06)	7.30 (±0.05)	7.36 (±0.04)
pO_2	20	35	53.3 (±15.8)	68.0 (±15.4)	70.3 (±13.9)
pCO_2	45	40	46.1 (±7.6)	35.4 (±6.0)	34.4 (±6.7)
Base	—	—	10.5 (±2.9)	7.9 (±2.9)	4.2 (±2.3)

* Adapted with permission from James, L. S.: In Fanaroff, A. A., Martin, R. J., and Merkatz, I. R. (eds.): Neonatal-Perinatal Medicine. Diseases of Fetus and Infant, 3rd ed. St. Louis, The C. V. Mosby Co., 1983; and Mondaanlou, H. D.: Contemp. Obstet. Gynecol. 4:37, 1974.
† Sea level, room air, minutes after birth.

NALOXONE

The need for naloxone in the ED is rare, but it can save lives. Narcotic depression may be seen in the neonate whose nonaddicted mother received narcotic analgesics within 60 to 90 minutes of delivery. In truly narcotic-depressed neonates, 1-minute Apgar scores are usually normal, but 5-minute and 10-minute Apgar scores are depressed because of inadequate respirations. Naloxone may be necessary to reverse narcotic-induced respiratory depression.[36]

Infants of narcotic-addicted mothers are addicted themselves and should not be acutely withdrawn with naloxone. Acute narcotic withdrawal in addicted neonates can have severe consequences. In addition, naloxone administration in nonaddicted neonates may not be innocuous because β-endorphins may play a role in transition to neonatal life,[37–39] and naloxone may block these beneficial effects.[40]

RESUSCITATION

EVALUATION

As stated at the beginning of this chapter, the emergency physician may commonly face three situations requiring resuscitation of a neonate: (1) precipitous delivery in the ED, (2) unexpected delivery on the way to the hospital, and (3) planned home delivery with unexpected complications.[40a] In any of these situations, the infant should be evaluated immediately with the Apgar score—the universal tool for the assessment of the newborn developed by Dr. Virginia Apgar in 1953 (Table 59-5).[41] Although the Apgar score is usually awarded at 1 and 5 minutes, this evaluation should be made whenever the baby is first seen. If the first

TABLE 59-5. THE APGAR SCORING SYSTEM

Assessment Parameter	Physical Sign	Scoring		
		0	1	2
Appearance	Color	Blue, pale	Acrocyanosis	All pink
Pulse	Heart rate	Absent	< 100	> 100
Grimace	Reflex activity*	No response	Faint cry	Active cry
Activity	Muscle tone	Flaccid	Flexion of arms and legs	Active motion
Respirations	Respiratory activity	Absent	Slow, irregular	Regular

* Reflex activity is tested by rubbing the back or flicking the heel.

Apgar score awarded is 7 or less, the infant should be re-evaluated and additional Apgar scores awarded at 5-minute intervals throughout the resuscitation. Keep in mind that premature babies may have lower Apgar scores than term infants because of decreased muscle tone and reflex irritability.

The following sections describe resuscitation procedures, based on the initial Apgar score awarded, then discuss techniques needed for resuscitation. Because the latest development, prophylactic intratracheal surfactant therapy,[16a] is so new, each ED should meet with the Obstetrics and Pediatrics Departments to develop a protocol for its use in out-of-hospital or ED delivery.

PROCEDURES

Note: If the amniotic fluid is meconium-stained and the baby has not yet been delivered, follow the procedure outlined in the meconium section (which follows under Special Problems) before proceeding to further resuscitation.

All babies, regardless of Apgar score, must first be dried off and kept warm. Hypothermia can severely compromise the newborn, causing acidosis, reduced perfusion, and increased oxygen consumption.

The principles of resuscitation—airway, breathing, circulation—are the same for the neonate as for the older child or adult. In the asphyxiated infant, good ventilation is critical and can be more difficult to attain than in larger humans. Earlier in this chapter, we discussed primary and secondary apnea. *Keep in mind the length of time that can be required to establish adequate respiratory effort in the asphyxiated newborn and the surprisingly good prognosis for survivors if adequate ventilation can be established.*

If the Apgar score is 8 to 10, suction the nose and oropharynx with a bulb syringe, towel the baby dry, keep him or her warm, return him or her to the mother (wrapped in a warm blanket), and observe.

If the Apgar score is 5 to 7, suction the nose and oropharynx with a bulb syringe. Stimulate breathing by vigorously rubbing the back. Toweling the baby dry is excellent for stimulating breathing. If the baby is slow to respond, or does not maintain regular respirations after stimulation is stopped, initiate bag-and-mask ventilation until good respirations are estab-

lished. Continue ventilation until the baby is pink. After withdrawal of respiratory support, observe carefully for deterioration. If the infant is stable, return the baby to the mother in warm blankets and continue to observe.

If the Apgar score is 0 to 4, suction the nose and oropharynx and quickly rub dry. Insert an orogastric tube, begin bag and mask ventilation immediately, and assess heart rate. As resuscitation begins, one individual should review the history, especially for acute blood loss. At 1 minute, if the heart rate is below 60 or if the infant is making no respiratory effort, prepare to intubate while continuing bag and mask ventilation. Once the baby is intubated and good air exchange is achieved, reassess the heart rate. If it is above 60, continue vigorous bagging at 40 to 60 breaths per minute until the baby is pink and the heart rate is above 100 and stable. Watch for the onset of gasping.

Most infants respond well to ventilation alone. If, however, the heart rate remains below 60 after good air exchange has been established, begin cardiac compressions at a rate of 120, with a ventilatory rate of 40. Administer 0.1 mL per kg of 1:10,000 epinephrine either through the endotracheal tube or into the sublingual tissue. Never inject epinephrine subcutaneously in an asphyxiated infant. If the heart rate is still below 60, insert an umbilical venous catheter (UVC). Then, through the UVC, administer 1 to 2 mEq/kg, of $NaHCO_3$, diluted as shown in Table 59-3. Bicarbonate must never be given undiluted because of its high osmolality. No bicarbonate should be given until adequate ventilation is established, and bicarbonate should be given only with extreme caution in premature infants. Flush the line with 3 to 4 mL of D5W. Inject a dose of epinephrine and flush the line again. If the heart rate does not respond, administer calcium gluconate, 100 mg per kg (1 mL/kg of a 10% solution diluted 1:3 with sterile water). Then, infuse 20 mL/kg of 5% human serum albumin (one part 25% albumin to 4 parts normal saline). Because calcium and bicarbonate precipitate if mixed together, the IV line must be adequately flushed between these medications.

After an initial trial of these measures, reassess the baby. If the baby's heart rate has not responded to resuscitation, the most common reason is inadequate ventilation. Recheck the adequacy of ventilation and all oxygen delivery equipment. Absent or decreased breath sounds on the left may be from intubation of the right main stem bronchus. If the endotracheal tube is in proper position and breath sounds are still unequal, consider the possibility of a tension pneumothorax. Perform needle aspiration if necessary. Try to obtain arterial blood gases, either through an umbilical artery catheter (if an experienced person is present to insert one) or peripherally. Blood gases document the adequacy of ventilation and show whether additional bicarbonate is necessary. Obtain an x-ray film if possible. Continue the resuscitation with atropine (0.1 mL IV for all neonates), then repeat the epinephrine, calcium gluconate, and sodium bicarbonate. If a reasonable history of acute blood loss is obtained, give additional volume expanders or blood, if available.

SPECIAL PROBLEMS

MECONIUM

Adequate DeLee suctioning of the trachea and nasopharynx before delivery can effectively prevent meconium aspiration syndrome.[42] If meconium is noted in the amniotic fluid before delivery, the baby's nasopharynx should be suctioned with a DeLee suction trap (see Fig. 59-6). After delivery of the head, but before delivery of the body, thread the suction catheter through the nostrils and use mouth suction to clear the meconium from the nasopharynx. If moderate to heavy meconium is present after delivery, visualize the vocal cords with a laryngoscope. Intubate with a 3.0 endotracheal tube, then place a 4 × 4 gauze pad or face mask over the end of the tube and use mouth suction as the tube is withdrawn. If meconium is found below the cords, repeat. After this procedure, the baby usually needs brief bag-and-mask ventilation to help inflate the lungs. Although the procedure outlined here can cause bradycardia and should not be continued for extended periods, it has been demonstrated to prevent meconium aspiration syndrome, a potentially devastating illness.[43]

THE PREMATURE BABY

The pediatrician should be called as soon as possible for all expected premature deliveries. These babies are more susceptible to all stresses surrounding birth. They lose heat quickly; therefore great care must be taken to keep them warm. Air exchange can be more difficult to achieve with bag and mask, especially for very low-birth-weight babies, and they must be intubated quickly if chest expansion is not adequate with bagging or if they do not respond to bag-and-mask ventilation. The ED, especially during an unexpected precipitous delivery, is not a good place to make a decision about the potential viability of a very premature baby. All babies should be supported if possible until a person experienced in the evaluation of premature infants can arrive and make any necessary decisions about viability and further care. Intratracheal surfactant can make a difference in survival of the most premature infants. Suitable protocols for its use should be prepared.

TECHNIQUES

BAG-AND-MASK VENTILATION

If assisted ventilation is needed, bag-and-mask ventilation should have continuous positive airway pressure (CPAP) capability and should allow interposition of an aneroid manometer to monitor the pressure delivered to the infant. A No. 8 French (Fr) feeding tube should be placed into the stomach during CPAP or bag ventilation to prevent abdominal distention, which can interfere with adequate ventilation. Adjust the CPAP valve to deliver 5 cm H_2O pressure, with enough flow to quickly reinflate the bag. Place the mask over the baby's nose and mouth. Cup two or three fingers under the baby's chin and extend the head slightly to obtain a good seal. Allow the bag to fill, and check the CPAP pressure on the manometer. Begin bagging at about 40 to 60 breaths per minute, watching the manometer to keep inflating pressure at 20 to 24 cm H_2O. Look at chest wall movement and listen to breath sounds to assess the adequacy of ventilation. If chest wall movement or breath sounds are inadequate, increase inflating pressures slightly. If ventilation is still inadequate, intubate the baby instead of using higher pressures with bag and mask ventilation.

Because of their small size, premature babies may be difficult to ventilate with bag and mask. One technique that may help is to turn the face mask around 180 degrees and cover the infant's entire face. Proceed quickly to intubation if bag-and-mask ventilation does not result in adequate ventilation.

ENDOTRACHEAL INTUBATION

A laryngoscope with a No. 0 Miller blade (see Fig. 59-6) allows good visualization of the glottis (Fig. 59-8). General guidelines for endotracheal tube size are shown in Table 59-6. Babies can vary from these guidelines. The tube should slide through the cords easily. Too large a tube can cause pressure necrosis, and a tube that is forced through the cords can cause significant trauma. A flexible Teflon introducer, or stylet, can be used to give stability to the endotracheal tube. Care must be taken that the introducer does not protrude from the end of the endotracheal tube.

Oropharyngeal intubation is the procedure of choice in emergency situations. Nasopharyngeal intubation can be more difficult and more time-consuming and should be considered an elective rather than an emergency procedure.

The baby's neck should not be hyperextended. The baby may lie flat or a towel or diaper may be placed under the head to bring it forward into the "sniff" position. A feeding tube placed into the stomach can help by identifying the esophagus. The laryngoscope is introduced into the right side of the baby's mouth

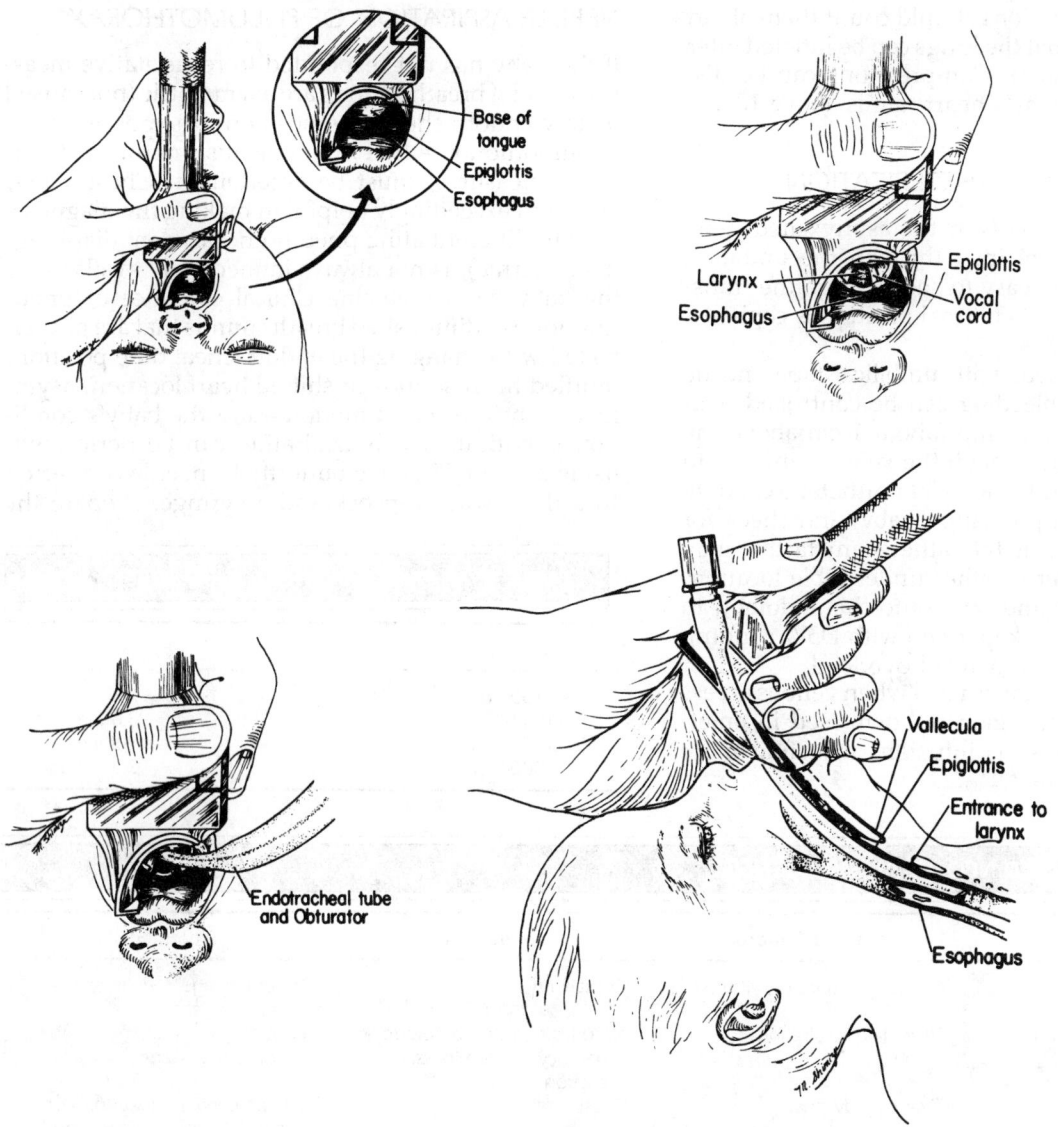

FIG. 59-8.   Neonatal intubation. With permission from Klaus, M., and Fanaroff, A. (Eds.): Care of the High-Risk Neonate, 2nd ed. Philadelphia, W. B. Saunders Company, 1979, p. 33.

and brought across the tongue as it is advanced, sweeping the tongue out of the way. The side of the hand can be held against the baby's cheek to stabilize the laryngoscope. The fourth and fifth fingers can be held under the baby's chin for additional stabilization and, if necessary, can provide slight pressure on the cords to bring them into view. The laryngoscope is frequently inserted down the esophagus past the vocal cords. If the cords are not initially visualized, the laryngoscope should be withdrawn slowly. When the cords drop into view, the laryngoscope is advanced into the vallecula, and the endotracheal tube is inserted 1 to 2 cm below the cords. To avoid uncertainty about the success of the intubation, visualize the cords *after* the tube has been inserted. The tube can be palpated at the sternal notch and advanced about 1 cm farther for correct placement. Ventilate at pressures of 20/4, increasing as necessary to 30/4. Adequacy of

air exchange and quality of breath sounds should be ascertained and the tube taped firmly into position.

HEART MASSAGE (CHEST COMPRESSIONS)

Although the principles behind heart massage in the infant are the same as those in older children and adults, the procedure requires modification because of the neonate's smaller size. The force used for compressions must be decreased, and the number of compressions per minute must be increased. Both hands are placed around the baby's chest, and the thumbs are positioned on the midsternum. The baby's chest should not be squeezed by the hands; instead, the fingers should act as a backboard while the thumbs apply force to the sternum. The presence of a femoral pulse indicates adequacy of compressions. Compressions should be about 120 per minute. The person doing cardiac compressions should count them aloud (i.e., 1,2,3; 1,2,3) so that the lungs can be inflated after every third compression. Compressions can be discontinued after the baby's heart rate is above 100.

UMBILICAL VENOUS CATHETERIZATION

Emergency vascular access in the asphyxiated newborn is most easily obtained through the umbilical vein, which is usually easy to see through the translucent umbilical cord. Its normal position is cephalad to the umbilical arteries.

Encircle the umbilicus with umbilical tape and tie loosely so that any bleeding can be controlled. Cut through the umbilical stump (about 1 cm above the skin) only far enough to open the vein, trying not to disturb the arteries. Advance a 5 Fr catheter 5 cm only (even less in a small premature baby) and check for blood return. Advancing the catheter any farther may position it in the liver or other undesirable location. Suture into position and tape onto the abdomen to secure. The line can be kept open with D5W running slowly (2 mL per hour) to avoid overload.

Intraosseous infusion can be used when venous access is difficult. The tibial region is often used in emergencies, and intraosseous infusions may find more use in prehospital care.[44]

NEEDLE ASPIRATION OF PNEUMOTHORAX

If the baby has not responded to resuscitative measures, and if breath sounds are asymmetric (not caused by low endotracheal tube position), the possibility of pneumothorax, either spontaneous or from resuscitative measures, must be entertained. Chest x ray, although exceedingly helpful in making the diagnosis (and in differentiating pneumothorax from diaphragmatic hernia), is not always immediately available. If the baby has convincing clinical evidence of pneumothorax—diminished breath sounds that are not corrected with changing the endotracheal tube position, muffled heart sounds or shifted heart location, asymmetric chest or chest motion—and the baby's condition is critical, needle aspiration can be performed, using a 23- or 25-gauge butterfly IV needle connected to a three-way stopcock and a syringe. Prepare the

TABLE 59-6. ENDOTRACHEAL TUBE SIZES

Weight	Size
< 1000 g	2.5 mm
1000–2000 g	3.0 mm
2000–3000 g	3.5 mm
> 3000 g	3.5–4.0 mm

TABLE 59-7. SELECTED NEONATAL EMERGENCIES

Condition	Signs and Symptoms	Evaluation	Treatment
Pneumothorax	Cyanosis, respiratory distress	Chest x ray	Tube drainage, needle aspiration
Upper airway obstruction	Struggling respirations	Nasogastric tube to determine patency of nasal passages, suction	Oropharyngeal airway, intubation if necessary
Diaphragmatic hernia	Cyanosis, dyspnea	Chest x ray	Endotracheal intubation, nasogastric tube, surgical consultation
Esophageal atresia, tracheal-esophageal fistula	Copious secretions, choking spells	Insert catheter through nose	Suction, surgical consultation
Congenital lobar emphysema	Progressive respiratory distress	Chest x ray	Emergency lobectomy
Intestinal obstruction	Vomiting, abdominal distention, failure to pass meconium	Abdominal x rays, barium enema	Surgery
Malrotation volvulus	Intermittent bilious vomiting, bloody stools	Abdominal x rays, upper GI series	Surgery
Necrotizing enterocolitis	Abdominal distention, bilious vomiting, bloody stools	Abdominal x rays	NPO, IV hyperalimentation antibiotics, surgery if necessary
Hirschsprung's disease (congenital megacolon)	Abdominal distention, bilious vomiting, no stools	Barium enema, rectal biopsy	Surgery
Congenital omphalocele	Herniation of bowel or liver in umbilical cord region	Cover with sterile dressing, NG suction	Surgery
Gastroschesis	Intestinal tract herniation through defect in abdominal wall	NG suction, cover intestinal tract with sterile plastic bag or polymer	Surgery
Respiratory failure hyaline membrane disease meconium aspiration fetal circulation persistence	Respiratory distress, cyanosis	Blood gases, chest-abdominal x rays	Respirator treatment, extracorporeal oxygenation in severe, nonresponsive cases, surfactant
Sepsis	Rapid deterioration after birth, respiratory distress, granulocytopenia, shock	Chest x ray, blood gases, cultures for meningitis	Immediate use of antibiotics; ampicillin and gentamicin can be started empirically Prophylactic surfactant

chest wall midway between clavicle and nipple and insert the needle in the nipple line, maintaining suction with the syringe. A tension pneumothorax is immediately evident, and release of air should improve the baby's appearance. If a collection of air is found, withdraw air until a physician experienced in chest tube insertion in neonates arrives. If no air is found, withdraw the needle while continuing to maintain suction with the syringe.

OTHER NEONATAL EMERGENCIES

The chief role of the emergency physician in other neonatal emergency conditions is recognition and suitable referral. Table 59-7 lists the most common conditions encountered and can serve as a brief guide to their evaluation. Any of these conditions can be associated with an urgent need for resuscitation based on the principles discussed earlier in this chapter.

REFERENCES

1. Paneth, N., and Fox, H.E.: The relationship of Apgar score to neurologic handicap: A survey of clinicians. Obstet. Gynecol. *61*:547, 1983.
2. Dweck, N.S., Huggins, W., Dorman, L.P., et al.: Developmental sequelae in infants having suffered severe perinatal asphyxia. Am. J. Obstet. Gynecol. *119*:811, 1974.
3. Gottfried, A.W.: Intellectual consequences of perinatal anoxia. Psychol. Bull. *80*:231, 1973.
4. Low, J.A., Galbraith, R.S., Muir, D., et al.: Intrapartum fetal asphyxia: A preliminary report in regard to long term morbidity. Am. J. Obstet. Gynecol. *130*:525, 1978.
5. Mulligan, J.C., Painter, M.J., O'Donoghue, P.A. et al.: Neonatal asphyxia. II. Neonatal mortality and long term sequelae. J. Pediatr. *96*:903, 1980.
6. Neigan, G., Prudham, D., and Steiner, H.: The Formative Years: Birth and Development in Newcastle-upon-Tyne. London, Oxford University Press, 1974.
7. Scott, H.: Outcome of very severe birth asphyxia. Arch. Dis. Child. *51*:712, 1976.
8. Stiener, H., and Neigan, G.: Perinatal cardiac arrest: Quality of the survivors. Arch. Dis. Child. *50*:696, 1975.
9. Thomson, A.J., Searle, M., and Russell, G.: Quality of survival after severe birth asphyxia. Arch. Dis. Child. *52*:620, 1977.
10. Nelson, K.B., and Ellenberg, J.H.: Apgar scores as predictors of chronic neurologic disability. Pediatrics *68*:36, 1981.
11. Broman, S.: Perinatal anoxia and cognitive development in early childhood. In Infants Born At Risk. Edited by Field, T., Sostek, A.M., Goldberg, S., et al. New York, Spectrum, 1979.
12. Finer, N.N., Robertson, C.M., Richards, R.T. et al.: Hypoxic-ischemic encephalopathy in term neonates: Perinatal factors and outcome, J. Pediatr. *98*:112, 1981.
13. Volpe, J.J.: Hypoxic-ischemic encephalopathy: Neuropathology and clinical aspects. In Neurology of the Newborn. Philadelphia, W.B. Saunders Co., 1981, pp. 180–238.
14. Wilson, A.L., Wellman, L.R., Fenton, L.J., et al.: What physicians know about the prognosis of preterm newborns. Am. J. Dis. Child. *137*:551, 1983.
15. Koops, B.L., Morgan, L.J., and Battaglia, F.C.: Neonatal mortality risk in relation to birth weight and gestational age: Update. J. Pediatr. *101*:969, 1982.
16. Drew, J.H.: Immediate intubation at birth of the very-low-birth-weight infant. Am. J. Dis. Child. *136*:207, 1982.
16a. Kendig, J.W., et al.: A comparison of surfactant as immediate prophylaxis and as rescue therapy in newborns of less than 30 weeks gestation. N. Engl. J. Med. 324:865, 1991.
16b. Long, W., et al.: A controlled trial of synthetic surfactant in infants weighing 1250 grams or more with respiratory distress syndrome. N. Engl. J. Med. 325:1696, 1991.
17. Smith, C.A., and Nelson, N.M.: The Physiology of the Newborn Infant. Springfield, Ill., Charles C Thomas, 1976.
18. Scarpelli, E.: Pulmonary Physiology of the Fetus, Newborn and Child. Philadelphia, Lea and Febiger, 1975.
18a. Notter, R.H., and Shapiro, D.L.: Lung surfactants for replacement therapy: Biochemical, biophysical and clinical aspects. Clin. Perinatol. *14*:433, 1987.
19. Rudolph, A.M., and Yuan, S.: Response of the pulmonary vasculature to hypoxia and H+ ion concentration changes. J. Clin. Invest. *45*:399, 1966.
20. Rudolph, A.M., Itskowitz, J., Iwamato, H., et al.: Fetal cardiovascular response to stress. Semin. Perinatol. *5*:109, 1981.
21. Karlburg, P., Cherry, R.B., Escardo, F.E., et al.: Respiratory studies in newborn infants. II: Pulmonary ventilation mechanics of breathing in the first minutes of life, including the onset of respiration. Acta Pediatr. Scand. *51*:212, 1962.
22. Phibbs, R.H.: Delivery room management of the newborn. In Avery, G.B. (ed.): Neonatology: Pathophysiology and Management of the Newborn, Philadelphia, J.B. Lippincott Co., 1981.
23. Epstein, M.F.: Resuscitation of the newborn. In Management of Labor. Edited by Cohen, W.R., and Friedman, E.A. Baltimore, University Park Press, 1983.
24. James, L.S.: Emergencies in the delivery room. In Neonatal-Perinatal Medicine. Diseases of Fetus and Infant, 3rd ed. Edited by Farnaroff, A.A., Martin, R.J., and Merkatz, I.R. St. Louis, The C.V. Mosby Co., 1983.
25. Bacsik, R.D.: Meconium aspiration syndrome. Pediatr. Clin. North Am. 24:463, 1977.
26. Adamsons, K., Jr., Behrman, R., Dawes, G., et al.: Resuscitation by positive pressure ventilation and tris-hydroxy-methyl-amino-methane of rhesus monkeys asphyxiated at birth. J. Pediatr. 65:807, 1964.
27. Dawes, G.: Foetal and neonatal physiology. Chicago, Year Book Medical Publishers, 1968.
28. Klaus, M., Fanaroff, A., and Martin, R.J.: The physical environment. In Care of the High Risk Neonate, 2nd ed. Edited by Klaus, M., and Fanaroff, A. Philadelphia, W.B. Saunders Co., 1979.
29. Perlstein, Ph. H.: Physical environment. In Neonatal-Perinatal Medicine Diseases of the Fetus and Infant, 3rd ed. Edited by Fanaroff, A., Martin, R.J., and Merkatz, I.R. St. Louis, The C.V. Mosby Co., 1983.
30. Hill, J.R.: The oxygen consumption of newborn and adult mammals. Its dependence on the oxygen tension in the inspired air and on the environmental temperature. J. Physiol. *149*:346, 1959.
31. Dawkins, M.J.R., and Hull, D.: Brown adipose tissue and the response of newborn rabbits to cold. J. Physiol. *172*:216, 1964.
32. Bland, R.D., Clarke, T.L., and Harden, L.B.: Rapid infusion of sodium bicarbonate and albumin into high-risk premature infants soon after birth: A controlled prospective trial. Am. J. Obstet. Gynecol. *124*:263, 1976.
33. Cross, K.W., Hey, E.N., Kennaird, D.L., et al.: Lack of temperature control in infants with abnormalities of the central nervous system. Arch. Dis. Child. *46*:437, 1971.
34. Adamsons, K., Jr., Gandy, G.M., and James, L.S.: The influence of thermal factors upon oxygen consumption of the newborn human neonate. J. Pediatr. *G6*:495, 1965.
35. Simmons, M.A., Adock, E.W., III, Bard, H., et al.: Hypernatremia and intracranial hemorrhage in neonates. N. Engl. J. Med. *291*:6, 1974.
36. Corbet, A.J., Adams, J.M., Kenny, J.D., et al.: Controlled trial of bicarbonate therapy in high risk infants. J. Pediatr. *91*:771, 1977.
37. Mondaanlou, H.D.: The high risk fetus: A biochemical profile. Contemp. Obstet. Gynecol. *4*:37, 1974.
38. Gerhardt, T., Bancalari, E., Cohen, H., et al.: Use of naloxone

to reverse narcotic respiratory depression in the newborn infant. J. Pediatr. *90:*1009, 1977.

39. Shaaban, M.M., Hung, T.T., Hoffman, D.I., et al.: β-endorphin and β-lipotropin concentrations in umbilical cord blood. Am. J. Obstet. Gynecol. *144:*560, 1982.

40. Wardlaw, S.I., Stark, R.I., Baxi, L., et al.: Plasma β-endorphin and β-lipotropin in the human fetus at delivery. Correlation with arterial pH and Po₂. J. Clin Endocrinol. Metab. *49:*888, 1979.

40a. Brunette, D.D., and Sterner, S.P.: Prehospital and emergency department delivery–Review of eight years experience. Ann. Emerg. Med. *18:*1116, 1989.

41. Apgar, V.: A proposal for a new method of evaluation of the newborn infant. Curr. Res. Anesth. *32:*260, 1953.

42. Carson, B.S., Losey, R.W., Bowes, W.A., Jr., et al.: Combined obstetric and pediatric approach to prevent meconium aspiration syndrome. Am J. Obstet. Gynecol. *126:*712, 1976.

43. Gregory, G.A., Gooding, C.A., Phibbes, R.H., et al.: Meconium aspiration in infants—a prospective study. J. Pediatr. *85:*848, 1974.

44. Miner, W.F.: Prehospital use of intraosseous infusions by paramedics. Pediatr. Emerg. Care *5:*5, 1989.

BIBLIOGRAPHY

Advanced Pediatric Life Support. American Academy of Pediatrics, American College of Emergency Physicians, 1989.

American Heart Association Textbook of Pediatric Advanced Life Support. American Heart Association, 1988.

Boehm, J.J.: Resuscitation of the newborn in prevention of asphyxia. *In* Gynecology and Obstetrics, Vol. 3. Maternal-Fetal Medicine, rev. ed. Edited by Schiarra, J.J., and Eschenbach, D.A. Philadelphia, Harper & Row, 1983.

Bonitz, W.E., and Sunshine, P. (Eds.): Neonatal resuscitation. *In* Current Therapy of Neonatal-Perinatal Medicine. Philadelphia, B.C. Decker, 1986, p. 360.

Bruck, K.: Temperature regulation in the newborn infant. Biol. Neonate *3:*65, 1981.

Collaborative European Multicenter Study Group: Surfactant replacement therapy for neonatal respiratory distress syndrome. Pediatrics *82:*683, 1988.

Dahm, L., and James, L.: Newborn temperature and calculated heat loss in the delivery room. Pediatrics *49:*504, 1972.

Fisher, D.E., and Paxton, J.B.: Resuscitation of the newborn infant. *In* Care of the High Risk Neonate, 2nd ed. Edited by Klaus, M.H., and Fanaroff, A.A. Philadelphia, W.B. Saunders Co., 1979.

Gandy, G.M., Adamson, K., Cunningham, N., et al.: Thermal environment and acid-base homeostasis in human infants during the first few hours of life. J. Clin. Invest. *43:*751, 1964.

Goland, R.S., Wardlaw, S.I., Stark, R.I., et al.: Human plasma β-endorphin during pregnancy, labor, and delivery. J. Clin. Endocrinol. Metab. *52:*74, 1981.

Goodlin, R.C.: Naloxone and its possible relationship to fetal endorphin levels and fetal distress. Am. J. Obstet. Gynecol. *139:*16, 1981.

Hallman, M., and Sluck, L.: Development of the fetal lung. J. Perinatol. Med. *5:*1, 1977.

Inselman, L.S., and Mellins, R.B.: Growth and development of the lung. J. Pediatr. *98:*1, 1981.

MANAGEMENT OF THE PEDIATRIC AIRWAY

Thom A. Mayer

CAPSULE

The most important aspect of the management of the critically ill or injured child is appropriate and aggressive treatment of the airway.

In children, the primary reason to initiate resuscitation is primary respiratory failure, followed by secondary cardiac arrest. For this reason, it is essential that emergency physicians and nurses be well trained in the evaluation and management of the pediatric airway. This is important not only in children who suffer cardiorespiratory arrest, but also in all critically ill or injured children.

In critically ill or injured children, the most important aspect of management is appropriate and aggressive treatment of the airway. In adults, the major cause of cardiac arrest is myocardial infarction. Resuscitating patients from such arrests requires working knowledge of the physiology of acute cardiac failure, as well as management of cardioactive drugs. In children, however, the primary reason to initiate resuscitation is primary respiratory failure; the next reason is secondary cardiac arrest. This has given rise to the dictum, "Adults *drop* dead—children *droop* dead." This simply reflects the fact that most children have a progression of respiratory failure that results in hypoxia and acidosis, with secondary cardiac arrest as a result of their primary respiratory arrest. For this reason, it is essential that emergency physicians and nurses be well trained in the evaluation and management of the pediatric airway, not only in children who suffer cardiorespiratory arrest, but also in all critically ill or injured children.

PEDIATRIC AIRWAY ANATOMY

There are numerous differences between the anatomy of the airway in the child and the adult. To begin with, proper positioning of the airway differs in adults and children because of anatomic features. In children, the head is larger and occupies a larger total body surface area and mass than in adults. In addition, the occiput is more prominent in children. The larynx in the child is both more anterior and more cephalad than in adults. The epiglottis is more cartilaginous and sits at roughly a 45-degree angle, effectively obscuring the vocal cords unless appropriate airway maneuvers are undertaken. The epiglottis is also more "spoon-shaped" than in the adult, which can make intubation and interpretation of lateral neck x rays more difficult.[1]

Although the narrowest portion of the adult airway is at the level of the vocal cords (or glottis), the limiting area of the pediatric airway up until the age of 10 to 12 years is the cricoid cartilage.[2] The cricoid cartilage is also the site of abundant, loose areolar columnar epithelium in the child, which is quite sensitive to both traumatic injury and infection. The columnar epithelium is also reactive, so that it is far more prone to the development of subglottic scarring than in adults. In addition, because the child's airway is smaller, narrowing of the airway causes a significant increase in airway resistance.

Particularly in young children, the chest wall is far more compliant than in adults, and is less well protected by muscle and fat, rendering it more susceptible to injury. Also, forces applied to the chest wall are more likely to be transmitted to the underlying pulmonary parenchyma. The diaphragm in children is also more compliant, and inserts at more of a horizontal angle. In cases in which the stomach or bowel is distended, this can cause significant respiratory compromise because the diaphgrams distend up into the chest more easily in children. Children also use their abdominal musculature for the mechanics of breathing to a far greater extent than do adults. For that reason, any forces that cause splinting of the abdominal muscles may also cause respiratory compromise.

EVALUATION OF THE PEDIATRIC AIRWAY

Regardless of how acutely ill or injured a child is, one of the first things that an emergency physician does is an initial evaluation of the patient's airway. In critically ill or injured patients, this is a distinct part of the evaluation. All good clinicians, however, spend the first few moments of examination determining how hard it is for the child to breathe, whether the examination is done in a tacit or explicit fashion. Even in the first few seconds, as the nurse or physician walks toward the patient, it is easy to begin to assess the rate and depth of respiration, as well as the amount of work that the patient is having to do to move air.

The most classic example of this is in the asthmatic patient, in whom experienced clinicians can usually tell a great deal about the severity of the attack during the first 20 to 30 seconds of the examination, often before arriving at the patient's bedside. The first assessment to make is the *overall rate* of respirations, which varies according to a child's age. In most cases, children in respiratory distress are tachypneic, although those with major trauma or prolonged hypoxia may be apneic. An attempt should also be made at the same time to assess the *depth* of respirations. Hyperpnea may indicate significant respiratory disease or underlying acidosis. Shallow respirations may reflect splinting of the chest or abdominal wall, or simply inability to move air.

Following the initial determination of the rate and depth of respirations, a clinician should next determine the *overall work of breathing*. This involves numerous factors, all of which result in the overall sense of how difficult it is for the patient to move air. In patients with significant respiratory compromise, a cascade of events occurs that basically reflects the body's attempt to recruit additional respiratory muscles to assist in the work of breathing. One of the earliest signs is *nasal flaring*, manifesting as widening of the nostrils on inspiration. This is particularly noticeable in young children with airway compromise, but also may be seen in older children as well.[3]

Retractions are the visible reflection of the use of additional airway muscles required to move air. This includes suprasternal, infraclavicular, subdiaphragmatic, and intercostal muscles. Although intercostal retractions have traditionally been discussed most extensively, in fact suprasternal, infraclavicular, and subdiaphragmatic retractions are also common. Most ominous is the simultaneous presence of all forms of retractions, reflecting the extreme amount of work that the child must do to move air effectively.[4]

After assessing the overall work of breathing, care should be taken to determine that there is *bilateral, symmetric chest wall rise* with inspiration. Failure of one side of the chest wall to move may mean that the child has a pneumothorax, hemothorax, tension pneumothorax, chest wall splinting, or airway obstruction.

Auscultation of the chest should always be undertaken, but can be notoriously inaccurate in children, particularly if done with an adult stethoscope. For example, it is common for a child to have a pneumothorax, yet breath sounds can be heard over each hemithorax. Similarly, even in children with complete lobar consolidation from pneumonia, it may be extremely difficult to hear rales or adventitial sounds. This is simply because the child's chest wall transmits sounds so easily that airway movement through normal segments often transmits through to the chest wall, obscuring what might normally be heard in adult patients. This problem can be obviated somewhat by the use of pediatric stethoscopes, but it is still difficult to rely solely on auscultation to determine the extent or presence of pulmonary disease in children.[1]

When present, *wheezing* is an important finding, although some children with extensive bronchospastic disease move so little air that wheezing is not present. In addition, in normal children and young adults, the narrowness of the pediatric airway can cause minor amounts of wheezing with forced inspiration and expiration, which can sometimes be mistaken for bronchospastic diseases.[5] Although some pediatric pulmonologists feel that *egophony* can be an important finding in children, it is difficult to reproduce reliably in the emergency department (ED) setting and therefore has limited utility.

The presence or absence of *cyanosis* is an important finding indicating significant desaturation of hemoglobin. When prehospital care and ED triage personnel see cyanosis, oxygen should be started on the patient immediately. As a result, this is a finding that physicians see less commonly because of appropriate field interventions.

Pulse oximetry is an extremely important adjunct in the management of the pediatric patient with a potentially compromised airway, and should be used on virtually all patients with suspected or confirmed respiratory failure. This allows for real-time data which can be extremely helpful in the management of the pediatric patient. Further, pulse oximetry should be used as a monitoring device in any child in whom either sedation or significant radiographic imaging is undertaken.[6]

AIRWAY INTERVENTION

AIRWAY POSITIONING

Failure to put the child in the proper position to allow adequate ventilation is one of the most common problems seen in both adult and pediatric EDs. As indicated, there are significant differences between the airway in the child and the adult. The prone position usually assumed by a child precludes the ability to maintain an open airway. Under these circumstances, the "mandibular block" of tissue, comprising the mandible, tongue, and associated muscle structures falls posteriorly producing near total airway obstruction. Instead, patients should first be placed in the "sniffing position," which consists of a slight amount of flexion of the neck on the long axis of the body and a slight amount of extension of the head on the neck. This can be produced by placing either a towel or the physician's hand under the occiput of the child. At the same time, a jaw thrust maneuver should be done to elevate the mandibular block of tissue. From a practical standpoint, this results in a position in which the nares and the tip of the mandible are at the same level. Even when endotracheal intubation is performed, it is still imperative to maintain the child in the sniffing position because the relatively soft tubes used in children can be compressed by failure to maintain an adequate position of the airway.

OXYGEN THERAPY

Oxygen should properly be considered a drug in ill or injured pediatric patients, but it is a drug with an extremely wide tolerance and few or no side effects in pediatric emergency patients. One of the most common failings of EDs is the failure to provide adequate oxygen therapy to the patient in a rapid fashion. Virtually any child who is undergoing any form of respiratory distress whatsoever should have oxygen provided to them immediately. This includes providing oxygen at the triage station. Theoretic concerns in adult patients such as chronic hypercapnia decreasing the oxygen drive are not a factor in pediatric patients except in extremely rare circumstances.[7] For this reason, humidified oxygen at high flow rates should be administered to any child in respiratory distress.

FOREIGN BODY OBSTRUCTION

Fortunately, complete foreign body obstruction in children is relatively uncommon. Partial airway obstruction caused by foreign bodies, however, is a common problem in the ED setting. In such circumstances, the child should be rapidly placed in the sniffing position and the pharynx should be suctioned and digitally swept for potential foreign bodies. Attempts should be made to ventilate the child by the bag-and-mask technique. If airway obstruction persists, the procedure should be repeated.

With significant foreign body obstructions in children under 1 year, the child may be turned upside down and four sharp back blows should be delivered, in an attempt to dislodge the foreign body.[8] In older children, the Heimlich maneuver may be used.

If these measures fail, direct visualization of the airway and removal of foreign bodies may be attempted with Magill forceps. Significant care should be taken during such manipulations, however, because inexperienced operators may simply drive the foreign body deeper into the airway. Nonetheless, careful attempts to visualize and extract the foreign body should be undertaken.

BAG-AND-MASK VENTILATION

The easiest form of assisted ventilation in a child is bag-valve-mask ventilation. This technique can be difficult in adults, owing to the difficulty in obtaining a proper airway seal and sufficient pressures to generate tidal volume. These are of far less concern in children.

Obtaining a proper airway seal in a child is usually easy with an appropriate-sized mask. These masks can be chosen either by use of the length-based resuscitation system or by ensuring that the mask fits snugly from the bony bridge of the nose to the midpoint of the symphysis of the mandible. Because of the child's smaller size, it is easier to obtain an adequate seal with minimal air leak in the child. Similarly, automatic-refilling resuscitation bags generate sufficient pressure to deliver adequate tidal volume of 15 cc per kg to the child. From a practical standpoint, this simply means that there should be bilateral, symmetric chest wall rise with each ventilation. Because of the possibility of gastric distention a nasogastric tube should be placed in all patients undergoing assisted ventilation so that the stomach can be decompressed.[1] This prevents potential distention of the diaphragms and airway compromise.

Even in cases in which there is relatively high-grade airway obstruction, bag-and-mask ventilation can usually be used to oxygenate the patient. Even in significant epiglottitis, it is possible to temporize with bag-and-mask ventilation until endotracheal intubation can be accomplished. In high-grade obstruction from epiglottitis, it may be necessary to use an anesthesia bag to allow for generation of higher peak airway pressures to overcome such obstruction. Unfortunately, most EDs are not equipped with anesthesia bags, but rather rely on some form of self-filling bag.

ENDOTRACHEAL INTUBATION

Indications for endotracheal intubation in the ill or injured pediatric patient include:

Inability to ventilate the child by bag-and-mask methods
The need for prolonged control of the airway, including prevention of aspiration
Maximization of oxygen and ventilation in children in shock
Need for controlled hyperventilation in head-injured patients[9]

Regardless of the reason chosen for endotracheal intubation, ventilation with high-flow oxygen is recognized as the most important aspect of this procedure. The child should be aggressively preoxygenated through bag-and-mask technique before *any* attempt at endotracheal intubation. Because bag-and-mask ventilation is virtually always successful as a temporizing measure in the ED, it should always be done before attempts at endotracheal intubation. Second, the child should be placed in an appropriate airway position, as indicated previously. Third, the appro-

priate equipment should be selected and prepared for intubation. Length-based resuscitation systems allow selection of an adequate-sized tube, although some EDs prefer to use either anatomic indicators or tables or charts. A stylet should be placed in the airway, but care should be taken to see that it does not extend past "Murphy's eye" because perforation of the trachea can occur if the stylet is allowed to advance outside the end of the endotracheal tube. The laryngoscope blade and light should be tested quickly to ensure that it is functioning. Adequate suctioning equipment, including a rigid tonsillar or Yankauer suction tip, should be provided.

Because of the differences in the pediatric airway, most experienced intubators prefer to use a straight blade in children because it allows easier visualization of the vocal cords. When "standard" adult technique is used with a curved blade, the tip of the blade lodges in the vallecula. When the laryngoscope blade is elevated in the same way as in the adult patient, the epiglottis is not sufficiently elevated to visualize the vocal cords. For intubators who prefer using a curved blade in children, it is usually preferable to use the tip of the blade to elevate the epiglottis itself, similar to the technique that would be used with a straight blade.

If length-based resuscitation systems or tables are not used, a simple way of choosing the appropriate tube size is to select a tube that is the same size as the child's external naris or the distal tip of the fifth finger. Both of these anatomic sites approximate the size of the cricoid ring until approximately 10 years of age.[10]

Care should be taken to advance the tube gently, but firmly past the cords once they have been visualized. The tube should be positioned so that there is bilateral, symmetric chest wall rise with appropriate ventilation, once the stylet has been removed. Tube position should be verified by chest x ray, but it is essential to continue to watch for bilateral symmetric chest wall rise throughout the child's resuscitation. While breath sounds are often used in the adult patient, they can be strikingly deceiving in the pediatric patient. It is not uncommon to have the tube placed in the esophagus and yet hear breath sounds. Similarly, it is possible to have the tube down the right main stem bronchus, and yet hear breath sounds on the left-hand side. This is simply because of the ability of the child's chest wall to transmit sound easily, as mentioned previously.

ORAL VERSUS NASOTRACHEAL INTUBATION

In the adult trauma patient in whom intubation is required and cervical spine injury has not been excluded, blind nasotracheal (NT) intubation is the preferred initial airway procedure.[11] In adult patients who are also apneic, either surgical cricothyroidotomy or careful oral intubation with in-line immobilization may be used. Does this logic extend to children? Understanding of several points is critical in developing a systematic approach to this problem in pediatric patients.

First, although cervical spine injuries are less common in children, they are still a major consideration, inasmuch as two thirds of patients with documented spinal cord injury have no radiographic abnormality.[12] Further, certain injuries predispose the child to risk of cervical spine injury, including auto-pedestrian collisions, falls, and motor vehicle accidents involving high speed collisions or unrestrained children. Second, for these reasons, maintenance of adequate cervical immobilization and avoidance of further cervical spine trauma during airway manipulation is critically important to all patients at risk for cervical spine injury. Third, *atraumatic* oral intubation in the crying, struggling child with an altered level of consciousness is impossible, even with adequate restraint. Atraumatic oral intubation of the flaccid patient with serious depression of the level of consciousness can be performed in experienced hands, but these patients constitute a small percentage of the airway problems seen in children.

Fourth, blind nasotracheal intubation in the non-apneic pediatric patient can be performed, but is much more difficult unless the intubator clearly understands the important anatomic differences between adults and children. Principal among these differences is the previously mentioned fact that the larynx is both more anterior and more cephalad and that the child's "floppy" epiglottis sits at nearly a 45-degree angle. Because of this, blind nasotracheal intubation in the child requires firm cricoid pressure to ensure that the nasotracheal tube is able to reach the level of the vocal cords without having to bend at a relatively acute angle in the hypopharynx. Unless this firm cricoid pressure is applied during the NT intubation, it is extremely difficult to place the tube successfully without direct visualization. An additional complicating factor in the child is the presence of highly vascular adenoidal tissue in the nasopharynx. Unless the tube is lubricated copiously and passed gently, significant bleeding may occur during nasotracheal intubation, which can greatly impair chances of visualizing the cords if intubation fails.

How, then, should the physician approach the child in need of endotracheal intubation but in whom the possibility of cervical spine injury has not been excluded? In all trauma patients, firm in-line cervical immobilization should be maintained, using rigid cervical collars, sandbags and tape, and/or pressure exerted by a nurse or assistant. Initial attempts at ventilation should be given by means of the bag-and-mask procedure. In some cases, bag-and-mask ventilation can be successfully maintained until the possibility of cervical spine injury has been more carefully evaluated. When *immediate* endotracheal intubation is required, bag-and-mask ventilation should still be used to preoxygenate the patient. Even when direct laryngeal injury or significant epiglottitis is present, bag-and-mask ventilation can usually be performed as a temporizing measure until the airway can be secured.

Surgical management of the airway should be reserved for the rare cases in which bag-and-mask ventilation cannot be performed and endotracheal intubation is not possible. (See subsequent text.)

In trauma patients in whom bag-and-mask ventilation can be adequately maintained, cervical spine radiographs should be obtained and a neurologic examination performed to assess the possibility of spinal cord injury. If the radiographs are normal, the neurologic examination shows *no* signs of cervical cord injury, and the history of injury is not suggestive of possible cervical spine injury, *cautious* oral intubation with adequate cervical immobilization should be performed where indicated.[13,14]

If cervical spine injury is highly suspected or intubation is required before adequate radiographs and definitive neurologic examination, *careful* nasotracheal intubation may be performed by those experienced in this technique. The intubator should copiously lubricate the endotracheal tube and have an assistant deliver firm cricoid pressure during the attempted intubation. No more than one to two attempts at blind nasotracheal intubation should be performed. If blind intubation fails and the patient is in need of immediate provision of an airway, rapid-sequence intubation can be performed. In most cases, the patient can be preoxygenated by the bag-and-mask technique, and rapid sequence intubation can be completed. Needle or surgical cricothyroidotomy is rarely necessary.

In patients with epiglottitis, it is commonly stated that elective nasotracheal intubations should be performed.[15] This should be performed in the operating suite by an experienced anesthesiologist, however, with someone capable of providing a surgical airway standing by in the same room. In the ED, the vast majority of patients with epiglottitis are able to maintain their own airway, with humidified supplemental oxygen provided by the least invasive means possible. Even in cases of epiglottitis with significant obstruction, however, these patients can usually be maintained by positive-pressure ventilation by bag and mask while they are being taken to the operating suite or intubated in the ED.

RAPID-SEQUENCE INTUBATION (TABLES 59-6A THROUGH 59-6C)

In most EDs, rapid-sequence intubation is commonly used to ensure that the airway is handled in an efficient, rapid, and atraumatic fashion in both adult and pediatric patients. The goals of rapid sequence intubation are:

Rapid airway control with minimal physical and psychological trauma
Prevention of regurgitation and aspiration
Prevention of rises in intracranial pressure in head-injured or ischemic patients

The technique itself consists of using a muscle relaxant to induce paralysis and cricoid pressure to prevent

TABLE 59-6A. RAPID SEQUENCE INTUBATION: PARALYZING AGENTS

Agent	Mechanism	Dose	Onset	Duration
Succinylcholine	Depolarizing	1.5 mg/kg	1–2 min	7–8 min
Vecuronium	Nondepolarizing*	0.15 mg/kg	1½–2 min	25–60 min
Pancuronium	Nondepolarizing*	0.1–0.15 mg/kg	1–5 min	30–80 min

* Nondepolarizing agents can be reversed with edrophonium, 0.5–1.0 mg/kg.

TABLE 59–6B. RAPID SEQUENCE INTUBATION: ADJUNCTIVE AGENTS

Agent	Mechanism	Dose	Comments
Thiopental	Sedative–barbiturate	2–4 mg/kg IV	Potential myocardial depression, hypotension
Etomidate	Sedative–imidazole	0.3 mg/kg IV	No cardiovascular side effects
Fentanyl	Synthetic narcotic High Potency	0.5–5 mg/kg slow IV	Respiratory depression Not ideal for rapid sequence Reversible with naloxone
Diazepam	Benzodiazepine	0.3 mg/kg IV	Less frequent cardiovascular effects than barbiturates
Midazolam	Benzodiazepine	0.1–0.2 mg/kg IV	Less frequent cardiovascular effects than barbiturates
Ketamine	Dissociative anesthetic	1–4 mg/kg IM	Raised intraocular, intracranial pressure Increased secretions Not ideal for rapid sequence
Atropine	Vagolytic	0.01–0.03 mg/kg IV	Decreases secretions
Lidocaine	Decreases ICP	1 mg/kg IV	Pretreatment on head-injured patients

TABLE 59-6C. MEDICATIONS FOR RAPID SEQUENCE INTUBATION

	Option 1 (Elective)	Option 2 (Elective)	Option 3 (Crash)
Vagolytic	Atropine	Atropine	
Sedation/amnesia	Thiopental	Etomidate	
Neuromuscular blockade	Succinylcholine or vecuronium	Succinylcholine or vecuronium	Succinylcholine or vecuronium

regurgitation (Sellick's maneuver).[16] In many cases, additional adjunctive agents are used to perform rapid-sequence intubation. These include sedatives to produce unconsciousness, vagolytic agents to decrease airway secretions, and lidocaine to decrease intracranial pressure. In many cases, however, the need for *immediate* control of the airway is such that a muscle relaxant to paralyze the patient is the only pharmacologic intervention possible. Nonetheless, the use of additional adjunctive agents is discussed in this section.

Two caveats are critical to remember throughout this procedure. First, it must be assumed that the patient has a full stomach and that aspiration is imminent unless adequate precautions are taken. Both nasogastric intubation and aspiration of gastric air, secretions, and particulate matter should be undertaken whenever possible. Sellick's maneuver, consisting of firm cricoid pressure with additional pressure lateral to the larynx against the spinal column, may prevent regurgitation and aspiration and should be used whenever rapid sequence intubation is performed. Care should be taken to avoid occluding the carotid arteries during this procedure, and the maneuver should be released if the patient is actively vomiting, to avoid tears of the esophagus. Second, in patients with suspicion of or clear evidence of cervical spine injury, the pharmacologic paralysis induced during this procedure relaxes the physical splinting offered by cervical muscular spasm and therefore extreme caution should be used to maintain adequate in-line cervical immobilization during this procedure. Because of these factors, rapid-sequence intubation always involves at least a two-rescuer approach. Ideally, three rescuers are used: one to intubate the patient, one to maintain cervical immobilization, and one to apply Sellick's maneuver.

MUSCLE RELAXANTS FOR INTUBATION

In selecting an agent to induce paralysis for rapid-sequence intubation, such agents should ideally have rapid onset and short duration, be reversible, and have the fewest possible side effects. Such agents may be either depolarizing or nondepolarizing muscle relaxants. The muscle relaxant with which there has been the most experience in the ED setting is succinylcholine, a depolarizing muscle relaxant, which acts by combining with the neuromuscular endplate, producing widespread fasciculation that proceeds predictably.[17] These fasciculations begin over the chest and abdomen, proceed to the neck, arm, and leg, and are followed by facial, pharyngeal, and laryngeal fasciculations. Finally, the intercostal and diaphragmatic muscles fasciculate before complete paralysis. Succinylcholine's onset of action occurs at approximately 1 minute and peaks at $1\frac{1}{2}$ to 2 minutes with a duration of action of approximately 7 to 8 minutes. To induce paralysis, a dose of 1 to 1.5 mg per kg should be given.[18]

There are several potential problems with neuromuscular blockade by means of succinylcholine. This drug causes a rise in intraocular, intragastric, and intracranial pressure, although it is not contraindicated in head-injured patients. Because of the rise in intraocular pressure seen with succinylcholine, it should never be used in penetrating eye injuries. With use of a prophylactic nasogastric tube and Sellick's maneuver (cricoid pressure), the rise in intragastric pressure (presumably caused by fasciculations of the gastric smooth muscle) can be obviated. Although succinylcholine does cause a brief and transient rise in intracranial pressure, it is still commonly used in rapid sequence intubation in patients with severe head injuries.[19] Succinylcholine should not be given in patients with neuromuscular diseases, crush injuries, paraplegia, or burns of more than one week's duration. Nonetheless, the drug can be safely used in patients immediately after the onset of either burns or spinal cord injury. Although bradycardia and excessive bronchial secretions have been reported with succinylcholine, this can be prevented by premedicating the patient with atropine.

The nondepolarizing muscle relaxants include pancuronium, vecuronium, and atracurium. Atracurium, however, has been shown to cause significant histamine release, resulting in profound hypotension, and is rarely used in either the ED or the operating suite.[20] Vecuronium has an intermediate onset and duration. Onset times vary from 90 seconds to 2 minutes, with a duration of action of 25 to 60 minutes. There are few cardiovascular side effects with this drug, and it has a low risk for histamine release. Because it is a nondepolarizing muscle relaxant, it is reversible with cho-

linergic agonists such as edrophonium. Vecuronium is available only as a powder, and must be reconstituted at the time of use, although it does not have to be refrigerated, as does the preconstituted form of succinylcholine.[21]

Pancuronium bromide is a longer-acting nondepolarizing agent with an onset of action from 1 to 5 minutes and a duration from 30 to 80 minutes.[22] The prolonged paralysis produced by the drug limits its usefulness in the immediate airway control of the pediatric patient in the emergency department, particularly when ongoing neurologic examinations must be performed. It is primarily used in those patients in whom succinylcholine or vecuronium is contraindicated, intubated patients who are fighting the ventilator, or patients requiring computed tomographic (CT) scans in whom patient movement is a problem and prolonged duration of action is not a problem.

Selection of a muscle relaxant depends on the individual patient's needs, as well as the experience of the physician with each of the drugs. In most cases, immediate airway control can be easily provided with either succinylcholine or vecuronium. By far the most experience has been with succinylcholine, and the list of potential complications, although extensive, has been shown to be infrequent in practical experience. For this reason, as well as its rapid onset and short duration, it is a common choice among experienced emergency physicians providing rapid sequence intubation. Because of its potential side effects, however, an increasing number of physicians have used vecuronium, even though it must be constituted at the time of its use. Because it does not need to be refrigerated, it is often used by helicopter flight crews for rapid-sequence intubation. The side effects with this agent are extremely limited, and it is likely to see increasing use as emergency physicians become more familiar with it. Pancuronium bromide is usually given only to patients in whom long-term paralysis for airway control is indicated. In most cases, this limits its usefulness in the ED.

ADJUNCTIVE MEDICATIONS FOR INTUBATION

When elective intubation is performed in the operating suite, it is common for the anesthesiologist to use some form of sedative agent to induce unconsciousness. These agents should ideally have a rapid onset, short duration, and limited side effects. The most commonly used agent is *thiopental*, a short-acting barbiturate with an onset of action in 10 to 20 seconds. Thiopental may reduce intracranial pressure and has the potential of decreasing metabolic and oxygen demands. In addition, like all barbiturates, it may cause hypotension from myocardial depression and peripheral vasodilation.[23] For this reason, its usefulness in the ED is somewhat limited because many patients needing emergency airway control also have some element of cardiovascular instability. It is also important to remember that thiopental is an extremely poor analgesic and therefore does not ensure that the patient will be pain-free during procedures.

An excellent alternative to thiopental is *etomidate,* imidazole derivative that rapidly produces unconsciousness. A dose of 0.3 mg per kg is well tolerated, even in patients with potential cardiovascular instability. There are minimal side effects from this agent and it has become popular with pediatric anesthesiologists and pediatric emergency physicians.[24]

Fentanyl is a short-acting, synthetic narcotic analgesic, with a high degree of potency. The duration of action varies from 30 minutes to approximately $3\frac{1}{2}$ hours, depending on the dose given. Compared with morphine sulphate, it produces less hypotension, hypertension, and less complete amnesia. Fentanyl does produce postrespiratory depression, and may not be the ideal agent for induction of unconsciousness during rapid sequence intubation.[25]

Both *diazepam* and *midazolam* are benzodiazepine derivatives producing sedation of somewhat slower onset than the previously mentioned agents. Although cardiovascular and respiratory side effects are infrequent compared with barbiturates, the degree of unconsciousness produced is somewhat irregular. Midazolam produces a faster onset of unconsciousness and a shorter duration of action, and is also considerably more amnestic. Although it has not been widely used, it may have a role in rapid-sequence intubation.

Ketamine is a highly disassociative anesthetic that produces rapid sedation and amnesia. In patients with documented hypovolemia, it causes a mild increase in systemic blood pressure through its sympathomimetic action. It also, however, produces intracranial pressure elevation, intraocular pressure elevation, and may produce excessive airway secretions. Because of its disassociative effects, it is usually not the agent of choice in awake and alert patients. Because it causes excessive secretions, premedication with atropine is recommended.[26]

Atropine is a vagolytic agent familiar to all emergency physicians, which is useful in blocking vagal stimulation during laryngoscopy. This helps prevent bradycardia and excessive secretions; however, to be effective, it must be given several minutes before the induction of muscle relaxation.

Given this armamentarium of agents, what is the most effective way to proceed with rapid sequence intubation? To begin with, the emergency physician should use the agents with which he or she has attained the most familiarity. Numerous agents can be used, in various different combinations. It is generally important to be able to induce muscle relaxation in an extremely rapid fashion, without dependence on adjunctive agents to produce unconsciousness or decrease secretions. Because of the nature of pediatric emergency medicine, there is often simply no time to do a semi-elective rapid sequence intubation, and it truly becomes a situation in which it is a crash induction. Under these circumstances, either succinylcholine or vercuronium is a reasonable alternative.

Because succinylcholine can be preconstituted in a refrigerated form, it is often the agent of choice in many EDs because it is a simple matter to draw it up and give it by intravenous push. Nonetheless, vecuronium is also a reasonable choice under such circumstances, provided that the nurses are adequately instructed in reconstituting the solution in a rapid and timely fashion. (See Tables 59-6A through 59-6C.)

It is also critical to ensure that not only the emergency physicians, but the respiratory therapists and nurses in the ED are familiar with performing Sellick's maneuver to prevent regurgitation and aspiration. All of the details of emergency airway management in children should be discussed in educational programs for the ED staff.

Under circumstances in which time allows a semi-elective rapid-sequence intubation, thiopental, etomidate, or other agents may be helpful in inducing unconsciousness. In a patient with status asthmaticus, in whom intubation is required because of impending respiratory failure, it is important to render the patient unconscious before intubation. In such circumstances, etomidate, ketamine, diazepam, and midazolam are reasonable alternatives because thiopental is contraindicated in status asthmaticus. If there is time to produce unconsciousness by any of the mentioned agents, it is also reasonable to assume that the patient may be pretreated with atropine also. In addition, patients with severe head injuries in whom intracranial pressure may be elevated may be treated with lidocaine in a dose of 1 mg per kg to attempt to help prevent rises in intracranial pressure and decrease the incidence of laryngospasm. This agent, however, must be given 3 to 5 minutes before airway manipulation to have its maximum effect.

Regardless of what agents are chosen to provide rapid sequence intubation, it is essential that the patient be effectively preoxygenated and suctioned before any attempt at airway manipulation. Although all EDs caring for ill or injured children should be capable of providing rapid-sequence intubation, effective instruction should be given to all staff members to ensure that they are familiar with this technique and the need for maintenance of appropriate maneuvers during airway manipulation.

SURGICAL MANAGEMENT OF THE AIRWAY

In rare circumstances, children may have direct injury to the larynx or trachea as a result of bicycle accidents, snowmobiling accidents, or simply running into a fixed object that strikes them in the larynx. These injuries, however, are unusual in children, rendering cricothyroidotomy or tracheostomy a rare necessity. Tracheostomy *per se* has no place in the ED, and should be performed only as an elective procedure by personnel trained and experienced in pediatric surgical airway management. The dictum "Ventilate—don't operate!" applies best to children.[27] Almost all children can be adequately ventilated and oxygenated without surgical intervention of any type. In rare patients with direct laryngeal injury, the preferred surgical method for airway control is needle cricothyroidotomy, which can provide up to 30 minutes of airway control when used with jet ventilation.

Needle cricothyroidotomy should be performed with the patient's head in a neutral position with adequate in-line cervical immobilization. After preparing the neck with antiseptic solution, one finger should be used to palpate the cricothyroid membrane in the midline, between the thyroid and the cricoid cartilage. It is critical to stay precisely in the midline during this procedure to ensure that the airway is appropriately cannulated and significant bleeding is avoided. An assistant should always be present to hold the child's head and neck and facilitate this midline position. Once the cricothyroid membrane has been identified, a 10 cc syringe should be attached to a large, 14 gauge catheter. While palpating the cricothyroid cartilage in the midline, the rescuer should insert a catheter just below the midpoint of the cricothyroid membrane, with a needle angled 45 degrees caudally. Rapid aspiration of air into the syringe indicates entry into the tracheal lumen. The stylet should be carefully withdrawn while the plastic catheter is advanced caudally into the trachea, taking care not to perforate the posterior tracheal wall. The position of the catheter should be rechecked by aspirating on the syringe. The hub of the catheter should be attached to a 3.5 millimeter pediatric endotracheal tube adapter. Bag ventilation can be delivered by this means or by connecting a high-flow oxygen source with a wide connector between the oxygen and cannula. Intermittent ventilation can be delivered by occluding the open port of the wide connector with the thumb. This technique allows 30 to 45 minutes of airway control under duress, and an additional 14-gauge needle may be placed adjacent to the initial one to allow for venting of the airway and blowing off carbon dioxide.

Surgical cricothyroidotomy should not be performed in children. In addition, it should be re-emphasized that needle cricothyroidotomy is also a procedure that is rarely indicated in children.[28]

PREHOSPITAL CARE

The most important aspect of prehospital care of the pediatric patient is to ensure that all prehospital care providers are adequately instructed in assessment of the pediatric airway, as well as bag-and-mask ventilation. Although endotracheal intubation of children is an important skill for paramedics, it is too often the case that prehospital care providers are not adequately trained in assessment and initial management of the airway bag and mask ventilation.

Nonetheless, paramedics can be taught to intubate children easily, assuming that the precepts of pediatric airway management mentioned in this chapter are followed carefully. In fact, endotracheal intubation of pediatric patients is in many respects simpler than in combative adult patients. In cases in which endotracheal intubation is performed in pediatric patients, paramedics should be cautioned regarding the ease of dislodgement of the tube and its placement into the right main stem bronchus. Caution should also be taken in ensuring that the patient is not given excessive airway pressures because this may convert a pneumothorax to a tension pneumothorax in a child.

HORIZONS

The use of length-based resuscitation equipment should help ensure that children have the appropriate-sized equipment and medication dosages. As this technique becomes more widespread, there will be increasing standardization of appropriate care to children. In addition, it is quite likely that additional helpful agents and pharmacologic manipulation of the children before airway control will be developed. For example, more specific muscle relaxants with fewer side effects and easier reconstitution will probably be available over the next 5 to 10 years. In addition, as experience increases with agents such as etomidate and midazolam, it is likely that they will have more widespread ED usage.

See Addenda for Chapter 59 (pp. 3361–3362) for illustrations.

REFERENCES

1. Mayer, T.: Emergency Management of Pediatric Trauma. Philadelphia, W.B. Saunders Company, 1985.
2. Mayer, T.: Initial evaluation and management of the injured child. *In* Emergency Management of Pediatric Trauma. Edited by Mayer, T. Philadelphia, W.B. Saunders Company, 1985.
3. Cohen, D.E., and Broennle, A.M.: Emergency department anesthetic management. *In* Textbook of Pediatric Emergency Medicine. 2nd ed. Edited by Fleisher, G.R., and Ludwig, S.L. Baltimore, Williams & Wilkins, 1988, pp. 53–65.
4. Backofen, J.E., and Roger, M.C.: Emergency management of the airway. *In* Textbook of Pediatric Intensive Care. Edited by Roger, M.C. Baltimore, Williams & Wilkins, 1987.
5. Steuart, R.D.: Endotracheal Intubation. *In* Current Therapy in Emergency Medicine. Edited by Hallaham, M.L. Toronto, B.C. Decker, 1987, pp. 11–21.
6. Kulick, R.M.: Pulse Oximetry. Pediatr. Emerg. Care, 3:127, 1987.
7. Hedges, J.R., Amsterdam, J.T., Cionni, D.J., et al.: Oxygen saturation as a marker for admission or relapse with acute bronchospasm. Am. J. Emerg. Med. 5:196, 1987.
8. Bushore, M., Fleisher, G., Siedel, J., and Wagner, D.: Advanced Pediatric Life Support Course. Dallas, American College of Emergency Physicians, 1990.
9. American College of Surgeons-Committee on Trauma: Advanced Trauma Life Support Course. Chicago, American College of Surgeons, 1988.
10. Yamamoto, L.G., Yim, G.K., and Britten, A.G.: Rapid sequence anesthesia induction for emergency intubation. Pediatr. Emerg. Care 6:200, 1990.

11. Stoetling, R.K.: Endotracheal Intubation. *In* Anesthesia, 2nd ed. Edited by Miller, R.D. New York, Churchill Livingstone, 1986, 523–552.
12. Pang, D., and Wilberger, F.: Spinal cord injury without radiographic abnormality in children. J. Neurosurg. *57*:114, 1982.
13. Dripps, R.D., Echenhoff, J.E., and Vandam, L.D. (eds): Introduction to Anesthesia: The Principles of Safe Practice. Philadelphia, W.B. Saunders Company, 1988, p. 190.
14. Weiskoph, R.B., and Fairley, H.B.: Anesthesia for major trauma. Surg. Clin. North Am. *62*:31, 1982.
15. Gennarelli, T.A.: Emergency department management of head injuries. Emerg. Med. Clin. North Am. *2*:749, 1984.
16. Sellick, B.A.: Cricoid pressure to control regurgitation of stomach contents during induction of anesthesia. Lancet 2:404, 1961.
17. Roberts, D.J., Clinton, J.E., and Ruiz, E.: Neuromuscular blockade for critical patients in the Emergency Department. Ann. Emerg. Med. *15*:152, 1986.
18. Thompson, J.D., Fish, S., and Ruiz, E.: Succinylcholine for endotracheal intubation. Ann. Emerg. Med. 1982; *11*:526, 1982.
19. Minton, M.D., Grosslight, K., Stirt, J.A., et al.: Increases in intracranial pressure from succinylcholine: Prevention by prior non-depolarizing blockade. Anesthesiology *65*:165, 1986.
20. Lennon, R.L., Olson, R.A., and Gronert, G.A.: Atracurium or vecuronium for rapid sequence endotracheal intubation. Anesthesiology *64*:510, 1986.
21. Casson, W.R., and Jones, R.M.: Vecuronium induced neuromuscular blockade: The effect of increasing dose on speed of onset. Anesthesia *41*:354, 1986.
22. Shanks, C.A.: What's new in skeletal muscular relaxants and their antagonists? Anesth. Clin. North Am. *6*:335, 1988.
23. Hudson, R.J., Stanski, D.R., and Burch, P.G.: Pharmacokinetics of methohexital and thiopental in surgical patients. Anesthesiology *59*:215, 1983.
24. Capan, L.M., Miller, S.M., and Turnborg, H. (eds.): Trauma Anesthesia and Intensive Care. Philadelphia, J. B. Lippincott, 1991.
25. Shudnofsky, C.R., Wright, S.W., Dronen, S.C., et al.: The safety of fentanyl use in the Emergency Department. Ann Emerg. Med. *18*:635, 1989.
26. White, P.F., Way, W.L., and Trevor, A.J.: Ketamine—Its pharmacology and therapeutic uses. Anesthesiology *56*:119, 1982.
27. Mayer, T.: Initial Evaluation and Management of the Injured Child. *In* Emergency Management of Pediatric Trauma. Edited by Mayer, T. Philadelphia, W.B. Saunders Company, 1985.
28. Mayer, T.A.: Emergency Pediatric Tracheostomy: A technique in search of an indication. Ann. Emerg. Med. *16*:606, 1987.

PEDIATRIC CARDIOPULMONARY RESUSCITATION

Paula Fink

CAPSULE

A child in severe cardiopulmonary distress presenting to an emergency physician can provoke panic in an otherwise prepared and organized emergency department (ED). This chapter includes guidelines and protocols to help the practitioner adequately approach, diagnose, and treat the child in "in extremis." The differences between adult and pediatric resuscitation and the general causes of pediatric cardiopulmonary arrests are reviewed.

INTRODUCTION

A common misconception is that children are "just little adults," and this fallacy can be evident in emergent cardiopulmonary resuscitation. Adults commonly have primary cardiac arrest secondary to coronary artery disease, whereas children have cardiac arrest secondary to respiratory failure. Pediatric respiratory failure can be from such varied causes as airway obstruction, primary pulmonary failure, or septic shock.

The size differences in children make a big difference in medication doses, whereas they make a minimal difference in adults. Doses must be determined by weight rather than by standard size or age. Some approximation may be necessary, though, in estimating the child's weight when only the age is known (Table 59-8), or the "length-based" system (Broselow) may be used. The pharmacologic differences in children also need special consideration because, for example, hepatic function may not be optimal at certain ages. Size and age differences also directly affect the cardiac compression rate and the ventilation volume and rate. (See Addenda, Fig. 59A–6.)

CLINICAL PRESENTATION AND EXAMINATION

The presentation of a child in frank cardiopulmonary arrest is obvious; however, the child in impending arrest may have a more confusing clinical presentation. With the exception of trauma and a few other catastrophic events, cardiopulmonary arrest in children is not sudden but is usually the result of a progressive deterioration of the respiratory and circulatory systems. Unlike cardiac arrest in adults, it is usually preceded by respiratory failure. The key to preventing arrest is in recognizing the signs and symptoms of respiratory distress in a child and intervening to stop the progression to cardiopulmonary failure.

TABLE 59-8. ESTIMATED WEIGHT (KG) BY AGE	
Newborn	3
1 month	4
3 months	5.5
6 months	7.0
1 year	10.0
2 years	12.0
3 years	14.0
4 years	16.0
5 years	18.0
6 years	20.0
7 years	22.0
8 years	25.0
9 years	28.0
10 years	34.0

HISTORY

The history of the illness is paramount in diagnosis and treatment, and should be tailored to the specific age of the patient.

INFANT

An infant can deteriorate rapidly within 8 hours, and the pertinent history should reflect this short time course. Feeding patterns should be determined. Did the child refuse to drink? What has he been fed: formula or water? Has he been given honey or any "home remedies"? What medications is the child taking? Has he been irritable, vomiting, or febrile? The past medical history, though short, is also important. The perinatal history regarding the gestational age at birth and the length of time the child needed to stay in the hospital after birth is valuable information. Did the child require advanced medical care after birth? A family history is important in specific areas. Has there been a sudden infant death syndrome (SIDS) victim in the family? Are there any congenital illnesses or syndromes in the family, including sickle cell disease, Down syndrome, or congenital heart disease? Is anyone in the family currently ill or hospitalized?

CHILDREN

The specific concerns of the toddler and young child's history address the fact that this age group has mobility but minimal judgment. Information concerning possible toxins and exposures can hold the key to the cause of cardiopulmonary arrest. Drowning and near-drowning are a major cause of arrest at this age, and the time under water, water temperature, and the care given at the scene are important information that can help in the approach to treatment of the arrest. Again, a past medical history may be helpful in treating or evaluating an arrest. A child with a history of asthma

on chronic steroids has a different response to stress than a previously healthy child.

ADOLESCENTS

Trauma is the major cause of death in adolescents, primarily from automobile accidents. The history surrounding the accident is of vital importance because mechanisms of injury increase the suspicion of certain internal or neurologic injuries. Adolescents, in their assertion of independence, may not tell the examiner details about ingestions or illicit drug use, and the examiner should consider obtaining drug screens. Offering privacy and confidentiality often helps to develop a rapport with a teenager and supply the physician with valuable information.

CLINICAL PRESENTATION

Shock, or imminent shock, in infants and children has certain clinical features. Defined at the cellular level as the failure to deliver adequate substrates to and remove waste from the cell, shock can result from many conditions. Usually, in children, it is the direct result of inadequate oxygenation of vital organs. The clinical manifestations of hypoxia begin subtly with air hunger and increased respiratory and heart rate. The child then exhibits lethargy, a decreasing level of consciousness, and confusion. The skin becomes peripherally cyanotic, then progresses to central cyanosis, mottling, and prolonged capillary refill. If the condition remains unchecked, there is further deterioration, with bradycardia, apnea, hypotension, and finally asystole and death. Because of the poor glucose stores in infants and children, hypoglycemia secondary to sepsis and stress can also cause deterioration and eventual cardiopulmonary arrest. Like hypoxia, hypoglycemia has a profound effect on the central nervous system (CNS), producing confusion, lethargy, and progression to coma.

Pure circulatory failure without respiratory failure is uncommon but can be seen in some patients with cardiac abnormalities. In this case, the patient may have a rapid heart rate but be hypotensive.

Respiratory failure can also be caused by the mechanical obstruction of the airway by foreign body aspiration, epiglottitis, or croup, but, if appreciated early, this type of respiratory arrest can be avoided.

LABORATORY TESTS

Laboratory values, with a few exceptions, are usually not helpful in the diagnosis of cardiopulmonary arrest because of the delay in getting the results and the blatant physical signs of the patient. A few "bedside" tests can be performed that can affect treatment. The dextrostick glucose level, which can be obtained in 2 minutes, is of great value in diagnosing hypoglycemic seizures, DKA, and complications of ethanol ingestions. The pulse oximetry monitor has improved pediatric acute care, but is useless in patients with hypotension or poor digital perfusion. The dipstick urinalysis can detect hematuria or ketonuria. A tabletop hematocrit centrifuge allows for a fast estimate of circulating red cell mass. Occult blood testing of the feces in the rectum can also inform the physician of gastrointestinal bleeding. Emergent laboratory values to obtain and have run "stat" include an arterial blood gas, complete blood count, blood glucose, and electrolytes. Appropriate drug levels and toxicologic screens should be drawn. Emergent radiographs of the cervical spine in trauma and chest are of great value as long as they can be obtained without obstructing the care of the patient and are of good quality.

INITIAL STABILIZATION

In 1966, the National Academy of Sciences-National Research Council, with the encouragement of the professional medical community and the lay public, recommended training health care givers in cardiopulmonary resuscitation (CPR) according to the standards set up by the American Heart Association (AHA). It was recommended that basic life support (BLS) be taught to the lay public in 1973, and the first advanced cardiac life support (ACLS) course was taught by the AHA in 1975. Little instruction in these courses was directed toward the resuscitation of infants or children. Because of this oversight, an outcry from pediatric care givers was heard, and in 1985 the National Conference revised the standards for pediatric BLS, neonatal resuscitation and, developed pediatric advanced life support (ALS) guidelines. The protocols in Figures 59-9 and 59-10 are based on guidelines that have evolved from this conference.

SEQUENCE OF CARDIOPULMONARY RESUSCITATION

Impending cardiopulmonary arrest symptoms, as described in the previous part of this chapter, can identify a child as being in need of emergent supportive care, but CPR should not be instituted until unresponsiveness is demonstrated (Table 59-9). The level of consciousness can be determined by gently shaking the child, being careful to keep the head and neck aligned in case of cervical injury. If there is no response to touch or verbal stimulus, one must assume that the victim is unconscious, and an assessment of the airway, breathing, and circulation should be done with speed and accuracy.

PROTOCOL FOR BRADYCARDIA

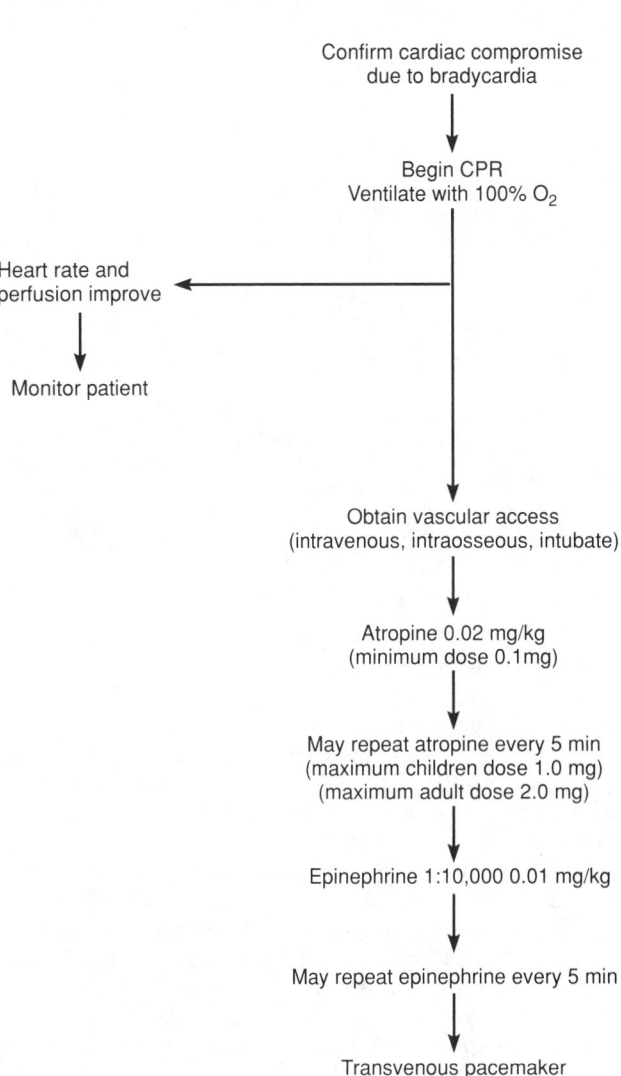

FIG. 59-9.   Protocol for bradycardia.

AIRWAY

Please refer to the section on pediatric airway management for a detailed discussion of this topic. The simplest solution to cardiopulmonary distress caused by an obstructed airway is to remove the obstruction. In pediatrics, this is especially important because most pediatric arrests are the result of respiratory compromise. Often the obstruction is caused by the tongue falling back and blocking the oropharynx. Positioning the patient to open the airway is the first procedure to be performed. If trauma is known to be the cause of the arrest, or the mode of injury is not known, manual in-line cervical immobilization must to be maintained until the neck is stabilized. If the mode of injury is known *not* to involve trauma, "head tilt" without hyperextension of the neck can open the airway.

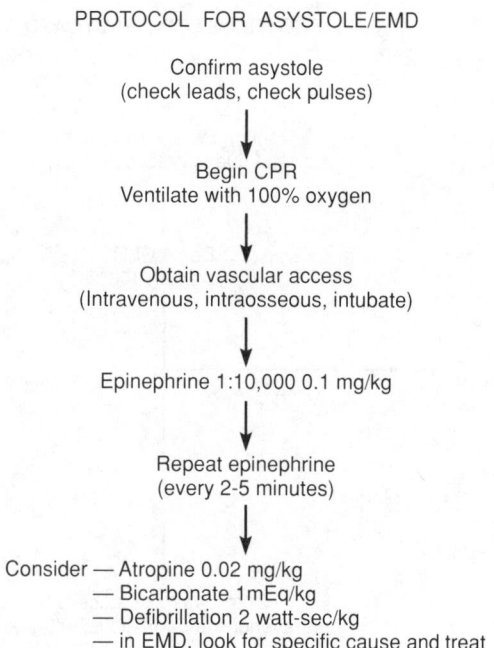

PROTOCOL FOR ASYSTOLE/EMD

Confirm asystole
(check leads, check pulses)

↓

Begin CPR
Ventilate with 100% oxygen

↓

Obtain vascular access
(Intravenous, intraosseous, intubate)

↓

Epinephrine 1:10,000 0.1 mg/kg

↓

Repeat epinephrine
(every 2-5 minutes)

↓

Consider — Atropine 0.02 mg/kg
— Bicarbonate 1mEq/kg
— Defibrillation 2 watt-sec/kg
— in EMD, look for specific cause and treat

FIG. 59-10. Protocol for asystole/EMD.

BREATHING

If the victim does not respond with spontaneous breathing, artificial respirations must be started. In the field, mouth-to-mouth ventilation is appropriate. In a health care facility, the rescuer should use bag-mask equipment supplying 100% oxygen. Pocket masks have been a boon to resuscitation, allowing the rescuer to be protected from communicable diseases while still being able to supply emergent ventilations to patients, but masks must be appropriate for the facial size of the patient.

The first assisted ventilations should be two slow breaths to allow the rescuer to assess the patency of the airway, determine the pressure required to raise the chest of the victim, and oxygenate the victim. If the chest does not rise, the rescuer should reposition the airway and repeat the ventilations. If this still does not allow good ventilation, obstruction secondary to a foreign body should be suspected.

Ninety percent of deaths from aspiration occur in children younger than 5 years, and the most commonly aspirated material is food. Airway obstruction from a foreign body should be suspected in infants and children who exhibit a sudden onset of respiratory distress. Unconscious patients who are difficult to ventilate or cannot be ventilated should be evaluated for foreign-body airway obstruction. Aid to the conscious patient with foreign-body aspiration may be attempted if the measures the patient is using to relieve the obstruction are ineffective or respiratory fatigue is evident.

Relief of airway obstruction in an infant can be attempted by holding the infant straddling the rescuers arm, lying on its abdomen, and the rescuer supporting the infant's head with one hand, holding the head lower than the body. The rescuer then delivers four forceful blows to the back between the shoulder blades with the heel of the hand. If the obstruction is not relieved, the child is turned over and placed between the rescuer's arm supporting the infant's head, neck, and back and the opposite hand placed on the infant's chest. Four chest thrusts are delivered in the same position as CPR chest compressions but at a slower rate. These maneuvers are repeated with frequent assessment of airway patency until the obstruction is relieved. Subdiaphragmatic abdominal thrusts (Heimlich maneuver) may be used for older children with choking or airway obstruction. Please refer to the subchapter on pediatric airway management for details.

The rate of respiration depends on the age of the child and the cause of the arrest. The normal rate of respiration in infants is 20 to 24 breaths per minute; in children it is 16 to 20 breaths per minute; and in adolescents and adults it is 12 to 16 breaths per minute. If the cause of the arrest is respiratory failure and it is likely that the victim has accumulated carbon dioxide, or is thought to have increased intracranial pressure, the patient should be hyperventilated.

CIRCULATION

After airway and breathing have been established, the absence of cardiac contractions or their efficacy must be evaluated. In an infant, the precordial impulse can often be felt on the chest, but without peripheral pulses, the circulation is ineffective. Pulses easily palpated in an infant or young child are the brachial or femoral arteries because the carotid is often obscured by fat. In older children and adults, the carotid is the best pulse to use to determine adequate circulation. Hypothermia, cyanotic heart disease, and methemoglobinemia can produce an ashen color in a patient with adequate circulation. Poor peripheral circulation as indicated by an ashen color and cyanosis can be misleading, and CPR should not be started if the patient has strong pulses but poor color.

Without palpable peripheral pulses, external cardiac compressions must accompany the artificial respirations. Before starting CPR, an attempt to get more help should be made. If you are out in the field, emergency medical services should be called, and in a hospital, the cardiac arrest team should be notified.

The infant or young child should be placed on a firm surface and support to the upper thoracic cage

---

TABLE 59-9. SIGNS OF CARDIOPULMONARY ARREST
Patient unresponsive
Agonal respiratory efforts
No organized respiratory motion of the chest wall
No blood pressure
No palpable pulse
Inaudible heart sounds

should be given by a towel to remove dead space and allow for effective compressions.[1] Finger placement for the compressions is just below the intermammary line where it intersects with the sternum. The rescuer should use two to three fingers and compress to a depth of 0.5 to 1 inch at a rate of 100 times per minute. The compressions should be smooth and in a steady rhythm with full release of the pressure on the chest without removing the fingers from the chest so as not to lose the landmarks.

In a child older than 1 year, the heel of the hand is used for compressions. Positioning is found by following the costal margins of the ribs to the sternum; two fingerbreadths above their intersection on the sternum is the position for compressions. Compressions should again be smooth and rhythmic to a depth of 1 to 1.5 inches and a rate of 80 to 100 times per minute.

When the child is older than 8 years or is the size of an adult, adult CPR procedures should be used. The positioning for compressions is the same as in a child, using the heel of the hand and compressing the lower third of the sternum rostral to the xiphoid process. Compressions should be to a depth of 1.5 to 2.0 inches and at a rate of 80 to 100 times per minute.

Coordination with breathing in the infant should be with a minimal pause in compressions at a ratio of five compressions to one breath. In older children, there can be a slight pause at the end of every fifth compression (1 to 1.5 seconds). Evaluation of the child by assessing the pulse and looking for spontaneous breathing should be done every 10 cycles. Refer to Table 59-10 for CPR ventilation and compression rates.

INTRAOSSEOUS (IO) INFUSIONS

Circulatory support often requires fluid administration, and intravenous line placement is often technically difficult and time-consuming. Intraosseous infusions were used extensively in the 1940s and subsequently fell out of favor with improvements in intravascular catheters.[2] The procedure has lately been rediscovered as a means of providing vascular access within the first 5 minutes to pediatric patients with vascular collapse. It has been shown that injections into the bone marrow are absorbed almost immediately into the circulation. The rates of infusion compare favorably with central line delivery and are faster than peripheral intravenous and intratracheal administration.

No medications have been found to be absolutely contraindicated by intraosseous infusion; however, there is a risk of fluid extravasation into the subcutaneous tissue, and medications that can cause tissue damage such as phenytoin, sodium bicarbonate and chemotherapeutic medications should be given with care. Because these lines are usually placed during resuscitation efforts and sterile technique often is not used, infection is a rare but possible complication. Absolute contraindications include osteogenesis imperfecta and an ipsilateral fracture of the bone because of fluid extravasation through the fracture.

TECHNIQUE

The choice of the site of infusion should be made with consideration of the patient's age, size, and illness. Limbs with cellulitis or major burns should be avoided to reduce the chance of infection. As stated above, a broken bone or a bone that had a previous attempt at IO placement should also be avoided. The optimal site in children is the proximal tibia, with the distal tibia and distal femur in infants as other choices. In adults, the sternum is an alternate site, but in children under 3 years the sternal marrow space is thought to be too small. That site may also inhibit chest compressions during resuscitation. Complications from sternal puncture have included mediastinitis, hydrothorax, and injury to the heart. Care must be taken with long bone IO placement to avoid damaging the growth plate by directing the needle away from the growth plate at about 10 to 15 degrees.

Currently, 15 and 18 gauge disposable bone-marrow aspiration needles are available. These should have a stylet to keep the bone cortex from plugging the needle, an adjustable screw guard to vary the needle length, a flange guard to allow the needle to be secured to the skin, and short length to allow for ease in placement. Any bone marrow needle or 18 gauge spinal needle can be used in an emergency.

To place the needle in the proximal tibia, the anteromedial surface of the tibia is sterilely prepared about 1 to 3 cm below the tibial tuberosity (Fig. 59-11). The needle is inserted at an angle of 10 to 15 degrees from vertical slanting away from the growth

TABLE 59-10. CARDIOPULMONARY RESUSCITATION GUIDELINES			
	Ventilation Rate (Breaths per Minute)	Compression Rate (Compressions per Minute)	Depth of Compression (Inches)
Infant (< 1 year)	20 to 24	100 or >	½–1
Child (1 to 8 years)	16 to 20	80–100	1–1½
Adult	12 to 16	80–100	1½–2

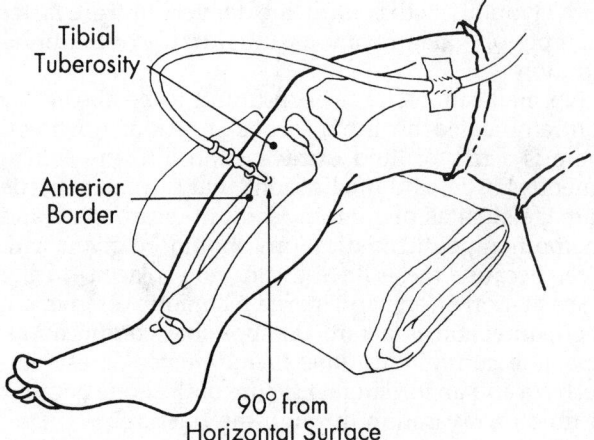

FIG. 59-11. Technique for infusion into proximal tibia.

plate with a boring, rotary motion. If the angle is vertical to the growth plate, the needle has less chance of glancing off the cortex of the bone and missing the marrow. The needle entry into the bone marrow is indicated by a sudden lack of resistance, the upright standing of the needle without support, and the free flow of fluid without extravasation into soft tissue. One may not be able to aspirate bone marrow into the needle because of the narrow gauge of the needle, but the needle should be flushed with saline before attachment to an intravenous line. Once the vascular volume has improved to allow conventional vascular access, the IO should be removed. The longer it is allowed to stay in place, the higher the risk of infection.

POSTARREST CARE

Once the patient has been resuscitated, care must be taken to prevent a recurrent arrest. Specific therapy maintained should reflect the probable cause of the initial arrest. Constant attention to the ABCs of CPR, however, often maintains the patient until transport to an adequate care facility.

Maintaining the airway is paramount, and care in securing the endotracheal tube, if placed, is key. A chest radiograph should be obtained to check for tube placement. Sedation may be needed if the patient is agitated. If the patient appears highly agitated and has good respiratory effort, you may consider extubation, but reintubation may be difficult in the face of airway edema. Ventilation can be continued by bag-mask in the nonbreathing patient, and a ventilator should be considered.

Cardiac perfusion should be constantly monitored by blood pressure and peripheral circulation assessment. Often the postarrest patient has an intravascular fluid deficit and may need volume. The injured heart may not be able to support circulation without a vasopressor like dopamine or dobutamine, and their administration should be considered. If the patient had an arrhythmia, the antiarrhythmic used to correct it may have to be given as a constant infusion.

FLUIDS AND MEDICATIONS

FLUIDS

Cardiopulmonary arrest from hypovolemic shock is common in pediatrics and can result from medical causes or trauma. In the treatment of these conditions, fluid therapy should resemble the fluids lost. Shock from dehydration should be treated with boluses of an isotonic crystalloid solution, shock from hemorrhage should be treated with blood transfusions after an initial crystalloid bolus, and shock from sepsis may be treated with colloids. In an emergent situation, the exact fluid given does not matter as long as it is isotonic.

The initial dose of fluid is 20 mL per kg given as soon as vascular access is obtained and "pushed" in manually by syringe. The patient should then be reassessed for signs of improvement because subsequent boluses may be necessary. A decrease in heart rate, improvement of peripheral circulation or increased level of consciousness are signs of response to fluid therapy. One should be aware that a patient in hypovolemic shock may need a total of 60 mL per kg of fluid to stabilize. Boluses of dextrose-containing fluids should be avoided because hyperglycemia may result and produce an osmotic diuresis.

MEDICATIONS AND DEFIBRILLATION

The following paragraphs describe the differences in dosage and use of resuscitation medications in pediatrics. Please refer to the other sections in the text for the pharmacology of these medications and Table 59-11 for pediatric doses and concentrations.

EPINEPHRINE

Epinephrine is a catecholamine with both alpha- and beta-adrenergic receptor stimulating actions. The alpha action is primarily vasoconstriction and causes a rise in systolic and diastolic blood pressure. Beta action produces an increase in myocardial contractility and heart rate. Epinephrine is indicated for treatment of asystole and electromechanical dissociation (EMD), and to render the heart more susceptible to defibrillation.

Infants and children seem to be sensitive to epinephrine, and it is safe, with few side effects. The current recommended dose is 0.01 mg per kg of a 1:10,000 solution. This can be given intravenously, intraosseously, or intratracheally. Often a child with hypotension responds to epinephrine, and administration as an infusion is indicated. The infusion rate for this is 1 μg per kg per minute, increasing as nec-

TABLE 59 11 PEDIATRIC CARDIOPULMONARY ARREST MEDICATIONS

Drug	Dose	Concentrations
Epinephrine hydrochloride	0.01 mg/kg 0.1 mL/kg	1:10,000 (0.1 mg/mL)
Sodium bicarbonate	1 mEq/kg 1 mL/kg	1 mEq/mL (84% soln)
Atropine sulfate	0.02 mg/kg 0.2 mL/kg Minimum dose of 0.1 mg(1 mL) Maximum dose: infants and children = 1.0 mg; adolescents 2.0 mg	0.1 mg/mL
Glucose	0.5–1.0 g/kg	0.5 g/mL D$_{50}$W 0.25 g/mL D$_{25}$W
Lidocaine hydrochloride	1 mg/kg	10 mg/mL (1%) 20 mg/mL (2%)
Bretylium tosylate	5 mg/kg	50 mg/mL
Infusions		
Epinephrine infusion	0.1–1.0 μg/kg/min	1 mg/mL 1:1,000
Dopamine hydrochloride infusion	10–20 μg/kg/min	40 mg/mL
Isoproterenol infusion	0.1–1.0 μg/kg/min	1 mg/5 mL
Lidocaine infusion	20–50 μg/kg/min	40 mg/mL (4%)

essary. Work has been done on using higher doses of epinephrine in arrest situations; 0.2 mg per kg is the dose suggested.[3] Currently no optimal dose has been determined for use in pediatric arrests, and until it is determined, 0.01 mg per kg is the suggested dose.

SODIUM BICARBONATE

Retention of carbon dioxide results from respiratory arrest and causes respiratory acidosis. This can best be treated with adequate ventilation. If the arrest is allowed to continue with lack of circulation, cell death occurs, producing lactic acid, which results in a metabolic acidosis. Sodium bicarbonate can correct this acidosis by combining with hydrogen to form carbon dioxide, which can be eliminated by ventilation.

When the circumstances surrounding the arrest indicate metabolic acidosis (a long period of inadequate ventilation or prolonged arrest), the administration of sodium bicarbonate is indicated as guided by arterial blood gas results. The indiscriminate use of bicarbonate may cause hypernatremia or a metabolic alkalosis, and large boluses of bicarbonate infused into the central circulation of infants can produce a hyperosmolar state that can cause intraventricular hemorrhage.

If there is clinical indication of a metabolic acidosis or if the blood gas shows a metabolic acidosis, the use of bicarbonate is indicated. The dose is 1 to 2 mEq per kg. Calcium salts precipitate out if given with bicarbonate, and catecholamines are inactivated if given with them. Being hyperosmolar, sodium bicarbonate can sclerose small veins and cause chemical burns if it extravasates into subcutaneous tissue. Therefore it cannot be given intratracheally.

ATROPINE

Atropine is a parasympatholytic drug with central and peripheral actions. Its central action is to stimulate the medullary vagal nucleus and, with low doses of atropine, this produces bradycardia. The peripheral effects of blocking the vagal nerve and increasing the heart rate are desired when giving atropine. Low doses should be avoided to avoid the paradoxic bradycardia. Atropine should be given at a dose of 0.02 mg per kg, with a minimum dose of 0.2 mg. The maximum total dose for a child is 1.0 mg, and that for adolescents and adults is 2.0 mg.

DEFIBRILLATION

The largest possible electrode that will not lose contact with the chest wall but will not touch the other electrode should be used. In small infants, the paddles may be placed on either side of the chest to ensure

TABLE 59-12. CAUSES OF ELECTROMECHANICAL DISSOCIATION (EMD)

Hypovolemia
Acidosis
Cardiac tamponade
Tension pneumothorax

TABLE 59-13. CAUSES OF PEDIATRIC CARDIAC ARREST

Respiratory
Asthma
Laryngotracheobronchitis
Bronchiolitis
Pneumonia
Epiglottitis
Apnea
Mechanical/anatomic obstruction
Foreign body aspiration
Developmental anomalies
Pulmonary edema
Congestive heart failure
ARDS
Aspiration
Metabolic
DKA
BPD
Cystic fibrosis
Gastrointestinal
Gastroesophageal reflux
Swallowing disorders
Congenital malformations of the esophagus
Bowel obstruction
Tracheal fistula
Cardiac
Congenital heart disease
Arrhythmias
Myocarditis
Hematology
Sickle cell disease
Cancer
Neurology
Seizure
Tumor
Acute hydrocephalus
Infectious
Meningitis
Dehydration, hypo/hypernatremic
Septic shock
Toxicologic
Anticholinesterase inhibitors
Infant botulism
Histamine-releasing agents
Trauma
Burns
Hemorrhagic shock
Closed head injury
Bowel perforation
Drowning
Other
SIDS
Prematurity

TABLE 59-14. EPIDEMIOLOGIC FACTORS ASSOCIATED WITH SIDS

Low birth weight
Prematurity
Low Apgar scores
Recent viral illness (especially RSV)
Young maternal age
Unmarried status of mother
Low maternal education level
Inadequate prenatal care
Maternal smoking during pregnancy
Maternal use of addictive drugs

TABLE 59-15. HIGH-RISK GROUPS FOR SIDS

Apparent life-threatening event survivors
Siblings of SIDS victims
Premature infants
Infants of drug-dependent mothers

is not successful, the voltage should be doubled and the shock repeated. If there is no response again, CPR should be continued and the patient evaluated for adequacy of oxygenation and ventilation before a repeat attempt of defibrillation.

CARDIAC RHYTHM ABNORMALITIES

The cardiac rhythm abnormalities of a child with impending cardiopulmonary arrest are much less complicated than those in adults. Myocardial damage from coronary artery disease, the cause of most adult cardiac arrests, is rarely the cause of a child's abnormal rhythms. In all arrhythmias, the patient must be evaluated to determine if the rhythm is compromising the cardiac output or could degenerate into a lethal rhythm. If there is no compromise or risk of degeneration, no treatment of the rhythm abnormality is indicated, and the patient should be observed for complications.

The response of the heart to the causes of a child's cardiopulmonary arrest is usually an attempt to increase cardiac output by increasing its heart rate. This can cause tachyarrhythmias, which compromise the diastolic filling and reduce stroke volume. The most common tachyarrhythmias found in children are sinus, supraventricular, and ventricular tachycardia. Once the heart begins to fail because of toxins or hypoxia, bradyarrhythmias may result. These also reduce cardiac output by reducing the heart rate. Finally, when the heart has failed, asystole occurs. Please refer to the subchapter on pediatric cardiac emergencies for normal heart rate ranges and discussions of the pathophysiology and pharmacologic treatment of some arrhythmias (AV block, SVT, atrial flutter and fibrillation, ventricular tachycardia and fibrillation).

EMD can cause cardiopulmonary arrest in children

optimal chest contact. There are infant paddles with a diameter of 4.5 cm and paddles for children of 8.0 cm and 13.0 cm in diameter available. Two joules per kg is the initial dose to be used. The voltage is delivered with firm pressure on the paddles and, if defibrillation as in adults. The heart has normal electrical activity, but its mechanical function is ineffective for circulation. The causes of EMD are the same in children and adults, with special emphasis on hypoxia, acidosis, and hypovolemia in children. Treatment of this rhythm requires the diagnosis of the cause and then specific directed treatment (Table 59-12).

CAUSES OF PEDIATRIC CARDIOPULMONARY ARREST

The annual incidence of cardiac arrest in children and adolescents is about 12 in 100,000.[4] The most common cause in infants is usually respiratory in origin rather than cardiac as in adults. As the child ages, the causes change from disease-oriented to trauma. The leading cause of death in children aged 1 to 14 years is trauma, with over 23,000 deaths per year.[5] In all children under 18, the leading cause of cardiac arrest is sudden infant death syndrome (SIDS), followed by trauma, including drowning and motor vehicle accidents. Table 59-13 lists the most common causes of cardiac arrest.

SIDS, the leading cause of cardiac arrest and death in infants, is defined as "the sudden death of any infant or young child which is unexpected by history and in which a thorough postmortem examination fails to demonstrate an adequate cause of death."[6] Incidence of SIDS peaks between 2 and 4 months of age, with 80% occurring before 5 months. Approximately 1.5 to 2 in 1000 infants in the United States are victims of SIDS, accounting for about 6000 to 7000 deaths per year.[7] Tables 59-14 and 59-15 list the associated epidemiologic factors and the high risk groups for SIDS. Those conducting studies have had a difficult job in determining risk factors for unexpected deaths, and these two lists still have a weak correlation.

REFERENCES

1. Orlowski, J.P.: Optimum position for external cardiac compression in infants and young children. Ann. Emerg. Med. 15:667, 1986.
2. Heinild, S., and Sondergaard, T. T.: Bone marrow infusions in childhood: Experiences from a thousand infusions. J. Pediatr. 30:400, 1947.
3. Goetting, M.G., and Paradis, N.A.: High dose epinephrine in refractory pediatric cardiac arrest. Crit. Care Med. 17:1258, 1989.
4. Eisenberg, M., et al.: Epidemiology of cardiac arrest and resuscitation in children, Ann. Emerg. Med., 12:672, 1983.
5. Bushore, M.: Children with multiple injuries, Pediatr. Rev. 10:49, 1988.
6. Bergman, A.B., Beckwith, J.B., and Ray, C.G.: Sudden Infant Death Syndrome: Proceedings of the Second International Conference on Causes of Sudden Death in Infants, Seattle, University of Washington Press, 1970, p. 18.
7. Goyco, Pedro G., Beckerman, Robert C., Sudden Infant Death Syndrome, Curr. Probl. Pediatr. 20:299, 1990.

BIBLIOGRAPHY

Fiser, D.H.: Intraosseous infusion. N. Engl. J. Med. 322:1579, 1990.

Fleisher, G., and Ludwig, S.: Textbook of Pediatric Emergency Medicine, Baltimore, Williams and Wilkins, 1988.

Glaeser, P.: Intraosseous needles: New and improved. Pediatr. Emerg. Care 4:135, 1988.

Kulick, R.: Pulse oximetry. Pediatr. Emerg. Care 3:127, 1987.

National Conference on Cardiopulmonary Resuscitation and Emergency Cardiac Care, Standards and Guidelines for Cardiopulmonary Resuscitation and Emergency Cardiac Care, JAMA 255:2905, 1986.

Perkin, R.M., and Anas, N.G.: Resuscitation and stabilization of the child with respiratory disease. Pediatr. Ann. 15:34, 1989.

Rosetti, V.A., et al.: Intraosseous infusion: An alternative route of pediatric intravascular access. Ann. Emerg. Med. 14:885, 1985.

Smith, R.J. et al.: Intraosseous infusions by prehospital personnel in critically ill pediatric patients. Ann. Emerg. Med. 17:491, 1988.

Textbook of Advanced Cardiac Life Support, American Heart Association, 1987.

Textbook of Pediatric Advanced Life Support, American Heart Association, 1988.

APPROACH TO THE PEDIATRIC EMERGENCY PATIENT

Thom A. Mayer, Robert C. Luten, and Michael F. Altieri

CAPSULE

Pediatric patients comprise nearly a third of all Emergency Department (ED) visits nationwide, accounting for nearly 30 million annual visits to EDs. Of these 30 million visits, only one to two million are seen at children's hospitals.[1] Therefore, the vast majority of pediatric patients are seen in general EDs around the country. The majority of these children have relatively minor illnesses and injuries and do not require referral to specialty institutions. Even in cases in which specialty referral is required, however, the initial, life-saving care and stabilization is provided by emergency physicians and their colleagues in a community setting. For that reason, it is essential that *all* emergency physicians in general EDs be well trained in immediate recognition and effective life-saving and stabilizing therapy for ill and injured children.

Although other chapters in this section address specific clinical entities seen in pediatric emergency medicine, it is critical to have an overall sense of the approach to evaluation and management of ill and injured children. This chapter provides that prospective by looking at pediatric emergency medicine from the perspective of the provider, patient, and process.

THE PROVIDER

The earliest training programs in pediatric emergency medicine were developed at children's hospitals, exclusively for training physicians who had completed pediatric residencies in the evolving specialty of pediatric emergency medicine. Most graduates of these programs worked at children's hospitals or academic institutions with EDs committed exclusively to children. Shortly after these training programs began, however, strong interest in pediatric emergency medicine developed among physicians with backgrounds in both pediatrics and emergency medicine. As of 1990, approximately 30 postgraduate fellowships in pediatric emergency medicine were available.[2] An increasing number of applicants for these postgraduate fellowships come from residency training programs in emergency medicine. The Section of Pediatric Emergency Medicine of the American Academy of Pediatrics was the first effort of an organized body to deal with the problems of pediatric emergency medicine. Shortly thereafter, additional specialty societies were developed, including the Society for Pediatric Emergency Medicine, the Society for Pediatric Trauma, and the American College of Emergency Physicians Section of Pediatric Emergency Medicine.[3] As of 1991, these combined organizations accounted for several thousand physicians who were providing pediatric emergency medicine on a day-to-day basis in both children's hospitals and general ED settings.

As it became recognized that specific skills and expertise were necessary to best care for ill and injured children, training courses were also developed to as-

sist in their care. The Advanced Pediatric Life Support course, jointly developed by ACEP and AAP, was the best example of a program designed to expose physicians to the broad range of problems with which children may present in the emergency setting. The Pediatric Advanced Life Support (PALS) course developed by the American Heart Association was a more narrow course, focusing on the initial resuscitation of the pediatric emergency patient. Training programs in pediatric emergency medicine have also seen significant development. The American Board of Emergency Medicine (ABEM) and the American Board of Pediatrics (ABP) in 1990 approved joint residency training programs comprising 5 years of training in pediatrics and emergency medicine, from which graduates emerge board-qualified in both emergency medicine and pediatrics.[4] In addition, subspecialty boards in pediatric emergency medicine are also being developed jointly between ABEM and ABP, which will presumably lead to subspecialty status or Certificates of Special Competence.

As the specialty of pediatric emergency medicine has grown, a wide body of literature has delineated the nature of pediatric emergency medicine in regard to pharmacology, pathophysiology, anatomy, physiology, toxicology, etc. One of the clearest horizons for pediatric emergency medicine in the future is the extension of this level of expertise to *all* EDs across the country. As indicated subsequently, the vast majority of skills and expertise necessary for the evaluation and resuscitation of pediatric patients do not require extensive commitment of physical resources, but rather depend on the training and expertise of a core group of physicians. One laudable goal for EDs is to ensure that at least one emergency physician is present who is specifically trained in and dedicated to pediatric emergency medicine.

The two types of physicians who have traditionally served as the primary caretakers of children, pediatricians and emergency physicians, differ markedly in their training and background regarding the care of pediatric emergency patients. For example, emergency physicians are well trained and extensively skilled in caring for extremely ill and injured adults. They are trained in managing the airway in an aggressive fashion, whether in the form of cardiopulmonary resuscitations for myocardial infarctions or advanced trauma resuscitation in injured patients, ensuring that shock therapy is handled rapidly and expeditiously, and performing procedures necessary to address the patient's life and limb threats. There is, however, some question as to the extent to which they are exposed to the recognition skills often critical to the evaluation and care of children.[5] Although large numbers of children present in the emergency setting, it is extremely unusual for any given ED (and therefore any given emergency physician) to gain an extensive amount of experience in the evaluation and resuscitation of critically ill and injured children.

Pediatricians are traditionally well trained in developmental aspects of the young patient, as well as in using recognition skills to delineate the sometimes subtle distinctions between the mildly ill and severely ill child. Although some have argued vehemently as to who is the best provider of pediatric emergency care, such debates miss the point that the vast majority of children are seen in general ED settings. If a central goal of pediatric emergency medicine is to extend the best possible care to children across the country, it is essential that emergency physicians and pediatricians work together to ensure that these skills and the recognition and treatment of children be extended to all EDs in the country. Significant success has been achieved when emergency physicians have worked closely with their pediatric colleagues to ensure that the child is the focus of care, without turf battles between specialities.

THE PATIENT: RECOGNITION OF SERIOUS ILLNESS

Most pediatric patients presenting to emergency departments have benign and often self-limited illnesses, most often of an infectious nature. This has given rise to the false dictum that "Children will get better no matter what you do." In emergency medicine, this is a misleading concept because the distinction among the mildly, moderately, and severely ill children is critical to ensuring that the best possible care is given to all children. One of the earliest premises of emergency medicine was that the response to the patient was geared not by the patient's initial presentation itself, but by the *potential* life and limb threat present.[6] For example, when a 50-year-old man presents with chest pain, the approach to the patient assumes that deterioration could take place. In most cases, patients in that age category are initially screened and treated as if they had a myocardial infarction or dissecting aneurysm, even though most such patients do not have these life-threatening conditions. Nonetheless, the patient is evaluated and treated to ensure that deterioration from these life-threatening illnesses does not occur. Similarly, the initial approach to the major trauma victim is likewise geared to the potential life-or-limb threat. Proceeding on the idea that most of the children seen in EDs will get better anyway can lead to disaster. Of the thousands of children that an emergency physician sees each year, the primary task is to pick out the children with potentially serious disease from this otherwise undifferentiated group of patients. Equally important, emergency physicians must be able to recognize when specific pediatric patients are beginning to deteriorate into shock or respiratory failure, requiring immediate intervention to stop the progression toward cardiopulmonary arrest.

Shock and respiratory failure are the primary syndromes responsible for death or permanent disability of children.[7] Through courses such as Advanced Pediatric Life Support and educational chapters such as the ones in this section of the textbook, large numbers of emergency physicians are now extremely skilled in the recognition and management of these two syndromes. It is equally important, however, to recognize children who risk progression of their illness or injury toward the shock or respiratory distress syndromes. Only when children are recognized early in the course of their therapy can this progression be stopped.

THE "AT-RISK" CHILD

The "at-risk" child is one who has an illness or injury of such nature or magnitude that it has the potential for progression to a serious outcome if left untreated. For example, most patients presenting to the ED with diarrhea and dehydration are not critically ill. Some, however, present with such severity or duration of symptoms that they fall into the category of "at-risk" children because their disease can progress further toward a shock syndrome.

Several types of children can easily be excluded from the at-risk category. Children with minor illnesses or injuries who are active, alert, and interacting appropriately with their parents are one example. At the opposite end are children who are obviously critically ill and may in fact be moribund. These children not only do not present a recognition problem, but usually have appropriate early interventions because of the severity of their illnesses or injuries. An additional group that can be excluded from the at-risk category are patients who might initially appear well, but are at risk because of serious diseases or risk factors. In most cases, these children can be easily recognized on the basis of their history or clinical presentation. For example, a child with Factor VIII deficiency who falls several feet onto his or her side is clearly at risk regardless of how active and alert he or she may be during the course of the initial clinical presentation. Similarly, whatever the level of activity or dehydration, a child under 6 weeks of age with even a low-grade fever is widely recognized as being at risk, regardless of the initial clinical presentation.[8]

The key to this concept is recognizing that *any disease process in a child is a part of a natural progression.* Although most children with infectious diseases, including gastroenteritis, appear only mildly ill, the potential progression of the patient and the duration and severity of the symptoms are such that these children may develop frank shock or respiratory failure, or even progress to cardiopulmonary arrest.

In general, patients who are categorized by emergency physicians as at risk generally fall into one of three categories. Children in the first category have a relatively common, usually benign disease, such as gastroenteritis, that can progress to a more severe form with severe dehydration and shock. For these patients, early recognition of the disease is critical with appropriate interventions to interrupt the disease cycle and its further progression. The emergency physician must be well trained in the early recognition of the natural progression of dehydration.

The second group of patients have an early form of a potentially serious disease. The child appears ill from a clinical standpoint and requires further diagnostic efforts to clarify whether a potentially serious disease is present. For example, patients with meningitis fall into this category, in which observation and specific diagnostic tests, in this case a lumbar puncture, are necessary. An additional example are patients considered at risk because of an early form of a serious disease, including the group with so called "occult bacteremia." A subsequent section of this chapter discusses the evaluation and treatment of these children in some detail. A certain subgroup of patients under 2 years with temperature elevations above 104 degrees Fahrenheit and no specific symptoms are at risk for the development of further disease.[9]

The final category of children who are at risk are those who initially appear clinically ill, but in whom the possibility of a serious disease can be ruled out by further evaluation. Examples of such children would be those who initially appear fussy or lethargic, and therefore receive a lumbar puncture to rule out meningitis. An additional example includes children with inspiratory stridor, in whom a lateral neck x ray is necessary to rule out epiglottitis. In general, the more experienced a clinician is with children, the more easily he or she can decide, on the basis of clinical observation, whether or not a child needs additional evaluation to ensure that a more serious disease is or is not present. For example, it is commonly recognized that physicians who are not familiar with children perform significantly larger numbers of laboratory and radiographic examinations than those with extensive experience in pediatric emergency medicine.[10] Nonetheless, this does not represent a "diagnostic nihilism" on the part of the pediatric emergency physician, it simply recognizes that the extensive clinical experience of one trained in pediatric emergency medicine can help reduce unnecessary laboratory and x-ray procedures. It is critical to state that the size of this third group of patients, although often smaller among specially trained emergency physicians, is still one that is always present, because further evaluation may be necessary in these patients. For example, even among physicians with significant training and experience in pediatric emergency medicine, there are still large numbers of negative lumbar punctures and lateral neck films. Thus, negative examinations can be brought down to a minimum number, but never fully eliminated.

One concept that is essential to the evaluation of ill and injured children is ensuring that a systematic approach is taken to every pediatric patient. For example, experienced pediatric emergency physicians are well aware that a careful observation of the vital signs in the initial evaluation of the patient can be critical. The dictum that "It takes evaluation of 1000 normal children to recognize one abnormal child" is valid for the emergency physician.[11] By performing a systematic and complete evaluation of all pediatric patients, regardless of the severity of illness or injury, the emer-

gency physician begins to "fill his data bank" in developing a strong sense of normal and abnormal findings in children. Because the vast majority of emergency physicians see large numbers of children during their daily work, adopting this thorough and systematic evaluation of each child is important.

Further, judicious observation of children can be extremely helpful in distinguishing children at risk from otherwise undifferentiated pediatric patients in the ED. McCarthy has described a technique referred to as "optimal observation," in which febrile infants are given antipyretics to lower temperature and then placed in the lap of the mother and re-evaluated. The scale developed by McCarthy et al. allows the clinician to quantify the interaction of the patient with the environment. This has been found to correlate strongly with the risk of severe infectious diseases, including occult bacteremia and meningitis.[12-13]

THE PROCESS: ROLE OF OBSERVATION

Although there are many similarities in evaluation of the adult and pediatric ED patient, there are also significant differences. Two of the most important differences are related to the role of observation in the care of the pediatric emergency patient and the fact that children require different medication dosages and size of resuscitation equipment.

History is important in any ED patient, including children, but its value somewhat different in the pediatric patient. This is particularly true in infants, in whom the history of many diseases is so nonspecific that it can be of limited use unless the clinician maintains a high index of suspicion regarding the relationship of subtle signs and symptoms. Thus, although the history is extremely valuable, in many cases it must be carefully related to the evaluation of the pediatric patient. For example, in adult patients with chest pain, risk factors for myocardial infarction, previous cardiac history, cardiac medications, and related illnesses are all extremely important information that must be evaluated early in the course of care. Conversely, in pediatric patients with infectious disease, two studies have shown that observation of the acutely ill child is more predictive of serious disease than are historical variables.[13-14] In addition, studies have also indicated that if a child is assessed as appearing well to the experienced eye, in most of cases the child does not have serious disease.[15]

More importantly, continued observation and re-evaluation of the pediatric patient is *essential* in providing optimal care to ill and injured children. Although this is also true in adult patients, the degree to which ongoing observation is necessary for pediatric emergency care is much more dramatic than in adult emergency medicine. Thus, the observation process in pediatric emergency medicine is concurrent, but discrete from elements of the history, physical examination, and laboratory tests.

In addition, it is essential to recognize that the role of follow-up care for patients discharged from the ED is accentuated in pediatric patients, particularly in those who are on the "borderline" between undifferentiated pediatric patients and those "at risk." For example, if a mildly dehydrated child presents to the ED and tolerates oral fluids well, defervescing through the course of the stay in the ED, it is entirely appropriate to discharge the child home for close observation. The ongoing observation and response to therapy in such a child is critical, however, because the dehydration may progress if the child is unable to tolerate oral fluids at home. For this reason, close telephone follow-up and ensuring that the family understands the need for follow-up medical care during the next 24 to 48 hours is essential.

An additional aspect of pediatric emergency care that differs from that of adults are the equipment needs necessary for optimal care of the child. It has long been recognized that pediatric patients require medication dosages on a weight or per kilogram basis. This is true for virtually all medications, including those used during an acute cardiopulmonary resuscitation. Although the dosages for these medications have been well known for many years, their application, particularly in emergency situations, has been variable. In addition, the size of equipment used during a cardiopulmonary resuscitation depends on the child's age and/or size. For that reason, Broselow and colleagues sought an alternate way to ensure appropriate medication dosages and equipment sizes during the acute care of children. Recognizing the correlation between length and lean body mass, a multicenter study was taken to compare the correlation in pediatric emergency patients between length and the child's total mass. This correlation was found to be highly significant, and paved the way for the development of the Broselow length-based resuscitation system.[16] Simply stated, the correlation between lean body weight and length allows calculation of appropriate drug dosages based on the child's overall length. In addition, appropriate equipment sizes can also be calculated based on the child's overall length, with considerable overlap among children of the same general size. Application of this logic in the operating suite setting has shown a strong correlation between the tube size selected by the Broselow system and that that would be selected by an experienced anesthesiologist.[17] Further, initial data from field and ED resuscitations indicate a high correlation between the Broselow length-based system and the medication and equipment that would be selected if there were sufficient time to allow weights and measurements to be taken.[18]

Because of its simplicity and accuracy, the length-based resuscitation system should be used in all general EDs, and should probably be used in prehospital settings by EMS providers. It is particularly important to have such a system available for EDs in which pediatric resuscitations are infrequent because it is un-

likely that the providers will be able to calculate drug dosages and equipment sizes quickly if they are not done on a routine basis.

In addition to using the length-based resuscitation system, other equipment needs are essential in pediatric emergency medicine. Appendix 59A summarizes these needs. In addition, policies and procedures should be described for the care of the pediatric emergency patient, including conscious sedation, use of topical anesthetics for suturing, and protocols for the management of pediatric multiple trauma, seizure disorders, intraosseous infusion, etc. Appendix 59B lists examples of such policies and procedures.

MEDICOLEGAL PEARLS

Pediatric emergency medicine represents an extremely important risk management problem in the ED. Although general ED visits by pediatric patients (one third of all ED visits) generally have a low rate of lawsuits associated with them, the devastating consequences that can result from misdiagnosis and mistreatment of a pediatric patient represent a serious problem for any ED group. In the ACEP closed claims experience, misdiagnosis of pediatric patients with meningitis was among the top four entities responsible for lawsuits.[19] Other errors such as missed fractures and failure to find a foreign body are also common in pediatric patients and therefore are an important area for professional liability claims. How can the emergency physician avoid such cases? Although the answer to this question is beyond the scope of this chapter, and Chapter 89 addresses risk management concerns in some detail, it is important to summarize several aspects of the risk management of pediatric emergency cases.

First and foremost, the medical record of a pediatric emergency patient should be scrutinized with extreme care. It is not uncommon to see a 10-month-old child who comes for the evaluation of fever with vital signs as follows:

Temperature equal to 103.4 (rectal)
Blood pressure not taken
Respirations 45 (crying)
Pulse 162

On the basis of these vital signs, it would not be unreasonable to assume that the child is potentially critically ill. In fact, experience tells us that most children with such vital signs on the triage note are in fact patients with benign and self-limited acute infectious diseases, such as upper respiratory infections or acute otitis media. Although the fever reading is accurate, the facts that the blood pressure was not taken and that the pulse and respirations are often taken while the child is crying are not noted on the triage sheet. In such circumstances, it is *essential* that the emergency physician note the change in vital signs during the course of the stay in the ED. It is extremely common for the emergency physician to walk into the room with such a patient and then find that, in fact, the fever has come down as a result of antipyretics being given at the triage station, and that the child is sleeping in the arms of the mother with a pulse rate of 100 and a respiratory rate of 20, without difficulty in breathing. All of this should be noted on the medical record, to ensure that an accurate estimation of the child's actual appearance is present. If, during evaluation by the physician, it becomes apparent that abnormal vital signs are both persistent and accurate, the child should be considered seriously ill until proven otherwise.

As indicated, the role of observation in the pediatric emergency patient is more important than in adults. For this reason, the emergency physician's medical record, as well as the nursing notes, should indicate the results of this observational period, including repeated physical examinations, especially in appendicitis. In addition, discharge instructions should be written out carefully for all pediatric patients. Many EDs use preprinted discharge instructions for pediatric patients with fever, minor trauma, diarrhea and dehydration, etc. In addition to these preprinted instructions, detailed instructions should be written on the discharge note regarding when and where the patient should go for follow-up care, including the circumstances under which he or she should return to the ED. Although protocols and procedures for the care of the pediatric emergency patient can be helpful, it is important to ensure that all emergency physicians, emergency nurses, and other members of the health care team are aware of these protocols and procedures. Any deviations from these protocols and procedures should be specifically noted in the medical record because plaintiff's attorneys delight in unexplained deviations from written protocol.

HORIZONS

Emergency medicine has truly improved the care of patients nationwide, including their access to quality medical care in a timely fashion. Over the next decade, it is likely that pediatric emergency patients will see an improved standard of care in EDs throughout the country, as the specialty develops further. The extension of pediatric emergency medicine to general EDs seems to be occurring fairly rapidly. It is likely that most EDs will have at least one emergency physician committed to promoting the standards of care for pediatric emergency patients, even if that physician is not specifically fellowship-trained in pediatric emergency medicine. The turf battles that traditionally characterize the development of a specialty are rapidly evolving to a spirit of close cooperation among pediatricians, emergency physicians, pediatric surgeons, and pediatric emergency physicians as the clarion call becomes the needs of the pediatric patient rather than the territorial imperatives of the providers.

REFERENCES

1. National Association of Children's Hospitals and Related Institutions: Annual Report-1990; Alexandria, Virginia.
2. Foltin, G., and Fuchs, S.: Advances in pediatric emergency medical service system. Emerg. Med. Clin. North Am. 9:475, 1991.
3. Luten, R.C.: Recognition of the sick child. In Problems in Pediatric Emergency Medicine. New York, Churchill Livingstone, 1988, pp. 1–12.
4. Clinton, J.E.: Growing pains. ACEP News 9:3, 1990.
5. Ludwig, S., Fleisher, G., Henretig, F., et al.: Pediatric training in emergency medicine programs. Ann. Emerg. Med. 114:170, 1982.
6. Rosen, P., and Honigman, B.: Life and death. In Emergency Medicine: Concepts in Clinical Practice. Edited by Rosen, P., Baker, F.J., Barkin, R.M., et al. St. Louis, C.V. Mosby, pp. 5–26.
7. Mayer, T.A.: Diagnosis and treatment of hemorrhagic shock. In The Clinical Practice of Emergency Medicine. Edited by Harwood Nuss, A., Linden, C., Luten, R.C., et al. Philadelphia, J.B. Lippincott, 1991, p. 814.
8. McLellan, D., and Giebink, G.S.: Perspectives on occult bacteremia in children. J. Pediatr. 109:18, 1986.
9. Teele, D.W., Marshall, R., and Klein, J.O.: Unsuspected bacteremia in young children. Pediat. Clin. North Am. 26:773, 1979.
10. Simon, J.: Problems in the use of the laboratory. In Problems in Pediatric Emergency Medicine. Edited by Luten, R.C. New York, Churchill Livingstone, 1988, p. 13.
11. Mayer, T.A.: Approach to the pediatric multiple trauma patient. In The Clinical Practice of Emergency Medicine. Edited by Harwood Nuss, A., Linden, C., Luten, R.C., et al. Philadelphia, J.B. Lippincott, 1991, p. 800.
12. McCarthy, P.L., and Jekel, J.F.: Further definition of history and observation variables in assessing febrile children. Pediatrics 67:5, 1981.
13. McCarthy, P.L.: Controversies in pediatrics: What tests are indicated for the child under two with fever? Pediatr. Rev. 1:2, 1979.
14. McCarthy, P.L., Sharpe, M.R., Spiesel, S.Z., et al.: Observation scales to identify serious illness in febrile children. Pediatrics 70:802, 1982.
15. McCarthy, P.L., Lembo, R.M., Fink, H.D., et al.: Observation, history, and physical examination in diagnosis of serious illness in febrile children ≤ 24 months. J. Pediatr. 110:26, 1987.
16. Lubitz, V.S., Seidel, J.S., Chameides, L., et al.: A rapid method for estimating weight and resuscitation drug dosages from length in the pediatric age group. Ann. Emerg. Med. 17:576, 1988.
17. Luten, R.C., Wears, R.L., Broselow, J., et al.: Length-based endotracheal tube size for pediatric resuscitation. (Abstract) Ann. Emerg. Med. 19:476, 1990.
18. Mayer, T.A.: Unpublished data, 1991.
19. Henry, G.L. (Ed.): Emergency Medicine Risk Management: A comprehensive review. Dallas, American College of Emergency Physicians, 1991.

EQUIPMENT NEEDS IN PEDIATRIC EMERGENCY MEDICINE

PEDIATRIC EQUIPMENT CHECKLIST

AIRWAY

Endotracheal Tubes

Uncuffed{ } 2.5{ } 3.0{ } 3.5{ } 4.0{ } 4.5{ } 5.0{ } (2 each)

Cuffed{ } 5.5{ } 6.0{ } 6.5{ } 7.0{ } 7.5{ } (2 each)

Stylets

{ } Stylets for endotracheal tube:
   Infant (2)
   Child (2)

Laryngoscope Blades

{ } Straight or Miller: No. 0 (Premature), 1 (Infant), 2 (Child)

{ } Curved Macintosh: No. 1 (Infant), 2 (Child), 3 (Medium Adult)

Pediatric Laryngoscope Handle

{ } Small handle (AA Cell)
{ } Large handle
{ } Spare bulb small
{ } AA cell set

Airways: Oral-Nasal

{ } Oral airways: No. 0–Infant, 1–Small Child, 2–Child, 3–Small Adult

{ } Nasopharyngeal Airways: Sizes: 12F, 14F, 16F, 20F, 24F

Masks and Cannula

{ } Nonrebreathing Masks: Infant, Child
{ } Pediatric Nasal Cannula (1)

CIRCULATION

Blood Pressure

{ } Newborn/Infant/Child BP Kit
{ } PASG: Child Size (1)

Intravenous Materials

{ } Jelco or Angiocath Catheters:
   Size spectrum
   16, 18, 20, 22, 24 GA (4 of each size)

{ } LR or NS 250 cc and 500 cc Bags (1 Each)
{ } D_5 1/2 NS
{ } Pediatric Tourniquets: Rubber bands for infants (6), Small Penrose Drains for Children (2).

{ } Tape (waterproof), 1/2 and 1 inch (2 rolls of each)

{ } Armboards: Infant and Child (2)
{ } "T" Connectors

{ } Alcohol and Betadine preps
{ } Macro IV tubing (1)
{ } Micro IV tubing (2)
{ } Buretrol IV set (1)
{ } IV infusion pump

Alternative Vascular Access

{ } Intraosseous needles: Illinois sternal iliac bone marrow needles: Gauges 15, 18 (2 each)

{ } Intraosseous needle kit (bone marrow needles, betadine swabs, tape, gauze, syringe 20 cc)

{ } Feeding tubes (endotracheal administration) 3.5 Fr, 5 Fr (1 each)

{ } Tuberculin syringes, 1 cc (2): Rectal administration of anticonvulsant medication

Monitoring

{ } Cardiac monitor, defibrillator, cardioverter, recording capability (infant and pediatric paddles)

{ } Pediatric monitor adhesive pads
{ } Defibrillation/monitor electrodes: (if hands-off option available with equipment)

Drug Administration

{ } Broselow Resuscitation Tape
{ } Pediatric drug dosage Rapid Reference Card

Telephone Numbers

{ } Air/helicopter transport
{ } Children's Hospital Emergency Department
{ } Poison Control Center

Suction Devices

{ } Yankauer suction
{ } Large bore suction
{ } De Lee suction with connector
{ } Bulb suction

Alternative Airway Equipment

{ } 10 or 12 gauge catheter-over-the-needle (2) or 14

Miscellaneous

{ } Tongue blades (3)
{ } Lidocaine jelly (2%)
{ } Neosynephrine nose spray (1/4%)

Cervical Spine

{ } Stifneck Baby-No-Neck, Stifneck Pediatric Collar (Entire series of sizes should be carried)

{ } Pediatric head immobilization system
{ } Shoulder pad support to align head and neck

BREATHING

Stethoscope

Pediatric stethoscope

Ventilation Equipment

{ } Bag-valve-mask
   resuscitator, self-inflating: Infant and Child
   sizes (1 Each) 250 cc/500 cc/1000 cc
{ } Masks: Clear disposable resuscitation masks;
   Neonate, Infant, Child, Adult
{ } Oxygen connecting tubing
{ } Peep valve
{ } Pediatric transcutaneous pacer

DISABILITY AND IMMOBILIZATION

{ } Hare-type child traction splint (1)
{ } Splinting materials of choice
{ } Pediatric backboard (1)

EXPOSURE AND PRECAUTIONS

Temperature Regulation

{ } Space Rescue Blanket, Silver Swaddler, heat
   blankets, etc.
{ } Overhead radiant warmer

Infection Control

{ } Disposable gloves
{ } Masks (surgical) (1 Box)

MISCELLANEOUS

{ } Obstetrics pack
{ } Multiple trauma dressings (pediatric Sc Size)
{ } Nasogastric Tube (10 or 12 Fr)
{ } Chest Tubes #8, 10, 12, 20, 28
{ } Pediatric ALS equipment organizer
{ } Penlight to check pupils
{ } Syringes 5 cc (2), 3 cc (2), 10 cc (1)
{ } 3-way stopcock
{ } Band-Aids (Children's colorful)
{ } Hypodermic needles, 18 gauge (5)

REFERENCES

Scoring Tables

{ } Pediatric Trauma Score Reference
{ } Glasgow Coma Scale Reference
{ } Croup Score

EXAMPLE OF ED POLICIES AND PRACTICES FOR PEDIATRIC PATIENTS

Fairfax Hospital—Emergency Department

Conscious Sedation for the Pediatric Patient

Effective Date: 10/25/90   Revised:

_____   _____
(Name)   (Name)
Chairman, Emergency Medicine   Chief, Pediatric Emergency Medicine

_____
(Name)
Director, Emergency Department

Purpose:

To develop a protocol to be followed when children require conscious sedation in the Emergency Department for reasons which include, but are not limited to, sedating the uncooperative patient, sedating the pediatric patient in order to perform a plastic repair, sedating the pediatric patient to perform a complicated suture repair, sedating and giving analgesics to the pediatric patient prior to performing a painful procedure, and sedating the pediatric patient for a procedure which requires a minimum of movement and a maximum of cooperation such as a CT scan.

Definitions:

Pediatric patients include all patients who are infants, children, and adolescents less than the age of majority.

Conscious Sedation:

Conscious sedation is a minimally depressed level of consciousness that retains the patient's ability to maintain a patent airway independently and continuously and respond appropriately to physical stimulation and/or verbal command. The caveat that loss of consciousness should be unlikely is a particularly important part of the definition of conscious sedation, and the drugs and techniques used should carry a margin of safety wide enough to render unintended loss of consciousness unlikely.

Goals of Conscious Sedation:

The goals of conscious sedation should include, but not be limited to:

1. Patient Welfare
2. Control of the Patient's Behavior
3. Production of Positive Psychological Response to treatment
4. Return to Pretreatment Level of consciousness by the Time of Discharge

Protocol:

1. Patients:

   Any pediatric patients who require sedation for the above-mentioned reasons and in whom there exists no contraindication for the administration of the specific sedating agent.

2. Rooms in which conscious sedation may be administered:

   Conscious sedation of the pediatric patient may take place in any of the rooms on the Acute side and in rooms 14 and 22 on the Non-Acute side.

3. Equipment available at patient's bedside:

   The following equipment must be available at the patient's bedside prior to the administration of conscious sedation:

   A. A positive-pressure oxygen delivery system that is capable of administering greater than 90% oxygen, at least five liters per minute for at least 60 minutes. This positive pressure delivery system should include bag-valve-mask, as well as a complete pediatric intubation set up.

B. An emergency or crash kit that would include IV materials and fluids, resuscitation drugs, and narcotic antagonists such as Narcan. These drugs and equipment must be checked and maintained on a regular basis.

4. Monitoring:

The patient undergoing conscious sedation should be monitored by an Emergency Department staff member who is skilled in the maintenance of the pediatric airway and is able to ventilate the pediatric patient in an emergency situation. All patients undergoing conscious sedation should have a 1) cardiorespiratory monitor in place, as well as a 2) pulse oximeter. These monitors should be in clear view of the personnel manning the nurses' station.

5. Documentation:

The Emergency Department record should contain documentation of the procedure done under sedation, as well as the administration and dosages of the drugs used for conscious sedation. Vital signs should be obtained and recorded at regular intervals while the patient is undergoing conscious sedation. These intervals should not exceed 30 minutes.

Discharge:

The patient should be fully awake and alert upon discharge and an evaluation of the patient's level of consciousness as well as vital signs should be documented on the chart at the time of discharge.

Agents for Conscious Sedation:

The following agents are recognized as acceptable to produce conscious sedation:

1. Demerol/Phenergan/Thorazine at the dose of 2 mg per kg of Demerol combined with 1 mg per kg of Phenergan combined with 1 mg per kg of Thorazine. This delivered via the IM route.

2. Demerol/Versed at the dosage of 1.5 mg per kg of Demerol and 0.15 mg per kg of Versed delivered via the IM route.

3. Versed alone delivered via the IV route at the dosage of 0.1 mg per kg.

4. Cloral hydrate at 50 to 100 mg per kg given via the oral route.

5. Ketamine at the dosage of 2 to 4 mg per kg given via the IM route.

6. Nitrous oxide delivered via inhalation in combination with oxygen (50% = 50% at sea level).

7. Fentanyl in a dose of 1 to 5 μg per Kg via the IV route.

Bibliography:

1. The American Academy of Pediatrics: Committee on Drugs and Section on Anesthesiology. Guidelines for the Elective Use of Conscious Sedation, Deep Sedation, and General Anesthesia in Pediatric Patients. Pediatrics 76:317–321, 1985.

2. Conscious Sedation of the Pediatric Patient for Suturing: A Survey. Authors: Hawk, Crockett, Ochsenschlager and Klein. Pediatric Emergency Care, Volume 6, Number 2, June 1990, pages 84–88.

PEDIATRIC CARDIAC EMERGENCIES

Karen S. Rheuban

CAPSULE

Evaluation and treatment of infants and children with known or suspected congenital or acquired heart disease requires an understanding of the pathophysiology of cardiovascular disease in the young. Although some similarities exist between adults and children with heart disease, children should not be treated as "little adults," and their evaluation and treatment should be tailored to their age and individual needs. This chapter reviews congenital and acquired heart disease in children and treatment of dysrhythmias.

CONGENITAL HEART DISEASE

STRUCTURAL

Structural congenital cardiovascular abnormalities may become hemodynamically significant in the neonatal period and often require early intervention. The transition from fetal life to that of the normal newborn is a complex process, and derangements in cardiovascular anatomy and physiology may not become apparent for hours to days after birth, when the ductus arteriosus closes and the pulmonary vascular resistance begins to drop.[1]

When faced with a sick infant or child, the clinician must carefully evaluate the patient's overall status. Is this infant in distress, well or poorly perfused, cyanotic or fully saturated?

The initial assessment should include complete vital signs, with both pulse and respiratory rate and temperature and blood pressure determinations in the right arm and a lower extremity. The presence of a murmur may indicate cardiac pathology, although significant heart disease may be present without a murmur. Murmurs may occur in systole or diastole, or be continuous (Table 59-16). Hepatomegaly and rales may be noted in the child with congestive heart failure. Careful attention should be paid to the quality of distal pulses. Diminished pulse amplitude may be noted in patients with left heart obstructive lesions, and bounding pulses are often found in patients with lesions manifested by diastolic runoff (such as patent ductus arteriosus or aortic insufficiency).

Laboratory studies include chest radiograph (preferably in the upright position), electrocardiogram (ECG) (for normal values, see Table 59-17), and oxygen saturation in cases with respiratory distress or cyanosis. The chest radiograph of the neonate may show a falsely elevated cardiothoracic ratio when the x ray is obtained in the recumbent position. Additionally, the thymic shadow may obscure the cardiac silhouette. The pulmonary vasculature may be increased, decreased, or even normal in patients with congenital heart disease. Echocardiography, when performed by an examiner experienced with children with heart disease, is usually sufficient to diagnose most cardiovascular disease in pediatric patients.

CYANOTIC HEART DISEASE

When asked to evaluate an infant for possible cyanotic congenital heart disease, the clinician must first determine that systemic arterial desaturation is present. Acrocyanosis, or cyanosis of the extremities, may be present in normal neonates, and is caused by vasomotor instability in response to cold stress, with an increase in oxygen extraction from that extremity. The arterial oxygen saturation is normal. True central cyanosis is characterized by cyanosis of the mucous membranes in addition to cyanosis of the extremities,

TABLE 59-16. CLASSIFICATION OF CARDIAC MURMURS

Systolic	Diastolic	Continuous
Pulmonic stenosis	Pulmonic insufficiency	Patent ductus arteriosus
Tricuspid regurgitation	Tricuspid stenosis	Venous hum
Atrial septal defect	Tricuspid rumble	Aorticopulmonary window
Aortic stenosis	Aortic insufficiency	Arteriovenous fistula
Ventricular septal defect	Mitral rumble	Bronchial collaterals
Mitral regurgitation	Mitral stenosis	Previous surgical shunt
Aortic coarctation		
Still's murmur		

TABLE 59-17. ELECTROCARDIOGRAPHIC CRITERIA IN CHILDREN*

Age Group	*Heart Rate (BPM)	Frontal Plane QRS Vector (degrees)	PR Interval (sec)	**Q III (mm)§	**Q V6 (mm)	RV1 (mm)	SV1 (mm)	R/S V1	RV6 (mm)	SV6 (mm)	R/S V6	**SV1 + RV6 (mm)	**R + S V4 (mm)
Less than 1 day	93–154 (123)	+59 to −163 (137)	.08–.16 (.11)	4.5	2	5–26 (14)	0–23 (8)	.1–U (2.2)	0–11 (4)	0–9.5 (3)	.1–U (2.0)	28	52.5
1–2 days	91–159 (123)	+64 to −161 (134)	.08–.14 (.11)	6.5	2.5	5–27 (14)	0–21 (9)	.1–U (2.0)	0–12 (4.5)	0–9.5 (3)	.1–U (2.5)	29	52
3–6 days	91–166 (129)	+77 to −163 (132)	.07–.14 (.10)	5.5	3	3–24 (13)	0–17 (7)	.2–U (2.7)	.5–12 (5)	0–10 (3.5)	.1–U (2.2)	24.5	49
1–3 weeks	107–182 (148)	+65 to +161 (110)	.07–.14 (.10)	6	3	3–21 (11)	0–11 (4)	1.0–U (2.9)	2.5–16.5 (7.5)	0–10 (3.5)	.1–U (3.3)	21	49
1–2 months	121–179 (149)	+31 to 113 (74)	.07–.13 (.10)	7.5	3	3–18 (10)	0–12 (5)	.3–U (2.3)	5–21.5 (11.5)	0–6.5 (3)	.2–U (4.8)	29	53.5
3–5 months	106–186 (141)	+7 to +104 (60)	.07–.15 (.11)	6.5	3	3–20 (10)	0–17 (6)	.1–U (2.3)	6.5–22.5 (13)	0–10 (3)	.2–U (6.2)	32	61.5
6–11 months	109–169 (134)	+6 to +99 (56)	.07–.16 (.11)	8.5	3	1.5–20 (9.5)	.5–18 (4)	.1–3.9 (1.6)	6–22.5 (12.5)	0–7 (2)	.2–U (7.6)	32	53
1–2 years	89–151 (119)	+7 to +101 (55)	.08–.15 (.11)	6	3	2.5–17 (9)	.5–21 (8)	.05–4.3 (1.4)	6–22.5 (13)	0–6.5 (2)	.3–U (9.3)	39	49.5
3–4 years	73–137 (108)	+6 to +104 (55)	.09–.16 (.12)	5	3.5	1–18 (8)	.2–21 (10)	.03–2.8 (.9)	8–24.5 (15)	0–5 (1.5)	.6–U (10.8)	42	53.5
5–7 years	65–133 (100)	+11 to +143 (65)	.09–.16 (.12)	4	4.5	.5–14 (7)	.3–24 (12)	.02–2.0 (7)	8.5–26.5 (16)	0–4 (1)	.9–U (11.5)	47	54
8–11 years	62–130 (91)	+9 to +114 (61)	.09–.17 (.13)	3	3	0–12 (5.5)	.3–25 (12)	0–1.8 (.5)	9–25.5 (16)	0–4 (1)	1.5–U (14.3)	45.5	53
12–15 years	60–119 (85)	+11 to +130 (59)	.09–.18 (.14)	3	3	0–10 (4)	.3–21 (11)	0–1.7 (.5)	6.5–23 (14)	0–4 (1)	1.4–U (14.7)	41	50

* With permission from Garson, A.: The Electrocardiogram in Infants and Children. Philadelphia, Lea & Febiger, 1983, p. 404.
* 2%–98% (mean)
** 98th percentile
§ mm at normal standardization
U undefined (S wave may equal zero)

and is the result of a reduced arterial oxygen saturation from either intracardiac right to left shunting or pulmonary disease. Pulmonary venous saturation is usually normal in patients with intracardiac right-to-left shunts, whereas pulmonary venous saturation is reduced in patients with lung disease. The administration of oxygen is helpful in differentiating these patients because oxygen saturation does not rise in infants with an obligatory intracardiac right-to-left shunt, and rises in patients with lung disease.[2] Congenital cardiovascular lesions that produce cyanosis in infancy include those characterized by reduced pulmonary blood flow, parallel pulmonary and systemic circulations, admixture lesions, and defects whose manifestations include acute pulmonary edema.

When a reduced systemic arterial oxygen saturation is documented, an arterial blood gas should be obtained. Many infants with extreme hypoxemia (PaO_2 < 40 torr) may also show evidence for metabolic acidosis. An elevated pCO_2 generally reflects respiratory disease, but may be seen in patients with severe pulmonary edema. Institution of an intravenous prostaglandin E_1 infusion (0.05 to 0.1 μg per kg per minute) may be life-saving for the infant with extreme hypoxemia secondary to congenital heart disease because it dilates the ductus arteriosus and increases pulmonary blood flow and/or mixing of pulmonary and systemic blood as in cases with transposition of the great arteries.[3] Complications of prostaglandin therapy include profound apnea, which may occur any time after institution of therapy, and hyperthermia. Personnel capable of intubating infants should

be readily available when an infant is begun on a prostaglandin infusion. If at all possible, the infant should be transferred to a facility with pediatric cardiology services as soon as possible.

All patients with cyanotic congenital heart disease are at risk for central nervous system (CNS) complications such as a brain abscess or a cerebrovascular accident. These complications should always be considered in the child with cyanotic disease and CNS symptoms (seizures, headaches, hemiparesis, aphasia, etc.). Polycythemia is a common finding in cyanotic infants and children, and is a significant risk factor in the development of cerebrovascular accidents. Caution should be taken to filter intravenous lines to prevent an inadvertent air embolus.

Patients with tetralogy of Fallot are at risk for the development of hypercyanotic spells when systemic vascular resistance drops during exercise or at other times when oxygen requirements increase.[4] Right-to-left shunting acutely increases during a hypercyanotic spell, and extreme hypoxemia and death may ensue quickly unless the spell is interrupted. The treatment of the infant or child with a hypercyanotic spell is outlined in Table 59-18. Maneuvers that increase systemic vascular resistance (such as placement in the knee-chest position and/or the administration of alpha-adrenergic agents by intravenous infusion) and increase ventricular filling by slowing the heart rate (beta-adrenergic blocking agents) are routinely used in terminating a hypercyanotic spell.[5] Surgical therapy, either placement of a systemic to pulmonary shunt or intracardiac repair, should be performed once

TABLE 59-18. TREATMENT OF HYPERCYANOTIC SPELLS

TABLE 59-18. TREATMENT OF HYPERCYANOTIC SPELLS

1. Placement in the knee-chest position
2. Morphine sulfate, 0.1–0.2 mg/kg SC or IM
3. Treat metabolic acidosis with NaHCO₃, 1 mEq/kg/IV
4. Oxygen has limited usefulness because of obligatory intracardiac right to left shunt
5. Alpha-adrenergic agents may be started to increase systemic vascular resistance, such as phenylephrine, 0.01 mg/kg IV
6. Propranolol helps by slowing the heart rate and increasing diastolic filling of the right ventricle. It may be given orally in mild cases at a dosage of 0.5–0.75 mg/kg PO or intravenously, at 0.01–0.1 mg/kg IV over 5 minutes

the patient develops a hypercyanotic spell, or sooner if significant arterial desaturation is present.

ACYANOTIC HEART DISEASE

LEFT-TO-RIGHT SHUNTS

Patients with lesions characterized by large left-to-right shunts (such as ASD, VSD, and PDA) usually do not become symptomatic until the pulmonary vascular resistance drops. Symptoms, when present, generally reflect pulmonary volume overload with increased work of breathing secondary to diminished pulmonary compliance. Tachypnea, tachycardia, and diaphoresis are the usual symptoms of infants with large shunts. Fluid retention may be significant, secondary to catecholamine excess and stimulation of the renin-angiotensin-aldosterone system.[6] Ventricular function is usually normal in infants with significant shunts, and because symptoms are related to pulmonary volume overload rather than myocardial dysfunction, treatment should be geared toward achieving diuresis rather than digitalization. Furosemide may be given intravenously (1 mg per kg) or orally in dosages of 1 to 4 mg per kg per day. Caution should be taken to preserve potassium balance by replacing potassium losses, either with KCl supplementation or by adding spironolactone in dosages of 1 to 4 mg per kg per day. When an infant with a large left-to-right shunt presents with severe respiratory distress, positive pressure ventilation may be necessary to improve gaseous exchange. A coincident pneumonitis must be considered in these infants as well. Early cardiac catheterization and surgery should be considered in symptomatic infants when medical therapy is suboptimal.

LEFT HEART OBSTRUCTIVE LESIONS

In contrast to infants with left to right shunts, those with left heart obstructive lesions may develop congestive heart failure secondary to the increased afterload against which the left ventricle must perform. In severe cases, such as hypoplastic left heart syndrome, severe coarctation of the aorta, severe aortic stenosis, or an interrupted aortic arch, a metabolic acidosis may develop secondary to diminished systemic perfusion. In these cases, prostaglandin E₁ therapy may be lifesaving because it dilates the ductus arteriosus and augments systemic blood flow. Most extreme cases also have severe respiratory distress secondary to acute pulmonary edema, and positive pressure ventilation and inotropic support may significantly improve symptoms. Diagnosis may be confirmed by echocardiography and/or cardiac catheterization, and surgical therapy tailored to the needs of the infant.

Older patients with hemodynamically significant aortic stenosis (left ventricular outflow tract gradient >50 mm Hg) are at risk for arrhythmias, syncope, and even sudden death during periods of increased cardiac output. Chest pain or syncope in a patient with aortic stenosis should never be disregarded, and mandates thorough evaluation.[7]

Patients with coarctation of the aorta may not present in early infancy, and indeed are often asymptomatic. Hypertension in the upper extremities is usually present, accompanied by a diminished blood pressure in the lower extremities. This hypertension is generally chronic, and thus does not require acute antihypertensive therapy, but rather surgical resection of the obstruction on an elective or semi-elective basis.

RIGHT HEART OBSTRUCTIVE LESIONS

Right heart obstructive lesions include valvular, infundibular, supravalvular and peripheral pulmonic stenosis. In general, unless the pulmonary stenosis is severe (i.e., right ventricular pressures at systemic or suprasystemic levels), most patients have few symptoms. Patients with severe pulmonary stenosis may develop systemic arterial desaturation secondary to right-to-left shunting across the foramen ovale, exercise intolerance, and heart failure.

CONGESTIVE HEART FAILURE

Congestive heart failure, when it occurs in children, may occur secondary to structural congenital heart disease, primary myocardial disease, rheumatic heart disease, bacterial endocarditis, Kawasaki disease, and dysrhythmias.

Heart failure in children with large left-to-right shunts generally reflects a volume overloaded state rather than myocardial dysfunction, and treatment should be directed at a reduction in total body water, using diuretics such as furosemide or the thiazide diuretics.[8,9] Attention to potassium balance is obligatory, and patients may either receive potassium supplementation or be treated with potassium-sparing diuretics such as spironolactone. Digitalization gen-

TABLE 59-19. PEDIATRIC CARDIOVASCULAR DRUG DOSAGES		
Drug	Oral Dose	Intravenous Dose
Diuretics:		
Furosemide	1–4 mg/kg/day (in 2–3 doses)	1 mg/kg
Chlorothiazide	10–20 mg/kg/day (in 2 doses)	
Spironolactone	1–4 mg/kg/day (in 2–3 doses)	
Digoxin	Total digitalizing dose (TDD)	$^2/_3$ po dose
	Prematures: 0.02 mg/kg	
	Others: 0.03 mg/kg	
	Give $^1/_2$ TDD, then in 6–8 hours	
	$^1/_4$ TDD, then in 6–8 hours $^1/_4$	
	TDD, then in 12 hours begin $^1/_8$	
	TDD PO BID	
Inotropes:		
Epinephrine		0.1 cc kg bolus of
		1:10,000 solution
		0.1–1.5 µg/kg/min
Dopamine		3–20 µg/kg/min
Dobutamine		3–20 µg/kg/min
Isoproterenol		0.05–1.0 µg/kg/min
Vasodilators:		
Sodium nitroprusside		0.5–10 µg/kg/min
Nitroglycerin		0.5–10 µg/kg/min
Hydralazine	1 mg/kg/day (in 2–3 doses)	0.15 mg/kg/dose
Diazoxide		3–5 mg/kg bolus
Enalapril	0.1 mg/kg/day (1–2 doses)	0.01 mg/kg bolus
Other drugs:		
Calcium chloride (10% solution)		0.3 ml/kg bolus
Atropine sulfate (0.1 mg/mL)		0.01 mg/kg bolus
Amrinone		0.5 mg/kg bolus then 5–20 mcg/kg/min

erally does not improve symptoms unless myocardial function is impaired.

Patients with impaired myocardial function usually respond well to inotropic agents. Digitalis, in the form of digoxin, remains the most widely used pharmacologic agent in the treatment of myocardial dysfunction in children. Digoxin may be administered orally or intravenously. Intravenous administration of digoxin should be reserved for infants and children who cannot be fed, or for patients whose cardiac output is so low that gastrointestinal perfusion (and thereby absorption) is significantly reduced. Patients with congestive heart failure and evidence of low cardiac output should be treated with intravenous inotropic agents, as outlined in Table 59-19. Dopamine, a natural precursor of norepinephrine, is a potent beta-adrenergic agonist that, at low doses (3 to 5 µg per kg per minute) has inotropic effects and augments renal perfusion. At high doses (>10 µg per kg per minute), marked vasoconstriction may develop. Dopamine should be administered through a central line after a central venous pressure confirms adequate ventricular filling pressures. Dobutamine, a sympathomimetic agent with predominant B_1 activity, may be administered through a peripheral intravenous line and has inotropic effects without significant vasoconstrictor effects. Isoproterenol, a sympathomimetic agent with both B_1 and B_2 effects, increases cardiac output by both inotropic and chronotropic effects. Unfortunately, the chronotropic effects are often excessive, and require termination of use of this agent. Epinephrine may also be used for constant infusion, although the chronotropic effects often outweigh the benefits of its use as an inotrope.

Vasodilator therapy of congestive heart failure has been used to alter preload (agents that dilate venous capacitance vessels such as nitroglycerin) or to decrease afterload (agents with direct arterial vasodilatory properties such as sodium nitroprusside, or hydralazine, or agents that inhibit angiotensin-converting enzyme, such as captopril or enalapril).[10] A careful assessment of fluid status is necessary before institution of vasodilator therapy; these agents should not be administered to patients who are volume-depleted.

ACQUIRED HEART DISEASE

Previously healthy infants and children whose presenting symptoms include fever and who are also found to have cardiomegaly and evidence of congestive heart failure should be evaluated for acute myopericarditis, bacterial endocarditis, acute rheumatic fever, and Kawasaki disease.

ACUTE MYOPERICARDITIS

Although the child with acute myocarditis generally presents with chest pain, fever, and dyspnea, the clinical features of myocarditis may be subtle. Tachycardia in excess of the fever or an arrhythmia or subtle gallop rhythm may be the only clinical finding. Etiologic agents that have been implicated in the development of myocarditis in the pediatric patient include viruses (most commonly the enterovirus family), rickettsia, fungi, and parasites. In addition to a high index of suspicion, supporting laboratory data may include an elevated erythrocyte sedimentation rate, an abnormal CPK-MB, electrocardiographic changes (such as decreased amplitude of the QRS complexes, an arrhythmia, or ST-T wave changes), cardiomegaly on the chest radiograph, and evidence of reduced ventricular function on the echocardiogram.

Acute therapy should be directed at stabilizing the patient. All patients should be admitted for observation and monitoring. After such lesions as rheumatic fever, Kawasaki disease, and bacterial endocarditis have been ruled out, therapy with anti-inflammatory agents should be initiated. Low cardiac output states should be treated as described in the section on congestive heart failure.

Acute pericarditis constitutes a true emergency, with pericardial tamponade a major complication of involvement of the pericardium. The finding of a pericardial friction rub in a patient with chest pain and fever indicates involvement of the pericardial space in an inflammatory process. Pulsus paradoxus, or an inspiratory decrease in systolic blood pressure greater than 10 mm Hg accompanied by chest pain, fever,

and cardiomegaly, should be cause for urgent echocardiographic assessment and therapy.[11] Electrocardiographic findings include diminished amplitude of the QRS complex and ST-T wave abnormalities. Pericardiocentesis may be both diagnostic and therapeutic and should be performed whenever there is evidence of pericardial tamponade. Agents that cause infectious inflammatory disease of the pericardium include bacteria, viruses, mycobacteria, and fungi. Blood cultures should be obtained before institution of antibiotic therapy when the pericardial fluid appears purulent. Acute bacterial pericarditis may be secondary to Staphylococcus aureus, Streptococcus pneumoniae, Neisseria meningitidis, and Hemophilus influenzae in children. Initial therapy should include antimicrobial agents that cover these organisms, pericardiocentesis, and surgical drainage to effect continued drainage of infected pericardial fluid.

KAWASAKI DISEASE

Kawasaki disease, an acute febrile illness of childhood, is characterized by high fever for more than 4 days, a generalized exanthem, lymphadenopathy (with at least one large lymph node greater than 1.5 cm in diameter), oropharyngeal changes (cracking and fissuring of the lips, erythema of the tongue), and changes in the extremities (with erythema and induration of the hands and feet and periungual desquamation). Kawasaki disease is characterized by an acute panvasculitis, with involvement of the heart in at least 50% of affected children and coronary artery aneurysms as documented by echocardiography and angiography in at least 20%.[12] Congestive heart failure may develop early in the course of Kawasaki disease, and the complications of myocardial infarction and pericardial tamponade from rupture of a coronary aneurysm may occur as well. No diagnostic test is now available to confirm the diagnosis of Kawasaki disease; hence, the diagnosis depends on a high index of suspicion on the part of the examiner. Initial treatment currently consists of hospitalization, supportive care, salicylate therapy, and high-dose intravenous gammaglobulin therapy, administered daily over 4 days.[13] Long-term therapy with antiplatelet agents is recommended for children with Kawasaki disease and coronary artery aneurysms.

ACUTE RHEUMATIC FEVER

Rheumatic fever is the most common cause of acquired heart disease in children worldwide. Although the incidence of rheumatic fever declined dramatically from 1910 to 1977, there was a resurgence in the 1980s.[13a] The reason is unknown, and many of the patients could not identify a "sore throat." Acute rheumatic fever occurs as a sequela of untreated group A streptococcal pharyngitis. The most important complication of rheumatic fever is carditis, seen in 50% of

---

TABLE 59-20. REVISED JONES CRITERIA FOR ACUTE RHEUMATIC FEVER

Major Manifestations	Minor Manifestations
Carditis	Fever
Polyarthritis	Arthralgia (cannot be used with arthritis)
Sydenham's chorea	Laboratory evidence for inflammation (ESR, C reactive protein)
Erythema marginatum	First degree AV block
Subcutaneous nodules	History of rheumatic fever

PLUS:
Evidence for streptococcal infection (positive throat culture, elevated ASO titer, scarlet fever)
The patient must demonstrate either ONE major manifestation and TWO minor manifestations, or TWO major manifestations with evidence of recent streptococcal disease.

affected individuals. Analysis of seven recent outbreaks of acute rheumatic fever demonstrated a range of carditis in 30 to 73% of patients.[13a] Rheumatic carditis is a pancarditis, involving the endocardium (causing valvular insufficiencies acutely and stenoses after many years), the myocardium (causing congestive heart failure) and the pericardium (leading to the development of a pericardial effusion). The most commonly affected valves are the mitral and aortic valves, which may become insufficient several days after the onset of illness. Other symptoms of rheumatic fever include an acute migratory polyarthritis, erythema marginatum, Sydenham's chorea, and subcutaneous nodules. Diagnostic criteria for the diagnosis of acute rheumatic fever have been described and are outlined in Table 59-20. Therapy consists of the administration of anti-inflammatory agents, penicillin, and treatment of dysrhythmias and congestive heart failure. Erythromycin is the usual alternative to penicillin, but resistance of group A streptococci to erythromycin has been increasing.[13b]

BACTERIAL ENDOCARDITIS

Infective endocarditis is one of the most significant complications of congenital or acquired heart disease. Bacterial pathogens frequently implicated in the cause of endocarditis include alpha-hemolytic streptococci and enterococci, which tend to produce a less acute course than the beta-hemolytic streptococci and staphylococci. The clinical features vary with the site of the infection, and the diagnosis may be missed for weeks. Unexplained fever, persistent splenomegaly, the appearance of a new murmur, evidence for peripheral embolization (Roth spots, splinter hemorrhages) all suggest the diagnosis of bacterial endocarditis. Diagnosis may be made with serial blood cultures, evidence for microscopic hematuria, depressed serum complement levels, and a high clinical index of suspicion. Echocardiography, although helpful when positive, may be negative for several weeks after onset of fever. Treatment should consist of broad spectrum antibiotic therapy, careful monitoring of the patient, and surgical intervention if hemodynamic instability or significant embolization occurs.

Prophylaxis against bacterial endocarditis is the key in the management of any patient with congenital heart disease (with the exception of the patient with an atrial septal defect) or acquired valvular disease. The current recommendations for prophylaxis against bacterial endocarditis are outlined in Table 59-21.

DYSRHYTHMIAS

In the era of extensive cardiovascular surgery and long-term survival of patients with congenital heart disease, the incidence of dysrhythmias in pediatric patients has increased dramatically.[14] Our enhanced suspicion of and capability to diagnose cardiac dysrhythmias in children has led to a greater number of children identified to be at risk for cardiac arrhythmias. Although knowledge of the adult ECG is useful in interpreting the pediatric ECG, developmental changes throughout infancy and childhood account for significant differences between the two.

BRADYDYSRHYTHMIAS

Normal heart rate varies with the age of the patient, as does the definition of bradycardia (see Table 59-21). A heart rate of 60 may be normal for a healthy, conditioned 10-year old, but is grossly abnormal for a newborn and may be associated with a severe reduction in cardiac output. Conversely, a heart rate of 200 may be normal for a crying infant, but is abnormal for an older child.

SINUS BRADYCARDIA

Sinus bradycardia may occur in states of increased vagal tone, hypoxia, or after surgery in the atrium. Asymptomatic sinus bradycardia generally requires no therapy, although it is prudent to treat the cause of the bradycardia whenever possible (for example, apnea, hypoxia, or elevated intracranial pressure).

DISORDERS OF ATRIOVENTRICULAR CONDUCTION

Isolated first-degree AV block is rarely of clinical significance other than its association with acute rheumatic fever. When first-degree AV block is associated with a right bundle branch block and/or left anterior hemiblock, concern is raised as to the possibility of potential progressive conduction abnormalities within the heart. Children should be followed for the development of progressive abnormalities in atrioventricular conduction, with 24-hour monitoring and, in some cases, electrophysiologic testing.

Mobitz type I second degree AV block (Wenckebach rhythm) is occasionally seen in normal hearts, and requires no intervention. Mobitz type II AV block, however, is more significant, and requires electrophysiologic evaluation to evaluate the location of the block in conduction, and thus the risk of complete heart block, syncope, and/or sudden death.

Complete heart block, or third degree AV block, may occur on a congenital basis, may be acquired secondary to myocarditis or electrolyte imbalance (hyperkalemia), or may develop after cardiac surgery. Congenital complete heart block may cause symptomatic low cardiac output in the neonatal period or later in life, when the escape rhythm slows progressively. The asymptomatic infant with complete heart block and a ventricular rate greater than 55 beats per minute may be followed closely with ambulatory electrocardiography and frequent evaluations. The symptomatic patient, the asymptomatic infant with a heart rate below 55, and the child with an awake heart rate less than 45 should undergo placement of a permanent pacemaker. The child with heart block secondary to hyperkalemia should undergo aggressive therapy to reduce the serum potassium, using such agents as calcium, insulin plus glucose, plus potassium-binding resins. Temporary pacemaker therapy should be instituted if there is evidence of hemodynamic compromise and an inadequate response to such agents as atropine and or isoproterenol.

TACHYDYSRHYTHMIAS

Tachydysrhythmias affect cardiac output by reducing diastolic filling times of the ventricles. Sinus tachycardia may occur during periods of stress, fever, hypovolemia and in association with myocarditis.

SUPRAVENTRICULAR TACHYCARDIA

Supraventricular tachycardia (SVT) is a common dysrhythmia in infancy and childhood, and should be considered a medical emergency in infancy. SVT may be manifest by low cardiac output with poor peripheral perfusion, and often signs of shock. This dysrhythmia is a narrow QRS tachycardia, with rates in the 200 to 300 range. As opposed to sinus tachycardia, this dysrhythmia generally starts and stops abruptly with little variation in the R-R interval.

Treatment of supraventricular tachycardia depends on the condition of the infant. Treatment is outlined in Table 59-22. Infants with evidence for low cardiac output and poor peripheral perfusion should be treated with synchronized direct current cardioversion, 0.5 watt-second per kg. R-wave synchronization is mandatory to prevent discharge on the T wave, and

subsequent ventricular fibrillation. Vagal maneuvers, often effective in older children and adults with supraventricular tachycardia, are generally not effective in infants. The diving reflex has been used to terminate supraventricular tachycardia in infants by placing an ice pack on the infant's face for a few seconds. Caution should be taken to prevent hypothermia; profound apnea may occur in selected infants.

Pharmacologic therapy of supraventricular tachycardia includes the use of a new agent, adenosine, a naturally occurring hormone that, when administered intravenously, causes a brief profound vagal effect on the AV node, and thus terminates supraventricular tachycardia with a reentrant mechanism involving the AV node.[15] It should be administered in emergency situations at doses of 37.5 µg/kg by rapid intravenous push. If unsuccessful, the dose may be doubled and repeated every minute.

Verapamil, widely used in adults with supraventricular tachycardia, has been shown to have disastrous side effects in infants, specifically, profound low cardiac output. We do not recommend the use of this drug in infancy. Once successfully cardioverted, the infant may be begun on oral digoxin, receiving half of a total digitalizing dose, followed by one quarter of the total digitalizing dose 8 hours later, another quarter of the total digitalizing dose in another 8 hours, and then, in 12 hours, beginning one eighth of the digitalizing dose bid. Propranolol may be used, at an oral dosage range of 1 to 4 mg per kg per day in 3 to 4 divided doses. The infant with poorly controlled supraventricular tachycardia should be treated with intravenous procainamide, administered as a bolus of 1 mg per kg every 3 to 5 minutes up to a total dose of 15 mg per kg. Once the tachycardia terminates, the patient may be treated with a continuous procainamide infusion of 20 µg per kg per minute until digitalization is complete. Hypotension may develop on

TABLE 59-21. PROPHYLAXIS AGAINST BACTERIAL ENDOCARDITIS*

Recommended Standard Prophylactic Regimen for Dental, Oral, or Upper Respiratory Tract Procedures in Patients Who Are at Risk*

Drug	Dosing Regimen†
	Standard Regimen
Amoxicillin	3.0 g orally 1 h before procedure; then 1.5 g 6 h after initial dose
	Amoxicillin/Penicillin-Allergic Patients
Erythromycin or	Erythromycin ethylsuccinate, 800 mg, or erythromycin stearate, 1.0 g orally 2 h before procedure; then half the dose 6 h after initial dose
Clindamycin	300 mg orally 1 h before procedure and 150 mg 6 h after initial dose

* Includes those with prosthetic heart valves and other high-risk patients.
† Initial pediatric doses are as follows: amoxicillin, 50 mg/kg; erythromycin ethylsuccinate or erythromycin stearate, 20 mg/kg; and clindamycin, 10 mg/kg. Follow-up doses should be one half the initial dose. Total pediatric dose should not exceed total adult dose. The following weight ranges may also be used for the initial pediatric dose of amoxicillin: <15 kg, 750 mg; 15 to 30 kg, 1500 mg; and >30 kg, 3000 mg (full adult dose).

TABLE 59-21. CONTINUED

Alternate Prophylactic Regimens for Dental, Oral, or Upper Respiratory Tract Procedures in Patients Who Are at Risk of Endocarditis

Drug	Dosing Regimen*
Patients Unable to Take Oral Medications	
Ampicillin	Intravenous or intramuscular administration of ampicillin, 2.0 g, 30 min before procedure; then intravenous or intramuscular administration of ampicillin, 1.0 g, or oral administration of amoxicillin, 1.5 g, 6 h after initial dose
Ampicillin/Amoxicillin/Penicillin-Allergic Patients Unable to Take Oral Medications	
Clindamycin	Intravenous administration of 300 mg 30 min before procedure and an intravenous or oral administration of 150 mg 6 h after initial dose
Patients Considered High Risk and Not Candidates for Standard Regimen	
Ampicillin, gentamicin, and amoxicillin	Intravenous or intramuscular administration of ampicillin, 2.0 g, plus gentamicin, 1.5 mg/kg (not to exceed 80 mg), 30 min before procedure; followed by amoxicillin, 1.5 g, orally 6 h after initial dose; alternatively, the parenteral regimen may be repeated 8 h after initial dose
Ampicillin/Amoxicillin/Penicillin-Allergic Patients Considered High Risk	
Vancomycin	Intravenous administration of 1.0 g over 1 h, starting 1 h before procedure; no repeated dose necessary

* Initial pediatric doses are as follows ampicillin, 50 mg/kg, clindamycin, 10 mg/kg; gentamicin, 2.0 mg/kg; and vancomycin, 20 mg/kg. Follow-up doses should be one half the initial dose. Total pediatric dose should not exceed total adult dose. No initial dose is recommended in this table for amoxicillin (25 mg/kg is the follow-up dose).

Regimens for Genitourinary/Gastrointestinal Procedures

Drug	Dosage Regimen*
Standard Regimen	
Ampicillin, gentamicin, and amoxicillin	Intravenous or intramuscular administration of ampicillin, 2.0 g, plus gentamicin, 1.5 mg/kg (not to exceed 80 mg), 30 min before procedure; followed by amoxicillin, 1.5 g, orally 6 h after initial dose: alternatively, the parenteral regimen may be repeated once 8 h after initial dose
Ampicillin/Amoxicillin/Penicillin-Allergic Patient Regimen	
Vancomycin and gentamicin	Intravenous administration of vancomycin, 1.0 g, over 1 h plus intravenous or intramuscular administration of gentamicin, 1.5 mg/kg (not to exceed 80 mg), 1 h before procedure; may be repeated once 8 h after initial dose
Alternate Low-Risk Patient Regimen	
Amoxicillin	3.0 g orally 1 h before procedure; then 1.5 g 6 h after initial dose

* Initial pediatric doses are as follows: ampicillin, 50 mg/kg; amoxicillin, 50 mg/kg; gentamicin, 2.0 mg/kg; and vancomycin, 20 mg/kg. Follow-up doses should be half the initial dose. Total pediatric dose should not exceed total adult dose.

* With permission from Dajani, A.S., et al.: Prevention of bacterial endocarditis—Recommendations by the American Heart Association. JAMA 264:2919, 1990.

administration of procainamide, and should be treated with fluid administration.

Supraventricular tachycardia in children may be treated initially with vagal maneuvers such as the Valsalva maneuver, the diving reflex, or brief gagging of the patient. Intravenous adenosine may be used safely in older infants and children, and verapamil may be administered intravenously in the patient without congestive heart failure. The dose of verapamil is 0.1 to 0.2 mg per kg IV push over 1 minute. The physician treating any child with verapamil should have calcium, atropine, and isoproterenol available to combat any extreme bradycardia that may ensue. This class of drugs should not be given to any patient who has

TABLE 59-22. TREATMENT OF ARRHYTHMIAS IN CHILDREN

A. Supraventricular tachycardia in infancy
   1. If the patient is hypotensive or poorly perfused, synchronized DC CARDIOVERSION 0.5 watt-sec/kg, followed by oral digitalization (see Table 59-19)
   2. If the patient is stable, the diving reflex may be tried (see text)
   3. Intravenous adenosine, 37.5 µg/kg rapid IV bolus. The dosage may be doubled every few minutes
   4. Intravenous procainamide, 1 mg/kg IV every 3–5 minutes up to a total dose of 15 mg/kg. A continuous infusion of procainamide of 20 µg/kg/min may be started while digitalization is performed
   5. Oral propranolol may be given in lieu of or in addition to digoxin, 1–4 mg/kg/day in 3 doses
B. Supraventricular tachycardia in children
   1. Vagal maneuvers (Valsalva, gagging, carotid sinus massage)
   2. Adenosine (see A3)
   3. Verapamil, 0.1–0.2 mg/kg IV push over 1 minute
   4. DC countershock for any hemodynamically unstable patient (see A1 above)
   5. Patients with pre-excitation should be treated with oral beta-blockers such as Atenolol, 1–2 mg/kg/day in a single dose after cardioversion.
C. Atrial flutter
   1. DC cardioversion if hemodynamically unstable
   2. Digitalization (see Table 59-19)
   3. Propranolol, 1–4 mg/kg/day in 3 doses PO
   4. Atenolol, 1–2 mg/kg/day, po
   5. Quinidine gluconate, 10–30 mg/kg/day in 2–3 doses PO (monitor initially for torsades de pointes)
   6. Amiodarone, 3–6 mg/kg/day po in one dose
D. Ventricular tachycardia
   1. DC cardioversion when associated with hemodynamic instability
   2. Lidocaine, 1 mg/kg bolus, and 20–50 µg/kg/min IV
   3. Propranolol, 0.01–0.1 mg/kg IV over 5–10 minutes
   4. Phenytoin, 3–5 mg/kg IV over 5 minutes
E. Ventricular fibrillation
   1. DC cardioversion 2 watt-sec/kg
   2. Ensure optimum pH balance with $NaHCO_3$
   3. Ensure adequate oxygenation
   4. Add bretylium tosylate, 5 mg/kg IV bolus
   5. Lidocaine as in D2

received beta-adrenergic blocking agents within the previous 48 hours.

Synchronized DC cardioversion should be performed on any child with evidence of low cardiac output or severe congestive heart failure secondary to supraventricular tachycardia. After cardioversion, older children with evidence of pre-excitation on the surface ECG should be treated with beta-blockers because a small number of children may shorten the antegrade refractory period of the accessory connection with digoxin therapy, placing them at risk for the development of life-threatening ventricular arrhythmias if they develop atrial flutter or fibrillation.

ATRIAL FLUTTER OR FIBRILLATION

Atrial flutter is a supraventricular dysrhythmia seen in children who have undergone surgery within the atria, in infants and children with dilated atria, and occasionally in otherwise healthy neonates. It is characterized electrocardiographically by flutter waves in lead II and varying degrees of AV block, with any-where from 1:1 conduction to 4:1 block. Direct current cardioversion is the fastest mode of conversion to normal sinus rhythm, and the patient is digitalized to prevent recurrences and block the AV node. If recurrent flutter is a problem, the patient may be treated with quinidine or, in refractory cases, amiodarone.

Atrial fibrillation is less common in children, and is generally characterized by an irregular ventricular response with a coarse to fine pattern of atrial activity, best seen in lead II on the ECG. Treatment consists of digitalization with the addition of propranolol when the ventricular rate is rapid. Caution should be taken NOT to treat patients with pre-excitation secondary to the Wolff-Parkinson-White syndrome with digoxin, to avoid the complication of augmented conduction through the accessory connection and ventricular fibrillation.

VENTRICULAR TACHYCARDIA

Defined as three or more premature ventricular beats in a row, ventricular tachycardia is an uncommon finding in patients without pre-existing heart disease. It may be seen in children with complex congenital heart disease, in patients following corrective cardiac surgery, and in patients with hypertrophic cardiomyopathy, intracardiac tumors, or the long QT syndrome. Syncope or sudden death may be the first presenting symptom. The evaluation of children with ventricular tachycardia should include an electrocardiogram, 24-hour ambulatory monitoring, an echocardiogram, and in some cases electrophysiologic testing. Patients with ventricular tachycardia and evidence of low cardiac output should be treated with DC cardioversion when hemodynamics are poor. Drug therapy of ventricular tachycardia includes lidocaine as a bolus of 1 mg per kg intravenously, and 20 to 50 μg per kg per minute as a continuous infusion. Other drugs that have been used in children with ventricular tachycardia include propranolol, phenytoin for postoperative tetralogy of Fallot associated with ventricular ectopy, procainamide, or bretylium.

VENTRICULAR FIBRILLATION

Ventricular fibrillation is a chaotic acute ventricular rhythm associated with no discernible cardiac contraction. Treatment is external cardiac massage and DC countershock, 2 watt-seconds per kg, as well as epinephrine, lidocaine, and bretylium as needed. After successful defibrillation, pharmacologic therapy with lidocaine, propranolol, or bretylium should be instituted.

REFERENCES

1. Rudolph, A.M., and Heymann, M.A.: Circulatory changes during growth in the fetal lamb. Circ. Res. 26:289, 1970.
2. Kafer, E.: Blood gases. In Long's Fetal and Neonatal Cardiology, 1st Ed. Edited by Long, W.A. Philadelphia, W.B. Saunders, 1990.
3. Clyman, R.I., and Heymann, M.A.: Pharmacology of the ductus arteriosus. Pediatr. Clin. North Am. 28:77, 1981.
4. Morgan, B.C., Guntheroth, W.G., and Mullins, R.S.: Physiologic studies of paroxysmal hyperpnea in cyanotic congenital heart disease. Circulation 31:70, 1965.
5. Park, M.K.: Cyanotic congenital heart defects. In Pediatric Cardiology for Practitioners. Chicago, Year Book Medical Publishers, 1984.
6. Baylen, B.G., Johnson, G., Tsang, R., et al.: The occurrence of hyperaldosteronism in infants with congestive heart failure. Am. J. Cardiol. 45:305, 1980.
7. Hossack, K.F., Neutze, J.M., Lowe, J.B., and Barratt-Boyes, B.G.: Congenital valvular aortic stenosis: Natural history and assessment for operation. Br. Heart J. 43:561, 1980.
8. Alpert, B., Barfield, J., and Taylor, W.: Reappraisal of digitalis in infants with left to right shunts and heart failure. J. Pediatr. 106:66, 1985.
9. White, R.D., and Lietman, P.S.: Commentary: A reappraisal of digitalis with left to right shunts and "heart failure." J. Pediatr. 92:867, 1978.
10. Shaddy, R.E., Teitel, D.F., and Brett, C.: Short term hemodynamic effects of captopril in infants with congestive heart failure. Am. J. Dis. Child. 142:100, 1988.
11. Noren, G.R., Staley, N.A., and Kaplan, E.L.: Nonrheumatic inflammatory diseases. In Moss' Heart Disease in Infants, Children and Adolescents, 4th ed., Edited by Adams, F. Baltimore, Williams and Wilkins, 1989.
12. Fujiwara, H., and Hamashima, Y.: Pathology of the heart in Kawasaki disease. Pediatrics 61:100, 1978.
13. Newburger, J., Takahashi, M., Burns, J.C., et al.: The treatment of Kawasaki syndrome with intravenous gamma globulin. N. Engl. J. Med. 315:341, 1986.
13a. Bisno, A.L.: Group A streptococcal infections and acute rheumatic fever. N. Engl. J. Med. 325:783, 1991.
13b. Seppala, H., et al.: Resistance to erythromycin in group A streptococci. N. Engl. J. Med. 326:292, 1992.
14. Gillette, P.C., Garson, A., Crawford, F., et al.: Dysrhythmias. In Moss's Heart Disease in Infants, Children and Adolescents, 4th ed. Edited by Adams, F. Baltimore, Williams and Wilkins, 1989.
15. Overholt, E.D., Rheuban, K.S., Gutgesell, H.P., et al.: Usefulness of adenosine for arrhythmias in infants and children. Am. J. Cardiol. 61:336, 1988.

ACUTE RESPIRATORY EMERGENCIES IN CHILDREN

Michael F. Altieri and Thom A. Mayer

CAPSULE

Acute respiratory emergencies are the most frequent cause of pediatric visits to Emergency Departments (EDs) across the country. The spectrum of these illnesses ranges from minor upper respiratory infections to life-threatening episodes requiring acute intervention.

INTRODUCTION

It is extremely important that the emergency physician approach each patient with a potential respiratory problem according to a protocol-oriented approach designed to assess whether the patient is stable, unstable, or potentially unstable. One of the most important factors is an assessment of the child's overall work of breathing. This involves ensuring that a combination of factors is assessed, including the respiratory rate, the respiratory depth, the effort of respiration, the use of accessory muscles, and the presence or absence of inspiratory or respiratory stridor.

In addition to ensuring that the emergency physicians approach such patients in a format that allows them to assess the overall potential severity of illness of the child, it is also important to educate the nursing staff, particularly the triage nurses, regarding differences between adults and children with respiratory diseases. Similarly, emergency physicians must educate prehospital care personnel as to the numerous ways in which children can present with respiratory illnesses, as well as specific treatment for the clinical entities with which children may present.

CROUP (LARYNGOTRACHEOBRONCHITIS)

Croup is a viral illness that usually affects children from 6 months to 3 years of age.[1] It is usually a non-life-threatening illness, but can become severe enough to require airway support when airway inflammation is significant enough to cause respiratory compromise. Croup is usually seen between November and March, but may occur in other months as well. The most common etiologic agent is the parainfluenza virus or respiratory syncytial virus (RSV).[2]

PATHOPHYSIOLOGY

Croup infects the vocal cords and the mucosa of the subglottic area. It causes edema of the mucosa and an increase in secretion of mucus. The edema and secretions inhibit the flow of air through the vocal cords and the subglottic area. Because the inflammation may variably affect the airway from the level of the vocal cords down to and including the bronchi, the term "laryngotracheobronchitis" is technically more accurate than "croup." In general, the severity of the illness can be closely correlated with the degree of airway narrowing caused by the combination of edema and an increase in mucus production.[3]

CLINICAL PRESENTATION

Croup usually begins with an upper respiratory infection type of prodrome, including low-grade fever and runny nose. A cough soon develops, then becomes increasingly severe and sounds like the barking of a seal. The child then develops stridor with sternal, suprasternal, and substernal retractions. The illness usually peaks between the third and fifth days.[4]

A second entity, called spasmodic croup, may be seen independently of infectious croup (laryngotracheobronchitis) or in conjunction with it. It is caused by spasm of the larynx. In spasmodic croup, there is a sudden onset of stridor with a croupy cough, and fever may or may not be associated with this. It is typically seen in the child with mild infectious croup, who becomes acutely worse when put to bed. Spasmodic croup often responds dramatically to exposure to humidity and/or the cool night air. The child's symptoms often resolve before presentation to the ED.

PHYSICAL EXAMINATION

Children with croup usually present as generally nontoxic in appearance, with mild rhinorrhea, variable degrees of inspiratory stridor, and a characteristic barking cough. Depending on the degree of inflammation and mucus secretion, the child may have different degrees of tachypnea, sternal or substernal retractions, and inspiratory stridor. Most children present with low-grade fever. There is a two to one (2:1) male-to-female ratio at an occurrence rate of approximately 50%.[6] In general, stridor does not become audible until approximately 75 to 90% of the airway has become occluded. Cyanosis only occurs in extremely severe cases, in which the airway has become significantly compromised.

PREHOSPITAL MANAGEMENT

Prehospital management should include the following:

1. Humidified oxygen; pulse oximetry if available. Call results to ED.
2. Consider 0.5 cc of racemic epinephrine in 2.5 cc of normal saline by nebulization.
3. Transport
   A. If the child has severe respiratory distress and shows signs of respiratory failure, assist with bag-valve-mask ventilation.
   B. Severe cases may need intubation or needle cricothyroidotomy.

EMERGENCY DEPARTMENT MANAGEMENT

EVALUATION

The initial evaluation of the ED patient presenting with croup should be an overall assessment of the child's

TABLE 59-23. CLINICAL CROUP SCORE*

	0	1	2
Inspiratory breath sounds	Normal	Harsh with rhonchi	Delayed
Stridor	None	Inspiratory	Inspiratory and expiratory
Cough	None	Hoarse cry	Barking cough
Retractions/flaring	None	Flaring, suprasternal retractions	As in 1 plus subcostal/intercostal retractions
Cyanosis	None	On room air	On 40% O_2
or			
PaO_2 (mm Hg)	70–100	<70	<70
CNS function	Normal	Depressed/agitated	Coma

* Modified from Downes, J.J., and Raphaely, R.: Pediatric intensive care. Anesthesiology *43*:242, 1975.

difficulty in breathing. The clinical croup score is helpful in this regard because it assesses inspiratory breath sounds, stridor, cough, retractions, cyanosis, and CNS function in a numeral fashion (Table 59-23).

CHEST X RAY

In cases in which the clinical diagnosis is evident based on the history and physical findings, a chest x ray may not be needed. In cases in which there is a question regarding involvement of the lower airway, a chest radiograph is appropriate. Croup can often be associated with a concomitant pneumonia, usually viral.[7]

LATERAL NECK X RAY

In the past, portable lateral neck x rays were generally restricted to patients in whom the diagnosis of epiglottitis or foreign body was being seriously considered. Although this is generally still an acceptable practice, the pressures of medical legal considerations often result in lateral neck x rays being taken on patients in whom the diagnosis of croup is virtually ensured by the history and physical findings, as well as by response to treatment. Lateral neck films in patients with croup typically show "ballooning" of the airway above the level of obstruction on the lateral film, and "steepling" at the level of obstruction on the AP film (Fig. 59-12). (See Radiologic Diagnosis of Epiglottitis, subsequently in this chapter section.)

PULSE OXIMETRY MONITORING

Pulse oximeter readings should be obtained on all patients in whom there is potential airway compromise, including those with croup. It is generally wise to continue to monitor the patient throughout his or her course of therapy in the ED because partial airway obstruction may progress during the ED stay.

ARTERIAL BLOOD GAS

Arterial blood gases are usually restricted to patients in whom significant respiratory failure is suspected. Even patients to be hospitalized because of severe illness may not need arterial blood gases, unless impending respiratory failure is suspected or there are signs of CO_2 retention or deterioration.

TREATMENT

Humidified oxygen should be provided to all children presenting to the ED with clinical signs or symptoms consistent with laryngotracheobronchitis. In patients with minimal signs of disease, humidified room air still allows better liquefaction and mobilization of secretions and decreased threat of airway obstruction. In cases in which cyanosis is present or the croup score indicates significant disease, high-flow oxygen should be provided. In patients in whom the croup score in the clinical evaluation indicates relatively mild disease, overall assessment of the patient and improvement of the hydrational status, both with humidified oxygen and through the gastrointestinal tract, may be all that is required in the ED management phase. Parents should be given specific discharge instructions regarding continuation of mist-vaporization treatments, close observation, and appropriate follow-up.

Racemic epinephrine (Vapo-Nephrine) should be considered for children with croup scores in the 4 to 5 range. These are usually children with significant respiratory compromise, often those with either sufficient severity of illness or duration of symptoms to require relief of airway obstruction. The medication is usually given in a dose of 0.5 cc in 2.5 cc of normal saline given by nebulized mist.[8] Significant controversy exists as to whether children who have been given racemic epinephrine require admission to the hospital. Generally, all such children should be admitted to the hospital because racemic epinephrine should be restricted to children whose clinical evaluation and croup score place them in a significant at risk category. In addition, a "rebound" phenomenon has been described in children receiving racemic epinephrine. In this phenomenon, clinical symptoms may dramatically worsen once the medication has worn off, resulting in what can present as dramatic airway compromise after an initial response to therapy. This response has been described as occurring as long as 6 hours after the initial treatment. Because of these considerations, most children who receive

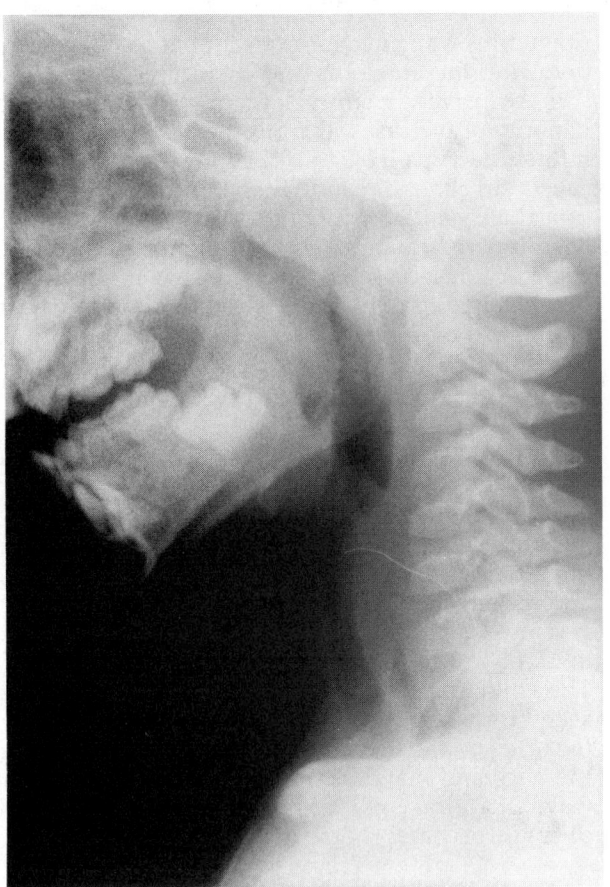

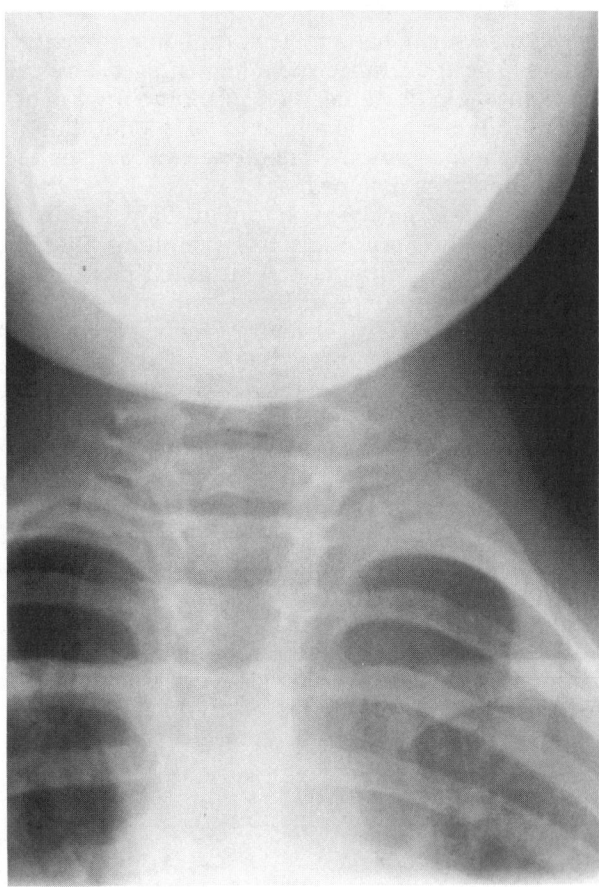

FIG. 59-12.   A. Lateral neck x ray in a child with croup demonstrates a normal epiglottis, a deep air shadow anterior to the epiglottis, indicating no inflammation, and "ballooning" of the hypopharynx above the level of obstruction at the cricoid cartilage. B. AP radiograph in a child with croup demonstrates "steepling" of the airway, reflecting narrowing in a concentric and progressive fashion that mimics that of a church steeple. This reflects the narrowing of the cricoid cartilage from inflammation.

racemic epinephrine require admission to the hospital, even if only overnight.

In all cases in which racemic epinephrine has been used, the patient's private pediatrician or the pediatrician on call should be consulted regarding such a decision. Rarely, a pediatrician or a gatekeeper physician for a managed care program may recommend discharge after suitable patient evaluation. Although this practice should be discouraged, no such patient should ever be discharged from the ED without at least 6 hours of observation.

Recent literature suggests that steroids may be of significant benefit in laryngotracheobronchitis if given early in the course of the disease. The effect seems to be independent of the degree of severity of the illness. In general, patients seen within the first 3 to 4 days of illness probably benefit from administration of steroids. These may be given by mouth (prednisone 2 mg/kg per dose every 8 hours times three doses) or as dexamethasone (0.6 mg/kg in a single intramuscular dose).[9]

WHEN TO HOSPITALIZE THE CHILD WITH CROUP

Hospitalization should be considered in any patient who has received racemic epinephrine or in whom clinical deterioration occurs despite therapy in the ED. In rare circumstances, intubation may be required to maintain the airway in a child with croup. In these cases, it is critical to remember that the cricoid area of the child's airway is both the narrowest portion of the airway and the site of active inflammation in croup. For this reason, it is usually necessary to select a tube size that is somewhat smaller than the child could normally accommodate, which helps to ensure minimal trauma to the mucosa of the cricoid cartilage while the endotracheal tube is in place.

In all children who are discharged from the ED, careful discharge instructions should be given, including specific instructions to return if airway obstruction worsens during therapy.

DIFFERENTIAL DIAGNOSIS

Epiglottitis usually has a more abrupt onset, results in a more toxic appearance and a higher fever, and produces supraglottic, rather than subglottic airway compromise. In any case in which there is a question regarding the diagnosis, a lateral neck x ray (see Fig. 59-12) should be obtained.

Upper airway foreign body can usually be distinguished by the abrupt onset of symptoms after the child has placed something in his or her mouth. Foreign bodies may lodge at any point in the airway, either above or below the level of the vocal cords. In many cases of airway foreign bodies, wheezing is present on a unilateral basis, which assists in making the diagnosis. Radiographs of the airway may also be helpful in identifying the foreign body, including inspiratory and expiratory radiographs.

Tonsilar hypertrophy can usually be readily distinguished on physical examination. In cases in which there is some question, lateral neck x rays and a chest x ray usually distinguish croup based on the findings listed previously.

Posterior pharyngeal abscesses can usually be readily distinguished, either on physical examination or by radiographs and CT scans (Figs. 59-13 and 59-14).

PITFALLS

Consider admission for any child who needs racemic epinephrine because a significant rebound phenomenon can be seen anywhere from 2 to 6 hours after administration of racemic epinephrine. Any child with a croup score of greater than 4 in the first 3 days of the illness should probably also be considered for admission because this child will probably get worse before he or she gets better. Antibiotics are not necessary with croup unless there is a concomitant pneumonia, and even at this time the pneumonia is probably viral. Blood count may be useful in this determination.

EPIGLOTTITIS

Epiglottitis is a life-threatening infection that carries the potential of complete and sudden airway obstruction. It is a rapidly progressing illness, usually seen in the preschool age group (between 2 and 5 years). Epiglottitis can clearly be seen at any age, however, from infancy to adulthood.[10] Unlike croup, it has no seasonal propensity.

PATHOPHYSIOLOGY

Epiglottitis is an infection of the upper respiratory tract involving the epiglottis and the aryepiglottal tissue. It is exclusively a supraglottic infection. In the vast majority of the cases, the infection is by Hemophilus influenzae Type B (80 to 90%). Other agents that may cause this illness include Staphylococcus aureus, N. catarrhalis, and Pneumonococcus, which have also been isolated from patients with epiglottitis.[11,12] This bacterial infection causes massive swelling and edema of the epiglottis and the entire supraglottic area. This swelling in the airway of a small child can rapidly lead to complete airway obstruction.

CLINICAL PRESENTATION

Unlike croup, epiglottitis has no prodrome phase. The child presents acutely ill, with a body temperature often elevated to 104° Fahrenheit, is toxic-appearing, and usually has significant stridor. Because of the severe dysphagia of epiglottitis, the child is often drooling and will not swallow his or her own secretions. The child speaks with a muffled voice and is often seen "tripoding," sitting on the edge of the bed with the arms on the bed behind him or her and throwing the neck and mandible forward to maximize the airway. Often the child refuses to lie down because the dyspnea becomes worse in a supine position.

PHYSICAL EXAMINATION

Children with epiglottitis usually have a high fever, appear toxic, and have stridorous respirations. If the epiglottis is visualized, it is enlarged and cherry red in color. *Attempts at visualization of the epiglottis should be done cautiously, only by a physician, and the anterior part of the tongue only should be instrumented with a tongue blade.* Even with extreme care, respiratory obstruction may occur, and in contemporary emergency medical practice, such examination is discouraged. Physicians should rely instead initially on clinical findings and the lateral neck radiograph (see Fig. 59-15) for diagnosis.

Physical examination may also demonstrate concomitant otitis media or pneumonia, but attention must first be directed to the cause of respiratory distress.

PREHOSPITAL MANAGEMENT

Prehospital management should include the following:

1. Keep the child calm.
2. Do not instrument the oral pharynx.
3. Use caution in starting an IV.

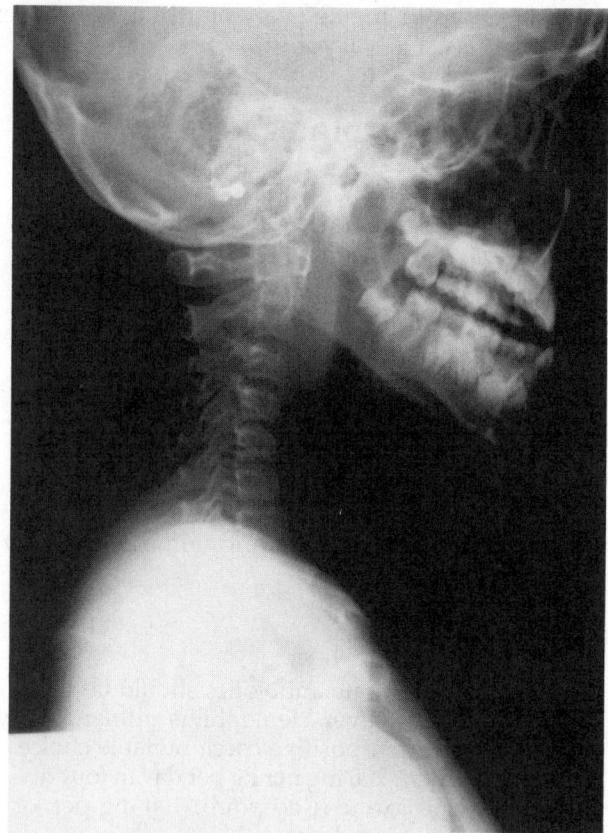

A

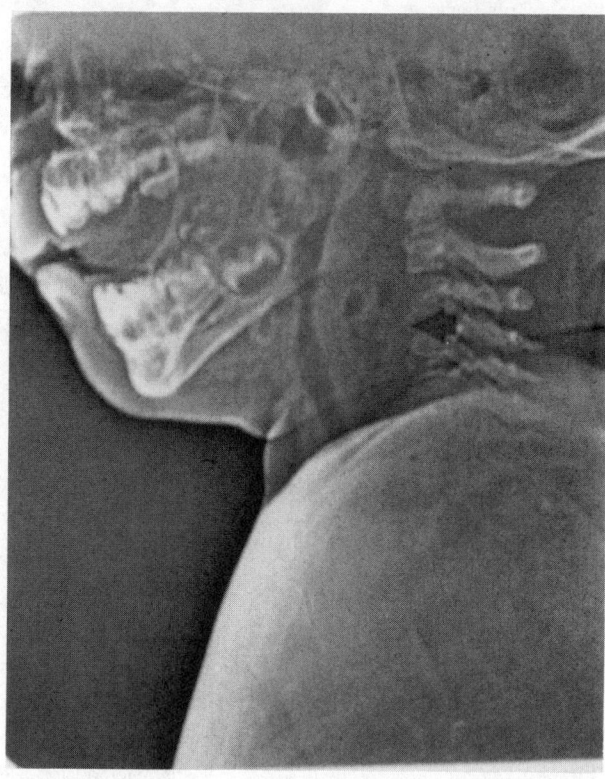

B

FIG. 59-13.   A. Lateral neck radiograph in a child with a posterior pharyngeal abscess shows straightening of the cervical spine, increased diameter in the retropharyngeal space, and loculation of fluid. B. Xeroradiograph of child with posterior pharyngeal abscess.

4. Transport the child in the sitting position. Do not force him or her to lie down because the respiratory distress will become worse.
5. Supplemental oxygen by blow-by or mask is advised.
6. If the child suffers complete airway obstruction during transport, the following three methods are recommended to establish an airway:
   A. Oral tracheal intubation
   B. Needle cricothyroidotomy
   C. A bag-valve-mask using high pressure and occluding the pop-off valve

   When complete airway obstruction occurs during transport, the prehospital care provider is faced with an extremely difficult situation. In all cases, an initial attempt should be made to ventilate the child through bag-valve-mask ventilation. Even in patients with a high degree of airway obstruction, it is sometimes possible to generate enough pressure through appropriate airway seal to oxygenate or ventilate the child until he or she can be transported to the hospital. In all such cases, there should be evidence of bilateral chest wall rise during ventilation. If this cannot be obtained, a single cautious attempt at intubation may be attempted if the prehospital care provider has the experience and technical expertise to intubate and the esti-

mated time to arrival at the hospital is more than a few minutes. Manipulation of the inflamed epiglottis, however, may cause significant laryngospasm, and this should be done only by experienced intubators and in the most extreme circumstances. If these techniques fail, needle cricothyroidotomy may be necessary to ensure that oxygenation and ventilation can be performed until an airway can be established in the hospital.
7. Notify the receiving hospital before the patient's arrival.

EMERGENCY DEPARTMENT MANAGEMENT

EVALUATION

If the diagnosis of epiglottitis is in doubt, i.e., if croup or foreign body aspiration is a serious consideration, airway films and chest x rays are indicated. These films should initially be done in the ED, where the emergency physician is available to handle endotracheal intubation and/or provision of a surgical airway. *Equipment for endotracheal intubation and cricothyrotomy should be kept at the bedside.*

As soon as the ED is aware of the potential of receiving a child with epiglottitis, the support services

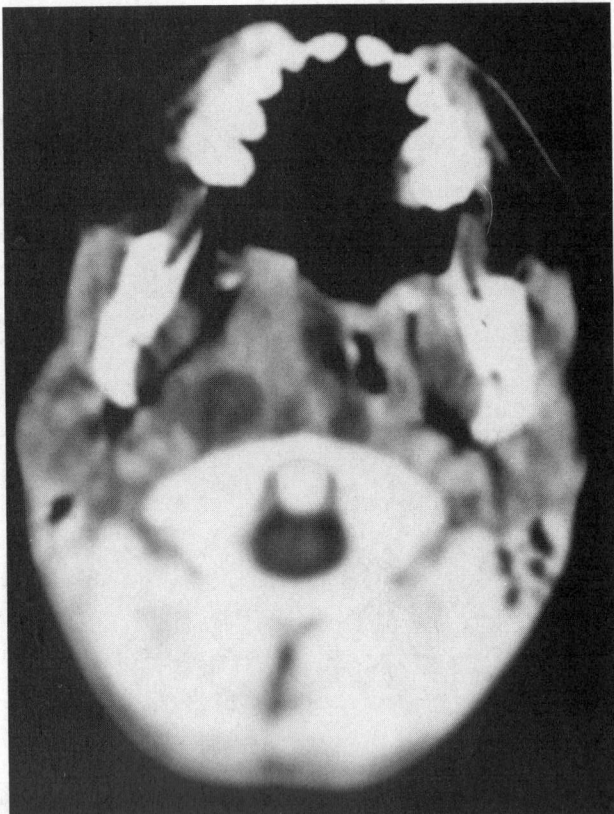

FIG. 59-14. CT scan of the head and neck, showing a large retropharyngeal abscess, just in front of the spinal column. Loculated areas are well visualized in several areas.

of Anesthesiology and ENT should be mobilized. If at all possible, an Operating Room (OR) should be prepared so that the patient may be transported there for intubation. Subsequently, the child should be monitored in an intensive care unit.

SECURING THE AIRWAY

Optimally, the person in the institution most experienced in endotracheal intubation should be summoned to perform the intubation. This is usually an anesthesiologist. Preferably, the intubation should be done in the OR, using halothane/nitrous oxide anesthesia. A person capable of supplying a surgical airway should be standing by. In an emergency situation of sudden respiratory obstruction, however, there should be no delay in attempting to provide even a temporary airway.

If the airway is obstructed in the ED, endotracheal intubation, needle cricothyrotomy and bag-valve-mask ventilation are the three methods that can be used to attempt emergency ventilation of the patient.

After the airway is secured, an intravenous line should be placed, the patient should be kept sedated (midazolam 0.1 to 0.3 mg/kg and/or morphine infusion 0.1 to 0.2 mg/kg per hour). In some cases, paralysis

vecuronium (0.1 mg/kg every hour) needs to be employed (with a ventilator in use).

DIFFERENTIAL DIAGNOSIS

The differential diagnosis of epiglottitis should include:

1. Croup
2. Upper airway foreign body
3. Tracheitis
4. Diphtheria
5. Tonsillar hypertrophy
6. Peritonsillar/retropharyngeal abscess

In general, children with epiglottitis have more severe airway obstruction than those with croup, a more rapid onset of illness, and higher fevers, and do not respond to efforts at humidification of the airway.

ANTIBIOTICS

The most appropriate antibiotics should be given immediately IV to cover Hemophilus influenzae (type B) as well as gram-positive cocci. Suitable choices include ampicillin, 200 mg per kg per day in four divided doses, or ceftriaxone (Rocephin), 100 mg per kg per day in two divided doses.

RADIOLOGIC DIAGNOSIS OF EPIGLOTTITIS

Soft tissue lateral neck radiographs can play an important role in subacute diagnosis. CT and MRI scanning have limited use because of time delays and need for isolation.

Interpretation of standard lateral neck radiographs may be difficult, but certain findings can be useful:

1. Ballooned hypopharynx
2. Increased epiglottic and aryepiglottic fold widths
3. Narrowed tracheal air column
4. Prevertebral soft tissue swelling
5. Obliteration of the vallecula and pyriform sinuses

Figures 59-15 and 59-16 demonstrate findings on lateral neck x rays. Interpretation is often difficult. Future developments in CT and MRI scanning will be welcome in assisting in diagnosis of these conditions.

A study by Rothrock et al.[13] attempted to define objective radiologic parameters on soft tissue lateral neck radiographs. Ratios of soft tissue structures of children with known epiglottitis were compared to those of children without it but with pharyngitis or croup. These investigators found that accuracy of diagnosis was enhanced with the following ratios:

$$\frac{\text{Epiglottic width}}{\text{Third vertebral body}} = \text{more than } 0.5$$

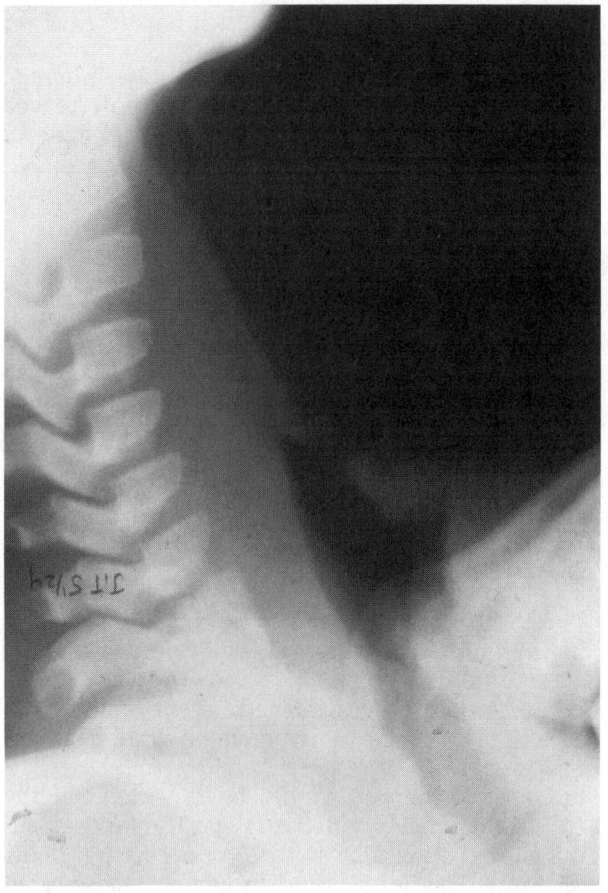

FIG. 59-15. Lateral neck x rays taken in a patient with epiglottitis show a classic "thumbprint"-shaped epiglottis, minimal to no airway shadow anterior to the epiglottis, and hyperaeration of the area proximal to the epiglottis.

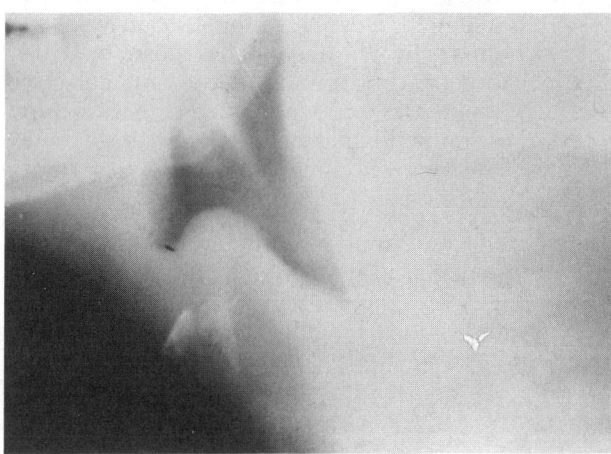

FIG. 59-16. Close-up view of the lateral airway in a child with epiglottitis shows the classic findings of a large epiglottis and a minimal shadow anterior to the epiglottis.

$$\frac{\text{Aryepiglottic width}}{\text{Third vertebral body}} = \text{more than } 0.35$$

$$\frac{\text{Epiglottic width}}{\text{Epiglottic height}} = \text{more than } 0.60$$

In the acute situation, such measurements may prove difficult.

More reliable direct information can come through the CT scan. The time delays and need for longer periods of positioning, however, are impediments to the use of this tool in the acute diagnosis of epiglottitis.

The primary use of radiologic evaluation is in patients in whom the diagnosis is not clinically obvious or if the condition has not progressed to an extreme state.

Some cases of epiglottitis never progress to complete respiratory obstruction, particularly when diagnosis and treatment are started early.

BRONCHIOLITIS

Bronchiolitis is a viral infection of the lower airways, usually caused by the respiratory syncytial virus (RSV). It can be caused by influenza virus, parainfluenza virus, and adenovirus.[14] Bronchiolitis is usually seen in children under 2 years, but is mostly seen in those under 1 year. It has a seasonal propensity and is mostly seen in the winter months (between November and March) when RSV is at its peak.

PATHOPHYSIOLOGY

This viral infection of the lower airway (bronchioles) produces edema of the mucosa and significantly increases the mucus-like secretions. It also causes spasm of the peribronchiolar muscles, which are underdeveloped, but nonetheless present in young children. In most cases of bronchiolitis, there is actual mucus over the epithelium, which not only decreases the airway's ability to offer a normal defense mechanism, but may also cause plugging of the airway. Fortunately, the epithelium of the airway usually regenerates in a brief time, usually 2 to 3 days, although the functional capacity of the cilia may take up to 2 weeks to return.[15]

CLINICAL PRESENTATION

The degree of symptoms present in children with bronchiolitis depends on the extent of pathophysiologic changes present in the ciliated epithelium. The child usually starts with symptoms of an upper respiratory infection, including nasal congestion, nasal discharge, and fever. Lower respiratory symptoms such as a tight cough and wheezing usually develop over a day or two (slower than in asthma).

The child can then develop varying degrees of respiratory distress. The symptoms include tachypnea, retractions (mainly intracostal), nasal flaring, and signs of hypoxia such as cyanosis and pallor. *Caution: young babies infected with the respiratory syncytial virus can develop periods of apnea along with the symptoms of bronchiolitis.*[16] Bronchiolitis usually lasts for 1 to 2 weeks, although improvement can be noted within several days, mirroring the cellular changes and regeneration mentioned previously.

PHYSICAL EXAMINATION

The examination of a child with bronchiolitis usually reveals a low-grade fever (101 to 102°F), tachypnea, nasal flaring, intercostal retractions, expiratory wheezes, and rales. In severe cases, the child may be noted to be cyanotic. The degree of respiratory difficulty depends on the combination of involvement of bronchiolar smooth muscular involvement, airway inflammation, mucus production, and mucus plugging. In young children, apnea may be present as well. The increased respiratory rate and inability to take fluids by mouth because of the tachypnea often results in clinical dehydration.

PREHOSPITAL MANAGEMENT

Prehospital management should include the following:

1. Administer humidified oxygen.
2. Nebulization treatments as per standing orders and on-line medical control.
   A. Albuterol—Weight less than 10 kg, 1.25 mg; weight over 10 kg, 2.5 mg, or
   B. Terbutaline by nebulization—≤ 10 kg of weight, 2 mg; weight over 10 kg, 4 mg, or
   C. Metaproterenol by nebulization (5% Solution)—weight ≤ 10 kg, 0.15 cc; weight over ≥ 10 kg, 3 cc; or
   D. Subcutaneous epinephrine (1 to 1000 Dilution)—0.01 cc per kg, max 0.3 cc
3. Assist ventilation with bag-valve-mask or endotracheal intubation if necessary.

EMERGENCY DEPARTMENT MANAGEMENT

EVALUATION

The ED evaluation should include:

1. Overall assessment of difficulty in breathing
2. Pulse oximetry
3. Arterial blood gases (if there are signs of respiratory decompensation)
4. Chest x ray
5. CBC
6. Electrolyte and BUN, as well as routine "chemistries," if the patient has had a history of decreased oral intake or vomiting, or if there are signs of dehydration
7. A nasal smear for RSV

TREATMENT

Treatment in the ED is based on clinical evaluation of severity and should include:

1. Humidified oxygen.
2. Beta-adrenergic drugs such as albuterol, terbutaline, metaproterenol, or epinephrine, as detailed previously.[17]
3. Consider the use of theophylline intravenously (bolus of 6 mg per kg over 20 to 30 minutes, then begin a theophylline drip of approximately 0.75 mg per kg per hour).
4. The use of steroids can also be considered, using methylprednisolone 1 mg per kg per dose given every 4 hours.[18]
5. Fluids should be encouraged, given orally if tolerated; if not, by intravenous hydration at approximately 1½ times maintenance.
6. Bolus fluid therapy should be considered if the child is significantly dehydrated. The boluses administered should be 10 to 20 cc per kg per bolus of normal saline solution. In general, slow rehydration is preferable, guided by electrolytes and renal function measures.
7. Assist ventilation if necessary by endotracheal tube.
8. Ribavirin, an antiviral agent used for the treatment of respiratory syncytial virus infection, can be used, but is usually not administered in the ED. It is usually administered to inpatients.[19]
9. The etiologic agents in bronchiolitis are invariably viruses. In children with areas of opacity on the chest radiograph, however, the clinician is faced with a dilemma. Does this represent atelectasis or pneumonia? In all likelihood, these opacities, which are not uncommon, represent atelectasis caused by mucus plugging. Some clinicians, however, recommend that antibiotic coverage be instituted whenever such abnormal chest radiographs are noted.

All children under 6 months should be tested for respiratory syncytial virus (RSV). If they test positive, they are at greater risk for apnea episodes with bronchiolitis, and require hospitalization.

DIFFERENTIAL DIAGNOSIS

The differential diagnosis of bronchiolitis should include asthma, congestive heart failure secondary to any congenital heart disease, cystic fibrosis, chronic or acute aspiration, pneumonia, and lower airway foreign body.

PITFALLS AND MEDICOLEGAL PEARLS

A patient should be considered for admission if: (1) there is severe respiratory distress necessitating assisted ventilation, (2) periods of apnea are noted, (3) a pulse oximeter data shows oxygen saturation consistently below 90% on room air or arterial blood gases show a po_2 of less than 60 on room air, and (4) intolerance is shown to fluids by mouth. If there is any doubt, a period of observation is warranted, with close monitoring.

PNEUMONIA

Pneumonia is an infection of the lung parenchyma that can involve the alveoli or be an interstitial process. It is a common infection in children, and the etiologic agents vary according to the age of the patient. These agents are discussed in the following paragraph.

PATHOPHYSIOLOGY

Table 59-24 categorizes the infectious etiologic agents by the age of the patient.[20]

Several organisms are much less commonly found in pediatric pneumonia. These include pertussis, mycobacterium tuberculosis, pseudomonas aeruginosa, Klebsiella pneumoniae, and anaerobes such as peptostreptococcus.[21]

CLINICAL PRESENTATION

Pneumonia usually presents as a febrile illness with tachypnea and cough and signs of lower respiratory illness (nasal flaring, intracostal retractions). In severe cases, cyanosis and pallor can be seen. Lower lobe pneumonia often presents in a young child as abdominal pain and vomiting and is often confused with gastroenteritis. The young infant may present with only irritability and poor feeding. Chlamydia pneumoniae is often seen in conjunction with conjunctivitis. The child is often afebrile, but usually has a severe cough and tachypnea.

PHYSICAL EXAMINATION

Physical examination should assess the following:

1. Fever
2. Tachypnea
3. Toxic appearance (variable)
4. Nasal flaring
5. Retractions (mainly intercostal)
6. Cyanosis or pallor
7. Rales and wheezes in the lung fields (difficult to hear in children)
8. Decreased breath sounds or egophony
9. Conjunctivitis (infants with chlamydia)
10. Otitis media (seen in children with Hemophilus influenzae pneumonia)

PREHOSPITAL MANAGEMENT

Prehospital management should include the following:

1. Supplemental oxygen by mask, nasal prongs, or blow-by
2. Assist with ventilation if necessary
3. Transport

EMERGENCY DEPARTMENT MANAGEMENT

EVALUATION

Laboratory tests should include CBC, arterial blood gas, pulse oximetry, chest x ray, blood culture, chlamydial culture if indicated, and sputum culture (difficult to obtain in a small child—can be obtained through ET suctioning if child is intubated) (Figs. 59-17 and 59-18).

TABLE 59-24. INFECTIOUS AGENTS IN RELATION TO AGE

Infant (1–2 Months of Age)	Young Child (2 Months–7/8 Yrs.)	Older Child (> 8 Yrs.)
1. Group B streptococcus	Streptococcus pneumoniae	Streptococcus pneumoniae
2. Staphylococcus aureus	Hemophilus influenzae	Mycoplasma
3. Chlamydia trachomatis	Staphylococcus aureus	Viruses
4. Streptococcus pneumoniae	Mycoplasma species	Staphylococcus aureus (rare)
5. Viruses	Viruses	

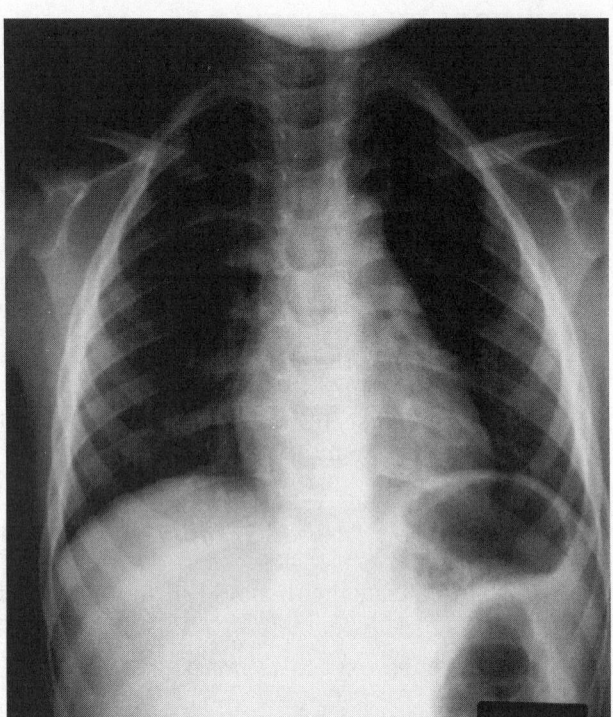

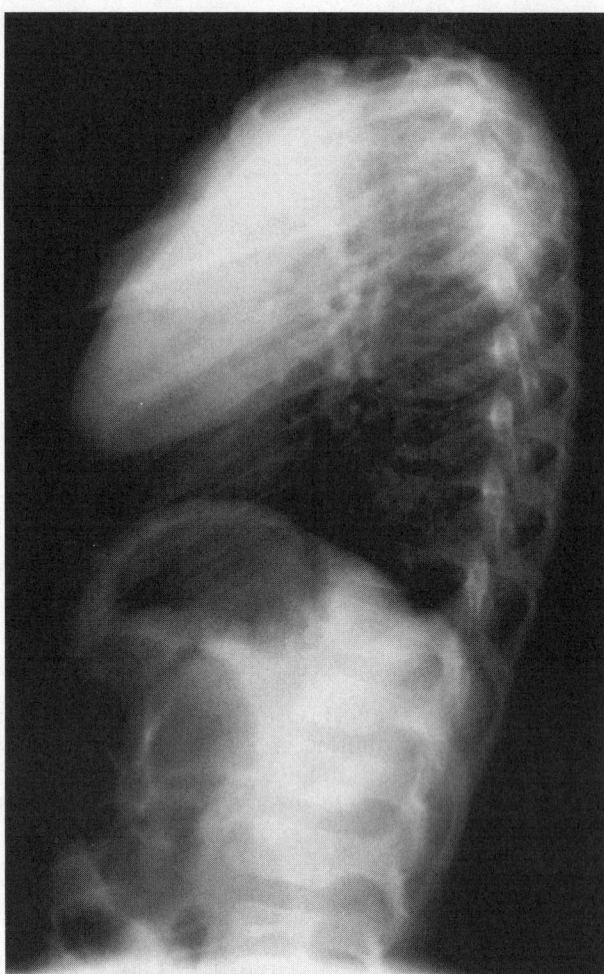

FIG. 59-17. A. PA radiograph of the chest in a patient presenting with cough and tachypnea shows an extremely ill-defined area in the right upper lobe, opposite the area of the aortic knob, which is difficult to visualize on the PA film. B. Lateral radiograph in the same patient shows a well-defined round pneumonia posteriorly just behind the thoracic spine.

TREATMENT

Treatment should be by supplemental oxygen mask, nasal prongs, or blow by. Assist ventilation if necessary by endotracheal intubation.

ANTIBIOTICS

Table 59-25 lists antibiotic dosages. For severe pneumonias that need supplemental oxygen ventilatory support, or close observation with IV antibiotics, admission is required and respiratory isolation is recommended.

DIFFERENTIAL DIAGNOSIS

Differential diagnosis should include lower airway foreign body, reactive airway disease, congestive heart failure, and aspiration.

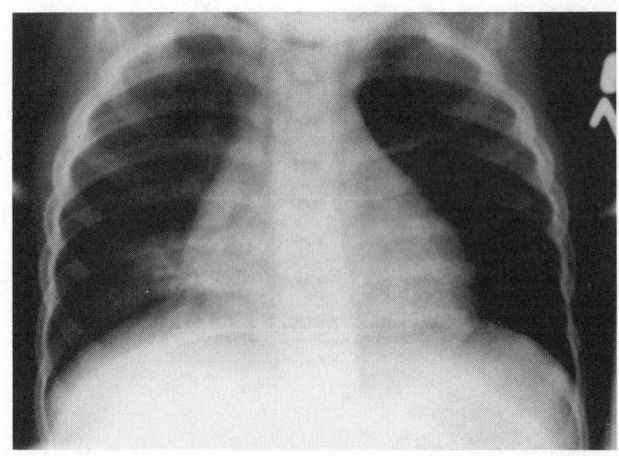

FIG. 59-18. PA radiograph in a child presenting simply with fever and tachypnea shows a discrete right middle lobe infiltrate. As is typical of children, the chest was totally clear to auscultation, including the right middle lobe.

TABLE 59-25. ANTIBIOTIC DOSAGES IN PEDIATRIC PNEUMONIA

A. Infant
   1. Oral Antibiotics
      a. Amoxicillin—30–40 mg per kg per day divided tid for 10 days
      b. Pediazole (if chlamydia is considered)—calculate on basis of erythromycin component—
        30–50 mg per kg per day for 10–14 days divided qid
   2. IV Antibiotics
      a. Ampicillin—200 mg per kg per day divided qid plus gentamicin—5 mg per kg per day
        divided tid
      b. Cefotaxime—50 mg per kg per dose q 8 h
B. Toddler to 8 Years
   1. Oral Antibiotics
      a. Amoxicillin—30–40 mg per kg per day divided tid for 10 days.
      b. Augmentin (calculate on the Amoxicillin dose)—30–40 mg per kg per day divided qid
        for 10 days.
      c. Cefaclor—30–50 mg per kg per day divided tid for 10 days
   2. IV Antibiotics
      a. Ampicillin—200 mg per kg per day (4 doses)
      b. Cefotaxime—50–100 mg per kg per day divided q 8 h
      c. Ceftriaxone—100 mg per kg per day divided bid (can be given IM).
C. Over 8 Years of Age
   1. Oral antibiotics
      a. Erythromycin—30–50 mg per kg per day for 10 days divided qid.
   2. IV Antibiotics
      a. Ampicillin—200 mg per kg per day. Plus oral erythromycin if mycoplasma is suspected.
        Dose 30–50 mg per kg per day. If staphylococcal pneumonia is suspected, nafcillin 100
        mg per kg per day divided qid is added to the ampicillin

DISPOSITION

Not all children who present to the ED with pneumonia necessarily require admission to the hospital. In fact, most can be discharged under close supervision of the parents and follow-up with the pediatrician within 1 to 2 days. For example, in a child who is mildly ill in appearance, but well hydrated, active, and able to take oral fluids, antibiotics by mouth, continued hydration, fever control, and close observation at home are appropriate therapy, with follow-up by the pediatrician within 24 to 48 hours.

In a moderate to severely ill child with significant respiratory distress and evidence of hypoxia on pulse oximetry, however, hospitalization and intravenous hydration and antibiotic therapy are required.

REFERENCES

1. Hen, J., Jr.: Current management of upper airway obstruction. Pediatr. Ann. *15*:274, 1986.
2. Goldhagen, J.L.: Croup: Pathogenesis in management. J. Emerg. Med. *1*:3, 1984.
3. Battaglia, J.D.: Severe croup: The child with fever and upper airway obstruction. Pediatr. Rev. *7*:227, 1986.
4. Davis, H.W., Gartner, J.C., Galvis, A.G., et al.: Acute upper respiratory obstruction: Croup and epiglottitis. Pediat. Clin. North Am. *28*:859, 1981.
5. Westley, C.R., Cotton, E.K., and Brooks, J.G.: Nebulized-racemic epinephrine by IPPB for the treatment of croup. Am. J. Dis. Child. *132*:484, 1978.
6. Adair, J.C.: Ten year experience with IPPB in the treatment of acute laryngotracheobronchitis. Anesth. Analg. *50*:649, 1971.
7. Stankiewicz, J.A., and Bowes, A.K.: Croup and epiglottitis: A radiologic study. Laryngoscope *95*:1159, 1985.
8. Barkin, R.M., and Rosen, P. (eds.): Emergency pediatrics: A Guide to Ambulatory Care. St. Louis, C.D. Mosby, 1990, p. 644.
9. Kairys, S.W., Olmstead, E.M., and O'Conner, G.T.: Steroid treatment of laryngotrachitis: A meta-analysis of the evidence from randomized trials. Pediatrics *83*:683, 1989.
10. Vernon, D.D., and Sarnaik, A.P.: Acute epiglottitis in children: A conservative approach to diagnosis in management. Crit. Care Med. *14*:23, 1986.
11. Lazoritz, S., Sanders, B.S., and Bason, W.M.: Management of acute epiglottitis. Crit. Care Med. *7*:285, 1979.
12. Brilli, R.J., Benzing, G., and Cotcamp, D.H.: Epiglottitis infants less than two years of age. Pediatr. Emerg. Care *5*:16, 1989.
13. Rothrock, S.G., Pignatello, G.A., and Howard, R.M.: Radiologic diagnosis of epiglottitis: Objective criteria for all ages. Ann. Emerg. Med. *19*:978, 1990.
14. Wright, P.F.: Bronchiolitis. Pediatr. Rev. *7*:219, 1986.
15. Wolfram, R.W.: Bronchiolitis. *In* The Clinical Practice of Emergency Medicine. Edited by Harwood-Nuss, A., Linden, C., Luten, R.C., et al.: Philadelphia, J.B. Lippincott, 1991, 730.
16. Burhn, F.W., Mokrohisky, S.T., and McIntosh, K.: Apnea associated with RSV infection in young infants. J. Pediatr. *3*:382, 1987.
17. Shuch, S., Canny, G., Reisman, J.J., et al.: Nebulized albuterol and acute bronchiolitis. J. Pediatr. *117*:633, 1990.
18. Atwater, K.M., and Crone, R.K.: Management of respiratory failure in infants with acute viral bronchiolitis. Am. J. Dis. Child. *138*:1071, 1984.
19. Taber, L.H., Knight, V., Gilbert, B.E., et al.: Ribavirin aerosol treatment of bronchiolitis associated with RSV infection in infants. Pediatrics *72*:613, 1983.
20. Turner, R.B., Lande, A.E., Chase, P., et al.: Pneumonia in pediatric outpatients. Cause and clinical manifestations. J. Pediatr. *111*:194, 1987.
21. Denny, F.W., and Clyde, W.A.: Acute lower respiratory tract infections in non-hospitalized children. J. Pediatr. *108*:635, 1986.

PEDIATRIC ASTHMA

Robert Bolte

CAPSULE

For the physician providing acute care for children, a knowledge of the optimal management of pediatric asthma is essential. Asthma, characterized by bronchial hyperreactivity and reversible airway obstruction,[1] is one of the most common chronic diseases of childhood, affecting 9% of the pediatric population.[2] Acute exacerbations are frequently encountered by physicians in the Emergency Department (ED). According to data for the United States, asthma is the cause of more than 10 million outpatient hospital visits per year in children under 15 years. In this same age group, asthma accounts annually for nearly 400,000 hospitalizations, with an average stay of 3.9 days.[3]

New developments in the physiologic understanding and pharmacologic treatment of pediatric asthma have occurred in recent years.[4]

1. The emergence of nebulized beta-adrenergic agonists in the treatment of bronchospasm.
2. A recognition of the role of cholinergic-mediated airway obstruction.
3. An understanding of asthma as an inflammatory disease, not simply bronchospasm.

This chapter discusses the clinical applications of these concepts in the emergency management of pediatric asthma.

NEBULIZED BETA-ADRENERGIC AGONISTS

For the past 40 years, epinephrine injections have been the mainstay of acute asthma treatment in children.[5] Some clinicians use subcutaneous epinephrine. Epinephrine, however, is a nonselective adrenergic agonist with potent a, β_1, and β_2 effects. Adverse effects such as nausea, vomiting, palpitations, tremor, and headache occur in 50% to 76% of children receiving injected epinephrine.[5,6] Because of epinephrine's nonselectivity and relatively short duration of action, alternative adrenergic agents were developed.

For more than a decade, inhaled long-acting β_2-selective agonists (e.g., albuterol) have been used in Europe, Canada, and Australia. In these countries, these agents have replaced epinephrine as the mainstay of acute asthma therapy.[7,8] Many of these drugs have become available in the United States.

Over the past few years, inhaled β_2-agonists have been frequently evaluated in the medical literature. There is an emerging consensus that:

1. The inhaled β_2-agonists produce bronchodilation at least as effectively as injectable epinephrine or terbutaline.[6,8–16]
2. In general, side effects are less with the inhaled β_2-agents than with injectable agents.[6,13,17]
3. The margin of safety of the newer β_2-selective agonists is wide.[6,18–22]
4. Failure of self-administered β_2-agonists to reverse an acute asthma attack does not predict the ED response to this class of agents.[15]
5. In the initial treatment of asthma, β_2-agonists produce more rapid and potent bronchodilation than does intravenous theophylline.[14]
6. In cases of acute asthma, if β_2-aerosol therapy is optimized, the additional use of theophylline (oral or intravenous) increases side effects but not bronchodilation.[23,24]

PHYSIOLOGY AND PHARMACOLOGY

An understanding of the adrenergic receptor classification system is fundamental to the discussion of the newer, more selective β_2-agents. Adrenergic receptors are characterized as α or β. Stimulation of the α-receptor results in vasoconstriction, bronchial mucosa decongestion, and possibly bronchoconstriction. The β receptors are further subdivided into β_1 and β_2. Beta$_1$-receptor stimulation results in positive chronotropic and inotropic effects on the heart. β_2-receptor stimulation leads to bronchodilation, enhanced mucociliary clearance (increased ciliary beat and decreased mucus viscosity), inhibition of mast cell degranulation, vasodilation, bronchial mucosa decongestion, and skeletal muscle tremor. The response to any given adrenergic agent depends on the predominant receptor type in the tissue and the selectivity of the agent.

On the molecular level, stimulation of the β_2-adrenergic receptor on the cell membrane activates the enzyme adenyl cyclase, which converts intracellular adenosine triphosphate to cyclic adenosine monophosphate. It is thought that cyclic adenosine monophosphate mediates smooth muscle relaxation and inhibition of mast cell degranulation by enhancing the binding of intracellular calcium to the cell membrane and endoplasmic reticulum. This bound intracellular calcium is unavailable for the cellular processes of smooth muscle contraction and secretion.[25,26]

Three classes of β-adrenergic agonists are currently available to the clinician for nebulization: the catecholamines, the saligenins, and the resorcinols.[27,28] The specific pharmacologic action of these agents is directly related to their chemical structures. The catechol nucleus determines the ability to activate adenyl cyclase and the susceptibility to catechol-O-methyl-transferase and sulfatase degradation. Alteration to a resorcinol or saligenin nucleus decreases the agent's susceptibility to degradation and therefore increases the duration of action. The ethanolamine side chain determines to a great extent the adrenergic selectivity of the drug. Furthermore, increasing the size of the amino group decreases susceptibility to monoamine oxidase degradation.[25,26] The chemical structures of the β-adrenergic agents are shown in Figure 59-19. The clinical pharmacologic properties of the nebulized β-adrenergic agonists are detailed in Table 59-26.

An analysis of the nebulized β-adrenergic agonists with regard to their relative utility in the treatment of acute asthma suggests that:

1. Although isoproterenol is a potent bronchodilator, it has a short duration of action and possesses significant β_1-adrenergic (cardiac) side effects.[29]
2. Isoetharine compares unfavorably in all parameters (potency, duration, and selectivity).[30]
3. Metaproterenol is a fairly potent agent with significant advantages in duration and selectivity when compared with isoproterenol and isoetharine.[29,31,32]
4. Terbutaline, albuterol (salbutamol), and fenoterol have comparable clinical effects. They may represent an improvement over metaproterenol in potency, duration, and selectivity.[29,33–35]

With the newer nebulized β_2-selective agents, an exacting dosing scheme based on the patient's body weight may not be necessary. Less than 10% of the inhaled drug is actually retained in the lungs.[36–38] Moreover, these agents possess a wide safety margin.[10,18,19,22] In addition, for a given volume of nebulized agent, the amount of drug actually inhaled may be directly proportional to the size[31] and therefore the tidal volume[39] of the child. Thus, a less precise but more practical dosage schedule based on age is acceptable. Table 59-27 details a suggested dosing and administration regimen. Dosage should be individually adjusted on the basis of clinical response and side effects.[40] All β-adrenergic agents should be used with caution in patients with cardiovascular disorders (particularly outflow tract obstructions of the left ventricle) and in patients receiving tricyclic antidepressants or monoamine oxidase inhibitors.

No respirator solution form of terbutaline is widely available in the United States; however, the parenteral solution of terbutaline has been used safely and effectively for nebulization,[9,12,13,16] and suggested dosage guidelines have been published.[7,9,12,26] The respirator solution form of albuterol became available in the United States in early 1987. Albuterol is considered by many authorities to be the drug of choice for the treatment of acute asthma.[6,7,18,28] Albuterol has been used in asthma therapy in Europe, Canada, and Australia for more then 15 years. It has been shown to be effective and safe, with minimal cardiovascular response, when delivered by inhalation. Fenoterol is an excellent agent with pharmacologic effects similar to those of albuterol,[41] but there is less reported experience on the use of fenoterol in acute severe pediatric asthma.[7]

For any suggested therapeutic regimen, cost considerations are always an important factor. At our institution, the total cost (including equipment) to the patient of nebulized β_2-agonist treatment is $13.25. This amount is comparable with the total cost of an epinephrine injection followed with an injection of Sus-Phrine ($12.40). Inhalation therapy becomes even more cost-effective when one considers that relapse and failure rates may be lower.[8]

DISCUSSION

A growing body of evidence indicates that β_2-selective agents delivered by nebulization should be cornerstones in the emergency treatment of pediatric asthma. Inhalation delivers the agonist directly to the target organ. Thus, only a relatively small amount of the drug is required to achieve the desired therapeutic effect. As a result, side effects are substantially minimized. Even the more β_2-selective agents, however, can produce cardiovascular effects at higher doses.[40,42] The duration of bronchodilation depends on the dose administered[40] as well as on the initial physiologic state of the smooth muscle. If the baseline smooth muscle tone is increased, the intensity and duration of bronchodilation is decreased.[43,44] It has been demonstrated in children that frequent administration of a nebulized β_2-agent at relatively low doses is a superior method of achieving early maximal bronchodilation with minimal side effects.[18,45]

Delivery by nebulization is preferred over intermittent positive-pressure breathing, which provides no additional bronchodilation[46,47] and increases the likelihood of pneumothorax and pneumomediastinum.[48] Nebulization also has several advantages over the use of metered-dose inhalers, particularly in the ED or office setting. Nebulization does not require respiratory coordination and therefore can be used in the young, uncooperative, or dyspneic child; however, because of technical aspects of delivery, about eight times as much agent is required to achieve equiv-

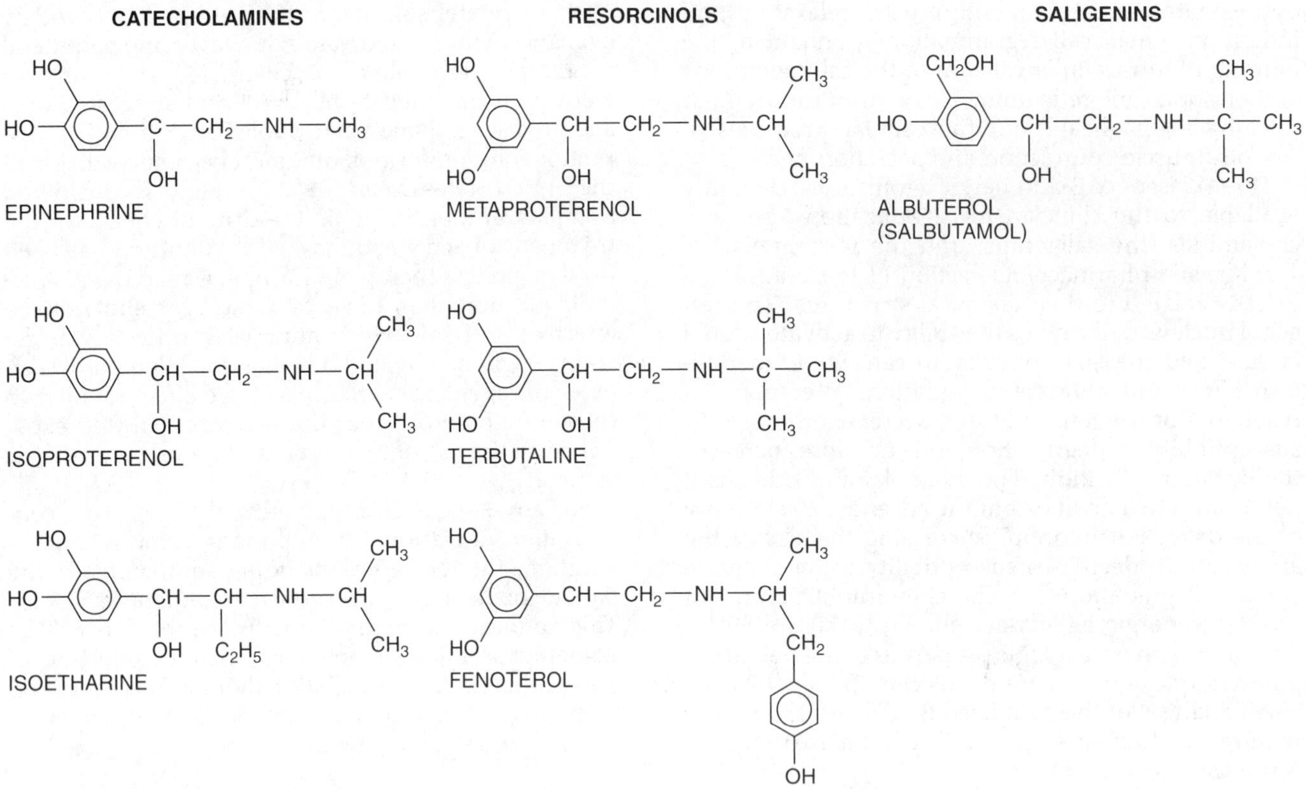

CATECHOLAMINES   RESORCINOLS   SALIGENINS

EPINEPHRINE   METAPROTERENOL   ALBUTEROL
                                                 (SALBUTAMOL)

ISOPROTERENOL   TERBUTALINE

ISOETHARINE   FENOTEROL

FIG. 59-19. Chemical structures of β-adrenergic agents.

alent bronchodilation.[49] Moreover, the prolonged duration of the nebulization treatment may allow delivery of the agonist to parts of the airway that were initially obstructed.[39,50] In addition, oxygen-driven nebulization minimizes the problem of ventilation-perfusion mismatch.

Nebulization should be powered by a continuous flow of oxygen at 6 L per minute.[18] This helps to correct the hypoxemia frequently associated with acute asthma. Clinical assessment often underestimates the degree of hypoxemia present,[51] and pulse oximetry can be a useful adjuvant.[52] The hypoxemia is primarily related to ventilation-perfusion mismatch.[53] Inhaled adrenergic agents,[54,55] aminophylline, and epinephrine[56,57] can aggravate the ventilation-perfusion mis-

match. This effect is seen frequently with the inhaled β₂-selective agents. Paradoxically, this decrease in oxygen saturation occurs despite improvement in pulmonary functions (peak expiratory flow rate) and can last up to 30 minutes.[58] The suggested mechanism involves a relative increase in perfusion to the hypoventilated lung because of either pulmonary vasodilation (β₂-effect) or increasing cardiac (β₁-effect) output.[59] This complication can be avoided by increasing the fraction of inspired oxygen. During the nebulization treatment, most children can use the hand-held mouthpiece. For infants and uncooperative children, a face mask is appropriate. It should be noted that a tight seal for the face mask is not needed and only serves to further upset the child.

**TABLE 59-26. CLINICAL PHARMACOLOGY OF THE
β-ADRENERGIC AEROSOLS***

Agent	Relative Potency†	Duration (Hours)	β-Selectivity
Isoproterenol	4	1–2	$\beta_2 = \beta_1$
Isoetharine	2	2–3	$\beta_2 \geq \beta_1$
Metaproterenol	3	3–4	$\beta_2 > \beta_1$
Terbutaline	4	4–6	$\beta_2 \gg \beta_1$
Albuterol	4	4–6	$\beta_2 \gg \beta_1$
Fenoterol	4	4–6	$\beta_2 \gg \beta_1$

* Adapted with permission from Stiell and Rivington,[7] Kelly[25] and Galant.[26]
† 4 = highest potency.

TABLE 59-27. PEDIATRIC DOSING AND ADMINISTRATION GUIDELINES FOR NEBULIZED ALBUTEROL

Albuterol (Salbutamol), 0.5 Respiratory Solution, 5 mg/ml

Patient Age (Years)	Dosage (mL)
<2	0.15
2–9	0.3–0.4
>9	0.5

- Dilute to a total volume of 3 mL with normal saline.
- Deliver by nebulizer, not intermittent positive-pressure breathing, with a continuous flow of oxygen at 6 L/min.
- May repeat every 20 to 30 minutes, depending on the clinical response. Unresponsiveness to three frequent treatments constitutes status asthmaticus.
- Adjust dosage on the basis of clinical response and the development of side effects.
- All β-adrenergic agents should be used with caution in patients with cardiovascular disease and in patients receiving tricyclic antidepressants or monoamine oxidase inhibitors.

Some have felt that inhaled agents may not be effective in the treatment of the asthmatic patient with a severely obstructed airway. Evidence suggests, however, that the inhaled β2-selective agonists provide bronchodilation comparable with that produced by injectable agents, regardless of the severity of the airway obstruction.[8,14] There was also some initial concern about the relationship between inhaled β-adrenergic agents and the increasing death rate among asthmatic persons; however, closer analysis implicated undertreatment rather than overtreatment as the major cause of asthmatic mortality.[60,60a] Nebulized β2-agents possess the advantages of increased duration of action and decreased incidence of side effects over injectable adrenergic agonists, while avoiding the pain of injections. The cost is roughly comparable with that of injectable regimens.

Albuterol has an extensive published history of pediatric use, excellent pharmacologic characteristics, a respirator solution dosage form, and a published history of its frequent low-dose administration in children. It is currently the nebulized β-adrenergic drug of choice in the treatment of acute pediatric asthma.

Avoidance of treatment-induced pain is a particularly important consideration in a child with a common chronic disease. The asthmatic child has many medical encounters because of acute exacerbations of his or her disease. As physicians, we should be concerned with minimizing the fear and discomfort of the child during these encounters. This approach may lead the patient to seek treatment earlier in the asthma attack because the physician is then seen as a provider of relief rather than as a source of additional pain. On both a physiologic and psychological basis, nebulized β2-selective agents are the treatment of choice in acute pediatric asthma, with epinephrine secondary.

NEBULIZED ANTICHOLINERGIC AGENTS

Inhalation therapy with pharmacologically active anticholinergic agents originated thousands of years ago in India. Various plants were prepared as combustible powders, and their smoke was inhaled for relief of respiratory distress. These practices were incorporated into Western medicine in the early nineteenth century. As epinephrine and ephedrine became available in the first half of the twentieth century, however, anticholinergic drugs for the treatment of asthma fell into disuse.[61] Advances in the understanding of the role of parasympathetic bronchomotor tone and the recent development of less toxic anticholinergic agents have renewed interest in inhaled anticholinergic drugs as therapeutic agents in the treatment of asthma.

PHYSIOLOGY AND PHARMACOLOGY

The baseline level of bronchomotor tone (airway caliber) is predominantly controlled by the parasympathetic nervous system.[62] Increased vagal stimulation leads to increased intracellular concentrations of cyclic guanosine monophosphate within smooth bronchial muscle, resulting in bronchoconstriction. This cholinergic-mediated bronchoconstriction can be blocked by atropine and ipratropium, which competitively antagonize acetylcholine at its receptor sites. Anticholinergic drugs may also inhibit acute airway obstruction by interfering with the release of inflammatory mediators from the mast cell.[63] In contrast to inhaled β-adrenergic agonists, which exert their bronchodilating effect mainly on the small airways, anticholinergic agents were believed to exert their effect predominantly on large- and intermediate-sized airways.[62] Some investigators,[64,65] however, suggest that there are also significant anticholinergic effects on the small airways.

Atropine is classified as a tertiary ammonium compound. It is absorbed well from the gastrointestinal tract and crosses the blood-brain barrier. Atropine decreases mucus secretion but does not significantly affect viscosity. Mucus transport rates and ciliary activity (beat frequency) are reduced.[62] The bronchodilating effect of nebulized atropine begins 5 to 15 minutes after administration, plateaus at 45 to 60 minutes, and lasts for approximately 4 hours.[66]

Ipratropium is a synthetic derivative of atropine. It is classified as a quaternary ammonium compound and has been used clinically as a bronchodilator in Europe since the mid-1970s.[62] It is a much more selective bronchodilator than atropine because it is poorly absorbed from the gastrointestinal tract and does not cross the blood-brain barrier. Therefore, the therapeutic margin for ipratropium administration is wide.[62] The lack of gastrointestinal absorption is significant because at least 90% of the dose of an inhaled drug is deposited in the oropharynx and then swallowed.[67] Quaternary compounds such as ipratropium do not affect mucus secretion, viscosity, or transport rates. The onset of bronchodilation and the peak of action are similar to those of atropine; however, ipratropium's duration of action is longer (up to 6 hours).[68]

CLINICAL STUDIES

Over the past 10 to 15 years, the role of anticholinergic drugs, particularly atropine and ipratropium, has been evaluated in the treatment of asthma.

In the chronic asthmatic child, nebulized atropine has been shown to be effective in improving pulmonary functions without causing significant cardiovascular effects.[69–71] Nebulized atropine has been shown to improve bronchodilation without causing adverse side effects in adults with acute asthma already being treated with multiple antiasthmatic agents.[72] Another study in acute asthmatic adults, however, failed to show additive bronchodilation.[73] The systemic side effects of atropine are dose-related. When it is administered by nebulization, serum levels are negligible after a single treatment but can become significant after multiple doses.[74] With nebulized atropine, dry mouth is a frequently occurring side effect.[70] Anisocoria,[75] flushing of skin,[70] urinary retention,[76] and prolongation of gastric emptying[77] are occasionally seen. Tachycardia, although a potential problem, is generally not of clinical significance.[62]

Clinical experience with the use of inhaled atropine in acute pediatric asthma is limited. Nebulized atropine at a dosage of 0.05 mg/kg of body weight (maximal dose of 1.5 mg) every 4 to 6 hours[62,70] may however, be useful in the management of acute asthma in the child who is resistant to conventional therapy, particularly in children with impending respiratory failure when other modalities with significant known morbidity (IV administration of isoproterenol,[78,79] mechanical ventilation) are being considered.

Ipratropium has been extensively studied[64,68,80–90] and has wide clinical use in Europe, Canada, and Australia. Its safety and efficacy in the treatment of the asthmatic child have been well documented.[64,80,81,83,85,89] In a randomized double-blind study involving 148 adults with acute asthma,[90] the combination of nebulized ipratropium with a nebulized β_2-selective agent was significantly more effective than either agent alone in relieving acute airway obstruction. Significantly, the added benefits of combination therapy were most pronounced in patients with the most severe degree of airway obstruction at presentation. In a randomized double-blind study in children with severe acute asthma (initial forced expiratory volumes in one second were 30% of predicted values),[89] after maximal bronchodilating effect was achieved with frequent low-dose albuterol nebulizations, nebulized ipratropium produced significant additive bronchodilation. This added bronchodilation resulted from the reversal of residual cholinergic-mediated bronchospasm.

Because of its poor gastrointestinal absorption and lack of central nervous system effects, nebulized ipratropium produces no significant systemic toxic effects, even at doses many times those required for maximal bronchodilation.[91] Dry mouth is a complaint in about 10% of patients,[90] and pupillary dilation with the use of nebulized ipratropium (presumably a direct topical effect) has been infrequently reported.[92] The recommended pediatric dose for nebulization is 250 µg. Currently, ipratropium is available in the United States only in a metered-dose inhaler.

Ipratropium will probably not supplant the β_2-adrenergic agents in the initial treatment of acute pediatric asthma. When the respiratory solution becomes available in the United States, however, ipratropium will probably become a significant adjuvant in the treatment of severe acute pediatric asthma in the ED.

CORTICOSTEROIDS

Corticosteroids have been used in the treatment of asthma for over 35 years.[93] Although they were initially hailed as miracle drugs, significant side effects became evident with their chronic use. Studies have helped to clarify the role of corticosteroids in the management of acute asthma; however, this is still an area of some controversy. This new information has definite implications for the ED management of the child presenting with an acute exacerbation of asthma.

PHYSIOLOGY AND PHARMACOLOGY

Although the exact mechanisms through which corticosteroids exert their antiasthmatic effects are not entirely clear, several theories have been advanced. An underlying principle is that corticosteroids do not interact directly with receptors on the cell surface; rather, they exert their effects by modifying protein synthesis at the nuclear level. The postulated mechanisms of action have been reviewed in the literature.[94]

1. Interference with synthesis and release of inflammatory mediators
2. Enhanced response to catecholamines:
   a. Stimulation of cyclic adenosine monophosphate metabolism
   b. Restoration or increased synthesis of β-adrenergic receptors

c. Inhibition of catechol-O-methyltransferase
d. Inhibition of phosphodiesterase
3. Diminished effects of cholinergic stimulation through inhibition of cyclic guanosine monophosphate
4. Improved mucociliary clearance
5. Stabilization of lysosomes
6. Alteration in leukocyte number and activity.

Extensive clinical experience with short courses of corticosteroid administration has shown that adverse effects are infrequent and generally clinically insignificant.[95] Pituitary adrenal recovery after high-dose short-term corticosteroid therapy occurs within 5 days.[96] A consensus of opinion, however, suggests that if high-dose corticosteroids are administered for longer than 10 days, the risk of pituitary-adrenal suppression must be considered for up to 1 year.[97]

Recommendations for short-course administration of oral corticosteroids include prednisone[1,95] or prednisolone,[98] 1 to 2 mg per kg of body weight per day, given every 12 hours for 5 to 7 days. Tapering the doses is generally not necessary.[2,95] For intravenous use, methylprednisolone is a reasonable choice on the basis of its short duration of pituitary-adrenal suppression and minimal effects on sodium retention. A reasonable dosage schedule is an initial 2 mg per kg of body weight intravenous bolus followed by a 1 mg per kg of body weight per dose every 6 hours.[99–102] Ratto et al.[103] demonstrated that, if the patient is able to tolerate an oral regimen, oral methylprednisolone is a safe and effective alternative in the treatment of status asthmaticus.

CLINICAL STUDIES

Since 1981, the American Academy of Pediatrics' Section on Allergy and Immunology has recommended the use of intravenous high-dose corticosteroids for hospitalized children in status asthmaticus.[1] Moreover, in the same statement, the Academy suggests their use in the ambulatory child with an acute exacerbation of asthma: "Corticosteroids should be considered when response to optimal bronchodilator therapy is inadequate. The physician should be prudent in the use of corticosteroids, but he/she should not wait until the child's symptoms are so severe that hospitalization may be necessary." This approach to the use of short courses of high-dose corticosteroids has in fact been widely adopted in clinical practice. Past clinical studies on the efficacy of corticosteroids in acute asthma, however, have arrived at conflicting conclusions.[104–109] More recent work supporting the value of corticosteroids in acute asthma suggests that the discrepancies among previous reports may have resulted from unintentional bias in patient selection[95] or differences in the specific parameters of pulmonary function (small versus large airway parameters) that were measured.[102]

As suggested by the Academy's 1981 statement, prevention of hospitalization and repeated emergency care is a major goal in the management of a child with an acute asthmatic exacerbation. This goal assumes even more importance in the current era of cost containment. Corticosteroids have been widely used in an effort to achieve this. In that context, four recent studies are of particular interest to the emergency physician.[95,101,110,111]

Two of the studies[101,110,111] involved adults seen in EDs for acute exacerbations of asthma. Patients with chronic obstructive pulmonary disease were specifically excluded in both studies. One study[110] evaluated a short course of high-dose oral corticosteroids in patients discharged after an acute asthmatic attack. This study demonstrated a decreased need for repeated emergency care (5.9% versus 21% for the placebo group) and fewer respiratory symptoms (15.6% versus 36.4% for the placebo group) in patients receiving corticosteroids during 7 to 10 days of follow-up. Another study[101] evaluated the use of an intravenous bolus of methylprednisolone, in addition to conventional therapy, in asthmatic persons presenting to the ED. Despite an average length of stay of only 4 hours, there was a 60% lower admission rate to the hospital in the corticosteroid group (19% versus 47% for the placebo group). In patients discharged from the ED, there was no difference between the groups in the need for repeated emergency care or early hospital readmission.

The use of a short course of high-dose oral corticosteroids was evaluated in a study of ambulatory pediatric asthmatics with acute exacerbations that were not completely responsive to bronchodilators.[95] All 22 patients in the group on corticosteroids improved during the week of treatment. Of the 19 patients who received placebo, eight (42%) required rescue intervention with oral corticosteroid administration because of persistence or worsening of symptoms or deterioration of pulmonary function.

Brunette et al.[111] studied a group of preschool asthmatic children with a history of repetitive emergency care and hospitalizations whose exacerbations were apparently induced by viral upper respiratory tract infections. High-dose oral corticosteroids were begun in half the patients at the onset of symptoms consistent with a viral respiratory infection, before overt symptoms of asthma were observed. Although this study was neither blinded nor placebo-controlled, the results were striking, with a 90% decrease in hospitalization rate during a 1-year observation period in the group aggressively treated with corticosteroids.

Studies suggest a significant role for corticosteroids in the management of acute exacerbations of asthma.[95,101,102, 107–110] If the child is not completely responsive to bronchodilator therapy, a short course of high-dose oral corticosteroids should be considered. If hospitalization is necessary, high-dose systemic corticosteroids are indicated.

REFERENCES

1. American Academy of Pediatrics, Section on Allergy and Immunology: Management of asthma. Pediatrics 68:874, 1981.
2. Cropp, G.J.A.: Special features of asthma in children. Chest 87(Suppl):55, 1985.
3. National Center for Health Statistics (Division for Health Interview Statistics). Vital and health statistics; 1980 and 1981 surveys. Unpublished data.
4. Konig, P.: Asthma: A pediatric pulmonary disease and a changing concept. Pediatr. Pulmonol. 3:264, 1987.
5. Ben-Zvi, Z., Lam, C., Spohn, W.A., et al.: An evaluation of repeated injections of epinephrine for the initial treatment of acute asthma. Am. Rev. Respir. Dis. 127:101, 1983.
6. Becker, A.B., Nelson, N.A., and Simons, F.E.R.: Inhaled salbutamol (albuterol) vs injected epinephrine in the treatment of acute asthma in children. J. Pediatr. 102:465, 1983.
7. Stiell, G., and Rivington, R.N.: Adrenergic agents in acute asthma: Valuable new alternatives. Ann. Emerg. Med. 12:493, 1983.
8. Ben-Zvi, Z., Lam, C., Hoffman, J., et al.: An evaluation of the initial treatment of acute asthma. Pediatrics 70:348, 1983.
9. Uden, D.L., Goetz, D.R., Kohen, D.P., et al.: Comparison of nebulized terbutaline and subcutaneous epinephrine in the treatment of acute asthma. Ann. Emerg. Med. 14:229, 1985.
10. Schwartz, A.L., Lipton, J.W., Warburton, D., et al.: Management of acute asthma in childhood. Am. J. Dis. Child. 134:474, 1980.
11. Elenbags, R.M., Frost, G.L., Robinson, W.A., et al.: Subcutaneous epinephrine vs nebulized metaproterenol in acute asthma. Drug Intell. Clin. Pharm. 19:567, 1985.
12. Pancorbo, S., Fifield, G., Davies, S., et al.: Subcutaneous epinephrine vs nebulized terbutaline in the emergency treatment of asthma. Clin. Pharm. 2:45, 1983.
13. Baughman, R.P., Ploysongsang, Y., James, W.: A comparative study of aerosolized terbutaline and subcutaneously administered epinephrine in the treatment of acute bronchial asthma. Ann. Allergy 53:131, 1984.
14. Rossing, T.H., Fanta, C.H., Goldstein, D.H., et al.: Emergency therapy of asthma: Comparison of the acute effects of parenteral and inhaled sympathomimetics and infused aminophylline. Am. Rev. Respir. Dis. 122:365, 1980.
15. Rossing, T.H., Fanta, C.H., and McFadden, E.R.: Effect of outpatient treatment of asthma with β-agonists on the response to sympathomimetics in an emergency room. Am. J. Med. 75:781, 1983.
16. Tinkelman, D.G., Vanderpool, G.E., Carroll, M.S., et al.: Comparison of nebulized terbutaline and subcutaneous epinephrine in the treatment of acute asthma. Ann. Allergy 50:398, 1983.
17. Pliss, L.B., Gallagher, E.J.: Aerosol vs injected epinephrine in acute asthma. Ann. Emerg. Med. 10:353, 1981.
18. Robertson, C.F., Smith, F., Beck, R., et al.: Response to frequent low doses of nebulized salbutamol in acute asthma. J. Pediatr. 106:672, 1985.
19. Lee, H., and Evans, H.E.: Lack of cardiac effect from repeated doses of albuterol aerosol. Clin. Pediatr. 25:349, 1986.
20. Bohn, D., Holtby, H., Mullins, G., et al.: The management of status asthmaticus with intravenous salbutamol in children. Am. Rev. Respir. Dis. 129:A206, 1984.
21. Prior, J.G., Cochrane, G.M., Raper, S.M., et al.: Self-poisoning with oral salbutamol. Br. Med. J. 282:1932, 1981.
22. Moler, F., Hurwitz, M., and Custer, J.: Improvement of clinical asthma scores and PCO_2 in children with severe asthma treated with continuously nebulized terbutaline. Am. Rev. Respir. Dis. 135:A380, 1987.
23. Fanta, C.H., Rossing, T.H., McFadden, E.R., Jr.: Emergency room treatment of asthma. Relationships among therapeutic combinations, severity of obstruction and time course of response. Am. J. Med. 72:416, 1982.
24. Siegel, D., Sheppard, D., Gelb, A., et al.: Aminophylline increases the toxicity but not the efficacy of an inhaled beta-adrenergic agonist in the treatment of acute exacerbations of asthma. Am. Rev. Respir. Dis. 132:283, 1985.
25. Kelly, H.W.: Controversies in asthma therapy and the $β_2$-adrenergic agonists. Clin. Pharm. 3:386, 1984.
26. Galant, S.P.: Current status of β-adrenergic agonists in bronchial asthma. Pediatr. Clin. North Am. 30:931, 1983.
27. McFadden, E.R.: Clinical use of β-adrenergic aerosols. J. Allergy Clin. Immunol. 76:352, 1985.
28. Turcios, N.: β-adrenergic agents in asthma. Pediatr. Rev. 7:12, 1985.
29. Choo-Kang, Y.F., Simpson, W.T., Grant, I.W., et al.: Controlled comparison of the bronchodilator effects of three β-adrenergic stimulant drugs administered by inhalation. Br. Med. J. 2:287, 1969.
30. Peerless, A.G., Rachelefsky, G.S., Mickey, M.R., et al.: Bronchodilator characteristics of nebulized metaproterenol sulfate, isoetharine, and atropine in chronic asthma. J. Allergy Clin. Immunol. 72:702, 1983.
31. Garra, B., Shapiro, G.G., Dorsett, C.S., et al.: A double-blind evaluation of the use of nebulized metaproterenol and isoproterenol in hospitalized asthmatic children and adolescents. J. Allergy Clin. Immunol. 60:36, 1977.
32. Freedman, B.J., and Hill, G.B.: Comparative study of duration of action and cardiovascular effects of bronchodilator aerosols. Thorax 26:46, 1971.
33. Beardshaw, J., MacLean, L., Chan-Yeung, M.: Comparison of bronchodilator and cardiac effects of hydroxyphenylorciprenaline and orciprenaline. Chest 65:507, 1974.
34. Blackhall, M.I., Dauth, M., Mahoney, M., et al.: Inhalation of fenoterol by asthmatic children. A clinical comparison with salbutamol, orciprenaline and isoprenaline. Med. J. Aust. 2:439, 1976.
35. Carmichael, J., Bloomfield, P., and Crompton, G.K.: Comparison of fenoterol and terbutaline administered by intermittent positive-pressure breathing. Br. J. Dis. Chest. 74:268, 1980.
36. Brain, J.D., Valberg, P.A.: Deposition of aerosol in the respiratory tract. Am. Rev. Respir. Dis. 120:1325, 1979.
37. Newman, S.P., Pavia, D., Moren, F., et al.: Deposition of pressurized aerosols in the human respiratory tract. Thorax 36:52, 1981.
38. Newhouse M.T., Dolovich, M.B.: Current concepts, control of asthma by aerosols. N. Engl. J. Med. 315:870, 1986.
39. Pavia, D., Thomson, M., and Shannon, H.S.: Aerosol inhalation and depth of deposition in the human lung. Arch. Environ. Health 16:131, 1977.
40. Reilly, P.A., Yahav, J., Mindorff, C., et al.: Dose-response characteristics of nebulized fenoterol in asthmatic children. J. Pediatr. 103:121, 1983.
41. Svedmyr, N.: Fenoterol: A beta-adrenergic agonist for use in asthma. Pharmacotherapy 5:109, 1985.
42. Walters, E.H., Cockroft, A., Griffiths, T., et al.: Optimal doses of salbutamol respiratory solution: Comparison of three doses with plasma levels. Thorax 36:625, 1981.
43. Pain, M.C., Read, J.: Patterns of response to bronchodilator in young patients with asthma. Aust. Ann. Med. 12:216, 1963.
44. Rebuck, M.B., Read, J.: Assessment and management of severe asthma. Am. J. Med. 51:788, 1971.
45. Beck, R., Robertson, C., Galdes-Sebaldt, M., et al.: Clinical and laboratory observations: Combined salbutamol and ipratropium bromide by inhalation in the treatment of severe acute asthma. J. Pediatr. 107:605, 1985.
46. Loren, M., Chai, H., Miklich, D., et al.: Comparison between simple nebulization and intermittent positive-pressure in asthmatic children with severe bronchospasm. Chest 72:145, 1977.
47. Smelzer, T.H., and Barnett, T.B.: Bronchodilator aerosol, comparison of administration methods. JAMA 223:884, 1973.
48. Karetsky, M.S.: Asthma mortality associated with pneumo-

thorax and intermittent positive-pressure breathing. Lancet *1*:828, 1974.

49. Weber, R.W., Petty, W.E., and Nelson, H.S.: Aerosolized terbutaline in asthmatics: Comparison of dosage strength, schedule, and method of administration. J. Allergy Clin. Immunol. *63*:116, 1979.

50. Shim, C., and Williams, M.H.: Bronchial response to oral versus aerosol metaproterenol in asthma. Ann. Intern. Med. *93*:428, 1980.

51. Hurwitz, M.E., Burney, R.E., Howatt, W.F., et al.: Clinical scoring does not accurately assess hypoxemia in pediatric asthma patients. Ann. Emerg. Med. *13*:1040, 1984.

52. Kulick, R.M.: Pulse oximetry. Pediatr. Emerg. Care *3*:127, 1987.

53. McFadden, E.R., and Lyons, H.A.: Arterial-blood gas tension in asthma. N. Engl. J. Med. *278*:1027, 1968.

54. Gazioglu, K., Condemi, J.J., Hyde, R.W., et al.: Effect of isoproterenol on gas exchange during air and oxygen breathing in patients with asthma. Am. J. Med. *50*:185, 1971.

55. Chick, T.W., Nicholson, D.P., and Johnson, R.L.: Effects of isoproterenol on distribution of ventilation and perfusion in asthma. Am. Rev. Respir. Dis. *107*:869, 1973.

56. Jezek, V., Ourednick, A., Stepanek, J., et al.: The effect of aminophylline on the respiration and pulmonary circulation. Clin. Sci. *38*:549, 1970.

57. Hales, C.A., Kazemi, H.: Hypoxic vascular response of the lung. Effect of aminophylline and epinephrine. Am. Rev. Respir. Dis. *110*:126, 1974.

58. Tal, A., Pasterkamp, H., and Leahy, F.: Arterial oxygen desaturation following salbutamol inhalation in acute asthma. Chest *86*:868, 1984.

59. Harris, L.: Comparison of the effects on blood gases, ventilation, and perfusion of isoproterenolphenylephrine and salbutamol aerosols in chronic bronchitis with asthma. J. Allergy Clin. Immunol. *49*:63, 1972.

60. Sly, R.M.: Effects of treatment on mortality from asthma. Ann. Allergy *56*:207, 1986.

60a. Molfiro, N.A., et al.: Respiratory arrest in near-fatal asthma. N. Engl. J. Med. *324*:285, 1991.

61. Gandevia, B.: Historical review of the use of parasympatholytic agents in the treatment of respiratory disorders. Postgrad. Med. J. *51*:13, 1975.

62. Gross, N.J., and Skorodin, M.S.: Anticholinergic, antimuscarinic bronchodilators. Am. Rev. Respir. Dis. *129*:856, 1984.

63. Kaliner, M.: Human lung tissue and anaphylaxis: The role of cyclic GMP as a modulator of the immunologically induced secretory process. J. Allergy Clin. Immunol. *60*:204, 1977.

64. Davis, A., Vickerson, F., Worsley, G., et al.: Clinical and laboratory observations: Determination of dose-response relationship for nebulized ipratropium in asthmatic children. J. Pediatr. *105*:1002, 1984.

65. Molho, M., Benzaray, S., Lidji, M., et al.: Salbutamol versus atropine. Site of bronchodilatation in asthmatic patients. Respiration *51*:26, 1987.

66. Peerless, A.G., Rachelefsky, G.S., Mickey, M.R., et al.: Bronchodilator characteristics of nebulized metaproterenol sulfate, isoetharine, and atropine in chronic asthma. J. Allergy Clin. Immunol. *72*:702, 1963.

67. Davies, D.S.: Parmacokinetics of inhaled substances. Scand. J. Respir. Dis. *103*:44, 1979.

68. Gross, N.J.: Sch 1000: A new anticholinergic bronchodilator. Am. Rev. Respir. Dis. *112*:823, 1975.

69. Cropp, G.J.A.: The role of the parasympathetic nervous system in the maintenance of chronic airway obstruction in asthmatic children. Am. Rev. Respir. Dis. *112*:599, 1975.

70. Cavanaugh, M.J., and Cooper, D.M.: Inhaled atropine sulfate: Dose response characteristics. Am. Rev. Respir. Dis. *114*:517, 1976.

71. Hemstreet, M.P.B.: Atropine nebulization—Simple and safe. Ann. Allergy. *44*:138, 1980.

72. Fairshter, R.D., Habib, M.P., and Wilson, A.F.: Inhaled atropine sulfate in acute asthma. Respiration *42*:263, 1981.

73. Karpel, J.P., Appel, D., Breidbart, D., et al.: A comparison of atropine sulfate and metaproterenol sulfate in the emergency treatment of asthma. Am. Rev. Respir. Dis. *133*:727, 1986.

74. Kradjan, W.A., Smallridge, R.C., Davis, R., et al.: Atropine serum concentrations after multiple inhaled doses of atropine sulfate. Clin. Pharmacol. Ther. *38*:12, 1985.

75. Jannun, D.R., Mickel, S.F.: Anisocoria and aerosolized anticholinergics. Chest *90*:148, 1986.

76. Pak C.C.F., Kradjan, W.A., Lakshminarayan, S., et al.: Inhaled atropine sulfate—Dose-response characteristics in adult patients with chronic airflow obstruction. Am. Rev. Respir. Dis. *125*:331, 1982.

77. Botts, L.D., Pingleton, S.K., Schroeder, C.E., et al.: Prolongation of gastric emptying by aerosolized atropine. Am. Rev. Respir. Dis. *131*:725, 1985.

78. Matson, J.R., Loughlin, G.M., and Strunk, R.C.: Myocardial ischemia complicating the use of isoproterenol in asthmatic children. J. Pediatr. *92*:776, 1978.

79. Mikhail, M.S., Hunsinger, S.Y., and Goodwin, S.R.: Myocardial ischemia complicating therapy of status asthmaticus. Clin. Pediatr *26*:419, 1987.

80. Lin, M.T., Lee-Hong, E., and Collins-Williams, C.: A clinical trial of the bronchodilator effect of Sch 1000 aerosol in asthmatic children. Ann. Allergy *40*:326, 1978.

81. Yeung, R., Nolan, G.M. and Levison, H.: Comparison of the effects of inhaled Sch 1000 and fenoterol on exercise-induced bronchospasm in children. Pediatrics *66*:109, 1980.

82. Ward, M.J., Fentem P.H., Smith, W.H.R.: Ipratropium bromide in acute asthma. Br. Med. J. *282*:598, 1981.

83. Groggins, R.C., Milner, A.D., and Stokes, G.M.: Bronchodilator effects of clemastine, ipratropium bromide, and salbutamol in preschool children with asthma. Arch. Dis. Chld. *56*:342, 1981.

84. Kreisman, H., Frank, H., Wolkove, N., et al.: Synergism between ipratropium and theophylline in asthma. Thorax *36*:374, 1981.

85. Mann, N.P., and Hiller, E.J.: Ipratropium bromide in children with asthma. Thorax *37*:72, 1982.

86. Rebuck, A.S., Gent, M., and Chapman, K.R.: Anticholinergic and sympathomimetic combination therapy of asthma. J. Allergy Clin. Immunol. *71*:317, 1983.

87. Leahy, B.C., Gomm, S.A., and Allen, S.C.: Comparison of nebulized salbutamol with nebulized ipratropium bromide in acute asthma. Br. J. Dis. Chest *77*:159, 1983.

88. Bryant, D.H.: Nebulized ipratropium bromide in the treatment of acute asthma. Chest *88*:24, 1985.

89. Beck, R., Robertson, C., Galdes-Sebaldt, M., et al.: Clinical and laboratory observations—Combined salbutamol and ipratropium bromide by inhalation in the treatment of severe acute asthma. J. Pediatr. *107*:606, 1985.

90. Rebuck, A.S., Chapman, K.R., Abboud, R., et al.: Nebulized anticholinergic and sympathomimetic treatment of asthma and chronic obstructive airways disease in the emergency room. Am. J. Med. *82*:59, 1987.

91. Cugell, D.W.: Clinical pharmacology and toxicology of ipratropium bromide. Am. J. Med. *81*:18, 1986.

92. Malani, J.T., Robinson, G.M., and Seneviratne, E.L.: Ipratropium bromide induced angle closure glaucoma (letter). N.Z. Med. J. *95*:749, 1982.

93. Carryer, H.M., Koelsche, G.A., Prickman, L.E., et al.: Effects of cortisone on bronchial asthma and hay fever occurring in subjects sensitive to ragweed pollen. Mayo Clin. Proc. *25*:482, 1950.

94. Fiel, S.B.: Should corticosteroids be used in the treatment of acute, severe asthma? I. A case for the use of corticosteroids in acute, severe asthma. Pharmacotherapy *5*:327, 1985.

95. Harris, J.B., Weinberger, M.M., Nassif, E., et al.: Early intervention with short courses of prednisone to prevent progression of asthma in ambulatory patients incompletely responsive to bronchodilators. J. Pediatr. *110*:627, 1987.

96. Streck, W.F. and Lockwood, D.H.: Pituitary adrenal recovery following short-term suppression with corticosteroids. Am. J. Med. *66*:910, 1979.

97. Chamberlin, P., and Meyer, W.J., III: Management of pituitary-adrenal suppression secondary to corticosteroid therapy. Pediatrics 67:245, 1981.
98. Landau, L.I.: Outpatient evaluation and management of asthma. Pediatr. Clin. North Am. 26:581, 1979.
99. Harfi, H., Hanissian, A.S., and Crawford, L.V.: Treatment of status asthmaticus in children with high doses and conventional doses of methylprednisolone. Pediatrics 61:829, 1979.
100. Haskell, R.J., Wong, B.M., and Hansen, J.E.: A double-blind, randomized clinical trial of methylprednisolone in status asthmaticus. Arch. Intern. Med. 143:1324, 1983.
101. Littenberg, B., and Gluck, E.H.: A controlled trial of methylprednisolone in the emergency treatment of acute asthma. N. Engl. J. Med. 314:150, 1986.
102. Younger, R.E., Gerber, P.S., Herrod, H.G., et al.: Intravenous methylprednisolone efficacy in status asthmaticus of childhood. Pediatrics 80:225, 1987.
103. Ratto, D., Alfaro, C., and Sipsey, J., et al.: Are intravenous corticosteroids required in status asthmaticus? JAMA 260:527, 1988.
104. Pierson, W.E., Bierman, C.W., and Kelley, V.C.: A double-blind trial of corticosteroid therapy in status asthmaticus. Pediatrics 54:282, 1974.
105. McFadden, E.R., Kiser, R., deGroot, W.J., et al.: A controlled study of the effects of single doses of hydrocortisone on the resolution of acute attacks of asthma. Am. J. Med. 60:52, 1976.
106. Kattan, M., Gurwitz, D., and Levison, H.: Corticosteroids in status asthmaticus. J. Pediatr. 96:596, 1980.
107. Loren, M.L., Chai, H., Leung, P., et al.: Corticosteroids in the treatment of acute exacerbations of asthma. Ann. Allergy 45:67, 1980.
108. Shapiro, G.G., Furukawa, C.T., and Pierson, W.E.: Double-blind evaluation of methylprednisolone versus placebo for acute asthma episodes. Pediatrics 71:510, 1983.
109. Fanta, C.H., Rossing, T.H., and McFadden, E.R.: Glucocorticoids in acute asthma—A critical controlled trial. Am. J. Med. 74:845, 1983.
110. Fiel, S.B., Swartz, M.A., Glanz, K., et al.: Efficacy of short-term corticosteroid therapy in outpatient treatment of acute bronchial asthma. Am. J. Med. 75:259, 1983.
111. Brunette, M.G., Lands, C., and Thibodeau, L.P.: Childhood asthma: prevention of attacks with short-term corticosteroid treatment of upper respiratory tract infection. Pediatrics 81:624, 1988.

SHOCK IN THE PEDIATRIC PATIENT

Thom A. Mayer

CAPSULE

It is difficult to overstate the importance of early recognition and treatment of shock in pediatric patients. Nearly a third of all patients seen in general Emergency Departments (EDs) are pediatric patients, and the care and treatment of children is common to virtually all EDs. Although most of these patients are not in shock, it is nonetheless important to ensure that all emergency physicians are well trained in the recognition and management of shock in children. There are significant differences between adults and children in regard to the diagnosis and treatment of shock, but virtually all aspects of recognition and management can be mastered by any well trained emergency physician.

INTRODUCTION

The pathophysiology and treatment of shock in adult patients are well described in Chapters 3 and 7. The purpose of this chapter is to highlight differences between the adult and pediatric patients regarding pathophysiology, recognition, and treatment.

Although the term "shock" is commonly used in both lay and medical terminology, it is one of the most overused and least understood terms. The best definition of shock is *a generalized state of inadequate tissue perfusion resulting in impaired cellular respiration*. The definition of shock does not rely on blood pressure, pulse rate, blood loss, or other factors. It is specifically related to impaired tissue perfusion. Chapter 3 offers a detailed explanation of the pathophysiology of shock, but it is perhaps best to rely for practical purposes on a mechanical definition for the proper maintenance of tissue perfusion, despite the fact that numerous circulatory, neurohumoral, endocrine, and other factors are present. Maintaining tissue perfusion requires a properly functioning pump (heart) pushing an appropriate amount of fluid (blood) through appropriate-sized and configured tubes (blood vessels) without obstruction to flow. This analogy helps to classify shock properly according to the cause of impaired tissue perfusion, which may come as a result of a failure of the pump, fluid, tubes, or obstruction to flow. From a hemodynamic standpoint, shock can therefore be classified as cardiogenic, hypovolemic, distributive, or obstructive. Table 59-28 summarizes some of the specific clinical states that may cause shock in each of these categories. This classification has extreme practical importance because the clinician should choose the appropriate therapy for the type and degree of shock which is present.

Hypovolemic shock is most commonly caused by acute blood loss (hemorrhagic shock) because acute trauma accounts for over 50% of all deaths in the pediatric age group. Further, most bench and clinical research on shock in both adult and pediatric patients involves studies using the model of acute blood loss. Hypovolemic shock, however, can also be caused by burns, peritonitis, diarrhea/dehydration, and heat loss. Whether the fluid lost is blood itself (acute hemorrhage), plasma (burns and peritonitis), or extracellular fluid (vomiting and heat loss), the pathophysiology of hypovolemic shock is still essentially the same, and the emergency physician should recognize the disease processes as similar in these clinical presentations.

The pathophysiology of *cardiogenic shock* is essentially the same in adults and children, but occurs less frequently, owing simply to the fact that serious, life-threatening cardiac disease is far less common in children than in adults. For example, myocardial infarction is extremely common in adults but extremely rare in children, limited essentially to those with anomalous left coronary artery, Kawasaki's disease, or severe congenital heart disease. Similarly, arrhythmias, valvular heart disease significant enough to cause cardiac failure, congestive heart failure, and cardiomyopathy are also extremely rare in children. Thus, primary cardiogenic shock is uncommon in the pediatric population. In extremely late cases of septic shock, acute cardiac failure may occur, but is relatively un-

common. Most cases of cardiogenic shock in children are a result of major underlying congenital heart disease, and many have undergone surgical reconstruction in an attempt to restore normal anatomy.

Obstructive shock is also extremely uncommon in children, with most cases caused by the development of tension pneumothorax or cardiac tamponade. Other causes of obstructive shock in adults include flail chest, pulmonary embolus, and massive hemothorax. All of these diagnoses are uncommon in children. Tension pneumothorax, however, develops relatively easily in those with serious chest trauma, so that obstructive shock does occur in the pediatric population. Unfortunately, the rising tide of urban violence has also resulted in an increasing number of cases of cardiac tamponade secondary to penetrating chest trauma.

By far the most common cause of *distributive shock* in the pediatric age group is sepsis. The other causes of distributive shock include spinal cord injury, anaphylaxis, drug reactions, and anesthesia, but all of these are far less common than shock caused by sepsis.

DIFFERENCES BETWEEN ADULT AND PEDIATRIC SHOCK

One of the most significant differences between adult and pediatric patients with shock is related to the types of shock seen in each population (Table 59-29). In adults, many patients develop shock as a result of cardiogenic factors, specifically as a result of myocardial infarction. In pediatric patients, hypovolemic and distributive shock are the most common causes of inadequate tissue perfusion. Because trauma accounts for 50% of all deaths in children, hypovolemic shock is the most common type seen by most clinicians. Distributive shock from sepsis as a result of acute infectious diseases is the second most common type.

A second, extremely important difference between adults and children relates to the child's response to acute adrenergic stimulation. One of the earliest findings in shock is a massive outpouring of catecholamines, resulting in predictable changes throughout the body. In children, however, there is a much more dramatic response to the norepinephrine surge, particularly in regard to heart rate and increases in total peripheral resistance.

Although the heart rate increases in all patients who undergo adrenergic stimulation, children seem to be much more sensitive to this endogenous catecholamine surge, with heart rates more markedly elevated than those seen in adults.

A second consequence of children's response to catecholamines is a rapid and dramatic increase in both peripheral and central vasomotor tone. This increase in vasomotor tone is particularly noticeable in the large venous beds (in which up to 50% of the total blood

TABLE 59-28. CLASSIFICATION AND CAUSES OF SHOCK*

Class	Clinical Cause
Hypovolemic	Hemorrhage
	Dehydration
	Burns
	Heat loss
	Peritonitis
Cardiogenic	Congenital heart disease
	Congestive heart failure
	Myocardial infarction
	Kawasaki's disease
	Anomalous right coronary artery
Obstructive	Tension pneumothorax
	Cardiac tamponade
	Hemo/pneumothorax
	Hypertension
	Flail chest
	Pulmonary embolus
Distributive	Sepsis
	Anaphylaxis
	Drugs
	Spinal cord injury
	Anesthesia

* Adapted with permission from Mayer, T. (ed.): Emergency Management of Pediatric Trauma. Philadelphia, W.B. Saunders Co., 1985.

volume resides in the resting state) and in the skin. This results in a massive "autotransfusion" of blood into the effective circulation in response to endogenous catecholamines. From a clinical standpoint, this results in an extremely effective "clamping down" of the peripheral blood vessels, accounting for the extremely mottled skin appearance that is a classic finding in children early in the stages of hemorrhagic shock. In addition, the dramatic response to norepinephrine is a rapid and important increase in the total peripheral resistance.

For all of these reasons, children are able to maintain what might appear to the uninitiated observer as a relatively normal homeostatic state until late in the development of shock. *The well-trained emergency physician, however, recognizes the fact that children can maintain normal systolic blood pressures until they have lost nearly 30% of their total blood volume.* This ability to maintain the systolic blood pressure is caused largely by the child's sensitivity to the norepinephrine surge. For this reason, emergency physicians and trauma surgeons should be well trained in the early recognition of shock in children (see subsequent text).

A third difference between adults and children in shock is the extremely thin margin for error in children. For example, if a child and an adult each fall from a height of 3 feet and strike their heads, both may sustain similar-sized scalp lacerations and similar amounts of blood lost. The amount of blood, however, accounts for perhaps 5% of the adult's total blood volume but may constitute as much as 20 to 25% of the child's blood volume. Similarly, because children are able to maintain their systolic blood pressures through a wider range of blood loss than adults, it is extremely important for health care providers to recognize the thin margin for error for recognition and aggressive treatment of shock in children.

A fourth difference between adults and children in shock relates to the types of traumatic injury that children undergo and the resultant pathophysiologic consequences. As is detailed in Chapter 44, children with head trauma have markedly different pathophysiology than do adults. In addition, liver and splenic injuries are far more common in children than in adults, partially due to the fact that their abdomens are less well protected by muscle and fat. All of these differ-

ences must be kept in mind during the treatment of the child in shock.

A fifth difference between adults and children is the well-known growth and developmental factor in pediatric patients. Medications are most frequently given to children on a "per-kilogram" basis because their age and relative size are important considerations. Similarly, although the Broselow length-based pediatric resuscitation system (see subsequent text) largely addresses this problem, until it is uniformly used in EDs and EMS systems across the country, the growth and developmental changes will continue to be worthy of consideration.

The sixth difference between adults and children in shock is related to the homeostatic thermoregulatory mechanisms, particularly in infants and small children. These patients are unable to regulate their core body temperatures as well as older children and adults, and this may vastly complicate the development of shock. It is not uncommon to find children who are otherwise well resuscitated, including appropriate airway management and fluid management, but with persistent acidosis and refractoriness to treatment. In many cases, these children are found to be hypothermic because they are unable to regulate their temperatures as well as adults. For this reason, warming of intravenous fluids and appropriate steps to warm the patient should be undertaken. (See subsequent text.)

Finally, even among children, differences in the treatment of shock are based on age. Infants are different from adults in many ways that result in important changes in treatment for these patients. The specific ways in which these differences manifest themselves are addressed in a later section.

RECOGNITION

It is essential that all emergency physicians be extremely well versed in recognition of shock in pediatric patients. To attain this familiarity, it is important to understand normal baseline values for pulse, respiratory rate, circulating blood volume, and systolic and diastolic blood pressure (Fig. 59-20). All of these factors vary according to the age and size of the child. For defining upper limits of normal in the emergency department, these pulse and respiratory rates are helpful. In general, it is easy to remember that the pulse rates should be less than 140 in infants, less than 120 in preschool children, and less than 100 in school age children. Similarly, the respiratory rate should be less than 30 for infants, less than 20 for preschoolers, and less than 15 for school age children.

The circulating blood volume in a child is approximately 85 cc per kilogram, which is well above the levels of 70 cc per kilogram in adult men and 75 cc

---

TABLE 59-29. DIFFERENCES BETWEEN ADULT AND PEDIATRIC SHOCK

1. Types of shock differ (Pediatric: Hypovolemic; Adult: Cardiogenic)
2. Increased response to catecholamine surge in children
3. Thin margin for error in children
4. Pathophysiologic response to injury
5. Growth and developmental factors
6. Irregular homeostatic thermoregulatory response in children
7. Special care of infants

per kilogram in adult women. Although many studies have attempted to delineate the normal systolic and diastolic blood pressures in children, from a practical standpoint it is easiest to remember that the minimal systolic blood pressure in a child should be 80 plus twice the child's age in years. For example, in a 10-year-old child, the minimum acceptable systolic blood pressure is 100 mm Hg (BP = 80 + (2 × 10)). The diastolic blood pressure should be approximately two thirds of the systolic blood pressure.

Because of the child's sensitivity to the norepinephrine surge that occurs early in shock, the first finding in shock is an increase in the pulse rate, out of proportion to that normally seen in adults. For this reason, any child with pulse rates exceeding those mentioned should be considered to be in shock until proven otherwise, particularly if either traumatic or infectious causes are present that would predispose them to shock. The natural tendency of emergency physicians and emergency nurses is to attribute tachycardia in pediatric patients in the ED to pain, anxiety, or parental stimulation. Although this is sometimes the case, if an appropriate mechanism of illness or injury is present and tachycardia persists for more than a few minutes in the ED, the child should be assumed to be in shock until proven otherwise.

Additional findings depend on the degree of fluid deficit. Although additional information is presented subsequently on specific findings in distributive, obstructive, and cardiogenic shock, most children have some element of either acute blood loss or fluid sequestration. For this reason, hypovolemic shock is an excellent model in the recognition of shock in pediatric patients. Table 59-30 lists the clinical findings most often seen with various degrees of blood loss. Until about 15% of the total blood volume is lost, the only findings are slightly increased heart rate and local swelling and bleeding. Between 15 and 30% blood loss, the heart rate increases, often dramatically, and a generalized increase in total peripheral resistance occurs. Two specific findings are correlated with this

increase in total peripheral resistance: increased diastolic blood pressure and prolonged capillary refill. Prolonged capillary refill may be helpful in adult patients in determining the presence of blood loss. This finding, however, occurs extremely early in the course of the development of hypovolemic shock in children because of the child's dramatic response to the norepinephrine surge. For this reason, capillary refill occurs early in the course of shock and is not as helpful in distinguishing early from later phases of blood loss.

Blood Pressure Changes. A somewhat more sensitive indicator of the development of shock in children is an increase in the diastolic blood pressure, such that it exceeds two thirds of the systolic BP. Unfortunately, in many EDs, the physician and nursing staffs do not routinely obtain diastolic blood pressures on children. It is not uncommon to note on the triage vital signs that a child's blood pressure is listed as "100/palp," indicating that the systolic blood pressure was palpated at 100, but the diastolic blood pressure was not auscultated. Although some maintain that obtaining both a systolic and diastolic blood pressure is not necessary in children with simple infectious diseases such as otitis media and upper respiratory infections, it is only by routinely obtaining a complete set of vital signs in children that physicians and nurses are able to become well skilled at obtaining and interpreting vital signs in seriously ill or injured children. *For that reason, accurate pulse rates, respiratory rates, and systolic and diastolic blood pressure should be obtained routinely on all children presenting to the ED.*

Because the child has such a dramatic response to norepinephrine and the inherent autotransfusion effect that occurs with the increase in peripheral vascular resistance, children are able to maintain their systolic blood pressure at a normal level until they have lost up to 30% of their total blood volume. It should be

---

Non-Age-Dependent

Systolic blood pressure = 2 × (Age in years) + 80
Diastolic blood pressure = ⅔ systolic BP
Circulating blood volume = 85 cc per kilogram
Tidal volume = 15 cc per kilogram

Age-Dependent

Maximum Pulse Rate		*Maximum Respiratory Rate*
Infants	140	30
Preschool	120	20
School Age	100	16

FIG. 59-20. *Normal cardiopulmonary parameters in children. Although complicated tables exist for calculating pulse, respiratory rates, blood pressure and blood volume, these parameters are more easily remembered, or can be posted in the ED resuscitation area.*

TABLE 59-30. CORRELATION OF CLINICAL FINDINGS WITH DEGREE OF BLOOD LOSS

Percent Blood Loss	Clinical Findings
0–15	Increased heart rate
	Localized bleeding and swelling
15–30	Increased heart rate
	Increased peripheral resistance:
	Increased diastolic blood pressure
	Prolonged capillary refill
	Tachypnea
30–50	Hypotension (decreased systolic BP)
	Tachypnea/hyperpnea
	Decreased urine output
	Decreased cerebral perfusion
	Acidosis
>50	Refractory hypotension
	Refractory acidosis
	End-organ damage

clearly understood, however, that the "cost" of maintaining the blood pressure is at the expense of the full recruitment of compensatory mechanisms, so that children in whom blood loss is extensive enough to cause a decrease in the systolic blood pressure are gravely ill.

Once the blood loss exceeds approximately 30%, the systolic blood pressure often falls dramatically. Children then develop a deadly spiral of hypotension, acidosis, and decreased central nervous system (CNS) and renal perfusion, and die unless extremely aggressive treatment is undertaken.

Degree of Blood Loss. When the emergency physician encounters a child who is potentially at risk for shock, he or she should correlate the physical findings carefully with the possible degree of blood loss. For example, if a child presents after a bicycle collision with an increase in the heart rate and diastolic blood pressure, he or she should be assumed to have lost at least 15 to 30% of blood volume (Table 59-30). On the other hand, if the child has an increase in the heart rate but a normal diastolic and systolic blood pressure, it is more likely that he or she has lost 10 to 15% of blood volume. Because the appropriate therapy is guided by an understanding of the amount of blood loss (or fluid sequestered), emergency physicians and nurses must understand how to correlate the physical findings with the degree of blood loss.

In patients with over 50% blood loss, there is both profound and often refractory hypotension and acidosis. These children routinely require aggressive intervention, including both transfusion and, in most cases, surgery.

Distributive Shock. These factors are helpful in both recognizing shock early and correlating it with the amount of blood loss or fluid loss in cases of hypovolemic shock. In *distributive shock*, additional findings are often present. In patients with sepsis, it is common to find that the extremities are warm and flushed early in the course of the patient's disease, although this progresses to more classic pale and mottled extremities late in the course of sepsis. Pediatric patients with sepsis often have extremely marked tachycardia, out of proportion to what might normally be expected based on other physical findings. Depending on the site of infection, source-specific findings may also be present (e.g., meningeal or neurologic findings in CNS disease). In septic shock, it is also common to find both tachypnea and hyperpnea, reflecting both an increased CNS drive and the degree of acidosis present. Examination of the skin in septic shock may be normal or show flushed extremities early in the course of the disease, although pale, mottled extremities may occur later. The presence of petechiae reflects the presence of vasculitis, and is not necessarily predictive of outcome; however, purpura usually reflects a serious underlying disease.

Obstructive Shock. Findings in *obstructive shock* usually reflect the cause of the obstruction itself. For example, in tension pneumothorax, distention of the affected thorax, hyperresonance, and tracheal deviation may occur. Similarly, in cardiac tamponade, one expects to see profound hypotension in conjunction with neck vein distention, with or without muffled heart tones. In both of these instances, some form of blunt or penetrating injury is usually present.

Cardiogenic Shock. Although *cardiogenic shock* is extremely uncommon in pediatric patients, most cases are caused by severe underlying congenital heart disease and present with congestive heart failure. In some patients with either prolonged hypovolemic or distributive shock, however, an element of cardiogenic shock also intervenes, and appropriate therapy with inotropic agents may have to be undertaken.

Urine Output. Regardless of the type or cause of shock, if it is severe enough or persists for a sufficent time, decreased perfusion to the renal bed and CNS may cause symptoms. One of the best ways of following the progression of shock is by urine output. Children should produce approximately 1 cc per kg per hour of urine, and infants produce 1 to 2 cc per kg per hour. If fluid resuscitation does not result in this amount of urine output, increased fluid boluses may be necessary. It is important, however, to recognize that urine output is a *dynamic*, not a *static* means of following the progression of shock. In patients with significant shock, an indwelling urinary catheter should be placed and appropriate renal studies undertaken. Although CNS changes including confusion and altered mental status may result from shock, an extremely large percentage of injured patients in the pediatric age group have CNS injury, and it is often difficult to distinguish decreased perfusion to the brain caused by shock from the brain injury itself.

Laboratory findings in shock should be strictly confirmatory, as opposed to being used to diagnose shock. The emergency physician and emergency nurse should be able to diagnose shock and institute treatment long before it is confirmed by laboratory findings. Certain laboratory tests, however, may be helpful in establishing the *degree* or *extent* of shock. For example, the emergency physician should have significant clinical suspicion of acidosis based on findings of tachypnea and hyperpnea, although arterial blood gases are helpful in confirming the degree of acidosis present. One exception to the strictly confirmatory role of the laboratory in patients in shock is related to infants. In some cases, hypoglycemia may be the earliest manifestation of impending shock in infants. In all patients in whom shock is suspected, a baseline set of laboratory studies should be obtained, including a blood count, electrolytes, blood urea, glucose, arterial blood gases, urinalysis, and clotting studies (including prothrombin time, partial thromboplastin time, platelet count, and fibrin split products).

TREATMENT

When the physician or nurse makes the diagnosis of shock, treatment should begin immediately. It is also important, however, to recognize what type of shock the patient is likely to have. In most cases, it is fairly clear whether the patient suffers from hypovolemic, distributive, obstructive, or cardiogenic shock. Because shock consists of a generalized state of inadequate tissue perfusion resulting in impaired cellular respiration, *the primary goal of shock therapy is to restore normal perfusion as quickly as possible to prevent impaired cellular respiration, as well as damage to the cells, organs, and body systems.* The more rapidly and aggressively shock treatment is undertaken, the more likely it is that the patient will survive with minimum morbidity.

From a pathophysiologic standpoint, the Fick equation (Fig. 59-21) is helpful in understanding the relationship among oxygen consumption, blood flow, fractional unloading of hemoglobin, and hemoglobin concentration. It is important to remember that any increase in blood flow itself is helpful in re-establishing a more normal physiologic state in patients with shock. Similarly, it is also helpful to remember that the cardiac output represents a simple product of the heart rate and the stroke volume. Because heart rate is maximally stimulated in children, even in the early stages of shock, improving the stroke volume becomes critical to the success of shock therapy.

Figure 59-22 illustrates the relationship between stroke volume and pre-load, myocardial contractility, and after-load. In the vast majority of cases of shock, initial therapy is directed toward maximizing the preload by ensuring that appropriate fluid therapy is undertaken as aggressively as possible. In all cases of hemorrhagic shock and most cases of distributive shock, there is either an absolute or relative decrease in circulating blood volume, so that rapid fluid infusion is an important part of optimizing preload. In most hypovolemic shock and early distributive shock, the child's myocardial contractility is normal and demonstrates substantial cardiac reserve because most children have a normal functioning myocardium. In late stages of septic shock, however, and in patients with congenital heart disease, it may be appropriate to stimulate myocardial contractility with the use of inotropic agents.

Although afterload reduction is an important part of shock therapy in adults with cardiogenic shock, it is far less commonly used in pediatric patients. In some cases of distributive and cardiogenic shock, however, afterload reduction may be necessary.

Because hypovolemic shock is the most common type of shock seen in children, treatment for this entity is discussed as the basic format for shock therapy, although distributive, obstructive, and cardiogenic

$$VO_2 = Q + 1.39\ Hgb \times (SaO_2 - SVO_2)$$

VO_2 = Oxygen consumption
Q = Blood flow
Hgb = Hemoglobin concentration
$SaO_2 - SVO_2$ = Fractional unloading of O_2

FIG. 59-21.   The Fick equation. This equation describes the relationship between oxygen consumption and blood flow, hemoglobin concentration, and fractional unloading of oxygen from the hemoglobin molecule. When conceptionalized in this manner, it is apparent that increases in blood flow will improve oxygen consumption, thereby demonstrating the importance of increasing blood flow in patients in shock.

Cardiac output = heart rate × stroke volume
- Preload
- Myocardial contractibility
- Afterload

FIG. 59-22.   Conceptual basis of pediatric shock therapy. Cardiac output is the product of heart rate and stroke volume. In children, the heart rate is already maximally stimulated because of the child's response to the catecholamine in shock. Therapy to improve cardiac output is therefore primarily aimed at increasing stroke volume. Because myocardial contractility and afterload are usually normal in children except in distributive (septic) shock, primary emphasis is placed on maximizing preload.

shock are discussed as well. The goals of therapy and treatment of hypovolemic shock are to:

1. Restore effective circulatory volume (maximize preload)
2. Maximize oxygen delivery
3. Decrease ongoing blood loss

RESTORING EFFECTIVE CIRCULATORY VOLUME

Restoring the circulatory volume basically reflects an attempt to maximize preload. This can be done by infusion of colloids or crystalloids, transfusion of blood, or blood products by autotransfusion. The mainstay of effective fluid therapy in children is infusion of crystalloid solutions. Although some pediatric intensive care physicians use colloid solutions in the intensive care unit (ICU), these play virtually no role in the ED. Crystalloid solutions that may be selected include lactated Ringer's solution or 0.9% sodium chloride, with or without 5% dextrose. Lactated Ringer's is the solution of choice in most EDs, although the potential hypoglycemia that may occur in the late stages of shock have caused some experts to recommend the use of lactated Ringer's with 5% glucose. Others argue that glucose in the initial stages of fluid resuscitation may be excreted in the urine, producing an osmotic diuretic effect. Although 0.9% sodium chloride is an effective alternative, scattered reports have indicated that large-volume infusions with this agent may produce hyperchloremic acidosis. For all practical purposes, isotonic crystalloid solutions are probably equally effective, whether in the form of lactated Ringer's, lactated Ringer's with glucose, or sodium chloride.

Ensuring appropriate fluid infusion requires a systematic approach to vascular access of the child (Fig. 59-23). One of the mainstays of vascular access in children up to the age of 5 years is intraosseous infusion, a safe and effective technique originally pioneered in the 1920s and widely used throughout the 1940s. The advent of intravenous cannulas at that time, however, caused the intraosseous technique to fall into disuse until recently. Large-bore (13 gauge to 16 gauge) bone marrow needles can be placed in the anterior surface of the tibia easily and with minimal training. This technique can be used by field personnel as well as emergency department physicians and nurses. Both clinical and bench research indicate that large volumes of intravenous fluid and a wide array of medications can be given by the intraosseous route. Although most needles used are 13 gauge needles placed by firm pressure against the bony cortex, the Melkerneedle (Cook Critical Care) can be placed by means of a screw-in technique, which may allow use in older children. In general, the technique is successful in children up to about 5 years, although it has been placed on occasion in elderly adults.

All EDs will be well served by establishing a protocol for vascular access in children. In most cases, this includes an initial attempt at percutaneous peripheral IV cannulation for a brief time, usually 1 to 2 minutes. If a peripheral intravenous cannula cannot be placed in this time, an intraosseous needle should be attempted in all children under 5. Once this has been secured, more controlled attempts at central venous cannulation or cutdown may be attempted. Canter and colleagues in Syracuse demonstrated the efficacy of such a protocol in a large series of pediatric patients; this experience has been duplicated elsewhere.

Table 59-31 lists important factors in obtaining peripheral percutaneous venous access. Among the most important of these is ensuring that the emergency care provider obtains and maintains skill in placing

such catheters. The emergency physician should ensure that he or she has the skill to place such catheters and will be able to do so under the stressful situations of a resuscitation when necessary. Because some EDs do not see a large number of acutely ill or injured patients, it may be necessary to rotate through the pediatric or neonatal ICU to develop and maintain such skill. The emergency physician should be aware of certain constant and fixed sites of veins in children, including the greater saphenous vein, the external jugular vein, and the fifth interdigital vein on the dorsum of the hand.

One technique that is particularly helpful to remember in children is to puncture the skin with a needle one size larger than the intravenous cannula to be used *before* threading the intravenous cannula through the skin. For example, if a 20-gauge catheter is being placed, pierce the skin first with an 18-gauge needle, after which the 20-gauge catheter can be threaded through the hole created by the larger needle. In effect, this helps prevent shearing of the catheter tip as it goes through the skin and allows much easier threading of the catheter once the vein is entered.

Although many EDs stress the utility of central venous catheter placement in children, the techniques used are fraught with difficulty, particularly if the subclavian technique is chosen. Ectopic placement of the catheter occurs commonly, and the length of the central venous catheters themselves restrict the amount of flow of crystalloid solution through the catheter because Poseuille's Law reflects the fact that length is a major determinant of flow through a catheter.

Peripheral venous cutdown is a safe and effective technique for placement of relatively short, large-bore cannulas. Unfortunately, fewer physicians are trained in this technique than was once the case. When used at the greater saphenous vein, the catheter can usually be placed in a relatively short period of time and has few complications, all of which are minor.

Whether central venous cannulation or peripheral venous cutdown is used, each of these techniques should be recognized as second-line techniques, to be used only after peripheral venous cannulation has failed and an intraosseous line has been placed.

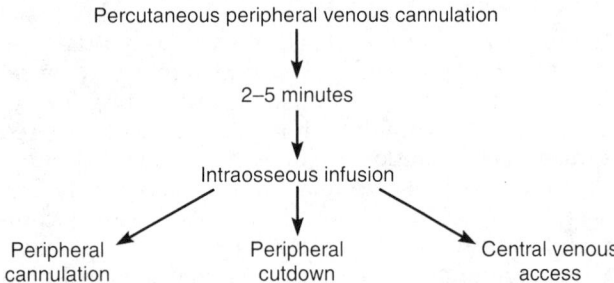

FIG. 59-23.   *Intravenous access protocol. Emergency physicians and their patients are well served by adherence to a time-dependent protocol to guide intravenous access. In this example, peripheral venous cannulation is attempted for a period not exceeding 2 to 5 minutes. If access has not been obtained, an intraosseous line is placed, after which more controlled attempts at either peripheral percutaneous cannulation, peripheral venous cutdown, or central venous access may be attempted, depending on the skill and preference of the physician.*

TABLE 59-31. PERCUTANEOUS INTRAVENOUS ACCESS IN CHILDREN

1. Attain and maintain skill
2. Puncture skin with needle before catheter placement
3. Enter vein bevel up—rotate 180 degrees after entry
4. Familiarize with constant, fixed sites
   —Greater saphenous vein
   —External jugular vein
   —Fifth interdistal vein
   —Median cephalic and basilica veins
5. Observe these sites in normal children
6. Flush catheter before puncture
7. Use of high-intensity "cold" transillumination

Once vascular access has been established, all children with shock (including persistent tachycardia in the face of an appropriate mechanism of illness or injury) should receive an *immediate* bolus infusion of 20 cc per kilogram of crystalloid. This infusion should occur over no more than 5 minutes, which may require manually pushing the fluid in after a small catheter has been placed. In patients with signs of more significant blood loss, such as profound tachycardia, an increase in the diastolic blood pressure, and a fall in the systolic blood pressure, it may be necessary to push as much as 40 cc per kilogram. Once the initial fluid infusion has occurred, strict attention should be paid to how the patient's vital signs change after the bolus infusion. If either 20 or 40 cc per kilogram have been infused and the patient's vital signs deteriorate, even more aggressive fluid therapy should be undertaken. In children with less than 25% blood loss, early initiation of appropriate fluid therapy may preclude the need for transfusion. In patients with more than 25% blood loss, however, transfusion with packed red blood cells is often necessary (Table 59-32). In patients with massive hemorrhage who present with hypotension and acidosis, immediate infusion of crystalloids should be undertaken, but most of these patients require transfusion and surgery to stop their blood loss. For example, a patient with a massively shattered spleen or liver can often be initially stabilized with aggressive crystalloid therapy, but many require surgery to control the source of bleeding. Patients with more isolated tears of the liver or spleen, however, can often be managed nonoperatively (see Chap. 44).

Autotransfusion helps restore the effective circulatory volume, but is less commonly used in pediatric patients than in adults. It is largely restricted to patients with penetrating chest injuries, although it has occasionally been used in patients with blunt abdominal trauma in which there has been no colonic injury. It was originally thought that military antishock trousers (MAST) had some effect in autotransfusion. This has since been shown to be inaccurate, however, particularly because children are so sensitive to the noradrenergic effects, which massively increase total peripheral resistance, effectively allowing a "physiologic autotransfusion." For this reason, MAST have little or no role in the management of pediatric shock, except perhaps to stabilize pelvic or femoral fractures.

It is essential to ensure that the physician and the nurse closely monitor the patient's response to fluid therapy. Treatment decisions depend on how the child's pulse, respirations, and systolic and diastolic blood pressure respond to the initial fluid infusion.

MAXIMIZING OXYGEN DELIVERY

Table 59-33 lists elements of pediatric shock therapy designed to maximize oxygen delivery. By far the most important is aggressive airway management to ensure oxygenation, ventilation, and humidification. Details

TABLE 59-32. GUIDELINES FOR INFUSION/TRANSFUSION IN PEDIATRIC SHOCK

% Blood Loss	Infusion/Transfusion
<25	LR* (3 cc LR per 1 cc blood loss)
25–50	½ volume LR (3 cc LR per 1 cc blood loss)
	½ volume PRBC† (1 cc PRBC per 1 cc blood loss)
>50	O negative or type-specific Blood LR Surgical hemostasis

* LR = Lactated Ringer's Solution
† PRBC = Packed Red Blood Cells

of pediatric airway management are listed in a previous subchapter, but it is important to recognize that all patients in shock should have 100% oxygen delivered to them through the most appropriate means. Transfusion of blood and blood products not only increases the effective circulatory volume, but also helps to maximize oxygen delivery by increasing oxygen-carrying capacity.

Measures to improve myocardial contractility are more often used in adult patients, but may be necessary in certain pediatric patients. This is particularly true of cases with massive hemorrhagic shock or late distributive (septic) or cardiogenic shock. In these cases, either isoproterenol, dopamine, or dobutamine may be used. Most pediatric emergency and intensive care physicians, however, use dopamine in such situations, except in infants (see subsequent text). The easiest means of providing dopamine therapy is by the "Rule of Sixes." Dopamine, 6 mg per kg, is placed in a metriset, after which appropriate fluid is added so that there are a total of 100 cc in the metriset. With this technique, the number of cc per hour on the volume infusion pump equals the number of micrograms per kilogram per minute of dopamine delivered to the patient. This technique greatly simplifies dopamine infusion in the ED because it is a simple mattner to increase the infusion as necessary to improve cardiac output.

An additional means of improving oxygen delivery is to decrease the patient's oxygen demands. For example, in patients with seizures or who are agitated or struggling against ventilation, sedation may be helpful in decreasing their oxygen consumption. Similarly, patients with fever should be treated because increasing the temperature by 1° Centigrade (Celsius) increases oxygen consumption by nearly 10%.

Theoretically, oxygen can be delivered in many ways, although few have found widespread use in the clinical setting. This includes the use of steroids, glucose-potassium-insulin preparations, ATP-magnesium and naloxone. Ongoing research into shock, however, indicates the complex interaction of a number of agents, including cytokines, eicosanoids, amines, opioid neurotransmitters, hormones, super-

TABLE 59-33. STEPS TO MAXIMIZE OXYGEN DELIVERY

1. Aggressive airway management
    Oxygenation with humidified 100% oxygen
    Ventilation
2. Transfusion of hemoglobin (when indicated)
3. Improving myocardial contractility
    Dopamine
    Dobutamine
    Isoproterenol
4. Decrease oxygen demands
    Appropriate sedation
    Treat fever
    Treat seizures
5. Potential Future Therapies
    Steroids
    Naloxone
    Glucose-potassium-insulin
    ATP-magnesium
    Eicosanoids
    Cytokines
    Fibronectin
    Superoxide radical modulators
    Immunotherapy

oxide radicals, fibronectin, and other agents. As this research progresses, additional means of manipulating these axes may find clinical efficacy.

DECREASING ONGOING BLOOD LOSS

The primary means of decreasing ongoing blood loss is surgery, although general measures to decrease obvious blood loss from the skin should also be undertaken. Pressure should be placed on any external bleeding points, and these should be elevated. In pediatric patients with head injuries and external hemorrhage, a pressure dressing should be placed on the head before elevation to prevent the possibility of air embolus in patients with dural venous sinus tears. Surgical control of external bleeding points with hemostats should be undertaken only on the scalp and extremities, and only when the vessel can be clearly seen before clamping. The vascular and neurologic bundles on the extremities are usually in close proximity, and blind clamping of vessels may inadvertently cause neurologic damage.

An additional means of decreasing ongoing blood loss is with specific blood component therapy. For example, in patients who develop bleeding diatheses, therapy with platelets, fresh frozen plasma, or cryoprecipitate may be necessary.

DISTRIBUTIVE SHOCK

Most cases of distributive shock in pediatric patients are caused by sepsis. Although acute blood loss may not be a factor in such patients, most patients in septic shock have a relative decrease in effective circulating blood volume caused by fluid sequestration and altered capillary permeability. For this reason, the vast majority of these patients also require aggressive fluid bolus therapy, usually with crystalloids. Although some pediatric intensive care physicians use colloid therapy in such patients in the ICU, the initial infusion in the ED should be with a crystalloid solution, usually lactated Ringer's. Stabilization of the cardiorespiratory system is essential because these patients often present with markedly abnormal clinical findings on the basis of their shock. Aggressive airway management and vascular access should be undertaken and an initial fluid bolus with at least 20 cc per kilogram of lactated Ringer's should be provided.

Once the cardiovascular system has been stabilized as well as possible, however, it is important to recognize and treat the underlying source of shock. Antibiotic therapy should be undertaken after appropriate cultures have been taken. In some cases of fulminant sepsis, such as those seen in patients in meningococcemia, however, it may be necessary to begin antibiotic treatment before obtaining cultures, particularly those of the cerebrospinal fluid. As additional generations of antibiotics are developed, therapy is likely to change over the coming years.

In some patients with distributive shock, a so-called myocardial depressant factor may be circulating, causing a decrease in myocardial contractility. In such patients, inotropic therapy with dopamine is indicated and should begin in the ED, but only after the patient has received appropriate fluid infusion. Providing inotropic stimulation when preload has not been maximized can be extremely dangerous.

Although steroids have been suggested as a possible course of treatment in septic shock, their usefulness has never been convincingly demonstrated in either adult or pediatric patients, except for children with bacterial meningitis or adrenal insufficiency. Because peripheral vascular resistance may be significantly altered in patients in the late stages of septic shock, it may be necessary to manipulate the vascular resistance to maximize cardiac output. In most cases, this requires the use of appropriate hemodynamic monitoring to ensure that calculations of cardiac output and systemic vascular resistance can be obtained.

In the future, it is likely that some form of immunotherapy, including the use of monoclonal antibodies will prove helpful in septic shock in children. Although there is some theoretic advantage to the use of naloxone in septic shock, it is not completely free of side effects, including hypotension, ventricular arrhythmias, and acute pulmonary edema. In most cases, use of naloxone is considered investigational or a last-ditch effort to save the patient. Although fibronectin and cryoprecipitate have been used in some adult patients and have improved target organ dysfunction, their use is not routinely recommended in patients with septic shock.

OBSTRUCTIVE SHOCK

The goal of therapy in obstructive shock is simply to remove the source of obstruction. In pediatric patients this is usually tension pneumothorax or cardiac tamponade. In either case, immediate decompression of the chest or pericardium, respectively, should be undertaken by the emergency physician. After needle decompression of a tension pneumothorax, an appropriate-sized chest tube should be placed. In most pediatric patients with cardiac tamponade, needle pericardiocentesis can be performed, although definitive surgical therapy is required. In rare cases, pediatric patients may present with hypertension of such a degree that obstructive shock may ensue. Although this is extremely uncommon, aggressive therapy should be undertaken with nitroprusside to lower the blood pressure to acceptable levels. In the past, diazoxide was used in these settings, but most emergency physicians and pediatric intensivists now prefer to use nitroprusside. Other, far rarer causes of obstructive shock include flail chest and pulmonary embolus. These are extremely uncommon in children, however, and rarely produce obstructive shock.

CARDIOGENIC SHOCK

Most cases of cardiogenic shock in pediatric patients are caused by significant congenital heart disease. Most of these are recognized at or shortly after birth and do not primarily present to the ED in cardiogenic shock. When they do, however, appropriate aggressive therapy should be undertaken.

MONITORING PEDIATRIC PATIENTS IN SHOCK

The most important reason for monitoring patients in the ED with shock is to ensure that their vital signs are reassessed on a continuing basis, every 5 minutes during initial resuscitation. *The child's response to fluid therapy is the most important predictor of eventual outcome.* This rarely requires the use of invasive hemodynamic monitoring in the ED. Even when the blood pressure is low, it can usually be determined accurately through the use of Doppler ultrasound, which should be available in all EDs. Indwelling arterial catheters are rarely needed in the ED, but may be placed in the pediatric ICU or operating room. Central venous catheters have extremely limited use in initial fluid therapy for pediatric patients, but are sometimes used to monitor ongoing fluid therapy, as a reflection of the right atrial pressure. Because the right atrial pressure correlates somewhat better with left atrial pressure in children than it does in adults, CVP lines are sometimes used

to determine the adequacy of fluid resuscitation. They should not routinely be used in the ED, however, and most pediatric intensive care physicians prefer a pulmonary artery catheter because additional information on cardiac output and systemic vascular resistance can be obtained from such a catheter.

In all patients with suspected or impending shock, an indwelling bladder catheter should be placed. It should be recognized that the initial urine drained from the bladder was present at the time of the initial injury or insult, and this should be measured and drained immediately. After that, children should produce at least 1 cc per kilogram per hour of urine, although infants may produce as much as 2 cc per kilogram per hour.

An extremely helpful way of monitoring ongoing therapy in children is by use of the pulse oximeter. This provides an excellent means of determining changes in oxygenation, despite the fact that decreased peripheral perfusion is present in most pediatric patients with shock. Although it may be difficult to interpret the results when perfusion is radically decreased, pulse oximetry is an important adjunct in monitoring pediatric patients in the ED.

THE SPECIAL CARE OF INFANTS

Infants who present in shock do so in ways that are substantially different from those seen in older children. In many cases, the first manifestation of shock in an infant may be decreased activity or lethargy. The ventricles of infants are far more noncompliant or "stiff" than those of older children, making manipulation of the stroke volume more difficult in these patients. For this reason, the use of cardioactive medications such as dobutamine or dopamine is undertaken earlier in the course of therapy than in older children. It is extremely common in infants for blood glucose to drop rapidly in response to shock, and this should be monitored and treated appropriately. Most cases of shock in infants are caused by sepsis or underlying congenital heart disease, and treatment should be geared toward this specific entity.

PREHOSPITAL CARE

Prehospital care providers should be trained by ED personnel in the early recognition and treatment of shock. The importance of airway and vascular access should be stressed, and prehospital care providers should be capable of providing appropriate airway management and intraosseous infusion. Both of these techniques have been widely used by paramedics with excellent results.

It is particularly important to ensure that paramedics understand the importance of providing 100% oxygen at the earliest possible time. In addition, they should be trained to infuse fluid at appropriate bolus amounts over extremely short time periods.

MEDICOLEGAL PEARLS

Whether shock in pediatric patients is from hypovolemic, distributive, obstructive, or cardiogenic factors, any child who may die or suffer significant morbidity is a potentially serious risk management problem. To avoid such problems, and to provide the best possible care for pediatric patients, all EDs should undertake an aggressive protocol-oriented approach to the care of pediatric shock victims. This is particularly true in departments where pediatric patients are infrequently seen because it is more difficult to maintain expertise when it is infrequently exercised. The use of the Broselow length-based resuscitation system is an excellent way to ensure that the appropriate-sized equipment and appropriate medication dosages are used. Continuing in-service education should be provided to nurses and paramedics within the ED and the EMS system to ensure that they are familiar with the presentations and treatment of pediatric shock.

When children present to the emergency department in shock, it is extremely important to ensure that the ED medical record and nurses' notes reflect accurately the therapy that was undertaken, as well as the patient's response to therapy. In most cases, it is advisable to dictate a note detailing the patient's course in the ED, regardless of whether the outcome is favorable or not. This simply ensures a more detailed and accurate record of the patient's care if there is later legal action.

HORIZONS

The advent of length-based resuscitation systems provides an important and elegantly simple way to ensure that the dosages of medication and size of equipment are appropriate. As the system becomes more widely used in the prehospital and ED phases of care, variations in therapy will be greatly reduced.

As experience increases with the use of intraosseous infusion, it is likely that this technique will become even more widespread, as will the number of medications given by this route.

Research on the use of hypertonic saline-dextran solution is promising in the adult population, and there will undoubtedly be studies to evaluate its use in pediatric patients. Should

hypertonic saline-dextran prove useful, it will probably be used in both the prehospital and ED settings.

Exciting research on the manipulation of thromboxanes, eicosanoids, leukotrienes and superoxide radicals may well result in forms of therapy that can be applied in both the prehospital and ED settings. It is likely that immunotherapy, including the use of monoclonal antibodies, will become an important mainstay in the therapy of patients with septic shock.

BIBLIOGRAPHY

Baley, J.E.: Neonatal sepsis: The potential for immunotherapy. Clin. Perinatol. *15:*755, 1988.

Berg, R.A.: Emergency infusion of catecholamines into bone marrow. Am. J. Dis. Child. *138:*810, 1984.

Bone, R.C., Fisher, C., Clemmer, T.P., et al.: A controlled clinical trial of high dose methylprednisolone in the treatment of severe sepsis and septic shock. N. Engl. J. Med. *317:*653, 1987.

Border, J.R.: Hypothesis: Sepsis, multiple organ failure in the macrophage. Arch. Surg. *123:*285, 1988.

Boyd, J.I., Stanford, G.C., and Chernow, B.: The pharmacotherapy of septic shock. Crit. Care Med. *5:*133, 1989.

Carcillo, J.A., et al.: Role of early fluid resuscitation in pediatric septic shock. JAMA *266:*1242, 1991.

Frye, D.E.: Multiple system organ failure. Surg. Clin. North Am. *68:*107, 1988.

Groeger, J.S., and Inturrisi, C.E.: High dose naloxone: Pharmacokinetics in patients in septic shock. Crit. Care Med. *15:*751, 1987.

Hesselvic, F., Brodlin, B., Carlsson, C., et al.: Cryoprecipitate Infusion fails to Improve organ function in septic shock. Crit. Care Med. *15:*475, 1987.

Jacobson, M.A., and Young, L.S.: New developments in the treatment of gram-negative bacteremia. West. J. Med. *244:*185, 1988.

Kanter, R.K., Zimmerman, J.J., Strauss, R.N., et al.: Pediatric emergency intravenous access: Evaluation of a protocol. Am. J. Dis. Child. *40:*132, 1986.

Karakusis, P.H.: Considerations in the therapy of septic shock. Med. Clin. North Am. *70:*933, 1986.

Lebel, M.H., et al.: Dexamethasone therapy for bacterial meningitis. Results of two double-blind, placebo-controlled trials. N. Engl. J. Med. *319:*964, 1988.

Mayer, T.A.: Diagnosis and treatment of hemorrhagic shock. *In* The Clinical Practice of Emergency Medicine, Edited by Harwood, Nuss, A., Linden, C., Luten, R.J., et al. Philadelphia J.B. Lippincott, 1991.

Mayer, T.: Emergency pediatric vascular access: Old solutions to an old problem. Am. J. Emerg. Med. *4:*98, 1986.

Mayer, T.: Management of Hypovolemic shock. *In* Emergency Management of Pediatric Trauma. Edited by Mayer, T. Philadelphia, W.B. Saunders, 1985.

Mayer, T.A., Walker, M.L., Matlak, M.E., and Johnson, D.G.: Causes of morbidity and mortality in severe pediatric trauma. JAMA *245:*719, 1981.

Miner, W.: Pre-hospital use of intraosseous needles by paramedics. Pediatric Emerg. Care 5:5, 1989.

Orlowski, J.P.: My kingdom for an intraosseous line. Am. J. Dis. Child. 38:803, 1984.

Orlowski, J.P.: The safety of intraosseous infusions: Risks of fat and bone marrow emboli to the lungs. Ann. Emerg. Med. 18:1062, 1989.

Parrish, G.A.: Intraosseous infusion in the Emergency Department. Am. J. Emerg. Med. 4:59, 1986.

Perkin, S., and Levin, L.: Shock in the pediatric patient. Part I.J. Pediatr. 101:163, 1982.

Quilligan, J.J., and Turkel, H.: Bone marrow infusion and it's complications. Am. J. Dis. Child. 71:457, 1946.

Rowe, M.I.: Shock in resuscitation. In Complications in Pediatric Surgery. Edited by Welch, C. Philadelphis, W.B. Saunders, 1984.

Schwartz, J.A., and Koenigsberg, M.D.: Naloxone-induced pulmonary edema. Ann. Emerg. Med. 16:142, 1987.

Serra, F.B.: The multiple organ failure syndrome. Hosp. Prac. 25:169, 1990.

Simmerman, J.J., and Dietrich, K.A.: Current perspective on septic shock. Pediatr. Clin. North Am. 34:131, 1987.

Sprung, C.L., Caralis, P.V., Marcial, E.H., et al.: The effect of high dose corticosteroids in patients with septic shock: A perspective controlled study. N. Engl. J. Med. 311:1137, 1984.

The Veteran Administration Systemic Sepsis Cooperative Study Group: Effect of high dose glucocorticoid therapy on mortality in patients with clinical signs of systemic sepsis. N. Engl. J. Med. 317:659, 1987.

PEDIATRIC INFECTIOUS DISEASES

Thom A. Mayer, Kathleen Kelly, George R. Schwartz, and Barbara K. Hanke

CAPSULE

This chapter covers pediatric infectious diseases, including those of the eyes, ears, mouth, and sinuses, and the lymph node drainage of those areas. These are the most common presenting complaints in the emergency department (ED) involving children. The topics reviewed include otitis media, otitis externa, periorbital cellulitis, sinusitis, cervical lymphadenitis, conjunctivitis, and gingivostomatitis.

OTITIS MEDIA

INTRODUCTION

Otitis media (OM) is one the most common infections in children. It occurs at least once in 85% of children. It is seen most frequently in children 3 to 36 months old but can also be present in neonates.

Otitis media is characterized by an effusion in the middle ear. Otolaryngologists have divided OM into purulent and serous, based on the quality of the effusion. They have further divided the diagnoses into acute and chronic, depending on the duration of symptoms and clinical findings. The emergency physician is primarily concerned with the diagnosis and treatment of acute purulent otitis media (APOM) and differentiating this from serous otitis media (SOM). Persistent SOM should be managed by an otolaryngologist.

The difficulty in diagnosing and treating OM is caused by overlap in the appearance of the serous and purulent OM. Serous OM usually follows an episode of APOM. A serous effusion can be present up to 12 weeks following APOM. This effusion can be contaminated again and a new infection may begin. Early in an acute infection the two processes can appear the same. In addition cultures of effusions from patients with SOM have grown organisms in 25% of patients with chronic SOM. These effusions were previously thought to be sterile. If there is a question as to whether the middle ear process represents an acute bacterial infection, it is best to treat the patient.

A careful history and physical examination with diligent use of the pneumatic otoscope should aid the emergency physician in the diagnosis and treatment of otitis media. A middle ear process that is not improving under conventional therapy should be referred early to an otolaryngologist.

PATHOPHYSIOLOGY AND ANATOMY

Malfunction of the eustachian tubes plays a significant role in the development of otitis media in children. The eustachian tubes of infants and young children are wide, short, and horizontal in relation to the pharynx. This allows reflux of nasopharyngeal secretions, which does not occur in the narrower, longer, and more acutely angled tubes of the adult. Hypertrophy of lymphoid tissue located at the pharyngeal opening of the eustachian tube can obstruct the tube, leading to stasis of middle ear secretions and subsequent bacterial proliferation. Lymphoid tissue becomes reactive and edematous in most upper respiratory infections. Most cases of APOM consequently follow an upper respiratory infection. Intrinsic malfunction of the eustachian tube has also been implicated.

The most common organisms cultured from APOM are Streptococcus pneumoniae, Hemophilus influenzae and, to a lesser extent, Group A B-hemolytic streptococcus. There is increasing prevalence of Moraxella catarrhalis (up to 13 to 20%), most of which produce β-lactamase. In the newborn period (under 4 weeks of age), Staphylococcus aureus and enteric pathogens predominate. Blood cultures are rarely positive in children with APOM. Most children should be treated empirically to cover the most common organisms in their age group unless complications have occurred or they are unresponsive to conventional therapy. In these cases, tympanocentesis should be done, preferably by an otolaryngologist, to identify the causative organism. Any child with APOM and spontaneous perforation of the tympanic membrane should have the drainage cultured for identification before antibiotic use.

CLINICAL PRESENTATION AND EXAMINATION

APOM usually accompanies an upper respiratory infection, but may also occur as an isolated entity. The child may present with complaints associated with an upper respiratory infection, such as fever, congestion and cough, as well as gastrointestinal disturbances. Depending on the child's age, he or she may complain of ear pain, decreased hearing or fullness. Infants and younger children may be more irritable and rub or pull at the involved ear. Many of the findings can vary. The absence of fever should not exclude the diagnosis because only 35% have an elevated temperature.

On physical examination, APOM is characterized by effusion, with a bulging tympanic membrane. The drum should be examined for color, quality of the effusion and, most importantly, its mobility. Examination with a pneumatic otoscope can most accurately diagnose otitis media in the child. The color of the drum is least important because it varies with crying and fever and is subjective. The drum in APOM may appear bright red or opaque yellow/white depending on the stage of infection. The light reflex is an unreliable indicator because it persists until late in the infection. The drum in APOM is convex, bulging toward the examiner. It has decreased mobility with positive and negative insufflation.

The presence of drainage from the ear with perforation of the tympanic membrane indicates APOM. The time from onset of symptoms to perforation can be rapid. Ear pain diminishes after perforation.

In SOM, the only complaint may be decreased hearing or fullness. SOM is the leading cause of hearing loss in children. Patients do not complain of pain and are not acutely ill. A history of previous APOM should be sought because most have a persistent effusion for many weeks after the acute episode. If the effusion persists beyond 4 weeks, the child should be evaluated by an otolaryngologist.

On examination, the patient with SOM has a retracted tympanic membrane from the negative pressure within the middle ear. The tympanic membrane is not hyperemic and the effusion is translucent. The presence of air bubbles on an air-fluid level behind the TM is diagnostic for SOM. The tympanic membrane also has decreased mobility with insufflation. Insufflation is often the only way that SOM can be diagnosed outside the otolaryngologist's office.

Again, the distinction between the two entities is often not clear, particularly when fever and other URI symptoms are present. If a bacterial infection is in question, it is best to treat with antibiotics.

DIFFERENTIAL DIAGNOSIS (TABLE 59-34)

The differential diagnosis in the well child complaining of ear pain is quite short. There may be an otitis externa, a furunculitis of the ear canal or a traumatic perforation of the tympanic membrane present. Less commonly and in the more acutely ill child ear pain may be the presenting complaint of a mastoiditis.

In infants and children who are febrile and ill-appearing, the diagnoses of sepsis, meningitis, and intracranial infection must be considered before the infectious process can be localized solely to the middle ear.

MANAGEMENT

ACUTE PURULENT OTITIS MEDIA

The antibiotic therapy for APOM (Table 59-35) is diverse and often tailored by the pediatrician to the individual child. The pediatrician has the advantage of knowing how the patient has responded in the past to a particular regimen as well as the regional population's resistance to certain treatments. Amoxicillin is still a reasonable starting regimen in the patient with a first time infection or who has been known to respond well in the past. The dose is 50 mg per kg per day in three divided doses. If the area is known to have high Hemophilus influenzae resistance, either erythromycin/sulfasoxazole (40 mg per kg per day of erythromycin in 4 divided doses) or amoxicillin fortified with clavulonic acid (50 mg per kg per day amoxicillin in 3 doses) is effective. Cefaclor in a dose of 50 mg per kg per day in 3 doses is slightly more effective than amoxicillin in some patients. Cefoxime is a newer cephalosporin still reserved for patients who are unresponsive to most conventional therapies, and is active against organisms producing β-lactamase. The dose is 8 mg per kg per day given as a once-a-day dose. Severe cases may require initial parenteral medication, particularly in the presence of nausea and vomiting.

Parents should be told of the importance of antipyretics in addition to antibiotics, not only to make the child more comfortable but to reduce seizure risk and decrease water losses. They should also be advised that the fever will persist until the child has received approximately 48 hours of therapy.

Analgesics may be necessary if the child is significantly uncomfortable. Caution should be used not to sedate the child. It is important to follow mental status closely to prevent a missed meningitis. Acetaminophen and topical analgesics are best.

Local heat may ease some of the discomfort. This is done best by the older child who can control the application of the hot compress and avoid burns.

The child with APOM on antibiotic therapy should be reevaluated in 48 to 72 hours. If he or she is not significantly improved, the antibiotic should be changed. The child should again be evaluated in 14 days after the course of the antibiotic. At this point, if an acute infection remains, the child requires referral to ENT for tympanocentesis and culture.

SEROUS OTITIS MEDIA

After an episode of APOM, it is common to have a persistent middle ear effusion. If the effusion is persistent 4 weeks after completion of the antibiotic and the child is complaining of diminished hearing, he or she should be seen by an otolaryngologist. Antihistamines and decongestants have not been shown to be effective. Prophylactic antibiotics may be used if the patient has recurrent episodes of APOM on a chronic SOM. Because this therapy is controversial,

TABLE 59-34. DIFFERENTIAL DIAGNOSIS IN OTITIS MEDIA

Otitis externa
Folliculitis
Traumatic perforation of the tympanic membrane
Mastoiditis

TABLE 59-35. ANTIBIOTICS FOR ACUTE PURULENT OTITIS MEDIA

Antibiotic	Dose
Amoxicillin	50 mg/kg/day in 3 doses
Erythromycin/sulfasoxazole	50 mg/kg/day (erythromycin) in 4 doses
Cefaclor	50 mg/kg/day in 3 doses
Amoxicillin/clavulanate	50 mg/kg/day in 3 doses
Trimethoprim/ sulfamethoxazole	8 mg/kg/day (trimethoprim), 40 mg/kg/day (sulfamethoxazole) in 2 doses
Cefoxime	8 mg/kg/day once daily

it should be initiated only after consulting with the otolaryngologist or pediatrician caring for the child. Myringotomy tubes may be indicated if the middle ear drainage is poor and language development is at risk.

INDICATIONS FOR HOSPITALIZATION

Children who require hospitalization for APOM are the febrile infant under 1 month of age, the ill-appearing child who is failing conventional therapy, and any child with significant complications associated with APOM (see subsequent text).

COMPLICATIONS (TABLE 59-36)

LOCAL COMPLICATIONS

The most benign complication is perforation of the tympanic membrane secondary to APOM. The drum usually heals normally without residual hearing deficits. Facial paralysis may result from facial nerve inflammation. This too is reversible if antibiotic therapy and ear drainage are prompt. Mastoiditis is a more serious local complication requiring debridement and having significant morbidity. Recurring infections can lead to the development of cholesteatoma in the middle ear with permanent hearing loss. Hearing loss and language delays are also associated with chronic serous otitis media. It is important to follow closely young children who have a significant number of infections.

Chronic infection may include perforation and mastoiditis with chronic discharge from the ear. This condition is not easily treated and requires referral to an otolaryngologist. Bacteria involved include Pseudomonas aeruginosa and Staphylococcus aureus. Anaerobic organisms (e.g., Bacteroides sp., anaerobic streptococci) may be involved as well. In the future, ciprofloxacin may be useful in this condition, although it is not yet established. Parenteral anti-Pseudomonas treatment with otic irrigation should be tried before surgery (Kenna et al., 1986).

TABLE 59-36. COMPLICATIONS OF OTITIS MEDIA	
Local Complications	Intracranial Complications
Tympanic membrane perforation	Meningitis
Facial paralysis	Lateral sinus thrombosis
Mastoiditis	Epidural abscess
Cholesteatoma	Brain abscess
Hearing loss	Subdural empyema
Other: Septicemia with distant septic foci	

INTRACRANIAL COMPLICATIONS

Children with otitis media can develop lateral sinus thrombosis, meningitis, subdural empyema, epidural abscess or brain abscess. They may seed these areas hematogenously or infection may spread locally. Children with purulent otitis media should be treated aggressively if meningeal signs or lethargy develop.

PITFALLS

- Failure to refer chronic otitis media can lead to permanent hearing loss and delay in language skills.
- Be aware of antibiotic resistance in your region.
- Recognize potential for complications.
- All patients should be re-evaluated 14 days after treatment.
- Be aware that some children may not tolerate antibiotics initially and must be started on parenteral medication in the ED.
- Refer cases of chronic suppurative otitis media for generalized treatment.

OTITIS EXTERNA

INTRODUCTION

Otitis externa is an infection of the external auditory canal caused by an excessively moist environment in the ear canal. It may be difficult to differentiate from otitis media, especially otitis media in which the tympanic membrane has perforated. Meticulous cleaning of the canal should be done in the ED both to ensure proper diagnosis and to aid in treating the infection.

Otitis externa is a frequent ED diagnosis, particularly in the summer months. It usually responds quickly to appropriate treatment. The physician should be aware of the potential complications of this normally benign disease process, especially in immunocompromised patients, and refer patients early who do not respond to conventional therapy.

PATHOPHYSIOLOGY AND ANATOMY

Otitis externa arises from excessively damp conditions in the ear canal. The dampness leads to maceration of the thin layer of skin overlying the bony inner two thirds of the canal. The macerated skin is pruritic, often leading the patient to put something in the canal to scratch the inner surface. With this maceration and scratching, the normal inhabitants of the ear canal (Pseudomonas species, Staphylococcus epidermidis, Staphylococcus aureus, Corynebacterium, and Streptococcus viridans) are able to invade the tissues. As the bacteria proliferate, the normally acidic pH of the canal is alkalinized. This new alkaline environment encourages further growth and spread of the bacteria. If the infection is extensive, cellulitis can develop. In addition, some infections are complicated by a folliculitis, which often requires incision and drainage.

As otitis externa progresses, the canal develops an exudative appearance not dissimilar to the purulent drainage seen after tympanic membrane rupture in cases of otitis media. It is important to suction debris from the canal to visualize the tympanic membrane. If the tympanic membrane cannot be seen, the patient should be treated as if otitis media is present.

Otitis externa often causes significant edema of the auditory canal, at times blocking the canal entirely. It is important to place a wick into this edematous canal to ensure delivery of the topical antibiotics to the inner canal.

Pseudomonas causes one half to two thirds of all external ear infections, followed by Staphylococcus species. Only 10% of otitis externa is fungal in origin. Aspergillus species cause 90% of the fungal infections. Clinical examinations in these cases may reveal hyphae or spores. Chronic seborrhea can involve the ear canal as well. Patients with this type of dermatitic otitis externa no doubt have other areas of involvement that are key to the diagnosis.

CLINICAL PRESENTATION AND EXAMINATION

Initially, the patient describes an itchy ear canal but by the time he or she presents to the emergency department, earache is the chief complaint. The pain is reproduced by touching the external surface of the ear, especially by moving the pinna or the tragus or by lying on the ear. As infection progresses, drainage from the ear develops, pain extends behind the ear and down the neck, and hearing decreases as the canal becomes increasingly edematous. If cellulitis is present, the patient may have low-grade fever and the pinna may be elevated, giving an asymmetric appearance to the ears.

On examination, a grayish-white exudate covers the canal walls. If edema is significant, the canal may be completely closed. At times, a tender, well localized folliculitis is visible. If it is not spontaneously draining, incision and drainage may have to be performed to hasten the resolution of the infection.

DIFFERENTIAL DIAGNOSIS (TABLE 59-37)

The differential diagnosis includes otitis media with or without tympanic membrane perforation, mastoiditis, trauma to the ear canal or tympanic membrane, foreign body in the canal, and malignant otitis externa in severely ill patients who are known or suspected to be immunocompromised. Malignant otitis externa is rarely seen in children compared with adults, but should be thought of in older children who may be compromised.

Most of these disorders can be differentiated by careful history taking and a thorough physical examination.

MANAGEMENT (TABLE 59-38)

Management of otitis externa should begin with the examination, at which time all exudate should be meticulously cleaned from the canal. This may be most easily done using Calgi swabs or suction if it is tolerated by the patient. Once the canal is cleaned, the patient or the parents should be instructed about the importance of keeping the canal dry. Dry the canals with a blowdryer not only in acute infection but also to prevent recurrences. Solutions containing alcohol/ boric acid combinations serve as drying agents, which also help maintain appropriate ear canal pH. With acute infections, topical eardrops containing antibiotic/steroid combinations (i.e., neomycin-steroid suspensions) should be used. A wick may aid in delivery of the drops to the internal canal. One-quarter-inch sterile packing works well. The patient should be fastidious about keeping the ear canals dry for at least 6 weeks after an acute infection.

TABLE 59-37. DIFFERENTIAL DIAGNOSIS OF OTITIS EXTERNA
Otitis media
Mastoiditis
Trauma
Foreign body in the ear canal
Malignant otitis externa (immunocompromised)

TABLE 59-38. MANAGEMENT OF OTITIS EXTERNA
Clean canal/suction exudate
Antibiotic/steroid otic drops
Insert wick if canal is closed
Culture canal if cellulitis is present
Fungal otitis externa requires 2% acetic acid solution
Admit patients with extensive cellulitis
Keep water out of ears at least 6 weeks

If cellulitis or significant edema of the auditory canal is present, give systemic antibiotics as well. A cephalosporin or erythromycin may be used initially. Culture the canal with a Calgi swab if the cellulitis is significant.

Fungal otitis externa is best treated with cleaning and a 2% acetic acid solution to restore canal pH to normal.

INDICATIONS FOR HOSPITALIZATION

Admit to the hospital patients who develop excessive cellulitis. Patients who are diabetic or immunocompromised and have evidence of cellulitis require admission and intravenous antibiotics.

COMPLICATIONS

Most of the complications of otitis externa involve delay in treatment with infection spreading locally and producing significant cellulitis. These patients respond well to IV antibiotics.

As mentioned, malignant (necrotizing) otitis externa is rare in children and has never been shown to occur in young children. As children approach young adulthood, the diagnosis should be considered. It occurs only in diabetic or immunocompromised patients. It is caused by an invasive Pseudomonas infection that leads to local vasculitis with small vessel thrombosis and tissue necrosis. There may be bony extension leading to facial nerve paralysis. Malignant otitis externa carries a high mortality rate. It requires aggressive antibiotic therapy and surgical debridement.

PITFALLS

- Always try to visualize the tympanic membrane. Treat with oral antibiotics if you are unable to do so.
- Clean the canals to aid initial antibiotic effectiveness.
- Tell patients to keep ears as dry as possible for 6 weeks.
- Insert a wick if the canal is closed.
- Be wary of immunocompromised patients with otitis externa.

PERIORBITAL CELLULITIS

INTRODUCTION

Periorbital cellulitis is a diagnosis frequently made when referring to any infection involving the structures of the orbit. There are five distinct infectious processes involving the orbit, of which periorbital or preseptal cellulitis is just one. It is important that emergency physicians understand the differences between these orbital infections and know how to recognize them, because their treatment varies (Table 59-39).

PATHOPHYSIOLOGY AND ANATOMY

Periorbital cellulitis is an inflammatory process limited to the eyelid. It is also known as preseptal cellulitis. The orbital septum acts as a barrier to spread of infection into the orbit. This septum encircles the orbit. The preseptal cellulitis is confined to the anterior structures of the eyelid. It does not affect vision or eye movements.

Orbital cellulitis involves an infection of the orbital fat. The infection has spread beyond the septum and the child has proptosis and limitation of eye movement associated with pain.

Subperiosteal abscess, as the name implies, is a collection of pus that accumulates between the periosteum and the bony wall of the orbit, usually on the medial aspect. Visual impairment is present, and there is lateral displacement of the globe.

Orbital abscess occurs when a collection of pus develops within the orbital fat. At this point, there is usually total ophthalmoplegia, visual loss, proptosis, and chemosis.

Cavernous sinus thrombosis is rarely seen since the advent of antibiotics. Infection spreads easily from the orbit to the cavernous sinus because of the lack of valves in the veins draining the area. Finding of extraocular muscle palsies in the contralateral eye of a patient with an orbital infection is pathognomonic.

Periorbital cellulitis is the most frequent orbital infection in young children. It is often associated with ethmoidal or maxillary sinusitis and with simple upper respiratory infections, acute or chronic otitis media, and overlying skin infections in this age group. Hemophilus influenzae type b is the leading pathogen, followed by Staphylococcus aureus, Staphylococcus epidermidis, and Streptococcus pneumoniae. Blood cultures of children with periorbital cellulitis are fre-quently positive, leading one to believe that the infection develops primarily by hematogenous spread rather than by direct local extension.

Orbital cellulitis seems to be a separate disease process from periorbital cellulitis, as are subperiosteal abscess, orbital abscess, and cavernous sinus thrombosis. These infections are rare in young children in comparison to periorbital cellulitis. These infections are almost always associated with a sinusitis. It is believed that orbital involvement results either from direct extension through the thin lateral wall of the ethmoidal sinus or by septic thrombophlebitis from valveless ethmoidal veins extending into the orbit. The organisms involved are usually Staphylococcus aureus or Streptococcus pneumoniae. The incidence of complications with these infections is much higher than with periorbital cellulitis.

CLINICAL PRESENTATION AND EXAMINATION

Children with periorbital cellulitis present with varying degrees of erythema and edema of the eyelids. There is tenderness of the lids, and conjunctivitis may be present. There may be an accompanying upper respiratory infection, otitis media, or purulent rhinorrhea secondary to a sinusitis. The degree of toxicity of the child's appearance can vary often and is related to the length of the illness. Vision and extraocular movements are normal.

Children with orbital cellulitis and abscesses are toxic, with varying degrees of ophthalmoplegia, proptosis, and visual loss. The frequently associated sinusitis may not be evident on examination. Fever is normally present. As complications such as meningitis or intracranial abscesses develop, lethargy and meningeal signs may be present.

Cavernous sinus thrombosis carries a high morbidity and mortality. Fortunately, it is rarely seen since the era of antibiotics began. The findings are similar to those of orbital abscess but seen in the contralateral eye as well. The children are universally toxic.

		TABLE 59-39. TYPES OF ORBITAL INFECTIONS		
Infection	Appearance	Eye Movements	Vision
---	---	---	---
Periorbital cellulitis	Erythema, edema of lids	Normal	Normal
Orbital cellulitis	Erythema, edema of lids, proptosis	Decreased	May be diminished
Subperiosteal abscess	Erythema, edema of lids, proptosis, lateral globe displacement	Decreased	Diminished
Orbital abscess	Erythema, edema of lids, proptosis, pupil unreactive	None	None
Cavernous sinus thrombosis	Same as orbital abscess but contralateral eye also involved	Decreased, both eyes	Diminished, both eyes

DIFFERENTIAL DIAGNOSIS (TABLE 59-40)

The differential diagnosis of the red, swollen eyelid in addition to periorbital cellulitis or the more serious intraorbital infections includes insect bite, trauma, conjunctivitis with reactive lid edema, allergy, retro-orbital tumors, renal disease with protein loss, and thyroid disease. These processes can usually be differentiated by good history taking and physical examination.

MANAGEMENT (TABLE 59-41)

The key to management of periorbital cellulitis and the intraorbital infections is first to identify which entity is present. If this cannot be done by history and examination a CT scan of the orbit is indicated. Most children with periorbital cellulitis should be admitted. Blood cultures should be obtained before treatment with intravenous antibiotics. Sinus films should be obtained. If the child is toxic, a lumbar puncture is indicated. If the possibility of a brain abscess is entertained, a CT scan should precede the LP. Children under 5 should be treated with cefuroxime (100 mg per kg per day) or oxacillin (150 mg per kg per day) and chloramphenicol (100 mg per kg per day). Children over 5 should be treated with oxacillin (150 mg per kg per day) or vancomycin (40 mg per kg per day) if they are penicillin-allergic. Occasionally a child can be treated as an outpatient if he or she is well-appearing and close follow-up is ensured. Outpatient treatment is with cefaclor (40 mg per kg per day) or amoxicillin/clavulanate (40 mg per kg per day). The child should be re-evaluated in 24 hours.

Children with orbital cellulitis or abscesses frequently require medical and surgical treatment. Surgery is required to drain the abscess and decompress the globe to relieve pressure on the optic nerve. Sinus drainage is often performed concurrently because sinus infection is often the cause of the infection. Nafcillin or oxacillin (150 mg per kg per day) and chloramphenicol (100 mg per kg per day) or an aminoglycoside is the current recommended intravenous therapy. These patients require 2 to 3 weeks of intravenous antibiotic therapy.

TABLE 59-40. DIFFERENTIAL DIAGNOSIS OF THE RED, SWOLLEN EYE

Conjunctivitis
Allergic reaction
Insect bite
Trauma
Tumor
Hyperthyroidism
Renal disease

TABLE 59-41. MANAGEMENT OF ORBITAL INFECTIONS

Hospitalization for intravenous antibiotics
Sinus x rays
Blood cultures before treatment
CT scan of orbit if abscess suspected
Surgical drainage of orbit and sinuses if indicated

MICROBIOLOGY

The microbiology of such infections includes Streptococcus pneumoniae, Hemophilus influenzae, and Moraxella catarrhalis. The latter two may be β-lactamase producers. Less commonly, Staphylococcus aureus or anaerobic organisms are involved. Hospital outbreaks from a resistant organism sometimes occur. Rapid dissemination of β-lactamase-producing, aminoglycoside-resistant strains of enterococcus and methicillin-resistant staphylococci has been reported.

INDICATIONS FOR HOSPITALIZATION

Virtually all patients with periorbital or orbital infections require inpatient management. Only the mildest cases of periorbital cellulitis with excellent follow-up can be managed with outpatient therapy.

PITFALLS

- Failure to recognize intraorbital from preseptal infections can delay definitive surgical treatment.
- Do CT scan and lumbar puncture on any child with lethargy and an orbital infection.
- If you are unsure of the diagnosis, see the child in 24 hours or arrange for close follow-up.

SINUSITIS

INTRODUCTION

Sinusitis in children is more prevalent than has been previously recognized. It can be present in young children as well as newborns. Although the incidence

TABLE 59-42. AGE OF SINUS DEVELOPMENT	
Sinus	Age
Maxillary	First trimester
Ethmoid	Second trimester
Sphenoid	First months of life
Frontal	Preschool age

does not compare with that in adults, it is a diagnosis that should be considered because the complications in childhood are much more severe.

The definition of sinusitis can vary among clinicians. It may refer to any inflammation of the paranasal sinuses which is present in most viral upper respiratory infections. For our purposes, sinusitis means any suppurative infection of the paranasal sinuses marked by fever, purulent rhinorrhea, irritability, or pain.

Chronic sinusitis is also seen in children, but these children require management by an otolaryngologist. Chronic sinusitis is usually the result of inadequate treatment of an acute infection. These children usually do not appear ill.

PATHOPHYSIOLOGY AND ANATOMY

Clinicians are often unsure of the presence of sinusitis in infants and children because they are unfamiliar with the age at which the various sinuses develop. Some knowledge of the development of the sinuses is necessary (Table 59-42).

The ethmoidal and maxillary sinuses are present at birth. The maxillary sinus begins initially in the first trimester. The ethmoidal sinus develops at about the fifth month of gestation. The sphenoid sinus appears shortly after birth; the frontal sinuses do not appear until 5 or 6 years of age.

The most frequently seen sinusitis in infants and toddlers involves the ethmoid sinus. The ostia draining the ethmoids are relatively large in comparison with the sinus chambers at this age, and contaminated secretions from the nasopharynx can freely enter the sinus. Once the mucus becomes inspissated or mu-

cosal edema develops, organisms are trapped in the sinus. This stagnant pool is an excellent culture medium for bacteria, and sinusitis develops.

Newborns are also at risk of ethmoidal sinusitis, either secondary to maternal contamination during delivery or, more commonly, secondary to the cleaning of their nares with cotton wool pledgets by nursery personnel.

Maxillary sinusitis is still the most frequently infected sinus in childhood. Most children with acute maxillary sinusitis are over 10 years of age, whereas those with ethmoidal sinusitis are in the 3-to-5-year group. There is a rise in the incidence of sinusitis as children attend school.

The frontal and sphenoid sinuses usually do not become infected until later childhood. Children with these infections require admission because they frequently develop intracranial complications.

Sinusitis develops when the normal flow of mucus in the sinus is obstructed and bacteria proliferate. Obstruction can occur if the mucus becomes thick and inspissated due to dehydration and fever or if mucosal edema obstructs the ostia. In addition, any foreign body, nasal polyp, tumor, or septal deformity can block normal sinus drainage. Any child found to have sinusitis secondary to a nasal polyp should be investigated for cystic fibrosis. Ten percent of children with cystic fibrosis have nasal polyps.

Children with allergic rhinitis can have chronic edema with obstruction of mucus flow leading to acute or chronic sinusitis.

Dental abscesses do not cause maxillary sinusitis in children as they do in adults. The maxillary bone is much thicker between the sinus and dental roots at this age.

CLINICAL PRESENTATION AND EXAMINATION

Symptoms of sinusitis vary according to age group (Table 59-43). In infants and toddlers, rely on parental history as well as the examination. The history usually reveals a recent upper respiratory infection marked by increasing nasal discharge. Parents often say that, although the discharge was initially clear, it is now

TABLE 59-43. SIGNS AND SYMPTOMS OF SINUSITIS			
Infants and Toddlers		Older Children	
History	Physical	History	Physical
URI	Fever	Headache	Facial tenderness
Congestion	Nasal crusting	Facial Pain	Purulent nasal discharge
Cough	Mucosal edema	Stuffy nose	Fever (less common)
Snoring	Irritability	Cough	
	Otitis media	Swimming/Diving	
	Pharyngitis		

greenish-yellow and often copious. Fever is present. Cough is present in 70%. There may be a history of snoring or increased mouth breathing.

On physical examination, the child may appear severely ill, depending on the length of illness. The child is febrile. Crusting about the nares is seen bilaterally. In addition, bilateral mucosal edema is seen. If findings of edema and crusting are unilateral, a nasal foreign body should be considered. Frequently sinusitis occurs together with otitis media or pharyngitis.

Older children are able to complain of the characteristic headache or facial pain associated with sinusitis. The history of fever is not as universal as with younger children. They often complain of a stuffy nose. Nasal discharge may or may not be present. Again, many in this group also have cough as one of their chief complaints. Children who dive or swim a great deal frequently develop sinusitis. A history of these activities should be sought.

The physical examination of the older child with sinus infection is not as revealing as in the toddler. Tenderness over the involved sinus may be the only finding. Maxillary sinusitis produces tenderness over the cheeks. Ethmoidal sinusitis leads to pain with palpation of the medial orbits. Frontal sinusitis causes pain with forehead percussion. Although the sphenoid sinus cannot be examined directly, patients complain of a severe vertex headache and are often toxic.

DIFFERENTIAL DIAGNOSIS (TABLE 59-44)

In younger children, the differential diagnosis includes simple upper respiratory infection with rhinorrhea, nasal foreign body, cystic fibrosis if polyps are present, sepsis, and intracranial infectious process if the child appears toxic.

The differential diagnosis is similar for the older child except that the incidence of foreign bodies is less and the possibility of a dental abscess increases as the child approaches the teen years. Older children frequently have allergy as an underlying problem as well.

DIAGNOSTIC EVALUATION

Transillumination may be difficult in young children, but can be quickly useful in diagnosis. For the maxillary sinus, the light source is placed over the midpoint of the inferior orbital rim and, with the child's mouth open, the physician assesses the transmission of light through the hard palate. Placing the light below the supraorbital ridge and evaluating symmetry reveals the frontal sinus. Absence of transillumination is evidence of a sinus cavity filled with fluid or tissue.

X rays can confirm sinusitis, particularly when the possibility of a frontal or sphenoid sinusitis exists. An

TABLE 59-44. DIFFERENTIAL DIAGNOSIS
Simple upper respiratory infection
Nasal foreign body
Cystic fibrosis
Sepsis
Intracranial infections
Dental abscesses (older children)

air-fluid level or sinus opacification is consistent with an acute infection. Mucosal thickening indicates chronic inflammation. CT scans are useful if one is looking for an orbital or intracranial abscess or if a tumor is suspected, but should not be needed in children with uncomplicated sinusitis.

Blood cultures should be done on any child with complications or toxic appearance. They are not necessary before antibiotic therapy if the child is well-appearing.

The blood count offers little information and is not necessary in most patients. It is elevated with acute infection and can be high in the otherwise nontoxic-appearing child. The presence of an elevated eosinophil count can indicate an underlying allergic cause.

The indications for lumbar puncture are the same for any toxic-appearing child. If meningeal signs are present of the possibility of meningitis is entertained, it should be done. If there is concern about an intracranial abscess, however, the lumbar puncture should be preceded by a CT scan.

Sinus aspiration can be used in severe cases, but such a procedure requires sedation and sometimes general anesthesia in young children. Severe facial pain with orbital complications is an indication for ENT referral for this procedure. Gram stain can then further guide parenteral treatment, with one organism or more per high-power field being good evidence of infection.

MANAGEMENT (TABLE 59-45)

Amoxicillin is still the drug of choice for uncomplicated outpatient treatment of sinusitis. Streptococcus pneumoniae, Hemophilus influenzae, moraxella catarrhalis, and beta-hemolytic streptococcus remain the predominant cause of acute sinusitis. In addition to amoxicillin, cefaclor, trimethoprim-sulfamethoxazole, erythromycin-sulfasoxazole, amoxicillin/potassium clavulanate and cefuroxime are also used. Diabetics and immunocompromised patients may have fungal infections or other opportunists. Cultures of the nasopharynx have not been shown to be useful. Outpatient treatment is recommended to be for 2 to 3 weeks, although for cases showing rapid relief, 10 days are sufficient.

TABLE 59-45. ANTIBIOTIC THERAPY

Antibiotic	Dose
Amoxicillin	50 mg/kg/day in 3 doses
Cefaclor	50 mg/kg/day in 3 doses
Erythromycin–sulfasoxazole	50 mg/kg/day in 4 doses
Trimethoprim–sulfamethoxazole	8 mg/kg/day and 40 mg/kg/day Sulfamethoxazole in 2 doses
Amoxicillin–potassium Clavulanate	50 mg/kg/day in 3 doses
Treat for 3 weeks minimally	

In addition to antibiotic therapy, attempts should be made to improve drainage. Hydration, mist, mucolytics, and decongestants improve sinus drainage. Decongestants should be limited to 4 to 5 days and should not be used in young children. Antihistamines should be avoided because they thicken mucus, unless the underlying cause has definitely been shown to be allergy-related. Topical steroids may also help the patient with underlying allergy problems.

The patient who is not demonstrating improvement after 48 to 72 hours of therapy should be referred to the otolaryngologist for possible antral lavage.

INDICATIONS FOR HOSPITALIZATION

The diagnosis of frontal or sphenoidal sinusitis is a criterion for admission to the hospital. The proximity of these infections to the intracranial cavity places patients at risk of intracranial abscesses. These patients require aggressive therapy with intravenous antibiotics and possibly surgical drainage.

Any patient with complications (see following paragraphs) requires hospitalization, as do children with severe pain and evidence of systemic infection.

TABLE 59-46. COMPLICATIONS OF SINUSITIS

Orbital Complications
Periorbital cellulitis
Orbital cellulitis
Subperiosteal abscess
Orbital abscess
Cavernous sinus thrombosis

Intracranial Complications
Meningitis
Epidural abscess
Subdural abscess
Brain abscess

Local Complications
Mucoceles
Osteomyelitis

COMPLICATIONS OF SINUSITIS (SEE TABLE 59-46)

ORBITAL COMPLICATIONS

Infection spreads easily to orbital contents from the ethmoid sinus because of the absence of valves in the ophthalmic veins. The open sutures about the orbit allow infection to spread easily to the intracranial area.

Periorbital cellulitis is the least serious of the orbital infections. It is inflammatory edema of the upper lid. There is no proptosis or limitation of eye movement. Intravenous antibiotics prevent further spread. Some patients can be treated with oral antibiotics.

Orbital cellulitis refers to edema of the entire orbital contents. Proptosis, chemosis, and limitation of extraocular movement are present. Aggressive antibiotic therapy is curative.

Subperiosteal abscess is a more serious orbital infection which, as the name implies, refers to a collection of pus between the sinus and the periorbita. The symptoms are the same as with orbital cellulitis, but these patients also have decreased visual acuity. Incision and drainage are necessary.

An orbital abscess develops when there is necrosis and then abscess formation within the periorbital fat. The globe is firm. There is total ophthalmoplegia, visual loss, and proptosis. These must be promptly drained.

Cavernous sinus thrombosis is the most dreaded complication of sinusitis. Patients present with proptosis, fixed globe, visual loss, and meningitis. Orbital signs occur in the opposite eye as well. The treatment is IV antibiotics, anticoagulation, and sinus drainage. There is a 15% mortality as well as significant morbidity.

INTRACRANIAL COMPLICATIONS

Meningitis, epidural abscess, subdural abscess, and brain abscess are all potential complications of sinusitis. Children frequently have an orbital infection as well. Any child with sinusitis or orbital infection suspected of having intracranial spread of infection requires a CT scan.

LOCAL COMPLICATIONS

Mucoceles are epithelial-lined cysts within the sinus cavity. They can be caused by ostia obstruction, chronic allergy or chronic infection. These lesions can expand and distort the sinus cavity and eventually cause swelling of the inner canthus.

Osteomyelitis of the maxilla as a complication of sinusitis is rarer since the advent of antibiotics but still more common in children than in adults. Children have more cancellous bone. Infection from bone spreads rapidly to overlying soft tissue producing a cellulitis. If facial cellulitis is present along with sinusitis, a bone scan is necessary. These patients need prolonged antibiotic therapy.

PITFALLS

- Always consider possibility of nasal foreign bodies.
- Refer children to otolaryngologist if not responding to treatment after 48 to 72 hours.
- Remember to consider the possibility of sinusitis in infants and newborns.
- Admit any patients with complications of sinusitis and those with frontal or sphenoidal sinusitis.
- Work up children with sinusitis and nasal polyps for cystic fibrosis.

CERVICAL LYMPHADENITIS

INTRODUCTION

Cervical lymphadenitis is a bacterial infection of the lymph nodes of the neck. It should not be confused with the normally palpable nodes common to prepubertal children or with the reactive lymphadenopathy associated with head and neck infections. Also, one must differentiate lymph nodes with bacterial infections from the similar-appearing lymph nodes of mononucleosis.

Most of the infections are caused by Staphylococcus aureus or Group A streptococcus and respond well to antibiotics. If the node becomes abscessed, incision and drainage may be necessary.

Mycobacterium infections and neoplasms can also present as enlarged cervical lymph nodes. Children who do not respond in a timely fashion to antibiotic therapy should be referred to rule out these possibilities. Recent evidence shows an increase in tuberculosis and lymphadenitis from other mycobacteria.

PATHOPHYSIOLOGY AND ANATOMY

Cervical lymphadenitis develops when bacteria proliferate in one of the nodes of the neck, evoking an inflammatory response. The bacteria arrive in the gland by way of lymphatics, which drain the head and neck. These areas have been colonized by bacteria but have not developed a localized infection. Cervical lymphadenitis usually affects one node at a time, un-

like the response seen with reactive lymphadenopathy. As the inflammatory response progresses, an abscess may develop.

CLINICAL PRESENTATION AND EXAMINATION

Children present initially with a firm, tender cervical lymph node at least 2 cm in diameter. There may be some refusal to turn the head to the right or left. In the chubby child, this may be the parents' first indication that something is wrong. Fever may or may not be present. The parents give a history of a rapidly enlarging mass. As the adenitis progresses, it may quickly become fluctuant, and the overlying skin may develop erythema. The white blood count is normal to slightly elevated. A history of a preceding upper respiratory infection, recent travel, cat scratches, or exposure to tuberculosis should be sought. Although attention is drawn to the neck area, each child should be examined for evidence of generalized lymphadenopathy or hepatosplenomegaly.

DIFFERENTIAL DIAGNOSIS (TABLE 59-47)

Reactive lymphadenopathy to a local infection of the oral cavity or pharynx is the most common cause of cervical lymph node enlargement. These areas should be inspected for infection.

Mycobacterium infections often present as cervical adenitis in young children rather than as primary pulmonary infections. Children who are suspected of having had tuberculosis exposures or who are not responding to antibiotic therapy should have PPD skin tests. Mycobacterium avium/intracellulare complex (MAIC) have also been found to cause adenitis in children. A common infection in immunocompromised patients, it can also infect the normal population. The importance of its detection is that it normally requires surgical excision. It is detected by PPD skin testing.

Cat scratch disease is among the differential diagnoses for cervical node enlargement. It is often difficult to diagnose because it is not considered. Symptoms may range from a mild flu-like illness to seizures. A specific cat scratch antigen can detect the disease. It is usually a self-limited infection.

Cervical masses are more likely to be inflammatory

TABLE 59-47. DIFFERENTIAL DIAGNOSIS OF CERVICAL LYMPHADENITIS

Reactive lymphadenopathy
Mycobacterium infection
Cat scratch disease
Neoplasm
Branchial cleft cyst

TABLE 59-48. MANAGEMENT OF BACTERIAL ADENITIS
Oral antibiotics to cover staphylococcus and streptococcus species
Needle aspiration (on all children under 6 weeks old, immunocompromised, toxic, or unresponsive to therapy)
Incision and drainage if abscessed
Place PPD skin test on children who are not improving
Place PPD skin test on initial visit if the child may be immunocompromised or has had tuberculosis exposure
Refer for excisional biopsy children with a large, firm, nontender lymph node

than neoplastic in young children. The older child or young adult who presents with a neck mass is more likely to have a malignancy and should be immediately referred for excisional biopsy.

A branchial cleft cyst with abscess formation can also present as a tender neck mass. These children require definitive excision of the cyst by an otolaryngologist.

MANAGEMENT (TABLE 59-48)

Most cases of cervical adenitis respond to antibiotics. Antibiotics should be chosen to cover staphylococcal and streptococcal infections. Dicloxacillin or cephalexin, both at doses of 50 mg/kg/day in 4 divided doses, is effective.

Needle aspiration culture and sensitivity is indicated if the child is toxic and febrile, under 6 weeks of age, not improving on conventional therapy, or suspected to be immunocompromised. The healthy child usually does not require needle aspiration before treatment.

Incision and drainage are required if an abscess develops. Antibiotics alone cannot completely treat the infection in these cases.

A PPD skin test should be placed on any child not improving on antibiotics. If the incidence of tuberculosis is high in a particular region or the child has a history of TB exposure or is immunocompromised, a PPD test should be placed on the initial visit. Once the PPD is placed, the physician must ensure good patient follow-up for interpretation of the results.

Any child with a persistent firm, nontender, enlarged lymph node that is unresponsive to antibiotics should be referred for possible excisional biopsy. CT scan can help delineate the extent of the mass.

INDICATIONS FOR HOSPITALIZATION

Any child with adenitis who appears toxic or is under 3 months of age should be admitted to the hospital, as should any child with a positive PPD skin test who has not improved on antibiotics.

PITFALLS

- Consider mycobacterium infections and place PPD skin tests when indicated. If this is done ensure followup.
- Refer older children for biopsy.
- Consider cat scratch disease.
- Aspirate and culture if indicated.
- Check for mononucleosis.

CONJUNCTIVITIS

INTRODUCTION

Pediatric conjunctivitis is divided into infections that occur in the newborn ("ophthalmia neonatorum") and those that occur in older children. This distinction is made because the pathogens and management differ between the two groups. In children, as in adults, conjunctivitis may be the result of a viral or bacterial infection, exposure to an allergen or chemical irritation, or associated with a dermatitis. In the emergency department we often see patients early in an infection before all the symptoms and physical findings have developed. It is best to err on the side of treatment with antimicrobials if a bacterial source is suspected (see also Chap. 55).

PATHOPHYSIOLOGY AND ANATOMY

Newborns acquire eye pathogens during vaginal delivery from the mother. Chlamydia trachomatis, Neisseria gonorrheae, Escherichia coli, and Herpes simplex are all capable of producing neonatal conjunctivitis. Neisseria gonorrheae is the most serious of these. Untreated, this infection can cause corneal perforation in just a few days. Any newborn with conjunctivitis

TABLE 59-49. MANAGEMENT OF CONJUNCTIVITIS IN NEWBORN OPHTHALMIA NEONATORUM
Chlamydia trachomatis
Oral erythromycin, 50 mg/kg/day for 3 weeks, as well as topical erythromycin
Neisseria gonorrheae
Intravenous penicillin or ceftriaxone
Topical antimicrobials
Pneumococcus, Staphylococcus, aureus, Escherichia coli
Topical erythromycin
Herpes simplex
Managed by ophthalmology with topical antiviral agents

should have Gram stain, Giemsa stain, and culture of the discharge performed.

In the older child, most conjunctivitis is a result of a viral infection, but the bacterial conjunctivitis that does develop results from the bacteria that normally inhabit the eyelashes. Staphylococcus epidermidis and Staphylococcus aureus comprise 65 to 90% of these organisms, followed by Corynebacterium, pneumococcus, and hemophilus. Prophylactic antibiotics given to children with severe viral conjunctivitis prevent superinfection with these organisms.

OPHTHALMIA NEONATORUM (TABLE 59-49)

CHLAMYDIA TRACHOMATIS

Clinical Presentation and Examination. Most cases of ophthalmia neonatorum are now caused by Chlamydia trachomatis infection acquired from the mother. It is a bilateral infection with purulent discharge seen in the second week of life. The follicular response on the underside of the eyelids normally seen in chlamydial infections is absent in the newborn. The cornea is clear. Diagnosis is made by Giemsa staining for intracellular inclusions and also by culture.

Chlamydia conjunctivitis is a self-limited infection without serious sequelae to the eye. The significance in its diagnosis is the associated pneumonia that develops in 10 to 20% of exposed infants. Chlamydia trachomatis is responsible for 30 to 40% of the pneumonias that occur in the first 6 months of life. The prevention of pneumonia is the reason treatment is necessary. If a diagnosis of chlamydia conjunctivitis is made, both the mother and her sexual partner should also be treated.

Management. Newborns with chlamydia conjunctivitis should be treated with topical and oral erythromycin (50 mg/kg/day) for 3 weeks. Newborns with suspected chlamydia pneumonia require admission for intravenous antibiotics, hydration and supplemental oxygen.

NEISSERIA GONORRHEAE

Clinical Presentation and Examination. Gonococcal conjunctivitis causes a severe bilateral infection marked by copious purulent discharge. The onset is in the first 3 days of life. The cornea may appear cloudy. If left untreated, the infection causes corneal perforation in less than a week. Diagnosis is made by culture and Gram stain.

Management. Infants with gonococcal conjunctivitis require admission for intravenous penicillin and topical antimicrobials. Ceftriaxone may be used if the organism is resistant to penicillin.

OTHER BACTERIA CAUSING CONJUNCTIVITIS IN THE NEWBORN

Clinical Presentation and Examination. Pneumococcus, Staphylococcus aureus, and Escherichia coli are among the other bacteria that can cause conjunctivitis in the newborn period. These infections may be unilateral and present in the first 2 weeks. They do not have any long-term sequelae.

Management. Most of these infections respond to erythromycin topicals. Cultures, Gram stain and Giemsa stain should be done on these infants as well.

VIRAL CONJUNCTIVITIS IN THE NEWBORN

Clinical Presentation and Examination. Viral infections of the eye are uncommon in the neonatal period. Primary herpetic conjunctivitis is the only viral infection at this time. This is acquired during delivery. The eye is reddened, tearing but without purulent drainage. Fluorescein staining of the cornea may only reveal what appears to be an abrasion or the characteristic dendritic appearance of the herpes infection may be obvious. Any newborn examined and felt to have a corneal abrasion should be evaluated in 24 hours to

---

TABLE 59-50. MANAGEMENT OF CONJUNCTIVITIS BEYOND THE NEWBORN PERIOD

Viral
Symptomatic relief with cool compresses

Epidemic Keratoconjunctivitis
(Adenovirus 8 and 19)
Broad spectrum topical antibiotics
Cool compresses
Strict hand-to-eye hygiene
Steroids may be needed but should only be given after ophthalmology evaluation

Herpes simplex
Corneal staining and slit lamp examination
Patch eye
Require immediate ophthalmology evaluation

Herpes zoster
Ophthalmology evaluation

Bacterial Infections
Topical 10% sodium sulfacetamide, erythromycin, gentamicin, tobramycin or polysporin (avoid neomycin)
Culture if patient returns within 24 hours with worsening symptoms.
If conjunctivitis is present over 2 weeks or discharge is copious, do Gram stain, Giemsa stain, and culture.

Allergic Conjunctivitis
Oral antihistamines
Topical antihistamine/vasoconstrictors
Cool compresses

Contact Lens Conjunctivitis
Clean lenses thoroughly
Replace soft lenses with new ones
Stop using soft lenses altogether

ensure normal healing. Patients at risk of a herpes infection should be managed by ophthalmology.

CONJUNCTIVITIS BEYOND THE NEONATAL PERIOD (TABLE 59-50)

VIRAL INFECTIONS

Clinical Presentation and Examination. Viral infections cause most of the pediatric conjunctivitis seen in our EDs. Viral conjunctivitis usually accompanies other upper respiratory symptoms but may also occur in isolation. The eye is reddened and irritated. There may be tearing but no purulent discharge. These mild infections are self-limited and need not be treated except for symptomatic relief with cool compresses.

Epidermic keratoconjunctivitis is the true contagious "pink eye," which spreads rapidly through families and schools. It is caused by adenovirus types 8 and 19. It causes the most severe conjunctivitis. Infection normally begins in one eye but soon the other becomes involved, often to a lesser extent. The eye is injected, with heavy tearing. There may be minimal mucopurulent discharge. Eyelids are swollen and ecchymotic, giving the appearance of trauma. A keratitis often develops between the fifth and twelfth days, causing intense pain, photophobia, and foreign body sensation. Subepithelial infiltrates develop after the tenth day, leading to diminished vision. Corneal staining with fluorescein reveals fine punctate uptake of stain. The patient also often has preauricular adenopathy and associated viral illness with sore throat, fever, and myalgias. The course of the infection is long, lasting up to 4 weeks. A similar but less severe infection is seen with Adenovirus 3 and 7.

Management. Treatment of epidemic keratoconjunctivitis consists of prophylactic broad spectrum topical antibiotics, cool compresses, and strict hand-to-eye hygiene. Referral to ophthalmology is necessary because steroids may help to improve the subepithelial infiltrates and subsequent diminished vision.

HERPES SIMPLEX

Clinical Presentation and Examination. Herpex simplex conjunctivitis is a unilateral infection. The eye is injected with slight mucoid discharge. The patient complains of pain and photophobia. Herpetic vesicles on the eyelid margin may be seen. The cornea should be stained looking for the characteristic dendritic appearance of the herpes lesions. Slit lamp examination should be performed if the patient is able to cooperate.

Management. Patch the eye and refer to ophthalmology immediately. The ophthalmologist will use topical antiviral agents and follow these patients closely because they may eventually require corneal transplants. Oral acyclovir is warranted in some cases.

HERPES ZOSTER

Clinical Presentation and Examination. Herpes zoster can also involve the cornea. It is not seen on a primary exposure, only with an outbreak of shingles confined to the first branch of the trigeminal nerve. The conjunctivitis is often mild. If the tip of the nose is involved in the outbreak, the cornea is involved.

Management. Herpes zoster involving the cornea, like herpes simplex, requires management by an ophthalmologist immediately.

BACTERIAL CONJUNCTIVITIS IN THE CHILD

Clinical Presentation and Examination. The organisms that cause bacterial conjunctivitis are the normal inhabitants of the patient's eyelashes. The infection begins with a unilateral purulent discharge, which may or may not become bilateral. Eyes are irritated and injected. Eyelids are swollen. Lashes are matted with dried discharge. The infection is often less severe than some of the viral infections and resolves on its own in 2 weeks if left untreated. Topical antimicrobials improve symptoms, and the course of the infection is often reduced to 3 or 4 days. Cultures are not necessary in the older child.

Management. Treat with topical 10% sodium sulfacetamide, erythromycin, gentamicin, tobramycin or polysporin combinations. Avoid topicals containing neomycin because these have a higher incidence of allergic reaction.

Cultures should be done if the patient returns within 24 hours with worsening discharge. Patients who are not improving on topical antibiotics should be seen by an ophthalmologist. Gram stain, Giemsa stain, and cultures should be done if the conjunctivitis is chronic (over 2 weeks), discharge is copious, or corneal injury is evident.

CHLAMYDIA CONJUNCTIVITIS IN THE OLDER CHILD

Clinical Presentation and Examination. Chlamydia infections may also be seen in the eyes of young adults in addition to newborns. In this case, it is transmitted from the genitourinary tract. It can be acquired in an inadequately chlorinated swimming pool. The eye is reddened, with a watery, mucoid discharge, and the characteristic follicular response is present on the underside of the eyelids. The infection may be unilateral or bilateral.

Management. The treatment is oral doxycycline in children over 8 and in young adults. In young children, oral erythromycin is still the treatment of choice. Topical erythromycin should be also used in both.

ALLERGIC CONJUNCTIVITIS

Clinical Presentation and Examination. Many allergies can cause conjunctival inflammation. In some cases, these symptoms are seasonal and recurrent, others are chronic and associated with multiple atopic symptoms, and others occur in isolation after exposure to a certain food, airborne allergen, or chemical substance. These patients complain of itching primarily. Tearing is present, the eye is reddened, and patients may describe a gritty sensation. Eyelids are often swollen and chemosis may be present.

Management. The patient with symptoms of chronic allergic conjunctivitis requires referral to an allergist. Some immediate relief may be attained by recommending use of oral antihistamines, topical antihistamine/vasoconstrictors, and cool compresses. Antibiotics are not indicated.

CONTACT LENS CONJUNCTIVITIS

Clinical Presentation and Examination. Giant papillary conjunctivitis is a recently described abnormality associated with soft contact lens use. It occurs in healthy patients with no history of previous problems. It is an immunologic reaction caused by proteins that have adsorbed to the soft lens. It is characterized by hyperemia, mucoid discharge, and papillary hypertrophy. Everting the upper lid reveals huge papillae.

Management. The patient with giant papillary conjunctivitis has three options. The treatment is to clean the lenses and try again, replace them, or stop wearing soft lenses. The papillary hypertrophy is completely reversible.

INDICATIONS FOR HOSPITALIZATION

Admit any newborn with suspected gonococcal conjunctivitis, herpes conjunctivitis, or chlamydial conjunctivitis and respiratory symptoms. In children beyond the newborn period, admit the child with severe epidemic keratoconjunctivitis who requires significant pain management.

DIFFERENTIAL DIAGNOSIS (TABLE 59-51)

The differential diagnosis of the red eye in children, in addition to the infections mentioned, includes corneal abrasion, corneal foreign body, acute glaucoma, traumatic iritis and uveitis. Corneal abrasions and conjunctivitis cause most the red eyes in the pediatric population. The physician should always determine whether trauma is a possibility. A thorough history

TABLE 59-51. DIFFERENTIAL DIAGNOSIS

Corneal abrasion
Foreign body
Acute glaucoma
Traumatic iritis
Uveitis

and physical examination including slit-lamp examination where indicated should help in making the correct diagnosis. If there are doubts or the child is too young to be adequately assessed in the ED, an immediate ophthalmologic consultation should be obtained. (See Chap. 55.)

PITFALLS

- Failure to recognize a herpetic corneal lesion
- Always obtain a culture, Gram stain, and Giemsa stain on all newborns with conjunctivitis
- Beware of prescribing steroids from the ED
- Young adults may also get chlamydia conjunctivitis
- Refer all patients who are not responding to initial therapy to ophthalmology

GINGIVOSTOMATITIS

INTRODUCTION

Gingivostomatitis is a herpes simplex infection of the oral cavity. It is often the primary herpes infection seen in young children. It recurs later as cold sores into adulthood. Herpes simplex virus antibodies are present in 70 to 90% of people by the time they reach adulthood.

PATHOPHYSIOLOGY AND ANATOMY

The Herpes simplex virus invades the oral cavity through direct contact with someone with the active virus or something with the virus on its surface. The characteristic painful vesicles develop on the lips, tongue, and buccal mucosa. Unlike herpangina (Coxsackie virus), which involves the posterior pharynx, gingivostomatitis affects the anterior oral cavity more severely.

Most cases of gingivostomatitis are self-limited and without complication. The main problems are pain control and maintaining hydration. There have been several reported cases of the virus spreading locally to involve the epiglottis and aryepiglottic folds.

TABLE 59-52. DIFFERENTIAL DIAGNOSIS
Herpangina
Stevens-Johnson syndrome
Kawasaki disease
Aphthous ulcers
Pharyngitis

CLINICAL PRESENTATION AND EXAMINATION

Gingivostomatitis occurs in children aged 1 to 4. Symptoms include fever and painful oral ulcerations. Cervical lymphadenopathy is common. The child may appear dehydrated from fever and poor oral intake. The lesions in the oral cavity can extend to the area surrounding the lips and can be severe.

DIFFERENTIAL DIAGNOSIS (TABLE 59-52)

The differential diagnosis includes herpangina, Stevens-Johnson syndrome, Kawasaki disease, aphthous ulcers, and severe viral or streptococcal pharyngitis. Herpangina, as mentioned earlier, involves the posterior pharynx with characteristic small ulcerations with white centers. There may be similar lesions on the palms of the hands and soles of the feet. It is caused by Coxsackie virus, and the children generally appear less toxic and better hydrated than children with gingivostomatitis. Children with Stevens-Johnson syndrome are toxic, and although their oral findings may appear similar to a severe gingivostomatitis, they also have a characteristic diffuse rash. Kawasaki disease, like Stevens-Johnson syndrome, is associated with a severe rash as well as swelling of the hands and feet and a conjunctivitis, and the children again appear more toxic. Aphthous ulcers and pharyngitis normally have localized findings and are easily distinguishable from a gingivostomatitis.

MANAGEMENT (TABLE 59-53)

Gingivostomatitis is a self-limited infection. Parents should be encouraged to push fluids. Popsicles are soothing and a good source of fluids. Hot or irritating foods should be avoided. An oral mixture of liquid antacid and benadryl mixed 1:1 provides significant relief. Parents must be advised of dose and frequency, however, to avoid overdosing the child. Oral xylocaine is not recommended in young children because of seizure risk. Additional analgesics and antipyretics may be necessary.

INDICATIONS FOR ADMISSION

Children who are significantly dehydrated and unable to take oral fluids should be admitted to the hospital.

TABLE 59-53. MANAGEMENT OF GINGIVOSTOMATITIS
Analgesics
Antipyretics
Antacid/diphenhydramine solution (mixed 1:1)
Encourage fluids
Admission for IV hydration if indicated

If there is doubt as to the diagnosis and the child appears toxic, he or she should be admitted to the hospital for further work-up.

PITFALLS

- Misdiagnosis of Kawasaki Disease or Stevens-Johnson syndrome as gingivostomatitis
- Failure to admit children who are dehydrated and unable to take oral fluids
- Failure to provide adequate analgesia

REFERENCES

OTITIS MEDIA

Bluestone, C.D.: The ear and mastoid infections. *In* Infectious Diseases. Edited by Gorbach, S.L., and Bartlett, J.G. Philadelphia, W.B. Saunders Co., 1992.

Cotton, R.T., and Myer, C.M., III: A Practical Approach to Pediatric Otolaryngology. Chicago, Yearbook Medical Publishers, Inc., 1988.

Fleisher, G.: Infectious disease emergencies. *In* Textbook of Pediatric Emergency Medicine. Edited by Fleisher, G., Ludwig, S., et al., Baltimore, Williams and Wilkins, 1988.

Handler, S.D., and Potsic, W.P.: Otolaryngology Emergencies. *In* Textbook of Pediatric Emergency Medicine. Edited by Fleisher, G., Ludwig, S., et al., eds,: Baltimore, Williams and Wilkins, 1988.

Jazbi, B.: 1980. Otitis media in infants and children. *In* Pediatric Otolaryngology: a Review of Ear, Nose and Throat Problems in Children. Edited by Jazbi, B. New York, Appleton-Century-Crofts, 1980.

Kenna, M.A., et al.: Medical management of chronic suppurative otitis media (without cholesteatoma) in children. Laryngoscope 96:146, 1986.

Klein, J.R., Rubin, J., and Balkany, T.J.: Otitis Media. *In* Clinical Pediatric Otolaryngology. Edited by Balkany, T.J., and Pashley, N.R.T. St. Louis, C. V. Mosby Co., 1986.

OTITIS EXTERNA

Balkany, T.J., Pashley, N.R.T., and Prina, D.M.: Otitis externa. *In* Clinical Pediatric Otolaryngology. Edited by Balkany, T.J., Pashley, N.R.T. St. Louis, C. V. Mosby Co., 1986.

Fleisher, G.: Infectious disease emergencies. *In* Textbook of Pediatric Emergency Medicine. Edited by Fleisher, G., Ludwig, S., et al. Baltimore, Williams and Wilkins, 1988.

PERIORBITAL CELLULITIS

Capoot, G.D., et al. Nose and sinus surgery. *In* Clinical Pediatric Otolaryngology. Edited by Balkany, T.J., and Pashley, N.R.T., St. Louis, C.V. Mosby Co., 1986.

Diamond, G.: Ophthalmic emergencies. *In* Textbook of Pediatric Emergency Medicine. Edited by Fleisher, G., Ludwig, S., et al. Baltimore, Williams and Wilkins, 1988.

Israel, V., and Nelson, J.D.: Periorbital and orbital cellulitis. *Pediatr. Infec. Dis. J.* **6**:404, 1987.

Jackson, K.J., and Baker, S.R.: Periorbital cellulitis. *Head Neck Surg.* **9**:227, 1987.

Jazbi, B.: Sinusitis in infants and children. *In Pediatric Otorhinolaryngology: a Review of Ear, Nose and Throat Problems in Children.* Edited by Jazbi, B. New York, Appleton-Century-Crofts, 1980.

Jazbi, B., and Hamtil, L.: Pediatric otorhinolaryngology and ophthalmology. *In Pediatric Otorhinolaryngology: a Review of Ear, Nose and Throat Problems in Children.* Edited by Jazbi, B.: New York, Appleton-Century-Crofts, 1980.

Maloney, J.R., et al.: The acute orbit-preseptal (periorbital) cellulitis, subperiosteal abscess and orbital cellulitis due to sinusitis. J. Laryngol. Otol. (Suppl.) *12*:1, 1987.

Meyer, C.M., III, and Cotton, R.T.: A Practical Approach to: Pediatric Otolaryngology. Chicago, Yearbook Medical Publishers, Inc., 1988.

Molarte, A.B., and Isenberry, S.J.: Periorbital cellulitis in infancy. J. Pediatr. Ophthalmol Strabismus *26*:232, 1989.

Rhinehart, E., et al.: Rapid dissemination of a β-lactamase-producing aminoglycoside-resistant Enterococcus fecalis among patients and staff on an infant-toddler ward. N. Engl. J. Med. *323*:1815, 1990.

Sinnott, J.T., et al.: Is this orbital or periorbital cellulitis? Postgrad. Med. *85*:267, 1989.

SINUSITIS

Capoot, G.D.J. and Blakeman, A.G.J. Nose and sinus surgery. *In* Clinical Pediatric Otolaryngology. Edited by Balkany, T.J., and Pashley, N.R.T. St. Louis, C.V. Mosby Co., 1986.

Fleisher, G.: Infectious disease emergencies. *In* Textbook of Pediatric Emergency Medicine. Edited by Fleisher, G., Ludwig, S., et al. Baltimore, Williams and Wilkins, 1988.

Jazbi, B.: Sinusitis in infants and children. *In* Pediatric Otorhinolaryngology: a Review of Ear, Nose and Throat Problems in Children. Edited by Jazbi, B. New York, Appleton-Century-Crofts, 1980.

Kennedy, D.W., et al.: Functional endoscopic sinus surgery. Arch. Otolaryngol. *111*:576, 1985.

Myer, C.M. III, and Cotton, R.T.: A Practical Approach to Pediatric Otolaryngology. Chicago, Yearbook Medical Publishers, Inc., 1988.

Shopfner, C.E., and Rossi, J.D.: Roentgen evaluation of the paranasal sinuses in children. Am. J. Roent. Rad. Ther. *118*:176, 1973.

Wald, E.: Sinusitis in children. N. Engl. J. Med. *326*:319, 1992.

CERVICAL LYMPHADENITIS

Cotton, R.T., and Myer, C.M., III: A Practical Approach to: Pediatric Otolaryngology. Chicago, Yearbook Medical Publishers, Inc., 1988.

Fleisher, G.: Infectious disease emergencies. *In* Textbook of Pediatric Emergency Medicine. Edited by Fleisher, G., Ludwig, S., et al. Baltimore, Williams and Wilkins, 1988.

Iseman, M.O.: Nontuberculosis Mycobacteria infections. *In* Infectious Diseases. Edited by Gorbach, S.L., et al. Philadelphia, W.B. Saunders Co., 1992, p. 1246.

Kinsella, J.P., Culver, K., et al.: Extensive cervical lymphadenitis due to Mycobacterium avium-intracellulare. Pediatr. Infect. Dis. J. *6*:289, 1987.

CONJUNCTIVITIS

Diamond, G.: Ophthalmic emergencies. *In* Textbook of Pediatric Emergency Medicine. Edited by Fleisher, G., Ludwig, S., et al. Baltimore, Williams and Wilkins, 1988.

Howes, D.S.: The red eye. Emerg. Med. Clin. *6*:43, 1988.

Lewis, L.S., et al.: Gonococcal conjunctivitis in prepubertal children. Am. J. Dis. Child. *144*:546,

Mannis, M.J.: Allergic blepharo-conjunctivitis—avoiding misdiagnosis and mismanagement. Postgrad. Med. *86*:123, 1989.

Reed, D.B.: Viral and bacterial conjunctivitis—prevention of disastrous results. Postgard. Med. *86*:103, 107, 1989.

Schacter, J.: Why we need a program for the control of Chlamydia trachomatis. N. Engl. J. Med. *320*:802, 1989.

GINGIVOSTOMATITIS

Bogger-Goren, S. 1987. Acute epiglottitis caused by herpes simplex virus. Pediatr. Infect. Dis. J. *6*:1133, 1987.

Feldman, H.L., and Aretakis, D. Herpetic gingivostomatitis in children. Pediatr. Nursing *12*:111, 1986.

White, J.D., and Scholl, P.D.: Hard and soft tissue lesions of the oral cavity. *In* Clinical Pediatric Otolaryngology. Edited by Balkany, T.J., and Pashley, N. St. Louis, C. V. Mosby Co., 1986.

INFECTION AND BACTEREMIA: MANAGEMENT OF THE FEBRILE CHILD UNDER 2 YEARS

Paul N. Seward

CAPSULE

Perhaps nothing in emergency medicine is quite so alarming as a febrile child. Surely for the anxious or angry parents who appear at the Emergency Department (ED) with the child at midnight, it is a difficult time. Considering the diagnostic uncertainties and the devastating outcome of missing the diagnosis of sepsis or meningitis, even the most experienced and courageous of clinicians may occasionally reach past the chart of a febrile toddler for the next chart in the stack.

All is not hopeless, however. There are good ways to approach this problem. Moreover, unlike much of the medicine we practice today, the approach to the febrile child is not fundamentally technologic. Instead, it is one that emphasizes the human qualities of medicine: basic clinical skills, communication with parents and families, and the integration of the patient into systems for continuity of care. Finally—to reassure the hesitant clinician—there is good evidence that, even if no technique can identify all bacteremic children, a good history and physical examination, accompanied by appropriate laboratory testing, can identify virtually all bacteremic children whose condition would otherwise have a bad outcome.[1,2]

Fever in infants under 3 months or with sickle cell disease, immunodeficiency, neutropenia, or similar conditions is often serious, and such children should be evaluated and possibly treated for sepsis, usually as hospital inpatients.

DEFINITIONS

Pascoe and Grossman, in their terse and excellent textbook, define the critical terms as follows:

Bacteremia: The presence of bacteria in the blood.
Septicemia: The presence and persistence of bacteria and their toxins in the blood, associated with systemic symptoms of fever and prostration.[3]

These definitions emphasize a critical and sometimes overlooked point: bacteremia and septicemia are not the same.

Septicemic children are sick. They are always in danger and usually appear significantly ill. These are the children who represent the bulk of the potentially poor outcomes and whose clinical presentation is generally suspicious.

Bacteremic children, on the other hand, may appear transiently ill only during the acute showering of bacteria and otherwise may appear relatively well. Also, it is probable that many of these children might cope with their infection and do well. An unknown number of them, however, if untreated, may develop focal infections, septicemia, or meningitis. These children represent the principal diagnostic problem that renders this area of pediatrics so particularly challenging.

EPIDEMIOLOGY

Usually, one of the best ways to approach diagnostic problems is to know, even before entering the room, whom one needs to worry about. Unfortunately, except to tell us that the younger the child, the greater the risk, the epidemiologist has little to offer.

First of all, it does not matter where one practices: there is no socio-economic predilection for bacteremia. The child of the suburbs has the same likelihood of problems and presents the same diagnostic dilemmas as the child of the inner city:[4-6]

1. Two to eight percent of febrile children between 3 and 24 months have blood cultures that test positive for bacteria.[3,5,7-9]
2. Of these bacteria, 50% to 60% are Streptococcus pneumoniae, whereas 20% to 30% are Haemophilus influenzae.[3,8] The remainder are Neisseria meningitidis, group A Streptococcus, and others.[8] Pneumococcus is commonly an occult infection, whereas H. influenzae is more likely to be associated with demonstrable infections.[3] Staphylococcal bacteremia is most commonly associated with bone or joint infections.[3]
3. Four to ten percent of these children develop meningitis, even if the result of the lumbar puncture at initial presentation was negative.[3] This is particularly true if the child's temperature is 41.1°C (106°F) or more.[10] Children with fevers above

40.0°C (104°F) have an increased risk of having bacteria in the cerebrospinal fluid.[3]

CLINICAL PRESENTATION

Even though a systematic history (including parental observations) and physical examination by an experienced clinician are the best tests available to identify the bacteremic child, they are nonetheless unreliable predictors of who is sick and who is not.[8,11]

Some studies may clarify this point. On the one hand, there are studies such as those of Crocker and associates, who in 1985 examined 201 febrile infants of ages 6 months to 2 years, 21 of whom had blood cultures positive for the presence of bacteria. They noted *no* correlation between bacteremia and increasing temperature or parental perceptions of "irritability" or "lethargy."[12] Similarly, Dershewitz and colleagues found in 1983 that no level of training enabled a practitioner to identify bacteremic children clearly.[6] And Soman, in his review of the literature of 1982, found no study in which the history and physical examination were completely reliable.[7]

Even so, a number of studies such as that of Schwartz and Wientzen[4] also exist. They examined 52 children between 2 and 36 months who appeared to the pediatrician to have toxic symptoms and who had temperatures higher than 38.8°C (106.8°F). Six of the toxic infants but *none* of the nontoxic infants had culture-positive bacteremia.[4] Similarly, in 1981, Waskerwitz and Berkelhamer studied 25 pediatricians at all levels in a pediatric training program and their evaluations of 292 febrile children under 24 months of age. They showed that no single finding was absolutely predictive of bacteremia and that combining findings did not improve predictive accuracy. The physician's assessment, however, was the *most* useful factor in prediction. Most important, the physician's assessment reliably identified *all* patients with serious *complications*. Finally, no bacteremic children were included in the group of patients whose doctors judged them not to be bacteremic, whose functioning at home (as determined by parental history) did not indicate illness, and who had no localized evidence of focal infection. In closing their report, the researchers comment, "This study supports the notion that a good history and physical examination are essential components of the evaluation of each child. No other procedures should be considered 'routine.' "[1]

Given that the examination is critical, if unreliable, what factors in the examination are the most useful? These are described in the following paragraphs.

AGE

Children in the first 2 to 3 months of life who have fevers above 38°C (100.4°F) must all be suspected of having bacteremia.[7,13]

VITAL SIGNS

Any child under 2 years with a temperature above 40°C (104°F), even one who does not appear particularly ill, must be evaluated carefully. Although no age-specific standards exist for heart and respiratory rates in febrile children, tachycardias and tachypneas that seem out of proportion to the degree of fever require close evaluation and management.

"GENERAL APPEARANCE"

This item is in quotes because it is both the most important and least quantifiable factor considered in the examination. Regardless of temperature, febrile children who appear ill *must* be watched with concern. Moreover, their appearance should be assessed, not only in an initial examination but also during a period of "optimal observation."[3,5,7] During this observation, the most important considerations are:

- Appearance: Color, tone, presence of respiratory difficulty, grunting, or flaring of the nostrils.
- Behavior: Does the child interact normally with the parents? Is the child interested in toys or a bottle? Does the child interact normally with the examiner? Most important, if irritable or unhappy, can the child be consoled by the parents?[3,8,10]
- Fever control: Were antipyretics previously given? On one hand, these may render the examination somewhat unreliable,[10] but on the other hand, some

TABLE 59-54. COMMON INFECTIOUS AGENTS

Infection	Age	Predominant Organism
Pneumonia	<2 years	Respiratory syncytial virus Haemophilus influenzae (Staphylococcus aureus) Pneumococcus
	>2 years	Pneumococcus Mycoplasma pneumoniae Viruses
Bacterial meningitis	Neonatal	Enteric organisms Group B Streptococcus
	>8 years	Haemophilus influenzae Pneumococcus (Neisseria meningitidis)
	8 years to adult	Neisseria meningitidis Pneumococcus
Otitis media	<8 years	Respiratory virus Pneumococcus Haemophilus influenzae
	>8 years	Pneumococcus Respiratory virus
Enteritis	<2 years	Virus Enteropathogenic Escherichia coli
	>2 years	Virus Salmonella sp. Shigella sp.

information may also be obtained from the quality of the patient's response to the lowering of the fever.

SOURCE OF INFECTION

Is there an otitis, a pharyngitis, an upper respiratory infection? Is there evidence of pneumonia or urinary tract infection? Although the presence of these infections does not rule out the development of sepsis or meningitis, it may do much to explain an uncertain clinical picture or to guide subsequent evaluation and care. Similarly, the absence of a focus of infection in a significantly febrile or ill-appearing child requires further evaluation.[3] Table 59-54 lists infectious agents that may be found in certain conditions.

LABORATORY EVALUATION

Given the need for further evaluation, the clinician must now embark on the second great paradox of pediatric bacteremia: although the laboratory examination is even more unreliable than the physical examination and cannot be used as a screening modality, it is nonetheless an essential part of the evaluation of the child in whom bacteremia is suspected. What laboratory tests are useful, and what are the values that should raise a suspicion? These are described in the following paragraphs.

WHITE BLOOD CELL COUNT

In most studies, approximately three fourths of children with Streptococcus pneumoniae bacteremia and one half of children with Hemophilus influenzae infection have a white blood cell count of more than 15,000 per mm^3.[3,5,7,8,12] or a polymorphonuclear neutrophil count of more than 9000 per mm^3.[12] In addition, Crain and Shelov studied 175 *infants* under 8 weeks of age and found that the clinical impression of sepsis, a white blood cell count of more than 15,000 per mm^3, or an erythrocyte sedimentation rate of 30 or more identified all infants with bacteremia and excluded 82% of those without.[2] Other laboratory indicators, including erythrocyte sedimentation rate and absolute polymorphonuclear neutrophil count, have seemed helpful in some studies, but none are absolute predictors.[7]

On the other hand, Murray and coworkers studied 80 children under 3 years of age who presented with acute fever of unknown origin (higher than 39.7°C, 103.5°F) and no localizing signs. Of this group, three proved to have bacteremia, and two had viremia. Twenty-seven of 58 children seen on follow-up in 2 days were completely well. No differences could be identified in age, sex, or initial white blood cell count.[9] Similarly, in 1979, Morens reviewed 328 consecutive inpatient admissions to a pediatric communicable disease service. Using a white blood cell count of 10,000

per mm^3 as a cutoff value for the diagnosis of bacteremia, he found a 69% false-positive rate and a 25% false-negative rate. Raising the criteria to 15,000 per mm^3 raised the sensitivity to 48% but decreased the selectivity. He felt that no criterion or combination of criteria was sufficiently predictive to be considered reliable, and he recommended using caution in the handling of all cases of fever in this age group.[14] Finally, Bausher and Baker note that patients who prove to have meningococcemia with low white blood cell counts and no meningeal signs may have a worse prognosis than those with more abnormal findings.[15]

BLOOD CULTURE

In a sense, the blood culture remains the gold standard for diagnostic tests—not so much a test that is immediately useful, but the test with which others are compared. It is worth noting, however, that beyond simply defining disease, there is some evidence that the blood culture may be useful in quantifying it. Sullivan and associates studied the relationship between the degree of clinical disease that eventually developed and the organism count on initial blood culture. They found that, for Streptococcus pneumoniae and Hemophilus influenzae, 92% of 25 patients with initial bacterial counts greater than 100 organisms/mL went on to develop meningitis or epiglottitis; however, only 10% of 42 patients with lower counts developed serious disease. No difference was noted for Neisseria meningitidis.[16]

Also, it is important to know how long blood cultures must be observed. Over a 3-year period in Children's Hospital of Pittsburgh, Rowley and Wald reviewed 268 blood cultures yielding positive results; they noted that only four specimens became positive after 48 hours and that all of these were from patients with a previously identified infective focus. They concluded that empiric antibiotic therapy may be discontinued in immunocompetent patients without a focus of infection and with blood cultures that are negative after 48 hours.[17]

OTHER TESTS

Other tests, including complement-reactive protein, have also been studied as possible screening methods. The results of these have been inconclusive at best, however, and they are not mandatory and may not even be useful.[7,8,12] Investigations are also continuing with such tests as leukocyte vacuolization, toxic granulation,[18] and examinations of the buffy coat.[19]

HOSPITAL MANAGEMENT

Even in the best of hands, the diagnosis of the febrile child is far from exact. The basic rule of emergency medicine must always come into play; in situations of diagnostic uncertainty, the worst possible scenario must be considered and measures taken to protect the patient from its likely outcome. At the same time, performing a sepsis work-up on every warm child is untenable. Therefore, the fundamental guidelines are:

For all children under 3 months of age with a temperature of 38.0°C (100.4°F) or higher:

Regard as septicemic and evaluate, treat, and admit to the hospital.[3,7,8,10,13]

For the febrile child between 3 months and 2 years of age:

1. Clinical observation by a skilled observer is more reliable than laboratory screening.[3,8]
2. Clinical observation includes both a thorough history and physical examination and a period of observation before the child is discharged. This observation period is the *most critical diagnostic test* and may be extended as long as necessary to resolve diagnostic uncertainty.[3,8]
3. Screening laboratory tests include at best only a white blood cell count and differential count. This should probably be done in any child under 2 years with a temperature of 40°C (104°F) or higher and without an identified focus of infection. Any such patient with a white blood cell count of 15,000 per mm^3 or more should have a blood culture, and empirical antibiotic therapy should be instituted. Urinalysis and chest radiography should also be considered, as these infections, though focal, may be occult.[7] All other tests should be regarded as part of a work-up for clinically suspected illness.[3,8,20]
4. This laboratory evaluation is not done to determine who should be admitted to the hospital; it is done to determine who of the mildly ill or apparently well children may be safely sent home without treatment and close follow-up.[3,8] Children who appear acutely ill must be evaluated for sepsis (with blood cultures and a lumbar puncture), treated, and admitted.
5. Similarly, any identified illness should be treated. It must be remembered, however, that the discovery of a specific focus of infection does not rule out a more disseminated infection as well.[3,8] Moreover, preexisting illness, including sickle-cell disease, neoplasms, immunosuppression from steroid use, immunodeficiency, or significant cardiac, pulmonary, or neurologic disease, may require treatment of any fever as suspected sepsis.[10]
6. A blood culture may be part of discharge planning for significantly febrile children or children whose illness, though not requiring hospital admission, is more severe than might be expected from the identified infection. All such children, however, should be treated with appropriate antibiotics and re-evaluated within 12 to 24 hours.[3,8]
7. Antibiotic coverage for children to be discharged should be instituted in the ED, preferably parenterally. It should include coverage for Streptococcus pneumoniae and Hemophilus influenzae at a minimum. When the antibiotic is selected, the relative prevalence of penicillinase-producing organisms in the locale should be considered. For example, the microbiology of sinus infections in children demonstrates increased Hemophilus influenzae and Moraxella catarrhalis organisms resistant to amoxicillin, but sensitive to cefuroxime.[22] Each ED should have weekly updates on bacterial isolates and antibiotic sensitivities.
8. All children whose blood cultures yield positive results must be reevaluated. If S. pneumoniae is the infecting organism and if there is significant improvement, the patient may continue on antibiotics with close outpatient follow-up. If any other organism (particularly H. influenzae or Neisseria meningitidis) is found or if there is no improvement, the patient should be admitted to the hospital for further evaluation and treatment, including a work-up for sepsis.[3,8]
9. The possibility of reliably following up the patient must play a major role in treatment decision making.[3,8]
10. In neutropenic children, fever must be considered as having a likelihood of bacteremia requiring aggressive treatment on an empiric basis.[21]

CONCLUSION

The febrile infant or toddler presents a problem that will always concern the physician who treats sick children. In the midst of diagnostic uncertainties, however, some basic principles of medical care hold true:

- Good clinical evaluation is the mainstay of diagnosis.
- Err on the side of caution.
- When possible, a combination of preventive therapy and close follow-up should be a sufficient safeguard for patients who are well enough to go home but still present diagnostic uncertainty.

MEDICOLEGAL PEARLS

- Insidious presentations of meningitis should be watched for, particularly in children under 1 year.
- Extremely high fever (e.g., 106°F or 41.1°C) has a high correlation with serious illness.
- Purpural skin rashes can be an early sign of the Waterhouse-Friderichsen syndrome caused by meningococcemia.
- Interhospital transfers of severely ill children should not be made by private vehicles. Suitable personnel should be available in case of complications.

REFERENCES

1. Waskerwitz, S., Berkelhamer, J.E.: Outpatient bacteremia: Clinical findings in children under two years with initial temperatures of 39.5°C or higher. J. Pediatr. *99*:231, 1981.
2. Crain, E.F., and Shelov, S.P.: Febrile infants: Predictors of bacteremia. J. Pediatr. *101*:686, 1982.
3. Grossman, M.: Bacteremia in the febrile child. *In* Quick Reference to Pediatric Emergencies. Edited by Pascoe, D.L., and Grossman, M. (eds.). Philadelphia, J.B. Lippincott Co., 1984, pp. 417–418.
4. Schwartz, R.H., and Wientzen, R.L.: Occult bacteremia in toxic-appearing, febrile infants. Clin. Pediatr. *21*:659, 1982.
5. Brook, I., and Gruenwald, L.D.: Occurrence of bacteremia in febrile children seen in a hospital outpatient department and private practice. South. Med. J. *77*:1240, 1984.
6. Dershewitz, R.A., Posner, M.K., and Paichel, W.: Comparative study of the prevalence outcome, and prediction of bacteremia in children. J. Pediatr. *103*:352, 1983.
7. Soman, M.: Diagnostic workup of febrile children under 24 months of age: A clinical review. West. J. Med. *137*:12, 1982.
8. Fleisher, G.R., and Ludwig, S.: Textbook of Pediatric Emergency Medicine. Baltimore, Williams & Wilkins Co., 1984, pp. 356–358.
9. Murray, D.L., Zonana, J., Seidel, I.S., et al.: Relative importance of bacteremia and viremia in the course of acute fevers of unknown origin in outpatient children. Pediatrics *68*:157, 1981.
10. Barkin, R.M., and Rosen, P.: Emergency Pediatrics. St. Louis, CV Mosby Co., 1984, pp. 180–182.
11. McCarthy, P.L., Lembo, R.M., Baron, M.A., et al.: Predictive value of abnormal physical examination findings in ill-appearing and well-appearing febrile children. Pediatrics *76*:167, 1985.
12. Crocker, P.J., Quick, G., and McCombs, W.: Occult bacteremia in the emergency department: Diagnostic criteria for the young febrile child. Ann. Emerg. Med. *14*:1172, 1985.
13. Berkowitz, C.D.: Fever in infants less than two months of age: Spectrum of disease and predictors of outcome. Pediatr. Emerg. Care *1*:128, 1985.
14. Morens, D.M.: WBC count and differential: Value in predicting bacterial disease in children. Am. J. Dis. Child. *133*:25, 1979.
15. Bausher, J.C., and Baker, R.C.: Early prognostic indicators in acute meningococcemia: Implications for management. Pediatr. Emerg. Care *2*:176, 1986.
16. Sullivan, T.D., LaScolea, L.J., and Neter, E.: Relationship between the magnitude of bacteremia in children and the clinical disease. Pediatrics *69*:699, 1982.
17. Rowley, A.H., and Wald, E.R.: The incubation period necessary for detection of bacteremia in immunocompetent children with fever. Clin. Pediatr. *25*:485, 1986.
18. Liu, C.H., Lehan, C., Speer, M.E., et al.: Early detection of bacteremia in an outpatient clinic. Pediatrics *75*:827, 1985.
19. Reik, H., and Rubin, S.J.: Evaluation of the buffy-coat smear for rapid detection of bacteremia. JAMA *245*:357, 1981.
20. Carrol, W.L., Farrell, M.K., Singer, J.I., et al.: Treatment of occult bacteremia: A prospective randomized clinical trial. Pediatrics *72*:608, 1983.
21. Shenep, J.L., Hughes, W.T., Roberson, P.K., et al.: Vancomycin, Ticarcillin and Amikacin compared with ticarcillin-clavulanate and amikacin in the empirical treatment of febrile neutropenic children with cancer. N. Engl. J. Med. *319*:1053, 1988.
22. Wald, E.R.: Sinusitis in children. N. Engl. J. Med. *326*:319, 1992.

BIBLIOGRAPHY

Crocker, P.J.: Occult bacteremia in the emergency department. Ann. Emerg. Med. *13*:45, 1984.

Callaham, M.: Inaccuracy and expense of the leucocyte count in making clinical decisions. Ann. Emerg. Med. *15*:774, 1986.

McLellan, D., and Giebink, G.S.: Perspectives on occult bacteremia in children. J. Pediatr. *109*:18, 1986.

EVALUATION AND MANAGEMENT OF CHILD ABUSE

Garrett E. Bergman

CAPSULE

Outbursts of parental defensiveness and hostility may generate anger in physicians. This anger, in turn, affects the physician's ability to manage child abuse injuries. This chapter outlines the spectrum of child abuse and neglect and offers practical approaches for positive intervention. Characteristic features of the victim and of the abusing parents or other offenders and some of the characteristic interaction dynamics between them are described. Some typical injuries are delineated, although the pathologic creativity of parents precludes a comprehensive listing of all the possible means of inflicting injury and pain on children. Finally, the measures for a physician to take when abuse or neglect is suspected and suggested specific answers for accusatory, defensive parents are given. The physician in the Emergency Department (ED) is in a critical position to identify and provide intervention for a common condition with a high morbidity and occasional mortality.

DEFINITION

Child abuse and neglect are defined legally, not medically, by Federal Public Law 93–247, The Child Abuse Prevention and Treatment Act of 1974. To receive Federal support in the implementation of this law, most states have followed with similar laws defining child abuse and neglect to mean "the physical and mental injury, sexual abuse, negligent treatment or maltreatment of a child under the age of 18 (years) by a person who is responsible for the child's welfare under circumstances which indicate that the child's health and welfare is harmed or threatened thereby." Some states add the vague descriptive "serious physical injury"; most states *require* physicians and others to report their suspicion, and most grant immunity from civil and criminal liability to physicians who report their suspicion in good faith. In many states, acts of omission as well as acts of commission are included; parents are expected to act responsibly in protecting their child from injury as well as not directly inflicting injury on their child.

One difficulty in deciding whether or not to be suspicious is the physician's own definition of "abuse." The scope of this definition depends on personal upbringing and societal tolerances, which vary over time and with locale. In some Scandinavian countries, any form of physical punishment is illegal. Recent state referenda in the United States have reaffirmed our society's expectation that schoolteachers as well as parents should be permitted to use corporal punishment on certain misbehaving students. Surely, the manner of punishment used by our parents in raising each of us influences our acceptance of physical discipline with the hand, a flat board, a "hickory stick," a belt, a lead pipe, a baseball bat, or a looped wire "switch." A parental act that leads to mild physical injury in a child may represent an extreme but socially acceptable form of discipline in one neighborhood, but may be a sign of serious intrafamilial discord in another.

Distinctions useful for recognizing and understanding the underlying dynamics of the abusers are usually made among several types of abuse. These categories are as follows:

1. Physical abuse.
2. Neglect.
3. Emotional abuse.
4. Sexual abuse.

Each is discussed separately, although each represents a serious breakdown in homeostasis in a functioning family unit. For statistical purposes, all categories are collectively counted as child abuse.

PHYSICAL ABUSE

EPIDEMIOLOGY

Accurate incidence figures of child abuse and neglect have been difficult to establish for several reasons. Most reports to central registries are generated by physicians in EDs or in inner-city hospital pediatric units,

rather than by physicians in private offices. As a result, the urban population is relatively overrepresented in the statistics, leading some to make erroneous conclusions. One estimate, however, based on studies of physical injury in several states and countries is a yearly incidence of serious inflicted physical injury of 400 cases per million population, or about 20 times the incidence of childhood leukemia. Members of all ethnic, religious, racial, and socioeconomic groups have been identified as abusers, perhaps with a true higher incidence in groups with greater frequency of life stresses, such as unemployment, incomplete schooling, and unplanned children.

Most cases of children with inflicted life-threatening physical injuries had been treated in an ED previously for injuries of suspicious origin. Most injuries to young children are inflicted by their mothers (who must supervise most of the child's day), although injuries inflicted by the father tend to be more serious. Injured children who are returned to their homes without intervention following an episode of abuse are thought to have a high likelihood of sustaining additional, more serious injuries, with permanent disabilities, and even an estimated 10% chance of being killed. Prospective statistics from several emergency units now document that, of the injuries in preschool children brought for treatment of trauma, about 10% are purposefully inflicted injuries.

Following the passage of federal and state child abuse reporting laws, the number of recognized cases rose rapidly for about a decade, leveling off in the late 1970s. These statistics probably reflect an increased awareness, a raised consciousness of physicians, and an increased ease of reporting. There is still great variability in the physician's willingness to recognize and report child abuse.

RECOGNITION OF PHYSICAL ABUSE

Any injury not fully explained by the history should raise the suspicion of abuse. A reasonable depth of experience in evaluating trauma is necessary in determining possible abuse, although it may be obvious that some injuries are deliberately inflicted by others. Pattern burns from heating coils, irons, or branding rods; wounds from belt buckles and whips; or bite marks from other humans are obvious (Fig. 59-24). Fractures, abrasions, and bruises may be more subtle, but often the child will provide necessary and valuable information if separated and questioned in a supportive manner.

The earliest recognition of willfully inflicted injuries was described by Caffey in 1946.[1] He identified "cupping"—x-ray evidence of repeated trauma to the growing ends of the long bones—and observed the association of a subdural hematoma with long bone fractures. In 1962 Kempe first used the term "battered child syndrome" to bring attention to this entity.[2] Now multiple fractures in various stages of healing are felt to be pathognomonic evidence of child abuse (Fig. 59-25). Any injuries a child could not possibly self-inflict

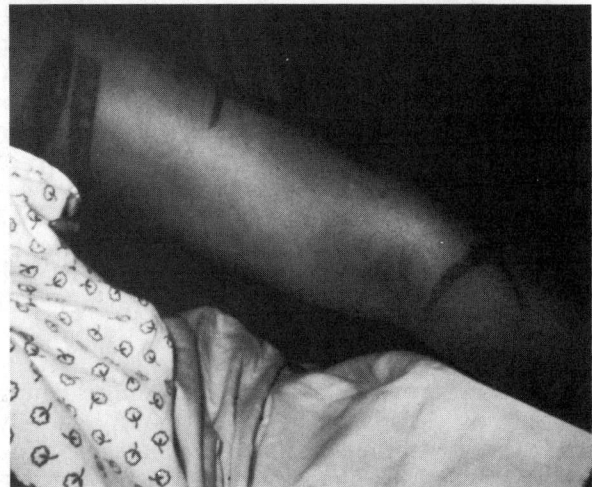

FIG. 59-24. *Multiple burns on the arm of a teen-age girl, inflicted by a steam iron.*

are highly suspicious, such as a spiral fracture of the femur in a 3-month-old who allegedly caught his leg between crib slats.

Some injuries that are highly suggestive of abuse and that should alert the physician to consider abuse as their causes are:

1. Head injuries, including skull fractures and subdural hematoma.
2. Limb injuries.
3. Burns, particularly immersion.
4. Some fractures in preschool-age children.
5. All perianal and perineal injuries.

Particularly vulnerable targets are children under 3 years old, and those who are handicapped (with cerebral palsy, retardation, deafness, or physical deformities). *Any serious injury* in a child under 1 year of age should be suspect because the children are not independently ambulatory. Children who roll out of

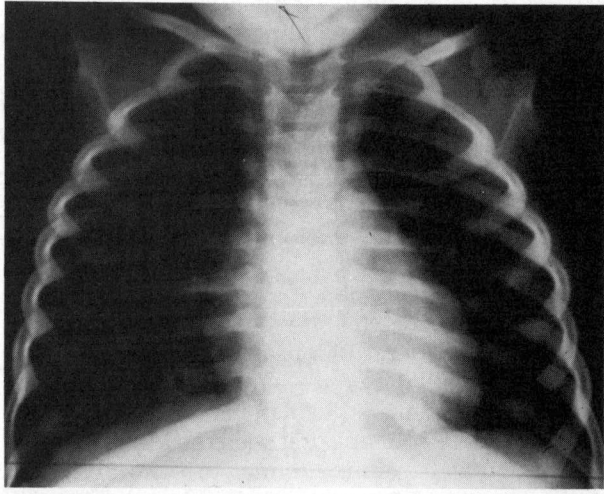

FIG. 59-25. *This child's x-ray findings demonstrate the concurrent appearance of a new fracture of the left clavicle with healing fractures of three ribs posteriorly, of different ages.*

bed onto a floor, even from waist height or higher, rarely sustain significant injury; that history would not adequately explain the combination of skull fracture, limb fracture, and multiple abrasions.

Critical to one's ability to assess whether the history given would satisfactorily explain the child's injury is a knowledge of developmental abilities of children at different ages. The physician should ask himself or herself: Could the child have reasonably performed the tasks attributed to him or her to create the injury? Also, an injury may be attributed to acts performed by siblings. Although siblings can and do inflict injuries on each other, the physician should be certain that the sibling really could have physically performed the act attributed to him or her. Is he or she strong enough? Coordinated enough? Is this an age-appropriate task? And lastly, should the parent have anticipated and prevented its injury?

The physical mechanisms of injury must be explored carefully in history-taking. A transverse fracture is caused by a direct blow at that site; a spiral fracture is caused by a twisting or rotary (torque) force; epiphyseal disruptions are caused by direct trauma to the limb; and greenstick or torus fractures are caused by a force directed along the longitudinal axis of the bone, most often as in falling on an outstretched arm. In each case of a fracture, does the proposed mechanism of injury fully explain the findings? If not, abuse should be suspected. Parents sometimes offer no explanation; for example, "the child woke up from her nap and now won't bear weight on her legs." In a case such as this, a fractured femur is almost surely caused by abuse.

RADIOLOGIC SIGNS

Occasionally, the radiologist suggests the diagnosis on the basis of characteristic x-ray findings. To reiterate, the presence of epiphyseal separations, multiple old fractures at different stages of healing, healing periosteal new bone formation reactions, skull fractures, multiple fractures at distant sites, evidence of deep soft-tissue injuries, or intraperitoneal air from a perforated viscus can be very suggestive. Additionally, splitting of the cranial sutures as a result of a subdural hematoma or recovery growth of the brain, widening of the distal anterior ends of ribs owing to costochondral separations, and callus at the site of tendon avulsions may be seen. The radiologist can often determine the age of a healing fracture to document multiple episodes of injury over time.

Although the child's age, nutritional status, state of anabolism or catabolism, and location of the fracture all influence the rate of bone healing, stages of healing can be recognized and roughly dated. Callus usually forms after 1 week, by which time the deep soft-tissue swelling at the fracture site has resolved. Complete resolution may take several months, with remolding of the deformed bone for a year or more. The presence of fractures at various stages of healing is evidence of repeated episodes of significant trauma.

To assess a child in whom abuse is suspected, the use of both plain roentgenograms and radioisotope bone scans is recommended. Using both of these imaging modalities together maximizes the ability to demonstrate acute and chronic skeletal injuries.

EXAMINATION

When examining the child, the physician should take careful note of the child's dress and grooming, behavior, and attitude toward him and the parent. Although not seen exclusively in children, the following behavioral characteristics can suggest that the child was raised in an unsafe or hostile environment:

1. The child does not cry aloud when examined, even when subjected to a painful procedure, such as a venipuncture.
2. The child is constantly looking around at the individuals and his environment, distrustful or wary of all adults, always alert for danger.
3. The child does not respond to the medical staff's offering of toys, food, or playthings because of his suspiciousness; he or she interacts little with adults and is apprehensive when they approach.
4. The child may suddenly show inappropriate behavior, such as extreme aggressiveness, diffidence, or regression; he or she may assume an adult role and attempt to "parent" others, particularly his own parent.
5. The child is often developmentally delayed, particularly in the area of speech, and will avoid expressing affect.
6. The child is often quiet and withdrawn, guarding against asserting himself or herself, and often sits passively for a long time if being watched.

When talking to the parents, taking a history and discussing the additional testing required, or reviewing the findings, the physician should carefully observe the parents and their reactions. The following behavioral characteristics support a milieu conducive to abuse:

1. The parent has either an inappropriate degree of overconcern or total lack of concern for the child's injury and its consequences.
2. The parent may justify the injury as an unfortunate outcome of punishment that not only was necessary but also was *obligated* by a parental mandate to raise the child to do the "right thing."
3. The parent may be critical toward the injured child and angry that the child is injured.
4. The parent offers little or no physical or verbal reassurance or comfort to the tearful child, touching him or her little, if at all.

Further discussion with the parents may reveal that they are immature and impulsive, acting out their frustrations through violence directed at the child. They may view the child as capable of nurturing and reassuring them and meeting their emotional needs.

Most abusive parents have experienced from their own parents only physical means of expressing anger and frustration. Drug and alcohol abuse are common but not necessary concomitants of child abuse; however, other antisocial behavior may be evident. In general, the perpetrator is isolated, socially alone, having never developed positive social ties with any relatives or friends.

Parents with little tolerance for frustration, who are unable to seek support from others, or who have poor self-esteem are easily threatened and fearful of authority. Perceived accusations or threats tend to elicit immediate defensiveness and hostility, precluding meaningful communication and often impeding information-gathering attempts. For this reason, personality characteristics and the details of a family's means of problem solving often are not elicited in the emergency setting, but revealed after a period of supportive social service or psychiatric intervention.

In summary, the recognition of child abuse depends on the physician's willingness to consider it as the cause of injuries, accidents, and ingestions. The physician must be vigilant to the possibility that parents fabricate histories and that the "facts" presented may not be true. Using any definition, the physician is expected to report his *suspicion* of abuse to the appropriate child protective or law enforcement agency, whose mandate it is to investigate further. A physician is not expected to perform the duties of a police officer, lawyer, social worker, district attorney, judge, therapist, or parent, despite the image occasionally portrayed in the media. The medical professional is expected to assess the congruence of the injury with the history offered to explain it, to satisfy himself or herself that the injury was, in fact, accidental.

PHYSICAL FINDINGS

Almost any injury can be the result of abuse. The most common physical findings are those associated with a *fracture, head trauma,* or *skin lesions.* Less common findings referable to injury of the thoracic or abdominal organs can be seen.

FRACTURE

Physical findings from any fracture can vary from pain, guarding, deformity, and resistance to passive movement to none, when an asymptomatic fracture is found incidentally on x-ray examination. When one suspicious fracture is found, a skeletal survey or radioisotope bone scan may demonstrate additional sites of fractures at different ages. Metaphyseal avulsion fractures are often caused by abuse. Skull fractures, rib fractures (especially if bilateral), and transverse fractures of the shaft of a long bone (especially multiple) are highly suggestive of abuse. Midshaft fracture of the clavicle, spiral fracture of the tibia (toddler's fracture), dislocation (with or without fracture) of the radial head (nursemaid's elbow), or fracture of the distal radius from falling on an outstretched arm

(Colles' fracture or variant) are commonly seen in young children and are *not* suggestive of abuse.

HEAD TRAUMA

Head trauma in abused children may be manifested by coma, seizure, subgaleal hemorrhage, alopecia, scalp contusions, or any other sign of cranial or intracranial trauma. A subdural hematoma in a young child may not evoke localizing signs. Nonspecific signs such as irritability, increasing head circumference, or failure to grow may be the only indications of intracranial injury, but hemiparesis and seizures can also result. The usual evaluation for stupor or coma may lead to diagnostic tests, such as a computed tomography (CT) scan, to demonstrate intracerebral bleeding, cerebral contusion, or subarachnoid bleeding. One child in our unit had experienced a contusion of his midpons with transient cardiopulmonary arrest as a result of being thrown and striking the base of his occiput on the floor. Head injuries are the primary cause of death in fatal cases of abuse.

Another recently described form of intracranial injury to a child is caused by the parent holding the child's arms or chest and shaking the child back and forth. The child's head, relatively large and heavy compared with that of an adult is alternately hyperextended and hyperflexed, causing multiple intracerebral hemorrhages, contusions, and infarcts, often with no external sign of injury. This *whiplash shaken-baby syndrome* causes serious long-term morbidity in the form of mental retardation and seizures. Analysis of cases of fatal child abuse reveals the major cause of death to be head injury.

CUTANEOUS INJURY

The most common physical signs of abuse are cutaneous: *bruises, burns,* and *abrasions.*

Bruises. The age of a bruise or hematoma can be estimated by changes in its appearance as the enclosed hemoglobin is metabolized and absorbed. A fresh superficial bruise is red or reddish blue; after 1 to 3 days the familiar "black-and-blue mark" appears and fades through green, green-yellow, then yellow-brown colors over a week to 10 days. Caution must be exercised, however, because the rate of color change (and hence the estimated age) does depend somewhat on the depth of the hemorrhage in the skin and subcutaneous tissues; i.e., an extensive hematoma may show all gradations of color simultaneously as the thinner areas of skin bleeding peripherally resolve quicker than the thicker central area.

Burns. Cutaneous burns are common manifestations of abuse. A child may present with a well-demarcated immersion pattern of feet, legs, hands, head, or buttocks having been purposefully scalded by being placed into hot water (Fig. 59-26). The extent of the burn depends on the temperature of the water and

the duration of exposure. Hot tap water (130 to 145°F) causes extensive skin burns with 15 to 30 seconds of exposure; freshly boiled water (180 to 200°F) can cause second-degree burns with only a few seconds of contact. Splashed or spilled hot liquids cause an interrupted nonconfluent pattern. Clothing tends to hold hot liquids in contact with the skin longer, predisposing to more extensive burns.

Children have also had their hands held over the open flames of a stove to warn them of the dangers of fire, resulting in extensive third-degree burns in a circumscribed area. Burns inflicted by hot objects often leave a pattern "branded" in the skin, such as from a heating coil, heated grate, electric iron, or hot bent wire (Fig. 59-27). Cigarette burns caused by deliberate pressing of the glowing tip into the skin often cannot be distinguished from the almost ubiquitous lesion of impetigo unless ashes are present or the history is clear, as it was for the child in Figure 59-28.

Abrasions. Abrasions are often self-inflicted from the child's daily activities. The location of the injury and its specific appearance may suggest its origin to be nonaccidental. Loopshaped abrasions are caused by the parent's whipping a child with a looped electric cord or rope (Fig. 59-29). Linear abrasions are found if a belt or wooden board has been used. Human bites, lead pipes, metal rods, or leather straps yield characteristic skin marks that can be matched to the instrument used, occasionally only after a visit to the home by a social worker.

ADDITIONAL PHYSICAL FINDINGS

INTRA-ABDOMINAL INJURY

Except in fatal or near-fatal cases, intra-abdominal injury is not common in child abuse. When it does occur, blunt trauma is the usual mechanism of injury. Laceration of the liver, laceration or rupture of the spleen, duodenal intramural hemorrhage, and traumatic pancreatitis are the most common consequences. Signs of

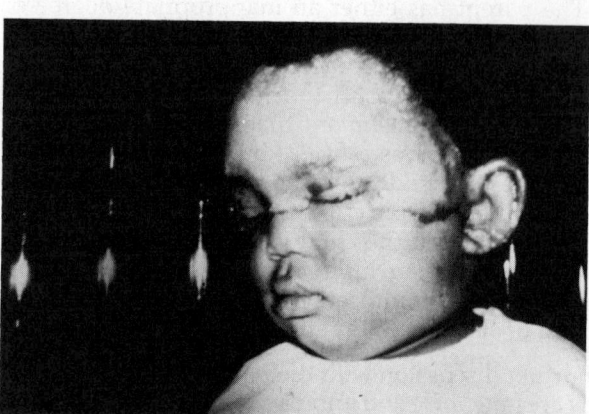

FIG. 59-26. A 15-month-old boy whose mother purposely poured hot water on his head and face.

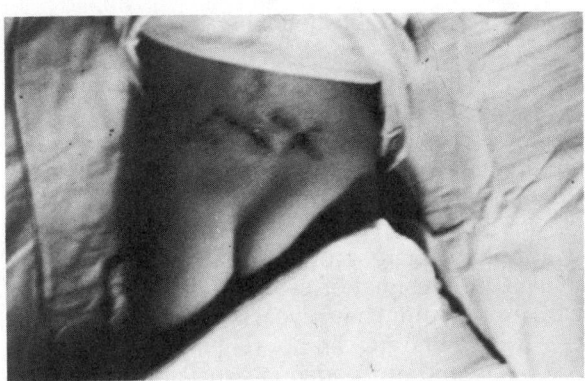

FIG. 59-27. The burned back of a 2-year-old girl whose mother held her against a space heater as punishment.

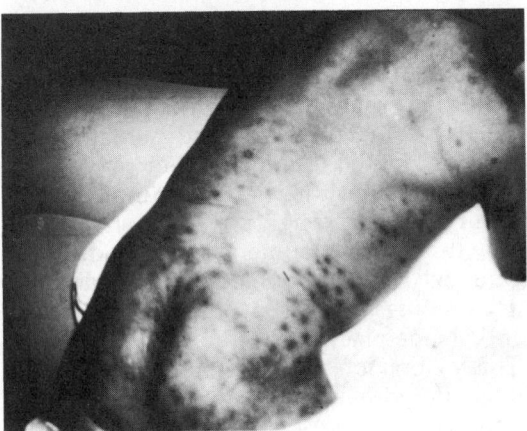

FIG. 59-28. Multiple healed cigarette burns in a 10-month-old who was the victim of his uncle's sadism.

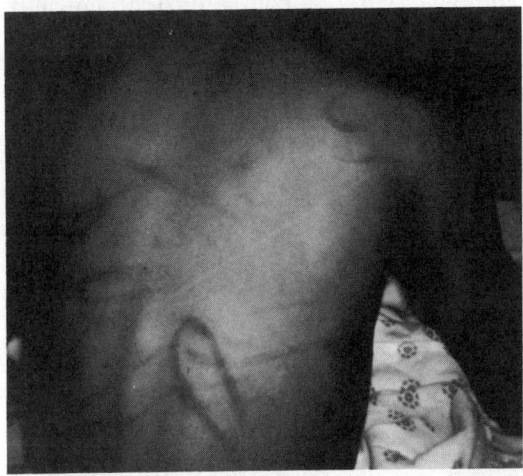

FIG. 59-29. Multiple loop-shaped whip marks on the back of a teenage boy who was being punished for not cleaning his room.

hypovolemic shock, peritonitis, severe abdominal pain, or high intestinal obstruction could suggest these diagnoses with little or no external evidence of trauma. Shock from massive occult intra-abdominal bleeding subsequent to liver or spleen trauma is second only

to brain injuries as a cause of death in child abuse. Hematuria can result from indirect renal trauma, with or without hypertension. (Extensive muscular injury with hemorrhage and muscle necrosis may rarely lead to myoglobinuria, with dark red or brown urine that tests positive for blood on standard dipstick tests but with no red cells.)

INTRATHORACIC INJURY

Injuries of the *intrathoracic* contents occur uncommonly and usually only concomitant with extensive additional injuries. The usual physical findings of cardiac tamponade, hemothorax, pneumothorax, or ruptured great vessel are evident and must be recognized and managed immediately.

TOXIC INJURY

Any signs or symptoms of an ingestion, particularly in a preambulatory child, could suggest abuse because children have been purposefully poisoned by their parents with all varieties of prescribed and street drugs, chemicals, toxins, and plants. These parents are usually severely psychiatrically disturbed, unlike the usual parent who, in a fit of rage, loses impulse control and physically injures the child. Severely disturbed or psychotic parents have also murdered their children by suffocation (indistinguishable in an infant, even on autopsy, from sudden infant death syndrome), by drowning, or by ritual exorcism.

DIFFERENTIAL DIAGNOSIS OF PHYSICAL ABUSE

Occasionally, an underlying bleeding disorder is suggested by the parent's history of the child's bruising very easily. Children with hemophilia should demonstrate hemarthroses and have an abnormal partial thromboplastin time. Von Willebrand's disease variably yields a prolonged bleeding time and lowered factor VIII level; a family history and the presence of other forms of mucocutaneous bleeding are usually present. Ecchymoses, petechiae, and abrasions have erroneously suggested abuse in a 5-year-old with Ehlers-Danlos syndrome, with abnormalities of subcutaneous connective tissues, and ligamentous laxity. The Vietnamese folk medicine custom of rubbing coins on the child's warmed skin to treat fever (C'ao Gio) can mimic the abrasions of a beating (Fig. 59-30).

Recurrent fractures can occur in rare instances in children with osteogenesis imperfecta, but strikingly blue sclera suggest the diagnosis; the history usually provides a feasible explanation, although the degree of trauma may seem trivial. The severest forms may begin with fractures caused by birth trauma; it is never acquired, with recurrent multiple fractures first appearing later in life. As with any uncertain diagnosis, the advice of an expert with more experience with

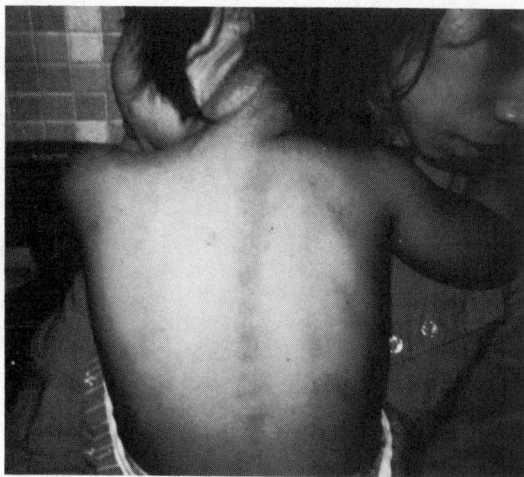

FIG. 59-30. Multiple abrasions from "coin-rubbing" over warm oiled skin, to draw out fever due to herpetic gingivostomatitis in a 2-year-old Vietnamese girl. *C'ao Gio* should not be considered abuse.

child abuse can be helpful in deciding whether any injury is of a suspicious nature and should be reported.

CHILD NEGLECT

RECOGNITION

Society expects parents to provide a minimum of the necessities of life to their offspring: food, water, clothing, shelter, education, and medical care for illness or injury. Any parent who does not fulfill these functions is considered neglectful and guilty of child neglect. Even more than in the case of physical abuse, however, uncertain definitions hinder the procuring of necessary interventions. Is an unimmunized 5-year-old, who is otherwise well, a victim of neglect? What if the 5-year-old has contracted tetanus? Few would argue against identifying and reporting a 5-year-old who has been locked in his room his whole life, who has been fed once daily, and who now weighs 26 pounds. One extreme is easy to recognize; the other is not.

The intra- and interpersonal dynamics of physical child neglect are different from those of physical abuse. The parents usually do not purposefully withhold basic needs from their child. Rather, they are oblivious that the child has needs. No explanation can be offered for the child's poor state of health or delayed development or unattended illness; the condition is unrecognized. Rather than viewing themselves as neglectful, the parents view themselves as "unlucky" and impotent to change their lot. Unresponsive to both their own needs as well as the needs of others, they lack both the motivation and means to help themselves; life to them is futile. Rarely could they generate enough energy to externalize their frustration and directly injure the child. Nevertheless, neglect can be fatal, and it must be recognized and treated. Nonfatal

patterns that are established may be repeated in a following decade.

Children with deprivation dwarfism, or *failure to thrive* have been inadequately fed for a long enough time that their weight (more than their height or head circumference) is below the third percentile for children of their age. History from the parent and physical examination of the child reveal no clues to an organic cause for inadequate growth, such as findings of chronic gastrointestinal or cardiorespiratory disease. Physical examination may reveal lack of subcutaneous tissue, an apathetic appearance (Fig. 59-31), self-stimulatory behaviors, and inadequate socialization. There may be physical signs of poor skin hygiene, unattended rashes, developmental delay, and dirty clothing that is inadequate for the weather. Frequently the child exhibits bizarre behavior when under observation in the hospital, such as drinking from a toilet bowel or picking through trashcans looking for food. After a couple of weeks of controlled adequate feeding, these children regain weight, although they may be permanently stunted physically and mentally. Failure to thrive presents in the first year or two of life, often at an incidental visit to the ED for intercurrent illness or injury. The thorough physician should assess the growth and development of all children he treats to recognize this condition early. Physical signs of neglect can occasionally be observed as being caused not by inadequacy of the parent but by abject poverty. This distinction must be made because the interventions offered may be different.

Is noncompliance to prescribed medical regimens to be considered *medical neglect*? The answer is *probably*, only as measured by the effect of this noncompliance on the child. For example, few physicians, let alone patients, complete a 10-day course of oral penicillin for documented Group A streptococcal pharyngitis, and few suffer any consequence. A child with an arrhythmia or diabetes mellitus, however, may suffer serious consequences as a result of parental noncompliance with prescribed administration of digitalis or insulin. In weighing whether simple and common noncompliance with recommended treatment should

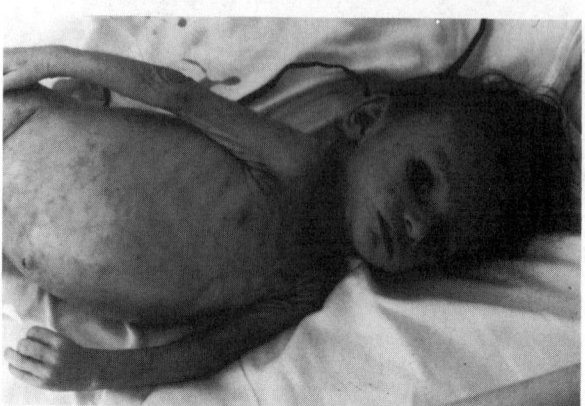

FIG. 59-31. This neglected child demonstrates severe inanition and loss of all subcutaneous fat, in the presence of an apathetic but hyperalert facial expression.

be considered neglect, the adverse effects of the omission relative to the gains possible with compliance must be considered.

ABANDONMENT

Abandonment is a special category of neglect, legally defined in each jurisdiction. When a young child is left at home unattended by a responsible adult or older child, or when a 5-year-old is left to care for two infants all day, the parent should be considered guilty of abandonment and the child welfare agency should be notified. In some areas, local fire safety regulations stipulate the age at which a youngster becomes capable of "babysitting" responsibly and may even specify the length of time permitted. Generally, an average 10- to 12-year-old can be expected to be responsible for one other youngster. Occasionally a neighbor reports crying, unattended children to the police. When brought by police or neighbors to the ED, these children may be hungry or thirsty or manifest a variety of injuries or illnesses that need medical attention. If parents cannot be located to provide consent for necessary medical treatment, the local child welfare agency may have to seek temporary legal custody of the child and then grant permission to treat.

EMOTIONAL ABUSE

Emotional abuse is difficult to define precisely, but it has profound effects on the emotional growth and stability of a growing child. In the young child, the lack of appropriate and adequate emotional support and stimulation lead to motor and developmental delays, cognitive dysfunction, and disturbed behaviors. Very young children, under 6 months, can be observed to be listless, withdrawn, and unresponsive as a result of depression. In the older child and adolescent, repeated admonitions such as "you're no damned good" in its various forms often lead to severe acting-out behaviors, running away, or depression and suicide attempts. The problems inherent in proving causality in mental and emotional disturbances, as well as difficulties in predicting the outcomes of specific interventions, make this category of child abuse difficult to substantiate. Consequently, intervention by child protective agencies is uncommon, and emotional abuse without concomitant physical abuse is rarely reported.

SEXUAL ABUSE

Most state laws are clearer and stricter about sexual abuse than about other physical abuse and neglect.

There is a lack of clear agreement, however, about what constitutes "sexual abuse of children" as defined by physicians, social workers, lawyers, police, and lawmakers. As a result, a broad, functional definition is more useful to the physician in an ED. Sexual abuse occurs when an adult or knowledgeable adolescent involves a child who is too young to comprehend or consent in activity designed to generate sexual gratification for the adult. Various forms of child sexual abuse include, but are not limited to:

1. *Molestation*—the physical fondling of the child's breasts, anus, genitals, or buttocks with the perpetrator's fingers or sometimes mouth; may include exhibitionism, or the showing of pictures.
2. *Sodomy*—contact between the penis and the victim's anus, or oral-genital contact.
3. *Prostitution*—encouraging or forcing the child to have intercourse or other sexual activity with another for some gain.
4. *Incest*—sexual activities between relatives either defined legally or by societal taboos, which may include intercourse; may be defined to include sexual activity between any adult and child residing in the same household.
5. *Rape*—attempted or successful forceful penetration of the vagina by the perpetrator's penis with or without ejaculation.
6. *Statutory rape*—intercourse with a girl younger than a legally defined age, perhaps by a man older than a certain age.

Sexual abuse of children is common, but accurate statistics are difficult to collect because much goes unreported. Some have suggested that, although girls are four to ten times more likely than boys to be victims of sexual abuse, this may represent a cultural bias toward girls that permits "sex play" among boys. Probably ten times as many children are sexually abused as are seriously physically abused, but many instances go unreported because no violence was involved and little physical evidence exists. Children of all ages have been sexually abused; indeed, oral fondling of an infant's genitals has been quietly condoned by some cultures in our society.

Most sexual abuse is committed by a relative, friend, or acquaintance of the victim, often in the victim's own house. The "dirty old man," or the sinister stranger who offers candy to entice a child to come with him, is uncommon. In some studies and numerous anecdotes, parents (when not perpetrators themselves) have condoned the abuse or have not tried to prevent it; for instance, despite her suspicions about a 17-year-old male cousin, one mother left him to care for her 2-year-old daughter for 4 hours, finding on her return that her crying child had sustained genital abrasions and ecchymoses.

Epidemiologic studies have clearly supported the distinction proposed by Gil in 1970[3] between physical abuse and sexual abuse. The average age of physically abused boys and girls, who are victimized at the same rate, is the same. The average age of a girl who is sexually abused is early adolescence, 9 to 13 years, whereas boys tend more often to be younger, in the 5- to 9-year-old age group. Whereas men and women are equally likely to be perpetrators of physical abuse, over 95% of known perpetrators of sexual abuse are men. In one study, stepfathers were overrepresented in both (24% of sexual abuse, 13% of physical abuse), and stepmothers more likely to live in the house where physical abuse occurred. Over 50% of the perpetrators of sexual abuse live in the same household or are first-order relatives of the victim. Sexual abuse is more often confirmed than physical abuse when investigated, and this confirmation more often leads to court action. One questionnaire study of primary care physicians demonstrated that, although over half reported seeing at least one case of sexual abuse of a child annually, only a third of these urged the family to report the incidence to welfare or legal agencies.

The dynamics of sexual abuse of a child differ from those of physical abuse and neglect and are extremely variable. Perpetrators of sexual abuse are not socially isolated, frustrated people with poor self-esteem, poor impulse control, or a need to be nurtured. They may appear to be successful, well-adjusted, and even loving relatives, but they are blatantly exploitive, taking advantage of the victim's loyalty. Usually there is a threat, expressed or implied, admonishing the child not to reveal the episode for fear of reprisals or emotional rejection. The child may be confused, anxious, suspicious, and uncertain where to turn for help.

Signs and symptoms of sexual abuse are protean, depending on the nature of the abuse and the age and developmental stage of the child victim. The verbal child may accurately describe the episode to the parents, who then bring the victim to the ED for verification and treatment. The child might present a somatic complaint to be brought for medical care and only then reveal a history of sexual abuse in confidence. As part of a physical examination for another reason, signs of genital trauma or venereal disease might be observed.

Genital trauma is not pathognomonic of abuse; girls can sustain laceration or abrasions of their labia from accidents in which they fall onto their vulva, such as when straddling a boy's bike; a boy can injure his penis or scrotum by catching it in his zipper or having a toilet seat fall on it. Rectal lacerations and bruises, vulvovaginitis, bruises on the upper thighs or buttocks, and genital trauma of any kind should, however, suggest the possibility of sexual abuse; any sexually transmissible disease in a preadolescent should be considered the result of sexual abuse.

Victimized children are often secretive and confused, unable to comprehend why their relative or acquaintance abused them, and afraid to ask. Numerous nonspecific behavioral or psychosomatic symptoms may result that may not immediately suggest sexual abuse. Some children with excessive anxiety, fears, nightmares, masturbatory activity, encopresis or enuresis, or who ask surprisingly sophisticated questions about specific sexual activities, may be struggling to deal with a single episode or continuing series of episodes of sexual abuse. Chronic abdominal pain in adolescent girls has been a common, totally nonspecific, symptom of incest. School performance also suffers in children with an unrevealed episode. Often a long period of building a trusting relationship with a physician is necessary before children reveal that they have been molested. In some centers, even in the ED, a therapeutic play session with anatomically accurate dolls has been extremely revealing.

ACUTE MANAGEMENT OF ABUSE

GOALS OF TREATMENT

Each ED should develop and have available for reference guidelines and procedures for personnel to follow when child abuse, neglect, or sexual abuse is suspected. A multidisciplinary approach to this problem, involving the primary physician, nursing personnel, social workers, and possibly consultant pediatricians or psychiatrists, can facilitate a comprehensive approach. The goals of acute management are threefold:

1. Identification and acute treatment of physical illness, injuries, malnutrition and psychologic sequelae in the child.
2. Protection of the child to ensure prevention of further injury or neglect.
3. Long-term psychosocial intervention to treat the pathologic family dynamics that led to abuse.

REPORTING OF ABUSE

When the history, physical examination, and laboratory assessment of the child's problem suggest abuse, neglect, or sexual abuse, the physician is morally as well as legally obligated to report the situation to the local community child welfare and/or law enforcement agencies. The physicians may be required to file a form or place a telephone call to provide the details of the situation. After receipt of such a report, the designated agencies will visit the home to investigate the circumstances of the injury or episode.

Parents must be told that a report of suspected child abuse and neglect is being filed. The physician, although uncomfortable in explaining his or her action to the parents, must convey his primary concern for the child's well-being, even if he or she wants to add that he or she is under a legal mandate to report. Following is a suggested explanation by the physician to the parents:

I'm sure you are good parents and want to do what is best for your Billy. I'm not sure how he could have sustained this injury from the accident you describe. We need to do some tests and will need help in gathering more information to ensure that Billy gets the best care. This report will set in motion a mechanism to help us to help Billy, and a social worker will visit you tomorrow. I'm sure this is upsetting to you, but I feel that with your help we can find out how he was injured and work out a good plan for you.

Often all the pertinent information is not available in the ED and will come to light later.

HOSPITALIZATION

Emergency hospitalization of the child may be necessary to treat injuries medically or to provide an interim safe environment while further investigations proceed. The following are situations in which hospitalization of the child should be considered:

1. When the injury is of a potentially serious nature, such as a fracture or head trauma.
2. When the child is too young to defend himself or run away, under 5 or 6 years old.
3. When the parents show no remorse, only anger, or persist in injuring the child.
4. When evidence suggests a repeated pattern of loss of impulse control by the parents and recurrent injuries.
5. When parents present evidence of social deviance in terms of severe isolation, drug or alcohol abuse, or any criminal behavior.
6. When the hostility and defensiveness of the parents appears to preclude the possibility of a positive intervention.

CONSULTATION

Rosenfeld and Newberger[4] have delineated the divergent approaches one must be prepared to take to effectively address the needs of a specific situation. Some parents benefit best from compassion, and others need external controls on their behavior. Consultation with one or more professionals experienced in child abuse in the acute situation can aid the decision-making process.

DOCUMENTATION

Chart documentation is essential. Studies have demonstrated that emergency physicians document the specifics of acute otitis media more completely than they do the specifics of a suspected case of child abuse. The child's explanation as well as that of the parents, should be recorded in exact words. Physical findings must be described as completely and accurately as possible and supported whenever possible by photographs. Direct observations of physical or behavioral action are more meaningful than overall impressions or conclusions. Handwriting must be legible. Dictated charts are preferable.

STAFF INTERVENTION

Just as the hospital staff of physicians, nurses, and social workers are expected to report merely their *sus-picions* of child abuse, they must be reminded that they see only a small fraction of the family dynamics. Regardless of the outcome of the investigations or legal proceedings on a single case, whether the child is returned to the home or placed in foster care, it is imperative that the staff realize they have performed an essential service for the community as well as for the child and family by recognizing abuse and intervening. Follow-up, often unemphasized, is important in protecting abused and neglected children.

SEXUAL ABUSE

Special problems in management of sexual abuse include the collection of evidence useful for legal procedures to prosecute the perpetrator. "Rape data collection kits" are available in most jurisdictions. Protocols to ensure proper collection, sealing, labeling, delivering, and processing of specimens of vagina secretions, saliva, rectal swabs, and pubic hairs should be established and made available. The reaction of a child to sexual molestation depends greatly on the reactions of his or her parents and other adults. Referral of all cases to the professionals at centers for treatment of victims of sexual abuse is desirable. If these centers are not available, close supervision, supportive counseling, and follow-up by a social worker are essential. Many children, even after a visit to such a crisis center, develop sleep disturbances, phobias, psychosomatic complaints, emotional regression, and personality changes, and feel anger, anxiety, sadness, guilt, and vulnerability. These changes are more severe in children whose episode of abuse was not reported immediately or who were victims of repeated episodes.

Treatment for possible gonorrheal infection must be given within 2 days after appropriate cultures are taken from children abused in a manner that could produce gonorrheal urethritis, vaginitis, proctitis, or pharyngitis. Standard Centers for Disease Control (CDC) recommendations or an equivalent should be followed. To prevent pregnancy, give two tablets of Ovral initially and repeat in 12 hours. (See Chap. 57.)

The management of incest requires the long-term intervention of mental health professionals experienced in family dynamics and often requires external motivation in the form of court-mandated services. The outcome is variable, but most families will remain intact. Effects on young female victims may not be resolved for decades.

COURT TESTIMONY

Occasionally, the emergency physician is called on to testify in a court proceeding regarding a case of child abuse, neglect, or sexual abuse. A well-documented record will help him or her remember details; he or she is expected to provide to the court a medical assessment of the injury and a medical assessment of the child's reactions. If the physician is designated as an "expert witness," he or she can also provide an interpretation, opinions, and impressions. He or she should provide the court with facts and avoid alignment with either the child, the family, or the state to maintain the value of his or her contributions to the proceedings.

A disturbing trend has been the surfacing of child abuse accusations in divorce proceedings and custody hearings. Such allegations can wreak havoc in the accused person's life and may, in fact, be a legal "tactic" of intimidation. Although protecting the child is the first concern, careful, impartial analysis of each case is essential.

Professionals in the courts, law enforcement and social service agencies, and medical fields all have some difficulty in dealing objectively with abused children and their families. Children's rights are being redefined and re-formed daily, and our expectations of parents' care for their children are being revised. As society recognizes that some parents need external assistance and restraints in their child rearing, mechanisms will be established to provide support for them before the tragic result appears in the ED. Until then, it is essential that the physician be willing to acknowledge, recognize, diagnose, and report any suspicion of child abuse to provide an access for constructive intervention on behalf of the child.

REFERENCES

1. Caffey, J.: Multiple fractures in long bones of infants suffering from subdural hematomas. AJR 56:163, 1946.
2. Kempe, C.H., Silverman, F.H., Steele, B.F., et al.: The battered child syndrome. JAMA 181:17, 1962.
3. Gil, D.G.: Violence Against Children: Physical Abuse in the U.S. Cambridge, Mass., Harvard University Press, 1970.
4. Rosenfeld, A.A., and Newberger, E.H.: Compassion and control: Conceptual and practical pitfalls in the broadened definition of child abuse. JAMA 237:2086, 1977.

BIBLIOGRAPHY

Ellerstein, N.S.(ed.): Child Abuse and Neglect: A Medical Reference. New York, John Wiley & Sons, Inc., 1981.
Green, F.C. (ed.): Incest and sexual abuse. Pediatric Annals S. No. 5, May 1979.
Helfer, R.E., and Kempe, C.H.: Child Abuse and Neglect: The Family and the Community. Cambridge, Mass., Ballinger Publishing Co., 1976.
Jellinek, M.S., et al.: Protecting severely abused and neglected children—An unkept promise. N. Engl. J. Med. 328:1628, 1990.
Ludwig, S.: Child abuse. In Fleisher, G., and Ludwig, S. (eds.): Textbook of Pediatric Emergency Medicine. Baltimore, Williams & Wilkins, 1983.
Newberger, E.(ed.): Child Abuse. Boston, Little, Brown, & Co., 1982.
Showers, T., Apolo, T., Thomas, J., and Beavers, S.: Fatal child abuse: A two-decade review. Pediatr. Emerg. Care 1:66, 1985.

OTHER PEDIATRIC EMERGENCIES: ASPHYXIATION, SUDDEN INFANT DEATH SYNDROME, AND HYPERPYREXIA

George R. Schwartz

CAPSULE

The pediatric emergencies discussed in this section are asphyxiation caused by food and foreign bodies, sudden infant death syndrome (SIDS), and hyperpyrexia.

FOOD AND FOREIGN BODY ASPHYXIATION

An analysis of data collected from 41 states over the years showed a total of 703 reported childhood deaths from asphyxiation. Food obstruction was the cause of 200 of these deaths. Nearly 89% occurred in children younger than 4 years. The age of highest risk is birth through 48 months, with a peak incidence at 12 months.

Foods involved have included nuts, seeds, hard candies, sausage-like meat products, raw carrots, peanut butter, and grapes. Prevention, of course, is of paramount importance. Some asphyxiations were associated with numbing anesthetics applied during teething. Because of their smoothness or shape, certain foods easily pass into the trachea (e.g., peanuts, grapes, seeds, hot dogs).

A choking infant should be placed upside down and given four measured blows with the heel of the hand between the shoulder blades. Then four chest compressions are delivered. If breathing is not subsequently regained, manual foreign body removal is attempted by forceps. The Heimlich maneuver can also be attempted. In most cases, foreign body obstruction can be managed by clearing the airway and using bag-valve-mask ventilation.

If obstruction persists, however; a cricothyrotomy may be needed. In small children, a simple 14-gauge needle can provide a sufficient lumen for respiration on a temporary basis. Jet insufflation can also be used as a temporary measure. (See section of this chapter on management of the pediatric airway.) In some cases of foreign body aspiration, the material is taken farther down the respiratory tract. The symptoms are at first reduced until pneumonia occurs, related to the obstruction, with wheezing and possible hyperresonance. If air is trapped, x ray on full inspiration and expiration may reveal the foreign body, which by this time requires endoscopic removal under anesthesia.

SUDDEN INFANT DEATH SYNDROME

Sudden infant death syndrome (SIDS) is the sudden and unexpected death of any infant or young child that is not explained by a thorough postmortem examination. As many as 7000 infants die of SIDS in the United States each year, with death usually occurring during sleep. Current therapy and pathologic findings in the brain suggest immaturity of the brain stem.

Clinical abnormalities that may be present before death include prolonged sleep apneas, frequent short apneas during sleep, excessive periodic breathing, hypoventilation, and a diminished ventilatory response to carbon dioxide accumulation. There appears to be a familial predisposition, so that a sibling of a child who suffered SIDS may be at greater risk. Although the incidence peaks in infants between 2 and 4 months, cases have been found, albeit rarely, at 12 months of age. Other risk factors include low birth weight, maternal smoking, maternal drug taking (particularly

opiates), and winter months. There is a higher incidence as well in multiple births and in boys.

The role of the emergency physician is to detect infants who may be at higher risk and to arrange for hospitalization with continuous monitoring for apnea and bradycardia. In some cases, respiratory syncitial virus (RSV) infection can also be accompanied by periods of apnea. The role of viruses in SIDS is unknown. In the hospital, EEG, ECG, electromyogram, and even transcutaneous oxygen monitoring can be used. Infants at risk for SIDS can be continuously monitored at home with an apnea and bradycardia monitor. If it is determined that an infant is at risk, the parents and guardians should be versed in pediatric CPR.

The most common situation that brings these children to the emergency facility is a parent's complaint that the child has stopped breathing or suddenly does not look well. Parents may describe frightening episodes in which they had to institute artificial ventilation or vigorous stimulation. After these episodes, the child in the Emergency Department (ED) usually appears lively and well. Such warning signs must not be overlooked, however.

A full neurologic examination should be done as well as tests to rule out pulmonary, cardiac, or CNS pathology. Sepsis may also be present with respiratory impairments, and if this is suspected, it must be evaluated through laboratory studies and blood cultures. Arterial blood gas values are not usually helpful unless they are taken shortly after an apneic episode—or during such a period. Previous reports suggested a possible elevated fetal hemoglobin as a risk factor, but this association could not be confirmed in subsequent tests (Zielke et al., 1989). Electrolytes should be checked, because low calcium and magnesium as well as high potassium levels can cause respiratory irregularities. Hypoglycemia may also produce a confusing clinical presentation. A toxicologic screen may be necessary if there is a possibility of accidental ingestion of drugs. Botulism is also a diagnosis that is often not considered because of its apparent rarity. Some authorities, however, believe that infant botulism is more common than generally appreciated—not only in children who have ingested honey. Once an apneic episode is documented, work-up should proceed in the hospital to rule out treatable causes.

Occasional concerns have surfaced regarding a connection between DPT immunization and SIDS. Multiple studies have not confirmed this suspicion.

If SIDS has occurred, the psychologic toll upon the parents is usually heavy, and they require much support and counseling. Most communities have a local chapter of the National Sudden Infant Death Foundation, and this support group can be valuable in helping parents cope with the sudden death of their child. In some instances later felt to be SIDS, parents have been accused of child abuse and brought to trial. Resuscitative measures that a parent may take on finding a child lifeless in bed can include rib fractures and shaking, the results of which can suggest child abuse.

Suitable investigations should be undertaken before accusations through the legal system.

Most important in emergency medicine is the sensitive detection of the infant at risk and instituting preventive measures.

The pathologic findings in suffocation and in sudden infant death syndrome (SIDS) are indistinguishable. When infants are found with their faces straight down there is a need to reassess the cause of death. Some deaths may be caused by rebreathing of expired gases, and there has been some increased concern recently about the safety of infant bedding, particularly polystyrene-filled cushions.

There have been previous observations that sleeping prone (face down) seems to increase the risk of SIDS. This face-down position, however, may in fact be causing the rebreathing and suffocation, which may be mistaken for SIDS.

Death from suffocation is certainly far more preventable and emergency medicine professionals can become involved with preventative education about avoidance of porous and polystyrene filled pillows and avoiding total face-down positioning.

CAVEATS AND CONSIDERATIONS REGARDING HYPERPYREXIA

Fever is not a disease, it is a symptom of disease process, usually respiratory, elsewhere in the body. Yet there are general considerations that can be isolated and discussed briefly.

First, take rectal temperatures. Particularly in the presence of tachypnea, oral temperatures can be misleading. Axillary temperatures can be erratic with environmental temperature changes.

In children between the ages of 3 and 24 months with a temperature over 39.4°C (103°F) hacteremia is present in approximately 5% of cases. As the temperature rises, however, the incidence of bacteremia also rises. Above 40.6°C (105°F), there is almost a 25% chance of finding bacteremia. Fever in infants younger than 8 weeks old is usually lower than 39.3°C, but bacteremia is more common and rapidly progressing fulminant sepsis is more frequent. There is no consensus of opinion regarding hospitalization criteria in infants 4 to 8 weeks old. Long-acting cephalosporin antibiotics (e.g., ceftriaxone intramuscularly, 50 mg/kg/day) have allowed some facilities to provide outpatient management with close follow-up and high cure rates.

High fevers are relatively frequently seen in children. Above 40.6°C (105°F), however, the incidence of serious, life-threatening disease increases markedly. Beware particularly of masked CNS infections, sepsis, poisoning with atropine or other anticholinergics, heat stroke, bulbar poliomyelitis, salicylate poisoning, or Waterhouse-Friderichsen syndrome.

A fever greater than 40.6°C (105°F) is unusual, and the underlying condition should not be left undiagnosed or untreated even if the fever abates with measures such as sponging, aspirin, etc. Viral conditions rarely result in such high fevers.

Periods of observation without intervention in such cases of uncommon temperature elevation can be dangerous, and early diagnosis is urgent. Waterhouse-Friderichsen's syndrome is associated with a mortality rate that increases markedly if left untreated for several hours. Similarly, early meningitis can progress rapidly and lead to convulsions and even status epilepticus.

Children who have undergone general anesthesia may be stricken with malignant hyperthermia, characterized by fever greater than 40.6°C (105°F), acidosis, muscle rigidity, and a greater than 50% mortality rate. It must be rapidly treated. Malignant hyperpyrexia has also been described in children who have not had anesthesia but who have a susceptibility related to pre-existent myopathy or neuropathy. Some success in treating this condition has been achieved using general measures to maintain respiration, external cooling, correction of electrolyte imbalances and acidosis, and the drug dantrolene (to prevent calcium release).

BIBLIOGRAPHY

Bonadio, W.A., Lehrmann, M., Hennes, H., et al.: Relationship of temperature pattern and serious bacterial infection in infants 4 to 8 weeks old 24 to 48 hours after antibiotic treatment. Ann. Emerg. Med. 20:1006, 1991.

Bosma, J.F.: Mechanisms of choking liability during transitional feeding. In Food and Choking in Young Children. Conference Proccedings, American Academy of Pediatrics, August 1983.

Dershewitz, R.A., Wigder, H.N., Wigder, C.M., and Nadelman, D.H.: A comparative study of the prevalence, outcome, and prediction of bacteremia in children. J. Pediatr. 103:352, 1983.

Food and Foreign Body Asphyxiation. FDA Drug Bulletin, Volume 14, Number 1, pp. 8–9, April 1984.

Kemp, J.S., and Thach, B.T.: Sudden death in infants sleeping on polystyrene-filled cushions. N. Engl. J. Med. 324:1858, 1991 (44 references).

Mittleman, R.E.: Examples of fatal choking in children. In Food and Choking in Young Children. Conference Proceedings. American Academy of Pediatrics, August 1983.

National Institute of Child Health and Human Development: Cooperative (epidemiological) study of SIDS risk factors. Pediatrics 79:598, 1987.

Oren, J., Kelly, D., and Shannon D.: Familial occurrence of sudden infant death syndrome and apnea of infancy. Pediatrics 80:355, 1987.

Rosenberg, N, Uranesich, P., and Cohen, S.: Incidence of serious infections in infants under age two months with fever. Pediatr. Emerg. Care 1:54, 1985.

Smialek, J.E., and Lambros, Z.: Investigation of sudden infant deaths. Pediatrician 15:191, 1988.

Teele, D.W., et al.: Bacteremia in febrile children under 2 years of age. J. Pediatr. *87*:227, 1975.

Welliver, R.C., and Ogra, P.L.: Respiratory syncytial virus. *In* Infectious Diseases. Edited by Gorbach, S.L., et al. Philadelphia, W.B. Saunders Co., 1992.

Zielke, H.R., et al.: Normal fetal hemoglobin levels in the sudden infant death syndrome. N. Engl. J. Med. *321*:1359, 1989.

DEHYDRATION, GASTROINTESTINAL, GENITOURINARY, HEMATOLOGIC, AND NEUROLOGIC EMERGENCIES

Garrett E. Bergman and Ellen B. Bishop

CAPSULE

This section discusses miscellaneous emergencies in children that have not been covered previously in this chapter. Included are dehydration, gastrointestinal and genitourinary emergencies, hematologic emergencies (idiopathic thrombocytopenic purpura, anemia, and sickle cell anemia), and neurologic emergencies (seizures, meningitis, and Reye's syndrome).

DEHYDRATION

In the normal state of homeostasis, there is a balance between intake and loss of water and electrolytes maintained by specific regulatory mechanisms. When losses exceed intake and the body is unable to compensate for these losses, the deficit that develops can produce serious consequences. Children are more prone to dehydration than adults for many reasons.

Excessive fluid losses from diarrhea, vomiting, or intestinal pooling compromise the small infant's intracellular and intravascular volumes sooner than in the older child or adult because of the following:

1. Insensible water losses are greater because of a greater surface area/body weight ratio in the infant.
2. The usual renal homeostatic mechanisms of acidifying and concentrating the urine are not yet fully developed, so there is less ability to compensate for alterations in fluid and electrolyte balance.

The more rapid development and progression of dehydration in children make its recognition and treatment critical because it is potentially a life-threatening emergency.

Most increased losses consist of hypotonic fluids; a relative excess deficit of water over electrolytes develops in the patient. The resulting state, however, depends not only on the quantity and quality of the losses but also on the nature of the concomitant intake. Boiled milk formula given to a baby with diarrhea is likely to cause a hypernatremic dehydration, whereas plain water (or other nonelectrolyte solution) replacement is likely to cause a hyponatremic dehydration.

The three types of dehydration differ in their pathogenesis, in the physical findings in the patient, and in the recommended treatment. By definition, isotonic dehydration is isonatremic, with serum sodium between 130 and 150 mEq/L; hypotonic (hyponatremic) if serum sodium is lower; and hypertonic (hypernatremic) if serum sodium is higher than 150 mEq/L.

To determine the magnitude and type of deficit a patient is suffering, the physician must know the duration of illness, the kind and amount of intake during this period, the nature and amount of abnormal losses, weight changes, the presence of any underlying renal, pulmonary, or central nervous system disease, and any drugs that were taken during this time. The amount of acute body weight loss is the best indication of the magnitude of the water losses. Beyond infancy, a 3% weight loss represents mild dehydration, 6% loss is considered moderate, and 9% or more severe. In infants, a larger percentage of the body weight is extracellular fluid, so a 5% weight loss would represent mild dehydration, 5 to 10% moderate dehydration, and above 10% severe dehydration.

In *isotonic* dehydration, losses of water are almost exclusively from the extracellular compartment with fairly well-maintained intracellular water. In *hypertonic* dehydration, there are approximately equal losses from both compartments; intracellular fluid shifts out of the cells to maintain the intravascular volume. In *hypotonic* dehydration, fluid shifts from the extracellular compartment (intravascular space) to the intracellular compartment, leading to poor maintenance of intravascular volume and the *earlier onset of shock*. Table 59-55 lists clinical findings of dehydration.

Therapy for dehydration consists of supplying the required maintenance fluids and electrolytes and correcting the deficits. Because of impending shock from volume depletion, it is often necessary to begin fluid replacement before the initial blood electrolyte determinations are completed. A solution containing 5% dextrose and 0.9% sodium chloride can be given as a bolus of 20 mL/kg over 15 minutes to reverse impending circulatory collapse. In all forms of dehydration, the fluid given after the initial bolus should contain sodium in a concentration between 0.3 and 0.9%, regardless of the patient's serum sodium, such a fluid will begin to correct the abnormality toward isonatremia. Under no circumstances should a child beyond the first day of life be given intravenous fluids that do not have sodium because seizures from water intoxication can quickly result. Various balanced salt solutions containing lactate, bicarbonate, and other electrolytes in addition to sodium chloride have been used effectively as initial therapy; potassium supplements should be withheld until renal function is demonstrated. Hyponatremic and isotonic dehydration can be easily corrected within 24 to 36 hours; hypernatremic dehydration is treated over a 2- to 3-day period because of the risk of convulsions if the serum sodium is decreased rapidly.

In milder cases, oral rehydration fluids, usually containing glucose and electrolytes, have been used widely. A rice-based electrolyte-containing solution has become available, with reports of improved fluid retention and decreased diarrhea (Pizarro et al., 1991).

GASTROINTESTINAL EMERGENCIES

One of the most common reasons for a child's visit to the Emergency Department (ED) is development of symptoms due to gastroenteritis. As already described, fluid loss may lead to significant dehydration earlier in the course of disease in infants than in older children and adults. In addition, home remedies for diarrhea and vomiting such as boiled milk, weak tea, and enemas do not meet the infant's needs for water and electrolytes and may accelerate the pathologic process. Most gastroenteritis in children is viral and needs no specific treatment. Diarrhea and vomiting without significant dehydration may be managed by restriction of oral intake to frequent small feedings of clear liquids for 24 to 36 hours, followed by a gradual return to the regular diet as tolerated. A prolonged clear-liquid diet may lead to the development of "starvation stools," which are green in color and watery in consistency. Diarrhea may also be caused by bacterial pathogens such as enteropathogenic Escherichia coli in young infants and Salmonella, Shigella, Campylobacter, and Yersinia in all age groups. High fever, blood and mucus in the stools, the characteristic green stools of Salmonella, and known exposure suggest to the physician that bacterial diarrhea may be present,

TABLE 59-55. EFFECTS OF TYPE OF DEHYDRATION ON PHYSICAL SIGNS

	Isonatremic Dehydration (Proportionate Loss of Water and Sodium)	Hyponatremic Dehydration (Loss of Sodium in Excess of Water)	Hypernatremic Dehydration (Loss of Water in Excess of Sodium)
*ECF Volume**	Markedly decreased	Severely decreased	Decreased
*ICF Volume**	Maintained	Increased	Decreased
Physical Signs			
Skin			
Color†	Gray	Gray	Gray
Temperature	Cold	Cold	Cold or hot
Turgor‡	Poor	Very poor	Fair
Feel	Dry	Clammy	Thickened, doughy
Mucous membrane	Dry	Slightly moist	Parched§
Eyeball	Sunken and soft	Sunken and soft	Sunken
Fontanelle	Sunken	Sunken	Sunken
Psyche	Lethargic	Coma	Hyperirritable
Pulse†	Rapid	Rapid	Moderately rapid
Blood pressure†	Low	Very low	Moderately low

* ECF = extracellular fluid; ICF = intracellular fluid.
† Signs of shock rather than of dehydration itself.
‡ Reflects magnitude of fluid loss from ECF.
§ Tongue often has shriveled appearance from loss of cellular fluid.
(From Behrman, R.E., and Vaughan, V.C.: Nelson Textbook of Pediatrics. 12th ed. Philadelphia, W.B. Saunders Co., 1983.)

and stool or rectal swab cultures should be obtained. A marked shift to the left in the white blood cell differential count and numerous polymorphonuclear leukocytes in the stained stool specimen would suggest enteroinvasive organisms. (See Food Poisoning, Chapter 86.)

Congenital anomalies such as atresia or stenosis of any part of the gastrointestinal tract will usually present with signs of obstruction early in the newborn period. Anomalies such as malrotation with volvulus or Hirschsprung's disease with toxic megacolon may present later in life. Pyloric stenosis evolves over the first few weeks of life to projectile, nonbilious vomiting. A pyloric "olive" may be palpable.

Idiopathic intussusception, usually seen in the second year of life, may be a cause of intermittent or sustained abdominal pain. Within 12 hours after the initial event, stools may appear like "currant jelly." A sausage-shaped mass may be felt in the right side of the abdomen. Barium enema may be therapeutic, reducing the intussusception with hydrostatic pressure. If barium enema is not successful, surgery should be performed without delay.

Gastroesophageal reflux is becoming a recognized cause of vomiting in young infants. Medical management consists of positioning the child upright after feedings, thickening feedings, and administering bethanechol, 8.7 mg/m²/day in three doses. Apneic episodes, recurrent pneumonia, and growth failure may be indications for more aggressive therapy.

PEDIATRIC APPENDICITIS

Appendicitis, still the most common childhood surgical emergency, shares a pathophysiology with the adult disease (Chap. 49). The natural history of the disease in children, however, is of far more rapid progression from obstruction to perforation. Also, the vague symptom complex is often masked in children. *Therefore all emergency physicians must assume that a child with abdominal pain or symptoms has appendicitis until proven otherwise.* If the disease is thoughtfully considered in all such children, failure to diagnose before perforation drops dramatically. Infants under 1 year have the highest perforation rate.

In addition to a careful history and a high degree of suspicion, a detailed and careful physical examination on all children with abdominal complaints is essential. Tenderness over McBurney's point is a cardinal finding, but far less common in children. The diagnostic value of a rectal examination in children cannot be overemphasized. In most patients, if a careful and reasoned approach to the rectal examination is followed, the pelvic rim can be swept easily with the finger and may reveal either point tenderness or fullness in the right lower quadrant. This examination should be done after explanation to the child and the parents, with a well lubricated glove, taking care to explain that the examiner's small finger is no larger in diameter than a normal bowel movement in the child. If such an examination is performed on all children with abdominal complaints, the examiner can obtain significant expertise in distinguishing the subtle findings of appendicitis on rectal examination. Look for vomiting, fever, irritability, diarrhea, and flexion of the thighs. Later there is abdominal distention.

The differential diagnosis includes acute mesenteric lymphadenitis, gastroenteritis, intussusception, UTI, Meckel's diverticulitis, Henoch-Schoenlein purpura, and other diseases.

Screening examinations should include a careful history and physical examination, a white blood cell count and differential, a urinalysis, and repeated physical examinations. The value of plain abdominal films is questionable, but often requested by the surgeon. The diagnosis can often be confirmed, when it is not clinically obvious, by barium enema.

URINARY TRACT INFECTIONS

Infants with urinary tract infection (UTI) frequently have no symptoms or signs except fever. There may be poor weight gain, poor feeding, vomiting, irritability, or jaundice. Diagnosis requires an uncontaminated urine specimen if a routinely collected specimen is highly suspicious. UTI presents significant diagnostic problems in children because symptoms are difficult to localize, particularly in infants and young children. There is a tendency to assume that UTI is a mild entity, but significant evidence suggests that most infections in infancy and up to 3 months involve the renal parenchyma. Older children may localize symptoms such as flank pain, dysuria, frequency, urgency, and suprapubic pain, but this is usually limited to school age children. In the preschool child and infant, these traditional symptoms are less frequently encountered. Instead, nonspecific fever, generalized abdominal pain, loose stools, enuresis, vomiting, failure to thrive, and poor feeding may all be symptoms. For these reasons, obtaining an adequate urine sample should be a part of the workup of any febrile child without localizing signs of disease within the infant or preschool age group. Uncircumcised male infants under 3 months have more frequent UTI.

The diagnosis of UTI is confirmed by obtaining an adequate urine sample. In school-age children, it is possible to obtain adequate samples by careful instructions to the child and the parent. Obtaining an uncontaminated urine specimen in the preschool child and infant represents a more difficult problem. Voided specimens obtained using a urine bag may be helpful at screening procedures, but result in extremely high false positive rates. In cases in which a UTI is suspected in an incontinent patient, the urine specimen should be obtained by suprapubic aspiration with a 22 gauge, 1½ needle or by catheter.

The two absolute criteria for a positive UTI are bacteria seen under the high-powered field examination, or growth of 100,000 csu/mL from the specimen. The presence of pyuria at a test for UTI is not sensitive, but in general, the presence of greater than 5 white blood cells per high-powered field in a catheterized or suprapubic specimen is considered presumptive evidence of UTI.

In afebrile patients over 3 months, outpatient therapy with sulfisoxazoles, amoxicillin, trimethoprim-sulfamethoxazole, or cephalosporins is acceptable, with a 10-day course recommended. The organism is Escherichia coli in 80 to 90% of cases. In mixed or complicated infections, Staphylococcus aureus may be involved. In children under 3 months, it is impossible to determine whether the child has upper or lower tract disease; therefore the assumption must be made of pyelonephritis. These children should be admitted for parenteral antibiotics including an aminoglycoside and ampicillin or another alternative. Similarly, in children with significant fever, regardless of age, upper tract disease must be assumed and the child should be admitted for initial management by parenteral antibiotics.

Radiographic evaluation of children with UTI has undergone significant change. Boys of any age and infants of both sexes should undergo radiographic evaluation by ultrasound or IVP as rapidly as feasible, to detect obstructive processes or underlying renal disease. Follow-up evaluation with voiding cystourethrogram is also recommended. Because younger children are most likely to have renal damage as a result of UTI, girls under 3 years with their first UTI should also have radiographic evaluation.

HEMATOLOGIC EMERGENCIES

Acute hemorrhage with circulatory collapse is clearly a life-threatening emergency. Treatment of impending shock by volume expansion must be instituted quickly. Most episodes of bleedings are not so dramatic but do require immediate care. Nosebleeds usually occur in normal children with trauma directly to the nasal mucosa during an upper respiratory infection or by their distal digit. If bleeding does not stop with local pressure, cauterization may be indicated. In all children with a bleeding problem, history should be obtained of previous episodes of bleeding and of anyone in the family with bleeding problems. Prothrombin time, partial thromboplastin time, and Ivy bleeding time screen for symptomatic congenital and acquired bleeding diatheses.

After volume replacement has been given to prevent or delay shock, 7 mL/kg of fresh, frozen, type-specific plasma can be given to correct any deficit of coagulation factors to safe levels. For soft tissue hematomas and hemarthroses in children with known deficiency of coagulation factors, specific preparations can be given according to the recommended schedules of administration outlined in Chapter 53.

IDIOPATHIC THROMBOCYTOPENIC PURPURA

Idiopathic (autoimmune) thrombocytopenic purpura is the most common cause of symptomatic thrombocytopenia seen in children. It is generally a well-tolerated, self-limited disease; most children recover spontaneously in a few months. The presentation is usually the acute development of cutaneous bleeding, petechiae, and ecchymosis, and often mucous membrane bleeding and epistaxis in an otherwise well child. Diagnosis is made by exclusion of other causes of thrombocytopenia, specifically drug or live virus vaccine exposure and marrow failure or replacement.

Most serious bleeding normally occurs in the first few days of the disease; corticosteroids may have a therapeutic role in the treatment of serious bleeding manifestations but are not indicated on a routine basis. Platelet transfusions are not effective because they too are affected by the circulating antibodies that cause the thrombocytopenia. Life-threatenting hemorrhage, such as intracranial bleeding is an indication for immediate splenectomy, which removes a major site of antibody production and the site at which "sensitized" platelets are removed from circulation. Most children demonstrate an immediate rise in platelet count postoperatively. Other forms of thrombocytopenia may respond well to platelet transfusions, 1 unit of platelet concentrate per 5 kg of body weight.

ANEMIA

The subacute development of anemia such as autoimmune hemolytic anemia, acute hemolysis in a G6PD-deficient patient, or an aplastic crisis in a child with any chronic hemolytic anemia (see discussion of sickle cell anemia) usually causes symptoms for a few days before high-output heart failure develops. With a more indolent progression of anemia, as can be seen in children who develop severe iron deficiency anemia, no change in activity level or physical condition may be noted until the child presents with heart failure or develops pneumonia or until the hemoglobin level falls below 3 to 4 g/dL. Rapid correction of severe anemia in a child can also precipitate heart failure as a result of fluid overload; partial exchange transfusion, administration of rapid-acting diuretics intravenously just prior to transfusion (furosemide, 1 mg/kg) and correcting anemia in stepwise fashion (up to 5 or 6 g/dL first day, 8 g/dL second day, 11 g/dL if necessary, on the third day) may prevent this complication. Except for volume replacement in acute hemorrhage, only cross-matched and prepared packed red blood cells should be used to treat anemia when transfusion is indicated. The volume of packed red blood cells to be given should be calculated by the following formula: $4 \times$ patient's weight (kg) $\times$ desired change in hemoglobin concentration. Generally, a transfusion is indicated in a self-limited anemia only to treat frank or incipient heart failure; it is rarely indicated in iron-deficiency anemia. In the presence of any anemia, an assessment of responsive reticulocytosis and a platelet and white blood cell count are indicated to rule out aplastic anemia.

SICKLE CELL ANEMIA

The patient with *sickle cell anemia*, whether homozygous (SS), hemoglobin S-C, or hemoglobin S-thalassemia, can present a life-threatening emergency in several ways. Specific organ involvement, such as pulmonary infection or infarction, or sudden large-vessel cerebrovascular occlusion can create problems of significant consequence. An unusual complication seen in young children and in pregnant women with sickle cell anemia is a sequestration crisis. For unknown reasons, the red blood cells suddenly become sequestered in the spleen or liver, causing severe anemia, massive splenomegaly (or hepatomegaly), and shock within minutes or a few hours. Immediate simple transfusion or exchange transfusion with nonsickling packed red blood cells is required.

Splenic hypofunction, even in the presence of palpable splenomegaly, can predispose a patient with sickle cell anemia to sudden overwhelming sepsis with all the associated complications. Streptococcus pneumoniae is most often involved; Staphylococcus, Hemophilus influenzae, and Salmonella may also be responsible. Fever and signs of infection in a child with sickle cell anemia must be considered potentially lethal, and antibiotics should be used with perhaps less restraint than in immunologically competent patients.

Sudden severe anemia with impending high-output heart failure can occur in patients with sickle cell disease from a hyperhemolytic crisis and from an aregenerative crisis; transient marrow failure can be associated with drugs, infection, or vitamin deficiency. These complications are usually short-lived and correctable; transfusion may be required. (See Chap. 53.)

NEUROLOGIC EMERGENCIES

SEIZURES

Although the causes of generalized seizures in children are varied, the commonest cause by far is the simple febrile convulsion caused by elevated body temperature. Characteristics of such benign generalized seizures are their association with extracranial febrile illness, occasionally familial incidence, peak occurrence between ages 6 months and 4 years (although children up to age 5 or 6 years can develop such a seizure), and a short duration, generally of less than 5 minutes. It is necessary to determine that the site of infection is not the central nervous system; many advocate routine examination of the cerebrospinal fluid in *all* children presenting with their first febrile convulsion, especially children under 18 months old when signs of meningitis are not reliable. Treatment, after the convulsion stops, consists of simply treating the underlying cause of fever, lowering the body temperature (acetaminophen and sponging with tepid water), and one intramuscular dose of phenobarbital, 5 to 10 mg/kg. Occasionally, children have a second short convulsion within 12 to 24 hours. An underlying convulsive disorder, precipitated by fever, should be suspected if the seizure lasts longer than 10 minutes, has any atypical features such as lateralizing signs, or is the third or fourth such episode. In all children who have a febrile convulsion, an electroencephalogram should be obtained at least 1 week after the seizure.

On the basis of these evaluations, daily maintenance anticonvulsant therapy may be necessary. Intermittent oral phenobarbital given to prevent a seizure concomitant with subsequent episodes of fever is not effective because therapeutic serum concentrations (10 to 30 mg/liter) are achieved only after several days or weeks of administration. It is important to stress that the normal child with an uncomplicated febrile convulsion has little likelihood of developing recurrent nonfebrile seizures or brain damage because parents may anticipate the worst.

Recurrent and nonfebrile seizures rarely present any life-threatening risk as long as certain precautions are observed. During the acute convulsive episode, an adequate airway must be maintained. Loosen the clothing around the child's neck, turn him on his side so that oral secretions can drain, minimize unnecessary stimulation, and give oxygen by mask if the convulsion is of long duration. Do not attempt to place any object in his mouth, even a plastic airway, because these may cause more local trauma and may obstruct the patient's breathing. The only other precaution necessary is to protect the patient from harming himself, as he might if he fell off the examining bed or litter. Oxygen administration by mask may be required in prolonged seizures.

STATUS EPILEPTICUS

Status epilepticus (SE) in children is defined as the presence of continuous seizures (grand mal, petit mal, or mixed) for 20 minutes or longer or the presence of refractory seizures so that clinical recovery between episodes is not evident. This entity, despite current therapy, may have a 10 to 15% mortality if not treated aggressively and appropriately.

Causes of status epilepticus include:

Primary seizure disorder
Neonatal seizures
Traumatic seizures
Subarachnoid hemorrhage
Hypoxic-ischemic seizures
Metabolic abnormalities, including:
1. Hypoglycemia
2. Hyponatremia
3. Hypernatremia
4. Hypocalcemia
5. Hypomagnesemia
Toxic ingestions
Febrile seizures (rarely)
Primary CNS infections

The general management of patients in SE includes aggressive control of the airway, which is *essential* to management. As indicated previously, rapid sequence intubation may be necessary. Basic life support, high-flow oxygen, and proper positioning are the first steps in prehospital care.

The choice of anticonvulsant agents in SE may be somewhat controversial and is under revision as new agents become available. Nonetheless, the best generally accepted knowledge concerning the use of anticonvulsants is reflected in Figure 59-32. The primary intent, following stabilization to the airway, is to ter-minate the seizures as rapidly as possible, because cellular ischemic changes begin within 10 to 15 minutes of the onset of continuous seizures.

Appropriate laboratory samples should be drawn for electrolyte, calcium, magnesium, and toxicologic studies. Standard therapy for potential metabolic and toxicologic problems should be undertaken, including Naloxone 0.1 mg/kg up to 2 mg IV and parenteral glucose. Glucose should be given according to the following guidelines:

1. Preterm infants D_{10} 2–4 mL/kg
2. Infants-3 years D_{25} 0.5–1.0 g/kg
3. Over 3 years D_{50} 0.5–1.0 g/kg

Anticonvulsants should be given as indicated in Figure 59–32.

In an occasional child, hypocalcemia, hypoglycemia, pyridoxine dependency, uremia, hypertension, or metabolic encephalopathy (Reye's syndrome, lead intoxication, electrolyte disturbance) can precipitate a generalized convulsion. These conditions may or may not be suggested by the clinical evaluation, and appropriate evaluations would be indicated.

MENINGITIS (SEE ALSO CHAP. 50)

Table 59-57 indicates organisms that are likely to be associated with different infections.

Meningitis can be a rapidly progressive infection

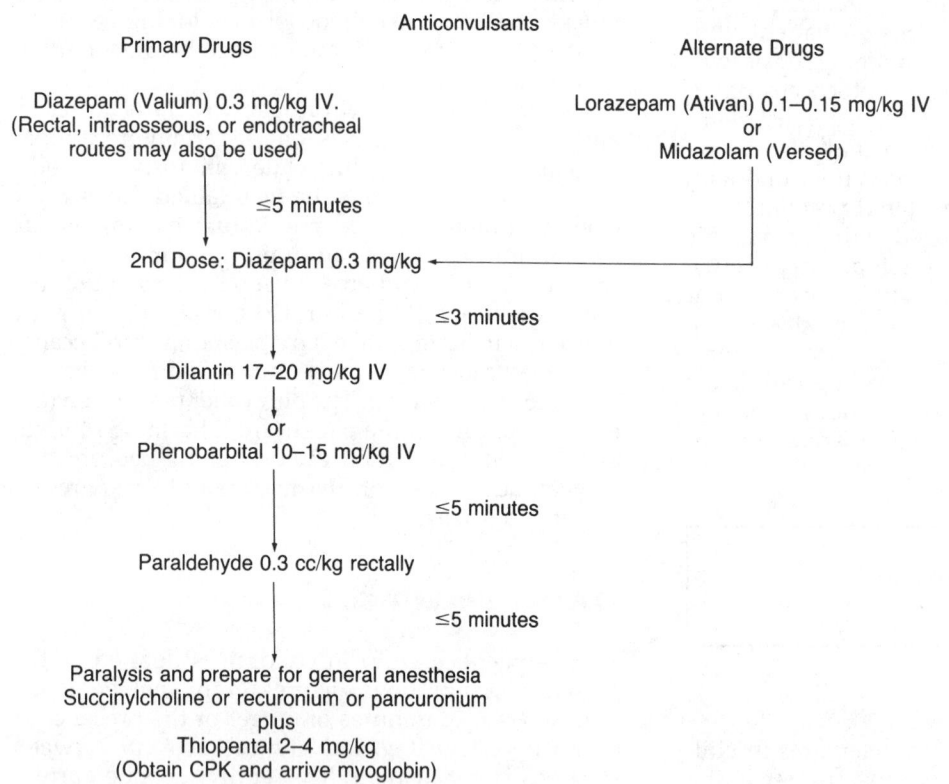

FIG. 59-32.   *Anticonvulsant use in status epilepticus.*

TABLE 59-56. CEREBROSPINAL FLUID FINDINGS

	Normal	Bacterial Meningitis	Viral Meningitis	Mycobacterial Meningitis	Brain Abscess	Subarachnoid Hemorrhage	Lead Encephalopathy
Appearance	Clear, colorless	Cloudy	Clear	Clear	May be clear or cloudy	Bloody, xantho-chromic	Clear
Opening pressure	70–180 mm. H$_2$O	Elevated	Normal to elevated	Elevated	Normal to elevated	Elevated	Elevated
White blood cells/mm^3	0–5 (0–10 in neonates)	500–40,000	5–2000 (usually less than 500)	50–500	Normal to elevated	Increase in proportion to red blood cells	Normal to elevated
Predominant cell type	Mononuclear	Polymorpho-nuclear	Mononuclear (polymorpho-nuclear early)	Mononuclear	Mononuclear	As in blood	Mononuclear
Glucose mg dL	Greater than 40 (⅔ serum glucose)	Low	Normal	Low	Normal	Low in proportion to white cells	Normal
Protein mg dL	Less than 40 (up to 100 in neonates)	Elevated	Elevated	Elevated	Elevated	Elevated	Elevated

causing death within hours of onset. In older children, presenting complaints of fever, headache, vomiting, and stiff neck are the same as in adults. The physician's index of suspicion must be raised significantly in young infants who may have nonlocalized, vague, nonspecific symptoms. Irritability, poor feeding, high-pitched cry, or "not acting right" may be the presenting symptom of an infant with meningitis. On physical examination, an older child may have classic signs of meningeal irritation present (Brudzinski's and Kernig's signs), whereas infants may have fever or hypothermia, irregular respirations, a staring expression, or a bulging fontanelle as the only clue that meningitis is present. The younger the child, the more liberal must be the criteria for performing a diagnostic lumbar puncture. One must accept a higher rate of negative lumbar punctures so as not to miss true cases of meningitis. Examination of cerebrospinal fluid must include cell count and differential, Gram stain, determination of sugar and protein content, and counterimmunoelectrophoresis, or later antigen agglutination, for suspected organisms. Streptococcus pneumoniae particularly may be present in the spinal fluid in large numbers before the expected neutrophil pleocytosis occurs. Table 59-56 summarizes cerebrospinal fluid findings of bacterial, viral, and mycobacterial meningitis as well as several other entities that must be differentiated from meningitis. If bacterial meningitis is suspected, treatment with intravenous antibiotics should begin in the ED. Table 59-57 indicates organisms that are likely to be associated with different infections. Neonates should have coverage for gram-negative organisms. If lumbar puncture results are equivocal and viral cause is suspected, benign results on a repeat lumbar puncture done 6 to 12 hours later may confirm that admission is unnecessary. It should be re-emphasized that early in the course of

TABLE 59-57. COMMON INFECTIOUS AGENTS

Infection	Age	Predominant Organism
Pneumonia	<2 years	Respiratory syncytial virus Haemophilus influenzae (Staphylococcus aureus) Pneumococcus
	>2 years	Pneumococcus Mycoplasma pneumoniae Viruses
Bacterial meningitis	Neonatal	Enteric organisms Group B Streptococcus
	>8 years	Haemophilus influenzae Pneumococcus (Neisseria meningitidis)
	8 years to adult	Neisseria meningitidis Pneumococcus
Otitis media	<8 years	Respiratory virus Pneumococcus Haemophilus influenzae
	>8 years	Pneumococcus Respiratory virus
Enteritis	<2 years	Virus Enteropathogenic Escherichia coli
	>2 years	Virus Salmonella sp. Shigella sp.

meningitis in children, symptoms can be vague. A high fever may be the only early sign, and the physician must evaluate it thoroughly to determine the site of infection. In unclear cases, CT scan can be used to assess the presence of structural causes. Evidence confirms that early dexamethasone administration (0.15 mg/kg every 6 hours) is beneficial in infants and children with bacterial meningitis.

TABLE 59-58. CLINICAL STAGING IN REYE'S SYNDROME

Stage 0:	Alert, wakeful (later development of evidence of encephalopathy)
Stage I:	Difficult to arouse, lethargic, sleepy, can obey commands
Stage II:	Delirious, combative, hyperreflexive, disoriented, responsive to noxious stimuli
Stage III:	Unarousable, predominantly flexor motor responses, decorticate
Stage IV:	Unarousable, predominantly extensor motor responses, decerebrate
Stage V:	Unarousable, flaccid paralysis, areflexia, pupils unresponsive, seizures

REYE'S SYNDROME

Reye's syndrome is fatty infiltration of the liver with encephalopathy and occurs primarily in children 1 to 16 years of age. History reveals a viral syndrome, usually either influenza or varicella, occurring 1 to 2 weeks before the onset of pernicious vomiting. The child becomes combative and delirious, and an altered sensorium may progress to coma. Recent controversial epidemiologic studies suggest that ingestion of aspirin or phenothiazines during the preceding viral illness may increase the risk of developing Reye's syndrome. Clinical staging (Table 59-58) helps determine therapy and predict outcome. Laboratory studies show hyperammonemia, elevated serum transaminases, prolonged prothrombin time and partial thromboplastin time, hypoglycemia, and unremarkable cerebrospinal fluid. Increased intracranial pressure can be treated in the ED with hyperventilation and intravenous mannitol (0.25 to 1.0 g/kg). Patients should be admitted to a pediatric intensive care unit, where monitoring of intracranial pressure can be carried out. Further therapy may include hypothermia, barbiturate coma, and continued osmotic diuresis to protect the brain from injury. With early recognition, good supportive care, and control of intracranial pressure, the mortality rate has decreased from 41% (1974) to under 20%. Children who present in advanced stages (e.g., stage V), however, still have a mortality rate of over 50%, and require early intubation, mannitol, diuretics, and vitamin K, as well as seizure control.

SELECTED READINGS

Alpert, J.J., and Reece, R. (eds.): Symposium on pediatric emergencies. Pediatr. Clin. North Am. 26:707, 1979.

Behrman, R.E., and Vaughan, V.C.: Nelson Textbook of Pediatrics. 12th ed. Philadelphia, W.B. Saunders Co., 1983.

De Nicola, L.K.: Reye's syndrome. In The Clinical practice of Emergency Medicine. Edited by Harwood-Nuss, A., et al. Philadelphia, J.B. Lippincott, 1991, p. 765.

Eichenwald, H.F.: Pneumonia syndromes in children. Hosp. Pract. Vol. 89, May 1976.

Field, M., et al.: Intestinal electrolyte transport and diarrheal disease. N. Engl. J. Med. 321:879, 1989.

Fleisher, G., and Ludwig, S. (eds.): Textbook of Pediatric Emergency Medicine. Baltimore, Williams and Wilkins, Co., 1983.

Graef, J.W., and Cone, T.E. (eds.): Manual of Pediatric Therapeutics. Boston, Little, Brown and Co., 1974.

Grosfeld, J.L. (ed.): Symposium on childhood trauma. Pediatr. Clin. North Am. 22:267, 1975.

Gruskin, A.B.: Fluid therapy in children. Urol. Clin. North Am. 3:277, 1976.

Herzog, L.W.: Urinary tract infections and circumcision. Am. J. Dis. Child. 143:348, 1989.

Hurwitz, E.S., Nelson, D.B., et al.: National surveillance for Reye's syndrome: A five year review. Pediatrics 70:895, 1982.

Leventhal, J.M.: Clinical predictors of pneumonia as a guide to ordering chest roentgenograms. Clin. Pediatr. 21:730, 1982.

McCarthy, P.L., Jekel, J.F., and Dolan, T.F.: Temperature greater than or equal to 40°C. in children less than 24 months of age: a prospective study. Pediatrics 59:663, 1977.

McCarthy, P.L., Sharpe, M.R., Spiesel, S.Z., et al.: Observation scales to identify serious illness in febrile children. Pediatrics 70:802, 1982.

McMillan, J.A., Stockman, J.A., and Oski, F.A.: The Whole Pediatrician Catalog: A Compendium of Clues to Diagnosis and Management. Vol. 3. Philadelphia, W.B. Saunders Co., 1982.

Odio, C.M., et al.: The beneficial effects of early dexamethasone administration in infants and children with bacterial meningitis. N. Engl. J. Med. 324:1525, 1991.

Orr, R.A., Dimand, R.J., Venkataraman, S.T., et al: Diazepam and intubation in emergency treatment of seizures in children. Ann. Emerg. Med. 20:1009, 1991.

Pizarro, D., et al.: Rice-based oral electrolyte solutions for the management of infantile diarrhea. N. Engl. J. Med. 324:517, 1991.

Rowe, D.S.: Acute suppurative otitis media. Pediatrics 56:285, 1975.

Scheuer, M.L., and Pedley, T.A.: The evaluation and treatment of seizures. N. Engl. J. Med. 323:1468, 1990.

Smith, C.A. (ed.): The Critically Ill Child—Diagnosis and Management. 2nd ed. Philadelphia, W.B. Saunders Co., 1977.

Telford, G.L., and London, R.E.: Appendicitis. In Infectious diseases. Edited by Gorbach, S.L., et al. Philadelphia, W.B. Saunders Co., 1992.

Wolf, S.M., et al.: The value of phenobarbital in the child who has had a single febrile seizure: a controlled prospective study. Pediatrics 59:378, 1977.

Wright, F.H., and Beem, M.O.: Diagnosis and treatment: management of acute viral bronchiolitis in infancy. Pediatrics 35:334, 1965.

Part VIII

Geriatric Emergencies

Chapter 60

GERIATRIC EMERGENCY MEDICINE

GENERAL CONSIDERATIONS

George R. Schwartz

CAPSULE

Our older population represents a substantial (12%) and ever-increasing portion of the patients who present in emergency departments (EDs). Even in 1976, elderly patients used one third of hospital beds and almost one third of each health care dollar.[1] This number has now increased and is closer to 40%. Sensitivity to the problems and needs of older people is vital as we witness an increasingly vigorous longevity and the general aging of our population. It is amazing that emergency medical units are still often planned without the elderly as a prime consideration despite the projections that within 50 years one of every five persons will be over 65. Even now, more than 11% of the population is 65 or older, up from 4% in 1900. Of the 65 and older group, those aged 75 or older rose from 29% in 1900 to 38% in 1970; it is expected to reach over 40% by the year 2000.[2]

Care of elderly patients in the ED requires changes in emphasis. A particular pitfall is focusing too closely on the patient's presenting problem without exercising sufficient vigilance in identifying possible underlying conditions, both social and medical, that may have caused the acute medical problem or injury. Elderly persons in particular require this type of attention. For example, falls are a major source of morbidity and mortality in the elderly and often have treatable causes, both medical (e.g., underlying diseases) and environmental (e.g., clothing, rugs, poor lighting, etc.)[3]

As with persons of any age group, elderly individuals frequently need active medical intervention that must be based on limited information. Life-saving actions might have to be taken even before a patient's identity is known: bleeding stopped, shock treated, fractures diagnosed and splinted, respiratory arrests or obstructions immediately alleviated, and lacerations sutured. Often the patient is not known by the staff, and there is little history on which to proceed, but prompt medical decisions must be made with attention to the known physiologic differences and response to trauma.

For a physician to stop treatment after the life-threatening problem has been controlled, however, or the obvious presenting symptom cared for, is to lose a substantial opportunity to evaluate problems that may have precipitated the accident or illness. Such considerations often directly influence the responses to treatment. Nutrition, drugs, and underlying medical problems are important factors in the development of emergency medical problems and are discussed in the sections that follow.

FOOD AND NUTRITION

Many older people live alone and are on fixed, low incomes. Loneliness, decreased sensitivity to taste, physical infirmity, and decreased vision all act to reduce the motivation to shop for fresh food items. Thus, there is a tendency to rely on processed foods and food that will keep on the shelf. Numerous studies have demonstrated that elderly patients frequently consume less than the minimum daily requirement of most vitamins. In addition, malabsorption can cause or compound nutritional deficiencies. Poor dentition reduces mastication, and frequent hypochlorhydria, as well as decreased intestinal secretions, further tend to reduce absorption.[4] Additionally, many processed and prepackaged foods have sufficient doses of monosodium glutamate (MSG) to produce or add to symptoms of dizziness, edema, and depression.

The use of supplemental vitamins does not solve

what is usually an overall problem with diet, not just insufficient intake of vitamins. Overall nutritional inadequacy is more prevalent than is usually appreciated. Vitamin deficiencies may cause weakness and a tendency to be accident-prone. In fact, there is a likelihood that we are not diagnosing underlying nutritional conditions by recognizing early presenting symptoms. Symptoms of early niacin deficiency, for example, include incapacity for mental and physical effort, loss of appetite, poor sleeping patterns, dizziness, syncope, paresthesias, palpitations, and depression. These symptoms appear well before the classic symptoms of diarrhea, dermatitis, and dementia. Also, mental changes caused by vitamin B_2 deficiency may appear before anemia.

Early scurvy represents another example of vitamin insufficiency. Vitamin C in food deteriorates when the food is kept for a prolonged time, stored without refrigeration, or exposed to light. Scurvy does not just suddenly appear; there is a slow and insidious progression of subtle signs and symptoms before the classic clinical manifestations occur. Infection or other stress may precipitate rapid development of signs and symptoms.

Common symptoms in early scurvy include joint pains, stiffness and pain with motion, unsteadiness of gait, and signs of confusion. Later, of course, there are problems of bleeding gums, skin changes, hair changes, overall depression and lassitude, and eventually death. The point, again, is not to promote supplemental vitamin use, but to emphasize that emergency problems in the elderly can appear against a background that may include nutritional inadequacy.

Another example of vitamin insufficiency may be seen in older people who have intermittently used alcohol to excess. When seen in an ED, these individuals might not have used alcohol for weeks; however, a chronic thiamine deficiency might cause or aggravate dizziness, memory lapses, or syncope, which could be related to the acute problem.

Poor nutrition over a period of months can lead to anemia with confusion and weakness.[5] In addition, osteoporosis is a frequently encountered problem that may lead to an increase in fractures. Hip fractures in women are particularly serious in mortality and morbidity and may be reduced through diet and estrogens.[6]

PHYSIOLOGIC CONSIDERATIONS

Clinically, evaluation of elderly persons is affected by the "normal" changes of aging. Studies, however, have shown that there are no changes in hemoglobin and hematocrit and few changes in fasting blood glucose, serum electrolyte concentration, and blood gas values in the absence of disease. There are age-related functional reduction in renal, pulmonary, and immune functions as well as reduced ability to maintain homeostasis after trauma. Suffice it to say, however, that physiologic changes should not be ascribed to "normal aging" until a thorough investigation or suitable referral is made.

MEDICATION PROBLEMS

It is not always possible to obtain a detailed history of medications that the patient is taking, but it may be these medications that have caused acute injury. Examples of such medications are phenothiazines, diuretics (with inadequate potassium replacement), tranquilizers, and antihypertensive medications (which can cause orthostatic hypotension). Falls may also be associated with weakness caused by anorexia or dehydration. Syncope may result from digitalis or diuretic use. In addition, drug interactions with nutritional factors are just beginning to be understood. Isoniazid-type drugs can result in symptoms of vitamin B_6 deficiency, Dilantin can precipitate folic acid deficiency anemia, and colchicine may reduce vitamin B_{12} absorption.

Older people tend to suffer from degenerative disorders, are more susceptible to various diseases, and frequently are taking several medications. Confusion, vision impairment, and forgetfulness can add to a medication problem.

About 3% of all hospital admissions are related to drug-induced illnesses. Of the drugs implicated in adverse reactions by Caranosus and colleagues,[7] four led the list and accounted for 75% of these problems: aspirin, digoxin, coumarin, and diuretics. Of hospital admissions for drug reaction, more than 35 to 40% are usually for people over 60.

It is also possible that reactions to medications are more easily overlooked in elderly persons because of the overall increase in medical disorders in this age group and the common habit of ascribing unclassifiable symptoms to aging in general.

Thus, a general principle of geriatric medicine as practiced in the ED is to be highly aware of medication problems as a cause of disease. In prescribing any medications, those with the fewest side effects should be given priority. In addition, if family members or friends are available, they should be made aware of the treatment plans.

Absorption dynamics and renal and hepatic metabolism may be impaired in elderly persons, leading to decreased excretion and metabolism. Drug distribution is altered because of changes in body composition (lean mass decreases, fat increases), and plasma binding through lowered albumin may cause increased free-drug actions. Thus, the concept of "standard doses" has to be re-evaluated, and doses must be more individualized for people over the age of 60.

A fall, resulting in lacerations or other injuries, may be caused by syncope caused by cardiac disease or various drugs (e.g., antihypertensives, vasodilators, tranquilizers, antiarrhythmic agents, antidepressants, aminophylline, beta-adrenergic agents, nitroglycerin, calcium antagonists) that can also cause syncope.

In an emergency department geriatric practice, overall emphasis has to be on detecting treatable problems or disorders that may underlie the acute presenting symptoms.

SYMPTOMS IN THE ELDERLY

Although a usual approach is to focus on diagnosis, it is worthwhile to consider overlooked diagnoses to alert the emergency practitioner to frequently unrecognized disorders. One such study[8] points out the need to evaluate for anemia, tuberculosis, and thyroid disease with myxedema coma and sensory alterations. Most cases of myxedema coma are in patients over 70. Also, psychiatric conditions may often be undiagnosed, particularly depressive states. The possibility of AIDS should not be overlooked. It may present a confusing clinical picture, with dementia and pneumonia as well as malignancies. Cases in the elderly usually result from blood transfusions (generally from transfusions before 1985, when blood bank testing was instituted), although sexual transmission is also possible.

Experienced clinicians recognize atypical presentations as being common in elderly persons (e.g., painless myocardial infarction, sepsis without fever, asymptomatic bacteriuria, or pneumonia presenting as confusion). Thyrotoxicosis in the elderly often presents not as a hyperkinetic syndrome but as a nonspecific clinical picture with weight loss, constipation, apathy, and other mental changes. Another example is hyponatremia, probably caused by oversecretion of antidiuretic hormone. This syndrome can cause marked mental status changes and is much more common in elderly individuals.

Appendicitis in the elderly may also present with fewer localized symptoms, and fever response can be diminished. Even when symptom presentation is completely typical, there is still a faster progression of the disease to perforation and peritonitis. Reported perforation rates range from 32 to 77%.[9] There is a mortality rate of 23% in patients over 80.[10]

The significance of these observations from an emergency medicine standpoint is that the index of suspicion must be higher and use of observation more liberal if we are to reduce mortality and morbidity in the elderly patient.

A further important consideration must be "sleep apnea," which can result in life-threatening cardiovascular and respiratory disorders.[11] This condition, present to some extent in one third of all elderly persons, is another reason to exercise particular care with medications.

DEMENTIA IN THE ELDERLY

Dementia is a commonly encountered symptom in the elderly, ascribed frequently to changes of aging. The purpose of an emergency evaluation of a demented elderly patient, however, is foremost to determine if there is a treatable or reversible cause. The neurologist undertakes a detailed and comprehensive evaluation to define prognosis, limitations, and need for assistance. These can be useful for the patient and family, but the role of the emergency physician is to determine if there are treatable conditions. Such conditions can be related to either overall systemic disease or specific neurologic causes.

For example, some metabolic or endocrine disorders, such as Addison's disease or hypothyroidism, can present with marked mental changes. Electrolyte abnormalities, such as low serum sodium, can produce markedly abnormal mental functioning. Nutritional causes include vitamin deficiencies, which should be particularly suggested if there is a prior history of alcoholism. In such cases, thiamine deficiency is far more common. Pernicious anemia, associated with inadequate vitamin B_{12}, can produce marked nervous system impairment, even without anemia or other characteristic signs. Usually there are paresthesias to help in the diagnosis.

Situations of pre-existing dementia may also be markedly worsened through various disease states. Through correction of such states, the individual's mental function may improve substantially. For example, hypoxia associated with chronic pulmonary disease, or in some cases, either hypercarbia associated with pulmonary disease or neurodegenerative disease, such as ALS with respiratory impairment, can result in inadequate pulmonary exchange with cerebral changes. Similarly, cardiac disease can lead to a decrease in cerebral blood flow, particularly when the patient is hypotensive. Chronic congestive heart failure with pulmonary edema can cause marked impairment of central nervous system (CNS) functioning, as may other conditions with arrhythmias which result in decreased blood flow to the brain. Bradyarrhythmias, or tachyarrhythmias such as atrial fibrillation with rapid ventricular response, can result in markedly diminished blood flow. In such cases, cardiac impairment, if present, must be corrected before the CNS can be fully evaluated. Occasionally, a severe depression can lead to worsening of a chronic dementia or result in a confusional state. The patient may present with profound apathy and withdrawal.

The principles of geriatric emergency medicine state that there are frequently multiple causes in the elderly patient. For example, an older person may have some CNS degeneration along with effects from cardiac causes, pulmonary causes, occasionally medications, or even infection. Thus, ascribing a condition to a single cause without carefully investigating the possibility of other causes, can lead to a partial or incomplete diagnosis. Dementia, for example, can also occur after trauma associated with hydrocephalus or subdural hematoma. These may present with nonspecific findings. Chronic infections may also provide nonspecific symptoms and may be diagnosed as a degenerative CNS disease. In such cases, one might miss a chronic fungus infection that is highly treatable. In addition, CNS tuberculosis, rising with the AIDS epidemic, is increasing. In this context, always be aware of the possibility that AIDS may be a possible cause of dementia.

In the ED, toxic causes should always be evaluated, whether the mental status change is caused by medication overdose, which could be deliberate or accidental, or a toxic substance in the environment, which may be highly treatable. For example, in one ED, repeated visits by an elderly person with confusion was not diagnosed as carbon monoxide poisoning associated with a faulty heater until the third return visit. In cases when this may be suspected, a carboxyhemoglobin level can be useful.

Benzodiazepines such as Halcion (triazolom) and Versed can produce confusion, memory loss, and even amnesia at "therapeutic" doses. Sleeping medications, widely used in nursing homes, can produce "pseudodementia."

DIAGNOSTIC CONSIDERATIONS

A study of diagnoses in people over 60 in one ED over a 6-month period is presented in Table 60-1. A comparison with the most common diagnoses in general practice (Table 60-2) shows the tremendous difference in the nature of conditions seen on an emergency basis from those treated in general office practice. For example, hypertension was the basis for 15% of visits in one large study; however, it was involved on an emergency basis with less than 2% of ED admissions. On the other hand, pulmonary and respiratory symptoms accounted for 2% or less of office visits. Putting all respiratory tract diagnoses together, there are 65 of 517 or 13%. When bronchitis, influenza, and upper respiratory infections (URIs) are added to this total, almost 17% of the emergency diagnoses refer to disorders within the respiratory system.

Particularly important are aspirations, which may occur chronically in the debilitated elderly.[11a] Predisposing factors are neurologic disorders that alter gag reflex, strokes, chronic conditions such as Parkinson's disease, swallowing disorders, and sedative and hypnotic medications. The result may be chronic bronchitis, unexplained recurrent pneumonia, sudden total or partial airway obstruction, or sudden onset of

TABLE 60-1. EMERGENCY DEPARTMENT DIAGNOSES IN PATIENTS OVER 60: 6-MONTH RETROSPECTIVE COMPILATION

Diagnosis	No. of Patients
Abdominal pain	24
Alzheimer's disease, dementia, confusion	12
Anal or rectal hemorrhoids (nonbleeding)	3
Anemia	11
Arrhythmia	14
Asthma	7
Back pain	7
Bronchitis	10
Cancer complications	6
Cardiopulmonary arrest	2
Chest pain (myocardial infarction)	11
R/O (myocardial infarction)	46
Angina	18
Chronic obstructive pulmonary disease	9
Congestive heart failure (CHF)	33
Diabetes mellitus	13
Diverticulitis	5
Dizziness/weakness	6
Drug overdose	2
Electrolyte imbalance/dehydration	21
Epididymitis or prostatitis	4
Fever (to be worked up)	6
Gallbladder (specific diagnosis)	5
Gastroenteritis	6
Gastrointestinal bleeding	10
Hypertension	8
Influenza	6
Infection, soft tissue	6
Intestinal obstruction	10
Liver disease	2
Musculoskeletal pain	6
Parkinson's disease	6
Pleural effusion	4
Pneumonia	40
Pyelonephritis/urinary tract infection	9
Pulmonary edema	5
Pulmonary embolus	3
Psychiatric diagnosis	4
Renal impairment	3
Renal stone/colic	5
Respiratory failure	4
Rheumatic heart disease	3
Sepsis or R/O	12
Stroke	16
Syncope	9
Trauma	43
Ulcer	4
Urinary retention	4
Upper respiratory infection	5
Vomiting	3
Miscellaneous (dermatologic, neurologic, zoster, etc.)	8
Total	519

TABLE 60-2. MOST COMMON DIAGNOSES IN THE ELDERLY (65 YEARS AND OVER)

U.S. California Study (1977)	% of all Diagnoses	Wisconsin Study (1978)	% of all Diagnoses
Hypertension	15.1	All cardiovascular disorders	14.4
Ischemic heart disease	9.8	Hypertension	8.9
General medical examination	8.1	Diabetes	5.5
Degenerative joint disease	6.5	Arthritis of all types	4.8
Diabetes	5.0	General medical examinations	3.1
Depression/anxiety	2.9	Surgical aftercare	2.8
Soft tissue injuries	2.3	Neuroses, etc.	2.0
Urinary tract infection	2.2	Obesity	1.8
Emphysema	2.0	Emphysema	1.3
Acute upper respiratory infection	1.9	Cerebrovascular disorders	1.3
Fractures/dislocations	1.5		
Acute sprains/strains	1.3		
Dermatitis/eczema	1.2		
Acute lower respiratory infections	1.0		
Bursitis, etc.	1.0		
Total	61.8%	Total	45.9%

bronchopneumonia. Lipid substances such as oil-based laxatives can cause severe pneumonitis. Sudden unexplained asthma or wheezing or chronic unexplained cough or bronchitis may provide a clue to the aspiration syndrome.

POST-EMERGENCY DEPARTMENT CARE

Elderly patients often need post-treatment care that may require wheelchairs, aids, special diets, physical therapists, or medical-surgical devices. Return for care by a primary physician may be delayed in a patient with such immediate needs. Emergency units that serve older patients must have resource information and personnel to arrange for the special care for the patient (e.g., home care, visiting nurses). Such care is often available, at least on a short-term basis, but requires experienced personnel to circumnavigate what is, to the uninitiated, a bewildering maze of bureaucracy.

HOME HEALTH CARE

The emphasis in the provision of health care to the elderly must be on maintaining functional capability. In the rush to diagnose and "work up" some conditions, this goal is occasionally forgotten. A prolonged hospitalization

and subsequent intermediate care facility stay for an elderly person may render him or her unable to return home. The defects in home health care add to this dilemma. These latter issues are in the early stages of review through the U.S. Congress,[12] but currently there are marked deficiencies in our ability to offer home care after an acute episode.

A review of Table 60-1 shows many groups seen in emergency facilities who could benefit from long-term home health care (e.g., those with Parkinson's disease, Alzheimer's disease and other states of dementia, stroke victims, and some of those disabled from trauma). At least 15 to 20% of those seen in emergency facilities would benefit from home health care. Katz and his colleagues[13] demonstrated that, for independent people between 65 and 69 years living in a community, the total life expectancy was 16.5 years, but, for 6.5 of these years, the elderly person required assistance because of substantial major functional impairment. After age 85, 60% of patients in the remaining years require substantial assistance.

An important issue for emergency health workers is to help provide medical and social care to maximize independent life. Sometimes, a small intervention (e.g., restoring electrolyte balance or helping to provide a visiting nurse) can result in major functional improvement. As our aging population gains more political power, we will see an increase in our ability as health care providers to offer needed home care services.

We are seeing not only an increase in the longevity of our population, but an increase in elderly citizens who are vocal and politically active. Aided by the substantial financial base of many pensioners, organizations of senior citizens and retired people are exerting unprecedented political and economic power.

NURSING HOME CARE

It can be useful for EDs to establish links with nursing homes in the community. Such relationships allow easier evaluation and management of medical problems that develop in nursing home residents. In addition, with our increasing elderly population, the use of nursing homes has increased. Estimates based on current projections indicate that, for people who have become 65 in 1990, approximately 43% will enter a nursing home before they die. Of these who enter nursing homes, more than half will be using such facilities for more than one year.[14]

The implications of this trend for emergency medicine includes increasing referrals from nursing homes and concomitantly discharging treated patients back to their nursing home facilities.

As was pointed out by Kane and Kane,[15] seeing these trends should encourage us to prompt a re-examination of the entire system of long-term care and exploring creative approaches for possible alternatives. Because medical care is frequently the determining factor in nursing home versus home health care, emergency physicians can assist in community development of options through enhancing available medical care for the elderly.

GERIATRIC EVALUATION UNITS

With the complex array of social factors, physical impairments, nutritional considerations, polymedications, an increased need for rehabilitation and follow-up care, a specialized focus on older patients is needed. Such an approach is demonstrably superior.

The patients in one geriatric evaluation unit had markedly lower mortality and were less likely to be in a nursing home after hospitalization. Moreover, the control group patients underwent substantially more acute hospitalization. Mental improvement in the geriatric units was superior, as was functional status.[16–18]

The results from this randomized trial of effectiveness were so conclusive that the geriatric evaluation unit should be considered a superior manner of caring for our acutely ill elderly and, overall, a financially responsible method for so doing. Initial investment in personnel, facilities, and equipment "pays off" in overall savings.

The problem arises when federal Medicare, which pays for the hospitalization, cannot provide the financial assistance to reduce hospitalization in the future. The development of health maintenance organizations (HMOs) is one answer to this dilemma,

although strong profit motives have put this into question. Long-term solutions are probably governmental and political.

Although the advances in geriatric evaluation units have primarily been in patient facilities with intensive multidisciplinary efforts, the following basic lessons can be applied to emergency facilities.

1. Impaired elderly patients can respond dramatically to treatment.
2. Specific attention to problems peculiar to, or found more frequently in, elderly populations is the simplest and least expensive approach (e.g., nutrition, physical therapy and rehabilitation, polypharmacy, social and living conditions).
3. The first step in focusing on such problems requires a basic checklist to be used with all patients over 65 that can be readily implemented in an ED. Such a checklist could uncover areas of need that can be addressed by home health care services, visiting nurses, and senior centers. For example:
   Living conditions
   Meals, nutrition
   Sensory changes (e.g., eyes, ears, touch)
   Medications—total (i.e., over-the-counter, herbal cures, and related types)
   Past medication problems (e.g., falls, dizziness, low potassium)
   Husband's or wife's health (If not living, when did he or she die?)
   Presence of depression or sleep disorders
   Home care needed

This is not meant to substitute for a regular history and physical examination. It is an attempt to highlight particular, often overlooked areas.

THE VERY OLD

The human life span is close to 115 years, although it is still extremely rare to find a person older than 105. As the geriatric population increases, there must be clearer distinctions between disease and disability—that is, some disease conditions (e.g., arthritis) account for much more disability than others (e.g., chronic lung disease or high blood pressure).

One study evaluated disability[19] and discovered that arthritis and rheumatism accounted for 34% of the total disability, followed by stroke, visual impairment, heart disease, and dementia.

The continued focus of geriatric emergency medicine is to learn to treat the acute disease or acute manifestation of a chronic disease process with concern for minimizing the concurrent disability. This is most relevant with the very old, who may have a diagnostic listing of many diseases, of which only one results in substantial disability.

We have tended to consider the field of geriatrics as a whole rather than paying attention to the special problems of each subgroup. Clear delineations such as neonate, adolescent, etc., which are found in the field of pediatrics, are not readily forthcoming in the older population. As the geriatric population becomes larger and the old and very old are studied more closely, it is likely that we will see clearer physiologic subgroups.

ETHICAL CONSIDERATIONS

Already there are many new concerns in treating the very old, ranging from the philosophic (what is human) to more specific concerns about quality of life.[20] For example, the heightened concerns about "dying with dignity" relate to the advent of machines and procedures for sustaining organs and prolonging life. This increases the pressure felt by physicians and caregivers, whose rule must be fervently prolife. One actual case illustrates what can happen when this orientation is not maintained.

An 81-year-old man was brought into the hospital after being discovered comatose at home. He had been depressed and living alone and had a history of cirrhosis and hypertension. On physical examination, he had no response to pain and showed persistent hypotension with dilated, nonreactive pupils. His respirations were poor, and he needed ventilatory support. The working diagnosis was "acute stroke," with the mechanism being central nervous system bleeding. When he did not improve and, in fact, deteriorated after 12 hours, the family was advised of his serious preterminal state. The decision was made to follow his wishes—that his life not be prolonged through extraordinary means. He was disconnected from his life support systems after a little more than 12 hours of hospitalization so that he could die with dignity. Subsequently, a blood test revealed toxic levels of Doriden. In the rush to assist the elderly in dying, the presence of treatable acute problems can be overlooked. The pressures of prepaid health plans and competition for resources such as hospitals and nursing homes have added to this dilemma.[21]

On the other hand, there is a rational time to withhold treatment in some cases, particularly when the decision has been made well before the acute episode. For example, a 74-year-old man with rapidly progressive amyotrophic lateral sclerosis, weighing less than 90 pounds, reached the point where he could move only his eyes. While on board an airplane, he stopped breathing shortly after he had been given supplemental oxygen in an effort to improve his comfort. His respiratory arrest was probably caused by the fact that his oxygen level was suddenly raised in the presence of long-standing hypercarbia and hypoxia. This caused a loss of his hypoxic stimulus to respiration.

Few, if any, could argue that intubation, ventilation, and tracheostomy would have been suitable at that time. There, indeed, comes a time to die.

The decision to withhold possible life-saving treatment (e.g., intravenous fluids, ventilators, adrenaline, cardiopulmonary resuscitation) is difficult to make in the emergency setting. In almost all cases, treatment should be given to avoid making the more serious error of not acting, which can result in the patient's death; after treatment, the patient's status can be reviewed. (See Chap. 5.)

In the field of geriatric medicine, the number of issues concerning biomedical ethics has grown rapidly. Analysis of ethical dilemmas, however, requires factual data, clarity, and examination of motives and consequences in addition to application of established rules and principles.

With this level of complexity, the acute care physician or nurse is rarely in any position to assess such issues adequately unless the situation has been previously reviewed and a decision made.[22]

"The geriatric demographic imperative," as described by gerontologist John Rowe, is leading to increasing attention to the myriad problems of the aging population. This includes not only needed research and treatments but an enhanced focus on early detection and prevention. To some extent, this imperative leads to increased awareness of health issues such as cholesterol in all age groups.

Geriatric emergency medicine has the additional mission of rapidly assessing and treating acute medical or surgical emergency conditions and restoring patients to their former level of stability, or providing the needed treatment and referral to enhance their functional abilities. The ultimate goal is to increase an individual's life expectancy with the least disability.

In the following sections of this chapter, we focus on common geriatric problems: chest pain, sepsis, falls, syncope and mental status, and the social and medical issues in family dynamics of acutely ill patients.

REFERENCES

1. Butler, R.N.: Testimony before the U.S. Senate Special Committee on Aging. October 1, 1976.
2. Ford, A.B.: The aged and their physicians: the practice of geriatrics. Philadelphia, W.B. Saunders Co., 1986.
3. Tinetti, M.E. and Speechly, M.: Prevention of falls among the elderly. N. Engl. J. Med. 320:1055, 1989.
4. Gupta, K.L., Dworkin, B., and Gambert, S.R.: Common nutritional disorders in the elderly: atypical manifestations. Geriatrics 43:87, 1988.
5. Morgan, A.G., et al.: National survey in the elderly. Int. J. Vitam. Nutr. Res. 43:465, 1973.
6. Dequeker, J. and Geusens, P.: Contributions of aging and estrogen deficiency to postmenopausal bone loss. N. Engl. J. Med. 313:453, 1985.
7. Caranosus, G.J.: Drug reactions. In: Schwartz, G., et al.: Principles and Practice of Emergency Medicine. 2nd Ed. Philadelphia. W.B. Saunders Co., 1986.

8. Geboes, K., Hellemans, S., and Bossaert, H.: Is the elderly paitent accurately diagnosed? Geriatrics 34:91. 1979.
9. Shamburek, R.D., and Farrar, J.T.: Disorders of the digestive system in the elderly. N. Engl. J. Med. 322:438, 1990.
10. Smithy, N.B., Wexner, S.D., and Dailey, T.H.: The diagnosis and treatment of acute appendicitis in the aged. Dis. Colon Rectum 29:170, 1986.
11. Shepard, J.W.: Cardiorespiratory changes in obstructive sleep apnea. In Kruger, M.H., Roth, T. and Dement, W.C. (editors): Principles and practice of Sleep Medicine. Philadelphia. W.B. Saunders Co. 1989, p. 537.
11a. Demeter, S.I., and Cordasco, E.M.: Problematic pulmonary syndromes in the elderly. In Geriatric Emergency Medicine, edited by Bosker, G., Schwartz, G.R., et al.: St. Louis, C.V. Mosby Co., 1990, p. 233.
12. House Bill 3436: The Medicare Long-Term Care Catastrophic Protection Act, 1988.
13. Katz, S., et al.: Active life expectancy. N. Engl. J. Med. 309:1218, 1983.
14. Murtaugh, C.M., and Kemper, P.: Lifetime use of nursing homes. N. Engl. J. Med. 324:595, 1991.
15. Kane, R.L., and Kane, R.A.: A nursing home in your future? N. Engl. J. Med. 324:627, 1991.
16. Rubenstein, L.Z., Abrass, I.B., and Kane, R.L.: Improved care for patients on a new geriatric evaluation unit. J. Am. Geriatr Soc. 29:531, 1981.
17. Rubenstein, L.Z., et al.: Effectiveness of a geriatric evaluation unit: a randomized clinical trial. N. Engl. J. Med. 311:1664. 1984.
18. Rubenstein, L.Z., et al.: The Sepulveda VA geriatric evaluation unit: data on 4-year outcomes and predictors of improved patient outcomes, J. Am Geriatr. Soc. 32:503, 1984.
19. Ford, A.B., et al.: Health and function in the old and very old. J. Am. Geriatr. Soc. 36:187, 1988.
20. Thomas, J.E.: Indicators of humanhood and the care of aging, chronically ill patients. Clin. Geriatr. Med. 2:3, 1986.
21. Thomasma, D.C.: Quality-of-life judgements, treatment decisions, and medical ethics. Clin. Geriatr. Med. 2:17, 1986.
22. Wanzer, S.H., et al.: The physician's responsibility toward hopelessly ill patients. N. Engl. J. Med. 320:844, 1989.

GENERALIZED CHEST PAIN IN THE ELDERLY

Dennis P. Price and George R. Schwartz

CAPSULE

The elderly patient with chest pain may represent one of the more challenging diagnostic problems. Some basic assumptions regarding such pain should be made.

First, until an initial, even brief, evaluation of the patient is made by a physician, assume the worst possible cause for the pain. Knowing the severity, duration, and location is only a small part of the evaluation. Some seemingly minor pains have dangerous causes. Consequently, the patient should be seen immediately. This necessity for speed has been accentuated because of the widespread use of thrombolytic agents and reperfusion strategies.[1] There is a compelling need for early therapy when indicated.

Second, after your initial evaluation, even if you feel there is no life-threatening cause for the patient's pain, assume that the potential exists and still maintain a high index of suspicion for the possibility of myocardial infarction.

Third, all complaints in some way represent a change in the pattern of the elderly patient's health, regardless of how chronic they may sound initially. For instance, the patient may have been having exertional pain for years, and initially you may see no change in its pattern. You then find that the patient has been more short of breath lately, experiences more dyspnea with exertion, and is unable to perform daily activities because of fatigue. The patient's pain pattern has not changed, but superimposed upon it is an angina equivalent. Understanding your elderly patient and the disease process, and assuming that a change has occurred in the patient's health pattern, will help you make the diagnosis.

DISEASE CLASSIFICATION— SPECIFICITY VERSUS URGENCY

The number of diseases associated with chest pain is great. Emergency evaluation is largely clinical; laboratory and other tests, however, may be helpful. We sometimes treat before obtaining a complete history or physical examination (i.e., impending cardiac or respiratory arrest, life-threatening arrhythmias, tension pneumothorax).

It follows that a more useful method of classification

TABLE 60-3. DEGREE OF URGENCY IN TREATING CHEST PAIN		
Most Urgent	**Urgent**	**Nonurgent**
Acute myocardial infarction	Pneumothorax (nontension)	Musculoskeletal pain
Aortic dissection	Pneumonia	Herpes zoster
Aortic transection	Pleurisy	Esophagitis
Tension pneumothorax	Pericarditis	
	Pulmonary embolism	

would be based on urgency (see Table 60-3). For instance, conditions that should be diagnosed immediately (i.e., within minutes) are myocardial infarction, acute aortic dissection, transection of the aorta (usually a history of severe injury), and tension pneumothorax. Others can be diagnosed within minutes to a few hours: pericarditis, nontension pneumothorax, pneumonia, and pulmonary embolism. Finally, there are conditions that need no specific diagnosis urgently, such as myofascial pain, rib fracture, esophagitis, and so forth.

RE-EVALUATION AND REASSIGNMENT OF RISK

The patient often requires more than just a history and physical examination to determine the risk associated with his or her pain. After an initial evaluation and assignment of risk, early, aggressive eliciting of other important facts must occur if the patient is to receive effective and efficient care.

Old charts, Emergency Department (ED) records, x rays, and electrocardiograms (ECGs) are helpful, as well as clinical information accompanying such materials, such as previous complaints, blood pressures, and medicines.

THE PATIENT'S FAMILY

A candid talk with the family may not only further define the patient's symptoms but may also shed light on nonmedical factors. The patient may have recently lost a spouse or may be worried about or seeking separation from the family because he or she feels like a burden to them. On the other hand, the family may have fears about the older patient's failing health.

THE PHYSICAL EXAMINATION

The physical examination must focus on the vital signs.

VITAL SIGNS

If there is any question of irregularity, the pulse should be taken apically. Both atrial and potentially troublesome ventricular premature beats may be missed if only the radial pulse is palpated because the ejection fraction of the premature beat is usually small. This is particularly true of atrial fibrillation. It is not uncommon to have a radial pulse of 80 or 90 recorded and then to find, when you examine the patient, that the apical rate is between 130 and 150.

Blood pressure should be recorded in both upper extremities; marked differences may be your first clue to serious central pain syndromes. Differences may be your earliest clue to an aortic dissection.

The respiratory rate and pattern are likewise helpful. Inspiration is usually longer than expiration, and the rate is somewhere between 12 and 14. Tachypnea is commonly seen in moderately advanced states of shock, early in myocardial infarction, and often in vasovagal states with severe pain. This sign is a highly sensitive indicator of severe abnormalities, although unfortunately not specific.

The patient's temperature should be obtained per rectum. It is not uncommon to find a 2° to 3°C difference between oral and rectal temperatures. Smoking, techniques in taking the temperature, tachypnea, and states of hydration may all lead to errors in taking oral temperatures.

The physical examination should also make note of sweating (anticholinergic activity), color (oxygenation and hematocrit), and temperature of the skin (perfusion). Abnormalities of any of these usually indicate serious disease and the need for measures such as placing the patient on a cardiac monitor, doing an ECG, and measuring arterial blood gases. In the elderly patient, try to perform these studies quickly and calmly so as not to add to the patient's general anxiety.

The rest of the examination starts from the neck down and includes five key points.

1. *Neck.* Examine the neck for jugular venous distention. The internal jugular venous system is probably the most reliable evidence of abnormality but the most difficult to read. If one is attempting to read elevated right ventricular filling pressures, however, it is acceptable to read the external jugular system. Carotid pulses should be palpated bilaterally for equality, upstroke (ejection fraction), and strength (core perfusion) and auscultated for murmurs. Be careful not to massage the carotid excessively because this may inadvertently cause bradycardia.
2. *Lungs.* The lungs should be auscultated for rales and wheezes, which, if present, must be interpreted in relation to the cardiac examination. If rales and wheezes are associated with an S_3 gallop, they usually indicate elevated left ventricular pressure and primary cardiac disease. If no S_3 gallop is heard, rales and wheezes usually indicate intrinsic lung

disease or congestive heart failure. One must also evaluate for signs of consolidation and effusion.

3. *Heart.* Probably the most important part of the cardiac examination is feeling for the apex beat. Lateral displacement indicates an enlarged or a displaced heart. You should also listen for adventitious sounds such as rubs. Murmurs should be noted as well, both for presence and absence.

4. *Abdomen.* The abdominal examination must be thorough. Note areas of tenderness, bowel sounds, size of the liver (tenderness of the liver may indicate congestive heart failure), abnormal masses and pulsations, and, most importantly, femoral pulses.

5. *Neurologic examination.* The neurologic findings associated with serious cardiovascular disease are usually not subtle. One should pay particular attention to mental status, the content of consciousness, the strength in the extremities, and the deep tendon reflexes. Usually, changes in these result from the effects of serious cardiovascular disease and sometimes from thyroid disease, which is mentioned elsewhere as a sometimes unsuspected cause of geriatric emergencies.

MYOCARDIAL ISCHEMIC SYNDROMES

MYOCARDIAL INFARCTION

The pain of myocardial ischemia represents the most urgent pain to which physician must respond (Table 60-4). The onset of infarction may be associated with bradyarrhythmias and tachyarrhythmias with secondary hypotension and its complications. These rhythms may also deteriorate to complete heart block or ventricular fibrillation. The first few hours after the infarction are the most dangerous in terms of arrhythmias and sudden death, and the most fertile for reperfusion therapies.[23]

The pain of myocardial infarction is usually localized in the center of the chest anteriorly and is described as squeezing, pressure-like, or choking. The classic patient may even give Levine's sign, which is a clenching of the fist in front of the sternum (though this is rare, occurring in fewer than 1% of patients).

The elderly patient may not present such a classic picture. Previous somatic diseases, such as cervical arthritis, shoulder bursitis, and dental disease, may cause a referral of cardiac pain to different areas.[4] This is thought to occur through a mechanism of facilitation, whereby pain impulses follow previous pathways established by somatic pain stimulations. Previous somatic pain thus alters the pattern of visceral (cardiac) pain.

Atypical symptoms may also cause myocardial infarction to go unrecognized in the elderly. In a retrospective study, Uretsky and colleagues studied patients with documented myocardial infarctions admitted to the Boston City Hospital and found that 26 of the 102 patients did not present with symptoms of chest pain. The mean age of these patients was 69.1 years as compared to 58.7 years for the more typical group. The most frequent complaints were dyspnea, seen in 14 patients; abdominal or upper gastric distress, seen in 5 patients; and fatigue, seen in 4 patients. This group had a significantly greater median delay between the onset of symptoms and (1) arrival at the hospital, (2) examination by a physician in the ED, (3) diagnosis of possible myocardial infarction, and (4) transfer from the ED to the intensive care unit. Mortality in this atypical myocardial infarction group was 50%, compared with 18% in the group with chest pain.[5]

The history of the patient just before the onset of symptoms is also helpful. Had he become increasingly tired? Had she been having more shortness of breath? Had paroxysmal nocturnal dyspnea increased? All of these changes may indicate ischemic disease.

One should also look for associated symptoms of infarction such as nausea, vomiting, sweating, lightheadedness, eructation, and syncope. Of course, as with patients of all ages, the traditional coronary disease risk factors such as hypertension, abnormal lipid profile, and positive family history of coronary disease should be determined.

On physical examination, one must pay careful attention to the blood pressure. Frequently, it is elevated during the early stages of myocardial infarction; however, it may also be low. If the patient is driven by a predominantly catecholamine response, the pulse will be elevated. If the patient is exhibiting a vasovagal reaction to myocardial ischemia, the blood pressure and pulse may be low. Make note of jugular venous distention, the pulses in both carotids and the patient's extremities, murmurs, and the presence of an S_3 or S_4 gallop.

If you think a patient has sustained a myocardial infarction, the first laboratory study to do is an ECG. In many cases of myocardial infarction, abnormalities on an ECG may develop only during the course of the patient's hospital stay. If the patient is a candidate for thrombolytic therapy, a complete laboratory examination, including tests of clotting ability and liver function, is needed.

Pain can be treated with intravenous morphine sulfate if there are no contraindications. Enough morphine should be administered to reduce the individual's pain by 80 or 90%. Allow the patient to titrate his or her own morphine dose; that is, it should be reduced to the level where the patient's anxiety is decreased. This allows easier evaluation and is easily reversed with naloxone hydrochloride (Narcan).

Administer intravenous lidocaine (Xylocaine) even in the absence of signs of ventricular irritability; the drug is safe and effective in reducing the incidence of ventricular fibrillation.[6,7] This is particularly important because classic warning arrhythmias may not occur

TABLE 60-4. DIFFERENTIAL DIAGNOSIS OF CHEST PAIN

Disease	Characteristics	Physical Findings	Laboratory Evaluation
Myocardial ischemia	Pressure-like pain; risk factors may be present	Nonspecific	ECG* normal or ST-T wave changes
Aortic dissection Aortic transection Tension pneumothorax	Sudden onset of ripping pain; hypertensive history; no good response to morphine	Pulse defects common in proximal dissection; aortic regurgitation if valve ring deformed; look for signs of pericardial tamponade	Normal ECG Widened mediastinum on chest x ray; aortic arteriography confirms diagnosis
Pericardial or pleural diseases	Stabbing-like chest pain; circumstances surrounding case aid in specific diagnosis	Pleural rub; pericardial three-component friction rub	Chest x ray may show effusion, infiltrate, enlarged cardiac silhouette; ECG may show ST-T wave elevations diffusely
Pneumonia	Teeth-chattering chill; productive cough	Fever; signs of consolidation	Chest x ray with suggestive infiltrate
Pulmonary embolism with hemorrhage	Sudden onset of dyspnea; correct clinical setting and predisposing factors	Tachypnea Right ventricular heave or S_3 gallop	Low PO_2; ECG with right ventricular strain pattern; chest x ray may show infiltrate if hemorrhage is present
Pneumothorax	Sudden onset of pain and dyspnea	Decreased breath sounds over involved lung	Chest x ray shows collapsed lung especially in expiratory film
Gastrointestinal	Past history usually suggestive; relationship to eating usually elicited	Examination may be normal; may show signs of peritoneal irritation or volume instability	Stool guaiac may be positive; oral cholecystogram, upper gastrointestinal series, endoscopy may be indicated to aid in diagnosis
Musculoskeletal	Pain diffused or localized; may be related to activity level	Areas of tenderness often found	X ray may disclose abnormal calcifications, unsuspected fracture, and osteoporosis

* ECG = electrocardiogram.

before all episodes of ventricular fibrillation, or they may occur almost concurrently with the onset of ventricular fibrillation.[8]

The loading dose of lidocaine should be adjusted so that the patient receives a bolus of 1 mg/kg. Also start a continuous drip with the first dose of lidocaine at 2 to 3 mg per minute. In cases of congestive heart failure, shock, and liver disease and in patients over 70, the loading dose should be reduced by 50%, and infusion rates should be between 1 and 2 mg per minute.

UNSTABLE ANGINA

The elderly patient with angina who presents with chest pain must be evaluated carefully. Any change in the pattern of the patient's angina must be sought. This includes both frequency and duration of the attacks, the level of activity bringing on the attacks, dyspnea associated with the angina, and increasing fatigue.

Other precipitating causes of ischemic pain must be sought, such as low-output states as seen with arrhythmias, hypovolemia from various causes, uncontrolled hypertension with concomitant increase in the afterload to the left ventricle, and worsening congestive heart failure.

AORTIC DISSECTION

Chronic stress placed on the aortic wall, perhaps from long-standing hypertension and age, causes changes in the aorta wall. These changes consist of deterioration of the collagen and elastic tissue with cystic changes. These changes are seen in some degree in all people as they age, but are usually marked in people with aortic dissection.

An aortic dissection begins with a tear of the intimal lining of the aorta and subsequent bleeding into the medial layer or sometimes just from spontaneous bleeding into the media.

The patient commonly presents with pain that is immediately severe, in contrast to that of an acute myocardial infarction, which has a slightly longer initial course. The patient may describe the pain as tearing or ripping. He or she may have nausea, vomiting, sweating, and a syncopal episode. If the dissection is proximal, just distal to the aortic valve, most of the pain is anterior. If distal dissection occurs, the pain may be felt in the upper back. Characteristically, the pain is not relieved with the usual doses of morphine.

The physical examination usually discloses hypertension and tachycardia. Hypotension with this disease usually indicates pericardial tamponade or rupture through the adventitial layer of the aorta with subsequent hypovolemia. With proximal dissection, pulse losses may occur as the hematoma dissects along through the aorta. Careful palpation of carotid, brachial, radial, and femoral pulses should be done repeatedly and recorded. This is most accurately done by taking the blood pressure in the extremity. Special attention should be paid to murmurs, especially aortic regurgitation secondary to deformation of the valve ring by the hematoma. A friction rub may be caused by blood leaking into the pericardial sac.

The ECG may show signs of hypertension such as left ventricular hypertrophy. Classically, there are no signs of acute infarction unless the coronary os has become obliterated by dissection. The chest x ray may show a widened mediastinum and abnormalities of the aortic silhouette, and a left pleural effusion may be found, indicating blood in the left pleural space. The diagnosis is confirmed by aortic arteriography.

PERICARDITIS

The causes of pericarditis are numerous: viral, bacterial, fungal, parasitic, neoplastic, and uremic. It may be secondary to drug use, trauma, connective tissue disease, or irradiation of the chest for tumors. In addition, it may be caused by hemorrhage resulting from anticoagulant therapy and is often seen 2 to 4 weeks after an acute myocardial infarction (Dressler's syndrome).

The pain may be pleuritic—stabbing in nature and varying with respiration—or similar to that of myocardial infarction. It may be intermittent and is often accentuated or alleviated by positional changes. Classically, it is improved by leaning forward.

Hypotension may indicate decreased filling of the cardiac chambers secondary to cardiac tamponade. The physician should be on the alert for signs of pulsus paradoxus. This is easily determined by having the patient breathe normally and listening for the Korotkoff sounds. In the normal individual, they will initially be interrupted during inspiration for about 5 mm Hg before being heard continuously during inspiration and expiration. The difference between the discontinuous and continuous Korotkoff sounds is the pulsus paradoxus. A difference of more than 10 mm Hg is considered abnormal. Abnormalities may be seen with cardiac tamponade, asthma, and congestive heart failure. Pericarditis that produces a large amount of fluid in a short time is more likely to cause problems with tamponade than an effusion that develops slowly; the latter gives the pericardium time to compensate and stretch. Jugular venous distention may

be noted if an effusion is interfering with cardiac filling.

A three-component friction rub is often heard when the patient sits forward during either forced inspiration or expiration, and the stethoscope is pressed firmly on the chest. When there is only one component to the rub, it may indicate a short systolic murmur and not a rub at all. The rub may be transient, which is quite characteristic of the disease.

The ECG shows diffuse ST-T wave elevation in a nonfocal distribution. The chest x ray may show pleural effusions or infiltrates if the pleura is involved as well. The cardiac silhouette may be enlarged if an effusion is present.

PLEURITIC PAIN

The causes of pleuritic pain are similar to those of pericardial pain. There are, however, two—namely, pneumonia and pulmonary embolism—that deserve particular attention in the elderly.

Most pleuritic pain is sharp, stabbing, and surprisingly localized. The patient may describe shortness of breath rather than pain; however, careful questioning may reveal that pain is causing him or her to avoid taking a deep breath. True dyspnea suggests involvement of the pulmonary parenchyma or impingement on the parenchyma such as from an effusion. Chills and productive cough suggest an infection. Sudden onset of dyspnea suggests pulmonary embolism.

Pulmonary embolism with hemorrhage (hence the pleuritic pain) is usually seen in individuals who have been on bed rest, have incompetent valves in the venous system of their legs, are postoperative, or have hemiplegia, sustained local trauma, or heart failure.

The physical examination may reveal a temperature elevation suggesting a viral or bacterial pneumonia. The lung examination may disclose signs of consolidation such as increased breath sounds, localized, wet rales, and dullness to percussion over the involved area. You may also find signs of pleural effusion, namely, decreased breath sounds at the bases, e to a changes above the effusion, and dullness over the effusion.

Laboratory tests are essential in working through the differential diagnosis of pleuritic chest pain. The chest x ray should be obtained in both the posterior-anterior and lateral projections; if an effusion is present or suspected, decubitus films are needed. Arterial blood gases may not only aid in the differential diagnosis but indicate the need for oxygen therapy; thus, tests should be obtained early in the course of the patient's evaluation. If the patient is coughing up sputum, a Gram stain may reveal a predominant organism that would dictate antibiotic therapy. A ventilation/

perfusion scan is indicated if a pulmonary embolism is suspected.

PNEUMOTHORAX

Normally, a negative atmospheric pressure in the intrapleural space holds the lung adjacent to the parietal pleura. When air enters the pleural space, secondary to rupture of an emphysematous bleb, or trauma, the lung tends to collapse. The amount of collapse correlates with the amount of air that has entered the space.

The symptoms are generally dyspnea and pleuritic pain over the involved lung field. In the elderly, however, pneumothorax may present as an acute respiratory decompensation. Blood pressure and pulse are generally normal. The diagnosis is confirmed by chest x ray done in both a posterior-anterior and lateral projection. The posterior-anterior film must be done in both inspiration and expiration. The latter is important so that a subtle pneumothorax is not missed. An expiration film makes the pneumothorax easier to see because the vasculature is more prominent in a less expanded lung. Also, there is less negative intrapleural pressure at the end of expiration.

ESOPHAGITIS

Esophagitis presents as retrosternal pain described as burning and may be associated with a sour taste in the mouth. The pain may radiate, starting in the epigastric area and moving upwards. The condition is usually made worse by bending over or lying down and may be more common after a heavy meal.

The physical examination is generally unrewarding. Characteristically, pain is immediately relieved by antacids. Using a mixture of antacids and 2 to 3 mL of 2% viscous lidocaine has been successful. Of course, a history must be highly suggestive of esophagitis before relying on the information obtained from an antacid challenge because of the possibility of the placebo effect.

PEPTIC ULCER

Gastric ulcers increase in incidence in the older population, reaching a peak at about the sixth decade. The symptoms are less well defined than with duodenal ulcer. Duodenal ulcer symptoms typically improve after eating and with antacids. Gastric ulcers, on the other hand, may actually be worsened by eating. The pain is usually in the epigastric region and described as burning and gnawing.

In uncomplicated disease, the physical examination generally reveals normal vital signs and, at times, some mild epigastric tenderness. The rectal examination, which should be done in all cases when peptic ulcer is suspected, will sometimes reveal heme-positive stool and, in severe cases, melena.

Tachycardia or orthostatic blood pressure changes with assuming the upright position—that is, a pulse rise of 30 or greater or systolic blood pressure drop of 20 to 30 mm Hg after 1 minute of standing—suggest volume depletion and serious bleeding.[9]

GALLBLADDER DISEASE

The incidence of gallstones increases with age and must be considered as a cause of chest pain in the elderly patient. The pain of gallbladder disease is caused by obstruction of either the cystic or the common duct. The pain is sudden in onset, reaches its maximum intensity quickly, and is often associated with nausea and vomiting. If the stone passes or falls back into the gallbladder, the pain subsides. The physical examination at that time may reveal only mild or no right upper quadrant tenderness. If the stone stays impacted in the cystic duct or the common bile duct, the pain continues. On examination, you may be able to feel tenderness or a mass in the right upper quadrant.

MUSCULOSKELETAL PAIN

Various musculoskeletal conditions are associated with chest pain, such as bursitis and arthritis of the shoulders. Fractures resulting from osteoporosis are another source of pain. If the pain is caused by a fracture, the onset is abrupt; arthritis and bursitis are more vague in onset.

The physical examination may disclose tenderness in an area. Of course, finding such an area does not rule out cardiac disease, so if the history is suggestive of other causes, further evaluation is warranted.

SKIN

The incidence of herpes zoster, another disease commonly seen in the elderly, increases with age. The pain is burning or aching and usually in a dermatome distribution. The rash may occur along with the symptoms or as late as 4 to 5 days after the onset of the symptoms. The pain, which may be extremely severe, may occur days, weeks, or months after the rash (postherpetic neuralgia). Acyclovir, 400 to 800 mg q.i.d., treats the chronic condition and may reduce complications.

REFERENCES

1. Grines, C.L., and O'Neill, W.W.: Emergency treatment and triage strategies for acute myocardial infarction in the reperfusion era. *In* Emergency Medicine: The Essential Update, Edited by Schwartz, G.R. Philadelphia, W.B. Saunders Co., 1989, p. 17.
2. Simons, M.L., et al.: Improved survival after early thrombolysis in acute myocardial infarction. Lancet *2*:578, 1985.
3. Gruppo Italiano per lo Studio della Streptochinasi nell Infarcto Miocardico (GISSI): Effectiveness of intravenous thrombolytic treatment in acute myocardial infarction. Lancet *1*:397, 1986.
4. Henry, J.A.: Cardiac pain referred to site of previously experienced somatic pain. Br. Med. J. *2*:1605, 1978.
5. Uretsky, B.F., et al.: Symptomatic myocardial infarction without chest pain: prevalence and clinical course. Am. J. Cardiol. *40*:498, 1977.
6. Lie, K.L., Wellens, H.J., and Durrer, D.: Lidocaine in the prevention of primary ventricular fibrillation: A double-blind randomized study of 212 consecutive patients. N. Engl. J. Med. *291*:1324, 1974.
7. Harrison, D.C.: Should lidocaine be administered routinely to all patients after acute myocardial infarction? Circulation *58*:581, 1978.
8. Lie, K.L., Wellens, H.J., and Durrer, D.: Characteristics and predictability of primary ventricular fibrillation. Eur. J. Cardiol. *1*:379, 1974.
9. Knopp, R., Claypool, R., and Leonardi, D.: Use of the tilt test in measuring acute blood loss, Ann. Emerg. Med. *9*:72, 1980.

BIBLIOGRAPHY

Alonzo, A.A., Simon, A.B., and Feinleib, M.: Prodromata of myocardial infarction and sudden death. Circulation *52*:1056, 1969.

Baughman, D.J.: Pain of myocardial infarction reproduced by precordial palpation. JAMA *241*:1328, 1979.

Dallen, J.E., et al.: Pulmonary embolism, pulmonary hemorrhage and pulmonary infarction, N. Engl. J. Med. *296*:1431, 1977.

Darsee, J.R.: Eructonesius without inferior myocardial infarction. N. Engl. J. Med. *298*:221, 1978.

Solomon, H.A., Edwards, A.L., and Killip, T.: Prodromata in acute myocardial infarction. Circulation *52*:463–471, 1969.

Stowers, M., and Short, D.: Warning symptoms before major myocardial infarction. Br. Heart. J. *32*:833, 1970.

SEPSIS IN THE ELDERLY

George R. Schwartz

CAPSULE

Although bacteremic infections in any age group are serious, in the elderly they are more common and more frequently life-threatening. Esposito and his colleagues[1] found a case-fatality rate of 26% in patients 65 or older with bacteremic infection. Smith[2] reports that patients aged 65 and older make up about 50% of all people with septicemia. Of these people, one half have a severe underlying disease.

For this discussion, bacteremic infection and sepsis are used interchangeably and distinguished from a transient bacteremia without infection. In the elderly, however, even a transient bacteremia associated, for example, with dental work or medical instrumentation may lead to more serious consequences such as endocarditis or abscess.

INTRODUCTION

There are alterations in immune function in the elderly. These immunologic reductions are related to aging, the environment (e.g., malnutrition, alcoholism), and underlying diseases, with the influences of each often difficult to separate. For example, the monocytes and macrophages undergo changes[3] in various disease states associated with aging, such as diabetes mellitus. An overall trend toward decreasing immunologic reactivity in the aged is compounded by medications that may be used for treatment. For example, corticosteroids or anticancer chemotherapy medications can markedly reduce the normal defense mechanisms. Splenectomy also predisposes to sudden overwhelming septicemias, particularly with the pneumococcus organism. Although overall antibody response may be less in the elderly, immunization is still effective and reduces mortality from infections such as influenza.[4] The immunologic deficiency in those over 80 has prognostic significance and underscores the need for early recognition and rapid treatment in this age group. When tests were made of cellular and humoral immunity in the elderly, patients over 80 who were hyporesponsive had a higher mortality rate over the subsequent 2 years than a similar group of octogenarians with more responsive immunologic systems.[5]

Smith[6] points out that the heightened sensitivity of the elderly to infection is not just related to decreasing immunologic function. He notes that there can be less ciliary activity in the respiratory tract, fewer digestive (and bacteria-killing) enzymes in the intestinal tract, and even reduced protection from natural barriers such as the skin.

Any sort of medical device or procedure heightens the risk of infection, from administration of a simple IV to placement of a urinary catheter or gastrostomy tube. With the heightened immunologic risk, a mild infection with bacteremia can rapidly progress to an overwhelming life-threatening infection with sepsis.

The overall approach to sepsis in the elderly is early recognition of the infection, identification of the source, suitable cultures for microorganism identification, and rapid institution of suitable antimicrobial agents.

Each of these areas is discussed subsequently.

EARLY RECOGNITION

In the late nineteenth and early twentieth centuries, physicians began to increasingly describe a clinical "shock" syndrome associated with bacteria in the blood.[7,8] Because of the lack of effective treatment, such cases were almost uniformly fatal. The introduction of effective antimicrobial drugs has, of course, completely changed this situation but underscores the importance of early recognition because the shock syndrome is a late phenomenon and difficult to treat even in a healthy younger person. With the decreased immunologic capability and less physiologic reserve in the elderly, early recognition is imperative to reduce mortality from sepsis. Findings of myocardial depressant substances causing early cardiac dysfunction in septic shock underscore the need for early treatment.[9]

CLINICAL MANIFESTATIONS

REDUCED FEVER

Although fever and chills are characteristic symptoms of sepsis, the elderly patient may present with confusing symptoms. Rather than fever, the elderly patient may present with hypothermia. Smith[2] reports that 20 to 30% of elderly patients present atypically. He notes that fever is absent in 12% of the elderly versus only 4% of younger patients.

Gleckman and Hilbert[10] reported on 27 patients who had afebrile bacteremia. Of this group, 25 (93%) were 65 years or older.

The reduced fever response is associated with aging but can also result from medications used to treat underlying chronic diseases. For example, salicylates, corticosteroids, and other antiinflammatory agents can markedly reduce the fever response. In addition, a study we conducted in our Emergency Department (ED) demonstrated that oral temperatures were often inaccurate, and a rectal temperature is mandatory in the elderly when infection is suspected. Mouth breathing, tachypnea, low ambient temperature, and difficulty in placing the oral temperature gauge may all give a falsely low and misleading reading.

MENTAL STATUS CHANGES

Mental status changes are also more common in the bacteremic septic elderly person. With pre-existent mental changes in older people, the deterioration caused by sepsis may be masked. Also, with temperature elevation, symptoms of a recent stroke can be reproduced, and unless a detailed evaluation occurs, symptoms caused by sepsis can be misdiagnosed as "stroke." Sometimes the presenting symptoms may be unexplained confusion or nonspecific malaise. Anorexia, vomiting, and diarrhea are also common nonspecific signs. The value of taking blood cultures and having a high index of suspicion is stressed and, if there are signs of infection, beginning antibiotics presumptively is recommended.

SKIN LESIONS

Also be particularly aware of skin lesions in the elderly. Not only can they cause a toxic shock-like syndrome,[11] but they can rapidly spread throughout nursing homes and hospitals.[12] Because of the readily treatable nature of these conditions (penicillin for Streptococcus infections, oxacillin or methacillin for staphylococcal along with adequate fluids, vasopressors, and supportive treatment), they must not be overlooked. Also, skin lesions such as the purpura associated with meningococcal infection, an ominous finding, could be ascribed in the early stages to easy bruisability. Diagnosing meningococcal sepsis early is essential because there are effective treatments early in the course of the disease (e.g., penicillin), but the prognosis can rapidly worsen as fulminant sepsis with hypotension develops.[13]

Decubitus ulcers or pressure sores are frequently found in the frail elderly, particularly those with neuromuscular diseases. When septicemia develops from decubiti, the mortality rate approaches 50%.[14] Because of the polymicrobial nature of this sepsis (Proteus species, Escherichia coli, Klebsiella, Pseudomonas, and gram-positive cocci), broad-spectrum antibiotic treatment is needed.[15]

OTHER EARLY SIGNS AND SYMPTOMS

The early signs of sepsis might refer to the source or infected organ. In one study of 190 febrile elderly patients, respiratory infections accounted for 58% and urinary tract infections for 15%—together, almost 75%.[16] Respiratory symptoms (cough, sputum, chest pain) and urinary tract infection (UTI) symptoms (flank pain, dysuria) should alert the physician to check further if there is even the slightest suspicion of bacteremia.

Although this study followed patients with fever, it must be stressed that the presentation in a septic elderly patient may be a hypothermic state.

Reviewing backward from a known septic state, Esposito and his colleagues[1] determined that the urinary tract led the list as a cause (34%), followed by the biliary system (20%), the respiratory system (13%), other abdominal infection such as diverticulitis or appendicitis (8%), endocarditis (7%), and meningitis (4%). These categories are covered in detail in subsequent sections.

The elderly patient with symptoms and signs of gallbladder infection, abdominal pain in the right upper quadrant, and tenderness must be evaluated for sepsis.

Other nonspecific effects of sepsis are on the gastrointestinal system, particularly in elderly patients with frequent vomiting and diarrhea.

LATER SIGNS OF SEPSIS

Shock, hypotension, circulatory collapse, and intense vasoconstriction (early vasodilation) are ominous and require immediate aggressive resuscitation, fluids, and antibiotics. One main objective in the elderly is to diagnose and begin treatment before reaching this often preterminal state. During the early "hyperdynamic" stage of septic shock, the skin is warm and dry. Treatment is easier and mortality much lower.

There is usually marked hyperventilation with a respiratory alkalosis and severe mental status changes early in this state. The mental changes (delirium) are partly from the infection, and when the individual is

in a shock state, they can be caused or increased by hypoperfusion. The persistent shock state may lead to hepatic impairment and renal failure, along with a marked acidosis.

The most common organisms responsible for bacteremic shock are Escherichia coli, Klebsiella, and Streptococcus. Staphylococcus is rising in importance. Broad-spectrum antibiotic coverage is essential until the culture is returned. The organisms are, of course, somewhat different, depending on the source of the infection. E. coli is the most common organism from biliary tract sepsis, whereas pneumococcus and Klebsiella are more common from the lungs, and Streptococcus and Staphylococcus are common from skin and soft tissue sources. If Pseudomonas aeruginosa is involved, newer antibiotics with anti-Pseudomonas activity are needed (e.g., piperacillin, mezlocillin, carbenicillin).

MENINGOCOCCAL SEPSIS

Meningococcal septicemia, although rare, deserves mention because this condition must be recognized early to reduce the high fatality rate. People over 60 have double the mortality rate when compared to that of all age groups combined.[17] Fever, chills, weakness, nausea, vomiting, and headache are nonspecific signs. The skin rash, which is petechial in nature, should be searched for. There is usually a marked leukocytosis, although the presence of leukopenia and thrombocytopenia indicates a worse prognosis. Patients may progress to a severe shock state with marked hypotension. Once this state develops, mortality in all groups becomes 50% or greater, even with intensive treatment and suitable antibiotic use. Penicillin and ampicillin, sometimes combined with chloramphenicol, have been the antibiotic choices for the last two decades. Sulfonamide-resistant meningococci have rendered the sulfa drugs of less use in this disease, and their use as "first-line" treatment is no longer recommended unless combined with other antibiotics. Some authorities recommend initiation of treatment with a third-generation cephalosporin (e.g., ceftriaxone).

LABORATORY EVALUATION

Standard tests that are available on an emergency basis can be useful. Testing for electrolytes and blood urea nitrogen (BUN) is important for fluid replacement. The arterial lactate levels may indicate severity.

The complete blood count (CBC) may show leukocytosis or leukopenia in some cases. Usually the presence of leukopenia carries a poorer prognosis. Thrombocytopenia may be evident. Abnormal clotting factors compatible with disseminated intravascular coagulation are seen in about 10% of cases.[19] Abnormalities of bilirubin or hepatic enzymes may point to the biliary system as the cause or can be nonspecific signs of cellular injury.

When neutropenia is present (often associated with treated cancer), the defenses are markedly impaired (particularly with a neutrophil count below 1000/mL). Infections in patients with neutropenia are usually bacterial, with gram-negative rods being most common, followed by Staphylococcus as the most common gram-positive organism. There may be few or no local symptoms[20] and, in skin/soft tissue infections, almost no pus. Because of the common staphylococcal organisms, treatment while awaiting cultures should include an antistaphylococcal antibiotic.

Other laboratory examinations reveal any skin lesions or organ system abnormality (e.g., liver enlargement, flank or biliary pain, cardiac arrhythmias or murmurs, central nervous system symptoms), which can help to focus the evaluation. The urine should be checked because it is so common a source, and there may be few symptoms. Sputum, cerebrospinal fluid, ascitic fluid, and any drainage should be cultured.

BLOOD CULTURES

Blood cultures are the cornerstones of evaluation and offer later guidance for treatment.

Three cultures at different times give the highest positive yield in sepsis because bacteremia can be intermittent. *It is unwise, however, to withhold antibiotics from a septic patient.* One or two blood cultures must suffice and treatment must be started, recognizing that even if a negative culture is returned, there is a 20% chance it is in error. The greatest error, of course, is to allow the patient to remain untreated when sepsis is suspected. Antibiotic treatment should rapidly follow the culture. The easiest method of culture is to take 30 mL of blood from a single site and divide it into three culture bottles. This can be repeated in 15 minutes. Later, after treatment is initiated, further cultures may be taken. This may prove valuable if the organism is unusual or insensitive to the antibiotic chosen.

X RAYS/SCANS

A chest x ray can be important in the diagnosis of pneumonia or an occult malignancy. Clinical signs and symptoms should guide x ray examination. Gallbladder studies may be indicated based on clinical symptoms, and computerized tomography (CT) and magnetic resonance imaging (MRI) scans can be useful if the central nervous system is involved or if an abscess is suspected.

Essential time should not be spent on time-consuming studies, however, in a septic elderly patient who requires, first, stabilization and treatment initiation, after which further testing may be done.

SOURCES OF INFECTION

The most common sources of infection in the elderly that lead to septicemia are:

1. Urinary tract
2. Gallbladder/biliary system
3. Respiratory system
4. Intra-abdominal infection
5. Endocarditis
6. Meningitis

Each is dealt with here only from the vantage point of sepsis with some caveats and tips. They are covered well in other chapters of this book.

URINARY TRACT INFECTIONS

Indwelling catheters, recent instrumentation, prostate enlargement with obstruction, and pelvic relaxation are all risk factors for infection. For sepsis to develop, the kidney must generally be involved in infection (pyelonephritis), although urinary tract symptoms may be scanty.

When sepsis arises from the urinary tract, the leading organisms are E. coli, followed by Proteus, Klebsiella, and Pseudomonas.[21] A Gram stain of sediment can be helpful.

When gram-negative rods are seen or suspected, an aminoglycoside (e.g., gentamicin) should be instituted, coupled with an agent for gram-positive cocci (e.g., ampicillin). Some of the newer antibiotics have been used as well as ceftriaxone (if Pseudomonas is unlikely). Discussion of the range of newer antibiotics is beyond the scope of this chapter but can be found in specific discussions throughout this book.

SEPTICEMIA FROM BILIARY TRACT INFECTION

As the second most common cause of sepsis in the elderly, biliary tract disease stands out because of the frequent need for surgery, although advances in antibiotics and supportive care have shown that good recovery can occur in some cases with only medical treatment.

Of 19 patients with sepsis from bacterial cholangitis, 15 recovered without operation.[22] Five refused surgery, three were considered unacceptable surgical risks, two were uncertain diagnoses, and five were between 82 and 90 years of age and responded to treatment.

Of the 76 bacteremic episodes cultured, the organisms were E. coli (48%), followed by Klebsiella (22%), Streptococcus (15%), and Proteus (10%). Nineteen of the 76 episodes had more than two bacteria cultured—of which streptococci were found in 14 of the 19 as the second or third organism.

In biliary tract infection, an effective antibiotic combination has been gentamicin and ampicillin. As empiric therapy, this is recommended; although some authors suggest other choices such as the acylureidopenicillin antibiotics, for example, piperacillin or mezlocillin.[23] With the wide choice of suitable antibiotics now available, the clinician should become comfortable with use of a particular regimen.

RESPIRATORY TRACT INFECTIONS

The most common cause of sepsis arising from the respiratory tract is pneumonia. There are usually preexistent lung diseases (e.g., COPD, emphysema) that predispose to infection. The organisms usually associated with community-acquired broncho-pneumonia in the elderly are Streptococcus pneumoniae and Haemophilus influenzae,[24] although Klebsiella is seen more frequently in debilitated or alcoholic patients.

The physician should not overlook the occasional extremely severe Legionnaires' disease, however, caused by a gram-negative bacillus. (This requires erythromycin or rifampin for antibiotic treatment.)

Sepsis caused by pneumonia is complicated by marked respiratory impairment, which frequently requires advanced ventilator management, treatment of respiratory failure, and management of sepsis.

Pneumonia remains a major cause of death in the elderly. At an extended-care facility, 41% of 1696 postmortem examinations of patients 65 or older showed evidence of terminal pneumonia, although as the primary cause of death pneumonia was only 15%.[25] Sepsis due to pneumonia can be fulminant and with the respiratory impairment can rapidly lead to death.

Antibiotic management depends on a Gram stain of the sputum. If there is a clear gram-positive diplococci pattern, penicillin is sufficient. If H. influenzae (small gram-negative coccobacilli) is involved, ampicillin is indicated. If there is concern about ampicillin resistance, a third-generation cephalosporin can be used. A mixed infection in a severely ill patient can usually be well treated with an ampicillin-gentamicin combination.

In general, gram-negative bacteria play a minor role in community-acquired pneumonias. In institutional settings where the patient is bedridden, however, coliform bacteria and Pseudomonas are more common.[26] Aspiration is also more frequent, and the achlorhydria that may be found allows bacterial colonization of the stomach contents.

Klebsiella pneumoniae (Friedländer's bacillus) is more common in the debilitated elderly and carries a high mortality rate (25 to 50%).

INTRA-ABDOMINAL INFECTION

The major considerations involve diverticulitis, intestinal perforation, appendicitis with peritonitis, and mesenteric ischemia and infarction.

In these cases, the condition may require surgical intervention (with perforation and appendicitis). Diverticulitis, however, may be treated with aggressive medical management unless perforation has occurred that necessitates surgery. Because of the anaerobic intestinal bacteria, preoperative antibiotic treatment should include clindamycin for Bacteroides infection in cases of spillage of large bowel contents into the peritoneal cavity.

BACTERIAL ENDOCARDITIS

Valvular abnormalities are far more common in the elderly and result in a surface and crevices that can lead to endocarditis. The clinical picture is that of septicemia with an added finding of signs of embolization: petechiae in the subconjunctiva, subcutaneous hemorrhages in the hands. Osler's nodes, or Janeway's lesions. Embolism to the kidneys can result in hematuria. Central nervous system (CNS) emboli can cause confusion and paralysis.

Examination must focus on signs of emboli and careful listening for a cardiac murmur. Misdiagnoses are common but can be lethal because the development of septic shock rapidly leads to congestive heart failure.

MENINGITIS

Diagnosis of bacterial meningitis is easy in the febrile patient with a stiff neck and other meningeal signs and symptoms. In the elderly patient who may be confused, obtunded, or have a multisystem disease, the diagnosis is difficult, particularly when sepsis supervenes.

If specific organisms are seen in the cerebrospinal fluid (e.g., pneumococcal or meningococcal meningitis), treatment can be focused using high doses of penicillin. Ceftriaxone has become a widely used cephalosporin because of its wide spectrum, low toxicity, and effective penetration of the cerebrospinal fluid.

Knowing the likely organism is of greatest importance in focusing specific therapy, as well as the clinician's experience with the newer antibiotics.

ANTIBIOTIC CONSIDERATIONS

In an analysis of data from 207 patients, the bacteria most commonly causing sepsis are E. coli (43%), Streptococcus pneumoniae (17%), Staphylococcus aureus (10%), Klebsiella pneumoniae (7.7%), beta-hemolytic streptococci (7.2%), Proteus (5.3%), Streptococcus viridans (2.8%), and Pseudomonas aeruginosa (1.4%). This information may serve to guide presumptive therapy before culture results are available.

The enormous range and variety of antibiotics now available to the clinician can be confusing. Libke's work[18] can help clarify the field. Often, it is best to gain familiarity with a few antibiotics and know how to use them well. Then, if one is dealing with an infection outside of this range, it is easier to get a specific consultation from an infectious disease specialist.

Any physician who may be called to treat sepsis in an elderly patient should have a basic regimen he or she knows how to use and be prepared to institute treatment without delay. Many of the broad-spectrum, third-generation cephalosporins were designed as less toxic alternatives to the aminoglycosides. In severely ill patients infected by undefined organisms, however, many clinicians are reluctant to replace the ampicillin-gentamicin or cephalosporin-aminoglycoside combinations with which they have become familiar and which have demonstrated efficacy. Certainly, after culture and sensitivity reports become available, it is always prudent to select the narrowest spectrum, least toxic effective antibiotic.

In the emergency setting, rapid decisions must be made, often without the benefit of culture material or even Gram stains of infected fluids. In such cases, the clinician must make some rapid assessments to determine the need for additional antibiotic coverage.

For example:

1. Is Pseudomonas infection likely?
2. Could the infecting organism be a penicillin-resistant staphylococcus?
3. Is Bacteroides infection (most likely from intestinal spillage) a problem?
4. Is Haemophilus influenzae infection resistant to ampicillin likely?
5. Is there a possibility of Legionella sepsis (requiring erythromycin or rifampin)?
6. Is the patient immunocompromised or granulocytopenic caused by preexistent disease, malnutrition, or possible treatment for cancer, an organ transplant, or another condition? In such cases anti-Pseudomonas treatment should be added.

7. Does severe renal or hepatic impairment mandate use of the least potentially toxic antibiotic available?
8. Does known allergy necessitate use of only certain antibiotic classes?

PATHOPHYSIOLOGY OF SEPTIC SHOCK: IMPLICATIONS FOR TREATMENT

Septicemic shock is caused by the damaging actions of exotoxins and endotoxins on a cellular level. Microthrombus formation leads to tissue necrosis and hemorrhage. The kidney can be involved with cortical or tubular necrosis. Necrosis can also occur in the liver. The lungs undergo marked change with edema and increased permeability of cells. Hyaline membrane formation occurs. Respiratory failure may occur. The heart, intestines, and glands (pancreas and adrenal) can undergo hemorrhage and necrosis.

TREATMENT CONSIDERATIONS

The major cause of death in septicemia is shock, which raises the mortality rate in the elderly. One study showed a 60% mortality,[27] another greater than 70%,[28] and this figure increases with advancing age. The pathologic and physiologic changes of septic shock are well covered elsewhere.[29]

For this discussion, we need focus only on the essential need to (1) reduce the damaging actions of exotoxins and endotoxins at a cellular level, (2) rapidly restore adequate perfusion and oxygenation to maintain the organ systems and cardiac and pulmonary function, and (3) correct the metabolic defects, primarily involving a severe metabolic acidosis. Septic shock can result in renal tubular necrosis, as well as adult respiratory distress syndrome (ARDS). Endotoxins may initiate disseminated intravascular coagulation.

Intensive intravenous fluid resuscitation with careful monitoring is critical. Avoid inotropic agents (e.g., dopamine) unless fluid resuscitation is unsuccessful. If used, dopamine is usually mixed as 400 mg in 500 mL of 5% dextrose and water, or saline solution, and the infusion is titrated. The physician should avoid vasoconstrictors (e.g., norepinephrine) because the profound vasoconstriction can reduce kidney and other organ flow.

Corticosteroids, although they are widely used and have theoretic benefit and efficacy in some laboratory animals, are of unproven benefit in this condition. High-dose steroids had no conclusive benefit in one study.[30] It should be remembered, however, that Addison's disease or acute adrenal insufficiency can be precipitated or worsened by the stress of infection. Naloxone has been used experimentally, but its benefit is unproved. The objective of these treatments is to correct the abnormalities in tissue perfusion so that cellular metabolism can be restored. The cornerstone of sepsis treatment, however, must be to treat the infection.

The elderly patient may have pre-existent renal or liver abnormalities, which can reduce excretion and metabolism. The reduced muscle mass requires adjustment in medication dosage. The presence of chronic biliary tract abnormalities or the acute biliary tract infection may also reduce hepatic metabolism. These considerations, however, pale in comparison to the urgency with which sepsis must be addressed in the elderly patient. With mortality rates over 70% (and even higher in the over-80 group), focus must be on fluid resuscitation and intravenous instillation of appropriate antibiotics.

LEGIONELLA PNEUMONIA

This disease is probably far more common than realized. Often called Legionnaires' disease after the American Legion Convention at the Bellevue Stratford Hotel in Philadelphia (1977), where an outbreak was first recognized, the condition is more serious in the elderly. More than 50% of the deaths are in the over-60 age group.

Overall mortality may range from 16%[31] to 47%.[32] Bacteremia is present in almost 40% of cases,[33] and deaths are caused by pulmonary insufficiency, sepsis, and circulatory collapse.[34]

The elderly are at higher risk because the condition has a predilection for patients with underlying pulmonary, cardiac, renal, or malignant disease.[35] Transplant patients are also at high risk, most likely because of immunosuppression.

The organism (Legionella pneumophila) lived in the stagnant water of the hotel's air conditioning system in the original outbreak, but has since been found in aerosols from portable humidifiers. Tap water may be contaminated with the organism.[36] *This condition should be considered in the septic elderly patient because the mortality is high, bacteremia and sepsis are frequent, and diagnosis is difficult.*

A Gram stain of the sputum shows neutrophils but usually no organisms. Chest x ray shows pneumonia, usually of one or two lobes, although a pleural effusion may be the only sign.[37] Blood tests are generally abnormal but nonspecific. There is an elevated white blood cell count, and serum sodium may be low.

Definitive diagnosis rests on specialized tests to detect the organisms. These include the following:

1. Direct fluorescent antibody (results available within a few hours when the lab is equipped).
2. Culture—Legionella pneumophila do not grow on standard bacteriology media (one of the principal reasons for the great puzzlement during the first carefully studied outbreak). Special media for culture are required.[38] Most laboratories are now equipped to detect this organism when requested. The geriatric emergency medicine practitioner, however, must be alert to this possibility; with cultures of blood or other material, he or she should specifically ask for this analysis. Radioimmunoassay of the Legionella antigen in the urine is not widely available and involves delay.

Erythromycin given intravenously (1 g every 6 hours) is the treatment of choice in the severely ill Legionella-septic patient.

REFERENCES

1. Esposito, A., et al.: Community-acquired bacteremia in the elderly; analysis of one hundred consecutive episodes. J. Am. Geriatr. Soc. 7:315, 1980.
2. Smith, I.M.: Prevalence, diagnosis and treatment of infectious diseases. In The Practice of Geriatrics, Edited by Calkins, E., Davis, P.J., and Ford, A.B. Philadelphia, W.B. Saunders Co., 1986.
3. Johnston, R.B.: Current concepts: immunology monocytes and macrophages, N. Engl. J. Med. 318:12, 1988.
4. Howells, C.H.L., et al.: Influenza vaccination and mortality from bronchopneumonia in the elderly, Lancet 1:381, 1975.
5. Roberts-Thompson, I.C., et al.: Aging, immune response and mortality, Lancet 2:368, 1974.
6. Smith, I.A.: Host resistance impairment and protection against infection. In The Practice of Geriatrics. Edited by Calkins, E., Davis, P.J., and Ford, A.B. Philadelphia, W.B. Saunders Co., 1986.
7. Brill, N.E., and Libman, E.: Pyocaneus bacillaemia, Am. J. Med. Sci. 118:153, 1899.
8. Felty, A.R. and Keefer, C.S.: Bacillus coli sepsis: Clinical study of 28 cases of bloodstream invasion by the colon bacillus. JAMA 82:1430, 1924.
9. Dhainaut, J.F.: Myocardial depressant substances as mediators of early cardiac dysfunction in septic shock. J. Crit. Care 4:1, 1989.
10. Gleckman, R., and Hilbert, D.: Afebrile bacteremia: A phenomenon in geriatric patients. JAMA 248:1478, 1982.
11. Cone, L.A., et al.: Clinical and bacteriologic observations of a toxic shock-like syndrome due to *Streptococcus pyogenes*, N. Engl. J. Med. 317:3, 1987.
12. Ruben, R.L., et al.: An outbreak of *Streptococcus pyogenes* infections in a nursing home. Ann. Intern. Med. 101:494, 1984.
13. Swartz, M.: Meningococcal disease. In Cecil Textbook of Medicine Edited by Wyngaarden, J.B., and Smith, L.H. Philadelphia, W.B. Saunders Co., 1988.
14. Galpin, J.E., et al.: Sepsis associated with decubitus ulcers. Am. J. Med. 61:346, 1976.
15. Allman, R.M.: Pressure ulcers among the elderly. N. Engl. J. Med. 320:850, 1989.
16. Brown, N.R. and Thomson, D.J.: Non-treatment of fever in extended care facilities. N. Engl. J. Med. 300:1246, 1979.
17. Anderson, B.M.: Mortality in meningococcal infections, Scand. J. Infect. Dis. 10:277, 1978.

18. Libke, R.D.: Use of newer antibiotics. *In* Emergency Medicine: The Essential Update. Edited by Schwartz, G.R., et al. Philadelphia, W.B. Saunders Co., 1989.
19. Jacobs, R.A.: Sepsis in adults. *In* Current Therapy in Emergency Medicine. Edited by Callaham, M. St. Louis, C.V. Mosby Co., 1987.
20. Pennington, J.E.: Fever, neutropenia and malignancy: a clinical syndrome in evolution. Cancer 39:1345, 1977.
21. Sanderson, P.J. and Denham, M.J.: Antibiotic practice in elderly patients. *In* The Treatment of Medical Problems of the Elderly. Edited by Denham, M.J. Baltimore, University Park Press, 1980.
22. Siegman-Ingra, Y., et al.: Septicemia from biliary tract infection. Arch Surg. 123:366, 1988.
23. Blenkharn, J.I., and Blumgart, L.H.: Streptococcal bacteremia in hepatobiliary operations. Surg. Gynecol. Obstet. 160:139, 1985.
24. Garb, J.L., et al.: Differences in etiology of pneumonias in nursing home and community patients. JAMA 246:2169, 1978.
25. Gerber, I.E.: Terminal pneumonia in the aged. Mt. Sinai J. Med. 47:166, 1980.
26. LaForce, F.M.: Hospital acquired gram-negative rod pneumonias: an overview. Am. J. Med. 70:644, 1981.
27. Wardle, N.: Bacteremia and endotoxic shock. Br. J. Hosp. Med. 21:223, 1979.
28. Sheagren, I.N.: Shock syndromes related to sepsis. *In* Cecil Review of General Internal Medicine, Edited by Smith, L.H. and Wyngaarden, J.B. Philadelphia, W.B. Saunders Co., 1985.
29. Williams, R.K.T., and Denham, M.J.: Septicemia and infective endocarditis. *In* Infections in the Elderly. Edited by Denham, M.J. Lancaster, England, MTP Press, Ltd., 1986.
30. Bone, R.C., Fisher, C.F., Clemmer, T.P., et al.: A controlled clinical trial of high dose methylprednisone in the treatment of severe sepsis and septic shock. N. Engl. J. Med. 317:653, 1987.
31. Galpin, J.E., et al.: Legionnaires disease: Description of an outbreak of pneumonia. N. Engl. J. Med. 297:1189, 1977.
32. Yu, V.L., et al.: Legionnaires disease: new clinical perspective from a prospective pneumonia study. Am. J. Med. 73:357, 1982.
33. Rihs, J.D., et al.: Isolation of *Legionella pneumophila* from blood using the BACTEC: A prospective study yielding positive results. J. Clin. Microbiol. 22:422, 1985.
34. Band, J.D. and Fraser, D.W.: Legionellosis. *In* Infectious Disease and Microbiology, 2nd ed. Edited by Braude, A.I., Davis, C.E., and Fierer, J. Philadelphia, W.B. Saunders Co., 1986.
35. Kirby, B.D., et al.: Legionnaires disease: Report of 65 nosocomially acquired cases and a review of the literature. Medicine 59:188, 1980.
36. Kundsin, R.B. and Walter, C.W.: Legionella prosthetic-valve endocarditis. N. Engl. J. Med. 9:58, 1988.
37. Munder, R.R., Yu, V.L., and Parry, M.F.: The radiographic manifestations of *Legionella* pneumonia. Semin. Respir. Infect. Dis. 2:242, 1987.
38. Vickers, R.M., et al.: Culture methodology for the isolation of *Legionella pneumophila* and other Legionellaceae from clinical and environmental specimens. Semin. Respir. Infect. Dis. 2:274, 1987.

EVALUATION OF FALLS AND THEIR TRAUMATIC CONSEQUENCES

Clark Chipman and George R. Schwartz

CAPSULE

Falls in the elderly are a common problem that the emergency physician or primary care physician must be prepared to manage. Discovering the cause of the fall or initiating investigative efforts to this end may ultimately be more valuable to the patient than treating the injuries suffered as the result of the fall.

The physician is more successful in caring for an elderly patient who has fallen if he or she has an understanding of the general priorities of care in an injured patient, the injuries that are most likely to occur in an elderly patient, who has fallen, and special considerations in therapy because of the patient's age. The most common significant injuries likely to occur with falls in the elderly are hip fracture, fracture of the surgical neck of the humerus, and Colles' fracture of the distal radius and ulna.

EMERGENCY EVALUATION OF FALLS AND THEIR CONSEQUENCES

Persons aged 65 or older comprise 10% of the population of our country, but experience 25% of all fatal injuries or some 28,000 deaths per year. Falls are the single largest cause of accidental death in the elderly and account for over half of all deaths in this age group. Falls are the second leading cause of accidental death in the United States, with almost three quarters of all falls occurring among the aged. The death rate from falls rises significantly for those aged 65 or older.[1] In individuals over age 65, deaths resulting from falls are more common than deaths from all other causes of accidents combined.[2]

Most elderly patients who fall do not sustain fractures. The Metropolitan Life Insurance Company, however, states that in the United States 10,000 persons die annually as a result of falls in and around the home, and 7 million are injured.[3] In Emergency Departments (EDs), it is common to treat an elderly person who has fallen. Thus, it behooves both the practitioner of emergency medicine and the physician who cares for aged patients to be familiar with falls and their possible complications. The morbidity from falls is alarming and often forces the older individual to enter a nursing home or make major living changes.[4] Yet most falls are preventable and require strategies for avoidance.[5]

An elderly individual who has fallen is more likely to be a woman. In a study of nursing home patients who fell, most falls (79%) occurred among women.[6,7] And in a large prospective study of falls occurring in the home, approximately three times as many women as men were involved.[3]

Although it is advisable for the examining physician to follow a systematic approach, ruling out more serious injuries initially, most elderly patients who fall do not present with injuries that are an immediate threat to life. Most patients are all too well aware of what has happened to them and, for them, the fall may be a devastating event. The physician's approach should be gentle and unhurried, and he or she must make every attempt to be aware of, and to administer to, the elderly patient's psychologic needs.

Many elderly patients are part deaf, and the strange surroundings and turmoil of the ED engender confusion, particularly if the patient fails to hear what is said. Great attention must be paid to making sure that patients hear and understand what is to be done.[8] Some elderly patients may become bewildered, frightened, or hostile if treated by the physician in an abrupt or intolerant manner. A sympathetic and cautious response to the patient's questions and needs may make a large difference in allaying fears and gaining cooperation. Patients are unhappy and distraught by being handicapped and in new surroundings, and although they may not have been disabled before hospitalization, they now may well be completely dependent on others for their care. From the first encounter, every attempt must be made to make the hospital experience one of the greatest possible dignity and comfort.[9]

TABLE 60-5. CAUSES OF FALLS IN THE ELDERLY

1. Common changes of age
2. Orthostatic hypotension
3. Cardiac arrhythmias
4. Poor footwear
5. Vertebrobasilar insufficiency
6. Dizziness, balance difficulties
7. Occult blood loss
8. Poor vision
9. Drugs (particularly barbiturates)
10. Depression
11. Others (syncope, transient ischemic attack, epilepsy, electrolyte imbalance, neurologic disorders)

WHY THE ELDERLY FALL

A patient, while walking, may feel her legs give and then falls. She doesn't recall any warning or symptoms; she did not trip or slip, and she did not lose consciousness. When seen in the ED, she may say, "I must have slipped," but this means "I don't know what happened, so I must have slipped." These falls should be investigated carefully because a treatable cause may be found. It is particularly important to discover the circumstances of the fall by asking the patient what she was doing at the time of the fall—her exact activity, exactly how she felt, and exactly how she fell.

A study has demonstrated that falls in the elderly are often serious and may represent a dangerous underlying process that is independent of the trauma caused by the fall.[10] Patients may be labeled with "generalized cerebral atherosclerosis," "vertebrobasilar insufficiency," "senility," or "chronic ear disease" in an attempt to define the nature of their disability. Often this occurs without a careful look at potentially treatable conditions. Perhaps this occurs because it is more direct and easier to treat the injury that has occurred, because these patients are poor historians, or because the possible causes are many.

Causes of falls can be divided into extrinsic or environmental causes resulting in the opportunity to fall, and intrinsic causes resulting in the liability to fall.[11] If the cause of the fall is wholly or partially extrinsic—i.e., something in the patient's environment—of course this should be corrected. Additionally, perhaps, an informed and concerned family member should survey the elderly patient's surroundings for other extrinsic possibilities so that falls may be avoided in the future. Such things as improper hand railings, steep steps, slippery rugs, and slippery bathtub surfaces should be corrected without delay.

The physician must also consider intrinsic causes for falls. If a patient has had a severe fall, and has been fortunate enough not to suffer a fracture or other serious injury, the examining physician should at least consider the possibility of admission to the hospital where a complete workup can be done in an attempt to discover the reason for the fall. On one hand, this might be labeled an "inappropriate admission"; on the other hand, the alternative may be an "appropriate admission" several days later when the same patient returns after sustaining a serious injury from a fall that was potentially preventable. Table 60-5 lists some of the intrinsic causes of falls in the elderly.

COMMON CHANGES OF AGE

The spinal, subcortical, and cortical reflexes that maintain posture are highly susceptible to the changes of aging. As patients become older, their tendency is to assume a more stooped posture and a broader-based gait and to propel themselves with shuffling steps as they watch closely in front in an effort to avoid stumbling over obstacles. Rather than preventing a fall, however, this "gait of the elderly" seems to ensure it. When one begins to fall, he or she prevents this by reflexly taking a larger step and preventing the fall. But in the elderly patient, not only is the broad-based shuffling gait a poor position from which to stabilize oneself, but slowed reflexes and weaker muscles make prevention of the fall even more unlikely. It has been noted that elderly patients tend to sway more than younger patients when attempting to stand absolutely still with both feet together. The amount of sway can be measured by an instrument attached to the patient's chest that records sway over a period of time. It is thought that the greater the tendency to sway, the greater the tendency to fall. Finally, the mental confusion and faulty judgment of some elderly patients can cause them to fall.[12]

ORTHOSTATIC HYPOTENSION

As a person becomes older, he or she usually has decreased muscle mass in the lower extremities. This, along with other changes of aging, leads to diminished vascular tone and increased venous pooling in the lower extremities. A drop of 20 mm Hg or more, either systolic or diastolic, has been reported in between 17 and 25% of apparently healthy older people.[12] If the elderly patient arises suddenly, often vasoactive reflexes are not quick enough to prevent a significant orthostatic drop in blood pressure and a fainting episode. In addition, many of the medications that elderly patients take (diuretics, antihypertensives, and antidepressants) may induce orthostatic hypotension.

CARDIAC ARRHYTHMIAS

As many as 26% of falls in the elderly may be associated with acute changes in cardiac status. Elderly patients often are not aware of the changes in cardiac rhythm, especially if they are at the same time experiencing temporary cerebral dysfunction. When other causes have been ruled out, Holter monitoring may be helpful.[13]

POOR FOOTWEAR

A large percentage of the elderly population has misshapen and poorly functioning feet from decades of improper footwear. In addition, pedal edema or other disorders may make the patient's current supply of footwear more ill-fitting and encourage the wearing of bedroom slippers. This may seem a mundane problem but certainly can cause falls in the elderly.

VERTEBROBASILAR INSUFFICIENCY

This should be suspected as a cause of the fall if the fall occurred when the patient was reaching overhead

or hyperextending his or her head to look at something at a higher elevation.

DIZZINESS

This in itself has been the topic of numerous lengthy and well-written articles. If the elderly patient is complaining of a recent onset of dizziness for which no cause is readily apparent, he or she should be referred for complete laboratory, neurologic, acoustic, and other appropriate testing.

OCCULT BLOOD LOSS

Any patient who has an unexplained fall should at least have postural pulses and blood pressures examined, a rectal examination with stool guaiac, and a hematocrit determined. Occult gastrointestinal bleeding is almost always unrecognized by the elderly patient.

POOR VISION

Often an elderly patient accepts or has lived with a diminution of vision for such a long time that he or she seems to forget that it is a fact. Diminished vision caused by cataracts, diabetes mellitus, or other disorders can predispose an elderly patient to falls, and is a particular risk factor for hip fractures.[7]

DRUGS

Elderly people on medication fall more often than those in a control group. Drugs given for complaints such as insomnia and mild psychologic disturbances contribute more to accidents than medications prescribed for more specific symptoms. The avoidance of overprescribing in the elderly is one of our most significant contributions to the reductions of falls and fractures in older patients.[14]

Unfortunately, alcohol intoxication is not an infrequent cause of falls in the elderly. It may affect the most innocent-appearing victim. The examining physician must keep this possibility in mind and specifically ask relatives or neighbors if alcohol is a problem.

DEPRESSION

This is a common and commonly unrecognized problem of the elderly patient. An episode of depression may cause the patient to take chances that he or she ordinarily would not, or to avoid necessary medication. It may also lead to other behaviors that might promote a fall.

OTHERS

Syncope caused by vasovagal attacks (increased carotid sinus sensitivity), cough syncope, micturition syncope, and defecation syncope should be considered. Transient ischemic attacks may be the culprit. Epilepsy has a second peak in incidence in old age caused by cerebrovascular disease or occasionally cerebral tumors. Electrolyte imbalance may result from improper diuretic therapy.

This list is by no means complete. Most readers, on examining it, will be able to add two or three other causes for falls in the elderly. What should be remembered is that determining the cause of the fall may in many instances be more important to the patient than caring for the injuries that have occurred. No patient has been treated completely until this question has been asked and answered sufficiently.

TRAUMATIC INJURIES FROM FALLS

Consider yourself for a brief moment in the following circumstances: you are the first physician called to see an 85-year-old woman who has been brought to the ED after a fall in her home. The emergency medical technicians who have transported the patient do not know the particulars of the fall. They were called by the woman's neighbors who became concerned because they had not seen her for several days and peered in the window of her house to see her lying on the floor. When you first see the patient, she is struggling, terrified, and disoriented as to where she is and how she got there. As you attempt to question her further, it is clear that she is confused and somewhat hostile, and complains bitterly of pain in her hip and in the back of her head.

As you imagine yourself beginning to care for the elderly woman, what are your priorities for treatment? How should you begin your approach to this patient, and what are the most likely possibilities for injury? What other pieces of information are important for this patient's care? What special considerations might be important in managing an elderly, confused, and potentially seriously injured patient?

TABLE 60-6. PRIORITIES IN THE MULTIPLE TRAUMA PATIENT*

Airway maintenance
Breathing (including control of the cervical spine)
Control of circulation and cardiac dysrhythmias
Control of hemmorrhage
Treatment of shock
Splinting of fractures
Evaluation of further injuries
Continuous monitoring

From American College of Surgeons: Advanced trauma life support course provider's manual, American College of Surgeons Committee on Trauma, 1980.

This section of the chapter discusses the topic of falls by first reviewing initial considerations and priorities in traumatized patients, emphasizing unique considerations in the elderly patient. It will then discuss specific problems in each of the anatomic areas, with emphasis on the more common orthopedic injuries sustained in falls.

The initial considerations are the same as for any injured patient—airway, breathing, and circulation (Table 60-6). In most EDs, as the physician is assessing these "ABCs," the nursing personnel are completely undressing the patient and obtaining the initial vital signs. Along with pulse, blood pressure, and respirations, the initial vital sign in an elderly patient who has fallen that may be of utmost importance is temperature. A patient who lives alone and falls without being found for several hours may suffer from hypothermia, which will not be recognized unless a rectal temperature is taken.[8] The physician should also be aware that, in a very elderly patient, a fall may herald the onset of serious disease and subsequent death. Often, on initial examination, the only indication of this may be a drop in blood pressure. This may be followed by rapid deterioration and subsequent manifestations of an acute underlying illness.[15] On the other hand, hyperthermia may indicate serious infection or sepsis.

CERVICAL SPINE

As he or she assesses the ABCs in a patient who has fallen, the physician must make every effort to protect the cervical spine. A patient who is alert, complains of no pain in the cervical region, has no tenderness to palpation over the dorsal spinous processes of the cervical spine, and can move his or her neck with no pain may be reasonably safely presumed to have an intact cervical spine. On the other hand, in managing a patient who is comatose, or is alert and has positive findings, the cervical spine must be immobilized with sandbags until a portable cross-table lateral x ray reveals it to be stable. It should be recalled that a severe injury to the spinal cord can occur without fracture or dislocation of the cervical spine. Hyperextension injuries are especially common in older individuals who fall forward and sustain trauma to the forehead or face. Such hyperextension can "pinch" the spinal cord between the posterior ligamentum flavum (which tends to become thickened with age) and posterior osteophytes, which are especially common in the elderly population.[16]

In a severely injured patient who needs intubation before the status of the cervical spine is determined, this should be accomplished by the blind nasotracheal route if the patient is breathing spontaneously or by the oral route if there are no spontaneous respirations. In both instances, intubation should be done with an assistant providing immobilization on the head and preventing any significant amount of extension or flexion of the cervical spine.

TORSO INJURIES

Any major bleeding point should be controlled with direct pressure, and the physician should auscultate and palpate the chest and abdomen. Elderly patients who fall fairly frequently fracture ribs or the sternum,[3] but during this initial rapid primary survey, the physician is attempting to detect more serious thoracic injuries. Although usually of no major consequence, such injuries to the bony thorax may cause respiratory decompensation in patients with such conditions as chronic obstructive pulmonary disease.

Likewise, in examining the abdomen, the physician attempts to diagnose a major intra-abdominal injury. In falls, the organs most likely to be injured are the encapsulated ones—specifically, the liver, spleen, bladder, and kidneys. If there is any doubt about the possibility of intraperitoneal hemorrhage, a peritoneal lavage should be performed. Surgical recommendations[17] also state that one should perform peritoneal lavage on a patient who has suffered significant injury if he or she is unconscious or intoxicated to a degree at which the physician cannot have adequate confidence in the abdominal examination. Finally, although it is of less urgency, it should be mentioned that (particularly with hip fractures) the patient may have a distended bladder with retention. In these circumstances, a catheter should be passed with full aseptic precautions, and the bladder emptied entirely. In either circumstance, a urine specimen should be sent to the laboratory for testing.[8]

In a seriously injured patient, as the physician is performing these initial steps in the primary examination, nursing personnel will be inserting large-bore intravenous lines and placing a nasogastric tube and Foley bladder catheter. The next step the physician will want to perform is to splint all obvious fractures. The physician's attention will then turn to a brief neurologic examination in an attempt to more accurately define the patient's neurologic status.

HEAD INJURIES

Although elderly patients who suffer head injuries have relatively fewer severe cerebral contusions than do younger patients, they have a higher incidence of subdural and intraparenchymal hematomas. Subdural hematomas are nearly three times as frequent in the elderly as in younger persons. On the other hand, epidural hematomas are rare.[18] It should be remembered that a subdural hematoma may produce a rather gradual onset of neurologic decline. In fact, a subdural hematoma resulting from an earlier fall may be the cause of the fall for which the physician is currently examining the patient! This possibility should always be kept in mind.

ORTHOPEDIC INJURIES: GENERAL CONSIDERATIONS

Osteoporosis, which occurs with increasing age, is the condition that most significantly increases the risk of fracture in the elderly skeleton. Osteoporosis should not be viewed as a pathologic process; rather, it is a change of the natural aging process that, unfortunately, makes the skeleton more susceptible to fractures. Compared with a 30-year-old, a 70-year-old woman has lost 25 to 30% of her bone density: a 70-year-old man loses 15 to 20%.[19] These changes can be confirmed both pathologically and radiographically. In a study designed to test osteoporosis by radiographic criteria, it was estimated that the incidence of osteoporosis of the spine of women between the ages of 45 and 79 years was approximately 29%, whereas only 18% of elderly men of a similar age were affected.[20] Perhaps this increased incidence of osteoporosis partially explains the higher incidence of fractures in elderly women.

Osteoporosis does not occur equally throughout the elderly skeleton. The areas most profoundly affected are the distal radius, the lumbosacral spine, and the neck of the femur. This has some interesting correlations in the incidence of sites fractured in elderly patients. If one considers the age distribution of fractures in general, it is noted that fractures of the upper limb have a bimodal age distribution with peaks in the young and the elderly. On the other hand, fractures of the lower limb have a J-shaped distribution, increasing as age increases. The rate of all fractures for both men and women increases progressively as a function of age. At age 35 to 44, the rate is higher in men. At age 45 to 54, the rates are approximately equal. From age 55 on up, the fracture rate in women is progressively higher than that of men.[21] The most common orthopedic injuries from falls are fractures of the neck of the femur, the radius and/or ulna, and the humerus.[3]

Treatment and rehabilitation of the elderly patient with skeletal injuries should start as soon as possible. Sterile dressings should be gently applied to open soft tissue injuries. Too often, fractures are left unsplinted until x rays are obtained, and such delay only tends to cause more pain and distress.[9]

In the fit adult, conservative treatment of some fractures is often considered a "safe and sure" method. The reverse is often true in the elderly. Morbidity from lying in bed far outweighs the morbidity of properly performed orthopedic surgery. As a rule, if operation is indicated, a reasonable goal is that surgery should take place within 24 hours. If a patient is felt to be unstable from other medical causes (i.e., diabetes mellitus or congestive heart failure), perhaps 48 hours is a reasonable period for a stabilization.[8]

Finally, the physician must ask about the tetanus immunization status in any patient who has an open wound, however small. Because most older individuals are not adequately protected against diphtheria and tetanus, if there is any question, the patient should receive appropriate immunization.[22]

SPECIFIC SITES

FRACTURES OF THE HIP

Femoral fractures are the most common type seen in the elderly. Annually 2% of women and 1% of men aged 85 or older have a femoral fracture.[23]

A patient with a fractured hip is, with rare exceptions, unable to walk. Usually, the patient is unwilling to sit, even partially upright on a gurney, and usually prefers not to be moved at all because this causes excruciating pain. Grossly, the affected extremity is externally rotated, abducted, and usually somewhat shortened. The patient usually localizes pain in the area of the greater trochanter or anterior pelvis and is tender to palpation or compression over the area of the greater trochanter. Occasionally, however, a patient with a hip fracture presents only with pain referred to the knee. Particularly in elderly patients this possibility must be considered, and, when hip fracture is suspected, radiograms of the hip on the side of the painful knee should be obtained. Occasionally, a patient with a fractured hip has little or no pain at the hip, but the possibility is considered by the examining physician. In these instances, a test that may be performed is to lift the patient's extended leg off the stretcher and gently "bump" the patient on the plantar surface of the foot. In this instance, the shock wave is transmitted up the tibia through the femur to the affected femoral neck, and the patient often feels pain in that area. Of course, one would not perform such a test on a patient who had acute pain with any motion of the affected hip. Pulses, sensation, and function should be assessed, compared with those of the unaffected extremity, and recorded on the patient's chart.

Usually, elderly patients with isolated femoral neck fractures have stable vital signs and are not clinically in shock. If there is any doubt about hemodynamic status, however, an intravenous line should be established before proceeding further.

After total assessment of the patient is completed as described, and if the physician is assured that no other significant injury has occurred, the patient should be made as comfortable as possible before proceeding further. Meperidine (Demerol) is usually sufficient to control muscle spasm and pain. Pain may also be relieved by proper positioning of the hip in gentle flexion with some support under the knee with pillows and sandbags. Should severe pain continue, however, simple traction is necessary. For emergency care, a Hare traction splint or Thomas half-ring splint is probably the best device to provide the necessary traction. No attempt should be made to try to reduce the fraction by traction, and often a small amount of tension reduces the patient's pain.[8]

If the patient is otherwise stable, he or she may go to the radiology department for appropriate x rays. The patient with a suspected hip fracture should have x rays of the affected hip and pelvis and a routine chest x ray. The latter, of course, is part of a routine surgical admission; this saves the elderly patient from having to make a second trip to the radiology department. The most helpful radiologic view for the primary practitioner in examining for hip fracture is a straight AP view of the pelvis that includes both femoral necks and trochanters.

There are several facts in interpreting this radiogram that can help the clinician to find what might otherwise be an occult fracture. First, one should be aware that the neck of the femur forms an inferior angle of approximately 135 degrees with the shaft of the femur, and the angle of the affected side should be compared with the nonaffected side. These should be nearly equal if the patient has not been rotated during the radiographic examination. Second, the clinician should follow Shenton's line. This is merely to remind one that, in a straight AP view, the smooth line formed by the inferior border of the neck of the femur appears to be almost continuous and unbroken with the line formed by the superior margin of the obturator foramen. Third, the physician should look for faint shadows around the neck of the femur superiorly and inferiorly formed by the iliopsoas muscles, bilaterally. These shadows appear to be distended or budging if a patient has suffered a fracture that has caused bleeding into the capsule surrounding the neck of the femur. Fourth, and most important, the physician must carefully examine all of the cortex of the femoral neck, both superiorly and inferiorly and along both trechanters. If this cortical line appears to be broken or not contiguous in any portion, additional views should be obtained. Finally, the clinician may wish to note the relative absence or presence of trabecular patterns through the femoral neck. The greater the degree of absence of these trabecular patterns, the more likely it is that the affected bone is osteoporotic. The greater the amount of osteoporosis, the greater is the likelihood of a complication with fixation of this particular fracture.[24]

Fractures of the hip in the elderly patient usually occur in one of four areas (Fig. 60-1). As one moves from superior to inferior, these fractures are termed subcapital, transcervical, intertrochanteric, and subtrochanteric. Intertrochanteric fractures are most common, followed by transcervical fractures.[25]

One must always seek orthopedic consultation for elderly patients with hip fractures. It is generally agreed that the minimal tests necessary for this patient, other than the aforementioned x rays, include electrocardiogram, CBC, electrolytes, BUN, blood glucose, and a urinalysis. Any other tests that seem appropriate for the patient's clinical condition or other medical conditions should also be ordered. Because most of these patients are destined for surgery, it is most important to note the time when the last meal was consumed and to withhold anything by mouth except for perhaps an occasional ice chip.

FRACTURES OF THE HUMERUS

The classic instance for this injury is the elderly person carrying a bag of groceries who slips while crossing a street. Often, when an individual falls, particularly if he or she is carrying something and has somewhat slowed reflexes, much of the force of the fall is absorbed on the deltoid area, the "point of the shoulder." In younger patients (this is also a common mechanism of injury in football players), this sort of injuring force usually leads to an acromioclavicular injury. In an elderly patient, the injury that commonly occurs is a fracture of the surgical neck of the humerus (Fig. 60-2). Because of force transmitted to the humeral shaft, the same sort of fracture often occurs in the elderly patient even if the force of the fall has been taken on the outstretched hand. In the younger patient, a shoulder dislocation is more likely to occur.

The elderly patient with this injury usually presents with pain and tenderness in the shoulder or upper humeral area. Frequently, even early after the injury, there is a surprisingly large bruise in the area of the fracture. This bruise may later include much of the upper arm, spread into the pectoral area, and may be alarming in appearance. The nature and spread of this bruise should be explained to the patient to prevent undue concern. After a thorough examination of the

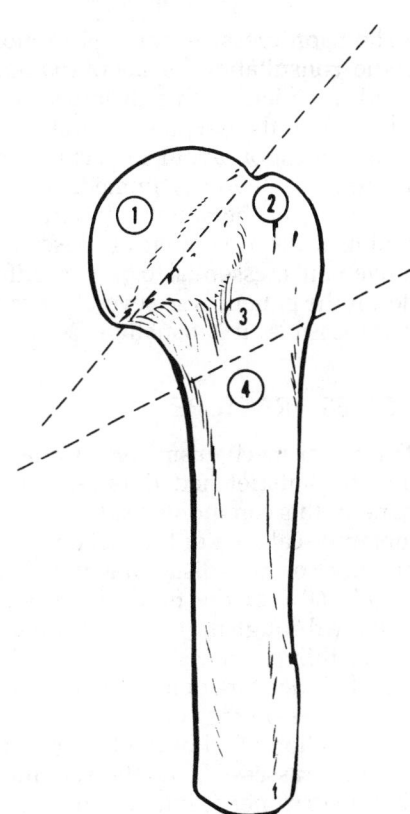

FIG. 60-2.   Humeral neck fractures occur between two or more segments. 1. Head. 2. Lesser tuberosity. 3. Greater tuberosity. 4. Shaft.

neurovascular status of the entire affected arm, radiographs of the painful area should be obtained. The physician should be aware that this injury is not infrequently accompanied by dislocation of the shoulder, and if any suspicion of this accompanying injury is present, additional confirming radiologic views should be obtained. Fracture-dislocations may be difficult to recognize, especially if the dislocation is posterior.

Once a diagnosis of fracture of the cervical neck of the humerus has been made, the important clinical determination that must be reached is whether or not the fracture is impacted or disimpacted. This is usually simply done. First, no fracture segment may be displayed more than 1.0 cm or angulated more than 45 degrees. The patient is merely instructed to bend forward from the waist about 20 to 30 degrees and to allow the affected arm to dangle dependently from the shoulder. When a patient has an impacted fracture, the arm can be moved gently while dangling from the shoulder without undue pain: the patient with a disimpacted fracture has exquisite pain with motion in this position. With impaction, no sense of false motion is detected by the examiner who palpates the humeral head with one hand and gently rotates the humeral shaft with the other hand at the bent elbow. This determination is important because a patient with an impacted fracture may be treated with

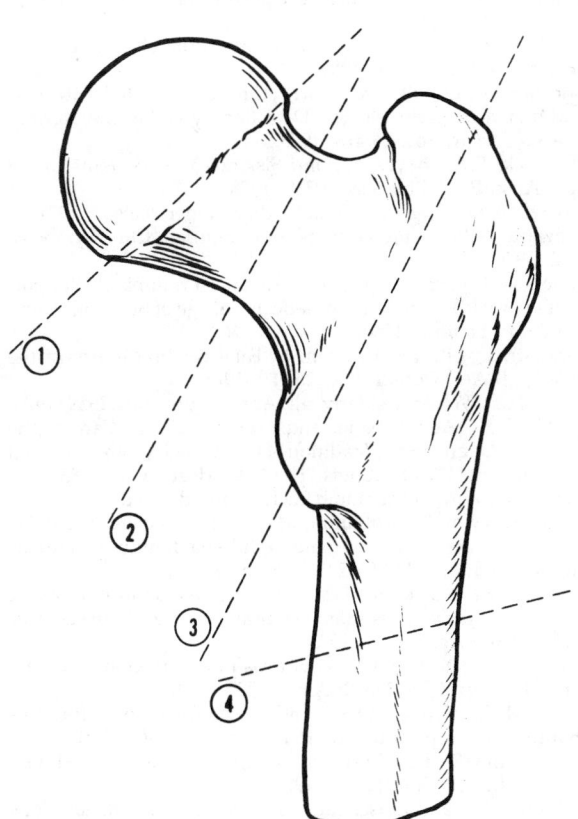

FIG. 60-1.   Common areas of hip (femoral) fracture in the elderly. 1. Subcapital. 2. Transcervical. 3. Intertrochanteric. 4. Subtrochanteric.

a sling, progressive range of motion, and an orthopedic consultation as an outpatient. On the other
hand, a patient with a disimpacted fracture must be
admitted to the hospital for probable surgery. If there
is any question about impaction or disimpaction or
appropriate therapy, immediate orthopedic consultation should be sought. In either instance, it is an
axiom in the treatment of these fractures that early
movement is essential to prevent stiffness of the shoulder. If the patient is so severely incapacitated that this
is impossible, it is usually wise to operate.[8]

COLLES' FRACTURE

The usual mechanism for a Colles' fracture is a fall
onto the outstretched, dorsiflexed hand. In the elderly
patient, this commonly leads to a fracture through the
metaphyseal area of the distal radius with dorsal an-
gulation of the distal fracture fragment. Approximately 60% of the time, there is an accompanying
fracture through the base of the ulnar styloid.[26] In most
cases, this produces an obvious deformity—the so-
called dinner-fork deformity, with a dorsal depression
and fullness in the volar aspect of the wrist. Sensation
and function of all of the fingers on the affected side
should be assessed, and the examiner should be aware
that median nerve injury and, less frequently, flexor
tendon injury at the wrist may be accompanying findings.

The minimal x-ray examinations include anteroposterior and lateral views of the affected wrist. The
films must also be carefully reviewed to rule out an
accompanying carpal fracture. If the fracture line goes
either into the distal radioulnar joint or into the radial
articular surface, the incidence of complication is
higher.[26] If there is any tenderness or swelling at the
elbow or if there is severe displacement of the distal
radial fracture fragment, accompanying radiograms of
the elbow should also be obtained to rule out concomitant elbow fracture.

Perhaps the most important message regarding
Colles' fractures in the elderly is that often this is not
a simple injury. Various degrees of malunion are not
uncommon, patient dissatisfaction with the final result
is not unusual, and often it takes a year or more for
the injured wrist to reach its final degree of repair.
Although some primary care practitioners might think
differently, it is a good idea to refer all Colles' fractures
in the elderly patient to an orthopedic surgeon. This
being the case, no attempts at reduction need be made
until the orthopedist arrives. The wrist should merely
be splinted in the position of maximum comfort, and
an analgesic given as necessary.

Because of the marked morbidity associated with
falls, it is worthwhile to educate patients and caregivers as to home safety measures and prevention of
falls.[5] Particularly, hip fractures are so common in
elderly women that risk factors have been identified,
including lower limb dysfunction, neurologic conditions, barbiturate use, and visual impairment.[7] Other

sedative medications and alcohol have been associated
with falls in some studies.

REFERENCES

1. Metropolitan Life Insurance Company: Mortality from leading types of accidents. Statistical Bulletin 59:10, 1978.
2. U.S. Department of Health, Education, and Welfare: U.S. Public Health Service Pub No. 1459 1:27, 1978.
3. Lucht, L.: A prospective study of accidental falls and resulting injuries in the home among elderly people. Acta Socio Medica Scandinavica 2:105, 1971.
4. Tinetti, M.E., Speechley, M., and Ginter, S.F.: Risk factors for falls among elderly persons living in the community. N. Engl. J. Med. 319:1701, 1988.
5. Tinnetti, M.E., and Speechley, M.: Geriatrics: prevention of falls among the elderly. N. Engl. J. Med. 320:1055, 1989.
6. Kalchthaler, T., Bascon, R.A., and Quintos, V.: Falls in the institutionalized elderly. J. Am. Geriatr. Soc. 26:424, 1978.
7. Grisso, J.A., Kelsey, J.L., Strom, B.L., et al.: Risk factors for falls as a cause of hip fracture in women. N. Engl. J. Med. 324:1326, 1991.
8. Devas, M.: Orthopedics. In Care of the Geriatric Patient: in the Tradition of E.V. Cowdry, 6th ed. Edited by Steinberg, F.U. St. Louis, The CV Mosby Co., 1983.
9. Freehafer, A.A.: Injuries to the skeletal system of older persons. In Working with Older People: A Guide to Practice, Vol. IV. U.S. Public Health Service Pub No. 1415. Edited by Chinn, A.B. Washington, D.C., July 1971.
10. Gryfe, C.I., Amies, A., and Ashley, M.H.: A longitudinal study of falls in the elderly population. Age Ageing 6:201, 1977.
11. Stout, R.W.: Falls and disorders of postural balance. Age Ageing 7(suppl):134, 1978.
12. Brocklehurst, J.C.: Postural instability in the elderly. Consul-tant, pp. 208–214, June 1980.
13. Bordon, M.: Occult cardiac arrhythmias associated with falls and dizziness in the elderly: Detection by Holter monitoring. J. Am. Geriatr. Soc. 26:418, 1978.
14. Whitlock, F.A., Boyce, L., and Siskind, V.: Accidents in old age. Aust. Fam. Physician 7:389, 1978.
15. Howell, T.H.: Premonitory falls. Practitioner 206:667, 1971.
16. Cloward, R.B.: Acute cervical spine injuries. Clin. Symposia 32:2, 1980.
17. American College of Surgeons: Advanced trauma life support course provider's manual. American College of Surgeons Com-mittee on Trauma, 1980.
18. Kirkpatrick, J.B. and Pearson, J.: Fatal cerebral injury in the elderly. J. Am. Geriatr. Soc. 25:489, 1978.
19. Witte, N.S.: Why the elderly fall. Am. J. Nurs. Nov:1959, 1979.
20. Avioli, L.V.: Aging, bone, and osteoporosis. In Care of the Geriatric Patient: In the Tradition of E.V. Cowdry, 6th ed. Edited by Steinberg, F.U. St. Louis, The C.V. Mosby Co., 1983.
21. Garraway, W.M., et al.: Limb fractures in a defined population. I. Frequency and distribution, Mayo Clin. Proc. 54:701, 1979.
22. Crossley, K., et al.: Tetanus and diphtheria immunity in urban Minnesota adults, JAMA 242:2298, 1979.
23. Brocklehurt, J.C., et al.: Fracture of the femur in old age: A two-centre study of associated clinical factors and the cause of the fall. Age Ageing 7:7, 1978.
24. Laros, G.S.: The role of osteoporosis in intertrochanteric frac-tures. Orthop. Clin. North Am. 11:525, 1980.
25. Laskin, R.S., Gruber, M.A., and Zimmerman, A.J.: Intertro-chanteric fractures of the hip in the elderly. In: Clinical Ortho-paedics and Related Research. Edited by Urist, M.R. Phila-delphia, J.B. Lippincott Co., 1979.
26. Dobyns, J.H., and Linscheid, R.L.: Fractures and dislocations of the wrist. In Fractures, Edited by Rockwood, C.A., and Green, D.P. Philadelphia, J.B. Lippincott Co., 1975.

SYNCOPE AND MENTAL STATUS CHANGE IN THE ELDERLY

Dennis P. Price and George M. Schwartz

CAPSULE

In younger individuals, one is frequently able to identify one disease process or pathophysiologic mechanism to explain a symptom, whereas in elderly persons a combination of disease processes and mechanisms, may contribute to the final common problem—inadequate oxygen delivery to the central nervous system. In elderly patients, brain perfusion may already be decreased by atherosclerosis and low cardiac output associated with cardiac and pulmonary disease. Anemia associated with another disease or caused by nutritional inadequacy may further limit the blood's oxygen-carrying capacity. Eating a large meal may also result in postprandial hypotension.

Elderly individuals may no longer possess adequate reserve to deal with seemingly minimal insult. Homeostatic mechanisms such as the ability to develop tachycardia, increase cardiac ejection fraction, and increase vasomotor tone may be hampered by age-related physiologic changes. Lack of exercise, poor nutritional states, concomitant disease, and prescribed and over-the-counter drugs may all contribute to dampening these homeostatic mechanisms.

SYNCOPE

CLASSIFICATION

The cause of syncope in elderly persons is often multifactorial. Thus a classification system listing all possibilities would render the system too diffuse to be helpful. Listed in Table 60-7 are the most common precipitating events or disease states associated with syncope in the elderly.

HISTORY

Because syncope is a symptom, only a careful history can dictate which direction and with what urgency an

evaluation should proceed. One must determine from the onset if syncope or presyncope characterizes the symptom with which the patient presents. Patients may use terms such as "dizzy," "lightheaded," or "passed out," but further questioning may actually disclose vertigo or weakness. The patient usually describes vertigo as "the room spinning." At the time of evaluation, the symptom may still be present. Weakness, if abrupt and transient, may be a syncope equivalent. Weakness, when subacute or chronic and persistent, is more likely to represent a nonspecific symptom of another disease state.

The circumstances surrounding the event should be determined. If the event is clearly related to assuming the upright position and is relieved by lying down, hypovolemic or vasomotor instability is suggested.

One should determine if the symptom began after starting a new drug or is temporally related to taking a drug (e.g., nitroglycerine). Was the patient urinating, defecating, or coughing before the episode?

Chest pain, palpitations, and dyspnea pose a special problem when dealing with syncope in elderly persons. These symptoms may be related to the cause of the syncope (i.e., myocardial infarction, arrhythmia), but such symptoms may also be secondary to poor coronary perfusion pressure caused by a hypotensive state from other causes. Hospitalization is usually necessary to establish a cause-and-effect relationship. A patient who appears confused or inattentive may be postictal. A witness to the event may then be able to fill in details. Short-lived tonic-clonic activity usually consisting of only a few jerks may accompany nonneurologic causes of syncope. History of previous seizures, prolonged seizure, and postictal state suggest a primary neurologic cause for the seizure. Vertebrobasilar insufficiency associated with loss of consciousness is usually associated with other neurologic symptoms such as hemiparesis or cranial nerve dysfunction symptoms.

PHYSICAL EXAMINATION

In the absence of ongoing symptoms, the examination is usually not helpful in establishing the cause of syncope. A few key points are helpful and should be assessed in all patients presenting with syncope.

The blood pressure and pulse should be checked for postural differences if the patient can tolerate the procedure, if the history suggests an orthostatic cause,

TABLE 60-7. CONDITIONS ASSOCIATED WITH SYNCOPE

Cardiac
Arrhythmia
  Tachyarrhythmia
  Bradyarrhythmia
  Sick sinus syndrome
  Pacemaker failure
Structural
  Aortic stenosis
  Idiopathic hypertrophic subaortic stenosis
  Myxoma
Negative cardiac inotropy
  Acute myocardial infarction
  Angina equivalent
  Drug effect
Hypovolemic States
Gastrointestinal hemorrhage
Vomiting or diarrhea
"Third spacing" (bowel infarction or obstruction, peritonitis)
Ruptured abdominal aortic aneurysm
Addison's disease
Diuretic use
Altered States of Cardiac or Vasomotor Reactivity
Carotid sinus syncope
Autonomic insufficiency
  Peripheral neuropathy (diabetes, alcoholic, syphilitic)
  Shy-Drager syndrome
Drug-induced
  Beta-blockers
  Calcium channel blockade
  Phenothiazines
  Antihypertensives
  Vasodilators
Vasovagal
Micturition, cough, Vasalva syncope
Pulmonary Embolism
Neurosyncope
Seizure
Vertebrobasilar insufficiency
Basilar migraine

and if no clear cause has been identified. Blood pressure and pulse should be taken first in the supine position, then compared with that in the standing position if the patient can tolerate the procedure and is not symptomatic or hypotensive in the sitting position.

One should always look for evidence of trauma that may have resulted from or caused the syncopal event. If the patient is not fully alert and shows evidence of head trauma, do not manipulate the neck until radiologic evaluation of the cervical spine has taken place.

LABORATORY TESTS

Although the history and physical examination suggest suitable laboratory tests in most younger patients, elderly patients pose special diagnostic problems. They may present with atypical symptoms, and the cause of syncope may be multifactorial. Consequently,

unless the cause is readily apparent most patients require a more elaborate screen, including ECG; chest x ray; evaluation of arterial blood gases, serum electrolytes, blood urea nitrogen, glucose levels, and stool guaiac; and a complete blood count.

Special procedures such as continuous portable cardiac monitoring, ventilation-perfusion pulmonary scanning. CAT scan of the head, MRI, and EEGs may be helpful in selected cases as part of an in-hospital evaluation.

CHANGE IN MENTAL STATUS

An acute change in mental status is a common reason why an elderly patient is brought to the emergency department. The patient may be acutely agitated, confused, or withdrawn. He or she may be mildly lethargic, inattentive, or have difficulty with recent memory. His or her overall level of daily performance may have deteriorated. He may be unable to walk unassisted or perform acts requiring complex motor skills. The family or patient may not be fully able to appreciate or verbalize the specific problem other than to say that there has been a change in the baseline status or functioning of the individual. Acute changes are often superimposed on chronic deficiencies.

Alteration in the elderly patient's functional ability is the likely reason he is brought to the emergency department (ED). To function adequately, an individual must have an *adequate level of consciousness, the willingness to function,* and the *ability to function.* Determining at what point the difficulty exists is essential to the evaluation.

Alterations in function characterized by a decrease in mental status may result from either metabolic or structural abnormalities of the central nervous system. Decreasing level of consciousness or awareness occurs only when the cortex of both cerebral hemispheres or upper brain stem structures with their reticular activating system are not functioning adequately. Metabolic processes affect all of these areas. Structural processes such as an intracerebral hemorrhage that are going to involve both cerebral hemispheres usually affect first one cortex then the other as the process continues. Consequently, function is initially lost, followed by decreasing level of awareness as the opposite cerebral cortex becomes involved. With structural lesions involving the upper brain stem, consciousness may be lost from the onset.

Clinically, metabolic causes of decreased mental status are thus characterized by diffuse non-lateralizing neurologic findings. They are unlikely to be associated with a new hemiparesis, hypesthesia, or aphasia.

Structural causes are characterized by new lateralizing neurologic findings. Exceptions to these general principles exist. Some metabolic comas (e.g., hypoglycemia) may cause lateralization, or metabolic insult may be superimposed on previous subtle structural pathology. Likewise, some structural pathology may be devoid initially of lateralizing findings (e.g., chronic subdural hematoma or frontal lobe pathology).

HISTORY

Attempts to define exactly in what ways the family feels there is a change in the mental status of the patient are important. Is the patient lethargic, inattentive, confused, or sleeping more than usual? These symptoms may be associated with many of the metabolic causes of mental status change. Other, more subtle changes may include poor concentrating ability, minor changes in usual dress and self-care, or, paradoxically, slight agitation and hyperreactivity. When asked, these patients may be disoriented to time and place, but rarely to person.

Similar symptoms may appear initially to be diffuse and metabolic, yet have a structural basis. With aphasia, the patient may not talk or may appear withdrawn. He or she may not be able to feed himself properly if suffering from weakness of the dominant hand. He or she may appear unkempt or inattentive to his left side with right cortical strokes. The symptoms may be subtle and not a dramatic change from baseline in the elderly individual with pre-existing central nervous system disease.

The ambulance crew can be helpful in describing the circumstances in which the patient was living, medications, potential toxins nearby, the odor of fumes, the temperature of the room, or other relevant factors. The decreased sense of smell in the elderly is probably an important factor in the increased accidental gas poisonings in this group.

The duration of the symptoms is likewise important. Those symptoms of identifiable onset and shorter duration are more likely to have a specific, potentially correctable cause.

Social, environmental, and psychological factors are generally more important in elderly individuals. Acute deteriorations in functional capabilities are seen in patients moved from a home in which they lived for a long time, as well as in patients recently hospitalized or institutionalized for other reasons. These patients with mild impairment may have been able to function adequately because of their familiarity with their surroundings. They may have developed coping mechanisms dependent on routine and familiarity to help them deal with mild impairment. When they are put into an unfamiliar setting, they must be given particular attention to avoid falls and other accidents.

The recent loss of a spouse may greatly impair an elderly individual. In addition, he or she may become so depressed and withdrawn after such an event as to appear organically impaired. Physicians must address this topic skillfully because it may be diagnostic.

Therapeutic intervention may include support systems and the myriad available services that need to be tapped. The issue of suicide in the patient must always be considered, both as a cause of the deterioration and as a potential risk. After the ED, good medical care of the elderly must extend into the community.

POLYPHARMACY

Drugs that the patient claims to be taking should be evaluated for the correct dose and frequency. Some patients may consciously take more drug than prescribed to alleviate a symptom, not realizing the potential for toxicity. Confused patients may be overmedicating or undermedicating themselves. For instance, a patient may be taking digoxin for shortness of breath resulting from heart failure. If the patient is experiencing progressive shortness of breath, he or she may take additional doses, which could become toxic.

Patients and family may not consider over-the-counter drugs, herbal cures, or home remedies as medicines and may not volunteer that they have been taking them. Many are cough and insomnia remedies that contain varying amounts of antihistamines and anticholinergic-type drugs. These alone or in combination with similar prescription drugs can be overly sedating or can lead to confusion.

Many of the drugs used by elderly persons for chronic disease have adverse central nervous system sedating qualities that are additive. The drugs may also contribute to decreased mental state because of their effects on body chemistries or fluid balance.

New drug therapy (both prescription and over-the-counter) should always be suspect in acute mental changes. Because hepatic, renal, and cardiac function may vary, however, even drugs that have been taken for a long period may accumulate and become intoxicants.

TREATMENT

Treatment is directed at the underlying cause. All comatose or semicomatose patients should receive naloxone (opiate antagonist), thiamine, and glucose. If the patient's blood can be tested immediately for glucose with one of the bedside dipstick methods and an elevated glucose level is found, glucose can be withheld.

Determining serum drug levels may be helpful with certain drugs to confirm a clinical suspicion.

Most patients have their illness diagnosed in the ED. In patients in whom a cause cannot be found, an in-hospital evaluation is indicated, but the patient's social or physical environment must not be overlooked in the hospital evaluation.

The advantage of geriatric evaluation units must be considered in view of their proven efficacy. Emergency medicine can be at the forefront of helping the elderly patient by adapting such innovations to the emergency unit.

BIBLIOGRAPHY

Black, Peter McL.: Brain Tumors: Medical review of progress. N. Engl. J. Med. *324*:1555, 1991.

Day, S.C., et al.: Evaluation and outcome of emergency room patients with transient loss of consciousness. Am. J. Med. *73*:15, 1982.

Graffagnino, C., Hachinski, V: Ischemic cerebrovascular disease. *In* Rakel, R. Ed.: Current Therapy. W.B. Saunders 1992, p. 809.

Kapoor, W.N., et al.: Syncope of unknown origin. JAMA *247*:2687, 1982.

Larson, E.B., et al.: Dementia in elderly outpatients: A prospective study. Ann. Intern. Med. *100*:417, 1984.

Lipsitz, L.A.: Syncope in the elderly. Ann. Intern. Med. *99*:92, 1983.

Ouslander, J.G.: Drug therapy in the elderly. Ann. Intern. Med. *95*:711, 1981.

Plum, F., and Posner, J.B.: Diagnosis of stupor and coma, 2nd ed. Philadelphia, F.A. Davis Co., 1972.

Purdie, F.R., Honigman, B., and Rosen, P.: Acute organic brain syndrome: A review of 100 cases. Ann. Emerg. Med. *10*:455, 1981.

Silverstein, M.D.: Patients with syncope admitted to medical intensive care units. JAMA *248*:1185, 1982.

HEAD PAIN IN THE OLDER PATIENT

Joel R. Saper

CAPSULE

Hundreds of illnesses are capable of inducing severe head pain requiring Emergency Department (ED) evaluation and treatment. Space limitations prevent mentioning even most of these. The following is a brief description of several selected organic presentations of particular relevance in older adults, in which intervention may be important or life-saving. Diagnostic procedures and overall approach to headache are covered in Chapter 16.

GLAUCOMA

Acute glaucoma may provoke a pattern of pain not entirely different from that of ocular migraine. Clouding of the cornea, altered pupillary response, and increased intraocular pressure are usually present, as are conjunctival injection, optic disc edema, and visual loss (often confused with classic migraine). Attacks may be precipitated by anticholinergic medications, some of which are used to treat acute migraine. In principle, then, it is possible that a patient with an acute migraine attack might precipitate a secondary glaucoma attack by using these drugs. A patient with glaucoma should not be given these medications, but subtle or undiagnosed cases of glaucoma may be pres-

ent. Ophthalmologic evaluation is essential when this diagnosis is suspected.

CEREBROVASCULAR DISEASE

OCCLUSIVE DISORDERS

Occlusive vascular disease provokes headache in 10 to 40% of cases. The distinction between the aura of classic migraine and transient events of a transient ischemic attack (TIA) is not always apparent clinically because the headache is often nonspecific and can be pulsatile. As in migraine, the headache of ischemic occlusive vascular disease can be worsened by bending, straining, or jarring, and tenderness of the superficial temporal or external arteries on the side of the diseased vessel is reported.

Fisher[1] has described a condition called transient migraine accompaniments (TMA). This condition, seen in patients over age 50 and also called late life migraine, is characterized by neurologic events similar to those occurring in TIA and migraine with aura (classic migraine). Visual phenomena with absence of headache constitute the most common presentation. A history of typical migraine earlier in life is common. On clinical grounds, the illness is difficult to distinguish from TIAs, and thus a complete evaluation (which might include arteriography) is required to rule out ischemic disease before the diagnosis of TMA can be established.

VASCULITIS

Vasculitis, particularly temporal arteritis (giant cell arteritis), is described elsewhere in this text. The diagnosis can occur in the absence of a significantly elevated sedimentation rate. This is especially true in patients who might have used aspirin or nonsteroidal anti-inflammatory drugs for pain control. The condition should be suspected in any patient over 40 who develops late-life onset of head pain in the presence of one of the following: joint symptoms, mild fever, jaw claudication, anemia, visual disturbances, or other "rheumatic" complaints.

HYPERTENSION

The relationship between chronic hypertension and headache remains uncertain, except in cases of aneurysm. Headache does not generally occur as a consequence of hypertension below 180//120 mm Hg. Mild to moderate hypertension may result from a migraine attack.

PHEOCHROMOCYTOMA

Acute paroxysmal headache, often on awakening from sleep or during or after exertion, may occur in up to 80% of patients with pheochromocytoma. In addition to hypertension, the triad of headache, tachycardia, and perspiration is present in most patients. The headache usually lasts less than an hour.

HYPERTENSION ASSOCIATED WITH MAOI TREATMENT

The use of monoamine oxidase inhibitor (MAOI) therapy has increased during the past several years for the treatment of psychiatric conditions and some painful diseases such as headache. During MAOI treatment, intake of sympathomimetic medications (including cold/decongestant preparations)[2] or the ingestion of food containing tyramine or active amines within 18 hours of the last dose of MAOI (approximate duration of gut MAO inhibition) can result in acute hypertensive reactions and head pain. The head pain can occur for a longer time than the hypertension and therefore cannot always be correlated on examination. A detailed medication history revealing MAOI therapy should lead to this consideration.

CAROTID ARTERY DISSECTION

Acute neck or head pain may be the presenting symptom in a patient with spontaneous carotid dissection. The pain is ipsilateral to the side of the dissection, and the head pain is most commonly localized to the forehead, orbit, retro-orbit, and cheek. Anterior or posterior neck pain, mastoid pain, and pain in the angle of the jaw are encountered. Transient ischemic attacks or stroke occur in one-third of patients. Oculosympathetic palsy, subjective bruit, and visual scintillations are noted in many patients. The syndrome can be confused with carotidynia (see next section), idiopathic carotiditis, and/or migraine or cluster headache. MRI, ultrasound imaging, and if necessary angiography, establish the diagnosis.

ACUTE CAROTIDYNIA

Acute carotidynia is an acute, idiopathic, painful affliction involving the carotid artery and is characterized by constant or repetitive short attacks of pain. Neurologic findings and other organic disease are absent. Carotidynia is frequently a component of migraine or cluster headache and can be confused with giant cell arteritis, spontaneous carotid dissection, or carotid atherosclerosis. Tenderness to palpation is characteristically present. The treatment is similar to that of migraine and cluster headache. MRI and ultrasound imaging assist in the diagnosis.

SUBARACHNOID HEMORRHAGE (SAH)

Approximately 28,000 people suffer from rupture of intracranial aneurysms each year in North America, and according to Edmeads,[3] approximately 25% of these have warning signals that are either ignored, misdiagnosed, or sent to surgery too late for beneficial outcome. "Sentinel headache," a warning headache before the actual catastrophic bleeding, occurs in up to 50% of patients and may be characterized by the so-called "thunderclap" head pain, presumably caused by a "warning leak." Features of this headache are generally nonspecific and can be provoked by exertion, including intercourse. Sudden onset of headache, stiff neck, nausea and vomiting, autonomic changes, and progression with or without neurologic deficits are compatible with subarachnoid hemorrhage. The following guidelines may be useful in distinguishing this illness from migraine and determining the nature of the diagnostic workup.

THE RELATIONSHIP OF HEADACHE TO EXERTION

Although migraine and effort-induced benign headache ("coital cephalgia," etc.) can occur after exertion, when moderate to severe headaches occur in this manner, SAH should be suspected.

ALTERED AWARENESS

Although migraine patients and those with benign headache may have transient alterations in mental function, the presence of confusion, obtundation, or other altered mental states should raise concern.

OCCIPITAL RADIATION OF PAIN

Benign headaches frequently involve the occipito-cervical region, but cervical pain radiating to between the shoulders or lower back in conjunction with frontal headache should suggest the possibility of hemorrhage or infectious tracking along the spinal theca.

AGE OF ONSET

Severe head pain in a patient aged 40 or older without a previous history of headache must be taken as a potentially serious indicator.

The reader is referred to the excellent review of this subject by Edmeads.[3]

A CT scan without contrast and an LP are appropriate studies to rule out subarachnoid hemorrhage. The value of these tests, however, is lowered after the first week following the acute event because evidence of previous bleeding could be absent. In such cases, angiography may be the only valid way to pursue a highly suspicious acute headache event.

Day and Raskin[4] have reported a patient with three severe headaches within a week, with normal results from two LPs and CT scans. The patient was subsequently shown to have an aneurysm. The authors conclude that there is a need for the more liberal use of angiography. Subsequent reports in the literature counter this recommendation, suggesting that long-term studies do not support the need for more aggressive use of angiography when an LP and CT scan are normal immediately after the headache.

The reader is encouraged to carefully consider each case individually. If the acute "thunderclap" headache has occurred more than 1 week to 10 days prior to the evaluation, less reliance can be placed on the LP and CT scan results than is possible if performed within hours of the acute headache.

BRAIN HEMORRHAGE

Although hemorrhage into the brain, as distinct from subarachnoid hemorrhage, is usually accompanied by neurologic symptoms, these symptoms may be subtle. In addition, we have reported two cases, and others appear in the literature, documenting the presence of brain hemorrhage in patients with prolonged and protracted migraine. Subtle neurologic symptoms, particularly mental dullness, may be the only early evidence in frontal hemorrhage. CT scanning is necessary when brain hemorrhage is suspected.

PSEUDOTUMOR CEREBRI

Benign increased intracranial pressure can occur without neurologic findings. Although disc swelling is present in over 95% of cases, several cases have been reported in which papilledema is absent. Headache of pseudotumor cerebri is nonspecific and sometimes not distinguishable from migraine. The condition is most often encountered in obese women, frequently those who have recently encountered hormonal disturbance or therapy. Increased size of the physiologic "blind spot" during visual field examination and delayed visual evoked responses may be helpful diagnostically. The diagnosis can be established with certainty only by lumbar puncture, demonstrating increased intracranial pressure. This test should not be performed until CT scan or MRI shows the absence of space-occupying lesions, particularly those of the posterior fossa.

POSTCONCUSSION SYNDROME

Up to 60% of patients suffering head trauma experience head pain for 2 months or longer following the seemingly minor assault. Flexion extension injury of the neck may also cause prolonged head pain.

The postconcussion syndrome is a constellation of several symptoms arising as a consequence of mild to moderate head or neck injury. True loss of consciousness does not necessarily occur, although a momentary "dazed" feeling is common. Additional symptoms comprising the syndrome include mental confusion or dulling of mentation, decreased concentration, memory impairment, dizziness (sometimes with vertigo), personality change, reduced sexual interest, and sleep disturbance. The syndrome may not develop for days, sometimes weeks, or occasionally months after the traumatic event and therefore may not be clearly evident when the patient is evaluated in the ED shortly after the injury. It may progressively worsen, spontaneously improve, or have a waxing and waning course. In geriatric patients, such symptoms are often ascribed to changes of aging or cerebral degeneration.

The headache associated with post-traumatic syndrome following mild to moderate head injury can be of several patterns. Daily global headache with occipitocervical areas of tenderness and aggravated by movement and exertion is the most common. Post-traumatic migraine and cluster-like headache are also possible. Focal trigger point tenderness around the head or neck occurs in most patients.

Because emergency physicians are most concerned with serious consequences of head injury (subdural hematoma, major neurologic deficits, skull fractures, etc.), adequate documentation of the specific details of the injury itself or of subtle neurologic changes does not always occur. Neurologic changes do not always occur when mild trauma is reported. Moreover, patients may not experience symptoms immediately after the trauma, and may not be immediately aware of amnesia for immediate events or momentary loss of consciousness. These may become more clearly evident later, long after the ED evaluation and documentation have taken place.

Current studies regarding the cause of these phenomena after mild to moderate head or neck injury suggest immediate or delayed neuronal sequelae, perhaps related to neuroreceptor/transmitter dysfunction within the central nervous system, although in some cases small areas of bleeding are apparently the cause, which can be detected on MRI scan more easily than on CT scan. The clinician is encouraged to precisely document the events of the trauma and to take note of even the most minor "momentary" alteration of consciousness, since this is important. A detailed assessment of mental function is encouraged. If not carried out, it should be documented as not performed rather than assumed to be normal, an assumption that can have significant adverse implications later on.

CONCLUSION

Little doubt exists that attitudes toward head pain are shifting. Most knowledgeable clinicians no longer consider head pain and its many presentations to reflect diseases rooted simply in emotional travail. Instead, data strongly support the likelihood that most older patients with recurring head pain suffer from a neurobiologic disturbance, usually inherited or acquired following an organic process that assaults or "perturbs" normal neuronal physiology. Patients with a genetic predisposition may be more vulnerable to secondary classes of head pain than those without a family history, a phenomenon seen in epilepsy and other illnesses.

REFERENCES

1. Fisher, C.M.: Late life migraine accompaniments as a cause of unexplained transient ischemic attacks. Can. J. Neurol. Sci. 7:9, 1980.
2. Harrison, W.M., et al.: MAOIs and hypertensive crises: The role of OTC drugs. J. Clin. Psychiatry 15:64, 1989.
3. Edmeads, J.: Emergency management of headache. Headache 28:675, 1988.
4. Day, J.W., and Raskin, N.H.: Thunderclap headache: Symptoms of unruptured cerebral aneurysm. Lancet 2:1247, 1986.

FAMILY DYNAMICS IN GERIATRIC CRISES

George R. Schwartz and Sally S. Garrigan

CAPSULE

Few elderly persons or their families prepare for a crisis. When a crisis, either physical or social, occurs, they present to the Emergency Department and bring with them a history of family interactions and influence. Those who work in this setting do not have the advantage of a detailed history or the luxury of time to obtain one. Some general knowledge about family dynamics and families in crisis, however, may enable us to better understand, accept, and serve our geriatric patients.

GENERAL CONSIDERATIONS

Under stressful conditions, such as acute illness and injury, family members tend to regress to earlier behavior, reawaken authority conflicts, and renew long-buried sibling rivalries. The Talmud says, "Do not judge a man (or woman) in his time of grief," which is wise counsel.

Looking at family dynamics, one must be as nonjudgmental as possible. Conflicting human emotions are part of the human condition. Physicians must encourage children of the elderly to openly discuss questions and concerns. Support for family members is often needed and, occasionally, outside counseling can be of benefit, although not as a rule. The acute care physician or nurse can often be the most helpful of the medical team. Family consultations or conferences with total freedom of expression can be helpful in dealing with the emotions and feelings of hopelessness and despair involved in caring for the elderly patient. On the other hand, professional concern and advice can give hope in these difficult times.[1] This involvement is in keeping with the "Family Sensitivity Concept"[2,3] or the family epidemiologic model. This context model is an attempt to rekindle the flame of broader perspective that has been partly extinguished through extensive subspecialization. Cultural differences must also be recognized.

Scheduled follow-ups for a surviving spouse should be mandatory to address the changes in eating and sleeping habits, as well as the depression that frequently occurs. *Such changes may occur while the spouse is in an acute care hospital or nursing unit as well as after a spouse's death.* Most studies, though not all, show an increased risk of mortality among bereaved spouses.[4]

Levav and his colleagues discuss the elderly patient and his or her spouse's reactions. They contrast the increased mortality in the elderly spouse with their findings that loss of a child was not associated with increased short- or long-term mortality in married parents.[5]

Though one may not get full agreement as to increased mortality, there is unanimity as to increased morbidity and disturbance in vegetative functions (e.g., eating, sleeping) associated with the illness or death of an elderly spouse. The oft-suspected increase in cancer risk associated with bereavement, however, has been questioned.[6]

The reasons for the increased morbidity and probably mortality may involve more than the feelings of grief and dissolution. The reason can include exposure to similar environmental risks and possible increases in suicide and life-endangering behaviors. Regardless, these studies clearly indicate that acute illness and death in an elderly person sometimes has marked effects on the family and the survivors.

Severe illness in a loved family member brings every member closer to facing his or her own mortality and carries to a personal level the time-limited nature of our physical life and our relative helplessness against aging. Certain emotional dynamics are particularly common: grief, guilt, fear, and anger. By understanding some of the dynamics discussed here as well as being sensitive to other family dynamics in individual cases, the acute geriatric care team can help maintain family cohesiveness.

GRIEF

Even when the elderly person is acutely ill or injured and has not died, severe illness reinforces death as a possibility and can cause a sudden, acute sense of loss. Grieving within the family may begin with an acute illness. In some cases, when the person who is not expected to survive makes a dramatic recovery, family members who have started grieving find themselves emotionally confused.

If the person does not survive the health crisis, the survivors usually go through a grieving process, which in the acute care setting often begins with denial. Emotional blunting is common in these circumstances and can lead to family misperception (e.g., he or she "didn't care" because he or she did not cry).

In some instances family members are directly involved in decision making about matters such as withholding of life support and "do not resuscitate" orders.[7] In such instances intrafamilial conflicts may be awakened as well. Physicians involved in caring for such patients need to recognize the frequently conflicting emotions experienced in such decision making.

GUILT

Regardless of the medical condition, there are some family members who retrospectively berate themselves for not seeing early signs or symptoms and for not bringing the patient to the hospital sooner, or not visiting more or being more attentive. These retrospective feelings of guilt tend to be greater when there have been mixed feelings about the ill person.

For example, in Case 1, a 76-year-old man was admitted into the hospital in a comatose state. Though cerebrovascular accident (CVA) was the initial working diagnosis, eventually a Doriden overdose was found to be the cause.

The children knew of their father's depression after the loss of their mother several years before and had seen his deterioration for several months before he attempted suicide. Despite their attempts to comfort him, the children had great guilt that they had not earlier recognized the seriousness of the situation.

In this case, the self-inflicted damage brought the severity of his problems rapidly into medical awareness while complicating the treatment. On the other hand, the elderly tend not to seek medical assistance, partly because of fear (of cost, of hospital, and diagnostic tests). Also, this delay in seeking care is caused by an expectation of and an increased tolerance for symptoms as just part of aging, as well as the frequent lethargy and depression that are too often considered part of "normal aging." Underreporting of illness or serious symptoms in elderly persons can be dangerous when coupled with our primarily passive health care system.[8]

FEAR

This stage includes both the fear that the parent or family member might die and concern about the care the patient might need in the future. Although the acute care is, of course, hospital-based, impaired elderly patients most frequently receive care from other family members when they leave the hospital.[9] Although the care might require a relatively minor commitment (e.g., a 70-year-old woman after a mild "stroke"), in some cases the care required can be all-encompassing (e.g., a 73-year-old man with rapidly progressive amyotrophic lateral sclerosis).

Added to this, also, is an element of fear about financial arrangements for the care of the elderly patient. The elderly patient with an acute illness may manifest great fear of hospitalization, often equating it with pain, suffering, or death, as well as fear about becoming ill and dependent and being forced to relocate.

ANGER

Often, family members who see their elderly parent or sibling with a serious acute illness may become very angry at the person for their contributions to the illness. For example, in Case 1, the children were feeling both guilty and angry at their father for this act of his own doing. Other manifestations can be seen in Case 2. In this situation, a 66-year-old woman had a 40-year history of smoking two packs of cigarettes per day. She was admitted into intensive care after suffering an acute myocardial infarction. The family members expressed great anger because they had re-

peatedly told her of the dangers of smoking. Thus anger may be used to help relieve feelings of guilt.

Other forms of anger might be related to the deteriorating medical course and the patient's eccentricity, stubbornness, and personality change. For example, Case 3 illustrates personality change in an elderly woman that created feelings of anger and hurt in her spouse. This case also illustrates other aspects of the family's dynamics.

After years of struggling with hypertension, Mrs. Y, 82 years old, began suddenly to lose her vision. Her 83-year-old husband drove her to the nearest medical facility for testing. After one hospital admission of several days, and intensive testing, Mrs. Y checked herself out against the advice of her physician. Questionable masses had been found in a CT scan, and biopsies had been done of her lungs and her arteries, both of which were negative.

Refusing to be readmitted to the hospital for further testing, Mrs. Y returned, with her husband, to their home in a small town. Their two sons, both living with their families out-of-state, were upset. The oldest son and his wife visited frequently and tried to convince Mrs. Y to return for more diagnostic testing. Her husband said the choice was her own to make, and although he would prefer that she return to the hospital, he would not make her go against her will. The younger son, very religious, said she should do as she wished and let God's will decide her course.

Mrs. Y steadily declined over the next few months, gradually losing all of her vision. She lost large amounts of weight and was bedridden. She became terribly angry and unreasonable with her spouse and, finally, demanded to be placed in a nursing home. Although demanding to be hand-fed, she refused to eat for anyone except one nurse. When the family visited, she would not respond to their questions and often told them to "go away."

The spouse was terribly hurt and angry and, eventually, visited her only twice a day for a few minutes at a time. Mrs. Y died without her husband at her bedside. The older son immediately went to help his father. The younger brother and wife arrived several days later. Their purpose was to attend the funeral and retrieve the jewelry that was to be left to them by prior agreement. (Mrs. Y kept a well-known list of who would receive her jewelry.)

The husband refused to view the body at the funeral home. He did attend the funeral, although he confided to a granddaughter that he would never again go to the cemetery to visit the grave site. He became unable to sleep because of nightmares and removed all of his wife's personal belongings.

The spouse in this case was reacting to his wife's illness and the behavior induced by her condition as if she were in a pre-illness state; the resultant anger, hurt, and probable guilt prevented a suitable grief reaction.

It becomes the physician's and the nurse's responsibility to help the family to cope when the illness, or possibly the treatment, results in marked personality or mental changes.

GREED AND MATERIAL CONCERNS

The elderly are different from younger people in their concerns. For example, frequent topics may be wills, living trusts, and inheritance patterns. The 82-year-old woman in Case 3 began keeping a list of all her possessions, with the name of a relative after each one. This sort of behavior may possibly contribute to the avarice and material concerns of family members that often surface when an elderly person becomes acutely ill.

Regardless of the cause, it is apparent that some family members have enormous concern about what they will inherit and "jockey" themselves to secure their position.

Occasionally, this behavior may cloud medical judgment. In Case 1, for example, there was pressure from the family members to remove artifical life support systems when the patient did not respond rapidly. In retrospect, the patient's wealth appeared to be a factor in this situation.

In general, the range of family dynamics is rarely openly explored, and often family members are left with hostility against each other, reawakening sibling rivalries, and feelings of insufficient love and abandonment if their inheritance is not up to their expectations.

The increased longevity of our population is more and more accompanied by chronic disease, frailty, and dependency. These problems pose an urgent challenge to the health care professionals working with the acutely ill patient in the context of his or her family.

A critical element of sensitivity and judgment is to know when to intervene and when the most intelligent and compassionate course is that of minimal interference as the family finds their own support, care, and social arrangements. Even when the patient is receiving the finest medical attention and home care, attention must still be focused upon the caregiver(s), who may be experiencing too great a burden or signs of distress. Sensitivity to caregiver distress has been the subject of recent reports[10-12] as well as increased attention to concepts and attitudes of filial obligation toward aging parents and siblings.[13,14] The greater stress on caregivers today has multiple roots. A study[15] has clearly demonstrated that, because of changing governmental guidelines and payments, elderly patients are being discharged earlier and sicker, still requiring treatment that would previously have been provided in a hospital. These conditions, coupled with frequently inadequate home health care assistance, result in families having to take up the slack. The increased role may strain the coping abilities of

caregivers, lead to family bitterness, and increase the risk of elderly abuse. It is the responsibility of the geriatric emergency medicine team to be aware of all available community resources, so that maximum care and assistance can be provided to the patient and family after discharge.

Attention to family dynamics in acute illness and injury will be an increased focus of concern as our society slowly learns how to effectively care for and interact with our growing elderly population. Some specific considerations are explored in the remainder of this section.

EMERGENCY GERIATRIC INTERVENTION

While gathering information about the presenting illness, it is usually helpful to include any accompanying family members in the interview. Skillful questioning can help determine who the family spokesperson is and, more importantly, who the decision maker is. Discovering how the family has coped with prior problems gives clues as to whether this family system has closed or open boundaries. A closed family system is going to be resistant to a plan that includes outside help. The decision to accept outside help is something with which families eventually have to struggle because their willingness and capacity to provide care at home usually erodes over time. The family's capacity to provide home care depends on such resources as time, health, availability, and, most importantly, the pattern of reciprocity established over the years. Many elderly whom we assess as having no support system have alienated their biologic families.[15] It is helpful to keep in mind that the trip to the Emergency Department (ED) may be viewed by the family as a crisis that may, in fact, reawaken many old family issues.

Crisis can also be a catalyst for new issues and feelings. Elderly spouses, in particular, may feel guilty for being healthy. Children can make unwise decisions to avoid feeling guilty. Guilt may also be related to events that occurred years ago. Spouses may be enraged by the loss of a partner and unfulfilled plans. Children may feel hostile toward a parent they remember as being abusive or neglectful. Old feelings of sibling rivalry may also erupt as one family member accuses others of being unresponsive to the present crisis. Relatives, on the other hand, may be too responsive. They may be overprotective and exaggerate limitations and underestimate capabilities of elderly family members. Some adult children, who may themselves be in their sixties or seventies, are unable to respond appropriately because of their own health and physical limitations. It is often difficult for elderly parents to accept the fact that their children cannot care for them because they frequently perceive those children as still young and ageless.[16]

Few people understand their Medicare benefits, and many have inadequate insurance coverage. For some partners, there is despair as savings reserved for retirement are depleted.[17] Few individuals or families make concrete plans for caregiving, and many elderly arrive in the ED in a state of crisis because of their inability to care for themselves.

CULTURAL CONSIDERATIONS

Because of the broad range of elderly patients using emergency care, an awareness is needed of the impact of cultural heritage on some families. None of these examples are absolute givens but rather possibilities to consider.

Southeast Asian families, for example, may struggle with the concept of filial piety (honoring their elders) versus the reality of the demands of life in today's society. For these people, family business is a private affair, and the process of seeking information for an assessment is invasive. Family business is so private that acceptance of outside help may be accompanied by shame. Crisis may precipitate family role changes; a black or Mexican or Native American man may not perceive himself to be a provider of personal care to a parent or spouse. The elderly patient may possibly be homosexual, in which case the family may try to exclude his or her life partner from long-term care decisions.

CRISIS INTERVENTION

It is important to be aware that, in the ED, most patients perceive themselves to be in a state of crisis. Simply put, a crisis is a perturbation in the patient's steady state, not a pathologic state. It may occur to anyone at any stage of life. Not only do roles change in crisis, but behaviors and attitudes change as well. Adult children who are close to their parents when things are going well may feel overwhelmed at times of illness, and people who are warm and caring may be neutral or even hostile when tired and faced with a crisis. The intensity of the crisis determines how long it takes for a person to reorganize.

It is helpful for the emergency staff to be aware of the stages of crisis and to recognize that not all people go through it in the same manner. The first stage is *shock*, followed by a *defensive retreat*, a period during which the elderly patient and/or the family attempts to keep things the same and in balance. Help is not seen as beneficial, and an attempt to maintain control is made by refusing assistance. The reality of the situation is accepted during the *acknowledgment* stage, and only at the point of *adaptation* are new responses and coping patterns formed.[18]

Crisis resolution and intervention are designed to offer immediate emotional-environmental first aid, us-

ing reassurance and encouragement. Although allowing some time for the patient and family to ventilate, crisis intervention in an ED setting is no time for psychologic interpretation but, rather, a time for mobilizing significant others, creating action, and accomplishing practical things.[19] It is during this process of mobilization that one of the most detrimental of family dynamics occurs: families and staff, in their attempt to respond to the present situation, may exclude the patient from any decision making.

SELF-DETERMINATION ISSUES

The legal and civil rights of older people are not always considered or respected. When a memory-impaired relative can no longer make rational decisions, families may act on his or her behalf, but must be legally empowered to do so.[20]

In addition to the legal aspects, self-esteem issues come into play. Assistance must be compensatory in nature but also contribute to the maintenance of self-worth. Assistance and decisions about providing assistance must be balanced between doing what is needed and doing more than what is actually required. Professionals, especially, fall into the trap of taking over, which, in fact, infantilizes aged persons. Professionals also have the added problem of meeting institutional needs. Value conflicts arise when obligation to the hospital conflicts with needs of the patient and family. Tight guidelines for admission criteria and length of hospital stay contribute to the conflict. Complicating the issue is a paucity of community resources. Having few alternatives erodes self-determination and limits patient decision making.[21] Patient advocacy, assistance with access to community resources, and family assessment are areas in which an ED social worker may be especially helpful.

Medical social workers operate in consultative, collaborative roles. They are enablers, assessing the situation and enhancing the problem solving and coping capacities of families. They are brokers who link patients with a number of systems. Finally, they are patient advocates, never losing sight of the patient's decision-making rights.

REFERENCES

1. Medalie, J.H., Kitson, G.C., and Zyzanski, S.T.: A family epidemiologic model. J. Fam. Pract. 12:79, 1981.
2. Culpepper, L., Murphy, J., and Fretwell, B.: Biology, primary care and community: A basis for rational geriatric care. Clin. Geriatr. Med. 2:1, 1986.
3. Maddox, G.L.: Families as context and resource in chronic illness. In Long Term Care. Edited by Sherwood, S. New York, Spectrum Publishers, 1975.
4. Kaprio, J., Koskenvvo, M., and Rita, H.: Mortality after bereavement. Am. J. Pub. Health 77:283, 1987.

5. Levav, I., et al.: An epidemiologic study of mortality among bereaved parents. N. Engl. J. Med. *319:*457, 1988.

6. Jones, D.R., Goldblatt, P.O., and Leon, D.A.: Bereavement and cancer. Br. Med. J. *289:*461, 1984.

7. Smedira, N.G., et al.: Withholding and withdrawal of life support from the critically ill. N. Engl. J. Med. *322:*309, 1990.

8. Rowe, J.W.: Health care of the elderly. N. Engl. J. Med. *13:*827, 1985.

9. Ouslander, J.G., and Beck, J.C.: Defining the health problems of the elderly. Annu. Rev. Pub. Health *3:*55, 1982.

10. Pearson, J., Verma, S., and Nellett, C.: Elderly psychiatric patient status and caregiver perceptions and predictors of caregiver burden. Gerontologist *28:*79, 1988.

11. Gilhooly, M.L.: The impact of caregiving on caregivers. Br. J. Med. Psychol. *57:*35, 1984.

12. Sanford, J.F.A.: Tolerance of debility in elderly dependents by supports at home: its significance for hospital practice. Br. Med. J. *3:*471, 1985.

13. Finely, N.J., Roberts, M.D., and Banahan, B.F.: Motivators and inhibitors of attitudes of filial obligation toward aging parents, Gerontologist *28:*73, 1988.

14. Houser, B.B., Berkman, S.L., and Bardsley, P.: Sex and birth order differences in filial behavior. Sex Roles *13:*641, 1985.

15. Silverstone, B., and Weiss, A.: Social work practice with the frail elderly and their families. Springfield, Ill. Charles C Thomas, 1983.

16. Hancock, B.: Social work with older people. Englewood Cliffs, N.J. Prentice-Hall, Inc., 1987.

17. Pilisuk, M., and Parks, S.H.: Caregiving: where families need help. Social Work *33:*436, 1980.

18. Hubschman, L.: Hospital social work practice. New York, Praeger Publishers, 1983.

19. Dougherty, A.B.: Emergency room: Fighting a stage of crisis. Nurs. Management *15:*11–13, 1984.

20. Powell, L.S., and Courtice, K.: Alzheimer's disease: A guide for families. Reading, Mass. Addison-Wesley, 1983.

21. Blayzk, S., and Canavan, M.M.: Therapeutic aspects of discharge planning. Social Work *88:*489–494, 1985.

BIBLIOGRAPHY

Cox, E.O., Parsons, R.J., and Kimboko, P.J.: Social service and intergenerational caregivers, Soc Work *33:*430, 1988.

Golan, N.: Treatment in crisis situations, New York, The Free Press, 1978.

Hepworth, D.H., and Larson, J.A.: Direct social work practice. Chicago, IL., The Dorsey Press, 1986.

Part IX

Psychiatric and Behavioral Emergencies

Chapter 61

INTRODUCTION TO PSYCHIATRIC AND BEHAVIORAL EMERGENCIES

Stephanie von Ammon Cavanaugh and William S. Gilmer

CAPSULE

A psychiatric emergency is a disturbance of affect, behavior, and/or thought that is judged by the patient, medical staff, family, or friends to require prompt intervention because the patient is: (1) potentially or actively suicidal or homicidal; (2) displaying acute or alarming psychiatric symptoms (for example, psychotic symptoms); or (3) experiencing acute subjective psychologic distress. Most commonly, patients who require emergent care are severely depressed, suicidal, psychotic, violent, or in a state of panic. The cause of these psychiatric disorders may be an identifiable organic factor and/or a psychiatric disturbance.

Emergently, the patient must be prevented from hurting himself or herself and others, and from leaving the hospital (eloping). An adequate evaluation must be performed, including a psychiatric and medical history from the patient and, because many patients are unable to give an accurate history, from family and friends. If a family member does not accompany the patient, a collateral history should be obtained over the phone. A mental status examination, physical examination, and appropriate laboratory tests should be performed. Finally, a provisional diagnosis is formulated, and a treatment and/or disposition plan outlined.

This and the next two introductory subchapters outline the basics of this process. First, we consider the psychiatric history and mental status examination. We then discuss the common psychiatric problems seen in the Emergency Department (ED). Differential diagnosis and emergent clinical considerations are reviewed. Finally, we deal with the issues in management of the psychiatric emergency, including psychotropic medications, restraints, disposition, commitment, and other medicolegal problems. The remaining chapters in this section discuss in depth the more common psychiatric problems seen in the emergency setting.

EARLY TRIAGE ASSESSMENT AND MANAGEMENT

Before a more thorough evaluation by the emergency physician, several factors must be considered by triage personnel when a patient with disturbance of affect, behavior, and/or thought presents to the ED.

Significant data may be obtained in the first step of the triage process by observing or "eyeballing" the patient. This step may seem self-evident, but is essential for efficient assessment and appropriate emergency management. First, the patient's *level of consciousness* should be assessed. An impaired level of consciousness alerts emergency personnel to the emergent need for more attentive medical and neurologic evaluation. The patient should be observed for signs of *psychosis*. Is the patient conversing with nonexistent others? Does he or she appear extremely suspicious or paranoid? Are the patient's verbalizations entirely out of touch with reality? Such a patient is psychotic and should be attended to more quickly. Signs of *agitation* on initial presentation should be noted. This behavior, if ignored or handled inappropriately, may escalate and pose a serious threat to the patient and others in the ED. The patient with a profound *depressive stance*, characterized by slumped and dejected posturing, sad facies, and downcast gaze, may be suicidal. Asking about suicidal ideation is an immediate priority.

The next obvious step in the early triage assessment is initial inquiry into the concerns that brought the patient to the ED: *What is the chief complaint?* This is followed by focused questioning regarding the following items: *recent drug ingestion or overdose, current thoughts of self-harm, recent illicit substance use, pertinent medical illness and allergies, history of psychiatric illness,* and *current medications.*

Following the above triage questioning, the patient's vital signs should be recorded. The patient then should be assisted into a hospital gown. Always ask a psychiatric patient, "May I take your vital signs?," "May I help you into your hospital gown?" because some paranoid patients may interpret such action as a physical threat. A hospital gown not only facilitates the physical examination but also protects the patient and others in the ED from harm inflicted by concealed weapons. It may also discourage a potentially dangerous patient from abruptly leaving before full assessment and disposition. Further, a hospital gown may assist in the detection of a patient who elopes from the ED. Separating the patient from his or her belongings also protects the patient and personnel from concealed weapons and elopement. If a patient adamantly refuses to change into a hospital gown or to be separated from his or her belongings, triage personnel should be alerted to the possibility that the patient may be carrying illicit substances and/or concealed weapons or suffering from a mental disorder with paranoid features. In emergent cases presenting with severe disorganization, disorientation, suspected overdose, or possible danger, it may be necessary to search personal belongings without the patient's permission to obtain identifying information, telephone numbers of family members and friends for collateral history, clues to ingested substances, and concealed weapons.

Placement of the patient in a room where he or she can be readily observed and heard by hospital personnel is imperative. Ideally, the room should be physically separate from other medical evaluation areas to enhance privacy and minimize overstimulation of the agitated patient. Care must be taken not to place the potentially violent or suicidal patient in an evaluation room with access to medical instruments or other injurious objects. Also, one-to-one supervision must be provided for such patients and those so confused or agitated that they may leave the ED before evaluation. If a separate room is available for psychiatric emergencies on an ongoing basis, it should be painted pale pink, the color suggested as most calming to the agitated patient.[1]

Security personnel should be alerted to the possibility of violent behavior and asked to report to the emergency area. They should be given specific instructions regarding their role with the patient, and if not already consistent with hospital policy, told to remove exposed weapons before assisting with the potentially violent patient. When a patient's behavior threatens to pose harm to himself or herself and others, placement in physical restraints is required. Triage personnel trained in applying restraints should instruct security and other personnel without experience in assisting in the restraining process. Emergent use of psychotropic medication (e.g., chemical restraints) before at least a brief evaluation by the emergency physician is rarely warranted.

Triage personnel should ask people accompanying the patient to the ED to wait until they have spoken to the evaluating emergency physician. In many cases, family and friends can provide comfort for the patient while waiting for evaluation and disposition. They may also deter the more disturbed patient from eloping from the ED or disturbing other patients, provide collateral history, and support the physician in his or her treatment plan or disposition. Family and friends, however, should not replace the role of security in monitoring the potentially violent patient. Further, in some cases, those accompanying the patient may cause him or her to be more agitated or psychotic. When this occurs, family and friends should be asked to wait in an area separate from the patient.

STRUCTURING THE PHYSICIAN'S ASSESSMENT

A SAFE ENVIRONMENT FOR THE INTERVIEW

Eyeballing the patient, triage information, and collateral history help to establish whether or not it is safe for the physician to interview the patient alone in a room with the door closed. Patients who are confused, paranoid, psychotic, agitated, or angry, or who have a history of violence, may be of risk to the examiner. Further, some patients evoke a gut feeling in the physician of fear or uneasiness. Such a feeling or intuition is valuable in suggesting that the examiner may not be safe with the patient. There is never any place for heroics on the part of the emergency physician interviewing a psychiatric patient. If the physician does not feel safe, a safe environment for the interview must be provided. In addition to protecting the physician from danger, a safe environment is reassuring for the disorganized or potentially violent patient. The physician may wish to leave the door open, be a safe distance from the patient, or have a security guard or other staff member present during the interview. In some cases, after a brief evaluation, psychotropic medication is administered to decrease agitation and the interview continued after the patient is calmer. Finally, physical restraints may be required before the interview can be safely conducted.

With all patients, it makes good sense to ask: "Is it all right if we sit down and talk?" "Are you comfortable in this room?" "Would it be all right if I closed the door?" The physician should always sit by the door and have a clear means of escape. If the examiner miscalculates and the patient threatens or attempts to harm the interviewer, the physician should stay out of the patient's reach. Because the violent patient is frightened by his or her loss of control, the physician should reassure the patient that he or she is safe and will not be harmed or allowed to harm others. The physician should immediately get help. To ensure quick access, each ED should have a prearranged system for requesting security and other personnel to assist in dealing with the violent patient. Five additional people are needed to restraint the patient, one for each limb and one to apply the restraints. Often a show of force calms the patient, who can then be verbally brought under control and restraints applied without using physical force.

COLLATERAL HISTORY

A collateral history is vital to the assessment of the psychiatric patient in the ED. Interviewing family and friends before interviewing the patient can help focus the interview, particularly with the more disturbed patient. It is important, however, to remember that history from those accompanying the patient may be biased and should be evaluated for accuracy like all other data. Although the initial assessment should be conducted with the patient alone, conducting the interview with trusted family members or friends can often facilitate the interview with the paranoid, confused, psychotic, or nonconversant patient. Further, a joint interview can elucidate family or interpersonal problems and supports. Valuable information from family and friends includes onset and progression of symptoms, recent stress, past personal and family psychiatric and medical history, drug abuse, medications, and the reasons why the patient was brought to the ED. Occasionally, a psychiatric patient refuses to allow the evaluating physician to talk with family or friends. Such a refusal may often be the product of the patient's psychiatric disorder. In these circumstances, the emergent need for collateral history may warrant its acquisition regardless of the patient's wishes. On the other hand, doctor-patient communication is privileged. Unless the patient is threatening to harm those accompanying him or her, information obtained from the patient should not be communicated to family or friends without the permission of the patient.

If no one accompanies the patient to the ED, every attempt should be made to obtain a collateral history from family or friends over the phone. Physicians, therapists, and facilities who have previously treated the patient may also provide valuable collateral history. Permission must be obtained from the patient to obtain such collateral history over the phone. If the patient refuses, again the emergent nature of his or her psychiatric condition may warrant acquisition of this information. The emergency nature of the need for collateral history obtained against the patient's wishes should be documented on the chart.

THE PATIENT INTERVIEW

The emergency physician who develops a positive relationship with a psychiatric patient is more likely to obtain accurate data and compliance with disposition and treatment. Being willing to listen and understand the patient's experience accurately (empathy) assists in this process. In the busy ED environment, listening attentively for a few minutes to the reason why the patient came to the ED, without interrupting or structuring the interview, helps the patient feel understood. Also, such unstructured time allows the physician to observe the patient's mood, behavior, patterns of speech, and/or disorganized or psychotic thinking that may not be evident when the interview is structured.

Although many patients readily answer questions from the psychiatric history and mental status examination in an organized fashion, some require other approaches. The patient who is overly detailed, circumstantial, tangential, disorganized, and/or psychotic often requires a structured interview, first focusing on the history of the present illness. Such patients need to be brought back to the question asked in a tactful, empathetic manner until it is satisfactorily answered with such statements or questions as: "I realize that what you were discussing is important to you, but I was wondering if we could return to what I was asking you?" "Excuse me for interrupting you, but . . ." "Have you noticed that it is difficult for you to stay on the topic?" Specific questions often yield more data than open-ended questions with such patients. Sometimes the patient has such severe psychopathology that a history and complete mental status examination is difficult to obtain. In such cases, a collateral history is essential. A severely disturbed patient should never be left alone while the examiner is obtaining a collateral history.

Severely depressed patients may also present a challenge to the psychiatric interviewer. They may have a long latency time before answering questions, and answer in single sentences without elaboration, or make little effort to answer questions. Gentle persistence and repetition of unanswered questions is helpful in interviewing such patients. "I know you are feeling very depressed (hopeless, discouraged, etc.), but it is important that I understand what you've been going through."

Understanding and following the patient's affective state or feelings is important during the psychiatric interview. The patient's feelings should be clarified. "Tell me what you were (are) feeling." "What was the experience like for you?" "Were (are) you depressed (anxious, angry, confused, etc.)?" Following the patient's affect during the interview gives valuable data about emotionally charged areas for the patient. Some patients become overwhelmed by their feelings and are unable to convey this experience to the examiner. Providing support, structure, or later returning to the emotionally charged subject are useful techniques: "I know this is terribly painful for you." "Let me ask you some specific questions so that it's easier for you to tell me about this." "Maybe we can return to this later." With the anxious, psychotic, or cognitively impaired patient, overwhelming affect may be evidenced by increased disorganization. Specifically clarifying the affect at such a point is helpful. "Was what you were just talking about upsetting you?" "Tell me how you felt." Psychotic patients in many cases, however, are unable to elucidate the affect, and disorganization is the only clue to the emotionally charged area.

In addition to understanding feelings, it is essential

to follow other leads in the psychiatric interview. Vague statements should be clarified. If a patient stops talking suddenly, ask what happened. If connections in a patient's thinking are not clear, the examiner might state, "I'm not sure that I understand the connection between the police and your mother. Could you explain that, please?". If a statement seems peculiar, the interviewer should attempt to understand the meaning. If a patient appears preoccupied or hallucinating, the examiner should ask him or her what is going on. The interviewer should not challenge the patient's psychotic thinking but attempt to understand his or her distorted perception of reality. This is accomplished by listening with as few comments as possible except those that clarify the patient's hallucinations or delusions. On the other hand, some patients who are delusional and hallucinating may need to be reassured that they are safe (e.g., "the FBI cannot hurt you here," "There is no poison gas coming through the window."). Interpreting reality to the patient should be differentiated from arguing with his or her psychotic view of the world, which only increases agitation.

During the interview, the examiner must set firm limits on inappropriate behavior (e.g., "It is better not to wander around because it disturbs other patients." "Maybe it would be better to talk first before you call the President."). Seductive behavior is dealt with by putting physical distance between the interviewer and the patient, setting limits on the behavior, and redirecting the conversation. "Exposing yourself is inappropriate. Please cover yourself up so we can get on with the interview." Conversely, there are situations in which allowing certain behaviors facilitates the psychiatric interview. For example, a nonpsychotic but agitated patient may be better able to tolerate the interview while pacing the room.

If a patient has difficulty communicating in English, translation into the primary language is essential for the psychiatric evaluation. Medical personnel are preferred for translation. If they are unavailable, the evaluator should assess the reliability of the family member or friend assisting in translation. The examiner should always ask the translator to repeat questions exactly and to translate the patient's responses verbatim.

The specifics of the psychiatric history and mental status examination are outlined in Tables 61-1 and 61-2, respectively.

THE PHYSICAL EXAMINATION AND OTHER DIAGNOSTIC TESTS

Organic factors that could cause or contribute to psychiatric symptoms must be ruled out. Lack of identification or proper treatment of an organic brain syndrome, particularly delirium, can cause significant medical morbidity and mortality. A physical examination (including a focused neurologic examination) and appropriate laboratory evaluation should be per-

formed. As with other procedures, the psychiatric patient should always be asked, "May I examine you?" "May I draw your blood?" An organic cause for psychiatric symptoms should be considered until proven otherwise in patients who are older, have a medical illness, are taking prescribed medications known to cause behavioral symptoms, have a history of drug and/or alcohol abuse, and/or have no previous psychiatric history.[2-4] A person with a receptive or fluent aphasia, particularly acute, may be confused with one whose communication is hampered by psychotic thinking. A patient who shows inattention; clouding of consciousness; or deficits in orientation, memory, and intellectual functioning has in most cases an organic brain syndrome. Patients who *for any reason* (e.g., psychosis, agitation, depression, mania) are unable to complete the portion of the mental status examination that tests intellectual functioning warrant careful organic evaluation. Even a patient who is oriented and has a clear sensorium may have an organic cause for psychiatric symptoms, as demonstrated by the following case history.

A 35-year-old hyperreligious mother of 16 was brought to the ED because of religious and paranoid delusions. She was 5 weeks postpartum, and the delusions, according to her husband, had begun 2 weeks earlier after the death of her premature baby and intensified since then. She had no previous psychiatric history. Although she communicated little with the examiner, the husband reported that her orientation, memory, and intellectual functioning were intact. Her temperature was 98.6°F, pulse 100, blood pressure 150/110 (she had a history of hypertension), and respirations 36. Although these vital signs could have been consistent with the agitation associated with her psychotic thinking, a physical and neurologic examination were performed. Significant cardiomegaly and a mild right hemiparesis were noted. On medical hospitalization, further evaluation revealed postpartum cardiomyopathy and a large ventricular thrombus, with secondary embolization to the right frontal, parietal, and occipital regions.

Finally, it must be remembered that a known psychiatric patient may also have serious medical illness, the signs and symptoms of which cannot be accurately communicated because of the psychiatric disturbance. The following case history is such an example.

A middle-aged chronic schizophrenic male presented to the ED because "snakes were gnawing at his innards." Even this presenting complaint was difficult to identify because of his severe communication difficulties, including looseness of associations, other delusions, and hallucinations. The patient's temperature was 101°F and pulse 90, but he appeared to be in no acute distress. He had right lower quadrant pain with rebound tenderness. His white blood cell count was 18,500 with a significant shift to the left. Subsequent abdominal surgery revealed an abscessed appendix, which was removed. After surgery, the patient said that he felt much better and was pleased to be rid of the snakes in his abdomen.

TABLE 61-1. PSYCHIATRIC HISTORY

Informants (if other than the patient)
  Who are they?
  Relationship to patient
  Interest/reason for coming with patient
  Estimate reliability of informant(s)
  Expectations for ED treatment
Patient Identification
  Name, age, sex
  Religion, race/nationality, primary language
  Marital status, children, or dependents
  Current living situation (where, with whom, how long?)
  Occupation (If employed or when patient last worked)
  Financial support
Chief Complaint
  Presenting problem
  Why does patient present now?
  What type of help is desired by the patient?
History of Present Illness
  When did the symptoms of the present episode begin?
  Course of symptom progression
  What life events, stresses, conflicts, or losses are related to
    the episode?
    (common problem areas: marriage, significant others, chil-
    dren, parents, job, finances, housing, neighborhood
    safety, changes in mental health care, legal difficulties)
  Changes in or lack of compliance with psychiatric medica-
    tions or other medications with psychoactive effects (e.g.,
    steroids, antihypertensives)
  Use of intoxicants (alcohol, marijuana, cocaine, PCP, heroin,
    other illicit drugs, other prescribed medications)
  Changes in health status
  Effects of patient's symptoms on family, coworkers, neigh-
    bors, and environment
  What interventions have been tried in this episode? What
    interventions were effective? Which were not? Why?
  Level of functioning before episode; present level of func-
    tioning
Psychiatric Review of Systems (if not covered previously)
  Mood
  Sleep alterations
  Appetite alterations
  Weight gain or loss
  Change in energy level
  Change in activity level
  Social withdrawal
  Change in interest in activities
  Changes in occupational/vocational functioning

  Delusions
  Hallucinations
  Somatic preoccupation
  Disorganized or bizarre behavior
  Behavior suggesting poor judgment
  Disorientation
  Memory deficits
  Self-destructive or suicidal thoughts or behavior
  Violent or destructive thoughts or behavior
Medications
  Record all medications (prescription and over-the-counter)
  Specifically ask about "nerve pills," sleeping pills, "diet
    pills," pain pills
  Inquire about medication taken belonging to others
  Psychopharmacologic agents: dose, duration, response,
    compliance, recent additions or changes
Past Psychiatric History
  Prior episodes, duration
  Past psychiatric treatment: names of psychiatrist or other
    caregiver, location, phone number (including permission
    to contact if indicated)
  Hospitalizations: location, length, types of treatment (ECT,
    psychopharmacologic agents, psychotherapy)
  Previous psychopharmacologic treatments: doses, duration,
    response; compliance
  Suicide attempts
  Aggressive behavior, arrests
  History of past alcohol or other illicit substance use (include
    route of administration); past treatment for alcohol or
    other substance abuse
Family History of Psychiatric Illness
  "Has anyone in your family ever had any emotional, ner-
    vous, or psychiatric problems?"
  "Has anyone in your family ever had symptoms similar to
    yours?"
  Diagnosis (ask specifically about depressive illness, alcohol
    and drug abuse, schizophrenia, anxiety) or description of
    behaviors if diagnosis is not known.
  "Has anyone in your family ever received or been advised
    to receive treatment or hospitalization for emotional or
    psychiatric concerns?"
  "What types of treatment were used? What was the re-
    sponse?
  "Has anyone in your family ever made a suicide attempt?
    Committed suicide?"
Present and Past Medical History
  Use standard questions for medical history.

TABLE 61-2. MENTAL STATUS EXAMINATION[5–10]

Mental Status Feature	Definition and Assessment	Mental Status Feature	Definition and Assessment
1. General Appearance Physical appearance and grooming	Compare appearance of age to stated actual age (e.g., chronic alcoholic may appear older than stated age) Well groomed Appropriately attired for weather and situation Unkempt, dirty, malodorous Bizarre (e.g., disorganized schizophrenic may wear heavy winter coat in		summer; manic may have exaggerated facial makeup) Physical abnormalities: scars (e.g., self-inflicted cigarette burns or wrist lacerations), tattoos, needle tracks
		Level of consciousness and attention	Alert Lethargic Semicomatose Fluctuations in state of consciousness

TABLE 61-2. CONTINUED

Mental Status Feature	Definition and Assessment	Mental Status Feature	Definition and Assessment
	Dysattention—Reduced ability to maintain attention to external stimuli (e.g., questions must be repeated because attention wanders) and to appropriately shift attention to new stimuli	2. *Emotionality* Mood	The predominant emotional state that is sustained over a period of time may be described by the patient upon questioning or inferred by the interviewer based on observation of the patient's behavior and content of thought. Note discrepancies.
Manner	Passive, withdrawn Effusive, seductive Grandiose, domineering Guarded, suspicious Hostile		*Ask:* "How are your spirits?" "How have you been feeling emotionally?" Common moods include: Depressed—Sad, down, blue, anhedonia (inability to experience pleasure)
Relationship to interviewer	Eye contact Patient's ability to appropriately relate and interact with interviewer (e.g., synchronization of nonverbal interaction with interviewer) Cooperative/Uncooperative		Euphoric—Great, high, up, never better Anxious Angry Apathetic
Motor behavior level of activity	Hyperactivity (as in mania) Hypoactivity (as in depression, dementia, delirium) Psychomotor retardation Includes decreased rate of motor activity, decreased rate of thought, and increased latency in speech production (as in depression) Agitation or restlessness (Increased frequency of nongoal-directed motor activity): pacing hand wringing finger or foot tapping head scratching frequent shifting of body position	Affect	The observable, more transient expression of an individual's emotional state. *Note:* range—Refers to variability of affect (e.g., depressed individuals often exhibit constricted range of affect) Amplitude—Refers to amount of energy expended in expressing an affect; may be described as intense, blunted, flattened, (as in some schizophrenics may show flattened affect)
Unusual movements	Tremors Tics Stereotyped movements Lip smacking Tardive dyskinesia		Stability—Observe for frequent or abrupt changes in affect during short period (as in PCP-intoxicated patients who may exhibit labile affective fluctuations)
Gestures	Note amount and appropriateness		Appropriateness—Observe for matching of affective expression with the content of verbal expressions, underlying mood and/or behavior (e.g., schizophrenics may show inappropriate affect that is discordant with content of speech)
Body positioning	Depressive posture— Slumped, leaning forward (as in depression) Posturing—Positioning of body parts in unusual manner (as in psychosis) Grimace—Form of facial posturing Echopraxia—Patient imitates movements of the interviewer (as in catatonia) Waxy flexibility—Patient allows the examiner to place his limbs in unusual positions (as in catatonia) Note: Catatonia may have organic as well as psychiatric causes.	3. *Thought Process*	Thought process is assessed by observation of how a patient is talking, i.e., the form of his speech; hence abnormalities are sometimes described as formal thought disorders.

TABLE 61-2. CONTINUED

	Definition and Assessment	Mental Status Feature	Definition and Assessment
Amount	Hyperverbal (as in mania) Poverty of speech (as in depression)		Claus has a sleigh pulled by "deinreer" (as in psychosis)
Rate of production	Increased rate of thoughts suggested by pressured speech (as in mania) *Ask:* "Have your thoughts been going fast? Racing?" Decreased rate of thought *Ask:* "Has your thinking slowed down?" (as in depression, dementia, delirium)	Clanging	Word approximations—Example: moving staircase for elevator Word associations are made by sounds rather than by meaning. Example: Now the cow to Mao somehow (as in mania)
Continuity	Assess linkage between associations expressed in patient's speech Circumstantial—Overinclusive detail but tight linkage of associations with attainment of goal Tangential—Goal in verbalization is missed because of associations that go off on tangents Flight of ideas—Repeated, abrupt shifts in topic, usually with an underlying thread of association (as in mania) Loosening of associations— Disruptions of meaningful associations (idiosyncratic associations, not consensually validated) between words or phrases (as in schizophrenia) Incoherence—Global loosening of associations Poverty of content of speech—Speech adequate in amount but conveys little information Word Salad—Words or phrases that are meaningless to the interviewer and the patient producing them (as in schizophrenia) Blocking—Sudden interruption and cessation of thought manifested as a break in speech (as in schizophrenia) Derailment—disruption of one train of thought and beginning on another, often associated with word blocking	Echolalia Perseveration 4. *Thought Content* Ideas of reference Paranoid/persecutory ideation Delusion	Patient repeats parts of the interviewer's words or phrases (as in catatonia) Persistent repetition of words or phrases (as in psychosis) or repetition of answers not related to successive questioning (as in, brain damage or dysfunction) *Ask:* "Does it seem that people are referring to you when they speak with others?" "Do you find yourself being referred to when you listen to the television or radio or when you read the newspaper?" If the answer is affirmative, always ask "How so?" Ask for examples. Ideation based on misinterpretation of actual circumstances; feelings of being harassed, persecuted, or unfairly treated A fixed false belief engendered without appropriate external stimuli, maintained in spite of evidence to the contrary, and not accepted by the person's subculture Follow up any positive responses with questions to determine how the individual came to have such a belief. "How did you find this out?" Paranoid delusion—False belief that one is being conspired against, cheated, followed, imprisoned, poisoned, maliciously maligned, etc. *Ask:* "Does it seem that anyone is deliberately trying to harm you or is out to get you in any way?" "How so?" "What gives you that feeling?" Grandiose delusion—Delusion involving exaggera-
Aphasia	Inability to understand or produce language (as in stroke)		
Paraphasias	Neologisms—Idiosyncratic word use or manufacture of new words by incorrect use of the sounds in a word. Example: Santa		

TABLE 61-2. CONTINUED

Mental Status Feature	Definition and Assessment	Mental Status Feature	Definition and Assessment
	tion of one's sense of importance, power, knowledge, or identity *Ask:* "Do you have any special relationship with God?" "Tell me about any special powers or abilities that you may have." "Is there any special mission that you have in life?" Somatic delusions—Subjective report that the body is disordered or disturbed; patient falsely believes he or she is ill, ugly, malodorous, deformed, or has body cavity filled with vermin (as in psychotic depression, schizophrenia) Delusions of sin and guilt—Belief of persecution because of moral transgression or personal inadequacy Delusions of poverty—False belief that one is poor Delusion of nihilism or nonexistence—Delusion of not being or nonexistence of the self Delusions of jealousy—Delusion that spouse or lover is unfaithful Delusion of love—Delusion that one is falsely loved by another Delusion of being controlled or influenced—Feelings, thoughts or impulses that are not one's own but imposed by an external source *Ask:* "Does it ever seem that others can control your thoughts, feelings, or actions?" Thought insertion—thoughts that are not one's own are inserted into one's mind *Ask:* "Can people put thoughts into your head?" Thought withdrawal—thoughts are removed from one's mind *Ask:* "Can people take thoughts out of your head?" Thought broadcasting—Thoughts broadcast from one's mind so that others can hear them *Ask:* "Do you think people can read your thoughts?" "Do your	Suicidal ideation/thoughts of self-harm	thoughts leak out of your head?" "Can your thoughts intersect with others?" *Ask:* "Sometimes when people feel (discouraged, hopeless, depressed, frightened, so nervous they can't stand it) they find themselves thinking about death." "Have you had thoughts about death." "Now?" "In the past?" "Have you ever had thoughts about ending your life or harming yourself?" "Now?" "In the past?" "Is there anything that could cause you to have such thoughts?" What is your plan for ending your life or harming yourself?" "Do you have the means to carry it out?" Also separately inquire about self-mutilation. *Ask:* "Does cutting yourself decrease the anxiety?" "Make you feel better?" (as in nonsuicidal self-mutilation commonly seen with borderline personality)
		Homicidal ideation/ thoughts of harm to others	*Ask:* "Have you ever had thoughts of seriously harming or ending the life of someone?" (If yes, details?) "Do you currently have any such thoughts?" "How might you do that?" "When might you do that?"
		Obsessions	Persistent, senseless, or irrational thoughts or impulses not experienced as voluntarily produced that invade consciousness *Ask:* "Do you have any thoughts or worries that recur over and over and you can't keep from intruding into your consciousness?"
		Compulsions	Repetitive or stereotyped activity in response to an obsession (e.g., repeatedly checking locks, stove, etc.; repeated needless counting; frequent, excessive washing of hands) *Ask:* "Do you have any activities you engage in to

TABLE 61-2. CONTINUED

Mental Status Feature	Definition and Assessment	Mental Status Feature	Definition and Assessment
Phobias	try to control these thoughts or worries?" Irrational fear of objects or situations (e.g., crowds, heights, elevators, going outdoors) *Ask:* "Are there any specific objects or situations that you avoid because they cause you extreme anxiety?"		*Ask:* "Do you ever experience any unusual sense on your skin or in your body?" *Note:* Visual, gustatory, olfactory, tactile, and visceral hallucinations often indicate an organic basis for the hallucination
5. *Perception* Derealization	Feeling estranged from one's environment *Ask:* "Do things around you seem strange or different?" "Like a movie?" (as in substance-intoxicated states, depression, extreme anxiety, severe stress)	6. *Intellectual Functioning* Orientation	Time: *Ask:* "Day of week?"* "Date?"* "Month?"* "Season?"* "Year?"* (1 point for each correct answer. Total 5) "How long have you been here?" "When did you arrive?" "What time is it now?"
Depersonalization	Alteration in perception of self, self-estrangement, perceiving self from a distance. *Ask:* "Do you feel unreal?" "Distanced from yourself?" (as in anxiety, schizophrenia)		Place: *Ask:* "Where are you?" "Location?" "Name of hospital?"* "Where in hospital?"* "City?"* "County?"* "State?"* (1 point for each correct answer. Total 5)
Illusions	Misinterpretation of a real external stimulus. Example: A shadow misinterpreted as an intruder, folds in the bedclothes as snakes (as in delirium, severe sleep deprivation)	Attention	Person: *Ask:* Names, relationships, and roles of people in patient's environment. Patient's full name. Note patient's general ability to remain focused on the interview process Digits span forward
Hallucinations	A disordered sensory perception occurring without stimulus. Auditory hallucination: *Ask:* "Do you ever seem to hear voices talking when no one is around?" "Coming from where, whom?" "Content? When? Do you ever hear your thoughts spoken aloud?" "Do you ever hear voices commenting on your behavior?" Command hallucination: *Ask:* "Are you ever commanded to harm yourself, others, or do a particular act?" Visual hallucination: *Ask:* "Do you ever seem to have visions or see things that other people could not see?" Details? Gustatory or olfactory hallucination: *Ask:* "Do you ever experience any unusual tastes or smells?" Tactile or visceral hallucination:	Concentration	*Ask:* "Please repeat these digits forward." Begin with 3 digits forward Increase to 6 digits or until patient fails Normal performance is 6 digits forwards (also tests immediate memory) *Note:* Impairments of attention and concentration may be seen in organic mental syndromes, depression, severe anxiety, and psychotic states Digits span backwards *Ask:* "Please repeat these numbers backwards" Begin with 2 digits Increase to 4 digits or until patient fails Normal performance is 4 digits backwards (also tests immediate memory) *Ask* the patient to spell the word world forwards

TABLE 61-2. CONTINUED

Mental Status Feature	Definition and Assessment	Mental Status Feature	Definition and Assessment
	and then backwards (dlrow) Serial 7s* (see arithmetic calculation) or serial 3s for patient with poor educational background. (Stop after 5. Alternate: spell world backwards. 1 point for each correct answer. Total 5 points.)		Differences and Similarities Apple and orange Train and motorcycle Child and dwarf Have patient describe a local or world event and explain the significance. Proverbs The patient should be familiar with the proverb; cultural differences may contribute to variability of the response. "People in glass houses shouldn't throw stones." "A stitch in time saves nine." "Don't cry over split milk." "You can catch more flies with honey than vinegar." Concrete response (e.g., organic brain disease, educational deficits) Idiosyncratic response (e.g., psychosis)
Memory	Immediate memory: Three unrelated objects— *Ask* the patient to immediately repeat the unrelated objects.* (1 point for each correct answer. Total 3) Then ask for recall of the items after 5 minutes.* (1 point for each correct answer. Total 3) Informally note if patient recalls details or facts discussed within past 15 minutes of interview (although impairment may actually be in realm of attention and/or concentration) Recent Memory: *Ask* for details of various activities within the past few days. Items must then be verified. *Ask* what time the patient went to bed last night, what clothing was worn yesterday, which was eaten for breakfast, lunch, earlier in the day. Remote past: *Ask* verifiable personal past details such as dates of birthdays and anniversaries, birthplace, past addresses. Also assess by inquiring about past presidents, significant historical events in patient's lifetime. Confabulation The patient makes up (falsifies) responses to questions not known or recalled (as in amnestic syndrome, dementia)	General intellect	Note patient's use of vocabulary and ability to conceptualize and express ideas in comparison to their educational level. If impairment is suspected, further assess patient's knowledge of general information. Example: name 10 countries other than the U.S.
		General cortical functioning	*Ask* the patient to name objects such as a pencil or watch.* (1 point each correct answer. Total 2) *Ask:* the patient to repeat "no ifs, ands, or buts." (1 point) *Ask:* "Take this paper in your right hand, fold in half, and put it on the floor."* (1 point each correct answer. Total 3.) *Ask:* patient to write a sentence.* (1 point) *Ask:* patient to read and obey the following: "close your eyes."* (1 point) *Ask* patient to copy the outline of simple geometric shapes (e.g., intersecting pentagons) (1 point)
Arithmetic calculation	Serial 7s *Ask* the patient to subtract 7 from 100, and then to continue making subsequent substractions by 7. This also tests concentration. *Ask* the patient to calculate a few simple problems such as making change.		
Abstract thinking	Patient's ability to abstract tests frontal lobe functioning		

TABLE 61-2. CONTINUED

Mental Status Feature	Definition and Assessment	Mental Status Feature	Definition and Assessment
Judgment	Ability to correctly perceive data from environment, process that data on previous experience and knowledge, and make a decision or act in a fashion that is culturally appropriate This is best determined by recent history and from observations made throughout the assessment From source other than patient, inquire about recent unusual or inappropriate behaviors or activities	Insight	Was patient adequately clothed when brought to the ED? Is patient able to make appropriate decision based on the environment? Is the patient aware of any impairment or difficulties that he or she is having? Does the patient have insight into the illness? How does he or she explain its cause? How does the patient see his or her condition impacting upon others?

* These questions are from the Mini Mental Status examination,[11] a screening examination for general intellectual functioning. A perfect score is 30. A score of less than 23 (less than 21 for those with an eighth-grade education) shows evidence of cognitive dysfunction.

REFERENCES

1. Schauss, A.G.: Tranquilizing effect of color reduces aggressive behavior and potential violence. Orthomolecular Psychiatry 8:218, 1979.
2. Wells, C.E.: Dementia. Contemporary Neurology Series. Philadelphia, F.A. Davis, 1972.
3. Plum, F., and Posner, J.B. (eds.): Diagnosis of Stupor and Coma. Contemporary Neurology Series. Philadelphia, F.A. Davis, 1966.
4. Lipowski, Z.J.: Organic mental disorders. In Comprehensive Textbook of Psychiatry. 3rd Ed. Edited by Kaplan, H.I., Freedman, A.M., and Saddock, B.J. Baltimore, Williams & Wilkins, 1980.
5. Leigh, H.: Mental status examinations: Systemic observation of the patient. In Psychiatry in the Practice of Medicine. Edited by Leigh, H. Menlo Park, California, Addison-Wesley, 1983.
6. Strub, R.L., and Black, F.W.: The Mental Status Examination in Neurology. Philadelphia, F.A. Davis Company, 1977.
7. American Psychiatric Association's Psychiatric Glossary. Washington, D.C., American Psychiatric Press, Inc., 1980.
8. Folstein, M.F., Folstein, S., and McHugh, P.R.: The mini mental status examination. J. Psychiatric Res. 12:180, 1975.
9. Glossary of Technical Terms. In Diagnostic and Statistical Manual of Mental Disorders. 3rd Ed, revised. Washington, D.C., American Psychiatric Press, Inc., 1987.
10. Taylor, M.A.: The Neuropsychiatric Mental Status Examination. New York, Pergamon Press, 1981.
11. Anthony, J.C., et al.: Limits of the "Mini-Mental Status" as a screening test for dementia and delirium among hospital patients. Psychol. Med. 12:397, 1982.

BIBLIOGRAPHY

Bassuk, E.L., and Birk, A.W.: The concept of emergency care. In Emergency Psychiatry, Concepts, Methods, and Practices. Edited by Bassuk, E.L., and Birk, A.W., New York, Plenum Press, 1984.

Bassuk, E.L., and Skodol, A.E.: The first few minutes: Identifying and managing life-threatening emergencies. In Emergency Psychiatry, Concepts, Methods, and Practices. Edited by Bassuk, E.L., and Birk, A.W. New York, Plenum Press, 1984.

Cavenar, J.O., Jr., Cavenar, M.G., Hillard, J.R., and Kahn, E.M.: Basic concepts of emergency care. In Psychiatric Emergencies, Intervention and Resolution. Edited by Walker, J.I., Philadelphia, J.B. Lippincott, 1983.

Leigh, H., Feinstein, A.R., and Reiser, M.F.: Systemic approach to comprehensive care: The patient evaluation grid. In Psychiatry in the Practice of Medicine. Edited by Leigh, H. Menlo Park, California, Addison-Wesley, 1983.

MacKinnon, R.A.: Diagnoses and psychiatry: Examination of the psychiatric patient. In Comprehensive Textbook of Psychiatry. 3rd Ed. Edited by Kaplan, H.I., Freedman, A.M., and Saddock, B.J., Baltimore, Williams & Wilkins, 1980.

MacKinnon, R.A., and Michels, R. (Eds.): The Psychiatric Interview in Clinical Practice. Philadelphia, W.B. Saunders Company, 1971.

Scheiber, S.C.: Psychiatric interview, psychiatric history and mental status examination. In Textbook of Psychiatry. Edited by Talbott, J.A., Hales, R.E., and Yudofsky, S.C., Washington, D.C., American Psychiatric Press, Inc., 1988.

Slaby, A.E., Lieb, J., and Tancredi, L.R. (Eds.): Handbook of Psychiatric Emergencies. 3rd Ed. New York, Medical Examination Publishing Co., 1986.

Tomb, D.A.: Assessment. In Psychiatry for the House Officer. 3rd Ed. Edited by Tomb, D.A., Baltimore, Williams & Wilkins, 1984.

OVERVIEW OF COMMON PSYCHIATRIC EMERGENCIES

Stephanie von Ammon Cavanaugh and William S. Gilmer

CAPSULE

The most common psychiatric problems seen in patients who present to the Emergency Department (ED) include: (1) organic brain syndromes, (2) psychosis, (3) suicidal ideation or attempt, (4) potential or actual violent behavior, (5) acute subjective psychologic distress such as depressed or anxious mood, and (6) somatic complaints with-

out demonstrable physical illness which are linked to psychologic factors. This subchapter reviews the differential diagnosis of these common psychiatric emergencies, followed by a brief discussion of their clinical management. Tables 61-3 and 61-4 outline the mental status features of common organic brain syndromes and common nonorganic psychiatric syndromes, respectively.

TABLE 61-3. MENTAL STATUS FEATURES IN COMMON ORGANIC BRAIN SYNDROMES[1,2]

	Delirium	Dementia	Amnestic Syndrome
General appearance/behavior	Fluctuating level of consciousness Hyper- or hypoalertness to stimuli May be agitated or slowed down	May be normal, disheveled, or unkempt Activity slowed down or, if psychotic, agitated	May be normal or disheveled
Mood/affect	Irritable, anxious, fearful, labile, or depressed	Normal, irritable, or, if psychotic, as in delirium	Normal
Speech/thought process	Increased or decreased rate Circumstantial Tangential Incoherent	Normal or slowed Circumstantial, tangential, or rambling Aphasia If psychotic, incoherent	Normal Circumstantial or tangential Confabulation
Thought content	May have: Ideas of reference Paranoid ideation Somatic delusions	Normal or, if psychotic, as in delirium	Normal
Perception vivid	Illusions Vivid visual hallucinations Less commonly, olfactory or gustatory hallucinations	Normal or, if psychotic, same as delirium	Normal
Orientation	Order in which impairment may be seen: time, place, person May fluctuate	Impairment depends on degree of dementia Order in which impairment occurs: time, place, person Does not fluctuate	Disorientation to time, place, and often person
Attention and concentration	Poor	Normal or decreased	Normal or decreased
Memory			
Immediate	Poor	May be normal or decreased	Normal
Recent	Poor	Poor	Poor
Remote	Impaired in severe delirium	Impaired in severe dementia	Impaired
General intellectual functioning	Depends upon severity of delirium Fluctuates	Depends upon degree of dementia May have difficulty with calculations, abstract thinking (concrete), constructional ability, apraxia, agnosia	Normal Normal

TABLE 61-4. MENTAL STATUS FEATURES OF COMMON PSYCHIATRIC SYNDROMES

	Schizophrenia	Mania	Depression	Anxiety and Panic Attacks
Appearance/behavior	Unkempt Bizarre, odd, or eccentric Suspicious Peculiar relatedness May be agitated	Exaggerated appearance, possibly bizarre Agitated, hyperactive, or boisterous Hyperacute to stimuli Relates well unless psychotic	Head lowered May look sad or tearful Movement slowed or may be agitated	May be agitated Appears anxious Evidence of autonomic hyperactivity
Mood/affect	Flat, bizarre, odd, or inappropriate	Euphoric, expansive, or irritable May be labile or hostile	Depressed Blunted or constricted range	Anxious Fearful
Speech/thought process	Vague, lacking in content Looseness of associations Thought blocking Derailment Neologisms	Pressured speech Flight of ideas Rhyming	Unless agitated, may have decreased production or increased latency If psychotic, may have illogical speech	Rapid, pressured speech May be overly inclusive of trivia or details
Thought content	Occasional suicidal ideation (related to command hallucinations and delusions) Elaborate, often fragmented delusions (paranoid, somatic nihilistic, control) Thought broadcasting Thought insertion Thought withdrawal	Suicidal ideation possible in dysphoric manics Grandiose or paranoid delusions	Suicidal ideation Ideas of guilt, worthlessness, hopelessness, helplessness If psychotic, delusions of sin, guilt, poverty, nihilism, or disease	Fears of going crazy or dying Preoccupation with somatic complaints
Perceptions	Frequent auditory hallucinations (two voices commenting on behavior) Visual hallucinations accompany the auditory hallucinations	Frequent auditory hallucinations Visual hallucinations accompany auditory hallucinations	Auditory hallucinations (usually self-deprecating)	None
Orientation	Disorientation is not from memory deficits, but delusions, hallucinations, and inattention to the environment		Intact (unless profoundly depressed or psychotic, then as in schizophrenia and mania)	Intact
Attention and concentration	Decreased	Variable	Decreased	Decreased
Memory	Problems with memory are not from true memory deficits, but related to hallucinations, delusions, or inattention to the environment			
General intellectual functioning	Intact if testable Abstraction may be concrete or personalized	Intact unless psychotic; then may not be testable	Slowed but intact	Intact (errors from poor attention and concentration)

ORGANIC BRAIN SYNDROMES

Diagnostically, it is essential to distinguish patients with an organic brain syndrome from those with a psychiatric disorder. An organic brain syndrome is an impairment of mental functioning secondary to structural or functional abnormalities of brain tissue which is "evidenced from history, physical examination or laboratory tests"[1] to be causally related to specific organic factors. Failure to identify and treat an organic brain syndrome, particularly a delirium, may be life-threatening, cause increased morbidity (i.e., brain damage), and result in harmful, inappropriate, or inadequate treatment. Patients who are more likely to have an organic cause for psychiatric symptoms are those: (1) without a previous psychiatric history, (2) over 45, (3) taking medications with central nervous system effects, (4) abusing drugs or alcohol, (5) with concurrent medical illness, or (6) who have sustained trauma. As mentioned previously, a good history, including a collateral history, vital signs, a physical examination, a focused neurologic examination, and appropriate screening laboratory tests assist in identifying the organic causes of psychiatric syndromes.

Memory deficits are present in delirium, dementia, and amnestic syndrome. In a *delirium*, there is evidence of dysattention, clouding of consciousness, memory impairment, incoherent speech, delusions, and visual hallucinations[1] (Table 61-3). Memory deficits and deterioration of higher intellectual functions (poor abstraction, aphasia, apraxia, agnosia) are present in *dementia*[1] (Table 61-3). Memory difficulties and confabulation without dysattention, clouding of consciousness, or deterioration of intellectual functioning are characteristic of the *amnestic syndrome*[1] (Table 61-3). Organic mood disorder, organic delusional disorder, organic hallucinosis, and organic personality syndrome can mimic psychiatric disorders. Patients with these disorders have no dysattention, little memory impairment, and minimal difficulties with higher intellectual functioning. In *organic delusional disorder,* the most prominent feature is delusions; in *organic hallucinosis,* hallucinations. Those with an *organic mood disorder* have a depressed, expansive, or euphoric mood, and those with an *organic anxiety disorder,* signs and symptoms of a generalized anxiety or panic disorder.[1] Those with *organic personality disorder* have changes in personality.[1]

PSYCHOSIS

Patients who are psychotic are out of touch with reality. They display one or more of the following: (1) inappropriate or bizarre appearance or behavior, (2) inappropriate, bizarre, flat, euphoric, or depressed affect, (3) illogical thinking manifested by abnormalities in the form of speech (i.e., poverty of speech, pressured speech, flight of ideas, loosening of associations, incoherence, and paraphasias), (4) delusions and/or (5) hallucinations. Psychotic patients are brought to the ED by family, friends, or those in the community because the patient's behavior is alarming to those around them. These patients may present themselves to the ED because they are frightened or perplexed, or at some level realize their psychotic symptoms warrant medical evaluation and treatment. Chronically mentally ill patients who are psychotic may also attempt to use the ED as an outpatient clinic to receive referrals, refills in prescriptions, or medication dosage changes. The differential diagnosis of psychosis includes psychotic organic brain syndromes (including psychoactive substance intoxication or withdrawal), mania, depression with psychotic features, schizophrenia, schizophreniform disorder, brief reactive psychosis, and delusional disorder. Psychotic organic brain syndromes include delirium, dementia with superimposed hallucinations or delusions, organic hallucinosis, organic delusional disorder, and psychotic organic mood disorders. See the previous section for characteristics of organic brain syndromes.

After ruling out an organic cause for the psychotic process, nonorganic psychiatric disorders may be considered. A patient with a *major depressive episode*[2] may develop psychotic symptoms. In a psychotic depression, the signs and symptoms of a major depressive episode usually precede the psychotic symptoms. These symptoms include at least five of the following for a 2-week period: depressed mood, marked diminished interest or pleasure in activities, significant weight gain or loss, decreased or increased appetite, insomnia or hypersomnia, fatigue or loss of energy, diminished ability to think or concentrate or indecisiveness, psychomotor agitation or retardation, feelings of worthlessness or inappropriate guilt, and/or suicidal ideation or attempt. Delusions or hallucinations are consistent with depressive themes of guilt, punishment, persecution, disease, death, or nihilism. The patient may have a personal or family history of depressive and/or manic episodes (Table 61-4). The average age of onset of a depressive illness is the mid-20s, but the onset may be at any age. A patient with a *manic episode*[2] often develops psychotic symptoms. The signs and symptoms of a manic episode include elevated, expansive, or irritable mood, inflated self-esteem, grandiosity, decreased need for sleep, pressure of speech, flight of ideas, subjective experience of racing thoughts, distractability, increase in goal-directed activity, unrestrained buying sprees, sexual indiscretion, or foolish business investments. The symptoms may precede the psychotic symptoms or occur simultaneously. Delusions or hallucinations associated with a manic episode are consistent with themes of inflated power, worth, knowledge, identity, or special relationship to a famous person or deity. Paranoid delusions, although less common, may also be present (Table 61-4). The patient may have a previous personal and/or family history of depressive and/or manic episodes. The onset of bipolar disorder is usually in the 20s, is rare after 45, but can occur at any age. Between depressive or manic episodes, patients with a major mood disorder usually return to their previous level of functioning.

With *schizophrenia,*[3] psychotic symptoms rather than a disorder of mood are primary. During the prodromal period (days to weeks), the patient may manifest: (1) inappropriate or flat affect; (2) social withdrawal; (3) impairment in social role; (4) peculiar behavior; (5) odd, overelaborate, vague, circumstantial speech; (6) odd "magical" thinking; and/or (7) unusual perceptual experiences. The patient most commonly comes to the ED during the psychotic phase. In this acute phase, the patient may show: (1) inappropriate, bizarre flat affect; (2) bizarre, inappropriate, or stereotyped behavior; (3) agitation or withdrawal; (4) looseness of association, paraphasias, incoherent speech; (5) bizarre fragmented delusions (thought broadcasting, delusions of being controlled); and/or (6) auditory hallucinations (a voice keeping up a running commentary on the patient's behavior or thoughts or two or more voices conversing with each other). Catatonic symptoms may also be present, including: (1) marked lack of reactivity to the environment, (2) reduction in spontaneous movements, (3) mutism, (4) catatonic negativism, motiveless resistance to all instructions, rigidity against attempts to be moved, and positioning of the body in inappropriate or bizarre postures, (5) waxy flexibility, and/or (6) echopraxia. It is important to note that catatonia is more frequently caused by organic pathology (hallucinogens, amphetamines, frontal lobe lesions, general paresis, diabetic ketoacidosis, porphyria, hyperparathyroidism, lupus erythematosus, viral encephalitis, and Wernicke's encephalopathy[4] than by schizophrenia, psychotic depression, or mania. The onset of schizophrenia is usually in adolescence or young adulthood and almost never after age 45. Patients with schizophrenia never return to their premorbid level of functioning between episodes. Symptoms of the prodromal, acutely psychotic, or residual phase (same symptoms as described for the prodromal phase) must last for 6 months (see Table 61-4). A *schizophreniform* disorder[5] differs from schizophrenia only in that the duration is less than 6 months.

A *brief reactive psychosis*[5] usually follows a stressful event, has an abrupt onset, and shows rapid shifts from one affect to another and/or overwhelming confusion. The psychotic symptoms are rarely as bizarre as in schizophrenia. The episode lasts a few days to a few weeks and never more than a month. After the psychotic episode, the person can be expected to return to his or her previous level of functioning. In a *delusional disorder*,[6] circumscribed nonbizarre delusions occur, with themes of erotomania, grandiosity, persecution, jealousy, love, or disordered bodily function, but no bizarre, peculiar, or odd affect, speech, or behavior.

In psychotic depression, mania, schizophrenia, schizophreniform disorder, delusional disorder, and brief reactive psychosis, there is no clouding of consciousness, disorientation, or memory deficits as seen in delirium and dementia. Significant impairments in attention and concentration caused by a disordered affective state, psychotic thinking, hallucinations, and/or delusions, are often present, however, and make assessments of intellectual functioning difficult to impossible. Delirium and psychotic dementia classically present with vivid visual hallucinations, whereas the nonorganic psychotic disorders present primarily with auditory hallucinations.

Psychotic patients may harm themselves or others or elope. As a result, the psychotic patient should be closely observed until evaluation by the emergency physician. Triage management, a safe environment for the interview and evaluation, and structuring the interview with a psychotic patient has been discussed previously. The use of restraints and psychotropic medication with the psychotic patient is discussed subsequently. *If a psychotic organic mental disorder is suspected, the use of psychotropic drugs should be carefully evaluated because level of consciousness may be an important indicator of deteriorating physical condition and is altered by psychotropic medication.* Psychotic patients, except in rare instances, require hospitalization. Commitment and hospitalization are reviewed subsequently. Chapter 62 provides an in-depth discussion of the diagnosis and management of psychotic patients.

SUICIDALITY

Patients with suicidal ideation, a suicide attempt, or other self-inflicted harm commonly present to the ED. Patients with various psychiatric problems may be suicidal, but not express these thoughts without being asked. Suicide risk should be assessed in all patients who present to the ED with psychiatric problems, regardless of whether the clinical situation seems to warrant it. The patient should be asked about present and past suicidal ideation and attempts, and attempts and completed suicides in family members. Chapter 22 outlines in detail the assessment of suicidal patients.

Men commit suicide three times as often as women, whereas women attempt suicide two to three times as often as men.[7-9] For men, the suicide rate increases up to the seventh decade, then declines; for women, the suicide rate peaks between ages 55 and 65.[10,11] Whites and American Indians are at higher risk than blacks.[7,11] People living alone, who feel no one cares, are without friends, and have limited social supports, are at greatest risk for suicide.[7,10,12] Those who are single, widowed, separated, or divorced, married without children, married with children over 18, and married with children under 18 are in descending order for risk of suicide.[7,10,12] Regardless of marital status, children under the age of 18 have a decreasing risk of suicide. A past history of suicide attempts increases the risk.[10-12] Ten percent of those who attempt suicide go on to kill themselves. The risk of suicide is higher for those who have a family history of completed or attempted suicides.[10] Sense of hopelessness and inability to see into the future are highly correlated with future suicide.[13,14] Suicidal ideation with paranoid ideation or hallucinations commanding the patient to harm himself or herself increases the risk of suicide. The patient whose suicide threat or attempt was to manipulate or punish someone in the environment is at a lesser risk than one whose wish to die is self-directed. Depression with severe agitation increases suicide risk.[12] Certain stresses are statistically associated with increased suicide risk: recent loss within 6 months, severe financial difficulties, job loss, severe family stress, childbirth, recent surgery, chronic severe illness, and intractable pain.[6,9,12] It is crucial to note that a patient without any of these risk factors can be acutely suicidal.

Seventy percent of patients who commit suicide have a major depressive disorder, mixed bipolar disorder, schizophrenia, psychotic organic mental disorder, alcoholism, drug abuse, and/or a borderline character disorder.[11,14,15] In the ED, these diagnostic categories are also likely to present with suicidal ideation, a suicide attempt, or self-inflicted injuries. Patients with depressed mood regardless of diagnosis often have suicidal ideation. The following depressed patients are at significant risk for suicide: those who are hopeless, agitated, or psychotic; those with previous attempts; those with recent loss of a loved one; those with a plan and a means to carry it out; and those with a suicide in the family. Patients who are manic can sometimes also display depressed features (mixed bipolar disorder) with suicidal ideation, which can be missed if not specifically asked for.

Psychotic patients of all diagnostic categories discussed in the last section can be of risk for self-harm and should be asked about suicidal ideation. Those with suicidal ideation are at significant risk. Psychotic patients may be driven to harm themselves because of delusions and hallucinations. Paranoid delusions can drive a patient to self-harm. "I took an overdose (or attempted to jump out the window) because I was so frightened and wanted to get away from the people who were trying to harm me." Delusions of guilt or worthlessness may drive a patient to a suicide attempt. "I am such a horrible person, I must die." Patients with command hallucinations that suggest self-harm are at risk. "The voice commanded me to take the overdose (or jump in front of the train)." "God told me to stab myself so I could join him in heaven." Psychotic thinking can at times inadvertently result in self-harm. "I poured gasoline on myself and lit it to purify my thoughts." Finally, psychotic persons may be of harm to themselves because of poor judgment or inability to accurately assess the environment. A schizophrenic may walk without a coat or shoes in subzero weather in a dangerous neighborhood, or a delirious patient may pull out an endotracheal tube.

Patients with severe character disorder may develop a pattern of suicide attempts to deal with anger, interpersonal rejection, loss of self esteem, or anxiety. Further, some severely character-disordered patients superficially cut themselves to relieve anxiety or to "feel real" without suicidal intent. These patients are not at severe risk, but may miscalculate and seriously harm or kill themselves. Patients with a severe character disorder may sometimes become so disordered that suicide attempts become bizarre and potentially lethal. Inquiry into the nature of past self-destructive attempts helps to identify this group.

Another group of patients with less severe or no character pathology may become suicidal or make a suicide attempt under severe environmental stress. Most commonly seen are suicide attempts that occur after a disagreement or rejection by a parent, spouse, or significant other. Such suicidal ideation or attempt is usually a cry for help, or a way to punish or get the attention of the significant other. On the other hand, adolescents who lose self-esteem and also experience the rupture of a valued relationship may impulsively make a lethal attempt.

Alcohol or drug abuse alone or combined with depression, psychosis, character pathology, and/or environmental stress greatly increases the risk of suicide. Drugs and alcohol alter mood, weaken defenses, impair judgment, and may result in marked increase of the dysphoric mood and suicidal ideation. For example, the mildly depressed man with passive suicidal ideation, marital stress, and job difficulties may become severely depressed and make a lethal suicide attempt under the influence of alcohol. Patients with an organic mental disorder secondary to intoxication or withdrawal from alcohol may also harm themselves. Finally, patients with alcohol and/or drug abuse may miscalculate drug intake and inadvertently overdose.

Patients who are actively suicidal can be extremely creative in carrying out a suicide attempt in the ED or during transfer to a medical, surgical or psychiatric facility. For this reason, the patient must be separated from medical equipment or belongings that could be used for self-injury. Further, one-to-one supervision (not by a family member) for the patient is mandatory in the ED and during transfer to a medical, surgical, or psychiatric facility. If a patient requires leather restraints because of active attempts at self-harm, one-to-one supervision is also required. Full leather restraints should never be used in lieu of one-to-one supervision. Evaluation of suicidal intent is a complex process. As a rule, a suicidal patient should never be sent home without evaluation by a psychiatrist or mental health professional. A patient who has made a suicide attempt should be given emergency medical or surgical care. If medically unstable, the patient should be transferred to a medical or surgical unit with one-to-one supervision (not by a family member) until a psychiatric consultant decides that the supervision is no longer necessary. If medically stable, the patient should be admitted to a psychiatric unit. Patients who have made a suicide attempt should be observed for 24 hours and evaluated by a psychiatrist or mental health professional before being discharged home. A patient who has made a suicide "gesture," for example, an overdose of 3 acetaminophen tablets, should also be evaluated by a psychiatrist or mental health professional before he or she is sent home because the severity of the suicide attempt does not necessarily correspond with the severity of the patient's future risk for suicide. A patient who has made a suicide attempt may tell the emergency physician that he or she is no longer suicidal. Patients may feel fine in the protected environment of the ED, only to deteriorate when they return to their home environment. Also, acutely suicidal patients may lie so that they may return home to complete the suicide. The emergency physician should never make a contract with a patient not to commit suicide and then discharge the patient home because the emergency physician does not have an ongoing relationship with the patient. The emergency physician should be suspicious of the patient who "accidentally" overdoses. Patients with an "accidental" overdose should never be sent home when medically stable until they can be assessed for suicidality and every attempt has been made to corroborate the patient's story with a collateral history.

VIOLENCE

Patients who are psychotic, paranoid, manic, under the influence of drugs or alcohol, character-disordered with poor impulse control, or have structural or functional abnormalities of brain tissue resulting in an organic brain syndrome may be of harm to others.[16] Occasionally, a suicidal patient may attempt to kill others, usually family members, before his or her own suicide. Consequently, all suicidal patients should be asked about homicidal ideation. Harm directed toward others is of two types. First, patients may have thoughts of harming a specific person within their environment, usually a family member or a person with whom they perceive they have a significant or special relationship. Second, patients may be violent to anyone in their environment as the result of agitation, poor impulse control, or psychotic disorganization. The best predictor of danger, whether specifically or more generally directed, is a past history of violent behavior.[16]

In psychiatric patients, harm directed at a specific person is often the result of paranoid delusions or command hallucinations. Paranoid patients may have thoughts of inflicting harm on a specific individual in the environment to protect themselves. "My mother is heading the conspiracy. I must stop her." Paranoid patients may also harm loved ones to protect them from supposed harm. For example, a woman with a postpartum psychosis killed her baby so that he could be protected by God and not harmed by the Devil, who she felt was threatening the baby's safety. A command hallucination may tell a patient to harm a specific person. "God told me to kill my husband because he is evil."

ED personnel must also be alert to patients who may escalate to more generally directed violence in the ED. An extremely agitated, disorganized, psychotic patient may become assaultive, at times with minimal warning. Manic patients who are extremely irritable and hyperactive may become combative if they feel that ED personnel are interfering with their activities. Paranoid patients may fear that ED personnel will harm them and become violent to protect themselves. Command hallucinations may direct patients to harm those in the ED. Patients with organic mental disorders may become agitated and combative because they are unable to process the environment accurately because of memory deficits, inability to abstract, poor impulse control, delusions, and hallucinations. Those with alcohol and drug intoxication or

withdrawal may become violent for similar reasons. Patients with character disorders and poor impulse control may become violent when angry, hurt, anxious, stressed, criticized, or prevented from doing what they wish. Patients with poor impulse control are even more dangerous when under the influence of drugs or alcohol.

We previously discussed the importance of putting all psychiatric patients in a hospital gown and separating them from their belongings to prevent access to weapons, and providing a safe environment for those assessing the potentially violent patient. The severely agitated psychiatric patient without an organic mental disorder can often be prevented from becoming violent by decreasing agitation with psychotropic medication. Patients who threaten to escalate to violence must be physically restrained, as discussed subsequently. Patients who are of harm to others must be hospitalized. Duty to protect the specific person to whom violent intent is directed is discussed subsequently.

ACUTE PSYCHOLOGIC DISTRESS

Patients may present to the ED because of severe psychologic distress associated with depression, mania, anxiety, panic, or overwhelming environmental stressors. Depressive moods can be associated with a major depressive disorder, a mixed bipolar disorder, dysthymia, an adjustment disorder with depressed mood, a life circumstance problem, or a grief reaction. The criteria for a major depressive disorder have been defined earlier in this chapter. Less severe depressive disorders may come to the ED with depressed affect. Patients with a *dysthymic disorder*[2] have had a depressed mood almost every day for at least 2 years with two of the following: poor appetite or overeating, insomnia or hypersomnia, low energy or fatigue, low-self-esteem, poor concentration or difficulty in making decisions, and/or feelings of hopelessness. Various stresses or losses in the environment can result in a depressed mood, which brings the patient to the ED. A patient with an *adjustment disorder* and *depressed mood* has had an identifiable stress within 3 months and demonstrates impairment in occupation, social or interpersonal functioning with symptoms of depressed mood, tearfulness, and/or hopelessness in excess of a normal and expectable reaction to stressors.[17] A *life circumstance problem* presents with a depressed mood, which is understandable or expectable in response to a stressor(s) and/or loss(es) in the environment.[18] Patients with a *grief reaction* present with sadness or depressed mood, diminished ability to think and concentrate, indecisiveness, fatigue, poor appetite, and/or insomnia. Guilt, if present, deals with things not done by the survivor. Thoughts of death are confined to feelings that the patient would be better off dead or wishes that he or she had died with the loved one. Preoccupation with worthlessness or marked psychomotor retardation usually suggests that the grief reaction is complicated by a major depressive disorder.[18]

The emergent use of psychotropic medication with depressed patients is discussed subsequently. Patients with a major depressive episode and suicidal ideation, severe agitation, and/or psychotic symptoms must be hospitalized; those with no suicidal ideation or mild psychotic symptoms, mild treatable agitation, an excellent support system, and referral to a psychiatrist within a short period of time may often be sent home. Patients with a dysthymic disorder are rarely hospitalized unless they are suicidal, and because they may respond to antidepressants, should be referred to a psychiatrist for evaluation. Patients with an adjustment disorder, life circumstance problem, or grief reaction often improve after a discussion of their difficulties. Referral to a mental health or pastoral care facility is appropriate. Patients who are suicidal in response to stress or loss should be hospitalized.

Manic patients, the criteria for whom was described previously, may initially experience euphoria. As the manic episode becomes more severe, however, they may experience a markedly unpleasant irritability, drivenness, or hyperactivity that causes them to seek help in the ED. Psychotropic medication may be helpful acutely to take the edge off the unpleasant feeling in the ED. Hospitalization is usually necessary. Patients with a mixed bipolar disorder may have signs and symptoms of both a major depressive disorder and a manic episode and require hospitalization.

Patients with an anxiety or panic disorder often visit the ED because of overwhelming anxiety and panic. Patients with a *panic disorder*[19] have discrete episodes of panic that, for the most part, come "out of the blue." The patient has four of the following symptoms:

1. Shortness of breath or smothering sensations
2. Dizziness, unsteady feelings or faintness
3. Palpitations or accelerated heart rate
4. Trembling or shaking, sweating, choking
5. Nausea or abdominal distress
6. Depersonalization or derealization
7. Numbness or tingling sensations
8. Flushes or chills
9. Chest pain or discomfort
10. Fear of dying
11. Fear of "going crazy" or doing something uncontrolled (see Table 61-4)

Patients with a panic attack should be treated with psychotropic medication as discussed subsequently. Patients with a panic attack need reassurance that the episode will subside, and that the disorder is highly treatable with psychotropic medication.[20] Patients should be given a referral to a psychiatrist before discharge from the ED.

A patient with an *anxiety disorder* visits the ED when the anxiety has become unbearable. An anxiety disorder[19] is defined as excessive worry, fear, apprehension, and/or anticipation of misfortune to self or others for 6 months and 6 of the following 18 symptoms:

Motor tension as manifested by

1. Trembling, twitching, feeling shaky
2. Muscle tension, aches, or soreness
3. Restlessness
4. Easy fatigability
   Autonomic activity as manifested by
5. Shortness of breath or smothering sensations
6. Palpitations or accelerated heart rate
7. Sweating, cold clammy hands
8. Dry mouth
9. Dizziness or lightheadedness
10. Nausea, diarrhea, or abdominal distress
11. Hot flushes
12. Frequent urination
13. Trouble in swallowing or "lump in throat"
    Vigilance and scanning as demonstrated by
14. Feeling keyed up or on edge
15. Exaggerated startle response
16. Difficulty in concentrating or "mind going blank" because of anxiety
17. Trouble in falling or staying asleep
18. Irritability (see Table 61-4).

It is important to differentiate an anxiety disorder from agitated depression, in which the patient experiences internal anxiety or agitation with a full-blown depressive disorder. Patients with an anxiety disorder should be treated with psychotropic medications, as described subsequently. Patients whose anxiety or panic continues to be intolerable may need hospitalization.

An *adjustment disorder with anxious mood*[17] is a reaction to an identifiable stressor with impairment in occupational, social, or interpersonal functioning with symptoms of anxiety, worrying, and/or jitteriness in excess of a normal or expectable reaction to the stressor. Patients with a life circumstance problem may respond to stress or loss with understandable anxiety. Patients with an adjustment disorder or life circumstance problem often respond with reduction of symptoms after discussing their problems with the emergency physician. Referral to a mental health or pastoral care facility is appropriate.

A patient who has been acutely stressed by a horrible event such as rape, spousal abuse, traumatic or violent injury, death of a loved one, or a serious threat to his or her life or integrity may present to the emergency room with intense psychologic distress. Some patients and families who have experienced a severe trauma respond to empathy, reassurance, support, structure, and an outpatient referral. Patients who are so traumatized that they continue to be uncontrollably upset, unable to communicate, unable to provide for basic functions for themselves, and have no support system that can manage their emotional state may need hospitalization for a day or two until psychologic reintegration begins to occur. A medical or surgical unit, particularly if the patient has physical injuries, is a supportive environment for such a patient. A psychiatric consultation on a medical/surgical unit is usually preferable to psychiatric hospitalization for the severely traumatized patient.

SOMATIC COMPLAINTS WITHOUT DEMONSTRABLE ORGANIC DISEASE

The emergency physician must always keep in mind that physical complaints that do not appear to have a demonstrable organic disease may represent undiagnosed physical illness. Additionally, patients with somatic complaints as a result of a psychiatric illness can develop co-existent physical illnesses.

Patients with panic disorder and anxiety disorder often present to the ED with complaints suggesting physical illness from overwhelming autonomic arousal. Patients with panic and anxiety disorders are frightened by these symptoms. Reassurance that the symptoms are real but not indicative of physical illness and that the disorder is highly treatable with psychotropic medication is comforting to these patients.[20]

Depressed patients, particularly the elderly, can present with somatic complaints with the signs and symptoms of a depressive illness. It is important to remember that there are many organic causes of depressive illness and that physical complaints plus a depressive illness may be the result of physical disease. Disposition should allow for work-up of possible organic causes of depression and also provide appropriate psychiatric treatment.

Patients with acute or chronic psychosocial stresses commonly present to the ED with physical complaints. There is often a psychophysiologic basis for these complaints, as with tension headache or gastrointestinal disturbance. Other patients may falsely perceive or amplify familiar or normal sensations. These patients are often unaware of the relationship between the stress and the physical symptoms. When physical symptoms appear to be related to stress, discussion of this possible link with the patient, symptomatic treatment such as ibuprofen for headache or antacids for gastrointestinal distress, and reassurance that no serious physiologic disorder exists are useful interventions. Follow-up with the primary care physician and, if the stress is severe or long-term, with a minister or a mental health professional should be suggested. It is important to note that patients who have been sexually or physically abused may present with vague somatic complaints. The management of these problems is discussed elsewhere in this text.

Somatoform disorders include somatization disor-

der, hypochondriasis, psychogenic pain disorder, and conversion disorder. The somatic symptoms of these disorders are "real" to these patients, and their psychologic origin out of their awareness. The symptoms are not feigned by the patient, but unconsciously produced. The evaluation and ED treatment of this group of interesting and difficult disorders is discussed in Chapter 62. *Somatization disorder*,[21] which has also been called Briquet's syndrome or hysteria, is a disease with somatic complaints in multiple systems for which no pathophysiologic mechanism can be found for the symptoms. The patient, however, has taken medication, seen a doctor, or altered his or her life style as a result of the symptoms. The onset of this disorder is before age 30, but usually begins earlier in adolescence or young adulthood. The patient's female family members are more likely to have somatization disorder and their male relatives, sociopathy. Drug abuse and depression are also common in relatives. To meet criteria for this disorder, the patient must have 13 of the following symptoms:

Gastrointestinal symptoms:

1. Vomiting (other than during pregnancy)
2. Abdominal pain (other than when menstruating)
3. Nausea (other than motion sickness)
4. Bloating (gassy)
5. Diarrhea
6. Intolerance of (gets sick from) several different foods
   Pain symptoms:
7. Pain in extremities
8. Back pain
9. Joint pain
10. Pain during urination
11. Other pain (excluding headaches)
    Cardiopulmonary symptoms:
12. Shortness of breath when not exerting oneself
13. Palpitations
14. Chest pain
15. Dizziness
    Conversion or pseudoneurologic symptoms:
16. Amnesia
17. Difficulty in swallowing
18. Loss of voice
19. Deafness
20. Double vision
21. Blurred vision
22. Blindness
23. Fainting or loss of consciousness
24. Seizure or convulsion
25. Trouble in walking
26. Paralysis or muscle weakness
27. Urinary retention or difficulty in urinating
    Sexual symptoms for the major part of the person's life after opportunities for sexual activity:
28. Burning sensation in sexual organs or rectum (other than during intercourse)
29. Sexual indifference
30. Pain during intercourse

31. Impotence

Female reproductive symptoms judged by the patient to occur more frequently or severely than in most women:

32. Painful menstruation
33. Irregular menstrual periods
34. Excessive menstrual bleeding
35. Vomiting throughout pregnancy. This psychiatric disorder is suspected when review of systems is positive in every system.

The patient usually has a history of seeing multiple physicians during the course of the illness. Because collateral history and old medical records are often not available, it may be difficult to make a definitive diagnosis in the ED. The somatic symptoms of somatization disorder are stable over time and respond poorly to psychiatric treatment. Intervention is directed toward preventing the patient from having unnecessary procedures and surgery and inappropriately using health care services. A referral should be made to a primary care physician or psychiatrist who can help prevent this inappropriate use of health care services. These patients may also have alcohol and drug abuse, depressive and anxiety symptoms, conversion disorders, and suicidal ideation and attempts. When patients present with these psychiatric symptoms, a psychiatric referral should be made.

Hypochondriasis is another disorder that presents with somatic complaints and is difficult to treat. The patient is preoccupied with the fear of having a serious illness, unsupported by physical evaluation. Despite reassurance that there is no medical illness, the patient continues to have the fear or belief that he or she is ill.[21] The onset of the illness may occur any time from young adulthood to the 50s and is chronic. Hypochondriasis must be differentiated from a depressive disorder with somatic complaints and a psychotic disorder with somatic delusions. While the patient with somatization disorder is usually interpersonally pleasant, although time-consuming, the patient with hypochondriasis can be demanding and unpleasant. These patients resist a referral to a psychiatrist because they view themselves as physically ill. As with somatization disorder, these patients have frequently seen many physicians. The relationship often ends when the physician becomes exasperated with the patient's angry demanding stance and the patient becomes dissatisfied with the physician's care. These patients should be referred to a tolerant and understanding primary care physician or psychiatrist who is able to maintain an ongoing relationship with these patients by listening to their complaints, doing minimal diagnostic tests, and seeing the patient in frequent but controlled visits. With such treatment, inappropriate use of health care services is controlled, and some patients may have an improvement of somatic complaints.

Patients with *somatoform pain disorder* are another group who have had multiple work-ups, seen many physicians, and may be unpleasant in their ED demands for pain medication and admission to the hospital. Either these patients have no organic cause for their pain, or if there is an underlying organic pathology, the complaint of pain or social or occupational impairment is in gross excess of the organic pathology.[21] These patients also resist referral to a psychiatrist, and are best referred to a primary care physician or, if available, a pain center with a multidisciplinary team.

Conversion disorder is a rare and highly treatable psychiatric illness. The symptoms are in the voluntary or sensory nervous system and mimic neurological disease. The neurologic examination or work-up is not consistent with neurologic disease. Symptoms are acute in onset and related to a psychosocial stressor. Because symptom production is unconscious, the patient is usually unaware of the relationship between the conversion symptoms and the stressor.[21] Hemianthesia, hemiparesis and "hysterical" blindness, deafness, aphonia, seizures, movement disorders, and difficulties in walking are common presentations. Neurologic work-up and psychiatric evaluation are essential with this disorder. Conversion-like symptoms are common with undiagnosed neurologic disease like multiple sclerosis. Further, a "true" conversion disorder can become chronic without psychiatric treatment.

Patients with *malingering* are seen commonly in the ED. These patients feign physical illness[18] for narcotics, shelter, financial compensation, and to evade criminal prosecution. The environmental goals become obvious with careful questioning by the examiner. Ascertaining what malingering patients want is essential to preventing inappropriate use of the ED. For example, homeless patients who feign illness to obtain a hospital bed are best given referrals for an emergency shelter. Too-solicitous treatment, however, encourages use of the ED on a routine basis for this problem. Patients who feign illness for drugs should never be given the drugs they desire but be referred to a drug rehabilitation program. Inquiry into recent job loss, job-related injuries, lawsuits, or consultation with a lawyer can uncover the patient who feigns illness for financial compensation. The patient's history and lack of positive physical findings should be documented on the ED record. Patients who malinger and, after evaluation, do not receive what they want from the ED personnel, may become angry and threaten a malpractice suit or physical harm. The patient should be asked firmly to leave the ED and, if necessary, be escorted by security personnel. The patient's behavior and the emergency physician's intervention should be documented on the chart.

Factitious disorder is a rare psychiatric disorder in which the patient feigns illness because of a psychologic need to assume the patient role.[22] This is the sole reason for feigning illness, whereas in malingering, there is an obvious recognizable environmental goal (i.e., shelter, monetary compensation, or avoidance of jail). Although patients with factitious disorder may secondarily demand narcotics, the compulsive need to feign illness and adopt the patient role is the primary psychologic motivation. Patients with this disorder subject themselves to extreme risk in producing these symptoms, such as by ingesting massive amounts of anticoagulants, injecting bones with feces, or instrumenting the urethra or anus to produce hematuria or rectal bleeding. These patients happily undergo invasive, dangerous, or painful medical procedures. As a result of their creative symptom production and subsequent medical care, these patients have self-inflicted or iatrogenically produced physical pathology. They have often worked in hospitals, have encyclopedic familiarity with medical jargon, and demonstrate pseudologica fantastica in which they elaborately spin falsehoods about occupations, family background, and illness in a fascinating, engaging, and often grandiose manner. In the extreme form of this disorder (Munchausen's syndrome), the patient spends all of his or her time going from city to city and hospital to hospital. Often EDs in the area have seen a patient with similar symptoms. Patients with factitious disorders may have a number of aliases. Once they are admitted to the hospital, they usually have an extensive, expensive work-up, are demanding and uncompliant, and when confronted with a negative work-up or discovered in voluntary symptom production, sign out against medical advice. Seasoned ED personnel are often suspicious of the elaborate, inconsistent, fantastic history, dramatic presentation, and questionable identification, insurance cards, and places of residence. The ED physician who suspects factitious disorder is often successful in preventing such a patient from being admitted to the hospital. Unfortunately, these are clever patients who often voluntarily produce symptoms for which admission to the hospital is mandatory. When these patients must be admitted, "rule out factitious disorder" should be written on the ED record to alert the ward physician.

Somatic delusions may be present in psychotic disorders. Psychotically depressed patients have the signs and symptoms of depression with delusions that they are physically ill, defective, or disordered. Patients who have an acute schizophrenic episode often have bizarre somatic delusions. Medicated schizophrenic patients, however, may present with less bizarre delusions. For example, a schizophrenic who felt that thoughts pressed on her eye presented to the emergency room with severe eye pain. On careful questioning, the delusion behind the pain became obvious. Patients with a paranoid disorder often present with no symptoms other than a delusion of physical disease, defect, or disorder. The ED physician usually quickly recognizes a somatic delusion. The difficulty arises when a psychotic misperception of actual physical phenomena is thought to be purely a somatic delusion. The example of the schizophrenic with acute appendicitis who presents with "snakes in the abdomen" illustrates this.

REFERENCES

1. Organic brain syndromes and disorders. *In* Diagnostic and Statistical Manual of Mental Disorders. 3rd Ed. Revised. Washington, D.C., American Psychiatric Press, Inc., 1987.
2. Mood disorders. *In* Diagnostic and Statistical Manual of Mental Disorders. 3rd Ed. Revised. Washington, D.C., American Psychiatric Press Inc., 1987.
3. Schizophrenia. *In* Diagnostic and Statistical Manual of Mental Disorders. 3rd Ed. Revised. Washington, D.C., American Psychiatric Press Inc., 1987.
4. Other neurobehavioral syndromes and neurological aspects of psychiatric disease. *In* Organic Brain Syndromes. Edited by Strab, R.L., and Black, F.W., Philadelphia, F.A. Davis Company, 1981.
5. Psychotic disorders not elsewhere classified. *In* Diagnostic and Statistical Manual of Mental Disorders. 3rd Ed. Revised. Washington, D.C., American Psychiatric Press Inc., 1987.
6. Delusional disorder. *In* Diagnostic and Statistical Manual of Mental Disorders. 3rd Ed. Revised. Washington, D.C., American Psychiatric Press Inc., 1987.
7. Hyman, S.E. (ed.): The suicidal patient. *In* Manual of Psychiatric Emergencies. Boston, Little, Brown and Company, 1984.
8. Tomb, D.A.: Psychiatry for the House Officer. 2nd Ed. Baltimore, Williams & Wilkins, 1984.
9. Weisman, M.M.: The epidemiology of suicide attempts. Arch. Gen. Psychiatry 30:737, 1974.
10. Hillard, J.R.: Emergency management of the suicidal patient. *In* Psychiatric Emergencies: Intervention and Resolution. Edited by Walker, J.I., Philadelphia, J.B. Lippincott, 1983.
11. Shader, R.I.: Assessment of suicide risk. *In* Manual of Psychiatric Therapeutics. Edited by Shader, R.I., Boston, Little, Brown & Company, 1975.
12. Roy, A.: Risk factors for suicide in psychiatric patients. Arch. Gen. Psychiatry 39:1089, 1982.
13. Beck, A.T.: Hopelessness and eventual suicide: A 10-year prospective study of patients hospitalized with suicidal ideation. Am. J. Psychiatry 142:559, 1985.
14. Fawcett, J.A.: Clinical assessment of suicidal risk. Postgrad. Med. 55:85, 1974.
15. Pokorny, A.D.: Predictions of suicide in psychiatric patients. Arch. Gen. Psychiatry 40:249, 1983.
16. Monahan, J. (ed.): The Clinical Prediction of Violence. Washington, DC, Government Printing Office (National Institute of Mental Health), 1981.
17. Adjustment disorders. *In* Diagnostic and Statistical Manual of Mental Disorders. 3rd Ed. Revised. Washington, DC, American Psychiatric Press, Inc., 1987.
18. V codes for conditions not attributable to a mental disorder that are a focus of attention or treatment. *In* Diagnostic and Statistical Manual of Mental Disorders. 3rd Ed. Revised. Washington, D.C., American Psychiatric Press Inc., 1987.
19. Anxiety disorders. *In* Diagnostic and Statistical Manual of Mental Disorders. 3rd Ed. Revised. Washington, D.C., American Psychiatric Press Inc., 1987.
20. Pollard, C.A., and Lewis, L.M.: Managing panic attacks in emergency patients. J. Emerg. Med. 7:547, 1989.
21. Somatoform disorders. *In* Diagnostic and Statistical Manual of Mental Disorders. 3rd Ed. Revised. Washington, D.C., American Psychiatric Press Inc., 1987.
22. Factitious disorder. *In* Diagnostic and Statistical Manual of Mental Disorders. 3rd Ed. Revised. Washington, D.C., American Psychiatric Press Inc., 1987.

MANAGEMENT OF PSYCHIATRIC EMERGENCIES

Stephanie von Ammon Cavanaugh, William S. Gilmer, and
Mark McClung

CAPSULE

This final introductory section discusses critical issues in the management of psychiatric emergencies including medication, restraints, medicolegal problems (commitment, elopement, confidentiality, duty to protect, and the right to refuse treament), and disposition.

PSYCHOTROPIC MEDICATION

AGITATION AND PSYCHOTIC DISORGANIZATION

Benzodiazepines and neuroleptics are used either separately or together to control agitation and psychotic disorganization in the Emergency Department (ED). Lorazepam and haloperidol are used most commonly because of their efficacy and safety. Lorazepam has a half-life of 10 to 20 hours and few active metabolites. It decreases anxiety and agitation, is useful for withdrawal from alcohol, barbiturates, and benzodiazepines, but does not control psychotic symptoms. It may cause paradoxic excitement, particularly in patients with brain damage. The most serious side effect is respiratory depression when it is given in respiratory disease, in combination with other sedatives, in large amounts, or by rapid intravenous push. Lorazepam may be given orally, intramuscularly, or intravenously. Haloperidol decreases agitation and psychotic disorganization. It has minimal effects on the cardiovascular system, causes minimal orthostatic hypotension (except when given intravenous push), and has few anticholinergic side effects. It may lower the seizure threshold slightly. Finally, haloperidol may cause extrapyramidal side effects (dystonia, pseudoparkinsonian symptoms, and akathisia), which can be controlled by benztropine, trihexyphenidyl, diphenhydramine, and amantidine. When haloperidol is given orally, elixir, rather than tablets, is suggested to prevent "cheeking" of pills. Also, elixir is more rapidly absorbed. Intramuscular doses are usually half the oral dose. Intravenous haloperidol is never given in more than a 2 mg bolus at one time. Neuroleptics other than haloperidol are also used in the ED. Haloperidol and lithium have been reported rarely to cause irreversible brain damage in sensitive individuals. As a result, the more potent phenothiazines—fluphenazine, trifluperizine, and the slightly more sedating perphenazine—are often used with lithium. These neuroleptics have a side effect profile similar to that of haloperidol. Less potent neuroleptics such as thioridazine, chlorpromazine, and mesoridizine cause fewer extrapyramidal reactions and are useful in patients with a previous history of severe extrapyramidal side effects and Parkinson's disease. These less potent neuroleptics, however, have more sedative, anticholinergic, and hypotensive side effects than the more potent neuroleptics. Molindone does not lower the seizure threshold but cannot be given intramuscularly. Fluphenazine, which lowers it only slightly, can be given intramuscularly. Fluphenazine, which lowers it only slightly, can be given intramuscularly. These two neuroleptics are preferred for patients with uncontrolled seizures. Those with a history of neuroleptic malignant syndrome should be given benzodiazepines to avoid the risk of the syndrome's recurring. *The risk/benefit ratio of using lorazepam and haloperidol to control agitation and psychotic symptoms in the patients suspected of having an organic brain syndrome, particularly delirium, should be evaluated. Sensorium is a sensitive indicator of deteriorating physical condition. Consequently, psychotropic medications should be avoided in conditions in which the level of consciousness is diagnostically critical.*

The goal of medicating the agitated and/or psychotic patient is adequate control of the symptoms so that assessment and disposition can be achieved. If a patient is transferred to a psychiatric facility, it is important not to overmedicate him or her. The patient should be medicated to ensure safe transfer, but not so that symptoms are obscured for evaluation by the receiving facility. In some state or county facilities, the patient may be inadvertently discharged if symptoms are obscured, only to reappear several hours later in the ED. If, in the emergency physician's judgment, the patient requires an amount of medication that obscures symptomatology, the clinical picture before medication should be documented, as should the reasons for the medication. Further, active treatment with lithium or antidepressants should not be initiated by the emergency physician before transfer. Such medications may also obscure the clinical picture and/or interfere with the treatment strategy of the receiving facility.

ANXIETY, PANIC, AGITATED DEPRESSION, AND MANIA

Overwhelming affects are also treated in the ED. Patients with hypomania and mania, who are not psychotic, are often given lorazepam and/or a neuroleptic for control of the agitation, irritability, and hyperactive behavior. Patients with panic attacks, severe anxiety, or agitated depression should be treated with lorazepam or alprazolam every half hour until the overwhelming affect subsides. A patient who has panic, anxiety, or an agitated depression that responds to benzodiazepines and is discharged from the ED should be given a 2- or 3-day supply of benzodiazepines for symptom control until the follow-up appointment.

MEDICATIONS FOR PATIENTS DISCHARGED FROM THE ED

Patients who are discharged from the ED should never be given more than a few days' supply of psychotropic medications. Those who require psychotropic medication should have ongoing outpatient psychiatric care, and the need for medication will encourage the patient to obtain or continue this care. Further, patients should never be given enough medication that an overdose could cause significant medical morbidity and mortality. As a rule, a few days of benzodiazepines are indicated for those with panic, anxiety, or agitated depression who might withdraw without them. Additionally, a few days of neuroleptics may be indicated for those with chronic psychotic illness. Antidepressants, lithium, or carbamezapine should never be started in the ED, because of the danger of overdose and the difficulty of monitoring side effects. Patients presently on psychotropic medications may come to the ED for refills when the medication runs out. The emergency physician may refuse to dispense these medications unless he or she is able to contact the mental health provider and confirm the present use of the medication requested. The ED is not an outpatient psychiatric clinic, and repeated availability of psychotropic drugs in the ED encourages its use for this purpose and discourages appropriate outpatient mental health care.

RESTRAINTS

Restraints are used when ED personnel assess a patient as potentially violent or demonstrating violent behavior. State mental health codes dictate that a patient may not be restrained before he or she begins to threaten or show violent behavior. Ideally, a patient should be restrained when he or she begins to threaten violence or show "imminent signs of impending violence" and before violent behavior occurs. Liberal interpretation of "threatening or violent behavior" may be needed to ensure protection of the patient and those in the ED. The mental health code states that restraints should never be used when less restrictive methods, such as one-to-one supervision, will suffice. Psychotropic medication (chemical restraints) should be used before physical restraints in the hyperactive, agitated, nonviolent patient. In many cases, however, the agitation and disorganization are so severe that the emergency physician feels that the safety of the patient and those in the ED is best served by first restraining and then medicating the patient.

Once a decision is made to restrain a potentially violent patient, at least five additional personnel are needed, one for each limb and one to apply the restraints. A strong or larger patient may require more personnel in the application of restraints. The goal is to have enough people to prevent both patient and staff from being harmed. Often an adequate show of force calms the patient, and he or she can be brought verbally under control while the restraints are applied without need of force.

In restraining a patient, as in cardiopulmonary resuscitation, one person should be in charge. This person should be familiar with the restraining process and tell those assisting exactly what to do. Security guards should be instructed to remove all harmful weapons and to stay out of the patient's vision until the restraining team is assembled. When the restraining team is ready, the team leader should move calmly, quickly, and with authority. This attitude is reassuring to the restraining team, who may be anxious or frightened, and to the patient, who is out of control. The person in charge should tell the patient in a calm voice: "You are out of control and need to be put in restraints for your protection and ours. No one will harm you." The patient may attempt to negotiate or threaten at this point to stop the restraining process. Nonetheless, the team must continue with the restraining process regardless of what the patient says. The restraints should be secured to the solid portions of the cart or bed, not the siderails. The restraints should be tight enough that the patient cannot escape, but not so tight as to compromise circulation or respiration. After all four limbs are secured, pulses should be checked. Some violent patients may also need a chest restraint. It is important to remember that restrained patients can still bite. The restraining team should not leave the patient until the team leader is sure that the patient is securely and safely restrained. An ED policy mandating that restraining personnel may not leave the patient until the team leader tells them to do so is advised.

Triage personnel or a physician may initiate the restraining process, but an order for restraints must

2624   Psychiatric and Behavioral Emergencies

be written by the emergency physician. The reason must be documented on the chart by the person initiating the restraints, and also by the physician writing the restraining order. Although hospital guidelines may vary for observing a patient in restraints in the ED, the standard of practice for a psychiatric unit is recommended both clinically and medicolegally. The patient should be checked every 15 minutes. A flow sheet documenting this observation is recommended. After a reasonable period (2 to 4 hours), the physician should redocument the need for restraints.

The patient in four-point leather restraints should never have an arm or leg restraint removed. Such removal can result in harm to the patient or others. If the patient cannot be completely taken out of leather restraints safely, all four restraints should remain in place. Water with a straw, a urinal, or a bedpan can be given to a patient in full leather restraints. When a patient stays in a 24-hour holding area, he or she may need to be fed. This is easily accomplished by putting up the head of the bed or cart and feeding the patient. If, for any reason, the patient must have one arm removed from the restraints, he or she requires one-to-one supervision until returned to all four leather restraints. Personnel should be instructed that patients in leather restraints may use any persuasive argument or threat to be released, and should not release them until they are no longer potentially dangerous. An ED policy requiring a physician's order to release a patient from full leather restraints is advised.

COMMITMENT

INVOLUNTARY

A patient may be involuntarily committed to the hospital for psychiatric treatment when he or she, because of a mental illness or defect, is imminently dangerous to himself or herself or others or is incapable of self-care. Mental health codes vary slightly from state to state, and the emergency physician should be familiar with the mental health code of his or her state. In most states, "mental illness or defect" is usually not defined by the mental health code. Harm to oneself or others is uniformly defined as "harmful threats or acts." The time period for "imminent harm" to self or others varies from state to state, but is typically 24 to 48 hours. A patient who is "unable to care for himself or herself" is unable to provide for basic needs such as food, water, and shelter, or demonstrates such poor judgment that he or she puts himself or herself at extreme risk. Examples include refusal to eat or drink for a protracted period of time, catatonic stupor, disorganization so great that the patient is unable to provide for basic needs, or behavior such as wandering in subzero weather without adequate clothing in a dan-

gerous neighborhood. It is best to err on the side of safety in uncertain or borderline situations. Further psychiatric evaluation during the 3 to 5 days of the patient's detention before the commitment hearing allows a more certain evaluation of danger to self or others. If the patient is not considered dangerous, he or she can be released before the commitment hearing. For example, a schizophrenic patient may have a documented history of attempting to kill his mother during a previous similar episode. The patient may evade any questions pertaining to thoughts of harming his mother and refuse hospitalization. In this instance, the emergency physician is safer in committing the patient for more thorough evaluation because the risk for harm to the mother is potentially high if the patient is released.

To commit a patient, the family, the hospital administrator, or the emergency nurse may petition the court for involuntary commitment. Every attempt should be made to have the family be the petitioner. Any licensed physician or, in many states, "qualified examiner" (i.e., licensed clinical psychologist) may fill out the first certificate. The examiner should write legibly and carefully document the reasons for commitment without medical jargon. For example, "the patient took 20 acetaminophen in an attempt to end his life and is of harm to himself." "The patient threatened to kill his wife and is of harm to others." "The patient was found in her own excrement, playing with a doll, and had not eaten for a week. She is unable to care for herself." The second certificate must be filled out by a psychiatrist, who may still be in training, but must be licensed in the state. In some states, a "qualified examiner" may fill out the second certificate.

VOLUNTARY

A patient may voluntarily commit himself or herself to a hospital for psychiatric treatment by signing a voluntary commitment form. Voluntary commitment is always preferable to involuntary commitment because a court hearing is not necessary. Once a patient has signed a voluntary commitment, he or she is committed to the hospital for at least 5 days, unless the treating physician feels that he or she can be released. When a patient wishes to leave the hospital, he or she signs a 5-day notice and may be released from the hospital no later than 5 days afterward. During this period, if the treating physician feels that continued hospitalization is necessary and the patient meets criteria for involuntary commitment, proceedings for the latter may be initiated. Patients who are not committable but need psychiatric hospitalization may be required to sign a voluntary commitment to be considered for admission to many psychiatric facilities. Other psychiatric facilities (usually open units) may allow a patient to sign an informal admission, which allows the patient to leave the treating facility at any time.

Patients who are not committable, but require psychiatric hospitalization and refuse admission, must sign out of the ED against medical advice (AMA). The need for psychiatric hospitalization should be carefully explained to the family with the patient present, and this documented on the chart. If the family is not present, they should be called and the patient asked to wait until their arrival. Family members who feel that the patient needs psychiatric hospitalization are often successful in persuading the recalcitrant patient to sign a voluntary commitment and enter the hospital. Providing the patient with appropriate psychotropic medication and time with the family often assists in this process. If the patient still insists upon leaving, other options should be presented to the patient and family and documented on the ED record. These options include inpatient hospitalization in the near future and/or an immediate outpatient referral. A noncommittable patient who needs hospitalization requires careful supervision at home. Often a psychotic patient is amenable to psychiatric hospitalization after 24 to 36 hours of appropriate psychotropic medication. Regardless of whether the patient seeks hospitalization at a later time, the importance of immediate outpatient care should be emphasized. Before the patient leaves the ED, an AMA form should be prepared and the patient asked to sign it. If the patient refuses, this should be documented on the record.

ELOPEMENT

Waiting in a busy ED can be particularly stressful for a patient with a psychiatric disturbance. Careful supervision and prompt evaluation, treatment, and disposition can help prevent the emotionally disturbed patient from eloping from the ED. Putting the patient in a hospital gown also deters the patient from leaving the emergency area and makes identification easier if elopement does occur. If a patient who has been evaluated elopes from the ED, the action taken depends on the patient's mental state. If the patient was committable, commitment papers should be initiated. Hospital security, the police, and the family should be informed, and every effort made to return the patient to the ED. These efforts should be recorded on the chart. If the patient was not committable but required psychiatric care, this AMA departure should be documented on the chart. Family members should be notified of the AMA departure. If the patient was not in need of psychiatric care, no further action is necessary.

A significant problem occurs when a patient who has not been evaluated elopes from the ED. If there is any concern that the patient may be of harm to himself or herself or others or be unable to care for himself or herself, hospital security and the police must be called and every attempt made to return the patient to the ED. If possible, the family must be notified. Collateral history often helps establish how serious the patient's mental disorder is. In some EDs, a patient who elopes is assumed to be committable until after psychiatric evaluation has taken place, and elopement is handled accordingly. In conclusion, the best way to handle elopement is to prevent it. Good triage information, careful supervision, prompt evaluation, and a hospital gown are the best deterrents.

CONFIDENTIALITY AND DUTY TO PROTECT

Doctor-patient communication is privileged and permission to telephone family or friends for a collateral history requires consent from the patient. If the patient is suicidal, homicidal, or unable to communicate for any reason, the emergency nature of the situation allows this privilege to be set aside. The reason for this breach of confidentiality must be documented on the chart.

The discussion of clinical information obtained from the patient with family and friends again requires permission from the patient. Confidentiality may be disregarded in only one instance: when a patient makes a *specific* threat against a *specific* individual. In this case, the physician has the duty to protect this individual. Because most mentally ill patients who make such threats are hospitalized, this constitutes adequate protection. Additionally, this warning may be communicated to the potential victim by the emergency physician or later by the subsequent treating psychiatrist. Because information is often lost in transfer to psychiatric facilities and patients prematurely discharged, the emergency physician must assess the seriousness of the threat. If the evaluating physician feels that the threat is serious, the individual to whom the threats are directed should be warned by telephone or letter and this documented in the chart. Similarly, if a patient elopes from the ED and has made specific threats against a specific individual, that individual must be warned.

A controversy exists about whether suicidal thoughts and actions should be communicated to family or friends without the patient's permission. Most suicidal patients readily grant such permission and are often hospitalized, so that family knowledge of suicidality is not required for safety of the patient. In some instances, patients have suicidal ideation but are not actively suicidal, and are sent home with family supervision and outpatient care. If such a patient refuses to allow the physician to discuss his or her suicidal thoughts with the family, hospitalization is necessary.

RIGHT TO REFUSE TREATMENT

A mentally ill patient has the right to refuse diagnostic tests and treatments, even if involuntarily committed and awaiting transfer to a psychiatric facility. If a psychiatric patient refuses medical treatment as a result of a mental disorder, this treatment may be provided against the patient's wishes if significant morbidity or mortality would occur without it. For example, a hypoglycemic, schizophrenic patient who feels that intravenous glucose will poison his system and kill him may have glucose administered to him. Likewise, a delirious patient who refuses life-saving treatment may be treated. The need for emergency medical treatment should be carefully documented on the chart. Additional documentation by another physician or medical personnel supporting the need for emergency treatment provides further legal protection for the treating physician. If a psychiatric patient is imminently dangerous to himself or herself or others and refuses psychotropic medications, the physician may initiate treatment on an emergency basis. Before emergency treatment is begun, commitment should be initiated and the emergency need for such treatment documented. Again, documentation by other medical personnel of the emergency need for psychotropic medication provides further support for the emergent treatment.

DISPOSITION

The disposition of a patient who presents with an emotional disturbance depends on the patient's psychiatric disorder, coexistent medical illness, insurance, social supports, and community resources. Disposition includes hospitalization, 24-hour hold, or outpatient referral.

HOSPITALIZATION

The first decision that the emergency physician must make is whether the patient needs hospitalization or not. Patients who are of harm to themselves or others or unable to care for themselves because of a mental disorder are routinely hospitalized. Most psychotic patients are hospitalized. Exceptions include chronically psychotic patients who have a stable living environment, no change in psychiatric symptomatology, stable appropriate outpatient care, and optimal treatment with psychotropic drugs with which they are compliant. Patients with a depressive disorder, agitated depression, or mania are most always hospitalized. Patients who have a severe anxiety disorder or panic disorder are often hospitalized if the anxiety or panic cannot be adequately controlled by anxiolytics in the emergency room. Patients with a disturbance of affect, cognition, or behavior thought to be secondary to an organic cause are hospitalized (e.g., delirium; dementia with agitation, onset or worsening of organic psychotic symptoms, or deterioration of cognitive functioning; an amnestic disorder that is acute, untreated, or of unknown cause; severe organic anxiety or depressive disorders; and unmanageable organic personality disorder).

The second decision of the emergency physician is where to hospitalize the patient. The patient with an acute medical problem and a psychiatric disturbance either as a result of the medical problem or coexistent with it should be hospitalized on an appropriate medical or surgical unit. Although medical or surgical units may be reluctant to accept medically or surgically ill patients with an emotional disturbance, most patients can be psychiatrically maintained during medical or surgical treatment with psychotropic medication, restraints, close supervision, and psychiatric consultation. There is significant risk in hospitalizing a medically or surgically unstable patient on a psychiatric unit without the appropriate resources to competently manage the patient's physical problem. A patient with a possible organic cause for the mental disturbance or a coexistent medical problem that requires treatment should be hospitalized where competent medical diagnostic and treatment facilities are available. For example, the elderly patient, the patient with significant but stable medical problems, and the patient with an initial or atypical episode of a psychotic or mood disorder are best hospitalized on a psychiatric unit in a general hospital. Patients who do not require a general hospital setting may be hospitalized in a psychiatric facility, but must be *medically cleared* before being transferred. A physical examination and focused neurologic examination must be performed. In addition, a toxicology screen, CBC, glucose, BUN, creatinine, electrolytes, and liver profile should be obtained for all psychotic patients being transferred to a psychiatric facility. All patients who are over 45 or have a history of cardiac disease should have an ECG, since many psychotropic medications have cardiovascular effects.

Insurance, bed availability, proximity of significant others, the site of previous psychiatric hospitalization, and severity and type of psychiatric disturbance also determine where the patient is hospitalized. The ED should maintain a list of psychiatric facilities in the area with the name, address, area served, telephone number, contact person, transfer policies, type of patient accepted, and insurance reimbursement required. Insurance or lack thereof plays a major part in where a patient can be hospitalized. If a patient has private insurance, it is essential to check psychiatric benefits, which have become increasingly poor over the past decade. Health maintenance organizations or preferred provider organizations reimburse only certain providers and psychiatric facilities. Patients with public aid or Medicaid must usually be hospitalized in a state or county psychiatric facility. The patient's address usually determines what state or county facility he or she should be sent to. Occasionally, private or university settings have beds set aside for public aid or Medicaid patients. If possible, patients should be hospitalized where they have been previously hospitalized or are receiving outpatient care. The severity and type of psychiatric disorder also determine what kind of psychiatric facility is required. For example, a suicidal patient should be hospitalized on a locked unit, a violent patient on a unit with a seclusion room, and a patient with primary alcoholism and secondary depression on a unit that specializes in alcohol-related problems.

Because transfer to the psychiatric facility within the hospital where the ED is located is not always possible, maintaining good relationships with the hospitals to which psychiatric patients are transferred is essential. A patient should never be sent to another psychiatric facility *without calling* the institution to check on bed availability and discuss the patient's condition. Although any of the emergency staff may call to determine bed availability, the physician should speak directly to a physician or mental health worker of that facility about the patient's condition. A legible record of the physician's psychiatric and medical assessment, laboratory tests, and treatment should be sent with the patient to the receiving psychiatric facility. EDs that routinely give inaccurate information, send patients without a transfer call, or inadequately clear transferred patients medically may receive poor cooperation from that facility in the future when a psychiatric bed is needed.

Preparing the patient for transfer is important. As mentioned previously, patients should be adequately medicated to ensure safe transfer without obscuring the clinical picture. Patients who have required full leather restraints should be transferred in restraints. Agitated, potentially combative patients who have not required restraints may have to be restrained before transfer if there is any concern for the patient's or transferring person's safety. Suicidal patients must have one-to-one supervision. Further, even if a patient is not of harm to himself or herself or others, it is wise never to leave a psychiatric patient alone during transfer. The need for restraints or one-to-one supervision should be documented on the clinical record and explained to those transferring the patient. All committable patients must be sent by ambulance. Patients who are not committable are most safely transferred by ambulance, and this should be explained to the patient and family. If the patient or family refuses to comply with ambulance transfer, this should be documented on the chart. Most ambulances require a petition and a commitment form (voluntary or involuntary), which mandates the need for further evaluation and allows the ambulance crew to detain the patient if he or she tries to escape from the ambulance.

BRIEF HOLDING

Some EDs have an area to hold patients who cannot be safely discharged and may need up to 24 hours of observation and treatment before appropriate disposition can be made. These holding areas are most often used for patients who are intoxicated with alcohol or drugs or present with impending withdrawal states.

OUTPATIENT REFERRAL

The emergency physician should bear in mind several facts when he or she discharges a patient with an emotional problem from the ED with an outpatient referral. First, if a definite appointment with a mental health care provider is not made during the ED visit, the patient may not be seen for several days to several weeks. Second, a patient who leaves the ED may choose not to get follow-up mental health care. Third, the emergency physician will have no ongoing relationship with the patient. Fourth, the emergency physician may have little accurate information about the patient's psychiatric difficulties. Finally, the emergency physician may have little formal psychiatric training. Many EDs have psychiatrists or mental health care professionals who consult with the ED staff to evaluate and decide on disposition for psychiatric patients. If a psychiatrist or competent mental health care professional is not available, the ED physician should err on the side of safety. An outpatient disposition for the patient who has overdosed, threatens suicide or harm to others, has a serious mood disorder, or is acutely psychotic is always a risk. When the emergency physician is unsure of the proper disposition and has no psychiatric consultant available, a psychiatric evaluation is often best obtained by transferring a patient to a psychiatric facility where a psychiatrist or trained mental health care professional is available to evaluate the patient.

Financial resources, proximity to residence, site of previous outpatient care, and the psychiatric problem determine the outpatient referral. As with inpatient facilities, it is important to maintain a list of outpatient facilities with the name, address, telephone number, contact person, fee schedule, type of problem treated, availability of psychiatric and medical services, and time to outpatient visit. Many private insurance policies poorly reimburse outpatient psychiatric care. As a result, a portion or all of the outpatient expense is borne by the patient. Health maintenance organizations or preferred provider organizations have designated health care providers. Medicare provides reasonable outpatient psychiatric reimbursement. Private psychiatrists or private clinics in private general hospitals, university hospitals, private psychiatric hospitals, or the community are reasonable referrals for patients with adequate financial resources or reimbursement from Medicare or private insurance. Patients under 65 on public aid or Medicaid often need to be cared for within the state or county system, although many private clinics have available allotted space for patients without reimbursement. State mental health clinics usually serve a particular area, and information regarding these clinics can be obtained from the county or mental health system. If a patient has previously been cared for by a psychiatrist or clinic, it is best to refer the patient back to the previous site of care. If the patient or family found this care unsatisfactory, the reasons for this dissatisfaction should be determined and another referral made. A patient who has a mood disorder, anxiety disorder, panic disorder, or psychotic disorder should be referred to a psychiatrist for evaluation because medication may be indicated in many cases. If an organic cause for the psychiatric symptomatology is suspected and this can be worked up safely on an outpatient basis, an appropriate medical as well as psychiatric referral should be made.

Patients are more likely to follow up with the outpatient referral if the emergency physician is able to make a follow-up appointment with the mental health care provider. Some clinics and mental health facilities provide 24 hour services for follow up appointments. Patients are also more likely to keep an outpatient appointment if they or their family or friends are familiar with or have been treated by the site or provider, or if the site or provider is in their neighborhood or in the same hospital as the ED. The patient should be given a card with the name, address, telephone number, contact person, and if possible, the time of appointment. If the emergency physician is unsure whether the mental health care provider is accepting outpatient referrals, two referrals should be made. As with in-hospital referrals, the patient's clinical state, physical examination, laboratory tests, and treatments should be legibly recorded and sent with the patient to the outpatient referral site.

SPECIAL PROBLEMS

THE PSYCHIATRIC TELEPHONE EMERGENCY

Families with a psychiatrically disturbed member may call the ED for advice. Although a brief history may be obtained over the telephone, the main goal is to get the patient to an environment in which assessment and treatment can be provided. If the patient will cooperate with the family, the family should be told to take the patient to the nearest ED or psychiatric facility that can deal with the problem. Patients with no previous psychiatric disorder should be taken to an ED that can rule out organic causes for the mental disturbance. A patient with an acute exacerbation of an

ongoing psychiatric illness and no physical illness or alcohol or substance abuse should be taken to the facility where he or she previously received care. If the patient refuses to cooperate, a family member must go to mental health court and fill out a petition, which is then presented by the state's attorney to the court. The judge may then order a 24-hour evaluation under emergency detention. With this emergency order, the police can either bring the patient to the nearest ED or assist in putting the patient in an ambulance for transfer to a psychiatric facility.

Psychiatric patients often call the ED for assistance. The name, address, and telephone number of the patient should be obtained first. After listening briefly to the problem, the listener should advise the patient to come to the ED or be referred to another facility where the patient's psychiatric difficulties can be assessed and treated. The psychiatric patient who calls to discuss problems over the telephone should be advised that it is impossible to deal with his or her difficulties over the telephone and told to come to the ED where proper assessment and treatment can take place. In most states, the police pick up a patient who is homicidal or suicidal and from whom identifying information can be obtained and bring him or her to the nearest ED for assessment. Patients who state that they are acutely suicidal and refuse to give identifying information, come to the ED, or get assistance within the environment are the most disturbing. "I am about to (or have just taken) an overdose, but wanted to talk to someone before I die." The emergency physician should *briefly* try to assess the type and amount of medication ingested, and why the patient has reached this point in his or her life, and then say "I know you've had a difficult time (paraphrase what the patient says). I know you are frightened. I want you to come to the Emergency Department now so that I can help you. Give me your name and address so I can get someone to bring you to see me (get a cab and we will worry about paying for it later) (find a friend or family member and have them bring you here)." "If you don't think I can help you, perhaps you will let me call someone who you think can." If, after a reasonable period, the patient refuses to give identifying information, get help, or come to the ED, the emergency physician is faced with the difficult decision of continuing to talk or hanging up. Referral to a suicide hotline is a reasonable option. The most annoying call is from the character-disordered patient who is lonely and wants reassurance. Such patients may threaten suicide if the emergency physician does not spend indeterminate periods of time on the telephone. The patient should be told firmly that he or she must come to the ED, and the telephone call ended promptly.

"REGULARS" IN THE ED

Chronic mentally ill patients often develop a relationship with an institution and its ED. Patients who visit an ED on a regular basis may do so because the clinic they attend does not provide consistent care with one mental health professional and/or the patient's psychopathology prevents the patient from using non-emergency room services appropriately. Some character-disordered patients become lonely, depressed, and anxious at night and during weekends, when there is no access to nonemergency mental health care. When a chronic psychiatric patient becomes a "regular," it is important to understand why the ED is being used inappropriately for psychiatric care. A plan should be devised to encourage the patient to obtain more appropriate care. Discussion with the family and treating mental health professionals can greatly assist in this process.

Another group of regulars in the ED include those with somatic complaints with no demonstrable organic cause. Patients with somatization disorder, hypochondriasis, and psychogenic pain disorder (briefly discussed in the previous section) are often unable to find a primary care physician with whom they can maintain an enduring therapeutic relationship. Because these patients view themselves as physically ill, a long-term relationship with a psychiatrist is equally problematic. As a result, the ED may become their health care provider. Every attempt should be made to refer these "regulars" to a clinic or physician who can develop an ongoing relationship with the patient. If, after this referral, the patient continues to visit the ED regularly, a plan should be worked out with the ongoing health provider to limit ED use.

BIBLIOGRAPHY

Bacani-Oropilla, G., and Lippmann, S.B.: When to use psychiatric referral in the ED. Hosp. Physician *30*:42, July, 1989.

Beyer, H.A.: Legal issues in a psychiatric emergency. *In* Emergency Psychiatry: Concepts, Methods, and Practices. Edited by Bassuk, E.L., and Birk, A.W. New York, Plenum Press, 1984.

Brackel, S.J.: The Mentally Disabled and the Law. 3rd Ed. Edited by Brackel, S.J., Perry, J., and Weiner, B. Chicago, American Bar Foundation, 1985.

Citrome, L., and Green, L.: The dangerous agitated patient: What to do right now. Postgrad. Med. *87*:231, 1990.

Monahan, J. (ed.): The Clinical Prediction of Violence. Washington, D.C., Government Printing Office (National Institute of Mental Health), 1981.

Pollard, C.A., and Lewis, L.M.: Managing panic attacks in emergency patients. J. Emerg. Med. *7*:547, 1989.

Shader, R.I. (ed.): Manual of Psychiatric Therapeutics: Practical Psychopharmacology and Psychiatry. Boston, Little, Brown and Company, 1981.

Soreff, S.M.: Management of the Psychiatric Emergency. New York, John Wiley and Sons, 1981.

Stoudemire, A., Fogel, B.S.: Pharmacology in the medically ill. *In* Principles of Medical Psychiatry. Edited by A. Stoudemire. New York, Grune and Stratton, 1987.

Walker, J.I. (ed.): Psychiatric Emergencies: Intervention and Resolution. Philadelphia, J.B. Lippincott, 1983.

Chapter 62

CLINICAL EVALUATION OF PSYCHIATRIC AND BEHAVIORAL EMERGENCIES

THE EMERGENT PSYCHOTIC PATIENT

Christos S. Dagadakis

CAPSULE

The onset and manifestation of psychosis are frightening and alarming to both the individual experiencing the psychosis and his or her family and friends. This alarm is frequently present in caregivers in emergent assessment and treatment settings. Providing a safe, structured environment and an unambiguous setting helps in the assessment and stabilization of the psychosis. Data gathered about the onset, past history, and course are essential to accurate assessment and optimal outcome. Frequently people accompanying the patient can give useful information that it may not be possible to obtain from the patient. The rapidity of onset and lack of past history of psychosis point toward ruling out medical causes for the disorder. Chronic psychotic illnesses presenting in an acute fashion frequently represent stopping of antipsychotic medicine, increase in life stresses, concomitant medical problem, use of street drugs, and/or exacerbation of the underlying condition for unclear reasons, often the natural course of illness.

INTRODUCTION

Psychosis is defined as a "major mental disorder of organic or emotional origin in which a person's ability to think, respond emotionally, remember, communicate, interpret reality, and behave appropriately is sufficiently impaired so as to interfere grossly with the capacity to meet the ordinary demands of life."[1] Often the patient has regressive behavior, inappropriate mood, decreased impulse control, and delusions and hallucinations. Severity and duration of the presentation and illness can range widely. The treatment varies with the diagnosis, level of impairment, risk to self or others, compliance of the patient, and availability of treatment options and referral sources.

PATHOPHYSIOLOGY

The pathophysiology of psychosis varies from the most definite causes related to toxic states, metabolic abnormality, neurologic abnormalities, infections, trauma, anoxia, use of psychoactive street drugs, and adverse medication reaction to states that justify the diagnosis of "psychosis nos" (not otherwise specified). The final pathway for much psychotic thinking, especially in schizophrenia, is related to multiple neurotransmitter pathways with a major influence of the dopamine transmission system.[2] Antipsychotic drugs are frequently developed based on the level of dopamine receptor blockade ability. Psychosis is frequently diminished by this dopamine receptor blockade, whether the illness is, for example, schizophrenia, organic delusional disorder, or postpartum depression. The short-term evaluation of acute schizophrenia, bipolar disorder, psychosis secondary to amphetamine-like drugs, and occasionally psychotic depression is difficult because the presentation may be similar. History is important in the differentiation of these psychoses. The psychosis that develops in withdrawal states may represent the result of the organism's attempt to return to a homeostasis with an increased release of neurotransmitters, increased sensitivity of receptors of the transmitters, or both.[3]

The physiology of the effectiveness of lithium salts and carbamazepine in the treatment of manic episodes and later prevention of the mania and depression is felt to involve multiple receptor systems, neurotransmitters, and enzymatic processes[4,5] to be related to the alteration of the neural cell membrane and a change in sodium transport with an eventual change in neurotransmitter release, sensitivity, or both. Sedative hypnotics help to decrease the agitation and anxiety of the psychotic process by decreasing neuronal transmission and appear to be helpful as adjuncts in schizophrenia and other psychoses.[6] These hypnotics do not have the dopamine-blocking effect of neuroleptics and are less useful when used alone in schizophrenia.[7]

ASSESSMENT AND STABILIZATION

The first concerns are safety and the creation of a nonagitating and supportive atmosphere. The chapter on the agitated patient outlines the safety, stabilization, and restraint issues. With the psychotic patient, it is particularly important to understand the individual's concerns and perceptions of the situation. This helps to establish rapport and structure the interview and process in the emergent setting. For example, an individual with persecutory delusions and much paranoid ideation requires the least ambiguity possible to minimize misinterpretations. Similarly, efforts must be made to minimize stimulation of the paranoia. In an individual with paranoia about government surveillance, questionnaires and documents that must be signed should be carefully explained and the number minimized. It is important to have a staff member or the actual evaluator talk to people who bring the psychotic patient in. Police, relatives, and friends frequently leave after dropping off the patient. These people may have crucial information and may be difficult to find later. They may also be needed to provide supplementary evidence for civil commitment.

Current and past history is as important as the clinical presentation and the mental status examination. At the minimum, vital signs, medicines and drugs taken in the last few days, and history of current active medical problems must be obtained early in the contact. Once some of the acute history is obtained from the patient or other sources, it will be clearer what laboratory tests should be done immediately and what immediate or subsequent parts of the physical examination are needed. The individual with no past history of mental disorder and a recent onset of symptoms is most likely to have a nonpsychiatric disorder with organic cause. The physical examination should focus on general medical screening, head injuries, and neurologic impairment. Frequently, psychotic individuals are poor historians and may not cooperate in a physical examination. The patient may have to be restrained to allow physical examination when (1) an organic cause for the psychosis is likely and physical examination is essential to assess this cause; (2) the individual is at significant risk for harm to himself or herself or others; or (3) the patient is not able to take care of his or her basic human needs. The crucial need for the physical examination should be explained whether the patient appears to understand it or not.

In the mental status examination, orientation, memory questions (especially about immediate and recent items) have the most validity in identifying organic disorder. All psychotic patients should be asked about suicidal and homicidal ideation and intent if present. Some individuals do not tell whether they have suicidal or homicidal thoughts or plans unless they are asked specifically. Asking about sensitive areas is often best left to the last part of the interview because rapport may require time, and patients share more as they trust the interviewer more. If sensitive questions are asked too early, the patient may stop talking completely, and even nonthreatening data may not be collectible. The mental status examination can first help to clarify whether psychosis exists and the nature of the psychosis, and can be a yardstick to measure the level of impairment and change over the course of time.

CLINICAL PRESENTATION

Psychosis must be considered whenever an individual is acting in a bizarre manner, appears to be preoccupied, is agitated, has unusual somatic complaints, refuses to talk, makes statements that are highly unusual or out of touch with reality, or has an emotional response beyond that which appears to be appropriate to the situation. Psychotic individuals may also have a concomitant physical illness, and in fact frequently do because of poor self-care. The medical illness may exacerbate the psychotic disorder. Certain "post" states are associated with occasional psychotic reactions (e.g., postpartum psychosis).

DIFFERENTIAL DIAGNOSIS

The range of causes of psychosis covers many body systems and causes. It is important that medical cause be considered when there is an apparent psychosis

---

TABLE 62-1. MEDICAL PROBLEMS WITH PSYCHIATRIC SYMPTOMS HAVING PSYCHOTIC FEATURES

Adrenal Cortical Insufficiency (Addison's disease): Thought disorder, suspiciousness, confusion, markedly fluctuating affect and behavior

Brain Damage (from trauma, circulatory abnormalities, and/or anoxia): Confusion, disorientation, irritability, affective lability, hallucinations, delusions

Hyperadrenalism (Cushing's disease): Somatic delusions, irritability, emotional lability, hypervigilance, referential thinking

Hyperthyroidism: Clouded sensorium, paranoia, agitation, delusions

Hyperparathyroidism and Hypoparathyroidism: Hyperactivity, irritability, confusion, disorientation, clouded sensorium

Hepatolenticular degeneration (Wilson's disease): Rapid mood swings, hallucinations, irritability, memory problems

Hypoglycemia: Agitation, confusion, anxiety

Hypoxia: Visual hallucinations, disorientation, confusion, memory problems

Infections (especially of the CNS): Confusion, irritability, disorientation, hallucinations, agitation

Intracranial Tumors: Clouding of consciousness, hallucinations (especially visual, gustatory, and olfactory), rapid shifts in mental state

Porphyria (acute intermittent type): Mood swings, confusion

Postpartum Psychosis: Confusion, mood lability, irritability, delusions, hallucinations

Seizures: Affective lability, paranoia, confusion, disorientation, visual, gustatory, olfactory, auditory hallucinations, automatic behaviors, and/or anger outbursts. Postictal states may have confusion, combativeness, and affective lability

Systemic Lupus Erythematosus: Thought disorder, confusion, elation, affective lability, paranoia, confusion, disorientation

---

(Table 62-1). A crucial part of the differential diagnosis is the past history of the current problem and presentation. An individual who comes in with paranoid delusions and who hears voices and is alternately agitated and labile could have schizophrenia, bipolar disorder (manic state), cocaine psychosis, or amphetamine psychosis. Beyond laboratory testing for drug use, the primary differential is based on detailed longitudinal history. If the patient is in the late teens or early twenties at first onset and experiences deterioration from episode to episode, the likelihood is that the patient has schizophrenia. If the onset is in the late thirties, the patient functions well between episodes, and there is no evidence of amphetamine-like drug use, bipolar disorder is more likely. Diagnostically, the overlap of polysubstance abuse and various psychiatric disorders can make the final diagnosis difficult. A person can have both schizophrenia and amphetamine abuse, for example. The cause of the emergent symptoms is not totally determinable. The differential diagnosis of most psychoses generally classified as psychiatric is summarized in Table 62-2. Psychoses from prescription drugs are summarized in Table 62-3.

INITIAL STABILIZATION

Stabilization beyond that required for agitation and immediate risk of harm is usually accomplished during the interview and assessment process. The anxiety and/or dysphoria fostered by the disorganization and distortions in thought can be moderated by structure, minimizing ambiguity, showing concern and respect, and clarifying the patient's concerns. The goals of the interaction and questions should be clarified. Once the patient's concerns are elicited, the interview can become more directed and the patient kept on track with the area of inquiry. The process of trying to understand the problem with respect can in itself help to decrease the sense of helplessness that is frequently part of the psychosis. Making statements about what the patient may be experiencing can establish both rapport and clarification; for example, "it seems like it must be frustrating when people don't understand your sense of being controlled by radio waves." If your assessment or observation is incorrect, the patient can correct you. Throughout this interview process, the patient must be observed carefully for areas of inquiry that are upsetting and for increasing agitation and stimulation. The interview can be modified to lower the stimulation.

Neuroleptic medications are often the drugs of choice for acute psychosis, whether the diagnosis is schizophrenia or a less clearly defined psychosis.[8,9] Haloperidol is used frequently because of its ease of administration, effectiveness, and relative safety. A usual first dose is 5 mg PO or IM. The liquid concentrate version is preferred over tablet form because it cannot be easily "cheeked" (not swallowed), and is absorbed more quickly. The concentrate is tasteless and colorless. The 5 mg dose can be repeated every ½ to 1 hour. For an extremely agitated or large person, an initial dose may be 10 mg. For an elderly or brain-damaged individual, a small dose such as 0.5 to 1 mg may be appropriate because sedation is frequent at higher doses. One should be ready for extrapyramidal symptoms with the use of neuroleptics, especially when the blood level is dropping, because some such as haloperidol have an antiextrapyramidal effect of their own at higher blood levels. Other neuroleptics can be equally effective in controlling schizophrenia, other psychoses, and agitation, but have different benefits and side effect profiles.[10] Although droperidol is approved primarily for use in anesthesia, it is a neuroleptic that can cause sedation and rapid control of agitation. Doses can range from 2.5 to 10 mg IM. Alternative neuroleptic antipsychotic options and sedating medications are described in this chapter's subsection on drugs for psychiatric disorders.

If sedation is indicated to help in decreasing the agitation, higher doses of neuroleptic or a sedating

TABLE 62-2. DIFFERENTIAL DIAGNOSIS OF EMERGENT PSYCHOTIC DISORDERS

Disorder	Onset	Presentation	Course	Prognosis	Treatment
Schizophrenia	Teens and 20s, rare in 40s	Hallucinations Delusions (especially bizarre ones) Social withdrawal Loose association Signs of disturbance for at least 6 months	For most, gradual deterioration	25% remit 50% improve with treatment 25% do not significantly improve Most have significant impairment in interpersonal relations and work function	Emergent Neuroleptics, with possible addition of lorazepam for help with agitation and sedation. Long-term: neuroleptics and monitoring of behavior
Schizophreniform disorder	As in schizophrenia	As in schizophrenia, but difficulties for less than 6 months	By definition, lasts for 6 months or less. If symptoms persist, the diagnosis is schizophrenia	Remission or progression to schizophrenia or other psychosis	Treatment as in schizophrenia
Schizoaffective disorder	Before 40s	Symptoms of both schizophrenic and affective disorder (usually manic)	Affective symptoms are cyclic. Delusions and/or hallucinations must be present for 2 weeks without affective symptoms	Variable, but usually similar to schizophrenia	As with schizophrenia in emergent state, subsequent addition of lithium carbonate or carbamazepine if cycles are frequent and a problem (an antidepressant may be added if depression is prominent).
Depression with psychosis	All ages, especially after 50 (rare in children)	Delusions, especially of decay and illness Hallucinations Negative symptoms (decreased energy, appetite, sleep disturbance, weight loss, constipation)	Episodic or intermittent—2 weeks of depressive mood are required at a minimum	Generally improves with treatment	Neuroleptic and antidepressant or electroconvulsive treatment (often an antidepressant or lithium is given after ECT for preventive of relapse)
Brief reactive psychosis	Any age	Delusions Hallucinations Emotionally coherent turmoil (presence of above after stressful events)	Few hours to one month	Full recovery	Neuroleptic and/or lorazepam or sedation with a benzodiazapine such as lorazepam structure and support
Bipolar disorder (manic)	Late 20s to early 30s; teens to 70s possible but less frequent	Distinct period of abnormal and persistently elevated, expansive, or irritable mood Hyperactivity Distractibility Flight of ideas Talkativeness Grandiosity Delusions Hallucinations	Cyclic (can have remission of episode of mania and usual subsequent depression)	General recovery and prophylaxis with lithium or carbamazepine	Lorazepam for sedation initially Lithium or carbamazepine (takes about 5 days to have antimanic effect) Neuroleptics can be used if psychosis is prominent
Delirium	All ages Acute onset (hours to days)	Reduced ability to maintain attention to external stimuli Disorganized thoughts Reduced level of conscientiousness Perception disturbance Disturbed sleep cycle	Variable	Generally short term Increased morbidity, long term	Treating the underlying organic disturbance and maintain homeostasis Neuroleptic especially haloperidol or droperidol to decrease agitation when present Lorazepam can be added to haloperidol

TABLE 62-2. CONTINUED

Disorder	Onset	Presentation	Course	Prognosis	Treatment
Psychosis not otherwise specified	Variable	Disorientation Psychomotor disturbance Many of the features of the above disorders but inadequate information is present to make a specific diagnosis	Variable	Variable	Neuroleptic and possibly lorazepam for sedation

TABLE 62-3. PSYCHOSES FROM PRESCRIPTION DRUGS

Antidepressants (mainly tricyclics and tetracyclics): Disorientation, confusion, paranoia, hallucinations

Atropinic action medications: Anticholinergic psychosis ("dry as a bone, red as a beet"), disorientation, confusion, visual hallucinations, agitation

Bromides: Emotional lability, delusions, hallucinations, confusion, disorientation, irritability

Cimetidine: Psychosis, paranoia, agitation, delirium

Digoxin: Psychosis with visual hallucinations

L-Dopa: Hypomania, hallucinations, paranoid delusions, delirium, agitation

Lidocaine: Psychosis with visual hallucinations

Penicillin (intravenous): Agitation, hallucinations, anxiety, and/or convulsions

Phenylbutazone (in large doses): Delirium and/or hallucinations

Podophyllin (oral and cutaneous): Visual hallucinations, sedation, paranoia, nausea

Propranolol: Psychosis with visual hallucinations, delirium, psychotic depression

Quinidine: Psychosis with visual hallucinations

Reserpine: Psychotic depression, nondepressed psychosis, catatonia

Salicylates (high doses): Confusion, agitation, delirium, hallucinations

Steroids (prednisone): Affective instability, manic-like state, schizophreniform state, confusion, disorientation

neuroleptic can be used, or a sedative hypnotic can be used by itself or in combination with the neuroleptic. If an individual has been taking a sedative hypnotic substance, additional use of a sedative hypnotic such as a benzodiapine may cause oversedation and/or respiratory depression. Lorazepam is an excellent hypnotic for emergent settings because it can be given IM with good absorption and has a shorter half-life than, for example, diazepam. The usual dose is 1 to 2 mg, with the dose repeated every $\frac{1}{2}$ to 1 hour with a usual maximum dosage of 10 mg in 24 hours. Diazepam has more erratic im absorption (best absorption from the deltoid). It is used both orally and in-

travenously. Diazepam may be more rapid in its oral effectiveness than lorazepam. The usual dose for diazepam is 5 to 10 mg every hour with a 60 mg maximum in 24 hours. Intravenous use is frequently difficult in an extremely agitated person because the intravenous site must be held steady if no IV is in place and a slow infusion of either diazepam or lorazepam is required (2 mg of lorazepam or 5 mg of diazepam over 1 minute). Haloperidol and lorazepam have been used together effectively with less haloperidol required over the course of stabilization.[11] Individuals who have PCP or phencyclidine psychosis can appear to improve with the use of benzodiazepine sedation, but when the sedation decreases, the symptoms are likely to return. Sedative hypnotics generally do not remove psychotic symptoms, but can modify their expression. If the psychotic symptoms are the target, a neuroleptic is generally necessary.

LABORATORY AND PROCEDURES

If emergent psychosis has an acute onset, the most useful tests are electrolytes, glucose, blood urea nitrogen, and creatinine to screen for metabolic abnormality; complete blood count to assess blood loss, infection, and nutritional deficiency; and a toxicology screen to help determine any contribution from drugs of abuse (Table 62-4). If meningitis is suspected, a lumbar puncture is indicated. If an electroencephalogram is available emergently and the patient can cooperate, it can help screen for a seizure disorder and occasionally for encephalopathy. In individuals in whom head injury is suspected, a computed tomographic (CT) scan and a screening neurologic examination are necessary. A skull x ray is indicated if a skull fracture is suspected. Pregnancy testing may be necessary for at-risk individuals before giving psychotropic medications. Some teratogenic risk may exist, especially with benzodiapines.[12]

TABLE 62-4. SCREENING LABORATORY TESTS FOR EMERGENT PSYCHOSIS

Laboratory Test	Indications	Pitfalls
Complete blood count	Elevated temperature History or appearance of poor self-care Possible trauma Substance abuse history Question of hypoxia	White blood cell counts are elevated in high stress states
Electrolytes, glucose, and blood urea nitrogen	Rule out hypoglycemia Assess dehydration and metabolic abnormality Possible delirium	Abnormalities may not be causative of psychosis but a result of poor self-care
CT scan	Focal neurologic signs History of recent head injury Unexplained delirium	Paranoid patients may be agitated by CT scan apparatus
EEG	Loss or alteration of consciousness before confusion or psychosis Signs of encephalopathy	Agitated or uncooperative patients preclude an EEG because the head must be held relatively still to connect electrodes, and attempts at sedation may mask abnormality
Alcohol level	Apparent alcohol use Alcohol on breath, staggering, and/or slurred speech History of recent alcohol use	Negative alcohol level does not preclude psychosis secondary to withdrawal
Toxicology screen	History of drug ingestions Apparent signs and symptoms of drug use	Presence of drugs may be in addition to underlying psychosis and not causative Negative screen does not preclude psychosis secondary to past drug use or current withdrawal
Skull x ray	Suspected skull fracture or penetrating wound	Rarely useful except in head trauma, and then the utility is for medicolegal reasons
Pregnancy test (hCG in serum or urine)	Before use of psychotropic emergent medications, especially benzodiazepines in women at risk for pregnancy	If urine is too dilute (less than 10 specific gravity), test is unreliable Inaccurate histories in psychotic individuals

MANAGEMENT AND INDICATIONS FOR ADMISSION

Indications for outpatient treatment:

1. Patient is not suicidal nor homicidal
2. Psychosis intensity has decreased with intervention in the emergency setting
3. Agitation has decreased
4. Outpatient living arrangement with observation is possible by others
5. Patient is willing to cooperate with treatment and take medications
6. Patient is able to provide self-care
7. Outpatient treatment and follow-up options are available

Indications for inpatient treatment:

1. Active suicidal or homicidal ideation
2. Agitation level of psychosis is unchanged by interventions
3. Ambivalence about medications and/or treatment
4. Self-care abilities are in doubt
5. No structure or outpatient option is available for immediate future
6. Treatment regimen requires continual observation and adjustment
7. Risk to self or others exists and patient is unwilling to obtain care (civil commitment is necessary)
8. Grave disability exists (inability to take care of basic human needs—usually civil commitment is necessary)

The above criteria apply to most of the diagnostic categories that could result in emergent psychosis. Bipolar individuals who are manic can have rapid changes in the level of psychosis and agitation. Unless the initial presentation was mild in severity, hospitalization is the safest course. Individuals who have taken phencyclidine have significant changes in level of sedation from medication. The same intense level of agitation can appear suddenly on discharge.

PITFALLS

- Missing a medical cause for the psychotic symptoms secondary to inadequate or cursory physical evaluation.
- Not looking for concomitant medical illness that does not cause the psychosis but may exacerbate it or be present in an individual with poor self-care.
- Not taking seriously physical complaints presented in a psychotic framework, such as a statement of "demons in my belly" which may represent abdominal pain.
- Not obtaining data from people who bring the patient in or who have had frequent contact and/or know the history.
- Not spending enough time to establish rapport and gather data.
- Treating agitated patients with a benzodiazepine before a history or laboratory result is obtained about recent use of other sedative hypnotics with resulting potential for respiratory depression.
- Making referrals for follow-up care when the availability for emergent care is not known.
- Giving too much neuroleptic to patients over age 60.
- Not giving a patient who has been stabilized on neuroleptics a warning about possible extrapyramidal symptoms and a plan to deal with them.
- As stated previously, not recognizing that variability of mania and types of psychosis may slow transient improvement but then worsen (e.g., PCP-induced psychosis).

MEDICOLEGAL PEARLS

- Civil commitment does not usually give permission to treat nonpsychiatric problems involuntarily.
- In some states, a specific level of risk and a subsequent court hearing about medications alone are required to treat involuntarily, even when the person is civilly committed.
- An individual who is psychotic may still be legally competent to make decisions about his or her medical care and finances. A court decision is necessary to declare legal incompetence.

HORIZONS

- Positron emission tomography (PET) scanning may become a useful tool in making a differential diagnosis in an emergent setting, especially between the psychosis of schizophrenia and mania.
- A multicenter study can clarify the relative utility of using haloperidol, lorazepam, or a combination of the two in agitated and psychotic patients.

NATIONAL CONTACTS

American Psychiatric Association, 202-682-6000.

REFERENCES

1. The American Psychiatric Association Psychiatric Glossary. Washington, DC, American Psychiatric Press, Inc., 1984, p. 114.
2. Creese, I., Burt, D.R., and Snyder, S.H.: Dopamine receptors binding predicts clinical and pharmacological potency of antischizophrenic drugs. Science 192:481, 1976.
3. Roy-Byrne, P.P., and Hommer, D.: Benzodiazepine withdrawal: Overview and implications for treatment of anxiety. JAMA 184:1041, 1988.
4. Baraban, J.M., Worley, P.F., and Snyder, S.H.: The second messenger systems and psychoactive drug action: Focus on the phosphoinositide system and lithium. Am. J. Psychiatry 146:10, 1989.
5. Post, R.M., and Weise, S.R.B.: Sensitization, kindling and anticonvulsants in mania. J. Clin. Psychiatry 50:12, 1989.
6. Cohen, S., and Khan, A.: Adjunctive benzodiazepine in acute schizophrenia. Neuropsychobiology 18:9, 1987.
7. Lingjaerde, O.: Benzodiazepines in the treatment of schizophrenia. In From Molecular Biology to Clinical Practice. Edited by Costa, E. New York, Raven Press, 1983.
8. American Psychiatric Association Task Force on Treatment of Psychiatric Disorder, Vol. 3. Washington, DC, American Psychiatric Association, 1989, p. 2584.
9. Dubin, W.R.: Rapid tranquilization: Antipsychotic or benzodiazepine? J. Clin. Psychiatry 49:12, 1988.
10. American Psychiatric Association Task Force on Treatment of Psychiatric Disorder, Vol. 2. Washington, DC, American Psychiatric Association, 1989, p. 1503.
11. Cohen, B.M., and Lipinski, J.F.: Treatment of acute psychosis with non-neuroleptic agents. Psychosomatics 27:7, 1986.
12. Hauser, L.A.: Pregnancy and psychiatric drugs. Hosp. Community Psychiatry 36:817, 1985.

BIBLIOGRAPHY

American Psychiatric Association Task Force on Treatment of Psychiatric Disorder. Washington, DC, American Psychiatric Association, 1989.

Hall, R.C.W. (ed.): Psychiatric Presentations of Medical Illness: Somatopsychic Disorders. New York, SP Medical & Scientific Books, 1980.

Hyman, S.E.: Manual of Psychiatric Emergencies. Boston, Little, Brown, and Company, 1988.

Hyman, S.E., Arana, G.W.: Handbook of Psychiatric Drug Therapy. Boston, Little, Brown, and Company, 1987.

Slaby, A.E., Lieb, J., and Trancredi, L.R.: The Handbook of Psychiatric Emergencies. 3rd Ed. New York, Medical Examination Publishing Company, 1986.

THE ASSAULTIVE PATIENT

Christos S. Dagadakis and Roland D. Maiuro

CAPSULE

The most important risk factors for immediate assaultive behavior are a recent history of serious assault, a general history of impulsivity, past physical violence toward others, intoxication or toxicity (or withdrawal with delirium), antisocial personality disorder, and psychosis associated with anger and the perception of a personal threat. Some risk of assault should be considered with all patients. A formal management plan for assaultive patients must be in place. This plan should include a protocol for calling personnel to aid in assaultive patient management, criteria for physical restraint of patients, and a policy and approach to medication management. Ambiguity should be minimized. Efforts to establish rapport and re-establish self-control and self-responsibility are essential once immediate safety is established. Developing alternative solutions to perceived patient problems can help decrease the risk of harm. There are many potential medicolegal consequences for not dealing with assaultive risk in the Emergency Department (ED), as well as in discharging a violence-prone patient without making a reasonable effort to decrease the risk of danger.

INTRODUCTION

Interpersonal violence has been identified as a public health problem of major proportion.[1] Physicians and health care providers frequently have contact with victims and perpetrators of violence. Health care providers are held accountable increasingly by the public to recognize cases at risk for assault and to make reasonable efforts to intervene. Effective strategies for dealing with the assaultive patient are of interest to health care providers because of personal safety issues. The identified patient, vulnerable family members, other patients in the treatment setting, and potential victims in the general community must also be protected from physical and emotional harm. The goal is to assess the likelihood of such behavior and manage the risk of harm.

PATHOPHYSIOLOGY

Assaultive behavior is determined by many factors and does not simply arise out of physiology. Violence is part of the social fabric of our society and is, in fact, sanctioned in areas such as sports and self-protection. It is often provoked by social and environmental events such as interpersonal conflict with intimate family members, territorial disputes between strangers, and, in some cases, authority figures who are viewed as domineering or unjust. It also involves a host of psychologic factors such as attitudes toward aggression, expectations regarding certain types of relationships, sentiments toward subgroups of people, and learned responses to stress and challenge.

Identifiable biologic conditions, however, greatly increase the likelihood that assaultive behavior will occur. These conditions may result in decreased cognitive control, as in the case of brain damage or temporary disinhibition caused by alcohol abuse, toxicity, and/or "fight or flight" survival reactions. Generally, the risk of assault is positively correlated with physiologic arousal. An individual with increased secretion of epinephrine, increased heart rate, increased blood pressure, sweating, dilated pupils, and muscle tension is ready to act. Usually the arousal is a response to perceived threat or frustration.

The physiologic basis for aggression can be seen most clearly in cases of brain damage, particularly those involving the frontal and temporal areas and certain hypothalamic damage. With brain damage, the individual may have limited ability to assess a situation accurately, especially in regard to threat. Comcomitant to impairment in receptive areas, one often sees expressive deficits whereby fewer response options are generated to deal with the perceived situation. These deficits are usually a direct function of fewer brain cells and/or impaired neural circuits.

With cortical damage, there is less neural or cognitive capacity to stand between the perceived threat or irritant and a response of anger and counteraggression. In some brain-damaged individuals, impulsivity is increased, causing poorly-thought-out responses. Associative learning between behavior and consequences may also be impaired. Brain-damaged individuals have more susceptibility to mind-altering substances such as alcohol and drugs, and are more vulnerable to fatigue. In some relatively rare cases, seizure disorders can elicit violent action (e.g., temporal lobe or partial seizures). This type of violent behavior, however, is usually blind, disorganized, and stereotyped in quality.[2] More risk is present in the postictal state, in which there may be confusion and less neural capacity to manage the disordered perceptual input.

A temporary state of brain disorder exists in toxic states and conditions of delirium. Alcohol and the sedative hypnotics decrease the quality and quantity of incoming information and impair the existing neural circuit function, especially of the cerebral cortex. The parts of the brain that evolved last seem to be affected first and then down the line to deeper or more primitive structures. Electrical activity and synaptic efficiency generally decrease and new learning is impaired. With amphetamines and similar drugs, there is an overactivity of norepinephrine neural pathways. These activating substances either directly stimulate neurons or prolong the effect of intrinsic neurotransmitters. In effect, there is an overload of multiple circuits as well as development of physiologic fatigue because of overactivity and lack of sleep with prolonged use. The likelihood of violent action may be related to resulting irritability and hypersensitivity to stimuli on the behavioral and neural levels. Temporary states of brain disorder share features of impaired input of information and impaired processing of the information, resulting in a higher risk of violent action.

CLINICAL PRESENTATION AND EXAMINATION

DETERMINATION OF RISK FOR IMMEDIATE ASSAULT OR VIOLENCE

The current consensus among mental health professionals is that it is beyond the expertise and capability of any professional to predict violence *absolutely* in the individual case.[3] It is important, however, for all clinicians to be familiar with the factors that increase or decrease the likelihood or *probable risk* of such acts. The risk of assault or violence can best be determined by assessing the presence or absence of factors such as the most recent history of assault or violence, past history of assault, current intoxication, antisocial personality disorder, brain damage, toxicity, delirium, psychosis, intense need to be in control, and cultural backgrounds associated with the acceptance of violence.

CLINICAL HISTORY

A recent history of violence is one of the best predictors of the potential for violence. Individuals who have violent episodes are frequently brought in by police,

family, institutional staff, or friends. It is crucial that data be gathered from these individuals about the episode and any available history. In the emergency or hospital setting, clinical protocols are typically directed at identifying risk factors for serious forms of injury. It is important to ask questions focused on the frequency, severity, and nature of previous assaultive behavior, injuries associated with such acts, apparent or expressed intent to harm, and the availability of weapons. A pattern of recent escalation on the part of the patient should lead the clinician to consider the case to be in the high risk category for immediate or future violence. All instances in which a previous or potential victim expresses acute concern about his or her safety should be taken seriously.

There is some evidence that a developmental triad of fire-setting, cruelty to animals, and bed-wetting increases the risk of impulsivity and violence, although all three are required to reliably enhance the risk. One of the strongest historical factors is the patient's own history of abuse and victimization within the family of origin, particularly for men. Many investigators have also found similarities in the profile of suicidal and homicidal men, indicating the need to ask about the history of suicide in the family, personal attempts, threats, and ideation.[4] It is also important to establish contact with the spouse or family members to assess and monitor danger. Although they are overlooked by many clinicians and researchers, persons who are violent toward intimates and family members probably represent the largest category of potentially dangerous individuals in our culture.[5]

If available, family members must give information if civil commitment is necessary. Such information often requires a signed affidavit to proceed. Despite their potential endangerment, family members may be reluctant to provide information under these circumstances. The care provider should be prepared to adopt a supportive and educative posture in such instances. Ambivalent feelings should not be interpreted as "uncooperative" but a natural response to a serious, out-of-control situation in which personal rights and freedoms must be carefully weighed against the risk of harm. It is often helpful for the care provider to realize that the "routine" matter of hospitalization may be traumatic and intimidating to family members. A consumer-oriented review of the benefits and common discomforts that attend involuntary hospitalization can often enhance cooperation in these cases.

Because of pressing schedules and other responsibilities, police and institutional informants frequently leave the scene quickly and assume that the health care provider will handle the situation. The assessment process can be facilitated by getting the data through a brief structured interview or questionnaire and making sure that you have a way to reach the referring parties if more information is needed. It is important to realize that the patient's version of the event may vary considerably from those provided by the informants, and in some cases may not be given at all. Some clinicians believe that the memory of perpetrators may be impaired or limited during periods of extreme rage and that this adds to the risk of underreporting already present because of psychologic defensiveness and social undesirability.[6] All the versions need to be considered to determine the risk.

SITUATIONAL AND CONTEXTUAL ISSUES

The specific targets of the patient's assault and threats, the emotional and legal consequences that have ensued, the availability of personal resources, and the level and quality of social support are useful in assessing current risk. If the violence was directed to a specific target for personal and unique reasons, the risk is somewhat less for the care provider. In the same case, however, the risk may be high for the identified personal target, particularly if it is an easily accessed and vulnerable family member. As a general rule, the greater the number of incidents and targets, the higher the risk. Any previous history of hitting caregivers, authority figures, or being violent in health care facilities, however, indicates a significant risk of immediate assaultiveness in the clinical setting.

It is important to know what has happened as a consequence of previous instances of assault or violence. If the patient has experienced serious consequences, both emotional and legal, yet appears to be unable to constrain his or her behavior, the prognosis is more guarded. In some cases, consequences can be helpful in defining reality limits for a patient. In other cases, the negative experiences may simply aggravate and alienate the patient further because they follow a downward spiral.

Generally, the greater the personal resources (e.g., socioeconomic status, employment, stable residence), the lower the risk. The availability of a supportive social network, whether it be family or friends, usually demonstrates some level of social responsibility and helps mitigate risk. An alienated or conflicted support system, however, may not mitigate risk at all and, in some cases, can increase it.

INTOXICATION AND TOXICITY

Intoxication with alcohol or sedatives increases the risk of violence. The risk is highest when the patient also appears noncooperative, makes angry verbal statements or behavioral postures, and is perceptually slow or disorganized. In some instances, patients who are on benzodiazepines can become violence-prone, especially with the ingestion of minute amounts of alcohol. Careful history taking regarding current prescriptions, as well as nonprescribed drugs, can help detect potential chemical interactions and diagnose atypical reactions.

Abuse of drugs such as cocaine, LSD, amphetamines, and phencyclidine hydrochloride (PCP) increases the risk of violence secondary to increasing arousal, irritability, and possible induction of psychosis and paranoia. PCP has a track record of inducing out-of-control behavior of particularly high intensity. It can also return to circulation from fat stores in the body and precipitate a toxic state after the patient has been stabilized.

Individuals who are intoxicated, whether it be from medical conditions, toxic substances, drugs, or alcohol, are at a higher risk for violent action. These individuals are frequently disoriented and have distorted perceptions of sensory and interpersonal stimuli and less cognitive capacity to process the information they gather. They may misperceive a situation as a threat to them and act accordingly. The toxic substances may lower their threshold for anger and increase the likelihood of impulsive behavior.

BRAIN DAMAGE

Brain-damaged individuals as a group have a higher risk for violence for many reasons. First, many individuals who have received brain injuries as a result of trauma were at a high risk for violence and impulsivity *before* their brain damage. For example, a person with a history of antisocial personality disorder, alcohol abuse, and frequent fights may have been injured in one of his or her fights. The brain damage then contributes an added risk for impulsivity, a tendency to get frustrated and angry, fewer cognitive faculties to solve problems and modify anger states, and increased vulnerability to the effects of drugs and alcohol. People with brain damage frequently have a higher level of social discord, financial problems, and diminished social support options and resources. People with developmental disabilities (mental retardation) also have fewer cognitive abilities to solve problems and may respond to frustrating situations with outbursts. Individuals who do not have the appearance of the overt behavior of a mentally retarded individual but who have a low IQ can get into frustrating situations when other people's expectations are too high.

PSYCHIATRIC DISORDER

In evaluating well over 1000 cases of interpersonal violence, Maiuro and his colleagues at the Harborview Anger Management Program have reported a broad spectrum of diagnosable profiles.[7] In accord with the findings of previous investigators, they have found many cases meeting criteria for personality disorders, various types of depression, impulse control disorder, unresolved learning disabilities or attention deficits, alcohol abuse, cyclic mood or arousal disorders, adjustment reactions, organic personality syndromes, and formal thought disorder.[8]

Psychosis, paranoia, manic-depressive conditions, and antisocial personality disorder have received special attention for their association with violence.[9] The psychotic individual whose reality testing is impaired may misinterpret a situation and perceive a threat and act accordingly. The individuals with paranoia and manic states are at highest risk for violence among patients with mental illness. People who are paranoid or have paranoid delusions of threat see others as likely to injure them. It is important to minimize the ambiguity of statements or actions to minimize their perception of threat. People who are manic frequently exhibit irritability, hyperactivity, and impaired reasoning, and occasionally are paranoid and psychotic. All of these characteristics increase the risk for violence. For example, a manic person who decides during the interview to help rearrange the furniture may become angry and strike out if he or she is stopped from this activity or an attempt is made to restrain him or her. Frequently, when people are psychotic, manic, anxious, or even depressed, they are physiologically aroused and agitated. This physiologic substrate increases the risk of violence and anger outbursts.

PERSONALITY AND CULTURAL DETERMINANTS

The overall violence risk increases as the number of risk factors increases. Individuals who have a strong need to be in control have an increased risk of violence when that control is threatened. An individual who has a "macho" style may respond violently when physically restricted or restrained in an attempt to maintain a sense of self and self-esteem. It is almost as if the patient is thinking, "They can't make me do this without a fight." The macho person may respond violently when his access to a friend or family member who may be in treatment in the facility is blocked. His sense of control is lowered by the illness of the friend or family member and his not being there to help. He may act violently in an ill-conceived attempt to "protect" the friend or family member. Violent action is possible when the person perceives that his "right" to something is denied or he feels wrongly accused or is physically impeded. Such individuals may abuse alcohol to "take the edge off" their agitation, only to find their self-control lowered in the face of stress. Individuals who have had difficulties with authority figures in their past may respond to caregivers in a similar fashion.

Risk of violence is increased for individuals with cultural backgrounds in which violence is sanctioned. For example, members of a street gang may have an ethos of acting violently and perceiving health care providers as agents of social control. Questions that imply a legal sanction or are perceived to threaten their sense of self and group identity may cause a violent outburst, especially when physiologically aroused or on a substance of abuse.

CLINICAL PRESENTATION OF THE ASSAULTIVE RISK PATIENT

The differential diagnosis of the potentially assaultive patient involves: (1) determining whether the person has a specific behavioral-emotional and situational profile associated with violence, and (2) determining whether a predisposing condition exists. The assaultive risk patient usually presents with features that help in his or her identification. No one aspect is definitive except for actual assaultive behavior in the assessment setting. The refusal to cooperate, including refusal to talk, is frequently associated with volatile behavior. Such individuals must be handled carefully because they may become explosive if pressed too vigorously for some desired action. Providing the patient with choices of action and time and space to deliberate can sometimes enhance the patient's sense of control and cooperation in such instances.

Motor agitation, including pacing, frequent shifts in the chair or stretcher, angry facial expressions, clenching of fists, and biting down with intensity are signs of risk. Recent and old scars on the patient's face and/or knuckles suggests that the individual deals with frustration by becoming violent. Other signs of past conflicts, such as a broken nose or black eye, may also be clues. The individual who is yelling loudly or whose volume of speech is increasing needs close monitoring. One who sits in the corner of the room with his or her back protected and scans the room is looking for threats and may respond to ambiguous situations as attacks. The individual who has a disheveled appearance or ripped clothing may have limited self-awareness and be at risk, especially if disoriented. As stated earlier, those who have signs of intoxication, especially from alcohol, have a higher propensity to violent behavior.

The individual who is threatened or angry may try to leave the treatment setting. Trying to stop this exit physically may result in physical confrontation. Any attempts to stop an individual in a physical rather than verbal fashion should involve readiness for a physical restraint procedure.

In toxic states and delirium, the character of the problem depends on the nature of the medical problem or toxic substance. The vital signs can be abnormal; the individual can have signs of an infective process or signs and history of an illness that has exacerbated; laboratory values can be abnormal; signs and symptoms of a metabolic disorder may be present; and a history of recent ingestion of a drug or toxic substance may be present. Personality disorder diagnoses are made primarily on the basis of history and, to a lesser extent, the interaction with staff and behavior in the emergent setting. Personality disorders represent behaviors or traits present in the recent past and long-term functioning. The behaviors and traits cause significant impairment in social or occupational functioning or subjective distress. The behaviors or traits that are limited to episodes of illness are not considered in making a diagnosis of personality disorder.[10] Antisocial, borderline, and paranoid personality disorders are the most likely to be associated with risk for violence.

People with antisocial personality disorder have had a history of behavior before age 15 such as truancy, frequent physical fights, theft, lying, physical cruelty, and fire setting. This is coupled with a pattern of irresponsible and antisocial behavior before 15. These individuals are influenced less by social rules and concern for others, increasing the risk for physical violence.

People with borderline personality disorder frequently have impulsive behavior, unstable and intense social relationships, intense anger, and irritability. People with paranoid disorder are at risk because unrealistic threats are perceived and may be acted on.

Individuals with intermittent explosive disorder have discrete episodes of loss of control of aggressive impulses. No signs of generalized impulsiveness or aggressiveness are seen between the episodes. History is the prime diagnostic tool with this disorder.

PROCEDURES AND LABORATORY TESTS

UNIT ASSAULT RISK MANAGEMENT PLAN

Each treatment unit needs a formal plan for the management of the range of risks. A continuum from heightened awareness and observation of an individual to maximal physical restraint is necessary.[11] In addition to planning, education of staff and periodic practice of potential events or scenarios are necessary to make the procedures effective and minimize the risks. A plan requires an estimate of the level of response required, a protocol for calling for help and the response, and the restraining procedure.

The options for level of response include one staff member periodically observing an at-risk person, two staff members present when interacting with an at-risk person so that one can call for help if needed, five people who are physically capable and willing to be involved for restraint, and maximal show of force with five or more staff members. Specially trained personnel may be necessary to disarm a patient with a weapon. Usually only police have had sufficient training to deal with a lethal weapon such as a gun or knife, and health care staff should be advised against heroic actions in such circumstances.

A written and readily available plan for calling for help needs to be in place. Telephone numbers for help should be near the telephone. It should be made clear what the facility's operators or receptionist will do when a call for help is made. An estimate should be made of the response time necessary to minimize the risk of harm and what is feasible in the institution. A plan needs to be developed for calling the police, and what to expect as a response. Some institutions have a specific physical restraint team that is sent by an overhead paging system or portable pagers with specifics of where to go on the pager. Some available alarm devices are the size of a pen and activate sensors in the ceiling. Alarms can be placed on walls. Codes can be developed for help. When an individual is interviewing a violence-prone patient, alerting other staff members of the risk and asking them to go by the office or work area is frequently useful. When staff members are stressed, their response may not be quick or efficient, and therefore overlearning of protocols and ready availability of plans can minimize the delay. Temporary staff must be oriented early about protocols and what their role should be.

STEPS FOR INITIAL STABILIZATION

1. People who are out of control should be physically restrained when the safety of the individual, other patients, and staff is at significant risk.
2. Establishment of rapport is essential if possible. Listening to the patient's concerns and acknowledging his or her difficulty helps rapport. Concern about the patient's physical comfort, such as providing a blanket if the person is cold, helps to reinforce a positive doctor-patient relationship. Attention to shared experiences and verbal attempts at bonding can sometimes help ("I see you're from Montana; I grew up in Butte"). Separating the good and bad encounters in the emergency setting can help maintain rapport. One staff member can assume the role of the "bad guy" and say, for example, that the patient cannot smoke, while another can be the "good guy" and focus on the person's concerns. Making accurate empathetic statements helps to give the patient the sense of understanding. An example of an empathetic statement could be: "It must really be upsetting to you that your gun was taken away." If recommendations are made, their impact is enhanced if the statement is put in the context of the patient's concerns and language. For example, if you are recommending an antipsychotic medication to an individual who has paranoid delusions, say something like, "It sounds like you are worried about disturbing thoughts and would like to have a clear head. There is a medicine that can help reduce your agitation and help you organize your thoughts so you can deal with things at home." This is more likely to be effective than: "I want to give you a medicine that will take away your delusions that

people are trying to harm you." (The patient is convinced that the delusions are true.)

3. Decrease anxiety by decreasing ambiguity. The more ambiguity in a situation, the more anxiety there is for both patient and health care giver. Telling the patient about who will examine him or her and a little about the time frame helps lower ambiguity. In paranoid individuals, telling the patient what you would like to do next when you are doing a physical examination lowers anxiety and the possibility of misinterpretation.

4. Have the person sit down. The level of intensity often decreases when both patient and staff person sit down.

5. Take consideration of physical space and territorial issues. A person who is agitated, paranoid, and/or angry has an expanded physical comfort zone. People who are not paranoid, agitated, or angry have a comfort zone of hand-shaking distance in most United States cultures. The zone can be doubled or tripled for the disturbed person. When a staff person gets too physically close, the patient may feel threatened and have a higher risk of violence. Touching should be limited to minimize the likelihood of misinterpretation.

6. At-risk individuals should be interviewed only in safe settings where help can be called, and there is sufficient space for safe physical restraint of the patient if necessary. At times, the hall is the safest place for interviewing. The staff member and the patient should have equal access to the door, so that each can get out quickly if the need arises and will not have to go over the other. The door can be left open if risk is expected.

7. Consider a clinical situation again if "your tummy tells of its unease." Subjective sense is frequently accurate about the risk in a situation, and it needs to be considered as one factor in the risk determination.

8. Alert coworkers to your concerns about the at-risk person. They can come to your help more quickly if there is a commotion. This also helps them to be careful when they interact with the individual, as in drawing blood or getting a blood pressure reading.

RESTRAINING PROCEDURES

A safe restraining procedure requires at least five staff members who are physically able and willing to participate. It also requires one staff member to take charge and direct it. Most restraining efforts can be briefly planned before they are implemented. Only in rare clinical situations is an absolutely imminent response necessary. In the planning process, assignments should be made to staff members for all four limbs and the head, one person for each point of restraint. In a practiced team, the first two people go for the arms and the second two for the legs. It is important to have a stretcher ready with restraints, if possible, to minimize the time required to personally hold the person. It is particularly important that one individual control the head because biting by the patient is a major risk for staff in restraining. Grabbing a large clump of hair is a relatively safe way to control the head (if the hair is grasped close to the scalp, there are few negative sequelae). Leather restraints are preferred because they are less likely to compromise circulation and abrade skin. Cloth restraints tend to be easier to escape from and can restrict circulation.

The minimum level of physical restraint is one arm and one leg, preferably on opposite sides (two-point). A one-point restraint allows a person to get off or fall off the stretcher. Three-point restraint restricts three limbs and four-point restraints, four limbs. Five-point restraint involves a leather belt circling the waist with the two arms attached to it. Note that the waist restraint is attached to the stretcher, as are the legs. Alternately, one arm can be attached to the stretcher above the head and the other at the waist. This latter approach makes trunk movement difficult. The arms should be alternated in the above-and-below-the-head position every half hour to minimize discomfort.

The individual who is restrained should have the need for restraint explained to him or her early on in the process; e.g., "We are going to put you in restraints to help you to control your behavior and for safety." The restrained individual should be checked frequently (every 15 to 30 minutes) and comfort measures offered such as asking about the need for a urinal or bedpan, water, food, or blankets. Restrained patients (mainly women) have been sexually assaulted while in the restrained state. Adequate observation is required, and the use of a locked room should be considered. Observation by video camera monitoring is an option. An individual who is likely to vomit can be restrained on his or her abdomen to minimize aspiration.

The restrained individual should be searched for sharp objects, matches, lighters, and other dangerous objects. If an individual is actively moving his or her torso, he or she may possibly overturn the stretcher, and a method for attaching the stretcher to a fixed object may be necessary. There is much more medicolegal risk in not restraining an individual at risk who subsequently harms himself or herself or others than in restraining the person when a reasonable basis for restraint can be documented and it is done in a competent fashion.

If an individual cannot be safely restrained with the staff available and help cannot arrive in time, letting the individual go may be safer for patient and staff. One period of special concern is when an individual has been brought to the emergency setting in restraints and these are taken off. This must be done carefully and with enough staff members to control behavior. One cannot necessarily depend on the actions of the individuals who have brought the person in. Frequently, nontreatment staff (e.g., police, security officers) do not know the procedures of the unit and may assume that all the controls will be taken over by the treating staff when the restraints are off. There is danger in the ambiguity. How the transfer is done should be discussed before it is done. Efforts at verbal restraint are discussed subsequently, and chemical restraint is discussed in the chapter on medication management of psychosis.

LABORATORY TESTS

The laboratory tests that seem most useful in assessing individuals at risk for violence are alcohol levels, toxicology screens; general screening tests such as complete electrolytes, glucose level, and complete blood counts; CT scans; and lumbar punctures. With alcohol and toxicology screens, one is determining the presence or absence of a psychoactive substance. With alcohol, the level of disinhibition must be quantified. Ability to walk and be relatively coherent at higher alcohol levels than 200 mg/dL usually indicates a long-standing alcohol abuse problem.

The presence of street drugs or medicines that correlate with disordered thinking can suggest a cause to the behavior observed and some prognostic assessment based on the pharmacokinetics of the drug. For example, with PCP, a diminution of agitated symptoms may not mean that the risk of violent behavior is past because the PCP can recirculate and decompensation can recur. In an individual who was disruptive when the alcohol level was high and later became much more cooperative, the odds are that the behavior correlated with the blood level of alcohol. Screening tests are useful in identifying abnormalities that may be contributing to the disordered behavior. A low blood glucose could explain transient agitation in an individual. An individual with a recent history of violence is more likely to have had an injury and loss of blood; thus a CBC is useful. Sometimes infections, especially of the central nervous system (CNS), can cause agitated or violent behavior. A CBC and/or a lumbar puncture, especially if a stiff neck is present and the behavior represents a marked change over baseline, may be useful. CT scans are most useful when there are neurologic abnormalities, especially new ones indicating a head injury or CNS infection.

CLINICAL MANAGEMENT AND DRUG TREATMENT

After initial stabilization, continue to decrease or minimize ambiguity to decrease anxiety. Monitor level of restraint and adjust it as the clinical situation changes. When psychosis is present, antipsychotic medications are indicated if the patient agrees or state law allows emergent involuntary treatment. Most neuroleptic medications are effective in decreasing the psychosis, but several are preferred in emergent settings because of ease of use and favorable side effect profile.[12]

Haloperidol is an antipsychotic that is frequently used because it is available in injectable, liquid concentrate, and tablet forms and has fewer cardiovascular effects.[13] In injectable form the volume is low (1 cc per 5 mg), and in liquid form it is colorless and relatively tasteless. Five to 10 mg every hour until control is established is the usual dose. Beyond 30 mg, little further antipsychotic effect is obtained in most patients, and the effect of further doses is sedation and decrease of agitation. An alternative for the sedation and agitation after 30 mg is the use of lorazepam, 0.5 to 1 mg every hour up to 10 mg in 24 hours.

Haloperidol's upper limit is 100 mg in a 24-hour period. Intramuscular haloperidol is most rapidly absorbed and may have a pharmacologic effect in 15 to 30 minutes. Liquid haloperidol is absorbed more rapidly than the pill form and has the advantage of little likelihood of being "cheeked" or retained in the mouth and later discarded. Both oral forms require at least 30 minutes for effects to appear. An alternative to haloperidol is thiothixene. It has a slower metabolism and should be given every 2 to 4 hours. It is more sedating than haloperidol. Two mg of thiothixene is equivalent to approximately 1 mg of haloperidol. The maximum for 24 hours is 100 mg. In injectable form, the thiothixene must be combined with sterile water and has a greater injection volume than haloperidol, which makes frequent injection more problematic. Droperidol is a highly sedating antipsychotic that may be indicated in psychotic patients requiring rapid stabilization. It may be given every 30 to 60 minutes at a rate of 2.5 to 5.0 mg, either IM or IV. Onset is 3 to 10 minutes with full effect in 30 minutes. A maximum of 15 mg for 24 hours is suggested, although more is probably safe as used in surgical anesthesia. Note: Droperidol is not approved by the Federal Drug Administration (FDA) to control psychosis and agitation. The dosage must be significantly reduced for the elderly (for example, haloperidol at 0.5 to 1 mg rather than 5 mg).

When anxiety and agitation are the major components and the person is not intoxicated, toxic, or metabolically disordered, lorazepam, 1 to 2 mg IM or PO every hour up to 10 mg can be used. It is relatively short-acting and has no active metabolites, and with its route of metabolism, glucuronidation is more likely to be intact in the elderly and in patients with liver disease. Lorazepam can be used IV, but should be administered slowly to avoid peak levels and minimize the risk of respiratory arrest. Equipment for resuscitation should be available when giving IV benzodiazepines, especially in medically unstable patients. IM absorption can be enhanced by giving lorazepam in the deltoid. In patients with severe respiratory problems, haloperidol can be used IM or PO or droperidol IV. Tegetol and propanalol have been used for longer-term treatment.

The presence of and seriousness of intent of verbal threats to harm or kill someone must be clarified. This is useful in determining the need for civil commitment and the need to warn the threatened people (see Medicolegal Pearls section). In cases in which vulnerable family members are victimized or at risk, the clinician should educate the family as to available shelter programs and victim advocacy services.

Whenever possible, alternative solutions to the patient's concerns should be developed. For example, if a patient is anxious and agitated secondary to feeling threatened when alone, an arrangement can be made for the patient to stay with someone and the agitation will decrease. Another patient's psychosis and voices can be decreased if a stressor such as no place to stay is ameliorated by a possible placement. For an alternative solution to be effective, it must be seen as a viable and helpful solution by the patient.

Use family, friends, and treating sources to develop a treatment and follow-up plan. Frequently, people who know the patient can suggest options and solutions that were not initially evident. They may know what has worked and what has not worked in the past, and may be useful in determining the individual risk.

HOSPITALIZATION CRITERIA

If the individual continues to be assaultive and has psychosis, admit for stabilization (voluntary or involuntary), usually on a psychiatric unit. If the patient has delirium, metabolic disorder, or toxic state and the symptoms of agitation continue, admit for stabilization and further diagnosis, usually on a medical floor. If the patient has no clear psychiatric or medical illness, referral can be made to the police authorities. Individuals who have brain damage that is stable but continued agitation can be admitted for behavior control and possible medication management, usually on psychiatric or neurologic services. Patients who are intoxicated with alcohol and agitated after other problems are ruled out can be sent to detoxification facilities if possible.

PITFALLS

- Not searching a patient for sharp objects. This is especially important for patients who are in restraints. Patients cut themselves out of restraints regularly.
- Touching patients to "calm" them. Frequently a physical contact is perceived as a threat or intrusion.
- Not listening to your "tummy." Subjective feelings are frequently accurate in alerting the clinician to possible risk. When your "body speaks," use it in concert with your head to determine a systematic course of action.

- Trying to restrain or stop the patient physically from leaving with insufficient staff to do it safely. The risk for injury for staff and the patient is high in these instances.
- Using too much force in a restraining procedure. Staff members can get carried away and hurt a patient, especially a highly provocative patient who is spitting, swearing, or attacking them.
- Forgetting to perform clinically warranted assessment and tests in an individual who is obnoxious or who has assaulted a staff member or other person. There is a tendency to get a loud or difficult patient out of the care setting as soon as possible, and parts of the physical or laboratory examination may be omitted.
- Forgetting to screen for assaultive risk or to establish rapport when the load of patients goes up in an emergency setting. Safety should always be considered primarily, and even minimal efforts toward rapport enhance safety.
- Missing multiple contributions to behavioral disorder: There is a tendency to oversimplify assessments of violence-prone patients or engage in "either/or" thinking when confronted with a difficult and challenging case. For example, an individual with a history of schizophrenia can *also* be toxic from PCP or metabolically disordered.
- Focusing exclusively on the well-being of the identified patient to the exclusion of family members. A risk assessment must not only incorporate the management needs of the emergency setting but also those of family members and intimates.
- Ensure adequate re-evaluation to detect subtle CNS disorders, infections, seizure problems, and metabolic disorders.

MEDICOLEGAL PEARLS

During the past decade, court decisions have underscored and broadened the treatment provider's duty to protect potential victims from violence-prone patients.[14] Tarasoff versus The Regents of the University of California established the need to act in cases in which a specific threat is made toward an identifiable victim. Jablonski versus Loma Linda Veterans Administration extended this duty to include situations in which the patient *behaves* dangerously or is judged to be potentially dangerous regardless of a specific threat. The need to protect was further expanded to include unintended victims who might be situationally at risk by virtue of proximity to a potential victim, such as children, other family members, and friends in the case of Hedlund versus the Superior Court of Orange County.

Although these rulings have stirred considerable debate among care providers regarding the practical limitations and therapeutic complications associated with such decisions, they have been generally supported by various legal and ethical statutes.[3] The net result is that the privilege of patient confidentiality is limited and, in cases where it is indicated, the clinician is obliged to take various actions to help safeguard potential victims.

Knowledge of state statutes regarding civil commitment, involuntary use of medications, and permission to treat emergent conditions is essential to minimizing subsequent medicolegal risk.[15] Civil commitment laws in some states give permission to treat only mental disorders and not other physical conditions involuntarily. Legal guardianship may be required to provide comprehensive health care.

GENERAL SUGGESTIONS FOR THE PRACTITIONER

When an explicit and credible threat to seriously harm or kill an identifiable person is made, and civil commitment and/or arrest by the police is not possible, an attempt should be made to locate and inform the potential victim or victims.[16]

If a strong historical basis exists for detaining or restraining a known violence-prone patient, and a current assessment is not safe or feasible, the practitioner should err on the safe side and take action to restrain the patient. If no attempt is made to hold the person, the staff and institution may be liable for his or her subsequent actions. Few, if any, health care professionals have been successfully sued for restraining a violence-prone patient when a reasonable basis and good faith effort can be demonstrated.

If the individual at risk for assault cannot be restrained safely with the staff available, and it is not possible to get sufficient staff to hold the person, realistic limitations to act should be acknowledged. In this instance, the clinical staff members are not obliged to try to stop the violence-prone individual if he or she tries to exit. Rather, the police and/or commitment officials should be called.

Information about an individual's alcohol and/or other substance abuse treatment is protected by Federal statute. Caution should be exercised in the release of such information. Giving information even to relatives may put the clinician and the institution at risk for up to $10,000 in fines.

HORIZONS

Research has shown that low cerebrospinal fluid (CSF) 5-hydroxyindoleacetic acid (5-HIAA) is associated with increased risk for violent action, suicide, and impulsive behavior.[17] Building on this research, less invasive laboratory tests (not involving a lumbar puncture) may be developed to provide similar information to the diagnostician. In addition, future research may show that serotonin metabolism, of which 5-HIAA is a measure, can be modified with medications and/or diet with a resulting reduction of risk for impulsiveness or violence.

Specialized clinical programs for anger management and violence are being developed, and multidisciplinary research on assaultive behavior continues to expand.[7,18] The use of cognitive, behavioral, and environmental interventions can help some individuals at risk to control their behavior. As the technology, experience, and use of these services grow, earlier intervention should be possible, decreasing the frequency with which violence-prone individuals come into emergent settings. This technology can also offer staff members in emergency settings better approaches for effective case management and follow-up care.

Risk checklists and indices are available,[19,20] but are not in widespread use. As their usefulness and predictive power are demonstrated, implementation in practice should increase. Such indices can provide a systematic and objective format to evaluate and screen assaultive risk, as well as develop institutional data bases for tracking interventions for assaultive behavior.

NATIONAL CONTACTS

American Psychiatric Association, 1400 K Street NW, Washington, DC, 20005. Telephone 202-682-6000.

American Association of Emergency Psychiatry, Mail Local 559, University of Cincinnati, Cincinnati, Ohio 45267

National Coalition Against Domestic Violence, P.O. Box 7032, Huntingwoods, Michigan 48070. Telephone 800-333-7233

Violence and Victims, Springer Publishing Company, 536 Broadway, New York, N.Y. 10012–3955. Telephone 212-431-4370

REFERENCES

1. Public health problem of violence receives epidemiologic attention. JAMA 254:881, 1985.
2. Delgado-Escueta, A.V., Mattson, R.H., King, L., et al.: The nature of aggression during epileptic seizures. N. Engl. J. Med. 305:3, 1981.
3. APA Committee of Legal Issues: White paper on duty to warn. Englewood Cliffs, NJ, Prentice-Hall, 1985.
4. Maiuro, R.D., O'Sullivan, M.J., Michael, M.C., and Vitaliano, P.P.: Anger, hostility, and depression in assaultive versus suicide attempting males. J. Clin. Psychol. 45:531, 1989.
5. Straus, M.A., Gelles, R.J., and Steinmetz, S.: Behind closed doors: Violence in the American family. New York, Doubleday/Anchor, 1980.
6. Elliot, F.A.: The neurology of explosive rage: The dyscontrol syndrome. Practitioner 217:51, 1976.
7. Helping angry and violent people manage their emotions and behavior. Hosp. Community Psychiatry 38:1207, 1987.
8. Maiuro, R.D., Cahn, T.S., Vitaliano, P.P., et al.: Anger, hostility, and depression in domestically violent versus generally assaultive men and nonviolent control subjects. J. Consult Clin. Psychol. 56:17, 1988.

9. Tardiff, K. (Ed.): The Psychiatric Uses of Seclusion and Restraint. Washington, DC, American Psychiatric Press, 1984.
10. American Psychiatric Association: Diagnostic and Statistical Manual of Mental Disorders, 3rd ed, revised. Washington, DC, American Psychiatric Association, 1987.
11. Wong, S.E., Woolsey, J.E., Innocent, A.J., et al.: Behavioral treatment of violent psychiatric patients. Psychiatr. Clin. North Am. *11*:569, 1988.
12. Brizer, D.A.: Psychopharmacology and the management of violent patients. Psychiatr. Clin. North Am. *11*:551, 1988.
13. Neborsky, R., Janowsky, D., Munson, E., et al.: Rapid treatment of acute psychotic symptoms with high- and low-dose haloperidol. Arch. Gen. Psychiatry *38*:195, 1981.
14. Gross, B.H., Southard, M.J., Lamb, H.R., and Weinberger, L.E.: Assessing dangerousness and responding appropriately: Hedlund expands the clinician's liability established by Tarasoff. J. Clin. Psychiatry *48*:9, 1987.
15. Appelbaum, P.S.: The right to refuse treatment with antipsychotic medication: Retrospect and prospect. Am. J. Psychiatry *145*:413, 1988.
16. Appelbaum, P.S.: Tarasoff and the clinician: Problems in fulfilling the duty to protect. Am. J. Psychiatry *142*:425, 1985.
17. Brown, G.L., Ebert, M.H., Goyer, P.F., et al.: Aggression, suicide, and serotonin: Relationship to CSF metabolites. Am. J. Psychiatry *139*:741, 1982.
18. Maiuro, R.D., and Eberle, J.A.: New developments in research on aggression: An international report. Violence and Victims *4*:3, 1989.
19. Maiuro, R.D., Vitaliano, P.P., and Cahn, T.C.: A brief measure for the assessment of anger and aggression. J. Interpersonal Violence *2*:166, 1987.
20. Yudofsky, S.C., Silver, J.M., Jackson, W., et al.: The overt aggression scale for the objective rating of verbal and physical aggression. Am. J. Psychiatry *143*:35, 1986.

BIBLIOGRAPHY

Hall, H.V.: Violence Prediction: Guidelines for the Forensic Practitioner. Springfield, IL, Charles C Thomas, 1987.

Hyman, S.E., and Arana, G.W.: Handbook of Psychiatric Drug Therapy. Boston, Little, Brown, and Company, 1987.

Hyman, S.E.: Manual of Psychiatric Emergencies. Boston, Little, Brown, and Company, 1988.

Slaby, A.E., Lieb, J., and Trancredi, L.R.: The Handbook of Psychiatric Emergencies, 3rd ed. Medical Examination Publishing Company, New York, 1986.

Tardiff, K.: Concise Guide to Assessment and Management of Violent Patients. Washington, DC, American Psychiatric Press, Inc., 1989.

ORGANIC BRAIN SYNDROMES AND DISORDERS

Stephanie von Ammon Cavanaugh

CAPSULE

The organic brain syndromes, delirium, and dementia are the most common mental disorders seen in the Emergency Department (ED) setting. Less common are organic amnestic syndrome, organic delusional syndrome, organic hallucinosis, organic mood disorder, organic anxiety disorder, and organic personality disorder. Ninety-five percent of all deliriums are reversible once the underlying cause is treated.[1] Many of the causes of delirium are life-threatening, and 25% of patients with delirium die.[2,3] Likewise, 35 to 40% of all patients with dementia require medical intervention; 15% have correctable disorders if treated before brain damage occurs, and for 20 to 25% with noncorrectable disorders, intervention improves cognitive functioning.[1,3,4] Although similar figures are not available for the other organic brain syndromes, many of the causes of these disorders are treatable. Because these less common organic brain syndromes mimic psychiatric disorders, an organic cause for psychiatric symptoms should be considered in all patients presenting with psychiatric complaints.

Once a diagnosis of an organic brain syndrome is made, the emergency physician must diagnose and treat all life-threatening conditions and/or those that could result in brain damage. Further, timely follow-up care must be provided for diagnosis and treatment of less emergent causes. Finally, patients with an organic brain syndrome who are severely or irreversibly impaired and unable to care for themselves must be ensured of a disposition that provides adequate custodial care.

DEFINITION

An organic brain syndrome is an impairment of mental functioning secondary to structural or functional abnormalities of brain tissue "evidenced from the history, physical examination, or laboratory tests" to be causally related to a specific organic factor.[5] Differences in clinical presentation of an organic brain syndrome are related to the underlying pathophysiology, duration, and localization of the abnormalities in the brain.

The Diagnostic and Statistical Manual of Mental Disorders, Third Edition, Revised (DSM-III-R) differentiates organic brain syndrome from organic mental disorder.[5] Organic brain syndromes are like constellations of signs and symptoms without reference to cause (e.g., delirium, dementia), whereas organic brain disorders have a known cause (e.g., alcohol withdrawal delirium, multi-infarct dementia).

Patients with delirium, dementia, and the amnestic syndrome have memory deficits. Patients with delirium have dysattention (reduced ability to maintain attention to external stimuli and appropriately shift attention to new stimuli), deficits in orientation and memory, difficulties in communicating, and perceptual disturbances (illusions, hallucinations). Patients with dementia have memory deficits and evidence of deterioration of higher intellectual functioning. Patients with the amnestic syndrome have recent and remote memory difficulties, without dysattention or impairment of general intellectual functioning. Patients with organic delusional disorders, organic hallucinosis, organic mood disorders, organic anxiety disorders, and organic personality disorders have no dysattention, little memory impairment, and no difficulties with higher intellectual functioning. Rather, these disorders mimic psychiatric disorders. In organic delusional disorder, the most prominent feature is delusions; in organic hallucinosis, hallucinations. Those with organic mood disorder have a depressed, expansive, or euphoric mood, and those with organic anxiety disorders have signs and symptoms of generalized anxiety or panic attacks. Those with organic personality disorders have changes in personality.

ASSESSMENT

A collateral history is essential (if obtainable) for patients with dysattention, memory deficits, difficulties in higher intellectual functioning, difficulties in communicating, delusions, hallucinations, and personality changes. A careful history of the onset and progression of the affective, cognitive, and behavioral and/or psychotic symptoms should be obtained. Possible organic causes should be elicited in the history and an attempt made to relate these causes temporarily to the mental symptoms. Careful inquiry should be made as to the onset and course of physical illness; trauma; the addition, discontinuation, or change in a prescription or over-the-counter medication with central nervous system effects; illicit drug and alcohol abuse; food and fluid intake; and/or environmental toxins or poisons. A careful review of systems often helps identify the cause of an organic brain syndrome. Past personal and family history of medical illness, surgeries, medications, and illicit drug and alcohol use may provide valuable clues to present causes of the organic mental disorder. A previous psychiatric illness does not rule out an organic cause for present psychiatric symptoms. For example, a patient with a bipolar disorder may develop hypothyroidism as the result of prolonged lithium use and present with an organic mood syndrome with depression. After the history, a mental status examination should be performed. Vital signs and a physical examination should be followed by a focused neurologic examination (cranial nerves, meningeal signs, limb strength, reflexes, Babinski's sign). The medical work-up depends on the specific organic brain syndrome and the possible causes and is discussed in detail under each organic brain syndrome.

DELIRIUM

Delirium is present in 10% of all patients admitted acutely to medical and surgical wards.[4]

CLINICAL FEATURES

The clinical features of delirium develop over a short period, hours to days. The signs and symptoms of delirium fluctuate during the day. Many patients may have a "lucid interval" or a period in which there appear to be no obvious symptoms of delirium. Delirium is often better during the day and worse at night. For the most part, delirium is caused by functional rather than structural changes in brain tissue and, as a result, is almost totally reversible if the causes of the delirium are treated before brain damage occurs. Table 62-5 lists common causes of delirium.

In delirium, there is evidence of wide nervous system dysfunction with disordered responsivity to sensory stimuli, dysfunction of the reticular activating system, and an inability to organize information at cortical levels.[4,6] Delirious patients demonstrate changes in level of consciousness, altered awareness of the environment, and reduced capacity to shift, focus, and sustain attention to environmental stimuli.

TABLE 62-5. CAUSES OF DELIRIUM

Metabolic (acidosis, alkalosis, electrolyte imbalance, hypercalcemia)
Hypoxia and anoxia
Hypoglycemia
Nutritional deficiency (thiamine, niacin, B_{12})
Endocrine (hypothyroidism, hyperthyroidism, Addison's disease, parathyroid disease, Cushing's syndrome)
Hepatic encephalopathy
Uremic encephalopathy
Hypertensive encephalopathy
Cerebral infarct
Cerebral hemorrhage
Central nervous system (CNS) vasculitis
CNS trauma
Space-occupying lesions (tumor, epidural hematoma, subdural hematoma, abscess)
Increased intercranial pressure
Epilepsy and postictal states
CNS infections (meningitis, encephalitis)
Systemic infection with sepsis and fever
Drugs, heavy metals, toxins, poisons
  Antimicrobials (acyclovir, amphotericin, cephalexin, cloroquine, isoniazid, rifampicin)
  Aminophylline, theophylline
  Anticholinergic drugs (antidepressants, neuroleptics, scopolamine, atropine-like drugs, diphenhydramine, benztropine, thihexyphenidyl)
  Anticonvulsant drugs (phenytoin, valproic acid)
  Bromide
  Baclofen
  Cardiac drugs (digitalis, quinidine, procainamide, lidocaine, beta-blockers, clonidine, methyldopa)
  Cimetidine, ranitidine
  Chemotherapeutic agents (5-fluorouracil)
  Drug intoxication (alcohol, benzodiazepines, barbiturates, glutethimide, phencyclidine, hallucinogens, tetrahydrocannabinol, amphetamines, cocaine)
  Drug withdrawal (alcohol, benzodiazepines, barbiturates, glutethimide)
  Disulfiram
  Lithium carbonate
  Levodopa
  Narcotics
  Nonsteroidal anti-inflammmatory agents
  Oral hypoglycemics (chlorpropamide)
  Steroids
  Heavy metals, toxins, poisons (carbon monoxide, lead, mercury, manganese, pesticides, solvents)
Multifactorial—the most common cause of a delirium results from a combination of these factors.

Clinically, these changes may be demonstrated by difficulty in obtaining or maintaining the patient's attention during the interview. The patient may preferentially attend inappropriately to internal or external stimuli, or fall asleep while talking and need to be aroused to continue on the interview. The severity of the delirium and changes in the EEG are directly related to the severity of the changes in awareness and dysattention.[6]

Delirious patients may have a retarded or agitated delirium. Examples of a retarded delirium include patients with severe renal or liver failure. Alcohol withdrawal is the prototype of the agitated delirium.

Patients evidence decreased responsivity to environmental stimuli in a retarded delirium and increased responsivity to stimuli in an agitated delirium. Further, there is disruption of the sleep-wake cycle with hypersomnia in a retarded delirium and insomnia in an agitated delirium.

The delirious patient shows difficulty with memory. Most commonly, immediate and recent memory are impaired. The amount of immediate and recent memory loss is related to the severity of the delirium. In mild delirium, this memory loss may be variable, whereas in severe delirium, it is severe. Immediate and recent memory loss are caused by impaired registration and retention of new memories, resulting from dysattention to environmental stimuli and disturbance in higher cortical functioning. Mild to significant lacunae in remote memory, occurring before the onset of the delirium, are often present. The severity of the remote memory loss covaries with the severity of the delirium.

Orientation is a memory function. Disorientation to time is common, even in mild delirium. Disorientation to place is frequent in moderate to severe delirium. Disordered perceptual experiences, as well as memory impairment, may also contribute to disorientation. For example, a patient in the ED may hallucinate being at home, at work, or in a social situation. Disorientation to person is also seen in delirium. In mild delirium, the names of newly introduced people are forgotten. In moderate delirium, the patient may misidentify the relationship of newly introduced people. In severe delirium, the names and relationships of familiar people may be forgotten.

Delirious patients may manifest various psychologic states, often with rapid changes. Although these symptoms are not essential for diagnosis, delirious patients may demonstrate fear, anxiety, lability of affect, anger, irritability, or depression. The delirious patient may have difficulty in communicating coherently, evidenced by inability to answer questions appropriately and disorganized thinking with rambling, irrelevant, or incoherent speech.

The delirious patient may have perceptual disturbances. Illusions and misperceptions of sensory stimuli are common in delirium. These perceptual disturbances are classically visual but often auditory. Shadows may be misinterpreted as an intruder, or a slammed door as a gunshot. Hallucinations may range from simple perceptions without relevant sensory stimuli to more complex ones. Shapes, light, animals, insects, or complex situations may be hallucinated. Somatic delusions in which the patient experiences bugs or vermin on the skin are common. Delusions usually arise in response to distorted or inaccurate perceptions. For example, a delirious patient may erroneously feel that the doctor in the ED is trying to kill or harm him or her with diagnostic procedures.

Several neurologic findings are seen in delirium. An irregular, rapid 8 to 10 cycles per minute fine to gross intention tremor may be seen.[4,6] Asterixis and multifocal clonus may also be present.[4,6] The DSM-III-R criteria for delirium are listed in Table 62-6.

TABLE 62-6. DSM-III-R CRITERIA FOR DELIRIUM*

A. Reduced ability to maintain attention to external stimuli (e.g., questions must be repeated because attention wanders) and to shift attention appropriately to new external stimuli (e.g., repeats answer to a previous question).

B. Disorganized thinking, as indicated by rambling, irrelevant, or incoherent speech.

C. At least two of the following:
   1. Reduced level of consciousness, e.g., difficulty in keeping awake during examination
   2. Perceptual disturbances: misinterpretations, illusions, or hallucinations
   3. Disturbance of sleep-wake cycle with insomnia or daytime sleepiness
   4. Increased or decreased psychomotor activity
   5. Disorientation to time, place, or person
   6. Memory impairment, e.g., inability to learn new material, such as the names of several unrelated objects, after 5 minutes, or to remember past events, such as history of current episode of illness

D. Clinical features develop over a short period (usually hours to days) and tend to fluctuate over the course of a day.

E. Evidence from the history, physical examination, or laboratory tests of a specific organic factor (or factors) judged to be etiologically related to the disturbance

* Reprinted with permission from Organic Mental Syndromes and Disorders. *In* Diagnostic and Statistical Manual of Mental Disorders, 3rd Ed., Revised. Washington, DC, American Psychiatric Press, Inc., 1987.

DIFFERENTIAL DIAGNOSIS

Delirium may be confused with mania or schizophrenia. It is rare for a patient over age 45 to develop schizophrenia or mania. Thus, those over 45 without a previous psychiatric history are more likely to have a delirium. The young, healthy-appearing patient more frequently has mania, schizophrenia, or a drug-related delirium, whereas the older, ill-appearing patient more commonly has a delirium. The manic patient has a history of depressive and manic episodes with periods of intact functioning between episodes, and often a euphoric mood. Irritability, however, may be seen in both mania and delirium. The distractibility of mania may be confused with the dysattention of an agitated delirium. If memory and other intellectual functions are testable, these are intact in the manic patient. Patients with delirium rarely have the grandiose delusions seen in mania. The schizophrenic has a history of schizophrenic episodes with a deterioration of social and occupational functioning between episodes. The level of consciousness is not impaired in schizophrenia. The acutely psychotic schizophrenic patient, however, may have difficulty in focusing and attending to the environment. This is sometimes confused with the dysattention of the delirium. Patients with schizophrenia often have a flat affect, bizarre delusions, and most frequently auditory hallucinations. Vivid visual hallucinations classically seen in delirium are less common in schizophrenia. Again, if testable, memory is intact in schizophrenia. Finally, asterixis and myoclonus are not symptoms of mania or schizophrenia. It is sometimes impossible to differentiate clearly between mania and delirium, or schizophrenia and delirium. In this situation, the emergency physician should proceed as if the patient is delirious, because the morbidity and mortality in untreated delirium are high.

The patient with dementia does not have dysattention or changes in the level of consciousness. Memory impairment and deterioration of higher intellectual functions are classically present. If a demented patient shows clouding of consciousness, dysattention, or psychotic symptoms, a superimposed delirium should be suspected. Demented patients can much more easily develop a delirium with a less severe physical stressor than those without dementia. For example, urinary retention, pneumonia, anticholinergic drugs, and mild dehydration can cause delirium in the demented patient.

MANAGEMENT

Once a diagnosis of a delirium is made, the emergency physician is committed to finding the cause of the delirium and treating all conditions that are life-threatening and/or could lead to irreversible brain damage. The brain is a sensitive indicator of systemic dysfunction, and most causes of delirium listed in Table 62-5 are life-threatening or could lead to irreversible brain damage. It is important to reiterate that the most common cause of delirium is multifactoral, and a systematic search for all possible causes of delirium is essential. Drug withdrawal should always be considered as a cause of delirium and is often missed in the emergency setting. Because a delirious patient is unable to give an accurate history, a collateral history (if possible) should be obtained. A physical and neurologic examination should be performed. A CBC, glucose, BUN, creatinine, electrolytes, liver profile, urinalysis, drug screen (blood and urine), chest x ray, and ECG should be obtained. If the patient appears clinically hypoxic, blood gases should be drawn. If a localizing lesion is found on neurologic examination, and life-threatening central nervous system (CNS) insult is suspected, skull films, computerized cranial tomography scan, and/or magnetic resonance imaging (MRI) should be ordered emergently.[4,6] The delirious patient is usually admitted to a medical or surgical service. Delirious patients with drug or alcohol intoxication or withdrawal may be admitted to the hospital or treated in the ED or 24-hour holding area. The evaluation and treatment of the specific medical abnormalities that underlie delirium is beyond the scope of this chapter, but is covered in detail in their respective sections of this textbook.

Because delirious patients are unable to understand accurately the environment and are often agitated and psychotic, they may be of harm to themselves or others and/or unable to cooperate with the medical work-up. Further, the delirious patient is usually severely medically ill. As a result, the patient should be placed where close supervision can be provided by nursing personnel. If possible, a family member whom the patient trusts should stay with the patient. The family member should be instructed to prevent the patient from harming himself or herself (i.e., pulling out intravenous lines, falling out of bed), wandering away, or disturbing others. Because the delirious patient has dysattention, memory deficits, delusions, and hallucinations, the environment should be interpreted to the patient. Medical personnel should introduce themselves and explain who they are and what they plan to do. The patient should be oriented to time and place. Patients who are hallucinating and delusional should be assured that these symptoms are the result of their medical illness and that no harm will come to them. Patients with an agitated delirium are hyperacute to stimuli. When possible, visual and auditory stimuli should be kept to a minimum.

In addition to these environmental interventions, physical restraints or psychotropic medications may be required to proceed with the diagnostic work-up and prevent the patient from harming himself or herself or others. Level of consciousness may be an important indicator of deteriorating physical condition, particularly in patients with acute central nervous system injury. As a result, the use of psychotropic drugs should be avoided in conditions in which the level of consciousness is critical diagnostically. In these instances, physical restraints may be preferable to psychotropic drugs during the diagnostic phases. If it becomes impossible to proceed with the medical work-up without psychotropic medication, the lowest possible dosage should be used to continue with the medical work-up. After the diagnosis is made and the patient's medical condition is stable, larger doses of psychotropic medications may be used to provide adequate sedation.

MEDICATIONS IN DELIRIUM

Benzodiazepines and/or neuroleptics[4,6,7] are used most commonly to treat the agitation and psychosis of delirium. Short-acting benzodiazepines, such as midazolam, are useful in isolated instances, but require individualized dosage, constant patient supervision, and careful attention to respiratory status. Further, most delirious patients become more confused and agitated when midazolam is metabolized. Lorazepam is an anticonvulsant; may be given orally, intramuscularly, or intravenously; has a half-life of 10 to 20 hours; and is, for the most part, safe in the medically ill. Lorazepam does not require oxidation for metabolic degradation (a process slowed by age, commonly used medications, and liver dysfunction) but only glucuronide conjugation (a process minimally affected by the factors that affect oxidation).[8] Oxazepam is similar to lorazepam but cannot be given intramuscularly. Other benzodiazepines that require

both oxidation and conjugation may result in many active metabolites with prolonged half-lives in the elderly and medically ill. Patients with moderate to severe respiratory disease, however, are at risk for CO_2 retention even at low doses of benzodiazepines because benzodiazepines reduce the ventilatory response to hypoxia.[9] Further, if lorazepam is given too rapidly IV, laryngospasm can result. This can be avoided by proper, slow IV administration. Finally, benzodiazepines are synergistic with other CNS depressants such as barbiturates, opiates, and alcohol. Oral, intramuscular, or intravenous lorazepam 0.5 to 2 mg is useful to control agitation. The dose depends on the age and weight of the patient and the severity of the delirium. For mild agitation, lorazepam, 0.5 to 1 mg, is recommended; for moderate agitation, lorazepam 1 to 2 mg; and for severe agitation, lorazepam 2 mg. Route of administration affects onset of action. Onset of action is 45 to 60 minutes orally, 30 to 90 minutes intramuscularly, and immediately intravenously. Thus, intramuscular or intravenous administration is preferable for more severe deliriums. If the patient is not adequately sedated, the previous or a lower dose may be administered 30 minutes later. In rare cases, lorazepam may cause paradoxic excitement in the delirious patient when not administered with haloperidol.

Haloperidol has also been used extensively to treat the delirious patient and is the safest of the neuroleptics in the medically ill. Haloperidol, a butyrophenone, is a potent neuroleptic, with few anticholinergic side effects; it causes almost no orthostatic hypotension orally or intramuscularly, and has almost no cardiovascular side effects. Haloperidol does cause extrapyramidal side effects. In practice, dystonias are rare when the delirious patient is given several doses of haloperidol to provide emergency tranquilization. Dystonic reactions that may involve the tongue, jaw, neck, buccofacial movements with salivation, torticollis, oculogyric irises, and opisthotonus most rapidly respond to benztropine, 1 to 2 mg intramuscularly (IM) or diphenhydramine 50 mg by intravenous push. If the dystonia does not remit within 30 minutes, the dose may be repeated. Benztropine is highly anticholinergic and diphenhydramine less so. Amanditine HCl 100 mg by mouth, although less rapidly acting, is less anticholinergic. Patients with Parkinson's disease may be made significantly worse by haloperidol. Haloperidol should not be used with epinephrine, because haloperidol blocks the vasopressor effect of the latter drug and may paradoxically further lower blood pressure; metaraminol, phenylephrine, or norepinephrine should be used. *Neuroleptic malignant syndrome*, which has been reported as a consequence of haloperidol administration, is rare during rapid tranquilization in the ED setting. Patients with a previous history of a neuroleptic malignant syndrome should never receive a neuroleptic. Haloperidol may lower the seizure threshold and should be used in combination with lorazepam in patients with risk for seizures. Haloperidol further depresses the sensorium when used with other CNS depressants. Finally, the half-life of haloperidol is 24 hours, and this should be taken into account when administering the drug. Oral elixir or IM dosages of haloperidol, depending on the patient's age and weight and the severity of the symptoms are useful for controlling the agitation and psychotic symptoms in the delirious patient. Elixir is more rapidly absorbed than capsules. Orally, for a mild delirium, haloperidol, 1 to 2 mg is suggested; for a moderate delirium, haloperidol, 2 to 5 mg; and for a severe delirium, haloperidol, 5 to 10 mg. Intramuscularly, for a mild delirium, haloperidol, 0.5 to 2 mg is useful; for a moderate delirium, haloperidol 2 to 5 mg; and for a severe delirium, haloperidol 5 mg. The same or a lower dosage may be repeated in 30 to 45 minutes if the desired effects have not been achieved. Although the Physicians' Desk Reference (PDR) does not recommend IV haloperidol, in practice 0.5 to 2 mg by slow IV push over 2 minutes is useful for severe agitation and psychotic symptoms. The intravenous line should always be cleared with a bolus of normal saline before intravenous haloperidol administration. Hypotension can be a side effect of this route of administration. Droperidol, 0.5 to 2 mg, a butyrophenone used in anesthesia that is more potent than haloperidol, can be given intravenously and is approved by the PDR for this route of administration. Intravenous droperidol can cause more orthostatic hypotension than haloperidol. It is important to note that the onset of action of an intravenous butyrophenone may not be as immediate as with lorazepam. More than a total of 2 mg given by intravenous push of haloperidol or droperidol is rarely needed, particularly if combined with intravenous lorazepam 1 to 2 mg.

Haloperidol and lorazepam are perscribed increasing in combination for the agitated psychotic, delirious patient. Lorazepam is an anticonvulsant, whereas haloperidol possibly lowers the seizure threshold. Lorazepam is more sedating than haloperidol, and in combination with haloperidol poses no risk of paradoxic excitement. Finally, haloperidol controls psychotic symptoms. Dosages of lorazepam, 0.5 to 2 mg orally, IM, or IV in combination with haloperidol, 0.5 to 5 mg orally, intramuscularly, or 0.5 to 2 mg intravenously are recommended depending on patient age and weight and the severity of the symptoms of delirium. For mild delirium, lorazepam, 0.5 to 1 mg and haloperidol, 0.5 to 2 mg orally or IM are useful. For moderate delirium, lorazepam, 1 to 2 mg and haloperidol, 05. to 5 mg orally or IM are recommended. For a severe delirium, lorazepam, 2 mg and haloperidol, 5 to 10 mg orally, 2 to 5 mg IM, or 2 mg intravenously is suggested. This or a lower dose can be repeated in 30 to 45 minutes if adequate sedation is not achieved.

Agitation associated with alcohol or benzodiazepine withdrawal is preferentially treated with benzodiazepines. Agitation associated with barbiturate withdrawal is best treated with barbiturates. The agitation associated with seizures is most appropriately treated with anticonvulsants. The agitation associated with Wernicke's encephalopathy (discussed under the amnestic syndrome) is first treated with intravenous thiamine and, if alcohol withdrawal coexists, benzodiazepines.

DEMENTIA

Approximately 4 to 15% of patients over 65[4] have evidence of at least a mild dementing process, and approximately 2 to 5%[10] have a severe dementing process requiring continuous custodial care. The prevalence of severe dementia increases to 15 to 20% in those over 80, half of whom have Alzheimer's disease.[10,11]

As with delirium, dementia is a common finding when a patient is brought to the ED for emergent medical problems. Often a patient is brought to the ED by the family or sent from the nursing home with "mental status changes." Less often, a demented patient is brought to the ED by the police or concerned others because the patient is unable to care for himself or herself or is found wandering in the streets or other public areas.

CLINICAL FEATURES

The signs and symptoms of dementia develop over months to years and are relatively stable, without the rapid fluctuations seen in delirium. A more rapid deterioration of the clinical picture can occur when the patient is ill, on medications with CNS effects, fatigued, stressed, moved from a familiar environment, or when visual, auditory, or sensory stimuli input is altered or diminished.[1,4] Although a dementia-like picture is more likely to be caused by structural changes of brain tissue, and is therefore irreversible, approximately 15%[1,3,4] have functional changes in brain tissue which are correctable if treated before brain damage occurs. Table 62-7 lists the common medical causes of dementia.

The hallmarks of dementia are memory deficits and deterioration of general intellectual functioning. In mild dementia, the patient has difficulty with recent memory. Impairment in registration of new memories results in diminished ability to retain new information. Immediate memory usually remains intact until the person is more severely demented. In moderate dementia, recent memory loss is more severe, and remote memory is also impaired. In severe dementia, the patient neither understands the present nor remembers the past.

Orientation is a memory function. The mildly demented patient may forget the day of the week or the date. Moderately demented patients may forget the

---

TABLE 62-7. MEDICAL CAUSES OF DEMENTIA

Degenerative disease (Alzheimer's disease, Pick's disease, Huntington's disease, Parkinson's disease,* Wilson's disease*)
Anoxia and hypoxia*
Hypoglycemia*
Nutritional deficiencies* (B$_{12}$, folate)
Endocrine dysfunction (hypothyroidism,* parathyroid disease,* Addison's disease,* Cushing's disease,* panhypopituitarism*)
Hepatic encephalopathy
Uremic encephalopathy*
Multi-infarct dementia
Cerebral infarct
Central nervous system vasculitis*
Multiple sclerosis*
Central nervous system trauma
Space-occupying lesions* (tumors, abscess, subdural hematoma)
Hydrocephalus—communicating* or noncommunicating
Epilepsy*
CNS infections (HIV,* Jakob-Creutzfeldt disease, cryptococcal meningitis,* neurosyphilis,* encephalitis,* meningitis*)
Drugs and Toxins*
   Alcohol (chronic use)
   Anticonvulsants (phenytoin, carbamezapine)
   Anticholinergic drugs (antidepressants, neuroleptics, scopolamine, atropine-like drugs, diphenylhydramine, benztropine, trihexylphenidyl)
   Barbiturates
   Benzodiazepines
   Bromide
   Cimetidine, ranitidine
   Cardiac drugs (digitalis, quinidine, beta-blockers, clonidine, methyldopa)
   Chemotherapeutic agents (5-fluorouracil)
   Disulfiram
   Levodopa
   Lithium carbonate
   Narcotics
   Nonsteroidal anti-inflammatory drugs
   Steroids
Heavy metals, toxins, and poisons (carbon monoxide, aluminum, arsenic, lead, mercury, manganese, pesticides, solvents)

---

* Reversible if treatment occurs before brain damage.

season and year. Moderately to severely demented patients may assume that they are at an earlier time in their lives and switch from period to period during the interview. Severely demented patients often have no time orientation.

Mildly demented patients properly identify familiar places but are unable to identify a new environment (i.e., the ED) without repeated orientation. In moderate dementia, familiar places are recognized but new places such as the hospital may be misidentified as home or the nursing home. In moderate to severe dementia, the person routinely misidentifies his or her environment. The patient may assume that he or she is at a place where he or she was earlier in his or her life (i.e., home, work). A severely demented patient no longer recognizes the environment.

In a mildly demented patient, newly introduced individuals are forgotten and those familiar to the patient remembered. In moderate dementia, the relationship of newly introduced people will be confused. For example, with an elderly patient, the young house physician may be misidentified as the friend of the patient's grandchild. The relationships and names of familiar family members and friends, however, continue to be remembered. With severe dementia, names and relationships of familiar people are forgotten or misidentified. In end-stage dementia, the patient no longer knows his or her own name.

The demented patient also experiences deterioration of general intellectual functioning. Abstract reasoning is impaired. The demented patient has difficulty in conceptualizing. Early in dementia, this may be manifested by an inability to deal conceptually with new tasks, while familiar conceptual tasks are easily accomplished. For example, assembling a new household item may be impossible, whereas cooking a meal is accomplished easily. In moderate dementia, difficulty with abstraction and conceptualizing becomes obvious on mental status testing. The patient may be unable to tell how an apple and an orange are different. Proverbs that the patient previously could interpret abstractly are interpreted concretely (i.e., "Obviously a rolling stone doesn't gather moss. It is rolling down the hill."). Conceptual misunderstanding of world events and personal events occurs. The ability to calculate becomes impaired. Digit span forward remains intact until the dementia has progressed considerably, although the ability to reverse digits will be impaired. Likewise, the patient has difficulty in spelling WORLD backwards. In severe dementia, abstraction may be so impaired that a patient is unable to understand simple tasks such as using a knife to cut meat, running a bath, or flushing the toilet.

Other disturbances in higher cortical functioning become evident in moderate dementia and are severely impaired in severe dementia. The patient may exhibit various disorders in language. Aphasic difficulties become evident. The ability to use language to express or conceptualize ideas becomes impaired. Speech may be tangential, circumstantial, or rambling because of memory impairment. Apraxia, the inability to carry out motor activities despite intact comprehension and motor function, may develop. The patient may display agnosia, the failure to recognize or identify objects despite intact sensory function. Finally, the patient may have constructional difficulty, and be unable to copy three-dimensional figures.

Judgment (the ability to correctly perceive data from the environment, process that data on previous experience and knowledge, and make decisions and act in a culturally appropriate manner) is impaired in dementia. In mild dementia, judgment is generally intact. In moderate dementia, judgment is impaired. For example, a demented patient may give away large sums of money to relative strangers. In severe dementia, judgment is severely impaired. A severely demented patient may go outside in nightclothes and no shoes in subzero weather.

Although the patient with mild to moderate dementia may have total preservation of social graces, changes in personality may become evident. There may be an accentuation or change of premorbid personality traits. A previously meticulous patient may be dirty or slovenly and not care about personal hygiene. A person who was energetic may become apathetic and show decreased interest and responsiveness to the environment. In moderate to severe dementia, the patient may show evidence of poor social judgment. The dignified elderly gentleman may make sexual advances to a stranger. The modest older woman may show no concern over showing her naked body to strangers. The patient may urinate or defecate in the bed. The previously good-natured patient may become irritable. Lability of affect (abrupt changes in affect) may also occur. Rarely, a personality change may be the presenting symptom of dementia and occur before deterioration of memory and higher intellectual functioning.

Misinterpretations are common in patients with memory dysfunction and deterioration of intellectual functioning. A patient who has misplaced glasses may accuse others of stealing them. A patient whose hearing aid is not working may feel that others are talking about him or her, only to find that they are not when the hearing aid is repaired. Agitation and confusion are common when the patient cannot understand or deal effectively with the environment. Illusions, hallucinations, and delusions can accompany this agitation and occur more commonly at night. Patients with multi-infarct dementia present with night-time agitation[12] earlier in the dementing process than those with Alzheimer's disease. Although 25 to 30%[4] of patients with dementia have delusions or visual hallucinations, the acute onset of hallucinations and delusions, particularly during waking hours, should alert the clinician to a superimposed delirium.[13] The DSM-III-R criteria for dementia are presented in Table 62-8.

The exact presentation of the dementia depends on whether it is progressive, stable, diffuse, localized, and/or primarily cortical or subcortical. Patients with a degenerative process such as Alzheimer's or Pick's disease have a diffuse progressive process. Patients with multi-infarct dementia will present with a stepwise deterioration.[12] Intellectual functioning controlled by areas not damaged by the infarcts is preserved. In a stable dementia, there may be improvement of cognitive functioning for 6 months to 2 years after the structural damage as the patient adapts to the deficits. The progression of symptoms seen in subcortical dementia (Parkinson's disease, Huntington's chorea, and HIV infection) is different from that seen in cortical dementia. In early subcortical dementia,[14] the memory loss is primarily related to retrieval of information rather than faulty registration. Recent memory loss may therefore appear "patchy." The inability to organize a task may occur before there is any deterioration of general intellectual functioning. Apathy or decreased motivation occurs early in sub-

cortical dementia. In moderate subcortical dementia, recent and remote memory losses are more severe, although inconsistent, again because of deficits in retrieval rather than registration. Organizational, spatial, and constructional difficulties are more evident than difficulties with language. Apathy is marked and is often confused with that of a depressive illness. Eventually, because subcortical structures project extensively to cortical areas, cortical functioning is severely impaired; severe subcortical dementia presents with the memory deficits and deterioration of general intellectual functioning found in cortical dementia. Judgment is poor, and the patient requires supervision for medical care and self-care.

No *specific* neurologic signs or symptoms are associated with dementia.[4] The causes of the dementia determine the neurologic findings, as do coexisting

---

TABLE 62-8. DSM-III-R CRITERIA FOR DEMENTIA*

A. Demonstrable evidence of impairment in short- and long-term memory. Impairment in short-term memory (inability to learn new information) may be indicated by inability to remember 3 objects after 5 minutes. Long-term memory impairment (inability to remember information that was known in the past) may be indicated by inability to remember past personal information (e.g., what happened yesterday, birthplace, occupation) or facts of common knowledge (e.g., past presidents, well-known dates).
B. At least one of the following:
　1. Impairment in abstract thinking, as indicated by inability to find similarities and differences between related words, difficulty in defining words and concepts, and other similar tasks
　2. Impaired judgment, as indicated by inability to make reasonable plans to deal with interpersonal, family, and job-related problems and issues.
　3. Other disturbances of higher cortical function, such as aphasia (disorder of language), apraxia (inability to carry out motor activities despite intact comprehension and motor function), agnosia (failure to recognize or identify objects despite intact sensory function), and "constructional difficulty" (e.g., inability to copy three-dimensional figures, assemble blocks, or arrange sticks in specific designs)
　4. Personality change, i.e., alteration or accentuation of premorbid traits
C. The disturbance in A and B significantly interferes with work or usual social activities or relationships with others.
D. Not occurring exclusively during the course of delirium.
E. There is evidence from the history, physical examination, or laboratory tests of a specific organic factor (or factors) judged to be etiologically related to the disturbance.

Criteria for severity of dementia:

Mild: Although work or social activities are significantly impaired, the capacity for independent living remains, with adequate personal hygiene and relatively intact judgment.
Moderate: Independent living is hazardous, and some degree of supervision is necessary.
Severe: Activities of daily living are so impaired that continual supervision is required, e.g., patient is unable to maintain minimal personal hygiene; largely incoherent or mute.

* Reprinted with permission from Organic Mental Syndromes and Disorders. In Diagnostic and Statistical Manual of Mental Disorders, 3rd Ed. Revised. Washington, DC, American Psychiatric Press, Inc., 1987.

neurologic conditions not contributing to the dementia. The neurologic examination may be normal, or with more advanced cortical dementia there may be evidence of frontal lobe release signs. Patients with multi-infarct dementia or dementia from brain trauma or space-occupying lesions may have focal neurologic signs. Patients with normal-pressure hydrocephalus may have incontinence and ataxia. The physical examination may be normal or abnormal, depending on the cause of the dementia or coexisting medical conditions. For example, a hypothyroid patient may present with dementia, thick edematous skin, husky voice, decreased body temperature and pulse, and hyporeflexia.

DIFFERENTIAL DIAGNOSIS

A depressed patient, because of psychomotor retardation and problems with attention and concentration, often complains of difficulties with memory. If the interviewer is persistent with the depressed patient, the mental status examination can be completed. As a rule, patients with depression complain of problems with memory, whereas patients with dementia are often unaware of memory difficulties unless confronted directly with observed deficits. Depressed patients emphasize their cognitive disabilities and draw attention to mistakes and failures. Demented patients attempt to cover cognitive deficits. Finally, although the onset of the memory deficits covaries with depressive symptoms, the onset of memory loss is gradual in demented patients.[15]

Delirium is differentiated from dementia by sudden onset, clouding of consciousness, dysattention, and acute onset of psychotic symptoms. As mentioned previously, patients with dementia and acute mental status changes should be assumed to have a superimposed delirium.

MANAGEMENT

When dementia is diagnosed, the emergency physician is committed to seeing that all reversible causes of dementia[16] *are identified and treated,* either in the ED, on a medical floor, or through referral to a primary care physician. *Further, any medical conditions or drugs that could be contributing to impaired cognitive functioning should be diagnosed and treated.* Because the patient's history may be unreliable, a collateral history, if possible, is essential. A patient who presents with dementia or is brought to the ED with mental status changes should have a physical and neurologic examination, CBC, glucose, BUN, creatinine, electrolytes, liver profile, urinalysis, chest x ray, and ECG. Thyroid battery, B_{12}, folate levels, computerized cranial tomography, or MRI may be obtained in the ED or later during the work-up in a nonemergency setting. Hypothyroidism, nutritional deficiencies, dehydration, electrolyte im-

balance, failure to take medications properly, and systemic illness are common causes of deteriorating mental status in the demented patient.[16] Patients with dementia are exquisitely sensitive to drugs with CNS effects, particularly those with anticholinergic effects.

In addition to organic causes, other nonmedical stresses may cause deterioration of cognitive functioning and should be identified. Sensory isolation, altered visual, auditory, or sensory stimuli; fatigue; stress; an unpredictable environment; change from a familiar environment; or the loss of an important relationship can cause deterioration of cognitive functioning in the demented patient. The emergency physician can provide useful recommendations for families caring for the demented patient at home. Sensory isolation should be avoided. Hearing aids, glasses, and dentures should be in good working order and used by the patient throughout the day. If possible, the patient should not be left without human contact for long periods. A television or radio left on in the demented person's room provides sensory stimulation. If a patient becomes confused at night, his or her hearing aid and glasses should be left on. A night light and soft music also decrease sensory isolation at night. Night-time psychotropic medications prescribed and monitored by the demented patient's primary care physician also help to control confusion. Stimuli in the demented patient's environment should be constant, predictable, and simplified to a level the patient can cope with. Families should orient the patient to time and provide a clock or watch and calendar in the patient's room. Meals and activities should be scheduled at the same time and the same place every day. Abrupt changes in the environment should be minimized when possible.

Likewise, demented patients may be confused and agitated by the ED setting, tests, and procedures. As a result, all ED personnel should orient the patient to who they are and what they are doing. Because immediate memory is impaired, plans and procedures must often be explained repeatedly to the patient. Given the decrease in the ability to abstract, simple concrete explanations of procedures are helpful for the demented patient. Patients are often reassured by the presence of a family member who interprets the environment to them. Agitated demented patients who are unable to cooperate with the medical work-up may need psychotropic medication as described under the treatment of delirium.

Families may bring their demented family member to the ED because the patient has become too difficult to manage at home, or the families need additional help or a vacation from the care of the patient. Such families may be skilled at leaving the demented family member in the ED or giving a history of medical problems that require inpatient medical care. If the emergency physician sends such a demented patient home to prevent "inappropriate" use of acute medical services, the problem is not solved. Family members who are overwhelmed by the care of a demented family member may abuse or neglect the patient. At the least, the severe stress of caring for the demented patient may be detrimental to the family or the primary caregiver. If the patient is returned home, the family must be given a referral that will immediately provide help in caring for the demented family member. Referral to a nursing home, which may take months, is not adequate. The emergency physician should be aware of the resources in his or her communities to assist such overburdened families. The ED must know all possible routes of assistance, including visiting nurse services and home health care availability.

AMNESTIC SYNDROME

The most common treatable presentation of the amnestic syndrome is as part of Wernicke-Korsakoff's syndrome in chronic alcoholics with thiamine deficiency.

CLINICAL FEATURES

The onset of the amnestic syndrome depends on the cause. The amnestic syndrome may result from any factor that causes bilateral damage to diencephalic or medial temporal structures of the brain.[17] Examples of acute onset include anoxia,[18] head trauma,[19] cerebrovascular accidents (occlusion of the postcerebral artery),[20] herpes simplex encephalitis, and temporal lobectomy.[18]

The onset of the amnestic syndrome (Korsakoff's syndrome) as the result of thiamine deficiency is subacute (a few weeks to a few days), and usually follows Wernicke's encephalopathy in 50 to 90% of cases.[21] Wernicke's encephalopathy is a delirium that presents with opthalmoplegia, ataxia, and peripheral neuropathy. With clearing of the delirium, the amnestic syndrome (Korsakoff's syndrome) becomes evident. Thiamine deficiency is seen in chronic alcoholism and is caused by poor absorption of thiamine. Alcohol interferes with the absorption of thiamine, and the lack of availability of thiamine is further impaired by poor nutritional status. Occasionally patients with vitamin-deficient diets or malabsorption may develop Wernicke-Korsakoff's syndrome. Patients with a deficiency of the enzyme tranketolase, for which thiamine is a cofactor, may be at greater risk of developing Wernicke-Korsakoff's syndrome. Intravenous glucose administration may use all available thiamine stores in the thiamine-deficient patient, resulting in an acute Wernicke-Korsakoff's syndrome.

The major deficit in the amnestic syndrome is in recent and long-term memory. Immediate memory is intact. Short-term memory is the most severely affected. This recent memory loss is also referred to as anterograde amnesia. Anterograde amnesia refers to

TABLE 62-9. DSM-III-R CRITERIA FOR AMNESTIC SYNDROME*

A. Demonstrable evidence of impairment in both short- and long-term memory; with regard to long-term memory, remote events are remembered better than more recent events. Impairment in short-term memory (inability to learn new information) may be indicated by inability to remember 3 objects after 5 minutes. Long-term memory impairment (inability to remember information that was known in the past) may be indicated by inability to remember past personal information (e.g., what happened yesterday, birthplace, occupation) or facts of common knowledge (e.g., past presidents, well-known dates).

B. Not occurring exclusively during the course of delirium, and does not meet the criteria for dementia (i.e., no impairment in abstract thinking or judgment, no other disturbances of higher cortical function, and no personality change).

C. There is evidence from the history, physical examination, or laboratory tests of a specific organic factor (or factors) judged to be etiologically related to the disturbance.

* Reprinted with permission from Organic Mental Syndromes and Disorders. In Diagnostic and Statistical Manual of Mental Disorders, 3rd Ed. Revised. Washington, DC, American Psychiatric Press, Inc., 1987.

difficulty in laying down new memories (registration) after the etiologic insult occurred. Because orientation is a memory function, amnestic patients may be disoriented. Remote memory loss or retrograde amnesia refers to the inability to retrieve memories that were laid down before the onset of the illness. Confabulation, in which the patient makes up events or haphazardly pieces fragments of the past together to fill gaps in memory, is also common. In the amnestic syndrome, there is no dysattention, clouding of consciousness, as in delirium, or deterioration of general intellectual functioning as in dementia. The DSM-III-R criteria for the amnestic syndrome are listed in Table 62-9.

MANAGEMENT

The clinical management depends on the cause of the amnestic syndrome. The amnestic syndrome caused by trauma, infarction, or anoxia is usually not reversible. Acyclovir may be useful in reversing the amnestic syndrome seen in herpes simplex encephalitis if the treatment is begun early enough.

Wernicke's encephalopathy, if not treated immediately, can lead to irreversible brain damage. If Wernicke's encephalopathy is suspected, the patient should be given thiamine,[4] 100 mg intravenously and 50 mg intramuscularly immediately. Additionally, 50 mg intramuscularly daily or 100 mg orally three times a day should be given for 7 days. Once the amnestic syndrome (Korsakoff's syndrome) has emerged, thiamine is less successful in reversing the syndrome. After treatment, Victor et al.[21] found that 20% of patients with the amnestic syndrome recovered fully after 5 years, 28% were significantly improved, and 25%

slightly improved; the remainder were the same or worse. Hence, when the amnestic syndrome is thought to be caused by thiamine deficiency, the patient should be given thiamine as described. **In practice, every alcoholic who comes to the ED should be given thiamine to prevent the reversible brain damage associated with untreated Wernicke-Korsakoff's syndrome.**

ORGANIC SYNDROMES THAT MIMIC PSYCHIATRIC DISORDERS

The emergency physician who carefully evaluates affective, cognitive, and behavioral symptoms is unlikely to miss delirium, dementia, or the amnestic syndrome because of the characteristic dysattention, memory deficits, and/or difficulties with general intellectual functioning. Organic delusional disorder, organic hallucinosis, organic mood disorder, organic anxiety disorder, and/or organic personality disorder can mimic psychiatric disorders. Consequently, the potentially reversible causes of these organic mental syndromes can be missed and the patient referred into the psychiatric system with an incomplete medical work-up. Patients who are referred into a psychiatric system are often felt to be "cleared medically," even after a brief ED evaluation. Finally, many psychiatric facilities have minimal resources for medical evaluation. Therefore, a patient who presents with a psychiatric syndrome should be considered to have an organic cause until it is proven otherwise. Undiagnosed physical illness, prescribed or illicit drugs, or alcohol should be considered as causes. Special attention should be paid to patients who have no previous personal history of psychiatric illness, particularly if the condition appears for the first time after age 45. Sudden changes in personality are most often the result of organic causes.

TABLE 62-10. DSM-III-R CRITERIA FOR ORGANIC DELUSIONAL SYNDROME*

A. Prominent delusions
B. There is evidence from the history, physical examination, or laboratory tests of a specific organic factor (or factors) judged to be etiologically related to the disturbance
C. Not occurring exclusively during the course of delirium

* Reprinted with permission from Organic Mental Syndromes and Disorders. In Diagnostic and Statistical Manual of Mental Disorders, 3rd Ed. Revised. Washington, DC, American Psychiatric Press, Inc., 1987.

TABLE 62-11. DSM-III-R CRITERIA FOR ORGANIC HALLUCINOSIS*

A. Prominent persistent or recurrent hallucinations.
B. There is evidence from the history, physical examination, or laboratory tests of a specific organic factor (or factors) judged to be etiologically related to the disturbance.
C. Not occurring exclusively during the course of delirium.

* Reprinted with permission from Organic Mental Syndromes and Disorders. In Diagnostic and Statistical Manual of Mental Disorders, 3rd Ed. Revised. Washington, DC, American Psychiatric Press, Inc., 1987.

ORGANIC DELUSIONAL SYNDROME

Delusions caused by a specific organic factor are the prominent clinical feature of this disorder. Affective changes, personality changes, psychotic behavior, and psychotic speech patterns may also accompany the delusions. Hallucinations are less prominent, although in some clinical situations the clinician may have difficulty in deciding whether organic delusional disorder or organic hallucinosis is a more appropriate diagnosis. There may be mild cognitive impairment in an organic delusional disorder. Dysattention and clouding of consciousness as seen in delirium, obvious memory deficits as seen in the amnestic syndrome and dementia, and deterioration of general intellectual functioning as seen in dementia are not present in this syndrome. The DSM-III-R criteria for delusional syndrome are presented in Table 62-10.

Amphetamines, cocaine, cannabis, and hallucinogens are the most common causes of organic delusional disorder.[5] With amphetamine and cocaine abuse, the picture may be indistinguishable from that of schizophrenia, paranoid disorders, and other nonorganic psychotic disorders.[4] Patients with temporal lobe seizures may develop an interictal schizophrenia-like syndrome with paranoid and religious delusions one or two decades after onset of the seizures; the psychosis is inversely related to the number of seizures, and is found most commonly in women with left-sided foci.[22,23] Huntington's chorea can present with a paranoid delusional picture. Cerebral lesions, particularly nondominant lesions, may present with an organic delusional disorder.[5] Management depends on the underlying cause of the syndrome. Symptomatic relief may be provided with haloperidol alone or combined with lorazepam, as described previously. Patients with temporal lobe seizures are not helped by neuroleptics.[4]

ORGANIC HALLUCINOSIS

The principal feature of this organic syndrome is hallucinations from an organic cause. The hallucinations are not part of a delirium or dementia and may be in any sensory modality, but are most commonly visual or auditory. The hallucinations in this syndrome may be simple or unformed to highly complex and organized. Some patients may be aware that the hallucinations are not real, whereas others may believe them to be real. Delusions, although not prominent, may further elaborate the hallucinations. Less commonly, patients may have associated symptoms, including affective changes, psychotic speech patterns, and psychotic behavior. The DSM-III-R criteria for organic hallucinosis are presented in Table 62-11.

Hallucinogens are among the most common causes of organic hallucinosis. Hallucinogens cause vivid visual hallucinations. With chronic use of hallucinogens, the patient may develop a persistent hallucinosis, even when the drug is no longer being used. The patient may have a schizophrenia-like picture[4] even though the capacity for human interaction remains intact.

Other drugs such as levodopa,[18] bromocriptine, amantadine, ephedrine, clonidine, pentazocine, propranolol, and methylphenidate can cause hallucinations. Discontinuing or decreasing the dosage of the medication is the treatment of choice.

Alcohol is another common cause of hallucinosis.[24] In contrast to delirium tremens, in which vivid visual hallucinations are common, alcohol hallucinosis most commonly presents with vivid auditory hallucinations. Organic hallucinosis, as in delirium tremens, occurs when there is cessation or marked reduction in alcohol intake. The onset of hallucinations can begin a few hours to 2 weeks after cessation of alcohol intake, but usually occurs within 48 hours after the last drink. After acute alcoholic hallucinosis, one in 10 patients develops chronic hallucinosis as the acute hallucinosis clears. Alcoholic hallucinosis can begin before delirium tremens and may also present after recovery from the delirium tremens. In alcoholic hallucinosis, there are no memory deficits, clouding of consciousness, or dysattention. Delirium tremens, the onset of which is during the same time frame as alcohol hallucinosis, presents with an agitated delirium and the autonomic signs and symptoms of withdrawal (increased temperature, pulse, blood pressure, and reflexes). If the emergency room physician is unable to differentiate alcohol hallucinosis from delirium tremens, the patient should be treated as if he or she has an alcohol withdrawal syndrome because untreated delirium tremens is associated with morbidity and mortality. Others may feel safer in treating all hallucinations during the alcohol withdrawal period with benzodiazepines because of the coexistence of alcoholic hallucinosis and delirium tremens in some alcoholic patients. If hallucinations persist after adequate benzodiazepine treatment, haloperidol may be added. Chronic alcoholic hallucinosis should be treated with neuroleptics. Haloperidol, 2 to 20 mg orally daily, is useful in treating alcoholic hallucinosis.

Sensory deprivation is a common cause of hallucinosis. The hallucination is usually in the modality in which there is sensory deprivation. For example, visual hallucinations are common after cataract surgery.[25,26] Treatment includes reversing, if possible, the sensory deprivation and/or increasing sensory stimuli.

Visual hallucinations[26] can result from any injury or disease that affects the visual pathway from the occipital cortex to the optic nerve. Visual hallucinations related to disease of the eye are unformed, whereas those related to abnormalities of deeper structures are complex.

Seizure foci in the temporal or occipital areas may cause hallucinations. The modality or complexity of the hallucination is determined by the location of the foci. Anticonvulsants to control the seizure foci are the treatment for this hallucinosis.

ORGANIC MOOD SYNDROME

The distinguishing feature of this syndrome is persistent depressed, elevated, or expansive mood from an organic cause. The severity of the mood syndrome may be mild to severe. Mild cognitive impairment may also be present. The diagnosis is not made if the mood disorder is part of a delirium. Table 62-12 outlines the DSM-III-R criteria for organic mood disorder.

A patient with an organic mood disorder with depressed features may also report one or more of the other symptoms associated with depressive disorders: decreased interest or pleasure in all or almost all activities, significant weight loss or gain when not dieting, a decrease or increase in appetite, insomnia or hypersomnia, psychomotor agitation or retardation, fatigue or loss of energy, feelings of worthlessness or excessive or inappropriate guilt, diminished ability to think or concentrate or indecisiveness, recurrent thoughts of death, or suicidal ideation. Delusions, although less commonly present, have depressive themes (delusions of personal inadequacy, punishment, guilt, nihilism, or disease).

Organic mood syndrome may be indistinguishable from a depressive syndrome without an identifiable organic cause. As a result, common organic factors causing or contributing to depression should be ruled out in all patients presenting to the ED with depression. Because patients with a family or personal history of depression may be more likely to develop depression with an organic stressor (i.e., hypothyroidism, alpha-methyldopa), a previous history of depression does not rule out an organic cause. If the emergency physician is unable to rule out organic

---

TABLE 62-12. DSM-III-R CRITERIA FOR ORGANIC MOOD SYNDROME*

A. Prominent and persistent depressed, elevated, or expansive mood
B. There is evidence from the history, physical examination, or laboratory tests of a specific organic factor (or factors) judged to be etiologically related to the disturbance
C. Not occurring exclusively during the course of delirium

---

* Reprinted with permission from Organic Mental Syndromes and Disorders. *In* Diagnostic and Statistical Manual of Mental Disorders, 3rd Ed. Revised. Washington, DC, American Psychiatric Press, Inc., 1987.

<table>
<tr><th colspan="2">TABLE 62-13. ORGANIC CAUSES OF DEPRESSION</th></tr>
</table>

Metabolic (hypercalcemia, hypocalcemia)
Hypovitaminosis (low B$_{12}$, low folate)
Endocrine (hypopituitarism, Addison's disease, hypothyroidism, hypoglycemia)
Uremia
Oat cell carcinoma of the lung
Gastrointestinal neoplasms and disease (cancer of the pancreas, inflammatory bowel disease)
Stroke (particularly nondominant)
Systemic lupus erythematosus
Parkinson's disease
Multiple sclerosis
Frontal lobe tumors
Viral infections (viral encephalitis, hepatitis, Epstein-Barr, infectious mononucleosis)
Drugs
  Common
    Antihypertensives (clonidine, guanethidine, hydralazine, methyldopa, propranolol, reserpine)
    Benzodiazepines
    Barbiturates
    Withdrawal from psychostimulants
  Less common
    Anticonvulsants
    Antimicrobials (ampicillin, cycloserine, dapsone, griseofulvin, isoniazid, metronidazole, nalidixic acid, nitrofurantoin, procaine penicillin, streptomycin, sulfanilamides, tetracyclines, trimethoprim sulfa)
    Disulfiram
    Digitalis
    Cimetidine, ranitidine
    Chemotherapeutic agents
    Immunosupressant drugs
    Levodopa
    Nonsteroidal anti-inflammatory drugs
    Steroids

<table>
<tr><th>TABLE 62-14. ORGANIC CAUSES OF MANIA</th></tr>
</table>

Degenerative diseases (Huntington's disease, Pick's disease, Wilson's disease)
Hypothyroidism
Uremia with progressive dialysis dementia
Carcinoid
Cerebral infarct (right hemisphere damage, temporal)
Postsurgery (right hemispherectomy, thalamotomy)
Post-traumatic encephalopathy
Space-occupying lesions (frontal, diencephalic, hypothalamic, parasaggital, spheno-occipital neoplasms)
Multiple sclerosis
Klinefelter's syndrome
Klein-Leven syndrome
Idiopathic calcification of the basal ganglion
Temporal lobe seizures
Infections (HIV, cryptococcal meningitis, Q fever, infectious mononucleosis, post-St. Louis Type A encephalitis, influenza, neurosyphilis, post-encephalitic Parkinson's)
Drugs
  Aminophylline
  Antidepressants
  Isoniazid
  Levodopa
  Procainamide
  Psychostimulants (amphetamines, cocaine, phencyclidine)
  Thyroid preparations
  Steroids

causes of depression in a depressed patient, this should be communicated to the physician to whom the patient is referred. Numerous illnesses and drugs have been associated with depressive symptoms.[27–30] Table 62-13 outlines the common organic causes of depression.

An organic mood disorder with elevated or expansive mood can present with one or more of the following associated features: irritable mood, inflated self-esteem or grandiosity, decreased need for sleep, pressured speech, racing thoughts, flight of ideas, distractibility, increased goal-directed activity, psychomotor agitation, excessive involvement in pleasurable activities with a high potential for painful consequences (e.g., unrestrained buying sprees, sexual indiscretions, or foolish business investments). If delusions or hallucinations are present, the content is consistent, with manic themes of inflated worth, power, knowledge, identity, or special relationship to a deity or famous person.

Clinically, hypomania or mania as the result of an organic cause may be indistinguishable from bipolar disorder. Also, patients with bipolar disorder may more quickly develop a hypomanic or manic picture when stressed by an organic factor. Furthermore, a manic episode must be differentiated from delirium (the differential diagnostic features of mania and delirium are discussed under the section on delirium). Thus, organic causes must be ruled out in all patients presenting with a hypomanic or manic episode. Again, as with the depressed patient, if organic factors are not ruled out, the emergency physician must convey this to the follow-up physician. Table 62-14 lists the organic causes of mania.[28,31,32]

The course of an organic mood disorder depends on the underlying cause. Treatment includes identifying the cause, removing the offending drug, or treating the underlying medical condition. Patients with an organic depressive disorder may be agitated. This agitation is best treated symptomatically with benzodiazepines, as discussed in the section on organic anxiety syndrome. Suicidal ideation may be present and carries the same risk as in the patient with a unipolar or bipolar depressive disorder. Patients exhibiting hypomanic or manic symptoms with an organic basis are best managed in the ED with a combination of lorazepam and haloperidol, as discussed under Delirium.

ORGANIC ANXIETY SYNDROME

The cardinal features of this syndrome are prominent, recurrent panic attacks or generalized anxiety caused

TABLE 62-15. DSM-III-R CRITERIA FOR ORGANIC ANXIETY SYNDROME*

A. Prominent, recurrent panic attacks or generalized anxiety

Panic Attacks:

At some time during the disturbance, one or more panic attacks (discrete periods of intense fear or discomfort) have occurred that were (1) unexpected, i.e., did not occur immediately before or on exposure to a situation that almost always caused anxiety, and (2) not triggered by situations in which the person was the focus of others' attention.

At least four of the following symptoms developed during at least one of the attacks:
1. Shortness of breath (dyspnea) or smothering sensations
2. Dizziness, unsteady feelings, or faintness
3. Palpitations or accelerated heart rate (tachycardia)
4. Trembling or shaking
5. Sweating
6. Choking
7. Nausea or abdominal distress
8. Depersonalization or derealization
9. Numbness or tingling sensations (paresthesias)
10. Flushes (hot flashes) or chills
11. Chest pain or discomfort
12. Fear of dying
13. Fear of going crazy or of doing something uncontrolled

Generalized anxiety:

At least 6 of the following 18 symptoms are often present when anxious (do not include symptoms present only during panic attacks):

Motor tension
1. Trembling, twitching, or feeling shaky
2. Muscle tension, aches, or soreness
3. Restlessness
4. Easy fatigability

Autonomic hyperactivity
5. Shortness of breath or smothering sensations
6. Palpitations or accelerated heart rate (tachycardia)
7. Sweating, or cold clammy hands
8. Dry mouth
9. Dizziness or lightheadedness
10. Nausea, diarrhea, or other abdominal distress
11. Flushes (hot flashes) or chills
12. Frequent urination
13. Trouble swallowing or "lump in throat"

Vigilance and scanning
14. Feeling keyed up or on edge
15. Exaggerated startle response
16. Difficulty concentrating or "mind going blank" because of anxiety
17. Trouble falling or staying asleep
18. Irritability

B. There is evidence from the history, physical examination, or laboratory tests of a specific organic factor (or factors) judged to be etiologically related to the disturbance.
C. Not occurring exclusively during the course of delirium.

* Reprinted with permission from Organic Mental Syndromes and Disorders. In Diagnostic and Statistical Manual of Mental Disorders, 3rd Ed. Revised. Washington, DC, American Psychiatric Press, Inc., 1987.

TABLE 62-16. ORGANIC CAUSES OF ANXIETY

Endocrine (hyperthyroidism, hypoparathyroidism, Cushing's syndrome)
Hypoglycemia
Pheochromocytoma
Chronic obstructive pulmonary disease
Cardiac arrhythmias
Mitral valve prolapse
Recurrent pulmonary embolism
Tumors of the third ventricle
Seizures (partial complex seizures, third ventricle seizure foci, diencephalic or temporal lobe seizures)
Drugs
    Withdrawal of central nervous system depressants (alcohol, barbiturates, benzodiazepines)
    Caffeine
    Psychostimulants (cocaine, amphetamines)
    Sympathomimetics
    Thyroid preparations
    Any drugs with anxiety or jitteriness as a side effect (i.e., lidocaine, procainamide, L-dopa, aminophylline, theophylline, steroids, fluoxetine, desipramine, tranylcypromine)

by an organic factor. Table 62-15 presents the criteria for this disorder. Mild cognitive impairment may be present, usually associated with difficulties in attention and concentration. The diagnosis is not made if the panic or anxiety is part of a delirium. The syndrome may be mild to severe. The course of the syndrome depends on the cause. The etiologic factors causing organic anxiety syndrome[28,33,34] are listed in Table 62-16.

Because organic anxiety syndrome may be indistinguishable from panic attacks or generalized anxiety, organic factors must be ruled out in any patient presenting to the ED with anxiety symptoms. Hypoxia, hypoglycemia, hyperthyroidism, intoxication with stimulants (caffeine, cocaine, amphetamines) and withdrawal from sedative drugs (barbiturates, benzodiazepines, alcohol) must be diagnosed and treated in the ED. Drugs that have anxiety and jitteriness as a side effect may be temporarily discontinued if there are no medical contraindications. Other causes that involve more extensive work-up must be carried out by the follow-up physician.

Symptomatic relief can be provided with benzodiazepines, except in those patients with lung disease. Benzodiazepines reduce ventilatory response to hypoxia when the respiratory center is no longer driven by hypercapnia. Lorazepam, 1 to 2 mg orally, may be repeated every hour until the anxiety or panic remits. Slow IV administration of lorazepam, 1 mg, is useful in severe anxiety or panic. Alprazolam, 0.25 to 1 mg orally, repeated every 45 minutes to 1 hour, is also useful in aborting organic anxiety or panic attacks. The patient may then be discharged with a benzodiazepine dosage of lorazepam, 0.5 to 2 mg orally 3 times a day to 4 times a day or alprazolam, 0.25 to 1 mg orally 3 to 4 times a day.

ORGANIC PERSONALITY SYNDROME

The major feature of this disorder is a change or accentuation of previous personality characteristics as a

TABLE 62-17. DSM-III-R CRITERIA FOR ORGANIC PERSONALITY SYNDROME*

A. A persistent personality disturbance, either lifelong or representing a change or accentuation of a previously characteristic trait, involving at least one of the following:
1. Affective instability, e.g., marked shifts from normal mood to depression, irritability, or anxiety
2. Recurrent outbursts of aggression or rage that are grossly out of proportion to any precipitating psychological stressors
3. Markedly impaired social judgment, e.g., sexual indiscretions
4. Marked apathy and indifference
5. Suspiciousness or paranoid ideation
B. There is evidence from the history, physical examination, or laboratory tests of a specific organic factor (or factors) judged to be etiologically related to the disturbance.
C. Not occurring exclusively during the course of delirium, and does not meet the criteria for dementia.

* Reprinted with permission from Organic mental syndromes and disorders. In Diagnostic and Statistical Manual of Mental Disorders, 3rd Ed. Revised. Washington, DC, American Psychiatric Press, Inc., 1987.

result of an organic factor. The personality change does not occur as part of a delirium or dementia. The DSM-III-R criteria for organic personality syndrome are listed in Table 62-17.

Organic personality disorder is most commonly caused by structural damage to brain tissue. The location of the lesion and the type of pathophysiologic process determine the type of personality disturbance. Head injuries involving the frontal and temporal lobes are the most frequent cause of a personality disturbance, particularly bilateral frontal lobe injuries. Two syndromes have been described with bifrontal lobe injury. The first is characterized by emotional lability, impulsivity, socially inappropriate behavior and hostility, and the second by apathy, indifference, and social withdrawal.[35,36] Frontal lobe tumors and cerebrovascular accidents involving the middle cerebral artery are a less common cause of personality changes.[4,28] These changes may also be seen with temporal lobe epilepsy, multiple sclerosis, lupus erythematosus, and Huntington's chorea. Degenerative dementia may present with personality changes before deficits in memory and general intellectual functioning occur.[16] Chronic cannabis, amphetamine, or cocaine abuse can present with personality changes.[5] Finally, heavy metal[28] poisoning can present with personality changes.

Patients are rarely brought to the ED with the presenting complaint of an organic personality disturbance unless the personality change is acutely disturbing to the family. For example, a patient with head trauma may become aggressive and unmanageable or demonstrate severe lability of affect. Aggressive behavior and severe lability of affect may be controlled on an acute basis with neuroleptics, although the response is highly variable. Less potent, more sedating

neuroleptics are often more efficacious than haloperidol but have more anticholinergic and orthostatic hypotensive effects than the more potent neuroleptics. Chlorpromazine, 25 to 100 mg orally or 25 to 50 mg intramuscularly; mesoridazine, 10 to 50 mg orally or 12.5 to 25 mg IM; or thiothixene, 2 to 10 mg orally; or 2 to 5 mg IM may be useful for aggressive behavior and severe lability of affect.

More commonly, a patient may present with other physical symptoms, and a change in personality is mentioned as part of the history. In this instance, the personality change gives an important clue to the cause of the physical illness.

INFORMED CONSENT

A patient with an organic brain syndrome may be unable to give informed consent; that is, to understand the risks and benefits of a medical procedure or treatment. If the patient does not cognitively understand these, written consent is not valid. Informed consent is less important when the benefits are great and the risk low, but critical if the risk is high,[37] even if the risk is at the benefit of saving the patient's life or preventing significant morbidity. In an ED, benign procedures are often performed on a cognitively impaired patient without rigorous informed consent. The emergency physician, however, is presented with medicolegal difficulties when a patient with an organic brain syndrome cannot understand the risks and benefits of a procedure with significant risk or refuses diagnostic tests or treatment that are imperative to prevent morbidity and mortality. In such cases, it is essential for the emergency physician to document the emergency nature of the diagnostic tests and treatment on the chart. If the procedure or treatment carries a significant risk, another consulting physician should also document the need on the chart. If the family is present, the emergency physician should carefully explain the procedure to the family and obtain their verbal and written informed consent. Such a signature is not legal unless the family member is the legal guardian, but is an extra safeguard in a malpractice suit. In summary, if a patient cannot give informed consent (even if he or she has signed the release form in the emergency area), the following should be documented on the ED record: (1) the patient was unable to understand the risks and benefits of the procedure because of the symptoms (list) of an organic brain syndrome; (2) the medical procedure(s) were explained to the family and the family agreed verbally and in writing, (3) the procedure(s) were performed on an emergency basis and the reasons why they were emergently necessary. If a family member is not available, (1) and (3) should be documented.[38]

COMPETENCY AND GUARDIANSHIP

A patient with an organic brain syndrome may become so mentally incompetent that a guardian, usually a family member, is appointed by the court to make medical and/or legal decisions. A patient's incompetence to consent to medical procedures or manage his or her legal affairs is always a legal decision, not a medical one, although medical evidence may be used in the court's determination. Guardianship may be for legal affairs, medical decisions, or both. Guardianship may be for a limited period of time (i.e., for an acute serious illness) or for an indefinite period of time (i.e., a severe dementia). If a patient has a legal guardian for medical decisions, that person must sign the consent form in the ED.[38]

REFERENCES

1. Detre, T., Jerecki, H.: Organic brain syndromes. *In* Modern Psychiatric Treatment. Edited by Detre, T. and Jerecki, H. Philadelphia, J.B. Lippincott Co., 1971.
2. Weddington, W.W.: The mortality of delirium: An underappreciated problem. Psychosomatics 23:1232, 1982.
3. Guze, S.B., and Cantwell, D.P.: The prognosis in organic brain syndromes. Am. J. Psychiatry 120:878, 1964.
4. Wells, C.E.: Organic syndromes: Delirium. *In* Comprehensive Textbook of Psychiatry. Edited by Kaplan, H.I., and Saddock, B.J. Baltimore, Williams & Wilkins, 1985.
5. Organic mental syndromes and disorders. *In* Diagnostic and Statistical Manual of Mental Disorders. 3rd Ed. Revised. Washington, DC, American Psychiatric Press, Inc., 1987.
6. Wise, M.G.: Delirium. *In* Textbook of Neuropsychiatry. Edited by Hales, R.E., and Yodofsky, S.C. Washington, DC, The American Psychiatric Press, Inc., 1987.
7. Slaby, A.E., and Cullen, L.O.: Dementia and delirium. *In* Principles of Medical Psychiatry. Edited by Stoudemire, A., and Fogel, B.S. New York, Grune & Stratton, 1987.
8. Greenblatt, D.J., and Shader, R.I. (eds.): Pharmacokinetics and Clinical Practice. Philadelphia, W.B. Saunders Co., 1985.
9. Lakshiminarawan, S., Sahn, S.A., and Hudson, L.D.: Effects of diazepam on ventilatory responses. Clin. Pharmacol. Ther. 20:173, 1976.
10. Thompson, T.L.: II. Psychosocial and psychiatric problems of the aged. *In* Clinical International Medicine in the Aged. Edited by Schrier, R.W. Philadelphia, W.B. Saunders Co., 1982.
11. Terry, R.D., and Katzman, R.: Senile dementia of the Alzheimer's type. Ann. Neurol. 14:497, 1983.
12. Cummings, J.L.: Multi-infarct dementia: Diagnosis and management. Psychosomatics 28:117, 1987.
13. Lipowski, Z.J.: Differentiating delirium from dementia in the elderly. Clinical Gerontologist 1:3, 1982.
14. Huber, S.J., Paulson, G.W.: The concept of subcortical dementia. Am. J. Psychiatry 142:1312, 1985.
15. Wells, C.E.: Pseudodementia. Am. J. Psychiatry 136:895, 1979.
16. Wells, C.E.: Diagnostic evaluation and treatment in dementia. *In* Dementia. 2nd Ed. Edited by Wells, C. Philadelphia, F.A. Davis Co., 1977.
17. Victor, M.: The amnestic syndrome and its anatomical basis. Can. Med. Assoc. J. 100:1115, 1969.
18. Lipowski, Z.J.: Organic mental disorders, introduction and review of syndromes. *In* Comprehensive Textbook of Psychiatry. Volume 2, 3rd. Ed. Edited by Kaplan, H.I., Freedman, A.M., and Sadock, B.J., Baltimore, Williams & Wilkins, 1980.
19. Kwentus, J.A., et al.: Psychiatric complications of closed-head trauma. Psychosomatics 26:8, 1985.
20. Mathew, R.J., and Meyer, J.S.: Pathogenesis and natural history of transient global amnesia. Stroke 5:303, 1974.
21. Victor, M., Adams, R.D., and Collins, G.H.: The Wernicke-Korsakoff Syndrome. Contemporary Neurology Series. Volume 7. Philadelphia, F.A. Davis, 1971.
22. Blumer, D., and Benson, D.F.: Psychiatric manifestations of epilepsy. *In* Psychiatric Aspects of Neurological Disease. Volume 2. Edited by Benson, D.F., and Blumer, D. New York, Grune & Stratton, 1982.
23. Bear, D., et al.: Interictal behavioral changes in patients with temporal lobe epilepsy. *In* Annual Review, Volume 4. Edited by Hales, R.E. and Francis, A.J. Washington, DC, American Psychiatric Press, Inc., 1985.
24. Surawicz, F.G.: Alcoholic hallucinosis, a missed diagnosis: Differential diagnosis and management. Can. J. Psychiatry 25:57, 1980.
25. Weisman, A.D., Hackett, J.P.: Psychosis after eye surgery. N. Engl. J. Med. 258:1284, 1958.
26. White, N.J.: Complex visual hallucinations in partial blindness due to eye disease. Br. J. Psychiatry 136:284, 1980.
27. Stoudemire, A.: Depression in the medically ill. *In* Psychiatry. Edited by Cavenar, J. New York, Basic Books, 1985.
28. Stoudemire, A.: Selected organic mental disorders. *In* Textbook of Neuropsychiatry. Edited by Hales, R.E., and Yudofsky, S.C. Washington, DC, The American Psychiatric Press, Inc., 1987.
29. Katerndahl, D.A.: Nonpsychiatric disorders associated with depression. J. Fam. Pract. 13:619, 1981.
30. Whitlock, F.A., and Evans, L.E.F.: Drugs and depression. Drugs 15:53, 1978.
31. Krathammer, C., and Klerman, G.L.: Secondary mania: Manic syndromes associated with antecedent physical illness or drugs. Arch. Gen. Psychiatry 35:1333, 1978.
32. Larson, E.W., and Richelson, E.: Organic causes of mania. Mayo Clin. Proc. 63:906, 1988.
33. Dietch, J.T.: Diagnosis of organic anxiety disorders. Psychosomatics 22:661, 1981.
34. MacKenzie, T.B., Popkin, M.K.: Organic anxiety syndrome. Am. J. Psychiatry 140:342, 1983.
35. Blumer, D., and Benson, D.F.: Personality changes with frontal and temporal lobe lesions. *In* Psychiatric Aspects of Neurological Disease, Volume 1. Edited by Benson, D.F., and Blumer, D. New York, Grune & Stratton, 1975.
36. Alexander, M.P.: Traumatic brain injury. *In* Psychiatric Aspects of Neurologic Disease, Volume 2. Edited by Benson, D.F., and Blumer, D. New York, Grune & Stratton, 1982.
37. Drane, J.F.: Competency to give informed consent. JAMA 252:925, 1984.
38. Perr, I.: Many faces of competence. *In* Law and the Mental Health Professions. Edited by Barton, W.E., and Sandborn, C.J. New York, International University Press, 1978.

THE DEPRESSED PATIENT

Jean-Pierre Lindenmayer

CAPSULE

Depression is a basic human emotion as well as a physiologic reaction with social communicative value and adaptive functions. The boundary between depression as a human affect and depression as a pathologic symptom is gradual. Once it has been established that the depressive symptom is a clinical state and not within the range of human mood, the clinician is faced with many possible causes underlying the depressive syndrome. These may range from the purely biologic to the psychologic and social, but most often represent a combination of these factors. A carefully taken history may provide clues as to these factors. The history of a clear major life event, such as a loss of a loved one, preceding the depression; several previous depressive episodes; or the use of reserpine as antihypertensive therapy are important causes. In an emergency situation, it is most valuable to determine why the patient presents himself or herself to the physician at this time. This not only helps to clarify cause, but also helps to direct initial therapeutic interventions at the most urgent issue. Predisposing factors for depression provide helpful clues for further causes and interventions. Alcohol dependence and chronic physical illness may predispose to depression and are important clinical states to be aware of.

PATHOPHYSIOLOGY

The original catecholamine hypothesis of affective disorder postulated that depression is characterized by a deficiency of functional norepinephrine. More recent studies have refined and enlarged the number of underlying pathophysiologic mechanisms of depression. These studies suggest a reduction in central α-adrenergic receptor responsiveness contributing to a dysregulation of norepinephrine release/metabolism that may underlie the vegetative and anxiety-related symptoms.[1] In addition, there is strong evidence of a disturbed serotonergic neurotransmission based on decreased serotonergic activity in subgroups of depressions. It has also been suggested that dysregulation in acetylcholine and dopamine metabolism are involved in the pathophysiology of depression. Further, a high number of depressed patients show a protracted elevation in plasmacorticosteroids, pointing to an overactive hypothalamic-pituitary adrenocortical system. This finding is related to the observation of cortisol nonsuppression by dexamethasone (DST) in about 44% of cases with major depressive illness. The DST is specific enough to have some diagnostic utility. Rates of nonsuppression are lower in schizophrenia and anxiety disorders than in psychotic affective disorders.

RECOGNITION

Depressed patients seen by the physician on an emergency basis usually suffer from rather severe states of depression that are not difficult to recognize. Their sad melancholic expression and either retardation or agitation are practically pathognomonic of depression. They complain of feeling sad and hopeless and of a reduced or absent capacity for enjoyment (anhedonia). They show a gloomy outlook on life and suffer from slowed-down thinking and indecisiveness. Their depressive ruminations often show ideas of self-accusation that sometimes can assume psychotic proportions with delusions of worthlessness. The patient may think that he or she has committed a terrible crime for which he or she deserves punishment. Rarely, the patient also may report hallucinations, particularly of an auditory nature, such as voices accusing him or her of various sins. In elderly patients, delusions of poverty or the belief that they have some fatal somatic disorder are observed frequently. In milder states, hypochondriac preoccupations are common. Suicidal ideation is almost always present in more severe depressions and must be evaluated carefully. Suicide threats, gestures, or attempts are probably the most frequent emergencies encountered in association with depression. Vegetative signs are also present in almost every depression. Easy fatigability, loss of appetite, and insomnia, particularly early awakening, are frequently reported. Loss of libido and constipation also are common complaints.[2] At times, the physical symptoms are so predominant that the depression is overlooked. Such "masked depressions" were first de-

TABLE 62-18. DIFFERENTIAL DIAGNOSIS OF DEPRESSION

1. *Acute Grief Reaction*
   Follows acute loss; lacks ideas of worthlessness, helplessness and hopelessness.
2. *Organic Affective Disorder with Depression*
   Caused by systemic illness, direct CNS disease, or treatment of physical disorder, such as hypothyroidism, hyperthyroidism, hypoparathyroidism, hyperparathyroidism, Cushing's disease, Addison's disease, pernicious anemia, hyperglycemia, hypoglycemia, diabetes, hypopituitarism, brain trauma, intracranial tumor, pancreatic carcinoma, lymphoma, systemic lupus erythematosus, viral infections, chronic obstructive lung disease, and reserpine toxicity.
3. *Primary Degenerative Dementia*
   Memory loss, disorientation and gradual loss of cognitive functions are predominant.
4. *Schizophrenia*
   Usually accompanied by poor premorbid and interepisode functioning. Lack of family history of affective disorder. Poor response to antidepressants.

scribed about 30 years ago. The agitated depressive patient may be more difficult to recognize. Motor restlessness, pacing, wringing of hands, and severe anxiety are prominent. The patient tends to be both demanding and clinging. The agitation can be so severe as to lead to physical exhaustion, which itself represents an emergency. The patient, when first seen, may have been anorexic for several weeks and may have lost a great deal of weight, leading to malnutrition. Occasionally, he or she may hide his or her feelings behind a cheerful facade that requires careful interviewing to reach the underlying depression.

DIFFERENTIAL DIAGNOSIS (TABLE 62-18)

ACUTE GRIEF REACTION

A typical depressive syndrome may follow after acute loss from the death of a loved one. Ideas of worthlessness, hopelessness, and helplessness together with marked decrease of functioning during a prolonged period of time are rarely present, however. This reaction usually occurs within the months after the loss, and its duration can vary, but does not usually exceed 6 to 8 months.

ORGANIC AFFECTIVE SYNDROME WITH DEPRESSION

A clear organic cause, such as reserpine or an infectious disease, may produce a depressive syndrome.

A careful history and physical examination establish the diagnosis.

PRIMARY DEGENERATIVE DEMENTIA

In elderly patients with dementia, symptoms of depression may be confused with manifestations of dementia, such as psychomotor retardation, loss of interest, and difficulties in concentrating with complaints of memory loss and disorientation. At times a major depressive syndrome can present primarily cognitive impairment, suggesting a pseudodementia, which resolves once the depression is treated.

SCHIZOPHRENIA

Catatonic schizophrenia may present with marked withdrawal, mutism, and psychomotor retardation, and may look like a depressive syndrome. Good premorbid adjustment, previous depressive episodes with good recovery, and a family history of affective disorders may help distinguish it from schizophrenia. Schizophrenic episodes may sometimes be followed by an episode of depression and is referred to as post-psychotic depression.

INITIAL STEPS

Contact with the patient may often be difficult because of his or her withdrawal and state of inhibition. The physician must first attempt to create an empathetic rapport between himself and the patient to be able to assess the nature, conditions, and severity of the depression. He or she must be tolerant and willing to wait for the patient's responses, and must avoid any critical statements. There should be an attempt to identify what brought the patient to the Emergency Department (ED) at this time. Possible precipitating events should be explored, such as the recent or threatened loss of a loved one. One of the most important aspects of the initial assessment is evaluation of the suicide risk. If a patient has attempted suicide, the question must be asked whether he or she still has suicidal wishes. If this is denied, one must examine carefully whether the suicide attempt has produced any change in the patient's environment. If the situation that precipitated the attempt is unchanged, the suicide risk is still high. Another important initial step is to evaluate the patient for psychotic features, such as delusions and hallucinations. The patient's ideas of guilt may be of delusional proportions and accompanied by misrepresentations of reality. The patient's relationship to the people with whom he or she is in closest contact should be examined to determine how much support the patient can get from them. The presence or absence of social support, particularly for the psychotically depressed patient, may be the determining factor in whether or not to hospitalize the patient.

EVALUATION OF THE SUICIDAL PATIENT

All states of depression may be accompanied by various degrees of suicidal preoccupation and action. The patient may express these in active or passive terms. A lesser suicide risk may be indicated by wishes expressed in a passive way, such as the wish "not to wake up in the morning," the wish to be killed by an accident, or ambivalence about the wish to die. A severe risk is represented by the patient who has thought out suicide plans, who has the instruments of destruction (pills, gun, etc.) or who reports impulsive suicidal wishes. The physician should also be alert to pick up indirect suicidal communications. The patient who reports with little affect that he has been driving his car recklessly, or that he has begun to put his financial affairs in order, communicates serious suicidal intention. In retarded depressions, suicidal preoccupation may be constant, but patients are too inhibited by their retardation to carry out the suicide attempt. The physician should ask every depressed patient directly about his or her suicidal thoughts and intentions during the initial assessment; more often than not, he or she gives accurate answers. All too frequently, physicians are uneasy or hesitant to ask questions like these because of the erroneous belief that this may "give the patient the wrong ideas." Actually, the opposite is true; most patients are relieved to discuss their thoughts because many who attempt to commit suicide do so ambivalently and allow life-saving interventions.[3] Although there is no exact way to predict a patient's suicidal intentions, several factors can be isolated during an interview that contribute to the suicide potential of a patient:

1. Age and sex. At high risk in terms of age are older men and young adults of both sexes. Men commit suicide more often, but women more often make unsuccessful attempts.
2. Marital status. Among divorced and widowed persons, suicide rates are four to five times higher than those reported for married individuals.
3. Previous suicide attempts and completed suicides in the family.
4. Recent suicide of a famous person given newspaper and television publicity. A detailed suicide plan that the patient describes.
5. Stressful precipitating events that have not been resolved. Most of these involve loss of persons close to the patient or of important material goods. The widowed are at their greatest risk during the first year of bereavement. Reactions may occur on the anniversary of the loss of a loved person.
6. Provocative statements about how much the patient will be missed, how others will be sorry or angry or glad.
7. Abrupt lessening of the depression, with a sudden feeling of relief when the decision has been made to go through with the suicide.
8. Auditory hallucinations giving the patient self-destructive orders.
9. Concomitant severe or chronic medical illness that the patient feels has totally exhausted his or her physical and psychologic resources or a condition that the patient judges to be fatal, whether it is or not, regardless of reassurances from the patient's physician.
10. Seriousness of suicide attempt: The more lethal the previous attempt, the greater the suicide risk. Conversely, the more rescue is available after a suicidal attempt, the lower the suicide risk.
11. Substance abuse: If the patient is intoxicated by alcohol or central nervous system (CNS) depressants, the higher the risk of suicide.

MANAGEMENT AND DISPOSITION

PSYCHOLOGIC MANAGEMENT

The physician should offer his help in a noncritical and emphatic fashion because the patient perceives his need for help as a blow to his self-esteem.[4] It is therefore important to convince the patient that coming to see a physician is not a sign of weakness but rather a sign of strength. Statements exhorting him to "straighten out" and "pull himself together" should be avoided because they are liable to increase the patient's guilt or hostility.[4]

During the interview, the physician should help the patient to express and ventilate some of the pent-up feelings, particularly anger, and possibly identify the loss that precipitated the depression, if it is of psychologic origin. In some depressions, the origin appears to be biochemical, and there is no specific environmental or psychologic "cause." A brief explanation of the illness and its basically favorable prognosis contribute toward relieving some of the patients anxieties and building up his or her trust in the physician. If the basis of the depression is an acute grief reaction to loss of a loved one, it is important to point out that this is normal.[5] The patient should be given support and encouraged to ventilate some of his or her feelings of sadness over the loss. The physician should explore with the patient other possible sources of emotional support and help him to accept them. Bland reassurance often has a negative effect because the patient may perceive it as indifference.

DISPOSITION

If the suicide risk has been evaluated as high, someone should be with the patient constantly, preferably a nurse. The decision must be made as to whether psychiatric consultation and hospitalization are necessary. As a rule, every patient admitted to an ED after an attempted suicide should be seen by the psychiatric consultant as soon as the patient is medically cleared. If the suicide risk is only minor, the patient can be discharged home with psychiatric follow-up. The family, however, should be made aware of the risk, and somebody should monitor the patient at home constantly. They should be asked to remove from ready access all available medication and dangerous objects in the house. Prescribed medication may have to be given in a quantity that cannot be used for suicidal purposes. The patient also should be told that he or she can call the physician day or night, if he or she should feel that suicidal urges are not under control. If the suicide risk is considerable, immediate hospitalization is indicated, directly through psychiatric referral. This decision is best explained to the patient and the family as a protective measure against the patient's suicidal urges. Other indications for hospitalization include lack of suitable social support, previous history of prolonged depression and lack of response to ambulatory antidepressant medication, drug intoxication and psychosis. If no real suicide risk appears to be present, psychiatric referral is indicated to have treatment instituted and possible future suicide risks monitored. In addition, in depressions with vegetative signs, psychotic symptoms, or both, patients should be placed on antidepressant medication (Table 62-19). The physician should explain the rationale of the treatment and that the positive effects will not appear before 2 weeks. The most frequent side effects to be anticipated should also be explained briefly. For retarded depressive syndromes, the patient should be treated with tricyclic antidepressants at sufficiently high dosages (150 mg or more, or 20 to 30 mg of protriptyline) on an increasing dosage schedule. To minimize sedative side effects during the day, one may administer the major part of the daily dosage to the patient before he or she retires. This also helps to treat any sleep disturbance present. Patients who have not responded to tricyclics in the past can be treated by a newer tetracyclic antidepressant (maprotiline, 50 to 300 mg) or by MAOIs in similarly adequate amounts (30 to 60 mg per day), provided that the patient can adhere to the necessary dietary restrictions. For agitated depressive syndromes, when adequate sedation is needed, we recommend an effective minor tranquilizer such as lorazepam in combination with a sedative tricyclic antidepressant (doxepin, amitriptyline, or the triazolopyridine, trazodone). In some cases, phenothiazines can be used. High doses of tricyclic antidepressants, if necessary in combination with a nonsedative antipsychotic drug in lower dosages, should be used in depressed patients with delusions and hallucinations. In addition, social supports should be rallied around the patient. The kind of treatment and disposition on which the physician has decided should be briefly discussed with the patient and his or her family. There should be an opportunity for them to ask any questions about the further course of action. Their response to the treatment plan and referral can be checked, and possible complications can be prevented in this fashion.

COMPLICATIONS

SUICIDE

As already noted, suicidal preoccupation is to a greater or lesser degree a constant feature of depressive states.

TABLE 62-19. ANTIDEPRESSANTS		
Amitryptiline	50	50–300
Nortryptiline	25	30–150
Imipramine	50	50–300
Desipramine	50	50–300
Protryptiline	10	50–60
Doxepin	50	50–300
Maprotiline	50	50–250
Amoxapine	100	50–400
Trazodone	50	150–400
Fluexetine	20	20–80
Bupropion	100	100–300

The careful appraisal of suicide risks is therefore particularly important. This is necessary not only at the initial evaluation of the patient but also later on, when the psychomotor retardation starts to lift. This is a particularly dangerous phase because the patient begins to become more active and is now able to put suicidal thoughts into action. When hospitalization and drug therapy are insufficient to remove the imminent and severe danger of suicide, electroconvulsive therapy may be indicated. A short series of shocks (up to eight) may be sufficient to lift the worst part of the depression so that the constant danger of suicide is eliminated.

REFUSAL OF HOSPITALIZATION

Occasionally depressed patients may refuse hospitalization once this course has been chosen by the physician. It is important not to try to convince the patient immediately but rather to try to explore his or her fears of hospitalization. Most often, it is regarded as another blow to the patient's self-esteem, generating guilt, particularly about his or her failure to fulfill the usual role in the family. Psychiatric hospitalization may also be feared because of the real and imagined stigmas attached to it by the patient's family and social environment. It may also mean to the patient that he "must be crazy" and that he will never be able to leave the hospital if the doctor recommends his going there. If the physician explores these various fears and remains firm in his decision, he is usually successful in his approach. In some situations, however, involuntary commitment is necessary. In any event, it is important for the physician to explain his rationale for hospitalization and possible commitment openly rather than be vague or secretive about it. In our experience, it is most helpful to have the cooperation of the family in this matter and to gain their support. If the family is also undecided as to the value and need for hospitalization, it is almost impossible to convince the patient. If, despite all discussion, hospitalization is still refused, the physician should insist on discharging the patient if he or she fails to comply. Usually, this threat is sufficient to persuade the patient and the family to follow the recommendations. Failure of the patient to follow recommendations regarding hospitalization is not essentially different from the situation in which a patient has a myocardial infarction. If the physician continues to care for the patient outside the hospital, he is assuming a medicolegal responsibility of which he should be aware. At the least, an immediate psychiatric consultation should be insisted on.

PHARMACOLOGIC COMPLICATIONS

Patients with glaucoma, prostatic hypertrophy, and pharmacologic complications present a partial contraindication to the use of tricyclics because of the anticholinergic properties of these agents. If the decision is made to use a tricyclic, the patient should be checked regularly. Also, patients with serious cardiac disease should be followed carefully because of possible arrhythmias and ECG changes. The newer antidepressants, trazodone and fluoxetine, have few anticholinergic effects and lower cardiovascular toxicity. Patients may report excessive initial sedation, dryness of mouth, sweating, and constipation. Postural hypotension also is not uncommon. More detailed discussion of the side effects and contraindications for each of the compounds can be found elsewhere.[6]

HORIZONS

The area of affective disorder is involved in major future developments promising helpful clinical tools:

- Research is under way to clarify the role and indications of psychotherapy in the treatment of depression.
- Further biochemical classification of subsyndromes within depressions will help to develop an individual biochemical profile for each depressed patient.
- Newer antidepressant medications are becoming more neurotransmitter-specific and freer of side effects.

REFERENCES

1. Siever, L.: Role of noradrenergic mechanisms in the affective disorders. In Psychopharmacology: The Third Generation of Progress. Edited by Meltzer. New York, Raven Press, 1987.
2. Beck, A.T.: The Diagnosis and Management of Depression. Philadelphia, University of Pennsylvania Press, 1967.
3. Greaves, G., and Small, L.: Comparison of accomplished suicides with persons contacting crisis intervention clinic. Psychol. Res. 3:390, 1972.
4. Bellak, L., and Small, L.: Emergency Psychotherapy and Brief Psychotherapy. New York, Grune and Stratton, 1965.
5. Lindemann, E.: Symptomatology and management of acute grief. Am. J. Psychiatry 101:141, 1944.
6. Bernstein, J.G.: Handbook of Drug Therapy in Psychiatry. Boston, J. Wright, 1983.

ACUTE GRIEF REACTIONS

Jean-Pierre Lindenmayer

CAPSULE

Acute grief reactions are commonly encountered in the Emergency Department (ED). These reactions may involve patients with symptoms of bereavement or, unexpectedly, emergency patients in critical condition and their families. Certain interventions may help with the natural process of adjustment to loss.

RECOGNITION

Acute grief reaction is the normal but painful process that individuals must experience after having lost a close relative or, to a lesser degree, after divorce, separation, or breakup with a lover. The bereavement process has been characterized by Lindemann[1] as having five distinct features:

1. Sensations of somatic distress with a lack of strength, feelings of exhaustion, anorexia, and insomnia.
2. Intense preoccupation with the image of the deceased.
3. Feelings of guilt, with the individual accusing himself of negligence and exaggerating minor omissions.
4. Feelings of hostility, often displaced onto the physician.
5. A change in conduct pattern such as restlessness, moving about aimlessly, or the feeling that all customary activity has now lost its significance.

The acute grief reaction usually lasts for 4 to 6 weeks, but its duration depends on the success with which an individual resolves this ultimate separation from the lost person and readjusts to the environment and the changes brought on by the loss. The individual first attempts to deny the reality of the loss but ultimately must accept the disappearance of the deceased. The separation process is painful and strains the individual's usual coping mechanisms considerably. If this process is avoided, or if the coping mechanisms of the individual fail, pathologic grief reactions are encountered. It is important that the physician be able to recognize pathologic grief reactions as differentiated from depression (Table 62-20) because, if these are

---

TABLE 62-20. DIFFERENTIAL DIAGNOSIS
1. PATHOLOGIC GRIEF REACTION: Intense anger toward lost object; sense of overwhelming helplessness; phobic avoidance of situations reminiscent of the lost person or taking on symptoms of deceased person; severe depression, apathy. 2. DEPRESSION: Sense of helplessness, worthlessness and hopelessness; vegetative signs; lasts much longer than grief reaction.

treated adequately, he or she can help prevent prolonged and serious social and psychologic maladjustments.

Examples of pathologic grief reactions are:

1. Bland acceptance of the loss with delayed grief reaction, the delay ranging from weeks to months, or sometimes occurring at an anniversary of the death.
2. Overactivity without a sense of loss, sometimes resembling activities formerly carried out by the deceased.
3. Taking on the symptoms belonging to the last illness of the deceased.
4. Progressive social isolation, with lack of initiative and inactivity.
5. Strong hostility against persons in the patient's environment, such as the physician who is accused of having neglected the deceased.
6. Self-punitive behavior, such as becoming involved in poor business transactions and other actions detrimental to the patient's economic existence.
7. Agitated depression.

Several factors determine the kind of grief reaction an individual will show. Certainly, the quality of the relationship with the deceased is important. The sex and age of the bereaved, the age of any surviving children, the timeliness of the loss, other crises occurring at the same time, and the presence of supportive relatives are other factors affecting the grief reaction.[2]

MANAGEMENT

The steps in the management of an individual who is experiencing an acute grief reaction are as follows:

1. The patient should first be allowed to ventilate his or her feelings about the suffered loss. Through empathetic listening, the physician can evaluate the quality of the grief reaction. Overreaction or the lack of an appropriate emotional response to the loss should warn the physician of possible difficulties later on. The nature of the loss and its meaning to the patient should be explored, as well as its circumstances. Patients with pathologic grief reactions should be referred for psychiatric consultation.
2. The suicide risk of the bereaved person should be evaluated. If the lost relative has provided the patient's only rewarding and important relationship, or if the latter feels responsible for the death of the relative, suicidal risk can be particularly high. Under these circumstances, psychiatric consultation is mandatory, and hospitalization may be indicated.
3. The bereaved should be encouraged to seek support from relatives. If the patient is alone, relatives or friends should be encouraged to stay with him during the first few days after the loss of the deceased.
4. If the death of the relative occurred in an accident, the bereaved and the family should be given the opportunity to view the body. This is also important for mothers who lose a child pre- or postnatally. *Preventing the bereaved from viewing the body fosters a state of partial denial.*[3]

5. A hypnotic medication may be given for the first few nights to combat insomnia (e.g., Dalmane, 15 to 30 mg, by mouth when retiring). Antidepressant medication should be given only for pathologic grief reaction such as agitated depression.
6. Follow-up appointments should be made so that the physician can continue to support the patient and help him to accept the pain of the bereavement and ultimately resolve it. If pathologic grief reactions appear subsequently, psychiatric referral should be instituted. In addition, the physical health of the bereaved should be monitored carefully during the year after the bereavement because there is often a tendency for marked deterioration of health following the loss of a close relative.

REFERENCES

1. Lindemann, E.: Symptomatology and management of acute grief. Am. J. Psychiatry *101*:141, 1944.
2. Greaves, C., and Chant, L.: Comparison of accomplished suicides with persons contacting crisis intervention clinic. Psychol. Res. *3*:390, 1972.
3. Kubler-Ross, E.: Crisis management of dying persons and their families. *In* Emergency Psychiatric Care. Edited by Resnick, H.L.P., and Ruben, H.L. Bowie, MD, Charles Press, 1975.

ANXIETY OR PANIC DISORDERS

Wayne J. Katon

CAPSULE

Anxiety disorders are among the most frequent problems physicians are called upon to diagnose and treat. A recent study found that, in 11% of visits to several thousand physicians in the United States, the patient's chief complaint was anxiety or nervousness.[1] This high prevalence of complaints of anxiety and nervousness is undoubtedly an underestimate because many patients present with one of the somatic symptoms of anxiety such as rapid heartbeat or chest tightness, or a psychophysiologic symptom caused by autonomic system arousal (diarrhea or epigastric pain).[2] In addition to the overt complaint of nervousness, another large subset of medical patients develop pathologic anxiety as a reaction to a serious medical disorder. This secondary anxiety often leads to amplification of symptoms of that disorder.[3]

One of the major advances in psychiatry in the last 10 years has been the change in the concept of anxiety as a common, unidimensional symptom necessitating treatment with minor tranquilizers to that of a component of several specific, clearly delineated syndromes, each with operationally defined symptoms, time course, and treatment. These syndromes include panic disorder, generalized anxiety disorder, social phobia, agoraphobia, simple phobia, post-traumatic stress disorder, and obsessive-compulsive disorder. This chapter focuses on panic disorder, the syndrome that is most likely to be associated with use of Emergency Department (ED) services. Because of the sudden, severe autonomic nervous system arousal associated with panic disorder, many patients with this disorder seek ED treatment, focusing on one of the frightening somatic components of the disorder.

INTRODUCTION

Patients with panic disorder frequently present to the Emergency Department (ED) because of the episodic, frightening nature of their symptoms. Cardiac, neurologic, and gastrointestinal complaints are common, and associated medical problems include labile hypertension, sinus tachycardia, hyperventilation, peptic ulcer disease, and mitral valve prolapse. Careful questioning about the history of autonomic symptoms of panic disorder, phobic behavior, and depressive symptoms usually allows the physician to make an accurate diagnosis. Specific psychopharmacologic treatments are effective in ameliorating anxiety, somatization, psychophysiologic symptoms (labile hypertension), and decrements in social and vocational functioning.

EPIDEMIOLOGY

Panic disorder is manifested by discrete periods of apprehension and fear and at least four of the following symptoms: palpitations; chest pain or tightness; choking or smothering sensations; dizziness; dyspnea; paresthesias; hot or cold flashes; sweating; faintness; trembling or shaking; derealization or depersonalization experiences; and a fear of dying, going crazy, or doing something uncontrolled during an attack.

Recent community studies have estimated that 1.6 to 2.9% of women and 0.4 to 1.7% of men have panic disorder.[4] Primary care studies have found that these patients are overrepresented in medical clinics, with approximately 6% of primary care patients suffering from panic disorder and/or agoraphobia.[5]

In clinical samples, panic disorder is significantly more common in women than men, with a ratio between 2.5 and 3.0.[4] The highest 6-month prevalence is in the 25-to-44 age group.[4]

Panic disorder tends to be a relapsing, remitting illness. Overall, in follow-up studies of patients with panic disorder and agoraphobia, approximately 50 to 70% of patients show some degree of improvement.[6]

There are three stages in the development of panic disorder. First, several controlled studies have determined that patients with panic disorder have experienced a higher frequency of stressful life events in the 6 months before the development of the syndrome than controls.[4] These stressful events are especially likely to have been perceived as threatening, uncontrollable, and likely to lead to a decrease in self-esteem. After a single or series of stressful events, the patient develops one or a flurry of panic attacks. These first attacks are frightening and often described by the patient as the worst experience of his or her life. With accurate diagnosis and reassurance, some of these patients may not go on to have further attacks. More likely, however, the patient's attacks increase in frequency, and as the patient has more attacks, he or she begins to associate specific environments with these autonomic episodes and may begin to actually avoid specific situations. Thus, if the patient has an attack while driving on a freeway, he or she may begin avoiding freeway driving. These phobias tend to be of social situations, especially situations in which the patient feels that escape would be difficult because of embarrassment or humiliation. Phobias of crowds, eating in public, and riding public transportation are all common.

In this second stage, patients increase their use of medical care, and often present to the physician focusing on one of the specific somatic accompaniments of a panic episode. Physicians try to reassure these patients with statements like, "It's just anxiety, stress, or your nerves." The patient, however, has often experienced significant stress and anxiety before but never had such a severe autonomic episode. These patients often perceive their anxiety or nervousness as secondary to the autonomic symptoms, and unless the diagnosis of panic disorder is made and the physician takes the time to provide careful explanation about the psychobiology of this autonomic disorder, the patient will seek consultation elsewhere.

Finally, some patients move into a third stage of the disorder, agoraphobia. The patient may be fearful of going out of the house unless accompanied by a significant other. These patients are fearful of crowds and many other social situations and often become dependent on their spouses or other companions because of decrements in social and vocational functioning.

DIFFICULTY IN DIAGNOSIS OF PANIC DISORDER

Patients with panic disorder have cognitive, affective and somatic symptoms, and the attacks have social consequences (increased dependency on spouse or other companion, vocational impairment). Because of the severe episodic autonomic symptoms associated with panic disorder, most patients selectively focus on the somatic component of the episode and present with one or more of these complaints.[2,7] In a study of 55 patients referred to psychiatric consultation by primary care physicians, who met DSM-III criteria for panic disorder, three clusters of presenting symptoms were seen.[2] These presenting symptoms included cardiac symptoms (chest pain and tachycardia), gastrointestinal symptoms (epigastric distress and left lower quadrant pain), and neurologic symptoms (headache, dizziness, paresthesias).

The presentation of cardiologic complaints is especially common in panic disorder because the primary symptoms (chest tightness or pain, tachycardia and dyspnea) are cardiorespiratory. These cardiac complaints are especially likely to provoke costly and sometimes invasive medical testing. Three recent studies have documented patients with chest pain and negative angiography testing as having a significantly higher prevalence of panic disorder than patients with chest pain with evidence of coronary artery disease (CAD) on angiography.[8–10] Bass and Wade studied 99 patients with chest pain undergoing coronary angiography.[8] Twenty-eight (61%) of the 46 with insignificant disease had a psychiatric diagnosis, compared to 23% of the 53 with significant obstruction. The most common diagnosis was panic disorder, and 52% of the patients with negative angiograms exhibited polyphobic behavior. Katon and colleagues studied 74 patients with chest pain who were referred to angiography.[9] Using structured psychiatric interviews blind to the angiography results, 43% of the 28 patients with chest pain and normal arteriography results met criteria for panic disorder, compared to 5% of the 46 patients with chest pain who were found to have coronary artery stenosis. Patients with chest pain and normal coronary arteries were found to have significantly more autonomic symptoms (dizziness, tachycardia, shortness of breath) associated with chest pain and were significantly more likely to have atypical chest pain. Beitman and colleagues also found that 43 (58%) of patients with chest pain and negative cardiac studies had panic disorder.[10]

In the first ED study, Wulsin and colleagues have also documented a high prevalence of panic disorder in patients with atypical chest pain.[11] Forty-nine ED patients with atypical chest pain were screened with a short panic disorder screen and 43% were found to meet criteria for panic attacks.

Several other cardiorespiratory symptoms are prominent in patients with panic disorder. These include tachycardia, shortness of breath, and labile hypertension. Patients with panic disorder frequently have higher basal heart rates than controls and episodic tachycardia associated with their anxiety attacks.[4] These patients may be misdiagnosed as having paroxysmal atrial tachycardia (PAT) and started on cardiac medications such as digoxin or a beta-blocker. Careful review of electrocardiograms reveals sinus tachycardia with lower rates than reported in PAT.

Patients with panic can also present with subjective dyspnea but actually are hyperventilating. Blood gas studies have revealed that a large subset of patients with panic disorder are chronically hyperventilating with lower carbon dioxide, bicarbonate, and phosphorus levels than controls.[4] Because of the chronic hyperventilation, slight stresses may lower carbon dioxide levels enough to provoke symptoms such as paresthesias, dizziness and faintness, which frighten the patient and lead to more anxiety. Thus, a vicious cycle of physiologic symptoms, fear, and catastrophic cognitions may be provoked secondary to these somatic symptoms and the subsequent worsened physiologic state.

ASSOCIATED MEDICAL ILLNESS AND PANIC DISORDER

Noyes and colleagues studied the interaction between panic disorder and physical illness by following patients with panic disorder and an outpatient control group over a 6-year period.[12] They found that patients with panic disorder had a significantly higher rate of hypertension and peptic ulcer disease over this period. Katon also found a significantly higher prevalence rate of hypertension in patients with panic disorder compared to primary care controls.[4]

Patients with panic disorder frequently develop labile hypertension with their anxiety attacks. Once these attacks are blocked by psychopharmacologic treatment, the labile hypertension usually subsides. Untreated patients with panic disorder and secondary labile hypertension may develop chronic hypertension that necessitates specific antihypertensive treatment.

Patients with panic disorder have been found to have an increased prevalence of mitral valve prolapse (MVP).[4] A recent review of 17 studies found that 18% of patients with panic disorder or agoraphobia met definite criteria for MVP and 27% met probable criteria for MVP versus an average rate of definite MVP of 1% in normal controls and probable MVP in 12%.[13] These studies must be understood in the context of new research on MVP. Recent studies have suggested that there are two groups of patients with MVP.[14] The first consists of persons in whom the disorder is primarily an echocardiographic finding. These patients are no more symptomatic than controls and have no more arrhythmias and a low risk of complications. The echocardiographic findings in this group are probably anatomic normal variants and reflect the technologic advances in defining valve motion but emphasize the difficulty in differentiating variants of normal valve mobility.[14] The second group consists of patients who typically have not only evidence or prolapse on echocardiography but also clinical findings of mitral valve regurgitation. These people have symptoms related to valvular insufficiency and appear to have an increased risk of infective endocarditis and progressive mitral regurgitation. Two useful markers have been identified to help differentiate between the first group (with trivial MVP) and the second group (with important MVP): (1) the degree of redundancy of the valve, a finding that can be defined echocardiographically; and (2) the presence of mitral regurgitation on physical examination.[14] Nishimura and colleagues recently found that almost every patient with a complication of MVP had redundant valves as indicated by an increase of mitral valve leaflet thickness of 5 mm or more.[15]

Recent evidence has determined that the MVP in patients with panic disorder is generally mild and not associated with thickened mitral valve leaflets (the high-risk group of MVP patients). Patients with panic disorder and MVP have also been found to respond as well as patients with panic disorder alone to treatment with imipramine.[17] The overall findings suggest that panic disorder is associated with an increased prevalence of MVP, but this seems to be a mild type that is principally an echocardiographic finding of little relevance for treatment and not necessitating prophylactic antibiotic treatment.

MEDICAL DIFFERENTIAL DIAGNOSIS

In medical patients with severe panic disorder, the physician should initially focus on any chronic medical illness that may precipitate panic (congestive heart failure, asthma) and review all pharmacologic agents that the patient is taking that could cause panic as a side effect.[18] For instance, a diabetic with a hypoglycemic episode, an asthmatic with a high serum level of aminophylline, and a cardiac patient with a supraventricular arrhythmia may all suffer from anxiety symptoms.

Medical illnesses that can cause symptoms resembling panic attacks include temporal lobe epilepsy, pheochromocytoma, hyperthyroidism, hypoglycemic episodes, mitral valve prolapse, cardiac arrhythmias, caffeinism, pulmonary embolus, electrolyte abnormalities, Cushing's syndrome, and menopausal symptoms.

Screening for illicit drug use is also essential. Both cocaine and marijuana have been implicated in causing panic disorder, and withdrawal from central nervous system depressants (e.g., alcohol, barbiturates, benzodiazepines) and opiates may cause autonomic hyperactivity and mimic panic disorder.[4]

At times, panic disorder occurs concomitantly with a chronic medical illness such as angina pectoris, hypertension, or asthma. Because of the excessive autonomic nervous system activity associated with panic disorder, the physician may see physiologic worsening of a chronic illness secondary to the anxiety attacks.[3] These patients frequently present with increasing resistance to medications that had formerly controlled their medical symptoms.

PSYCHOBIOLOGY OF PANIC DISORDER

Recent psychiatric research has suggested that panic disorder is associated with a biophysiologic abnormality, as demonstrated by the observed familial predisposition, the positive treatment response to specific psychopharmacologic agents, and the specificity of response to provocative agents (lactate, CO_2, clonidine, yohimbine, isoproteronol, and caffeine).[4]

Both normal fear and abnormal anxiety responses involve deep brain structures more than the cerebral cortex specifically; (1) the limbic system (hypothalamus, septum, hippocampus, amygdala, and cingulum); (2) other neuronal bodies including the thalamus, locus ceruleus, median raphe nuclei, and dental/interposital nuclei of the cerebellum; and (3) connections between these structures.[19] Recent research using PET scan, magnetic resonance imaging (MRI) brain imaging techniques and brain electrical activity mapping have implicated temporal lobe abnormalities in panic disorder as well as temporal lobe blood flow changes during normal fear.[4]

Recent research has postulated several competing theories about the genesis of panic attacks, including (1) the locus ceruleus theory; (2) the benzodiazepine-GABA model; (3) the lactate theory; and (4) the CO_2 theory.

LOCUS CERULEUS THEORY

The locus ceruleus (LC) is located in the dorsolateral tegmentum of the pons and contains nearly half of the noradrenergic neurons of the brain. The locus ceruleus is believed to control the sympathetic nervous system and to represent the area of the brain that is associated with alarm reactions to external threatening stimuli.[4] Activation of the LC has been associated with alarm and fear reactions in monkeys, and bilateral lesions of the LC were associated with failure to show normal cardiorespiratory responses to threatening stimuli.[20]

Recent provocative challenge tests with clonidine (which decreases LC activity) and yohimbine (which increases LC activity) have demonstrated an increased oscillatory range in noradrenergic activity in patients with panic disorder compared to controls.[21] These medications are agonists (clonidine) and antagonists (yohimbine) of the inhibitory alpha-2 adrenergic receptory of the LC, leading several researchers to postulate that patients with panic disorder may have abnormalities of their alpha-2 noradrenergic receptor system.[21]

GAMMA-AMINOBUTYRIC ACID-BENZODIAZEPINE HYPOTHESIS

Researchers have discovered brain benzodiazepine receptors that are linked to a receptor of the inhibitory neurotransmitter (GABA).[22] Binding of a benzodiazepine (Bz) to the Bz receptor facilitates the action of GABA, which is known to increase the permeability of chloride ions through the chloride ion channel. The heightened permeability of the cell to chloride ions decreases neuronal excitability by hyperpolarizing the neuronal membrane. These diffuse, inhibitory short GABA-ergic circuits and associated Bz receptors are present throughout the brain and spinal cord. GABA and benzodiazepines have inhibitory effects on the locus ceruleus and may also act to decrease anxiety by modulating the ascending activating systems (serotonergic, noradrenergic, and probably dopaminergic) that are implicated in the expression of fear.[4]

There also appear to be endogenous anxiogenic compounds that act on Bz receptors.[23] Thus, these receptors may mediate both increases and decreases in anxiety. Recent research has found that panic disorder patients may be less sensitive to the catecholamine-reducing effects of anxiolytic Bzs and more sensitive to the effect of Bzs with anxiogenic properties.[23] These results suggest that an abnormality of the Bz receptor may be present in some patients with panic disorder.

LACTATE AND CARBON DIOXIDE THEORIES

Early research in the 1940s and 1950s found that patients with panic disorder could be distinguished from controls by their higher oxygen consumption with vigorous exercise and greater serum lactate production.[4] This finding led to speculation that patients with panic attacks were more sensitive to the effects of lactate than controls. Subsequently, patients with panic disorder have been repeatedly shown to be more sensitive to infusions of 10 mg per kg of 0.5 molar sodium lactate infusions than controls.[24] About 75% of panic disorder patients have anxiety attacks provoked by these infusions, compared to 5% of controls. Interpretation of these findings in explaining an overall theory of the genesis of panic attacks remains controversial, however.[24] One theory suggests that sodium lactate produces nonspecific arousal and uncomfortable bodily sensations in all patients, but that

patients with panic disorder overreact to these stimuli because of their hypervigilance. A biologic explanation postulates that lactate is converted in the body to bicarbonate and CO_2. The CO_2, unlike bicarbonate, crosses the blood-brain barrier, producing a transient intracerebral hypocapnia (causing stimulation of the brain stem chemoreceptors).[25]

CARBON DIOXIDE THEORY

Panic attacks with CO_2-provocative tests are associated with exaggerated ventilatory responses and increases in plasma norepinephrine and diastolic blood pressure.[26] Patients with panic disorder have been postulated to have hypersensitive CO_2 receptors or CO_2 receptors with low set points. When triggered by increasing CO_2, these receptors evoke a subjective anxiety attack associated with an exaggerated ventilatory response and subsequent hypocapnic alkalosis. Patients may "learn" to hyperventilate to maintain low levels of CO_2 and avoid triggering their CO_2 sensors, thus explaining the repeated finding that many patients with panic disorder are chronic hyperventilators.[26]

It is not yet clear which of these theories is correct. Brain neurophysiologic research in the next decade, aided by innovations in brain imaging, promises to help unravel the enigmatic cause of severe anxiety.

TREATMENT

In the context of the ED, where the patient has often presented with a frightening somatic complaint such as tachycardia or chest pain, the first step in treatment is education and negotiation of differing explanatory models.[4] It is often helpful for the physician to describe panic attacks as caused by dysfunction of the autonomic nervous system in which a burst of catecholamines is released into the peripheral circulation, causing symptoms such as tachycardia, chest pain, dyspnea, and dizziness. A further analogy about panic attacks being similar to the flight-or-fight response may help. The patient can be provided with the following explanation: "If you were walking down a dimly lit street and heard a sudden sound behind you, your heart would begin to race, your breathing rate increase, you would feel warm, tense, and shaky and would be prepared to either flee or fight for your life. These attacks that you are having are caused by dysregulation of the same area of the brain that controls the fight-or-flight response, but you are having this alarm or danger response at inappropriate times when there is no danger." This explanation also leads naturally into a discussion of medications that dampen or alleviate the dysregulation of the autonomic nervous system.

Recent double-blind, placebo-controlled studies have documented that three pharmacologic classes of medication are equally effective and significantly more effective than placebo in the treatment of panic disorder:

1. The tricyclic antidepressants
2. The high-potency benzodiazepines
3. The monoamine oxidase inhibitors[27]

In medical patients, the first-line treatment of panic disorder should be the tricyclic antidepressants. These medications are safe, and studies of primary care patients have demonstrated that 50% of patients with panic disorder also have a major depression. Imipramine is the best-studied medication in the treatment of panic disorder, with at least 10 double-blind controlled studies demonstrating its efficacy.[27] Recent studies have also documented that other tricyclics such as desipramine, nortriptyline, amitriptyline, clomipramine, doxepin, and fluoxetine are also effective.[27]

Patients with panic disorder can be started on 25 mg of imipramine or desipramine, with an increase of 25 mg every 2 to 3 days. The endpoint of treatment should be when the patient's panic attacks are completely ameliorated. This usually requires a 100 to 300 mg dosage.

A subgroup of patients with panic disorder develop intolerable side effects on all tricyclic antidepressants. Some of these patients can be treated with minute dosages of tricyclics, 5 to 10 mg initially, with a gradual increase in dosage. Another alternative is to add a low dosage of alprazolam, lorazepam, or clonazapam with the tricyclic, which often decreases the initial anxiety and jitteriness that can be transient side effects of tricyclics. A small subgroup of patients, however, do not tolerate tricyclic antidepressants, and the high-potency benzodiazepines represent an effective second line of treatment. Alprazolam, lorazepam, and clonazepam have all been demonstrated to be more effective than placebo in the treatment of panic disorder. Patients should be started on 0.5 mg of alprazolam bid, with a gradual increase by 0.5 mg increments every 2 to 3 days until panic attacks cease. Equivalent dosages of lorazepam and clonazepam to 0.5 mg. of alprazolam are 1.0 mg of lorazepam and 0.25 mg of clonazepam.[4] One caveat is that patients with prior histories of polydrug or alcohol abuse, personality disorder, or chronic benign pain probably should not be treated with benzodiazepines because of potential problems with abuse.

Monoamine oxidase inhibitors are potentially the most effective medications for panic disorder, but the lack of familiarity of most physicians with these medications and the potential "hypertensive crisis" that can ensue when the patient does not follow a low-tyramine diet preclude their regular use in primary care. In a patient who has not responded to a tricyclic antidepressant or benzodiazepine, psychiatric consultation may be helpful.

REFERENCES

1. Schurman, R.A., Kramer, P.D., and Mitchel, J.B.: The hidden mental health network: Treatment of mental illness by non-psychiatrist physicians. Arch. Gen. Psychiatry 42:89, 1985.
2. Katon, W.: Panic disorder and somatization: A review of 55 cases. Am. J. Med. 77:101, 1984.
3. Katon, W., and Roy-Byrne, P.P.: Panic disorder in the medically ill. J. Clin. Psychiatry 50:299, 1989.
4. Katon, W.: Panic Disorder In the Medical Setting. Rockville, MD, U.S. Department of Health and Human Services, Public Health Service, Alcohol, Drug Abuse and Mental Health Administration, 1989.
5. Katon, W., Vitaliano, P.P., Russo, J., et al.: Panic disorder: Epidemiology in primary care. J. Fam. Pract. 23:233, 1986.
6. Reich, J.: The epidemiology of anxiety. J. Nerv. and Ment. Dis. 176:300, 1988.
7. Clancy, J., and Noyes, R.: Anxiety neurosis: A disease for the medical model. Psychosomatics 17:90, 1976.
8. Bass, C., and Wade, C.: Chest pain with normal coronary arteries: A comparative study of psychiatric and social morbidity. Psychosom. Med. 14:51, 1984.
9. Katon, W., Hall, M.L., Russo, J., et al.: Chest pain: Relationship of psychiatric illness to coronary arteriographic results. Am. J. Med. 84:1, 1988.
10. Beitman, B.D., Basha, I., Flaker, G., et al.: Atypical or non-anginal chest pain: Panic disorder or coronary artery disease. Arch. Intern. Med. 147:1548, 1987.
11. Wulsin, L.R., Hillard, J.R., Geier, P., et al.: Screening emergency room patients with atypical chest pain for depression and panic disorder. Int. J. Psychiatry Med. 18:315, 1988.
12. Noyes, R., and Clancy, J.: Anxiety neurosis: A 5-year follow-up. J. Nerv. Ment. Dis. 162:200, 1976.
13. Margraff, J., Ehlers, A., and Roth, W.T.: Mitral valve prolapse and panic disorder: A review of their relationship. Psychosom. Med. 40:93–113, 1988.
14. Wynne, J.: Mitral valve prolapse. N. Engl. J. Med. 314:577, 1986.
15. Nishimura, R.A., McGoon, M.D., Shub, C., et al.: Echocardiographically documented mitral-valve prolapse: Long-term follow-up of 237 patients. N. Engl. J. Med. 313:1305, 1985.
16. Gorman, J.M., Geotz, R.R., Fyer, M., et al.: The mitral valve prolapse-panic disorder connection. Psychosom. Med. 50:114, 1988.
17. Gorman, J.M., Fyer, A.F., Gliklick, J., et al.: Effect of imipramine on prolapsed mitral valves of patients with panic disorder. Am. J. Psychiatry 138:977, 1981.
18. Rosenbaum, J.F.: The drug treatment of anxiety. N. Engl. J. Med. 7:401, 1982.
19. Marks, I.M.: Fear, Phobias and Rituals: Panic, Anxiety and Their Disorders. New York, Oxford University Press, 1987, pp. 190–191.
20. Svensson, T.H.: Peripheral, autonomic regulation of locus coeruleus noradrenergic neurons in brain: Putative implications for psychiatry and psychopharmacology. Psychopharmacology 92:1, 1987.
21. Charney, D.S., and Heninger, G.R.: Abnormal regulation of noradrenergic function in panic disorders. Arch. Gen. Psychiatry 43:1042, 1986.
22. Insel, T.R., Ninan, P.T., Aloi, J., et al.: Bz receptors and anxiety in non-human primates. Arch. Gen. Psychiatry 41:741, 1984.
23. Roy-Byrne, P.P., and Cowley, D.: Panic disorder: Biological aspects. Psychiatric Annals 18:457, 1988.
24. Margraf, J., Anke, E., and Roth, W.T.: Sodium lactate infusions and panic attacks: A review and critique. Psychosom. Med. 48:23, 1986.
25. Carr, D.B., and Sheehan, D.V.: Panic anxiety: A new biological model. J. Clin. Psychiatry 45:323, 1984.
26. Gorman, J.M., Fyer M.R., Goetz, R., et al.: Ventilatory phys-

iology of patients with panic disorder. Arch. Gen. Psychiatry 45:31, 1988.

27. Lydiard, R.B.: Panic disorder: Pharmacologic treatment. Annals of Psychiatry 18:468, 1988.

PSYCHIATRIC EMERGENCIES IN SEVERELY ILL MEDICAL, SURGICAL, OR OBSTETRIC PATIENTS

Jean-Pierre Lindenmayer and Nathan S. Kline

CAPSULE

Severe medical, surgical, or obstetric illness presents a major psychologic and physical stress for the patient and requires the mobilization of a maximum of coping abilities. The patient must adapt to the loss of function that results from the illness, the demands of confinement in a hospital, and the demands of multiple diagnostic or surgical procedures. Although cooperation with the treatment recommended by the physician is not always easy, it is essential. If these coping strategies are called on too abruptly, or if the patient fails to respond to these many demands, an emergency situation can result wherein the patient's psychologic or physical health is acutely endangered.

In addition, other factors associated with the patient's lack of coping abilities may lead to emergency situations. The attitudes and reactions of the physician, and also those of the family, may contribute to creating an emergency, and therefore must be considered as well.

PSYCHOLOGIC RESPONSES TO PHYSICAL ILLNESS

REACTIONS TO THE ILLNESS

Disruption of somatic well-being causes anxiety in every normal human being and brings about various degrees of feelings of helplessness, particularly when the condition occurs suddenly, reactions tend to be more severe. To cope with this anxiety, the patient may demonstrate less mature forms of behavior that can be more or less adaptive. The main reaction is in the area of dependency, with some patients reacting in an overly dependent fashion. Others, fearful of dependency, feel that they may be made helpless by their illness and therefore try to minimize its reality and the need for treatment. Other reactions may be depression, denial, lack of cooperation, agitated anxiety, exaggerated pain reactions, prolonged convalescence, and drug dependence. The degree with which these forms of behavior appear depends on the severity and nature of the illness, the patient's pre-existing level of psychologic functioning, and the psychosocial environment (including the medical staff and the patient's family). All these reactions are used by the patient to reduce anxiety about his or her physical illness and what it represents. Sometimes illness can pose a major threat to the patient's self-image as an independent, self-sufficient individual, or it may revive strong underlying wishes to be taken care of. The physician is then seen as a protective, omnipotent authority who will take care of the patient.

The anxieties related to illness are obviously greatest when the patient is threatened by a life-threatening disease (e.g., terminal cancer). Such patients are brought to emergency departments (EDs) as the progression of the disease results in severe pain or a medical crisis. The prospect of death, a universal fear, can be overwhelming to the patient, producing a helpless and lonely feeling, particularly if his family and physician shy away from him because of their own fear of death. Patients cope with this fear in various ways, often in a manner similar to the way they have handled previous separation experiences. Doctor-patient relationships in these circumstances are particularly important.

The difficulties related to illness also are significant when they force the patient to adjust to radical changes in lifestyle. A patient with myocardial infarction compelled to reduce activities may develop a depression. A patient in chronic renal failure who has to reorganize life around frequent dialysis may respond by neglecting his diet.

Other factors influencing the patient's reaction to illness are his expectations and anticipations about treatment. These attitudes may include both negative and positive aspects. This applies particularly to surgical procedures for which the patient may have unrealistic expectations that can lead to disappointment and more severe reactions.

REACTIONS TO THE HOSPITAL

Anxieties also determine, in part, reactions to the hospital environment and the medical procedures related to the illness. The two extreme reactions are (1) the patient who wants to sign out against medical advice; and (2) the patient who tries to postpone discharge in direct or indirect ways. Both reactions are extreme positions on the spectrum of dependence: In the former, the patient cannot tolerate dependence and is afraid of losing his personal freedom; in the latter, the patient's dependency needs are satisfied by the hospital, and he does not want to give up this gratification. All other reactions can be placed between these two extremes. Some patients make continuous special demands, and are easily annoyed and critical of the staff, picking fights with them in every available situation. Other patients may be overly clinging and dependent, exaggerating their physical complaints without clear organic causes, and may turn the staff against them through their excessive demands and overutilization of available services. Other factors that contribute to anxieties regarding hospitalization can be the temporary separation from family and the newness and strangeness of the environment of the hospital, with its particular and peculiar pattern combining sensory deprivation and overstimulation.

REACTIONS TO SURGERY

Anxieties related to a surgical experience are certainly common and appropriate, but if they provoke an exaggerated emotional response or are handled by the patient inappropriately, they can lead at times to emergency situations, necessitating intervention by the physician. These anxieties are usually related to the real or symbolic meaning of the particular organ involved in surgery, to the loss of control resulting from anesthesia, or to other underlying fantasies and expectations. The reactions can be classified into (1) preoperative and (2) postoperative syndromes.

PREOPERATIVE SYNDROMES

These can range from utter and supreme calmness to panic and overt psychosis.[1] Such reactions are related to the anticipation the patient feels about the surgery, usually a mixture of hope and despair.[2]

POSTOPERATIVE SYNDROMES

These consist of a heterogeneous group of reactions, such as depressions, anxiety states, paranoid states, and postoperative delirium. Accurate prognosticators for postoperative psychiatric complications are the patient's unrealistic expectations of surgery, the major use of denial, and excessive preoperative anxiety.[3] Other factors involved are age (patients over 65 years are more susceptible), the duration and depth of anesthesia, the type of surgical intervention, and the degree of organic impairment caused by the surgery as well as the preoperative degree of organic brain disturbance.

FAMILY'S REACTION TO PATIENT'S ILLNESS

The patient's illness also represents an additional stress for the family, for whom this new situation can create various problems. If the family's coping abilities fail in dealing with these, the result can certainly provoke an emergency situation for the patient. These problems depend on the nature of the relationship of the patient with his family, the nature and duration of the illness, and the family's cohesiveness. Frequent reactions of family members are feelings of guilt for not having sent the patient earlier for medical attention or feelings of resentment for being deprived of the patient's support and help. Even the inconvenience of hospital visits sometimes can produce considerable irritation, leading the family to minimize the patient's complaints, possibly leading to premature discharge from the hospital. The withdrawal of family support can contribute to exacerbations of the illness or create emergency situations. In one case, a young woman with lupus erythematosus had been stabilized successfully with appropriate medical treatment. When her discharge was planned, it became clear that her mother did not want to take her back into her family because of various negative feelings she had about her daughter and the illness. The daughter subsequently developed an acute psychotic reaction that required psychiatric intervention.

PHYSICIAN'S REACTION TO PATIENT'S ILLNESS

An emergency situation may be a result not only of the nature of the patient's condition and the ways he deals with it but also of some sudden reaction or change in the physician's attitude toward the patient or his or her illness. A particularly dependent and demanding patient, turned away by an impatient physician, may resort to bizarre behavior to gain the physician's attention. Another chronically ill patient may react with intense depression and withdrawal after his or her house staff physician has been rotated to another floor or has taken an unannounced vacation. At times, it is actually the physician who determines whether an emergency situation will or will not result. For example, a 23-year-old woman with chronic renal failure had been treated on a medical floor for several weeks. Her hospital course was punctuated by several minor psychotic episodes, during which she would wander off the floor, show severe paranoid ideation, and cause considerable disruption in ward routine. Unwisely, psychiatric consultation was delayed and finally requested on an emergency basis only when she attempted suicide.

GENERAL PRINCIPLES OF MANAGEMENT

PSYCHOLOGIC MANAGEMENT

The most important factor is the quality of the doctor-patient relationship. The physician should be compassionate and understanding toward the patient, showing that he is an ally, not an antagonist. Communications should be in terms the patient can understand. It may be necessary to repeat to the patient several times *who* the physician is, *where* the patient is, and *what* the purpose of the examination is. This is particularly important if the patient is paranoid or delirious.

Once initial contact has been established, the physician should discuss some of the facts relevant to the present illness and gradually inquire about the patient's feelings toward the illness and how it has affected or will affect his or her present and future life. Realistic and unrealistic expectations about the illness and its treatment should be discussed. This is especially important for patients involved in surgical procedures. If the patient shows excessive denial of underlying feelings of anxiety, *this should be left untouched*. In other words, the patient should *not* be forced to "face" his or her illness if he or she chooses to deal with the problem by denial.

In contrast, other patients may wish to know all the details. In any case, questions that the patient may ask about diagnostic and therapeutic procedures should be answered, whenever possible and appropriate, in a straightforward and open fashion, because this often helps reduce his anxiety considerably. Throughout the interview, the physician will be able to gather data in this more or less "unstructured" fashion to judge the patient's mental status. Questioning should also include inquiries into the possibility of suicidal ideation and in all cases should be directed toward an assessment of the patient's state of orientation. This last point, together with the evaluation of the patient's memory function, may help establish the presence of an organic brain syndrome.

In addition to gathering information from the patient, the physician should ask the nursing staff for their observations of the individual's behavior. Because the nurses are in constant contact with the patient, they usually have valuable information to contribute. It may be important to interview the family if the emergency has been precipitated by some change in the domestic situation.

DISPOSITION

Evaluation of the patient's medical and mental status leads to a decision about disposition. The physician may decide that additional support and clarification, together with sedative medication, are sufficient to bring the situation under control. In some cases, however, psychiatric consultation may be required.

If suicide risk is prominent, precautions must be taken, such as 24-hour nursing, removal of sharp objects, and locking of windows. A patient who is violent or who wanders off the ward may have to be restrained. It should be kept in mind, however, that restraints sometimes increase, rather than decrease, the agitation. Often, when restraints are required, they can be discontinued after a relatively brief period in certain patients. The patient should be evaluated after a half hour or so to determine whether restraints must be continued. A patient with "acute brain syndrome," or delirium, should have his environment simplified as much as possible. It is helpful to have one nurse, familiar to the patient, take care of him, rather than rotate nurses automatically according to hospital routine.

CONSIDERATIONS IN PSYCHIATRIC CONSULTATION

When requesting a psychiatric consultation, it is imperative that the physician be clear about the following two points so that both the physician and the patient may receive maximal benefit: (1) What are the reasons for psychiatric consultation, and are they spelled out clearly for the psychiatrist? (2) Has the physician adequately prepared the patient to be seen by a psychiatrist?

INDICATIONS FOR PSYCHIATRIC CONSULTATION

It is important that the physician decide what the objectives of such a consultation should be and what kind of problems he wants solved by the psychiatrist, who otherwise might focus on aspects with which the physician is less concerned. The major indications for such a request, limited to the context of emergency care, are as follows:

1. A mental condition that substantially interferes with necessary medical treatment.
2. An acute pre- or postoperative syndrome that interferes with proper surgical treatment (e.g., pulling out transfusion needles).
3. Suicidal or homicidal tendencies.

4. Acute psychosis in a patient who presents major management problems on the ward, such as wandering off the floor, going into other patients' rooms, and picking fights with the staff.

PREPARATION OF PATIENT FOR CONSULTATION

Adequate preparation is important for several reasons. Usually, the consultation is requested by the physician and therefore is an involuntary procedure for the patient. The latter may have various ambivalent feelings about seeing a psychiatrist, ranging from indifference to anxiety to total refusal to speak to the consultant. These feelings should be clarified as much as possible by discussing them with the patient and by informing him of the purpose of the consultation.

PSYCHOPHARMACOLOGIC MANAGEMENT

If severe panic and agitation are present, sedation with a psychotropic agent may be necessary. Acute psychotic productions, such as delusions and hallucinations, should be controlled by medication. In the use of these drugs, the patient's medical condition and possible side effects must be taken into careful account. In addition, the patient's vital signs and neurologic status should be as stable as possible when such treatment is instituted.

Low doses of phenothiazines of the sedative type, such as chlorpromazine, should be given parenterally. If the medical status permits it, a dosage schedule beginning with 25 mg administered intramuscularly every 4 hours should be established, with the dose increased, if necessary, by 25-mg steps every 4 hours until the patient is sufficiently sedated yet fully arousable. Because of the hypotensive effect of chlorpromazine, the blood pressure should be taken before and between each dose, and the next dose should be withheld if there is a significant drop in blood pressure. Once the dose that gives the required effect is reached, the physician should give that dose orally on a 6-hour basis. If there are reasons to anticipate seizures, paraldehyde can be administered intramuscularly instead of a phenothiazine. With elderly patients and those with cerebrovascular problems for whom hypotensive effects are particularly undesirable, a butyrophenone like haloperidol can be given, starting with 0.5 to 1.0 mg administered orally four times daily or 0.5 to 1 mg given intramuscularly every 30 to 60 minutes. In elderly patients, one must use sedating medications with caution, beginning with the lowest dose and increasing only as needed. Benzodiazepines such as chlordiazepoxide are suitable for short-term use: 10 mg given intramuscularly every 2 to 4 hours usually is sufficient in the acute stage, with transfer to oral dose as soon as the patient is stabilized.

The more frequent side effects of the phenothiazines are extrapyramidal symptoms, such as dyskinesia, pseudoparkinsonism, and akathisia. An antiparkinsonian agent (benztropine, procyclidine, or biperiden) effectively helps control these effects. Postural hypotension is another frequent side effect, although this usually does not constitute a problem because patients with this condition are kept at bed rest. Occasionally, more severe hypotension can develop, particularly with high doses of intramuscular medication. For a patient with cardiovascular disease, the doses should be increased more slowly, and the blood pressure should be monitored more frequently. If a hypotensive episode develops, vasopressor medication such as norepinephrine may be indicated. *Epinephrine, however, is contraindicated* because it may accentuate the hypotension.

No specific teratogenic effects arising from the use of phenothiazines during pregnancy have been reported. These medications, therefore, can be used during pregnancy when essential. Both an extrapyramidal and a postnatal depression syndrome, followed by agitation in the newborn, have been noted, however.[4]

SYNDROMES AND THEIR MANAGEMENT

ACUTE REACTIONS IN INTENSIVE CARE UNITS

Medical and surgical intensive care units (ICUs) present for most patients a rather new and frightening environment: isolation from familiar persons as well as sensory monotony with transient overstimulation and sleep deprivation because of the constant activity of staff and the various monitoring devices. Stabilizing natural day and night patterns are similarly altered, particularly when there are no windows in the ICU. Patients usually react to these new demands with anxiety and, to a greater or lesser degree, with denial.[5] The effect of confinement in such units, together with the physiologic defects arising from the underlying illness, can lead to acute psychiatric emergencies. In addition, ICU staff may contribute to patient problems through overconcern with technical aspects and avoidance of interpersonal contact with the patient.

The most severe reaction is delirium (acute organic brain syndrome), which is characterized by disorientation with respect to time, place, and person; fluctuating states of consciousness; and disturbed mood, ranging from severe agitation to depression. These syndromes occur particularly after cardiac surgery and in the elderly patient.

Other acute reactions include paranoid reactions in which the patient may feel that the staff and the physician are against him or that the treatment he is receiving is actually detrimental to him (e.g., medication is poisoned, food is contaminated, and he is "being experimented with"). At times, this may lead the patient to refuse necessary procedures or treatment and to want to sign out against medical advice. Acute states of depression and anxiety states are also encountered frequently. If the patient is not in contact with reality, the physician must help him appraise the situation more correctly by reducing overstimulation, explaining carefully and simply whatever is being done, and providing appropriate information and reassurance. When agitation and high levels of anxiety are present, tranquilizing medication and night-time sedation should be used carefully. In such situations, the drugs of choice are the benzodiazepines. Sudden decreases in such agitation may result in excess physiologic depression because formerly adequate doses of medication now become excessive. If the patient's mental state interferes in a major way with his or her medical or surgical treatment, psychiatric consultation should be requested.

ACUTE REACTIONS TO RENAL DIALYSIS AND TRANSPLANTATION

RENAL DIALYSIS

For patients with progressive end-stage kidney disease, maintenance hemodialysis is usually the major treatment modality that will prolong life. Adaptation to both the disease itself and the treatment can be demanding and difficult for the patient as well as for the family. The treatment usually requires that the patient spend 6 to 8 hours, two or three times a week, attached to the dialysis machine. This invariably leads to feelings of intense dependence on the machine, which the patient perceives on one hand as a lifesaving and sustaining apparatus yet on the other hand as a severe limitation to freedom and a constant reminder of his or her extreme fragility. The illness and treatment also require from both patient and family drastic changes in their usual life pattern so that all concerned can adjust to the new situation. In addition, there is the constant hope for an eventual kidney transplant or, if this has already been done, the continuous fear of possible rejection. If adaptation to these multiple demands and stresses fails, various acute psychiatric problems can develop that may aggravate the already difficult situation significantly, such as: (1) delirium (acute organic brain syndromes); (2) depressive states; and (3) anxiety states.[6]

Delirium (Acute Organic Brain Syndromes). The patient presents states of confusion of various degrees that alternate with more lucid intervals and that usually are accompanied by cognitive impairments, such as problems in orientation, reduced attention span, and difficulties in recognizing familiar faces and environments. In more severe forms there are hallucinations, mainly of the visual type, and delusions, often of the persecutory type. There is always some lability of affect, ranging from agitated perplexity to absent-minded withdrawal.

Renal and extrarenal factors, such as infections or cardiac and pulmonary decompensations, can lead to this syndrome. It is important to recognize the underlying organic cause and correct it because this syndrome is usually reversible. In his approach to these patients, the physician should help them appraise reality correctly by, for example, repeating *where* the patient is, *who* the physician is, and *what* his function is. Reassurance, structure, and support should be provided for the patient. If agitation is severe and prevents proper medical treatment, a phenothiazine or benzodiazepine may be indicated and should be used as described in the previous section.

Acute Depressive States. These states are seen most commonly in association with acute medical and social problems.[6] Patients express feelings of hopelessness and helplessness, and sometimes anger at the physician or the staff, because of the need to endure chronic dialysis and to lose their autonomy. Suicidal preoccupation, with actual direct or indirect suicide attempts, is particularly frequent among patients on maintenance dialysis.[7]

The physician should attempt to clarify, in a supportive fashion, some of the underlying reasons for the patient's depression, because there are often real family, social, and financial difficulties. The physician should also carefully explore suicidal preoccupations that may be indirect, such as the deliberate neglect of dietary restrictions. For continuous supportive treatment, psychiatric consultation is usually required. Antidepressant medication can be used to alleviate some of the symptoms of the depression.

Anxiety States. Acute anxiety reactions or panic states are often related to the sense of danger produced by the dialysis procedure, in which the patient sees his blood continually flowing out and back again through a complex system of machinery.[6] The physician can be of great help to the patient by identifying such fears in a supportive fashion and correcting them through appropriate information if they are a result of distortions of reality. Also, speaking to other patients who have adapted to the procedure successfully can help reduce the anxieties of the patient. Minor tranquilizers can also contribute to overcoming a transiently difficult situation. If the fears and anxieties continue to be manifested, psychiatric consultation is indicated.

RENAL TRANSPLANTATION

Acute reactions after the transplantation procedure are rather infrequent, particularly compared with reactions after cardiac transplantation. Occasionally, depressive states can be observed related to a constant concern over possible rejection or ambivalence over accepting the donor's kidney (living or cadaver transplant). These depressive states can be particularly severe and accompanied by suicidal ideation in patients who have rejected their transplant and, while awaiting new ones, are thus forced to resume chronic dialysis.[8] Another factor that can affect the patient's adaptation to the transplant is steroid medication used for immunosuppression, which may produce a steroid psychosis or the typical Cushing "moon face."

If such difficulties arise, psychiatric consultation is usually indicated to help the patient achieve better psychologic acceptance of his or her transplant. This is especially important if the patient has to go back on chronic dialysis.

ACUTE REACTIONS TO HEART SURGERY

PREOPERATIVE REACTIONS

Cardiac surgery, with its threat to life and its symbolic implications, represents a major challenge to the patient's coping abilities. The heart certainly occupies a central position in the patient's conception of his or her body and is directly related to his or her very existence. Particular coping mechanisms are mobilized by the patient so that he or she can deal with the stress related to cardiac surgery. Immobilization, hysterical amnesia or depersonalization, belligerence, excitement, and denial are used.[9] Other reactions, such as preoperative depression and anxiety states, have been correlated with the postoperative course. The highest mortality has been found among preoperatively depressed patients, and the greatest morbidity has been observed among preoperatively anxious patients.[10]

Adequate preoperative preparation of the patient is important to reduce the intensity and frequency of these reactions. A good patient-doctor relationship is vital. The physician should help clarify some of the patient's preoperative expectations. Psychiatric intervention may be needed if the reaction is severe and endangers the postoperative course.

POSTOPERATIVE REACTIONS

The most severe psychiatric complication after cardiac surgery is a postoperative psychosis, usually delirium (acute organic brain syndrome). It is characterized by impairment of orientation, memory, intellectual function, and judgment, and by lability of affect.[11] Sometimes a schizophrenia-like psychosis can be observed; these states are related etiologically to a number of factors, ranging from organic factors causing CNS dysfunction to the particular ICU environment, factors related to the intensive anxiety of having an operation on the heart, and the fear of death. Most of these states are transient and usually clear up after a few days.

Another postoperative reaction resembles a "catastrophic" response, with the patient lying immobile with an affectless mask, cooperating passively with the staff, and responding monosyllabically to questions.[10] These reactions clear after 4 to 5 days, with the patient experiencing amnesia regarding the episode.

The physician must provide reassurance and support during this difficult period. If the patient is disoriented, it is helpful to indicate where he is, what the purpose of the medical procedures is, and who the physician is. It is also important to keep the environment as simple and constant as possible, because the patient's cognitive capacities are greatly impaired. If suicidal ideation is present, precautions should be taken to protect the patient, and psychiatric consultation should be requested. Psychotropic medication should be used cautiously and sparingly, in view of the delicate cardiovascular and pulmonary situation.

REACTIONS TO PLASTIC SURGERY

Acute psychologic reactions after plastic surgery are not infrequent, particularly after interventions that involve the face. Acute psychotic states of a schizophrenic type and depressions with feelings of hopelessness may be encountered. These reactions can be understood as resulting from abrupt changes in the body image that the patient cannot tolerate. In some cases, the patient may have had unrealistic expectations about the results of the surgery, hoping that it would solve all his interpersonal problems. As a rule, the less prominent the preoperative disfigurement and the more it is used to cover severe personality difficulties, the greater is the likelihood of adverse psychologic reactions.[12]

In most cases, psychiatric consultation is necessary. This is especially important if further plastic surgical interventions are contemplated.

REACTIONS TO AMPUTATION

The loss of a body part through amputation can occasionally result in psychologic reactions similar to those seen with other significant losses. These patients can present the physician with postoperative depressions characterized by feelings of hopelessness and helplessness, preoccupation with death, and not infrequently with suicide.[13] This syndrome is seen particularly in elderly patients for whom amputation "seems to symbolize the encroachment of death."[13] Other reactions to amputation include defiance, regression, and fears resulting from nonacceptance.[14] Later, patients commonly report phantom sensations or the perception of a phantom limb. These phenomena are related to the persistence, after the amputation, of the mental representation of the intact model of the body. Such patients are rarely seen on an emergency basis unless pain is a component of their sensation.

The depressive reactions are caused partly by unrealistic preoperative expectations; patients have either tended to minimize the effect of the amputation or hoped that the amputation would be a total cure for their illness. It is therefore important, if possible, to clarify the expectations of the patient preoperatively and to rectify them in a nontraumatic way. In handling postoperative reactions, the physician should support and repeatedly point out that the reality of the situation does not correspond with the gloomy picture the patient may paint. Antidepressant medication, such as doxepin, amitryptyline, or imipramine, also may be indicated. If the depression interferes with the proper postoperative progress, or if suicidal ideation is present, psychiatric consultation should be requested.

ACUTE REACTIONS TO COLOSTOMY

After colostomy, a patient experiences serious changes in body form and function that cause new, often stressful challenges to his or her coping abilities. He or she must adapt to the loss of a psychologically valued organ; to the loss of a basic body control function; to a radically changed body image; and to the colostomy training, with its possible restrictive family and social implications. These stresses can threaten or disrupt the patient's usual coping abilities and lead to acute psychiatric difficulties.

The most frequent acute reaction is a postoperative depression, characterized by feelings of personal inadequacy and helplessness and by disturbances of eating and sleeping patterns and of sexual function. It often is precipitated by the initial sight of the colostomy, which is perceived as a mutilation and disfigurement.[15] The patient becomes concerned and fearful about possible spillage and other problems related to the colostomy, and how the environment will react to it; he also may show suicidal ideation. Later on, a marked sense of weakness out of proportion to the patient's physical state can be found and may lead to severe restrictions of activities and social withdrawal.[15]

If possible, time should be spent by the surgeon in the preoperative phase—establishing a supportive and trusting patient-doctor relationship. The patient should be helped with verbalizing preoperative expectations and fears about the surgery, and accurate information should be given when appropriate. Fears and distorted preoccupations expressed in a postoperative depression should be corrected in a supportive fashion by the physician. The effect of the colostomy on the patient's family, work situation, and other social involvements must also be explored. Other staff members can help the patient regain some degree of self-esteem through bowel control by colostomy training. If the depression continues in spite of these supportive approaches, psychiatric intervention is necessary. After the initial crisis has been resolved, the patient also may benefit from participation in colostomy clubs, which provide continuous support on a long-term basis.

ACUTE REACTIONS TO EYE SURGERY

A patient whose eyes have been bilaterally bandaged after some form of eye surgery not infrequently presents a postoperative psychosis ("black patch delirium"). He or she appears restless, anxious, and suspicious. He or she is disoriented with regard to time and place and may misidentify people around him or her and replace them with familiar figures from the home or work environment. Sometimes there may be delusions with persecutory content, auditory and visual hallucinations, and (rarely) suicidal ideation. This syndrome usually begins early in the postoperative period and is often worse at night, when auditory cues that helped the patient orient himself or herself are less available. Elderly patients are particularly susceptible.

In the management of such a syndrome, the quality of the doctor-patient relationship is of central importance.[16] The physician should offer some of the correct appraisal of the visual reality that the patient is unable to provide for himself any longer owing to his temporary blindness. He can begin by explaining preoperatively to the apprehensive patient both the operative procedures and what is to be expected once the bilateral masking has been applied. Postoperatively, the physician must help the patient in a literal sense to reorient, because reality orientation is temporarily severely limited. This can be done by using other perceptual channels that are not impaired and by providing the patient with auditory, gustatory, tactile, and olfactory perceptual cues.[16] It should be pointed out repeatedly to the patient where he or she is and who the people are around him or her and the room and surroundings should be described. If possible, arrangements should be made to have a family member stay at the bedside. It also is helpful to have the same nurse take care of the patient, as far as possible.

ACUTE REACTIONS TO MASTECTOMY

RECOGNITION

Women who undergo mastectomy for carcinoma of the breast have to adjust to the loss of an important organ that has various meanings to them; to a significant change of their body image; and to the frightening possibility of having a deadly disease. These adjustments are difficult and can lead at times to acute psychiatric problems. A frequent reaction is a postmastectomy depression, characterized by anxiety, insomnia, feelings of shame and worthlessness, and occasional ideas of suicide or actual attempts.[20] Underlying themes to this depression are mainly twofold: (1) the mourning over the loss of the breast, which is the most visual and most valued evidence of the woman's sexuality; and (2) the fear of having lost major attributes of the mothering role, since the breast represents the nurturing function. The younger woman still in her childbearing years is more prone to this syndrome than is the older, postclimacteric woman. For the latter, the difficulties lie more in adjusting to the possible malignant disease and the threat of death. The depression is most extreme in women who have invested irrational, disproportionate pride or shame in their breasts.[20]

MANAGEMENT

The proper management of the surgeon-patient relationship is of great importance. The surgeon must take time to discuss with the patient some of her anxieties and fears with regard to her perceived loss of femininity and to the presence of a possible malignant tumor. He should approach the patient with support and understanding, pointing out the reality when the patient appears to distrust it. If he does not feel comfortable in doing this, a psychiatric consultation may be more appropriate. In addition, antidepressant medication can be helpful at times.

The patient's husband also should be involved if he is available. He should be told about the pre- and postoperative feelings his wife will have to deal with, particularly that she may be afraid that he may reject her because of her mastectomy. He should be encouraged to focus, in his interactions with his wife, on her past and still-present feminine achievements. He also should be instructed and prepared for the sight of the operative scar and should learn to treat it in a casual way.

The other major issue for the mastectomy patient is coping with the prognosis of her illness, which in turn depends on how far it has progressed when treatment is begun. If the prognosis is compromised, the question of how to deal with terminal illness will involve both patient and physician. This is discussed in the preceding section of this chapter.

REACTIONS TO DEATH AND DYING

ATTITUDES TOWARD DEATH AND DYING

Facing and, to the extent possible, accepting death is a difficult and frightening task for the terminally ill patient and all those involved in his or her care. How it is accomplished is determined largely by the attitude toward death of the patient, the family, and the physician as well as the surrounding staff. These attitudes, to a large extent, are related to the underlying fear of death present in every human being and to the meaning a given individual attaches to death. For some patients it may mean isolation and loneliness, for some it may represent a punishment, and for others it may awaken repressed childhood fears of abandonment. The intensity of the fear of death and the pre-existing personality traits together determine the way each individual deals with death and dying. One of the chief coping mechanisms is denial. By stating, "this doesn't happen to me, only to my neighbor," by be-

coming feverishly busy with medical machinery around dying patients, by avoiding talk with terminally ill patients, some physicians and nurses attempt to deny their own fear of death and the finality of the end of life.

Other attitudes toward death and dying may include the view that death represents a reunion with beloved ones in a world after death and that it represents a relief, a reward, or an act of cosmic retribution.[17] It is important that the physician first examine his own attitudes toward death when dealing with terminally ill patients. This, in turn, will help him better understand his patients' attitudes and fears and will allow him to assist them through their terminal illness and to death with dignity. Ignoring these issues and avoiding the patient only increase the latter's despair and sense of isolation, sometimes to the point of precipitating a crisis situation.

REACTIONS TOWARD DEATH AND DYING

Kübler-Ross[18] has described a sequence of five stages that can be seen as typical coping mechanisms of patients dealing with death. They can occur in sequence or may be present to various degrees at the same time. After an initial temporary state of shock, the patient attempts to deny his fatal illness and then may postpone seeking help. This denial is replaced by feelings of anger, rage, envy, and resentment over the fatal, uncontrollable course that life is taking. This anger often is projected on the outside, on family and staff, which may increase the patient's isolation. This is followed by the "bargaining" stage, in which patients try to have some special favor fulfilled by God, usually some extension of life, in return for good behavior. Depression is the next stage, with feelings of sadness regarding the impending loss of loved ones and everything achieved in life. During this phase of genuine mourning, the patient should be allowed to express his sorrow and should be given support rather than encouraged superficially to "cheer up." Finally, if the patient has been able with some help from the outside to work through the previous stages, he reaches the stage of acceptance. This should not be confused with a hopeless "giving up"; it is rather a stage characterized by acceptance of fate without anger or depression.

DEALING WITH THE DYING PATIENT

How to Tell the Patient. In an extreme emergency situation, patients often ask whether they are going to die. Usually they should be reassured that this will not happen, even when the situation, in fact, is grave. The family, however, should be informed of the critical nature of the illness. In contrast, it is important to realize that most patients with terminal illness actually know the truth without being told. A relative or someone else in the patient's environment will give the nonverbal message that there is something seriously wrong by the way he deals with the patient. Therefore, the question "whether or not to tell" is less of an issue. The question, "How do I share this knowledge with my patient?" is really the crucial one.[18] The physician must devote some time to deciding how ready and willing his patient is to hear the truth. If the patient indicates verbally or nonverbally that he is ready, the physician should present the facts in a simple but emphatic way, pointing out any hopeful aspects of the treatment and particularly stressing that everything possible will be done to provide the best and most appropriate treatment. It is important to let the patient know that he will not be "dropped." The physician should take enough time to stay with the patient for a while after he or she has been told the facts about his or her illness to give support and evaluate reactions. Preferably, he or she should communicate all this to the patient in a place where some degree of privacy is ensured, rather than in the hallway with a group of medical students around him.

Helping the Patient Cope with Terminal Illness. Weisman[17] has listed a few guidelines to help the physician deal with the terminally ill. Patients of this sort are frequently seen on an emergency basis when home care becomes difficult or sudden deterioration occurs.

1. *Adequate relief of pain.* The patient should be given sufficient and appropriate pain-relieving medication and sedation if he or she desires it, but not to the point where he or she is dehumanized. Customary concerns about addiction dangers are no longer relevant.
2. *Open and candid communication with patient and family.* Diagnosis and treatment should be dealt with as already described. The patient should be involved as much as possible in important decisions about his or her treatment. The physician should also be available to the family and open to their needs for information, advice, and support.
3. *Preservation of self-esteem and autonomy.* The physician can support and stress the aspects of the patient's functioning that are still intact or still rewarding to the patient. He or she can also try to give the patient control over daily functions and routines, so far as this is medically and practically feasible.
4. *Genuine courage to accept what cannot be changed.* The patient does not expect superficial reassurance but rather wants to know that the physician is willing and ready to share his or her concern about the inevitable and to provide help in accepting it.

Psychiatric consultation may be required if some of the aforementioned reactions become excessive and destructive. This may be the case if the patient's depression becomes severe or even of psychotic proportions or if his or her anger regarding the terminal illness alienates all those around him or her, staff and family included.

Helping the Dying Patient in the ED. Critically ill or injured patients seen in the ED present a particular problem because there is typically little time or leisure available to give attention to their emotional needs. The various members of the medical team have to concentrate first on attempting to stabilize the vital functions and to save the patient's life. If the patient is conscious, however, he or she is usually anxious, possibly in a state of emotional shock, or at times even aware of the seriousness of the situation. Once the patient's vital functions are stabilized, it is important for the physician or a member of the treatment team to communicate with the patient to allay his anxieties. A few guidelines should be followed:

1. The patient should be told where he is, who the physician and the people around him are, and what is being done to him.
2. If the patient was brought alone, assurance should be given that all efforts will be made to notify his family and that they will be asked to come immediately.
3. The patient should be informed about his state in a simple and honest way, but only if he appears to be ready for this. Hope should always be included in any such statement. If a patient asks if he is dying, he should *not* be told so. Instead, he can be told that the physician does not know, but that everything possible will be done to save his life and that he should not give up.[19]
4. If the patient is conscious, he or she should be involved in important decisions related to treatment. This is particularly true for necessary major surgical interventions. If the patient is not conscious, his family will have to be involved.
5. If other family members or companions of the patient have been killed in the same accident, this should not be communicated to the patient until his vital functions are well stabilized or his critical condition is under control. The moment to communicate further bad news should be chosen with great care because the patient is already in emotional shock concerning his own injuries.
6. Once initial care has been given to the patient and his medical needs have been temporarily met, family members or friends should be allowed to see him for a short time and in a restricted number. This is particularly important if the patient is dying. The family or the patient, if conscious, may want to exchange last concerns, give some last reassurance, or ask for forgiveness.[19]

Helping the Family of the Patient. The family, in anticipating loss, also goes through phases similar to those of the patient. Their initial reactions are denial and disbelief regarding the fatal outcome. Later on, they may show anger at the doctor for not having diagnosed the illness earlier, and they may have a guilty feeling that in some ways it is their fault that the patient is going to die. The family will also have to cope with practical problems such as changed and possible increased financial demands or the care and raising of children in the case of a dying parent. Loneliness will have to be faced. To be able to deal with these many demands, the family should maintain a balance between serving the patient and respecting their own needs. Once death has occurred, the family become involved in the mourning process and have to work through their feelings of loss, anger, and guilt to acceptance of the loss. During the anticipatory grief phase and during the mourning phase, the physician can be helpful in providing support and understanding. He also can spot and identify particular difficulties the family may have in dealing with the terminal illness, and he can initiate appropriate professional contacts, such as psychiatric consultation, referrals to the social worker, and contacts with the chaplain.

Some special problems arise for families who have a member admitted to an ED in critical condition. They may themselves be in a state of emotional shock and may need support from the staff, and the chance to ventilate their feelings. Because they want to remain close to a critically ill or dying patient, family members should be able to wait in a place not too far from the patient where some privacy is assured. The hospital chaplain or another person trained in dealing with grief-stricken relatives can help greatly by staying with the family. If the patient is dead on arrival or dies during emergency procedures, the family should have the opportunity to see the body if they request it.[19] This can help them face, and ultimately accept, the reality of the death of their relative.

PATIENTS WHO REFUSE TREATMENT

Severely ill patients who refuse lifesaving treatment or necessary diagnostic procedures present a major challenge and frequently create feelings of frustration and helplessness in the physician and staff. Because of these feelings, both the physician and patient often become entrenched in their mutually opposed opinions, and communication breaks down completely, preventing further discussion that might have helped change the patient's mind. There are ways of handling such situations of refusal that can help the patient change his or her position and accept treatment.

Fear is one of the most important contributing factors in the patient's refusing procedures or wishing to leave the hospital. Lack of communication between patient and doctor or disorganized thinking caused by some organic process may be other factors. In handling individuals who refuse treatment, it is helpful to distinguish two types of patients: (1) those with psychopathology, and (2) those without psychopathology.[21]

REFUSAL WITH COEXISTING PSYCHOPATHOLOGY

Patients may refuse treatment because of irrational fears related to an underlying psychosis with an active delusional system. Other patients may be in a state of panic and may refuse treatment because their cognitive capacities are severely impaired by an acute organic brain syndrome.

REFUSAL WITHOUT COEXISTING PSYCHOPATHOLOGY

In this situation, a patient may refuse treatment because he or she has not been adequately involved by the staff in important decisions concerning treatment or because his or her family has been avoided by the physician and has not been informed appropriately about the procedures. Divergent opinions among the staff regarding the advisability of a particular procedure can also contribute to the patient's refusal. Religious or philosophic beliefs can be the reason for refusing certain types of treatment. In the emergency setting, the patient has not had time to prepare and often is fearful of unfamiliar physicians. Also, he may deny the seriousness of the problem. Bringing in familiar physicians or staff members when possible is of utmost help.

MANAGEMENT

It is important to realize that the patient's refusal is not necessarily final. It is therefore helpful to take time to listen to the patient's reasons for his refusal. The physician should inquire into possible underlying fears of real or imaginary dangers about the procedures and particularly should ensure that the patient understands the purpose and nature of the treatment or procedure. One of the crucial questions to be answered through this investigation is whether there is significant psychopathology and, if so, how it interferes with the patient's adjustment. For example, if the patient has an acute organic brain syndrome, attention and treatment must be focused on its cause, which in turn will ameliorate the patient's mental status. Psychiatric consultation is indicated in most cases in which psychopathology is present.

Other steps to be taken involve family and staff. If possible, the family should be informed about what is at stake and about the nature of the procedure. This is obligatory in the case of children or adolescents because in such cases the parents' attitudes may have a significant influence on the patient's acceptance or refusal of procedures. The position of the staff should also be examined briefly in terms of the agreement of different staff members on the course of treatment. Especially with a large staff in which there are various hierarchical levels, any disagreement about the treatment or procedures planned is communicated to the patient and increases his ambivalence.

Finally, the physician must be able to review his treatment plan[21] and determine whether an alternative, more acceptable approach is available or whether a postponement of the procedure to a more appropriate time might be feasible.

If, despite all efforts, the patient continues to refuse the procedure and wants to leave the hospital, the physician should carefully record on the chart (1) the treatment or procedure indicated; (2) the fact that the patient has refused all advice; and (3) the action taken to help him or her accept the physician's recommendation. If the patient is intoxicated or otherwise mentally incapacitated, attempts should be made to keep him or her in the hospital until the altered state of consciousness clears. Actual physical restraint, however, is dangerous and has legal implications that must be considered. Police may have to be involved if the patient presents indications that he or she might hurt himself or herself or others.

REFERENCES

1. Abram, H.S.: Psychiatry and surgery. In Freedman, A.M., Kaplan, H.T., and Sadock, B.J. (eds.): Comprehensive Textbook of Psychiatry, II. Baltimore, Williams & Wilkins Co., 1981.
2. Hackett, T.P., and Weisman, A.D.: Psychiatric management of operative syndromes. The therapeutic consultation and effect of non-interpretive intervention. Psychosom. Med. 22:267, 1960.
3. Abram, H.S., and Gill, B.F.: Predictions of postoperative psychiatric complications. N. Engl. J. Med. 265:1123, 1961.
4. Appleton, W.S., and Davis, J.M.: Practical Clinical Psychopharmacology. New York, Medcom, Inc., 1973.
5. Hackett, T.P., Cassem, N.H., and Wishnie, H.A.: CCU: appraisal of its psychologic hazards. N. Engl. J. Med. 279:1365, 1968.
6. Levy, N.B.: Coping with maintenance hemodialysis—psychological considerations in the care of patients. In Massry, S.G., and Sellers, A.L. (eds.): Aspects of Uremia and Dialysis. Springfield, Ill., Charles C Thomas, Publisher, 1976.
7. Abram, H.S., Moore, G.L., and Westervelt, F.B.: Suicidal behavior in chronic dialysis patients. Am. J. Psychiatry 127:1199, 1961.
8. Abram, H.S.: The psychiatrist, the treatment of chronic renal failure, and the prolongation of life. III. Am. J. Psychiatry 128:1534, 1972.
9. Fox, H.M., Rizzo, N.D., and Gifford, S.: Psychological observations of patients undergoing mitral surgery. Psychosom. Med. 16:186, 1954.
10. Kimball, C.P.: Psychological responses to the experience of open heart surgery. I. Am. J. Psychiatry 126:348, 1969.
11. Blachly, P.H., and Star, A.: Post-cardiotomy delirium. Am. J. Psychiatry 121:371, 1964.
12. Taylor, B.W., Litin, E.M., and Litzow, T.J.: Psychiatric considerations in cosmetic surgery. Mayo Clin. Proc. 41:608, 1966.
13. Caplan, L.M., and Hackett, T.P.: Emotional effects of lower-limb amputation in the aged. N. Engl. J. Med. 269:1166, 1963.
14. Kelham, R.L.: Some thoughts on mental effects of amputation. Br. Med. J. 1:334, 1958.
15. Sutherland, A.M., et al.: The psychological impact of cancer and cancer surgery. Cancer 5:857, 1952.
16. Weisman, A.D., and Hackett, T.P.: Psychosis after eye surgery. N. Engl. J. Med. 258:1284, 1958.
17. Weisman, A.D.: Thanatology. In Freedman, M., Kaplan, H.T., and Sadock, B.J. (eds.): Comprehensive Textbook of Psychiatry. II. Baltimore, Williams & Wilkins Co., 1975.
18. Kübler-Ross, E.: On Death and Dying. London, Macmillan, 1969.
19. Kübler-Ross, E.: Crisis management of dying persons and their families. In Resnik, H.L.P., and Ruben, H.L. (eds.): Emergency Psychiatric Care. Bowie, Md., Charles Press, 1975.
20. Rennecker, R., and Culter, M.: Psychological problems of adjustment to cancer of the breast. JAMA 148:833, 1952.
21. Himmelhoch, J.M., et al.: Butting heads: patients who refuse necessary procedures. Psychiatr. Med. 1:24, 1970.

BIBLIOGRAPHY

Castelnuovo-Tedesco P.: Psychiatric Aspects of Organ Transplantation. New York, Grune & Stratton, 1971.

Kemph, J.P.: Renal failure, artificial kidney and kidney transplant. Am. J. Psychiatry 122:1270, 1966.

Pasternak, S.A.: When a patient wants to sign himself out. Hosp. Physician 5:120, 1969.

SOMATOFORM DISORDERS

Beverly Fauman

CAPSULE

The somatoform disorders are often complex and difficult to confirm. They may occur in combination with other physical illnesses, can be exacerbated by emotional stress, and often occur in patients who at other times have serious physical illnesses (leaving the physician unsure and uncomfortable about the diagnosis). Also, confrontation is not curative. The best prognosis is associated with early detection and aggressive treatment. If the emergency physician suspects one of the somatoform disorders and has no evidence of a significant, life-threatening illness, he or she should refer the patient to (or *back* to) a primary care physician.

INTRODUCTION

Somatoform disorders are illnesses in which the patient's symptoms and idea of what is wrong are physical, but responsible and thorough physical, laboratory, and psychiatric evaluation determine that the illness originates in the patient's psyche. There are four major categories of somatoform disorders defined in the standard psychiatric diagnostic manual[1]: conversion reaction, somatization disorder, hypochondriasis, and psychogenic pain disorder. It is often difficult to distinguish these categories from one another, and patients with somatoform disorders frequently have a history of significant physical illness as well. In some disorders, the patient complains of or feigns symptoms that are under his or her voluntary control. These are called factitious disorders. Somatoform disorders are not under the patient's voluntary control.

A conversion reaction is commonly thought to be the conversion of a psychologic idea, wish, or fantasy that is uncomfortable for the patient into a physical symptom that accomplishes the dual purpose of expressing the conflicting wish and relieving the psychologic conflict.

Somatization disorders are much less discrete episodes of illness than conversion disorders; rather, they occur in sequences involving various organ systems, appear less bizarre than conversion symptoms, and frequently lead the physician to do expensive diagnostic tests or operations. Because a patient who is prone to somatization disorder generally has different somatic complaints at different times, and therefore may consult multiple specialists, it may take some time for one physician to pull the whole picture together.[2]

Hypochondriasis differs from somatization disorder in the following ways: commonly, the patient focuses on only one organ system, and has a persistent, almost delusional conviction that something is wrong with that system. The hypochondriac appears to misinterpret or exaggerate normal bodily sensations. Thus, although a patient with somatization disorder may consult physicians in multiple specialties, the hypochondriac patient is more likely to consult, for example, a succession of cardiologists. Occasionally, one can identify a family member from whom the patient has "inherited" the symptom. A parent or grandparent may have died of colon cancer or myocardial infarct, and the patient demands repeated barium studies or electrocardiograms for reassurance about normal variations in stool or pulse.[3]

Psychogenic pain disorder is the term for complaints of chronic, unremitting pain for which thorough evaluation cannot provide an explanation. A patient who has had an organic cause for the pain, but for whom the pain still persists long after it should, is also diagnosed as having psychogenic pain disorder. These patients are difficult to treat because they may become addicted to narcotics and are fearful of the recurrence of pain. Thus, they become demanding, and prompt caretakers to feel that they are being manipulative. Many of these patients have lawsuits pending related to the original injury that caused the pain, lending further suspicion that the patient is "faking." Some authors believe that psychogenic pain disorder is a manifestation of depression, particularly because some of these patients respond to antidepressants.

PATHOPHYSIOLOGY AND ANATOMY

The somatoform disorders may affect any part of the body or any organ system. That is why it can be so problematic to diagnose. A patient who is prone to somatoform disorder may have different somatic complaints at different times.

Somatization disorder, by definition, is diagnosed when a patient has recurrent complaints of symptoms over time, beginning before age 30, and involving many organ systems. Many of these complaints suggest serious illness, but occur in a patient who simply does not look that sick. Common complaints in somatization disorder include difficulty in swallowing, fainting, nausea, menstrual pain that the patient believes is more frequent or more severe than most women experience, pain during intercourse, shortness of breath, palpitations, and dizziness.[4] These are not pathognomonic for somatization disorder, nor are they the only symptoms. The diagnosis is made from the whole picture.

Often, one clue to conversion reaction or psychogenic pain disorder is a discrepancy between the described symptom and what we know about physiology and anatomy; the symptom "just cannot be." A conversion symptom must be related to a "perceived" sensation to be able to serve as a conversion. Thus, gastric secretions, blood pressure, or other silent physiologic processes are not generally part of a conversion disorder. The conversion symptom may, however, give rise to corresponding motor and physiologic changes, which some have called "conversion complications."

The hypochondriac patient, as mentioned previously, appears to be exquisitely sensitive, or to overreact to ordinary physiologic functions. This patient may regularly check his or her own blood pressure, pulse, stool, or urine stream for reassurance. As with somatization disorder, certain organ systems are more likely than others to be the focus of the hypochondriac's concern, but any fixed, chronic concern with an organ system or body site may occur. In the Emergency Department (ED), the physician who used to see the patient who is convinced he has an occult cancer now sees the patient with the conviction that he has been exposed to AIDS.

PREHOSPITAL ASSESSMENT AND STABILIZATION

Somatoform disorders are difficult to diagnose in the field, particularly if they present as emergencies. Instructions to the field should be to believe that the patient is really organically ill, and to stabilize him or her as one would for the symptoms and vital signs of the apparent illness. The important thing to remember is that these patients are best managed over the long term by a single primary care physician, and that unusual or invasive diagnostic tests or procedures should be kept to a minimum. If possible, the patient's primary care provider should be contacted before any invasive or risky diagnostic or therapeutic measures are undertaken.

CLINICAL PRESENTATION AND EXAMINATION

The somatoform disorders present much like regular medical illnesses. The patient generally believes that he or she has an organic and probably serious disorder, and is unlikely to volunteer the information that would lead the physician to recognize the emotional basis of the symptoms.

In general, certain presentations are more suggestive of one of the somatoform disorders. These include serious or worrisome symptoms without accompanying signs; the fact that the patient is under age 30 or has had recurrent or ongoing symptoms starting before age 30; and the fact that the symptoms often revolve around breathing, urination, eating, elimination, or activity of the voluntary muscles. Palpitations, neurologic symptoms, or symptoms related to the sexual organs are also common.

The onset of a conversion reaction is sudden, usually in reaction to a particular event and in an emotionally charged setting. The patient appears healthy and less concerned about the symptom than one would expect. The family does not appear insightful, and is often oversolicitous, in contrast to the patient's lack of concern. There is often a history of a curious undiagnosed illness in the past that subsided spontaneously or even "miraculously." Recurrence is not unusual, and it may or may not be manifested by the same symptom. Conversion symptoms are culture-bound, and thus today we rarely see the dramatic, discrete, "obvious" conversions described by Freud, Janet, and Charcot.

A good history and physical examination, a thorough neurologic examination, and the physician's ability to recognize an ill patient are the best diagnostic tools. The sooner a conversion reaction is identified, the more amenable it is to treatment. Conversely, multiple laboratory tests, specialty consultations, and other delays in defining the illness make it more entrenched and harder to treat.

Conversion symptoms typically involve voluntary muscles, although they may take virtually any form. Pain is not a common conversion symptom. The most frequent complaints are motor disturbances and sensory abnormalities. The symptoms may either mimic physical illness or complicate existing physical illness. The patient experiencing a conversion reaction is not faking; that is, he or she does not have conscious control over the symptom, did not choose it, and is not aware or willing to accept the idea that it is psychologic. Questioning must proceed gently, for the purpose of gathering information and not to confront the patient or to try to get him or her to admit what is happening. The physician is trying to determine what psychologic conflict might be resolved by the patient's symptom. Conversion can exist when a conflict cannot be discovered, but the diagnosis cannot be established with confidence. Questions should focus on what was happening when the symptoms began, and what the symptom prevents the patient from doing.

The conversion symptom serves an adaptive function for the patient. The conversion process is believed to spare the patient the anxiety, guilt, or shame that would otherwise have been engendered by the unacceptable idea, which constitutes the "primary gain." Secondary gain is achieved by the sick role.

The patient with hypochondriasis, psychogenic pain disorder, or somatization disorder has an extensive history of physician contact[5]; the patient with conversion reaction may have much more episodic medical intervention. Although the conversion disorder patient is often relatively unconcerned about his or her symptoms, the other disorders carry with them a great deal of worry and concern, as well as outrage if the complaints are not taken seriously.

The hypochondriac has developed a fixed, almost delusional preoccupation with a body part or body function. He or she has not been well for some time, and may have suffered real illness between hypochondriac episodes. These real illnesses have two effects: they relieve the hypochondriac complaints for weeks to months, and confirm for the patient that he or she was justified to be concerned. The hypochondriac may be a man or woman, usually middle-aged or older. His or her relationship with family, friends, and physicians is characterized by his or her focus on symptoms, medications, and illness. In contrast to the other disorders discussed here, the malady is usually relatively constant, and the patient may stay with one physician, even though all treatment efforts have been ineffective.[3,5]

As noted previously, signs and laboratory findings do not correspond to the patient's symptoms. The physician should not proceed with any invasive or

TABLE 62-21. THE SOMATOFORM DISORDERS: DIFFERENTIAL DIAGNOSIS IN THE EMERGENCY DEPARTMENT

Myocardial infarct
Pulmonary embolism
Hypoglycemia
Cerebral vascular accident
Hyperglycemia
Hyperventilation
Panic disorder
Depression
Domestic violence or child abuse
Schizophrenia

risky diagnostic tests that are not dictated by good clinical judgment. Whenever possible, a single primary care provider should be identified for these patients to oversee and determine the necessary diagnostic and therapeutic measures indicated.

DIFFERENTIAL DIAGNOSIS

The primary diagnoses to exclude are relatively imminently life-threatening ones (Table 62-21): myocardial infarct, stroke, hyperglycemia, hypoglycemia, or pulmonary embolism. Depression, hyperventilation, panic disorder, and conversion disorder may respond to rapid intervention, so a psychiatric consultation in the ED may be useful. An early manifestation of a schizophrenic disorder may be bizarre or obsessive concerns about bodily functions; here also, a psychiatric evaluation may establish the correct diagnosis. It is apparent that patients who are victims of domestic violence, or who are themselves abusive parents, may sometimes present to an ED with vague, unusual, or hypochondriac complaints, often between episodes of violence. It is not clear whether this is a conscious cry for help, a manifestation of depression, or an unconscious wish to be discovered or stopped. The physician should make it a practice to evaluate all patients who appear to have a somatoform disorder for a domestic violence history. Other disorders that may be considered should be evaluated only to the extent needed to rule out acute illness. The patient should then be referred to a primary care physician.

INITIAL STABILIZATION

The patient with a somatoform disorder stabilizes initially with reassurance that the physician is taking the complaints seriously and will evaluate them. Vital signs should be obtained, and any deviation explored. Remember that ketoacidosis may present only as slightly rapid respirations and hypothyroidism can present as only slightly depressed temperature, blood pressure, or heart rate.

LABORATORY AND OTHER PROCEDURES

To facilitate appropriate treatment of a patient with any of the somatoform disorders, the ED should limit involvement and evaluation to the symptoms and signs that suggest acute physical illness. If the patient is knowledgeable or insistent about some obscure or risky test or treatment, make a note of it; this is probably not a naïve patient or one without a medical history. In the ED, you should not order tests for rare or unlikely disorders that are not imminently serious. Refer the patient instead to a primary care physician.

Patients with somatoform disorders experience much of their morbidity from procedures and laboratory tests, often unnecessary ones.

MANAGEMENT AND INDICATIONS FOR ADMISSION

Reassurance is necessary but short-lived. Perform the laboratory tests needed to confirm the absence of significant acute illness. Consult other physicians and further evaluate or hospitalize the patient if you have significant concerns, but not if you are merely feeling pressured by the patient to do more. A patient with conversion disorder may need to be hospitalized because the symptoms greatly impair function, although conversion reactions are often treated effectively in the ED. A psychiatric consultation may be useful to help with management or a decision to admit.

PITFALLS

The problems that arise when the patient with somatoform disorder is misdiagnosed or mismanaged in the ED are frustrating at best and life-threatening at worst. The frustration comes from feeling that you have been manipulated by the patient. Frustration can be minimized by: (1) relying on your medical judgment and objective findings to determine the need for further tests or treatment; (2) obtaining a consultation or second opinion when you are uncertain; and (3) recognizing that the patient is really helpless to control his or her symptoms and the accompanying anxiety.

Potential life-threatening problems are addressed by: (1) not ordering or performing risky tests or procedures that can be postponed, and (2) referring the patient to a primary care physician who can oversee and coordinate further management.

MEDICOLEGAL PEARLS

Patients who eventually seem to have a psychologic basis for their symptoms are likely to anger the physician, who is eager to identify and treat "real" diseases. There is the potential for at least two adverse outcomes: first, the physician may do or say something to express this anger, which may provoke a lawsuit subsequently; and secondly, the physician may do or say something to ensure that no diagnosis is overlooked, leading to excessive testing with its inherent costs and risks.

There are several steps to follow to minimize the legal risks. Most importantly, realize that the patient does not have conscious control over his or her symptoms and is not trying to take advantage of the system or harass you. This is the patient's rather poor adaptation to life, and the patient is helpless. Many patients with psychogenic pain disorder are involved in lawsuits, and the pain may actually disappear when the lawsuit is settled. This does not prove that the pain was factitious, or under the patient's willful control.

If the patient comes in with a complaint that suggests serious illness, be sure to indicate in your note how you explained that symptom, or why you do not believe the patient is experiencing a stroke, myocardial infarct, or other life-threatening disease. Avoid the use of pejorative or derogatory descriptions in the record, but explain *in the chart* your reasons for not performing particular laboratory tests.

HORIZONS

Patients with somatoform disorders accumulate a hefty medical record. They have recurrences or are chronically ill. They rarely appreciate their physician's efforts, and tend to distrust them. The emergency physician does not reap the rewards of correct diagnosis and management. On the other hand, the primary care physician who gets to know the somaticizing patient well over time may get satisfaction from long-term successful management, which includes recognizing episodes of "real" illness and minimizing the diagnostic procedures and consequent morbidity. The patient with hypochondriasis often feels significantly better for long periods after a serious physical illness.

REFERENCES

1. Diagnostic and Statistical Manual of Mental Disorders, 3rd Edition, Revised. Washington, DC, American Psychiatric Association, 1987.
2. Monson, R.A., and Smith, Jr., G.R.: Somatization disorder in primary care. N. Engl. J. Med. *308*:1464, 1983.
3. Brown, H.N., and Vaillant, G.E.: Hypochondriasis. Arch. Intern. Med. *141*:723, 1981.
4. Quill, T.E.: Somatization disorder. JAMA *254*:3075, 1985.
5. Adler, G.: The physician and the hypochondriacal patient. N. Engl. J. Med. *304*:1394, 1981.

BIBLIOGRAPHY

Fauman, B.J., and Fauman, M.A.: Emergency Psychiatry for the House Officer. Baltimore, Williams & Wilkins, 1981.

Ford, C.V.: The Somatizing Disorders—Illness as a Way of Life. New York, Elsevier Scientific Publishing Co., Inc., 1983.

Tomb, D.A.: Psychiatry for the House Officer, 3rd Ed. Baltimore, Williams & Wilkins, 1988.

PSYCHIATRIC EMERGENCIES IN CHILDREN AND ADOLESCENTS

EVALUATION, DEFINITIONS, AND GENERAL APPROACH

Harris Rabinovich

CAPSULE

The essential element in the management of psychiatric emergencies in children and adolescents is the ability to make a correct diagnosis. Many conditions have overlapping symptoms and resemble each other superficially. A general method of evaluation is presented that maximizes the reliability of symptom data. All the major psychiatric disorders of children and adolescents that produce emergencies are reviewed in detail, and methods to evaluate them are presented.

INTRODUCTION

At one time, a chapter or section like this would have been introduced with the caveat that psychiatric disorders were functional and that organic disorders had to be ruled out before psychiatric causes, evaluations, and treatments were considered. Many disorders once viewed as functional are now known to be at least partly organic, and therefore the caveat should be changed. All psychiatric emergencies in children and adolescents should be screened medically to make sure that they are not the province of the pediatrician or the pediatric neurologist. The evaluation should include a medical history, physical examination, and appropriate laboratory examinations when indicated. It is sometimes difficult to determine whether a psychiatric emergency in a child or adolescent should be cared for by the child psychiatrist, pediatrician, or pediatric neurologist, who may have to collaborate closely until a clear determination can be made. A good example of such an emergency are pseudoseizures, which have been reported with incest, learning disability, and existing epilepsy.[1,2] Fortunately, newer diagnostic techniques such as CT scan, MRI, and EEG telemetry have improved diagnosis considerably.[3]

Therefore every effort should be made initially in a psychiatric emergency involving a child or adolescent to resolve diagnostic uncertainty and all appropriate diagnostic studies used.

The presence or absence of a psychologic precipitant has not proved as useful in distinguishing medical and psychiatric disorders as was thought previously. For example, studies of major depressive disorder show that there may or may not be a psychologic precipitant. Similarly, the time course of the onset of symptoms has not proved helpful in distinguishing medical from psychiatric conditions. A good example is post-traumatic stress disorder, the complex of physical and psychologic symptoms that can develop after a "psychologically distressing event that is outside the range of human experience."[4] Reactions can be acute, chronic, or delayed. The delayed reaction may follow an incident that reminds the child or adolescent of the original psychologically traumatic event. Thus we begin the evaluation of any emergency situation in a child or adolescent by using any and all diagnostic methods to distinguish between medical and psychiatric emergencies. We recognize that the process of distinguishing is not always straightforward, and at any point in the evaluation and treatment planning process, diagnostic questions may re-emerge and should be addressed and not ignored.

TYPES OF EMERGENCIES

What constitutes a psychiatric emergency (Table 62-22) in a child or adolescent? The definition depends on whose perspective we take. From the perspective of the treating professional, an emergency arises whenever there is a serious risk to the child or adolescent's well-being through the development of dangerous symptoms or behavior. The symptoms or behavior may develop because of a child or adolescent's internal psychologic conflicts, conflicts with the environment, or as part of a disorder with a biologic cause. The child or adolescent's environment may contain a direct risk such as incest and physical or sexual

TABLE 62-22. PSYCHIATRIC EMERGENCIES IN CHILDREN AND ADOLESCENTS

1. Dangerous symptoms or behavior
2. The environment represents a risk
3. People in the environment cannot manage the child or adolescent

abuse, or an indirect risk such as inadequate care and supervision. Because we describe some environmental risks as indirect, this should not diminish the perception that they are extremely dangerous. From the parental, familial, or environmental perspective, a psychiatric emergency exists whenever a child or adolescent is unmanageable in that setting. An emergency may involve an infant who will not stop crying and sleep, a retarded child who bites people, or an adolescent who stays out all night. A section such as this cannot possibly address all the psychiatric emergencies of children and adolescents, but presents some general methods of assessing these emergencies, some comments on the more common ones and their related psychiatric disorders, and some general ideas about intervention.

METHODS OF EVALUATION

The evaluation of a psychiatric emergency in a child or adolescent must include the evaluation of principal environments, including: immediate family, extended family, foster home, school camp, jail, hospital, or any environment within which the patient spends significant periods of time. In each of these environments it is important to identify principal caretakers, which could be parents, grandparents, teachers, counselors, social workers, or even siblings. A principal caretaker has a significant amount of interaction with the child or adolescent and thereby gains intimate knowledge. In the case of a younger child, a principal caretaker can supply information that the younger child cannot, such as the duration and course of some disorder or the medical history. In the case of adolescents, a principal caretaker can provide information that the adolescent might withhold because of psychologic conflict, such as patterns of drug use or history of prior difficulty with authorities. In both children and adolescents, a principal caretaker's report is required for a complete evaluation.

The history taking starts with the principal caretaker for children and may or may not start with the principal caretaker for adolescents. It may be important to start with the adolescent to gain confidence and form a therapeutic alliance. A thorough history of the chief complaint and symptom inventory is required from both patient and principal caretaker. If there are any significant discrepancies between the reports of the patient and the caretaker, it is important to confront both and resolve the discrepancies.

INTERNAL AND EXTERNAL SYMPTOMS

Some symptoms are best described as internal. These include suicidal ideas, suicidal plans, moods, auditory and visual hallucinations, and delusional ideas. These symptoms may or may not have been shared with caretakers. But characteristically, internal symptoms are best known to the patient. In any discrepancy between patient and caretaker reports involving internal symptoms, greater weight should probably be given to the patient's report. External symptoms are those best known or observed by a caretaker, and may include social withdrawal, appetite changes, irritability, and difficulties with rules and limits. In any discrepancy between patient and caretaker reports involving external symptoms, greater weight should probably be given to the caretaker's report.

There is a risk of serious errors in evaluation if the history taking involves only the dangerous symptoms, behavior, or chief complaint. Every effort must be made to make a complete diagnosis, which requires a full symptom inventory. A good example of a potential pitfall is suicide attempts. Suicide attempts can be part of an adjustment disorder, major depressive disorder, or psychosis. In serious gestures or attempts, the intervention is hospitalization. In nondangerous gestures or attempts, however, diagnosis is a major factor in deciding whether or not to hospitalize. The lack of insight and poor judgment consistent with psychosis certainly suggest hospitalization because there is no way of knowing whether the psychotic child or adolescent could control the suicidal behavior. It is not necessary to ask about every psychiatric symptom. Each disorder or group of disorders has one or more principal symptoms that must be present if the diagnosis is to be made. For example, a depressed or irritable mood or loss of interest or pleasure must be present for a diagnosis of depressive disorder. Questions about mood and anhedonia can be used as screening questions to check for the presence or absence of such a disorder. If mood changes and anhedonia are not present by both patient and caretaker reports, this diagnostic category can safely be skipped.

All history taking must include cognizance of the child or adolescent's cognitive abilities. Questions must be asked in a way that the patient understands. The examining clinician may be called upon to examine children and adolescents with cognitive impairments secondary to neurologic disorders or with diminished mental capacity, and should not make any assumption on how much the patient understands based on physical size alone. Some of the questions may contain concepts beyond the understanding of young children and limited adolescents, and must be asked in such a way that they translate the concept into terms the patient will understand. For example, young children and limited adolescents do not understand the concept of mood states and are unable to respond to questions about being depressed in any informative way. They can tell, however, if they are as happy as other children or cry more than other children. In this way, a younger child or limited adolescent can be asked about depressed moods. In special circumstances, information must be obtained from younger children by nonverbal methods. These circumstances include young age (under 6) and severely traumatic experiences like rape, kidnapping, or witnessing murder or other forms of extreme violence. For the younger child, it may be necessary to use puppets or dolls to play out the appropriate scenario and have the child play himself or herself and give characteristic responses. For the severely traumatized child, Pynoos and Elk have developed a nonverbal method that involves introducing dangerous elements into a child's drawings and examining the response.[5] With the exception of these two circumstances, every effort should be to examine the child or adolescent verbally.

HALLUCINATIONS AND DELUSIONS

Hallucinations and delusions are necessary but not sufficient to make a diagnosis of psychosis; however, they are so important in the evaluation of psychiatric emergencies that their evaluation is carefully reviewed here. These symptoms are a major source of diagnostic variance in child psychiatric evaluations. The diagnosis of psychosis will be missed unless it is remembered that these symptoms are internal. The child or adolescent must be asked explicitly about the various kinds of hallucinations and delusions. Most of the time, the caretaker has no knowledge of these symptoms. On occasion, a caretaker may witness a younger child conversing with no one, or a frightened adolescent may share a delusion, but these are exceptions rather than the rule. Several phenomena (Table 62-23) that get confused with psychotic symptoms, and false-positive psychotic diagnoses can occur in these cases. For a symptom to be considered indicative of psychosis, it must occur in full consciousness. Symptoms that occur when the child or adolescent is falling asleep, waking, febrile, or under the influence of medication or abused substance cannot be considered diagnostic of anything. Younger children experience only hallucinations. Imaginary friends, elaborate fantasies, eidetic imagery, derealization, and depersonalization, however, have to be distinguished from true hallucinations. The older child can display ideas of reference, but fully formed delusions are seen in adolescence. To ask the younger child about the presence of hallucinations, it may be important to ask, "Do your ears play tricks on you?" In this way, the concept of perceptual distortions and hallucinations are introduced. The same method can be used for visual and tactile hallucinations. If voices are present, it is important to know if they are commenting, com-

TABLE 62-23. PHENOMENA THAT ARE CONFUSED WITH HALLUCINATIONS

1. Hypnogogic and hypnopompic phenomena
2. Febrile hallucinations
3. Imaginary friends
4. Elaborated fantasies
5. Eidetic imagery
6. Derealization

manding, or conversing. Delusions of thought control, thought insertion, broadcasting, or withdrawal are pathognomonic of schizophrenia. Hallucinations can also occur in children and adolescents in nonpsychotic disorders of conduct and emotions.[6] The presence of hallucinations or delusions that are temporal and thematically congruent with affective symptoms suggests an affective psychosis. The presence of bizarre delusions, commenting or conversing hallucinated voices, thought disorder, disturbance in social functioning, and absence of affective symptoms suggest a schizophrenia-like psychosis. Hallucinations in a child with symptoms of emotional or conduct disorder do not suggest psychosis.

SUICIDE

Adolescent suicide is uncommon; the rate in 1984 for all 15- to 19-year-olds was 9 per 100,000 population.[7] Although the rates for younger adolescents and children are considerably less, it has been estimated that there are from 100 to 1000 adolescent suicide attempts for each successful adolescent suicide. Therefore adolescent suicide attempts are the commonest pediatric psychiatric emergency presented to clinicians.[8] The recent documentation that suicide completion and attempt rates increase after telecasts of shows dealing with adolescent suicide suggests that this can be a group phenomenon.[9] The clinician must not only be able to manage the individual suicidal adolescent but may also be called upon to help manage the group phenomenon. Suicidal attempts have pejoratively been described as manipulative. Although failed teenage romances or parent-child conflict are a common antecedent of suicidal gestures, they can also occur as a response to rape, physical and sexual abuse, and drug and alcohol dependence. Although suicidal attempts may have an environmental change as their objective, they have the potential of being lethal. All suicidal behavior should be considered seriously and should never be dismissed or treated casually because it seems manipulative.

Once the child or adolescent who has attempted suicide has been medically cleared, the evaluation begins. The aim of the evaluation is to decide whether or not the patient must be hospitalized or can return home and be treated on an outpatient basis. The evaluation begins with a history of events that led up to the suicide attempt and is taken from both patient and principal caretaker. Considerations peculiar to the evaluation of a suicide attempt include lethality of method, degree of social isolation, efforts to avoid discovery, statements about premeditation, intention to die, and current suicidal intent. Studies of successful adolescent suicide attempts have revealed certain risk factors that should be kept in mind during the evaluation.[10]

Risk factors for adolescent boys, in order of descending importance, are prior suicide attempt, major depression, substance abuse, antisocial behavior, and family history of suicide. Risk factors for adolescent girls in order of descending importance are major depression, prior suicidal attempt, antisocial behavior, family history of suicide, and substance abuse. From the same studies of successful suicide attempts for adolescent boys, it has been estimated that a prior suicide attempt increases the odds of a successful suicide 22 times and for adolescent girls, a major depression increases the risk of successful suicide 49 times.

Suicide and Major Depressive Disorder. A review of the small number of follow-up studies of suicidally depressed teenagers reveals that their suicide rate is even greater than that projected from psychologic autopsy studies of successful adolescent suicide completers. In addition, most of the suicide factors mentioned previously are frequently associated with major depression disorder, such as substance abuse, family history of suicide, and prior suicide attempt. Therefore the evidence points to the need to hospitalize the child or adolescent with major depressive disorder who has made a suicide attempt. The need is even more compelling for the suicidal child or adolescent with major depressive disorder with psychotic features. The principal or required symptoms to make a diagnosis of major depressive disorder (Table 62-24) are depressed mood and anhedonia (markedly diminished interest or pleasure in activities). The associated symptoms include appetite change, insomnia or hypersomnia, psychomotor agitation or retardation, fatigue, excess or inappropriate guilt, diminished ability to think or concentrate, and recurrent thoughts of death or suicide. A total of five symptoms must be present for at least 2 weeks to make the diagnosis of major depressive disorder.

A child or adolescent who has made a serious suicide attempt, however, and has the principal symptoms and less than the required number of associated symptoms, should be treated for major depressive disorder.

Inpatient versus Outpatient Treatment. The behavior of the treating clinician can influence whether or not the child or adolescent's parents or caretakers will accept hospital admission. Specifically, clinicians who introduce the need for admission to a family or caretaker suddenly, without warning, at the end of an examination do not make as many successful referrals for inpatient hospitalization as those who raise the possibility of admission early in the examination. The clinician can document the need for admission by reviewing the symptoms with the child or adolescent's

TABLE 62-24. DIAGNOSTIC CRITERIA FOR MAJOR DEPRESSIVE DISORDER

1. Principal symptoms (At least one is required to make the diagnosis)
   a. Depressed mood
   b. Anhedonia or loss of pleasure
2. Associated symptoms (The total of principal and associated symptoms must equal five)
   a. Appetite change (increase or decrease)
   b. Sleep disturbance (insomnia or hypersomnia)
   c. Disturbance of psychomotor activity level (agitation or retardation)
   d. Fatigue or loss of energy
   e. Inappropriate guilt
   f. Impaired concentration
   g. Suicidal thoughts, plans, or attempts

parents or caretaker and commenting on the dangerousness of the symptoms. The alternative outpatient treatment for major depressive disorder involves having the family or caretaker monitor the child or adolescent around the clock for possibly some 4 to 6 weeks. We estimate that time span because that is how long antidepressant medication would have to be taken before one could reasonably expect full symptom relief. The decision to manage and treat the suicidal depressed or nondepressed child or adolescent at home places a lot of stress on the family. Rates of psychiatric disturbance of up to 50%, including substance abuse, have been reported in the parents of children and adolescents who have attempted suicide. The ability of parents or family to protect and follow through with outpatient treatment must be taken into account when making recommendations about hospitalization to the family.

Suicide and Other Factors. Several other important factors have been found in adolescent suicide attempts (Table 62-25). Adolescent suicide attempters have been found to have higher rates of physical illness than age-matched peers. The rates run some 30 to 50% higher than those of control groups.[12] In adolescent boys who attempt suicide, physical illness has also been associated with multiple adverse family factors, poor school achievement, and previous suicide attempts. In adolescent girls, pregnancy or fear of pregnancy has often been associated with suicide attempts. The association between drugs and alcohol and adolescent suicide attempt is well established. As a group, drug- and alcohol-abusing adolescents have

TABLE 62-25. FACTORS ASSOCIATED WITH SUICIDE ATTEMPTS IN ADOLESCENTS

1. Physical illness (boys)
2. Pregnancy
3. Drug and alcohol abuse
4. Parent conflict

higher rates of attempted suicide than their non-abusing peers.[13] The most important external factor in emotional disturbances of children and adolescents who attempt suicide is conflict with parents or caretakers. The patients see their parents or caretakers as hostile, indifferent, overly demanding, critical, rigid, and overcontrolling. It is much too easy to see the patient's point of view and blame the parents, especially when the patient has just made a suicide attempt. It is much more difficult in these situations to see how the patient's temperament or personality contributes to the conflict. Thus, evaluation should include a careful medical history, a careful drug and alcohol history, and an evaluation of the patient's functioning in the family. In the end, the clinician must weigh all the factors and decide whether it is safe for this child or adolescent to go home and be treated as an outpatient. All children and adolescents who make suicide attempts require follow-up psychiatric care. For adolescents for whom an accidental overdose in an intoxicated state can be distinguished from a suicide attempt, referral to a drug detoxification program may be the optimal disposition. Studies of adults who attempt suicide suggest that an individual given an actual follow-up appointment rather than a name and number is more than likely to keep the appointment.[14] Therefore, any time the child or adolescent is sent home from the evaluation and referred for outpatient treatment, a follow-up appointment should be made rather than simply giving the parent or caretaker a name and number to call the next day.

PSYCHOSIS AND SCHIZOPHRENIA IN CHILDREN AND ADOLESCENTS

Psychotic children and adolescents with nonaffective psychosis are rarely referred to the clinician as emergencies; they are estimated to average 1% of outpatient referrals and 5% of inpatient referrals. Although many of these children and adolescents turn out to have schizophrenia as adults, there has been considerable controversy over how to make the diagnosis in children. In adolescents, the clinical picture resembles adult schizophrenia or a schizophreniform disorder, depending on the duration of the disorder. The diagnosis of schizophrenia requires 6 months of continuous disturbance with at least 1 week of an active phase. Active-phase symptoms include delusions, prominent hallucinations, incoherence or marked loosening of associations, catatonic behavior, and flat or grossly inappropriate affect.[4] Because this is a chronic disorder, many children and adolescents referred as psychiatric emergencies have been diagnosed previously and may be in current treatment. They are extremely sensitive to conflict and the expression of negative emotion, both within their fam-

ilies and in their social environments outside the family. These environmental stresses may produce a return of active-phase symptoms. In this case, the clinician has the choice of intervening pharmacologically or hospitalizing the patient. The ability of those in the home environment to manage the acutely disturbed schizophrenic child or adolescent is usually the deciding factor in whether or not hospitalization is required. Pharmacologic intervention is not difficult because most of these children and adolescents are usually taking neuroleptic medication, and some increase in the current regimen is all that is required. The adolescent with onset of illness during adolescence usually responds better to neuroleptic medication than the adolescent with childhood onset or the child with schizophrenia.

DIAGNOSIS OF SCHIZOPHRENIA IN CHILDREN

Although the use of the diagnosis of schizophrenia in children is in dispute because there are no agreed-upon diagnostic criteria, a clinical description is possible. These symptoms occur in the absence of any neurologic disorder. These children have long-standing hallucinosis. The voices comment, give commands, converse, and are permanent. There is marked disturbance in social functioning, particularly in school and with peers. Peculiar behavior, impairment in personal hygiene and grooming, circumstantial speech, and lack of interest may all be seen. Children under 6 do not describe hallucinations, but display gross failures in reality testing. For example, they might be unable to understand why television cartoon characters cannot come out of the television set and play, or that Mickey Mouse is fictional. They are active and may require neuroleptic medications. Their parents may describe these children as having complete lack of insight and judgment as to what is dangerous. These children have been known to set fires, run into traffic, jump out of windows, and try to injure peers and siblings. In these cases, hospitalization is required to perform the evaluation and stabilize the child. All children and adolescents with an initial presentation of psychotic symptoms should be hospitalized for evaluation and treatment. A small number of these children turn out to have organic brain disease and the remainder have "formes frustes" of schizophrenia. They will probably require neuroleptic medication, and the introduction of neuroleptics is best accomplished in the hospital.

CONDUCT DISORDER

The clinician responsible for evaluating psychiatric emergencies in children and adolescents sees many patients with conduct disorders. Typical symptoms include violent acts, fire-setting, cruelty to animals, truancy, lying, running away from home, and anti-social behavior. Conduct-disordered children and adolescents must have a cluster of symptoms that have existed for 6 months or longer. Individual conduct disorder symptoms or similar symptoms are also characteristic of other psychiatric disorders of children and adolescents. Truancy, which must be distinguished from school refusal or phobia, is characteristic of conduct disorder. School refusal or school phobia is characteristic of emotional disorders. In truancy, the child or adolescent does not experience difficulty in leaving home for school, never arrives at school, and spends the school day in some pleasurable alternative activity. Conduct disorder seldom coexists with emotional disorders except for depression. In fact, there is one report of the successful treatment of conduct and depression symptoms with antidepressant medication.[15] With few exceptions, the caretakers of conduct-disordered children and adolescents decide to seek emergency psychiatric consultation because they have decided that the patient is a danger to himself or herself or others in the current living environment. Many of these children have long histories of conduct symptoms, but the symptom that is beyond the threshold of tolerance for most caretakers is fire-setting. A caretaker's perception that fire-setting is a symptom of serious psychiatric disorder has been confirmed by research studies. In comparison to non-fire-setting conduct-disordered children, fire-setters are more destructive, more antisocial and aggressive, and have greater disturbances in relationships. Fire-setting children are responsible for more dangerous domestic fires than older fire-setters. Behaviorally, fire-setting children are clinically similar to young children who soil themselves, smear and destroy food and furnishings, and wander dangerously from home. These children often come from the most chaotic and violent homes. Parents or caretakers are frequently psychiatrically disturbed, alcoholic, or drug-addicted, and unable to care for these children.[16] Fire-setting identifies one of the most seriously disturbed subgroups of conduct-disordered children, who usually require inpatient evaluation once they come to the clinician's attention. The conduct-disordered adolescents who are at the greatest risk are those with symptoms of suicide and depression as well as conduct disorder. As mentioned previously, antisocial behavior has been found to be an important risk factor in the successful suicide of adolescents, both boys and girls. Therefore any adolescent with conduct disorder should be carefully evaluated for symptoms of suicide and depression. If symptoms of conduct disorder and suicide or depression are found, the adolescent should be considered for inpatient referral or, at the least, intensive outpatient treatment.

EMERGENCIES REQUIRING RESPITE CARE

One other group of children and adolescents that might need emergency intervention and or hospitalization are those with severe neurodevelopmental delays or mental retardation and severe behavioral difficulties. Although they may not have psychiatric disorders, they can develop dangerous behavioral symptoms under stress. Assaultive and self-injurious behavior in a mentally retarded or neurodevelopmentally delayed child or adolescent is a bona fide psychiatric emergency and should be treated accordingly. Every effort should be made to control the symptom in the home environment because the alternative of hospitalization and the loss of familiar surroundings and people is an additional stressor. In the home, pharmacologic and behavioral interventions are usually available. Much stress and tension accompany the day-to-day care of these children and adolescents, and sometimes the parents or caretakers of these patients need a respite. Temporary hospitalization of the patient may allow the parents and caretakers to resume the care of these difficult children and adolescents with renewed vigor and more positive attitudes. Respite hospitalization may also enable a neurodevelopmentally delayed or mentally retarded child or adolescent to remain in the home and avoid chronic institutionalization.

REFERENCES

1. Goodwin, J., Simms, M., and Bregman, R.: Hysterical seizures: A sequel to incest. Am. J. Orthopsychiat. 49:697, 1979.
2. Silver, L.B.: Conversion Disorder with pseudoseizures in adolescence: A stress reaction to unrecognized and untreated learning disabilities. J. Am. Acad. Child Psychiat. 21:508, 1982.
3. Holmes, G.L., Sackellares, J.C., McKiernan, J., et al.: Ragland, M., Dreifuss, J. Evaluation of childhood seizures using EEG telemetry and video tape monitoring. J. Pediatr. 97:554, 1980.
4. American Psychiatric Association: Diagnostic and Statistical Manual of Mental Disorders, Third Edition, Revised. Washington, DC, American Psychiatric Association, 1987, pp. 247–251.
5. Pynoos, R.S., and Elk, S.: Witness to violence: The child interview. J. Am. Acad. Child Psychiat. 25:300, 1986.
6. Garralda, M.I.: Hallucinations in children with conduct and emotional disorders. J. Study Child. Psychol. Med. 14:589, 1984.
7. Mortality Statistics Branch. Division of Vital Statistics. National Center for Health Statistics, 1986.
8. Hawton, K., and Goldacre, M.: Hospital admissions for adverse effects of medicinal agents (mainly self-poisoning) among adolescents in the Oxford, Oregon. Br. J. Psychiatry 141:106, 1982.
9. Gold, M.S., and Davidson, L.: Suicide contagion among adolescents. In Advances in Adolescent Mental Health Volume III Depression and Suicide. Edited by Stillman, A.R., and Feldman, R.A. Greenwich, CT, JAI Press, 1988, pp. 106–109.

Clinical Evaluation of Psychiatric and Behavioral Emergencies **2695**

10. Shaffer, D., Garland, A., Gould, G., et al.: Preventing teenage suicide. A critical review. J. Am. Acad. Child Adol. Psychiat. 27:675, 1988.
11. Shaffer, D.: Suicide in childhood and early adolescence. J. Child Psychol. Psychiat. 15:275, 1974.
12. Garfinkel, B.D., Froese, A., and Hood, J.: Suicide attempts in children and adolescents. J. Psychiat. 139:1257, 1982.
13. Harjanic, B.: Adolescent suicide. Adv. Behav. Pediatr. 1:195, 1980.
14. Rogawski, A.B., and Edmundson, B.: Factors affecting the outcome of psychiatry interagency referral. Am. J. Psychiatr. 127:925, 1971.
15. Puig-Antich, J., and Weston, B. The diagnosis and treatment of major depressive disorder in childhood. Ann. Rev. Med. 34:231, 1983.
16. Stewart, M.A., and Calver, K.W.: Children who set fires: The clinical picture and follow-up. Brit. J. Psychiat. 140:35, 1982.

SELECTED SPECIFIC ISSUES IN THE EMERGENCY DEPARTMENT

Gary J. Grad, Jean-Pierre Lindenmayer, and Nathan S. Kline

CAPSULE

Some specific conditions that might bring children and adolescents with psychiatric disorders to the Emergency Department (ED) are discussed in this section.

DEFINITION AND CONCEPTS

As with adult patients, emergencies in children or adolescents can be seen as sudden behavioral or emotional responses to overwhelming anxiety. The child's or adolescent's usual coping mechanisms have broken down or are inadequate to deal appropriately with the anxiety. Much more than with adult patients, however, the parents define what constitutes a "psychiatric emergency" for their child because children and adolescents seldom seek out physicians when acutely anxious or upset. The parents are the ones who are presented with the child's distress, and they request treatment when their own anxiety over their child's unusual behavior has become so overwhelming that they feel helpless. Also, again much more than with the adult patient, the parents' presentation of the child as an "emergency" actually may be an expression of internal family distress, not of the child's pathology. It is therefore particularly important in these situations to explore carefully how the "emergency" came to be labeled as such and by whom.

Psychiatric emergencies in children and adolescents differ in another major way from those in the adult.

The child or adolescent patient is limited in his or her ability to register complaints about upset feelings and situations in affects or words, unlike the adult. Distress is most often manifested by action and changes in behavior that are either developmentally deviant or disordered for the given child. The younger patient, for example, may begin to play with much younger children, or an adolescent may react by running away from home rather than expressing his or her depression. As children become older, they differentiate along developmental lines, and the ways in which they express their reactions to stress become more like those of adults. Therefore, specific syndromes differ more among adolescents than among younger children, whose abnormal behavior is more difficult to recognize and diagnose correctly.

Another aspect that differentiates young patients from adult patients is represented by acute difficulties related to the lack of mastery of a developmental step. The normal psychologic development of children can be seen in the context of the mastery of new and more complex situations. If difficulties in handling these situations arise, they should be resolved as quickly as possible, because they may otherwise lead to further developmental problems. One example of such a situation is that of the school-phobic child (often afraid of separation from his mother), who warrants emergency care.

Another feature that distinguishes young patients from adult patients who show acute behavior difficulties is reflected in the frequent overlapping of organic and functional difficulties. It may be difficult to differentiate the effects of underlying "soft" neurologic signs or of a seizure disorder from the effects of psychologic problems related, for example, to a disturbed family situation. Generally, these aspects must be explored through specialized consultations once the immediate emergency situation has been handled.

INTERVIEWING IN THE EMERGENCY SETTING

In interviewing both the parents and the child, the following three important questions should be answered:

1. *Why did the crisis occur now?* Recent changes in the child's environment should be noted (including recent moves, changes in the composition of the household, death or illness of close relatives or friends, changes in school) because the child may be sensitive to these, and the problem may be directly related to such occurrences.
2. *Who labeled the situation as a crisis?* The physician should explore here whose anxiety tolerance has been overtaxed—the child's or the parents'—or was the situation identified by community agencies? Once this has been clarified, the physician must address himself or herself specifically to the main participant in the emergency situation.
3. *What are the expectations of the patient and the parents?* This is particularly important with children and families, as already noted. The physician should take these expectations into account when formulating the management plan.
4. Finally, careful attention should be paid to the *psychologic and physical developmental history* because this will give the physician an idea of the acuteness and extent of the problem as well as of the possibility of an underlying organic basis. Comparison by the physician with childhood norms will aid this process. (See previous section.)

If a physical examination is indicated, it must be geared to the presenting complaints. Physical findings, developmental anomalies, and hard and "soft" neurologic signs[1] as well as an evaluation of mental status indicating cognitive deficits, help point to organic factors in the cause of the physical or behavioral complaint. After the presenting situation has been fully evaluated, constellations of symptoms and signs may point to specific diagnoses, lead to further evaluations through specialized consultations, or both.

HANDLING THE PARENTS

The parents of the child with an organic deficit, especially if it is severe and irreversible, may feel that some deficit in themselves caused the disorder. In most instances, this is not true, and the doctor should indicate this to the parents through a complete and thoughtful presentation. When organic deficits exist, the parents may withdraw from the child, deny the existence of the organic problem, or both. These reactions tend to perpetuate the difficulties of the child, who has already been compromised in his adaptive ability. Parents can be counseled that organic deficits do not place an absolute limit on a child's development and that there are many agencies that can help them and their child. Finally, the parents may not want to believe the physician and may seek further consultation with other experts. This may be necessary and cannot be denied to the family, but the sooner accurate and adequate treatment for the child begins, the greater is the possibility that he or she will be helped. Continuous consultations may maintain unreasonable hopes and stave off feelings of guilt, fear, and depression—but not really help the family or the child.

If the difficulty is seen as primarily psychologic, the parents may again be prone to react with withdrawal and denial. The physician may reassure them that not all psychologic problems indicate severe or long-term illness in the child or themselves and that they are not necessarily to blame. They may want to find some organic disease to reassure themselves and may attempt to do so through additional consultations rather than through appropriate psychiatric help. Again, this may delay help for the child and lead to a worsening of the situation.

We have focused on the reactions of the parents, but the physician should also explain his findings to the child in an age-appropriate, nonpatronizing way that should help enlist the child's cooperation in the management of his problem.

PSYCHOPHARMACOLOGIC MANAGEMENT

Many times, the physician uses a psychotropic medication to help alter the situation. Medication use should be target-symptom–directed, and the physician should be familiar with the medication used. Patients placed on medication for behavioral problems should be referred for follow-up evaluation at frequent intervals. Initial emergency management may require medication, but because the child's problem may be situational or caused by some resolving developmental issue, it is useful to reduce medication, discontinue it after 3 to 6 months, and reevaluate the problem (except in a very few syndromes). If the problem still exists, psychiatric consultation should be sought. A basic notion about medication use is that, although it may be the treatment of choice for specific syndromes and indispensable for certain emergency situations, "psychiatric complaints in children require psychological methods of management to a greater or lesser degree and drugs do not cure, educate, or unlearn the basic causes of the disorder but only alleviate the most prominent symptoms."[2] This, however, may often be sufficient to induce a significant improvement.

DESTRUCTIVE AND BIZARRE BEHAVIOR

The child who is brought on an emergency basis because he or she has manifested bizarre actions or destructive behavior or both deserves a careful evaluation. Causes of such behavior are many and varied, ranging from the organic to the psychologic. The behaviors differ also from the younger child to the adolescent.

THE PRESCHOOL CHILD

The preschool child may show self-preoccupation, lack of communicative skills, lack of relatedness to others, stereotyped affect and activities, mutilation of self and others, and sleep disturbances. He or she often has a history of developmental lag and, if without mental retardation and physical abnormalities, may be suffering from one of the variants of childhood psychosis.

THE SCHOOL-AGE CHILD

The school-age to pre-teenage child may present destructive behavior together with periods of lack of awareness of his or her surroundings, destruction of property, continuous fighting, homicidal threats and attempts, learning problems, clumsiness, accident-proneness, and destruction of pets. The most frequent cause here may be an underlying hyperactive syndrome, which is discussed in detail subsequently.

THE ADOLESCENT

The adolescent may manifest eating disturbances, severe weight fluctuations, panic states, and somatic symptoms, as well as symptoms similar to those of the depressed or psychotic adult. Most frequently, the underlying cause is an incipient schizophrenic process.

Other causes for destructive behavior less related to the patient's age can be central nervous system disorders, such as a seizure. This should be investigated, particularly if the bizarre or destructive behavior includes alterations of consciousness or involuntary motor movements not preceded by emotional upsets. Also, a child with acute lead poisoning may present with symptoms of irritability and agitation; lead poisoning has also been associated with the hyperkinetic syndrome.[4]

If firm limit-setting by the physician and the parents has not brought the acute destructive and agitated behavior under control, medication is needed to remedy, at least temporarily, the loss of control. Effective medications include diphenhydramine, 5 mg. per kg per 24 hours in three or four doses, but not to exceed 300 mg. each day; chlorpromazine, 50 to 100 mg. and 200 mg. daily in divided doses in younger and older children, respectively; and thioridazine in doses similar to those recommended for chlorpromazine (but not in children under 2 years). The piperazine group of phenothiazines and butyrophenones are not indicated for general use because the incidence of dyskinesias is high in children. Minor tranquilizers, specifically chlordiazepoxide and diazepam, may lead to "paradoxic" reactions, including rage and temper tantrums, especially in those under 6 years and in children with "soft" signs of neurologic damage.[2,5] Generally, medications should be begun at low doses and maintained at the lowest doses necessary to alleviate symptoms. The major side effect of note associated with diphenhydramine is tiredness. Parkinsonian syndromes as a consequence of phenothiazines may be corrected with antiparkinsonian drugs, as in adult patients. Tardive dyskinesia is manifested in children more often in the trunk, arms, and legs than periorally, as in adults. It should be remembered that other commonly used medications may also lead occasionally to psychiatric emergencies in children (e.g., the aggressive behavior seen in children who are placed on barbiturates, cold or allergy medications, or methylphenidate and amphetamine).

Depending on the severity and degree of the destructive and agitated behavior as well as on how much it inhibits the child in school, leads to familial unhappiness, and stops him or her from having normal peer relationships, child psychiatric consultation must be sought. Supportive counseling for the parents, with emotional support for the child (as provided through the family, school counselor, or religious affiliate), may be adequate in the instance of a family crisis, as long as serious injury to the child or others is not threatened. The child also requires increased supervision. This not only helps control the situation but also increases the attention the child receives from his parents, which probably was decreased as a result of the crisis. If the situation is dangerous and under insufficient control, or if the child is homicidal, psychiatric hospitalization will be necessary.

THE HYPERACTIVE SYNDROME

School-age children who present with variations of the aforementioned dangerous behaviors in addition to learning difficulties may be suffering from the hyperactive syndrome. A history of birth difficulties, injury to the central nervous system, and/or lead intoxication, as well as parental and school reports of excessive activity, distractability, restlessness, and short attention span, strengthen this diagnosis. Once environmental factors (situational reactions, food dyes, monosodium glutamate in foods, etc.) have been ruled out, these children are often referred for medication, for example, amphetamine sulphate (Benzedrine), dextroamphetamine sulphate (Dexedrine), or methylphenidate hydrochloride (Ritalin), 2.5 mg twice a day in those under 5 years or 5 mg twice a day in older children. This medication can be doubled weekly until 60 mg daily is reached for Ritalin and 40 mg daily for the amphetamines. Behavioral alterations should occur rapidly if the medication is effective. Side effects other than the toxic ones, but not dose-related, include anorexia and insomnia, which can be reduced by giving the medication before school and at lunch time on school days only, and only during the school year. Pemoline (Cylert) has also more recently been used for this syndrome. The range of dosage is 18.75 to 75 mg per day given in the morning (not recommended for children under 6 years). This medication has been related less often to anorexia and insomnia than have methylphenidate and dextroamphetamine. Phenothiazines and imipramine also have been used for this syndrome. Often, parents are not willing to have their children placed on medications for long periods; the physician should elicit the parents' feelings about medication use so that their negative reactions do not lead to persistence of the child's symptoms through parental noncompliance. The physician may decide to seek child psychiatric or neurologic consultation if the amphetamines and methylphenidate do not control the symptoms.

FIRE-SETTING AND RUNNING AWAY FROM HOME

Fire-setting by a young child, especially if it does not endanger property or the child, may be seen as natural curiosity about exciting natural phenomena. Education by the parent may be adequate to handle the situation. A nonpunitive approach may be suggested. Fire-setting by the school-age child may be part of a syndrome including enuresis and hyperkinesis.[6] The medications indicated for hyperkinesis may be used, but child psychiatric consultation is more appropriate. In the adolescent, it may be part of vengeful, group antisocial, or homosexual activity, which again requires psychiatric consultation. In other children, however, fire-setting can be a sign of severe underlying psychologic disturbance.

Often, running away from home is not serious because usually the child is easily found and not absent long. This may not even come to the attention of the physician unless he or she specifically asks, although the child's feelings of rejection by the parent may be involved. When the child endangers himself or herself or does not seem to intend to be found, severe family conflict or rejection should be suspected, and child psychiatric consultation is recommended.

SCHOOL PHOBIA

School phobia is most common in kindergarten and in the first grade, in the third to fourth grades, and in junior and senior high school.[7] In the first few years of school, it usually is related to the child's concerns about leaving home and also to the mother's anxiety about separation from her child. Later on, it can be related to greater learning demands on the child.

The child may present to the physician at the point of entering school with multiple, minor physical complaints that lead to his or her inability to attend school. When the physician notices this, he should reassure the mother that the child is not ill (usually the case), limit his examinations unless illness is quite probable, and help set a date with the school for the child's return. The father may be brought in more actively to provide support, especially for his wife. If school attendance still does not proceed, more severe pathology may be suspected, and psychiatric consultation should be sought. The third- to fourth-grade child who will not go to school should have adequate psychologic tests to rule out retardation or other causes of school failure. A hyperactive syndrome may be discovered, for which the medication previously indicated is necessary. The child who will not attend high school after successful previous attendance should receive psychiatric consultation, especially because more severe psychopathology can be suspected.

ANOREXIA

The anorexic child may present at times as a true medical emergency requiring immediate hospitalization. More frequently, however, the patient will come to the attention of the physician because of severe weight loss, requests for special diets to lose weight, amenorrhea, or concerns by the parents for their child's dieting or food fads. The patient is usually a girl and may be a young teenager, although the syndrome is most common in young women in their late teens and early 20s.

The syndrome is best treated, if noticed very early, before the point of medical emergency or before a severe, overt family conflict over eating develops. Psychiatric consultation is necessary. The treatment approach may include the physician, psychiatrist, and other professionals who attempt to intervene through the family's patterns as well as the individual's problems. Antidepressants, and especially the monoamine oxidase inhibitors, have been claimed to be useful, although prolonged administration for several months usually is needed.

SEXUAL PROMISCUITY AND PREGNANCY

Promiscuous behavior is difficult to define. The physician's role may be to intervene only when the adolescent is being self-destructive. Parental reactions may be extremely punitive and nonproductive. The physician may be of help in modulating parental responses, noting the adolescent's behavior, and developing a working relationship with the parents and teenager that will allow them to seek psychiatric help. The physician should be aware of punitive attitudes on his or her part also, which could drive the patient away from professional help.

The adolescent who becomes pregnant does so for a variety of reasons, ranging from being in love to wanting to be loved through the baby. She may consult the physician and show tremendous ignorance about her body and about pregnancy. A variety of issues may arise, including adequate care of the pregnant woman, decisions about termination of the pregnancy, the desire for and possibility of marriage, keeping or giving up the child, and parental responses of anger and withdrawal from the adolescent. The physician can be most helpful in preliminary counseling of the parents and their daughter, and in locating adequate gynecologic, pediatric, and (if necessary) psychiatric facilities.

RAPE AND INCEST

The raped child or adolescent presents the physician with multiple problems and issues. He must first determine whether rape has occurred and, if so, determine the extent of any bodily damage and the possibility of pregnancy or infection. Rapport should be established with the victim and her parents. If penetration has occurred, examination should proceed only after parental consent has been obtained. Vaginal aspirate can be examined for sperm and can be used for bacterial culture. Treatment for gonorrhea may be necessary, and an anti-implantation pill may be used. A VDRL is necessary several weeks after the rape. Adequate records for police use are appropriate, if they are to be informed. In some areas this is not an automatic procedure but depends on the parents' decision.

The parents may be as upset and angry as the victim, who may feel angry, violated, and guilty. The physician should help the patient in a supportive way to ventilate her upset feelings about this extremely frightening experience. Immediate psychiatric help may be indicated by the degree of upset experienced by the victim or parents or both. In some instances, more

severe psychologic reactions may occur some time after the rape. Contact should be maintained for up to 3 months, and psychiatric help should be made available if and when necessary.[8,9] Hospitalization may be needed for very young victims. Often the rapist is known to the family, and they must be counseled against any attempt at retribution other than through legal channels.

Incest is probably more common than suspected. It may come to the attention of the physician on routine examination of a child patient with frequent vaginal infections or as part of a pattern of parental abuse or neglect. In some states it must be reported and legally constitutes abuse. The most common pattern is father-daughter incest. Surprisingly often, the mother knows of the incestuous relationship. Its existence is greatest in disturbed families in which the daughter has, in a sense, taken the mother's place or in which there is severe psychopathology in family members. Psychiatric consultation is imperative if the physician has proof of the existence of incest.

ABUSE AND NEGLECT

The abused or neglected child comes to the attention of the physician when presented for medical care following the abuse. The infant may not be developing at a normal rate and may show failure to thrive without renal, cardiac, or CNS defects. The child may have injuries that cannot be explained adequately by the parents, such as multiple skin lesions, old and new fractures, and retinal hemorrhages. There also may be delay in seeking medical attention. The abused child is often the one in the family who is seen as "different": the youngest, the oldest, the only one of a particular sex, one having physical deformities, one who creates a nuisance, or one who has any combination of these features. The parents are often immature, have problems controlling their anger, are not gratified in their own lives (unemployed or drug or alcohol users), and cannot satisfy a wide variety of their partner's needs in the marital relationship. Patterns of abuse may have been present in their own parents' homes.

The physician's role in situations of child abuse and neglect is well defined. He documents the possibility of abuse and begins the attempts necessary to guarantee the child's future safety. If the physician suspects abuse and if the child is under 5 years and in possible danger if allowed to go home, the child should be hospitalized.[10] Necessary laboratory tests and specialty consultations should be obtained, both to treat the child and to document the abuse as accurately as possible. This should be done in either the inpatient or outpatient situation. The home circumstances and the parents should be evaluated as soon as possible. This is usually accomplished through the child welfare agency that is designated to do so in each area. It is advisable to obtain psychiatric consultation for the parents. In situations of possible abuse, it is often difficult to maintain a neutral, helpful attitude toward the parents. They must be advised of the physician's suspicions and that welfare agencies will be involved. The physician may have to wait before discharging the hospitalized child until he or she is notified by these agencies as to whether the child will be placed or allowed to be sent home. Most of the responsibility falls on social agencies and psychiatric facilities after the diagnosis is made, but physical care of the child may continue to be the responsibility of the physician.

SITUATIONAL REACTIONS

Throughout the discussion of emergency situations in childhood and adolescence, we have mentioned the possibility of symptoms demanding emergency treatment stemming from the child's reaction to stressful situations. In this section, several situations will be briefly mentioned that are particularly stressful to the child and may warrant special attention. In all these situations, the child may regress in his behavior. Additional support and appropriate concern for the child can be helpful in mastering these periods of stress.

The first of these is the death of a close relative (parent or sibling). The child should be gently informed of the death and allowed to ask questions. These are determined by the attachment of the child to the dead person, the child's level of cognitive development, and his or her ongoing personality patterns. It should be made clear to the child that he is not responsible for the death. Severe behavioral symptoms should lead to psychiatric consultation.

Children, especially 5- and 6-year-olds, are particularly sensitive to the separation necessitated by hospitalization. Parents should be allowed as much contact as possible with the child through visiting. The child should be stimulated by ward staff through play, books, and so forth. The older child may react to hospitalization or chronic illness with antitherapeutic behavior. In all instances, the child should be told as much as possible in advance about the hospitalization, when this can be anticipated, and the treatment of the illness should be explained in terms the child can understand.

ADOLESCENT DRUG USE

Adolescent drug use is common today. Patterns include occasional experimentation, addiction, attempts at self-medication, psychologic distress, and suicide attempts. It is most important for the physician to attempt to discover why drug use is occurring. If the adolescent patient presents himself or herself, it may be because of acute intoxication or overdose, for which emergency measures will be indicated. The adolescent may also consult a physician in an attempt to find out what effect a medication will have, with physical symptoms from chronic drug use, or as a method of informing parents, physician, or both of his or her drug use to get help or to create a difficult situation. The physician should attempt to determine the patterns of use as well as the reasons that the patient is presenting at that time. The patient with an addiction problem who seeks help voluntarily should be directed to appropriate, nonpunitive agencies. A psychologically distressed youth may require psychiatric consultation. The informed physician can educate the adolescent about drugs, their effects, and their use.

A most important aspect of adolescent drug use is the handling of the patient's parents. The latter may present as if an emergency exists, and if so they may be reassured that the adolescent (if he or she is willing, and the physician feels competent) will be seen by the physician and the situation evaluated. The occasional use of nonaddicting drugs should not be viewed as an emergency but still should be evaluated. Such occasional use, if nonprogressive and occurring without antisocial behavior or psychiatric disturbance, may best be handled nonpunitively. The most important aspects of the consultation are the maintenance of trust with the adolescent and his or her parents and the avoidance of involvement in a family argument. If there is severe mistrust between parents and child or severe family discord (especially with the occurrence of violence), psychiatric—most probably child psychiatric—consultation should be recommended.

In the emergency setting, it is particularly important to evaluate the young person in the context of his or her environment. Frequently, if the adolescent is brought in by the police, the officers apply pressure on the physician not only to take blood and urine tests, but also to provide details regarding former usage. Naturally, this sort of action destroys all confidence. Furthermore, bearing in mind the highly variable child detention facilities and the possibilities of extreme psychic trauma for an adolescent placed in such a holding facility, the physician may find it best to defer discussion or to seek psychiatric opinion without actually referring the patient. It is difficult to counsel in a crisis environment.

It is essential that the emergency physician have a broad perspective of drug use in our society to evaluate the individual patient and differentiate between adolescents who are simply experimenting with drugs and those who are already addicted or are becoming addicted.

REFERENCES

1. Chamberlain, H.R.: Mental retardation. *In* Pediatric Neurology. Edited by Farmer, T.W.: Hagerstown, Md., Harper & Row, 1975, pp. 90–117.
2. Conners, C.K.: Organic therapies. *In* Comprehensive Textbook of Psychiatry. II. Edited by Freedman, A., Kaplan, H.T., and Sadock, B.J.: Baltimore, Williams & Wilkins Co., 1975, pp. 2240–2246.
3. Prugh, D.G., and Kisley, A.J.: Psychosocial aspects of pediatrics and psychiatric disorder. *In* Pediatric Neurology. Edited by Farmer, T.W.: Hagerstown, Md., Harper & Row, 1975, pp. 564–596.
4. David, O.: Personal communication, 1973.
5. Conners, C.K.: Psychopharmacological treatment of children. *In* Clinical Handbook of Psychopharmacology. Edited by DiMascio, A., and Shader, R.I.: New York, Science House, 1970, pp. 281–287.
6. Linn, L.: Other psychiatric emergencies. *In* Comprehensive Textbook of Psychiatry. II. Edited by Freedman, A.M., Kaplan, H.T., and Sadock, B.J.: Baltimore, Williams & Wilkins Co., 1975, pp. 1785–1798.
7. Berlin, I.N.: Psychiatry and the school. *In* Comprehensive Textbook of Psychiatry. Edited by Freedman, A.M., Kaplan, H.T.,
and Sadock, B.J.: Baltimore, Williams & Wilkins Co., 1975, pp. 2251–2262.
8. Lewis, M., and Lewis, D.O.: Pediatric management of psychologic crises. Curr. Probl. Pediatr. 3:12, 1973.
9. Burgess, A.W., and Holstrom, L.L.: Rape trauma syndrome. Am. J. Psychiatry, *131*:981, 1974.
10. Helfer, R.E.: Child Abuse and Neglect: The Diagnostic Process and Treatment Programs. Department of Health, Education and Welfare Publication No. (OND) 75–69, U.S. Government Printing Office, 1975.

BIBLIOGRAPHY

Morrison, G.C., and Smith, W.R.: Emergencies in child psychiatry: a definition. *In* Emergencies in Child Psychiatry. Edited by Morrison, G.C.: Springfield, Ill., Charles C Thomas, 1975, pp. 13–20.

Weiner, J.M.: Organic therapies. *In* Comprehensive Textbook of Psychiatry. III. Edited by Freedman, A., Kaplan, H.T., and Sadock, B.J.: Baltimore, Williams and Wilkins Co., 1980, pp. 2679–2685.

THE ABUSED, ASSAULTED ADULT

Susan V. McLeer and Rebecca A.H. Anwar

CAPSULE

Each year over 20,000 people die from interpersonal violence in the United States. For each reported death there are at least 100 nonfatal assaults.[1] Because of underreporting, official crime statistics do not begin to reflect the extent of violence in our society. Hospitals, and specifically emergency departments (EDs), however, see larger numbers of patients presenting with injuries caused by such assaults.[2] The medical evaluation and care provided for abused and assaulted adults must extend beyond the specific presenting medical and/or surgical problems. It is essential for physicians to determine if injuries were caused by a mode of assault or abuse that is highly likely to recur, as in adult domestic violence and abuse of the elderly. If recurrence appears likely, the ED staff must determine the patient's need for protection against further assault or abuse. It is additionally important that emergency physicians understand the behavioral, cognitive, and neurophysiologic changes that can be precipitated by severe stress to provide the patient with guidance as to when he or she should seek treatment for the probable psychologic sequelae of assault and/or abuse.

INTRODUCTION

Adult domestic violence, by far the most prevalent of the recurrent forms of assault or abuse, is defined as the use of physical force by one partner against the other in an intimate relationship, regardless of marital status or cohabitation. Elder abuse is the willful infliction of physical pain or injury, debilitating mental anguish, or financial exploitation of an older person. It also includes active and passive neglect. Active neglect is the failure of a caretaker of an older person to intervene or resolve a significant need despite the awareness of available resources; passive neglect includes unintentional neglect.

Although some studies have indicated that physical force is used against men as often as, if not more than, against women,[3,4] the physical abuse of men does not appear to be a widespread clinical problem.[5] Three factors account for this phenomenon: (1) the strength differential between men and women is sufficiently great that men are less apt to be injured, (2) the means of physical force used by women has been demonstrated to be less serious than those used by men (hitting and throwing things versus use of fists and weapons), (3) the study indicating that women use physical force against men frequently does not address the issue of motivation, e.g., the use of physical force in self-defense during a battering episode. Physical abuse of women, on the other hand, has become a problem of crisis proportion, with 20 to 25% of adult women in the United States having been abused at one time or another by a male intimate.[3]

Data from regional studies, including a random sample survey of 2000 older persons in the Boston metropolitan area, indicate a prevalence rate for elder abuse of 32 per 1000.[6] Although a national study is yet to be done, it is estimated that about 4% or about 1.1 million older Americans are victims of elder abuse each year, with women being at greatest risk.[7]

CLINICAL PRESENTATION

Domestic violence perpetrated against women may be the single most common cause of injuries presented by women to the health care system, accounting for more injury episodes than automobile accidents, muggings, and rapes combined.[8] As many as 30 to 40% of injured women seeking care in ED settings may have injuries caused by battering.[9–12] Moreover, battering is a chronic problem, with the severity and frequency of beatings increasing over time.[13–15] Seventy-five percent of those first injured continue to experience ongoing abuse.[10]

Battering accounts for 1 out of every 5 women seeking medical care,[8] with most battered women not seeking care for injuries, but presenting with general medical, behavioral and/or psychiatric problems. Women are more likely to be battered during pregnancy; hence, as many as 25% of obstetric patients may be battered.[11] Battered women as compared to nonbattered women are more likely to present with depression, anxiety, family/marital, or sexual problems (19% versus 8%) or vague medical complaints (12% versus 3%).[10] Drug and alcohol abuse is even more prevalent, with battered women having 16 times the risk of abusing alcohol and 9 times the risk of drug abuse, compared to nonbattered women.[10] One out of 10 battered women who seek care in medical settings attempts suicide, and of those who do, 50% will do so again.[10] In 1984, 1310 women and 806 men were killed during acts of domestic violence.[16] Clearly, domestic violence is a source of great morbidity and significant mortality in our society.

Although it is unknown how many older abuse victims seek emergency care, it is known that older persons are in more frequent contact with health care providers than younger persons because of the greater likelihood of both chronic and acute illness.[17] Symptomatology of elder abuse is often contributed to normal aging changes (e.g., "old people bruise easily") or health problems more common in older persons (e.g., hip fracture).

INITIAL IDENTIFICATION

Studies have demonstrated that, if asked, battered women almost always admit to having been battered.[8] In spite of this fact, the necessary questions are infrequently asked by health care providers. Without systematic use of protocols designed to identify and diagnose victims of domestic violence, physicians have been found to identify only one abuse victim in 35.[10,18] Mental health professionals, charged with asking rather intimate questions of clients, identify only one abuse victim out of 30.[19]

It has been demonstrated that health professionals can be easily trained to identify victims of domestic violence through the use of brief protocols.[12,20–22] Unless an institutionalized system exists for ensuring the use of such protocols, however, it appears that professionals will continue not to systematically diagnose battering. In a study conducted in a Philadelphia teaching hospital, introduction of an ED protocol designed to detect injuries caused by battering increased the identification of battered women from 5.6% of female trauma patients to 30%. An 8-year follow-up study in the same hospital found that, without continued monitoring and use of protocols, the identification of battering decreased to preprotocol levels.[23]

Similarly, there is gross underreporting of elder abuse.[24,25] The absence of written protocols has been identified as a major barrier for health care professionals in the detection of elder abuse.[26] EDs of hospitals that have implemented elder abuse protocols have found a substantial improvement in the way elder abuse cases are processed and documented.[27–29] There is also much better long-term follow-up.[26,31]

Children in violent families suffer considerably. At least 26 to 33% of all children who witness parental violence demonstrate significant behavioral and/or emotional problems.[19,32] One study has demonstrated that 75% of boys who witnessed battering scored above standardized norms for behavioral dysfunction on well validated rating scales.[33] No systematic studies have been conducted on the effects of witnessing violence on girls.

In addition to the indirect effects of witnessing parental violence, children are at heightened risk for being physically abused themselves. In fact, there is a 129% greater chance of child abuse in families where a husband has hit his wife.[3] One third of families in which the husband-wife violence was severe enough to be considered wife abuse also evidenced child abuse.[34] The implications of these findings are significant for health providers. Whenever a child is identified as being abused, one should ask if the child's mother is being battered. Likewise, whenever a battered woman is identified, one needs to determine if there are children in the family and if they are also being abused.

CLINICAL EVALUATION

The emergency physician's role with adult victims of assault or abuse is a complex one, and given limited time, certain tasks must be delegated to other health care professionals to meet the minimal requirements of providing adequate care. The emergency physician bears the ultimate responsibility for the quality of the medical care provided, and so must ensure that necessary protocols are followed. A seven-step protocol has been found useful in providing care to adult victims of abuse or assault (Table 62-26).

STEP 1. OBTAIN TRAUMA AND PSYCHOSOCIAL HISTORY

ADULT VICTIMS OF DOMESTIC VIOLENCE

Establishing that the woman's injuries are secondary to battering is the first task. Of female trauma patients, 16 to 30% report that they have been battered when asked directly about how the injury occurred. Some women, however, do not admit that they have been battered. Any trauma or burn that seems incompatible with a history of the injury suggests battering and indicates the need for gentle probing as to how things are at home, the presence of undue stress, frequent disagreements, etc. Asking more about disagreements and whether they have escalated to shouting, loss of temper, slapping, etc. aid in eliciting a history of bat-

TABLE 62-27. STRUCTURED INTERVIEW FOR VICTIMS OF DOMESTIC VIOLENCE*

How were you hurt?
Has this happened before?
When did it first happen?
How badly have you been hurt in the past?
Was a weapon involved?/Is there a weapon in the house?
What kind?
Who lives in the home?
What are the children's ages?
Are the children in danger?
Have they been hit or hurt by him?
How badly have they been hurt?
Have you ever told anyone about this before? If so, who?
What have you done in the past to protect yourself?
What have you done in the past to get help?
Have you ever called the police?
If yes, when, and what did they say/do?
Did you report this incident to the police? If not, why not?
If yes, what precinct?
What did they say?
Have you obtained a protective order?
Have you ever tried to press charges this time or before?
Does your boyfriend/husband have a criminal record?
Has he beaten up or hurt other people?
Has he threatened to kill you?
What did he do?
Are you afraid to go home?
Where can you go?
Have you ever called Women Against Abuse, Women in Crisis, etc?
If yes, do you have a contact there? Who?

* With permission from McLeer, S.V., and Anwar, R.A.H.: The role of the emergency physician in the prevention of domestic violence. Ann. Emerg. Med. *16*:1156, 1987.

tering. Information must be collected to facilitate a comprehensive assessment of the battered woman's needs, resources, and priorities to develop immediate and long-range plans designed to minimize and/or eliminate future abusive episodes. A structured interview that can be used to obtain the necessary information for treatment planning is outlined in Table 62-27.

TABLE 62-26. SEVEN STEP PROTOCOL FOR ADULT VICTIMS OF ASSAULT AND ABUSE*

Obtain trauma history		X
Diagnose and treat medical/surgical problems	X	±X
Evaluate emotional status		X
Determine risk to woman and children		X
Determine need for legal information		X
Develop follow-up plan		X
Document status in medical record	X	±X

* With permission from McLeer, S.V., and Anwar, R.A.H.: The role of the emergency physician in the prevention of domestic violence. Ann. Emerg. Med. *16*:1159, 1987.

TABLE 62-28. CLASSIFICATION OF TYPES OF ELDER ABUSE*

Physical or Sexual Abuse
   Bruises (bilateral and at different stages of healing)
   Welts
   Lacerations
   Punctures
   Fractures
   Evidence of excessive drugging
   Burns
   Physical constraints (tying to beds, etc)
   Malnutrition and/or dehydration
   Lack of personal care
   Inadequate heating
   Lack of food and water
   Unclean clothes or bedding
   Lack of needed medication
   Lack of eyeglasses, hearing aids, false teeth
   Difficulty in walking or sitting
   Venereal disease
   Pain or itching, bruises or bleeding of external genitalia, vaginal
      area, or anal area
Psychologic Abuse (vulnerable adults react by exhibiting resignation, fear, depression, mental confusion, anger, ambivalence, insomnia)
   Threats
   Insults
   Harassment
   Withholding of security and affection
   Harsh orders
   Refusal on the part of the family or those caring for the adult
      to allow travel, visits by friends or other family members,
      attendance of church
Exploitation
   Misuse of vulnerable adult's income or other financial resources
      (victim is best source of information), but in most cases has
      turned management of financial affairs over to another person; as a result, there may be some confusion about finances)
Medical Abuse
   Withholding or improper administration of medications or necessary medical treatments for a condition, or the withholding of aids the person would medically require such as false teeth, glasses, hearing aids
   May be a cause of
      Confusion
      Disorientation
      Memory impairment
      Agitation
      Lethargy
      Self-neglect
Neglect
   Conduct of vulnerable adults or others that results in deprivation of care necessary to maintain physical and mental health
   May be manifested by
      Malnutrition
      Poor personal hygiene
      Any of the indicators for mental abuse

* With permission from Council on Scientific Affairs, American Medical Association: Elder abuse and neglect. JAMA *257*:468, 1987.

The initial identification of battered women can be achieved by a triage nurse. A more detailed history takes 30 to 40 minutes and may require the availability of a social worker or trained domestic violence volunteer.

TABLE 62-29. RISK FACTORS FOR ELDER ABUSE

1. Lives with family and has needs that exceed or will soon exceed family's resources
2. High frustration and stress levels among primary caretakers
3. Family has history of family violence
4. Drug or alcohol abuse by caretakers or elderly patient
5. Family system is under severe external stress, e.g. illness or job loss

VICTIMS OF ELDER ABUSE

The elderly person who is at risk for abuse is frequently dependent on the abuser for basic needs such as food, shelter, clothing, medical care, and social stimulation. Consequently, the abused older person may be terrified of disclosing that abuse is occurring. Studies have indicated that elder abuse is recurrent in up to 80% of cases.[36] The abuser is a relative 86% of the time and lives with the elderly person in 75% of cases.[36] Of the abusers, 50% are children or grandchildren, and 40% are spouses.

In a study on elder abuse presenting in an ED, only 33% of abuse victims stated outright that they were being abused, and 6% were reported by neighbors and nonabusive relatives. Another 61% were detected by medical professionals during the course of evaluation and/or hospitalization. This underscores the need for clear protocols for identifying victims of elder abuse.[37] In most cases, abuse was inferred from the physical appearance of the patient (42%) and findings from the social service evaluation of the patient's living conditions (19%). For classification of types of elder abuse, see Table 62-28.

Several risk factors have been identified as associated with elder abuse and underscore the need to obtain historic information from multiple sources (Table 62-29). These risk factors indicate that abuse is apt to occur in families where there is a history of violence and/or substance abuse or a discrepancy between family needs and resources. Hence, it is of utmost importance to gather clinical data regarding the living circumstances of the elderly patient and those of the caretaker and his or her family.

As with other forms of domestic violence and abuse, a history of previous injuries and/or physical deterioration suggests abuse and/or neglect. Likewise, because evidence of physical trauma is found in 50% of elder abuse cases, a careful physical and functional assessment is of utmost importance. Protocols have been developed for EDs to aid in the clinical assessment of the elderly patient. A particularly useful protocol that can be used and modified according to institutional needs is the Elder Assessment Instrument (EAI) developed at the Beth Israel Hospital in Boston (Fig. 62-1).

Date_____ Person completing form _____
Payment status (check one)_____ Blue Cross/Blue Shield
_____ Medicaid _____ Medicare _____ Private Payment
_____ Other _____
Residence (check one): _____ Home
_____ Name of nursing home
_____ Other (e.g., son's/daughter's)

Accompanied by _____ Family _____ Friend _____ Alone
_____ Nursing home personnel
Reason for visit _____ Cardiac _____ Changed mental status
_____ Fall _____ GI _____ Orthopedic
_____ Other (specify) _____
Current mental status: _____ Oriented
_____ Confused _____ Unresponsive

1) General Assessment

	Very Good	Good	Undecided	Poor	Very Poor	No basis for Judgement
a) Clothing						
b) Hygiene						
c) Nutrition						
d) Skin integrity						

Additional comments:_____
_____
_____
_____
_____
_____

2) Physical Assessment

	Definite Evidence	Probable Evidence	Uncertain	Probably no Evidence	No evidence	No basis for judgement
a) Bruising						
b) Contractures						
c) Decubiti						
d) Dehydration						
e) Diarrhea						
f) Impaction						
g) Lacerations						
h) Malnutrition						
i) Urine burns, excoriations						

Additional comments:_____
_____
_____
_____
_____

3) Usual Lifestyle

	Totally Independent	Mostly Independent	Uncertain	Mostly Dependent	Totally Dependent	No basis for Judgement
a) Administration of medication						
b) Ambulation						
c) Continence						
d) Feedings						
e) Maintenance of hygiene						
f) Maintenance of finances						
g) Family involvement						

Additional comments:_____
_____
_____
_____
_____
_____

4) Social Assessment

a) Narrative statement regarding patient identified
social problems: _____
_____

b) Family nursing home perception of problem: _____
_____
_____
_____
_____

	Very Poor quality	Good quality	Uncertain	Poor quality	Very poor quality	No basis for judgement
c) Financial situation						
d) Interaction with family						
e) Interaction with friends						
f) Interaction with nursing home personnel						
g) Living arrangement						
h) Observed relationship with care provider						
i) Participation in daily social activities						
j) Support systems						
k) Ability to express needs						

Additional comments: (recent changes in life situation: _____
_____
_____
_____

FIG. 62-1. Elder Assessment Instrument (EAI). With permission from Fulmer, T., and Wettle, T.: Elder abuse screening and interventions. Nurse Pract. 13:35, 1986).

5) Medical Assessment

	Definite Evidence	Evidence	Possibility	Probably no Evidence	No evidence	No basis for Judgement
a) Duplication of similar medications (e.g., multiple laxatives, sedatives)						
b) Usual doses of medication						
c) Alcohol/substance abuse						
d) Greater than 15-percent dehydration						
e) Bruises and/or fractures beyond what is compatible with alleged trauma						
f) Failure to respond to warning of obvious disease						
g) Repetitive admission due to probable failure of health care surveillance						

(Attach description of any additional physical findings). Additional comments (Note: if either 5a or 5b has been answered in the affirmative, please elaborate and be as specific as possible).

_____

_____

_____

FIG. 62-1. continued

6) Summary Assessments

	Definite Evidence	Evidence	Possibility	Probably no evidence	No evidence	No basis/not applicable
a) Evidence of financial possession abuse						
b) Evidence of physical abuse						
c) Evidence of psychological abuse						
d) History of recent life crisis						

Additional comments:_____

_____

7) Disposition

	Yes	No
a) Referral to elder assessment team		
b) Referral to clinical advisor		

8) General comments: (Nursing home contact person and today's date _____

_____

_____

_____

_____

STEP 2: DIAGNOSE AND TREAT MEDICAL AND/OR SURGICAL PROBLEMS

This step becomes the first priority when a patient is severely injured and/or medically compromised. In doing an assessment for both battered women and victims of elder abuse, however, careful attention must be paid to the patterns of injury and signs of physical neglect because these may support the diagnosis of assault and/or abuse. Dehydration and malnutrition, inappropriate or soiled clothing, poor hygiene, old, uncared-for injuries, or other signs of medical neglect are particularly indicative of elder abuse. Both battered women and abused elderly patients may show physical signs of sexual abuse or rape, and all should be asked whether sexual assault has occurred. A body map of injuries is particularly helpful for both abused elderly patients and for other victims of domestic violence (Figure 62-2).

STEP 3: EVALUATE THE EMOTIONAL STATUS OF THE ASSAULTED OR ABUSED PATIENT

The emotional status of all assaulted or abused adults needs determination. Studies have indicated that assaulted adults, particularly sexually assaulted adults, are at extreme risk for the development of post-traumatic stress disorder (PTSD).[38] PTSD is an anxiety disorder caused by exposure to an event that is outside the range of usual human experience. Patients with PTSD undergo behavioral and cognitive changes as well as neurophysiologic changes. Studies have demonstrated that the autonomic nervous system is hyperreactive, with peripheral evidence of heightened adrenergic activity. In the early phase of PTSD, there is an additional increase in the release of adrenal corticosteroids, but as a more chronic course develops, the adrenal activity decreases, resulting in a reverse

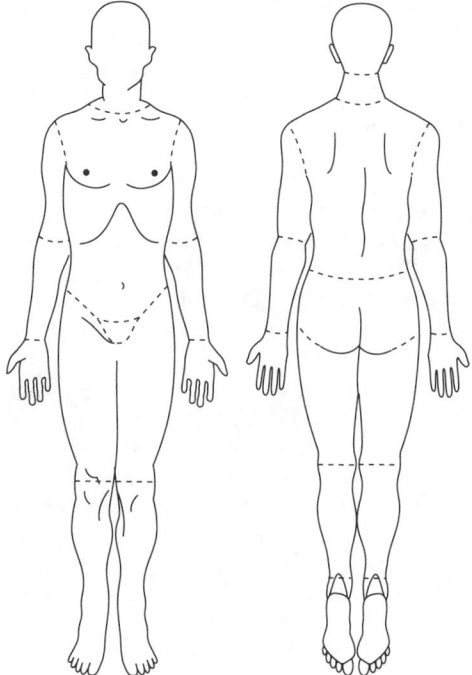

FIG. 62-2.   Body map and indications of elder abuse. With permission from James, J., Dougherty, D., Schelble, D., and Cunningham, W.: Emergency department protocol for the diagnosis and evaluation of geriatric abuse. Ann. Emerg. Med. *17*:1012, 1988.

Indicators
Head Injuries
   Absence of hair
   Hemorrhaging below scalp
   Broken teeth/Eye Injuries
Unexplained bruises:
   Face, lips, mouth
   Torso, back, buttocks
   Bilaterally or upper arms
   Clustered, forming patterns
   Morphologically similar to striking object
   In various stages of healing
Unexplained burns:
   Cigar or cigarette burns
   Immersion burns
   Friction from ropes or chains
   Patterned like electric iron, burner
Sprains/dislocations
Lacerations or abrasions: Mouth, lips, gums, bite marks

ratio of peripheral markers of adrenergic activity and adrenal cortical activity. The behavioral and cognitive components of the post-traumatic stress response are organized around efforts to cope with or avoid increased anxiety. Stimuli that are reminiscent of the original trauma can precipitate severe anxiety attacks. Consequently, patients develop behavioral patterns designed to avoid places, persons, and situations that are reminiscent of the trauma. Diagnostic criteria for PTSD are listed in Table 62-30.

Of patients who initially give evidence of the development of PTSD following assault, many develop persistent post-traumatic stress symptoms. These

TABLE 62-30. DIAGNOSTIC CRITERIA FOR POST-TRAUMATIC STRESS DISORDER*

A. The individual has experienced an event that is outside the range of usual human experience and is psychologically traumatic, e.g., serious threat to one's life or physical integrity; serious threat or harm to one's children, spouse, or other close relatives and friends; involves destruction of one's home or community, or involves seeing another person who is mutilated, dying or dead, or the victim of physical violence.

B. The traumatic event is persistently re-experienced in at least one of the following ways:

Recurrent and intrusive distressing recollections of the event.

Recurrent distressing dreams of the event.

Sudden acting or feeling as if the traumatic event were recurring (includes a sense of reliving the experience, illusions, hallucinations, and dissociative [flashback] episodes, even those that occur upon awakening or when intoxicated) (in young children, repetitive play in which themes of aspects of the trauma are expressed).

Intense psychologic distress at exposure to events that symbolize or resemble an aspect of the traumatic event, including anniversaries of the trauma.

C. Persistent avoidance of stimuli associated with the trauma or numbing of general responsiveness (not present before the trauma), as indicated by at least three of the following:

Deliberate efforts to avoid thoughts or feeling associated with the trauma.

Deliberate efforts to avoid activities or situations that arouse recollections of the trauma.

Inability to recall an important aspect of the trauma (psychogenic amnesia).

Markedly diminished interest in significant activities (in young children, loss of recently acquired developmental skills such as toilet training or language skills).

Feelings of detachment or estrangement from others.

Restricted range of affect, e.g., unable to have loving feelings.

Sense of a foreshortened future, e.g., child does not expect to have a career, marriage, children, or a long life.

D. Persistent symptoms of increased arousal (not present before the trauma) as indicated by at least two of the following:

Difficulty in falling or staying asleep.

Irritability or outbursts of anger.

Difficulty in concentrating.

Hypervigilance.

Exaggerated startle response.

Physiologic reactivity at exposure to events that symbolize or resemble an aspect of the traumatic event (e.g., a woman who was raped in an elevator breaks out in a sweat when entering any elevator).

E. The symptoms in criteria B, C, and D co-occurred during a period of at least 1 month.

* With permission from American Psychiatric Association: Diagnostic and Statistical Manual of Mental Disorders. Third Edition—Revised. Washington, DC, American Psychiatric Association, 1987, p. 250.

symptoms may meet partial or full criteria for PTSD and can be most disruptive to normal life. They may persist for months, if not years, after the original assault. Patients with PTSD experience difficulties in interpersonal, intimate relationships and may develop a variety of phobic behaviors, including agoraphobia, which prevent participation in many job-related activities as well as social activities that were once experienced as enjoyable. The possibility of an intense and prolonged stress response should be discussed with the assaulted patient so that he or she may understand different signs and symptoms of stress and seek appropriate help when needed.

The development of a post-traumatic stress response is something that needs evaluation and discussion with all victims of assault and/or abuse, including stranger assault. In forms of assault that are recurrent, e.g., domestic violence and elder abuse, the evaluation of emotional status is somewhat more complicated. Three additional areas must be evaluated: (1) specific coping mechanisms being used, (2) the presence or absence of a serious psychiatric disorder, and (3) the potential for suicidal or homicidal behaviors. Each of these provides vital information in the assessment of a person's functional ability as well as the intensity of the strain on coping skills. The assessment of coping skills in victims of assault or abuse is relatively simple and can be determined during the collection of the basic clinical history with the addition of a few extra questions (Table 62-31). The other two categories require assessment by a mental health professional who is knowledgeable about the adaptive and psychologic sequelae following chronic victimization and battering.

The need to use a mental health professional with clinical experience and familiarity with the research in the field of domestic violence and elder abuse cannot be overestimated. Victims' emotional responses are all too frequently misinterpreted using standard psychologic and psychiatric techniques without considering what would be a normative response to the most serious stress of chronic victimization.

Research has demonstrated that battered and abused people respond to domestic stress much like other individuals in life-threatening situations. Studies with both civil disasters and war victims have indicated that, during the impact phase, when the threat of danger is perceived as a reality, victims respond with feelings of shock, denial, disbelief, and fear. Confusion and dazed apathetic behaviors are not uncommon. Theorists have offered the explanation that, as the level of danger increases, new defensive strategies are used that increasingly involve an internal focus with decreased external activity and appearance of extreme apathy. This phenomenon has been repeatedly noted in crime victims. Adult victims of domestic violence and elder abuse also demonstrated most, if not all, of these same reactions. In the absence of a clear history and clinical experience with disaster victims, however, victims of domestic violence and elder abuse are most often misdiagnosed and improperly treated.

Victims of domestic violence and elder abuse must be evaluated for suicidal and homicidal potential. One out of every ten battered women attempts suicide. Of those, 50% try more than once. Another way of expressing the risk of suicide among victims of domestic violence is that 26% of all female suicide attempts are preceded by physical abuse. This is even higher among black women, for whom 50% of all suicide attempts are preceded by abuse. Although empiric studies have not been carried out regarding the likelihood of suicidal and/or homicidal behavior amongst victims of elder abuse, it should be noted that the age group at highest risk for successful suicide is the elderly population (over 65 years of age). Hence, this becomes a most important area of assessment in elderly patients.

Both adult victims of domestic violence and elder abuse can also have serious psychiatric disorders independent of the experience of having been clinically abused. It is important to diagnose and treat these major psychiatric disorders in this population because appropriate treatment will aid the individual in gaining more control and enhanced coping abilities. Nonetheless, one cannot overemphasize the need to be careful regarding specific psychiatric diagnoses because in the assaulted and abused adult it is easy to misinterpret symptoms that occur secondary to the severe stress of chronic, unremitting battering and/or abuse and attribute them to other disorders.

TABLE 62-31. ASSESSMENT OF COPING SKILLS*

Is the woman able to function at home and at work?
What efforts has she made in the past to cope with battering?
  Whom has she contacted?
  How often?
  What has been the response?
Has her behavior or mental status changed?
  Is she more aware of the danger of harm, or less?
  Is she reaching out, or withdrawing?
  Does she seem in a fog or emotionally dulled?

* With permission from McLeer, S.V., and Anwar, R.A.H.: The role of the emergency physician in the prevention of domestic violence. Ann. Emerg. Med. *16*:1156, 1987.

INITIAL STABILIZATION AND MANAGEMENT

STEP 4: DETERMINE RISK TO THE ABUSED AND/OR ASSAULTED PATIENT

In recurrent forms of abuse and/or assault, it is essential to assess the patient's need for protection from further abuse. For women who are being battered in the home, it is essential not only to assess the risk for the woman herself, but also to determine if she has children and if they are at heightened risk for physical

TABLE 62-32. RISK FACTORS FOR ESCALATING VIOLENCE*

Children in the home
Batterer threatens to kill spouse
Presence of a weapon
Threat of retaliation
Isolation
Pathologic jealousy in spouse
Use of drugs and/or alcohol
Escalation of violence
Failure of multiple support systems

* With permission from McLeer, S.V., and Anwar, R.A.H.: The role of the emergency physician in the prevention of domestic violence. Ann. Emerg. Med. 16:1158, 1987.

TABLE 62-33. ASSESSMENT OF LEGAL NEEDS*

Has the battered woman ever sought legal help in order to stop the battering?
Is she familiar with the Protection Against Abuse Act?
    Has she used it in the past?
    Was it effective in decreasing her contact with the battering spouse?
    If no, were the police called to enforce the court order?
    Did the police provide adequate protection?
Has the battered woman filed a criminal complaint against the batterer?
    Was the case heard?
    If yes, what was the outcome?
    If no, why? Did the battered woman drop charges?
Does the woman want to pursue either the criminal or civil legal procedures at this time? If yes, give her specific written instructions of what needs to be done.
Regardless of her answer to the question above, give her the name and phone number of a contact person for legal help.
In states that do not have a Protection Against Abuse Act, a criminal complaint can be filed with the District Attorney's permission.

* With permission from McLeer, S.V., and Anwar, R.A.H.: The role of the emergency physician in the prevention of domestic violence. Ann. Emerg. Med. 16:1158, 1987.

abuse. Risk factors that are associated with increased injury and/or death are indicated in Table 62-32.

The most immediate need for the battered woman and/or her children may be for an immediate safe shelter providing protection from the batterer. The fact of revealing to health care professionals that she has been battered may increase her risk of being severely battered on return to her home. The woman herself is the best judge of how dangerous it would be for her to return immediately. Most community organizations working with adult victims of domestic violence maintain shelters at undisclosed locations. Hotline workers can aid the woman in gaining access to a shelter. Unfortunately, there are insufficient shelters in the United States; hence, if the shelters are filled, one should not overlook the battered woman's friends and relatives as potential resources. Hotel rooms can also be used to provide temporary shelter for women at high risk.

With elderly patients who are being abused or neglected, it is essential to involve the social service department in the hospital to assess the patient's need for removal from the current living situation and placement in a safer environment.

STEP 5: DETERMINE THE NEED FOR LEGAL INFORMATION

The legal systems for providing aid to adult victims of domestic violence and elder abuse have developed independent of each other. The systems relating to battered women are targeted toward protecting the woman against further abuse, but do not involve mandated reporting in most states. The protocol for determining the need for legal information for victims of domestic violence is outlined in Table 62-33.

Almost all states in the United States have responded aggressively and enacted legislation designed to protect victims of domestic violence. The battered woman can use the civil laws for protection against abuse or institute criminal action. Alternatively, she can initiate both civil and criminal actions.

The Protection Against Abuse Laws provide the opportunity for a woman to obtain a court order stating that the abuser cannot come near her or her property. It can be designed also to indicate that the batterer stay away from her place of work also. The court order does not give the batterer a criminal record. Violation of the order does. Should the batterer appear at the woman's home or directly threaten her, she can call the police, who theoretically can then arrest the batterer and file criminal charges. A Protection Against Abuse Order is sufficient to provide the necessary structure to protect the battered woman in some instances. In other instances, it helps not at all. The batterer may be so violent that he escalates his attack on finding out that a court protection order has been obtained. He may break through doors or windows, hide in closets with weapons, etc., to gain access to the woman. Needless to say, when a woman is under such direct attack, it is not possible for her to call the police. In such instances, it is helpful for the battered woman to speak to neighbors and ask them to call the police if the batterer is seen near the property or trouble is feared.

Assault is a crime whether it occurs in the street or in the privacy of a person's home. Hence, battered women can choose to petition the District Attorney's office to initiate criminal charges against the batterer. This can be done in tandem with a Protection Against Abuse Order. The risk to the battered woman, however, may be great unless the batterer is held in jail pending trial. The more frequent scenario, however, is a pretrial hearing, bail set, and the man released on bail. Hence, the batterer once again has access to the woman. The batterer's rage over facing criminal

TABLE 62-34. STATES WITHOUT ELDER ABUSE REPORTING LAWS*

TABLE 62-34. STATES WITHOUT ELDER ABUSE REPORTING LAWS*

Indiana	Mississippi	New York
Kansas	New Jersey	Pennsylvania
Maryland	North Dakota	South Dakota

* With permission from Fulmer, T., and Wettle, T.: Elder abuse screening and interventions. Nurse Pract. 11:35, 1986.

TABLE 62-35. FOLLOW-UP PLANNING FOR VICTIMS OF DOMESTIC VIOLENCE*

Determine the need for emergency shelter and work with woman in analyzing whether the plan for emergency shelter is adequate.

Develop a concrete plan for mobilizing help when violence erupts at home.

Design long-term planning process with scheduled follow-up visit within the week.

Give woman the name and phone number of a contact person with the local group working with battered women (e.g., Women Against Abuse, Women in Crisis, etc).

Give woman the name and phone number of a contact person who can help her navigate through the legal process when necessary.

If children are at risk, involve the Child Neglect/Abuse Team in the institution and file an official report of suspected child abuse.

* With permission from McLeer, S.V., and Anwar, R.A.H.: The role of the emergency physician in the prevention of domestic violence. Ann. Emerg. Med. 16:1159, 1987.

charges may be great, and hence the woman's risk may be significantly increased. The decision to initiate criminal charges against a batterer should be discussed with community experts on domestic violence, and activity should be carefully coordinated to ensure that the woman will be safe from harm.

Regarding elder abuse, most states have passed laws requiring mandatory reporting of elder abuse. In a review by Thobaben et al.,[39] seventeen states were identified as having laws which specifically covered the elderly, 21 states included the elderly under disabled adult laws and 4 states provided for "voluntary" reporting. Nine states did not have provisions for the reporting of elder abuse at the time of the review. Table 62-34 indicates those states without elder abuse reporting laws as of 1985.

In states in which there are systems for mandated reporting, the burden on the hospital system for evaluating the status of the abused elderly patient is somewhat relieved by an initiated investigation by Adult Protective Services. In states without mandated reporting, hospital social service departments must attend to the issue of evaluating the status of the patient and his or her living situation and develop plans that will provide a safe and healthy environment on release from the hospital.

For all adult victims of domestic violence, the value in providing the patient with concrete information, including names and phone numbers, cannot be overemphasized. Most communities have staff members associated with Women Against Abuse, Women in Crisis, and community agencies working with the abused elderly, who can provide legal counseling and advocacy. These resources are of enormous value to abused patients who might not use the resource immediately after an ED visit, but may find a need for services later.

STEP 6: DEVELOP A FOLLOW-UP PLAN

This process takes considerable time in the ED setting and yet is essential if a serious effort is to be directed toward interrupting the cycle of violence and minimizing, if not preventing, future violence. The essential tasks are outlined in Table 62-35. In cases of elder abuse, it may also be necessary to mobilize adult protective services to provide periodic home visits tar-

geted at assessing the ongoing well-being and safety of the patient.

As has been previously noted, there is an interrelationship between a woman's being battered in the family system and a heightened risk of child abuse in the home. This means that there must be a coordinated effort between the ED team working with battered women and the institutionalized system for reporting and intervening in cases of suspected child abuse.

PITFALLS

1. Avoid blaming the victim. Battered women are a heterogeneous group and do not have a characteristic profile of psychologic features leading to the seeking of victimization. Batterers, on the other hand, are extremely violent people, with 60% having past records of criminal charges and/or convictions. Batterers, unlike victims, have past histories that are heavily filled with experiences of witnessing severe domestic violence or being recipients of physical abuse during childhood.

2. Do not assume that the situation is less serious if the woman abuses drugs or alcohol. Battered women are at 16 times the risk of abusing alcohol and have 9 times the risk of abusing drugs of nonbattered women. The abuse of substances by battered women is most frequently a secondary problem precipitated by chronic battering and victimization. The abuse of alcohol and drugs is not the cause of the battering.

3. Do not expect a "quick fix." The entrapment by the batterer is considerable from both an emotional and an economic point of view. The presence of children in the home may make it even more difficult for the battered woman to ex-

tricate herself from the situation. Early in the process, the woman experiences shock and disbelief that the man who loves her could do such things to her. Coping skills during this phase of the relationship are hence directed toward decreasing the violence while preserving the relationship. This coping strategy is doomed to fail because the victim has no control over the batterer's violence. At a point when the woman perceives that she cannot control the batterer's violence, her coping strategy shifts toward the development of escape skills.

Battered women have been found to be at greatly increased risk for injury and/or death when they decide to leave the batterer once and for all. The persistence and violence of the batterer's effort to maintain contact with the woman makes leaving a most difficult task. Health care professionals should not give up if the battered woman does not leave immediately. The process of leaving is difficult, dangerous, and frightening. Continued support through the escape phase is essential, and women who do not leave immediately should not be viewed as noncompliant patients.

4. Do not dismiss signs of elder abuse as evidence of the aging process. Poor nutrition, multiple bruises, and injuries may well be physical markers suggesting that the patient is receiving inadequate and abusive care. Patterns of injury as well as patterns of medical relapse should be examined carefully to ensure that abuse and/or neglect are not the cause. Frequent exacerbations of medical illness may indicate that the patient is not being provided with needed medication. These findings in the elderly do not definitively "prove" the presence of abuse, but should be signals for initiating a thorough and careful social service evaluation to determine if there are patterns of abuse and/or neglect in the elderly person's life.

MEDICOLEGAL PEARLS

STEP 7: DOCUMENT FINDINGS AND RECOMMENDATIONS IN THE MEDICAL RECORD

The medical record is an invaluable document for all adult victims of assault and/or abuse. It provides a basis for documenting damages and emotional status at the time of the assault for individuals who are prosecuting the alleged perpetrator of the abuse. Additionally, for those who are victims of adult domestic violence, the medical record provides a document of great importance in obtaining a Protection Against Abuse Order. Likewise, the medical record can be helpful when victims of elder abuse are seeking financial help through court activity to have adequate resources for housing, food, and medical care.

NATIONAL CONTACTS

National Coalition Against Domestic Violence
P. O. Box 15127
Washington, D.C. 20008-0127
202-293-8860

National Aging Resource Center on Elder Abuse
810 1st Street, N.E., Suite 500
Washington, DC 20002-4205
202-682-2470

REFERENCES

1. U.S. Department of Justice, Federal Bureau of Investigation: Uniform Crime Reports—Crime in the United States, 1986. Washington, DC, United States Department of Justice, 1987.
2. Center for Disease Control: Surgeon General's Workshop on Violence in Public Health: Source Book. Leesburg, Virginia, October 27–29, 1985. Atlanta, Center for Disease Control, 1985, p.H.1.
3. Straus, M.A., Gelles, R.J., and Steinmetz, S.K.: Behind Closed Doors: Violence in the American Family. Garden City, New York, Doubleday, Anchor Press, 1980.
4. Straus, M.A., and Gelles, R.J.: Societal change and changes in family violence from 1975 to 1985 as revealed by two national surveys. Journal of Marriage and the Family 48:465, 1986.
5. Steinmetz, S.: "The battered husband syndrome." Victimology: An International Journal 2:499, 1977.
6. Pillemer, K., and Finkelhor, D.: The prevalence of elder abuse: A random sample survey. Gerontologist 28:51, 1988.
7. Kosberg, J.I.: Preventing elder abuse: Identification of high risk factors prior to placement decisions. Gerontologist 28:43, 1988.
8. Stark, E., and Flitcraft, A.H.: "Spouse Abuse" in Surgeon General's Workshop on Violence and Public Health Source Book. Leesburg, Virginia. October 27–29, 1985. Washington, DC, National Center on Child Abuse and Neglect, 1985.
9. Flitcraft, A.: Battered Women: An Emergency Room Epidemiology. M.D. Thesis, New Haven, Connecticut, Yale School of Medicine, 1977.
10. Stark, E., and Flitcraft, A.H.: Wife Abuse in the Medical Setting: Introduction for Health Personnel. Monograph #7, Washington, DC, Office of Domestic Violence, 1981.
11. Stark, E.: The Battering Syndrome: Social Knowledge, Social Theory and the Abuse of Women. Ph.D. Dissertation. Department of Sociology, SUNY, Binghamton, New York, 1984.
12. McLeer, S.V., and Anwar, R.: A study of battered women presenting in an emergency department. Am. J. Public Health 79:65, 1989.
13. Dobash, R.E., and Dobash, R.P.: The case of wife beating. J. Fam. Issues 2:439, 1981.
14. Synder, D.K.: Differential patterns of wife abuse: A date based topology. J. Consult. Clin. Psychol. 40:878, 1981.
15. Walker, L.E.: The Battered Woman's Syndrome. New York, Springer Publishing Company, 1984.
16. Browne, A.: When Battered Women Kill. New York, MacMillan/Free Press, 1987.
17. Capezuti, E.: Preventing Elder Abuse and Neglect. *In* Practicing Prevention for the Elderly. Edited by Lavizzo-Mourey, R., Day, S., Diserens, D., and Griso, J.A. Philadelphia, Hanley and Belfus, 1989.
18. Stark, E., Flitcraft, A., and Frazier, W.: Medicine and patriarchal violence: The social construction of a private event. Int. J. Health Serv. 9:461, 1979.

19. Hilberman, E., and Munson, K.: Sixty battered women. Victimology: An International Journal 2:460, 1978.
20. Kurz, D.: Emergency department response to battered women. A case of resistance. Social Problems 34:501, 1987.
21. Flaherty, E.W., Kurz, D., Olson, K., et al.: Identification and Intervention with Battered Women in Hospital Emergency Departments. Final Report (Grant #R01 MH37180). Bethesda, Maryland, National Institute of Mental Health, 1989.
22. Bain, J., Finkel, K., Hargot, L., and Lent, B.: Wife assault: A medical prospective. In Ontario Medical Review. Edited by Ontario Medical Association. Toronto, Ontario, November 1987.
23. McLeer, S.V., Anwar, R.A.H., Herman, S., and Maquilling, K.: Education is not enough: A systems failure in protecting battered women. Ann. Emerg. Med. 18:651, 1989.
24. Callahan, J.J.: Elder abuse: Some questions for policymakers. Gerontologist 28:453, 1988.
25. Appleton, W.: Elder abuse—diagnose, treat, cure. Ann. Emerg. Med. 17:1104, 1988.
26. Rathbone-McCuan, E., and Voyles, B.: Case detection of abused elderly parents. Am. J. Psychiatry 139:189, 1982.
27. Carr, K., et al.: An elder abuse assessment team in an acute hospital setting. Gerontologist 26:115, 1986.
28. Fulmer, T., and Ashley, J.: Toward the development of a social policy statement on elder abuse. OASIS 5:1, 1988.
29. Jones, J., Dougherty, J., Schelble, T., and Cunningham, W.: Emergency department protocol for the diagnosis and evaluation of geriatric abuse. Ann. Emerg. Med. 17:1006, 1988.
30. Fulmer, T., and Wetle, T.: Elder abuse. Screening and intervention. Nurse Pract. 11:33, 1986.
31. Fulmer, T., and O'Malley, T.: Inadequate Care of the Elderly—a Health Care Perspective on Abuse and Neglect. New York, Springer Publication Company, 1987.
32. Levine, M.: Interparental violence and its effect on the children: A study of 50 families in general practice. Med. Sci. Law 15:172, 1975.
33. Jaffe, P., Wolfe, D., Wilson, S., and Zak, L.: Similarities in behavioral and social maladjustment among child victims and witnesses to family violence. Am. J. Orthopsychiatry 56:142, 1986.
34. Straus, M.A.: Family Patterns and Child Abuse in a Nationally Representative American Sample. Paper presented at the 2nd International Congress on Child Abuse and Neglect. London, 1978.
35. McLeer, S.V., and Anwar, R.A.H.: The role of the emergency physician in the prevention of domestic violence. Ann. Emerg. Med. 16:1155, 1987.
36. AMA Council on Scientific Affairs: Elder abuse and neglect. JAMA 257:966, 1987.
37. Jones, J., Dougherty, J., Scheible, D., and Cunningham, W.: Emergency Department Protocol for the Diagnosis and Evaluation of Geriatric Abuse. Ann. Emerg. Med. 17:1006, 1988.
38. American Psychiatric Association: Diagnostic and Statistical Manual of Mental Disorders. 3rd Edition—Revised. Washington, DC, American Psychiatric Association Press, 1987.
39. Thobaben, M., and Anderson, L.: Reporting elder abuse: It's the law. Am. J. Nurs. April, 1985, pp. 371, 1985.

BIBLIOGRAPHY

U.S. Department of Justice, Federal Bureau of Investigation: Uniform Crime Reports—Crime in the United States 1986. Washington, DC, United States Department of Justice, 1987.

Center for Disease Control: Surgeon General's Workshop on Violence in Public Health: Source Book. Leesburg, Virginia, October 27–29, 1985. Atlanta, Center for Disease Control, p.H.1., 1985.

McLeer, S.V., Anwar, R.A.H., Herman, S., and Maquilling, K.: Education is not enough: A systems failure in protecting battered women. Ann. Emerg. Med. 18:651, 1989.

Kurz, D.: Emergency department response to battered women. A case of resistance. Social Problems 34:501, 1987.

McLeer, S.V., and Anwar, R.A.H.: The role of the emergency physician in the prevention of domestic violence. Ann. Emerg. Med. 16:1155, 1987.

Pillemer, K., and Finkelhor, D.: The prevalence of elder abuse: A random sample survey. Gerontologist 28:51, 1988.

Capezuti, E.: Preventing elder abuse and neglect. In Practicing Prevention for the Elderly. Edited by Lavizzo-Mourey, R., Day, S., Diserens, D., and Griso, J.A. Philadelphia, Hanley and Belfus, 1989.

Jones, J., Dougherty, J., Schelble, T., and Cunningham, W.: Emergency department protocol for the diagnosis and evaluation of geriatric abuse. Ann. Emerg. Med. 17:1006, 1988.

Fulmer, T., and Wetle, T.: Elder abuse. Screening and intervention. Nurse Pract. 11:33, 1986.

AMA Council on Scientific Affairs: Elder abuse and neglect. JAMA 257:966, 1987.

Jones, J., Dougherty, J., Schelble, D., and Cunningham, W.: Emergency department protocol for the diagnosis and evaluation of geriatric abuse. Ann. Emerg. Med. 17:1006, 1988.

MEDICATIONS FOR PSYCHIATRIC DISORDERS

Christos S. Dagadakis

CAPSULE

Major advances in pharmacotherapy and diagnosis for mental illnesses since the 1950s have made mental disorders more treatable and improved the quality of life for many. The five types of psychotropic medications often used in psychiatric disorders are the neuroleptic antipsychotics, antimanic drugs, antidepressants, antianxiety drugs, and antiextrapyramidal symptom agents. Antipsychotic and antianxiety medications are more nonspecifically effective for symptom configurations across diagnostic groups. Antimanic and antidepressant medications have more diagnostic specificity. Antiextrapyramidal agents are effective in controlling side effects mainly of neuroleptics. Effective treatment requires tailoring the medication to the diagnosis, target symptom, and clinical situation.

INTRODUCTION

Neuroleptic antipsychotic medications began to be used in the early 1950s with the introduction of the phenothiazines, which contributed to a revolution in the care of the acutely psychotic and the chronically mentally ill with periodic psychosis. The antidepressant medications began to be developed and have clinical utility in the late 1950s with the use of the tricyclics and monoamine oxidase (MAO) inhibitors. Barbiturates had been used for anxiety before, and meprobamate during the 1950s, but these were displaced by benzodiazepines in the 1960s. Benzodiazepines continue to be one of the most likely prescribed classes of medications. Lithium also began to be used widely mainly to prevent and treat mania in the late 1960s and early 1970s. In the 1980s, anticonvulsants, especially carbamazepine, have been used effectively

with bipolar disorder. Neuroleptics have continued to be frequent treatment for psychosis.[1] Almost all the neuroleptics have similar therapeutic effectiveness and similar limitations.[2] One new neuroleptic, clozapine, appears to have antipsychotic effect and is useful in treating the negative symptoms of schizophrenia with little or no risk for tardive dyskinesia, a major problem with other neuroleptics. It has its own risks, especially agranulocytosis. It has a special role for mainly schizophrenic patients who are resistant to treatment with the other neuroleptics or have problems with tardive dyskinesia or dystonia.[3]

A second generation of antidepressants has shown much promise, especially buproprion, trazodone, and fluoxetine. The latter two have little lethal risk even when taken in an overdose. Antidepressants have been found helpful in panic disorder and post-traumatic stress disorder in addition to depression.

Benzodiazepines have been useful in treating anxiety and, in some individuals, panic disorder. They are also helpful in managing acute psychosis, usually in combination with a neuroleptic. Benzodiazepines have a risk for withdrawal with long term use and for abuse. The use of benzodiazepines must be carefully considered in patients prone to substance abuse. There is a particular risk of respiratory depression when these drugs are combined with alcohol or other sedative hypnotics.

The use of lithium and carbamazepine to treat acute mania usually does not bring about immediate attenuation of symptoms. Frequently, 5 days to several weeks are required. Thus they are less useful in the emergent setting. More rapid improvement in manic symptoms is likely with benzodiazepines, especially lorazepam or clonazepam. The benzodiazepines can be combined with a neuroleptic when psychosis is present.

Antiextrapyramidal symptom (antiparkinsonian) drugs are indicated with dystonias, tremors, drooling, and in some patients, akathisia. Benztropine mesylate, trihexyphenidyl, and diphenhydramine are frequently used and effective. Akathisia is less responsive than the other symptoms. Amantadine and propranolol have been found helpful in akathisia. Benzodiazepines may also help with the symptoms. Tardive dyskinesia is not usually responsive to medication management. Some of these agents are helpful in some individuals but may worsen symptoms in others.

ANTISPYCHOTIC MEDICATIONS (NEUROLEPTICS)

PHYSIOLOGY

Neuroleptic medications are felt to decrease psychotic symptoms by blocking dopamine (D_2) receptors.[4] Although the research is substantial and convincing that dopamine blockade correlates with antipsychotic effect, the actual mechanism of the decrease in psychosis is unknown. One relatively new antipsychotic, clozapine, appears to have a different type of dopamine blockade with more selectivity for receptors in the limbic area of the brain. Other antipsychotics appear to affect receptors more in the striatal areas. In addition, clozapine does not increase serum prolactin and cause prolactin-related side effects as do other neuroleptics. All neuroleptics except clozapine can bring on extrapyramidal symptoms such as acute dystonias, akathisia, and tardive dyskinesia.

INDICATIONS

Neuroleptic medications are primarily indicated for acute psychosis and for ongoing treatment and prevention of relapse for chronic psychosis. The effectiveness of all of the neuroleptics except clozapine is similar. The main differences are in side effects, especially level of sedation and types of preparations (oral, IM, and long-acting IM products). Clozapine has been effective in some individuals with chronic schizophrenia who have been unresponsive or intolerant to other neuroleptics. To date, response predictors to clozapine have not been determined, and the main indications are refractoriness to standard neuroleptics or with the presence of severe extrapyramidal symptoms or tardive dyskinesia.[1] Clozapine is unlikely to be started in emergency settings because its distribution is through the manufacturer, with an elaborate protocol of monitoring because of the frequency of blood dyscrasias.

Because of the risk of tardive dyskinesia in 20 to 40% of patients taking neuroleptics chronically, these medicines have limited use in individuals without psychosis. Some individuals with refractory anxiety or obsessive-compulsive, bipolar, or borderline personality disorder may benefit from neuroleptics. Other treatment modalities should be tried first with these nonpsychotic individuals.

The choice of a neuroleptic in the emergent setting usually depends on the level of acuity, past success with particular neuroleptics in a particular patient, the patient's preference, mode of delivery required, history of medication compliance, dispositional options, likelihood of adverse side effects with doses given to stabilize, and presence of other medical problems and/or use of other medications. It is generally useful to limit the number of neuroleptics used in an emergent setting except in patients in whom a specific one has been helpful. This results in staff familiarity with the use, dosages, and side effect profiles. A useful option is "at-hand" medications in the emergent setting, e.g., haloperidol, 1 mg or 5 mg PO liquid concentrate, or IM preparations; thiothixene, 5 mg PO and IM preparations; thioridazine 50 mg PO; and fluphenazine decanoate and haloperidol decanoate for long-acting use. This combination allows one to treat most acute psychoses with haloperidol with the least risk for adverse immediate outcome except for extrapyramidal symptoms, which are a possibility with most neuroleptics; to use a more sedating neuroleptic thiothizene available po and IM or thioridazine PO. Thioridazine minimizes the dystonia and parkinsonian symptoms but has some greater orthostatic effect than the haloperidol and thiothixene when sedation is desired. It is useful to have readily available the two most widely used long-acting depot neuroleptics for patients already on them who have missed their last dose or in special situations to start someone who is relatively noncompliant with medications and has taken the parent compound in the recent past with little difficulty. Depot medication treatment may be more effective once the individual is first stabilized on oral neuroleptics. There is some increased risk in starting a patient on depot neuroleptics without a PO trial with the shorter-acting version. If the person has an idiosyncratic reaction or allergy to it, he or she will have a serum level for many weeks to months with a depot decanoate preparation. In some clinical situations, the risk is worth the benefit of having a neuroleptic on board for the individual for enough time to help the psychosis. You may have an individual who is agreeable to a medication while in the emergent setting but has shown ambivalence about continuing medication because of his or her psychosis. If the psychosis is improved, he or she may choose to continue the medication because it aids clearer thinking. With the depot decanoate preparations, a po version of the medication must be given until adequate blood levels are present from the depot. For fluphenazine decanoate, the period when adequate blood levels are achieved is 1 to 3 days. For haloperidol decanoate, it is from 3 to 6 days up to several months. Haloperidol decanoate may be taken for 3 to 4 months to reach steady state, and the oral medication may be continuous and decreased as the long-acting contribution increases. For most patients, the dosage period for fluphenazine is every 2 to 3 weeks and for haloperidol every 4 weeks after the steady state is reached. Plans must be developed for follow-up because an isolated decanoate injection usually does not bring about stabilization. Generally, many studies support a chlorpromazine equivalent of 400 to 600 mg/day to be adequate for psychosis treatment for most patients.[1] Table 62-36 gives equivalent dosages for a range of standard neuroleptics used in emergent settings and their characteristics.

TABLE 62-36. EMERGENT NEUROLEPTIC MEDICATIONS

Drug	Equivalent Dose Per Day (mg)	Dose	Mode	Target Symptoms	Frequent Side Effects
Haloperidol (Haldol)	8–12	0.5–1 mg (elderly, brain-damaged, or extremely small people) 5 mg (average-size people) 10 mg (extremely large or extremely agitated people)	IM or PO (liquid 2 mg/mL concentrate preferred over pills); 10 mg usual dose	Psychosis or psychosis and agitation	EPS + +
Droperidol (Inapsine)	Usually not used on a daily basis	25–100 mg	IM or IV (IM almost as rapid in effect as IV)	Psychosis, especially with agitation and need for sedation	Sedation + + EPS +
Loxapine (Loxitane, Daxolin)	40–60	25–50 mg	IM or concentrate capsule	Psychosis, with or without agitation	EPS + + Sedation +
Thiothixene (Navane)	16–24	4–10 mg	IM (4 mg/2 mL) po, concentrate (5 mg/mL) or pills (1, 2, 5, 10, 20)	Psychosis, with or without agitation	EPS + +
Fluphenazine HCL (Prolixin, Permitril)	8–12	0.5–5 mg	IM (2.5 mg/mL) concentrate (5 mg/mL) or pills (0.25, 1, 2.5, 5, 10)	Psychosis	EPS + +
Chlorpromazine (Thorazine)	400–600	25–100 mg	IM (25 mg/mL, 10 mg/mL), liq. concentrate (30 mg/mL, 100 mg/mL), pills (30, 75, 100, 200, 300)	Psychosis and insomnia	Sedation + + anticholinergic effect + + Orthostatic hypotension + Extrapyramidal symptoms + Cardiac problems with high dose given rapidly (especially IM)
Mesoridazine (Serentil)	200–300	50–100 mg	IM (25 mg/mL) Concentrate (25 mg/mL) Pills (10, 25, 50, 100)	Psychosis	Sedation + + Orthostatic hypotension + Anticholinergic effect + Cardiac problems with high dose given rapidly (especially IM)
Thioridazine (Mellaril)	400–600	50–100 mg	Pills (10, 15, 25, 50, 100, 150, 200)	Psychosis and insomnia	Sedation + + Anticholinergic effect + + Orthostatic hypotension + +

SIDE EFFECTS

Most studies of neuroleptic use in emergent settings show that the incidence of side effects is less than 10%, with sedation, hypotension, and extrapyramidal symptoms being the most frequent of these.[5] Sedation, when present, generally occurs in the first few days of treatment. It may be modified by decreasing the dose, moving most or all of the dose to bedtime, or moving to a less sedating neuroleptic. Sedation correlates with less potent neuroleptics (higher mg doses to get similar antipsychotic effect). Orthostatic hypotension also occurs more frequently in the first few days of treatment and has moderate improvement for many patients over time. It is more frequent with the use of the IM mode and with lower-potency neuroleptics. The blood pressure drop is probably caused by the alpha-1 blocking aspect of neuroleptics. The management of orthostatic hypotension may involve lowering the doses, changing to a less hypotensive drug, educating the patient about getting up suddenly and maintaining good hydration, and use of support hose or abdominal binders in some patients. Extrapyramidal symptoms are more common in the high-potency neuroleptics; a lower mg dose achieves an antipsychotic effect similar to that of other "low-potency, higher mg" drugs. The effect can be decreased by lowering the dose, changing to a lower-potency neuroleptic, or using an antiparkinsonian agent. These agents can frequently be tapered after a few weeks to months of use without return of extrapyramidal symptoms. Although clozapine is different from most neuroleptics in having few extrapyramidal and parkinsonian symptoms, it can cause orthostatic hypotension and tachycardia in higher doses. The dose can be lowered or started more slowly. In patients with cardiac disease, electrocardiograms (ECGs) can be monitored. Generally, most changes such as increases in Q-R intervals and changes in T waves have not had great clinical importance. Individuals with poor cardiac function should be placed on high-potency neuroleptics to avoid hypotensive episodes. Each neuroleptic's side effect profile should be reviewed before use and the significance of the side effect should be considered in each individual patient. For example, a young man may become reluctant to use thioridazine because it may have more effect on male sexual function with decreased erectile potential and retrograde ejaculation than other drugs. At a minimum, these potential side effects should be discussed with the patient if the clinical state warrants. The risk of tardive dyskinesia should be discussed with patients who are likely to continue with the neuroleptic at some time during the first few days of treatment when the psychosis is improved. There is little evidence that tardive dyskinesia develops with brief use of neuroleptics. Multiple episodes of use may result in a higher risk.

ANTIDEPRESSANT MEDICATIONS

PHYSIOLOGY

As with the phenothiazines, the use of antidepressants became an effective clinical modality before the neurotransmitters involved and the mechanism of action were well understood. All of the currently used antidepressants have multiple modes of action, and many involve multiple neurotransmitters. An antidepressant effect may result from monoamine oxidase inhibition, increase in norepinephrine uptake, increase in serotonin uptake, downregulation of beta-norepinephrine receptors, blockage of norepinephrine uptake, blockage of serotonin uptake, reuptake inhibition of dopamine, and multiple other modalities. Few have a pure effect.[6] The antidepressants can best be divided into monoamine oxidase inhibitors (MAOIs) and non-MAOIs, which include tricyclic antidepressants (TCAs) and heterocyclics (HCAs).[7] Two relatively new antidepressants—fluoxetine, which is a pure serotonin reuptake inhibitor, and buproprion, which inhibits the reuptake of dopamine—do not fit well into the latter two categories.[6,8] Others such as methylphenidate and lithium, which are used infrequently primarily as antidepressants, differ significantly pharmacologically. The MAOIs increase the availability of neurotransmitter, primarily by decreasing their destruction by monoamine oxidase. The TCAs and HCAs generally cause norepinephrine uptake inhibition (except trazodone) and/or serotonin uptake inhibition.

INDICATIONS

The appropriateness of starting antidepressants in an emergent setting is limited because of the lack of immediate response, complications of change in treatment of subsequent outpatient treatment source, risk of suicide by providing increased energy for an attempt before outpatient follow-up is available, and the provision of the means for a successful suicide with an overdose of the treating drug with most of the antidepressants.

It frequently takes several weeks for antidepressants to have their full effect. A subsequent treating source may have significantly limited therapeutic options once an antidepressant has been started; for example, once fluoxetine is started, many weeks (5 is a conservative number) may be required to switch to a monoamino-oxidase inhibitor because of interactional problems and the long half-life of fluoxetine. If it may take many weeks for a patient to be seen in an outpatient follow-up setting, starting an antidepressant in the emergent setting may make sense when suicide is a lower risk and provisions are made for care if difficulties develop. If the person has a significant risk of suicide, starting an antidepressant with a low risk for overdose may not prevent suicide by other means if no timely follow-up care is available because the antidepressant effect may not have occurred. Some anergic individuals may have more energy to carry out a suicide attempt when the depression begins improving. There have been reports of a few individuals who were not previously suicidal becoming intensely so with fluoxetine.

MAOIs are primarily indicated in individuals who have an atypical depression with features such as hypersomnia, hyperphagia, and social sensitivity.[9] The MAOIs are used as second-line drugs by most clinicians when the patient has been unresponsive to the non-MAOI drugs. MAOIs have been used effectively to treat panic disorder. MAOIs have dietary restrictions and have side effect profiles that frequently make them less tolerated than the other antidepressants. TCAs and HCAs are effective in the treatment of major depression and other depressive disorders, especially when vegetative symptoms are present consistently. Some are also useful in treating panic disorder. Most TCAs and HCAs cause some sedation and anticholinergic symptoms. Desipramine tends to be more activating, and amitriptyline is among the most sedating drugs. Several antidepressants (including trazadone and amoxapine) have a more rapid onset of action, but ultimately their effectiveness after 1 to 2 months tends to be no greater than that of TCAs or other HCAs. If a patient is particularly unlikely to continue treatment without a rapid response, these two could be more useful. Alprazolam, a benzodiazepine, has been found to have some antidepressant effect but is generally not used as a primary antidepressant, partly because of the risk for addiction and the availability of generally more effective drugs. It is useful primarily in panic disorder and may be useful for the depressive symptoms that may coincide with the disorder. Lithium is used primarily as a preventive agent for mania and subsequent depression and for preventing isolated depression in the bipolar patient. Lithium alone is less effective as a primary antidepressant, even in bipolar disorder. In some medically compromised elderly patients, methylphenidate has been used to treat depression, but is generally avoided in others because of the abuse potential, development of tolerance, and a mixed picture of effectiveness. Table 62-37 lists commonly used antidepressants with their doses, particular indications, and side effects.

SIDE EFFECTS

Most of the TCAs and HCAs cause some sedation and anticholinergic symptoms (desipramine in lesser

TABLE 62-37. ANTIDEPRESSANTS ENCOUNTERED FREQUENTLY IN EMERGENT SETTINGS

Drug	Usual Daily Adult Dose (mg)	Special Indications (Beyond Depression)	Frequent Side Effects
Tricyclics* *(most sedation)*			
Amitriptyline (Elavil, Edep)	150–200	Pain management (most research and use for pain) (25–75 mg)	Sedation and orthostatic hypotension, anticholinergic effects (especially dry mouth)
Clomipramine (Anafranil)	100–200	Obsessive-compulsive disorder (with or without depression)	Sedation and orthostatic hypotension, anticholinergic effects (especially dry mouth)
Doxepin (Sinequan, Adapin)	150–250	Pain management (25–100 mg) H_2 receptor blocker (gastric acid decrease)	Sedation and orthostatic hypotension, anticholinergic effects (especially dry mouth)
Imipramine (Tofranil, Janimine)	150–200	Panic disorder, phobias (usual depressive dose); enuresis (less than depressive dose)	Sedation and orthostatic hypotension, anticholinergic effects (especially dry mouth)
Amoxapine (Asendin)	150–200	Rapid onset, dopamine blocking effect may help psychosis; short half-life	Greater risk for tardive dyskinesia than other TCAs
Nortriptyline (Pamelor)	75–100	Pain management (25 mg) best reliability and research for blood level test, lowest hypotensive effect of TCAs	Therapeutic window on blood levels, less intense anticholinergic effects
Desipramine (Norpramin, Pertofrane) *(least sedation)*	150–250	More activating, least anticholinergic of TCAs	Tremor, less intense anticholinergic effects
Heterocyclics* *(most sedation)*			
Trazodone (Desyrel)	150–400	Low lethality with overdose; little anticholinergic effect; rapid onset; short half-life	Sedation, orthostatic hypotension, priapism in men
Maprotiline (Ludiomil)	100–150		Sedation, long half-life, anticholinergic symptoms, seizure risks, especially with rapid increase of dose
Fluoxetine (Prozac) *(least sedation)*	20–40	Little or no weight gain; activating helpful in panic disorder and obsessive-compulsive disorder, long half-life, low lethality with overdose; no hypotension	Nervousness, insomnia, nausea, long half-life
MAOIs			
Phenelzine (Nardil)	45–60	Anxiety, phobias, panic disorder	Orthostatic hypotension and tyramine containing, food prohibition
Tranylcypromine (Parnate)	30–40	Non-anxious, low energy, withdrawn patients, rapid onset, less orthostatic hypotension than phenelzine	Orthostatic hypotension and tyramine containing, food prohibition, insomnia if taken in evening
Other			
Buproprion (Wellbutrin)	300	Activating (different effect from other antidepressants); possibly lower risk to induce mania	Anxiety, tremor, seizure risk with history of brain injury on rapid increase or high dose

* Ranked in order of sedation.

amount and amitriptyline the most). The most frequent side effect of the TCAs is dry mouth. Most TCAs and HCAs have some cardiac effects, generally orthostatic hypotension, and some conduction decrease (little if any with trazodone). Myocardial contractility may be decreased and/or tachycardia may develop. Except in individuals with major conduction difficulties or other major cardiac pathology, most of the TCA and HCA antidepressants are tolerated well, but monitoring with electrocardiograms (pretreatment, first few weeks, and intermittently) is indicated in at-risk individuals. There is a small risk of seizures with HCAs and TCAs, especially with maprotiline. Buproprion has a significant seizure risk in patients with a history of head injury or seizure disorders, and in higher or combined doses. Many of the anticholinergic symptoms of dry mouth, urinary retention, sinus tachycardia, blurred vision, constipation, and sedation can be improved by decreasing the dose. The sedating antidepressants can be given partly or totally at bedtime.

The constipation can be helped with hydration or bulking agents such as psyllium preparations or stool softeners such as docusate sodium. Urinary retention can be often helped with bethanechol chloride. Mania can be precipitated by any of the antidepressants and is a significant possibility in those with bipolar disorder or a risk of it. The risks are lowered with concomitant use of lithium or carbamazepine. The main side effect risk for trazodone and fluoxetine, the two antidepressants with the least risk for lethal overdose, are sedation, orthostatic hypotension, and priapism (rarely) in men with trazodone; and anxiety, agitation, insomnia, nausea, tremor, and possibly rare suicidal ideation in patients who had no such ideation before treatment with fluoxetine.

Most antidepressants cause weight gain, but fluoxetine can cause weight loss and decreased appetite. Again, the symptoms can be helped by decreasing the dose (for fluoxetine, this may involve going to every-other-day doses). MAOIs cause frequent orthostatic hypotension and occasional insomnia, and promote anxiety in some patients. The major risk with MAOIs is ingestion of tyramine-containing foods or sympathomimetic medication, which may cause severe hypertension. The hypotension can be managed with increased fluid intake, increased dietary salt, care in arising from chairs and beds, support hose, and/or abdominal binders. If a hypertensive episode occurs, sublingual nifedipine or IV phentolamine can be used along with stimulus decrease. Antidepressants can be combined or potentiated by medications such as lithium, but a discussion of this is beyond the scope of this chapter and of limited use in emergent settings. It is best left to ongoing care providers.

ANTIANXIETY AGENTS

PHYSIOLOGY

Antianxiety medications range from sedative hypnotics to beta-blockers, with each class having different physiologic effects. Sedative hypnotics are the most widely used class. The whole class causes central nervous system (CNS) depression. Both barbiturates and benzodiazepines mediate some of their antianxiety effect through gamma aminobutyric acid (GABA) effects on neural transmission. Benzodiazepines also appear to affect norepinephrine and serotonin turnover and acetylcholine systems. For benzodiazepines, much of the decrease in anxiety is separate from the CNS sedation. Benzodiazepines affect the cortex less than barbituates.[10] Barbiturates also may affect acetycholine and noradrenergic transmission.[11] Beta-blockers modify the physical manifestation of anxiety by blocking sweating, tachycardia, tremor, palpitations, and the "butterflies in the stomach" feeling. The mechanism is blockade of beta-adrenergic receptors. For some individuals, their observation of the physical symptoms of anxiety results in increased autonomic arousal in a vicious cycle, which is prevalent in performance anxiety. Antihistamines and meprobamate appear to produce their effect by sedation and decrease of CNS arousal. Similarly, antidepressants and phenothiazines that have some anxiolytic effect may manifest it partly by their sedative properties. Neuroleptics have an arousal-decreasing effect. Buspirone, a relatively new anxiolytic agent, causes little sedation. It does not attach to the benzodiazepine receptors. It appears to block presynaptic dopamine receptors and affect serotonin activity.[12] The treatment of anxiety appears to involve multiple diverse pathways and neurotransmitters.

INDICATIONS

People with anxiety present in emergent settings with somatic complaints, subjective discomfort and/or physiologic arousal, or a combination of these. The form of medication often depends on the underlying diagnosis; frequency, duration, and intensity of the symptoms; medication use history; and the patient's perception of what would help. If the anxiety is an outgrowth of psychosis or depression, treating the underlying disorder makes the most sense on a long-term basis, but some added lowering of the subjective discomfort and/or arousal by benzodiazepines is frequently helpful. There is little evidence that one benzodiazepine is more effective than another for anxiety control, and their main differences are in rapidity of absorption and duration of action. For example, diazepam has a rapid achievement of peak plasma level orally (½ to 2 hours) and a long half-life (20 to 50 hours), and lorazepam has an oral plasma peak in 1 to 6 hours and a half-life of 10 to 18 hours. If a rapid response to an oral benzodiazapine is desirable, diazepam is a better choice; and if there is concern about continuous presence of a sedating compound, lorazepam is preferable. In an individual who has an isolated increase in somatic symptoms with no clear cause and appears to have autonomic arousal, short-term benzodiapines or buspirone may help. If the individual's history of somatic concerns is long-term, the initiation and management of pharmacologic treatment is best left to an ongoing treatment source because dependence is a possibility with benzodiazepines and impact on anxiety is not rapid with buspirone. Buspirone has the advantage of not being sedating or addicting. Similarly, for brief periods of intense subjective anxiety in response to a meaningful event, brief treatment with a benzodiazepine or antihistamine-like hydroxazine may help and have little abuse potential. If the subjective anxiety or the combination with somatic complaints is ongoing, the same risk exists for dependence, and intermittent interventions in emergent settings with drugs are less effective.

Individuals who meet the criteria for panic disorder may benefit from the use of alprazolam or antidepressants, especially imipramine or MAOIs. Alprazolam often has a more rapid effect on the anxiety, and on a longer-term basis helps the panic disorder. Imipramine or MAOIs are less likely to have an immediate effect. If these latter two are considered, referral to a follow-up source for starting these makes more sense because more ongoing support may be necessary to deal with the side effect profiles and dose titration. Using alprazolam in a person with a history or predilection to addiction or drug abuse is not wise because it can be addictive in longer-term use, which is likely with panic disorder. Individuals who appear in emergent settings with hyperventilation but no panic disorder and no chronic history of anxiety usually do not require medications. Their symptoms during and after the hyperventilation frequently indicate to them that they are out of control. Teaching them to control their breathing and environment and thus their symptoms is often more useful than transferring

TABLE 62-38. EMERGENT ANTIANXIETY MEDICATIONS

Drug	Emergent Dose	Usual Dosage Range (mg/day)	Peak Pulse/ Onset Level (po) in Hours	Half-Life (Hours)	Indications and Cautions
Benzodiazepines					
Lorazepam (Ativan)	1–2 mg po or IM every 1–2 hrs to maximum of 10 mg in 24 hours	2–6 po	1–6 (intermediate) 1–1.5 (IM)	10–18	Severe anxiety, agitation especially in psychosis, mania, and ETOH withdrawal; sedation with other sedative disinhibition
Diazepam (Valium)	5–10 mg po or 5 mg IV	5–40 mg	0.5–2 (fast)	20–50	Need for rapid onset, erratically absorbed IM, best absorption in deltoid (and as with lorazepam)
Alprazolam (Xanax)	0.25–0.5 mg po	0.75–4	1–2 (intermediate)	12–15	Panic disorder as in lorazepam, addictive potential
Chlordiazepoxide (Librium)	5–25 mg	15–100	0.5–4 (intermediate)	5–30	Anxiety; ETOH withdrawal as in lorazepam
Clonazepam (Klonopin)	0.5–1 mg	1.5–20	1–2 (intermediate)	18–50	Mania as in lorazepam
Beta-Blockers					
Propranolol (Inderal)	20–40 mg po	60–120 mg (bid– tid dosing)	< 1	3–6	Somatic symptoms (tremor, shaking, etc.) can cause depression, additive blood pressure reduction with other drugs such as neuroleptics and antidepressants
Antihistamine					
Hydroxyzine (Vistaril, Atarax)	50–100 mg po	100–400 mg	1 approx.	4–6	Nonaddicting and sedation; dry mouth
Others					
Buspirone (Buspar)	(Note: symptom control is not immediate). The initial dosage is 5 mg tid	20–30 mg	1–3	10–12	Dizziness, nervousness, no cross-tolerance with benzodiazepines (does not block withdrawal if benzodiazepine is stopped)

the control to a medication. Patients who have post-traumatic stress disorder usually require psychotherapy and often antidepressant medications which are not started immediately unless depression is a major component. Benzodiazepines have been less helpful with post-traumatic stress disorder because of addictive risk and because the disorders tend to be chronic and disinhibition may be troublesome. Individuals with phobic disorders, including agoraphobia, may improve on antidepressants. In grief reactions, blunting the experiencing of the feelings of loss may prolong the reaction. Use of a sedative-hypnotic for sleep can be helpful for short-term use in these individuals. Table 62-38 lists antianxiety agents with their doses and the characteristics that influence their appropriateness in various forms of anxiety.

In the emergent setting the ready availability of a few antianxiety agents allows staff members to become familiar with their use. The availability of parenteral lorazepam is useful. In general, diazepam has erratic absorption if given IM, but IM lorazepam is well absorbed. If IM diazepam is used, its absorption is best from the deltoid. Oral diazepam, 5 mg, lorazepam, 1 mg, hydroxyzine, 25 mg, and propranolol, 20 mg are useful dosages to have in the emergent setting. Most often, antianxiety medication can be given through prescriptive sources.

SIDE EFFECTS

For benzodiazepines, the most frequent side effects are sedation, dizziness, disorientation, and/or ataxia. Occasionally some patients can be disinhibited or agitated with these drugs. A risk exists for addiction with long-term use in higher doses. The short-acting and intermediate-acting drugs have more addictive risk. Tolerance does not usually develop in usual clinical practice. Hydroxyzine can cause sedation and/or anticholinergic symptoms. Buspirone can cause dizziness, nervousness, headache, and/or nausea and does not prevent withdrawal from rapid decrease of benzodiazepines. Propranolol can cause depression, decreased exercise tolerance, and hypotension, especially when taken with other hypotensive medications. Often the side effects can be decreased for all of the above medications by decreasing the dose. Changing to a long-acting benzodiazepine such as diazepam or clonazepam can lower the risk for withdrawal and decrease the frequency of dosage and the link between anxiety decrease and pill taking.

ANTIMANIC MEDICATIONS

PHYSIOLOGY

The two main antimanic medications, lithium and carbamazepine, are felt to have different mechanisms of action. Lithium changes norepinephrine and serotonin effects. It also alters sodium transport in neuronal cells and may alter the metabolism of catecholamines. The actual antimanic effect is unclear. Similarly, the antimanic effect of carbamazepine is obscure and its mechanism of action unknown.[10] One hypothesis of the effect of carbamazepine and other anticonvulsants used to prevent and treat mania is decrease of sen-

---

TABLE 62-39. ANTIMANIC DRUGS

Drug*	Dose	Serum Level Peak (Hours)	Half-Life (Hours)	Side Effects
Lithium —carbonate, capsules & tablets (Eskalith, Lithane, Lithobid) —citrate (syrup) (Cibralith-S)	Acute manic: Starting 300 mg. tid, then frequently to 1300 mg until blood level of 0.8–1.2 mEq/L is reached. Maintenance: Frequently 900–1200 mg with blood levels of 0.6–0.8 mEq/L	1—3	18–20 (up to 36 in elderly)	Tremor, nausea, diarrhea, leukocytosis, renal changes, hypothyroidism, polydipsia, polyuria
Carbamazepine (Tegretol)	Initial 200 mg bid, increase weekly by 200 mg/day until therapeutic blood level is reached (4–12 mg/ml) Maintenance dose: 800–1200 mg/day	4–5	Initially, 25–65; after repeated doses, 12–17	Sedation, dizziness, nausea, unsteadiness. Rarely, aplastia, aremia (10–16/million) and agranulocytosis (30–48/million)
Lorazepam (Ativan)	1–2 mg every 1–2 hrs IM or po to 10 mg maximum/day	1–2 (oral) 1–1.5 IM	10–18	Sedation (disinhibition in some)
Clonazepam (Klonopin)	0.5–1 mg	1–2	18–50	As in lorazepam, but more sedating

* Valproic acid has been used experimentally for prevention in bipolar disorder. Calcium channel blockers have been used experimentally for acute mania but are rarely used in usual clinical practice.

sitization and "kindling" of transmission in neural pathways.[13] The other anticonvulsants tried with bipolar disorders are valproic acid and clonazepam. These may have similar effects, although clonazepam may be effective only in the acute manic phase. Clonidine and calcium channel blockers have been used experimentally in acute mania. The mechanism of action in mania is unknown. The neural changes from lithium and carbamazepine have been felt by some to decrease explosive behavior and anger outbursts, but the mechanism is unclear. Lithium has been used to prevent relapse of alcohol use, but its effectiveness for this is being questioned and its physiologic effect is unknown.

INDICATIONS

Generally, antimanic drugs (Table 62-39) are used in the treatment of mania and the prevention of mania and subsequent depression as well as recurrent depression in bipolar patients. Both lithium and carbamazepine do not have a major immediate effect to decrease mania and frequently need augmentation in the acute phase with benzodiazepines (especially lorazepam or clonazepam) and/or neuroleptics when psychosis is present. Lithium carbonate is a naturally occurring salt that is well absorbed and eliminated by renal excretion. Although lithium is not particularly effective as an antidepressant in unipolar depression, it is useful as an augmenting agent for antidepressants such as imipramine, fluoxepine, and tranylcypromine.

Carbamazepine is related to tricyclic antidepressants and is usually a second-line drug in the treatment of bipolar disorder because it has sedative qualities and a risk of leukopenia and aplastic anemia. When lithium has not been effective or tolerated in bipolar patients, carbamazepine is often helpful. In some individuals, the combination of lithium and carbamazepine has helped, although neither has been useful separately.

In individuals who are poor in medication compliance, have a major imminent risk for suicide, and/or are unwilling to have frequent monitoring and blood tests, the risk with lithium and carbamazepine may be greater than the potential benefit. Both must be taken regularly, and blood levels must be maintained at therapeutic ranges to achieve an effect. Episodic use, which some patients desire, is of little clinical use because the primary effect is prevention of mania and depression in bipolar disorder. Neither may be absolutely effective, even in the most compliant patients, and should be seen as decreasing the frequency of mood change episodes rather than total prevention.

The usual therapeutic blood levels for lithium in acute mania are 0.8 to 1.2 mEq/mL and from 0.6 to 0.8 mEq/mL for maintenance. These levels should be drawn 10 to 12 hours after the last dose (usually with the last dose at night and blood drawing in the morning). Occasionally, when a lithium level is drawn soon after a dose of lithium has been ingested, the level is elevated, e.g., 1.5 mEq/mL may be seen as a toxic level and attempts are made to treat for an overdose or toxicity. This level usually represents neither. The symptoms of toxicity (ataxia, confusion, vomiting, weakness and drowsiness) should be present. The history and clinical picture of an overdose should be present before lavage is done. A starting dose of lithium, 300 mg tid, is usual; frequently 1800 mg per day is required in acute mania (with blood level monitoring). Frequent maintenance levels are in the 900 to 1500 mg per day range. Lithium levels on inpatients are taken several times per week until the patient is stable and the blood level consistent. For outpatients in acute phases, one-time-per-week levels may be sufficient. For maintenance levels, 3 to 4 times per year are common.

Lithium can have renal toxicity, suppress thyroid function, and deplete sodium. Baseline thyroid screen, electrolytes, creatine levels, complete blood count, and urinalysis and electrocardiogram in people over 40 or with cardiac pathology are necessary. These blood tests can be repeated quarterly to semiannually if stable. An increasing lithium level with no changes in dose, life style, or mood may indicate toxicity, and kidney function testing, especially creatinine, can be obtained.

Carbamazepine levels are also monitored (therapeutic range: 4 to 12 μg per mL) and complete blood count (CBC) taken before use and several weeks after beginning therapy. Once a patient is stabilized, CBCs every 3 to 4 months are generally adequate.

The less frequent use of lithium and carbamazepine for explosive disorder and disturbed behavior is usually in the context of multiple effort to change the behavior. Dosages are similar to bipolar prevention levels.

Individuals who have schizoaffective disorder with both features of schizophrenia or ongoing psychosis and affective cycles are frequently treated with neuroleptics and lithium or carbamazepine.

SIDE EFFECTS

With lithium, the most frequent side effects are tremor, nausea, diarrhea, leukocytosis, and renal changes. The tremor can be helped with propranolol and the nausea minimized by taking lithium with meals. Occasionally, slow-release lithium products can minimize the symptoms. With carbamazepine, sedation, dizziness and nausea are the most frequent side effects. Usually, with time, many of these improve. The rare aplastic anemia and agranulocytosis requires monitoring of white blood cell (WBC) count, hematocrit, and occasionally platelet count.

<table>
<tr><td>

ANTIEXTRAPYRAMIDAL SYMPTOM–ANTIPARKINSONIAN MEDICATIONS

</td></tr>
</table>

PHYSIOLOGY

The most frequent extrapyramidal effects of neuroleptics are dystonias, parkinsonian symptoms, and, with long-term use, tardive dyskinesia. Generally, all symptoms but the last can improve on lowering the dose of the neuroleptic. When acute dystonia occurs, chronic parkinsonian symptoms develop, or akathisia appears, antiextrapyramidal symptom medications can help (Table 62-40). These are usually not helpful in tardive dyskinesia. Extrapyramidal symptoms are felt to result from an imbalance between dopamine and acetylcholine in the striatum. This imbalance appears to be altered in medications with an anticholinergic effect (e.g., benztropine or diphenhydramine) or a dopaminergic drug (e.g., amantadine). Studies have shown little difference in effectiveness between amantadine and anticholinergic agents.[14]

INDICATIONS

ACUTE DYSTONIAS

Acute dystonias involve rigidity of muscles and cramping, usually in the tongue, face, neck, and back. Occasionally, in oculogyric crisis, the eye muscles tense and the eyes roll back. Acute dystonias usually occur during the first week of neuroleptic treatment, especially with high potency agents such as haloperidol and in young men. These symptoms are usually uncomfortable and upsetting for the patient, and require quick treatment. The two most frequent treatments are benztropine, 1 to 2 mg IM, or diphenhydramine, 25 to 50 mg IM. Diphenhydramine can be more rapid if given IV, but benztropine is usually just as rapid in IM as IV. IM use of either benztropine or diphenhydramine results in improvement within 30 minutes. One advantage of benztropine (and disadvantage if it is not well tolerated) is its long half-life of between 12 and 15 hours. Diphenhydramine needs to be repeated every 6 hours because its half-life is 4 to 6 hours. Intravenous treatment is rarely necessary except in extraordinary discomfort and agitation from the symptoms. In the rare instance of laryngeal dys-

---

TABLE 62-40. ANTIEXTRAPYRAMIDAL SYMPTOMS AND ANTIPARKINSONIAN DRUGS FOR NEUROLEPTIC-INDUCED SYMPTOMS

Drug	Indications	Usual Dose (mg/Day)	Emergent Use	Half-Life (Hours)	Side Effects/Comments
Dopamine-releasing Amantadine (Symmetrel)	Akathisia, EPS resistant to anticholinergic drugs	100–300 po (divided dose)	Infrequent	10–28	Confusion, hallucinations, restlessness, may exacerbate schizophrenia slowly over months (dopamine-releasing)
Anticholinergics Benztropine (Cogentin)	EPS, especially dystonia	1–4 po	1–2 mg IM or po	12–15	Dry mouth, blurred vision, urinary retention (cholinergic blockade symptoms), abuse potential, can decrease blood levels of phenothiazines and possibly other neuroleptics
Biperiden (Akineton)	EPS	2–6 po	Infrequent: 2 mg IM 8 mg maximum in 24 hours	Approximately 4–6	As with benztropine
Procycyclidine (Kemadrin)	EPS	5–20	Infrequent: 2.5–5 mg po	Approximately 6–8	As with benztropine
Trihexyphenidyl (Artane)	EPS	5–15	Infrequent 2 mg po	3–4	As with benztropine
Antihistamine (with anticholinergic effects) Diphenhydramine (Benadryl)	EPS, especially dystonia	20–100	25–50 mg (usually 50 mg) po or IV	4–6	As with benztropine, also sedation
Beta-blocker Propranolol (Inderal)	Tremor Akathisia	30–160	Infrequent	4–6	May add to hypotension from neuroleptic

tonia, as much as 4 mg of IM benztropine should be given in the first 10 to 15 minutes. If this is not successful, 1 to 2 mg of IV lorazepam can be given. If anticholinergic agents are not effective in dystonia, 1 to 2 mg of lorazepam can be given IM.

NEUROLEPTIC-INDUCED PARKINSONISM

In neuroleptic-induced parkinsonism, the patient has muscular rigidity, mask-like facies, akinesia, hypersalivation, drooling, and/or tremor. It usually appears 5 to 20 days after beginning neuroleptics, and is more frequent in women than men.[15] The frequency of parkinsonism with neuroleptic use is higher in the elderly, as is the risk of confusion and severity of other anticholinergic side effects with the antiextrapyramidal agents. Anticholinergic agents are frequently helpful (Table 62–39). A change to a low-potency neuroleptic, especially one with a strong anticholinergic effect such as thioridazine may also decrease parkinsonian symptoms.

AKATHISIA

Akathisia involves a sense of restlessness and a need to walk or pace. It is usually experienced as unpleasant and begins within 5 to 40 days of starting neuroleptics.[15] It is sometimes difficult to distinguish from agitation and anxiety. The fidgety motor movements may be confused with dyskinesias. It is more frequent with the depot neuroleptics and may be more prevalent near the end of the injection cycle. Decreasing the dose of neuroleptic may be the most effective treatment. A response often occurs within 2 hours of starting propranolol. Anticholinergics, amantadine, and benzodiapines have been helpful with some patients. Changing to a low-potency neuroleptic such as thioridazine may also help.

TARDIVE DYSKINESIA

Tardive dyskinesia often involves involuntary movements of the tongue, mouth, face, extremities, and spine. These movements are usually slow and sometimes stereotyped. For some, the only effective treatment is to stop neuroleptics. Often the symptoms worsen with decrease or cessation of neuroleptics. For many, the symptoms are permanent. Generally, antiparkinsonian medications are not helpful with this disorder. There is no consistently effective medication. Sometimes when neuroleptics are stopped suddenly, a transitory dyskinesia develops; this is not tardive dyskinesia. Usually no medication is necessary, and the symptom can be avoided by gradual decrease of neuroleptics when possible.

SIDE EFFECTS

Amantadine's main side effects or adverse reactions include anticholinergic effects, confusion, insomnia,

and worsening of psychosis. The anticholinergics can cause blurred vision, dry mouth, constipation, urinary retention, and difficulty in swallowing. In large doses, or when the patient is particularly sensitive to anticholinergics, they can cause hyperthermia, dry mouth, confusion, disorientation, and hallucinations. Diphenhydramine often causes sedation and sleepiness, and can cause anticholinergic symptoms as described previously. Propranolol can cause bronchospasm, hypoglycemia, depression, and less exercise capability.

LABORATORY TESTS

Each class of medications and each individual medication has differing laboratory tests required for safety and optimal performance. These are summarized in Table 62-40. Pregnancy tests are indicated for all of the medications discussed in at-risk women. Frequently an individual with a mental disorder, especially psychosis, is not a reliable informant about her pregnancy status. If there is any question as determined in the clinical evaluation, a serum or urine human chorionic gonadotropin pregnancy test is prudent. In situations in which an individual's life is in danger or the person cannot be managed in any other way, treatment without pregnancy testing may be indicated. In the competent individual who does not wish pregnancy testing and can understand the risks to her fetus, medications may be given, with good documentation in the chart or informed consent and the basis for assessing the patient's competency.

PITFALLS

1. Starting neuroleptic medications in an agitated nonpsychotic patient because there is significant risk of tardive dyskinesia with long-term use.
2. Getting a lithium level soon after a usual dose and assuming that the level obtained (1.2 to 2.0 mEq/L) indicates toxicity and/or an overdose and lavaging the patient. (Levels are elevated soon after a usual dose.)
3. Giving antidepressant medications without a definite follow-up that is likely and feasible.
4. Giving 1000 mg or more of tricyclics in a prescription (lethal amount for most TCAs).
5. Not warning patients about, and management of, the orthostatic hypotension and sedation common to many antidepressants and neuroleptics.
6. Not recognizing that extrapyramidal symptoms often appear when the blood level of some neuroleptics is dropping and the internal anticholinergic effect is decreasing (e.g., haloperidol).

TABLE 62-40. LABORATORY TESTS WITH USE OF PSYCHIATRIC DRUGS IN EMERGENT SETTINGS

Pregnancy Tests
Pregnancy test for all at-risk women (serum HCG or urine HCG)
Benzodiazepines and Sedative Hypnotics
ETOH and/or toxic screen in people with high index or suspicion of sedative or ETOH use
Tricyclic and Heterocyclic Antidepressants
ECG if cardiac pathology is present or likely. QT prolongation is often present in higher doses of tricyclics. Serum levels to assess absorption and dosage (nonemergent)
Lithium
Prelithium Evaluation—CBC, urinalysis (UA), thyroid screen (T_3, T_4, TSH), electrolytes, blood urea nitrogen (BUN), creatinine, ECG if over 40 or with cardiac pathology
Monitoring of lithium—Therapeutic level .6–1.2 mEQ/l
Subsequent Evaluation in Emergent Setting
1. Lithium level to see if patient is taking lithium or is toxic
2. Electrolytes, BUN, creatinine, and UA if there is evidence of poor self-care or dehydration
3. Thyroid screen if patient is depressed
Carbamazepine
CBC initially, repeat hematocrit and WBC count if 3–4 months, carbamazepine level 4–12 μg/mL
Clozaril
CBC (laboratory tests monitored weekly by clozaril project management system)

7. Giving a sedating antianxiety agent to a patient who has ingested another sedating agent, usually alcohol.
8. Giving large quantities of benzodiazepines in prescriptions from emergent settings, which may result in the "word hitting the street" and multiple drug abusers appearing in the setting.
9. Patients who "cheek" medications (liquid forms are more reliable).
10. Giving usual doses of neuroleptics and other psychotropic medications to elderly and/or brain-damaged patients (lower doses are often indicated).
11. Giving chlordiazepoxide or diazepam IM with resultant erratic absorption, (absorption best in the deltoid); better still, using lorazepam.

MEDICOLEGAL PEARLS

1. Explain risks and benefits of medications to patients and document doing so, especially to paranoid and angry patients and those with histories of lawsuits.
2. Determine if the patient can understand treatment options and is competent to agree to medications. If he or she is competent, treatment alternatives must be discussed. If you give one alternative, and an adverse outcome occurs and there were other viable alternatives, there is some legal exposure.
3. Give written instructions, to be signed by the patient and a copy kept by the treatment setting.
4. Know the local requirement about giving medications involuntarily.

HORIZONS

1. Clozaril-like medications with low risk for tardive dyskinesia and other major side effects such as agranulocytosis are being developed.
2. More site-specific neurotransmission-altering drugs are also under development.

NATIONAL CONTACTS

American Psychiatric Association
1400 K Street N.W.
Washington D.C. 20005
202-682-6000

American Association for Emergency Psychiatry
Mail Location 55A
University of Cincinnati
Cincinnati, OH 45267
513-558-4870

REFERENCES

1. Kane, J.M.: The current status of neuroleptic therapy. J. Clin. Psychiatry 50:323, 1989.

2. Cohen, B.M., and Lipinski, J.F.: Treatment of acute psychosis with non-neuroleptic agents. Psychosomatics 27:7, 1986.

3. Lieberman, J.A., Kane, J.M., and Johns, C.A.: Clozapine: guidelines for clinical management. J. Clin. Psychiatry 50:329, 1989.

4. Snyder, S.H.: Dopamine receptors, neuroleptics, and schizophrenia. Am. J. Psychiatry 138:460, 1981.

5. Dubin, W.R.: Rapid tranquilization: Antipsychotics or benzodiazepines. J. Clin. Psychiatry 49:12, 1988.

6. Davis, J.M., and Glass, A.H.: Antidepressant Drugs in Comprehensive Textbook Psychiatry. 5th Ed. Edited by H.I. Kaplan and B.J. Sadock, Baltimore, Williams & Wilkins, 1989.

7. Berstein, J.G.: Handbook of Drug Therapy in Psychiatry, 2nd Ed. Littleton, Mass., 1988.

8. Golden, R.N., et al.: Brupropion in depression: I. Biochemical effects and clinical response. Arch. Gen. Psychiatry 45:139, 1988.

9. Klein, D.F., et al.: Diagnosis and Drug Treatment of Psychiatric Disorders: Adults and Children. 2nd Ed. Baltimore, Williams & Wilkins 2:1643, 1980.

10. Olin, B.R., et al.: Drug Facts and Comparisons. St. Louis, Facts and Comparisons, J.B. Lippincott Co., 1990.

11. Harvey, S.C.: Hypnotics and sedation. In Goodman and Gilman's The Pharmacological Basis of Therapeutics. 7th Ed. Edited by A.G. Gilman and L.S. Goodman. New York, Macmillan Publishing Company, 1985.

12. Eison, A.S., and Temple, D.L.: Buspirone: Review of its pharmacology and current perspective on its mechanism of action. Am. J. Med. 38:1, 1986.

13. Post, R.M., and Weiss, P.B.: Sensitization, kindling, and anticonvulsants in mania. J. Clin. Psychiatry 50:23, 1989.

14. Klaus, J.R., and Israel, M.: Drug Consults: Amantadine-Therapy of anticholinergic resistant extrapyramidal symptoms. Micromedex Inc., 65, 1990.

15. Slaby, A.E., Lieb, J., and Tancredi, L.R.: Handbook of Psychiatric Emergencies. 3rd Ed. New York, Medical Examination Publishing Co., 1986.

BIBLIOGRAPHY

American Psychiatric Association Task Force on Treatment of Psychiatric Disorders. Washington, DC, American Psychiatric Association, 1989.

Bernstein, J.G.: Handbook of Drug Therapy in Psychiatry, 2nd Ed. Littleton, Mass., P.S.G. Publishing Co. Inc., 1988.

Hyman, S.E., and Arana, G.W.: Handbook of Psychiatric Drug Therapy. Boston, Little, Brown and Company, 1987.

Kaplan, H.I., and Sadock, B.J.: Comprehensive Textbook of Psychiatry. 5th Ed. Baltimore, Williams & Wilkins, 1989.

Slaby, A.E., Lieb, J., and Tancredi, L.R.: Handbook of Psychiatric Emergencies. 3rd Ed. New York, Medical Examination Publishing Co., 1986.

Part X

Environmental Emergencies

Chapter 63

HIGH ALTITUDE ILLNESS

James R. Tryon

CAPSULE

The term "high altitude illness" includes many specific clinical syndromes. To be inclusive, one would have to consider any pathologic state resulting from increasing altitude. This includes illnesses caused by harsh environmental factors such as decreased ambient temperature and increased exposure to solar radiation, in addition to those associated with decreased barometric pressure.

In this section we discuss clinical entities specifically associated with decreased barometric pressure, i.e., a decrease in pO_2. These illnesses include acute mountain sickness (AMS), high altitude pulmonary edema (HAPE), high altitude cerebral edema (HACE), and high altitude retinal hemorrhage (HARH). Although they have been labeled as separate clinical syndromes, these conditions probably represent a variation in target organ responses to a common pathologic stimulus.

INTRODUCTION

Acute mountain sickness is the prototypic high altitude illness. In the classical Chinese history, the Qian Han Shu, written about 30 BC, the author describes the route from western China to the Hindu Kush crossing as the "Great Headache Mountain" and describes "men's bodies become feverish, they lose colour, and are attacked with headache and vomiting; the asses and cattle being all in like condition." An even more graphic description of symptoms was given by the Jesuit missionary Jose de Acosta as he accompanied the Spanish conquistadors in Peru in the 16th century. While traveling over a high mountain, Acosta recorded that he "was suddenly surprised with so mortall and strange a pang, that I was ready to fall from the top to the ground. . . . I was surprised with such pangs of straining and casting, as I though to cast up

my heart too; for having cast up meate, fleugme, and choller, both yellow and greene; in the end I cast up blood, with the straining of my stomacke. . . . I therefore perswade myselfe, that the element of the aire is there so subtile and delicate, as it is not proportional with the breathing of man, which requires a more grosse and temprate aire."

The understanding of altitude-related illnesses has accelerated over the past century or so, largely because of experience gained from mountain climbing and ballooning. It is now clear that the reduced partial pressure of oxygen is the primary pathogenic stimulus for the development of the illness. Rate of ascent also appears to be a contributing factor. High altitude is usually considered to begin at 8000 feet. At this altitude, most visitors from lower altitudes have an arterial oxygen saturation below 90%. Normal physiologic response to altitude includes adjustments to hypoxia and hypocapnia. There is a wide degree of variation in individual response to these physiologic conditions, and although it is incompletely understood, altitude-related illness appears to be related to a blunted response in affected individuals.

HIGH-ALTITUDE PHYSIOLOGY

The partial pressure of inspired oxygen at sea level is about 149 torr, giving a partial pressure of alveolar oxygen of about 100 torr. At 15,000 feet (4570 m), the partial pressure of inspired oxygen drops to 80 torr, giving a partial pressure of alveolar oxygen of 43 torr, less than half that at sea level. (To put 15,000 feet into perspective, Pike's Peak in Colorado is 14,110 feet, Mt. McKinley is 20,320 feet, and Mt. Everest is 29,028 feet. One can surmise how low the alveolar pO_2 was in Reinhold Messner and Peter Hubeler when they reached the summit of Mt. Everest in May, 1978 without supplemental oxygen!) The resulting tissue hypoxia may impair function at the cellular level by interfering with cellular oxidative metabolism.

Individuals respond to the hypoxic environment with both short- and long-term compensatory mechanisms. The immediate reflex physiologic mechanisms are hyperventilation and hyperperfusion. The increase in minute ventilation is mediated by the aortic and carotid bodies in response to arterial hypoxemia, causing an increase in depth as well as rate of ventilation. The pCO_2 falls as the individual tries to defend the alveolar pO_2. Respiratory alkalosis results, and it can be profound. The calculated pH of a human subject on Mt. Everest was reported to be about 7.70. Initially, this respiratory alkalosis acts as an inhibitory force on ventilation; but renal compensation partially corrects the alkalosis and, along with CSF pH changes, enhances the ventilatory drive within a few days. The alkalosis also causes a left shift in the oxygen hemoglobin dissociation curve, but compensation brings it back to the right. Alterations in hemoglobin-oxygen affinity seem to play a small role in the adaptation to altitude, however.

The hypoxemia of altitude is exacerbated by exercise because of increased tissue demands for oxygen. It is also worsened by ventilatory depression during sleep. Individuals tend to develop a periodic breathing pattern similar to Cheyne-Stokes respirations during sleep. This results in greater fluctuations in resting O_2 saturation. The cause is not known, but even awake subjects exhibit a more cyclical breathing pattern.

The cardiovascular system responds to hypoxemia in many ways. There is an initial increase in heart rate that serves to increase the cardiac output. The stroke volume remains unchanged, however. After a few days at high altitude, the cardiac output begins to fall despite the persistence of the tachycardia. It is believed that a decrease in stroke volume occurs because of hypoxic depression of the myocardium. Eventually, the relationship of cardiac output to minute ventilation returns to normal except in extreme altitudes, where cardiac output remains increased.

In general, hypoxia tends to cause vasodilation in the coronary and cerebral circulation. In the cerebral circulation, this occurs in the face of a competitive tendency towards vasoconstriction from the hypocarbia of hyperventilation. Hypoxic chemoreceptor reflexes in the skeletal muscles and splanchnic bed produce vasoconstriction. The overall effect, then, is to maintain blood pressure and increases in coronary and cerebral blood flow. The pulmonary vasculature responds by increasing pulmonary vascular resistance. The stress of exercise at high altitude causes an increase in cardiac output, which further exacerbates the pulmonary artery pressure. There is a regional redistribution in pulmonary blood flow and perhaps overperfusion of some of the pulmonary capillary beds.

Most people experience some volume loss during the first few days at altitude. The various mechanisms include increases in insensible loss from hyperventilation that of itself can be as much as 3 liters per day, fluid shifts between the intravascular and intracellular compartments, the effects of exercise, and the variable loss from the cold- or hypoxia-induced diuresis. There seems to be a significant difference among individuals in volume regulation, and this may be important in identifying people who are more susceptible to high altitude illness. Mountaineering lore has long held that individuals who urinate freely on exposure to altitude have little trouble with mountain sickness; this is referred to as the Hohendiurese in Alpine literature. The diuresis is thought to be a marker of effective adaptation to high altitude. In fact, the renal effects of altitude include bicarbonate excretion to compensate for the initial respiratory alkalosis, so the diuresis may therefore partly reflect the adequacy of that compensation. The exact effect of altitude on the renal system and the relative contribution of the various systems involved in fluid balance remain to be defined.

Long-term compensation to altitude includes stimulation of 2,3-diphosphoglycerate production, development of polycythemia, and tissue adaptation with increased capillary and mitochondrial density.

ACUTE MOUNTAIN SICKNESS

PRESENTATION AND SYMPTOMS

The signs and symptoms of acute mountain sickness (AMS) develop over the first 8 to 24 hours at high altitude. The incidence, severity, and duration of the illness depend on: (1) the rate of ascent, (2) the altitude, and (3) the susceptibility of the individual. Abrupt ascent to an altitude of 9800 ft (3000 m) causes symptoms in approximately 30% of subjects. In one study, about 67% of climbers on Mt. Ranier developed at least mild symptoms in ascending to 14,400 feet (4392 m) in 33 hours. Other reports confirm a variable but significant percent of patients developing symptoms at as low as 8200 feet (2500 m). American ski resorts in the western United States range from approximately 8000 to 10,000 feet, and one may anticipate an incidence of AMS of about 10%. No sex difference in response has been reported, and it appears that children are susceptible as well. The most common symptoms are headache, insomnia, fatigue, and anorexia. Less common are nausea and vomiting. The headache described is throbbing in nature, usually worse in the morning and in the supine position, and aggravated by exercise. The appetite is generally poor, but nausea occurs less frequently, and actual vomiting is not typically seen despite Jose de Acosta's dramatic description. Children may experience nausea and vomiting more commonly than adults. Fatigue is prominent, but the quality of sleep is poor and may aggravate symptoms because of relative hypoventilation. Although some authors list dyspnea as a symptom, it is difficult to separate this out as a feature of mild AMS as opposed to a physical expectation of being at higher altitude for all individuals; however, as the severity of AMS increases, it is likely that dyspnea becomes a more prominent symptom. Symptoms may vary significantly between individuals, but tend to be constant for any individual from one exposure to the next. Physical findings point to a state of fluid imbalance and altered vascular integrity. They include rales, peripheral and periorbital edema, oliguria, petechiae, and retinal hemorrhages. There is some variability in duration according to the literature, but generally symptoms tend to worsen on the second and third day, then abate, with resolution after the fourth to seventh day.

A chronic form of mountain sickness develops rarely, with symptoms persisting for a month or longer. It occurs more frequently in men, usually over 30. Characteristic symptoms are severe headache and mental confusion. Hematocrit may exceed 60%.

Although the setting probably lends credence to the diagnosis of AMS, other illnesses are possible. Pneumonia should be considered as part of the differential. Climbers may be more susceptible to deep vein thrombosis because of venous stasis and hyperviscosity aggravated by dehydration. The occurrence of pulmonary embolism is well documented. These problems become more difficult to sort out as the severity of AMS increases, and pulmonary or central nervous system dysfunction becomes more prominent.

TREATMENT

Acute mountain sickness is usually a self-limited disorder, although in severe cases it can be fatal. In the mild to moderate form, it can be treated symptomatically, with rest, aspirin, acetaminophen, or ibuprofen for headache, and avoidance of alcohol and other depressants until acclimatization has occurred. In the more severe forms, descent remains the most unequivocally successful treatment. Modest descents of about 1000 feet have been associated with dramatic improvement. Unfortunately, descent is not always an immediate option. Other mechanism-directed therapies include oxygen, respiratory stimulants, diuretics, and corticosteroids.

Oxygen therapy seems to be a logical choice for the hypoxia. By increasing the inspired pO_2, the alveolar pO_2 increases, lowering pulmonary artery pressure, improving ventilation/perfusion mismatching, improving PaO_2, and reducing cerebral blood flow. Clinically, it is helpful in relieving dyspnea, tachycardia, and sometimes headache. It is said to be particularly effective for AMS when administered at low flow, i.e., 1 to 2 L/min during the night. Severe AMS may not be readily reversible with oxygen alone, however, and oxygen is usually not available in adequate amounts in field situations.

Acetazolamide has been used to treat AMS as a respiratory stimulant. Acetazolamide is a sulfonamide that inhibits renal carbonic anhydrase, causing bicarbonate diuresis and extracellular acidosis. Respirations are stimulated by the acidosis. It has been reported to be variably effective in established AMS, and its role is probably more important as a prophylactic agent in prevention.

Fluid retention and evidence of edema provide the rationale for using diuretic therapy. The theory is that enhanced diuresis may modify the fluid shift into the intracellular space. Furosemide in a dosage of 80 mg twice a day for 2 days was reported to be effective in treating established AMS in 446 soldiers at high altitude in one report. Studies with other diuretics are limited and preclude judgment about their effectiveness. Use of diuretics including furosemide have not proven effective as prophylactic agents.

Dexamethasone appears to be the only drug so far that is beneficial in treating AMS, as well as in prophylaxis. In paired and unpaired studies in the field, and under simulated conditions, it appears to be effective in treating patients with established AMS and also in reducing the symptoms if started before ascent. The presumed mechanism is reduction of brain edema which is thought to contribute to the syndrome.

Adverse side effects seem to be uncommon, but symptoms of AMS or adrenal insufficiency have been observed after abrupt discontinuation of the drug. The dosage is 8 mg initially, followed by 4 mg every 6 hours by mouth.

PREVENTION

Current prevention strategies for AMS include (1) identifying susceptible individuals, (2) acclimatization, and (3) drug therapy. It is well known that there is a wide variation among individuals in their susceptibility to altitude illness. The cause of this variation is not well understood, but basically it appears that there are substantial interindividual differences in the strength of the hypoxic ventilatory response. These differences appear to be partly familial, possibly genetic, and may reflect differences in hypoxic sensitivity of the carotid body. Individuals with the ability to climb to high altitudes seem to have high hypoxic ventilatory responses, and manifest fewer symptoms of AMS. It is interesting to note in this regard that athletes who excel in endurance running tend to have relatively low hypoxic ventilatory responses, which seems to imply an increased sensitivity to AMS. Thus it appears that preascent ventilatory sensitivity to hypoxia may be a determinant of adaptation to the hypoxia of high altitude. Individuals who have experienced significant AMS or other altitude-related illness are likely to develop similar symptoms on repeat exposure to altitude.

There are also acquired changes in sensitivity to hypoxic exposure as well. The exact mechanism of adaptation is unclear, but ventilatory sensitivity to hypoxia appears to increase over time. This is the principle that underlies the concept of acclimatization. Acclimatization can be accomplished by staging, which is the process of remaining at an intermediate altitude for 2 or 3 days before climbing to the intended altitude. Recommended staging altitudes are between about 7000 to 10,000 feet (about 2000 to 3000 m). Alternatively, a plan of gradual ascent of not more than 1000 feet (300 m) per day is recommended. Guidelines are generalized because of the variation in susceptibility to the illness.

Drug therapy may include acetazolamide or dexamethasone. Both drugs have been demonstrated to be effective in reducing the frequency of AMS. Their use in combination may be more effective than single drug therapy. Several dosage schedules have been recommended for acetazolamide. In general, it seems advisable to start with 500 mg per day, either bid or every day with a sustained release preparation, 24 hours before ascent. Side effects are common but minor. The dosage of dexamethasone has been empirically established at 4 mg every 6 hours, starting 24 to 48 hours before ascent.

Generally, the mainstay of prevention is a sensible rate of ascent. Drug therapy should be considered for people who must make an emergency ascent or who have previously suffered acute symptoms at reasonable ascent rates.

HIGH ALTITUDE PULMONARY EDEMA (HAPE)

High altitude pulmonary edema is a noncardiogenic pulmonary edema thought to be caused by hypobaric alveolar hypoxia. It is considered a severe, potentially life-threatening form of AMS. Until recently, it was characterized and treated as a form of pneumonia or congestive heart failure despite its occurrence in young, otherwise healthy patients. Charles Houston is credited with describing the first clear account of the illness in the English language in 1960, when a 21-year-old cross-country skier developed symptoms after crossing a 12,000-foot pass near Aspen. It has now been clearly delineated as a separate clinical entity related to high altitude exposure, and not to cardiac failure. The exact pathophysiologic mechanism remains to be determined, but it seems to bear some similarity to adult respiratory distress syndrome (ARDS).

HAPE occurs in a setting of rapid ascent to altitudes between 8000 and 12,000 feet, and is not exclusively limited to extreme altitudes. It usually occurs in young, physically active patients within the first 1 to 4 days of ascent and is more common in men. Possible risk factors include pre-existing upper and lower respiratory tract infection, sedation at altitude, familial susceptibility, cold, previous episodes, physical exertion, and individuals in the pediatric age range. Women in the premenstrual, water-retaining phase may be more vulnerable to all forms of AMS. There

is also a descent/reascent form of the disease, which may affect highlanders. The exact incidence is difficult to extract from the literature because of cross-reporting of individuals at altitude with rales, and the characterization of a so-called subclinical form of the illness. It is reported to occur in 1 to 2% of climbers who attempt to climb Mt. McKinley, and that incidence has remained stable over the past decade. Higher incidences have been described elsewhere.

HAPE has been classified as type I or type II. Type I affects individuals from lower altitude who visit elevations above 8000 feet. Type II is the resident-reascent form of the illness. It affects highlanders who descend to lower altitudes for 2 to 7 days and then return. Children and young adults appear to be more susceptible.

High altitude bronchitis (HAB) is a common entity above 14,000 feet. Clinically, it presents with symptoms typical of acute bronchitis. It may represent a form of sterile bronchial inflammation brought on by a high minute volume of cold, dry air. No direct association has been made with HAPE, but the similarities are obvious, and individuals with HAB should be watched for further respiratory problems.

PRESENTATION

In addition to the symptoms of AMS, patients develop a dry cough, dyspnea, increasing fatigue, decreased exercise tolerance, and confusion. The cough may become productive of clear to frothy sputum. In more severe cases, the dyspnea worsens, and mental status worsens either as a consequence of hypoxia or concomitant cerebral edema. Coma and death may ensue within 6 to 12 hours if treatment is not begun.

Physical findings include observable tachypnea, tachycardia, fever, and central cyanosis. The fever is characterized as low grade, but may reach 104°F. On auscultation of the lung fields, rales develop, initially in the region of the right middle lobe, but then progress diffusely.

PREVENTION AND TREATMENT

The best treatment, of course, is prevention. As with AMS, proper acclimatization and reasonable ascent rates significantly reduce the incidence of HAPE. Ascent rates of 1000 feet per day at elevations between 10,000 and 14,000 feet, and 500 feet per day above 14,000 feet, are recommended. Close monitoring of susceptible individuals and early recognition of the signs and symptoms of the illness are important. The mainstay of treatment for established HAPE is oxygen administration and descent. Modest descents of 1000 or 2000 feet may bring about significant clinical improvement. It has been speculated that acetazolamide may be helpful in prevention, but has not been adequately studied. No studies have documented its effectiveness in established HAPE. Use of adjuvant treatment modalities such as CPAP masks and light-weight hyperbaric chambers have been more recently used as temporizing measures. Successful application of other drug regimens such as morphine, naloxone, furosemide, and nifedipine are anecdotal or controversial.

HIGH ALTITUDE CEREBRAL EDEMA

High altitude cerebral edema (HACE) is the least common but most severe form of AMS. Unlike the other altitude-related illnesses, it can cause permanent injury. It has been reported to have occurred at as low as 9000 feet, but usually presents at altitudes above 12,000 feet. The exact mechanism of injury is not clear, but it is hypothesized that a vasogenic cerebral edema caused by hyperperfusion or a cytotoxic cerebral edema caused by hypoxia is responsible.

PRESENTATION

Severe headache is the hallmark symptom. Patients experience an early truncal ataxia that progresses to severe gait disturbance. Mental status deteriorates as confusion, emotional lability, and impaired judgment develop. Auditory and visual hallucinations may occur. Physical findings include demonstrable neurologic defects, papilledema, retinal vessel engorgement, and probably retinal hemorrhages. Seizures are an uncommon complication. Progression to obtundation, coma, and death may occur without proper intervention.

PREVENTION AND TREATMENT

As with all forms of severe AMS, rapid descent and oxygen administration are critical. Prophylactic use of dexamethasone in AMS may have an impact on the incidence of HACE as well as on the acute course of the illness, but this has not been proven. Acclimatization is considered a key factor in prevention, although HACE has been documented in individuals who limited their rate of ascent to 1000 feet per day.

HIGH ALTITUDE RETINAL HEMORRHAGE

High altitude retinal hemorrhage (HARH) is a condition characterized by increased dilation of retinal veins and arteries, diffuse or punctate preretinal hem-

orrhage, papillary hemorrhage, and papilledema. It has a reported incidence of about 4% at 13,900 feet, greater than 50% at 17,000 feet, and almost 100% at 21,000 feet. The condition is associated with heavy physical exertion and rapid ascent. It is usually asymptomatic, although macular involvement is said to occur about 5% of the time, in which case a visual field defect may be present. The characteristic finding is a flame-shaped hemorrhage, although other findings such as cotton wool exudates and vitreous hemorrhage have been described. Intraocular pressure remains unchanged at high altitude. After returning to lower altitudes, most individuals have a spontaneous resolution of hemorrhage and no residual visual change. The significance of HARH is that it may be an early warning sign of HACE. Its pathogenesis is unclear, but it may share the same defect in vasoregulation hypothesized for other forms of altitude-related illness. Acclimatization may be helpful in reducing the rate of occurrence, but not necessarily the overall risk.

RECOMMENDATIONS FOR EMERGENCY DEPARTMENT EVALUATION AND TREATMENT

It would be a mistake to consider acute mountain sickness as an esoteric group of illnesses unrelated to the mainstream of practice of emergency medicine in the United States. The incidence of AMS among skiers in the mountain states is significant, and one author estimates that it results in annual lost revenues between $50 and $75 million to the tourist industry. Its clinical relevance increases when it is considered in the context of other pre-existing illness and the lifestyles of "type A" vacationers.

The evaluation in the Emergency Department (ED) centers around being able to accurately include AMS as part of the differential diagnosis by history. The physical examination may show only a mild tachypnea and tachycardia, and the patient may appear somewhat anxious. In my experience, it may be difficult to distinguish AMS from a hyperventilation syndrome, except that there is no discernible psychogenic motive. Additional findings such as hemoptysis, sputum production, rales, fever, calf tenderness, heart rates above 140, or headache out of proportion to other symptoms help to direct the physician's efforts. Relevant laboratory data may be obtained from oximetry, arterial blood gases, chest x-ray, ECG, and rhythm monitoring. In general, laboratory results may be normal for the altitude, or perhaps, a mild respiratory alkalosis may be demonstrated.

When the clinical presentation is mild and the workup is otherwise negative, the patient can be reassured and treated symptomatically. In my opinion, use of mild sedation during the brief acclimatization phase may be acceptable, depending on the patient. This is more applicable to patients at the lower ranges of high altitude, where exacerbation of respiratory depression during sleep is less likely to complicate the symptoms. Short-acting, short half-life benzodiazepines in low doses appear to be safest.

In patients with more acute symptoms, a brief period of observation may be necessary to secure the diagnosis. This is especially relevant in older patients or those with significant pre-existing illness such as COPD. Hospitalization and consultation are a reasonable option in patients with persistent respiratory difficulty, or in whom the chest x ray indicates the possibility of HAPE. In milder forms, the x ray may show unilateral focal infiltrates, most often in the right middle lobe. In more severe forms, bilateral focal infiltrates appear, and pleural effusions may be present. Hospitalization is also necessary in patients in whom the diagnosis is uncertain and other possibilities such as pulmonary embolism are considered. The possibility of HACE mandates hospitalization, although treatment is empirical, with dexamethasone, cautious diuresis, and descent. In the ED, acute mountain sickness is, in the final analysis, a diagnosis of exclusion.

BIBLIOGRAPHY

Dickinson, J.G.: Acetazolamide in Acute Mountain Sickness. Br. Med. J. *295*:1161, 1987.

Ellsworth, A.J., et al.: Acetazolamide or dexamethasone use versus placebo to prevent acute mountain sickness on Mount Rainier. West. J. Med. *154*:289, 1991.

Foulke, G.E.: Altitude-related illness. Am. J. Emerg. Med. *3*:217, 1985.

Hackett, P.H., and Roach, R.C.: Medical therapy of altitude illness. Ann. Emerg. Med. *16*:980, 1987.

Hart, L.E., and Sutton, J.R.: Environmental considerations for exercise. Cardiol. Clin. *5*:245, 1987.

Jacobson, N.D.: Acute high-altitude illness. Am. Fam. Phys. *38*:135, 1988.

Johnson, T.S., and Rock, P.B.: Acute mountain sickness. N. Engl. J. Med. *319*:841, 1988.

Katz, I.R.: Is there a hypoxic affective syndrome? Psychosomatics *23*:846, 1982.

Moore, L.G.: Altitude-aggravated illness: Examples from pregnancy and prenatal life. Ann. Emerg. Med. *16*:965, 1987.

Rabold, M.: High altitude pulmonary edema: A collective review. Am. J. Emerg. Med. *7*:426, 1989.

Schoene, R.B.: High altitude pulmonary edema: Pathophysiology and clinical review. Ann. Emerg. Med. *16*:987, 1987.

Staub, N.C.: Pulmonary edema due to increased microvascular permeability. Annu. Rev. Med. *32*:291, 1981.

Weil, J.V.: Lessons from high altitude. Chest *97*:70S, 1990.

West, J.B.: High points in the physiology of extreme altitude. Adv. Exp. Med. Biol. *227*:1, 1988.

Zell, S.C., and Goodman, P.H.: Acetazolamide and dexamethasone in the prevention of acute mountain sickness. West. J. Med. *148*:541, 1988.

Chapter 64

TRAUMA FROM ENVIRONMENTAL PRESSURE ALTERATIONS

DIVING AND ALTITUDE EMERGENCIES

George R. Schwartz and Barbara K. Hanke

CAPSULE

Several decompression diseases will be discussed: the "bends," nitrogen narcosis, injuries from diving equipment, and air embolism.

NITROGEN-RELATED DISEASE STATES (THE "BENDS")

PATHOPHYSIOLOGY

Humans exposed to gaseous environments containing physiologically inert gases (i.e., air containing approximately 80% nitrogen) distribute these gases through the body in proportions that depend on the partial pressure of the inert gas and its solubility in water, body fluids, and fat. Generally, we are concerned with nitrogen, but in some artificial environments, helium is used to replace nitrogen.

If environmental pressure suddenly decreases, nitrogen tends to come out of solution. If the pressure is much lower and the change is rapid, bubbles form. *Pain in the joints* is an early symptom, owing to joint sensitivity to internal pressure changes. Nitrogen bubbles may occlude the blood vessels of the lungs or brain. Bubbles within fat cells can cause bursting and release of fat into the circulation, compounding the problem with *fat embolism*. *Air embolism* (discussed subsequently) may also occur if the pressure changes cause disruption of the lung, and in such instances the nitrogen bubbles are of much less consequence than the lung damage and resulting air embolism, which may be rapidly fatal.

The degree of bends symptoms depends predominantly on the rapidity of decompression, the number and size of the bubbles, and the areas in which they lodge. A small amount of bubble development can occur with no symptoms. Physical activity increases the symptoms in both severity and speed of onset. This is probably related to increasing vascular turbulence and formation of vacuum cavities by muscle and joint movement. Individual susceptibility depends primarily on body build. Poorly perfused fatty tissues in which nitrogen has a higher solubility support bubble growth well. Therefore, individuals with more fat are more susceptible and develop more severe symptoms.

Venous gas emboli may also cause arterial embolization by intrapulmonic shunts.

PREDISPOSING SITUATIONS

Several factors predispose to acquiring the bends:

1. Scuba diving with too rapid ascent.
2. Flying in aircraft after scuba diving.
3. Rapid ascent or decompression in an airplane.
4. High-altitude flying with inadequate pressurization of cabin and inadequate denitrogenation.
5. Too-rapid ascent by tunnel workers (caisson disease).

SYMPTOMS

Most symptoms appear within 1 hour, with onset in some cases within minutes and in others more delayed (Table 64-1). After 3 hours, few individuals acquire new symptoms or develop initial symptoms. If exposure to depth is followed by exposure to reduced atmospheric pressure, however, symptoms may develop as late as 12 hours after the dive. If initial symp-

TABLE 64-1. TIME COURSE OF SYMPTOM DEVELOPMENT IN BENDS*	
Minutes	Percentage with Symptoms
30	50
60	85
180	95
360	99

* With permission from U.S. Navy Divers' Manual 8:32, Navy Department, Washington, D.C., 1973.

TABLE 64-2. TYPE OF SYMPTOMS (BENDS)	
Type	Percentage Manifesting
Local pain—legs or joints	90
Dizziness (staggers), neurologic symptoms	20–50%
Paralysis	2
Chokes (shortness of breath)	2
Collapse	0.5–1

toms are seen after 24 hours, the condition almost certainly is not decompression sickness. Sometimes symptoms can be relatively mild, however, and patients may present many hours and even days after the onset. Even so, recompression may be successful in aiding recovery. For classification, it has become customary to indicate type I as a milder insult and type II as more severe and including CNS involvements.

In divers, symptoms differ somewhat from those developing in aviators, owing to the increased dissolved nitrogen in the diver's blood and tissues in relation to the greatly increased pressure under water, as well as to the greater physical work usually being performed. Decompression sickness thus is generally more severe in divers, and permanent sequelae are more common. In divers, the latent period before clinical symptoms develop depends primarily on depth of dive, rate of ascent, and physical activity. Other factors are also important, e.g., whether earlier dives had occurred that day and the amount of "surface time" between dives. Divers' manuals contain tables that coordinate the various factors and indicate safety limits. Particularly useful are *The New Science of Skin and Scuba Diving*,[1] the *U.S. Navy Divers' Manual*,[2] and the *National Oceanic and Atmospheric Diving Manual*.[3]

The characteristic symptoms (Table 64-2) involve pain in joints and bones, worsening with movement, and usually not confined to a single site. The pain is usually described as deep and gnawing. Exposure to cold increases the symptoms. The pains disappear rapidly on descent, and return on immediate reascent.

PROTECTION

In situations of known predicted rapid ascent, protection against bends can come from denitrogenation before diving or flying. For example, exposure to 100% oxygen for 16 hours or more reduces the incidence of bends to zero. Even prebreathing with oxygen for 1 hour, however, can reduce the chance of symptoms by almost 50%.

DIAGNOSTIC TESTS

The history is of greatest importance in diagnosis. There may, however, be some x-ray findings, includ-ing bubbles in joints, bursae, tendon sheaths, or muscles. One quick diagnostic test is to inflate a blood pressure cuff around the joint to > 200 mm. The increased pressure may result in rapid relief of symptoms in that joint.[4] If there has been increased pulmonary pressure during ascent, mediastinal emphysema may be present and pneumothorax may occur. Ultrasound apparatus may detect bubbles in the vascular system. If rupture of the lung occurs, air embolism may result, with possible disastrous consequences as large amounts of air are released into the vascular space. MRI imaging can be used in detecting CNS and spinal cord damage. CT is of less use. The time required for MRI takes time from treatment and is of little use in the acute situation.

CHOKES

Chest pain, cough, and variable degree of dyspnea are seen. The cough may be paroxysmal and is nonproductive. The pain may be pleuritic in nature. Sometimes it is described as burning, substernal pain. In advanced stages, cyanosis and syncope may occur. An additional finding is a fiery red pharynx. These symptoms are believed to reflect nitrogen "bubble" pulmonary emboli with pulmonary irritation and reflex cough responses. The possibility of fat embolization contributing to the clinical picture has been suspected on histologic grounds.[5] If there is no evidence of lung damage (e.g., pneumothorax), air embolism is not a factor.

Chest x ray, the electrocardiogram (ECG), and auscultation are inconsistent aids. Rales may be heard and right heart dilation may occur, although even with severe symptoms, these findings may not be present. A "crunching" sound synchronous with the heartbeat may be audible. Chest x-ray findings during an acute episode have demonstrated right heart enlargement. Arterial blood gases may demonstrate hypoxia and hypocarbia with mild acidosis.

SKIN LESIONS

A pruritic, warm, painful, blotching red rash may occur, usually on the torso, resulting from nitrogen bubble emboli in the distal vessels of the skin. During descent, the lesions disappear. Once they are present, however, the areas again may become tender and edematous 5 to 6 hours after ascent. Small skin blebs that produce a burning sensation are a slightly different manifestation. These are thought to be from nitrogen gas trapped in the glands of the skin. Pruritus may be an early symptom. The skin manifestations are themselves harmless, but if widespread may be a sign of impending chokes, central nervous system (CNS) involvement, or cardiovascular irregularity.

CENTRAL NERVOUS SYSTEM MANIFESTATIONS

The CNS symptoms may range from mild headache to "staggers," delirium, and coma. Convulsions and transient loss of vision may occur, as well as signs of spinal cord impairment. The type of symptoms produced depends on the site of embolization and any reflex spasm that occurs. Some neurologic symptoms may take days or weeks to disappear. Permanent sequelae are not common in aviators, but they occur more frequently in divers. On the electroencephalogram (EEG), irregular slowing has been seen when focal deficits from cerebral gas embolization are present. Severe CNS involvement may lead to convulsions and death.

CARDIOVASCULAR SYMPTOMS

Cardiovascular symptoms include hypotension, bradycardia, syncope, arrhythmias, and even coronary occlusion. The presence of cardiac symptoms or signs requires continuous monitoring. *When death occurs early in decompression sickness, it is almost always from cardiovascular disturbances.*

DELAYED SHOCK SYNDROME

Hypotension may occur, and in 1 to 3 hours circulatory collapse and pulmonary edema can develop. This is believed to be associated with loss of intravascular volume and secondary hypovolemic shock, coupled with increased pulmonary endothelial permeability and pulmonary hypertension. The proposed mechanism involves widespread nitrogen gas and fat emboli, causing ischemia and increased capillary permeability. Local hypoxia causes release of kinins, histamine, and other vasoactive substances. The result is loss of fluid from the vascular compartment into the lung parenchyma and systemic vascular "pooling."

EMERGENCY TREATMENT

The best treatment for decompression sickness is to transport the patient immediately to a decompression chamber, where the total decompression regimen may take 24 to 28 hours.[2] The patient should be kept at total rest with 100% oxygen by mask, at 5 liters per minute, in a *slight* Trendelenburg position, lying on the left side to reduce chances of gas bubbles forming a "lock" in the heart, which if present can seriously reduce cardiac output. Some authorities recommend the use of an inert gas such as helium with the oxygen to avoid oxygen toxicity, although some experiments have suggested that the nitrogen bubbles may enlarge during the breathing of the oxygen-helium mixture.[6]

In contrast to earlier recommendations of a marked Trendelenburg positioning, some authorities now suggest a supine position to reduce cerebral pressure and ease respirations.[4] There are, unfortunately, no good research data available to support either position. Particularly when delays or prolonged transport might occur, marked alterations in positioning should be avoided.

Supportive treatment includes intravenous fluids monitored by a central venous pressure (CVP) catheter if a shock state is present. A vasopressor can be used to correct the hypotension resulting from widespread vasodilation, but replacement of fluids is essential in view of "third-space losses." Urine flow, blood pressure, and pulse should be monitored. Intermittent positive pressure breathing (IPPB) should be used if pulmonary edema is present. Morphine and diuresis offer little effectiveness in this form of pulmonary edema. If an unpressurized plane is used to transport the patient, it should be flown as low as possible and continuous oxygen should be supplied. A cardiac monitor should be used during transport to detect potentially lethal arrhythmias. A pressurized airplane should ideally be at one atmosphere. (Commercial aircraft are usually pressurized to the equivalent of 5000 feet, but pressure can be increased.)

If a decompression chamber is not available, the patient should be kept at complete bed rest, breathing oxygen by nasal cannula, and should remain in slight Trendelenburg position on the left side. Sedation usually is necessary. Mannitol may also be used, but should not delay or replace the primary treatment, which is recompression. Corticosteroids are usually given intravenously as well, although their benefit has not yet been proven. Unless symptoms are confined to joints and are mild, a cardiac monitor is advisable and respiratory function should be monitored by serial arterial blood gas determinations. Hyperbaric oxygenation may also help.

Each emergency department should have the 24-hour telephone number of the nearest decompression chamber. If questions arise, the Air Force School of Aerospace Medicine in San Antonio will provide 24-hour consultation. In addition, a National Diving Accident Network with a 24-hour "hot line" has been established at Duke University. The telephone number is (919) 684-8111 and a knowledgeable physician will be paged on request.

NITROGEN NARCOSIS

Owing to the high pressure with underwater descent, increased nitrogen is dissolved in the blood. The effects of the nitrogen have been termed "rapture of the depths," descriptive of the development of an apathetic, slightly euphoric mental state. Mild effects may be seen at depths as shallow as 50 feet, and below 200 feet most individuals experience significant impairment of logical thought. The phenomenon of nitrogen narcosis has led to the growth of helium-oxygen environments for prolonged sojourns under water, since a similar effect is not found with helium.

When nitrogen narcosis is present, suitable action should include direct assistance of the diver by a companion and the return of both to the surface using suitable decompression schedules. If possible, another diver should be sent to assist.

DANGERS FROM DIVING EQUIPMENT

There are two major types of diving units in use: the "open-circuit" and the "closed-circuit."

1. The closed-circuit unit uses 100% oxygen, and the exhaled gas goes through a canister where carbon dioxide is absorbed. It is dangerous because of the inefficient carbon dioxide removal with aging of the material in the canister, and the limitations on depth from high-concentration oxygen under pressure, which can result in lung damage.
2. The open-circuit unit uses a tank of compressed air, a valve, and a regulator, which can be inspiration-triggered or a forced-air type. These units need routine inspection and should be used only by those familiar with their limitations. Rarely, a high level of carbon monoxide may be introduced into the compressed air inadvertently through a malfunctioning compressor. The subsequent symptoms of carbon monoxide poisoning may present a diagnostic dilemma resolved by a carboxyhemoglobin level.

Although fear is often voiced about equipment failure, almost all catastrophes in fact result from human error, e.g., inattention to well-known safety procedures, fatigue, lack of attention to time, and inadequate familiarity with the equipment. The most serious problems in diving arise from air embolism.

AIR EMBOLISM

When a person is "skin diving," a lungful of air is inhaled and the diver heads for the bottom or as far as he or she can go. The increasing pressure on descent decreases the volume of air within the lungs, and the volume increases on ascent. However, the volume is not at any time greater than the original inspired volume. As a result, *air embolism is not a danger in skin diving*.

When one is diving with a *scuba tank*, however, a lungful of air can be taken well beneath the surface, and with volume increase upon ascent, rupture of the lungs can occur, resulting in rapidly fatal air embolism. A quantity of air at 100 feet under water occupies four times the volume at the surface. Thus, when a diver ascends, it is essential that he or she exhale continuously. The actual rate of volume expansion becomes more rapid as the surface is approached. Once the lungs are at full expansion, an additional volume change from only an additional 4-foot ascent is sufficient to rupture a portion of the lung. This phenomenon accounts for the occasional reports of air embolism occurring during scuba training in swimming pools. The exact damage can vary from a minimal pneumothorax and mediastinal emphysema to a total hemopneumothorax, with air in the arterial tree leading to cerebral air embolism and rapid loss of consciousness. The air bubbles also may lodge in the visceral organs. Ischemia to the bowel can result from mesenteric artery occlusion. Direct embolization to the coronary arteries can result in sudden death. (See next section on diving injuries for more details.)

TREATMENT

Treatment involves prompt recompression, as well as the other methods mentioned for air in the vascular compartment. A tension pneumothorax may develop and require immediate thoracostomy, or at least insertion of a needle to release the trapped gas. A simple, nonprogressive pneumothorax, however, responds well to needle aspiration. The needle can be inserted into the second intercostal space at the midclavicular line. A tube thoracostomy, however, is the safest procedure in all cases and eliminates the need for repeat chest x rays at frequent intervals.

EBULLISM

Ebullism is a syndrome of air embolism caused by exposure to altitude where the total ambient pressure approaches 47 mm Hg (63,000 feet) or less. The result is not only acute hypoxia, but "evaporation" or "boiling" of body fluids, with widespread air bubble formation. Animal studies demonstrate vaporization at the entrance of the great veins into the heart, which causes blockage of venous return and a fall in cardiac output. Bubbles are widespread throughout the heart and arterial system.[7] This is rapidly fatal, owing primarily to cardiac and cerebral hypoxia. Lung rupture may not occur if the airway is open.

The ebullism syndrome is essentially untreatable unless it happens accidentally in a vacuum test environment and unless treatment is instituted within 1 to 2 minutes. The treatment includes rapid recompression to hyperbaric levels. The body, as for any air in the intravascular compartment, should be in a slight Trendelenburg, left lateral position. Artificial ventilation may be necessary, and chest tubes must be inserted if pneumothorax has occurred. Aspiration of gas is feasible from the right heart and can be done through a CVP catheter.

EXPLOSIVE DECOMPRESSION INJURIES

Explosive decompression injury occurs almost exclusively in conditions of extremely high altitude flight or space flight, where the change in pressure is extremely large and rapid. Time of useful consciousness is less than 10 seconds.

TYPE OF INJURY

Explosive decompression can cause internal injuries to the gas-containing organs, owing to rapid expansion. Pulmonary damage, with hemorrhage and air emboli, can result. Tympanic membranes may rupture, and sinus pressure can cause extreme pain. The gastrointestinal (GI) tract probably would not be damaged significantly, however, because severe lesions are difficult to produce experimentally. There is also danger of injury from flying objects in this sort of decompression, and individuals have even been pulled out of aircraft through small portholes when a window was lost.

BLAST INJURY

High-pressure *blast injuries* are produced by explosions or rapid decompression. The effects are primarily those of direct trauma related to the intensity of the blast wave.

Death results chiefly from disruption of the vascular structures of the lungs, with hemorrhage, hemoptysis, air embolism, and respiratory failure. Nonlethal blast injury causes damage to the tympanic membrane and pressure damage to the hearing apparatus, producing hearing loss that may be permanent.

Injuries to abdominal viscera have been reported. Hypoxia and cardiac contusion can result in arrhythmias.

Brain injuries secondary to blasts have been reported with hemorrhage into the brain substance. Air embolism from the lung also may be involved in CNS abnormalities.

Injuries to the bony skeleton from blast waves through air or water are rare, unless contact is made through solid structures transmitting the blast pressure.

Treatment of blast injuries should focus on the lungs and heart. Blood pressure and oxygenation should be supported. Chest tubes are frequently required because of hemopneumothorax. Hemorrhage into the GI tract should be expected on the basis of animal experiments, and CNS hemorrhage may occur depending on the degree of blast pressure.

Hyperbaric therapy may be needed if air embolism is a concern.

PRESSURE DISORDERS OF THE EAR

Two types of pressure disorders of the ear are presented: *aerotitis media (barotitis media)* and *delayed otitis media*.

AEROTITIS MEDIA

This is a noninfectious condition caused by a pressure differential between the air in the tympanic cavity (middle ear) and that of the surrounding atmosphere.

Ordinarily, the pressure is equalized in the middle ear through the eustachian tube. With altitude increase of approximately 500 feet, the air in the middle ear expands, and sufficient pressure develops to open the eustachian tube and allow exit of air. On descent, air must pass into this cavity through the eustachian tube. If there is edema of the tube, as may occur with upper respiratory infections or a mechanical obstruction, the air may not be able to pass back through the eustachian tube on descent. The problem almost always occurs on descent, as the positive pressure from the expanding gas in the middle ear generally can push through even an edematous eustachian tube. The anatomy of the eustachian tube is such that air passage from the nasopharynx into the middle ear cavity is opposed in the resting anatomic position. Contraction of the dilator muscles occurs with swallowing, yawning, or a Valsalva maneuver, allowing opening of the normal eustachian tube. If this tube is obstructed, however, negative pressure occurs, and with altitude change symptoms of pain, vertigo, and tinnitus develop. If the altitude change without equalization is 2000 to 3000 feet, the tympanic membrane may rupture.

As a result of the relative negative pressure produced by deficiencies in middle ear ventilation on descent, negative pressure trauma to the tissue occurs with hyperemia, mucosal edema, and petechiae. There is outpouring of fluid transudate within the middle ear, which may be mixed with blood.

Acute barotitis media may occur when an individual has a respiratory infection, if altitude change is very rapid, or occasionally if he or she is asleep during descent. Once a substantial negative pressure has developed within the middle ear, the usual procedures (yawning, Valsalva, swallowing) are ineffective in opening the eustachian tube.

Because children often experience difficulty and discomfort on the descent of an airplane, vigorous measures can allow equalization of pressure and prevent several weeks of ear difficulties. Such techniques include (1) having the child chew gum, suck ice, or swallow; (2) inducing a Valsalva maneuver (clamp nose and hold mouth closed); and (3) encouraging crying. In severe difficulty, the flight attendant can be informed and the pilot can reduce rate of descent in certain instances or otherwise modify the landing approach.

CLINICAL SYMPTOMS

In acute barotitis media, one or both ears may be affected. Symptoms begin during or immediately after descent from altitude, and pain can be mild or intense. If the tympanic membrane ruptures, a sharp pain occurs, often accompanied by a loud noise and vertigo. Once rupture occurs, the acute pain subsides because this disruption allows equalization of pressure and the membrane is no longer being stretched. Hearing loss of a temporary nature is present, usually first affecting the lower frequencies. There are initial sensations of "ear fullness" and pain; tinnitus and vertigo are less common unless the membrane has ruptured.

Otoscopic observation demonstrates changes ranging from mild hyperemia to redness and retraction of the entire tympanic membrane. A fluid level frequently can be seen that may appear dark because of blood. Blood in the external canal indicates tympanic membrane rupture.

In divers, there may be pain on descent as external pressure increases (so-called "ear squeeze"). In this case, ascent usually provides rapid relief. The tympanic membrane may rupture on descent if the eustachian tube is blocked or if descent is too rapid.

TREATMENT

Use these measures:

1. Nasal vasoconstriction (with oxymetazoline hydrochloride (Afrin) or phenylephrine hydrochloride (Neo-Synephrine) drops).
2. Antihistamines (one to two Actifed tablets every 3 to 4 hours).
3. Attempts at Valsalva maneuver (if the tympanic membrane is still intact).
4. Inflation of the eustachian tube (politzerization) if such a device is available. Begin pressure at 20 mm Hg and raise with 5 or 10 mm increments. This is usually ineffective, however.
5. Myringotomy; drain any gross blood, because there is a danger of healing with fibrosis if a clot forms in the middle ear.
6. Antibiotics may be used, although their efficacy has not been demonstrated. If the purpose is to prevent secondary infection, an antibiotic with good sinus penetration and a broad spectrum (such as ampicillin) should be used. The basic condition, however, is noninfectious initially.
7. The presence of a ruptured tympanic membrane requires no additional treatment, although the patient should be advised against putting anything in the ear canal, and swimming is interdicted until healing occurs (usually three weeks). In rare instances or with large defects, the membrane may not heal. In large tears of the tympanic membrane, otolaryngologic consultation is necessary and a repair can be performed. The morbidity, however, from a chronic perforation may be minimal, and in fact, when there is congenital narrowing of the eustachian tube, a persistent perforation offers sustained relief. This, of course, is the basis for tube insertion in children with chronic otitis media.

DELAYED OTITIS MEDIA

Delayed otitis media usually occurs after breathing oxygen, which fills the middle ear cavity. As the oxygen is absorbed, negative pressure is produced and fluid accumulates in the middle ear. This normally occurs after sleep and is felt to be related to decreased swallowing during sleep and a consequent reduced tendency to equalize pressure. Treatment is similar to that for aerotitis media.

SINUS DISORDERS

Two sinus disorders—*aerosinusitis* (*barosinusitis*) and barodontalgia—are discussed.

AEROSINUSITIS

Aerosinusitis is caused by the differential in pressure between the sinuses and the external environment when sinus ostia are obstructed, and it usually affects the frontal or maxillary sinuses. Because air cannot leave or enter, pain may occur on both ascent and descent. Radiographic diagnosis can be made with a Waters view of the maxillary sinus showing an air-fluid level in the antrum. Frontal sinusitis may also be seen on this film, and if present, it requires more vigorous therapy owing to the rare, but lethal, situation of extension of infection and cavernous vein thrombosis. Pre-existing sinus infection is commonly present. Initial symptoms include pain over the sinus and severe headache, often accompanied by increased lacrimation. Occasionally, tooth pain may be the presenting symptom, and sinusitis must be differentiated from barodontalgia in such instances.

For purposes of definition and therapy, sinusitis has come to be classified as grades I, II, or III.[8] Grade I is mild and transient, grade II is characterized by more severe pain lasting up to 24 hours with radiographic evidence of sinusitis, and grade III patients have prolonged pain which continues for days and radiologic evidence of severe sinusitis with air-fluid levels, sinus clouding, or opacity. Although the basic treatment is the same for all cases of frontal sinusitis, the presence of severe (grade III) sinusitis in an aviator can be treated by reascent to altitude (in either an airplane or an altitude chamber) and then use of decongestants along with slow descent to attempt to permit equilibration. If this is successful, the course will be prolonged and flying should be proscribed for at least 3 weeks and longer in some cases.

Several treatments are recommended:

1. Use of vaporizer.
2. Antihistamines.
3. Nasal vasoconstrictor (Neo-Synephrine or Afrin).
4. Antibiotics systemically (broad-spectrum).
5. Control of pain.

If infected fluid persists in the sinus, a drainage procedure is needed and otolaryngologic consultation is necessary.

BARODONTALGIA

Barodontalgia is acute dental pain that occurs more on ascent than descent, and is related to trapped air expanding in the tooth. This symptom indicates pre-existing dental disease. It may occur soon after a filling is inserted, or it may indicate other problems such as a periapical abscess.

The following treatments are recommended:
1. Analgesia.
2. Incision and drainage of abscess if present.
3. Dental consultation.

DISEASES WORSENED BY ALTITUDE CHANGES

Some diseases may be aggravated by altitude and pressure changes, and rapid changes can precipitate a severe life-threatening crisis.

For example, in bullous emphysema, increase in altitude can lead to rupture of a bleb and pneumothorax. After any procedure that allows air into a closed space (e.g., abdominal surgery, pneumoencephalography, cytoscopy), reduced pressure causes expansion of the air, with symptoms of pain and signs of distention.

Abdominal cramps are common with ascent because of the expansion of colonic gas. Generally, relief occurs with passage of flatus or redistribution of gas in the colon.

A rare occurrence involves air in a closed space abscess (e.g., amebic), and symptoms are produced by increasing altitude.

REDUCED PRESSURE DISEASES RELATED TO OXYGEN

Any pulmonary difficulty may be worsened by altitude (even at 5000 or 10,000 feet), and marginally compensated patients can become cyanotic. Treatment is the same as for acute respiratory failure. Oxygen should be given with caution at low flow (2 to 3 liters per minute by mask). Arterial blood gases are a valuable guide to further use of oxygen. If decompensation is severe, the patient should be transported to a sea level environment accompanied by medical personnel who can provide supplemental oxygen during the trip; when there is insensitivity to carbon dioxide, as in severe chronic lung disease or alveolar hypoventilation, artificial ventilation may be needed to maintain adequate oxygenation. Patients with severe neuromuscular conditions (e.g., amyotrophic lateral sclerosis) may have chronic carbon dioxide retention. If they become short of breath during an aircraft flight, giving 100% oxygen may result in apnea. If a patient has a gastrostomy tube, it should be unclamped during ascent to avoid gaseous expansion in a closed space, which can lead to respiratory difficulty.

HIGH-ALTITUDE PULMONARY EDEMA

This is a poorly understood condition involving the development of pulmonary edema 12 to 48 hours after ascent usually greater than 10,000 feet. Characteristic signs of pulmonary edema appear: cough, dyspnea, possibly hemoptysis, and reduced exercise tolerance. Chest radiographs demonstrate fluffy infiltrates with a heart that appears to be of normal size. Arterial blood gases demonstrate hypoxemia.

Although probably ineffective, the usual treatment measures for pulmonary edema are often employed (e.g., digitalis, morphine, diuretics), but the most important aspects of treatment are oxygen, bed rest, and return to a lower altitude. Healthy young men are more likely to develop this condition. In severe cases, rapid cerebral swelling may also develop, requiring immediate osmotherapy to avoid death.

ACUTE MOUNTAIN SICKNESS

The syndrome of acute mountain sickness occurs generally with ascent to greater than 10,000 feet in an individual acclimatized to sea level. Symptoms can range from mild headache, fatigue, and mild dyspnea to a more serious syndrome with pulmonary or cerebral edema. Use of diuretics (e.g., furosemide or acetazolamide) may prevent or reduce the symptoms. Severe cases should prompt immediate return to a lower altitude with supplemental oxygen. Dexamethasone and acetazolamide may provide a preventive treatment in susceptible individuals.[9]

ACUTE AIR SICKNESS

Air sickness ("motion sickness," "seasickness") generally is not caused by barometric pressure changes, although it may be worsened by pressure within the ear. The problem stems from the labyrinth, and individual susceptibility is variable.

The best treatment is removal of the stimulus. If this is not possible, a substance such as dimenhydrinate (Dramamine), 50 mg orally, may be used. Military testing for the space program showed that, in the absence of organic disease, the most effective motion sickness remedy was scopolamine, 0.3 mg or 0.6 mg, taken with dextroamphetamine, 5 mg or 10 mg, an hour before flight.

NATIONAL CONTACTS

Divers Alert Network, 919-684-4544. Naval Medical Research, 301-295-1839.

School of Aerospace Medicine
Brooks Air Force Base, San Antonio, Texas.

REFERENCES

1. Association Press: The New Science of Skin and Scuba Diving. Association Press, New York, 1988.
2. U.S. Navy Divers' Manual: Navy Department, Washington, D.C., 1985.
3. National Oceanic and Atmospheric Administration Diving Manual. U.S. Govt. Printing Office, No. 003-017-00468, 1979.
4. Kizer, K.W., and Neuman, T.S.: Meeting the challenge of SCUBA diving emergencies: Recognition, resuscitation and recompression. Emerg. Med. Reports 12:17, 1991.
5. Clay, J.R.: Histopathology of experimental decompression sickness. Aerosp. Med. 34:1107, 1963.
6. Strauss, R.H., and Kunkle, T.D.: Isobaric bubble growth: A consequence of altering atmospheric gas. Science 186:443, 1974.
7. Dunn, J.E., II, et al.: Experimental animal decompressions to less than 2 mm. Hg absolute (pathologic effects). Aerosp. Med. 36:725, 1965.
8. Rodenberg, H.: Severe frontal sinus barotrauma in an airline passenger—case report and review. J. Emerg. Med. 6:113, 1988.
9. Zell, S.C., Goodman, P.H.: Acetazolamide and dexamethasone in the prevention of acute mountain sickness. West. J. Med. 148:541, 1988.

BIBLIOGRAPHY

Arthur, D.C., Margulies, R.A.: A short course in diving medicine. Ann. Emerg. Med. 116:689, 1987.

Bassett, B.: Diving casualties. In Emergency Medicine. Edited by Greenberg, M., and Roberts, J. Philadelphia, F. A. Davis Co., 1982.

Bassett, B., and Roberts, J.: Altitude exposure. In Emergency Medicine. Edited by Greenberg, M., and Roberts, J. Philadelphia, F. A. Davis Co., 1982.

Bayne, C.G.: Acute decompression sickness. J. Am. Coll. Emerg. Physician 7:351, 1978.

Beard, S.E., et al.: Comparison of helium and nitrogen in production of bends in simulated orbital flights, Aerosp. Med. 38:331, 1961.

Behnke, A.R.: Decompression Sickness Following Exposure to High Pressures. In Fulton, J.G. (ed.): Decompression Sickness. Philadelphia, W. B. Saunders Co., 1951, pp. 53–89.

Boettinger, M.L.: Scuba diving emergencies: Pulmonary overpressure accidents and decompression sickness. Ann. Emerg. Med. 12:563, 1983.

Burkhardt, W.L., Adler, H., and Thonetz, A.T.: A roentgenographic study of bends and chokes at altitudes. J. Aviation Med. 17:462, 1946.

Clamann, H.G.: Decompression sickness. In Aerospace Medicine. Edited by Armstrong, H.G. Baltimore, Williams & Wilkins Co., 1961, pp. 175–188.

Cockett, A.T.K., et al.: Pathophysiology of bends and decompression sickness. Arch. Surg. 114:296, 1979.

Cryssanthou, C., et al.: Studies on dysbarism influence or bradykinin and bradykinin antagonists on decompression sickness in mice. Aerosp. Med. 35:741, 1964.

Degner, E.A., Ikels, K.G., and Allen, T.H.: Dissolved nitrogen and bends in oxygen-nitrogen mixtures during exercise at decreased pressures. Aerosp. Med. 36:418, 1965.

Divers Alert Network: Report on Fatalities, 1989. Durham, NC, 1991.

Flinn, D.E., and Womack, G.J.: Neurologic manifestations of dysbarism: A review and report of a case with multiple episodes. Aerosp. Med. 36:418, 1965.

Garges, L.M.: Maxillary Sinus Barotrauma Aviat. Space Environ. Med. 56:796, 1985.

Green, R.D., and Leitch, D.R.: Twenty Years of Treating Decompression Sickness. Aviat. Space Environ. Med. 58:322, 1987.

Gribble, M.DeG.: A comparison of the "high altitude" and "high pressure" syndromes of decompression sickness. Br. J. Ind. Med. 17:181, 1960.

Haake, R., et al.: Barotrauma—Pathophysiology, risk and prevention. Chest 91:608, 1987.

Harvey, E.N.: Decompression sickness and bubble formation in blood and tissues. Bull. N.Y. Acad. Med. 21:505, 1965.

Haymaker, W., and Johnson, A.D.: Pathology of decompression sickness: A comparison of the lesions in airmen with those in caisson workers and divers. Milit. Med. 117:285, 1965.

Jones, H.B.: Gas exchange and blood-tissue perfusion factors in various body tissues in decompression sickness. *In* Decompression Sickness. Edited by Fulton, J.F. Philadelphia, W. B. Saunders Co., 1951, pp. 278–321.

Kim, T.S.: High altitude pulmonary edema. Illinois Med. J. *154*:409, 1978.

Kizer, K.W.: Disorders of the deep. Emerg. Med. *16*:18, 1984.

Kiżer, K.W.: Dysbaric cerebral air embolism in Hawaii. Ann. Emerg. Med. *16*:535, 1987.

Lewis, S.T.: Decompression sickness in USAF operation flying, 1968–1971. Aerosp. Med. *43*:11, 1261, 1972.

Millen, E.J., et al.: Circulatory adaptation to diving in the freshwater turtle. Science *145*:591, 1964.

Nims, L.F.: Environmental factors affecting decompression sickness. *In* Decompression Sickness. Edited by Fulton, J.F. Philadelphia, W. B. Saunders Co., 1951, pp. 192–222.

Powell, M.R.: Gas phase separation following decompression in asymptomatic rats. Visual and ultrasound monitoring. Aerosp. Med. *43*:1240, 1972.

Rait, W.L.: The etiology of post decompression shock in air-crewmen. Armed Forces Med. J. *10*:790, 1959.

Robin, D.E.: Of seals and mitochondria. N. Engl. J. Med. *275*:646, 1966.

Roth, E.M.: Space Atmospheres. NASA Sp-117. NASA, Washington, D.C., 1966.

Roth, E.M.: Gas physiology in space operations. N. Engl. J. Med. *275*:3, 144, 1966.

Rumbaugh, D.M., and Ternes, J.W.: Learning set performance of squirrel monkeys after rapid decompression to vacuum. Aerosp. Med. *36*:8, 1965.

Schreiner, H.R., and Kelley, P.L.: Underwater Physiology. *In* Third Symposium on Underwater Physiology, March, 1966. Edited by Lambertson, C.J. Baltimore, Williams & Wilkins Co., 1967, pp. 275–299.

Stapczynski, J.S.: Blast injuries. Ann. Emerg. Med. *11*:687, 1982.

Stewart, T.W.: Common Otolaryngologic Problems of Flying. Am. Fam. Physician *19*:113, 1979.

Whilten, R.H.: Scotoma as a complication of decompression sickness. Arch. Ophthalmol. *36*:220, 1946.

Womack, G.J.: Evidence for the cerebral vasoconstrictor effects of breathing 100% O_2. Aerosp. Med. *32*:328, 1961.

SPECIAL PROBLEMS OF UNDERWATER DIVING

Jeffrey Sipsey

CAPSULE

The popularity of scuba diving continues to grow in the United States. There are an estimated 3 million certified scuba divers, and 300,000 newly trained divers enter the ranks each year. Compounding the thrill, excitement, and exhilaration of diving are risks to humans in the hyperbaric environment. Humans have adapted to life in a rather narrow range of ambient pressure. As they venture beyond these limits, they must be aware of the physical changes and their effects on the body. The diver needs to be trained to understand and respect the laws of physics and his or her limitations in the undersea environment.

In 1988, the Divers Alert Network (DAN) reported approximately 600 treated scuba diving injuries in the United States. This actually represents an underreporting of the number of "diving accidents" because of (1) the failure of divers to recognize symptoms, (2) a diver's denial of symptoms in seeking treatment for diving-related illnesses, and (3) financial reservations in pursuing recompression treatment.

Physicians in all communities across the country should be knowledgeable in the clinical recognition of diving-related illnesses. Scuba (compressed air) diving is done in oceans, lakes, ponds, swimming pools, quarries, and caves. Air travel can carry the sport scuba diver to dive locations around the world in a matter of hours. It is not unusual for a diver to complete his or her last dive hours before boarding a flight home from some tropical resort and present to the Emergency Department (ED) with signs and symptoms of barotrauma or decompression sickness. (See Table 64-3 for guidelines for flying after diving.)

The diagnosis of these diving-related emergencies depends on a thorough dive history, an understanding of the pathophysiology of dysbaric injuries, a high level of suspicion for these conditions, and a thorough physical (neurologic) examination.

TABLE 64-3. GUIDELINES FOR FLYING AFTER DIVING

Dive Schedule	Surface Interval before Flying at 8000 Ft.
Nondecompression dives	
1. Less than 2 hours total dive time in last 48 hours	12 hours
2. Multi-day, unlimited diving	24 hours
Dives requiring decompression stops	24–48 hours

PHYSICS

To understand the physical principles of diving and the pathophysiology and treatment of diving accident victims, some basic elements of physics must be reviewed and understood.

The hyperbaric environment is one of increased pressure. Numerous disciplines are pursuing work and studies related to hyperbaric conditions, and different terminology is used to describe and measure the units of pressure.

Atmospheric pressure is the force exerted by the weight of the total column of air in the atmosphere at a specific location. At higher elevations, because the column of air is shorter, the atmospheric pressure is less.

Hydrostatic pressure refers to the force exerted on a body by the weight of any liquid into which it is immersed. Because liquids are not compressible, the depth/pressure relationship is linear and directly proportional, doubling the depth with double the pressure.

Pressure is measured with gauges, which are usually calibrated to indicate zero at normal atmospheric pressure. Gauge readings are normally indicated as such, i.e., atmospheres gauge, ATG versus atmospheres absolute, ATA (Table 64-4). The total pressure to which a diver is exposed at any particular depth is the absolute pressure: the sum of the gauge pressure measured on the depth gauge and the ambient atmospheric pressure at the dive site.

The physical behaviors of gases of most concern to a diver are their compressibility and solubility.

TABLE 64-4. Pressure Conversion

1 atmosphere (ATA) = 33 feet of sea water (fsw)
= 33.9 feet of fresh water (ffw)
= 14.696 psi
= 1.013 bars
= 760 mm Hg

Boyle's law states that (if the temperature is constant and the mass is fixed), the volume of a gas is inversely proportional to the pressure exerted on that gas.

$$P1 \times V1 = P2 \times V2$$

As the ambient pressure increases, the volume of a gas decreases (Table 64-5). The ear discomfort experienced by travelers when flying or when driving over mountain passes is a common example of gas volume changes occurring in a closed gas-containing structure. The discomfort (and sometimes pain) results from the distortion of the tympanic membrane by the pressure differential across the membrane.

If a diver descends from the ocean's surface to 33 feet of sea water (fsw) (from 1 atmosphere of pressure [ATA] to 2 ATA) with an inflated balloon, the volume of the balloon decreases by 50% from its original volume. If the diver descends an additional 33 fsw (to 3 ATA), however, the final volume of the balloon is $33\frac{1}{3}$% of the original volume. The change in volume of a gas is greatest in the shallower depths of a dive.

BAROTRAUMA IN DIVING

Because the body is composed mostly of water, the effects of pressure are equally applied over the entire body, and there are negligible effects of compression. Any gas-containing structures, however, are affected by pressure changes as defined by Boyle's law. Most of the anatomic structures (middle ear, sinuses, lungs) have developed with channels for communication with the ambient atmosphere to allow for pressure equilibration. When these passages are obstructed, either functionally or pathologically, the tissues surrounding the closed air space can be injured by the generated pressures.

To adapt to the underwater environment, humans have developed equipment to improve their functionality and survival. Human vision is based on the refraction of light waves through the air-cornea interface. Diving masks and helmets have been developed to maintain this interface underwater. Loss of

TABLE 64-5. BOYLE'S LAW RELATIONSHIPS

Depth	Absolute Pressure	Volume	Gas Volume	Bubble Diameter	Percent Change
0 fsw	1 ATA	1	100%	100%	
33 fsw	2 ATA	1/2	50%	79%	−21%
66 fsw	3 ATA	1/3	33%	69%	−10%
99 fsw	4 ATA	1/4	25%	63%	− 6%
132 fsw	5 ATA	1/5	20%	58%	− 5%
165 fsw	6 ATA	1/6	16.6%	55%	− 4%

body heat is avoided by the use of diving suits, wet or dry. The wet suit allows a thin layer of water to surround the body. Warmed by the body, this layer enhances the thermal insulation of the neoprene suit. The dry suit insulates the body with a cocoon of air. Both are attempts to minimize conductive heat loss.

The functional diver is neutrally buoyant, not having to expend additional energy to maintain a constant depth. Analogous to the swim bladder of fish, the diver uses a buoyancy compensator, which he or she inflates with air or deflates, to balance his or her weight (body weight, dive tanks, weight belt, camera, game bag and catch, etc.) at any depth.

All these anatomic structures and mechanical devices are subject to Boyle's law and all can be associated with significant injury (barotrauma). (See Table 64-6.)

DIVING TRAUMA

MASK SQUEEZE

The diver's mask has a rigid faceplate and a flexible rubber or latex body which conforms to the shape of the diver's face. During the descent phase of the dive, the air within the mask is compressed and the mask volume decreases. The diver should release air through his or her nose into the mask to increase the volume of gas and equalize the pressure. Anxious, novice divers sometimes fail to follow this normal procedure. The negative pressures within the mask are applied directly to the soft tissues of the face and produce edema and subcutaneous and subconjunc-

tival hemorrhage in the enclosed periorbital skin and conjunctiva.

The patient presents complaining of facial and periorbital ecchymosis and may complain of significant eye pain and visual discomfort. Evaluation should include examination for corneal injuries. Treatment is symptomatic.

EAR SQUEEZE

The most common injury in the hyperbaric environment is barotrauma to the tympanic membrane (an "ear squeeze").

The middle ear is a closed air space with a flexible membrane as one of its walls. The eustachian tube provides a channel to introduce or remove air from the middle ear and equalize pressure during the descent or ascent phases of a dive.

All divers must learn to "clear" their ears every few feet (equalize pressure) by one of several mechanisms: (1) gently blowing against a closed glottis with closed lips and a pinched nose (Toynebee), (2) blowing with an open glottis against closed lips and pinched nose (Valsalva), or (3) swallowing with a closed glottis, lips, and nose (Frenzel). If there is any sensation of ear fullness, discomfort, or pain, the diver should stop the descent, and even ascend slightly to increase the gas volume (decrease the pressure) in the middle ear, to help equalize the pressures on both sides of the tympanic membrane.

The degree of injury to the tympanic membrane (TM) has been categorized in the Teed classification, a graduated scale of the degree of injury.

   Grade 0—Normal
   Grade 1—Mild erythema of the TM
   Grade 2—Erythema, injection of the entire TM
   Grade 3—Vesicles of the TM
   Grade 4—Some hemorrhage of middle ear, + TM perforation
   Grade 5—Hemorrhage filling the middle ear

EXTERNAL CANAL SQUEEZE (REVERSE EAR SQUEEZE)

In temperate and arctic diving environments, it is necessary for the diver to wear some type of thermal protection (wet suit or dry suit). The wet suit includes a neoprene hood, which covers the head to retain body heat. If this fits too tightly over the ear and occludes the external auditory meatus, it creates a closed air space in the external auditory canal with a neoprene diaphragm on one end and the tympanic membrane on the other. During the descent phase of the dive, as the volume of gas in this space decreases, the diver is able to increase the gas volume only in the middle ear on one side of the tympanic membrane, but unable to introduce any air into the external auditory canal. If the diver does not ascend and adjust the hood, the pressure generated may rupture the tympanic membrane. A ruptured tympanic membrane will exclude the diver from any further diving activities for months.

Many swimmers wear ear plugs, but these should never be worn by scuba divers because they cause a reverse ear squeeze on descent. Other workers in the hyperbaric environment (tunnel workers, chamber attendants) who require noise suppression should ensure that their ear protectors are vented to provide communication between the external auditory canal and the ambient atmosphere.

Reverse ear squeeze may also occur if the extended ear canal is blocked by cerumen. Treatment consists of keeping the ear canal dry and giving antibiotics if the tympanic membrane is perforated. Referral to an otolaryngologist should be made if there is a perforation.

BAROSINUSITIS (SINUS SQUEEZE)

Bloody sputum has classically been described as a sign of air embolism, but is most commonly caused by a sinus squeeze with drainage of the blood from the hemorrhagic mucosa through the ostia and mixing with the expectorated sputum—a blood-streaked sputum. A frothy, blood-tinged sputum is characteristic of the pulmonary edema, like the sputum from a drowning or near-drowning victim. The barotraumatized lung from a pulmonary overpressurization accident is not grossly hemorrhagic.

CRANIAL NERVE BAROTRAUMA (ALTERNOBARIC FACIAL PARALYSIS)

Barotrauma to the sixth and seventh cranial nerves have been reported. These nerves pass through or near sinuses, where they can be exposed to increased pressure in the sinuses and produce a compression neuropraxia. The patient presents with a Bell's palsy or facial numbness, but not necessarily with pain referred to any of the sinuses. The symptoms may be of short duration or require several months to resolve.

PERILYMPH FISTUAL (ROUND WINDOW TEAR)

Many divers have difficulty in "clearing their ears" during the descent phase of a dive. Instead of stopping and ascending slightly, they perform the Valsalva maneuver repeatedly with increasing intensity. Some may complain of sensing a "pop" during the episode; however, any ear pain is not relieved. A diver can generate significant pressures during a strong Valsalva maneuver and cause inner ear barotrauma resulting in a tear to the round window.

The patient may complain of fullness in the affected ear, muffled sounds, ringing, tinnitus, and possibly vertigo. The onset of symptoms may occur shortly after the dive, but more typically develops after several hours or in the morning after the diving. During the delay, the leakage of endolymph from the cochlea progresses to produce symptoms.

Audiometry is essential and typically shows high frequency sensorineural loss in the affected ear. Emergency referral to an experienced otolaryngologist is necessary.

Some otolaryngologists support immediate surgery with placement of a fascial or perichondral graft to seal the defect in the membrane. Others manage the patient conservatively with bed rest and head elevation for several days. If there is no resolution of symptoms by that time, they proceed to surgical repair.

Round window rupture is a contraindication to any further diving. The usual injury is unilateral, but the risk of a subsequent rupture of the contralateral round membrane is high and would leave the patient partially deaf.

Remembering that the biggest gas volume changes occur closest to the surface (the first 30 feet of a dive), these injuries can occur in training dives in local swimming pools.

ALTERNOBARIC VERTIGO (ABV)

If a diver is unable to clear one ear, and the middle ear pressure exceeds that of the opposite side by 50 mm or more, he or she will develop vertigo and possibly nausea and vomiting. The increased middle ear pressure compromises blood flow to the middle ear and the asymmetric function of the vestibular end organs presents as vertigo. ABV can occur both on descent and, more commonly, on ascent, but through different mechanisms.

The symptoms of vertigo, tinnitus, and fullness in the affected ear are usually short-lived, resolving spontaneously within minutes of surfacing. A "hiss" as the pressure releases accompanies the symptom resolution. Audiometry is required to evaluate the transient inner ear ischemia for sensorineural damage. The differential diagnosis includes otologic decompression sickness, inner ear barotrauma with perilymphatic fistula, or round window rupture. ABV may result in underwater disorientation caused by vertigo, with resultant drowning.

PULMONARY BAROTRAUMA

Pulmonary overinflation syndrome occurs if the air inside the lung does not equilibrate during the diver's ascent.

The lungs are the largest air-containing structure in the body. With each breath, the diver fills them with a given volume of air; however, the gas density varies with the depth of the dive. During the ascent phase of a dive, as the gas expands in volume with the decrease in ambient pressure, normal airways allow the free flow of air. Flow can be obstructed voluntarily by the diver or produced functionally by degenerative pulmonary disease, or air can be "trapped" in poorly ventilated regions of the lung. The expanding air overpressurizes the lung, and if this pressure exceeds the 80 mm Hg structural elastic limits of the lung. The three possible outcomes of a pulmonary overpressure problem are: (1) pneumothorax, (2) pneumomediastinum, or (3) cerebral arterial gas embolism.

PNEUMOTHORAX

As a result of the pulmonary overpressurization, air is forced through the lung tissues and through the pleura into the pleural cavity, causing a pneumothorax. The patient complains of chest pains and/or dyspnea. Management in the ED is similar to that for spontaneous pneumothorax, with tube thoracostomy for significant pneumothorax.

If the diver has developed a pneumothorax before reaching the surface, during the remaining ascent the pneumothorax will also expand according to Boyle's law and could present as a tension pneumothorax, requiring immediate field intervention. A patient requiring recompression therapy for any condition but also having a pneumothorax must have a tube thoracostomy to prevent the development of a tension pneumothorax during treatment.

A detailed neurologic examination is essential to evaluate for possibly related comorbid air embolism with either unrecognized or denied symptoms.

The diver should be restricted from diving until he or she has had pulmonary function testing and consultation with a diving medicine specialist.

PNEUMOMEDIASTINUM AND SUBCUTANEOUS EMPHYSEMA

The air driven by the excessive intrapulmonic pressure may follow a path of less resistance and dissect through the interstitial tissues into the mediastinum and cephalad into the neck. The diver may sense a clicking sound in the chest or complain of swelling in the neck, a crinkling in the skin, or voice changes. The examiner should be particularly attentive to palpation of crepitus in the soft tissues of the neck and ascultation of a Hamman's crunch in the chest (the heart motion compressing the air blebs in the mediastinum).

Treatment is conservative. Mild cases may be discharged home. Moderate to severe cases should be admitted for bed rest and 100% oxygen administration to enhance resolution of the subcutaneous air. Massive pneumomediastinum may produce airway compromise, and recompression therapy would be of benefit.

A detailed neurologic examination is essential to evaluate for possibly related comorbid air embolism with either unrecognized or denied symptoms.

The diver should be restricted from diving until he or she has had pulmonary function testing, possibly including dilutional studies and body plethysmography and consideration of ventilation scanning.

CEREBRAL ARTERIAL GAS EMBOLISM

Cerebral arterial gas embolism is a life-threatening risk of scuba diving. As a result of pulmonary overinflation during ascent, air is forced through the alveolar and capillary walls into the bloodstream. Carried in the pulmonary vein to the left side of the heart, the gas is embolized systemically. Buoyancy of the gas in the blood, the diver's head-up position on ascent, and the large percentage distribution of circulation to the brain predisposes most of the gas bubbles to be carried to the brain. The bubbles are distributed systemically, and the second most critical organ of involvement is the heart.

The typical clinical history is of a diver making an emergency free ascent because he has run out of air in his tanks. As he ascends, he feels that he is running out of air and decides to hold his breath until reaching the surface. This is usually done in a panic situation, and the rationale is not objective. Divers are taught that, because of the expansion of air in the lungs during ascent, they have enough air in their lungs to reach the surface, and they must continuously exhale during an emergency ascent. They must also flare their bodies to decrease their rate of ascent as they near the surface, because the expansion of the gas increases within 30 feet of the surface, increasing their buoyancy and their rate of ascent.

Breaking the surface, the diver may immediately call for help, and frequently reaches the surface and indicates that he is "OK." Within seconds and up to 10 minutes later, he may develop acute neurologic symptoms. These can range from speech problems and upper extremity weakness, through hemiparesis and aphasia, to seizures, unconsciousness, or cardiac arrest. The diver may even lose consciousness before reaching the surface.

The gas embolized to the brain mechanically obstructs arterial blood flow, causing areas of localized ischemia. Immediately surrounding areas lose their autoregulation and dilate further. There is injury to the blood-brain barrier and development of vasogenic cerebral edema. With significant embolization there is global, transient cessation of areas of brain function.

The victim recovered in cardiac arrest may have arrested secondary to near-drowning, or the arrest may be a primary event. There can be direct embolization of the coronary arteries, and evolution of a myocardial infarction or the arrest may be an arrhythmic event secondary to the systemic hypertension and the catecholamine release associated with the cerebral injury. The air bubbles may also lodge in the visceral organs, and bowel ischemia may result from mesenteric artery ischemia.

The immediate aid to the embolism victim is to establish the ABCs. Many of the victims in full arrest respond to basic life support (BLS) resuscitation and recover spontaneous respirations and pulse, but remain in a deep coma.

Trendelenburg and left lateral decubitus positioning place the aortic outflow tract at the lowest point of the ventricular wall and decrease the release of additional gas into the system. It is difficult, however, to manage a patient requiring resuscitation in this position. The victim should be placed minimally in a supine position. In the immediate postaccident phase, the Trendelenburg position is most efficacious. Controversy has developed regarding the effectiveness of the Trendelenburg position in prevention of embolization to the brain and the deleterious effect of increased intracranial pressure when the cerebral circulation has lost its autoregulation.

The patient should be transported to the nearest recompression chamber as soon as possible. With cerebral air embolism, complications may include cardiac arrhythmias, seizures, and air embolisms to other areas of the body. Standard management should be initiated. Corticosteroids are frequently given, although their efficacy is unproven. Persistent neurologic defects are found in approximately one third of survivors. Mortality is less than 5%, but complications are more severe in the patient who presents comatose.

CNS OXYGEN TOXICITY

High levels of oxygen can be toxic to tissues. Long-term exposure of the lungs to 100% oxygen produces epithelial injury. If the FIO_2 is maintained less than or equal to 0.5 ATA, there is no risk of pulmonary oxygen toxicity.

There is also CNS oxygen toxicity, which manifests as grand mal seizures. This occurs when the FIO_2 approaches 280 to 300, and can be seen in the dry hyperbaric treatment chamber when oxygen is used as the treatment gas in a hyperbaric environment.

Oxygen as a breathing gas in diving is used only in closed breathing systems (a small volume of recirculating breathing gas in a system that injects oxygen into the system to replace it as it is consumed and removes CO_2 as it is produced) at rigid depth restrictions, and essentially the realm of military diving. Some commercial fisheries divers who perform decompression diving, however, have begun to use ox-

ygen in water at depths of 40 to 50 FSW to decompress and eliminate nitrogen from their bodies more effectively. The high likelihood of an unattended grand mal seizure under water makes this an extremely dangerous practice.

SHALLOW WATER BLACKOUT

Divers may experience a sudden loss of consciousness under water without panic or warning. Its most common cause is cerebral hypoxia from hyperventilation. "Free divers" (snorklers, swimmers, swimming pool underwater racers) frequently attempt to extend their time underwater by hyperventilating before submerging. The fallacy is that there is minimal increase in the oxygenation of the blood, and the critical effect is that hyperventilation lowers the arterial pCO_2. This decreased pCO_2 reduces the usual stimulus for the diver to breathe.

At depth, the increased pressure provides an apparent increased FIO_2 to the body and increases the arterial pO_2. The diver, having lowered his starting arterial pCO_2, has extended the time until his normal respiratory drive responds. He may stay under water long enough for the PO_2 to decrease to low levels. Either hypoxic drive or the eventual response to CO_2 levels drives the diver to surface, but as the pressure decreases as the diver ascends, so does his FIO_2 (of the air in his lungs), precipitously. If this level should fall below 0.16, the diver blacks out (syncope).

NATIONAL CONTACTS

Divers Alert Network
24 Hour Hotline
919-684-4544

U.S. Navy Diving Unit
Panama City, Florida
904-234-4351

U.S. Navy Medical Research Institute
Bethesda, Maryland
301-295-1839

HYPERBARIC MEDICINE

Barbara K. Hanke

CAPSULE

Hyperbaric oxygen therapy (HBOT) is the delivery of 100% oxygen at greater than one atmosphere of pressure (usually two to three atmospheres) in a hyperbaric chamber unit to therapeutically increase the level of dissolved oxygen in the blood and decrease the partial pressure of other dissolved gases (i.e, nitrogen). It has traditionally been used to treat decompression sickness, but may have an increasing role in toxicology and in trauma (Table 64-7). HBOT may promote wound healing by inducing capillary proliferation and epithelialization.

HYPERBARIC THERAPY

There are relatively few hyperbaric units because they are costly to maintain, and local Poison Centers can be consulted for the location of the nearest one. Various types of recompression chambers are in use, and HBOT is administered according to established protocols for each unit. The benefits versus risks should be weighed for each patient because side effects of HBOT include pulmonary oxygen toxicity, cerebral oxygen toxicity (i.e., seizures within a few hours of three ATA and FIO_2 at 1.0), fires, explosions, and decompression sickness on decompression. The medical director of each unit is available for guidance and should be consulted before any patient transfer.

In addition to the obvious indications for diving accidents with decompression sickness or air embolism, HBOT has been recommended for some carbon monoxide-poisoned patients. The usual indications are a level of carboxyhemoglobin greater than 30% or the presence of symptoms of CO poisoning in patients with lower levels. Of course, the location of the nearest hyperbaric unit and the transport time should be taken into consideration, especially if the indications are borderline. Although no human clinical trials have ever proven that HBOT prevents the late neuropsychiatric sequelae of CO poisoning, it does provide more rapid resolution of acute effects and decrease mortality if the patient presents with severe neurologic impairment, cardiovascular involvement, significant metabolic acidosis, or combined carbon monoxide and hydrogen cyanide poisoning in the setting of smoke inhalation.

HBOT may also be indicated for cyanide poisoning (along with sodium nitrite and thiosulfate), on the basis of animal data that it decreases morbidity and mortality. The medical director of the nearest hyperbaric unit can be consulted to weigh the risks and benefits of any proposed HBOT intervention in a specific patient.

TABLE 64-7. INDICATIONS FOR HYPERBARIC OXYGEN THERAPY

Air or gas embolism
Decompression sickness
Carbon monoxide poisoning
Clostridial myonecrosis (gas gangrene)
Crush injury, compartment syndrome, other acute traumatic ischemias
Exceptional blood loss, anemia
Necrotizing soft tissue infections
Brown reclose spider bites
Osteomyelitis (refractory)
Osteoradionecrosis
Compromised skin grafts and flaps
Thermal burns
Poisoning with cyanide, hydrogen sulfide, or carbon tetrachloride; methemeglobinemia

BIBLIOGRAPHY

Bakker, D.J.: Clostridial myonecrosis. *In* Problem Wounds: The Role of Oxygen. Edited by Davis, J.C., and Hunt, T.K. New York, Elsevier, 1988.

Hyperbaric Oxygen Therapy Undersea and Hyperbaric Medical Society, 1986.

Kizer, K.W., and Neuman, T.J.: Meeting the challenge of scuba diving emergencies: Recognition, resuscitation, and decompression. Emerg. Med. Reports *12:*17, 1991.

Nemiroff, P.M., and Langu, A.P.: The influence of hyperbaric oxygen and irradiation on vascularity in skin flaps. Surg. Forum *37:*565, 1987.

Chapter 65

MAMMALIAN BITES

Edward Newton

CAPSULE

Mammalian bites are a common presenting complaint in Emergency Departments (EDs), and emergency physicians should develop a systematic approach to these injuries. Dog bites are common and capable of inflicting severe soft tissue damage, although they are the least likely to result in infectious complications. Conversely, cat bites rarely cause severe soft tissue injury but frequently become infected. Human bites are intermediate in both respects, although the "closed-fist injury" is notorious for its high rate of infectious complications and poor functional result.

The treatment of bite wounds is controversial, although there is a consensus regarding the importance of thorough debridement and irrigation in preventing infection. With the exception of hand wounds, cat bites, and bites in patients with increased risk for infection, prophylactic antibiotics are not indicated, and low-risk wounds may be sutured. Penicillin is the drug of choice for cat bite prophylaxis. A combination of penicillin and dicloxacillin or a first-generation cephalosporin and dicloxacillin or amoxicillin-clavulanate are all acceptable choices for human bite prophylaxis.

Wounds showing early signs of infection may be treated on an outpatient basis with debridement, splinting, elevation, and oral antibiotics, providing that careful followup care is available. More advanced infections and infected human bites of the hand should be admitted for surgical debridement and parenteral antibiotics. The choice of antibiotic in these cases is controversial, but many successful regimens have been described.

A multitude of systemic diseases may be transmitted by mammalian bites, although rarely. The most serious of these is rabies. Guidelines for rabies prophylaxis are provided.

INTRODUCTION

Mammalian bites are among the most ancient afflictions of man, but only relatively recently have they come under scientific scrutiny. Even so, despite the accumulation of large amounts of data, many areas of controversy and confusion remain regarding the management of mammalian bites. From a medical perspective, there are three main areas of concern regarding these bites. The most immediate concern is the soft tissue damage inflicted by the bite which may have significant functional and cosmetic implications, and may even result in death. Secondly, bites present a risk of local infection and sepsis. Finally, there is a risk of transmission of several potentially devastating diseases from animals to humans, including rabies.

Mammalian bites fall into three broad categories: domestic animal bites, which are by far the most common, wild animal bites, and human bites. Each of these categories is distinguished not only by cause but also by epidemiologic pattern, pathophysiology, and potential for causing infection. The exact distribution of offending species varies from region to region, depending on the animal population and the customs of the inhabitants. In North America, the vast majority (>90%) of reported bites are inflicted by dogs, followed by humans and cats. Most of the reported literature deals primarily with dog bites, and much less information is available regarding bites by other species.

EPIDEMIOLOGY

The true incidence of mammalian bites is unknown because most victims never seek medical attention. Public Health surveillance for rabies has generated a reporting mechanism for those seeking medical attention, which reveals that at least one million persons per year sustain animal bites in the United States.[1] Other studies have shown that less than half of animal bites are reported, and some authors estimate as many as 3.5 million animal bites per year in the U.S.[2] Accurate data are lacking in respect to human bites, and wild animal bites are rare. Nevertheless, up to 0.5% of the U.S. population sustains an animal bite every year,[3] and these injuries may constitute 1% of all ED visits.[4]

The annual cost of mammalian bites to society is similarly difficult to define precisely. Apart from the medical costs pertaining to treatment of the injury, additional costs accrue through the need for reporting, quarantine of animals, and police costs.[5] Up to one third of victims undergo some form of disability,[6] 1% are admitted to hospital,[7] and 32% of bites result in some form of litigation.[8] Estimated costs in 1979 amounted to $30 million.[9] Present estimates would no doubt greatly exceed this amount.

Fatalities from animal bites are rare, although there are approximately 15 fatal dog bites per year in the U.S. A review of 157 fatal dog bites from 1979 through 1988 revealed that 70% occurred in children under 10, and a further 10% in persons over 69.[10] Although they represent only 1% of the AKC registered dogs,[11,12] pit bull terriers were involved in 20% of these fatalities in 1979 and in 62% of fatal bites in 1988, reflecting the inherent aggressiveness and increasing popularity of this breed.[10] Overall, family or neighborhood dogs, not strays, account for the vast majority of dog bite injuries. Other species of large dogs are also capable of inflicting great damage and death, particularly in the vulnerable populations of children, the aged, and the disabled.

The population at risk for each type of bite varies somewhat. Dog bites are the most common in children between the ages of 2 to 15, with a male preponderance of 2:1. The incidence peaks in warm weather and late afternoon.[2] It has been estimated that 20% of children will be bitten at some point in their lives. Children are at greater risk because their small size makes them less intimidating to animals, they are more likely to be engaged in inadvertently provocative behavior such as running and bicycling, and they may, from lack of experience, fail to recognize and avoid threatening behavior in animals. For similar reasons, bites tend to be more severe in children because they are less able to defend themselves against an aggressive animal. Because of their small stature, small children are especially vulnerable to disfiguring facial bites and even intracranial penetration.[13] Older victims are most typically bitten on the extremities while fending off attacks.

Cat bites and scratches, on the other hand, are twice as common in women and occur mainly on the upper extremities. Significant soft tissue injury is rare, and the overriding concern in cat bites is the risk of infection.

Human bites are of two types. Occlusional bites may occur at any age but are particularly common in preschool children. The most common sites of injury are the distal phalanges, ears, nose, and genitalia. The second type of human bite occurs almost exclusively in young adult men and occurs when a clenched fist is lacerated against an opponent's teeth during a fist fight. The resultant innocuous-appearing laceration over the metacarpal phalangeal joint may result in devastating infection and loss of function in the hand unless proper care is obtained. Self-inflicted human bites, such as tongue biting during a seizure, are common but rarely cause severe infections.

Wild animal bites are rare in the U.S. and include primarily wild animals kept as pets or laboratory animals such as chimpanzees, rats, ferrets, and large felines. True wild animal bites are generally inflicted by smaller species such as rats, raccoons, bats, squirrels, and skunks. Apart from the usual concerns with soft tissue injury and infection, the possibility of rabies must be seriously entertained in these bites.

PATHOPHYSIOLOGY OF INJURY

Although the vast majority of mammalian bites are usually not life-threatening, they may occasionally be severe enough to require urgent intervention. Large animals may generate up to 450 lbs per square inch of occlusional pressure,[14] which can easily crush the larynx and trachea, lacerate major vessels, and fracture bones, including the skull in small children. Soft tissue injuries range from trivial abrasions and superficial scratches to massive avulsion of skin, muscle, and neurovascular tissue. In rare cases, blood loss may be sufficient to produce shock.

In the more common situation, the victim presents with one or several lacerations that are not immediately life-threatening but require timely assessment.

Dog bites tend to be a combination of tearing lacerations and crush injuries resulting in triangular flaps, often surrounded by areas of devitalized and necrotic tissue. Vascular insufficiency in an extremity may result from direct laceration or crushing of a vessel, or from subsequent development of a compartment syndrome. Edema and necrosis of crushed tissue surrounding the bite produce a higher susceptibility to infection in these wounds by organisms inoculated from the animal's mouth. Despite this, the incidence of infection in dog bites is surprisingly low. In various studies, the infection rate has ranged from 1.6 to 16%,[2,7,15-17] but averages approximately 4%, which is comparable to the rate for lacerations in general.[18]

Infection in bite wounds is a complex and controversial subject. Apart from the species of animal involved, a host of other factors determine whether an individual bite becomes infected and which organisms are involved as the principal pathogens. Risk factors

TABLE 65-1. RISK FACTORS FOR INFECTION FOLLOWING MAMMALIAN BITES

Species Factors	Wound Factors	Victim Factors
Cat (50%)	> 12 hours old	Age > 50 years
Human (16%)	Location on hand or foot	Chronic alcohol abuse
Dog (2–5%)	Closed fist injury	Diabetes
	Puncture wound	Malignancy
		Immunocompromise from:
		radiotherapy
		chemotherapy
		medication
		asplenism

for wound infection include wound characteristics, victim factors, type of treatment, and time elapsed before treatment is rendered (Table 65-1).[7]

Infection is more likely to occur in wounds of the extremities than in facial bites, presumably because of better blood supply to the face. Nonbite lacerations to the hands result in an infection rate of 1.1% to 8.5%, whereas dog-bite wounds of the hand become infected in up to 36% of cases.[7] Infection of facial dog bites is unusual.[8,17,18]

The same holds true for bites by other species, including humans. Reviews of human bite wounds reveal overall infection rates from 15-50%.[7,18-20] These data, however, are skewed by the disproportionate number of "closed-fist injuries" (CFI) in this group because patients with these injuries tend to present only after infection occurs. Bites of the face and bites inflicted by children have infection rates of less than 4%[17] because they tend to be more superficial, are located more often on areas other than the hand, and

receive earlier medical care. Such bites do not appear to be at high risk for infection. In CFI, however, the reverse is true. Patients tend to be older, do not seek medical care until their wounds are clinically infected, and by definition have wounds of the hands, which are more prone to infection. Clinical infection occurs in approximately 50% of these wounds.[21]

The typical CFI occurs when the closed fist of the patient has struck the tooth of his opponent, resulting in a laceration overlying the metacarpophalangeal joint (Fig. 65-1). Occasionally an associated fracture of the metacarpal head, foreign bodies in the wound including fragments of teeth, laceration of the extensor tendon, and penetration of the joint capsule also occur. Once the hand is returned to its resting position, the inoculum of bacteria is tracked into relatively avascular areas of the hand and effectively sealed, preventing the essential drainage of the wound. Inoculation of organisms into the MCP joint space has a tenfold increase in infection compared to other soft tissues.[21] CFI results in the notoriety of human bites as being especially prone to infection (Fig. 65-2).

Cat bites and scratches are also notorious for pro-

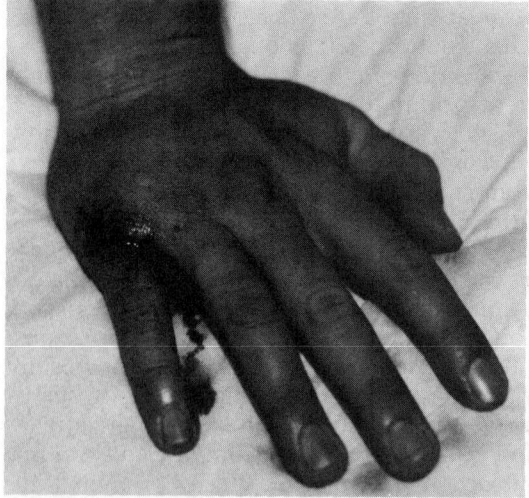

FIG. 65-1. "Fight-bite." Striking someone in the teeth often results in serious injury to the tissue overlying the metacarpal head (closed-fist injury).

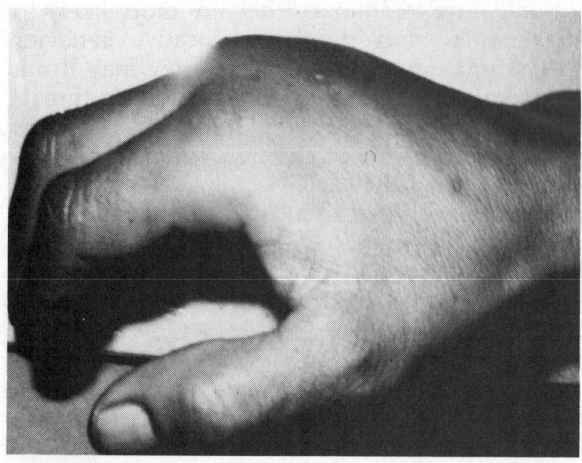

FIG. 65-2. Human bite to the hand. This patient waited until obvious infection was present to seek care.

ducing infection for somewhat the same reasons. Because of the needle-like-structure of their teeth, deep puncture wounds are typical, but often initially appear benign. Because of deep inoculation of bacteria into the avascular spaces of the hand and the resultant inability to adequately debride and irrigate the wounds, a high rate of infection results. As many as 30 to 50% of cat bites become infected, and most patients with cat bites present to physicians with established infections.[7,21,22] Because of cats' habit of frequently licking their paws, deep cat scratches tend to show the same propensity for infection as bites and share the same bacteriologic spectrum. Involvement of the eye is common in cat scratches and potentially serious.

Bites by other animals can usually be related to one of the above groups in terms of the soft tissue damage produced and the risk of infection. For example, bites by primates other than humans show a 15% infection rate.[14] Large herbivores such as cows and horses tend to produce severe crush injuries, which may not break the skin but often cause massive swelling, compartment syndrome, and neurovascular injury.[7] Bites by rodents tend to be minor in terms of soft tissue injury and cause infection approximately 2 to 10% of the time.[14,23]

The type of wound also influences the incidence of infection. Paradoxically, larger wounds are less likely to become infected than small puncture wounds for several reasons. First, patients with large wounds tend to present for medical care earlier than those with minor punctures. Second, avulsions and lacerations are more accessible than puncture wounds for debridement and irrigation, which has been clearly shown to decrease infection rates. Puncture wounds are often deep, with inoculation of bacteria into relatively poorly draining, avascular spaces. Consequently, puncture wounds are almost twice as likely to become infected as lacerations resulting from animal bites.[24]

Victim factors are also important in terms of the prognosis for infection. Any degree of immunocompromise can result in a much higher incidence of infection, both local and systemic. Patients with diabetes, chronic alcohol abuse, malignancy, asplenism, and undergoing treatment with immunosuppressive medication must be considered at higher risk and followed with particular care.

Probably the most critical statistical variable in terms of infection is the time elapsed from the time of the bite until the patient seeks medical care. This is somewhat misleading, however, because patients with relatively minor wounds do not seek medical care until their wounds become infected, generally 12 hours or more after the bite was sustained. Patients presenting immediately after being bitten tend to have more severe or cosmetically significant soft tissue injuries, or are concerned with the possibility of rabies, tetanus, or other infections.[25] Nevertheless, older wounds are no doubt more likely to develop significant infection simply from the lack of adequate local wound care and the uninterrupted multiplication of bacteria in the wound.

BACTERIOLOGY

DOG BITES

The oral flora of dogs has been carefully studied and reveals that up to 64 species of bacteria may be present, many of which are potential human pathogens.[17] The role of individual species in producing clinical infection is less clear, however, and no single species accounts for a majority of infections. Many infections contain multiple organisms, and the importance of each species in these cases has yet to be determined. Finally, up to 48% of cultures show no growth,[26] which probably represents infection with anaerobic or other fastidious organisms.

The most common isolates from infected dog bites include staphylococcal species (10 to 25%), streptococcal species (24 to 46%), Pasteurella multocida (0 to 50%), Pseudomonas species (10 to 20%), other gramnegative aerobes (25%), and anaerobic species (13 to 76%).[7,14,25-28] The role of anaerobic species is controversial in part because of the difficulty in culturing these organisms from wounds; however, it seems clear that they are frequently isolated when proper techniques are used.

Additional poorly characterized species may occasionally be isolated and have been known to produce devastating systemic infection, particularly in immunocompromised hosts. These include the CDC o-numeric strains II-J, EF-4, M-5, and DF-2. II-J can be cultured as part of the normal mouth flora from 90% of dogs and has caused several reported cases of sepsis, meningitis, and death from renal failure and DIC in humans.[29-32]

CAT BITES

The bacteriology of cat bites is simpler in that the vast majority of infections are due to Pasteurella multocida, a facultative anaerobic gram-negative organism that is part of the normal mouth flora in most felines. Infection with this organism produces cellulitis and often lymphangitis and lymphadenitis soon after the bite. The wound typically shows a serosanguinous or grayish purulent exudate. Infection is apparent within 24 hours in 70% of cases and within 48 hours in 90%.[18] This helps to distinguish Pasteurella from some other pathogens that take longer to produce clinical infection. In addition to local wound infection, Pasteurella can also produce serious systemic complications, including septicemia, endocarditis, meningitis or brain abscess from direct inoculation, osteomyelitis, tenosynovitis, and septic arthritis.[21,33-36] Once infection is established, up to 25% of patients require admission for parenteral antibiotics and wound debridement. Cat bites may also become infected with a variety of other organisms, including primarily Staphylococcus, Streptococcus, and less commonly, enteric gram-negative rods.

Cat scratches and bites can produce the syndrome known as "cat scratch disease," in which a tender raised papule occurs at the site of inoculation, followed by local lymphadenitis in the region draining the site of the cat scratch after a 3- to 10-day incubation. Usually only a single node is involved, and the patient complains of low-grade fever and malaise. Symptoms resolve quickly without treatment in most cases, although lymph nodes may remain swollen for up to 6 months and occasional serious complications such as encephalitis occur. The causative agent is unknown, although there have been many suggested candidates. There is no specific treatment, although tetracycline or erythromycin are often given with unproven efficacy.[42-44]

HUMAN BITES

The human mouth may harbor 42 species of bacteria when healthy but up to 190 species in the presence of gingivitis or periodontal disease.[17] Almost half of human bite infections contain mixed gram-positive and gram-negative bacteria, and the incidence of gram-negative infection may predominate in diabetics.[17] Anaerobes are found in 50 to 60% of infected human bites, always in conjunction with other bacteria.[14,37,38] The most common isolates on culture from these wounds are streptococcal species (43 to 95%), particularly Streptococcus viridans; staphylococcal species (25 to 50%); and Eikenella corrodens (10 to 33%).[7,14,17,21,22,38] The latter organism is a slow-growing facultative anaerobic gram-negative bacterium, also found in dog bite infections.[21] It acts synergistically with Streptococcus viridans to produce more fulminant infection.[39]

A multitude of other human pathogens may also be transmitted, depending on the species and medical condition of the source. Human bites are capable of transmitting hepatitis B virus, actinomycosis, Hemophilus influenzae, Neisseria species, syphilis, tuberculosis, scarlet fever, and theoretically, rabies.[14,21,40,41] The risk of HIV transmission by a human bite is certainly present because 44% of HIV-infected patients shed the virus into their saliva. There are no clearly documented cases of transmission of HIV through human bites, however, and these wounds are considered by the CDC to be at low risk for transmission of HIV.[17,38,40,41] Nevertheless, patients bitten by HIV-infected persons should be offered prophylaxis with AZT and followed closely with serologic testing for up to 2 years after such exposure. Unusual

and multiply resistant organisms may cause infection when the source is a previously hospitalized patient. This is not a rare occurrence among medical personnel, and such wounds should be cultured to determine the antibiotic susceptibility of the infecting agents.[21]

WILD ANIMAL BITES

Other rare infectious complications that may result from small wild animal bites include leptospirosis, bubonic plague,[45] rat bite fever,[46] tularemia,[47] Herpes simiae virus,[48] brucellosis,[49] Erysipelothrix, and tetanus[2] (Table 65-2).

RABIES

One of the most feared consequences of animal bites is rabies. Although human cases of rabies are currently rare in the U.S., rabies remains a significant cause of death in certain underdeveloped nations in which vaccination of domestic animals is not practiced. Over the past 20 years, there has been an average of only two cases per year of human rabies in the U.S.,[50] and many of these have resulted from corneal transplantation[6] and inhalation of rabies-contaminated aerosols.[3,51]

Rabies may be transmitted when the saliva of an infected animal comes into contact with the abraded or lacerated skin or mucosa of another mammal. It is not necessary for a bite to occur. In fact, many patients with rabies deny any high-risk contact with animals.[50] The incubation period may range from 10 days to as long as 1 year. Even when bitten by a rabid animal, only 50 to 60% of untreated victims develop rabies.[3]

In the past, domestic animals were the primary vector for the transmission of rabies to humans. Since the policy of vaccinating domestic animals has become routine, the main reservoir for rabies in the U.S. has shifted to wild animals. Currently the species most commonly found to be rabid are skunks (40%), rac-

---

TABLE 65-2. DISEASES TRANSMITTED BY MAMMALIAN BITES

Animals	Humans
Rabies	Hepatitis B virus
Bubonic plague	Tuberculosis
Tularemia	Actinomycosis
Leptospirosis	Scarlet fever
Rat bite fever	Syphilis
Erysipelothrix	Gonorrhea
Herpes simiae virus	Rabies*
Tetanus	HIV*
Pasteurellosis	
Cat scratch fever	

*Theoretic concern only, no cases recorded.

coons (35%), bats (20%), and foxes (3%). Rodents and lagomorphs rarely harbor rabies virus, with an incidence range from 0.16 to 0.6%.[51,52] Other animals are sporadically found to be rabid, including cattle, horses, wolves, coyotes, weasels, and ferrets.[51] There are significant regional differences in the incidence and animal vectors involved, and clinicians should acquaint themselves with the pattern in their vicinity.

The primary issue when managing a patient bitten by a potentially rabid animal is whether or not to administer active and passive rabies prophylaxis. Knowledge of the local pattern of rabies is helpful but, when there is doubt, public health authorities should be consulted. Up to 25,000 patients per year are appropriately treated for high-risk exposure with Human Rabies Immune Globulin (HRIG) and Human Diploid Cell Vaccine (HDCV).[53] Unlike previous regimens using Duck Embryo Vaccine (DEV), this treatment has minor and self-limited side effects, and because the current vaccine has greater antigenic potency, only five injections are required compared to 25 with the previous vaccine. Table 65-3 illustrates an algorithmic approach to the use of HRIG and HDCV.[53] Bites by rats, mice, squirrels, chipmunks, rabbits, hamsters, gerbils, etc. do not generally require rabies prophylaxis.

HRIG is given up to 8 days after exposure in a dose of 20 IU per kg. One half of the serum is infiltrated around the wound (except mucosal wounds) and the remainder injected intramuscularly. The immunoglobulin has a half-life of 21 days and is effective in binding the rabies virus before it can reach the central nervous system (CNS). It is necessary to use immunoglobulin because active immunization with HDCV does not produce significant antirabies titers for at least 1 week.[51] Vaccination is performed by injecting 1 ml of HDCV intramuscularly on days 0, 3, 7, 14, and 28. The combination of immunoglobulin and vaccine is extremely effective in preventing clinical rabies. Of 511 proven rabid bites in humans in which this combination has been used, no cases of rabies have been reported.[51]

Potential side effects of the vaccine include allergic reactions (which are rare with the HDCV), fever, headache, chills, diarrhea, malaise, and local reactions at the site of injection (redness, swelling, and pain).

TABLE 65-3. PROPHYLAXIS PROTOCOL FOR RABIES EXPOSURE*

TABLE 1. Rabies postexposure prophylaxis guide—July 1984

The following recommendations are only a guide. In applying them, take into account the animal species involved, the circumstances of the bite or other exposure, the vaccination status of the animal, and presence of rabies in the region. Local or state public health officials should be consulted if questions arise about the need for rabies prophylaxis.

	Animal species	Condition of animal at time of attack	Treatment of exposed person*
DOMESTIC	Dog and cat	Healthy and available for 10 days of observation	None, unless animal develops rabies†
		Rabid or suspected rabid	RIG§ and HDCV
		Unknown (escaped)	Consult public health officials. If treatment is indicated, give RIG§ and HDCV
WILD	Skunk, bat, fox, coyote raccoon, bobcat, and other carnivores	Regard as rabid unless proven negative by laboratory tests¶	RIG§ and HDCV
OTHER	Livestock, rodents, and lagomorphs (rabbits and hares)	Consider individually. Local and state public health officials should be consulted on questions about the need for rabies prophylaxis. Bites of squirrels, hamsters, guinea pigs, gerbils, chipmunks, rats, mice, other rodents, rabbits, and hares almost never call for antirabies prophylaxis.	

* All bites and wounds should immediately be thoroughly cleansed with soap and water. If antirabies treatment is indicated, both rabies immune globulin (RIG) and human diploid cell rabies vaccine (HDCV) should be given as soon as possible, regardless of the interval from exposure. Local reactions to vaccines are common and do not contraindicate continuing treatment. Discontinue vaccine if fluorescent-antibody tests of the animal are negative.

† During the usual holding period of 10 days, begin treatment with RIG and HDCV at first sign of rabies in a dog or cat that has bitten someone. The symptomatic animal should be killed immediately and tested.

§ If RIG is not available, use antirabies serum, equine (ARS). Do not use more than the recommended dosage.

* Reproduced with permission from Centers for Disease Control: MMWR 33:393–403, 1984.

EVALUATION AND TREATMENT

The goals of treatment of mammalian bites are to stabilize life-threatening injuries, preserve neurovascular function, restore acceptable cosmesis, and prevent infection.

Treatment must begin with a rapid assessment of the patient to address airway patency, volume status, and neurovascular integrity. Fractures and limbs with severe soft tissue injury should be splinted. In the more common and less drastic scenario, wounds should be assessed for potential complications and pertinent historical information elicited. Significant history should include the time and circumstances surrounding the bite, the type of animal involved, its apparent state of health, and whether it is available for observation. Truly unprovoked attacks by stray or wild animals should be considered at high risk for rabies, depending on the local incidence of animal rabies. Any medical condition of the victim that might place him or her at higher risk for infection should be specifically sought out. Accurate history is often unavailable because of the patient's age, state of intoxication, or outright denial in the case of human bites.

The wound should be examined to detect foreign bodies, tendon laceration, joint penetration, and neurovascular injury. All lacerations over the metacarpophalangeal area should be considered possible closed-fist injuries, even if another mechanism is suggested by the patient. These wounds must be carefully explored under suitable conditions of lighting, local anaesthesia, and hemostasis. It may sometimes be necessary to extend small wounds to adequately visualize underlying structures. Saline or contrast arthrograms may be required to prove joint capsule integrity. Patients with suspected vascular injury or compartment syndrome should undergo arteriography and have compartment pressures measured. If either study is positive, prompt consultation with a vascular surgeon is indicated.

Although most lacerations do not require radiographic evaluation, radiographs of closed-fist injuries may be positive in up to 70% of cases and should be obtained.[54] Positive early findings include fractures, radio-opaque foreign bodies, and air within the joint capsule (Fig. 65-3). Late findings in established infections may demonstrate subperiosteal or periarticular resorption of bone, periostitis, and narrowing of the joint space.

The approach to treatment of bite wounds differs significantly, depending on whether or not the wound appears clinically infected at the time of presentation. The presence of fever, induration, swelling, erythema, tenderness, foul odor, pain, adenopathy, or evidence of lymphangitis should be elicited.

Routine culture and sensitivity of fresh, uninfected bite wounds is not indicated because many of the organisms inoculated into the wound do not ultimately cause infection. There is little predictive value and much unnecessary expense in obtaining such cultures. Similarly, gram stains of uninfected wounds do not yield any helpful information. Both studies, however, are of some value in the patient presenting with a clinically infected wound, especially if he or she has failed a course of antibiotic treatment. Given the wide variety of potential bacterial pathogens, aerobic and anaerobic culture and sensitivity should be taken from purulent wound material, and blood cultures should be obtained in patients who appear septic. Gram stains of infected wounds are helpful if they demonstrate one predominant organism that may help guide initial antibiotic therapy, but not if either no organisms are seen or the stain reveals multiple organisms.

WOUND CARE

Much of the recent controversy surrounding treatment of mammalian bites has centered on the relative

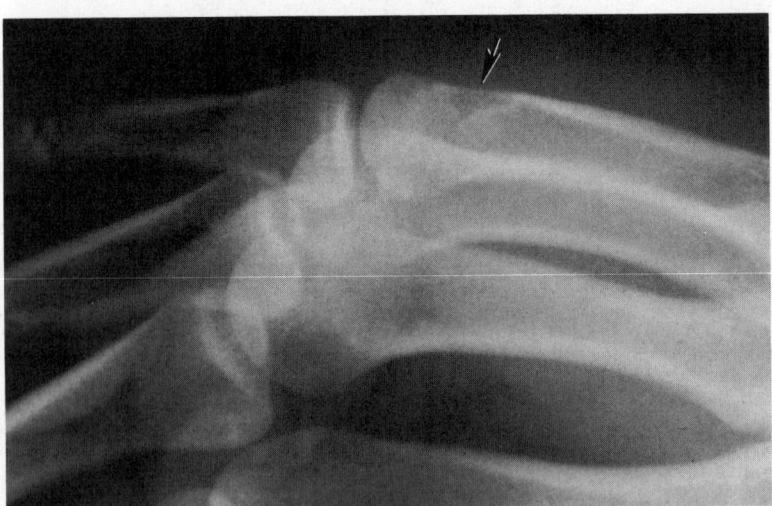

FIG. 65-3.   An x-ray film of a human bite wound may show a fracture (as in this case); foreign bodies or air in a joint space may also be discovered.

merits of one antibiotic versus another. As a result, some physicians may be misled into thinking that bite wounds are best treated with antibiotics. In fact, meticulous local wound care has repeatedly been demonstrated to be much more effective in preventing infection than any combination of antibiotics.

Local care of apparently uninfected wounds includes debridement of devascularized tissue and foreign material. Wound edges may be excised to produce clean margins, which not only reduce the incidence of infection but also improve the cosmetic result. After this, the wound should be irrigated with at least 200 cc of normal saline or a 1% povidone solution under pressure, with either an 18-gauge plastic intravenous catheter attached to a 20 cc syringe or a commercial irrigation set. Stock povidone solution (10%) and povidone scrub solution should not be used because they are too irritating to tissue. Irrigation with benzalkonium chloride 1% solution is viricidal but is also irritating to tissues. Its use should be reserved for wounds in which transmission of HIV, rabies, or other serious viral diseases is thought to be possible.[55-57] Antitetanus vaccination status should be verified and toxoid administered if indicated. Most bite wounds are not highly tetanus-prone unless contaminated by soil, but tetanus immunoglobulin should be given to patients with inadequate primary immunization (Table 65-4).

Several studies have examined the efficacy of debridement, irrigation, and excision of wound margins on the incidence of infection. Debridement reduced the infection rates from 62% to 2% in one study,[28] although less dramatic results have been obtained in other studies, which show a 2.5 times increase in infection when debridement is omitted.[57] Similarly, irrigation of the wound as described previously decreases the infection rate 6 to 10 times.[28,57] One of the reasons why puncture wounds are infection-prone is that it is difficult to perform debridement and irri-

gation on this type of wound. Irrigation is sometimes successful if the plastic cannula can be introduced into the puncture wound and irrigation performed. If the surrounding soft tissues begin to swell, however, the process should be terminated. It is imperative that universal precautions be taken when irrigating these wounds because the return spray is unpredictable and may be laden with serious pathogens.

SUTURING OF BITE WOUNDS

There is a continued reluctance among clinicians to suture bite wounds regardless of the location and source, for fear of promoting infection. Several studies have addressed this issue, with contradictory results.[7,8,16,17,24,39,49,65] At least 10% of bite wounds require suturing for cosmetic or functional reasons, and these wounds, in some studies, have a significantly lower rate of infection than nonsutured bites.[16] Callaham found infection rates of 3% in sutured wounds versus 25% in nonsutured wounds in one study, and 10% versus 21% in another.[1,28] Part of the explanation for this paradox is that high-risk wounds such as punctures of the hand are never sutured, whereas intrinsically low-risk wounds are more likely to be sutured. When puncture wounds are excluded, a slightly higher incidence of infection has been found. Nevertheless, it does demonstrate that low-risk wounds can be sutured without inviting undue complications.

Wounds that demonstrate signs of infection, however early, should not be sutured. Similar constraint applies to high-risk wounds such as punctures, wounds that cannot be adequately debrided and irrigated, cat or human bites of the hand, particularly the "closed-fist injury," and bites in patients with risk factors for infection and poor healing. Other wounds may be sutured if seen within 12 hours of occurrence. This includes virtually all fresh dog bite wounds, human bites of the face and torso, and bites of the ears, nose, genitalia, and neck. Regardless of whether the bite is sutured or not, the area should be dressed, elevated if an extremity is involved, and rechecked within 48 hours. Patients should be instructed to return at the first sign of fever, purulent drainage, cellulitis, or lymphangitis.

CRITERIA FOR ADMISSION

Admission for parenteral antibiotics and careful wound care should be considered for patients with established infections, especially of the extremities, tendon lacerations, open joints, fractures, or tenosynovitis. Patients at high risk for infection, including diabetics and other immunocompromised bite victims, should be considered candidates for admission on an individual basis. Obviously, those with established serious infections such as osteomyelitis, sepsis, meningitis, septic arthritis, and aggressive cellulitis should be admitted for parenteral antibiotics and de-

---

TABLE 65-4. INDICATIONS FOR TETANUS IMMUNIZATION IN BITE WOUNDS

Previous Immunizations	Tetanus Toxoid	Tetanus Antitoxin
No previous immunizations or uncertain	Yes	Yes
One previous injection of DT or DTP	Yes	Yes
Two previous injections of DT or DTP	Yes	Yes
Three or more previous injections of DT or DTP	No*	No

* Unless more than 5 years have elapsed since the last booster.
  Abbreviations: DT = Diphtheria and tetanus toxoids; DTP = diphtheria and tetanus toxoid and pertussis vaccine.
  Source: Data from Centers for Disease Control: Ann. Intern. Med. 95:723, 1981.[18]

bridement of their wounds. Reliable patients presenting with fresh human bites, even of the closed fist injury (CFI) variety, may be treated as outpatients with oral antibiotics if there are no significant associated injuries and no increased risk factors for infection. Some physicians give parenteral antibiotics because time delays may increase infection risk.[17a]

ANTIBIOTIC USE IN BITE WOUNDS

The discussion regarding antibiotic usage in bite wounds is controversial and has been extensively reviewed by Callaham.[17] Two separate categories of wounds need to be considered: fresh, uninfected bite wounds and wounds that are clinically infected at the time of presentation. The indications, drug selection, and route of administration vary according to various factors. These include the nature and age of the wound, the species involved, and the presence of increased risk factors in the individual patient (e.g., immunosuppression, chronic illness).

CLINICALLY UNINFECTED WOUNDS

One of the major controversies in the care of bite wounds is related to the role of prophylactic antibiotics for uninfected animal bites. As stated, too often a prescription for an antibiotic is substituted for thorough local wound care. Nevertheless, there is unquestionably a role for antibiotics in certain injuries. At issue, then, is which patients should receive antibiotics and which antibiotic they should receive.

No single antibiotic can be expected to be effective against every possible pathogen that can contaminate bite wounds. The rapid emergence of resistant strains of familiar organisms further complicates the search for the antibiotic panacea. Also, in vitro susceptibilities of certain organisms may not correlate well with the clinical effectiveness of the antibiotic, which may not be well absorbed or penetrate well into tissue.[17]

In fact, many bite wounds have never shown any benefit from antibiotics. Fresh, uninfected *dog bites* have been studied several times, and no statistical difference has been noted between patients receiving antibiotics and those receiving placebo, although one study[28] showed a beneficial trend with penicillin compared to placebo. Other studies of dog bites have shown virtually identical infection rates with oxacillin,[58] penicillin,[59] and oxacillin or erythromycin.[60] In all cases, wounds of the hands showed greater benefit from antibiotic treatment than wounds elsewhere, and many clinicians treat these wounds with a short course of antibiotics. Fresh dog bite wounds of the face rarely require antibiotics when adequate wound care is provided.

Cat bites, on the other hand, do appear to benefit from antibiotic prophylaxis. Oxacillin has been shown in a small study to greatly reduce infection rates in cat bites from 67% to 0%.[61] Because the only isolate from infected wounds in the placebo group was Pas-

teurella multocida, penicillin prophylaxis is expected to be equally efficacious. Penicillin-allergic patients may be treated with cephalosporins if the previous reaction to penicillin was minor. Patients with severe penicillin allergy should receive a course of tetracycline if they are nonpregnant adults, or erythromycin if tetracycline is contraindicated. Several treatment failures have occurred with erythromycin in Pasteurella infections, and patients treated with erythromycin should be closely followed.

Human bites are intermediate in their tendency to become infected, although the CFI is notoriously prone to severe infection. Consequently, most physicians use prophylactic antibiotics in treating these wounds. The high frequency of Staphylococcus aureus (46%) resistant to penicillin[60] as well as Eikenella corrodens and anaerobes resistant to oxacillin[39] presents a dilemma regarding which antibiotic is most suitable. A reasonable choice in this instance is to administer a first-generation cephalosporin with good activity against penicillinase-producing Staphylococcus and reasonably good activity against Eikenella and other Gram-negative organisms. Good results in human bites have been obtained with cephalosporins in several studies.[17,19]

Penicillin alone is not a good choice for human bite prophylaxis because the vast majority of Staphylococcus species are resistant. Resistance has also been increasing among anaerobes, and in one study, up to 47% of human-source Bacteroides fragilis were resistant because of the production of B-lactamase, although 100% of anaerobic animal isolates remained sensitive to penicillin.[37] A combination of dicloxacillin and either ampicillin or penicillin is advocated for prophylaxis by some authors with good results obtained.[4] This combination provides adequate coverage for the vast majority of possible infections (including Staphylococcus, Streptococcus, Pasteurella, Eikenella, and most anaerobes, but compliance suffers when so many pills are prescribed. An untested alternative might be to administer intramuscular long-acting penicillin, followed by a course of oral dicloxacillin.

Patients with previous mild or questionable allergic reactions to penicillin can be treated with cephalosporins. Those with severe reactions should receive a course of erythromycin or ciprofloxacin, which provides better coverage for Staphylococcus aureus, although at much greater expense.

Amoxicillin clavulanate (Augmentin-R) is theoretically attractive for use as prophylaxis in any bite wound because it has good in vitro activity against virtually all bite pathogens. In the single study in which it was compared to penicillin with or without dicloxacillin,[62] however, no significant advantage was demonstrated, and a significant number of patients in the Augmentin group developed diarrhea.[17] Further studies are needed to clarify the advantages, if any, provided by amoxicillin/clavulanate in bite wound prophylaxis although it may prove to be an acceptable alternative.[37]

INFECTED WOUNDS

Patients presenting with infected wounds should receive antibiotics. There is a considerable advantage in these cases in administering the antibiotic parenterally to achieve adequate and sustained serum levels as quickly as possible. The ideal choice of antibiotic for initial use is debatable, however (i.e., when the infecting agent or agents are unknown), because many conflicting results and opinions have been published.

Bite wounds, particularly *cat bites*, that show early (less than 24 hours) signs of cellulitis can be treated with penicillin on the presumption that Pasteurella multocida is the responsible agent. Tetracycline is acceptable as an alternative in penicillin-allergic patients because treatment failures are not uncommon with erythromycin. Late-onset infections should be treated for potential staphylococcal and streptococcal causes as well. There is disagreement regarding the usefulness of first-generation cephalosporins in both cat and dog bite wounds that may be infected with Pasteurella multocida. Pasteurella has been found resistant to oral cephalosporins, erythromycin, and oxacillin in vitro.[63] Despite this finding, patients treated with any of these medications tend to get well clinically, although treatment failures have been reported.[17]

Patients presenting with infected *dog bites* can be treated as outpatients with a combination of penicillin and dicloxacillin providing the infection is minor. This combination is effective against Staphylococcus, Streptococcus, Pasteurella, and Eikenella, the most common pathogens. An oral form of cefuroxime (cefuroxime axetil) and oral ciprofloxacin are available and show good in vitro activity against most organisms involved.[37] Their efficacy has not been clinically studied in this regard, but they may prove to be useful alternatives for outpatient therapy of minor infections, particularly in penicillin allergy.

More serious infections require parenteral coverage with broad-spectrum antibiotics until culture and sensitivity results are available. Cefuroxime, cefotaxime, and ceftriaxone are all effective against the vast majority of pathogens typically involved and should be part of the inpatient regimen.[37]

Patients presenting with infected *human bites* generally require admission to the hospital and parenteral antibiotic coverage. The combinations of cefoxitin and gentamicin,[14] cefuroxime, cefotaxime, or ceftriaxone,[37] cefalothin and gentamicin,[17] imipenem-cilastin sodium,[17] amoxicillin clavulanate,[14] and oxacillin and gentamicin,[64] have all been described. Consideration should be given to the addition of ceftazidime or ticarcillin if Pseudomonas is suspected or cultured, or if the patient is immunocompromised or does not respond to other regimens. Diabetic patients with severe infections should be well covered for gram-negative organisms. The addition of clindamycin should also be considered in penicillin-allergic patients, or when anaerobic infection is suspected or proven.

Because of the complexity and potentially devastating consequences of bite wound infections, infectious disease consultation should be obtained in all severe or complicated cases.

PITFALLS

No doubt the most common single error made in the treatment of bite wounds is the failure to adequately debride and irrigate the wounds. As stated above, local wound care is the most effective means available to reduce subsequent infection. Although provision of adequate wound care is time-consuming, the resultant benefits make it cost-effective.

In addition to reducing infection rates, local wound care allows careful exploration of the wound, which often reveals significant and otherwise unsuspected complications. The detection of joint capsule penetration, partial or complete tendon lacerations, intracranial penetration, violation of bone cortex, and vascular injury are crucial to the patient's full recovery and may be best demonstrated on wound exploration.

Similarly, bite wounds should be dressed in bulky dressings and elevated for 24 to 48 hours if an extremity is involved. This is not only more comfortable for the patient, it diminishes the amount of swelling and improves circulation in the extremity. Hand wounds should be splinted in the position of function to avoid later stiffness of finger joints, a common adverse result in hand bites.

The classic "pitfall" in dealing with bite wounds is failure to recognize a CFI as a human bite. Patients who sustain such injuries may be intoxicated, and often have other injuries that may take precedence in terms of treatment. In addition, they often deny the mechanism of injury if they are able to provide a history, out of a sense of embarassment. Consequently, any wound overlying the metacarpophalangeal joints should be considered a possible CFI, and should be explored carefully. Failure to consider this cause can have devastating results. Also, genital area wounds may be human bites.

The final pitfall is the failure to recognize wounds that are not responding to oral antibiotics and to obtain cultures to direct further antibiotic therapy. Although the vast majority of bite wounds heal well with or without antibiotics, occasionally a smoldering infection develops because of either impaired immunity in the victim or an unusual infecting organism or some retained material. Such wounds should be cultured and admission considered if the patient is deteriorating.

MEDICOLEGAL PEARLS

Virtually all states require that animal bites be reported to public health authorities. The purpose of this reporting is primarily to detect cases of rabies, but it is also useful when an individual animal repeatedly bites humans. Repeated offenses by the same animal may form a legal basis for having the animal destroyed.

Because animal bites so frequently result in civil litigation, it is essential to document thoroughly all injuries. Photographs or videotapes are a useful adjunct in this regard and can assist the treating physician if he or she is called to testify in subsequent legal proceedings.

The issue of culpability for transmitting disease by means of a human bite is complex and as yet largely unresolved. Patients with serious transmissible diseases such as AIDS, who knowingly inflict a bite on another person with the intention of infecting that person, have been charged with attempted murder, even though no infection has occurred in the bite recipient. To date, there have been too few cases to develop a legal standard.

REFERENCES

1. Callaham, M.L., Treatment of common dog bites: Infection risk factors. JACEP 7:83, 1978.
2. Kizer, K.W. Epidemiologic and clinical aspects of animal bite injuries. JACEP 8:134, 1979.
3. MMWR 29:265, 1980
4. Lieth, G.D. Bite wounds. Am. Fam. Physician 11:93, 1975.
6. Pinckney, L.E., and Kennedy, L.A.: Human deaths induced by dog attacks in the United States. Pediatrics 69:19, 1982.
7. Callaham, M.L.: Topics in Emergency Medicine April 1982, 1-13.
8. Shultz, R.C., and McMaster, W.C.: The treatment of dog bite injuries, especially those of the face. Plast. Reconstr. Surg. 49:494, 1972.
9. Maetz, H.M.: Animal bites, a public health problem in Jefferson County, Alabama. Public Health Rep. 94:528, 1979.
10. Sacks, J.J., Sattin, R.W., and Bonzo, S.E.: Dog bite-related fatalities from 1979 through 1988. JAMA 262:1489, 1989.
11. Viegas, S.F., Calhoun, J.H., and Mader, J.: Pit bull attack: A case report and literature review. Texas Med. 84:40, 1988.
12. Back, B.R., Kucan, J.O., Demarest, G., and Smoot, E.C.: Mauling by pit bull terriers: Case report. J. Trauma 29:517, 1989.
13. Karlson, T.A.: The incidence of facial injuries from dog bites. JAMA 251:3265, 1984.
14. Goldstein, E.J.C., and Richwald, G.A.: Human and animal bite wounds. Am. Fam. Physician 36:101, 1987.
15. 1986 Case records. N. Engl. J. Med. 315:241, 1986.
16. Callaham, M.L.: Dog bite wounds. JAMA 244:2327, 1980.
17. Callaham, M.L. Controversies in antibiotic choices for bite wounds. Ann. Emerg. Med. 17:1321, 1988.
17a. Classen, D.C., et al.: The timing of prophylactic antibiotics and the risk of surgical wound infection. N. Engl. J. Med. 326:281, 1992.
18. Aghababian, R.V., and Conte, J.E.: Mammalian bite wounds. Ann. Emerg. Med. 9:79, 1980.
19. U.Bite, Human bite injuries of the hand. Can. J. Surg. 27:616, 1984.
20. Lindsey, D., et al.: Natural course of the human bite wound: Incidence of infection and complications in 434 bites and 803 lacerations in the same population. J. Trauma 27:45, 1987.
21. Galloway, R.: Mammalian Bites. J. Emerg. Med. 6:325, 1988.
22. Rest, J.G., and Goldstein, E.J.C.: Management of human and animal bite wounds. Emerg. Med. Clin. North Am. 3:117, 1985.
23. Ordog, G.J.: Rat bites: Fifty cases. Ann. Emerg. Med. 14:126, 1985.
24. Brown, C.G., and Ashton, J.J.: Dog bites: The controversy continues. Am. J. Emerg. Med. 3:83, 1985 (editorial).
25. Brook, I.: Human and animal bite infections. J. Fam. Pract. 28:713, 1989.
26. Ordog, G.J.: The bacteriology of dog bite wounds on initial presentation. Ann. Emerg. Med. 15:1324, 1986.
27. Goldstein, E.J.C., Citron, D.M., and Finegold, S.M.: Dog bite wounds and infection: A prospective clinical study. Ann. Emerg. Med. 9:508, 1980.
28. Callaham, M.L.: Prophylactic antibiotics in common dog bite wounds: A controlled study. Ann. Emerg. Med. 9:410, 1980.
29. Bracis, R., Seibers, K., and Julien, R.M.: Meningitis caused by Group II-J following a dog bite. West. J. Med. 131:438, 1979.
30. Findling, J.W., Pohlmann, G.P., and Rose, H.D.: Fulminant Gram-negative bacillemia (DF-2) following a dog bite in an asplenic woman. Am. J. Med. 68:154, 1980.
31. Check, W.: An odd link between dog bites, splenectomy. JAMA 241:255, 1979.
32. Butler, T., et al.: Unidentified gram-negative infection. Ann. Intern. Med. 86:1, 1977.
33. Johnson, R.H.: Unusual infections caused by Pasteurella multocida. JAMA 237:146, 1977.
34. Francis, D.P., Holmes, M.A., and Brandon, G. Pasteurella multocida: Infections after domestic animal bites and scratches. JAMA 233:42, 1975.
35. Klein, D.M., and Cohen, M.E.: Pasteurella multocida brain abscess following perforating cranial dog bite. J. Pediatr. 92:588, April 1978.
36. Arons, M.S., and Polayes, I.M.: Pasteurella multocida: The major cause of hand infections following domestic animal bites. J. Hand Surg. 7:47, 1982.
37. Goldstein, E.J.C., and Citron, D.M.: Comparative activities of cefuroxime, enoxacin, and ofloxacin against aerobic and anaerobic bacteria isolated from bite wounds. Antimicrob. Agents Chemother. 32:1143, 1988.
38. Goldstein, E.J.C. Management of human and animal bite wounds. J. Am. Acad. Dermatol. 21:1275, 1989.
39. Schmidt, D.R., and Heckman, J.D.: Eikenella corrodens in human bite infections of the hand. J. Trauma 23:478, 1983.
40. Hamilton, J.D., Larke, B., and Qizillbaah, H.: Transmission of Hepatitis-B by a human bite: An occupational hazard. Can. Med. Assoc. J. 115:439, 1976.
41. MacQuarrle, M.B., Forghani, B., and Wolochow, D.A.: Hepatitis-B transmitted by a human bite. JAMA 230:723, 1974.
42. Torres, J.R., Sanders, C.V., Strub, R.L., and Black, F.W.: Cat-scratch disease causing reversible incephalopathy. JAMA 240:1628, 1978.
43. Carithers, H.A., Carithers, C.M., and Edwards, R.O.: Cat-scratch disease: Its natural history. JAMA 207:312, 1969.
44. Steiner, M.M., and Vuckovitch, D.: Cat scratch disease with encephalopathy. J. Pediatr. 62:514, 1963.
45. Ordog, G.J., Balasubramanian, S., and Wasserberger, J. Rat bites: 50 cases. Ann. Emerg. Med. 14:126, 1985.
46. McHugh, T.P., Bartlett, R.L., and Raymond, J.I. Rat bite fever: Report of a fatal case. Ann. Emerg. Med. 14:1116, 1985.
47. Evans, M.E., and Hunter, P.T.: Tularemia and the tomcat. JAMA 248:1343, 1981.
48. Lancet, Sept. 3, 1983: 553. Animal bites and infection.
49. Robertson, M.G. Brucella infection transmitted by dog bite. JAMA 225:750, 1973.
50. Human rabies—Oregon, 1989. MMWR 38:335, 1989.
51. Kauffman, F.H., and Goldmann, B.J. Rabies. Am. J. Emerg. Med. 4:525, 1986.
52. Morrison, A.J., and Wenzel, R.P.: Rabies: A review and current approach for the clinician. South. Med. J. 78:1211, 1985.
53. CDC Rabies prevention—United States, 1984. MMWR 33:393, 1984.
54. Dreyfuss, U.Y., and Singer, M.: Human bites of the hand: A study of 106 patients. J. Hand Surg. 10:884, 1985.
55. Hawkins, J., Paris, P.M., and Stewart, R.D.: Mammalian bites: Rational approach to management. Postgrad. Med. 73:52, 1983.
56. Stevenson, J., et al.: Cleaning the traumatic wound by high pressure irrigation. JACEP 5:17, 1976.

57. Callaham, M.L.: Treatment of common dog bites: Infection risk factors. JACEP 7:83, 1978.

57a. Callaham, M.L.: When an animal bites. Emerg. Med. 23:105, 1991.

58. Ellenbaas, R.M., McNabey, W.K., and Robinson, W.A.: Prophylactic oxacillin in dog bite wounds. Ann. Emerg. Med. 11:248, 1982.
phylactic oxacillin in dog bite wounds. Ann. Emerg. Med. 11:248, 1982.

59. Boenning, D.A., Fleisher, G.R., and Campos, J.M.: Dog bites in children: Epidemiology, microbiology, and penicillin prophylactic therapy. Am. J. Emerg. Med. 1:17, 1983.

60. Rosen, R.A. The use of antibiotics in the initial management of recent dog bite wounds. Am. J. Emerg. Med. 3:19, 1985.

61. Ellenbaas, R.M., McNabey, W.K., and Robinson, W.A.: Evaluation of prophylactic oxacillin in cat bite wounds. Ann. Emerg. Med. 13:155, 1984.

62. Goldstein, E. J. C., et al.: Outpatient therapy of bite wounds: Demographic data, bacteriology, and a prospective, randomized trial of amoxicillin clavulanic acid versus penicillin +/− dicloxacillin. Int. J. Dermatol. 26:123, 1987.

63. Goldstein, E. J. C., Citron, D. M., and Richwald, G.A.: Lack of in vitro efficacy of oral forms of certain cephalosporins, erythromycin, and oxacillin against Pasteurella multocida. Antimicrob. Agents Chemother. 32:213, 1988.

64. Mann, R.J., Hoffeld, T.A., and Farmer, M.D.: Human bites of the hand: Twenty years experience. J. Hand Surg. 2:97, 1977.

Chapter 66

THE DIAGNOSIS AND TREATMENT OF SNAKEBITE

James R. Roberts

CAPSULE

Venomous snakebites are uncommon events that should be approached with great clinical respect. Envenomation can cause significant morbidity and even mortality if left untreated or mismanaged. The clinical course of a poisonous snake bite is dynamic and often unpredictable because of the complex pathophysiology of venoms, which can produce clinical effects ranging from local tissue loss to coagulopathies and multisystem failure. Ill-conceived heroic first-aid measures, such as a vascular tourniquet, ice, and aggressive incision and suction, should be avoided. The early use of adequate amounts of antivenin, coupled with sound clinical judgment and aggressive supportive care, usually brings about a favorable outcome.

INTRODUCTION

Snakes are among the most interesting and most feared reptiles on the earth, yet little is known about the mysterious poisons they inject into animals and humans, and even less is known about the specific pathophysiology that results from their venoms. Therefore, the medical literature is filled with myths, misunderstandings, folklore, anecdotal treatments, contradictions, and false conclusions about the treatment of poisonous snakebites. A well-documented, controlled, prospective, double-blind study has yet to be completed for the treatment of snakebite in humans. Although the diagnosis and treatment of snakebite infrequently cause problems, they test the emergency physician's ability to act quickly and rationally in a situation in which time is of the essence and patient anxiety is great.

The number of species of snakes in the world is estimated to be between 2500 and 3000. Of these, fewer than 15% are poisonous to humans, and probably fewer than 200 species are actually dangerous. Considering that almost all of the 20,000 species of spiders are venomous and that the number of venomous terrestrial arthropods ranges into several tens of thousands, snakes pose a comparatively small threat to humans.

The coral snakes, cobras, kraits, and mambas are members of the family Elapidae. The rattlesnakes, copperheads, and water moccasins (cottonmouth) are members of the family Crotalidae and are also called pit vipers. Pit vipers possess a heat-sensing organ, which occupies a pitlike depression on both sides of the head between the eyes and the nostrils. These highly sensitive organs enable snakes to strike prey with great accuracy, even in total darkness, based on the body heat of the victim.

Like other reptiles, snakes are poikilothermic and seek shelter when temperatures fall below approximately 12°C (55°F) and rise above 38°C (100°F). Hence, they hibernate in the winter, are often nocturnal, and seek shelter in caves and under logs. They lack external ears and moveable eyelids, have a top crawling speed of 2 to 4 miles per hour, eat their food whole, commonly eat other snakes, and attack humans only when threatened.

The mysterious flicking tongue of the snake picks up particles from the ground and air. The tiny forked tips are then inserted into pits in the palate that are lined with sensitive cells, called Jacobson's organs, which serve to identify the particles. Snakes have a well-developed sense of smell and can track their prey over terrain that would dumbfound a bloodhound.

RANGE

Snakes range from the Arctic circle to the southern tip of South America and are found in trees, deserts, the ground, fresh water, and sea water. Only Iceland, Ireland, New Zealand, and a few small islands lack snakes completely. Poisonous snakes are found in

America in all the states except Hawaii, Alaska, and Maine, but only two families and four species need concern the practicing physician in the United States. To make a sound clinical decision about therapy and prognosis of a snakebite, it is important that the physician be familiar with the specific poisonous species in the immediate surrounding areas. This information is obtained by calling a local zoo or herpetology society.

There are about 30 kinds of rattlesnakes (genera: *Crotalus* and *Sistrurus*) throughout the United States. They are found mainly in the southwest, Texas, and Florida. The diamondback rattlesnake is considered the most deadly snake in the United States.

Copperheads (*Agkistrodon contortrix*) are found in the eastern and southern United States and into New England and usually inhabit dry, rocky areas. The water moccasins (*Agkistrodon piscivorus*), called "cottonmouth" because of the cotton-white interior of their mouths, are semi-aquatic and inhabit the swampy areas in marshes and bayous of the eastern and southeastern states.

Two species of brightly colored coral snakes inhabit the United States. Eastern coral snakes (*Micrurus fulvius* and *Micrurus tenere*) range from coastal North Carolina and Florida to Texas; the less poisonous Arizona coral snake (*Micruroides euryxanthus*) is found in the southwestern United States.

Although not native to the United States, cobras, kraits, mambas, and other exotic species may be found in zoos and in the private collections of herpetologists and other collectors.

INCIDENCE AND MORTALITY

Although the actual figures are difficult to obtain, it is estimated that there are about 8000 poisonous snakebites per year in the United States. Rattlesnakes account for about 55% of these bites, copperheads 34%, cottonmouths 10%, and coral snakes 1%. Fewer than 1% of the victims die of snakebite poisoning, with rattlesnake bites accounting for more than 70% of reported deaths. Only 10 to 15 persons die each year in the United States from the bites of poisonous snakes. The majority of these deaths occur in Texas, Georgia, Florida, Alabama, and South Carolina. Bites by poisonous snakes in the New England states are extremely rare. Death or serious morbidity from a copperhead bite is rare. About one-half of all copperhead bites result in no systemic symptoms at all, producing only mild local reactions.

Rattlesnake bites are the most destructive, resulting in a much higher incidence of tissue necrosis and permanent, serious damage to the bitten area. Mortalities from coral snakebites are low. Only about 30 coral snakebites are reported each year throughout the country. In one series,[1] there were no deaths in 33 cases of coral snakebites, and in another report,[2] only one death in 11 cases. Eastern coral snakes are more dangerous than the Arizona variety.

Most bites occur when the victim is within 1 mile from home, often in his own yard. Those most frequently bitten are children and young adults. Victims are often intoxicated or participating in a dare or other dangerous behavior. Snakebite often occurs in those involved in collecting and marketing snakes. Most bites occur in the daylight hours of the summer months, but bites by poisonous snakes are not uncommon after dark. Almost all bites occur on the extremities, approximately one third on the upper extremities and two thirds on the lower extremities; most are on the hands and fingers, lower legs, and feet. Bites of the head, neck, and trunk account for only 1 to 2% of bites.

Death from bites by venomous snakes in the United States is not instantaneous. However, of 133 deaths reported,[3] approximately 38% occurred in the first 12 hours after the bite, and slightly over 90% in the first 48 hours; delay in treatment was the most important factor contributing to mortality.

IDENTIFICATION OF POISONOUS SNAKES

Poisonous snakes can be distinguished from nonpoisonous snakes by a variety of methods (Fig. 66-1). Pit vipers have an identifiable pit in front of the eye and a slit-like or vertical elliptical pupil. In addition to numerous small teeth, two well-developed fangs, up to 1 inch long, protrude from the maxilla on a hinge mechanism. The undersurface of a pit viper has a single row of subcaudal plates or scales. Nonpoisonous snakes, on the other hand, have round pupils, lack definite fangs but have small teeth arranged in rows, and possess a double row of ventral scales. Poisonous coral snakes are an exception because they lack pits and have round pupils similar to those of nonpoisonous snakes.

Venom is produced in glands behind the eyes, and muscle contractions force it through the long, hollow fangs, like the action of a hypodermic needle.

CHARACTERISTICS OF THE BITE

Pit vipers produce a characteristic bite when they inject venom into a victim. Most people, however, are bitten by an unidentified snake, usually a nonpoisonous variety. Nonvenomous snakes have four rows of small,

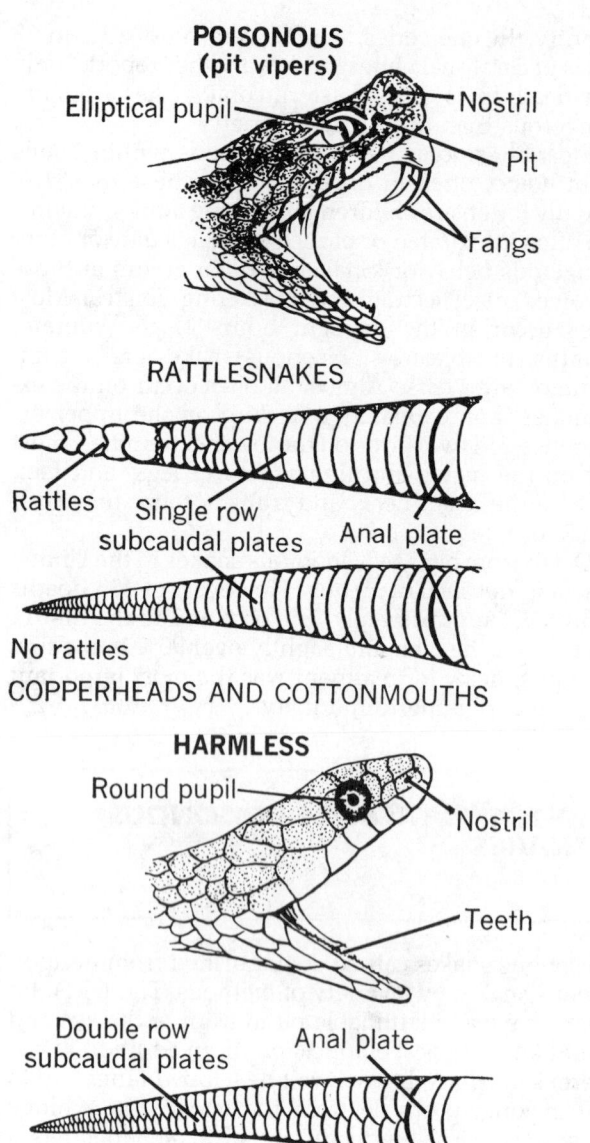

FIG. 66-1. Features of pit vipers and harmless snakes. With permission from Parrish, H.M., and Carr, C.A.: *JAMA 201:*927, 1967; copyright © 1967. American Medical Association.

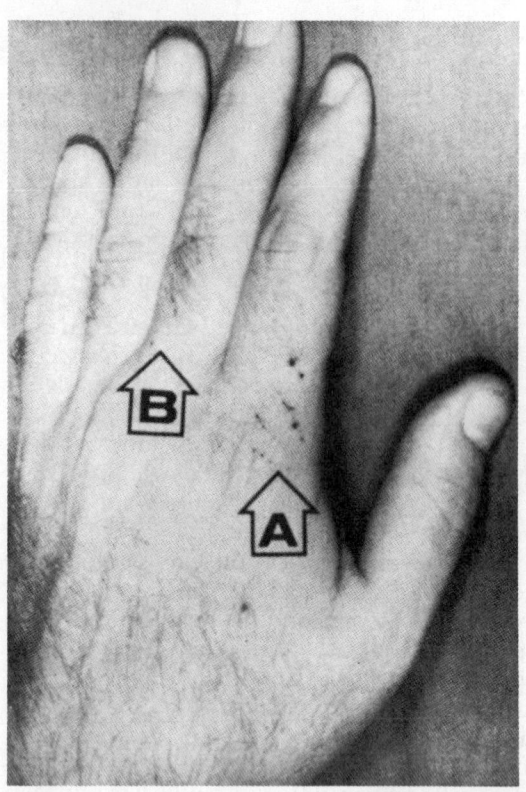

FIG. 66-2. Typical marks on a hand bitten by a nonpoisonous snake. Four rows of teeth marks (A) on the victim's index finger; two rows of teeth marks (B) on the middle finger. Venomous snakes may also produce teeth marks in addition to fang marks. With permission from Parrish, H.M., et al.: *South. Med. J. 66:*1413, 1973.

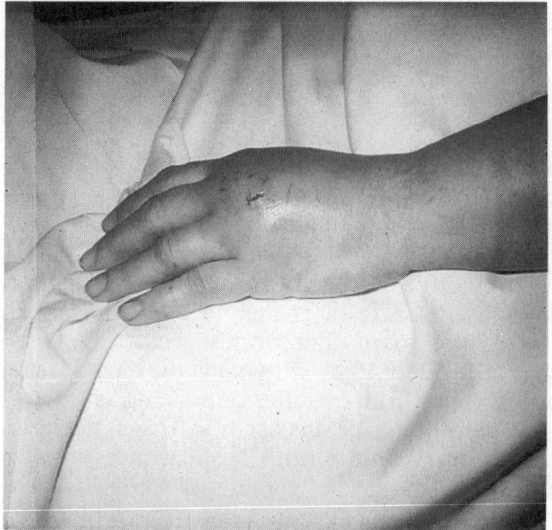

FIG. 66-3. This bite from a nonpoisonous boa constrictor produced significant soft tissue injury and a wound infection.

curved, needlelike teeth on the upper jaw and two rows on the lower jaw. An example of the bite they produce is shown in Figure 66-2. The bite is similar to the scratches made by a blackberry bush. There is little local swelling with only slight discomfort and itching around the teeth marks. A small ooze of blood may be seen, but there are no systemic effects. Importantly, venomous snakes may also leave small tooth marks in addition to fang marks. Larger nonvenomous snakes, such as boa constrictors and pythons, may fracture bones with their powerful jaws or produce lacerations with their sharp teeth (Fig. 66-3). In the absence of bony injury or significant soft tissue injury, the proper treatment for bites by nonvenomous snakes consists of wound cleansing and administration of tetanus toxoid. Although there are

reports of coagulopathies resulting from bites of some foreign species of so-called nonpoisonous snakes,[4] serious problems do not result from bites of the nonpoisonous snakes found in the United States.

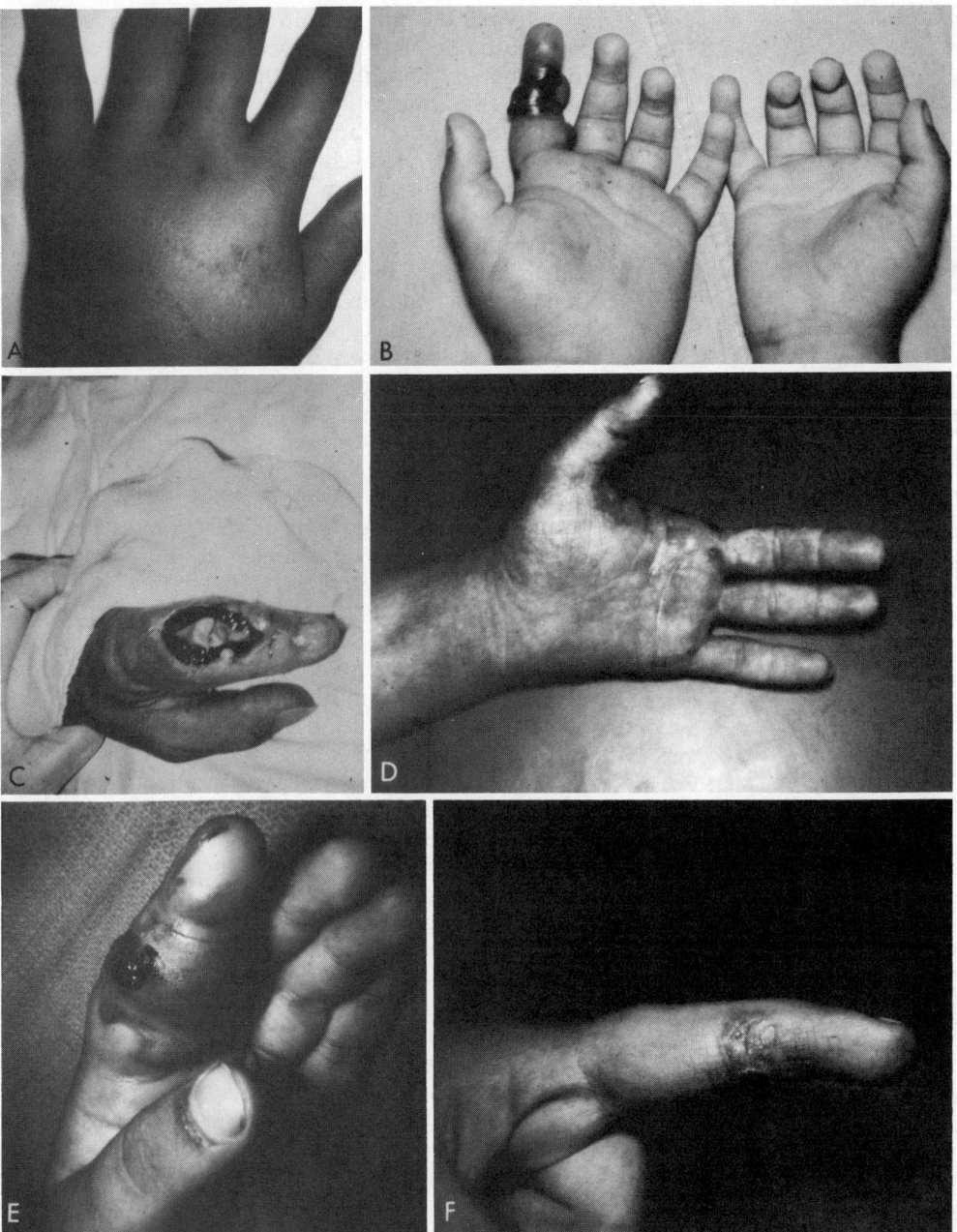

FIG. 66-4.   Appearance of hands bitten by poisonous snakes.

A. Snakes rarely bite a person more than once, but this hand was bitten three times (twice on the dorsum of the hand and once on the palmar surface of the index finger) by a pygmy rattlesnake.

B. Left index finger one hour after being bitten by a cottonmouth moccasin. The envenomation has produced asymmetry and edema, hemorrhagic transudate, bleb formation, and early necrosis.

C. Bite of timber rattlesnake three weeks after envenomation. There was loss of extensor tendon and the dorsal capsule of the PIP joint, with complete immobility and anesthesia of the finger.

D. Final result in the patient shown in C after filleting the finger and using the available skin over the thumb webspace.

E. Left index finger two hours after rattlesnake bite.

F. Final result of patient shown in E, utilizing local surgical treatment.

Not all bites by poisonous snakes result in envenomation, and a "dry bite" may be encountered. Although is is commonly stated that about one third of venomous bites are "dry," in my experience the vast majority of patients bitten by pit vipers experience some envenomation. When the bite of a rattlesnake does cause envenomation, there is almost instantaneous pain in the area bitten ranging from excruciating to mild. The amount of pain is probably related to the amount of venom that is injected. Within a matter of minutes, the injured tissue may become swollen and ecchymotic and, in a short time, necrotic (Fig. 66-4).

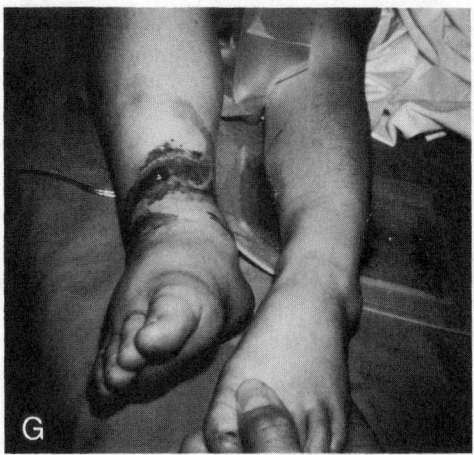

FIG. 66-4. *Continued.* G. Swelling and ecchymosis developed within 3 hours following the bite of a western diamond-back rattlesnake in a 6-year-old child. There were no systemic complications. With permission from Snyder, C.C., Straight, R., and Glenn, J.: Plast. Reconstr. Surg. *49:*275, 1972; © 1972, The Williams & Wilkins Co., Baltimore.)

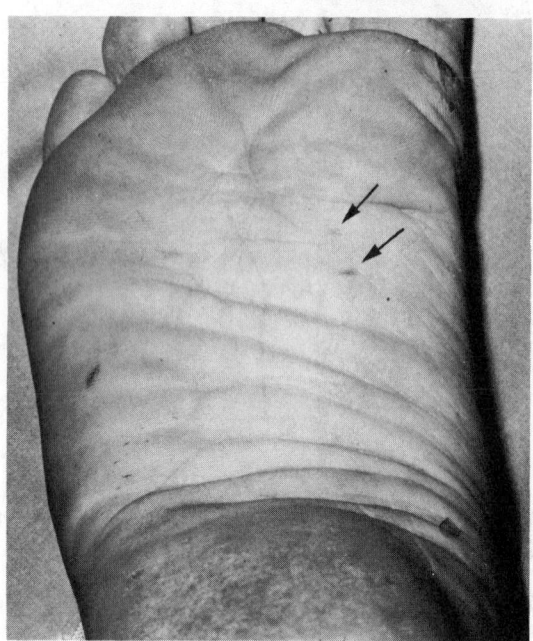

FIG. 66-5. Typical puncture-type fang marks on a foot bitten by a poisonous pit viper. Two fang marks 1 cm apart were found in the sole of the right foot. The skin around the fang marks was numb to the touch. With permission from Huang, T.T., et al.: Ann. Surg. *179:*598, 1974.

Occasionally, there is anesthesia around the bite. Systemic symptoms can develop rapidly, often in a matter of minutes, depending on the location of the bite. A notable exception to this scenario, however, is the bite from the Mojave rattlesnake, which may produce a neurologic form of systemic envenomation in the absence of significant pain or soft-tissue damage at the bitten area.

The pain from a copperhead bite or the bite from some rattlesnakes such as the Mojave rattlesnake may be minimal despite envenomation. Pain from a cottonmouth bite has been described as less severe than the extremely painful bite of the diamondback, timber, prairie, or Pacific rattlesnake, and more severe than that of the copperhead.

The actual physical characteristics of the fang marks of a venomous snake may vary considerably, but an identifiable pattern is often present. The fangs may merely produce scratch marks, but usually distinct puncture marks can be identified (Fig. 66-5). Only one puncture may be seen if a glancing blow has occurred or if the snake has lost a fang. Multiple puncture wounds may be present if multiple bites are involved, or if the snake has developed more than two fangs. In addition to fang marks, venomous snakes may also inflict bite marks with their short, sharp teeth, producing a bite pattern that may lead the uninformed to think that this was the bite of a nonvenomous snake. The distance between fang marks from rattlesnakes may vary from a few millimeters to more than 4 cm. The depth of penetration is variable but may be estimated as equal to the distance between the fang marks on the skin. Russell[5] states that a rattlesnake almost always envenomates only the subcutaneous tissue and that intramuscular penetration is rare. The deepest bites are inflicted by the larger diamondback and timber rattlesnakes.

The thorns of plants and cacti and the bites of other animals such as nonpoisonous snakes, rats, mice, and lizards have been mistaken for venomous snake bites. Therefore a careful search for puncture wounds is required. Fang marks may be subtle and may escape identification by inexperienced observers.

Only minor scratch marks may be seen at the site of envenomation by a coral snake. The fangs of coral snakes are less than 6 mm long and may fail to penetrate the skin, especially if heavy clothing is worn. The distance between coral snake fang marks may vary from 2 to 8 mm. Coral snakes may strike and hold on to a victim and exert a "chewing" motion, producing more than one wound. A history of a snake's retaining its bite for a few seconds suggests a coral snake as the culprit.

The amount of venom injected with each bite varies considerably, and not all bites involve true envenomation. This is an important point, and many patients are subjected to needless treatment in cases in which either the offending snake was nonpoisonous or no actual envenomation occurred. The snake seems able to control the amount of poison released and injects up to three-fourths of its supply per bite. An immediate second strike may also be dangerous. Because bites by poisonous snakes may involve no venom at all, it is not surprising that the home remedies often used as treatment, such as mud, chicken fat, and whiskey, are often deemed successful. Basically, larger and older snakes inject a greater amount of more toxic venom, but even newborn snakes are a threat.

INFLUENCE OF THE BITE LOCATION

The area bitten greatly influences the prognosis. Direct blood envenomation is probably rare and may account for the majority of rapid deaths. Snyder[6] found that a lethal dose of venom injected directly into a vein in a dog leads to death in less than 1 minute. Bites of the face and neck are particularly dangerous because of the vascularity of this region. When injected into subcutaneous tissue, venom spreads mostly by lymphatic rather than venous flow. Deeper envenomation probably results in some uptake of venom by the venous system. Life-threatening airway obstruction, necessitating intubation or cricothyrotomy, may result from a pit viper bite to the tongue.[7]

Because most bites occur in the extremities and actual mortality is low, the main concerns for the emergency physician are (1) distinguishing a bite by a poisonous snake from that by a nonpoisonous snake, (2) deciding if envenomation actually has occurred, (3) preventing or limiting severe tissue damage, and (4) life support in cases of severe envenomation.

CLINICAL PRESENTATION

VENOMS AND THEIR EFFECTS

Venom is an extremely complicated substance that varies greatly, not only from species to species, but also among different varieties of the same species and even from time to time in the same snake. Dried snake venom is a remarkable substance that may retain its deadly properties up to 26 years when stored under proper conditions. No venom has been analyzed completely, and it is this complexity that has hampered advances in treatment. In general, pit vipers' venom possesses mainly tissue toxins and hemotoxins. All organs and tissues may be affected by crotalid venom, and the venom of the Mojave rattlesnake can alter neuromuscular transmission. Coral snake venom contains mainly neurotoxins, producing neuromuscular blockade and nerve conduction, although this is not absolute and may be misleading in some instances, causing errors in clinical judgment. The age, size, and individual sensitivity of the patient alter responses to envenomation.

LOCAL REACTIONS

Rattlesnakes, Copperheads, and Water Moccasins. At the site of crotalid (pit viper) envenomation, tissue destruction is greatest. There is direct necrosis of tissue almost immediately. Blood and fluid extravasate, and

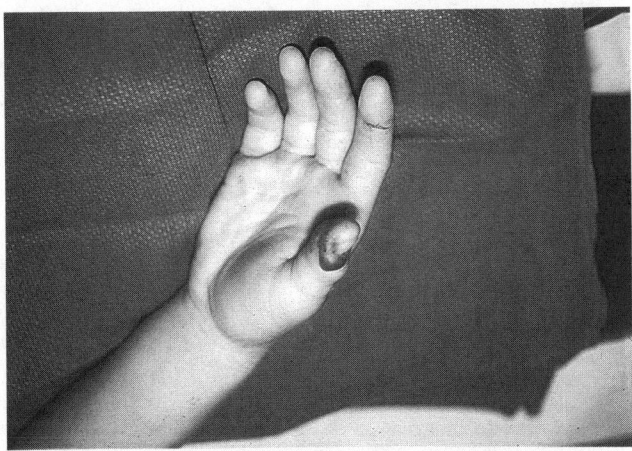

FIG. 66-6. Copperhead envenomation producing only local ecchymosis and blistering and minimal soft tissue swelling. Most bites from this snake do not require antivenin.

tissue pressure increases and obstructs circulation, producing ischemic damage that compounds the direct effects of venom.

Ecchymosis develops rapidly, and blebs and blisters may appear. The skin assumes a gangrenous appearance, and there may be local sloughing. An entire extremity may become swollen in a matter of minutes. Pain is often severe. The only exception to this is the bite from the Mojave rattlesnake (described earlier).

Bites from all North American crotalids produce edema. Edema is greatest after envenomation from the diamondback rattlesnake. Less swelling may be encountered after envenomation from other types of rattlesnakes.

The major morbidity following envenomation from rattlesnakes consists of functional joint stiffness, loss of sensibility, and contracture. In one series,[8] such complications occurred in 23% of patients envenomated by rattlesnakes in the southwestern United States. Amputation or death following envenomation is rare if adequate medical treatment is available.

Copperhead bites often cause mild local reactions and minor tissue injury (Fig. 66-6), but except in rare cases, serious local or systemic reactions do not occur.

Coral Snakes. Bites by coral snakes produce little or no local reaction. Pain is usually mild and confined to the immediate bite area, but numbness and weakness in the affected limb may be experienced within a few hours. Fatal envenomation may have occurred without significant local tissue reaction.

SYSTEMIC MANIFESTATIONS

Pit Vipers (Crotalids). Systemic signs of pit viper envenomation are varied. In mild cases, there may be general weakness, fatigue, anxiety, and nausea. Abnormal tastes (metallic, rubbery) in the mouth and tingling of the tongue and lips are curious symptoms of envenomation that may occur before significant lo-

TABLE 66-1. SIGNS AND SYMPTOMS IN 100 RATTLESNAKE BITES

Sign or Symptom	Frequency*
Fang marks	100/100
Swelling and edema	74/100
Pain	65/100
Ecchymosis	51/100
Vesiculations	40/100
Changes in pulse rate	60/100
Weakness	72/100
Sweating and/or chill	64/100
Numbness or tingling of tongue and mouth, or scalp or feet	63/100
Faintness or dizziness	57/100
Nausea, vomiting, or both	48/100
Blood pressure changes	46/100
Change in body temperature	31/100
Swelling regional lymph nodes	40/100
Fasciculations	41/100
Increased blood clotting time	39/100
Sphering of red blood cells	18/100
Tingling or numbness of affected part	42/100
Necrosis	27/100
Respiratory rate changes	40/100
Decreased hemoglobin	37/100
Abnormal electrocardiogram	26/100
Cyanosis	16/100
Hematemesis, hematuria, or melena	15/100
Glycosuria	20/100
Proteinuria	16/100
Unconsciousness	12/100
Thirst	34/100
Increased salivation	20/100
Swollen eyelids	2/100
Retinal hemorrhage	2/100
Blurring of vision	12/100
Convulsions	1/100
Muscle contractions	6/100
Increased blood platelets	4/25
Decreased blood platelets	42/100

* Times symptoms or sign was observed per total number of patients. With permission from Russell, F.E.: Snake Venom Poisoning. Philadelphia, J.B. Lippincott, 1980.

cal responses are noted. More severe cases are marked by vomiting, sweating, tachycardia, tachypnea, paresthesias, blurred vision, slurred speech, salivation, defecation, epistaxis, hematuria, hematemesis, muscle fasciculations, convulsions, coma, and death. Acute anaphylactic reactions or urticaria may rarely occur with systemic envenomation.[9] Table 66-1 lists the comparative frequency of a wide variety of clinical signs and symptoms noted in 100 cases of rattlesnake bites. It is difficult to attribute the effects to specific moieties in the venom, although kinins, slow-reacting substance, histamine, phospholipase-A, and serotonin have been implicated. Pit viper venoms have been reported to contain unidentified proteolytic enzymes, nonenzymatic proteins, lecithinase, adenosine triphosphatase, ribonuclease, desoxyribonuclease, L-amino acid oxidase, cholinesterase, and hyaluronidase. Proteases catalyze the breakdown of tissue proteins and phospholipids by altering membrane permeability, whereas thrombin-like enzymes alter blood coagulability. Various unidentified cardiotoxins, neurotoxins, and hemotoxins abound in venom, making it a most complex substance to deal with clinically.

Coral Snakes. Coral snake venom is different from viper venoms in its effect (Table 66-2). It is mainly neurotoxic. It is often difficult initially to evaluate the severity of a coral snakebite. Systemic effects usually occur within 1 to 7 hours, although delays of up to 18 hours have been reported. Symptoms may develop suddenly and precipitously, and progress rapidly.[10] Paralysis of cranial nerves may occur in 2½ hours, and complete respiratory paralysis has occurred within 4 hours of envenomation. Systemic signs and symptoms that have been reported after bites by coral snakes include drowsiness, severe anxiety, dilated or pinpoint pupils, dyspnea, weakness, fasciculations and tremor, dysphagia, headache, blurred vision, and generalized seizures. It may take weeks for weakness or paresthesias from a coral snake bite to disappear.

CARDIOVASCULAR AND RESPIRATORY EFFECTS

Rattlesnake Venom. Intravenous injection of lethal amounts of rattlesnake venom in dogs produces a precipitous drop in blood pressure and peripheral vascular resistance. This potent vasodilator activity works directly or indirectly on arterioles or precapillary sphincters. An electrocardiographic pattern of myocardial damage or ischemia can be seen, and premature ventricular contractions and sinus tachycardia are noted. Respiratory activity is decreased, leading to apnea, and intestinal activity is increased, producing vomiting and defecation. There is almost immediate leakage of plasma into the intravascular space, with a rise in the hematocrit. Ownby[11] noted the direct lysis of endothelial cells and immediate extravasation of blood and attributes this to the direct action of venom on blood vessels, rather than an effect secondary to necrosis. Clinically, pulmonary edema, vascular collapse, and irreversible shock can occur. These symptoms may be accentuated in pregnancy.

Copperhead Venom. The venom from a copperhead is similar to that of a rattlesnake with the potential to produce similar pathology. Most bites from copperheads, however, do not produce serious systemic reactions and usually do not require administration of crotalid antivenin.

Coral Snake Venom. Coral snake venom has fewer cardiovascular effects, but the venom does depress myocardial and skeletal muscle. Death usually results from respiratory arrest or cardiac collapse. Although respiratory paralysis may be complete, it is ultimately reversible. The venom has an inhibitory effect on neuromuscular transmission by a blocking action on acetylcholine receptor sites that is not affected by neostigmine or edrophonium. A direct interference of axonal transmission has also been demonstrated.[12] Clinically, the first signs of this may be ptosis, strabismus, slurred speech, dilated pupils, dysphagia, and muscle weakness.

HEMATOLOGIC EFFECTS

The hematologic effects of crotalid envenomation are commonly seen and can be most dramatic. The pathophysiology has been studied in some detail. Clotting mechanisms, red cell morphology, platelet count and function, and bleeding tendencies have all been reported as markedly abnormal, but the literature is confusing in many cases. Complex coagulopathies commonly develop after severe envenomation from pit vipers and are most pronounced after envenomation from rattlesnakes. The abnormalities have been attributed to a variety of anticoagulants, procoagulants, fibrinolysins, hemorrhagins, and hemolysins.[13] A thrombin-like activity appears to be the most prominent effect.[14] Importantly, the coagulopathy may be severe in the absence of impressive local symptoms.

Disseminated intravascular coagulation (DIC) (defibrination syndrome, consumption coagulopathy, intravascular coagulation-defibrinolysis syndrome), in its strict definition,[15] is probably rare following envenomation. A true case of DIC has been reported in the bite of the saw-scaled viper (*Echis carinatus*), a snake not found in the United States. The venom of this snake appears to activate prothrombin directly, convert it to thrombin, and cause platelet aggregation. This syndrome may respond dramatically to heparin treatment when other forms of therapy have failed to correct the hypofibrinogenemia and thrombocytopenia.

Hasiba[16] has reported a DIC-like syndrome after the bite of the American timber rattlesnake (*Crotalus horridus horridus*). In this case, the patient developed petechiae, gingival bleeding, and ecchymosis with hypofibrinogenemia, thrombocytopenia, and the production of fibrin degradation products, and was treated with heparin. In vitro tests, however, suggested that heparin probably had little therapeutic effect. Other studies have failed to demonstrate a beneficial effect of heparin in envenomation.[17,18] Pit viper envenomation results in local platelet consumption at the site of injury.[19] Clinically, this results in an initial drop in the platelet count of up to 60%, but platelet counts lower than 10,000/mm³ may be seen within a few hours. A rebound in the platelet count occurs within 6 to 24 hours.

The documentation of true DIC after the bite of an American snake is lacking in the literature.

Other hematologic syndromes have been reported in cases of bites from snakes not native to the United States. Among them are (1) hypofibrinogenemia without thrombocytopenia or fibrinolysis caused by the Malayan pit viper and (2) hypofibrinogenemia without

TABLE 66-2. SIGNS AND SYMPTOMS IN CORAL SNAKE ENVENOMATION*	
Sign or Symptom	**%**
Fang marks	85
Local swelling	40
Paresthesia	35
Nausea	30
Vomiting	25
Euphoria	15
Weakness	15
Dizziness	10
Diplopia	10
Dyspnea	10
Diaphoresis	10
Muscle tenderness	10
Fasciculations	5
Confusion	5

* n = 20.
With permission from Kitchens, C.S., and Van Mierop, H.S.: Envenomation by the eastern coral snake (Micrurus fulvius fulvius): A study of 39 victims. JAMA *258*:1615, 1987.

thrombocytopenia but with fibrinolysis caused by the saw-scaled viper.

The blood of patients bitten by poisonous snakes has been observed to remain unclotted for days, but with minimal to no clinical hemorrhage. Complete afibrinogenemia has been reported as early as 1 hour after a bite. Fatal intracerebral hemorrhage has occurred, but bleeding tendencies seem to be related to platelet count and prothrombin time rather than to absolute fibrinogen levels.

Often, the prothrombin time and the partial thromboplastin time are prolonged after envenomation. A complete series of coagulation studies must be ordered, and clinical improvement can be monitored closely with these parameters.

Spherocyte transformation, acanthocytosis, increased red cell osmotic fragility, false-positive direct Coombs' tests, Heinz body formation, intravascular hemolysis, and burring of erythrocytes may occur (Fig. 66-7). Venom also interferes with routine procedures in cross-matching blood for transfusions, and cross-matching and typing should be considered early in the management of patients bitten by poisonous snakes.

RENAL COMPLICATIONS

Snake venom has a variety of complex nephrotoxic effects. Renal failure is rare after poisonous snake bites; however, when it does occur, it is usually the result of either tubular necrosis or cortical necrosis. Glomerulonephritis and proliferative nephritis, presumably on a hypersensitive basis, have been reported, as well as nephrotic syndrome and renal infarction.

Hemoglobinuria, probably secondary to intravascular hemolysis, and myoglobinuria may occur.

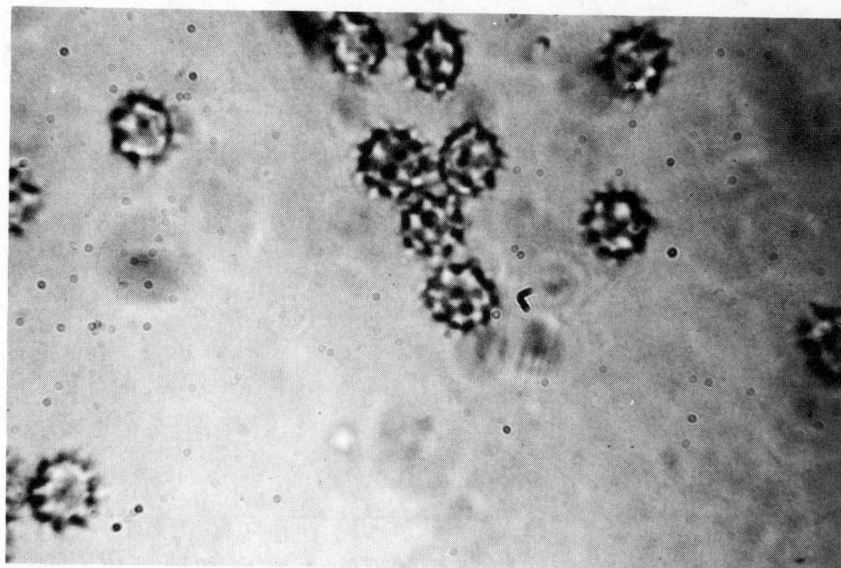

FIG. 66-7.   Burred erythrocytes readily elicited by snake venom are observed in the peripheral blood of patients bitten by poisonous snakes. With permission from Huang, T.T., et al.: Ann. Surg. *179:598, 1974.*

INFECTION

Infection does not seem to be a major complication of snakebite, but it is often difficult to differentiate infection from envenomation. Many authors suggest the routine parenteral use of broad-spectrum antibiotics when envenomation results in devitalized tissue.

Positive cultures have been found for both aerobic and anaerobic organisms in the oral cavity of rattlesnakes. Of the gram-negative bacteria, Aerobacter, Proteus, and Pseudomonas are the most common; less frequently found are strains of Salmonella. The gram-positive organisms are enterococcus, Streptococcus viridans, and histotoxic clostridia. In most studies, no *Clostridium tetani, Bacteroides,* or coagulase-positive staphylococci have been isolated. Deaths have been reported from tetanus following snakebite, although the tetanus organism has not been cultured in the oral cavity of snakes in the United States.

TREATMENT

The specific treatment of snakebite is a subject of extreme controversy. The medical literature is often biased, contradictory, and anecdotal. Conclusions are drawn from animal studies or uncontrolled clinical trials. Many authors are staunch advocates of their particular therapeutic regimen and fail to acknowledge results of varying treatments.

Two distinct therapeutic approaches are advocated. One is that of high-dose antivenin therapy, a regimen that eschews the need for and condemns the use of surgical therapy. The other school is that of an immediate surgical approach without the use of anti-venin therapy in all patients except those with severe systemic symptoms. It is probable that no single technique or therapeutic intervention is adequate for all cases, and a combination of therapeutic modalities is necessary.

The controversy is partly because of the tremendous variation in the composition of snake venoms and in individual susceptibility to their effects, leading to a variety of clinical presentations and pathophysiology. All authorities do, however, agree that the more rapidly treatment is instituted, the better are the results.

When a patient is suspected of having been bitten by a poisonous snake, it is important to establish if the offending snake truly was poisonous and if envenomation occurred. The characteristic fang marks and severe local and systemic reactions described can be helpful in deciding. In doubtful cases, observation in the emergency department (ED) is justified. In confirmed cases, the patient should avoid all unnecessary exercise, such as walking to the hospital, and no alcohol should be consumed. Both increase the escape of venom from the injection site. In cases of severe systemic reactions, first priority must be given to establishing an adequate airway and ensuring proper ventilation and cardiovascular integrity.

PREHOSPITAL ASSESSMENT AND STABILIZATION

FIRST AID AND FIELD TREATMENT

The most important aspect of field treatment of a poisonous snakebite is rapid transfer to the nearest hospital. Undue emphasis has been placed on the value of the immediate field treatment of bites by poisonous snakes. Because of the excitement generated in both the patient and the observer, there is a compelling urge to intervene quickly and definitively, hoping to stave off certain amputation or death (Fig. 66-8). As noted, mortality following snakebite in the United States is extremely rare, and even in fatal cases, death does not occur for many hours after envenomation. Misguided attempts to limit soft-tissue injury or offer a quick cure in the field may compound tissue loss, produce serious neurovascular or tendinous injury, or delay proper medical therapy. Basic first aid should include placing the patient at rest, immobilizing the extremity below the level of the heart, removal of rings, and rapid transport to a medical facility. (See also Surgical Treatment.)

The following section discusses the various approaches to therapy and details the applicability of each regimen to field treatment.

CONSTRICTION BAND (TOURNIQUET, LIGATION)

The use of a tourniquet (or, more correctly, a constriction band) is the most common recommendation for the initial treatment of a bite by a poisonous snake.[20] Although there is a theoretic disadvantage of concentrating the venom in an extremity with the use of a tourniquet and thereby increasing the amount of local necrosis, there is convincing evidence that a wide constricting band loosely applied 4 to 6 inches proximal to a bite decreases systemic absorption of venom. In the absence of systemic symptoms, or if a medical facility is less than 1 hour away, a tourniquet is not recommended. If systemic symptoms develop, however, or if the hospital is more than 1 hour away, most authors suggest applying a tourniquet. A sudden onset of systemic envenomation after removal of a tourniquet in a victim who had been asymptomatic for 2 hours after the bite of a poisonous snake has been documented.[21] The systemic symptoms paralleled a rise in the level of venom in the serum and urine after removal of the tourniquet.

With subcutaneous envenomation, venom spreads slowly by lymphatics, unless direct intravascular envenomation has occurred. You should be able to insert a finger under a properly applied tourniquet, which occludes lymphatic circulation and leaves arterial flow intact. A tourniquet that produces ischemia or venous obstruction is contraindicated. Most venom remains in the subcutaneous tissues for a considerable time, and a tourniquet, once placed, should not be removed prematurely because this may perpetuate the spread of venom by a milking action.

The constricting band should be released after antivenin is administered or if surgery is performed. As edema increases, the tightness of the band should be reassessed. If the band becomes too tight because of the advancement of edema, it may act as a venous obstruction and should be removed. There is some

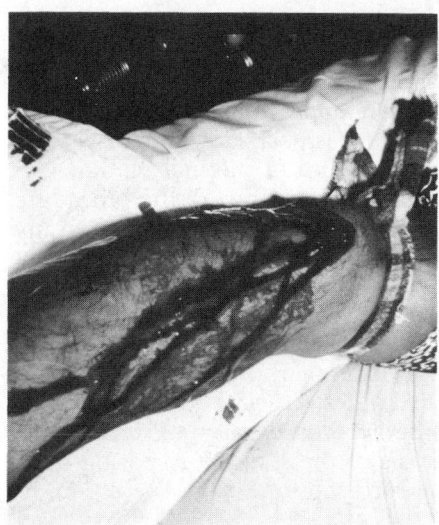

FIG. 66-8. *Inappropriate first aid treatment of this snakebite included a tight venous tourniquet and deep incision marks. Little or no envenomation had occurred.*

evidence that a broad compression bandage, such as an Ace bandage, wrapped on the bitten area to include and compress the entire extremity, offers some advantage over the traditional tourniquet.[21]

COOLING AND CRYOTHERAPY

There is no scientific rationale for the use of cryotherapy in the treatment of snakebite, although in the past its use had been recommended. There is no evidence that venom is inactivated by cooling, and attempts to decrease the temperature of the bitten area are often disastrous. Such methods as packing the extremity in ice are to be strongly condemned because this aggravates tissue loss and may result in needless amputation. Although minor cooling for a few hours is not deleterious, the use of any form of cold treatment should not be recommended as a first aid measure.

INCISION AND SUCTION

The time-honored practice of incision and suction over the fang marks is of minimal value in removing venom from the subcutaneous tissue. The technique should be applied only if the patient is more than a few hours from the hospital; its routine use is discouraged. It is probably of value only if performed within the first 5 to 15 minutes after envenomation, and it is never recommended in the ED or if antivenin is readily available. The early use of incision and prolonged suction can remove 50% of the venom in dogs experimentally envenomated. It is estimated, however, that even under ideal field circumstances, only about 10% of venom can be expected to be removed. In field conditions, a single vertical incision through and beyond each fang mark may be made. The depth of the incision should not exceed 1 cm. A knowledge of anatomy is essential to perform this procedure safely so that nerves, arteries, or tendons are not inadvertently severed. Continuous suction should be applied over the incisions. A mechanical suction apparatus is preferred, but mouth suction may be used safely. Venom does not penetrate the intact mucosa of the mouth, and it is inactivated by the stomach. Although the procedure has not been scientifically evaluated in humans to any great extent, some authors recommend the use of Sawyer's extraction device (Sawyer Products, Long Beach, CA 90807), a suction apparatus that delivers one atmosphere of negative pressure. The device is placed directly over the incision marks and applied continuously for 30 to 60 minutes. Cruciate or cross-hatching incisions should be avoided because such incisions may lead to necrosis of the skin flaps, posing difficulties on surgical correction.

MANAGEMENT OF THE ENVENOMATION

Even if asymptomatic, all patients suspected of having been bitten by a posionous snake should be observed for 6 to 8 hours. Delayed toxicity has been reported as long as 12 to 18 hours after the bite, but this is extremely rare. Figure 66-9 presents an overview of treatment.

LABORATORY EVALUATION

If evidence of envenomation exists, a baseline complete blood count, fibrinogen level, platelet count, prothrombin time, partial thromboplastin time, blood urea nitrogen, blood for type and crossmatch (or hold), and electrolytes should be obtained. These studies should be repeated every 2 to 8 hours, depending on the clinical course. A peripheral smear for the changes in red cell morphology may help in estimating the severity of the bite. In the case of coral snakebites, serial arterial blood gas determination helps to monitor pulmonary function. The urine should be examined for hemoglobin and myoblogin, and stools should be examined for occult blood.

Coagulopathies are seen on laboratory evaluation of surprisingly moderate crotalid envenomations. It is prudent to evaluate any envenomated patient for coagulation defects, but the totally asymptomatic patient need not be treated with anything more than local wound care and observation.

ANTIVENIN

The mainstay of medical therapy is the expeditious use of adequate amounts of antivenin. Antivenin is a suspension of venom-neutralizing antibodies that is prepared from the serum of horses hyperimmunized against the venom of specific snakes. Two types are commercially available. The Crotalidae polyvalent antivenin (Wyeth) is active against the venom of rattlesnakes, cottonmouths, and copperheads, and the pit vipers native to Central and South America. It is concentrated preparation of serum globulins obtained by fractionating blood from horses immunized with the venom of the Eastern and Western diamondback rattlesnake, the tropical rattlesnake, and the "fer-de-Lance." An antivenin is also available for the Eastern and Texas coral snakes (Micrurus fulvius, Wyeth). No antiserum is available against the less virulent Arizona coral snake, Micruroides euryxanthus. Antivenin for the exotic snakes found in zoos, e.g., cobras, is not commercially available in the United States, although some zoos have a supply on hand prepared in foreign countries.* The antivenin is supplied in the dry state, which must be reconstituted and used immediately. The unconstituted form has a shelf-life of 5 years, is rarely stocked in hospital pharmacies, and is presently of equine origi only. A 1-mL vial of one-tenth dilution of horse serum accompanies each vial of antivenin and can be used as a skin test for sensitivity. A negative skin test is no guarantee that a hypersensitivity reaction will not occur when antivenin is administered.[22] Less allergenic antivenin derived from sheep may be available in the future.

Immediate hypersensitivity reactions to antivenin are frequent. Anaphylactic shock may occur but is rarely fatal and is treated in the usual fashion. Antivenin therapy also results in the subsequent development of serum sickness in almost all cases if more than 10 vials are used. Serum sickness, characterized by skin rashes, fever, malaise, lymphadenopathy, and articular pains, usually appears 7 to 21 days after antivenin has been administered, and a negative sensitivity test does not mean that serum sickness will not develop. Children and small adults need relatively more antivenin than do large adults. A protocol for the treatment of patients sensitive to antivenin, in cases in which its use is deemed necessary, is found in the drug information insert accompanying each vial of antivenin. A history of sensitivity to horse serum and other allergic conditions should always be sought, and antivenin should be used with extreme caution when the possibility of immediate sensitivity exists. In life-threatening situations, antivenin may be warranted even when a sensitivity by skin testing or history has been shown (Fig. 66-10).

---

* The *Antivenin Index* is a catalog of available foreign antivenins that are stored in the United States. It may be helpful in the treatment of bites by exotic snakes. This publication contains the names of exotic snakes, names and addresses of manufacturers of antivenin, and data on the specific antivenins. (Antivenin Index in Tucson: 602-626-6061)

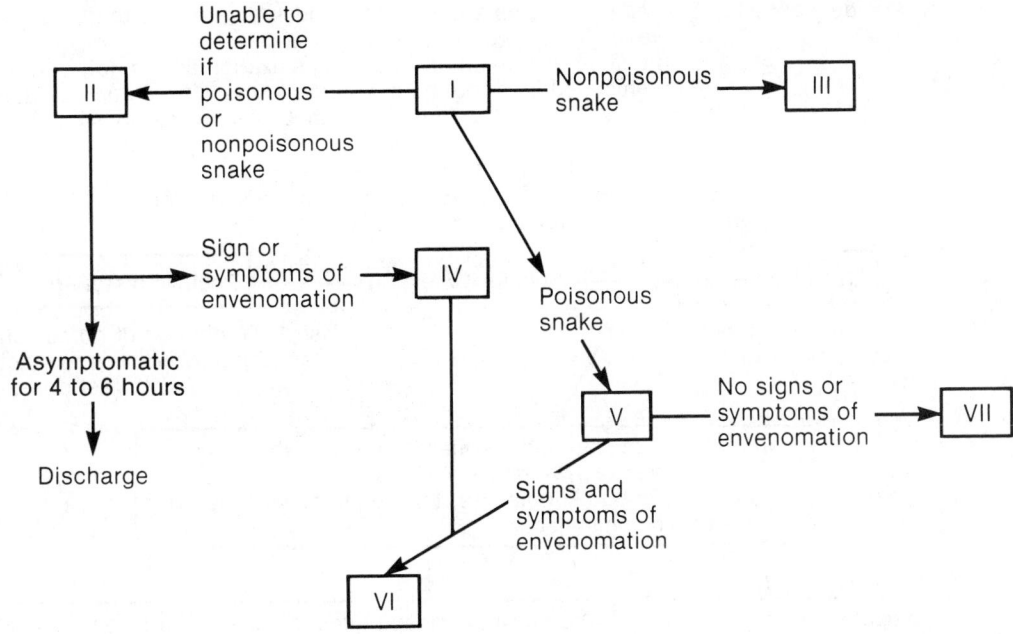

I. Initial evaluation
   1. Determine if snake was poisonous or nonpoisonous (character of bite, local or systemic reaction, snake identification)
   2. Initial history and physical examination with attention to underlying medical problems, allergies, circumstances of bite
   3. Begin record of vital signs
II. 1. NPO/monitor vital signs—strict bed rest—immobilize bitten area
   2. Large-bore IV, blood work—draw baselines and hold
   3. Obtain antivenin for possible use
   4. Tetanus prophylaxis
   5. Observe in emergency department for 4–18 hours
III. 1. Tetanus prophylaxis
   2. Clean wound and assess for bony injury
   3. Check wound in 48–72 hours
IV. 1. Begin ECG monitoring, test for sensitivity to antivenin if its use is deemed necessary
   2. Send baseline blood to lab
   3. Intubation equipment, respirator in room
   4. Obtain antivenin
V. 1. NPO/strict bed rest
   2. Large-bore I.V.
   3. Draw and send baseline blood work
   4. Monitor vital signs and ECG
   5. Tetanus prophylaxis
   6. Obtain antivenin for possible use and test for sensitivity to horse serum if antivenin will be used
   7. Intubation equipment and respirator at bedside
   8. Immobilization of bitten area
VI. 1. Call for help if available after skin testing, antivenin immediately if severe or deemed necessary or patient is pregnant
   2. Reassess airway, breathing, cardovascular status—admit to intensive care unit
   3. Evaluation for early fasciotomy
   4. Central venous pressure or Swan-Ganz catheter if shock occurs
   5. Foley catheter and urine for studies, forced diuresis if urine positive for hemoglobin or myoglobin
   6. Medication for relief of pain as needed
   7. Antibiotics after aspiration for culture
VII. 1. Observe for 24 hours
   2. Discharge if asymptomatic

FIG. 66-9.   A systematic approach to the treatment of bites by poisonous snakes.

INDICATIONS FOR ANTIVENIN

Crotalids. Figure 66-11 is a guide for grading the degree of envenomation from crotalids based on physical findings and clinical symptoms. This method of grading bites solely on the basis of *initial* pain, edema, and ecchymosis is merely a clinical guide. Strict adherence to this guide may be misleading and may lead to disastrous consequences. A poisonous snakebite is a dynamic, ever-evolving process that can suddenly and precipitously change, often with unexpected severity. Patients require repeat evaluation and reassessment of the degree of envenomation, and you cannot solely rely on the initial grade of envenomation when spec-

General guidelines:
1. Test *all* patients as soon as it has been determined that antivenin is required.
2. Skin testing may result in future sensitization and is not recommended as a routine procedure in non-envenomated patients.
3. A negative history for allergy does not rule out the possibility of a severe reaction or development of serum sickness.
4. Use normal saline as a control when testing.
5. ***Weigh the risk of withholding antivenin against the risk of death from envenomation.***

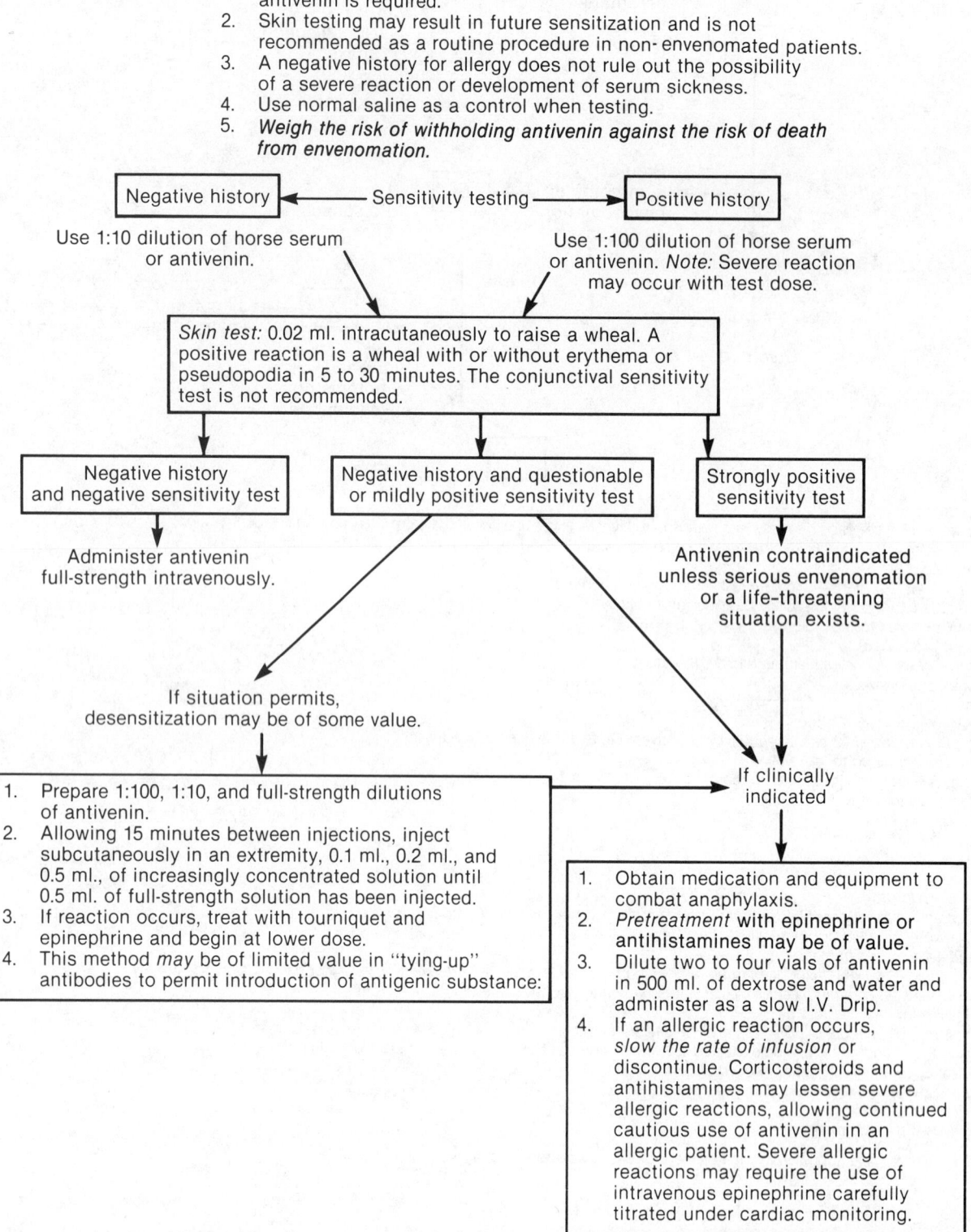

| Negative history | ←— Sensitivity testing —→ | Positive history |

Use 1:10 dilution of horse serum or antivenin.

Use 1:100 dilution of horse serum or antivenin. *Note:* Severe reaction may occur with test dose.

Skin test: 0.02 ml. intracutaneously to raise a wheal. A positive reaction is a wheal with or without erythema or pseudopodia in 5 to 30 minutes. The conjunctival sensitivity test is not recommended.

| Negative history and negative sensitivity test | Negative history and questionable or mildly positive sensitivity test | Strongly positive sensitivity test |

Administer antivenin full-strength intravenously.

Antivenin contraindicated unless serious envenomation or a life–threatening situation exists.

If situation permits, desensitization may be of some value.

1. Prepare 1:100, 1:10, and full-strength dilutions of antivenin.
2. Allowing 15 minutes between injections, inject subcutaneously in an extremity, 0.1 ml., 0.2 ml., and 0.5 ml., of increasingly concentrated solution until 0.5 ml. of full-strength solution has been injected.
3. If reaction occurs, treat with tourniquet and epinephrine and begin at lower dose.
4. This method *may* be of limited value in "tying-up" antibodies to permit introduction of antigenic substance:

If clinically indicated

1. Obtain medication and equipment to combat anaphylaxis.
2. *Pretreatment* with epinephrine or antihistamines may be of value.
3. Dilute two to four vials of antivenin in 500 ml. of dextrose and water and administer as a slow I.V. Drip.
4. If an allergic reaction occurs, *slow the rate of infusion* or discontinue. Corticosteroids and antihistamines may lessen severe allergic reactions, allowing continued cautious use of antivenin in an allergic patient. Severe allergic reactions may require the use of intravenous epinephrine carefully titrated under cardiac monitoring.

FIG. 66-10.   Guide to sensitivity testing and the use of equine serum (antivenin). Consult your local poison control center for expertise in your locale.

ulating on prognosis. Serial laboratory studies may also be helpful in assessing the changing spectrum of envenomation.

Antivenin is not recommended as prophylaxis in dry bites. The use of antivenin in grade I envenomation is the subject of some debate, and it is generally not recommended in minor envenomations. If pain is minimal, if minor swelling is confined to the bitten area, and if no blisters or ecchymoses develop, antivenin should be withheld. Although two to four vials of antivenin are recommended for grade II envenomation by the manufacturer, Russell[5] recommends a minimum of 5 to 8 vials for such bites. There is little evidence to support the use of 1 to 3 vials of antivenin under any circumstances. Larger doses (10 to 50 vials) of antivenin are recommended in the early treatment of severe envenomation of life-threatening magnitude (grades III and IV) and in this instance may be life-saving. The actual amount of antivenin administered should be individualized to reflect the evolving clinical course. In the case of a bite from a Mojave rattlesnake, a particularly venomous snake, it has been suggested that antivenin in amounts up to twice the normal recommended dose be administered (when envenomation has been proved).

The actual efficacy of antivenin in preventing tissue necrosis, myolysis, or hematologic abnormalities has been questioned,[23] although studies demonstrate an increased survival rate in dogs when antivenin is used. There is also evidence that, if given soon enough, antivenin reduces the amount of local tissue destruction in rabbits.[8] Antivenin alone may not reverse the hypotension seen with severe envenomation, and the concomitant use of intravenous fluids and vasopressors may be required. Antivenin may be useful in the treatment of coagulopathies associated with envenomation,[24] but the degree of its efficacy is unclear.

When antivenin is used, it should be administered *intravenously* as soon as possible. The initial dose of reconstituted antivenin should be diluted in 250 to 500 mL of 5% dextrose in water and given as a slow intravenous drip over the first 30 to 60 minutes. Allergic reactions are often related to the rate of infusion, and some reactions may be minimized by slowing the infusion rate.

In serious envenomation, the use of antivenin is warranted even if the skin test is positive or if a reaction to horse serum occurs during therapy. It may be necessary to give antihistamines or epinephrine to ameliorate immediate hypersensitivity reactions. Loprinzi described titrating an intravenous epinephrine infusion to control serious allergic reactions in a patient concurrently being treated with an antivenin infusion.[25] The intramsucular and intra-arterial routes are not indicated, and the bitten area should not be injected locally.

It is important to remember that children require more antivenin than adults. The clinical course in children may be precipitous and exaggerated.

Grade O—No evidence of envenomation. History of suspected snakebite. Fang wound(s) may be present. Minimal pain, less than 1 inch of surrounding edema and erythema. No systemic manifestations during first 12 hours after bite.

Grade I—Minimal envenomation. History of suspected snakebite. Fang wound(s) usually present. Moderate pain or throbbing localized at fang wound(s), surrounded by 1 to 5 inches of edema and erythema. Minor swelling, erythema, and ecchymosis, limited to the immediate bitten area. Laboratory findings are normal. No evidence of systemic involvement after 12 hours of observation.

Grade II—Moderate envenomation. The signs and symptoms of Grade I rapidly progress during first 12 hours, with severe and more widely distributed pain; edema spreading toward the trunk; petechiae and ecchymoses limited to area of edema. Nausea, vomiting, giddiness, and mild temperature elevation usually present. Minor coagulation defects may be present. Other laboratory tests demonstrate only minor abnormalities.

Grade III—Severe envenomation. May resemble Grade I or II when brought under observation, but course rapidly progressive. May arrive in shock within a few minutes of bite. Within 12 hours, edema spreads up extremity and may involve part of trunk. Petechiae and ecchymoses may be generalized. Systemic manifestations may include rapid pulse, shock-like state, subnormal temperature. Coagulopathy present by both laboratory parameters and clinical observations.

Grade IV—Very severe envenomation.[6] Seen especially after envenomation by large rattlesnakes. Characterized by sudden pain, rapidly progressive swelling, which may reach and involve trunk within a few hours, with ecchymoses, bleb formation, and necrosis. Systemic manifestations, often commencing within 15 minutes of bite, usually include weakness, nausea and vomiting, vertigo, numbness or tingling of lips or face. Muscle fasciculations, painful muscular cramping, pallor, sweating, cold and clammy skin, rapid and weak pulse, incontinence, convulions, and coma also may be observed; death may occur.

FIG. 66-11. Grading of Crotalid envenomation by the manufacturer of antivenin polyvalent (Wyeth Laboratories). There is little evidence to support the use of one or two vials in minor envenomations.

Authors who advocate routine early use of antivenin are often staunch opponents of surgical therapy. Russell[5] claims that in his experience with the use of antivenin in more than 650 cases of snake venom poisoning over 25 years, not a single fasciotomy was required.

Coral Snakes. Because of possible delayed reactions to coral snake envenomation, all suspected victims should be hospitalized and closely observed. There is little clinical experience with severe envenomation by coral snakes, but approximately three quarters of persons bitten by a coral snake are envenomated.[10] It has been recommended that three to five vials of antivenin be given prophylactically if a person has definitely been bitten by a coral snake.

FLUID THERAPY

Severe envenomation may cause cardiovascular collapse, and hypotension after a poisonous bite may be severe. In the first hour, it may result from a direct

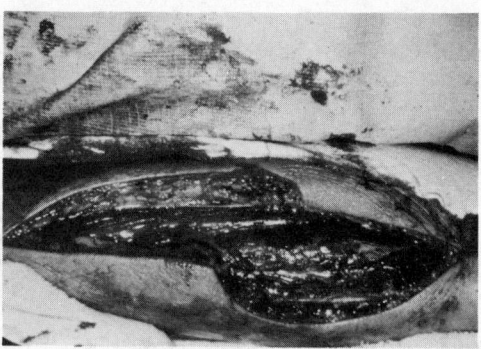

FIG. 66-12. A fasciotomy was performed because of the development of a compartment syndrome following envenomation by a western diamondback rattlesnake. There is necrosis of the muscles, indicating subfascial injection of venom.

toxic effect of venom on the myocardium and peripheral vascular system and may respond to fluids. After the first hour, fluid shifts into the area of envenomation may produce a profound hypovolemia. Large amounts of lactated Ringer's solution and packed red cells may be required to correct this defect. Occasionally, careful use of vasopressors may be required initially. A central venous pressure reading and a record of hourly urine output can be useful in monitoring fluid balance. If the urine is discolored (by hemoglobin or myoglobin), attempts to ensure a urine output of at least 1.5 mL/kg/hour in adults are suggested. In children over the age of 5 years, 30 to 50 mL per hour is suggested; for children aged 2 to 5, 20 to 30 mL per hour; and for children under 2, 10 to 20 mL per hour. This urine output may be accomplished with intravenous fluids if the cardiovascular system can handle the fluid load, or with the use of osmotic diuretics such as mannitol. Acute renal failure can probably be prevented, and this should be a priority early in the treatment of snakebite. All patients so treated or observed should have a large (No. 16 to 18) intravenous line routinely inserted. For more serious cases, a Swan-Ganz catheter or central venous line is indicated.

ANTIBIOTICS

Although *Clostridium tetani* organisms have not been found in the fangs or mouths of snakes, tetanus prophylaxis is recommended. The value of routine antibiotics is unclear, but secondary infection of necrotic tissue and osteomyelitis of fingers and toes have occurred. Moreover, bacteria have been cultured from snake venom. After aspiration of material for Gram stain and aerobic and anaerobic cultures in infected or highly contaminated bites, broad-spectrum antibiotics should be started parenterally. Cultures at the time of initial envenomation are of no value in predicting future infection. A first- or second-generation cephalosporin at a dose of 1 or 2 g intravenously every 6 hours is a good initial choice. If sepsis occurs, an

antibiotic effective against anaerobes (e.g., chloramphenicol or Cleocin) should be added. Tetracyclines should not be used in children, and penicillin alone is probably inadequate.

BLOOD PRODUCTS

Packed red blood cells may occasionally be needed to correct the hemolytic anemia associated with snakebite. One should draw blood immediately to type and cross-match, because hemolysis may interfere with subsequent attempts. Although clotting abnormalities are often seen, they usually regress spontaneously. In severe crotalid envenomation, coagulopathies are common, and fibrinogen, fresh frozen plasma, or platelets are required for bleeding problems.

CORTICOSTEROIDS

Most studies fail to prove a beneficial effect of steroids in the acute phase of snake venom poisoning. Steroids have not been of consistent value in reducing swelling, necrosis, or bleeding tendencies or increasing survival rate. There is some evidence that corticosteroids may be harmful.

Corticosteroids are of benefit in treating allergic reactions to horse serum, and the addition of 100 mg of hydrocortisone to each vial of diluted antivenin to avert possible reactions has been advocated.

The efficacy of corticosteroids in reversing the shock-like state induced by severe envenomation has not been studied. At present, the routine use of corticosteroids is not recommended.

HEPARIN

Coagulopathies following snakebite are extremely complex. There is no evidence that the routine use of heparin is of value, and its use at this time is discouraged. Coagulopathies are best managed with component therapy using platelets and fresh frozen plasma as indicated by laboratory tests.

ANTIHISTAMINES

Antihistamines may be synergistic with snake venom and therefore should not be used, except to manage acute hypersensitivity reactions to antivenin.

SURGICAL TREATMENT

It is generally accepted that surgical intervention is *not indicated* to assess the extent of tissue damage or to excise the bitten area. Routine fasciotomy has met with great criticism and has been discouraged by most authors. Despite extensive edema following crotalid envenomation, vascular compromise is rare. Fasciotomy has gained acceptance as a beneficial surgical treatment of a documented compartment syndrome and should be considered early in the management (Fig. 66-12). With the introduction of noninvasive arterial studies[26] and the wick catheter to measure compartment pressures directly, fasciotomy should be considered only on the basis of objective criteria. Marked elevation of compartmental pressure may compound tissue damage through ischemia and may limit circulation enough to prevent the local perfusion of antivenin. Fasciotomy itself does not prevent the necrosis, which is caused by the activity of venom, but may minimize the effect of elevated tissue pressure. Fasciotomy has been advocated as a prophylactic therapy in bites of the digits because of the limited capacity of the fingers and toes to swell, but even in these areas is usually unnecessary.

SNAKEBITE DURING PREGNANCY

Little is known about snakebite during pregnancy. Parrish[27] describes four pregnant patients bitten by pit vipers. Three delivered normal infants; one patient aborted 24 hours after envenomation. Possible mechanisms accounting for abortion may be (1) anoxia associated with shock, (2) bleeding into the placenta and uterine wall, and (3) uterine contractions initiated by venom. It is advisable to institute aggressive therapy in pregnant patients bitten by poisonous snakes.

Entman et al reported a death of an infant delivered by a mother who was bitten 6 weeks before delivery by a copperhead.[28] The mother had developed anaphylaxis during antivenin therapy that was treated with epinephrine, and the authors suggest that the resultant vasoconstriction may have contributed to the fetal demise. If was further suggested that ephedrine (25 to 50 mg IV bolus) should be the first-line therapy of anaphylaxis during pregnancy to bypass the uterine hypoxia that may result from epinephrine use. Snakebite, like other injuries, may increase fetal loss.[29] If slowing of fetal movements occurs, antivenin should be given to the mother.[30]

IMMUNIZATION

Attempts at producing active immunization by a toxoid have not been successful, mainly because the methods used for detoxifying venom have led to production of a poorly immunogenic substance.

Encouraging results have been reported recently in this field, however, with the poisonous Habu snake in Japan. Apparent successful immunization in humans has been reported sporadically following mul-

tiple injection of small amounts of snake venom in people intimately involved in snake handling.

Persons who are repeatedly envenomated by the same snake do not develop immunity to the venom and may actually develop allergy (hypersensitivity) to subsequent bites.[31]

PITFALLS

Common errors in the management of a poisonous snake bite include the following:

1. Overaggressive first-aid treatment, such as improper incision and the use of a constricting tourniquet and ice.
2. Underestimating the potential severity of the bite based on initial evaluation and failure to periodically re-evaluate the clinical situation and need for additional therapy.
3. Delay in administering antivenin and failure to administer proper amounts. Underdosing is the usual error.
4. Premature discharge (before 6 to 8 hours of observation) of the patient with signs of a bite (puncture marks) but no systemic or local symptoms.
5. Failure to administer antivenin in a documented coral snake bite, even in the absence of systemic symptoms.
6. Failure to consider fasciotomy as an uncommon but useful adjunct in selected cases.
7. Relying on a skin test to rule out a subsequent allergic reaction.
8. Skin testing on a routine basis, even when antivenin is withheld. This may sensitize the patient to future horse serum exposure.
9. Failure to administer antivenin in the case of life-threatening envenomation because of an allergic reaction to the antivenin.
10. Failure to use the resources of the regional poison center, local experts, or the antivenin index for exotic antivenins.

MEDICOLEGAL PEARLS

From a medicolegal standpoint it is important to adequately observe patients and avoid premature discharge. Whenever possible, expert consultation should be obtained because snakebite is so uncommon that few physicians have extensive clinical experience. Patients should be apprised of the risks and benefits of antivenin therapy, including the subsequent development of serum sickness. All physicians should be familiar with the poisonous snakes in their area and treatment resources before the snakebitten patient arrives for treatment. In one case, a snakebite victim with few symptoms was discharged early and later died. There was a lawsuit.

REFERENCES

1. Sowder, W.T., and Gehres, G.W.: Snakebite myths and misinformation, J. Fla. Med. Assoc. 55:319, 1968.
2. Parrish, H.M., and Khan, M.S.: Bites by coral snakes. Report of 11 representative cases. Am. J. Med. Sci. 253:561, 1967.
3. Parrish, H.M.: Analysis of 460 fatalities from venomous animals in the U.S. Am. J. Med. Sci. 245:129, 1963.
4. Mandell, F., Bates, J., Mittleman, B., et al.: Major coagulopathy and nonpoisonous snake bites. Pediatrics 65:314, 1980.
5. Russell, F.E.: Snake Venom Poisoning. Philadelphia, J.B. Lippincott Co., 1980.
6. Snyder, C.C. et al.: A definitive study of snakebites. J. Fla. Med. Assoc. 55:330, 1968.
7. Gerkin, R., Sergent, K.C., Curry, S.C., et al.: Life-threatening airway obstruction from rattlesnake bite to the tongue. Ann. Emerg. Med. 16:813, 1987.
8. Grace, T.G., and Omer, G.E.: The management of upper extremity pit viper wounds. J. Hand Surg. 5:168, 1980.
9. Hogan, D.E., Dire, D.J., and Hoot, F.: Anaphylactic shock secondary to rattlesnake bite. Ann. Emerg. Med. 19:814, 1990.
10. Kitchens, C.S., and Van Mierop, L.H.S.: Envenomation by the eastern coral snake (micrurus fulvius fulvius). JAMA 258:615, 1987.
11. Ownby, C.L., et al.: Pathogenesis of hemorrhage induced by rattlesnake venom. Am. J. Pathol. 76:401, 1974.
12. Rosenberg, P.: Effects of venoms on the squid giant axon. Toxicology 3:125, 1965.
13. DeVries, A., and Cohen, I.: Hemorrhagic and blood coagulation disturbing action of snake venom. In Poller, L. (ed.): Recent Advances in Blood Coagulation. Boston, Little, Brown & Co., 1969.
14. Gaffney, P.J., Marsh, N.A., and Talaiak, P.: Snake venom and hemostasis: Some suggested mechanisms of action. Southeast Asian J. Trop. Med. Pub. Health 10:258, 1979.
15. Wintrobe, M.M., et al.: Clinical Hematology. 7th ed. London, Henry Kimpton, 1974, pp. 1211–1224.
16. Hasiba, U., et al.: DIC-like syndrome after envenomation by the snake Crotalus horridus horridus. N. Engl. J. Med. 292:505, 1975.
17. Ruiz, C.E., Schaeffer, R.C., Weil, M.H., and Carlson, R.W.: Hemostatic changes following rattlesnake venom in the dog. J. Pharmacol. Exp. Ther. 213:414, 1980.
18. Warrell, D.A., Pope, H.M., and Prentice, C.R.M. Disseminated intravascular coagulaton caused by the carpet viper: Trial of heparin. Br. J. Haematol. 33:335, 1976.
19. Simon, T.L., and Grace, T.G.: Envenomation coagulopathy in wounds from pit vipers. N. Engl. J. Med. 305:443, 1981.
20. Stewart, M.E., Greenland, S., and Hoffman, J.R.: First aid treatment of poisonous snake bite: Are currently recommended procedures justified? Ann. Emerg. Med. 10:331, 1981.
21. Pearn, J., Morrison, J., Charles, N., et al.: First aid for snakebite—Efficacy of a constrictive bandage with limb immobilization in the management of human envenomation. Med. J. Aust. 2:293, 1981.
22. Jurkovich, G.J., Luterman, A., McCullar, K., et al.: Complications of crotalidae antivenin therapy. J. Trauma 28:1032, 1988.
23. Stahnke, H.L.: The Treatment of Venomous Bites and Stings. Tempe, Arizona, Arizona State University Press, 1966.
24. Reid, H.A., Thean, P.C., and Martin, W.J.: Specific antivenin and prednisone in viper bite poisoning: Controlled trial. Br. Med. J. 2:1378, 1963.
25. Loprinzi, C.L., et al.: Snake antivenin administration in a patient allergic to horse serum. South Med. J. 76:501, 1983.
26. Curry, S.C., Kraner, J.C., Kunkel, D.B., et al.: Noninvasive vascular studies in management of rattlesnake envenomations to extremities. Ann. Emerg. Med. 14:1081, 1985.
27. Parrish, H.M., and Khan, M.S.: Snakebite during pregnancy. Obstet. Gynecol. 27:468, 1966.
28. Entman, S.S., and Moise, J.J.: Anaphylaxis in Pregnancy. South. Med. J. 77:402, 1984.
29. Ellenhorn, M.J., and Barceloux, D.G.: Medical Toxicology. New York, Elsevier, 1988, p. 143.
30. James, R.F.: Snakebite in pregnancy. Lancet 12:731, 1985.
31. Parrish, H.M., and Pollard, C.B.: Effects of repeated poisonous snakebite in man. Am. J. Med. Sci. 247:277, 1990.

BIBLIOGRAPHY

Brown, J.H.: Toxicology and Pharmacology of Venoms from Poisonous Snakes. Springfield, Ill., Charles C Thomas, 1973.

Chavarria, A.P., Villarejos, V.N., and Zomeo, M.: Clinical importance of the prothrombin time determination in snake venom poisoning. Am. J. Trop. Med. Hyg. 19:342, 1970.

Danzig, L.E., and Abels, G.H.: Hemodialysis of acute renal failure following rattlesnake bite with recovery. JAMA 175:136, 1961.

Dvilansky, A., and Biran, H.: Hypofibrinogenemia after Echis cholorata bite in man. Acta Haematol. Kbh. 49:123, 1973.

Furtado, M.A., and Lester, I.A.: Myoglobinuria following snakebite. Med. J. Aust. 1:674, 1968.

Gill, K.A.: The evaluation of cryotherapy in the treatment of snake envenomization. South. Med. J. 63:552, 1970.

Glass, T.G.: Early debridement in pit viper bite. Surg. Gynecol. Obstet. 136:774, 1973.

Henderson, B.M., and Dujon, E.B.: Snakebites in children. J. Pediatr. Surg. 8:729, 1973.

Huang, T.T., et al.: The use of excisional therapy in the management of snakebite. Ann. Surg. 179:598, 1974.

Jimenez-Porras, J.M.: Biochemistry of snake venoms. Clin. Toxicol. 3:389, 1970.

Ledbetter, E.O., and Kutscher, A.E.: The aerobic and anaerobic flora of rattlesnake fangs and venom. Arch. Environ. Health 19:770, 1969.

Parrish, H.M., and Carr, C.A.: Bites by copperheads in the U.S. JAMA 201:927, 1967.

Parrish, H.M., et al.: Clinical features of bites by non-venomous snakes. South. Med. J. 66:1412, 1973.

Russell, F.E., and Emery, J.A.: Effects of corticosteroids on lethality of Ancistrodon contortrix venom. Am. J. Med. Sci. 241:507, 1961.

Sitprisa, V., et al.: Further observations on renal insufficiency in snakebite. Nephron 13:396, 1974.

Snyder, C.C., and Knowles, R.P.: Snakebite! Consultant (SKF) 3:44, 1963.

Snyder, C.C., Straight, R., and Glenn, J.: The snakebitten hand. Plast. Reconstr. Surg. 49:275, 1972.

Weiss, H.J., et al.: Afibrinogenemia in a man following the bite of a rattlesnake (Crotalis adamantus). Am. J. Med. 47:625, 1969.

CHAPTER 67

TOXIC BITES AND STINGS

Loren Johnson

CAPSULE

The victim of a bite or sting by a venomous animal may give a specific history of direct experience with the injury; often, however, the opposite is true. A patient presents with a lesion from an unknown source, and the clinician is left to his or her own devices based on an understanding of the natural history of venom syndromes.

Four categories of injury by venomous animals can occur. These include direct mechanical injury, poisoning by the venom, hypersensitivity reactions to the venom, and the transmission of disease or infection through the skin.

Management objectives for all envenomations can be outlined as follows: assessment of local and systemic toxicity to confirm and quantify the envenomation; identification of the offending organism, whenever possible; removal of venom from the wound and the use of measures to retard absorption; the neutralization of venom and the administration of agents to counteract its effects; and the treatment of secondary and late toxic effects.

INTRODUCTION

Few subjects in medicine have inspired as many superstitions, phobias, and harmful cures as the bites and stings of venomous animals. Snakes have been regarded as products of satanic transformation, "cursed above every beast" (Genesis 3:14). Along with other venomous land and sea creatures, they have been thought to be endowed with great supernatural power in aboriginal as well as modern cultures. This lore has led to a tendency toward anxiety and hysteria among victims and overaggressive treatment by providers. Advances in the scientific understanding of animal venoms in the past few decades have led to much more rational approaches to treatment and re-ferral, so that proper attention can be given to the most serious cases.

As the self-appointed custodians of our native planet, we are extremely fortunate to be blessed with a domain of enormous biologic diversity. The variety of venomous species in all the regions of the world is exceeded only by the ways that humans find to encounter these animals in their habitats. A comprehensive review of this subject is therefore beyond the scope of this chapter, which is intended to be a brief review of the representative classes of animals and their venom syndromes with an emphasis on indigenous species of North America. The reader may find more thorough reviews by consulting the general references at the end of this chapter. For injuries by nonindigenous species, one can obtain advice and antivenom information from research institutions and zoological gardens by referral through regional poison control centers. Snakebites are discussed extensively in the previous subchapter.

OCCURRENCE

In his classic survey of county coroners throughout the United States between 1950 and 1959, Parrish reported 460 deaths caused by venomous animals: 50% from insect stings, 30% from snakebites, 14% from spider bites, and 6% from a variety of others.[1]

Research in the chemistry and biology of venoms has led to numerous medical and scientific advancements. For example, many useful enzymes have been identified, and purified neurotoxins have become important research tools to study the selective effects of stimulation or blockade of various types of synaptic channels involved in nerve transmission.

A 1985 nationwide survey of Poison Control Centers in the United States summarizing 30,938 animal bite calls reported no mortality and only 10% significant morbidity, with 43% of the total calls on victims 17 years of age or younger.[2] Approximate percentages of these calls relating to venomous injuries were as follows: bees, wasps and hornets, 17.5%; scorpions,

TABLE 67-1. TREATMENT OF ARACHNID BITES

Treatment Objectives	Brown Spider Bite	Black Widow Spider Bite	Scorpion Sting*	Centruroides sculpturatus or C. gertschi†
		Type of Bite		
Confirm and quantitate envenomation. Look for signs of local and systemic toxicity	*Local:* Vesicle with expanding ischemic center. Marked swelling and erythema *Systemic:* Occasional hemolytic reactions and renal failure	*Local:* Burning pain spreads regionally *Systemic:* Muscle spasms, hypertension and neurotoxicity, over 12 hours; adrenergic and cholinergic crisis	*Local:* Pain and slight swelling *Systemic:* Generally none	*Local:* Minimal reaction *Systemic:* Cholinergic and adrenergic crisis
Identify offending organisms by species	More aggressive therapy required for bite of *Loxosceles reclusa* than for other brown spiders	Antivenin is available		In Mexico, antivenin may be lifesaving
Remove venom from wound and retard absorption	Cleanse wound; if *L. reclusa,* excise area of central discoloration	Applying constricting band; cleanse and cool topically	Cleanse and cool topically	Apply constricting band; cleanse and cool topically
Neutralize venom or counteract its effects	May elect to give corticosteroids and antihistamines to reduce inflammation	Calcium and muscle relaxants as needed. Antivenin,‡ single vial IV or IM, for severe reactions, if not allergic		Antivenin is available in Mexico for severe reactions, if patient is not allergic to horse serum
Treat secondary and late toxic effects	Repeated débridement of ischemic tissue; germicidal soaks; late physiotherapy and reconstructive surgery as needed	Monitor and treat for hypertensive crisis and neurologic sequelae; antivenin in severe reactions particularly children, elderly, and medically compromised patients		Support airway, ventilation and perfusion. Treat convulsions; monitor for shock, arrhythmias

* In the United States except Arizona.
† Small scorpions in Arizona and Mexico.
‡ Lyovac (Merck Sharp & Dohme).
Abbreviations: IV = Intravenous; IM = intramuscular.

7%; other insects, 4%; black widow spiders, 1%; brown spiders, 0.3%; unknown spiders, 11%; fish and coelenterates, 0.5%; rattlesnakes, 0.2%; copperheads, 0.1%; unknown snakes, 0.9%; and nonpoisonous snakes, 0.8%.[3] These data reflect the fact that the large majority of injuries are from arthropod stings and that any inflammatory lesion of unknown source is likely to be labeled as a spider bite.

ARTHROPOD INJURIES: SPIDERS, SCORPIONS, CENTIPEDES (CLASS ARACHNIDA); STINGING INSECTS (ORDER HYMENOPTERA); ECTOPARASITES; AND CATERPILLARS

TYPICAL PRESENTATIONS

- A house painter enters the emergency department 8 hours after being bitten by a plain brown spider. There is a small ischemic plaque with surrounding pain, itching, and erythema.
- A middle-aged housewife presents after being bitten on the neck by a black spider. There is right-sided neck pain and swelling, and myalgias and spasms of the abdominal muscles. Her blood pressure is 260/140 mm Hg, and she has no prior history of hypertension.
- A child is brought in 2 hours after being stung on the hand by a scorpion. She has marked local edema, excessive salivation, and opisthotonos.
- A hiker with a past history of Hymenoptera allergy presents with facial swelling, stridor, cyanosis, and a blood pressure of 60/40 mm Hg.

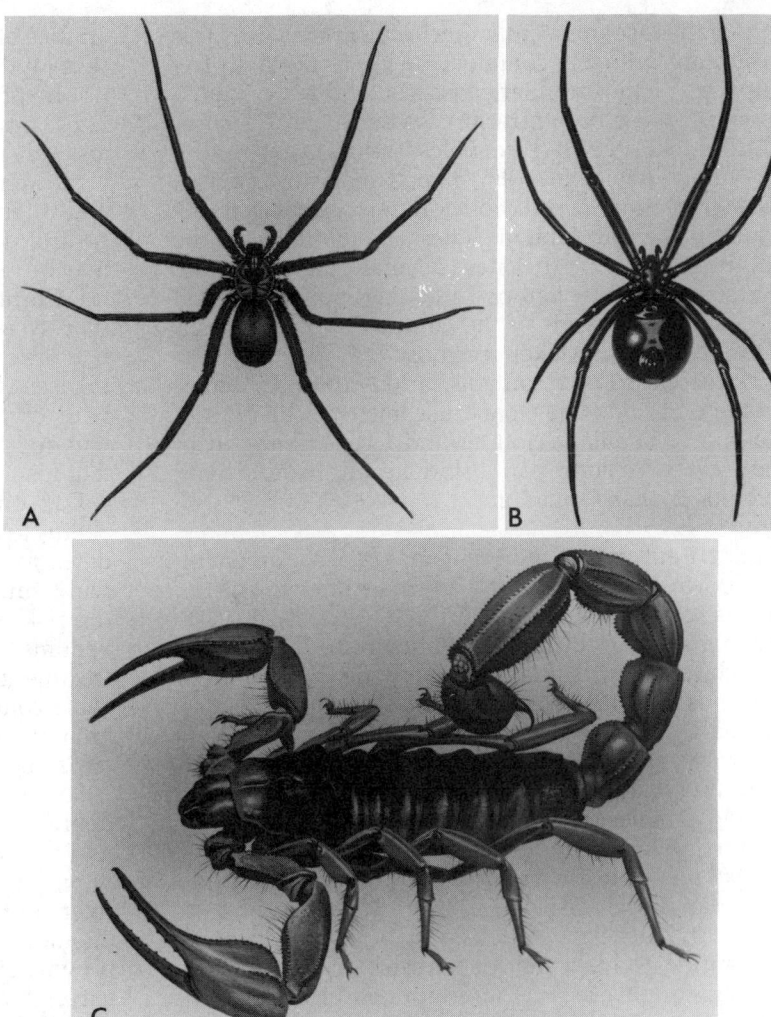

FIG. 67-1.   Arachnids. A. Brown recluse spider, *Loxosceles reclusa* (violin on dorsal surface; × 1.5). B. Black widow spider, *Latrodectus mactans* (hourglass on ventral surface; × 1.5). C. Hairy scorpion, *Hadrurus arizonensis* (shown actual size). (Courtesy of Frazier, C.A.; reproduced by permission of Merck Sharp & Dohme, Division of Merck & Co., Inc.)

- A child enters with multiple wheal formations and retained honeybee stingers.
- A gardener walks into the emergency department with a swollen hand.

The phylum arthropoda consists of "bugs" with multijointed legs and includes a wide variety of venomous forms, including spiders and scorpions (Class Arachnida), stinging insects (Order Hymenoptera), biting and blood-feeding insects, and many others. Several are important disease vectors in humans and animals.

For the typical arthropod bite or sting, the difference between primary toxicity, local hypersensitivity, and local infection may be ill-defined, and the suspect arthropod may go unseen or incorrectly identified. When taking a history of an unknown venomous injury, one must consider the setting of the injury, the behavior pattern of suspect organisms, and the clinical presentation and pattern of lesions; and perform a careful search for retained arthropod parts. Even after this search for a rational diagnosis, one is often left with "arthropod envenomation" as the only label available.

Table 67-1 outlines the general treatment of arachnid bites and stings.

SPIDER BITES—CLASS ARACHNIDA (Fig. 67-1)

All spiders are carnivorous and most are venomous. Some have neurotoxic venoms and many have necrotizing venoms, but most are timid, seldom capable of penetrating the skin with their fang-like chelicerae, and seldom bite unless squeezed or threatened.

NECROTIZING SPIDER BITES

Brown spiders of the genus Loxosceles are hunter spiders with venom containing digestive enzymes, which are used to help them devour their prey. They are common to outbuildings and storage areas throughout the warmer parts of the United States, and low-grade cases of necrotic arachnidism caused by this group are probably common, owing to the high frequency of exposure. Serious cases tend to be limited to bites by the brown recluse spider (Fig. 67-1A), or fiddle-back special (Loxosceles reclusa), a spindly, drab spider with a violin-shaped marking oriented backward on its dorsal cephalothorax, endemic to the southern central United States and portions of the southeastern United States. Several other less toxic but somewhat dangerous Loxosceles species inhabit the warmer portions of the United States, and their bites are often mistaken for those of L. reclusa.

Loxosceles venom contains various potent cytotoxic and lipolytic enzymes that cause microvascular injury leading to capillary clotting and local infiltration of leukocytes,[4] resulting in a slow-healing wound with necrotic eschar formation.

Clinical Features.   A mild sting may be associated with the brown spider bite; however, more often the victim is unaware of the bite until the development of regional pain after the first few hours. Pruritus, malaise, and chills and sweats are common. The wound itches, becomes red with a blanched center, and forms a hemorrhagic vesicle. It may stabilize at this stage or show impending necrosis, with central ecchymosis and surrounding blanching, overlying a firmly indurated plaque. The lesion has been characterized as having a halo or bullseye appearance. In addition, there may be extensive erythema, regional lymphadenitis, and a scarlatiniform rash. By 5 days, the expanding ecchymosis blackens in a stellate shape; by 2 to 4 weeks, the entire necrotic area demarcates and the central eschar sloughs, leaving an indurated ulcer with undermined edges. Areas with a thick subcutaneous fat pad are prone to the formation of large ulcers and microabscesses and poor healing.

Systemic toxicity can occur at any time during the development of the ischemic injury. Headache, fever, weakness, chills, nausea, malaise, and leukocytosis are common. Purpura may occur. Hemolytic reactions may take place within 24 hours and lead to jaundice and renal tubular necrosis.[5] Occasionally fatal reactions may result from disseminated intravascular coagulation.[6] Convulsions and heart failure have been reported in children.

Management.   Treatment of Loxosceles reclusa bites is highly controversial. Early excisional removal of skin and subcutaneous tissue sites containing venom was favored by several investigators; however, subsequent experience has shown that this does not limit or prevent necrotic eschar formation or speed wound healing.[7-9] This is probably based on the fact that by the time victims present to the Emergency Department (ED), venom has been absorbed into subcutaneous lymphatics, where most of the damage occurs. For the rare patient who presents within a few minutes of a known L. reclusa bite, it may be reasonable to consider excision of the central site; however, comparative studies of early excision versus elevation, ice, and expectant therapy have shown that excision is generally not helpful.[10]

Basic treatment includes cleansing of the bite site and elevation and immobilization of the affected area. Continuing ice compresses are recommended initially, and intermittent ice compresses are helpful for pain control during the first 2 to 3 days. Antihistamines may be given for pruritus, but are otherwise not helpful. Corticosteroids have not been found effective, either systemically or intradermally, and most investigators recommend that corticosteroids be given only in cases of serious systemic toxicity. Antibiotic therapy with erythromycin, 250 mg PO qid is also recommended.[10,11] All victims should be immunized against tetanus.

Dapsone, 100 mg bid has been advocated for its ability to suppress the leukocyte response.[10] Candidates for treatment must undergo G6PD screening, and hematocrits must be followed closely because of the risk of hemolysis with this drug. Research antivenoms have also been studied. Combinations of both treatments have been thought to be helpful;[11] however, comparative clinical experience has been very limited and critics have contended that the benefit of dapsone does not outweigh the risk.[12]

For large ulcerative lesions, necrotic skin should be debrided and enzymatic debridement ointments such as Travase may be applied for 7 to 10 days until the wound is clean and ready for skin grafting.[10] An antivenom for the treatment of Loxosceles laeta envenomation is available in South America, where this large brown spider is known to cause serious systemic toxicity.

Hyperbaric oxygen therapy (HBO) has been shown to be beneficial on the basis of preliminary studies. This is based on the well-known properties of HBO in the promotion of neurovascularization and increased fibroblast activity in wound healing.

OTHER INFLAMMATORY SPIDER BITES

Tarantulas are known to bite when handled carelessly, but North American varieties are generally not dangerous. Contact with the hair of some of these animals causes minor inflammation.

Other North American spiders that inflict inflammatory bites include the running spider, Chiricanthium; the jumping spiders, Phidippus; and the golden orb spider, Argiope.[10]

NEUROTOXIC SPIDER BITES

Black Widow Spider Bites.   Black widow spiders of the genus Latrodectus are widespread throughout temperate and tropical regions and are noted for their potent neurotropic toxins. They are trapping spiders who catch insects in elaborate webs and use their venom to immobilize their prey for a later meal. The

North American black widow spider (Latrodectus mactans) is representative of this group. The female is a large, shiny black spider with a characteristic red hourglass marking on the ventral surface of its globular abdomen (See Fig. 67-1B). It is widespread throughout most of the United States, but most have been reported from the southern half, with the highest frequency in the central valley of California. Other North American widow spiders include the red widow spider, Latrodectus bishopi of central Florida; the brown widow spider, Latrodectus geometricus, of south Florida; and Latrodectus variolus, of the Eastern United States.

Latrodectus spiders tend to spin webs and trap their prey. They are generally not aggressive and bite defensively when encountered in their own habitat. Human encounters usually occur outdoors in warm weather around homes and gardens where spiders tend to nest in debris-covered areas. Bites on the buttocks and genitalia, common in the early part of this century, are much less common since the advent of the flush toilet and the decline of the outdoor privy.[13] Epidemics of spider bites and spider phobia have been known to occur near the Mediterranean and elsewhere, owing to cyclic expansions of the Latrodectus population.

Black widow spider venom is among the most potent neurotoxic substances known. It contains protein fractions that bind to calcium channels in synaptic endplates to permit massive release of acetylcholine and norepinephrine. The venom action is partially calcium-dependent, but is not affected by calcium or sodium channel blocking drugs. This is thought to be the reason for the effectiveness of calcium infusion as a transient specific inhibitor of venom toxicity.

Unlike the venom of most other spiders, black widow spider venom contains no inflammatory or cytotoxic agents and causes only minimal localized inflammation at the site of the bite.

Clinical Features. Once a victim is bitten, there is an immediate pinprick sensation, and local dull pain and numbness develop in a few minutes. Redness and swelling may appear around a focal site. Within 1 to 2 hours, pain spreads to regional lymph nodes and muscle spasms occur in abdominal and upper truncal muscles. Anxiety, nausea, vomiting, dizziness, and headache are common. In most cases toxicity resolves at this point; however, in serious cases, severe pain, anxiety, paresthesias, dyspnea, expiratory grunting, dysphagia, ptosis and edema of eyelids, low-grade fever, and skin rash may develop. A burning sensation may involve the soles of the feet. Sweating, lacrimation, salivation, and bronchorrhea may occur. Arterial and cerebrospinal fluid pressures may be elevated, especially with head and neck bites. Hypertensive crisis is not uncommon in elderly patients and those with preexisting hypertension. Within 48 hours, the neurologic dysfunction resolves. Weakness, myalgias, and malaise may persist for longer periods, especially in untreated cases. Fatalities are rare, and life-threatening reactions are usually seen only in small children, aged persons, and those with unstable medical conditions.

Generalized muscle spasms tend to mimic heat cramps. The occurrence of pain, rigidity and vomiting may mimic peritonitis; however, with peritonitis, the victim tends to remain still and exhibit signs of rebound tenderness between episodes of vomiting, whereas the victim of black widow spider envenomation tends to writhe in severe pain.

Management. Initial treatment includes topical cleansing, ice application, and analgesic administration. Calcium gluconate, 10% 0.1 mL per kg given slowly intravenously (IV) at 2-to-4-hour intervals[14] is the mainstay of therapy. Muscle relaxants such as methocarbamol, up to 1 g, may be given parenterally and provide additional relief, but are not as effective as calcium gluconate. Hypertensive crisis can be treated with nifedipine, or with an infusion of Labetalol, sodium nitroprusside, or hydralazine. When symptom onset is precipitous and envenomation appears severe, ventilatory support may be required and vital signs should be monitored carefully during the first several hours.

The use of horse serum antivenin (Lyovac) may be justified, particularly in children, the elderly, and patients with unstable medical conditions. One ampule is given IM or diluted in normal saline and given intravenously after the appropriate sensitivity testing, in accordance with package insert instructions.[15] Rarely, a second ampule may be necessary. All victims should be immunized against tetanus.

Other Neurotoxic Spider Bites. There is a great deal of experience with the use of horse serum antivenom for bites of the red back spider, Latrodectus hasselti, in Australia. Antivenom is given to victims in all age groups and provides rapid relief of symptoms within 30 minutes. Skin testing and preadministration of antihistamines and epinephrine are routine and the frequency of anaphylaxis is minimal, with no reports of fatalities from allergic reactions.[16]

Funnel web spiders of the genus Atrax are a particularly aggressive group of large spiders, indigenous to Australia and the Indo-Pacific, which cause potentially lethal neurotoxic envenomation resulting in severe cholinergic and adrenergic discharge. Immobilization and lymphatic compression of the affected extremity are recommended as first aid. Antivenom, which is available in indigenous areas, may be lifesaving.[10]

Phoneutrea is a genus of large, aggressive spiders found in South America with marked neurotoxicity for which antivenom is likewise available.

OTHER INFLAMMATORY ENVENOMATIONS

A wide variety of terrestrial animals may inflict painful and inflammatory bites and stings. The offending agent is frequently not seen, and these injuries tend to be mistakenly identified as spider bites. Bites by spiders, centipedes, millipedes, caterpillars, biting flies, fleas, reduvid bugs, ants, venomous ticks, and reptiles, and stings and irritations by stinging insects, ants, beetles, caterpillars, and amphibians can all be considered. Topical treatment includes cleaning, ice, elevation, and application of soothing compresses such as baking soda, vinegar, Burrow's solution, or papain (Adolph's Meat Tenderizer), as recommended by local medical authorities. Local infection is common and should be treated with early antibiotic administration. Allergic reactions are likewise not uncommon and may be severe enough to require treatment. Patients with severe systemic reactions should be referred for immunotherapy.

SCORPION STINGS

Scorpions (Fig. 67-1C) are among the most ancient terrestrial animals, with a fossil record of 400 million years. They are widespread in desert and temperate zones and are successful predators, using their stings to immobilize their prey. They are nocturnal and tend to sequester themselves upside down under debris.

Old-World scorpion stings are potentially lethal, particularly those by members of the family buthidae, which are common in Asia, Africa and South America. In the United States, the relatively common members of the family vejovidae may inflict a locally painful sting only.

Special species of the family buthidae, genus Centruroides in Mexico and one species in the southwestern desert portions of the United States possess a potentially dangerous neurotoxic sting. Centruroides exilicanda, also known as the bark scorpion, is a small yellow scorpion common to Arizona, New Mexico, and portions of Southern California and is representative of this group.

Human encounters with scorpions in the United States number more than 2000 per year, with only a small percentage requiring treatment.[17] They tend to occur in the summer, when night-time temperatures exceed 70°F.[18] A typical scenario involves stings by scorpions hiding in clothing or chance encounters with children playing in debris-covered areas.

Clinical Features. Scorpion venom consists of peptide mixtures. Those of non-Centruroides species and most Centruroides species in North America may cause local pain, erythema and nausea, then release of kinins. These effects usually develop over the first hour and resolve within 4 hours. The neurotoxicity caused by Centruroides exilicanda arises from sodium channel stimulation of nerve endings resulting in increased cholinergic and adrenergic activity. Toxins of some other scorpions have also been studied for their ability to inhibit potassium channel activity.[19-21]

Sympathetic symptoms of C. exilacanda envenomation include tachycardia, hypertension, mydriasis, perspiration, and piloerection. Parasympathetic symptoms are transient and may include increased salivation, lacrimation, urination, defecation, and gastrointestinal distress. Other neurologic sequelae may include numbness, hyperesthesia, headache, and local cramping. Opisthotonos seizures and visual defects may also occur. Hyperactivity is common in children. Principal effects occur during the first 4 hours and resolve over 24 hours.[22]

Serious cardiac toxicity has been well documented in children with old-world scorpion envenomation and is thought to be caused by adrenergic stimulation. Echocardiography may show evidence of congestive cardiomyopathy, and the ECG may show evidence of myocardial injury and arrhythmias.[23-27]

Management. Wound cleansing, cool compresses and mild analgesics, and tetanus prophylaxis constitute adequate management for most scorpion stings. For C. exilicanda stings, the parasympathomimetic effects may be blocked with atropine, but this is usually unnecessary because of the transient nature of these effects. Deaths have been reported from overaggressive use of narcotic analgesics and phenobarbital,[28] but more recent experience suggests that narcotics and benzodiazepines are safe for controlling pain and hyperactivity when titrated in appropriate doses.

A goat serum antivenom for C. exilicanda is available in Arizona only and is reported to be effective; however, its safety and efficacy have not been thoroughly determined.[20]

HYMENOPTERA STINGS

BEE, WASP, HORNET, AND YELLOWJACKET STINGS

Hymenopterids (Fig. 67-2) are prevalent in all 50 states. Hypersensitivity to their stings occurs in nearly 1% of cases and accounts for the greatest mortality rate from any group of venomous animals in the United States, with 50 deaths reported annually. Only 25% of allergic patients have a known history of hypersensitivity, and the severity of reactions increases as a function of repeated exposure.

Classification and Differentiation. There are four families of Hymenoptera of special significance to insect allergy. These include (1) the Apidae, or honeybees; (2) the Bombidae, or bumblebees; (3) the Vespidae, or wasps, hornets and yellowjackets; and (4) the Formicidae, or ants (discussed in another section).

Bumblebees are relatively docile and rarely sting humans. The Vespidae pose the greatest individual danger of hypersensitivity, and, because they are scavengers, their stings are more likely to cause bacterial infection. The common honeybee accounts for more stings and deaths than any other species and triggers swarm attacks by releasing an alarm odor known as

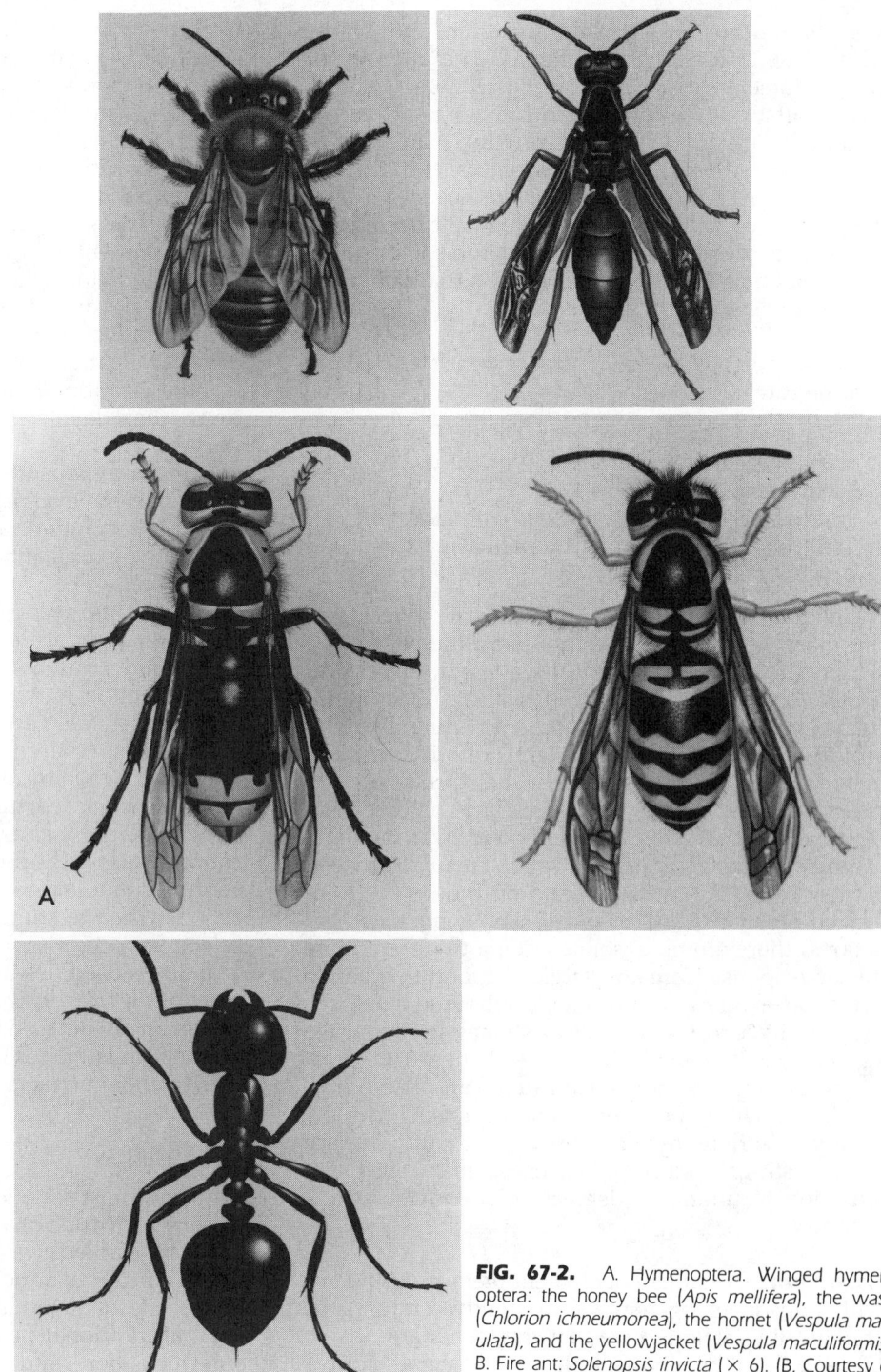

FIG. 67-2. A. Hymenoptera. Winged hymenoptera: the honey bee (*Apis mellifera*), the wasp (*Chlorion ichneumonea*), the hornet (*Vespula maculata*), and the yellowjacket (*Vespula maculiformis*). B. Fire ant: *Solenopsis invicta* (× 6). (B, Courtesy of Frazier, C.A.; A and B reproduced by permission of Merck Sharp & Dohme, Division of Merck & Co., Inc.)

a pheromone. This is the only species that leaves its barbed stinger and venom sac in situ. Thus, the presence of the stinger is an accurate diagnostic clue, and its absence makes a specific diagnosis difficult. An aggressive tropical variety of the honeybee, known as the African killer bee, is no more toxic than the domestic bee, but it is prone to swarm attacks and is expected to expand its range to the southern United States.

Signs and Symptoms. Honeybee venom contains basic polypeptides, spreading factors, histamine, serotonin, and nonenzymatic proteins, with nine identifiable antigens. Wasp venom is similar and contains large amounts of acetylcholine, serotonin, and kinins, with 12 to 13 identifiable antigens. The quantity of venom injected in single stings is minuscule, and swarm attacks with fewer than 500 stings are rarely fatal in the absence of hypersensitivity, but they typically cause lethargy, nausea, abdominal cramps, and hypertension, and may cause severe headache, convulsions, fever, and sepsis. Intravenous calcium gluconate provides some relief of symptoms. Parenteral antibiotics may be essential in many situations of infected stings with bacteremia.

Allergy. Allergic reactions to Hymenoptera stings may be categorized as:

1. Immediate-local, with inordinate local swelling;
2. Immediate-mild-generalized, with diffuse swelling or urticaria;
3. Immediate-severe-generalized, with anaphylaxis;
4. Delayed, with serum sickness-like reactions and atypical reactions.

Generally, the more rapid the onset of the reaction, the more severe it is, with most fatalities occurring within the first hour from airway obstruction and shock. Stings about the face, neck, and mucous membranes are prone to cause life-threatening swelling around the airway. Delayed allergic reactions usually include arthralgias, gastrointestinal disturbances, and fever; however, unusual responses have occurred, including blood dyscrasias, kidney and liver damage, cerebrovascular accidents, peripheral neuropathy, serum sickness-like reactions, and birth defects. In localized reactions, and even in some generalized reactions, there are no absolute criteria to differentiate a toxic response from an allergic one, and the degree of response to a sting is no index to subsequent degrees of reactivity. Cross-sensitivity exists among all species, especially with Vespidae exposure. Antigens are present in body parts and sensitization can arise by inhalation of wind-borne contaminants, raising the possibility of serious hypersensitivity without a history of prior stings. Indeed, other insects may cause sensitization to unknown degrees of specificity in this manner.

Treatment. Treatment of Hymenoptera stings begins with nonsqueezing removal by gently scraping the stinger away, taking care that fragments are not retained. Clean the wound with soapy water and apply ice. Early topical coverage with a paste of meat tenderizer containing papain is soothing and is said to have a detoxifying effect. Allergy-prone patients, or those who manifest the slightest allergic response, should apply a lymph-constricting band proximal to the sting and seek the nearest source of epinephrine and medical attention. In the event of anaphylaxis, aqueous epinephrine in a 1:1000 solution is given subcutaneously. The initial requirement usually is 0.4 to 0.5 mL, and the injection site is massaged vigorously to hasten absorption. For severe anaphylaxis, epinephrine may be given IV in a 1:10,000 solution, injected slowly with caution. The patient is observed closely in case a repeated dose is needed in 20 to 30 minutes. If shock occurs, begin oxygen and apply military antishock trousers (MAST). Intravenous fluid therapy is essential, and if there is severe glottal edema, tracheotomy may be required. Both antihistamines and steroids have delayed effectiveness and are recommended as adjuncts to therapy. Beginning with a daily total dose equivalent to prednisone, 40 mg initially, oral steroids are given twice daily with phased reduction by 5 mg each morning over 5 to 7 days. Thereafter, total resolution of symptoms may justify discontinuation of steroid therapy by the second or third day. In all cases, explicit cautionary advice must be given.

For future exposure, a sting kit should be prescribed for hypersensitive patients, including a lymph-constricting band, injectable and inhalant forms of epinephrine, an oral antihistamine, and detailed written instructions. The patient should carry medical identification tags; wear shoes and light, drab, smooth clothing; apply an insect repellent containing diethyltoluamide; and avoid the use of scented toiletries. Outdoor travel and work around endemic areas such as gardens and garbage collection sites should be avoided, especially in the summer. In addition, the American Academy of Allergy Committee on Insects[29] has recommended that patients who have had systemic or large local reactions be given hyposensitization therapy during risk periods. Ninety-five per cent of individuals so treated have shown lesser reactions when re-stung. Skin testing can be helpful in selecting species specific hyposensitization mixtures and dose schedules at least 3 weeks after a previous reaction; however, it is unreliable, potentially sensitizing, and ill-advised for diagnosis, which should rest on the history alone. To confirm the diagnosis, freeze-dried venom extracts (Pharmalgan) are effective.[30]

ANT STINGS

Stings by most varieties of ants (Fig. 67-2B) cause itching and formation of a wheal and vesicle. Occasionally there are marked swelling and hypersensitivity. Stings by two species of imported fire ants of the southeastern United States have a unique alkaloidal necrotizing factor that additionally causes intense burning pain, pustule formation, and scarring, and may cause retrosternal pain, dyspnea, hypertension, and hemolysis. Fire ants average about 5 mm in length and may be brown or black. They are aggressive inhabitants of agricultural areas, and attack humans or livestock in swarms.

Treatment consists of early wound cleansing and the application of ice, followed by a topical anti-inflammatory agent. Special attention and full-scale precautionary measures are directed toward the treatment and prophylaxis of hypersensitivity reactions. Death, although rare, has been increasingly reported.

ECTOPARASITE AND MISCELLANEOUS INFESTATIONS AND INJURIES

A wide variety of arthropod parasites infest humans and act as vectors for the spread of communicable diseases. Discussion here ·is limited to the diagnosis and treatment of toxic and direct manifestations.

TICK PARALYSIS AND BITES

In addition to being vectors for tularemia and Rocky Mountain spotted fever, all varieties of pregnant female hard ticks (Fig. 67-3) can cause progressive neurologic impairment through a toxic salivary gland factor that is thought to interfere with synaptic transmission in the spinal cord and peripheral nerves. Rarely, there is brain stem dysfunction. In most cases, the tick's attachment in a hair-bearing area has gone unrecognized for several days while the victim develops ataxia, impaired coordination and areflexia, and ascending motor weakness, similar to that seen with Landry-Guillain-Barré syndrome. The typical occurrence, in a child during summer, raises suspicion of anterior poliomyelitis; however, fever, pain, selective muscle spasms, and spinal fluid abnormalities are absent and the victim is apathetic. In the absence of respiratory embarrassment, the effects are entirely reversible with careful search for and detachment of ticks. Intact removal can be accomplished by smothering the tick with petrolatum or gasoline. In a few minutes, the tick releases its hold and can be extracted whole. Otherwise, mouth parts must be excised. When a tick bite is followed within 1 to 12 days by a rash, headache, nausea, vomiting, myalgias, and stomach pains, consider the diagnosis of Rocky Mountain spotted fever. Early therapy with tetracycline can avert later severe complications. Various diagnostic serologic tests are available (e.g., Weil-Felix, complement fixation, latex agglutination). However, these tests are not useful for early diagnosis in the emergency department, which rests on clinical detection. Lyme disease, caused by the deer tick, is covered extensively in the next section of this chapter.

Bites by the venomous pajaroello tick, common to coastal areas of southern California, may cause vesicle formation, necrosis, and a painful, superficial ulcer that heals slowly.

MOSQUITO AND FLY BITES

Mosquitos, deer flies, black flies, and sand flies are all blood-sucking insects among the order Diptera, a group responsible for the transmission of several viral, bacterial, and parasitic diseases. Bites cause focal pain, itching, and swelling, and treatment is palliative. In the case of mosquitoes, there may be urticaria, lethargy, headache, and nausea, but anaphylaxis and death are rare. In the case of black flies, the bite can be extremely painful. It should be cleansed, and a topical anti-inflammatory cream should be applied.

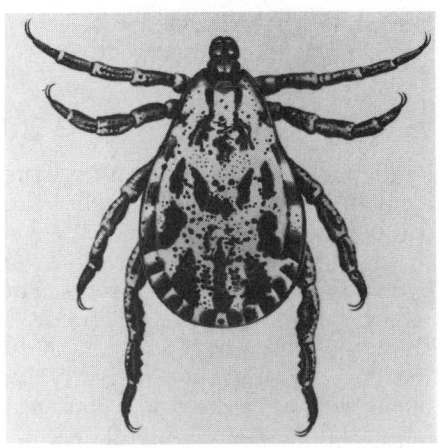

FIG. 67-3.   Rocky Mountain wood tick, *Dermacentor andersoni* (× 6). (Courtesy of Frazier, C.A.; reproduced by permission of Merck Sharp & Dohme, Division of Merck & Co., Inc.)

Oral steroids may be needed for systemic reactions, which are rare. In cases of known allergy, hyposensitization therapy may be justified; however, the application of a diethyltoluamide insect repellent is the best preventive measure.

If the mosquito bites occur in an area where malaria is endemic, primaquine can be administered for 14 days unless the patient has glucose-6-phosphatase deficiency. If fever, chills, myalgias, and signs of malaria are present, diagnosis can be made on a blood smear and suitable chemotherapy started with chloroquine. Chloroquine phosphate, 500 mg/by mouth once weekly, is also the usual regimen for malaria chemoprophylaxis.

LOUSE INFESTATION

Lice are small, gray, crablike parasites that are readily transferred through personal and clothing contact.

Body lice (Pediculus humanus linnaeus) are important vectors of disease, particularly typhus, trench fever, and louse-borne relapsing fever. They cause severe itching, excoriation, pustule formation, and puncta and lichenification along lines of scratching.

Head lice (Pediculus humanus capitis) are found most commonly in scalp hair of women and children, where they deposit prominent nits, or ova. Excoriations, pustule formation, and posterior cervical adenopathy are common, and the hair is usually lusterless and dry.

Pubic lice (Phthirus pubis linnaeus) infest human pubic hair and may migrate to the armpits, eyelashes, and eyebrows, from which they must be meticulously debrided. Recognition is usually delayed until intense itching develops. Small irregular bluish macular eruptions may appear about the trunk and thighs.

Treatment of all lice infestation consists of eradication by thorough shampooing and fine combing of the involved areas, and by applying an ectoparasiticide such as gamma benzene hexachloride. The patient should be instructed to boil clothing and to refer sexual partners for treatment.

BEDBUG AND REDUVIID BUG BITES

Bedbugs are reddish-brown nocturnal blood-feeders averaging 4 to 5 mm in length. They are prevalent throughout the world, and cause itching and erythematous wheals with central red puncta, which may evolve to itching purpuric spots. Local swelling and rare systemic reactions can occur. Bed sheets may show the brown or black spots of blood digested by the bug. Kissing bugs or reduviid bugs are larger blood-sucking arthropods that cause hemorrhagic papules, bullae, and painful urticarial lesions. Treatment is palliative, and prevention requires eradication from sleeping quarters.

MITE INFESTATION

Chigger mites are tiny (0.4 to 0.6 mm) arthropods, harbored in green vegetation in hot temperate areas, which burrow into the skin of their host in the larval stage, creating papular lesions that itch intensely and occasionally look hemorrhagic. Papules about the waist are common because the organism may crawl about until it meets the resistance of clothing. Topical astringents such as camphor and phenol ointment, or a layer of clear fingernail polish, asphyxiate the mite and reduce itching. Oral antihistamines may be helpful.

Itch mites or scabies cause a similar infestation from indoor sources of contact. Outbreaks can be epidemic, most patients showing typical raised itching puncta of burrows, and some showing a diffuse, crusting, nonitching rash that resembles exfoliative dermatitis. Gamma benzene hexachloride is still effective, although there are indications of mild resistance to the drug, which must be applied two or three times initially, and again in one week to cover eggs that may have hatched during the interval. Clothing and bedding must be cleansed thoroughly, and those sharing housing must be referred for treatment.

FLEA BITES

Fleas are small, wingless, blood-sucking insects that infest specific animal hosts, including humans. Bites result in grouped, itching, papular eruptions. Outbreaks are especially common in children in summer. The patient must be thoroughly bathed, and infested rooms must be decontaminated. Fingernail trimming and antipruritic drugs help prevent excoriations.

IRRITATING CATERPILLAR STINGS

Some caterpillars, such as the gray furry pus caterpillar (*Megalophyte opercularis*), are protected by tiny fragile spines that have an urticating effect on contact, and may cause respiratory irritation on inhalation. There is immediate, intense rhythmic pain that may spread regionally. Local swelling, regional lymphadenopathy, nausea, fever, muscle cramps, headaches, and numbness can occur. A gridlike contact lesion develops rapidly and desquamates within hours or days. Spines can be removed with adhesive tape application. Calcium gluconate, given IV, and antihistamines may provide relief.

BLISTER BEETLES

The extruded hemolymph or the crushed-out coelomic fluid of certain beetles may have a powerful urticating and vesicating effect on the skin and eyes on contact. The toxic substance is cantharidin, sometimes prepared as "Spanish fly" and taken orally under the erroneous assumption that it is an aphrodisiac. In this form, it is highly nephrotoxic, and the fatal dose is less than 60 mg. Cutaneous blisters may benefit from topical treatment with magnesium sulfate and methyl alcohol packs.

MARINE ANIMAL BITES AND STINGS (JELLYFISH, STINGRAY, STINGING FISH, SEA URCHINS, STINGING CORAL, OCTOPI, AND CONE SHELLS)

TYPICAL PRESENTATIONS

- A bather enters the ED with painful, whiplike, urticarial eruptions after contact with a large jellyfish.
- A surfer is brought in with a large puncture wound of the calf after stepping on a stingray.
- A fisherman enters with pain and slight swelling of his thumb after handling a sculpin.

Only a handful of the world's venomous marine species (Fig. 67-4) inhabit coastal waters of the United States, but in some areas, the above-mentioned presentations are fairly common. Hundreds of persons each year are injured by stingrays in warmer coastal waters. On the Pacific Coast, sculpin stings requiring treatment are estimated at 300 annually and jellyfish stings are common among surf bathers and fishermen (Fig. 67-4A). In Atlantic and Gulf Coast waters, the Portuguese man-of-war (*Physalia physalis*), a hydroid with trails of tentacles several yards long, poses a significant threat to bathers.

Most venomous marine species are sedentary or slow-swimming and use their venom apparatus defensively. Injuries arise from inadvertent contact. Stinging marine vertebrates, such as stingrays (Fig. 67-4B) and spiny fish (including catfish), possess remarkably similar thermolabile venoms; *thus, heat application rather than ice application is the primary mode of therapy*. As a whole, marine animal venoms are simpler

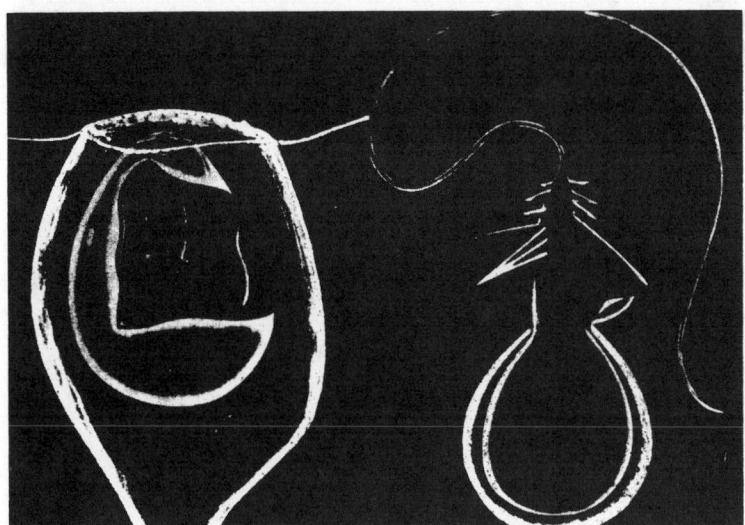

A

FIG. 67-4.   Marine animals. A. Diagrammatic sketch of the undischarged and discharged nematocysts of a jellyfish. (From Findlay, E.: Marine toxins and venomous and poisonous marine animals. *In* Russell, F.A. (ed.): Advances in Marine Biology, Vol. 3. New York, Academic Press, 1965, p. 275. Fig. 2; reproduced by permission.) B. Stinging action of the round stingray. C. Stonefish: *Synanceja horrida.* (Reprinted by permission. From Halstead, B.W.: Dangerous Marine Animals. Cambridge, Md., Cornell Maritime Press, Inc., 1959.)

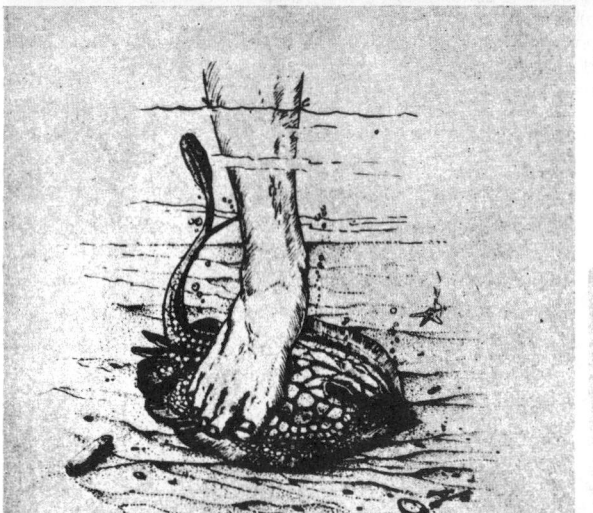

B

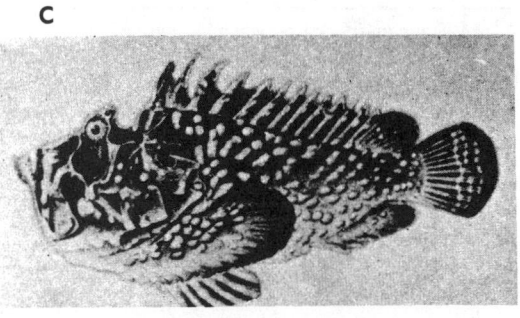

C

and shorter-acting than those of terrestrial animals. Deaths are rare except when caused by drowning or anaphylaxis; however, the "stonefish," found in the Indo-Pacific area, can cause hypotension and cardiovascular collapse (Fig. 67-4C). Although no venomous marine animals have been suspected of harboring tetanus spores, bacterial contamination is not uncommon, and tetanus prophylaxis is therefore advisable.

Table 67-2 outlines the basic treatment for marine animal bites and stings.

JELLYFISH AND HYDROID STINGS

Jellyfish and hydroid tentacles (Fig. 67-4) carry an abundance of capsular stingers with springlike microscopic barbs that trigger when mechanically or histochemically stimulated. The venom contains a number of quaternary ammonium compounds, histamine, and low-molecular weight proteins that effect paralysis through cholinergic neurons.

Tentacle contact produces localized edema, erythema, vesiculation, itching, and pain in a whiplike urticarial pattern. The pain may spread regionally, and weakness, nausea, headache, truncal muscle spasms, increased lacrimation, perspiration, vertigo, violent twitching, and dyspnea can occur. Collapse and cardiac arrest have been reported. The anaphylaxis phenomenon was discovered during studies with these toxins, and the risk is significant.

Treatment is directed at preventing nematocyst discharge by stabilization, fixation, and removal of tentacles. The area should be rinsed with sea water, and large fragments should be teased away. Medicinal alcohol, drinking alcohol, or meat tenderizers can be used as fixatives. Next, a drying agent, such as dry sand, flour, or talc, helps coalesce the tentacles so that they can be scraped away with a blade. Rinsing with a dilute basic solution such as baking soda or ammonium hydroxide helps neutralize the acidic venom. Antihistamines, topical corticosteroids, and opiate analgesics may be needed. Systemic complications are treated symptomatically. One should never stimulate

TABLE 67-2. GENERAL TREATMENT OF JELLYFISH, STINGRAY, AND SPINY FISH STINGS

	Jellyfish Stings	Stingray Sting	Spiny Fish Stings
Confirm and quantitate envenomation; look for signs of local toxicity	*Local:* Wheal and flare, burning pain *Systemic:* Allergic reactions, shock, cardiac arrhythmias	*Local:* Puncture wound with severe pain *Systemic:* Shock, cardiac arrhythmias	*Local:* Severe pain with minimal reaction *Systemic:* Shock, cardiac arrhythmias
Identify offending organism by species			
Remove venom from wound and retard absorption	Remove tentacles gently; rinse with sea water or scrape away with beach sand; *do not apply fresh water;* do not touch with bare hands; apply alcohol topically	Remove all foreign material and irrigate wound; anesthetize locally as needed; rule out retained spine by x-ray	Cleanse and cool topically
Neutralize venom or counteract its effects	Baking soda mixture followed by topical anti-inflammatory creams	Immerse extremity in tap water as hot as patient can tolerate before débridement; continue immersion up to 60 minutes	Immerse extremity in tap water as hot as patient can tolerate before débridement; continue immersion up to 60 minutes
Treat secondary and late effects	Monitor and treat for anaphylaxis; support airway, ventilation, and perfusion; support blood pressure with repeated doses of epinephrine and colloidal fluids IV; consider MAST garment	Monitor for shock and cardiac arrhythmias until pain resolves	Monitor for shock and cardiac arrhythmias until pain resolves

Abbreviations: MAST = Military antishock trousers; IV = intravenous.

nematocyst discharge by rubbing the area or applying fresh water.

STINGRAY INJURY

Stingrays (Fig. 67-4B) impale their victims with a sheathed spine, up to 30 cm in length, carried on the whiplike tail. Most punctures and lacerations occur in the calf when the victim treads on the animal; however, penetrations of the thorax or abdomen can occur.

As the sting penetrates the skin, the integumentary sheath is ruptured, releasing the venom. Portions of the sheath and, rarely, portions of the spine remain in the wound. The venom contains thermolabile proteins and serotonin. It depresses respiration and causes reversible repolarization and atrioventricular conduction changes in mammalian hearts. Locally, the intense pain is maximal by 90 minutes and may persist for several hours. Wounds are jagged and may have surrounding discoloration, erythema, and edema, which are slow to resolve. Pain is severe, and weakness, nausea, syncope, sweating, regional muscle cramping, and lymph node pain are common. Severe envenomation may cause vomiting, diarrhea, sweating, respiratory distress, and arrhythmias.

Treatment begins with removal of accessible pieces of the integumentary sheath and irrigation with salt water. A lymph-constricting band is applied intermittently above the wound site, and the extremity is submerged for up to 90 minutes in a bath of water as hot as the victim can tolerate. This treatment significantly alleviates the pain and systemic complications. The wound is then injected with a local anesthetic and inspected directly; radiographs should be studied for evidence of retained material. Debridement, suturing, and systemic analgesia may be required. Individualized antibiotic therapy should be considered, and the patient should be protected against tetanus.

FISH STINGS

Pacific Coast sculpins and bullheads, together with the notorious stonefish (Fig. 67-4C), of the South Pacific, are members of the scorpionfish family. All are slow-moving bottom dwellers with spines located dorsally and in the anal and pelvic areas. Integumentary sheaths around some of the dorsal spines form the venom apparatus.

Envenomation arises from shallow punctures that have a surrounding ischemic appearance and cause excruciating pain, hyperesthesia, paresthesias, swelling, and blister formation. Severe envenomations by the stonefish and other extremely toxic species may cause dyspnea, hypotension, collapse, and death within 1 hour. Continuous immersion of the affected part, in water as hot as the patient can tolerate, is clearly the most effective treatment. In addition, infiltration of the wound with a solution of emetine hydrochloride may be beneficial.

Other stinging fish, including surgeonfishes, toadfishes, ratfishes, weaverfishes, and catfish, cause similar intoxications with their stings. All of their venoms are thermolabile and respond well to the detoxifying effects of hot water immersion.

SEA URCHIN PUNCTURES

Both the brittle calcareous spines and the tiny pincerlike pedicellaria of some sea urchins are venomous. Punctures, arising when bathers step on the animal, pose a difficult problem for foreign body removal and give rise to granulomatous tracts. There is immediate, intense burning pain at the site, and generalized weakness, numbness, paresthesia, muscle atonia, dyspnea, and arrhythmis may occur. Even mild cases can cause dizziness, poor coordination, and localized pain. Driving can be very hazardous after such a sting. Spines of Diadema, a Caribbean genus, may be up to a foot long and may cause dark staining in the puncture tract.

For this group, debridement is advised because spines are not absorbed readily. Spines of most other sea urchins are resorbed within days, and debridement is seldom worthwhile.

CORAL STINGS

Fire coral and stony coral are tropical species that cause pain, itching, and papular lesions on abrasive contact. Pustules may form and desquamate or ulcerate. Secondary infections are common, and wounds must be scrubbed and soaked thoroughly. A commonly used name is "devil's reef." Symptoms are severe within hours and usually clear in 3 days. Some patients experience generalized weakness, dizziness, and burning local pain. These corals are found around the Mexican coastline in particular.

OCTOPUS BITE

Octopi, with their powerful jaws shaped like an inverted parrot's beak, can inflict deep punctures, with pain, tingling, itching, and profuse bleeding from the wound. Swelling may be marked. Central nervous system dysfunction and fatalities have been reported from bites by tiny cephalopods, found along Australia's Great Barrier Reef, but those along the Pacific Coast of North America, although among the largest in the world, are relatively docile and less toxic.

CONE SHELL STING

Cone shells, including Californian and Hawaiian coastal varieties, extend the proboscis and impale the victim with a harpoon-like disposable radular tooth.

The injury usually occurs when the attractive shell is scraped by an unwary collector. There is immediate intense pain about the ischemic-looking wound, which heals slowly. Numbness, tingling, and muscular irritability are common. Incoordination, aphonia, dysphagia, visual disturbances, chest pain, and coma can occur, and, rarely, death from cardiac failure or respiratory paralysis may ensue.

SEA SNAKE BITE

Sea snakes inhabit tropical waters across the Indo-Pacific area from the Red Sea to Mexico's Sea of Cortez. Their venom is specifically toxic to striated muscle, releasing myoglobin between 30 minutes and 8 hours after the bite. There is marked weakness, ptosis, and muscular rigidity. Pain is excruciating, and death may occur early from cardiac failure, or later from renal tubular necrosis. Treatment is directed at maintaining renal output by means of supporting the blood pressure and alkalinizing the urine.

NONVENOMOUS BITES

Treatment of shark and other nonvenomous marine bites is straightforward. Wound infections are common, and prophylactic antibiotic therapy and tetanus immunization are advised.

REFERENCES

1. Parrish, H.M.: Death from bites and stings of venomous animals in the United States. Arch. Intern. Med. *104*:198, 1959.
2. Litowitz, T.L., Normann, S.A., and Veltri, J.C.: 1985 Annual Report of the American Association of Poison Control Centers National Data Collection System. Am. J. Emerg. Med. *4*:427, 1986.
3. Banner, W., Jr.: Bites and stings in the pediatric patient. *In* Current Problems in Pediatrics. Edited by Lockhart, J.D., vol. XVIII:1–69, 1988.
4. Wasserman, G.S., and Anderson, P.C.: Loxoscelism and Necrotic arachnidism, J. Toxicol. Clin. Toxicol. *2*:451, 1983.
5. Chu, J., Rush, C.T., and O'Connor, D.M.: Hemolytic anemia following brown spider (Loxosceles reclusa) bite. Clin. Toxicol. *12*:531, 1978.
6. Vorse, M., et al.: Disseminated intravascular coagulopathy following fatal brown spider bite. J. Pediatr. *80*:1035, 1972.
7. Auer, A.T., and Hershey, F.B.: Surgery for necrotic bites of the brown spider. Arch. Surg. *108*:612, 1973.
8. Arnold, R.E.: Brown recluse spider bites: Five cases with a review of the literature. JACEP *4*:262, 1976.
9. Fardon, D.W., Wingo, C.W., and Robinson, D.W.: The treatment of brown recluse spider bite. Plast. Reconstr. Surg. *40*:482, 1967.
10. Rees, R.S., et al.: Management of the brown recluse spider bite. Plast. Reconstr. Surg. *68*:768, 1981.
11. Rees, R.S., et al.: The diagnosis and treatment of brown recluse spider bites. Ann. Emerg. Med. *6*:945, 1987.
12. Berger, R.S.: A critical look at therapy for the brown recluse spider bite. Arch. Dermatol. *107*:298, 1973.

13. Rauber, A.: Black widow spider bites. J. Toxicol. Clin. Toxicol. 21:473, 1983–84.
14. Key, G.A.: A comparison of calcium gluconate and methoxcarbamal (Robaxin^R) in the treatment of latrodectism. Am. J. Trop. Med. Hgy. 301:273, 1981.
15. Report: Antivenin (Latrodectus Mactans), West Point, PA, 1975. Marck, Sharp & Dohme, 1975.
16. Sutherland, S.K., and Trinca, J.C.: Survey of 2144 cases of redback spider bites. Med. J. Aust. 2:620, 1978.
17. Litovitz, T.L., Normann, S.A., and Veltri, J.C.: 1985. Annual Report of the American Association of Poison Control Centers National Data Collection System. Am. J. Emerg. Med. 4:427, 1986.
18. Yaron, R.: Scorpion venom: A tutorial review of its effects in men and experimental animals. Clin. Toxicol. 3:561, 1970.
19. Moczydlowski, E., Lucchesi, K., and Ravindran, A.: An emerging pharmacology of peptide toxins targeted against potassium channels. J. Mem. Biol. 105:95, 1988.
20. Curry, S.C., et al.: Envenomation by the scorpion Centruroides sculpturatus. J. Toxicol. Clin. Toxicol. 21:417, 1983.
21. Carbone, E., et al.: Selective modification of the squid axon Na currents by Centruroides noxius Toxin II-10. J. Physiol. (Paris) 79:179, 1984.
22. Likes, K., Banner, W., and Chavez, M.: Centruroides exilicauda envenomation in Arizona. West J. Med. 141:634, 1984.
23. Amitai, Y., Mines, Y., and Aker, M., Goitein, K., Scorpion sting in children: A review of 51 cases. Clin. Pediatr. 24:136–140, 1985.
24. Brand, A. et al.: Myocardial damage after a scorpion sting: Long-term echocardiographic follow-up. Pediatr. Cardiol. 9:59–61, 1988.
25. Gueron, M., et al.: Hemodynamic and myocardial consequences of scorpion venom. Am. J. Cardiol. 45:979, 1980.
26. Gueron, M., and Weizmann, S.: Catecholamines and mycardial damage in scorpion sting. Am. Heart. J. 75:715, 1968.
27. Ismail, M., Osman, O.H., Detkovic, D.: electrocardiographic studies with scorpion venom. Toxicon 14:79, 1976.
28. Stahnke, H.L.: Arizona's lethal scorpion. Ariz. Med. 29:490, 1972.
29. Insect Allergy Committee of the American Academy of Allergy: Insect sting allergy. JAMA, 193:109, 1965.
30. Food and Drug Administration: FDA approves insect venom products. FAD Drug Bull. 9:15, 1979.

BIBLIOGRAPHY

SPIDER BITES (GENERAL)

Rees, R.S., and Campbell, D.S.: Spider Bites in Management of Wilderness and Environmental Emergencies (2nd ed.). Edited by Auerbach, P.S. and Geehr, E.C. St. Louis, C.V. Mosby Co., 1989.

BROWN SPIDER BITES

Atkins, J.A., Wingo, C.W., Sodeman, W.A., et al.: Necrotic arachnidism. Am. J. Trop. Med. Hyg. 7:165, 1958.

Dillaha, C.J., Jansen, C.T., et al.: North American loxoscelism. JAMA 1988:33, 1964.

Hershey, F.B., and Aulenbacher, C.E.: Surgical treatment of brown spider bites, Am. Surg. 170:300, 1969.

Nance, W.E.: Hemolytic anemia of necrotic arachnidism. Am. J. Med. 31:801, 1961.

Russell, F.E., Waldron, and Mandon, M.B.: Bites by the brown spiders Loxosceles unicolor and Loxosceles arizonica in California and Arizona. Toxicon 7:109, 1969.

BLACK WIDOW SPIDER BITES

Britos, S.A., Orsincher, O.A., and Fulginiti, S.: Effects of venom gland extract of the black widow spider on rat brain and heart levels of noradrenaline, 5-hydroxytryptamine and acetylcholine. Toxicon 16:393, 1978.

Frontali, N.: Catecholamine-depleting effect of black widow spider venom on iris nerve fibers. Brain Res. 37:146, 1972.

Howard, B.D., and Gunderson, C.B., Jr.: Effects of mechanisms of polypeptide and neurotoxins that act presynaptically. Ann. Rev. Pharmacol. Toxicol. 20:307, 1980.

Pintos, J.E.B., et al.: Peripheral adrenergic effect of latrodectus mactans venom on smooth muscle. Toxicon 11:395, 1973.

HYMENOPTERA STINGS AND ALLERGY

Barclay, W.R.: Emergency treatment of insect sting allergy. JAMA 240:2735, 1978.

Barr, S.E.: Allergy to Hymenoptera stings—review of the world literature: 1953–1970. Ann. Allergy 29:49, 1971.

Bonner, J.R.: Stinging insect allergy—what to do for the patient. Consultant 18:49, 1978.

Feingold, B.E.: Allergic reactions to hymenoptera stings. J. Asthma Res. 9:55, 1971.

Hoffman, D.R., Miller, J.S., and Sutton, J.L.: Hymenoptera venom allergy. Ann. Allergy 45:276, 1980.

Hunt, K.J., et al.: A controlled trial of immunotherapy in insect hypersensitivity. New Engl. J. Med. 299:157, 1978.

Lichtenstein, L.M.: Allergic responses to airborne allergens and insect venoms. Fed. Proc. 36:1727, 1977.

Miller, H.E., and Ward, W.A.: Heparin treatment of bee and wasp stings. JACEP 3:168, 1974.

Muller, U., Spiess, J., Roth, A.: Serological investigations in hymenoptera sting allergy. Clin. Allergy 7:147, 1977.

Ortel, T.O., and Loehr, M.M.: Bee sting anaphylaxis: use of M.A.S.T. Ann. Emerg. Med. 13:459, 1984.

Passero, M.A., Dees, S.C.: Allergy to stings from winged things. Am. Fam. Physician 7:74, 1973.

Pearn, J.H.: Bee stings in operational theaters. Milit. Med. 137:241, 1972.

Reisman, R.E.: Treating patients with insect sting allergy. Consultant 19:23, 1979.

TICK PARALYSIS

Cherington, M., and Snyder, R.D.: Tick paralysis. New Engl. J. Med. 78:95, 1978.

Faust, E.C., and Russell, P.F.: Clinical Parasitology, 7th ed. Philadelphia, Lea and Febiger, 1964. pp. 986–987.

Haller, J.S., and Fabara, J.A.: Tick paralysis: A case report with emphasis on neurological toxicity. Am. J. Dis. Child. 124:915, 1970.

Rose, I.: A review of tick paralysis. J. Can. Med. Assoc. 70:175, 1954.

MARINE ANIMAL BITES AND STINGS

Bitseff, E.L., Garoni, W.J., Hardison, C.D., Thompson, J.M.: The management of stingray injuries of the extremities. Southern Med. J. *63*:417, 1970.

Halstead, B.W.: Poisonous and Venomous Marine Animals. Washington, D.C., U.S. Government Printing Office, 1965.

Russell, F.E.: Marine Toxins and Venomous and Poisonous Marine Animals. London, Academic Press, 1965.

ADDITIONAL BIBLIOGRAPHY

Anderson, P.C.: What's new in loxoscelism? Mo. Med. *70*:711, 1973.

Auerbach, P.S. and Geehr, E.C. (eds.): Management of Wilderness & Environmental Emergencies (2nd ed.), St. Louis, C.V. Mosby Co., 1989.

Banner, W., Jr., Spiders. *In* Management of Wilderness and Environmental Emergencies (2nd ed.), St. Louis, C.V. Mosby Co., 1989.

Frazier, C.A.: Insect Allergy. St. Louis, Warren H. Green, Inc., 1969.

Frazier, C.A.: Allergic responses to biting and stinging insects. J. Asthma Res. *10*:3, 1972.

Insect Allergy Committee of the American Academy of Allergy: Insect sting allergy. JAMA *193*:109, 1965.

Marsden, P.D.: Coleptera (Beetles). *In* Beeson, P.B., and McDermott, W. (eds.): Textbook of Medicine. Philadelphia, W. B. Saunders Company, 1975.

McConnell, J.G., et al.: Alkaloid from fire ant venom. Science *168*:840, 1970.

McHugh, T.P., Ruderman, A.E., and Gibbons, T.E.: Rocky Mountain spotted fever. Ann. Emerg. Med. *13*:1132, 1984.

Rose, I.: A review of tick paralysis. J. Can. Med. Assoc. *70*:175, 1954.

Schaeffer, R.C., Carlson, R.W., Puri, V.C., et al.: Effects of colloidal and crystalloidal fluids in rattlesnake venom shock in the rat. J. Pharm. Exper. Ther. *206*:687, 1978.

Stair, T., Ricci, R., Pedicano, J., and Kane, J.: Malaria in the emergency department. Ann. Emerg. Med. *12*:422, 1983.

TICK-BORNE DISEASES

Mary Anne Mangelsen

CAPSULE

Although recognized as vectors of disease since 1893, ticks have been given more attention since the 1980s, when they were indicted as the vectors of Lyme disease. It has been known for years that human vector ticks are capable of transmitting bacterial, viral, rickettsial, and protozoan diseases as well as harming man by the mechanical injury of their bites and the production of their own toxins (Table 67-3). About 300 species are bloodsucking ectoparasites of mammals, birds, reptiles, and amphibians and nearly all are capable of biting man. Emergency medicine includes the necessity of recognizing the vector (which may vary from a speck to almost a centimeter in size), the method of removing it properly from the skin, the bite, and the disease syndromes. This section of the chapter reviews Lyme disease, Rocky Mountain spotted fever or tick-borne typhus, babesiosis, Colorado tick fever, Ehrlichiosis, tick-borne encephalitis and tick paralysis, Q fever, relapsing fever, and tularemia.

THE LIFE OF A TICK

Although the 1- to 2-year life cycle of a tick may vary according to species, a typical female hard tick increases greatly in size after an engorgement of blood for 5 to 13 days, drops off the host to deposit in 14 to 41 days 2000 to 8000 small, oval, brown eggs, and then dies 3 to 36 days after oviposition. After 2 to 7 weeks, larvae with three pairs of legs emerge from the eggs, attach themselves to small animals for a blood meal, drop off, and molt into nymphs with eight legs. Nymphs may hibernate over the winter and, after one or more blood meals, molt into adults on the ground. The same or different species of mammals (deer, dogs, mouse, raccoon, rabbits, birds) may serve as hosts for the various stages. The mature unengorged tick may be about the size of a large freckle; the immature nymph may be as small as the head of a pin.

The tick's mouth (borne on a capitulum) with its transverse rows of recurrent file-like teeth anchors the parasite to the host. Glands secrete a tenacious fluid during feeding that, after a few hours, aids the tick in burying its head in the skin. Body fluids, feces, and

TABLE 67-3. MOST COMMON TICK-BORNE DISEASES OF NORTH AMERICA

Disease	Pathogen	Vector	Common Locations
Babesiosis	Babesia microti	Ioxdes dammini (deer tick) (Figure 67-5)	Islands and coastal areas of Massachusetts and New York
Colorado tick fever	Orbivirus	Dermacentor andersoni (wood tick)	Rocky Mountains
Ehrlichiosis	Ehrlichia canis	Rhipicephalus sanguineus	Southern United States and East Coast
Lyme disease	Borrelia burgdorferi	I. dammini pacificus Amblyomma americanum	Throughout United States, greatest in New England and Minnesota and Wisconsin
Q fever	Coxiella burnetii	D. andersoni A. americanum	Ubiquitous in the United States
Relapsing fever	Borrelia hermsii	Ornithodoros hermsi	Western United States
Rocky Mountain spotted fever	Rickettsia rickettsii	D. andersoni Dermacentor variabilis (dog tick)	Predominantly southeastern United States
Tick-borne encephalitis	Flavivirus	Ixodes marxi Ixodes cookei	Canada and northern United States
Tick paralysis	Neurotoxin	D. andersoni D. variabilis	
Tularemia	Franciscella tularensis	D. variabilis A. americanum	Deep South and Utah

the engorged blood may all be carrying microbes. Typically, however, ticks salivate copiously during feeding, the saliva serving as the most obvious vehicle for transmission.

TICK REMOVAL

Forcible removal of the tick is likely to tear the body away from the capitulum, which remains embedded in the skin. I can personally attest to the fact that using a hot match on the dorsum of the tick does not usually induce it to budge; neither does the application of vaseline, fingernail polish, polish remover, or alcohol. In fact, these methods can cause the thin wall of the engorged tick to rupture and spill its engorged blood. The most effective method known to date is to grasp the tick (with gloves) as close as possible to its head with a blunt forceps and slowly pull upwards with steady, even pressure. Then kill the tick in disinfectant and disinfect the bite site.

LYME DISEASE

DNA hybridization studies of nine strains of the Lyme disease spirochete indicates that these organisms constitute a new species of Borrelia.[1] Most patients with

this disease have no memory of tick exposure because the nymph form of Ixodes dammini (Fig. 67-5) is too small. Other vectors may be indicted in the future.

This Borrelia disease causes a systemic, immune-mediated inflammatory disorder characterized by the rash erythema chronicum migrans (ECM) (Fig. 67-6) which may be followed by involvement of the joints, heart, and nervous system. Typically, the symptoms appear for the first time in the summer. The disease follows a chronic, relapsing course and, during the later stages, arthritis is the principal clinical manifestation. All age groups are affected.

CLINICAL PRESENTATION

The first stage begins several weeks after the tick bite and is characterized by erythema chronicum migrans (ECM) (Fig. 67-6) at the site of the bite, a low-grade fever, chills, malaise, stiff neck, arthralgias, and myalgias. Some patients report nausea, vomiting, sore throat, lymphadenopathy, and occasionally conjunctivitis. Additional annular lesions may develop. Kernig and Brudzinski's signs are usually absent.

In the untreated patient, the second stage develops within weeks to months of the rash, and involves the heart and central nervous system (CNS). Headache of fluctuating intensity, lack of concentration, and a Bell's palsy or bilateral facial palsies are common. A combination of meningoencephalitis, radiculoneuritis, and myelitis may be present, but coma does not occur. Treatment can resolve the meningoencephalitis within 2 weeks. Dysesthesias, weakness, and loss of deep tendon reflexes usually resolve in 7 to 8 weeks with or without antibiotic therapy. Neurologic syndromes in which Lyme disease has been implicated are shown in Table 67-4. As noted, Lyme disease is the new "great imitator." In its various stages, it can masquerade as a flu-like syndrome, syphilis, multiple sclerosis, or presenile dementia.

Myocarditis with conduction system abnormalities most commonly develop in young men. Cardiac valves are spared. First, second, or complete heart block may continue for up to 6 weeks and has not been helped by antimicrobial therapy. Cardiac monitoring is recommended for patients with a PR interval of 0.3 seconds or more. A temporary pacemaker may be indicated. Stage three is the development of frank arthritis weeks to years after ECM. Other forms of arthritis that might be confused with Lyme disease include (1) periarticular juvenile rheumatoid arthritis; (2) Reiter's syndrome; (3) psoriatic arthritis; (4) gonococcal arthritis; (5) reactive arthritis associated with Salmonella, Shigella or Yersinia infections; (6) postinfectious or infectious arthritis; or (7) temporomandibular joint syndrome (TMJ).[3] Early treatment with antibiotics may or may not prevent this stage.

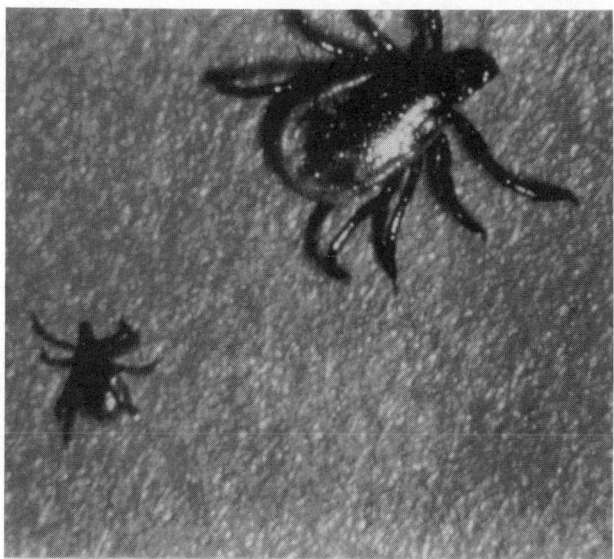

FIG. 67-5. *Lyme disease vector, Ixodes dammini tick. Courtesy of Dr. Andrew Spielman, Department of Tropical Public Health, Harvard School of Medicine, Harvard University, Boston, Massachusetts.*

DIAGNOSIS

The diagnosis of stage 1 rests on the recognition of ECM since blood cultures and serologic testing identify Borrelia burgdorferi less than 50% of the time.[4] Nonspecific tests include an increased erythrocyte sedimentation rate and increased serum glutamic oxaloacetic transaminase level. Serum IgM is elevated. Spinal fluid typically reveals a normal opening pressure, a lymphocytic pleocytosis, an elevated protein level, and normal glucose values. The organism is rarely recovered. Computerized tomography (CT) of the head is negative. Enzyme-linked immunosorbent assay (ELISA) is the currently preferred procedure, with better sensitivity and specificity for all stages of the disease, but in the first weeks of infection even ELISA lacks the desired level of sensitivity.[5]

Because even the skin manifestations of this disease may be subtle, clinical suspicion of Lyme disease should be aroused by a young patient with arthritis or negative rheumatoid and antinuclear antibody factors, in combination with cardiac conduction abnormalities or lymphocytic meningitis. Although serologic assays remain the best tests, a small percentage of patients with Lyme disease may be seronegative and require an assessment of T-cell blastogenesis.[6] Even so, immunologic tests indicate exposure and do not by themselves prove that the patient has an active infectious process.[7] Neither should they form the sole basis for administration of antibiotic therapy.

Patients with a negative serologic test and presumptive or definite signs and symptoms of Lyme disease should receive prompt antibiotic therapy without a delay for laboratory confirmation on convalescent specimens. Early administration of antibiotics is likely, however, to abrogate the antibody response.

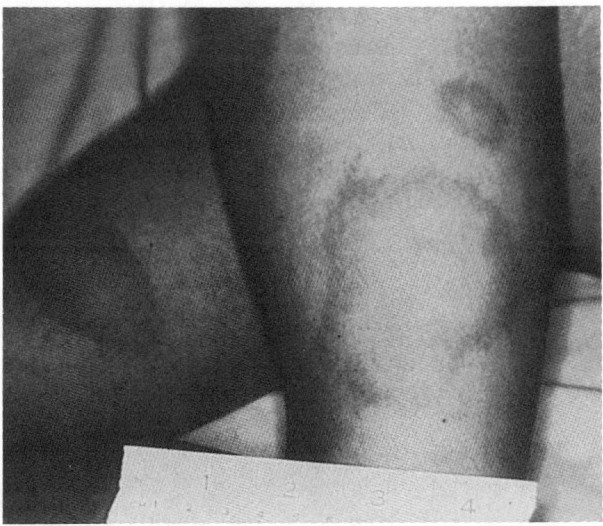

FIG. 67-6. *Example of erythema chronicum migrans (ECM) lesion. With permission from Steere, A.C., et al.: The clinical evolution of Lyme arthritis. Ann. Intern. Med. 86:685–698, 1977.*

TREATMENT

Table 67-5 lists the treatment regimens for Lyme disease, but these recommendations are based on limited data and are subject to future changes.

Aspirin therapy (3.6 g per day in divided doses) or prednisone (40 to 60 mg per day in divided doses) has been recommended for adults with complete heart block and cardiomegaly.[9] The appropriate treatment for Lyme disease during pregnancy is unclear. Some physicians choose to give high dose intravenous pen-

TABLE 67-4. NEUROLOGIC SYNDROMES IN WHICH LYME DISEASE HAS BEEN IMPLICATED

Clearly established association	Meningitis Encephalitis Cranial and spinal nerve palsies Radiculitis Peripheral neuropathy
Possible association	Acute transverse myelitis Guillain-Barré syndrome (with oligoclonal banding) Neuropsychiatric syndromes Severe incapacitating fatigue Optic neuritis Spastic paraparesis Ataxia Carpal tunnel syndrome Epilepsy Chorea Amyotrophy
Unlikely to be associated	Multiple sclerosis Presenile dementia

icillin to all pregnant women with Lyme disease. No vaccine is available.

ROCKY MOUNTAIN SPOTTED FEVER (RMSF, TICK-BORNE TYPHUS)

Originally identified in the Rocky Mountain states, RMSF occurs predominantly in the southeastern United States, although an increase in the number of cases has been observed in several eastern states in the past few years. The wood tick (Dermacentor andersoni) in the west and the dog tick (Dermacentor variabilis) in the southeast are vectors as well as reservoirs of Rickettsia rickettsii, the gram-negative obligate intracellular microorganism. In Connecticut, an endemic area, three species of ticks were found positive for this rickettsial organism. The skin rash appears 2 to 3 days after the abrupt onset of headache,

TABLE 67-5. TREATMENT REGIMENS FOR LYME DISEASE

Manifestation	Regimen*
Early infection* 　Adults	Tetracycline, 250 mg orally 4 × daily, 10–30 days† Doxycycline, 100 mg orally 2 × daily, 10–30 days†‡ Amoxicillin, 500 mg orally 4 × daily, 10–30 days
Children (≤8 yr)	Amoxicillin or penicillin V, 250 mg orally 　3 × daily or 20 mg/kilogram of body weight/day in 　divided doses, 10–30 days In case of penicillin allergy: Erythromycin, 250 mg orally 3 × daily or 　30 mg/kilogram/day in divided doses, 10–30 　days‡
Neurologic abnormalities (early or late)* 　General	Ceftriaxone, 2 g intravenously 1 × daily, 14 days§ Penicillin G, 20 million U intravenously, 6 divided 　doses daily, 14 days§ In case of ceftriaxone or penicillin allergy: Doxycycline, 100 mg orally 2 × daily, 30 days§ Chloramphenicol, 250 mg intravenously 4 × daily, 　14 days§
Facial palsy alone	Oral regimens may be adequate
Cardiac abnormalities	
First-degree atrioventricular block 　　(PR interval <0.3 sec)	Oral regimens, as for early infection
High-degree atrioventricular block	Ceftriaxone, 2 g intravenously 1 × daily, 14 days§ Penicillin, 20 million U intravenously, 6 divided 　doses daily, 14 days§
Arthritis (intermittent or chronic)	Doxycycline, 100 mg orally 2 × daily, 30 days Amoxicillin and probenecid, 500 mg each orally 　4 × daily, 30 days Ceftriaxone, 2 g intravenously 1 × daily, 14 days Penicillin, 20 million U intravenously, 6 divided 　doses daily, 14 days
Acrodermatitis	Oral regimens for 1 month usually adequate

* Treatment failures have occurred with all these regimens, and retreatment may be necessary.
† The duration of therapy is based on clinical response.
‡ The antibiotic has not yet been tested systematically for this indication in Lyme disease.
§ The appropriate duration of therapy is not yet clear for patients with late neurologic abnormalities, and it may be longer than two weeks.

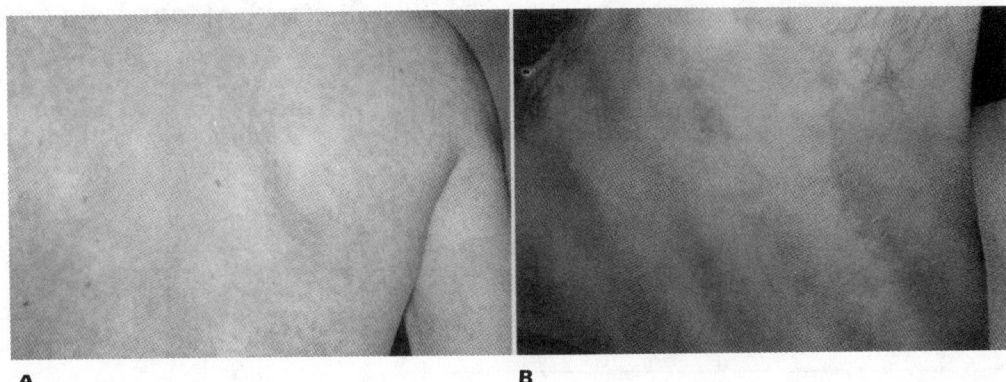

FIG. 67-7.   Rocky Mountain spotted fever. Courtesy of Howard M. Simons, M.D.

fever, chills, myalgia, nausea, and vomiting. It consists of 1 to 4 mm blanching macules which become petechial and usually start on the distal extremities and spread to the trunk, palms, and soles. Eventually the neck and face are involved (Fig. 67-7). Because the rash is frequently confused with the rash of viral exanthems, measles, and drug eruptions, delay in treatment is common. The disease has even presented as thrombotic thrombocytopenic purpura.[10] Fatal cases present most commonly in stupor or coma.

DIAGNOSIS

Thrombocytopenia is present in about 30% of the cases and hyponatremia in 25%. Chest x rays may demonstrate alveolar or interstitial infiltrates. Once the rash develops, the diagnosis can be confirmed by immunofluorescence of skin biopsies of fresh macules using fluorescent antibodies to Rickettsia rickettsii. Indirect hemagglutination (IHA) and indirect fluorescent antibody tests (IFA) appear to be the most sensitive serologic tests currently in use for the diagnosis of RMSF.[11]

TREATMENT

Oral tetracycline, 500 mg every 6 hours, or 25 mg per kg loading dose, with the same dose divided daily thereafter, or chloramphenicol, 50 mg per kg loading dose followed by the same dose divided in four doses per day is the antimicrobial therapy of choice. Chloramphenicol has the advantage of treating meningococcemia when the latter is included in the differential diagnosis in a patient with fever and rash.

BABESIOSIS

Spread by the same deer tick that is a vector for Lyme disease in New England, the protozoan Babesia mi-

croti may cause a mild self-limited illness or produce no symptoms. Asymptomatic parasitemia makes the incubation period unknown and the disease acquirable through blood transfusions. The illness develops insidiously, with fever, myalgias, chills, and malaise. In splenectomized patients, overwhelming sepsis can develop and a persistent infection has been reported in a patient infected with human immunodeficiency virus (HIV).

The diagnosis is made by a blood smear that demonstrates intraerythrocytic ring forms of the parasite. The ring form of B. microti is distinguished from the ring form of Plasmodium falciparum by the lack of intraerythrocytic pigment. Clindamycin, 1.2 gm intravenously every 12 hours combined with quinine, 650 mg orally three times daily is the treatment of choice for the adult.

COLORADO TICK FEVER

The Colorado tick fever orbivirus is spread to humans by the wood tick Dermacentor andersoni. This self-limited disease is confined to the Rocky Mountain area. Not associated with a rash, the disease is characterized by the sudden onset of fever, chills, headache, retro-orbital pain, myalgias, nausea, and vomiting. An afebrile interval of one to two days interrupts the febrile illness. Frequently, leukopenic patients are diagnosed more definitively by the detection of antibodies to the virus or by virus isolation from red blood cells. Convalescence of longer than 3 weeks is common. Treatment is symptomatic.

EHRLICHIOSIS

The brown dog tick (Rhipicephalus) is presumed to be the vector of the rickettsia Ehrlichia canis. Ehrlichiosis is rare but can be distinguished from Rocky Mountain spotted fever by the lack of a rash. Most patients have a sudden onset of fever, rigors, headache, myalgias, nausea, and vomiting. Lymphopenia, leukopenia, thrombocytopenia, and abnormal liver function tests are most frequently found. Inclusion bodies (the rickettsiae) are seen in atypical lymphocytes on peripheral blood smears. Latex agglutination tests are negative for Rickettsia rickettsii antibodies. Tetracycline, 500 mg every 6 hours is a reasonable dose for adults.

TICK-BORNE ENCEPHALITIS AND TICK PARALYSIS

Spread by the Ixodes species, tick-borne encephalitis is a rare disease caused by the Powassan virus (Flavivirus). The virus is found in the Ixodes species from Ontario, Canada, and the eastern United States. The diagnosis of meningoencephalitis is based on the demonstration of the viral antibodies in the serum or by the isolation of the virus in brain tissue. Treatment is supportive.

Tick paralysis, on the other hand, is a progressive paralysis with loss of tendon and superficial reflexes caused by a neurotoxin in tick saliva. Symptoms may not be present until a few days after the tick attachment. Local skin change around the site of the bite and a morbilliform rash has been reported. Sensory loss is rare. Providing that paralysis is not far advanced, removal of the tick can bring about rapid and complete recovery. Dermacentor andersoni and D. variabilis in the Rocky Mountains and Ixodes holocyclus in Australia are responsible. The emergency physician should be alerted to the travel history of patients, especially young patients with long hair.

Q FEVER

Caused by Coxiella burnetii, an obligate intracellular rickettsia, Q fever is infrequently found in the U.S. and is rarely transmitted by tick bites. Individuals are usually infected through inhalation of dust heavily contaminated by the excreta, placentas, and uterine discharges of domesticated reservoirs: cattle, sheep, and goats. Extremely resistant, the organism can live in dried organic matter for up to 18 months and in tap water or milk for up to 42 months.

Less common sources of infection are infected hides, clothing, straw, and droplet spray from one person to another.

CLINICAL PRESENTATION

After an incubation period of 9 to 20 days, most patients complain of an abrupt onset of fluctuating fever, chills, headache, and myalgias. Neck stiffness may suggest meningitis. There is no rash. In about half the cases, there is x-ray evidence of a pneumonitis, manifested clinically by a nonproductive cough developing in the second week of fever. Other symptoms may include arthralgias, nausea, vomiting, pleuritic chest pain, and diarrhea. Hepatomegaly and splenomegaly may be prominent.

DIAGNOSIS

Q fever should be suspected in anyone with a febrile illness in which there is no obvious cause, or whose occupation involves direct or indirect contact with animals, animal products, or ticks. A differential diagnosis includes viral pneumonia, psitticosis, primary atypical pneumonia, or pulmonary mycotic disease.

Definitive diagnosis is based on organism isolation, direct fluorescent antibody staining of the organism in tissue, and/or an increase in specific antibody titer.

Although the disease is usually self-limited, complications have included endocarditis, hepatitis, thrombophlebitis, pulmonary embolus, hemolytic anemia, arteritis, thromboangiitis obliterans, pleuropericarditis, pericardial effusion, and myocarditis.

TREATMENT AND PROPHYLAXIS

Doxycycline, 100 mg bid usually prompts a quick response and is believed to prevent relapse. Chloramphenicol has also been used with success.

Vaccines are available for persons who come into direct contact with livestock or their products.

RELAPSING FEVER

Relapsing fevers are transmitted by body lice and ticks, although head lice, bedbugs, and fleas have also been implicated as vectors. A night feeder, the tick Ornithodoros is most prevalent in the western and central western states around the Rocky Mountains. It attaches itself to the host for a short time, taking up blood and leaving its infected saliva or excreta.

The spirochetes that cause relapsing fever are classified under the genus Borrelia. When the organisms are circulating in the peripheral blood, patients present with rigors, headache, fever, myalgias, and arthralgias. The untreated disease continues similarly for about 4 days, remits for 10, and then recurs. Usually there are two relapses. Relapse is related to the antigenic variation occurring on the surface of the spirochete. Physical examination reveals abdominal tenderness, hepatophenomegaly, or an occasional ill-defined macular, papular, or petechial rash. Leukocytosis and an elevated erythrocyte sedimentation rate are common. Spirochetes may be seen on peripheral blood smears during the febrile episodes 70% of the time[12] and can be cultured from the blood.

The antimicrobial treatment of choice is the same as for Rocky Mountain Spotted Fever.

TULAREMIA

Caused by the bacillus Franciscella tularensis, tularemia was originally spread most frequently by infected rabbits. It is now believed to be spread predominantly by ticks: the dog tick, Dermacentor variabilis, and the Lone Star tick, Amblyomma americanum. Although the infection occurs throughout the U.S., it is most common in Oklahoma, Missouri, Arkansas, Texas, and Utah.

Tularemia can be transmitted to humans by ticks or deer flies, handling or ingestion of infected animal tissue, or inhalation of infected aerosols. The disease is characterized by sudden fever, chills, malaise, and fatigue about a week after contact with the infective agent. Tick-borne tularemia causes a painful skin ulcer at the site of the bite and painful regional lymphadenopathy. Lung involvement occurs in all forms of tularemia after the bacteremia, and an enteric form follows ingestion of infected animal tissues. The latter follows a fulminant and fatal course unless treated properly. Tularemia is treated with 1 g of intramuscular streptomycin daily for 7 to 10 days. Tetracycline with chloramphenicol is an alternate regimen but may cause a relapse if not initiated within 10 to 12 days after the onset of illness. Relapses are frequent in this regimen, and another dose is given during the first week.

PROPHYLAXIS

At present knowledge, prophylactic antibiotics are not indicated for patients who present after sustaining a tick bite. In the case of RMSF, the antibiotics are only bacteriostatic and their use before the development of an immune response may only delay an infection. Although most tick bites are innocuous (for example, about 1 in 1000 to 2000 ticks in an endemic area may be carrying the rickettsiae that cause RMSF), patients who report such bites should be advised to check their temperature regularly and report any elevations to a physician.[13]

MEDICOLEGAL PEARLS

Every patient entering an emergency facility with an unknown neurologic problem in an area endemic for Lyme disease should be tested for the presence of anti-Borrelia burgdorferi antibody. Similarly, the emergency physician must develop a high index of suspicion for any symptoms that may be attributable to a tick-borne disease prevalent in the area in which he or she is working or in an area from which the patient came.

HORIZONS

The capacity of other ticks as well as other arthropods to transmit disease is poorly defined, as is the role of various mammals and birds as reservoirs. Even the control of tick-borne diseases as we know them depends on judicious integration of management, vector control, chemotherapy, and immunization. Yet the relative efficacy of different control measures and their potential impact on disease, epidemiology, and the environment, along with the logistics and financial implications, have not been resolved. The possibilities of deriving synthetic vaccines by genetic engineering are present now, but the reality is in the distant future.

REFERENCES

1. Schmid, G.P., et al.: DNA Characterization of Lyme Disease Spirochetes. Yale J. Biol. Med. 57:539, 1984.
2. O'Neill, P.M., and Wright, D.J.: Lyme disease. Brit. J. Hosp. Med. 40:284, 1988.
3. Steere, A.C., Schoen, R.T., and Taylor, E.: The clinical evolution of lyme arthritis. Ann. Intern. Med. 107:725, 1987.
4. Shrestha, M., Grodzicki, R.L., and Steere, A.C.: Diagnosing early Lyme disease. Am. J. Med. 78:235, 1985.
5. Petri, W.A., Jr., and Farr, B.N.: Lyme disease. Current opinion. Infect. Dis. 1:188, 1988.
6. Dattwyler, R.J., et al.: Seronegative Lyme disease. N. Engl. J. Med. 319:1441, 1988.
7. Duffy, J., Mertz, L, et al.: Diagnosing Lyme disease: The contribution of serologic testing. Mayo Clin. Proc. 63:1116, 1988.
8. Steere, A.: Lyme Disease. N. Engl. J. Med. 321:586, 1989.
9. Olson, L.J., et al.: Cardiac involvement in Lyme disease: Manifestations and management. Mayo Clin. Proc. 61:745, 1986.
10. Turner, R.C., Chaplinski, T.J., and Adams, H.G.: Rocky Mountain spotted fever presenting as thrombotic thrombocytopenic purpura. Am. J. Med. 81:153, 1986.
11. Kaplan, J.E., and Schonberger, L.B.: The sensitivity of various serologic tests in the diagnosis of Rocky Mountain Spotted Fever. Am. J. Trop. Med. Hyg. 35:840, 1986.
12. Boyer, K.M., Munford, R.S., Maupin, G.O., et al.: Tick-borne relapsing fever: An interstate outbreak originating at Grand Canyon National Park. Am J. Epidemiol. 105:469, 1977.
13. Hornick, R.: Tick-borne diseases. N. Y. State J. Med. 1036, 1983.

Chapter 68

NEAR-DROWNING

Barbara K. Hanke, Alan I. Fields, James E. Gerace, and George R. Schwartz

CAPSULE

Submersion injuries are a tragic and preventable cause of major morbidity and mortality in children and young adults. This chapter presents a rational approach to the treatment and prevention of drowning and near-drowning in these patients and reviews management priorities in both the prehospital phase and the emergency department (ED). Ascertaining the degree of anoxic brain insult secondary to hypoxemia is perilous on initial presentation and difficult to predict for an individual patient, and therefore aggressive resuscitation should be performed in all cases.

INTRODUCTION

The term "drowning" is defined as death by suffocation in water or other liquid and thus has a lethal connotation. Near-drowning is the term used for submersion from which an individual survives at least 24 hours, irrespective of the eventual outcome.

Drowning ranks as the second leading cause of death in the 1- to 4-year-old age group and as the third leading cause of accidental death in the United States, accounting for over 8000 deaths annually. Although all ages are affected, there is a trimodal distribution of near-drowning incidence with peaks in the toddler age group, at 8 to 10 years old, and in the adolescent period. Public education should be aimed at these greatest subgroups of individuals at risk because most drownings are preventable. Drowning occurs most frequently in rivers and canals, with lakes ranking second and the ocean third. The incidence of near-drowning is unknown but is thought to be greater than that of drowning. Submersion accidents in residential pools account for 3000 annual ED visits in children under 5.

PATHOPHYSIOLOGY

Hypoxemia is the single most important consequence of near-drowning. Its degree and duration depend on the duration of submersion and, if fluid was aspirated, the volume of the fluid. Approximately 10 to 20% of victims do not aspirate water because of laryngospasm and/or breath-holding. This has been referred to as "dry drowning." Although the P_{O_2} can rapidly decrease to tensions incompatible with life, early resuscitation can result in rapid and complete recovery. With aspiration of fluid, hypoxemia occurs almost immediately and is more severe and more difficult to treat. Hypoxemia occurs because of shunting of blood through perfused but nonventilated alveoli. The major underlying mechanism of nonventilation of alveoli following fresh water aspiration is thought to be alteration of the normal surface tension properties of surfactant, with collapse of the alveoli. With seawater aspiration, hypoxemia results from fluid in the alveoli, preventing ventilation. Reflex airway closure and a decrease in compliance occur in both fresh water and seawater aspiration and may contribute to hypoxemia. Thus, although seawater and fresh water drownings may involve different causes for the subsequent lung pathology, they are not clinically different, and both cause an increase in intrapulmonary shunting, ventilation, perfusion abnormalities, and hypoxemia.

Acidosis is common after a significant near-drowning and may be respiratory, metabolic, or a combination. The p_{CO_2} can rise rapidly during periods of apnea or hypoventilation, and the hypoxemia that frequently occurs may result in the excess production of lactate. Usually the patient has been resuscitated and is either breathing spontaneously or being ventilated when blood gases are first drawn. Thus, the P_{CO_2} is often normal or low, whereas the pH remains low because the metabolic component persists longer.

Pulmonary edema is common in near-drowning, being reported in up to 75% of cases with either fresh water or seawater aspiration. With *seawater aspiration*, pulmonary edema is thought to be caused by hypertonicity, which results in a movement of fluid or plasma from the vascular system into the alveoli. Following *fresh water aspiration*, pulmonary edema appears to result from injury of the alveolar capillary membrane and alteration of surfactant, both of which allow exudation of protein-rich plasma.

Although blood volume changes have seldom been measured in human near-drowning victims, clinical experience and laboratory observations indicate that seawater near-drowning can sometimes produce hypovolemia and even shock as fluid passes from the vascular system into the alveoli if large volumes of extremely saline water are aspirated. Although fresh water near-drowning can produce hypervolemia, it is usually transient because of a redistribution of fluid into other body compartments, including the lungs. Thus, either type of near-drowning may lead to hypotension or shock, especially if CPR was needed.

Cardiac function in near-drowning is influenced by hypoxemia, changes in blood volume and serum electrolytes, and acidosis. Atrial fibrillation and premature ventricular contractions are the most frequently observed arrhythmias. Ventricular fibrillation is a probable cause of death in some victims who die shortly after submersion, but is uncommon in subjects who reach a hospital. It most often correlates with the severity of the hypoxic-ischemic insult and the need for CPR.

Electrolyte changes are seldom sufficient to be of clinical significance. Although profound changes may occur acutely, spontaneous recovery is usually so rapid that, by the time the patient reaches the hospital, the derangements are mild or nonexistent. More caution, however, should be exercised in patients with renal impairments.

Hematocrit and hemoglobin values are usually normal in both fresh- and seawater near-drowning victims, suggesting that most victims do not aspirate large quantities of fluid. Hemolysis, resulting in hemoglobinuria and hemoglobinemia, can occur after either type of aspiration, although it is more common with fresh water accidents, but rarely clinically significant.

Renal abnormalities have been observed in both fresh water and seawater near-drownings. These most commonly consist of proteinuria and/or cylindruria; however, transient azotemia and acute renal failure have been reported. It appears most likely that hypoxemia, hypotension, and lactic acidosis are the major factors producing renal abnormalities; however, hemoglobinuria and myoglobinuria should always be considered and treated if present.

PREHOSPITAL ASSESSMENT AND STABILIZATION

Near-drowning victims require prompt and vigorous therapy, and on-scene treatment may be the most important determinant of patient outcome. Survival is approximately 70% if a trained resuscitator is present and approximately 40% if one is not. The physiologic derangements present and the type of therapy required are remarkably similar in fresh-water and seawater near-drowning victims. The most significant include lack of spontaneous respiration, hypoxemia, acidosis, and pulmonary edema. Oxygenation and fast transport are the absolute priorities in pre-hospital care.

The single most important immediate requirement of all near-drowning victims is the restoration of effective ventilation and strict attention to the ABCs. A delay in initiating resuscitation of only a few seconds may mean the difference between recovery and death. Mouth-to-mouth resuscitation should begin as soon as possible; i.e., in the water for rescuers who are able to do so, and on shore for those who are not. External cardiac compressions are started on land once pulselessness has been established. Elaborate "lung draining" procedures are contraindicated because they waste valuable time, are ineffective, and may induce vomiting. Most near-drowning victims do not aspirate large volumes of fluid and therefore do not have "fluid-filled lungs." The mouth and upper airway, however, must be patent, and dentures, secretions, and debris should be rapidly removed. Obstructed airways should be treated appropriately and quickly. Cervical spine immobilization may be necessary if there is a suspicion of cervical spine trauma (e.g., from diving), or if the accident was unwitnessed.

Airway control is paramount, including endotracheal intubation if available. Because near-drowning patients tend to swallow water, their airways should be isolated from the GI tract to prevent vomiting and aspiration. With bag-mask ventilation, cricoid pressure should be applied to prevent stomach overdistention. The patient who is breathing on his or her own should be placed in the left lateral decubitus position with suction apparatus available.

If there is cardiac arrest, closed cardiac massage must be done in addition to mouth-to-mouth resuscitation. Oxygen by mask should be administered as soon as available and in as high a concentration as possible. Mechanical devices, preferably hand-operated or controlled, can be used as soon as they are on the scene. Treatment of cardiac arrhythmias should proceed per ACLS protocols, and the patient should have continuous cardiac monitoring.

Therapy must be continued en route to the hospital. Remember that cold water immersion with resultant hypothermia may have a protective effect on the brain. Even after 20 to 40 minutes of cardiac arrest, full CPR is warranted along with rewarming, particularly in children. Resuscitation should always be attempted in the field until further ED evaluation.

The return of consciousness and of spontaneous respiration should not lull one into a false sense of security. Although ventilatory assistance may no longer be required, hypoxemia may still be present. Thus, all patients who have lost consciousness or have aspirated water should be treated with oxygen and transferred to an ED where a more complete evaluation can be performed.

Paramedic personnel should also try to get as accurate a history as possible (time in water, temperature of water, etc.) before leaving the scene.

EMERGENCY DEPARTMENT EVALUATION AND MANAGEMENT

CLINICAL PRESENTATION

The predominant clinical features are related to the lungs and the nervous system. Respiratory signs and symptoms vary considerably in type and severity and include apnea, shallow rapid breathing, a substernal burning sensation, pleuritic chest pain, inability to take a deep breath, rasping cough, expectoration of pink frothy sputum, dyspnea, cyanosis, rales, rhonchi, and dullness of the lung fields. Pyrexia and leukocytosis are common and do not necessarily indicate the presence of infection. The chest roentgenogram is frequently abnormal, often correlating poorly with signs and symptoms, ranging in severity from patchy infiltrates to extensive pulmonary edema.

The most common neurologic findings after a mild insult are restlessness and lethargy, usually transient. Seizures occasionally occur shortly after the acute insult. Unconsciousness is fairly common although usually of brief duration, responding to the initial resuscitative measures and improvement of oxygenation. In patients with mild hypoxia, recovery is usually rapid and complete.

With severe hypoxia, prolonged residual neurologic deficits may occur.

LABORATORY EVALUATION

Arterial blood gases constitute the most important test following near-drowning and should be performed in all victims as soon as possible. They should be used not only for management in severe cases of submersion but to reveal subtle abnormalities in an otherwise normal-appearing patient. A chest radiograph may be a valuable method of following the course of the patient, although it may not reflect functional abnormalities. A worsening of the chest x ray or the persistence of an infiltrate after several days may indicate the presence of a bacterial pneumonia superimposed on the aspiration. The electrocardiogram (to look for evidence of ischemia due to a hypoxic insult, or a long QT syndrome or evidence of electrolyte abnormalities), serum electrolytes, complete blood count, plasma hemoglobin, creatinine, blood urea nitrogen, urinalysis, and sputum for smears and cultures should be obtained as early as possible and repeated as indicated. If clinically relevant, a toxicology screen, blood alcohol level, or level of serum anticonvulsants should be sent. Cervical spine x rays should be done in the setting of possible trauma.

EMERGENCY DEPARTMENT MANAGEMENT

Initial evaluation and therapy should be aimed at intensive respiratory care to prevent anoxic brain injury. The requirement for ventilatory assistance and oxygen is governed by the clinical status of the patient and the results of arterial blood gas analysis. Ventilatory assistance is generally required if the patient is not breathing, if the P_{CO_2} is greater than 50 mm Hg, or if the P_{O_2} is less than 50 mm Hg on maximum concentrations of oxygen. This should be accomplished initially by means of a mask. Prolonged ventilation or inadequate oxygenation with other initial measures, however, requires endotracheal intubation. If the airway is not well protected (e.g., poor gag reflex, altered state of consciousness), an endotracheal tube should be inserted.

After resuscitation, hypoxia usually becomes the most pressing clinical problem. Oxygen should be administered to raise the P_{O_2} to 60 to 80 mm Hg or to a saturation of about 85%. This may require only a simple nasal cannula or a nonrebreathing mask or possibly, after intubation, a volume respirator and positive end-expiratory pressure (PEEP). PEEP should be used with caution until neurologic and cardiac functions have been assessed for increased intracranial pressure or myocardial dysfunction. CPAP may also be used (Table 68-1).

Respiratory acidosis is treated by ventilation. When metabolic acidosis is severe (i.e., pH below 7.10), bicarbonate (1 μg/kg) can be administered slowly. The treatment for lactic acidosis is hemodynamic support to improve perfusion. Hyperventilation for the purpose of cerebral resuscitation is controversial, but lowering the P_{CO_2} by hyperventilation improves the pH.

Cardiac arrhythmias usually respond to correction of hypoxemia, hypothermia, and acidosis; if not, they should be treated by standard methods. If shock is present, vasopressors and volume expanders may be needed, and invasive monitoring is indicated.

Pulmonary edema usually responds well to bed rest, oxygen, and diuretics. In the presence of hypovolemia the effect of diuretics may be limited. In the presence of profound pulmonary edema with severe respiratory embarrassment, it may be necessary to apply positive pressure ventilation and PEEP.

Shock may be caused by hypervolemia, hypoxia, or spinal injury. Central venous pressure and urinary output should be followed. The combination of pulmonary edema and shock presents a difficult clinical problem. In this situation, treatment with colloids such as albumin or plasma is recommended to increase the intravascular osmotic pressure and draw fluid into the vascular system from the lungs. This therapy, however, is not without hazard; as in the presence of injury to the alveolar capillary membrane this material may pass from the pulmonary capillaries into the alveoli. Volume expansion (with either colloid or crystalloid) is critical. Inotropic agents such as dopamine or dobutamine may be added to maintain adequate perfusion.

Electrolyte abnormalities are seldom of clinical significance, and the routine administration of saline in all fresh water near-drownings and the use of water solutions in all seawater near-drownings is not recommended. Treatment should be given only when significant derangements exist.

Convulsions and restlessness usually respond to reoxygenation of the patient. Should that prove ineffective, 5 to 10 mg of diazepam given slowly intravenously or barbiturates can be used as required with suitable precautions in case of apnea.

Mild azotemia and proteinuria do not require treatment. Acute tubular necrosis is managed by standard means. Hemoglobinuria is best treated by maintaining an adequate urine flow.

Extensive hemolysis, though rare, may lead to severe anemia and is best treated with packed cells.

Bronchospasm, if present, may be treated with a bronchodilator such as nebulized isoetharine or metaproterenol. Intravenous aminophylline may also be used. A rectal temperature with a glass thermometer should be obtained in any patient with a history of significant submersion. If the patient is hypothermic (body temperature less than 28°C.), aggressive passive and active rewarming techniques should be instituted. Ventricular fibrillation may not respond to defibrillation attempts at a body temperature less than 30°C, and spontaneous cardiac activity may be inhibited at these lower temperatures. Therefore resuscitation efforts should be continued until the core temperature reaches at least 30°C. For a low body temperature to be protective rather than a poikilothermic response to death, it should also be secondary to an ice water immersion (water temperature less than or equal to 10°C).

Bacterial pneumonia may occasionally occur in near-drowning victims, especially if heavily polluted water is aspirated. Although transient fever and leukocytosis are common, bacterial pneumonia is not. Thus the routine use of broadspectrum antibiotics in all near-drowning victims is not generally recommended. Antibiotics may be started if the aspirated fluid is contaminated with dirt or sewage, or if there is pre-existent lung disease. The clinical course should dictate use of antibiotics. Hot tub near-drownings are frequently colonized with Pseudomonas, and initial treatment with antibiotics may be indicated

TABLE 68-1. RESPIRATORY MANAGEMENT

In the nonbreathing patient:
—Endotracheal intubation as early as possible
—Ventilate with 100% oxygen
In the patient with spontaneous ventilation:
—Start supplemental oxygen to keep Po_2 60–80 mm/Hg by nasal cannula or nonrebreathing mask
—if patient is still hypoxic or hypercarbic, or if there is an unprotected airway:
   • Endotracheal intubation
   • Ventilate with 100% oxygen
   • Consider PEEP or IMV with CPAP

pending culture results if the chest x ray is positive.

Although corticosteroids have been used in the treatment of near-drowning because of the inflammatory reaction that may be present in the lungs and because some victims aspirate gastric contents, to date there is no evidence that these hormones are of value in the treatment of water aspiration. Thus, in the absence of gastric aspiration or possible adrenocortical insufficiency, there is no clear indication for the administration of corticosteroids.

The stomach should be decompressed by means of nasogastric tube as early as possible in the resuscitation because most near-drowning victims vomit, with the attendant risk of aspiration of gastric contents. A Foley catheter should also be placed in critical patients to monitor urine output which presents as a delayed onset of lung pathology.

CEREBRAL RESUSCITATION

With improved methods of treatment of cardiopulmonary complications (invasive monitoring, PEEP, etc.), the hypoxic/ischemic insult resulting in brain damage or brain death is now the major cause of most morbidity and mortality in submersion injuries. Except for ice water near-drownings (body temperature below 28°C), the outcome is poor if the Glasgow Coma Scale is less than 5 on admission to the hospital. Treatment of increased intracranial pressure seems to have no effect in preventing severe neurologic sequelae. Furthermore, some attempts at brain resuscitation (including barbiturate coma and moderate postarrest hypothermia) have been unsuccessful. (See Chap. 4.)

Several new techniques have recently been helpful in the laboratory setting, but have yet to have controlled human clinical trials in asphyxial cardiac arrest. These include postarrest mild hypothermia (to 34°C), a postanoxic hypertensive bout or "brain flush" with a mean arterial pressure of 120 to 140 mm Hg for up to 5 minutes, and the use of calcium channel blockers.

Until the appropriate protocols have been established and proven, cerebral resuscitation measures continue to be controversial.

LATE COMPLICATIONS

The major complication of near-drowning is "secondary drowning," which presents as a delayed onset of lung pathology. This may result from aspiration pneumonitis, superimposed bacterial pneumonia, or inhalation of foreign material. This has been reported in individuals who appear to recover from the acute insult and are allowed to go home. Respiratory symptoms usually begin within a few hours and are profound. The syndrome is most likely to occur following near-drowning in seawater or heavily polluted water and is commonly associated with secondary infections. This is usually prevented by admitting to the hospital for at least 24 hours of observation all near-drowning victims who have aspirated water or lost consciousness. These patients should have their vital signs and arterial blood gases monitored and should receive a chest x ray and prompt treatment as previously outlined. When this syndrome occurs, the patients are usually sicker and have a lower survival rate than those who are immediately admitted to the hospital. With this syndrome, vigorous therapy with all the modalities mentioned above, including antibiotics, is recommended.

OUTCOME AND PROGNOSIS

Ascertaining the degree of anoxic insult is perilous initially and depends on many factors, including ef-

TABLE 68-2. NEUROLOGIC OUTCOME OF NEAR-DROWNING VICTIMS

Neurologic Response to Painful Stimuli at 1 Hour Postresuscitation with Body Temperature Above 28°C	Prognosis
Purposeful withdrawal from pain	Excellent
Decorticate posturing	Good—generally all have a good recovery
Decerebrate posturing	Good—most recover; a few have neurologic deficits
Flaccid (in absence of cervical spine injury)	Poor—some recover; most have severe neurologic deficit or brain death

fectiveness of initial resuscitation, duration of submersion, and water temperature. Because one cannot predict the outcome for an individual patient at the time of presentation to the ED, aggressive resuscitation should be performed in all cases.

The primary determinant of the ultimate prognosis in near-drowning victims is the duration of hypoxia, as modified by hypothermia. Although the common pathway for injury to various organ systems in all victims of near-drowning is hypoxemia, acidosis, and hypoperfusion, important physiologic differences between a young child and an adult affect the prognosis. First, young children may become hypothermic more rapidly than adults. This hypothermia may be significant in view of documented cases of complete recovery of pediatric patients who sustained prolonged submersion, in one case up to 66 minutes. The protective effect of hypothermia generally involves submersion in ice water less than or equal to 10°C resulting in a body temperature less than or equal to 28°C. Vigorous resuscitative efforts and rewarming are warranted even in cases that initially seem hopeless.

In addition, some authors feel that the diving reflex may play an important role. This reflex, which allows air-breathing mammals to submerge for prolonged periods, consists of bradycardia and redistribution of blood flow to the heart and brain, affording a greater protection for these organs against hypoxia. More recently, however, experiments tend to cast doubt on the role that this reflex may play in the pediatric population, and it seems unlikely that it contributes significantly to the prolonged resuscitability of children who are victims of cold water near-drownings. Hypothermia may thus confer substantial protection to the child's central nervous system against the hypoxic insult resulting from a near-drowning episode, but the diving reflex may not make a significant difference in long-term prognosis.

Several factors have been identified as predictive of poor patient outcome: submersion for more than 5 minutes, a serum pH of less than 7 at time of ED presentation, need for CPR in the ED, and a poor initial neurologic examination upon resuscitation (Table 68-2). There are, however, some good reported outcomes despite the presence of some of these factors, and obtaining accurate submersion times and temperatures of the water and the patient make comparing different studies difficult. More aggressive treatment of some patients may also have improved the outcome in certain cases.

CRITERIA FOR ADMISSION

The criteria for hospital admission include a history of apnea, cyanosis, loss of consciousness, or CPR. If the patient has had an abnormal chest x ray, hypoxemia, acidosis, or abnormal physical examination, he or she should obviously also be admitted. If the patient has no clinical findings of respiratory or neurological abnormalities, does not have a history of a significant submersion injury and has a normal arterial blood gas, chest x ray, and physical examination, he or she should be observed in the ED for at least 4 to 6 hours. If all three (chest x ray, physical examination, and arterial blood gas) are still normal at the end of that period, the patient may be discharged home with well-documented patient discharge instructions, including the possibility of delayed pulmonary complications. If the patient has any of the noted risk factors in terms of history, abnormal physical examination, or abnormal laboratory findings, the patient should be admitted for observation at least overnight.

PREVENTION

Prevention is paramount to prevent drowning and near-drowning incidents, and public education should involve both lay and paramedical personnel, including babysitters and parents of young children. Children who recover from a submersion accident may have no fear of water, and parents have often noted no change in behavior of these children at pools and beaches or in the bathtub. Thus, parents must take care to avoid a second immersion accident. A significant number of parents of a child involved in a near-drowning episode do not take effective measures to prevent such an accident from recurring, and all children in these families remain at an increased risk.

Prevention in the toddler age group, when children are recently mobile but have no judgment or fear of water, should be aimed at parent education. Safety barriers should be placed around any water hazard (e.g., swimming pools, spas) and should be consistently kept locked. It appears that the most effective way to institute barriers is through legislation. Three-sided barriers, in which the house is the fourth barrier side, have been historically unreliable in preventing near-drowning accidents. In most instances, an adult is home when the near-drowning occurs, but is either distracted or believes that someone else is supervising the child. One third of the time, the episode occurs in a neighbor's or relative's pool. Training in CPR should be mandatory for owners of pools. If effective CPR is not carried out at the scene, any chance of reasonable outcome may be lost.

Another major source of submersion accidents involving infants and children is bathtubs. Usually an older sibling in a large family is supervising a younger child when the accident occurs. Children should also not be allowed to play with 5-gallon buckets of water; several submersion accidents have been reported.

Child abuse or neglect should be considered in evaluating submersion injuries.

Children with seizure disorders, who have a 4 to 5 times increased risk of drowning and near-drowning accidents, should be closely supervised in the bathtub and at swimming pools and the beach.

In the case of the 8-to-10-year-old age group, the children have often been left to swim alone. These children may be overconfident and attempt to swim long distances or "show off." Risk-taking behavior, possibly influenced by alcohol or drugs, is generally involved in teenage drownings.

PITFALLS

- Always attempt resuscitation in near-drowning victims.
- Cervical spine immobilization and evaluation should be instituted in all diving injuries or shallow water submersion injuries.
- Get arterial blood gases in all patients with a significant submersion injury by history, even though they may have a normal chest x ray and physical examination.
- A rectal temperature with a glass thermometer should be obtained in any patient with a history of a significant submersion.
- Treat hypoxia aggressively, with early endotracheal intubation when necessary.

MEDICOLEGAL PEARLS

Documentation of resuscitation measures, body temperature of the patient, and reasons for termination of the resuscitation are of paramount importance. Patient discharge instructions should include the possibility of delayed pulmonary complications and detail worrisome signs and symptoms requiring repeat ED evaluation.

BIBLIOGRAPHY

Burrichter, M.A., and Layon, J.L.: Drowning and near-drowning. Hospital Medicine, August 1991, p. 77.

Conn, A.W.: Near-drowning and hypothermia. Can. Med. Assoc. J. *120*:397, 1979.

Conn, A.W., et al.: Cerebral resuscitation in near-drowning. Pediatr. Clin. North Am. *26*:691, August 1979.

Conn, A.W., et al.: Cerebral salvage in near-drowning following neurological classification by triage. Anaesth. Soc. J. *27*:201, 1980.

Dean, J., et al.: Prognostic indicators in pediatric near-drowning: The Glasgow coma scale. Crit. Care Med. *9*:536, 1981.

Fandel, I. and Bancalari, E.: Near-drowning in children: Clinical aspects. Pediatrics 58:573, 1976.

Fields, A.I.: Drowning and Near-drowning, Life Threatening Episodes in Infants and Children. Symposium, Upjohn Company, 1983.

Fields, A.I., and Holbrook, P.R.: Near-drowning in the pediatric population. *In* Textbook of Critical Care. 2nd ed. Edited by Shoemaker, W.C., Ayers, S., Grenvik, A., Holbrook, P.R., and Thompson, L. The Society of Critical Care Medicine, 1989, pp. 67–69.

Fleetham, J.A., et al.: Near-drowning in Canadian waters. Can. Med. Assoc. J. 118:914, 1978.

Fuller, R.H.: Drowning and the post-immersion syndrome. A clinicopathologic study. Milit. Med. 128:22, 1963.

Giammona, S.T., and Modell, J.H.: Drowning by total immersion: Effects on pulmonary surfactant of distilled H_2O, isotonic saline, seawater. Am. J. Dis. Child. 114:612, 1967.

Giammona, S.T.: Drowning: Pathophysiology and management. Curr. Probl. Pediatr. 1:1, 1971.

Gooden, B.A.: Drowning and the diving reflex in man. Med. J. Aust. 2:583, 1972.

Grausz, H., et al.: Autorenal failure complicating submersion in seawater. J.A.M.A. 217:207, 1971.

Griffin, G.C.: Near-drowning. Its pathophysiology and treatment in man. Milit. Med. 131:12, 1966.

Hoff, B.H.: Multisystem failure: A review with special reference to drowning. Crit. Care Med. 7:310, 1979.

Knopp, R.: Near drowning. J. Am. Coll. Emerg. Phys. 7:249, June 1978.

Lerner et al.: Mild cerebral hypothermia during and after cardiac arrest improves neurologic outcome in dogs. J. Cerebral Blood Flow Metab. 10:57, 1990.

Levin D.L.: Near-drowning. Crit. Care Med. 8:590, 1980.

Martin, C.M., and Barrett, O.N.: Drowning and near-drowning: A review of ten years' experience in a large Army hospital. Milit. Med. 136:439, 1971.

Martin, T.G.: Near-drowning and cold water immersion. Ann. Emerg. Med. 13:263, 1984.

Modell, J.H., et al: Blood gas and electrolyte changes in human near-drowning victims. J.A.M.A. 203:337, 1968.

Modell, J.H.: The pathophysiology and treatment of drowning and near-drowning. Springfield, Ill. Charles C Thomas, 1971.

Modell, J.H. and Moya, F.: Effects of volume of aspirated fluid during chlorinated fresh water drowning. Anesthesiology 27:662, 1966.

Modell, J.H., Graves, S.A., and Kuck, E.J.: Near-drowning: Correlation of level of consciousness and survival. Can. Anaesth. Soc. J. 27:211, 1980.

Moser, R.H.: Drowning: A seasonal disease. J.A.M.A. 229:563, 1974.

Orlowski, J.P.: Drowning, near-drowning, and ice-water submersions. Pediatr. Clin. North Am. 34:75, 1987.

Pearn, J., and Nixon, J.: Prevention of childhood drowning accidents. Med. J. Aust. 1:616, 1977.

Pearn, J.: Neurological and psychometric studies in children surviving freshwater immersion accidents. Lancet 1:7, 1977.

Pearn, J.: Survival rates after serious immersion accidents in childhood. Resuscitation 6:271, 1978.

Pearn, J.H.: Secondary drowning in children. Br. Med. J. 281:1103, 1980.

Peterson, B.: Morbidity of childhood near-drowning. Pediatrics 59:304, 1977.

Ramey, C.A., Ramey D.N., and Hayward J.S.: Dive response of children in relation to cold-water near-drowning. J. Appl. Physiol. 63:665, 1987.

Reulet, J.B.: Hypothermia pathophysiology, clinical settings, and management. Ann. Intern. Med. 89:519, 1978.

Rivers, J.E., et al.: Drowning. Its clinical sequelae and management. Br. Med. J. 2:157, 1970.

Rowe, M.I., Arango, A., and Allington, G.: Profile of pediatric drowning victims in a water-oriented society. J. Trauma 17:587, 1977.

Rutledge, R.R., and Flor, R.J.: The use of mechanical ventilation with positive end-expiratory pressure in the treatment of near-drowning. Anesthesiology 38:794, 1973.

Safar, P.: Cerebral resuscitation after cardiac arrest: A review. Circulation 74:IV-138, 1986.

Shaw, K.N., et al.: Submersion injuries: drowning and near-drowning. Emerg. Med. Clin. North. Am. May 7(2), 355, 1989.

Sterz et al.: Stroke. December, 1990.

Young, R.S.K., et al.: Neurological outcome in cold water drowning. J.A.M.A. 244:1233, 1980.

Chapter 69

HYPOTHERMIA AND FROSTBITE

HYPOTHERMIA

Loren Johnson

CAPSULE

Hypothermia is body chilling caused by impaired heat production or accelerated heat loss. The degree and duration of chilling and the patient's underlying physiologic state are important determinants of prognosis and treatment.

Management consists of preventing heat loss, rewarming the patient, and treating underlying disorders. Intravenous dextrose and naloxone are given initially and thiamine is given as soon as possible in the Emergency Department (ED). Passive rewarming by covering the patient with blankets and preventing further heat loss is the safest course in patients who are capable of shivering and have a core temperature of 30°C (86°F) or more. Active external rewarming by applying a heat source to the torso may be reasonably safe in patients with moderately severe hypothermia of short duration; however, this rewarming method has been associated with rewarming shock and lethal ventricular fibrillation. Active internal rewarming using heated humidified oxygen, heated fluid exchange, or extracorporeal circulation is the standard of care for patients with a core temperature of 28°C (82.4°F) or less, and is considered stabilizing treatment for prevention and conversion of cold-induced ventricular fibrillation.

Severely hypothermic victims can be safely intubated; however, jaw rigor may make nasotracheal intubation the preferred approach. Rough handling must be avoided to minimize risk of ventricular fibrillation.

Drugs are generally ineffective in the severely hypothermic patient. Overly aggressive sodium bicarbonate administration and hyperventilation are to be avoided because of the risk of causing alkalosis-induced ventricular fibrillation. Electrical defibrillation is generally not successful until core temperature exceeds 28°C. Bretylium tosylate has been shown to decrease the fibrillatory threshold in hypothermic animals and may be protective in humans.

Hypothermia reduces metabolic demands and has a protective effect on the brain and other vital organs in victims who have experienced circulatory collapse in the presence of rapid chilling, such as from immersion in cold water. The moribund hypothermic patient may therefore be viable in the absence of vital signs and should be given the benefit of resuscitation and rewarming to near-normal temperatures before declaration of death.

INTRODUCTION

Accidental hypothermia is a spontaneous decrease in core temperature to less than 35°C (95°C) as the result of chilling. It is an abnormal physiologic and pathologic condition. Its severity is indicated by the degree to which core temperature is lowered, and can be classified as mild hypothermia (32 to 35°C), moderate hypothermia (28 to 32°C) or severe hypothermia (less than 28°C). It occurs in one of three clinical settings:

1. Cold water immersion
2. Cold weather exposure
3. Subacute cold stress in persons with impaired thermoregulatory function.

Physiologic compensation is acutely brought about by peripheral vasoconstriction, which reduces heat loss, and by shivering, which increases heat production. When the duration of cold stress is prolonged, endocrine mechanisms may be invoked to increase heat production. Continued chilling, however, may suppress physiologic processes to a degree sufficient to make a person appear lifeless. The deeply hypothermic individual is comatose and may appear dead. It is therefore of utmost importance that emergency personnel maintain a high degree of suspicion for this condition and that accurate core temperatures, either rectal or tympanic, be obtained in all patients exposed to cold.

The choice of methods for rewarming the hypothermic patient is influenced by the degree and duration of the heat deficit, the presence of underlying or complicating conditions, and the techniques and equipment available.

HISTORY AND INCIDENCE

Ever since half of Napoleon's army succumbed to the winter cold during the retreat from Moscow in 1812, hypothermia and local cold injury have been known as a great scourge of war.

Civilian interest in hypothermia was aroused in the late 1960s, when the British noted the epidemic occurrence of hypothermia among elderly persons who lived in poorly heated homes.[1,2] At about the same time, observations of mountain rescue teams indicated that young and healthy people can also experience rapid demise when exposed to wet, windy, and cold conditions.[3-5] During the past decade, several investigators have recognized differences between "urban" hypothermia among elderly and physiologically impaired individuals and that occurring in victims of exposure. The pathophysiology of hypothermia has become more widely understood, and various new techniques for internal rewarming have been developed which hold promise for reducing mortality.

An annual mortality of over 700 cases related to excessive cold has been reported by the Centers for Disease Control (CDC); however, the overall mortality of hypothermia in the United States is not known.[6] Mortality in treated victims is reported to be between 0 and 50% in various series and appears to depend on risk factors such as age extremes, the presence of intoxicants, and the victim's state of health and nutrition. With the increased numbers of aged, homeless, and disabled persons nationwide, as well as the increasing cost of fossil fuels, hypothermia could easily become a disastrous public health problem in the United States.

PHYSIOLOGY OF TEMPERATURE REGULATION

In accordance with the Van't Hoff law and the Arrhenius equation, the logarithm of biochemical reactions varies directly with changes in absolute temperature. Mammals developed as homeotherms to maintain an optimal functional state. Humans evolved in the tropics between the 70°F isotherms. Migration to cooler climatic areas became possible with the invention of clothing, shelter, and agriculture.

Human core temperature varies within a narrow normal range of 36.4 to 37.5°C (97.5 to 99.5°F). The thermoregulatory center in the anterior hypothalamus integrates input from peripheral skin temperature receptors and adjacent central blood temperature receptors, and effects compensatory adjustments in heat production and retention. Increased heat production is accomplished by increasing the basal metabolic rate and by shivering, which is the involuntary contraction of truncal muscles. Heat retention is accomplished by effecting peripheral vasoconstriction and, on a conscious level, heat is retained by the intelligent use of shelter and warm clothing.

Basal thermogenesis approximates 50 kcal per hour per square meter of body surface, or about 100 kcal per hour in average adults. Intense exercise or shivering can yield 500 kcal per hour, but generally cannot be maintained for more than a few hours. Animal experiments have shown that depletion of glycogen stores in the liver can be a rate-limiting factor for maintaining high levels of heat production during cold stress.[7] Although shivering increases heat production, its occurrence impairs peripheral vasoconstriction and may result in a minimal net heat gain.

Clothing reflects heat and retains a warm-air envelope known as the "private climate." Its insulating value is measured by the unit "clo," which is equal to that of a standard suit of clothing that keeps the average person warm at an ambient temperature of 15.56°C (60°F).[8] Unfortunately, standard clothing provides little protection from wind and wetness. To protect the body from excessive heat loss during foul weather, clothing is worn in closely fitting layers with outer garments that shed wind and water, wool or synthetic garments that retain insulative value when wet, and inner garments that release moisture and keep warm air close to the body. Footwear should insulate and be nonconstrictive. Hands should be covered with a mitten shell that reduces the surface area for radiant heat loss. Above all, the head and neck must be covered to reduce radiant heat loss from this highly vascular area.[4,6,8] Advanced materials technology has enabled the development of wet and dry diving suits and self-contained environment suits that have greatly expanded the range of human operation from deep water to outer space.[8,9]

MECHANISMS OF HEAT LOSS

Body heat is lost through conduction, convection, evaporation, and radiation. Conductive heat loss is rapid during immersion in cold water or contact with cold ground. Convective and evaporative heat loss are the most important mechanisms in persons exposed to wind and moisture. With the body clothed, radiant heat loss is primarily from the unprotected head. It may equal half of the body's total heat production when ambient temperature is 4°C (39.2°F).[6]

The body has three concentric layers that regulate heat loss and gain:[10]

1. The outer layer consists of skin and subcutaneous adipose tissue, which protect against heat loss.
2. The intermediate layer consists of skeletal muscles, which are responsible for shivering.
3. The inner layer consists of vital organs and viscera, which must be kept warm at all costs.

Cold reflex vasoconstriction severely limits blood flow to the skin, thus limiting the rate of heat exchange. Additionally, subcutaneous fat has one third the thermal conductivity of muscle and, along with the skin, creates an insulating shell to conserve heat by separating the deeper core from the environment.[10,11]

The anatomic arrangement of the arteries and veins within the extremities allows their function as a countercurrent heat exchanger. Arterial blood flow to the extremities rewarms venous blood returning through the accompanying venae comitantes. This minimizes heat loss from the core. Rhythmic waves of cold-induced vasodilation, known as the "hunting phenomenon," occur in an attempt to economically conserve the cold extremity. Central neural modulators control this response as well as the shivering response.[5] With prolonged exposure to temperatures below 15°C (59°F) blood flow increases intermittently in the extremities. This response, however, provides an inadequate supply of oxygen in the presence of generalized hypothermia. Thus, unless internal body warmth is restored, the limb may be "sacrificed" to ischemia in deference to preservation of core organs.[12]

After a few weeks of moderate exposure, most people can acclimatize to cold by developing improved vasomotor tone and neuroendocrine control of nonmuscular thermogenesis.[7,11] Some persons fail to acclimatize and appear to be more susceptible to cold injury. Some individuals have a specific vulnerability to local cold stress, such as those with Raynaud's phenomenon and cold-induced hypersensitivity. Elderly persons, newborns, and patients with drug intoxication or neuroendocrine disorders may be nonadaptive to cold stress because of underlying impairment of thermoregulatory responses.

DEVELOPMENT OF HYPOTHERMIA

With the initial chill and subsequent fall of the body core temperature to 35°C (95°F), peripheral and central thermoreceptors induce cutaneous vasoconstriction and a systemic catecholamine response. As a result, blood pressure, heart rate, and respiratory minute volume increase. In addition, the shivering mechanism is activated and intermittent vasodilation occurs in skeletal muscles. If chilling continues over a period of hours, there is a gradual stimulation of basal thermogenesis by means of endocrine mechanisms, causing an increase up to three times normal.[13,14]

A further decline in temperature below 30°C (86°F) is associated with progressive suppression of metabolism, mental function, and cardiorespiratory function (Table 69-1). Additionally, central temperature regulation is grossly impaired, and the victim becomes essentially poikilothermic, with the basal metabolic rate declining 6% for each 1° reduction in core temperature.

At 28°C (82.4°F), the heart rate and basal metabolic rate fall to 50% of normal. Shivering ceases and is replaced by muscle rigidity. There is a direct depression of cardiac pacemaker activity and a prolongation of conduction time. Bradyarrhythmias, atrial fibrillation, and atrial flutter are common. T-wave inversion and prolongation of the P-R and S-T intervals may occur. The presence of a J wave, or Osborne wave, occurs in approximately one third of patients with hypothermia. It appears as a slow positive deflection or hump at the end of the QRS complex (Fig. 69-1).[15] This may be an injury current or a slowing of depolarization, but it is entirely reversible when the heart is rewarmed.[16,17]

Below 28°C (82.4°F), there is a significant risk of ventricular fibrillation, the major cause of death in victims with accidental hypothermia.[11,18] It may occur spontaneously and has been reported to occur with physical manipulation such as CPR and rough handling.[48] Endotracheal intubation has been shown not to induce arrhythmias in a large multicenter hypothermia survey.[19] Prehospital CPR is contraindicated in severely hypothermic patients with a weakly palpable pulse and spontaneous respiration or those with an organized rhythm with or without a pulse. The fibrillatory threshold may also be lowered by hypocapnia and alkalosis secondary to excessive ventilation and excessive sodium bicarbonate administration. Cold-induced ventricular fibrillation may be difficult if not impossible to cardiovert, and it is therefore recommended that, after an initial attempt at electrical defibrillation, CPR should be started and maintained while aggressive attempts at rewarming are under-

TABLE 69-1. PROGRESSIVE SUPPRESSION OF SYSTEMIC FUNCTION DURING BODY CHILLING

Temperature (°C)	Neurologic	Cardiovascular	Pulmonary	Skeletal Muscles	Metabolic
37°	Agitation	Increased pulse and blood pressure; peripheral vasoconstriction	Increased respiratory rate	Shivering begins	Autonomic excitation
35°	Confusion and apathy	Intense peripheral vasoconstriction	Marked increase in respiratory minute volume	Shivering becomes most intense	BMR three to six times normal
30°	No response to verbal stimuli	Supraventricular arrhythmias	Decrease in respiratory minute volume; gag and cough decreased	Shivering alternates with rigor	Metabolic exhaustion
25°	No response to painful stimuli	Risk of ventricular fibrillation	Gag absent	Sustained rigor	BMR 50% of normal
20°	No EEG activity	Ventricular fibrillation	Apnea	Sustained rigor	Minimal thermogenesis
15°	No EEG activity	Asystole	Apnea	Sustained rigor	Minimal thermogenesis

Abbreviations: BMR = Basal metabolic rate; EEG = electroencephalogram.

taken.[20] Pretreatment with antiarrhythmic drugs such as lidocaine and procainamide has not been shown to be effective in preventing ventricular fibrillation. Bretylium tosylate has been reported to prevent ventricular fibrillation in pretreated animals; however, its effectiveness in converting the rhythm during rewarming has been variable in controlled studies.[21–23] Thoracotomy, heated mediastinal lavage, and open cardiac massage have occasionally been performed with limited success.[24,25]

Although respirations are stimulated early in the development of the hypothermic state, there is definite depression of respiratory function as temperature falls below 30°C (86°F). Hypothermia depresses the cough reflex and may cause direct injury to the lungs, resulting in noncardiogenic pulmonary edema. Cold-induced bronchorrhea can result in aspiration of tracheobronchial secretions and cause pneumonia in conjunction with atelectasis.

Below 25°C (77°F), marked respiratory depression is common and frank apnea may occur. In addition, the reduction in temperature shifts the oxyhemoglobin dissociation curve to the left, making less oxygen available to the tissues. Lactic acidosis arises from anaerobic metabolism because of decreased availability of oxygen and poor perfusion. Concomitant respiratory depression causes combined respiratory and metabolic acidosis.

Below 20°C (68°F), asystole may occur. Central nervous system (CNS) responses to hypothermia include progressive depression of the mental status. At 30°C (86°F), most persons are comatose. At 20°C (68°F), the electroencephalogram is a straight line. Cerebral blood flow is decreased by 6 to 7% for every 1°C below normal. Neuronal metabolism is reduced at the same rate, however, so that the brain is somewhat protected from damage at low temperatures.[18]

The combination of poor fluid intake, plasma leakage, and cold diuresis makes hypovolemia and relative circulatory failure a common underlying feature of hypothermia.[26,27] Prolonged acidemia and cold-induced diuresis may also contribute to significant hypokalemia. Urine output continues to be an important monitor of organ perfusion in later stages of hypothermia.

Circulatory failure may prevent mobilization and excretion of organic acids, augmenting the metabolic acidosis when the patient is rewarmed.

The leukocyte and platelet counts may be reduced as a result of splenic and intravascular sequestration, and disseminated intravascular coagulation has been reported.[28–30]

Profound hyperkalemia and elevated serum ammonia levels indicate cell lysis, and these markers, combined with significant hypofibrinogenemia, predict a dire prognostic outcome.[3] Insulin secretion may be inhibited, leading to hyperglycemia. Conversely, glycogen levels may become depleted from the liver, leading to hypoglycemia.[7,31] Unless there is preexisting deficiency, plasma cortisol and thyroid hormone levels are generally above normal.[14]

Drugs given during the hypothermic state tend to be biologically ineffective and poorly detoxified by the liver. Thus they may be present in the circulation and tissues long after their pharmacologic effect is desired.

At 20°C (68°F), the patient is apneic, gray, and rigid, and appears dead. Recovery, however, has been reported in a patient with a temperature as low as 17°C (62.6°F). *Therefore, no hypothermic patient should be declared dead until resuscitation has been shown to be futile after the patient has been rewarmed to near normal temperatures.*[20,32]

IMMERSION HYPOTHERMIA

Immersion hypothermia is usually the result of a brief, but overwhelming exposure of an otherwise healthy individual to water less than 15.56 to 21.11°C (60 to 70°F)). Conductive heat loss, the primary cause of death in boating accidents, occurs 26 to 32 times faster in water than in air. It results in uniform fatality within seconds to minutes at −1.11°C (30°F) and 50% mortality within 1 hour at 4.44°C (40°F).

The **H**eat **E**scape **L**essening **P**osition (HELP) is an arms-crossed, knee-chest position that can be assumed by persons with a flotation device in cold water. This reduces heat loss by lessening exposed surface areas, including the groin and chest.

Immediate submersion is common after falling into cold water, perhaps because of brainstem hypothermia or aspiration caused by gasping after sudden exposure to cold water.[36,37] Many near-drowning victims have been resuscitated without neurologic sequelae following submersion in cold water for several minutes. Rapid occurrence of hypothermia with gradual slowing of cerebral blood flow protects the brain in this setting.[36,38,39]

The application of advanced rewarming techniques, such as extracorporeal rewarming, has expanded the limits of recoverability for immersion hypothermia. A 2½-year-old child with a core temperature of 19° has been resuscitated with ECR, resulting in complete neurologic recovery, after 66 minutes of submersion.[40]

COLD WEATHER HYPOTHERMIA

Hypothermia from cold weather exposure occurs in healthy victims who may be exposed for long periods to adverse conditions. Convective heat loss or wind chill may be the most significant factor of heat loss in a windy environment. Under normal circumstances, radiation of body heat is responsible for 70% of heat loss, half of which is lost from the uncovered head. Exhaustion after heavy exercise in the outdoors has been observed to cause hypothermia in mountaineers and marathoners. Wet clothing and inadequate carbohydrate intake are common predisposing factors.[4,14] Healthy persons may shiver intensely for several minutes to hours before succumbing to cold stress, and may develop considerable dehydration, metabolic acidosis, and hepatic glycogen depletion in the process.[7,14] In addition, their illness may be complicated by frostbite or immersion injury to locally exposed tissues.

Typical behavioral complications of hypothermia during cold weather exposure include apathy, mental instability, and poor judgment.[4] The most striking example of this problem is paradoxic undressing in the

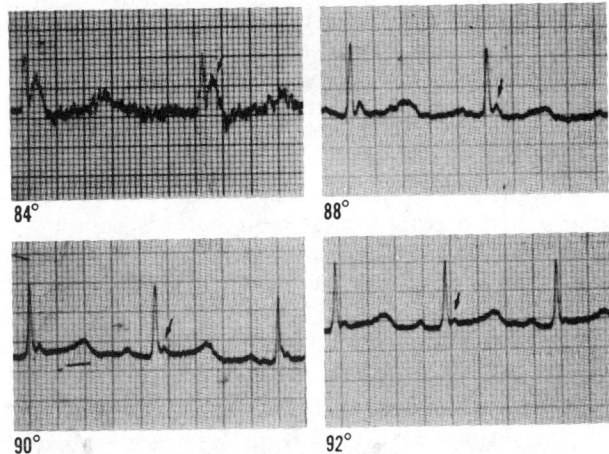

FIG. 69-1. Serial lead II electrocardiograms taken during the rewarming process, showing bradycardia, skeletal muscle tremor, and the prominent J or Osborne waves, which are pathognomonic of hypothermia. With rewarming, there is a gradual emergence of P waves and a gradual increase in the heart rate. (With permission from Fernandez, J.P., et al.: Accidental hypothermia. JAMA *212*:153, 1970.)

presence of severe cold, which may lead rescuers to suspect that the victim has been assaulted sexually.[41]

HYPOTHERMIA FROM THERMOREGULATORY IMPAIRMENT

Hypothermia in persons with thermoregulatory impairment is a more complex problem. Mortality in this group is higher than in healthy individuals suffering the same amount of heat loss. The elderly are at risk because of decreased thermogenesis, an inadequate vasoconstrictor response, decreased muscle mass, and decreased behavioral response to cold.[1] Small children and neonates are particularly at risk because of impaired thermoregulation, an increased surface-to-mass ratio, a deficiency of subcutaneous fat, and a reduced ability to shiver.[42]

In the United States, hypothermia is most frequently seen in alcoholic persons.[19,41,43,44] Alcohol causes vasodilation, reducing the effectiveness of the normal cutaneous vascular response to cold. Additionally, alcohol is a CNS depressant; its anesthetic properties reduce a victim's ability to sense cold and it alters the behavioral response to cold stress.

Hypothermia also occurs in persons intoxicated with other drugs; barbiturates and phenothiazines, cyclic antidepressants, parasympatholytics, benzodiazepines, and narcotics have all been implicated. These drugs impair both shivering and peripheral vasoconstriction.

Endocrinopathies such as hypopituitarism, hypothyroidism, and hypoadrenalism may cause hypothermia. Eighty per cent of patients with myxedema have been found to have subnormal temperatures, and the degree of heat deficit is clearly related to mortality in this condition.[45] Hypothermia is said to occur in as many as 50% of patients with hypoglycemia and, as with other endocrinopathies, may be the only clue to the diagnosis.[18,31] Hypothalamic disorders caused by trauma, tumors, and degenerative neurologic diseases such as Wernicke's encephalopathy may also cause thermoregulatory impairment.[46,47]

In addition, hypothermia may occur with exfoliative dermatitis, erythrodermas, and burns secondary to impairment of cutaneous thermoregulatory mechanisms. In sepsis, hypothermia may result from alteration of hypothalamic set point and has been associated with a poor prognosis.[48]

DIAGNOSIS AND CLINICAL FEATURES

Shivering, ataxia, and confusion are the warning signs of exposure hypothermia. Failure to recognize these symptoms at their outset can lead to tragic errors in the outdoor setting.

Patients with hypothermia may present in an awake, confused, or comatose state. If the patient is awake and shivering, the diagnosis may be obvious. If he or she is comatose, a palpably cold abdomen and muscle rigidity may be the only physical findings that help differentiate this diagnosis from other causes of coma. Thus, recognition depends on adequate clinical suspicion and diagnosis depends on accurate measurement of the rectal temperature using a low-reading thermometer. The best device for temperature measurement and monitoring is a continuous-reading thermistor probe (scale range of 20 to 42°C or 68 to 107.6°F) inserted at least 5 cm into the rectum. Few EDs have such a device, but most hospitals keep one with the hydraulic heating and cooling pad, or in the operating suite.

Correlates of poor survival include low body temperatures, prolonged cold stress, the presence of associated underlying conditions, poor response to rewarming therapy, and the development of associated complications.[3,11,16,19,41,43,49–52] Although it is difficult to make valid comparisons of the safety of various rewarming methods, in one study mortality appeared to be significantly higher among patients treated with active external rewarming methods than among those treated with passive rewarming methods.[53] Nevertheless, the choice of rewarming methods is still a controversial issue even among experts.

PREHOSPITAL STABILIZATION

For the conscious patient who is shivering, all wet clothing should be removed immediately and the vic-

tim surrounded with warm blankets or a sleeping bag. IV access should be obtained with a normal saline solution, and 50% dextrose, 25 g, should be given, along with naloxone in the appropriate clinical context. Heated humidified oxygen should be given when available.

For the obtunded patient who is shivering or rigid and spontaneously breathing, the airway should be protected and the cardiac rhythm monitored. A heated saline IV solution at 40 to 45°C should be administered in a 300 to 500 cc bolus and in volumes up to 20 cc per kg over the first hour. Dextrose and naloxone should be given. Cardiac monitoring may be difficult in this circumstance because of the presence of muscle tremor artifact.

For the patient who is apneic and pulseless and extremely stiff or rigid, treatment should include the aforementioned IV fluids and drugs. An endotracheal tube should be placed as gently as possible. Jaw rigor may make orotracheal intubation impossible, and in this case blind nasotracheal intubation can usually be accomplished. Assisted ventilation and heated humidified oxygen should be administered at physiologic rates and at a gas delivery temperature of 45°C. If the cardiac rhythm is supraventricular, CPR should be withheld until the temperature is determined. If the core temperature exceeds 28°C and the patient remains pulseless, CPR should be administered and the patient treated as for electromechanical dissociation. If the rhythm is ventricular fibrillation, CPR should continue in concert with aggressive core rewarming and advanced cardiac life support modalities, including the administration of bretylium tosylate when available.

MANAGEMENT

SUPPORTIVE MEASURES

Successful resuscitation of the hypothermic patient depends on good supportive care, prevention of further heat loss, and application of a safe method for rewarming and treatment of the underlying cause.

Hypothermic patients should have frequent vital sign determinations and be evaluated for associated underlying disorders. Laboratory evaluation should include complete blood count, arterial blood gas, serum glucose, electrolyte, BUN, creatinine, magnesium, calcium, amylase, prothrombin time, partial thromboplastin time, platelet count, and fibrinogen level. Toxicologic evaluation should be considered, depending on clinical circumstances.

To avoid dysrhythmias, patients with core temperatures below 32°C (89.6°F) should be handled gently. The electrocardiogram should be continuously monitored (Fig. 69-1). A thermistor probe should be placed in the rectum. A central line can be established for central venous pressure (CVP) determination and heated IV fluid administration. Swan-Ganz catheter placement is unnecessary and should be avoided because of the risk of inducing ventricular fibrillation. The bladder should be catheterized and urine output monitored. Patients with prolonged hypothermia are moderately hypovolemic, and their fluid deficit should be replaced during the first 1 or 2 hours with a crystalloid solution heated to a temperature not to exceed 44°C (111.2°F).[11] An initial volume of 20 cc per kg is recommended, followed by additional amounts to be guided by the results of CVP and urine output determination.

If the gag reflex or ventilation is inadequate, an endotracheal tube should be placed as gently as possible to gain control of the airway. If jaw rigor makes orotracheal placement impossible, blind nasotracheal tube placement can be accomplished. Assisted ventilation and heated, aerosolized, supplemental oxygen should be provided as needed. The patient should be suctioned whenever necessary to remove tracheobronchial secretions. Following tracheal intubation, the stomach should be emptied by means of gentle placement of a nasogastric tube.[11]

Additional doses of 50% dextrose can be given, depending on bedside or laboratory glucose determinations. Dextrose, 5% in normal saline, is the IV resuscitation fluid of choice in the hospital setting. Thiamine should be given and additional naloxone considered, depending on the clinical setting.

The interpretation of arterial blood gases in the hypothermic patient may pose a confusing dilemma to the clinician. The blood gas machine warms the patient's blood to 37°C and indicates values that would correspond to the patient's at that temperature. This is known as the uncorrected blood gas as opposed to corrected values, which are derived from correction factors applied to account for temperature effects on gas pressure solubility and hemoglobin dissociation curves. Cold temperature decreases the pH and increases the pCO_2 and pO_2 as reflected in the Severinghaus nomogram (Table 69-2).[54-56] Advocates of the use of uncorrected blood gas results in the resuscitation of hypothermia victims cite the importance of maintaining alveolar ventilation at physiologic rates rather than rates which might induce a relative respiratory alkalosis and increase the risk of ventricular fibrillation.[54]

Metabolic acidosis should be corrected cautiously because the patient's metabolic picture changes rapidly on rewarming and alkalosis could easily result.[57] Sodium bicarbonate should be reserved for only the well-ventilated, seriously acidotic patient. Overcorrection with excessive doses can lead to alkalemia, which might predispose to arrhythmias.[54] Lidocaine may be given for treatment of ventricular irritability, but bretylium is the only drug that has been shown to be effective for this purpose in laboratory animals.

TABLE 69-2 CORRECTION FACTOR FOR ARTERIAL BLOOD GASES BASED ON BODY TEMPERATURE		
	Above 37°C Change/ °C > 37	Below 37°C Change/ °C < 37
pH (unit)	− 0.015 unit	+ 0.015 unit
pCO_2 (mm Hg)	+ 4.4%	− 4.4%
pCO_2 (mm Hg)	+ 7.2%	− 7.2%

Example: Body temperature = 35°C. Measured at 37°C:
$pH = 7.15$; $pO_2 = 104$ mm. Hg; $pCO_2 = 53$ mm. Hg. True "effective" values:

$$pH = 7.15 + 0.015 (37-35) = 7.18$$
$$pO_2 = 104 - [.044 (37 - 35)] 104 = 95$$
$$pCO_2 = 53 - [0.72 (37-35)] 53 = 41$$

Levothyroxine and corticosteroids may be given if myxedema and pituitary or adrenal failure are suspected. Other drugs, including pressors and insulin, should be avoided because they have little biologic activity in the presence of hypothermia and may have undesired activity after the patient is rewarmed.[21]

Fluid and electrolyte repletion and correction of acidosis are particularly important in patients who have been hypothermic for prolonged periods. As a result of cold-induced diuresis, prolonged hypothermia can lead to marked fluid and electrolyte depletion. Potassium should be given in replacement doses only and may be necessary in the dehydrated acidotic patient. It is not uncommon, however, for the serum potassium level to be normal initially and rise into the toxic range during rewarming.[3]

Hypothermia may be associated with aspiration pneumonia and pulmonary edema. It may be important to obtain a chest x ray early in the workup. Cervical spine x rays should be obtained in any patient in whom trauma is a possibility, and abdominal x rays should be obtained to rule out free air, especially if heated peritoneal dialysis is to be performed.[11]

REWARMING TECHNIQUES

Safe rewarming is geared to the prevention and early recognition of life-threatening arrhythmias and the avoidance of the well-known phenomenon of central temperature "afterdrop" and "rewarming shock." These may occur during rewarming when blood flow through cold peripheral tissues increases the return of chilled blood from the extremities to the central circulation, producing a fall in core temperature. This afterdrop may further chill the heart and cause myocardial failure, decreased cardiac output, and a reduction in systemic blood pressure (rewarming shock). Additionally, myocardial cooling may increase the risk of cold-induced ventricular fibrillation.

Three types of rewarming methods can be considered for hypothermic patients (Table 69-3).

TABLE 69-3. REWARMING METHODS	

Passive	Warm blankets at room temperature
Active external	Heating pad
	Warm water bath
Active internal	Heated humidified oxygen by mask or endotracheal tube
	Heated intravenous fluids
	Heated gastric balloon lavage and heated enemas
	Heated peritoneal dialysis
	Heated mediastinal lavage
	Heated extracorporeal circulation and hemodialysis

PASSIVE REWARMING

The patient is insulated (e.g., with blankets) at room temperature to prevent further heat loss. This method depends on basal thermogenesis, which may produce up to 70 kcal of heat per hour at normal temperatures and 30 kcal per hour at 28°C (82.4°F).[58] The rate of rise of body temperature varies between 0.3 and 2.0°C per hour, depending on the patient's overall clinical status.[14] Proponents of this method contend that it is the most physiologic approach for elderly patients who have developed hypothermia over periods longer than 12 hours. They maintain that it reduces the incidence of core temperature afterdrop and rewarming shock, which tend to occur when heat is applied externally.[14] Failure to rewarm and the occurrence of dysrhythmias are poor prognostic signs and may indicate that a more aggressive approach is necessary.

ACTIVE EXTERNAL REWARMING

A heating pad is applied externally, or the trunk is immersed in a warm water bath maintained at a temperature of 45°C (113°F). This method depends on conductive heat transfer through the skin, the rate of which varies as a function of body surface area, vasomotor activity, and the thickness of the subcutaneous fat pad. Calculated heat gain in a nonobese individual with a temperature of 28°C (82.4°F) is 600 kcal per hour but occurs much faster in the presence of vasodilation.[58] Hydraulic pads at 45°C (113°F) can be expected to raise the temperature 1 to 2°C per hour; however, overaggressive use of a heating pad may injure the skin. Warm water immersion raises the temperature even faster; however, submersion of the patient in water makes monitoring and resuscitation almost impossible. Proponents of active external rewarming cite the advantages of more rapid rewarming in reducing the degree of core temperature after a drop in the incidence of rewarming shock or overall mortality has been demonstrated.

ACTIVE INTERNAL REWARMING

With this method, heated fluid or humidified gas is delivered or exchanged internally. One liter of IV fluid heated to 44°C (111.2°F) provides only 17 kcal to the patient with a temperature of 28°C (82.4°F), and 1 hour of heated humidified oxygen administration provides only about 30 kcal through the airway.[58] These heat gains are helpful, but may be inadequate to raise the deep body temperature quickly. Heated enemas, nasogastric lavage, and chest tube lavage have all been proposed or tried with mixed reports of success.[11,24,25,32]

Heated peritoneal lavage using 2 L of dialysate at 44°C, exchanged every 30 minutes, can accomplish 68 kcal of heat gain per hour.[58] Two catheter-wire guided trochars can be placed through the midline into the right and left abdominal gutters and can be used as afferent and efferent exchange lines to accomplish exchanges of up to 6 L per hour. Barring contraindications this technique is reasonably safe, simple, and readily available for emergency department use in any community hospital.[11,53,59] It also provides the potential to remove toxic dialysable drugs.[11,60] Minor bleeding is not uncommon, and severe intra-abdominal hemorrhage and disseminated intravascular coagulation during rewarming by peritoneal lavage have been reported.[30]

Heated cardiopulmonary bypass using the femoral-femoral bypass technique can be used to provide extracorporeal rewarming (ECR) and simultaneous circulatory support. This technique provides the most rapid and physiologic method of internal rewarming and is the rewarming method of choice for victims of severe hypothermia and those who require cardiopulmonary resuscitation or rapid rewarming for stabilization of arrhythmias.[11,12,40,58,61,62] The recent introduction of portable bypass machines now makes it possible to perform ECR in the ED in hospitals with this capability. Rewarming rates of up to 500 kcal per hour can be accomplished. The disadvantages of ECR include the risks of heparinization. Severe epistaxis, and gastrointestinal bleeding have been reported.[32]

Proponents of internal rewarming contend that it is the most physiologic approach because the core is rewarmed first, before perfusion of the chilled periphery. They cite a reduction in the incidence of core temperature afterdrop and rewarming shock; however, there is not enough overall experience to make the comparisons of mortality. Opponents contend that these techniques, with the exception of heated IV fluid administration and heated humidified oxygen delivery by mask, are unnecessarily invasive.

Obviously, no single rewarming method is best. It is advisable, however, to select a method or combination of methods to best suit the needs of each patient. Generally, patients with mild to moderate exposure hypothermia probably improve on their own, no matter what method is used. Although the experience with internal rewarming techniques is limited, heated humidified oxygen delivery and heated peritoneal dialysis appear to offer the safest and most effective means of restoring stable cardiovascular function in mild and moderately hypothermic patients.[12,51,59–61,63,64]

COMPLICATIONS AND SEQUELAE

Severe or prolonged hypothermia may cause noncardiogenic pulmonary edema, gastric submucosal hemorrhage, pancreatic necrosis, cerebrovascular accidents, and myocardial infarction. Pneumonia is exceedingly common because of the loss of protective cough reflexes, cold-induced bronchorrhea, and direct injury to lung tissue. It is the leading cause of death among patients who survive rewarming.

PITFALLS

Significant hypothermia may go unrecognized in the clinical setting when a standard thermometer or disposable device is used to determine the temperature and fails to register in the hypothermic range. This error may be compounded when an elderly or metabolically impaired patient fails to shiver and the physician fails to perform an adequate examination and recognize clues such as coolness of the abdomen to palpation.

Rough handling must be avoided, especially in patients with hypothermia of long duration or a core temperature below 28°C, who are vulnerable to ventricular fibrillation. Even with a nonpalpable pulse, CPR should be withheld initially in the presence of an organized rhythm on the cardiac monitor.

Drugs should generally be avoided because they are ineffective at low temperature ranges and may present unwanted side effects once the patient is rewarmed. Exceptions include oxygen, dextrose, naloxone, thiamine (which should be given to patients with a decreased level of consciousness), and bretylium tosylate, which may prevent ventricular fibrillation.

Aggressive correction of acidosis with bicarbonate administration or hyperventilation should be avoided because of the risk of causing alkalosis-induced ventricular fibrillation.

Patients with acute, severe hypothermia caused by rapid chilling or a specific metabolic defect such as hypoglycemia may appear nonviable, but should not be declared dead until they are rewarmed above 28°C and shown to be nonviable.

REFERENCES

1. Collis, K.J., Dore, C., Exton-Smith, A.N., et al.: Accidental hypothermia and imapired temperature homeostasis in the elderly. Br. Med. J. 1:335, 1977.

2. McNichol, M.W., and Smith, R.: Accidental hypothermia. Br. Med. J. 1:19, 1964.

3. Hauty, M.G., Esrig, B.C., Hill, J.G., and Long, W.B.: Prognostic factors in severe accidental hypothermia: Experience from the Mt. Hood tragedy. J. Trauma 2710:1107, 1987.

4. Lathrop, T.: Hypothermia: Killer of the unprepared. Portland, OR, Mazamas Mountain Club, 1975.

5. Pozos, R.S., Israel, D., McCutcheon, R., Wittners, L.E., Jr., and Sesler, D.: Human studies concerning thermal induced shivering, postoperative "shivering" and cold-induced vasodilation. Ann. Emerg. Med. 16:1037, 1987.

6. Centers for Disease Control (CDC): Hypothermia—United States. MMWR 32:46, 1983.

7. Fuhrman, F.A., and Crisman, J.M.: The influence of acute hypothermia on the rate of oxygen consumption and glycogen content of the liver and on the blood glucose. Am. J. Physiol. 149:552, 1947.

8. Burton, A.C., and Edholm, O.G.: Man in a cold environment. London, Edward Arnold Ltd., 1955.

9. Steinman, A.M., Hayward, J.S., Nemiroff, M.J.: Immersion hypothermia comparative protection of antiexposure garments in calm versus rough seas. Aviat. Space Environ. Med. 550, June 1987.

10. Cabanac, M.: Temperature regulation. Annu. Rev. Physiol. 37:415, 1975.

11. Danzl, D.F., Pozos, R.S., and Hamlet, M.P.: Accidental Hypothermia. In Management of Wilderness Environmental Emergencies (2nd ed.). Edited by Auerbach, P.S., and Geehr, E.C. St. Louis, C. V. Mosby Co., 1989.

12. Gregory, R.T., Patton, J.F., and McFadden, J.T.: Cardiovascular effects of arteriovenous shunt rewarming following experimental hypothermia. Surgery 73:561, 1973.

13. Maclean, D., and Emslie-Smith, D.: Accidental Hypothermia. Philadelphia, J. B. Lippincott Co., 1977.

14. Maclean, D., and Emslie-Smith, D.: Accidental Hypothermia. Oxford, Blackwell Scientific Publications, 1977, pp. 173–246.

15. Trevino, A., Razi, B., and Beller, B.M.: The characteristic electrocardiogram of accidental hypothermia. Arch. Intern. Med. 127:470, 1971.

16. Talman, K.G., and Cohen, A.: Accidental hypothermia. Can. Med. Assoc. J. 103:1357, 1970.

17. Witherspoon, J.M., Goldman, R.F., and Breckenridge, J.R.: Heat transfer coefficients of humans in cold water. J. Physiol. 63:459, 1971.

18. Wong, K.C.: Physiology and pharmacology of hypothermia. West. J. Med. 138:227, 1983.

19. Danzl, D.F., and Pozos, R.S.: Multicenter hypothermia survey. Ann. Emerg. Med. 16:1042, 1987.

20. Pugh, L.G.: Accidental hypothermia in walkers, climbers, and campers. Br. Med. J. 1:123, 1966.

21. Danzl, D., Sowers, M.B., Vicario, S.J., et al.: Chemical ventricular defibrillation in severe accidental hypothermia. Ann. Emerg. Med. 11:698, 1982.

22. Elenbaas, R.M., Mattison, K., Cole, H., et al.: Bretylium in hypothermia-induced ventricular fibrillation in dogs. Ann. Emerg. Med. 13:994, 1984.

23. Murphy, K., Nowak, R.M., and Tomlanovich, M.C.: Use of Bretylium tosylate as prophylaxis and treatment in hypothermic ventricular fibrillation in the canine model. Ann. Emerg. Med. 15:1160, 1986.

24. Coughlin, F.: Heart-warming procedure. N. Engl. J. Med. 228:326, 1973.

25. Linton, A.L., and Ledingham, I.M.: Severe hypothermia with barbiturate intoxication. Lancet 1:24, 1966.

26. Kanter, G.S.: Hypothermic hemoconcentration. J. Appl. Physiol. 214:856, 1968.

27. Moyer, J.H., Morris, G., and Debakey, M.E.: Hypothermia: 1. Effect on renal hemodynamics and on excretion of water and electrolytes in dog and man. Am. Surg. 145:26, 1957.

28. Chadd, M.A., and Grey, O.P.: Hypothermia and coagulation defects in the newborn. Arch. Dis. Child. 47:819, 1972.

29. Cohen, I.J.: Cold injury in early infancy. Relationship between

mortality and disseminated intravascular coagulation. Isr. J. Med. Sci. *13*:405, 1977.

30. Mahajan, S., Meyers, T.J., and Baldini, M.G.: Disseminated intravascular coagulation during rewarming following hypothermia. JAMA *245*:2517, 1981.

31. Curry, D.L., and Curry, K.P.: Hypothermia and insulin secretion. Endocrinology *87*:750, 1970.

32. O'Keefe, K.M.: Accidental hypothermia: A review of 62 cases. Ann. Emerg. Med. *6*:491, 1977.

33. Hayward, J.S., Erickson, J.D., and Collis, M.L.: Thermal balance and survival time prediction of man in cold water. Can. J. Physiol. Pharmacol. *53*:21, 1974.

34. McCance, R.A.: The hazards to men in ships lost at sea, 1940–1944. Medical Research Council, Special Reports Series 291, London, 1956.

35. Molnar, G.W.: Survival of hypothermia by men immersed in the ocean. JAMA *131*:1046, 1946.

36. Goode, R.C., Duffin, J., Miller, R., et al.: Sudden cold water immersion. Respir. Physiol. *23*:301, 1975.

37. Keatinge, W.R., Prys-Roberts, C., Cooper, K.E., et al.: Sudden failure of swimming in cold water. Br. Med. J. *1*:480, 1969.

38. Orlowski, J.P.: Drowning, near-drowning, and ice water submersions. Pediatr. Clin. North Am. *34*:75, 1987.

39. Nemiroff, M.J.: Science and the citizen: Reprieve from drowning. Sci. Am., August 1977, p. 57.

40. Bolte, R.G., Black, P.G., Bowers, R.S., Thorne, J.K., and Cornell, H.M.: The use of extracorporeal rewarming in a child submerged for 66 minutes. JAMA *260*:377, 1988.

41. Wedin, B., Vanguard, C., and Hirvonnen, J.: Paradoxical undressing in fatal hypothermia. J. Forensic Sci. *24*:543, 1979.

42. Koth, R.J., and Blackburn, M.G.: Temperature regulation in the neonate. Clin. Pediatr. *12*:634, 1973.

43. Hudson, L.D., and Conn, R.D.: Accidental hypothermia. Associated diagnosis and prognosis in a common problem. JAMA *227*:37, 1974.

44. Weyman, A.E., Greenbaum, D.M., and Grace, W.J.: Accidental hypothermia in an alcoholic population. Am. J. Med. *56*:13, 1974.

45. Forester, C.F.: Coma in myxedema. Arch. Intern. Med. *111*:734, 1963.

46. Ehrmantraut, W.R., Ticktin, H.E., and Fazurkas, J.F.: Cerebral hemodynamics and metabolism in accidental hypothermia. Eur. J. Intens. Care Med. *1*:65, 1975.

47. Philip, G., and Smith, J.F.: Hypothermia and Wernicke's encephalopathy. Lancet *2*:122, 1973.

48. Bryant, R.E., Hood, A.F., Hood, C.E., et al.: Factors affecting the mortality in gram-negative rod bacteremia. Arch. Intern. Med. *127*:120, 1971.

49. Duguid, H., Simpson, R.G., and Stowers, J.M.: Accidental hypothermia. Lancet *2*:1213, 1961.

50. Fitzgerald, F.T., and Jessup, C.: Accidental hypothermia: A report of 22 cases and review of the literature. Adv. Intern. Med. *27*:127, 1982.

51. Miller, J.W., Danzl, D.F., and Thomas, D.M.: Urban accidental hypothermia: 135 cases. Ann. Emerg. Med. *9*:456, 1980.

52. Reuler, J.B.: Hypothermia: Pathophysiology, clinical settings, and management. Ann. Intern. Med. *89*:519, 1978.

53. Gregory, R.T., and Doolittle, W.H.: Accidental hypothermia. II. Clinical implications of experimental studies. Alaska Med. *15*:48, 1973.

54. Delaney, K.A., Howland, M.A., Vassallo, S., and Goldfrank, L.R.: Assessment of acid-base disturbances in hypothermia and their physiologic consequences. Ann. Emerg. Med. *18*:72, 1989.

55. Kelman, G.R., and Nunn, J.F.: Nomograms for correction of blood PO_2, PCO_2, pH and base excess for time and temperature. J. Appl. Physiol. *9*:201, 1956.

56. Severinghaus, J.W.: Oxyhemoglobin dissociation curve correction for temperature and pH variation in human blood. J. Appl. Physiol. *9*:201, 1956.

57. Maclean, D., and Griffiths, P.D., Browning, M.C., et al.: Metabolic aspects of spontaneous rewarming in accidental hypothermia and hypothermic myxoedema. Q. J. Med. *43*:371, 1974.

58. Myers, R.A.M., Britten, J.S., and Cowley, R.A.: Hypothermia: Quantitative aspects of therapy. JACEP *8*:523, 1979.

59. Johnson, L.A.: Accidental hypothermia: Peritoneal dialysis. JACEP *6*:556, 1977.

60. Patton, J.R., and Doolittle, W.H.: Core rewarming by peritoneal dialysis following induced hypothermia in the dog. J. Appl. Physiol. *33*:800, 1972.

61. Lee, H.A., and Ames, A.C.: Hemodialysis in severe barbiturate poisoning. Br. Med. J. *1*:1217, 1965.

62. Zell, S.E., and Kurtz, K.J.: Severe exposure hypothermia: A resuscitation protocol. Ann. Emerg. Med. *14*:339, 1985.

63. White, J.D.: Hypothermia: The Bellevue experience. Ann. Emerg. Med. *11*:417, 1982.

64. Truscott, D.G., Firor, W.B., and Clein, L.J.: Accidental profound hypothermia: Successful resuscitation by core rewarming and assisted circulation. Arch. Surg. *106*:216, 1973.

FROSTBITE AND OTHER COLD INJURIES

Loren Johnson

CAPSULE

Frostbite and other forms of cold injury result from chilling of peripheral body parts. Frostbite consists of a freezing injury and subsequent ischemic and inflammatory insult from exposure to subfreezing temperatures. Immersion injury or trench foot is caused by an ischemic insult from prolonged exposure to cold water. Chilblains (also known as perniosis) are lesions caused by a nodular subcutaneous vasculitis, usually of the pretibial areas, feet, and lateral thighs, which occurs in the setting of prolonged and recurrent cold exposure. These injuries tend to occur in the same setting as hypothermia, wherein peripheral vasoconstriction is a normal physiologic response to preserve vital core organs at the expense of peripheral tissue.

Immediate rewarming in a warm water bath at 38 to 41°C (100 to 106°F) is the treatment of choice for frostbite. Once rewarmed, injured tissue must be handled carefully to protect intact blisters. Exposure to water heated above 43.3°C (110°F) and re-exposure to cold conditions must be avoided. After rewarming, injured parts should be protected with nonadherent dressings and should be splinted and elevated. Drainage of blister fluid, debridement of clear blisters, the application of aloe vera, and the administration of nonsteroidal anti-inflammatory drugs (NSAIDs) are considered to be helpful in the removal and inhibition of deleterious prostaglandins. A medical sympathectomy, with an intra-arterial injection of an alpha blocking agent such as reserpine, may be helpful during recovery. Antiseptic whirlpool immersion, careful delayed debridement, and physiotherapy assist in restoration of function.

OCCURRENCE

Local cold injury can occur by exposure to freezing and non-freezing temperatures. The extremities are most commonly affected, the feet more often than the hands. Facial injuries are not uncommon and injuries to the male genitalia have been reported.

Frostbite results from exposure of peripheral body parts to freezing temperatures. The degree and depth of injury depend on the severity and duration of the exposure. Most cases occur in ambient temperatures under −7°C (20°F) after a few hours of exposure.[1]

Immersion injury results from immersion in water less than 10°C (50°F) for more than 12 hours.[2] Immobility and dependency are predisposing factors. These injuries have caused millions of casualties during war, including the Napoleonic wars, the two World Wars, and the Korean war. Civilian casualties tend to involve accidental exposure in outdoor activities such as mountain climbing and winter sports, and occupational exposures.[3]

Our most basic understanding of prevention and treatment comes from the military experience, beginning with Baron Larrey, Napoleon's surgeon, who recognized the importance of gentle rewarming and protection of the frostbitten extremity from further cold exposure once it is rewarmed.[4] Since that time, advancements in management have largely been limited to the refinement of rewarming injury assessment and reconstructive surgical techniques.[5] Investigators have come to realize that severe frostbite is largely a fixed injury wherein the objective of treatment is to minimize complications, salvage as much tissue as possible, and the key public health objective must be education and prevention of injury.

PREDISPOSING FACTORS

The causative factors for frostbite are the same as those for hypothermia in cold weather exposure. These include cold ambient temperatures, wetness, wind chill (Table 69-4), exhaustion, and exposure at high altitude with its attendant hypoxemia and heat loss from hyperventilation. Tight, constrictive, or wet clothing is a causative factor.[6] Diabetes, peripheral vascular disease, and cigarette smoking are known to be risk factors.[7] Behavioral risk factors include mental illness and alcohol intoxication. Blacks and other persons of warm geographic origin have been shown to suffer a greater incidence of injury in military studies.[8–11] During the Korean war, the risk of cold injury was doubled in those with previous frostbite injury.[12]

PATHOPHYSIOLOGY

The frostbite injury has been characterized as a direct freezing injury and an indirect ischemic injury resulting from vascular damage and insufficiency. It has been divided into four phases: prefreeze or chilling, freeze-thaw, vascular stasis, and late ischemic.[13]

Freezing can damage tissue by disrupting enzyme function, denaturing proteins, and desiccating cells through ice crystal formation in the extracellular fluid, which becomes hyperosmotic in respect to the intracellular fluid. It is well known, however, that less specialized tissues can survive freezing.[14]

The rate of heat loss from the skin is a function of cutaneous blood flow, which is ordinarily much greater than necessary to support cellular function. Human extremities immersed in iced saline undergo maximal vasoconstriction as the deep limb temperature drops below 15°C (59°F). With further cooling, the vasoconstriction is interrupted by rhythmic bursts of vasodilation (the "hunting phenomenon").[15] This cold-induced vasodilation occurs three to five times per hour and is thought to be controlled by discrete neural oscillators.[16] As the deep limb temperature drops below 10°C (50°F), the skin freezes. Continued immersion results in cell wall damage to deep structures, including nerves, muscles, and arteries. Nonetheless, the skin is still salvageable at this stage as long as neurovascular function returns with rewarming. In

TABLE 69-4. WIND-CHILL INDEX*

Wind Speed		Cooling Power of Wind Expressed as "Equivalent Chill Temperature"																				
Knots	Mph	Temperature (°F)																				
Calm	Calm	40	35	30	25	20	15	10	5	0	−5	−10	−15	−20	−25	−30	−35	−40	−45	−50	−55	−60
		Equivalent Chill Temperature																				
3–6	5	35	30	25	20	15	10	5	0	−5	−10	−15	−20	−25	−30	−35	−40	−45	−50	−55	−60	−70
7–10	10	30	20	15	10	5	0	−10	−15	−20	−25	−35	−40	−45	−50	−60	−65	−70	−75	−80	−90	−95
11–15	15	25	15	10	0	−5	−10	−20	−25	−30	−40	−45	−50	−60	−65	−70	−80	−85	−90	−100	−105	−110
16–19	20	20	10	5	0	−10	−15	−25	−30	−35	−45	−50	−60	−65	−75	−80	−85	−95	−100	−110	−115	−120
20–23	25	15	10	0	−5	−15	−20	−30	−35	−45	−50	−60	−65	−75	−80	−90	−95	−105	−110	−120	−125	−135
24–28	30	10	5	0	−10	−20	−25	−30	−40	−50	−55	−65	−70	−80	−85	−95	−100	−110	−115	−125	−130	−140
29–32	35	10	5	−5	−10	−20	−30	−35	−40	−50	−60	−65	−75	−80	−90	−100	−105	−115	−120	−130	−135	−145
33–36	40	10	0	−5	−15	−20	−30	−35	−45	−55	−60	−70	−75	−85	−95	−100	−110	−115	−125	−130	−140	−150

| Winds above 40 have little additional effect | Little danger | Increasing danger (Flesh may freeze within 1 minute) | Great danger (Flesh may freeze within 30 seconds) |

Danger of freezing exposed flesh for properly clothed persons

* Courtesy of Plans and Training, USARAL. In Alaska Med. March 1973.

contrast, further cooling below −5°C (−23°F) damages skin irreparably.[17]

Prolonged cooling, with or without freezing, can also cause ischemic injury as a result of arteriospasm and microvascular stasis. Numerous animal studies have shown sequential arterial and arteriolar constriction; venular and capillary dilation; capillary leakage; arteriovenous shunting; platelet, fat, and red blood cell aggregation; and thrombosis in small veins, resulting in a zone of vascular insufficiency. When external warmth is applied, perfusion from deep vessels tends to return slowly in relation to the accelerated oxygen demand, exacerbating the ischemic insult. Rapid rewarming minimizes this discrepancy, and has been shown to be an effective measure for conserving tissue and promoting recoverability.[5,18] It is therefore the proven keystone for successful therapy, but the circumstantial delays usually encountered with the evacuation of frostbite victims often make rapid rewarming difficult.

Prevention of vascular damage is the key to recoverability and ability to support a skin graft.[19]

The inflammatory response also plays an important role in the ischemic injury, as evidenced by increased survival of rabbit ear tissue when antiprostaglandin and thromboxane A_2 inhibitors are used.[7] Analysis of white or clear blister fluid in human frostbite cases demonstrates increased levels of prostaglandins PGF_L and TxA_2. Clinical protocols that include debridement of white blisters, topical aloe vera application (Dermaide Aloe, Dermaide Research Corp., Chicago, Illinois) and orally administered ibuprofen have demonstrated marked improvement in tissue survival.[20]

CLINICAL FEATURES

Frostbite begins insidiously with paresthesias and numbness as an extremity or exposed area of tissue begins to freeze from its distal and outer surfaces. Freezing that reaches just into the epidermis usually appears as a shallow, blanched wheal formation on the nose or ears, known as frostnip or incipient frostbite, and disappears with contact rewarming, leaving only mild erythema. Freezing that penetrates more deeply into skin and underlying structures results in one of the four degrees of injury described in the following paragraphs from which one can determine the prognosis and therapy.

Superficial frostbite is a part- or full-thickness injury to the skin of an extremity, with additional damage to sensitive underlying structures such as nerves, muscles, and vasculature. It appears as a pale, waxy area with a doughy consistency to the touch, unless it is prolonged for several hours. The injury is nonnecrotizing, and the deep neurovascular dysfunction is usually reversible. Edema, itching, burning, deep pain, and return of coarse tactile sensation on rewarming are characteristic features.

The injury is defined as first-degree if the edema remains mild and the mottled cyanotic appearance changes to rubor without vesicle formation. Desquamation and transient swelling, erythema, and cold sensitivity can be expected over the next few weeks.

Second-degree frostbite is defined by the formation of

thick, clear, or pink vesicles extending dorsally down to the tips of the digits. The failure of return of distal neurovascular function and persistent cyanotic appearance with no vesicle formation or the development of small dark hemorrhagic vesicles that do not extend to the tips of the digits is an unfavorable prognostic sign. The edema gradually resolves and the vesicles contract and dry within 2 to 3 weeks, forming a dark eschar. The area looks necrotic, but the germinative layer of dermis is intact, so that sloughing of the eschar after 4 weeks reveals poorly keratinized skin, which is easily traumatized. Eventually complete healing occurs, with partial regeneration of toenails or fingernails. Late sequelae usually include paresthesias, hyperhidrosis, and transient or persistent cold sensitivity. The cold sensitivity is characterized by reactive vasodilation, tingling pain, and edema caused by even the most mild cold exposure.

Third-degree frostbite is a full-thickness necrotizing injury to the skin and soft tissues that may involve the more resistant connective tissue and bone. The injured part appears pale and lifeless, feels hard or woody in texture, and is devoid of movement or sensation. Deep neurovascular function is severely damaged or lost. On rewarming, the mottled cyanotic appearance persists, bordered by the vesicle formation of second-degree injury. Deep swelling and pain develop over the next several hours, and small dark vesicles form over the next few days. As the swelling resolves, a thick gangrenous eschar forms within 2 weeks, and deep aching and burning pain may occur for up to 5 weeks. Some functional regeneration and healing can be expected. The eschar or carapace protects the underlying fibrous healing, granulation and epithelialization processes, which usually require 2 to 3 months for completion. Pain, hyperhidrosis, and risk of moist gangrene are significant during this period. Trophic ulcerations, severe cold sensitivity, and arthritis may appear as late sequelae.

In *fourth-degree frostbite*, the entire thickness of the distal portions of the digits or extremity is devitalized and relatively painless after rewarming. There is mild to moderate edema, and gangrene is slow to develop once the edema resolves. Demarcation between living and dead tissue takes about 1 month, and spontaneous amputation takes at least another month.

Immersion injuries tend to be more diffuse than frostbite injuries, with ischemia involving the entire thickness of the limb. When the injury is severe, the prognosis is similar to that of deep frostbite, and the likelihood of amputation is high.

PREHOSPITAL STABILIZATION

Patients with frostbite injuries in the prethaw phase who can be transported for definitive treatment in 1 hour or less should be treated for intercurrent hypothermia and transported as expeditiously as possible. Rapid rewarming can then be accomplished in the Emergency Department (ED) or other definitive setting. Oxygenation, IV fluid resuscitation, and maintenance of body warmth are essential. The chilled extremity should be protected from further freezing or inadvertent slow rewarming by removing wet clothing, covering the patient with warm blankets, and insulating the injured extremities. Frozen mittens and boots should be thawed and then cut off.

The worst scenario for tissue salvage is rewarming and refreezing or rechilling. Any consideration to undertake field rewarming must take this risk into account and provide pain relief and supportive care of the disabled victim en route. There have been many cases of victims who have been able to walk to safety on frozen feet who would have been disabled if the injured part had been prematurely rewarmed.

For cases of prethaw injury with delayed transport in a setting where body heat can be maintained and rapid rewarming of the extremity can be accomplished at the scene or en route, this option should be considered and is preferred to prolonged spontaneous rewarming during transport. Warm water-soaked towels can be used as a substitute for warm water immersion; however, special care must be taken to avoid overheating, re-exposure to cold, or mechanical trauma to injured tissues.

MANAGEMENT

Presentation of frostbite injury to an ED in the prethaw phase is rare and presents an ideal opportunity for rapid immersion rewarming. This treatment is probably beneficial even in the partially rewarmed state of the freeze-thaw phase. The injured part should be immersed gently in a well agitated water bath at 38 to 41°C (100 to 106°F) for 20 minutes, or until there is erythematous flushing. Pain may be excruciating at this time, and narcotic analgesia and/or ketorolac may be required. Wet and constrictive clothing are removed while general body warmth is restored.

During the post-thaw vascular stasis phase, the injured surface should be cleansed gently with an antiseptic solution and the extremity should be elevated and cradled with pillows and fluff dressings. Clear vesicles should be drained or debrided and these areas should be covered with topical aloe vera (Dermaide aloe) every 6 hours.[20,21] Ibuprofen, 400 to 800 mg po twice daily, or a comparable systemic anti-inflammatory agent should be given as early as possible. Ketorolac, the potent antiprostanoid parenteral analgesic agent, appears to be an ideal choice for the treatment of pain; however, there is limited experience on which to base such a recommendation at this time. Smoking is prohibited because of its peripheral vasoconstrictive effects.

Various diagnostic imaging techniques have been used to assess the degree of vascular injury. These include thermography, angiography, digital plethysmography, and radioisotope vascular and bone scanning. These techniques have been advocated for early assessment of tissue viability and have advanced the ability of surgeons to make early decisions regarding amputation and rehabilitation; however, no technique is entirely reliable during the period of vascular instability, which lasts 2 to 3 weeks.

The frostbite injury presents a high risk of infection because of the presence of devitalized tissues, edema, and loss of skin barrier protection. Early parenteral penicillin therapy during edema formation has been advocated as a way to control streptococcal infection.[21] The patient should be immunized against tetanus.[22]

The injured surface should be bathed in an antiseptic solution and cradled gently in an open fashion, with sterile cotton between the fingers and toes. Clear vesicles are drained and ruptured vesicles should be debrided. Gentle whirlpool treatments with a dilute lukewarm antiseptic solution are begun early and continued twice daily. These reduce the risk of infection, aid debridement, soften the eschar, and give the patient a sense of progress in therapy. Physiotherapy should begin early, with frequent active mobilization of each involved joint; otherwise passive mobilization is required. Constricting eschars are bivalved, and the extremity is elevated frequently to minimize swelling.

Sympathectomy relieves arteriospasm, but is a major surgical procedure that is contraindicated during the acute phase of therapy because blood flow may be diverted preferentially to uninjured tissues. The intra-arterial injection of sympatholytic drugs obviates these problems because it can be performed easily and selectively. An intermediate alpha blocker, tolazoline hydrochloride, can be mixed with a long-acting alpha-blocking substance, reserpine, and injected with saline. The reserpine effect begins in 3 to 24 hours, and persists for 2 to 4 weeks.[23,24]

Nifedipine at a dose of 20 mg to 60 mg po daily has been shown to be effective in clearing the lesions of chilblains and preventing the occurrence of new lesions by way of its vasodilator effect.[16] It is likewise effective in preventing Raynaud's phenomenon and should be useful for the vascular instability of the post-thaw frostbite injury; however, there are no reports of its use for this purpose.

Several other measures have been used to enhance microvascular perfusion, but most, including intravenous heparin administration, systemic vasodilators, ethanol, enzymes, steroids, and flavenoids, have not proven useful. Dimethyl sulfoxide (DMSO), an experimental freely diffusing osmotic buffer, has been somewhat effective when applied topically to superficial frostbite lesions in animals; however, this substance is exothermic when mixed with water, and its therapeutic benefit may derive from earlier rewarming.[25] Antisludging agents, such as low molecular weight dextran and experimental nonionic surfactants, may prove helpful with more clinical experience.[19] Hyperbaric oxygen therapy has been recommended but has not been proven of value.[26]

In general, amputations, revisions, and dermatoplasties should be delayed until there is complete demarcation and separation of gangrenous tissue. In this way, large amounts of underlying tissue may be conserved, except when early liquefaction or the development of moist gangrene or infection necessitate early amputation. Surgeons usually amputate toes and feet much earlier than fingers and hands for functional and rehabilitation purposes. When given ample time for demarcation, injuries to the upper extremity tend to exhibit a surprising amount of tissue regeneration and sparing of extremity length. Advancements in diagnostic imaging and early assessment of vascular supply to bone and deep tissues have permitted much earlier application of amputation, debridement, grafting, and rehabilitation procedures with hopeful results.[27]

Late sequelae of frostbite injury are extremely common, including cold sensitivity, pigmentary changes, and hyperhidrosis in most cases and pain, hyperesthesia, and hyperkeratosis in few cases.[18] Epiphyseal damage and growth deformities are common in children, and postinjury arthritis is common in all age groups.[1,28–30]

PITFALLS

Premature rewarming and failure to protect the frostbitten extremity from physical jostling and thermal extremes must be avoided. Rescuers tend to focus on the obvious injury, such as the severely frostbitten extremity, and may fail to recognize hypothermia and the need for supportive care of vital functions, including oxygenation, hydration, and general body rewarming. It is not uncommon for mentally ill, homeless, and debilitated persons to present with frostbite injuries in the late ischemic phase, and these injuries should not be subject to premature amputation based on a presumption of full-thickness necrosis.

REFERENCES

1. Blair, J.R., Schatzki, R., and Orr, N.D.: Sequelae to cold injury in one hundred patients: Followup study four years after occurrence of cold injury. JAMA 163:1203, 1957.
2. White, J.C., and Scoville, W.B.: Trench foot and immersion foot. N. Engl. J. Med. 232:415, 1945.
3. Smith, D.J., Robson, M.C., and Heggers, J.P.: Frostbite and other cold-induced injuries. In Wilderness and Environmental Emergencies. Edited by Auerbach, P.S., and Geehr, E.C. St. Louis, C.V. Mosby Co., 1989.
4. Larrey, D.J.: Memoirs of military surgery, Vol. 2. Baltimore, Joseph Cushing, 1814.

5. Fuhrman, F.A., and Crissman, J.M.: Studies on gangrene following cold injury. VII. Treatment of cold injury by immediate rapid rewarming.

6. Washburn, B.: Frostbite—what it is—how to prevent it—emergency treatment. N. Engl. J. Med. 266:974, 1962.

7. Reus, W.F., et al.: Acute effects of tobacco smoking on blood flow in the cutaneous micro-circulation. Br. J. Plast. Surg. 37:213, 1984.

8. Hamlet, M.D.: An overview of medically related problems in the cold environment. Milit. Med. 152:393, 1987.

9. Miller, D., and Bjornson, D.R.: An investigation of cold-injured soldiers in Alaska. Milit. Med. 127:247, March 1962.

10. Rennie, D.W., and Adams, T.: Comparative thermoregulatory response to Negroes and white persons to acute cold stress. J. Appl. Physiol. 11:201, 1957.

11. Sumner, D.S., et al.: Host factors in human frostbite. Milit. Med. 139:454, June 1974.

12. Orr, K.D., and Fainer, D.C.: Cold injuries in Korea during winter of 1950–1951. Fort Knox, KY, Army Medical Research Laboratory, 1951.

13. Kulka, J.P.: Vasomotor microcirculatory insufficiency: Observations on non-freezing cold injury of the mouse ear. Angiology 12:491, 1961.

14. Merryman, H.T.: Mechanisms of freezing in living cells and tissues. Science 124:515, 1956.

15. Pozos, R.S., Israel, D., McCutcheon, R., Wittmers, L.E., Jr., and Sesler, D.: Human Studies Concerning Thermal Induced Shivering, Postoperative "Shivering" and Cold-Induced Vasodilation. Ann. Emerg. Med. 16:1037, 1987.

16. Rustin, M., et al.: The treatment of chilblains with nifedipine. Br. J. Derm. 120:267, 1989.

17. Keatinge, W.R., and Cannon, P.: Freezing point of human skin. Lancet 1:11, 1960.

18. Mills, W.J., Jr.: Frostbite. Alaska Med. 15:27, 1973.

19. Weatherly-White, R.C.A., Sjostrom, B., and Paton, B.C.: Experimental studies in cold injury. J. Surg. Res. 4:17, 1964.

20. Heggers, J.P., et al.: Experimental and clinical observations on frostbite. Ann. Emerg. Med. 16:1056, 1987.

21. McCauley, R.L., et al.: Frostbite injuries: A rational approach based on the pathophysiology. J. Trauma 23:143, 1983.

22. Didlake, R.H., and Kukora, J.S.: Tetanus following frostbite injury. Contemp. Ortho. 10:69, 1985.

23. Porter, J.M., et al.: Intra-arterial sympathetic blockage in the treatment of clinical frostbite. Am. J. Surg. 132:625, 1976.

24. Snider, R.L., and Porter, J.M.: Treatment of experimental frostbite with intra-arterial sympathetic blocking drugs. Surgery 77:557, 1975.

25. Wood, D.C., et al.: Some experimental studies with dimethyl sulfoxide (DMSO) in cold injury. Curr. Ther. Res. 12:97, 1970.

26. Okuboye, J.A., and Ferguson, C.C.: The use of hyperbaric oxygen in the treatment of experimental frostbite. Can. J. Surg. 11:78, 1968.

27. Gottlieb, L.J., Zachary, L.S., and Krizek, T.J.: Aggressive surgical treatment of frostbite injuries. Presented at Mid-western Association of Plastic Surgeons Meeting, May 1987.

28. Brown, F.E., Spiegel, P.K., and Boyle, W.E., Jr.: Digital deformity: An effect of frostbitten children. Pediatrics 71:955, 1983.

29. Carrera, G.F., et al.: Radiographic changes in the hands following childhood frostbite injury. Skeletal Radiol. 6:33, 1981.

30. Knize, D.M., et al.: Prognostic factors in the management of frostbite. J. Trauma 9:749, 1969.

CHAPTER 70

HEAT STRESS DISEASES

Audrey Urbano-Brown and
Robert P. Proulx

CAPSULE

All hyperthermic patients with altered mental status or neurologic deficits should receive rapid cooling measures along with initial general stabilization. Differential diagnosis will modify subsequent therapy. Because a cooling delay translates directly into increased morbidity and mortality, rapid prehospital transport is mandated. External evaporative cooling measures are the current standard of care. External evaporative cooling can be initiated en route to the emergency department (ED) and continued until signs of neurologic recovery at safe core temperatures are achieved. Iced saline peritoneal lavage, effective in the canine model, is under investigation. Prevention of heat stress disease through education should be a part of every discharge plan.

INTRODUCTION

Heat stress disorders span a spectrum from minor heat illnesses through heat exhaustion and heat stroke. Heat stroke is a true medical emergency that results from complete loss of thermoregulatory control. Once the body's cooling mechanisms are overwhelmed, accurate diagnosis, rapid cooling and supportive care are essential to reduce morbidity and prevent mortality.

PATHOPHYSIOLOGY

The important difference between minor heat illnesses and heat stroke is the maintenance of thermoregulation. In any animal, the core body temperature at any given moment is the result of internal and external factors that increase or lower temperature. In warm-blooded animals, internal homeostatic mechanisms are at work to maintain body temperature within relatively narrow limits. This is *thermoregulation*.

The body's heat production results from absorption of heat from sources external to the body (for example, sunshine, environmental temperature) and from internal heat-producing metabolic processes. Normal adult basal metabolic processes generate approximately 2000 to 4000 Kcal per day. Strenuous exercise can contribute an additional 600 to 900 Kcal per hour, and solar irradiation an additional 100 to 150 Kcal per hour, depending on ambient temperature.

Heat loss is continual and is effected by several mechanisms. *Radiation* of heat through space occurs when heat emanates from the body in rays, much like rays of heat from hot asphalt. *Convection*, the movement of air, transfers heat as cooler air passes over a warmer object; by this mechanism heat is blown off the body by cool breezes. Both radiation and convection are effective when air temperature is less than body temperature. Radiation accounts for approximately 60% of the total heat loss from the nude person at normal room temperature. Convection, at room temperature without gross air movement, accounts for an additional 12% of the body's heat loss. Although *conduction* transfers heat directly from the body to another cooler object, such as a chair, only 3% of the body's total heat is dissipated in this manner. In water, at comfortable temperatures, the rate of heat loss through conduction increases several fold. Once ambient air or water temperature exceeds body temperature, conduction becomes ineffective. *Evaporation* of water from the body as sweat and insensible water losses accounts for the final 25% of total heat loss from the nude individual at rest. Despite continual insensible water loss from the lungs, the respiratory evaporative heat loss component is clinically significant only in panting mammals, not in humans.

As ambient temperature climbs higher than 35° C (95° F), virtually all heat loss is accomplished by sweating. As ambient humidity exceeds 75%, the rate of evaporation decreases drastically and sweating becomes an ineffective means of dissipating heat. Without effective heat dissipation, body temperature rises.

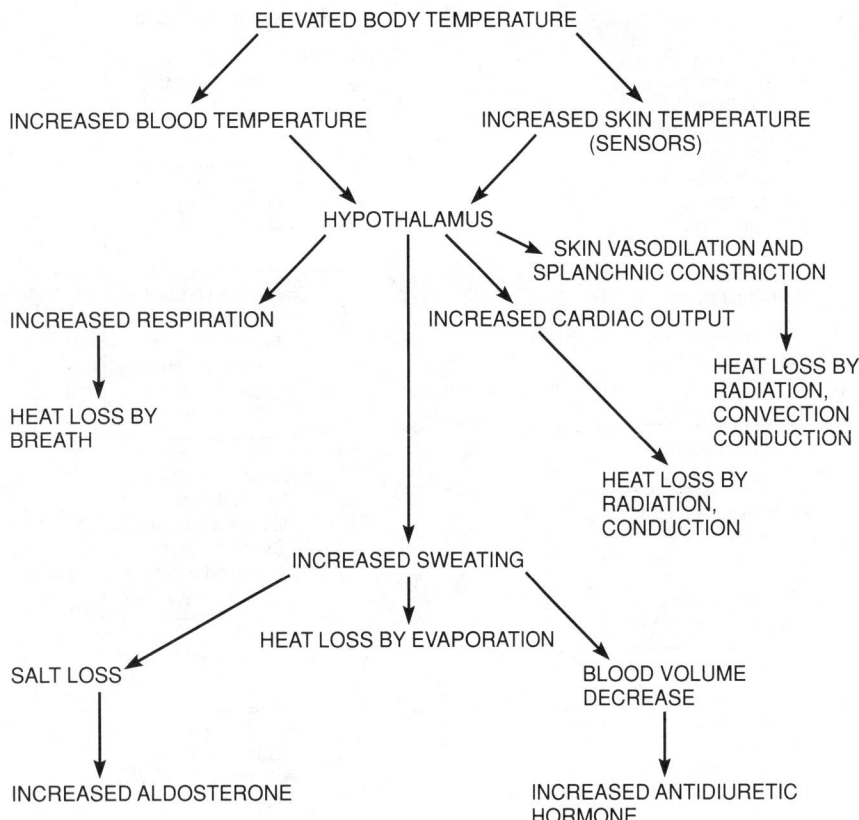

ELEVATED BODY TEMPERATURE

INCREASED BLOOD TEMPERATURE

INCREASED SKIN TEMPERATURE
(SENSORS)

HYPOTHALAMUS

SKIN VASODILATION AND
SPLANCHNIC CONSTRICTION

INCREASED RESPIRATION

INCREASED CARDIAC OUTPUT

HEAT LOSS BY
RADIATION,
CONVECTION
CONDUCTION

HEAT LOSS BY
BREATH

HEAT LOSS BY
RADIATION,
CONDUCTION

INCREASED SWEATING

HEAT LOSS BY EVAPORATION

SALT LOSS

BLOOD VOLUME
DECREASE

INCREASED ALDOSTERONE

INCREASED ANTIDIURETIC
HORMONE

FIG. 70-1.   *Physiology of temperature control.*

In summary, because of the mechanisms of heat dissipation, heat, humidity, and lack of wind are all conducive to heat stress disease.

Temperature control in human beings is accomplished both acutely and gradually through acclimatization. As core body temperature rises acutely, blood and skin temperatures rise. Skin sensors, along with the direct effect of warmed blood, stimulate the anterior hypothalamic heat-sensitive neurons to maintain a set-point temperature of approximately 37° (98.6° F). When the body's normal temperature range of approximately 97 to 99° F is exceeded, the autonomic nervous system is activated by hypothalamic neuronal output to bring about several changes, which maximize heat loss at the skin/air interface. Under autonomic control, skin vasodilation and splanchnic vasoconstriction occur, increasing the amount of blood shunted to peripheral blood vessels. Cardiac output increases up to four times baseline, allowing more warm blood to pass through these dilated skin vessels away from hyperthermic core organs. Respiratory rate increases to maximize evaporative heat loss through exhaled air. Cholinergic sympathetic nerve-fiber output controls the increased production of sweat. With increased losses of sweat, a hypotonic salt-containing solution, aldosterone, and antidiuretic hormone secretion are stimulated, resulting in sodium reabsorption and restoration of circulating blood volume. Fig-

ure 70-1 reviews the physiology of temperature control.

The process by which the human system gradually adapts to a variety of environmental conditions is *acclimatization*. Acclimatization occurs over several days to weeks when a person is exposed to continuing heat stress. A more efficient response to any given heat load develops gradually as sweat production increases to approximately two and one-half times its previous maximum within 6 weeks. Associated with the increase in sweat production is a decrease in sodium chloride concentration of the sweat itself, mediated by aldosterone secretion. As a result, an acclimatized runner loses from 3 to 4 L of fluid per hour and the losses of the unacclimatized athlete approximate 1 to 1½ L of fluid per hour. Increased hypotonic fluid losses decrease extracellular fluid volume and thereby renal blood flow. Aldosterone secretion is stimulated, sodium retention follows, and circulatory blood volume and cardiac output increase. As previously reviewed, cardiac output increases, along with hypothalamic-induced skin vasodilation, allow more effective heat loss.

The basic thermal range of cell viability extends from −1°C (formation of ice crystals occurs and disrupts the cell) to 46°C (114.8°F) at which protein damage is inevitable. When the thermal regulatory checks and balances are overwhelmed or broken down, the body

Increased Heat Production:

Decreased Heat Loss:

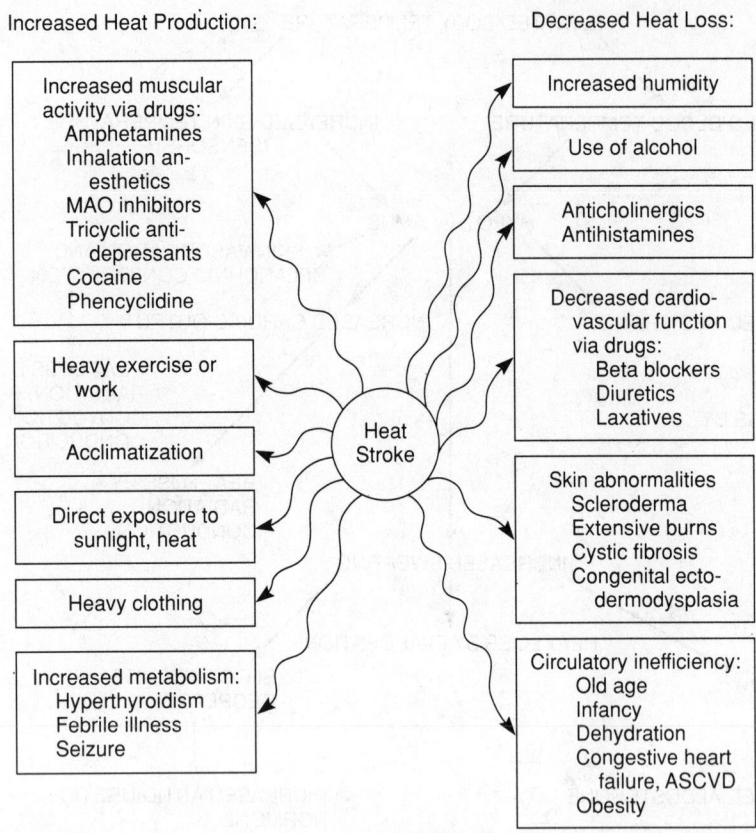

FIG. 70-2. *Factors predisposing to heat stroke.*

gets too hot. Central circulatory volume is then shunted to maintain heart, lung and brain function at the expense of peripheral vasoconstriction, and core temperature skyrockets. Such a breakdown in thermoregulatory control occurs with the increased endogenous heat production that accompanies strenuous activity, fever or seizures or by means of drugs known to increase metabolic heat production. Drugs known to increase metabolic heat production include amphetamines, monamine oxidase inhibitors, cocaine, phencyclidine (PCP), aspirin, and tricyclic antidepressants. Conversely, thermal regulatory control mechanisms may fail because of decreased heat loss from drug effects. Beta blockers, diuretics, laxatives, and sympatholytics blunt cardiac output increases. Antihistamines, phenothiazines, anticholinergics, and ethanol interfere with behavioral responses to heat stress and with the production of sweat. Further impaired ability to dissipate heat occurs in the elderly with atherosclerotic cardiovascular disease (ASCVD), the obese, and in states of dehydration in which cardiac output can be only marginally increased as core temperature increases. Inability to perspire effectively occurs with sweat gland and skin abnormalities such as scleroderma, cystic fibrosis, and previous burn wounds. Finally, survivors of heat stroke have permanently altered and inefficient thermoregulatory responses, placing them at great risk for subsequent heat

stress disease. The factors predisposing to the breakdown of thermoregulatory control are summarized in Figure 70-2.

CLINICAL PRESENTATION/ EXAMINATION

MINOR HEAT ILLNESSES (TABLE 70-1)

In minor heat illnesses, thermoregulation is maintained. Although little is known about diagnosis and treatment, definitions of several of these noncritical disorders have been established.

Heat edema is a self-limited swelling of the hands and feet (occasionally progressing to pitting ankle edema) which occurs on initial exposure to a hot environment. Resolution occurs after several hours in cooler surroundings.

Heat cramps are the painful contractions that follow exertion of commonly used skeletal muscles (usually the thighs and shoulders). The patient usually has normal vital signs. They are probably precipitated by mild hyponatremia resulting from the replacement of sodium and water losses of sweat with hypotonic fluids. Heat cramps occur more commonly in the fit, acclimatized individual who is able to sweat more profusely than in an unacclimatized counterpart. Treatment for this self-limited condition is to rest and stretch in a cool environment. Massage of the involved limbs generates heat and should be discouraged. Ingestion of whole salt tablets induces vomiting, gastritis, and cerebral dehydration. If cramps persist despite rest in a cool environment, oral rehydration with a 0.1% saline solution is recommended. This solution can be prepared by adding ¼ teaspoon of salt to 1 quart of water. Alternatively, intravenous rehydration with normal saline may be done and can provide dramatic relief, but should be monitored to avoid fluid overload. Heat cramps, a benign entity, must be distinguished from exertional rhabdomyolysis, in which muscle pain does not abate with rest and rehydration. Rhabdomyolysis, characterized by death of muscle cells, results in the release of creatine phosphokinase (CPK) and myoglobin. Myoglobinuria may be complicated by renal failure. When subjective complaints of muscle pain exceed objective findings on physical examination, consider screening CPK and a urinalysis before hospital discharge. Other entities in the differential diagnosis include hyperventilation, black widow spider bite, and hypokalemia.

Heat tetany is manifested by carpopedal spasm, probably secondary to hyperthermia-induced hyperventilation. Tetany is precipitated by rapid pH and body temperature changes. Consequently, on examination, hyperventilation may no longer be present despite cramping. Serum calcium is usually normal. Although Chvostek's sign may be positive, calcium and magnesium should be checked only if symptoms persist after resting and stretching in a cool environment.

Heat syncope occurs because of postural hypotension in unacclimatized individuals secondary to shunting of blood to peripheral tissues for cooling. Dehydration, if present at all, is usually mild. To treat heat syncope, place the patient supine, rehydrate if necessary, and instruct the patient to avoid prolonged or sudden standing in the heat.

Prickly heat is a maculopapular erythematous rash most common on clothed areas of the body. Prickly heat appears when maceration and infection block sweat-gland pores. Treatment involves exposing the rash to dry, cool air several hours a day.

Heat exhaustion is a nebulous but common problem characterized by volume depletion due to sweating. Fluid and electrolytes that are lost are not adequately replaced, resulting in illness. To understand the electrolyte losses, evaluate the electrolyte composition of sweat: primarily sodium (30 to 50 milliequivalents per liter), chloride (45 to 55 milliequivalents per liter) and potassium (5 milliequivalents per liter). Physiologic replacement requires approximately 300 mL of 0.9% NaCl and 700 mL of free water per liter of sweat lost. As a consequence of inadequate rehydration, signs

TABLE 70-1. MINOR HEAT ILLNESSES
Heat edema
Heat cramps
Heat tetany
Heat syncope
Prickly heat
Heat exhaustion

and symptoms of heat exhaustion reflect tissue hypoperfusion, although thermoregulation is maintained. The patient may present with anxiety, irritability, headache, dizziness or malaise, but cerebral function, i.e., mental status, is normal. Nausea, vomiting, anorexia, hyperventilation, tachycardia, and orthostatic blood pressure changes may be present. Signs of heat cramps, heat tetany, or heat syncope may accompany heat exhaustion also. No laboratory tests are diagnostic. BUN, creatinine, hematocrit, sodium, and chloride may reflect dehydration. Core temperature is usually below 39°C (102° F). Treatment consists of rest, removal of clothing, and removal from the hot environment. Volume replacement should be guided by objective evaluation (orthostatic blood pressure changes, BUN, creatinine, hematocrit, etc.), and overhydration should be avoided. In mild cases, oral 0.1% saline solution should suffice; more severe dehydration may require normal saline or 0.5 NS IV. Uncomplicated recovery can be expected within several hours.

HEAT STROKE

Heat stroke is a true medical emergency that results from the loss of thermoregulatory control. Heat stroke claims 5000 lives per year in the United States. Eighty percent of these deaths are in individuals older than 50 years of age. Mortality ranges from 20 to 70%.

Heat stroke is characterized by abnormal cerebral function with core temperature usually greater than 40°C (104°F). Although anhidrosis was historically considered an essential feature, now heat stroke is recognized in patients with normal or even extreme sweating. When sweat gland failure and anhidrosis do occur, the clinical entity of *classic heat stroke* is produced. Clinical presentation can therefore be divided into that of classic heat stroke, a problem of heat dissipation, and *exertional heat stroke*, a problem primarily of increased heat production.

Central nervous system (CNS) dysfunction is universal at core temperatures greater than 45°C (113°C). Intracranial edema occurs, especially in the cerebellum, with microhemorrhages demonstrated throughout the CNS. Mental status changes result and are evident as confusion, lethargy, agitation, seizures, or coma. Focal signs, including hemiplegia and decerebrate posturing, have been described. CNS changes are all potentially reversible, with reported cases of

TABLE 70-2. HEAT DISEASE SYNDROMES

Syndrome	Rectal Temperature	Central Nervous System	Skin	Acute Renal Failure	Rhabdo-myolysis	DIC	Treatment
Classic heat stroke exhaustion	Above 40°C (140°F)	Seizure, psychosis, coma	Hot and dry	Uncommon	Rare	Uncommon	Rapid cooling
Exertional heat stroke	Above 40°C (140°F)	Seizure, psychosis, coma	Sweating present	Common	Common	Common	Rapid cooling
Heat exhaustion	Under 39°C (102°F)	Headache, dizziness, nausea, other mild symptoms	Sweating present	—	—	—	Rest, re-hydration as needed

recovery in patients with fixed pupils and flat EEGs. The most common persistent deficits are those in cerebellar functions.

Heat stress stimulates hyperventilation and tachycardia. The resulting respiratory alkalosis induces increased cellular uptake of potassium as well as tetany and carpopedal spasm. Tachycardia occurs to maintain cardiac output in the face of profound vasodilation of cutaneous blood vessels. With the shunting of blood to the periphery and profuse sweating, hypovolemia can precipitate acute tubular necrosis in the kidney. Myoglobinuria, secondary to rhabdomyolysis (rare in classic heat stroke, more common in exertional heat stroke), further damages kidney tubules. In severe cases, skeletal muscle injury may raise creatine phosphokinase above 20,000 international units/(IU) per liter. In the liver, centrilobular necrosis occurs because of direct thermal injury, producing abnormal liver enzymes.

Thermal injury also occurs to vascular endothelium and causes increased platelet aggregation and changes in capillary permeability. Thermal deactivation of plasma proteins further depletes clotting factors. Disseminated intravascular coagulopathy (DIC) (more common in exertional heat stroke) may occur secondary to decreased production and activity of clotting factors combined with intravascular clotting factor consumption. These clinical presentations of classic and exertional heat stroke, as well as those of heat exhaustion, are contrasted in Table 70-2.

DIFFERENTIAL DIAGNOSIS

The differential diagnosis of hyperthermia with mental status changes or neurologic deficits includes:

1. Infectious diseases (meningitis, cerebral falciparum malaria)
2. Severe dehydration
3. Central anticholinergic syndrome
4. Cerebral vascular accident (intracerebral bleeding, stroke, or subarachnoid hemorrhage)
5. Neuroleptic malignant syndrome
6. Malignant hyperthermia
7. Monamine oxidase inhibitors (administered in conjunction with tyramine containing substances, narcotics, or tricyclic antidepressants)
8. Amphetamine toxicity
9. Salicylate toxicity
10. Idiopathic lethal catatonia
11. Thyroid storm
12. Drug withdrawal syndromes
13. Pheochromocytoma
14. Status epilepticus.

The *central anticholinergic syndrome* mimics atropine poisoning. It is precipitated by anticholinergics, including the neuroleptics (antipsychotics). Confusion, agitation, or coma may develop, associated with hyperthermia, tachycardia, and increased muscular tone. Poor motor coordination, ataxia, and dysarthria may be present in the awake patient. Treatment is with physostigmine (Antilirum), withdrawal of anticholinergic agents, and cooling.

The *neuroleptic malignant syndrome* (NMS), a lethal complication of neuroleptic medications, is discussed elsewhere in this text. The two most common offending agents are haloperidol (Haldol) and fluphenazine (Prolixin). This syndrome is characterized by hyperthermia, alternating levels of consciousness (agitation, coma, seizure), skeletal muscle rigidity, and autonomic nervous system instability. Autonomic nervous instability may include fluctuating blood pressure, marked ptyalism, urinary incontinence, and profound diaphoresis. When alert, patients may present with mutism. Hyperthermia similar to that of heat stroke, 39.4°C (103°F) to 42.2°C (106°F) may be present. The hot and sweaty victim of NMS, however, also demonstrates lead-pipe rigidity of skeletal muscles, distinguishing the two syndromes. NMS is higher in patients receiving neuroleptics and affects men five times more often than women. Eighty percent of the afflicted are under 40. The severe syndrome carries a 20% mortality, primarily from respiratory failure. Treatment is with bromocriptine (Parlodel), 2.5 to 10 mg orally every 8 hours, rapid cooling, antipyretics, and withdrawal of all neuroleptics. Promethazine (Phenergan), prochlorperazine (Compazine) and chlorpromazine (Thorazine) all have neuroleptic properties and can be offending agents. Anticholinergics, used to treat extrapyramidal dysfunction, are ineffective or only partially effective in NMS.

Malignant hyperthermia is an autosomal dominant metabolic disease that can cause sudden death if the individual is exposed to certain precipitating agents or conditions. Precipitating factors include depolarizing muscle relaxants such as succinylcholine (Anectine), gaseous anesthetics (halothane), or the physiologic stress of trauma, heat, strenuous exercise, and viral infections. Unlike NMS, malignant hyperthermia is peripheral or postsynaptic in origin, and neuromuscular blockade (as with bromocriptine) is ineffective. The heat generated in this disease is by generalized skeletal muscle contraction. Abnormal calcium influx occurs through mitochondrial and muscle sarcoplasmic reticulum inhibiting the normal contraction-relaxation mechanism. Although muscle biopsy and contracture tests can be diagnostic, no accurate chemical screening test is available. Malignant hyperthermia can be suspected in the asymptomatic patient with creatine phosphokinase levels elevated into the thousands or one who demonstrates exaggerated anxiety and muscle fasciculations after administration of depolarizing muscle relaxants. A subsequent unexplained rise in temperature heralds the disease. The malignant hyperthermic patient is rigid, hot, and dry, unlike the sweaty, rigid NMS patient or the patient with normal muscular tone in heat stroke. Complications of the prolonged generalized muscle contractions of malignant hyperthermia include rhabdomyolysis, hemolysis, and consumptive coagulopathy progressing to DIC. Treatment is by removal of the precipitating agent, cooling blankets, dantrolene sodium (2 mg per kg up to 10 mg per kg IV) and supportive care.

Amphetamine toxicity results in sympathetic overactivity with increased heart rate, respiratory rate, blood pressure, and temperature. Restlessness, fine tremor, and muscle twitching may progress to frank seizure. Mydriasis and diaphoresis are common. Treatment includes gastric lavage and activated charcoal instillation, aggressive cooling, and supportive care of arrythmias, seizures or hypertension.

Idiopathic lethal catatonia is a rare hyperthermic syndrome characterized by stupor, mutism, and waxy flexibility. This form of catatonia was described before the advent of neuroleptics and does not necessitate a diagnosis of schizophrenia or require neuroleptic treatment. Despite absence of autonomic dysfunction (with lack of diaphoresis or vital sign fluctuation), acute lethal catatonia may be clinically indistinguishable from the mental status changes of NMS. Catatonic

signs are nonspecific; therefore metabolic and intracranial disorders need to be excluded. Treatment is cooling and supportive care as needed.

PREHOSPITAL ASSESSMENT AND STABILIZATION

All hyperthermic patients with altered mental status or neurologic deficits should receive rapid cooling measures along with initial general stabilization. Differential diagnosis modifies subsequent therapy. In the field, every effort should be made to prevent heat load. The hot patient should be stripped of clothing and kept in air conditioning if available. Water can be sprinkled on the patient and evaporated by air conditioning, fanning, or open windows (or helicopter doors) during the ride to the ED. An intravenous line should be established and oxygen given. Seizure precautions should be undertaken and cardiac monitoring performed en route. Because effective cooling delay translates directly into increased morbidity and mortality, rapid transport is mandated.

In the wilderness environment or with prolonged transport times, recognition of the gravity of the situation is important. The victim must be transported as soon as possible to the nearest capable medical facility. In the meantime, every effort to reduce heat load must be made. All clothing should be removed and the patient placed in the shade. Tent flaps should be opened while awaiting transport. If water is available, a spray of water and fanning to evaporate it should be used. If a cold stream or lake is available, cautious immersion with ongoing extremity massage should be undertaken. If shaking chills occur, the patient should be removed from the water until they stop, then reimmersed. Treatment should be discontinued when CNS signs and symptoms disappear and the skin temperature appears equal to a normal control (yourself), using the back of the hand as a sensor. When transportation becomes available, it should take priority over makeshift cooling measures. In many situations, transport may have to be by ground to some point where more rapid air transport is available.

TREATMENT

INITIAL STABILIZATION AND PROCEDURES (FIG. 70-3)

The treatment of hyperthermia associated with mental status changes or neurologic deficits is rapid and aggressive cooling. Using 38.5°C (101.3°F), as an end

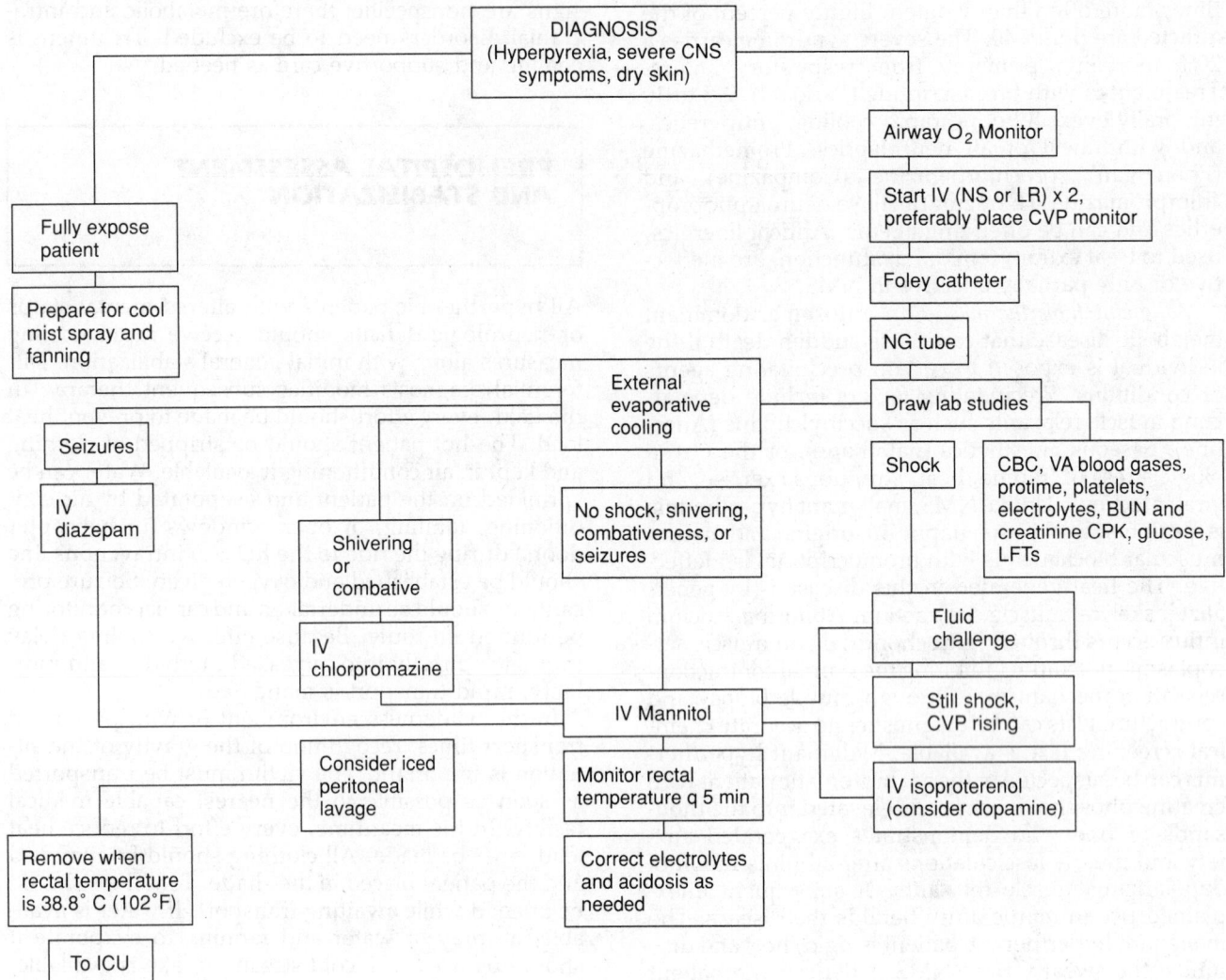

FIG. 70-3. Proposed plan for management of heat stroke in the emergency department.

point, heat stroke victims cooled within 1 hour suffer a 5% mortality. Mortality rose to 18% when cooling required more than 1 hour.

As with any other life-threatening condition, the ABCs of resuscitation must be attended to and supportive care administered. Airway support and effective ventilation must be ensured. Circulatory support may require two large-caliber intravenous lines with normal saline or Ringer's lactate solution, the IV fluids of choice. Central venous monitoring to avoid overhydration (especially in classic heat stroke, in which sweat gland dysfunction may prevent significant fluid losses) is recommended. A urinary catheter will aid in monitoring fluid status. If not already done, the patient must be fully exposed and transferred to a cool environment. Spontaneous cooling of the naked patient is known to occur at 0.03°C to 0.06°C per minute. A rectal probe for accurate measurement of core temperature is necessary. Glass or electric thermometers that do not register above 41°C (105.8°F) are inadequate.

The most rapid method of cooling remains controversial. Some centers advocate immersion in a tub of ice water to promote conduction of heat away from the body. Although this is an effective method of cooling, mechanical complications abound. An agitated, hallucinating patient in a tub is difficult to control or assess; electrical monitoring and defibrillation become hazardous and CPR, if needed, is difficult to perform. Obese patients are difficult to fit into a tub. Cutaneous vasoconstriction ensues with decreased heat loss if the extremities are not massaged during immersion. Seizures, pulmonary edema, and dysrhythmias have occurred as complications of this method of treatment.

External evaporation achieved by spraying the naked patient with cool mist while using fans to enhance air flow over the body reduces core temperature by 0.06°C to 0.16°C per minute. Electrical monitoring equipment can be kept water-free, CPR can be performed as necessary, and shivering and vasoconstriction are minimized by this technique. Evaporative cooling using warmed or room-temperature water is standard in most centers. A gurney equipped with drains along the sides, such as a radiation contamination unit, or a stretcher reinforced with rolled towels along all sides, can be used. Extreme care must be taken to avoid and dry up any leaks. A special bed, atomizer and fan unit, the Makkah Body Cooling Unit, has been developed and is used primarily in the Middle East for the thousands who experience heat stroke en route to Mecca. The average cooling rate of this unit is 0.087°C per minute for initial core temperatures greater than 42°C (107.6°F), with a best cooling rate of 0.175°C per minute achieved.

In the canine model, peritoneal lavage with fluid cooled to 6°C (42.8°F) has produced the most rapid cooling. Bynum et al. demonstrated a cooling rate of 0.56°C per minute in the liver, kidney, and brain of dogs cooled with iced peritoneal lavage. Rectal and skin temperature cooling in this dog model, however, did not exceed rates for external evaporative methods. Horowitz published a case report on the use of iced peritoneal lavage in a 58-year-old man presenting comatose with a rectal temperature exceeding 42.5°C (108.5°F). Core temperature fell to 41.5°C (106.7°F) after 20 minutes of iced water gastric lavage and external evaporative cooling (using room-temperature saline and a fan), but the patient remained comatose. Open peritoneal lavage with 2 L of iced saline instilled over 20 minutes was then performed. Core temperature dropped to 37.6°C (100°F) within 90 minutes, achieving a cooling rate of 0.11°C per minute. More importantly, the patient became verbally responsive after the lavage fluid had infused (core temperature 39.4°C approximately 103°F), suggesting, as in the dog model, that internal organs may cool more rapidly with this procedure than can be gauged by rectal temperature changes. Further controlled study of peritoneal lavage in heat stroke is required before concluding that there is an advantage of this method over external evaporative cooling.

Although commonly used, iced saline gastric lavage has been shown to be no more effective than external evaporation, with cooling rates up to 0.16°C per minute. Benefits of this adjunctive measure must be weighed against the risk of aspiration. If it is chosen, consecutive 200 to 300 mL aliquots of iced saline should be instilled by means of a 16 French (Fr) Salem sump nasogastric tube.

Ice packs placed along the groin, neck, and axillae increase cooling by 5%. Although more manageable than ice water tub immersion, vigorous simultaneous extremity massage must accompany this procedure to prevent loss of heat transfer with peripheral vasoconstriction and shivering. As adjunctive therapies, cold intravenous fluids and inhalation of cold helium are of questionable minimal benefit. Ice water enemas are ineffective and may result in water intoxication. High-frequency jet ventilation increases heat exchange in the lungs. The cooling rate achieved, however, is only 0.062°C per minute, the same as for exposure of the patient. So far, only panting mammals demonstrate significant respiratory evaporative heat loss.

During heat stroke, the hypothalamic temperature set point is normal. The body's mechanisms for heat loss are overwhelmed and this normal temperature cannot be achieved. As a result, antipyretics and pharmacologic agents that reduce fever by resetting an elevated set point are useless. Aspirin and Tylenol are ineffective. Dantrolene sodium appears to be no more effective than spontaneous cooling (cooling rate 0.036°C per minute), although it is still used in neuroleptic malignant syndrome. Figure 70-3 outlines a proposed plan for management of heat stroke in the ED.

LABORATORY EVALUATION AND MEDICAL TREATMENT (TABLE 70-3)

The most common complication of heat stroke is hypotension secondary to dehydration, peripheral vasodilation, or myocardial depression. Each pint of sweat lost is equivalent to one pound of fluid loss, and fluid replacement is necessary. Volume monitoring should accompany rehydration. Vasopressors that enhance vasoconstriction hamper cooling efforts. Persistent hypotension despite adequate cooling and CVP-monitored rehydration may necessitate the use of inotropic agents. Not extensively studied, Isuprel (isoproterenol) is recommended in older literature.

Shivering may result from cooling efforts, may be violent, and may progress to frank seizure. Chlorpromazine (25 to 50 mg IV) or diazepam IV can be used to control shivering. Chlorpromazine acts as a vasodilator also. Its hypothalamic effect to induce hyperthermia is not a significant factor with external evaporative cooling in progress. Seizures can be treated with diazepam or phenobarbital IV.

Acute renal failure may occur in up to 25% of heat stroke patients, but long-term dialysis is rarely necessary. Acute renal failure and rhabdomyolysis are

TABLE 70-3. LABORATORY PARAMETERS

Arterial blood gases (corrected for temperature) (unless corrected, expect errors in Po_2 and Pco_2)
Complete blood count
Urinalysis
Electrolytes
Blood glucose
Blood urea nitrogen, creatine
Prothrombin time, partial thromboplastin time
Platelet count
Fibrin degradation products
Liver function enzymes, including SGOT
Creatine phosphokinase
Calcium
ECG

common in exertional heat stroke and rare in classic heat stroke. Rhabdomyolysis presents with muscle tenderness, myoglobinuria, and hyperkalemia. Ischemic compartment syndromes result from huge plasma leaks into damaged muscle tissue. Exogenous and endogenous calcium is deposited into injured muscle tissue, causing serum levels to fall. When deposits of calcium in the muscle later dissolve, hypercalcemia occurs in the oliguric patient. Calcium replacement is recommended for CNS and respiratory symptoms only. Mannitol (12.5 to 25 g IV) and furosemide may be given to decrease cerebral edema and ensure urine flow adequate to prevent acute tubular necrosis.

Hypokalemia is corrected with cooling and resolution of respiratory alkalosis. Therefore it should be treated only if accompanied by metabolic acidosis. Hyperkalemia from excessive exertion with significant muscle damage may require dialysis when associated with renal failure.

Direct thermal injury to the liver is manifested as centrilobular necrosis with rising liver enzymes and falling prothrombin levels. Vitamin K therapy may be required. Frank DIC is treated with heparin and epsilon aminocaproic acid (EACA).

ECG changes occur commonly, requiring monitoring of the patient during treatment. Most changes resolve with the return of body temperature to normal. Sinus tachycardia at rates of 140 to 150 beats per minute corresponds to the severity of heat injury. Nonspecific T-wave flattening or inversion and conduction abnormalities (increased QT interval, bundle branch block patterns) have been described and are usually transient.

Rarely, a heat stroke victim is affected with progressive hepatic failure, persistent coagulopathy, or irreversible CNS changes (usually cerebellar). Prognosis is poor with the appearance of myocardial failure (falling cardiac output and cardiac index), SGOT levels greater than 1000 IU per liter or hypoglycemia. Coma persisting for more than 10 hours is associated with a high rate of mortality, as is an admission rectal temperature above 42.2°C (108°F).

INDICATIONS FOR ADMISSION

All patients with hyperthermia and altered mental status require hospital admission. Complications occurring within 6 hours to 3 days after admission include jaundice and falling PT levels, extensive rhabdomyolysis, renal failure, and DIC. Permanently altered and unstable thermoregulatory mechanisms in the survivor of heat stroke increase susceptibility to future heat illness. Prevention through education should be a part of every discharge plan.

PREVENTION

Despite multiple risk factors and the vagaries of the daily forecast, morbidity and mortality from heat-stress disease can be decreased with public education. Physicians, nurses, coaches, organizers of athletic events (military and civilian), and athletes should be familiar with the symptoms of heat stress and its treatment and predisposing factors.

Exertion should be limited when temperature and humidity are high. An environmental heat stress prediction is available from the meteorologic service as the Wet Bulb Globe Temperature (WBGT) index. This index measures three forms of heat load: humidity (by wet bulb thermometer), ambient dry air temperature (by dry bulb thermometer), and the sun's radiant heat (by black globe thermometer). The wet bulb globe temperature can be calculated:

$$WBGT = (0.7\ Twb) + (0.2\ Tg) + (0.1\ Tdb)$$

Twb = temperature (wet bulb thermometer)

Tg = temperature (black globe thermometer)

Tdb = temperature (dry bulb thermometer)

Of importance, 70% of the WBGT is determined by humidity.

The WBGT can also be calculated from the dry air temperature (Tdb) and environmental water vapor pressure (Pa), variables obtainable from the local weather stations:

$$WBGT = (0.567\ Tdb) + (0.393\ Pa) + 3.94$$

At a WBGT above 23 to 28°C (73 to 82°F), the risk of thermal injury is high, and heavy exertion should be avoided. Unacclimatized or heat-sensitive individuals should avoid strenuous activity (hiking, running, sports practice, etc.). At a WBGT above 28°C (82°F), athletic events should be rescheduled or delayed. Conversely, a WBGT less than 10°C (50°F) represents a low risk of hyperthermia but a possible risk of hypothermia. Portable heat stress monitors are available commercially or can be constructed. Additional information can be obtained from the American College of Sports Medicine and the Departments of the Army, Navy, and Air Force.

In addition to limiting exertion during periods of high temperature and humidity, activities in direct sunlight should be avoided. Summer events should be scheduled before 8:00 A.M. or after 6:00 P.M. and light, loose clothing should be worn to minimize solar irradiation. At least 2 weeks of acclimatization in a hot environment should be encouraged to allow maximum efficiency of heat control mechanisms. Despite gradual increases in the duration of vigorous activity, the body's thermoregulatory system may still be overwhelmed by extreme exertion or temperature. Therefore, all athletes should be advised of (and screened for) early symptoms of heat injury: headache, nausea, dizziness, clumsiness, stumbling, excessive sweating or lack of sweating, and hallucinations.

As little as 3 to 5% dehydration can affect performance and elevate rectal temperature. Adequate hydration before exertion (400 to 500 mL) should be stressed. During activity, 100 to 200 mL of water should be available and consumed every 2 to 3 km or approximately every 20 to 30 minutes. Fluid, along with electrolyte replacement, is appropriate after exertion, although argument exists over the optimal rehydration fluid. Rapid gastric emptying is known to occur with large volumes (500 to 600 mL) at cold temperatures (10 to 15.8°C). Solutions of greater than 200 mOsm/L are known to slow gastric emptying. Commercial rehydration fluids delivering approximately 0.2 g of Na and 2.5 g of glucose per 100 mL of water are good choices for rapid absorption. Salt supplements ingested without fluids can precipitate gastritis, vomiting, and cerebral dehydration. They are not only harmful but also unnecessary.

Finally, elderly people, small children, individuals with skin or sweat-gland abnormalities, and those who are ill, unacclimatized, or have a previous history of heat stroke should be cautious when attempting rigorous activity in a hot environment. They must be made aware of their potential for heat stress injury. Further detailed information on the prevention of thermal injuries can be obtained from the American College of Sports Medicine.

NATIONAL CONTACTS

American College of Sports Medicine, Position Statement: Prevention of Thermal Injuries during Long-Distance Running, 1985.

Etiology, Prevention, Diagnosis and Treatment of Adverse Effects of Heat. Departments of the Army, Navy and Air Force. Technical Bulletin No. 175, April, 1969.

BIBLIOGRAPHY

Adam, J.M.: Heat, health and holidays. Practitioner *206*:363, 1971.

American College of Sports Medicine, Position Statement: Prevention of Thermal Injuries during Distance Running, 1985.

American Physiological Society: Handbook of Physiology. Washington, D.C., American Physiological Society, 1964, pp. 259, 551, 625.

Austin, M.G., and Berry, J.W.: Observations on one hundred cases of heatstroke. J.A.M.A. *161*:1524, 1956.

Bass, D.E., et al.: Mechanisms of acclimatization to heat in man. Medicine *34*:323, 1955.

Brodeur, V.B., Bennet, S.R., and Griffin, L.S.: Exertional hyperthermia, ice baths and emergency care at the Falmouth Road Race. J Emerg. Nursing *15*:304, 1989.

Callaham, M.L.: Hyperthermia. *In* Emergency Medicine: A Comprehensive Review. Edited by Kravis, T., and Warner, C. Rockville, MD, pp. 419–427, 1983.

Clowes, G.H.A., Jr., and O'Donnell, T.F., Current concepts: Heat stroke. N. Engl. J. Med. *291*:557, 1974.

Costrini, A.M., et al.: Cardiovascular and metabolic manifestations of heat stroke and severe exhaustion. Am. J. Med. *66*:296, 1979.

Danzl, D.F.: Hyperthermic syndromes. Ann. Fam. Pract. *37*:157, June, 1988.

Darling, R.C.: Heat exhaustion, heatstroke and heat cramps: A textbook of medicine. *9*:517, 1955.

Devine, J.A.: Heat stroke in the aged. Am. J. Med. *47*:251, 1969.

Eichler, A.C., McRae, A.S., and Root, H.D., Heat stroke. Am. J. Surg. *118*:855, 1969.

Ferris, E.B., Jr., et al.: Heat stroke: Clinical and chemical observations on 44 cases. J. Clin. Invest. *17*:45, 1938.

Gauss, H., and Meyer, K.A.: Heat stroke: Report of one hundred and fifty-eight cases from Cook County Hospital, Chicago, Am. J. Med. Sci. *154*:554, 1917.

Gold, J. Development of heat pyrexia. JAMA *173*:1175, 1960.

Gottschalk, P.G., and Thomas, J.D.: Heat stroke. Proc. Mayo Clin. *41*:470, 1966.

Gronert, G.A.: Controversies in malignant hyperthermia. Anaesthesiology *59*:273, 1983.

Guyton, M.L.: Textbook of Medical Physiology, 5th edition. Philadelphia, W.B. Saunders Co., 1976.

Hartle, S.,Jr.: Environmental considerations for exercise. Cardiol. Clin. *5*:245, 1987.

Heat wave related mortality—United States: C.D.C. Morbidity and Mortality Weekly Report. *30*:357, 1980.

Henry, C.D.: The pathophysiology of heat stroke. Crit. Care Update *7*:5, 1980.

Hirsch, E.F., et al.: Biochemical changes observed in heat exhaustion under field conditions. Milit. Med. *135*:881, 1970.

Hoagland, R.J., and Bishop, R.H., Jr.: A physiologic treatment of heat stroke. Am. J. Med. Sci. *241*:415, 1961.

Horowitz, B.Z.: The golden hour in heat stroke: Use of iced peritoneal lavage. Am. J. Emerg. Med. *7*:616, 1989.

Hubbard, R.W., Matthew, C.B., Durkot, M.J., and Francescioni, R.P.: Novel approaches to the pathophysiology of heat stroke: The energy depletion model. Ann. Emerg. Med. *16*:1066, 1987.

Humphrey, M.J., and Blanck, T.J.J.: Malignant hyperthermia. Consultant *24*:61, 1984.

Kessinger, A., and Rigby, R.G.: Hemorrhage and heat stroke. Geriatrics *25*:115, 1970.

Kew, M.C., et al.: The effects of heat stroke on the function and structure of the kidney. Q. J. Med. *36*:277, 1967.

Khogali, M., and Weiner, J.S.: Heat stroke: Report on eighteen cases. Lancet *8163*:276, 1980.

Knochel, J.P.: Environmental heat illness. J. Appl. Physiol. *16*:869, 1961.

Koroxenidis, G.T., Shepherd, J.T., and Marshall, R.J.: Cardiovascular response to acute heat stress. J. Appl. Physiol. *16*:869, 1961.

Lazarus, A.: Differentiating neuroleptic related heatstroke from neuroleptic malignant syndrome. Psychosomatics *30*:454, 1989.

Lowance, D.: Heat injury: A possible association with lithium carbonate therapy. J. Med. Assoc. Ga. *69*:284, 1980.

Malamud, N., Haymaker, W., and Custer, R.P.: Heat stroke: A clinicopathologic study of 125 fatal cases. Milit. Surg. *99*:397, 1946.

Meikle, A.W., and Graybill, J.R.: Fibrinolysis and hemorrhage in a fatal case of heat stroke. N. Engl. J. Med. *276*:911, 1967.

Mehta, A.C., and Baker, R.N.: Persistent neurological deficits in heat stroke. Neurology *20*:336, 1970.

O'Donnell, T.F., Jr.: Medical problems of recruit training: A research approach. U.S. Navy Med. *568*:28, 1971.

O'Donnell, T.F., and Clowes, G.H.A., Jr.: The circulatory abnormalities of heat stroke. N. Engl. J. Med. *287*:734, 1972.

Oechsli, F.W., and Buechley, R.W.: Excess mortality associated with three Los Angeles September hot spells. Environ. Res. *3*:277, 1970.

Perchick, J.S., Winkelstein, A., and Shadduck, R.K.: Disseminated intravascular coagulation in heat stroke: Response to heparin therapy. JAMA *231*:480, 1975.

Rampertaap, M.P.: Neuroleptic malignant syndrome. South. Med. J. *79*:331, 1986.

Redfearn, J.A.,Jr., and Murphy, R.J.: History of heat stroke in a football trainee. JAMA *208*:699, 1969.

Robey, J.M., Blythe, C.S., and Mueller, F.O.: Athletic injuries application of epidemiologic methods. JAMA *217*:184, 1971.

Robinson, S., et al.: Rapid acclimatization to work in hot climates. Am. J. Physiol. *140*:168, 1943.

Schickele, E.: Environment and fatal heat stroke: An analysis of 157 cases occurring in the army in the U.S. during World War II. Milit. Surg. *100*:235, 1947.

Scott, J.: Heat related illnesses. Postgrad. Med. *85*:154, 1989.

Shapiro, Y., et al.: Heat intolerance in former heat stroke patients. Ann. Intern. Med. *90*:913, 1979.

Shibolet, S., et al.: Heatstroke: Its clinical picture and mechanism in 36 cases. Q.J. Med. *36*:526, 1957.

Slovis, C.M., Anderson, G.F., and Casolaro, A.: Survival in a heat stroke victim with a core temperature in excess of 46.5°C. Ann. Emerg. Med. *11*:269, 1982.

Sohal, R.S., et al.: Heat stroke: An electron microscopic study of endothelial cell damage and disseminated intravascular coagulation. Arch. Intern. Med. *122*:43, 1968.

Sorenson, J.B., and Ranek, L.: Exertional heat stroke: Survival in spite of severe hypoglycemia, liver and kidney damage. J. Sports Med. Phys. Fitness *28*:108, 1988.

Sprung, C.L., et al.: The metabolic and respiratory alterations of heat stroke. Arch. Intern. Med. *140*:665, 1980.

Stefanini, M., and Spicer, D.D.: Hemostatic breakdown, Fibrinolysis and acquired hemolytic anemia in a patient with fatal heatstroke. Pathogenetic mechanisms. Am. J. Clin. Pathol. *55*:180, 1971.

Stine, R.J.: Heat illness. JACEP *8*:154, 1979.

Strasser, A.L.: Prompt treatment of heat stress can reduce medical catastrophes. Occup. Health Saf. 21, 1988.

Tek, D., and Olshaker, J: Hyperthermia, Pulmonary edema and DIC in an 18-year-old military recruit. Ann. Emerg. Med. *19*:715, 1990.

Thompson, P.D., et al.: Death during jogging or running: A study of 18 cases. JAMA *242*:1265, 1979.

Tintinall, J.E., Krame, R.L., and Ruiz, E.: Emergency Medicine: A Comprehensive Guide, Second Edition, New York, McGraw-Hill, Inc., pp. 753–756.

Weber, M.D., and Blakely, J.A.: The hemorrhagic diathesis of heat stroke. Lancet *1*:1190, 1969.

Weiner, J.S., and Khogali, M.: A physiological body-cooling unit for treatment of heat stroke. Lancet *8167*:507, 1980.

Wilkinson, R.T., et al.: Psychological and physiological response to raised body temperature. J. Appl. Physiol. *19*:287, 1964.

Wilson, G.: The cardiopathology of heatstroke. JAMA *114*:557, 1940.

Wyndham, C.H., Strydom, N.B., and Morrison, J.F.: Fatigue of the sweat gland response. J. Appl. Physiol. *21*:107, 1966.

Yudis, M., et al.: Acute renal failure complicating heat stroke—A case report. Milit. Med. *136*:884, 1971.

Chapter 71

LIGHTNING AND ELECTRICAL INJURIES

LIGHTNING INJURIES

Edgar B. Billowitz

CAPSULE

Although they both involve exposure to intense electrical energy, lightning injuries and high voltage electric current injuries are so fundamentally different that they may be considered separate entities. Lightning injuries are characterized by exceedingly high voltages of remarkably short duration, whereas power line or household current injuries involve much lower voltage for more sustained periods of time. Lightning characteristically "flashes over" the surface of the body, tending to spare the deeper structures from severe damage, whereas power line current tends to traverse the less resistant deeper tissues (nerves, blood vessels, and muscles), causing occult, extensive, and progressive damage. Lightning tends to cause asystole and apnea; even after full cardiopulmonary arrest, lightning victims given appropriate resuscitation often have a good prognosis for functional recovery. Power line injuries, on the other hand, characteristically cause ventricular fibrillation, and even after resuscitation, these victims often have much more severe residua, namely, deep burns, muscle and nerve damage, amputations, renal failure, and central nervous system (CNS) deficits.

INTRODUCTION

Each year in the United States, several hundred people die from accidental electrocution by lightning, and three to four times this number are injured by it. Over 1000 people are killed annually by generated electric current.

Electrical injuries vary from the trivial to the fatal. These injuries are frequently deceptive in their initial presentation; the victim may in fact be worse or better than he or she appears. In lightning injury, for example, the scenario may be dramatic: a blinding flash, a deafening thunderclap, the victim at times propelled through the air and left senseless, and his or her clothing literally blown off. And yet, despite this ominous, surreal appearance, the victim may survive and do well. With high-tension power line trauma, on the other hand, the victim may present with only unimpressive entry and exit wounds, but this may belie the severity of deep tissue destruction, involving nerves, blood vessels, and muscles, and leading to a crush type injury complex. Lightning and electrical injuries are discussed separately in this chapter. Table 71-1 summarizes the differences between lightning and generated electric current.

PATHOPHYSIOLOGY OF LIGHTNING INJURIES

To understand the effects of lightning on the body, the clinician must understand the nature of lightning itself. Lightning is a complex electrical event, accompanied by blast, acoustic, thermal, magnetic, and light energies. In the initiating stage, static electricity is created in a cloud (generally cumulonimbus) by the friction of water molecules and ice particles.[1] When this electric charge, which is negative relative to the earth, achieves a potential difference greater than the insulating capacity of the intervening air (10^5 to 10^8 volts), a lightning discharge occurs.

This lightning discharge is more complicated than

TABLE 71-1. COMPARISON OF LIGHTNING AND GENERATED POWER CURRENTS

Parameter	Lightning	Power Line
Voltage	10 million–2 billion volts	110–70,000 volts
Amperage	20,000–200,000 amps	Less than 1,000 amps
Duration	1/1000–1/10 sec	Seconds to minutes
Pathway	Flashover (external)	Internal
Type of current	DC	AC
Cardiac effects	Asystole	Ventricular fibrillation
Burns	Superficial	Deep
Immediate cause of death	Prolonged apnea	Ventricular fibrillation

it appears to the naked eye. The initial downward stroke produces a branching, ionized pattern that is easily visible. This is called a *leader stroke*; it travels at 1/2000 the speed of light, and carries a charge of 100,000 to 1,000,000,000 volts. When this leader stroke is approximately 50 meters from the earth, a *pilot stroke* arises from the ground to complete the circuit. This is followed immediately by an earth-to-cloud *return stroke*, which follows the ionized pathway of super-heated particles already established. The return stroke is much faster and more powerful than the leader stroke (1/10 the speed of light and up to 2 billion volts), but is less visible than the leader stroke because of its speed. Following the return stroke, another cloud-to-earth discharge can occur, called a *dart leader*. This sequence can occur from 1 to 40 times, most commonly 4 to 7 times, and accounts for the flickering visibly perceived during a lightning flash.

Accompanying the lightning flash is the thunderclap. This is created as the cylinder of air surrounding the electrical charge is superheated to a temperature of 8000°C[2] to 20,000°C,[3] creating a rapid expansion and then contraction. The expanding column decays within a meter or two from a shock wave to a sound wave.[4] This thunderclap may produce acoustic damage to the ear as well as blast effect to other organs, e.g., shock lung.[5] The photic component has been implicated in the production of cataracts.

There are five basic pathways whereby lightning strikes a person:

1. Direct strike
2. Contact strike
3. Side flash, or "splash"
4. Stride potential, or step voltage
5. Ground current

Direct strike occurs when the individual is struck directly by a lightning discharge. Chance of direct strike is greatly enhanced when the victim carries a metal object, such as a golf club or umbrella, or is wearing something metallic on his or her head, such as a hairpin, metal buttons on a cap, or even a hearing aid.[6] Laboratory simulation experiments have demonstrated that lightning preferentially strikes one dummy with a hairpin over an identical dummy without a hairpin.[7]

Contact strike occurs when lightning strikes an object that the victim is touching, such as a tree, and the current is transferred to him or her. A certain amount of the energy is absorbed by the primary strike object.

Side flash (or *splash*) is a common mechanism of strike; the lightning first completes its circuit onto a nearby object, traverses a certain distance, and then jumps across the intervening lower-resistance air bridge to strike the victim. This often involves a person standing near a tree in a rainstorm. Multiple victims can be struck simultaneously by side flash.

Stride potential, or *step voltage*, occurs when a lightning discharge, radiating outward from the stroke epicenter, encounters a potential difference between the two legs of the victim. The current enters the closer leg and exits through the farther leg, primarily traversing the lower body. This may account for the phenomenon of *keraunoparalysis*, first described by Charcot in 1879.[8] Keraunoparalysis is characterized by paretic, cold, insensate, and pulseless legs for hours to days after a lightning strike, and generally resolves. It is thought to be caused by endogenous catecholamine release. Farm animals are more susceptible to being struck and killed by stride potential because the greater distance between their legs causes greater current potential, and because the heart in the quadruped lies in the current pathway.[9]

Ground current is created when a bolt hits the ground and is transferred to the victim with an amount of energy inversely proportional to the distance from the strike.

I was struck by lightning ground current while jogging. The current ran across the left foot, but because the other foot was off the ground at that instant, a true stride potential was not generated. The less harmful ground current caused only transient numbness and tingling.

A most important concept in understanding how lightning behaves once it strikes the body is the phenomenon of *flashover*. Just as electric current is known to flow over the outside of a metal conductor, lightning tends to flow over the surface of the body, with relative sparing of the deeper tissue. This explains how the body can withstand the magnitude of amperage sustained in a lightning strike.

The flashover current is enormously powerful and produces several clinically apparent sequelae. First, it instantly vaporizes surface moisture into superheated steam, which can cause burns in moist areas, especially the axillae and groin, and skin creases. This rapidly expanding steam causes the victim's clothing and shoes to be literally blown off his or her body. For this reason, victims of lightning have sometimes been mistaken for victims of crime, having been found dead with their tattered clothing nearby.[2]

The flashover also superheats metal objects on the victim such as packframes, necklaces, or coins. These may be melted, spot-welded, or actually vaporized, leaving marks of thermal skin burns.

Flashover is also responsible for the pathognomonic burns seen in lightning injuries; these burns, termed *keraunographic markings* or Lichtenberg figures, are described as a feathery, arborescent, or fernlike pattern. They are probably caused by a complex flow of electrons rather than by actual thermal trauma. They fade spontaneously within hours to days.[10,11]

Lightning can also injure through mechanisms other than electric:

1. There is a *blast effect* similar to that of an explosion. Moulson[5] reports a case of blast injury to the lungs in a patient who had no contact with the electrical discharge.
2. The sound waves cause acoustic injury. This is probably responsible for the ruptured tympanic membranes seen in one third to one half of lightning victims. In addition, for those struck while talking on the phone, 160 decibels (db) of sound energy have been measured.[12]
3. Blunt injury. The victim may fall or be struck by flying debris. Moreover, as the victim becomes momentarily electrically charged, he or she may be violently propelled some distance as he or she is attracted to, or repelled from, a nearby charge.
4. Thermal injury. The victim may be burned by atmospheric gases heated to 20,000°C,[3] by clothing caught on fire, or by objects on his or her person superheated by flashover.
5. Photic injury. The bright flash has been implicated in eye injury, including retinal damage and cataracts.

PREHOSPITAL ASSESSMENT AND STABILIZATION

In lightning disaster involving multiple victims, the rescuers should direct their initial attention to those who are apparently dead. This is in contradistinction to the normal triage situation; the reason for this re-versal is that individuals who are breathing will in all probability survive without immediate intervention, whereas those in cardiac arrest have a good chance at survival only with prompt cardiopulmonary resuscitation (CPR). Severe lightning strike tends to cause asystole and apnea; the inherent automaticity of the heart normally allows resumption of heartbeat within a brief period, but the centrally mediated apnea can be prolonged. Often the victim can be sustained by the simple measure of assisted ventilation. If ventilation is not promptly restarted, hypoxia develops, and *secondary* cardiac arrest occurs, often in the form of ventricular fibrillation. When cardiac monitoring is not available, the rescuer's best guess is that the early pulseless state is caused by asystole and that the late pulseless state by ventricular fibrillation.

The significantly injured patient should be handled like any patient with other major trauma. CPR is performed according to standard protocols, as is treatment of arrythmias. The victim does not carry any electric charge, but lightning may indeed strike twice in the same place, and so the team should move to a safer spot with expediency.

The possibility of blunt trauma should be considered and treated accordingly. Cervical spine (C-spine) precautions are prudent. Concomitant medical problems and drug or alcohol intoxication should also be sought.

CLINICAL PRESENTATION

The clinical presentation in lightning injury is most variable and unpredictable. Three general presentations have been described: minor, moderate, and severe.[2] The patient with minor injury has stable vital signs, a history of brief unconsciousness or confusion, is generally amnestic concerning preceding events, and often complains of muscle or sensory disturbance. The patient with moderate injury has a persistently decreased level of consciousness or disorientation, labile hypertension, arrythmias and ECG changes, and skin burns, and may have ruptured tympanic membranes as well as severe motor and sensory disturbances. The patient with severe injury presents with severe CNS and/or cardiac abnormality: coma, CNS bleeding, electrical destruction of brain tissue, hypoxic encephalopathy, apnea, asystole, or ventricular fibrillation. Prognosis is poor in severe injury.

Selected patients with severe injury may do well if they receive early CPR. It is recommended that CPR be continued for extended periods in these patients because full recovery has been reported even after prolonged arrest times.[1,13,14] This preservation of vital organs is attributed to the "no flow" theory, or instantaneous cessation of all cellular metabolism at the moment of strike.[13] Some dispute this theory.

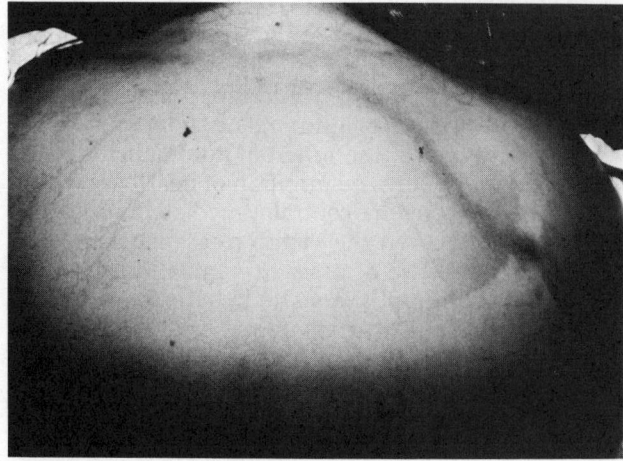

FIG. 71-1. Keraunographic markings on upper back of patient struck by lightning. (Courtesy of Robert Lowe, M.D.)

HISTORY

On presentation in the ED, a detailed history should be obtained from bystanders and/or rescue personnel. General patterns of injury exist, but individual situations are difficult to predict or reconstruct.

PHYSICAL EXAMINATION

A meticulous head-to-toe examination, including detailed neurologic examination, is absolutely mandatory, looking for occult injury and subtle neurologic deficits, establishing a baseline of normal functions to compare against possible delayed injury.

Areas of specific interest in the physical examination are described in the following paragraphs.

HEAD

Look for evidence of lightning strike in hairpins, metal buttons, etc., or for corresponding burns, that clue the examiner as to the electrical entry site.

EYES

Blindness may be transient or permanent,[8] and may result from retinal, optic nerve, or occipital lobe injury. Cataracts may develop early or be delayed for months or years; most commonly they are seen after a few months. Other injuries include corneal ulcer, iritis, ectopia lentis, iridocyclitis, vitreous hemorrhage, abnormalities of reaction and accommodation, and hyphema.[4,8,15] Baseline visual acuity should be recorded.

EARS

The ears are frequently involved. Tympanic membrane rupture has been reported at a rate of 30 to 50%.[16] Hearing impairment or deafness results from disrup-

tion or necrosis of the ossicles, complete ablation of the organ of Corti,[17] acoustic nerve damage, and other mechanisms. Labyrinthitis has been noted, with endolymphatic hydrops.[12]

NECK

Look for signs of occult C-spine injury or skin burns from metal necklaces.

LUNGS

Blast lung, aspiration, or ARDS may occur.

HEART

Lightning behaves like a massive DC countershock ("cosmic cardioversion"[4]), causing asystole and then resumption of rhythm with pulse. An impressive variety of cardiac abnormalities are routinely encountered, including atrial and ventricular arrythmias, ischemia, and myocardial muscle damage.[18-24] These generally have a favorable prognosis, however. PVCs may be delayed in onset, and prolonged monitoring has been recommended in selected cases.[23] ECG changes are commonly encountered, demonstrating ischemic or infarct patterns or nonspecific findings such as ST and T wave changes, axis changes, and P-wave inversion; these normally resolve.

VASCULAR SYSTEM

Hypertension, often to high levels, is frequently reported,[8] and treatment, when required, is with the usual agents. Rapid resolution is the rule. Keraunoparalysis, mentioned earlier, is apparently caused by intense vasospasm, and also resolves.

MUSCULOSKELETAL SYSTEM

Muscle damage may occur from passage of lightning electrical current, and may cause pain and swelling. Compartment syndrome and hemochromogen nephropathy, seen often in high voltage injuries, are rarely seen in lightning injuries. Shoulder dislocations, notably of the posterior variety, as well as spinal compression fractures, may result from seizure or muscle contractions.

SKIN

The classic burn pattern of lightning injury is termed keraunographic marking (Fig. 71-1). It has an arborescent, fern-like, or feathery configuration, and is evanescent, appearing at once or after a few hours and then disappearing over hours to days. *Linear burns* occur in areas of moisture such as skin folds, axillae, and groin, and result from instantaneous steam production during flashover. *Punctate burns*[8] have a pattern unique to lightning; they are discrete, circular, small, and may be full thickness. Ordinary thermal burns result from ignition of clothing or superheating of metal objects on the victim. Delayed healing with Marjolin's ulcer development has been reported.[1]

NERVOUS SYSTEMS

Lightning produces an unpredictable array of central and peripheral nervous system abnormalities with variable time of onset and duration. One may find unconsciousness, confusion, amnesia, seizures, motor or sensory deficits, paresthesias or dysesthesias, transverse myelitis, dysarthria, personality changes, hysteria, and keraunophobia. The clinician must always consider CNS hemorrhage.

A meticulous examination is often most rewarding. Frequent re-examinations are mandatory; the frequency is dictated by the patient's condition.

PREGNANCY

The fetus risks about a 50% chance of death when the mother is struck by lightning.[25,26] The amniotic fluid apparently serves as a preferential path for electric current flow.

DIFFERENTIAL DIAGNOSIS

The unwitnessed victim of lightning strike may indeed present difficulty with the diagnosis, particularly when the examining physician fails to consider this unusual entity. Most emergency physicians see few, if any, cases in their careers. The differential diagnosis includes the entities listed in Table 71-2.

The diagnosis can be established when the setting is compatible (victim outdoors, lightning present) and the individual displays features distinctive of, or unique to, lightning injury; e.g., ruptured tympanic membranes, punctate burns or keraunographic markings, thermal burns from superheated personal metal objects, or clothing and shoes blown off. Another interesting finding that may help to clinch the diagnosis is the magnetization of metal objects, which Erikssen states invariably occurs.[27]

INITIAL STABILIZATION

Standard care includes IV access, O₂, cardiac monitoring, nasogastric tube and Foley catheter as indicated, and frequent vital signs. If the patient has suffered cardiac or respiratory arrest, CPR is continued

TABLE 71-2. DIFFERENTIAL DIAGNOSIS OF LIGHTNING STRIKE

CVA
Myocardial infarction
Primary arrythmia
Acute intoxication
Hysteria
Saddle embolus of the iliac bifurcation
Aortic dissection
Pheochromocytoma
High tension electric injury
Pulmonary embolus
Assault victim
Sepsis

in the standard fashion. Despite the drama of the antecedent events, the physician must not forget the orderly sequence of the ABCs. Shock is not common; it may be from secondary trauma or posthypoxic organ system failure, and is again treated according to standard protocols. In general, fluid is given sparingly because cerebral edema is more common than shock.

LABORATORY TESTS AND PROCEDURES

Routine laboratory tests include CBC, electrolytes, BUN and creatinine, liver function tests, cardiac enzymes, urine for myoglobin, chest x ray, C-spine series, and 12-lead ECG. Toxicology, PT, PTT, type and cross, ABGs, and CT are obtained as clinically indicated.

MANAGEMENT, ADMISSION, AND PROGNOSTIC FACTORS

Mortality has been reported to be 20 to 30% overall in lightning injuries,[28] but because of the likelihood of underreporting nonfatal injuries, the actual mortality may be much less. Cooper[26] found that patients who have suffered cardiopulmonary arrest had a mortality of 77%, those with cranial burns had mortality of 38%, and those with leg burns had a mortality of 30%.

Management of complications in the lightning-struck patient follows established protocols. The stable patient generally remains so, although delayed arrythmias, delayed hypertension, and (rarely) delayed vascular thrombosis can occur. If the patient has suffered cardiac arrest, posthypoxic complications should be anticipated, such as multiple organ failure, sepsis, cerebral edema, corneal desiccation, pressure ulceration, etc.

Tetanus prophylaxis should not be neglected.

If significant myoglobin is found in the urine, which is rare, the kidneys are flushed with high fluid volumes, mannitol, and sodium bicarbonate.

For the unconscious patient, protocols involving dextrose, thiamine, and Narcan may be appropriate.

INDICATIONS FOR ADMISSION

The moderately or severely harmed patient clearly requires admission. Indications for admission of the patient with minor injuries are unclear at present. Selected patients with minor injuries might be safely observed in a holding area and discharged if stable.

PREVENTION

The risk factors for lightning strike are reasonably well defined. At the earliest sign of lightning threat, the individual should seek a safe haven, such as a house or car, avoid open areas and elevated structures, and should not seek shelter under a tree. Metal objects should be removed, even tiny items like hairpins. Groups should spread out to avoid multiple victims. If one is caught in the open, he or she should lie down in a depression, curled up, hands and feet together, preferably on some insulating material like a raincoat or plastic sheeting.[8] Houses are generally safe, but one should avoid talking on the phone,[29] stay away from chimneys, and turn off the radio and television.

PITFALLS

- Do not confuse lightning burns with power line burns.
- Do not confuse steam burns or superheated metal burns with entry/exit burns.
- Check tympanic membranes.
- Get baseline hearing and vision examinations.
- Consider the possibility of accompanying trauma.
- Remember tetanus immunization.
- Do not confuse keraunoparalysis with spinal cord injury, compartment syndrome of the legs, or saddle embolus.
- Do not do fasciotomy unless the diagnosis of compartment syndrome is firmly established—which is rare.
- Remember the reverse order of prehospital triage; i.e., begin with the apparently dead.
- Do not abandon resuscitative efforts too early.

MEDICOLEGAL PEARLS

Lightning injury has unpredictable, sometimes grave sequelae; 70% of survivors have permanent residuae,[26] and medicolegal issues may arise. The emergency physician must be meticulous in patient care, and must also provide sympathy and understanding to the family to help forestall malpractice claims. Appropriate specialists should be consulted early. Predictable complications should be anticipated. Patient and family should be advised of possible delayed complications, such as cataract formation, and should confirm that they understand this possibility before signing a medical release.

HORIZONS

The most common cause of death in lightning injury is prolonged respiratory arrest. It is theorized that, with prompt CPR, the 30% mortality could be greatly reduced and many of these victims restored to a productive life. The future of lightning injury treatment lies in testing this hypothesis, and this is being done as bystander CPR becomes more widely available.

REFERENCES

1. Apfelberg, D.B., et al.: Pathophysiology and treatment of lightning injuries. J. Trauma 14:6, 1974.
2. Cooper, M.A.: Lightning injuries. In Management of Wilderness and Environmental Injuries. Edited by Auerback, P., and Geehr, E. New York, Macmillan, 1989.
3. Plueckhahn, V.D.: Injury and death caused by lightning. Med. J. Aust. 144:673, 1986.
4. Epperly, T.D., and Stewart, J.R.: The physical effects of lightning injury. J. Fam. Pract. 29:3, 1989.
5. Moulson, A.M.: Blast injury of the lungs due to lightning. Br. Med. J. 289:270, 1984.
6. Tandberg, D.: Destruction of hearing aid by lightning strike. Am. J. Emerg. Med. 8:326, 1990.
7. Kitagawa, N., et al.: Discharge experiments using dummies and rabbits simulating lightning strokes in human bodies. Int. J. Biometeorol. 17:239, 1973.
8. Craig, S.R.: When Lightning Strikes. Postgrad. Med. 79:4, 1986.
9. Golde, R.H., and Lee, W.R.: Death by lightning. Proc. I.E.E., 1976; 123:10R, 1976.
10. Amy, B.W., et al.: Lightning Injury with Survival in Five Patients. JAMA 253:2, 1985.
11. McCrady-Kahn, V.L., and Khan, A.M.: Lightning burns. West. J. Med. 134:3, 1981.
12. Youngs, R., et al.: Severe sensorineural hearing loss caused by lightning. Arch. Otolaryngol. Head Neck Surg. 114:1184, 1988.
13. Ravitch, M.M., et al.: Lightning stroke. N. Engl. J. Med. 264:1, 1961.
14. Taussig, H.B.: "Death" from lightning—And the possibility of living again. Ann. Intern. Med. 68:6, 1968.
15. Abt, J.L.: The pupillary responses after being struck by lightning. JAMA 254:23, 1985.

16. Kristensen, S.T., and Veteras, K.: Lightning-induced acoustic rupture of the tympanic membrane. J. Laryng. Otol. *99*:711, 1985.
17. Bergstrom, L.V., et al.: The lightning damaged ear. Arch. Oto-laryngol. *100*:12, 1974.
18. Burda, C.D.: Electrocardiographic changes in lightning stroke. Am. Heart. J. *72*:4, 1966.
19. Chia, B.L.: Electrocardiographic abnormalities and congestive cardiac failure due to lightning stroke. Cardiology *68*:49, 1981.
20. Jackson, S.H.D., and Parry, D.J.: Lightning and the heart. Br. Heart J. *43*:454, 1980.
21. Kleiner, J.P., and Wilkin, J.H.: Cardiac effects of lightning stroke. JAMA *240*:25, 1978.
22. Kleinot, M.B., et al.: The cardiac effects of lightning injury. S. Afr. Med. J. 1141, 1966.
23. Kotagal, S., et al.: Neurological, psychiatric, and cardiovascular complications in children struck by lightning. Pediatrics *70*:2, 1982.
24. Palmer, A.B.D.: Lightning injury causing prolongation of the Q-T interval. Postgrad. Med. J. *63*:891, 1987.
25. Chan, Y.F., et al.: Lightning accidents in pregnancy. J. Obstet. Gynecol. *79*:761, 1972.
26. Cooper, M.A.: Lightning injuries: Prognostic signs for death. Ann. Emerg. Med. *9*:3, 1980.
27. Eriksson, A., and Ornehult, L.: Death by lightning. Am. J. Forensic Med. Pathol. *9*:4, 1988.
28. Cooper, M.A.: Lightning injuries. Emerg. Med. Clin. North Am. *1*:3, 1983.
29. Andrews, C.J., et al.: Telephone-mediated lightning injury: An Australian survey. J. Trauma *29*:5, 1989.

ELECTRICAL INJURIES

Edgar B. Billowitz

CAPSULE

Electric current causes complex, unique, and unpredictable injury patterns. Low-voltage currents, arbitrarily defined as less than 1000 volts, tend not to cause significant deep tissue damage, but may produce death secondary to ventricular fibrillation or apnea. Special cases include oral commissure injuries in children from chewing on an electric cord, and immersion (bathtub) electrocution. High-voltage current injuries, defined as involving currents greater than 1000 volts, are among the most devastating and tragic injuries sustained by human beings.

INTRODUCTION

High-voltage current injury has two general patterns: *surface burns* and *internal current flow* injury.

Surface burns are caused by (1) arcing, (2) flash burns, and (3) flame burns from ignition of clothing. These may be deep burns, third- or fourth-degree, because electrical arcs bear temperatures of 2500 to 20,000°C, and electric flash temperatures may be as high as 800°C.

Internal current flow injuries occur when the body acts as an electrical conductor; they are characterized by entry and exit wounds, occult destruction of deeper tissues similar to crush injury, and frequent need for escharotomy, fasciotomy, and amputation (Figs. 71-2 and 71-3). A periosseous core of necrotic muscle may be hidden beneath overlying healthy muscle.[2] Virtually all organ systems of the body may be involved. Concomitant major trauma is not uncommon, and two or more types of burns often occur in the same patient. Fluid requirements for internal current flow injury cannot be predicted by any burn formula; other parameters (urine output, CVP, etc) must be followed to ensure adequate resuscitation. Renal failure secondary to myoglobin pigment deposition, hypovolemia, or direct current injury is a definite threat. Early consultation and referral to a burn center are essential in major injury.

Electric current injuries remain a frequently misunderstood entity in many emergency departments (EDs). What are the hallmarks of major injury? When can the patient be safely discharged? Without a proper understanding of physics and pathophysiology, gross underestimation of severity may result or, alternatively, inappropriate admission may occur.

Electric current injuries cause 1000 to 1500 deaths per year and constitute about 2 to 5% of burn unit admissions. Mortality is about 20% overall,[3] and 2 to 5% in the burn unit. The first recorded death by generated electrical energy occurred in 1879, when a stagehand in France was killed while connecting the stage lights.[4] At present, the vast majority of high voltage injuries involve men injured at work: linemen, crane operators, construction workers, and farmers are the most frequently injured.[5-7] Installation of home TV antennas also constitutes a significant risk. Children are frequently the victims of low-voltage current injuries, particularly involving the classic oral commissure burn sustained while chewing on an electric cord.

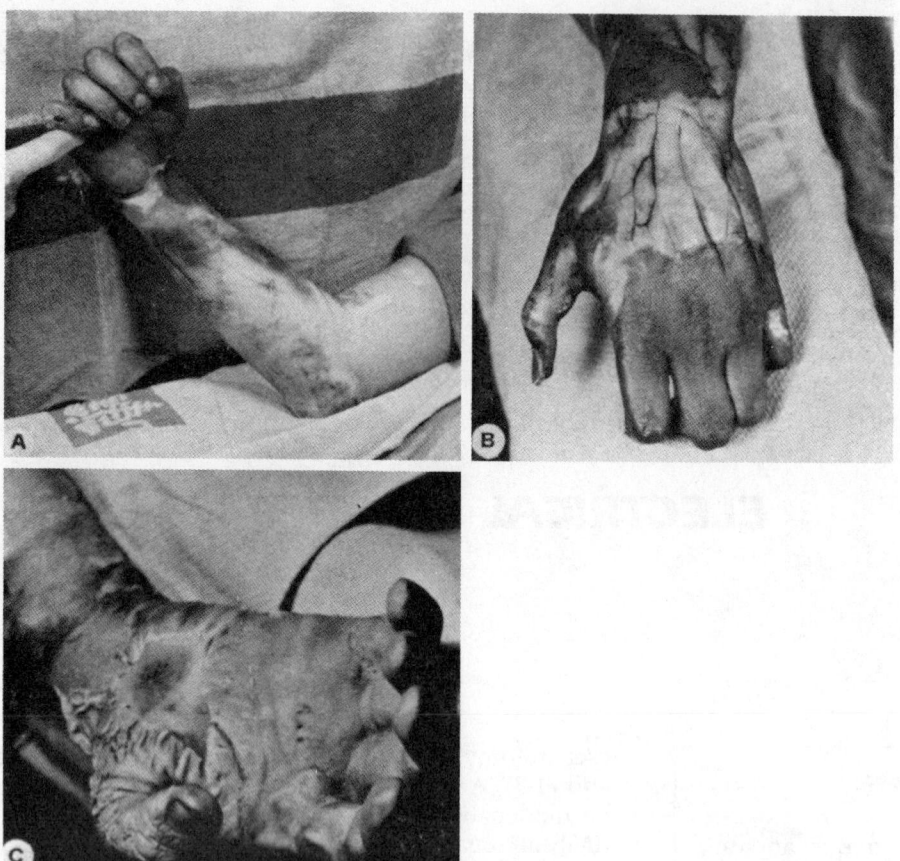

FIG. 71-2.   A,B,C. The gross tissue necrosis of these extremities necessitated amputation. With permission from Taylor, P.H., et al.: The intriguing electrical burn. J. Trauma 2:309, 1962.

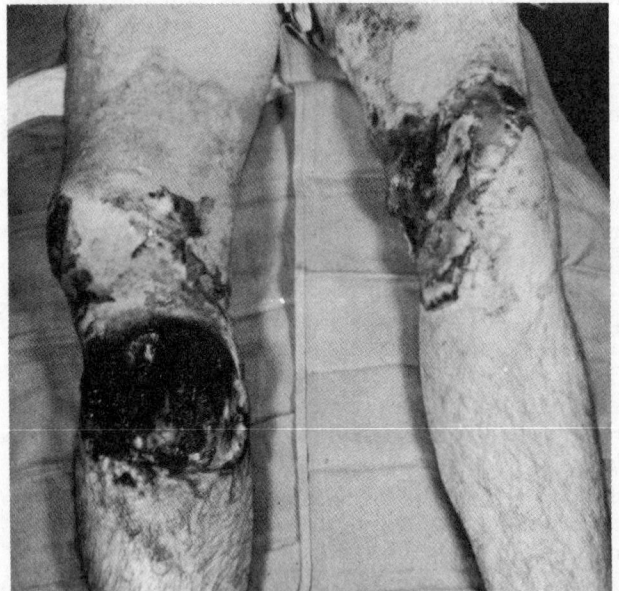

FIG. 71-3.   Destruction of the knee joints by the exploding force of the exiting current. With permission from Taylor, P.H., et al.: The intriguing electrical burn. J. Trauma 2:309, 1962.

Only about 50% of injured workers are able to return to their occupations. Many suffer blunt trauma, central nervous system (CNS) and peripheral nerve injury, orthopedic injury (with a 35 to 60% amputation rate),[3] vascular thrombosis or hemorrhage, disfiguring skin burns, surgical abdominal injuries or gastrointestinal (GI) bleeding, cardiac and lung injuries, sepsis, and psychiatric disturbances. Truly, these injuries are among the most challenging and demanding that the ED team can encounter.

PATHOPHYSIOLOGY

In surface burns, the pathophysiology of injury resembles that of burns from any heat source. In internal current flow injuries, there is controversy concerning the mechanism by which cells are damaged. Some investigators claim that there is a unique action of the current on the cells, or perhaps some alteration of macromolecules, whereas others, the majority, state that all damage is caused by the conversion of electrical energy into heat.

Heat production is quantified by the formula $P = I^2 R$, where P = heat, I = amperage, and R = resistance. In the clinical situation, only the voltage is normally known, and the following relationship applies: amps = volts/ohms.

Six factors determine the outcome of human contact with electrical current:

1. Volts
2. Amps
3. Resistance
4. Type of current
5. Duration
6. Pathway

Clinically, only the voltage and current type are definitely known; the pathway and duration are only roughly estimated; and the amperage and resistance are largely unknown.

VOLTAGE

In the United States, low voltage is defined as current of less than 1000 volts, and high voltage is current of more than 1000 volts. The voltage is the "driving force" of the current, like water behind a dam.[3] Low-voltage injuries rarely cause deep tissue destruction, but prolonged contact with the hand under special circumstances can cause injury sufficient to require amputation.

Low voltage, however, can cause sudden death.

When external resistance is low, the internal flow of current may be sufficient to cause ventricular fibrillation. This is the apparent mechanism of death when the victim suffers electrocution injury in the bathtub. In these cases, no sign of internal tissue damage is found on autopsy.[5,8]

Another special case of low-voltage current injury involves the oral commissure injury sustained when a child chews on a household electric cord (Fig. 71-4).[9] There are deep burns at the angles of the oral commissure, at times accompanied by lingual, dental, and palatal injury. The depth of injury is thought to be caused by arcing of the current in the mouth, as well as deep local contact burns facilitated by low resistance because of the saliva. These injuries frequently involve the labial artery, with typically delayed rupture and hemorrhage 3 to 7 days after injury. Cosmetic disfigurements and functional deficits commonly ensue. Remote injury does not tend to occur.

High-voltage injury produces different effects from those of low-voltage injury, and they are unique in the field of traumatology. Voltage varies from 1000 volts to 220,000 volts. High voltage can jump abut 1 inch per 20,000 volts; once the arc is formed, however, it can be drawn out to 10 feet before the contact is broken.[10]

AMPERAGE

Amperage is a measure of the flow of a volume of electrons per unit time. Greater amperage means

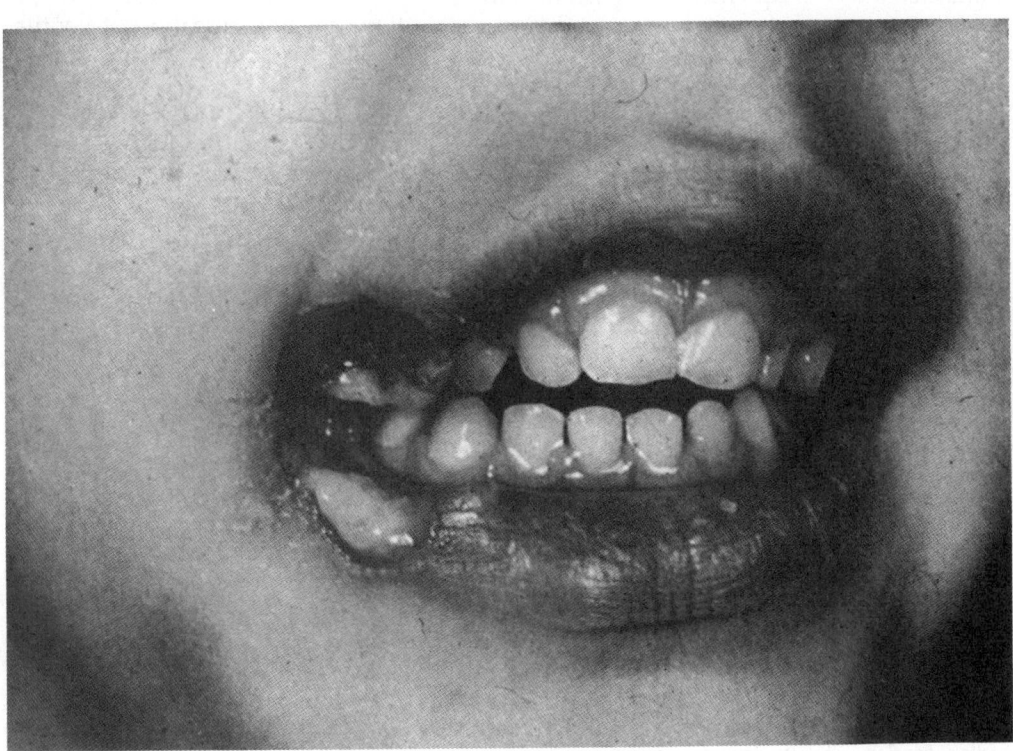

FIG. 71-4.   Destruction of oral commissure. With permission from Sturim, H.S.: The treatment of electrical injuries. J. Trauma *11*:11, 1971.

TABLE 71-3. TISSUE RESISTANCE FROM HIGHEST TO LOWEST
1. Bone
2. Fat
3. Tendon
4. Skin
5. Muscle
6. Artery
7. Nerve

greater damage. Two milliamperes can produce pain; 0.1 to 1 amps can induce respiratory arrest or ventricular fibrillation; 2 amps may produce burns; and 10 amps may produce asystole.

RESISTANCE

Resistance to electrical current is a complex process. Tissue resistance can vary widely under different circumstances. For example, a dry, heavily callused palm may measure 1,000,000 ohms of resistance, whereas a moist, thin palm may register only 100 ohms of resistance. Children have less tissue resistance because of their higher body water content and thinner skin.

Different body tissues exhibit a graded order of resistance (Table 71-3). It has been generally held that, once the skin has been breached, the electrical current travels preferentially along tissues of least resistance, namely, nerve, artery, and muscle, and consequently causes more damage to these tissues.

This is probably an oversimplification. First, Hunt[11] has concluded that living tissue acts as a volume conductor, and that once skin resistance has been overcome, all internal resistance, with the exception of bone, is uniform with regard to current flow. Moreover, if indeed the current does flow along tissues of least resistance, we must remember that heat production is directly related to resistance, and so, although more highly resistant tissue may have relatively less flow, there is still relatively greater heat production.

This accounts for the phenomenon of "core injury" (Fig. 71-5).[12] Because bone has the highest resistance, it tends to produce the greatest heat. After the current flow has stopped, the bone acts as a heat sink, continuing to heat the periosseous muscle. On surgical exploration, deep muscle is frequently found to suffer greater thermal injury than superficial muscle. When high internal resistance is combined with small cross-sectional area, such as in the arm, the heat production is concentrated, producing greater injury. Conversely, with greater cross-sectional area and less resistance, as in the trunk, the heat production is accordingly less.[2,12]

TYPE OF CURRENT

AC current creates more damage than equivalent amounts of DC current. AC current has a greater ability to produce ventricular fibrillation than DC current, at equal voltages. In addition, at household frequencies, AC current causes tetanic muscle contractions, so that the stronger flexor grip is often "frozen" to the electric source, prolonging contact. It is said that experienced linemen present the dorsal surface of the hand to electric wire when there is any remote chance of injury, so that if they should be shocked, the arm will flex away from the contact point. Low voltage AC current may also produce tetanic contraction of the muscles of respiration, causing cessation of ventilation.[4]

DURATION

The longer the duration of contact, the greater the damage. Low voltage tends to cause sustained contact

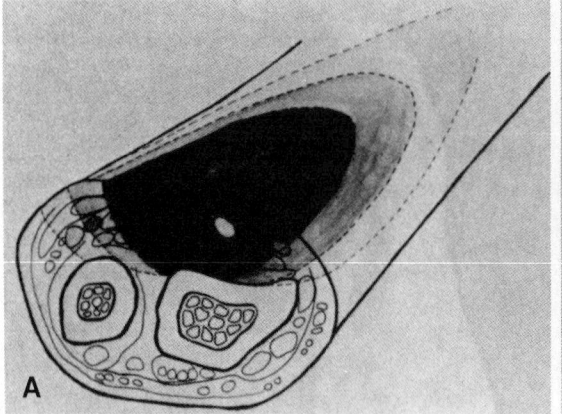
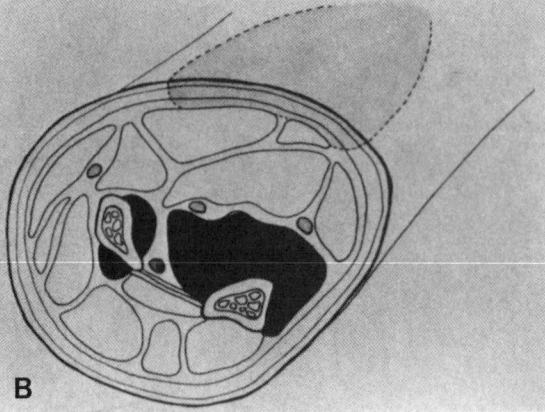

FIG. 71-5. A. Central area of total necrosis at entrance point of current. Surrounding zones of lesser degree of thermal tissue damage. B. Periosseus myonecrosis underlying a more peripheral zone as in A. With permission from Luce, E.A., et al.: High tension electrical injury of the upper extremity. Surg. Gynec. Obstet. *147*:38, 1978.

because of muscle contraction, whereas high voltage often knocks the victim away from the contact.

PATHWAY

The pathway may be inferred from the location of entry and exit wounds, which may be multiple. Hand-to-hand current flow carries a 60% mortality, whereas hand-to-foot pathway has a 20% mortality, because the hand-to-hand pathway involves the heart and the spinal cord from C4 to C8.[4,13]

PREHOSPITAL CARE

The initial extrication and resuscitation of the electrical injury victim may be dangerous and difficult, but ultimately rewarding.

The first rule dictates rescuer safety. The power must be cut off to ensure a safe rescue. If the injury current is still flowing, only those with expert knowledge should attempt to free the victim from the power contact. There are many myths describing the alleged safe modes of separating the victim from the power source, e.g., using long wooden handles, insulating gloves, belts, insulated tools, or fabrics, but none of these are absolutely safe.[14] Especially under wet conditions, rescuer safety cannot be ensured when the power is still flowing. The worst scenario involves multiplying the number of victims. If an arrest victim is still found to be on a pole, he must be lowered to the ground immediately for resuscitation because CPR is ineffective in the upright position.

After safe extrication, the resuscitation process begins. The victim should be considered a burn patient with blunt injury and crush trauma. Despite an often imposing and dramatic victim presentation, the orderly sequence of priorities must be followed. Airway, breathing, and circulation must be verified or established in the standard fashion. Cervical spine (C-spine) immobilization is frequently required. Two large-bore IVs, oxygen (O_2), and monitoring should be instituted promptly. A rapid assessment is performed, looking for signs of head injury, chest trauma, intra-abdominal hemorrhage, and orthopedic fractures and/or dislocations. Particular attention must be paid to peripheral pulses. Estimation of total surface body area burns is required. A careful search for entry and exit wounds is also important.

Fractures and dislocations should be splinted. A long spine board should be used. Constricting rings must be removed. Wounds are dressed using sterile technique.

Communication with the receiving hospital should be instituted early. If the victim has indeed suffered a high-tension burn, immediate transfer to a level I facility with a burn unit is optimal.

If cardiac arrest has occurred, cardioversion can be attempted if available in the field. If this is unsuccessful, repeated attempts after further oxygenation are warranted, with resuscitation per ACLS protocols.

CLINICAL PRESENTATION

The victim of electric current may present with a varied and often confusing clinical picture. At one end of the spectrum, there may be only trivial burns from low-voltage contact, often associated with great anxiety or hysteria. Or, at the other end of the spectrum, the victim may demonstrate grossly charred or mummified extremities, or gross scalp or even cranial tissue loss. He or she may exhibit only small entry and exit wounds, which belie hidden tissue destruction. Flame or arc burns may predominate. It must again be emphasized that there may be a combination of two or more types of electrical injury. CPR may be in progress, or the patient may initially appear to be stable, only to decompensate in a precipitous and unexpected manner. Occult intra-abdominal hemorrhage or CNS bleeding may manifest at any time.

Because of the suddenness of an electrical injury, the victim and his or her family are not prepared for such a potentially devastating and life-changing event. Consequently, extremes of psychologic reaction may be encountered.

A comprehensive physical examination is performed after the initial survey, and frequent reassessments are essential. Complications involving virtually every organ system occur. Table 71-4 portrays the incidence of complications in one study.

TABLE 71-4. COMPLICATIONS OF ELECTRICAL INJURY IN 182 PATIENTS*

Complication	No. of Patients
Neurologic	195
Cardiac	85
Sepsis	26
Ophthalmologic	19
Musculoskeletal	17
Scars and contractures	17
Auditory	14
Gastrointestinal	12
Pulmonary	11
Renal	11
Vascular	7
Other	12
Total	426

* With permission from Butler, E.D., and Gant, T.D.: Electrical injuries, with special reference to the upper extremities. Am. J. Surg. *134*:95, 1977.

SKIN

Cutaneous burns are carefully noted and charted; a burn diagram is helpful. A detailed search must be made for entry and exit wounds, which are often subtle and may be multiple. I examined a lineman struck by a high tension power line; the entry wound was in the hand, exposing bone and disarticulating several MCP joints. The exit wound was not initially evident; however, a careful search finally revealed a 4 cm round blowout exit wound hidden in the folds of the perineum. The patient did not survive.

Entry wounds are typically described as depressed, with a central area of necrosis and surrounding bullseye pattern of variable viability. Exit wounds tend to be larger and reflect the concentration of electrical energy that gathers before it blasts its way out through the resistance of the skin (Fig. 71-6).[15]

Other burns may be superficial or deep. When the electric current arcs across the skin, it tends to jump

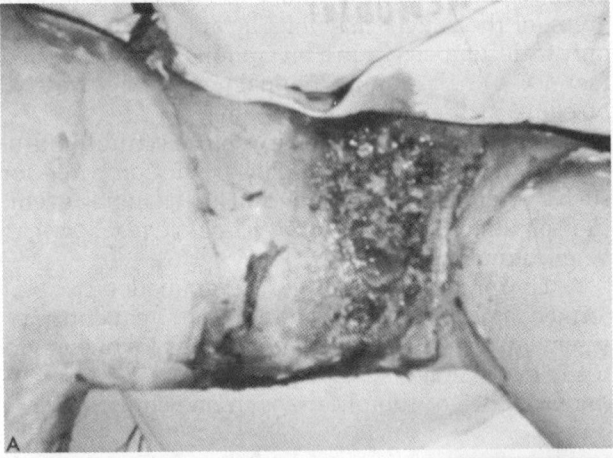
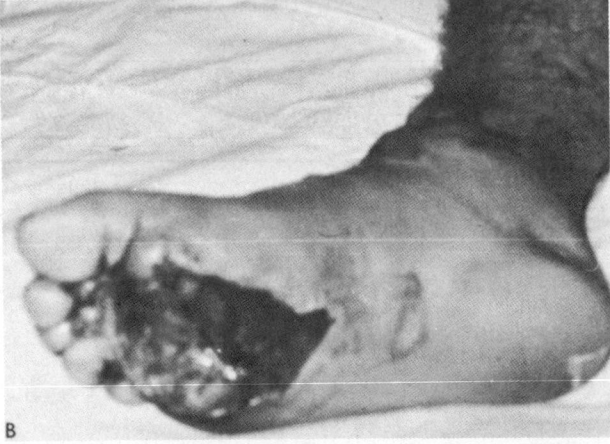

FIG. 71-6.   A. Electrical entry wound. The area of contact is hard, charred, centrally depressed, and leathery. Note extreme swelling proximal to the wound. B. Electrical exit wound. Usually rounded and charred, with depressed edges, exit wounds are more likely to "explode" externally as the charge exits. With permission from Baxter, C.R.: Present concepts in the management of major electrical injury. Surg. Clin. North Am. *50*:6, 1970.

across the flexor creases, producing typical "kissing" lesions. These are found most commonly at the flexor surfaces of the wrist, antecubital area, and axilla (Fig. 71-7).[12] Peculiar to the arc or flash burn is "metallization." Because of the extremely high temperature generated by the electric arc, metal particles become volatilized from the electrodes; these may be impregnated into the skin by the blast effect, producing a unique metallic sheen.[8]

Deep tissue emphysema has also been noted in deep burns, and apparently results from superheating of tissue fluids during electrical passage.[8]

NEUROLOGIC

The nervous system is the most commonly affected organ system in electric injury. From 33 to 100% of patients suffer from neurologic injury, depending on the criteria. Injury involves the central and peripheral nervous systems. Symptoms of central lesions involving the brain include unconsciousness, confusion, amnesia, depression, irritability, paralysis, paresis, sensory deficits, central vein thrombosis, hemorrhage, cerebral edema, necrosis of brain tissue, chronic headache, cognition impairment, and many others.

Spinal cord injury lesions may cause sclerosis, transverse myelitis, ascending paralysis, various complete or incomplete cord syndromes, acute spasticity, and other, often subtle lesions. Delayed lesions tend to be permanent.[16-18]

Peripheral nerve deficits are common. The median nerve is the peripheral nerve most commonly affected. Motor dysfunction appears to predominate over sensory loss. Causalgia and reflex sympathetic dystrophy are frequently noted, and often require sympathectomy.

Neurologic lesions are often subtle, and may appear after a delay of minutes to hours. Detailed neurological examination is mandatory, with frequent periodic re-examinations. Several authors have noted that some lesions were not evident for many days.

Cardiac abnormalities rank behind neurological lesions in frequency. No single pattern predominates. Arrythmias range from lethal to benign. ECG changes are frequent. Ischemia or infarct may occur, and septal rupture or pericarditis are also complications, although rare.[19-24]

MUSCULOSKELETAL SYSTEM

Musculoskeletal injury is common in victims of electrical injury. Coagulation necrosis of muscle has already been mentioned. Compression fractures of the thoracic spine must be excluded. Dislocation of the shoulder, generally posterior, is not uncommon. A particularly deceptive situation involves bilateral posterior shoulder dislocations; because there is no asymmetry, it may be overlooked initially. Osteomyelitis may develop, and sterile sequestrae of bone may

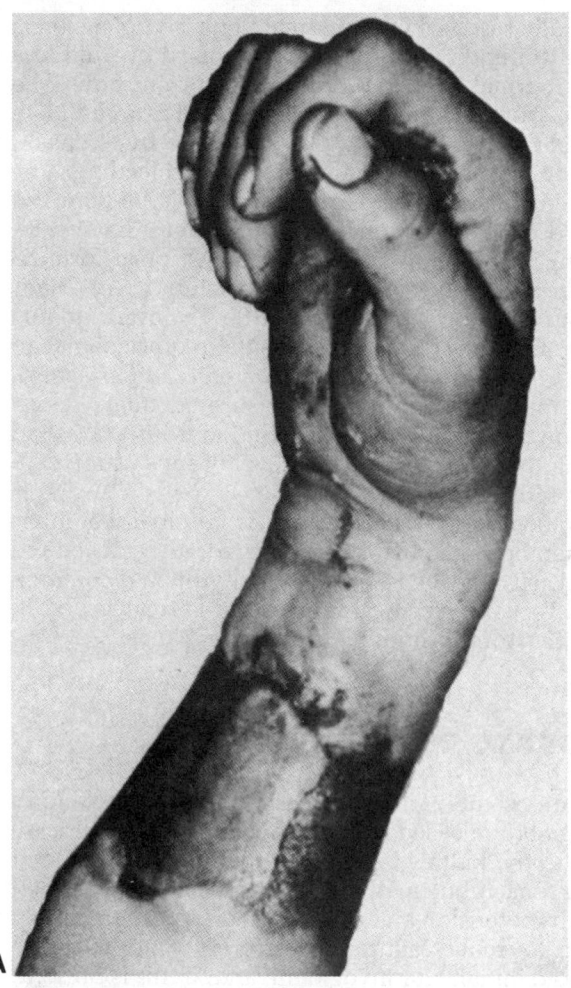

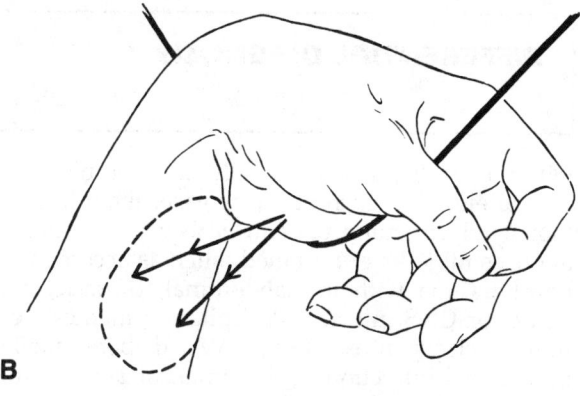

FIG. 71-7. A. Palmar and skip burn of the distal part of the volar aspect of the forearm from current arc. Totally ischemic hand. B. Arcing from current source to palm and volar aspect of wrist and forearm. With permission from Luce, E.A., et al.: High tension electrical injury of the upper extremity. Surg. Gynec. Obstet. 147:38, 1978.

form sinus tracts long after injury, requiring excision. Long bone fractures, particularly of the upper extremities, also occur with some frequency. Bilateral femoral neck fractures in a high voltage victim have been reported with delayed diagnosis.[40]

GASTROINTESTINAL SYSTEM

The gastrointestinal tract is particularly prone to injury in wounds involving the abdominal wall. Complications include peptic ulceration, Curling's ulcer, necrosis of the gallbladder, perforation or necrosis of any hollow viscus, pancreatitis, esophageal lesions,[25] liver abnormalities, splenic bleeding or infarct, and various functional complaints.

VASCULAR SYSTEM

Vascular problems include hemorrhage, thrombosis, vasospasm, thrombophlebitis, and aneurysm formation.

INFECTIONS

Infectious sequelae include clostridial myositis, osteomyelitis, pneumonia, cellulitis, superficial burn wound infection, and septic thrombophlebitis. Inapparent foci of infection have been described, such as paraspinatus or iliopsoas abscesses.[15]

PREGNANCY

The *pregnant patient* carries a significant risk of fetal death or postnatal morbidity/mortality. The amniotic fluid apparently provides a preferential path for current flow. Pregnant women should seek medical attention after any electrical shock, no matter how minor it appears.[26,27]

DIFFERENTIAL DIAGNOSIS

Differential diagnosis is usually not a problem in the typical electrical current injury case. Even in the obviously electrocuted patient, however, secondary diagnoses must be entertained, such as accompanying blunt trauma with intraabdominal, thoracic, orthopedic, or CNS injuries. Precipitating medical conditions such as intoxication, CVA, diabetes mellitus, myocardial infarction, arrhythmia, or suicidal intention should also be considered.

Occasionally, an unwitnessed case may present a dilemma in differential diagnosis. In low-voltage injury, the victim may have no external sign of electrical contact at all, as in bathtub electrocution, but may present with apnea or in cardiac arrest. The child who presents with oral burns from chewing on a cord may have an inaccurate history, causing the lesion to be confused with other types of trauma, but the characteristic pattern should establish the diagnosis.

In high-voltage injury, the differential diagnosis may occasionally be unclear, especially in unwitnessed cases, because the victim is frequently amnestic, confused, obtunded, or unconscious. In victims with only entry and exit wounds, the condition may be confused with snakebite, primary crush injury, assault, open fracture, venous occlusion, or infection. In high-voltage situations involving thermal burns, the clinician may consider lightning injury, simple thermal burns, or arterial occlusion.[28]

INITIAL STABILIZATION

The victim of electrocution may require intensive stabilization. Oxygen administration, cardiac monitoring, and at least two large-bore IVs are standard. When CPR is in progress, the resuscitation is continued according to established protocols.

The airway may be compromised by neck burns or thermally induced edema of the upper airway. An artificial airway should be established early, if it appears to be necessary, rather than the physician adopting an attitude of watchful expectancy.

Breathing may be compromised by chest wall burns, centrally induced apnea, blunt trauma (including pneumo- and/or hemothorax), blast lung, aspiration, or carbon monoxide intoxication when ignition occurs in an enclosed space. Therefore, escharotomy, intubation with assisted ventilation, high flow O_2, and chest tubes are used as the situation dictates.

Transient hypertension may occasionally be seen early, probably because of catecholamine release, and generally resolves without treatment. Hypotension is not uncommon, and is generally caused by fluid loss from thermal burn and/or internal current flow. The edema from true current damage is said to accumulate almost immediately.[15] Other causes of hypotension include occult hemorrhage or external bleeding.

When hypotension is present, two large-bore IVs should be started at once, using lactated Ringer's solution. For thermal burns, a standard burn formula may be used with lactated Ringer's solution (see Chap. 44, Burns.). For internal current flow injuries, no formula quantifies fluid loss, and fluid requirements are often grossly underestimated; therefore, other parameters must be monitored to ensure adequate resuscitation, including hourly urine output, CVP (in young, healthy individuals), level of sensorium, capillary refill, pulse, and BP.

For persistent hypotension, the possibility of internal hemorrhage must be considered, and packed red blood cells may be necessary. Arrhythmia is common in all types of electrical injury, and is treated no differently from arrhythmia from other causes.

AVOIDING RENAL FAILURE

An important early consideration is renal failure. Myoglobin released from damaged muscle is directly toxic to the kidney because the pigment is deposited in the renal tubules. When myoglobinuria is combined with hypotension and acidosis, there is a high danger of acute renal failure. Therefore, urine must be checked initially for myoglobin, and, if this is present, treated aggressively. Mannitol is given as a bolus of 1 g per kilogram (kg), and then continued as a drip of 12.5 g per hour. Alkalinization of the urine is accomplished by adding $NaHCO_3$ to the IV fluids. Urinary output should be maintained at a high level, approximately 1.5 cc per kg per hour to 2.0 cc per kg per hour or higher.[29] It must be emphasized that once mannitol is started, the urine output alone is no longer an adequate measure of tissue perfusion. Hemochromogens also can cause a paradoxic alkalinization of the urine.[15]

In selected cases, initial stabilization can be continued in the operating room.

LABORATORY AND OTHER EVALUATIONS

Standard laboratory and x-ray examinations required for major electrical injury include the following:

1. CBC
2. Ions

3. PT, PTT
4. Amylase
5. BUN, creatinine
6. UA
7. Serum and urine myoglobin
8. Cardiac enzymes
9. ABG
10. ECG
11. Chest x ray
12. C-Spine x ray

In selected cases, the following may also be used:

1. Carboxyhemoglobin
2. Type and crossmatch
3. Blood alcohol
4. Toxicology (drug screen)
5. Creatine kinase
6. CT of head and abdomen
7. Echocardiography
8. Cardiac Doppler
9. Technetium or xenon muscle scan

PROCEDURES

Constricting rings, which may have been previously neglected, should be removed. Escharotomy may be necessary on the chest wall when respiratory excursions are restricted. Extremities frequently require escharotomy. It is important to realize that, after escharotomies of extremities, fasciotomy may be required. Endoneurolysis may also be required to preserve peripheral nerve integrity.[5]

Peritoneal lavage or CT scans of the abdomen are employed in the search for occult hemorrhage.

Burns should be treated with great care because infection still constitutes a major source of mortality.

Foley catheterization may be necessary to monitor urine output, and nasogastric intubation is required for ileus or gastric distention, and also to check for upper GI bleeding.

MANAGEMENT

Burn specialists should be consulted as early as possible. Major burn cases require a team involving the burn specialist, orthopedic surgeon, trauma surgeon, plastic surgeon, internist, and sometimes the neurosurgeon. Crisis intervention or psychiatric counseling may also be required early. The ED physician plays a crucial, often decisive role in determining the patient's future. Much hinges on the crucial first hour. Potential problems must be anticipated, and a plan formulated.

Urine should be monitored on an ongoing basis. Persistently pigmented urine may indicate massive muscle necrosis and need for urgent amputation.

About 35 to 60% of all high-voltage injury patients eventually require amputation.[3] In five combined series, there were 112 amputations in 138 cases.[30-34] A major issue concerns how to accomplish early recognition of devitalized muscle. The timing and necessity of debridement, decompression, or amputation remain controversial. Early debridement and decompression may favorably alter the outcome of injured extremities, but much is still unknown, and controversy exists currently about evaluation in management. On initial exploration, it is often difficult to differentiate viable from nonviable muscle. If muscle bleeds when cut and contracts when stimulated, this is thought to be a sign of viability. Often, however, on re-exploration, such muscle may be found to be necrotic. A healthy reddish color is also thought to be a sign of viability, but the myoglobin released from damaged muscle may turn red when exposed to ambient oxygen, confusing the true picture.[15,35] Xenon or technetium scans may help clarify viability so that healthy tissue is not unnecessarily sacrificed or dead tissue allowed to release toxins or serve as a focus of infection. Tetanus prophylaxis must not be neglected. Clostridial myositis remains a distinct threat, and anticlostridial prophylaxis should be considered in consultation with the accepting physician.

Management of burns to the oral commissure in children must be planned in consultation with the oral surgeon. There are proponents of many different strategies.[9]

INDICATIONS FOR HOSPITAL ADMISSION

For high-voltage injuries, admission is indicated in virtually all cases. ICU or burn and trauma units are generally appropriate.

For low-voltage injuries, indications for admission are less clear (see Table 71-4). When cardiac or respiratory irregularities have occurred, the patient should be admitted. For burns to the oral commissure, admission policies vary, and the decision to admit must be made in consultation with the plastic surgeon. Bleeding of the labial artery has a peak occurrence at 3 to 5 days, and may be alarming but is not massive.

In a large percentage of the cases of low-voltage injury, the patient may be safely sent home, often after a period of 4 to 6 hours of observation.[36]

PROGNOSTIC FACTORS AND "POST-SYNDROME"

In low-voltage injury, the course tends to be predictable. Burns behave like burns from other thermal sources. If there has been cardiopulmonary arrest, as in bathtub electrocution or internal current flow mishaps that may occur in the hospital, the course is similar to that of postarrest syndrome from any cause, e.g., hypoxic encephalopathy, sepsis, renal failure, GI hemorrhage or perforation. Prognostic factors for oral commissural burns are more elusive, and depend on the patient's age, duration of contact, and other factors; initial examination may not accurately foretell the ultimate degree of functional and cosmetic deficit.

In high-voltage injuries, the course is more variable and uncertain. The ED physician must be prudent in making predictions to patients or their families. Mortality is relatively low in those who survive long enough to arrive at the hospital (2 to 5%) and is generally caused by sepsis or head injury.

Neurologic injury has been noted to fall into two general patterns. Interestingly, patients who present with deficit tend initially to improve, whereas those whose onset of neurologic injury is delayed (days to years) tend to have permanent lesions. Transverse myelitis commencing more than 2 years after injury has been reported.

Gastrointestinal problems may be subtle or gross, and may not be recognized early. Dysphagia is not uncommon and may persist for years.

Cataracts may appear early or be delayed for years, and initial or even repeated examinations may not detect clues to their subsequent formation.[37]

An initially normal ECG is probably a good indicator that no significant cardiac abnormality will ensue, although cases of delayed abnormality in the ECG have been noted.[24] Sudden death has been described after about 2 weeks, secondary to precipitous hypokalemia of unexplained cause.[15,38]

Delayed massive hemorrhage from a major artery is uncommon, but should be anticipated, particularly in deep burns involving the axillary artery.[39]

Seizure disorder may be initiated by electrical injury, and then become chronic.

PREVENTION

Numerous logical preventative measures have been postulated. Open sockets and outlets must be covered with "childproof" devices. Extension cords should be avoided when possible, but when used they should be in good condition and not frayed. When small chil-

dren are present, the cords should be covered. Plug-in electrical appliances should be kept away from the bathtub. In community planning, underground high tension lines are safer than exposed wires. Transformer stations must be secured from inadvertent or intentional access. Community education programs, particularly at the school level, are necessary to help prevent accidents.

Safety standards in industry must be constantly updated and enforced. Most electrical accidents are preventable.[8]

PITFALLS

- Multiple entry and/or exit wounds may coexist in one patient.
- More than one type of burn may be found in the same patient.
- Do not underestimate the potential devastation of deep current burns or their fluid requirements.
- Burn formulas do not estimate fluid requirements in deep current burns.
- Re-examine the patient frequently.
- Once mannitol is started, the urinary output no longer reflects adequacy of tissue perfusion.
- Major blunt trauma frequently accompanies electric current injury.
- The presence of peripheral pulses does not ensure viability of the extremity.
- Search carefully for dislocations, especially of the bilateral posterior shoulder.
- Consult with burn and trauma specialists early.
- Do not confuse subcutaneous emphysema from superheating of body fluids (early) with clostridial myositis (delayed).
- Do not forget about postburn hypokalemia.
- Perform early escharotomy and/or fasciotomy when indicated.
- Do not forget about paradoxic alkalinization of the urine and the consequent necessity to monitor arterial blood gases.
- Calculate the fluid requirements from the time of injury, not the time of presentation in the ED.
- Respect the unpredictability of electrical current coursing through the human body.

MEDICOLEGAL PEARLS

The field of electrical trauma is fraught with potential for malpractice, and tort claims against the party responsible for the offending electrical apparatus.

The best defense against malpractice resides in meticulous patient care based on solid understanding of pathophysiologic principles and sympathetic communication with the patient and his family from the outset. Bad results frequently occur, even in the best of hands. Accurate record keeping is a natural corollary of this situation. Baseline recording of normal findings is essential.

The physician must also act as a patient advocate. The patient must demonstrate that he or she understands the nature and course of present disabilities and the possibility of late-onset deficits such as cataract formation, chronic GI disturbances, neurologic deficits, and psychiatric maladjustments. The patient should be advised against premature signing of a medical release, which might preclude him or her from recovering just compensation for delayed medical injuries if they ensue. The physician must ensure that the patient be scheduled for appropriate periodic follow-up examinations, e.g., ophthalmologic, neurologic, gastroenterologic.

HORIZONS

Much research has been done on electrical injury, but much more is yet needed to answer basic questions. We must establish the optimum timing for exploration(s), the ability to better differentiate viable from nonviable muscle, the knowledge of how to avoid amputation or at least make it as distal as possible, and guidelines delineating the optimum timing and type of covering for burns. We must also elucidate more clearly the cause of progressive tissue destruction: whether it is ongoing thrombosis, slow manifestation of original irreversible muscle damage from the current itself, or perhaps some combination thereof.

Research has been done on the role of thromboxane, an arachidonic acid metabolite, in progressive tissue loss. The investigators postulate that thermal injury causes release of elevated amounts of thromboxane, which in turn causes microvascular vasoconstriction and platelet aggregation leading to thrombosis. Treatment with thromboxane blocking agents prevents development of anticipated muscle necrosis in laboratory animals. It is hoped that this can be extrapolated in the clinical situation, with improvement in patient outcome.[29]

REFERENCES

1. Taylor, P.H., et al.: The intriguing electrical burn. J. Trauma 2:309, 1962.
2. Hunt, J.L., et al.: Vascular lesions in acute electric injuries. J. Trauma 14:6, 1974.
3. Robinson, M. and Seward, P.N.: Electrical and lightning injuries in children. Pediatr. Emerg. Care 2:3, 1986.
4. Kobernick, M.: Electrical injuries: Pathophysiology and emergency management. Ann. Emerg. Med. 11:633, 1982.
5. Butler, E.D., and Gant, T.D.: Electrical injuries with special reference to the upper extremities. Am J. Surg. 134:95, 1977.
6. MMWR: Occupational electrocution—Texas, 1981–1985. MMWR 36:44, 1987.
7. Helgerson, S.D., and Milham, S.: Farm workers electrocuted when irrigation pipes contact power lines. Public Health Rep. 100:3, 1985.
8. Skoog, T.: Electrical injuries. J. Trauma 10:10, 1970.
9. Sturim, H.S.: The treatment of electrical injuries. J. Trauma 11:959, 1971.
10. Artz, C.P.: Changing concepts of electrical injury. Am J. Surg. 128:461, 1974.
11. Hunt, J.L., et al.: The pathophysiology of acute electric burns. J. Trauma 16:5, 1976.
12. Luce, E.A., et al.: High tension electrical injury of the upper extremity. Surg. Gynec. Obstet. 147:38, 1978.
13. Thompson, J.C., and Ashwal, S.: Electrical injuries in children. Am. J. Dis. Child. 137:231, 1983.
14. Cooper, M.A.: Electrical and lightning injuries. Emerg. Med. Clinic North America, 2:3, 1984.
15. Baxter, C.R.: Present concepts in the management of major electrical injury. Surg. Clin. North Am. 50:6, 1970.
16. Christensen, J.A., et al.: Delayed neurological injury secondary to high-voltage current with recovery. J. Trauma 20:2, 1980.
17. Levine, N.S., et al.: Spinal cord injury following electrical accidents: Case reports. J. Trauma. 15:5, 1975.
18. Farrell, D.F., and Starr, A.: Delayed neurological sequelae of electrical injuries. Neurology, 18:601, 1968.
19. Chandra, N.C., et al.: Clinical predictors of myocardial damage after high voltage electrical injury. Crit. Care Med. 18:3, 1990.
20. Homma, S., et al.: Echocardiographic observations in survivors of acute electrical injury. Chest 97:1, 1990.
21. Jensen, P.J., et al.: Electrical injury causing ventricular arrhythmias. Br. Heart J. 57:279, 1987.
22. Kinney, T.J.: Myocardial infarction following electrical injury. Ann. Emerg. Med. 11:11, 1982.
23. McBride, J.W., et al.: Is serum creatine kinase-MB in electrically injured patients predictive of myocardial injury? JAMA 25:6, 1986.
24. Purdue, G.F., and Hunt, J.L.: Electrocardiographic monitoring after electrical injury: Necessity or luxury. J. Trauma 26:2, 1986.
25. Flisak, M.E., Berman, S.: Electrical injury of the esophagus. Am J. Roentgenol. 150:103, 1988.
26. Lieberman, J.R., et al.: Electrical accidents during pregnancy. Obstet. Gyn. 67:6, 1986.
27. Jaffe, R., et al.: Case report: Fetal death in early pregnancy due to electric current. Acta Obstet. Gynecol. Scand. 65:283, 1986.
28. Burke, J.F., et al.: Patterns of high tension electrical injury in children and adolescents and their management. Am. J. Surg. 133:492, 1976.
29. Robson, M.C., et al.: A new explanation for the progressive tissue loss in electrical injuries. Plast. Reconstr. Surg. 73:3, 1984.
30. Solem, L., et al.: The natural history of electrical injury. J. Trauma. 17:7, 1977.
31. Rouse, R.G., and Dimick, A.R.: The treatment of electrical injury compared to burn injury: A review of pathophysiology and comparison of patient management protocols. J. Trauma 18:1, 1978.
32. Parshley, P.F., et al.: Aggressive approach to the extremity damaged by electric current. Am. J. Surg. 150:78, 1985.
33. Hunt, J.L., et al.: Acute electric burns. Arch. Surg. 115:434, 1980.
34. Mann, R.J., and Waltquist, J.M.: Early decompression fasciotomy in the treatment of high-voltage electrical burns of the extremities. South. Med. J. 68:9, 1975.
35. Wilkinson, C., and Wood, M.: High voltage electric injury. Am. J. Surg. 136:693, 1978.
36. Grube, B.J., et al.: Neurological consequences of electrical burns. J. Trauma 30:3, 1990.
37. Saffle, J.R., et al.: Cataracts: A long-term complication of electrical injury. J. Trauma 25:1, 1985.
38. Dixon, G.F.: The evaluation and management of electrical injuries. Crit. Care Med. 11:5, 1983.
39. Hartford, C.E., and Ziffren, S.E.: Electrical injury. J. Trauma 11:4, 1971.
40. Tompkins, G.S., et al.: Bilateral simultaneous fractures of femoral neck, case report. J. Trauma 30:1415, 1991.

Chapter 72

LASER AND MICROWAVE INJURIES

Leon Goldman

CAPSULE

Laser and microwave injuries are relatively rare. Laser injuries involve a nonspecific coagulation necrosis and can affect eye structures, skin, or the respiratory system. Initial considerations in microwave injuries are eye and testes exposure. The possibility of both types of injuries reinforces the need for prevention, and job safety is paramount.

APPLICATIONS OF THE LASER

Lasers are used extensively in industry for metal-working of many types, for information handling in many diverse fields including computer technology and video disk communications, and also for monitoring construction. In the military, lasers are used for ranging, communications, radar, and weaponry. An important use of lasers is the laser-induced thermonuclear fusion advanced as a partial answer (some years hence) to the energy crisis, and also for use in weaponry. Related to this is the recent development of uranium enrichment by lasers. The use of the laser is currently being extensively expanded to permit transmission through fiberoptics for all types of communication systems, whether in an aircraft, in the telephone system, or in a house. The medical and surgical use of lasers has grown tremendously.

These several applications mean increasing use of high- and higher-output laser systems or many types of lasers ranging from the x-ray region of the spectrum to far into the infrared zone. Increasing concern about exposure to operating personnel is therefore necessary as is, in some instances, exposure of the general public.

Fortunately, there is an awareness of the need for concern on the part of both industry and government. An example of cooperative work is the American National Standards Institute Manual on the Safe Use of Lasers.[1] A book is also available.[2]

DIAGNOSIS AND TREATMENT IN MEDICINE

Lasers are used for extensive analytic analyses with many different spectroscopic techniques. Spectroscopy may be useful in environmental pollution, detection of carcinogenic materials, or particle microanalysis with special microemission spectroscopy. In the field of immunology with fluorochromes, flow cytofluorometry is used for mass diagnoses of Pap smears and for detailed immunologic studies. Laser laboratory diagnostic instrumentation includes laser nephelometry for particle measurements of circulating immunoglobulins and rheumatoid factor.

There have been extensive developments in laser surgery with higher-output, flexible, safe instrumentation with good performance standards. In addition, attached microscopes are available for precise microsurgery. Laser angioplasty is still in its infancy.

There has been progressive development in gynecologic laser surgery, with excellent results in the treatment of intraepithelial neoplasia, both vaginal and cervical. With the increasing incidence of sexually transmitted disorders, lasers have become popular and effective in the treatment of condylomata acuminata in both men and women. The laser attached to a colposcope can be used to treat small infections and early lesions.

There is also considerable interest in the laser as a stimulating agent for treating chronic infections and ulcers that are slow to heal. These lasers are low-output, open systems with helium-neon, helium-cadmium, and krypton laser systems. More controls are needed to evaluate these stimulating effects of lasers and also to assess the benefits of laser acupuncture.

LASER REACTION IN TISSUE

The laser reaction in tissue is, in brief, a nonspecific coagulation necrosis similar to that of an electric burn.

In more than 14 years of research and clinical applications of the laser, there has been no evidence of carcinogenesis. Several organizations have developed laser standards and grading systems for laser hazards.[3,4]

OUTLINE OF THE TREATMENT OF LASER INJURIES

ACUTE EYE TRAUMA

1. Consultation with an ophthalmologist is necessary in laser injuries.
2. Topical and systemic steroids, including sodium sulfacetamide (Blephamide) ophthalmic suspension.
3. Fundus picture and detailed description of the current injuries, if these occur in a large laser facility.
4. Repeat examination at least once within 24 hours because most laser eye injuries usually do not appear severe at the outset.
5. Chronic eye problems may possibly occur from continued exposure to low-intensity impacts; detection is possible through frequent eye examinations.

SKIN INJURIES FROM ACCIDENTAL OR INTENTIONAL EXPOSURES

1. *Acute:* Treat as for electrical burns. Most are mild.
   a. Topical corticosteroids if injury is mild.
   b. Topical antibiotics as indicated.
   c. Débridement, excision, and graft replacement if injury is severe.
   d. For contaminated wounds (infections from materials processed; radioactive compounds), débride locally and irrigate with saline. If radioactive contamination has occurred, suitable steps should be instituted.
2. *Chronic:* Apply bland creams to prevent dryness. There is no evidence of carcinoma, as yet, from chronic laser radiation exposure (no data yet on ultraviolet lasers).

With the increasing interest in and development of high-output laser weaponry, it is necessary to develop procedures for the treatment of laser injury added to other trauma caused by bullet wounds, burns, nuclear weapons, chemical warfare, and infections.

RESPIRATORY SYSTEM

1. *Acute:* Evaluate the hazards of material processing regarding substances, industrial hygiene, and other factors. Therapy, local and systemic, should be directed toward the toxicity of substances inhaled.
2. *Chronic:* Evaluate the hazards with laboratory tests and analyses of materials, pulmonary function, and hematology.

PREVENTION OF LASER INJURIES

The following are important considerations in preventing laser injuries:

1. A definite program of laser safety.
2. Protection.
   a. Area control.
   b. Personnel.
      (1) Specific laser-protective glasses for eyes.
      (2) Skin protection.
      (3) Environmental protection in material processing.

As indicated for material processing, eye protection should be considered for open processes, and consideration also given to the production of pulmonary irritant or toxic materials such as phosgene from laser impacts on certain types of firebrick and beryllium from some alloys. Treatment should be given for inhalation of toxic substances. In addition to the acute treatment, the patient should continue to be watched for chronic changes. Pulmonary edema may occur in hours, depending on the nature of the substances inhaled.

If injuries from lasers occur in an establishment where there is an extensive laser facility, special forms must be used to record complete data in the emergency treatment. For example, in eye injuries the exact location and description of the lesions must be given. Here, a fundus picture helps considerably. For the skin also, if necessary, pretreatment and past-treatment photographs should also be taken to evaluate the type and location of the burn. In air pollution from laser processing, it is necessary again that the patient be examined repeatedly to determine any late effects of such atmospheric exposures.

Patients should always be reassured that the laser is not carcinogenic. Whether such promises can be made when there is more extensive use of ultraviolet laser systems and even x-ray laser systems cannot be determined yet.

MICROWAVE EXPOSURES

INITIAL CONSIDERATIONS

The immediate concern in an injury from microwaves is eye exposure. Lens damage could not occur in a human from acute-exposure microwave without severe facial burns.

The other area of concern in microwave injury is exposure of the testes.

Harmful effects of microwave therapeutic diathermy develop from exceeding the recommended doses for such therapy. This may occur through error, be intentional, or develop in a treated area with reduced pain sensitivity. It is necessary that rings, pins, other metal objects, and dentures be removed before these treatments are given. This precaution also includes metallic orthopedic prostheses. Microwave ovens, a spin-off from radar research, have few hazards if radiation is below the government standard of 10 milliwatts per square centimeter (mW cm^2) (to have 1 mW cm^2 5 cm: from the oven when new and 5 mW cm^2 after use). Eye injuries and secondary virus infections may develop, chiefly through misuse. Some microwave ovens have been implicated in pacemaker malfunctions.

With the increasing interest in cancer hyperthermia, there will be more applications of microwaves and need for more consideration about microwave burns of the skin. In cancer hyperthermia research, lasers have been used with microwaves and radiofrequency.

TREATMENT

Eye. The same precautions are used for immediate treatment and follow-up care as with the laser, described previously. Because of the danger of possible cataract formation from severe or unusual microwave exposure, the patient should be examined for a long period after exposure or accident, and the power density of exposure determined definitely. This subject of eye involvement, as indicated, is still controversial, especially in respect to occupational exposures.

Testes. If there has been some concern about exposure to high-output microwave, even without discomfort to the scrotal area, it is well that, after a period of some 3 to 4 weeks, detailed examinations of the sperm be performed to reveal any late sequelae. Burns may develop from metal contacts on the skin by absorption of microwave radiation.

Body Burns. The treatment is the same as for electrical burns.

ELECTROMAGNETIC FIELDS

Although problems have been few, concern has been raised about the relationship of electromagnetic fields to cancer risk and reproductive health. See Bibliography.

REFERENCE

1. Safety with Lasers and Other Optical Sources by David Sliney, U.S. Environmental Hygiene Agency, and Myron L. Wolbarst, Medical Center of Duke University.
2. Stiney, D.: Safety with Lasers and Other Optical Sources. New York, Plenum Press, 1980.
3. ANSI Standards for Safe Laser Use. New York, American National Standards Institute, 1986.
4. Krieger, G.R.: Lasers. In Hazardous Material Toxicology. Edited by Sullivan, J.B., and Krieger, G.R. Baltimore, Williams and Wilkins, 1992.

BIBLIOGRAPHY

American National Standards Institute: Safe Use of Lasers, 1973.

Appleton, B.: Microwave cataracts. JAMA 229:407, 1974.

Appleton, B.: Results of Clinic and Surveys for Microwave Ocular Effects. DHEW Publication No. (FDA) 73–8031, BRH/DBE73–3, 1973.

Bern, M.W.: Laser surgery. Sci. Am. 264:84, 1991.

Goldman, L., and Rockwell, R.J., Jr.: Lasers in Medicine. New York, Gordon and Breach Science Publishers, 1972.

Goldman, L.: Applications of the Laser. Cleveland, CRC Press, 1973.

Krieger, G.R., and Irms, R.: Nonionizing electromagnetic radiation (221 references). In Hazardous Material Toxicology. Edited by Sullivan, J.B., and Krieger, G.R. Baltimore, Williams and Wilkins, 1992.

Moore, W., Jr.: Biological Aspects of Microwave Radiation. HEW National Center for Radiological Health TSB4, July, 1968.

Peterson, R.C.: Bioeffects of microwaves: A review of current knowledge. J. Occup. Med. 25:103, 1983.

Rockwell, R.J., Jr. (Ed.): Laser Safety in Surgery and Medicine. 2nd Ed. Cincinnati, Rockwell, 1985.

Chapter 73

RADIATION INJURY

George L. Voelz

CAPSULE

The need for medical management of ionizing radiation cases has been infrequent—virtually nonexistent in most hospital emergency departments (EDs). This is in stark contrast to the high public interest and concern over radiation as an environmental hazard. Successful medical management of these cases, which can range from suspect exposures to major medical emergencies, depends on advance planning and trained personnel. Management of persons contaminated externally with radioactive materials is directed toward early recognition of the problem, avoidance of secondary spread of contamination within the hospital, and skin decontamination by washing or showering. The action is simple in concept but difficult to execute skillfully. Treatment of acute radiation effects from life-threatening doses of external radiation requires rigorous measures to prevent infection, hematologic support measures for bone marrow depression, and general patient care over a period of 6 weeks or more. Much more probable are the cases of lesser or only suspect exposures, which need assessment of the potential dose by a radiation dosimetry specialist and knowledgeable medical counsel on the potential of future biologic effects.

INTRODUCTION

Ionizing radiation is any radiation, as either particles or electromagnetic energy, with sufficient energy to produce ions in matter. When such radiations pass through tissue, ionization of molecules within cells produces immediate biochemical changes that can cause more visible biologic effects later, such as skin burns, cataracts, the acute radiation syndrome, chromosomal aberrations, genetic mutations, or cancer.

Ionizing radiations may be separated into two general classes: (1) *penetrating radiations* (x rays, gamma rays, and neutrons) and (2) *nonpenetrating radiations* (alpha and beta particles). Penetrating radiations can produce damage through the entire exposed portion of the body, either whole-body or localized exposures. Such exposures occur from sources outside the body, such as x-ray machines, accelerators, or gamma sources. These are termed *external* radiation and have produced most serious radiation exposure cases. The nonpenetrating radiations produce their damage by immediate contact of radioactive material (for example, beta emitters that can produce beta burns) on the skin or by internal deposition through inhalation, skin absorption, wounds, or ingestion. Alpha particles do not have sufficient penetrating power to cause external damage, even skin damage, but are serious internal contaminants. *Internal* contamination is an important concern in health protection of radiation workers, but has only rarely caused emergency medical problems. Accidental internal exposures do, however, require rapid evaluation so that preventive treatments can be given promptly to reduce exposure.

A report on radiation accidents from 1944 through February 1989 records 305 major events worldwide.[1] A listing of the "device" or source of radiation indicates that 18 accidents involved acute exposure from a critical (uncontrolled "chain reaction") accident, 217 resulted from radiation devices (e.g., sealed sources, x-ray machines, accelerators), and 70 occurred through internal exposure to radionuclides (e.g., transuranics, medical misadministrations, fission products). A total of 101 deaths resulted from 33 of these accidents. Not all deaths were from radiation. There were 50 acute radiation deaths, 40 delayed (>60 days) or associated radiation deaths, and 11 nonradiation deaths from blast, burns, or chemicals. Heavy contributors to the numbers are the 27 radiation deaths from the Chernobyl reactor accident in Russia in 1986 and 8 deaths from exposure to a lost high-level sealed source in Morocco in 1984. Deaths from radiation therapy, nuclear medical procedures, and medical misadventures numbered 28.

One source of radiation doses and/or radioactive contamination that is frequently overrated is the transportation of radioactive materials. Although accidents of commercial transport vehicles carrying such materials have occurred, they have not been responsible for significant radiation accidents. Of much more concern are sealed sources, such as radiography sources, which may be lost through careless transport or use by poorly trained technicians. Unknown and unannounced radiation cases entering the ED are most likely to arise from such mishandled radiography sealed sources.

Two systems are currently used for radiation dosimetry: conventional and SI (Système International) metric units. Conventional units are still frequently used in the U.S. The conventional unit of absorbed dose is the *rad;* one rad is 100 ergs of energy absorbed in one gram of material, such as tissue. One rad is equivalent to 0.01 *gray* (Gy), the similar SI unit. The rad is commonly used for acute external radiation exposures (see Table 73-1 for dose-effect relationships). To express a dose for all types of ionizing radiation on a common scale of biological effect, i.e., dose equivalent, the rad value is adjusted by a quality factor (QF) and sometimes other factors. The conventional unit of the calculated dose equivalent is the *rem.* One rem is equivalent to 0.01 *sievert* (Sv), the SI unit. The rem is commonly used to describe low doses or low dose rates, such as occur with most occupational or environmental exposures, because the QF is based on chronic effects, such as cancer induction, rather than acute effects. QF values commonly used are 1 for electrons, x rays, or gamma rays, 10 for neutrons, and 20 for alpha particles.

The basic measurement of radioactivity is the number of disintegrating atomic nuclei per second (dps). The *curie* is the conventional unit used to describe the quantity of activity; a curie is 3.7×10^{10} dps. The unit is frequently modified by the use of a prefix, such as (10^{-3}), micro (10^{-6}), nano (10^{-9}), or pico (10^{-12}). The comparable SI unit is the *becquerel* (Bq), which is de-

fined as one dps. Thus, one nanocurie (3.7×10^1 dps) equals 37 becquerel.

PREHOSPITAL ASSESSMENT AND STABILIZATION

Radiation accidents may occur at facilities with emergency plans to handle such accidents. These plans should be coordinated with local hospitals and EDs. An important detail in the plan is prompt notification by the facility to the hospital on details of the accident. The medical staff must know the number and condition of involved persons, nature of the radiation source, and whether significant radioactive contamination is present. The latter information determines if a planned set-up of decontamination supplies, equipment, and procedures should be activated (Table 73-2). Some plant facilities have decontamination facilities and trained personnel to perform the necessary clean-up before transporting the patient to the hospital. This procedure is preferable to immediate transport to the hospital if the condition of the patient permits.

Conventional first-aid and emergency medical treatment of serious physical injuries have priority over radioactivity considerations. Transportation to the hospital can be made by ambulance or air, depending on the urgency of the injuries. If radioactive contamination is present, wrapping the contaminated patient in a sheet or blanket (not plastic) during transport may reduce the spread of contamination. This problem is not serious, however, because the vehicle can be decontaminated successfully afterward. No special precautions for the attendants during transport is ordinarily required, although advice on this subject should

TABLE 73-1. DOSE-EFFECT RELATIONSHIPS AFTER ACUTE WHOLE-BODY IRRADIATION (X- OR GAMMA)

Whole Body* Dose (Rad)	Clinical and Laboratory Findings
5–25	Asymptomatic. Conventional blood studies are normal. Chromosome aberrations detectable.
50–75	Asymptomatic. Minor depressions of white cells and platelets detectable in a few persons, especially if baseline values are established.
75–125	Minimal acute doses produce prodromal symptoms (anorexia, nausea, vomiting, fatigue) in about 10–20% of persons within 2 days. Mild depressions of white cells and platelets in some persons.
125–200	Symptomatic course with transient disability and clear hematologic changes in most exposed persons. Lymphocyte depression of about 50% within 48 hours.
250–350	Serious, disabling illness in most persons with about 50% mortality, if untreated. Lymphocyte depression of about 75+% within 48 hours.
500+	Accelerated version of acute radiation syndrome with gastrointestinal complications within 2 weeks, bleeding, and death in most exposed persons.
5000+	Fulminating course with cardiovascular, gastrointestinal, and CNS complications resulting in death within 24–72 hours.

* Conversion of rad (midline) dose to radiation measurements in R can be made roughly by multiplying rad times 1.5. For example, 200 rad (midline) is equal to about 300 R (200 × 1.5).

be sought if a health physicist or radiation monitor is present at the scene.

CLINICAL PRESENTATION AND EXAMINATION

HISTORY

Persons exposed to ionizing radiations often present with a known history of exposure. The patient usually knows that he or she was exposed to a radiation-producing machine or a radioactive source. Thus the estimate of damage and need for treatment are likely to present more difficult problems than making the initial diagnosis or determining the nature of the insult.

There is always an exceptional case to disprove the rule. Here the presenting symptoms and course, rather than the history, must ultimately raise the question of radiation as a potential agent. Preliminary diagnoses of flu (nausea, vomiting), mumps (swollen parotid glands), skin ulcerations, burns, or bone mar-

row depression have been made when a history of radiation exposure was not immediately known or suspected.

ACUTE RADIATION SYNDROME

The acute exposure of the whole or a major portion of the body to a large amount (i.e., over 100 rad of x- or gamma rays) of penetrating radiation results in a progressive series of signs and symptoms known as the *acute radiation syndrome*. A summary of the principal characteristics of this syndrome after exposures of various magnitudes is shown in Table 73-1. Time relationships of the principal signs, symptoms, and hematologic changes are shown in Figure 73-1.

Initial symptoms of anorexia, nausea, vomiting, and fatigue occur within 2 to 6 hours after exposure. The severity of symptoms is variable, so that their intensity is not very meaningful. Absence of nausea and vomiting suggests exposure to a relatively low dose. The early presence of fever, diarrhea, delirium, or hypotension strongly suggests the possibility of exposure to a supralethal dose. Prodromal symptoms subside within a few hours to several days if supralethal doses are not involved. There follows a relatively symptom-

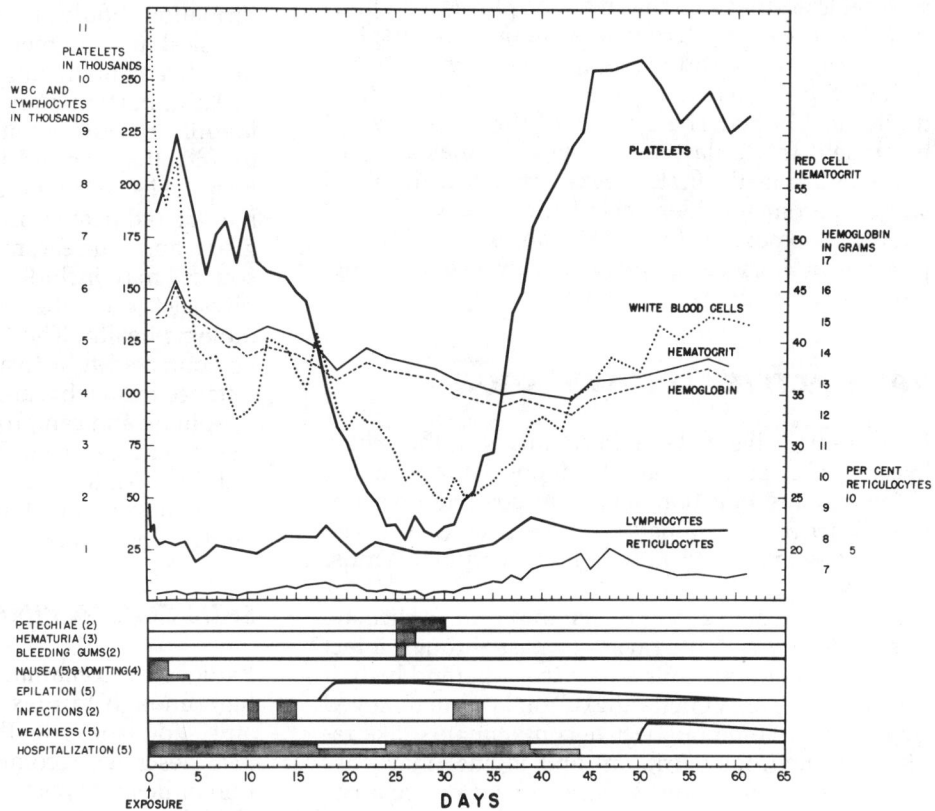

FIG. 73-1. Average hematologic values, clinical signs, and symptoms of five patients exposed to 236 to 365 rad in a criticality accident at the Y-12 plant in Oak Ridge, Tennessee, in June 1958. A fission "chain reaction" occurred when an enriched uranium solution inadvertently flowed into a large metal container, producing an unsafe geometry. All five exposed men recovered with supportive care. (From Andrews, G. A.: JAMA 179:191, 1962.)

free latent period for a week or more; shorter latent periods are present after higher exposures.

Skin erythema may appear within minutes to hours after a single large exposure, but it is not a reliable sign in evaluating the severity of exposure because of variations because of the energy (penetration power) of the radiation. If erythema is present from exposure to penetrating radiation, serious systemic injury is certain.

An early and important clinical indicator of damage is the response of the peripheral lymphocyte count. If there are 1200 or more lymphocytes per mm^3 at 48 to 72 hours after exposure, the likelihood of survival is excellent. Lesser counts at this time occur with more serious exposures; fewer than 500 lymphocytes per mm^3 at 48 hours suggests a poor prognosis. A fluctuating leukocytosis is usually present for the first few days after exposure.

LOCALIZED RADIATION SKIN BURNS

Radiation burns may occur in a localized area of skin as a result of direct contact with high-level radioactive source or exposure to an intense radiation beam. The possibility of a radiation burn may be recognized after exposure, but in the absence of such history, the presence of an area of burning pain without known cause is the presenting complaint. There may or may not be noticeable erythema in the area. The physical findings at the burn area are deceptively minor in the first few days compared with the possible future injury.

Radiation burns develop much more slowly than do thermal burns. The severity of the burn may not be evident for 10 days to 2 weeks. Erythema comes in waves during the first 2 weeks. Damage to the blood supply becomes evident about the third week, and after high exposures (over 3000 rad to the skin) may proceed to moist desquamation with ulceration, necrosis, and gangrene.

RADIOACTIVE CONTAMINATION

Loose radioactive material in contact with the skin is likely to cling and may also be deposited in wounds. If there is any question about the possible presence of radioactive contamination on the patient, a survey with beta-gamma and alpha survey instruments must be made.

Many radioactive contaminants are in particulate (insoluble) form, which will not pass through intact skin. They continue to irradiate the skin (and body if the radiations are penetrating) until they are removed by washing. Some radioactive contaminants, like radioactive hydrogen (tritium) and iodine, may pass through the intact skin. Wounds or burns are a potential source of entry into the body for all contaminants. Inhalation and ingestion of radioactive contaminants are common modes of exposure. All loose contamination may transfer to other people, clothing, or instruments on contact.

The most important initial action when radioactive contamination has occurred is simply to recognize its presence before the patient or attending medical personnel begin to move around the hospital and "track" the contamination to other parts of the building. Even if the levels are not harmful, such extension of the contamination makes the subsequent radiologic surveys and cleanup procedures unnecessarily difficult and expensive.

MANAGEMENT OF IONIZING RADIATION CASES

INITIAL CONSIDERATIONS

Evaluation of radiation injury requires an immediate assessment of the type of potential radiation exposure—external (whole-body, nonuniform, or local), radioactive skin contamination, internal emitters, and associated physical injuries. This information is gathered by history initially. If associated physical injuries are life-threatening, these should be treated first by conventional means. During these proceedings, information should also be gathered by both history and physical measurements to identify any significant radioactive contamination.

An important planned emergency procedure is to identify resources within the hospital and the community that can aid in radiologic assessments. The hospital list should include all individuals licensed to handle radioactive materials—pathologists, radiologists, and nuclear medical specialists. External resources may include local health physicists, medical physicists, or other specialists with training in radiologic health. The U.S. Department of Energy can be contacted to activate their regional radiologic assistance teams that are available for medical advice by telephone and can provide professional radiologic assistance at the scene if needed.

Table 73-2 lists important planning considerations for management of radioactively contaminated patients in hospitals.

SKIN CONTAMINATION

Radioactive contamination on the skin is usually not high enough to present a direct radiation hazard of any seriousness to the attending personnel. Table 73-3 describes recommended procedures for protection of hospital personnel and facilities in performing skin decontamination of a patient.

The patient cleanup is usually fairly simple: removal of contaminated clothing, showering (if patient is am-

TABLE 73-2. PLANNING CONSIDERATIONS FOR HOSPITAL MANAGEMENT OF THE RADIOACTIVELY CONTAMINATED PATIENT

1. Assemble hospital team of staff persons trained to manage contaminated radiation cases, including physicians, medical physicists, technicians, and nurses. Designate a team leader. Develop a list of consultants for advice—include physicians and health physicists experienced in handling such problems.
2. Use preselected area in hospital that is suitable for decontamination of patients—consider location of room in an area of the hospital having a nearby outside entry, showers, hot and cold water, floor drains, ease of room washdown, table suitable for washdown, and isolation of air movement through air-conditioning or heating system. Consider autopsy room, physiotherapy room, cast room, or regular emergency room as possible locations unless a special decontamination room is available.
3. Plan to evaluate the patient's medical condition immediately to determine priority of need for medical or surgical treatment, important diagnostic procedures, and decontamination procedures.
4. Plan to move patient within the hospital as little as possible so as to minimize hospital contamination. Keep patient in selected work area for medical and minor surgical treatment until loose contamination has been removed.
5. Arrange to have health physicist monitor area entrances and hallways after the patient is located in the room to prevent tracking to other hospital areas.
6. Be prepared to set up monitoring station(s) at exits from the work area. Personnel should not leave the room (area) unless monitored for radioactivity. Equipment or property should not be removed from the room unless monitored. Designate persons to perform these monitoring tasks at specific locations.
7. Prepare a list of decontamination room supplies and either store them in the room or identify where they are available for quick assembly.

National Council on Radiation Protection and Measurements: Management of Persons Accidentally Contaminated with Radionuclides, Report No. 65, Washington, D.C., 1980.

bulatory), or washing skin surfaces with detergent and water. After each washing, the skin is monitored with survey instruments to evaluate the progress. If washing does not remove contaminants satisfactorily in areas that are covered with hair, clipping or shaving may be helpful. Undiluted household bleach (5% sodium hypochlorite) can be used as a good decontamination solution if detergent and water do not do an adequate job. For use around the face or wounds, the bleach should first be diluted with five parts of water.

Skin wounds require special attention. Wash the contaminants away from the wound, if possible. Débridement or excision of the wound surfaces may be necessary if particles are embedded. If the contaminant is an alpha-emitting radioactive material, measurements should be made by experienced health physicists because alpha particles have such poor penetration power that they are masked by moisture, blood, or tissue. Special radiologic instrumentation may be necessary for proper evaluation in these cases.

TREATMENT OF RADIATION SKIN BURNS

No special therapy has been successful for local skin burns caused by ionizing radiation. These should be treated in a manner similar to that used for thermal burns, with bland ointments and protective dressings. In beta burns, as soon as the area can be delineated, surgical excision and full-thickness skin grafting are advisable because of the prolonged, painful nature of the burn and the poor healing of this type of lesion.

INITIAL MANAGEMENT OF ACUTE RADIATION INJURY

A difficult part of medical management of radiation exposure is the evaluation of the degree of exposure and the distribution of the dose throughout the body. During the first few days up to several weeks, diagnostic evaluation and preparation for later therapeutic measures are the main activities, unless the exposure has been excessively high (supralethal—1000 rad or more). In the latter case, a constellation of immediate symptoms including nausea, vomiting, diarrhea, and shock requires symptomatic, supportive, and palliative treatment during what will probably prove to be a relatively short course—perhaps 2 to 10 days. Treatment will generally require antiemetics, sedation, vasopressor agents, and fluids.

The mild-exposure case (less than about 125 rad whole-body exposure) requires evaluation to confirm the dose, but the patient generally requires only reassurance that no serious effects are anticipated and that treatment is not needed. If there is any concern that a higher dose might have occurred, the patient should be followed weekly on an outpatient basis for diagnostic hematologic changes during the first month after exposure. Chromosome analysis on peripheral lymphocytes can provide an important biologic assessment for doses above about 10 rad (x ray or gamma) and should be done as soon as possible after exposure. The study is best performed by a laboratory that has calibration studies available to relate the find-

---

TABLE 73-3. HOSPITAL DECONTAMINATION PROCEDURES FOR PROTECTION OF PERSONNEL AND FACILITIES

1. Personnel should wear surgical scrub suits, surgical caps and gowns, and rubber gloves (surgical, household, or industrial depending on duties).
2. The team leader should be trained to recognize the rare instance in which there may be a need for masks, respirators, or supplied airpacks because of the presence of high levels of alpha or beta radionuclides.
3. Rubber or plastic shoe covers are desirable. Those performing the actual decontamination with water should wear plastic or rubber laboratory aprons. Good temporary shoe covers for dry areas can be improvised from brown paper bags held on with adhesive or masking tape.
4. Air-conditioning and forced-air heating systems should be turned off so that radioactive particulates are not carried into ducts or to other rooms unless a special filter system has been designed for use under these conditions.
5. The floors should be protected with a disposable covering to reduce tracking by keeping cleaner surfaces and to aid the cleanup tasks. The covering should be changed when significant contamination is present. Brown paper rolls (36 inches wide, 60-pound weight) are ideal where water is not used. Plastic sheets are useful where spillage of liquids is a problem, although ribbed or nonskid types should be used to reduce the chance of slips and falls.
6. All contaminated clothing should be placed carefully into plastic or paper bags to reduce secondary contamination of area.
7. Avoid splashing solutions used in decontamination.
8. Patients and other potentially contaminated personnel may move to clean areas only after surveys show satisfactory decontamination.
9. All passage of persons and property between contaminated and clean areas must be surveyed and regulated by monitoring teams.
10. Supplies are passed through monitoring stations from clean areas to contaminated areas. Reverse flow must not occur unless supplies are monitored and found clean.
11. All individuals on the decontamination team must be trained in radiologic monitoring and decontamination techniques. Persons not working on the team should be excluded from the work area.
12. Fiberboard or steel drums with tight-fitting tops should be obtained for contaminated materials. Labels describing the contents should be affixed so that proper disposal can be carried out without reopening them. They may be sealed with masking tape or some other type of sealing tape.
13. Personal dosimeters (pocket chambers, film badge, or thermoluminescent dosimeters) should be supplied to all personnel working in the decontamination area. Personnel should be rotated after a dose of 5 rems (or less, if possible) is received.
14. The entry of all nonessential personnel including family, visitors, and administrative persons should be restricted.

National Council on Radiation Protection and Measurements: Management of Persons Accidentally Contaminated with Radionuclides, Report No. 65, Washington, D.C., 1980.

---

ings to a radiation dose. The individual can be advised that statistical increases in risk of late effects, such as cancer or leukemia, that have been identified in large population studies are relatively small incremental risks in any given individual case, but are believed to be proportional to the doses delivered to the various organs. On the other hand, it is prudent to advise men that initiation of birth control methods for several months is advisable to avoid any potential congenital defects in conceptions during this period. After several months, this potential risk is essentially returned to normal and further precautions are not needed.

Cases in the intermediate- to high-dose ranges (200 to 1000 rad whole-body doses) require close medical observation and probably active treatment during the period of peak bone marrow depression at about 20 to 30 days after exposure. The only initial treatment may be for symptomatic relief of nausea and vomiting. There is need for prompt planning for future thera-

peutic measures that may be required. The problem is simply one of keeping the patient alive for 5 or 6 weeks until bone marrow function begins to recover.

The therapeutic requirements fall into the following areas:

1. Control of infections—protection from exogenous infection by reverse isolation techniques or preferably "clean" room environments; sterilization of foods and personal items; bacterial monitoring by culture samples for potential endogenous sources of infection in the patient; use of antibiotics (especially prophylaxis against gastrointestinal tract bacilli), transfused leukocytes, and possibly immune globulin.
2. Control of bleeding—use of platelet transfusions or fresh whole blood and protection from trauma, and

3. Rest, psychologic support, and other supportive therapy as needed.

For immunosuppressed patients, it is recommended that all blood components be irradiated with 50 Gy (5000 rad) before transfusion.[2] This procedure diminishes immunogenicity and decreases prevalence of graft versus host disease later.

The above therapies are aimed at providing support with the expectation of recovery from the radiation-induced aplastic anemia. If this support fails, heroic efforts in suspected lethal exposures (900+ rads, whole body) might include the use of bone marrow transplantation, although its value is still uncertain and probably limited. Bone marrow transplants in 13 patients after the Chernobyl accident proved not to be useful.[3]

Fortunately, a period of a week or more is available to arrange for special consultation and advice on the necessary hospital services as well as time to move the patient to a hospital staffed to provide the necessary laboratory, bacteriologic, and hematologic services.

TREATMENT FOR INTERNAL CONTAMINATION

The treatment for internal assimilation of radioactive material is aimed at reducing the absorbed radiation dose and hence the risk of possible future biologic effects. Two general processes are used: (1) reduction of absorption and internal deposition, and (2) enhanced elimination or excretion of absorbed radionuclides. Both are most effective when begun at the earliest possible time after exposure.

The decision to treat internal contamination must be made early when limited information is available. There are usually no signs or symptoms from the exposure except those associated with physical injuries. The health physicist or radiation monitor may have information on the general level of contamination at the accident site. Measurements of activity on nasal swipes may be helpful if taken within a few minutes of the accident and before washing the face or showering. Nasal swipes are used primarily for alpha emitters, such as the transuranic elements (plutonium, americium, etc.). They cannot be expected to yield valid information by the time the patient is transported to the hospital. For some radionuclides, such as iodine, tritium, or cesium, intake may be estimated by the initial excretion in the urine samples. Whole-body counts in the first day or two are usually difficult to interpret because of the presence of skin contamination in these accidents. These counters are so sensitive that residual skin contamination that appears low or absent to conventional field survey instruments can still be misleading for assessing internal radionuclide deposition.

The decision to treat is most likely to be based on a qualitative judgment as to whether an exposure is high or low. Few internal exposures (except for medical misadministrations) have been high enough to cause acute effects. The decision to treat usually involves concerns about an increased risk of a late health effect, such as cancer.

Fortunately, most of the recommended therapies result in little or no risk to the patient. If a significant reduction in radiation dose is thought to be possible from treatment, it is probably best to proceed with treatment. The recommended treatments can reduce the dose by factors of about 2 to 10, certainly a worthwhile goal.

Preventive treatment to reduce absorption may include removal of gastric contents if the material was ingested. Fast-acting purgatives may be valuable in reducing the residence time of radioactive materials in the colon. Gastrointestinal absorption may be reduced for certain radionuclides by use of appropriate agents: 100 mL of an aluminum-containing antacid (aluminum phosphate gel is preferred) reduces uptake of strontium; magnesium sulfate or barium sulfate is useful for radium and strontium; 1 g three times daily of Prussian blue (potassium ferric ferrocyanide, which is not FDA-approved, but has been used safely for humans) is effective for cesium, thallium, and rubidium.

Blocking and diluting agents enhance elimination rates of certain radionuclides or reduce the quantity of radionuclide incorporated in tissue. The most important of these is the use of stable iodide (six drops of saturated solution of potassium iodide in a glass of water; or 300 mg of potassium iodide, crush tablet if enteric-coated) to block radioactive iodine uptake in the thyroid. Forcing fluids to 3000 to 4000 mL per day increases excretion of radioactive hydrogen (tritium).

The excretion of some radionuclides can be enhanced by use of a chelating agent that binds the nuclide in a soluble complex. Excretion occurs by way of urine and feces. The most useful drug for radionuclides is diethylenetriaminepenta-acetic acid* as either the zinc salt (ZnDTPA) or the calcium salt (CaDTPA). A typical daily treatment regimen is to give 1 g of DTPA intravenously in 250 mL of isotonic saline or 5% glucose. The drug is packaged in 4 mL vials containing 1 g of DTPA. It has also been given safely by injecting the 4 mL intravenously over a 5-minute period. Inhalation of 1 g of DTPA over a 15- to 30-minute period by means of a nebulizer is another convenient method of administration. Do not give more than one treatment per day. DTPA effectively chelates the transuranium metals (plutonium, americium, cu-

---

* Physicians needing this drug should contact the REAC/TS Center, Oak Ridge Tennessee (See National Contacts Section) for the drug protocol and permission to obtain the drug.

rium, and californium), the rare earths (such as cesium, yttrium, lanthanum, promethium, and scandium), and some transition metals (such as zirconium and niobium). Clinical use has been primarily for treatment of plutonium and americium.

There have been no serious side effects of this drug with normal clinical doses. Experiments in dogs have shown that divided doses (5 times per day) can produce serious gastrointestinal effects and possible death. Kidney irritation is recognized as a potential hazard, so routine clinical urinalysis is recommended before each administration. The ZnDTPA is preferred over the CaDTPA for women who may be pregnant.

DTPA is an investigational new drug and is not available through commercial sources. If it is not immediately available, the calcium salt of ethylenediaminetetra-acetic acid (CaEDTA, calcium disodium edetate, Versenate) may be used, but it is much less effective.

After inhalation of "insoluble" radioactive particulates, chelation therapy is not useful. Because solubility is usually not known, a clinical trial of chelation is usually warranted. Multiple lavages of the bronchopulmonary tree have been successful in removing 25 to 50% of inhaled insoluble radioactive particulates in dogs if treatment is initiated within the first week. This technique should be used only after careful consideration of the long-term risk of the exposure hazard against the immediate risk of procedures requiring general anesthesia. It must be performed by a team of specialists experienced in bronchopulmonary lavage.

PITFALLS

Written plans for decontamination of patients (such as Table 73-3) must be exercised periodically to be executed effectively. Because these procedures are not used frequently, the necessary training and knowledge of the staff will be found lacking unless such exercises are conducted.

Radiation accidents have proven of particular interest to the news media. An administrative arrangement must be made by the hospital to have some trained person(s) designated to be the public information officer.

Patients with combined injuries, i.e., serious burns or other trauma plus significant radiation exposures, have a much worse prognosis than would be expected from an assessment of the several injuries individually.[4] Animal studies indicate that infection control and antimicrobial therapy are particularly important in managing combined injuries. Débridement of all wounds must be meticulous, with the excision of all devitalized tissue to prevent any nidus for infection.

Do not underestimate the value of clinical assessment in acute radiation exposure cases. Accidental radiation doses are usually distributed unequally to different parts of the body. The position of the body relative to the source plus shielding factors, including shielding of interposed tissues of the body, results in nonuniform dose distribution to various tissues. After high, even potentially lethal doses, some areas of bone marrow receive relatively lower doses. It is from such areas that one hopes to see eventual recovery of the bone marrow. Measurements by personnel dosimeters do not take such differences into account. They can only estimate the dose at the location of the detector. Dosimetry mock-up studies of the accident can be helpful, but these may take a number of days to complete. In serious acute exposures, clinical evaluation of the patient certainly adds useful and important information to both dose assessment and biologic injury.

HORIZONS

Significant advances in the treatment of radiation injuries are unlikely in the forseeable future. Protective drugs or therapeutic agents that will change treatment importantly are not likely to appear. Exposure prevention must continue to be the major goal.

The clinical experience gained from the use of several thousands of bone marrow transplantations in cancer therapy provides technology that may yet prove useful for future treatment of near lethal accidental radiation exposures. The Chernobyl experience suggests that only HLA-identical transplantations should be performed and only when the whole body exposure exceeds 900 rads.[3] Transplantation at lesser doses may reduce the spontaneous recovery of the patient's viable marrow cells.

Colony stimulating factors (CSF) may be useful in stimulating myelopoiesis during recovery from radiation injury to the bone marrow. These factors include granulocyte-monocyte CSF (GM-CSF), granulocyte-CSF, and macrophage-CSF. Further investigation is needed into this use of CSF.

The clinical experience gained from the use of several thousands of bone marrow transplantations in cancer therapy provides technology that may yet prove useful for future treatment of near lethal accidental radiation exposures. The Chernobyl experience suggests that only HLA-identical transplantations should be performed and only when the whole body exposure exceeds 900 rads.[2] Transplantation at lesser doses may reduce the spontaneous recovery of the patient's viable marrow cells.

Colony stimulating factors (CSF) may be useful in stimulating myelopoiesis during recovery from radiation injury to the bone marrow. These factors include granulocyte-monocyte CSF (GM-CSF), granulocyte-CSF, and macrophage-CSF. Further investigation is needed into the use of CSF.

NATIONAL CONTACTS

Radiation Emergency Assistance Center/Training Site (REAC/TS), Oak Ridge Associated Universities,

Oak Ridge, TN 615-576-3131 (Office) 615-481-1000
Beeper 241 (24 hour)

Radiation Emergency Management Services (REMS) Corporation (F.A. Mettler, M.D.), 3004 La Mancha St., Albuquerque, NM 87104 505-243-0236

Radiation Management Consultants (R.E. Linnemann, M.D.) 5301 Tacony St., Box D5, Philadelphia, PA 19137 215-537-0672 (Office) 215-243-2990 (24 hour)

University of Pittsburgh (Niel Wald, M.D.), Dept. of Radiation Health, Graduate School of Public Health, Pittsburgh, PA 15261 412-624-2732

The E.L. Saenger Radiation Laboratory (E.L. Saenger, M.D.), University of Cincinnati Medical Center, Cincinnati, OH 45267 513-558-4282

REFERENCES

1. Lushbaugh, C.C., Fry, S.A., Sipe, A., and Ricks, R.C.: An historical perspective of human involvement in radiation accidents. *In* Radiation Protection Today—The NCRP at Sixty Years. Proceedings of the 25th Annual Meeting, April 5–6, 1989. Bethesda, National Council on Radiation Protection and Measurements, 1990.
2. Drum, D.E., and Rappeport, J.M.: Treatment of whole-body radiation accident victims. *In* Medical Management of Radiation Accidents. Edited by Mettler, F.A., Jr., Kelsey, C.A., and Ricks, R.C., Boca Raton, CRC Press, Inc., 1990, pp. 89–108.
3. Baranov, A.E.: Transplantation of bone marrow in victims of the Chernobyl accident. *In* Medical Aspects of the Chernobyl Accident. Report IAEA-TECDOC-516. Vienna, International Atomic Energy Agency, 1989.
4. Conklin, J.J., Walker, R.I., and Hirsch, E.F.: Current concepts in the management of radiation injuries and associated trauma. Surg. Gynecol. & Obstet. *156*:809, 1983.

BIBLIOGRAPHY

American Medical Association: A Guide to the Hospital Management of Injuries Arising from Exposure or to Involving Ionizing Radiation. Chicago, A.M.A., 1984.

Hubner, K.F., and Fry, S.A. (eds.): The Medical Basis for Radiation Accident Preparedness, North Holland, Elsevier, 1980.

Leonard, R., and Ricks, R.: Emergency department radiation accident protocol. Ann. Emerg. Med. *9*:462, 1989.

Mettler, F.A., Jr., Kelsey, C.A., and Ricks, R.C.: Medical Management of Radiation Accidents, Boca Raton, CRC Press, Inc., 1990.

National Council on Radiation Protection and Measurements: Management of Persons Accidentally Contaminated With Radionuclides, Report No. 65. Washington, D.C., 1980.

Pons, P., and Sullivan, J.B.: Radiation land radioactive emergencies. *In* Hazardous Material Toxicology. Edited by Sullivan, J.B., and Krieger, G.R. Baltimore, Williams and Wilkins, 1992, p. 441.*

Ricks, R.C.: Hospital Emergency Department Management of Radiation Accidents. Report ORAU-224. Oak Ridge, Oak Ridge Associated Universities, 1984.

Schleien, B.: Preparedness and Response in Radiation Accidents. Food and Drug Administration, National Center for Devices and Radiological Health. Washington, D.C., U.S. Government Printing Office, 1983.

Voelz, G.L.: Ionizing radiation. Chapter 26 in Occupational Medicine: Principles and Practical Application. Edited by C. Zenz. Chicago, Year Book Medical Publishers, Inc., 1988, pp. 426–462.

* Useful table on half-lives and suggested ED equipment.

Chapter 74

SMOKE INHALATION AND OTHER INHALATION INJURIES

SMOKE INHALATION

Dennis P. Price, Harvey Silverman, and George R. Schwartz

CAPSULE

Smoke inhalation is responsible for significant morbidity and mortality. The cause of smoke inhalation injuries, including carbon monoxide poisoning, and patient evaluation, diagnosis, and treatment are reviewed.

The two main causes of lung injury from acute smoke inhalation are direct thermal injuries and the inhalation of toxic gases and particulate matter. The frequent lag period between inhalation and symptom formation makes diagnosis difficult and emphasizes the need for follow-up and sequential testing.

INTRODUCTION

The problem of smoke inhalation (smoke poisoning, pulmonary burn, respiratory burn) has been generally recognized within the past two decades, but knowledge in this area is far from complete.

Reports in the 1960s by Phillips,[1,2] Stone,[3] and others pointed out that respiratory injury is a principal cause of mortality in patients with body surface burns. Moreover, respiratory injury can occur without body surface burns. Zikria and co-workers[4,5] reviewed the autopsies in deaths from fires in New York City over a 2-year period and did not find a consistent association of pulmonary pathology with the presence or absence of surface burns.

Smoke inhalation is a significant problem, both in incidence and in morbidity and mortality. For example, on November 21, 1980, 84 persons lost their lives at the MGM Grand Hotel fire in Las Vegas, Ne-

vada. Eighty persons died as a result of smoke inhalation at the scene of the fire. An additional 600 patients were seen at area hospitals for respiratory complaints. It is usually the emergency physician who is called upon to diagnose and to initiate treatment of the victim.

CAUSES

The precise causative factors of smoke inhalation are not known; however, several known factors are involved in producing inhalation injury. The two main causes of lung injury from acute smoke inhalation are: (1) thermal injuries and (2) the inhalation of toxic gases and particulate matter. They are described as follows.

HEAT AND HUMIDITY

In 1945, noting the uncertainty of the relative roles of thermal and chemical factors, Moritz and colleagues[6] published the results of investigations to determine the pathologic characteristics of uncomplicated thermal injury of the lungs and air passages and of the temperatures that are necessary for their production. Using, in dogs, an insulated transoral cannula that extended from outside the mouth to below the vocal folds of the larynx, the experimenters were surprised to find that dry air heated to 500°C was cooled to no more than 50°C by the time it reached the tracheal bifurcation, and no injury was noted, either of the lower trachea or more distally. It was necessary to force the inhalation of steam to produce significant pulmonary injury. The importance of this experiment was in showing that the upper airway is efficient in cooling inspired air and that the energy content of hot dry air is not sufficient to produce lower respiratory damage. Thermal burn of the respiratory tract is generally confined to the upper airway, where it may occasionally cause sufficient edema to obstruct the airway.

In 1967, Stone[3] reported the effects of various temperatures and humidities on the survival of experimental rats. Placing rats in drying ovens at various temperatures and standard humidity, they found that mortality for a given time of exposure increased with increased temperature. Keeping the temperature constant with varying humidity, it was found that increased humidity was associated with increased mortality for a given time of exposure.

SMOKE

Smoke is generally considered to be a combination of particulate matter, volatilized products of combustion, and various gases. Smoke particles consist principally of carbon, which may be coated with the condensed products of combustion. The particles vary in size, but many are less than 1 micron and are small enough to be inhaled deeply into the lungs.

In Stone's study,[3] the presence of cotton smoke significantly increased mortality and appeared to be a more important factor than humidity. Zikria and associates[4,5] compared the effects of wood smoke and kerosene smoke on dogs. Wood smoke produced significant pulmonary pathology and mortality, but kerosene smoke did not. Analysis of the two types of smoke revealed that wood smoke contained 10 times the quantity of carbon monoxide and 20 times the quantity of aldehyde gases. Cotton smoke also was shown to contain large quantities of aldehydes. Wood and cotton, as furniture, mattresses, and clothing, are usually burned in house fires. Newer synthetics can release hydrogen cyanide gas when burned, as well as gases that cause intense respiratory tract irritation.

Although aldehydes cause damage in laboratory conditions, other irritants such as acid anhydrides may be more significant under clinical conditions, because aldehydes tend to condense out of smoke before they are inhaled, whereas the acid anhydrides enter the lungs more readily. Other substances, such as oxides of nitrogen and sulfur, or the products of combustion of plastics, can also produce respiratory irritation.

Toxic substances (e.g., industrial solvents and insecticides) may be released from storage units damaged during fire and thus contribute to the clinical problem.

More recently, animal models have been developed that more closely mimic the disease encountered clinically. Welch[7] found that goats exposed to nitrogen tetroxide showed significant pulmonary dysfunction, as manifested by delayed clearance of inhaled [133]xenon isotope. Walker[8] showed the nonlethal injury in goats exposed to burning cotton towel waste to be a necrotic tracheobronchitis and bronchiolitis with pseudomembrane and respiratory epithelium cast formation.

Smoke inhalation is becoming an increasing problem that is related to increased use of synthetic materials in building products and furnishings. For instance, polyvinyl chloride, frequently implicated in smoke toxicity, is a plastic polymer used extensively in home and office in the production of electrical wire, telephone and cable coverings, and furnishings. It liberates large amounts of hydrogen chloride and carbon monoxide as well as phosgene gas. In addition, the fire retardants used on these combustible synthetic materials may also contribute to their toxicity.

Hydrogen cyanide generated during the combustion of products such as orlon, nylon, wool, acrylic fibers, polyurethane, and ureaformaldehyde may contribute to smoke toxicity.

Sublethal concentrations of hydrogen cyanide may by themselves or with various other factors such as low ambient oxygen concentration or carbon monoxide intoxication contribute to fire mortality.

SOOT

In Zikria's study,[5] kerosene soot and wood soot were blown into the distal trachea by bronchoscopy, and neither produced mortality nor significant pathology. Particulate matter, in and of itself, is probably not significant in the etiology of the clinical problem.

CARBON MONOXIDE

The role of carbon monoxide (CO) poisoning in the clinical spectrum of smoke inhalation has often been emphasized. In Zikria's review of autopsy results,[4] he noted that carbon monoxide levels greater than 50% were found in 24% of patients dying within the first 12 hours, making carbon monoxide poisoning the probable primary cause of death. Furthermore, another 34% had carbon monoxide levels between 11 and 49%. Carbon monoxide poisoning was found in 39% of those dying within the first 12 hours who did not have a body surface burn. Birky[9] found a lethal concentration of carbon monoxide in 60 percent of 530 deaths from fires.

Zarem and co-workers[10] reported on 13 patients who presented to the emergency department (ED) with smoke inhalation and had carbon monoxide levels from 8 to 40%. In retrospect, he was able to attribute some of the symptomatology to the carbon monoxide poisoning that had not been diagnosed on clinical grounds.

The ubiquitous nature of carbon monoxide makes it of great concern to the emergency physician because it can be lethal if the inspired air contains as little as 0.1 volume %. Carbon monoxide is tasteless, odorless, and nonirritating to the mucous membranes, so it can be inhaled without the victim's awareness. It is present in automobile exhaust, coal gas, water gas, exhaust from heat stoves and furnaces with inadequate ventilation, smoke from burning buildings, and coal mine fires.

There is sometimes a poor correlation between the carboxyhemoglobin level and clinical signs and symptoms. Part of this results from a combination of cyanide (from burning of nitrogen-containing compounds) poisoning with carbon monoxide toxicity. Also, a short exposure to high levels of carbon monoxide can produce a high carboxyhemoglobin level, but little acidosis or metabolic complications. On the other hand, chronic exposure to low carbon monoxide levels can have serious metabolic consequences with a lower carboxyhemoglobin level. The earliest symptoms of carbon monoxide poisoning are slight headache with muscular weakness, palpitations, dizziness, and mental confusion. Excitement and bizarre behavior may follow. These symptoms progress to coma when the carboxyhemoglobin level exceeds 40%. Level of consciousness, i.e., mental status, is the most important sign of severity of carbon monoxide poisoning. Effective initial treatment involves rapid maintenance of the airway and respiratory state and treatment of metabolic consequences (bicarbonate deficit with acidosis, possible hypokalemia). Administration of 100% oxygen (through intubation tube or tightly sealed nonrebreather face mask) is important. *A hyperbaric oxygen chamber is the most effective means of supplying oxygen to a victim of carbon monoxide poisoning* and should be used in severe cases when available after consultation with the hyperbaric unit medical director. The high oxygen pressures markedly shorten carboxyhemoglobin half-life and also reduce intracranial pressure and cerebral edema. Long-term aftereffects of severe CO poisoning are common—particularly neurologic and evidence of central nervous system (CNS) dysfunction. Rapid, effective treatment can reduce the delayed effects. When cyanide poisoning is also suspected, treatment is essentially the same, with the addition of amyl nitrate initially.

Carbon monoxide itself is not considered a pulmonary irritant, and clinical problems result from preferential combination with hemoglobin, producing carboxyhemoglobin, which cannot carry oxygen to the tissues. Carboxyhemoglobin levels greater than 50% usually are lethal, and levels above 10% are considered significant. Carbon monoxide combines with hemoglobin more than 200 times as readily as does oxygen. Besides decreasing the oxygen-carrying capacity of the blood by virtue of decreasing the amount of hemoglobin available to combine with oxygen, carboxyhemoglobin decreases the delivery of oxygen to tissues because of an effect wherein the dissociation of oxygen from hemoglobin is impaired.

HYPOXIA

Hypoxia is an important contributing factor to the syndrome of smoke inhalation. This appears to be the result of a low oxygen content in the environment secondary to oxygen consumption by the fire, as well as of the presence of carbon monoxide.

In summary, smoke inhalation is a highly lethal clinical condition resulting from irritating products of combustion, carbon monoxide poisoning, cyanide poisoning, and concomitant hypoxia and asphyxiation.

The manifestations of the syndrome of smoke inhalation range from a mild, short-lived cough to fulminant death within minutes. These manifestations are difficult to predict because of the many fire factors involved with its cause. Also, pre-existing disease and other injuries sustained in the fire, especially body surface burn, may alter the course of the disease. Particular factors in the history, findings, and laboratory investigations dictate appropriate therapy.

CLASSIFICATION

The inhalation injury may be classified on either *anatomic* or *temporal* grounds.

ANATOMIC GROUNDS

Anatomically, the injury may be classified as affecting the upper airway (primarily inflammation and edema of the larynx and trachea) or as affecting areas more distal (primarily inflammation, edema, profuse secretions and debris of the lower airways, and disruption of the alveolar capillary membrane).

TEMPORAL GROUNDS

Smoke inhalation injuries are more often classified on temporal grounds that conform to fairly distinct *clinical stages*. The classification most commonly referred to is that proposed by Stone,[3] consisting of three clinical stages, of which patients exhibit one or more to varying degrees:

Stage 1: Pulmonary or Respiratory Insufficiency. This stage generally occurs within the first 24 hours and is manifested by respiratory distress, often appearing as though it were caused by upper airway obstruction. An early symptom is pain on deep inspiration. True airway obstruction (from edema of glottic or supraglottic structures) usually develops in the first 6 hours. The early stages are often associated with a tracheobronchitis.

Stage 2: Pulmonary Edema. This occurs generally 8 to 36 hours after injury and may be of insidious or acute onset. In addition to being associated with the inhalation injury itself, it also may be related to cardiac disease, tracheostomy, overhydration, or a combination of these factors.

Stage 3: Bacterial Pneumonia. This occurs as early as 2 days after injury or as late as 2 weeks or more afterward. The earlier it occurs, the worse the prognosis. All patients with significant inhalation injury have a bacterial pneumonia to some degree. The recognition that fairly distinct temporal stages occur is of importance to the emergency physician, in that it emphasizes that the patient who initially appears well may develop significant symptomatology. Clinical findings must be correlated with time elapsed since the inhalation.

EVALUATION OF THE PATIENT

HISTORY

An attempt should be made to obtain information concerning the circumstances of the injury. It is important to know the location of the patient, the duration of exposure, the presence of toxic materials, and whether or not loss of consciousness took place.

The patient in an enclosed area is much more likely to suffer clinically significant smoke inhalation. Duration of exposure is of obvious importance, and many patients with brief exposure hold their breath while escaping, thus avoiding lower respiratory injury. Patients found unconscious, however, may have lower tract injury. Fires involving toxic substances should alert the emergency physician. Loss of consciousness may be caused by anoxia or carbon monoxide toxicity, or by an anesthetic effect of the substance inhaled.

The physician should also seek evidence of other conditions that might have contributed to exposure, such as head injury, alcohol or drug use, or myocardial infarction. If possible, a brief medical history should be obtained with special emphasis on pre-existent cardiac or pulmonary disease.

Inquiry should be made as to whether the patient took measures to protect the respiratory tract. The three survivors of the well-studied Coconut Grove nightclub fire in Boston in 1942 who did not sustain respiratory injury covered their mouths with wet cloths. This fire focused attention on the problem of smoke inhalation. The Massachusetts General Hospital received 114 casualties within a few hours. Within a few minutes of reaching the facility, 75 had died of "uncontrollable anoxia." Of the remaining 39 patients, 36 developed respiratory symptoms and seven died as a result of pulmonary complications.

SIGNS AND SYMPTOMS

The signs and symptoms in the victim of smoke inhalation who presents to the ED are variable, depending on the nature of the substance inhaled as well as the contribution of hypoxia and carbon monoxide poisoning to the clinical picture. It is worthwhile to repeat that the initial absence of signs and symptoms does not rule out significant pulmonary damage.

Those patients with signs and symptoms may complain of sore throat, hoarseness, dyspnea, or dysphagia. Frequently there is cough, which may produce carbonaceous sputum that may be blood-tinged. Secretions may be profuse. The patient may complain of headache or dizziness, may be restless and exhibit confused or irrational behavior, or may be comatose. There may be stridorous respirations, nasal flaring, a brassy cough, tachycardia, tachypnea, and suprasternal and intercostal retractions appearing similar to a croup-like state. The patient may be cyanotic or have the "cherry-red" appearance of carbon monoxide poisoning. In most published clinical studies, however, this cherry-red appearance has not been noted or has been overlooked in patients with documented carbon monoxide poisoning. Convulsions may occur.

Patients also may complain of nausea and may vomit, perhaps on the basis of swallowed particulate smoke originally deposited on the oral and nasal mucosa. Gastric dilation may occur.

The presence of facial burns, particularly about the mouth and nose—especially second- or third-degree burns—is often associated with smoke inhalation.

Erythema, or blistering of the nasal and oral mucosa, is associated with an increased incidence of respiratory injury. The presence of singed nasal hairs is also accepted as being associated with a greater likelihood of smoke inhalation injury.

Auscultation of the chest may initially be normal; it may reveal diminished breath sounds; or it may reveal rales, rhonchi, or wheezes. The presence of the latter, on admission, is a poor prognostic sign.

LABORATORY DATA

Arterial blood gases and carboxyhemoglobin levels are the most important laboratory determinations and should be obtained in all patients in whom the diagnosis of smoke inhalation is made or suspected.

The results of arterial blood gas studies are variable, but most often they reveal initially a normal or decreased pO_2, a slight decrease in pCO_2, and a near-normal pH. The findings of normal blood gases do not rule out the possibility of future deterioration, consistent with the previously noted latent period seen in many patients. Abnormal blood gases, decreased pO_2 being the most common, indicate the need for admission and treatment. An elevated pCO_2 usually indicates a more severe injury and a poorer prognosis. The arterial pH may be so low that the administration of bicarbonate will be considered.

Arterial blood gas studies should be obtained to provide baseline values and a guide for initial treatment, and frequent serial determinations are mandatory in management. Carboxyhemoglobin levels should be obtained. This is of major importance in initial diagnosis and therapy. The reported pO_2 may well be normal in the face of markedly elevated carboxyhemoglobin levels.

Other laboratory data, although usually less helpful in the early period, should be obtained: i.e., a complete blood count, serum electrolytes, blood urea nitrogen, and glucose. Elevated serum uric acid levels, the cause and significance of which are unclear, have been reported in smoke inhalation patients.

Although early sputum cultures have not been particularly reliable in predicting the pathogens in the pulmonary infections that often follow, one should be obtained initially, particularly if the patient has a productive cough.

OTHER INVESTIGATIONS

Although chest x-ray films usually do not show acute changes at first and therefore are not helpful in initial diagnosis and treatment, they should be obtained as a baseline study. A lateral neck film may be useful in helping to assess airway edema.

Myocardial infarction is not an uncommon complication of smoke inhalation, and all adult patients should have an electrocardiogram.

Laryngoscopy may be of great help in the early period. The finding of an acutely inflamed larynx in a patient with an uncertain diagnosis would be significant. Repeated laryngoscopy to follow the progress of laryngeal edema may indicate the need for tracheal intubation while it can still be done electively.

Although many patients have symptoms that appear to be caused by acute upper airway obstruction, the cause is most often tracheobronchitis. These patients, without true upper airway obstruction, do not benefit from, and may even deteriorate following, tracheostomy. Laryngoscopy, including transnasal fiberoptic laryngoscopy, can indicate which patients have upper airway obstruction and therefore might benefit from tracheal intubation or, perhaps, tracheostomy. In addition, laryngoscopy, being a fairly rapid procedure, may be useful in triage when mass smoke inhalation casualties are involved, indicating which patients are more likely to suffer acute deterioration.

Bronchoscopy may be performed, but it is more often a therapeutic procedure performed during the hospital course to remove crusts and debris. Emergency endoscopy may aid in diagnosis, but is rarely necessary.

Other diagnostic measures have been used to some extent, but are of questionable usefulness to the emergency physician at present. Spirometry, done acutely, has shown decreases in vital capacity, forced expiratory volume delivered in 1 second, and maximum breathing capacity. Measurements made on the second or third day have shown decreased pulmonary compliance, increased respiratory resistance, and increased work of breathing. Pulmonary scans (with ^{133}xenon) may show abnormalities as well.

Preliminary work with pulmonary cytology has shown a correlation between certain cytologic changes and subsequent clinical diagnosis.

DIAGNOSIS

The diagnosis of smoke inhalation, in any event a matter of controversy, may be difficult at first except in obvious cases. The emergency physician must maintain a high index of suspicion in view of the well documented latent period; if he or she seriously considers this diagnosis but is still uncertain after a few hours, the patient should probably be admitted for observation for 48 hours.

Stone has made the definite diagnosis of smoke inhalation on the basis of the presence of three factors:[3] (1) facial burns; (2) mucosal burns or singed nasal hairs; and (3) a history of burns having been suffered in a closed space. He considered the diagnosis probable if two of these criteria are met.

SIGNS AND SYMPTOMS

The diagnosis also should be made if wheezes, rales, or rhonchi are present, if the patient is in respiratory distress, or if there is a history of unconsciousness not attributable to other causes. Patients with abnormal arterial blood gases with no other apparent explanation, or those with mental status changes, require admission and treatment. Patients with elevated carboxyhemoglobin levels (above 15%) should be admitted even if there are no other signs and symptoms. Patients with initial levels of 50% or higher will probably sustain pulmonary damage from smoke inhalation. There is a direct correlation between carboxyhemoglobin levels and length of hospitalization.

The presence of significant cough, particularly if productive of copious secretions or carbonaceous material, dysphagia, hoarseness, or changes on chest x-ray films, should indicate admission with the presumptive diagnosis of smoke inhalation.

Reliable patients presenting with minimal symptoms of smoke inhalation (e.g., mild cough), absence of positive findings, and a questionable history of significant exposure can be observed for a few hours and discharged if there have been no increase in symptoms or changes in findings. All patients not admitted must be clearly warned of the possibility of development of symptoms and strongly advised to return in that event. A baseline chest x ray should be taken.

Table 74-1 indicates patient factors that increase risk of having sustained smoke inhalation.

TABLE 74-1. PATIENT FACTORS SUGGESTIVE OF SMOKE INHALATION

Historical Factors
Injury sustained in a closed space
Inhalation of noxious gases
Loss of consciousness

Physical Findings
Abnormal vital signs otherwise unexplained
Abnormal mental status otherwise unexplained
Wheezing, rales, rhonchi
Burns about head and neck
Erythema, blisters, soot in oropharynx
Carbonaceous sputum
Hoarseness or stridor

Laboratory Findings
Elevated carbon monoxide level
Hypoxia
Abnormal chest film with infiltrates or atelectasis
Abnormal electrocardiogram

DIAGNOSIS AND EVALUATION OF FIREFIGHTERS

Firefighters are sometimes patients in the ED, and their evaluation deserves special mention. They often present with a history of chronic production of carbonaceous sputum, so that its presence is not as significant as in the civilian patient.

Studies have shown that significant concentrations of carbon monoxide may still be present after a fire has been extinguished, or they may be present at fires that produce little visible smoke. Firefighters in those circumstances may remove or fail to wear protective masks and suffer subclinical carbon monoxide poisoning. Repeat exposure at another fire shortly thereafter may produce a cumulative effect, evident in mental confusion or poor judgment.

Finally, firefighters working in heavy protective garments in the heat produced by the fire may become dehydrated, and this should be borne in mind if a firefighter has collapsed at a fire. Firefighters are also exposed to myriad chemical fumes from products used in the home, including cyanide.[3a,3b]

TREATMENT

Because there are multiple variables, including density and composition of smoke, length of exposure, severity and clinical stage of injury, presence or absence of body surface burns, even certainty of diagnosis, and because animal models have been difficult to design, the treatment of smoke inhalation is controversial in many respects.

Steam insufflation has been used in rats and dogs to study some types of therapy, on the basis that there is a pathologic similarity with the clinical smoke inhalation injury. In the rat model, therapy with 40% *oxygen* and high humidity decreased mortality and pulmonary sepsis. Treatment should be individualized, and recognition of the clinical stage is helpful.

Initial therapy in the ED after initial assessment (ABCs) should be the administration of *high humidity* and *oxygen.* Adequate humidity cannot be achieved with the nasal oxygen apparatus and requires more advanced equipment, such as a heated *nebulizer* or *croup tent.* Arterial blood gas studies help to determine the proper oxygen concentration, keeping in mind the possibility of a normal pO_2 with carbon monoxide poisoning. This therapy alone may be sufficient for patients with mild or moderate distress. Patients in severe distress (e.g., with stridor, depressed mentation, and loss of gag reflex) require *intubation* and *oxygen* administration as an initial measure.

Carbon monoxide poisoning requires treatment with *100% oxygen*, which cannot be achieved with nasal or simple face mask apparatus. The half-life of carbon monoxide in the patient breathing room air is more than 4 hours, whereas it is less than 1 hour in a patient breathing 100% oxygen. If available, *hyperbaric oxygen* therapy is the treatment of choice.

BRONCHODILATORS

Should oxygen and humidity not be sufficient for the smoke inhalation patient, further treatment is indicated. Bronchodilators by means of aerosol and intravenous aminophylline may be given, but are often unsuccessful.

CORTICOSTEROIDS

The indications for, and dosage and duration of, therapy with steroids are controversial. Patients with respiratory distress who have not responded adequately to oxygen and humidity should be given a large intravenous dose of steroids over 1 to 5 minutes. The dose should be no less than 1 g of hydrocortisone or an equivalent drug, and larger doses have been recommended by some clinicians, with a repeat dose in 8 to 12 hours if needed. This therapy is particularly effective for wheezes that have not responded to these measures. Maintenance steroids should not be given routinely without clinical indications because they have been shown to be associated with virulent pulmonary infections. Steroids have been given in the hope of preventing or lessening the pulmonary edema phase, but there is no proof that they are effective. Asymptomatic patients should not be given ''prophylactic'' steroids.

OTHER MEASURES

Good pulmonary toilet is mandatory, with encouragement of deep coughing and proper suctioning as needed. Prophylactic antibiotics should not be given because not only have they been shown to be of no value, but also they are associated with pulmonary infections from resistant organisms. There is no evidence that detergents and proteolytic enzymes are of value. It is usually recommended that analgesia and sedation be used cautiously to avoid respiratory depression, although opiates can be reversed readily with naloxone. A nasogastric tube may be needed for decompression, and antacids may be given for gastric upset and perhaps to help prevent stress ulcers. Reports of elevated histamine levels have led to recommendations that antihistamines be given. As noted previously, bronchoscopy may be helpful in removing crusts and debris, but usually is not done acutely. Intermittent positive pressure breathing may help to loosen secretions.

FLUID THERAPY

Fluid therapy should be guided by usual parameters such as urine output and central venous pressure, without blind adherence to formulas. Recommendations have been made for both moderate fluid restriction, to try to lessen pulmonary edema, and fluid administration based on a consideration of the pulmonary injury as a 10 to 15% body surface burn. It can be helpful to weigh the patient daily.

Smoke inhalation may cause increased pulmonary vascular resistance leading to an increase in central venous pressure. In this case, central venous pressure may not be an accurate guide to fluid administration. In ill patients in whom accurate fluid administration is paramount, the Swan-Ganz catheter may be used as a more accurate guide.

INDICATIONS FOR INTUBATION AND TRACHEOSTOMY

Intubation or tracheostomy may become necessary. True upper airway obstruction, with increasing edema and immobility of the cords seen on repeated laryngoscopy, requires intubation. Other indications are:

1. Increasing stridor with a dropping pO_2. (Monitor also with pulse oximetry.)
2. Profuse tracheobronchial secretions unmanageable with nasotracheal suction.
3. Severe burns of the face, mouth, and nares with rapidly increasing edema. (This indication is not absolute if the patient has received large quantities of intravenous fluids free of colloids.)
4. To prevent aspiration in patients unable to swallow.
5. The need for ventilatory support.

Orotracheal or nasotracheal intubation is preferable to tracheostomy, and it may be used in the awake patient by the emergency physician, using topical anesthesia. Tracheostomy should be avoided if possible. It has been strongly criticized because of its complications, particularly life-threatening infections in the acute phase. In addition, pulmonary edema has been noted many times directly after tracheostomy. (It is

speculated that this is caused by an acute lowering of intra-alveolar pressure through loss of the glottic barrier.) Although this is not well documented, tracheal intubation may also lead to pulmonary edema.

If tracheostomy is elected, it should be done in the operating room under controlled circumstances, using a cuffed tube with a positive pressure apparatus immediately available.

Stone has reported a marked difference in mortality after some basic therapeutic changes.[3] During the first 5-year period, in which tracheostomy was performed almost routinely for the majority of patients suspected of having a pulmonary burn, and antibiotics were administered prophylactically in most cases, mortality was 65%. During the second 5-year period, oxygen, humidification, and steroids were used as the main treatment, with 22% mortality.

VENTILATORS

Intermittent positive pressure breathing may be used for administering drugs, for atelectasis, or for pulmonary edema. Caution must be taken to prevent infection of the patient from contaminated apparatus. Patients placed on a respirator should have the benefit of a volume cycle machine, perhaps with expiratory resistance or positive end-expiratory pressure.

PULMONARY EDEMA

The treatment of pulmonary edema in the patient with smoke inhalation depends on the cause. In cases caused by smoke inhalation alone, the most effective treatment is positive pressure ventilation. Digitalis, diuretics, and the other usual treatments for pulmonary edema are not effective. If cardiac disease or overhydration is contributing to the pulmonary edema, the usual therapeutic measures for these conditions should be used in addition to positive pressure ventilation. Similarly, the pulmonary edema associated with tracheostomy responds only to positive pressure ventilation. If there is progressive hypoxia with a near-normal pO_2 and a chest film showing pulmonary edema, this constitutes the "adult respiratory distress syndrome."

PNEUMONIA

The emergency physician may occasionally be called upon to diagnose and treat the pneumonia phase. Pneumonia that develops early, within the first 3 days, tends to include microabscess formation and is particularly lethal. There is often poor correlation of sputum culture results with the responsible pathogen in early pneumonia, but blood cultures are often positive and correlate well. The pathogen is often Staphylococcus aureus or Pseudomonas. Pneumonias that develop later tend to be less lethal and have better sputum culture correlation and (usually) negative blood cultures. The pathogens are usually gram-negative bacteria. The pneumonias, early and late, should be treated with specific antibiotics and good bronchopulmonary care.

ON-SITE TREATMENT

On-site treatment is limited by the availability of equipment. The suspected smoke inhalation victim should be moved to a site free of smoke, well away from the fire. Coughing should be encouraged. If available, oxygen should be administered to all suspected victims. Respiratory and cardiac arrest should be treated in the normal fashion, using whatever equipment is at hand. Patients should be removed to an emergency facility as soon as possible. A kit to treat cyanide poisoning is available from Eli Lilly Pharmaceutical Corporation.

PROGNOSIS AND COMPLICATIONS

Because of the variability of the severity of smoke inhalation injury, and because of changing therapeutic approaches, the prognosis is unclear. Mortality figures from series of the 1960s show mortality in the range of 50%. Using strict diagnostic criteria, in the period 1960 to 1969, Stone reported a total mortality of 41%. As noted, however, the figures were significantly improved with a change in therapeutic approach.

Stone's figures indicate that, the earlier symptoms occur, the greater the mortality. For the second 5-year period, Stone reported a mortality of 30% for pulmonary insufficiency, 23% for pulmonary edema, and 10% for pneumonia.

In general, it appears that most survivors eventually suffer no long-term symptomatology. Various complications have been reported, however, including bronchiectasis, chronic bronchitis, bronchiolitis obliterans, and bronchial and tracheal stenosis.

REFERENCES

1. Phillips, A.W., and Cope, O.: Burn therapy. II. The revelation of respiratory tract damage as a principal killer of the burned patient. Ann. Surg. 155:1, 1962.
2. Phillips, A.W., and Cope, O.: Burn therapy. III. Beware the facial burn! Ann. Surg. 156:759, 1962.
3. Stone, H.H., et al.: Respiratory burns: A correlation of clinical and laboratory results. Ann. Surg. 165:157, 1967.
3a. Lowery, W.T., et al.: Study of toxic gas production during actual fires in the Dallas area. J. Forensic Sci. 30:59, 1985.
3b. Large, A.A., et al.: The short-term effects of smoke exposure on the pulmonary function of firefighters. Chest 97:806, 1990.
4. Zikria, B.A., Ferrer, J.M., and Floch, H.F.: The chemical factors contributing to pulmonary damage in "smoke poisoning." Surgery 71:704, 1972.
5. Zikria, B.A., Weston, G.C., and Chodoff, M.: Smoke and carbon monoxide poisoning in fire victims. J. Trauma 12:641, 1972.
6. Moritz, A.R., Henriques, F.C., and McLean, R.: The effects of inhaled heat on the air passages and lungs. Am. J. Pathol. 21:311, 1945.
7. Welch, G.W., et al.: The use of steroids in inhalation injury. Surg. Gynecol. Obstet. 145:539, 1977.
8. Walker, H.L., McLeod, C.G., and McManus, W.F.: Experimental inhalation injury in the goat. J. Trauma 21:962, 1981.
9. Birky, M.M., and Clarke, F.B.: Inhalation of toxic products from fires. Bull. N.Y. Acad. Med. 57:997, 1981.
10. Zarem, H.A., Rattenborg, C.C., and Harmel, M.H.: Carbon monoxide toxicity in human fire victims. Arch. Surg. 107:851, 1973.

BIBLIOGRAPHY

Ambiavagar, M., Chalon, J., and Zargham, I.: Tracheobronchial cytologic changes following lower airway thermal injury. J. Trauma 14:280, 1974.

Beal, D.D., and Conner, G.H.: Respiratory tract injury: A guide to management following thermal and smoke injury. Laryngoscope 80:25, 1970.

Beal, D.D., Lambeth, J.T., and Conner, G.H.: Follow-up studies on patients treated with steroids following pulmonary thermal and acrid smoke injury. Laryngoscope 78:396, 1968.

Bergeaux, G., and Klein, R.C.: Hyperuricemia following smoke inhalation. Am. Rev. Resp. Dis. 109:145, 1974.

Burke, J.F.: The sequence of events following smoke inhalation. J. Trauma 21:721, 1981.

Clark, C.J., Campbell, D., and Reid, W.H.: Blood carboxyhaemoglobin and cyanide levels in fire survivors. Lancet, June 20, 1981, p. 1332.

Coburn, R.F.: Mechanisms of carbon monoxide toxicity. 8:310, 1979.

Cohn, A.M.: Concepts in management of burns of the respiratory tract. South. Med. J. 66:297, 1973.

Crapo, R.O.: Smoke inhalation injuries. JAMA 246:1694, 1981.

Demarest, G.B., Hudson, L.D., and Altman, L.C.: Impaired alveolar macrophage chemotaxis in patients with acute smoke inhalation. Am. Rev. Respir. Dis. 119:279, 1979.

DiVincenti, F.C., Pruitt, B.A., Jr., and Reckler, J.M.: Inhalation injuries. J. Trauma 11:109, 1971.

Donnellan, W.L., Poticha, S.M., and Holinger, P.H.: Management and complications of severe pulmonary burn. JAMA 194:155, 1965.

End, E.: Comment on smoke inhalation. Am. Fam. Physician 8:31, 1973.

Epstein, B.S., et al.: Hypoxemia in the burned patient. Ann. Surg. 158:924, 1963.

Faling, L.J., Medici, T.C., and Chodosh, S.: Sputum cell population measurements in bronchial injury: Observations in acute smoke inhalation. Chest 65:56S, 1974.

Fein, A., Leff, A., and Hopewell, P.C.: Pathophysiology and management of the complications resulting from fire and the inhaled products of combustion: Review of the literature. Crit. Care Med. 8:94, 1980.

Garzon, A.A., et al.: Respiratory mechanics in patients with inhalation burns. J. Trauma 10:57, 1970.

Harrison, H.N.: Respiratory tract injury, pathophysiology and response to therapy among burned patients. Ann. N.Y. Acad. Sci. 150:627, 1968.

Harrison, H.N., and Zikria, B.A.: Management of respiratory problems in burned patients. Mod. Treat. 4:1263, 1967.

Kenny, J.M.: Smoke inhalation: A therapeutic rationale. Connecticut Med. 42:300, 1978.

Kutsumi, A., Kuroiwa, Y., and Takeda, R.: Medical report on casualties in the Hokuriku Tunnel train fire in Japan with special reference to smoke-gas poisoning. Mount Sinai. J. Med. 5:469, 1979.

Landa, J., Avery, W.G., and Sackner, M.A.: Some physiologic observations in smoke inhalation. Chest 61:62, 1972.

Mayer, B.W., Smith, D.S., and Hayden, M.J.: Acute smoke inhalation in children. Am. Fam. Physician 7:80, 1973.

Mintz, A.A., et al.: Pediatric grand rounds: Smoke inhalation and respiratory burns. Tex. Med. 68:90, 1972.

Morse, L.H., and Pasternak, G.: Toxic hazards of firefighters. In Hazardous Materials Toxicology. Edited by Sullivan, J.B., and Krieger, G.R. Baltimore, Williams and Wilkins, 1992, p. 545.

Myers, R.A.M., et al.: Value of hyperbaric oxygen in suspected carbon monoxide poisoning. JAMA 246:2478, 1981.

Noe, J.M., and Constable, J.D.: A new approach to pulmonary burns: A preliminary report. J. Trauma 13:1015, 1973.

Perez-Guerra, F., Walsh, R.E., and Sagel, S.S.: Bronchiolitis obliterans and tracheal stenosis. JAMA 218:1568, 1971.

Phillips, A.W., Tanner, J.W., and Cope, O.: Burn therapy. IV. Respiratory tract damage (an account of the clinical, x-ray and postmortem findings) and the meaning of restlessness. Ann. Surg. 158:799, 1963.

Polk, H.C., Jr., King, N., and Weiner, L.J.: Respiratory burn injury (smoke inhalation). D.M. 229:10, 1973.

Polk, H.C., Jr., and Stone, H.H.: Contemporary Burn Management. Boston, Little, Brown & Co., 1971.

Reed, G.F., and Camp, H.L.: Upper airway problems in severely burned patients. Ann. Otol. Rhinol. Laryngol. 78:741, 1969.

Robinson, N.B., et al.: Ventilation and perfusion alterations after smoke inhalation injury. Surgery 90:352, 1981.

Stone, H.H., and Martin, J.D.: Pulmonary injury associated with thermal burns. Surg. Gynecol. Obstet. 129:1242, 1969.

Stone, H.H., Martin, J.D., and Claydon, C.T.: Management of the pulmonary burn. Am. Surg. 33:616, 1967.

Taylor, F.W., and Gumbert, J.L.: Cause of death from burns: Role of respiratory damage. Ann. Surg. 161:497, 1965.

Thom, S.R., Strauss, M.B., and Hart, G.B.: Use of hyperbaric oxygen therapy for patients with smoke inhalation injury. Hosp. Phys. 20:8, 1984.

Thomas, D.M., and Conner, E.H.: Management of the patient "overcome by smoke." J. Ky. Med. Assoc. 66:1051, 1968.

Wanner, A., and Cutchavaree, A.: Early recognition of upper airway obstruction following smoke inhalation. Am. Rev. Resp. Dis. 108:1421, 1973.

Webster, J.R., McCabe, M.M., and Karp, M.: Recognition and management of smoke inhalation. JAMA 201:287, 1967.

Wroblewski, D.A., et al.: The significance of facial burns in acute smoke inhalation. Crit. Care Med. 7:335, 1979.

Zikria, B.A., et al.: Respiratory tract damage in burns: Pathophysiology and therapy. Ann. N.Y. Acad. Sci. 150:618, 1968.

Zikria, B.A.: CO level measures smoke injury. Med. World News, p. 17, Sept. 21, 1973.

OTHER INHALATION INJURIES

James R. Ungar (with Contributions on Nitrogen Dioxide and Chlorine by Stephen Sahn)

CAPSULE

The human airway is exposed to a variety of gases and contaminants in the inspired air. Of these, carbon monoxide and chlorine cause most reactions seen in the Emergency Department (ED). Inhalation injury caused by ammonia, hydrogen chloride, sulfur dioxide, nitrogen dioxide, phosgene, formaldehyde, hydrogen cyanide, and hydrogen sulfide are encountered less frequently. Most gases induce airway damage by producing inflammation and edema of the epithelial mucosa. The location and extent of injury depend on the solubility, concentration, and duration of exposure to the noxious gases. For example, chlorine injury is associated with pulmonary edema, whereas sulfur dioxide is more commonly associated with cough, wheezing, and bronchospasm.

Initial evaluation of the patient should include a detailed history to allow the physician to identify the nature of the combustible material inhaled. Symptoms may be minimal at the onset of injury, but they may progress significantly over time: hence some patients require prolonged observation in the ED and possibly hospital admission.

Therapeutic strategies of most inhalation injuries are nonspecific and supportive. The initial step is securing airway patency by endotracheal intubation of patients with severe distress or refractory hypoxemia. Secretions are usually profuse, and therefore, the largest endotracheal tube should be used to facilitate tracheobronchial suctioning. Occasionally, as with ammonia inhalation, emergency tracheostomy will have to be performed because of severe upper airway edema. Correction of hypoxemia, when present, should be done early by oxygen administration. Hypoxemia may respond to oxygenation by means of face mask, but may occasionally require intubation, and mechanical ventilation with the addition of PEEP. Pharmacologic therapy may include bronchodilators for the treatment of bronchospasm and steroids for the treatment of nitrogen dioxide inhalation.

INTRODUCTION

The surface area of the pulmonary gas exchange surface has been estimated to cover 140 m^2. This is comparable to the gastrointestinal surface area and is some 50 times greater than the adult skin surface area. Thus, the pulmonary portal of entry represents a significant surface area for exchange of gases, vapors, and even particulates. The significance of the inhalation of toxic chemicals by the pulmonary route takes on added significance when one considers that undegraded noxious materials can be delivered directly to the brain and other vital organs without first passing through the liver, in which deactivation and detoxification might otherwise occur.

The degree of absorption of the inhaled chemical depends largely on the physical state of the material in question. Fumes, vapors, and gases are molecular in size or in the submicron range, and are absorbed into the pulmonary capillaries in accordance with established physicochemical laws. The site of action of these materials is a function of their solubility and the dosage presented to the respiratory tract.

Highly soluble vapors (such as ammonia) are usually trapped in the aqueous mucous lining of the turbinates and pharynx, so that little, if any, of the vapor reaches the lower respiratory tract unless the inhaled dosage is high. This would then effectively overwhelm the trapping mechanism of the upper airways and would allow sufficient quantities of the noxious material to reach the lower respiratory tract and alveoli and produce a chemical burn of the lungs, with subsequent development of pulmonary edema. High ammonia concentrations can cause severe burns of the cornea and upper airway. Decontamination must be rapid, with copious irrigation of exposed body parts.[2a] In contrast, gases of relatively low aqueous solubility

produce relatively little upper respiratory tract irritation, although they readily reach the lower respiratory tree, at which point they initiate inflammatory reactions of varying degree. For example, phosgene gas is relatively insoluble in water. Even if inhaled in small doses, it readily reaches the alveoli, at which point it slowly hydrolyzes to hydrochloric acid and causes delayed pulmonary edema. Thus, in general, gases or vapors of lower water solubility are more capable of inducing significant reactions in the lower respiratory tract than are those of higher water solubility.

The rate at which a gas or vapor diffuses depends on the partial pressure gradient between the alveolar air and the pulmonary capillary. The partial pressure in the blood is primarily a function of the solubility of the gas or vapor in what is, for all practical purposes, an aqueous medium. Nonpolar (slightly soluble) gases or vapors saturate the blood at a rate directly proportional to pulmonary blood flow. Because of the diminished solubility of nonpolar compounds in the blood, there is limitation of uptake, and they rapidly reach equilibrium with the vascular compartment. The net effect of establishing this equilibrium is to diminish the pressure gradient for diffusion between the alveoli and the capillaries and to reduce the effective driving force for absorption between the ambient air and the body tissues. For soluble gases or vapors, the rate of blood saturation is directly proportional to alveolar partial pressure because the rate of uptake is not hindered by solubility considerations.

The rate of absorption of gases or vapors can be altered by physical activity and disease states. The rate of absorption can be greatly increased by increasing capillary blood flow in the lungs because this tends to increase the volume of blood presented to the alveoli per unit time and allows more rapid uptake of the gas in question. In patients with impaired hepatic or renal function, a more rapid accumulation of toxicants occurs than in normal individuals.

INHALATION OF PARTICULATE MATTER

The large bulk of inhaled particulate matter is cleared and removed in the upper airway. The bronchi and bronchioles also play an important role in the removal of particulate matter. As repeated branchings take place with only a slight increase in cross-sectional area, the surface area of the walls is greatly increased. Owing to the increased surface area, particles are more likely to impinge on the mucous coat than on the upper air passages. This "bronchiolar filter" has inherent ciliary action that causes particles lodged on the mucous film to be swept to the oropharynx. Many of the smaller particles reach the alveoli, in which removal by ciliary action is not possible. Here, removal is accomplished by alveolar phagocytes, termed "dust cells" after the particulate matter they contain. Following phagocytosis of the particles on the alveolar walls, the debris is deposited in the pulmonary connective tissue or the lymphatics.

The ability of particulate matter to produce a local or systemic effect by the pulmonary portal of entry depends largely on the physical nature of the material. The chemical nature is of secondary importance because particles too large to reach the lower airways and alveoli have less pathologic potential, regardless of their chemical composition. It is particle size, density, and surface area that determine biologic activity.

Particles larger than 5 microns in diameter are usually not important factors in eliciting pulmonary inflammatory reactions or in permitting absorption. Mass is normally a function of size. Large particles, once set in motion, have more inertia than do smaller particles. Because of the numerous changes of air flow direction in the respiratory tree, particles with high kinetic energy and inertia are most likely to impinge on the upper airway, because they are relatively incapable of changing direction and follow the branches of the respiratory tract. Depth of pulmonary penetration is also a function of particle density—the greater the density, the less the probability of deep penetration. Another factor that inhibits larger particles from deeply penetrating the respiratory tract is their tendency to stay suspended in air for relatively short periods in comparison with smaller and lighter particles.

Once impingement occurs in the upper air-conduction passages, the particulates are removed as described previously. The chemical properties of the particulate become important in determining the nature of the biologic response in those particles that have deeply penetrated the lung.

CLINICAL PRESENTATION

In our modern industrialized age, a growing concern for the emergency physician lies in the early detection, management, and awareness of complications associated with the inhalation of pollutant gases and a wide variety of noxious industrial compounds.

Frequently encountered pollutant gases such as carbon monoxide, nitrogen dioxide, sulfur dioxide, and ozone are capable of inducing hypoxemia and increasing the susceptibility to infection by diminishing ciliary activity, and, by a direct action on alveolar macrophages, they can interfere with the macrophages' phagocytic properties and their subsequent lytic action. In addition, all these compounds are able, through oxidant-induced cellular and biochemical changes, to induce emphysematous changes in the lung.

One of the major toxic reactions associated with inhalation of toxic gases or fumes is that of acute pulmonary edema. The overall incidence of chemically induced pulmonary edema is relatively small, but the frequency is not at all negligible. The early recognition of this problem is important because therapy and prognosis differ in many respects from that for the pulmonary edema from heart failure observed in usual clinical practice.

"LAG PHASE" FROM TIME OF EXPOSURE TO DEVELOPMENT OF PULMONARY EDEMA

Frequently, a "lag phase" is encountered after inhalations; this represents an appreciable interval of as long as 10 to 12 hours between exposure and development of pulmonary edema. The emergency physician must be acutely aware of this possibility because close observation is indicated in all cases of exposure to industrial intoxicants that are capable of eliciting this phenomenon. Among the industrial agents known to produce delayed pulmonary edema are phosgene, phosphorus compounds, methyl bromide, cadmium fumes, and oxides of nitrogen, ozone, and dimethyl sulfate.

The mechanisms responsible for the development of acute pulmonary edema after exposure to these compounds have not been fully elucidated. In general, there is a working hypothesis that toxic agents produce direct toxic injury on the alveolar-capillary membranes, increase endothelial permeability, and induce the transudation of fluid from the capillary into the interstitial spaces and alveoli.

The mechanism of injury after exposure to nitrogen dioxide and dimethyl sulfate is believed to arise from the conversion of these agents to more chemically irritating substances at the cellular level; thus, nitrogen dioxide is converted to nitric acid, and dimethyl sulfate becomes sulfuric acid on inhalation.

Certain other agents, such as hydrogen fluoride, hydrogen sulfide, chlorine, ozone, and phosgene, also produce irritation of the bronchial tree and cause an acute chemical bronchitis.

TREATMENT OF PULMONARY EDEMA SECONDARY TO TOXIC INHALATIONS

The most effective therapy for chemically induced pulmonary edema calls for oxygen to be administered under controlled positive pressure, with judicious use of nebulized bronchodilators for the correction of attendant bronchospasm. Intravenous corticosteroids, followed by oral steroid supplementation for several days, have been found beneficial in more severe cases. Nebulized nonirritant fluids help to prevent secondary bacterial pneumonia. If superimposed bacterial pneumonitis is suspected, broad-spectrum antibiotic coverage is indicated pending definitive culture reports. In certain circumstances, tracheostomy is required, either for respiratory failure or to aid in the clearing of secretions. Morphine is contraindicated in certain intoxications, such as those arising from ozone and hydrogen sulfide, because both of these intoxicants act as central nervous system (CNS) depressants and profound respiratory depression can occur when morphine is used in conjunction with them.

CARBON MONOXIDE INHALATION (WITHOUT SMOKE OR FIRE)

The ubiquitous nature of carbon monoxide makes it of great concern to the emergency physician, because it can be lethal if the inspired air contains as little as 0.1 volume%. Carbon monoxide is tasteless, odorless, and nonirritating to the mucous membranes, so it can be inhaled without the victim's awareness. It is present in automobile exhaust, coal gas, water gas, exhaust from heat stoves and furnaces with inadequate ventilation, smoke from burning buildings, and coal mine fires.

In 1895, Haldane demonstrated that the detrimental effect of carbon monoxide in the inhaled air is a function of anoxia and that carbon monoxide in itself is not toxic. Carbon monoxide has an affinity some 210 times that of oxygen for hemoglobin, forming a relative stable compound (carboxyhemoglobin) that does not dissociate significantly during passage through the lung or tissue capillaries. Therefore, the fraction of the blood hemoglobin bound to carbon monoxide is functionally ineffective. Also, the remaining hemoglobin available for transport of oxygen develops an increased oxygen affinity, tending to reduce tissue capillary pO_2 and hamper oxygen unloading to the tissues.

SYMPTOMS OF CARBON MONOXIDE POISONING

The earliest symptoms of carbon monoxide poisoning are slight headache with muscular weakness, palpitations, dizziness, and mental confusion. Excitement and bizarre behavior may follow. These symptoms progress to coma when the carboxyhemoglobin level exceeds 40%. Carboxyhemoglobin has a cherry red color, which accounts for the frequency with which the lips of a carbon monoxide-poisoned individual are reported to be of this color. Levels of 10% may be found in smokers and tunnel workers, and mild symptoms can occur at this level. Carboxyhemoglobin level determination is the best guide as to how therapy should proceed.

TREATMENT

The goal of therapy is to drive the carbon monoxide off the hemoglobin molecule and at the same time maintain adequate oxygenation to the tissues. This usually requires the administration of 100% oxygen,

and sometimes even hyperbaric oxygen administration in the more severe cases. Treatment with oxygen will reduce the concentration of carboxyhemoglobin by 50% within 40 minutes of the initiation of therapy; without the use of oxygen, a similar drop in carboxyhemoglobin would require 4 hours.

NITROGEN DIOXIDE

It has been known since the early 1950s that nitrogen dioxide (NO_2) was present in high concentrations in silo gas and was predominantly responsible for lung damage in silo workers.[1] Nitrogen dioxide is also released in several industrial settings, which include electroplating, acetylene welding, combustion of cellulose film and plastics, detonation of explosives, and industrial reactions using nitric acid.[2] The present threshold limit for human industrial exposure to nitrogen dioxide has been set at 5 ppm.[3]

Nitrogen dioxide reacts with water in the respiratory tract to form nitric acid; the nitrates and nitrites that are formed by the dissociation of nitric acid cause extensive tissue damage. NO_2 is a powerful oxidant. Large concentrations cause acute pulmonary edema, whereas low concentrations cause acute inflammation and bronchospasm as well as alveolar epithelial and pulmonary capillary endothelial injury.[4]

CLINICAL PRESENTATION

Rarely, some individuals die after a short exposure to very high concentrations of nitrogen dioxide. This rapid course is probably secondary to marked hypoxemia and possibly methemoglobinemia. More commonly, after exposure to NO_2, there is a lag period of several hours before symptoms develop. Patients generally present with cough, dyspnea, and wheezing and may have associated nausea, headache, tachycardia and chest pain. Wheezing is a prominent feature of the acute phase. This increase in airway resistance appears to be mediated by histamine.[5] If higher levels of NO_2 are present, the patient may develop pulmonary edema.

If the patient survives the acute phase of pulmonary edema, a second phase of the illness begins several days later. This phase lasts from 2 to 5 weeks, with the patient remaining relatively asymptomatic or with minimal symptoms. The third phase begins after this time and is characterized by fever, progressive dyspnea, and cough. The chest radiograph, which may have been normal during the acute and subacute phase if no pulmonary edema was present, shows evidence of nodular interstitial lung disease. Arterial blood gases usually show hypoxemia, and the Pco_2 may vary over a wide range, depending on the degree of injury and underlying lung disease. The patients may go on to die in chronic respiratory failure or recover with evidence of obstructive airways disease.[6]

TREATMENT

A trial of corticosteroids in the acute phase is indicated. Methylprednisolone (0.5 to 1.0 mg per kg IV q 6 hrs.) or its equivalent should be given. The length of corticosteroid treatment depends on the intensity of exposure and the clinical course. The role of prophylactic antibiotics is unclear, but they probably should be withheld unless evidence of infection is documented. Methylene blue to reverse methemoglobinemia, dimercaprol (BAL), and hyperbaric oxygen probably should not be used in routine cases because these agents may have adverse affects. Hyperbaric oxygen used experimentally causes a worsening in pulmonary injury.

If pulmonary edema develops from NO_2 inhalation, treatment is similar to that for the adult respiratory distress syndrome. This includes careful fluid balance, supplemental oxygen, and intubation and mechanical ventilation with positive end-expiratory pressure if necessary.

CHLORINE

Chlorine is used commonly as a bleaching agent in the paper and textile industry and as a disinfectant of water and sewage.

Chlorine reacts with water to produce hydrochloric acid and a number of other products such as hypochlorous acid, perchloric acid, and other unstable oxidizing agents. This series of reactions, in which unstable oxidizing compounds form stable hydrates of organic chlorine, produces more tissue damage than is produced by equivalent amounts of hydrochloric acid.[7]

CLINICAL PRESENTATION

Following chlorine exposure, patients present with cough, dyspnea, and chest pain. The conjunctivae and mucous membranes of the mouth are often hyperemic. Chest examination usually reveals rales and wheezing. Pulmonary edema occurs after severe exposure and may occur either immediately or after several hours. Arterial blood gases usually show hypoxemia and hypocapnia. The chest radiograph shows pulmonary edema.

TREATMENT

The patient should be removed immediately from the area of the accident and supplemental oxygen administered. A solution of 2 cc 8.4% sodium bicarbonate and 2 cc normal saline by face mask nebulizer may reduce symptoms.[11] Endotracheal intubation may be needed if there is severe edema of the upper airway. In patients with severe pulmonary edema, intubation and mechanical ventilation with positive end-expiratory pressure (PEEP) may be needed.[8] The role of corticosteroids in the treatment of chlorine inhalation is not definitely established, although there has been a single report suggesting a beneficial effect.[9] If there is pulmonary edema, corticosteroids (methylprednisolone 1.0 mg per kg IV q 6 hrs. or its equivalent) should be given for 48 to 72 hours. When exposure is less, the patient has only mucous membrane symptoms, and the chest radiograph and the arterial blood gases are normal, corticosteroids probably should be withheld. If, however, there is a widening of alveolar-arterial oxygen gradient or abnormalities on chest radiograph, similar doses of corticosteroids probably should be given, as in patients with pulmonary edema. There is no proven role for prophylactic antibiotics with chlorine inhalation, and these drugs should be withheld until evidence of infection is documented. Although previous follow-up studies of nonlethal chlorine exposure were inconclusive, later studies suggest residual restrictive ventilatory impairment and decreased oxygen exchange.[12]

REFERENCES

1. Lowry, T., and Schuman, L.M.: "Silo filler's disease": a syndrome caused by nitrogen dioxide. JAMA 162:153, 1956.
2. Lakshminarayan, S.: Inhalation injury of the lungs. In Sahn, S.A. (ed.): Pulmonary Emergencies. New York, Churchill Livingstone, 1982, pp. 375–386.
2a. Balmes, J.R.: Acute pulmonary injury from hazardous materials. In Hazardous Materials Toxicology. Edited by Sullivan, J.B., and Krieger, G.R. Baltimore, Williams and Wilkins, 1992, p. 425.
3. Tabershaw, I.R., Ottoboni, F., and Cooper, W.C.: Oxidant: Air quality criteria based on health effects. J. Occup. Med. 10:464, 1968.
4. Buckley, R.D., and Balchum, O.J.: Acute and chronic exposures to nitrogen dioxide: effects on oxygen consumption and enzyme activity on guinea pig tissues. Arch. Environ. Health 10:220, 1965.
5. Guidotti, T.L.: The higher oxides of nitrogen: inhalation toxicology. Environ. Res. 15:443, 1978.
6. Becklake, M.R., Goldman, H.I., Bosman, A.R., and Freed, C.C.: The long-term effects of exposure to nitrous fumes. Am. Rev. Tuberc. 76:398, 1957.
7. Kramer, D.G.: Chlorine. J. Occup. Med. 9:193, 1967.
8. Conner, E.H., Dubois, A.B., and Comroe, J.H.: Acute chemical injury of the airway and lungs. Anesthesiology 23:538, 1962.
9. Chester, E.H., Kaimal, J., Payne, C.B., Jr., and Kohn, P.M.: Pulmonary injury following exposure to chlorine gas: possible beneficial effects of steroid treatment. Chest 72:247, 1977.
10. Weil, H.G., George, R., Schwarz, M., and Ziskind, M.: Late evaluation of pulmonary function after exposure to chlorine gas. Am. Rev. Respir. Dis. 99:374, 1969.
11. Hurlbut, R., et al.: Pharmacotherapy. In Hazardous Materials Toxicology. Edited by Sullivan, J.B., and Krieger, G.R. Baltimore, Williams and Wilkins, 1992, p. 405.
12. Schwartz, D.A., et al: Pulmonary sequelae associated with accidental inhalation of chlorine gas. Chest 97: 820, 1990.

Chapter 75

EMERGENCIES OF ATMOSPHERIC POLLUTION

Charles A. Riley

CAPSULE

This chapter discusses the health effects of meteorologic conditions that cause critically increased concentrations of "usual" pollutants. This excludes inhalation of known toxic fumes or causes of pneumoconiotic exposure. Categories include: (1) sulfur dioxide (SO_2), a particulate complex produced by combustion of coal and crude oil; (2) photochemical smog (principally ozone and NO_2); (3) carbon monoxide (CO), and (4) naturally occurring allergens. The particulate volcanic ash exposure from the Mount St. Helens eruption in 1980 is reviewed in detail.

INTRODUCTION

Climatic conditions have caused several well-known atmospheric catastrophes with significant morbidity and mortality. The best-known episode occurred in Donora, Pennsylvania, in October of 1948, with at least 20 attributed deaths. It was estimated that concentrations of SO_2 and particulate matter exceeded 1 mg per meter squared, as pollutants from a local zinc smelter were trapped in the steep-sided valley. An episode in November, 1953, in New York City killed at least 200 people. Exposures in London in December of 1952 (SO_2 greater than 1.5 ppm and total particulates 4.4 mg per meter squared) and December of 1962 were associated with 4000 and 700 deaths, respectively.

The first episode in London introduced the term "smog" (a journalistic contraction meaning smoke-polluted fog) because the offending pollutants were a complex mixture of coal smoke, sulfur dioxide, fog droplets, and possibly other unidentified and unsuspected even more active substances. The second episode 10 years later had identical meteorologic conditions, but the decreased mortality has been attributed to a reduction in the permitted level of coal smoke, increased patient education regarding exposure avoidance, and improved therapy for symptoms.

On May 18, 1980, an extremely high level of particulate exposure occurred after the eruption of the Mount St. Helens Volcano in Washington. This more recent event has been closely studied for immediate and long-term health effects.[1,2]

The morbidity and mortality from environmental pollutants generally involve exacerbation of common chronic pulmonary conditions including chronic bronchitis, asthma, emphysema, and bronchiectasis. Autopsy findings include changes consistent with tracheobronchitis, with congestion, desquamation and evidence of excessive production of mucus. Deaths are also caused by an exacerbation of cardiovascular conditions, although not to the same degree as pulmonary disease.[3]

The clinical presentation of patients reacting to environmental pollutants varies from mild cough to dyspnea and severe wheezing with respiratory failure or cor pulmonale. The appropriate treatment of these respiratory emergencies is detailed elsewhere.

PHOTOCHEMICAL SMOG

SULFUR DIOXIDE

In most major cities, components of photochemical smog regularly exceed the United States Environmental Protection Agency (EPA) standards for air quality. The most important component is sulfur dioxide, with an EPA air quality standard of 0.03 ppm. At this concentration, there is only a reduction in visibility distance and minor eye and upper respiratory effects.

Demonstrable decline in pulmonary function occurs at 0.04 ppm, and individuals with known pulmonary disease worsen at levels of 0.08 to 0.17 ppm. Epidemiologic studies have demonstrated excess hospital admissions and mortality at more than 0.17 ppm. The lower levels of exposure cause no significant harmful effects in normal individuals; however, people with known lung disease, particularly reactive airway disease or asthma, can experience a rapid decline in function. This phenomenon occurs most markedly in individuals who are exercising in such conditions. Exercise not only increases ventilatory exchange and therefore atmospheric exposure, but is also a known trigger for airway reactivity. Therefore, asthmatics who exercise in conditions of heightened sulfur dioxide concentration are at highest risk.

OZONE

Ozone is the second most important pollutant, with a primary air quality concentration of photochemical oxidants of 0.08 ppm for a maximal 1-hour average. At this level, there is increased frequency of eye irritation, cough, and chest discomfort. Lung function is reported to decrease at 2 hours of exposure at 0.25 to 0.74 ppm. Pathologic injuries are observed at exposures of 0.05 to 1.0 ppm. Ozone also induces edema of membranes and an increased susceptibility to bronchospasm, as much in normal individuals as in asthmatics. Exposure at 0.4 to 0.6 ppm for 2 hours has markedly increased polymorphonuclear leukocytes in bronchial lavage fluid, and controlled animal studies demonstrate alveolar injury. About 50% of U.S. population is in areas where ozone concentrations often exceed the National Air Quality Standard of 0.12 ppm (1 hour maximum),[2a] with increases predicted.[2b] Children and adolescents are most affected, particularly while exercising.

NITROUS OXIDE

Nitrous oxide (NO_2) has a primary air quality concentration of 0.05 ppm. At 0.1 ppm, bronchospasm is more easily provoked in asthmatics. Acute exposure probably accounts for relatively little acute disease save for minor respiratory illnesses in children. Chronic exposures are speculative in terms of development or worsening of chronic lung disease.

PREVENTION AND TREATMENT

The primary treatment is prevention. Patients with known lung disease should be educated to follow weather and pollution reports, usually published in local newspapers or television reports of atmospheric pollutant conditions. Emergency department (ED) staff would be wise to familiarize themselves with such information in the event of inquiries about such conditions and their health effects. Advice to persons with lung disease should be to stay indoors and avoid pollutant contact. Certain adverse atmospheric conditions might weigh more heavily in decisions for admission to the hospital rather than discharge to a more harmful environment. Those who must go outdoors should be requested to avoid exercise (particularly athletic competition) or wear masks to limit the exposure.

There is little information regarding the use of air filters in homes or work places. Hepa filters are felt to be the most efficacious and useful in these situations. Air conditioning has certainly reduced respirable contaminants and symptoms, as well as controlled environmental mold. Pretreatment with indomethacin has had limited success in partially blocking ozone effects.[2a] Pretreatment with atropine may prevent increases in airway resistance from high ozone concentrations.

Treatment of increased asthmatic or bronchitis symptoms should follow the usual regimen (bronchodilators, antibiotics for purulent sputum, and perhaps steroids to lessen the irritant or inflammatory effects). Boushey has proposed both a local histamine production and a reflex bronchospasm in respect to oxidant pollutants.[4,5] Therefore, antihistamines and antimuscarinic therapy in the form of aerosolized iprotroprium bromide would be effective.

CARBON MONOXIDE

Carbon monoxide is frequently elevated in areas near freeways. Aronow and others have repeatedly documented susceptibility to angina at exposures of 70 to 85 ppm over 1 hour and impaired cognitive function at 85 to 207 ppm reflecting a blood carboxyhemoglobin level of 3 to 6.5%. The carboxyhemoglobin level in chronic smokers is approximately 5%.[6]

PREVENTION AND TREATMENT

In respect to carbon monoxide exposure, individuals with known coronary or peripheral occlusive vascular disease should remain indoors and/or avoid exertion. Transient increase in vasodilator medication would seem reasonable, but has not been investigated. ED treatment of such individuals with increased symptoms includes high concentrations of oxygen therapy (i.e., 100% oxygen by nonrebreather mask) to displace CO from the carboxyhemoglobin and increase oxygen content of arterial blood until the CO has been eliminated. Hyperbaric oxygen therapy is an indicated treatment for severe carbon monoxide toxicity, but paucity of facilities and time involved in transport are probably the major limiting considerations.

ALLERGENS

Environmental allergens, or pollen exposure, also account for a great number of respiratory symptoms and are indirectly related to weather conditions. It is recognized, however, that there is no direct correlation between absolute pollen count and absolute intensity of allergic symptoms and requirements for treatment. Sensitization of airways to allergens may occur in the context of heightened SO_2 or ozone exposure.

PREVENTION AND TREATMENT

Allergic symptoms from increased pollen counts should be treated appropriately, again with advice to avoid exposure.

THE MOUNT ST. HELENS EXPERIENCE

The Mount St. Helens eruption was dispersed over a distance of 150 miles downwind. The known cause of death in 17 individuals (of 62 total deaths) was direct asphyxia by volcanic ash. Extensive occlusion of the upper airways with ash and excessive mucus was seen at autopsy, and purulent tracheobronchitis was noted as a contributing factor in two additional deaths. Thermal burns were the major cause of death in three patients and contributory in several others. These individuals did not have the pulmonary findings of those who died from asphyxia. A 4-year controlled follow-up of loggers working in the area has demonstrated a mild increase in cough and wheezing in the year after exposure, associated with a mild but significant decline in FEV_1 and forced vital capacity (FVC). This effect was noted most in nonsmokers, but the symptoms and decline in function equaled those of control subjects over the following year.[7]

The total suspended particulates in Yakima, 135 kilometers northeast of Mount St. Helens, averaged between 5.8 and 33.4 mg per meter squared, far exceeding the emergency levels of 0.875 mg per meter squared of the National Ambient Air Quality (NAAQ) standards. A major concern has been that 90% of the ash is "respirable" size (less than 10 micrometer) and contains 3 to 7% crystalline silica, which is fibrogenic to lung tissue. At the conclusion of the 4-year study, there was no evidence of pulmonary fibrosis in the exposed subjects, but surveillance is ongoing regarding the late effects of the ash exposure.[8]

PREVENTION AND TREATMENT IN VOLCANIC ERUPTIONS

In respect to volcanic ash events, immediate evacuation of the downwind area and restriction to indoors for any individuals who cannot be evacuated is important. Occupational Health and Safety Administration (OSHA)-approved respirators should be obtained before venturing into contaminated areas. The long-term consequences of remaining in a devastated area depend on the analysis of the ash and subsequent recommendations. In the event of apparent asphyxia, immediate intubation, respiratory support, and bronchoscopic removal of secretions once indicated. Antibiotic treatment of appropriate bacterial infection is necessary, but corticosteroids have not been evaluated.

REFERENCES

1. Martin, T.R., Wehner, A.P., and Butler, J.: Pulmonary toxicity of Mount St. Helens ash. Am. Rev. Respir. Dis. *128*:158, 1983.
2. Baxter, P.J., et al.: Mount St. Helens eruptions, May 18 to June 12, 1980. An overview of the acute health impact. JAMA *246*:585, 1981.
2a. Paulo, M., and Gong, H.: Respiratory effects of ozone: Whom to protect and how. J. Resp. Dis. *12*:482, 1991.
2b. Leaf, A.: Potential health effects of global climatic and environmental changes. N. Engl. J. Med. *23*:1577, 1989.
3. Goldstein, E., Hackney, J.D., and Rokaw, S.N.: Photochemical air pollution. West. J. Med. *142*:69, 1985.
4. Boushey, H.: Asthma, sulfur dioxide and the clean air act. West. J. Med. *136*:129, 1982.
5. Boushey, H.A., and Sheppard, D.: Air pollution. *In* Textbook of Respiratory Medicine. Edited by Murray, J.F., and Nadel, J.A. Philadelphia, W.B. Saunders, 1988.
6. Aronow, L.: Editorial: Effect of ambient level of carbon monoxide on cardiopulmonary disease. Chest *74*: pp. 1, 1978.
7. Buist, A.S.: Are volcanoes hazardous to your health? What haven't we learned from Mount St. Helens? West. J. Med. *137*:94, 1982.
8. Buist, A.S., et al.: A 4-year perspective study of the respiratory effects of volcanic ash from Mount St. Helens. Am. Rev. Respir. Dis. *133*:526, 1986.

Chapter 76

WILDERNESS AND TRAVEL MEDICINE

WILDERNESS MEDICINE

Kenneth V. Iserson

CAPSULE

Somewhat paradoxically, wilderness medicine is a direct outgrowth of the developments in modern medicine and the related biosciences and biotechnology. At one time in medicine's history, there was only one rather basic level of care that could generally be delivered. This level is now relegated to care delivered only in remote or isolated environments or during disasters. Yet, even in wilderness medicine, the limitations of care are being expanded. New forms of communication and transportation have opened up unexpected avenues of delivering medical information to wilderness medical practitioners and transporting patients to the source of that expertise. Simultaneously, scientific advances on many fronts including physiology, psychology, toxicology, epidemiology, and microbiology, have been applied to wilderness activities as well as to the prevention of injury and illness. Care for those who are acutely disabled in the wilderness environment is constantly improving.

INTRODUCTION

ENVIRONMENT

Test pilots describe going beyond the recognized capabilities of their airplane as "pushing the edge of the envelope." The limits of wilderness medicine are being expanded in three basic areas that are doing this: environment, knowledge, and people. Individuals are constantly pushing the edge of the commonly accepted environmental constraints on human activity. This results in a new awareness of the true physiologic limits on humans and the new medical problems that they encounter. As the environmental limits are pushed further and further, activities once thought daring and only for the most well-conditioned and hardy souls becomes common for the general populace.

Before World War II, venturing under the sea for prolonged period outside a submarine was performed only by men in hard diving helmets with air hoses linking them to the surface. These relatively few men, who dove for a living, were well conditioned to their environment and knew, at least as well as could be expected at the time, the risks and preventive measures needed in their work. Subsequently, SCUBA equipment and training became available and were disseminated to the general population. Sport diving became a popular pastime. With the influx of less well trained, poorly conditioned, and often careless divers, there was marked increase in the need for knowledge about and treatment for hyperbaric injuries. More recently, pushing the envelope even further, pregnant women, individuals with cardiac and pulmonary diseases, and elderly people are venturing into diving.

Similar scenarios can be sketched for mountain climbing and high altitude sickness, space travel and gravitational disorientation, spelunking and psychologic stress, winter and water sports and hypothermia, and even domestic or foreign remote travel and infectious diseases. The science of wilderness medicine is trying to catch up.

KNOWLEDGE

Scientific knowledge has kept pace in many areas with the explosion in wilderness activity. Although common medical problems in the wilderness, such as hypothermia and hyperthermia, have been studied for a long time and continue to produce new information, some new exciting areas of interest include studies on high altitude sicknesses, hyperbaric medicine, space medicine, and the epidemiology of wilderness medical problems.

Other specific areas of scientific exploration in wilderness medicine, in both basic science laboratories and the clinical setting, include prevention, recognition, and treatment of infectious diseases common to remote areas of the country or world; prevention and treatment of toxigenic diarrheas and the resulting acute dehydrations; the benefits and hazards of flora and fauna found in uncommon environments; the effect of stress reactions and substance abuse in the wilderness; and improvement in search and rescue techniques to assist those who become ill or injured in the wilderness.[1]

PEOPLE

Although there may be limits on human interaction with the environment, these limits have not yet been reached. As the envelope keeps getting pushed further and further, and more of the general populace finds interesting activities, or even their livelihood, lying within its expanded borders, the scope of wilderness medicine will itself continue to broaden.

An important new area of wilderness medicine is helping individuals whose disabilities previously prevented them from using wilderness areas for work or recreation to find acceptable methods of doing so.

ADVANCED MEDICAL TECHNIQUES IN THE WILDERNESS

Wilderness medical emergencies require distinctly different approaches, skills, and realizations from those used in ordinary medical emergencies.

ROLE OF WILDERNESS MEDICAL PERSONNEL

Individuals assuming the role of medical care provider, whether as physician, dentist, nurse, paramedic, physician assistant, or other medically trained person, must often use sketchy knowledge or even an "educated guess" in treating patients far from access to medical care. Even when a communication link exists, the on-site person may have to perform evaluations or procedures without the benefit of ever having done them before.

Credentials are not always an adequate guide to the success of a wilderness practitioner. Many people have advanced medical training, as affirmed by their licenses or certifications, and therefore think that they can operate successfully in a wilderness environment. The training that medical practitioners receive is normally in well-equipped facilities with backup and additional expertise readily available. Much of the training, especially for nurses and physicians, is often in narrow areas of medicine. Wilderness medical care is

distinctly different and can cover every discipline in medicine. Therefore, when either choosing a wilderness practitioner for a specific venture or volunteering to act in that capacity yourself, it is important to assess not only the formal training and degrees but also specific abilities.

WILDERNESS TRIAGE

An uncomfortable part of wilderness medicine for most people, including well-trained medical practitioners, is the frequency with which patients can die from diseases or injuries that might be treatable in an urban or sophisticated medical environment. This is not unique to the wilderness, but may also be found in medically poor regions of the world and during disaster situations anywhere. People can die in the wilderness of diseases and injuries that would cause only temporary disability in urban environments. Going into the wilderness is a risk, and most people do not realize this. The time and effort needed to locate injured or seriously ill patients can be enormous, not to mention the time needed to get trained medical personnel to the site and to move the patient to a suitable medical facility. Tough decisions may have to be made when balancing concerns for the safety of the maximum number of people involved in a deteriorating situation in the wilderness, including potential rescuers (see Search and Rescue, this chapter) against the chances of survival of an individual patient. Medical personnel in this setting are often called upon to make this type of decision. Anyone involved in wilderness medicine must be aware of this.[2]

REDUCING DISLOCATIONS

In the wilderness setting, dislocations should be reduced early if delay is expected in moving the patient. This is essential for the comfort of the patient, decreases the incidence of arthritis, and improves any neurovascular compromise. This course of action is approved by the Wilderness Medical Society for both physician and nonphysician care providers.[2] In settings that are not strictly wilderness and where emergency personnel fall under the purview of a base station, bureaucratic complications may arise if procedures are done without permission from the supervising authorities. Early reduction may be easy to perform without any analgesia. If analgesia is necessary or preferred, rather than commonly used general sedation that may not always be optimal or even practical in the specific wilderness setting, alternative methods of anesthesia are available, including hypnosis or regional blocks.[3]

SETTING FRACTURES

Most fractures are not set in the wilderness area. Bringing angulated fractures of long bones (femur, tibia-fibula, humerus, radius-ulna) into general alignment, however, often aids in extrication or splinting. It may also reduce neurovascular deficits. Splints are often easily made from available equipment or natural resources. It is important to stabilize the injured area as securely and comfortably as possible, but maintain maximal function if the injured person must also actively remove himself or herself from the wilderness setting.

CHEST TRAUMA

Pneumothorax is a common injury in either blunt trauma or overpressure injuries. Relief of a tension pneumothorax may often be life-saving. Needles, with or without a one-way Heimlich valve that can be fashioned by cutting a finger off of a rubber glove, can be used. A urethral catheter or endotracheal tube also works. The one-way valve, although useful, is not usually essential because patients are normally under positive pressure ventilation.

AIRWAY

If a controlled airway, rather than merely opening an airway by positioning, is needed, it can be quickly obtained in even the most adverse settings. There are few substitutes for an endotracheal tube. Although it is good to have a larynogoscope, and lightweight ones are now available, they are still usually not carried in the field even by larger expeditions. Alternatives include blind nasotracheal or digital intubation or cricothyrotomy. Digital intubations, using the index and middle finger to guide the endotracheal tube, have been used successfully in both the prehospital and wilderness settings.[4] A great benefit of this technique is that only the tube and your hand is necessary. An alternative, the cricothyrotomy, can be successfully accomplished in nearly any unconscious patient. A knife, a tube, and a knowledge of the landmarks are all that is required. In the wilderness setting, antisepsis is not the first concern, although materials for this purpose should be available.

MEDICAL KITS[2,5–13]

In deciding what to put into a medical kit for the wilderness, the first consideration is the skill level of the medical providers who will be using the kit. As the well-known medical axiom for choosing a stethoscope goes, it is what is between the ears, rather than what goes into the ears, that counts. Even the most well-provisioned kit cannot include equipment for *every* possible medical emergency. Knowledge of and practice in the basic skills is the most important factor.

Improvisation is always a large part of any type of wilderness medical care.

FACTORS TO CONSIDER IN DESIGNING A MEDICAL KIT

Assembling a medical kit that is appropriate to support a proposed trip requires assessing several factors:

PURPOSE OF THE TRIP

Selectivity is the key in choosing appropriate medical equipment. Groups intent only on providing self-treatment should consider the most common injuries they will sustain. On recreational trips, the medical kit displaces other equipment that might be wanted. Hikers, white water canoers, and climbers all need a different medical kit to meet their specialized environment.

Because search and rescue (SAR) team personnel must be equipped to handle the medical emergencies that they expect to encounter, they can justify carrying specialized medical gear. A medical kit for an SAR group varies somewhat with the environment. It is usually more complex than a wilderness trip kit because the SAR kit is carried when there is knowledge of or expectation that someone is injured. The key to developing a kit is knowing how to use one piece of equipment for multiple purposes.

LEVEL OF MEDICAL TRAINING

It is inappropriate to include medications and equipment that no trip member has the level of knowledge or experience to use safely. Trip members responsible for medical care of the group should have direct input into the contents of the medical kit. Levels of training and experience can differ widely among groups of physician, nurse, and EMS personnel. A degree or license may not guarantee knowledge in any specific area. Pretrip training to supplement the knowledge base of the providers may be required.

DESTINATION

The terrain, altitude, weather, propensity for endemic diseases, and other inherent dangers that could be encountered must be considered. Groups heading into remote areas in which local inhabitants may request medical help must consider this demand on their supplies if they plan to respond.

LENGTH OF TRIP

The total time during which the party must be supported from the kit affects its contents. Some problems are likely only during particular times; for example, the treatment of friction blisters is most important during the first few days of a hike. Sometimes, on a long trip, outside medical supplies can be easily obtained to restock the kit.

INTERVAL UNTIL OUTSIDE MEDICAL HELP CAN BE REACHED

Some trips progressively distance themselves from medical care by slowly penetrating a wilderness area. On other trips, time required to obtain help may be deceptive. A river raft trip into a canyon may last only hours; evacuation in the event of an accident may take many days of dangerous and laborious effort.

SIZE OF THE PARTY

Although an increase in the number of participants influences the quantity of some medications and bandaging materials, the increase is not linear. Frequently only minimal additions are needed to serve a larger group adequately. The size of the main medical kit for a large party can be reduced by equipping each member with a personal kit containing bandages, blister supplies, and personal medications.

BULK, WEIGHT, AND COST

Even if cost were not a factor, the weight and bulk of a kit are potential limiting factors. Because bandaging is bulky and splints may be awkward to pack, the use of extemporaneous materials (e.g., clothing for bandaging or local fabrication of splints) may be incorporated into plans for the medical kit. Medical equipment may also be reduced by using multifunctional components. If one piece of equipment or drug can be used for many different purposes (e.g., urethral catheters for bladder drainage, as a chest tube, posterior nasal pack, and foreign body remover; antihistamines for their antihistaminic, anticholinergic, local anesthetic, and sedative properties), weight can be significantly reduced. Knowledgeable medical team members are needed to optimize this tactic.

Some organizations and SAR groups use a modular approach to medical kits. Separate kits, with increasing sophistication and differing purposes are available for individuals and situations requiring more advanced equipment. Although the basic kit is designed for use by laymen, only specially trained individuals (e.g., physician, nurse, paramedic) can use the more advanced kits; and carry them into the field only when required.

CONTAINER

Containers for the medical kit must be chosen for maximal protection of contents and accessibility. Damage is to be expected, and may render materials useless when needed. In situations in which there is danger of the loss of equipment, such as on white water trips, the medical kit components should be split up into several kits so that all equipment would not be lost if an accident occurred.

The medical kit must be easily located when needed. This entails both making it visible (fluorescent orange), and placing it where it can be reached easily. Kits that unroll or open to display their components make selection of items convenient. For small kits, this is not usually a necessity. For large kits, those that are expected to have frequent use, or kits used frequently in urgent situations, rapid accessibility and easy identification of contents are important.

EQUIPMENT

The equipment for a wilderness medical kit may be considered in light of its function.

STOPPING BLEEDING

Although this can be accomplished with direct pressure using the bare hand, various pressure bandages are manufactured. Pneumatic splints and tourniquets fall into this category.

TREATING WOUNDS

Wound closures range from butterfly bandages and Steri-strips to suturing materials with surgical instruments or surgical staples. Cleansing materials, local anesthetics, and bandaging materials are also in this category. Material for blister treatment is the most commonly used item in this group.

SPLINTING

Prefabricated splints are now manufactured in lightweight designs but may be improvised in the field. Backboards and cervical collars are not usually needed except by SAR groups.

TAKING VITAL SIGNS

A watch to time a pulse or respirations is important. A thermometer is useful for most wilderness teams. A low-reading thermometer is essential for cold-weather expeditions. A stethoscope and blood pressure cuff are useful in some situations, but may be of no value to lay groups.

ADMINISTERING MEDICATIONS

Special equipment in addition to the medications is essential only if injectable medications or intravenous fluids are carried. Injectable medications are susceptible to damage not only from breakage, but also from light, heat, and cold. If an intravenous line is to be used, it is often difficult to keep it flowing during transport. Pressure on the system can be maintained by placing the IV bag under the patient, in a blood pressure cuff, in a blood pump (disposable), or wrapped in an elastic bandage.

PROVIDING LIFE SUPPORT

Airways, antishock trousers, chest tubes, and similar items are generally considered only by experienced medical rescue teams or prolonged remote expeditions. For experienced practitioners, a nasogastric tube, ballooned urethral catheter endotracheal tube, and scalpel can supply many needs. The nasogastric tube is useful not only to decompress the stomach, but also as a tourniquet, a suction catheter, and, if necessary, a urinary catheter. The urethral catheter with balloon is useful not only for bladder drainage, but also as a makeshift chest tube, especially in children when there is no hemothorax, as a nasal pack, and as a foreign body remover. The endotracheal tube can also be used for surgical airways and as a chest tube.

MEDICATIONS

Medications from any of the following groups or for application to any of the following problems can be added to a wilderness medical kit:

antibiotics	analgesics	anaphylactics
anti-inflammatories	antiemetics	antidiarrheals
	antiparasitics	antitussives
antipyretics	cardiovascular	decongestants
bronchodilators	medications	diabetes
dental preparations	dermatologic	medication
	medications	laxatives
hemorrhoidal	intravenous	otic medications
preparations	fluids	
muscle relaxants	ophthalmologic medications	vaginal medications
sedatives	snakebite antivenin	

The necessity for specific treatment must take into account that the ideal drug for each would increase the requirement for medical knowledge on the part of the user tremendously, and that the cost, bulk, and weight of the kit would similarly increase. The possibility of side effects or untoward reactions to administered medications must also be taken into account, because treatment of these conditions may be complex.

SEARCH AND RESCUE

PREPLANNING FOR SEARCH ACTIVITIES

PERSONNEL

Trained people are essential for a successful search effort. Even if only a line search is anticipated, trained and experienced leadership is necessary to ensure that the search is carried out with a high probability of detection. Wilderness searches are much more complex and require not only individual training in field search techniques, but also knowledgeable individuals to coordinate the search effort. Untrained volunteers can often obscure clues and hinder the search effort by encumbering the search teams and being a danger to themselves and others.

Search dogs may be useful, but require much advance training. Not only do they and their handlers need training in the specific type of search and environment in which they will be used, but the remainder of the search team, especially the leadership, must be experienced in using them in operations. They may be available through local agencies only in emergency situations.

EQUIPMENT

Both personal and group equipment should be adequate for the search effort. Personal equipment allows the searcher to remain in the field safely and effectively for the required time. Group equipment includes radios and other communication devices, transportation other than hiking (horses, four-wheel drive vehicles, helicopters), and major technical rescue equipment (ropes, haul and relay devices, stokes litters, backboards). The equipment must be compatible with the search effort, the personnel and leaders must be trained in the use of the equipment, and the equipment must be kept available and operational. The time to test the efficacy of equipment is not during an actual search effort. When more than one team is working together on a search, it is essential that they know in advance that their equipment, including communication channels, is compatible.

PREPLANNING FOR RESCUES

MEDICAL RESCUES

Personnel involved in rescue operations need medical skills for themselves, their team, and the victim. No matter how technically skilled a rescuer is, his or her effectiveness is markedly reduced if not accompanied by at least a basic knowledge (and willingness to apply that knowledge) of first aid. SAR groups should, as a minimum, require that all members have a current Advanced First Aid card or its equivalent. If SAR groups hold regular meetings, a few minutes at each meeting is the best method of "force-feeding" medical knowledge to reluctant SAR personnel.

Personal medical equipment should be carried by all team members. This includes equipment to take care of blisters, small cuts, and fractured fingers or toes, cactus removers (in the desert), and any individually needed medications. The team should have available and prepackaged for taking into the field specific splinting, bandaging, and airway equipment, fluids, and medications, depending on the rescue situation and the medical expertise of the rescue team. Advanced medical equipment (narcotics, IVs) may have specific restrictions, such as being only carried and used by paramedics, RNs, PAs, physicians, or other licensed individuals.

TECHNICAL RESCUES

Whether or not an SAR member is an expert at technical rescue, he or she must be well enough trained to support safely the more advanced technical members on a mission. This takes repeated training and practice. A mission is not the place for initial training. Even worse is to let an inexperienced person manage a rope system unsupervised. This is how accidents occur.

The equipment necessary for rescue must be available, in good working order, appropriate for the task required, and regularly used by the technical team. This includes communication gear. An actual operation is not the time to try out new and untested equipment. When more than one team is working together, it is essential than they have already checked out whether their equipment and systems are compatible.

SPECIAL RESCUES

Some SAR operations involve unusual environments, such as caves, mines, rivers, or the extremes of hot or cold environments. Even though an SAR group may encounter these environments rarely, it is essential that regular trainings be held to update and refresh the members on the skills needed if such an operation takes place. In each case, the leader must ensure that the individuals participating in operations in these environments, whether they be searchers or rescuers, are properly trained and equipped for such a mission. More mundane, checking to see whether all members are equipped with enough water (in the desert) or warm clothes (in cold environments) is often overlooked. Preparation by repeated practice in these environments can often make this less necessary.

Practice sessions have been stressed because they serve three purposes. First, they teach individual members and group leaders the skills necessary for actual operations. Second, they point out difficulties in operational management, equipment, or the approach to problems that can be worked out in advance. Finally, and most important, practices weld a team together. They instill a sense of camaraderie and trust that cannot be otherwise imbued.

INITIAL RESPONSE

NOTIFICATION

There are two elements to the notification process. The first is that of notifying the SAR command. This can be done by someone coming out of the field and calling the sheriff's office, a relative saying that the individual(s) had not returned as expected, or a patrol noticing an "abandoned" vehicle. Although often delayed, the manner of this notification process is a matter of circumstances, and certainly out of the purview of SAR teams. This step is essential, however, if SAR response is needed.

The second element is the manner in which individual SAR members are contacted. This must be expeditious and effective. A paging system works, but is too expensive for many groups. A phone tree also works, but is slower and not as effective. When two or more units must be contacted, the system can become confusing if not worked out in advance, practiced, and agreed to by all parties.

MANAGEMENT TEAM

If the situation is confusing (no need for a search, no haste needed, situation unclear) and a subsequent response will not be unduly slowed, a management team can be assembled. Usually consisting of the most experienced SAR members, the team determines the best plan of attack for the problem. Often this results in no response from the entire SAR team because it is deemed unjustified. It may also result in calling additional support teams (helicopters, dogs, horses). It should be understood, though, that the management team takes on a weighty responsibility by deciding whether or not, when, and how the SAR response should take place.

HASTY TEAM

A hasty team is just that—a rapid response team. Unlike the management team, the hasty team is generally part of the entire SAR response. The team is composed of a few individuals who can "fly down the trail" and report back on the condition of the victim, the situation that the remainder of the SAR team will encounter, and any special difficulties that should be anticipated. They should also, of course, be ready to provide initial medical care if needed.

LEADERSHIP

COMMAND SYSTEMS

Leadership is the most important element of any (successful) SAR operation. Not only does the success of the mission depend on solid leadership, but so does the safety of the SAR team members.

Leadership is commonly acknowledged by its *absence* in "pick-up" search or rescue efforts by untrained or unorganized groups. Even here, though, if one or a few individuals can demonstrate early that they have the expertise to guide the operation, some form of leadership can occur. Sadly, however, this rarely happens. This is perhaps the most dangerous of all SAR-type operations—a floundering body without a head.

Many SAR groups follow the *military system* of ranks. This works if the officers are both experienced and respected. Otherwise it does not work.

The *Incident Command System* (ICS), developed by the U.S. Forest Service and used by many SAR organizations, takes well-trained and experienced personnel from many areas and fits them into their particular jobs.[10] This system works well for the paid Forest Service. Direct application to mostly-volunteer SAR missions is difficult.

The ICS can be modified in several ways. Useful for SAR missions are on-site command "flows." In this type of leadership, there usually is an overall incident commander, designated by experience, rank, or however the group determines. As each element of the operation proceeds, however, the on-site SAR member most capable of directing that element (haul, lower, medical, evacuation, helicopter ground support) is placed in charge. As soon as that operation is completed, the command flows to the commander of the next operation. The difficulty in using this system is that the team members must know and trust one another. This takes many practices or actual operations to achieve.

Multi-organizational operations are the most difficult type of SAR system to lead, especially if there is no preeminent person or group. The easiest way to lead many organizations on one SAR operation is through a designated (sheriff) authority. If that is not possible, or if that individual does not have the required expertise, the operation often ends in frustration, if not disaster. The key here is to have multi-organizational practices in advance, so that leadership can be worked out successfully.[11]

PRIORITIZATION

One of the main jobs of SAR leadership is to determine the timing of the mission based on available information and the use of the available resources. Although SAR missions are always "an emergency," the nature of the problem, victim profiles, weather conditions, and other factors determine the speed and type of response. The leadership makes that decision. There is never enough personnel or equipment to do the "optimal" search, especially in large or wilderness areas. Therefore the leaders must use available resources in the most effective manner.

WITHDRAWING THE TEAM

The leaders also have the duty to withdraw the SAR team if this becomes necessary. This might occur if they are in danger, if the mission is seen to be futile, or because they are exhausted. This is often a difficult decision, but the safety and needs of the group must outweigh the needs of any one victim.

DECISION FOR NO RESPONSE

This is the often the most difficult decision that SAR leadership must make. It takes more expertise to make this decision than nearly any other. The decision is usually based on an unfavorable risk-benefit situation for the rescue team. Often there are enormous pressures on the leadership not to make this decision.

REFERENCES

1. Auerbach, P.S., and Geehr, E.C.: Management of Wilderness and Environmental Emergencies, 2nd ed. St. Louis, C.V. Mosby Co., 1989.
2. Iserson, K.V. (Ed.): Wilderness Medical Society Position Statements. Point Reyes, CA, Wilderness Medical Society, 1989.
3. Iserson, K.V.: Reducing dislocations in a wilderness setting: Use of hypnosis. J. Wild. Med. 1: , 1990.
4. Hudon, F.: Intubation without laryngoscopy. Anesthesiology 6:476, 1945.
5. Goodman, P.H., Kurtz, K.J., and Carmichael, J.: Medical Recommendations for Wilderness Travel—Part 3: Medical Supplies and Drug Regimens. Postgrad. Med. 78:107, 1985.
6. Auerbach, P.S.: Medicine for the Outdoors. Boston, Little Brown, 1986.
7. Darvell, F.: Mountaineering Medicine, 11th ed. Berkeley, Wilderness Press, 1985.
8. Forgey, W.: Wilderness Medicine, 3rd ed. Merrillville, IN, ICS Books, 1987.
9. Illingsworth, R.: Medical equipment for expeditions. Br. Med. J. 282:202, 1981.
10. National Association for Search and Rescue: Incident Commander Field Handbook: Search and Rescue. Fairfax, VA, NASAR, 1987.
11. Drabek, T.E., Tamminga, H.L., Kilijanek, T.S., and Adams, C.R.: Managing Multiorganizational Emergency Responses: Emergent Search and Rescue Networks in Natural Disaster and Remote Area Settings. Denver, University of Colorado, 1981.
12. Kizer, K.W.: Wilderness medicine and the backcountry medical kit. Res. Staff Phys. 37:79, 1991.
13. Kizer, K.W.: Wilderness emergencies: Be prepared. Emerg. Med. 23:89, 1991.

TRAVEL MEDICINE

David Gregory

CAPSULE

As many as one in six travelers to the tropics and subtropics returns with an acquired illness. Diseases acquired by travelers are of particular interest to the emergency physician, who is likely to be the first physician to confront the illness of the returning traveler. This chapter discusses the general approach to these illnesses and some of the specifics of the more common ones.

INTRODUCTION

Travelers' diseases range from the familiar and self-limited to the exotic and life-threatening. Diagnosis of the cause of fever is especially challenging. Some perspective on the incidence of the less common travelers' diseases is given by a study of 7886 Swiss short-term tourists traveling to developing countries in which no cases of typhoid fever, cholera, dengue, poliomyelitis, TB, or tetanus were reported.[1] In this case study, acute respiratory tract infections with fever, gastrointestinal infections (acute and chronic diarrheal disease and hepatitis), and sexually transmitted diseases accounted for 87% of illnesses acquired by short-term visitors to developing countries, with only 8% of illness diagnosed as malaria and 5% as helminthiasis.

Factors to be considered in arriving at the diagnosis of travelers' illness include: specific knowledge of the diseases endemic to the countries of travel, the incubation periods of the diseases being considered in a given patient, the mode of travel chosen by the patient, specific "risk" behavior (e.g., swimming in fresh water, sleeping in tents, sexual activity), immunizations and prophylactic drugs taken before and during the time of exposure, and details of medical care obtained during the trip as well as details of any over-the-counter medications taken. Many infectious diseases that are rare in developed countries may be contracted by travelers to developing countries, e.g., measles, brucellosis, listeriosis, anthrax, botulism, rabies, trichinosis, or tuberculosis.

Occasionally, illnesses presenting to the emergency department (ED) may be diseases of travel occurring in patients who have never left home. Scombroid poisoning and ciguatera poisoning from contaminated imported fish,[2] cholera imported in contaminated oysters,[3] and type E botulism from ungutted salted whitefish[4] are examples of these.

There are two general guiding principles in managing the illnesses of travel medicine: (1) most diagnoses are not made unless the specific disease is considered and sought, and (2) rare diseases, once found, should be promptly referred for expert management. Especially difficult to remember are diseases with long incubation periods, such as hydatid cyst disease or amoebic abscess, presenting months or even years after the initial infection.

Travel to the United States, Canada, Australia, New Zealand, and Western Europe is said to be associated with little or no risk of acquisition of a serious illness. Even travelers returning from parts of these relatively safe countries, however, may present to their hometown EDs with exotic illnesses: for example, plague or coccidioidomycosis acquired in the southwestern U.S., botulism acquired from sampling certain native Eskimo delicacies in Alaska, giardiasis from Rocky Mountain spring water, or hydatid cyst disease acquired from exposure to the sheepdog cycle.

Every ED should have the weekly Center for Disease Control (CDC) Morbidity and Mortality Weekly Report (MMWR). The MMWR provides current information on clusters of diseases reported from throughout the world and is invaluable as a source of continuing education and review of both common and rare diseases acquired by travelers. The CDC now also provides an international health requirements and recommendations hotline, available 24 hours a day by Touch-tone phone at 404-332-4559. Current information about vaccine and chemoprophylaxis recommendation, clinical information about diseases of travelers, and news of outbreaks of disease throughout the world are provided.

Advice for travelers preparing for a trip to developing countries is also provided in several publications with annual revisions and is not dealt with in detail in this chapter. The recommended publications are the CDC's Health Information for International Travel,[5] the World Health Organization's International Travel and Health,[6] The Medical Letter,[7] and the Scientific American Textbook of Medicine.[8]

It is worth emphasizing that tourists planning travel to developing countries should consult a physician who is skilled at giving travel advice 2 to 3 months before the trip so that plenty of time for gathering information about the specific area of travel and for administering needed vaccinations is available.

The remainder of this chapter does not attempt to duplicate detailed information found in textbooks of infectious disease.[9,10] but deals with the diagnostic approach to the ill returning traveler and considers the more common traveler's diseases.

DIARRHEAL DISEASE (SEE ALSO CHAP. 86)

Acute diarrheal disease is one of the most common illnesses acquired during travel, and may have any one of a large number of chemical, viral, bacterial, or parasitic causes. Enteropathogenic Escherichia coli, Shigella, Salmonella (including typhoid fever), and Campylobacter cause the large majority of cases of bacterial travelers' diarrhea. Cholera is rare, but may cause severe watery diarrhea requiring large volumes of replacement fluid and electrolytes.[10a] Type E botulism may present with diarrhea and should be considered in patients with an exposure history consistent with this disease. Viral diarrheas are generally as common as among nontravelers. Falciparum malaria may present as an afebrile illness resembling travelers' diarrhea. Plague may present as an afebrile or febrile gastroenteritis. Chronic diarrhea, acquired during travel, may be caused by Campylobacter (more common in one study of backpackers' diarrhea than giardiasis), Salmonella species, giardiasis, or Entomoeba coli. Chronic diarrhea in travelers to the tropics should be evaluated by stools collected both for culture and for ova and parasite examination, especially to detect amebiasis and thus avoid the long-term complications of liver abscess formation.

Preventive treatment regimens for travelers' diarrhea, including the use of bismuth subsalicylate, doxycyclines, trimethoprim-sulfamethoxaxole, and ciprofloxacin have been shown to be effective. Whether these regimens should be routinely used is somewhat controversial and is a decision best left to the patient and the consulting physician giving pre-travel advice.

Travelers' diarrhea, once acquired, can be effectively treated with loperamide or bismuth subsalicylate to help ameliorate symptoms. Trimethoprim alone, trimethoprim-sulfamethoxazole, or ciprofloxacin can be given as effective antibiotic treatment for travelers' diarrhea.

TYPHOID FEVER

Salmonella infections that persist beyond the diarrheal stage produce a clinical syndrome known as enteric fever; when specifically caused by Salmonella typhi, it is called typhoid fever. Usually the initial infection produces gastroenteritis with fever, nausea, vomiting, and diarrhea occurring within 6 to 48 hours after ingestion of contaminated foods. These symptoms clear within 2 to 7 days and, in the case of enteric fevers, are followed at 10 to 14 days by gradual onset of fever, headache, malaise, anorexia, and myalgias. Abdominal pain occurs in about one third of the patients, as does constipation. Hepatosplenomegaly is frequently seen; rose spots are seen as a transient blanching erythematous maculopapular rash in up to one half of patients. Confusion, lethargy, or coma may be seen in about 10% of patients. Sustained fever lasts 2 to 3 weeks in untreated cases.

Diagnosis of the enteric fever stage of illness is usually made by growth of the offending organism in blood culture. Stool cultures are frequently negative. The most efficient tissue for culture diagnosis is bone marrow aspirate, which may yield a positive culture even after partial treatment with chloramphenicol or other antibiotics. The differential diagnosis of typhoid fever is broad and includes malaria, miliary tuberculosis, brucellosis, lymphoma, endocarditis, meningoencephalitis, and causes of the acute surgical abdomen.

Treatment of the enteric fevers has been reported to be successful with the use of the new quinolones, including ciprofloxacin. Chloramphenicol may also be used, although it has been less successful in comparative trials. Septic complications of typhoid fever may require surgical drainage of abscesses or prolonged antimicrobial therapy.

HEPATITIS (SEE ALSO CHAP. 49)

Hepatitis A is endemic in developing countries; its acquisition by means of contaminated food presents considerable risk to the nonimmune traveler. Traveler's diarrhea and hepatitis A can be coinfections, and efforts to avoid the former help to avoid the latter. Further protection against hepatitis A can be offered by prophylactic administration of gamma globulin to travelers at particular risk, given as close to the time of exposure as possible.

Hepatitis B is endemic throughout the developing world. The visiting traveler may acquire this disease through sexual contact, blood transfusion, or contaminated needles (from IM injections, shared IV drug use, or acupuncture). Persons expecting to engage in high-risk behavior should be offered hepatitis-B vaccine before travel.

Non-A, non-B hepatitis may be enterically transmitted, and outbreaks have been reported from East Africa,[11] India, Nepal, Burma, Pakistan, and Russia. With a specific serologic assay available for this disease, more cases may be uncovered in the future.

SEXUALLY TRANSMITTED DISEASES

Careful questioning of the ill traveler about his or her sexual behavior during travel is important for several reasons. The risk of the acquisition of AIDS must be considered, especially in patients who have had sex with prostitutes. Sexual transmission of hepatitis B is common in Southeast Asia and Japan. The problem of penicillin-resistant gonorrhea acquired in foreign travel has been obviated somewhat by the availability of effective third-generation cephalosporins, but resistance must still be considered and follow-up cultures for test of cure are especially important in such circumstances. Lymphogranuloma venereum is more common in tropic and subtropic countries and should be considered in the traveler returning with inguinal buboes, mucopurulent or bloody rectal discharge with tenesmus and diarrhea, suppurative cervical lymphadenopathy, or primary genital ulcerative lesions.

MALARIA

Malaria is the most important disease to be considered in the ill traveler returning from the tropics. It is preventable, and recommendations for drug prophylaxis are summarized annually in the CDC's Recommendations for the Prevention of Malaria Among Travelers.[12] Advice is given concerning particular areas of travel, alternative drug regimens, clinical factors in choice of regimen such as age and presence of pregnancy, and the adverse effects of chemoprophylactic drugs. Detailed recommendations for the prevention of malaria are available 24 hours a day from the CDC Malaria Hotline at 404-332-4555. Failure of the traveler to carefully follow directions for malaria prophylaxis may result in acquisition of malaria.[13]

Malaria must always be considered in travelers returning from endemic areas with fever, and should always be searched for with thick film examinations of blood in such patients. It has also been seen in the U.S. in the Southwest and states along the Gulf of Mexico.[13a]Transmitted by the bite of mosquitoes, it presents after an incubation period of 10 days to 4 weeks with chills, high fever, sweats, and, especially during the height of the fever, with profound prostration. The patient may appear relatively well between paroxysms of parasitemia, but appear gravely ill at the height of the fever. Patients with malaria frequently complain of a feeling in their bones as though they had been "stashed in the freezer."

Four species of Plasmodium cause malaria: falciparum, vivax, ovale, and malaria. Initial injection of the malarial parasite by the mosquito bite is followed by travel of the parasite to the liver, where maturation occurs, followed by rupture of infected hepatocytes and invasion of red blood cells. Cycles of intracorpuscular maturation, rupture, and release cause paroxysms of chills and fever. (P. vivax and P. ovale can persist in the liver and may cause recurrent disease if not properly treated for the hepatic phase of the infection. P. falciparum and P. malaria are not maintained in hepatocytes.)

Plasmodium falciparum causes the most severe form of malaria, probably because it is able to infect all stages of the circulating erythrocyte; other species are limited to infections of the reticulocyte. About 150 U.S. travelers are diagnosed each year with P. falciparum, acquired from travel abroad. Most have visited subsaharan Africa. P. falciparum can obstruct the microcirculation and has protean clinical manifestations: pneumonia and/or ARDS; cerebritis with seizure and/or coma; abdominal pain, nausea, vomiting, and diarrhea; and acute intravascular hemolysis leading to profound anemia and hemoglobinuria with acute renal failure. Clinical manifestations other than fever may include jaundice (usually mild unless the disease is P. falciparum), hepatosplenomegaly, anemia, leukopenia, and thrombocytopenia.

The diagnosis of malaria is made by careful examination of stained thick and thin smears of peripheral blood, preferably by an experienced examiner. Malarial parasites must be distinguished from those of babesiosis in appropriate circumstances. The inexperienced examiner may misidentify platelets lying on red cells as malaria parasites, with disastrous consequences for the patient who actually has meningococcemia or typhoid fever.

Guidelines for the treatment of malaria change from year to year. In most parts of the malaria-endemic world, Plasmodium falciparum is resistant to chloroquine. The CDC's current publication recommendations for the prevention of malaria among travelers should also be consulted whenever a diagnosis of malaria has been made or is being considered, for advice concerning current treatment of established disease. The CDC hotline for international health information may also be consulted. The currently recommended drug for presumptive treatment of malaria is pyrimethamine-sulfadoxine (Fansidar). For adults, three tablets (75 mg pyrimethamine and 1500 mg sulfadoxine) are given orally as a single dose. For children weighing 5 to 10 kg, ½ tablet is given as a single dose; for children weighing 11 to 20 kg, 1 tablet is given as a single dose; for children weighing 21 to 30 kg, 2 tablets are given, and for children weighing more than 45 kg, the adult dose of 3 tablets given as a single dose is given. Cases of P. ovale or P. vivax should be treated also with primaquine, 15 mg daily for 2 weeks, to eradicate hepatic parasites. For patients with G6PD deficiency, 45 mg of primaquine given weekly for 8 weeks may minimize the risk of hemolysis, although the daily regimen is unlikely to cause any more than occasional, mild degrees of hemolysis. For treatment of severe malaria, parenteral quinidine by slow IV infusion is recommended.[13b] For details, call the Malaria Branch of the CDC at 404-488-4046.

DENGUE

Dengue is an acute febrile illness transmitted by Aedes aegypti, with a 5- to 8-day incubation period. It is endemic and at times epidemic in the tropical Americas, including parts of Mexico, and in Africa and Asia.[14] Fever with chills but no rigors, retro-orbital pain, headache, arthralgias, nausea and vomiting, cutaneous hyperesthesia, and altered taste sensation are seen. The fever lasts from 5 to 7 days, after which a maculopapular rash may appear with recurrence of fever. The rash lasts another day to 5 days and may desquamate. The palms and the soles are spared.

Severe hemorrhagic complications, with a mortality in untreated cases of 50%, may occur with dengue. Petechiae, gum bleeding, purpura, and epistaxis may occur. Circulatory failure may ensue. Lab abnormalities include thrombocytopenia, appearance of fibrin-split products, hyponatremia, decreased serum fibrinogen and clotting factors V, VII, IX, and X, and reduced serum complement. Mortality in treated dengue hemorrhagic shock syndrome is about 2%.

Diagnosis can be made by culture of the dengue virus from the blood during the first few days of illness, but dengue is more often diagnosed by acute and convalescent sera (at 7 to 14 days after onset of symptoms).

YELLOW FEVER

Yellow fever shares dengue endemicity in tropical areas of South America and Africa, but it has not been seen in Asia. Unlike dengue, however, yellow fever is a preventable disease, and yellow fever vaccine should be administered to all travelers to endemic areas except pregnant women and infants under 9 months.[15] Five percent of patients contracting yellow fever die. The liver, kidney, heart, and gastrointestinal tract are directly damaged by the virus; if sufficient liver damage occurs to cause jaundice, the case fatality rate rises to 20 to 50%.

A 3-to-6 day incubation period is followed by abrupt onset of fever, chills, headache, backache, nausea and vomiting, a flushed face with conjunctival injection, and leukopenia. After 3 days of illness, a brief remission (lasting several hours to a day) usually occurs,

followed by reappearance of fever, jaundice, hemolysis, hematemesis, oliguria, and albuminuria. Bradycardia inappropriate for the degree of fever, also seen in typhoid fever, is common in both phases of the disease. Death occurs 7 to 10 days after the onset of illness in fatal cases.

Diagnosis is made by virus isolation, detection of viral antigen by ELISA, or appearance of specific antibodies at 7 to 14 days into the illness.

MENINGOCOCCAL DISEASE

The incidence of endemic meningococcal disease in developed countries is about the same as the incidence of injury from lightning strikes. Travelers to areas of the world where meningococcal disease is hyperendemic or epidemic, however, should be considered at increased risk of having this disease as a cause of febrile illness on return. In recent years, equatorial Africa and Brazil have been particular areas of such risk.[16] The initial treatment of patients with fever who have returned from such areas should, of course, include penicillin or a cephalosporin active against the meningococcus. An effective vaccine available for most of the epidemic meningococcal groups should be offered to patients traveling to epidemic areas.

SCHISTOSOMIASIS

The flatworm human blood flukes cause significant morbidity and mortality throughout Africa, South America, and Asia.[17] Infection is acquired by swimming or wading in contaminated fresh water. The infective cercariae, derived from intermediate snail hosts, penetrate human skin. Initial infection is asymptomatic; subsequent exposures result in "swimmer's itch," a pruritic macular rash that occurs within 24 hours after penetration. The organisms then travel through lung and liver and assume habitation in the mesenteric blood vessels (for the species Schistosoma mansoni, S. mekongi, S. japonicum, and S. intercalatum) or in the urinary tract (S. hematobium). Egg-induced granuloma formation causes scarring with resulting portal hypertension from cirrhosis, pulmonary hypertension, or in the case of S. hematobium, ureteral obstruction.

The beginning of the release of eggs at 4 to 8 weeks after infection may produce an acute febrile illness (called Katayama fever), with fever, chills, headache, sweating, and cough. Hepatosplenomegaly, lymphadenopathy, and eosinophilia are found. The acute illness usually abates in a few weeks, but massive infection may progress to death.

Chronic interstitial schistosomiasis usually presents with fatigue, mild abdominal pain, and diarrhea (associated with chronic granulomas of the bowel wall). Hepatomegaly is first seen, followed by splenomegaly. Patients may present with bleeding esophageal varices years after the initial infection. Eosinophilia is usually present.

Urinary schistosomiasis usually presents with terminal hematuria and dysuria. IVP or ultrasound may demonstrate ureteral obstruction or renal or bladder filling defects.

Diagnosis depends on a travel history arousing suspicion followed by the demonstration of schistosome eggs in stool or urine, or by finding the organism in a biopsy of the rectum.

Treatment can be safely administered with a single dose of 40 mg per kg of praziquantel for S. mansoni or S. hematobium infection. For S. japonicum, 20 mg per kg is given 3 times a day for 1 day.

LEISHMANIASIS

The protozoan disease leishmaniasis, transmitted by sandfly bites, has an incubation period that averages 3 to 8 months, with a reported range of 10 days to 34 months. It may present as an acute febrile illness indistinguishable clinically from malaria, typhoid fever, acute schistosomiasis, or any one of many other febrile illnesses. It may also present as a chronic illness with prolonged fever, progressive weight loss, weakness, huge splenomegaly (the spleen is usually soft and nontender compared to the hard spleen of schistosomiasis), hepatomegaly, anemia, leukopenia, hypergammaglobulinemia, and hypoalbuminemia. The disease has been misdiagnosed as leukemia.[18] Infection may be asymptomatic or progress to full-blown kala-azar.

The diagnosis is made by a travel history arousing a high index of suspicion, followed usually by the demonstration of amastigotes in bone marrow aspirates. Splenic puncture is positive in 98% of cases but should be done only by experienced hands. Treatment is with pentavalent antimonial compounds given over at least 20 days and should be supervised by a physician experienced in the use of these drugs.

PLAGUE

Yersinia pestis infection occurs in the Southwestern United States, in South America, and the developing countries of Africa and Asia. Plague is transmitted by the bite of an infected flea or direct ingestion of contaminated meat (of rats, ground squirrels, rock squirrels, or prairie dogs). The bubonic form of the disease, with fever, chills, and a tender enlarged local lymph node, is the more common form. Septicemic plague without adenopathy accounts for a sizable minority of cases (up to 25%), and has a high case fatality rate because of the frequently missed diagnosis. Other forms of plague include meningitis, pharyngitis, pneumonia, and gastroenteritis.

Anyone with an unexplained febrile illness who has recently returned from an area endemic for plague (the incubation period is 2–8 days) should be treated with an antibiotic active against Y. pestis until this diagnosis has been ruled out with appropriate cultures.

Diagnosis is septicemic plague may be made by finding bipolar organisms in the routine Wright stain of peripheral blood, by culture of the blood, or retrospectively (in successfully treated cases) by demonstration of a four-fold or greater increase in hemagglutination titer, or presumptively by a single titer of greater than 1:16. Serology can be performed by the CDC. Diagnosis of bubonic plague can be made in the same way as for septicemic plague but is made more frequently by demonstrating bipolar staining organisms in an aspirate of the involved node, positive fluorescent antibody staining of a smear from the node aspirate, or positive culture of the node.

The usual drug of choice for plague is streptomycin, 30 mg per kg per day, in two divided doses, for 10 days for patients with normal renal function. For patients with hypotension and poor tissue perfusion, or with plague meningitis, chloramphenicol should be given intravenously (25 mg per Kg as the initial dose, followed by 60 mg per Kg per day in four divided doses; after the patient has improved sufficiently, oral chloramphenicol to finish a 10-day course may be given in a dose of 30 mg per Kg per day). For patients at the less ill end of the spectrum with buboes and mild disease, treatment with oral tetracycline or trimethaprim-sulfamethoxazole has been successful.

Patients with known or suspected plague should be placed in respiratory isolation for at least 48 hours after treatment has begun. Initial radiographs of the lung may be negative and cough may be absent. Contacts of patients with plague should be promptly placed on chemoprophylaxis with tetracycline or trimethaprim and sulfamethoxazole, preferably after prompt consultation with public health authorities.

POLIOMYELITIS

Paralytic poliomyelitis remains a problem in the developing countries of the world. Travelers to developing countries should have their polio vaccinations current. Acquisition of the virus can result in no symptoms at all in about 95% of cases, abortive poliomyelitis (associated with a nonspecific illness of a few hours to 2 to 3 days of fever, headache, anorexia, vomiting, and abdominal pain, with no specific features or clues to its diagnosis) in about 5% of cases, and rarely a frank paralysis in about 1 case in 1000. The incubation period for polio has a wide range, reported to be from about 1 to 7 weeks from virus acquisition to expression of symptoms.

PITFALLS

Illness in a traveler returning from the tropics or subtropics presents a considerable challenge to the emergency physician. Important principles of travel medicine to keep in mind are:

1. Many travelers' illnesses are preventable by proper planning, well in advance of travel, specifically geared toward the area of travel, with appropriate education regarding avoidance of vectors of disease, appropriate vaccination status attained before travel, and appropriate chemoprophylaxis.
2. Many travelers' illnesses are rarely seen in the ED. Careful history taking and physical examination must often be followed by early consultation with local infectious disease consultants or the CDC international travel 24-hour-a-day hotline 404-332-4559. Careful follow-up of returning travelers with early, seemingly minor complaints must be arranged.

REFERENCES

1. Steffen, R., Richenbach, M., Wilhelm, U.R.S., et al.: Health problems after travel to developing countries. J. Infect. Dis. 156:84, 1987.

2. CDC: Scombroid Fish Poisoning—Illnois, South Carolina. M.M.W.R. 38:140, 1989.
3. CDC: Toxigenic Vibrio Cholerae 01 Infection Acquired in Colorado. M.M.W.R. 38:19, 1989.
4. CDC: International outbreak of type E botulism associated with ungutted, salted whitefish. M.M.W.R. 36:812, 1987.
5. Centers for Disease Control (CDC): Health Information for International Travel, 1990. Write: Superintendent of Documents, U.S. Government Printing Office, Washington, DC 20402.
6. World Health Organization: International Travel and Health. Vaccination Requirements and Health Advice, 1990. Write: WHO Regional Office for the Americas, Regional Adviser, Epidemiology, Pan American Sanitary Bureau, 525 Twenty Third Street, N.W., Washington, DC, 20037.
7. Advice for travelers. Medical Letter 32:33, 1990.
8. Weller, P.F.: Health advice for international travelers. Sci. Am. Med., Curr. Top. Med. 4:1, 1989.
9. Hoeprich, P.D., and Jordan, M.C.: Infectious Diseases. Philadelphia, J.B. Lippincott Company, 1989.
10. Mandell, G.L.; Douglas, R.G., Jr., and Bennett, J.E.: Principles and Practices of Infectious Disease. New York, Churchill Livingstone, 1990.
11. CDC: Enterically transmitted non-A, non-B hepatitis—East Africa. M.M.W.R. 36:241, 1987.
12. CDC: Recommendations for prevention of malaria among travelers. M.M.W.R. (No. RR-3), 1990.
13. CDC: Malaria in travelers returning from Kenya; failure of self-treatment with pyrimethamine/sulfadoxine. M.M.W.R. 38:363, 1989.
13a. Cholera—New Jersey and Florida. M.M.W.R. 40:287, 1991.
13b. CDC: Treatment with quinidine gluconate of persons with severe Plasmodium falciparum infection: Discontinuation of parenteral quinine from CDC drug service. M.M.W.R. 40 No. RR-4, 1991.
14. CDC: Imported dengue fever—United States. M.M.W.R. 40:519, 1991.
15. CDC: Yellow fever vaccine: Recommendations of the immunization practices advisory committee (ACIP). M.M.W.R. 39 (No. RR-6), 1990.
16. CDC: Meningococcal disease among travelers returning from Saudi Arabia. M.M.W.R. 36:559, 1987.
17. CDC: Acute schistosomiasis in U.S. travelers returning from Africa. M.M.W.R. 39:140, 147, 1990.
18. London, O. Kill as Few Patients as Possible. Ten Speed Press, 1987, pp. 7–8.

WILDERNESS INFECTIOUS DISEASES

Sharon Kolber

CAPSULE

Wilderness-acquired zoonoses, although not new diseases, are affecting a new population.

Recreational activities are exposing more individuals to flea, tick, and other insect bites, contaminated surface water, animal bites, and animal fluids and tissues through handling. These infections are not common, but take their toll in lives lost each year. Education, adequate immunizations, and increased awareness among medical personnel will improve the diagnosis and treatment of these illnesses.

This chapter reviews leptospirosis, plague, rabies, tetanus, tick-borne diseases, tularemia, infectious diarrhea, and water disinfection and purification.

LEPTOSPIROSIS

Leptospirosis is caused by the spirochete Leptospira interrogans. This species is divided into two complexes: interrogans, which contains most of the pathogenic strains; and biflexa, which is a saphrophytic organism with no known living hosts.[1] There are 25 serogroups and 188 serotypes (serovars) known at this time.[2] The most common organism to infect humans is L. interrogans, serovar icterohaemorrhagiae.

These spirochetes are found throughout the United States and are common in tropical areas of the world. Most cases in the U.S. occur in the South.[3] Outbreaks are more common in summer and early autumn and most occur in men and boys of teen to middle age.

The reservoir hosts of leptospirosis are commonly rodents (rats, mice, moles), but a wide variety of animals have been found to be carriers. These include cattle, pigs, dogs, hedgehogs, foxes, jackals, mongooses, skunks, raccoons, bandicoots, bats, deer, and rabbits. Man is only accidentally involved in the chain of infection. Outbreaks in humans may be associated with epidemics among domestic animals, including cattle and dogs. The host animals carry *Leptospira* in their kidneys that can be excreted in the urine, contaminating fresh water, muddy soil, or food.

Transmission of the spirochete occurs through penetration of mucous membranes (i.e., nose, mouth, conjunctiva, genitalia) or skin barriers, especially abraded or diseased areas. Ticks can carry the organism but are of little importance in transmission of the disease. In past decades, leptospirosis was found predominantly in sewer workers, farmers, slaughterhouse workers, and other occupations with direct animal contact. In Thailand and Vietnam, cases are associated with work in rice fields. In the last decade, the rates of infection in these occupations have decreased, but an increasing rate has been found associated with recreational activities such as swimming, rafting, kayaking, and mountain biking through streams and puddles.

CLINICAL PRESENTATION

When obtaining the patient history, inquiries should be made about exposure to natural surface water, animals, and recent illnesses in the family.[4] The incubation period is 1 to 2 weeks after exposure. Symptoms are abrupt in onset in 75 to 100% of patients[5] and include fever, chills, myalgias, and headaches. Other findings include conjunctival injection, nausea, vomiting, diarrhea, abdominal pain, jaundice, nonproductive cough, petechiae, and photophobia. Less commonly seen are an injected pharynx, lymphadenopathy, maculopapular rash, and profound, cutaneous hyperesthesia.[5] Signs of meningitis or pneumonia may also be seen.

Weil's syndrome is the severe form of the disease, which includes complications of shock, hepatitis, renal failure, hemorrhage, aseptic meningitis, or rarely, myocarditis. The mortality of Weil's syndrome is up to 40%, whereas that of anicteric leptospirosis is around 1%.[6]

LABORATORY EVALUATION

A complete evaluation includes a CBC with platelets, liver function tests, electrolytes, BUN, creatinine, coagulation studies, blood cultures, sputum culture, urinalysis and culture, and chest x ray. Blood should also be collected for antibody titer.

Laboratory evaluation may reveal an elevated or decreased WBC count, but frequently with 75 to 90% neutrophils.[1] Sputum, if present, may be blood-tinged. Urinalysis often shows some red blood cells (RBCs) and white blood cells (WBCs) as well as protein. Hepatic involvement occurs in 50 to 59% of patients with leptospirosis, producing jaundice (10%) and/or moderate increases in hepatic transaminases.[4,6] Pulmonary involvement produces bilateral infiltrates, often with peripheral predominance.[7] Initial patchy lesions may progress to consolidation and ground-glass appearance on chest x ray.[4] Renal involvement has been found in 22% of patients,[4] with 7 to 8% developing acute renal failure. In Edward's series of 24 patients with leptospirosis, 54% were found to have thrombocytopenia.[8] In this group, both thrombocytopenic and nonthrombocytopenic patients had mildly increased fibrin degradation products with otherwise normal coagulation studies.[8]

Diagnosis of leptospirosis is made by positive blood, urine, or sputum culture or increased antibody titers. Leptospira may be isolated from blood or CSF cultures in the first 4 to 9 days of the illness. Antibody agglutination titers, however, may not increase until 6 to 12 days after onset of the illness, and if antibiotics are given early, the antibody titer may not increase at all. If antibiotics are started within 5 days of onset, peak antibody titers are low. If antibiotics are started within 1 to 2 days of onset, there may be no antibody reaction.[1] Darkfield microscopy may show organisms.

MANAGEMENT

Treatment includes supportive care, analgesia, and antibiotics. Historically, leptospirosis has been treated with penicillin, although controlled studies of its efficacy are unavailable. In England, amoxicillin, 500 mg t.i.d. for 5 days, is believed to be empirically successful. In vitro studies have suggested penicillin, tetracycline, and erythromycin as useful drugs. McClain et al. studied doxycycline versus placebo in the treatment of leptospirosis and found that doxycycline, 100 mg b.i.d., decreased the duration of illness by 2 days, decreased the fever, malaise, myalgias, and headache, and prevented leptospirosis if given in the first few days of the illness.[9] Jarisch-Herxheimer reactions have been reported 4 to 6 hours after treatment with antibiotics. This reaction has been noted to cause a sharp temperature spike, marked hypotension, and precipitation or aggravation of the common signs and symptoms.

Supportive care for hepatic, pulmonary, and renal involvement is necessary as mortality increases to 15 to 40% with these complications.[5]

PREVENTION

Prevention efforts such as rodent control, pet immunizations, and use of protective and waterproof garments have had a significant impact on outbreaks of leptrospirosis. Doxycycline, 200 mg per week, was used prophylactically in Panama and was 96% efficacious in preventing infection. The incidence of infection in the placebo group was 4.2% and 0.2% in the doxycycline group.[10]

Vaccines have been produced, but are serotype-specific and have limited utility with this organism's many serotypes. Pet immunizations are important for prevention, but leptospirosis has been found in pets with adequate immunization.

PLAGUE

Although plague presently has not the impact of previous epidemics, it is still a potentially fatal disease in the United States today. Between 1975 and 1984, an average of 20 cases per year were reported in this country. The fatality rate of these cases was 18%.[11] This disease is endemic to all continents except Australia. In the U.S., cases have been reported in 14 Western states, with most occurring in New Mexico, Arizona, Colorado, California, Oregon, and Nevada.[12]

Yersinia pestis, the causative agent of plague, is a gram-negative rod endemic to the western rodent population, including squirrels and prairie dogs.[13] Epizootics may include rabbits, field mice, and wood rats. Transmission of plague occurs most commonly by flea bite, but may also result from direct exposure to animal fluids (e.g., skinning infected animals) or aerosolization of bacteria from animals with pneumonic plague. Infected fleas may reside on pets that are allowed to roam and transport the bacteria into the home. Cats usually become ill when infected, but dogs show few symptoms. It is believed that a flea bite may discharge up to 100,000 organisms.

Studies of the transmission of plague have shown that 66 to 82% were caused by flea bites, 15 to 22% by direct contact with infected animals, and 11% by equivocal causes, and in one series, 3% were secondary to contact with domestic cats.[14-16] Since 1970, animal surveillance has included serosurveys of wild carnivores and dogs on U.S. Indian reservations because these seem to reflect plague epizootics in the rodent population. In 1983, 19 cases of plague were found among dogs on Navajo reservations in New Mexico.

Plague may present as bubonic, septicemic, or pneumonic disease or a minor syndrome. Bubonic plague presents with a bubo or lymphadenitis with high fever and constitutional symptoms. The mortality of untreated bubonic plague is 50–60%.[17] Septicemic plague is diagnosed by positive blood cultures with or without the lymphadenitis and presents as fever and abdominal symptoms, but may be complicated by septic shock, disseminated intravascular coagulation, thrombosis, and necrosis of internal organs.[18] Pneumonic plague may occur as the presenting infection or develop secondary to bubonic or septicemic plague. Pneumonic plague has a 100% mortality if untreated. Pestis minor presents with mild symptoms and lymphadenopathy.

CLINICAL PRESENTATION

The patient should be questioned about residence in a rural area or recent travel to an endemic area. In addition, inquiry should be made about pets in the home and outdoor activities such as hunting, trapping, hiking, or camping. Hull showed that the greatest risk factor in New Mexico is residence in a rural area. Of 84 cases between 1980 and 1985, 12% were related to hunting or trapping, 8% were associated with hiking, camping or picnicking, and 80% were related to fleas from epizootic outbreaks near home or work or transport by pet to the home.[19]

The classic symptoms of bubonic plague are fever and tender lymphadenitis usually occurring in inguinal, axillary, or cervical nodes. Fever, abdominal pain, and leukocytosis with a left shift are typical findings. Atypical presentations may include exudative pharyngitis, conjunctivitis, meningitis,[20] pneumonia, or an acute abdomen. Evidence of bites may or may not be present. Local cutaneous ulcers or pustular lesions may occur in 10% of patients.[17]

In a review of 71 cases of plague by Hull et al., 57% of patients had GI symptoms, and these symptoms were more common in septicemic than bubonic plague. Septicemic plague is difficult to diagnose because no specific symptoms differentiate it from other infections. Symptoms include fever, chills, malaise, headache, nausea, vomiting, diarrhea, and abdominal pain. Signs include tachycardia, tachypnea, and hypotension. The nonspecific signs and symptoms make the diagnosis difficult, and delayed diagnosis contributes to the morbidity and mortality. Untreated septicemic plague is invariably fatal. Patients over 40 years old have a greater risk of developing septicemic plague than bubonic plague, but the risk of death from septicemic plague is greater in those under 30 years old because more of the older patients receive empiric antibiotic treatment.[21]

Pneumonic plague presents as the primary manifestation of plague or following septicemic or bubonic plague. Patients appear acutely ill, with cough, dyspnea, and, in later stages, cyanosis. The sputum is frequently blood-tinged. Respiratory isolation must be maintained for 72 to 96 hours after treatment is started.

DIFFERENTIAL DIAGNOSIS

Septicemic plague is difficult to differentiate from any other severe systemic illness. Malaria, typhoid, and typhus should be considered in the differential. Pneumonic plague may be confused with any gram-negative pneumonia, mycoplasma, or streptococcal pneumonia. Bubonic plague may be confused with staphylococcal or streptococcal lymphadenitis, cat scratch fever, lymphogranuloma venereum, syphilis, or tularemia.[22]

LABORATORY PROCEDURES

Yersinia pestis appears as a gram-negative bacillus with a bipolar or "safety pin" appearance. Positive blood cultures are diagnostic of septicemic plague. Cultures may also be obtained by aspiration of the bubo. A fluorescent antibody stain may be performed on this aspirate. This test is sensitive and specific, and in some states may be available on the same day.[19] Serologic tests for antibodies may also be performed. A fourfold change in acute and convalescent passive hemagglutination titers over at least 10 days or a single convalescent titer of 1:16 or greater is diagnostic. Serum antibody is usually not detected, however, until day 8 to 14 of the disease.

IMMUNIZATION

A formalin killed vaccine is available and is recommended for people who are exposed to plague by their occupation or travel to endemic areas. Use is not widespread because plague is a rare disease, and frequent immunization is required.[12]

MANAGEMENT

Early treatment is essential when plague is suspected, especially septicemic or pneumonic plague. Streptomycin is the drug of choice, although tetracycline and chloramphenicol may also be used.

Streptomycin: Adults, 30 mg/kg/day in 2 to 4 divided doses IM for 10 days.[23,24] Children, 20 to 40 mg/kg/day IM in 2 to 4 divided doses for 10 days. Infants, 10 to 20 mg/kg/day IM in 2 to 4 divided doses for 10 days.[17]

Tetracycline: 12 to 20 mg/kg/day IV in divided doses for 10 days.[17] Oral = 15 mg/kg (maximum 1 g as loading dose) followed by 30 mg/kg/day in 4 divided doses.

Chloramphenicol: (indicated if meningitis or hypotension present): 50 to 75 mg/kg/day IV in 4 divided doses.[17,24]

TMP-SMX may be used if all other agents are contraindicated.[21]

Gentamicin is felt to be effective, although controlled trials are not available. The dosage is 5 mg/kg/day in 3 to 4 divided doses IV, then decrease to 3 mg/kg/day on clinical improvement.[17]

If the patient is treated empirically, blood cultures or acute and convalescent titers are needed to confirm the diagnosis.

Buboes can be treated with hot, moist packs. Incision and drainage are usually not indicated unless there is poor resolution with antibiotics and symptomatic treatment.

Patients should be kept in respiratory isolation for 48 to 72 hours and observed for respiratory signs and symptoms. If there is evidence of pneumonic plague, isolation should continue until the patient has received 96 hours of antibiotics.[25]

PROPHYLAXIS

Contacts of the patient should be examined for evidence of illness. Outbreaks are more likely to be secondary to exposure to the same transmitting organisms than from human-to-human transmission. Prophylaxis is not indicated for contacts of nonpneumonic cases, but patient contacts should be kept under surveillance. Prophylaxis for persons exposed to pneumonic plague consists of tetracycline 15 mg/kg/day orally, or TMP-SMX for 7 days if the patient is pregnant or under 8 years old.[17,23]

PITFALLS

Diagnosis of septicemic plague is difficult on initial presentation, yet this disease is rapidly progressive and may be fatal even with early initiation of therapy. In Hull's series in New Mexico from 1980 to 1984, only 17% of the patients with septicemic plague had the diagnosis suspected on admission. Inaccurate diagnosis of septicemic plague was present in 83% of the patients who died.[26] Nonendemic areas may have higher mortality rates secondary to delay in diagnosis because of less familiarity with this disease.[17] Early treatment is the key.

RABIES

Rabies must be considered among wilderness-acquired zoonoses because wild animals—skunks, bats, raccoons, and foxes—are responsible for 81% of the cases of rabies in the temperate zone of America. This differs from many of the Latin American countries, in which the majority of cases are from dogs, cats, and other domestic animals.[27]

The rabies virus is a neurotropic bullet-shaped rhabdovirus that produces fatal encephalitis. Transmission occurs by way of bites from infected animals, inhalation of aerosolized virus (e.g., in bat caves), or exposure to mucous membranes or broken skin. The incubation period is usually 1 to 2 months but can be as short as 10 days or up to 2 years. The virus replicates and travels up nerves to the spinal cord and brain.

Most (80%) of the patients present with classic symptoms of a nonspecific prodrome followed by excessive motor activity and brainstem dysfunction. Fever, chills, myalgias, malaise, headache, photophobia, mental status changes, and upper respiratory and GI symptoms may occur. These symptoms may progress to pharyngeal spasm, grimacing, opisthotonos, and seizures. SIADH, dysrhythmias, and hallucinations are not uncommon. Twenty percent of patients present with paralytic rabies, showing paresis, pain, and flaccid paralysis with progression. The differential diagnosis should include other viral causes of encephalitis, poliomyelitis, Guillain-Barré syndrome, and acute transverse myelitis.[28]

Management relies on early diagnosis. High-risk bites are those of bats, skunks, bobcats, badgers, wolves, coyotes, weasels, raccoons, and foxes. Moderate risk is attributed to stray dogs, cats, and pet skunks. Low risk is associated with pet dogs, cats, and farm animals. Negligible risk is present with rodents and rabbits. Many of animals are asymptomatic when they have rabies, and therefore behavior is not a reliable indicator of infection. If the biting animal can be safely caught, it can be examined for rabies. Wounds on the hands, arms, and head are at greater risk of rapid progression.

Treatment is with human rabies immunoglobulin, 20 IU/kg IM, with one half of the dose at the bite site and one half IM elsewhere. Human diploid cell vaccine is given, 1 cc. IM on 0, 3, 7, 14, and 28 days from injury. Tetanus prophylaxis and aggressive wound care are essential; cleansing the wound with 20% soap solution or 1% aqueous benzalkonium chloride followed by rinsing is effective.[29] These wounds should not be closed with sutures. Rabies is discussed further in Chapter 65, Mammalian Bites.

TETANUS

Tetanus still accounts for about 50 deaths per year in the U.S. in spite of our immunization program. People at increased risk include intravenous drug abusers and foreign-born and elderly people. In 1987 and 1988, 71% of patients with tetanus were over 50.[30] The case fatality rate is still 21 to 31%.[30,31] The vast majority (94%) of tetanus cases from 1985 to 1986 were in patients who had not received their primary series of vaccinations.[31]

Tetanus is caused by the exotoxin of Clostridium tetani, a gram-positive anaerobic spore-forming rod. The bacteria and spores are ubiquitous. The bacteria produce a toxin, tetanospasmin, which interferes with inhibitory neurotransmitters, causing spasm, tachycardia, sweating, and arrhythmias. The usual cause of death is the inability to ventilate because of paralysis.

A history of tetanus-prone wounds is found in 70% of cases.[31] Presentation may be generalized, local, or cephalic. Generalized cases present with trismus or spasm of the muscles of mastication. Opisthotonus, which is spasm of the stronger posterior back muscles causing lumbar lordosis and extension of the neck and legs with arm flexion, is common. Noise or light may trigger these spasms.

Localized tetanus presents with spasm only in a particular muscle group. This less common form may continue for weeks and be self-limited. Cephalic tetanus presents as trismus with paralysis of one or more cranial nerves.[32] Neonatal tetanus presents with restlessness and failure to nurse, progressing to tetany and sympathetic overactivity.

Management of tetanus includes supportive care, which may include mechanical ventilation with pharmacologic paralysis, plus excision or débridement of the wound, human tetanus immunoglobulin (3000 to 10,000 units IM) and penicillin G, 2 million units IV every 4 hours. Sedation and beta-blockers may be useful in controlling excess sympathetic activity. A dark and quiet environment decreases stimulation.

Prevention of tetanus would be easy if all patients were up to date on their vaccinations. Adequate immunization is 99% effective, yet many deaths occur yearly in the U.S. Increased attention to immunization status, especially in people over 50, and attention to wound care can decrease the incidence of tetanus.

TICK-BORNE DISEASES

Numerous diseases are spread by tick bites in the U.S., including Lyme disease, Rocky Mountain spotted fever, Colorado tick fever, relapsing fever, tick paralysis, and others. Most of these illnesses are associated with a particular region of the U.S. For example, Lyme disease occurs most often in the New England States, Minnesota, and Wisconsin, whereas Rocky Mountain spotted fever is most prevalent in the Southeastern U.S.

Commonly, tick-borne infections present with fever, chills, myalgias, headache, and sometimes a rash. Diagnosis is made by identification of the infecting organism or toxin, antibody titers, or cultures; treatment is specific to each organism.

TULAREMIA

Francisella tularensis is the causative gram-negative bacillus in tularemia. It is transmitted by the bite of ticks or deer flies, or by handling or ingestion of infected animals. F. tularensis has been found in rabbits, hares, rodents, moles, beavers, muskrats, squirrels, rats, and mice. Tularemia presents with fever, chills, malaise, and fatigue. Most cases are of the ulceroglandular type, exhibiting a painful skin ulcer and tender lymphadenopathy.

Diagnosis of tularemia is made by history and these symptoms and signs, often accompanied by hepatosplenomegaly or pneumonia. Skin testing and agglutination titers are used to provide laboratory diagnosis. Recommended treatment is with streptomycin, 30 to 40 mg/kg/day IM in two divided doses for 3 days, then one half the dose for 4 to 7 days more.

WILDERNESS-ACQUIRED DIARRHEA

Use of surface water as drinking water may lead to diarrhea if adequate disinfection is not performed. Surface water in the U.S. may be contaminated with many organisms. As with gastroenteritis, often the cause is viral and is not identified. In addition, enteric bacteria such as Shigella, Salmonella, and Campylobacter may be found in surface water. Giardia lamblia probably accounts for most of the identified causes of wilderness acquired diarrhea. Leptospira and Entamoeba histolytica may also be present.

WATER DISINFECTION IN THE WILDERNESS

Surface water in U.S. wilderness areas may be contaminated with chemicals, organic debris, bacteria, viruses, and parasites such as Giardia lamblia or Entamoeba histolytica. Ingestion by humans may result in gastroenteritis or diarrhea, and the risk of infection depends on the number of organisms ingested. Care must be taken to disinfect this water adequately before it is used for drinking.

Many products are available for disinfection and purification of water. Heat is probably the most effective way of killing all microorganisms in the water. Bacteria, viruses, Giardia, and other cysts are killed by boiling.[29] The disadvantage of this method is that it requires fuel and a fire or stove.

Filtration is an effective method of disinfection if the filter has a small enough pore size (i.e., 0.2 microns) to adequately filter bacteria and Giardia cysts. Filters are not recommended as the sole means of disinfection if viruses are a concern (i.e., in foreign travel).

Iodine and chlorine are used frequently and are easy methods of disinfection. Ongerth et al. found iodine more effective than chlorine in the disinfection of water contaminated with Giardia cysts.[33] Iodine is not recommended however, if the patient has unstable thyroid disease or previous reactions to iodine or may be pregnant. Chlorine or iodine doses may need to be doubled if water is cloudy. Use of charcoal or filters following adequate concentrations and exposure time to the halogens (chlorine, iodine) may make the water more palatable. Specific recommendations for use of each form of iodine may be obtained from manufacturers or the local health department.

REFERENCES

1. Turner, L.H.: Leptospirosis. Brit. Med. J. *1*:231, 1969.
2. Waitkins, S.A.: Leptospirosis as an occupational disease. Brit. J. Indust. Med. *43*:721, 1986.
3. Heath, C.W. et al.: Leptospirosis in the United States. N. Engl. J. Med. *273*:857, 1965.
4. Cacciapuoti, B., et al.: A waterborne outbreak of leptospirosis. Am. J. Epidemiol. *126*:535, 1987.

5. Sanford, J.: Leptospirosis—Time for a booster. N. Engl. J. Med. *310*:524, 1984.
6. Jevon, T.R., et al.: A point-source epidemic of leptospirosis. Postgrad Med. *80*:121, 1986.
7. Im, J., et al.: Leptospirosis of the lung. Am. J. Radiol. *152*:955, 1989.
8. Edwards, C.N., et al.: Thrombocytopenia in leptospirosis. The absence of evidence for disseminated intravascular coagulation. Am. J. Trop. Med. *35*:352, 1986.
9. McClain, B.L., et al.: Doxycycline therapy for leptospirosis. Ann. Intern. Med. *100*:696, 1984.
10. Takafuji, E.T., et al.: An efficacy trial of doxycycline prophylaxis against leptospirosis. *310*:497, 1984.
11. Barnes, A.M., et al.: Plague in the United States, 1984. MMWR. CDC surveillance summary. *34*:9SS, 1985.
12. Doll, J., et al.: Human plague—United States, 1988. MMWR. *37*:653, 1988.
13. Johnson, J.E.: *Yersinia (Pasteurella)* infections, including plague. *In* Harrison's Principles of Internal Medicine. Tenth Edition. Edited by Petersdorf et al., New York, McGraw-Hill, 1983, pp. 979–981.
14. Barnes, A.M., et al.: Plague in American Indians, 1956–1987. MMWR. CDC Surveillance Summary. *37*:11, 1988.
15. Eidson, M., et al.: Feline plague in New Mexico: Risk factors and transmission to humans. Am. J. Public Health *78*:1333, 1988.
16. Kaufmann, A., et al.: Trends in human plague in the United States. J. Infect. Dis. *141*:522, 1980.
17. Welty, T.K.: Plague. Am. Fam. Physician *33*:159, 1986.
18. Humphrey, M., et al.: *Yersinia pestis:* A case of mistaken identity. Pediatr. Infect. Dis. J. *7*:365, 1988.
19. Hull, H.F., et al.: Plague (letter). West. J. Med. *145*:393, 1986.
20. Becker, T.M., et al.: Plague meningitis—A retrospective analysis of cases reported in the United States, 1970–1979. West. J. Med. *147*:554, 1987.
21. Hull, H.F., et al.: Plague masquerading as gastrointestinal illness. West. J. Med. *145*:485, 1986.
22. Butler, T., et al.: Plague and tularemia. Pediatr. Clin. North Am. *26*:355, 1979.
23. Ganem, D.E.: Plasmids and pestilence—Biological and clinical aspects of bubonic plague. West. J. Med. *144*:447, 1986.
24. Leopold, J.C.: Septicemic plague in a 14 month old child. Pediatr. Infect. Dis. *5*:108, 1986.
25. Welty, T.K., et al.: Nineteen cases of plague in Arizona. West. J. Med. *142*:641, 1985.
26. Hull, H.F., et al.: Septicemic plague in New Mexico. J. Infect. Dis. 1987; *155*:113, 1987.
27. Steele, J.H.: Rabies in the Americas and remarks on global aspects. Rev. Infect. Dis. 1988; 10(Suppl.*10*): S595–S597, 1988.
28. Kauffman, F.H., et al.: Rabies. Am. J. Emer. Med. *4*:525, 1986.
29. Auerbach, P.S., and Geehr, E.C.: Management of Wilderness and Environmental Emergencies. St. Louis, MO, C.V. Mosby, 1989.
30. CDC: Tetanus—United States, 1987 and 1988. MMWR *39*:37, 1990.
31. CDC: Tetanus—United States, 1985–1986. MMWR *36*:477, 1987.
32. Jagoda, A., et al.: Cephalic tetanus. Am. J. Emerg. Med. *6*:128, 1988.
33. Ongerth, J.E., et al.: Backcountry water treatment to prevent giardiasis. Am. J. Public Health. December *79*:1633, 1989.

Chapter 77

SUN-INDUCED DISORDERS

David A. Kramer and Richard Steinmark

CAPSULE

The medical manifestations of solar radiation are myriad. Emergency physicians can expect to see more of these disorders as exposure increases. It is important to recognize a photosensitivity reaction so that the offending drug may be avoided. A handful of medications is implicated over and over again: sulfonamides, tetracyclines, thiazides, and phenothiazines. The most frequent of the sun-induced afflictions continues to be sunburn, which is by no means always benign and may at times warrant hospital admission. Several systemic conditions are dramatically worsened by sun exposure. Most important among these are the porphyrias and lupus erythematosus, with a few other congenital metabolic diseases being less common. Skin cancer is also clearly related to sun exposure. The mainstay of management for these conditions is prevention with topical sunscreens.

INTRODUCTION

Sun-induced maladies are increasing at an alarming rate, largely because of an increase in sun exposure, specifically exposure to ultraviolet radiation. Outdoor recreational activities and sunbathing continue to gain popularity. In the Victorian era, a suntan was usually the result of hard outdoor labor, and was therefore considered a blemish of the working class. Now a suntan signifies leisure time, is considered esthetic, and most ironically, is even thought of as a "healthy glow." To cater to these perceptions, an entire new industry has developed: tanning salons. But perhaps most concerning of all is atmospheric ozone depletion by halogenated hydrocarbons. Already, large holes have been formed in the polar regions of our most important filter for short wavelength ultraviolet rays. Despite United States bans on fluorocarbon-containing aerosol sprays, large amounts of these chemicals continue to spew forth, further jeopardizing the remaining ozone. These issues have not gone unnoticed by the scientific community. Over the past 10 years, a proliferation of medical literature has generated an awareness of the problems among lay persons as well as health workers. These concerns have prompted an onslaught of consumer products, both over-the-counter and prescription, aimed at sun protection.

The health consequences of solar radiation are numerous. Photosensitivity reactions are the most important of the acute disorders. Sunburn is the most common adverse effect of ultraviolet radiation on the human body. Polymorphous light eruption (PMLE) and solar urticaria are two additional acute cutaneous eruptions caused by sunlight. Several ocular conditions are caused by solar damage to the eye. Furthermore, some systemic diseases are greatly exacerbated by sun exposure, most notably lupus and the porphyrias. Finally, the long-term effects of solar radiation are significant, and include skin cancer and premature aging. These are currently major public health concerns. Emergency physicians are called on to recognize and treat many of these conditions and make specific recommendations for preventive measures.

PATHOPHYSIOLOGY AND ANATOMY

The sun emits electromagnetic radiation over a broad range of wavelengths. About 40% of this energy falls in the visible spectrum (400 to 700 nm). Fifty-one percent is infrared, and microwave, gamma ray, and charged particle emission together account for only 1% of the total. The remaining 9% of the energy is emitted as ultraviolet radiation (UVR), which is subdivided into UVA (320 to 400 nm), UVB (290 to 320 nm), and UVC (200 to 290 nm).[1] The UVR is responsible for almost all sun-induced disorders.

The primary determinant of UVR transmission through the atmosphere is its absorption by ozone. A 1% decrease in ozone allows 3% more UVB to reach the earth's surface.[1] Other factors influence UV penetration as well. These include altitude (4% increase per 1000 feet), reflection from snow, sand, and, to a lesser extent, water (but UVR penetrates 40% down to 50 cm of water). Of course, season (130 times more in summer than winter) and time of day (50% of UVR arrives between 11 AM and 1 PM) are also important in determining UV exposure.[2] UV light, in contrast to visible light, is blocked by window glass.

For electromagnetic radiation to invoke biologic damage, it must first be absorbed. The major light-absorbing molecules in human skin include melanin, keratins, porphyrins, aromatic amino acids, and peptide bonds. These are termed chromophores. The absorption of energy alters the chromophore and produces an excited state, which leads to either free radical formation, another chemical reaction, or simply liberation of heat or light (fluorescence). The wavelength that induces a particular disease manifestation is referred to as the action spectrum for that disease. For example, UVB is responsible for sunburn, whereas UVA is implicated in many phototoxic drug reactions. UVC, which is effectively absorbed by ozone, is generated by germicidal or mercury lamps and causes skin erythema and keratoconjunctivitis, even at low doses.[3,4]

The prototypical and best studied reaction to UVR is erythema, or the sunburn reaction. The smallest amount of energy required to produce erythema in a given individual is termed the minimal erythema dose (MED). The histologic changes of sunburn are maximal in the skin at 24 hours after exposure. Epidermal alterations consist of shrunken, dyskeratotic cells with unrecognizable or pyknotic nuclei, called sunburn cells. In addition, a mixed inflammatory infiltrate develops in the dermis. Dermal changes are primarily caused by UVA, which has greater tissue penetration, whereas epidermal changes are due to UVB, which is more erythrogenic. Melanin protects by acting as a filter, absorbing UVR, and probably trapping free radicals produced by UVR.[4]

CLINICAL CONSIDERATIONS

PHOTOSENSITIVITY

There are two types of photosensitivity reactions, phototoxic and photoallergic. A photosensitizing compound acts as a chromophore, absorbing light energy and causing tissue damage either directly or indirectly. Indirectly, the compound functions as a low molecular weight hapten that becomes photoactivated, enabling binding to a carrier protein. The hapten-protein complex then acts as a photoantigen that produces an immunologic reaction. This is referred to as photoallergy. When a direct, nonimmunologic process is involved, the phenomenon is referred to as phototoxicity. Phototoxic reactions are much more common

than photoallergic reactions.[5] Listed in Table 77-1 are drugs and chemicals clearly implicated in these processes.

Phototoxicity was originally thought of as an exaggerated sunburn response, and on the surface there are many similarities. Common to both are erythema and edema of sun-exposed skin. Later, hyperpigmentation and desquamation are noted. The mechanisms and evolution of the processes are, however, distinctly different. The action spectrum for photosensitivity reactions is almost always UVA; they may therefore occur without a sunburn (which is primarily caused by UVB). Classically, phototoxicity is seen after ingestion of medications; sulfonamides (Fig. 77-1),

TABLE 77-1. DRUGS AND CHEMICALS KNOWN TO CAUSE PHOTOSENSITIVITY REACTIONS*

Phototoxic Drugs
  Griseofulvin
  Nalidixic acid (bullous reaction)
  Phenothiazines, especially chlorpromazine
  Protryptaline
  Sulfonyureas (eczematous reaction)
    Chlorpropamide
    Tolbutamide
  Tetracyclines, especially demethylchlortetracycline
Thiazides
Dyes
  Anthraquinone
  Eosin
  Methylene blue
  Rose bengal
Coal tar derivatives
  Acridine
  Anthracene
  Phenanthrene
  Pyrene
Furocoumarins
  Psoralen
  8–Methoxypsoralen
  4,5,8—Trimethoxypsoralen
Photoallergic
  Halogenated salicylanilides
  Antifungal agents
    Multifungin
    Fentichlor
    Jadit
  Phenothiazines
  Sulfonamides
  Sunscreens
    PABA esters
    Digalloyltrioleate
  Whiteners
    Stilbenes
  Fragrances
    Musk ambrette
    6-methylcoumarin
  NSAIDs
    Piroxicam
  Others
    Pyrithiol hydrochloride
    Fluorouracil derivatives

* Modified with permission from Bickers, D.: Sun-induced disorders. Emerg. Med. Clin. North Am. 3:659, 1985.

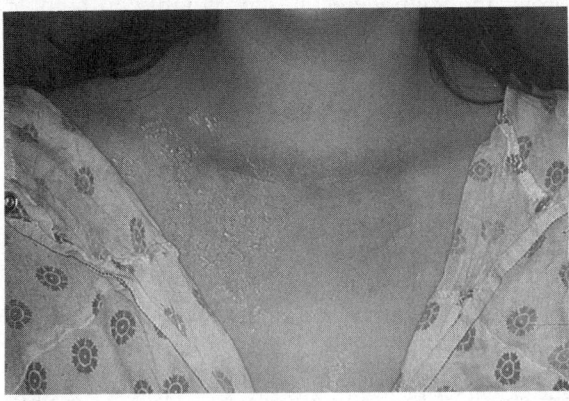

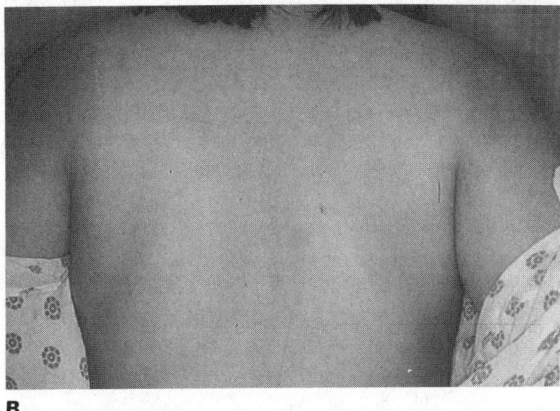

A   **B**

FIG. 77-1.   A and B. This photosensitivity reaction to trimethoprim/sulfamethoxazole occurred less than 24 hours after prolonged sun exposure. Note demarcation along clothing lines.

thiazides, tetracyclines, and phenothiazines are the most common offenders. A burning sensation typically occurs during sunlight exposure, followed by a rapid onset of erythema, edema, and in severe cases, vesiculation. These changes are prominent within 2 to 6 hours and resolve over 2 to 4 days. It should be noted that there is also a delayed phototoxicity response that more closely resembles sunburn in its time course. Usually this type is related to psoralen derivatives (found in certain plants and also used in combination with UVA radiation to treat psoriasis), with redness and swelling peaking at about 48 hours.[3] For unclear reasons, a small number of patients have continued disease even after stopping exposure to all suspected photosensitizers and decreasing sun exposure. These individuals are termed persistent light reactors.[5] Chlorpromazine has long been blamed for irreversible discoloration of sun-exposed areas of skin, but a recent study indicates that many affected patients may have resolution of skin changes after substitution of haloperidol for chlorpromazine.[6]

Clinical manifestations of photoallergy are of two types, immediate urticarial or delayed papular to eczematous rash. Antibody-dependent or cell-mediated responses are involved respectively. Less light energy is required than for phototoxicity reactions.[7] Halogenated salicylanilides, a common soap and cosmetic additive in the 1950s and 1960s, are the prototype photoallergens. Usually the affected skin is sharply delineated along sun-exposed lines (Fig. 77-1).[5]

Treatment of photosensitivity reactions consists primarily of elimination of the causative chemical. A thorough drug history is essential, with referral for diagnostic confirmation by photopatch testing often required. Most patients improve gradually after decreasing sun exposure and removing the offending agent. Severely affected persistent light reactors may require systemic steroids for flare-ups, and in some incapacitated patients, cytotoxic or immunosuppressive agents are used.[5]

SUNBURN

This most common solar-mediated afflictions can be conceptualized as cutaneous inflammatory responses to UVR-induced release of mast cell and keratinocyte mediators. Prostaglandins are probably the most important of these, with elevated levels of PgD_2, PgE_2, and arachidonic acid demonstrable in sunburned skin. Also implicated are histamine, serotonin, kinins, released lysosomal enzymes, and UVR-produced free radicals.[4,7]

The most effective wavelength for producing sunburn on typical Caucasian skin is 297 nm, with a logarithmic decrease in potency as the wavelength increases or decreases. Photosensitive meters capable of monitoring UVR have been in place at several U.S. National Weather Service stations since 1974. The data from these meters fortunately does not suggest an increase in UVB reaching the surface of the planet over the years 1974 to 1985, despite ozone depletion. This is presumably because the meters are located in the continental U.S., whereas ozone damage is greatest in the polar regions. In any case, the best currently available data do not yet show any alteration in UVR penetration in the U.S.[8]

Sunburn response varies markedly among individuals. It is determined by the thickness of the stratum corneum and the genetically influenced capacity for melanogenesis. Other factors are involved also. Elderly patients have a decreased sunburn response, which evolves more slowly.[4] Black persons sunburn more than is generally expected, although they are four to eight times less likely to burn than whites with the same solar exposure.[3] Six skin types have been described, based on susceptibility to actinic injury. This is defined as injury induced by electromagnetic radiation, especially from sunlight. Patients can be categorized into one of the six types based on their personal tanning and burning histories (Table 77-2). For skin type II, the minimal melanogenic dose (MMD,

TABLE 77-2. ASSESSMENT OF RISK OF ACTINIC INJURY*

Skin Type	History of Burns	Tans
I	Always	Never
II	Always	Sometimes
III	Sometimes	Always
IV	Rarely	Always
V	Darker pigmentation	
VI	Darkest pigmentation	

* Modified with permission from Bickers, D.: Sun-induced disorders. Emerg. Med. Clin. North Am. 3:659, 1985.

or tanning dose) is equal to the MED, so that tanning in sunlight cannot occur without burning. Patients with skin types III or IV have an MMD significantly less than their MED, and tanning may occur with suberythemal doses of UVR.[4]

People with sunburn frequently present to Emergency Departments (EDs) for treatment, generally because of marked pain or systemic symptoms. Three to eight MEDs produce moderate or severe sunburn. A two-phase response is seen. The first phase is an immediate or early erythema, which fades within 30 minutes. The second phase follows a latent period of up to 6 hours; it consists of a delayed erythema that peaks at 15 to 24 hours. Warmth, tenderness, and swelling occur at this stage. In severe cases, excruciating pain, vesiculation, fever, chills, nausea, and delirium may be present. Desquamation results after 4 to 7 days, as with other partial-thickness burns. Treatment is geared toward symptom relief. Cool topical soaks with water or Burrow's solution are generally helpful. Nonsteroidal anti-inflammatory drugs decrease prostaglandins and are useful, especially early in the course of treatment. Topical steroids have been found to be of minimal benefit, but systemic steroids are recommended. Prednisone, 40 to 60 mg po, with rapid tapering, seems to shorten the course and ease the discomfort. Steroids are contraindicated in severe second-degree burns because of the risk of infection, and in such a case transfer to a burn center must be considered. Other patients may require hospitalization with partial-thickness burns because of uncontrollable pain.[4,5]

A few words should be said about artificial tanning, which is usually attempted through use of tanning salons or photosensitizers. Tanning booths expose the user to variable amounts of radiation that further fluctuate with the age of the bulb. Many produce over 95% UVA, which causes actinic damage. Some have short-wave UVR in greater proportions than sunlight, causing more erythema and less tan. Reports of sunlamp overradiation are increasing. Another medical problem is brought up by the use of products containing oil of bergamot or 5-methoxypsoralen (5-MOP), which are promoted to stimulate a quick tan. The photosensitizer 5-MOP is not only cytotoxic and

phototoxic to melanocytes, it is also highly mutagenic and carcinogenic to keratinocytes and melanocytes.[4] It is probably wise to discourage the use of these products.

POLYMORPHOUS LIGHT ERUPTION

Polymorphous light eruption (PMLE) refers to an incompletely understood disorder that is clinically manifested as a delayed abnormal skin reaction to solar radiation. There is no clear agreement as to the action spectrum. Although most investigators feel that UVB is the chief offender, it has been demonstrated that at least some of the patients react to UVA or visible light, suggesting that more than one disease entity may be included under this heading. A moderate amount of circumstantial evidence points toward an endogenous photoallergic process in PMLE. No allergen has yet been identified, however, and the disease is still considered idiopathic.[5,7]

The clinical manifestations of PMLE, as implied by the term, are diverse. It occurs in all races.[3] The onset is often in the first or second decade of life, with recurring pruritic eruptions confined predominantly to exposed skin.[4] Lesions begin to appear anywhere from a few hours to several days after sun exposure. These skin changes range from eczema to small papules to plaques to large nodules; the first two types are more common. The eruption tends to be monomorphous in a given patient.[9] The lesions usually persist for several days before fading spontaneously. A useful point in the dagnosis is that the symptoms tend to be much more prominent on initial solar exposure in the spring (Fig. 77-2), and there is generally a decreased reaction with subsequent exposures. This phenomenon is known as hardening. Most patients have PMLE chronically, although in one third, the disease regresses spontaneously.[5] The main differential consideration is lupus, but photosensitivity, porphyria, solar urticaria, and lymphocytic infiltrates should also be con-

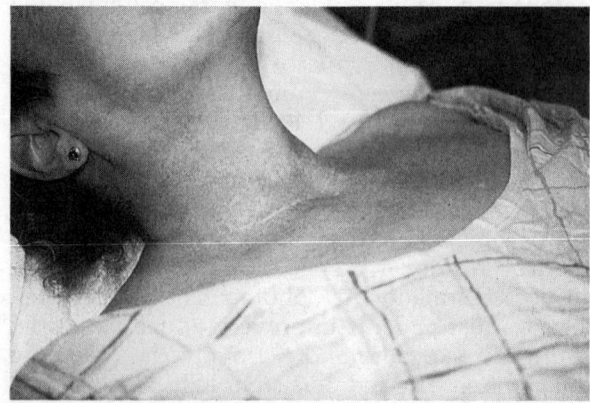

FIG. 77-2. This woman with previously undiagnosed polymorphous light eruption came to the ED with an unrelated problem. She had had this rash on initial sun exposure in the spring every year for 11 years.

sidered. Standard phototesting to provoke a lesion can suggest PMLE as the diagnosis.[2]

The mainstay of treatment is photoprotection with sunscreens and avoidance of sunlight. Antihistamines and topical corticosteroids provide some relief. In severe and persistent cases, antimalarial drugs have been of significant benefit. Also effective is artificial hardening with UVR.[5]

SOLAR URTICARIA

Solar urticaria is an uncommon condition. Patients report a pruritic rash that arises within seconds to minutes of sun exposure. The lesions are wheals, with or without flare, that fade within 1 hour. The action spectrum varies from patient to patient, and it may be UVA, UVB, or visible light. Most recent evidence points toward an immediate hypersensitivity reaction mediated by IgE, as might be expected from the urticarial nature of the response. Treatment is with antihistamines.[3,4,7]

THE PORPHYRIAS

Of the seven types of porphyria, cutaneous manifestations and solar sensitivity are prominent in four, and may occur in all except acute intermittent porphyria. These diseases result from overproduction of porphyrins or porphyrin precursors, secondary to hereditary enzyme deficiencies in the heme synthesis pathway. In addition to skin changes, many are also characterized by neurologic involvement. They are inherited as autosomal dominant, with the exception of erythropoietic porphyria, which is autosomal recessive. The porphyrias are traditionally divided into two groups, erythropoietic and hepatic, depending on whether the biochemical abnormality predominantly affects the bone marrow or the liver (Table 77-3).

Erythropoietic porphyria (EP) and erythropoietic protoporphyria (EPP) are the most likely of the porphyrias to present with acute cutaneous reactions to sunlight. In both of these conditions, porphyrin metabolites in the skin are phototoxic. The action spectrum lies within the visible range. This accounts for solar reactions that are not blocked by window glass, and also explains deeper cutaneous damage because of the greater penetrance of visible light. EP is a rare but devastating disease. Marked photosensitivity is apparent from infancy. The baby screams when in sunlight, then becomes erythematous, and blisters develop. Gradual scarring and ulceration of exposed body parts cause tissue destruction and gross disfigurement. Hirsutism also results, and patients become nocturnal. Uroporphyrin colors the nails and teeth a dirty brown. These features are believed to account for the legendary werewolf of the Middle Ages. Affected patients also have pink urine; diagnostic confirmation is elevated urinary porphyrins. EPP is one of the most common porphyrias. The photosensitivity is milder than with EP, although diagnosis is still usually made within the first decade of life. Burning, stinging, erythema, and edema result acutely from sun exposure. Chronic changes include scarring of prominent sites such as the bridge of the nose, purpura-like lesions, and premature aging. Urinary porphyrins are not elevated. Diagnosis is by elevated red blood cell protoporphyrin.[2,5,10]

Treatment of EP begins with rigorous avoidance of sunlight from the time of diagnosis. Splenomegaly (from hemolysis) may be present, and splenectomy may help the cutaneous photosensitivity. Frequent skin infections are treated as they occur. EPP patients are often helped by oral beta carotene. Perhaps because of its free radical scavenging and antioxidant effects, this medication may permit longer sun exposure with decreased symptoms.[5]

The hepatic porphyrias manifest with differing degrees of neurologic or cutaneous symptoms, depending on the specific disease. The neurologic derangements are episodic, with acute attacks consisting of neurologically mediated severe abdominal pain. Central nervous system (CNS) dysfunction may occur, ranging from seizures to psychosis to quadraplegia and death from respiratory paralysis. During the attack, urinary porphobilinogen is elevated, although this is not measured on a standard urine porphyrin screen. Among the hepatic porphyrias, porphyria cutanea tarda produces the most consistent cutaneous involvement, with virtually 100% of patients developing fragility and blistering of exposed skin. In other hepatic porphyrias, skin abnormalities are similar but less frequent. Toxic porphyria is the only disease in this group with a nonhereditary cause. The most significant epidemic occurred in Turkey in 1959 from mass ingestion of hexachlorobenzene, which was used as a fungicide on grain. The clinical and laboratory abnormalities are indistinguishable from those of porphyria cutanea tarda, and differentiation is made on epidemiologic grounds. Treatment is primarily supportive and symptomatic. Many drugs are known to exacerbate the porphyrias, and these should be discontinued. For acute neurologic attacks, the treatment

---

TABLE 77-3. CLASSIFICATION OF THE PORPHYRIAS*

Erythropoietic
    Erythropoietic porphyria
    Erythropoietic protoporphyria
Hepatic
    Acute intermittent porphyria
    Variable porphyria
    Hereditary coproporphyria
    Porphyria cutana tarda
    Toxic porphyria

*Modified with permission from Bissell, D. M.: Porphyria. In Cecil Textbook of Medicine, 17th Ed. Edited by Wyngaarden, J. B., and Smith, L. H., Jr. Philadelphia, W. B. Saunders Co., 1985.

is more involved. Hypoglycemia, pain, agitation, and tachycardia may all require treatment with glucose, meperidine, chlorpromazine, and propranolol, respectively. Intravenous hematin may be needed if these measures fail.[10]

LUPUS ERYTHEMATOSUS

Photosensitivity and cutaneous changes are common in lupus, and are occasionally the presenting complaint in a patient with no previous diagnosis of this condition. The action spectrum is UVB. Sunlight may exacerbate or induce discoid lupus erythematosus (DLE) and exacerbate the systemic form (SLE) in most patients, although photosensitivity is not an essential feature of the disease. The pathogenesis is felt to be related to the ability of UV light to greatly enhance the antigenicity of native DNA, resulting in endogenous photoallergy. The skin lesions are typically erythematous patches, which later progress to elevated scaly plaques. Chronically, scarring, atrophy, and hyperpigmentation may be seen. Commonly affected sites include the malar area (butterfly rash), the V of the neck, and the exposed areas of the arms. Hair follicle involvement leads to alopecia.[5,11] In some patients, sun exposure appears to cause progression of the disease from DLE to SLE.[3]

Sunscreens containing PABA to block UVB are recommended, as is the avoidance of potentially photosensitizing drugs. Steroids may be given, either topically or intralesionally. Antimalarials are used for severe unresponsive cases.[11]

SUN-INDUCED OCULAR DISORDERS

Although visible radiation from the sun enables human vision, neighboring wavelengths of electromagnetic radiation in the UV range can damage several parts of the eye. Photokeratoconjunctivitis, solar retinopathy, and cataracts are all linked to sun-gazing.

Snow blindness (photokeratoconjunctivitis) occurs in harsh radiant settings. These include the sea, sand, and snow. It is also seen in oxyacetylene or arc welders who wear inadequate UV eye protection. Symptoms begin after a latent period of about 8 hours. A gritty foreign body sensation with pain, photophobia, lacrimation, and severe blepharospasm are then noted. Objective findings may be scant. Conjunctival injection and chemosis, along with a dull cornea containing diffuse punctuate erosions on fluorescein staining, may be detected. Treatment is similar to that for a corneal abrasion. Topical antibiotics, mydriatic/cycloplegic patches, and oral analgesics are all useful. A recheck in 24 hours allows repeat treatment if pain persists.[4,12]

Other types of photophthalmia are less likely to present to the ED, but are mentioned briefly for the sake of completeness. Numerous studies have attempted to link cataract formation to sunlight exposure, and, despite difficulties in data interpretation, the evidence currently favors a causal role for UVR, although other factors appear important as well. The mechanism is probably UVA-induced alteration in lens tryptophan, causing damaged lens proteins that scatter rather than transmit light.[12-15] Solar retinopathy is a well-described entity that occurs acutely after sun-gazing and presents with central scotoma, decreased visual acuity, and macular edema. These changes may resolve partially, completely, or not at all. Severely affected patients with significant carotid artery stenosis may occasionally experience temporary blindness in one or both eyes as a result of bright light, usually sunlight. The cerebrovascular disease in these patients produces some degree of retinal ischemia, thereby delaying regeneration of the visual pigments necessary for vision. Symptoms last for minutes to hours; treatment is either with aspirin or carotid endarterectomy for the underlying condition.[16]

PEDIATRIC CONSIDERATIONS

Although any of the previously mentioned disorders may occur in children, certain problems are more likely to present in the pediatric population. Many of these are metabolic abnormalities, which cause altered photosensitivity.

In addition to the acute conditions, which will be discussed, recent studies indicate that childhood is a critical period for the development of skin cancer, so that adults with a history of severe sunburn as youngsters are at increased risk for cutaneous melanoma.[17]

Perhaps the most notorious of the congenital photosensitivity syndromes is xeroderma pigmentosum, a rare, autosomal recessive, progressive disease caused by defective DNA repair. Manifestations may begin as early as infancy, with skin erythema, bullae, and photophobia. If untreated, patients may die during childhood from internal malignancy or uncontrolled progression of the skin condition. Diagnosis is made by testing lymphocytes or skin fibroblasts for the DNA repair abnormality. Treatment consists of avoidance of sunlight, use of sunscreens, and application of fluorouracil topically on and around "changed" skin. The key to management is early diagnosis so that prevention of exposure can begin.[2,18]

Lupus is rare in children. Neonatal lupus can, however, present in infancy with skin lesions and photosensitivity. Cardiac involvement, usually AV block, is found in 50 to 60% of these babies, and most have autoantibodies. Although the disease frequently regresses before 1 year of age, the cardiac abnormalities are generally permanent.[2]

A disease similar to PMLE in all clinical respects except age of onset occurs commonly in American Indians. Manifestations are usually noted before age 10, and because of this difference from PMLE, some investigators prefer a separate term, "actinic prurigo."

It appears to be inherited as an autosomal dominant trait.[18]

Several other photodermatoses of childhood are rare but deserve mention. Ataxia telangiectasia is a progressive multisystem disease with symptoms of telangiectasias on sun-exposed areas, ataxia, and immunologic abnormalities leading to infection and neoplasia. Bloom's syndrome presents as photosensitivity and growth retardation, also with immunodeficiency and frequent leukemias. Hartnup's disease manifests between ages 3 and 9 as ataxia and pellagra-like symptoms caused by tryptophan malabsorption.[18]

The laboratory investigation of the photosensitive child frequently extends beyond the purview of the emergency physician, necessitating referral. Tests may include skin biopsy, cutaneous phototesting, porphyrin assays of red blood cells, plasma, urine, and feces, chromosome analysis, and assays for DNA repair if xeroderma pigmentosum is a consideration.[18]

LONG-TERM EFFECTS OF SOLAR RADIATION

Chronic sun exposure causes cutaneous malignancies as well as the familiar actinic changes of sun-aged skin. Evidence now clearly implicates UVR in the genesis of squamous cell cancer, basal cell cancer, and malignant melanoma. The incidence of malignant melanoma is 25,800 cases per year in the U.S., representing a steady increase over the last 50 years. In fact, the rate of development of new cases is doubling every 10 to 15 years, and the increase in mortality from malignant melanoma is greater than for any cancer except lung cancer in women. The current mortality rate is 10 to 20%, with no effective treatment available for metastases. Regular use of an effective sunscreen (sun protective factor 15 or more) has been shown to decrease skin cancer risk by 78%.[19]

The features of sun-aged skin include wrinkling, looseness, decreased elasticity, atrophy, dryness, and solar keratoses. The role of the sun in producing these changes can be dramatized by comparing the smooth, white, soft abdominal skin of an elderly patient with the same person's chronically sun-exposed, rough, leathery neck. The action spectrum for actinic aging is probably UVA.[4] Retinoic acid applied topically does not reverse severe actinic damage, but does help efface small wrinkles and shrink deeper ones.[20]

TREATMENT AND PREVENTION

Specific management of individual disorders has been outlined in the sections discussing those disorders.

General information, especially regarding sunscreens, is discussed in the following paragraphs.

Sunscreens are rated by the manufacturer with a sun protection factor (SPF) number as a measure of efficacy. The SPF is generally between 2 and 15, and it is the factor by which the MED is altered by using the product. For example, the MED is 8 times higher with SPF 8 lotion than with no lotion at all.

There are two categories of topical sunscreens, physical and chemical. The physical sunscreens are opaque, reflecting and scattering visible and UV light. Zinc oxide is the most familiar of the physical agents. Chemical agents absorb UVA; PABA-related compounds (padimate O, padimate A, or octyldimethyl PABA) or benzophenone derivatives (oxybenzone, dioxybenzone) are used frequently. PABA offers protection primarily from UVB. Adding a benzophenone in combination will extend the protective effect into the UVA range.[4] This is important and should be considered in conjunction with a knowledge of the action spectrum of the disease to be prevented.

Although a wide array of sun protection products is available, the American public, as a group, is unaware of their usefulness. A recent survey found that only 41% of individuals use sunscreens at all. Even more surprising is that 32% of sunscreen users and 61% of oil and lotion users use them with the false notion that they will promote a tan.[17]

MEDICOLEGAL PEARLS AND PITFALLS

- Assume a serious underlying disease in any infant with a history of easy sunburn.
- Skin erythema from sunlight through a window glass indicates visible light or UVA sensitivity, as with porphyria or phototoxic reactions.
- Possible skin cancer usually requires biopsy for diagnosis, and patients should be referred promptly, even for suspected nonmelanoma, because squamous cell cancer *can* metastasize.
- Consider child abuse in a child with diffuse erythematous markings.
- Documentation of a complete drug history is important in any patient with a rash.

REFERENCES

1. Loggie, B., and Eddy, J.: Solar considerations in the development of cutaneous melanoma. Semin. Oncol. *15*:494, 1988.
2. Kahn, G.: Photosensitivity and photodermatitis in childhood. Dermatol. Clin. 4:107, 1986.
3. Willis, I.: Photosensitivity reactions in Black skin. Dermatol. Clin. 6:369, 1988.
4. Gentile, D., and Aurbach, P.: The sun and water sports. Clin. Sports Med. 6:669, 1987.
5. Bickers, D.: Sun-induced disorders. Emerg. Med. Clin. North Am. 3:659, 1985.

6. Thompson, T., Lai, S., Yassa, R., and Gerstein, W.: Resolution of chlorpromazine-induced pigmentation with haloperidol substitution. Acta Psychiatr. Scand. *78*:763, 1988.

7. Epstein, J.: Phototoxicity and photoallergy in man. J. Am. Acad. Dermatol. *8*:141, 1983.

8. Scotto, J., et al.: Biologically effective ultraviolet radiation: Surface measurements in the United States, 1974 to 1985. Science *239*:762, 1988.

9. Horio, T.: Photoallergic reaction: Classification and pathogenesis. Int. J. Dermatol. *23*:376, 1984.

10. Bissell, D.M.: Porphyria. *In* Cecil Textbook of Medicine, 17th ed. Edited by Wyngaarden, J.B., and Smith, L.H., Jr. Philadelphia, W.B. Saunders Co., 1985.

11. Tuffanelli, D.: Discoid lupus erythematosus. Clin. Rheum. Dis. *8*:327, 1983.

12. Wittenberg, S.: Solar radiation and the eye: A review of knowledge relevant to eye care. Am. J. Optometry Physiol. Optics *63*:676, 1986.

13. Zigman, S.: Role of sunlight in human cataract formation. Surv Ophthalmol. *27*:327, 1982.

14. Dolezal, J., Perkins, E., and Wallace, R.: Sunlight, skin sensitivity, and senile cataract. Am. J. Epidemiol. *129*:559, 1989.

15. Campo, R., Sipperley, J., Hall, G., and Rappazzo, J.A.: Medjugorje maculopathy. N. Engl. J. Med. *318*:1207, 1988.

16. Eiebers, D., Swanson, J., Cascino, T., and Whisnant, J.: Bilateral loss of vision in bright light. Stroke *20*:554, 1989.

17. Hurwitz, S.: The sun and sunscreen protection: Recommendations for children. J. Dermatol. Surg. Oncol. *14*:657, 1988.

18. Ramsay, C.: Photosensitivity in children. Pediatr. Clin. North Am. *30*:687, 1983.

19. Deleo, V.: Prevention of skin cancer. J. Dermatol. Surg. Oncol. *14*:902, 1988.

20. Kligman, L.: Preventing, delaying, and repairing photoaged skin. Cutis *41*:419, 1988.

Chapter 78

NUTRITIONAL EMERGENCIES

George R. Schwartz

CAPSULE

The presence of anorexia nervosa and bulimia can be detected in the Emergency Department (ED) through careful evaluation and laboratory tests of urine and serum electrolytes. Deaths are believed to result from cardiac arrhythmias, although serious problems have resulted from gorging and vomiting, including gastric rupture and a Mallory-Weiss type of syndrome. Diet pills can cause hypertension and cerebral hemorrhage when taken in excess.

Vitamin deficiency and excess syndromes can also be detected in the ED. The deficiency syndromes are more common in the elderly, those with gastrointestinal disorders with vomiting, diarrhea and malabsorption, and those with chronic drug or alcohol addiction. Excess vitamin syndromes are usually associated with vitamins A, D, and E. These occur during fad diets, and when excess vitamins are given to self-treat a variety of conditions such as night blindness, mental deterioration, or sexual disorders.

Occasionally severe protein deficiency malnutrition is discovered, with rash, fatty liver, marasmus, anemia, ascites and debilitation.

Water intoxication syndromes with profound hyponatremia can be life-threatening because of seizures, coma, electrolyte imbalance and pulmonary edema. Slow reversal is necessary.

The eosinophilia-myalgia syndrome manifests as excess eosinophils along with fever, rash, fasciitis, and muscle pain caused by ingestion of the amino acid supplement, tryptophan. Eosinophil count is the easiest way to confirm the diagnosis.

RECOGNITION OF ANOREXIA NERVOSA, BULIMIA, AND THEIR COMPLICATIONS IN THE EMERGENCY DEPARTMENT

Anorexia nervosa is a syndrome of self-starvation found predominantly among adolescent and young adult women. It is characterized by a focus on food, body image, and being thin to the point where life-threatening emaciation and vitamin deficiency syndromes may develop.

Bulimia is an eating disorder characterized by eating binges frequently followed by prolonged fasting, self-induced vomiting, and laxative and/or diuretic abuse. Some patients with anorexia nervosa also manifest bulimia. Many patients with the "bulimia syndrome," however, are of normal weight or overweight. The incidence of these disorders appears to be increasing.

Of women between the ages of 13 and 20, 5 to 25% have a history of bulimia. Usually the act of self-induced vomiting is occasional and of little consequence. In some persons, however, it becomes a chronic pattern leading to serious electrolyte disorders, poor overall health, decreased muscle strength, rotten teeth, cardiac arrhythmias, and even death.

Many emotional and physical problems are associated with these difficult-to-treat disorders, and the emergency physician may be in a good position to recognize these individuals and to provide initial management and suitable referral.

CLINICAL SIGNS

Thin young women may present to the ED with muscle weakness, cramps, dizziness, or carpopedal spasm. Many initially deny any self-purging (e.g., vomiting, use of laxatives or diuretics). With laxative use, hypocalcemia may result in carpopedal spasm. Such patients usually give a history of weight loss and occasionally admit to the use of diuretics because of "edema." Blood pressure is generally normal or low (as opposed to that in a syndrome of mineralocorticoid excess, or even excess licorice ingestion, which can also cause severe hypokalemia and myopathy, but with elevated blood pressure).

The parotid glands are often enlarged, and tooth enamel may be eroded. Sometimes a history of hematemesis indicates severe vomiting that has resulted in a Mallory-Weiss syndrome (Table 78-1).

LABORATORY FINDINGS

Laboratory findings of hypokalemia and metabolic alkalosis (secondary to compulsive vomiting) are confirmatory. Sodium levels may also be decreased, and

		Disorders		
Behavior	Cardiovascular/ Pulmonary	Gastrointestinal	Electrolyte/ Renal	Other
Starvation	Heart failure, beriberi, heart disease	Constipation	Reduced glomerular filtration, tubular dysfunction	Amenorrhea, leukopenia, thrombocytopenia, hypothermia, hair loss, vitamin deficiency syndromes (see Table 78-4)
Eating binges	Heart failure, refeeding edema	Gastric dilation or rupture, pancreatitis, vascular compression		Electroencephalogram abnormalities
Self-induced vomiting	Aspiration pneumonitis, ipecac-induced myocarditis	Parotid enlargement, tooth enamel erosion, oral cavity trauma, Mallory-Weiss syndrome, esophagitis, esophageal rupture	Metabolic alkalosis, hypokalemia, hypochloremia	
Purgative abuse	Arrhythmias	Cathartic colon	Hypocalcemia, hypokalemia, kaliopenic nephropathy	Electrocardiogram abnormalities
Diuretic abuse	Cardiac arrhythmias, orthostatic hypotension	Constipation	Hypokalemia, hyponatremia, hypercalcemia, hyperuricemia	Electrocardiogram abnormalities

TABLE 78-1. COMPLICATIONS OF ANOREXIA NERVOSA AND BULIMIA*

* Adapted with permission from Harris, R. T.: The perils of gorging and purging. Acute Care Medicine 1:15, 1984.

the chloride level is usually below normal. In patients who abuse laxatives, but are not vomiting, the hypokalemia is associated with a metabolic acidosis caused by loss of bicarbonate in the diarrheal stool.

If diuretic abuse is coupled with bulimia, sodium and potassium levels are lowered and the uric acid and calcium levels raised. Laxative use lowers calcium levels. Urinary findings vary according to the syndrome and whether the condition is acute or chronic (Table 78-2).

Since ipecac has come into common use for inducing vomiting in cases of poisoning, it is now widely available. Ipecac-related deaths have been reported among bulimic individuals and are believed to be caused by emetine cardiotoxicity, probably in conjunction with electrolyte imbalances.

PROBLEMS OF GORGING

Occasionally, severe pain with acute gastric dilation can occur as a result of the massive quantities of food ingested by bulimics (sometimes as much as 15,000 calories in an hour). Gastric rupture has been reported, with sudden sharp pain and evidence of peritonitis. Postbinge pancreatitis may also occur, as may vascular compression of duodenal blood vessels.

OTHER PROBLEMS OF ANOREXIA

The effects of starvation include anemia, amenorrhea, infertility, constipation, and hepatic and renal dysfunction (Table 78-3). The insufficient protein intake

TABLE 78-2. URINE ELECTROLYTE VALUES IN HYPOKALEMIC METABOLIC ALKALOSIS ACCORDING TO CAUSE

Cause	Urine Electrolyte Value		
	Sodium	Potassium	Chloride
Conn's syndrome*	↑	↑	↑
Diuretic ingestion			
Recent	↑	↑	↑
Remote	↓	↓	↓
Vomiting			
Recent	↑	↑	↓
Remote	↓	↑	↓↓
Bartter's syndrome	↑	↑	↑

* Representative of primary states of mineralcorticoid excess. ↓ Indicates values of less than 10 mmol/l; ↑ indicates higher values.

can cause edema, such as in kwashiorkor, although this syndrome usually requires a low-protein diet in the presence of carbohydrate, and rarely affects adults.

Additional problems may be associated with the toxicity of products ingested. For example, use of "diet pills" bought over the counter can result in phenylpropanolamine and caffeine overdose with marked agitation, possible hypertension, and seizures. Deaths have been reported from cerebral hemorrhage. Amphetamine-containing diet preparations are far less common than they were years ago, but occasionally an individual presents after chronic amphetamine use with paranoia, agitation, sweating, and dilated pupils.

Occasionally, the use of laxatives (Ex-Lax, Correctol) results in phenolphthalein poisoning.

TABLE 78-3. ANOREXIA NERVOSA

Associated Conditions	Laboratory and X-ray Findings
Pericardial effusions	Abnormal serum and urinary electrolytes
Sinus bradycardia	Anemia
Hypotension	Normal cortisone, high aldosterone
Low voltage QRS complexes	
St-T wave abnormalities	
Pitting edema	Thyroid function often abnormal (low T3)
Muscle wasting	Follicle-stimulating hormone and luteinizing hormone reduced
Anemia	
Amenorrhea	
Hypothermia	Leukopenia
Dry skin	Coagulation defects
	Pneumothorax
	Pneumomediastinum
	Mallory-Weiss syndrome
	Gastric dilation and infarction

The osteoporosis often present in patients with anorexia nervosa is related to decreased food intake along with urinary and fecal calcium losses.

Sudden death during fasting has occurred, associated with cardiac causes. The liquid protein diet, formerly in wide use, was associated with rare prolongation of the Q-T interval and intractable ventricular arrhythmias. The exact cause is undetermined.

TREATMENT

Treatment of the more severe disorders generally requires intravenous saline with potassium supplementation, depending on serum electrolyte determinations. Because of the compulsive nature of the pattern of the laxative and diuretic abuse and self-induced vomiting, borderline patients may benefit more from intravenous therapy and an initial psychologic evaluation. Be aware that anorexia nervosa is a complex, potentially life-threatening condition, and a referral to someone with substantial experience in treating these disorders is mandatory.

ACUTE PRESENTATIONS OF VITAMIN DEFICIENCY SYNDROMES

Although extreme vitamin deficiency syndromes are rare because of food availability and social programs, particular subgroups of individuals may be at particular risk—for example, elderly persons; those with gastrointestinal disorders leading to excessive vomiting, diarrhea, or malabsorption; anorectic or bulimic patients; and those with drug- or alcohol-related problems. The onset of vitamin deficiency syndrome is often faster than generally expected (e.g., 3 to 4 weeks

for scurvy and 1 month for pellegra), although vitamin B_{12} deficiency (<80 μg/mL) generally takes substantially longer to develop (e.g., often years after a gastrectomy) and may present with neurologic disturbances and no anemia. Folic acid deficiency may occur more rapidly in persons on limited or fad diets, in pregnancy, or in persons with poor diet who chronically ingest large amounts of alcohol.

Vitamin B disorders (niacin, thiamine) can occur insidiously, although occasionally with a severe, life-threatening presentation (e.g., beriberi cardiomyopathy), with heart failure, pulmonary edema, and rapid demise unless treated.

The widespread "fad" diets, use of drugs and alcohol, the increased incidence of anorexia nervosa and bulimia, and the growing elderly population make vitamin deficiency syndromes more likely to be encountered.

Elderly patients frequently consume less than the "minimum daily requirement" of many vitamins,[1-8] and the symptoms that may result are frequently ascribed to other causes. Malabsorption, poor dentition, hypochlorhydria, and decreased intestinal secretions further tend to reduce absorption. Drugs and/or medications may also interact with nutrients.

As the mean age of the elderly population increases, these problems will tend to increase, despite some simple partial solutions (e.g., dental work, hearing aids, visual aids). Many of our elderly, either living independently or in institutions, are in states of malnutrition.

It is well known that severe chronic malnutrition is accompanied by marked physical and psychologic changes: apathy, emotional instability, retardation, memory impairment, and even psychotic illness. Some of our elderly are experiencing undiagnosed symptoms of these types.

Much of what we know of malnutrition has involved prisoners who have volunteered for studies, such as with Terris and Goldberger's classic studies on pellagra in the early years of the twentieth century.[9] Prisoners of war provided an unfortunate human testing ground for chronic malnutrition.[10]

Hunger Disease. A unique book in the annals of medicine, and a book extremely difficult to read without great emotion, contains scientific reports on hunger disease by Jewish physicians in the Warsaw ghetto in 1940.[11]

The Nazi troops had sealed several hundred thousand people off from the outside world, determined to starve their prisoners to death. Amidst this evil catastrophe, a group of physicians decided to undertake a careful investigation of the clinical, metabolic, and pathologic consequences of starvation. One physician survived to recover the manuscript and prepare it for publication so that the group's last wish before death was accomplished, *non omnis moriar*—"I shall not wholly die."

The relevance of this work in the present day, aside from the deep historical significance, is to demonstrate what may occur clinically in particularly vulnerable groups. Even where the general standard of nutrition is high, there are people prone to malnutrition—the mentally ill, the aged, alcoholics (particularly elderly alcoholics), as well as those with chronic gastrointestinal disease and malabsorption. Some of these patients present with acute signs and symptoms; other signs and symptoms remain in the shadowy background as "pre-existent" conditions unless they are recognized by the acute care physician or nurse.

One recent example clarifies this "background." In 1988, Dr. Lindenbaum and his colleagues published a remarkable study that demonstrated neuropsychiatric disorders caused by cobalamin deficiency (vitamin B_{12}) in the absence of anemia or macrocytosis.[12]

What made this study particularly important was the wide range of symptoms—paresthesias being most common, followed by ataxia, memory loss, weakness, and fatigue. With some of the patients, the diagnosis was not made for years because of the absence of anemia. This study revealed that 40% of the 141 patients had no anemia or macrocytosis; 25 of these were 60 or older (63%). This study underscores the underdiagnosis of hypovitaminosis syndromes despite our sophisticated medical care system.

In the late twentieth century, we should not make the mistakes that were made in the late eighteenth century. James Lind first published "A Treatise on the Scurvy" in 1753.[13] In this work, he clearly showed the benefits of using lemons and oranges to prevent scurvy, which had been responsible for millions of deaths. Yet, 100 years later, ships were still sailing without a supply of lemons and returning with scorbutic sailors, after having buried others at sea. It took almost 50 years for the British navy to take notice of his findings. Lind was bitter at the time of his death, feeling he had failed to convey his important conclusions.

When deficiency syndromes do arise, replacement of a single vitamin is usually inadequate because we are dealing with problems with the entire diet (including, usually, protein and trace minerals) as well as possible other problems already mentioned (e.g., malabsorption, poor dentition, depression, medications, alcoholism). In some cases, however, supplemental vitamins, zinc, iron, and iodine can reduce mortality in children.[13a,b,c]

The symptoms and signs in Table 78-4 represent "full-blown" syndromes. These conditions do not suddenly appear; there is a slow and insidious progression, although severe stress or infection may rapidly precipitate some signs or symptoms. Profound deficiencies may also occur in patients maintained for a considerable time on intravenous fluids, particularly after surgery for a gastrointestinal disorder.

Many chronic conditions (e.g., Wernicke's encephalopathy, dementia) do not respond well to dietary change because the physiologic future has given way to permanent anatomic change through deterioration and cell death. Similarly, chronic calcium deficiency

TABLE 78-4. SIGNS AND SYMPTOMS OF VITAMIN AND NUTRITIONAL DEFICIENCY

Protein-Calorie Malnutrition	Thiamine Deficiency
Pallor	Peripheral neuropathy
Fatigue	Paresthesias
Coldness	Weakness, muscle tenderness
Inanition	Mental confusion
Contractures	Memory changes
Anemia	Beriberi heart disease (severe cardiac failure)
Impaired immunity	Wernicke's encephalopathy
Hypoproteinemia and edema	Footdrop, wristdrop
Hypotension	Decreased deep tendon reflexes
Autonomic nervous system hyporesponsiveness	Pulmonary and peripheral edema
Organ wasting (including heart)	
Niacin Deficiency	**Ascorbic Acid Deficiency**
Dermatitis*	Petechial hemorrhage
Mental confusion	Follicular hyperkeratosis
Gastrointestinal disturbance (e.g., pancreatic disorders)	Aching limbs
Depression	Bleeding or swollen gums
Lethargy	Joint effusions, hemorrhages
Diarrhea	Dyspnea
Weight loss	Edema
B_{12} Deficiency	Neuropathy
Anemia (macrocytic)	Depression
Myelopathy	Confusion
Peripheral neuropathy	Ocular hemorrhages
Optic atrophy	Coiled hairs, hair loss
Impaired vibration sense	Dry eyes
Ataxia	Abdominal colic
Footdrop	**Folic Acid Deficiency**
Fatigue, difficulty concentrating	Macrocytic anemia
Exaggerated deep tendon reflexes	Diarrhea
Paresis, paresthesias	History of chronic medication (anticonvulsant use)
Limb pain, cramps	Anorexia
Disorientation and mental confusion	Irritability
Depression	Confusion
Memory impairment	Dementia
	Depression

* Hyperkeratotic hyperpigmentation on backs of hands, elbows, and neck.

in the elderly can lead to widespread osteoporosis and, although this condition is not easily reversed, treatment should certainly begin with calcium and estrogens as needed for women.

Despite the resistance of some symptoms, others may clear rapidly when the deficiency is corrected. For example, the confabulation and disorientation of Korsakoff's psychosis may respond to thiamine within hours. Ocular abnormalities are present in over 90% of cases (nystagmus, sixth nerve palsies, sluggish pupils) and will similarly respond rapidly, although nystagmus may be permanent.[14] The emotional abnormalities (anxiety, insomnia, later depression, some psychosis) usually respond well. Ataxia, on the other hand, takes a month or two for maximum resolution, and one fourth to one half of the patients have ongoing balance difficulties. The confusion states take weeks to clear, and some memory loss remains unless treatment is started immediately after a short illness.

Table 78-4 lists some vitamins and known symptoms of deficiency. Blood may be tested for vitamin levels, although there are usually unacceptably long delays in return of results. Signs and symptoms are often most important for diagnosis. In cases of questionable diagnosis, treatment can be initiated with little risk.

VITAMIN EXCESS SYNDROMES

With nutritional awareness and proliferation of health-food stores, vitamin excess syndromes are becoming more frequent. The general myth that "large doses of vitamins can't hurt" is usually true in the case of the water-soluble B vitamins and vitamin C, but there is substantial danger from excesses of vitamins A, D, or E.[15] Table 78-5 lists various vitamin A, D, and E syndromes and their treatment. Vitamin C, more than 1 g/day, may increase kidney stone incidence. Overdoses of niacin can cause glucose intolerance, hepatotoxicity, and other distressing symptoms.

WATER INTOXICATION SYNDROMES

Endocrine alterations are well addressed in other sections. Some mention of water-related syndromes, however, is appropriate here.

Episodic water intoxication, which is characterized by profound hyponatremia and diverse neurologic signs ranging from ataxia to irreversible coma, occurs in patients with chronic psychiatric disorders.[16] The cause of the polydipsia is unclear, although the prevailing view is that it is somehow related to the psychosis and dementia with cognitive dysfunction.

This condition has a marked abnormality in renal water excretion, probably because of increased sensitivity to the antidiuretic effects of vasopressin as well as to enhanced vasopressin secretion at a lower osmotic threshold.

Some elderly patients present with a similar electrolyte profile (e.g., hyponatremia), and this syndrome must be considered. Conditions that may mimic this include (1) polydipsia accompanied by excessive salt depletion through sweating or diuretics or (2) an inappropriate antidiuretic hormone (ADH) associated with an underlying condition such as cancer, chronic pulmonary infections, or CNS lesions or secondary to some drugs (e.g., vincristine, nicotine, narcotics, clofibrate, carbamazepine).

Water intoxication is diagnosed by taking a careful history along with evaluating laboratory tests that demonstrate low serum and urine sodium and low specific gravity. The presentation may be acute with seizures, coma, trismus, or opisthotonos.[17] The x ray may show pulmonary edema, and computerized tomography (CT) scan can show cerebral edema and symmetric compression of the ventricles.

TREATMENT

Respiratory impairment must be treated with intubation or a ventilator if needed. Fluid restriction is commonly ordered. Saline solution infusion can slowly clear symptoms, but if symptoms are refractory or life-threatening, hypertonic saline may be given cautiously. The basic condition is water excess, and too-rapid administration of hypertonic saline can be dangerous.[18] Nairns[19] suggests raising the serum sodium 2 mEq/L per hour to a level of 120 to 130 mEq/L.

CALORIE-PROTEIN MALNUTRITION

Kwashiorkor and marasmus, although uncommon, do occur in the United States population.[20,21] Kwashiorkor actually means "deposed child" because the child "deposed" from the breast by another is more likely to develop kwashiorkor when weaned to a diet of cereal grains, cassava, plantain, and sweet potato.

In another African dialect, kwashiorkor means "red boy," possibly referring to the red-orange hair of affected children. The condition is characterized by dry skin, rash, edema, ascites, fatty liver, diarrhea, anemia, weakness, and irritability.

In the United States, it has been associated with intestinal malabsorption and kidney disease. Occasionally, a patient with anorexia nervosa presents with edema and liver disease related to low protein intake.

Some extreme diets are too low in protein and, when they are coupled with diarrhea-causing foods, cause low serum protein and altered electrolyte balance. The "liquid protein" diet, on the other hand, is high in protein, and deaths reported on this diet are probably related to ketosis, acidosis, electrolyte imbalance (particularly potassium), and fatal cardiac arrhythmia.

EOSINOPHILIA-MYALGIA SYNDROME

The recently described eosinophilia-myalgia syndrome has affected 5000 to 10,000 individuals. The illness is characterized by severe muscle pain, weak-

TABLE 78-5. VITAMIN A, D, AND E SYNDROMES

Hypovitaminosis A

Symptoms:
   Associated with malabsorption, diarrhea,
      gastroenteritis, or protein deficiency with
      infection
   Night blindness
   Conjunctival xerosis
   Corneal xerosis, ulcers
   Keratomalacia (leading to blindness)
Treatment:
   If eye lesions are occurring, treatment is
      urgent. An intramuscular injection of
      100,000 units of water-miscible vitamin A
      will rapidly restore vitamin A levels. Oral
      supplementation is adequate in most
      cases. Oil-based vitamin A should not be
      given parenterally.

Hypervitaminosis A

Symptoms:
   Headache
   Malaise, anorexia
   Vomiting
   Pleural effusion, ascites
   Possible papilledema in adults
   Alopecia
   Weight loss
   Dermatitis
   Skeletal pain
   Liver enlargement, cirrhosis
Laboratory Findings:
   Elevated vitamin A levels
   Hypercalcemia
   Abnormal liver function tests
   Bone resorption on x-ray in chronic cases
Treatment:
   Simply eliminating the excessive vitamin is
      usually satisfactory. With hypercalcemia,
      however, normal saline intravenously
      over several days is effective.

Vitamin D Deficiency

   May be associated with decreased intake or
      can be related to anticonvulsant medica-
      tions (e.g., hydantoins, barbiturates)
Symptoms:
   Bone pain
   Hyperparathyroidism
   Senile osteomalacia and fractures
   Muscle weakness
Laboratory Findings:
   Low-serum vitamin D level (< 10 ng/mL),
      hypoparathyroidism, hypocalcemia

Vitamin D Intoxication

Symptoms:
   Metastatic calcification
   Hypercalcemia
   Renal insufficiency
   Anorexia
   Anemia
   Dermatitis
Laboratory Findings:
   Elevated serum calcium, increased calcium in
      urine
   Serum vitamin D elevated (usually above 50
      ng/mL)
   X-ray evidence of periosteal thickening or
      metastatic calcification
   Urine may show proteinuria
   ECG may show arrhythmias
Treatment:
   Fluids, saline diuresis
   Stop vitamin D intake
   Treat severe hypercalcemia with calcitonin
      or mithramycin
   Cholestryamine orally (8 g b.i.d.) may aid in
      decreasing hypercalcemia*

Vitamin E Excess

Long-term excess can cause:
   Nausea
   Vomiting, gastrointestinal upset
   Weakness and fatigue
   Creatinuria
   Visual blurring
Evaluation:
   Blood levels (normal 0.5 to 2.0 mg/dL)
Treatment:
   Simple discontinuance†

---

   * See Jibami, M., and Hodges, N. H.: Prolonged hypercalcemia after industrial exposure to vitamin D.
Br. Med. J. 290:748, 1985, for more information.
   † See Biereo, J. G., Corash, C., and Hubbard, U. S.: Medical uses of vitamin E. *N. Engl. J. Med.*
308:1063, 1983, for more information.

---

ness, mouth ulcers, and eosinophilia (>1000 cells/mm³). Other manifestations include fever, abdominal pain, respiratory symptoms, and skin rash. Eosinophilic infiltration is found in muscles and in the liver. At least ten deaths have been associated with the syndrome.[22,23]

The outbreak has been strongly linked to a single Japanese manufacturer of the food supplement L-tryptophan.[24] There was a change in the manufacturing practice in 1988. A new strain of genetically engineered bacteria (bacillus amyloliquefactens) was used for fermentation; filtration processes were also modified. Investigation has revealed a dimer (two tryptophan molecules joined as one) present in the implicated tryptophan preparation; however, a direct cause-effect relationship has not been established. Therefore, although a contaminant of some sort is suspected, it has not yet been identified. Some authorities believe a direct tryptophan effect is also involved.

Recognition of this syndrome is important in the emergency setting because, although L-tryptophan tablets have been removed from the market, bottles are still in homes, and tryptophan may also be a constituent of other amino acid supplements.

Treatment consists of supportive care and prednisone, which reduces the eosinophilia and may diminish muscle pain.

REFERENCES

1. Hughes, R.E., et al.: Clinical manifestations of ascorbic acid deficiency in man. J. Clin. Nutr. 24:432, 1971.
2. Hessov, I.B., and Elsborg, L.: Nutritional studies on long-term surgical patients with special reference to the intake of vitamin B$_{12}$ and folic acid. Int. J. Vitam. Nutr. Res. 46:427, 1976.
3. Morgan, A.G. et al.: Nutritional survey in the elderly. Int. J. Vitam. Nutr. Res. 43:465, 1973.
4. Roos, D.: Neurological symptoms and signs in a selected group of partially gastrectomized patients with particular reference to B$_2$ deficiency. Acta Neurol. Scand. 50:719, 1974.
5. Vir, S.C., and Love, A.H.G.: Nutritional evaluation of B groups of vitamins in institutionalized aged. Int. J. Vitam. Nutr. Res. 47:213, 1977.
6. Gupta, K.L., Dworkin, B., and Gambert, S.R.: Common nutritional disorders in the elderly: atypical manifestations. Geriatrics 43:87, 1988.
7. Munro, H.N.: Nutrition and the elderly: A general overview. J. Am. Coll. Nutr. 3:341, 1984.
8. Morley, J.E.: Nutritional status of the elderly. Am. J. Med. 81:679, 1986.
9. Terris, M., and Goldberg, O.N.: Pellagra. New Orleans, 1964. Louisiana State University Press.
10. Helweg-Larsen, P., et al.: Famine disease in German concentration camps: complications and sequels. Acta Psychiatr. Neurol. Scand [Suppl] 83, 1952.
11. Winick, M. (Ed.): Hunger disease: Studies by the Jewish physicians in the Warsaw ghetto. New York, John Wiley & Sons, 1979.
12. Lindenbaum, J., et al.: Neuropsychiatric disorders caused by cobalamin deficiency in the absence of anemia or macrocytosis. N. Engl. J. Med. 318:26, 1988.
13. Lind, J.: A treatise on the scurvy, ed 3, London, S. Crowder, D. Wilson, G. Nicholls, T. Cadell, T. Becket, & Co., 1772.
13a. Rahmathullah, L., et al.: Reduced mortality among children in southern India receiving a small weekly dose of vitamin A. N. Engl. J. Med. 323:929, 1990.
13b. Keusch, G.T.: Vitamin A supplements—Too good not to be used. N. Engl. J. Med. 323:985, 1990.
13c. Tonglet, R., et al.: Efficacy of low oral doses of iodized oil in the control of iodine deficiency in Zaire. N. Engl. J. Med. 326:236, 1996.
14. Victor, M., Adams, R.D., and Collins, G.H.: The Wernicke-Korsakoff syndrome. Oxford, Blackwell Scientific Publications, 1971.
15. Goldman, J.M., Ahn, Y., and Wheeler, M.F.: Vitamin D and hypercalcemia, JAMA 254:1719, 1985.
16. Goldman, M.B., Luchins, D.J., and Robertson, G.L.: Mechanisms of altered water metabolism in psychotic patients with polydipsia and hyponatremia. N. Engl. J. Med. 318:7, 1988.
17. Eisbruch, A., Lweinski, U., and Djaidett, M.: Severe opisthotonos and trismus associated with water intoxication. J.R. Soc. Med. 77:158, 1984.
18. Gill, G.: Treatment of hyponatremic seizures with intravenous 29.2% saline. Br. Med. J. 292:625, 1986.
19. Nairns, R.G.: Therapy of hyponatremia: does haste make waste? N. Engl. J. Med. 314:1573. 1986.
20. Van Duzen, J., et al.: Protein and calorie malnutrition among preschool Navajo children. Am. J. Clin. Nutr. 22:657, 1969.
21. Van Duzen, J., et al.: Protein and calorie malnutrition among preschool Navajo children: A follow-up. Am. J. Clin. Nutr. 22:132, 1969.
22. Hertzman, P.A., Blevins, W.L., Mayer, I., et al.: Association of the eosinophilia-myalgia syndrome with the ingestion of tryptophan. N. Engl. J. Med. 322:869, 1990.
23. Silver, R.M., Heyes, M.P., Maize, J.C., et al.: Scleroderma, fascitis, and eosinophilia associated with the ingestion of tryptophan. N. Engl. J. Med. 322:874, 1990.
24. EMS epidemic may be linked to single L-tryptophan manufacturer. Food Chemical News, June 25, 1990, p. 67.

BIBLIOGRAPHY

Altmeyer, R. B., et al.: Spontaneous pneumomediastinum as a complication of anorexia nervosa. W. Va. Med. J. 77:189, 1981.

Baher, et al.: Anorexia nervosa. Curr. Concepts Nutr. 11:139, 1982.

Baxi, S. C., and Dailey, G. E., III: Hypervitaminosis A: A cause of hypercalcemia. West. J. Med. 137:429, 1982.

Brotman, A. W., et al.: Case report of cardiovascular abnormalities in anorexia nervosa. Am. J. Psychiatry 140:1227, 1983.

Farris, W. A., et al.: Protracted hypervitaminosis A following long-term low-level intake. JAMA 247:1317, 1982.

Frank, A., et al.: Fatalities on the liquid-protein diet: An analysis of possible causes. Int. J. Obes. 5:243, 1981.

Halmi, K. A., Falk, J. R., and Schwartz, E.: Binge eating and vomiting: A survey of a college population. Psychol. Med. 11:697, 1981.

Harris, T.: The perils of gorging and purging. Acute Care Medicine, 1:15, 1984.

Hatoff, D. E., et al.: Hypervitaminosis A unmasked by acute viral hepatitis. Gastroenterology 82:124, 1982.

Herbert, V.: Toxicity of 25,000 IV vitamin A supplements in "health food" users [editorial]. Am. J. Clin. Nutr. 36:185, 1982.

James, M. B., et al.: Hypervitaminosis A: A case report. Pediatrics 69:112, 1982.

Johnson, C., et al.: Psychopharmacological treatment of anorexia nervosa and bulimia. J. Nerv. Ment. Dis. 1983.

Kaplan, A. S., et al.: Carbamazepine in the treatment of bulimia. Am. J. Psychiatry 140:9, 1983.

Katz, J. L., et al.: Anorexia nervosa in bulimia [letter]. Arch. Gen. Psychiatry 39:487, 1982.

Kay, J., et al.: Hematologic and immunologic abnormalities in anorexia nervosa. South. Med. J. 76:1008, 1983.

Mirkin, G. B., et al.: The Beverly Hills Diet: Dangers of the newest weight-loss fad. JAMA 246:2235, 1981.

Mitchell, J. E., et al.: Electrolyte and other physiological abnormalities in patients with bulimia. Psychol. Med. 13:273, 1983.

Niiya, K., et al.: Bulimia nervosa complicated by deficiency of vitamin K-dependent coagulation factors. *JAMA 250*:792, 1983.

Pentlow, B. D., et al.: Acute vascular compression of the duodenum in anorexia nervosa. Br. J. Surg. *68*:665, 1981.

Pyle, R. L., Mitchell, J. E., Eckert, E. D., et al.: The incidence of bulimia in freshman college students. Internat. J. Eating Disord. 2:75, 1983.

Ragauan, V. V., et al.: Vitamin A toxicity and hypercalcemia. Am. J. Med. Sci. *283*:161, 1982.

Rosenberg, H. K., et al.: Pleural effusion and ascites: Unusual presenting features in a pediatric patient with vitamin A intoxication. Clin. Pediatr. *21*:435, 1982.

Saul, S. H., et al.: Acute gastric dilatation with infarction and perforation: Report of fatal outcome in patient with anorexia nervosa. Br. J. Surg. *68*:665, 1981.

Silverman, J. A., and Krongrad, E.: Anorexia nervosa: A cause of pericardial effusion? Pediatr. Cardiol. *4*:125, 1983.

The enigma of anorexia nervosa. (editorial). Nutr. Rev. *41*:121, 1983.

Weber, F. L., Jr., et al.: Reversible hepatotoxicology associated with hepatic vitamin accumulation in a protein-deficient patient. Gastroenterology *82*:118, 1982.

Winick, M. (ed.): Hunger Disease; Studies by The Jewish Physicians in the Warsaw Ghetto. New York, John Wiley & Sons, 1979.

Part XI

Toxicology

Chapter 79

POISON CONTROL CENTERS

Martin J. Smilkstein

CAPSULE

The management of toxicologic emergencies is one of the most common and challenging problems in emergency medicine. The actual magnitude of the problem is unknown, but it appears certain that well over 2 million exposures to toxic substances occurred in the United States in 1987, resulting in several hundred thousand visits to emergency departments (EDs).[1] As a result, emergency physicians encountered patients in all age groups, thousands of different poisonous agents, routes of exposure including ingestion, inhalation, injection, dermal and ocular absorption, and bites and stings. With increasing awareness of the toxic hazards of the workplace and the environment, ongoing development of new drugs, new chemicals, and new uses for old agents, probably no other area of emergency medicine is as all-encompassing or dynamic. With recent major shifts in approaches to basic poison management and the development of new antidotes and treatment adjuncts, providing optimum care to the poisoned patient has become an even greater challenge to the emergency physician.

Fortunately, the evolution of a unique national network has provided a support system to assist in handling toxicologic exposures. The first poison control center was established in Chicago in 1953; since that time tremendous growth and organization have occurred.[2] Today the roster of the American Association of Poison Control Centers (AAPCC) includes over 100 centers, including 37 that meet more strict guidelines and have been designated regional poison control centers (Source: AAPCC membership directory 1988).

POISON CONTROL CENTER SERVICES

Poison control center services include provision of information accessible by telephone 24 hours a day, 365 days a year, to both consumers and health care providers. This is accomplished by the use of trained Certified Specialists in Poisoning Information, who may be nurses, pharmacists, or others with adequate health-oriented background and specialized training. The information they provide is derived from comprehensive poison information sources (e.g., Poisindex[3]), specialty texts, and required written treatment protocols, all designed to provide appropriate, consistent recommendations. In addition, backup staffing includes a medical director and specialty consultants knowledgeable in important related areas such as pediatrics, nephrology, and hyperbaric medicine.[2]

Other important functions include communication with 911 emergency services and responsibility for outreach educational programs for both medical professionals and the public. In some instances, in areas lacking a designated poison treatment center, poison control centers have been able to stock and supply a full range of antidotes and other adjuncts (e.g., hemoperfusion cartridges). At present, there is tremendous variability among poison control centers; emergency personnel should know the capabilities of the centers that they use.

PREHOSPITAL AND OUT-OF-HOSPITAL CARE

Undoubtedly, poison control centers have had the greatest impact outside of health care facilities, primarily by affecting the care of accidental poisoning in children. Of the 1,166,940 poison exposures reported in the AAPCC 1987 report, 731,625 (63%) involved children under 6.[1] Fortunately, most were not serious; in this age group only 22 fatalities occurred, and 538,973 (74%) of exposures caused either no effect or only a minor effect.[1] Instead of presenting to the ED, most of these cases comprised a portion of the 873,194 (75%) of those treated outside health care facilities. In New York state, the savings in health care costs from avoiding these unneeded ED visits was estimated at over 19 million dollars in 1985.[4]

Recommendations in these cases may include reassurance, dilution of ingested agents with milk or water, irrigation for skin or eye decontamination, induction of emesis with ipecac, or when available, home use of activated charcoal. Telephone follow-up is also provided to determine if further therapy or referral to a health care facility is needed.

In addition to cases managed at home or at the workplace, well over 130,000 patients were referred to health care facilities by poison control centers in 1987.[1] Generally, *all symptomatic patients, those with potentially dangerous exposures, potentially suicidal patients (including adolescents and adults with suspicious histories), and potential cases of child abuse or neglect are referred.* Many poison control centers also contact police or ambulance dispatchers when appropriate.

In addition to recommending ED care, the poison control center staff may initiate appropriate care by phone, advise prehospital care personnel on appropriate field management and data gathering (e.g., collecting pill containers, obtaining history from family or friends, recording unusual odors or other clues), and provide advanced notification and poison management information to the receiving ED. This comprehensive approach is in place at many poison control centers, and serves as a model for future development in other centers.

HAZARDOUS MATERIAL SPILLS

An area of increasing concern in prehospital care is the proper approach to hazardous material exposures. Some poison control centers have taken on active roles in the evaluation and management of hazardous material spills, actually dispatching personnel to the scene to work in conjunction with local officials. Most centers do not take on this role, but can be invaluable in facilitating communication by identifying and notifying the appropriate agencies.

HOSPITAL REFERRALS FROM POISON CONTROL CENTERS

A controversial area for future consideration is the role of the poison control center in destination policy in prehospital care. Because certain exposures may require specialized care such as pediatric intensive care, hemodialysis, or hemoperfusion, unusual antidotes, or hyperbaric oxygen, consideration of these issues may be important in deciding ambulance destination. Because many of these exposures may involve unusual agents or require specialized knowledge to determine appropriate care, it is unlikely that prewritten protocols can cover all contingencies. With comprehensive, rapidly accessible resources and specialist backup available, poison control centers may play a more important role in destination policy in the future.

EMERGENCY DEPARTMENT MANAGEMENT

The poison control center can be an invaluable resource when patients with potential toxicologic problems are seen in the ED. Even the most knowledgeable emergency specialist cannot be familiar with the manifestations and treatment of poisoning by each of the thousands of potential offending agents. The agents responsible for fatal poisonings in the 1987 AAPCC annual report dramatically illustrate this point. In addition to deaths from more common agents such as antidepressants and analgesics, deaths from boron tribromide, chloroform, oxalic acid, trichloroethane, sulfuryl fluoride, paraquat, water hemlock, colchicine, chloroquine, flecainide, merthiolate, and others were reported.[1] It is critical that clinically relevant information about these and other unusual exposures be rapidly available to the emergency physician. Even in common exposures, access to concise advice is often invaluable.

Another critical role of the poison control center is identification of agents potentially causing toxicity. In its simplest form, this involves identification of pills and capsules. Microfiche or computerized listings allow rapid identification by the letter or number encoded on many medications.[5] Other systems include product listings and ingredients by brand name, so that potentially toxic ingredients can be identified directly from the name on the label.[3] Other useful identification services include listing potentially causative agents on the basis of presenting signs or symptoms, identification of some foreign medications, translation of street slang terms for drugs of abuse, and identification of likely agents resulting from mixture of chemicals or those likely to be associated with a particular occupational setting. Identification of plants, mushrooms, spiders, or snakes can also often be facilitated by Certified Specialists in Poison Information, or through information sources readily accessed by them. Once identification of any of these agents is made, the poison control center can provide guidelines to the management of the patient.

The information sources used by poison control centers not only describe the likely toxicity of a given agent, but are uniquely designed to provide information on the dose likely to be toxic, the time course of toxicity, the value of laboratory assessment of toxicity, and other critical features. Even widely available information such as recommendations regarding basic poison management—including gastric emptying, activated charcoal, and antidotal therapy—are changing rapidly, and current, accurate information is beyond the scope of most texts. In addition to information specific to a given poison, concise guidelines for supportive care are also generally available as they relate to the agent involved. For these and many other reasons, emergency management of toxicologic patients is greatly facilitated by consultation with a poison control center.

PATIENT DISPOSITION

The information sources described previously also offer valuable information to assist in patient disposition decisions. Determining the likelihood of further decompensation, the need for ongoing treatment, intensive care monitoring, extracorporeal drug removal (e.g., hemodialysis, hemoperfusion), hyperbaric oxygen therapy, or outpatient follow-up requires detailed practical information, often most readily obtained from poison control center sources. In addition, poison control centers are often aware of the facilities that have these treatments and others, including antidotes and antivenoms, and are thus able to assist in determining appropriate transfer destinations when the treating hospital lacks a critical treatment modality. When transfer is indicated, the poison control center can also assist in communicating important patient and treatment information to the receiving facility.

TOXICOLOGY EDUCATION

Most poison control centers provide poison prevention and treatment information to the public, but they also play a critical role in the education of prehospital care personnel, nurses, and physicians. Toxicology is a required area of study in emergency medicine residency programs, and many residencies now require or offer full-time rotations at poison control centers. Because of increasing emphasis on toxicology and the recent increasing demand for academically oriented emergency physicians, many residents are participating in poison control center-based medical toxicology fellowships after residency.

EPIDEMIOLOGY AND DATA COLLECTION

A final important role of the poison control center is providing ongoing monitoring of trends in toxicology. Important information on the efficacy of poison prevention measures such as education, childproof containers, and others can be monitored by observing these trends. Moreover, additional factors are associated with those who contact poison control centers. For example, children aged 2 to 6 in families who have contacted poison control centers are at increased risk (1 to 6 times) for injuries.[6] Therefore such data can be used in injury prevention programs.

The emergence and disappearance of certain poisonings can be detected by data analysis, and tells us a great deal about the problems likely to be seen in the ED. Analysis of signs and symptoms associated with certain agents has served to dispel many myths and allow more rational treatment guidelines. An increasing number of poison control centers participate in the AAPCC annual data collection, but more participation is needed. Participating poison control centers are responsible for areas including 57% of the United States population, but even within those areas, reporting is never complete.[1] As increasing numbers of centers participate, and with increased reporting by health care personnel, it is hoped that analysis of these data will yield even more valuable information.

REFERENCES

1. Litovitz, T.L., Schmitz, B.F., Matyunas, N., and Martin, T.G.: 1987 annual report of the American Association of Poison Control Centers national data collection system. Am. J. Emerg. Med. 6:479, 1988.
2. Manoguerra, A.S., and Temple, A.R.: Observations on the current status of poison control centers in the United States. Emerg. Med. Clin. North Am. 2:185, 1984.
3. Rumack, B.H. (ed.): Poisindex volume 58. Denver, Micromedex, 1988.
4. Galizia, A., Weisman, R., and Fisher, L.: Cost/benefit analysis of regional New York State Poison Control Centers. Presented at the American Public Health Association meeting, October 1987. Am. J. Public Health, in press.
5. Rumack, B.H. (ed.): Identidex (TM). Denver, Micromedex, 1988.
6. Baraff, L.J., et al: The relationship of poison center contact and injury in children 2 to 6 years old. Ann. Emerg. Med. 21:153, 1992.

Chapter 80

PREHOSPITAL AND INTERHOSPITAL CARE OF THE POISONED OR OVERDOSED PATIENT

Theodore Benzer and Neal Flomenbaum

CAPSULE

Frequently, poisoned or overdosed patients are brought to the hospital by emergency personnel and paramedics, and occasionally they must be transferred from one facility to another for treatment available only at a specialized center. Although not always able to deliver *definitive* therapy for poisoned or overdosed patients, prehospital personnel are invaluable for securing the airway, stabilizing circulation, and instituting life-saving Basic Life Support (BLS) and Advanced Life Support (ALS) measures. Astute prehospital evaluation of both the patient and the environment is especially helpful in later making a specific etiologic diagnosis of the patient's clinical condition or identifying a specific causative drug or poison.

PREHOSPITAL MANAGEMENT

INFORMATION GATHERING

Probably one of the most important jobs of prehospital personnel in management of the toxic emergency is evaluation of the patient's environment to the extent permitted by the patient's condition. As an example, an elderly patient brought in unconscious from home may be suffering from disease as diverse as hyperosmolar coma, sepsis, poisoning, overdose, or intoxication. If, however, an astute emergency worker notices the unvented space heater in the corner of the room and reports this finding to the emergency department (ED) staff, the diagnosis of carbon monoxide poisoning can be pursued expeditiously. (This consideration is especially important because oxygen treatment en route may effectively treat the signs and

symptoms before the patient can be examined in the ED.

In addition to an obvious empty pill bottle, suicide note, or illicit drug paraphernalia found with a patient, prehospital personnel should be aware of unusual smells, sources of carbon monoxide, or evidence of toxic chemicals in the patient's environment. Chemicals in the workplace also present a challenge but may be a more obvious source of poisoning when only a few specific chemicals may be involved. A vomiting, diaphoretic patient in an insecticide factory would be quickly evaluated for organophosphate poisoning. A comatose infant with pinpoint pupils found on the floor of a kitchen, however, may be more of a diagnostic challenge unless the emergency worker sees a half-empty can of insecticide (organophosphates) on the floor or an open bottle of diphenoxylate (opioid) tablets under the dresser.

Prehospital evaluation should include transport to the ED of containers (labeled or not), pills and pill bottles, and any possible ingested plant material for definitive identification. If possible, animals at the scene that may be either sources or victims of the poisoning should be restrained and transported later by appropriate means (e.g., ASPCA).

AVOIDING DANGER TO RESCUE PERSONNEL

Any intoxication, intentional or not, poses risks to prehospital personnel. Emergency personnel and paramedics must protect themselves from intoxication or inhalation of toxic chemicals and fumes by using appropriate protective clothing and masks and providing adequate ventilation to enclosed spaces suspected of having high concentrations of carbon monoxide. Many toxic gases are colorless and odorless, and several toxic chemicals (such as organophosphates) can be absorbed through intact skin. Paramedics and emergency personnel must also be aware of the danger of mouth-to-mouth resuscitation in a patient suspected of having cyanide poisoning. Protocols written to cover the actions of prehospital personnel should include specific instructions, and ambulances must be adequately equipped to avoid intoxication and poisoning of the rescuer.

As with all patient interactions, care must be taken to avoid blood and body fluid contamination. Patients with illicit IV drug ingestions are especially prone to blood-borne infections (e.g., HIV and hepatitis), and great care must be taken to avoid contamination during treatment of the patients and handling of their drug paraphernalia.

INITIAL MANAGEMENT

Initial control of airway, breathing, and circulation is of prime importance in the toxic emergency, as in any emergency. Prehospital personnel must be aware that the patient's condition may deteriorate rapidly and unpredictably. Definitive control of the airway with endotracheal intubation and establishment of an intravenous line should be considered early in the management of an overdose. Decontamination of skin and eyes exposed to dangerous chemicals or caustics should also begin expeditiously with copious irrigation. Some consideration may be given to the administration of ipecac to alert patients with an appropriate recent oral ingestion. Control of the airway of a vomiting patient in the back of a moving ambulance can be difficult, however. There is also a potential loss of gag reflex in the patient before vomiting. On the other hand, because of time constraints, gastric lavage is almost never practical in the prehospital setting.

The New York State and New York City Life Support Protocols have been adapted to demonstrate approaches in cases of poisoning or drug overdose. These protocols appear at the end of this chapter.

INTERHOSPITAL TRANSPORT

Emergency physicians and hospitals must carefully weigh the benefits and risks of transferring a sick, poisoned or overdosed patient to a tertiary care center. Generally, a patient with a toxic emergency should be moved to another facility only if the primary hospital does not have the specialized therapy needed to treat poisoning or overdose requiring such treatment. Even in these instances, the risks of a patient experiencing seizures, dysrhythmias, or hypotension en route to another hospital must be carefully weighed against the deficiencies of the first hospital. Patients with overdose or poisoning with camphor, cyclic antidepressants, beta blockers, calcium channel blockers, Isoniazid (INH), cyanide, strychnine, and propoxyphene often deteriorate rapidly during the first hour after the ingestion.

Patients suffering from carbon monoxide poisoning and having specific indications for hyperbaric oxygen therapy should be transferred to a facility having this capability (see Guide to Identification of Hyperbaric Candidates, adapted from the New York City Operating Guide for Emergency Medical Service Hyperbaric Candidates, at the end of this chapter). Transfer of these patients should be with constant 100% oxygen therapy en route. Assisted ventilation should be used in patients who are not breathing spontaneously or those with COPD who may stop breathing with high-concentration oxygen therapy.

Patients should be transferred to facilities where specific antidote therapy is available, such as an Antivenin Center established for a geographic area. (See Approach to the Patient Suffering from Animal/Human Bites or Snakebite, at the end of this chapter.

Finally, transfer of a patient to a facility capable of hemodialysis or hemoperfusion may be required if the initial facility does not perform these procedures. Most commonly, poisoning with methanol or ethylene glycol and serious overdoses of salicylates, theophylline, and lithium may require such treatment. All other measures, such as the use of repetitive doses of orogastric charcoal for theophylline, and intravenous bicarbonate treatment for salicylates, should be instituted before and continued during the interhospital transport. Care should be taken to ensure that the patient is indeed a candidate for the specific modalities available only at a tertiary care center, and all potentially beneficial measures should be instituted while transport arrangements are being made.

As with any patient transfer between institutions, care must be taken to ensure that the patient has been medically stabilized as much as possible within the time frame dictated by the nature of the exposure. As always, it is important that the receiving physician and receiving hospital have agreed to accept the patient and assume care. It is also important that the transfer be made in an appropriate ambulance with Advanced Life Support available, along with all other necessary personnel (respiratory therapy, nurse, and/or physician) in accordance with accepted standards of interhospital transport described in ACLS and ATLS protocols (and in accordance with ACEP guidelines and the 1987 U.S. Federal COBRA legislation).

The following New York City Emergency Medical Service protocols are presented as examples of prehospital and interhospital protocols for the care of poisoned or overdosed patients.

LIFE SUPPORT PROTOCOLS

POISONING

GENERAL

CAUTION!

TAKE PRECAUTIONS NOT TO CONTAMINATE SELF OR OTHERS!

---

1. If possible, identify the product or substance ingested or inhaled by, or coming in contact with, the patient.
2. Estimate the amount of product or substance ingested, if applicable.
3. Estimate the duration of exposure to the product or substance.
4. If possible, bring the product or substance and container with the patient to the hospital.

PATIENT WHO IS CONSCIOUS AND ALERT

CAUTION!

SUCH PATIENTS MAY DETERIORATE RAPIDLY. BE ESPECIALLY ALERT FOR RESPIRATORY INSUFFICIENCY OR ARREST!

SWALLOWED POISONS

1. If possible, contact the Poison Control Center, local Medical Control, or Receiving Hospital for instructions for treatment, which may include the administration of milk, water, ipecac, the induction of vomiting, etc.
2. Transport, keeping the patient warm.
3. Obtain and record the vital signs, and repeat en route as often as the situation indicates.
4. Record all patient care information, including the patient's medical history and all treatment provided, on a Prehospital Care Report.

INHALED POISONS

1. Ensure that the scene is safe for entry. If danger of poisonous gases, vapors, or sprays or a low-oxygen environment is present, it may be necessary to obtain assistance from trained rescue personnel.
2. Remove the patient to fresh air.
3. Place the patient in a position of comfort.
4. Ensure that the patient's airway is open and that breathing and circulation are adequate.
5. Administer high-concentration oxygen.
6. Transport, keeping the patient warm.
7. Obtain and record the vital signs, and repeat en route as often as the situation indicates.
8. Record all patient care information, including the patient's medical history and all treatment provided, on a Prehospital Care Report.

SKIN OR EYE(S) CONTAMINATION

1. Refer to the *BURNS/CONTAMINATIONS (CHEMICAL/RADIATION)* PROTOCOL.

PATIENT WHO IS UNCONSCIOUS OR HAS
ALTERED MENTAL STATUS

1. Ensure that the patient's airway is open and that breathing and circulation are adequate, and suction as necessary.
2. Administer high-concentration oxygen.
3. Transport, keeping the patient warm.
4. Obtain and record the vital signs, and repeat en route as often as the situation indicates.
5. Record all patient care information, including the patient's medical history and all treatment provided, on a Prehospital Care Report.

APPROACH TO THE PATIENT WITH ALTERED MENTAL STATUS OR COMA OF UNKNOWN ORIGIN

DEFINITION: Altered mental status—any patient presenting with a mental status of less than alert and oriented × 3.

1. *Treatment*
   a. Maintain ABCs and intervene as required.
   b. Assist ventilation as necessary.
   c. Administer high concentration of oxygen. In children, humidified oxygen is preferred.
   d. Determine level of consciousness.
   e. Monitor vital signs as needed.
   f. If the patient is conscious, has a gag reflex, and is able to drink without assistance, provide glucose or a sugar solution with orange juice by mouth, then transport, keeping the patient warm.
   g. Place patient in left lateral recumbent position unless contraindicated.
   h. Assess and monitor Glasgow Coma Scale.
   i. If suspicion of poisoning, bring substance to the hospital.
   j. If the patient is **unresponsive** or **responds only to painful stimuli,** transport immediately, taking cervical and spinal precautions if indicated. Keep the patient warm enroute.
   k. Record all patient care information, including the patient's medical history, if available, and all treatment provided on the Ambulance Call Report.

APPROACH TO ALTERED MENTAL STATE

For patients presenting with altered mental status.

1. Administer oxygen.
2. Draw an SMA 6 for blood glucose level.
3. Begin an IV infusion of dextrose 5% in water (D_5W) to keep the vein open.

4. Administer dextrose, 25 g (50 cc of a 50% solution), IV bolus.*
5. In patients with diabetic histories in whom an IV route is unavailable, administer glucagon, 1.0 mg, IM. (Thiamine need not be administered to these patients).
6. Administer thiamine, 100 mg, IV bolus.
7. If there is no change in mental status, administer naloxone, up to 0.8 mg, IV bolus (restraints may be applied if appropriate). Naloxone may be administered at the same dosage IM if no IV route is available.
8. Administer a repeat dose of dextrose, 25 g (50 cc of a 50% solution) if the patient's mental state fails to improve significantly.
9. Administer repeat naloxone, up to 2.0 mg, IV bolus, if patient's respiratory status fails to improve significantly.

APPROACH TO THE VICTIM OF POISONING OR DRUG OVERDOSE

1. *Special Assessment Considerations*
   A. Survey the scene, note especially:
      1) Hazardous situations.
      2) Remnants of the poison or drug.
      3) Containers and/or drug paraphernalia.
      4) Vomitus.
   B. Determine the age and the weight of the victim.
   C. Attempt to determine the drug or poison.
      1) How was it taken?
      2) How long ago?
      3) How much of the substance was taken?
      4) Was it all at once or over a period of time?
   D. Determine the patient's present signs and symptoms.
   E. Determine the patient's medical history.
   F. Perform a Glasgow Coma Scale and record findings.
   G. Assess need for ALS assistance.

---

* If a drug overdose is strongly suspected, administer naloxone prior to dextrose and thiamine.

2. *General Treatment*
  A. Remove the patient from any hazards.
  B. Maintain ABCs.
  C. Administer appropriate oxygen.
  D. Assist ventilation as necessary by BVM with supplemental oxygen or demand valve resuscitator.
  E. Initiate appropriate subprotocol treatment.
  F. DO NOT ATTEMPT TO NEUTRALIZE POISON OR DRUG (with egg whites, lemon juice, baking soda, etc.).
  G. DO NOT FOLLOW DIRECTIONS ON CONTAINER LABELS.
  H. Be prepared to suction the patient.
  I. Treat for shock.
  J. Monitor the patient's condition and vital signs.
  K. Place the patient in the left lateral recumbent (coma) position.
  L. Transport any of the following with the patient:
    1) Remnants of substance.
    2) Containers of drug paraphernalia as appropriate.
    3) Vomitus.
  M. Transport to appropriate facility.
3. *Ingested Substances*
  A. If landline available, call Poison Control Center; follow their advice.
  B. Dilute substance with one to two glasses of water or milk.
  C. DILUTION IS CONTRAINDICATED IN UNCONSCIOUS OR CONVULSING PATIENTS.
  D. DO NOT ATTEMPT TO INDUCE VOMITING UNLESS DIRECTED BY THE POISON CONTROL CENTER.
  E. If the substance is a corrosive poison or petroleum product, transport the patient IMMEDIATELY to the appropriate facility.
4. *Injected Substances and Snakebites*
  A. Attempt to calm the patient.
  B. Remove jewelry from affected area if swelling begins to occur.
  C. Place injection site lower than the patient's heart if possible.
  D. Implement snakebite operating procedure.
5. *Inhaled Substances (Including Smoke Inhalation)*
  A. Remove patient from source as soon as this can be done safely.
  B. Administer appropriate humidified oxygen.
  C. If the patient is unconscious, assist ventilations and *hyperventilate patient* by BVM with supplemental oxygen or demand valve resuscitator.
6. *Surface Contact Substances*
  A. Remove patient from source as soon as this can be done safely.
  B. Remove all contaminated clothing.
  C. Rinse affected area thoroughly for 5 to 10 minutes.
  D. Bandage any substance burns with dry aseptic dressings.

APPROACH TO THE PATIENT SUFFERING FROM ANIMAL/HUMAN BITES OR SNAKEBITE

1. *Special Assessment Considerations*
  A. **Make sure that the scene is safe for entry.**
  B. Determine the source of the bite:
    1. type of animal.
    2. behavior of the animal (if known).

2. *Treatment*
  A. Dress and bandage as appropriate.
  B. Minor wounds may be washed with soap and water (when possible).

NOTE!
IF SNAKEBITE IS INVOLVED, THE PATIENT MAY REQUIRE THE USE OF A SPECIALTY REFERRAL CENTER.

3. *Special Assessment Considerations for Snakebite*
  A. Locate the bite.
  B. Remove any constricting items of clothing.

4. *Treatment for Snakebite*
  A. If the patient has been bitten by a pit viper, carry out the following steps:
    1. Calm and reassure the patient. This will decrease the spread of any venom through the system.
    2. Locate the bite area, clean gently with soap and water if possible.
    3. Place venous constricting bands above and below the bite site.

NOTE!
THE DISTAL PULSE IN THE EXTREMITY SHOULD NOT DISAPPEAR. THE PURPOSE OF THE VENOUS CONSTRICTING BAND IS TO LIMIT THE SPREAD OF THE VENOM.

    4. Immobilize the extremity with a splint if possible.
    5. Monitor vital signs as necessary.
    6. Be alert for the onset of shock.
    7. Place the patient on high concentration of oxygen.
    8. If possible, try to make identification of the offending snake so that the correct antivenom can be administered.
    9. Transport the patient promptly to the hospital or Speciality Referral Center and make the necessary notifications enroute.
    10. Be alert for vomiting.
    11. Do not give the patient any liquids.

CAUTION!
NEVER ATTEMPT TO SUCK THE VENOM FROM THE WOUND USING YOUR MOUTH!

APPROACH TO A PATIENT EXPOSED TO A RADIATION ACCIDENT

A. *Special Assessment Considerations*
   The following guidelines should be followed when treating a patient exposed to a radiation accident:
   1. **ALWAYS DO A 10-SECOND SCENE SURVEY!**
   2. Protect yourself from the dangers of exposure.
   3. Alert the Dispatcher to notify the Police, Fire, EMS HAZMAT Response Team, EPA and DEP.
   4. Before care can be administered, the patient must be decontaminated by HAZ MAT TEAM.
   5. Have the patient remove all jewelry, clothing and shoes.
   6. Administer appropriate patient care.
   7. Before transporting the patient, cover the ambulance stretcher mattress with a blanket.
   8. Wrap the patient in the blanket and fashion a head covering from a sheet.
   9. Only the patient's face should show when ready to transport.
   10. Make the necessary notification/standby to the hospital to which the patient is being transported prior to the arrival of the patient.
B. Treatment
   After the patient has been decontaminated, refer to the appropriate BLS protocol for the treatment of each patient.

ALL PATIENTS ARE TO BE TREATED SYMPTOMATICALLY AND TRANSPORTED IN THE USUAL MANNER!

APPROACH TO THE PATIENT EXPOSED TO A HAZARDOUS MATERIAL

A. *HAZARDOUS MATERIAL ACTION GUIDE*
   All personnel, regardless of training, should follow the guidelines listed below in regard to calls involving a hazardous material spill/incident:
   1. **ALWAYS DO A 10 SECOND SURVEY!**
   2. Never underestimate the size of the spill or incident.
   3. Establish and maintain proper communications with the Borough or Citywide Dispatcher.
   4. Stay upwind and upgrade at all times. Monitor weather and wind changes.
   5. Do not breathe any smoke, fumes, or vapors.

6. Do not touch or walk through any spilled materials. You will only increase the size of the incident.
7. Do not eat, drink, or smoke at the scene of the incident. These are all direct routes of entry into the body.
8. Do not touch your face, nose, mouth, or eyes.
9. Eliminate all sources of ignition such as flares, flames, sparks, smoking, flashes, flashlights, gas and diesel engines, and portable radios.
10. If your unit is the first on the scene, notify the Dispatcher and give a 10–12. Request the assistance of the EPA, DEP, Police, Fire, and the EMS HAZMAT Response Team.
11. Do not drive through any spilled materials. You are only increasing the size of the incident.
12. Identify the substance, if possible, using the **DOT EMERGENCY RESPONSE GUIDEBOOK.** Inform the Dispatcher of your findings.
13. Observe all safety precautions and directions as set forth by the On-Scene Commander, Police, Fire, EPA, DEP.
14. **ALL ORDERS SHOULD BE TAKEN FACE TO FACE!**
15. Remain clear of all restricted areas until declared safe by the On-Scene Commander.

GUIDE TO IDENTIFICATION OF HYPERBARIC CANDIDATES*

PURPOSE

To specify the criteria to be used to identify candidates for referral to a hyperbaric center.

SCOPE

This procedure applies to all members of the New York City Emergency Medical Service, the employees of voluntary hospitals who provide prehospital emergency medical care through the New York City Emergency Medical Service (NYCEMS) dispatch system, and to the personnel of other agencies participating in the 911 system.

POLICY

Hyperbaric center candidates will be transported to the nearest 911 Receiving Hospital for evaluation and stabilization.

---

* Example from New York City Operating Guide for Emergency Service Hyperbaric Candidates.

If the patient's condition warrants, after consultation and receiving approval for transfer from the Senior Emergency Department Physician of Bronx Municipal Hospital, the patient may be transported to Bronx Municipal Hospital Center (BMHC) or directly to the North American Hyperbaric Center (NAHC) for treatment.

PROCEDURE

A. The Emergency Department Physician at the 911 Emergency Receiving Hospital shall:
1. Evaluate and stabilize the patient(s).
2. Use the following criteria to identify candidates for treatment in a hyperbaric chamber:
   a. Carbon monoxide poisoning
   b. Smoke inhalation
   c. Cyanide poisoning
   d. Decompression sickness
   e. Gas gangrene
   f. Gas embolism
   g. Patients exposed to carbon monoxide who have been unconscious, or present with signs of central nervous system derangement, regardless of their carboxyhemoglobin level.
3. Consult with the Senior Emergency Department Resident at Bronx Municipal Hospital Center (212-430-5121 or 430-5104) to determine if the following carbon monoxide-exposed patients require hyperbaric oxygen therapy:
   a. Any symptom-free patient who has a carboxy-hemoglobin level of 25% or more.
   b. All pregnant patients who present with medical conditions as outlined in Section A, item #2.
4. Ascertain from the BMHC referring physician if the patient shall be transported to the BMHC emergency department *or* to NAHC.
5. In the event of the unavailability of NAHC, contact the Tour Commander.
6. Once the patient(s) are stabilized and acceptance of the patient(s) has been received, notify the Tour Commander for emergency transport arrangements giving the following information:
   a. number of patient(s);
   b. age and sex;
   c. condition of each patient (critical, on a stretcher, able to sit, etc.), other medical or surgical problems (i.e., burns, trauma, pregnancy, suffering from a communicable or infectious disease, protective isolation, or suffering from disorientation or an emotional disturbance);
   d. how each patient must be transported (i.e. sitting or on a stretcher);
   e. number of hospital personnel (and weight factor) accompanying the patient(s);
   f. type of monitoring or therapy equipment they will be using for each patient (weight factor);
   g. name of hospital or facility accepting the patient(s).
7. Contact the EMS Tour Commander if the request for transport is cancelled at any time. The name and title of person cancelling the request are required.

B. The Tour Commander Shall:
1. When it is determined by the 911 Emergency Department Physician that hyperbaric oxygen therapy is needed, coordinate the transfer of patient(s) from the emergency department to Bronx Municipal Hospital Center or the North American Hyperbaric Center.
   NOTE: NAHC has a total capacity of 6 patient's, 4 walk-in and 2 critical-multiplace chambers.
2. If the patient(s)' condition allows, have the patient(s) transported by ambulance. If the patient(s)' condition or circumstances necessitates, the Tour Commander may arrange for a MEDEVAC after consulting with the Medical Control Physician on duty.
3. Cancel all responding units if the request for transport is cancelled by the 911 Referring Facility.
4. Coordinate the transfer of patients from the Hyperbaric Chamber to BMHC for follow-up treatment, as directed by the BMHC staff.
   NOTE: If NAHC is unavailable, the Tour Commander shall follow the outlined procedures in the Division Memoranda which addresses Hyperbaric Center transfers.

C. Communications Dispatcher Shall:
1. Advise the Tour Commander if patient(s) are members of the New York City Police Department or Fire Department. Enter all appropriate information on the "Tracking Mask for NYPD/NYFD Patients" into the system.
2. As required, have a supervisor and a unit respond to the receiving hospital or helicopter landing site for the transport of the patient(s) to the hospital or Hyperbaric Chamber.
3. Make notifications as required.
4. After the unit turns the patient(s) over to the emergency department and completes the paperwork, advise the unit whether they are to stand by or go to a "10–97 or 10–98" status.

D. The Assigned Supervisor Shall:
1. Respond to the scene or hospital as requested.
2. If circumstances warrant that the patient(s) must be transported from the scene to BMHC or NAHC, notify the Tour Commander. Ensure that the Tour Commander is informed which EMS member is riding with the patient(s). The operator of the vehicle will drive the ambulance to the hospital.

3. When required, respond to the helicopter landing site for the transfer of the patient(s) and the hospital employees to the helicopter, or from the helicopter to the waiting ambulance for transport to BMHC or NAHC.

E. Members of the Service Shall:

1. Notify the dispatcher if they believe the patient(s) they are treating are possible hyperbaric candidates.

2. BLS and ALS units shall follow all EMS Patient Treatment and Transport Protocols. All units shall document on the ACR:

   a. How long the patient was exposed (i.e. carbon monoxide, smoke, cyanide, etc.) or has been experiencing symptoms (i.e. decompression sickness, gas gangrene, CNS derangement, etc.)

   b. How long the patient has been receiving oxygen therapy.

3. Transport the patient(s) to the nearest 911 Receiving Hospital. Complete the necessary paperwork associated with the assignment and, unless directed by the EMS dispatcher to stand by, return to a "10–97 or 10–98" status.

NOTE: *If a helicopter is required from the scene, notify the Tour Commander when a supervisor is not on the scene.*

BIBLIOGRAPHY

Agreement between the Emergency Medical Service and Bronx Municipal Hospital Center/North American Hyperbaric Center, dated March 3, 1985.

Agreement between the Emergency Medical Service and Mount Sinai Medical Center/Hyperbaric Center.

EMS Advisory No. 5A, "Hyperbaric Treatment for CO Poisoning and Smoke Inhalation," dated April 1986.

Memorandum from Cink Weitzel, Systems Specialist EMS, Re: Minutes from Ad Hoc Patient Triage Committee, dated August 26, 1983.

Memorandum from Starr L. Grimm, MSN, MPH, Associate Director (Acting), Re: Hyperbaric Patient Triage, dated September 30, 1983.

Protocol approved by the Hyperbaric Advisory Committee, dated April 21, 1983; "New York City Emergency Medical Service 911 System Hyperbaric Specialty Referral Center Standards."

Recommendations for Operating Procedures for Hyperbaric Patients, dated June 13, 1984.

Revised Recommendations for Operating Procedures for Hyperbaric Centers dated July 7, 1984.

Chapter 81

THE POISONED PATIENT

OVERVIEW AND GENERAL CONSIDERATIONS

George R. Schwartz

CAPSULE

The range of possible substances that can cause poisoning is vast. In fact, every substance is a potential poison if it is admitted into the body in large enough quantities. To provide a compendium of all possible poisons is therefore impossible for practical purposes. Chapter 83 lists substances commonly involved in poisonings and includes a synopsis of medical management in such cases. Moreover, throughout this book, the diagnosis and treatment of poisonings and drug overdoses are discussed in some detail. The index has been designed to allow ready reference to these discussions, which are listed under the general heading of "Poisonings."

The principal thrust of this chapter is:

1. To provide a brief historic introduction and review the basics of emergency toxicology.
2. To detail the method of evaluating a poisoned patient or one in whom poisoning is suspected.
3. To describe the sequence of good general medical management in cases of poisonings.
4. To describe the role of the laboratory in the poisoned patient.
5. To describe techniques involved in the management of poisonings and their indications and contraindications (e.g., emesis, lavage, dialysis).
6. To present an approach to symptom and sign analysis when poisoning is present or suspected but the actual substance involved is not known.
7. To present some of the controversies that exist among experts in poisoning management and the reasons for the differences of opinion (e.g., the management of the ingestion of petroleum distillates, the efficacy of dialysis, and other techniques).
8. To provide techniques and detailed evaluation of selected common patient presentations, including the unconscious patient; the hypo- and hypertensive patient; and patients with seizures, dysrhythmias, acid-base disorders, and perplexing clinical signs/symptoms.

HISTORIC SURVEY

The history of poisoning is as old as mankind. Earliest man had to contend with animal venoms and poisonous plants. In some instances this knowledge of poisons (e.g., curare) was used for hunting. Hippocrates mentions poisons in some detail, and the well-known draught of Socrates was hemlock, the state poison of the Greeks. Aristotle included information about poisonings in his writings. Dioscorides, a Greek physician in the court of Nero, classified poisons, and his classification into plant, mineral, and animal poisons is still a convenient format.

The early Romans developed deliberate poisoning into a profession. A cadre of experts sold their services, primarily for political assassination. Like the "contract killers" or "hit men" of our current day, however, they sold their knowledge of poisons and methods of poisoning to the highest bidder.

Dr. Lester Haddad provided technical assistance in developing this chapter.

Most early poisons were of plant origin, but there is evidence that there was also knowledge of arsenic poisoning. Arsenic was the likely agent used in the murder of Claudius, which resulted in Nero becoming emperor of Rome.

In the Middle Ages deliberate poisonings continued, and in the Renaissance such well-known families of poisoners as the Borgias became prominent in Italy.

The most powerful historic influence on the development of a science of toxicology was probably Phillipus Aureolus Paracelsus. Born Theophrastus Bombastus von Hohenheim, he assumed the name Paracelsus and lived throughout the 16th century in a peripatetic manner. Many of his ideas were new to his time, and he was often viewed as a maverick physician and was sometimes ridiculed. His major contribution in the field of poisonings was his visionary realization that poisoning is often a matter of dose and that the difference between the therapeutic and highly toxic effects of a substance is usually dose-related.

Until the 20th century, the major focus was on detection and description of poisonings rather than on treatment and antidotes. The tremendous advances in pharmaceuticals, along with new technology and an enhanced knowledge of the chemical nature and action of substances, have given impetus to more effective treatment. The growth of emergency medicine has served to focus more attention on applied toxicology because facilities are more advanced and time delays from the time of poisoning to that of treatment have been reduced. Skilled emergency physicians are extremely important in rapidly diagnosing and initiating suitable treatment.

EMERGENCY TOXICOLOGY

EVALUATION PLAN

The field of toxicology (the science of poisons) is broad and multidisciplinary. *Emergency toxicology is the application of toxicologic knowledge within a limited time frame and often limited data base in order to formulate the most effective treatment plan.*

To formulate such a plan, clinical information must be integrated with knowledge of the physiologic dynamics of the poisonous substance. Symptom and sign analysis (Table 81-1) may enable possible or presumptive identification of the poison when information is inadequate or the patient is unable or unwilling to provide it. Also, Tables 81-2 through 81-6 should be helpful in evaluation.

When dealing with the emergency situation, attention to supporting vital functions is first and foremost. The basic medical management will be reviewed in the next section. The following is an outline of the questions that should be kept in mind when evaluating a poisoned patient.

1. Nature of Poison and Route of Entry
   a. What is the chemical nature of the poison?
   b. Is the dose potentially lethal?
   c. Was the substance taken orally, parenterally, or through the skin, lungs, gastrointestinal tract, or rectum?
   d. Can the substance be rapidly eliminated (e.g., by emesis), or neutralized or counteracted? Is lavage or whole-bowel irrigation suitable? Is catharsis helpful?
2. Absorption Dynamics and Distribution in Body
   a. What is the time course of absorption or effect, or both? Is emesis or lavage likely to be effective? If delays have occurred or if the route of entry was other than oral, can the substance be bound? (In this context consider antidotes, antibodies, and binding agents.)
   b. Will activated charcoal be of value?
   c. What is the target organ of the poison? Where is the storage site in the body (e.g., fat storage, bound to plasma protein)? Which system will be compromised or injured by the poison? Can this organ injury be reduced or prevented?
   d. Will metabolism produce other products that might be hazardous?
3. Excretion Dynamics
   a. How is the substance excreted? Is it excreted in the urine or stool, through the lungs, by the liver, and biliary system, or other routes?
   b. Can elimination be hastened (e.g., with purgatives, with diuresis, through acidification or alkalinization of the urine, using dialysis or ion-exchange resins, through blood exchange?
4. The Role of the Laboratory
   a. Are there specific tests of poison level (e.g., carboxyhemoglobin, serum alcohol, barbiturate)?
   b. What tests are useful in evaluating the clinical status of the patient? Which tests allow determination of any baseline values as well as allow the course of organ injury to be followed?
5. What other problems might coexist, related or unrelated to the poisoning (for example, trauma, infection, hypothermia, or hyperthermia)?

METABOLISM OF TOXIC SUBSTANCES

Metabolic reactions within the body have evolved so that it can cope with limited quantities of almost any chemical substance. The metabolic reactions, however, are not basically programmed for detoxification, so that, when acting on a poison, some metabolic products may be as active chemically or even more dangerous than the original poison (for example, when methanol is metabolized to formaldehyde and formic acid). It is worthwhile to remember also that metabolic systems are often less developed in the young; thus in infants and children some toxicants

TABLE 81-1. SYMPTOM AND SIGN ANALYSIS TO ASSIST IN IDENTIFICATION OF CHEMICAL AGENT OR CLASS OF AGENT WHEN TYPE OF POISONING IS NOT KNOW

Agent	State of CNS	Convulsions	Pupils	Salivary Activity	Respirations	Heart Rhythm and Rate	Blood Pressure	Diarrhea	Skin Change
Atroprine-like or anticholinergic syndrome	Excitability, coma if severe	Possible	Dilated	Dry	Usually ↑	Tachycardia	↑ Slightly	No	Flushed
Cholinergic type	Excitability, coma if very severe	Usually not	Constricted	Secretions increased markedly	↓ If severe Possible wheezes; ↓ respirations in severe cases	Bradycardia	↓ If severe ↓	Yes	Flushed; may be in shock if severe
CNS tranquilizers, barbiturate type	Depressed	Not usual	Nystagmus, midpoint unless hypoxic—then dilated	No marked change	↓↓ Possible pulmonary edema	Tachycardia	↓	Possible	May be in shock state
CNS tranquilizers, nonbarbiturate (minor type)	Depressed	Not usual	Not changed unless very severe—then dilated	No marked change	↓	Tachycardia	↓	No	VS usually maintained unless very severe
CNS tranquilizers, phenothetazine type	Depressed	Possible	Either slightly constricted or no marked change	Dry	Slightly depressed unless very severe	Tachycardia	↓	No	Flushed
Aspirin	Usually depressed	Possible	No marked change	No marked change	↑ ↑	Tachycardia	↓ If severe	Possible	Not marked
Narcotic	Depressed	Not usual	Constricted	Tend to dry	↓↓ Possible pulmonary edema	Tachycardia	↓	No	Not marked
Carbon monoxide	Depressed	Possible if severe	No marked change	No marked change	↑	↑	↓	Possible	Red color
Neuromuscular blocking agent	No change until hypoxic	No	No change	No significant change	↓ ↓	↑	↓	Possible	Not marked
Cardiovascular—digitalis	Slightly depressed	If severe	No marked change	No marked change	No marked change	Slow rate arrhythmia	↓	Yes	Not marked
Adrenergic—e.g., amphetamine	Excited	No	Dilated	Dry	Increased	Tachycardia, possible arrhythmias	↑	No	Flushed
Alcohol	Depressed if severe	No	No marked change	Slightly increased	↓	Tachycardia	↓	Possible	Flushed
Cyanide	Depressed	Frequent	Not much change unless severely hypoxic—then dilated	Not much change	↓ ↓	Tachycardia and arrhythmias	↓	Possible	Cyanosis

TABLE 81-2. COMMON AGENTS CAUSING SEIZURES

Camphor	Organophosphate insecticides
Carbon monoxide	Phencyclidine
Chlorinated hydrocarbons	Phenol
Cocaine	Phenothiazines
Isoniazid	Propoxyphene hydrochloride
Lithium	Strychnine
	Tricyclic antidepressants

With permission from Haddad, L. M.: A general approach to the emergency management of poisoning. *In* Clinical Management of Poisoning and Drug Overdose. Philadelphia, W. B. Saunders Company, 1983.

TABLE 81-3. CAUSES OF A HIGH ANION GAP METABOLIC ACIDOSIS

Uremia
Diabetic ketoacidosis
Lactic acidosis
Salicylate toxicity
Methanol poisoning
Ethylene glycol poisoning
Nondiabetic alcoholic ketoacidosis
Paraldehyde toxicity

may be active at lower dose ranges and may remain active for a longer period of time. For example, some barbiturates—primarily, hexabarbital and secobarbital (phenobarbital less than the others)—depend on liver metabolism. The elderly are also at higher risk of metabolic impairment because of basic changes of aging in addition to the presence of disease.

There are four major types of enzymatic metabolic reactions: hydrolysis, oxidation, reduction, and conjugation. The precise metabolic fate of most poisons has not been described, and medical science has not progressed to such a point that any of these processes can be substantially hastened. As a result, metabolic treatment of poisoning is rudimentary at best, and technologic advances have been made in the direction of enhancing elimination by use of dialysis and hemoperfusion techniques, lavage, emesis, and charcoal. Specific antidotes are also being developed.

HEMODIALYSIS

Hemodialysis plays a definite role in the management of the toxicologic patient. As technologic advances provide simpler hemodialysis units, they will become available for use in EDs to a vastly greater extent. It is therefore important to understand some of the physicochemical and pharmacologic principles involved in hemodialysis of an ingested drug.

First, the basic principle underlying hemodialysis is that blood containing circulating drugs or metabolites of those drugs will be cleared of the poisonous chemicals through their passage via a semipermeable membrane into fluid containing none of the drug. Thus, effective dialysis requires a high enough plasma concentration of the drug to ensure that enough is removed to favorably influence the clinical course. If the poison has wide distribution in the body and toxic effects are related to tissue concentration, the amount of plasma tends to be only a fraction of the total, and lowering the plasma level might have no significance. Even if the substance is highly dialyzable, supportive treatment is indicated in the type of situation cited. For example, after distribution of the drug haloperidol, the plasma contains only 0.25% of the total amount of drug in the body. Conversely, if the drug is being actively absorbed from the small intestine and distribution has not occurred, dialysis during this period might be of much greater value. The next factor of importance is the molecular weight of the drug (which is generally assumed to bear directly on molecular size). Clearance through a dialysis membrane is directly proportional to the blood concentration and is related to the molecular weight. In fact, the relationship between molecular weight and clearance is such that doubling the molecular weight reduces clearance by greater than twofold. As the molecular weight approaches 350, and using the currently available membranes, the rate of drug permeation is reduced to such a low level that dialysis is unlikely to make any significant difference. Also, if the drugs are of low mo-

lecular weight but are bound to a carrier (e.g., plasma protein), dialysis efficacy is markedly reduced.

The use of hemodialysis is another area of controversy in poison management. The diverging opinions probably reflect the lack of large-scale, controlled studies, which are difficult to perform in the clinical practice of medicine, particularly for advocates of dialysis who face an ethical problem if they withhold the procedure that they believe will help the patient.

These principles regarding hemodialysis in management of poisoning are currently acceptable:

1. Dialysis should be considered when the drug is largely confined to the blood and is dialyzable. Some common agents in which dialysis has been employed include salicylates, phenylbutazone,

---

TABLE 81-4. COMMON TOXIC CAUSES OF CARDIAC ARRHYTHMIA

Amphetamine	Phenol
Arsenic	Phenothiazines
Carbon monoxide	Phenylpropanolamine
Chloral hydrate	Physostigmine
Cocaine	Propranolol
Cyanide	Quinine, quinidine
Digitalis	Succinylcholine chloride
Dinitrophenols	Theophylline
MAO inhibitors	Tricyclic antidepressants

Bradyarrhythmias
Anticholinesterase agents (including organophosphate insecticides)
Beta-adrenergic blockers (e.g., propranolol)
Cardiac glycosides
Physostigmine

Adapted with permission from Haddad, L. M.: A general approach to the emergency management of poisoning. *In* Clinical Management of Poisoning and Drug Overdose. Philadelphia, W. B. Saunders Company, 1983.

TABLE 81-5. CAUSES OF SEVERE MUSCLE WEAKNESS

Nicotine poisoning
Succinylcholine and curare-like substances
Neostigmine excess
Botulism

With permission from Haddad, L. M.: A general approach to the emergency management of poisoning. *In* Clinical Management of Poisoning and Drug Overdose. Philadelphia, W. B. Saunders Company, 1983.

TABLE 81-6. COMMON POISONINGS ASSOCIATED WITH HYPERTENSION

Phenylpropanolamine
Amphetamine
Ephedrine
Cocaine
Clonidine
MAO inhibitors (e.g. tranylcypromine, phenylzine)
Thyroid hormones

phenobarbital, sulfonamides, sulfonylureas, methanol, ethylene glycol, lithium, and theophylline.

2. Dialysis is of no use with irreversibly acting drugs once they have entered the body (e.g., cyanide, organophosphate, cholinesterase inhibitors).

3. Dialysis should not be used if effective pharmacologic or biochemical antagonists are available (for example, naloxone for narcotics).

4. Dialysis is of increasingly limited value as the molecular weight of the chemical substance approaches 350. This is because of the slowness of dialysis through available membranes.

5. Hemodialysis should be considered only when the amount ingested is dangerous to life and when the speed of elimination by hemodialysis is substantially greater than elimination through usual metabolic and excretory pathways.

6. Hemodialysis may be of value in severely intoxicated patients in whom the usual routes of elimination are impaired (e.g., renal impairment, liver disease, or cardiac disease resulting in impaired excretion).

7. Hemodialysis should be used only when the dangers have been assessed and when the benefits outweigh the dangers. The major dangers include hemorrhage, air embolism, infection, electrolyte abnormality, and circulatory overload.

8. *Peritoneal dialysis* may be used when hemodialysis is not available. Use of frequent gastric lavage with saline may also serve as a type of dialysis. Repeated doses of charcoal can also be used. Although generally less desirable, peritoneal dialysis and exchange transfusion may be more useful in small children. A new, useful innovation is a charcoal perfusion device or a polystyrene resin. These devices have been useful with long-acting barbiturates, salicylates, and theophylline. Only experienced personnel should undertake the use of these devices because of the complications that can occur.

9. If hemodialysis is required, there should be minimal delay. Prearranged protocols are of great use

and can be prepared in consultation with the renal service, ED, and Poison Control Center. Such prior "decision making" offers effective, decisive emergency care.

See also Addenda, p. 3347.

BASIC MEDICAL MANAGEMENT OF POISONINGS

The basic elements of the medical management of poisonings follow:

1. Support vital functions.
2. Identify agent (when possible).
3. Remove, neutralize, or reverse effects.
4. Hasten excretion.
5. Treat damaged or poisoned organs or systems. Prevent damage whenever possible.

INITIAL MANAGEMENT

When a patient has been poisoned, the immediate view must be to maintain life. The vital functions must be evaluated and supported as necessary. Most commonly this refers to the respiratory system. Many drugs and poisons act to depress the respiratory center. At times, however, maintenance of blood pressure and treatment of shock states are necessary. Any cardiac dysrhythmia must be identified and monitored. Potentially lethal arrhythmias must be treated rapidly. Occasionally, CNS depression may be life-threatening.

During the initial evaluation and support of vital functions, a member of the emergency team should make efforts to identify the poison. If the patient cannot or will not provide this information, all sources of history should be rapidly explored. Information from friends, knowledge of available drugs and poi-

---

TABLE 81-7. COMMON DRUGS THAT PRODUCE THE ANTICHOLINERGIC SYNDROME AND THE USE OF PHYSOSTIGMINE IN SUCH CASES

Drugs	Treatment
Atropine Ornade	Use physostigmine (side effects are those of cholinergic stimulation and can be reversed with atropine). If atropine reversal is necessary, use a dose half that of physostigmine.
Diphenhydramine hydrochloride (Benadryl) Bentyl	*Children:* 0.5 mg IV slowly. The dose may be slowly raised to a total of 2 mg or stopped before that if cholinergic symptoms (e.g., salivary glandular activity, diarrhea) becomes prominent.
Probantheline bromide (Probanthine) Methapyriline (Sominex)	*Adults:* Begin with 2 mg slowly IV—raise to a total of 4 mg if no effect. Repeat if anticholinergic symptoms again become prominent. With careful monitoring, the total dose should not exceed 4 mg in a half hour. The anticholinergic poisoning symptoms include CNS hyperactivity and seizures initially, but with marked overdosage, coma and medullary paralysis may occur. Tachycardia, mydriasis, and decrease in secretions are also prominent. *Caution: Physostigmine has potential severe side effects and should be reserved for severe poisonings.*

* With permission from Haddad, L. M.: A general approach to the emergency management of poisoning. *In* Clinical Management of Poisoning and Drug Overdose. Edited by Haddad, L. M., and Winchester, J. F. Philadelphia, W. B. Saunders Company, 1983.

TABLE 81-8. CHOLINERGIC SYNDROME	
Anatomic Site of Action	Physiologic Effects
Muscarinic Effects	
Sweat glands	Sweating
Pupils	Constricted pupils
Lacrimal glands	Lacrimation
Salivary glands	Excessive salivation
Bronchial tree	Wheezing
Gastrointestinal	Cramps, vomiting, diarrhea, tenesmus
Cardiovascular	Bradycardia, fall in blood pressure
Ciliary body	Blurred vision
Bladder	Urinary incontinence
Nicotinic Effects	
Striated muscle	Fasciculations, cramps, weakness, twitching, paralysis, respiratory embarrassment, cyanosis, arrest
Sympathetic ganglia	Tachycardia, elevated blood pressure
Central Nervous System Effects	Anxiety, restlessness, ataxia, convulsions, insomnia, coma, absent reflexes, Cheyne-Stokes respirations, respiratory and circulation depression

* With permission from Haddad, L. M.: A general approach to the emergency management of poisoning. *In* Clinical Management of Poisoning and Drug Overdose. Edited by Haddad, L. M., and Winchester, J. F. Philadelphia, W. B. Saunders Company, 1983.

sons, empty bottles, and previous treatments or physicians must be assessed. Table 81-1 illustrates a symptom and sign analysis. Using nine easily observed signs, one may possibly place an unknown poison in one of the drug categories shown. Such categorization is particularly important when large doses have been taken, and reversal should be undertaken when such treatment is possible. For example, the so-called anticholinergic syndrome can be produced by a large number of drugs, and physostigmine has occasional value in reversing some of the abnormalities. Table 81-7 indicates some compounds involved in the anticholinergic syndrome and the use of physostigmine in such instances. The trend in toxicology has been to limit the use of physostigmine markedly because of adverse side effects. In severe cases, identification as to class or type of drug may be extremely useful when dialysis is considered. On the other hand, acetylcholine-type symptoms can be seen with organophosphate insecticides (the most common insecticide poisoning). Absorption can occur through oral ingestion or transdermally. A cholinergic syndrome is produced (Table 81-8). Other cholinergic poisonings (neostigmine, physostigmine) present similarly.

Although identification or probable identification of the poison is important, excessive time must not be expended at this point on specific or class delineation. Frequently, overdoses with suicidal intent involve more than one drug, and the clinical picture can be confusing. The higher priority is to support vital functions, provide advanced life support, and remove the agent or reverse its action. If there is a possibility of a narcotic or opiate-like substance being involved, a trial of naloxone (Narcan) should be undertaken. Similarly, if insulin or an insulin-like substance is possibly

involved, a solution of 50% dextrose can be infused after blood has been taken for glucose determination. When glucose is infused, thiamine, 100 mg. intramuscularly (IM), should also be given.

Evaluation of level of consciousness is important in determining whether or not there are signs of CNS deterioration. The Glasgow Coma scale may be helpful. Grading coma from 0 (asleep but able to be aroused and to answer questions) to grade 4 (respiratory depression, circulatory decompensation, absence of stimulus response) is frequently used. A descriptive approach is usually most useful, particularly when multiple specialists will be involved in the clinical care of the patient.

Because alcohol is so often found associated with other drug overdoses, a breath analyzer can be useful in the initial evaluation. Blood alcohol levels are often unavailable for 1 to 2 hours, and a breath test can produce immediate results.

THERAPEUTIC, TOXIC AND LETHAL LEVELS OF PHARMACOLOGIC AGENTS

As hospital laboratories become more capable of rapidly providing blood levels of various drugs, the emergency physician can more effectively treat the patient using quantitative information as well as careful monitoring of the clinical state. Table 81-9 provides the therapeutic, toxic and lethal levels of well over 100

| | The Significance of Blood Level | | |
Compound	Therapeutic or Normal	Toxic	Lethal
Acetaminophen	3 mg%	4 hr.: 12 mg%	30 mg%
		12 hr.: 5 mg% or	12 mg%
		half-life in serum	
		> 4 hr.	
Acetazolamide	1–1.5 mg%	—	—
Acetohexamide	2.1–5.6 mg%	—	—
Acetone	—	20–30 mg%	55 mg%
Acetylsalicylic acid	see Salicylate		
Aluminum	0.03 mg%	—	—
Aminophylline	1–2 mg%	2–4 mg%	—
Amitriptyline	8–20 µg%	40 µg%	0.5–2.0 mg%
Ammonia	50–170 µg%	—	—
Amphetamine	2–3 µg%	> 10 µg%	0.005–0.2 mg%†
Arsenic	7 µg%	0.1 mg%	0.1–1.5 mg%
Aspirin	see Salicylate		
Aventyl	see Nortriptyline		
Barbiturates			
short-acting	0.2–0.4 mg%	0.7 mg%	1–3 mg%‡
intermediate	0.1–0.5 mg%	1–3 mg%	3–5 mg%‡
phenobarbital	1–2.5 mg%	4–6 mg%	8–15 mg%‡
barbital	ca. 3 mg%	6–8 mg%	10 mg%
Benadryl	see Diphenhydramine		
Benemid	see Probenecid		
Benzedrex	see Propylhexedrine		
Benzene	—	Any measurable	0.094 mg%
		amount	
Boric acid	0.08 mg%	4 mg%	5 mg%
Bromide	5 mg%	50 mg%	100–200 mg%
Brompheniramine	0.8–1.5 µg%	—	—
Butazolidin	see Phenylbutazone		
Cadmium	—	0.005 mg%	—
Caffeine	—	0.5 mg%	10–15 mg%
Carbamazepine	0.2 mg%	0.8–1 mg%	—
Carbon monoxide	0–13% carboxyhemoglobin	25–35%	60%
Carbon tetrachloride	—	2.5 mg%	—
Carisoprodol	1–4 mg%	—	—
Celontin	see Methsuximide		
Chloral hydrate	1 mg%	10 mg%	10–25 mg%‡
Chlordiazepoxide	0.1–0.3 mg%	0.55 mg%	2–3 mg%
Chloroform	—	7–25 mg%	39 mg%
Chloroquine	0.15 mg%	—	1 mg%
Chlorpheniramine		2–3 mg%	—
Chlorpromazine	0.05–0.1 mg%	0.1–0.2 mg%	0.3–1.2 mg%
Chlorpropamide	3–14 mg%	—	—
Chlorprothixene	0.004–0.03 mg%	—	—
Chlorzoxazone	1–2 mg%	—	—
Codeine	2.5 µg%		0.2 mg%
Copper	100–150 µg%	540 µg%	—
Compazine	see Prochlorperazine		
Cyanide	0.015 mg%	—	0.5 mg%
Darvon	see Propoxyphene		
DDT	1.3 µg%	—	—
Demerol	see Meperidine		
Desipramine	0.059–0.14 mg%	—	0.3–2 mg%
Dextropropoxyphene	see Propoxyphene		
Diabinese	see Chlorpropamide		
Diamox	see Acetazolamide		
Diazepam	0.1–0.25 mg%	0.5–2 mg%	2 mg%
Dieldrin	0.15 µg%	—	—
Digitoxin	1–3 µg%	—	3 µg%
Digoxin	0.07–0.2 µg%	0.2 µg%	0.4 µg%
Dilantin	see Diphenylhydantoin		
Dilaudid	see Hydromorphone		
Dimetane	see Brompheniramine		
Dinitro-o-cresol	—	3–4 mg%	7.5 mg%
Diphenhydramine	0.1–0.5 mg%	—	1 mg%
Diphenylhydantoin	0.5–2.2 mg%	3–5 mg%	5–10 mg%
Divinyl oxide	—	—	70 mg%

TABLE 81-9. CONTINUED*

The Significance of Blood Level

Compound	Therapeutic or Normal	Toxic	Lethal
Doriden	see Glutethimide		
Doxepin	—	—	1 mg%
Dymelor	see Acetohexamide		
Elavil	see Amitriptyline		
Ethanol	50 mg%	150 mg%	400 mg%
Ethchlorvynol	0.2–1.5 mg%	2 mg%	10–15 mg%
Ethinamate	0.5–1 mg%	—	—
Ethosuximide	10 mg%	>16 mg%	—
Ethyl chloride	—		40 mg%
Ethyl ether	90–100 mg%	—	140–189 mg%
Ethylene glycol	—	150 mg%	200–400 mg%
Fenfluramine	—	—	0.1–0.6 mg%
Flexin	see Zoxazolamine		
Fluoride	0–0.05 mg%	—	0.2–0.3 mg%
Fluothane	see Halothane		
Furadantin	see Nitrofurantoin		
Gantrisin	see Sulfisoxazole		
Gold	300–600 μg%	—	—
Glutethimide	0.02–0.75 mg%	1–8 mg%	3–10 mg%†
Halothane	15 mg%	—	20 mg%
Heroin	see Morphine		
Hexachlorophene	—	—	1 mg%
Hydrogen sulfide	—	—	0.092 mg%
Hydromorphone	—	—	0.01–0.03 mg%
Imipramine	0.005–0.016 mg%	0.06 mg%	0.2–0.4 mg%
Inderal	see Propranolol		
Isopropanol	—	—	80 mg%
Iron (serum)	0.04–0.2 mg%	0.5 mg%	1 mg%
Lactate	10–20 mg%	—	75 mg%
Lead	0.005–0.06 mg%	0.1 mg%	0.2 mg%
Librium	see Chlordiazepoxide		
Lidocaine	0.2 mg%	0.6–1 mg%	—
Liquiprin	see Acetaminophen		
Lithium	0.42–0.83 mg%	1.39 mg%	1.39–3.47 mg%
LSD	—	0.1–0.4 μg%	—
Madribon	see Sulfadimethoxine		
Magnesium	1.5–2.5 mEq/liter	—	5 mEq/liter
Manganese	0.015 mg%	0.46 mg%	—
Marijuana (as THC)	7 μg%	—	—
Mellaril	see Thioridazine		
Meperidine	60–65 μg%	0.2 mg%	0.5–3 mg%†
Meprobamate	0.5–3 mg%	3–10 mg%	10–20 mg%‡
Mercury	0.006–0.012 mg%	—	0.3–1 mg%
Methadone	48–86 μg%	—	0.1–0.4 mg%
Methamphetamine	—	0.01–0.5 mg%	0.1–4 mg%†
Methanol	—	20 mg%	89 mg%
Methapyrilene	0.2–0.4 mg%	3–5 mg%	5 mg%
Methaqualone	0.5 mg%	1–3 mg%	>3 mg%
Methemoglobulinemia	15%	30%	70% Hgb
Methsuximide	0.25–0.75 mg%	—	—
Methylene chloride	—	—	28 mg%
Methylene dioxyamphetamine	—	—	0.4–1 mg%
Methyprylon	1 mg%	3–6 mg%	3–10 mg%
Milontin	see Phensuximide		
Morphine	0.01 mg%	—	0.05–0.4 mg%†
Mysoline	see Primidone		
Nebs	see Acetaminophen		
Nickel	0.041 mg%	—	—
Nicotine	0.03 mg%	0.5–1 mg%	0.5–5.2 mg%
Nitrofurantoin	0.18 mg%	—	—
Noctec	see Chloral hydrate		
Noludar	see Methyprylon		
Norpramin	see Desipramine		
Nortriptyline	10–16 μg%	0.5 mg%	1 mg%
Orinase	see Tolbutamide		
Orphenadrine	—	0.2 mg%	0.4–0.8 mg%
Oxalate	0.2 mg%	—	1 mg%
Papaverine	0.1 mg%	—	—

2933

Table Continued on following page

TABLE 81-9. CONTINUED*

Compound	The Significance of Blood Level Therapeutic or Normal	Toxic	Lethal
Paramethoxy-amphetamine	—	—	0.2–0.4 mg%
Paraldehyde	5–8 mg%	20–40 mg%	50 mg%
Pentazocine	0.05 mg%	0.2–0.5 mg%	0.3–2 mg%†
Perphenazine	—	0.1 mg%	—
Phencyclidine	—	—	0.1 mg%
Phenmetrazine	—	—	0.4 mg%
Phensuximide	1–1.9 mg%	—	—
Phenylbutazone	5–15 mg%	—	—
Placidyl	see Ethchlorvynol		
Potassium (serum)	4–6 mEq/liter	6–8 mEq/liter	8 mEq/liter
Primidone	1–2 mg%	5–8 mg%	ca. 10 mg%
Probenecid	10–20 mg%	—	—
Procainamide	0.6 mg%	1 mg%	1.2 mg%
Prochlorperazine	—	0.1 mg%	—
Promazine	—	0.1 mg%	—
Propoxyphene	5–20 μg%	0.1 mg%	0.1–3 mg%‡
Propranolol	0.0025–0.02 mg%	—	0.8–1.2 mg%
Propylhexedrine	—	—	0.2–0.3 mg%
Quaalude	see Methaqualone		
Quinidine	0.3–0.6 mg%	ca. 1 mg%	3–5 mg%
Quinine	—	0.2 mg%	1 mg%
Rela	see Carisoprodol		
Salicylate	2–10 mg%	6 hr§: 50 mg%	90–120 mg%
	30 mg% for rheumatics	12 hr§: 40 mg%	70–100 mg%¶
		24 hr§: 25 mg%	50–65 mg%¶
		48 hr§: 10 mg%	20–30 mg%¶
Sinequan	see Doxepin		
Sodium	135–145 mEq/liter	160 mEq/liter	200 mEq/liter
Soma	see Carisoprodol		
Sparine	see Promazine		
Strychnine	—	0.2 mg%	0.9–1.2 mg%
Sulfadiazine	8–15 mg%	—	—
Sulfadimethoxine	8–10 mg%	—	—
Sulfaguanidine	3–5 mg%	—	—
Sulfanilamide	10–15 mg%	—	—
Sulfisoxazole	9–10 mg%	—	—
Talwin	see Pentazocine		
Taractan	see Chlorprothixene		
Tegretol	see Carbamazepine		
Theophylline	1–2 mg%	2–4 mg%	—
Thiocyanate	—	—	20 mg%
Thioridazine	0.10–0.20 mg%	—	0.5–2 mg%
Thorazine	see Chlorpromazine		
Tigan	see Trimethobenzamide		
Tin	0.012 mg%	—	—
Tofranil	see Imipramine		
Tolbutamide	5.3–9.6 mg%	—	—
Toluene	—	—	1 mg%
Tribromoethanol	—	—	9 mg%
Trichloroethane	—	—	10–100 mg%
Trilafon	see Perphenazine		
Trimethobenzamide	0.1–0.2 mg%	—	—
Tylenol	see Acetaminophen		
Uric acid	3–7 mg%	—	20 mg%
Valium	see Diazepam		
Valmid	see Ethinamate		
Warfarin	0.1–1 mg%	—	—
Xylocaine	see Lidocaine		
Zarontin	see Ethosuximide		
Zinc	68–136 μg%	—	—
Zoxazolamine	0.3–1.3 mg%	—	—

* Adapted with permission from Done, A. K.: Emerg. Med. 7:193, 1975.
† Higher level is for tolerant users.
‡ Lower level applies in presence of alcohol.
§ After single acute ingestion only.
¶ Lower figure indicates severe poisoning and death is possible; higher figure—almost certain lethality.
Note: Very few of these determinations can now be done by hospital laboratories, but with technologic advances in the future, such laboratory results may be available for physicians treating poisoned patients. Knowledge of the blood levels can be currently useful for clinical research.

drugs. Most such laboratory determinations are still not available in time to be clinically useful in the acutely poisoned patient, but increasing numbers are available. Even when results are returned many hours or even days later, the values can be useful for future clinical correlations, particularly with increasing concerns about chronic lead poisoning and mercury poisoning from paint in children.[1,2]

REFERENCES

1. Shannon, M., and Graef, J.: Hazards of lead in infant formula. N. Engl. J. Med. *326*:137, 1992.
2. Clarkson, T.W.: Mercury—An element of mystery. N. Engl. J. Med. *323*:1137, 1990.

BASIC MANAGEMENT

Lynn Augenstein and Ken Kulig*

CAPSULE

This subchapter is not meant to be a thorough overview on toxicology. Rather, certain specific topics are addressed in which recent advances may alter traditional concepts. In addition, current controversial areas in managing poisoned patients are addressed. Finally, newer drugs of abuse or overdose are highlighted.

GENERAL MANAGEMENT OF THE POISONED PATIENT

SUPPORTIVE CARE

An important rule in toxicology is to "treat the patient, not the poison." There are few agents for which a specific antidote dramatically reduces the patient's symptoms. More often, good supportive care with meticulous attention to supporting the patient's vital functions is all that is needed to ensure a good outcome. The ABCs should take top priority, with adequate assessment and support of a clear airway, breathing, and circulation. Endotracheal intubation should be considered if the patient is significantly obtunded or comatose, or has evidence of respiratory failure. IV access should be obtained in highly symptomatic patients; supplemental oxygen may be needed, and cardiac monitoring should be considered.

Any patient with an altered level of consciousness should receive naloxone (Narcan) and dextrose intravenously. The doses are:

Naloxone: Child—2.0 mg initially, up to 5–10 mg
Adult—2.0 mg initially, up to 10 mg

Dextrose: Child—0.5–1 g/kg body weight, IV (2–4 mL 25% dextrose in water per kg body weight)
Adult—50–100 mL 50% dextrose in water, IV

Note that naloxone may also be effective if given by means of an endotracheal tube or sublingually if intravenous access is impossible. Giving dextrose to a patient who is depleted of thiamine, such as an alcoholic, may precipitate a Wernicke's encephalopathy. Therefore, 100 mg of thiamine should be given intravenously or intramuscularly to alcoholic patients before dextrose administration.

Further supportive measures depend on the clinical status of the patient. For hypotension, the use of Trendelenburg's position, intravenous fluids, or pressor agents (e.g., dopamine or norepinephrine bitartrate [Levophed]) may be indicated. For hypertension, administration of agents appropriate for the severity of the hypertension may be necessary. Appropriate antiarrhythmic therapy may be necessary for the treatment of drug-induced cardiac arrhythmias.

SEIZURE CONTROL

Seizures deserve special mention because toxin-induced seizures may be difficult to control. For example, theophylline toxicity may induce seizures that are refractory to the usual anticonvulsant medications. Amoxapine, one of the newer cyclic antidepressant agents, also may produce refractory seizures. Certainly, if a specific antidote is available to counteract a toxin-induced seizure, it should be given. For example, isoniazid-induced seizures are difficult to control without the administration of pyridoxine, a specific antidote. For most causes of toxin-induced seizures, however, there are no specific antidotes, and in most cases, diazepam should be given intravenously to control the seizures. This should be followed

*Dr. Augenstein was the recipient of a McNeil Fellowship in Clinical Toxicology at the time of this writing.

by intravenous phenytoin, phenobarbital, or both in appropriate doses. If the seizures are refractory to the initial administration of these drugs, more aggressive measures should be taken. Prolonged seizures may lead to profound morbidity or even death. Sequelae of prolonged seizures include severe lactic acidosis caused by prolonged muscle activity, hypoxia, rhabdomyolysis with subsequent myoglobinuria and renal failure, and irreversible brain injury. The initial step for treating refractory seizures is to paralyze the patient with an agent like pancuronium (Pavulon). This stops the muscle activity that contributes greatly to the morbidity. The patient requires endotracheal intubation and ventilatory support if this is done. The brain seizure continues despite muscle paralysis, so inducing pentobarbital coma or utilizing general anesthesia is an appropriate step. Continuous electroencephalogram monitoring is necessary to assess the efficacy of this therapy because, in a paralyzed patient, it would otherwise be difficult to determine if the patient is still experiencing seizures.

LABORATORY (SEE NEXT SECTION OF THIS CHAPTER)

Appropriate use of the laboratory is important in managing poisoned patients. Too much emphasis is placed on using toxicology "screens" to make a diagnosis in a poisoned patient. The cause of a poisoned patient's

TABLE 81-10. SUBSTANCES WHOSE QUANTITATIVE DETERMINATIONS ARE IMPORTANT ON AN IMMEDIATE BASIS

Ethanol
Methanol
Ethylene glycol
Acetaminophen
Salicylates
Digoxin
Carboxyhemoglobin
Iron/Total iron-binding capacity
Theophylline
Anticonvulsants
Lithium

TABLE 81-11. CAUSES OF HIGH ANION GAP METABOLIC ACIDOSIS (PARTIAL LIST)

$$\text{Anion gap} = Na^+ - (Cl^- + HCO_3^-)$$
Normal is 12 mEq or less.

Salicylates	Isoniazid
Methanol	Paraldehyde
Ethylene glycol	Cyanide
Alcoholic ketoacidosis	Lactic acidosis
Uremia	(hypotension, seizures, etc)
Carbon monoxide	Hydrogen sulfide
Iron	Diabetic ketoacidosis

signs and symptoms is usually evident from a thorough and appropriate history taking and physical examination, and specific toxicology laboratory tests can then be used as adjuncts. Physicians should become familiar with the laboratory at their own institutions and know its capabilities and limitations. Under certain circumstances, the measurement of specific quantitative serum levels may be necessary to aid in management (Table 81-10). Acetaminophen levels should be considered in all multiple drug overdoses. Acetaminophen poisoning may have no initial symptoms.

General laboratory tests may be useful in managing toxicologic problems. An increased anion gap metabolic acidosis may be detected on assessment of serum electrolytes, perhaps aiding in the diagnosis of a poisoned patient (Table 81-11). Serum glucose determination should be done, especially in patients with altered levels of consciousness. Measurement of blood urea nitrogen and serum creatinine may be important both to assess baseline renal function in a patient exposed to renally excreted agents and to assess the renal toxicity of certain agents. Arterial blood gas sampling gives important information about the acid-base status and degree of oxygen saturation and, depending on the method used, indicates carboxyhemoglobin or methemoglobin levels.

RADIOGRAPHS

Certain drugs are radiopaque, and a plain abdominal x-ray film may provide useful information about how much of the drug is in the intestinal tract. Iron pills are a classic example of pills that are radiopaque; however, chewable children's vitamins with iron are not consistently radiopaque. Heavy metals, such as arsenic and lead, are also radiopaque. One study[1] demonstrated that potassium chloride, ferrous sulfate, and calcium carbonate were strongly radiopaque in a cadaver model. A multivitamin with iron (adult-sized) was moderately radiopaque. Several other substances were weakly radiopaque. Looking for pills in abdominal radiographs, therefore, has limited usefulness in assessing poisoned patients, unless the substance is known to be consistently radiopaque. The presence of radiopaque pills, however, may occasionally be reported by the radiologist in patients not being treated for overdose; one patient had an enteric aspirin bezoar. These can be very hazardous, since a breakup of the bezoar can result in marked toxicity.

Another possible use of plain abdominal radiographs is in the evaluation of so-called body packers, individuals who smuggle packets of illicit drugs such as heroin or cocaine by ingesting them and recovering them after passage through the intestinal tract. The packets are sometimes inserted directly into the rectum or vagina for recovery later. The packets may be made of latex balloons, condoms, or stronger grades of latex, securely tied at both ends. They may show up with varying densities on plain abdominal films.

PREVENTING ABSORPTION— CONTROVERSIES

An area of continuing controversy in the fields of emergency medicine and toxicology is the issue of gastrointestinal decontamination. Many studies have compared the efficacy of ipecac-induced emesis, gastric lavage, and charcoal administration in preventing drug absorption. Most of these studies do not address the issue of clinical outcome and are therefore difficult to interpret. One study did address clinical outcome in poisoned patients presenting at the Emergency Department (ED).[2] Emesis and gastric lavage followed by activated charcoal was compared with administration of activated charcoal alone, without gastric emptying. No advantage was found in inducing emesis, and gastric lavage improved outcome only if done within 1 hour of ingestion of the alleged toxin. These data corroborate other authors' findings that administering activated charcoal alone may be more advantageous than inducing emesis or performing gastric lavage in selected patients.[3–5] Removal of the ingested substance by lavage or emesis, however, is still the recommended procedure, followed by charcoal. Pills can be recovered many hours after ingestion. The issue of multiple-dose charcoal is one of ongoing evaluation and controversy. Few data support improvement, and adverse effects are reported.[5a,14] New products containing charcoal and cathartics, e.g., a sorbital-charcoal mixture (Actidose), require further evaluation.[5b]

EMESIS

Inducing emesis with syrup of ipecac is most effective within 30 minutes of ingestion of a poison. The main advantage of syrup of ipecac is its widespread availability in homes; therefore, it is often useful in accidental poisonings in children. Contraindications to its use are listed in Table 81-12. The doses are:

Adults and children over 12 years
   of age: 30 mL
Children 1–12 years of age: 15 mL
Children 6 months–1 year of age: 5–10 mL in a
                                  supervised
                                  setting

Besides the contraindications listed, induction of emesis with ipecac has another disadvantage. It prevents the administration of activated charcoal, usually for 2 to 4 hours, because of repeated emesis. Thus, in the ED, where lavage can be performed on charcoal administered immediately, ipecac has little utility. An exception might be its use in infants who have recently ingested a poison because lavage tubes may be too small to adequately allow passage of pills or pill particles.

Ipecac may also be used for substances not adsorbed by charcoal or when significant ingestion of sustained-release or enteric-coated tablets is suspected. The physician must also be aware of complications associated

---

TABLE 81-12. CONTRAINDICATIONS TO IPECAC-INDUCED EMESIS

Coma or possible rapid onset of coma
Seizures or possible rapid onset of seizures
Ingestion of acids, alkalis, or other caustics or corrosives
Ingestion of most petroleum distillates (consult a poison center)
Medical conditions that make emesis dangerous (e.g., anatomic abnormalities, recent surgery, hypocoagulable state)

---

with ipecac-induced emesis, such as aspiration pneumonitis, diaphragmatic rupture, and Mallory-Weiss tear with GI bleeding. Cardiotoxicity may also occur from emetine.

GASTRIC LAVAGE

If gastric lavage is to be performed, care must be taken to prevent tracheal aspiration of gastric contents. Thus, if the patient is comatose or convulsing, endotracheal intubation with a cuffed endotracheal tube should be performed before insertion of the lavage tube. As with ipecac, lavage should not be performed for ingestion of strong acids or alkalis or of most petroleum distillates. Lavage should be performed with the patient in the left lateral decubitus position and with the gurney in Trendelenburg's position. A large-bore orogastric or nasogastric tube, No. 36 to 40 French (Fr), should be used in adolescents and adults, with smaller tubes used in children. Tepid tap water or saline can be used as lavage fluid, with saline being preferable in infants. Aliquots of 200 to 300 mL should be instilled for adults and adolescents, and aliquots of 100 mL are used for infants. Lavage should be continued until the effluent is clear. After this, an adequate dose of activated charcoal should be instilled by means of the lavage tube before it is removed. Also, in severe ingestions requiring lavage, charcoal may be instilled before lavage, allowed to adsorb for 5 minutes, and removed with the lavage effluent. A second dose of charcoal should be given after lavage.

Gastric lavage is not an entirely benign procedure. Esophageal perforation and tracheal aspiration have been reported as complications, and the physician must take this into account before doing this procedure. Also, as mentioned before, gastric lavage may have little benefit when performed more than 1 hour after ingestion of a toxic agent has occurred. Sometimes, however, large quantities of ingested matter are retained in the stomach because of prior meals or adrenergic effects, and can be recovered hours after ingestion. Lavage may be useful in ingestions of substances not adsorbed by charcoal.

ACTIVATED CHARCOAL

Activated charcoal plays an important role in the treatment of poisoned patients. Most drugs and many chemicals are adsorbed to activated charcoal, making them unavailable for absorption into the bloodstream via the intestinal mucosa. Table 81-13 lists substances that probably are not adsorbed to activated charcoal to a significant degree. As mentioned previously, activated charcoal alone has been shown to be more effective than ipecac-induced emesis in preventing drug absorption in some studies. Activated charcoal will probably soon become more available in homes and in the prehospital medical care setting. Activated charcoal administration alone will probably replace many ED gastric decontamination procedures.

Activated charcoal should be given in a dose of 50 to 100 g in adolescents and adults. In children, 1 to 2 g/kg of body weight can be given up to a dose of 50 g. Activated charcoal should be given with a diluent, either water or a cathartic, with a minimum of 240 mL of diluent per 30 g of charcoal. The initial dose of charcoal should nearly always be given with a cathartic (except possibly if diarrhea is already present).

Newer, superactivated charcoal may be superior to regular charcoal. Multiple doses of activated charcoal are discussed subsequently. Complications with the use of activated charcoal are rare but can include constipation, aspiration, and intestinal obstruction.

CATHARTICS

Cathartics should be given in conjunction with activated charcoal to hasten gastrointestinal elimination of toxins. Doses usually recommended are

Sorbitol: Children—1 g/kg of body weight per dose of 35% solution; Adults—1–2 g/kg of body weight per dose of 70% solution
Magnesium sulfate: Children—250 mg/kg of body weight per dose; Adults—15–30 g/dose
Magnesium citrate: 4 mL/kg of body weight per dose (300 mL maximum)

Cathartics can be given either mixed with activated charcoal or separately, and some charcoal products are available premixed with cathartics. Magnesium-based cathartics should be avoided in patients with renal failure, and sodium-based cathartics should be avoided in patients with congestive heart failure.

When using multiple-dose charcoal regimens (discussed later), repeated doses of cathartics must be used with caution. For adults, a second dose of a cathartic may be given, with caution, 4 to 8 hours after the first dose. Further doses are usually not needed and may be dangerous. Hypermagnesemia has been reported with repeated doses of magnesium-based cathartics.[7,8] If more than two doses are used, magnesium levels should be monitored. If an ileus is present, repeated doses of cathartics should not be used. For infants and small children, repeat doses of cathartics are usually not needed and may cause significant fluid and electrolyte problems.[9]

WHOLE-BOWEL IRRIGATION

Evidence is increasing that whole-bowel irrigation has a role in certain ingestions, especially enteric-coated or sustained release preparations and toxins not adsorbed by charcoal (e.g., iron). A balanced electrolyte solution (Colyte, GoLYTELY) is given by NG tube (1 to 2 L/hr in adults, 400 mL/hr in children) until the rectal effluent is clear. Results are prompt because washout takes only a few hours. A large amount of the solution may distend the stomach, causing vomiting and pulmonary aspiration. It is unknown if whole-bowel irrigation interferes with concomitant charcoal administration.

ENHANCING ELIMINATION

MULTIPLE-DOSE CHARCOAL

Repeated doses of oral activated charcoal enhance the elimination of some drugs from the body, even after absorption of the drug has taken place. Even after administration of certain drugs intravenously (e.g., theophylline, phenobarbital), multiple-dose charcoal can hasten elimination.[10–12] Certain drugs probably undergo an enteroenteric circulation (i.e., they are secreted into the intestinal lumen and are then reabsorbed into the bloodstream). The presence of charcoal in the intestinal lumen probably interrupts this process by adsorbing the drug, preventing its reabsorption. The concept has been called gastrointestinal dialysis. Interrupting enterohepatic recirculation with charcoal may also play a role with some drugs. Table 81-14 lists drugs for which multiple-dose charcoal has been shown to enhance elimination. It may be helpful for many other agents, but the table lists only agents in which this modality has specifically been studied.

The optimal dosage of multiple-dose charcoal has not been established. Usually, an initial dose of activated charcoal of 50 to 100 g in an adult or 1 g/kg of body weight in a child (as mentioned previously) is given with a cathartic. Repeat doses of 20 to 50 g in an adult or one half the initial dose in a child is then given every 2 to 6 hours. The risks of multiple-dose charcoal therapy are the same as those previously described for single-dose therapy.[5a,5b] Multiple-dose charcoal should not be used if an ileus is present.

In adults, a repeat dose of charcoal with a cathartic may be used (see the cautions described in the section

TABLE 81-13. SOME AGENTS NOT SIGNIFICANTLY ADSORBED TO ACTIVATED CHARCOAL
Acids
Alkalis
Boric acid
Ethanol
Ethylene glycol
Iron tablets
Mercury
Lithium

TABLE 81-14. AGENTS OF OVERDOSE AGAINST WHICH MULTIPLE-DOSE CHARCOAL MAY BE HELPFUL	
Amitriptyline	Meprobamate
Atrazine	Methotrexate
Carbamazepine	Nadolol
Cyclosporine	Notriptyline
Dapsone	Phenobarbital
Desmethyldiazepam	Phenylbutazone
Dextropropoxyphene	Phenytoin
Diazepam	Piroxicam
Digitoxin	Proscillaridin
Digoxin	Salicylates
Doxepin	Sotalol
Glutethimide	Theophylline

(Data with permission from Rumack B. H.: POISINDEX Information System, 54th Ed. Denver, Micromedex, 1987; and Mauro L. S., Mauro V. F., Brown D. L., et al: Enhancement of phenytoin elimination by multiple-dose activated charcoal. Ann. Emerg. Med. 16:1132, 1987.)

on cathartics). In children, repeat doses of charcoal with cathartics are probably not indicated and should be used only with extreme caution.

The effectiveness of a charcoal preparation may relate to the surface area of the activated charcoal particles used. Once Super-Char (3150 m²/g) appeared to be the leader in reducing aspirin absorption.[13] Charcoal in multiple doses must be given carefully because of complications, particularly bowel obstruction and aspiration. These have been reported, suggesting a reappraisal of the widespread use of charcoal.[14]

DIURESIS

Forced diuresis is an overused and probably ineffective treatment of most poisonings. Alkaline diuresis is effective in enhancing the elimination of salicylates and phenobarbital. Maintaining an adequate output of alkaline urine, however, is probably as effective as forcing marked increases in urinary output and risking fluid overload. Acid diuresis may enhance elimination of certain drugs, but is rarely, if ever, indicated because it may increase the risk of renal failure should rhabdomyolysis and myoglobinuria occur.

HEMODIALYSIS

Hemodialysis is not a widely used tool in toxicology, but it can be effective in certain selected poisonings:

- Salicylate—severe, unresponsive to usual measures,
- Ethylene glycol and methanol—acidosis, high blood levels,
- Lithium—severe toxicity present,
- Theophylline—significant toxicity, serum levels higher than 60 to 100 μg/mL,
- Renal failure—in a poisoned patient in whom the main route of elimination of the toxin is renal,
- Severe fluid, electrolyte, or acid-base disturbances related to poisoning.

HEMOPERFUSION

Hemoperfusion over a charcoal or resin column may be an effective treatment in certain circumstances (e.g., theophylline or ethchlorvynol poisoning). The risks, however, are numerous, including the destruction of blood products, especially platelets.

If physicians have questions about the utility of certain modalities used in enhancing elimination of a specific poison, they should consult a regional poison control center for the latest information.

SPECIFIC ANTIDOTE THERAPY

Unfortunately, there are very few poisonings in which a specific antidote is useful in reversing toxicity. For this reason, meticulous attention must be given to the techniques previously mentioned. For most poisonings, good supportive care alone results in a good outcome. Table 81-15 lists agents for which a specific antidote may be indicated. Up-to-date dosing information and specific indications for these antidotes are available from poison control centers. Some of these antidotes are discussed in more detail in subsequent chapters, but a few of these antidotes deserve special mention here.

HYPERBARIC OXYGEN (HBO)

Hyperbaric oxygen therapy is the delivery of 100% oxygen at increased atmospheric pressure. This is done in a hyperbaric chamber, usually at a pressure

TABLE 81-15. SPECIFIC ANTIDOTE THERAPY	
Toxic Agent	**Antidote**
Acetaminophen	N-acetyl-L-cysteine
Anticoagulants (coumarin type)	Vitamin K
Anticholinergics	Physostigmine
β-Blockers	Glucagon
Calcium-channel blockers	Calcium
Carbon monoxide	Oxygen, hyperbaric oxygen
Carbon tetrachloride	Hyperbaric oxygen
Cholinesterase inhibitors	Atropine, pralidoxime
Cyanide	Sodium nitrite, thiosulfate, hyperbaric oxygen
Cyclic antidepressants	Serum alkalinization
Digitalis	Digoxin-specific antibodies
Ethylene glycol	Ethanol
Extrapyramidal crisis	Diphenhydramine, benztropine
Heavy metals	Dimercaprol, d-penicillamine, ethylenediamine tetra-acetic acid (EDTA)
Hydrofluoric acid, fluoride	Calcium
Hydrogen sulfide	Sodium nitrite, hyperbaric oxygen
Insulin, oral hypoglycemics	Dextrose
Iron	Deferoxamine
Isoniazid, hydrazines	Pyridoxine
Methanol	Ethanol
Methemoglobin inducers	Methylene blue
Opiates, opioids	Naloxone

of 2 to 3 atmospheres. Traditionally, these chambers have been used to treat decompression sickness associated with diving accidents, but they are playing an increasing role in toxicology.

Carbon monoxide poisoning is the main indication for HBO therapy, but not all patients with this poisoning need HBO. Various regimens exist for treating carbon monoxide poisoning with HBO; the usual indications are a carboxyhemoglobin level of higher than 30% or the presence of symptoms of carbon monoxide poisoning in patients with lower levels. Although hyperbaric chambers are becoming more commonplace, there are still many EDs that are several hundred miles from the nearest chamber. Poison control centers can provide information about the closest chamber to a particular hospital. Before transferring a patient for HBO therapy, the physician should consult with the medical director of the hyperbaric unit in the area.

Hyperbaric oxygen therapy may be indicated for the treatment of poisoning with cyanide (in conjunction with sodium nitrite and thiosulfate), hydrogen sulfide, and carbon tetrachloride and for the treatment of methemoglobinemia.[6] Again, consultation should

be obtained with the director of a hyperbaric unit when considering HBO for these poisonings.

GLUCAGON

Overdose with beta-blocking agents can produce severe toxicity, particularly to the cardiovascular system. Severe bradycardias, hypotension, and conduction disturbances can occur. Glucagon may reverse this toxicity, producing positive inotropic and chronotropic effects on the heart, probably because of stimulation of the synthesis of cyclic adenosine monophosphate.[6] Glucagon should be used in conjunction with other treatments, such as atropine or isoproterenol administration or cardiac pacing. The dose is 0.05 to 0.15 mg/kg of body weight (usually about 10 mg in adults) given IV over about 1 minute, followed by a continuous intravenous infusion of 1 to 5 mg/hr. Glucagon used for this purpose should be diluted with preservative-free saline or 5% dextrose instead of the diluent provided, which contains phenol.[6]

PHYSOSTIGMINE

Physostigmine is an acetylcholinesterase inhibitor that is sometimes used to reverse signs of anticholinergic poisoning. It is probably overused and can be dangerous, producing bradycardia, asystole, or seizures. In anticholinergic poisoning, the use of physostigmine may be indicated in treating myoclonic seizures, severe hallucinations, hypertension, or arrhythmias. It should not be used routinely as a therapeutic trial for patients with coma of unknown origin. Cyclic antidepressants may produce some of these same anticholinergic findings. The use of physostigmine may be indicated here, but only for the specific indications previously mentioned. In reality, physostigmine is rarely if ever needed in the management of cyclic antidepressant toxicity. Moreover, most patients who overdose on more specific anticholinergic agents can be managed without physostigmine.

UPDATE ON SPECIFIC COMMON POISONINGS

ACETAMINOPHEN

The current standard antidotal therapy in the United States for treating significant acetaminophen poisoning is oral N-acetyl-L-cysteine (NAC, Mucomyst). The plasma acetaminophen level should be measured 4 hours after an acute overdose, or as soon as possible after 4 hours, and plotted on the standard nomogram (Fig. 81-1). If the level is above the lower toxicity line on the nomogram, then oral NAC should be given and continued every 4 hours for 72 hours.

An area of controversy exists in that NAC is an oral

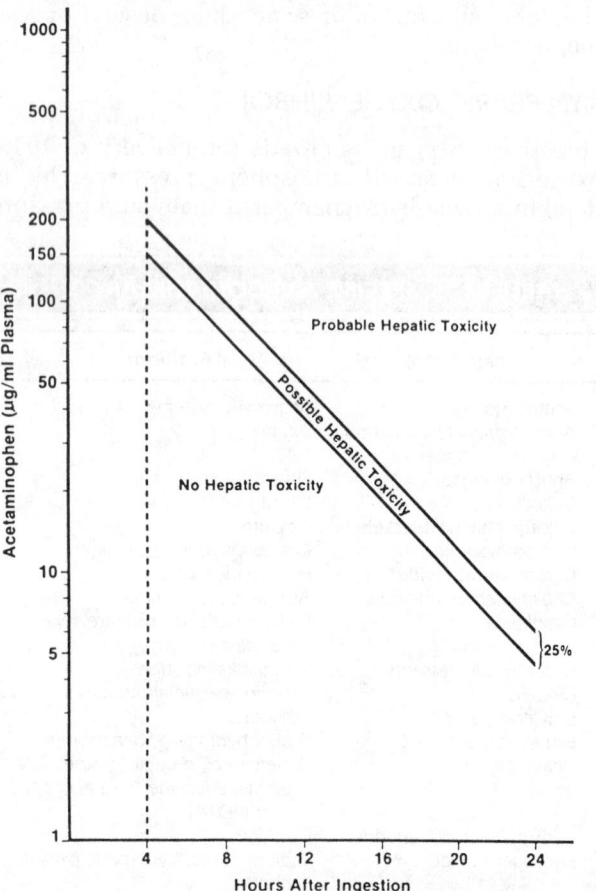

FIG. 81-1. Nomogram for acetaminophen poisoning. Cautions for the use of this chart:
1. The graph should be used only in relation to a single acute ingestion.
2. Serum levels drawn before 4 hours post-ingestion may not represent peak levels. (From Medindex, Micromedex, Englewood, Colorado, with permission.)

TABLE 81-16. RELATIVE TOXICITY OF CYCLIC ANTIDEPRESSANTS

Generic Name	Trade Name	Structural Classification	CNS Toxicity	Cardiovascular Toxicity
Amitriptyline	Elavil Amitid Endep Amitril	Tricyclic	+ + + +	+ + + +
Amoxapine	Asendin	Tricyclic	+ + + +	+
Clomipramine	*	Tricyclic	+ + + +	+ + + +
Desipramine	Norpramin Pertofrane	Tricyclic	+ + + +	+ + + +
Doxepin	Adapin Sinequan	Tricyclic	+ + + +	+ + + +
Imipramine	Tofranil Presamine SK-Pramine Janimine	Tricyclic	+ + + +	+ + + +
Loxapine	Loxitane	Tricyclic	+ + + +	+
Maprotiline	Ludiomil	Tetracyclic	+ + + +	+ + +
Mianserin	*	Tetracyclic	?	?
Nortriptyline	Aventyl Pamelor	Tricyclic	+ + + +	+ + + +
Protriptyline	Vivactil	Tricyclic	+ + + +	+ + + +
Trazodone	Desyrel	Miscellaneous	+	+
Trimipramine	Surmontil	Tricyclic	+ + + +	+ + + +
Viloxazine	*	Bicylic	?	?
Zimelidine	*	Bicylic	?	?

Scale of toxicity: + = least toxic, + + + + = most toxic.
* Investigational drug
(With permission from Rumack, B. H.: POISINDEX Information System, 54th Ed. Denver, Micromedex, 1987.)

antidote and activated charcoal given orally for the overdose may interfere with NAC absorption. In fact, in vitro studies have shown that NAC is significantly adsorbed to activated charcoal.[15] Two in vivo studies on human volunteers, however, have shown no significant difference in NAC absorption when given with or without activated charcoal.[16,17] Another factor to be considered is that there is no known correlation between serum NAC levels and NAC's efficacy in the treatment of acetaminophen overdose. Thus, even if part of a dose of NAC is adsorbed to charcoal, the remainder is probably effective in preventing toxicity.

Because of the discrepancy between in vivo and in vitro data, care should be taken when giving charcoal to a patient with an acetaminophen overdose, although charcoal does not seem to be contraindicated. The following guidelines are recommended for the use of charcoal in treating acetaminophen overdose.[6] Activated charcoal should be administered as soon as possible to prevent a subsequent toxic level of acetaminophen. Activated charcoal should not be used concomitantly with NAC. Charcoal should be removed by lavage if less than one hour has elapsed between charcoal and NAC administration.

Further care should be used if multiple-dose charcoal is indicated for the treatment of a substance ingested with acetaminophen for which this regimen has shown clinical efficacy (e.g., salicylates, theophylline, phenobarbital).[6] As soon as possible after the overdose, administer a dose of charcoal with a cathartic (perhaps after a gastric emptying procedure). Assess the plasma acetaminophen level. If the level is potentially toxic and less than 1 hour has elapsed since the charcoal was given, remove any charcoal in the stomach by way of a nasogastric tube, and administer oral NAC. Then, alternate charcoal and NAC every 2 hours and lavage residual charcoal before each NAC dose. This regimen should be reserved for a select group of patients.

Some of this controversy may be resolved if intravenous NAC becomes available in the United States. Currently, intravenous NAC is approved for use in Canada and several European countries. In the United States, studies are under way on the treatment of acetaminophen overdose patients with intravenous NAC. This is still an investigational drug, however, and for patients to receive intravenous NAC, they must be enrolled in the study and receive pyrogen-free NAC provided to the study centers. For the current status of intravenous NAC or for the location of the centers involved in the study, consult the local poison center.

CYCLIC ANTIDEPRESSANTS

Cyclic antidepressants remain a significant cause of morbidity and mortality. Some newer agents differ from the traditional tricyclic antidepressants. Table 81-16 lists both the older and newer agents along with their relative toxicities. Manifestations of toxic levels of cyclic antidepressants include lethargy, coma, seizures, respiratory depression, and hypotension. Cardiac toxicity is common, causing tachycardia, conduction delays, supraventricular and ventricular arrhythmias, and a prolonged Q-T interval. A prolonged QRS complex (greater than 0.10 seconds) is a good predictor of seizures and arrhythmias.[17]

AMOXAPINE, LOXAPINE

Amoxapine is a tricyclic agent that in overdose is associated with a higher incidence of seizures and a lower incidence of cardiovascular toxicity than are traditional tricyclic antidepressants.[18] Seizures may be very difficult to control and may require aggressive management.

Loxapine is a tricyclic antipsychotic agent with toxic effects similar to those of its metabolite, amoxapine.

MAPROTILINE

Maprotiline is a tetracyclic agent, dissimilar from traditional tricyclic antidepressants. Its toxic effects, however, are similar to those of traditional agents.[19] Coma, seizures, and significant cardiovascular toxicity occur with overdose of this agent. The treatment of toxicity from this agent is the same as for that from the classic tricyclic antidepressants.

TRAZODONE

Trazodone has a unique structure that is neither tricyclic nor tetracyclic.[19] Trazodone seems to be much less toxic than traditional tricyclic antidepressants, even in massive ingestions. Cardiac toxicity seems to be minimal and CNS depression mild.[19]

TREATMENT OF CYCLIC ANTIDEPRESSANT POISONING

Initial stabilization includes airway management, with endotracheal intubation if the patient is comatose or has lost the gag reflex. Ipecac should not be given, because the patient may rapidly become comatose or convulse. Gastric lavage should be done, followed by administration of activated charcoal with a cathartic. Multiple-dose charcoal may be helpful.

Serum alkalinization (to a pH of 7.45 to 7.50) may dramatically reverse some signs of toxicity.[20] This procedure is recommended for the treatment of hypotension, ventricular arrhythmias, and a prolonged QRS complex (greater than 0.10 seconds). Seizures should be treated with sodium bicarbonate to prevent the acidosis that usually accompanies them. This acidosis could rapidly lead to worsening cardiac toxicity. Diazepam should also be given for seizures, followed by administration of phenytoin and possibly phenobarbital.

Alkalinization can be accomplished in two ways. If the patient is intubated, hyperventilation, manually or with the ventilator, can be done. Otherwise, sodium bicarbonate (1 to 2 mEq/kg of body weight) can be given in a bolus IV. This could be followed by a continuous infusion of 2 to 3 ampules (88 to 132 mEq) of sodium bicarbonate in a liter of 5% dextrose in water. Arterial blood gases should be monitored with the goal of keeping the serum pH around 7.45 to 7.50.

For ventricular arrhythmias, besides alkalinization, the administration of lidocaine, phenytoin, or both may be indicated. If a prolonged QRS complex does not become narrower after alkalinization, phenytoin may help. For hypotension, if the patient does not respond to an intravenous fluid challenge or alkalinization, a vasopressor may be needed. Norepinephrine is preferred, as dopamine may not be effective.[20] Isoproterenol or a pacemaker may be needed for heart block or bradycardia. Torsades de pointes may occur with cyclic antidepressant poisoning. Isoproterenol or overdrive pacing may be needed to treat this arrhythmia.

Forced diuresis, hemodialysis, and hemoperfusion are not helpful in poisoning with cyclic antidepressants, because these agents have wide distributions and are highly protein-bound. Physostigmine is rarely if ever indicated in poisoning by these agents and may make the patient worse by inducing seizures, bradycardia, or asystole.

DIGOXIN, DIGITOXIN

A breakthrough in toxicology was the development of digoxin immune Fab (Digibind) for the treatment of severe digoxin or digitoxin toxicity. Digoxin immune Fab is a substance containing purified fragments, antigen-binding (Fab), of digoxin-specific antibodies obtained from sheep.[20] These antibody fragments bind molecules of digoxin, making them unavailable for binding at their site of action on cells in the body. The Fab-digoxin complex accumulates in the blood and thus is excreted in the kidney. Patients with signs of severe cardiac toxicity from digoxin usually respond dramatically with 30 minutes of an infusion of Fab.[21]

The signs of digitalis poisoning encompass a multitude of cardiac arrhythmias, including ventricular arrhythmias and varying degrees of heart block. Gastrointestinal symptoms and central nervous system symptoms are also common. Hyperkalemia can also occur and may be severe and life-threatening, because of the ability of digitalis preparations to inactivate the cell membrane sodium-potassium adenosine triphosphatase pump, resulting in a rise in extracellular potassium.[21] The hypokalemia present in patients on chronic digitalis therapy is usually due to the concomitant use of diuretics.

Indications for using Fab in digitalis toxicity are fairly specific. Most patients with digitalis toxicity can be managed successfully without Fab. Its use is indicated for digoxin or digitoxin toxicity that is manifested by life-threatening signs—severe ventricular arrhythmias, such as ventricular tachycardia or ventricular fibrillation, or severe bradydysrhythmias that are unresponsive to atropine. Severe hyperkalemia in the presence of digitalis toxicity is another indication for the use of Fab.

Digoxin immune Fab is given intravenously either as a bolus injection (for imminent cardiac arrest) or as an infusion over 30 minutes. It is available in most parts of the country. Information on the availability and use of Digibind can be obtained at any time by telephoning Burroughs Wellcome at 1–800–334–4828.

SALICYLATES

Salicylate poisoning remains a significant cause of morbidity and mortality in all age groups. The Done nomogram (Fig. 85-2) can be a useful tool in managing salicylate poisoning, but it must be used properly; it is useful only in cases of a single acute ingestion of aspirin.[22] It is not useful in ingestions of enteric-coated or slow-release aspirin preparations. In these cases, peak levels may be delayed for up to 24 to 36 hours. Nor is the nomogram useful for chronic salicylate poisoning; with chronic salicylism, patients can be extremely ill while having seemingly "low" serum salicylate levels. A further word of caution is that even though salicylate levels usually peak in overdoses of regular aspirin at about 6 hours after ingestion, continued absorption can occur after that time. Therefore, repeat determinations of salicylate levels should be done to ensure that absorption has stopped and that therapy is working.

The physician should not rely totally on serum salicylate levels to manage patients. Clinical findings, including vital signs, acid-base status, and fluid-electrolyte status, are more important. Administration of multiple-dose charcoal, urine alkalinization, and maintenance of good urine output are the mainstays of therapy. Hemodialysis may be indicated for severe cases: persistent acid-base or fluid-electrolyte problems; noncardiogenic pulmonary edema; central nervous system deterioration as manifested by seizures, obtundation, or cerebral edema; and renal failure.

NEWER DRUGS OF OVERDOSE

IBUPROFEN

The introduction of ibuprofen preparations as over-the-counter analgesics has led to an increase in poisonings from these agents in both children and adults. Hall and associates studied 126 cases of ibuprofen overdose and published their results along with a review of the literature.[23] Although ibuprofen overdose is often benign, serious signs and symptoms, even

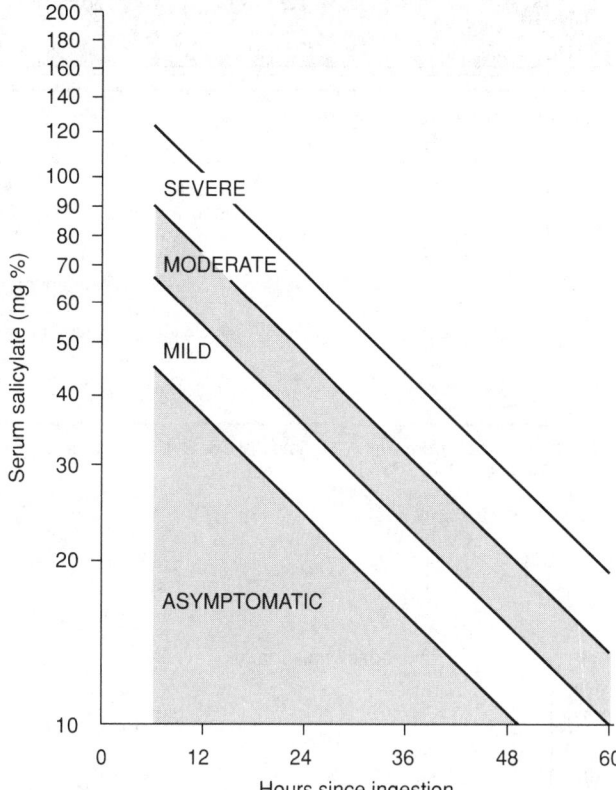

FIG. 81-2.   Nomogram for relating serum salicylate level to severity of intoxication at varying intervals after acute ingestion of single doses of aspirin. (With permission from Done A. K.: Salicylate intoxication: Significance of measurements of salicylates in blood in cases of acute ingestion. Pediatrics 26:800, 1960.)

death, can occur. Mild symptoms include gastrointestinal upset, lethargy, headache, rash, and blurred vision. More serious signs of toxicity include coma, seizures, apnea, renal failure, bradycardia, and metabolic acidosis.

In pediatric ingestions in Hall and associates' series, the milligrams of ibuprofen ingested per kilogram of body weight correlated well with symptoms. Table 81-17 shows their recommendations for managing pediatric poisonings if the amount ingested is known. For adults, the history of the amount ingested did not correlate with symptoms. Thus, for adults, any symptomatic patient or any patient in whom the ingestion was a suicide attempt requires evaluation by a physician. It should be noted that in Hall and associates' series, the onset of symptoms was always within 4 hours of ingestion.

The plasma levels of ibuprofen may help to predict the severity of toxicity in overdose. Hall et al.'s review included a nomogram relating the severity of symptoms to the plasma ibuprofen level (Fig. 81-3).

Treatment of ibuprofen overdose is supportive. Airway and ventilatory support may be needed. Hypotension may necessitate the administration of fluids or vasopressors. Significant metabolic acidosis may require the use of intravenous sodium bicarbonate,

Amount of Ibuprofen Ingested (mg/kg body weight)	Therapy
<100	Observe at home.
100–200	Induce emesis at home. Observe at home for 4 hrs. If symptoms develop, refer to health care facility.
200–400	Empty stomach immediately. Refer immediately to health care facility. Minimum of 4 hr of observation. Administer charcoal and cathartic.
>400	Refer immediately to health care facility. Greatest potential for seizures, so induced emesis may be risky. Observe for at least 4 hr. Administer charcoal and a cathartic.

TABLE 81-17. RECOMMENDATIONS FOR MANAGING CHILDREN 5 YEARS OLD OR YOUNGER WITH IBUPROFEN INGESTION

(With permission from Hall A. H., Smolinske S. C., Conrad F. L., et al: Ibuprofen overdose: 126 cases. Am. Emerg. Med. *15*:1308, 1986.)

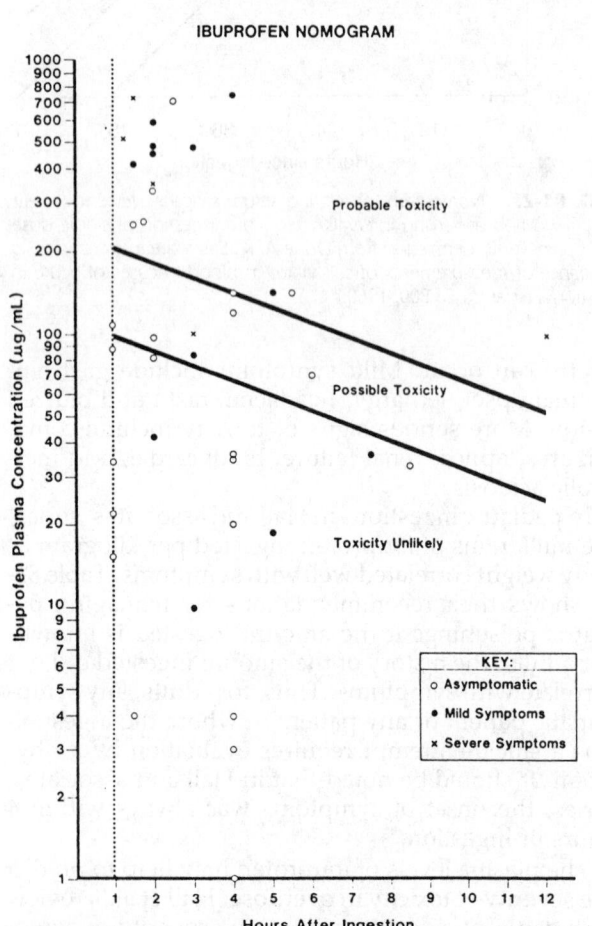

FIG. 81-3. Nomogram relating plasma ibuprofen level to severity of intoxication. *Severe symptoms* include seizures, apnea, bradycardia, hypotension, renal failure, coma. *Mild symptoms* include mild central nervous system depression, gastrointestinal upsets, rash, headache, nystagmus, blurred vision, muscle fasciculations (With permission from Hall, A. H., Smolinske, S. C., Conrad, F. L., et al: Ibuprofen overdose: 126 cases. Ann. Emerg. Med. *15*:1308, 1986.)

and atropine may be needed for symptomatic bradycardia. Gastric emptying procedures may be indicated, although caution must be used when syrup of ipecac is given because seizures may occur with large ingestions. Charcoal and a cathartic should be administered. Multiple-dose charcoal may be of benefit, but its use with ibuprofen has not been studied.

CALCIUM-CHANNEL BLOCKERS

Calcium-channel blockers have been introduced to the United States for the treatment of angina, hypertension, and certain arrhythmias. Currently, nifedipine, diltiazem, and verapamil are available in the United States. With their increased availability have come the expected increase in accidental exposures in children and suicide attempts in adults and adolescents. Toxicity varies slightly from agent to agent and with the amount ingested. Overdoses have resulted in severe toxicity and fatality. Major effects have included hypotension and bradydysrhythmias, including third-degree heart block and asystole.[6] Central nervous system depression, seizures, confusion, pulmonary edema, nausea, and vomiting have also been reported.

In treating calcium-channel blocker overdoses, inducing emesis may be contraindicated, because increasing vagal stimulation may worsen cardiac effects. Specific therapy for hypotension or significant bradycardia or heart block includes the administration of intravenous calcium salts, either calcium chloride or calcium gluconate.[18] For hypotension, intravenous fluids and dopamine may also be required. For heart block, atropine, isoproterenol, glucagon, or cardiac pacing may be required in addition to intravenous calcium. Diazepam, along with phenytoin or phenobarbital, may be required for seizures.

Not enough is known about overdose with these agents to predict toxicity on the basis of the amount of drug ingested or on plasma levels. Onset of symptoms from ingestion of these agents is within 4 to 6 hours, unless a slow-release preparation is ingested.

Hemodialysis and hemoperfusion should not be expected to be of benefit because of the high degree of protein binding and the wide distribution of these agents.

ETHYLENE GLYCOL POISONING

Ethylene glycol (antifreeze) is an important cause of toxin-induced renal failure and profound metabolic acidosis, CNS injury, and cardiovascular collapse. The reported use of 4-methylpyrazole,[24] an inhibitor of alcoholic dehydrogenase is an important treatment addition. Early detection and use of this substance may constitute effective treatment before serious renal impairment. If the kidneys are abnormal, dialysis is needed on an emergency basis.

REFERENCES

1. Savitt, D.L., Hawkins, H.H., and Roberts, J.R.: The radiopacity of ingested medications. Ann. Emerg. Med. 16:331, 1987.
2. Kulig, K., Bar-Or, D., Cantrill S.V., et al.: Management of acutely poisoned patients without gastric emptying. Ann. Emerg. Med. 14:562, 1985.
3. Curtis, R.A., Barone, J., and Giacona, N.: Efficacy of ipecac and activated charcoal/cathartic. Arch. Intern. Med. 144:48, 1984.
4. Neuvonen, P.J., Vartiainen, M., and Takola, O.: Comparison of activated charcoal and ipecac syrup in prevention of drug absorption. Eur. J. Clin. Pharmacol. 24:557, 1983.
5. Neuvonen, P.J., and Olkkola, K.T.: Activated charcoal and syrup of ipecac in prevention of cimetidine and pindolol absorption in man after administration of metoclopramide as an antiemetic agent. Clin. Toxicol. 22:103, 1984.
5a. Watson, W.A., et al.: Gastrointestinal obstruction associated with multiple-dose activated charcoal. J. Emerg. Med. 4:401, 1986.
5b. Keller, R.E., et al.: Contribution of sorbital combined with activated charcoal in prevention of salicylate absorption. Ann. Emerg. Med. 19:654, 1990.
6. Rumack, B.H.: POISINDEX® Information System, 54th Ed. Denver, Micromedex, 1987.
7. Smilkstein, M.J., Smolinske, S.C., Kulig, K.W., et al.: Severe hypermagnesemia due to multiple dose cathartic therapy (abstract). Vet. Hum. Toxicol. 28:494, 1986.
8. Jones, J., Heiselman, D., Dougherty, J., et al.: Cathartic-induced magnesium toxicity during overdose management. Ann. Emerg. Med. 15:1214, 1986.
9. Farley, T.A.: Severe hypernatremic dehydration after use of an activated charcoal-sorbitol suspension. J. Pediatr. 109:719, 1986.
10. Berlinger, W.G., Spector, R., Goldberg, M.J., et al.: Enhancement of theophylline clearance by oral activated charcoal. Clin. Pharmacol. Ther. 33:351, 1983.
11. Mahutte, C., True, R.J., Thurry, M.M., et al.: Increased serum theophylline clearance with orally administered activated charcoal. Am. Rev. Respir. Dis. 128:820, 1983.
12. Berg, M.J., Berlinger, W.G., Goldberg, M.J., et al.: Acceleration of the body clearance of phenobarbital by oral activated charcoal. N. Engl. J. Med. 307:642, 1982.
13. Krenzelok, E.P., and Heller, M.P.: Effectiveness of commercially available aqueous activated charcoal products. Ann. Emerg. Med. 16:1340, 1987.
14. Tenenbein, M.: Multiple doses of activated charcoal: Time for reappraisal? Ann. Emerg. Med. 20:529, 1991.
15. Klein-Schwartz, W., and Odera, G.M.: Adsorption of oral antidotes for acetaminophen poisoning (methionine and N-acetylcysteine) by activated charcoal. Clin. Toxicol. 18:283, 1981.
16. Renzi, P, Donovan, J.W., Martin, T.G., et al.: Concomitant use of activated charcoal and N-acetylcysteine. Ann. Emerg. Med. 14:568, 1985.
17. North, D.S., Peterson, R.G., and Krenzelok, E.: Effect of activated charcoal administration on acetylcysteine serum levels in humans. Am. J. Hosp. Pharm. 38:1022, 1981.
18. Boehnert, M.T., and Lovejoy, F.H.: Value of the QRS duration versus the serum drug level in predicting seizures and ventricular arrhythmias after an acute overdose of tricyclic antidepressants. N. Engl. J. Med. 313:474, 1985.
19. Kulig, K.: Management of poisoning associated with "newer" antidepressant agents. Ann. Emerg. Med. 15:1039, 1986.
20. Frommer, D.A., Kulig, K.K., Marx, J.A., et al.: Tricyclic antidepressant overdose—A review. JAMA 257:521, 1987.
21. Wenger, T.L., Butler, V.P., Haber, E., et al.: Treatment of 63 severely digitalis-toxic patients with digoxin-specific antibody fragments. J. Am. Coll. Cardiol. 5:118A, 1985.
22. Done, A.K.: Salicylate intoxication: Significance of measurements of salicylates in blood in cases of acute ingestion. Pediatrics 26:800, 1960.
23. Hall, A.H., Smolinske, S.C., Conrad, F.L., et al.: Ibuprofen overdose: 126 cases. Ann. Emerg. Med. 15:1308, 1986.
24. Galliot, M., Astier, A., Vu Bien, D., et al.: Treatment of ethylene glycol poisoning with intravenous 4-methylpyrazole. N. Engl. J. Med. 319:97, 1988.

USE OF THE TOXICOLOGY LABORATORY IN EMERGENCY MEDICINE

Mary Ann Howland
and Balkrishena Kaul

CAPSULE

The usefulness of the toxicology laboratory lies in its ability to perform three functions: (1) confirm a presumptive toxicologic diagnosis, (2) provide rapid quantitative information as dictated by the intoxicant, and (3) assess the contribution of drugs to the clinical status of the patient with an altered mental status, no history, and atypical physical findings.

The capabilities of the laboratory must be explored and these questions addressed:

1. Which analytic techniques are used?
2. What are the hours of operation?
3. Which drugs can be tested on an immediate basis?
4. Is there an alternative laboratory for analysis of substances not routinely analyzed by the first laboratory?
5. Do they perform a rapid screen; If so, which drugs are included?
6. Are positive findings confirmed by a second independent analytic technique?

ANALYTIC TECHNIQUES

Several analytic techniques are in common usage. A specific drug may be detected by a number of techniques, and laboratories differ as to which procedures are routinely used for specific identification.

CHROMATOGRAPHY

THIN-LAYER

Thin-layer chromatography (TLC) is most often used as a screening procedure on urine. Many drugs or their metabolites that are excreted in the urine are detected by TLC. At least 50 mL of urine should be submitted to the laboratory. The urine is prepared (extracted and concentrated), and a spot of the urine extract and a known standard are applied to the bottom of a chromatographic plate. A solvent, acting as the mobile liquid phase, is then allowed to migrate up the plate. As this solvent travels, it carries different compounds to characteristic distances. The plate is allowed to dry, and a chromogenic agent is applied. The distance moved by the compound is then compared to the standards. In addition, various chemicals are applied in sequence to see if confirmatory color reactions can be elicited visually or by inspection under various wavelengths of ultraviolet light. A presumptive identification is then made.

Thin-layer chromatography is fairly easy to perform and is the least expensive of the commonly used analytic techniques. The test requires 3 to 4 hours to complete and is done only on urine. Drawbacks to using TLC are that it is time-consuming, strictly qualitative, less sensitive, and sometimes the least specific. The exact identification of a specific drug depends somewhat on the expertise of the laboratory person-

nel, and often only the class of a drug, for example antihistamines or tricyclics, can be identified. Sometimes only metabolites of the parent drug are detected.

GAS AND HIGH-PRESSURE LIQUID

Gas chromatography (GC) and high-pressure liquid chromatography (HPLC) utilize the same basic principle as TLC. Instead of a plate, however, both GC and HPLC use columns that are packed with the stationary phase. In GC, the prepared test sample is injected and then heated to vaporization, and the gaseous sample moves through the column. A device at the end of the column detects the chemical, and a graphic representation results. Each particular substance transverses the column at a different speed. Therefore, the time it takes to reach the detector is noted and compared to standards, allowing accurate identification. The size of the peak on the graph allows quantification. HPLC is similar to GC except that a high-pressure pump moves the test sample with a mobile solvent through the column, avoiding the necessity of the test compound being volatile. GC and HPLC are sensitive, specific, both qualitative and quantitative, and available in most laboratories. These techniques can be used to analyze both blood and urine. The turnaround time is 2 to 4 hours.

IMMUNOASSAYS

The *enzyme multiple immunoassay technique* (EMIT), the *radioimmunoassay* (RIA), and the *fluorescent immunoassay* (FIA) are similar in principle. All three methods use labeled drug antibody complexes to which the unlabeled test drug is added. Identification and quantification are made by measuring the amount of labeled drug that was displaced and comparing it to a known standard curve.

EMIT

In the EMIT, the known drug antibody complex is labeled with an enzyme that, when *not* attached to antibody, causes lysis of bacterial cells. The reaction is carried out in a bacterial medium. A clear solution, resulting from bacterial lysis, reflects large displacement of labeled drug by unlabeled drug in the test specimen. The clarity of the solution is measured by means of optical density spectrophotometry, and the results are compared to a standard curve. Some of the newer EMITs do not rely on bacterial lysis, but use other enzymes. The principle is the same, however.

RIA

With RIA, the labeling is done using a radioactive isotope, and displaced labeled radioactive drug is counted after antibody-bound labeled and unlabeled drug have been precipitated. Again, the results are compared to a standard.

FIA

Fluorescent immunoassay is a relatively new technique that also uses competitive protein binding. A fluorogenic enzyme substrate is used. The fluorescence that is produced and measured is proportional to the drug level.

The EMIT, RIA, and FIA are qualitative and quantitative. The EMIT and FIA are faster than RIA and easier to perform. These techniques are intermediate in accuracy between the least accurate TLC and the most accurate GC and HPLC. The EMIT, FIA, and RIA are more sensitive than they are specific. For example, with the EMIT analysis, the blood and urine of a patient who has received naloxone before the specimens are sent for toxicologic analysis may be read as false-positive for opioids. One cannot, for example, differentiate the various barbiturates in the EMIT assay, but a total composite barbiturate level is given.

ACCURACY OF TECHNIQUES

Each analytic technique has strengths and weaknesses. For truly accurate results, each positive immunoassay (RIA, EMIT, FIA) finding must be confirmed by a second independent technique, preferably by a chemical procedure (TLC, HPLC, GLC). For forensic toxicology (testing in the workplace, postmortem examinations, and medical legal disputes) confirmation by GC-MS is the standard.

TOXICOLOGIC TESTS

Certain toxicologic tests should be available on an immediate basis. These include determinations for acetaminophen, carboxyhemoglobin, digoxin, ethanol, ethylene glycol, iron, lithium, methanol, methemoglobin, phenobarbital, salicylates, and theophylline. These 12 tests are listed because knowing the specific blood concentration may directly influence therapy. Many of these substances are not identified on a routine screen, and one must specifically request analysis for them. Lithium and iron, for example, are not usually detected unless a specific request is made, even though they may be present in high concentrations.

ACETAMINOPHEN

Toxic blood levels of acetaminophen require administration of N-acetyl-L-cysteine (Mucomyst) as an antidote. A case could be made here for not needing immediate acetaminophen blood level determination and instead treating every suspected case with N-acetyl-L-cysteine. This practice, however, would lead to gross unnecessary overtreatment of many patients and perhaps miss some unsuspected cases. Also, the useful Rumack-Matthew nomogram relies on quantitative determination. Many hospitals now routinely obtain acetaminophen levels in all suicidal patients.

CARBOXYHEMOGLOBIN

High carboxyhemoglobin levels in a symptomatic patient require administration of 100% oxygen and hyperbaric oxygen therapy. Note, however, that low carboxyhemoglobin levels with a convincing history would still lead one to treat with oxygen, and possibly even hyperbaric oxygen, if warranted because low blood levels may not accurately reflect tissue levels.

DIGOXIN

Toxic digoxin levels severe enough to cause refractory cardiac arrhythmias and hyperkalemia require therapy with Fab digoxin antibody fragments. A good history of digoxin use combined with the classic signs and symptoms, (even without a digoxin level) is reason enough to administer Fab. Interpretation of digoxin levels depends on the time drawn after ingestion. Digoxin has a long distribution half-life, and levels 6 hours after ingestion are most reflective of cardiac effects in the therapeutic setting. Endogenous digoxin-like substances have been measured in certain situations (pregnancy, renal failure, young children) and are another reason not to administer Fab to an asymptomatic patient or hemodynamically stable patient just because of an elevated digoxin level. The regional poison control center can assist in deciding if, when, and how Fab digoxin antibody fragments (Digibind) to use.

ETHANOL

Sometimes a negative or very low drug level can also be helpful, as with ethanol. A comatose patient with AOB (alcohol on breath) and a blood ethanol level of less than 100 mg/dL either has ingested one or more other drugs simultaneously or has a medical or surgical reason for this coma, and it should not be attributed to ethanol intoxication. Frequently, trauma and drug abuse occur in the same patient. The expected clinical effects from high levels of ethanol depend on the tolerance of the patient. A chronic alcoholic may be awake and walking with a level of 400 mg/dL, a level potentially fatal in the occasional drinker. Remember, however, that ethanol is metabolized at 15 to 30 mg/dL per hour, and within 4 to 6 hours enough ethanol should be metabolized to improve a mental status that is clouded solely on the basis of ethanol. If this fails to occur, more diagnostic testing should take place.

ETHYLENE GLYCOL AND METHANOL

Ingestion of ethylene glycol can lead to central nervous system (CNS) symptoms, an anion gap metabolic acidosis, and acute renal failure. Methanol ingestion produces a frequently latent anion gap metabolic acidosis and blindness. When levels of either substance exceed 25 mg% (earlier if an acidosis is already present) therapy with hemodialysis (using a two-catheter setup or a single double-lumen catheter, or any setup with minimal recirculation) and concurrent ethanol administration is required. High initial levels usually require a second 4- to 6-hour hemodialysis. In addition, a rebound of about 5 mg% may occur several hours after hemodialysis. Therefore, the hemodialysis catheters should not be removed until a methanol level close to 0 returns. The measurement of ethylene glycol is technically difficult to accomplish; it may not be available in most laboratories and therefore may be unavailable to most physicians. A word of caution: some laboratories have misread *propylene* glycol (found in Dilantin, and phenobarbital, and Valium) for ethylene glycol. Again, knowing ahead of time which facility is capable of performing this assay accurately is advisable. Other ancillary laboratory findings that may help diagnose an ethylene glycol ingestion are urinary calcium oxalate crystals, the presence of an osmolar gap, and hypocalcemia. The presence of an osmolar gap is helpful, but its absence is not confirmatory because a normal osmolar gap may now range from minus 5 to positive 10 with a significant standard deviation (see Additional Tests, p. 2949). Methanol is fairly easy to measure. With methanol poisoning, a thorough visual history and fundoscopic examination looking for hyperemic disks is mandatory.

IRON

Iron intoxication usually occurs when more than 20 mg per kg of elemental iron has been ingested. *Free iron* is the form that is most toxic and potentially fatal. The best way to test for free iron was thought to be simultaneously measuring serum iron and total iron binding capacity (TIBC); if the serum iron was greater than the TIBC, free iron was presumed to be present. We now recognize, however, that in the overdose setting the TIBC is falsely elevated because of the laboratory methodology and is therefore of no value in the overdose setting. Instead, the presence of signs and symptoms consistent with iron poisoning, and/or a serum iron greater than 350 μg/dL should be used to determine whether deferoxamine (Desferal) should be administered. Excretion of the deferoxamine-iron chelate (representing the presence of free iron) makes the urine an orange to reddish color. To properly evaluate the urine color change, however, it is necessary to obtain a baseline urine for comparison purposes before administration of deferoxamine. This also diminishes the possibility of diluting out the orange color in a full bladder before visualization. Because the half-life of deferoxamine is short (about an hour), the effects of deferoxamine by the intramuscular route are gone by 6 hours. Unless this is appreciated, the absence of a color change at 6 hours may be mis-

terpreted as negative. An x-ray film of the abdomen may be helpful in revealing the presence of iron tablets, which are radio-opaque, and again the measure of the effectiveness of gastric evacuation. Chewed iron tablets of the liquid formulation are less likely to be visualized on x ray.

LITHIUM

Intoxication with lithium can be life-threatening. Interpretation of lithium plasma levels depends on when they were drawn relative to the ingestion and whether the patient has taken an acute overdose or is chronically receiving therapeutic doses. In the chronic setting, levels above 2 mEq/L in conjunction with an altered mental status, hyperreflexia, and tremors may require hemodialysis. In the acute setting, it is more difficult to predict the patient's course: if the body can quickly eliminate lithium renally before distribution to the CNS system and other vital tissues can occur, the patient will do well. Levels of 6 to 8 mEq/L in a patient with a clear sensorium, no tremors, hyperreflexia or clonus and whose levels decrease to 1 mEq/L within a day, may do well without hemodialysis. In all other cases, the patient should be hemodialyzed to eliminate the lithium before further distribution to the brain occurs. Because the lithium can be cleared from the plasma more quickly than from the tissues, a significant rebound often occurs. This may necessitate a second hemodialysis if the rebound levels exceed 1 mEq/L and the patient is still symptomatic.

METHEMOGLOBIN

Levels of methemoglobin above 30 mg per dL usually require treatment with methylene blue. The diagnosis of methemoglobinemia should be suspected in a cyanotic patient with chocolate-brown-colored blood who does not respond to oxygen. Arterial blood gas determinations may show a normal pO_2. Levels here can confirm a presumptive diagnosis and guide repeated doses of methylene blue if they are required. Methemoglobin levels may also be helpful to guide therapy in cyanide poisoning.

SALICYLATES AND PHENOBARBITAL

The pKa and renal excretion of these drugs allow ion trapping and excretion by means of an alkaline urine. Knowing the levels can guide the administration of fluids and bicarbonate and can be of value in the decision to begin dialysis.

THEOPHYLLINE

Levels of theophylline above 90 to 100 μg/mL in an acute overdose put the patient at high risk for the development of life-threatening, intractable seizures.

The commonly used theophylline preparations with a substained-release action may not peak for 12 to 24 hours after ingestion. Repeated theophylline assays can assist in predicting the severity of the ingestion, the efficacy of gastric decontamination, and the need for possible charcoal hemoperfusion. Repeated oral doses of activated charcoal have been proven to both reduce measured serum levels of theophylline and decrease morbidity and mortality associated with significant theophylline overdoses. They are a good temporizing measure and should also be continued throughout the extracorporeal removal.

DRUG SCREENS

Many physicians order a "drug screen" on every patient suspected of ingesting drugs, with no consideration to signs, symptoms, or history. Frequently, only blood is sent for screening when the majority of drugs are better detected in the urine. It is impossible for the toxicology laboratory to test for every known drug, and a routine "screen" may fail to identify many toxic substances. Likewise, as the number of drugs assayed are increased, the longer it takes the laboratory to accomplish the task. This often means that the toxicology report comes back after the patient has been admitted to or discharged from the hospital, leading to poor use of the laboratory, not to mention the expense. The best policy, therefore, is to indicate which specific drugs—according to the history and the patient's signs and symptoms—are most likely to be causing the patient's problems. Even severe acetaminophen ingestions, however, may first be asymptomatic. These drugs can then be looked for first, speeding the process. Again, communication with the laboratory is vital. Blood is obviously the correct specimen for quantitative analysis; however, for qualitative identification, urine is usually superior. Sending both specimens (a minimum of 10 mL of blood and 50 mL of urine) is the best procedure. Note, however, that a screen for heavy metals is best accomplished with a *24-hour urine collection* in a special metal-free container obtained from the laboratory.

Toxicology "screens" are usually not necessary because they rarely alter management. Two large studies, one prospective and one retrospective, demonstrated a negligible impact on management. The use of stat quantitative blood tests for specific drugs or toxins (mentioned previously) is preferred. We consider it appropriate to send a drug screen in a sick patient with no history, a patient with a significantly altered mental status, one who has noncontributory physical findings, and one who does not improve in several hours. These screens are also used for medicolegal and psychosocial purposes, before a patient is declared brain dead, nonemergently to rule out drug-induced psychosis for psychiatric purposes, and routinely to rule out a hidden acetaminophen overdose in a suicidal patient.

There are several pitfalls to avoid. A negative drug screen means only that the drugs tested for were absent, and simply sending specimens for analysis does not ensure that a specific toxin or drug will be detected. The drugs specifically screened for should be listed. This allows recognition of the fact that drugs not tested for could nevertheless be present. Likewise, a positive drug screen indicates only the *presence* of a drug. Quantitative analysis in some cases may allow evaluation of that drug's impact. Trauma and other medical problems, however, frequently coexist with drug ingestion, and this must always be taken into consideration in assessing and treating the patient.

DRUG TOLERANCE

One common myth regarding serum levels is that there is always a direct correlation between the drug concentration and that drug's effect. For many drugs this is true, but there are many exceptions. Generally, with drugs that exhibit tolerance, the chronic abuser may have high serum levels and not be incapacitated, in comparison to the novice with an acute ingestion and identical serum levels who may be near death (example: ethanol and phenobarbital). The effects of drugs with a high volume of distribution secondary to extensive tissue binding often do not correlate with their serum levels (usually quite small) and in fact may not be identified because the assay may not be sensitive enough or the drug may be metabolized too quickly for the parent drug to be identified. Quantitative analysis of amphetamines, antihistamines, benzoidizepines, cocaine, opiates, phencyclidine, phenothiazines, and tricyclic antidepressants offers little clinical relevance.

ADDITIONAL TESTS

Although they are not usually considered toxicologic laboratory tests, the serum electrolyte, glucose, blood urea nitrogen (BUN), and arterial blood gas analyses are indispensable aids in diagnosing and treating any overdosed or poisoned patient. A recent change in electrolyte measurement technology has resulted in normal chloride values being higher and therefore altering interpretation of the anion gap. Therefore the technology in your laboratory should be investigated. The urinalysis is also necessary for any complete evaluation.

ISSUES IN DRUG TESTING IN THE WORKPLACE

There are many points to consider if an establishment is going to implement drug testing in the workplace. Key are the objectives of the testing, what drugs will be screened for, when the testing will be done (pre-employment, random, for cause) the implications of a positive test (rehabilitation, penalties, retesting), obvious and hidden costs, as well as moral, ethical, and legal ramifications. From the perspective of the test itself, considerations include the sensitivity and specificity of the test, cut-off values, confirmatory tests for a positive test (using GC-MS), quality control and proficiency, and prevalence of drug abuse in the workplace. Even if an employee tests positive for a drug and it is a true positive, consideration should be given to the following: a positive result may indicate drug exposure (not necessarily abuse); the possibility of passive exposure; timing of the exposure; tolerance; correlation of effect to level; and alternative explanations such as medical use, food (poppy seed cake), etc. Drug testing has become increasingly popular over the past decade without *any* studies that substantiate a favorable effect on drug deterrence. The lack of any demonstrable benefit is even more significant when one takes into account that there are many false positive results, and that many laboratories operate with poor quality control and no independent proficiency testing to ensure results.

People's lives can be significantly affected by drug testing in the workplace, and therefore extreme care should be taken to see that, when it is done, it is carried out with the utmost reliability and precision. For all of these reasons, nonmedical related requests for testing in the ED, whether by police, parents, employers, or even patients themselves, are difficult to justify and almost always inappropriate.

BIBLIOGRAPHY

Bailey, F.L.: Legal factors surrounding drug testing in the workplace. Pharmacotherapy 7:58, 1987.

Bailey, D.N.: The role of the laboratory in treatment of the poisoned patient: Laboratory perspective. J. Anal. Toxicol. 7:136, 1983.

Baselt, R.C.: Analytical Procedures for Therapeutic Drug Monitoring and Emergency Toxicology. California, Biomedical Pub., 1980.

Brett, A.: Implications of discordance between clinical impression and toxicologic analysis in drug overdose. Arch. Intern. Med. 148:437, 1988.

Council on Scientific Affairs: Issues in employee drug testing. JAMA 258:2089, 1987.

Done, A.K.: Solving the poison puzzle. In Back to Basics, Common Emergencies in Daily Practice. Edited by Cohen, J.J. New York, EM Books, 1979, pp. 253–262.

Dougherty, R.: Controversies regarding urine testing. J. Subst. Abuse Treat. 4:115, 1987.

Frings, C.S., Battaglia, D.J., and White, R.M.: Status of Drugs-of-Abuse Testing in Urine under Blind Conditions: An AACC Study. Clin. Chem. 35:891, 1989.

Hoyt, D.W., Finnigan, R.E., Noe, T., et al.: Drug testing in the workplace—Are methods legally defensible? A Survey of experts, arbitrators and testing laboratories. JAMA 258:504, 1987.

Kellerman, A., Fihn, S., LoGerfo, J., et al.: Impact of drug screening in suspected overdose. Ann. Emerg. Med. 16:1206–1216, 1987.

McBay, A., and Hudson, P.: Cost effective drug testing. J. Forensic Sci. p. 575–579.

McCarron, M.M.: The use of toxicology tests in emergency room diagnosis. J. Anal. Toxicol. 7:131, 1983.

Mowry, J.B., and Skoutakis, V.A.: The role of the toxicology laboratory. In Clinical Toxicology of Drugs: Principles and Practice. Edited by Skoutakis, V.A. Philadelphia, Lea & Febiger, 1982, pp. 19–36.

Rumack, B.H., and Matthew, H.: Acetaminophen poisoning and toxicity. Pediatrics 55:871, 1975.

Tilstone, W.U., and Lawson, D.M.: Laboratory diagnosis of the toxicologic patient. In Clinical Management of Poisoning and Drug Overdose. Edited by Haddad, L.M., and Winchester, J.E. Philadelphia, W.B. Saunders Co., 1983, pp. 41–50.

Weisman, R., and Howland, M.A.: The toxicology laboratory. Top Emerg. Med. 5:9, 1983.

Winchester, J.F., Gelfand, M.C., Knepshield, J.H., et al.: Dialysis and hemoperfusion of poisons and drugs-update. Trans. Am. Soc. Artif. Intern. Organs 23:762, 1977.

Winter, S.D., Pearson, R., Gabow, P., et al.: The fall of the serum anion gap. Arch. Intern. Med. 150:311, 1990.

Chapter 82

TOXICOLOGIC EVALUATION AND MANAGEMENT BY CLINICAL PRESENTATION

Neal Flomenbaum, Lewis Goldfrank, and James R. Roberts

CAPSULE

The clinical approach to the poisoned or over-dosed patient begins with the question, Is this patient's life in immediate danger, potential danger, or no danger?[1] The answer accordingly places the patient into one of several clinical management categories. One such clinical algorithm used for the past decade by the New York City Poison Control Center and participating hospitals divides all known or suspected overdosed and poisoned patients into three categories:

1. The unconscious patient.
2. The conscious but uncooperative or agitated patient.
3. The conscious and cooperative patient.[2]

Several key management decisions and procedures will depend on which of these categories is most applicable to the patient. The full algorithm is presented in Figure 82-1. The basic algorithm is supplemented by two questions:

1. Is there concomitant trauma?
2. Is there a treatable toxic syndrome?

Table 82-1 can be helpful in this evaluation. In addition, Table 82-2 is a compilation of syndromes associated with specific toxins. If a specific toxic syndrome can be identified, the treatment can be focused. Unfortunately, many drug ingestions involve several different drugs, and often alcohol as well. For these reasons, treatment must often be of a general type.

THE UNCONSCIOUS PATIENT

All unconscious patients should have a complete evaluation of each vital sign, including a rectal temperature at an appropriate time, early in the assessment. The initial treatment then includes:

1. *Neck stabilization*—if indicated.
2. *Airway stabilization—ventilation, oxygenation:* A bedside assessment is adequate initially, but should be followed by an arterial blood gas determination as soon as possible to accurately assess the patient's respiratory and acid-base status.
3. *Circulatory stabilization*—blood pressure, pulse rate and rhythm, intravenous access and electrocardiographic (ECG) monitoring. For the hypotensive patient, a fluid challenge should be initiated with normal saline or lactated Ringer's solution before the use of vasopressors. For the normotensive or hypertensive patient, an intravenous solution of D5W keeping the vein open (KVO) is adequate. Both a 12-lead ECG (for baseline and PR, QRS, QT interval abnormalities) and continuous cardiac monitoring (for dysrhythmias) are necessary.
4. *Temperature stabilization—life-threatening hyperthermia*—defined here as a rectal temperature of 40.5°C or higher (in the adult) must be treated immediately, regardless of the cause. After treatment, the temperature of the patient's environment must be carefully controlled to prevent further heat loss; many drug overdoses cause thermoregulatory instability, rendering the patient poikilothermic, resulting in the body assuming the temperature of the surroundings. Some drug-related causes for hyperthermia include phenothiazines, cyclic antidepressants, amphetamines, lithium, cocaine, any stimulant that produces severe agitation, ethanol, and sedative-hypnotic withdrawal.

True *hypothermia*, defined as a core temperature of less than 35°C, must also be *recognized.* Hypothermia can cause confusing clinical findings—altered mental status, hypotension, bradycardia—that can simulate or exacerbate the toxicity of an overdose or poison. The administration of many cardiac medications in hypothermia not only may be useless but also may actually result in lethal arrhythmias. Passive rewarming, D50W (50% dextrose in water), thiamine, and naloxone administration may be all that is necessary for mildly hy-

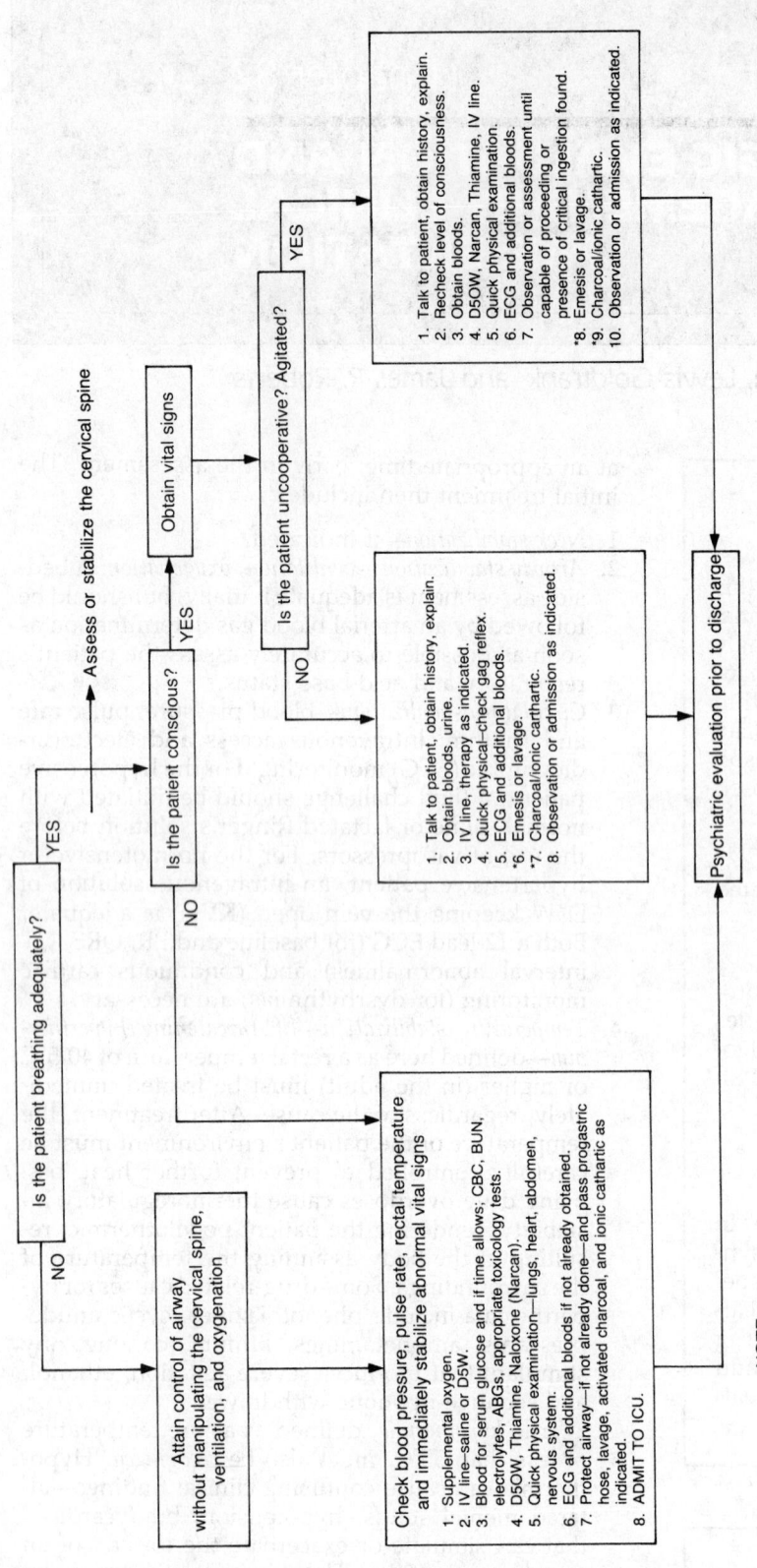

FIG. 82-1. Algorithm for managing the poisoned or overdosed adult without specific toxic syndromes. Whenever a toxic syndrome is identified, additional specific therapy may be added anywhere in the algorithm. With permission from Flomenbaum, N. Goldfrank, L, et al.: General management. *In* Goldfrank's Toxicologic Emergencies. Edited by Goldfrank, L, Flomenbaum, N., et al. 4th ed. Norwalk, Connecticut, Appleton-Lange, 1990, pp. 14–15.

NOTE:
*Unless contraindicated.

pothermic patients who are otherwise stable. One must interpret blood pressure, pulse rate, respiratory rate, and arterial blood gas results in light of the core temperature, because changes in such parameters may be physiologic as opposed to toxin-related.

5. *Diagnostic studies.* With the establishment of intravenous access, blood, urine, and gastric aspirate should be collected for toxicologic analysis; 20 mL of whole blood and 60 mL of urine should be submitted. (Gastric aspirates may be saved or sent with the initial blood and urine sample.) Only a single routine serum specimen need be drawn *before* initiation of basic therapy, and that sample should be sent for glucose, blood urea nitrogen (BUN), and electrolyte determinations. An appropriate drug-coma "screen" may be requested when a second specimen is obtained, but one must be familiar with the specific substances screened for and, more importantly, those drugs that are not assessed by the screen. For example, one cannot rule out methanol toxicity, an anticholinergic ingestion, or lithium toxicity with a standard coma panel. Contact the laboratory personally to ensure that the specific analysis is available, and then specify on the laboratory slip any particular substance that may have been ingested. Supplemental studies that may be useful include blood for osmolality by the freezing point depression method (to help diagnose ethanol, methanol, ethylene glycol poisoning), serum ethanol level, and an arterial blood specimen sent for carboxyhemoglobin and methemoglobulin determinations. A routine urinalysis is also mandatory for the initial evaluation.

6. *Initial routine therapy.* Few substances can or should be administered to an unconscious patient routinely on the basis that such substances may dramatically improve a patient's condition without causing harm. The following four medications are recommended (dosages are for adults): 50% *dextrose* (50 mL IV, 25% in infants at 2 to 4 mL/kg), repeated if indicated; *thiamine* 100 mg IV or IM in adults, to prevent Wernicke's encephalopathy from occurring if the dextrose depletes the patient's remaining thiamine stores;[3] supplemental *oxygen;* and *naloxone.*

NALOXONE INFUSIONS

Published dosage recommendations for naloxone range from 0.8 to 2 mg as the initial adult dose. For a comatose adult, however, particularly one with an abnormal breathing pattern or suspected drug overdose, the starting dose of naloxone should be 2 mg. Using this dose initially saves valuable time and perhaps obviates the necessity of repeating smaller doses several times. One should keep in mind that several synthetic and semisynthetic opioids, such as propoxyphene (Darvon), codeine, and pentazocine (Tal-

TABLE 82-1. DIAGNOSTIC ODORS*	
Odor	**Toxin**
Acetone (sweet, like Russet apples)	Lacquer, alcohol, isopropyl alcohol, chloroform; ketoacidosis
Acrid (pear-like)	Paraldehyde, choral hydrate
Alcohols (fruit-like)	Alcohol, isopropyl alcohol
Ammoniacal	Uremia
Bitter almonds	Cyanide (in choke cherry, apricot pits)
Carrots	Circutoxin
Coal gas (stove gas)	Carbon monoxide (odorless but associated with coal gas)
Disinfectants	Phenol, creosote
Eggs (rotten)	Hydrogen sulfide, mercaptans, disulfuram (Antabuse)
Fish or raw liver (musty)	Hepatic failure, zinc phosphide
Fruit-like	Amyl nitrite, alcohol, isopropyl alcohol
Garlic	Phosphorus, tellurium, arsenic (breath and perspiration), parathion, malathion, selenium, dimethyl sulfoxide (DMSO), thallium
Halitosis	Acute illness, poor oral hygiene
Mothballs	Camphor-containing products
Peanuts	RH-787 (Vacor)
Pungent, aromatic	Ethchlorvynol (Placidyl)
Shoe polish	Nitrobenzene
Tobacco (stale)	Nicotine
Violets	Urinary turpentine
Wintergreen	Methyl salicylate

* With permission from Flomenbaum, N., Goldfrank, L., et al.: *In:* Goldfrank's Toxicologic Emergencies. Edited by Goldfrank, L., Flomenbaum, N., et al. 4th ed. Norwalk, Connecticut, Appleton-Lange, 1990.

win), as well as fentanyl and its illegal "designer" congeners, though specifically antagonized by naloxone, may require much larger doses (10 mg or more of naloxone) than other opioids.

Naloxone is a pure antagonist, with no agonist properties. Administering naloxone will not add to central nervous system (CNS) depression if the patient has ingested a nonopioid CNS depressant, such as phenobarbital. The half-life of naloxone is relatively short—approximately 1 hour—and is almost certainly shorter than whatever opioid the patient may have used. If the initial dose of naloxone causes a severely agitated state, the method of choice to deal with the reaction is to prevent the patient from harming himself or the staff by the appropriate humane, nontraumatic application of light physical restraints. Any attempt to reverse the naloxone pharmacologically may result in greater CNS depression than was present initially. Although almost every part of an acute opioid withdrawal reaction ("cold turkey") can be precipitated by naloxone, seizures, fever, or hallucinations are clearly not part of pure opiate withdrawal; however, they may indicate concomitant sedative-hypnotic or alcohol withdrawal. One should never withhold naloxone because of the fear of producing life-threatening withdrawal. A potential danger of naloxone use is the pre-

TABLE 82-2. TOXICOLOGIC SYNDROMES (TOXIDROMES)

Toxin	Vital Signs	Mental Status	Symptoms	Clinical Findings	Laboratory Findings
Acetaminophen	Normal	Normal	Anorexia, nausea, vomiting	RUQ tenderness Jaundice	Abnormal LFTs
Amphetamines	Hypertension, tachycardia, hyperthermia	Hyperactive, agitated, toxic psychosis	Hyper-alertness	Mydriasis, hyperactive bowel sounds, flush, diaphoresis	—
Anticholinergics	Tachycardia, hypotension, hypertension, hyperthermia	Altered (agitation, lethargy to coma)	Blurred vision, confusion	Dry mucous membranes, mydriasis, diminished bowel sounds, urinary retention	ECG abnormalities, widened QRS complex
Arsenic (acute)	Hypotension, tachycardia, hyperthermia	Alert to comatose	Abdominal pain, vomiting, diarrhea, dysphagia	Dehydration, hair loss	Renal failure, abnormal abdominal x-ray, dysrhythmias
Arsenic (chronic)	Normal	Normal to encephalopathic	Abdominal pain, diarrhea	Melanosis, hyperkeratosis, sensory-motor neuropathy, hair loss, Mee's line, skin cancer	Leukopenia, thrombocytopenia, proteinuria, hematuria, abnormal LFTs
Barbiturates	Hypoventilation, hypotension, hypothermia	Altered (lethargy to coma)	Intoxication	Disconjugate eye movement, hyporeflexia, bullae	Abnormal ABGs
Beta blockers	Hypotension, bradycardia	Altered (lethargy to coma)	Confusion, dizziness	Cyanosis, seizures	Hypoglycemia, ECG
Botulism	Hypoventilation	Normal unless hypoxic	Blurred vision, dysphagia, sore throat, diarrhea	Ophthalmoplegia, mydriasis, ptosis	Normal Multiple patients with common or varied symptoms
Carbon monoxide	Often normal	Altered (lethargy to coma)	Headache, dizziness, confusion, nausea, vomiting	Seizures	Elevated carboxyhemoglobin, ECG abnormalities Multiple patients with common or varied symptoms
Clonidine	Hypotension, hypertension, bradycardia, hypoventilation	Altered (lethargy to coma)	Dizziness, confusion	Miosis	Normal
Cocaine	Hypertension, tachycardia, hyperthermia	Altered (anxiety, agitation, delirium)	Hallucinations	Mydriasis, tremor, perforated nasal septum, diaphoresis, seizures	ECG abnormalities, increased CPK
Cyclic antidepressants	Tachycardia, hypotension, hyperthermia	Altered (lethargy to coma)	Confusion, dizziness	Mydriasis, dry mucous membranes, distended bladder, flush, seizures	Prolonged QRS complex, cardiac dysrhythmias
Digitalis	Hypotension, bradycardia	Normal to altered	Nausea, vomiting, anorexia, visual disturbances, confusion	None	Hyperkalemia, ECG abnormalities, increased digoxin level
Disulfiram/Ethanol	Hypotension, tachycardia	Normal	Nausea, vomiting, headache, vertigo	Flush, diaphoresis, tender abdomen	Abnormal ECG (ventricular arrhythmias)
Ethylene glycol	Tachypnea	Altered (lethargy to coma)	Intoxication	—	Anion gap acidosis, osmolal gap, crystalluria, hypocalcemia, QTc prolongation, renal failure

TABLE 82-2. CONTINUED

Toxin	Vital Signs	Mental Status	Symptoms	Clinical Findings	Laboratory Findings
Iron	Hypotension (late), tachycardia (late)	Normal unless hypotensive, lethargy	Nausea, vomiting, diarrhea, abdominal pain, hematemesis	Tender abdomen	Hyperglycemia (child.), leukocytosis (child.), heme + stool/vomit, metabolic acidosis, ECG and x-ray abnormalities
Isoniazid	Often normal	Normal or altered (lethargy to coma)	Nausea, vomiting	Seizures, peripheral neuropathy ?	Anion gap, metabolic acidosis, abnormal LFTs
Isopropyl alcohol	Hypotension, hypoventilation	Altered (lethargy to coma)	Intoxication	Hyporeflexia, breath odor of acetone	Ketonemia, ketonuria, no glycosuria
Lead	Hypertension, hyperthermia	Altered (lethargy to coma)	Irritability, abdominal pain, nausea, vomiting, constipation	Tender abdomen, peripheral neuropathy, seizures	Anemia, basophilic stippling, radiopaque material on abdominal x ray
Lithium	Hypotension (late)	Altered (lethargy to coma)	Diarrhea, confusion	Weakness, tremor, ataxia, myoclonus, seizures	Leukocytosis (chronic therapy), ECG abnormalities, renal abnormalities
Meperidine	Hypotension, bradycardia, hypoventilation, hypothermia	Altered (lethargy to coma)	Intoxication	Mydriasis, absent bowel sounds, seizures	Abnormal ABGs
Mercury	Hypotension (late)	Altered (psychiatric disturbances)	Salivation, diarrhea, abdominal pain	Stomatitis, ataxia, tremor	Proteinuria, renal failure
Methanol	Hyperventilation, hypotension	Altered (lethargy to coma)	Blurred vision, abdominal pain, intoxication	Hyperemic disks	Anion gap metabolic acidosis, increased osmolal gap
Opioids	Hypotension, bradycardia, hypoventilation, hypothermia	Altered (lethargy to coma)	Intoxication	Miosis, absent bowel sounds	Abnormal ABGs
Organophosphates/carbamates	Bradycardia/tachycardia, hypotension, hyperventilation/hypoventilation	Altered (lethargy to coma)	Diarrhea, abdominal pain, blurred vision, vomiting	Salivation, diaphoresis, lacrimation, urination, defecation, miosis, seizures	Abnormal RBC and plasma cholinesterase activity
Phencyclidine	Hypertension, tachycardia, hyperthermia	Altered (agitation, lethargy to coma)	Hallucinations	Miosis, diaphoresis, myoclonus, blank stare, nystagmus, seizures	Myoglobinuria, leukocytosis, increased CPK
Phenothiazines	Hypotension, tachycardia, hypothermia/hyperthermia	Altered (lethargy to coma)	Dizziness	Miosis/mydriasis, decreased bowel sounds, tremor	Abnormal ECG, abnormal KUB
Salicylates	Hyperventilation, hyperthermia	Altered (agitation, lethargy to coma)	Tinnitus, nausea, vomiting, confusion	Diaphoresis, tender abdomen	Anion gap metabolic acidosis, respiratory alkalosis, abnormal LFTs & coagulation studies
Sedative-hypnotics	Hypotension, hypoventilation, hypothermia	Altered (lethargy to coma)	Intoxication	Hyporeflexia, bullae	Abnormal ABGs
Theophylline	Tachycardia, hypotension, hyperventilation, hyperthermia	Altered (agitation, lethargy to coma)	Nausea, vomiting, diaphoresis, confusion	Diaphoresis, tremor, seizures	Hypokalemia, hyperglycemia, metabolic acidosis, abnormal ECG

* With permission from Goldfrank, L., et al.: Vital signs and toxicologic syndromes. *In* Goldfrank's Toxicologic Emergencies. Edited by Goldfrank, L., Flomenbaum, N., et al., 4th ed. Norwalk, Connecticut, Appleton-Lange, 1990, pp. 66–7.

cipitation of withdrawal vomiting in a patient who is opioid-dependent, yet is in coma from a nonopioid overdose. The result is vomiting in an unconscious patient, and aspiration must be prevented.

Multiple boluses of naloxone may be indicated to achieve reversal of opioid-induced CNS depression. If the patient does respond initially to naloxone, an IV naloxone drip may be used to maintain the patient in an aroused but nonagitated state and to avoid the "peak and trough" response to boluses. In naloxone IV infusion, two thirds of the initial bolus dose that reversed respiratory depression is administered hourly by continuous infusion. It may be necessary to administer half of the initial loading dose at 30 minutes to prevent the decline of the initial naloxone plasma level. *Caution:* Assess the patient's state of consciousness no less than 1 hour after the drip is turned off to avoid discharging a patient who only *appears* alert and oriented because of the naloxone infusion.

MEDICATIONS NOT TO BE USED ROUTINELY IN COMATOSE PATIENTS

PHYSOSTIGMINE

Do not give physostigmine routinely to the comatose patient. The indications for its use are relatively few and specific. In a known anticholinergic overdose characterized by pupillary dilation, dry mucosa, absent bowel sounds, and *severe problematic agitation,* symptomatic supraventricular tachycardia, or a seizure that is unresponsive to diazepam or phenytoin, or both, the cautious, slow IV administration of 2 mg of physostigmine salicylate (in the adult) may be indicated. The reason for not administering physostigmine routinely to a comatose patient is that, in the absence of an anticholinergic poisoning, a *cholinergic* reaction will result from the physostigmine that is characterized by salivation, urination, and defecation, and possibly severe bradycardia or asystole. The sudden flooding of the airway with secretions may result in aspiration or "drowning" unless the patient is aggressively suctioned. Physostigmine is a general CNS stimulant, and although it may transiently arouse patients with benzodiazepine, or barbiturate, and alcohol induced coma, the indiscriminate use of this "antidote" is discouraged.

ANALEPTICS

Analeptics, such as amphetamines, doxapram, nikethimide, or picrotoxin, do not arouse a comatose patient reliably or predictably and may increase the risk of agitation.

PHYSICAL EXAMINATION

After the initial evaluation and therapy, the next step in management is to complete the initial physical ex-

amination, concentrating on breath sounds and heart sounds, and abdominal and neurologic examinations. One should approach even the most "obvious" overdose with the aim of ruling out other possible causes of altered mental status (see Table 82-2). Protean clinical manifestations of hypoglycemia and even focal neurologic findings may clear after the administration of dextrose.[4] Although focal findings and partial seizures may be manifestations of toxic-metabolic problems (e.g., lithium overdose), they obviously suggest the possibility of structural damage, which may need to be evaluated by a CT or MRI scan. CNS infections (meningitis, encephalitis) may also mimic a drug overdose, and if they cannot be ruled out by other means, lumbar puncture may be essential. The physical examination should also include frequent repeating of vital signs to assess the overall stability of the patient's physical condition.

THE PATIENT WHO REMAINS HYPOTENSIVE

If the patient remains hypotensive despite an adequate fluid challenge, several important, serious possibilities must be considered:

1. The patient may have ingested a potent vasodilator (e.g., phenothiazines or antihypertensive medication) and requires more fluid.
2. The patient may have ingested a myocardial depressant (e.g., antihistamines, phenothiazines, calcium channel blockers, or beta-blockers in massive quantities) and requires an inotropic medication, vasopressor, calcium, or glucagon.
3. There is concomitant trauma (e.g., ruptured spleen or liver from occult blunt abdominal trauma, neurogenic shock from head or spinal trauma, etc.)
4. The patient is suffering from septic shock.

It should be emphasized that few patients who abuse opioids present to the Emergency Department (ED) with hypotension from the opioid itself. Those who do almost never remain hypotensive after initial treatment with naloxone and IV fluid. If an opioid abuser remains hypotensive after initial treatment, trauma must be assumed to be the cause until proved otherwise. Neurogenic or septic shock may also occasionally be present with a drug overdose.

THE PATIENT IN HYPERTENSIVE CRISIS

A true hypertensive crisis secondary to drug ingestion is rare, but it may be seen with sympathomimetics such as amphetamines or cocaine. Hypertension may also occur secondary to phencyclidine (reportedly), massive anticholinergic overdoses, or as a result of a disulfiram (Antabuse) and alcohol reaction or as the initial manifestation of the interaction between an MAO inhibitor and a contraindicated food or medication. Phentolamine, given as a 5 mg IV bolus, has been recommended as a general therapeutic measure for drug-induced hypertension because of its short-acting alpha-blocking action, but it is not always effective. Sodium nitroprusside may be required in severe hypertension. For a patient with an unknown ingestion and severe hypertension, sodium nitroprusside is the drug of choice because of its potency and rapid onset of action, and the ability to titrate the infusion and to rapidly terminate its effect if necessary because of sudden hypotension or adverse reaction.

THE PATIENT WHO PRESENTS WITH SEIZURES

Seizures may occur secondary to almost any drug overdose. Other non–drug-related causes of seizure, such as hypertensive crisis, head trauma, hypoglycemia, or CNS infection, should always be considered. Seizures may be a direct toxic effect of the ingested drug, or secondary to hypoxia, hypotension, or hypertension. Seizures may also occur as a result of drug withdrawal (ethanol, sedative hypnotics). Drugs that frequently cause seizures in overdose include isoniazid, cocaine, carbon monoxide, camphor, caffeine, lithium, lead, theophylline, propranolol, cyclic antidepressants, phenothiazines, propoxyphene, and phencyclidine. Subarachnoid hemorrhage or meningitis may mimic a drug overdose; these may also present with an altered mental status and seizures.

Isolated seizures resulting from drug overdose may progress to life-threatening status epilepticus, hyperthermia, or metabolic acidosis, and must be treated aggressively. The initial treatment includes supplemental oxygen and the use of anticonvulsant medication. Diazepam or lorazepam is the initial drug of choice, but occasionally phenytoin, barbiturates, or even general anesthesia may be required. In selected cases, specific antidotes may be required to terminate seizures, such as pyridoxine for isoniazid-related seizures.

THE PATIENT WHO PRESENTS WITH CARDIAC ARRHYTHMIAS

DYSRHYTHMIAS

When a possible drug-overdose patient presents with a life-threatening dysrhythmia, the physician may be forced to manage the problem long before the responsible drug or toxin is identified. In this instance, the objective should be to manage the dysrhythmia without inadvertently administering a medication that will exacerbate the condition. For example, although Class I antiarrhythmics, such as procainamide, quinidine, and disopyramide, may be effective in managing ventricular tachycardia in certain situations, administering them to a patient who overdoses on a cyclic antidepressant may exacerbate the condition. For this reason, unless anticholinergic agents can be ruled out before the patient is treated, this class of antidysrhythmics should be avoided in favor of "safer" medications. (The use of phenytoin in the presence of a cyclic antidepressant overdose has become controversial.)

TACHYCARDIA

Sinus tachycardia is frequently encountered in drug overdose as a result of anxiety, hypotension, hyperthermia, direct myocardial stimulation, or as an anticholinergic effect.

"Fast" ventricular dysrhythmias, including (1) ventricular premature contractions, (2) ventricular tachycardia, and (3) ventricular fibrillation, may result from the following drugs:

1. Anticholinergics (antihistamines, antiparkinsonian drugs, antipsychotics, belladonna alkaloids).
2. Digitalis preparations.
3. Stimulants such as cocaine, amphetamines, or theophylline.

The differential diagnosis includes:

1. Myocardial ischemia, injury, infarction (possibly secondary to a drug overdose).
2. Hypoxemia of any cause (especially carbon monoxide, cyanide, CNS depressants).
3. Electrolyte abnormalities such as hypokalemia and hypercalcemia.
4. A mechanical irritant such as a central venous pressure (CVP) catheter irritating the endocardium.

To determine the cause, blood for BUN, glucose, electrolyte, and arterial blood gas determinations, a toxicology screen—as well as a specific request for anticholinergics, stimulants, and digitalis levels—are indicated. When a digitalis level is requested, one will probably get back a digoxin level (by radioimmunoassay) because most laboratories are able to routinely determine other digitalis preparations. In a patient who is *not* supposed to be on any form of digitalis, however, even a minute (cross-reacting) amount of "digoxin" detected in the presence of a typical digitalis–toxic dysrhythmia suggests the possibility of a massive ingestion of digitoxin, digitalis leaf, foxglove, or another cardiac glycoside.

The pharmacologic treatment of the "fast" ventricular dysrhythmia includes:

1. 100% oxygen and the normalization of blood pressure and electrolytes.
2. Lidocaine, 1 mg/kg IV bolus, followed by 1 to 4 mg kg/min IV drip (may repeat bolus to maximum of 225 mg total in an adult; lidocaine is relatively safe and often effective no matter what toxin one is dealing with).
3. Propranolol 1 mg over 5 minutes IV to total of 5 to 7 mg.
4. Phenytoin (Dilantin) IV at no more than 50 mg/min to 500 to 1000 mg total.

Bretylium is relatively *contraindicated* for digoxin overdoses and has not proved to be efficacious in other overdose situations. Specific antibodies (Fab-fragment) are now available for the treatment of life-threatening digitalis intoxication. The treatment of fast ventricular dysrhythmias secondary to an unknown overdose is often relegated to a trial and error method, because the response to specific antiarrhythmic medications may be unpredictable.

BRADYCARDIA

Sinus bradycardia is uncommon in drug overdose, but may be seen in patients with concomitant hypothermia, after an opioid overdose, organophosphate (or carbamate) poisoning, digitalis overdose, beta receptor blockade, calcium channel blockade, quinidine overdose, or in clonidine ingestion. "Slow" dysrhythmias include second-degree or third-degree heart block with (1) very slow ventricular rate, (2) "escape" ventricular contractions, (3) altered mental state, or (4) hypotension (absolute or relative). The differential diagnosis includes (1) myocardial ischemia, injury, or infarction, (2) increased intracranial pressure, and (3) electrolyte abnormalities. Treatment includes atropine, 0.5 mg IV repeated every 5 minutes as necessary to a total dose of 2 mg.

Although an isoproterenol (Isuprel) infusion is usually listed as the next step in the treatment of bradycardias, isoproterenol is extremely difficult to control and often results in a supraventricular or ventricular tachycardia. A pacemaker may be required in selected cases. Calcium chloride (5 to 10 mL of a 10% solution) has been advocated for the treatment of cardiovascular collapse secondary to calcium channel blocking medications, and glucagon (5 to 10 mg bolus) may be of value in reversing the myocardial depression secondary to beta-blocking and calcium channel-blocking medication.

THE PATIENT WHO PRESENTS WITH AN ACID-BASE DISORDER

The differential diagnosis of a metabolic acidosis with a widened anion gap contains several of the common severe drug overdoses requiring treatment in the intensive care unit. An algorithmic approach to diagnosis can be found in Figure 82-2. A discussion of possible *drug* causes of metabolic acidosis and other acid-base disturbances follows.

RESPIRATORY ALKALOSIS

Salicylate poisoning in adults causes a mixed disturbance—respiratory alkalosis and metabolic acidosis, with the respiratory alkalosis predominating in the early phase. Preterminally, or in association with a sedative hypnotic overdose, the respiratory alkalosis is replaced by a respiratory acidosis in addition to a severe *metabolic* acidosis. Patients with severe agitation from any stimulant may have a respiratory alkalosis, but continued hyperactivity may lead to a lactic (metabolic) acidosis.

RESPIRATORY ACIDOSIS

This may result from drugs and usually involves CNS depressants (sedative-hypnotics, especially barbiturates or opioids).

METABOLIC ACIDOSIS

An acidosis with widened anion-gap (lactic acidosis) commonly occurs after a seizure, but should clear within an hour after the seizures are controlled. Causative drugs and differential diagnosis of metabolic acidosis are both incorporated into the mnemonic "A MUD PILE."

> *A*—alcoholic ketoacidosis, aspirin
> *M*—methanol
> *U*—uremia
> *D*—diabetic ketoacidosis
> *P*—paraldehyde (and phenformin)
> *I*—isoniazid and iron
> *L*—lactic acidosis
> *E*—ethylene glycol and ethanol (as in alcoholic ketoacidosis)

Salicylates can also be a cause.

The treatment for metabolic acidosis is to treat the underlying cause. Sodium bicarbonate ($NaHCO_3$) is given only when necessary and should not be used routinely merely to obtain a normal pH. Bicarbonate is generally not required to treat the metabolic acidosis secondary to a seizure, but it is frequently required in the management of the severe acidosis that occurs with methanol or ethylene glycol poisoning. Alkalinization of the serum has been advocated for the treatment of the hypotension and cardiac dysrhythmias and conductance abnormalities that are seen with severe tricyclic antidepressant overdose. Alkalinization of the urine is useful to trap the ionized form of salicylates and phenobarbital in the renal tubule to prevent reabsorption, thereby enhancing excretion.

PERSISTENT UNCONSCIOUSNESS OR DETERIORATION IN MENTAL STATE

If a patient's state of unconsciousness does not resolve as expected, or if it initially resolves only to deteriorate again, the possibility of the existence of large concretions of medications that are inaccessible to lavage or emesis must be considered. This is particularly true of CNS depressants such as barbiturates and meprobamate. Flexible endoscopy, whole bowel irrigation, or gastrotonomy may be indicated in such situations. Other causes of unconsciousness should also be reconsidered, along with the possibility of obtaining a CT scan and/or neurologic consultation.

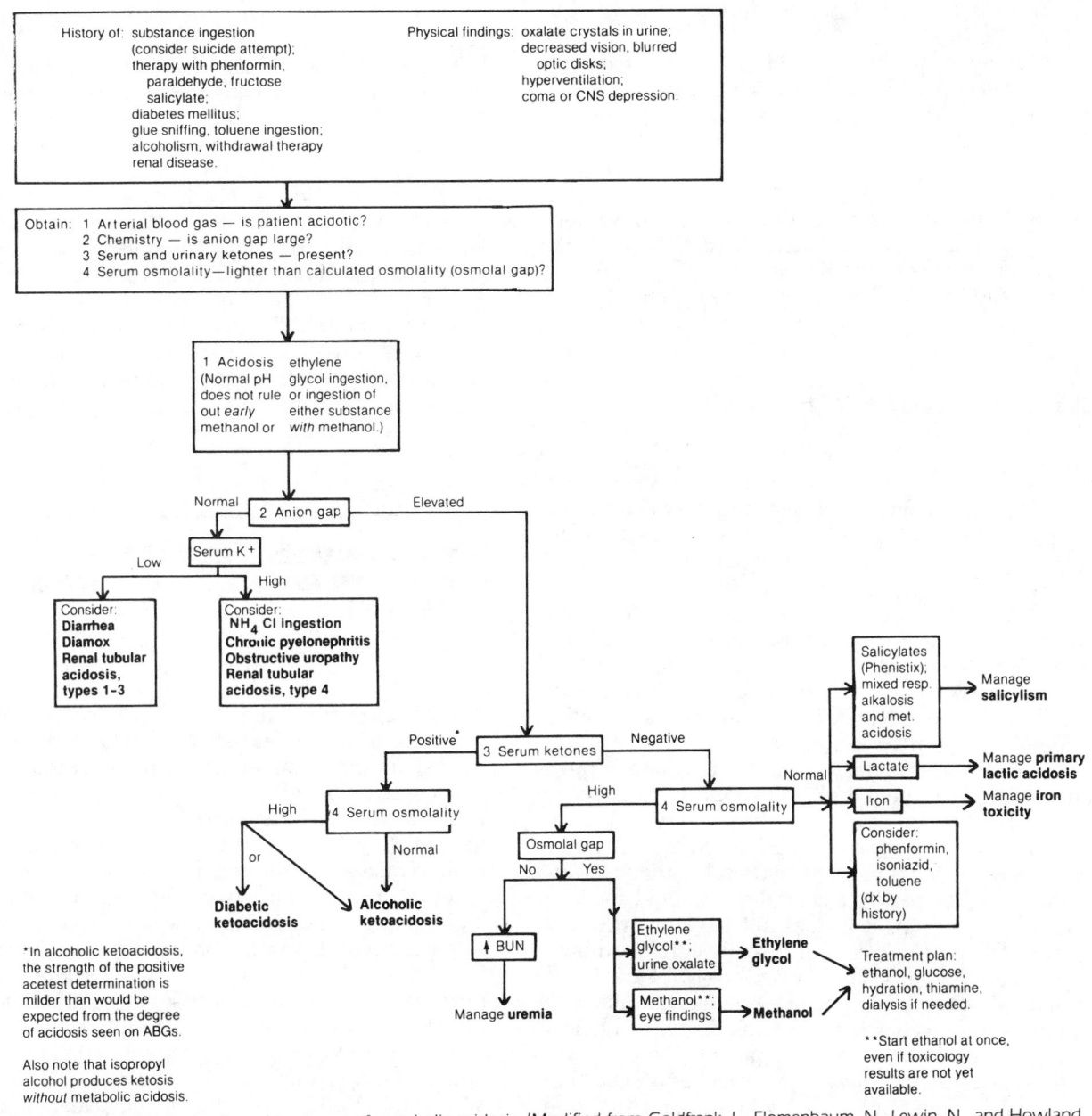

FIG. 82-2.   *Algorithm for diagnosis and treatment of metabolic acidosis. (Modified from Goldfrank, L., Flomenbaum, N., Lewin, N., and Howland, M. A. Methanol, ethylene glycol, and isopropanol. In Goldfrank's Toxicologic Emergencies. Edited by Goldfrank, L., Flomenbaum, N., et al., 4th ed. Norwalk, Connecticut, Appleton-Lange, 1990, p. 486.*

OVERDOSES

Pitfalls to avoid in managing the unconscious overdose patient include the following:

1. Not believing the history of a significant ingestion in the light of a relatively stable patient. Alternatively, allowing the history to guide treatment despite clinical findings to suggest an alternative poisoning.
2. Relying on history or physical findings to decide on the routine use of naloxone, D50W, and thiamine, rather than giving them to all unconscious patients.
3. Choosing vasopressors as the initial management of hypotension, rather than using adequate IV fluids and inserting a CVP or Swan-Ganz (to measure pulmonary wedge pressure) catheter first.
4. Not thinking about the possibility of concomitant trauma or infection, or, conversely, attempting to use the Glasgow coma scale inappropriately as a determinant for "aggressive" or "nonaggressive" therapy. Presumed CNS trauma cases may turn out to have non-existent or trivial head injury, in which

case the Glasgow Coma Scale has no prognostic significance.

5. Keeping the patient in the ED once the initial treatment has been completed, rather than admitting to ICU or failing to observe a seemingly minor ingestion for an adequate amount of time (for the toxic effect of an ingestion to become clinically evident).
6. Neglecting to perform gastric emptying or neglecting to administer activated charcoal because the patient comes to the hospital "too long" after the ingestion for the procedure to be beneficial.

COMA VERSUS "PSYCHOGENIC UNRESPONSIVENESS"

As a way of bridging two paths of the management algorithm—the comatose patient and the alert but uncooperative patient—it is worth considering a problem that frequently arises in the ED when the staff begins to suspect that a "comatose" patient is actually more awake and alert than he or she appears. When an overdose patient arrives "unconscious," but breathing and with stable vital signs, all of the initial procedures—D50W, thiamine, naloxone, and oxygen—can be administered safely if there is any doubt as to the patient's true level of consciousness.

As part of the physical examination, one should attempt to open the mouth and check the gag reflex. When the patient's jaw is clenched tightly and there is no other evidence of a seizure disorder, a psychogenic cause is possible. Other useful maneuvers include lifting the patient's hand directly above the face and letting it drop. If it does not fall straight down gently striking the face, but instead shifts gradually to the side as it falls, disobeying the law of gravity, a psychogenic cause is *suggested*. A somewhat noxious stimulus, such as pinching the shoulder once or twice, may also be useful to arouse a patient. *Noxious inhalants, such as spirits of ammonia, should be avoided*, because severe injury may result when an unresponsive patient is thought to be resisting the "correct" response to ammonia. Inserting pledgets in a patient's nostrils has caused alkali injury. Similarly, severe injury and death have resulted from accidentally pouring the solution down the patient's mouth or endotracheal tube. Standard neurologic maneuvers for assessing the level of CNS function, such as testing for a cold water caloric response, may be misleading or confusing in a drug overdose. Deviation from a strict rostral/caudal pattern of deterioration of neurologic function characterizes certain drug overdoses. Ultimately, no one neurologic test will decidedly resolve the issue of true versus feigned coma, and a combination of tests and tact is necessary. One should consider a computed tomographic (CT) scan of the head or lumbar puncture in any patient with an altered mental status when the diagnosis of drug ingestion is in question or the physical examination leads to doubt about cause.

One key to successfully managing the patient with psychogenic loss of consciousness is to avoid confronting the patient in full view of relatives, friends, or staff. Making it known to the patient that friends and relatives are waiting outside, that the (alleged) ingestion "should be wearing off about now," explaining what has to be done and why in a firm and nonemotional tone, and avoiding physical abuse or humiliation will often enable a "comatose" patient to regain consciousness over a period of a few minutes.

If the patient still resists further treatment and if one is dealing with a known ingestion that is harmless, it is probably better to leave the patient alone. If the ingestion is known, and is potentially dangerous, it must be removed.

THE CONSCIOUS BUT UNCOOPERATIVE OR AGITATED PATIENT

The patient who is conscious but uncooperative appears to be somewhat better off initially than the comatose or apneic patient, but one must immediately address the issue of why the patient is uncooperative or agitated. The possibilities that must be ruled out immediately include hypoxemia, hypotension, hypoglycemia—or other metabolic or electrolyte abnormalities, hypothermia, hyperthermia, or exposure to a CNS stimulant such as cocaine, amphetamines, LSD, or phencyclidine. Central nervous system infection or bleeding, sedative-hypnotic drug withdrawal, and head trauma are common causes of agitation that may mimic drug overdose. One should try to enlist the cooperation of the agitated patient by talking to him and reassuring him, but in many cases this is not successful. Within minutes of the patient's arrival, complete vital signs, including a rectal temperature (followed by arterial blood gas determination) should be obtained, and thiamine, D50W, oxygen, and naloxone routinely given.

The remainder of the assessment and interventions in the agitated patient are similar to those recommended for the unconscious patient with the following exceptions:

1. The patient's behavior must be dealt with in a humane, medically safe, and expeditious manner.
2. Emesis (Table 82-3) instead of lavage may be an option for removing unabsorbed toxin, although activated charcoal alone is adequate in many instances.

Because it is difficult to empty the stomach, maintain an endotracheal tube, or secure an intravenous line in a wildly agitated patient, uncooperative patients with unknown or life-threatening ingestions may require physical and chemical restraints. The agitated state can quickly result in hyperthermia, metabolic acidosis (see Fig. 82-2), rhabdomyolysis, and even skeletal or CNS trauma if the patient should fall off the stretcher.

Physical restraints, however, must be light enough that the patient does not inadvertently become hyperthermic because of the inability to dissipate the heat generated by his or her agitated state. For this same reason, in cases of large or life-threatening drug overdose, we would not recommend the use of any major tranquilizers (such as phenothiazines or haloperidol) that may produce anticholinergic effects or interrupt thermoregulatory control. If a pharmacologic agent is deemed necessary for sedation, we favor a benzodiazepine, regardless of the presence of any underlying psychiatric disorders. Intravenous diazepam and lorazepam, titrated in small doses, are acceptable chemical restraints. They act rapidly and are quite effective and free of many of the side effects of the phenothiazines (hypotension, lowering of the seizure threshold, extrapyramidal reactions). One must exercise extreme caution in using these agents, however, because one runs the risk of masking a sign (abnormal behavior) of a structural or metabolic problem that must be treated immediately (e.g., hypoglycemia, hypoxemia).

TABLE 82-3. EMESIS WITH SYRUP OF IPECAC*

Dose
  Adult
    30 mL (2 tbsp)
  Children
    6–12 months, 10 mL (2 tsp)
    1–5 years, 15 mL (1 tbsp)
    Over 5 years, 30 mL (2 tbsp)
    One additional dose (a second dose) may be given if the patient has not vomited within 30 min
Contraindications
  Child less than 6 months of age
  Nontoxic ingestion
  Comatose patient
  Patient experiencing seizures
  Any patient expected to rapidly deteriorate
  Ingestion of a strong acid or alkali
  When vomiting will delay administration of an oral antidote
  Compromised gag reflex
  Patient with a hemorrhagic diathesis (cirrhosis, varices, thrombocytopenia)
  Concomitant ingestion of sharp, solid materials (thermometer, glass, nails, razor blades)
  Evidence of significant vomiting prior to ipecac utilization
  Any patient with an accidental "pure" petroleum distillate or turpentine ingestion, or any patient who is symptomatic (pulmonary, neurologic, cardiac) following a hydrocarbon ingestion.

* With permission from Flomenbaum, N., Goldfrank, L., et al.: General management. *In* Goldfrank's Toxicologic Emergencies. Edited by Goldfrank, L., Flomenbaum, N., et al., 4th ed. Norwalk, Connecticut, Appleton-Lange, 1990, p. 16.

THE PATIENT WHO IS ALERT AND COOPERATIVE

As in the case of the alert but uncooperative or agitated patient, reassurance and establishing rapport are indicated in the alert and cooperative patient. In addition, a history should be obtained, a rapid physical examination should be performed, and blood and urine specimens should be obtained for laboratory analysis. Whether or not establishing an IV or obtaining an ECG is indicated in this subset depends on the ingestion, the reliability of the information or informant, or both, and the age and general health of the patient.

Here, too, emesis or lavage may be possible, and if indicated (as opposed to activated charcoal alone), perhaps patient preference should be allowed. The choice is presented in a firm, nonjudgmental manner, making it clear to the patient that further help and/or support (e.g., psychiatric) is available after care for the ingestion itself is rendered. The patient should be told to make up his mind quickly. Emesis or lavage, followed in either case by activated charcoal and cathartic (Tables 82-3 through 82-6), should then be instituted.

PSYCHIATRIC CONSULTATION

If at all possible, every person with an intended drug ingestion should be required to see a psychiatrist before being discharged. Even though the suicide risk may not appear to be as much of a concern in the case of a drug abuser who is seen repeatedly or frequently in the same ED, a "crescendo" pattern may escape notice by the staff. Similar to "crescendo angina," an established pattern of drug ingestion (such as one episode per week) suddenly changes, and within a week or two the patient is seen much more frequently than previously. Each time such a patient is discharged home after acute management in the emergency department, he or she is at an increased risk of a fatal overdose unless some of the underlying factors can be addressed and the cycle broken.

Miscalculated "suicide gestures" (particularly with salicylates, acetaminophen, digitalis, methanol, ethylene glycol) also sometimes result in death. It is impossible to differentiate gestures from true attempts with any certainty in a medical emergency service, and certainly in both cases psychiatric consultation is urgently needed.

TABLE 82-4. LAVAGE*

Tube
  Adult/Adolescent
    Large-bore orogastric Lavacuator hose, 36- to 40-French
  Children
    16- to 28-French orogastric-type tube
Procedure
  1. Endotracheal or nasotracheal intubation should precede gastric lavage in the unconscious or seizing patient, with or without an absent gag reflex.
  2. If the patient can tolerate intubation without trauma, the patient merits intubation. In any case, the airway must be meticulously protected. (Vomiting commonly follows lavage.)
  3. The proper length of the tube that will be passed is measured and marked before insertion. Once the tube is introduced, confirmation of position of the tube in the stomach is essential.
  4. The patient should be kept in the left lateral decubitus position.
  5. A saline lavage solution initiated with 200 mL aliquots should be instilled in an adult (or 50–100 mL aliquots in a child).
  6. This should be continued for at least several liters of lavage in an adult or until no particulate matter is seen and the lavage is clear.
  7. The tube should be used for instillation of activated charcoal and a cathartic.
Contraindications
  Strong acid or alkali ingestion
    Significant hemorrhagic diathesis (relative contraindication)
    Nontoxic ingestion

* With permission from Flomenbaum, N., Goldfrank, L., et al.: General management. In Goldfrank's Toxicologic Emergencies. Edited by Goldfrank, L., Flomenbaum, N., et al., 4th ed. Norwalk, Connecticut, Appleton-Lange, 1990, p. 9.

TABLE 82-5. ACTIVATED CHARCOAL*

Dose
  Adult and child
    Initial dose: 1 g/kg body weight or 10:1 ratio of activated charcoal:drug, whichever is greater. Following massive ingestions, 2 g/kg may be indicated; however, it may be difficult to administer doses in excess of 100 g.
Repetitive doses
  0.5 to 1 g/kg body weight every 2 to 6 h tailored to the dose and dosage form of drug ingested (larger doses and shorter dosing intervals may occasionally be indicated). Note: Do not use repetitive doses of cathartics or premixed charcoal-cathartic combinations.
Procedure
  1. Add 4–8 parts of water to chosen quantity of activated charcoal, if in powdered form. This will form a transiently stable slurry that the patient can drink or have placed down an orogastric hose.
  2. The activated charcoal can be given in a mixture with the chosen cathartic (if the cathartic is an appropriate one).
  3. If the patient vomits the dose, it should be repeated. Smaller, more frequent, or continuous nasogastric administration may be better tolerated. An antiemetic is sometimes needed.
  4. Repetitive doses are probably useful for drugs with a small volume of distribution, low plasma protein binding, biliary or gastric secretion, or active metabolites that recirculate.
Contraindications
  Caustic acids or alkalis (ineffective, and will accumulate in burned areas, making endoscopy difficult).
  Ileus (for repetitive dosing).
  Patients with a risk of aspiration and an unprotected airway.

* With permission from Flomenbaum, N., Goldfrank, L., et al.: General management. In Goldfrank's Toxicologic Emergencies. Edited by Goldfrank, L., Flomenbaum, N., et al., 4th ed. Norwalk, Connecticut, Appleton-Lange, 1990, p. 10.

REMOVAL OF AN EXTERNAL TOXIN

The chemicals that individuals are commonly exposed to externally include organophosphate or carbamate insecticides from crop dusting, gardening, or roach extermination accidents; caustic acids from exploding batteries; caustic alkalies such as lye (a common form of retribution in some inner city areas); and mace, which is again being used frequently in crowd control. In all cases, the principles of management are as follows:

1. Protect the staff by wearing gowns, gloves, shoe covers, and so on. Some cases of secondary poisoning have occurred because emergency personnel were exposed to toxins such as organophosphates merely by touching the victim or his clothing.
2. Remove all the patient's clothing and place it in a plastic bag.
3. Wash the patient with soap and copious amounts of water, *twice*, no matter how much time has elapsed since the exposure. Never attempt to neutralize an acid with a base or vice versa. The heat of neutralization (added to the heat of hydration) will only increase the thermal damage.

If the eye is involved, it must be irrigated with the lids fully retracted for no less than 20 minutes. A drop of proparacaine hydrochloride solution or other ophthalmic local anesthetic in the involved eye will facilitate irrigation. Lids may be held open with a special retractor or one fashioned from a paper clip. An adequate irrigation stream may be obtained by running a liter of normal saline through regular IV tubing held a few inches from the eye. Particulate matter is removed with a cotton-tipped applicator. Finally, checking the lid fornices with pH paper strips is important to ensure adequate irrigation. The eye is generally slightly acidic, and a strongly basic reaction after lye exposure means inadequate irrigation. Whenever pos-

TABLE 82-6. CATHARTICS*

Dose

Adults and children

Magnesium citrate	4 mL/kg to 30 mL per dose
Magnesium sulfate	250 mg/kg up to 30 g
Sorbitol	1 g/kg (0.5 g/kg in children, with a maximum 50 g of 35% concentrate in children over 1 year; maximum 150 g in adults)

Precautions

Not warranted in routine management of trivial ingestions in children.

Do not use Fleet's phospho-soda in children

Do not use repetitive doses of cathartics, especially in children; *never* repeat Mg^{++} containing cathartics.

Sorbitol administration in children should be used cautiously, with attention paid to fluid and electrolyte status.

Oil-based cathartics should not be used because of the risks of aspiration and enhanced toxin absorption.

Contraindications

Adynamic ileus

Diarrhea

Abdominal trauma

Intestinal obstruction

Renal failure (magnesium sulfate)

---

* With permission from Flomenbaum, N., Goldfrank, L., et al.: General management. *In* Goldfrank's Toxicologic Emergencies. Edited by Goldfrank, L., Flomenbaum, N., et al., 4th ed. Norwalk, Connecticut, Appleton-Lange, 1990, p. 10.

sible, eye irrigation must first be performed at the scene, *before transport.* By the time the patient arrives at the hospital irreversible caustic damage may have occurred. Serious alkali burns may occur within 15 to 20 seconds of initial exposure.

Avoid using any greases or creams; they will only keep the poison in close contact with the skin and make ultimate removal more difficult.

REFERENCES

1. Rumack, B., and Sullivan, J.: The treatment of poisoning: A systemic approach. *In* Rumack, B. (ed.): Poisindex. Denver, Micromedex, 1985.
2. Flomenbaum, N., Goldfrank, L., et al.: General management of the poisoned and overdosed patient. *In* Goldfrank's Toxicologic Emergencies, 4th ed. Norwalk, Ct., Appleton-Lange, 1990, pp. 5–20.
3. Reuler, J.B., Girard, D.E., and Cooney, T.G.: Wernicke's encephalopathy. N. Engl. J. Med. *312*:1035, 1985.
4. Andrade, R., Matthew, V., Gernsheimer, J., et al.: Hypoglycemic hemiplegic syndrome. Ann. Emerg. Med. *13*:529, 1984.

Chapter 83

TOXICOLOGIC EVALUATION AND MANAGEMENT BY SPECIFIC POISONINGS

QUICK REFERENCE GUIDE TO INITIAL TREATMENT OF COMMON POISONINGS

Howard C. Mofenson and Thomas R. Caraccio

CAPSULE

This chapter provides a guide to initial treatment of specific common poisonings. Antidotes, enhancement of elimination, and toxicokinetics are discussed, and common poisons and their respective treatments are enumerated.

THE USE OF ANTIDOTES

Antidotes are available for only a relatively small number of poisons. An available antidote should be administered only after the vital functions are established. Table 83-1 summarizes the commonly used antidotes and their indications and methods of administration. Most informational, so-called first aid measures and antidotes on commercial product labels are notorious for their inaccuracy; it is preferable to contact the regional poison control center rather than follow recommendations on these labels.

ENHANCEMENT OF ELIMINATION

The medical methods for elimination of the absorbed toxic substances are diuresis, dialysis, hemoperfusion, exchange transfusion, plasmapheresis, enzyme induction, and inhibition. The methods to increase urinary excretion of toxic chemicals and drugs are being studied extensively, but the other modalities have not been well evaluated.

Generally, these methods are needed in only a few instances and should be reserved for life-threatening circumstances or when a definite benefit is anticipated.

DIURESIS

Diuresis increases the renal clearance of compounds that are partially reabsorbed in the renal tubules. *Forced-fluid diuresis* is based on the principle that it will shorten exposure for reabsorption at the *distal* renal tubules. The risks of diuresis are fluid overload, with cerebral and pulmonary edema, and disturbances in acid-base and electrolyte balance. Failure to produce a diuresis may imply prerenal or renal failure. If renal failure is present, dialysis should be considered.

Osmotic diuresis is meant to increase the osmotic gradient and prevent reabsorption from the *proximal* loop and *distal* tubules. Mannitol is used to initiate this type of diuresis, and then fluids are added in sufficient amounts to produce a diuresis similar to forced-fluid diuresis.

Acid and alkaline diuresis is based on the principle that, to inhibit reabsorption of certain toxic agents, the urinary pH can be adjusted so that the substance is maintained in its ionized form, which interferes with its passage back into the blood. Electrolyte and acid-base monitoring is necessary. Hypokalemia and hypocalcemia are frequent complications. *Acid diuresis* is accomplished by using ammonium chloride (Antidote 2, Table 83-1). Ascorbic acid may be used as an adjunct.

TABLE 83-1. ANTIDOTES*

Medications	Indications	Comments
1. **N-Acetylcysteine** (NAC, Mucomyst), Bristol. Glutathione precursor that prevents accumulation and helps detoxify acetaminophen metabolites. **Dose:** *Adult,* 140 mg/kg PO of 5% solution as loading dose, then 70 mg/kg PO every 4 hr for 17 doses as maintenance dose. *Child,* same as adult. **Packaged:** 10 and 20% solution in 4, 10, and 30 mL vials.	Acetaminophen toxicity. Most effective within first 8 hr (to make more palatable, administer through a straw inserted into closed container of citrus juice) **AR*:** Stomatitis, nausea, vomiting. See Acetaminophen in text. The full course of therapy is required in any patient whose level falls in the toxic range.	IV preparation experimental. The dose of NAC should be repeated if the patient vomits within 1 hr after administration. Methods to stop vomiting of the NAC are: (a) placement of a tube in the duodenum, (b) slow administration over 1 hr, (c) one half hour before NAC dose use metoclopramide (Reglan) 1 mg/kg intravenously over 1–2 min (max dose 10 mg) every 6 hours or droperidol (Inapsine) 1.25 mg IV; for extrapyramidal reactions use diphenhydramine (see 18, Diphenhydramine).
2. **Ammonium chloride,** USP, usually given by nasogastric tube. **Dose:** *Adult,* 2 grams every 6 hr in 60 mL dose to maximum of 12 g/day or 1.5 g as 1–2% IV q 6 hr up to 6 g/day. *Child,* 75 mg/kg (2.75 mEq/kg) 4 times/day to maximum of 2–6 grams IV or PO. **Packaged:** 325, 500, and 1000 mg tablets: 2.14% in 500 mL, 21.4% in 30 mL, 26.75% in 20 mL.	Acidification of urine may enhance the elimination of phencyclidine and other weak bases (amphetamines and strychnine), but the danger of rhabdomyolysis and precipitation of myoglobin in the renal tubules in an acid milieu indicates this therapy is too dangerous to recommend routinely.	Goal in acid diuresis is to keep urine pH 4.5–5.5 and output 3–6 mL/kg/hr. Monitor blood pH, keep at 7.2–7.3. A diuretic may be used to enhance acid diuresis. Contraindications: weak acid drugs, rhabdomyolysis and myoglobinuria, liver dysfunction, renal dysfunction, closed head injury.
3. **Amyl nitrite.**	See 14, Cyanide kit.	
4. **Antivenin Black Widow Spider** (*Latrodectus mactans*) **Dose:** 1–2 vials infused over 1 hr. **Packaged:** 6000 units/vial with 2.5 mL sterile watering and 1 mL horse serum 1:10 dilution.	Black widow spider; all *Latrodectus* species with severe symptoms. Most healthy adults survive with supportive care. Used in elderly or infants or if underlying medical condition causing hemodynamic instability. **AR:** Same as antivenin polyvalent because derived from horse serum.	Preliminary sensitivity test. Supportive care alone is standard management.
5. **Antivenin Polyvalent** for Crotalidae (pit vipers), Wyeth. IV only. **Dose:** depends on degree of envenomation—minimal: 5–8 vials, moderate: 8–12 vials, severe: 13–30 vials. Dilute in 500–2000 ml of crystalloid solution and start IV at a slow rate, increasing after the first 10 min, if no reaction occurs. **Packaged:** 1 vial (10 mL) lyophilized serum, 1 vial (10 mL) bacteriostatic water for injection, 1 vial (1 mL) normal horse serum.	Venoms of crotalids (pit vipers) of North and South America. **AR:** (Shock anaphylaxis) Reaction occurs within 30 min. Serum sickness usually occurs 5–44 days after administration. It may occur in less than 5 days, especially in those who have received horse serum products in the past. Symptoms include fever, edema, arthralgia, nausea, and vomiting, as well as pain and muscle weakness.	Consider consulting with Regional Poison Control Center and herpetologist. Administer IV. Preliminary sensitivity test. Never inject in fingers, toes, or bite site.
6. **Antivenin,** North American coral snake. Wyeth. IV only. **Dose:** 3–5 vials (30–50 mL) by slow IV injection. First 1–2 mL should be injected over 3–5 min. **Packaged:** 1 vial antivenin, 10 mL. 1 vial bacteriostatic water 10 mL for injection.	*Micrurus fulvius* (Eastern coral snake); *Micrurus tenere* (Texas coral snake) **AR:** Anaphylaxis (sensitivity reaction). Usually 30 min after administration. Signs/Symptoms: Flushing, itching, edema of face, cough, dyspnea, cyanosis. Neurologic manifestations: Usually involve the shoulders and arms. Pain and muscle weakness are frequently present, and permanent atrophy may develop.	Same as for Antivenin Polyvalent: for Crotalidae. Does not neutralize the venom of *Micrurus euryxanthus* (Arizona or Sonoran coral snake).
7. **Atropine** (various manufacturers). Antagonizes cholinergic stimuli at muscarinic receptors. **Dose:** *Adult,* initial dose 2–4 mg IV. Dose every 2–5 min as necessary until cessation of secretions. Severe poisoning may require doses up to 2000 mg. *Child,* initial dose of 0.05 mg/kg to a max of 2 mg every 2–5 min as necessary until cessation of secretions.	Therapy in carbamate and organophosphate insecticide poisonings. Rarely needed in cholinergic mushroom intoxication (*Amanita muscaria, Clitocybe, Inocybe* spp.) Lack of signs of atropinization confirms diagnosis of cholinesterase inhibition. **AR:** Flushing and dryness of skin, blurred vision, rapid and irregular pulse, fever, and loss of neuromuscular coordination.	If cyanosis, establish respiration first because atropine in cyanotic patients may cause ventricular fibrillation. If severe signs of atropinization, may correct with physostigmine in doses equal to one-half dose of atropine. If symptomatic, administer until the end point of drying secretions and clearing of lungs. Hallucinations, flushing of the skin, dilated pupils, tachycardia, and elevation of body temperature are not end points

* See footnote at end of table.

TABLE 83-1. CONTINUED

Medications	Indications	Comments
Packaged: 0.3 mg/mL in 30 mL; 0.4 mg/mL in 0.5, 1, 20, and 30 mL vials; 1 mg/mL in 1 and 10 mL vials.		and do not preclude atropine administration. Atropinization should be maintained for 12 to 24 hours, then taper dose and observe for relapse. Atropine has successfully been administered by IV infusion, although this method has not received FDA approval. **Dose:** Place 8 mg of atropine in 100 mL D5W or saline. Conc. = 0.08 mg/mL Dose range = 0.02–0.08 mg/kg/hr or 0.5 mL/kg/hr. Severe poisoning may require supplemental doses of intravenous atropine intermittently in doses of 2–4 mg until drying of secretion occurs.
8. **BAL**	See 17, Dimercaprol	
9. **Bicarbonate**	See 35, Sodium bicarbonate	
10. **Botulism antitoxin,** Connaught Med. Research Labs. **Dose:** *Adult,* 1 vial IV stat then 1 vial IM repeat in 2–4 hr if symptoms appear in 12–24 hr. *Child,* Check with state health department.	Prevention or treatment of botulism.	Contact local or state health department for full management guidelines.
11. **Calcium disodium edetate** (EDTA), Versenate, Riker. **Dose:** *Adult,* Max 4 g. *Child,* 1g. Moderate toxicity, IM or IV, 50 mg/kg day for 3–5 days. Severe toxicity, IV or IM, 75 mg/kg day for 4–5 days, divided into 3–6 doses daily. Dilute 1 g in 250–500 mL saline or D5W, infuse over 4 hr twice daily for 5–7 days. Max 1 g. For lead levels over 69 µg/dL or if symptoms of lead poisoning or encephalopathy: Add BAL alone initially, 4 mg/kg, then combination BAL and EDTA at different sites. EDTA dose: 12.5 mg/kg IM. (See Lead in text for latest recommendations.) Modify dose in renal failure. **Packaged:** 200 mg/mL, 5 mL amps.	For chelation of cadmium, chromium cobalt, copper, lead, magnesium, nickel, selenium, tellurium, tungsten, uranium, vanadium, and zinc poisoning. **AR:** 1. Thrombophlebitis. 2. Nausea, vomiting. 3. Hypotension. 4. Transient bone marrow suppression. 5. Nephrotoxicity, reversible tubular necrosis (particularly in acid urine). 6. Fever 4–8 hr after infusion. 7. Increased prothrombin time.	Hydrate first and establish renal flow. Avoid plain sodium EDTA because hypocalcemia may result. Procaine 0.25–1 mL of 0.5% for each mL of IM EDTA to reduce pain. Do not use EDTA orally. Limit use to 7 days (otherwise loss of other ions and cardiac dysrhythmias may occur.) **MP*:** Calcium levels, urinalysis, renal profile, erythrocyte protoporphyrin, blood lead, and liver profile. Contraindicated in iron intoxication, hepatic impairment, and renal failure.
12. (A) **Calcium gluconate** (various manufacturers). **Dose:** *Adult:* 10 g in 250 mL of water PO or by NG tube. 30 g max daily dose. **Packaged:** 500, 650 mg, 1 g tabs.	To precipitate fluorides, magnesium, salts, and oxalates after oral ingestion.	
(B) **Calcium gluconate** 10%. **Dose:** IV 0.2–0.5 mL/kg of elemental calcium up to maximum 10 mL (1 g) over 5–10 min with continuous ECG monitoring. Titrate to adequate response. **Packaged:** 10% in 10 mL vial.	Calcium channel blocker poisoning, e.g., nifedipine (*Procardia*), verapamil (*Calan*), diltiazem (*Cardizem*). It improves the blood pressure but does not affect the dysrhythmias. Hypocalcemia as result of poisonings. Black widow spider envenomation.	Repeat dose as needed. Monitor calcium levels. Contraindicated with digitalis poisoning.
(C) **Calcium chloride.** **Dose:** IV 0.2 mL/kg up to maximum 10 mL (1 g) with continuous IV monitoring. Titrate to adequate response.	Hydrofluoric acid (HF) (if irrigation with cool water fails to control the pain). **AR:** IV bradycardia, asystole, necrosis with extravasation.	Infiltration with calcium gluconate should be considered if HF exposure results in immediate tissue damage and erythema and pain persists following adequate irrigation.
(D) **Infiltration of calcium gluconate.** **Dose:** Infiltrate each square cm of the affected dermis and subcutaneous tissue with about 0.5 mL of 10% calcium gluconate using a 30-gauge needle. Repeat as needed to control pain. **Packaged:** 10% in 10 mL vial.		

* See footnote at end of table.

TABLE 83-1. CONTINUED

Medications	Indications	Comments
(E) **Calcium Gel** 3.5 g USP, calcium gluconate powder added to 5 oz of KY jelly.	Dermal exposures of hydrofluoric acid less than 20%.	Gel must have direct access to burn area. If pain persists, a calcium gluconate injection may be needed.
13. **Chlorpromazine** (various manufacturers). Phenothiazine derivative. **Dose:** *Adult,* 1 mg/kg dose IV/IM or 0.5 mg/kg dose if taken with barbiturate. **Packaged:** 25 mg/mL in 1, 2, and 10 mL vials.	Only in *pure* amphetamine OD, with life-threatening manifestations. (Diazepam [Valium] is preferred.) Toxicity: CNS depression, coma, hypotension, extrapyramidal syndrome, agitation, fever, convulsions, dry mouth, cardiac arrhythmias, ECG changes.	Do not use if any signs of atropinization or ''street drug'' amphetamines are present. Watch for hypotension. In general it is safer to use diazepam (Valium) or haloperidol (Haldol).
14. **Cyanide antidote kit,** Lilly. Nitrite-induced methemoglobinemia attracts cyanide off cytochrome oxidase and thiosulfate forms nontoxic thiocyanate. **Doses:** *Adult,* amyl nitrite. Inhale for 30 sec of every min. Use a new ampule every 3 min. Reapply until sodium nitrite can be given. Then inject IV 300 mg (10 mL of 3% solution) of Na nitrite at a rate of 2.5 to 5 mL/min. Then inject 12.5 grams (50 mL of 25% sol) of Na thiosulfate. *Child,* use the following chart for children's dosage. **Packaged:** 2–10 mL ampules Na nitrite injection: 2–50 mL ampules Na thiosulfate injection; 0.3 mL amyl nitrite inhalant.	Cyanide poisoning. **AR:** Hypotension, methemoglobinemia.	*Note:* If a child is given the adult dose of Na nitrite, a fatal methemoglobinemia may result. *Do not use methylene blue* for methemoglobinemia in cyanide therapy. Observe for hypotension and have epinephrine available. Cyanide kit should have amyl nitrite changed annually. Administer oxygen 100% between inhalations of amyl nitrite. Monitor hemoglobin, arterial blood gases, methemoglobin concentration (nitrite given to obtain a methemoglobin of 25%). Some add cyanide ampule to resuscitation bag.

Hemoglobin	*Initial Child Dose of Sodium Nitrite 3% (do not exceed 10 mL)*	*Initial Child Dose of Sodium Thiosulfate (do not exceed 12.5 grams)*
8 g	0.22 mL/kg (6.6 mg/kg)	1.10 mL/kg
10 g	0.27 mL/kg (8.7 mg/kg)	1.35 mL/kg
12 g	0.33 mL/kg (10 mg/kg)	1.65 mL/kg
14 g	0.39 mL/kg (11.6 mg/kg)	1.95 mL/kg

If signs of poisoning reappear, repeat above procedure at one-half the above doses.

Medications	Indications	Comments
15. **Deferoxamine mesylate** (DFOM, Desferal), Ciba. Has a remarkable affinity for ferric iron and chelates it. **Therapeutic Dose:** *Adult,* 90 mL/kg IM or IV every 8 hr to a max of 1 g per injection, may repeat to maximum of 6 g in 24 hr. *Child,* same as adult. IM or IV. IV administration should be given by slow infusion at rate not exceeding 15 mg/kg/hr. **Packaged:** 500 mg/amp (powder).	DFOM is useful in the treatment of symptomatic iron poisoning or cases where the serum iron is greater than 500 μg/dL. A positive result of a DFOM challenge test is not a definite indication that therapy is necessary in the asymptomatic patient. Oral DFOM is not recommended. Iron intoxication. Therapeutic: see dose in left column. *Diagnostic trial.* Give deferoxamine, 50 mg/kg IM (up to 1 g). If serum iron exceeds TIBC, unbound iron is excreted in urine, producing a ''vin rose'' color of chelated iron complex in the urine (pink orange). However, may be negative with high serum iron exceeding TIBC. **AR:** Flushing of the skin, generalized erythema, urticaria, hypotension, and shock may occur. Blindness has occurred rarely in patients receiving long-term, high-dose DFOM therapy. Contraindicated in patients with renal disease or anuria.	Therapy is usually continued until urine color and/or iron levels are normal. Therapy is rarely required over 24 hr. Establish a good renal flow. To be effective DFOM should be administered in first 12–16 hr. In mild to moderate iron intoxication, IM or IV route. In severe intoxication or shock, IV route only. Monitor serum iron levels, urine output, and urine color.
16. **Diazepam** (Valium), Roche. **Dose:** *Adult,* 5–10 mg IV (max 20 mg) at a rate of 5 mg/min until seizure is controlled. May be repeated 2 or 3 times. *Child,* 0.1–0.3 mg/kg up to 10 mg IV slowly over 2 min. **Packaged:** 5 mg/mL, 2 mL, 10 mL vials.	Any intoxication that provokes seizures when specific therapy is *not* available, e.g., amphetamines, PCP, barbiturate and alcohol withdrawal. Chloroquine poisoning. **AR:** Confusion, somnolence, coma, hypotension.	Intramuscular absorption is erratic. Establish airway and administer 100% oxygen and glucose.

TABLE 83-1. CONTINUED

Medications	Indications	Comments
17. **Dimercaprol** (BAL), Hynson, Westcott, and Dunning. **Dose:** Recommendations vary, contact Regional Poison Control Center. Prevents inhibition of sulfhydryl enzymes. Given deep IM only. For *severe lead poisoning:* see 11, EDTA. For *mild arsenic or gold:* 2.5 mg/kg every 6 hr for 2 days, then every 12 hr on the third day, and once daily thereafter for 10 days. For *severe arsenic or gold:* 3–5 mg/kg every 6 hr for 3 days, then every 12 hr thereafter for 10 days. For *mercury:* 5 mg/kg initially, followed by 2.5 mg/kg 1 or 2 times daily for 10 days. **Packaged:** 100 mg/mL 10% in oil in 3 mL amp.	For chelation of antimony, arsenic, bismuth, chromates, copper, gold, lead, and mercury nickel. **AR:** 30% of patients have reactions: fever (30% of children), hypertension, tachycardia, may cause hemolysis in G6PD deficiency patients. Doses greater than recommended may cause various adverse effects: nausea, vomiting, headache, chest pain, tachycardia, and hypertension.	Contraindicated in hepatic insufficiency, with the exception of postarsenic jaundice. Should be discontinued or used only with extreme caution if acute renal insufficiency is present. Monitor blood pressure and heart rate (both may increase), urinalysis, qualitative urine excretion of heavy metal. Contraindicated in iron, silver, uranium, selenium, and cadmium poisoning.
18. **Diphenhydramine** (Benadryl), Parke-Davis. Antiparkinsonian action. **Dose:** *Adult,* 10–50 mg IV over 2 min. *Child,* 1–2 mg/kg IV up to 50 mg over 2 min. Maximum 24 hr 400 mg. **Packaged:** 10 mg/mL in 10 and 30 mL vials. 50 mg/mL in 1, 5, 10, and 30 mL vials. Caps, tab 25. 50 mg. Elixir, syrup 12.5 mg/5 mL.	Used to treat extrapyramidal symptoms and dystonia induced by phenothiazines and related drugs. **AR:** Fatal dose, 20–40 mg/kg Dry mouth, drowsiness.	Continue with oral diphenhydramine 5 mg/kg/day to 25 mg 3 times a day for 72 hr to avoid recurrence.
19. **EDTA**	See 11, Calcium disodium edetate	
20. **Ethanol** (ETOH). Competitively inhibits alcohol dehydrogenase. **Dose:** *Loading:* Administer 7.6–10.0 mL/kg of 10% ETOH in D5W over 30 min IV or 0.8–1.0 mL/kg 95% ETOH PO in 6 oz of orange juice over 30 min. While administering loading dose start maintenance. **Maintenance Dose:** Volume of 10% ETOH needed IV or 95% oral solution (not in dialysis). (See table of maintenance dose below.) If patient is on dialysis, add 91 mL/hr in addition to regular maintenance dose. See comments to prepare 10% solution if not commercially available. **Packaged:** 10% ethanol in D5W 1000 mL; 95% ethanol. May be given as 50% solution orally.	Methanol, ethylene glycol. Ethanol infusion therapy may be started in cases of suspected methanol and ethylene glycol poisoning presenting with increased anion gap and osmolal gap, or if the urine shows the crystalluria of ethylene glycol poisoning or the hyperemia of the optic disc of methanol intoxication. **AR:** CNS depression, hypoglycemia.	Monitor blood ethanol 1 hr after starting infusion and every 4–6 hr. Maintain a blood ethanol concentration of 100–200 mg/dL. Monitor blood glucose, electrolytes, blood gases, urinalysis, and renal profile at least daily. Continue infusion until safe concentration of ethylene glycol or methanol is reached. Ethanol-induced hypoglycemia may occur. Dialysis, preferably hemodialysis, should be considered in severe intoxication not controlled by ethanol alone. To prepare 10% ethanol for infusion therapy: Remove 100 mL from 1 L of D5W and replace with 100 mL of tax-free bulk absolute alcohol after passing through 0.22 micron filter. 50 mL vials of pyrogen-free absolute ethanol for injection are available from Pharm-Serve, 218–20 96th Avenue, Queen's Village, NY 11429. Telephone 718–475–1601.

Maintenance Dose: Patient Category	mL/kg/hr using 10% IV	mL/kg/hr using 50% oral
Nondrinker	0.83	0.17
Occasional drinker	1.40	0.28
Alcoholic	1.96	0.39

Medications	Indications	Comments
21. **Fab** (antibody fragment) (Digibind). **Dose:** The average dose used during clinical testing was 10 vials. Dosage details are specified by the manufacturer. It should be administered by the IV route over 30 min. Calculate on basis of body burden either by known amount ingested or by serum digoxin concentration. Calculation of dose of FAB: 1. Known amount ingested multiplied by bioavailability (0.8) = body burden. Body burden divided by 0.6 = number of vials.	Digoxin, digitoxin, oleander tea with life-threatening intoxications, refractory dysrhythmias, hyperkalemia. 40 mg binds 0.6 mg digoxin.	Contact Regional Poison Control Center. Preliminary sensitivity test. Administer through a 0.22 micron filter. It causes a rise in measured bound digoxin but a fall in free digoxin.

TABLE 83-1. CONTINUED

Medications	Indications	Comments
2. Known serum digoxin (obtained 6 hr postingestion) multiplied by volume distribution (5.6 L/kg) and weight in kg divided by 1000 = body burden. Body burden divided by 0.6 = number of vials.		
22. **Glucagon.** Works by stimulating production of cyclic adenyl monophosphate. **Dose:** 50–150 μg/kg over 1 min IV followed by a continuous infusion of 1–5 mg/hr in dextrose and then taper over 5–12 hr. **Packaged:** 1 mg (1 unit) vial with 1 mL diluent with glycerin and phenol; also in 10 mL size.	Propranolol and other beta blocker intoxication. **AR:** Generally well tolerated—most frequent are nausea, vomiting.	Do not dissolve the lyophilized glucagon in the solvent packaged with it when administering IV infusion because of possible phenol toxicity. Effects of single dose observed in 5–10 min and last for 15–30 min. A constant infusion may be necessary to sustain desired effects.
23. **Labetalol hydrochloride** (Normodyne) Schering; (Trandate) Glaxo. Nonselective beta and mild alpha blocker. **Dose:** IV 20 mg over 2 min. Additional injections of 40 or 80 mg can be given at 10 min intervals until desired supine blood pressure achieved. Max dose 300 mg. Alternative: Slow IV infusion: 200 mg (40 mL) is added to 160 or 250 mL of D5W and given at 2 mg/min. Titrate infusion according to response. **Packaged:** Solution 5 mg/mL in 20 mL.	Hypertensive crises secondary to cocaine. **AD:** GI disturbances, orthostatic hypotension, bronchospasm, congestive heart failure, A-V conduction disturbances, and peripheral vascular reactions.	Concomitant diuretic enhances therapeutic response. Patient should be kept in a supine position during infusion. **MP:** Monitor blood pressure during and after administration.
24. **Methylene blue,** Harvey and others. Physiologically transformed to reduced form, leukomethylene blue, which is then oxidized to methylene blue in the presence of methemoglobin. The methemoglobin is converted to hemoglobin. **Dose:** *Adult,* 0.1–0.2 mL/kg of 2% solution (1–2 mg/kg over 5 min IV). *Child,* Same as adult. **Packaged:** 1% 10 mL ampules. May repeat in 1 hr if necessary.	Methemoglobinemia **AR:** GI (nausea, vomiting), headache, hypertension, dizziness, mental confusion, restlessness, dyspnea when IV dose exceeds 7 mg/kg. Treatment is unnecessary unless methemoglobin is over 30% or respiratory distress.	Saliva, urine, and other body fluids may turn blue. *Contraindications:* Renal insufficiency, cyanide poisonings when sodium nitrite is used to induce methemoglobinemia in G6PD deficiency patients. Monitor hemolysis, methemoglobin level, and arterial blood gases. Avoid extravasation because of local necrosis.
25. **Naloxone** (Narcan). Pure opioid antagonist. **Dose:** *Adult,* 0.4–2.0 mg IV and repeat at 3-min intervals until respiratory function is stable. Before excluding opioid intoxication on the basis of a lack of naloxone response a minimum of 2 mg in a child or 10 mg in an adult should be administered. *Child,* Initial dose is 0.01 mg/kg IV. If no response, a subsequent dose of 0.1 mg/kg may be administered. **Packaged:** 0.02 mg/mL, 0.4 mg/mL ampule, and 10 mL multidose vial.	Narcotic, opiate, CNS depression. This drug is relatively free of adverse reactions. Rare report of pulmonary edema. Should be administered with caution in pregnancy. It is used only to reverse depression and hypoxia.	Naloxone infusion therapy should be used if a large initial dose was required, repeated boluses are necessary, or a long-acting opiate is involved. In infusion therapy the initial response dose is administered every hour and may need to be boosted in a half hour after starting. The infusion may be tapered after 12 hr of therapy. Naloxone infusion: calculate daily fluid requirements, add initial response dose of naloxone multiplied by 24 to the solution. Divide fluid by 24 to determine mL/hr of naloxone infusion. Dose not cause CNS depression. Routes: IV or endotracheal are preferred routes. Pentazocine (Talwin), dextromethorphan, propoxyphene (Darvon), and codeine may require larger doses.
26. **Nicotinamide** (various manufacturers). **Dose:** *Adult,* 500 mg IM or IV slowly, then 200–400 mg q 4 hr. If symptoms develop, the frequency of injections should be increased to every 2 hr (max 3 grams/day). *Child,* one half suggested adult dose. **Packaged:** 100 mg/mL; 2, 5, 10, 30 mL vials; 25 and 50 mg tablets.	Vacor poisoning: phenylurea pesticide intoxication. *Note:* Vacor 2% is now available only to professional exterminators. 0.5% Vacor is available to the general public and can be toxic to children if swallowed. **AR:** Large doses: flushing, pruritus, sensation of burning, nausea, vomiting, anaphylactic shock.	Nicotinamide is most effective when given within 1 hr of ingestion. Do not use niacin or nicotinic acid in place of nicotinamide. Monitor liver profile.

TABLE 83-1. CONTINUED

Medications	Indications	Comments
27. **Oxygen** 100%. **Dose:** *Adult,* 100% oxygen by inhalation or 100% oxygen in hyperbaric chamber at 2–3 atm. *Child,* same as adult.	Carbon monoxide, cyanide, methemoglobinemia. Any inhalation intoxication.	Half-life of carboxyhemoglobin is 240 min in room air 21% oxygen; if a patient is hyperventilated with 100% oxygen, half-life of carboxyhemoglobin is 90 min; in chamber at 2 atm, half-life is 25–30 min.
28. **Pancuronium bromide** (Pavulon). Nondepolarizing (competitive) blocking agent. **Dose:** *Adults and children,* initially, 0.1 mg/kg IV; for intubation, 0.1 mg/kg IV, repeated as required (generally every 40 to 60 minutes). **Packaged:** Sol 1 mg/mL in 10 mL; 2 mg/mL in 2 and 5 mL containers.	Neuromuscular blocking agent. Used for intubation and seizure control acts in 2 min, lasts 40–60 min. **AR:** Main hazard is inadequate postoperative ventilation. Tachycardia and slight increase in arterial pressure may occur owing to vagolytic action.	The required dose varies greatly and a peripheral nerve stimulator aids in determining appropriate amount. Should monitor EEG, since motor effect may be abolished without decreasing electrical discharge from brain.
29. **D-Penicillamine** (Cuprimine) Merck; (Depen) Wallace. Effective chelator and promotes excretion in urine. **Dose:** 250 mg 4 times daily PO for up to 5 days for long-term (20–40 days) therapy: 30–40 mg/kg/day in children. Max 1 g/day. For chronic therapy 25 mg/kg/day in 4 doses. **Packaged:** 125 and 250 mg capsules.	Heavy metals, arsenic, cadium, chromates, cobalt, copper, lead, mercury, nickel, and zinc. **AR:** Leukopenia (2%); thrombocytopenia (4%); GI; nausea, vomiting, anaphylactic shock, diarrhea (17%); fever, rash, lupus syndrome, renal and hepatic injury.	This is not considered standard therapy for lead poisoning after chelation therapy. May produce ampicillin-like rash, allergic reactions, neutropenia, and nephropathy. Contraindication: hypersensitivity to penicillin. **MP:** Routine urinalysis, white differential blood count, hemoglobin determination, direct platelet count, renal and hepatic profiles. Collect 24 hr urine, quantify for heavy metal.
30. **Physostigmine salicylate** (Antilirium), Forest. Cholinesterase inhibitor. A diagnostic trial is not recommended. **Dose:** *Adult,* 1–2 mg IV over 2 min: may repeat every 5 min to max dose of 6 mg. *Child,* IV, 0.5 mg over 2 min to a max dose of 2 mg. Once effect accomplished, give lowest effective dose every 30–60 minutes if symptoms recur. **Packaged:** 1 mg/mL 2 mL/amp.	Used if conventional therapy fails for coma, convulsions, severe cardiac dysrhythmias, severe hypertension, hallucinations secondary to anticholinergics, antihistamines, and anticholinergic plants. **AR:** Death may result from respiratory paralysis, hypertension/hypotension, bradycardia/tachycardia/asystole, hypersalivation, respiratory difficulties/convulsions (cholinergic crisis).	Do not consider for the following: antidepressants, amoxapine, maprotiline, nomifensine, bupropion, trazodone, imipramine. IV administration should be at a slow controlled rate, not more than 1 mg/min. Rapid administration can cause adverse reactions. Can be reversed by atropine. Lasts only 30 min. Contraindicated in asthma, cardiovascular disease, intestinal obstruction.
31. **Pralidoxime chloride** (2-PAM, Protopam), Ayerst. Cholinesterase reactivator by removing phosphate. **Dose:** *Adult,* 1 g IV at 0.5 g min or infused in 150 mL saline over 30 min. Repeat every 8–12 hr when needed; if severe, 0.5 g/hr infusion. *Child,* 25–50 mg/kg IV over 30 min, no faster than 10 mg/kg/min. **Packaged:** 1 g/20 mL vials.	Organosphosphate insecticide poisoning. Not usually needed in carbamate insecticide poisoning. Most effective if started in first 24 hr before bonding of phosphate. **AR:** Rapid IV injection has produced tachycardia, muscle rigidity, transient neuromuscular blockade. IM: conjunctival hyperemia, subconjunctival hemorrhage, especially if concentrations exceed 5%. Oral: nausea, vomiting, diarrhea, malaise.	Should be used only after initial treatment with atropine. Draw blood for RBC cholinesterase level before giving 2-PAM. The use of 2-PAM may require a reduction in the dose of atropine. **MP:** Monitor renal profile and reduce dose accordingly.
32. **Propranolol** (Inderal). Nonselective beta blocker. **Dose:** *Adult,* 0.1–0.15 mg/kg IV, administered in increments of 0.5–0.75 mg every 1–2 min with continuous ECG and blood pressure monitoring up to 10 mg. *Child,* 0.01–0.015 mg/kg dose slow IV with repeat dose every 6–8 hr as needed. **Packaged:** 1 mg/mL; tab: 10, 20, 40, 60, 80, 90 mg; cap: 20, 80, 160 mg.	Cocaine intoxication. Has not been scientifically proved to be safe and effective. Anecdotal reports only. Labetalol is theoretically preferred agent for cocaine intoxication. **AR:** Bradycardia, hypotension, pallor; neurologic effects include hallucinations, coma, and seizures.	Not a specific antidote; used for catecholamine storm and dysrhythmias. Increased mortality has been reported in animals that received propranolol for cocaine poisoning, and hypertension has occurred in humans following its use in cocaine intoxication.
33. **Protamine sulfate.** **Dose:** 1 mg neutralizes 90–115 units of heparin. Maximum dose = 50 mg IV over 5 min at 10 mg/mL. **Packaged:** 5 mL = 50 mg; 25 mL = 250 mg.	Heparin overdose. **AR:** Rapid administration causes anaphylactoid reactions.	**MP:** Monitor thromboplastin times. Doses of up to 200 mg have been tolerated over 2 hr in an adult.

TABLE 83-1. CONTINUED

Medications	Indications	Comments
34. **Pyridoxine (Vitamin B₆).** Gamma-aminobutyric acid agonist. **Dose:** *Unknown amount ingested:* 5 gm over 5 min IV. *Known amount:* Add 1 gram of pyridoxine for each gram of INH ingested IV over 5 min. **Packaged:** 50 and 100 mg/mL; 10, 30 mL.	Isoniazid (INH), hydrazine. **AR:** Unlikely owing to the fact that vitamin B₂ is water soluble. However, nausea, vomiting, somnolence, and paresthesia have been reported from chronic high doses.	Pyridoxine is given as 5–10% solution IV mixed with water. It may be repeated every 5–20 min until seizures cease. Some administer pyridoxine over 30–60 min. **MP:** Correct acidosis, monitor liver profile, acid-base parameters.
35. **Sodium bicarbonate.** **Dose:** IV 1–3 mEq/kg as needed to keep pH 7.5 (generally 2 mEq/kg every 6 hours). When alkalinization is desired to correct acidosis to a pH of 7.3, use 2 mEq/kg to raise pH 0.1 unit. **Packaged:** 50 mL, 44.6 mEq, 50 mEq ampule.	To promote urinary alkalinization for salicylates, phenobarbital (weak acids with low volume of distribution excreted in urine unchanged). To correct severe acidosis. To promote protein-binding and supply sodium ions into Purkinje cells in cyclic antidepressant intoxication. **AR:** Large doses in patients with renal insufficiency may cause metabolic alkalosis. In patients with ketoacidosis, rapid alkalinization with sodium bicarbonate may result in clouding of consciousness, cerebral dysfunction, seizures, hypoxia, and lactic acidosis.	Alkaline diuresis. The assessment of the need for bicarbonate should be based on both the blood and urine pH. Maintain the blood pH at 7.5. Keep the urinary output at 3–6 mL/kg/hr. May use a diuretic to enhance diuresis. Potassium is necessary to produce alkaline diuresis. Monitor electrolytes, calcium, pH of both urine and blood, arterial blood gases.
36. **Sodium nitrite.**	See 14, Cyanide kit	
37. **Sodium thiosulfate.**	See 14, Cyanide kit	
38. **Vitamin K** (AquaMEPHYTON) Merck. Promotes hepatic biosynthesis of prothrombin and other coagulation factors. Competitive antagonist of warfarin. It may be administered orally in the absence of vomiting. **Dose:** *Adult,* 2.5–10 mg IV, depending on potential for hemorrhage. Severe bleeding, 5–25 mg slow IV push. Rate 1 mg/min. Repeat every 4–8 hr depending on prothrombin time. *Child,* 1–5 mg IV may be given orally when vomiting ceases. **Packaged:** 2 mg/mL in 0.5 mL ampules. 2.5 or 5 mL vials.	Warfarin (coumarin), salicylate intoxication.	Fatalities from anaphylatic reaction have been reported following IV route. It takes 24 hr for vitamin K to be effective. The need for further vitamin K is determined by the prothrombin time test. If severe bleeding, fresh blood or plasma transfusion may be needed.

* This is for information purposes and is not intended to substitute for independent judgment. It is always advisable to review the package insert for the most up-to-date information. Contact Regional Poison Control Center for additional details on use.

AR = adverse reactions to antidotes. MP = monitor parameters.

It enhances the elimination of weak bases such as amphetamines and fenfluramine (Pondimin). Ammonium chloride is contraindicated if rhabdomyolysis is present. *Alkaline diuresis* with sodium bicarbonate can be used in the therapy of weak acids, such as salicylates, and long-acting barbiturates, such as phenobarbital (Antidote 35, Table 83-1).

DIALYSIS

Dialysis is the extrarenal means of removing certain toxins from the body and can substitute for the kidney when renal failure occurs. Dialysis is never the first measure instituted; however, it may be life-saving later in the course of the severe intoxication. It is needed only in a small minority of intoxications such as methanol, ethylene glycol, lithium, and salicylates. *Peritoneal dialysis* is only one twentieth as effective as hemodialysis. It is easier to use and less hazardous to the patient but also less reliable in removing the toxin. *Hemodialysis* is the most effective means of dialysis but requires experience with sophisticated equipment. *The patient-related criteria for dialysis* are anticipated prolonged coma and the likelihood of complications, renal impairment, and deterioration despite careful medical management.

HEMOPERFUSION

Hemoperfusion is the extracorporeal exposure of the patient's blood to an adsorbing surface (charcoal or resin). This procedure has extended extracorporeal removal to a large range of substances that were either poorly dialyzable or nondialyzable. *Hemoperfusion may be used for agents* with high protein binding, low aqueous solubility, and poor distribution in the plasma water. In these cases, hemodialysis is relatively ineffective. Hemoperfusion has proved useful in glutethimide (Doriden) intoxication, barbiturate overdose even with short-acting barbiturates, theophylline, cyclic antidepressants, and chlorophenothane (DDT). The commonly used types are activated charcoal and resin cartridges. In general, supportive care is all that is required. Analysis of studies with hemodialysis and hemoperfusion does not indicate that they reduce morbidity or mortality substantially except in certain cases.

TOXICOKINETICS FOR THE PRACTICING PHYSICIAN

Toxicokinetics is clinical pharmacokinetics from the viewpoint of the toxicologist. Pharmacokinetics is a mathematical description of what the body does to a drug. Knowledge of the toxicokinetics of a specific toxic agent allows the physician to plan a rational approach to the definitive management of the intoxicated patient after the vital functions have been stabilized.

The *LD*$_{50}$ (the lethal dose for 50% of experimental animals) and the *MLD* (the minimum lethal dose) are seldom relevant in human intoxications, but indicate the potential toxicity of the substance. *Protein-binding* of toxic agents influences the volume distribution, elimination, and action of the drug. Diuresis and dialysis are usually reserved for drugs with less than 50% protein binding. The *therapeutic blood range* is the concentration of any drug at which the majority of the treated population can be expected to receive therapeutic benefit. The *toxic blood range* is the concentration at which this majority are expected to have toxic manifestations. The range is not an absolute value. *Blood concentrations* are a quantitative aid in determining whether more specific measures need to be instituted in correlation with the clinical manifestations. The *apparent volume distribution (Vd)* is the percentage of body mass in which the drug is distributed. It is determined by dividing the amount absorbed by the blood concentration. When a substance has a large volume distribution, as in most lipid-soluble chemicals (above 1 liter per kg), and is concentrated in the body fat, it is not available for diuresis, dialysis, or exchange transfusion. *Elimination routes* of detoxification allow the physician to make therapeutic decisions, such as using ethanol to interfere with the metabolism of methanol and ethylene glycol into more toxic metabolites. *Urine identification* is qualitative and allows only the identification of an agent.

Never manage a poisoned patient solely by laboratory tests, and always treat according to the manifestations of poisoning, not the laboratory test results. The laboratory toxicology analyst should be given whatever historical information is available so that the agent can be sought and identified as rapidly as possible. Toxicologic analysis is like a miniresearch project, unlike most other laboratory tests. *Specimens* for toxicologic analysis require the patient's name, date, time of ingestion, time specimen was drawn, therapeutic drugs administered, patient's manifestations, and other relevant data. The toxicologic specimens that should be obtained for analysis are (1) vomitus or initial gastric aspiration, (2) blood, 10 mL (ask the analyst about the type of container and anticoagulant), and (3) urine, 100 mL.

COMMON POISONS AND THERAPY

Abbreviations Used in Following List of Common Poisons

t$\frac{1}{2}$ = half-life (time required for blood level to drop by 50 per cent of the original value)
Vd = volume of distribution (liter per kg)
TLV = threshold limit value in air
TWA = time-weighted average
PPM = parts per million in air and water

Conversion Factors

1 gram	= 1000 milligrams (mg)
1 milligram (mg)	= 1000 micrograms (μg)
1 microgram (μg)	= 1000 nanograms (ng)
Blood levels:	
1 microgram per mL	= 100 micrograms per dL
	= 1 milligram per liter
	= 1000 nanograms per mL
100 mg per dL	= 0.1 gram per dL
	= 1000 mg (1 gram) per liter
	= 1.0 mg per mL

ACETAMINOPHEN, APAP (TYLENOL)

Toxic dose: Child, 3 or more g; adult, 7.5 or more g. Liver toxicity, 140 mg per kg. *Toxicokinetics:* Absorption time, 0.5 to 1 hour. Vd, 0.9 liter per kg. Route of elimination by liver. Draw peak blood level after 4 hours in overdose. *Manifestations:* First 24 hours: malaise, nausea, vomiting, and drowsiness, followed by a latent period of 24 hours to 5 days; then hepatic symptoms, disturbances in clotting mechanism, and renal damage. *Management:* (1) Activated charcoal has been contraindicated when *N*-acetylcysteine is con-

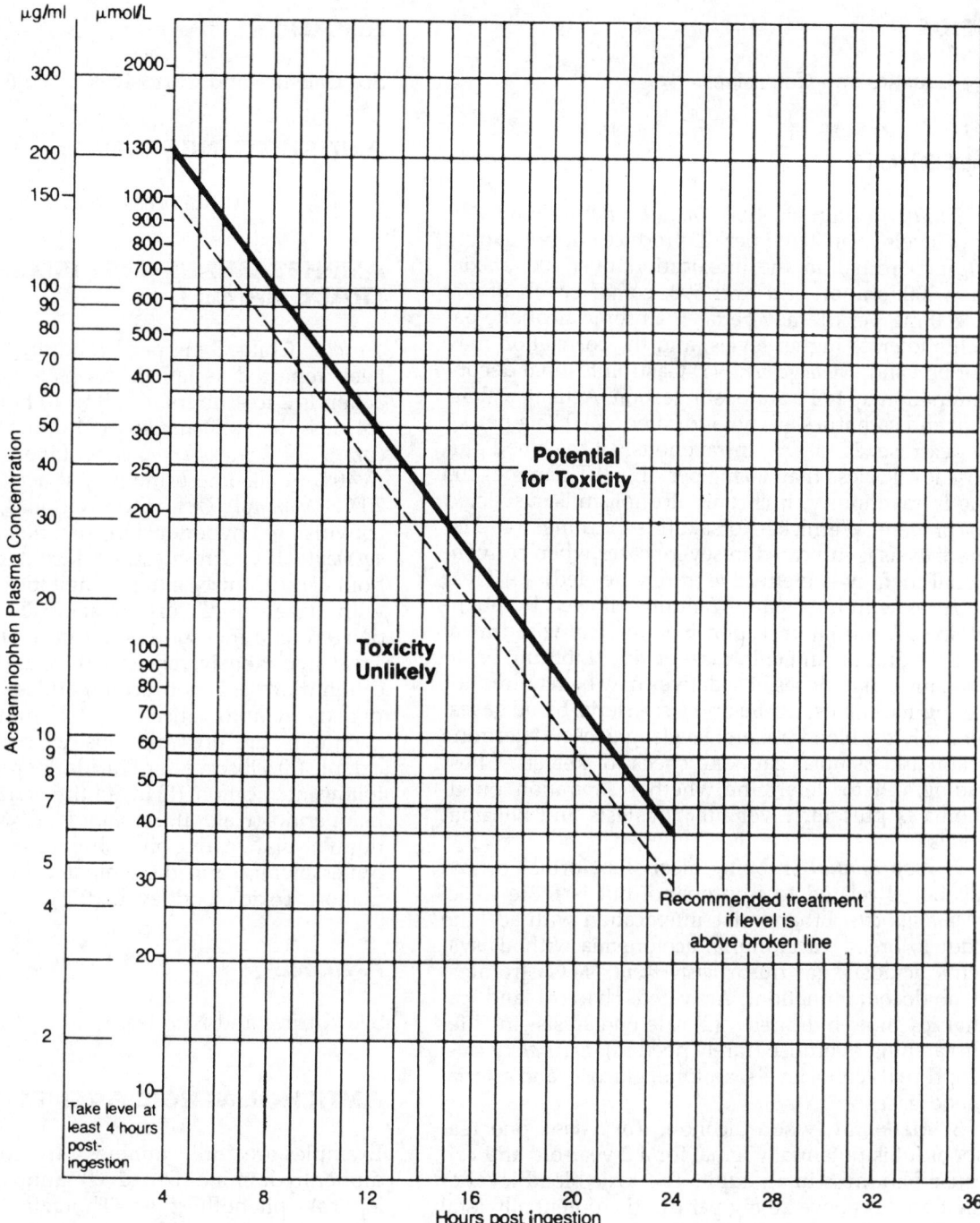

μg/ml   μmol/L

300   2000

200   1300
150   1000
       900
       800
       700
100   600
90
80   500
70
60   400
50   300
40   250
30   200

**Potential
for Toxicity**

20

       100
       90
       80   **Toxicity
       70   Unlikely**
10   60
9
8   50
7
       40

5   30
4
              **Recommended treatment
       20   if level is
              above broken line**

2

       10
Take level at
least 4 hours
post-
ingestion

4   8   12   16   20   24   28   32   36

Hours post ingestion

Acetaminophen Plasma Concentration

FIG. 83-1.   Nomogram for acetaminophen intoxication. Start N-acetylcysteine therapy if levels and time coordinates are above the lower line on the nomogram. Continue and complete therapy even if subsequent values fall below the toxic zone. The nomogram is useful only in acute, single ingestions. Serum levels drawn before 4 hours may not represent peak levels. (With permission from Rumack BH, Matthew H: Acetaminophen poisoning and toxicity. Reproduced by permission of Pediatrics 55:871, 1975.)

templated; use gastric lavage. More recently, however, activated charcoal may be given in the first few hours or alternated 2 hours after the N-acetylcysteine. (2) N-Acetylcysteine for toxic overdose (Antidote 1, Table 83-1). Start and give a full course if a toxic dose has been ingested or if blood concentrations are above the toxic line on the nomogram shown in Figure 83-1. (3) In this instance, a saline sulfate cathartic is preferred to sorbitol. *Laboratory aids:* APAP level, optimally at 4 to 6 hours. Plot levels on nomogram in Figure 83-1 as a guide for treatment. Monitor liver and renal profiles daily.

ACIDS

See Caustics and Corrosives.

ALCOHOLS

1. *Ethanol* (grain alcohol). *Manifestations:* Blood ethanol levels over 30 mg per dL produce euphoria; over 50, incoordination and intoxication; over 100, ataxia; over 300, stupor; and over 500, coma. Levels of 500 to 700 mg per dL may be fatal. Chronic alcoholic patients tolerate higher levels, and the correlation may not be valid. *Management:* (1) Gastrointestinal decontamination up to 1 hour postingestion. Activated charcoal and cathartics are not indicated. (2) 0.25 g per kg of dextrose, 25 to 50%, intravenously if the blood glucose level is less than 60 mg per dL, (3) Thiamine, 100 mg intravenously, if chronic alcoholism is suspected to prevent Wernicke-Korsakoff syndrome. (4) Hemodialysis is indicated in severe cases when conventional therapy is ineffective (rarely needed). (5) Treat seizures with diazepam (Valium) followed by phenytoin (Dilantin) if unresponsive. (6) Treat withdrawal with hydration and chlordiazepoxide (Librium) or diazepam. Large doses of sedatives may be required for delirium tremens. *Laboratory aids:* Arterial blood gases, electrolytes, blood ethanol levels, glucose, determine anion and osmolar gap, and check for ketosis. Chest radiograph to determine whether aspiration pneumonia is present. Liver function tests and bilirubin levels.

2. *Isopropanol* (rubbing alcohol). Normal propyl alcohol is related to isopropanol but is more toxic. *Manifestations:* Ethanol-like intoxication with acetone odor to breath, acetonuria, acetonemia without systemic acidosis, gastritis. *Management:* (1) Gastrointestinal decontamination. Activated charcoal and cathartics not indicated. (2) Hemodialysis in life-threatening overdose (rarely needed). *Laboratory aids:* Isopropyl alcohol levels, acetone, glucose, and arterial blood gases.

3. *Methanol* (wood alcohol). *Toxic dose:* one teaspoonful is potentially lethal for a 2-year-old and can cause blindness in an adult. The toxic blood level of methanol is above 20 mg per dL, the potentially fatal level over 50 mg per dL. *Manifestations:* Hyperemia of optic disc, violent abdominal colic, blindness, and shock. *Management:* (1) Gastrointestinal decontamination. Activated charcoal and cathartics are not indicated. (2) Treat acidosis vigorously with sodium bicarbonate intravenously. (3) Initiate ethanol therapy (Antidote 20, Table 83-1). (4) Folinic acid and folic acid have been used successfully in animal investigations. (5) Consider hemodialysis if the blood methanol level is greater than 50 mg per dL or if significant metabolic acidosis or visual or mental symptoms are present. *Note:* The ethanol dose has to be increased during dialysis therapy. (6) Ophthalmology consultation. *Laboratory aids:* Methanol and ethanol levels, electrolytes, glucose, and arterial blood gases.

ALKALI

See Caustics and Corrosives.

AMITRIPTYLINE (ELAVIL)

See Tricyclic Antidepressants.

AMPHETAMINES (DIET PILLS, VARIOUS TRADE NAMES)

Toxicity: Child, 5 mg per kg; adult, 12 mg per kg has been reported as lethal. *Toxicokinetics:* Peak time of action is 2 to 4 hours. t½, 8 to 10 hours in acid urine (pH less than 6.0) and 16 to 31 hours in alkaline urine (pH, 7.5). *Route of elimination:* Liver, 60%; kidney, 30 to 40% at alkaline urine pH; at acid urine pH, 50 to 70%. *Manifestations:* Dysrhythmias, hyperpyrexia, convulsions, hypertension, paranoia, violence. *Management:* (1) Gastrointestinal decontamination up to 4 hours. (2) Control extreme agitation or convulsions with diazepam. Chlorpromazine (Thorazine) may be dangerous if ingestion is not pure amphetamine. (3) Treat hypertensive crisis with diazoxide. (4) Acidification diuresis is not recommended. (5) Treat hyperpyrexia symptomatically. (6) If unusual neurologic symptoms are present, consider cerebrovascular accident. (7) Observe for suicidal depression that may follow intoxication. (8) In life-threatening agitation use haloperidol (Haldol). *Laboratory aids:* Monitor for rhabdomyolysis (creatine phosphokinase), myoglobinuria, hyperkalemia, and disseminated intravascular coagulation. Toxic blood level, 10 μg per dL.

ANILINE

See Nitrites and Nitrates.

ANTICHOLINERGIC AGENTS

Examples are antihistamines—hydroxyzine (Atarax), diphenhydramine (Benadryl); antipsychotics (neuroleptics)—phenothiazines (Thorazine); antidepressant drugs (tricyclic antidepressants)—imipramine (Tofranil); antiparkinson drugs—trihexyphenidyl (Artane), benztropine (Cogentin); over-the-counter sleep, cold, and hay fever medicine (methapyrilene); ophthalmic products (atropine); plants—jimsonweed (Datura stramonium), deadly nightshade (Atropa belladonna), henbane (Hyoscyamus niger); and antispasmodic agents for the bowel (atropine). *Toxicokinetics:* See Table 83-2. *Manifestations:* Anticholinergic signs—hyperpyrexia, dilated pupils, flushing of skin, dry mucosa, tachycardia, delirium, hallucinations, coma, and convulsions. *Management:* (1) Gastrointestinal decontamination up to 12 hours postingestion. (2) Control seizures with diazepam. (3) Control ventricular dysrhythmias with lidocaine. (4)

TABLE 83-2. TOXICOKINETICS OF ANTICHOLINERGIC AGENTS

Drug	Potential Fatal Dose	Peak Effect	Vd	t½	Excretion Route
Atropine	Child: 10–20 mg; adult: 100 mg	1–2 hours, may be prolonged in overdose	2.3 liters/kg	2–3 hr	Renal (30–50%) hepatic (50–70%)
Diphenhydramine	20–40 mg/kg; 2 oz has been fatal in 2-year-old	3–4 hours, may be prolonged in overdose	3–4 liters/kg	5–8 hr	Renal (some hepatic)

TABLE 83-3. ANTICONVULSANTS

Drug	Peak Time of Action/Hrs (steady state)	Vd (liters/kg)	t₁/₂ (hr)	Route of Elimination %	Protein-Binding %	Blood Level (µg/ml)	Comment*
Carbamazepine (Tegretol)	6–12 (2–4 days)	0.8–1.4	30–60	Liver (98)	70	Therapeutic, 5–12	Related to tricyclic antidepressants, can cause dysrhythmias
Ethosuximide (Zarontin)	24–48 (5–8 days)	0.6–0.8	24–56	Liver (80–90) Renal (10–20)	0	Therapeutic, 40–100	
Phenytoin (Dilantin)	Oral, 6–12 IV, 1 (5–10 days)	0.6–1.0	20–30; varies in toxic doses: zero order kinetics	Liver (95)	87–93	Therapeutic, 10–20; toxic, 20–30; nystagmus only, 30–40; ataxia, 40 +; coma, convulsions	Dysrhythmias with parenteral use only
Primidone (Mysoline)	3–4? (4–7 days)	0.6	Parent, 3–12; metabolites, 30–36	Liver	70–80	Therapeutic, 8–12 primidone and 10–25 phenobarbital (PB); toxic, over 50 primidone and over 40 PB (see Barbiturates)	Metabolized to active metabolites phenylethylmalonamide and PB; overdose gives white crystals in urine†
Valproic acid (Depakene)	? (1–4 days)	0.3–0.5	8–15	Liver (80–100)	20	Therapeutic, 60–100	Produces nausea and vomiting, changes in liver function
Clonazepam (Clonopin)	(4–12 days)		20–60	Liver (98)	90	Therapeutic, 20–70 ng/mL	

* Manifestations: The major manifestations of these agents are depression of consciousness and respiratory depression. Other significant manifestations are mentioned in this column.

† Primidone produces whorls of shimmering white crystals in the urine from precipitation of intact primidone in massive overdose.

Physostigmine (Antidote 30, Table 83-1) for life-threatening anticholinergic effects refractory to conventional treatments. (5) Treat urinary retention. (6) Treat cardiac dysrhythmias only if patient tissue perfusion is not adequate or if the patient is hypotensive.

ANTICONVULSANTS

See Table 83-3. *Toxic dose:* Specific anticonvulsant blood levels and the clinical manifestations will indicate toxicity. In general, the ingestion of five times the therapeutic dose is expected to have the potential for toxicity. *Management:* (1) Gastrointestinal decontamination up to 12 hours postingestion. (2) Monitor specific anticonvulsant blood levels. (3) The effectiveness of hemoperfusion and dialysis has not been established.

ANTIDEPRESSANTS

See Tricyclic Antidepressants.

ANTIFREEZE

See Alcohols (Methanol) and Ethylene Glycol.

ANTIHISTAMINES

See Anticholinergic Agents.

ARSENIC AND ARSINE GAS

Toxic dose: In humans, the inorganic arsenic trioxide toxic dose is 5 to 50 mg; the potential fatal dose is 120 mg. Organic arsenic is less toxic. The maximum allowable concentration for prolonged exposure is 0.05 PPM. See Table 83-4. Humans are more sensitive than rodents to arsenic. Acute poisoning results from accidental ingestion of arsenic-containing pesticides. (Ant traps sold in some states contain arsenic.) *Toxicokinetics:* Rapidly absorbed by inhalation and ingestion. Crosses placenta and can cause fetal damage. Distributes into spleen, liver, kidneys. *Excretion:* In

TABLE 83-4. COMPARATIVE ACUTE TOXICITIES OF SOME COMMON ARSENICALS

Arsenical	Oral LD$_{50}$ in Rats (mg/kg)	Estimated Mortality in Human Poisoning (%)
Arsenic trioxide	385	12
Sodium arsenite	42	65
Calcium arsenite	ca. 275	?
Lead arsenite	1500+	5
Ortho Crabgrass Killer*	3719	None known

* Product containing 8% each of only mildly toxic octyl NH$_4$ and dodecyl NH$_4$ methanearsonate.

With permission from Done, A. K.: . . . And old lace. Emergency Med. 5:246, 1973.

urine, 90%. Following acute ingestion, it takes 10 days to clear a single dose; after chronic ingestion it takes up to 70 days. *Arsine gas:* Forms when active hydrogen comes in contact with arsenic. This may occur when zinc, antimony, lead, or iron is contaminated with arsenic and comes in contact with acid. This causes arsine inhalation intoxication, characterized by a latent period of 2 to 48 hours and a triad of abdominal pain, jaundice (from hemolysis), and hematuria. *Manifestations:* Gastroenteritis, neurologic and cardiac abnormalities, subsequent renal involvement. A garlic odor on the breath may be a clue. Smaller doses and prolonged low-level exposure produce subacute (stomatitis) and chronic (peripheral neuropathy) symptoms.

Management: (1) Gastrointestinal decontamination. Follow with abdominal radiographs; arsenic is radiopaque. (2) Intravenous fluids to correct dehydration and electrolyte deficiencies. (3) Treat shock with oxygen, blood, and fluids as needed. (4) In severe cases, administer BAL (dimercaprol) (Antidote 17, Table 83-1). (5) In chronic poisoning, D-penicillamine (Antidote 29, Table 83-1) may be used to chelate arsenic. Therapy should be continued until the urine arsenic is less than 50 mg per liter. (6) Hemodialysis is effective in acute poisoning and can be used concurrently with chelation therapy in severe cases, especially if renal failure develops. (7) Arsine intoxication is treated by exchange transfusion and hemodialysis if renal failure occurs. BAL is ineffective. *Laboratory aids:* Blood arsenic and 24-hour urine arsenic levels. Excessive exposure is indicated by a level of 50 μg per liter of arsenic in urine, but persons whose diets are rich in seafood may excrete 200 μg per day. View values over 100 μg per day with suspicion. Monitor electrocardiogram (ECG) and renal function. Normal blood arsenic level is less than 7 μg per dL (false values occur in inexperienced laboratories).

ASPIRIN

See Salicylates.

ATROPINE

See Anticholinergic Agents.

BARBITURATES

See Table 83-5. *Management:* (1) Gastrointestinal decontamination up to 8 to 12 hours. Activated charcoal and a cathartic in repeated doses have been shown to reduce the serum half-life and increase the nonrenal clearance over 50%. Give every 4 hours while the patient is comatose. (2) Supportive and symptomatic care is all that is necessary in most cases. (3) Forced alkaline diuresis (if the patient is not in shock) for phenobarbital intoxication. Sodium bicarbonate, 44 to 88 mEq/liter, and potassium chloride, 20 mEq/liter, should be given at a rate to produce a urine flow of 3 to 6 mL per kg per hour and a urine pH of 7 to 8. Additional sodium bicarbonate (1 to 2 mEq/kg) and potassium chloride (20 to 40 mEq/liter) may be needed to achieve an optimal urine pH. Ensure adequate hydration and renal function before alkalinization. Not useful for other barbiturates (Antidote 35, Table 83-1). (4) In severe cases that do not respond to conservative measures, consider hemodialysis and hemoperfusion. (5) Treat any bullae as a local second degree skin burn. (6) Give intensive care monitoring to comatose patient. *Treatment of withdrawal: In an emergency,* use pentothal or diazepam intravenously. If the patient is stable, a pentobarbital tolerance test may be given; 200 mg of pentobarbital is given orally and the patient examined after 1 hour for signs of intoxication (nystagmus, slurred speech, and ataxia). If none are present, the dose is repeated every 3 hours until these signs develop. This is the stabilizing dose; the patient is maintained on this dose for 72 hours and then changed to phenobarbital, 30 mg substituted for each 100 mg of pentobarbital. The phenobarbital is tapered, decreasing by 10% or 30 mg every 3 to 5 days. *Laboratory aids:* Emergency plasma barbiturate concentrations rarely alter management.

TABLE 83-5. BARBITURATES: EXAMPLES AND ELIMINATION*

	Long-Acting		Intermediate*	Short-Acting	
Generic name	Barbital	Phenobarbital	Amobarbital	Pentobarbital	Secobarbital
Trade name	Veronal	Luminal	Amytal	Nembutal	Seconal
Slang name	—	Purple hearts	Blue heaven	Yellow jackets	Red devils
pK$_a$	7.74	7.24	7.25	7.96	7.9
Detoxification	Renal	Renal 30% Hepatic 70%	Hepatic 98%	Hepatic 90–100%	Hepatic 90–100%
Onset: IV	22 min	12 min	—	0.1 min	0.1 min
PO	Over 6 hr	3–6 hr (peak 12–18 hr)	Less than 3 hr (peak 3–4 hr)	10–15 min (peak 2–4 hr)	10–15 min (peak 2–4 hr)
Protein-binding (%)	5	29	—	35	44
Hypnotic dose (mg)	300–500	100–200	50–200	50–100	50–100
Fatal dose (grams)	10	8	5	3	3
Toxic dose (mg/kg)	8	8	3–5	3–5	3–5
Therapeutic level (μg/mL)	5–8	15–35	5–8	1–4	3–5
Toxic level (μg/mL)	Over 30	Over 40	10–30	Over 10	Over 10
Lethal level† (μg/mL)	Over 100	Over 100	Over 50	Over 35	Over 35
Duration of action	Over 6	Over 6	Less than 3	Less than 3	Less than 3
Half-life (hr)	58–96	24–96	16–24	36–50	25–50
Rate of metabolism (hr)	—	0.7	2.5	—	—
Volume distribution liter/kg	—	0.75	0.5–1.1	0.65–1.5	0.65–1.5

Manifestations

    Low dose: Euphoria, ataxia, incoordination, nystagmus on lateral gaze

    High dose: Flaccid coma, hypotension, respiratory depression, pulmonary edema (particularly with the short-acting barbiturates), subcutaneous bullae (6%), dermatographia

* Classification into long-acting, intermediate, and short-acting has no relationship to the duration of coma.

† These levels are not absolute, and tolerance occurs.

BENZENE

See Hydrocarbons.

BENZODIAZEPINES (BZP)

See Table 83-6. *Toxicity:* Low toxic potential. More than 500 mg has been ingested without respiratory depression. Benzodiazepines have an additive effect with sedatives such as alcohol and barbiturates. Most patients intoxicated with BZP alone recover within 24 hours. Many of these agents have active metabolites with a long plasma t$\frac{1}{2}$, so performance in skilled tasks such as driving may be impaired. Withdrawal may be delayed. *Manifestations:* Central nervous system depression. Deep coma leading to respiratory depression suggests presence of other drugs. *Management:* (1) Gastrointestinal decontamination. (2) Supportive and symptomatic care. (3) Withdrawal, if it occurs, is treated with a long-acting benzodiazepine on a tapering schedule. *Laboratory aids:* Document benzodiazepines in urine. Quantitative blood levels are not useful.

BLEACH

Household bleaches are 4 to 6% sodium hypochlorite. Commercial types are 10 to 20%. *Manifestations:* Difficulty in swallowing; pain in mouth, throat, chest, or abdomen. General household strength bleach does not produce burns; commercial strength bleach may. Inhalation of gases produced by mixing chlorine bleach with acids (toilet bowel cleaner and rust removers—chlorine gas) or with household ammonia (chloramine gas) is irritating to mucous membranes, eyes, and upper respiratory tract. *Management:* (1) Ingestion—Do not induce emesis. Dilute with water or milk. Avoid acids. (2) Esophagoscopy only if unusually large amounts have been ingested, the patient is symptomatic, or the product was stronger than the average household bleach. (3) Inhalation—Remove from contaminated area. Observe for pulmonary edema.

BOTULISM

See article on foodborne illnesses in Chapter 86.

BRAKE FLUID

See Ethylene Glycol.

CALCIUM CHANNEL BLOCKERS

Used in treatment of effort angina and supraventricular tachycardia. See Table 83-7. *Manifestations:* Hy-

TABLE 83-6. BENZODIAZEPINES (BZP)

Drug	Oral Dosage Range	Peak oral Plasma levels (*hr*)	Half-Life (*hr*)	Major Active Metabolites (*half-life in hr*)	Elimination Rate
ANXIOLYTICS					
Diazepam (Valium)	6–40 mg/day	1–2	20–50	Desmethyldiazepam (30–60)	Slow
Chlordiazepoxide (Librium, Libritabs, various others)	15–100 mg/day	2–4	5–30	Desmethylchlordiazepoxide, demoxepam, desmethyldiazepam	Slow
Clorazepate (Tranxene)	15–60 mg/day	—	30–60	Desmethyldiazepam	Slow
Prazepam (Centrax)	20–60 mg/day	6	78	3-Hydroxyprazepam, desmethyldiazepam	Slow
Halazepam (Paxipam)	60–160 mg/day	1–3	7	N-3-Hydroxyhalazepam, desmethyldiazepam	Slow
Oxazepam (Serax)	30–120 mg/day	1–2	5–10	None	Rapid to intermediate
Lorazepam (Ativan)	2–6 mg/day	2	10–20	None	Intermediate
Alprazolam (Xanax)	0.75–4 mg/day	0.7–1.6	12–19	α-Hydroxyalprazolam	Intermediate
HYPNOTICS					
Flurazepam (Dalmane)	15–60 mg	—	50–100	Desalkylflurazepam (50–100)	Slow
Flunitrazepam (Rohypnol—investigational Roche)	1—2 mg	< 1	—	7-Aminoflunitrazepam (23) N-Desmethylflunitrazepam (31)	—
Temazepam (Restoril)	15–30 mg	2–3	9–12	None	Intermediate
Triazolam (Halcion)	0.125–0.5 mg	0.5–1.5	2.3	α-Hydroxytriazolam	Rapid

TABLE 83-7. CALCIUM CHANNEL BLOCKERS

	Nifedipine	Verapamil	Diltiazem
Trade name	Procardia	Calan, Isoptin	Cardiazem
Onset of action	Oral: < 20 min sublingual: < 3 min IV: < 1 min	Oral: < 1 hr — IV: < 2 min	Oral: < 15 min — —
Peak effect	Oral: 1–2 hr	5 hr	30 min
Half-life (hr)	2.5–5	2–7	2–6
Route of elimination	Liver/kidney	Liver/kidney	Liver/kidney
Toxic level (ng/mL)	> 100	> 300	> 200

potension, bradycardia within 1 to 5 hours, central nervous system depression, and gastric distress. *Management:* (1) Gastrointestinal decontamination. (2) Treat hypotension and bradycardia with calcium gluconate or chloride. See Antidote 12B, Table 83-1. Dopamine may be used if necessary. (3) Heart block—may respond to IV calcium, atropine sulfate, 0.5 to 1 mg, or isoproterenol. (4) Ventricular pacing may be required in the severely intoxicated patient. (5) Patients receiving digitalis run the risk of toxicity and should be carefully monitored. *Laboratory aids:* Specific drug levels, blood sugar and calcium, ECG.

CAMPHOR

(External analgesic rubs, Vicks Vaporub 4.8%, Campho-Phenique, 11%). Many camphorated oil products were removed from the marketplace in September, 1982. Five milliliters of camphorated oil (20% camphor)

TABLE 83-8. CARBON MONOXIDE (CO)

CO in Atmosphere	Duration of Exposure	Saturation of Blood (%)	Symptoms
Up to 0.01	Indefinite	1–10	None
0.01–0.02	Indefinite	10–20	Tightness across forehead, slight headache, dilation of cutaneous vessels
0.02–0.03	5–6 hr	20–30	Headache, throbbing temples
0.04–0.06	4–5 hr	30–40	Severe headache, weakness and dizziness, nausea and vomiting, collapse, leukocytosis
0.07–0.10	3–4 hr	40–50	Above, plus increased tendency to collapse and syncope, increased pulse and respiratory rate
0.11–0.15	1.5–3 hr	50–60	Increased pulse and respiratory rate, syncope, Cheyne-Stokes respiration, coma with intermittent convulsions
0.16–0.30	1–1.5 hr	60–70	Coma with intermittent convulsions, depressed heart action and respirations, death possible
0.50–1.00	1–2 min	70–80	Weak pulse, depressed respirations, respiratory failure and death

equals 1 g of camphor. *Toxicity:* Adult, 5 g; child, 1 g has been fatal. *Toxicokinetics:* Onset of manifestations, 5 to 90 minutes. Readily and rapidly absorbed through the skin, mucous membranes, and gastrointestinal tract and crosses the placenta. Route of elimination: Rapidly metabolized in liver to the glucuronide form, which is excreted in urine. Pulmonary excretion causes a distinctive odor on the breath. *Manifestations:* Nausea, vomiting, and burning epigastric pain. Seizures may occur suddenly and without warning within 5 minutes of ingestion. Apnea and vision disturbances may occur. *Management:* (1) Induction of emesis is contraindicated because of early seizures. (2) Remove residual drug by gastric lavage. (3) Administer activated charcoal and a saline cathartic. Avoid giving oils or alcohol. (4) Treat seizures with IV diazepam. (5) Treat apnea with respiratory support.

CARBON MONOXIDE (CO)

This is an odorless gas produced from incomplete combustion; it is found also as an in vivo metabolic breakdown product of methylene chloride (paint removers). Observe for the symptoms described in Table 83-8. Contrary to popular belief, the skin rarely shows a cherry-red color in the live patient. *Toxicokinetics:* CO is rapidly absorbed through the lungs. The rate of absorption is directly related to alveolar ventilation. Elimination occurs through the lungs. The t½ in room air equals 5 to 6 hours; in 100% oxygen, 90 minutes; in hyperbaric oxygen, 20 minutes. The nomogram pictured in Figure 83-2 can be used to decide quickly whether serious CO intoxication is likely to have occurred and to select patients at high risk or who need early management in the intensive care unit or hyperbaric oxygen.

Management: (1) Remove the patient from contaminated area and expose to fresh air. Establish vital functions. (2) Give 100% oxygen to all patients until the carboxyhemoglobin level falls to 5 to 10%. Assisted ventilation may be necessary. (3) Monitor arterial blood gases and carboxyhemoglobin levels. Determine carboxyhemoglobin level at time of exposure by using nomogram. *Note:* A near normal carboxyhemoglobin level does not rule out significant CO poisoning. (4) Only if pH is below 7.1 after correction of hypoxia and adequate ventilation, give sodium bicarbonate to correct acidosis. (5) Consider hyperbaric oxygen for patients with carboxyhemoglobin over 25%, or over 15% if patient is pregnant, is a child, has cardiac or liver disease, or has a disturbance in mentation. (6) Treat seizures with intravenous diazepam. (7) Monitor electrocardiogram, chest radiograph and serum creatine phosphokinase (CPK), and lactate dehydrogenase (LDH) levels. (8) Treat cerebral edema with elevation of the patient's head, minimizing intravenous fluid, hyperventilation, and if needed, mannitol and intracranial pressure monitor. (9) Reevaluate after recovery for neuropsychiatric sequelae. *Laboratory aids:* Arterial blood gases show metabolic acidosis and normal oxygen tension but reduced oxygen saturation.

CARBON TETRACHLORIDE

See Hydrocarbons.

CAUSTICS AND CORROSIVES

Common acid substances are hydrochloric acid, sulfuric acid (battery acid), carbolic acid (phenol), nitric acid, oxalic acid, hydrofluoric acid, and aqua regia (mixture of hydrochloric and nitric acids). These are used as cleaning agents. Common alkali substances are sodium or potassium hydroxide (lye), sodium hypochlorite (Clorox) (bleach), sodium carbonate (nonphosphate detergents), potassium permanganate,

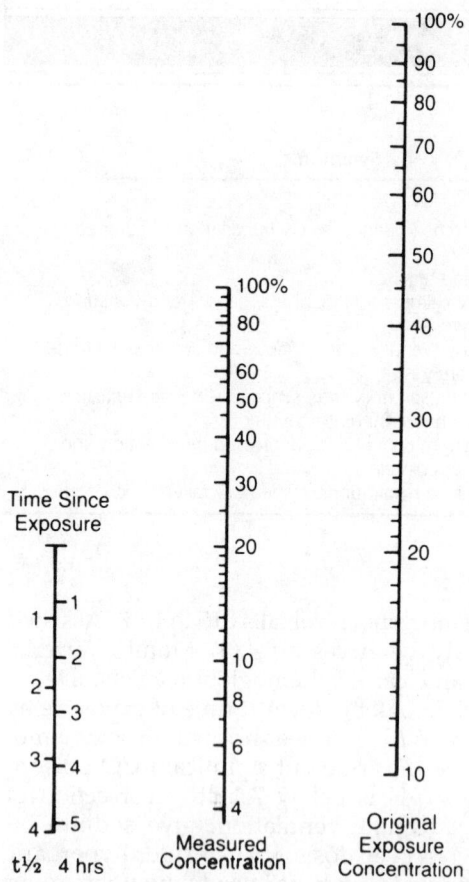

FIG. 83-2. Nomogram for calculating carboxyhemoglobin concentration at time of exposure. The time since exposure is given on two scales to allow for the effects of previous oxygen administration on the half-life of carboxyhemoglobin (left-hand scale assumes a half-life of 3 hours). *Note:* The nomogram assumes a half-life of carboxyhemoglobin of 4 hours in a subject breathing room air. Most patients have not received supplementary oxygen before admission, and at best this will have been administered by means of a face mask, giving a maximum fractional inspired oxygen concentration of 50 to 60% with little effect on carboxyhemoglobin elimination. The scale on the left side of the time column makes allowances for prior oxygen supplements by assuming a short half-life of 3 hours. The nomogram may help decide quickly whether serious carbon monoxide intoxication is likely to have occurred and may help select patients at high risk for early management in the intensive care unit. The nomogram may be an oversimplification because patients usually are not resuscitated with constant concentrations of oxygen, and many patients may hyperventilate, thus changing elimination characteristics. (Redrawn from Clark et al: Blood carboxyhemoglobin and cyanide levels in fire. Lancet 1:1332, 1981.)

ammonia, electric dishwashing agents, cement, and flat disk batteries. *Toxicity:* Acids produce mucosal coagulation necrosis. They usually do not penetrate deeply (exception: hydrofluoric acid). The gastric mucosa is the primary site of injury. Alkalis produce liquefaction necrosis and saponification and penetrate deeply. Oropharyngeal and esophageal damage by solids is more frequent than by liquids. Liquids are more likely to produce gastric damage. *Toxic dose:* Adult potential fatal dose of concentrated acid/alkali

is 5 mL. The absence of oral burns does not exclude the possibility of esophageal burns (10 to 15%).

Management: (1) Dilute with milk or water immediately, up to 30 mL in children or 250 mL in adults. Neutralization with acidic or alkaline agents is contraindicated. Dilute only if patient can swallow. (2) Gastrointestinal decontamination is contraindicated. In acid ingestions, however, some authorities advocate nasogastric intubation and aspiration in the early postingestion phase. Patients should receive only intravenous fluids following dilution until surgical consultation is obtained. Dermal and ocular decontamination should be carried out. (3) Esophagoscopy may be indicated postingestion to assess severity of burn. (4) Steroids are controversial. Some recommend administration of steroids if burns are found or esophagoscopy is not performed. (5) Antibiotics are not useful prophylactically. (6) Barium swallow may be necessary at 10 days to 3 weeks to assess severity of damage. (7) Esophageal dilation may need to be performed at 2- to 4-week intervals if evidence of stricture is found. (8) Intraposition of the colon may be necessary if dilation fails to provide an adequate-sized esophagus. (9) Inhalation management requires immediate removal from the environment, and clinical, x-ray, and arterial blood gas evaluation when appropriate. Oxygen and respiratory support may be required.

CHLORAL HYDRATE

See Sedative Hypnotics.

CHLORDANE

See Organochlorine Insecticides.

CHLORDIAZEPOXIDE (LIBRIUM)

See Benzodiazepines.

CHLORINE GAS

Chlorine gas is a yellow-greenish gas with an irritating odor, used in bleach, in manufacture of plastics, and for water purification. Exposure usually results from transportation mishaps, industrial accidents, chemistry experiments, the mixing of household cleaners with bleach containing hypochlorite, and accidental release around swimming pools. Its density is greater than that of air, and an odor is detected at concentrations of less than 0.5 PPM. Chlorine acts as an oxidizing agent and also acts with tissue water to form hypochlorite and hydrochloric acid and generate free oxygen radicals. *Toxic dose and management:* The threshold limit value is less than 1 PPM; 4 PPM is tolerated for 0.5 hour; 15 PPM immediately irritates mucous membranes of eyes, ears, nose, and throat; 30 PPM

TABLE 83-9. PHARMACO-TOXICOKINETICS OF COCAINE

Type	Route	Onset	Peak	Duration t½ (min)	Possible Fatal Dose (Adult)
Hydrochloride	Insufflation	1–5 min	20–60 min	60–75	750–800 mg
	Ingested	Delayed	30–90 min	60–75	1.4 grams
	IV	2–3 min	30–60 min	60–75	20–800 mg
Free base	Smoked	< 2 min	seconds	< 20	750–800 mg
Coca paste	Smoked			Not known	
Crack	Smoked	(Fastest) 4–6 sec	seconds	< 20 5–7	Not known

produces choking and chest pain; 60 PPM produces pulmonary edema; 400 PPM for 30 minutes is lethal; and 1000 PPM is fatal in a few minutes.

Management: (1) Remove the patient from contaminated environment and stabilize vital functions. Decontamination procedures for dermal and ocular contamination as indicated. Protect rescue personnel with breathing apparatus. Classification—If symptomless or with a cough that clears up in less than 1 hour, rest for 12 hours and report if symptoms occur; no vigorous exercise for 24 hours. If symptoms persist beyond period of exposure, admit to hospital and treat with bronchodilators (theophylline or albuterol, not epinephrine) and humidified oxygen. Noncardiac pulmonary edema is treated with positive end-expiratory pressure; corticosteroids are controversial; furosemide (Lasix) may be used. For conjunctival irritation, copious water irrigation and fluorescein stain for corneal damage. For dermal burns, copious water irrigation and conventional treatment of burns. *Laboratory aids:* Chest radiograph (may not reflect damage for 24 hours), arterial blood gases, cardiac monitor for dysrhythmias.

CHLORPROMAZINE (THORAZINE)

See Phenothiazines.

CLINITEST TABLETS

See Caustics and Corrosives.

COCAINE (BENZOYLMETHYLECGONINE

Toxic dose: The potential fatal dose is 1200 mg, but death has occurred with 20 mg parenterally. *Toxicokinetics:* See Table 83-9. *Manifestations:* Hypertension, convulsions, hyperthermia, and cardiac dysrhythmias. *Management:* (1) Supportive care. Cardiac and thermal monitoring. Phenytoin may be effective for ventricular dysrhythmias, whereas lidocaine may be ineffective and enhance toxicity. Control anxiety and convulsions with diazepam. Labetalol intravenously

(Antidote 23, Table 83-1) has been used to control life-threatening hypertension and tachycardia. A non-threatening environment to reduce all sensory stimuli and protect patient from injury is required.

CODEINE

See Opioids.

CORROSIVES

See Caustics and Corrosives.

CYANIDE

See Table 83-10. Hydrocyanic acid and sodium and potassium salts act rapidly and are extremely poisonous. The acid is extremely volatile, producing cyanide, which has a distinctive odor of bitter almonds and can produce death within minutes after inhalation. Cyanide interferes with the cytochrome oxidase system. *Classes of cyanides and derivatives:* (1) Hydrogen cyanide and simple salts in large doses act to produce death in 15 minutes. (2) Halogenated cyanides such as cyanogen chloride produce irritant and vesicant gases that may cause pulmonary edema. (3) Nitriles such as acrylonitrile and acetonitrile. Cyanides are used as fumigants (hydrogen cyanide), in synthetic rubber (acrylonitrile), in fertilizers (cyanamide), in metal refining (salts), and in the home in some silver and furniture polishes. Cyanide in the seeds of fruit stones is harmful only if the capsule is broken. *Manifestations:* Seizures, stupor, cardiac dysrhythmias, pulmonary edema, lactic acidemia, decreased arterial venous oxygen difference. Bright red venous blood.

Management: Attendants should not administer mouth-to-mouth resuscitation. (1) Immediately, 100% oxygen. If inhaled, remove patient from contaminated atmosphere. (2) Cyanide antidote kite (Antidote 14, Table 83-1). Use antidote only if certain of diagnosis and significant toxicity (impairment of consciousness). (3) Gastrointestinal decontamination by gastric lavage.

Toxicology

TABLE 83-10. FORMS OF CYANIDE AND THEIR TOXICITY

Common Forms	Toxicity
Hydrocyanic acid	PFD* = 50 mg (0.5 mg/kg)
Potassium/sodium cyanide	PFD = 150–300 mg (2 mg/kg)
Calcium and ferric or ferrocyanides	Low order of toxicity; PFD = 50 g
Sodium nitroprusside	5 mg/kg causes acute toxicity; PFD = 3–4 g (195–260 mg)
Bitter almonds	
Oil	2 oz kills immediately
Almonds	50–60 bitter almonds; each contain 0.001 gram of hydrogen cyanide
Pulp	240 grams
Peach seed	100 grams of moist seeds = 88 mg of cyanide
Apricot	
Wild	100 grams of moist seed = 217 mg of cyanide
Cultivated	100 grams = 8.7 mg of cyanide
Laetrile (amygdalin); cyanogenic glycoside in kernels of apricots	
Laetrile strengths:	HCN in mg/g
tablets: 250 mg	2.7
tablets: 500 mg	29–51.5
parenteral 10 mL, 3 g vial	23.2–27.9
Amygdaline, parenteral, 10 mL, 3 g vial	8.3–51.3
Hydrogen cyanide inhalation; acrylonitrile, cyanamide, cyanogen chloride, cyanides, nitroprussides (produced in fire involving polyurethane foams)	Maximum allowable concentration, 10 PPM TLV* = 5 mg/m³ in air for cyanide salts 0.2–0.3 mg/liter is immediately fatal 0.13 mg/liter (130 PPM) is fatal in 1 hour
Hydrogen cyanide liquid	Rapidly absorbed through skin

*PFD, Potential fatal dose; TLV, Threshold limit values.

TABLE 83-11. DIGITALIS PREPARATIONS

	Digoxin	Digitoxin
Trade name	Lanoxin	Crystodigin
Onset time po	1.5–6 hr	3–6 hr
Peak	4–6	6–12
Half-life	31–40 hr	4–6 days
Protein-bound (%)	25	90
Vd	7–8 liters/kg	0.6 liter/kg
Route of elimination	Renal, 75%	Liver, 80%
Toxic blood levels	2.4 ng/ml	> 30 ng/ml
Enterohepatic route	Small	Large

No syrup of ipecac. Activated charcoal not very effective (1 g binds only 35 mg of cyanide). (4) Treat seizures with intravenous diazepam. (5) Correct acidosis. (6) Other antidotes: In Europe, dicobalt edetate, 600 mg, is used intravenously, followed by 300 mg if the response is not satisfactory. Hydroxycobalamin (vitamin B_{12}) is a useful antidote but must be given immediately after exposure in very large doses. Dose: 1800 mg of vitamin B_{12} per dL of KCN is usually required (forms cyanocobalamin).

DDT AND DERIVATIVES

See Organochlorine Insecticides.

DESIPRAMINE (NORPRAMIN, PERTOFRANE)

See Tricyclic Antidepressants.

DIAZEPAM (VALIUM)

See Benzodiazepines.

DIGITALIS PREPARATIONS

See Table 83-11. *Manifestations:* Abdominal pain, nausea, vomiting, diarrhea, dysrhythmias, heart block, central nervous system depression, colored-halo vision. *Management:* (1) Gastrointestinal decontamination. Repeated doses of activated charcoal may interrupt enterohepatic recirculation. (2) Treat ventricular premature contractions, including bigeminy, trigeminy, quadrigeminy, ventricular tachycardia, and atrial tachycardia, with phenytoin. Lidocaine also may be administered for ventricular dysrhythmias. (3) Treat bradycardia and second and third degree AV block with atropine. External pacing may be needed. (4) Treat hyperkalemia (above 6 mEq/liter with intravenous glucose 5 to 10 per cent, intravenous sodium bicarbonate, intravenous insulin (insulin is not used in children), and Kayexalate retention enema (25% in sorbitol 25%) in severe cases. If hyperkalemia is present (ominous sign), insertion of a pacemaker should be seriously considered. Hemodialysis is the treatment of choice for severe or refractory hyperkalemia. (5) Direct current countershock may cause life-threatening dysrhythmias. (6) Specific Fab antibody fragments (Digibind) (Antidote 21, Table 83-1) have been used for life-threatening cardiac dysrhythmias, hyperkalemia, and cases refractory to conventional measures. *Laboratory aids:* Monitor ECG and potassium and digitalis levels. Draw digoxin levels 6 to 8 hours postingestion.

DIPHENHYDRAMINE (BENADRYL)

See Anticholinergic Agents.

DOXEPIN (SINEQUAN, ADAPIN)

See Tricyclic Antidepressants.

ETHCHLORVYNOL (PLACIDYL)

See Sedative Hypnotics.

ETHYL ALCOHOL

See Alcohols.

ETHYLENE GLYCOL (SOLVENT, ANTIFREEZE)

Toxic dose: Death has occurred after a 60 mL ingestion; fatal dose = 1.4 mL per kg of 100% solution. The threshold limit value (TLV) is 50 PPM. *Toxicokinetics:* Time of onset, 30 minutes to 12 hours for central nervous system and metabolic abnormalities to occur (Phase I). Twelve to 36 hours postingestion, cardiopulmonary depression (Phase II). In Phase III (2 to 3 days postingestion), renal failure occurs. The $t\frac{1}{2}$ is 3 hours (during ethanol therapy this is prolonged to 17 hours). *Management:* (1) Gastrointestinal decontamination up to 2 to 4 hours postingestion. Activated charcoal and cathartics are not indicated. (2) Treat seizures with intravenous diazepam. Exclude hypocalcemia. (3) Correct acidosis with intravenous sodium bicarbonate. (4) Initiate ethanol therapy to block metabolism (Antidote 20, Table 83-1). (5) Early hemodialysis is indicated if the ingestion was large; if the blood ethylene glycol level is greater than 50 mg per dL, if severe acid-base or electrolyte abnormalities occur despite conventional therapy; or if renal failure occurs. (6) Thiamine and pyridoxine have been recommended but not extensively studied. (7) Use of 4-methylpyrazole, an inhibitor of alcoholic dehydroxygenase, may be used early (before renal impairment). *Laboratory aids:* Complete blood count, electrolytes, urinalysis (look for oxalate crystals), and arterial blood gases. Obtain ethylene glycol and ethanol levels, plasma osmolarity (use freezing point depression method). Calcium, creatinine, and BUN studies. An ethylene glycol level of 100 mg per dL is usually toxic (levels are very difficult to obtain).

FLURAZEPAM (DALMANE)

See Benzodiazepines.

GLUTETHIMIDE (DORIDEN)

See Sedative Hypnotics.

HALLUCINOGENS

1. *LSD* (lysergic acid diethylamide). *Toxic dose:* ≥ 35 μg. Street doses are typically 50 to 300 μg. *Toxicokinetics:* Peak effect, 1 to 2 hours. Duration, 12 to 24 hours, $t\frac{1}{2}$, 3 hours. Route of elimination, bile.

2. *Morning-Glory Seeds* (*Rivea corymbosa* or *Ipomoea*). These have one-tenth the potency of LSD.

3. *Mescaline/Peyote* (trimethoxyphenylethylamine or *Lophophora williamsii*). *Toxic dose:* ≥ 5 mg per kg. Each button of mescaline contains 45 mg (4 to 12 produce symptoms). *Toxicokinetics:* Peak effect, 4 to 6 hours. Duration, 14 hours.

4. *Psilocybin.* Similar in effect to LSD but short-acting. Peak effect, 90 minutes. Duration, 5 to 6 hours.

5. *Nutmeg* (*Myristica*). *Toxic dose:* 5 to 15 grams (1 to 3 nutmegs). Peak effect, 3 to 6 hours. Duration, up to 60 hours.

6. *Marijuana* (*Cannabis sativa*) (δ-9-tetrahydrocannabinol, THC). One joint equals 500 mg of marijuana; when smoked, 50% is destroyed. *Toxicokinetics:* Time of onset, 2 to 3 minutes (smoked). Duration, 2 to 3 hours, $t\frac{1}{2}$, 28 to 47 hours (shorter for chronic user). *Note:* 1% of the metabolite can be detected in urine up to 2 weeks after use. *Manifestations:* Visual illusions, sensory perceptual distortions, depersonalization, and derealization. *Management:* "Talk-down" technique.

7. *Inhalants.* Nitrites (amyl and isobutyl nitrite)—act immediately; aromatic hydrocarbon in airplane model glues, plastic cements (benzene, toluene, xylene)—see hydrocarbons; *nitrous oxide* and *halogenated hydrocarbons.*

8. *Tryptamine Derivatives* (DMT, dimethyltryptamine; DET, diethyltryptamine; DPT, dipropyltryptamine). Rapid onset of action, but duration is only 1 to 2 hours.

9. *STP* or *DOM* (2,5-dimethoxy-4-methyl-amphetamine). Acts like LSD but lasts 72 hours or longer.

10. *MDA* (3-methoxy-4,5-ethylenedioxy amphetamine). Related to amphetamine, produces a mild LSD-like reaction lasting 6 to 10 hours (love pill).

See also Alcohols, Amphetamines, Anticholinergic Agents, Barbiturates, Cocaine, Opioids, Phencyclidine, Phenothiazines, and Tricyclic Antidepressants.

HALOPERIDOL (HALDOL)

See Phenothiazines.

HEROIN

See Opioids.

TABLE 83-12. COMMON EXAMPLES OF ALIPHATIC HALOGENATED HYDROCARBONS

	Estimated Fatal Dose (Ingested)	TLV-TWA (PPM)	Synonyms
Trichloroethane 1, 1, 1	5.7 g/kg	350	Methyl chloroform, Triethane, chlorethane, Glamorene Spot Remover, Scotchgard
Trichloroethane 1, 1, 2	580 mg/kg	10	Vinyl trichloride
Trichloroethylene	Controversial, 3–5 mL/kg	50	—
Tetrachloroethanene	Not known	5	Acetylene tetrachloride
Dichloromethane	25 mL	100	Methylene chloride
Tetrachloroethylene	5 mL	50	Tetrachloroethene Perchloroethylene
Dichloroethane	0.5 mL/kg	200	—
Carbon tetrachloride	3–5 mL	5	—

HYDROCARBONS

1. *Petroleum Distillates.* Gasoline (petroleum spirit), 2 to 5% benzene; kerosenes (coal oil, kerosene, jet aviation fuel No. 1, charcoal lighter fluid); petroleum naphtha (cigarette lighter fluid, ligroin, racing fuel); petroleum ether (benzene); turpentine (pine oil, oil of turpentine); and mineral spirits (Stoddard solvent, white spirits, varasol, mineral turpentine, petroleum spirit). *Manifestations:* Materials aspirated during the process of ingestion may produce pneumonitis. Hypoxia associated with aspiration is the cause of central nervous system depression, not absorption. It is *unlikely* that a child accidentally or an adult during siphoning would ingest a sufficient quantity to warrant the induction of emesis.

2. *Aromatic Hydrocarbons. Benzene,* a solvent used in manufacturing dyes, phenol, and nitrobenzene, has a threshold limit value (TLV) of 10 PPM by inhalation according to the Occupational Safety and Health Administration (OSHA). The National Institute for Occupational Safety and Health (NIOSH) value is 1 PPM. The adult ingested toxic dose is 15 mL. Chronic exposure may cause leukemia. Two hundred PPM is fatal in 5 minutes. *Toluene,* used in manufacturing TNT, has an OSHA TLV of 200 PPM by inhalation; the NIOSH figure is 100. The adult ingested toxic dose is 50 mL. *Styrene* has an OSHA TLV of 100 PPM by inhalation. *Xylene,* used in the manufacture of perfumes, has an OSHA TLV of 100 PPM by inhalation. The adult ingested toxic dose is 50 mL. *Manifestations:* Asphyxiation, central nervous system depression, defatting dermatitis, and aspiration pneumonitis. A bite into a tube of household plastic cement by a young child does not warrant the induction of emesis. Ingestion of hydrocarbon with a benzene fraction over 5% may warrant induction of emesis.

3. *Aliphatic Halogenated Hydrocarbons.* See Table 83-12 for common examples. *Manifestations:* Myocardial sensitization and irritability, hepatorenal toxicity, and central nervous system depression. Dichloromethane may be converted into carbon monoxide in the body. Trichloroethylene concentrates in the fetus (pregnant women should not be exposed) and causes a disulfiram (Antabuse) reaction ("degreaser's flush") when associated with ingestion of ethanol. The decision to induce emesis must be based on the toxicity of the agent.

4. *Dangerous Additives.* Dangerous additives to the hydrocarbons, such as heavy metals, nitrobenzene, aniline dyes, insecticides and demothing agents, may warrant the induction of emesis.

5. *Heavy Hydrocarbons.* These have high viscosity, low volatility, and minimal absorption, so emesis is unwarranted. Examples are asphalt (tar), machine oil, motor oil, (lubricating oil, engine oil), diesel oil (engine fuel, home heating oil), petrolatum liquid (mineral oil, suntan oils), petrolatum jelly (Vaseline), paraffin wax, transmission oil, cutting oil, and greases and glues.

6. *Products Treated as Petroleum Distillates.* Essential oils (e.g., turpentine, pine oil) are treated as petroleum distillates. Mineral seal oil (signal oil), found in some furniture polishes, is a heavy, viscous oil that *never* warrants emesis; it can produce severe pneumonia if aspirated. It has minimal absorption. *Management:* Dermal decontamination. Removal from the environment in inhalation.

First Aid Treatment. See Table 83-13. *The use of activated charcoal, oils, and cathartics is not advised in petroleum distillate ingestions. General management:* (1) In the asymptomatic patient: observe several hours for development of respiratory distress. (2) In the symptomatic patient: supportive respiratory care for respiratory distress. Bronchospasm may be treated with IV aminophylline or albuterol. Avoid epinephrine. Monitor ECG; arterial blood gases; liver, pulmonary, and renal function; serum electrolytes; serial radiographs. Observe for intravascular hemolysis and disseminated intravascular coagulation. If cyanosis is present that does not respond to oxygen or the arterial Pao_2 is normal, suspect methemoglobinemia that may require therapy with methylene blue. Steroids have not been shown to be beneficial. Antimicrobial agents are not useful in prophylaxis. (Fever or leukocytosis

TABLE 83-13. FIRST AID TREATMENT FOR HYDROCARBON INGESTION

Symptoms	Contents	Amount	First Aid
None	Petroleum distillate only	Less than 2 mL/kg	None
None	Heavy hydrocarbon	More than 2 mL/kg	None*
	Mineral seal oil		None
	Petroleum distillate	Minimum, 30 mL	Consider emesis induction†
None	Petroleum distillate with dangerous additive	Depends on toxicity of additive	Consider emesis induction†
	Aromatic and halogenated hydrocarbons	Depends on toxicity of hydrocarbon	Consider emesis induction†
Loss of protective airway reflex; convulsions	Petroleum distillate with dangerous additive	Depends on toxicity of additive	Consider endotracheal intubation prior to gastric aspiration and lavage
Breathing difficulty	Aromatic and halogenated hydrocarbons	Depends on toxicity of individual hydrocarbon	Consider endotracheal intubation before gastric aspiration and lavage

* Emesis may be necessary if machine oil contains triorthocresyl phosphate (TOCP), which causes weakness, sensory impairment, and "partially reversible damage to the spinal cord."
† Emesis induction is rarely indicated if the patient has already vomited. Emesis usually should be induced with proper positioning.

TABLE 83-14. IRON CONTENT OF SOME PREPARATIONS

Salt	Elemental Iron Content (%)	Average Tablet Strength (mg)	Iron Content per Tablet (mg)
Ferrous sulfate	20	300	60
Ferrous sulfate (dried)	29.7	200	65
Ferrous gluconate	11.6	320	36
Ferrous fumarate	33	200	67

may be produced by the chemical pneumonitis itself.) It is not necessary to treat pneumatoceles. Most infiltrations resolve spontaneously in 1 week except for lipoid pneumonia, which may last up to 6 weeks.

IMIPRAMINE (TOFRANIL)

See Tricyclic Antidepressants.

IRON

The iron content of some preparations appears in Table 83-14. *Toxic dose:* Range, 20 to 60 mg per kg or greater of elemental iron. Dose to induce emesis, ≥ 20 mg per kg. The potential fatal dose is 180 mg per kg (600 mg of elemental iron). *Toxicokinetics:* Absorption occurs chiefly in the small intestine. For excretion there is no normal route except blood loss or gastrointestinal desquamation. *Manifestations:* Phase I—Mucosal injury, possibly with hematemesis (1 to 6 hours postingestion). Phase II—patient appears improved (6 to 48 hours). Phase III—cardiovascular collapse and

severe metabolic acidosis. Phase IV—sequelae of intestinal stricture and obstruction or anemia (weeks to months). Patients asymptomatic for 6 hours rarely develop serious intoxication manifestations.

Management: (1) Gastrointestinal decontamination. Emesis should be induced in ingestions of elemental iron of over 20 mg per kg. Emesis should be followed by gastric lavage if large amounts have been ingested (over 60 mg per kg). The solution to be used for lavage is 1 to 1.5 per cent sodium bicarbonate to form ferrous carbonate salts, which are poorly absorbed. One hundred milliliters of this solution should be left in the stomach (prepared by dilution of a sodium bicarbonate ampule with saline). The use of deferoxamine (Desferal) in the gastrointestinal tract is controversial. The use of diluted Fleet's enema solution risks severe hypertonic phosphate poisoning. (2) Postlavage abdominal radiograph—if significant amounts of residual radiopaque material are present, consider removal by endoscopy or surgery because coalesced tablets have produced hemorrhagic infarction and perforation peritonitis. (3) Protect the mucosal surfaces with demulcents if damage is evident. (4) Diagnostic chelation test—deferoxamine not reliable. (5) Indications for chelation therapy with deferoxamine are serum iron greater than total iron binding capacity, or positive diagnostic chelation test; serum iron over 500 mg per dL; and systemic signs of intoxication independent of serum iron level. Chelation should be performed within 12 to 18 hours to be effective.

Laboratory aids: Serum iron levels correlate with the clinical course. Iron levels drawn at 2 to 6 hours that are below 350 mg per dL predict an asymptomatic course; levels of 350 to 500 are associated with mild gastrointestinal symptoms (rarely serious); and levels greater than 500 suggest the possibility of serious Phase III manifestations. White blood cell counts greater than 15,000 per μL, blood glucose levels over 150 mg per dL, radiopaque material present on abdominal radiograph, vomiting, and diarrhea predict iron levels greater than 300 mg per dL. Monitor complete blood counts, blood glucose, serum iron, stools, and vomitus for occult blood; electrolytes; acid-base balance; urinalysis and urinary output; liver function tests; BUN; and creatinine. Obtain type and match of blood in severe cases. Abdominal radiographs. Follow-up is necessary for sequelae in significant intoxications—gastrointestinal series for intestinal strictures and anemia secondary to blood loss. Patients who develop fever or toxic symptoms following iron overdose should have blood and stool cultures checked for *Yersinia enterocolitica*.

ISONIAZID (INH, NYDRAZID)

This is an antituberculosis drug frequently used in suicides by American Indians and Eskimos. *Mechanism of toxicity:* It produces pyridoxine deficiency (doubles excretion of pyridoxine). *Toxic dose:* 1.5 g, 35 to 40 mg per kg, produces convulsions; severe toxicity is seen at 6 to 10 g; 200 mg per kg is an obligatory convulsant. *Toxicokinetics:* Absorption is rapid, with a peak in 1 to 2 hours (clinical symptoms may start in 30 minutes). Volume distribution is 0.6 liter per kg. It passes the placenta and into breast milk at 50% of the maternal serum level. Not protein-bound. Elimination is by the liver, which produces a hepatotoxic metabolite, acetylisoniazid. The $t\frac{1}{2}$—slow acetylators (2 to 4 hours) may develop peripheral neuropathy (50% of blacks and whites). Fast acetylators (0.7 to 2 hours) may develop hepatitis (90% of Asians and most patients with diabetes). Excreted unchanged, 10 to 40%. *Major toxic manifestations:* Visual disturbances, convulsions (90% or more with one or more seizures), coma, resistant severe acidosis (from lactate secondary to hypoxia, convulsions, and metabolic blocks).

Management: (1) Control seizures with large doses of pyridoxine, 1 gram for each gram of isoniazid ingested (Antidote 34, Table 83-1). If the dose ingested is unknown, give at least 5 g of pyridoxine intravenously. (2) Correct acidosis with fluids and sodium bicarbonate (pyridoxine may spontaneously correct the acidosis). (3) Diazepam may be used as a supplement to control the seizures. (4) After the patient is stabilized or if asymptomatic, gastrointestinal decontamination procedures may be carried out, keeping in mind the rapid onset of convulsions. Asymptomatic patients should be observed for 4 hours. (5) Hemodialysis is rarely needed but may be used as an adjunct for uncontrollable acidosis and seizures. Hemoperfusion has not been adequately evaluated. Diuresis is ineffective. *Laboratory aids:* Isoniazid toxic levels are above 8 μg per mL. Monitor the blood glucose (often hyperglycemia), electrolytes (often hyperkalemia), bicarbonate, and arterial blood gases. Monitor the temperature closely (often hyperpyrexia).

ISOPROPYL ALCOHOL

See Alcohols.

KEROSENE

See Hydrocarbons.

LEAD

Acute lead poisoning is rare. *Acute toxic dose:* 0.5 g. *Management:* (1) Gastrointestinal decontamination. (2) Supportive care, including measures to deal with the hepatic and renal failure and intravascular hemolysis. (3) Ethylenediaminetetraacetic acid (EDTA) in all severe cases if lead levels confirm absorption. *Chronic* lead poisoning occurs most often in children 1 to 6 years of age who are exposed in their environment and in adults in certain occupations or from illicit whiskey. *Chronic toxic dose:* Determined by blood lead level and clinical findings. Over 25 μg per dL indicates excess body burden. A chronic dose of 0.6 mg a day increases the body burden, 2.5 mg a day results in toxicity in 4 years, and 3.5 mg a day causes toxicity in a few months. *Toxicokinetics:* Absorption—10 to 15% of the ingested dose is absorbed in adults; in children up to 40% is absorbed with iron deficiency anemia. Inhalation absorption is rapid and complete. Vd—95% present in bone. In blood, 95% is in red blood cells. $t\frac{1}{2}$, 35 days; in bone, 10 years. The major elimination route for inorganic lead is renal. Organic lead is metabolized in the liver to inorganic lead; 9% is excreted in the urine per day. *Manifestations of acute symptoms of chronic lead poisoning* (ABCDE): Anorexia, apathy, anemia; behavior disturbances; clumsiness; developmental deterioration; and emesis. Manifestations of encephalopathy are "PAINT:" *P*, persistent forceful vomiting; *A*, ataxia; *I*, intermittent stupor and lucidity; *N*, neurologic coma and convulsions; *T*, tired and lethargic. In adults one may see peripheral neuropathies and "lead gum lines."

Management: (1) Gastrointestinal decontamination with enemas if radiopaque foreign bodies are noted.

TABLE 83-15. CHOICE OF CHELATION THERAPY BASED ON SYMPTOMS AND BLOOD LEAD CONCENTRATION*

Clinical Presentation	Treatment	Comments
Symptomatic children		
Acute encephalopathy	BAL, 450 mg/M^2/day CaNa$_2$-EDTA, 1500 mg/M^2/day (EDTA) not used alone if blood Pb > 72 μg/dL or symptoms present	Start with BAL, 75 mg/M^2 IM every 4 hours After 4 hours start continuous infusion of CaNa$_2$-EDTA, 1500 mg/M^2/ day Therapy with BAL and CaNa$_2$-EDTA should be continued for 5 days Interrupt therapy for 2 days Treat for 5 additional days, including BAL if blood Pb remains high Other cycles may be needed depending on blood Pb rebound.
Other symptoms	BAL, 300 mg/M^2/day CaNa$_2$-EDTA, 1000 mg/M^2/day Monitor BUN, creatinine, AST, ALT, urine	Start with BAL, 90 mg/M^2 IM every 4 hours After 4 hours start CaNa$_2$-EDTA, 1000 mg/M^2/day, preferably by contin- uous infusion, or in divided doses IV (through a heparin lock) Therapy with CaNa$_2$-EDTA should be continued for 5 days BAL may be discontinued after 3 days if blood Pb < 50 μg/dL Interrupt therapy for 2 days Treat for 5 additional days, including BAL if blood Pb remains high (> 50 μg/dL) Other cycles may be needed depending on blood Pb rebound
Asymptomatic children		
Before treatment, measure venous blood lead		
Blood Pb > 70 μg/dL	BAL, 300 mg/M^2/day CaNa$_2$-EDTA, 1000 mg/M^2/day	Start with BAL, 50 mg/M^2 IM every 4 hours After 4 hours start CaNa$_2$-EDTA, 1000 mg/M^2/day, preferably by contin- uous infusion, or in divided doses IV (through a heparin lock) Treatment with CaNa$_2$-EDTA should be continued for 5 days BAL may be discontinued after 3 days if blood Pb < 50 μg/dL Other cycles may be needed depending on blood Pb rebound
Blood Pb 56 to 69 μg/dL	CaNa$_2$-EDTA, 1000 mg/M^2/day	CaNa$_2$-EDTA for 5 days, preferably by continuous infusion, or in divided doses (through a heparin lock) Alternatively, if lead exposure is controlled, CaNa$_2$-EDTA may be given as a single daily outpatient dose IM or IV Other cycles may be needed depending on blood Pb rebound
Blood Pb 25 to 55 μg/dL		
Perform CaNa$_2$-EDTA provocation test to assess lead excretion ratio		
If ratio > 0.70	CaNa$_2$-EDTA, 1000 mg/M$_2$/day	Treat for 5 days IV or IM, as above
If ratio 0.60 to 0.69		
Age < 3 years	CaNa$_2$-EDTA, 1000 mg/M^2/day	Treat for 3 days IV or IM, as above
Age > 3 years	No treatment	Repeat blood Pb and CaNa$_2$-EDTA provocation test periodically
If ratio < 0.60	No treatment	Repeat blood Pb and CaNa$_2$-EDTA provocation test periodically

* With permission from Piomelli, S., et al.: Management of childhood lead poisoning. J. Pediatr. *105*:523–532, 1984.

Do not delay therapy until clear. (2) Remove from exposure. For children, see Table 83-15. *Laboratory aids:* (1) Provocation mobilization test—50 mg per kg of EDTA intramuscularly for 1 dose and collect the urine for 6 to 8 hours. A ratio of micrograms excreted in the urine to milligrams of Ca-EDTA administered greater than 0.6 represents an increased lead body burden, and chelation should be administered. (2) Evaluate complete blood count, levels of serum iron, or ferritin; repeat blood lead levels and erythrocyte protoporphyrin. (3) Flat plate of the abdomen and long bone radiographs (knees usually). (4) Renal function tests. (5) Monitor electrolytes, serum calcium, phosphorus, blood glucose.

LINDANE

See Organochlorine Insecticides.

LITHIUM (ESKALITH, LITHANE)

Most cases of intoxication have occurred as therapeutic overdoses. The toxic dose is determined by serum levels, although intoxication has occurred with levels in the therapeutic range.

Toxicokinetics: Absorption is rapid, with complete peaking in 1 to 4 hours. Vd is 0.5 to 0.9 L per kg. It is not protein-bound. The t½ therapeutically is 18 to 24 hours. Eighty-nine to 98% is excreted by the kidney unchanged, one third to two thirds in 6 to 12 hours. Excretion is decreased in the presence of hyponatremia and dehydration. The cerebrospinal fluid concentration is one half the plasma concentration. The breast milk level is 50% of the maternal serum level—toxic to the nursling. *Manifestations:* The first sign of toxicity may be diarrhea. Fine tremor of hands, lethargy, weakness, polyuria and polydipsia, goiter and hypothyroidism, and fasciculations are side effects. Severe toxicity is manifested by ataxia, impaired mental state, coma, and seizures (limbs held in hyperextension with eyes open in "coma vigil"). Cardiovascular manifestations are dysrhythmias, hypotension, flat T waves, and increased QT interval.

Management: (1) Gastrointestinal decontamination may not be useful after 2 hours because of rapid absorption. In slow-release preparations, decontamination may be useful up to 24 hours postingestion. Activated charcoal is not indicated. (2) Hospitalize if intoxication is suspected because seizures may occur unexpectedly. (3) Restore normothermia and fluid and electrolyte balance, particularly sodium. If diabetes insipidus is present, an infusion of sodium may cause hypernatremia. Current evidence supports saline infusion as enhancing excretion of lithium. (4) Forced diuresis has no role, unless the glomerular filtration rate is low. Consider only when the lithium level is not above 2.5 mEq per liter and fails to fall below 1 mEq per liter within 30 hours. (5) Hemodialysis is the treatment of choice for severe intoxication. Lithium is the most dialyzable toxin known. Long runs of 12 hours or longer should be used until the lithium level is less than 1 mEq per liter because of extensive reequilibration rebound. Follow levels every 4 hours after dialysis. Dialysis may have to be repeated. Expect a time lag in neurologic recovery. If hemodialysis is not available or delayed, peritoneal dialysis can be used but is less effective. (6) Monitor ECG. Refractory dysrhythmias may be treated with magnesium sulfate and sodium bicarbonate. (7) Aminophylline may increase lithium excretion and decrease lithium reabsorption but has not been extensively studied. (8) Avoid thiazides and spironolactone diuretics, which increase lithium levels.

Laboratory aids: Lithium level determinations should be performed every 4 hours. Although they do not always correlate with the manifestations at low levels, they are predictive in severe intoxications. Levels of 0.6 to 1.2 mEq per liter are usually therapeutic. Levels over 4.0 mEq per liter are severely toxic. Other tests to be monitored are complete blood count (lithium causes leukocytosis), renal function, thyroid, ECG, and electrolytes. Factors that predispose to lithium toxicity are febrile illness, sodium depletion, concomitant drugs (thiazide and spironolactone diuretics), impaired renal function, advanced age, and fluid loss in vomiting and diarrheal illness.

LOMOTIL (DIPHENOXYLATE AND ATROPINE)

See Opioids and Anticholinergic Agents.

LSD (LYSERGIC ACID DIETHYLAMIDE)

See Hallucinogens.

MARIJUANA

See Hallucinogens.

MEPERIDINE (DEMEROL)

See Opioids.

MEPROBAMATE (EQUANIL, MILTOWN)

See Sedative Hypnotics.

MERCURY

Management: (1) Inhalation of elemental mercury—remove from exposure. (2) Ingestion of mercuric salt—gastrointestinal decontamination. A protein solution such as egg white or 5% salt-poor albumin can be given to reduce salt to mercurous ion (less toxic). Give activated charcoal and cathartic. (3) Chelating agents (do not use Ca-EDTA because of nephrotoxicity): Dimercaprol (BAL) enhances mercury excretion through the bile as well as the urine and would be the choice if there were renal impairment from the mercury (Antidote 17, Table 83-1). Penicillamine (Antidote 29, Table 83-1) or *N*-acetyl DL-penicillamine (investigational use). Use of BAL in methyl mercury intoxication increases the brain mercury and appears to be contraindicated; penicillamine and its analogue should be used (decreases mercury in brain). A new chelator, 2.3-dimercaptosuccinic acid, holds promise of less toxicity and more specific therapy and is now available under the Orphan Drug Program.* (4) Monitor fluid and electrolyte levels, renal function, hemoglobin levels. Obtain blood and urine mercury levels (consult the laboratory for proper collection technique and containers). (5) Hemodialysis early in the symptomatic patient is useful. (6) New but not established approaches are Polythiol resin to bind the methyl mercury excreted in the bile; heat and sauna treatment to increase mercury excretion through perspiration; and a regional dialyzer system using L-cysteine. (7) Surgical excision of *local injection sites.*

Laboratory aids: (1) Blood levels are below 2 to 4 μg per dL and urine levels below 10 to 20 μg per liter in 90% of adult population. Levels above 4 μg per dL in blood and 20 μg per liter in urine probably should be considered abnormal. Blood levels are not always reliable. Exposed industrial workers' urine levels are 150 to 200 μg. (2) In asymptomatic patients with urine levels under 300 μg per liter, a chelating challenge with BAL or penicillamine may bring a significant increase that may aid in establishing the diagnosis. (3)

---

*Inquiries can be made to the National Information Center for Orphan Drugs and Rare Diseases, 800–336–4797.

Approximately 150 μg per liter of mercury in urine is equivalent to 3.5 μg per dL in blood. (4) Methyl mercury is excreted mainly through the feces, so urine mercury would not be a reliable measurement. (5) Mercury is also excreted in the sweat and saliva. The parotid fluid level is approximately two thirds that of the blood. Because the hair is porous, it may absorb mercury from the atmosphere; however, hair concentrations of 400 to 500 μg are likely to be associated with neurologic symptoms.

METHADONE

See Opioids.

METHANOL

See Alcohols.

METHAQUALONE

See Sedative Hypnotics.

METHYPRYLON (NOLUDAR)

See Sedative Hypnotics.

NARCOTIC ANALGESICS

See Opioids.

NEUROLEPTICS

See Phenothiazines.

NITRITES (NO₂) AND NITRATES (NO₃)

These are readily available in both inorganic and organic forms. Organic nitrates used for angina pectoris are listed in Table 83-16. Inorganic nitrates have more toxicologic importance in natural foods and contaminated well water. *Potential fatal doses:* Nitrite, 1 g; nitrate, 10 g; nitrobenzene, 2 mL; nitroglycerin, 0.2 g; and aniline dye (pure), 5 to 30 g. *Toxicokinetics:* Onset of action of nitroglycerin sublingually is 1 to 3 minutes, with a peak action of 3 to 15 minutes and a duration of 20 to 30 minutes. Other routes have a slower onset (2 to 5 minutes) and longer duration of action (1.5 to 6 hours). Nitrites are potent oxidizing agents converting ferrous to ferric iron, which cannot carry oxygen. Normally, humans have 0.7% of methemoglobin, which is converted by methemoglobin reductase into oxygen-carrying hemoglobin. Liver detoxification by dinitration is the route of elimination. *Toxic manifestations* depend on the level of methemoglobinemia. At 10% "chocolate cyanosis" occurs; at 10 to 20%, headache, dizziness, and tachypnea occur; and at 50% mental alterations are present and coma and convulsions may occur. Headache, flush, and sweating are caused by the vasodilatory effect; hypotension, tachycardia, and syncope may also occur. Severe hypoxia may produce pulmonary edema and encephalopathy. Levels above 50% produce metabolic acidosis and ECG changes; cardiovascular collapse occurs at levels of 70%.

Management: (1) Dermal decontamination, if indicated. Aniline dyes may be removed with 5% acetic acid (vinegar). (2) Gastrointestinal decontamination if ingested. (3) Hypotension can be treated by the Trendelenburg position and fluid challenge. Vasoconstrictors (dopamine or norepinephrine) are rarely needed. (4) Methylene blue (Antidote 24, Table 83-1) is indicated for methemoglobin levels above 40%, dyspnea, metabolic acidosis (lactic acidosis), or an altered men-

TABLE 83-16. ORGANIC NITRATES FOR ANGINA PECTORIS

Drug and Route	Trade Name	Onset (min)	Duration (hr)
Nitroglycerin			
Oral	Many	Varies	4–6
Sublingual	Many	1–3	¼–½
2% ointment	Nitrobid Nitrol	Varies	3–6
Isosorbide dinitrate	Isordil		
Sublingual		1–3	1.3–3
Oral		2–5	4–6
Chewable		2–5	2–3
Timed release		Varies	—
Pentaerythritol tetranitrate, oral	Peritrate	2–5	3–5
Erythrityl tetranitrate, oral	Cardilate	2–5	4–6

TABLE 83-17. OPIOIDS (NARCOTIC OPIATES)

Drugs Generic	Trade	Equivalent IM Dose* (mg)	Oral* (mg)	Peak Action (hr)	Half-Life (hr)	Duration (hr)	Potential Toxic Dose (mg)
Alphaprodine	Nisentil	45	—	0.5	—	1–2	—
Butorphanol	Stadol	2	12	—	3	3–4	—
Camphorated tincture of opium	Paregoric		25 mL	—	—	4–5	—
Codeine	Various	120	200	—	3	3–6	800
Diacetylmorphine	Heroin	3.0	60	—	0.5	3–4	100
Dihydrocodeine	Hycodan	5–10	—	—	—	—	100
Diphenoxylate	Lomotil	40–60	—	Delayed by atropine	—	—	—
Fentanyl	Sublimaze	0.2	—	0.5	—	1–2	—
Hydromorphine	Dilaudid	1.5	6.5	0.5–0.75	2–3	4–5	100
Meperidine	Demerol	75–100	300	0.5–1	3	4–6	1000
Methadone	Dolophine	10.0	20	4	—	4–6	120
Morphine	Various	10.0	60	0.75–1	2–3	4–6	200
Nalbuphine	Nubain	10.0	60	—	5	3–6	—
Oxycodone	Percodan	15	30	—	—	3–4	—
Oxymorphone	Numorphan	1.0	6.5	1	2–3	4–5	—
Pentazocine	Talwin	60	180	0.75	2	4–7	—
Propoxyphene	Darvon	240	—	2–4	12–36	2–4	500

"Ts and blues" are a combination of pentazocine (Talwin) and tripelennamine (Pyribenzamine) used intravenously. Pentazocine now has naloxone added to it to counter this abuse. Innovar is fentanyl plus droperidol, used as an IV anesthetic.

* Dose equivalent to 10 mg of morphine.

tal state. (5) Oxygen, 100%, or a hyperbaric chamber should be used in symptomatic patients if methylene blue fails or is not effective, e.g., chlorate intoxication or G6PD deficiency. *Laboratory aids:* Methemoglobin levels, arterial blood gases. Blood has a chocolate-brown appearance and fails to turn red on exposure to oxygen.

NORTRIPTYLINE (AVENTYL, PAMELOR)

See Tricyclic Antidepressants.

OPIOIDS (NARCOTIC OPIATES)

See Table 83-17. The major metabolic pathway differs for each opioid but they are 90% metabolized in the liver. Patients should be observed for central nervous system and respiratory depression and hypotension. Pulmonary edema is a potentially lethal complication of mainlining (intravenous use). *Manifestations:* All opiate agonists produce miotic pupils (except meperidine and Lomotil early), respiratory and central nervous system depression, physical dependence, and withdrawal. *Management:* (1) Supportive care, particularly an endotracheal tube and assisted ventilation. (2) Gastrointestinal decontamination up to 12 hours postingestion, as opiates delay gastric emptying time, but this is of no benefit if overdose is by injection. Convulsions occur rapidly with propoxyphene (Darvon) and codeine overdose, and this may be an indication not to use an emetic for gastrointestinal decontamination in this drug overdose. (3) Naloxone (Narcan) (Antidote 25, Table 83-1) may be given in bolus intravenous doses and by continuous drip. Naloxone must be titrated against the clinical response and precipitation of withdrawal in narcotic addicts. It should be repeated as often as necessary because many opioids in overdose can last 24 to 48 hours, whereas the action of naloxone lasts only 2 to 3 hours. *Larger doses are needed for codeine, pentazocine, and propoxyphene.* (4) Pulmonary edema does not respond to naloxone and needs respiratory supportive care. Fluids should be given cautiously in opioid overdose, because these agents stimulate antidiuretic hormone effect and pulmonary edema is frequent. (5) *If the patient is comatose, give 50% glucose* (3 to 4 per cent of comatose narcotic overdose patients have hypoglycemia). (6) *If the patient is agitated,* consider hypoxia rather than withdrawal and treat as such. (7) *Observe for withdrawal* (nausea, vomiting, cramps, diarrhea, dilated pupils, rhinorrhea, piloerection). If these occur, stop naloxone.

Opioid Addict Withdrawal Score. Symptoms of withdrawal are diarrhea, dilated pupils, gooseflesh, hyperactive bowel sounds, hypertension, insomnia, lacrimation, muscle cramps, restlessness, tachycardia, and yawning. Each sign or symptom is given 0, 1, or 2 points, depending on the severity. A score of 1 to 5 is mild; 6 to 10, moderate; and 11 to 15, severe. Seizures are unusual with withdrawal. They indicate severity regardless of the rest of the score. *Management:* Mild withdrawal is treated with diazepam orally, 10 mg every 6 hours; moderate withdrawal, with intramuscular diazepam; and severe withdrawal, with diazepam and diphenoxylate (Lomotil) for the diarrhea. Methadone orally may be used, 20 to 40 mg every 12

TABLE 83-18. ORGANOCHLORINE PESTICIDES (DDT DERIVATIVES)

Chemical Name	Trade Name	Toxicity Rating	Elimination Time	Comment
Endrin	Hexadrin	Highest	hrs–days	Banned
Lindane	1% in Kwell; Benesan; Isotox; Gamene	Moderate to high	hrs–days	Scabicide; general garden insecticide
Endosulfan	Thiodan	Moderate	hrs–days	
Benzene hexachloride	BHC, HCH	Moderate	wks–mos	Banned, produces porphyria (cutanea tarda)
Dieldrin	Dieldrite	High	wks–mos	
Aldrin	Aldrite	High	wks–mos	
Chlordane (10% is heptachlor)	Chlordan	High	wks–mos	Restricted; termiticide
Toxophene	Toxakil Strobane-T	High	hrs–days	
Heptachlor	—	Moderate	wks–mos	Malignancy in rats
Chlorophenothane	DDT	Moderate	mos–yrs	Banned in 1972
Mirex	—	Moderate	mos–yrs	Banned; red anticide
Chlordecone	Kepone	Moderate	mos–yrs	Tidewater, Virginia, contamination
Methoxychlor	Marlate	Low	hrs–days	
Perthane	—	Low	hrs–days	
Dicofol	Kelthane	Low	hrs–days	
Chlorobenzilate	Acaraben	Low	hrs–days	Banned

hours, decreased by 5 mg every 12 hours. When 10 mg is reached, add Lomotil. Clonidine (Catapres), 6 μg per kg every 6 hours, can be used with informed consent. (This is an unlisted use of clonidine; the manufacturer states that relief from withdrawal symptoms has been reported with 0.8 mg/day.)

Propoxyphene (Darvon). *Manifestations:* Onset may be as early as 30 minutes after ingestion. Convulsions occur early. Patients may develop diabetes insipidus, pulmonary edema, and hypoglycemia. *Elimination:* Metabolism is 90% by demethylation in the liver. Peak plasma level of 1 to 2 hours after oral dose. Half-life is 1 to 5 hours. As little as 10 mg per kg has caused symptoms, and 35 mg per kg has caused cardiopulmonary arrest. Therapeutic blood level is less than 200 μg per mL. *Treatment* (in addition to the general management): (1) Emesis can be dangerous because of the rapid onset of seizures. (2) Indications for naloxone are respiratory depression, seizures, coma, and miotic pupils. Signs of naloxone effect are dilation of pupils, increased rate and depth of respirations, reversal of hypotension, and improvement of obtunded or comatose state. (3) Naloxone and intravenous glucose should be tried first to control seizures. If these fail, diazepam may be tried.

ORGANOCHLORINE INSECTICIDES (DDT DERIVATIVES)

See Table 83-18 for a listing of these agents. The *toxic dose* varies greatly. Chlorophenothane (DDT), 200 to 250 mg per kg, is fatal; 16 mg per kg causes seizures. Methoxychlor, 500 to 600 mg per kg, is fatal. Chlordane, 200 mg per kg, is fatal (chlordane house air

guidelines are below 5 μg per M^3; the occupational threshold limit value [TLV] is 500 μg per M^3). These insecticides interfere with axon transmission of nerve impulses. Metabolism varies; they resist degradation in human tissue and the environment. They accumulate in adipose tissue; the elimination route is by the liver. *Manifestations:* Central nervous system stimulation, convulsions, late respiratory depression, increased myocardial irritability. Endrin produces liver toxicity with guarded prognosis. Chronic exposure causes liver and kidney damage. *Management:* (1) Dermal decontamination, discard contaminated leather goods. Protect personnel. Gastrointestinal decontamination, no oils. Emesis can be dangerous owing to rapid seizures. Many are dissolved in petroleum distillates, presenting an aspiration hazard. (2) No adrenergic stimulants (epinephrine) should be used because of myocardial irritability. (3) Cholestyramine, 4 g every 8 hours, has been reported to increase the fecal excretion. (4) Anticonvulsants, if needed.

ORGANOPHOSPHATE INSECTICIDES (OPI)

These may cause (a) irreversible inhibition of cholinesterase, either direct (TEPP) or delayed (parathion or malathion), or (b) reversible inhibition of cholinesterase (carbamates). Examples of OPI are listed in Table 83-19. Absorption is by all routes. The onset of acute toxicity is usually before 12 hours and always before 24 hours. *Toxic manifestations:* Early, cholinergic crisis—cramps, diarrhea, excess secretion, bronchospasms, bradycardia. Later, sympathetic and nicotine effects occur—twitching, fasciculations, weakness, tachycardia and hypertension, and convulsions. Central nervous system effects are anxiety, confusion,

TABLE 83-19. EXAMPLES OF ORGANOPHOSPHATE INSECTICIDES (OPI)

Common Name	Synonym	EFD*
Agricultural Products (highly toxic; LD_{50} is 1–50 mg/kg)		
Tetraethyl pyrophosphate	TEPP, Tetron	0.05
Phorate	Thimet	
Disulfoton†	Di-Syston	0.2
Demeton†	Systox	
Terbufos	Counter	
Chlortriphos	Calathion	
Mevinphos	Phosdrin	0.15
Parathion	Thiophos	0.10
Methamidophos	Monitor	Delayed neuropathy
Monocrotophos	Azodrin	
Octamethyl-diphosphoramide	OMPA, Schradan	
Azinphosmethyl	Guthion	0.2
Ethyl–nitrophenyl thiobenzene PO_4	EPN	
Animal Insecticides (moderately toxic; LD_{50} is 50–500 mg/kg)		
DEF	DeGreen	
Dichlorvos	DDVP, Vapona	
Coumaphos	Co-ral	
Trichlorfon	Dylox	
Ronnel	Korlan	10.0
Dimethoate	Cygon, De-Fend	
Fenthion	Baytex	Long-acting
Leptophos	Phosvel	
Chlorfenvinophos (tick dip)	Supona, Dermaton	
Household and Garden Pest Control (low toxicity; LD_{50} is 500–1300 mg/kg)		
Malathion	Cythion	60.0
Diazinon‡	Spectracide, Dimpylate	25.0
Chlorpyrifos‡	Lorsban, Dursban	
Temephos	Abate	

* EFD, Estimated fatal dose (grams/70 kg).
† Most OPI degrade in the environment in a few days to nontoxic radicals. These are taken up by the plants and fruits.
‡ Some classify these as moderately toxic.

emotional lability, and coma. Delayed respiratory paralysis and neurologic disorders have been described.

Management: (1) Basic life support and decontamination with careful protection of personnel. (2) Atropine (Antidote 7, Table 83-1), if symptomatic, every 10 to 30 minutes until drying of secretions and clear lungs occur. Maintain for 12 to 24 hours, then taper the dose and observe for relapse. (3) Intravenous pralidoxime (2-PAM) may be required after atropinizaton (Antidote 31, Table 83-1). It should be given in the first 24 hours. It is used in the presence of weakness, respiratory depression, or muscle twitching. Its use may require reduction in the dose of atropine. (4) Careful dermal and gastrointestinal decontamination when stable. (5) Suction secretions until atropinization drying is achieved. Intubation and assisted ventilation may be needed. (6) *Do not* use morphine, aminophylline, phenothiazine, or reserpine-like drugs or succinylcholine. *Laboratory aids:* Draw blood for red blood cell cholinesterase determination before giving pralidoxime. Levels are usually more than 50% depressed for severe symptoms. Monitor chest radiograph, blood glucose, arterial blood gases, ECG, blood coagulation status, liver function, and the urine for the metabolite alkyl phosphate *p*-nitrophenol. *Note:* If the diagnosis is probable, do not delay therapy until it is confirmed by laboratory tests. Atropine is both a diagnostic and a therapeutic agent. A test dose of 2 mg in adults and 0.05 mg per kg in children may be administered parenterally. In the presence of severe cholinesterase inhibition, the patient fails to develop signs of atropinization.

It is not medically advisable to administer atropine or pralidoxime prophylactically to workers exposed to organophosphate pesticides.

Carbamates (esters of carbonic acid). Carbamates cause reversible carbamylation of acetylcholinesterase. Pralidoxime is usually not indicated in the management, but atropine may be required. The major differences from OPI are (1) toxicity is less and of shorter duration; (2) they rarely produce overt central nervous system effects because of poor penetration; and (3) cholinesterase returns to normal rapidly so that blood values are not useful in confirming diagnosis. Some common examples of carbamates are

Ziram, Temik (alkicarb) (taken up by plants and fruit), Matacil (aminocarb, carazol), Vydate (oxamyl), Isolan, furadan (Carbofuran), Lannate (methomyl, Nudrin), Zectran (mexacarbate), and Mesural (methiocarb). These agents are all highly toxic. Moderately toxic are Baygon (propoxur) and Sevin (carbaryl). Some of these agents may be formulated in wood alcohol and have the added toxicity of methyl alcohol.

PARADICHLOROBENZENE

See Hydrocarbons.

PARAQUAT AND DIQUAT

Paraquat is a quaternary ammonia herbicide rapidly inactivated in the soil by clay particles. Nonindustrial preparations of 0.2% are unlikely to cause serious intoxications. *Toxic dose:* Commercial preparations such as Gramoxone 20% are very toxic; one mouthful has produced death. Systemic absorption in the course of occupational use is apparently minimal. Paraquat on marijuana leaves is pyrolyzed to nontoxic dipyridyl. *Toxicokinetics:* "Hit and run" toxin. Less than 20% is absorbed. The peak is 1 hour postingestion. The route of elimination is the kidney. Most of the dose is eliminated in the first 40 hours; it is detected in urine for 15 days. Volume distribution is over 500 liters per kg. *Manifestations:* Local corrosive effect on skin and mucous membranes. Acute renal failure in 48 hours (often reversible). Pulmonary effects in 72 hours are progressive, and oxygen aggravates the pulmonary fibrosis. Diquat does not produce effects on the lungs but produces convulsions and gastrointestinal distention. Long-term exposure may cause cataracts. Chlormequat's target organ is the kidney.

Management: (1) Gastrointestinal decontamination despite corrosive effects should be done cautiously with a nasogastric tube; administer local adsorbent. Repeated doses of activated charcoal are recommended. Dermal and ocular decontamination as needed. (2) Hemodialysis and hemoperfusion may be carried out in tandem. Hemoperfusion with charcoal alone is the present choice; however, the results are still poor. Continue hemoperfusion until blood paraquat levels cannot be detected. (3) Diuresis may be of value but consider the risk of fluid overload. (4) Niacin and vitamin E have not been effective. (5) Avoid oxygen unless absolutely necessary (PaO$_2$ below 60 mm Hg) because this aggravates fibrosis. Some use hypoxic air, FiO$_2$ 10 to 20%. (6) Corticosteroids may help prevent adrenocortical necrosis. *Laboratory aids:* Blood levels above 2 μg per mL at 4 hours or above 0.10 μg at 16 hours are usually fatal. Blood level testing and advice may be obtained from ICI American, (800) 327–8633. Monitor renal, liver, and pulmonary functions and chest radiographs. Urine test for paraquat exposure: alkalinization and sodium dithionite give an intense blue-green color in exposure.

PARATHION

See Organophosphate Insecticides.

PENTAZOCINE (TALWIN)

See Opioids.

PERPHENAZINE

See Phenothiazines.

PETROLEUM PRODUCTS

See Hydrocarbons.

PHENCYCLIDINE (ANGEL DUST, PCP, PEACE PILL, HOG)

This is the "drug of deceit" because it is substituted for many other drugs, such as THC and mescaline. There are now at least 38 analogues. Smoking may give cyanide poisoning. Improper mixing has caused explosions. *Toxic dose:* Two to 5 mg smoked or "snorted" produces drunken behavior, agitation, and excitement. Five to 10 mg produces stupor, coma, and myoclonic convulsions. Ten to 25 mg smoked, snorted, or taken orally results in prolonged coma and respiratory failure. It is usually fatal over 25 mg (250 ng per mL blood concentration). *Toxicokinetics:* Weak base. Rapidly absorbed when smoked, snorted, or ingested and secreted into stomach gastric juice. Absorbed in alkaline intestine, but ion-trapping takes place in acid gastric media. Half-life is 30 to 60 minutes. Lipophilic drug with extensive Vd. The onset of action if smoked is 2 to 5 minutes (peak in 15 to 30 minutes); orally, 30 to 60 minutes. The duration at low doses is 4 to 6 hours and normality returns in 24 hours. At large overdoses coma may last 6 to 10 days (waxes and wanes). An adverse reaction in overdose occurs in 1 to 2 hours. *Route of elimination:* By liver metabolism (50 per cent). Urinary excretion of conjugates and free PCP. *Manifestations:* Sympathomimetic, cholinergic, cerebellar. Observe for violent behavior, paranoid schizophrenia, self-destructive behavior. Clues to diagnosis are bursts of horizontal, vertical, and rotary nystagmus, coma with eyes open.

Management (avoid overtreatment of mild intoxications): (1) gastrointestinal decontamination up to 4 hours postingestion, but this may not be effective because PCP is rapidly absorbed. Insert nasogastric tube into stomach for administration of activated charcoal every 6 hours, because PCP is secreted into the stomach even if it is smoked or snorted. (2) Protect patient and others from harm. "Talkdown" is usually ineffective. Low sensory environment. Diazepam (Valium) may be used orally or intramuscularly in the uncooperative patient. (3) For behavioral disorders and toxic psychosis—haloperidol (Haldol), 2 to 5 mg, or diazepam or both. (4) Seizures and muscle spasm—control with diazepam, 2.5 mg, up to 10 mg (Antidote 16, Table 83-1). (5) Dystonic reaction—diphenhydramine (Benadryl) intravenously (Antidote 18, Table 83-1). (6) Hyperthermia—external cooling. (7) Hypertensive crisis (dopaminergic)—diazoxide, 3 to 5 mg per kg intravenously up to 300 mg bolus, or nitroprusside. (8) Acid diuresis ion-trapping (controversial). Ammonium chloride use is not routinely recommended. If rhabdomyolysis occurs, myoglobin may precipitate in the renal tubules. (Antidote 2, Table 83-1): (9) No phenothiazines in the acute phase of intoxication because they lower the convulsive threshold. May be needed later for psychosis.

Laboratory aids: (1) CPK level is the clue to the amount of rhabdomyolysis occurring and the chance of myoglobinuria developing. Values up to 20,000 units have been reported. (2) Test urine for myoglobin and pigmented casts. Test urine with ortho-toluidine; a positive test without red blood cells on microscopic examination suggests myoglobinuria. (3) Monitor urine and blood pH and urinary output if acidifying patient. (4) Measure phencyclidine level. (5) Evaluate BUN, ammonia, electrolytes, blood glucose (20% have hypoglycemia) levels. (6) Test for PCP in gastric juice; levels are 40 to 50 times higher than in blood. *Complications:* Rhabdomyolysis, myoglobinuria, and renal failure. Dopaminogenic hypertensive crisis, cerebrovascular accident (CVA), encephalopathy, and malignant hyperthermia. Schizophrenic paranoid psychosis (induced in chronic users or precipitated in acute users). Loss of memory for months. Teratogenic cases have been reported. Children have been intoxicated from inhalation in a room where adults were smoking PCP. PCP-induced depression and suicide.

PHENOBARBITAL

See Barbiturates.

PHENOTHIAZINES AND OTHER MAJOR NEUROLEPTICS

Phenothiazines are represented by aliphatic compounds: chlorpromazine (Thorazine), promethazine (Phenergan), promazine (Sparine), triflupromazine (Vesprin), methoxypromazine (Tentone); piperazine compounds (dimethylamine series); acetophenazine (Tindal), fluphenazine (Prolixin), prochlorperazine (Compazine), perphenazine (Trilifon), trifluoperazine (Stelazine); and piperidine compounds: mepazine (Pacatal), mesoridazine (Serential), thioridazine (Mellaril), pipamazine (Mornidine). Nonphenothiazines are the thioxanthines: clorprothixene (Taractan), thiothixene (Navane); butyrophenones: haloperidol (Haldol), droperidol (Inapsine); dibenzoxazepines: loxapine (Loxitane, Daxolin); and dihydroindolones:

molindone (Moban, Lidone). These have pharmacologic properties similar to those of the phenothiazines. *Manifestations:* Clues to phenothiazine overdose are miosis, tremor, hypotension, hypothermia, respiratory depression, radiopaque pills on radiograph of abdomen, and increased QT waves in the ECG. Anticholinergic actions are also present. Major problems are respiratory depression, myocardial toxicity (quinidine-like), neurogenic hypotension (antidopaminergic), and idiosyncratic reaction, which may occur at therapeutic levels. Idiosyncratic reaction consists of opisthotonos, torticollis, orolingual dyskinesis, and oculogyric crisis (painful upward gaze) and can be mistaken for a psychotic episode. Extrapyramidal crisis is frequent in children and women. Death is usually from cardiac effects. Phenothiazines are metabolized by the liver into many metabolites. Some remain in the body longer than 6 months.

Management: (1) Gastrointestinal decontamination. Emesis induction may be useful if symptoms have not occurred. If symptoms are already present, many of these agents have antiemetic action, so lavage may be required. Always provide gastric lavage to comatose patients after the airway is protected regardless of the time of ingestion because of inhibition of gastric motility. (2) Extrapyramidal signs (idiosyncratic reaction) can be treated with diphenhydramine (Benadryl) (Antidote 18, Table 83-1), or benztropine (Cogentin), 1 to 2 mg intravenously slowly. Symptoms recur, and these drugs should be continued orally for 2 to 3 days. *This is not the treatment of overdose,* only of the idiosyncratic reaction. (3) Monitor ECG for dysrhythmias and treat with antidysrhythmic agents. (4) Hypotension is treated with the Trendelenburg position or fluid challenge or both. Vasopressors are used only if these fail. Dopamine (Intropin) should not be used to treat the hypotension because these drugs are antidopaminogenic. If a pressor agent is needed, use norepinephrine (Levarterenol, Levophed). (5) Physostigmine may be used for life-threatening anticholinergic symptoms. (6) A radiograph of the abdomen is useful to detect undissolved tablets, which may be radiopaque. (7) Treat hypo- or hyperthermia with external physical measures (not drugs).

Laboratory aids: A ferric chloride test of urine can confirm exposure to phenothiazines if there is a sufficient blood level. Blood levels are *not* useful in management.

PHENYLPROPANOLAMINE (PPA)

See Amphetamines.

PRIMIDONE

See Anticonvulsants.

PROPOXYPHENE

See Opioids.

TABLE 83-20. PROPRANOLOL AND BETA BLOCKERS

Drug	Solubility and Absorption (%)	Membrane Stabilizer	Relative Potency (Propranolol = 1)	Plasma Half-life	Elimination	Protein-Bound	Vd (liter/kg)
Atenolol (Tenormin) Dose: 50–100 mg MDD = 100 mg	Water (46–62)	no	1.0	6–9	95% renal	3–10	0.7
Metoprolol (Lopressor) Dose: 50–400 mg MDD = 450 mg	Fat (over 95)	no	1.0	3–4	Hepatic	10	5.6
Nadolol (Corgard) Dose: 40–320 mg MDD = 320 mg	Water (15–25)	+/−	1.0	17–23	70% renal	25	2.1
Pindolol* (Visken) Dose: 20–60 mg MDD = 60 mg	Fat (over 90)	no	6.0	3–4	Hepatic (40% renal)	57	2.0
Propranolol† (Inderal) Dose: 40–160 mg MDD = 480 mg	Fat (100)	+ +	1.0	2–3	Hepatic (less than 1% renal)	90–95	3.6
Timolol‡ (Blocadren) Dose: 20 mg MDD = 60 mg Ophthalmologic (Timoptic, 0.25–0.5%) Dose: 1 drop twice daily	Fat (over 90)	no	6.0	3	Hepatic (20% renal)	< 10	1.5

* Partial agonists.
† Substantial first pass.
‡ Mitochondrial calcium protection during ischemia.
MDD, maximum daily dose.

PROPRANOLOL AND BETA BLOCKERS

Some of these agents available in the United States at this time are listed in Table 83-20. *Toxic dose:* Varies considerably. *Toxicokinetics:* Peak action is 1 to 2 hours orally and lasts 24 to 48 hours. In drugs with long half-lives, e.g., nadolol, it may take many days to recover from overdose toxicity (Table 83-20). *Manifestations:* Observe for bradycardia and hypotension. Fat-soluble drugs have more CNS effects. Partial agonists may produce tachycardia and hypertension (oxprenolol, pindolol).

Management: (1) Gastrointestinal decontamination up to 2 hours postingestion. (2) Treat hypoglycemia (frequent in children) and hyperkalemia. (3) Control convulsions. (4) Cardiovascular manifestations: Bradycardia—if hemodynamically stable and asymptomatic, no therapy. If unstable (hypotension or atrioventricular block), use atropine, isoproterenol, glucagon, and pacemaker. Ventricular tachycardia or premature beats—use lidocaine, phenytoin, or overdrive pacing. Myocardial depression and hypotension—correct dysrhythmias, institute Trendelenburg positioning, and fluids. Monitor with pulmonary arterial wedge pressure (PAWP) catheter. If low cardiac output with low PAWP, give more fluids. If low cardiac output with normal PAWP, use glucagon (Antidote 22, Table 83-1). Avoid quinidine, procainamide, and disopyramide (Norpace). Glucagon is probably the drug of choice because it works through adenyl cyclase mechanism not affected by the beta blockers. It is given as a bolus and may be continued as an infusion (Antidote 22, Table 83-1). If bronchospasm is present, give aminophylline. Hemodialysis or hemoperfusion for low volume distribution drugs that are low protein binding and water-soluble (nadolol and atenolol), particularly with evidence of renal failure. If hypoglycemia is present, give intravenous glucose. *Laboratory aids:* Monitor blood glucose, potassium, ECG, PAWP. Fatal blood level of propranolol is 0.8 to 1.2 mg per dL (8 to 12 µg per mL).

QUINIDINE AND QUININE (ANTIDYSRHYTHMIC AND ANTIMALARIAL AGENTS)

Toxic dose in child is 1 g; in adult it is 2 to 8 g. There is 95 to 100% absorption, peak action in 2 to 4 hours. Half-life is 3 to 4 hours (quinidine gluconate, 8 to 12 hours). Large Vd. Metabolized predominantly by the liver. *Manifestations:* Cinchonism (headache, nau-

---

TABLE 83-21. QUANTITIES OF ASPIRIN INGESTED: DEPOSITION AND MANIFESTATIONS*

Category	Amount Ingested (*mg/kg*)	Toxicity Expected	Gastrointestinal Decontamination	Manifestations Anticipated
Nontoxic	< 150	No	No	None
Usually nontoxic	> 150	No	Yes (home)	None
Mild intoxication	150–200	Yes	Yes (ECF)	Vomiting, tinnitus, mild hyperventilation
Moderate intoxication	200–300	Yes	Yes (ECF)	Hyperpnea lethargy or excitability
Severe intoxication	300–500	Yes	Yes (ECF)	Coma, convulsions, severe hyperpnea
Very severe intoxication	> 500	Yes	Yes (ECF)	Potentially fatal

* See toxic dose indications for gastrointestinal decontamination.
ECF, emergency care facility.

TABLE 83-22. RECOMMENDATIONS FOR FLUID MANAGEMENT FOR MODERATE OR SEVERE SALICYLISM

Purpose	Rate (*mL/kg/hr*)	Duration (*hr*)	Na	K	Cl (*mEq/L*)	HCO$_3$	Glucose (%)
Volume expansion Administered as 0.45% saline with 23 mEq/L sodium NaHCO$_3$	20	0.5–1.0	100	0	77	23	5–10
Hydration Ongoing losses Alkalinization Administered as 0.33% saline and NaHCO$_3$ to obtain urine pH 7.5–8.0, blood pH 7.5	4–8	Until therapeutic BCS 30 mg/dL	56	40	56	1–2 mEq/kg child; 50–100 mEq adult	5–10
Maintenance	2–6	—	56	30	40 *(mEq/day)*	20	

For severe acidosis pH < 7.15 may require 1–2 mEq/kg every 1–2 hours. Usual fluid loss is 200–300 mL/kg, but carefully monitor for fluid overload. Potassium may be needed in excess of 40 mEq/L when alkalinizing.

---

sea, vomiting, tinnitus, deafness, diplopia, dilated pupils). Myocardial depression, dysrhythmias, ECG changes—prolongation of PR, QRS, and QT intervals. Skin rashes and flushing. Hemolysis in G6PD deficiency. Dementia reported. *Management:* (1) Gastrointestinal decontamination. (2) Monitor ECG and liver function. (3) May need antidysrhythmic drugs and pacemaker and alkalinization.

SALICYLATES

Toxic dose: See Table 83-22. Methyl salicylate (oil of wintergreen): 1 mL equals 1.4 g of salicylate. One teaspoonful equals 21 adult aspirins. *Toxicokinetics:* Plasma concentration is significant in 30 minutes and peaks in 1 to 2 hours. Half-life is 3 to 6 hours (therapeutic) to 12 to 36 hours (toxic). Urine pH influences urine salicylate elimination. *Manifestations of acute ingestion* (see Table 83-21): The metabolic disturbance in adults and older children is usually respiratory alkalosis; in children under 5 years of age, the initial respiratory alkalosis usually changes to metabolic or mixed metabolic acidosis and respiratory alkalosis with acidosis predominating within a few hours.

Management: (1) Gastrointestinal decontamination is useful up to 12 hours postingestion because some factors delay absorption (food, enteric-coated tablets, other drugs); pylorospasm may delay emptying; and concretions may form. Activated charcoal should be administered every 4 hours until stools are black. Concretions may be removed by lavage, endoscopy, or gastrostomy. (2) Intravenous fluid should be given as recommended in Table 83-22. Alkalinization enhances salicylate excretion. Potassium is essential to produce adequate alkalinization. Monitor *both* the urine and blood pH. Do not use the urine pH alone to assess the need for alkalinization (Antidote 35, Table 83-1). (3) Fluid retention can be treated with mannitol (20%), 0.5 gram per kg over 30 minutes, or furosemide, 1 mg per kg intravenously. (4) Hyperpyrexia should be treated with external cooling. (5) Abnormal bleeding or hypoprothrombinemia needs vitamin K, 10 mg intramuscularly, and, if bleeding continues, fresh blood or platelet transfusion (Antidote 38, Table 83-1). (6) Dialysis (hemodialysis) or hemoperfusion is indicated if there is persistent acidosis (pH <7.1) and lack of response to fluid or alkali in 6 hours; if serum salicylate levels are initially greater than 160 mg per dL or greater than 130 mg per dL at 6 hours postingestion (do *not*

TABLE 83-23. MANAGEMENT OF CHRONIC SALICYLATE INTOXICATION

Classification	Urine pH	Blood pH	Hydration	NaHCO₃ (mEq/L)	Potassium (mEq/L)
Mild	Alkaline	Alkaline	Yes	Yes	20
Moderate	Acid*	Alkaline	Yes	pH 7.5†	40
Severe	Acid	Acid	Yes	pH 7.5	40‡ 80§

* Paradoxic acid urine and alkaline blood indicate potassium depletion.
† Bicarbonate administered to keep blood pH 7.5 and urine pH 7.5–8.0.
‡ Normal serum potassium and ECG.
§ Low serum potassium and/or abnormal ECG indicating potassium deficiency.

use the salicylate level as the sole criterion for dialysis); or if there are coma and uncontrollable seizures, congestive heart failure, acute renal failure, or progressive deterioration despite good management. (7) Chronic toxicity is usually a more severe intoxication because of the cumulative pharmocokinetics of salicylates. Management needs are outlined in Table 83-23.

Laboratory aids: The metabolic acidosis of salicylism has a moderately elevated anion gap. Hyper- or hypoglycemia may exist. Serum salicylate levels used in conjunction with the Done nomogram (Figure 83-3) are useful predictors of expected severity after *acute single ingestions*. The Done nomogram is *not* useful in chronic intoxications, methyl salicylate, phenyl salicylate, or homomethyl salicylate ingestions. The salicylate level for use in the Done nomogram should be obtained 6 hours postingestion. Before 6 hours, levels in the toxic range should be treated, and patients with levels below the toxic range should be retested if a potentially toxic dose is ingested. Monitor urine output, urine pH, electrolytes, arterial blood gases, blood glucose, prothrombin time, renal function, serum salicylate level, and urine salicylate with the ferric chloride test. Arterial blood pH should be kept at 7.5. *Prognosis:* Persistent vigorous treatment of salicylate ingestion is essential, as recovery has occurred despite decerebrate rigidity.

SEDATIVE HYPNOTICS, NONBARBITURATE

See Table 83-24. *Management* is primarily supportive (especially intubation and ventilator therapy with continuous positive airway pressure (CPAP) for adult respiratory distress syndrome) and with the use of hemoperfusion or hemodialysis in patients who are severely intoxicated and fail to respond to good supportive care and whose intoxication is life-threatening. (1) *Chloral hydrate* management includes cautious gastrointestinal decontamination. Avoid the use of epinephrine and catecholamines that may produce dysrhythmias. Propranolol, 0.1 mg per kg in 1 mg increments, appears to be more effective than lidocaine for ventricular dysrhythmias. (2) *Ethchlorvynol*

management includes gastrointestinal decontamination up to 12 hours postingestion. Resin hemoperfusion (Amberlite XAD-4) is the best method of extracorporeal removal when other measures fail in a life-threatening situation (ingestion of over 10 g or 100 mg per kg, with serum levels of over 100 μg per mL in the first 12 hours or 70 μg per mL after 12 hours in patients with prolonged life-threatening coma). External rewarming if temperature is below 32° C. (3) *Glutethimide* management includes gastrointestinal decontamination up to 24 hours post-ingestion. Concretions may form. Resin hemoperfusion appears to

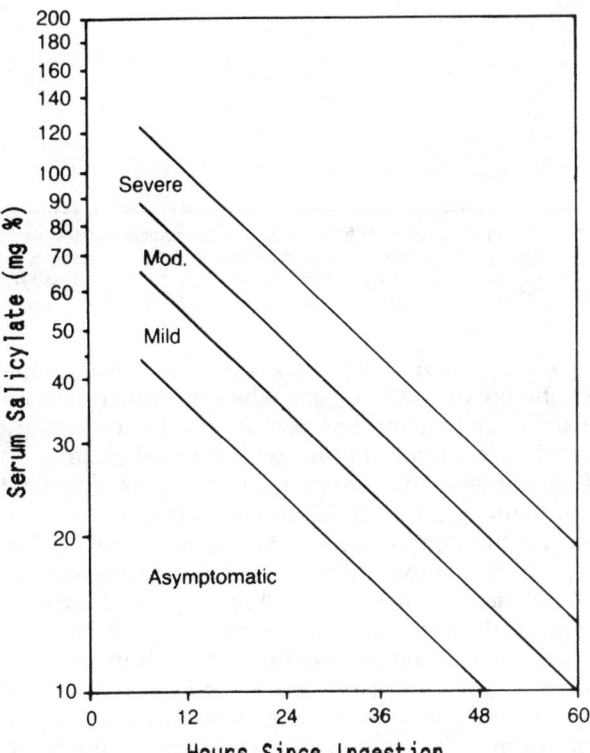

FIG. 83-3. The Done nomogram for salicylate intoxication. For limitations of use, see *Laboratory aids.* (Redrawn from Done, A: Salicylate intoxication: Significance of measurements of salicylate in blood in cases of acute ingestion. Pediatrics 26:800, 1960. © American Academy of Pediatrics, 1960.)

TABLE 83-24. NONBARBITURATE SEDATIVE HYPNOTIC DRUGS

	Absorption and Toxic Dose	Peak Hours	Vd (L/kg)	Protein-Bound (%)	Elimination Route	Serum Half-life (hr)	Toxic Level (µg/ml)	Manifestations and Comments*
Chloral hydrate (Noctec)	Rapid TD, 2 g FD, 4–10 g	1–2	0.6	40	Hepatic 90% to active metabolite trichloroethanol (TCE)	4–8	100 (80 TCE—very toxic)	Pearlike odor; dysrhythmias (especially ventricular), hepatotoxic, irritant to mucosa of GI tract; ARDS; radiopaque capsules
Ethchlorvynol (Placidyl)	Rapid TD, 2.5 g	2–4	3–4	35–50	Hepatic 90%	(1–6) 21–105 in toxic dose	20–80	Prolonged coma up to 200 hr, apnea, hypothermia, pulmonary edema, pink gastric aspirate, pungent odor
Glutethimide (Doriden) (highest mortality of all sedative hypnotics, 14%)	Slow, erratic TD, 5 g FD, 10 g	6	Large, 10–20	50	Hepatic 98% to toxic metabolite 4-hydroxyglutarimide (4HG)	10	120–80	Prolonged, cyclic coma up to 120 hr, anticholinergic signs, convulsions, recurrent apnea, hyperthermia
Meprobamate (Equanil, Miltown)	Rapid TD, 10 g	4–8	1.0	20	Hepatic 90%	6–16	30–100, 200	Coma, convulsions, pulmonary edema, apnea, concretions in stomach
Methaqualone (Quaaludes, "love drugs")	Rapid TD, 800 mg FD, 125 mg/kg	1–3	2–6	80	Hepatic 90%	10–40	8–10	Hypertonia, hyperreflexia, convulsions, apnea, acts "drunk," bleeding tendencies
Methyprylon (Noludar)	Rapid TD, 3 g	2–4	1–2		Hepatic 97%	3–6; over 8 in toxic dose	30	Hyperactive coma lasts 30 hr, miosis, persistent hypotension, pulmonary edema. Mortality rare

* Comment includes other features besides the typical manifestations of all these agents—coma, respiratory depression, psychologic and physiologic withdrawal, hypotension, hypothermia (except glutethimide hyperthermia).

TD, toxic dose; FD, fatal dose; ARDS, adult respiratory distress syndrome.

be the best method of extracorporeal removal in life-threatening protracted coma when the patient has ingested over 10 g and has a serum level of over 30 µg per mL. Treat hyperthermia with external cooling. (4) *Meprobamate* management includes gastrointestinal decontamination up to 12 hours postingestion, with charcoal hemoperfusion in prolonged coma with life-threatening complications. Concretions may form in the stomach and may require breaking up or surgical removal. (5) *Methaqualone* management includes gastrointestinal decontamination. Forced diuresis, dialysis, and hemoperfusion are not indicated. Fatalities are rare. (6) *Methyprylon* management includes gastrointestinal decontamination and may require treatment of the hypotension with vasopressors of the alpha adrenergic variety—levarterenol (Levophed). The hypotension usually does not respond to position or fluids alone. This is a dialyzable drug, but dialysis usually is not necessary. Fatalities are rare.

STRYCHNINE

Primarily available as a rodenticide and component of cathartics and "tonics." Adulterant of "street drugs," particularly marijuana and cocaine. *Toxic dose:* 5 to 10 mg; fatal in doses of 15 to 30 mg. *Toxicokinetics:* Rapid absorption. Manifestations may occur within 15 to 30 minutes. Low protein binding. Hepatic metabolism, which appears to be saturable. Twenty percent is excreted in urine. Has been found in the urine up to 48 hours after a 700 mg dose. *Manifestations:* Interferes with postsynaptic neurotransmitter inhibition by glycine. Hyperacusis is often the first sign. Mild cases—face stiffness (trismus and risus sardonicus). Moderate cases—extensor muscle thrusts. Severe cases—tetanic convulsions with opisthotonos. Death occurs within 1 to 3 hours after ingestion. The prognosis for survival improves if the patient survives beyond 5 hours. The complications of intoxication are lactic acidosis, hyperthermia, rhabdomyolysis and renal damage from precipitation of myoglobin in the renal tubules, and death from hypoxia. *Management:* (1) Emesis appears contraindicated because of rapid absorption and the early onset of seizures. Gastric aspiration and lavage may be used after the seizures are controlled. Activated charcoal should be given and repeated. (2) Control convulsions with diazepam or phenobarbital. (3) Supportive care for respiratory depression. (4) Acid diuresis and dialysis do not appear to be justified on the basis of available studies. (5) Paralysis with assisted ventilation is useful.

TEAR GAS (LACRIMATORS)

CS (chlorobenzylidine), "riot control;" CN powder (chloroacetophenone, 1%; Mace (chloroacetophenone). *Management:* Dermal and ocular decontamination. Protect attendants from contamination. Ophthalmologic evaluation. Oxygen therapy may be needed for dyspnea and respiratory distress.

THEOPHYLLINE

Toxic dose: Acute, single dose greater than 10 mg per kg yields mild toxicity. Greater than 20 mg per kg, moderate manifestations. *Toxicokinetics:* Absorption is complete. Peak levels occur within 60 to 90 minutes after ingestion of liquid preparations; 1 to 3 hours after regular tablets; and 3 to 10 hours after slow-release preparations. Vd. 0.3 to 0.7 L per kg. Protein-binding, 15 to 40%. Half-life varies: 3.5 hours average in a child and 4.5 hours in an adult (range from 3 to 9 hours). In neonates and young infants, the drug's half-life is much longer. Overdose increases the half-life. *Elimination:* Hepatic metabolism, 90% (demethylation and oxidation); 8 to 10% is excreted unchanged in the urine. *Manifestations:* Acute toxicity generally correlates with blood levels; chronic toxicity does not. Ten to 20 µg per mL is the therapeutic range, but some mild gastrointestinal toxicity may occur. Twenty to 40 µg per mL is moderate toxicity, with gastrointestinal and CNS stimulation. Over 50 µg per mL—seizures and dysrhythmias may occur, but they may also occur at lower levels and without gastrointestinal symptoms. Children tolerate higher serum levels. Chronic intoxication is more serious and difficult to treat. Many factors increase theophylline concentration.

Management: (1) Gastrointestinal decontamination in acute overdose, up to 4 hours with regular preparations and up to 8 to 12 hours with slow-release preparations. Test aspirate or vomitus for blood. Give activated charcoal every 4 hours. Do not induce emesis if hematemesis exists. (2) Monitor ECG, obtain theophylline levels every 4 hours until in the therapeutic range of 10 to 20 µg per mL. (3) Control seizures with diazepam. If coma, convulsions, or vomiting exists, intubate immediately. (4) Hypotension is treated with fluid challenge and if this fails, vasopressors. (5) He-

matemesis is managed with iced saline lavage and blood replacement if needed. (6) Charcoal hemoperfusion is the management of choice in life-threatening convulsions, dysrhythmias, hematemesis, or intractable vomiting refractory to conventional measures. Differences in slow release preparations from regular preparations: little or no gastrointestinal symptoms with high levels; peak concentration times may be 10 to 24 hours postingestion; and onset of seizures may occur 10 to 12 hours postingestion. *Laboratory aids:* Monitor theophylline levels, check for occult blood in vomitus and stools, monitor vital signs and hemoglobin and hematocrit (for hemorrhage). Monitor cardiac, renal, and hepatic function, electrolytes, blood glucose, arterial blood gases, and acid-base balance.

TOLUENE

See Hydrocarbons.

TRANQUILIZERS

See Sedative Hypnotics.

TRICHLOROETHYLENE

See Hydrocarbons.

TRICYCLIC ANTIDEPRESSANTS (TCAD)

These agents are generally rapidly absorbed from the gastrointestinal tract, but absorption may be prolonged in overdose owing to anticholinergic action. Their bioavailability has considerable variation among patients, and they are highly bound to plasma and tissue proteins. Protein-binding decreases with decreasing pH. The Vd is large, usually 10 to 20 L per kg. The TCAD are metabolized primarily in the liver. *N*-Demethylation of the tertiary amines yields the active secondary amine metabolites; hydroxylation gives rise to inactive metabolites. Forty per cent is excreted in the feces and only 3% in the urine unchanged. The $t\frac{1}{2}$ varies from 9 to 198 hours. In an overdose, the half-life may be much longer. Tricyclic tertiary amines (metabolized to active metabolites) are amitriptyline (Elavil), imipramine (Tofranil), and doxepin (Sinequan). Tricyclic secondary amines (metabolized to nonactive metabolites) are desipramine (Norpramin, Pertofrane), protriptyline (Vivactil), and nortriptyline (Aventyl). Tricyclic dibenzoxazepine (metabolized to a major metabolite) is amoxapine (Asendin).

Manifestations: The onset of action varies from less than 1 hour to 12 hours after ingestion. The phases of intoxication are (1) consciousness with dry mouth, mydriasis, ataxia, increased deep tendon reflexes, and changes in the ST segment; (2) Stages I and II coma with hypertension, tachycardia above 160, mydriasis, and supraventricular tachycardia; and (3) Stages III and IV coma with hypotension, heart rate under 120, respiratory depression, tonic-clonic seizures, and ventricular dysrhythmias. The central nervous system effects occur early, and seizures are common. *Cardiovascular toxicity* is frequent in the serious poisonings and results from anticholinergic effects, sympathomimetic activity (by blocking reuptake of catecholamines), quinidine activity, catecholamine depletion, and alpha adrenergic blockage. Cardiotoxic effects include cardiac dysrhythmias, hypertension, hypotension, and pulmonary edema.

Toxic dose: The TCAD have a narrow margin of safety. In a child, a 375-mg dose and in adults, as little as 500 to 750 mg has been fatal. The following dosages may serve as a guide to the degree of toxicity: Less than 10 mg per kg produces light coma, mydriasis, and tachycardia and has a good prognosis. At 20 mg per kg, Stage III manifestations are produced. At 30 mg per kg, fatalities may result. At 50 mg per kg, the mortality rate is increased. Over 70 mg per kg is rarely survived. Therapeutic blood levels are in the range of 50 to 170 ng per mL. If the QRS interval is less than 0.10 sec for 6 hours, the prognosis is good. If it is greater than 0.10 sec, seizures may occur, and if it is over 0.16 sec, serious dysrhythmia may occur.

NEWER ANTIDEPRESSANTS. Amoxapine (Asendin) allegedly has less cardiotoxicity. Patients with amoxapine overdose may develop the syndrome of seizures, rhabdomyolysis, and acute renal tubular necrosis. Recent reports indicate more fatalities with amoxapine than with TCAD. Maprotiline (Ludiomil) is a tetracyclic compound with cardiac toxicity similar to the existing tricyclic antidepressant drugs. Trazodone hydrochloric acid (Desyrel) is an antidepressant chemically unrelated to the other antidepressants. It produces less serious toxicity, although orthostatic hypotension, vertigo, and priapism have been reported. Bupropion (Wellbutrin) is a phenylaminoketone antidepressant that produces dose-related seizures. Nomifensine (Merital) was withdrawn in 1986 because of reports of hemolytic anemia associated with it.

Management: (1) Maintenance of vital functions. ICU care until there are no abnormalities in the ECG for 24 to 48 hours. (2) Gastrointestinal decontamination (omit emesis) if the patient is alert. Intact pills have been recovered by lavage up to 18 hours after ingestion. Suspected cases should have ECG monitoring. (3) Activated charcoal cathartic every 4 to 6 hours and continuous nasogastric suction for the first 48 hours may interrupt enterohepatic recycling of tricyclic antidepressants. (4) Control seizures with intravenous diazepam. Intravenous phenytoin (Dilantin) may be added for seizures not responding to diazepam alone. For refractory seizures, physostigmine may be used (Antidote 30, Table 83-1). (5) Life-threatening delirium and hallucinations can be treated with physostigmine. Physostigmine was the drug of choice, but recently its use has been advocated only when conventional therapy has failed. (6) All cardiovascular complications of TCAD should *first* be treated by alkalinization of blood with sodium bicarbonate to a pH of 7.5 to 7.55 (Antidote 35, Table 83-1). Serum potassium levels should be followed, as a sudden increase in blood pH can aggravate or precipitate hypokalemia. Specific cardiovascular complications should be treated as follows: *Hypotension*—norepinephrine (Levophed), a predominantly alpha-adrenergic drug, is preferred over dopamine. (Hypertension that occurs early rarely requires treatment.) *Serious conduction defects* are best managed with phenytoin, and patients may need a temporary transvenous pacemaker. *Sinus tachycardia* usually does not require treatment. If the tachycardia persists despite alkalinization and the patient is unstable, physostigmine may be used. *Supraventricular tachycardia* that does not respond to alkalinization alone may be treated with phenytoin, physostigmine, or synchronized cardioversion. *Ventricular tachycardia*—after alkalinization and phenytoin, intravenous lidocaine (for one dose only) may be required for persistent ventricular tachycardia. Synchronized cardioversion may be needed if lidocaine fails. *Ventricular fibrillation* should be treated with DC countershock. *Laboratory aids:* Arterial blood gases with blood pH, ECG, serum electrolytes, BUN and creatinine, serum phenytoin level, urine output, and, in severe cases, central venous pressure and/or pulmonary wedge pressure should be monitored.

TURPENTINE

See Hydrocarbons.

XYLENE

See Hydrocarbons.

Chapter 84

ALCOHOL AND ITS SUBSTITUTES

ALCOHOL-RELATED EMERGENCIES

John I. Ellis, Michael Whiting, and Martha Roper

CAPSULE

Alcoholism and alcohol abuse account for a tragically large amount of disease and disability in the United States. The number of acute and chronic problems associated with alcohol is vast, ranging from trauma to dementia to malnutrition. Many life-threatening disorders are caused by or associated with alcohol. Rapid recognition and treatment of these is vital. Treatment of most alcohol-related diseases remains nonspecific, consisting mostly of supportive care, adequate nutrition, and abstinence from alcohol.

Many diseases associated with alcohol are less than clinically obvious on casual examination. Although it may sometimes be distasteful, only careful and systematic attention to the alcoholic patient can avert potential disaster.

ALCOHOL ABUSE AND ALCOHOLISM

EPIDEMIOLOGY

Ethyl alcohol in all its various forms, hereafter referred to simply as "alcohol" or "ethanol," is the most widely used and abused recreational drug in the U.S. It is also one of the largest health and social problems in the world. It is responsible for more than 200,000 deaths annually in this country alone. Alcohol abuse and alcoholism cost America more than $60 billion a year.[1] Roughly 50% of traffic fatalities, 50% of deaths by fire, 67% of drownings, 67% of homicides and aggravated assaults, 40% of forced rapes, and 35% of suicides are related to alcohol.[2]

The definition of the term "alcoholism" has un-

dergone dramatic change over the last several decades. Originally considered mainly a defect of character, it is now generally recognized as a complex disease state involving psychiatric, genetic, neurochemical, and physical processes. The definition and concept of alcoholism have evolved to consider the multifactorial nature of the disease. Any patient who has a physiologic dependence on alcohol or in whom alcohol use adversely affects physical health, ability to function in society, or interpersonal relationships can be considered to suffer some degree of alcoholism. The pattern of abuse that an alcoholic engages in is of some importance because the diseases associated with periodic, heavy "spree" abuse differ from those seen with chronic, daily abuse.

Although of vital and arguably primary importance, the recognition and treatment of the basic state of alcoholism is well beyond the scope of this chapter in an Emergency Medicine text. Many local, regional, and national sources of information and resources exist to deal with this problem. This discussion concentrates mainly on acute, common, or life threatening problems directly associated with alcoholism and alcohol abuse likely to be seen in Emergency Departments (EDs).

ALCOHOL INTOXICATION

Acute alcohol intoxication may be defined as a state of physical and/or psychologic impairment caused by ingestion of ethyl alcohol. The patient with acute intoxication may present with any mental status, from seemingly normal through garrulous and "tipsy" to frankly comatose.

Alcohol is almost exclusively used by the oral route. It is rapidly absorbed from both the stomach and intestines, producing measurable rises in blood alcohol concentration (BAC) within 5 minutes.[3] Peak effects are seen within 1 to 1.5 hours of ingestion. Many factors influence the absorption of alcohol, including the presence of food or water in the stomach, habituation, and derangements or alterations of gastric and intestinal motility.[3,4] Because alcohol is both water-soluble and lipophilic, it rapidly enters cells. It diffuses rapidly into all aqueous body compartments; therefore BAC directly reflects concentrations throughout the body.[5]

Alcohol is eliminated from the body by various routes. The rate of elimination varies widely among individuals, and depends mainly on habituation. Approximately 10% of blood alcohol is excreted unchanged by the lungs and the kidneys, a fact that allows estimation of BAC by breath or urine tests. The remainder of blood alcohol is eliminated by metabolism in the liver. The rate-limiting step is the oxidation of alcohol to acetaldehyde by alcohol dehydrogenase in the hepatocyte. This process reduces large amounts of NAD to NADH, often dramatically altering cellular oxidation-reduction (redox) potential.[6]

In the nonhabituated individual, BAC can be expected to fall at the rate of approximately 15 mg/dL/hr.[3] Chronic drinkers may metabolize ethanol at a much greater rate, owing to induction of alcohol dehydrogenase in the liver.

Alcohol dehydrogenase is present in various genetically determined isoenzyme forms, each metabolizing at a different rate. Patients of Asian or Native American descent often possess elevated levels of a particular isoenzyme that produces acetaldehyde rapidly. This is believed to produce the "Oriental flush" often seen in these patients when intoxicated.[3,5]

PRESENTATION OF THE INTOXICATED PATIENT

The effects of drinking alcohol depend on genetic factors, the habituation of the drinker, the rate of consumption, and the rate of elimination. With continued consumption in excess of elimination, however, a typical progression of intoxication may be observed. Initially, alcohol produces a psychologic excitatory effect, with euphoria, garrulousness, and aggressive behavior. Fine motor control and concentration, however, deteriorate. With ongoing consumption, motor control continues to deteriorate. Ataxia of voluntary activities, speech, and gait predominate. The gaze may become disconjugate. Finally, with even higher BACs, all central nervous system (CNS) functions are depressed in a manner similar to that produced by ether or chloroform anesthesia. Loss of protective airway reflexes, coma, and death from respiratory depression may occur.

Although essentially all patients consuming enough alcohol move through the above sequence of events, the specific BACs associated with each stage of intoxication are difficult to predict. Chronic alcohol abusers tolerate much higher BACs with milder symptoms. Table 84-1 suggests rough guidelines. The LD_{50} in the nonhabituated patient is approximately 500 mg/dL,[4] although deaths have been reported with levels as low as 400 mg/dL,[5] and the authors have seen patients survive unintubated with levels as high as 780 mg/dL.

Some discussion of BACs in the context of the law is warranted. In the last few decades, more and more attention has been turned to the tragic effects of alcohol intoxication on automobile drivers and others engaged in hazardous activities requiring alertness and motor control. Most states now legally consider BACs of 100 mg/dL or greater to be presumptive evidence of intoxication, subjecting the offender to ever-increasing penalties. California recently lowered the "legally drunk" level to 80 mg/dL, and other states have followed. Many industries (such as aviation) have stricter standards. It is to be hoped that, with public education and enforcement of these laws, much alcohol-related morbidity and mortality from trauma will be averted.

MANAGEMENT OF THE INTOXICATED PATIENT

The intoxicated patient usually presents with an altered level of consciousness. This may manifest as anything from agitation to frank coma. Alcohol may

TABLE 84-1. SYMPTOMS ASSOCIATED WITH BLOOD ALCOHOL CONCENTRATIONS

Level (mg/dL)	Nonhabituated	Habituated
50–80	Euphoria, garrulousness	Often no effect
100	Incoordination, legally drunk in most states	Minimal to no effect
125–150	Agitation, emotional lability, some decrease in alertness	Euphoria, beginning incoordination
200–250	Decreasing alertness to lethargy	Incoordination, lability
300–350	Stupor to coma	Drowsiness, motor retardation
>500	LD_{50}	Coma

or may not be detectable on the breath. As with any patient in the ED, primary importance must be given to the ABCs. The airway should be ensured. Patients with obviously occluded airways or absent gag reflexes should be endotracheally intubated. Those with borderline gag reflexes or levels of consciousness should at least be placed in a lateral decubitus position with close continuous observation and suctioning; many of these patients are better managed by intubation. Breathing should be assisted with a bag-valve device or mechanical ventilation if inadequate. Blood pressure, pulse, and skin signs such as temperature, color, and diaphoresis must be rapidly assessed and any derangements corrected by proper use of IV fluids, oxygen, or pharmacologic agents.

Special care must be taken not to assume that alteration of consciousness in a patient with a history of alcohol consumption or alcohol on the breath is entirely caused by ethanol. Trauma, infection, other drug toxicity, or metabolic emergencies such as diabetic ketoacidosis, myxedema coma, or hypothermia must be ruled out. *Complete* initial vital sign determination, including core temperature measurement by rectal or tympanic membrane measurement, is mandatory. A rapid, thorough history and physical examination must be performed.

Any patient with significant alteration of consciousness should receive 100 mg thiamine and 2 mg of naloxone IV as a standard "ALOC cocktail." The routine administration of 50% glucose is somewhat controversial because evidence is mounting that high serum glucose levels may worsen ischemic events.[7] Perhaps a better course of action may be to assess the blood glucose concentration with one of the commonly available, quick, and accurate bedside glucose test strips before indiscriminately giving glucose, only giving it when indicated.

LABORATORY EVALUATION

Laboratory evaluation of the significantly "intoxicated" patient should begin with determination of the blood glucose and the blood alcohol concentration (BAC). Glucose may be rapidly and fairly accurately assessed at the bedside as mentioned previously. BAC measurement is commonly rapidly available in most laboratories; alternatively, it may be estimated by one of the breath or urine tests or estimated by the osmolar gap method (Fig. 84-1). If BAC is also measured directly, the osmolar gap may provide clues to possible intoxication with other substances or coingestions. *Any disparity between the BAC and the observed clinical status mandates further intensive investigation, as does failure of the patient's alteration of mental status or response to graded stimuli to improve smoothly during observation.*

A complete blood count should be obtained to assess possible infection or anemias. Serum electrolytes, including calcium, phosphorus, and magnesium in the patient with signs of chronic alcoholism, should be measured and any derangement or elevated anion gap must be investigated and treated. Blood urea nitrogen

Calculated Serum Osmolarity = 2(Na) + glu/18 + BUN/2.8

For every 100 mg/dL
ETOH raises Osm by 22.8 mOsm/kg
Isopropyl alcohol raises Osm by 17.6 mOsm/kg
Ethylene glycol raises Osm by 19.0 mOsm/kg

Osmolar Gap = Measured Osmolarity − Calculated Osmolarity.

Normal = less than 10 mOsm/kg.
Higher osmolar gaps suggest presence of other osmotically active substance in serum

FIG. 84-1. Calculation of osmolar gap.

(BUN) and creatinine may help in determining hydration status and renal function. Urinalysis should be done to check for infection, ketosis, or the presence of hemoglobin or myoglobin in the urine. Prothrombin time should be measured in patients with signs of liver disease.

Noncontrast CT scanning of the head should be considered in any patient suspected of sustaining head trauma to rule out possible subdural or epidural hematomas. This obviously includes patients with significant head trauma or focal neurologic findings on examination. Additionally, patients with disparity between their BACs and their clinical mental status or who fail to improve during observation should be scanned. It must be noted that alcoholic patients are more prone to intracerebral bleeding because of the coagulopathies that may occur with liver disease; therefore relatively minor head injuries may cause intracerebral bleeding. The threshold for computed tomographic (CT) scanning of the alcoholic patient should be low. Lumbar puncture should be performed in patients with altered mental status and unexplained fever or other signs of infection.

EMERGENCY TREATMENT

Emergency treatment of the acutely intoxicated patient is directed toward three areas: (1) supportive care, (2) recognizing and treating any potential or actual complications of alcohol abuse, and (3) referral as appropriate for further treatment of alcoholism and alcohol-related diseases.

Supportive care at a minimum should begin with attention to the ABCs, and then be aimed at preventing injury to the intoxicated patient. In the absence of complicating factors, a safe, quiet environment should be provided for the patient to metabolize his or her alcohol load. Restraint of the patient who is unable to adequately judge his or her condition or care for himself or herself because of alcohol intoxication is strongly advised. This is preferable to allowing the patient to leave the ED in a state of significant intoxication because the patient may cause injury to himself or others, leaving the physician and institution holding some liability.[10-12]

An IV line of a dextrose/saline solution containing a multivitamin preparation, with 1 mg of folate, 100 mg of thiamine, and 1 to 2 g of magnesium sulfate per liter is often administered to the intoxicated patient because many alcoholic patients are deficient in these vitamins and nutrients through both poor diet and direct effects of alcohol.[3,6,8,9]

After any life-threatening problems are identified and treated, a thorough history and physical examination focusing on both acute problems and chronic complications of alcohol abuse should be performed, with specific laboratory and x-ray examinations ordered as potential problems are identified.

REVERSING ALCOHOL INTOXICATION

Many techniques and agents have been advanced throughout history as having some effect in reversing alcohol intoxication or increasing elimination of alcohol. Nearly all of these, when subjected to controlled study, have proven valueless. In particular, aminophylline, amphetamine, naloxone, physostigmine, yohimbe, vitamin B-12, thyrotropin-releasing hormone, and propranolol have had no effect in reversing experimental alcohol intoxication in controlled studies.[13] The time-honored cup of black coffee usually yields only a somewhat more alert "drunk." The specific benzodiazepine antagonist, flumazenil, has been shown to reverse the effects of mixed benzodiazepine-ethanol ingestions to about the same degree as those of benzodiazepines alone.[14-16] Unfortunately, it has not been shown to have any predictable effect against ethanol alone.[13,17] Activated charcoal has no activity in lowering blood ethanol concentrations or area under the curve of BAC in humans.[18-19] Because ethanol, like other general anesthetic agents, acts on the lipid phase of cell membranes rather than on specific receptors such as the opiate or benzodiazepine receptors, it seems unlikely that a specific antidote for ethanol will be forthcoming.

ALCOHOL WITHDRAWAL

Alcohol withdrawal is a complex syndrome that ranges from the common morning hangover[20] to mild tremulousness, diaphoresis, and anxiety[21,22] to frank delirium tremens. Withdrawal is precipitated by declining alcohol levels; the severity is related to the rapidity of declining of alcohol level, duration of drinking, and amount of alcohol consumed.[23]

PATHOPHYSIOLOGY

Many mechanisms of alcohol withdrawal have been proposed and abandoned; several current theories partially explain the manifestations of withdrawal, but none provides a unifying explanation. The pathophysiology is multifactorial and represents the diverse and complex effects of alcohol on the CNS.

Ethanol, a small, weakly polar molecule, is widely distributed with body water,[21] acting on receptors of numerous neurotransmitters.[24] Because it is also highly lipid-soluble, it partitions into the lipid phase of cell membranes, as do the general anesthetics.[24]

Alcohol potentiates the effects of the inhibitory neurotransmitter GABA, through either cell membrane effects or direct stimulation of the GABA-benzodiazepine-chloride receptor.[25] In withdrawal, there is decreased GABA-ergic activity, perhaps accounting for the global hyperactivity and seizures typifying withdrawal.[25,26]

Considerable evidence demonstrates involvement of the adrenergic system in withdrawal. Inhibitory alpha-2 receptors are downregulated during chronic alcohol abuse; similarly, alcohol upregulates stimulatory beta receptors. During withdrawal, these effects are reversed, resulting in extreme sympathetic stimulation.[25] Elevated CSF, serum, and urine norepinephrine levels during withdrawal correlate well with the extensive stimulatory symptoms found in withdrawal.[27-29] Derangement of dopamine metabolism may also be related to alcohol withdrawal hallucinations.[25,26]

Recent studies also implicate involvement of the serotonin and opiate receptors in regulating the desire for alcohol. Also, the number of calcium channel receptor sites increases with chronic alcohol use, and calcium channel blockers may inhibit this increased effect.[30]

Successive withdrawal episodes may have a sensitizing effect, leading to withdrawal symptoms, especially seizure, after milder provocation.[31] This phenomenon, kindling, may be suppressed by adequate treatment of withdrawal episodes.[25]

MANIFESTATIONS (TABLE 84-2)

In a classic study, Isbell et al. maintained 10 former opiate addicts in an intoxicated state for up to 87 days.[32] After withdrawal of alcohol, all demonstrated tremulousness, nausea and/or vomiting, malaise, and diaphoresis. Those who continued drinking for 48 or more days developed tremor, hyperreflexia, hypertension, hallucinations, seizures, and delirium tremens. These changes are thought to occur in patients who have acquired tolerance to and physiologic dependence on alcohol, resulting in a generalized increase of CNS neuronal activity. When alcohol levels abruptly decline and depressant effects of alcohol are

	TABLE 84-2. MANIFESTATIONS OF ALCOHOL WITHDRAWAL			
Stages	Signs and Symptoms	Onset	Duration	Incidence
1	Anxiety, tremulousness, alcohol craving.	6–24 hours	Up to 48 hours	80%
2	Hallucinations	8 hours to 3 days	Hours to days	Up to 25%
3	Grand mal seizures	6–48 hours	Usually <6 hours	Up to 33%
4	Global disorientation and autonomic hyperactivity (delirium tremens)	3 days to 2 weeks	2–5 days	5–10%

absent, the previously appropriate compensating mechanisms result in hyperexcitability and inappropriately increased neurotransmitter release.[24]

There are numerous methods for classifying degrees of withdrawal,[21] but in the ED, clinical evaluation remains the most important. Generally, withdrawal is classified according to severity (major and minor) and chronology (early and late).[20] Some authors[23,33] have grouped the symptoms of withdrawal into stages; however, patients may exhibit some or all symptoms over time.

"THE SHAKES"

Stage One, commonly known as "the shakes," typically begins within 6 to 24 hours of cessation or reduction of alcohol intake. The alcoholic craves alcohol or other sedatives. Symptoms initially include tremulousness, anxiety, diaphoresis, mild agitation, anorexia, and insomnia. Further symptoms include tachycardia, hypertension, nausea, vomiting, and gross tremor. Electromyelography (EMG) demonstrates that the tremor represents an exaggeration of the physiologic tremor, occurring at 6 to 8 Hz.[20] Untreated, these symptoms peak at 24 to 36 hours and in mild withdrawal resolve by 48 hours.[34] Chronic heavy drinkers may have elevated blood alcohol levels at the onset of withdrawal symptoms. As many as 80% of alcoholics have mild withdrawal symptoms on cessation of drinking,[35] and most self-treat with further drinking.

HALLUCINATIONS

The second stage of withdrawal is an exacerbation of the first, typified by increased tremor and hyperactivity. Insomnia and nightmares are common, and hallucinations or illusions are present in approximately one fourth of patients.[33] This stage begins shortly after alcohol levels decline; without treatment, the hallucinations persist from several hours to several days. Hallucinations are not predictive of progression to seizures or delirium tremens (DTs).[34]

Illusions are usually misinterpretations of shadows or silhouettes and can be threatening or benign. Alcoholics are also well known for withdrawal hallucinations, which are most commonly visual, but can be auditory, tactile, olfactory, or multisensory. In spite of the hallucinations, the sensorium is otherwise clear, and the patient may answer orientation questions clearly. Conversely, in DTs, the sensorium is markedly altered. The EEG is usually normal during hallucinations.[20] Acute alcoholic hallucinosis should be distinguished from the chronic variety, which is indistinguishable from chronic paranoid schizophrenia.[36]

WITHDRAWAL SEIZURES

Generalized convulsions, the hallmark of stage 3 alcohol withdrawal, develop in up to one third of those with untreated withdrawal.[21] Withdrawal seizures or "rum fits" arise most often in the first 2 days of withdrawal but may occur much later. The entire convulsive episode seldom lasts longer than 12 hours.[37] Victor and Brausch show that convulsions are most frequently generalized and single or paired, but may be multiple; less than 5% result in status epilepticus. In the same study, the EEG was abnormal in only 16% of patients with alcohol withdrawal seizures, compared to 50% in patients with idiopathic epilepsy. Other studies have found fewer than 5% of alcohol withdrawal patients to have EEG abnormalities.[38] Patients having withdrawal seizures are at higher risk (up to 40%) for progressing to DTs.[23]

Treatment of Seizures. Alcohol withdrawal seizures are not epilepsy and do not require long-term anticonvulsant therapy because they are self-limited. The clinician, however, must distinguish alcohol withdrawal seizures from true epilepsy and seizures caused by head injury or other potentially reversible causes.

A study of first-time seizures in alcoholics without focal signs found that 6% had intracranial lesions.[40] Therefore patients with first-time seizures should have a complete evaluation, including head CT scan and neurologic referral. Patients who present with alcohol withdrawal and focal motor seizures (unless previously well documented) or status epilepticus also require a complete evaluation. In a retrospective study,

24% of alcohol withdrawal seizures were focal; of these, 15% had identifiable lesions.[41] Status epilepticus (SE) is rarer in alcohol withdrawal, comprising 3.3% of patients in the study by Victor and Brausch.[37] Of all patients in SE, only 15% of cases may be attributed to ethanol withdrawal.[42] If evaluation fails to show a fixed cause of seizure, these patients may require sedation for withdrawal symptoms, but do not need long-term anticonvulsant therapy. The diagnosis of alcohol withdrawal seizure is a diagnosis of exclusion, and should be withheld until the workup is complete.

Treatment of patients with known alcohol withdrawal seizures remains controversial. Many authors advocate oral or IV loading with phenytoin (Dilantin) to prevent further seizure activity,[20,34,43] but the studies have been poorly designed to assess the efficacy of such treatment. A recent prospective, randomized, placebo-controlled study of patients with alcohol withdrawal seizures found no difference in seizure incidence between the phenytoin and placebo groups.[44] *No other studies have convincingly demonstrated a beneficial effect of phenytoin in withdrawal seizures, and therefore its use is not routinely recommended.*

Patients with *known* epilepsy and alcohol withdrawal should have sedation as needed and serum anticonvulsant levels drawn; subsequently, appropriate loading and maintenance doses of the previously prescribed drugs should be administered. Patients in withdrawal who have no previous history of seizures should also be managed with sedatives and require no ongoing anticonvulsant therapy. Such patients should not be discharged from the ED unless satisfactory arrangements for detoxification, observation, and follow-up are made.

DELIRIUM TREMENS

Delirium tremens (DTs), the final and potentially life-threatening withdrawal stage, is marked by an increased severity of the autonomic symptoms, superimposed on global disorientation. Other symptoms include hypertension, tachycardia, fever (to 104°F or higher), and profound confusion. Extreme cases can result in rhabdomyolysis, hypotension, circulatory collapse, and death.[33] The DTs have variable onset, but typically appear on days 3 to 5 of withdrawal. DTs are found in 5 to 10% of patients in withdrawal, and the mortality has declined from as high as 25% to less than 5%.[21,34] In more than 80% of patients, the major symptoms resolve in less than 3 days.[23]

DTs are a medical emergency requiring aggressive evaluation and treatment. They are often precipitated by serious illness or injury, including gastrointestinal bleeding, pancreatitis, hypoxia, meningitis, pneumonia or other infection, and trauma; each must be excluded before making the diagnosis of delirium tremens.

ASSESSMENT AND INITIAL THERAPY

The initial assessment of a patient thought to have alcohol withdrawal requires a complete history and thorough physical examination. Although the history may be difficult to obtain because the patient is uncooperative or unable to answer questions, usually questions can be answered by interviewing paramedics, family, friends, and even the patient. Essential information includes amount of alcohol regularly consumed, type(s) consumed, time of last drink, history of previous withdrawal symptoms, and reasons for stopping drinking.

During the physical examination, search for signs of withdrawal, chronic illness, and accompanying disease or trauma. Particular attention should be given to observing signs of chronic alcohol abuse. A complete examination requires that the patient be completely undressed.

The history and examination should be a guide to intervention. A patient with "the shakes" who has stopped drinking for only a short time may require only mild oral sedatives, multivitamins, thiamine, and some food. More severe withdrawal requires more aggressive treatment; patients whose symptoms are not quickly quelled should be admitted. In any acutely ill patient, consider concomitant withdrawal from barbiturates or benzodiazepines, toxic ingestions, occult trauma, infection, or the myriad other problems to which alcoholics are predisposed.

Any patient with significant signs and symptoms of withdrawal needs immediate assessment of the ABCs and a complete set of vital signs (including a core temperature), followed by an IV, 50 to 100 mg of thiamine IV or IM, IV narcan, and a dextrostick or 25 g of D50. Breathalyzer or blood alcohol levels should be obtained. Further tests (CBC with differential, glucose, electrolytes, calcium, phosphorus, magnesium, amylase, liver enzymes, arterial blood gases, urinalysis, chest x ray, etc.) are ordered as clinically indicated. Fluids are also given as clinically indicated, with care taken to avoid fluid overload. *Serial examinations are essential; failure to improve appropriately warrants complete re-evaluation and more aggressive management.* During the period of observation, the patient should be in a high visibility area and placed in the lateral decubitus position to minimize the risk of aspiration.

BENZODIAZEPINES

Benzodiazepines are the current standard therapy for alcohol withdrawal. As a class, they are preferred for their relatively high therapeutic index, excellent sedative properties, and anticonvulsant activity.[24,34,45] Benzodiazepines bind at the GABA-benzodiazepine-chloride receptor in the CNS, which is thought to have decreased GABA stimulation during withdrawal.

Although many benzodiazepines have been studied, the most commonly prescribed are diazepam and chlordiazepoxide. Each is extremely long-acting and has active metabolites. Each is given IV or PO; IM doses are poorly and erratically absorbed. Typically, doses equivalent to diazepam 10 mg are given every 15 to 60 minutes until symptoms resolve, or until the patient is sedated. Treatment of withdrawal may require massive doses initially, which are then rapidly tapered. Usually doses are reduced 25 to 50% per day and the course continued for 4 to 7 days. Because of the long half-life, the patient is then afforded a gentle taper as the residual drug is metabolized.[34] Lorazepam has become popular because it is well absorbed IM and has no active metabolites. It may be used in patients with hepatic disease, although no evidence shows improved function with its use. In critically ill patients, IV infusions of midazolam have been used successfully, but require ICU monitoring and titration of effect.[25,46] *Numerous studies compare the efficacy of various benzodiazepines, but none has ever been proven superior.*[45] Because benzodiazepines have significant abuse potential and there is a modest street market for them, care should be taken in prescribing them for outpatient therapy.

BARBITURATES

In the past, barbiturates were used frequently for treatment of withdrawal because of their high degree of cross-tolerance with alcohol and their anticonvulsant activity. With the advent of benzodiazepines, barbiturate use has fallen because of perceived risks of hepatic enzyme induction, respiratory depression, and abuse.[24,34] There has been a resurgence of interest in barbiturate use based on two studies. The first, a double-blind, controlled study, found diazepam and barbital equivalent in treating mild withdrawal and barbital superior in treating delirium tremens.[47] The second, an uncontrolled prospective study, showed that phenobarbital given 260 mg IV followed by 130 mg IV every 30 minutes as needed for light sedation is effective in controlling seizures and other withdrawal symptoms without significant side effects.[48]

BETA-BLOCKERS

Several studies have examined the use of beta-blockers in treating the autonomic symptoms of withdrawal. Propranolol was found to be effective in reducing heart rate, blood pressure, and tremor during withdrawal.[49] Two prospective randomized double blind studies found that atenolol, 50 to 100 mg per day, resulted in a decreased number of patients requiring benzodiazepines and a decreased number of benzodiazepine doses required for patients needing sedation. The atenolol group also had significantly shorter hospital stays, decreased alcohol craving, and a lower treatment failure rate.[50,51] Some evidence suggests that propranolol has a greater CNS effect because of greater transport across the blood-brain barrier.[52] Further tri-

als will determine the extent to which beta-blockers are indicated and which is the most effective.

ALPHA-2-AGONISTS

Alpha-agonists have been shown to decrease the adrenergic symptoms of withdrawal, theoretically by suppressing norepinephrine over production during withdrawal.[21] Although clonidine is effective,[53] another trial found it less effective than chlormethiazole, with more associated side effects.[54] Lofexidine, available only experimentally, also appears promising; a prospective double blind study shows modestly decreased pulse and blood pressure as well as lower serum norepinephrine levels in the drug group.[55] Further experimentation is necessary to define alpha-agonist efficacy and dosages before general usage will be accepted.

PSYCHOTROPIC DRUGS

Phenothiazines and butyrophenones have been used successfully in treating alcohol withdrawal. Side effects, however, including increased seizure frequency, hypotension, extrapyramidal symptoms, hyperpyrexia, and death,[34,45] have virtually eliminated their use except for treatment of primary psychopathology persisting after withdrawal resolves.[56] A possible exception is low-dose haloperidol (a butyrophenone), which is used extensively at 0.5 to 2.0 mg without significant side effects.[20,25,34]

OTHER PHARMACOLOGIC AGENTS

In the past, ethanol, paraldehyde, and chloral hydrate have been used for withdrawal therapy based on their cross-tolerance with alcohol. Although effective in some ways, these agents have largely been abandoned.[24] Ethanol is still used as a treatment in some centers, but is limited to PO or IV administration; it does nothing to reverse the induced metabolic abnormalities, and the concentration that may be given IV can be inadequate in patients requiring large doses. The short half-life can make titration difficult. Paraldehyde also continues to have its proponents, although administration is difficult and complications frequent. Paraldehyde has a noxious odor and must be given in glass because it melts plastic. Local irritation after administration is common: gastritis, sterile abscess, and proctitis follow oral, intramuscular, and rectal administration respectively. Intravenous administration has been associated with pulmonary edema.[21] Nearly one fourth of patients receiving paraldehyde in one study became apneic.[57] Chloral hydrate can only be given orally and has a low therapeutic index.

Magnesium deficiency was once thought to be a prominent component of withdrawal pathophysiology, and administration of magnesium was thought to diminish withdrawal symptoms and complications.[58] A controlled double blind study of magnesium therapy, however, showed no benefit compared to placebo.[59] Hypomagnesemia, however, can result in tremor, hallucination, and seizures, and therefore should be treated.[23]

Two anticonvulsants, carbamazepine and chlormethiazole, have become popular in Europe for the treatment of alcohol withdrawal; each is considered by some to be a standard therapy for withdrawal.[21,54] Carbamazepine (Tegretol) is favored because of a theoretic advantage in suppressing "kindling" and kindled seizure foci.[60] Several studies, including a prospective double-blind trial by Malcolm et al.,[60] found carbamazepine to be safe and effective, with few side effects. When given in doses of 200 mg every 6 hours, carbamazepine was as effective as oxazepam. Although no parenteral form is available, possible advantages include lack of abuse potential and hepatotoxicity. Chlormethiazole, a sedative anticonvulsant, has been shown to be effective in treatment of withdrawal; however, it has not been approved for use in the U.S., and multiple deaths have been associated with its use in alcohol withdrawal.[21]

ALCOHOL-RELATED DISEASES

The acute and chronic diseases associated with the use of alcohol are myriad, ranging from trauma to dementia to malnutrition, as well as effects on the developing fetus in a pregnant woman. All organ systems may be affected through either direct toxic effects or the nutritional deficiencies that often accompany alcohol use.

The following sections offer a brief overview of alcohol-associated diseases, with more extensive discussion when the particular disease state is found exclusively or mainly in the setting of alcohol use or alcoholism. Because most of the disease states are more thoroughly covered elsewhere in the text, the reader is referred to the specific sections involved for details of management and in-depth discussion.

METABOLIC DISORDERS

ALCOHOLIC KETOACIDOSIS

In 1940, Dillon et al. described five patients with severe ketoacidosis and normal or only slightly elevated blood glucose levels.[61] All five either admitted to alcoholism or had presumptive evidence of chronic alcohol abuse. Since then, the distinct syndrome of alcoholic ketoacidosis (AKA) has been described and well documented.[62-64] Most patients with the disorder are heavy chronic alcoholics, classically with an in-

crease in their baseline consumption in the weeks before presentation. Because of gastrointestinal problems such as gastritis or pancreatitis, vomiting, or the exclusive consumption of alcohol, a decrease in food intake occurs in the days preceding presentation. It appears that cessation of carbohydrate consumption and depletion of body carbohydrate stores are a prerequisite to the onset of the syndrome. In this setting, fatty acids are increasingly utilized, leading to ketone production. This disorder recurs in patients who are predisposed and is not directly related to the amount of alcohol ingested.

Patients commonly present with complaints related to gastrointestinal distress or shortness of breath. Alteration of mental status, either with or without signs of withdrawal, is common. Physical examination uniformly demonstrates Kussmaul respirations. Other findings, such as ketotic breath, tachycardia, or specific abdominal findings, are variable. Often an infection such as pneumonia is present.

Laboratory findings are typical. A high anion gap metabolic acidosis with low, normal, or only slightly elevated serum glucose is pathognomonic in the setting of alcohol abuse. The pH may be normal because of metabolic alkalosis from protracted vomiting. Specifically measured serum ketones are markedly elevated, with a markedly elevated beta-hydroxybutyrate/acetoacetate ratio. Because of this, urinary or serum colorimetric tests, which measure only acetoacetate, may be misleadingly negative or only trace-positive. Serum lactate levels are usually only modestly elevated. Insulin levels are typically low-normal, whereas cortisol, growth hormone, and glucagon all tend to be elevated. Serum electrolytes, especially phosphate and magnesium, may be diminished. The arterial pH is usually in the range of 7.10 to 7.30, although profound acidemia may occur.

The differential diagnosis of AKA includes DKA, alcoholic gastritis with starvation, peptic ulcer disease, and pancreatitis. The differential diagnosis of an anion gap acidosis in an alcoholic includes AKA; DKA; uremia; lactic acidosis from hypoxia, hypertension, or sepsis; and ingestion of salicylates, INH, iron, methanol, or ethylene glycol.

The treatment of this syndrome, when recognized, is fairly straightforward. Replacement of fluids and carbohydrate stores usually reverses the abnormalities within 24 to 36 hours. Large amounts of IV 5% dextrose in saline, along with oral nutrition when this becomes possible, are necessary. Without adequate replenishment of carbohydrates, ketosis may recur. Any electrolyte abnormalities, with special emphasis on magnesium, potassium, and phosphate, should be corrected.[65] There is no place for insulin in the treatment of alcoholic ketoacidosis. Sodium bicarbonate may be considered in patients with severely depressed pH (less than 7.00), but, considering the prompt response usually seen to fluid and dextrose replacement, this is usually unnecessary and should be done cautiously. In uncomplicated cases, prognosis with proper therapy is excellent. Deaths do occur, usually in the setting of severe volume depletion or other concurrent illness.

ALCOHOLIC HYPOGLYCEMIA

This somewhat rare syndrome is seen exclusively in chronic, severe alcoholics. Several factors must exist before it can occur. First, hepatic glycogen stores must be depleted. This occurs mainly through the consumption of a diet severely deficient in carbohydrates for a prolonged period. Additionally, alcohol inhibits glycogenesis by numerous pathways, causing fat instead of glycogen to be deposited in hepatocytes.[6] With continued alcohol consumption, the liver becomes less and less able to engage in gluconeogenesis, leading to a gradual decline in serum glucose levels.[62] Profound hypoglycemia may result, with complications of coma, seizures, and death. Unlike other forms of hypoglycemia, the alcoholic type is unresponsive to glucagon.

The typical patient is a chronic "street alcoholic," usually found unresponsive. Physical examination may reveal the signs of hypoglycemia with diaphoresis, tachycardia, and tremulousness. In patients with alcoholic neuropathy or infection, these may be absent. Neurologic examination usually reveals a depressed level of consciousness and nonfocal neurologic motor examination, although transient focal neurologic findings in hypoglycemia are occasionally seen. The patient may have seizures.

If not treated promptly, hypoglycemia can lead to permanent brain injury. For this reason, again it must be emphasized that ALL patients with altered level of consciousness, even those with a strong odor of ethanol on the breath, should either have serum glucose evaluated with a rapid bedside test strip or receive IV dextrose immediately on presentation. Thiamine, 100 mg IV or IM, should be administered with the glucose because of the possibility of precipitating acute Wernicke's encephalopathy with the administration of glucose alone.[65,66] Serum glucose before dextrose administration should be measured immediately, preferably with one of the bedside glucose test strips, and serum should be sent to the laboratory for confirmation. Repeated IV boluses of 50% dextrose may be necessary. Because all patients with alcoholic hypoglycemia are in a starvation state, treatment is not complete even after the initial glucose is given and the level of consciousness normalizes. These patients should be continued on IV 10% dextrose until they can ingest adequate amounts of carbohydrates by mouth to create at least a partial glycogen buffer in the liver.

WATER AND ELECTROLYTE DISORDERS IN ALCOHOLICS

The effects of alcohol on body water and electrolyte balance are complex. Any generalization, such as "all

TABLE 84-3. SERUM ELECTROLYTE FINDINGS IN CHRONIC ALCOHOLISM

Electrolyte	Finding
Magnesium	Diminished
Calcium	Usually diminished
Phosphate	Diminished, may drop during treatment
Sodium	Variable
Potassium	Often diminished

alcoholics are dehydrated," is obviously false because the habits and nutritional patterns of alcoholics vary as widely as socioeconomic status or choice of beverage. Although most disorders of water and electrolytes in the alcoholic patient are variable and unpredictable, a few consistent observations have emerged (Table 84-3).

Alcohol ingestion produces an immediate increase in urine volume and fall in urine osmolarity, caused by suppression of ADH.[8] Alcohol administered by way of the carotid artery in animals produces the same response without a rise in blood alcohol levels.[67] This prompt but limited diuresis is reversed in the withdrawal phase by increased levels of ADH and antidiuresis yielding no net change in water balance in the well hydrated drinker.[68] The water balance seen in any particular patient therefore depends more on factors other than on the effects of ethanol itself.

Many chronic alcoholics have a poor diet and poor intake of nonalcoholic fluids. The consumption of distilled spirits, which contain relatively little water compared to beer and wine, contributes to volume contraction. This, along with the effects of withdrawal, vomiting, diarrhea, and possible infection, can cause severe intravascular and total body water depletion, at times presenting as hypovolemic shock.

On the other hand, severe chronic alcohol abuse can lead to water intoxication and hyponatremia. Patients with vomiting or diarrhea who replace the volume lost with hypotonic beer or wine, or those who drink massive quantities of beer, which is low in sodium, are prone to this. Water intoxication may cause seizures and altered sensorium, and has additionally been implicated in the syndrome of central pontine myelinolysis.[69]

Alcohol use is associated strongly with hypomagnesemia and total body magnesium depletion.[8,70] Poor dietary intake is a major factor in its development. Additionally, alcohol causes decreased gastrointestinal absorption and a direct renal leak of magnesium even on the first day of consumption.[8] Magnesium levels in alcoholics have been found to be diminished in serum, brain, cerebrospinal fluid (CSF), and muscle. Hypomagnesemia has been implicated in cardiac arrhythmias, seizures, tremors, and CNS irritability.

Hypophosphatemia is a common and significant derangement found in alcoholics. In addition to hypophosphatemia observed on presentation, serum phosphate commonly drops significantly after carbohydrate feeding, probably as a result of a shift of phosphate into hepatocytes.[8] Severe hypophosphatemia is associated with rhabdomyolysis, cardiovascular collapse, and hematologic abnormalities.

Although somewhat unpredictable, electrolyte and water abnormalities are common in alcoholics. As mentioned previously, an IV line with dextrose, sodium chloride, multivitamins, 100 mg thiamine, 1 mg folate, and 1 to 2 g of magnesium sulfate should be administered to alcoholic patients with evidence of chronic use. Additionally, serum sodium, potassium, chloride, bicarbonate, calcium, phosphorus, and magnesium should be measured. Special attention should be paid to serial measurement of the serum phosphate levels in hospitalized alcoholic patients to detect the sometimes severe drop in their serum phosphate levels often seen with resumption of adequate nutrition.

OTHER METABOLIC AND ENDOCRINE DISORDERS

Alcohol may be a factor in the cause of many disorders likely to present in the ED. Although many are chronic or multifactorial, ethanol abuse should be considered in the differential diagnosis of these conditions. Table 84-4 lists some of these.

NEUROLOGIC DISORDERS

WERNICKE-KORSAKOFF SYNDROME

Well known as one of the disorders most closely associated with chronic alcoholism, Wernicke's encephalopathy remains underdiagnosed in a large percentage of cases.[65,72–74] Its prevalence in autopsy studies is between 0.8 and 3% of the general population, depending on the geographic region involved.[72–77] Among alcoholics, the prevalence is as high as 12.5%.[75] Only about 20% of cases are diagnosed before death. This underdiagnosis is unfortunate because Wernicke's encephalopathy is a major reversible cause of dementia and if untreated, has 10 to 20% mortality.[65,72,75] Additionally, approximately 80% of patients who survive Wernicke's encephalopathy evidence some degree of Korsakoff's psychosis.[72,73] Increased awareness and treatment of this disorder are vital.

At its root, Wernicke's encephalopathy is a nutritional disorder caused by deficiency of thiamine, also

known as vitamine B_1. Thiamine as thiamine pyrophosphate is a coenzyme necessary for the metabolism of glucose in both the Krebs cycle and oxidative phosphorylation. Because the brain depends on glucose for its metabolism, it is particularly susceptible to the deranged glucose metabolism caused by thiamine deficiency. Important in the alcoholic patient is the fact that magnesium is necessary in the utilization of thiamine.[73]

Although the only prerequisite to the development of Wernicke's encephalopathy is a diet deficient in thiamine, it has been observed that not all thiamine-deficient alcoholics develop the disease. This is perhaps caused by an inherited difference of activity of thiamine-dependent transketolase.[73,78]

Wernicke's encephalopathy is associated with necrosis of both neurons and myelinated structures in a symmetric pattern involving the mammillary bodies, cerebellar vermis, hypothalamus, third and sixth cranial nerve nuclei, and areas of the tegmentum.[66,72–77] Petechial and, occasionally, gross hemorrhage is seen in these areas on gross pathologic examination. CT and magnetic resonance imaging (MRI) scanning can occasionally demonstrate characteristic changes in the diencephalon in patients with Wernicke's encephalopathy.[73,74,79]

Because laboratory and radiographic findings are nonspecific or only occasionally present, Wernicke's encephalopathy remains a clinical diagnosis. The abrupt onset of the triad of oculomotor abnormalities (nystagmus, gaze paresis, pupillary abnormalities, or ptosis), ataxia, and mental confusion comprise the classic description of Wernicke's syndrome. Ocular changes and ataxia may precede the confusional state by a few days.[74] The nystagmus typically seen is bilateral horizontal and upgaze-evoked nystagmus. Ataxia is cerebellar in nature and characterized by broad-based gait and truncal ataxia, with lower extremity involvement predominating over upper extremity ataxia. Disorientation, apathy, inattention, and drowsiness, described as a "generalized confusional state," constitute the classic mental status changes observed.

The classic presentation notwithstanding, many variants of the syndrome exist, contributing to underdiagnosis. The classic triad may be incompletely present. Importantly, coma or stupor may be the sole presentation. Hypothermia and hypotension from hypothalamic involvement are frequently seen.[65,66,72–77,80] The often extremely protean presentation of the disease mandates that Wernicke's encephalopathy be considered in the differential diagnosis of all alcoholic patients with mental status changes.

Wernicke's encephalopathy must be treated as a true medical emergency because delay or failure to treat it may result in long-term disability or death. Essentially, all alcoholic patients with abnormal mental status should receive at least 100 mg of thiamine intramuscularly or intravenously. Those in whom the

---

TABLE 84-4. OTHER METABOLIC AND ENDOCRINE EFFECTS OF ALCOHOLISM

Hyperlipidemia	Gynecomastia
Hyperuricemia	Menstrual irregularities (amenorrhea,
Hypogonadism	menorrhagia)
Impotence	Reversible Cushing's syndrome
Testicular atrophy	

diagnosis is strongly suspected or confirmed by examination should be admitted and receive at least 100 mg of thiamine intravenously for 5 days or more.

Ocular findings can be expected to resolve within hours to days with adequate therapy.[72–74,81] Indeed, it has been suggested that reversal of ocular findings be used as a criterion for "titrating" initial thiamine therapy, with up to 1000 mg being necessary in the first 12 hours.[74] Ataxia and confusion may be slower to resolve, gradually disappearing over weeks to months even with adequate therapy. Variable amounts of permanent disability may remain.

Resistance to thiamine therapy may be seen in patients with hypomagnesemia because magnesium is a necessary cofactor in thiamine utilization.[9,65,74,82] The many nutritional deficiencies seen in alcoholics argue strongly for the use of a standard IV solution in alcoholic patients seen in the ED to avoid inadvertently omitting any part of therapy. In our institution, a standing protocol exists for the administration to alcoholic patients of an IV solution consisting of one liter of D_5 0.45N saline with one ampule of a commercially prepared multivitamin solution, 100 mg of thiamine, 1 mg of folate, and 2 g of $MgSO_4$. The solution should be adjusted to correct other metabolic disorders as identified.

Korsakoff's psychosis, originally believed to be a distinct disorder, is now recognized as the chronic phase of the Wernicke-Korsakoff syndrome. It is characterized by various degrees of retrograde and anterograde amnesia, with often fanciful cofabulation appearing in early stages to cover for the patient's lapses in memory.[83] Later in the disease, the adaptive confabulation often disappears, and patients become severely disabled. Institutionalization is often the only recourse. Wernicke's and Korsakoff's syndromes often blend imperceptibly into each other. Treatment with thiamine early in the course of Korsakoff's syndrome may reverse or arrest some aspects of the disease, but in more than 50% of cases, recovery is incomplete.[74]

ALCOHOLIC CEREBELLAR DEGENERATION

This syndrome, characterized pathologically by degeneration of Purkinje cells in the anterior and superior cerebellar vermis and adjacent hemispheric areas, is encountered in up to 27% of the brains of alcoholic patients at autopsy.[74,75] Men are more frequently affected than women. Clinically, patients with this disorder evidence a wide-based stance with varying degrees of gait and truncal ataxia. As in Wernicke's syndrome, the lower extremities are affected much more than the upper extremities. Nystagmus, dysarthria, and tremor may be observed, but almost exclusively during acute episodes of intoxication, metabolic derangement, or withdrawal; with resolution of these acute states, the nystagmus, dysarthria, or tremor disappears.[73] Disorders of consciousness are absent in the pure syndrome of cerebellar degeneration. CT or MRI scanning may demonstrate atrophy of the midline cerebellar cortex.

The differential diagnosis of ataxia in an alcoholic includes phenytoin or barbiturate toxicity, heavy metal poisoning, subdural hematoma, CVA, hepatic encephalopathy, tumor, cerebellar hematoma, neuropathy, and carcinomatous cerebellar degeneration.

The cause of alcoholic cerebellar degeneration remains largely unknown. Although it is seen almost exclusively in chronic alcoholics with excessive consumption for at least 10 years, there is little evidence that alcohol itself causes the lesions. The similarity of the cerebellar lesions to those of Wernicke's syndrome suggest a nutritional component. Other experiments suggest that electrolyte abnormalities may play a role.[84]

The only treatment of this disorder involves alcohol abstention and adequate nutrition. With therapy, the symptoms may be arrested or even reversed. In the emergency setting, it becomes critical to *identify potentially treatable conditions* in alcoholics.

CENTRAL PONTINE MYELINOLYSIS

Central pontine myelinolysis (CPM) is a rare disorder that most commonly affects alcoholics, but is also seen in patients with other diseases complicated by electrolyte abnormalities or malnutrition such as burns, cancer, diabetes, or Addison's disease. The pathologic lesion is an area of pallorous demyelination in the base of the pons. Approximately 10% of patients also have symmetric extrapontine lesions in the striatum, thalamus, cerebellum, or cerebral white matter.[73] These lesions may often be seen on high-resolution CT or MRI scanning.

The cause of this syndrome is controversial. It is encountered almost exclusively in patients with hyponatremia. The first reports coincided with the beginnings of the widespread use of intravenous fluids for the correction of electrolyte abnormalities, leading to the hypothesis that this is an iatrogenic disorder caused by too-rapid correction of severe hyponatremia leading to water shifts within the brain.[73,74,85] Others have proposed that it is the brain edema caused by hyponatremia itself that is the root of the problem.[86] Clinical experience and recent investigations suggest that both factors play a role, but that higher rates of correction of hyponatremia are definitely associated with higher incidences of CPM.[87]

The signs and symptoms of CPM may be subclinical or obscured by other problems such as alcohol withdrawal. It may present in a vague, protean fashion. Classically, during treatment of hyponatremia, manifestations are the subacute onset of progressive quadriparesis, pseudobulbar palsies such as dysarthria or difficulty in swallowing, and paresis of horizontal eye movements. With more severe involvement, pupillary paresis, decerebrate posturing, respiratory failure, and stupor or coma may become prominent. The "locked-in" state can result. CPM is often fatal in 2 to

3 weeks, although rare cases of partial or complete recovery have been reported.

The cornerstone of treatment is prevention. In light of the increasing evidence that excessively rapid correction of hyponatremia plays a major role in the development of the syndrome, the careful, slow correction of hyponatremia to levels of not more than 120 to 130 mOsm/liter seems the only prudent course. A rate of correction of less than 12 mOsm per liter per day through the use of free-water restriction or isotonic saline infusion is probably safest.[88,89]

Once the syndrome has developed, the only treatment is general supportive care, ensuring adequate nutrition and maintenance of normal serum electrolytes.

CHRONIC DEMENTIA AND CEREBRAL ATROPHY

Studies have indicated that, matched for age, alcoholic persons have significantly increased incidence of cortical atrophy, low brain weight and volume, with dilation of the lateral ventricles and widening of the cerebral sulci, and impaired performance on neuropsychologic tests over control nonalcoholic patients.[1,72-75,90] With abstinence from alcohol, some of these changes may be reversible.[91]

The acute or subacute onset of dementia in an alcoholic patient, as in any other patient, may signal a metabolic encephalopathy, infection, or a post-traumatic lesion such as subdural hematoma. All patients with new-onset dementia deserve a thorough workup to identify potentially reversible causes of dementia.

ALCOHOLIC PERIPHERAL NEUROPATHIES

Alcoholic polyneuropathy is a commonly seen problem in the chronic alcoholic patient, most probably caused by nutritional deficiencies. Symptoms are usually related to burning, painful paresthesias or numbness in a "stocking-glove" distribution. Physical examination usually reveals deficits in light touch and vibratory sensation. Deep tendon reflexes, especially the Achilles reflex, are often diminished or absent. In severe cases, motor weakness, muscle atrophy, muscle changes, and loss of proprioception leading to ataxia are seen. Autonomic dysfunction, causing impotence, orthostatic hypotension, bladder and bowel control problems, or Argyll-Robertson pupils is occasionally encountered.[74] Treatment again involves nutritional support and abstention from alcohol.

Mononeuropathies, such as the well-known "Saturday night palsy," are usually the result of pressure damage to superficially located individual nerves. The usual scenario is that of an intoxicated individual lying in the same position without moving for a number of hours, then awakening with a wrist or ankle drop. Commonly involved nerves are the radial, ulnar, and common peroneal nerves. A dense deficit of both sensory and motor modalities in the distribution of the nerve in question is the rule on physical examination.

Recovery of function depends on the amount of damage suffered by the nerve and the general metabolic and nutritional status of the patient. Treatment involves splinting of the extremity in a position of function to avoid contracture and further damage to the often insensate limb, range-of-motion exercises, and referral to a neurologist for long-term care. Occasionally swelling around the nerve may be severe, with vascular compromise, requiring surgical decompression. The presence of fasciitis is an emergency that requires rapid decompression to save the function of the extremity.

ALCOHOL-RELATED MYOPATHIES

The muscles are affected by alcohol abuse to a larger extent than has previously been appreciated, through both direct toxic effects and the nutritional and metabolic derangements discussed previously. Two fairly distinct syndromes, the acute and chronic alcoholic myopathies, have been described.

ACUTE ALCOHOLIC MYOPATHY

This is a syndrome of acute muscle necrosis that occurs largely in binge drinkers. It may range in severity from an asymptomatic state or mild muscle achiness with transient, small rises in serum creatine kinase to frank rhabdomyolysis. Alcoholism is the most common cause of rhabdomyolysis.[92,93]

Numerous factors contribute to the pathogenesis of acute alcoholic myopathy. Alcohol itself has a direct toxic effect on skeletal muscle; administration of ethanol to well-nourished volunteers causes muscle damage.[73,94] Additionally, the hypophosphatemia common in alcoholics is well known to cause rhabdomyolysis. Ischemic muscle damage may result when a drunken person "passes out" and lies immobile on an extremity for a number of hours. Finally, the increased muscular activity associated with alcohol withdrawal may contribute to this condition.

The patient with acute alcoholic myopathy presents with complaints of muscle pain with or without swelling, usually after a heavy binge of drinking lasting 1 or more days. It commonly presents on awakening after the heavy binge, and is often accompanied by symptoms of alcohol withdrawal.[95] Involvement often predominates in the lower extremities, especially the calves. Involved muscle groups are usually tender and may be tense. Compartment symdromes may occur.

Laboratory examination always shows elevated serum levels of creatine kinase (CK) activity, usually greater than 10 to 20 times normal values. Myoglobinemia may be detectable, although this is often transient because of rapid renal clearance.[93] Serum potassium levels may be increased. In severe rhabdomyolysis, the main complication is the development of acute renal tubular necrosis. Elevated blood urea nitrogen (BUN) and creatinine and an active urine sediment are seen in these cases. The urine may be brown to red in color if myoglobin is being excreted. Urine ortholidine testing, the commonest test found on urinary dipsticks, does not distinguish between the heme in hemoglobin and myoglobin; therefore urine dipsticks show positive blood during myoglobinuria. An acellular urine sediment in with positive dipstick for blood is highly suggestive of myoglobinuria. Hemolysis, however, must be ruled out to positively diagnose myoglobinuria. The most sensitive and specific laboratory test remains elevated CK MM isoenzyme levels; when markedly elevated, this test is virtually pathognomonic for skeletal muscle injury.

As mentioned, the major risk of morbidity for patients with acute alcoholic myopathy is the development of acute renal tubular necrosis. Obviously, any alcoholic patient with complaints of acute muscle pain should be investigated further with measurement of serum CK, BUN, creatinine and urinalysis. Additionally, alcoholic myopathy should be considered in any binge-drinking alcoholic or patient in alcohol withdrawal. Patients with significantly elevated CK, BUN, or creatinine, or evidence of myoglobinuria should be considered for admission for observation and intravenous hydration to avoid renal damage. Specfic details of management of rhabdomyolysis and acute renal tubular necrosis may be found in the appropriate sections of this text.

CHRONIC ALCOHOLIC MYOPATHY

In contrast to the acute syndrome, chronic alcoholic myopathy is usually seen in the chronic, daily alcohol abuser. Notably absent are such acute markers of muscle injury as pain, swelling, and elevated CK or serum and urinary myoglobin. These patients often also have other chronic complications of ethanol abuse such as neuropathy, Wernicke's syndrome, or cirrhosis, and are usually seen for complaints and problems unrelated to their muscular disease. The cause of the chronic syndrome is thought to be mainly nutritional deprivation.[95]

The usual muscular-related complaint in these cases is a progressive, gradual muscle weakness, most prominent in the hips and shoulder girdle. Physical examination often reveals atrophy. Histologic studies have shown that this disorder selectively affects type I ("fast twitch") fibers, relatively sparing the type II myocytes.[96] These patients usually give no history of episodes of acute myopathy.

Treatment of this chronic syndrome, as with most other chronic alcoholic problems, consists of abstinence from alcohol and adequate nutrition.

ALCOHOL-ASSOCIATED GASTROINTESTINAL DISORDERS

The effects of ethanol on the gastrointestinal tract are diverse. Many of the common and life-threatening complaints encountered in the alcoholic patient in the ED are related to the effects of alcohol on various parts of the gastrointestinal system. A brief discussion of some of the most prominent problems is presented; the reader is referred to the more in-depth discussions of each specific problem elsewhere in the text for details of diagnosis and management.

ALCOHOLIC LIVER DISEASE

One of the major sources of morbidity and mortality in alcoholics, liver disease in alcoholism consists of three classic syndromes: fatty liver, alcoholic hepatitis, and cirrhosis. As many as 30,000 deaths per year occur from the complications of alcoholic liver disease.[1]

FATTY LIVER

A common clinical and biopsy finding in alcoholic patients, excessive fat deposition in hepatocytes may occur in persons who consume even the relatively moderate amount of 20 to 40 grams of alcohol per day.[97] Usually asymptomatic and merely an incidental finding on physical examination, the hepatic enlargement caused by hepatic steatosis may also cause mild jaundice or upper abdominal pain from capsular stretching. No specific treatment is necessary or available beyond abstinence from alcohol and adequate nutrition. Alcoholic fatty liver does not predispose to cirrhosis, and resolves in the absence of alcohol consumption in 4 to 6 weeks.[97,98]

ALCOHOLIC HEPATITIS

This is often the most difficult of alcoholic liver diseases to diagnose because of its variable, often vague presentation, which may range from totally asymptomatic to fulminant hepatic failure.

Classically characterized by insidious, slow onset of anorexia, vomiting, jaundice, low-grade fever and abdominal pain, it may be impossible to distinguish from other causes of hepatitis. Extrahepatic manifestations such as GI bleeding may predominate.

Emergency management is similar to that of other forms of hepatitis. Physical examination should concentrate on estimating the severity of hepatitis and on recognizing any potential life-threatening complications. Laboratory evaluation should include complete blood count, liver enzymes to estimate the severity of ongoing hepatic necrosis, and a prothrombin time. Viral serology should be considered to rule out other causes of hepatitis.

Treatment depends on the severity of the disease. Only patients with mild disease should be considered for discharge from the ED, with prompt follow-up with a gastroenterologist or internist. Indications for admission include intractable vomiting, significantly abnormal vital signs, any sign of encephalopathy, gastrointestinal bleeding, renal insufficiency, deep jaundice, or prolonged prothrombin time.

ALCOHOLIC CIRRHOSIS

Cirrhosis, the irreversible stage of alcoholic liver disease, develops in only 10 to 20% of chronic alcoholics, suggesting that other factors besides alcoholism per se contribute to its development.[97] Approximately 120 to 180 grams of alcohol per day for 15 years appears to be a critical "total dose" necessary for the development of cirrhosis.[99]

Usually presenting to the ED only when complications intervene, the cirrhotic patient may be asymptomatic or have vague chronic complaints relating to weight loss, fatigue, or abdominal discomfort. Advanced cirrhosis yields a fragile patient, at high risk for GI bleeding from esophageal varices or other sites, infection, encephalopathy, or frank liver failure.

Emergency management of the patient with cirrhosis should concentrate on the identification and treatment of complications. Gastrointestinal bleeding should be treated gently, because overhydration can increase bleeding rates from esophageal varices.[97] Abdominal pain or increased ascites may signal the development of spontaneous bacterial peritonitis, even with no fever, and mandates paracentesis for Gram's stain and culture. Coagulopathies predispose to intracranial and gastrointestinal bleeding; signs of these should be sought actively. Any relatively minor infection, GI bleeding, or use of alcohol or other sedative drugs may tip the patient over into encephalopathy. Additionally, patients with alcoholic cirrhosis are at significantly higher risk for hepatocellular carcinoma.

Cirrhosis is a chronic, end-stage disease characterized by a slow, gradual loss of function. Any acute or subacute change in the patient therefore probably signals a new problem or complication and mandates an intensive effort to identify and treat any of the multitude of complications that may accompany this disorder. Most patients with complications of cirrhosis should be admitted for inpatient care.

ALCOHOLIC PANCREATITIS

Although the exact pathogenesis of this disease is unclear, alcohol abuse is definitely associated with pancreatitis, both acute and chronic. The most common presenting complaints are related to epigastric abdominal pain radiating to the back and vomiting. History usually reveals an alcoholic binge immediately preceding the onset of pain and vomiting. The patient is usually lying still in bed, often curled on his or her side. Abdominal findings may vary from benign to board-like rigidity. A mass representing an inflamed, phlegmonous pancreas or a pseudocyst may be found. Bowel sounds are usually preserved.[51] Laboratory findings are nonspecific. Elevated serum amylase and lipase are often found, but their degree of elevation does not correlate with severity of the attack. Normal

levels may be encountered in chronic pancreatitis; alternatively, elevation of amylase may occur because of vomiting. Radiographic findings are variable: occasional calcifications in the pancreas area are seen, and a "sentinel loop" of localized ileus may be helpful. CT scan may be necessary to identify the severely edematous, hemorrhagic pancreas or pseudocyst.

Hypotension, tachycardia, and skin signs of shock are ominous findings, as are acidosis, decreased hematocrit and diminished serum calcium levels. Prognosis in acute pancreatitis is inversely proportional to the patient's age. Complications include shock, pseudocysts, abscess formation and sepsis, coagulopathies, diabetes mellitus, and malabsorption.

Management consists of fluid resuscitation of patients, control of vomiting, and pain control. Signs of infection and hemorrhage should be actively sought and treated. Only patients with relatively minor episodes, able to tolerate oral nutrition and hydration, and in whom outpatient pain control is possible should be considered for discharge. *All others necessitate admission.* Close follow-up is essential even in mild-appearing cases.

OTHER GASTROINTESTINAL DISORDERS

Excessive ethanol consumption is a well-known cause of esophageal reflux, hemorrhagic gastritis, esophageal and gastric carcinoma, and chronic diarrhea. The newly developed bacterium Heliobacter pylori (first cultured in 1982) may also be involved in alcoholic gastritis and ulcer, offering the possibility of more treatment options (e.g., bismuth and metronidazole with tetracycline or ampicillin).[51a] Gastrointestinal bleeding from Mallory-Weiss tears, esophageal varices, or gastric or duodenal bleeding is common and often life threatening. See Table 84-5 for a list of alcohol-related gastrointestinal problems. Patients with hematemesis, melena, marked anemia from bleeding, or any unstable vital signs mandate admission to the hospital.

HEMATOLOGIC DISORDERS (TABLE 84-6)

Alcohol affects all elements of the blood in complex ways. Many of these may have an impact on a patient's presentation to the ED.

Anemia of varying degrees is common among patients with severe alcoholism. Although ethanol itself

TABLE 84-5. GASTROINTESTINAL DISORDERS ASSOCIATED WITH ALCOHOLISM

Gastroesophageal reflux	Gastrointestinal Bleeding
Esophageal carcinoma	—Mallory-Weiss tears
Erosive gastritis	—Gastritis
Chronic diarrhea	—Esophageal varices
Steatorrhea	—Coagulopathies
Malabsorption	—Internal hemorrhoids

TABLE 84-6. HEMATOLOGIC DISORDERS ASSOCIATED WITH ALCOHOLISM
Red Cells—Anemias
Marrow suppression
Megaloblastic (folate deficiency)
Iron deficiency (blood loss)
Sideroblastic
Hemolytic
White Cells
Leukopenia
Depressed function
Reduced T cell number
Hemostatis
Thrombocytopenia
Platelet dysfunction
Disseminated intravascular coagulation
Coagulation factor deficits

has a myelosuppressive effect and causes vacuolization of erythrocyte precursors, most alcohol-related anemias appear to be mainly caused by malnutrition.[101] The most characteristic finding is macrocytosis, often with mean cell volumes over 100 cu μ. This is caused by folate deficiency in most cases. Disorders of iron metabolism are also common among alcoholics, giving rise to microcytic, hypochromic anemias and sideroblastic anemia. With cessation of alcohol abuse and adequate nutritional support, these anemias usually resolve. Chronic gastrointestinal bleeding may also cause hypochromic, microcytic anemia in the alcoholic.

Alcoholics with liver disease are also often predisposed to hemolytic anemia. The peripheral blood may show many bizarre erythrocyte forms. These anemias carry a poorer prognosis for resolution. Patients with profound or symptomatic anemia should be admitted. Other patients with anemia should be referred for appropriate evaluation and treatment.

Leukocyte cell lines are affected by alcohol also. Leukopenia may become profound if the alcoholic patient with nutritional deficiencies is further stressed by infection.[102] Additionally, leukocyte function is depressed by alcoholism, and may be responsible for the reduced resistance to infection seen in alcoholics.

Coagulopathies are common in alcoholics because of both platelet and humoral defects. Platelet number and function are both depressed by alcoholism. Contributing to this are nutritional deficiencies, especially of folate, splenic sequestration caused by portal hypertension, and a direct toxic effect of alcohol.[101] Additionally, patients with liver disease may manifest humoral coagulation deficiencies, usually decreased activity of the vitamin K-dependent clotting factors II, VII, IX, and X. Patients with prolonged prothrombin times should be given parenteral vitamin K. This may be expected to effect a variable decrease in prothrombin time, depending on the amount of hepatic dysfunction and the patient's nutritional status.

CARDIAC DISORDERS

Alcohol and alcohol abuse have diverse effects on cardiac structure and function. Although effects of lifestyle and other habits have been difficult to separate from the actual effects of alcohol, certain definite associations have been observed. Additionally, alcohol may exacerbate or uncover preclinical cardiac disease from other causes.

ACUTE EFFECTS OF ALCOHOL ON THE HEART

Acute alcohol consumption has a variable effect on cardiac function. Although it has been shown to have a direct negative inotropic effect, it also has a vasodilatory effect, often yielding no change or even a slight improvement in cardiac index.[1,103–104] Patients on beta blockers or other drugs that interfere with adrenergic tone may show a more pronounced decrease in cardiac function when acutely intoxicated.[103,105] Patients with already compromised left ventricular function may have exacerbations of their CHF caused by alcohol intoxication.

Arrhythmias, both supraventricular and ventricular, are well known to be a complication of alcohol abuse. Dubbed the "holiday heart syndrome" because it was originally observed in alcoholics increasing their consumption around the holiday season, this syndrome occurs in alcoholics during or immediately after a heavier-than-normal drinking binge.[106] Atrial fibrillation is by far the most commonly observed arrhythmia, but premature atrial contractions, atrial flutter, paroxysmal atrial tachycardia, premature ventricular contractions, and ventricular tachycardia are also seen.[103,104,106,107] A positive correlation between blood alcohol concentration and mean rate of ventricular premature contractions has been observed.[107] Organic heart disease, even subclinical, increases the risk of "holiday heart" many times.[103,104] Many epidemiologic studies have shown a positive correlation between alcohol abuse and sudden cardiac death.[103,104,108–110]

Electrocardiographic and electrophysiologic changes that have been observed during acute alcohol intoxication include P-R, QRS, and Q-T prolongation, varying degrees of heart block including third degree, bundle branch blocks, and prolonged H-V intervals.[103,104,107] It is not possible to make any generalization, however, because the effects of chronic alcoholism, electrolyte and nutritional abnormalities, and underlying heart disease are difficult to discriminate.

CHRONIC EFFECTS OF ALCOHOL ON THE HEART

Chronic alcohol consumption may lead to progressive cardiac dysfunction and eventual development of congestive heart failure with all its complications. Studies in which the various effects of the metabolic, nutritional, and lifestyle problems to which alcoholics are prone have been controlled and have demonstrated clearly that alcohol consumption itself can cause progressive myocardial damage leading ultimately to dilated cardiomyopathy.[103,104] It has been suggested that alcohol abuse is a contributing factor in up to 50% of cases of congestive cardiomyopathy.[111]

Alcoholic cardiomyopathy is impossible to distinguish clinically from dilated cardiomyopathy from any other cause; it is diagnosed in a patient with dilated cardiomyopathy by a history of alcohol abuse and exclusion of other possible etiologic factors. It is typically seen in men aged 30 to 55 with alcohol consumption comprising 30 to 50% of daily calories over a 10- to 15-year period.[104] Onset is usually insidious, with progressive complaints of dyspnea, fatigue, and palpitations. Overt CHF with orthopnea, paroxysmal nocturnal dyspnea, peripheral and pulmonary edema, and ascites often follows.

The treatment of alcoholic cardiomyopathy is essentially the same as treatment of dilated cardiomyopathy of any cause. Additionally, however, abstinence from alcohol is vital because it may arrest or slow progression of the disease. Many investigators have reported improved cardiac function after cessation of alcohol consumption, a process requiring up to a year.[112–115] Attention to nutrition, thiamine, and other B vitamins is also important.

ALCOHOL-RELATED PULMONARY DISEASES AND INFECTIONS

Alcoholics are prone to infections because of a life style of neglect, poor nutrition, decreased serum bactericidal activity, impaired phagocytosis, decreased cell mediated immunity, and abnormalities in migration and function of polymorphonuclear leukocytes.

Although alcohol is known to be toxic to pulmonary mucosa and cilia, there is no compelling evidence that alcohol itself causes any predictable effect on the lung in most patients.[116] In some patients of Asian or Native American descent, in whom alcohol also causes facial flushing, alcohol consumption is associated with bronchoconstriction and wheezing.[116] The mechanism for this is unclear, although some feel that an allergic response to ingredients in alcoholic beverages may be responsible.

The major impact of ethanol on the respiratory system is through the loss of airway protective reflexes which acute alcohol intoxication causes, including impaired cough reflex, decreased lung clearance, increased intolerance of smoking, and recurrent aspirations (secondary to intoxications and seizures). Alcoholics have significantly higher incidences of pneumonia caused by various organisms, most notably Klebsiella and pneumococcus.[116] Pneumonia in alcoholics tends to be more severe and has a poorer prognosis, probably because of associated nutritional factors. Persons acutely intoxicated by ethanol have

periodic aspiration of oral flora, leading to aspiration penumonias and pulmonary abscesses. Alcohol appeared to be the major cause of primary lung abscesses in several series.[116–118] Tuberculosis is also significantly more common in alcoholics.[119]

ACUTE ABDOMEN (SPONTANEOUS BACTERIAL PERITONITIS)

Alcoholic patients have an increased incidence of spontaneous bacterial peritonitis, unassociated with perforation within the intestinal tract. Possibly, microscopic perforation occurs and, with decreased immunologic response, overgrowth occurs. The condition is more common in alcoholics with cirrhosis and ascites. Diagnostic paracentesis can confirm the diagnosis and enable culture. Fluid resuscitation and intravenous broad spectrum antibiotic therapy (for aerobic and anaerobic organisms) is necessary until culture reports are returned.

The possibility of a perforated viscus causing peritonitis must be evaluated. Gastric perforation is increased in alcoholics as well.

FETAL ALCOHOL SYNDROME

Although the fetal alcohol syndrome is not an emergency problem, the physician should caution all women of child-bearing age on the possible effects of alcohol on a developing fetus. These include retardation, congenital abnormalities in appearance, and cardiac abnormalities. The ED can provide this information to patients who might not receive it otherwise.

MEDICOLEGAL PEARLS

- Never assume that a diminished level of consciousness is caused only by alcohol intoxication. Thorough evaluation of any patient with altered level of consciousness is mandatory.
- All comatose patients should receive 2 mg of naloxone IV and 100 mg of thiamine IV, and either have a rapid bedside glucose strip test performed or receive 25 g dextrose IV empirically.
- Indications for CT scanning include evidence of trauma, focal neurologic findings, a discrepancy between measured blood alcohol concentration and clinical status, or failure of the patient to improve in response to graded stimuli over time.
- In any alcohol-withdrawing patient, exclude trauma or medical catastrophe as the inciting event.
- Administer dilantin to patients in status epilepticus or with proven seizure foci. Guard against aspiration.
- Wernicke's encephalopathy may present with the classic signs of oculomotor dysfunction, ataxia, and clouding of consciousness. Alternatively, coma, hy-

- potension, or hypothermia may be the only presenting signs.
- Central pontine myelinolysis is associated with the rapid correction of hyponatremia. Serum sodium should be corrected slowly over days in the absence of life-threatening symptoms of hyponatremia.
- Any acute or subacute deterioration of function in the chronically demented patient may signal a new metabolic encephalopathy, infection, infarction, or subdural hematoma. These patients deserve thorough workup including CT and LP.
- Acute alcoholic myopathy is underdiagnosed and capable of causing death from acute renal tubular necrosis. Evidence of rhabdomyolysis should be sought in the binge drinker complaining of muscle pain, the patient in withdrawal, and in the drinker "found down."
- Alcohol use causes erosive gastritis, but has not shown an association with peptic ulcer disease. GI bleeding in alcoholics is common and may be immediately life-threatening.
- Do not overlook treatable causes of dementia in the chronic alcoholic who is not acutely intoxicated.
- Pancreatitis can be lethal in an alcoholic. Hospital admission and intensive treatment are indicated in all but the mildest cases.
- Signs of an acute abdomen may signal spontaneous bacterial peritonitis, which requires rapid diagnosis and initiation of treatment.
- Seizure-prone patients should be observed. Cases of seizures with aspiration in prison have led to deaths and resultant lawsuits.

REFERENCES

1. West, L.J. (Moderator): Alcoholism. Ann. Intern. Med. *100*:405, 1984.
2. Institute of Medicine, Division of Health Promotion and Disease Prevention: Alcoholism, Alcohol Abuse, and Related Problems: Opportunities for Research. Washington, D.C., National Academy of Sciences, 1980.
3. Kissin, B.: Alcohol abuse and alcohol-related illnesses. In Cecil's Textbook of Internal Medicine. Edited by Wyngaarden, J.B., and Smith, L.H., Philadelphia, W.B. Saunders Co., 1988.
4. Sellers, E.M., and Kalant, H.: Alcohol intoxication and withdrawal. N. Engl. J. Med. *294*:14, 1976.
5. Maling, H.M.: Toxicology of single doses of ethyl alcohol, International Encyclopedia of Pharmacology and Therapeutics. Sect 20, Vol II. Alcohols and Derivatives. Edited by Tremolieres, J. Oxford, Pergamon Press, 1970.
6. Lieber, C.S.: Metabolism and metabolic effects of alcohol. Med. Clin. North Am. *68*:1, 1984.
7. Browning, R.G., Olson, D.W., Stueven, H.A., and Mateer, J.R.: 50% dextrose: Antidote or toxin? Ann. Emerg. Med. *19*:1990.
8. Kaysen, G., and Noth, R.H.: The effects of alcohol on blood pressure and electrolytes. Med. Clin. North Am. *68*:1, 1984.
9. Fink, E.B.: Magnesium deficiency in alcoholism. Alcoholism: Clin. Exper. Res. *10*:683, 1986.
10. Carroll, P., and Maher, V.F.: Legal issues in the care of neurologically impaired patients. Adv. Clin. Care *4*:10, 1989.
11. Shindul, J.A., and Snyder, M.E.: Legal restraints on restraint. Am. J. Nurs. *81*:393, 1981.
12. Young, G.P.: The agitated patient in the emergency department. Emerg. Med. Clin. North Am. *5*:4, 1987.
13. Hatch, R.C., and Jernigan, A.D. Effect of intravenously administered putatative and potential antagonists of ethanol on sleep time in ethanol-narcotized rats. Life Sci. *42*:11, 1988.
14. O'Sullivan, G.F., and Wade, D.N. Flumazenil in the management of acute drug overdosage with benzodiazepines and other agents. Clin. Pharmacol. Ther. *42*:254, 1987.
15. Hojer, J., and Baehrendtz, S.: The effect of flumazenil (Ro 15–1788) in the management of self-induced benzodiazepine poisoning: A double-blind controlled study. Acta Med. Scand. *224*:357, 1988.
16. Prischl, F., Donner, A., Grimm, G., Smetana, R., and Hruby, K.: Value of flumazenil in benzodiazepine self-poisoning. Med. Toxicol. Adverse Drug Exp. *3*:334, 1988.
17. Fluckiger, A., Hartmann, D., Leishman, B., and Ziegler, W.H.: Lack of effect of the benzodiazepine antagonist flumazenil (Ro 15–1788) on the performance of healthy subjects during experimentally induced ethanol intoxication. Eur. J. Clin. Pharmacol. *34*:273, 1988.
18. Minocha, A., et al.: Activated charcoal in oral ethanol absorption: Lack of effect in humans. J. Toxicol Clin. Toxicol. *24*:225, 1986.
19. Katona, B.G., Siegel, E.G., Roberts, J.R., Fant, W.K., and Hassen, M.: The effect of "superactive" charcoal and magnesium citrate solution on blood ethanol concentrations and area under the curve in humans. J. Toxicol Clin. Toxicol. *27*:129, 1989.
20. Turner, R.C., Lichstein, P.R., Peden, J.G., Busher, J.T., Waivers, L.E.: Alcohol withdrawal syndromes: A review of pathophysiology, clinical presentation, and treatment. J. Gen. Intern. Med. *4*:432, 1989.
21. Adinoff, B., Bone, G.H.A., and Linnoila, M.: Acute ethanol poisoning and the ethanol withdrawal syndrome. Med. Toxicol. *3*:172, 1988.
22. Hilbom, M.: Binge versus chronic drinking and alcohol-withdrawal seizures. Epilepsia *29*:495, 1988.
23. Brown, C.G.: The alcohol withdrawal syndrome. Ann. Emerg. Med. *11*:276, 1982.
24. Sellers, E.M., and Kalant, H.: Alcohol intoxication and withdrawal. N. Engl. J. Med. *294*:757, 1976.
25. Rosenbloom, A.: Emerging treatment options in the alcohol withdrawal syndrome. J. Clin. Psychiatry *49*:28, 1988.
26. Airaksinen, M.M., and Peura, P.: Mechanisms of alcohol withdrawal syndrome. Med. Biol. *65*:105, 1987.
27. Hawley, R.J., Major, L.F., Schulman, E.A., and Linnoila, M.: Cerebrospinal fluid 3-methoxy-4-hydroxyphenyglycol and norepinephrine levels in alcohol withdrawal. Arch. Gen. Psychiatry *42*:1056, 1985.
28. Giacobini, E., Izikowitz, S., and Wegmann, A.: Urinary norepinephrine and epinephrine excretion in delirium tremens. Arch. Gen. Psychiatry *3*:289, 1960.
29. Carlsson, C., and Haggendal, J.: Arterial noradrenaline levels after ethanol withdrawal. Lancet *2*:889, 1967.
30. Meyer, R.E.: Prospects for a rational pharmacotherapy of alcoholism. J. Clin. Psychiatry *50*:403, 1989.
31. Ballenger, J.C., and Post, R.M.: Kindling as model for the alcohol withdrawal syndromes. Br. J. Psychiatry *133*:1, 1978.
32. Isbell, H., Fraser, H.F., Wikler, A., Belleville, R.E., and Eisenman, A.J.: An experimental study of the etiology of 'rum fits' and delirium tremens. Q. J. Stud. Alcohol *16*:1, 1955.
33. Benke, R.H.: Recognition and management of alcohol withdrawal syndrome. Hosp. Pract. *11*:79, 1976.
34. Guthrie, S.K.: The treatment of alcohol withdrawal. Pharmacotherapy *9*:131, 1989.
35. Victor, M., and Adams, R.D.: Effect of alcohol on the nervous system. Res. Publ. Assoc. Res. Nerv. Ment. Dis. *32*:526, 1953.
36. Diagnostic and Statistical Manual of Mental Disorders, Third

Edition, Revised. American Psychiatric Association, Washington, D.C., 1987, pp 131–132.

37. Victor, M., and Brausch, C.: The role of abstinence in the genesis of alcoholic epilepsy. Epilepsia 8:1, 1967.

38. Hauser, W.A., Ng, S.K.C., and Brust, J.C.M.: Alcohol, seizures, and epilepsy. Epilepsia 29:S66, 1988.

39. Simon, R.P.: Alcohol and seizures (editorial). N. Engl. J. Med. 319:715, 1988.

40. Earnest, M.P., Feldman, H., Marx, J.A., et al.: Intracranial lesions shown by CT scans in 259 cases of first alcohol-related seizures. Neurology 38:1561, 1988.

41. Earnest, M.P., and Yarnell, P.R.: Seizure admissions to a city hospital: the role of alcohol. Epilepsia 17:387, 1976.

42. Aminoff, M.F., and Simon, R.P.: Status epilepticus: Causes, clinical features and consequences in 98 patients. Am. J. Med. 69:657, 1980.

43. Sampliner, R., and Iber, F.L.: Diphenylhydantoin control of alcohol withdrawal seizures. JAMA 230:1430, 1974.

44. Chance, J.F.: Emergency department treatment of alcohol withdrawal seizures with phenytoin. Ann. Emerg. Med. 20:520, 1991.

45. Engle, J.P., Leoni, J.M., and Donnelly, A.J.: Management of alcohol withdrawal: Treatment controversies. American Pharmacy NS28:729, 1988.

46. Lineaweaver, W.C., Anderson, K., and Hing, D.N.: Massive doses of midazolam infusion for delirium tremens without respiratory depression. Crit. Care Med. 16:294, 1988.

47. Kramp, P., and Rafaelsen, O.J.: Delirium tremens: A double-blind comparison of diazepam and barbital treatment. Acta Psychiat. Scand. 58:174, 1978.

48. Young, G.P., Rores, C., Murphy, C., and Dailey, R.H.: Intravenous phenobarbital for alcohol withdrawal and convulsions. Ann. Emerg. Med. 16:847, 1987.

49. Sellers, E.M., Zilm, D.H., and Degani, N.C.: Comparative efficacy of propranolol and chlordiazepoxide in alcohol withdrawal. J. Stud. Alcohol 38:2096, 1977.

50. Kraus, M.L., Gottlieb, L.D., Horwitz, R.I., and Anscher, M.: Randomized clinical trial of atenolol in patients with alcohol withdrawal. N. Engl. J. Med. 313:905, 1985.

51. Horwitz, R.I., Gottlieb, L.D., and Kraus, M.L.: The efficacy of atenolol in the outpatient management of the alcohol withdrawal syndrome. Arch. Intern. Med. 149:1089, 1989.

51a. Peterson, W.L.: Heliobacter pylori and peptic ulcer disease. N. Engl. J. Med. 1043, 1991.

52. Lerner, W.D., and Fallon, H.J.: The alcohol withdrawal syndrome (editorial). N. Engl. J. Med. 313: 1985.

53. Baumgartner, G.R., and Rowen, R.C.: Clonidine vs chlordiazepoxide in the management of acute alcohol withdrawal syndrome. Arch. Intern. Med. 147:1223, 1987.

54. Robinson, B.J., Robinson, G.M., Maling, T.J.B., and Johnson, R.H.: Is clonidine useful in the treatment of alcohol withdrawal? Alcohol Clin. Exp. Res. 13:95, 1989.

55. Cushman, P., and Sowers, J.R.: Alcohol withdrawal syndrome: Clinical and hormonal responses to α2-adrenergic agonist treatment. Alcohol Clin. Exp. Res. 13:361, 1989.

56. Miller, S.J., Frances, R.J., and Holmes, D.J.: Use of psychotropic drugs in alcoholism treatment: A summary. Hosp. and Commun. Psychiatry 39:1251, 1988.

57. Thompson, W.L., Johnson, A.D., and Maddrey, W.L.: Diazepam and paraldehyde for treatment of severe delirium tremens. Ann. Intern. Med. 82:175, 1975.

58. Embry, C.K., and Lippman, S.: Use of magnesium sulfate in alcohol withdrawal. Am. Fam. Physician 35:167, 1987.

59. Wilson, A., and Vulcan, B.: A double-blind, placebo-controlled trial of magnesium sulfate in the ethanol withdrawal syndrome. Alcoholism: Clin. and Exp. Res. 8:542, 1984.

60. Malcolm, R., Ballenger, J.C., Sturgis, E.T., and Anton, R.: Double-blind controlled trial comparing carbamazepine to oxazepam treatment of alcohol withdrawal. Am. J. Psychiatry 146:617, 1989.

61. Dillon, E.S., Dyer, W.W., and Smelo, L.S.: Ketone acidosis of nondiabetic adults. Med. Clin. North Am. 24:1813, 1940.

62. Williams, H.E.: Alcoholic hypoglycemia and ketoacidosis. Med. Clin. North Am. 68: 1984.

63. Levy, L.J., Duga, J., Girgis, M., and Gordon, E.E.: Ketoacidosis associated with alcoholism in nondiabetic subjects. Ann. Intern. Med. 78: 1973.

64. Jenkins, D.W., Eckel, R.E., and Craig, J.W.: Alcoholic ketoacidosis. JAMA 217: 1971.

65. Lindberg, M.C., and Oyler, R.A.: Wernicke's encephalopathy. Am. Fam. Physician 41: 1990.

66. Watson, A.J., Walker, J.F., Tomkin, G.H., Finn, M.M., and Keogh, J.A.: Acute Wernicke's encephalopathy precipitated by glucose loading. Ir. J. Med. Sci. 150: 1981.

67. VanDyke, H.B., and Ames, R.G.: Alcohol diuresis. Acta Endocrinol. 7: 1951.

68. Eisenhofer, G., and Johnson, R.H.: Effect of ethanol ingestion on plasma vasopressin and water balance in humans. Am. J. Physiol. 242: 1982.

69. Burcar, P.J., Norenburg, M.D., and Yarnell, P.R.: Hyponatremia and central pontine myelinolysis. Neurology 27: 1977.

70. Flink, E.B.: Magnesium deficiency in alcoholism. Alcoholism: Clin. Exper. Res. 10: 1986.

71. Noth, R.H., and Walter, R.M., Jr.: The effects of alcohol on the endocrine system. Med. Clin. North Am. 68: 1984.

72. Reuler, J.B., Girard, D.E., and Cooney, T.G.: Wernicke's encephalopathy. N. Engl. J. Med. 312: 1985.

73. Charness, M.E., Simon, R.P., and Greenberg, D.A.: Ethanol and the nervous system. N. Engl. J. Med. 321: 1989.

74. Nakada, T., and Knight, R.T.: Alcohol and the central nervous system. Med. Clin. North Am. 68: 1984.

75. Torvik, A., Lindboe, C.F., and Rogde, S.: Brain lesions in alcoholics: A neuropathological study with clinical correlations. J. Neurol. Sci. 56: 1982.

76. Craviato, H., Korein, J., and Silberman, J.: Wernicke's encephalopathy: A clinical and pathological study of 28 autopsied cases. Arch. Neurol. 4: 1961.

77. Harper, C.: The incidence of Wernicke's encephalopathy in Australia—a neuropathological study of 131 cases. J. Neurol. Neurosurg. Psych. 46: 1983.

78. Mukherjee, A.B., Svoronos, S., and Ghazanfari, A.: Transketolase abnormality in cultured fibroblasts from familial chronic alcoholic men and their male offspring. J. Clin. Invest. 79: 1987.

79. Roche, S.W., Lane, R.J., and Wade, J.P.: Thalamic hemorrhages in Wernicke-Korsakoff syndrome demonstrated by computed tomography (Letter). Ann. Neurol. 23: 1988.

80. Ackerman, W.J.: Stupor, bradycardia, hypotension, and hypothermia—a presentation of Wernicke's encephalopathy with rapid response to thiamine. West. J. Med. 121: 1974.

81. Cole, M., Turner, A., Frank, O., Baker, H., and Leevy, C.M.: Extraocular palsy and thiamine therapy in Wernicke's encephalopathy. Am. J. Clin. Nutr. 22: 1969.

82. Traviesa, D.C.: Magnesium deficiency: A possible cause of thiamine refractoriness in Wernicke-Korsakoff encephalopathy. J. Neurol. Neurosurg. Psych. 37: 1974.

83. Sacks, O.: The lost mariner. In The Man Who Mistook His Wife for a Hat. New York, Harper and Row, 1987.

84. Kleinschmidt-DeMasters, B.K., and Norenberg, M.D.: Cerebellar degeneration in the rat following rapid correction of hyponatremia. Ann. Neurol. 10: 1981.

85. Kleinschmidt-DeMasters, B.K., and Norenberg, M.D.: Rapid correction of hyponatremia causes demyelination: relation to central pontine myelinolysis. Science 211: 1981.

86. Messert, B., Orrison, W.W., Hawkins, M.J., et al.: Central pontine myelinolysis. Neurology 29: 1979.

87. Brunner, J.E., Redmond, J.M., Haggar, A.M., Kruger, D.F., and Elias, S.B.: Central pontine myelinolysis and pontine lesions after rapid correction of hyponatremia: A prospective magnetic resonance imaging study. Ann. Neurol. 27: 1990.

88. Sterns, R.H.: Severe symptomatic hyponatremia: treatment and outcome: A study of 64 cases. Ann. Intern. Med. 107: 1987.

89. Laureno, R., Karp, B.I.: Pontine and extrapontine myelinolysis following rapid correction of hyponatremia. Lancet 1: 1988.

90. Harper, C.G., Kril, J.J., and Holloway, R.L.: Brain shrinkage in chronic alcoholics: A pathological study. Br. Med. J. *290:* 1985.

91. Carlen, P.L., Wilkinson, D.A., Wortzman, G., and Holgate, R.: Partially reversible cerebral atrophy and functional improvement in recently abstinent alcoholics, measured by MRI. Neuroradiology *30:* 1988.

92. Wrenn, K.D., and Slovis, C.M.: Sorting through rhabdomyolysis: an enigma made manageable. Emerg. Med. Reports *8:* 1987.

93. Gabow, P.A., Kaehny, W.D., and Kelleher, S.P.: The spectrum of rhabdomyolysis. Medicine. *61:* 1982.

94. Song, S.K., and Rubin, E.: Ethanol produces muscle damage in human volunteers. Science *175:* 1972.

95. Haller, R.G., and Knochel, J.P.: Skeletal muscle disorders in alcoholism. Med. Clin. North Am. *68:* 1984.

96. Hanid, A., Slavin, G., Mair, W., et al.: Fiber type changes in striated muscles of alcoholics. J. Clin. Pathol. *34:* 1981.

97. Pimstone, N.R., and French, S.W.: Alcoholic liver disease. Med. Clin. North Am. *68:* 1984.

98. Leevy, C.M.: Fatty liver: A study of 270 patients with biopsy proven fatty liver and a review of the literature. Medicine *41:* 1962.

99. Pequignot, G., Tuyns, A.J., and Berta, J.L.: Ascitic cirrhosis in relation to alcohol consumption. Int. J. Epidem. *7:* 1978.

100. Geokas, M.C.: Ethanol and the pancreas. Med. Clin. North Am. *68:* 1984.

101. Eichner, E.R.: The hematologic disorders of alcoholism. Am. J. Med. *54:* 1973.

102. Larkin, E.C., Watson-Williams, E.J.: Alcohol and the blood. Med. Clin. North Am. *68:* 1984.

103. Davidson, D.M.: Cardiovascular effects of alcohol. West. J. Med. *151:* 1989.

104. Segel, L.D., Klausner, S.C., Gnadt, J.T., and Amsterdam, E.A.: Alcohol and the heart. Med. Clin. North Am. *68:* 1984.

105. Child, J.S., Kovick, R.B., Levisman, J.A., et al.: Cardiac effects of acute ethanol ingestion unmasked by autonomic blockade. Circulation *59:* 1979.

106. Ettinger, P.O., Wu, C.F., De la Cruz, C., et al.: Arrythmias and the "holiday heart": Alcohol associated cardiac rhythm disorders. Am. Heart J. *95:* 1978.

107. Buckingham, T.A., Kennedy, H.L., Goenjian, A.K., et al.: Cardiac arrhythmias in a population admitted to an acute alcoholic detoxification center. Am. Heart J. *110:* 1985.

108. Rosengren, A., and Wilhelmsen, L.: Separate and combined effects of smoking and alcohol abuse in middle aged men. Acta Med. Scand. *223:* 1988.

109. Suhonen, O., Aromaa, A., and Reunanen, A.: Alcohol consumption and sudden coronary death in middle-aged Finnish men. Acta Med. Scand. *221:* 1987.

110. Gordon, T., and Kannel, W.B.: Drinking habits and cardiovascular disease: The Framingham study. Am. Heart J. *105:* 1983.

111. Brigden, W., and Robinson, J.: Alcoholic heart disease. Br. Med. J. *2:* 1964.

112. Schwartz, L., Sample, K.A., and Wigle, D.E.: Severe alcoholic cardiomyopathy reversed with abstention from alcohol. Am. J. Cardiol. *36:* 1975.

113. Kupari, M.: Reversibility of alcoholic cardiomyopathy. Postgrad. Med. J. *60:* 1984.

114. Agatston, A.S., Snow, M.E., and Samet, P.: Regression of severe alcoholic cardiomyopathy after abstinence of 10 weeks. Alcoholism *10:* 1986.

115. Baudet, M., Rigoud, M., Rocha, P., et al.: Reversibility of alcoholic cardiomyopathy with abstention from alcohol. Cardiology *64:* 1979.

116. Krumpe, P.E., Cumminskey, J.M., Lillington, G.A.: Alcohol and the respiratory tract. Med. Clin. North Am. *68:* 1984.

117. Bernhard, W.F., Malcolm, J.A., and Wylie, R.H.: Lung abscess: A study of 148 cases due to aspiration. Dis. Chest *43:* 1974.

118. Estrera, A.S., Platt, M.R., Mills, L.J., et al.: Primary lung abscess. J. Thorac. Cardiovasc. Surg. *79:* 1980.

119. Smith, F.E., and Palmer, D.L.: Alcoholism, infection, and altered host defenses: A review of clinical and experimental observations. J. Chron. Dis. *29:* 1976.

ALCOHOL TOXICODYNAMICS AND CLINICAL CORRELATIONS

Harold Osborn

Inflaming wine, pernicious to mankind, unnerves the limbs, and dulls the noble mind.
Homer: The Iliad VI: 261.

CAPSULE

The question of how to treat alcohol intoxication has plagued humanity for centuries. Not only the intoxication itself but its complicating medical, surgical, and psychiatric emergencies are the physician's challenge. A complete differential diagnosis and skillful management are necessary for individualized treatment. Commonly associated disorders, i.e., infection, trauma, and bleeding, must be sought and treated appropriately. This chapter reviews the pathophysiology, evaluation, and treatment of alcohol intoxication and its clinical effect on multiple organ systems.

INTRODUCTION

The term alcohol commonly implies ethanol (ethyl alcohol), although there are a large number of alcohols. Alcohols are hydroxy derivatives of the aliphatic hydrocarbons. Ethanol, with one hydroxyl group, is a member of the monohydroxy alcohol series (along with methanol, isopropanol, and others); ethylene glycol possesses two hydroxyl groups and, along with propylene glycol, is a member of the dihydroxy series. The ethanol in all alcoholic beverages results from the fermentation of a sugar by yeast. The sugars are derived from cereals, vegetables, or fruits. For example, barley, a cereal, is used as the raw material in the making of beer, ale, and whiskey.

Alcoholic drinks have been prepared since the earliest times. Records of ancient civilizations give evidence of the use of alcoholic beverages from as early as 6000 BC.[1] The oldest forms of alcohol were fermented beverages of low alcoholic content such as wine, which originated in the Middle East. The Old Testament describes Noah as planting the first vineyard on Mt. Ararat in present-day Turkey. The use of wine was widespread in Greek civilization by 1700 BC, and drinking became institutionalized in the worship of Dionysus, reputed to have brought the grapevine to Greece. The Romans adopted Dionysus as a deity, changing his name to Bacchus. Festivals associated with Bacchus celebrated the harvest and the origins of life and were associated with heavy drinking. Although the technique of distillation was probably known to the Greeks and Romans, distilled liquors were not introduced into Europe until around 1250 AD and did not become popular until the 18th century.

Alcohol was early held to have medicinal value. In the Sumerian city of Nippur, beer and wine were used for healing purposes as early as 2000 BC. Alcohol was once thought to be the elixir of life ("aqua vitae") and a cure for various ailments. The word whiskey comes from the Gaelic "usquebough" meaning "water of life." Today we know better.

It is estimated that 5 to 10% of all drinkers in the American population (10 million people) are alcohol-dependent.[2,3] The rate of alcohol consumption has increased by over 30% in the last 25 years. More than 200,000 Americans die annually of alcoholism, and 1 out of every 10 deaths is alcohol-related.[3] Alcohol is the leading killer of persons between 15 and 45 years. For untreated alcoholics, life expectancy decreases by 12 to 15 years as compared to the normal population.[2] Mortality from the regular use of alcohol begins to increase when 3 to 5 drinks are consumed per day and rises sharply with the consumption of 7 or more drinks a day.[4] Although the consumption of 2 drinks or less a day may be safe for most people, no amount is currently considered safe for pregnant women.

The problem use of alcohol exacts an economic as well as a human toll. Twenty percent of our total national expenditure for hospital care is alcohol-related, and 12% of our total national health expenditure for adults is for alcohol abuse.[3] In the United States alone, the cost of alcohol-related lost productivity and health expenses is estimated to be $117 billion per year.[5]

Alcohol adversely affects almost every organ system in the body (see subsequent text). It creates abnormalities in fetal development and increased mortality from cirrhosis, infections, cardiovascular disease, malignancies, and accidents. Two thirds of all incidents of domestic violence are alcohol-related, as is one third of all instances of child abuse.[3] Alcohol is associated with 50% of traffic fatalities, 50% of deaths by fire, 67% of drownings, 67% of homicides and aggravated assaults, 40% of rapes, and 35% of suicides.

In a country that has become increasingly preoccupied with drug use, excessive use of alcohol remains one of the most serious and pervasive problems we face. In the U.S. today, alcoholism constitutes a major health issue and presents a significant challenge to all facets of our society.

CHARACTERISTICS OF ALCOHOL

Alcohol (C_2H_5OH) is a colorless, odorless hydrocarbon composed of weakly charged molecules. It is fully miscible in water and, with a volume of distribution of 0.6L per kg (roughly equivalent to total body water), diffuses easily across cell membranes, and reaches all areas of the body. Ethanol has a molecular weight of 46 daltons and yields 7.1 Kcal per gram when oxidized (Table 84-7). Although the caloric yield of alcohol is high, its calories are "empty," lacking in nutrient value. Distilled spirits, for example, are devoid of protein and carbohydrates. Chronic drinkers can obtain over half their caloric intake from alcohol and become malnourished of proteins, minerals, and vitamins in the process.

Distilled liquors usually contain alcohol concentrations of 40 to 50% (80 to 100 proof). The alcohol in wines varies from 10 to 20% and averages approximately 12% by volume. The concentration in beers runs from 2 to 6% ethanol, with low-calorie/low alcohol content beers having the weakest concentration. Other products containing ethanol can sometimes cause intoxication. Mouthwashes contain up to 75% ethanol and colognes contain 40 to 60%.[6] Ethanol is an ingredient in over 700 medicinal preparations in the U.S. as a diluent or solvent, in concentrations ranging from 0.3% to 68%.[7] Congeners found in alcoholic beverages may contribute to toxicity in heavy drinkers. They include low-molecular-weight alcohols (methanol and butanol), aldehydes, esters, histamines, phenols, tannins, iron, lead, and cobalt.

TABLE 84-7. ETOH STATISTICS

1 g ethyl alcohol = 7.1 Kcal energy (~7.0)
Volume of distribution = 0.54 L/Kg (~0.6)
Specific gravity = 0.7939 gr/mL (~0.8)
Millimeters/fluid ounce = 29.9 (~30)
Proof = 2x percent ethanol by volume (e.g., 80 proof = 40% ethanol)
100 mg% = 100 mg deciliter = 0.1g/100 mL = 0.1%
100 mg% = 21.7 mmOl/L = 0.127% (vol/vol)
1 mL/kg of 100% ethanol (1 g/kg) produces a blood level of approximately 100 mg%.
One ounce of whiskey, glass of wine, or 12 ounce bottle of beer raises the blood alcohol approximately 25 mg% in an average-sized adult.
Metabolism of ethanol
Maximum rate = 100 – 125 mg/kg/hr. (chronic alcoholics 175 mg/kg/hr)
Average adult = 7 to 10 g/hr.
Average reduction in ETOH levels = 15–20 mg%/hr (chronic alcoholics 30 to 40 mg%/hr.)
Ethanol blood level (mg. %)

$$= \frac{dose\ (mg)}{VD\ (L/Kg) \times body\ weight\ (kg) \times 10}$$

Ethanol dose (mg) = ethanol ingested (mL) × ethanol concentration (%) × 800
Ethanol concentration = proof/2
Lethal dose = 5.8 gr/kg nontolerant adult
3 gr/kg child

Alcohol is a physically addicting drug. With chronic use, the degree of tolerance to alcohol is not as marked as for the opiates.[8] Withdrawal manifestations after abrupt termination or relative diminution in the intake of alcohol are much more severe, however. The consumption of 1 mL per kg of absolute ethanol (100%) raises the blood alcohol level to roughly 100 mg%. Each ounce of whiskey, glass of wine, or 12-ounce bottle of beer increases the blood alcohol by approximately 25 mg%. Lethal doses are reported to be 5 to 8 g per kg for adults and 3 g per kg for children. Alcohol is metabolized at around 10 to 20 mg% per hour (somewhat faster in chronic drinkers).

PHARMACOKINETICS

ABSORPTION

Ethanol, like the other aliphatic alcohols, is highly lipid-soluble and hence is rapidly and efficiently absorbed from the gastrointestinal (GI) tract (stomach, small intestine, and colon).[8] Vaporized alcohol can be absorbed from the lung through the pulmonary vascular bed. Although this is an unusual route of entry, fatal intoxication has occurred after *inhalation* of alcohol. The stomach extracts only about 20% of an orally ingested dose, and the small intestine extracts the rest.[6] Thus, because gastric absorption is rate-lim-

iting, anything that delays gastric emptying can affect absorption. High concentrations of alcohol can cause pylorospasm and delay absorption. Absorption also depends on the volume and character of the alcoholic beverage, the presence or absence of food, GI motility, the presence of GI disorders, co-ingestion of drugs, concentration of alcohol, the time taken to ingest the drink, and individual variations. Under optimal conditions, 80 to 90% of an ingested dose of alcohol is absorbed in 30 to 60 minutes. Depending on the above variables, however, complete absorption may take 2 to 6 hours. Increased absorption is seen with rapid gastric emptying, alcohol intake without food, the absence of congeners, dilution (maximum absorption occurs at concentrations of 20% by volume), and carbonation.

Women obtain higher blood alcohol levels than men after an equivalent dose of alcohol,[9] and are more susceptible than men to alcoholic liver disease. A possible explanation for these phenomena rests in the recent demonstration of local metabolism of ethanol in gastrointestinal tissue.[10] Alcohol dehydrogenase, located in the gastric mucosa, oxidizes a portion of the ingested ethanol and reduces the amount available for absorption. This phenomenon, labeled "first-pass metabolism," is more pronounced in men than in women and in nonalcoholics than in alcoholics.[11] Thus, the reduced gastric oxidation of alcohol and its greater bioavailability in women results in relatively greater absorption, increased alcohol levels, and presumably an enhanced susceptibility to liver disease.

DISTRIBUTION

Because it is both water- and lipid-soluble, after absorption, alcohol distributes through total body water. With a volume of distribution of 0.6 L per kg in adults (higher in men than women) and 0.7 L per kg in children, alcohol is uniformly spread throughout all tissues and fluids of the body. The placenta is permeable to alcohol, and thus the fetus is fully exposed. Because of the brain's abundant blood supply, the concentration of alcohol in the brain quickly approaches that of the blood. The alcohol concentration in the brains of people dying of alcohol intoxication varies from 300 to 600 mg per 100 g.[8]

When distribution is complete, alcohol is stored in every tissue and fluid of the body in a concentration proportional to the water content of the tissue or fluid. The alcohol concentration in blood is maintained by back diffusion, which occurs whenever the blood alcohol level falls below tissue concentrations.

ELIMINATION

Over 90% of the alcohol ingested is removed by enzymatic oxidation, and 5 to 10% is excreted unchanged by the kidneys and lungs. Oxidation proceeds in the

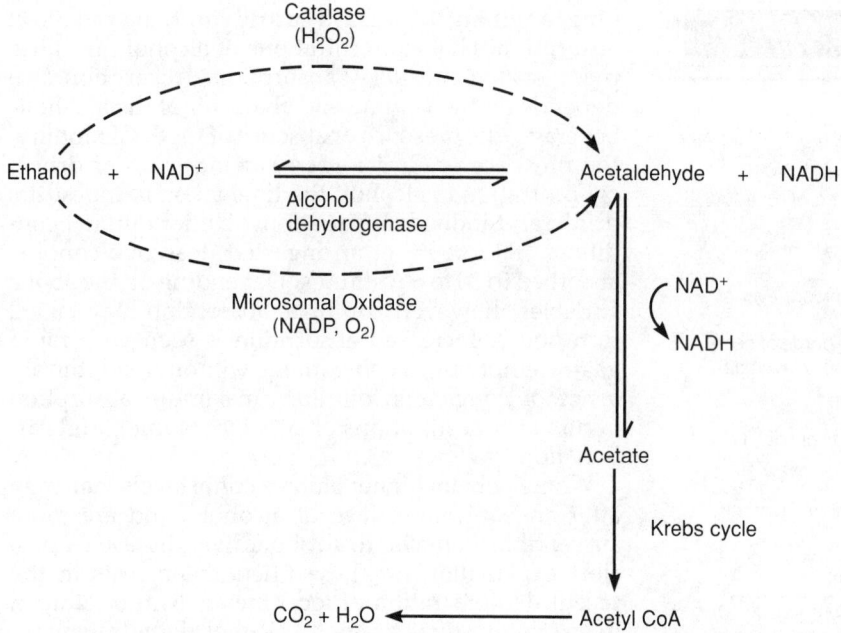

FIG. 84-2. *Principal pathways of ethanol oxidation.*

liver, and the hepatocytes contain three main ethanol-related metabolic pathways: an alcohol dehydrogenase pathway, located in the cytosol; a microsomal ethanol-oxidizing system (MEOS), located in the endoplasmic reticulum; and a peroxidase-catalase system, also derived from the hepatic microsomes[12] (Fig. 84-2).

The alcohol dehydrogenase system, located in the cytosol (cell sap), is the main pathway for alcohol metabolism in the body and constitutes the rate-limiting step. Alcohol dehydrogenase (ADH) is a zinc-containing enzyme with a molecular weight of 85,000 daltons that uses nicotinamide adenine dinucleotide (NAD) as a hydrogen acceptor. In the ADH-mediated pathway, hydrogen is transferred from the substates ethanol and acetaldehyde to NAD, converting it to its reduced form, NADH (Fig. 84-2). The oxidation of ethanol thus generates an excess of reducing equivalents in the cytosol in the form of NADH. Consequently, the NAD/NADH ratio is dramatically altered, which in turn shifts the oxidation reduction (redox) potential of the cell. This alteration in the oxidation state is responsible for various metabolic abnormalities associated with alcoholism such as the development of acidosis, inability to promote gluconeogenesis, and alterations in lipid metabolism. In the final steps of ethanol metabolism, acetate enters the Krebs cycle and is metabolized progressively to acetyl CoA and then to CO_2 and H_2O.

The MEOS pathway is normally responsible for little ethanol metabolism, but becomes more important as the ethanol concentration rises and with chronicity of drinking. The capacity of alcohol to stimulate and induce the MEOS forms the basis for the well-estab-lished interactions between alcohol and a host of other drugs metabolized by this system.

Alcohol is unique among CNS depressants because all others are primarily cleared by the hepatic microsomal enzyme system, whereas alcohol is metabolized principally by a cytosolic liver enzyme.

The capacity of the ADH enzyme system is saturated at relatively low alcohol levels. Although the metabolism of ethanol may technically be Michealis-Menten kinetics,[13] many characterize it as zero-order kinetics (a fixed amount rather than proportion of ethanol is metabolized per unit of time). The amount of alcohol metabolized is roughly proportional to body weight and liver weight. In adults, the average rate of alcohol metabolism is 100 to 125 mg per kg per hour in occasional drinkers and 175 mg per kg per hour in habitual drinkers. The average adult metabolizes 7 to 10 g per hour of alcohol and the blood alcohol level (BAL) falls 15 to 20 mg% per hour. Various dietary, hormonal, and pharmacologic factors can alter the metabolism of alcohol. For example, starvation decreases the rate of oxidation, although not appreciably. Chronic drinkers may reduce their alcohol levels by up to 30 to 40 mg% per hour because of the involvement of the MEOS system.[14] These facts become important in the interpretation of alcohol levels in the clinical situation (see subsequent text).

An appreciable but insignificant amount of alcohol is eliminated by respiration. This amount increases slightly after ingestion of large quantities of alcohol. The excretion of alcohol in the lungs obeys Henry's law: the ratio between the concentration of alcohol in the alveolar air and the blood is constant. Because the alveolar air/blood constant is 1:2100 (approximately

0.05%), little is excreted by this route. This relatively constant relationship, however, forms the basis for the use of breath samples to estimate blood alcohol levels. Errors can be induced by hyperventilation, however.

PATHOPHYSIOLOGY

The means by which ethanol exerts its pathologic action have not yet been completely elucidated. Alcohol may impair microtubular function or create changes in cell membrane structure and functions.[15] Alcohol increases the expansion and fluidity of membranes, and this in turn may lead to abnormalities in functions that are mediated by membrane-bound proteins. Ethanol may exert its intoxicating effect through a complex of membrane proteins containing a receptor for the inhibitory neurotransmitter GABA and an associated chloride ion channel. It now appears that ethanol modifies GABA-activated neurotransmission by stimulating ion flux through the chloride channel and potentiating GABA-activated inhibition of cerebral cortical neurons.[16–18]

In addition to the inherent toxicity of the ethanol moiety itself, the byproducts of the metabolism of ethanol can lead to additional toxicity. Some evidence suggests that acetaldehyde, the first product of the cytosol-mediated metabolism of alcohol, is inherently toxic to biologic systems.[19,20] According to Truit and Walsh, acetaldehyde stimulates the release of biogenic amines from neuronal storage sites and alters their metabolism, acts as a CNS depressant at higher concentrations and interferes with pyruvate-stimulated oxidative phosphorylation in mitochondria, inactivates coenzyme A, and inhibits myocardial protein synthesis.[21]

Korsten and coworkers showed that peak blood acetaldehyde levels were higher in chronic drinkers and that this effect dissipated with abstinence.[22] These higher levels are apparently the result of an acetaldehyde-induced impairment in mitochondrial function and inhibition of oxidation.

Despite these observations, there is as yet no unifying concept linking the oxidative metabolism of alcohol to the selective organ damage seen with alcoholism. It is still unclear why organs such as the heart, pancreas, and brain, which have minimal or no capacity to oxidize alcohol, are susceptible to alcohol-induced damage. It may be that other biochemical mediators are involved in addition to alcohol and acetaldehyde. Some work has suggested that non-oxidative metabolism of alcohol can occur in organs that lack oxidative metabolic pathways and that the fatty acid ethyl esters produced can mediate organ damage.[23]

In addition to the toxicity of ethanol and acetaldehyde, the oxidation of ethanol leads to an altered cellular environment characterized by a relative excess of NADH over NAD. This altered redox potential has negative consequences for many cell functions. Finally, the chronic use of alcohol can depress appetite and interfere with the absorption of amino acids, vitamins, and other nutrients essential for normal bodily functions.

CLINICAL EFFECTS OF ALCOHOL

Ethanol is the most commonly used intoxicant known to man. Acutely, ethanol ingestion results in flushed facies, tachycardia, increased sweating, mydriasis, dysarthria, muscular incoordination, altered consciousness, labile emotionality, increased gregariousness, occasional antisocial behavior, and nystagmus. The nystagmus must be distinguished from that associated with Wernicke's encephalopathy, a complication of chronic ethanolism. The odor of alcohol on the patient's breath may provide a useful clue but cannot be relied on. Some forms of alcohol create no odor and thus can be missed. Conversely, some patients may have an odor of alcohol on their breath but some other explanation for the alteration in their mental status. A diagnosis of inebriation must be confirmed by a blood alcohol level. The finding of an inappropriately low alcohol level or persistent impairment in mental status that fails to improve despite a declining alcohol level should prompt a search for other causes besides alcohol intoxication. Other causes of altered mental status in drinkers include the following: mixed overdose (alcohol substitutes like methanol and ethylene glycol, opiates, sedative-hypnotics, etc.), head injury, hypoglycemia, seizures, and sepsis.

Intoxication with alcohol is defined by the National Safety Council as a blood alcohol concentration of 100 mg% or more (a concentration of 100 mg% is equivalent to 0.127% (vol/vol) or 21.7 mOsm/liter). This recommendation has been adopted by most states. Levels as low as 47 mg% (10.2 mOsm per liter) are associated with an increased risk of motor vehicle accidents, however.

A "standard drink" is defined as 44 mL (1.5 oz) of distilled liquor (80 proof or 40% alcohol by volume), 360 mL (12 oz) of beer (5% alcohol), or 150 mL (5 oz) of wine (12% alcohol) and contains about 15 g of alcohol.[24] Ingestion of a standard drink by a 70 kg person results in a peak blood alcohol concentration of 4.3 to 8.7 mOsm per liter (0.02 to 0.04% or 20 to 40 mg%).

In nonalcoholic individuals, impairment of judgment and of recently learned skills can occur at blood alcohol levels as low as 5.4 mOsm per liter (0.025%). Gross motor control and orientation may be significantly affected at concentrations of 11 mmOl per liter (0.05%) and more.[25,26]

The degree of intoxication with alcohol is influenced by the speed of drinking (and hence the rate of rise of the blood alcohol level), the quantity of ethanol consumed, the presence or absence of tolerance, and whether the blood alcohol level is rising or falling. Acute tolerance may occur even within a single episode of drinking. Observations of people who have taken alcohol reveal a diminished physiologic and behavioral response to the same level on the descending portion of the blood alcohol curve (the Mellanby effect).[27]

In addition to acute tolerance, chronic tolerance may occur with sustained drinking. Chronic tolerance has a metabolic (pharmacokinetic) and a functional (pharmacodynamic) component.[28] Metabolic tolerance refers to changes in the absorption, distribution, metabolism, or excretion of a drug. In the case of ethanol, metabolic tolerance is based on enhanced metabolism through the MEOS system. Functional tolerance refers to resistance to the effects of a drug at the cellular level. With ethanol, this tolerance may be mediated by serotonergic and noradrenergic neurons.[29]

Ethanol is a selective CNS depressant at low doses and a general CNS depressant at high doses. Although ethanol stimulates animated behavior at lower levels, its depressant action is largely responsible. Ethanol depresses first the areas of the brain involved with the most highly integrated functions. The cortex is released from its integrating control. Mental processes based on training and experience, which govern sobriety and restraint, are adversely affected early. This leads to enhanced activity and boisterousness. This early phase, however, is succeeded by impairment of neural activity as the alcohol level increases, causing sedation and depression.

A blood alcohol level (BAL) to 30 to 120 mg% is characterized by euphoria, garrulous behavior, decreased attention span, and loss of judgment (Table 84-8). At a BAL of 180 to 300 mg%, one sees confusion, exaggerated emotions, decreased perception of pain,

TABLE 84-8. STAGES OF ACUTE ALCOHOLIC INFLUENCE/INTOXICATION*

Blood-Alcohol Concentration (% W/V)	Stage of Alcohol Influence	Clinical Signs/Symptoms
0.01–0.05	Sobriety	No apparent influence Behavior nearly normal by ordinary observation Slight changes detectable by special test
0.03–0.12	Euphoria	Mild euphoria, sociability, talkativeness Increased self-confidence, decreased inhibitions Diminution of attention, judgment, and control Loss of efficiency in finer performance tests
0.09–0.25	Excitement	Emotional instability, decreased inhibitions Loss of critical judgment Impairment of memory and comprehension Decreased sensitory response, increased reaction time Some muscular incoordination
0.18–0.30	Confusion	Disorientation, mental confusion, dizziness Exaggerated emotional states (fear, anger, grief, etc.) Disturbance of sensation (diplopia, etc.) and of perception of color, form, motion, dimensions Decreased pain sense Impaired balance, muscular incoordination, staggering gait, slurred speech
0.27–0.40	Stupor	Apathy, general inertia, approaching paralysis Markedly decreased response to stimuli Marked muscular incoordination, inability to stand or walk Vomiting, incontinence of urine and feces Impaired consciousness, sleep or stupor
0.35–0.50	Coma	Complete unconsciousness, coma, anesthesia Depressed or abolished reflexes Subnormal temperature Incontinence of urine and feces Embarrassment of circulation and respiration Possible death
0.45+	Death	Death from respiratory paralysis

* Adapted with permission from Dabrowski, K.M.: Alcohol determination in the clinical laboratory. Ann. J. Clin. Pathol. 74:749, 1980.

and impaired balance. A BAL of 270 to 400 mg% is characterized by stupor, muscular incoordination, nausea, and incontinence. Coma usually occurs at levels of 350 to 500 mg% and is accompanied by cardiovascular abnormalities, decreased reflexes, and anesthesia. Medullary depression and respiratory arrest usually occur at a BAL over 500 mg%. Although the LD_{50} has been reported to be 450 mg%, this depends on the presence or absence of tolerance. Chronic alcoholics may exhibit few signs of clinical intoxication despite BALs over 300 mg% and may survive levels above 500 mg%.[30,31] The average BAL in fatal cases is approximately 400 mg%.[8]

Factors that may influence the lethal dose of ethanol include age, the nutritional state of the individual, adrenal insufficiency, the presence of other depressants, and, of course, tolerance. An important point to remember is that for most patients there is a narrow margin between the anesthetic and fatal dose of ethanol. A person deeply intoxicated is near death, and a dose of alcohol slightly greater than that necessary to cause profound intoxication can be a fatal dose, particularly if combined with a sedative or hypnotic drug.

Ethanol is a vasodilator and can cause a decrease in preload, afterload, and systemic resistance.[6] It can lead to myocardial depression and can produce cardiac dysrhythmias (atrial fibrillation) in binge drinkers and chronic alcoholics.[32,33]

ALCOHOLISM

"Alcoholism is a disease, not a chronic state of moral turpitude."
Becker and Morrelli

According to the National Council on Alcoholism and the American Medical Society's Committee on Alcoholism, "Alcoholism is a chronic, progressive, and potentially fatal disease. It is characterized by tolerance and physical dependency or pathologic organ changes, or both—all the direct or indirect consequences of the alcohol ingested."[34]

Alcoholism denotes a pathologic dependence on alcohol. Alcohol is unlike the opiates in that a much smaller percentage (<10%) of those who regularly use alcohol become physiologically addicted. Although historically alcoholism was perceived as representing a defect in moral character, a more unified and enlightened view now conceives alcoholism as a multifactorial, genetically influenced disorder.[35,36]

Alcoholism should be suspected in any patient who presents with unexplained trauma, seizures, or bizarre behavior. Suggestive physical findings include flushed facies, bilateral parotid enlargement, liver enlargement, stigmata of cirrhosis (jaundice, palmar erythema, gynecomastia, spider angioma), fluctuating mild hypertension, peripheral neuropathy, nystagmus, and repeated infections. Some of the systemic effects of alcoholism are listed in Table 84-9.

Concern for early detection and intervention has led to attempts to create diagnostic screening systems. The Brief Michigan Alcoholism Screening Test (MAST)[37] and the Cage Questions[38] are two such devices. In 1972, a select committee assembled by the National Council on Alcoholism developed criteria for the diagnosis of alcoholism[39] (Table 84-10). Data supporting a diagnosis of alcoholism were separated into two tracks. These are Track I: Physiologic and Clinical and Track II: Behavioral, Psychological, and Attitudinal. Diagnostic levels 1 to 3 were developed for each sign and symptom, and these levels were weighted in terms of their predictive value for a diagnosis of ethanolism. Diagnostic level I represents a definite indication for the presence of alcoholism, Diagnostic Level II a probable indication of alcoholism, and Diagnostic Level III a possible indication. A diagnosis of alcoholism can be made if one or more of the major criteria or several minor criteria in *both* categories are fulfilled.

As can be seen from the MAST and National Council on Alcoholism questionnaires, the presence of physiologic tolerance and/or dependence is not essential for a diagnosis of alcoholism. Emphasis is placed on the social and behavioral concomitants of heavy drinking. According to Jaffe, "A preoccupation with the acquisition of alcohol, the compulsive use of alcohol, and a relapse to alcohol use are the most sensitive indicators that alcohol is a consistent problem of central importance."[40] In the Emergency Department (ED) setting, questions about the patient's ability to function physically and psychologically in the face of heavy drinking are just as appropriate as quantifying the amount of alcohol consumed per day.

Alcoholism is commonly associated with affective disorders, especially depression.[41,42] There is a higher rate of alcoholism among manic-depressives than in the general population.[43] An association between alcoholism and unipolar affective disorders has been described in men and women.[44,45]

Alcohol consumption affects mood, judgment, and self-control and creates a situation conducive to self-injury. Various studies report the risk of suicide as 6 to 30 times greater among alcoholics than in the general population.[46,47] Alcohol dependence is the second most important risk factor in suicide (next to age). From 25 to 37% of suicides involve the use of alcohol, as determined by autopsy.[48] Although many people drink alcohol in a misguided attempt to cure depression, all available evidence points to the fact that alcoholism adversely affects mood and cognitive ability.

Research has pointed to an increased incidence of alcoholism in families.[49-51] Twin studies also indicate that normal alcohol-drinking behavior is partly under genetic control.[52]

TABLE 84-9. SYSTEMIC EFFECTS OF ALCOHOLISM*

Integument
  Pellagra
  Signs of trauma
  Infestation
Head
  Fracture
  Subdural hematoma
Mouth
  Nutritional stomatitis
  Cheilosis
  Increased incidence of cancers
Eyes
  "Tobacco-alcohol" amblyopia
  Ophthalmoplegia (Wernicke-
    Korsakoff syndrome)
Gastrointestinal
  Esophagus
    Esophagitis
    Diffuse esophageal spasm
    Mallory-Weiss tear
    Rupture with mediastinitis
    Increased incidence of cancers
  Stomach and duodenum
    Acute erosive gastritis
    Chronic hypertrophic gastritis
    Peptic ulcer
    Hematemesis
    Increased incidence of cancers
  Bowel
    Malabsorption
    "Alcoholic diarrhea"
  Liver
    Steatosis
    Alcoholic hepatitis
    Cirrhosis
  Pancreas
    Acute pancreatitis
    Chronic recurrent pancreatitis
    Calcific pancreatitis
    Exocrine pancreatic
      insufficiency
      Pseudocyst

Respiratory and cardiovascular
  Atelectasis
  Pneumothorax
  Respiratory depression
  High prevalence of smoking
  Cardiovascular
    cardiomyopathy
  Beriberi
Genitourinary
  Hypogonadism (in men)
  Impotence (in men)
  Infertility (in women)
Endocrine and metabolic
  Decreased testosterone
  Hyperglycemia
  Hypoglycemia
  Hyperlactemia
  Hyperuricemia
  Metabolic acidosis
  Respiratory acidosis
  Alcoholic ketoacidosis
  Hypophosphatemia
  Hypermetabolism
  Hypokalemia
  Hypomagnesemia
  Hypercholesterolemia
  Hypertriglyceridemia
  Protein malnutrition
  Hypotransferrinemia
  Vitamin B deficiencies
Neurologic
  Acute intoxication
  Withdrawal syndromes
  Amblyopia (optic neuropathy)
  Wernicke-Korsakoff syndrome
  Cerebellar degeneration
  Polyneuropathy
  Pellagra
  Marchiafava-Bignami disease
  Central pontine myelinolysis
  Cerebral atrophy dementia
  Myopathy

* Adapted with permission from West, L.J., Maxwell, D.S., Nobel, E.P., et al.: Alcoholism. Ann. Intern. Med. *100*:412, 1984.

Moreover, linkage analysis has implicated chromosomes 4, 6, and 11 in the genetic risk for alcoholism.[53] The technique of restriction fragment length polymorphism (RFLP) has been used to demonstrate a structural mutation in the gene that codes for alcohol dehydrogenase. This altered gene is prevalent among Asians, and may explain the alcohol-flush syndrome that is common in this population.[54,55] Blum and coworkers reported the first allelic association of the dopamine D_2 receptor gene in alcoholism. In brain samples from alcoholics and nonalcoholics, the presence of the A1 allele of the dopamine D_2 receptor gene correctly classified 77% of alcoholics and its absence classified 72% of nonalcoholics.[56] Blum et al. suggest that this or a related gene could be responsible for susceptibility to at least one subtype of alcoholism. Although there is probably a genetic predisposition to alcoholism, it is not as clear-cut as other genetically determined diseases, and the basis for it is not yet completely understood. Epidemiologic studies suggest the following risk factors for alcoholism: a positive family history of alcoholism or total abstinence, a history of alcoholism or total abstinence in the spouse, coming from a broken home, being the last child in a large family, having female relatives over more than one generation with a history of recurrent depression, and heavy smoking.

Alcohol is unique among pharmacologic agents in that self-induced intoxication is socially accepted. A national survey has revealed that fewer than 20% of people questioned perceived alcoholism as a health problem.[57] This view is not limited to the lay public. Alcoholism is underdetected and underdiagnosed in our health care system. In one study, less than 10%

TABLE 84-10. MAJOR AND MINOR CRITERIA FOR THE DIAGNOSIS OF ALCOHOLISM*

Major Criteria Criterion	Diagnostic Level†
TRACK I. Physiologic and Clinical	
A. Physical Dependency	
1. Physiologic dependence as manifested by evidence of a withdrawal syndrome when the intake of alcohol is interrupted or decreased without substitution of other sedation. It must be remembered that overuse of other sedative drugs can produce a similar withdrawal state, which should be differentiated from alcohol.	
a. Gross tremor (differentiated from other causes of tremor)	1
b. Hallucinosis (differentiated from schizophrenic hallucinations or other psychoses)	1
c. Withdrawal seizures (differentiated from epilepsy and other seizure disorders)	1
d. Delirium tremens. Usually starts between the first and third day after withdrawal and minimally includes tremors, disorientation, and hallucinations	1
2. Evidence of tolerance to the effects of alcohol.	
a. A blood alcohol level of more than 150 mg/100 mL without gross evidence of intoxication.	1
b. The consumption of one fifth of a gallon of whiskey or an equivalent amount of wine or beer daily, for a period of 2 or more consecutive days, by a 180 lb. individual.	1
3. Alcoholic "blackout" periods.	
B. Clinical Major Alcohol-Associated illnesses. Alcoholism can be assumed to exist if major alcohol-associated illnesses develop in a person who drinks regularly. In such individuals, evidence of physiologic and psychologic dependence should be searched for.	
Fatty degeneration in absence of other known cause	2
Alcoholic hepatitis	1
Laennec's cirrhosis	2
Pancreatitis in the absence of cholelithiasis	2
Chronic gastritis	3
Hematologic disorders:	
Anemia: hypochromic, normocytic, macrocytic, hemolytic and stomatocytosis, low folic acid	3
Clotting disorders, prothrombin elevation, thrombocytopenia	3
Wernicke-Korsakoff syndrome	2
Alcoholic cerebellar degeneration	1
Cerebral degeneration in absence of Alzheimer's disease or arteriosclerosis	2
Central pontine myelinolysis (diagnosis only possible postmortem)	2
Marchiafava-Bignami's disease	2
Peripheral neuropathy (see also beriberi)	2
Toxic amblyopia	3
Alcoholic myopathy	2
Alcoholic cardiomyopathy	2
Beriberi	3
Pellagra	3
TRACK II. Behavioral, Psychologic, and Attitudinal	
The following behavior patterns shows psychologic dependence on alcohol in alcoholism:	
1. Drinking despite strong medical contraindication known to patient	1
2. Drinking despite strong, identified, social contraindication (job loss for intoxication, marriage disruption because of drinking, driving while intoxicated)	1
3. Patient's subjective complaint of loss of control of alcohol consumption.	2

* Adapted with permission from Criteria for the Diagnosis of Alcoholism. Am. J. Psychiatry *129*:127, 1972.
  † Diagnostic Levels:
    Level 1. Classical definite, obligatory. This criterion is clearly associated with alcoholism.
    Level 2. Probable, frequent, indicative. This criterion lends strong suspicion of alcohol; other corroborative evidence should be obtained.
    Level 3. Potential, possible, incidental. These manifestations are common in people with alcoholism, but do not by themselves give a strong indication of its existence. They may arouse suspicion, but significant other evidence is needed before the diagnosis is made.

TABLE 84-10. CONTINUED

Minor Criteria	
Criterion	Diagnostic Level

TRACK I. Physiologic and Clinical	
A. Direct Effects (ascertained by examination)	
1. Early:	
Odor of alcohol on breath at time of medical appointment	2
2. Middle	
Alcoholic facies	2
Vascular engorgement of face	2
Toxic amblyopia	2
Increased incidence of infections	3
Cardiac arrhythmias	3
Peripheral neuropathy (see also Major Criteria, Track I, B)	2
3. Late (see Major Criteria, Track I, B)	
B. Indirect Effects	
1. Early:	
Tachycardia	3
Flushed face	3
Nocturnal diaphoresis	3
2. Middle:	
Ecchymoses on lower extremities, arms, or chest	3
Cigarette or other burns on hands or chest	3
Hyperreflexia, or if drinking heavily, hyporeflexia (permanent hyporeflexia may be a residuum of alcoholic polyneuritis)	
3. Late	
Decreased tolerance	
C. Laboratory Tests	
1. Major—Direct	
Blood alcohol level at any time of more than 300 mg/100 mL	1
Level of more than 100 mg/100 mL in routine examination	
2. Major—Indirect	1
Serum osmolality (reflects blood alcohol levels), every 22.4 increase over 200 mOsm/liter reflects 50 mg/100 mL alcohol	2
3. Minor—Indirect	
Results of alcohol ingestion	
Hypoglycemia	3
Hypochloremic alkalosis	3
Low magnesium level	2
Lactic acid elevation	2
Transient uric acid elevation	3
Potassium depletion	3
Indications of liver abnormality	
SGPT elevation	2
SGOT elevation	3
BSP elevation	2
Bilirubin elevation	2
Urinary urobilinogen elevation	2
Serum A/G ratio reversal	2
Blood and blood clotting:	
Anemia (hypochromic, normocytic, macrocytic, hemolytic with stomatocytosis), low folic acid	3
Clotting disorders, prothrombin elevation, thrombocytopenia	3
ECG abnormalities	
Cardiac arrhythmias; tachycardia; T waves dimpled, cloven, or spinous; atrial fibrillation; ventricular premature contractions; abnormal P waves	2
EEG abnormalities	
Decreased or increased REM sleep, depending on phase	3
Loss of delta sleep	3
Other reported findings	3
Decreased immune response	3
Decreased response to Synacthen test	3
Chromosomal damage from alcoholism	3

TABLE 84-10. CONTINUED

	Minor Criteria	
	Criterion	Diagnostic Level
TRACK II. Behavioral, Psychologic, and Attitudinal		
A. Behavioral		
1. Direct effects		
Early		
Gulping drinks		3
Surreptitious drinking		2
Morning drinking (assess nature of peer group behavior)		2
Middle:		
Repeated conscious attempts at abstinence		2
Late:		
Blatant, indiscriminate use of alcohol		2
Skid Row or equivalent social level		2
2. Indirect effects		
Early:		
Medical excuses from work for variety of reasons		2
Shifting from one alcoholic beverage to another		2
Preference for drinking companions, bars, and taverns		2
Loss of interests in activities not directly associated with drinking		2
Late:		
Chooses employment that facilitates drinking		3
Frequent automobile accidents		3
History of family members undergoing psychiatric treatment; school and behavioral problems in children		3
Frequent change of residence for poorly defined reasons		
Anxiety-relieving mechanisms such as telephone calls inappropriate in time, distance, person or motive (telephonitis)		2
Outbursts of rage and suicidal gestures while drinking		2
B. Psychologic and Attitudinal		
1. Direct effects		
Early:		
When talking freely, makes frequent reference to drinking alcohol, people being "bombed," "stoned," etc., or admits to drinking more than peer group		
Middle:		
Drinking to relieve anger, insomnia, fatigue, depression, social discomfort		
Late:		
Psychologic symptoms consistent with permanent organic brain syndrome (see also Major Criteria, Track I, B)		
2. Indirect effects		
Early:		
Unexplained changes in family, social, and business relationships; complaints about wife, job, and friends		3
Spouse makes complaints about drinking behavior, reported by patient or spouse		
Major family disruptions, separation, divorce, threats of divorce		
Job loss (caused by increasing interpersonal difficulties) frequent job changes, financial difficulties		3
Late:		
Overt expression of more regressive defence mechanisms; denial, projection, etc.		3
Resentment, jealousy, paranoid attitudes		3
Symptoms of depression; isolated crying, suicidal preoccupation		3
Feelings of "losing his or her mind"		2

of alcoholics referred for inpatient treatment were referred by physicians.[58] Health providers tend to have an overly pessimistic view of the benefits of treatment for alcoholism. Clearly, success in the efforts to combat alcoholism will require increased efforts at public education and greater acceptance of alcoholism as a medical illness that is amenable to treatment.

CHRONIC EFFECTS OF ALCOHOLISM

Alcoholics have a mortality rate approximately double that of nonalcoholics.[59] This doubling derives from deaths caused by cirrhosis, infections, accidents, malignancies, and cardiovascular diseases. In one study, cirrhosis and violent deaths contributed approximately one half of the excess deaths in heavy drinkers.[59] The direct role of alcohol in violent deaths is hard to separate from the effect of personality traits in those who drink.

Alcoholism increases the risk of developing cancer of the tongue, mouth, oropharynx, esophagus, and liver.[3] Although it is debated whether alcohol exerts its carcinogenic effects through the associated use of tobacco, there appears to be a synergistic effect between alcohol and tobacco increasing the risk of cancer.[60] Finally, alcoholic cancer patients have a poorer chance of survival and a greater chance of developing another primary tumor than do nonalcoholic cancer patients.[51]

Excess cardiovascular mortality in heavy drinkers from myocardial infarction and other causes has been found in several studies.[59,61,62] Also of note is the improved cardiovascular mortality in mild drinkers compared to both heavy drinkers and total abstainers. The effect may be mediated through an alcohol-induced elevation of high-density lipoprotein.[63,64]

LABORATORY TESTS

Dietary deficiencies, acid-base disorders, and the diuretic effect of ethanol can create low levels of various electrolytes: potassium, magnesium, calcium, zinc, and phosphorus. Patients with alcoholic cirrhosis also may be hyponatremic, although their total body sodium stores are increased. Hypokalemia can lead to periodic muscle paralysis, motor weakness, and areflexia. Low magnesium levels can lead to mental status changes, arrhythmias, and inhibition of the action of parahormone releasing calcium stores. Hypokalemia can lead to tetany, motor weakness, and ECG changes (prolonged QT interval). Low levels of zinc are said to be the cause of gonadal dysfunction, impaired

wound healing, and depressed immune responsiveness. Finally, low phosphate levels can lead to myocardial failure, motor weakness, platelet dysfunction, and hemolysis.

Acid-base disturbances may exist in the alcoholic patient. The differential diagnosis of an anion gap metabolic acidosis includes diabetic ketoacidosis; alcoholic ketoacidosis; uremia; lactic acidosis (sepsis, hypotension, hypoxia, carbon monoxide, cyanide); and ingestion of iron, INH, methanol, ethylene glycol, or salicylates. In AKA (but not in DKA), the glucose level is low or only slightly elevated, the B-hydroxybutyrate levels are elevated over the levels of acetoacetate by as much as 11 or 12 to 1, and the condition responds to the administration of glucose and saline. A metabolic alkalosis may be seen in alcoholics with persistent vomiting from gastritis or those who are severely hypokalemic. Finally, a respiratory alkalosis may be seen in alcoholics with cirrhosis because of an increased central respiratory drive.

Hypoglycemia can occur from malnutrition, liver disease, and the inhibition of gluconeogenesis by alcohol. All alcoholics with any alteration in mental status must be immediately assessed for hypoglycemia with a fingerstick determination and a blood glucose.

Alcoholics who present with weakness and painful muscles may be manifesting an alcoholic myopathy. This diagnosis may be confirmed with a serum creatine phosphokinase level. Rarely, one can see the development of myoglobinuria, manifested by dark urine that is dipstick-positive for blood but negative for RBCs. Although hemolysis can create a urine with a similar appearance, in hemolysis the serum should be pink and in myoglobinuria the serum should be clear.

Alcoholic patients may also manifest the following abnormalities: an elevated MCV, gamma glutanyl transferase (GGT), uric acid, triglyceride, and slight anemia. Those with pancreatitis have elevated amylase and lipase levels. Those with liver disease may show elevations of aspartate aminotransferase (AST), alkaline phosphatase, bilirubin, leukocytes, prothrombin times and blood ammonia. One can also see low albumin levels and a hemolytic anemia.

Determination of alcohol levels in the blood is made indirectly and directly. Indirect tests involve the use of breath samples. Ethanol breath analyzers are portable and provide a rapid and simple estimate of blood alcohol levels based on a blood/breath ratio of 2100/1. This ratio varies among patients and within individuals over time.[65] Results are affected by recent use of alcohol (within 15 minutes), recent belching or vomiting, inadequate expiratory specimen, and presence of airway obstruction. Direct methods involve the assessment of whole blood alcohol levels, which are required for forensic purposes. Blood alcohol levels are measured by gas chromatography as well as enzymatic and chemical oxidation reactions. Gas chromatography is simple, inexpensive, and specific for ethanol and is the procedure of choice. Proper collection requires use of nonalcohol skin antiseptics, although their use, when studied, has not been found to influence the blood alcohol assay.[66,67]

Ethanol is one of several solvents that can be detected with measurements of serum osmolality. This is because these solvents can achieve a high level in the blood and have relatively low molecular weights. Osmolarity is best determined by freezing point depression, especially when dealing with alcohol and its substitutes. The other method, vapor pressure determination, involves heating and volatilizes the solvents, yielding erroneous results.

The osmometer measures osmolality (solute/kg of solvent) not osmolarity (solute/liter of solution). The normal serum osmolality is 280 to 295 mOsm. Normally, when there are no additional osmotically active substances in the blood serum, osmolality can be calculated as follows:

$$\text{Osmolality} = 2(\text{Na}) + \frac{\text{glucose}}{18} + \frac{\text{BUN}}{2.8}$$

In addition to ethanol, other hydrocarbons that can increase serum osmolality include: ethyl ether, isopropanol, methanol, acetone, and ethylene glycol.

The presence of these other osmotically active hydrocarbons in the blood can be indirectly assessed by measuring the osmolality directly and comparing it to the calculated value. The normal difference between measured and calculated values (osmolar gap) should be less than 10 mOsm/kg H_2O. A gap greater than 10 mOsm/kg/H_2O suggests the presence of some osmotically active substance. Lethal levels of these agents can cause significant changes in measured osmolality (Table 84-11). Some (e.g., ethylene glycol), however, may contribute only a small increase in serum osmolality despite obtaining a lethal concentration.

The amount that any of these agents contribute to serum osmolality can be determined by measuring the agent directly in the serum and dividing it by its molecular weight.

for ethanol:
$$\text{osmolality (mOsm/kg } H_2O) = \frac{\text{serum ethanol (mg \%)} \times 10}{46}$$

A rise of 4.6 mg% (roughly 5 mg%) in the blood alcohol level results in a rise of 1 mOsm in serum osmolality. Assessment of the osmolal gap can be used as a screening measure for the presence of certain selected solvents including ethanol.

TREATMENT

The therapeutic approach to the alcohol-intoxicated patient must begin with attention to the ABCs. Patients who are stuporous or comatose must have an assessment of the gag reflex. Any patient with a depressed gag reflex must be intubated to protect the airway. An intravenous line should be established with D_5W NS and bloods should be sent for CBC, electrolytes, Ca, Mg, alcohol level, glucose, BUN and creatinine. Additional tests such as amylase, ECG, ABG, serum ammonia, clotting studies, LFT's, serum osmolality, CPK, toxicology screen, KUB, and urinalysis may be ordered as needed. An immediate bedside fingerstick glucose determination should be performed in all cases.

If the fingerstick glucose is low or normal, the patient should receive 25 to 50 g of glucose IV as $D_{50}W$ followed by an intravenous infusion of $D_{10}W$. All alcoholics should receive thiamine, 100 mg IV or IM.

TABLE 84-11. TOXIC SUBSTANCES CONTRIBUTING TO SERUM OSMOLALITY AT THEIR LETHAL LEVELS*

Substance	Molecular Weight	Lethal Level (mg/dL)	Change in Osmolality mOsm/kg H_2O
Ethanol	46	350	80
Ethyl ether	26	180	70
Isopropanol	60	340 (toxic)	60
Methanol	32	80	27
Acetone	58	55	10
Trichloroethane	133	100	9
Paraldehyde	132	50	4
Ethylene glycol	62	21	4
Chloroform	119	39	3
Salicylate	180	50	3
Chloral hydrate	165	25	2
Ethchlorvynol	144	15	1

* Adapted with permission from Glasser, L., Sternglanz, P.D., Combie, J., et al.: Serum osmolality and its applicability to drug overdose. Am. J. Clin. Pathol. 60:698, 1973.

Patients who are malnourished, withdrawing from alcohol, or show signs of magnesium deficiency (e.g., tetany) should be given 2 g (16.2 meq) of magnesium sulfate IV at a rate not to exceed 150 mg/min.[68] Hypokalemia and hypophosphatemia can be corrected with the infusion of 20 to 40 meq of potassium phosphate per liter of intravenous fluid. Patients who are seizing and or withdrawing can be treated with intravenous diazepam (5 to 10 mg total dose) or lorazepam (2 to 4 mg total dose).

All alcoholic patients should be assessed carefully for signs of trauma, infection, hepatic failure, GI bleeding, neurologic disturbances, cardiac arrhythmias, and myopathies. Coma is rare with an alcohol level under 300 mg% , and alcohol-induced coma should steadily improve with time.[69] Any comatose alcoholic with a level less than 300 mg% or who fails to improve with observation should be evaluated for some other pathologic process. Patients in this category should receive blood cultures, paracentesis, head CT, and lumbar puncture as appropriate. Because alcoholic patients are more prone to both trauma and intracerebral bleeding caused by coagulopathies, the threshold for CT scanning in these patients should be low.

GUT DECONTAMINATION

Because the absorption of alcohol from the gastrointestinal tract is fairly rapid with alcohol, evacuation 1 hour or more after ingestion usually has little to offer. Exceptions include the coingestion of other highly toxic agents and the possibility of delayed gastric emptying as seen with ingestion of high concentration alcohol, food, and drugs that slow gut motility like opiates and anticholinergics.

Activated charcoal is of limited benefit in preventing the absorption of alcohols. When used in experimental ethanol intoxication, it failed to produce a difference in peak concentrations or time to peak concentrations in human volunteers.[70] Charcoal has, however, been reported to adsorb significant amounts of whiskey congeners, which may be responsible for the hangover syndrome.[71] Because many overdoses are mixed and alcohol is often ingested in conjunction with other agents, it is prudent to use activated charcoal and cathartic agents liberally when treating intoxicated patients.

ENHANCED ELIMINATION

Fructose given intravenously to inebriated patients can increase the metabolism of ethanol by 25%. The increase in metabolic rate, however, is outweighed by the serious side effects of fructose therapy: nausea and vomiting, abdominal pain, pruritus, lactic acidosis, and shock.[72]

Hemodialysis increases the clearance of ethanol dramatically. This increased clearance (as much as three- to four-fold) must be remembered and adjusted for when patients who are receiving therapeutic ethanol for ethylene glycol or methanol ingestions are placed on dialysis. Hemodialysis has no place in the routine treatment of ethanol intoxication because most patients do well with good supportive care.

MEDICAL TREATMENT

All deficits of fluids, electrolytes, and acid/bases should be treated in the ED. Clotting disorders should be corrected with vitamin K and fresh frozen plasma as needed. All alcoholic patients should receive intravenous preparations of multivitamins in addition to parenteral thiamine. Patients who are encephalopathic should be treated with cleansing enemas if bleeding is present, and lactulose, 15 to 30 mL every hour or neomycin 0.5 to 1 g by mouth as needed.

Febrile alcoholics should be worked up aggressively for infection. Fever should be attributed to withdrawal or to seizures only as a diagnosis of exclusion. If sepsis, meningitis, or peritonitis is suspected, the patient should be cultured and started on broad spectrum antibiotics.

Naloxone has been promoted from time to time as an antidote for ethanol-induced coma. No well-controlled studies exist, however, to confirm the beneficial effect of naloxone in the treatment of ethanol coma.[73] One study of severe alcohol intoxication failed to show any beneficial effect in reversing ethanol-induced CNS depression.[74]

CRITERIA FOR ADMISSION

Most uncomplicated patients intoxicated with alcohol can be successfully discharged from the ED after an evaluation and period of observation. No patient, however, should be discharged while still in an intoxicated state. Patients with altered mental status and a mixed overdose, those with severe trauma, those in moderate to severe alcohol withdrawal, and those with another disease state (e.g., pancreatitis, infection, GI bleeding, encephalopathy, etc.) should all be admitted.

Many chronic drinkers are poor and lack social support, and cannot follow through with treatment plans. Because of this, the threshold for admission should be lower for alcoholics who are homeless, medically indigent, or otherwise disadvantaged.

Alcoholics who are sober and desire alcohol detoxification can be admitted for "drying out" and rehabilitation. Reports of short-term (6 months) improvement rates of 80% and long-term (abstinence for more than 1 year) improvement rates of up to 50% from "good clinics" are encouraging.[3] The national average for improvement from treatment is probably around 25%.

Inpatient alcohol programs have an advantage over outpatient programs in that they enforce abstinence, provide more support and structure, and separate the patient from the social environment associated with drinking. For the patient who is highly motivated and has good social support, there may be no difference in cure rate between inpatient and outpatient treatment. Hospitalization should be considered in the following circumstances[75]:

1. The patient has additional medical problems
2. Depression, confusion, or psychosis might interfere with outpatient care
3. The patient is in the midst of a severe life crisis
4. Outpatient treatment has been tried and failed
5. It is impossible for the patient to get to the outpatient center.

Authorities recommend continued contact after abstinence is achieved for a period of at least 6 months. No matter what type of rehabilitation is planned, an alcoholic patient can always be referred to Alcoholics Anonymous (AA). AA is a self-help group of recovering alcoholics that offers support and crisis intervention and is available in almost every community.

Disulfiram (Antabuse) has been used with some success in the treatment of alcohol abuse. The drug inhibits aldehyde dehydrogenase leading to a build-up of acetaldehyde in the blood after the consumption of ethanol. The peak in levels of acetaldehyde usually occurs approximately $\frac{1}{2}$ hour after drinking, but this depends on the dose of alcohol ingested and the rate of intake. The disulfiram-alcohol reaction is manifested by: nausea and vomiting, tremor, diarrhea, and hypotension or hypertension. Disulfiram should not be prescribed to patients with hypertension, diabetes, heart disease, or history of stroke. Alcoholics are often given 250 mg of disulfiram a day for 6 to 12 months at a time. In addition to disulfiram, various other drugs including chlormethiazole, oral hypoglycemics, and metronidazole can cause a similar effect (Table 84-12).

TABLE 84-12. DRUG INTERACTIONS WITH ALCOHOL

Interacting Drugs	Adverse Effects (Probable Mechanism)	Comments and Recommendations
Acetaminophen	Severe hepatotoxicity with therapeutic doses of acetaminophen in chronic alcoholics (mechanism not established)	Incidence unknown; warn patients
Anticoagulants, oral	Decreased anticoagulant effect with chronic alcohol abuse (increased metabolism)	Monitor prothrombin time in chronic alcoholics
	Increased anticoagulant effect with acute intoxication (decreased metabolism)	Warn patients and monitor prothrombin time
Antidepressants, tricyclic	Increased toxicity of both drugs with amitriptyline or trazodone (decreased metabolism)	Avoid concurrent use; to some extent, desipramine may partly counteract deleterious effects of alcohol on cognitive functions; the combination with amitriptyline can cause additive euphoria, which has led to abuse
	Decreased imipramine and desipramine effect in alcoholics (mechanism not established)	Monitor imipramine and desipramine concentrations
	Decreased cognitive function (probably additive)	Avoid concurrent use
Barbiturates	Decreased sedative effect with chronic alcohol abuse (increased barbiturate metabolism)	Avoid barbiturates in alcohol abusers, if possible
	Increased CNS depression with acute intoxication (additive; decreased barbiturate metabolism)	
Benzodiazepines	Increased CNS depression (additive effects, possibly increased absorption and decreased metabolism of benzodiazepines)	Even small amounts of alcohol may impair driving ability in patients taking benzodiazepines; zopiclone may not interact
	Possible increased anxiety with lorazepam (mechanism not established)	Healthy volunteers had more anxiety than with either drug alone
	Anterograde amnesia with triazolam and possibly other benzodiazepines (mechanism not established)	Avoid concurrent use

TABLE 84-12. CONTINUED

Interacting Drugs	Adverse Effects (Probable Mechanism)	Comments and Recommendations
Beta-adrenergic blockers	May block signs of delirium tremens	Avoid beta-blockers in alcoholics
	Decreased beta-blockade with propranolol (increased metabolism)	Reported only with propranolol, but warn patients taking any beta-blocker; acebutolol, oxprenolol and metoprolol may not interact; dosage should not be changed after short-term increased use of alcohol
	Increased beta-blockade with sotalol (decreased elimination)	Monitor clinical status
Bromocriptine	Possible increased bromocriptine toxicity (mechanism not established)	Clinical evidence limited; warn patients
Caffeine	Caffeine may further decrease reaction time (synergism or antagonism)	Variable response
Cephalosporins	Disulfiram-like effect with cefamandole, cefoperazone, cefotetan or moxalactam (probably inhibition of intermediary metabolism of alcohol)	Avoid alcohol and alcohol-containing medications; cefonicid does not interact
Chloral hydrate	Prolonged hypnotic effect (synergism); adverse cardiovascular effects (mechanism not established)	Avoid concurrent use
Chlormethiazole	Increased chlormethiazole toxicity (decreased metabolism)	Avoid concurrent use
Cimetidine	Increased alcohol effect (possibly inhibition of acetaldehyde in ALDH-1 deficiency)	Small effect; clinical significance not established
Contraceptives, oral	Possible increased alcohol effect (decreased metabolism)	Caution patients
Cycloserine	Increased alcohol effect or convulsions (mechanism not established)	Avoid concurrent use; warn patients
Cytarabine	Aggravation of pain from acral erythema caused by cytarabine (mechanism not established)	Three case reports in patients receiving IV cyclosporine in an alcohol base; pain was controlled by slowing the infusion rate and giving analgesics
Digitoxin	Possible decreased digitoxin effect (competition for common enzyme)	In vitro studies; monitor digitoxin concentration in alcoholics
Digoxin	Possible decreased digoxin effect (competition for common enzyme)	In vitro studies; monitor digoxin concentration in alcoholics
Disulfiram	Abdominal cramps, flushing, vomiting, confusion, psychosis (inhibition of intermediary metabolism of alcohol)	Avoid alcohol and alcohol-containing medications; single report of dyspareunia and male discomfort, when woman taking disulfiram and man intoxicated
Guanadrel	Increased sedation and orthostatic hypotension (additive)	Avoid concurrent use
Heparin	Increased bleeding (additive)	Avoid large amounts of alcohol
Hypoglycemics, sulfonylurea	Decreased hypoglycemic effect with chronic alcohol abuse (increased metabolism)	Avoid large amounts of alcohol
	Increased or prolonged hypoglycemic effect with acute ingestion of alcohol, especially in fasting patients (suppression of gluconeogenesis)	
	Minor disulfiram-like symptoms, particularly with chlorpropamide (inhibition of intermediary metabolism of alcohol)	Inform patients; unlikely with small amounts of alcohol with meals

TABLE 84-12. CONTINUED

Interacting Drugs	Adverse Effects (Probable Mechanism)	Comments and Recommendations
Isoniazid	Increased incidence of hepatitis (mechanism not established)	Incidence of serious consequences unknown
	Possible decreased isoniazid effect in some alcoholics (increased metabolism)	Do not use isoniazid alone in alcoholics
Ketoconazole	Possible disulfiram-like reaction (mechanism not established)	Several case reports
Lithium	Possible increased lithium effect (mechanism not established)	Clinical significance not established; monitor lithium concentration
Maprotiline	Seizures, possibly due to maprotiline toxicity (mechanism not established)	Single case report
Meprobamate	Decreased sedative effect with chronic alcohol abuse (increased metabolism)	Avoid meprobamate in alcoholics
	Increased CNS depression with acute intoxication (additive and decreased metabolism)	Warn patients
Methaqualone	Increased CNS depression (probably decreased methaqualone metabolism)	Occurred after single dose of alcohol given 72 hours after single dose of methaqualone-diphenhydramine; avoid concurrent use
Methotrexate	Increased hepatotoxicity in chronic alcoholics (mechanism not established)	Monitor hepatic function
Metronidazole	Mild disulfiram-like symptoms (possibly inhibition of intermediary metabolism of alcohol)	Vomiting rare; nausea mild or absent; excitement, giddiness, and flush found pleasant by some, have led to abuse; may occur with IV drugs containing alcohol; single report with vaginal metronidazole
Mianserin	Increased toxicity of both drugs (decreased metabolism)	Avoid concurrent use
Nitroglycerin	Possible hypotension (additive)	Reported only when nitroglycerin was taken an hour or more after alcohol; warn patients
Nonsteroidal anti-inflammatory drugs	Increased bleeding (additive)	Avoid large amounts of alcohol
	Acute renal failure (mechanism not established)	Single case report
Phenformin	Lactic acidosis (synergism)	Avoid phenformin in alcoholics
Phenothiazines	Impaired motor coordination with chlorpromazine (probably additive); may occur with all phenothiazines	Warn patients, especially drivers
Phenylbutazone	Impaired motor coordination (probably additive)	Warn patients, especially drivers
Phenytoin	Decreased anticonvulsant effect with chronic alcohol abuse (increased metabolism)	Monitor phenytoin concentration in alcoholics
	Increased phenytoin toxicity with acute intoxication (decreased metabolism)	Warn patients
Ranitidine	Increased alcohol effect (mechanism not established)	Small effect; clinical significance not established
Salicylates	Increased bleeding (additive)	Avoid large amounts of alcohol
Tetracyclines	Decreased doxycycline effect in alcoholics (increased metabolism)	Tetracycline HCl does not interact
Triclofos sodium	Possible prolonged hypnotic effect (synergism)	Avoid concurrent use

* Adapted with special permission from The Medical Letter Handbook of Adverse Drug Interactions, 1991.

ALCOHOL-DRUG INTERACTIONS

Alcohol is responsible for various drug interactions with various agents.[76] (see Table 84-12). Depending on the agent involved and the duration of drinking, the results may be antagonistic, additive, or synergistic. Acute intoxication with alcohol can transiently increase levels of certain drugs (e.g., phenytoin) because of competition for shared metabolic pathways. In contrast, chronic ethanolism can cause increased drug clearance and lower drug levels because of enhancement of these same pathways.

When increased microsomal oxidation occurs, there is a spill-over stimulation to other microsomal oxidizing systems. This leads to accelerated metabolism of drugs sharing similar microsomal metabolic pathways. The half-lives of phenytoin, tolbutamide, INH, and warfarin are 50% shorter in abstaining alcoholics than in nondrinkers.[77] For a similar reason, the potential toxicity of acetaminophen can be enhanced by alcohol through the induction of hepatotoxic intermediates metabolized by way of the P450 system.[78]

Ethanol has additive effects when ingested with antihistamines, barbiturates, and other sedative-hypnotics, tricyclic antidepressants, glutethimide, phenothiazine, narcotics, and chloral hydrate ("Mickey Finn"). Alcohol can enhance the aspirin-induced increase in bleeding time.

Alcohol can cause a potentially serious reaction when combined with disulfiram (Antabuse). The reaction is thought to be caused by the inhibition of ADH and the build-up of acetaldehyde or the accumulation of some other toxic product. Symptoms include skin flushing, nausea and vomiting, palpitations, diaphoresis, vertigo, disorientation, headache, and chest and abdominal pains. This unpleasant interaction has been used clinically in an attempt to encourage patients to stop drinking.[79]

The "antabuse reaction" has also been described when alcohol is used in association with other agents: cephalosporin, chloramphenicol, griseofulvin, nitrofurantoin, sulfonamides, chlorpropramide, tolbutamide, chloral hydrate, metronidazole, coprinus atramentarius (mushroom), and industrial chemicals (amides, oximes, carbamates, dithiocarbamates, and thiuran derivatives). Treatment is symptomatic and involves gut decontamination (if appropriate), charcoal, IV hydration, antiemetics, and monitoring for seizures and arrhythmias.

Stimulants, including amphetamines and caffeine, do not reliably counteract the sedative effects of alcohol. Coffee is thus not an effective antidote to alcohol. In fact, coffee may antagonize the positive effect of *small* doses of alcohol on reaction time and coordination.

Many people who abuse illicit drugs do so in conjunction with alcohol. Alcohol is often consumed in combination with marijuana or opiates as well as legal drugs such as sedative hypnotics. This can result in serious medical consequences as well as trauma and suicide.

Alcoholic patients with cirrhosis and ascites have an increased incidence of spontaneous bacterial peritonitis (SBP). Patients with SBP present with fever and abdominal pain, with or without peritoneal signs. The diagnosis can be difficult to make clinically and often rests with the analysis of ascitic fluid obtained from

TABLE 84-13. PATTERN OF FETAL ALCOHOL SYNDROME*

Abnormality	Frequency
Growth	
Microcephaly	+ + +
Developmental delay	+ + +
Intrauterine growth retardation	+ + +
Craniofacial	
Short palpebral fissures	+ + +
Midfacial hypoplasia	+ + +
Maxillary hypoplasia	+ + +
Limb	
Palmar crease abnormalities	+ +
Joint abnormalities (mild to severe)	+ +
Miscellaneous	
Cardiac	
Atrial septal defect	+ +
Ventricular septal defect	+
Tetralogy of Fallot	+
Liver disease (hepatic fibrosis)	+

+ + + = common; + + = moderately frequent; + = occasional.
* Adapted with permission from Hill, L.M. and Kleinberg, F.: Effects of drugs and chemicals on the fetus and newborn (second of two parts). Mayo Clin. Proc. 59:755–765, 1984.

a paracentesis. Escherichia coli and streptococci are the most common organisms. Because of the difficulty in establishing the diagnosis and the high mortality associated with SBP, all patients with fever and ascites should receive a diagnostic paracentesis as part of their evaluation in the ED.[80]

Finally, alcoholic patients can develop fever secondary to seizures or withdrawal. It is not uncommon, however, for an infection to precipitate withdrawal in an alcoholic. All febrile alcoholic patients in withdrawal must be carefully evaluated for an infectious cause before a disposition is made.

ALCOHOL-RELATED FETAL EFFECTS

The fetal alcohol syndrome (FAS) was first noted in 1963 by French investigators.[81] The most common features include: retardation of prenatal and postnatal growth, low IQ, mild to moderate microcephaly, short palpebral fissure, maxillary hypoplasia, joint abnormalities, fine tremor, poor hand-eye coordination, and cardiac malformations (Table 84-13). CNS seems to be most susceptible to the in utero exposure to alcohol. The FAS has been reported in as many as one third of the infants born to mothers who consume 150 g or more of alcohol per day. Studies of pregnant women who drink but are not alcoholic have revealed an increased incidence of spontaneous abortion, low birth weight, and altered development, although the threshold is unknown.

It has been suggested that ethanol in the prenatal period is the leading cause of mental retardation in the U.S. and accounts for 59% of all congenital anomalies.[82] Prenatal exposure to more than three drinks a day triples the risk of a subnormal IQ (<85) at age 4. Although the ingestion of less than three drinks a day has not been demonstrated to cause fetal damage, the American Medical Association and the Surgeon General have recommended abstention from alcohol during pregnancy.

REFERENCES

1. Barbor, T.: Drinking throughout the ages. In Alcohol Customs and Rituals. Edited by Snyder, S. The Encyclopedia of Psychoactive Drugs. New York, Chelsea House Publishers, 1986, p. 23.
2. Lewis, D.C.: Diagnosis and management of the alcoholic patient. R.I. Med. J. 63:27, 1980.
3. West, L.J., Maxwell, D.S., Noble, E.P., and Solomon, D.H.: Alcoholism. Ann. Intern. Med. 100:405, 1984.
4. Becker, C.E.: Alcohol and drug use. Is there a "safe amount?" West. J. Med. 141:884, 1984.
5. Sixth Special Report to Congress on Alcohol and Health. Rockville, MD. Dept. of Health and Human Services, National Institute on Alcohol Abuse and Alcoholism, 1987, p. 21. (DHHS publication no. (ADM) 87–1519).
6. Ellenhorn, M.J., and Barceloux, D.G.: Alcohols and glycols. In Medical Toxicology. Edited by Ellenhorn, M.J., and Barceloux, D.G. New York, Elsevier, 1988, pp. 782–812.
7. Committee on Drugs, 1983–1984, American Academy of Pediatrics: Ethanol in liquid preparations intended for children. Pediatrics 73:405, 1984.
8. Ritchie, J. M.: The aliphatic alcohols. In The Pharmacological Basis of Therapeutics. Edited by Gilman, A.G., Goodman, L.S., Rall, T.W., and Murad, F. New York, Macmillan, 1985, pp. 372–387.
9. Jones, B.M., and Jones, M.K.: Male and female intoxication levels for three alcohol doses or do women really get higher than men? Alcohol Tech. Rep. 5:11, 1976.
10. Julkunen, R.J., DiRadova, C., and Lieber, C.S.: First pass metabolism of ethanol—a gastro-intestinal barrier against the systemic toxicity of ethanol. Life Sci. 37:567, 1985.
11. Frezza, M., DiPadova, C., Pozzato, G., et al.: High blood alcohol levels in women. The role of decreased gastric alcohol dehydrogenase activity and first pass metabolism. N. Engl. J. Med. 322:95, 1990.
12. Lieber, C.S.: Metabolism and metabolic effects of alcohol. Med. Clin. North Am. 68:3, 1984.
13. Wilkinson, P.K.: Pharmacokinetics of ethanol: A review. Alcoholism Clin. Exp. Res. 4:6, 1980.
14. Sidel, F.R., and Pless, J.E.: Ethyl alcohol: Blood levels and performance decrements after oral administration to man. Psychopharmacologia 19:246, 1971.
15. Williams, J.A., and Lee, M.: Microtubules and pancreatic amylase release by mouse pancreas in vitro. J. Cell Biol. 71:795, 1976.
16. Charness, M.E., Simon, R.P., and Greenberg, D.A.: **Ethanol and the nervous system.** N. Engl. J. Med. 321:442, 1989.
17. Nestros, J.N.: Ethanol specifically potentiates GABA-mediated neurotransmission in feline cerebral cortex. Science 209:708, 1980.
18. Suzdak, P.D., Schwartz, R.D., Skolnick, P., et al.: Ethanol stimulates GABA receptor mediated chloride transport in rat brain synptoneurosomes. Proc. Natl. Acad. Sci. USA 83:4071, 1986.
19. Isselbacher, K.J.: Metabolic and Hepatic Effects of Alcohol. New Engl. J. Med. 1977; 296:612–616.
20. Cederbaum, A.I., Lieber, C.S., and Rubin, E.: Effects of chronic ethanol treatment on mitochondrial functions: Damage to coupling site I. Arch. Biochem. Biophys. 165:560, 1974.
21. Kissin, B., and Degleiter, H.: The Biology of Alcoholism, Vol. I: Biochemistry. New York, Plenum Press, 1971, p. 630.
22. Korsten, M.A., Matsuzaki, S., Feinman, L., et al.: High blood acetaldehyde levels after ethanol administration. N. Engl. J. Med. 292:386, 1975.
23. Laposata, E.A., and Louis, L.G.: Presence of non-oxidative, ethanol metabolism in human organs commonly damaged by ethanol abuse. Science 231:497, 1986.
24. Modell, J.G., and Mounty, J.M.: Drinking and flying—The problem of alcohol use by pilots. N. Engl. J. Med. 323:455, 1990.
25. Modell, J.G.: Behavioral, neurologic, and physiologic effects of acute ethanol ingestion. In The Alcoholic Patient: Emergency Medical Intervention. Edited by Fassler, D. New York, Gardner Press, 1990.
26. Kalant, H.: Ethanol and the nervous system: Experimental neurophysiological aspects. Int. J. Neurol. 9:111, 1974.
27. Mellanby, E.: Alcohol: Its absorption into and disappearance from the blood under different conditions. Medical Research Council. Special Report Series. London 15:1, 1919.
28. Tabakoff, B., Cornell, N., and Hoffman, P.L.: Alcohol tolerance. Ann. Emerg. Med. 15:1005, 1986.
29. Khanna, J.M., Kalant, H., Le, A.D., et al.: Role of serotonergic and adrenergic systems in alcohol tolerance. Prog. Neuro-Psychopharmacol. 1981;5:459–465.
30. Davis, A.R., and Lipson, A.H.: Central nervous system depression and high blood ethanol levels. Lancet 1:566, 1986.
31. Linblad, B., and Olsson, R.: Unusually high levels of blood alcohol. JAMA 236:1600, 1976.

32. Lang, R.M., Borow, K.M., Newmann, A.G., et al.: Adverse cardiac effects of acute alcohol ingestion in young adults. Ann. Intern. Med. 102:742, 1985.

33. Thorton, J.R.: Arterial fibrillation in healthy non-alcoholic people after an alcoholic binge. Lancet 2:1013, 1984.

34. Seixas, F.A., Blumne, S., Cloud, L.A., et al.: A definition of alcoholism, Ann. Intern. Med. 85:764, 1976.

35. Goodwin, D.W.: Is Alcoholism Hereditary? New York, Oxford University Press, 1976, pp. 23–26.

36. Eckardt, M.J., Harford, T.C., Kaelber, C.T., et al.: Health hazards associated with alcohol consumption. JAMA 246:648, 1981.

37. Pokorny, A.P., Miller, B.A., and Kaplan, H.B.: A paper and pencil questionnaire. Ann. J. Psychiatry. 129:342, 1972.

38. Mayfield, D., McLeod, G., and Hall, P.: More detailed interview screening. Ann. J. Psychiatry. 131:1121, 1974.

39. Criteria Committee, National Council on Alcoholism: Criteria for the diagnosis of alcoholism. Ann. J. Psychiatry. 127:135, 1972.

40. Jaffe, J.H.: Drug and addiction abuse. In The Pharmacological Bases of Therapeutics, Ed. 7. Edited by Gilman, A.G., Goodman, L.S., Rall, T.W., and Murad, F. New York, Macmillan Publishing Co., 1985, pp. 532–581.

41. Schuckit, M.A.: Alcoholism and affective disorder: Diagnostic confusion. In Alcoholism and Affective Disorders. Edited by Goodwin, D.W., and Erickson, C.K. New York, SP Medical and Scientific Books, 1979, pp. 9–19.

42. Mayfield, D.G.: Alcohol and affect: Experimental studies. In Alcoholism and Affective Disorders. Ibid., pp. 99–107.

43. Winokur, G., and Clayton, P.: Family history studies: II. Sex differences and alcoholism in primary affective illness. Br. J. Psychiatry 113:973, 1967.

44. Mayfield, D.G., and Coleman, L.L.: Alcohol use and affective disorders. Dis. Nerv. Syst. 29:467, 1968.

45. Schuckit, M., Pitts, F.N., Reich, T., et al.: Alcoholism: I Two types of alcoholism in women. Arch. Gen. Psychiatry. 20:301, 1969.

46. Medhus, A.: Mortality among female alcoholics. Scand. J. Soc. Med. 3:111, 1975.

47. Goodwin, D.W.: Alcohol in suicide and homicide. Q.J. Stud. Alcohol. 34:144, 1973.

48. Day, N.: Alcohol and Mortality Report prepared for National Institute on Alcohol Abuse and Alcoholism under contract No. NIA 76–10CP, 1977.

49. Cotton, N.S.: The familial incidence of alcoholism: A review. J. Stud. Alcohol 40:89, 1979.

50. Goodwin, D.S.: Alcoholism and heredity. Arch. Gen. Psychiatry 36:57, 1979.

51. Cleninger, C.R., Bohman, M., and Sigvardsson, S.: Inheritance of alcohol abuse. Arch. Gen. Psychiatry 38:861, 1981.

52. Partanen, J.K., Bruun, T., and Markanen, N.: Inheritance of drinking behavior: a study on intelligence, personality, and the use of alcohol in adult twins. Helsinki, Finnish Foundation for Alcohol Studies, 1966.

53. Hill, S.Y., Goodwin, D.W., Cadoret, R., et al.: Association and linkage between alcoholism and eleven perological markers. J. Stud. Alcohol 36:981, 1975.

54. Agarwal, D.P., Garada, S., and Goedde, H.W.: Radical differences in biological sensitivity to ethanol. Alcoholism (NY) 5:12, 1981.

55. Yoshida, A., Yuang, I.-Y., and Ikawa, M.: Molecular abnormality of an inactive aldehyde dehydrogenase variant commonly found in Orientals. Proc. Natl. Acad. Sci. U.S.A. 81:258, 1984.

56. Blum, K., Noble, E.P., Sheridan, P.J., et al.: Allelic association of human dopamine receptor gene in alcoholism. JAMA 263:2055, 1990.

57. Institute of Medicine, Division of Health Promotion and Disease Prevention. Alcoholism, Alcohol Abuse, and Related Problems, Opportunities for research. Washington, D.C., National Academy of Sciences, 1980.

58. Mendelson, J.H., Miller, K.D., Mello, N.K., et al.: Hospital treatment of alcoholism: A profile of middle income Americans. Alcoholism (N.Y.) 6:377, 1982.

59. Klatsky, A.L., Friedman, G.D., and Sieglaub, A.B.: Alcohol and mortality. Ann. Intern. Med. 95:139, 1981.

60. Noble, E.P. (Ed.): Third Special Report to the U.S. Congress on Alcohol and Health, Rockville, MD. National Institute on Alcohol Abuse and Alcoholism, 1978.

61. Wilhelmsen, L., Wedel, H., and Tiblin, G.: Multivariate analysis of risk factors for coronary heart disease. Circulation 48:950, 1973.

62. Dyer, A.R., Stanler, J., Paul, O., et al.: Alcohol consumption, cardiovascular risk factors, and mortality in two Chicago epidemiological studies. Circulation 56:1067, 1977.

63. Hennekens, C.H., Willet, W., Rosner, B., et al.: Effects of beer, wine, and liquor in coronary deaths. JAMA 242:1973, 1979.

64. Barboriak, J.J., Rimm, A.A., Anderson, A.J., et al.: Coronary artery occlusion and alcohol intake. Br. Heart J. 39:289, 1977.

65. Jones, A.W.: Variability of the blood: breath alcohol ratio in vivo. J. Stud. Alcohol. 39:1931, 1978.

66. Goldfinger, T.M., and Schaber, D.: A comparison of blood alcohol concentration using non-alcohol and alcohol-containing skin antiseptics. Ann. Emerg. Med. 11:665, 1982.

67. Ryder, K.W., and Glick, M.R.: The effect of skin cleansing agents on ethanol results measured with the DuPont Automatic clinical analyzer. J. Forensic Sci. 31:574, 1986.

68. Linderman, R.D., and Pappen, S.: Therapy of fluid and electrolyte disorders. Ann. Intern. Med. 82:64, 1975.

69. McMicken, D.B.: Alcohol-Related Disease. In Emergency Medicine: Concepts and Clinical Practice, 2nd ed. Edited by Rosen, P., Baker, F.J., Barkin, R.M., Braen, G.R., Dailey, R.H., and Levy, R.C. St. Louis, C.V. Mosby Co., 1988, pp. 109–2072.

70. Minocha, A., Herold, H.A., Barth, J.A., et al.: Use of activated charcoal in ethanol overdose (Abstract). Vet. Hum. Toxicol. 28:318, 1985.

71. Damrau, F., and Goldberg, A.H.: Adsorption of whiskey congeners by activated charcoal. South. West Med. J. 52:179, 1971.

72. Lovejoy, F.H.: Ethanol intoxication. Clin. Toxicol. Rev. 4:1, 1981.

73. Naloxone for ethanol intoxication, editorial comment. Lancet 2:145, 1983.

74. Nuotto, E., Palva, W.E., and Lahdemanta, V.: Naloxone fails to counteract heavy alcohol intoxication. Lancet 2:167, 1983.

75. Schuckit, M.A.: Alcoholism and drug dependency. In Harrison's Principles of Internal Medicine. 11th edition. Edited by Brunwald, E., Isselbacher, K.J., Petersdorf, R.G., Wilson, J.D., Martin, J.B., and Fauci, A.S. New York, McGraw-Hill, 1987, p. 366.

76. Interactions of drugs with alcohol. Med. Lett. 23:33, 1981.

77. Kater, R.M.H.: Accelerated metabolism of drugs in alcoholics. Gastroenterology 56:412, 1969.

78. McClain, C.J.: Potentiation of acetaminophen hepatotoxicity by alcohol. JAMA 244:251, 1980.

79. Sellers, E.M., Naracho, C., and Peachey, J.E.: Drugs to decrease alcohol consumption. N. Engl. J. Med. 305:1255, 1981.

80. Conn, H.O., and Fessel, J.M.: Spontaneous bacterial peritonitis in cirrhosis: variations on a theme. Medicine 50:161, 1971.

81. Lemoine, P., Harousseau, H., Borteyou, J.P., et al.: Les enfants de parents alcooliques: Anomalies observees à propos de 127 cas. Quest. Med. 21:476, 1968.

82. Abel, E.L., Sokol, R.J.: Incidence of fetal alcohol syndrome and economic impact of FAS-related anomalies. Drug Alcohol Depend. 19:51, 1987.

ALCOHOL SUBSTITUTES

Harold Osborn

CAPSULE

This section discusses three substances often used as substitutes for ethanol. These substances are methanol, ethylene glycol, and isopropyl alcohol. Characteristics, pharmacokinetics, pathophysiology, clinical effects, laboratory tests, and treatment are described for each.

METHANOL

Methanol (wood alcohol, CH_3OH) is an alcohol made from the destructive distillation of wood pulp. It is used commercially as a solvent, antifreeze (especially in windshield washer solution), and paint remover. It is present in varying concentrations in these different forms: antifreeze (95%), windshield fluid (35 to 95%), and Sterno canned heat (4%). Methanol is found in shellacs, paints, duplicating fluid, gas additives, and nail polish removers and is used to adulterate ethyl alcohol prepared for industrial purposes.

CHARACTERISTICS

Methanol is a colorless, volatile liquid with a distinctive odor. It is fully miscible in water and has a molecular weight of 32 daltons. It penetrates body tissues easily and has a volume of distribution like that of ethanol, 0.6 to 0.7 L/Kg. Methanol is intoxicating, and epidemics of methanol toxicity have resulted from the consumption of contaminated whiskey.

PHARMACOKINETICS

Methanol is well absorbed from the GI tract, with peak levels occurring within 30 to 90 minutes.[2] Absorption can also occur from the skin and through the lungs and has occasionally been significant enough to result in toxicity.

After absorption, methanol is widely distributed throughout the body. Concentrations are highest in the kidney, liver, GI tract, vitreous humor, and optic nerve. Methanol is also found in brain, muscle, and fat. A small amount of methanol is found in the expired breath of normal subjects, possibly because of endogenous production.[3,4]

In humans, the liver is responsible for most of the metabolism of methanol. In poisoning situations, however, a significant amount is excreted in the breath. The kidneys excrete from 2 to 5% of unchanged methanol in the urine. Methanol is metabolized in the liver to formaldehyde in a reaction catalyzed by alcohol dehydrogenase, the enzyme common to the metabolism of ethanol as well (Fig. 84-3). Formaldehyde is quickly metabolized to formic acid by aldehyde dehydrogenase and formate is oxidized to carbon dioxide in a reaction in which folate serves as a cofactor. Folate deficiency in exposed individuals facilitates acidosis and may increase methanol toxicity. The variable rates of this folate-dependent pathway account for the variation in toxicity among species. Ethanol has 10 to 20 times greater affinity for alcohol dehydrogenase than methanol and thus ethanol is metabolized preferentially if both are present. This fact explains the efficacy of ethanol in the prevention of methanol toxicity.

The elimination of methanol from the blood is slow compared to that of ethanol. Study of the kinetics of methanol has been hampered by the fact that the elimination of methanol in human intoxications is usually altered by hemodialysis or the administration of ethanol. At low doses (0.08 g per kg) in three human volunteers, methanol was metabolized following first-order kinetics with a half-life of 3 hours.[5] Animal studies suggest that the elimination kinetics are "zero order" (saturation kinetics) at blood concentrations in the range encountered in many reported cases (i.e., 100 to 200 mg%).[6,7] Data obtained from cases before treatment indicate that methanol is metabolized at 8 to 9 mg% per hour in the setting of an overdose.[8]

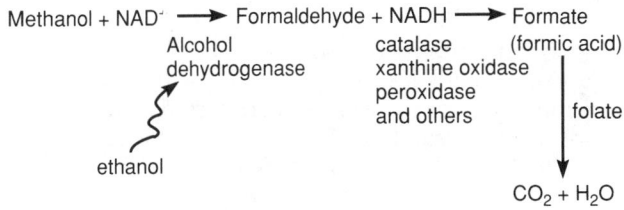

FIG. 84-3.   Principal pathways of methanol metabolism.

PATHOPHYSIOLOGY

Methanol, like ethanol, is a CNS depressant but is not harmful by itself. Rather, it is the accumulation of its two main metabolites, formaldehyde and formic acid, that accounts for its main toxicity.

Formaldehyde is quickly metabolized to formic acid by various enzyme systems: aldehyde dehydrogenase, xanthine oxidase, glyceraldehyde-3-phosphate hydrogenase, catalase, perioxidases, aldehyde oxidase, and a glutathione-dependent formaldehyde dehydrogenase. The formation of formic acid accounts for the bulk of the anion gap metabolic acidosis that appears in methanol poisoning. Lactate may be generated as well, secondary to a formate-induced inhibition of mitochondrial respiration and tissue hypoxia.[9] Clinical toxicity is said to correlate better with formic acid levels than with methanol levels, and this is why the latter, by themselves, cannot be totally relied on. Formate can also disturb axoplasm flow by inhibition of cytochrome oxidase.[10] The local production of formaldehyde in the retina accounts for the optic papillitis and retinal edema seen with methanol poisoning. Methanol can also be oxidized in the kidney.

CLINICAL EFFECTS

Patients appearing early with methanol intoxication appear inebriated but lack the euphoria seen with ethanol. Once the CNS sedating effect of methanol has dissipated, however, there may be a latent period of 1 to 72 hours. Presumably, this is the period during which methanol is metabolized and acidosis develops. The fatal dose of methanol is somewhere between 60 and 240 mL, but as little as 10 mL has proved toxic.[11]

Symptoms of methanol toxicity include vertigo, nausea and vomiting, diarrhea, abdominal pain, dyspnea, agitation, blurred vision, photophobia (often described as "flashes" or a "snowstorm"), and decreased visual acuity. Extremely ill patients may present with bradycardia, blindness, seizures, or coma. Physical examination sometimes, but not invariably, reveals constricted visual fields, fixed and dilated pupils, retinal edema, or hyperemia of the disk. Methanol, rarely, can cause pancreatitis or low grade hepatitis. Patients dying from methanol intoxication have developed respiratory apnea, opisthotonos, and seizures.[12]

LABORATORY TESTS

A frequent finding in methanol poisoning is the presence of an acidosis. Most patients with a serum bicarbonate under 18 meq/L were reported to have methanol levels over 50 mg%.[1] Mortality correlates best with the severity of acidosis. When formate levels exceed 20 mg%, ocular injury and acidosis are likely.[13]

A significant methanol ingestion creates an osmolar gap. For every increase of 3.2 mg% in the methanol level, the osmolar gap increases by 1 mOsm/kg H_2O. A lethal level of methanol (80 mg%) increases the serum osmolality by 27 mOsm/kg H_2O (see Table 84-11).

Methanol can cause hematologic abnormalities. The mean corpuscular volume of RBCs is elevated. Leucocytosis and anemia have also been reported. If the liver or kidney is affected, hyperamylasemia or elevated liver function tests may result. Methanol poisoning can also cause hypophosphatemia and an elevation in CPK.

Because of some endogenous production, normal serum methanol levels may be approximately 0.05 mg%. Levels under 20 mg% are usually not associated with toxicity, but patients with levels over 20 mg% are usually symptomatic. CNS symptoms correlate with levels above 20 mg%; ocular symptoms are seen with levels over 100 mg%. Levels above 50 mg% usually imply a serious poisoning. Concomitant ingestion of ethanol and significantly elevated alcohol levels have a protective effect in the face of methanol toxicity.

Laboratory evaluation of patients with suspected methanol intoxication should include the following: serum electrolytes, BUN, and creatinine; arterial blood gases; serum osmolality; blood levels of methanol, ethanol, ethylene glycol; liver function tests; amylase; and CBC.

TREATMENT

Basic treatment should proceed as for ethanol intoxication. Airway, breathing, and circulation should be assessed and stabilized. GI evacuation, glucose, thiamine, and naloxone should be provided as indicated. Because charcoal does not adsorb the alcohols well, it should be provided only if coingestion of other substances is suspected.

The aggressive treatment of acidosis is imperative. Sodium bicarbonate, 1 to 2 meq per kg, should be administered intravenously and a bicarbonate infusion begun whenever the arterial pH is less than 7.20. Years ago, before more modern treatment modalities were available, the treatment of methanol poisoning with bicarbonate alone occasionally improved visual acuity. Data from individual cases indicate that bicarbonate administration may enhance the elimination of formate.[8] Swartz, reporting on a prison epidemic of methanol poisoning, suggested that bicarbonate and ethanol sufficed for patients who were moderately intoxicated.[1] Thus bicarbonate and ethanol should be begun early in the treatment of suspected methanol poisoning.

Ethanol provides an alternative substrate for alcohol dehydrogenase and has greater affinity for the enzyme than does methanol. Its use is based on the assumption that competition for a shared metabolic pathway prevents the conversion of methanol to its toxic intermediates and allows time for its elimination.

Optimally, a blood ethanol of 100 to 150 mg% should be attained, although in practice it is often difficult to titrate precisely. A loading dose of 0.8 g per kg of 5 to 10% ethanol IV, followed by 130 mg per kg per hour should be provided. Oral loading with 20 to 40% ethanol is an acceptable alternative if no intravenous preparation of ethanol is available. Additional adjustments should be based on serial ethanol levels. When hemodialysis is performed, maintenance doses of 250 to 350 mg per kg per hour are advised because ethanol is dialyzed out with the methanol.

The following are indications for ethanol therapy.[14]

1. Methanol level > 20 mg%
2. Presence of symptoms, pending levels
3. Ingestions of over 0.4 mL/kg, pending levels
4. Acidosis
5. Any patients being considered for hemodialysis

Because folate is a cofactor in the conversion of formic acid to carbon dioxide, the administration of folate may assist in the detoxification of methanol metabolites. Folic acid, 30 mg, may be given IV every 4 hours for several days.[2] Leucovorin folinic acid, the active form of folate, may be given instead of folate.

A compound that can inhibit the activity of the enzyme alcohol dehydrogenase in both animals and humans is 4-methyl pyrazole.[15,16] In animal studies, it has been shown to reduce the toxic effects of both ethylene glycol and methanol.[8] Usually the administration of 20 mg per kg 4-MP inhibit the formation of formic acid for 24 hours.[17]

Hemodialysis, but not hemoperfusion, is effective in removing methanol and its toxic metabolites. Indications for hemodialysis include:[19]

1. Methanol level > 20 to 50 mg%
2. Metabolic acidosis unresponsive to bicarbonate
3. Formate levels > 20 mg%
4. Visual impairment
5. Renal failure

Because rebound rises in methanol after dialysis have been reported, patients with methanol poisoning should be dialyzed until the methanol levels approach 0 mg% and the metabolic acidosis clears.

ETHYLENE GLYCOL

Ethylene glycol (1,2 ethanediol, $(CH_2)_2(OH)_2$) is structurally similar to ethanol but possesses two hydroxyl groups. It is a nonvolatile, water-soluble liquid discovered originally as a substitute for glycerine. It is used commercially in paints, lacquers, pharmaceuticals, polishes, cosmetics, and as a deicer and antifreeze. Its viscosity and sweet taste may have made it popular as a poor man's substitute for alcohol.

CHARACTERISTICS

Ethylene glycol is a colorless, odorless liquid with a boiling point of 197°C. It is completely miscible in water and has a low freezing point. Its volume of distribution is 0.8 L per kg, and it has a molecular weight of 62 daltons. The minimum lethal dose is approximately 1 to 1.5 mL per kg or 100 mL in a normal-sized adult. Survival after ingestions of 240 to 2000 mL has been described, however.[20,21] Ethylene glycol is estimated to cause 40 to 60 deaths each year in the U.S.[22] Like methanol, it is not the parent compound but rather its metabolites that are toxic to the body.

PHARMACOKINETICS

Ethylene glycol is rapidly absorbed from the GI tract with peak levels occurring within 1 to 4 hours post ingestion. Inhalation is not usually associated with toxicity, although cases of chronic poisoning have been reported in factory workers exposed to vapors of ethylene glycol.[23]

The kidneys filter and then passively reabsorb most of the ethylene glycol that is absorbed. Approximately 20% of a dose of 1 mg per kg is excreted unchanged.[19] Metabolism occurs principally in the liver, where ethylene glycol is oxidized to glycoaldehyde by alcohol dehydrogenase (Fig. 84-4). Glycoaldehyde is oxidized to glycolate and then to glyoxylate. Glyoxylate, in turn, can be metabolized in several ways: a reversible transamination to glycine, an irreversible oxidation to oxalate, and conjugation to oxalomalate, alpha-hydroxy-alpha beta ketodipate and gamma-hydroxy alpha ketoglutarate. Ethylene glycol metabolism increases the NADH/NAD ratio and produces lactic acid. Various cofactors are required for the metabolic reactions described: NAD, pyridoxal phosphate, thiamine pyrophosphate, and various amino acids. The plasma half-life of ethylene glycol is approximately 3 hours.

PATHOPHYSIOLOGY

Like ethanol, ethylene glycol is a CNS depressant, and as with methanol, its metabolites, not the parent compound itself, are toxic. Of the metabolites, glyoxylate is more toxic than glycoaldehyde.[24] Glycolate and glyoxylate interfere with the Krebs cycle and mitochondrial metabolism. Aldehyde production inhibits oxidative phosphorylation, respiration, and glucose metabolism. Aldehydes also interfere with protein synthesis, DNA replication, and ribosomal RNA synthesis.[25,26] They react with enzymes requiring sulfydryl groups for activity, collagen, and amino groups on proteins. The prominent CNS symptoms that occur after the ingestion of ethylene glycol coincide with the greatest amounts of aldehyde production.[22] Glycoaldehyde, glycolic acid, and glyoxylic acid all contribute to CNS depression.

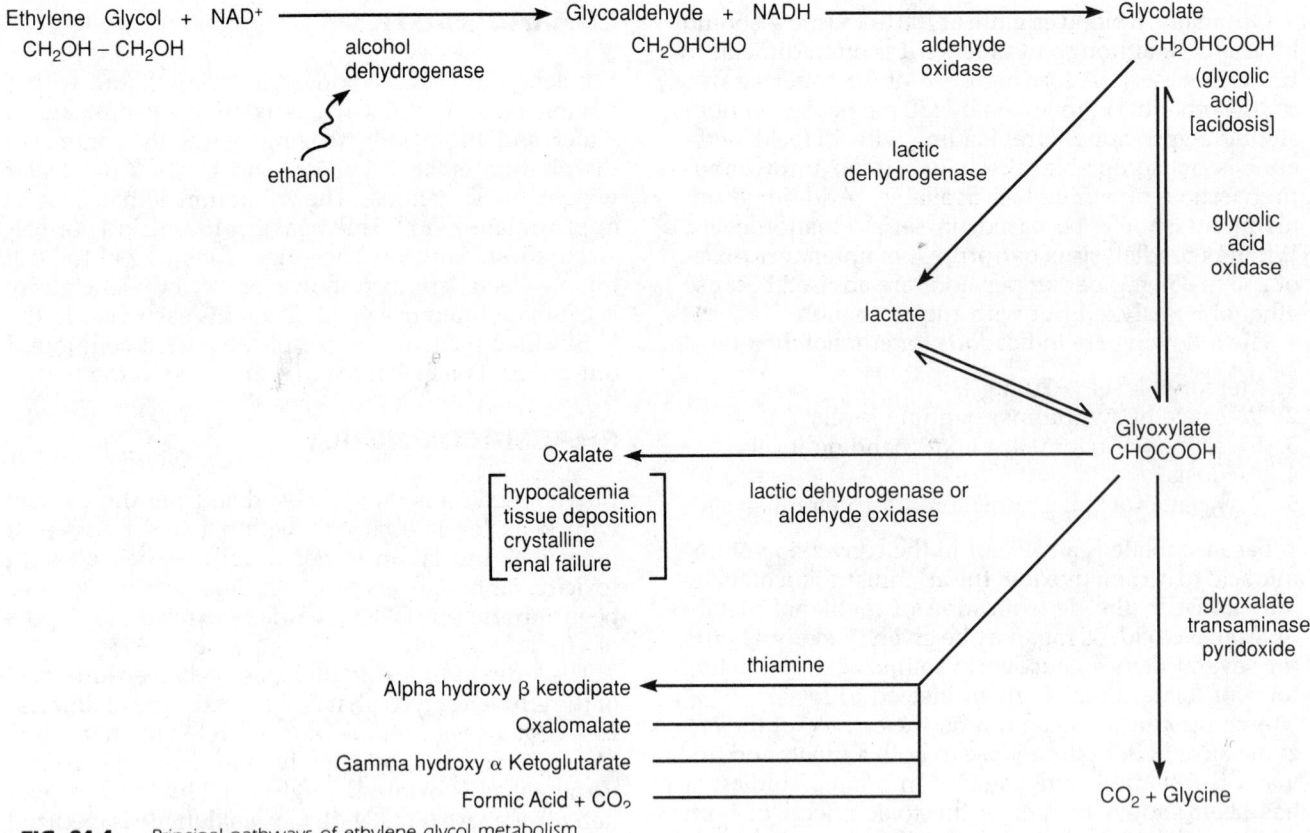

FIG. 84-4. Principal pathways of ethylene glycol metabolism.

The metabolic acidosis that follows significant poisoning with ethylene glycol is caused by the accumulation of glycolic acid and (to a lesser extent) lactic acid.[27] Oxalate accumulation in ethylene glycol poisonings can lead to extensive renal damage and myocardial depression. Hypocalcemia may result from the complexing of calcium with oxalate.

CLINICAL EFFECTS

Ethylene glycol poisoning was first described by Pons and Custer as occurring in three stages.[28] In the first stage (1 to 12 hours after ingestion), CNS depression can occur. Patients may appear inebriated without the odor of alcohol or acetone and may develop hallucinations, stupor, coma, meningismus, and focal or generalized seizures.[29,30] Ocular findings include decreased visual acuity, papilledema, optic atrophy, opthalmoplegia, and nystagmus.

The second stage of poisoning (12 to 24 hours after ingestion) is characterized by cardiovascular changes including CHF, hypertension, tachycardia, and arrhythmias.

In the third stage (24 to 72 hours after ingestion), acute renal failure may be seen. Renal failure may present with oliguria and flank pain and is caused principally by proximal renal tubular damage. The deposition of oxalate crystals and the direct toxic effects of the metabolites of ethylene glycol contribute to CNS and renal damage.

LABORATORY TESTS

Because oxalate is a product of the metabolism of ethylene glycol, calcium oxalate crystals may be identified in the urine, although not invariably. Hypocalcemia may occur and may be manifested by tetany and prolongation of the QT interval on the ECG. CPK levels may be elevated, and frequently there is an anion gap metabolic acidosis.

With severe ingestions, there may be an anion gap. Because the molecular weight is greater than ethanol and methanol, however, a significant osmolal gap may not appear. Serum osmolality may be measured by vapor pressure method with ethylene glycol because it possesses such a high boiling point. A rise in the blood level of ethylene glycol by 6 mg% raises the serum osmolality 1 mOsm per kg of H_2O. The diagnosis of ethylene glycol poisoning should be suspected in an inebriated patient with or without an odor of alcohol who presents with calcium oxalate crystals in the urine. The diagnosis may be confirmed with a blood level for ethylene glycol (although levels will probably not be available for days or weeks because few laboratories are able to measure ethylene glycol). Levels of 50 mg% or more are associated with serious toxicity and suggest the need for dialysis. As with methanol, because metabolites are the toxic elements, blood levels of ethylene glycol, even if readily available, are not a precise way to assess toxicity. Glycolic acid and bicarbonate levels correlate better with the clinical picture.

TREATMENT

Basic treatment should proceed as for ethanol intoxication. Supportive care, including airway stabilization, GI evacuation, glucose, thiamine, naloxone, and charcoal, should be provided as needed.

Acidosis should be treated with an infusion of bicarbonate when the pH is less than 7.20.

As in methanol poisoning, ethanol is an alternate substrate for alcohol dehydrogenase. It has an affinity for the enzyme 100 times that of ethylene glycol and thus can prevent metabolism of the latter. A loading dose of 0.8 g per kg of a 5 to 10% ethanol solution IV should be followed by 130 mg per kg per hour in an effort to maintain the serum ethanol level at 100 to 150 mg%. As in methanol poisoning treated with hemodialysis, maintenance doses of 250 to 350 mg per kg per hour may be necessary once the patient is on hemodialysis.

Indications for ethanol therapy are:

1. Ethylene glycol level > 20 mg%
2. Presence of symptoms pending levels
3. Ingestions of over 0.5 mL per kg pending levels
4. Acidosis
5. Any patient being considered for hemodialysis

Pyridoxine and thiamine are cofactors for the metabolism of ethylene glycol and should be given as follows: pyridoxine, 50 mg IM Q4H for 2 days, and thiamine, 100 mg IM Q4H for 2 days. Magnesium is also a cofactor and should be provided, especially in alcoholic patients. As mentioned previously, 4-methyl pyrazole can inhibit the activity of alcohol dehydrogenase.[15,16] Recently it has been demonstrated to be successful in the treatment of a patient with a serious ethylene glycol ingestion.[31] Because its inhibition of alcohol dehydrogenase is far more predictable than that seen with ethanol, it may well have a place in the future treatment of ethylene glycol poisoning.

Lastly, hemodialysis at present remains the treatment of choice for ethylene glycol poisoning. Dialysis enhances the elimination of the metabolites of ethylene glycol as well as the parent compound itself.

Indications for hemodialysis include:

1. Ethylene glycol level > 20–50 mg%
2. Metabolic acidosis unresponsive to bicarbonate
3. Crystalluria
4. Renal failure
5. Deteriorating vital signs

The end point of dialysis should be an ethylene glycol level approaching 0 mg% and clearance of the

metabolic acidosis. When hemodialysis is being performed, maintenance doses of ethanol should be raised to 250 to 350 mg per kg per hour or 95% ethanol should be added to the dialysate.

ISOPROPYL ALCOHOL

Isopropyl alcohol (2-propanol, isopropanol, $CH_3CH_0HCH_3$) is an aliphatic alcohol used as a solvent and disinfectant. It is widely used in rubbing alcohol, skin lotion, hair tonic, after-shave lotion, and window cleaning fluid. Like ethanol, isopropyl alcohol is a CNS depressant, although it lacks many of the toxic and metabolic effects of ethanol. Isopropanol is the second most commonly ingested alcohol, after ethanol.[32]

CHARACTERISTICS

Isopropanol is a clear, volatile hydrocarbon with a bitter taste and aromatic odor. As a CNS depressant, it has twice the potency of ethanol. The toxic dose is estimated to be 1 mL per kg of a 70% isopropanol solution, although as little as 0.5 mL per kg can cause symptoms. The lethal dose in an adult is said to range from 2 to 4 mL per kg or roughly 200 mL or more.[19] Adults, however, have survived ingestions of many times this amount.

PHARMACOKINETICS

Isopropanol is rapidly and efficiently absorbed from the GI tract. Eighty percent of an ingested dose is absorbed within 30 minutes, and absorption is usually complete within 2 hours.[6] Although ingestion is the major route of poisoning, toxicity can occur secondary to inhalation during sponge bathing of febrile patients.[33] Dermal absorption after prolonged contact may contribute to the toxicity as well.

Isopropanol, like ethanol and methanol, distributes in body water and has a volume of distribution of 0.6 to 0.7 L per kg. The kidney excretes 20 to 50% of an absorbed dose in its unchanged form. Isopropyl alcohol is metabolized to acetone by alcohol dehydrogenase, and acetone is, in turn, eliminated by the lungs and kidneys. Acetone can, however, be further metabolized to acetate, formate, and carbon dioxide. In the metabolism of isopropanol to acetone, few related ketoacids are formed and thus, in contrast to methanol and ethanol ingestions, acidosis is rarely seen.

The kinetics of isopropanol metabolism are first-order (concentration-dependent).[34] The metabolic half-life is estimated to be 2.5 to 3.2 hours.[35] By contrast, the elimination of isopropanol's metabolite, acetone, is much more prolonged, and therefore clinical effects are longer-lasting than those seen in ethanol intoxication.

PATHOPHYSIOLOGY

Isopropanol is a powerful CNS depressant and can depress the cardiovascular system as well. Although acids are generated in the metabolism of isopropanol, in practice acidosis is rarely a significant clinical problem. The first step in its metabolism is catalyzed by alcohol dehydrogenase and requires NAD as a cofactor. As a consequence, the ratio NAD/NADH is shifted to the reduced form and, as seen with ethanol intoxication, gluconeogenesis can be blocked and hypoglycemia can occur.

CLINICAL EFFECTS

One typically sees intoxication within 30 to 60 minutes of ingestion. With isopropanol ingestions, the euphoria seen with ethanol is lacking. The sweet, pungent odor of acetone is often on the breath. The duration of CNS depression is more prolonged than with ethanol because of the biologic activity of isopropanol metabolites. Significant ingestions can result in coma, hypotension, and respiratory arrest.

Patients may develop nausea, vomiting, and dehydration. Hematemesis from a hemorrhagic gastritis has been described. Hemorrhagic tracheobronchitis may also occur. Hypotension, when it occurs, is secondary to peripheral vasodilation but can be exacerbated by fluid and blood loss. CNS effects include dizziness, headache, confusion, and coma. The depressive effects can last up to 24 hours. Pupillary myiosis and nystagmus may be present.[19] Acute tubular necrosis, hepatocellular damage, myoglobinuria, and hemolytic anemia have been described.[36]

LABORATORY TESTS

In the absence of dehydration, routine blood studies are within normal limits. Unless there is a concomitant ingestion of ethanol, the alcohol level is not elevated. Rarely, GI bleeding or hemolytic anemia results in a low hematocrit. Acetone levels are elevated and should be quantitated with dilutions to assess the amount of acetone present in the blood. Hypoglycemia can occur and should be ruled out initially with a fingerstick assessment.

Being an alcohol, isopropanol can contribute to the osmolal gap. With a molecular weight of 6 daltons, a rise in the isopropanol blood level of 6 mg% raises the serum osmolality by 1 mOsm per kg of H_2O and contributes to the generation of an osmolal gap (see Table 84-11).

A toxic level of 50 mg% produces an elevation in serum osmolality of 8 to 9 mOsm per kg of H_2O and a lethal level of 200 mg% produces a change of 34 mOsm per kg of H_2O. Acetone itself can elevate serum osmolality, and this must be considered when attempting to correlate serum osmolality with isopropanol levels. Thus, a serious isopropanol ingestion should be diagnosable by assessing the osmolal gap. As with all alcohols, the serum osmolality must be measured by freezing point depression and not by vapor pressure methodology.

The hallmark of an isopropanol ingestion is the presence of inebriation, a negative or low alcohol level, an elevated osmolar gap, and a ketosis without acidosis. A given isopropanol level (which must be determined by gas chromatography) is roughly twice as toxic as a similar ethanol level. Blood levels of 50 mg% are associated with intoxication in nontolerant patients, whereas blood levels of 150 mg% should produce coma. Levels of 200 to 400 mg% and more are considered lethal. This may, however, be tempered by the provision of treatment. Survival with dialysis has been reported with isopropanol levels as high as 560 mg%.[37]

TREATMENT

The basis of treatment of an overdose of isopropanol is good supportive care. Like ethanol and methanol, isopropanol is well absorbed from the GI tract and gut evacuation has little to offer more than 2 hours after ingestion unless gastric emptying is delayed or a coingestion has occurred. Children who ingest more than 0.5 mL per kg of a 70% solution should undergo GI evacuation. Because CNS depression comes within 30 minutes of ingestion, ipecac should not be used for evacuation. As with the other alcohols, isopropanol is not well adsorbed by charcoal, although charcoal should be given for suspected polydrug ingestion.

Severe isopropanol overdoses have been successfully treated with peritoneal dialysis and hemodialysis.[38,39] Indications for dialysis include:

1. Ingestions of more than 3 to 4 mL per kg of a 70% solution
2. Blood levels over 400 mg%
3. Hypotension unresponsive to fluids and pressors
4. Prolonged coma
5. Complicating underlying diseases
6. Renal failure.[19]

REFERENCES

1. Swartz, R.D., Millman, R.P., Billi, J.E., et al.: Epidemic methanol poisoning: Clinical and biochemical analysis of a recent episode. Medicine 60:373, 1981.
2. Becker, C.E.: Methanol Poisoning. J. Emerg. Med. 51–58, 1933.
3. Eriksen, S.P., and Kulkarni, A.B.: Methanol in normal human breath. Science 141:639, 1963.
4. Axelrod, J., and Daly, J.: Pituitary gland: Enzymatic formation of methanol from 5-methyl adenosine. Science 150:892, 1965.
5. Leaf, G., and Zatman, L.J.: A study of the conditions under which methanol may exert a toxic hazard in industry. Br. J. Ind. Med. 9:19, 1952.

6. Clay, K.L., Murphy, R.C., and Watkins, D.W.: Experimental methanol toxicity in the primate: Analysis of metabolic acidosis. Toxicol. Appl. Pharmacol. *34*:49, 1975.

7. McMartin, K.E., Makao, A.B., Martin-Amat, G., et al.: Methanol poisoning I: The role of formic acid in the development of metabolic acidosis in the monkey and the reversal by 4-methylpryrazole. Biochem. Med. *13*:319, 1975.

8. Jacobsen, D., Webb, R., Collins, T.D., et al.: Methanol and formate kinetics in late diagnosed methanol intoxication. Med. Toxicol. *3*:418, 1988.

9. Jacobson, D., and McMartin, K.E.: Methanol and ethylene glycol poisonings: Mechanisms of toxicity, clinical course, diagnosis, and treatment. Med. Toxicol. *1*:309, 1986.

10. National Institutes of Health: Use of folate analogue in treatment of methyl alcohol toxic reactions is studied. JAMA *242*:1961, 1979.

11. Winchester, J.F.: Methanol, isopropyl alcohol, higher alcohols. *In* Clinical Management of Poisoning and Drug Overdose. Edited by Hadded, L.M., and Winchester, J.F. Philadelphia, W.B. Saunders, 1983, pp. 393–407.

12. Bennet, I.L., Cary, F.H., Mitchell, G.L., et al.: Acute methyl alcohol poisoning: A review based on experiences in an outbreak of 323 cases. Medicine *32*:431, 1953.

13. Osterloh, J.D., Rond, S.M., Grady, S., et al.: Serum formate concentrations in methanol intoxication as a criterion for hemodialysis. Ann. Intern. Med. *104*:200, 1986.

14. Ekins, B.R., Rollins, D.E., Duffy, D.P., et al.: Standardized treatment of severe methanol poisoning with ethanol and hemodialysis. West. J. Med. *142*:337, 1985.

15. Li, T.K., and Theorell, H.: Human liver alcohol dehydrogenase: Inhibition by pyrazole and pyrazole analogs. Acta Chem. Scand. *23*:892, 1969.

16. Pietrusko, R.: Human liver alcohol dehydrogenase—Inhibition of methanol activity by pyrazole, 4-methylpyrazole. Biochem. Pharmacol. *24*:1603, 1975.

17. McMartin, K.E., Hedstrom, K.G., Tolly, B.R., et al.: Studies on the metabolic interactions between 4-methylpyrazole and methanol using the monkey as an animal model. Arch. Biochem. Biophys. *199*:606, 1980.

18. McCoy, H.G., Cipolle, R.J., Ehlers, S.M., et al.: Severe methanol poisoning: application of pharmacokinetic model for ethanol therapy and hemodialysis. Am. J. Med. *67*:804, 1979.

19. Ellenhorn, M.J., and Barceloux, D.G.: Alcohols and glycols. *In* Medical Toxicology. Edited by Ellenhorn, M.J., and Barceloux, D.G. New York, Elsevier, 1988, pp. 782–812.

20. Scully, R., Galdabini, J., McNealy, B.: Case records of the Mass.

21. Gen. Hosp. Case *38*:1979. New Engl. J. Med. *301*:650, 1979.

21. Stokes, J.B., and Averon, F.: Prevention of organ damage in massive ethylene glycol ingestion. JAMA *243*:2065, 1980.

22. Parry, M.F., and Wallach, R.: Ethylene glycol poisoning. Am. J. Med. *57*:143, 1974.

23. Troisifn, F.M.: Chronic intoxication with ethylene glycol vapor. Br. J. Ind. Med. *1*:65, 1950.

24. Beasley, V.R., and Buch, W.B.: Acute ethylene glycol toxicoses: A review. Vet. Hum. Toxicol. *22*:255, 1980.

25. Kun, E.: A study on the metabolism of glyoxal in vitro. J. Biol. Chem. *194*:603, 1952.

26. Klamerth, O.L.: Influence of glycoxal on cell function. Biom. Chin. Biophys. Acta *155*:271, 1968.

27. Clay, K.L., and Murphy, R.C.: On the metabolic acidosis of ethylene glycol intoxication. Toxicol. Appl. Pharmacol *39*:39, 1977.

28. Pons, C.A., and Custer, R.P.: Acute ethylene glycol poisoning. Am. J. Med. Sci. *211*:544, 1946.

29. Brown, C.G., Trumbull, D., Klein-Schwartz, W., et al.: Ethylene glycol poisoning. Ann. Emerg. Med. *12*:501, 1983.

30. DaRoza, R., Henning, R.J., Sunshine, I., et al.: Acute ethylene glycol poisoning. Crit. Care Med. *12*:1003, 1984.

31. Galliot, M., Astier, A., Bien, D.V., et al.: Treatment of ethylene glycol poisoning with intravenous 4-methylpyrazole. N. Engl. J. Med. *319*:97, 1988.

32. Litovitz, T.L., Normann, S.A., and Veltri, J.C.: 1985 annual report of the American Association of Poison Control Centers National Data Collection System. Am. J. Emerg. Med. *4*:427, 1986.

33. Gosselin, R.E., Hodge, H.C., Smith, R.P., et al.: Isopropyl alcohol. *In* Clinical Toxicology of Commercial Products, 4th ed. Baltimore, Williams and Wilkins, 1976, p. 185.

34. Lacouture, P.G.: Isopropyl alcohol. Clin. Toxicol. Rev. *3*:3, 1980.

35. Daniel, D.R., McAnally, B.H., and Garriott, J.C.: Isopropyl alcohol metabolism after acute intoxication in humans. J. Anal. Toxicol. *5*:110, 1981.

36. Chguin, M.A.: Isopropyl alcohol poisoning with acute renal insufficiency. J. Maine Med. Assoc. *40*:288, 1949.

37. Alexander, C.B., McBay, A.S., and Hudson, R.P.: Isopropanol and isopropanol deaths—ten years experience. J. Forensic Sci. *27*:541, 1982.

38. Depner, T.A., and Mecikalski, M.B.: Peritoneal dialysis for isopropanol poisoning. West. J. Med. *137*:322, 1981.

39. Freireich, A.W., Unique, T.J., Xanthaky, G., et al.: Hemodialysis for isopropanol poisoning. N. Engl. J. Med. *277*:699, 1967.

ALCOHOL WITHDRAWAL MANAGEMENT ISSUES: DIFFERENTIAL DIAGNOSIS AND EMERGENCY TREATMENT

David B. McMicken

CAPSULE

Previous sections of this chapter have gone deeply into the toxicity of alcohol, alcohol substitutes, and conditions worsened or caused by excessive alcohol, including alcohol withdrawal.

Management problems in the ED usually involve assessment of the seriousness of the alcohol-related state, initiation of suitable treatment for intoxication or withdrawal, and a decision as to hospitalization. Although the alcoholic patient usually does not invoke sympathy, proper emergency attention and consideration of psychosocial factors may have an enormous impact on outcome. Guidelines for treatment and therapy are provided.

INTRODUCTION

The emergency physician sees the tragic effects of alcohol abuse daily. Motor vehicle accidents, drownings, suicides, homicides, divorce, violent crime, child abuse, unemployment, and disruption of the family are often either directly or indirectly associated with excessive alcohol consumption. One study determined that 40% of all patients entering the ED in the evening had been drinking, and 32% had blood alcohol levels greater than 80 mg/dL (0.08%).[1]

PATHOPHYSIOLOGY

The neuropharmacology of alcohol withdrawal is complex and not fully understood. Chronic alcohol consumption has a depressant effect on the central nervous system (CNS). The hallmark of alcohol withdrawal is the sudden exhibition of CNS excitation with increased cerebrospinal fluid (CSF), plasma, and urinary catecholamine levels.[2,3]

Two phenomena have been described in alcoholics with importance in the emergency situation. "Kindling" suggests that, as alcoholics have more and more withdrawal episodes, they become sensitized, and future withdrawals become progressively more severe. "Reinstatement" is a phenomenon whereby alcoholics progressively enter cycles of loss of control and withdrawal after shorter and shorter intervals of drinking.[3-5]

DIFFERENTIAL DIAGNOSIS IN THE EMERGENCY UNIT

The alcohol withdrawal syndrome can be confused with:

1. Acute schizophrenia
2. Encephalitis
3. Drug-induced psychosis
4. Thyrotoxicosis
5. Anticholinergic poisoning
6. Withdrawal from other sedative-hypnotic type drugs.

It may even be difficult to differentiate immediately between alcohol withdrawal and alcohol-induced hypoglycemia.

Acute schizophrenia usually has its onset in adolescence or early adulthood. Manifestations include multiple bizarre delusions and a flat affect with the patient otherwise oriented. The patient in alcohol withdrawal is usually older (20s or 30s), hyperactive, and possibly disoriented.

Encephalitis can produce headache, confusion, fever, and seizures. Thyrotoxicosis is more common in women, and its features include irritability, insomnia, tremor, weight loss despite a good appetite, palpitations, and frequent stools. Physical examination may reveal lid lag, tachycardia, and a bruit over the thyroid. There is no relationship between the onset of encephalitis or thyrotoxicosis and alcohol consumption.

Anticholinergic poisoning can occur with many different drugs or plant ingestion. The classic clinical picture is a patient with dry mouth, dry eyes, dry skin, hypoactive bowel sounds, urinary retention, and delirium. Amphetamine and cocaine intoxication produce anorexia and insomnia, with physical signs of CNS sympathetic overactivity.

In opioid withdrawal, the mental status is usually normal, the patient is afebrile, and seizures are uncommon except with meperidine. In contrast, patients with alcohol withdrawal are usually disoriented and febrile, and may have seizures.[6]

Signs of alcohol withdrawal usually begin 6 to 24 hours after the decrease in the patient's usual intake of alcohol. If a patient manifests withdrawal 3 or more days after his or her last drink, one should consider drugs with a longer half-life. The barbiturate and benzodiazepine withdrawal syndromes usually progress more slowly and have a higher frequency of seizures, which appear later (7 days instead of 2 days), and status epilepticus is more common.[6,7]

Glucose (25 g of dextrose IV) produces a dramatic response in hypoglycemic patients. Unlike hypoglycemia from other causes, alcohol-induced hypoglycemia is unresponsive to glucagon because of depleted liver glycogen stores.[8] Thiamine (50 mg IV followed by 50 mg IM) should be given to prevent the precipitation of Wernicke's encephalopathy by the dextrose solution depleting the last of the patient's thiamine stores. Although Wernicke's encephalopathy is a medical emergency, alcohol-induced hypoglycemia is much more common and has serious and permanent morbidity if left untreated. Thiamine should be given in a timely fashion, but glucose therapy should never be delayed.[9]

CLINICAL PRESENTATION

Isbell's classic study in 1955 confirmed the relationship between alcohol and the withdrawal syndrome.[10] He documented the fact that the severity of signs and symptoms depend on both the dose and duration of ethanol consumption. The withdrawal syndrome may occur any time after the blood alcohol level starts to fall. Therefore only a reduction, not the abrupt cessation of ethanol intake, may precipitate withdrawal.[10,11]

The withdrawal syndrome develops 6 to 48 hours after the reduction of ethanol intake and lasts from 2 to 7 days. The alcohol withdrawal state constitutes a wide spectrum, ranging from mild withdrawal with insomnia and irritability to major withdrawal with diaphoresis, fever, disorientation, and hallucinations. The syndrome also includes anxiety, insomnia, irritability, tremor, anorexia, tachycardia, hyperreflexia, hypertension, fever, decreased seizure threshold, auditory and visual hallucinations, and finally delirium.[12]

Minor alcohol withdrawal occurs less than 24 hours after the cessation or significant decrease in alcohol intake. It is characterized by mild autonomic hyperactivity: nausea, anorexia, tremor, tachycardia, hypertension, hyperreflexia, insomnia, and anxiety.

Major alcohol withdrawal occurs more than 24 hours, and occasionally up to 5 days, after the decline or termination of drinking. Major withdrawal is characterized by more pronounced hyperactivity in addition to disorientation, hallucinations, diaphoresis, and fever.

Delirium tremens, seldom appearing before the third post-abstinence day, is the extreme end of the spectrum and consists of gross tremor, profound confusion, fever, incontinence, frightening visual hallucinations, and mydriasis. Only 5% of patients hospitalized for alcohol withdrawal go on to develop delirium tremens.[13-15]

True delirium tremens is rare.[16] Alcohol withdrawal and delirium tremens are not synonymous. The mortality rate for delirium tremens is frequently quoted at 15 to 20% based on a 1953 study by Victor. Today, patients managed aggressively in the intensive care unit have mortality rates much lower than 15%.[15,17,18] The relationship between the withdrawal states is unclear. Seizures can occur in both minor and major withdrawal.

Alcoholic hallucinosis, still a controversial and poorly understood entity, is a unique disorder of the chronic alcoholic consisting of auditory hallucinations in an otherwise clear sensorium. These auditory hallucinations are often threatening and are most prominent at night. It is sometimes difficult to distinguish between this disorder and schizophrenia, and indeed a few of these patients eventually prove to be schizophrenic. Most authorities, however, now disagree with Bleuler, who originally thought that alcoholic hallucinosis could be a syndrome of schizophrenia induced by alcohol.[19,20] In schizophrenia, the age of onset of the hallucinosis is earlier, there is no temporal relation of psychotic symptoms to the cessation of alcohol use, and the course is chronic.[21]

Alcoholic hallucinosis should also be differentiated from the auditory hallucinations of acute alcohol withdrawal. The latter are usually visual, whereas the former are usually auditory. Patients with auditory hallucinations from alcohol withdrawal do not have a clear sensorium and usually have other signs of withdrawal such as fever, tachycardia, tremor, delusions, or confusion. Although most patients present after abstinence, alcoholic hallucinosis can occur without change in a patient's drinking habits.[22]

PREHOSPITAL CARE AND ASSESSMENT

The alcohol-dependent patient may have withdrawal, a mixed alcohol-drug ingestion, occult head trauma, or cervical spine injury. Patients who are unable to sit without assistance or have an altered mental status require an intravenous line. Naloxone (0.8 mg) and glucose (dextrose 25 g) with thiamine (50 mg) are given by IV push. The airway must be maintained and respirations supported. The emergency medical technician should monitor the patient's vital signs and neurologic status. The cervical spine should be immobilized if trauma is suspected.

It is usually best to withhold treatment with benzodiazepines until the patient can be evaluated in the ED. The emergency medical technician should be alert for other medical disorders that accompany alcoholism, such as pneumonia, sepsis, gastrointestinal bleeding, hepatic failure, heart failure, and intracranial hemorrhage.

EMERGENCY DEPARTMENT CARE AND PHYSICAL EXAMINATION

Family, friends, bystanders, or paramedics may give more reliable historical data than the patient. Accurate vital signs are essential, including rectal or core temperature. Hyperthermia, hypothermia, tachypnea, or tachycardia may indicate serious disorders that frequently accompany the alcohol-dependent patient (Table 84-14). Rapid, thorough examination should be performed with attention to the level of consciousness, signs of hepatic failure, renal failure, or coagulopathy. It is important to be alert for signs of trauma such as subcutaneous emphysema, ecchymosis, subconjunctival hemorrhage, Battle's sign, or fractures. The neurologic examination should search for focal findings: central facial palsy, hemiparesis, asymmetry of reflexes, upgoing toes, or asymmetry of pupillary response. When errors occur in the management of the inebriated patient, it is usually because trauma is not recognized.

TABLE 84-14. DISORDERS ASSOCIATED WITH ABNORMAL VITAL SIGNS IN THE ALCOHOL-DEPENDENT PATIENT

Hyperthermia
  Sepsis
  Drug ingestion (phenothiazine, aspirin)
  Anticholinergic poisoning
  Heat stroke
  Intracranial hemorrhage
  Alcohol withdrawal
Hypothermia
  Sepsis
  Drug ingestion (phenothiazine, sedative-hypnotic)
  Hypoglycemia
  Diabetes
  Exposure
  Wernicke's encephalopathy
Tachypnea
  Sepsis
  Hypoxia
  Acidosis
  Cerebral insult
  Pulmonary insult
Tachycardia
  Sepsis
  Shock
  Anticholinergic, cocaine, amphetamine poisoning
  Alcohol withdrawal
  Drug withdrawal

MANAGEMENT

The alcohol withdrawal syndrome must be promptly recognized and treated. Treatment is necessary to provide relief from anxiety and hallucinations, halt progression to major withdrawal, allow detection of a treatable primary psychiatric illness, prepare the patient for long-term alcohol abstinence with minimal risk of new drug dependence, and prevent withdrawal seizures (see first section of this chapter.). Treatment is also necessary to calm the patient and allow adequate examination to detect medical illnesses frequently accompanied or precipitated by alcoholism, such as pancreatitis, pneumonia, and hepatitis. Restraints may be necessary. Theoretic liability for detention by reasonable restraint is inconsequential compared to the potential injury the patient may inflict on himself or herself or the hospital staff.

NONPHARMACOLOGIC INTERVENTION

A growing body of data indicates that supportive care (reassurance, reality orientation, personal attention, and general nursing care) can be effective in patients with mild alcohol withdrawal. This requires frequent monitoring of signs and symptoms. Supportive care does not appear to prevent hallucinations, seizures, or arrhythmias. Therefore, patients in moderate to severe withdrawal should receive pharmacologic intervention in addition to supportive care.[23–25]

PHARMACOLOGIC INTERVENTION

Over the years, more than 150 different drug and drug combinations have been reported in the literature for the treatment of alcohol withdrawal. Treatment regimens have used alcohol, alpha-adrenergic agonists, antihistamines, barbiturates, benzodiazepines, beta-blockers, butyrophenones, calcium channel blocking agents, carbamazepine, chloral hydrate, clomethiazole, dopamine agonists, lithium carbonate, magnesium sulfate, meprobamate, phenothiazines, paraldehyde, and valproic acid.

BENZODIAZEPINES

Although no benzodiazepine has shown clear superiority, lorazepam (Ativan) is becoming more widely used. It is important that the emergency physician become familiar with a particular regimen and be aware of side effects, dosage ranges, and risks. As with antibiotics of similar spectrum, the physician must develop his or her own plan of use. The following discussion provides some basis for these decisions.

Benzodiazepines are currently the mainstay of treatment. They have equal efficacy or superiority to other agents. The benzodiazepines have superior anticonvulsant activity and minimal respiratory and cardiac depression in comparison with other CNS depressants, and can be given parenterally in the uncooperative patient.[24,26] Numerous benzodiazepines, including alprazolam (Xanax), chlordiazepoxide (Librium), chlorazepate (Tranxene), diazepam (Valium), flurazepam (Dalmane), halazepam (Paxipam), lorazepam (Ativan), midazolam (Versed), and oxazepam (Serax) have been studied. There is no evidence of clear superiority of any one benzodiazepine.[15,24,27–30]

The ideal benzodiazepine would have rapid and complete absorption from an intramuscular injection site; an intermediate elimination half-life; an elimination process unaffected by liver disease, renal insufficiency, or aging; and no active metabolite. Although no one benzodiazepine has all these characteristics, lorazepam (Ativan) comes the closest.

Lorazepam has good bioavailability with oral, intramuscular, and intravenous routes. It is rapidly and completely absorbed from intramuscular sites in agitated patients with no intravenous access. Lorazepam's half-life is intermediate (14 ± 5 hours) and reaches a steady state in 36 to 48 hours without extensive accumulation.[31] It is metabolized (conjugated) in the liver, yielding inactive products.[32] Although lorazepam's half-life increases in patients who have cirrhosis and liver failure, it is much less than the increase with chlordiazepoxide. Its elimination is altered only minimally in renal failure and in the elderly. In contrast, chlordiazepoxide has the following disadvantages. Its half-life is significantly prolonged in liver failure and renal failure. Parenteral chlordiazepoxide has to be refrigerated and reconstituted, and is poorly absorbed from intramuscular injections.[26,27,33–35]

Lorazepam may be given intravenously in a dose of 0.5 mg to 4.0 mg, depending on the severity of the withdrawal. Dosing can be repeated at 15- to 30-minute intervals for patients in severe withdrawal. An intramuscular dose of 0.07 mg/kg can be used.[36] The oral dosage schedule for moderate withdrawal is 6 to 7 mg per day in three divided doses, tapering the amount 20 to 28% per day over 4 days.[37,38] If lorazepam is not available, diazepam (Valium) can be given (5 mg IV every 5 minutes) until the patient is calm.[39]

For the critically ill patient in the ICU, the short-acting midazolam can be considered. The onset of action is rapid (minutes). Infusions of 20 to 75 mg per hour of midazolam have been reported.[27,28]

The dosage of benzodiazepines required for alcohol withdrawal is highly variable. The dose should always be titrated to the patient's agitation. Massive doses have been required in patients with delirium tremens: 2335 mg of diazepam in 48 hours, 2640 mg of diazepam and 35 mg haloperidol over 48 hours, 75 mg of midazolam in one hour, and 2850 mg of midazolam over 5 days.[27,28,40,41] Such large dosages are hazardous and require Intensive Care Unit admission for close monitoring.

BUTYROPHENONES

Haloperidol, a dopamine blocker, should be considered in patients with major withdrawal or delirium tremens not responding to intravenous benzodiazepines. Haloperidol is more potent than chlorpromazine, has lower anticholinergic properties, and has less propensity to cause cardiovascular side effects or lower the seizure threshold. Haloperidol has little effect on myocardial function or respiratory drive.[15,42]

The safety and efficacy of haloperidol by the IV, IM, or oral route in the ED have been reported.[42] Haloperidol and lorazepam in combination are safe and may be synergistic. Safe use in extremely high doses in patients with serious underlying medical illness has been documented in several studies: 240 mg of haloperidol and 480 mg of lorazepam given over 24 hours in a patient[43] and 485 mg of haloperidol over 8 hours in another patient without significant adverse effects.[15,44] Adams et al. have advocated an aggressive protocol with escalating doses of the combination of haloperidol and lorazepam[43] (Table 84-15). Such high dosages must be accompanied by extremely careful monitoring because of respiratory impairment, seizures with aspiration, and cardiac changes. Pulse ox-

TABLE 84-15. ESCALATING DOSAGE PROTOCOL FOR COMBINA-TION HALOPERIDOL/LORAZEPAM TREATMENT OF PSYCHOTIC PATIENTS WITH SERIOUS UNDERLYING MEDICAL ILLNESS*†

Time	Haloperidol (mg) IV	Lorazepam (mg) IV
0 min	3	0.5–1
20 min	5	0.5–2
40 min	10	0.5–10
Every hour	10	0.5–10

* Adapted with permission from Adams, F., Fernandez, F., and Anderson, B.S.: Emergency pharmacotherapy of delirium in the critically ill cancer patient. Psychosomatics 27:33, 1986.
† Haloperidol dose based on degree of agitation; lorazepam dose based on desired level of sedation. Stop at any point that achieves adequate control and set dose and interval as determined by patient requirements (e.g., return of agitation). At 12 to 18 hours, stop lorazepam, increase haloperidol dosage interval, and allow sedation to lighten. Resedate if agitation returns.

imetry is advised when large doses are used. (See first section of this chapter.)

BETA BLOCKERS

Propranolol and atenolol have been studied in alcohol withdrawal.

Beta-blockers should be considered as an *adjunct* by the emergency physician in mild to moderate alcohol withdrawal. Contraindications include insulin-dependent diabetes, hypotension, lung disease that may lead to bronchospasm, and congestive heart failure.

ALPHA AGONISTS

The alpha-adrenergic agonist clonidine has proved effective in opiate withdrawal.[17] Clonidine is not a controlled substance and has little or no addictive or abuse potential. It can be useful in mild or outpatient cases.

Whether clonidine prevents seizures, hallucinations, or delirium in severe cases has not been determined, and use in the ED is not advised except in the mildest cases. It may be a promising treatment agent in mild alcohol withdrawal patients who are candidates for an outpatient program.

CARBAMAZEPINE

Several studies from Scandinavia have used carbamazepine as the primary drug therapy for alcohol withdrawal. These studies were generally not well controlled.[45,46]

Theoretic advantages of carbamazepine include its anticonvulsant effects, low abuse potential, lack of interaction with disulfiram, antidepressant or mood-enhancing properties, and metabolism not affected by advanced liver disease. Carbamazepine is not available for IV administration and is not without significant side effects. Carbamazepine has no advantages over benzodiazepines.

CALCIUM CHANNEL BLOCKING AGENTS

Recent studies have examined calcium channel activity in alcohol dependency and withdrawal seizures. Caroverine (group B calcium channel blocking agent not available in the United States) appeared to be equal to meprobamate in one preliminary study.[47] Further investigation of calcium channel blocking agents is required.

SUMMARY OF PHARMACOLOGIC INTERVENTION

Rapid, aggressive control of alcohol withdrawal is crucial. The cornerstone of treatment is a benzodiazepine. Lorazepam is preferable because of the previously discussed qualities. Midazolam is a reasonable alternative in the ICU.

TRIAL USE OF MEDICATIONS IN THE ED

In mild cases, an initial test dose of 1 to 2 mg of lorazepam or 50 to 100 mg of chlordiazepoxide can be given orally to the patient in the emergency department. The patient is observed for 3 to 4 hours, which guides the emergency physician as to doses required for subsequent treatment.[48] Outpatient treatment consists of chlordiazepoxide, 25 to 100 mg three times a day, or lorazepam, 1 to 2 mg three times a day in a tapering dose for 3 to 6 days, depending on the severity of symptoms. Patients should be observed until it is clear that their withdrawal will not progress and require hospitalization. Adequate diet, abstinence, and participation in a rehabilitation program in the community are also necessary. Any patient requiring 300 mg of chlordiazepoxide per day to control his withdrawal should be considered for admission. Approximate equivalent doses relative to chlordiazepoxide, 100 mg are diazepam, 20 mg; oxazepam, 120 mg; and lorazepam, 5 mg.[24]

Haloperidol should be considered in major withdrawal not responding adequately to benzodiazepines. In stable, admitted patients, beta-blockers should be considered as an adjunct to benzodiazepine therapy if there are no contraindications. Combination therapy makes pharmacologic sense in alcohol withdrawal; benefits include the reduction of the risks associated with prolonged and heavy sedation, faster symptom resolution, and quicker recovery.[26]

ADJUNCT THERAPY

Patients being treated for alcohol withdrawal should receive thiamine (50 mg IV) and glucose (dextrose, 25 g IV). Multivitamin preparations are usually added to the patient's IV fluid because of chronic malnutrition. Two preparations are available: MVI (5 mL), which contains vitamins A through E, and MVI-12, which adds folic acid, vitamin B_{12}, and biotin. Serum folate and cobalamin (vitamin B_{12}) levels should be drawn before MVI-12 is used if the patient has a significant anemia. Serum folate levels, however, are of limited usefulness in alcoholics because low levels are common in the absence of morphologic changes of folate deficiency and normal levels are not infrequent in the presence of megaloblastic change.[49]

Volume depletion can be corrected with normal saline. Reversal of electrolyte and metabolic disorders (hypomagnesemia, hypophosphatemia, hypokalemia, and acidosis) is discussed in another chapter. Although treatment of electrolyte disorders and acidosis benefits the patient, it does little to abate the withdrawal syndrome.

Paraldehyde, ethyl alcohol, and phenothiazines no longer have a place in the treatment of alcohol withdrawal.[13,39] Paraldehyde is limited to oral and rectal administration because intramuscular and intravenous use are associated with the development of sterile abscesses and pulmonary edema. Because oral paraldehyde is impractical in a patient with major withdrawal, a rectal oil-retention enema is used for treatment. Rectal administration may cause proctitis and does not allow titration of the drug to the patient's condition. Paraldehyde is frequently given in inadequate doses, which produce lengthy delays before the patient is calmed. Overdose can produce respiratory arrest. Treatment with ethyl alcohol continues to exacerbate the patient's preexisting metabolic disorders caused by alcoholism.[37,39] Phenothiazines are usually undesirable because they can, in the dosages required to calm patients in alcohol withdrawal, produce hypotension, lower seizure threshold, disturb central temperature regulation, and cause extrapyramidal effects.[37,39,50,51]

RADIOGRAPHS AND LABORATORY TESTING

Blood samples should be taken to determine electrolytes, BUN, CBC, creatinine, glucose, prothrombin time, calcium, phosphate, magnesium, and serum levels of any anticonvulsants the patient may be taking. Arterial blood gases should be considered if there is a suspicion of acidosis or pulmonary compromise. Chest x ray should be obtained in patients with temperature elevation, tachypnea, or abnormal findings on physical examination of the chest.

It is well known that alcohol withdrawal itself is capable of producing fever.[10] Over half of febrile patients in withdrawal, however, have an infectious cause (usually pneumonia) of their fever.[52] Fever in an alcoholic should be considered to result from an infectious cause until proven otherwise.

Although fever may indicate meningitis, it may also occur with intracranial hemorrhage, brain abscess, alcohol withdrawal, toxic ingestions, and infections outside the CNS. If meningitis is suspected but increased intracranial pressure is possible, the patient should have blood cultures and be empirically started on antibiotics. Not without hazard in a subarachnoid hemorrhage or brain abscess, the lumbar puncture may be delayed until an intracerebral lesion can be ruled out with computed tomography (CT) or magnetic resonance imaging (MRI) scanning.[53–55]

The only benefit of skull radiography would be the determination of occult head trauma not previously appreciated, such as a depressed fracture. There is little relationship between significant intracranial sequelae and the presence of a skull fracture.[56] Focal findings on neurologic examination or patients with signs of head trauma and seizures should be considered for CT scan (Table 84-16).

ADMISSION GUIDELINES AND DISPOSITION

Because of the alcoholic's inability to care for himself or herself, satisfactory outpatient treatment is difficult to obtain. Optimal outpatient therapy includes a concerned family member or friend to ensure that the patient takes medications properly, appears at follow-up appointments, abstains from alcohol, and maintains an adequate diet. Alcoholic patients who undergo outpatient treatment need close supervision;

TABLE 84-16. INDICATIONS FOR URGENT CT SCAN IN THE ALCOHOL-DEPENDENT PATIENT

1. Partial (focal) seizures
2. Signs of increased intracranial pressure or focal findings on neurologic examination
3. Evidence of acute head trauma and seizure
4. New onset seizures
5. Unimproved or deteriorating level of consciousness

therefore a follow-up appointment within 24 to 48 hours should be considered.

The problem of when to hospitalize the alcoholic and on what service is a constant dilemma for the emergency physician. Most of these patients have medical, psychiatric, and social problems. Hospitalization is frequently necessary to adequately diagnose and treat these multiple problems. Moreover, with the alcoholic who is no longer able to care for himself or herself, hospitalization is often dictated for this reason alone.

The following are suggested guidelines for admission for detoxification of alcohol-dependent patients. In choosing medical or psychiatric admission, medical illness always takes priority.

ACUTE INTOXICATION

Acute intoxication alone seldom requires admission. Combined alcohol-drug overdose or associated medical, psychiatric, or social problems may necessitate hospitalization. *Acute intoxication is a diagnosis of exclusion.* Hypoglycemia, hypoxia, carbon dioxide narcosis, carbon monoxide poisoning, mixed alcohol-drug overdose, ethylene glycol and methanol poisoning, hepatic encephalopathy, psychosis, severe vertigo, and psychomotor seizures can manifest in a manner similar to that of ethanol intoxication. Blood alcohol level and breath alcohol determination can help to support this diagnosis. Beware of the person who has a relatively low blood alcohol level (e.g., 100 mg%), but has substantial mental changes. These patients must be observed and further evaluated. Also, children may have lower blood alcohol levels but more pronounced physiologic effect.

ALCOHOL WITHDRAWAL

Patients with signs of major withdrawal (fever, hallucinations, confusion, extreme agitation) always require admission. Patients with mild alcohol withdrawal can be observed in the ED. After 6 hours of observation, the alert, oriented patient whose vital signs, physical examination, suggested laboratory analysis, and chest x ray are within normal limits may be released from the ED. Nevertheless, the patient requires treatment for the underlying alcoholism and should be advised or referred accordingly. Other guidelines for hospitalization are helpful (Table 84-17). Also see the first section of this chapter for treatment of alcohol withdrawal seizures.

SEIZURES

Patients with their first seizure are usually admitted. This allows initiation of drug therapy, diagnostic evaluation, and continuous monitoring of patient status. Patients with partial seizures or focal neurologic findings on physical examination require admission unless

---

TABLE 84-17. GUIDELINES FOR HOSPITALIZATION FOR DETOXIFICATION*

The presence of a medical or surgical condition requiring treatment (hepatic decompensation, infection, dehydration, malnutrition, cardiovascular collapse, cardiac arrhythmias, or trauma)
Hallucinations, tachycardia > 100 min, severe tremor, extreme agitation, or a history of severe alcohol withdrawal symptoms
Fever > 38.5° C
Wernicke's encephalopathy
Confusion or delirium
Recent history of head injury with loss of consciousness
Social isolation

* Adapted with permission from Jacob, M.S., and Sellers, E.M.: Emergency management of alcohol withdrawal. Drug Ther. *24*:28, 1977.

these findings have been previously documented. Patients with seizures associated with head trauma or with mixed alcohol-drug withdrawal seizures are admitted. Status epilepticus or recurrent seizures during observation in the ED indicate a lack of seizure control necessitating hospitalization. (See the first part of this chapter for treatment.) As of the latest information from double-blind studies (1991),[56a,56b] dilantin is of little, if any, use in preventing alcohol withdrawal seizures unless there is a pre-existent seizure disorder.

PSYCHIATRIC AND SOCIAL PROBLEMS

Alcoholic patients requiring admission with acute intoxication, withdrawal, seizures, or medical/surgical disorders are best managed on acute care floors and should not be initially admitted to a general psychiatric service. Many hospitals today have Chemical Dependency Units that combine the advantage of the acute care floor and a secure psychiatric unit. Some psychiatric and social conditions in the alcoholic can still be better handled on a general psychiatric unit: psychosis, exacerbation of schizophrenia, depression with suicidal tendencies, any patient who is a danger to himself or herself or others, or alcoholic hallucinosis with an otherwise clear sensorium. Any patient who is no longer able to care for himself or herself also requires admission. Although this patient's ultimate destination is a rehabilitation center or a board-and-care program, hospitalization is necessary to rule out medical or psyciatric illness and adequately treat impending withdrawal symptoms. Patients who wish to stop drinking are usually admitted to a hospital or detoxification unit to treat impending withdrawal.[57-60] Be aware of depression and suicide risk in all alcoholics.

REHABILITATION

Most communities have either an Alcoholics Anonymous chapter or a treatment center for anyone who desires help with alcohol. In small communities, clergy or social workers can usually arrange rehabilitation.

Whatever medical, psychologic, or social problem brings the alcoholic to the ED, the underlying problem is alcoholism. The ultimate goal is abstinence. Abstinence can be attained, even in the most difficult patient. This disease will surely progress if we do not first recognize alcoholism and then make sure that the patient has the opportunity to participate in a rehabilitation program.[57,61,62]

The emergency physician can play a pivotal role in identifying the alcoholic, treating concomitant conditions and withdrawal, and ensuring suitable follow-up care and aftercare arrangements.

REFERENCES

1. Holt, S., et al.: Alcohol and the emergency service patient. Br. Med. J. *281*:638, 1980.
2. Hawley, R.J., Major, L.F., Schulman, E.A., et al.: Cerebrospinal fluid 3-methoxy-4-hydroxyphenylglycol and norepinephrine levels in alcohol withdrawal. Arch. Gen. Psychiatry *42*:1056, 1985.
3. Linnoila, M., Mefford, I., Nutt, D., et al.: Alcohol withdrawal and noradrenergic function. Ann. Intern. Med. *107*:875, 1987.
4. Ballenger, J.C., and Post, R.M.: Kindling as a model for the alcohol withdrawal syndromes. Br. J. Psychiatry *133*:1, 1978.
5. Edwards, G.: The alcohol dependence syndrome: A concept as stimulus to enquiry. Br. J. Addict. *81*:171, 1986.
6. Goldfrank, L.R.: Alcohol withdrawal. Emerg. Med. *18*:24, 1986.
7. Sellers, E.M.: Alcohol, barbiturate and benzodiazepine withdrawal syndromes: Clinical management. Can. Med. Assoc. J. *139*:113, 1988.
8. Freinkle, N., et al.: Alcohol hypoglycemia. I. Carbohydrate metabolism in patients with clinical alcohol hypoglycemia and the experimental reproduction of the syndrome with pure ethanol. J. Clin. Invest. *42*:1112, 1963.
9. Marx, J.A.: The varied faces of Wernicke's encephalopathy. J. Emerg. Med. *3*:411, 1985.
10. Isbell, H., Franser, H.R., Wikles, A., et al.: An experimental study of the etiology of "rum fits" and delirium tremens. Q.J. Study Alcohol *16*:1, 1955.
11. Brown, C.C.: The alcohol withdrawal syndrome. Ann. Emerg. Med. *11*:276, 1982.
12. Victor, M., and Adams, R.D.: The effect of alcohol on the nervous system. Res. Publ. Assoc. Nerv. Ment. Dis. *32*:526, 1953.
13. Jacob, M.S., and Sellers, E.M.: Emergency management of alcohol withdrawal. Drug Ther. *24*:28, 1977.
14. Nordstrom, G., and Berglund, M.: Delirium tremens: A prospective long-term follow up study. J. Stud. Alcohol *49*:178, 1988.
15. Sellers, E.M., and Kalant, H.: Alcohol intoxication and withdrawal. N. Engl. J. Med. *294*:757, 1976.
16. Victor, M.: Treatment of alcoholic intoxication and the withdrawal syndrome: A critical analysis of the use of drugs and other forms of therapy. Psychosomatics *28*:636, 1966.
17. Adinoff, B., Bone, G.H., and Linnoila, M.: Acute ethanol poisoning and the ethanol withdrawal syndrome. Med. Tox. *3*:172, 1988.
18. Olbrich, R.: Alcohol withdrawal states and the need for treatment. Br. J. Psychiatry *134*:466, 1979.
19. Schuckit, M.A., and Winokur, G.: Alcoholic hallucinosis and schizophrenia: A negative study. Br. J. Psychiatry *119*:549, 1971.
20. Gross, M.M., Halpert, E., and Sabot, L.: Some comment on Bleuler's concept of acute alcoholic hallucinosis. Q.J. Stud. Alcohol *24*:54, 1963.
21. Diagnostic and Statistical Manual of Mental Disorders. American Psychiatric Association, Third Edition, Revised, 1987.
22. Surawicz, F.G.: Alcoholic hallucinosis: a missed diagnosis. Can. J. Psychiatry *25*:57, 1980.
23. Naranjo, C.A., Sellers, E.M., Chater, K., et al.: Nonpharmacologic intervention in acute alcohol withdrawal. Clin. Pharmacol. Ther. *34*:214, 1983.
24. Sellers, E.M., and Naranjo, C.A.: New strategies for the treatment of alcohol withdrawal. Psycho. Pharm. Bull. *22*:88, 1986.
25. Whitfield, C.L., Thompson, G., Lamb, A., et al.: Detoxification of 1,024 alcoholic patients without psychoactive drugs. JAMA *239*:409, 1978.
26. Rosenbloom, A.J.: Optimizing drug treatment of alcohol withdrawal. Am. J. Med. *81*:901, 1986.
27. Rosenbloom, A.J.: Emerging treatment options in the alcohol withdrawal syndrome. J. Clin. Psychiatry *49*:12, 1988.
28. Lineaweaver, W.C., Anderson, K., Hing, D.N.: Massive doses of midazolam infusion for delirium tremens without respiratory depression. Crit. Care Med. *16*:294, 1988.
29. Linnoila, M.: Benzodiazepines and alcoholism. *In* Benzodiazepines Divided. New York, Edited by Trimble, M.R. John Wiley & Sons Ltd., 1983, p. 291.
30. Mendels, J., Wasserman, T.W., Michaels, T.J., et al.: Halazepam in the management of acute alcohol withdrawal syndrome. J. Clin. Psychiatry *46*:172, 1985.
31. Hollister, L.E., Greenblatt, D.J., Rickels, K., et al.: Benzodiazepines 1980: Current update. Psychosomatics *21*:1, 1980.
32. Kyriakopoulous, A.A., Greenblatt, D.J., and Shade, R.I.: Clinical pharmacokinetics of lorazepam: a review. J. Clin. Psychiatry *39*:16, 1978.
33. Kraus, J.W., Desmond, D.V., Marshall, J.P., et al.: Effects of aging and liver disease on disposition of lorazepam. Clin. Pharmacol. Ther. *24*:411, 1978.
34. Perry, P.J., et al.: Absorption of oral and intramuscular chlordiazepoxide by alcoholics. Clin. Pharm. Ther. *23*:535, 1978.
35. Verbeeck, R., Tjandramaga, T.B., Berberckmoes, R., et al.: Biotransformation and excretion of lorazepam in patients with chronic renal failure. Br. J. Clin. Pharmacol. *3*:1033, 1976.
36. Hosein, I.N., DeFreitas, R., Beaubrun, M.H.: Intramuscular and oral lorazepam in acute alcohol withdrawal and incipient delirium tremens. Curr. Med. Res. Opin. *5*:632, 1978.
37. Miller, W.C., McCurdy, L.: A double-blind comparison of the efficacy and safety of lorazepam and diazepam in the treatment of the acute alcohol withdrawal syndrome. Clin. Ther. *6*:364, 1984.
38. Solomon, J., Rouck, L.A., and Keopke, H.H.: Double-blind comparison of lorazepam and chlordiazepoxide in the treatment of the acute alcohol abstinence syndrome. Clin. Ther. *6*:52, 1983.
39. Thompson, W.L., Johnson, A.D., and Maddrey, W.L.: Diazepam and paraldehyde for treatment of severe delirium tremens: A controlled trial. Ann. Intern. Med. *82*:175, 1974.
40. Nolop, K.B., and Natow, A.: Unprecedented sedative requirements during delirium tremens. Crit. Care Med. *13*:246, 1985.
41. Woo, E., and Greenblatt, D.J.: Massive benzodiazepine requirements during acute alcohol withdrawal. Am. J. Psychiatry *36*:821, 1979.
42. Clinton, J.E., Sterner, S., Stelmachers, Z., et al.: Haloperidol for sedation of disruptive emergency patients. Ann. Emerg. Med. *16*:319, 1987.
43. Adams, F., Fernandez, F., and Anderson, B.S.: Emergency pharmacotherapy of delirium in the critically ill cancer patient. Psychosomatics *27*:33, 1986.
44. Teaser, G.E., Murray, G.B., and Cassem, N.H.: Use of high-dose intravenous haloperidol in the treatment of agitated cardiac patients. J. Clin. Psychopharmacol. *5*:344, 1985.
45. Butler, D., and Messiha, F.S.: Alcohol withdrawal and carbamazepine. Alcohol *3*:113, 1986.
46. Ritola, E., and Malinen, E.: A double-blind comparison of carbamazepine and clomethiazole in the treatment of alcohol withdrawal syndrome. Acta Psychiatr. Scand. *64*:254, 1981.

47. Koppi, S., Eberhardt, G., Haller, R., et al.: Calcium channel blocking agent in the treatment of acute alcohol withdrawal—caroverine vs. meprobamate in a randomized double-blind study. Neuropsychobiology 17:49, 1987.

48. Lewis, J.: Washington report. J. Stud. Alcohol 40:539, 1979.

49. Savage, D., and Lindenbaum, J.: Anemia in alcoholics. Medicine 65:322, 1986.

50. Golbert, T.M., et al.: Comparative evaluation of treatments of alcohol withdrawal syndromes. JAMA 201:113, 1967.

51. Sellers, E.M., and Kalant, H.: Alcohol withdrawal and delirium tremens. In The encyclopedic handbook of alcoholism. Edited by Pattison and Kaufman, New York, Gardner Press, 1982, pp. 147–166.

52. Rose, H.D., et al.: Fever during acute alcohol withdrawal. Am. J. Med. Sci. 2650:112, 1970.

53. Duffy, G.P.: Lumbar puncture in spontaneous subarachnoid hemorrhage. Br. Med. J. 285:1163, 1982.

54. Pettito, F., and Plum, F.: The lumbar puncture. N. Engl. J. Med. 290:225, 1974.

55. Talan, D.A.: Role of emperic parenteral antibiotics prior to lumbar puncture in suspected bacterial meningitis: State of the art. Rev. Infect. Dis. 10:365, 1988.

56. Masters, S.J.: Evaluation of head trauma: efficacy of skull films. J. Roentgenog. 135:539, 1980.

56a. Chance, J.F.: Emergency department treatment of alcohol-withdrawal seizures with phenytoin. Ann. Emerg. Med. 20:520, 1991.

56b. Allredge, B.K., et al.: Placebo-controlled trial of intravenous diphenylhydantoin for short-term treatment of alcohol withdrawal seizures. Am. J. Med. 87:645, 1989.

57. Guidelines for admission of alcohol-dependent patients to general hospital. JAMA 210:121, 1969.

58. Leery, C.M.: When to hospitalize the patient with cirrhosis. Hosp. Pract. 3:40, 1968.

59. Twerski, A.J.: When to hospitalize the alcoholic. Hosp. Pract. 1:47, 1969.

60. Lewis, D.C., and Femino, J.: Management of alcohol withdrawal. Rational Drug Therapy 16:1, 1982.

61. Kane, G.P.: Helping the alcoholic into treatment. Hosp. Phys. 15:55, 1979.

62. Smith, J.W.: Rehabilitation for alcoholics. Postgrad. Med. 64:143, 1978.

Chapter 85

DRUG AND SUBSTANCE ABUSE EMERGENCIES

DRUG ABUSE

James R. Ungar, George R. Schwartz, and David G. Levine

CAPSULE

Alcohol and drug abuse are responsible for various acute reactions requiring prompt medical intervention. *Drug abuse refers to the use, generally by self-administration, of psychoactive substances in a manner that adversely affects medical, psychosocial, or economic well-being.* So defined, the term encompasses alcohol abuse, which affects more people than all other forms of drug abuse combined. The need for emergency services for alcohol-related medical behavioral problems has long been recognized. The expanding use of other mind-affecting substances has created additional demands for skilled treatment of drug-induced crises.

INTRODUCTION

The term "addict" is derived from the Latin *addictus*, literally "given over," describing an individual who is awarded to another as a slave. In common parlance, addiction denotes an established pattern of compulsive drug abuse generally occurring at the expense of all non—drug-related activities. It is the extreme form of drug dependence. *Psychologic dependence* is characterized by variable degrees of obsessive preoccupation with drugs, preference for the intoxicated state, and chronic or recurrent abuse. *Physical dependence* is an altered physiologic state produced by repeated drug use and requiring continued drug use to prevent the emergence of withdrawal symptoms. This vulnerability to abstinence phenomena is often included in the concept of addiction. *Tolerance* is manifested by a diminished response to a constant dose of a drug,

reflecting changes in pharmacodynamic and cellular mechanisms. Cross-tolerance is observed between different drugs of the same class.

Drugs of abuse are commonly categorized as follows: narcotics, sedatives, stimulants, psychedelics, inhalants, and alcohol. Clinically significant physical dependence occurs only with narcotics (morphine-type drug dependence) and with sedatives and alcohol (CNS depressant drug dependence). Psychologic dependence is seen in connection with all these agents.

WHO ARE THE ABUSERS?

Alcohol and drug abusers are a heterogeneous group who represent a spectrum of subcultures ranging from extreme deviance to unalloyed conventionality. Skid-row derelicts and inner-city junkies compose only a small fraction of the affected population, which extends deeply into the working and affluent classes. These individuals are subject to an increased risk of both acute and chronic medical problems. Chronic ill health results as much from poor nutrition and hygiene as from direct drug toxicity. Frequent and recurrent use of the intravenous route also contributes significantly to addicts' morbidity. Diseases of long standing may retard recovery from alcohol-and drug-related emergencies.

Crises occur during intoxication and withdrawal. Intoxication may lead to adverse physiologic or psychologic reactions and, in cases of severe overdose, to coma and death. Withdrawal phenomena also require timely assessment and may, in certain circumstances, progress to a fatal outcome. "Polydrug abuse," which refers to the habitual abuse of a variety of drugs, depending primarily on availability, has become increasingly prevalent and seriously complicates both the clinical presentation and proper management of drug abuse emergencies. It is conservatively estimated that 2 million Americans are chronic polydrug users. Nonusers, including children, are also subject to accidental intoxication.

Conducting an orderly and systematic history and physical and laboratory examinations is frequently impractical in patients with acute alcohol and drug reactions. More often, diagnosis and treatment must proceed concurrently. Coma, delirium, convulsions, and psychoses are common presenting symptoms. Differential diagnostic possibilities must include exogenous poisons of all varieties; metabolic disorders; infections, injuries, and other diseases of the central nervous system (CNS); and psychiatric disorders. Historical data should be obtained from the patient whenever possible, as well as from family, friends, and others, concerning the drugs involved, dose, route of administration, and time of last use. Particularly in the case of illicit drug abuse, reliable histories may be unobtainable. Occasionally, alcohol, drugs, prescriptions, or paraphernalia may be found among the patient's possessions, providing clues to the agents involved. Physical examination should be directed toward evaluating (1) the patient's status and requirements for support of vital functions, (2) diagnostic signs suggesting specific intoxication or withdrawal syndromes, (3) sequelae of chronic alcoholism or drug abuse, and (4) evidence of concurrent illness or injury.

The constellation of historical and physical findings determines which laboratory and radiographic examinations are appropriate. Gross metabolic, hepatic, and renal diseases may be revealed by routine screening tests. Serum electrolytes should be monitored in patients requiring intravenous hydration. Serial measurement of arterial blood gases is necessary for precise evaluation and control of respiratory status. Toxicologic analysis may finally confirm the diagnosis, although the results are generally unavailable during the initial management of the patient. Samples of blood, urine, vomitus, and other specimens should be saved for future toxicologic study.

NARCOTIC ANALGESICS

The narcotic analgesics comprise naturally occurring, semisynthetic, and synthetic substances with pharmacologic properties similar to those of morphine, the principal alkaloid of opium. All drugs in this group have CNS effects, including analgesia, sedation, mental clouding, and mood changes. Other effects are suppression of the cough reflex and suppression of gastrointestinal motility. In addition, narcotics regularly produce a dose-related centrally mediated respiratory depression. Commonly abused narcotics are listed in Table 85-1.

ABUSE PATTERNS

An estimated 500,000 Americans are addicted to heroin, the preferred drug for most narcotics users. Heroin addiction is most prevalent among the urban poor, and a significant heroin-related subculture exists in the ghettos. The illicit status of this drug subjects the addict to adverse social and toxicologic consequences. Heroin is commonly adulterated with quinine, lactose, and mannitol, and occasionally with barbiturates.

Habitual users typically experience a profound euphoria after a "fix." The acute state is characterized by satiation of motivating drives. Repeated use leads to tolerance, requiring higher doses to achieve the desired effects and in many cases simply to prevent withdrawal—doses in the lethal range for nontolerant individuals. An invariable concomitant is the development of a morphine-type physical dependence. Psychologic dependence is manifested by compulsive drug-seeking behavior that often remains undiminished even after prolonged abstinence.

Depending on the particular preparation, narcotics may be used in many ways. Smoking, sniffing ("snorting"), ingesting, and injecting subcutaneously ("skin popping"), intramuscularly or intravenously ("shooting up") are all common practices. Intravenous injection is the preferred method in most parts of the world because the high cost of narcotics dictates an efficient method of administration. Furthermore, the intravenous technique produces a sudden "rush" of intensely pleasant sensations in addition to the drowsy euphoria that follows.

Physicians, nurses, and other health professionals engage in illicit narcotics use with a higher frequency than occurs among the general population. In such cases, meperidine (Demerol), pentazocine (Talwin), fentanyl, and other legitimate pharmaceutical products are diverted for self-administration. Pentazocine is a synthetic analgesic with properties of both narcotics agonists and antagonists. When administered to an opiate-dependent individual, pentazocine evokes withdrawal symptoms. Psychotomimetic effects, such as visual hallucinations, depersonalization, and dysphoria occur at high doses.

Methadone is an orally effective long-acting synthetic narcotic used as a maintenance narcotic in rehabilitation programs for heroin addicts. Inevitably, some methadone is diverted into illicit channels. Methadone's longer duration of action, 24 to 48 hours, is an important consideration during both intoxication and withdrawal. An even longer-acting congener, acetylmethadol, has a duration of 72 to 96 hours.

COMMON MEDICAL PROBLEMS

Except for their addictive properties, narcotic analgesics are relatively innocuous when administered in nontoxic doses. The physiologic and psychologic hazards of chronic narcotic use are not well understood. Nevertheless, addicts are subject to an increased prevalence of a variety of maladies. Much of the morbidity is a result of hypodermic needle use, particularly needle sharing, unsterile technique, and injection of particulate matter. Hepatitis is endemic among addicts. AIDS is becoming a serious hazard from intravenous drug use and needle sharing. Pulmonary hypertension may result from emboli representing accumulations of cotton fibers and undissolved debris. Bacterial endocarditis may occur in both left and right heart valves. Tetanus appears with increased frequency where heroin is "cut" with quinine (eastern United States), and malaria is transmitted by needle where quinine is not used (western United States). Cellulitis and skin abscess are common, especially among "skin poppers." Some unusual cases of Guillain-Barré syndrome (acute polyneuritis) have also been observed that were believed to be related to intravenous opiate abuse. Other factors contributing to the ill health of narcotics addicts are the substandard nutrition, hygiene, and medical care prevalent among the lower socioeconomic strata.

INTOXICATION

The syndrome of narcotic overdose, particularly after intravenous injection of heroin, is a puzzling phenomenon that cannot be explained solely in terms of an excessive intake of the drug. Analyses of body fluids and residual drug samples usually do not point to an actual pharmacologic overdose. One addict may "OD" while another sharing the same syringe is unaffected. Death may occur suddenly—sometimes immediately after injection. Fulminant pulmonary edema is often evident. Such observations have led to considerable speculation concerning the mechanisms underlying the overdose syndrome. Acute hypersensitivity reactions, effects of quinine and other adulterants, and synergism with alcohol and barbiturates may contribute significantly to its genesis. At present, the evidence for any of these hypotheses is inconclusive. The latest insights have come through epidemiologic studies of epidemic heroin-related deaths. Through detailed studies of hundreds of drug-related deaths, Ruttenber and Luke discovered that risk factors for heroin-related deaths included the use of ethanol (which might make individuals more vulnerable to the toxic effects of heroin). Also, the authors noted an increase in the quantity of quinine adulteration of heroin packets during the initial stages of an epidemic.

The typical presentation of heroin overdose is (1) depressed level of consciousness, (2) depressed respiration, and (3) constricted pupils. In severe cases, the patient is comatose and apneic. Frothy pulmonary edema is present on initial examination in more than half the cases. Temperature may be normal, elevated,

TABLE 85-1. COMMONLY ABUSED NARCOTICS
Opium
Morphine
Codeine
Heroin
Fentanyl, sufentanyl
Hydromorphone (Dilaudid)
Oxymorphone (Numorphan)
Levorphanol (Levo-Dromoran)
Oxycodone (Percodan)
Meperidine (Demerol)
Methadone (Dolophine)
Pentazocine (Talwin)

or subnormal. Vomiting often occurs. The clinical picture is variable, depending in large measure on the degree and duration of hypoxia. With severe hypoxia, the skin changes from pale to cyanotic, the pulse becomes weak and slow, hypotension advances to shock, and grave neurologic signs appear: depression of deep tendon reflexes; emergence of pathologic reflexes; and paralytic dilatation of the pupils.

The first consideration in the treatment of narcotic overdose is the maintenance of adequate respiration. The physician must evaluate an obtunded or comatose patient to determine the frequency and depth of spontaneous respirations, the degree of pulmonary congestion, and the presence of cyanosis. When there is evidence of respiratory failure, a patent airway must be established, preferably by endotracheal intubation with a cuffed tube, and positive-pressure ventilation with an oxygen-rich mixture must be instituted. Patients with pulmonary edema are at high risk and require careful management. Diuretics, digitalis preparations, corticosteroids, and antihistamines are of dubious efficacy in combating this complication. Assisted ventilation with oxygen administration is crucial, and in advanced cases when secretions cannot be cleared sufficiently, tracheostomy is indicated.

Along with the institution of respiratory support, cardiovascular status should be assessed. Hypotension and cardiac arrhythmias frequently improve when hypoxia and acidosis are corrected. Severe hypotension may require volume expansion, administration of vasopressors, and measures used in treating shock from other causes.

Samples of blood, urine, and other fluids should be obtained for toxicologic analysis. A diagnosis of heroin intoxication is confirmed by detection of morphine, its major metabolite. Tests for other narcotics are available in most laboratories and should be requested in appropriate cases. Analysis for CNS depressants and alcohol are indicated when clinical findings suggest multiple drug abuse. Gastric lavage should be performed after intubation, and stomach contents should be saved for subsequent analysis. Routine laboratory data should be supplemented by liver function tests. After blood is drawn, 50 cc of 50% glucose solution should be given intravenously because hypoglycemia may be present. Thiamine, 100 mg IM, should be given also. Analysis of arterial blood gases in stuporous or comatose patients assists in evaluation of respiratory depression and monitoring of treatment effectiveness. Chest films provide a gauge of the extent of pulmonary congestion. A CT of the head should be obtained in comatose patients and when trauma is suspected.

NARCOTIC ANTAGONISTS

Narcotic antagonists provide specific treatment for narcotics poisoning. The antagonist of choice is naloxone (Narcan). In the recommended dosage range, naloxone has no morphine-like activity and cannot further depress respiration. Other antagonists, such as nalorphine (Nalline) and levallorphan (Lorfan), have agonistic properties as well and are for that reason less desirable for treating respiratory depression when the cause is uncertain. Naloxone has the additional advantage of effectively counteracting the depressant activity of other narcotic antagonists, including pentazocine.

The usual initial dose of naloxone is 0.4 mg. to 0.8 mg. administered intravenously. If the ingested substance is possibly codeine, pentazocine, or propoxyphene, however, much larger initial doses (up to 2.0 mg.) are needed for desired effects. This has been of particular importance in small children. If the diagnosis of narcotic intoxication is correct, an improvement in respiratory rate and depth should be observed after ½ to 2 minutes. Recovery is often dramatic, but care is required at this point. Patients may emerge from a narcotic-induced coma into an agitated state characterized by delirium and combativeness. Hypoxia, pulmonary edema, polydrug intoxication, and the precipitation of an opiate withdrawal syndrome may all contribute to the problem. Attendants must be prepared to control a confused and struggling patient. It is important to bear in mind that the *target symptom is respiratory depression.* Treatment with antagonists should be restricted to the lowest dose that effectively corrects respiratory inadequacy. They should not be used to facilitate the return to consciousness of a patient who is breathing adequately without assistance. An antagonist-induced withdrawal syndrome cannot be treated with narcotics until the antagonist has been eliminated from the body.

If the patient fails to respond to the administration of an antagonist, one or two additional doses should be given at 5-minute intervals. Unresponsiveness to repeated doses casts doubt on the diagnosis and requires further evaluation for other causes of coma and respiratory depression (see Chapter 11.) Patients who demonstrate a satisfactory response should remain under close observation, ideally on an in-patient basis for 24 hours. Severe respiratory depression may recur within several hours, necessitating further treatment with antagonists, because they are eliminated more rapidly than most opiates. In poisoning with methadone and other long-acting narcotics, antagonist administration every 2 to 3 hours must continue until recovery is complete. A more efficient means may be a continuous naloxone infusion in such difficult cases.

Patients who have been resuscitated from a narcotic overdose should be hospitalized for further observation and general medical assessment—particularly when pulmonary edema, fever, or convulsions complicate the acute episode. Pulmonary edema may be a late development, especially in intoxication with long-acting opiates. Pneumonia, often secondary to aspiration, is another frequent pulmonary complication. Many other causes of fever must be considered, and body fluids should be cultured to identify the pathogen. Staphylococcal infections are common. Seizures may result from codeine, pentazocine, and meperidine toxicity. Meperidine poisoning is characterized by respiratory depression, pupillary dilation, tremor, hyperactive reflexes, and convulsions. Concurrent intoxication with stimulants or withdrawal from depressants may account for seizures in this setting. In cases of severe poisoning, catheterization of the bladder may be indicated to relieve urinary retention. Rarely, myoglobinuria, acute renal failure, and transverse myelitis occur.

Before discharge, recovered patients should be encouraged to enroll in a rehabilitation program. Some addicts are more receptive to referral after an overdose experience, and the opportunity should not be lost.

WITHDRAWAL

An interruption of regular narcotic administration in an individual who has a morphine-type physical dependence leads to the development of an abstinence syndrome. The rapidity of onset of symptoms depends primarily on the particular narcotic and the usual daily dose. Drugs with short durations of action, such as heroin and meperidine, are associated with brief and intense withdrawal syndromes. Withdrawal from methadone and other long-acting preparations is milder but more prolonged.

The narcotics abstinence syndrome is a stereotyped physiologic reaction characterized by autonomic disturbances, CNS hyperexcitability, and emotional lability, generally accompanied by persistent drug-seeking behavior. In heroin withdrawal, the first symptoms appear about 8 hours after the last dose and include lacrimation, rhinorrhea, diaphoresis, yawning, and sneezing. As the syndrome unfolds, the addict experiences malaise, restlessness, irritability, depression, insomnia, and anorexia. Gastrointestinal symptoms may include nausea, vomiting, abdominal cramps, and diarrhea. Myalgias, arthralgias, tremors, and twitches are often prominent. Pupils are moderately dilated. Episodes of pilomotor erection are seen (the term "cold turkey" denoting the untreated syndrome derives from this sign). Mild "rebound phenomena" such as hyperpnea, hyperpyrexia, and hypertension regularly occur. All but the most inexperienced addicts are aware that the administration of a narcotic promptly and completely suppresses the symptoms of withdrawal. If they remain abstinent, their symptoms peak in 2 or 3 days and then gradually subside in a week or so. Subtle physiologic abnormalities can be detected for many months after withdrawal, but the significance of these protracted abstinence phenomena is unclear.

In general, emergency services should not assume responsibility for detoxification of narcotic addicts but should refer them to specialized facilities. Medically supervised detoxification is directed toward reversing physical dependence while minimizing the discomfort and drug-craving experienced during withdrawal. The common methods of detoxification involve a stepwise reduction in daily opiate intake until abstinence is achieved. Because of cross-tolerance, any narcotic other than one with antagonist properties may be used for this purpose. Substitution of methadone is recommended because of its longer duration of action and its reliable gastrointestinal absorption. Withdrawal may be carried out slowly over many months or rapidly in several days. Acceptance of the regimen is increased when the addict has some control over the pace of detoxification. Unpleasant symptoms, primarily the flu-like illness of early withdrawal, are less prominent when the dosage reduction is gradual. Symptomatic treatment of the abstinence syndrome is an alternative to gradual detoxification. Sedatives may be prescribed to reduce irritability and insomnia. Mild analgesics provide some relief from muscle and joint pains. GI symptoms may respond to non-narcotic remedies. *Detoxification by any method is followed in most cases by a return to regular narcotics use.*

In narcotic abuse, the tendency has been toward the shorter-acting high-potency narcotics, fentanyl (20 times as potent as morphine) or sufentanyl (2000 times morphine potency). Various derivatives are being synthesized (e.g., "China white," alpha-fentanyl), resulting in increased deaths from overdose, particularly on the United States West Coast.

SEDATIVE-HYPNOTICS

The sedative-hypnotics (Table 85-2) include the barbiturates and various other substances with general CNS depressant activity. Antianxiety agents (minor tranquilizers) are considered under this heading because of numerous similarities in pharmacologic properties and patterns of abuse. Cross-tolerance occurs among most of the sedatives. By these criteria, ethyl alcohol is also a member of this class, but because of its unique significance as a drug of abuse, it will be considered separately. Barbiturates and other de-

TABLE 85-2. COMMONLY ABUSED CNS DEPRESSANTS (SEDATIVE-HYPNOTICS)

Barbiturates
  Pentobarbital (Nembutal)
  Amobarbital (Amytal)
  Secobarbital (Seconal)
  Secobarbital plus amobarbital (Tuinal)
Nonbarbiturate sedatives
  Chloral hydrate (Noctec)
  Paraldehyde
  Ethchlorvynol (Placidyl)
  Glutethimide (Doriden)
  Methyprylon (Noludar)
  Methaqualone (Quaalude) (withdrawn from market in USA)
Antianxiety agents
  Meprobamate (Miltown)
  Chlordiazepoxide (Librium)
  Diazepam (Valium)
  Oxazepam (Serax)

pressants can produce relaxation, somnolence, stupor, and coma. In sufficient doses, all cause respiratory depression. Sedatives are used in the treatment of a variety of psychiatric disturbances and convulsive disorders and as adjuncts to anesthesia.

Methaqualone (Quaalude, Parest, etc.) abuse has become prominent. The amount of abuse became so high that the drug has been removed from the formulary. Major hazards have been associated with overdose of methaqualone with alcohol and severe CNS depression leading to death, primarily from respiratory depression. As few as six methaqualone tablets with alcohol can lead to serious hazard. The relative unavailability of methaqualone has substantially decreased its use.

ABUSE PATTERNS

Although the true extent of abuse of barbiturates, tranquilizers, and other sedatives is unknown, there is no doubt that these substances constitute a public health problem of the highest magnitude. Abuse patterns vary from occasional episodes of self-medication to entirely drug-oriented life styles. Habitual use of sedatives frequently begins iatrogenically, especially among individuals who have no identification with drug-using subcultures. Prescribed for their tension-reducing or sleep-inducing properties, these drugs are often ingested in increasing doses, until physical dependence develops. Recreational use of sedative drugs by adolescents and young adults resembles in may respects periodic binges of alcohol intoxication. The desired effect is a "disinhibition euphoria." Some users indulge in the hazardous practice of intravenous injection of barbiturates. With this technique, the addict experiences a "rush" of sensations not obtained when the drugs are taken by mouth.

Barbiturate abusers characteristically prefer the short-acting compounds, such as amobarbital, pentobarbital, and secobarbital. These drugs may be taken orally or parenterally, either alone or in combination with other drugs and alcohol. Intermediate- and long-acting barbiturates such as butabarbital and phenobarbital do not produce a comparable degree of euphoria and consequently are rarely sought for this purpose. As with the barbiturates, certain nonbarbiturate sedatives are favored above others by virtue of their effects, reputation, and availability. Chloral hydrate, glutethimide, methyprylon, and methaqualone are among the more commonly abused drugs in this group. Meprobamate and the benzodiazepines, particularly chlordiazepoxide, diazepam, and alprazolam (Xanax) also have abuse potential. Diazepam is a favored drug of some youthful abusers as well as many of their more conventional elders. The tranquilizers by themselves rarely cause fatal reactions but may contribute to acute polydrug toxicity.

COMMON MEDICAL PROBLEMS

Chronic intoxication with sedative-hypnotics appears to be considerably more deleterious than addiction to opiates when measured in terms of impairment of mental and physical function. The habitual user often neglects his personal hygiene and nutrition, with adverse consequences to health maintenance. The risk of automotive and industrial accidents is increased as well. Barbiturate addicts who use hypodermic needles are subject to the same serious health hazards as are heroin "mainliners." In addition, because of their alkalinity, barbiturate solutions are extremely irritating if inadvertently injected intra-arterially. In such instances, a prolonged, intensely painful vasoconstriction is precipitated that can cause severe ischemic damage to the affected extremity. Immediate hospitalization for anticoagulant treatment is necessary.

INTOXICATION

Acute barbiturate or other sedative poisoning is most often a consequence of deliberate ingestion of an overdose, although accidental poisoning clearly occurs also. Tolerance to the euphoric effects of barbiturates is not accompanied by a proportionate elevation in the lethal dose. This reduction in the margin of safety, along with the common practice of ingesting multiple CNS depressants including alcohol, probably accounts for most cases of accidental overdose. "Drug automatism," in which intoxication leads to confusion and repeated ingestion, does not appear to be a significant cause of barbiturate poisoning.

Intoxication with sedative-hypnotics resembles alcoholic inebriation and may include dysarthria, ataxia, emotional lability, and a clouded sensorium. Sustained horizontal and vertical nystagmus usually are demonstrable. Severe intoxication is characterized by a progressive depression of consciousness along with respiratory and cardiovascular failure. Respirations may be slow or rapid and shallow. Ventilation is often further compromised by pulmonary edema, atelectasis, or pneumonitis. Blood pressure drops as a result of a centrally mediated vasomotor depression and direct cardiac and peripheral vascular effects and secondarily as a result of hypoxia. Renal failure may develop if adequate perfusion is not maintained. Pupils may be constricted or dilated with advanced hypoxia. Deep tendon reflexes are often depressed, and pathologic reflexes may appear. Glutethimide has also been reported to cause sudden apnea and acute laryngeal spasm, not associated with other sedatives.

Treatment is primarily supportive. Good nursing care is essential and may be all that is required if cardiopulmonary functioning remains relatively normal. When spontaneous respirations are inadequate and gag and cough reflexes are suppressed, an airway should be established with an endotracheal tube. Insufficient respiratory exchange is treated with mechanical ventilation and oxygen administration and monitored by arterial blood gas analysis. Tracheostomy may be necessary when coma is profound and prolonged. Severe hypotension and shock generally respond to volume expansion with intravenous fluids. Prompt correction is required to avoid renal failure and other sequelae. Vasopressors and fluids may be administered to support blood pressure at about 90/60 mm Hg, and central venous pressure should be monitored. Induction of vomiting should not be considered except for fully conscious patients. Because of the dangers of aspiration in obtunded patients, gastric lavage should be undertaken only after endotracheal intubation. The value of lavage depends on how soon it is performed after drug ingestion. Gastric half-life (when half of an ingested substance passes through the pylorus) is approximately 30 to 45 minutes, although the presence of food in the stomach can change this considerably. Activated charcoal should be administered.

Body fluids should be analyzed for barbiturates and other CNS depressants as indicated. Lethal blood levels of the commonly abused CNS depressants are generally in the range of 1 to 3 mg per dL, although tolerance and other factors account for considerable variability from case to case. Baseline values for serum electrolytes should be obtained, along with other routine laboratory determinations. Measurements of body weight and fluid balance are important in comatose patients.

Forced diuresis accelerates the elimination of longer-acting barbiturates. Excretion of short-acting barbiturates and of most nonbarbiturate sedatives is only slightly enhanced. If renal function is adequate, mannitol infusion at a rate of 1 L per hour, with sodium bicarbonate and potassium chloride added to the solution, should produce optimal output of urine. Alkalinization minimizes the tubular reabsorption of weak acids, particularly phenobarbital. Close monitoring of fluid and electrolyte balance, including potassium and magnesium levels, is required for periodic adjustment of the composition of the infusate. Hemodialysis is rarely indicated, but in extreme cases or when renal failure supervenes, it may be life-saving. Virtually all sedative-hypnotics are dialyzable, although short-acting barbiturates, benzodiazepines, and glutethimide are less efficiently removed. Consultation with a dialysis team should be sought when clinical deterioration continues in the face of sound medical management.

Analeptics are generally not helpful in the treatment of sedative poisoning, and may have adverse effects. Only clinicians experienced with their use should consider administering stimulants in this setting.

Whenever possible, the physician should evaluate recovered patients to assess the extent of their drug abuse, suicidal intent, and psychologic instability. Appropriate referral for follow-up care can then be made.

WITHDRAWAL

Drug dependence of the barbiturate type is associated with a charateristic abstinence syndrome that, in its severest form, can be fatal. Following an initial period of apparent improvement, which may last for 8 to 16 hours as the intoxication clears, symptoms of withdrawal emerge. Anxiety, tremulousness, insomnia, and weakness intensify as the syndrome progresses. These symptoms are often accompanied by nausea, vomiting, abdominal cramping, and anorexia. Postural hypotension is typically present. Coarse tremors, muscular twitches, excessive blinking, exaggerated startle responses, and hyperactive deep tendon reflexes indicate a heightened degree of neurologic irritability that generally reaches a peak in 2 to 3 days. Convulsions of the grand mal type are most likely to occur at this time, although they may appear as much as a week after withdrawal, particularly in the case of long-acting substances.

Improvement may begin as the seizures subside, or a slowly progressive delirium may develop. This organic brain syndrome is characterized by disorientation, vivid visual and auditory hallucinations, paranoid delusions, and overwhelming anxiety. In the course of the delirium, which may continue for several days, most patients display hyperventilation, tachycardia, hypertension, and fever. Marked hyperthermia can lead to cardiovascular failure and death. Usually, however, even the untreated syndrome clears in about a week.

Recognition of the sedative-hypnotic withdrawal syndrome is important. It must be remembered that withdrawal can begin shortly after recovery from an overdose. Because of the potential severity of the syndrome and the large doses of barbiturates that must be administered to treat it, detoxification should be performed on an inpatient basis.

Addicts may be stabilized on an adequate dose of a barbiturate and then receive decreasing daily doses until a drug-free state is achieved. Stabilization doses are estimated from the history and from the clinical response to trial intoxicating doses. Pentobarbital may be substituted for any barbiturate and for most other CNS depressants (including alcohol). Phenobarbital substitution is based on the same principles, but the longer duration of action allows for a smoother decline in blood levels. Withdrawal from lesser known sedatives should be done without substitution. Generally, the dose cannot be reduced by more than 10% daily without the emergence of symptoms. Close observation for signs of excessive or inadequate dosing is necessary throughout the course of detoxification, which may require several weeks to complete.

Seizures should be treated with a short-acting barbiturate. Diphenylhydantoin and other nonbarbiturate anticonvulsants are ineffective in this instance. Delirium, once developed, is generally refractory to further barbiturate administration, although aggressive treatment with parenteral sedatives may shorten the duration and decrease the intensity of the reaction.

CNS STIMULANTS

The central nervous system (CNS) stimulants are sympathomimetic substances that elicit states of heightened alertness, elevated mood, and enhanced psychomotor activity. The principal drugs of abuse in this group are the amphetamines and cocaine. Amphetamines have powerful stimulant effects that last for several hours. Appetitie suppression and respiratory stimulation are centrally mediated. Peripheral effects include blood pressure elevation and bronchial dilation. Cocaine is a local anesthetic obtained from leaves of the South American plant, *Erythroxylon coca*. Cocaine has systemic and central nervous system effects similar to those of the amphetamines. It is covered in detail subsequently. Table 85-3 presents some commonly abused CNS stimulants.

TABLE 85-3. COMMONLY ABUSED CNS STIMULANTS

Amphetamines
  Amphetamine (Benzedrine)
  Dextroamphetamine (Dexedrine)
  Methamphetamine (Desoxyn, Methadrine)
  Methamphetamine plus pentobarbital (Desbutal)
Phenmetrazine (Preludin)
Methylphenidate (Ritalin)
Cocaine

AMPHETAMINES, PHENMETRAZINE, AND METHYPHENIDATE

ABUSE PATTERNS

Amphetamines are taken by mouth, absorbed through the nasal mucosa, and injected intravenously. Habituation may occur after the prescription of amphetamines for obesity or mild depressions. In other cases, the drug is self-administered to allay fatigue and to improve performance of arduous tasks. Recreational use of amphetamines specifically for their energizing effects occurs primarily among polydrug abusers. The transition from intermittent to sustained use marks the emergence of psychologic dependence. Tolerance develops with repeated use, necessitating substantial increases in dosage. Intravenous injection of methamphetamine is a particularly destructive practice in which the primary goal is to experience the intense "rush" following injection. "Speed freaks" typically repeat these injections every few hours for several days until supplies run out or exhaustion and paranoia supervene. Such "runs" are followed by a prolonged sleep. Subsequently, symptoms of lethargy and depression may persist until another "run" begins. The latest drug problem is inhalation of methamphetamine crystals, which may also be smoked like "crack." This substance has been called "ice." Its increased hazards are the result of rapid absorption and high serum levels of the drug.

Phenmetrazine, methylphenidate, and other stimulants have similar effects and are subject to similar patterns of abuse. Users of CNS stimulants often seek relief from the agitation they produce by using opiates, barbiturates, and alcohol. These drugs may be taken alternately or simultaneously, evoking complicated psychophysiologic responses.

Over-the-counter stimulants (usually containing propanolamine, caffeine, and ephedrine) have been marketed to look like amphetamines. Deaths (caused apparently by hypertensive crises with cerebral hemorrhage or by cardiac arrhythmias) have been reported from use of "over-the-counter speed."

COMMON MEDICAL PROBLEMS

Chronic stimulant abuse is associated with nervousness, tremulousness, sleeping difficulties, anorexia, and weight loss. Common cardiovascular side effects are arrhythmias and impaired blood pressure regulation. A variety of gastrointestinal, respiratory, and dermatologic symptoms are seen in connection with abuse of these drugs. Signs of mental deterioration such as memory impairment, shortened attention span, and emotional instability have been observed among long-term high-dose users.

Intravenous use of stimulants carries with it the morbidity resulting from injection of allergens, par-

ticles, and pathogens. An additional hazard of intravenous methamphetamine use is a generalized necrotizing angiitis resembling polyarteritis nodosa that produces hypertension, pulmonary edema, pancreatitis, and renal failure. Bacterial endocarditis and septic emboli occur with higher frequency in these groups, particularly when tablets are ground and mixed with water before injection. Subacute bacterial endocarditis occurs more commonly with methylphenidate injection, owing to insoluble components in the tablets. "Speed freaks" characteristically neglect their personal hygiene and nutrition to an alarming degree, even in comparision with other drug abusers. Inhalation of amphetamines or methamphetamine (ice) can result in pulmonary irritation or pneumonia, as well as problems with high dose levels.

OVERDOSE MANAGEMENT

Acute overdose reactions reflect an accentuation of the usual pharmacologic effects of stimulants; anxiety, irritability, tachycardia, other arrhythmias, hypertension, headache, chest pain, and abdominal cramps. The skin is often moist and flushed. Bruxism and gnawing at the lips also are commonly seen. Pupils are dilated. Confusion and panic frequently lead to assaultive or self-destructive behavior. A toxic psychosis may develop, manifested by delirium, auditory and visual hallucinations, and paranoia. Life-threatening doses produce hyperthermia, convulsions, and cardiovascular collapse. Sudden deaths presumably are the result of acute cardiac arrhythmias. Toxicologic studies can detect amphetamines or other stimulants in the body, but the findings are usually not available until after the acute reaction has passed.

In less severe intoxications, calm surroundings and mild sedation with a short-acting barbiturate or a benzodiazepine may be sufficient treatment. With more extreme reactions, chlorpromazine or thioridazine may be useful for their antipsychotic and sedative effects. In addition, phenothiazines counteract the peripheral adrenergic effects of amphetamines, tending to reduce temperature, pulse, and blood pressure, although an occasional paradoxic hyperthermia has been reported. Anticholinergic reactions requiring physostigmine treatment occasionally result from synergistic reacitons between common adulterants and the phenothiazines. Haloperidol is also useful for controlling acute psychotic symptoms and has been advocated as the pharmacologic agent of choice in amphetamine poisoning owing to its dopaminergic activity. If the drugs have been taken by mouth, induced vomiting or gastric lavage may be of value, because stimulants tend to delay gastric emptying.

Severe hypertension occasionally develops and can cause intracranial bleeding. Sustained systolic pressure above 200 mm Hg should be brought under control with an alpha-adrenergic blocking agent such as phenoxybenzamine or phentolamine. Hyperthermia should be controlled when temperatures rise above 102°F. Phenothiazines can be used to suppress shivering and reduce fever. Convulsions tend to occur in connection with a rapid rise in body temperature. Seizures may reflect stimulant toxicity, sedative withdrawal, or both conditions simultaneously. Intravenous barbiturate administration is indicated and should be continued as needed to suppress seizure activity. In extreme cases, status epilepticus develops, and vigorous treatment is required.

AMPHETAMINE PSYCHOSIS

Amphetamine psychosis is a distinctive paranoid psychosis that develops in a setting of chronic amphetamine abuse. Similar psychophysiologic reactions are associated with abuse of cocaine, methylphenidate, phenmetrazine, and other CNS stimulants. The syndrome may include paranoid thinking, often with persecutory delusions; auditory, visual, or haptic hallucinations, the latter sometimes leading to excoriation of the skin from attempts to remove imagined parasites; hyperactivity, especially stereotyped compulsive behavior; and labile affective state in which anxiety and hostility generally predominate. In the typical presentation, there is no confusion, disorientation, or memory impairment, distinguishing this syndrome from most toxic psychoses. Amphetamine psychosis should be considered in the differential diagnosis of acute paranoid schizophrenia, for which it is frequently mistaken on initial evaluation. A history of stimulant abuse, physical sequelae such as emaciation, or signs of acute intoxication strongly suggest the diagnosis. Toxicologic analysis of body fluids provides confirmation.

A tranquil and reassuring environment is vital in the management of amphetamine psychosis and may be all that is required in some cases. An accompanying acute intoxication should be treated as already described. Benzodiazepines or other sedatives may be administered for agitation; phenothiazines or haloperidol should be used for more extreme paranoid behavior. Hospitalization is advisable if the psychosis persists or progresses. The symptoms abate as the drug is excreted. Hallucinations rarely continue for more than 1 to 2 days after cessation of amphetamine use. Patients usually sleep excessively for several days and manifest a confused, dreamlike state while awake. If there is no further use of stimulants, the psychosis generally clears within a week.

Chronic "speed" users commonly undergo a progressive psychosocial disintegration. Referral for supportive services is often necessary.

WITHDRAWAL

Although CNS stimulants do not induce physical dependence of a degree comparable to that seen with narcotics and sedatives, withdrawal is not symptom-free. Hypersomnia occurs for the first few days. Depression, fatigue, and apathy are typical and may persist for weeks or months, depending partly on the extent of drug abuse preceding withdrawal. These symptoms may reflect the unmasking of an underlying exhaustion resulting from chronic overstimulation. Relief is often sought through renewed use of stimulants. Emergency treatment is not required. Referral for psychiatric evaluation and counseling is appropriate. In addition, some clinicians recommend prescription of a brief course of tricyclic antidepressants.

COCAINE

Cocaine is now the most abused major stimulant in America. A naturally occurring alkaloid found in the leaves of the plant *Erythroxylon coca*, it has been used since the sixth century to relieve such varied conditions as malaise, fatigue, and depression. It is reported to have been the first hunger suppressant among the ancient nobles and was used extensively by lower classes and slaves to increase work endurance and cold tolerance.

Despite the fact that Nicholas Monardes alluded to the medicinal and illicit use of coca leaves in the sixteenth century, it was not until 1857 that Niemann isolated cocaine from the coca leaf and thus introduced it to the "civilized world." Cocaine was first used medicinally in 1884 by Kohler as a topical anesthetic for opthalmologic surgery. That same year, Halsted performed the first nerve block, using cocaine as the anesthetic. Halsted expanded the use of cocaine to include mind-altering experiments (none of which were published in the literature) and eventually became the first cocaine-impaired physician on record. Freud advocated the use of cocaine in the treatment of asthma, alcoholism, opiate addiction, and diminished libido. Freud also fell prey to chronic cocaine dependency.

The original formulation of Coca-Cola by John Styth Pemberton contained cocaine from Peruvian coca leaves and caffeine from African cola nuts. The passage of the Pure Food and Drug Act in 1906 took the cocaine out but left the caffeine in. With the Harrison Tax Act of 1914, overt cocaine use diminished. Accurately labeled a dangerous drug but erroneously dubbed a "narcotic," its use has become strictly controlled under the comprehensive Drug Abuse Prevention and Control Act of 1970.

Cocaine is transported from South America to the United States, where it enters in the form of its hydrochloride salt—the end product of numerous refinement steps from the original coca leaf. The hydrochloride salt is relatively pure (80% to 87%), water-soluble, white, and crystalline. It is either nasally insufflated (snorted) or injected (slammed) by abusers to achieve a stimulant state. It is estimated that 10 million Americans have used cocaine in this form, 5 million use it regularly, and 5000 use it for the

TABLE 85-4. COMMON STREET NAMES OF DRUGS OF ABUSE

Stimulants (amphetamines unless otherwise noted)

Bennies	Double cross	Roses
Blue angels	Flake (cocaine)	Snow (cocaine)
Chris	Footballs	Speed
Christmas trees	Gold dust (cocaine)	Speedball (heroin + cocaine)
Coast to coast	Green and clears	Truck driver
Coke (cocaine)	Hearts	Uppers
Crystal	Lip poppers	Whites
Dexies	Meth	

Analgesics

Heroin		Other
Boy	Scat	Black (opium)
Brown	Shit	Blue velvet (paregoric + antihistamine)
H	Skag	Dollies (methadone)
Horse	Smack	M (morphine)
Junk		Microdots (morphine)
		Perks (Percodan/Percocet)
		Pinks and greys (Darvon)
		Poppy (opium)
		Tar (opium)
		Terp (terpin hydrate)

Cannabinols

Marijuana-like		Hashish-like
Acapulco gold	MJ	Bhang
Brick	Muggles	Charas
Grass	Pot	Gage
Hay	Reefer	Ganja
Hemp	Roach	Hash
Jive	Rope	Rope
Joint	Sativa	Sweet Lucy
Key	Stick	
Lid	Tea	
Locoweed	Weed	
Mary Jane	Yesca	

Phencyclidine (PCP)

Angel dust	Hog	Shermans
Aurora	Jet	Sherms
Busy bee	K	Special A coke
Cheap cocaine	Lovely	Superacid
Cosmos	Mauve	Supercoke
Criptal	Mist	Supergrass
Dummy mist	Mumm dust	Superjoint
Goon	Peace pill	Tranq
Green	Purple	Whack
Guerilla	Rocket fuel	

Hallucinogens

Acid (LSD)	Cube (LSD)	Mescal (mescaline)
Blue dots (LSD)	D (LSD)	Owsleys (LSD)
Cactus (mescaline)		Pearly gates (morning-glory seeds)

first time every day. Unfortunately, the potential adverse effects of "pure" cocaine are exponentially compounded by the practice of adding adulterants (stepping on) to the original product to increase the pusher's profit margin significantly. Thus, cocaine can be "cut" with local anesthetics (procaine, lidocaine, tetracaine), other stimulants (amphetamine, caffeine, methylphenidate, strychnine), hallucinogens (lysergic acid and diethylamide [LSD], PCP, marijuana, hashish), opioids (codeine, heroin), and a wide variety of other substances (quinine, talc, cornstarch, lactose, mannitol, inositol, sucrose, maltose).

Cocaine goes by about as many names (Table 85-4) as there are ingredients with which it is cut. Thus, the emergency physician can expect to hear such terms as toot, blow, nose-candy, her, she, lady, flake, rock, and coke all used to describe cocaine. Speedball is a combination of cocaine and heroin, which is administered intravenously, with potentially lethal effects (reputed to have killed comedian John Belushi). In 1987, speedballing accounted for one third of all cocaine-related emergency visits in Miami. The price of cocaine varies significantly, as does its purity. Drug Enforcement Administration statistics show that nationally the price of cocaine varies between $80 and $120 per gram and $1200 and $2500 per ounce, with purity ranging from 20% to 70%. The Drug Enforcement Administration reports a trend toward a reduction in price, with an increase in purity; thus, cocaine is no longer just a drug for the rich. Incidentally, pharmaceutical cocaine for the medical industry sells for about $200 per ounce. Used medically, it is the topical anesthetic of choice for procedures in the nose, throat, and oral cavity. Its onset is immediate, with a duration of action up to one hour. In addition to its anesthetic effects, it is a potent vasoconstrictor and decongestant, making it an ideal adjunct in nasal packing for epistaxis and nasotracheal intubation. After nasotracheal intubation with a 10% cocaine solution, blood levels of the drug are less than 150 ng/mL.

Besides its local anesthetic properties, cocaine is a potent CNS stimulant. Its exact mechanism of action is unknown but may be related to depression of inhibitory pathways. Cocaine prevents the uptake of norepinephrine and dopamine by the adrenergic nerve terminals and also prevents the uptake of exogenously administered epinephrine, resulting in increased levels of circulating catecholamines. The result is increased adrenergic symptoms.

There are numerous ways in which cocaine can be introduced into one's system. Nasal insufflation remains the most common route of abuse. Cocaine, in its crystalline hydrochloride form (water-soluble and permeable through mucous membranes) is arranged in columns (called lines) on a hard nonporous surface (usually a mirror or smooth glass top). A typical line measures one eighth of an inch by two inches. This is inhaled into the nostrils with any convenient hollow cylindrical device (a straw, rolled-up currency, or a special cocaine insufflator purchased for nominal cost at any modern "head shop.") "Coke spoons" hold from 5 to 10 mg of powder, and one spoonful is snorted per nostril (a "one on one"). Some of the commerically produced cocaine insufflators are ingeniously camouflaged to resemble trade-name inhalers (Vicks and Afrin nasal decongestants); thus, their use in public is anything but rare. Typically, 1 g of cocaine yields about 40 lines.

FREE BASE

The trend in the late 1980s was to get higher faster, using less of the drug. Significant fervor was created in the news media (stemming from the untimely deaths of several youthful sports celebrities) over an alleged new form of cocaine called crack, reputed to be pure cocaine at one third of the cost. In reality, crack is simply cocaine that has been free-based—a process in which the hydrochloride molecule is removed from the cocaine, leaving the basic cocaine molecule free, by itself (hence the term free base). The process is simple and is performed with little cost and expertise. Of the two processes currently used, the more sophisticated of the two utilizes crystalline cocaine, alkali, and ether.

Cocaine hydrochloride is water-soluble. Thus, a solution of cocaine is created by dissolving a fixed amount (usually a gram) of cocaine in water. To this solution is added a small amount of an industrial strength alkali (sodium or ammonium hydroxide), which forms a chloride precipitate and leaves free cocaine (water-insoluble but petroleum-soluble) in suspension above it. To this suspension is added a given amount of anhydrous diethyl ether, and the resultant is shaken vigorously. Because of the differentials in specific gravity, the solution of cocaine and ether floats to the top, where it is then drawn off and set on an evaporating dish for about 5 minutes. Because of the extreme volatility of the ether, evaporation is completed during this time, leaving behind a dry, crystalline version of the cocaine known as "free base." The free base is then scraped up, placed in a water pipe or rolled in a cigarette, and smoked. Free base is not water-soluble; therefore it cannot be snorted or injected (without consequences). Anhydrous diethyl ether is *extremely* flammable; thus the process is not without risk of fire and explosion. The safer, though reputedly less refined, way to produce free base is by placing the powder hydrochloride into aqueous solution, adding a predetermined amount of standard baking soda, and heating the resulting mixture to boiling. The free base congeals at the bottom and hardens into a rock-like consistency when the mixture cools. It is extracted from the water and smoked.

The effects of smoking free base are rapid and profound. Being absorbed directly through the alveoli, cocaine is rapidly introduced into the systemic circulation and delivered to the brain in amounts almost comparable with those achieved through parenteral administration, despite the fact that a typical inhalation on the pipe (a "hit") involves a dose less than one fiftieth of a gram. This immediate CNS stimulation is described as a "head rush" and typically lasts no longer than 5 to 10 minutes. The user, in an effort to recapture this initial sensation of euphoria, takes repeated doses of the drug, without a satisfactory end point being achieved. The assault is escalated until the user runs out of drug, money, or life. After the assault, the user is usually exhausted and markedly depressed.

The rapid rise of plasma cocaine levels associated with free-basing has profound effects on the cardiovascular system. There is an almost immediate surge in heart rate and blood pressure because of overstimulation of the adrenergic nervous system, and at extremely high doses, cocaine has a direct toxic action on the myocardium, causing cardiac failure and sudden death. Clear-cut evidence is emerging of a causal relationship between increasing dosage of cocaine and onset of angina pectoris and even acute myocardial infarction. The mechanism of the latter is thought to be mediated by a combination of tachycardia, marked increase in afterload, and increases in myocardial oxygen demand, and direct cocaine-induced coronary artery vasospasm (Lange, 1989). This is certainly hazardous for those with underlying fixed coronary artery disease, but it also places otherwise normal subjects at increased risk of cardiac damage in the face of cocaine abuse. In fact, the occurrence of acute myocardial infarction in any young patient (under 40) without a history of risk factors should raise the suspicion of coronary spasm related to cocaine abuse until proved otherwise.

Cocaine abuse has been implicated in the cause of cerebrovascular accidents in otherwise young, normotensive patients; the adrenergic stimulation causes a rapid surge in blood pressure that precipitates intracerebral hemorrhage, especially in persons with underlying arteriovenous malformations and cerebral aneurysms.

Cocaine (pKa = 8.6) is rapidly hydrolyzed in the stomach but poorly absorbed in the alkaline environment of the duodenum. Because of its vasoconstrictive properties, cocaine alters its own absorption after first-order kinetics; its half-life when intranasally administered is 75 minutes, compared with 48 minutes for oral administration. When it is parenterally administered, the half-life increases to nearly 3 hours.

Cocaine is metabolized by enzymatic hydrolysis to several detectable urinary byproducts, including benzoylecgonine (the basis of the urinary drug screen for cocaine abuse), ecgonine, norbenzoylecgonine, and norecgonine. The hydrolysis occurs within the liver and by means of pseudocholinesterases in the plasma. N-demethylation occurs within the liver. A portion of the cocaine introduced into the system is excreted unchanged in the urine in an amount dependent inversely on the pH of the urine (the lower the urinary

pH, the greater the amount of *unmetabolized* drug excreted). This phenomenon is not helpful in the elimination of the drug because only a very small percentage is excreted unchanged, regardless of urinary pH.

The median lethal dose of cocaine by oral administration is about 500 mg. Deaths by oral administration are usually secondary to rupture of packets concealed within a smuggler's gastrointestinal tract ("body packer" syndrome). By contrast, deaths after parenteral (including free-basing) administration have been reported with as little as 20 mg of cocaine. Because a portion of the metabolic breakdown of cocaine depends on pseudocholinesterases within the plasma, individuals with a deficiency of this enzyme are at greater risk of toxic and lethal reactions from standard use of the drug. Concomitant use of drugs that affect neurotransmitters, such as monoamine oxidase inhibitors, reserpine, methyldopa, and tricyclic antidepressants, has been associated with the precipitation of catecholamine crisis in the cocaine abuser.

The manifestations of **cocaine overdose** involve mainly the central and autonomic nervous system. After low doses, symptoms of excitement, euphoria, and restlessness occur that quickly progress to apprehension and anxiety. Low doses increase motor activity, initially manifested by twitching of small muscles in the fingers and face. With higher doses, hyperreflexia and tonic-clonic seizures may occur.

Further stimulation is followed by CNS depression: paralysis of motor activity, hyporeflexia and eventual areflexia, stupor progressing to coma, loss of vital functions, and death. This biphasic response (stimulation followed by depression) to cocaine abuse has been called the caine reaction (Table 85-5).

Cocaine initially stimulates and then depresses the medullary respiratory center. It also has direct effects on the lungs and can precipitate noncardiogenic pulmonary edema when high doses are administered parenterally. The cardiovascular and neurovascular sequelae have already been discussed. In addition, cocaine has been implicated in the initiation of many cardiac dysrhythmias, including sinus tachycardia, ventricular ectopic impulses, ventricular tachycardia

TABLE 85-5. THE CAINE REACTION

Phase	Central Nervous System	Circulatory System	Respiratory System
Early stimulation	Excitement; apprehension; emotional instability; sudden headache; twitching of small muscles, especially in the face and fingers	Pulse varies, usually slows; possible elevated blood pressure; pallor	Increased rate and depth
Advanced stimulation	Convulsions (tonic-clonic), resemble grand mal epilepsy	Increase in both heart rate and blood pressure	Cyanosis, dyspnea, gasping, irregular respiration
Depression	Paralysis, areflexia, coma, loss of vital signs, death	Circulatory failure, pulseless death	Respiratory failure, ashen gray appearance, cyanosis, death

or fibrillation, and asystole. Hyperthermia secondary to direct hypothalmic stimulation, vasoconstriction, and increased muscular activity may be a contributing factor in cocaine-related deaths.

EMERGENCY MANAGEMENT OF COCAINE TOXICITY

The Drug Evaluation Handbook of the American Medical Association suggests a maximal safe dose of clinically administered cocaine to be 1 mg per kg of body weight. Realistically, the maximal dose recommended by standard textbooks of anesthesiology and pharmacology is 3 mg per kg of body weight.

The fatal dose varies with the route of administration, being about 1.4 g by insufflation in a 70 kg individual and 700 to 800 mg by intravenous, subcutaneous, or respiratory routes. The fatal dose is much higher on a milligram-by-milligram basis by the oral route because cocaine is rapidly hydrolyzed in the stomach. Perhaps because of idiosyncratic reaction as much as direct toxicity, fatalities from as little as 25 mg applied to mucous membranes have been reported.

The human body has been shown capable of detoxifying one lethal dose of cocaine per hour or more than 10 g per day, but individual variations is so great as to make this fact of academic importance only. It is far more important to remember that cocaine has low therapeutic ratio and margin of safety.

It is interesting that a bona fide case of cocaine-induced anaphylaxis has never been recorded; subsequently, the toxic effects of cocaine have been attributed to overdose (actual or relative), rapid intravascular absorption, or allergy (theoretically). Thus systemic toxicosis from cocaine is thought to be caused by an overwhelming adrenergic stimulation of the central nervous, cardiovascular, and respiratory systems, as manifested in the caine reaction. These signs are listed in the order in which they are expected to occur clinically, and the physician should make every attempt to assess by clinical signs the patient's progression into the caine reaction and to institute appropriate therapy immediately. Usually, these signs are easily observed. The progression need not be extensive, and resolution typically occurs within 20 minutes.

In fatal cases, however, an *accelerated* onset and progression of symptoms through the caine reaction are observed. Convulsions and death are likely to occur within 2 to 3 minutes (although they can be delayed for up to 30 minutes). If a patient survives the first 3 hours of an accelerated caine reaction, recovery is likely. If recovery does occur, it is likely to be complete in 1 to 3 hours, or there might be persisting headache or malaise for several days. Those cases with severe circulatory collapse or respiratory failure have a high incidence of brain damage caused by cerebral hypoxia.

TREATMENT

The management of cocaine intoxication depends on the patient's progress through the caine reaction. Obviously, the fundamentals of resuscitative efforts must always be kept in mind, and during the depression phase, ventilation may be inadequate, necessitating endotracheal intubation and assisted ventilation.

Seizures may be controlled with diazepam and, if necessary, phenobarbital. Status epilepticus is best treated with a muscle relaxant, such as pancuronium bromide, with control of the airway, with or without an ultra-short-acting barbiturate, such as thiopental. If the patient is hyperthermic, succinylcholine should not be used because muscle fasciculations induced by this drug could make the situation worse.

The cardiovascular effects of hypertension and tachycardia are managed according to their severity: mild forms require only supportive care and observation; significant tachycardia (more than 150 beats/per minute) and hypertension (higher than 180/120 mm Hg) can be treated by nonselective β-adrenergic blockade (with propranolol) alone or in combination with either phentolamine (α-adrenergic blockade) or sodium nitroprusside. The rationale for the use of α-adrenergic blockade in the treatment of cocaine-induced hypertension is that the elevation in blood pressure is caused not only by β-adrenergic stimulation (tachycardia with increased cardiac output) but also by vasoconstriction associated with α-adrenergic overdrive. The use of propranolol by itself in the hyperkinetic, tachycardiac, hypertensive cocaine-intoxicated patient can be dangerous in that it may result in unopposed α-adrenergic-mediated vasoconstriction and aggravate existing hypertension. A rational and viable alternative to the above regimen is the use of labetalol, an adrenergic receptor blocking agent that has *both* α_1-and nonselective β-adrenergic actions. It has been used successfully in the treatment of significant hypertension and tachycardia in cocaine intoxication and theoretically is the *single* drug of choice.

Hypotension is treated with parenteral fluids and, if necessary, pressors such as dopamine or preferably norepinephrine. Complications of ventricular ectopy, tachycardia, and fibrillation are treated by standard advanced cardiac life support (ACLS) protocols. Hyperthermia is treated supportively. Table 85-6 outlines the treatment of cocaine intoxication.

PHENCYCLIDINE

Phenylcyclohexylpiperidine (phencyclidine, PCP) is a drug of increasing abuse. According to the United States Department of Health and Human Services, its primary abusing population is young black and Hispanic men. Emergency Department (ED) visits related

TABLE 85-6. TREATMENT OF COCAINE INTOXICATION

Symptoms	Treatment
Respiratory depression	Endotracheal intubation/assisted ventilation
Convulsions	Diazepam
	children 0.1–0.3 mg/kg body weight IV
	adults 2–10 mg IV
	If necessary: phenobarbital
	children 5 mg/kg body weight IV
	adults 60–100 mg IV
	If necessary: thiopental
	+
	Succinylcholine 40–100 mg IV
	or
	Pancuronium 0.05 mg/kg body weight IV
Cardiovascular effects	
Tachycardia	Observation
	If necessary: propranolol 1 mg IV—dose may be repeated to total of 5 mg
Hypertension	Observation; avoid hypertonic fluids
	If necessary:
	propranolol
	phentolamine
	nitroprusside
	labetalol
Hypotension	Hypertonic fluids
	dopamine
	epinephrine bitartrate (preferred)
Ventricular ectopy	Lidocaine 1 mg/kg body weight stat followed by ½ bolus q 10 min until every ectopy suppressed or until total dose of 3 mg/kg body weight administered; then drip at 2–4 mg/min
Ventricular fibrillation	Standard advanced cardiac life support protocols
Hyperthermia	Generalized cooling measures

to PCP use increased by 82% in 1987, with PCP-related deaths up nearly 95%. To compound the problem, clandestine PCP laboratories are emerging nationwide, with capabilities of manufacturing massive quantities of this illicit substance. In 1985, for example, two PCP labs were located in Michigan, manufacturing 2.75 million doses of PCP per month. One gallon of PCP sells on the street for about $13,000, and wholesale quantities of PCP solution for dipping "joints" or cigarettes are available at $300 per fluid ounce.

In 1957, PCP was developed as a general anesthetic (Sernyl). Although it produced satisfactory anesthesia, many patients experienced severe, frightening postanesthetic reactions that could persist for several days. Subsequently, PCP was not clinically used in humans but instead was marketed as a veterinary anesthetic (Sernylan). Veterinary use was soon discontinued as well.

In 1967, an oral form of PCP emerged in California, but its unpredictable side effects discouraged its use until the late 1970s. It has slowly but steadily grown in popularity since. Smoking is the most common dosing route, with users mixing powdered or liquefied PCP with tobacco, marijuana, parsley, mint, or oregano.

Few other drugs are described by so many names as PCP (see Table 85-4), and frequently it is misrepresented as other drugs such as tetrahydrocannabinol (THC), LSD, cocaine, or psilocybin, resulting in inadvertent overdose and mixed overdose involving PCP.

Phencyclidine is an arylcyclohexylamine related to ketamine. It is a weak base with a pKa of 8.5. Markedly lipophilic, is has a wide distribution throughout the body and is rapidly absorbed through any route of administration. It is metabolized by conjugation in the liver, where both conjugated and free forms are excreted in the urine.

EFFECTS

Phencyclidine has a varied mechanism of action, which in turn results in diverse clinical presentations among its users. By modifying association pathways linking the cerebral cortex to deeper brain tissue, it alters the user's ability to process sensory stimuli and respond appropriately. The result is psychotic behavior, anesthesia, and sedation. In addition, PCP can have both cholingeric (salivation, bronchorrhea, and bronchospasm) and anticholinergic/adrenergic (tachycardia, hyporeflexia, hypotension) effects. Dopaminergic activity is manifested by athetosis, although dopaminergic antagonism can prevail, as evidenced by localized dystonia. When all these confusing symptoms are combined with drug impurity, a variable half-life of 7 to 46 hours, and polydrug ingestions, we begin to appreciate the varied clinical presentations of the PCP abuser.

Nonetheless, the hallmarks of the PCP intoxication syndrome are nystagmus and hypertension, with 57% of affected persons exhibiting one or both. Hypertension tends to be mild. Thirty percent of patients have a mild tachycardia (100 to 120 beats/min). Surprisingly, 46% of patients are alert and oriented. Because 37% present with some form of acute organic brain syndrome, it is not surprising that these patients tend to be poor historians, and the emergency physician must look to friends or significant others to elicit a meaningful history. Abnormal behavior is common, and includes violence, agitation, bizarre actions, hallucinations, mutism, and staring (listed according to decreasing frequency of occurrence). The anesthetizing effects of PCP may prevent the intoxicated patient from responding appropriately to pain and can increase the risk of accidental or intentional injury. Death by drowning or jumping from heights has also been reported.

Despite the fact that PCP is readily detected in the urine through thin-layer or gas chromatography, it should be kept in mind that not all toxicology screens detect PCP and that there is a poor correlation between urine PCP levels and clinical severity of intoxication. Elevated serum levels of uric acid and creatine kinase are ominous signs in PCP intoxications because as they imply PCP-induced rhabdomyolysis with the potential for renal failure. A quick method of screening rhabdomyolysis is dipping the urine for blood. A positive result from the dip in the face of a negative result from microscopic examination for red blood cells is strong presumptive evidence for the presence of myoglobinuria secondary to rhabdomyolysis (hemoglobinuria and large doses of ascorbic acid can also mimic this finding).

Therapeutic priorities in treatment of PCP intoxication are determined by the degree of intoxication, which is arbitrarily divided into major and minor intoxications.

MAJOR INTOXICATIONS

The complications from PCP intoxication are directly proportional to its severity. Acute brain syndrome is the most common presentation of major intoxication and is manifested by poor judgment, inappropriate affect, decreased attention span, and inability to concentrate. Severely intoxicated patients may rapidly progress to coma or be comatose on arrival. Compounding this problem are the concomitant injuries frequently found in the phencyclidine-intoxicated person, so that altered level of consciousness may be caused by drug effects, head injury, or both. Computed tomography (CT) is often required to distinguish between the two.

Catatonic patients characteristically display catalepsy, posturing, mutism, rigidity, staring, and negativism, all of variable duration from a few hours to several days. Patients intoxicated with PCP may be erroneously diagnosed as being purely psychotic, because they frequently exhibit characteristics of hallucinations, mania, paranoia, and homicidal or suicidal behavior. Residual psychosis may persist for several weeks.

MINOR INTOXICATIONS

With minor PCP intoxications, patients may exhibit any of the findings of major intoxications but to a much diminished degree. Sedation is common, with the patient responding to verbal and tactile stimuli but becoming stuporous on withdrawal of stimuli. The symptoms mimic sedative-hypnotic overdose. Agitation is frequently seen, with increased psychomotor activity and irritability. These patients tend to be alert and oriented. Violence, manifested both verbally and physically, is a common presentation in the ED. Bizzarre behavior without overt thought disorders is seen in some alert and oriented patients. Some intoxicated individuals are happy, if not euphoric, without any untoward effects.

TREATMENT

The treatment of PCP intoxication remains a subject of controversy and ranges from intervention in all cases to close observation and supportive care, which avoid the potential morbidity of vigorous therapy. Intervention should focus on life support, elimination of the drug, behavior modification, and treatment of motor abnormalities.

LIFE SUPPORT

These measures are reserved for patients exhibiting a need for this type of intervention. Classically, life support is required primarily in the major intoxications, but because of premorbid conditions, polydrug abuse, and other extenuating factors, it can be called on at any time, and treatment plans must be individualized. Complications include cardiovascular dysfunction, respiratory distress, CNS abnormalities, rhabdomyolysis, urinary retention, and metabolic and temperature derangements.

The most common cardiovascular abnormalities are tachycardia and hypertension. These are usually seen in conjunction with agitation and require no specific treatment unless they are hemodynamically significant. Nonetheless, continuous cardiac and blood pressure monitoring is indicated. Sedatives of the benzodiazepine variety are remarkably effective in reducing agitation and subsequently tachycardia and hypertension; seldom are antihypertensives or cardiac drugs required.

Respiratory distress may occur in the catatonic patient because of pooling of upper airway secretions; comatose patients should have endotracheal intubation to maintain and protect the airway. Respiratory arrest is rare (3% of patients) in PCP intoxications. Naloxone (Narcan) is given intravenously as an adjunct to therapy because many patients have mixed PCP and opiate overdoses. Serial arterial blood gas sampling is used to assess the adequacy of ventilation and to monitor acid-base derangements.

Although seizures are rare (3% of patients) in PCP overdoses their presence should be treated vigorously to prevent complications of hypoxemia and rhabdomyolysis. Intravenous diazepam is the drug of choice for uncomplicated seizures. Prolonged seizures should be treated with pancuronium or some other curarelike agent because rhabdomyolysis and acute renal failure should be avoided at all cost in PCP overdose with seizures. Close monitoring of urinary output and blood urea nitrogen and creatinine concentrations are imperative once rhabdomyolysis has occurred. Peritoneal dialysis or hemodialysis may be required in patients with acute renal failure. Acidification of the urine to enhance renal excretion of PCP by ion trapping is contraindicated in the presence of rhabdomyolysis because acidfication decreases renal excretion of myoglobin with subsequent precipitation of acute renal failure. Acute urinary retention secondary to PCP use is easily handled by bladder catheterization.

DRUG ELIMINATION

In the past traditional therapy has been to enhance clearance of PCP by gastric lavage to diminish absorption and by acidification of the urine to enhance excretion.

Gastric lavage followed by the administration of activated charcoal is indicated in the treatment of PCP intoxication, regardless of the route of PCP use; the rationale here is that PCP is absorbed in the enterohepatic circulation and re-excreted into the gut. Thus, serial administrations of activated charcoal should be considered, especially in patients with persistent symptoms.

The practice of trapping ions of PCP to promote their excretion in the urine by acidification with ascorbic acid or ammonium chloride has sound theoretic indications. It probably should not be used however for several reasons:

1. 90% of PCP clearance is hepatic.
2. As alluded to above, urine acidification reduces myoglobin clearance and can precipitate acute renal failure.
3. Probably less than 11% of unbound PCP in intoxicated patients is renally excreted and therefore clinically insignificant.
4. Acidification techniques tend to worsen pre-existing metabolic acidosis.

BEHAVIOR MODIFICATION

Abnormal behavior, such as lethargy, withdrawal, stupor, euphoria, or bizarre acts, is usually not harmful to the patient or others and resolves spontaneously. Behavioral abnormalities are frequently exacerbated by external stimuli (loud noises, bright lights), and close observation in a video-monitored room is the best form of management.

For *extreme* violence or agitation, the patient should be restrained. "Mummification" is preferred to four-point restraints for patient safety, comfort, and reduction of potential for rhabdomyolysis, but is easier said than done with a struggling, agitated patient. Haloperidol (5 to 10 mg administered intramuscularly every hour, as needed) is a tremendous adjunct in treating these patients. Phenothiazines should not be used in PCP overdoses, for they reduce seizure threshold, precipitate hypotension, and accentuate anticholinergic effects.

TREATMENT OF ADVERSE MOTOR REACTIONS

In addition to seizures, the common motor findings in PCP intoxication are generalized rigidity (5% of patients) and dystonia and athetosis (1% to 3% of patients). Diphenhydramine (25 to 50 mg administered intramuscularly or intravenously) is effective for dystonia. Athetosis is usually transient and requires no specific treatment.

HOSPITAL DISCHARGE

Minor intoxications can usually be adequately handled with 4 to 6 hours of ED observation. Psychiatric or social service consultation, or both, is indicated for management of acute cases and to decrease the likelihood of recurrence. The patient should be discharged from the ED in the company of a responsible adult who understands the rationale for follow-up care and who has been counseled about the possibility of post-intoxication confusion, anxiety, or depression. Favorable results have been achieved in the treatment of depression secondary to chronic cocaine and PCP abuse with the tricylic antidepressant desipramine.

Major intoxications with PCP should be handled in an intensive care unit until stabilization has occurred. In complicated cases, the patient may require weeks of in-house recovery.

DESIGNER DRUGS

Designer drugs include a number of compounds that produce effects similar or identical to those of currently illegal street drugs (or controlled substances). "Designer" describes the attempt to chemically modify a scheduled drug so that it becomes legal under the definition of current narcotic legislation. In California, considered to be the home of the designer cult, the major drugs encountered are analogues of fentanyl and meperidine.

Fentanyl analogues have the *potential* for causing fatal overdose. About 100 overdoses have been recorded in the past 5 years. It is estimated that fentanyl analogues are available to about 10% of narcotic users in California. With over 200 *fatal* heroin overdoses recorded annually in the state, 100 overdoses over a 5-year period is certainly not a very striking number. There exist no hard and fast scientific data as to whether the fentanyls are actually more dangerous than heroin. The other big problem with researching adverse effects of designer drugs is that they are difficult to detect, and there is no national surveillance program to determine where and how intensively they are distributed. Recent increases in fentanyl use in the eastern United States with reported deaths (Martin et al, 1991) may portend a widening evidence of use.

Meperidine analogues rose to scientific prominence in 1982 when Langston discovered cases of parkinsonism caused by the neurotoxin methyl-phenyltetrahydropyridine (MPTP), a compound produced during the synthesis of the meperidine analogue methylphenylpropenylpiperidinol propanoate (MPPP). The production of MPPP is an equilibrium reaction and *always* produces some MPTP.

The Centers for Disease Control and the National Institute of Drug Abuse began work with William Langston at the Santa Clara Valley Medical Center in January 1985 to identify people exposed to MPTP in 1982. Several people reported *recent* use of a drug that produced symptoms similar to those noted in 1982.

The best data available at present on the availability of meperidine analogues come from law enforcement intelligence information. In a raid on a clandestine PCP laboratory in Brownsville, Texas, in late 1984, it was learned that this laboratory was also producing a new meperidine analogue named PEPAOP. It is similar to MPPP and also contains a contaminant, PEPTP, an analogue of MPTP. A link was also established between the operators of this laboratory and the original MPPP/MPTP manufacturers in California. Other evidence includes data from two methamphetamine laboratories raided in San Diego in late 1984. Both had "cookbook" recipes for the production of MPPP.

The only way to confirm the presence of meperidine analogues in urine or street samples is to send them to the Langston laboratory or the Drug Enforcement Administration's Special Testing Laboratory.

Until adequate analytic techniques are developed, screening for the *acute symptoms* of meperidine analogue exposure remains the only means of determining the presence of these drugs in a given patient. Additionally, the emergency physician can focus on the chronic symptoms of what has come to be called MPTP-induced parkinsonism in deciding whether a given patient has been exposed to a meperidine an-

alogue. The sequence of symptoms now being seen in most cases is different from those observed by Langston et al. in their original study. These patients were characterized by severe symptoms of irreversible parkinsonism. Most people exposed to meperidine analogues have not shown these severe symptoms but have subtle manifestations of early parkinsonism.

CLINICAL PRESENTATIONS

In general, there appear to be three stages of clinical presentations produced by meperidine analogues:

The Acute Phase. The patient experiences the psychotropic effects of the drug. Unless the clinician is able to get a sample of the drug or a urine sample from the patient within 24 hours of ingestion, the diagnosis must be made by inference from the clinical presentation. The two cardinal symptoms are the history of drug use that produced an atypical disorienting "high" that was strikingly different from that of opioids, and the complaint of an intense burning that travels from the injection site along the course of the afferent vein. Other common but less diagnostic symptoms include blurred vision, metallic or medicine-like taste in the mouth, tics, myoclonic jerks, athetoid movement, hyperhydrosis, and muscle rigidity.

The Subacute Phase. This is observed in patients who continue to use meperidine analogues over the course of several days. During periods of continuous use, adverse symptoms may persist long after the attenuation of psychotropic effects.

The Chronic Phase. Prolonged use results in symptoms of pain and stiffness in the muscles and joints, tremors of the limbs, blurred vision, bradykinesia (slow and effortful movement), oiliness of the skin, hyperhydrosis, memory loss, and dysarthria.

TREATMENT

Acute overdosage is treated the same as other narcotic toxicities. Antiparkinson drugs may be useful in controlling Parkinson-like, extrapyramidal symptoms. Chronic brain damage can respond partially to removal of the drug, good nutrition, and overall change in lifestyle.

HALLUCINOGENS AND CANNABIS

The hallucinogens are a heterogeneous group of substances that produce characteristic "psychedelic" alterations in perception, thought, and affect. Although

| TABLE 85-7. COMMONLY ABUSED PSYCHEDELICS |

Indole group
  Lysergic acid diethylamide (LSD)
  Psylocybin, psylocin
  Dimethyltryptamine (DMT)
  Diethyltryptamine (DET)
  Dipropyltryptamine (DPT)
  Iboga alkaloids
  Harmala alkaloids
  Myristicin compounds, morning glory seeds
Phenylethylamine group
  Peyote, mescaline
  Dimethoxymethylamphetamine (DOM, STP)
  Methylene dioxyamphetamine (MDA)
  Methoxymethylene dioxyamphetamine (MMDA)
Miscellaneous
  Phencyclidine (PCP)
  Nutmeg
  Cannabis, tetrahydrocannabinol (THC)

there are differences in potency, route of administration, somatic side effects, and duration of action, all these agents produce similar CNS effects. The term "cannabis" encompasses the various preparations derived from the Indian hemp plant Cannabis sativa and other Cannabis species. Marijuana and related drugs have some effects similar to those of the sedatives and, particularly in higher doses, to the hallucinogens. See Table 85-7 for commonly abused psychedelics.

ABUSE PATTERNS

The use of hallucinogens is most prevalent among educated, affluent young people who smoke marijuana more or less regularly. The usual pattern is an occasional "trip" separated from other episodes by several weeks or months. Physical dependence does not occur. A temporary tolerance to the effects of these drugs rapidly develops after a few daily doses. For most users, a feeling of satiety follows intoxication, resulting in longer intervals between doses than dictated by the tolerance phenomenon. In addition, there is a tendency toward diminished hallucinogen use with time, so that long-term chronic abuse is rarely encountered.

Lysergic acid diethylamide (LSD) is the most potent hallucinogen known. The major effects of LSD ingestion are referrable to the CNS and are considerably influenced by the expectations of the user. The subjective experience is multifaceted and may include feelings of transcendence, hyperemotionality, novelty of perception, and various ineffable alterations in consciousness. Most effects subside within 8 to 10 hours. Use of LSD in the United States has undergone a resurgence and has increased in the past several years.

Phencyclidine hydrochloride (PCP) has come to public attention owing to its gaining prominence among adolescents. Bizarre deaths (some caused by drowning and jumping from rooftops) have occurred. The "angel dust," "THC," or "hog" is occasionally smoked or snorted or mixed with marijuana. Muscular incoordination, nystagmus, loss of judgment, and feelings of weightlessness occur even with small doses of PCP and is probably related to the deaths from falls and drownings. Serious overdosage itself is far less common than injury resulting from the drug's effects on judgment. (See previous detailed discussion.)

Marijuana smoking is extensively practiced in the United States. It is estimated that 26 million Americans have tried it, that 13 million smoke regularly, and that 2.5 million do so daily. The use of more potent preparations such as hashish ("hash"), hashish oil, THC, and other cannabinoids is less widespread. Smoking produces effects within a few minutes that persist for several hours. Oral ingestion has a longer onset and duration, and the intensity of intoxication is less controlled by the user. Cannabis intoxication produces mood changes, typically mild euphoria; perceptual changes, particularly altered time sense; and various changes in thought processes. With higher doses, disturbances of perception may be marked.

COMMON MEDICAL PROBLEMS

Hallucinogen abuse has been associated with severe depression, paranoia, and prolonged psychosis. Pre-existing psychiatric disorders may be of primary significance in these cases. It appears likely that for certain vulnerable individuals the intense drug experience is sufficient to disrupt psychologic equilibrium.

Information concerning the effects of long-term marijuana use on health is accumulating rapidly. Habitual smokers are subject to an increased risk of bronchitis and other pulmonary diseases. There is conflicting evidence concerning other effects on physical and mental health. The possible psychologic consequences of chronic intoxication are the subject of much controversy.

INTOXICATION

Adverse reactions to hallucinogens are primarily psychologic and behavioral. A "bad trip" is characterized by diminished cognitive control, sensory overload, dysphoria, and panic. Fear of persistence of the reaction is common. Judgment is impaired and behavior is unpredictable. Somatic effects are sympathomimetic: pupillary dilatation, hyperthermia, tachycardia, hypertension, nausea, tremor, and hyperreflexia. "Flashbacks" are recurrences of elements of the drug-induced state subsequent to a period of known pharmacologic activity. Most of these reactions occur within a few days of hallucinogen use and consist of transient episodes of subtle perceptual and affective alterations. In some cases the experience is an intense repetition of an unpleasant aspect of the acute state. Frequent "tripping" is associated with an increased frequency of flashbacks.

Adverse reactions to cannabis are rare in view of the extensive use of these preparations. Intoxication, especially with the more potent forms, can lead to toxic psychosis, paranoia, confusional states, and unpleasant emotional reactions. Perceptual distortions and hallucinations occur. Severe anxiety may be prominent. Physical findings are generally limited to conjunctival injection, tachycardia, hypertension, and dryness of the mouth. Deaths from cannabis overdosage are virtually unknown. Toxicologic determinations are available for most of these substances but are rarely necessary for diagnosis or treatment.

Most adverse reactions to hallucinogens and cannabis are handled uneventfully without medical assistance. Individuals who do seek treatment generally go to neighborhood facilities well known in the drug-using community. Those seen at conventional emergency services tend either to be experiencing more prolonged and intense emotional reactions or to be novices in drug abuse. Finding an understanding person in a serene environment reassures most individuals on a "bad trip," "stoned," or having flashbacks. Characteristically, the user is in a highly suggestible state and responds readily to "talkdown" techniques. Drug-induced panic can be dispelled by a therapist with a benevolent interest in the patient and a confident, deliberate manner. For patients who do not regain their composure, minor tranquilizers and sedatives have value as adjuncts to a supportive environment. Chemotherapy with phenothiazines carries the risk of anticholinergic reactions. Hospitalization is unnecessary except in extreme cases when psychosis or dysphoria persists.

WITHDRAWAL

Withdrawal phenomena are not pronounced after discontinuation of hallucinogen use. Interruption of regular use of cannabis products can lead to irritability, sleeping difficulties, and disturbed gastrointestinal function. These symptoms are generally mild and usually subside without specific treatment. Support groups and counselling can, however, be useful during this period.

INHALANTS

A variety of substances including anesthetics and solvents may be inhaled to produce brief episodes of intoxication. The use of volatile and gaseous anesthetics for such purposes actually antedates their medical applications. Organic solvents are mixtures of petroleum distillates and are found in houshold products such a varnishes, paint thinners, cleaning and lighter fluids, and glues. These chemicals enter the bloodstream through the pulmonary alveoli and rapidly induce alterations in consciousness. See Table 85-8 for commonly abused inhalants.

TABLE 85-8. COMMONLY ABUSED INHALANTS

Anesthetics
  Gases: Nitrous oxide, ethylene, cyclopropane, halothane
  Volatile liquids: Diethyl ether, chloroform, ethyl chloride
Organic solvents
  Gasoline, kerosene, toluene, benzene, carbon tetrachloride
Miscellaneous
  Aerosols: Freon and other fluorocarbon propellants
  Amyl nitrite
  White correction fluid (used in typing)

ABUSE PATTERNS

Anesthetics are diverted for recreational use by health professionals and others who have access to these agents. Gases are administered from the tank, generally with the use of a face mask or other device. Volatile liquids are poured over a cloth that may be held up to the face or placed in the mouth. The intoxication is brief, and inhalation is repeated periodically. Simultaneous intoxication with marijuana or other drugs is common.

Organic solvents are ubiquitous. Intentional sniffing of their vapors is primarily a phenomenon of childhood and adolescence. Youngsters who might have difficulty in obtaining other mind-affecting substances find these to be readily available. Paraphernalia for solvent inhalation include moistened cloths, bags, balloons, and atomizers. Aerosol abuse follows essentially the same pattern.

Inhalants induce a rapidly reversible organic brain syndrome that is similar in most respects to acute alcohol or sedative intoxication. A dreamy euphoria is typical. In some cases, hallucinations accompany the acute state. Drowsiness is a common aftermath. Tolerance and dependence are usually not seen with abuse of inhalants.

Amyl nitrite, which is administered by inhalation in the treatment of angina pectoris is occasionally used for nonmedical purposes. Its reputation for enhancing the duration and intensity of sexual orgasm is responsible for perpetuation of its use in the drug culture. Hypotension is the major adverse effect.

COMMON MEDICAL PROBLEMS

The hazards of inhalation have not been firmly established. Damage to the brain, lungs, heart, liver, kidneys, and bone marrow occurs in some cases, although most of the evidence is drawn from studies of industrial exposure, which may not be comparable to the occasional deliberate sniffing of vapors.

INTOXICATION

Inhalers do not frequently receive emergency medical treatment because the effects of inhalants are generally short-lived. Adverse effects may include agitation, incoordination, confusion, disorientation, delirium, convulsions, and coma. Usually, the inhaler stops before these symptoms emerge. Anoxia occurs with the use of hazardous inhalation techniques. In addition, some agents have direct respiratory depressant effects. Pulmonary edema may develop, further compromising oxygenation. Cardiac arrhythmias and hypotensive episodes are common. This cardiovascular toxicity may be aggravated by anoxia. Cases of sudden death after sniffing of aerosols have been reported and are believed to result from acute arrhythmias.

Removal of the causative agent and exposure of the patient to fresh air are often sufficient to reverse the toxic effects. For more severe reactions, respiratory assistance and oxygen administration may be required. Hypotensive episodes should not be treated with sympathomimetics because of the dangers of precipitating an arrhythmia in a sensitized myocardium.

Supportive medical treatment usually leads to prompt recovery. Patients should be maintained under observation until cardiopulmonary functions have stabilized. Follow-up care in severe poisoning should include assessment of hepatic and renal status. Psychiatric evaluation is indicated after acute symptoms have subsided, particularly in children.

WITHDRAWAL

Withdrawal syndromes do not occur with most of these substances. Habitual use of ether can produce physical dependence and subject the user to a withdrawal syndrome similar to that seen with alcohol.

BIBLIOGRAPHY

Baselt, R.C., Wright, J.A., and Cravey, R.H.: Therapeutic and toxic concentrations of more than 100 toxicologically significant drugs in blood, plasma, or serum: a tabulation. Clin. Chem. 21:44, 1975.

Bourne, P.G. (ed.): A Treatment Manual for Acute Drug Abuse Emergencies. Washington, D.C., National Clearing House for Drug Abuse Information, Publication No. 16, 1974.

Brecher, E.M., and the editors of Consumers Reports: Licit and Illicit Drugs. Boston, Little, Brown & Co., 1972.

Cogen, F.C., Rigg, G., Simmons, I.L., et al.: Phencyclidine associated acute rhabdomyolysis. Ann. Intern. Med. 88:210, 1978.

Corales, R.L., Maull, K.I., Becker, D.P.: Phencyclidine abuse mimicking head injury. JAMA 243:2323, 1980.

Cregler, L.L. and Mark, H.: Cardiovascular dangers of cocaine abuse. Am. J. Cardiol. 57:1185, 1986.

Dailey, R.H.: Fatality secondary to misuse of TAC (tetracaine, adrenaline, cocaine) solution. Ann. Emerg. Med. 17:159, 1988.

Ellenhorn, M.J., and Barceloux, D.G.: Medical Toxicology, New York, Elsevier, 1988.

Fish, F. and Wilson, W.D.C.: Excretion of cocaine and its metabolites in man. J. Pharm. Pharmacol. 32:1355, 1969.

Foster, B., et al.: Pathogenesis of coronary artery disease and the acute coronary syndromes. N. Engl. J. Med. 326:310, 1992.

Freed, E.F.: Drug abuse by alcoholics: a review. Int. J. Addictions 8:451, 1973.

Gawin, F.H., Ellinwood, E.H.: Cocaine and other stimulants: Actions, abuse, and treatment. N. Engl. J. Med. 318:1173, 1988.

Gay, G.R.: Clinical management of acute and chronic cocaine poisoning. Ann. Emerg. Med. 11:562, 1982.

Giannini, A.J., Malone, D.A., Giannini, M.C., et al.: Treatment of depression in chronic cocaine and phencyclidine abuse with desipramine. J. Clin. Pharmacol. 26:211, 1986.

Goldfrank, L., Flomenbaum, N., and Weisman, R.: General management of the poisoned and overdosed patient. Hospital Physician, July 1981.

Handal, K.A., Schauben, J.L., and Salamone, F.R.: Naloxone. Ann. Emerg. Med. 12:438, 1983.

Itkonen, J., Schnoll, S. and Glassroth, J.: Pulmonary dysfunction in freebase cocaine users. Arch. Intern. Med. 144:2195, 1984.

Kogan, M.J., Verchey, K.G., DePace, A.C., et al.: Quantitative determination of benzoyl-ecgonine and cocaine in human biofluids by gas-liquid chromatography. Anal. Chem. 49:1965, 1977.

Lange, R.A., et al.: Cocaine-induced coronary artery vasospasm. N. Engl. J. Med. 23:1557, 1989.

Martin, M., et al.: China white epidemic—An eastern U.S. Emergency Department experience. Ann. Emerg. Med. 20:158, 1991.

McCarron, M.M., Schulze, B.W., Thompson, G.A., et al.: Acute phencyclidine intoxication: Incidence of clinical findings in 1,000 cases. Ann. Emerg. Med. 10:237, 1981.

Moore, R., Rumack, B., Conner, C., and Peterson, R.: Naloxone. Am. J. Dis. Child. 134:156, 1980.

National Institute on Drug Abuse Research Monogram Series 64:1, 1986.

National Institute on Drug Abuse: PCP: Update on Abuse. Rockville, MD, October, 1980.

Pasternack, P.F., Colvin, S.B., and Baumann, F.G.: Cocaine-induced angina pectoris and acute myocardial infarction in patients younger than 40 years. Am. J. Cardiol. 55:847, 1985.

Patel, R., Ansari, A., and Hughes, J.I.: Myoglobinuric acute renal failure associated with phencyclidine abuse. West. J. Med. 131:244, 1979.

Pope, H.G., Jr., Ionescu-Pioggia, M., and Cole, J.O.: Drug use and life-style among college undergraduates. Arch. Gen. Psychiatry 38:588, 1981.

Rich, J.A., and Singer, D.E.: Cocaine-related symptoms in patients presenting to an urban Emergency Department. Ann. Emerg. Med. 20:616, 1991.

Ruttenber, A., and Luke, J.: Heroin-related deaths. New epidemiologic insights. Science, 226:14, 1984.

Sapira, J.D.: The narcotic addict as a medical patient. Am. J. Med. 45:555, 1969.

Schlaadt, R.D., Shannon, P.T.: Drugs of Choice—Current Perspectives on Drug Use, 2nd Ed. Englewood Cliffs, New Jersey, Prentice-Hall, 1986.

Schuckit, M.: Drug and Alcohol Abuse. A Clinical Guide

to Diagnosis and Treatment, 2nd Ed. New York and London, Plenum Press, 1985.

Segar, D.L.: Topics in Emergency Medicine: Substances of Abuse. Rockville, Maryland, Aspen Publications, 1985, p 7.

Shearer, R.J., ed.: Manual on Alcoholism. Chicago, American Medical Association, 1968.

U.S. Department of Health and Human Services: Patterns and Trends in Drug Abuse; A National and International Perspective. June 1985, pp. I-1–IV-28.

U.S. Department of Health, Education, and Welfare. First Special Report to the U.S. Congress on Alcohol and Health. Publication No. (HSM) 72-9099, Washington, D.C., 1971.

Waldron, V., Klimt, E., and Seibel, J.: Methodone overdose treated with naloxone infusion. JAMA 225:53, 1973.

Wesson, D.R., and Smith, D.E.: A conceptual approach to detoxification. J. Psychedel. Drugs. 2:161, 1974.

Wyler, D.J.: Malaria—resurgence, resistance, and research. N. Engl. J. Med. 308:934, 1983.

Zimmerman, J.L., et al.: Cocaine-associated chest pain. Ann. Emerg. Med. 20:611, 1991.

SUBSTANCE-INDUCED, PSYCHIATRIC DISORDERS

Michael S. Easton

CAPSULE

Over the past decade, extensive information has accumulated about the rate of drug abuse in our population. In an NIMH epidemiologic catchment area study, the 1-month, 6-month, and lifetime prevalence of drug abuse disorders were reported as 1.3%, 2%, and 5.9% respectively. Alcohol, the most widely abused drug, had prevalences of 2.8%, 4.7% and 13.3%. Of the individuals with an alcohol disorder, 28.5% had a comorbid drug abuse in their lifetime. This is six times greater than in the general population. Almost 50% of those who abused drugs had a lifetime prevalence of alcohol abuse. In people who abused alcohol and drugs, the risk of experiencing a mental disorder was two to four times greater than that of the nonabusing general population. Given the extensive number of individuals suffering from these illnesses, emergency physicians must be prepared to adequately diagnose and treat substance abuse disorders. Although the treatment of acute psychoactive substance intoxication and overdose has been clearly delineated in the previous chapter section, the overall dependency problem has not been given adequate attention. This is partly because the medical profession continues to view addiction as a social or behavioral problem rather than a multifactorial pathophysiologic and psychosocial disorder. As a result, we tend to overlook the ramifications these disorders have on individuals in perpetuating their drug use, altering their behavior, and affecting their psychologic state. Often the severity of an addiction and its comorbid psychiatric or medical problems is overlooked, or when recognized is not viewed as a primary problem or adequately addressed. Emergency Departments (EDs) are often the means by which such patients enter the health care system.

The object of this chapter is to provide a general understanding of the pharmacokinetics and addictive properties of various abused drugs along with their comorbid psychiatric and medical complications. With a better understanding of the psychotropic and addictive qualities of these substances, emergency physicians can make better treatment and follow-up recommendations.

The "problem" or "drug-seeking" patient is commonly seen in the ED. Many such patients are only mildly addicted; others are deeply addicted. In either case, the ED is probably the best location from which to identify problems and refer such patients.

PSYCHOSTIMULANTS

At one time, stimulants (cocaine and amphetamines) were not viewed as physically addicting or having high abuse potential in humans. Yet animal models always demonstrated that chronic stimulant use led to neurochemical changes regulating mood, behavior, and the experience of pleasure, and produced both a physiologic addiction and a withdrawal syndrome. These studies predicted many of the problems we are presently experiencing with humans. A quick review of some of this information will help us to understand the clinical sequelae seen in humans.

Abuse liability is generally determined by a drug's

reinforcing properties and toxicity, following either acute or chronic administration. Stimulants are extremely strong reinforcers because of their euphorogenic effects on the mesocortical/mesolimbic dopamine "pleasure" pathways. When animals are given unlimited access to stimulants, they rapidly escalate drug self-administration, resulting in compulsive use at the exclusion of all other reinforcers (e.g., water, food, socialization and sex). Thirty-day mortality rates in rats given unlimited access to stimulants can be as high as 90% (two to three times greater than with opiates). Only when access to these substances is limited will animals regulate their use. Studies also demonstrate how stimulants can impair the acquisition of new behavior, disrupt normal behavior, and produce disruptive social behaviors. Similar correlations can be seen in the human stimulant-abusing population. Long-term chronic use of stimulants also produces two phenomena: tolerance (decreased response to a given dose) and sensitization (increased response to a given dose). Animal models have demonstrated tolerance to the cardiovascular and euphorogenic properties of stimulants, without change in their reinforcing properties. Sensitization produces increased stereotypic, compulsive, and locomotor behavior in response to repeated single doses. The human correlate of this is an increasing need for more frequent and greater doses to produce euphoria in exclusion of all other needs. At the same time, smaller doses have produced greater degrees of abnormal behavior, and may increase susceptibility to various psychiatric symptoms. Finally, acute high doses and/or chronic administration have been shown to cause neurotoxic effects in animals, ranging from temporary decreases in monoamine levels to permanent decreases in dopamine levels. Such effects in humans have been hypothesized to result in depression, anhedonia (inability to experience pleasure), and intense drug craving, all of which are frequently associated with stimulant abusers.

MECHANISM OF ACTION

Both cocaine and amphetamines, although chemically different, have sympathomimetic properties and exhibit similar neuropharmacologic and behavioral effects when administered in high doses. The effects of both are to increase monoamine (norepinephrine, dopamine and seratonin) transition by either blocking reuptake or increasing release and/or direct agonistic properties. Cocaine may have a slight preferential effect on the dopamine system compared to amphetamines.

PHARMACOKINETICS

Cocaine is used in a variety of forms. The hydrochloride (HCL) salt, a water-soluble white crystalline powder, is used intranasally or intravenously. For smoking, cocaine HCL is converted to its free base by neuralizing the salt with aqueous bicarbonate and then

extracting the alkaloid in ether (see previous chapter section). Coca paste, which is also smoked, is a partially purified extract of the coca leaf and is an impure, less potent form of "free base."

Cocaine, an ester of benzoic acid has a significantly short plasma half-life (approximately 90 minutes) and requires more frequent ingestion than the amphetamines.

The various routes of administration markedly influence the effects of stimulants by altering the rates and magnitude of peak plasma levels.

Bioavailability for the oral or nasal route of ingestion is around 20 to 30%. When chewed (in the form of coca leaf) or inhaled (cocaine HCL), it is absorbed directly through mucous membranes in the nose or mouth and the GI track after swallowing. Blood levels are detected in 3 to 5 minutes after nasal or oral absorption (nasal being somewhat quicker) and 10 to 15 minutes following gastric absorption. Plasma levels tend to remain low (especially with chewing), and peak slowly. The effects, although less intense, last longer than with other routes of administration.

After intravenous injection, subjective and physiologic effects can occur within 30 seconds. Their intensity varies according to the dose and speed of injection (quick low-dose injections have greater effects than multiple larger doses given slowly). Subcutaneous or intramuscular injections are not popular because cocaine induces vasoconstriction and thereby self-limits its rate of absorption.

Pulmonary inhalation (cocaine smoking) and rapid intravenous injection provides the quickest and greatest drug delivery to the CNS. The large capillary/alveolar surface is exposed, resulting in rapid absorption of a large volume or drug. There is also an approximate transit time from the lung-heart-carotid artery to the brain of 7 to 10 seconds. This results in a quick and intense drug effect.

TOXICOLOGY

Cocaine is quickly metabolized by esterases in the liver and serum into several water-soluble substances, which are then excreted in the urine. The major metabolite in the urine is benzoylecgonine. This is usually measured in most standard urine toxicology screens. After average doses, urine toxicology remains positive for cocaine for approximately 24 hours. Heavy freebasing or large-dosage use may lead to positive tests for 7 to 10 days after use and, rarely, even longer. Amphetamines, because of their longer half-lives, produce positive urine toxicology for 2 to 3 days following chronic use.

PSYCHIATRIC ASPECTS OF ACUTE INTOXICATION

The acute effects of psychostimulants consist of the following: euphoria, disinhibition, grandiosity, impulsiveness, hypersexual behavior, hypervigilance, decreased judgment, psychomotor agitation, and compulsive rituals. With sporadic exposure to lower doses, many of these symptoms are mild and do not become problematic, but in some individuals, higher doses or chronic use can cause a wide range of serious psychiatric symptoms.

PSYCHIATRIC COMPLICATIONS AND TREATMENT

Stimulant-induced agitation or hypomania can occur even after acute low-dose use. Hyperactivity, restlessness, rapid speech, and irritability are dominant symptoms. In more severe cases, inflated self-esteem, grandiosity, decreased need for sleep, disorganized thinking, and flight of ideas are present.

Toxic psychosis can also occur after acute exposure, but is probably more common after chronic high dose administration. It is speculated that, after CNS sensitization stimulants may cause certain individuals to become more susceptible to these symptoms. Hallucinations can be visual or auditory but are more commonly tactile, with patients feeling as though they have insects crawling under their skin (formicaria). In some instances, they may self-inflict severe skin lesions from compulsive scratching. More severe psychosis can result in hyperarousal, hypervigilance, suspiciousness, and paranoid or persecutory delusions.

Agitation or hyperarousal, if mild, can probably be treated acutely in the ED over a few hours with low doses of shorter-acting benzodiazepines (lorazepam, 2 mg PO or IM every 2 to 4 hours until sedation is achieved). More severely psychotic, agitated, or assaultive patients should be restrained and carefully treated with adequate doses of high-potency antipsychotic (e.g., haloperidol, 5 to 10 mg PO or IM every hour until sedation is achieved). Careful clinical evaluation can help distinguish these episodes from other psychiatric conditions. Individuals who do not respond to conservative treatment in the ED may need extended observation (12 to 24 hours) or hospitalization. Most cocaine-induced symptoms resolve within 12 hours to 1 week if the patient remains abstinent.

Chronic stimulant abuse can induce symptoms similar to *generalized anxiety disorder*. Once it is clear that stimulants are the cause of this condition, the treatment is abstinence. *Panic attacks* are also not infrequent. It is unclear if these episodes are more common in predisposed individuals. There is some speculation that stimulants may cause CNS sensitization, resulting in panic attack disorder. Again, the treatment is abstinence. If panic attacks or generalized anxiety persist, they should be referred for follow-up and treated with nonaddicting psychotropic antidepressants (tricyclics, MAO inhibitors, buspirone). Benzodiazepines generally should not be used because of their high abuse potential.

MEDICAL COMPLICATIONS

Stimulants can induce a considerable variety of medical complications. Their main adverse effects involve the respiratory, cardiac, and central nervous systems. Toxic reactions are probably related to the route of administration and dose, although their toxic range may be wide.

Stimulants produce characteristic sympathomimetics effects such as tachycardia, increased blood pressure, pupillary dilation, hyperthermia, increased blood glucose, and increased blood flow preferentially to skeletal muscle and brain. Tachycardia and cardiac sensitization can cause arrythmia, fibrillation, or myocardial infarction. Hypertension and hypertensive crisis have also been reported. Peripheral vasoconstriction can lead to decreased heat transmission, resulting in hyperthermia. Increased rapid respiration can result in hypoxia, CO_2 retention, respiratory depression, and pulmonary edema. Forceful inhalation has been reported to result in pneumomediastinum, pneumopericardium, or pneumothorax. Exhaustion from lack of sleep, poor physical condition, malnutrition, and dehydration are common. Lack of judgment, increasing the risk of accident and/or violent behavior, also results in a variety of medical problems (e.g., trauma).

Several medical complications are related to these drugs and their route of administration. Nasal inhalation leads to localized vasoconstriction, resulting in damage to the mucous membranes. Chronic use may induce episodes of epistaxis or nasal septum perforation. Rebound vasodilation can result in chronic rhinitis. Inhaled particles carrying bacteria can lodge in the sinuses or lungs, causing chronic infections. Intravenous use, usually associated with lack of sterility, can cause numerous systemic bacterial or fungal infections such as endocarditis, pneumonia, or CNS abscess. Materials used to "cut" these substances frequently result in the formation of granulomas in various organs. The skin is frequently affected, resulting in cellulitis and abscess formation at the sites of injection. The sharing of dirty needles leads to a risk of viral transmission (e.g., hepatitis A, B, non-A, and non-B; Epstein-Barr; and HIV). Cocaine smoking has been shown to cause damage to the alveolar surface of the lung, impairing gas diffusion.

FATALITIES

Death from cocaine use was reported as early as 1891, but was not taken seriously by the medical community until recently. The increasing nationwide statistics reporting sudden death probably underestimate its prevalence. Its cause is unclear, but it may be the result of cardiac toxicity, convulsions, and/or respiratory suppression. The findings on autopsy are usually nonspecific. This is an acute phenomenon and is believed to be the result of overdose and/or an acute toxic reaction. Its occurrence is not necessarily related to the magnitude or chronicity of drug exposure because deaths from cocaine have been reported from a variety of dosages (less than 200 mg to over 1000 mg). Toxicity may also be potentiated by other sympathomimetics, antihypertensives, and antidepressants, many of which are used or abused by these patients (see previous chapter section).

ABSTINENCE (WITHDRAWAL) SYNDROME FROM STIMULANTS

The most common problem encountered in chronic users is the abstinence (withdrawal) syndrome. It has been described by numerous authors as being divided into two phases: first, the "crash" experienced the first few hours after stimulant use and, second, the withdrawal, which may follow over the next 1 to 14 days.

The Crash immediately follows a binge (the usual pattern of stimulant abuse). Although it is most severe in chronic users, it is also experienced following a single binge. Individuals exhibit depression, mild agitation, or anxiety associated with increased stimulant craving followed by hypersomnia. Alcohol or sedative hypnotics are frequently used during this period to achieve sleep. Patients tend to become hyperphagic (they are usually anorexic while binging) and exhibit normal or dysphoric mood.

The Withdrawal is frequently seen in chronic abusers and consists of anergia (decreased energy), anhedonia (decreased pleasure), and depressed mood. These symptoms may gradually increase over 1 to 8 days after abstinence. Along with depressive symptoms, intense stimulant craving is also noted. Animal studies have substantiated the physiologic nature of this syndrome because behavioral depression and craving can be induced in animal models after chronic stimulant administration. The symptoms of withdrawal usually subside after 6 to 18 weeks, but can be longer in chronic high-dose users.

TREATMENT OF STIMULANT ABSTINENCE SYNDROME

The combination of marked anhedonia and intense craving make it difficult for individuals to abstain from these drugs, creating a great obstacle in treating these addicts. Several pharmacologic agents have been investigated to minimize these symptoms during the first weeks or months of treatment (when chance of relapse tends to be the greatest). It is hypothesized that these symptoms result from dopamine and or norepinephrine depletion after chronic use. Dopaminergic agents (methylphenidate, bromocriptine and amantadine) have been evaluated in a small number of clinical studies (most of which had small sample size, were open studies, and lacked controls). Studies with some positive results indicated that improvement occurred after a few weeks of treatment; however, to date there is minimal scientific support for efficacy of these dopamine agonists. Several studies have also looked at tricyclic antidepressants. Again, the studies are limited and poorly controlled but are slightly more

positive, indicating that these medications may have some efficacy in cocaine-induced anhedonia. Because it is believed that stimulants induce euphoria by way of specific dopamine tracks, some investigations have looked at the efficacy of dopamine-blocking agents (depot neuroleptics) in extinguishing the reinforcing properties of stimulants, thereby leading to a decrease in their use. Although animal studies show such an approach to be effective, these agents produce dysphoria and a host of other side effects, making them impractical in this patient population. Such treatments should be administered as part of an overall drug treatment program that also includes family and social issues.

PHENCYCLIDINE

Phencyclidine (PCP) was originally developed in 1956 as a unique anesthetic agent producing a dissociative, amnestic analgesia without typical CNS depression at clinical doses. It was never generally introduced because patients frequently suffered prolonged and bizarre behavior during emergence. It was used for some time as a veterinary anesthetic, but is no longer marketed in the U.S.A.

MECHANISM OF ACTION OF PCP

The current interest in PCP is a result of its rise in abuse (first described in 1969) and a recent understanding of its unique psychotropic properties, in that it produces a toxic psychosis very similar to acute schizophrenia. Animal and pharmacologic studies have demonstrated that, although PCP has a variety of qualities similar to those of other drugs of abuse, it clearly qualifies as a unique psychotropic agent. Many of its effects are produced only by PCP, its chemical analogues, sigma-agonist opiates, and a few unrelated chemicals with PCP-like effects. Its properties appear to be mediated by a specific CNS receptor (sigma receptor) postulated to exist for an endogenous PCP-like substance.

In addition to its sigma receptor effects, PCP demonstrates the behavioral characteristics of dopaminergic agonists and CNS depressants. Although PCP is associated with aggressive behavior in humans, animal studies have not demonstrated this. Reinforcing properties, tolerance, and dependence have been exhibited in animal models. Marked withdrawal symptoms, also noted in animals following cessation of chronic high doses, include hyperactivity, diarrhea, sedation, tremors, and bruxism.

PHARMACOKINETICS OF PCP

PCP is usually administered by smoking. It is often mixed with cannabis. Less frequently, intranasal or intravenous routes are used. Its serum half-life is short following single low doses (45 minutes) with peak blood levels occurring over 1 to 4 hours after inhalation. Because it is highly lipid-soluble, PCP is sequestered into adipose tissue, resulting in an increased half-life following chronic administration (up to 3 days). Because PCP is a weak base, acidification of the urine may increase PCP excretion.

TOXICOLOGY OF PCP

PCP is typically identified in most standard urine toxicology screens. Because it is lipid-soluble, these tests may be positive for up to a week after abstinence in chronic users.

ACUTE INTOXICATION

At low doses (5 mg or less), PCP exerts CNS depressant effects, analgesia, a dissociative state, impaired perceptions, euphoria, and anxiety. On physical examination, one notes vertical and horizontal nystagmus, miotic or normal reactive pupils, and absent corneal reflex. With higher doses (5 to 10 mg), one notices nystagmus, hyperreflexia, increased muscle tone, ataxia, and slurred speech. Overdose (over 20 mg) may result in severe CNS and respiratory depression, muscular rigidity, coma, and death. Most of our knowledge of PCP concerns its acute administration and resulting complications.

ACUTE PSYCHIATRIC COMPLICATIONS

Individuals experiencing complications from acute intoxication usually end up in the ED as a result of strange or assaultive behavior. The hallmarks of PCP intoxication are bizarre behavior, nystagmus, and fluctuant mental status. Of the psychoactive substance-induced psychosis, PCP may be the easiest to mistake for acute schizophrenia. Patients are frequently confused and disoriented, and exhibit posturing and catatonia. Unfortunately, we know little about the effects of chronic use on humans. Although acute intoxication is a frequent problem in some EDs, PCP is abused by a small segment of the population, making adequate studies difficult.

TREATMENT OF ACUTE PSYCHIATRIC COMPLICATIONS

Mildly dysphoric or agitated individuals can be treated with low doses of short-acting benzodiazepines (e.g., lorazepam 2 mg PO or IM prn every 2 to 4 hours until sedation is achieved and may be discharged for the ED after 3 to 6 hours of observation. Frequently, many of these individuals are agitated or extremely aggressive, needing restraints and careful treatment with a high-potency antipsychotic. Most individuals can be adequately sedated with 5 to 10 mg of haloperidol, but higher doses may be occasionally needed (5 to 10 mg/IM PRN every hour). If symptoms are not controlled with 10 to 20 mg of haloperidol after 2 to 3 hours, the differential diagnosis should be expanded to ensure that no additional factors are involved. Most patients should be re-evaluated after 8 to 12 hours. If altered mental status persists, hospitalization for further observation and treatment is necessary. If improved, patients can be safely discharged from the ED. Because PCP may have an extended half-life and effect, some physicians advocate a 7-day course of low-dose haloperidol treatment (5 mg HS) with follow-up. Such a practice may be questionable, considering the noncompliance seen in this patient population. As with other chemical dependencies, these patients should be given appropriate referrals to specialized treatment programs.

These individuals should not be treated with low-potency antipsychotics (e.g., chlorpromazine), which can enhance autonomic dysfunction, lower the blood pressure, and reduce the seizure threshold. Although benzodiazepines may be effective in mildly agitated individuals, they may also enhance lack of control over behavior.

MARIJUANA

Marijuana (Cannabis sativa) and related compounds are probably the most frequently used illicit drugs in our society. Although use is reportedly declining, it is being used by an increasingly younger population in which the consequence of its abuse may be greatly underestimated.

PHARMACOKINETICS

Over 400 compounds have been identified in the cannabis plant and over 150 in its smoke following incineration. With such a wide variety of known and unknown substances, it is difficult to identify which compounds are responsible for its psychoactive properties in vivo. Delta tetrahydrocannabinol (THC) is most commonly identified as the major psychoactive compound, consisting of between 5 to 20 mg per marijuana cigarette, with concentrations up to 100 mg in the more potent strains. Hashish, made from the concentrated resin of the cannabis plant, can contain 8 to 12% THC, and hashish oil can have concentrations as high as 25 to 60%.

Cannabis products are most commonly used by smoking, but ingestion (in the form of cookies or brownies) is not infrequent. Because THC and its metabolites appear to be the largest psychoactive component of cannabis, they have been the most studied. Oral ingestion results in slow and erratic absorption, with peak plasma levels over 1 to 6 hours. These can become high if large doses are ingested. Bioavailability by this route is low (10 to 20%), mostly due to rapid hepatic metabolism. Smoking causes immediate but low peak plasma levels, with an overall bioavailability ranging from 13 to 40% (probably caused by various smoking techniques; dose of smoke; and rate, depth, and duration of inhalation).

THC is quickly metabolized to its major metabolite 11-nor delta 9-THC-9-carboxylic acid (THCA). Its half-life varies from 58 hours in infrequent users to 24 hours in chronic users. Because of its high lipid solubility, tissue sequestration, and accumulation, it may persist in the body for an extended time. THCA is excreted mostly in the feces (60%) and the urine (only 25%). It difficult to correlate the behavioral effects of cannabis to THC blood levels. Because of the multitude of compounds and metabolities and tissue accumulation, their pharmacokinetics are unclear and their psychologic effects do not appear to be related to peak plasma level (as with other drugs).

TOXICOLOGY

THC is rapidly metabolized but may be identified in urine up to 30 days in chronic users, 7 to 10 days in once- or twice-weekly users, and 3 to 4 days following sporadic use.

TOLERANCE AND DEPENDENCE

Animal studies clearly demonstrate that, after chronic exposure to higher doses of THC, tolerance and dependence develop. An abstinence syndrome has been demonstrated in animals and reportedly in some humans. It typically consists of anorexia, anxiety, insomnia, agitation, depression, restlessness, dysphoria, tremors, sweating, hyperreflexia, and lateral gaze nystagmus. Onset may be within 10 hours after a large decrease in exposure or abstinence. It may peak in 48 hours and continue, to a lesser degree, for more than 7 days. There is no clear treatment for this syndrome, which may contribute to relapse in the early stages of abstinence. It is usually mild, so that supportive measures are sufficient and hospitalization does not appear to be needed unless it is indicated for a drug treatment plan. Drugs with high abuse potential (e.g., benzodiazepines) should not be used in these patients unless under close medical supervision.

ACUTE INTOXICATION

Cannabis induces, along with a sense of euphoria, a host of perceptual and cognitive changes in its users.

Studies have demonstrated distorted perception in terms of object size, distance, object tracking, color discrimination, auditory signal detection, and reaction time. A unique phenomenon seen with marijuana is a distortion of time sense. Cognitive tests demonstrate impairments consisting of decreased understanding of new information and decreased short-term memory. These changes are dose-related and may last up to 2 hours after ingestion. The degree to which these impairments contribute to automobile and work-related injury has long been overlooked. Toxicology screening of the trauma patient, for example, reveals that alcohol and marijuana are the drugs most commonly found (alcohol in 55%, marijuana in 24%).[*]

PSYCHIATRIC COMPLICATIONS

ACUTE

The most frequent reactions leading to ED visits include cannabis-induced panic attacks and severe anxiety. Moderate anxiety can usually be treated with reassurance and a quiet room. Sometimes low doses of short-acting benzodiazepines (lorazepam 2 mg PO or IM) may be useful. A brief toxic delirium consisting of cognitive disorganization, paranoia, auditory hallucinations, derealization, depersonalization, changes in perception of body image, manic-like symptoms, or severe depression may also be seen after ingestion of large doses of marijuana. It appears to be self-limited and resolves within a few hours, but can last up to a few days. If patients are extremely agitated or psychotic, they may need antipsychotics (haloperidol, 2 to 5 mg IM every 2 to 4 hours until sedation is achieved and/or hospitalization for further evaluation and treatment).

CHRONIC

The existence of an amotivational syndrome, although still controverial as a unitary cause, is often seen in marijuana users. This manifests as a loss of interest in conventional social goals, decreased ambition, decreased personal habits, dulled cognitive function, impaired attention span, distractibility, poor communication skills, apathy, withdrawal, decreased socialization, and lack of insight. This may be of greatest concern in adolescents who demonstrate diminished school performance, emotional lability and outbursts, and subtle personality changes. These symptoms tend to resolve slowly with abstinence, and usually reflect multifaceted dysfunction with chronic marijuana use seen as one of a host of behaviors.

---

[*] Clark, R.F., and Harchelroad, F.: Toxicology screening of the trauma patient. Ann. Emerg. Med. 20:151, 1991.

MEDICAL COMPLICATIONS

Because cannabis smoking is common, the degree to which it may contribute to a variety of health hazards is probably underestimated. Chronic users frequently exhibit respiratory disorders such as rhinitis, dyspnea, decreased exercise tolerance, increased risk of chronic cough, and bronchitis. Pulmonary functions show decreased ventilatory function, decreased vital capacity, and impaired gas diffusion. Pulmonary disease caused by chronic marijuana smoking may be similar to that seen with cigarettes (e.g., emphysema, pulmonary cancer, etc.). Cardiovascular effects consist of tachycardia, elevation of S-T segments, increased amplitude of P wave and inversion, or flattening of T wave on ECG. High doses can induce PVCs. Blood pressure changes, if present, are variable. Chronic use can cause changes in the male reproductive system consisting of decreased sperm count and motility, abnormal sperm cell morphology, and a possible decrease in plasma testosterone. Effects on the female reproductive hormones may lead to menstrual abnormalities, can adversely affect pregnancy, and increase the probability of fetal abnormalities and low birth weight.

OPIATES

Opiates (opium) have been used for their analgesic properties since the first century and have been abused throughout history. Although they are the most effective treatment for pain, they also possess high abuse potential. There is an ongoing search for a dependence-free opiate analgesic, but this has not yet been achieved.

Opiates can be divided into: (1) natural alkaloids derived from the opium poppy (opium, morphine, codeine); (2) semisynthetic derivatives of morphine (e.g., diacetylmorphine [heroin], oxycodone, and hydromorphine [dilaudid]); (3) pure synthetics (e.g. meperidine [Demerol], methadone, and propoxyphene [Darvon]); and (4) preparations containing opiates (e.g., paregoric). Both the semisynthetic and the pure synthetics are the most commonly abused.

MECHANISM OF ACTION

The means by which opiates exert their full effect remain unclear. Although they bind stereospecifically to multiple opiate receptors, this does not explain their full spectrum of action in animal models. Opiates decrease the release of acetylcholine, increase the synthesis and turnover of catecholamine, and act as direct agonists at dopamine receptors.

PHARMACOKINETICS

Opiates are readily absorbed by way of the gastrointestinal and other mucosa. Parenteral administration leads to more rapid elevation of blood levels and effect, although the duration of action tends to be shorter than with oral administration. Morphine and most of its congeners have similar durations of action (3 to 4 hours), do not accumulate in tissue, and are almost completely excreted after 24 hours. Morphine is metabolized by means of hepatic conjugation, 90% of which is excreted in the urine over 24 hours. Heroin is rapidly metabolized to monoacetylmorphine and then morphine. Codeine and oxycodeine are more effective orally than parenterally and are metabolized in the liver, where a small portion is desmethylated to form morphine.

TOXICOLOGY

These drugs are identified in most urine toxicology screens as morphine or codeine. Because of their short half-lives, they are rarely located in the urine for more than 24 to 36 hours. Street heroin if frequently mixed with quinine, which has a longer half-life, and may be identified in the urine of heroin addicts 5 to 7 days after its use.

TOLERANCE AND DEPENDENCE

Opiates demonstrate typical reinforcing properties in animal self-administration studies. Unlike consumption of psychostimulants, consumption of opiates gradually rises over a period of weeks, followed by a steady rate of self-administration, avoiding grave toxicity or withdrawal.

Tolerance to the different effects of opiates varies. There is characteristically decreased duration and intensity of analgesia, euphoria, and CNS depression, along with a marked elevation of the lethal dose. Dependence and mild withdrawal symptoms develop after 1 or 2 weeks of multiple daily dosing, although naloxone can induce moderate withdrawal after only 3 or 4 days of opiate use. Although dependence almost always results with opiate administration, its relationship to compulsive use is unclear and complex. There is probably a large number of individuals who are not using illicit drugs but are mildly addicted to prescription medications for the treatment of chronic pain syndromes. Many of these individuals demonstrate little or no dose escalation and mild drug-seeking behavior. Not all dependent individuals go on to lose control over their opiate use, and sometimes opiates are effectively used in chronic medical conditions. This is substantially relevant in EDs because of the need to differentiate the chronic stable user of narcotics for a medical need from the addiction-prone patient who is escalating drug use and losing control of his or her intake.

ACUTE INTOXICATION

After IV administration, opiate users experience flushing of the skin and an intense "rush" (described as a sense in the lower abdomen similar to sexual orgasm) lasting 30 to 60 seconds. This is followed by a brief period of euphoria and then a sense of tranquility which may last for a few hours. The pharmacologic characteristics of heroin make it the most abused of the opiates. Its lipid solubility results in a rapid effect because of easy passage across the blood-brain barrier and CNS metabolism to morphine (which does not readily cross this barrier). Intoxication produced analgesia, mental clouding, drowsiness, poor concentration, decreased mentation, apathy, motor retardation, lethargy, and dysphoria in some individuals. In addition, opiates induce central respiratory depression and stimulate brain stem chemoreceptors, causing, in some, nausea and vomiting. Decreased gastrointestinal secretions and inhibition of smooth muscle contractions are common, leading to decreased gastric motility, decreased uterine and bladder tone, and pupillary constriction. Their cardiovascular effects are minimal, but peripheral vasodilation can contribute to hypotension.

ACUTE OVERDOSE AND TREATMENT

Exact toxic doses in various individuals are difficult to quantify because of the rapid development of tolerance and varying individual sensitivity. Because the quality of opiate available on the street is variable (heroin is usually diluted with other active and inactive substances), accidental overdoses resulting from ingestion of high-grade heroin, pure pharmaceutical opiates, and "designer" opiates is not uncommon. In nontolerant subjects, 40 to 60 mg of methadone or 120 mg of oral morphine (>30 mg IV) can cause serious toxicity.

Overdosed patients present with the triad of stuporous mental status or coma, depressed respiration, and pinpoint pupils. Prolonged decreased respiratory rate can cause cyanosis, hypotension, and shock. Pupils may be dilated after extended hypoxia. Decreased urine production, hypothermia, skeletal muscle flaccidity, and pulmonary edema may also be seen. Death is usually the result of respiratory failure. Polysubstance abuse is common in these patients, and sedative hypnotics may contribute to complicating the clinical picture.

Treatment consists of supportive measures and the use of pure narcotic antagonists to reverse severe respiratory and CNS depression. Naloxone, 0.4 mg IV every 5 minutes, should produce a quick response. If it does not do so after administration of 10 mg, this usually indicates complication by other medications (e.g., sedative hypnotics or alcohol, frequently abused by this patient population) or an erroneous diagnosis. Naloxone should be administered with care because,

if given in excess, it can quickly precipitate opiate withdrawal, which is not easily treatable during its period of action. The depressant effects in opiate overdose can last 24 to 72 hours. Because naloxone's half-life is shorter than this, careful monitoring is needed so that patients do not slip back into a coma.

OPIATE ABSTINENCE (WITHDRAWAL) SYNDROME

Symptoms of opiate withdrawal represent hyperexcitability of the organs previously depressed by chronic opiate abuse. Their severity varies according to the potency of opiate used, degree of tolerance developed, and time since the last dose. The abstinence syndrome is expressed by both behavioral and physiologic symptoms. The former consist of purposefully goal-oriented actions directed at getting more drug, such as complaints, demands, or manipulations, and are highly dependent on the environmental surroundings. Early withdrawal from heroin (6 to 10 hours after the last dose) produces yawning, lacrimation, rhinorrhea, anxiety, and increasing drug-seeking behavior. Over the next 12 to 14 hours, the patient experiences piloerection, pupillary dilation, anorexia, hot and cold flashes, muscle cramps (both skeletal and abdominal), tremors, and insomnia. As the syndrome further progresses, nausea, vomiting, diarrhea, hypertension, tachycardia, tachypnea, and increased temperature can occur. With morphine and heroin, these symptoms reach their peak within 48 to 72 hours. Leukocytosis is common, and ketosis and electrolyte imbalance may result from dehydration. The syndrome usually abates within 7 to 10 days. Methadone, because of its longer half-life, displays a slower onset of symptoms (24 to 48 hours) and is generally less dramatic, but resolves over a longer period (3 to 7 weeks).

MANAGEMENT OF OPIATE WITHDRAWAL

In the past, methadone was the treatment of choice for narcotic withdrawal because of its longer half-life and a duration of action lasting from 24 to 36 hours, making once-a-day oral administration possible. Withdrawal can usually be prevented by 10 to 40 mg/day in most opiate-dependent individuals, and these doses should not produce the euphoria associated with opiate abuse. Because it is often impossible to know the dose of street drug used or the degree of tolerance developed by an individual, the minimal dose of methadone needed to block withdrawal should be titrated over a 24-hour period. At the onset of measurable symptoms, administer 10 mg of oral methadone. Some degree of symptom abatement should be noted within the next hour. This dose can be repeated over the next 24 hours as needed. One should remember that more than 40 mg of methadone is rarely needed in 24 hours. This stabilization dose should be administered over the next day or two (preferably b.i.d.), followed by a daily decrease of methadone by no greater than 5 mg/day. In individuals dependent on short-acting opiates, detoxification can be achieved in 7 to 21 days. In patients who have been chronically dependent on methadone (e.g., greater than 1 year), the time needed for successful detoxification is generally much longer. Chronic methadone patients should have their dosage decreased once every 7 to 10 days. Twenty-one day detoxification for chronic methadone patients is probably too short and may precipitate abstinence syndrome. Typically, once the methadone dosage is decreased below 15 mg/day, many individuals experience increasing difficulty with withdrawal, and detoxification may need to be dramatically slowed (e.g., 2 mg every 10 to 14 days). Most chronic opate abusers tend to have low tolerance to discomfort. In light of this, it is important for them to understand that, although symptoms can be minimized, most individuals experience some degree of discomfort.

Recently the use of clonidine (Catapres) has become a popular and effective way to treat opiate withdrawal in detoxification programs. Clonidine, an alpha-2-adrenergic autoreceptor agonist, acts to decrease output from the locus ceruleus, thereby decreasing the noradrenegic drive associated with withdrawal. Doses of 0.1 mg can be administered orally 3 to 4 times a day, provided that hypotension does not result. The dose can be increased daily until symptoms abate (0.6 to 1 mg/day in divided doses should be sufficient). Transdermal clonidine patches, along with oral supplements, are now being used by many inpatient detoxification centers. Clonidine alone is usually not sufficient to suppress all the withdrawal symptoms. Adjunctive quinine (for muscle cramps) and Bentyl (for GI hypermotility) are frequently added to this treatment. Clonidine should be continued for 7 to 10 days to prevent heroin or morphine withdrawal and longer for methadone. Clonidine should be withdrawn slowly to prevent rebound hypertension. Although extremely effective, clonidine can produce serious hypotension and needs to be monitored closely. Although it is relatively safe, its use has, until recently, been limited to inpatient settings. Experienced clinicians are using clonidine patches more frequently in highly monitored outpatient detoxification programs.

MEDICAL COMPLICATIONS

As with other serious drug addictions, patients on opiates suffer from a variety of medical, psychologic, and socioeconomic difficulties. The death rate among addicts may be as high as 1% per year, much of which is attributed to overdose, accidents, violence, and (to a lesser degree) medical complications.

At present, the most serious complication of IV heroin abuse is the transmission of HIV. In addition, hepatitis B is frequent among these individuals. Staphylococcus aureus endocarditis is not uncommon, along with other systemic bacterial infections. The IV drug abuser commonly presents with other complications such as foreign body emboli and pulmonary fibrosis, abscess, or tuberculosis. Injection sites are frequently the location of fibrosis, abscess formation, infection, ulceration, and occasionally gangrene.

REHABILITATION FOR OPIATE ADDICTION

Presently there are two different approaches to the long-term rehabilitation of opiate addicts: methadone maintenance and drug-free treatment. Methadone treatment evolved from the clinical observation that certain individuals are unable to abstain from opiate use. This led to the hypothesis that long-term opiate use induces long-lasting neurophysiologic changes, causing addicts to experience craving or symptoms months or years after withdrawal. It was theorized that methadone can alleviate these symptoms, releasing patients from persistent need to seek and use these drugs and enabling them to rehabilitate their lives. Although, in the past, individuals were chronically maintained on doses up to or greater than 80 mg/day of methadone, it is now understood that 20 to 40 mg/day is sufficient. Although treatment for almost all other substance-abuse disorders advocates total abstinence from addictive psychotropics as a prerequisite to recovery, methadone maintenance stands out as the only treatment recommending continued exposure to such substances for rehabilitation. The efficacy of methadone maintenance has never been adequately evaluated, and has not been proven superior to drug-free treatment.

An increasing number of centers are choosing to treat these patients with quick methadone or clonidine detoxification followed by drug-free treatment approaches (e.g., Narcotics Anonymous, therapeutic communities). In addition to this, narcotic antagonists, (e.g., naltrexone), following adequate detoxification, are also being used in some programs. These agents block the euphoria and reinforcing properties of opiates, thereby causing diminished drug-seeking so that the individual gives up on trying to get "high."

HALLUCINOGENS

Hallucinogens (Table 85-9) are a group of pharmacologically similar agents that, when ingested, induce a state of marked perceptual alterations consisting of illusions, marked sensitivity to internal and external stimuli, euphoria, and a sense of introspection and

TABLE 85-9. HALLUCINOGENIC DRUGS

Drug	Source	Duration of Action
D-lysergic acid-diethylamide (LSD)	Synthetic	6–12 hours
Dimethyltryptamine (DMT)	Synthetic	30–90 minutes
Dimethoxymethyl-amphetamine (DOM, "STP")	Synthetic	6–24 hours
Psilocybin	Mushroom	4–8 hours
Mescaline	Peyote cactus	6–12 hours

profound insightfulness. In more severe cases, delusions and hallucinations are also present. Because of their "reality-altering" psychotropic properties, they have been used for spiritual or religious purposes by many cultures throughout time.

Pharmacologically, these psychotropics can be divided into two groups: (1) The indolealkylamines, which resemble the neurotransmitter 5-hydroxytryptamine [D-lysergic acid diethylamide (LSD), psilocybin, and dimethyltryptamine (DMT)] and (2) the phenylethylamines, which are similar to the monoamines [mescaline and the phenylisopropylamines (STP)]. Because these drugs are similar in many of their aspects, we shall primarily refer to LSD because it is the most studied and best understood of this class of psychotropics.

LSD ("acid") is a synthetic derivative of the ergot fungus. It is extremely potent and is effective at doses as low as 50 µg. It is ingested orally or through other mucous membranes (sublingual, rectal, corneal) and is administered in various forms such as drops on sugar cubes or paper (blotter), pills, or celluloid squares (window panes).

PHARMACOKINETICS

LSD is well absorbed through the mucous membranes and quickly distributed through body tissues, although only a small amount reaches the CNS, where it apparently inhibits midbrain serotonin neurons. Its half-life is 2 to 3 hours, but its duration of action following a usual dose is 6 to 12 hours. LSD is metabolized by conjugation in the liver into inactive substances.

TOXICOLOGY

LSD and other hallucinogens are identified on most standard urine toxicology screens. Because of their short half-lives, the tests are rarely positive 24 to 36 hours after ingestion.

TOLERANCE AND DEPENDENCE

After repeated administration, tolerance is quickly developed to these substances, leading to the ingestion of larger doses or decreased frequency of use. Cross-tolerance also appears to exist among the various hallucinogens. In animal studies, these substances appear to have weak reinforcing properties and do not produce the same compulsive use as other abused drugs. This is also evident in humans, in whom chronic "compulsive" use is uncommon. Chronic regular users are more apt to exhibit other forms of severe psychopathology and to abuse other psychotropics as well. Physical dependence has not been demonstrated in animals or humans, nor has a withdrawal syndrome been demonstrated.

ACUTE INTOXICATION

Effects usually begin between 20 and 60 minutes after ingestion, the intensity of which depends on the amount ingested and the tolerance of the individual. Physiologic symptoms consist of tachycardia, increased blood pressure and temperature, pupillary dilation, hyperreflexia, and nausea. Psychologic effects include visual illusions, perceptual changes, hallucinations, mood lability, increased sensory awareness, alteration in sense of time, and feelings of depersonalization.

ACUTE PSYCHIATRIC COMPLICATIONS

Although most people experience the reality-distorting properties of hallucinogens as a pleasant or exciting experience, others find it disorienting and frightening. The most common problem is a "bad trip," an episode of extreme anxiety with a sense of loss of self-control. The probability of such an experience is multifactorial, depending on the individual's state, the environment in which the drug is used, and the dose ingested. These reactions are transient and limited to the duration of action of the drug. Pharmacologic treatment is usually unnecessary. Reassurance and a calm, supportive environment are frequently sufficient to alleviate anxiety. When conservative treatment is not effective, high-potency benzodiazepines (e.g., lorazepam 2 mg) may be useful. These patients rarely need antipsychotic medication.

A toxic delirium consisting of agitation, disorientation, hallucinations, delusions, and paranoia may be experienced by some patients. In such states, injuries or accidental suicides can occur (jumping from a window in an attempt to fly). This is a transient condition and clears within 24 hours without sequelae. In these cases, supportive treatment may not be sufficient and high-potency benzodiazepines (lorazepam, 2 mg IM every 1 to 2 hours until sedation is achieved) or, in more severe cases, haloperidol (5 to 10 mg IM every 1 to 2 hrs until sedation is achieved) may be necessary.

SEQUELAE OF HALLUCINOGEN USE

In some individuals, a drug-precipitated psychosis may continue after hallucinogen use. It is speculated that this occurs in patients with underlying psychiatric conditions (schizophrenia, manic-depressive illness). Many of these individuals may have been previously symptomatic and used these drugs in an attempt to self-medicate. Follow-up treatment includes pharmacotherapy of the underlying illness. Although there is no evidence that these drugs can cause chronic psychiatric conditions, many families and patients find it easier to blame the condition on the use of hallucinogens than to face the stigma of suffering from a psychiatric illness.

Flashbacks or brief spontaneous recurrences of perceptual changes such as those experienced while using a hallucinogen have been reported days, months, or years after drug use. They may last from a few minutes to a few hours and can be precipitated by various environmental or emotional cues and/or other drug use. The exact cause and validity of this phenomenon has not been adequately studied. It is unclear whether or not these events are from some chronic effect of these drugs. The generally accepted view is that they are a learned conditioned response causing cognitive recollection of the hallucinogenic experience in certain conditions. Their treatment consists of reassurance that the episodes will pass and evaluation of the possible existence of other comorbid psychiatric syndromes that may need treatment.

MEDICAL COMPLICATIONS

Medical sequelae from the hallucinogens are not well defined. There are some reports of chromosomal damage, along with increased rates of stillbirths and deformities in animal-administered high doses of LSD. Controlled studies have demonstrated no associated phenomena in humans.

SEDATIVE-HYPNOTICS

The sedative-hypnotics consist of a large number of chemically different substances, all of which induce, to varying degrees, central nervous system depression. Benzodiazepines (BZs) are presently the most commonly prescribed sedative hypnotic, followed by the barbiturates. Numerous other chemically unrelated substances (meprobamate, chloral hydrate, paraldehyde, etc.) are less frequently prescribed but nonetheless continue to be seen in the abusing population.

MECHANISM OF ACTION

These drugs act by a number of mechanisms in the CNS. Benzodiazepines have a specific action on certain GABA receptors (BZ-GABA-cloride ion channel complex) and exhibit a low toxicity profile. The barbituartes and other agents act on the same receptor complex, but in a nonspecific manner, and exhibit greater toxicity profiles.

TOLERANCE AND DEPENDENCE

The sedative-hypnotics demonstrate dispositional tolerance (increased metabolism), pharmacodynamic tolerance (cellular adaptation) and, because of their actions on similar receptor systems, develop cross-tolerance with other sedative hypnotics. BZs and barbiturates are easily interchangeable, although cross-tolerance may not be as complete between BZs and other sedative hypnotics.

Tolerance to the sedative properties of these drugs develops quickly. There is only moderate tolerance to the lethal effects of these drugs (in contrast to the opiates). Induction of their metabolism also leads to a decreased intensity and duration of their effect, resulting in more frequent use of higher quantities of drug. This, in turn, increases the likelihood of overdose and/or organ (e.g., brain) damage. Benzodiazepines appear to be safer in this regard because they do not produce severe CNS or respiratory depression.

Following chronic administration of therapeutic doses, physical dependence is apparent with all of these agents. Short-acting barbiturates can produce clinically significant withdrawal after weeks of mild intoxication, or following 10 to 12 days of heavy daily intoxication. Typically, the clinical use of benzodiazepines produces dependence after weeks or months of daily administration. With the increasing use of high-potency, short-acting benzodiazepines, the clinician needs to be aware that these substances carry a greater risk of severe sedative-hypnotic withdrawal when quickly discontinued after chronic use of therapeutic doses.

The relationship between tolerance or dependence and drug-seeking behavior (abuse) is complex and unclear. Many individuals chronically use these substances for medical purposes and develop dependence but do not go on to exhibit compulsive abuse.

ABUSE

Sedative-hypnotics are probably among the most widely abused medications available. They are frequently used with other drugs (e.g., opiates, cocaine, alcohol), resulting in severe intoxication and complicated overdoses in the ED. A large number of patients do not use illicit drugs but are addicted to prescription medications for the treatment of anxiety or insomnia. Many of these individuals demonstrate little or no dose escalation and only mild drug-seeking behavior, making it easy to overlook their addiction. In addition, it is not uncommon for an alcoholic to use these medications because of their cross tolerance.

BENZODIAZEPINES

These are the most commonly prescribed medications for anxiety and insomnia. They are classified by their length of action (short-acting [e.g., triazolam], intermediate-acting [e.g., alprazolam, lorazepam], and long-acting [e.g., diazepam]); their receptor affinities (high or low potency); the presence of active or inactive metabolites; their method of metabolism (hepatic conjugation or oxidation); their lipid solubilities, and their duration of action. All of these characteristics contribute to their preferential use in various conditions, their side effect profiles, their degree of abuse (some BZs produce greater degrees of euphoria than others), and the severity of withdrawal symptoms that they may produce.

TABLE 85-10. SIGNS AND SYMPTOMS OF SEDATIVE-HYPNOTIC INTOXICATION

Drowsiness
Slurred speech
Confusion
Agitation
Disorientation
Impaired concentration
Nystagmus
Tremor
Ataxia
Hyporreflexia
Respiratory depression
Hypotonia

BARBITURATES

These are less commonly prescribed since the development of the benzodiazepines. They are typically used as ultra-short-acting anesthetic agents (methohexital, thiopental), short- or intermediate-acting sedative-hypnotics (amobarbital, pentobarbital), or long-acting antiseizure medications (phenobarbital). The long-acting agents are also commonly used in the treatment of sedative-hypnotic withdrawal. The other CNS depressants such as chloral hydrate (Noctec), glutethimide (Doriden), ethchorvynol (Placidyl) or meprobamate (Miltown) are less frequently prescribed but are encountered sporadically in sedative-hypnotic-dependent patients.

TOXICOLOGY

These agents can be easily identified in standard urine toxicology screens. Depending on the agent abused and its frequency of use, they can continue to appear in the urine from 24 hours to 7 to 10 days after cessation of the drug. Plasma levels are also available for many of these substances and are useful in monitoring the recovery of individuals experiencing sedative-hypnotic overdose.

ACUTE INTOXICATION AND OVERDOSE

Individuals may use these medications to make suicide attempts, take accidental overdoses, or abuse them with or without alcohol, leading to intoxication or overdose.

Sedative-hypnotic intoxication resembles that seen with alcohol and may present with drowsiness, slurred speech, cognitive impairments, confusion, or disorientation (Table 85-10). Physical examination reveals impaired coordination, tremors, ataxia and vertical and horizontal nystagmus. Behaviorally, these patients may be disinhibited, labile, irritable or agitated. If severely agitated or assaultive, these individuals are best restrained and, if necessary, treated with low doses of haloperidol (5 to 10 mg IM over 60 to 90 minutes should be sufficient).

Severe overdose leads to signs of CNS depression, consisting of clouded or obtunded consciousness, decreased corneal, gag and deep tendon reflex, or coma. Cardiovascular and pulmonary functions can be depressed, leading to hypoxia, respiratory acidosis, and shock. Severe overdose is usually seen with the nonbenzodiazepines, but any of these agents when combined with alcohol can be lethal. Such cases need aggressive and careful treatment in the ED. Treatment consists, in general, of adequate pulmonary, cardiac, and renal support until blood levels drop below lethal levels. When possible, techniques to increase metabolism and excretion of these agents may be useful.

ABSTINENCE (WITHDRAWAL) SYNDROME

After chronic administration, all of these agents produce a potentially lethal withdrawal syndrome, the severity of which is related to the dose, the chronicity of its administration, and the half-life of the particular agent. The more rapidly it is withdrawn or the shorter its half-life, the more severe the abstinence symptoms can be. After chronic use, even gradual detoxification produces some degree of withdrawal in most individuals. After cessation of short-acting agents, symptoms may begin within 4 to 6 hours and can peak in 3 to 4 days. With longer-acting agents, symptom onset is slower, and the course of withdrawal may be prolonged. Early manifestations of withdrawal consist of irritability, anxiety, nausea, tachycardia, and diaphoresis, which progress to labile vital signs, hyperactive reflexes, tremors, and agitation. Generalized seizures may occur 3 to 4 days after cessation of the short-acting agents and 1 to 2 weeks after that of the longer-acting agents. Patients can also go on to develop delirium, which, as in alcohol withdrawal, may last for 7 to 10 days, is not easily treatable, and has a high rate of morbidity and mortality.

MANAGEMENT OF SEDATIVE-HYPNOTIC WITHDRAWAL

These patients are generally unreliable historians and tend to be unable or unwilling to give an accurate history regarding their drug use habits. Detoxification, as with alcohol and opiates, consists of carefully titrating a cross-tolerant medication over 24 hours to block withdrawal symptoms. The pentobarbital challenge test is a well-documented technique for this purpose. Individuals are given 200 mg of pentobarbital and, within an hour, are examined for signs of intoxication. If they are mildly intoxicated, a dose of 800 mg/day (100 to 200 mg every 6 hours) or less should be adequate to stabilize these individuals over the following 24 hours. If signs of intoxication are not noted after the initial dose, additional 100 mg doses should be administered every 2 hours until intoxication is observed. The total dose to induce intoxication is then calculated and given up to every 6 hours over the next day. Once the patient is stable, the dose is decreased by 100 mg/day or as tolerated until the individual is completely detoxified. Once the patient is stabilized, phenobarbital, a longer-acting, less intoxicating barbiturate with greater antiseizure efficacy, can be substituted (30 mg phenobarbital = 100 mg pentobarbital) and reduced by 25% per day. Another option is to give lorazepam, 2 mg every 1 or 2 hours for signs of withdrawal and calculate the total daily dose given to control abstinence symptoms. When the patient is stable, this can then be replaced by a long-acting benzodiazepine such as diazepam (10 mg diazepam = 2 mg lorazepam) and decreased over the next 4 to 5 days. There is some evidence that agents such as carbamazepine (400 to 800 mg/day) or valproic acid (250 to 1000 mg/day) may reduce or block benzodiazepine withdrawal. Their use, along with traditional detoxification protocols, may necessitate the need for lower doses of sedative-hypnotic to block withdrawal and may expedite detoxification.

DESIGNER DRUGS

Designer drugs refer to analogues of controlled substances in which slight chemical alterations create new drugs with similar pharmacologic and behavioral effects. These techniques have been widely used in the pharmaceutical industries for years to produce many of the synthetic psychotropics presently on the market. In this context, these "bootleg" street drugs are being produced to avoid federal regulations and control. The major concern with these drugs is that they are clandestinely manufactured, typically are poorly produced, and contain a variety of impurities that may themselves be toxic. The most frequently encountered designer drugs are the opiate and phenylisopropylamine (amphetamine) analogues.

OPIATE ANALOGUES

Morphine has long been used to produce analogues with a wide range of both agonistic and antagonistic activity (e.g., heroin, nalorphine). Meperidine (Demerol) has been a template for the production of MPPP, a look-alike drug sold on the street as a synthetic heroin. Unfortunately, its production at times is contaminated with byproducts that are potent neurotoxins. Small quantities of these impurities have been reported as causing severe parkinsonism in young IV drug abusers because of its neurotoxic effects on the dopamine-producing cells in the substantia nigra. Fentanyl is another extremely potent opiate that has been templated for a number of look-alike drugs. It has led to the clandestine production of designer opiates 100 to 1000 times more potent than morphine. These Fentanyl-like drugs may be responsible for the recent increase in opiate-related overdoses and death.

PHENYLISOPROPHYLAMINE ANALOGIES (HALLUCINOGENIC AMPHETAMINES)

The two most common designer drugs in this class are methylenedioxyamphetamine (MDA) and methylenedioxymethamphetamine (MDMA or ecstasy). They are chemically similar to catecholamine and probably have similar actions. They are reported to induce euphoria and altered mental status to a lesser degree than seen with other more powerful hallucinogens (e.g., LSD). MDA has been shown to cause serotonin nerve termination degeneration in rat brains, although so far its acute toxicity in man appears to be low. Toxic manifestations of MDA overdose have been reported as restlessness, agitation, sweating, rigidity, convulsions, hypertension, tachycardia, and hyperpyrexia. Although MDA is an amphetamine derivative, its pyschoactive properties in man appear to be distinct and it may actually represent a unique pharmacologic agent.

PHARMACOLOGIC INTERVENTION FOR DRUG-INDUCED AGITATION AND PSYCHOSIS

(see Table 85-11.)

BENZODIAZEPINES

These psychotropics are extremely effective in reducing mild to moderate states of drug-induced anxiety and/or agitation. Lorazepam (Ativan) is perhaps best suited for ED use. It is a high potency BZ, is well absorbed in IM form (unlike most other BZs), has a short to intermediate half-life (15 hours) and has no active metabolites. Dosing usually consists of 2 mg IM or PO (IM having a more rapid onset of action) and can be repeated every 1 to 2 hours if necessary. For most cases, 2 to 4 mg should be adequate to control the target symptoms. If much higher doses are needed, the patient should either be treated with a neuroleptic and/or have his or her differential diagnosis re-examined (e.g., a primary psychiatric condition or another CNS organic syndrome).

NEUROLEPTICS (ANTIPSYCHOTICS)

These medications are extremely effective in the treatment of drug-induced agitation, psychosis, and delirium. Haloperidol (Haldol) is probably the most commonly used neuroleptic in the ED setting. It is a high-potency antipsychotic, can be given IM, has approximately a 24-hour half-life and has only one known active metabolite. Unlike low- or moderate-potency neuroleptics, it has minimal anticholinergic and/or cardiovascular effects. Haloperidol does have a higher propensity to induce extrapyramidal side effects (EPS), e.g., dystonia, akathisia, than some of the other neuroleptics. This is not a frequent problem because low doses are used in this patient population. When EPS does occur, Benadryl (25 to 50 mg PO/IM PRN every 4 to 6 hours), Cogentin (1 to 2 mg PO/IM PRN every 6 to 8 hours) or Ativan (2 mg PO/IM PRN every 4 to 6 hours) are effective. One must be careful in giving Benadryl and Cogentin because of their anticholinergic side effects. Ativan, on the other hand, exaggerates the sedative properties of haloperidol and other drugs that patients may be abusing. There is a body of literature claiming that, because of a synergistic effect, the combinations of IM Ativan (2 mg) and IM Haldol (5 mg) PRN every 1 to 4 hours may be the most effective treatment for various forms of acute agitation and/or psychosis. Large, well-desgined stud-

---

TABLE 85-11. DRUG-INDUCED PSYCHIATRIC SYNDROMES AND THEIR TREATMENT

Drug	Syndrome	Treatment
Cannabis	Anxiety	Support/Ativan
	Toxic psychosis	Ativan or Haldol
	Chronic psychosis	Antipsychotic
	Amotivational syndrome	Abstinence
PCP	Mild agitation	Ativan
	Psychosis/Delirium	Ativan or Haldol
Psychostimulants	Anxiety	Ativan
	Agitation/psychosis	Ativan or Haldol
	Panic attack or generalized anxiety	Abstinence and appropriate follow-up
Opiates	Overdose	Naloxone and support
	Withdrawal	Detoxification (Methadone or Clonidine)
Sedative-hypnotics	Agitation	Haldol
	Overdose	Supportive therapy
	Withdrawal	Barbiturate or benzodiazepine Detoxification
Hallucinogens	Agitation/anxiety	Support and/or Ativan
	Toxic psychosis	Haldol
	Drug-precipitated psychosis	Follow-up and treatment of underlying illness

ies have not yet been done to clearly demonstrate this claim.

The low-potency antipsychotic chlorpromazine (Thorazine) probably should not be used in these already compromised individuals because of its ability to induce dramatic hypotension or an atropine-like delirium (caused by its strong anticholinergic side effects).

NONPHARMACOLOGIC TREATMENT OF ADDICTIVE DISORDERS

BASIC GUIDELINES

The best approach to the treatment of addictive disorders (see Table 85-12 for signs and symptoms) appears to be by using a disease model (e.g., addiction is a chronic illness that causes multiple psychologic and social problems). The causes of various addictions are multifactorial and the population is heterogeneous. Therefore, treatment must be approached with an open mind because many individuals do not respond to the more accepted forms of therapy.

GOALS OF TREATMENT

Detoxification from the abused drug is the first step in any treatment. Not all patients exhibit signs of withdrawal or need medical treatment when terminating the use of an abused drug. Those who do should be treated in a medically supervised setting.

Abstinence, or the act of not indulging in the abused drug, is begun only after a successful detoxification and is the mainstay of treatment for most addictive disorders. The most effective way to achieve abstinence and how long it must be maintained is the subject of heated debate. At present it is believed that, at least initially, self-help groups such as Alcoholics Anonymous (AA), Cocaine Anonymous (CA), and Narcotics Anonymous (NA) may be the most effective means of maintaining abstinence over extended periods.

Sobriety is the ultimate goal in individual recovery. Drug use is the central factor in the existence of most of these patients (in a psychologic and social sense). Once removed, drugs must be replaced by major changes in the patient's habits and life style. It is these changes that constitute sobriety and are paramount to successful rehabilitation. Without accomplishing this, individuals may be abstinent from drugs but tend to be dissatisfied with the quality of their lives. The best way to achieve sobriety is unclear but, at present, it is believed that a combination of self-help group participation and some form of psychotherapy is necessary to achieve this goal.

TABLE 85-12. SIGNS AND SYMPTOMS OF DRUG USE

PSYCHOSTIMULANTS:
Elevated BP, increased pulse, hyperreflexia, moist skin, dilated pupils, dry mouth, tremors, hyperactivity, paranoia, altered sensorium, possible hallucinations
PCP:
Euphoria, hypertension, tachycardia, hyperreflexia, diaphoresis, decreased responsiveness to pain, fluctuating mental status, may progress to stupor or coma, convulsions, arrhythmias, hypertensive crisis
CANNABIS:
Postural hypotension, tachycardia, conjunctival injection, distortion of time and space perception, anxiety, paranoia, possible hallucinations
HALLUCINOGENS:
Hypertension, tachycardia, hyperreflexia, mild hyperthermia, flushed skin, dilated pupils, euphoria, hallucinations, depersonalization, possible severe anxiety and paranoia
NARCOTICS:
Hypotension, hyporreflexia, mild hypothermia, constricted pupils, possible cyanotic skin with overdose, depressed respirations, patient possibly obtunded or comatose
SEDATIVE-HYPNOTICS:
Hypotension, hyporreflexia, mild hypothermia, possible cyanotic skin with overdose, possible constricted pupils, lateral gaze nystagmus, depressed respirations, ataxia, slurred speech, confusion, disinhibition, drowsiness to coma

TREATMENT PROGRAMS

The role of the ED is to have available the community resources for referral. Additionally, two main forms of treatment are available for the substance abuser/addict: self-help groups, AA being the largest of these, and professionally run chemical dependency programs, which tend to follow a disease model of addiction. It is generally accepted that individuals seeking abstinence should attend self-help groups regardless of the other forms of therapy they may be receiving. It is less clear which individuals need to attend professional programs and, if they do, whether inpatient or outpatient treatment is indicated. The following guidelines may be helpful in matching individuals to treatment programs.

1. Inpatient treatment, following detoxification, is usually indicated for patients with medical or severe concurrent psychiatric problems (e.g., depression, anxiety disorders, dementia); those with frequent heavy use, and those who have not been successfully treated in outpatient settings. The trend, until recently, has been to initiate treatment with 21- to 30-day hospitalizations. It is unclear whether extended inpatient stays have an overall significant (or any) impact on the long-term outcome of these disorders. Therefore there has been a shift toward shorter stays or no inpatient treatment for the less seriously ill, with the main focus on outpatient programs and self-help groups.

2. Many individuals may find that self-help groups alone are not sufficient for them to stop abusing drugs and or improve the quality of their lives. These individuals can benefit from attending professionally run outpatient programs for psychotherapy and education. The best of the programs treat families, based on the realization that addicts are enmeshed in complex networks and that the entire family and extended family must be involved.

3. Lastly, it is becoming increasingly recognized that a percentage of these individuals suffer from non-drug-related psychiatric syndromes that will threaten their abstinence. In many instances, such syndromes need treatment administered by professionals knowledgeable in addictive disorders.

SELF-HELP GROUPS

Self-help groups, which all addicts should attend, are an important part of the lifelong process of recovery. These are nonprofessional organizations that constitute the cornerstone of treatment for most addicts. They view addiction as a disease and the treatment as based on "12 steps," which the patient needs to follow for recovery. An important therapeutic aspect of these programs is that the group setting is used as a powerful method to confront the addict's denial of his or her illness. Individuals are educated about the signs, symptoms, and effects of addictive disorders. Addicts are taught that they are individually unable to control their drug use and need the group and treatment to help them maintain abstinence. Finally, these groups provide an abstinent social support system, role models, and a place to learn new behaviors and coping skills to aid addicts in rehabilitating their lives.

BIBLIOGRAPHY

GENERAL

Kozel, N.J., and Adams, E.H.: Epidemiology of drug abuse: An overview. Science 234:970, 1986.

Mirin, S.M., and Weiss, R.D.: Substance abuse. *In* The Practitioner's Guide to Psychoactive Drugs. Edited by Bussuk, E.L., Schoenover, S.C., and Gelenberg, A.J., New York, Plenum Medical Book Comapny, 1983, pp 221–290.

Redda, K.K., Walder, C.A., and Barnett, G. (eds.): Cocaine, Marijuana, Designer Drugs: Chemistry, Pharmacology, and Behavior. Florida, CRC Press, 1989.

COCAINE

Clegler, L.L., and Mark, H.: Medical complications of cocaine abuse. N. Engl. J. Med. 315:1495, 1986.

Ficshman, M.W.: Cocaine and the amphetamines. *In* Psychopharmacology: The Third Generation of Progress. Edited by Meltzer, H.Y. New York, Raven Press, 1987, pp. 1543–1552.

Gawin, F.H., and Ellinwiid, E.H.: Cocaine and other stimulants: Actions, abuse and treatment. N. Engl. J. Med. 318:1173–1182, 1988.

Kleber, H.D., and Gawin, F.H.: Cocaine. *In* APA Annual Review. Edited by Frances, A.J., and Hales, R.E. Washington, DC, American Psychiatric Press, 1986, vol. 5, pp. 160–85.

Millman, R.B.: Evaluation and clinical management of cocaine abusers. J. Clin. Psychiatry 49:27, 1988.

O'Brien, C.P., Childress, A.R., Arndt, I.O., et al.: Pharmacological and behavioral treatment of cocaine dependance: Controlled studies. J. Clin. Psychiatry 49:2(suppl): 1988.

PHENCYCLIDINE

Allen, R.M., and Young, S.J.: Phencyclidine-induced psychosis. Am. J. Psychiatry 135:1081, 1978.

Blaster, R.L.: The behavioral pharmacology of phencyclidine. *In* Psychopharmacology: The third generation of progress. Edited by Meltzer, H.Y. New York, Raven Press, 1987, 169:1573–1578.

Clover, D.H. (eds): Phencyclidine: An Update: NIDA Res. Monograph 64, DHHS Publ. No. (ADM) 86–1443, U.S. Gov. Printing Office, Washington, 1986.

Yesavage, J.A., and Freeman, A.M.: Acute phencyclidine intoxication: Pscyhopathology and prognosis. J. Clin. Psychiatry 39:664, 1987.

MARIJUANA

Ehrenkranz, J.R.L., and Hembree, W.C.: Effect of marijuana on male reproductive function. Psychiatric Annals 16:243, 1986.

Estroff, T.W., and Gold, M.S.: Psychiatric presentation for marijuana abuse. Psychiatric Annals 16:221, 1986.

Halikas, J.A.: Marihuana use and psychiatric illness. *In* Miller LI (ed); Marihuana: Effects on Human Behavior. New York, Academic Press, 1974, pp. 265–302.

Jones, R.T., Benowitz, N.L., and Herning, R.I.: Clinical relevance of cannabis tolerance and dependence. J. Clin. Pharmacol. 21:1435, 1981.

McDonald, D.I., and Czechowicz, D.: Marijuana: A pediatric overview. Psychiatric Annals 16:215, 1986.

Mendelson, J.H.: Marijuana. *In* Psychopharmacology: The Third Generation of Progress. Edited by Meltzer, H.Y. New York, Raven Press, 1987, 168:1565–1569.

OPIATES

Charney, D.S., Sternberg, D.E., Kleber, H.D., et al.: The clinical use of clonidine in abrupt withdrawal from methadone. Arch. Gen. Psychiatry 38:1273, 1981.

Gold, M.S., Pottash, A.C., Sweeney, D.R., et al.: Opiate withdrawal using clonidine. JAMA 243:343, 1980.

Jaffe, J.H., and Martin, W.R.: Opioid analgesics and antagonists. *In* Goodman and Gilman's The Pharmacological Basis of Therapeutics. Edited by: Gilman, A.G., Goodman, L.S., and Rall, T.W. New York, Macmillan, 1985, pp. 491–531.

Wesson, D.R., and Smith, D.E.: A conceptual approach to detoxification. J. Psychedelic Drugs 6:161, 1974.

HALLUCINOGENS

Bowers, M.B.: Acute psychosis induced by psychotomimetic drug abuse: I. Clinical findings. Arch. Gen. Psychiatry 27:437, 1972.

Bowers, M.B.: Acute psychosis induced by psychotomimetic drug abuse. II. Neurochemical findings. Arch. Gen. Psychiatry 27:440, 1972.

Brawley, P., and Duffield, J.C.: The pharmacology of hallucinogens. Pharmacol. Rev. 24:31, 1972.

Jaffe, J.H.: Drug addiction and drug abuse. *In* Goodman and Gilman's The Pharmacological Basis of Therapeutics, ed 7. Edited by Gilman, A.G., Goodman, L.S., and Rall, T.W. New York, Macmillan, 1985, pp 535–584.

Tucker, G.J., Quinlan, D., and Harrow, M.: Chronic hallucinogenic drug use and thought disturbance. Arch. Gen. Psychiatry 27:443, 1972.

SEDATIVE-HYPNOTICS

Allgulander, C.: Dependence on sedative and hypnotic drugs. Acta Psychiatr. Scand. 270(suppl):1, 1978.

Busto, U., Sellars, E.M., Naranjo, C.A., et al.: Withdrawal reaction after long term therapeutic use of benzodiazepines. N. Engl. J. Med. 315:854, 1986.

Epstein, R.S.: Withdrawal symptoms from chronic low-dose barbiturates. Am. J. Psychiatry 137:107, 1980.

Harvey, S.C.: Hypnotics and sedatives. *In* Goodman and Gilman's The Pharmacological Basis of Theraputics, ed 7. Edited by Gilman, A.G., Goodman, L.S., and Rall, T.W. New York, Macmillan, 1985, pp. 339–371.

Wesson, D.R., and Smith, D.E.: Barbiturates: Their Misuse and Abuse. New York, Human Sciences Press, 1977.

Wikler, A.: Diagnosis and treatment of drug dependence of the barbiturate type. Am. J. Psychiatry 125:158, 1968.

Chapter 86

FOOD POISONING

George R. Schwartz

CAPSULE

"Food poisoning," following the ingestion of certain foods, has multiple causes.

It may be caused by bacterial *toxins* that are ingested preformed or elaborated in the intestine by bacteria contaminating the particular food. For example, the ingestion of food (such as salads, ham and cold meat products, and cream-filled desserts) contaminated with enterotoxin is responsible for staphylococcal food poisoning. Botulism, staphylococcal food poisoning, cholera (Vibrio cholerae), and food poisoning from Clostridium perfringens and Bacillus cereus are considered true intoxications, because clinical illness is produced in each case by a toxin.

Food poisoning may also be caused by a direct *infection* or "invasion" of the intestine by bacteria, as classically occurs in salmonella food poisoning after ingestion of contaminated food—particularly poultry, milk and dairy products, egg products, and water. Other causes of food poisoning by direct bacterial infection include shigellosis (bacillary dysentery), Campylobacter fetus (enteritis), Streptococcus faecalis, and Yersinia enterocolitica.

Escherichia coli produces gastroenteritis both by elaboration of an enterotoxin, as the cause of E. coli "traveler's diarrhea," and by direct bacterial invasion. Furthermore, in certain bacterial infections, it is unclear whether the acute gastrointestinal symptoms are caused by toxin or by direct infection, as with Vibrio parahemolyticus.

Food poisoning may also be caused by viruses (an example is rotavirus in children) and protozoa, such as Entamoeba histolytica, the etiologic agent in amebiasis, and Giardia lamblia. Food poisoning produced by marine organisms, plants, and mushrooms is discussed later in this chapter. Food poisoning may also occur from toxic contaminants (PCBs, heavy metals, radioactivity) or from natural toxic substances (akee fruit).

This chapter is divided into three sections discussing (1) food poisoning caused by botulism, (2) food poisoning caused by microorganisms, and (3) food poisoning caused by chemicals naturally present in foods and plants.

FOOD POISONING CAUSED BY BOTULISM

Botulism is a serious disease caused by the toxin elaborated by the spore-forming anaerobic bacillus Clostridium botulinum. The toxin is generally conceded to be the most poisonous substance yet discovered. As an example of its toxicity, as few as 950 molecules of toxin can be lethal for white mice, and the amount that can cause human death has been estimated to be between 0.1 and 1 μg. The toxins are good antigens, but natural immunity in people rarely occurs because the lethal dose is less than that needed to elicit antibody production. Botulism is considered a rare disease, and outbreaks must be reported to the Centers for Disease Control (CDC) in Atlanta, Georgia.

From 1899 to 1977, 766 outbreaks involving 1961 cases were reported in the United States. There were 99 deaths. The Canadian experience from 1919 through 1973 was reported by Dolman. He found 62 authenticated outbreaks involving 181 persons, with 83 deaths. The incidence of fatality has been substantially reduced over the past 2 decades from greater than 60% to less than 20%. This reduction is primarily because of better respiratory care of victims, although it is possible that milder cases are being recognized. Prompt administration of antitoxin is probably also a factor. There is good reason to suspect that botulism is far more common than is generally realized and is underdiagnosed.

The following form the basis for this statement:

1. The diagnosis is difficult to make, particularly in isolated cases. One analysis of eight cases of botulism caused by contaminated smoked fish showed that the attending physicians failed to reach the diagnosis initially in each instance. An outbreak of botulism occurred in New Mexico in 1978, and more than half the affected group were not correctly diagnosed initially in the Emergency Department (ED) (see subsequent text). Because death may occur rapidly from respiratory paralysis, cases unassociated with a large outbreak are likely to be unrecognized. Conversely, because there is a range of disease—from very mild to lethal, the very mild cases associated with only a slight headache and perhaps some malaise and nausea—mild weakness may never come to medical attention.

2. Recent studies have demonstrated the syndrome of infant botulism. In fact, only since 1976 has there been intensive investigation of this syndrome; it was then realized that intestinal production of the toxin by the Clostridium botulinum organism was probably occurring chronically within the affected infant. Infant botulism is not new. It is, however, finally being recognized, and estimates of its frequency have been rising yearly. Intestinal infection and botulism have been reported in adults.

MODE OF TOXIN ACTION

The action of the toxin prevents the release of the neurotransmitter acetylcholine at the neuromuscular and other cholinergic junctions. The botulinum toxin is protein in nature, and there are at least seven immunologically distinct types. In human beings, almost all disease results from the types identified as type A, type B, and type E, although there have been recent reports of type "F." It is impossible to determine in the acute situation the type of toxin involved in a case of botulism. As a result, the initial treatment requires use of a trivalent (A, B, and E) anti-serum, which will be described in more detail in the section on treatment. Because of the potent functional denervation of muscle by the toxin, injections have been used in dystonias (Jankovic, 1991).

GEOGRAPHIC CONSIDERATIONS

Despite the difficulty in differentiating toxin type, some epidemiologic information is of interest and might perhaps have increasing relevance in the future. Of the outbreaks reported in the United States, approximately 40% were tested for type of toxin; 26% were type A, 7.8% were type B, and 4.2% were type E. Although outbreaks were reported from 44 states, 5 states (California, Oregon, Washington, Colorado, and New Mexico) accounted for more than half the cases. This may relate to the altitude, particularly in Colorado and New Mexico. A large part of these two states has an altitude greater than 5000 feet, with a resultant reduction in the temperature at which water boils. At 5000 feet, water boils at approximately 95°C (203°F) as compared with 100°C (212°F) at sea level. Any chef can tell you this difference is important in food preparation. At 10,000 feet, water boils at about 90°C. (194°F.). Temperature makes a substantial difference when it comes to killing spores of C. botulinum in foods. A large-scale test demonstrated that type A and type B spores can be totally destroyed by boiling for 6.5 hours at 100°C. At 95°C, the time required for killing spores is doubled (13 hours). Using a pressure cooker can make a substantial difference. Heating to 120°C. (248°F.) resulted in spore death within 3 minutes. Although spores are resistant to heat, toxin is readily inactivated by heat. Boiling for 5 minutes, even at high altitude, ensures destruction of the toxin.

More than 90% of reported botulism outbreaks caused by type A occurred west of the Mississippi River. Two thirds of the reported type B outbreaks occurred in eastern states. Most of the type E outbreaks in the United States occurred in Alaska or in the Great Lakes region. No type A or type B has been reported from Alaska.

TYPES OF FOOD IMPLICATED

Botulism is much more likely to result from home-processed foods—particularly those that are smoked, pickled, or home-canned—than from commercially processed foods. Despite the widely publicized outbreaks that have resulted from commercially prepared foods, of 766 outbreaks in the United States over a 78-year period, only 66 could be traced to commercial foods. The CDC reports have been confusing in this statistic. In a report by a CDC representative in 1969, the statement appears that "since 1910 . . . only a few outbreaks have been ascribed to commercially prepared foods." In a 1977 report, the figure is given of 66 such outbreaks. This seems larger than "a few." No definitions of "commercially prepared foods" are given that might account for this apparent difference. Home-canned vegetables (e.g., tomatoes, beans) have been frequently implicated. If the pH of the food is lower than 4.5, toxin formation is unlikely, although there have been some reports of toxin production from pickled herring kept at a pH of 4 to 4.2. Cases have been reported from smoked fish and from ham and other meats. The word botulism actually arises from the Latin *botulus*, which means sausage. In Alaska, a recent outbreak involved stored beaver tail and beaver flippers. The incidence of botulism appears to be higher among Eskimos because of their storage and ingestion of uncooked seal and whale meat.

Spoilage of the food may be obvious, but relying on gross signs is inadequate because of the lethality of very small amounts of the toxin. Although toxin-containing foods are the principal cause of the clinical syndrome of botulism, it has been demonstrated that infants who ingest spores may develop botulism through formation of toxin within the gut. Although uncommon, wound botulism has been reported in association with soil-contaminated deep wounds suitable for growth of the anaerobic C. botulinum.

All age groups may be affected by botulism. The observation has been made that, in an outbreak, children fare better than adults. This is believed to be related to lesser food intake by children.

INFANT BOTULISM

Infant botulism is a newly identified condition that may be more common than currently diagnosed. It was first recognized in 1976, and 58 cases were reported in 1976 and 1977. By 1980, there were 139 laboratory-confirmed cases, and 815 by 1988.

About one third of all reported cases of infant botulism in 1976 were associated with ingestion of honey containing C. botulinum spores. In a recent analysis of 90 different jars of honey, nine (10%) were contaminated by C. botulinum spores. It is theorized that the spores elaborate small amounts of toxin in the infants' intestines. As of 1977, all cases except one so far reported were in infants under 6 months old. Because of these findings, honey is not recommended for children under 1 year of age. The sole case in 1977 of an older child was a patient aged 35 weeks. More reports of infant botulism at ages greater than 6 months have been made as physicians look for such cases.

Symptoms in children are more insidious and may be chronic. The children seem lethargic and flaccid. They have a poor cry and problems with eating. Heretofore, they would have been diagnosed as having "failure to thrive" or "infection." Constipation is the most common presenting symptom. Loss of head control is a particularly striking symptom. Weakness may progress to respiratory paralysis and death. Some physicians have wondered whether botulism might be one cause of the sudden infant death syndrome (SIDS). In 139 cases of infant botulism reported by 1980, there were 3 deaths. Respiratory arrest was the cause of death in two children, and infection was the cause of death in the third child. The low fatality rate might indicate deficiencies in case detection.

Diagnosis rests on identification of C. botulinum or botulinum toxin in the child's feces. Of 58 cases reported, 90% had botulinum toxin in the feces. Differential diagnosis includes sepsis, myasthenia, heavy metal poisoning, muscular dystrophy, hypothyroidism, poliomyelitis, diseases of metabolism, and nonspecific syndromes. The only other clinical test that showed consistent alteration in infant botulism was the electromyogram, which demonstrated a peculiar pattern of brief duration, small amplitude, and overly frequent motor unit action potential.

WOUND BOTULISM

The syndrome of botulism following infection of a wound by C. botulinum was first reported in 1943.

Neurologic signs and symptoms develop within 1 to 2 weeks following a wound that has been contaminated with C. botulinum. The wound is usually one that has significant tissue injury, such as an open fracture, crush injury, or amputation. In all three of the recent cases, treatment with cephalosporin antibiotics failed to be prophylactic against the colonization of the bacteria in the wound. Wounds infected with C. botulinum may appear innocuous, without induration, crepitus, or lymphadenopathy. The neurologic picture is indistinguishable from that which occurs following ingestion of the toxin, and treatment with antitoxin is advised as soon as this rare syndrome is suspected. Perhaps physicians should inquire as to previous wounds when investigating patients with neurologic complaints. Unlike cases of food-borne botulism in which a certain amount of toxin is ingested, wound botulism results in ongoing production of toxin. Delays in diagnosis may make a substantial difference in the clinical course.

THE 1978 NEW MEXICO OUTBREAK

In April 1978, there was an outbreak of botulism resulting from individuals eating contaminated food in a country club in Clovis, New Mexico. The 34 cases were found to be type A. The outbreak could not be traced definitely to any food. However, there was some evidence implicating canned three-bean salad. Two people died. This was the second largest outbreak of botulism to occur in the United States since 1899 and the largest caused by type A botulinum toxin. Attention to prompt respiratory care and antitoxin use is credited with the low fatality rate. Careful case findings also might have detected the milder cases.

The following clinical cases illustrate common presentations of botulism.

Case 1: A 36-year-old female school teacher in excellent health ate a buffet on April 13, 1978 between approximately 6:00 and 8:00 P.M. She went to bed that night feeling fine and the next day appeared normal. At approximately 8:00 P.M.—24 hours after the ingestion of food now known to have been contaminated with spores and botulinum toxin—she complained of blurred vision. She had a difficult time making an image remain constant. Over the next hour, this symptom waxed and waned, then at 9:00 P.M. she became dizzy and lightheaded and developed a slight headache and slurred speech.

At approximately 1:00 A.M. the following morning (30 hours after ingestion), she went to an emergency facility and a diagnosis of "flu syndrome" was made. By the next morning, however, after other cases had surfaced, she was called back and admitted to the hospital. On admission, her vital signs were stable, and her blood gases were within normal limits. While in the hospital, she was treated with 1 million units of penicillin intravenously, four times daily, and she received one ampule of trivalent antitoxin intravenously and one ampule of trivalent antitoxin intramuscularly after 24 hours.

Her course deteriorated slightly over the next weeks, and 4 days after admission a loss of the gag reflex was noted, as well as diminution of vital capacity from 1900 to 1400 cc. Her condition stabilized, however, and began to improve, and she was discharged 2 weeks after admission. Six months later, she still had decreased salivation, some difficulty in swallowing, and a decreased overall energy level. On admission, her only abnormal laboratory examination was elevation of the white blood cell count to 12,000 with 79 segmented cells. Over the next several days, this count rose to 15,000 and returned to normal in a week.

Case 2: A 49-year-old man in good health had a complete dinner at the same buffet on the night of

April 13, 1978. He slept well that night and on the next day decided to return to Albuquerque by automobile. As he was driving, he noticed his eyes were "more tired than usual." By approximately 6:00 P.M. (24 hours after ingestion), he noticed he had some blurring of vision and a slight staggering of gait. He went to bed that night feeling generalized malaise and weakness, and at 5:30 A.M. (35.5 hours after ingestion), he awakened with nausea and vomiting. At that point, he had difficulty in speaking and poor respirations and generalized weakness. He went to a hospital ED, and the initial suspicion was that he had suffered a stroke. On the next day, however, his condition was recognized as botulism.

Examination showed an obese man with a slight tachycardia of 108, normal temperature, and normal blood pressure. His extraocular muscles showed weakness of the third, fourth, and sixth cranial nerves, and his deep tendon reflexes were decreased. His arterial blood gases showed a PO_2 of 55, a PCO_2 of 25, and a pH of 7.48. His white blood cell count was 7000, with 36 segment cells and 36 bands.

Over the next 24 hours, he had progressive respiratory difficulty and required intubation and later tracheostomy and ventilator support. Initial treatment included penicillin, 4 million units per day for 1 week, and he received two ampules of multivalent antitoxin. Subsequently, the type of botulinum toxin was identified as type A.

After a stormy hospital course, he began to improve and was discharged on July 15, 1978 after a total hospitalization of 3 months. Five days after discharge, he was found dead in a chair. The cause of death was officially listed as cardiovascular disease, although the postmortem examination was inconclusive.

Case 3: A 52-year-old man had eaten at the buffet on the evening of April 13, 1978 at approximately 6:00 to 8:00 P.M. On April 14, at approximately 3:00 A.M.— 8 to 9 hours after the meal—he began getting blurred vision that progressed to double vision. By early morning, he had slurred speech and swallowing problems, and he was stumbling. At an ED, the suspicion was that he had had a "stroke." Subsequently, as the word spread about botulism, the diagnosis was established. Over the next 12 hours (18 to 30 hours after ingestion), he had increasing respiratory distress, and was intubated and put on ventilator treatment the evening of April 14. At this time, he had diffuse weakness (proximal muscles weaker than distal). He also was constipated and had urinary retention. His initial treatment was 4 million units of penicillin per day for 5 days, and one vial of multivalent antitoxin intravenously and another intramuscularly. He was discharged after 2 months. More than 6 months later, however, he still had some muscle weakness and occasional difficulty in swallowing.

Case 4: The patient, an 11-year-old boy, also ate at the buffet that evening. On Friday morning, 36 hours after ingestion, he had blurred vision and trouble in walking. He was nauseated, vomited three times, and developed a mild, persistent frontal headache. Although he did not complain of shortness of breath, his arterial blood gases showed a pH of 7.42, PCO_2 of 32, and PO_2 of 59. His white blood count was 9000, with 72 segmented cells and 5 bands. His pulmonary function tests demonstrated 46% of what would be expected at his age and weight. He was treated with penicillin and antitoxin, and his condition did not worsen. He was discharged after 1 week.

Case 5: The mother of the preceding patient, a 37-year-old woman in good health, also ate at the buffet and 40 hours afterward complained of "weird eyes," which "sometimes saw double." She had a dry mouth but no initial dysphagia. After a week she did complain of some problems in eating and swallowing. She also complained of mild shortness of breath, but her blood gases were normal. She was hospitalized and treated with two ampules of antitoxin and penicillin. Her condition improved, and she was discharged after 5 days. All laboratory studies were normal.

SUMMARY OF CLINICAL SIGNS AND COURSE

The following facts have been noted concerning botulism outbreaks:

1. In many outbreaks, initial cases are incorrectly diagnosed as "flu," "viral syndrome," or "stroke." Early recognition and diagnosis are most difficult. It is important to note that in none of the preceding cases was the correct diagnosis made on initial physician contact.
2. Symptoms usually appear within the first 24 hours but may be delayed as long as 48 hours or even longer than 72 hours. My experience with the New Mexico outbreak exhibited a range of 8 to 80 hours for patients to develop initial symptoms.
3. Earliest symptoms involve vague malaise, headache, weakness, dizziness, blurred vision, and sometimes dry mouth. In the largest series of botulism patients from a single outbreak (in Michigan, 1977), dry mouth was found in all those affected, and 86% had difficulty with focusing or diplopia. This outbreak was type B in origin.
4. Progression is variable, but most commonly initial symptoms appear, and in severe cases progression over the subsequent 6 to 8 hours leads to respiratory paralysis. Of 34 cases studied in New Mexico, 11 required mechanical ventilation. Botulism can be mild; symptoms may rarely progress beyond nausea and mild visual problems, or perhaps fatigue. Mild cases usually clear in 1 week.
5. An important early symptom is blurring of vision. Patients usually do not complain of classic "diplopia." Instead, they say "Everything is blurred," or "I can't get the image into focus," or "My eyes are tired or wandering."

6. Progression of more severe cases includes increasing problems with vision, slurred speech, dryness of mouth, diffuse weakness, difficulty in swallowing, and difficulty in walking, usually described as "staggering." The rapidity of the course is highly individual over a 24-hour period. Most significantly, the sensorium and intellectual functioning remain intact, and memory is not impaired. The neurologic symptoms are usually bilateral and symmetric and are motor, not sensory. The cerebrospinal fluid is normal.

7. Nausea and vomiting may occur, but large studies have demonstrated that in only 30 to 40% of cases of botulism were nausea and vomiting prominent. With detailed questioning, nausea was found as a symptom in 60 to 70% of patients. In contrast, visual difficulty was reported in more than 90% of the patients. Constipation and urinary disturbance was found in less than 50% of the patients. The visual disturbance results from abducens nerve palsy.

8. More severe cases show early third cranial nerve involvement. Pupils may become fixed and dilated.

9. *As a general rule, the earlier the onset, the more severe the case.*

CLINICAL DIFFERENTIATION IN ADULTS

Early cases are difficult to diagnose, as are mild cases that do not progress. No laboratory test can readily be used to diagnose botulism in the ED. Common conditions that figure in the differential diagnosis include Guillain-Barré syndrome, cerebrovascular accident or transient ischemic attack, tick paralysis, heavy metal poisoning (particularly lead), psychiatric conditions, drug abuse, alcohol intoxication, untoward reaction to anticholinergic medication, myasthenia gravis, dilantin toxicity, atropine poisoning, encephalitis, carbon monoxide poisoning, electrolyte abnormalities, and amyotrophic lateral sclerosis.

Diagnosis in adults rests on clinical grounds. Confirmation comes from observing botulism in a mouse (sensitive to 900 molecules) that has been injected with toxin from the patient's serum or with the suspected food. It is worthwhile to test for toxin even weeks after the onset of clinical illness because of the high sensitivity of the mouse to the toxin as well as the reports of circulating toxin even 2 weeks after onset. Clostridium botulinum and toxin also may be identified in the patient's feces.

Put all specimens in *leakproof* containers, and remember that botulinum toxin is the most powerful toxin known. In case of a spill, neutralize with a strong alkaline solution if available. Suitable specimens may include serum, stool, vomitus, food samples, food containers, or wound material. The specimens should be refrigerated. Label carefully! Include in particular any drugs the patient is taking. Call the CDC for further information.

MEDICAL TREATMENT

IMMEDIATE CARE

Immediate attention must be given to airway and respiratory function. When deaths occur initially, they almost always result from respiratory paralysis. Careful gastric lavage should be performed. Emesis can be initiated if there is a good gag reflex. In addition, charcoal should be instilled through the tube after emesis and lavage. A cathartic is unlikely to be helpful but can be used and may speed the flow of the charcoal. Similarly, colonic enemas can be used.

If there is difficulty with breathing and arterial blood gases and vital capacity deteriorate or initially show hypoxia, hypercapnia, or a vital capacity of less than 1000 mL, tracheostomy should be considered. Certainly, with borderline cases, a trial of ventilatory assistance can be instituted before any surgical procedure. In the large 1977 Michigan outbreak of type B botulism, the presence of ptosis, dilated and sluggishly reacting pupils, and paresis of the medial recti was associated with the need for artificial ventilatory support in 8 of 11 patients. These aspects of third nerve dysfunction became apparent after approximately 12 hours. Tracheostomy is best performed as a slow, careful procedure under ideal conditions because a ventilator may be necessary for months.

ANTITOXIN THERAPY

Trivalent antitoxin is available from the CDC and should be administered to all patients with suspected botulism. Each vial of equine antiserum contains 7500 IU of type A, 5500 IU of type B, and 8500 IU of type E antitoxins. One to two vials are administered intravenously initially and again in 4 hours. One vial of antiserum may be given intramuscularly in 24 hours; repeated injections may be indicated, depending on the clinical condition. Desensitization may be necessary because the antitoxin is a horse serum derivative. In cases of known reactions to horse serum, 100 mg. of hydrocortisone can be injected before the use of antiserum. Allergic reactions can be treated with antihistamines or steroids, or both. Of 30 patients in the 1978 New Mexico outbreak who received antitoxin, one developed serum sickness. Antitoxin of human origin (from people who received muscle injections for dystonia) has been used in infant botulism with some reported success (Hathaway, 1992), but must be given early in the course.

PENICILLIN

Penicillin is indicated in the management of infant botulism and patients with wound botulism, because these two forms of botulism are caused by active infection with C. botulinum. Because botulinum food poisoning is caused by toxin and not by the organism, penicillin probably serves no role in management of these patients; however, it is often used on an empiric basis. Penicillin therapy is usually continued for 1 week. Penicillin also may be indicated in the event of aspiration pneumonia, and can play a role if there is intestinal infection by C. botulinum.

GUANIDINE HYDROCHLORIDE

Guanidine hydrochloride has been used experimentally to compete chemically with the toxin. No dramatic results have been observed with guanidine, and its use is no longer routinely recommended.

RESPIRATORY FUNCTION

Continued meticulous maintenance of respiratory function is a most important aspect of treatment. A patient's improvement is best followed by periodic assessment of vital capacity and arterial blood gases off ventilatory support. In pre-existing pulmonary disease, the baseline state may require estimation. Pulse oximetry can be used in the ED.

HOSPITALIZATION

In severe cases, patients may be hospitalized for as long as 3 to 6 months. Weaning from the ventilator may be difficult. With long-term hospitalization, release from the hospital must follow a graded rehabilitation program. Muscle wasting, lack of conditioning, orthostatic hypotension, and syncope frequently follow prolonged bed rest and muscle inactivity. There may be some minor dysphagia or malaise 6 to 12 months after the onset of illness.

MORTALITY

The use of antitoxin and supportive therapy can reduce the mortality rate from 50 to 70% in untreated cases to 10 to 25%.

FOOD POISONING CAUSED BY MICROORGANISMS

SHIGELLA (SHIGELLOSIS)

The Shigella species are aerobic, gram-negative, non-motile bacteria. There are four main species, all of which can cause human disease. Asymptomatic carriers are common. Differentiation as to type is done serologically with type-specific antisera. The invading organisms produce Shiga-toxin.

When bacillary dysentery occurs, the cause can be the ingestion of as few as 200 organisms. If a "suboptimal" number of bacteria are ingested, or if there is some immunity, an individual can have a subclinical infection or a nonsymptomatic carrier state. The range of clinical illness is broad. Children between the ages of 1 and 10 years are more susceptible to severe illness.

Although the condition is found more often in the tropics, it is endemic throughout the world. Epidemics have been traced to a variety of foods contaminatd by feces, but most commonly milk, eggs, and dairy products are implicated.

The incubation period is usually about 48 hours, but may be as short as 8 hours, or symptoms can be postponed for a week. It appears that there is some small intestinal colonization, but the large intestine is the preferred area. Bacterial growth depends on factors of immunity and existing flora, as well as the number of shigella organisms. Usually, within 1 week after recovery, the organism is not found in the feces.

Occasionally sequelae are reported, including neuropathy, arthritis, and skin eruptions. Sepsis in the acute stage is rare, but serious.

SYMPTOMS AND SIGNS

Following are features of Shigella poisoning:

1. Severe diarrhea: mucus, bloody stool.
2. Abdominal colic and tenderness.
3. Tenesmus.
4. Fever to 40°C. (104°F.) and malaise.
5. Pain often relieved by defecation.
6. Bowel sounds active and high pitched.
7. Possible syncope and hypotension with Shigella dysenteriae; if this species is responsible for the illness, it is usually more severe.
8. Outpouring of polymorphonucleocytes into the intestines and stool; sometimes sheets of white blood cells can be seen microscopically.
9. Rise in fever and white blood cell count.
10. Possible convulsions, particularly in younger children with higher peak temperature and a family history of seizures; sometimes sheets of white blood cells can be seen microscopically.
11. Hypotension and shock (more common in the elderly).

DIAGNOSIS

Table 86-1 shows a differential diagnosis of shigellosis with a comparison of amebic dysentery. The following features are helpful in diagnosis:

1. Stool culture.
2. A rise in serum agglutinin titer in 50% of the cases; however, this is not useful in diagnosis or treatment because of the delay.
3. White blood cell count usually greater than 10,000 with a left shift.

TABLE 86-1. ACUTE DIFFERENTIATION OF SHIGELLOSIS FROM AMEBIC DYSENTERY IN ELDERLY PATIENTS*

Amebic Dysentery	Shigella
Usually slower in progression, with mild to moderate diarrhea	Rapid onset, often with severe explosive diarrhea, with cramps and tenesmus
Temperature usually less than 101°F	Temperature usually more than 101.5°F (although hypothermia may be present)
Usually moderate symptoms that tend to wax and wane (only rarely presenting with a fulminant course with explosive diarrhea)	Rapid dehydration can lead to hypotension and shock (which is the reason for the estimated 10 to 20% mortality rate in the elderly)
Blood in stool on microscopic examination	Gross blood in stool
Fecal smear shows mononuclear cells and trophozoites	Fecal smear shows many leukocytes
Other systemic manifestations outside of the gastrointestinal tract (e.g., amebic liver abscesses, lung abscesses, central nervous system [CNS] symptoms, intestinal perforation, peritonitis)	Some systemic manifestations (e.g., meningitis, pyelonephritis, and osteomyelitis) have been reported, but are rare. Other manifestations—e.g., arthritis or Reiter's syndrome—occur days to weeks after the acute syndrome. Abdominal pain is common, however.

* A therapeutic trial with antibiotics is necessary if shigellosis is suspected because the mortality is so much higher in the elderly.

TREATMENT

For managment of shigellosis, give supportive treatment by preventing dehydration and maintaining electrolytes. The diarrheal condition is usually self-limited. Shock with dehydration and acidosis may occur, however, particularly in infants and the elderly. Convulsions respond to titrated diazepam or lorazepam.

Antibiotics are useful in moderate to severe cases for shortening the clinical course. *Possible choices* include, for adults, *ampicillin*, 1 g intravenously every 6 hours in the severe cases; otherwise, ampicillin 500 mg. orally four times daily for 5 days. This has been the accepted treatment for the past 8 to 10 years. Drug-resistant strains have resulted, however. Thus, selection of an antibiotic is more difficult. *Other choices* include *cephalothin*, or its derivatives, 1 g four times a day. *Chloramphenicol* was the old "standby," but risk of toxicity and bone marrow suppression has made it a less desirable choice. Fluoroquinolone antimicrobials have gained use in this condition, using norfloxacin or ciprofloxacin, given early in the course, and as prophylaxis.

Antidiarrheal agents (e.g., diphenoxylate hydrochloride and atropine [Lomotil], paregoric, or opiates) must be used cautiously because they may prolong the clinical course. Nonproductive tenesmus would be the best indication for using such agents.

For amebic colitis, antimicrobial therapy is needed—usually metronidazole followed in 1 week by diiodohydroxyquin (to eradicate cysts) (Table 86-1). Hospitalization and intensive treatment may be needed in infants and elderly patients.

SALMONELLA FOOD POISONING

The salmonellae, named for Dr. Salmon who described them in 1885, are gram-negative motile bacteria. The most common form of salmonella-induced human disease is the syndrome of Salmonella gastroenteritis. The range of gastroenteritis can be mild to severe, with the latter being associated with abdominal pain, colitis, and signs of a systemic inflammation (fever, elevated white blood cell count, malaise, etc.).

Typhoid fever is caused by Salmonella typhosa and differs from the common gastroenteritis primarily by its severity, prolonged course, and hematogenous dissemination of the bacillus with accompanying diffuse manifestations. A persistent carrier state can result.

The primary reservoir is the vertebrate intestine, and the passage is from person to person by fecal contamination of foodstuffs. Most commonly, meat, poultry, dairy, and egg products have been implicated. Other items, however, including creamy foods and prepared salads, have been implicated. Sterilization of contaminated foods is not always achieved by cooking, especially in large stuffed turkeys and in cooked eggs. Disease may also come by way of pets, because salmonellae can cause disease in animals, commonly dogs, cats, birds, and turtles.

To produce clinical disease in humans, at least 100,000 to 1 million bacteria of the nontyphoid salmonellae are usually required. To achieve these levels, a growth medium (i.e., food) is necessary, because simple contamination usually does not involve transfer of so many organisms. Subsequently, intestinal multiplication occurs. The need for a "minimum dose" makes direct fecal-oral transmission uncommon except with infants and children, and in the United States waterborne transmission is uncommon because of overall water sanitation.

The clinical disease results from an infection. There appears to be no production of toxin. Thus, prevention must focus on overall sanitation and identification of asymptomatic carriers. Prevention is important not only in terms of human comfort but also in view of studies that have demonstrated that salmonellosis costs at least $500 to $1000 per case for diagnosis, treatment, and follow-up.

Because Salmonella bacteria are killed at a pH level of 2, antacid use may increase susceptibility, as do conditions of reduced stomach acidity (including subtotal gastrectomy, vagotomy, and gastroenterostomy).

Salmonella gastroenteritis is a reportable infectious disease. Estimates have been made that the incidence reported by the CDC (10 cases per 100,000 population) represents one tenth to one hundredth of the actual incidence. The incidence is highest in the summer, and although all age groups may be affected, children under 5 years have the highest rate of infection.

Increased intercountry tourism, as well as intercountry trade involving foods, has resulted in increased risks of acquiring Salmonella gastroenteritis. There are more than 2500 species of Salmonella, some of which are found in one country and not in another. The mass tourism tends to make a more uniform distribution (one of the aspects of a "world community"). The largest outbreak of Salmonella food poisoning in recorded history occurred in the United States in 1985. This situation demonstrates the impact of large companies with wide food distribution. Over 14,000 cases were reported (almost all confirmed) with at least four associated deaths. The source was a large dairy, and contaminated low-fat milk was the vehicle for transmission of the Salmonella typhimurium. Lawsuits involving at least $100 million have been filed. In 1987, the New York State Department of Health investigated a hospital outbreak involving almost 1000 cases traced to raw eggs. This led to attempts by some states to regulate the cooking of eggs. At least 9 deaths occurred in this outbreak. The median age of 77.5 emphasizes the increased severity in the elderly and immunocompromised.

Some epidemiologists believe Salmonella infections are increasing, in part, because of the widespread use of antibiotics in animal feed and the development of drug-resistant bacteria. These can be passed widely by contaminated beef or chicken.

SYMPTOMS AND COURSE OF ILLNESS

Following are general features of Salmonella gastroenteritis:

1. General incubation period is 8 to 48 hours.
2. Complaints of general malaise, headache, mild abdominal pain, and fever of 37.78 to 38.33°C. (100° to 101°F.) are common initially.
3. Despite some nausea and vomiting that may occur, major symptoms are cramps and diarrhea; tenesmus is common and may help in diagnosis.
4. Rarely, the presence of bloody diarrhea; shigellosis and amebic dysentery are more often associated with bloody stools.
5. Occasionally, abdominal symptoms so severe as to suggest appendicitis or some other acute intra-abdominal process.

Although most acute symptoms subside within 2 to 5 days, occasionally a prolonged course of weeks occurs. Death from Salmonella gastroenteritis is uncommon and occurs primarily in infants, the aged, and persons with severe underlying disease.

Although arbitrary divisions have been made between a "gastroenteritis" and the systemic disease "typhoid fever," the division may not be clinically clear-cut. Salmonella bacteria other than S. typhosa (the cause of typhoid fever) may produce gastrointestinal symptoms, as well as sustained fever, and even positive blood cultures. In addition, it is possible to be infected by Salmonella bacteria and have few gastrointestinal signs and symptoms, but manifest chills, fever, and anorexia, and even some hepatosplenomegaly or respiratory symptoms. Spiking fever, headache, abdominal cramps, and rose spots on the torso are useful diagnostically.

The presence of bacteremia may result in a localized internal abscess, and even endocarditis, septic arthritis, or osteomyelitis can occur. Newborns and infants may develop meningitis. Such severe infections usually show striking signs and a marked leukocytosis, though in typhoid fever leukopenia occurs after the first 1 to 2 weeks.

DIAGNOSIS

Diagnosis and differentiation from shigellosis, enterotoxic E. coli, and amebic dysentery may be difficult. Other less common causes of acute diarrheal disease, such as that produced by Vibrio parahaemolyticus or viral agents, can also cause difficulty in diagnosis.

Definitive diagnosis clinically rests on isolation of the organism from the stool. If the contaminated food is available, it can be cultured. Excretions from pets can be tested as well if they appear to be possible sources.

A fecal smear may show inflammatory leukocytes, but usually somewhat less than with shigellosis and amebic dysentery. Bloody diarrhea is uncommon in Salmonella enterocolitis.

If there are systemic signs, blood cultures may show bacteremia. Although immunologic tests of various titers may show increases, the time delays usually render such tests of limited value.

TREATMENT

The cornerstone of treatment is prompt correction of dehydration and fluid and electrolyte imbalances. Intravenous fluids may be necessary, depending on clinical symptoms.

Antimotility agents (e.g., Lomotil and similar agents) that inhibit activity of the bowel substantially may also increase the severity of the disease. Experimental animals pretreated with antimotility agents showed increased susceptibility to Salmonella infection. If symptoms are severe and no contraindications are present, a low dose of morphine or atropine can be used to partially relieve symptoms.

If the patient shows high fever, chills, or other evidence of severe systemic infection, antibiotics are indicated. Chloramphenicol (50 to 60 mg/kg/day in four to six doses) may be used, but because of toxicity, third-generation cephalosporin or ampicillin (100 to 200 mg/kg/day in four divided doses) is recommended. Ciprofloxacin and other fluoroquinolone antibiotics have been highly effective against Salmonella, even eliminating carrier states. The trend is to use these antibiotics early to shorten clinical course and decrease carrier states. The course of antibiotics is for 10 days to 2 weeks. In cases in which there is evidence of an abscess, endocarditis, osteomyelitis, or other evidence of persistent internal infection, antibiotics may have to be continued for 4 to 6 weeks, and surgical drainage may be needed.

ENTEROPATHIC ESCHERICHIA COLI (TRAVELER'S DIARRHEA)

METHOD OF ACQUISITION

Dairy and meat products and contaminated water are common vehicles for infection. There is some suggestive evidence that bismuth salicylate may be effective prophylactic therapy against traveler's diarrhea (30 to 60 mL every 4 hours). Other prepared foods (salads, sauces) may harbor bacteria from fecal contamination. A general rule is to eat cooked foods shortly after preparation and to thoroughly wash raw fruits and vegetables and peel them thoroughly.

SYMPTOMS AND COURSE OF ILLNESS

Acute diarrhea may begin 8 to 12 hours after ingestion of contaminated food or water, though there may be a delayed onset of up to several days. Common symptoms include abdominal cramps, tenesmus, and profuse watery diarrhea, though there is a wide range of clinical illness.

There are two types of E. coli associated with food poisoning. One type does not produce a toxin, and symptoms result from intestinal infection. The other type is more commonly associated with the epidemic diarrhea of travelers, and this type does produce an enterotoxin. In the latter type, symptoms result from infection as well as from the effect of one of the toxins upon the colon. In general, E. coli produces a clinical disease that is usually milder than Salmonella disease or shigellosis, but in severe cases it may be indistinguishable from them. In fact, one strain of E. coli can cause severe hemorrhagic colitis and produce a toxin similar to one produced by Shigella dysenteriae. E. coli hemorrhagic colitis can be particularly severe in institutional settings. In one situation, 55 of 169 residents of a nursing home were affected. Of the residents, older age and previous gastrectomy increased the risk of acquiring the infection. Of the 55 affected residents, 19 (35%) died from the following causes: hemolytic-uremic syndrome (12 patients), acute colitis (1), cardiorespiratory failure (1), and nonspecific causes (5). This study also highlights the increased susceptibility in the elderly—55 of 169 residents versus 18 of 137 staff members—and the much higher morbidity and mortality. Of the total, 35% of the residents died from their infection, whereas none of the staff died.

E. coli diarrheal disease is of particular concern in infants and young children and the aged, who have limited tolerance to electrolyte imbalance because of overall condition, underlying illness, or medications that can affect electrolytes (e.g., diuretics).

DIAGNOSIS

Diagnosis may be possible by isolation of the organism in food or water and by culture of stool. Serologic diagnosis through testing for rises in titer against E. coli can be done, but such tests are not readily available. Smear of stool is important. Polymorphonucleocytes can be present, usually less than with shigellosis. Bloody diarrhea is also much less common.

TREATMENT

Supportive treatments are generally satisfactory, although the trend is to begin antibiotics early in the course. The disease generally lasts in its acute form for only 2 or 3 days. Nonspecific symptoms and malaise, however, usually continue for at least 1 week when untreated.

Doxycycline (100 mg by mouth daily) has shown a demonstrable benefit when used prophylactically, as has ciprofloxacin. Doxycycline or tetracycline should be used in severe cases when there is evidence of high fever. Bactrim (trimethoprim-sulfamethoxazole) and ciprofloxacin have also been used successfully. In the usual case, however, the disease is treated effectively with *clear liquids* and intravenous fluids if the diarrhea is severe enough to produce dehydration or electrolyte imbalance, but antibiotic use shortens the clinical course and reduces symptoms.

OTHER CAUSES OF "TRAVELER'S" DIARRHEA

While E. coli is the most common cause, "traveler's" diarrhea may also be caused by other microorganisms including Rotavirus (up to 10% of cases), Salmonella or Shigella (15 to 20%) and parasites (0 to 5%).

Rotavirus infection is generally self-limiting. Infants who are breast-feeding have some resistance. A woman traveling an endemic area with an infant should breast-feed if possible, since infants can rapidly become dehydrated from the diarrhea.

Giardia lamblia infection generally occurs days to weeks after the exposure and is characterized by foul-smelling, water stools. A stool smear and culture will help in diagnosing this parasite. This condition is usually not severe, but it occasionally requires treatment with metronidazole (250 mg three times daily for 5 days). Quinacrine may also be used. Pregnant women should not generally be treated because of dangers of the drugs to the fetus. In severe cases, the amino-glycoside antibiotic paromomycin has been given orally after the first trimester. It has poor absorption from the gastrointestinal tract and high fecal concentrations.

Entamoeba histolytica is a parasite that invades the mucous membranes of the intestines, causing ulcerations, hemorrhage and diarrhea. In severe cases, the parasite may cause perforation of the intestines or may invade other organs—particularly the liver or lung. Diagnosis rests on physical examination, stool examination, and possibly liver function tests and liver scan. Treatment of confirmed cases is mandatory and should include metronidazole and iodoquinol.

Although antibiotic treatment can reduce the clinical course of traveller's diarrhea, the growing problem of antimicrobial resistance must be emphasized. In Operation Desert Shield (1990–1991), numerous outbreaks of diarrhea occurred among U.S. forces. Stool cultures were positive in almost half of the 400 cases analyzed. Of 125 E. coli infections, 39% were resistant to trimethoprim-sulfamethoxazole (Bactrim), 63% to tetracycline, and 48% to ampicillin. Of 113 Shigella infections, 85% were resistant to Bactrim, 68% to tetracycline, and 21% to ampicillin. Importantly, all bacterial isolates were sensitive to ciprofloxacin and norfloxacin, newer antibiotics to which significant resistance has not yet developed.*

CLOSTRIDIUM PERFRINGENS CONDITIONS

Clostridium perfringens is a nonmotile gram-positive spore-forming rod. Disease is caused by growth of bacteria and toxin formation. It is now considered to be one of the most common types of food poisoning.

METHOD OF ACQUISITION

Meat and poultry products are commonly implicated, as are gravies and creamy (dairy or mayonnaise-containing) foods.

---

* Hyams, K.C., et al.: Diarrheal disease during Operation Desert Shield. N. Engl. J. Med. 325:1423, 1991.

SYMPTOMS AND COURSE OF ILLNESS

Because large numbers of organisms (usually greater than 10^6 organisms per gram) are generally necessary to cause signficant disease, most food poisoning resulting from C. perfringens is relatively mild. The incubation period is more than 8 hours and usually less than 24 hours. The disease is associated with cramps and diarrhea. Diarrhea is generally not as profuse as that found with Shigella, Salmonella or E. coli; characteristically, it is not bloody. There may be mild nausea, but vomiting is uncommon.

DIAGNOSIS

Diagnosis is made by detection of organism in food and stool.

TREATMENT

Symptomatic therapy is generally all that is required.

BACILLUS CEREUS CONDITIONS

Bacillus cereus is a slightly curved gram-positive rod found singly and in chains. It is motile. Disease arises from infection and some toxin production.

METHOD OF ACQUISITION

Food, particularly meat, dairy, and poultry products, has been discovered to be contaminated with this organism. Dried foods (e.g., mixes, potatoes) may be contaminated. Fried rice has been the source of some outbreaks. Growth does not ordinarily occur until hydration.

SYMPTOMS AND COURSE OF ILLNESS

Average incubation period is 8 to 12 hours. Average duration of illness is approximately 24 hours. Symptoms in order of magnitude are diarrhea, abdominal cramps, nausea, and vomiting. Fever is generally absent or is below 37.78°C (100°F). The clinical course may resemble that of staphylococcal food poisoning, with vomiting as the dominant symptom.

TREATMENT

Supportive therapy with intravenous fluids is usually sufficient even for relatively severe cases. Antinauseants may be given. There is no evidence that antibiotics are of value.

CHOLERA

Cholera is caused by Vibrio cholerae, a curved, motile, gram-negative rod. This condition is included because it can be rapidly fatal. Fortunately, however, it is rare in the United States at this time. During worldwide cholera pandemics, the United States has had many cases, e.g., 150,000 deaths in 1832 and 1849 and 50,000 deaths in 1866. In the United States, cholera is still endemic along the Gulf Coast with cases being reported particularly from Texas and Louisiana, where association with contaminated water and seafood has been found. The organism produces a proteinaceous toxin that can be activated by heat and acids.

METHOD OF ACQUISITION

In the epidemic form, the vibrio are usually waterborne or come from seafood. Person-to-person transmission is usual in the nonepidemic form. Occasionally, it may come from a restaurant in which a worker is infected. The food can also become contaminated, particularly when "night soil" (human excrement) is used as a fertilizer.

SYMPTOMS AND COURSE OF ILLNESS

The illness develops usually within 8 to 48 hours after ingestion with a severe enteritis associated with passage of copious amounts of non-foul-smelling diarrhea usually containing mucus and occasionally blood. The disease arises in association with an exotoxin that causes a severe disorder of the intestinal tract and results in marked intestinal secretions. Frequently the first stool is more than 1000 mL with a characteristic appearance of "rice water." The symptoms arise directly from the gastrointestinal fluid and electrolyte losses. Prostration and a shock-like state may occur rapidly. The patient may die within 12 to 24 hours if intravenous fluids or oral electrolytes are not provided. The illness characteristically lasts 1 to 7 days. With adequate fluid and electrolyte repletion, recovery is rapid. Hypokalemia is a particular problem in children, because the stool contains a higher potassium level than it does in adults.

DIAGNOSIS

Clinical suspicion of cholera is important, particularly in endemic or epidemic areas. Persons with decreased stomach acidity (because of surgical operations and antacids) are at higher risk. Also those with type 0 blood are at higher risk for unknown reasons.

The organism may be identified by culture, and one may look for the organisms on a Gram-stain slide. At medical centers familiar with cholera, a fluorescent antibody technique may identify the organism positively within 1 hour.

TREATMENT

The patient in a shock state must be treated with intravenous fluids. Oral fluids may be used when intravenous fluids are not available. A glucose-containing electrolyte solution may be given orally.

Generally acidosis, severe potassium losses, and dehydration occur. Those experienced in treating cholera use weight as a measure of dehydration and consider the case to be severe if there is greater than 10% body weight loss and mild if the loss is less than 5%.

In severely ill patients, the use of tetracycline has caused a highly significant reduction in total stool volume and duration of diarrhea and has resulted in more rapid disappearance of the organism from the stool. The dose administered should be approximately 1 g of tetracycline by mouth initially, then at least 500 mg every 6 hours for a total of 3 days. The usual stool composition per liter in adults is sodium (135 mEq), potassium (15 mEq), bicarbonate (45 mEq), and chloride (100 mEq); in children it is sodium (105 mEq), potassium (25 mEq), chloride (90 mEq), and bicarbonate (30 mEq). In children and pregnant women, treatment with furazolone (Furoxone) has been used successfully and avoids tetracycline risks.

Cholera may be prevented by cooking all foods thoroughly, boiling water, and immunization, which seems to offer up to 75% protection for up to 18 months. Even when clinical disease develops, cholera appears to be less severe in the vaccinated patient.

CAMPYLOBACTER ENTERITIS

METHOD OF ACQUISITION

Raw milk most frequently has been implicated in the transmission of Campylobacter enteritis.

DIAGNOSIS

Diagnosis rests on isolating the organism (*Campylobcater fetus* subspecies *jejune*) from a fecal specimen.

The common symptoms include diarrhea (in more than 90%), abdominal pain (in more than 80%), frequently with fever, headache, nausea, or vomiting. Bloody diarrhea is less common, but blood in the stool is present in about one fourth of cases.

TREATMENT

Treatment is supportive, but must include identification and stopping the offending food. For severe illness (particularly in the elderly or young children), tetracycline, Bactrim, or erythromycin can be used, as well as ciprofloxacin, which has been shown to shorten the clinical course.

LISTEROSIS

Caused by the gram-positive bacillus Listeria monocytogenes, listerosis can result in septicemia and meningitis as well as focal infectious symptoms. Milk and cheese products have been increasingly involved in its spread throughout the population. There is an increased susceptibility in immunocompromised patients and pregnant women. Ampicillin is usually the antibiotic of choice in treatment.

STAPHYLOCOCCAL FOOD POISONING

Enterotoxic staphylococci are found widely on the skin and mucous membranes of many individuals. Most staphylococci (a gram-positive, clustered coccus) cannot elaborate this particular toxin.

When foodstuffs are contaminated, lack of refrigeration and warm environment are ideal for bacterial growth and toxin elaboration. Foods usually implicated are those with a high fat content such as creamy cakes, custards, creamed soups, mayonnaise, and so on. Cases, however, have been reported from meat products as well. Milk has rarely been implicated. The ideal food as a culture medium is pancake batter, which has a pH close to 7 and a high moisture content and is frequently left without refrigeration for hours. Also beware of turkey stuffing and cooked and dressed turkey too large to fit into a refrigerator and caressed by many persons during its preparation.

Staphylococcal food poisoning is common. The toxin is preformed and is remarkably "heat stable." Therefore, even if food is subsequently cooked, a period of hours is necessary for toxin destruction. In fact in one test, autoclaving for 15 minutes did not result in substantial reduction in potency.

There are at least four different types of toxin, but all may be elaborated by the same organism and, with minor variation, all have the same unfortunate effect.

SYMPTOMS AND COURSE OF ILLNESS

Symptoms usually begin with $\frac{1}{2}$ hour to 6 hours after ingestion and may begin slowly or violently. Severe nausea and vomiting are common. The affected individual vomits repeatedly, then has dry heaves and may even vomit blood—probably representing a vomiting-induced Mallory-Weiss syndrome. After vomiting, abdominal cramps may become severe and diarrhea may develop. The diarrhea, however, is usually relatively mild, and the individual scarcely notices this symptom.

Patients appear markedly "gray" and severely ill. Severe dehydration can occur, and intravenous therapy should be started. Although the acute stage usually lasts less than 12 hours, many patients complain of severe nausea and malaise for 1 to 2 days.

Milder cases do occur and may not be diagnosed as staphylococcal food poisoning unless a careful history is taken.

Initial studies were conducted with paid volunteers. Despite increased pay, few, if any, would volunteer again. Thus, current studies are done with primates, but monkeys are far less susceptible than humans. Toxin is not formed in appreciable amounts below 12.78°C. (55°F.) or above 48.89°C. (120°F.) If the food is acidic, toxin is produced slowly, depending on temperature and acidity. If there is contaminated food with a pH of 7, or greater than 30% moisture content, appreciable amounts of toxin are produced in $4\frac{1}{2}$ hours at 32.22°C. (90°F.). Given the same food, but changing the temperature, the same amount of toxin

was produced in 10 hours at 18.33°C. (65°F.) and in 9 hours at 46.11°C. (115°F.). Thus, the conclusion is that to prevent staphylococcal food poisoning, "keep it hot, keep it cold, or eat it within 2 hours."

Simple diagnosis can be made by a Gram stain of the suspected food, which shows abundant staphylococci if contaminated (although this, of course, is not a test for the toxin). A culture can verify type, but the time necessary for culturing renders the findings primarily of scholarly interest.

TREATMENT

To manage staphylococcal food poisoning, give intravenous fluids. To prevent retching, Compazine, 10 mg. intramuscularly, can be used. Also, propantheline bromide, 15 mg or 30 mg intramuscularly, is effective. H_2 blockers (e.g., cimetidine or ranitidine) can be given intramuscularly or intravenously. Monitor electrolytes and urine output.

Fatalities have been reported in young children owing to mineral imbalance and dehydration. In the elderly, the severe retching may worsen existing heart disease and myocardial infarction has been reported, as has a Mallory-Weiss type of bleeding. Basically, simple supportive treatment results in a satisfactory outcome in the vast majority of patients.

Because the disease is caused by a preformed toxin, antibiotics are of no value. No suitable antitoxin is available for routine use.

Physicians should document their findings carefully; many restaurant outbreaks result in legal action.

Although the acute stage is over generally within 2 days, weakness and malaise can continued for 2 weeks in some cases.

TRICHINOSIS

The worm Trichinella spiralis enters the body through pork or other meat that has been inadequately cooked. For many reasons, the United States does not routinely inspect for trichinosis, although an enzyme assay being developed will allow such testing in the future—a necessity for exporting pork to many countries.

Trichinosis in humans causes weakness, swelling, and muscle pain along with general malaise and a low-grade fever. The duration of the acute illness is usually 3 weeks, although chronic indolent cases have been reported as well as rapidly developing cases leading to death.

According to the CDC, only 60 cases were reported in 1984. Autopsy studies have demonstrated that up to 4% of Americans harbor trichinella worms in their muscles. Thus, few cases are actually diagnosed. Symptoms are usually ascribed to "flu." The condition is rarely progressive. More often, the worms become encapsulated and do not cause later clinical disease.

FOOD ADDITIVES (Table 86-2)

There are well over a thousand food additives generally recognized as safe (GRAS), most of which are benign. Certain substances may trigger reactions in sensitive people. For example, sulfites are commonly added to fruit and vegetable salads and to potatoes to prevent darkening. Acute attacks of asthma have been triggered by such substances. Because of their dangers, sulfites have been removed from the "GRAS" list for use in restaurants and salad bars. Another substance widely used is monosodium glutamate (MSG), which acts as a flavor enhancer. Depending on dosage, many people develop tingling, flushing, diaphoresis, nausea, vomiting, balance difficulties, diarrhea, or headache. Some more sensitive individuals respond with behavioral changes includ-

ing anger and depression. Diuresis (best through sweating) can help to eliminate MSG, and patients should be told to avoid it in the future.

The subject of additives is generally beyond the scope of emergency medicine unless reactions occur that bring people to emergency facilities. Migraine headache caused by MSG is an example often seen in EDs.

When outbreaks of food poisoning or food reactions occur, however, the emergency facility is often in the best position to detect early "epidemics." It is prudent then to be in touch with the CDC through their reports and the state health department. When there are oc-

TABLE 86-2. OTHER FOOD POISONINGS AND THEIR TREATMENTS*

Name	Food Involved	Symptoms/signs	Treatment
Chinese restaurant syndrome (MSG syndrome)	Monosodium glutamate	Flushing, diaphoresis, weakness, headaches, pruritus, lethargy, depression, hypotension, arrhythmias, asthma, balance difficulties, vomiting	No specific treatment: IV fluids as needed
Cyanide poisoning	Pits from apricots, cherries, cassava, unripe millet, bitter almonds	Metabolic poisoning, loss of consciousness, cyanosis, convulsions	Amyl nitrite, oxygen
Cycad poisoning	Cycad starch and leaves (eaten in Philippines, Malay)	Neurologic symptoms, weakness, paresthesias	No specific treatment
Diascorism	Toxic yam with diascorine	Convulsions, deaths have occurred	Anticonvulsants
Ergotism	Grain with ergot fungus	Hypertension, vasoconstriction, CNS symptoms	Vasodilation by amyl nitrite inhalation or papaverine infusion
Favism	Fava bean	Glucose-6-phosphate dehydrogenase deficiency (inherited) produces hemolysis, severe anemia	Supportive: monitor urinary output, transfusions as needed: deferoxamine may arrest hemolysis
Fish poisoning (ichthyosarcotoxism) (ciguatera toxin)	Ciguatera (sea bass, snapper, barracuda)	Fish usually good as food contains a toxin that causes weakness, paresthesia, GI symptoms, hypotension, and, in fatal cases, respiratory paralysis (probably formed due to ingestion of dinoflagellate by the fish)	Gastric lavage, respiratory support as needed; charcoal
	Puffer fish	Far Eastern fish contains a neurotoxin that can cause paralysis (tetrodotoxin) and death	
	Tuna, mackerel, mahi mahi, (scombroid)	Bacteria act on histidine in flesh, producing a toxin with GI symptoms; headache and allergic manifestation (histamine-like)	Antihistamines, cimetidine, supportive and symptomatic treatment
Hemagglutination	Castor bean, partially cooked bean flakes, kidney bean flour, legume seeds	Nausea, vomiting, respiratory impairment, anemia; deaths reported from castor beans	No specific treatment
Lathyrism	Some beans, peas	Muscular weakness, partial paralysis, spinal cord impairments	No specific treatment
Licorice poisoning	Licorice	Weakness, myopathy, hypokalemia	IV treatment for fluid-electrolyte imbalance
Paralytic shellfish poisoning	Mussels and clams, usually along Pacific coast June to October—associated with "red tides"	Paresthesias, neurologic symptoms, respiratory paralysis	Supportive, particular attention to respiratory function
Sulfite sensitivity	Added to foods as antioxidant, found in mixes, wines	Asthma, urticaria	Bronchodilators
Tartrazine (Yellow dye #5) sensitivity	Orange-yellow colored foods	Urticaria, asthma, anaphylaxis	Supportive and symptomatic

* Of the food poisonings listed, the fish and shellfish contain poisons generally not present in a dangerous amount (the puffer fish is an exception). Ergotism is due to a fungus contaminant. In contrast, yam poisoning, cyanide poisoning, hemagglutination reaction, cycad poisoning, lathyrism, and favism result from chemicals that are natural constituents of the foods.

casional toxicities (e.g., heavy metal contamination, polybromophenols [PCBs]), special testing can be initiated in the ED.

FOOD POISONINGS CAUSED BY CHEMICALS NATURALLY PRESENT IN FOODS AND PLANTS (Tables 86-3 through 86-5)

As has been previously discussed, the difference between what is therapeutic and what is toxic may be just a question of dosage. Foods are composed of many chemical substances that are essential for life, such as carbohydrates, proteins, minerals, and vitamins. Many foods, however, contain chemical substances that are part of their nature but do not appear to be involved in nutritional processes. In many cases, the chemicals exert modest effects, and even ingestion of large quantities will not exert apparent toxic effects. For example, lettuce contains the chemical lactucin, which exerts sedative effects when it is concentrated. Another example is spinach which has a high oxalic acid content; however, even with larger ingestions, which might produce feelings of malaise and bloating, a spinach overdose would only rarely present as a clinical problem. Conversely, there are common foods that can cause severe poisoning because of their being underripe, because too much has been eaten, or because the patient has been taking a pharmacologic agent that interacts in some way with a chemical or chemicals in a food. For example, the "vomiting sickness" of Jamaica has been traced to eating the unripe akee fruit. The toxic substance has been termed "hypolycin" because it acts to rapidly lower blood sugar.

The common potato plant ordinarily has leaves that contain belladonna-type actions. When some potatoes are unripe, belladonna poisoning can occur. In fact, deaths have been linked to eating potatoes.

Alcohol is an example of toxicity of a common food in which overdosage may be lethal. However, there are many more. Severe toxicity with sympathomimetic effects can come from an overdose of nutmeg because of the content of myristin, and a prized fish of Japan called "fugu" contains a toxin that exerts cholinergic effects. Overdose can cause cholinergic poisoning.

As an example of food-drug interactions, the presence of tyramine in aged cheese, pickled herring, chianti wine, and some other aged foods can cause hypertensive crises in patients who are taking monoamine oxidase inhibitors for treatment of depression.

See the References for further information.

MUSHROOM POISONING

Although the Psilocybe mushroom has gained notoriety, poisoning from ingestion of these mushrooms can induce severe vomiting, abdominal cramps, and marked hallucinations, but the poisoning is relatively benign because of a large tolerance of the body to psilocybin. The mushroom Amanita muscaria has also been eaten for its hallucinatory effects, and the Vikings were said to have consumed them before going into battle because of the rage-like reaction induced. With overdose, muscarine causes parasympathomimetic symptoms that occur usually within one-half hour after ingestion and cause profuse salivation, lacrimation, bradycardia, and other cholinergic responses. Treatment involves atropine, which can be given at a dose of 0.5 to 1 mg. intramuscularly or intravenously (when symptoms warrant). This dose can be repeated every 30 minutes.

Important questions in the assessment of mushroom poisoning are:

1. When were the mushrooms eaten, and when did symptoms appear (time course)? *Rationale:* Symptoms that begin immediately or within the first hour usually herald a relatively minor poisoning. Emesis, charcoal, and a cathartic should be used. Delayed symptoms are characteristic of the amatoxin-containing mushrooms. The nature of the symptoms may indicate seriousness of the ingestion (e.g., hallucinations, muscarinic effects, sweating, delirium).
2. How many mushrooms were eaten, and what types were they? *Rationale:* If different types were ingested, it is difficult to arrive at identification by symptoms. In addition, of course, there is a dose-related effect.
3. Did anyone who ate the mushrooms not get sick? *Rationale:* People often blame mushrooms because the widespread awareness of their toxicity, whereas another food poisoning or virus might be the cause of symptoms.

TABLE 86-3. POISONOUS PLANTS AND THEIR CHEMICAL ACTIONS IN THE BODY

Plant	Chemical Action
Jimson weed	Atropine-like action
Larkspur	
Nightshade	
Tomato and potato leaves	
Morning glory seeds	LSD (lysergic acid diethylamide)
Crocus	Colchicine-like effects
Foxglove	Cardiac glycosides (digitalis-like)
Oleander	
Lily-of-the valley	
Christmas rose	
Mistletoe	Sympathomimetic amines
Poinsettia	Parasympathomimetic (cholinergic effects)
Hemlock	Strychnine-like
Mountain laurel	Curare-like
May apple	Irritating resin-like podophyllin
Wisteria	

TABLE 86-4. SIGNS AND SYMPTOMS OF COMMON AND /OR SERIOUS PLANT INTOXICATIONS*

	Dieffenbachia/Philodendron	Colchicum/Gloriossa	Euphorbia/Hippomane	Actaea/Anemone/Ranunculus	Convallaria/Digitalis/Nerium	Aconitum	Solanum	Pieris/Rhododendron/Veratrum	Conium/Laburnum/Nicotiana/Sophora	Cicuta	Taxus	Gelsemium	Brugmansia/Datura	Amaryllis/Narcissus/Wisteria	Ilex	Abrus/Ricinus	Prunus	Phytolacca	Podophyllum	Karwinskia
Mouth and Throat																				
Burning/irritation	++	++	D	++	+	+	D	+	+											
Increased salivation	+		D	++		+		D	+	+	D									
Dry mouth												+	++							
Dysphonia/dysphagia	+		D			±					+	+	+							
Gastrointestinal tract																				
Nausea		+			+	±		D	+	+	D			+	+	DD				
Vomiting		+	+	+	+	±		D	+	±	D			++	++	DD	D	++	+	
Diarrhea		++	+	+	+	±	D	D						±	±	DD		D	+	
Abdominal pain		++	++	+	+		D	D			D			+			D	+		
Decreased bowel sounds									+				++						±	
Cardiovascular																				
Tachycardia													+							
Bradycardia					+			++			D									
Arrhythmias					±	++					D									
Conduction defects					++															
Hypertension													+							
Hypotension								++			D									

Nervous and Neuromuscular																	
Dizziness			+		+	+		+	+								
Weakness/lethargy	±		+		+	+		D						D			
Syncope	±																
Delirium/psychosis	±									+							
Tremors/convulsions	±				D±	D±			±					D±		±	
Depression/coma					D	+		D						D±			
Headache					+	±			+								
Paresthesias			++		D												
Muscle weakness/paralysis	±				D	+			+					D±		±	DD
Visual																	
Mydriasis			+			±		+		+							
Visual disturbances			+		D	+			+	+							
Cutaneous																	
Increased sweating					+	+								D	++		
Dry skin										++				D			
Flushing/rash								D		+							
Cyanosis								D						D±			
Miscellaneous																	
Hyperthermia				+						+							
Painful/bloody micturition	+																

Key: + = Commonly occurs; ++ = pronounced or persistent; ± = occasionally reported; D = delayed onset; DD = occurrence significantly delayed.

TABLE 86-5. COMMON DANGEROUS HERBAL REMEDIES*

Botanical Name of Plant Source	Common Names	Remarks
Arnica montana L.	Arnica, Arnica Flowers. Wolf's-bane. Leopard's Bane. Mountain Tobacco. Flores Arnicae.	Aqueous and alcoholic extracts of the plant contain choline, plus two unidentified substances that affect the heart and vascular systems. Arnica, an active irritant, can produce violent toxic gastroenteritis, nervous disturbances, change in pulse rate, intense muscular weakness, collapse and death.
Atropa belladonna L.	Belladonna. Deadly Nightshade.	Poisonous plant that contains the toxic solanaceous alkaloids hyoscyamine, atropine and hyoscine.
Solanum dulcamara L.	Bittersweet twigs. Dulcamara. Bittersweet. Woody Nightshade. Climbing Nightshade.	Poisonous. Contains the toxic glycoalkaloid solanine; also solanidine and dulcamarin.
Sanguinaria canadensis L.	Bloodroot. Sanguinaria. Red Puccoon.	Contains the poisonous alkaloid sanguinarine and other alkaloids.
Cytisus scoparius (L) Link.	Broom-top. Scoparius. Spartium. Scotch Broom. Irish Broom. Broom.	Contains toxic sparteine, isosparteine and other alkaloids; also hydroxytyramine.
Aesculus hippocastanum L.	Buckeye. Aesculus. Horse Chestnut.	Contains a toxic coumarin glycoside, aesculin (esculin). A poisonous plant.
Acorus calamus L.	Calamus. Sweet Flag. Sweet Root. Sweet Cane. Sweet Cinnamon.	Oil of calamus, Jammu variety, is a carcinogen (causes cancer). FDA regulations prohibit marketing of calamus as a food or food additive.
Heliotropium europaeum L.	Heliotrope.	A poisonous plant. It contains alkaloids that produce liver damage. Not to be confused with garden heliotrope (*Valeriana officinalis* L.).
Conium maculatum L.	Hemlock. Conium. Poison Hemlock. Spotted Hemlock. Spotted Parsley. St. Bennet's Herb. Spotted Cowbane. Fool's Parsley.	Contains the poisonous alkaloid conine and four other closely related alkaloids. Often confused with water hemlock (*Cicuta maculata* L.). Not to be confused with the conifer hemlock, hemlock spruce, etc. (*Tsuga canadensis* [L.]. Carr.)
Hyoscyamus niger L.	Henbane. Hyoscyamus. Black Henbane. Hog's Bean. Poison Tobacco. Devil's Eye.	Contains the alkaloids hyoscyamine, hyoscine (scopolamine) and atropine. A poisonous plant.
Exagonium purga (Wenderoth) Bentham, *Ipomoea jalapa* Nutt, and Coxe. *Ipomoea purga* (Wenderoth) Hanye. *Exagonium jalapa* (Wenderoth) Baillon.	Jalap Root. Jalap. True Jalap. Jalapa. Vera Cruz Jalap. High John Root. (Possibly also known as High John the Conqueror. John Conqueror. St. John the Conqueror Root. Hi John Conqueror.)	A large twining vine of Mexico, this plant has undergone many name changes. The drug is a powerful, drastic cathartic. Purgative powers of jalap reside in its resin. In overdoses, jalap may produce dangerous hypercatharsis.
Datura stamonium L.	Jimson Weed. Datura. Stamonium. Apple of Peru, Jamestown Weed. Thornapple. Tolguacha.	Contains the alkaloids atropine, hyoscyamine and scopolamine. Illegal drug for nonprescription use. A poisonous plant.
Convallaria majalis L.	Lily of the Valley. Convallaria. May Lily.	Contains the toxic cardiac glycosides convallatoxin, convallarin and convalamarin. Poisonous plant.
Lobelia inflata L.	Lobelia. Indian Tobacco. Wild Tobacco. Asthma Weed. Emetic Weed.	A poisonous plant that contains the alkaloid lobeline plus a number of other pyridine alkaloids. Overdoses of the plant or extracts of the leaves or fruits produce vomiting, sweating, pain, paralysis, depressed temperatures, rapid but feeble pulse, collapse, coma, and death.
Mandragon officinarum L.	Mandrake, Mandragora. European Mandrake.	The plant is a poisonous narcotic similar in its properties to belladonna. Contains the alkaloids hyoscyamine, scopolamine, and mandragorine.
Podophyllum peltatum L.	Mandrake. May Apple. Podophyllum. American Mandrake. Devil's Apple. Umbrella Plant. Vegetable Calomel. Wild Lemon. Vegetable Mercury.	A poisonous plant, it contains podophyllotoxin, a complex polycyclic substance, and other constituents.
Phoradendron flavescens (Pursh.) Nutt. *Viscum flavescens* (Pursh.)	Mistletoe. Viscum. American Mistletoe.	Poisonous. Contains the toxic pressor amines β-phenylethylamine and tyramine.
Phoradendron juniperinum Engelm.	Mistletoe. Viscum. Juniper Mistletoe.	May be poisonous. Little is known about its properties.
Viscum album L.	Mistletoe. Viscum. European Mistletoe.	Poisonous. Contains the toxic pressor amines β-phenylethylamine and tyramine.
Ipomoea purpurea (L) Roth	Morning Glory.	Contains a purgative resin. In addition, morning glory seeds contain amides of lysergic acid but with a potency much less than that of LSD.
Vinca major L. and *Vinca minor* L.	Periwinkle, Greater Periwinkle. Lesser Periwinkle.	Contains pharmacologically active, toxic alkaloids such as vinblastine and vincristine that have cytotoxic and neurological actions and can injure the liver and kidneys.
Hypericum perforatum L.	St. Johnswort. Hypericum. Klamath Weed. Goatweed.	A primary photosensitizer for cattle, sheep, horses and goats. Contains hypericin, a fluorescent pigment, as a photosensitizing substance.

TABLE 86-5. CONTINUED

Botanical Name of Plant Source	Common Names	Remarks
Euonymus europaea L.	Spindle-tree.	Violent purgative.
Dipteryx odorata (Aubl.) Willd. *Coumarouna odorata* (Aubl.) and *Dipteryx oppositifolia* (Aubl.) Willd. *Coumarouna oppositifolia* (Aubl.)	Tonka Bean. Tonco Bean. Tonquin Bean.	Active constituent of seed is coumarin. Dietary feeding of coumarin to rats and dogs causes extensive liver damage, growth retardation, and testicular atrophy. FDA regulations prohibit marketing of coumarin as a food or food additive.
Euonymus atropurpurea Jacq.	Wahoo Bark. Euonymus. Burning Bush. Wahoo.	The poisonous principle has not been completely identified. Laxative.
Eupatorium rugosum Houtt. *E. ageratoides* L.f. and *E. urticae-folium*	White Snakeroot. (Also called Snakeroot, Richweed.)	Poisonous plant. Contains a toxic, unsaturated alcohol called *tremetol* combined with a resin acid. Causes "trembles" in cattle and other livestock. Milk sickness is produced in humans by ingestion of milk, butter, and possibly meat from animals poisoned by this plant.
Artemisia absinthium L.	Wormwood. Absinthium. Absinth. Absinthe. Madderwort. Wermuth. Mugwort. Mingwort. Warmot. Magenkraut. Harba Absinthii.	Contains a volatile oil (oil of wormwood) that is an active narcotic poison. Oil of wormwood is used to flavor *absinthe*, an alcoholic liqueur illegal in this country because its use can damage the nervous system and cause mental deterioration.
Corynanthe yohimbe Schum. *Pausinystalia yohimbe* (Schum.) Pierre	Yohimbe. Yohimbi.	Contains the toxic alkaloid yohimbine (quebrachine) and other alkaloids.

* Prepared by the Food and Drug Administration, Washington, D.C.

4. Did the patient consume alcoholic beverages? *Rationale:* Some mushrooms have a disulfiram-type effect with added alcohol. As with Antabuse, there can be extreme nausea, vomiting, and headache.

The most severe mushroom poisoning comes from those containing peptide toxins (phallotoxins or amatoxins). They can be deadly at low doses. Symptoms may be delayed several hours to as long as 24 hours after ingestion. Severe abdominal pain, diarrhea, and vomiting are present. Amatoxins cause liver, brain, and renal tubule cell injury, which may lead to death. Early treatment consists of the following:

1. Supportive treatment, with monitoring of vital signs and urine output. Renal failure may occur. Urine output must remain high. Early diuresis may be necessary.
2. Large doses of steroids have been used empirically.
3. Hemodialysis or peritoneal dialysis should be used early, when available, because of the small molecular size of the peptide toxins. Dialysis may have substantial benefit if used early.
4. Penicillin, chloramphenicol, and sulfamethoxazole have been used in animals to decrease binding of the toxin to albumin. This might be of value if dialysis is used subsequently. Thioctic acid (50 to 150 mg every 6 hours) has been used in Europe, but is not well tested.

If severe poisoning has occurred, all of these measures should be instituted as early as possible, along with activated charcoal and catharsis.

The characteristic course has been divided into three stages: (1) the first 24 hours (*Acute Symptoms*), (2) some remission (24 to 36 hours), and (3) severe stage (with clinical liver damage, renal failure, and seizures), which can lead to death in up to 80% of cases.

A specimen of the ingested mushroom can prove valuable in identification. For quick ED testing, rub some of the mushroom cap over newsprint and allow to dry. A drop of concentrated hydrochloric acid is applied to the paper. A bluish-green color indicates amatoxins. The mushroom should then be sent for chemical analysis. A negative "newsprint" test does not mean that amatoxins may not be present. Only a positive test is useful.

MISCELLANEOUS FOOD POISONS

Table 86-2 summarizes some other food poisonings and their treatment.

OTHER FOOD TOXINS ("TOXIDROMES")

Types of Food Toxins. There are several ways in which food toxins find their way into the foods we eat. They may be produced by organisms found in the food, such as microorganisms (e.g., botulism, staphylococcal food poisoning, or scombroid); algae (e.g., neurotoxic mussel poisoning); or dinoflagellates (e.g., ciguatera). They may be natural chemical constituents of substances not safe to ingest, such as poisonous mushrooms or unripe fruits and vegetables (e.g., the unripe Jamaican akee fruit contains a substance that causes hypoglycemia; the green potato contains toxic solanine alkaloids). They may even be the result of the inadvertent inclusion of animal glands during the preparation of a food product. For example, a large outbreak of thyrotoxicosis occurred after neck trimming that contained a large amount of bovine thyroid hormone were inadvertently included during the preparation of ground beef.

Some cases of illness from food toxins occur as the result of ingestion of excessive amounts of substance that is tolerated in smaller doses. For example, ingestion of large amounts of nutmeg can cause toxicity from the sympathomimetic effects of myristin, a natural constituent of the spice. "Fugu," a culinary delicacy highly prized by the Japanese, is a fish that contains tetrodotoxin, a cholinergic neurotoxin, which can cause respiratory paralysis and rapid death if ingested in excessive amounts. Specially licensed chefs learn how to prepare the fugu with an apparently "desirable" small amount of the tetrodotoxin, which is tolerated by fugu devotees. Overdose causes respiratory paralysis. Alcohol is yet another example of a foodstuff that is well tolerated in small amounts, but can cause serious illness, and even death, if consumed in excess. Some food "toxins" cause illness as a result of interactions with medications. Tyramine, present in aged cheese, pickled herring, chianti wine, and some other aged foods, can cause headaches and hypertension in patients taking monamine oxidase inhibitors for treatment of depression. Similarly, the "broad bean" can cause illness through the formation of derivatives of dihydroxyphenalaline and dopamine. Some patients with genetic deficiencies of enzymes may have illness precipitated by the ingestion of foods not toxic to other individuals (e.g., some patients with a variety of glucose-6-phosphate dehydrogenase (G6PD) deficiency may develop severe hemolysis after the ingestion of fava beans).

Examples of some of these types of toxic food ingestion will be covered in depth; others are summarized in Table 86-2.

Diagnosis of food toxin-related illness is often difficult, especially in the ED. The clinical history is often confusing and toxin identification difficult. One important clue from the history is the determination of whether the case is isolated or one of a large group. Epidemiologic assessment may be difficult, however, if the outbreak is small or if a multitude of possible foods are involved. Although some food toxins have highly characteristic symptom complexes and are, therefore, relatively easy to diagnose (e.g., staphylococcal, MSG, ciguatera poisonings), others, such as botulism, are notoriously difficult to diagnose.

SCOMBROID FOOD POISONING

As in botulism and staphylococcal food poisoning, scombroid is the result of the ingestion of a toxin produced by bacterial contaminants of the foodstuff, in this case fish contaminated by Proteus morgani. These bacteria cause a breakdown of histadine in the fish with chemical decarboxylation and production of a histamine-like toxin. The fish associated with this poisoning are of the scombroid variety, such as tuna, albacore, mackerel, and skipjack. Contaminated fish may smell foul (ammonia-like) and have an unpleasant metallic taste.

Most laboratories cannot test for histamine. The normal histamine level of fish flesh is less than 6 mg per 100 grams. Over 10 mg signifies likely bacterial contamination (usually with proteus or achromobacter). Severe illness generally requires a level greater than 100 mg per 100 g.

Clinical Signs and Symptoms. The symptoms begin within 10 minutes to 1 hour after the ingestion of the contaminated fish and resemble those of a histamine reaction (flushing and pruritus). Other symptoms include nausea, headache, thirst, chest pain, diarrhea, skin blotches, and sometimes mouth blisters. Symptoms can be severe.

Treatment consists of intravenous antihistamines, such as benadryl or chlorpheniramine. Cimetidine and other H-2 blockers have also been reported to have been used successfully in this condition.

Production of the toxin is prevented by proper refrigeration of fresh-caught fish.

CIGUATERA FISH POISONING

Ciguatera poisoning results primarily from the ingestion of contaminated barracuda, snapper and groups from warm waters such as in the Caribbean or the Gulf of Mexico and near Hawaii. Larger fish tend to be more implicated as they ingest smaller fish with toxin. A dinoflagellate (the green algae *Lyngbia majuscula*) becomes concentrated in the organs of these fish and elaborates an unpleasant neurotoxin that is not readily inactivated by heat or cold. This toxin causes paresthesias (especially of the lips, tongue and throat), pruritus, a feeling of hot-cold reversal, and a variety of gastrointestinal symptoms, including nausea, vomiting, and diarrhea. Encephalopathy and respiratory failure, as well as shock, may occur. Symptoms usually begin within 12 hours after fish ingestion, but may be delayed up to 30 hours. Gastrointestinal symptoms, often delayed up to 30 hours, are often the initial presenting complaints, and the neurologic symptoms may present insidiously.

Treatment is supportive, and there is no specific antidote. Severe cases may benefit from the use of IV mannitol. IV fluids, oxygen, and pain relief are all important. IV calcium has reportedly been of some benefit. Laboratory tests are usually normal. An immunoassay is available to confirm the presence of this toxin and a sample of the possibly contaminated fish can be sent for assay. The time delay for confirmation, however, requires that diagnosis and treatment of ciguatera poisoning be based on clinical grounds.

TOXIC ENCEPHALOPATHY FROM MUSSEL POISONING

Intoxications associated with the ingestion of shellfish include paralytic shellfish poisoning, neurotoxic shellfish poisoning, and a recently described toxic encephalopathy associated with the ingestion of mussels contaminated by the neuroexcitatory amino acid, domoic acid. Only the latter is discussed here.

In Canada in late 1987, an outbreak of more than 250 cases of mussel-associated poisoning occurred. Reported symptoms included vomiting (75%), abdominal cramps (50%), diarrhea (42%), headache (43%), and short-term memory impairment (25%). Encephalopathy, coma, mutism, seizures, and purposeless chewing and grimacing also occurred. The more severe neurologic symptoms occurred primarily in older patients and patients with coexistent medical problems. Treatment was supportive and included intubation for airway protection, management of unstable blood pressure, cardiac arrhythmias, and seizures. Cognitive deficits that had not resolved more than two years after the ingestion were described.

The illness was associated with the production of domoic acid, a neuroexcitatory amino acid similar to glutamic acid, which is believed to be produced by an algae (Nitzschia pungens), which lodges in the digestive glands of mussels. In Canada, where this outbreak occurred, mussels are tested for the presence of domoic acid before commercial distribution. No new cases have been reported there since testing was instituted.

PLANT POISONINGS

The number of plants that can exert toxic actions is vast. For emergency treatment, it is useful to identify the major type of chemical actions caused by the poisoning. Table 86-3 identifies common plants and their chemical actions. Table 86-4 offers symptoms and signs associated with plant intoxications, and Table 86-5 was prepared by the Food and Drug Administration (FDA) to alert health professionals and consumers to some herbal remedies that can be dangerous.

BIBLIOGRAPHY

BOTULISM

Arnon, S.S.: Infant botulism. Ann. Rev. Med. *31*:57, 1980.
Arnon, S.S., Midura, T.F., Damus, K., et al.: Honey and other environmental risk factors for infant botulism. J. Pediatr. *94*:331, 1979.
Botulism from wounds (editorial). Br. Med. J. p. 214, Feb. 1974.
Centers for Disease Control: Botulism in the United States 1899–1977. Handbook for Epidemiologists, Clinicians, and Laboratory Workers, issued May 1979.
Cherington, M., and Ginsberg, S.: Type B botulism: Neurophysiologic studies. Neurology *21*:43, 1971.
Cherington, M.: Botulism: Ten-year experience. Arch. Neurol. *30*:432, 1974.
de Jesus, V., Slater, R., et al.: Neuromuscular physiology of wound botulism. Arch. Neurol. *29*:425, 1973.
Dolman, C.E.: Human botulism in Canada (1919–1973). Can. Med. Assoc. J. *110*:191, 1974.
Donta, S.T.: Food poisoning. *In* Medical Microbiology and Infectious Diseases. Edited by Braude, A.I. Philadelphia, W.B. Saunders Co., 1981, p. 1034.
Field, M., et al.: Intestinal electrolyte transport and diarrheal disease. N. Engl. J. Med. *321*:879, 1989.
Fullerton, P., Gogna, N.K., and Stoddart, R.: Wound botulism. Med. J. Aust. *28*:662, 1980.
Haaland, K.Y., and Davis, L.E.: Botulism and memory. Arch. Neurol. *37*:657, 1980.
Hatheway, C.F.: Clostridium botulinum. *In* Infectious Disease. Edited by Gorbach, S.L., et al. Philadelphia, W.B. Saunders Co., 1992.
Hauschild, A.H.: Clostridium botulinum in food-borne pathogens. New York, Dekker, 1989.
Hill, O.W., and Chesney, J.: Botulism—An ever-present menace: A report of three simultaneous cases due to type E. Review of the pediatric aspects and treatment. Clin. Pediatr. *5*:554, 1966.
Infant botulism in 1931: Discovery of a misclassified case. Am. J. Dis. Child. *133*:580, 1979.
Jankovic, J., and Brin, M.F.: Therapeutic uses of botulinum toxin. N. Engl. J. Med. *324*:1187, 1991.
Jensen, L.B.: Poisoning Misadventures. Springfield, Ill., Charles C Thomas, 1970, p. 65.
Johnson, R.O., Clay, S.A., and Arnon, S.S.: Diagnosis and management of infant botulism. Am. J. Dis. Child. *133*:586, 1979.
Jurwitz, S., Jacobs, M.R., Lichter, J., et al.: Botulism: A case report. S. Afr. Med. J. *47*:1003, 1980.
Koenig, M.G., Drutz, D.J., Mushlin, A.J., et al.: Type B botulism in man. Am. J. Med. *42*:208, 1967.
Lagos, J.C., and Hagwood, K.W.: Flaccid paralysis of acute onset in children. South Med. J. *63*:451, 1970.
Lecour, H., Ramos, H., Almeida, B., et al.: Food borne botulism: A review of 13 outbreaks. Arch. Intern. Med. *148*:578, 1988.
Mayer, R.F.: The neuromuscular defect in human botulism. Electroenceph. Clin. Neurophysiol. *25*:397, 1968.
Merson, M.H., Hughes, J.M., Dowell, V.R., et al.: Current trends in botulism in the United States. JAMA *229*:1305, 1974.
Midura, T.F., Snowden, S., Wood, R.M., and Arnon, S.S.: Isolation of *Clostridium botulinum* from honey. J. Clin. Microbiol. *9*:282, 1979.
Neff, T.A.: Total management of botulism. N. Engl. J. Med. *282*:816, 1970.
Nelson, K.E.: The clinical recognition of botulism. Editorials. JAMA *241*:503, 1979.
Oh, S.J.: Botulism: Electrophysiologic studies. Ann. Neurol. *1*:481, 1977.

Polin, R.A., and Brown, L.W.: Infant botulism. Pediatr. Clin. North Am. 26:345, 1979.

Ryan, D.W., and Cherington, M.: Human type A botulism. JAMA 216:513, 1971.

Schantz, E.J., and Sugiyama, H.: Toxic proteins produced by Clostridium botulinum. J. Agr. Food Chem. 22:26, 1974.

Schuck, P.H.: Botulism and nitrites. Science 180:1322, 1973.

Seals, J.E., Snyder, J.D., Edell, T.A., Hatheway, C.L., et al.: Restaurant-associated type A botulism: Transmission by potato salad. Am. J. Epidemiol. 113:436, 1981.

Sonnabend, D., Sonnabend, W., Heinzle, R., Sigrist, T., et al.: Isolation of Clostridium botulinum type G and identification of type G botulinal toxin in humans: Report of five sudden unexpected deaths. Department of Pathology, Institute of Medical Microbiology, Kantans Hospital, St. Gallen, Switzerland, 1980.

Stuart, P.F., Wiebe, J.D., McElroy, R., et al.: Botulism among Cape Dorset Eskimos and suspected botulism at Frobisher Bay and Wakeham Bay. Can. J. Public Health 61:509, 1970.

Terranova, W., Breman, J.G., Locey, R.P., and Speck, S.: Botulism type B: Epidemiologic aspects of an extensive outbreak. Am. J. Epidemiol. 108:150, 1978.

Terranova, W., Palumbo, J.N., and Breman, J.G.: Ocular findings in botulism type B. JAMA 241:475, 1979.

Tsunenari, S., Uchimura, Y., Kanada, M.: Puffer poisoning in Japan—A case report. J. Forensic Sci. 25:240, 1980.

Wand, M., and Mather, J.A.: Diphenylhydantoin intoxication mimicking botulism. N. Engl. J. Med. 286:88, 1972.

Wound botulism—Texas, California, Washington: Morbid. Mortal. Weekly Rep., January 25, 1980.

FOOD POISONING AND CHEMICALS IN FOODS AND PLANTS

Auerbach, P.S.: Marine envenomations. N. Engl. J. Med. 325:486, 1991.

Balandrin, M.F., et al.: Natural plant chemicals: Sources of industrial and medicinal materials. Science 228:1154, 1985.

Carter, A.O., et al.: A severe outbreak of Escherichia coli 0157:H7: associated hemorrhage colitis in a nursing home. N. Engl. J. Med. 317:24, 1987.

Chia, J.K., Clark, J.B., Ryan, C.A., et al.: Botulism in an adult associated with food borne intestinal infection with Clostridium botulinum. N. Engl. J. Med. 315:239, 1986.

Drusco, G.M., and Serrao, E.: Healthy carriers of positive staphylococcal coagulase and the prevention of food poisoning in aircraft catering. Minerva Med. 14:11:1991, 1980.

DuPont, H.L., Sullivan, P., Evans, D.G., et al.: Prevention of travelers diarrhea (emporiatric enteritis). JAMA 243:237, 1980.

Eastaugh, J., and Shepherd, S.: Infection and toxic syndromes from fish and shellfish consumption. Arch. Intern. Med. 149:1735, 1989 (96 refs.).

Fleming, D.W., et al.: Pasteurized milk as a vehicle of infection in an outbreak of listerosis. N. Engl. J. Med. 312:404, 1985.

Goruzzo, E., et al.: Use of norfloxacin to treat chronic typhoid carriers. J. Infect. Dis. 157:1221, 1988.

Gross, R.L., and Newberne, P.M.: Naturally occurring toxic substances in foods. Clin. Pharmacol. Ther. 22:680, 1978.

Hedbert, C.W., Fishbein, D.B., Janssen, R.S., et al.: An outbreak of thyrotoxicosis caused by the consumption of bovine thyroid gland in ground beef. N. Engl. J. Med. 316:993, 1987.

Holmberg, S.D.: Cholera and related illnesses caused by Vibrio species. In Infectious Diseases. Edited by Gorbach, S.L., et al. Philadelphia, W.B. Saunders Co., 1992.

Hooper, D.C., and Wolfson, J.S.: Fluoroquinolone antimicrobial agents. N. Engl. J. Med. 324:385, 1991.

Kolata, G.: Testing for trichinosis. Science 227:621, 1985.

Lee, C.: Fish poisoning with particular reference to ciguateria. J. Trop. Med. Hyg. 83:93, 1980.

Loewenstein, M.S.: Epidemiology of Clostridium perfringens food poisoning. N. Engl. J. Med. 286:1026, 1972.

McMillan, M., and Thompson, J.G.: An outbreak of suspected solanine poisoning in schoolboys. Quart. J. Med. 48:227, 1979.

Merson, M.H., Morris, G.K., Sack, D.A., et al.: Travelers' diarrhea in Mexico. N. Engl. J. Med. 294:1299, 1976.

Morris, J.G., and Black, R.E.: Cholera and other vibrioses in the United States. N. Engl. J. Med. 312:343, 1985.

Morrow, J.D., Margolies, G.R., Rowland, J., and Roberts, L.J.: Evidence that histamine is the causative toxin of scombroid fish poisoning. N. Engl. J. Med. 324:716, 1991.

Munro, L.C.: Naturally occurring toxicants in foods and their significance. Clin. Toxicol. 9:647, 1976.

Netchvolodoff, C.V., and Hargrove, M.D.: Recent advances in the treatment of diarrhea. Arch. Intern. Med. 139:813, 1979.

Olson, K.R., et al.: Amanita phalloides-type mushroom poisoning. West. J. Med. 137:282, 1982.

Perl, T.M., Bedard, L., Kosatsky, T., et al.: An outbreak of toxic encephalopathy caused by eating mussels contaminated with domoic acid. N. Engl. J. Med. 322:1775, 1990.

Schwartz, G.R.: In Bad Taste: The MSG Syndrome. Santa Fe, Health Press, 1988.

Sours, H.E., and Smith, D.G.: Outbreaks of foodborne disease in the United States, 1972–1978. J. Infect. Dis. 142:122, 1980.

Sundaram, M.B., and Swaminathan, R.: Body potassium depletion and myopathy due to chronic licorice ingestion. Postgrad. Med. J. 55:48, 1981.

Taylor, D.N., Porter, B.W., Williams, C.A., et al.: Campylobacter enteritis: A large outbreak traced to commercial raw milk. West J. Med. 137:365, 1982.

Teitelbaum, J.S., Zatorre, R.J., Carpenter, S., et al.: Neurologic sequelae of domoic acid intoxication due to the ingestion of contaminated mussels. N. Engl. J. Med. 322:1781, 1990.

Telzak, F.E., et al.: A nosocomial outbreak of Salmonella enteritidis due to the consumption of raw eggs. N. Engl. J. Med. 323:395, 1990.

Tolle, S.W., and Elliot, D.L.: Evaluation and management of diarrhea. West. J. Med. 140:293, 1984.

Wistrom, J., et al.: Short-term self-treatment of traveller's diarrhea with norfloxacin—A placebo-controlled study. J. Antimicrob. Chemother. 23:905, 1989.

Yolken, R.H., et al.: Antibody to human rotavirus in cow's milk. N. Engl. J. Med. 312:605, 1985.

Part XII

Emergency Medical Services (EMS) Systems

SECTION ONE. OPERATIONAL ASPECTS OF EMS

EMS SYSTEMS DEVELOPMENT IN THE UNITED STATES

Alexander Kuehl

CAPSULE

The influence of experienced physicians on the development of prehospital care has ebbed and flowed over the years. Because Emergency Medical Services (EMS) appear to be entering a period of both consolidation and change, it is critical that physicians, especially emergency physicians, interact at every level of EMS systems.

INTRODUCTION

Throughout the world, for the 150 years before 1950, physicians were involved both conceptually and operationally in the provision of ambulance services; however, during World War II, physician involvement waned. Simultaneously, rapid changes in the structure and delivery of health care, reflecting differences in basic health care philosophy and in the integration of new methodologies among the various countries, accentuated the international differences in approach to prehospital care.[1]

In the United States, two major patterns of ambulance services evolved in the 20 years immediately after World War II. In the larger cities, uncoordinated hospital-based ambulances gradually coalesced into more centrally coordinated citywide programs, usually administered by the municipal hospitals or the fire departments. In rural areas, the traditional funeral home "ambulances" gave way to volunteer fire department or rescue squad models. In both urban and rural areas, a few for-profit providers continued to deliver transport services, occasionally contracting with local government to provide emergency prehospital and transport services. Unfortunately, there was minimal coordination among the providers and little integration of prehospital services with medical facilities.[2]

Before the mid-1960s, there existed little legislation or regulation applicable to ambulance services; ambulance providers usually had relatively limited formal training; and physician involvement at any level was minimal. Although change probably would have come eventually, several factors intersected in the late 1960s to cause a revolution in prehospital care.

The first of these factors grew out of the requirements of the 1966 National Highway Act for the individual states to develop rudimentary programs addressing highway trauma.[3] The report by the National Academy of Science/National Research Council, "Accidental Death and Disability: The Neglected Disease of Modern Society," identified accidental death and disability as a serious and unrecognized medical epidemic; it focused attention specifically on problems with the delivery of prehospital care.[4] Partly as a result of that report, the Nixon Administration was lobbied to fund EMS demonstration projects; the result was that, in 1971, the Department of Health, Education, and Welfare (DHEW) funded several EMS demonstration projects and the Department of Transportation (DOT) began the development of national training and ambulance standards.[5] Later, in 1972, the Robert Wood Johnson Foundation developed a grant program for the establishment of regional EMS systems.[6]

Ultimately, in 1973, the Emergency Medical Service System Act (P.L. 93–154), largely based on the activities of the various demonstration projects and grant programs, was adopted.[7] The thrust of the law was to encourage the development of multicounty comprehensive EMS systems. The 15 "essential" components emphasized by the act were a usable but somewhat defective template for the initial EMS system design efforts.[8] Although medical involvement was not formally addressed in the legislation, the medical director of the DHEW program recognized and encouraged the need for local physician leadership.

To develop the individual multicounty regions necessary to secure federal funding through the EMSS Act, state EMS legislation was often necessary. The resulting state laws varied tremendously, especially in regard to the issues of responsible medical control, overall authority, and financing. In some states, physician direction was required; in others, medical control was not addressed. Often, the responsibility for "coordinating" the regional activities was assigned to a regional council composed of physicians, prehospital providers, and consumers; commonly, medical interest was limited to physicians somewhat removed from the medical mainstream. Currently, all but four states have an EMS Director, but only a handful have a physician in that position.

Because the Federal regulations were relatively flexible, a timely series of innovations directed at prehospital medicine during the late 1960's were able to influence the initial designs of the regional programs.[2,9] Several physician-directed prehospital cardiac response programs and the Vietnam War experience with organized trauma care were publicized.[10] Gradually, it was accepted that prehospital care could be delivered by trained nonphysicians such as individuals educated as Emergency Medical Technicians (EMTs) through the use of DOT-approved curriculum. Although the EMT concept did not require physician input at any level, the paramedics who grew directly out of the physician-directed cardiac response programs were essentially extensions of the physician.[11] These two diverse categories developed more or less independently, with EMT becoming a nationally standard level, whereas the paramedic category differed markedly from locality to locality. The practice of the EMT was commonly called Basic Life Support (BLS) and the practice of the paramedic (usually first trained as an EMT) was labeled Advanced Life Support (ALS). Because of the relatively great differences in initial training requirements between the two levels, many jurisdictions introduced intermediate levels, which quickly blurred the distinctions between the two. By 1980, prehospital care providers existed at virtually every level of training between 70 and 2000 hours; the degree of required medical supervision was almost as variable.[7,9]

The decade of the 1970s was a period of rapid EMS innovation; some concepts grew and others faded from the scene. Unfortunately, subsequent amendments to the EMSS Act of 1973 did not address the absence of required medical direction in the original. Although some of the state legislative efforts mandated medical control, most neglected to address the issue, both because of lack of physician input and the failure of the authors to recognize the need.

In 1978, the National Academy of Sciences released a report finding "EMS in the United States in midpassage urgently in need of midcourse corrections but uncertain as to the best direction and degree." The committee then recommended "research and evaluation directed both to questions of immediate importance to EMS system development and to long range questions. Without adequate investment in both types of research, EMS in the United States will be in the same position of uncertainty a generation hence as it is today."[9] Those sentiments are probably as true today as they were in 1978.

In the 1980s, the Federal Government involvement in EMS ended.[2] As the various states attempted once again to update EMS legislation and as physicians took a greater interest in prehospital care, formal medical control trickled down from the paramedic level to the intermediate levels and ultimately to the BLS level.[12] Transiently, in the early 1980s, it appeared that independent licensure for ALS providers might emerge; however, this trend peaked and then diminished as the medical community began to exert influence to the contrary. Currently, physician direction is a relatively standard nationwide requirement for intermediate and advanced providers, whereas medical direction for EMTs is growing, especially regarding the use of the MAST garment and the automatic defibrillator.[13]

Unfortunately, in most jurisdictions, the vagueness of the initial law has created a confused situation regarding medical control authority. While many EMS regions have either a formally designated regional medical director or a physician advisory committee, the authority varies from absolute to nil. In the latter case, the individual ambulance service medical directors retain both the authority and the accountability. More enlightened and often newly developing EMS regions have established a relatively powerful medical director selected by a medical advisory committee. Such system medical directors delegate significant responsibility to the individual service medical advisors. State laws, however, remain the determining factors as to authority, and in many cases they remain unclear or even contradictory, effectively preventing the local delegation of medical control authority.[14] In some parts of the country, medical control is contracted from a local medical school or teaching hospital by the ambulance agency.

PERSONNEL AND TRAINING

Currently, there are five general levels of training for prehospital providers; the borders between them are vague. Although there are now national curricula for each of the provider levels, the DOT curriculum for EMT-Ambulance is the only one that approaches universal use.

1. Citizen CPR and First Aid (Initial Responder)
2. First Responder
3. Basic Emergency Medical Technician (EMT-Ambulance)
4. Intermediate Emergency Medical Technician (EMT-Intermediate)
5. Advanced Emergency Medical Technician (EMT-Paramedic)

"First responder" was originally the generic name for these providers, often police officers or firemen trained in CPR and first aid.[9] Many jurisdictions have now expanded the role of first responders to include many of the skills traditionally taught to EMTs, and in a growing number of jurisdictions, the use of the automatic defibrillator. The specific term First Responder is now used to describe individuals trained to the DOT national standard. The descriptive term "initial responder" is recommended for emergency personnel who are not educated to a formal First Responder level.

The EMT-Ambulance (EMT) curriculum was originally standardized in 1970. The program has since expanded to over 100 hours and now includes training in the use of the MAST garment. Some states have added additional training modules to allow the use of epinephrine for anaphylaxis and the use of the automatic defibrillator. Obviously the need and requirement for physician involvement expands as the EMT activities become more medically sophisticated.[15,16]

The first "intermediate" providers were EMTs with added training modules in advanced airway management, intravenous cannulation, drug use, arrythmia recognition, and/or defibrillation. Initially, the intermediate EMTs were originally thought to be on a progressive ladder to paramedic. It became quickly obvious that further progress up the ladder to paramedic was difficult and perhaps unnecessary.[9] Consequently, today it is possible for intermediate EMTs trained for 200 hours to effectively duplicate the clinical interventions done in other areas by paramedics with 500 or more hours of training. This discrepancy developed because the initial paramedic programs put a heavy emphasis on teaching the scientific basis of prehospital care, whereas more recently developed intermediate programs have de-emphasized those basic science requirements. The significant financial cost of training and of refreshing traditional paramedics is pushing many local programs and medical directors away from the paramedic level toward the intermediate levels; concurrently, the demand for prehospital services beyond the basic level is pushing systems to upgrade EMT-A's to the intermediate level. In spite of the thrust of the 1978 "midpassage" recommendation, only recently have researchers started to rigorously compare the clinical success of various types of interventions, providers and system models.[9,17,18] When the EMT-A moves up to intermediate, a void is created, which partly explains the growing interest in the use of upgraded first responders on ambulances. No matter which provider is used in a given system, physicians must be involved in the choice of the provider level, the training, and the operations.[13,19]

Recently, it has been suggested that, unless additional expanded health care roles can be developed for the more highly educated paramedics, many programs may revert to intermediate levels as more cost-effective, yet medically satisfactory prehospital care providers.[20] Certainly, in the more rural areas of the United States and in developing countries, the focus of prehospital training is at the basic and intermediate levels. Where there is a relative surplus of physicians or nurses, they are used effectively as the ALS element of prehospital systems.

COMMUNICATIONS

Approximately 50% of the United States ambulance services are accessed through dialing 911, although some areas still use a seven-digit telephone number. Universal use of 911 and ultimately "enhanced" 911 must be encouraged across the country.[9]

As EMS systems developed, the organization and operation of the dispatching of ambulances was usually left as the responsibility of administrators. Gradually, the awareness of the need for medically prioritizing responses, rather than "first in-first out," became obvious. Although organization structure and ambulance distribution remain, for the most part, outside the direct domain of medical control, the caller questioning sequences for medical priority determinations and the algorithmic determinations of which level unit to dispatch to a given call have fallen under increased medical scrutiny. In the early 1980s, many medically developed prioritization/dispatching systems independently evolved. Recently, a state level emergency medical dispatch (EMD) course was implemented in Utah and is expanding nationally. Such programs make it much easier for local medical directors to develop successful EMD programs for their localities.[21,22]

Generally, ultra-high level radio frequencies (UHF) are used for medical control and transmission of medical information, and very high level frequencies

(VHF) are used for dispatch. Increasingly, telephone lines and cellular phone networks are being used in EMS communications; the danger is that in disaster situations, these modes will be inoperative.

OPERATIONS

If one uses Stout's definition that "an EMS System is a network of organizations generating a comprehensive, coordinated response to a patient's need for on-scene medical care, medical transportation, and en-route support," various prehospital providers can be integrated into a system in dozens of ways.[8] Urban systems are increasingly multitiered with first responder, BLS and ALS components. Rural systems tend to use a variety of levels, usually with an intermediate EMT level as the most sophisticated; however, several rural and suburban systems have a formal nurse or physician response built in as the ALS component.

Other unsolved operational issues are whether non-transport response vehicles should be used by the initial providers with another tier transporting, what is the optimal response time target, which type of transport vehicle design is most safe and efficient, and how aeromedical responses should be integrated in the system.[8,23,24]

Generally, the combination of a smoothly functioning EMS system and a plan to augment and expand its function is the underpinning of medical disaster preparedness for all but the most extensive disasters. Because the first 12 hours are critical for medical disaster response, medical resources from distant areas need to arrive within that time frame. The National Disaster Medical System is developing in the United States with the dual purposes of bringing medical resources to the disaster victims and of transporting patients to distant hospital facilities within an acceptable time frame.[25,26]

MEDICAL CONTROL

When ALS providers first began to deliver medical care in the field, the physician community expressed strong concerns as to how well care could be provided and the impact on the practice of medicine. Consequently, extensive direct medical control was required in most early paramedic programs. Gradually, it became apparent that prehospital ALS was both relatively safe and not threatening to the day-to-day practice of medicine; the requirements for concurrent

direction by physicians gradually waned. In some areas, physician surrogates, such as nurses, actually replaced the physicians; in others, the ALS providers operated under expanded standing orders.[9,27] Originally, cardiac telemetry had been regularly transmitted from prehospital scenes to medical control physicians; this practice is much less commonly used currently because physician concerns about the ability of ALS providers to interpret rhythm strips have diminished.

The aggressive retrospective call review that marked the early days of prehospital ALS have also become more routine and perfunctory. Only recently has the need for more thorough concurrent and retrospective quality assurance of prehospital care reappeared as a critical task for medical directors.[13,27,28]

HORIZONS

Arguably, the most significant modern advance in prehospital care has been the gradual development of comprehensive organized EMS systems. Because the initial impetus for the regional organization of EMS systems was the EMSS Act of 1973, many of the resulting systems were organized around the trauma center concept central both to that law and the subsequent regulations.[2,7,29,30] Although the regional organization of EMS systems has varied significantly, a few general future trends can be identified.

First, EMS is in transition from being a relatively unimportant cottage industry to being a significant force in health care delivery. Initially perceived as a relatively inexpensive and insignificant facet of health care, EMS is now a medically, politically, and economically influential partner. As both physicians and hospitals increasingly recognized that EMS systems can have a profound impact on many aspects of health care delivery, no longer are a few visionary individuals allowed to direct, within a vacuum, the provision of prehospital care. Because the medical and economic impact is potentially great, virtually every national health care association has developed a committee on EMS affairs. The citizens and governments of most cities, counties, and states have come to view EMS with the same attitudes and expectations as they do police and fire protection.

Second, the cost of providing contemporary prehospital care has accelerated even faster than health care costs in general. With the universal diminution of volunteerism and the rapid growth in sophistication and accountability for prehospital medicine, those responsible for funding EMS are starting to ask logical and penetrating questions concerning the efficiency and quality of prehospital and disaster medicine.[17,26] As costs and accountability grow, the public will demand the end of the traditional EMS fiefdoms in jurisdictions where fully integrated and efficient systems do not yet exist.

Third, eventually those reponsible for the development of regional EMS systems must cross the prehospital-hospital interface and actually influence hospital design, designation, and operation. Needless to say, such a new direction captures the attention and concern of the entire health care industry.

Fourth, sooner or later EMS provision in a jurisdiction becomes a politically charged topic. Because it has a high profile, EMS is a highly visible element of government, a service that is vulnerable to criticism because of both the relative frequency of its need and the high cost of its failure. It is increasingly common to observe EMS administrators and medical directors caught in the media spotlight, buffeted by political agendas, financial cutbacks and expanding needs.

Finally, the rapid growth and innovative, if unproven, development marking the adolescence of EMS is coming to an end. Indeed, the normal evolutionary trend of gradual growth and consolidation may have been overtaken by a "hypermaturity." In a sense, EMS development is rapidly being trapped in the *status quo*, a sort of equilibrium where evolutionary change is either not acceptable or too expensive for the existing powerful players. Although little doubt exists that new medical and technical advances applicable to the prehospital environment will eventually be integrated into our EMS systems, the resistance to change is great. For example, in New York City, the training of EMS first responders within the department initially met with great resistance from that department, the EMS, and the budget office. The program was ultimately approved by the city administration during an election year and then was effectively cancelled as soon as the votes were counted.

When a developmental stalemate is reached, cataclysmic change is likely. As greater efficiency and professionalism are demanded of EMS and as volunteerism and funding decline, it may be necessary to expand the scope of prehospital services to keep EMS as an affordable public service. It is not surprising that many countries have chosen to view prehospital care more broadly as a public health activity rather than as a sibling of the fire or police services. Nor is it surprising that the privatization of prehospital care is often promoted as an essential next step. Physicians must continue to influence the direction of EMS evolution both organizationally and personally.

NATIONAL CONTACTS

American College of Emergency Physicians
PO BOX 619911
Dallas, TX 75261
800-798-1822

National Association of EMS Physicians
230 McKee Place, Suite 500
Pittsburgh, PA 15213
800-228-3677

National Disaster Medical System
5600 Fishers Lane
Rockville, MD 20857

REFERENCES

1. Kuehl, A.E. (Editor): The NAEMSP Medical Directors' Handbook, St. Louis, C.V. Mosby, 1989, pp. 3–27.
2. Boyd, D.R., Edlich, R.F., and Miak, S.H.: Systems Approach to Emergency Medical Care. Norwalk, CT, Appleton, Century-Crofts, 1983.
3. Law of the 89th Congress, Highway Safety Act of 1966, Washington, DC, 1966.
4. Accidental Death and Disability, the Neglected Disease of Modern Society. Washington, DC, Division Medical Sciences—National Academy of Sciences, 1966.
5. Hanlan, J.J.: Emergency Medical Services. New program for old problem. Health Services Reports 88:205, 1973.
6. Special Report on Emergency Medical Service Systems. Princeton, Robert Wood Johnson Foundation, 1973.
7. Law of the 93rd Congress, Emergency Medical Services System Act of 1973, Washington, DC, 1973.
8. Stout, J.L.: High Performance EMS Systems. Miami, The Fourth Party, Inc., 1989; pp. 8–12. (in press)
9. Emergency Medical Services at Midpassage. National Research Council—National Academy of Sciences, Washington, DC, 1978.
10. Pantridge, J.F., and Geddes, J.F.: A mobile intensive care unit in the management of myocardial infarction. Lancet 2:271, 1967.
11. Page, J.O.: Paramedics. Morristown, NJ, Backdraft Publications, 1979.
12. American College of Emergency Physicians: Position Paper on Emergency Medical Services, Dallas, 1986.
13. Pepe, P.E., and Stewart, R.D.: Role of the physician in the prehospital setting. Ann. Emerg. Med. 15:1480, 1986.
14. Braun, O., McCallion, R., and Fazackerly, J.: Characteristics of midsized urban EMS Systems. Ann. Emerg. Med. 16:490, 1986.
15. Eisenberg, M., Bergner, L., and Hallstrom, A.: Paramedic programs and out-of-hospital arrest. I. Factors associated with successful resuscitation. Am. J. Public Health, 69:30, 1979.
16. Stults, K.R., Brown, D.D., Schug, V.L., et al.: Prehospital defibrillation performed by emergency medical technicians in rural communities. N. Engl. J. Med. 310:219, 1984.
17. Eisenberg, M.S., Horwood, B.T., Cummins, R.O., et al.: Cardiac arrest and resuscitation: A tale of 29 cities. Ann. Emerg. Med. 19:179, 1990.
18. Hargarten, K.M., Stueven, H.A., and Waite, E.M.: Prehospital experience with defibrillation of coarse ventricular fibrillation: A ten-year review. Ann. Emerg. Med. 19:157, 1990.
19. Eisenberg, M., Copass, M., Hallstrom, A., et al.: Treatment of out-of-hospital cardiac arrests with rapid defibrillation by emergency medical technicians. N. Engl. J. Med. 302:1379, 1980.
20. Kuehl, A.E.: Perspectives on international EMS system development. Emerg. Med. Services, 18:37, 1989.
21. Clawson, J.J.: Dispatch priority training strengthening the weak link. J. Emerg. Med. 6:32, 1981.
22. Eisenberg, M.S., Carter, W., Hallstrom, A., et al.: Identification of cardiac arrest by emergency dispatchers. Am. J. Emerg. Med. 4:299, 1986.
23. Baxt, W.G., and Mordy, P.: The impact of rotocraft aeromedical emergency care service on trauma mortality. JAMA 249:3047, 1984.

24. Brismar, B., Alveryd, A., Johnson, O., et al.: The ambulance helicopter is a prerequisite for centralized emergency care. Acta Chir. Scand. (Suppl) 530:89, 1986.
25. Cowan, M., Butman, A.M., and Bosner, L.V.: Mass casualty planning: Model for in-hospital disaster response. JWAEDM 2:83, 1986.
26. Jacobs, L.M., Ramp, J.M., and Breay, M.J.: An emergency medical system approach to disaster planning. J. Trauma 19:157, 1979.
27. Holroyd, B.R., Knopp, R., and Kallgen, G.: Medical control quality assurance in prehospital care. JAMA 256:1027, 1986.
28. Medical Control of Emergency Medical Services: An overview for Emergency Physicians. Dallas, American College of Emergency Physicians, 1984.
29. Cales, R.H., and Helig, R.W.: Trauma Care Systems. Rockville, MD, Aspen Publications, 1986.
30. West, J.G., Trunkey, D.D., and Lim, R.C.: Systems of trauma care. A study of two counties. Arch. Surg. 114:455, 1979.

EMS SYSTEMS FACTORS AND SURVIVAL OF CARDIAC ARREST

Mickey S. Eisenberg

"In the industrially developed countries, sudden cardiac death is the leading cause of death. It was recognized at the dawn of recorded history and even depicted in Egyptian relief sculptures from the tomb of a noble of the sixth dynasty approximately 4,500 years ago. Sudden cardiac death has left no age untouched; sparing neither saint nor sinner, it has burdened man with a sense of uncertainty and fragility. The enormity of this problem demands attention. In the United States sudden cardiac death claims about 1,200 lives daily or approximately one victim every minute."

Bernard Lown[1]

CAPSULE

Sudden cardiac death is defined as "death caused by underlying heart disease occurring without symptoms or with symptoms of less than an hour's duration."[2] Almost all sudden cardiac deaths occur before the patient can reach hospital care. Sudden cardiac death is a major subset of the larger problem of coronary artery disease. Coronary artery disease is the leading cause of death among adults, and according to the National Center for Health Statistics accounts for over half a million deaths per year.[3] Well over half of the deaths from coronary artery disease occur suddenly, with little or no warning, often in adults without known heart disease.[4] The average age for sudden cardiac death is 64 years (in men 63, in women 68). It is three to four times more likely to occur in men than women.

Because sudden cardiac death is a prehospital emergency for which emergency medical service (EMS) systems and emergency departments (EDs) are the primary source of care, it is important that emergency physicians understand the factors associated with successful resuscitation to help increase the likelihood that a patient can be resuscitated. Physicians should ask themselves, "What is the likelihood of resuscitation from sudden cardiac arrest in my community? How can this likelihood increase?"

PATHOPHYSIOLOGY OF SUDDEN CARDIAC ARREST

CAUSE

Although the causes of sudden cardiac death are many and include valvular heart disease, cardiomyopathy, myocarditis, coronary artery spasm, the most common cause, accounting for 80 to 90% of all sudden cardiac deaths, is coronary artery disease. Autopsy studies of patients with sudden cardiac death demonstrate that 80% have underlying coronary artery disease, usually involving major pathologic changes in two or more arteries.[5,6]

RISK FACTORS

The risk factors for sudden cardiac death are identical to those associated with coronary artery disease, namely cigarette smoking, hypercholesterolemia, hypertension, and diabetes.[7,8] Since males are more prone to coronary artery disease, males have more sudden cardiac deaths. Cobb and associates[9] have shown that a history of myocardial infarction, angina, congestive heart failure, or hypertension was present in three quarters of patients who were resuscitated from out-of-hospital cardiac arrest. For the remainder, cardiac arrest was the first manifestation of cardio-vascular disease.

Numerous clinical risk factors have been identified that place individuals at higher risk of sudden cardiac death. These include ventricular ectopy, especially complex ventricular premature depolarizations in patients with underlying cardiovascular disease, electrocardiographic abnormalities such as prolonged QT intervals or repolarization abnormalities, extensive coronary artery narrowing, and abnormal left ventricular function (as manifested by a decreased ejection fraction).[10,11] These predictors have been determined from studies of selected high-risk populations. The sensitivity and specificity of these predictors throughout the general population are not well characterized, and thus their applicability to the general population is poorly defined. In addition, the invasiveness and cost of some of these studies limit widespread use. There is, regrettably, no unique or practical combination of risk factors, signs, symptoms, or studies that can accurately identify patients at immediate risk of sudden cardiac death. Although high-risk factors can be shown, there is no way to identify the imminent likelihood of a sudden cardiac arrest episode.

SYNDROMES OF SUDDEN CARDIAC ARREST

Numerous triggers for sudden cardiac death have been postulated. These include ischemia, electrolyte imbalances, platelet abnormalities, psychologic stress, and neurochemical transmitters. Unfortunately, the precise mechanism for sudden cardiac death is not well characterized. Data from Cobb and associates[9] demonstrate that approximately 20% of patients who were resuscitated and admitted to the hospital after an out-of-hospital episode of ventricular fibrillation had electrocardiographic evidence of transmural myocardial infarction, a smaller percentage had a myocardial infarction of indeterminate age, almost half had ST-T wave changes, and approximately 25% had no ECG changes at all.

The lack of consistent pathologic, electrocardiographic, or other findings among patients with sudden cardiac death suggests that several pathophysiologic syndromes may exist. Based on prodromal symptoms, pathologic findings and prognosis, it is possible to suggest three syndromes (Table 87-1). As causes are better understood, it may be possible to be able to identify more syndromes.

PREVENTION

Prevention is the only means to deal decisively with the problem of sudden cardiac death. Unfortunately, at this time, prevention is not realistically possible. Although reduction of risk factors may reduce the incidence of coronary artery disease, and thus the incidence of sudden cardiac death, it is unlikely that there will be a dramatic community-wide lowering of risk factors. Furthermore, some risk factors cannot be lowered, such as male sex or the presence of diabetes. Although prevention remains an elusive dream, the only practical solution at present is the treatment of the acute event.

FACTORS ASSOCIATED WITH SUCCESSFUL RESUSCITATION

Every cardiac arrest event is associated with a unique set of circumstances related to the patient and the events surrounding the cardiac arrest. These factors can be grouped into fate and system factors. Fate factors include patient characteristics or chance events, such as the prior medical condition of the patient, the cardiac rhythm at the time of collapse, and whether the collapse was witnessed. System factors include characteristics of the EMS system such as the type of service, whether or not a bystander initiates CPR, and the various time intervals from collapse to CPR and

TABLE 87-1. SYNDROMES OF SUDDEN CARDIAC DEATH*

	Infarction	Ischemia	Electrical
Pathophysiology	Infarcted area causes pump failure or may lead to rhythm disturbance	Ischemic area may trigger rhythm disturbance	Rhythm disturbance triggered by poorly understood mechanisms
SCD percentage	20%–30%	Unknown	Unknown
Autopsy	Coronary artery occlusion with resultant myocardial infarction	Evidence of ischemia	"Normal" heart—usually evidence of underlying coronary artery disease
Most common	Ventricular fibrillation and other rhythms	Ventricular fibrillation	Ventricular fibrillation
Warning before collapse	Minutes to hours	Minutes	None or seconds
Mortality within 1 year after discharge	5%	Unknown	30%

* With permission from Eisenberg, M.S.: Sudden cardiac death and resuscitation: The results. In Critical Care: State of the Art, Vol 8. Edited by Cerra, F.B. Fullerton, CA, Society of Critical Care Medicine, 1978.

TABLE 87-2. CARDIAC RHYTHM AND OUTCOME FOR PARAMEDIC-TREATED CASES*

Rhythm (on Arrival)	Number	%	Discharged	%
Ventricular fibrillation	1238	58%	385	31%
Ventricular tachycardia	50	2%	23	46%
Asystole	576	27%	11	2%
Idioventricular	162	8%	5	3%
Other or unknown	125	6%	19	15%
Total	2151	101%†	443	21%

* With permission from Center for Evaluation of Emergency Medical Services, Division of Emergency Medical Services, King County Health Department, Seattle, Washington.
† Does not equal 100% because of rounding out of figures.

TABLE 87-3. CONTROLLED STUDIES OF SURVIVAL (DISCHARGED ALIVE) FROM OUT-OF-HOSPITAL CARDIAC ARREST: BYSTANDER CPR COMPARED TO LATE CPR*

Location/System (reference)	Witnessed Arrest	Rhythm	Number of Patients	Discharged Alive (N)	Odds Ratio†
1. Oslo, Norway EMTs only	Not reported	Not reported	BYS CPR = 75	36% (27)	6.7
			LATE CPR = 556	8% (43)	
2. Birmingham Paramedics only	Implied yes	VF or VT	BYS CPR = 7	86% (6)	6.0
			LATE CPR = 12	50% (6)	
3. SEATTLE EMTs and Paramedics	76% overall witnessed	VF only	BYS CPR = 109	43% (47)	2.9
			LATE CPR = 207	21% (43)	
4. Winnipeg EMTs only	Not reported	VF or VT	BYS CPR = 65	25% (16)	6.2
			LATE CPR = 161		
5. Iceland EMTs only	Not reported	All rhythms	BYS CPR = 38	42% (16)	11.5
			LATE CPR = 84	2%	
6. Vancouver EMTs and Paramedics	77% overall witnessed	All rhythms	BYS CPR = 43	21% (9)	4.0
			LATE CPR = 272		
7. Los Angeles Paramedics	41% overall witnessed	All rhythms	BYS CPR = 93	22% (20)	5.6
			LATE CPR = 150	5% (7)	
		VF only	BYS CPR = 45	27% (12)	6.0
			LATE CPR = 70	6% (4)	
8. King County EMTs and Paramedics	Not reported	All rhythms	BYS CPR = 108	23% (25)	2.2
			LATE CPR = 379	2% (45)	
9. Pittsburgh Paramedics	Not reported	VF/VT only	BYS CPR = 25	24% (6)	4.3
			LATE CPR = 59	7% (4)	
10. Milwaukee EMTs and Paramedics	Witnessed only	All rhythms	BYS CPR = 1248	15% (182)	1.0
			LATE CPR = 252	15% (38)	
		Coarse VF	BYS CPR = 628	24% (148)	1.0
			LATE CPR = 151	23% (35)	
11. Michigan/Ohio communities (EMTs and paramedics)	Not reported	All rhythms	BYS CPR = 472	13% (56)	2.7
			LATE CPR = 1367	5% (64)	
12. King County EMT-Ds and Paramedics	Both	All rhythms	BYS CPR = 726	27% (196)	2.4
			LATE CPR = 1317	13% (177)	
	Witnessed only	All rhythms	BYS CPR = 579	32% (186)	1.7
			LATE CPR = 718	22% (158)	
13. York/Adams, Pa EMTs and Paramedics	Witnessed only	VF only	BYS CPR = 157	22% (34)	4.5
			LATE CPR = 225	6% (13)	
14. Tucson, Arizona EMTs and Paramedics	Witnessed only	All Rhythms	BYS CPR = 65	20% (13)	2.5
			LATE CPR = 130	9%	

* Adapted with permission from Cummins, R.O., and Graves, J.: Clinical results of standard CPR: Prehospital and in-hospital. *In* Cardiopulmonary Resuscitation. Edited by Kaye, W., and Bircher, N.G. New York, Churchill Livingston, 1989.
† "Odds ratio" of survival is calculated as follows: the product of the number of patients discharged alive in the bystander CPR group, and the number who died in the late CPR group, divided by the product of the number discharged alive in the late CPR group and the number who died in the bystander CPR group.

TABLE 87-4. DISCHARGE RATES FOLLOWING OUT-OF-HOSPITAL CARDIAC ARREST RELATED TO THE TIME UNTIL INITIATION OF CPR AND DEFINITIVE CARE*

Time from Collapse to CPR	Time from Collapse to Definitive Care		
	8 min	8–16 min	16 min
4 min	43%	19%	10%
4–8 min	27%	15%	6%
8 min		7%	0%

* Adapted with permission from Eisenberg, M.S., Bergner, L., and Hallstrom, A.: Cardiac resuscitation in the community: The importance of rapid delivery of care and implication for program planning. JAMA *241*:1905, 1979.

collapse to defibrillation and definitive care. System factors most predictive of outcome are the time from collapse to CPR and the time from collapse to defibrillation and definitive care.[12]

FATE FACTORS

Age, sex, and prior medical condition are the predominant fate factors associated with successful resuscitation from sudden cardiac death. For patients discharged alive after out-of-hospital arrest, the average age is 61 compared to 66 for nonsurvivors. There is no relationship of sex to admission or discharge. Patients with a prior history of congestive heart failure have a lower likelihood of survival. Another strong predictor of successful or unsuccessful resuscitation is whether the collapse was witnessed.[12] If the collapse is seen or heard directly, the patient has a much higher likelihood of survival compared to one with an unwitnessed cardiac arrest. Another important predictor is the rhythm associated with the cardiac arrest episode. Patients with ventricular fibrillation or ventricular tachycardia have the highest likelihood of admission and discharge after cardiac arrest. Patients with asystole, idioventricular, and other rhythms have a much poorer likelihood of resuscitation. Table 87-2 illustrates the survival rates for patients in various rhythms who were treated by paramedics in King County, Washington.

SYSTEM FACTORS

Characteristics of the system are also strongly associated with the likelihood of survival. An important system factor, CPR initiated by bystanders, is associated with an increased likelihood of survival in patients compared to those who do not receive bystander-initiated CPR. In a review of articles reporting controlled studies of prehospital CPR, Cummins demonstrated that bystander CPR has a dramatic effect on the likelihood of resuscitation.[13,14] Table 87-3 shows the results of 14 controlled studies comparing patients with early bystander CPR versus those with late CPR.

In all of the studies, except for one, the odds ratio for the probability of survival from an out-of-hospital cardiac arrest was significantly greater than 1.0.

A single study from Milwaukee did not demonstrate a beneficial effect of bystander CPR,[15,16] probably because of an extremely rapid aid unit response time. In Milwaukee, the average response time for the first arriving emergency vehicle is 2.1 minutes. There is little discrepancy between the time from collapse to CPR by bystanders and the time from collapse to CPR by aid unit personnel. In King County, Washington, where the average aid unit response is approximately 5 minutes and in other communities with response times longer than those in Milwaukee, there is a greater opportunity to perform bystander CPR and a longer duration of bystander CPR. In all these other cities, a beneficial effect of bystander CPR has been shown.

Other important system factors include the time from collapse to provision of defibrillation and definitive care. The two critical system factors of time from collapse to CPR and time from collapse to defibrillation and definitive care appear to be intimately related. Previous studies suggest that the early initiation of CPR prolongs the duration of VF and therefore prevents deterioration from coarse VF to fine VF and ultimately asystole. This increases the likelihood that VF will last longer and that the response to defibrillation will be positive.[17] When CPR is delayed or the time to defibrillation is greater than 10 to 12 minutes after the start of CPR, it is more likely the patient will be in fine VF and a defibrillatory shock will convert the rhythm to asystole.[18] Shown in Table 87-4 is the relationship of time from collapse to CPR and time from collapse to definitive care.

The term definitive care encompasses all advanced life support (ALS) interventions, including defibrillation, intravenous medications, and endotracheal intubations. Although some studies have demonstrated the independent benefit of defibrillation,[19–21] no studies have quantified the individual benefit of medications or intubation. It would be difficult to conduct such studies since the combination of all these treatments define the standard of care for cardiac arrest.

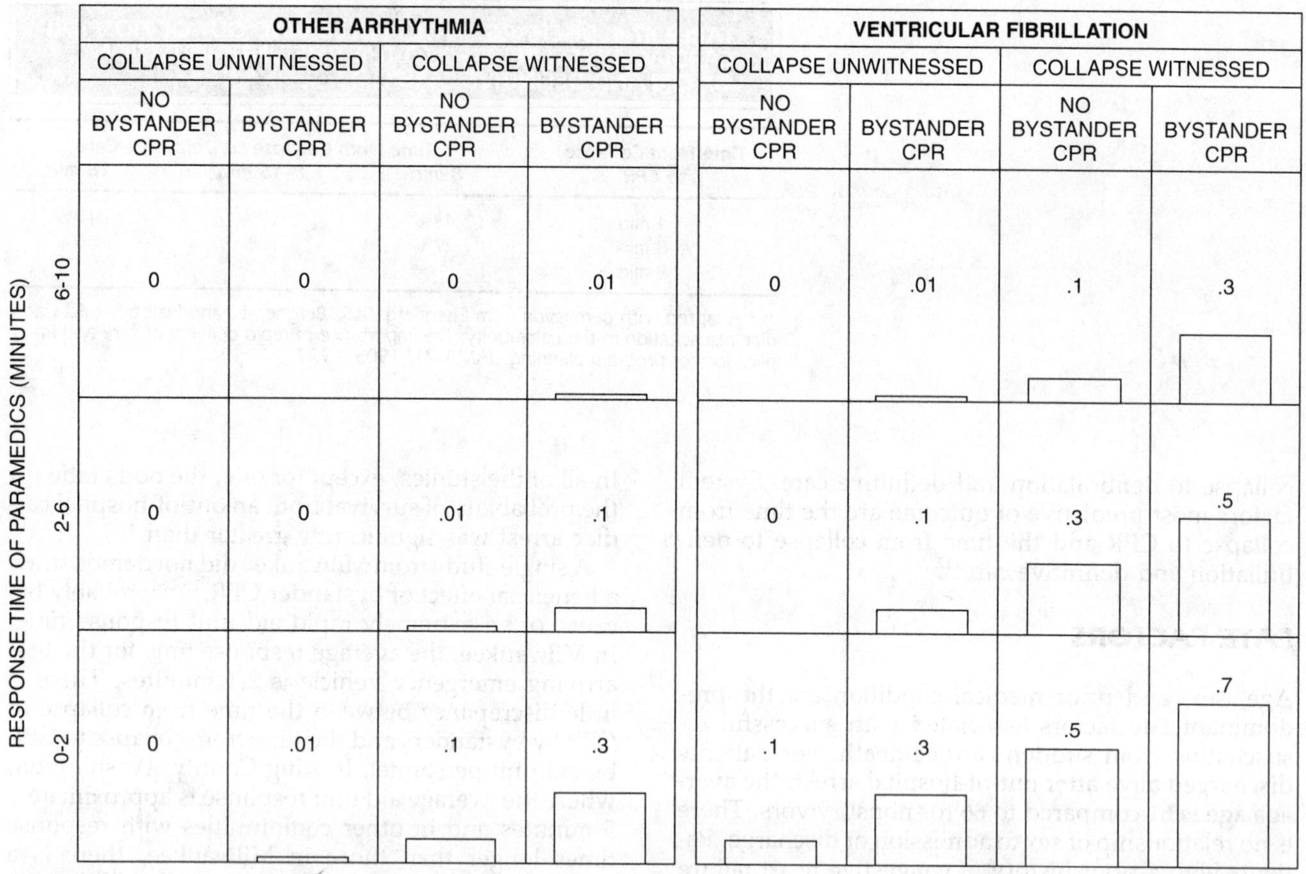

	OTHER ARRHYTHMIA				VENTRICULAR FIBRILLATION			
RESPONSE TIME OF PARAMEDICS (MINUTES)	COLLAPSE UNWITNESSED		COLLAPSE WITNESSED		COLLAPSE UNWITNESSED		COLLAPSE WITNESSED	
	NO BYSTANDER CPR	BYSTANDER CPR	NO BYSTANDER CPR	BYSTANDER CPR	NO BYSTANDER CPR	BYSTANDER CPR	NO BYSTANDER CPR	BYSTANDER CPR
6–10	0	0	0	.01	0	.01	.1	.3
2–6	0	0	.01	.1	0	.1	.3	.5
0–2	0	.01	.1	.3	.1	.3	.5	.7

FIG. 87-1. Chance of successful resuscitation (*colored bars*) from sudden cardiac death depends critically on the particular circumstances surrounding the cardiac arrest and on the speed with which definitive care can be provided by paramedics or physicians. The nature of the arrhythmia that results in the victim's loss of circulation and the presence of bystanders who witness the victim's ensuing collapse cannot be controlled. The response time of paramedic units and the likelihood that a bystander will be able to perform CPR can be improved by increasing the number of emergency-cardiac-care vehicles and personnel and educating the public in CPR. With permission from Eisenberg, M.S., Bergner, L., Hallstrom, A.P., and Cummins, R.O.: Sudden cardiac death. Sci. Am. *254*:37, 1986.

The probability of successful resuscitation is determined by the combination of fate and system factors associated with the cardiac arrest event. This relationship is shown in Figure 87-1. Only when there is a combination of "good" fate and system factors is there any reasonable likelihood of survival. For example, if the rhythm is ventricular fibrillation, the collapse is witnessed, bystander CPR occurs, and the paramedic response time is 2 to 6 minutes, there is a 50% probability of successful resuscitation and discharge from hospital.

DEVELOPMENT OF PREHOSPITAL EMSs

As recently as the early 1960s, prehospital EMSs were inadequate and ineffective. Care was predominantly provided by private ambulance and mortuary companies, with the ambulance often doubling as a hearse. The vehicles were staffed with attendants with variable training in first aid. The National Highway Safety and Traffic Act, enacted in 1966, encouraged the development of EMS at the local level. Although the motive for the passage of this act was the desire to reduce mortality from traffic accidents, it stimulated general improvements in emergency care. Furthermore, the act developed the standardized emergency medical technician (EMT) 81-hour training course, which has subsequently been increased to 110 hours. The course provides instruction for firefighters, ambulance personnel, and first responders in basic life support (BLS) techniques including patient assessment, cardiopulmonary resuscitation, control of external hemorrhage, management of airway problems, and immobilization of patients with musculoskeletal injuries. By the mid 1980s, there were over 400,000 certified EMTs in the United States.

The late 1960s and early 1970s saw the development of a more sophisticated form of emergency medical prehospital service. The first prehospital advanced

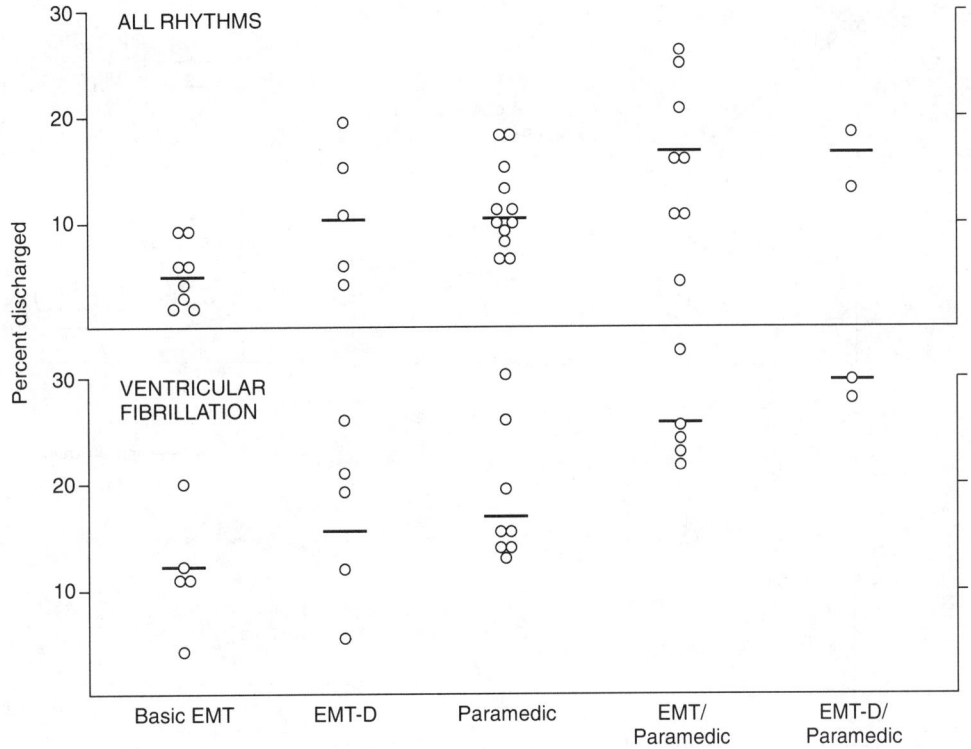

FIG. 87-2. Percent discharged from out-of-hospital cardiac arrest in all rhythms (top panel) and ventricular fibrillation (bottom panel) from five emergency medical service systems. The circles represent the percent discharged from individual communities, and the horizontal line represents the weighted mean discharge rate. With permission from Eisenberg, M.S., et al.: Cardiac arrest and resuscitation: A tale of 29 cities. Ann. Emerg. Med., in press 1991.

unit was started in 1966 in Belfast, Ireland by Drs. Pantridge and Geddes. Their unit, known as a mobile intensive care unit (MICU), was staffed by a physician and nurse and provided early treatment, primarily anti-arrhythmic drugs for suspected acute myocardial infarction.[22] These early units were able to successfully defibrillate a small number of patients who went into cardiac arrest after arrival of the unit. The first MICUs in the United States, patterned after the Belfast model, were started in the late 1960s by Grace in New York City, Crampton in Charlottesville, Virginia and Warren in Columbus, Ohio. Shortly thereafter, Nagel in Miami, Cobb in Seattle, Criley in Los Angeles, and Warren in Columbus, pioneered the concept of substituting paramedics for physicians. MICUs were initially concerned with delivering emergency coronary care, but soon began to encompass all types of prehospital emergency care.

FIVE TYPES OF SYSTEMS

Virtually all prehospital EMS systems in the U.S., whether privately or publicly run, can be characterized as one of five types:

1. Basic EMT: Ambulance or aid response unit staffed with personnel trained in basic cardiac life support.
2. EMT-D: Basic EMTs also trained in the use of defibrillators.
3. Paramedic: Personnel trained in advanced cardiac life support and able to provide definitive care, defibrillation, medication, and endotracheal intubation.
4. Basic EMT/Paramedic: a double-response system with the first responding unit staffed with basic EMTs and the second responding unit staffed with paramedics.
5. EMT-D/Paramedic: A double-response system with the first responding unit staffed with EMT-D trained personnel and the second responding unit staffed with paramedics.

Several dozen communities represented by one of these five types of prehospital systems have published their survival experience for managing sudden cardiac arrest. The range of discharge rates within the five systems for all rhythms and ventricular fibrillation is shown in Figure 87-2. The respective adjusted discharge rates for VF for the five systems were 12%, 16%, 17%, 24%, and 29%.[23]

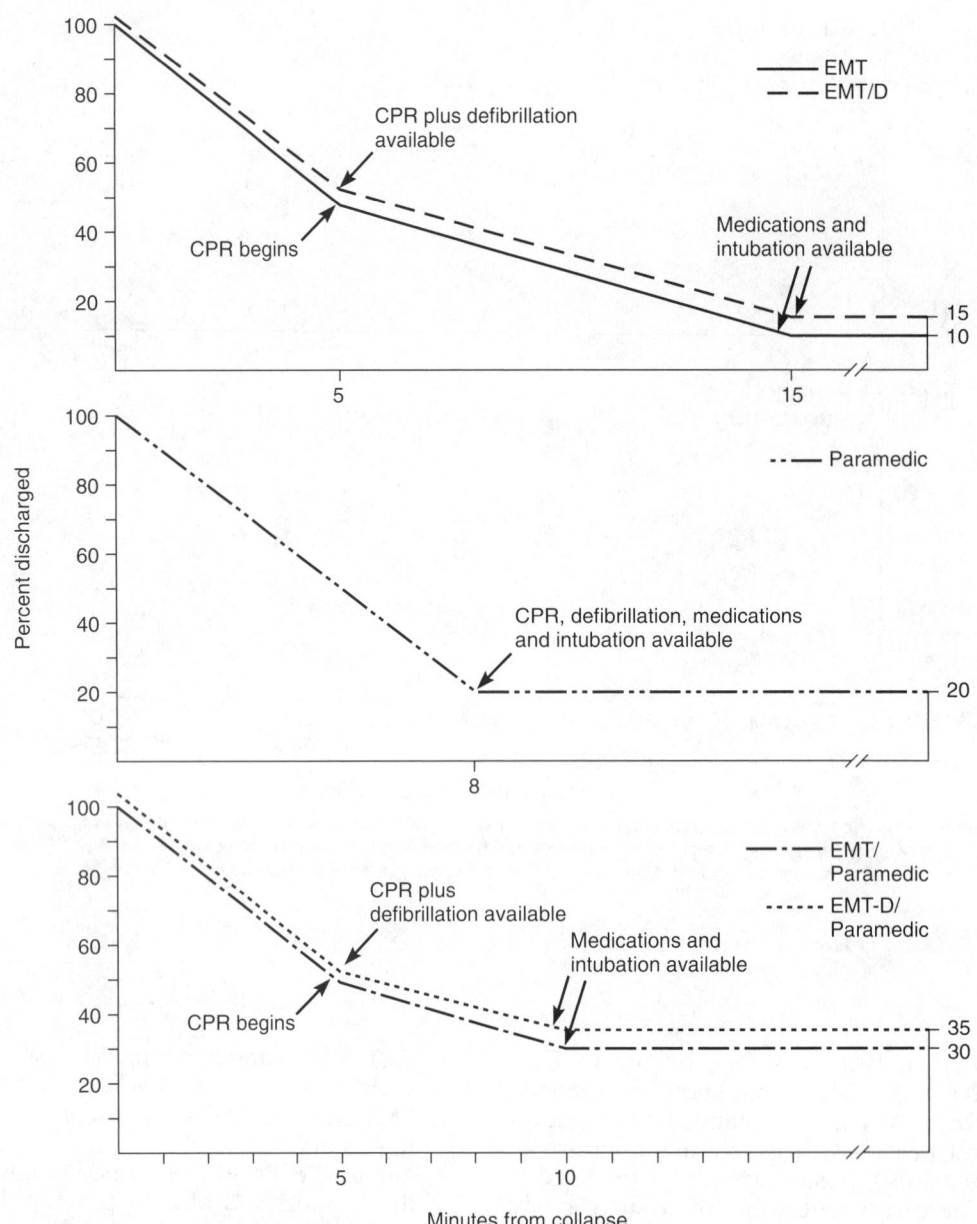

FIG. 87-3. Hypothetical survival curves for out-of-hospital cardiac arrest treated by five types of emergency medical survival systems. Basic emergency medical technician (EMT) and EMT-defibrillation (EMT-D) services are depicted in the top panel, paramedic services in the middle panel, and EMT/paramedic and EMT-D/paramedic services in the bottom panel. CPR denotes cardiopulmonary resuscitation. With permission from Eisenberg, M.S., et al.: Cardiac arrest and resuscitation: A tale of 29 cities. Ann. Emerg. Med., in press.

BASIS FOR OUTCOMES FROM THE FIVE TYPES OF SYSTEMS

The upward trend in survival among the five EMS systems suggests a strong correlation between the type of system and survival. There is a general improvement in survival as the type of EMS system increases in sophistication. The largest increase occurs between single-response and double-response sys-

tems. What is the explanation for this improvement in survival? The most obvious difference between the systems is in the times required to provide cardiopulmonary resuscitation, defibrillation, intravenous medications, and endotracheal intubation. Conceptually, these therapeutic interventions can be considered to alter the survival curve after cardiac arrest. Physicians think of survival curves in months or years. The survival curve for cardiac arrest, however, is defined in minutes. It can be argued that the natural history of cardiac arrest without intervention is biologic death within minutes. If, however, various interventions can be brought to the scene of the cardiac arrest, the survival curve can be altered, and if definitive care can be provided, the survival curve can reach a plateau. The hypothetic cardiac arrest survival curves for the five EMS systems, which display the effects of various interventions on survival, are shown in Figure 87-3.

EMT SYSTEM

The survival curves, while hypothetic, correspond with the actual survival experience of these five types of systems. The curves propose that the ability to resuscitate an individual is a function of time and type and sequence of therapy. The curves display a series of interventions occurring at different times—CPR, defibrillation, intubation, and medication. In presenting these hypothetic curves, several assumptions are made. The first is that the probability of survival following cardiac arrest falls linearly with time and varies according to the therapeutic intervention. The slope of the survival curve is steepest without intervention; the probability of survival is zero after 10 minutes without CPR. In all systems the survival curves start at 100% because at that moment there is a theoretic 100% chance of resuscitation. The slope of the curves improves after CPR and defibrillation and stabilizes after medication and intubation are provided. In the EMT system, the survival curve improves when EMTs arrive at the scene (assuming an average interval of 5 minutes). Survival still continues to fall, but at a slower rate. The ultimate result, however, is still poor because of the long time required to reach the hospital, where definitive care can begin. The few lives that are saved are those with rapid response and close location to the hospital. Basic EMT systems are found in many rural parts of the country.

EMT-D SYSTEM

The EMT-D system demonstrates the same initial fall in survival as that of the EMT system. In an EMT-D system, however, CPR and defibrillation are brought to the patient simultaneously. The survival curve is shifted with a flatter slope than with CPR alone. The slope still continues downward because medications and intubation are not available at the scene and must await arrival to a hospital. In King County, Washington, EMT-D systems can save almost 20% of patients with out-of-hospital cardiac arrest.[19]

PARAMEDIC SYSTEM

In most communities, paramedic systems have slower average response times than basic EMT systems. In single-response paramedic systems, the reported response times in the literature range from 6 to 8 minutes on the average. CPR is administered later, and defibrillation is delayed compared to EMT-D systems. Although this should theoretically decrease survival rates, they are in fact often equal to or better than EMT-D systems. This is probably because of the earlier medications and intubation provided by paramedics compared to EMT and EMT-D systems. The probability of survival initially falls lower than that of EMT and EMT-D systems because of the longer response time. Once paramedics arrive at the scene, however, definitive care is provided, stabilizing survival at that point.

EMT/PARAMEDIC SYSTEM

In this system, the EMTs start CPR early, and paramedics provide defibrillation and definitive care several minutes later. The EMTs provide CPR at approximately 5 minutes, thus altering the slope of survival, and paramedics arrive approximately 5 minutes later, providing definitive care and stabilizing survival.

EMT-D/PARAMEDIC SYSTEM

In an EMT-D/paramedic system, the best situation exists. EMTs arrive at the scene providing both CPR and defibrillation, again improving the slope of the survival curve. Paramedics arrive approximately 10 minutes after collapse and are able to stabilize the patient, achieving survival rates of up to 35%.

OPTIONS TO IMPROVE SURVIVAL

SHORTENING THE TIME FROM COLLAPSE TO CPR

It is clear that any measure that can allow CPR to occur sooner is likely to increase survival from out-of-hospital cardiac arrest. This assumes, however, that defibrillation and advanced care will also arrive in a reasonable time. CPR alone does not save sudden cardiac arrest patients. One way to shorten the time from collapse to CPR is to increase the number of emergency vehicles. There are, however, practical and financial limits to this approach. In many communities, the average response time of EMT vehicles is already extremely short. Further improvements in response time may require substantial investments in equipment and personnel with little likelihood of gain. For example, King County, Washington currently has an average response time of 4 minutes, an achievement utilizing 100 fire department EMT vehicles scattered throughout 500 square miles. To lower the response time by 30 seconds would require an additional 31 new vehicles. Response time is proportional to the square root of the area in square miles divided by the number of vehicles. In other communities, geography and physical structures such as high-rise buildings may impose a practical limit on response times that may be difficult to improve.

Another way to improve the time from collapse to CPR is to improve access to the emergency system. Emergency telephone numbers (911) have done much to speed response to the setting of the cardiac arrest.

Efforts to train the public in CPR have been successful and have contributed to increasing rates of bystander CPR. Citizen CPR programs were first initiated by Cobb and his colleagues in 1971.[24] Citizen CPR programs have become an important part of many EMS systems. Training is usually provided by local fire departments or public agencies, often free or for a small fee. The American Red Cross and the American Heart Association have actively endorsed and supported the concept of citizen CPR training. Both organizations provide training programs ranging from 3 to 9 hours. In addition, these training courses afford the opportunity to teach students emergency telephone numbers, risk factors for coronary artery disease, and the warning signs of myocardial infarction. Efforts to target CPR training to individuals more likely to perform it may offer an even more effective use of public education dollars.

The mass media may play an important role in educating the public in CPR. CPR demonstrations have been shown during nationally televised baseball games, and several public service spots have been shown on evening news programs. Other potential instructional options include placing CPR instructions in telephone books and on shopping bags.

Another approach to provide CPR quickly is for the emergency dispatcher to provide telephone instructions in CPR to the individual reporting a cardiac arrest. In 1974, the Phoenix Fire Department implemented a telephone instruction program. Reports suggested that it was possible to give instruction over the telephone. Based upon the Phoenix experience, a CPR message was developed by Carter and colleagues in King County, Washington.[25,26] The telephone CPR message is presented in two parts; first the bystander is instructed to perform ventilations and then to return to the telephone to receive the second part of the instructions, which involves instructions on chest compressions. Since the program began in 1981, the rate of bystander CPR has increased from 32% to 54%.

SHORTENING THE TIME FROM COLLAPSE TO DEFIBRILLATION

Although defibrillation is only one component of definitive care, it appears to be the most important, and when provided rapidly may be all that is necessary to convert the heart to a self-perfusing rhythm. A way to provide defibrillation rapidly is to train EMTs or first responders, such as firefighters or police of-

ficers, to perform defibrillation. Programs involving EMT defibrillation have demonstrated the benefit of this procedure. Defibrillation can occur with manual or automatic defibrillators. The use of automatic defibrillators lowers the training time and studies have demonstrated that its sensitivity and specificity is comparable to that of EMT's using manual defibrillators.[27]

Automatic external defibrillators have also been placed in public places and lay responders trained to attach the device to victims of cardiac arrest. Studies have demonstrated the benefit and limitations of such strategies.[28–30]

IMPROVING SURVIVAL FROM CARDIAC ARREST: THE CHAIN OF SURVIVAL

Effective prehospital emergency care for out-of-hospital cardiac arrest involves a sequence of steps which, if provided rapidly enough, can result in successful resuscitation. These steps are linked in a chain that has been termed "The Chain of Survival." The four links are early access, early basic CPR, early defibrillation, and early advanced cardiac life support. For prehospital EMS programs to be successful, each link in the chain must receive special attention. An emergency service is literally only as good as its weakest link. Concentration on one link to the exclusion of the others results in programs that have little impact on improving cardiac arrest survival rates. Improvements in each of the links can shave valuable seconds and minutes in the management of cardiac arrest, particularly when drugs are involved.[31]

A keener understanding of the factors associated with successful resuscitation and the role prehospital EMS systems play in cardiac resuscitation has done much to improve survival from otherwise fatal events.

ACKNOWLEDGMENTS

The content of this chapter is based in part on research activities conducted by the Center for Evaluation of Emergency Medical Services, Division of Emergency Medical Services, Seattle—King County Department of Public Health, Seattle, Washington. Research by the Center for Evaluation of Emergency Medical Services is supported by grants from the National Center for Health Services Research, the Laerdal Medical Corporation, and the Physio-Control Corporation.

REFERENCES

1. Lown, B.: Sudden cardiac death: the major challenge confronting contemporary cardiology. Am. J. Cardiol. 43:313, 1979.

2. Cobb, L.A., and Werner, J.A.: Predictors and prevention of sudden cardiac death in the heart. Edited by Hurst, W. New York, McGraw-Hill, 1982.
3. Advanced data from vital and health statistics of the National Center for Health Statistics. No. 172, August 24, 1989, U.S. Department of Health and Social Services.
4. Kuller, L.H.: Sudden death: Definition and epidemiologic considerations progress. Prog. Cardiovasc. Dis. 23:1, 1980.
5. Reichenbach, D.D., Moss, N.S., and Meyer, E.: Pathology of the heart in sudden cardiac death. Am. J. Cardiol. 39:865, 1977.
6. Weaver, W.D., Lorch, G.S., Alvarez, H.A., and Cobb, L.A.: Angiographic findings and prognostic indicators for patients resuscitated from sudden cardiac death. Circulation 54:895, 1976.
7. Friedman, G.D., Klatsky, A.L., and Siegelaub, A.B.: Predictors of sudden cardiac death. Circulation 52:164, 1975.
8. Kuller, L.H., Perper, J., and Cooper, M.: Demographic characteristics and trends in arteriosclerotic heart disease mortality: Sudden death and myocardial infarction. Circulation 52:1, 1975.
9. Cobb, L.A., Werner, J., and Trobough, G.: Sudden cardiac death: 1. A decade's experience with out-of-hospital resuscitation. Mod. Concepts Cardiovasc. Dis. 49:31, 1980.
10. Ruberman, W., et al.: Ventricular premature beats and mortality after myocardial infarction. Circulation 64:297, 1981.
11. Haynes, R.E., Hallstrom, A.P., and Cobb, L.A.: Repolarization abnormalities in survivors of out-of-hospital ventricular fibrillation. Circulation 57:654, 1978.
12. Eisenberg, M.S., Bergner, L., and Hallstrom, A.: Sudden cardiac death in the community. New York, Praeger, 1984, p. 34.
13. Cummins, R.O., and Eisenberg, M.S.: Prehospital cardiopulmonary resuscitation: Is it effective? JAMA 253:2408, 1985.
14. Cummins, R.O., and Graves, J.: Clinical results of standard CPR: Prehospital and inhospital. In Cardiopulmonary Resuscitation. Edited by Kaye, W., and Bircher, N.G. New York, Churchill Livingston, 1989.
15. Stueven, H., et al.: Bystander first responder CPR: Ten years experience in a paramedic system. Ann. Emerg. Med. 15:707, 1986.
16. Thompson, B.M., et al.: Comparison of clinical CPR studies in Milwaukee and elsewhere in the United States. Ann. Emerg. Med. 4:750, 1985.
17. Cummins, R.O., Eisenberg, M.S., Hallstrom, A.P., et al.: Survival of out-of-hospital cardiac arrest with early initiation of cardiopulmonary resuscitation. Am. J. Emerg. Med. 3:114, 1985.
18. Weaver, W.D., et al.: Improved neurologic recovery and survival after early defibrillation. Circulation 69:943, 1984.
19. Eisenberg, M.S., et al.: Treatment of out-of-hospital cardiac arrest with rapid defibrillation by emergency medical technicians. N. Engl. J. Med. 302:1379, 1980.
20. Stults, K.R., Brown, D.D., Schug, V.L., and Bean, J.A.: Prehospital defibrillation performed by emergency medical technicians in rural communities. N. Engl. J. Med. 310:219, 1984.
21. Cummins, R.O., et al.: Automatic external defibrillators used by emergency medical technicians: A controlled clinical trial. JAMA 257:1605, 1987.
22. Pantridge, J.F., and Geddes, J.S.: A mobile intensive care unit in the management of myocardial infarction. Lancet 2:271, 1967.
23. Eisenberg, M.S., et al.: Cardiac arrest and resuscitation: A tale of 29 cities. Ann. Emerg. Med. In press.
24. Cobb, L.A., and Hallstrom, A.P.: Community-based cardiopulmonary resuscitation: What have we learned? N. N.Y. Acad. Sci. 382:330, 1982.
25. Carter, W.B., et al.: Development and implementation of emergency CPR instruction by telephone. Ann. Emerg. Med. 13:695, 1984.
26. Eisenberg, M., et al.: Emergency CPR instruction via telephone. Am. J. Public Health 75:47, 1985.
27. Cummins, R.O., and Eisenberg, M.S.: Automatic external defibrillators: Clinical issues for cardiology. Circulation 73:381, 1986.
28. Eisenberg, M.S., et al.: Use of the automatic external defibrillator in homes of survivors of out-of-hospital ventricular fibrillation. Am. J. Cardiol. 63:443, 1989.
29. Cummins, R.O., Schubach, J.A., Litwin, P.E., and Hearne, T.R.: Training lay persons to use automatic external defibrillators: success of initial training and one year retention of skills. Am. J. Emerg. Med. 7:143, 1989.
30. Weaver, W.D., Sutherland, K., Wirkus, M., and Bachman, R.: Emergency medical care requirements for large public assemblies and a new strategy for managing cardiac arrest in this setting. Ann. Emerg. Med. 18:155, 1989.
31. Weiss, L.D., et al.: Non-traumatic prehospital sudden death in young patients—An urban EMS experience. Prehosp. Disaster Med. 6:315, 1991.

THE EFFECT OF EMS SYSTEMS FACTORS ON TRAUMA SURVIVAL

C. Gene Cayten and Jane G. Murphy

CAPSULE

Seriously injured patients benefit from an organized system of care. Because definitive resuscitation can frequently be accomplished only in the operating room (OR), the time from injury to the OR should be minimized. Advanced life support (ALS) and helicopter use have value under carefully defined circumstances. Medical control is necessary to ensure appropriate system function. Endotracheal intubation has the greatest life-saving potential among prehospital procedures. Triage to trauma centers of the most severely injured patients results in fewer preventable deaths. The immediate availability of

Supported by the Division of Injury Epidemiology and Control of the Centers for Disease Control.

an appropriately staffed emergency department (ED), a fully trained and equipped trauma team, and an OR and intensive care unit (ICU) are critical. The importance of the numbers of hospital beds and of major trauma patients treated in a hospital each year are less clear.

INTRODUCTION

The general consensus is that more emphasis is needed on preventing trauma, reconfiguring emergency medical service systems, and improving the clinical management of hospitalized trauma patients.[1-3] Changes in any one of these factors could improve survival rates and decrease levels of disability among patients suffering traumatic injuries.

This chapter reviews the effects of emergency medical service (EMS) systems factors on the process and outcomes of trauma patient care. Such a review is complicated because any given EMS system is complex and made up of many interrelated components. These include manpower, communications, equipment, system procedures, and trauma center designation, as well as triage and treatment and transfer protocols.

Three major areas are addressed:

1. The effects of variation in time factors in the prehospital care of patients

2. The effects of configurations of prehospital care (the role of physicians, of basic life support (BLS) versus advanced life support (ALS), and of procedures performed by ALS-trained paramedics)

3. The effects of hospital characteristics such as trauma center designation, number of beds, and number of major trauma patient admissions.

Issues of patient triage—decisions regarding the sorting of patients with respect to "disposition, destination, or priority"—cut across all three areas.[4] As Champion points out, triage determines the kind of scene-to-hospital transport used, levels of prehospital

and hospital care, and the timing of therapies. Because triage decisions are made many times in a given patient's treatment, the potential effects of specific triage decision points are highlighted and summarized throughout the chapter.

TIME FACTORS

Time factors are generally grouped into six categories: time from injury to initial ambulance response (response time); time spent by the ambulance crew at the scene of the injury (scene time); time spent transporting the patient from the scene of the injury to the receiving hospital (transport time); total prehospital time (the sum of response time, scene time, and transport time); time spent in an emergency department (ED time) and time from injury to operative intervention (time to OR).

RESPONSE TIME

Time from injury to initial ambulance response is most critical in rural areas, where distances between patients and ambulances often are great and therefore response times are often long. In a Florida study, Alexander et al. found that 60.5% of calls were answered in less than 5 minutes in urban counties served by ALS crews, while the corresponding proportion in rural counties was 36.7%.[5] Baker found an inverse relationship between county population density and county mortality rates for victims of motor vehicle accidents[6]; at least part of this relationship is presumably attributable to differences in response time.

SCENE TIME

The time spent by EMS personnel at the scene varies according to the type of injury (penetrating or blunt), whether ALS procedures are used, and whether helicopter transport is used.

TABLE 87-5. MEAN TIMES AT SCENE FOR PENETRATING TRAUMA

City	Year	Author	Time (min.)	Type of Responder
Milwaukee, WI[35]	70–81	Aprahamian	21.0	ALS
San Francisco, CA[63]	81–82	Mackersie	6.5*	ALS
Charleston, SC[64]	81–85	Clevenger	33.5	ALS (Stabilize)
Denver, CO[12]	82–84	Pons	9.8	ALS
Bronx, NY[9]	83–84	Cayten	19.0	BLS
Houston, TX[28]	83–86	Pepe	15.8	ALS
Charleston, SC[64]	86	Clevenger	8.3	ALS (Scoop and run)

* Includes blunt

TABLE 87-6. MEAN TIMES AT SCENE FOR BLUNT TRAUMA				
Geographic Area	**Year**	**Author**	**Time (min.)**	**Type of Responder**
Olympia, WA[24]	80	Hedges	25	ALS
Denver, CO[11]	82–84	Cwinn	14	ALS
Bronx, NY[9]	83–84	Cayten	20	BLS
			27	ALS
South Carolina[8]	83	Reines	18.9	BLS
			24.8	ALS
Sydney, Australia[65]	84	Potter	13	ALS*
Brisbane, Australia[65]	84	Potter	17	BLS*

* Excludes entrapped patients.

TYPE OF INJURY

Times at the scene for penetrating injuries tend to be relatively brief. Most such injuries occur in urban environments, in which distances to hospitals, where definitive care is available, are short. In fact, Eastman et al. call field stabilization for penetrating trauma patients an invalid concept.[7] Table 87-5 summarizes the results of studies of times at the scene for penetrating trauma. The effect of field stabilization versus "scoop and run" is seen in Clevenger's data: mean scene times were reduced from 33.5 to 8.3 minutes when the policy for the care of patients requiring resuscitative thoracotomy was changed. The general triage decision rule for patients with penetrating injuries is to get them to hospitals as quickly as possible.

On the other hand, times at the scene for patients with blunt injuries tend to be longer because extrication and axial splinting are often required. Reines found that extrication increased mean scene times from 20.5 to 31.1 minutes.[8] Similar results are summarized in Table 87-6. The need for extrication is also frequently accompanied by the need for other procedures such as intravenous (IV) line insertions, endotracheal intubations, and MAST. Studies have attempted to show a relationship between shorter scene times for blunt trauma patients and survival.[9] Their small samples sizes, however, have not provided sufficient power to test this hypothesis. Although there are no clear triage guidelines with respect to the optimal time frames for the care of these patients in the field, it is generally agreed that on-line medical control is essential when scene times for blunt trauma are delayed by extrication or patient inaccessibility.

ADVANCED LIFE SUPPORT

It has been argued that ALS procedures unnecessarily extend scene time. Aprahamian, however, showed that the combination of IV and endotracheal tube insertion resulted in scene times of no more than 22 minutes.[10] Cwinn[11] and Pons[12] found that mean scene times for patients receiving both IVs and MAST were not longer than were times for those patients receiving only IVs. Triage decisions regarding the use of advanced life support procedures must be taken, weighing the potential benefit of the procedures against the possible lengthening of scene time.

HELICOPTER TRANSPORT

On the average, helicopter transport requires crews to spend longer times at the scene because time is required for the helicopter to reach the injury site. In a series of studies, average scene times ranged from 18.5 minutes in San Diego[13] to 61.8 minutes for entrapped patients in a study in Danville, PA.[14] Seriously injured patients in rural areas far from trauma centers generally benefit most from helicopter transport. The triage decision to call for a helicopter is easiest in cases in which extrication is required because the already lengthy scene time gives the helicopter time to arrive.

MEDICAL CONTROL

Some trauma experts have emphasized the need for medical control in minimizing scene times,[15,16] whereas others have questioned whether on- and off-line medical control causes unacceptable delays in transporting patients.[17,18] Although there have been no controlled studies comparing prehospital trauma care with and without medical control, the appropriateness of helicopter triage to a trauma center has been found to improve with physician medical control.[19]

TRANSPORT TIME

The critical issues regarding transport times are (1) whether or not the additional time needed to bring patients to Level I trauma centers is detrimental for patients with some types of injuries, and (2) whether helicopters can effectively diminish transport time in rural areas, thereby increasing patient survival rates.

LEVEL I TRAUMA CENTERS VERSUS NEAREST HOSPITAL

Trauma center experts feel strongly that the relatively small amount of time lost in urban areas in bypassing the nearest hospital is more than compensated for by the continuous readiness of a trauma center to care for severely injured patients.[20-22] Lowe, for example, documented delays of 1 to 2 hours in the provision of definitive care at nontrauma centers.[23] In response, many urban areas have regionalized trauma systems in which prehospital caregivers use criteria including Trauma Scores and location and mechanism of injury to triage patients to trauma centers versus nearby hospitals.[4]

The issue is less clear in rural areas. In the semirural areas of Thurston County, Washington, Hedges found ground transport times to average 19.4 minutes,[24] and in South Carolina, Reines found average transport times to be 14.8 minutes.[8] How much these times would have been increased by requiring trauma victims to be transported to trauma centers, and the effects of such increases, remain to be explored. In most rural communities, especially where helicopter transport is not readily available, patients should be taken to the nearest appropriate hospital. Initial stabilization should be performed and transport to a trauma center should then be considered.

HELICOPTER TRANSPORT IN RURAL AREAS

Decreases in military evacuation times have been associated with improved survival rates. Studies of helicopter transport in civilian settings relate improved survival rates more closely to the presence of physicians on helicopters than to shorter transport times.[25-27] Studying patients injured in motor vehicle crashes in rural San Diego County, Baxt compared the survival rates of patients transported by ambulances with those transported by helicopters.[25] Although transport times were longer for those transported by helicopters, the average survival rate was higher. Baxt concluded that survival was improved because physicians on the helicopters frequently performed advanced resuscitative procedures not available in am-

bulances staffed by paramedics. Thus, helicopters apparently are most useful in rural areas when scene times are not unduly prolonged by waiting for transport, and when physicians staff them.

TOTAL PREHOSPITAL TIME

Total prehospital time is considered the time from injury (or call for ambulance dispatch) to arrival at the hospital. Prehospital times are generally longer in rural than in urban settings.[7]

The relationship between total prehospital time and survival has been studied (Table 87-7). In general, the research supports the view that prehospital times of up to 50 minutes to trauma centers do not adversely affect mortality. For example, Pepe studied 498 consecutive patients suffering penetrating injuries who were hypotensive and brought to a regional trauma center rather than local hospitals in Houston.[28] Patient survival was not significantly related to total prehospital time in the first hour except for a slight trend toward decreased survival in patients with trauma scores of 2 or 5, and when total prehospital time was longer than 40 minutes.

TIME IN THE EMERGENCY DEPARTMENT

Once a patient has reached an ED, survival often depends on the receipt of prompt and definitive treatment. For many patients, particularly those with penetrating injuries, this means rapid triage from the ED to the OR. To expedite this process, some trauma centers have developed operating rooms in their EDs.[29,30] In other EDs, such as that at the University of Minnesota, selected patients are taken directly to the OR, bypassing the ED entirely. Survival rates using these methods have shown improvement over those of historical controls.

TABLE 87-7. TOTAL PRE-HOSPITAL TIME

Geographic Area	Year	Author	Pre-Hospital Time (min)	Type of Responder	Types of Patients
Seattle, WA[43]	32–81	Fortner	43.0	ALS	Surviving bridge jumpers
Bronx, NY[9]	83–84	Cayten	32.2	BLS	Blunt & penetrating
			41.1	ALS	
South Carolina[36]	82	Reines	50.0	Surv	All ALS
			46.0	Non-Surv	
Denver, CO[12]	82–84	Pons	20.5	ALS	Penetrating wounds requiring laparotomy or thoracotomy
Denver, CO[11]	82–84	Cwinn	27.5	ALS	Blunt injuries requiring laparotomy or thoracotomy
South Carolina[66]	83	Reines	42.1	BLS	MVA with BP < 80
			46.6	ALS	
Mobile, AL[15]	83–84	Jurkovich	24.1	ALS	
				BLS	
Houston, TX[28]	83–86	Pepe	32.6	ALS	Hypotensive penetrating trauma

TIME FROM INJURY TO OPERATIVE INTERVENTION

Although Cowley's data[31] and some military casualty data suggest that trauma patient survival varies inversely with the length of time between injury and definitive care, relatively few studies relate patients' outcomes to time elapsed between injury and operative intervention. Not only is the actual time of injury often unknown, the relationship between survival and time to OR is made problematic by the intervention of events in the prehospital care and ED care systems.

Nevertheless, some neurosurgical conditions, by virtue of their pathophysiology, are expected to be sensitive to lengthy times from injury to operative intervention. For example, Sielig and Decker found higher mortality rates and diminished functional recoveries among patients with subdural hematomas who were operated on more than 4 hours after their injuries.[32] Prompt triage of patients with injuries sensitive to definitive care to appropriately staffed hospitals and from EDs to ORs should enhance survival.

CONFIGURATION OF PREHOSPITAL CARE

Three issues concerning the optimal prehospital configuration of care are important: the role of physicians, the use of BLS versus ALS, and use of procedures performed by ALS-trained paramedics.

THE ROLE OF PHYSICIANS

Most prehospital care provided by physicians in the United States has been carried out in programs using helicopters. In San Diego, Baxt and Moody showed that, despite prolonged field times in their helicopter program, the presence of physicians to perform advanced life support techniques resulted in better-than-expected survival rates.[33] Other authors, however, have reported that only a relatively small percentage of advanced interventions performed by physicians are not normally performed by paramedics.[14,27] These results suggest that improved survival rates among patients on helicopters staffed by physicians may be attributable to physician judgment more than to technical skill.[34] A protocol to guide the sending of physicians when their skill and judgment have a high likelihood of having an impact remains to be developed.

BLS VERSUS ALS CARE

The relationships between patients' outcomes and the use of BLS care (provided by emergency medical technicians (EMTs)) versus ALS care (provided by paramedics) for trauma patients has been studied. Researchers have noted an improvement in blood pressures among trauma patients cared for by ALS crews.[35,36] Reines et al., however, did not find blood pressure increases to be predictive of patients' survival.[36] Other studies purporting to show the value of ALS in the care of trauma patients have been difficult to interpret. For example, Jacobs compared ALS with BLS care in Boston.[37] He found that patients cared for by paramedics showed significantly more improvement in trauma scores between the field and the ED. He also found improvement in trauma score to be significantly correlated with survival; however, there was no significant direct correlation between paramedic care and survival. Studies by Reines et al.[36] and Cayten et al.[9] tend to confirm that prehospital stabilization procedures carried out by ALS crews extend scene time. The effects of stabilization, however, are unclear.[20,38]

Despite the controversies, most major urban areas and regionalized trauma systems have protocols to guide the dispatch of BLS versus ALS crews. Apparent cardiac arrest patients and major trauma patients are generally triaged to ALS crews when these are available. In addition, a BLS crew may request assistance from an ALS crew if it seems likely that the patient's prehospital condition could be improved by ALS procedures.

PROCEDURES USED BY ALS-TRAINED PARAMEDICS

Several stabilization procedures are used by ALS-trained paramedics. Their efficacy is a matter of debate.

ENDOTRACHEAL INTUBATION

Successful endotracheal intubation by paramedics is a well established ALS procedure,[39,40] and is considered by some to be the prehospital procedure with the greatest life-saving potential. Triage criteria for endotracheal intubation are a standard part of most ALS systems. As Table 87-8 shows, however, the proportion of patients in whom intubation is attempted and successful varies widely across types of injuries and EMS systems. In a comprehensive study of field endotracheal intubation by ALS personnel, Stewart et al. found that paramedics have the most difficulty in intubating trauma patients in cardiac arrest and deep coma.[41] The successful intubation rate of 78.8% for all trauma patients was significantly lower than the comparable rate of 90.6% for patients with nontraumatic cardiac arrests.

The question of the usefulness of intubation also has been raised. Rhee recently studied the use of bag-mask ventilation in semiconscious patients.[42] He found that the method often provides inadequate ventilatory support for injured patients.

TABLE 87-8. USE OF ENDOTRACHEAL INTUBATION FOR TRAUMA

City	Year	Author	No. of Pts.	% of Patients Intubated	Types of Patients
Seattle, WA[43]	32–81	Fortner	27	15 (55%)	Surviving bridge jumpers
Pittsburgh, PA[41]	80–82	Stewart	33	26 (79%)	Cardiac arrest or deep coma from trauma
Seattle, WA[67]	80–83	Copass	30	29 (97%)	Surviving patients requiring CPR
			101	66 (65%)	Nonsurviving patients requiring CPR
Milwaukee, WI[10]	81–82	Aprahamian	95	81 (85%)	Traumatic cardiac arrest
Denver, CO[12]	82–84	Pons	203	27 (13%)	Penetrating wounds requiring laparotomy or thoracotomy
South Carolina[8]	83	Reines	435	50 (12%)	MVA pts and BP < 80
San Diego, CA[13]	84–85	Shackford	88	57 (65%)	Surviving patients TS ≤ 8
			155	103 (53%)	Nonsurviving patients TS ≤ 8

INTRAVENOUS FLUIDS

As with endotracheal intubation, triage criteria for IV insertions vary among EMS systems, and thus the proportions of patients in whom IV insertions are attempted and successful vary widely. Results of 11 studies of the issue are summarized in Table 87-9. The proportion of attempts that were successful ranged from 74% in Aprahamian's study[10] to 100% in Fortner's Seattle research.[43] Mean amounts of fluid infused also vary. With most series reporting infusions of less than 1000 mL before ED arrival, the value of such administration is questionable, particularly if extra scene time is required to place the line. Lewis used a computer simulation model to relate rate of fluid loss to rate of fluid replacement.[44] He showed that there is no significant benefit to the patient for any rate of bleeding when prehospital times are shorter than 30 minutes.

Complications have also been reported with the prehospital insertion of IV lines. Lawrence and Lauro reported that IV lines started in the field have significantly higher complication rates than do those started in the ED.[45] Despite these problems, IV lines remain a standard ALS procedure.

DRUGS

There are few indications for the use of prehospital medications among trauma patients. The only accepted use of prehospital medication for trauma patients is to treat an underlying medical condition which may have precipitated the injury, i.e., arrythmias, hypoglycemia, seizure, etc.

HOSPITAL CHARACTERISTICS

The relationships between three hospital characteristics and survival rates of trauma patients are important. The hospital characteristics are trauma center designation, number of beds and number of major trauma admissions per year.

TRAUMA CENTER DESIGNATION

The American College of Surgeons Committee on Trauma (ACSCOT) has suggested three levels of hospital resource commitment for trauma care. Trauma center designations (level I, level II, and level III) are related to resources committed. Level I trauma centers (the highest level) have the resources required to deal with the most severely injured trauma patients. Much research has focused on whether Level I trauma center designation is related to improved survival rates.

The results of a series of studies support the conclusion that trauma centers improve survival.[13,46–48] West and Trunkey compared Orange County, where MVA patients were brought to the nearest hospital, to San Francisco County, where the severely injured were brought to the level I trauma center at San Francisco General Hospital.[48] They found significantly more preventable deaths among younger and less severely injured patients in Orange County. This study, however, compared only one trauma center with several community hospitals, and there is reason to believe that San Francisco General is unusual among trauma centers in terms of its high level of expertise in trauma care.

Several studies using the preventable death method have found fewer deaths among potentially salvageable patients in trauma versus nontrauma centers.[21,36,44,49,50] For example, Reines and Duffy performed a preventable death study in eastern South Carolina and found 43% of non-CNS deaths to be potentially salvageable at nontrauma centers compared to 12.5% at a newly organized trauma center.[36] Studies using the preventable death method, however, have come under suspicion. Salmi pointed out that the method does not take into account patients who would have died but survived because of high quality care, and that it invites selection bias in the choice of hospitals for evaluation and of criteria against which to assess care.[30]

TABLE 87-9. USE AND SUCCESS OF IVS FOR TRAUMA PATIENTS

City	Year	Author	No. of Patients in Study	No. of Patients with IV Inserted/ (% Total)	% of Success in Attempts	Mean Amount Infused in Patients with IVs
Seattle, WA[43]	70–81	Fortner	23[a]	23/(100%)	100%	1200
Milwaukee, WI[68]	76	McManus	236	154/(65%)	——	475
Milwaukee, WI[35]	78–81	Aprahamian	48[b]	39/(81%)	——	< 1000
San Francisco, CA[63]	81–82	Mackersie	97	——	86%	——
Milwaukee, WI[10]	81–82	Aprahamian	95[c]	70/(100%)	74%	860
Seattle, WA[67]	81–83	Copass	30[c,i]	30/(100%)	100%	2200
Boston, MA[37]	80–81	Jacobs	101[c,j]	70/(78%)	70% TS 1–3	625
					TS 4–13	1050
					TS 14–16	650
Sacramento, CA[69]	82–83	Smith	52[f]	41/(79%)	79%	669
South Carolina[8]	83	Reines	435[f]	325/(76%)	88%	——
Denver, CO[12]	83–84	Pons	203[g]	108/(53%)	——	——
San Diego, CA[13]	84–85	Shackford	88[h,i]	76/(86%)	86%	——
			195[h,j]	158/(81%)	81%	

a = Survivors of Aurora bridge falls, b = Major open intra-abdominal falls, c = Traumatic cardiac arrests, d = In 33 patients data were available, e = Patients with BP of 100 mm Hg at scene or ED, f = Victims of MVA's with BP of < 80 and complete data, g = Patients with penetrating wounds of chest and abdomen undergoing emergency laparotomy or thoracotomy, h = Patients with trauma score ≤ 8, i = Survivors, j = Nonsurvivors, k = Two IVs inserted.

On the other hand, some studies have shown significant improvements in trauma patients' survival without the implementation of trauma centers.[5,51–54] Ornato reported a 23.9% decline in the number of trauma deaths in Nebraska from the period 1969–1972 to 1979–1982.[53] Trauma center designation had taken place in Nebraska, but the plan covered only two of six regions and the differences found were not explainable in terms of center designation. Ornato attributed improved trauma survival rates to better prehospital EMS, physician education with advanced trauma life support, and the establishment of three helicopter transport services. Alexander et al. used a mileage population death index (MPDI) to compare death rates from MVAs in Florida.[5] Counties with large metropolitan teaching hospitals had significantly lower MPDIs than other counties. The better results were attributed to prompt access to definitive care.

Based on these studies, it has become generally accepted that optimal survival is based on the adequacy of the initial resuscitation and the early recognition of serious injuries.[55] This usually requires the timely availability of a trauma surgeon, a fully-trained and equipped trauma team, an operating room, and intensive care capability. Whether level I trauma center designation per se further improves patient outcome is difficult to assess. Official designation probably has its greatest impact in upgrading hospital capabilities for trauma care.

It is certain that level I trauma center designation is frequently used as a triage criterion for the transport of trauma patients. In many EMS systems, trauma scores or Glasgow coma scores are used to determine whether patients should be taken to the nearest hospital or to a trauma center. The ongoing readiness of trauma center personnel and equipment to treat se-

verely injured patients is widely considered to offset any small delay caused by bypassing the nearest hospital.

NUMBER OF HOSPITAL BEDS

Number of hospital beds has been related to the appropriateness of a hospital to be a trauma center. Although the original ACSCOT guidelines stated that a level I trauma center "will most likely be a hospital of over five hundred beds. . . ,"[56] later versions have dropped any reference to precise numbers of hospital beds. Several studies, however, have found number of beds to be directly related to trauma patient survival.[1,23,57] For example, a study in northwest Oregon conducted in the early 1980s found that hospitals with fewer than 200 beds had higher mortality rates for MVA patients than hospitals with more than 200 beds.[23] The difference was attributed to the reduced ability of some small hospitals to manage multisystem trauma quickly. A 1971 study by Strauch in Connecticut, however, found no relationship between number of beds and trauma patient survival, although there was no control for severity of injury.[58]

As with trauma center designation, the apparent relationship between number of hospital beds and survival is probably an artifact of the true relationship between number of beds and availability of the staff and equipment needed quickly to manage trauma patients, and the relationship between the early definitive management of injuries and survival. Number of hospital beds is generally not used directly in patient triage, although trauma centers are usually larger hospitals than are nontrauma centers.

NUMBER OF MAJOR TRAUMA ADMISSIONS

The ACSCOT suggested that, besides having a critical mass of equipment, staff, and beds, trauma centers also must care for a minimum number of "major trauma" patients each year.[56] The Committee recommended that each level I trauma center should see 600 major trauma patients each year. Although the ACSCOT provided a triage algorithm indicating which patients should be taken to trauma centers, they did not specifically define "major trauma." This has led to the development of many different definitions.

Various cut-offs of ISS scores have been suggested as definitions of major trauma.[7,59–61] For example, Schwab has defined patients with ISSs of 16 to 25 as "severely" injured[61] and Detmer considered patients with an ISS of 15 or greater to have "high severity" injuries.[59] Eastman et al. also point out that an arbitrary probability of death (calculated using the TRISS method) of 5% or greater could be used to define major trauma,[7] whereas Champion considered patients to have major trauma if they had trauma scores of less than 12 on arrival to the hospital.[4]

Given that there is no consensus regarding what constitutes major trauma, how did the ACSCOT decide that 600 such patients per year would be required for Level I designation? The number was apparently based on studies showing that, for certain surgical procedures, operative mortality is inversely correlated with the frequency with which the surgery is performed.[62] Although there have been no studies relating frequencies of specific trauma-related surgeries to patients' outcomes, it seems reasonable to assume that similar relationships hold.

As with beds, number of trauma admissions is generally used only indirectly as a triage criterion in that these are weighted in trauma center designation decisions.

PITFALLS

- Prolonged scene times when trauma centers are in close proximity
- Lack of medical control
- Helicopter programs without specific protocols for use
- Trauma center designation without enforceable triage protocols

HORIZONS

- Mechanisms for earlier access to definitive care in sparsely populated areas

- Fluids providing greater resuscitative effect per cc, improving the rationale for starting IV lines in the field
- Reimbursement policies to foster triage of appropriate patients to trauma centers
- Improved prehospital triage to better direct appropriate patients to trauma centers

REFERENCES

1. Moylan, J.A., Detmer, D.E., Rose, J., and Schulz, R.: Evaluation of the quality of hospital care for major trauma. J. Trauma 16:517, 1976.
2. National Academy of Sciences National Research Council. Accidental Death and Disability: The Neglected Disease of Modern Society. Public Health Service Publication 1071:A-13, 1966.
3. Trunkey, D.D.: Trauma care at mid passage—a personal view point: AAST Presidential Address, 1987.
4. Champion, H.R.: Triage. In Trauma Care Systems. Edited by Cales, R.H., and Heilig, . Rockville, MD, 1986, pp. 79–108.
5. Alexander, R.H., Pons, P.T., Krischer, J., and Hunt, P.: The effect of advanced life support and sophisticated hospital systems on motor vehicle mortality. J. Trauma 24:486, 1984.
6. Baker, S.P., Whitfield, R.A., and O'Neill, B.: Geographic variations in mortality from motor vehicle crashes. N. Engl. J. Med. 316:1384, 1987.
7. Eastman, A.B., Lewis, F.R., Champion, H.R., and Mattox, K.L.: Regional trauma system design: Critical Concepts. Am. J. Surg. 154:79, 1987.
8. Reines, H.D., Bartlett, R.J., Chudy, N.E., et al.: Is advanced life support appropriate for victims of motor vehicle accidents; The South Carolina Highway Trauma Project. J. Trauma 28:563, 1988.
9. Cayten, C.G., Longmore, W., Keuhl, A., et al.: BLS versus ALS for trauma in an urban setting (abstract). Ann. Emerg. Med. 15:23, 1986.
10. Aprahamian, C., Darin, J.C., Thompson, B.M., et al.: Traumatic cardiac arrest: Scope of paramedic services. Ann. Emerg. Med. 14:583, 1985.
11. Cwinn, A.A., Pons, P.T., Moore, E.E., et al.: Prehospital advanced trauma life support for critical blunt trauma victims. Ann. Emerg. Med. 16:399, 1987.
12. Pons, P.T., Honigman, B., Moore, E.E., et al.: Prehospital advanced trauma life support for critical penetrating wounds to the thorax and abdomen. J. Trauma 25:828, 1985.
13. Shackford, S.R., Mackersie, R.C., Hoyt, D.B., et al.: Impact of a trauma system on outcome of severely injured patients. Arch. Surg. 122: , 1987.
14. Anderson, T.E., Rose, D.W., and Leicht, M.J.: Physician-staffed helicopter scene response from a rural trauma center. Ann. Emerg. Med. 16:58, 1987.
15. Jurkovich, G.J., Campbell, D., Padrta, J., and Luterman, A.: Paramedic perception of elapsed field time. J. Trauma 27:892, 1987.
16. McSwain, N.: Medical control of prehospital care. J. Trauma 24:172, 1984.
17. Gold, C.: Prehospital advanced life support vs. "scoop and run" in trauma management. Ann. Emerg. Med. 16:797, 1987.
18. Luterman, A., Ramenofsky, M., Berryman, C., et al.: Evaluation of prehospital emergency medical service (EMS): Defining areas of improvement. J. Trauma 23:702, 1983.
19. Champion, H.R., Sacco, W.J., Gainer, P.S., and Patow, S.M.: The effect of medical direction on trauma triage. J. Trauma 28:235, 1988.
20. Border, J.R., Lewis, F.R., Aprahamian, C., et al.: Panel: Prehospital trauma care—stabilize or scoop and run. J. Trauma 23:708, 1983.
21. Cales, R.H.: Trauma mortality in Orange County: The effect of implementation of a regional trauma system. Ann. Emerg. Med. 13:1, 1984.

22. Certo, T.F., Rogers, F.B., and Pilcher, D.B.: Review of care of fatally injured patients in a rural state: Five-year follow-up. J. Trauma 23:559, 1983.
23. Lowe, D.K., Gately H.L., Frey, C.L., et al.: Patterns of death, complications and error in the management of motor vehicle accidents: Implications for a regional system of trauma care. J. Trauma 23:503, 1983.
24. Hedges, J.R., Sacco, W.J., and Champion, H.R.: An analysis of prehospital care of blunt trauma. J. Trauma 22:989, 1982.
25. Baxt, W.G., and Moody, P.: The impact of rotocraft air medical emergency service on trauma mortality. JAMA 249:3047, 1983.
26. Baxt, W.G., Moody, P., Cleveland, H.C., et al.: Hospital-based rotocraft aeromedical emergency care services and trauma mortality: A multicenter study. Ann. Emerg. Med. 14:859, 1985.
27. Fischer, R.P., Flynn, T.C., Miller, P.W., and Duke, J.H.: Urban helicopter response to the scene of injury. J. Trauma 24:946, 1984.
28. Pepe, P.E., Wyatt, C.H., Bickell, W.H., et al.: The relationship between total prehospital time and outcome in hypotensive victims of penetrating injuries. Ann. Emerg. Med. 16:3, 1987.
29. Dove, D.B., Stahl, W.M., and Del Guercio, L.R.M.: A five year review of deaths following urban trauma. J. Trauma 20:760, 1980.
30. Salmi, L.R., Williams, J.I., Guibert, R., et al.: Preventable deaths and the evaluation of trauma programs: Flawed concepts and methods. 30th Annual Proceedings American Association for Automotive Medicine, October 6–8, Montreal, Quebec, 1986.
31. Cowley, R.A., Hudson, F., Scanlan, E., et al.: An economical and proved helicopter program for transporting the emergency critically ill and injured patient in Maryland. J. Trauma 13:1029, 1973.
32. Seelig, J.M., Becker, D.P., Miller, D., et al.: Traumatic acute subdural hematoma: major mortality reduction in comatose patients treated within four hours. N. Engl. J. Med. 304:1511, 1981.
33. Baxt, W.G., and Moody, P.: The differential survival of trauma patients. J. Trauma 27:602, 1987.
34. Rhee, K.J., Strozeski, M., Burnery, R.E., et al.: Is the flight physician needed for helicopter emergency medical services? Ann. Emerg. Med. 15:174, 1986.
35. Aprahamian, C., Thompson, B.M., Towne, J.B., and Darin, J.C.: The effect of a paramedic system on mortality of a major open intra-abdominal vascular trauma. J. Trauma 23:687, 1983.
36. Reines, H.D., and Duffy, K.H.: Survivability of victims of traumatic injuries in Eastern South Carolina. Am. Surg. 49:203, 1983.
37. Jacobs, L.M., Sinclair, A., Beiser, A., and D'Agostino, R.B.: Prehospital advanced life support: Benefits of trauma. J. Trauma 24:8, 1984.
38. Trunkey, D.D.: Is ALS necessary for pre-hospital trauma care? J Trauma 24:86, 1984.
39. Jacobs, L.N., Berribeitra, F.D., and Bennett, B.: Endotracheal intubation in the pre-hospital phase of emergency medical care. JAMA 250:2175, 1983.
40. Smith, J.P., and Bodai, B.I.: The urban paramedic's scope of practice. JAMA 253:544, 1985.
41. Stewart, R., Paris, P., Winter, P., et al.: Field endotracheal intubation by paramedical personnel. Chest 85:341, 1984.
42. Rhee, J., O'Malley, R.J., Turner, J.E., and Ward, R.E.: Field airway management of the trauma patient: the efficacy of bag mask ventilation. Am. J. Emerg. Med. 6:333, 1988.
43. Fortner, G.S., Oreskovich, M.R., Copass, M.K., and Caprico, C.J.: The effects of prehospital trauma care on survival from a 50 meter fall. J. Trauma 23:976, 1983.
44. Lewis, F.R., Jr.: Prehospital intravenous fluid therapy: Physiologic computer modeling. J. Trauma 26:804, 1986.
45. Lawrence, D.W., and Lauro, A.J.: Complications from I.V. therapy: Results from field-started and emergency department-started I.V.'s compared. Ann. Emerg. Med. 17:314, 1988.
46. Baker, C.C., DeGutis, L.C., De Santis, et al.: Impact of a trauma service on trauma care in a university hospital. Am. J. Surg. 149:453, 1985.
47. Clemmer, T.P., Orme, J.F., Thomas F.O., and Brooks, K.A.: Outcome of critically injured patient treated at Level I trauma centers versus full service community hospitals. Crit. Care Med. 13:861, 1985.
48. West, J.G., Trunkey, D.D., and Lim, R.C.: Systems of trauma care: A study of two counties. Arch. Surg. 114:455, 1979.
49. West, J.G.: Validation of autopsy method for evaluating trauma care. Arch. Surg. 117:1033, 1982.
50. West, J.G., Cales, R.H., and Gazzaniga, A.B.: Impact of regionalization, the Orange County experience. Arch. Surg. 118:740, 1983.
51. Civil, I.D., Ross, S.E., and Schwab, C.W.: Major trauma in an urban New Zealand setting: resource requirements. Aust. N.Z. J. Surg. 57:543, 1987.
52. Gertner, H.R., Jr., Baker, S.P., and Rutherford, R.B.: Evaluation of the management of vehicular fatalities secondary to abdominal injury. J. Trauma 12:425, 1972.
53. Ornato, J.P., Craren, E.J., Nelson, N.M., and Kimball, K.F.: Impact of improved emergency medical services and emergency trauma care on the reduction in mortality from trauma. J. Trauma 25:575, 1985.
54. Ottoson, A., and Krantz, P.: Traffic fatalities in a system with decentralized Trauma Care. JAMA 251:2668, 1984.
55. Roy, P.: The value of trauma centers: a methodologic review. Can. J. Surg. 30:17, 1987.
56. American College of Surgeons Committee on Trauma. Field Categorization of trauma patients and hospital trauma index. Bulletin of the American College of Surgeons 65:28, 1980.
57. Houtchens, B.: Major trauma in the rural mountain West. JACEP 6:343, 1977.
58. Strauch, G.O.: Major abdominal trauma in 1971: A study of Connecticut by the Connecticut Society of American Board Surgeons and the Yale Trauma Program. Am. J. Surg. 125:413, 1973.
59. Detmer, D.E., Moylan, J.A., Rose, J., et al.: Regional categorization and quality of care in major trauma. J. Trauma 17:592, 1977.
60. Knudson, P., Frecceri, C.A., and DeLateur, S.A.: Improving the field triage of major trauma victims. J. Trauma 28:602, 1988.
61. Schwab, C.W., Peclet, M., Zackowski, S.W., et al.: The impact of air ambulance system on an established trauma center. J. Trauma 25:580, 1985.
62. Luft, H.S., Bunker, J.P., and Enthoven, A.C.: Should operations be regionalized? The empirical relation between surgical volume and mortality. N. Engl. J. Med. 301:1364, 1369, 1975.
63. Mackersie, R.C., Christensen, J.M., and Lewis, F.R.: The prehospital use of external counterpressure: Does MAST make a difference? J. Trauma 24:882, 1984.
64. Clevenger, F.W., Yarbrough, D.R., and Reines, H.D.: Resuscitative thoracotomy: The effect of field time on outcome. J. Trauma 28:441, 1988.
65. Potter, D., Goldstein, G., Fung, S.C., and Selig, M.: A Controlled trial of pre-hospital advanced life support in trauma. Ann. Emerg. Med. 17:582, 1988.
66. Reines, H.D., and Duffy, K.H.: The effect of EMS transit time on mortality from major trauma. (Abstr.) J. Trauma 24:679, 1984.
67. Copass, M.K., Oreskovich, M.R., Bladergroen, M.R., and Carrico, C.J.: Prehospital cardiopulmonary resuscitation of the critically injured patient. Am. J. Surg. 148:20, 1984.
68. McManus, W.F., Aprahamian, C., and Darin, J.C.: Prehospital advanced emergency care: A potential pitfall. J. Trauma 18:305, 1978.
69. Smith, P., Bodai, B.I., Hill, A.S., and Frey, C.F.: Prehospital stabilization of critically injured parents: A failed concept. J. Trauma 25:65, 1985.

BIBLIOGRAPHY

National Research Council and the Institute of Medicine. Injury in America. Washington, D.C., National Academy Press, 1985.

Rhodes, M.: Direct transport to the operating room for resuscitation of trauma patients. J. Trauma 28:1095, 1988.

LEVELS OF CARE IN THE PREHOSPITAL ARENA: PERSONNEL AND TRAINING

Lawrence Mottley

CAPSULE

There are four nationally recognized levels of prehospital care providers: Certified First Responder (CFR), Emergency Medical Technician—Basic (EMT), Emergency Medical Technician—Intermediate (EMT-I), and Paramedic. These four are discussed in this section. There are other combination and hybrid levels in some jurisdictions, which are not uniform across the country. Indeed, some states permit a modular increment to the EMT that allows single skill addition to the scope of EMT practice, such as EMT-MAST or EMT-I.V. Nevertheless, the four provider levels discussed here provide an understanding of the concepts underlying prehospital care.

CERTIFIED FIRST RESPONDER

In 1985, this newest level of recognized Emergency Medical Services (EMS) responders was formalized by the development of a 40-hour national standard curriculum. CFR is designed for nonmedical emergency response agencies such as fire and police departments, whose members are often first to arrive at the scene of a medical emergency. The curriculum content of the Department of Transportation CFR course is controversial. The course is essentially a "mini-EMT" course containing information on such topics as the differential diagnosis of diabetic emergencies, cardiac problems, types of epilepsy, and a host of other interesting but difficult topics that are difficult to master in a 40-hour course, and not obviously needed for a true First Responder (FR). Thus, the EMS community has two approaches to the CFR course based on differing philosophies of the role of the FR. The DOT approach has just been outlined. Other agencies, such as New York State, have seen the CFR course as more of a "what to do until the ambulance comes" course, focusing the limited course time on only the most urgent medical emergencies: Airway, cardiopulmonary resuscitation (CPR), cervical-spine immobilization, bleeding control, vital sign and shock, and emergency childbirth. The New York State curriculum specifically states that it is not intended for ambulance personnel. The CFR is trained only in the techniques immediately necessary to prevent the loss of a life or the occurrence of a preventable disability.

Given the extremely short time available for the CFR course, it seems logical to focus only on the practical skills and knowledge that are most time-critical. If the CFR can perform CPR, prevent further injury, and administer oxygen, the patient will be far better served than if the CFR attempts inadequate treatment of all emergencies. Other illnesses and injuries that are less urgent can and should await the arrival of EMT level personnel.

EMERGENCY MEDICAL TECHNICIAN

The EMT is the foundation on which is built the structure of prehospital medical care. A system cannot offer meaningful Advanced Life Support (ALS) without solid Basic Life Support (BLS). The EMT course, originally an 81-hour course first offered in 1972, remains the backbone of the training prehospital curriculum.[1] There has been substantial change in this course since its inception, not necessarily for the better. Originally designed as a basic program to allow the EMT to quickly treat broad classes of medical illnesses and to safely splint and rapidly transport injuries, this course has often been subverted by well-intentioned but non-"streetwise" physicians into a much longer course that teaches EMTs the differential diagnoses of the various common medical emergencies which, while interesting, have no practical value to the street EMT. Not only do such additional minutiae not improve patient care, they detract from it.

The attempt to elucidate the differential diagnosis of bronchospastic versus cardiac asthma is difficult enough in an orderly, well-lit Emergency Department (ED); it is usually impossible in a field situation and is moot because the EMT treatment is oxygen in either case. Similarly, the inordinate amount of time spent on the salient identifying characteristics of "blue bloaters" versus "pink puffers" has caused many an oxygen starved patient to be sacrificed on the altar of "No Oxygen For Emphysema." This knowledge may be relevant if the transport time to the hospital exceeds 2 hours, but is of no practical use; it is the rare hypercarbic blue bloater who is found hiking in the wilderness. *Attempts to make diagnoses in the field that do not change field treatment result in unnecessarily prolonged field treatment times and a consequent greater chance of an adverse event occurring before arrival at a hospital.*

EMS physicians and instructors must look critically at the EMT curriculum to ensure its relevance to the field situation. We do a disservice to our students when we train them to a level beyond their ability to treat, especially because physicians are often the first to criticize when field times are prolonged.

The current EMT course has now expanded to 121 hours from the original 81 with little change in the practical skills. Such an overemphasis on the rote memorization of medical terms and impractical knowledge has resulted in the loss of many highly motivated skills-oriented people from EMT classes, to the detriment of our patients.

Paradoxically, although knowledge of marginal benefit is allowed to consume precious course hours, proven lifesaving equipment such as the semi-automatic defibrillator is not yet a standard part of the standard EMT armamentarium. It is rare indeed that advances in technology allow the EMT to perform safely techniques that have previously required ALS training; it is rarer still that the advance is an effective and time-critical modality.[2,3] Most critical studies indicate that the cardiac arrest survival rate with BLS only is negligible.[4] EMT defibrillation has been available since at least 1985, yet is still not part of the EMT course. Soon, American Red Cross-trained corporation employees or restaurant personnel will be able to offer a higher level of care to the cardiac arrest victim than an EMT.

In summary, the fundamental direction of the curriculum is to emphasize knowledge that can cause a change in field therapy, use of effective time-critical technology, and elimination of extraneous information that can delay patient care as well as prolong the EMT course to the extent that EMS volunteers are discouraged from taking it.

EMERGENCY MEDICAL TECHNICIAN—INTERMEDIATE

The EMT-I was proposed in the early 1980s to reflect the reality that the majority of prehospital care in the United States is provided by volunteers. Given the time and training requirements, the restriction to only EMT and paramedic levels essentially guaranteed that there would be no ALS in areas served by volunteers.

EMT-I is a subset of the paramedic program. It focuses on the most emergent illnesses and those for which simple prehospital treatment is available. Its

curriculum, of several hundred hours, is designed to allow the EMT-I to recognize and treat cardiac arrest and arrhythmias, hypoglycemia, asthma/COPD, and anaphylaxis. To accomplish this, the EMT-I must be able to eliminate from consideration the other diseases which may manifest similar symptoms from a different cause. Wheezing, for example, may be caused by asthma, COPD, anaphylaxis, CHF, and a host of other causes. While the paramedic has sufficient didactic training to make this differential diagnosis more often, the EMT-I does not and must rely much more heavily on direct medical control. This need for closer on-line medical supervision, rather than the available range of practical skills, is the primary difference between the EMT-I and the paramedic.

The DOT curriculum does not mandate the skills of either endotracheal intubation or defibrillation. With the advent of semiautomatic defibrillation, however, there is no rationale for withholding the latter. Intubation clearly requires both initial education and ongoing experience. The lack of opportunities to use this skill in low call volume areas has led many jurisdictions not to approve endotracheal intubation for EMT-I. This is an issue with no clear resolution. There are major disadvantages to both approaches. The underlying issue is the lack of a safe and effective device to maintain a secure airway for use by BLS personnel.

PARAMEDIC

The Paramedic level was deemed at the outset to be the gold standard of prehospital care. Although the DOT curriculum sets 400 hours as the minimum course length, many programs add hundreds of hours to teach locally approved skills above the DOT minimum or to meet local medical control standards.[5]

Paramedics are best used for the acute medical illness, in which their training allows them to intervene to reverse or slow the progress of the acute episode. In contrast, the treatment of choice for the vast majority of trauma patients is BLS only. If paramedics are used for the treatment of trauma, strict medical oversight must ensure that unnecessary ALS procedures do not delay transport. It makes little sense to spend even 3 minutes starting an IV when the hospital is only 20 minutes away.

Some assumptions underlie the decisions as to the extent of the paramedic's role: (1) the treated illnesses should be life-threatening, acute, and able to be treated by paramedics with an acceptable risk-benefit ratio; (2) treatment modalities must be relatively easy to learn and perform, given the time constraints of the course. Paramedics, by virtue of their more extensive didactic training, are usually given much more latitude in their patient care. Early paramedic programs required paramedics to contact Medical Control before initiating any treatment, even for patients "in extremis." This led to both delayed patient care and circumvention of protocols. As experience was gained with paramedic care, it became clear that trained and well-supervised paramedics could reliably diagnose and treat acute, life-threatening diseases, and equally as important, identify cases in which direct Medical Control was needed to initiate treatment when the diagnosis was in doubt. Paramedics now typically operate under standing orders which permit them to take the initial steps in the ALS treatment of most acute illnesses without contacting Medical Control. Such an approach expedites patient care, minimizes pre-hospital time, and adds to the efficiency of the overall EMS system.

The scope of practice of the Paramedic varies widely. The minimum medications are those for ACLS, altered mental status, and respiratory compromise. Some jurisdictions authorize the use of thrombolytic agents, steroids, and plasma expanders. Practical skills minimally include IV access, endotracheal intubation, manual defibrillation, and electrocardiogram interpretation; however, in some areas central venous and intraosseous lines, cardioversion, and even cricothyrotomy are included. In most states, the paramedic may perform any procedure authorized by the Medical Director as long as the paramedic has been adequately trained.

Any discussion of paramedic training would be incomplete without emphasizing the axiom that BLS comes before ALS. Yet paramedics show more skill decay in BLS skill than in ALS skills.[6,7] The temptation to focus solely on advanced skills to the detriment of basic skills must be avoided.

> ## UNMET TRAINING NEEDS FOR ALL EMT LEVELS

INFECTIOUS DISEASE

Despite good evidence that hepatitis is an occupational hazard,[8] it has taken the regulatory authority of the Occupational Safety and Health Administration (OSHA) to mandate vaccination protection from hepatitis B, and to require education for all levels of EMT in proper precautions to protect themselves from these diseases.[9] Perhaps because these regulations may apply only to paid EMS employees, many EMS providers remain ignorant of the mechanisms of disease transmission. Even when knowledgeable, almost two thirds report that they do not always wear gloves—the most basic protection—when treating a bleeding patient.[10] Perhaps such training could reduce the attrition caused by concerns with AIDS and other infectious diseases.[11]

PREHOSPITAL TRAUMA CARE

A standardized rapid approach to the assessment and care of a trauma victim has a beneficial effect on patient outcome. Courses such as BTLS, PHTLS, and the New York State Critical Trauma Care course (for EMTs) have had widespread acceptance as CME, but must be adopted into the appropriate standard curricula, preferably in lieu of some of the less useful medical information described previously. These skills are easily learned and translated into direct patient benefits such as reduced on-scene time.[12]

GERIATRIC CARE

This requires additional emphasis in the future because our population over 65 is increasing rapidly. Observing for all medications, checking environments, providing EMS cards to identify people with chronic conditions, etc. require relatively little time, but are not yet being done on a widespread basis.

AMBULANCE ACCIDENT PREVENTION

Too little attention has been paid to the mechanics of emergency vehicle operation, despite entire textbooks dedicated to this issue. Local protocols for the use of lights and sirens in response and transport modes must be part of the basic EMT curriculum, along with the risks and benefits to the patient. Because most ambulance accidents occur in daylight at intersections,[14] and most injuries in ambulance accident injuries are easily avoidable by seat belt use,[15] application of this basic EMT knowledge is essential to safe EMS operations.

> ## REFERENCES

1. NHTSA: Emergency Medical Technician—Ambulance. U.S. Gov't Printing Office,
2. Eisenberg, M.S., and Cummins, R.O.: Defibrillation performed by the EMT. Circulation 74:IV9,
3. Cummins, R.O., et al.: Automatic External defibrillators used by EMTs. A controlled clinical trial. JAMA 257:1605, 1987.
4. Olson, D.W., et al.: EMT defibrillation: the Wisconsin experience. Ann. Emerg. Med. 18:806, 1989.
5. NHTSA: Emergency Medical Care, A Manual for the Paramedic in the Field. U.S. Government Printing Office,
6. Zautcke, J.L., et al.: Paramedic Skill Decay. J. Emerg. Med. 5:505, 1987.
7. New York City EMS Division of Training (personal communication).
8. Pepe, P., et al.: Viral hepatitis risk in urban EMS personnel. Ann. Emerg. Med. 15:454, 1986.
9. OSHA: CFR 1910. 1030. May 30, 1989.
10. Smyser, M., et al.: AIDS-related knowledge, attitudes, and precautionary behaviors among emergency medical professionals. Public Health Rep. 105:496, 1990.

11. Thompson, M.E.: Prehospital providers' AIDS knowledge and attitudes. Maryland Med. J. *38*:1027, 1989.
12. Werman, H.A., et al.: Basic trauma life support. Ann. Emerg. Med. *16*:124, 1987.
13. Koin, D., and Eie, K.: Prehospital emergency care. *In* Geriatric Emergency Medicine. Edited by Bosker, G., Schwartz, G., et al. St. Louis, C.V. Mosby Co., 1990.
14. New York State EMS (personal communication).
15. Auerbach, P.S., et al.: An analysis of ambulance accidents in Tennessee. JAMA *258*:1487, 1987.

EMS SYSTEM DESIGN

Jack L. Stout

CAPSULE

Of all the forces influencing an EMS system's ability to convert available dollars into clinical performance and response time reliability, system design is by far the most powerful.

DEFINING THE EMS SYSTEM

For each individual patient, the "EMS system" includes individuals and organizations from whom action is required, either before or after the EMS incident, to produce a timely, coordinated, and clinically effective response sufficient to ensure the best possible chance of survival without disability. Although EMS systems meet the needs of noncritical patients, many EMS systems fail to meet the more demanding requirements of the critically ill and injured.

"System design" refers to the EMS system's underlying legal, organizational, and financial infrastructure. System design determines:

- Which organizations play which roles within the EMS system
- How an organization is selected to serve a given role within the system
- How dollars flow into and within the system
- If and how organizations are rewarded for carrying out their roles within the system
- If and how organizations are penalized or replaced for failure to carry out their roles within the system

ECONOMIC EFFICIENCY AND ITS SIGNIFICANCE TO PATIENT CARE

In the EMS industry, economic efficiency (Fig. 87-4) is the ability of an organization (or "system" of or-

ganizations) to convert dollars into service—i.e., clinical and response time performance. Every EMS system falls into one of the categories in Table 87-10.

A common mistake is to confuse "price" (i.e., user-fee schedule) with "cost" (i.e., dollars consumed in the process of producing the service, regardless of how such cost is recovered). More heavily subsidized EMS systems often generate higher costs and lower prices than less heavily subsidized systems.

Economic efficiency among EMS systems varies by more than 300%. That is, when compared in terms of *total system cost per patient transport* or *total system cost per capita of service area population*, some EMS systems require three times more money to produce clinical and response time performance equal to that of more efficient systems.

In affluent communities willing and able to subsidize the higher costs of less efficient system designs and production methods, economic efficiency is not essential to quality patient care. (As used here, this term includes both clinical performance and response time reliability—i.e., the timely delivery of clinically sound patient care.) Macro-level economic forces of long-term duration, however, are increasing competition for local tax dollars in cities and counties across the nation. *Thus, in a large and growing number of communities, the quality of prehospital care available is directly related to the system's proficiency in converting dollars into service.* Dollar for dollar, more efficient EMS systems produce better patient care. And more than any other

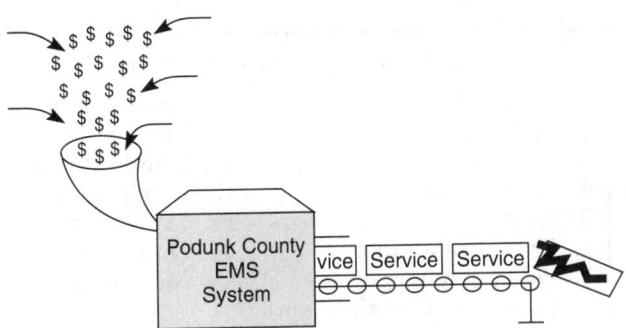

FIG. 87-4.   Efficiency. *Is this the best we can do with the money we have?*

factor, EMS system design determines the levels of efficiency at which the systems operate.

ELEMENTS OF AN EMS SYSTEM

The federal EMS Act of 1973 named 15 components of an EMS system (Fig. 87-5), and required that they be addressed as a prerequisite to federal funding. The implication was that if all 15 components were present, a "system" could be declared, and if all 15 components were in order, the "system" must be a good one. Propelled with the force of more than $300 million in federal EMS grants, this 15-component view of EMS and its effects remain with us today—e.g., EMS laws on the books in several states still incorporate the 15 components.

Unfortunately, the 15-component perspective was poorly thought out, and failed to provide a productive framework for designing, developing, managing, evaluating, and ultimately comparing EMS systems. For example, *finance* was not among the 15 components. Nor were *management* and *medical direction*. The *legal foundation* needed to create and sustain organizational roles and relationships within the system was not among the 15 components. Some experts believe that the 15-component system perspective actually inhibited EMS progress, and others argue that it was useless but harmless. Few, if any, believe it was helpful.

The "EMS System Matrix" shown in Figure 87-6 has proven useful for designing, developing or improving, managing, evaluating, and comparing EMS systems. Complete and accurate information for every "cell" of the matrix constitutes a reasonably comprehensive description of how an EMS system is organized, financed, and controlled. Completing the matrix also makes clear the roles and responsibilities of the various organizations that make up the system, and the legal structure that ensures (or fails to ensure) that the system functions as planned.

Notice that the matrix allows documentation of both low-cost and expensive systems, single-jurisdiction and regional systems, privatized and socialized systems, single-tiered and multi-tiered systems, efficient and inefficient systems, well-organized and poorly-organized systems, subsidized and unsubsidized systems, clinically sound, and deadly systems. In short, any system can be documented using the matrix and can be compared with any other, regardless of how differently the systems may be organized, financed, and managed. (In most cases, the act of documenting a system, using the matrix format, brings to light flaws and oversights in the system's basic design.)

TABLE 87-10. EMS SERVICE AND COST

Quality and Cost*	Efficiency
Substandard service at below-average cost	Average
Superior service at above-average cost	Average
Substandard service at above-average cost	Poor
Superior service at below-average cost	Superior

* A common mistake is to confuse "price" (i.e., user-fee schedule) with "cost" (i.e., dollars consumed in the process of producing the service, regardless of how such cost is recovered). More heavily subsidized EMS systems often generate higher costs and lower prices than less heavily subsidized systems.

The "15 Components" from the EMS Act of 1973

1. Manpower
2. Training
3. Communications
4. Transportation
5. Facilities
6. Critical care units
7. Public safety agencies
8. Community participaion
9. Accessibility to care
10. Transfer of patients
11. Standard medical recordkeeping
12. Public information
13. Evaluation
14. Disaster planning
15. Mutual aid agreements

FIG. 87-5.   The 15 components of an EMS system.

EMS System Structure Matrix

Process Elements	Input Elements									Diagnosis Specific* Output Specifications
	A. Organization & Management	B. Personnel	C. Equipment	D. Communications	E. Facilities	F. Information System	G. Finance	H. Legal	I. Off-line Medical Control	
1. Demand/ Prevention										
2. Bystander Action/ System Access										
3. Complaint-taking Function										
4. Telephone Protocols/ Pre-arrival Instructions										
5. 1st Responder Dispatch										
6. Ambulance Dispatch										
7. 1st Responder Services ("Rescue")										
8. Ambulance Services										
9. On-line Medical Control										
10. Receiving Facility Interface										
11. Off-line Medical Control										

*Note: Diagnosis Specific refers to chief complaint, presenting problem, or presumptive diagnosis, depending upon stage of response.

FIG. 87-6. EMS System Structure Matrix. Included by permission of the author. For a more detailed discussion of its elements and its use, see Chapter 2, *High Performance EMS* (*HPEMS*) by Jack L. Stout, scheduled for release in 1991 by JEMS Publishing Company, Solana Beach, CA.

MAJOR PROCESS ELEMENTS

A complete discussion of all system elements is beyond the scope of this chapter. The following discussion of important process elements, however, provides a solid foundation for understanding the basic EMS system design.

PUBLIC EDUCATION AND CPR TRAINING

This includes prevention, such as seat belt awareness and the "feet first, first time" water safety program, programs to combat drunk driving, citizen CPR training, and programs to encourage the proper use of 911 access. Indicators of effectiveness include percentage of witnessed cardiac arrest with CPR in progress when help arrives, length of time cardiac symptoms were experienced before the system was contacted, and similar measures. In many EMS systems, including some that are otherwise excellent, this component is loosely organized, operates without clear objectives or effectiveness measures, and is ineffective.

CONTROL CENTER OPERATIONS

These include the splitting of 911 "complaints" into police, fire, and medical categories; the giving of prearrival instructions to persons at the scene; the use of priority-dispatch protocols governing, among other things, the use of first-responder units, and the dispatching of air and ground ambulances to emergency and routine calls; and, in advanced urban systems, the aggressive use of system status management (SSM) to simultaneously improve productivity and response time reliability. SSM is an increasingly sophisticated technology for maximizing response time reliability using available resources. Its major elements are: flexible scheduling to match around-the-clock production capacity to patterns of demand for service; geographic deployment and event-driven redeployment to precision-allocate whatever production capacity is remaining at any point in time; and, systematic elimination of causes of delayed calls resulting from factors other than the number and locations of vehicles.

In more advanced EMS systems, BCLS instructor certification is often required of control center personnel, as are Emergency Medical Dispatch (EMD) and EMT or paramedic certification. In the most advanced EMS systems, persons responsible for handling telephone requests for medical assistance are experienced paramedics with additional training in use of priority-dispatch protocols, prearrival instructions, and system status management.

Ideally, a certified medical dispatcher completes telephone interrogation using physician-approved telephone algorithms, providing prearrival instructions when appropriate (e.g., Clawson protocols). System response is governed by physician-approved priority dispatch protocols. Not longer than 20 seconds into the caller-interrogation process (i.e., 30 seconds after initial call-receipt in 911 systems), the call is automatically electronically "shipped" to a fire service dispatcher for first-response alert (usually on about 40% of 911 calls, as determined by protocol), and a paramedic ambulance is dispatched. To facilitate complete coordination of system resources, medical dispatchers handle all requests for emergency response (i.e., 911 medical), routine transport (7-digit access), inter-facility transport, long distance transport, and helicopter scene response.

FIRST-RESPONDER SERVICES

These include the rapid delivery of initial basic life support (BLS) procedures and, in some systems, advanced life support (ALS) services, but exclude transportation. When needed, first-responders also provide additional trained manpower to assist during transport. Medium and heavy rescue and extrication services are also included under first-responder services.

First-responder services operate at various levels of clinical capability including sub-EMT, EMT, EMT-D, intermediate ALS levels, and paramedic first-response. The most cost-effective level of first-responder

service is the EMT-D level (automated defibrillator). Because of declining demand for fire suppression service, the most common and cost-effective method of delivering first-responder services is the use of already-existing firefighter personnel responding on firefighting apparatus. A common mistake is to assume that it costs more to send a large and expensive engine than a smaller "rescue" unit. In fact, the marginal cost (i.e., the additional cost in excess of already-budgeted fire department expenditures) of fire engine first-response is only about $27 per transport, while the cost of operating a separate rescue system is a minimum of several hundred dollars per response. Even amortized capital equipment and maintenance costs are surprisingly similar.[1] The most costly method is to use separate "rescue" crews responding on special "rescue" vehicles. (The difference in annual marginal cost per unit is several hundred thousand dollars.) In light-duty fire stations, the same crew may man either a fire truck or a rescue unit, depending on the nature of the call.

Most first-responder programs are single-tiered. That is, all first-response units are staffed and equipped to deliver the same level of care. Some systems, however, use more than one level of first-response capability—i.e., a "multi-tiered" first-responder program. The use of the term "tiered" has caused considerable confusion within the EMS industry, and among members of the press, elected officials other non-EMS public officials. A given EMS system may employ a single-tiered, multi-tiered, or no first-response component *and* a single-tiered or multi-tiered ambulance service component. Some people refer to a system using single-tiered first-response and single-tiered ambulance response as a "two-tiered system." Others refer to the same combination as "single-tiered." To avoid confusion, it is always best to identify the component being described. When physician-developed priority dispatch protocols are used by appropriately training personnel, first-response units are sent out on from 35 to 45% of 911 medical requests.

AMBULANCE SERVICES

These include BLS or ALS delivered at the scene and en route, as well as emergency and routine medical transportation to, from, and between health care facilities. In some EMS systems, emergency and routine transport services are treated as organizationally, functionally, and financially separate systems. In more efficient EMS systems, these services are dealt with as an integrated continuum of care. This difference in orientation is a critical aspect of EMS system design. Ambulance response time standards commonly used by well-respected systems are given in Table 87-11.

The use of "average response times" has been abandoned in more advanced systems because average response times reveal only what happened on about

TABLE 87-11. AMBULANCE RESPONSE TIME STANDARDS		
Area	Life-Threatening	Non-Life-Threatening
Metropolitan areas*	90% within 8 min.	90% within 12 min.
Outlying suburbs	90% within 12 min.	90% within 15 min.
Rural areas	90% within 15 min.	90% within 20 min.
Wilderness areas	90% within 60 min.	90% within 60 min.

* Response times among various districts or neighborhoods (often election districts) within major cities must also be reasonably equal in many systems.

one-half of all calls (i.e., the median and the mean are very similar in ambulance response time distributions). Impressive-sounding average response times are sometimes deliberately reported to both public and private agencies to mask life-threatening response time deficiencies.[2]

Ambulance services are delivered using either the "specialized production strategy" (e.g., nonemergency ambulances for routine patient transport, BLS ambulances for non-life-threatening emergency calls, with ALS ambulances reserved for only the most serious calls) or the "flexible production strategy" (i.e., all ambulances in the system, emergency and routine, staffed and equipped to operate at the paramedic level). Once again, the term "tiered" is used and creates confusion. When every patient (emergency and nonemergency) is transported by a paramedic ambulance, the ambulance component is clearly "single-tiered." When paramedic units transport critical patients, BLS units transport non-life-threatening emergencies, and "invalid coaches" transport nonemergency patients, the ambulance component is clearly three-tiered. Several communities, however, use government-operated paramedic ambulances to transport 911 patients and allow multiple private firms to transport nonemergency patients in BLS ambulances, and refer to their ambulance component as "single-tiered."

Although the "specialized production" strategy was widely assumed to be the more efficient production method throughout most of the 1970s, the track record experience of several all-paramedic, full-service systems (i.e., systems using paramedic ambulances for emergency, nonemergency, and interfacility transports) clearly shows that, at any given level of response time reliability, the all-paramedic, full-service system is considerably less expensive. In fact, as of this writing, every EMS system in the U.S. that is capable of placing a paramedic ambulance on the scene of 90% or more of all presumptively-classified life-threatening emergencies within 8 minutes or less (roughly equivalent to an average response time of less than 5 minutes), at a per capita per year subsidy cost of less than $3, uses the flexible production strategy.

Some ALS systems operate with two paramedics on every ambulance; others operate with one paramedic and one EMT. Although well-credentialed experts hold strong opinions in favor of and against both staffing methods, no patient outcome studies lend facts to the debate. Even the proponents of "one and one" staffing, however, agree that pairing an EMT and paramedic on an ALS unit does not produce adequate team performance unless the EMT is specifically trained to function as an integral part of an ALS team. Similarly, EMT-level first-responders must also be given "paramedic-assist" training if they are to function effectively as part of the ALS team.

Patterns of consumer demand for emergency service in a community of approximately 200,000 people are shown in Figures 87-7 and 87-8. The days shown are Tuesdays and Sundays. On each chart, the second line from the top shows the "average peak demand" during each hour of the day for that day of the week over a 1-year period. The "average peak demand" is calculated by averaging the 10 highest demand levels experienced for a given hour of the day/day of the week during the entire year. In other words, to reach the 90% level of response time reliability, ambulances must be staffed to cover "average peak demand."

Note that the shape of consumer demand for EMS is not a flat line. Furthermore, demand patterns differ and tend to recycle by day of week. (For example, compare Tuesday with Sunday.) *In every EMS market, the pattern of EMS demand is unique, more or less predictable (depending on volume of demand), and never flat.* Peak-load staffing to better match "supply" (i.e., coverage) with "demand" (i.e., call volume) is an essential first step in improving response time reliability without increasing cost. Furthermore, by using income earned from performing nonemergency and interfacility transports (using paramedic units) to fund additional peak-load paramedic production capacity, response time reliability, disaster readiness, and system productivity can be improved, while substantially reducing the system's dependence on local tax support. Productivity is measured by the unit hour utilization ratio (U/UH). A "unit hour" is one hour of on-duty time by a fully staffed and equipped ambulance. Dividing the number of patients transported (not total responses) during a given period by the number of unit hours produced during the same period yields the U/UH ratio. High U/UH ratios and poor response times are common. Low U/UH ratios and good response times are also common. The challenge is to simultaneously produce higher U/UH ratios *and* good response time reliability. Among all-paramedic, full-service systems meeting the 8 minute/90% standard,

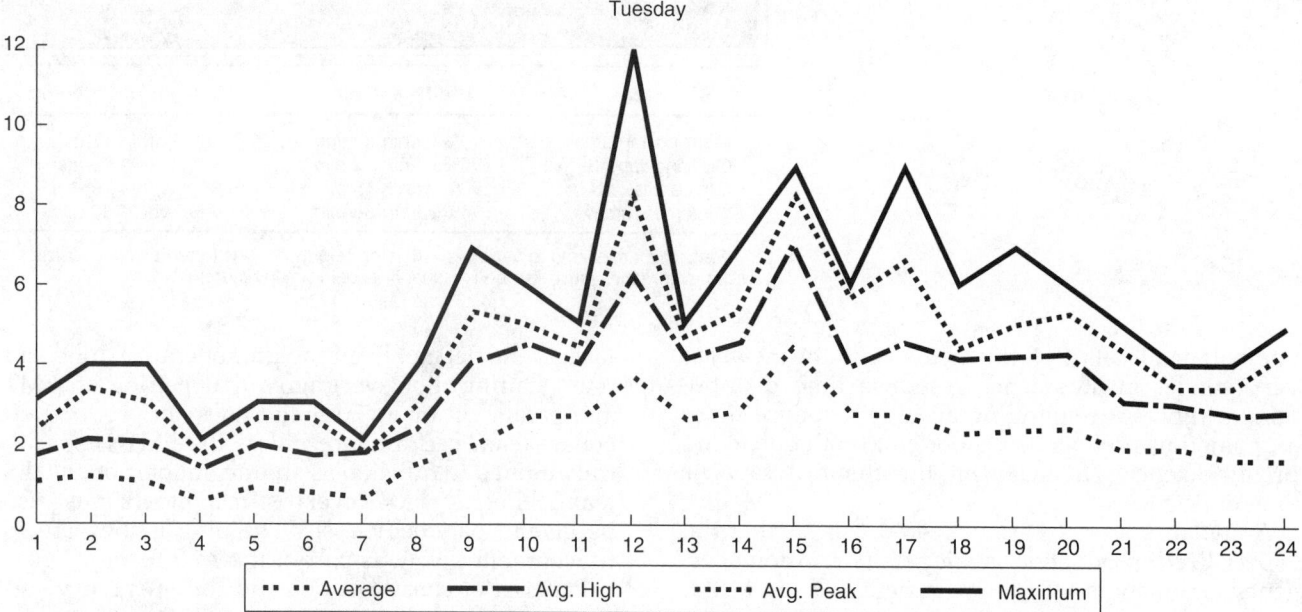

FIG. 87-7. Consumer demand for emergency services on Tuesday.

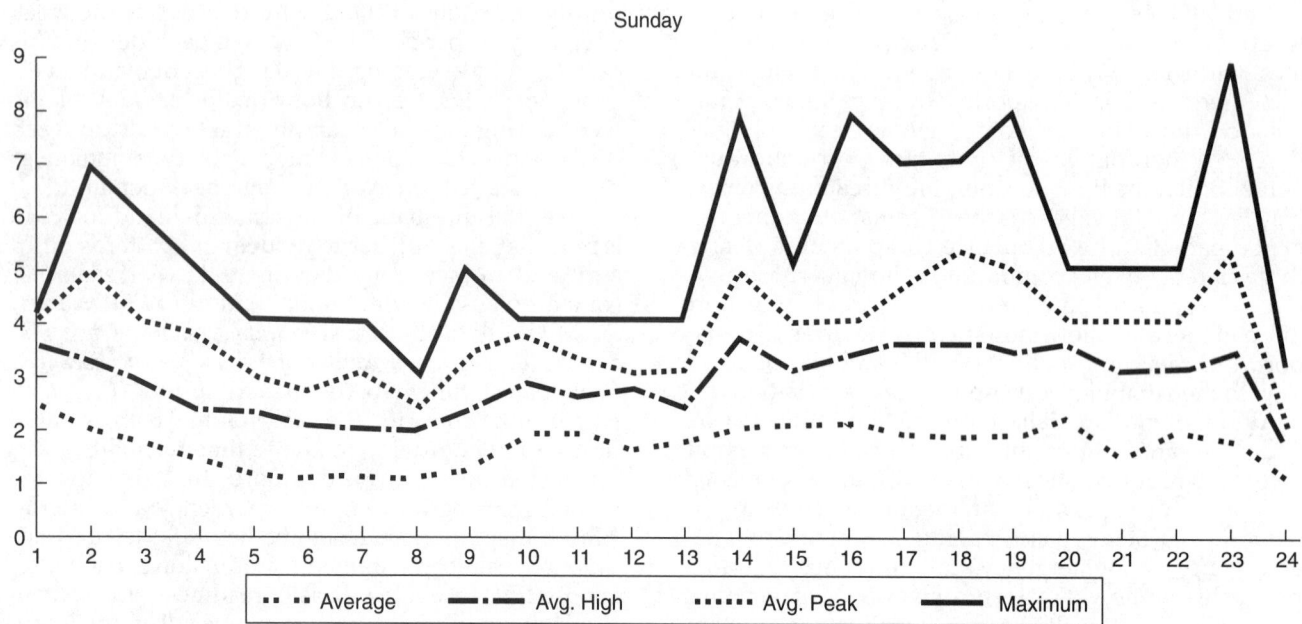

FIG. 87-8. Consumer demand for emergency services on Sunday.

U/UH ratios range from 0.32 to 0.45. Among tiered ambulance systems meeting the same response time standard, U/UH ratios of 0.11 to 0.15 are common, and ratios above 0.20 are extremely rare.

Although local tax subsidies of ambulance services range from zero to $26 per capita per year, subsidy levels in excess of $5 per capita per year appear to be unnecessary in metropolitan areas. No positive correlation has been found between the level of local tax subsidy and the quality of ambulance service deliv-

ered. For example, two of our industry's most beleaguered systems (i.e., those serving Washington, D.C. and Detroit) enjoy more than ten times as much subsidy (per capita per year) as ambulance systems internationally recognized for their quality of care and response time reliability (e.g., Tulsa, Fort Wayne, Kansas City, Las Vegas, Syracuse, and others).

Per capita per year ambulance service subsidies ranging from zero to $5 are considered low; those from $5 to $10 are considered average; and subsidies from

```
                    Tulsa System—1989 Data

        Number Full-Time Field Personnel.................. 77
                       Population Served............ 450,000
                  Annual Patient Transports ............ 33,000

      Current Annual Wage, 3 yr. Paramedic
          Excluding Extraordinary Overtime........... $23,500

                       Current Subsidy Level ............. zero

   Paramedic wage at $0 per capita/per year subsidy.................. $23,500
   Paramedic wage at $1 per capita/per year subsidy.................. $29,344
   Paramedic wage at $2 per capita/per year subsidy.................. $35,188
   Paramedic wage at $4 per capita/per year subsidy.................. $46,876
   Paramedic wage at $6 per capita/per year subsidy.................. $58,565
   Paramedic wage at $8 per capita/per year subsidy................. $70,253
   Paramedic wage at $10 per capita/per year subsidy................ $81,941
   Paramedic wage at $15 per capita/per year subsidy............... $111,162
```

FIG. 87-9.   Compensation for paramedics (3 years of employment).

$10 to $15 are considered high. Subsidy levels in excess of $15 per capita per year do exist but are rare (and probably cannot be justified in metropolitan areas). In rural areas, poor economies of scale induce both higher costs and longer response times.

While higher subsidy levels may be justified in rural areas, stand-alone monojurisdictional minisystems are much less efficient than economically powerful multijurisdictional regional EMS systems. Two excellent examples of multijurisdictional rural EMS systems are the Acadian System, serving approximately one third of the entire State of Louisiana, and the recently expanded EMSA system, which now accounts for approximately one half of all patient transports in the State of Oklahoma.

Although a small subsidy may be needed to support adequate paramedic wages, the amount of subsidy required for this purpose in metropolitan area should rarely exceed $2 to $3 per capita per year. Figure 87-9 shows compensation for paramedics after 3 years of employment in the Tulsa system (1989 figures), and how compensation would be affected if subsidies were made available at various levels to fund increased compensation. (A clinically advanced system meeting the industry's most stringent response time standards, Tulsa's ambulance system receives no local tax support whatsoever). As the figures show, $1 to $3 in subsidy is easily sufficient to fund highly desirable paramedic wages in metropolitan systems, provided that the money is not wasted on inefficient production methods.

The primary effect of tax subsidy is to reduce price below cost. For example, the Tulsa system (i.e., EMSA) currently receives no local tax subsidy and thus must charge user fees based on the full cost of service, plus losses from uncollectibles. In 1989, EMSA's total system cost per patient transport was $185.50; and EMSA's total average bill for ambulance service was $324.30. The average total bill includes base rate, mileage, and all add-on charges. Comparisons of base rates alone are usually misleading, sometimes intentionally. Like many ambulance services, EMSA also offers a subscription membership program allowing residents to fix price and prepay uninsured portions of ambulance service fees.[3] As Figure 87-10 shows, if subsidies were made available to EMSA, the average total bill could be reduced by about $24 for each $1 of subsidy per capita per year. Given a subsidy of $13.61 per capita per year, EMSA could do without fee-for-service income.

Figure 87-10 also provides comparable information for the Kansas City and Reno systems. All three of these systems are all-ALS, full-service ambulance systems required by local ordinance to meet the 8-minute/90% standard of response time reliability. In addition, all are single-provider systems in which a single private firm has been granted (by bid competition) exclusive rights to provide both emergency and nonemergency service throughout the respective service areas.

DIRECT MEDICAL CONTROL

This includes assistance provided by a physician in radio contact with field personnel. Such assistance may involve consultation in assessing the patient's condition and/or authorization to perform certain advanced procedures in the field. *It is important to understand that, during the time when field personnel are in contact with such a physician, the care being rendered in the field is actually an extension of that physician's personal practice of medicine.*

Subsidy/Price Tradeoffs — 1990 Data

Underlying Data:

Tulsa: average bill @ zero subsidy = $324.30; system cost per capita/yr. = $13.61
Reno: average bill @ zero subsidy = $404.00; system cost per capita/yr. = $13.22
Kansas City: average bill @ zero subsidy = $391.60; system cost per capita/yr. = $18.74

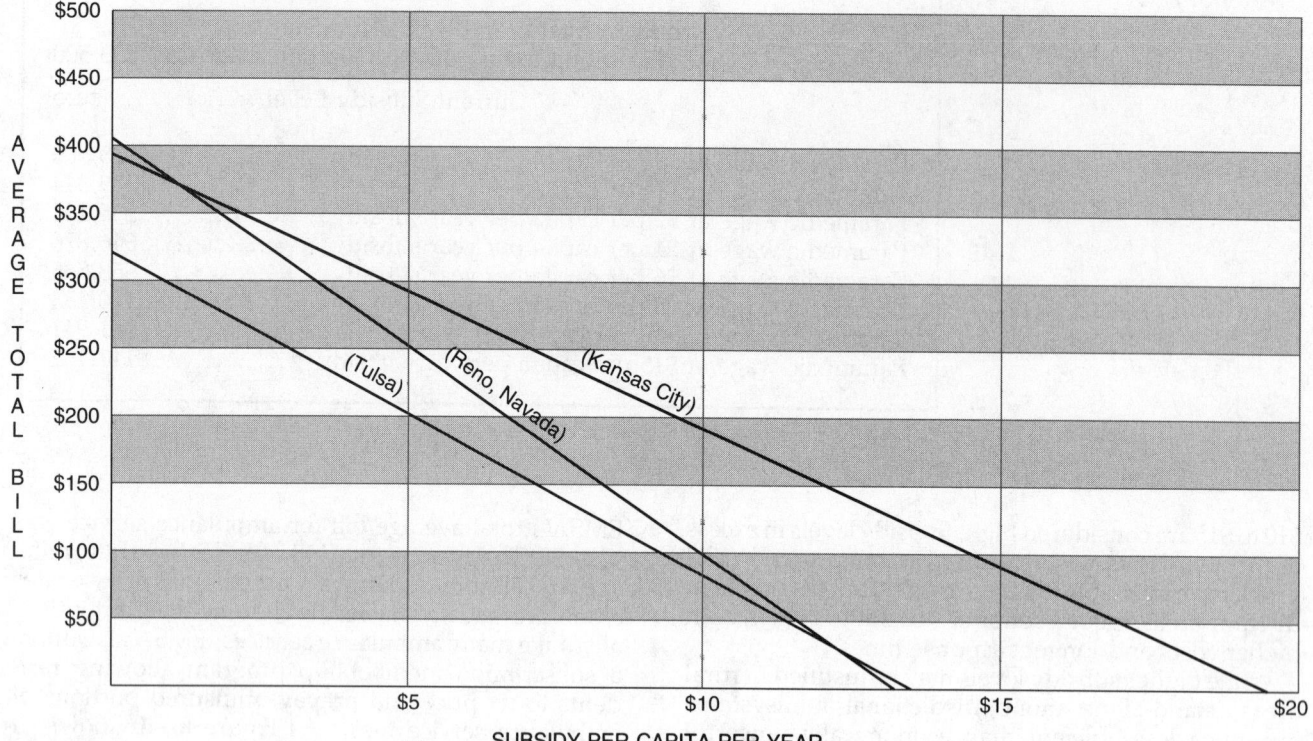

FIG. 87-10.   Subsidy/price trade-offs.

In well-designed systems, physicians participating in direct medical control receive special instruction and certification, participate in the quality-assurance program, and periodically ride ambulances to become familiar with the conditions under which prehospital care is actually rendered.

Some experts strongly advocate a fully-centralized system of direct medical control—i.e., direct control from a single receiving facility. Others advocate shared responsibility by all acute care receiving facilities in the system's service area. Both positions have merit. Centralized control makes it easier to ensure quality and consistency; decentralized control allows emergency physicians throughout the service area to become more familiar with and supportive of the prehospital care system, and allows each physician to direct personally the prehospital care of the patients he or she receives.

Because control comes from a remote location in either case, the real issue is not location. To the paramedic in the field, it would make no difference if the direct control physician were speaking from a location deep within a sand trap on the thirteenth hole. (The amortized communications system cost per patient served would not be different either.) Whether direct control is centralized or not, the physicians involved must understand the prehospital care environment and be familiar with the prehospital care system, its protocols, and its people. Any system of direct medical control that achieves these aims works well. Beyond that, it is a matter of personal preference.

INDIRECT MEDICAL QUALITY ASSURANCE

This includes the establishment, and monitoring of compliance with, standards and protocols governing all aspects of the system's operations affecting patient care. Among these are personnel qualifications (e.g., for control center personnel, first responders, ambulance personnel, and on-line medical control physicians), operating protocols (e.g., priority-dispatching protocols, transport/destination protocols, and medical protocols including standing orders), the ongoing external medical quality assurance process, and the conduct of prehospital care research.

In most well-designed EMS systems, some sort of "Medical Control Board" is established, made up of emergency physicians from acute care receiving facilities throughout the service area. This Board controls the establishment and monitoring of standards governing every aspect of the system affecting patient care, and appoints the system's medical director. The system's quality assurance staff reports directly and solely to the medical director. Funding is provided, usually from user fees, for quality control purposes at the rate of $3–$4 per patient transport. The quality assurance process encompasses prearrival phases of care, including prevention, bystander action, system access, telephone inquiry, priority dispatch, and prearrival instructions (when appropriate), as well as first-responder care, ambulance service, and on-line medical control components.

Indirect medical control can be "internal" or "external." Good systems have both. "Internal" medical control is the process conducted and controlled by the agencies or firms who provide the services in question. For example, a "medical director" hired by a private ambulance company or local fire department is part of an "internal" medical control process. In contrast, a medical director hired by a medical control board is part of the "external" quality control process. The dif-

ference is that an internal medical director serves at the pleasure of the very organization(s) whose work he is supposed to oversee, whereas an external medical director is organizationally (and financially) independent of the organizations whose work he evaluates. Objectivity, perceived or real, is the primary difference.[4]

MAJOR POLICY ISSUES

Figure 87-11 summarizes the most significant policy questions affecting EMS system design. Because clinical performance is the purpose of prehospital system development, the structure and funding of medical oversight are listed first.

Once the medical oversight issues have been resolved, policies affecting the delivery of first-response and ambulance services can then be addressed. Al-

The Most Important Policy Questions

I. Medical Oversight (i.e., Purpose and Performance)
  A. Objectivity: Internal vs. External Q/C
  B. Makeup: Physician Board, Single Physician, Other
  C. Power: Advisory vs. Authoritative
  D. Scope: Component vs. Systemwide
  E. Funding: Level and Source

II. 1st Response:
  A. Method: Engines, Rescue Units, Other, or None
  B. Dispatch: All 911, Priority Dispatch, or Other
  C. Level: Basic, EMT-D, Paramedic

III. Ambulance:
  A. Level: Basic vs. Paramedic
  B. Form of Competition:
    1. *For* the Market: Periodic vs. "Triggered"
    2. *Within* the Market: Emergency, Routine, or Both
    3. No competition
  C. Production Strategy: Flexible vs. Specialized
  D. Staffing: Static vs. Variable
  E. Deployment: Static vs. Event-Driven
  F. Scope of Service: Full-Service vs. Emergency-only
  G. Business Structure (Enterprise, Franchise, or Other)
  H. Service Area: Mono- vs. Multi-Jurisdictional
  I. Performance Required: Ordinance, Contract, or Faith
  J. Consequences of Failure to Perform:
    1. Chronic Major Default: Termination vs. Acceptance
    2. Minor Default: Fine vs. Acceptance

IV. Method of Finance:
  A. Level of Funding } Effect
  B. Source(s) of Funding

(CAUSE — bracketing items II and III)

FIG. 87-11. *Policy questions affecting EMS design.*

though standards of quality and response time reliability do affect dollar requirements, the way in which the system is structured affects funding requirements even more. For example, if the decision is made to use separate rescue units (rather than existing fire department personnel and vehicles) for first-response delivery, dollar requirements will be greatly increased.

Similarly, if the decision is made to use the "specialized production strategy" for ambulance services delivery (rather than the "flexible production strategy"), subsidy requirements will be greater. And when the decision is made to use paramedic-level first response, in conjunction with BLS ambulances, third-party recovery of ALS costs is reduced nearly to zero. Level staffing (rather than peakload staffing) forces a choice between poor response time reliability during peak periods of demand and the extra expense of wasted production capacity during off-peak periods. Compared with the financial implications of these structural policies, clinical and response time requirements have limited effect on funding needs and sources.

Because system design and production methods greatly affect funding requirements, and because funding limitations often exist independent of other concerns, it is often advantageous to begin by establishing policies governing medical oversight, funding levels, and funding sources, and then adopt production methods that are capable of achieving the desired levels of service within the already-established funding constraints. Thus, patients are assured of receiving the best care possible from the dollars available.

REFERENCES

1. Stout, J.L., and Carter, J.: Fire vs. private EMS. J. Emerg. Med. Serv. (June) 1987.
2. Stout, J.L.: Measuring response time performance. J. Emerg. Med. Serv. (September) 1978.
3. Stout, J.L.: Why subscription programs? J. Emerg. Med. Serv. (October) 1986.
4. Stout, J.L.: Organizing quality control in EMS. J. Emerg. Med. Serv. (March) 1988.

MEDICAL CONTROL

Alexander Kuehl, T. MacClean, and Paul E. Pepe

CAPSULE

Direct and indirect medical control both require formal authority, and both must come together into a system with neither gaps nor overlaps. The precise legal foundations of medical control of prehospital care and the logical operating superstructure were neither well described nor developed as Emergency Medical Services (EMS) grew in the 1970s. Today legislators, physicians, EMS and care providers are still attempting to mold the accumulated experience of the last decade and the political forces of the moment into workable, legitimate medical control constructs for the future.

INTRODUCTION

EMS providers and medical directors have learned a great deal over the last two decades about the need

for medical control in prehospital care. Unfortunately, the necessity for defined medical direction was not fully appreciated in 1973, when the first major federal legislation concerning EMS was written.[1] As a consequence, subsequent state EMS legislation usually either did not address medical control at all or was limited in scope. In states where the original EMS legislation was limited but flexible, modifications to EMS in general and EMS medical control in particular were more easily accomplished than in states where the laws were either rigidly written or required legislative rather than regulatory amendment. This impediment was especially daunting when modifications of medical control activities or authority threatened politically potent organizations and institutions.[2]

In most areas of the United States, the original development of medical control constructs reflected the relative interests and strengths of the medical community, EMS regional council, and individual ambulance providers. With neither clear legislative direction nor well established models, it is not surprising that the philosophy and mechanics of medical control varied tremendously. Over the past decade, a philosophic and scientific basis for medical direction has gradually evolved. Now the major problem is to mesh these developing principles of prehospital medical control into EMS systems that have evolved to varying degrees without them.[3]

This chapter attempts to describe the elements of medical control as they have evolved. It is beneficial to remember that the regulatory language surrounding the 1973 legislation (P.L. 93–154) made provision for "off-line" project medical directors, who were to coordinate the activities of the existing "on-line" medical directors. The local medical directors who existed before the initiation of the regional federal EMS program generally functioned in both capacities.[4,5]

ELEMENTS OF MEDICAL CONTROL

The two traditional elements of medical control are direct (on-line) and indirect (off-line). From time to time, other adjectives have been used, such as prospective, immediate, retrospective, clinical and administrative. Because systems of EMS medical control are not uniform, a universal terminology remains elusive.[6]

In 1978, medical control was defined as "the direction of patient care by a physician . . . remote from the ambulance attendant and his patient. Some degree of indirect medical control through the use of treatment protocols that are in effect such as standing orders is commonly practiced. It is not certain at this time what degree of authority or responsibility is appropriate to delegate."[2]

Today, direct medical control normally refers to either radio supervision or the actual on-scene presence and direction of prehospital personnel by a physician or a designated surrogate. Indirect medical control can be provided prospectively, concurrently, or retrospectively. Prospectively, it includes the medical design of the EMS system, the creation of clinical protocols, and the education and certification of the providers; concurrently, it consists of the observational monitoring of prehospital patient care; and retrospectively, it includes quality assurance, risk management, continuing education, and remediation activities. In summary, direct medical control physicians are usually surrogates for the indirect medical control physician, on whose license a provider may be thought to function.

Before the wide use of the Military Antishock Trousers (MAST) as a basic life support (BLS) adjunct, neither first responders nor EMT-As (see Ground and Air Emergency Transport, this chapter) had significant medical input in their education, operation, or quality assurance. The apparent need and logic for the BLS use of MAST led to increased interest by local medical directors into other aspects of BLS care; thus the widespread use of MAST by BLS providers and the formal introduction of MAST into the EMT-A curriculum

brought most EMT-As into the sphere of medical control. When EMT-As were upgraded to the intermediate levels through education in traditional advanced life support (ALS) interventions such as advanced airway control and IV cannulation, they almost always came under medical control.[7]

The original national EMT-A curriculum and the subsequent state regulations regarding BLS care essentially created independent practitioners; the simultaneous development of paramedic programs created physician extenders. The first paramedic programs began with intense medical input and supervision, which often ebbed as the ability of the paramedics to carry out traditional physician tasks in the field became more obvious.[6] Several authors, however, have indicated that the concurrent on-scene presence of a physician and intense quality assurance improves patient outcomes at all provider levels.[8]

PROSPECTIVE INDIRECT MEDICAL CONTROL

Most EMS systems developed with a significant degree of prospective medical input, mainly concerning the choices of system configurations and provider levels; the development of training programs and protocols; the expansion of emergency medical dispatch (EMD); and disaster medicine preparedness.

During the 1970s, as local EMS systems evolved, few physicians took an active role. Depending on the specific clinical interests and expertise of those few physicians, the foci of the individual programs were defined. For example, in Maryland and Illinois, leadership by surgeons led to the development of renowned trauma systems, whereas in Seattle, internists created a program unsurpassed in the area of cardiac emergencies. Usually, several physicians became prominent members of the local EMS governing body or regional council; often, a single physician became the project medical director.[4] In recent years, a growing public demand for better and more accountable prehospital emergency care has encouraged local political leaders to recruit and appoint physicians to paid, occasionally full-time regional medical director roles.[9]

One of the first prospective medical requirements that must be addressed is the determination of the emergency medical requirements of the community. These determinations, along with an analysis of all existing medical resources, often define the initial system design in regard to the choice of provider levels. Other than medical need, the major influence on provider level decisions is the ability of the jurisdiction to educate and maintain the skills of the field providers. Individual state laws may limit the choice of level of provider to those defined by the state EMS regulations; however, there is usually significant flexibility for local variation and innovation, especially in the area of ALS protocols.[5]

The development of treatment protocols for intermediate EMTs and paramedics was originally the domain of either the individual service medical director or a local medical advisory committee. Gradually, other involved medical providers requested and were usually given the opportunity to participate in the development of local treatment and transport protocols. Some states, however, developed universal protocols that mandated, with various degrees of local flexibility, the treatment options to be used across the state.[10]

The structure and operation of call receiving, patient questioning, and call priority determination have become the aspects of prospective medical control into which medical influence is most rapidly expanding. Second only to the conceptualization of a comprehensive EMS system, the tasks of optimally prioritizing and responding to patient request are critical factors in providing satisfactory patient care.[11]

The first attempts at developing priority EMD were made locally by medical directors who faced the dilemma of getting the right unit to the right patient at the right time, all in the face of overwhelming demand. Clawson, in Salt Lake City, developed both a program and an accompanying text that combined and refined many of the evolving dispatch concepts. When modified for local differences, the resulting EMD program can be used effectively in most EMS systems.[11]

As medical control physicians have become more knowledgeable and sophisticated about the operation of EMS systems, they have begun to realize the medical importance of operational issues such as ambulance placement strategies, work schedules, and staffing patterns. In most jurisdictions, long and complex political and economic histories influence these decisions. Physicians, however, should not be reticent about suggesting or even mandating medically appropriate changes.

Originally, the education of prehospital care providers, especially at the intermediate and advanced levels, was service-specific. As the various states adopted standardized training curricula, many of the differences within states disappeared. Still, marked differences exist among the states because of the lack of a universally accepted national curriculum above the EMT-A level and the variations in certification mechanisms. Because most curricula have been developed at minimal levels, local physician input is critical to the refinement of standard state education requirements. Some states, however, do not allow care providers to practice skills beyond those taught in the standardized statewide programs.[12]

Obviously, the development of treatment and transport protocols should reflect the system's choice of provider levels, the individual philosophies of the responsible physicians, and, hopefully, solid clinical studies of the myriad existing approaches. Treatment protocols are divided between standing orders, which

may often be performed without concurrent physician input, and medical control options, which require concurrent medical direction. There is then a continuum, ranging from all standing orders to no standing orders at all; in the latter case direct medical control is required for every action. The exact point chosen on the continuum depends on local operational factors, physician preferences, and state law. Most protocols are clinically initiated on identification by the prehospital care provider of either a presumptive diagnosis or a constellation of symptoms. Logically, more highly trained and/or experienced prehospital care providers would operate with less direct medical control; however, other factors influence these decisions. For example, in urban environments, the need for extensive and time-consuming prehospital treatment options is less than in rural environments. In reality, the attitude of the responsible physician is the single most influential factor in the determination of the degree of clinical independence allowed the prehospital care provider.

CONCURRENT INDIRECT MEDICAL CONTROL

Indirect medical control, performed concurrent with patient care, is generally limited to process-oriented quality assurance, such as observation of prehospital care or EMD function by either physicians or physician surrogates such as senior-level providers or specially trained nurses.

Despite the 1978 expectations of the Committee on EMS of the National Academy of Sciences to the contrary, some authors have emphasized the critical importance of concurrent quality assurance, usually linked to direct patient care by the physician or a senior surrogate.[2,8,13] Concurrent process-oriented quality assurance has many advantages over retrospective run review, but is obviously much more expensive and difficult, especially in larger systems.

RETROSPECTIVE INDIRECT MEDICAL CONTROL

Currently, the vast majority of retrospective indirect medical input into prehospital care is focused on call review, documentation- and outcome-related quality assurance, remedial education, and risk management. The most confusing aspect of retrospective medical control is related to the imprecise and arbitrary division between medical quality assurance and employee discipline.[14]

DIRECT MEDICAL CONTROL

Direct medical control traditionally describes the concurrent interaction between care providers at the scene and a physician.[15] As indicated earlier, the extent of direct medical control reflects the degree to which the physician-director wishes to maintain "hands-on" authority over the actions of the providers. Clearly, there is a dearth of research as to how much direct medical control is appropriate; in fact, the best answer probably varies with the individual prehospital provider.[2] As long as the "physician extender" model is applied to paramedics, there is likely to be a trend toward less, rather than more, concurrent direct medical control for paramedics. With less educated care providers undertaking more sophisticated interventions, a greater degree of direct and indirect medical control is probably indicated; however, the availability of devices such as the automatic defibrillator allows providers to deliver interventions traditionally reserved for paramedics, with considerably fewer hours of education.

The provision of direct medical control by radio, with or without the transmission of medical telemetry, has been the usual exposure of most physicians to prehospital care. But the reader should realize that, originally, direct medical control was provided by physicians responding with the providers, and that model is once again growing in popularity.[8]

During the time following the initiation of the original prehospital programs, telemetry sent from the field, along with direct communication between the ALS provider and a physician, was generally thought essential for the appropriate operation of an ALS system. The usefulness and necessity of telemetry indirect medical control, however, are being questioned.[16] The apparent success of prehospital personnel in providing ALS, linked with the overwhelming number of ALS calls, may have led to overreliance on standing orders. Rather than simply reinstating the use of the traditional standbys such as medical options, telemetry, and radio contact, however, several authors have recommended the increased presence on the scene of an EMS physician acting as a practitioner, evaluator, and educator.[8]

The challenge of the 1990s is to find the economic and medical balance that best serves the needs and budget of the public. Obviously, each jurisdiction must make its own decision, but it is hoped that there will be more clinical and educational research on which to make the decisions.

Currently, myriad configurations are used for the provision of direct medical control, ranging from systems in which one physician trains the care provider, provides radio medical control, and treats the patient, to systems in which the physician gives the orders over the radio but never sees either the patient or the care provider[3] (base station medicine). The base station is the site designated by an EMS to provide direct medical control over care providers in the prehospital setting. Although some large, mature systems have removed direct medical control from emergency departments (EDs), most base stations still remain in hospitals. They may be staffed either by specially trained nurses or paramedics acting as physician surrogates or by physicians. The latter may be attending staff or residents. If the station is staffed by physician surrogates, a physician should be available for consultation.

The practice of base station medicine is a unique experience, unlike others in medicine. Traditionally, no courses in base station medicine are taught either in medical school or in most residencies. When practicing medicine "over the air," one must conceptualize the patient to make the appropriate therapeutic decisions. Because health care providers rely heavily on visual stimuli to perform patient assessment, they may have difficulty in talking someone at a remote location through a procedure or resuscitation.

Ideally, the staff of a base station should have firsthand knowledge of the prehospital environment, participation in ED patient care, and interest in prehospital research and education.[6] By virtue of the specialty, emergency physicians have an interest in, or at least an exposure to, prehospital care. Within the specialty, there is knowledge of and participation in curriculum development and training of prehospital care providers. Emergency physicians should be exposed to street medicine and the prehospital working environment. The working environment of emergency physicians gives day-to-day experience in triage. For instance, exposure to toxicology allows the emergency physician to better inform the prehospital provider about what to anticipate with a particular poison. During an emergency medicine residency, most of the training period is spent in the ED. Therefore, after a period of orientation, residents generally become comfortable with base station operation and can provide continuity. Training in emergency medicine, however, does not guarantee adeptness in practicing medicine "over the air." Continued exposure to both the base station and the streets is necessary to maintain the requisite expertise.

Realistically, there are not enough emergency physicians to staff all base stations. Therefore greater emphasis should be placed on selecting and training residents or staff from other specialties who have an interest in prehospital care. Adequate training should be provided so that the highest level of prehospital care is delivered. Formal national courses that focus on the diverse aspects of providing medical control are now available for neophyte physicians. Preparation should include ride-alongs, exposure to the medicolegal aspects of prehospital care, curriculum preparation, management problems, and a supervised probationary period. The predictable medical, ethical, and administrative problems can be presented in the form of case scenarios, allowing the trainee to act as the base station physician in a benign environment. Each scenario can then be structured to illustrate a principle of management. With these prerequisites and education techniques, physicians will be prepared as well as possible to provide direct medical control.

HORIZONS

A major problem facing regional EMS systems as they evolve into the 1990s is codifying and clarifying medical control. As the significant players of the recent past leave the arena, many new physicians with innovative ideas are preparing to lead, but because mechanisms for choosing the future directors are often not defined, optimal constructs have not been universally accepted, and high legal and social visibility makes the risks significant, smooth transition to new procedures may be difficult.

No matter who provides medical control in the future, it is crucial to recall that we may be on the verge of technologic revolutions that may alter the way in which medical control physicians view clinical, educational, and supervisory problems in the future. The logical and economical solutions of the future may place the medical community in direct conflict with strongly established provider groups and demanding consumers.

The design of the EMS medical control construct for a single crew, a service, a region, or a state must be crafted while taking into account the existing medical, economic and political environments. Authority for the various aspects of medical control must be established, and the medical community, care providers, and society at large must know who is medically responsible. The direct and indirect facets of medical control must be carefully fitted together, with neither overlaps nor gaps.

NATIONAL RESOURCES

American College of Emergency Physicians
P.O. Box 619911
Dallas, TX 75261
800-798-1822

National Association of EMS Physicians
230 McKee Place, Suite 500
Pittsburgh, PA 15213
800-228-3677

National Disaster Medical System
5600 Fishers Lane
Rockville, MD 20857

REFERENCES

1. Stout, J.L.: High Performance EMS Systems. Miami, The Fourth Party, Inc., 1989, pp. 8–12 (in press).
2. Emergency Medical Services at Mid-Passage, National Research Council—National Academy of Medicine. Washington, DC, 1978, p. 41.
3. Braun, O., and Callaham, M.: Direct Medical Control. In EMS Medical Directors' Handbook, Edited by Kuehl, A.E. St. Louis, C.V. Mosby, 1989, pp. 175–211.
4. Boyd, D.R., Edlich, R.F., and Micik, S.H. (Editors): Systems Approach to Emergency Medical Care. Norwalk, CT, Appleton-Century-Crofts, 1983.
5. Fowler, R.L.: Emergency medical services legislation. In EMS Medical Directors' Handbook. Edited by Kuehl, A.E.: St. Louis, C.V. Mosby, 1989, pp. 15–27.
6. Medical Control of EMS: An Overview for Emergency Physicians. Dallas, ACEP, 1984.
7. Eisenberg, M.S., Bergner, L., and Hallstrom, A.: Paramedic programs and out-of-hospital cardiac arrest: I. Factors associated with successful resuscitation. Am. J. Public Health 69:30, 1969.
8. Pepe, P.E., and Stewart, R.D.: Role of the physician in the prehospital setting. Ann. Emerg. Med. 15:1480, 1983.
9. Reines, D.: The emergence of medical control. In Kuehl AE: EMS Medical Director's Handbook. Edited by Kuehl, A.E. St. Louis, C.V. Mosby, 1989, pp. 155–161.
10. Emergency Medical Services Systems Program Guidelines. Publications No. (MSA) 75–2013, Department of Health, Education and Welfare. Washington, DC, 1975.
11. Clawson, J.J., and Dernocoeur, K.B.: Principles of Emergency Medical Dispatch. Englewood Cliffs, NJ, Brady/Prentice, Hall, 1989.
12. Lewis, R.P., Stang, J.M., Fulkerson, P.K., et al: Effectiveness of advanced paramedics in a mobile coronary care system. JAMA 214:1902, 1979.
13. Dinerman, N., Rosen, P., Pons, P.: Medical control in prehospital care. Curr. Top. Emerg. Med. 2:1,1988.
14. Ryan, J.: Quality assurance in Emergency Medical Service Systems. In Kuehl AE: EMS Medical Directors' Handbook. Edited by Kuehl, AE. St. Louis, C.V. Mosby, 1989, pp. 213–229.
15. Rousch, A.: Principles of EMS Systems, A Comprehensive Text for Physicians. Dallas, ACEP, 1989.
16. Cayten, C.G., et al.: The effect of telemetry in urban prehospital cardiac care. Ann. Emerg. Med.: 14:976, 1985.

THE ROLE OF THE HOSPITAL AND CATEGORIZATION IN THE EMS SYSTEM

Alan R. Dimick

CAPSULE

In the years before the concept of prehospital Emergency Medical Services (EMS) was conceived, the hospital Emergency Department (ED) was viewed by patients with anxiety and concern as the last resource in a medical crisis or accidental injury. Today, the ED is viewed by the community as a service responsibility of the hospital, providing care ranging from that for the patient with a medical or surgical emergency to nonemergent care, resolution of social and behavioral problems, and comprehensive stabilization of all medical conditions. The ED is now the focal point of all EMS in the community and serves as the key element for medical control in an EMS system.

INTRODUCTION

In 1984, Riggs and Cross published a landmark book, *The Hospital's Role in Emergency Medical Services Systems*, and detailed in it the role of the hospital in providing prehospital EMS as well as the relationships within the hospital of the ED to the various clinical services and departments. They also included chapters in design, staffing, organization, management, and finance. Their chapter on ED categorization provides an excellent historical review of the development of the various categorization systems up to 1983.

Because the categorization of hospital emergency services is so important to the provision of emergency medical care, it is felt that a brief historical review of the development of such categorization is pertinent. In 1971, the American Medical Association (AMA) Commission on Emergency Medical Services published its *Guidelines for the Categorization of Hospital Emergency Capabilities*, providing the basis for numerous state and regional programs. Two years later, the American Hospital Association (AHA) recommended a similar approach, followed shortly thereafter by the Joint Commission on the Accreditation of Hospitals standards for hospital emergency services, which paralleled the AMA and AHA efforts.

The primary purpose of classification of hospital emergency services is to identify the readiness and capability of a hospital and its staff to provide optimal care. With advance knowledge of hospital emergency capabilities, emergency medical services personnel and patients should be better able to make informed choices regarding hospital destination. This concept is of prime importance in delivering effective emergency care.

At the outset in 1971, the Commission stated that its intention was to evaluate overall hospital capability to respond to a wide variety of emergency conditions rather than to provide definitive treatment for specific types of medical emergencies. This approach, termed horizontal categorization, defined four levels of care capability for any and all emergencies. Titled Comprehensive, Major, General, and Basic, these levels signified capabilities ranging from advanced care at one extreme to basic resuscitation and stabilization at the other.

Although continuing to support the need for a classification scheme, the Commission soon recognized that the 1971 guidelines did not provide sufficient information regarding hospital capabilities for handling specific types of emergencies. The Commission further noted that the original guidelines did not address the realities of rural areas, where a broad range of emergency capabilities was not routinely available, and that even some urban areas had experienced difficulty in meeting requirements for comprehensive hospital emergency services.

By 1975, an alternative known as vertical categorization became the focus that, for a time, appeared likely to replace the horizontal approach. Vertical categorization defines the capability of an emergency care facility to care for specific groups of critically ill patients such as those with behavioral, burn, cardiac, pediatric, and traumatic emergencies. Thus, the vertical approach could be used to address more appropriately such questions as "can Hospital 'A' adequately manage a critical cardiac patient?" rather than the horizontal approach that asks, "does Hospital 'A' offer comprehensive, major, general or basic care for all emergency patients?"

This more flexible approach to categorization was also viewed as more cost-effective because a hospital could choose to maintain or upgrade to a given level of service for one critical care area without committing additional resources across the spectrum of emergency services. For instance, under a vertical categorization scheme, it is both conceivable and appropriate for a hospital to be categorized at one level for burn care, the same or another level for the treatment of trauma, yet another level for cardiac care, and perhaps not any level for the remaining areas.

In its effort to refine the categorization concept further, in 1980 the AMA and AHA cosponsored an invitational conference of 100 EMS physicians and administrators. One year later, the Commission published the proceedings as the *Provisional Guidelines for the Optimal Categorization of Hospital Emergency Capabilities*, which described criteria for vertical categorization of nine critical care areas, including acute medical, behavioral, burn, cardiac, neonatal/prenatal/ pediatric, obstetric/gynecologic, poisoning/drug, spinal cord, and trauma emergencies.

Experience with horizontal and vertical categorization has led to several important conclusions. First, only 5% of EMS patients present with critical conditions, another 15% are characterized as serious, and the remaining 80% have medical problems that do not necessitate distinguishing among hospital capabilities. Second, as the isolated process of hospital emergency services categorization has evolved to an integrated process of EMS system development, the terminology surrounding classification has expanded to include additional implementation methods, including verification, accreditation and designation.

To provide consistency throughout the guidelines, the Commission adopted the following definitions: A *medical emergency* is an actual or perceived disorder of vital systems caused by illness or injury, presenting as an immediate or potential threat to life or function. A *qualified specialist* is a physician with special competence in that specialty. Factors suggesting special competence in that area include, but are not limited to, residency or fellowship training, board certification, and direct experience.

A hospital may provide tertiary, secondary, or a lesser level of care. The highest level, represented by tertiary care services is termed level I (except for perinatal care, which has historically been termed level III), and the lowest is level III (Table 87-12). Not all services recognize all three levels and not all describe only clinical capabilities; others additionally include education and research.

According to this scheme, classification refers to the minimal criteria for hospital resources and categorization, verification, accreditation and designation address the process for their implementation. Although categorization has previously been used to describe both standards and process, the Commission endorses using classification to describe the former and categorization as an alternative method for the latter.

Finally, all hospitals identified by EMS systems as providing specialized emergency care must recognize their obligation to provide equal access to care for all patients, regardless of ability to pay.

As EMS technology matures, emphasis is increasingly focusing on a systems approach. EMS systems are composed of components such as training, triage, transportation, and treatment, and of special care capabilities such as those described in this chapter. Indicative of this maturation process are the *Guidelines for EMS Systems* developed by the American College of Emergency Physicians (ACEP), which describe the relationship between system components and special care capabilities, including hospital emergency facilities. A companion ACEP document, *Guidelines for Trauma Care Systems,* describes individual components of a system for trauma care.

The 1989 AMA guidelines, developed by their respective medical specialties, define the current state of the art for hospital emergency capabilities. Although some have been published previously elsewhere, others have been developed at the invitation of the Commission and appear in the document for the first time. The Commission acknowledges that, as updated guidelines are published by individual specialties, they will supersede those appearing in this document.

Although these 1989 AMA Guidelines on categorization have broadened the scope and increased the depth for critical care guidelines, capabilities for managing emergencies arising from exposure to radiation and to hazardous materials remain to be defined. Additionally, because some guidelines are new and others are pending revision, not all references are current. The Commission intended to address these changes in future editions, which were planned for publication every 3 to 4 years, but the Commission was abolished by the AMA Board of Trustees in October, 1989.

TABLE 87-12. LEVELS OF CARE

Classification	Categorization	Verification	Accreditation	Designation
Level III:				
Limits hospital participation	No	No	No	Yes
Level II:				
Accommodates system need	No	No	No	Yes
Level I:				
Requires external evaluation	No	Yes	Yes	Yes

The 1989 edition of the guidelines assumes a new approach to classification of hospital emergency capabilities that combines aspects of both the horizontal and vertical approaches. Unlike previous editions, which incorporated ED criteria into each of the individual specialty guidelines, this document now recognizes a single, separate ED guideline. Also, where possible, the guidelines include criteria for prehospital and interhospital triage, thereby indicating which patients should be treated in specialized facilities.

These guidelines do not constitute standards of care, and should be viewed as describing essential or minimal criteria to be used to facilitate optimal care. Thus, as individual facilities evaluate their capability to care for various types of emergency patients, this ideal may not be entirely achievable in some areas because of geographic location, hospital size, or other reasons. Nevertheless, hospitals should still demonstrate their commitment to patient care by attempting to achieve at least some of the specified items.

BIBLIOGRAPHY

American College of Emergency Physicians: Guidelines for Emergency Medical Services Systems. Ann. Emerg. Med. *17:*742,1988.

American College of Emergency Physicians: Guidelines for Trauma Care Systems. Ann. Emerg. Med. *16:*459,1987.

American College of Emergency Physicians: Categorization of Emergency Services. Ann. Emerg. Med. *13:*546,1984.

American Medical Association: Guidelines for the Categorization of Hospital Emergency Capabilities. Chicago, American Medical Association, 1989.

American Medical Association: Provisional Guidelines for the Optimal Categorization of Hospital Emergency Capabilities. Chicago, American Medical Association, 1981.

American Medical Association: Guidelines for the Categorization of Hospital Emergency Capabilities. Chicago, American Medical Association, 1971.

Cross, R.E., Jr., and Riggs, L.M., Jr.: Emergency Department Categorization in the Hospital's Role in Emergency Medical Services Systems. Chicago, American Hospital Association, 1984, pp. 31–57.

Hellig, R.W., Jr., and Whalen, E.: Hospital Care. *In* Emergency Medicine: A Comprehensive Review. Edited by Kravis, T.C., Warner, C.G., Benson, D.R., et al. Rockville, MD, Aspen Publishers, 1986.

National Research Council: Regionalization and Categorization: An Approach to Change in The Emergency Department: A Regional Medical Resource. Washington, DC, National Academy Press, 1980, pp. 37–41.

National Research Council: Accidental Death and Disability: The Neglected Disease of Modern Society. Washington, DC, US Department of Health, Education and Welfare, 1966, pp. 18–23.

Neely, K.W., et al.: Analysis of hospital ability to provide trauma services—Comparison between teaching and community hospitals. Prehosp. Disaster Med. *6:*455, 1991.

Riner, R.M., Collins, K.M., Foulke, G.E., et al.: Categorization of hospital emergency services—Developing valid criteria. West. J. Med. *147:*602,1987.

GROUND AND AIR EMERGENCY TRANSPORT

Sheryl G.A. Gabram, Lenworth M. Jacobs, and Ralph R. Garramone

CAPSULE

Prehospital transport can use both ground and air to transfer patients rapidly to hospitals. The concept of prehospital care of the trauma patient originated in the military, but the positive effect on patient outcome caused the military experience to be extrapolated to the civilian environment. Trauma was the impetus to the development of basic prehospital medical care and improved care for trauma patients was appreciated in the civilian setting. The concept of expanding prehospital care was then extrapolated to the cardiac patient. Prehospital advanced medical care was developed as a result of treating critical cardiac patients.

Well developed ground and air prehospital systems have decreased mortality in cardiac and trauma patients. Ground transport offers accessibility of prehospital care in various weather conditions. Because many patients taken to hospitals do not require advanced medical care, different levels of care are available in ground transport. Helicopter transport should be reserved for the most critically ill or injured patients. Air medical transport offers three advantages over ground transport: the highest level of medical expertise, the most sophisticated medical equipment in the prehospital setting, and rapid transfer to a tertiary care hospital.

This chapter discusses ground and air emergency transport in two sections. Both sections begin with a historical perspective on the development of each type of transport. Other subjects include legislative efforts to establish the ground system, composition of prehospital medical teams and their skill capabilities, types of equipment and characteristics of the transport vehicle, helicopter demograhics and economics, aeromedical safety, and the impact of both types of transport on medical care.

GROUND EMERGENCY TRANSPORT

HISTORICAL PERSPECTIVE

The Emergency Medical Services System (EMSS) is a comprehensive, multicomponent system designed to respond promptly to both medical and surgical emergencies within a community and deliver high-quality emergency care.[1,2] The system has been in evolution since it was originally conceived in response to military conflicts and the care of the trauma patient. The victim of sudden medical illness, however, is the primary recipient of today's advanced services.

One of the earliest descriptions of organized trauma care was recorded in the *Iliad*. Homer described soldiers wounded in the battle of Troy being carried off the battlefield and treated in nearby barracks and ships. By the first century A.D., wounded Roman soldiers were taken to hospitals along the border of the Roman empire.

In the 19th century, Baron Dominque Jean Larrey, the chief surgeon in Napoleon's army, made two innovative changes in the care of wounded soldiers that have endured until today. First, he used horse-drawn ambulances to transport injured soldiers off the battlefield within hours of being injured. Second, he concentrated the wounded soldiers in one area, close to the front lines, where he and other medical personnel initiated initial medical treatment.[3]

Military conflicts have continued to be a source of innovation and improvement in the development of patient care and transport systems. During World War I, there was a 12-to-18-hour average time lag between injury and definitive treatment. The overall mortality rate was 8.5%. During World War II, this time lag was reduced to between 6 and 12 hours, and the mortality rate fell to 5.8%. It was during the Korean conflict that the United States Army employed the mobile army surgical hospital (MASH). This further reduced the time from injury to definitive surgical care to between 2 and 4 hours. The overall mortality was reduced to 2.4%. This concept was further improved in Viet Nam, where the average time required to remove an injured soldier from the field was 65 minutes and the mortality rate fell to 1.7%.[4]

This decrease in both mortality and transit time has been attributed to a systems approach to trauma patients. It must be realized that, during this same period, improved surgical techniques, methods of anesthesia, antibiotics, and knowledge of antisepsis, as well as the importance of nutrition, all contributed to the lower mortality rates. The most important advance, however, was creating an organized response to the trauma patient and realizing that trauma is a time-related disorder.[4] The more rapidly hemorrhage is controlled, the patient transported, and definitive care administered, the better the outcome.

Ischemic heart disease is the leading cause of death in the United States. Over 650,000 deaths occur each year from ischemic heart disease, and approximately half of these patients reach a hospital by activation of a local EMS system. Trauma is the fourth leading cause of death in America and the leading cause of death in people between the ages of 1 and 44.[5] For people up to age 75, motor vehicle accidents are the leading mechanism of accidental death. Twenty-five percent of all injury victims are in the pediatric age group. More childhood deaths result from trauma than from all other causes combined. Head injury accounts for approximately half of the deaths in most trauma series. Spinal cord injuries affect over 10,000 Americans each year. Each year approximately 2 million people are burned seriously enough to require medical attention. Of these, 500,000 require Emergency Department (ED) visits and 70,000 require hospitalization.[3,6]

LEGISLATION

Before the establishment of the present EMS system and the realization that trauma and acute medical emergencies are time-related, transportation of patients to hospitals was performed by volunteers driving ambulances in their spare time. Frequently the patient was given little, if any, care en route to the hospital because the driver had no First Aid training; in fact, the patient might even have been transported unattended.[7]

In 1966, differences in prehospital care of both medically ill and injured patients were brought to the attention of the public and policy makers in a document entitled "Accidental Death and Disability: The Neglected Diseases of Modern Society." This was published by the National Academy of Sciences' National Research Council (NAS NRC).[8] In addition to outlining the magnitude of the trauma problem in the United States, this report cited 30 recommendations in an effort to reduce trauma deaths and disability. The report cited the need for a National Council on Accident Prevention. It cited deficiencies in ambulance service, including diverse or nonexistent standards for vehicles and equipment, inadequate training standards for ambulance attendants, inadequate certification standards, limited data on current services, insufficient research toward improvement of existing ambulance service and toward adoption of helicopters as a future method of transport. The report made recommendations to correct these and other deficiencies. The report also recommended the institution of a Trauma Registry and Hospital Trauma Committees to establish standards of care, Cardiopulmonary Resuscitation (CPR) training and evaluation of pre-hospital care.

In 1973, passage of the EMS systems Act, Public Law 93–154, was accomplished as part of the Public Health Services Act. The administration of the EMSS Act came under the responsibility of what would later be known as the Department of Health and Human Services (DHHS) in 1975. These laws created authority for an organized framework at the national, state, regional, and local levels within which a sophisticated EMS system could be developed. Specifically, it divided the states into 300 geographic regions for the purpose of EMS planning and funding.[2]

EMERGENCY MEDICAL TECHNICIANS

Today the EMS program is part of the Reconciliation Act of 1981, and part of the Health Prevention Block Grant which is included in Public Law 97–35.[2] These changes encouraged a shift in responsibility for EMS funding from Federal to state government. Considerable attention has been placed on training and certification of Emergency Medical Technicians (EMTs) and paramedics, establishing vehicular standards for ambulances and developing communications systems. Currently, in the United States there are two levels of training for EMS personnel:

1. Basic Life Support (BLS): ". . . provides pre-hospital, non-invasive emergency patient care designed to optimize the patients' chances of surviving the emergency situation."[2]
2. Advanced Life Support (ALS): ". . . provides both noninvasive and invasive emergency patient care designed to optimize the patients' chances of surviving the emergency situation."[2]

Basic standards of training for EMTs, as well as requirements for certification and licensure are specified by state law. Essentially, four levels have been determined based on degree of training.

EMT-A   The EMT-A is trained in BLS and is also certified in cardiopulmonary resuscitation, basic airway management using a bag-valve mask, control of external hemorrhage, splinting and bandaging, and extrication and emergency driving.

EMT-I   The EMT-I Is trained in the skills described for EMT-A's plus ALS, advanced airway management, and administration of intravenous fluids. In addition, the EMT-I has training in patient assessment, shock management, and physiology.

EMT-D   The EMT-D is trained in all of the skills described for both EMT-A and EMT-I plus use of automated electrocardioversion.

EMT-P   The EMT-P is trained in all of the skills described for the other levels, plus cardiac monitoring and defibrillation, administration of medications for resuscitation, and limited invasive therapeutic techniques including endotracheal and nasotracheal intubation and needle thoracostomy.

In 1966, the National Highway Safety Act gave the Department of Transportation (DOT) the authority to provide funds for the development of basic EMS programs. This led to the development of a standard curriculum for the training of ambulance personnel. Before this, the American Academy of Orthopaedic Surgeons was in the forefront in providing training programs for emergency care providers. In fact, in 1971, the Academy published *Emergency Care and Transportation of the Sick and Injured,* then the only readily available textbook that defined the knowledge and skills required of ambulance personnel in meeting the needs of their patients.[1]

Basic emergency medical technology is now part of a 120-hour curriculum authorized by individual states. The National Registry of EMTs, the leading certifying and testing agency in the country, reports a total of approximately 160,000 EMTs in the United States and 8 other countries. Recertification of EMTs certified by the National Registry is required every 2 years and includes a 20-hour refresher course, yearly CPR recertification and 48 hours of continuing education.[2]

As the benefits of emergency medical services were realized, several states proceeded to train individuals to provide a more advanced level of prehospital care. This had clearly been in effect in other countries before its inception here in the United States. Pantridge in Belfast, Ireland and Grace in New York City in the late 1960s devised a mobile intensive care unit (MICU) equipped with defibrillation, cardiac pacing, and antiarrhythmic drug capability.[9,10]

Just as the trauma patient served as the focus for improving basic emergency medical care, the acutely ill cardiac patient provided the impetus for advanced emergency medical care. Advanced ambulance services in the early 1970's were usually initiated by a single physician, were locally based, and varied greatly from state to state. In 1977, however, the University of Pittsburgh Emergency Medical Technician–Paramedic National Training Course was developed.

This course outlined 15 specific areas and formed the foundation on which a national standard could be established:

1. The role of the EMT-paramedic
2. Human systems and patient assessment
3. Shock and fluid therapy
4. Pharmacology
5. Respiratory Emergencies
6. Cardiovascular emergencies
7. Central nervous system
8. Soft tissue injuries
9. Musculoskeletal emergencies
10. Medical emergencies
11. Obstetric/gynecologic emergencies
12. Pediatric and neonatal emergencies
13. Behavioral emergencies
14. Rescue techniques
15. Telemetry and communications

A national standard has not yet been achieved. Not all states currently use the National Registry EMT-P examination, and most states continue to use state-approved exam or programs. Recertification of paramedics certified by the National Registry is required every 2 years and includes a 48-hour refresher course, 24 hours of continuing education, and advanced cardiac life support (ACLS) certification by the American Heart Association, as well as acknowledgement of satisfactory field performance by a medical director. There are an estimated 22,000 advanced EMTs in the United States, with 50% located in California, New York, Illinois, Florida, and Ohio.[2]

Since the nationwide adoption of the principles of BLS and ACLS, there has been an improvement in hospital morbidity and mortality in cardiac patients, as well as a reduction in the incidence of cardiac arrest en route to the hospital.[11-13]

VEHICLES AND EQUIPMENT

Along with advances in the training of EMT's came advances in ground transportation vehicles. Recommendations for the new vehicles was made on the national level in 1974 with the adoption of the DOT General Services Administration KKK-A-1822 specifications.[14] This was supplemented by the American College of Surgeons' "Essential Equipment for Ambulances," which established recommendations for ambulance equipment.[15] Most vehicles are modified from a standard van chassis. The patient compartment is large enough to permit transport of two patients plus personnel.

For airway management, oropharyngeal and nasopharyngeal airways are used to support the tongue anteriorly and prevent the most common cause of upper airway obstruction, posterior displacement of the tongue.[4] Endotracheal and nasotracheal tubes are used if the patient cannot maintain an adequate airway or if there is concern about imminent respiratory arrest. These represent the definitive method of airway management and should be available in sizes for pediatric to aged patients.

A laryngoscope equipped with either a conventional or fiber optic light source and an assortment of blade sizes and shapes is essential. A bag-valve-mask apparatus with transparent masks in adult, pediatric, and infant sizes should be available. A portable suction device is necessary. A battery-powered unit is preferred with the capacity for adjustment of vacuum and flow for use with infants. Portable oxygen is essential, with the capacity for 5 to 15 liters per minute of flow. A humidification system is beneficial, especially for the long-term administration of oxygen, and particularly if used with an endotracheal or tracheostomy tube.

Intravenous supplies, including cannulas, tubing, and fluids together with intravenous medications for arrythmia control should be available. Portable ECG telemetry equipment with defibrillator capability is essential. For both more advanced and future transportation teams, transcutaneous oxygen saturation monitors and end tidal CO_2 monitors should be available.[16]

INTERVENTION IN THE FIELD

Many of the changes in both the education of EMT's and evolution of the MICU came from the recognition that the trauma patient, as well as the critically ill medical patient, requires rapid care. Controversy exists, however, as to whether to "scoop and run" or stabilize the patient in the field. Some physicians advocate little or no treatment in the field, but rather quick and efficient transport of the patient from the site of injury or illness to a facility where definitive care can be delivered. Others, however, recommend performing initial resuscitative measures in the field followed by rapid transport to a hospital facility.

The first priority of resuscitation of the multisystem-injured trauma patient is airway management. This may involve the administration of oxygen and close observation to ensure that the patient's airway is patent and remains so. It may also involve the placement of an endotracheal tube and assisted ventilation. The degree of management involves proper assessment by prehospital personnel and medical control as well as the level of training of the EMT.

The second priority is control of external hemorrhage with direct pressure and treatment of shock. A controversy exists as to when intravenous access should be obtained: in the field, while en route to the hospital, or in the ED of the receiving hospital. The problem centers on how much prehospital time is consumed by this practice. If intravenous access adds one minute or less to the prehospital time, it should be done in the field; otherwise it should be performed in the ambulance.[7] Again, the decision depends on the experience and training of the prehospital personnel. With this there is no controversy.

The third priority is vertebral column stabilization. Because definitive diagnosis of injury to the vertebral column requires radiographic analysis, any patient with suspected injury to the spinal column should be immobilized in the field. The cervical spine should be addressed first. Cervical traction can be applied manually until a cervical collar can be applied. The rigid two-piece Philadelphia collar and the one-piece polyethylene Stiffneck collar minimize flexion, extension, and rotation. The anterior portion of the Philadelphia collar is easily removed for inspection of the neck, and the Stiffneck collar has a large opening in the anterior aspect for this purpose. A long spinal board is used in conjunction with a rigid cervical collar to immobilize the entire vertibral column.

For the patient suffering from cardiac arrest, congestive heart failure, diabetic ketoacidosis, drug overdose, or other acute medical emergency; intervention may be provided by EMTs on arrival, provided that there is recognition of a potentially treatable problem. The trauma patient, on the other hand, may require management of intra-abdominal, intrathoracic, or intracranial hemorrhage. The treatment of these injuries is best accomplished in a hospital facility, and all efforts of the EMT should be focused on the expedient transport of the patient to such a facility.

Although an exhaustive review of the literature and thorough discussion of field intervention are beyond the scope of this chapter, it is essential that such intervention be considered. Endotracheal intubation by qualified prehospital personnel has proven to be a safe and efficacious method of providing definitive airway management and guarding against aspiration. In 1983, Jacobs et al.[17] reported a prospective review of 178 endotracheal intubations performed in the field by paramedics during a 9-month interval. This represented a success rate of 96.6%. There were no reported complications. The application of the Pneumatic Antishock Garment (PASG), although in itself a subject of controversy, is one method of treatment that can be quickly implemented. The application of a PASG may have some use in the treatment of hypovolemic shock by increasing peripheral vascular resistance, splinting fractures and tamponading hemorrhage from extremity and pelvic fractures.[7] More controversial is the subject of intravenous access.

Various reports in both the trauma and medical literature have discussed the topic of intravenous access in the field.[4,7,18–21] These reports cite the length of time required to establish an intravenous line, the relatively small volume of fluid infused during transport, and the minimal if any improvement in overall outcome as reason to limit this practice. Most data suggest that intervention in the field beyond assessment, extrication, airway management, control of hemorrhage, and fracture stabilization has not proven useful in the trauma patient.[7,17,18,20,21] This is supported by the report by Gervin et al.,[21] in which patients with penetrating cardiac injuries were studied. No patient with this injury survived if an attempt was made at prehospital resuscitation with concomitant prolongation of prehospital transport time. In contrast, there was an 80% survival in patients in whom transport delays were minimal. The general recommendation by most trauma surgeons is that multisystem-injured patients require definitive care as quickly as possible. Transport time should not be prolonged by attempting procedures in the field that could be accomplished more expeditiously either en route or at the hospital.

In patients suffering an acute myocardial infarction, it has been estimated that approximately half of the overall mortality occurs in the prehospital period, usually within the first 2 hours after onset of symptoms.[22] Intuitively, it would seem beneficial to provide these patients with oxygen, pain relief, treatment of pulmonary edema, and interpretation and correction of hemodynamically compromising dysrythmias as soon as possible. Large communities with many individuals trained in BLS and rapidly responding paramedics report a 40% success rate in the resuscitation of patients with documented ventricular fibrillation, provided that CPR is instituted within 4 minutes and followed by ACLS within 8 to 10 minutes.[22]

Eisenberg et al. considered variables that were believed to be associated with improved outcome in patients experiencing out-of-hospital cardiac arrest. A paramedic program was compared to the already existing EMT service in the Seattle, Washington area. Rapid time to initiation of CPR and rapid time to definitive care were determined to be most predictive of successful outcome from out-of-hospital cardiac arrest. The significance of bystander-initiated CPR was considered, but was felt to reflect the significance of early initiation of CPR. Similarly, the type of service reflects the time to definitive care. Because paramedics provide definitive care with defibrillation, intubation, and administration of intravenous medications, care is provided earlier than with EMTs, who must transport the patient to a hospital facility where definitive care can be instituted.[23] In support to Eisenberg, a prospective study by Dean et al. has shown defibrillation to be beneficial in the prehospital treatment of patients suffering an acute myocardial infarction and out-of-hospital ventricular fibrillation.[18] These patients should be transported by mobile units capable of defibrillation and advanced airway management, to a hospital rapidly where definitive treatment with thrombolysis, pacemakers, invasive monitoring, and angioplasty are available.

After initial assessment and extrication of the trauma patient, rapid transport to definitive treatment at a hospital facility is paramount. Second, for both trauma patients and medically ill patients, rapid and accurate airway management must be accomplished. Third, for trauma patients, the PASG (the utility of which is still controversial) can be quickly applied, especially if it is already in place on the stretcher before the patient is moved. For the cardiac patient, defibrillation in the case of ventricular fibrillation is of documented benefit. Intravenous access, although useful, should not delay transport.

Improvements in EMS Systems have increased both the availability of prehospital services and the number of patients who arrive in the ED in extremis. Not infrequently, the EMT responds to a patient who is dead. Local EMS systems protocol must have specific directions in this regard. The generally accepted criteria for the presumption of death in the field have been developed by the American College of Surgeons Committee on Trauma.[6] The presumption of death at the scene is made by a physician in radio contact with EMTs.

The EMT must have sufficient training and equipment to assess the patient adequately. In the field, this may range from physical examination to electrocardiographic monitoring. The Trauma Score, as described by Champion et al., has proven to be instrumental in helping to identify patients for whom resuscitation is futile.[24] The information obtained by applying the Truama Score, however, must supplement the clinical information gathered at the scene. The physician in command must have sufficient information, knowledge, and judgment to direct the EMTs. The question of presumption of death in the field involves ethical, legal, and economic considerations at once. Rapid transport of such patients creates an unnecessary risk to EMS personnel, the occupants of other motor vehicles, and pedestrians. A 40% increase in the emergency vehicle accident rate occurs when the vehicle is running under lights and siren.[7] In addition, rapid transport of a dead patient interferes with the dispatch of personnel and equipment to aid patients who are potentially salvageable.

AIR EMERGENCY TRANSPORT

HISTORICAL PERSPECTIVE

The use of the helicopter for transport of critically injured patients originated in the military conflicts. Airlifting patients to appropriately equipped hospitals began during World War I,[25] and increased further during World War II.[26] Use of rotor-wing aircraft, i.e., helicopters, as rapid transport vehicles began during the Korean War.[27] Both the irregular terrain and the distances to the Mobile Army Surgical Hospitals (MASH) favored the use of the helicopter instead of fixed wing transport. The MASH units were strategically located to receive the incoming wounded who were secured on litters outside the helicopter.[28] The use of helicopters contributed to the reduction in time to definitive medical care, from 6 to 12 hours during World War II to 2 to 4 hours during the Korean War. This reduction in time was thought to be a major contributor to the decrease in mortality that also occurred, from 5.8 to 2.4%.[27]

The number of injured soldiers transported by helicopter increased tenfold during the Vietnam War. Approximately 200,000 soldiers were airlifted by helicopter to surgical hospitals.[29] The configuration of the helicopter was altered, allowing the patient to be transported inside the helicopter attended by an ALS-trained flight crew. Instead of only a transport vehicle, the helicopter now allowed for earlier medical interventions enroute to the definitive care hospital. Time to definitive care decreased further to 35 minutes. This, coupled with other technologic advancements, further decreased mortality to 1.7%.[29]

Civilian helicopter use began in the 1960s when the concept of rapid transport to definitive care hospitals evolved.[30] Originally, police and fire departments provided helicopter services for search and rescue operations and "scoop and run" medical transports. The Chicago Fire and Police Departments cooperated in medical missions, transporting rescued patients to Cook County Hospital. The "Hover Jumpers," the flight crew employed by the Los Angeles Fire Rescue Units, actually jumped out of the helicopter when the terrain prohibited landing.[31]

Federal funding by the National Highway Traffic Safety Administration (NHTSA) of several helicopter aeromedical programs, using public service or military equipment, allowed evaluation of helicopters in the civilian environment.[32] The NHTSA actually concluded that, for the predicted usage, helicopters were economically prohibitive, had a questionable role in urban transfers, and were of limited use because of nonmedical configurations. Even if all these factors were addressed, they would require integration into the current EMS systems to be effective.

Although cognizant of the negative environment at that time, St. Anthony's Hospital in Denver, Colorado instituted the first continuously operating civilian hospital-based helicopter program, "Flight for Life," in October of 1972.[33,34] Helicopters Unlimited was contracted to provide a single engine Alouette 316 helicopter. Denver, although an urban area is located close to mountainous terrain that is inaccessible to medical ground transport. The possibility of the 1976 Winter Olympics being held in Denver, Colorado prompted consideration of a hospital-based emergency medical helicopter service dedicated to medical transports in the event of serious injury. Although Denver did not obtain the bid for the Winter Olympics, plans for developing a civilian hospital-based helicopter program proceeded. Strong medical leadership of the program was advocated by NHTSA. With this proviso, the Director of the Intensive Care Service selected and trained the early medical flight crews. The aircraft was medically configured and had a goal of less than 5 minute liftoff from time of request for service. The hospital made a commitment to expand their services to care for the increasing number of critically injured patients. Integration with the EMS system was accomplished by establishing a helicopter communications center to coordinate flights and to disseminate information to first responders, emergency medical technicians (EMTs), and law enforcement and public safety agencies.[33] Radios were installed in the aircraft, enabling flight crew members to communicate with ground personnel en route to the scene of an accident. As the program developed, the helicopter served as a backup to counties around Denver lacking ground services. This eliminated the need to remove local services out of their communities for long transports into the city of Denver.[34] Gradually, with time the medical expertise of the flight crew and rapid transport times were acknowledged by prehospital care providers who increased the use of the program.[33] As of 1989, "Flight for Life" operated two helicopters and transported over 27,000 patients (personal communication, "Flight for Life" program).

DEMOGRAPHICS AND ECONOMICS

Over the past 17 years, the civilian emergency medical helicopter industry has grown beyond expectation. Predictions of the number of hospital based programs made in 1985[35] have been exceeded. As of July 1989, 165 hospital programs operated 213 helicopters in 136 cities around the country.[36] The 108,900 patients transported by the hospital-based programs in 1988 represented an 11.2% increase over the previous year.[37] Hospital-based programs include those operated by a single hospital, the most common type of program, and those operated and directed by a group of hospitals, known as a consortium. An example of a consortium program is the Boston MED FLIGHT helicopter service, directed by a board representing four Boston hospitals. The helicopter is based at the Boston City Heliport. It is a consortium by strict definition, in that all four hospitals not only provide financial support but are also involved in medical policy decision making (personal communication, S. Wedel, MD Medical Director, Boston MED FLIGHT).

Approximately 10% of transports are performed by public use programs, i.e., those directed by police and fire departments.[38] Military medevac services also exist throughout the country. One of the most developed public service systems is the Maryland State Police aviation program, operating seven helicopter bases serving the entire state of Maryland.[39] The Miami Fire rescue aeromedical program operating in Florida involves the Fire department as well as Police aviators. Medical control is provided from Jackson Memorial Hospital.[40]

Historically, helicopter emergency programs placed a large economic burden on the sponsor hospital.[41] To be competitive with ground services, the early programs set the charge for transports well below the costs of the program. With increases in technology, level of training of the flight crew, and expansion from single- to twin-engine helicopters, costs have increased. Matching charges and costs is the only financial way for programs to survive. Acceptance of this concept over the years has allowed increases in transport charges to balance total costs. In 1988, the average transport charge for a 100-mile round trip flight, with the helicopter departing and returning to the sponsor hospital, was $1433.[42] Connecticut's critical care helicopter service has its rates established by the Office of Emergency Medical Services, a state agency. The total cost of the program, including the vendor contract, medical flight crew salaries, fuel charges, equipment, taxes, and insurance rates is divided by the projected number of flights per year, and this figure establishes the fee. Fee composition varies and may consist of a base charge plus hourly or mile charges and equipment and/or medical service charges. The overall goal is to match charges with actual expenses. In an attempt to curb health care costs, in the future it may be more financially feasible for a sponsor hospital to expand services to a two- or three-helicopter program as dictated by need rather than instituting a new service at another hospital. In this way, the cost of the facilities such as the helipad, hangar, and specialized tools need not be duplicated, and overall health care costs may be kept lower.

AIRCRAFT AND SAFETY

For emergency medical helicopters to be used for urgent medical transport, several characteristics are essential to the safe and effective completion of a medical mission. Dependable performance is an absolute necessity. The aircraft must be airborne quickly, respond within a large radius, cruise at a high speed, and be conveniently accessible for patient loading and unloading.[38] It must have the power to make a vertical ascent from a scene while fully loaded with one or two patients, a medical flight crew, and medical equipment; and be able to clear any obstacles. Lighter, less expensive, single-engine helicopters were used exclusively until 1980, when the larger twin-engine helicopters were introduced for EMS use.[43] In hospital-based programs, the twin-engine helicopter far exceeds the number of single-engine helicopters in use today.

Currently, the most popular hospital-based EMS helicopter is the MBB Twin engine BK-117, considered the state-of-the-art EMS aircraft.[38] Manufactured jointly by West Germany's Messerschmitt-Bolkow-Blohm and Japan's Kawasaki companies, its rigid rotor system provides a highly maneuverable aircraft requiring a landing zone of only 60×60 ft in area. The minimal landing zone requirement lends itself well to accident scene responses. With a cruising speed of 155 miles per hour and a 150-mile radius, distant interhospital transports are also achievable. The 200 cubic foot cabin space, which is separated from the aviation compartment, allows maximal double patient transport. This additional space may accommodate such devices as the neonatal isolette, portable intra-aortic balloon pump, and other sophisticated medical equipment. In an emergency circumstance, the BK-117 has the best single-engine performance of all twin-engine helicopters.[44]

Safety is an integral part of all aeromedical programs. Aeromedical helicopter accidents peaked in the early 1980s as providers with limited experience instituted new programs. The aeromedical helicopter accident rate at that time was more than double that of the rest of the helicopter industry.[45] The Aviation Safety Institute analyzed 84 aeromedical helicopter accidents from 1975–1986 to make recommendations to decrease the high accident rate.

Several changes have occurred during the evolution of helicopter EMS. The number of mechanical failures causing accidents has dramatically decreased as stricter maintenance schedules have been enforced.[46] Rocky Mountain Helicopters, the largest medical helicopter vendor in the country, employs one mechanic per helicopter.[38] On a full-time basis, this mechanic's sole responsibility is to maintain the aircraft and ensure that it is flightworthy at all times. Adverse weather conditions and night flying were found to be major factors in pilot error-attributable accidents. This is significant because 40% of helicopter EMS flying occurs at night.[47] As a result of the accident trend, three industry organizations, the Association of Air Medical Services (AAMS), Helicopter Association International (HAI), and the National Emergency Medical Service Pilots Association (NEMSPA) refined and improved Visual Flight Rule weather minimums for EMS helicopters, depending on the time of day and length of flight.[38] Most helicopter emergency medical services operate under visual flight rule (VFR) minimums, meaning that the pilot must have visual contact with the ground during all phases of flight. For day local flying, NEMSPA recommends a 500-foot ceiling with a 1-mile visibility compared to the night cross country flying guidelines of a 1000 foot ceiling and 3-mile visibility. To reduce pilot fatigue, the Federal Aviation Administration (FAA) now restricts the number of consecutive hours and the number of flying hours per shift.[48] To fulfill these rest requirements, a busy program needs a minimum of four pilots.

In Connecticut's critical care helicopter service, LIFE STAR, the pilot is blinded to the type of patient to be transported to avoid an emotional influence on the decision-making process. The pilot is given only the information necessary to make a weather decision before liftoff. This avoids acceptance of a transport for emotional reasons in marginal weather circumstances and enhances safety.

In general, a change of the thought pattern in aviation has occurred. The original expectation was to justify flight cancellation; however, the modern concept is to justify a flight acceptance.[47] Continuous monitoring of these aviation aspects is an ongoing process and encourages changes in the system, which will guarantee continued emphasis on safe flight operations.

MEDICAL FLIGHT CREW

Hospital-based emergency medical helicopter services provide ALS-trained flight crews, and many programs offer higher additional skill levels. Throughout the country, more than 50% of flight crews consist of a flight nurse and a paramedic.[49] Physicians, emergency medical technicians, and respiratory therapists are also used as flight crew members.

To date, no national flight nurse training course exists. In 1986, the National Flight Nurses Association printed national practice standards for flight nurses.[50] It was the intention of the association to ensure a high level of expert care offered by flight nurses across the country at the scene of an accident and during the transport of critically ill patients. An air medical crew national standard curriculum has been developed jointly by the U.S. Department of Transportation, Samaritan Air Evac, and the Association of Air Medical Services.[51] It provides a guideline for the training of flight crew members; however, standardized certification has not been established. Many hospital-based programs construct their own educational training courses. The 4-month flight nurse course for the critical care helicopter service for the State of Connecticut addresses the pathophysiology and treatment of disease processes.[41,52] The flight nurses rotate through the operating room, cardiac, surgical, neonatal, and pediatric intensive care units, accumulating expertise. The advanced skills that are perfected by the flight nurses before completion of the program are oral and nasotracheal intubations, cricothyroidotomies, insertion of central (subclavian or femoral) lines, needle thoracostomies, chest tube insertion, and intraosseous cannulations. Paramedic certification is also a standardized part of the course. To date, many different hospital programs require different courses, which may change if a national course is provided.

Quality assurance of the medical management at the scene or during transport is important to guarantee a high level of medical care. In Connecticut's critical care helicopter program, the medical director and the chief flight nurse review all flight run forms every other week in preparation for the biweekly morbidity/mortality conference. At these conferences, attended by all medical flight crew members, all deaths, complications, and difficult or interesting cases are presented by the flight nurse responsible for the transport. Scientific literature related to the case presented is distributed for discussion. This continuing education and skill assessment contributes to the higher level of medical care offered on emergency medical helicopters.

The impact of a physician as a medical flight crew member was studied by Baxt et al.[53] In a prospective randomized trial, a statistically significant reduction in mortality of bluntly injured patients treated aboard a medical helicopter emergency care service by a flight nurse and a flight physician was demonstrated when compared to a flight nurse-paramedic medical team. The small number of patients affected by this raises the question of availability and real need for this limited resource, the physician. Schwartz et al.[54] identified a subgroup of transports that benefitted from physician attendance. The objective measurement used was intubation success rate, which was found to increase on the scene transports when a physician was present with an experienced flight nurse. Critical interhospital transports did not objectively benefit from the presence of a physician. It is possible that, as a flight crew matures with experience, the impact of physician skills and judgment may decrease.

Some hospital-based programs offer specific teams of trained individuals depending on the medical diagnosis of the patient. A cardiac transport team staffed by a cardiologist, nurse, and two paramedics was formed to transfer critically ill cardiac patients to a university hospital by ground or air mode of transport.[55] The group of patients transported by this team were critically ill cardiac patients in that the majority, 62%, underwent significant hospital procedures. The benefit of the team in terms of improving patient outcome, however, was not studied. Other unique cases involve the transport of high-risk neonatal patients often accompanied by a neonatologist in addition to the regular flight crew. In terms of resources, the specific indications for these specialized teams has not been clearly defined.

EQUIPMENT

All hospital-based helicopter EMS offer advanced life support skills and are therefore equipped with the paramedic level equipment. This consists of pediatric and adult intubation equipment, intravenous peripheral catheters, intravenous fluids, advanced cardiac life support medications, and a cardiac monitor with defibrillation capability. In addition, many EMS helicopters, because of the higher level of medical care offered, carry more sophisticated equipment and medications such as automated blood pressure cuffs, infusion pumps for various vasoactive medications, chest tube and central line equipment, heated humidified oxygen, end tidal CO_2/pulse oximeter, neuromuscular blocking agents, and nebulized respiratory treatments.

The use of neuromuscular blocking agents, paralytics, for intubation by a flight crew has been reported.[56] Paralytics were used by a physician-flight nurse medical crew in intubating 24 patients at the scene of an accident. The intubation success rate for patients requiring paralytics was 100%, and no early complications were found. The overall success rate of intubating trauma patients in the field was 92.6% (n = 136). Another study compared the use of paralytic agents administered by a physician-flight nurse team to a control group. The control group consisted of patients transported from another hospital ED who were given a paralytic for the helicopter flight.[57] Intubation success rates and complication rates were similar for both groups of patients. This study concluded that paralytic agents could be safely used at accident scenes by a physician-flight nurse team. In the absence of physicians, some programs have protocols for the administration of these medications if necessary.

Hospital-based programs have the advantage of testing and incorporating pieces of equipment aboard the helicopter that are routine in intensive care units (ICUs) or operating rooms. The end tidal CO_2/pulse oximeter is such a device. This monitor measures respiratory rate, amount of exhaled carbon dioxide, and oxygen saturation of the blood. The end tidal CO_2 correlates well with pCO_2 levels and may be used as an aid to hyperventilation and endotracheal tube placement.[58] The monitor also has a graph displaying the depth of ventilation. Pulse oximetry allows oxygen saturation monitoring and is often a good predictor of respiratory failure. A sensor is placed on a patient's finger or nose (in pediatric patients, the sensor may be placed on a toe or around a foot). The sensor emits a light that is transmitted through the blood, where a portion of red and infrared light is absorbed by the blood.[59] The sensor detects the amount of light that is not absorbed, converts this to the oxygen saturation, and counts the pulse. A distinct reading occurs with each pulsation, allowing the crew to increase the amount of oxygen being delivered to the patient if necessary. A sudden decrease in the oxygen saturation may indicate some acute pulmonary process such as a tension pneumothorax. Because endotracheal intubation is frequently performed in critically ill or injured patients, monitoring changes in oxygenation and ventilation may prevent unexpected catastrophes. The availability and use of such pieces of equipment contributes to providing a more intense level of medical management.

Another piece of useful equipment was tested by a flight crew aboard a helicopter and reported by Schwartz et al.[60] In a prospective randomized trial, a "tube tamer" device used for securing endotracheal tubes was compared to the usual taping procedure. The tube holder is a fabricated device with a Velcro piece that attaches to the tube. In this crossover study, the tube tamer was found to be significantly better than tape and benzoin in terms of speed and success rate of application. Although it was tested in an aeromedical program, its use was recommended in all prehospital intubations.

Long, in Portland, Oregon, has organized a cardiac transport team specifically for patients requiring intra-aortic balloon pump therapy during transport. The cardiac transport team is responsible for the insertion of the balloon at the referring hospital and the patient is transported by "Life Flight," Emmanuel Hospital's helicopter program, using a portable balloon pump device. Organized teams, available from the sponsor hospital for helicopter missions, enable innovative therapies to be extended outside the tertiary care center. This allows therapy to begin earlier in the disease process.

IMPACT ON MEDICAL CARE

Aeromedical helicopter transport affects medical care by offering several advantages. Flight crews, because of the concentrated experience in transporting only critically ill patients coupled with a higher level of medical expertise, may improve patient outcome by treating disease earlier. The speed of the helicopter provides rapid transport without the problem of obstructed traffic or terrain. Patients transported by EMS helicopters are generally taken only to higher levels of hospital care. Improving the survival of critically ill patients with the use of helicopter transport probably is the result of the three advantages.

Trauma patients account for a large proportion of EMS helicopter transports. The American College of Surgeons has published guidelines on triage to Level I Trauma Centers from the scene of an accident and interhospital transfers.[15] Appendix D of these guidelines lists indications for interhospital helicopter transport for trauma, burn, neonatal, high-risk pregnancy, cardiac, and acute medical patients. Appendix F describes the triage decision scheme for scene trauma patients. These indications should be used in educational programs for all individuals involved in transferring patients to tertiary care facilities.

One of the first papers reporting the effect of helicopter transport on trauma patient outcomes was published by Baxt and Moody in 1983.[61] Trauma patient outcome was predicted using the TRISS methodology for ground and air transported trauma patients.[62-64] TRISS combines calculation of the trauma score,[65] a physiologic index of severity, and the injury severity score,[66] an anatomic index of severity. Based on these two numbers, the outcomes of patients are compared to the probabilities of survival in a large trauma patient population to determine any effect of the variable being studied. In Baxt's study,[61] the TRISS methodology demonstrated that the outcome of the ground transported patients was statistically no different from that of a large trauma patient population treated at a major trauma center. A statistically significant 52% reduction in predicted mortality for the helicopter transported group was found, however. This was attributed to a highly trained medical crew (flight nurse/physician team) capable of performing a wide variety of procedures.

The concept of air versus ground ambulance transport of trauma patients has been extensively studied.[61,67-76] A review of this literature demonstrates an advantage of rotorcraft in air medical transport except in the area of urban transport, where controversery does exist. Schiller et al.[75] compared ground transports to helicopter transports in an urban environment, Phoenix, Arizona. The two groups were similar in trauma score and the number of patients with head injuries. No statistically significant mortality differences were found between the two groups. Injury severity scores were not calculated in the two populations, and therefore probability of survival could not be compared using the TRISS methodology. This is important because the two groups may in fact have been different on the basis of severity of injury. When considering air transport for urban patients, the level of care and availability of ground transport in the area is an important factor. Pheonix has a well developed and integrated ground prehospital system with accessible trauma centers. This may not be true for other urban areas in the country, and therefore care must be taken when extrapolating this data. The Houston program, an urban setting, reviewed 577 flights to the scene of an accident over a 1-year period.[68] Because the overall mortality rate was 35.7%, it was determined that the helicopter was called appropriately. The benefit of air transport could not be established, however, because a ground cohort group was not identified. This study concluded that, in the large metropolitan area of Houston, with poor freeway systems limiting rapid access to trauma centers, aeromedical transport is indicated. As in rural transports, the benefit of aeromedical transport of trauma patients injured in an urban environment depends on accessibility to the trauma centers and level of prehospital care available.

The advantages of helicopter transport in rural communities are much more obvious. Some of the reasons accounting for the differences when compared to the urban setting include longer transport times, longer distances to trauma centers, and a generally lower level of prehospital care available in less densely populated areas. In 1966, the National Academy of Science published a study on accidental death and disability.[8] They reported that 70% of fatal accidents occurred in rural regions. At that time, a patient was four times more likley to die from injury in a rural than an urban environment. Boyd[76] studied rural interhospital transfers of trauma patients, comparing ground versus helicopter modes of transport. Using two similar cohorts, which differed only in the method of transport, he calculated the probability of survivals based on the TRISS methodology. The patients transported by ground had the same mortality as predicted by TRISS calculations. The aeromedically transported patients had a 25% reduction in predicted mortality. The reduction in mortality had the greatest impact in the group with a greater than 10% chance of dying (i.e., probability of survival less than 90%). In this rural area of Georgia, time to definitive care at a Trauma Center was statistically greater in the ground-transported group. The rapid aeromedical transport may have contributed to the survival differences. The role of a helicopter in rural transport has been clearly established.[57,70–72,76]

Although time is an important factor in the treatment of trauma patients, improved survival of trauma patients transported by hospital-based helicopter services may be from other factors. Baxt et al.[74] reported the lowest mortality rate, 32%, for head-injured patients with a Glasgow Coma Score less than or equal to 8 who were transported by an aeromedical crew consisting of a physician and a nurse. In this study, a comparable ground-transported group was identified. Time to intubation, number of patients intubated and hyperventilated during transport, and time to the trauma center were similar in both groups. The better survival rate in the aeromedically transported group was speculated to be caused by a better communication system and integration of the helicopter service with the trauma center. Immediate head computed tomography (CT) scans were performed in 46% of the air-transported patients as compared to 3% of the ground-transported patients. Aeromedical programs are often considered extensions of the trauma center, providing the highest available level of prehospital care directly at the scene of the accident.

The benefit of aeromedical transport to the nontrauma patient is difficult to quantify. Trauma patients are categorized based on objective measures, trauma score and injury severity score, which are predictive of survival. For example, in the cardiac patient, the Killip classification[77] applies only to patients with acute myocardial infarction. Its use in predicting complications during transport and therefore outcome may be questioned because it does not include magnitude of chest pain and arrhythmias. In the cardiac literature, the patient populations of the transported patients may be dissimilar, and therefore the impact of the mode of transport is difficult to determine.[78] Complication rates for the transport of cardiac patients vary in the literature from 0% to 32%, dependent on the patient population transported and the definition of complication.[78–81] Aeromedical transport of the cardiac patient has been determined to be safe; however, the added benefit of helicopter transport cannot be substantiated because of the difficulty in performing comparison studies. Work is needed to standardize cardiac patient populations and other nontrauma patient populations to better define appropriate helicopter use.

FUTURE ISSUES

In the next generation of helicopter emergency medical services, several changes may occur. Safety, flight crew training, equipment, research, and quality assurance are most likely to be affected.

Currently, certain additional safety features for helicopter use are being tested. Regulation regarding the mandatory use of these features, such as helmets, night vision enhancement devices, and fireproof suits may occur in the near future.

No national certification exists for medical flight crew members. The introduction of a national curriculum[51] may eventually lead to national certification. Hospitals, however, may prefer to continue to offer their own educational training programs to flight crew members, tailoring them to the specific needs of their programs. Quality assurance has already infiltrated the medical aspect of helicopter programs. The Association of Air Medical Services, an organization representing emergency air medical services, has recently introduced standards specifically relating to quality assurance of dispatch centers.[82] Accountability from all segments of a medical aviation program is a trend for the future.

More sophisticated devices are expected to be developed for routine helicopter transport use. The use of a portable intra-aortic balloon pump has increased in several helicopter programs. A portable high ultra-frequency jet ventilator, developed by Gluck from Hartford, Connecticut and Advanced Pulmonary Technologies of Glastonbury, Connecticut, has been used in fixed-wing transports and is expected to be evaluated in helicopter medical transportation. The close integration and high medical expertise of flight programs with their sponsor hospital allows ease in testing new technology compared to ground ambulance services.

Research efforts involving earlier treatment protocols for trauma as well as nontrauma patients may occur as scene transports increase. The opportunity to study early metabolic and hormonal changes of injured patients, which may impact on ultimate survival, is becoming possible. The identification of these early factors may lead to changes in treatment modalities, which may be instituted at the scene of the accident. Because helicopter programs are associated with tertiary care centers, alteration of care through well-designed prospective research studies is achievable. Providing the best care and at the same time the most appropriate care are goals of tertiary care centers.

Health care costs are rising, and therefore a continued audit of helicopter programs should be conducted to ensure appropriate transfers. A paper published by Schwartz, et. al.[83] documented a significantly decreased length of hospital stay and charges for patients transported directly from the scene of an accident to the trauma center compared to transfer from a small community hospital. These patients were matched for injury severity. The differences in charges for both groups was more pronounced for air- as opposed to ground-transported patients. The initial charge for helicopter services may be offset by the savings in length of stay and hospital charges. More research is needed to document any functional changes in patients transported rapidly by helicopter services.

CONCLUSION

Ground and air prehospital transport in the civilian arena have developed substantially during the past 30 years. Each mode has specific indications for use, and together they have contributed to the success of prehospital care. As technology increases, quality assurance will become more important to document appropriate use of each component of the system. Prehospital medical care has been shown to save lives. Identifying the positive and negative aspects of the system to improve medical care even further while controlling health care costs is a challenge for the next decade.

REFERENCES

1. Rockwood, C.A., Mann, C.M. Farrington, J.D., et al: History of Emergency Medical Services in the United States. J. Trauma 16:299, 1976.
2. Jacobs, L.M., and Bennett, B.R.: Emergency Medical Services. In The MGH Textbook of Emergency Medicine. Edited by Wilkins, E. Baltimore, Williams & Wilkins, 1983.
3. Trunkey, D.D.: Trauma. Sci. Am. 249:28, 1983.
4. Jacobs, L.M.: Initial management and evaluation of the multisystem injured patient, Part 1. J. Nat. Med. Assoc. 79:361, 1987.
5. Committee on Trauma Research Commission on Life Sciences National Research Council and the Institute of Medicine: Injury in America—A continuing Public Health Problem. Washington, DC, National Academy Press, 1985.
6. American College of Surgeons Committee on Trauma: Hospital and Pre-Hospital Resources for Optimal Care of the Injured Patient. February, 1987.
7. McSwain, N.E., and Timberlake, G.A.: Controversial Issues in Pre-Hospital Care. Top. Emerg. Med. 9:1, 1987.
8. National Academy of Sciences' National Research Council: Accidental Death and Disability: The Neglected Disease of Modern Society. Washington,DC, National Academy Press, 1966.
9. Pantridge, J.F., and Geddes, J.S.: Cardiac Arrest After Myocardial Infarction. Lancet 1:807, 1966.
10. Grace, W.J., and Chadbourn, J.A.: The mobile coronary care unit. Dis. Chest. 55:452, 1969.
11. Pantridge, J.F.: The effect of early therapy on the hospital mortality from acute myocardial infarction. Q.J. Med. 39:621, 1970.
12. Grace, W.J., and Chadbourn, J.A.: The first hour in acute myocardial infarction. Heart Lung 3:736, 1974.
13. Lambrew, C.T.: The experience in telemetry of the electrocardiogram to a base hospital. Heart Lung 3:756, 1974.
14. Federal Specifications—Ambulance—Emergency Medical Care Vehicle. USGSA, January 2, 1974. KKK-A-1822.
15. American College of Surgeons Committee on Trauma: Essential Equipment for Ambulances. Bull. Am. Coll. Surg. 1970; 55:7, 1970.
16. Stohler, S., and Jacobs, B.B.: Interhospital Transfer of the Critical Patient. Emerg. Care Q. 4:66, 1989.
17. Jacobs, L.M., Berrizbeitia, L.D., Bennett, B., and Madigan, C.: Endotracheal intubation in the pre-hospital phase of emergency medical care. JAMA 250:2175, 1983.
18. Dean, N.C., Haug, P.J., and Hawker, P.J.: Effect of mobile paramedic units on outcome in patients with myocardial infarction. Ann. Emerg. Med. 17:1034, 1988.
19. Jacobs, L.M., Sinclair, A., Beiser, A., and D'Agostino, R.B.: Pre-hospital advanced life support: Benefits in trauma. J. Trauma 24:8, 1984.
20. Shuster, M., and Chong, J.: Pharmacologic intervention in prehospital care: a critical appraisal. Ann. Emerg. Med. 18:192, 1989.
21. Gervin, A.S., and Fischer, R.P.: The importance of prompt transport in salvage of patients with penetrating heart wounds. J. Trauma 22:443, 1982.
22. Lambrew, C.T., Carveth, S.W., and McIntyre, K.M.: Advanced cardiac life support (ACLS) in perspective. In Textbook of Advanced Cardiac Life Support. Edited by McIntyre, K.M., and Lewis, A.J., 1983, pp. 3–10.
23. Eisenberg, M., Bergner, L., and Hallstrom, A.: Paramedic programs and out-of-hospital cardiac arrest: I. Factors associated with successful resuscitation. Am. J. Public Health 69:30, 1979.
24. Champion, H.R., Gainer, P.S., and Yackee, E.: A progress report on the trauma score in predicting fatal outcome. J. Trauma 26:927, 1986.
25. Dolev. E.: The first recorded aeromedical evacuation in the British Army—The true story. J.R. Army Med. Corps 132:34, 1986.
26. Barger, J.: Strategic aeromedical evacuation: The inaugural flight. Aviat. Space Environ. Med. 57:613, 1986.
27. Neel, S.: Helicopter Evacuation in Korea. U.S.A.F. Med. J. 6:681, 1955.
28. Pons, P.T.: Advances in prehospital care: The technology of Emergency Medical Services. Med. Instrum. 22:143, 1988.
29. Neel, S.: Army aeromedical evacuation procedures in Vietnam. JAMA 204:309, 1968.
30. Felix, W.R.: Metropolitan aeromedical service: State of the art. J. Trauma 16:873, 1976.
31. Stapleton, K: The Hover Jumpers. Rotoways 2:11, 1970.
32. Helicopters in Emergency Medical Service, NHTSA experience to date. Washington, DC, U.S. Government Printing Office DOT H5820231, 1972.
33. Cleveland, H.C., Bigelow, D.B., Dracon, D., and Dusty, F.: A civilian air emergency service: A report of its development, technical aspects and experience. J. Trauma 16:452, 1976.
34. Thomas, F.: The development of the nation's oldest operating civilian hospital-sponsored aeromedical helicopter service. Aviat. Space Environ. Med. 59:567, 1988.
35. Cowart, V.S.: Helicopter, other air ambulances: Time to assess effectiveness. JAMA 253:2469, 1985.
36. Collett, H.M.: Mid year report. Hosp. Aviat. 8:26, 1989.
37. Collett, H.M.: Annual Transport Statistics. Hosp. Aviat. 8:3, 1989.
38. Hodges, J.: Aeromedical transport. Emerg. Care Q. 4:1, 1989. 1–12
39. Ramzy, A.I.: The Maryland EMS System. Emerg. Care Q. 6: (In press)
40. Gomex, G.A.: The emergency medical services of Dade County Florida. Emerg. Care Q. 6: (In press)
41. Jacobs, L.M., Bennett-Jacobs, B.B., and Schwartz, R.: A medical helicopter transportation system for Connecticut. Conn. Med. 49:489, 1985.
42. Collett, H.M.: 1989 Transport Charge Survey. Hosp. Aviat. 8:19, 1989.
43. Jensen, D.: More room at the top. Rotor Wing Int 1986; 20:26, 1986.
44. Negrette, A.J.: Pilot Report: BK117 A-3 Agility Joining Function. Rotor Wing Int. November, 1987.
45. Analysis of 84 Aeromedical Helicopter Accidents for the Period 1975 to 1986. Aviation Safety Institute. Worthington, OH 1986 H614–885–4242.
46. Manningham, D.: The EMS Safety Dilemma. Bus. Comm. Aviat., May 1987.
47. Collett, H.M.: Risk management and the aeromedical helicopter. Emerg. Care Q. 2:31, 1986.
48. CFR 14 Part 135. Office ot the Federal Register. National Archives and Records Administration. Washington, DC. Revised January, 1989.
49. Association of Hospital Based Emergency Air Medical Services: 1988 Membership Directory. Pasadena, California.

50. National Flight Nurse Association: Practice Standards for Flight Nursing. Columbia, MO, Waters Printing Company, 1986.
51. U.S. Department of Transportation, NHTSA: Air Medical Crew National Standard Curriculum. ASHBEAMS, Pasadena, California, 1988.
52. Jacobs, B.B., and Jacobs, L.M.: An educational program for flight nurses. *In* Proceedings of the International Aeromedical Evacuation Congress. Zurich, Switzerland, International Aeromedical Evacuation Congress, 1985, pp. 223–4.
53. Baxt, W.G., and Moody, P.: The impact of a physician as part of the aeromedical prehospital team in patients with blunt trauma. JAMA *257*:3246, 1987.
54. Schwartz, R.J., Jacobs, L.M., and Lee, M.: The role of the physician in a helicopter emergency medical service. Prehospital and Disaster Medicine *5*:31, 1990.
55. Gore, J.M., et al.: Evaluation of an emergency cardiac transport system. Ann. Emerg. Med. *12*:675, 1983.
56. Gabram, S.G., Jacobs, L.M., Schwartz, R.J., and Stohler, S.S.: Airway intubation in injured patients at the scene of an accident. Conn. Med. *53*:633, 1989.
57. Syverud, S.A., Barron, S.W., Storer, D.L., and Hedges, J.R.: Prehospital use of neuromuscular blocking agents in a helicopter ambulance program. Ann. Emerg. Med. *17*:236, 1988.
58. Gemmel, C., and Jacobs, L.M.: The use of end tidal CO2/pulse oximeter on an EMS helicopter. Presented at the Association of Hospital Based Emergency Air Medical Services Meeting, Milwaukee, Wisconsin, 1987.
59. Cohen, M.J., and Jacobs, L.M.: Transcutaneous and transconjunctival Oximetry. Emerg. Care Q. *3*:72, 1987.
60. Schwartz, R.J., Salonia, R., and Jacobs, L.M.: Prospective evaluation of methods to secure endotracheal tubes. Hosp. Aviat. *8*:6, 1989.
61. Baxt, W.G., and Moody, P.: The impact of a rotorcraft aeromedical Emergency care service on trauma mortality. JAMA *249*:3047, 1983.
62. Champion, H.R., Frey, C.F., and Sacco, W.J.: Determination of national normative outcomes for trauma. J. Trauma *24*:651, 1984.
63. Major trauma outcome study. Bull. Am. Coll. Surg. *68*:40, 1983.
64. Boyd, C.R., and Tolson, M.: Evaluating trauma care: The TRISS Method. J. Trauma *27*:370, 1987.
65. Champion, H.R., et al.: Trauma Score. Crit. Care Med. *9*:672, 1981.
66. Baker, S.P., O'Neill, B., Haddon, W., and Long, W.B.: The injury severity score: A method for describing patients with multiple injuries and evaluating emergency care. J. Trauma *14*:187, 1974.
67. Urdaneta, L.F., et al.: Evaluation of an emergency air transport service as a component of a rural EMS system. Am. Surg. *50*:183, 1984.
68. Fischer, R.P., Flynn, T.C., Miller, P.W., and Duke, J.H.: Urban helicopter response to the scene of injury. J. Trauma *24*:946, 1984.
69. Baxt, W.B., et al.: Hospital-based rotorcraft aero medical emergency care services and trauma mortality: A multicenter study. Ann. Emerg. Med. *14*:859, 1985.
70. Leicht, M.J., et al: Rural interhospital helicopter transport of motor vehicle trauma victims: Causes for delays and recommendations. Ann. Emerg. Med. *15*:450, 1986.
71. Urdaneta, L.F., et al.: Role of an emergency helicopter transport service in rural trauma. Arch. Surg. *122*:992, 1987.
72. Anderson, T.E., Rose, W.D., and Leicht, M.J.: Physician-staffed helicopter scene response from a rural trauma center. Ann. Emerg. Med. *16*:85, 1987.
73. Baxt, W.G., and Moody, P.: The impact of a physician as part of the aeromedical prehospital team in patients with blunt trauma. JAMA *257*:3246, 1987.
74. Baxt, W.G., and Moody, P.: The impact of advanced prehospital emergency care on the mortality of severely brain-injured patients. J. Trauma *27*:365, 1987.
75. Schiller, W.R., et al.: Effect of helicopter transport of trauma victims on survival in an urban trauma center. J. Trauma *28*:1127, 1988.
76. Boyd, C.R., Corse, K.M., and Campbell, R.C.: Emergency interhospital transport of the major trauma patient: Air versus ground. J. Trauma *29*:789, 1989.
77. Killip, T., and Kimball, J.T.: Treatment of myocardial infarction in a coronary care unit. Am. J. Cariol. *20*:457, 1967.
78. Schneider, S., et al.: Critical cardiac transport. Air versus ground? Am. J. Emerg. Med. *6*:449, 1988.
79. Kaplan, L., Walsh, D., and Burney, R.E.: Emergency aeromedical transport of patients with acute myocardial infarction. Ann. Emerg. Med. *16*:55, 1987.
80. Bellinger, R.L., et al.: Helicopter transport of patients during acute myocardial infarction. Am. J. Cardiol. *61*:718, 1988.
81. Gabram, S.G., Piacentini, L., and Jacobs, L.M.: The risk of aeromedical transport for the cardiac patient. Emerg. Care Q. *5*:72, 1990.
82. Association of Air Medical Services. Safety Standard Guidelines, Pasadena, California, 1988.
83. Schwartz, R.J., Jacobs, L.M., and Yaezel, D.: Impact of pretrauma center care on length of stay and hospital charges. J. Trauma *29*:1611, 1989.

DISASTER PLANNING AND OPERATION IN THE EMERGENCY DEPARTMENT

Eric K. Noji

CAPSULE

This chapter addresses issues related to medical planning and response to disasters and mass casualty events with a particular emphasis on Emergency Department (ED) disaster protocols. Key elements in hospital disaster planning are described, including community hazard analysis, community disaster agencies and organizations, disaster training, roles and responsibilities for those reponsible for disaster operations, supply, manpower and equipment logistics, requirements of the Joint Commission on the Accreditation of Healthcare Organizations, and the purposes, responsibilities, and principles of triage.

INTRODUCTION

Natural disasters such as earthquakes, cyclones, tsunamis (tidal waves), and volcanic eruptions have claimed about 3 million lives worldwide during the past 20 years, adversely affecting the lives of at least 800 million more people, and have caused property damages exceeding $23 billion.[1] Although past disasters have produced their share of massive casualty situations, the future appears to be even more bleak. Increasing population density in flood plains and in seismic and hurricane-prone areas, the development and transportation of thousands of toxic and hazardous materials, the potential risks that can occur from incidents at fixed-site nuclear and chemical facilities, and the catastrophic possibilities from massive fires and explosions, all point to the probability of large mass casualty occasions in the future.[2,3] Recent catastrophes have included the Bhopal chemical accident in 1984, the Mexico City earthquake in 1985, the Chernobyl nuclear power plant accident in 1986, the Armenian earthquake and Hurricane Gilbert in 1988, and most recently, Hurricane Hugo in 1989.

Because of these recent events, much international attention has become focused on the problem of effectively dealing with natural and technological disasters.[4-7] In fact, the United Nations General Assembly has recently designated the 1990s as The International Decade of Natural Disaster Reduction (IDNDR), during which a concerted international effort will be made by the world's scientific community to reduce the loss of life and damage caused by natural disasters.[8]

The purpose of this chapter is to discuss disaster planning and operations with particular emphasis on the ED. Despite efficient field management of disaster victims, a rapid flow of victims from a disaster scene can quickly overwhelm a hospital emergency department.[9-11] The point at which the ED becomes overwhelmed often varies according to the time of day, the nature of the injuries, and the amount of preparation time before the arrival of victims.[12-16] When it appears that normal procedures will be overwhelmed, EDs must have a specific set of protocols that direct the mobilization of personnel and equipment outside of the ED and permit rapid assessment, stabilization, and triage to definitive care of victims of a mass casualty incident.[17-26]

DEFINITION OF DISASTER

Before discussing how to manage disasters, we must first define what is meant by a disaster. A situation that overwhelms the resources of a small rural community hospital may be a rather routine event at a large university teaching medical center.[19,27-29] Examples are a multivehicle accident involving 4 or 5 seriously injured persons, or a case of a family presenting with carbon monoxide poisoning. On the other hand, more than 25 patients at one time overwhelm even the best staffed trauma center.[11] According to the World Health Organization, a disaster can be defined as a sudden ecologic phenomenon of sufficient magnitude to require external assistance.[4,5] At the community level, this can be defined operationally as any community emergency that seriously affects people's lives and property and exceeds the capacity of the community to effectively respond to that emergency.[30]

From the standpoint of the ED, a disaster exists when the number of patients and/or severity of illness or injury are such that normal daily ED operations are no longer possible. In other words, a situation exists in which the number of patients presenting in a given time are such that the ED cannot offer even minimal care for them without external assistance.[13,14,31] Disasters characterized by the production of large numbers of deaths and injuries are also referred to as "mass casualty incidents."[12,32,33] On the other hand, disasters certainly cannot be defined simply by a given number of victims. Large university hospitals may not have the facilities to manage even two chemically contaminated patients.[34-37] The arrival of one important political person with severe injuries (e.g., President of the United States, the Pope) can completely disrupt normal operations of even the most efficient ED.[38,39]

Regardless of how a disaster is defined numerically or situationally for a given institution, there is a point at which it is impossible for any ED to continue normal operations.[14,40-42] At this point, it is imperative that the hospital and, more specifically, the ED institute a pre-established protocol for effectively dealing with such an extraordinary situation. These new protocols (e.g., mobilization of appropriate outside assistance) must be instituted rapidly to reduce potential morbidity and mortality.

In many hospitals in the United States, disasters are often divided further into external or internal events.[43] External disasters are events that occur physically outside the hospital (e.g., transportation accidents, terrorist actions, etc.). As a result of this external event, patients are brought to the hospital from the outside, usually to the ED. Unless the outside disaster was a chemical accident with contaminated patients, the hospital and its staff, patients, and visitors are in no immediate physical danger.[44]

Internal disasters are events that occur within the physical plant of the hospital itself (e.g., fire, laboratory accident involving radioactive material) that severely compromise the ability of the hospital to function.[45,46] Of course, a disaster may be both internal and external, for example, an earthquake that severely damages the hospital.[47,48] Such events may damage the infrastructure of the hospital and its equipment as well as injure or kill hospital staff, patients, and visitors.

TYPES OF DISASTER

Disasters can be classified into natural and man-made.[49] Natural disasters include earthquakes, hurricanes, floods, tsunamis, fires, tornadoes and extremes of temperature. Man-made events include transportation accidents, chemical or nuclear power plant accidents, and civil disturbances.[3] Of course, a technologic disaster may result from a natural disaster, for example, a chemical plant accident resulting from an earthquake.

CHARACTER OF MASS CASUALTY EVENTS INVOLVING EDs

Extensive disaster research over approximately the past 30 years has shown that EDs experience great difficulty coping with even moderate numbers of patients following a disaster.[50-52] The reasons for this difficulty include confusion, lack of planning, and lack of emergency training. Hospitals are often not well integrated into overall community disaster planning.[53] Hospital disaster plans often exist only on paper and are rarely referred to, let alone carried out during a real disaster. Shortcomings of disaster plans include:

1. Delayed or improper notification
2. Poor delineation of command structure
3. Overloaded or broken communications networks
4. Improper or incomplete identification
5. Lack of supplies
6. Lack of public relations

What usually happens in the ED when a disaster occurs in the community? Transportation of patients to the ED is usually uncoordinated with no thought to equitable distribution of patients.[54] As a result, nearby hospitals are usually overwhelmed with the majority of severely injured patients, while those further away see few patients.[55] There is also a pattern to ED patient flow during a disaster. Most casualties are transported to the hospital over a relatively short period, i.e., most patients arrive at the ED within 1½ hours after the disaster has occurred.[10] On the whole, most of the patients presenting to an ED in a disaster have minor injuries and do not require advanced trauma services.[55]

Victims of mass casualty events may arrive at hospitals by various means, including ambulances, private automobiles, police vehicles, cabs, and on foot.[56-59] As a result, hospitals may receive patients in all sorts of unplanned ways, and the patient flow is essentially not under the control of the formal EMS system.[10] Interestingly, ambulatory patients and those with relatively minor injuries may arrive at the ED before the more serious cases. This is because they are able to leave the disaster site in taxis, buses, private cars, vans, and police vehicles. The more severely injured, who often need extrication, arrive at a later stage. The result is that less severely injured patients often tend to be treated before the more seriously injured.[10] A large number of ambulatory cases arriving early can create serious problems in that the ED may become badly overcrowded early, resulting in confusion in the efforts to provide treatment. Similarly, when attention is being paid to early arrivals at a hospital, it is easy for the more seriously injured cases brought in later not to be noticed immediately or to be given delayed treatment.

Because of this phenomenon, announcements of numbers of patients to be brought to the ED by the local emergency communications center or by the on-site command post may greatly underestimate the total number of patients who actually arrive at the ED's door. Under normal circumstances, an ED is prepared to manage a few critically ill or injured individuals at one time. When confronted by large numbers of patients simultaneously, and especially when patients begin arriving with little or no advance warning, the resulting disruption of operations may severely impair an otherwise efficient department.[60]

Under these circumstances, walk-in or highly vocal patients may be examined before critically injured or unconscious victims. The established triage process is abandoned. Rescuers, emergency technicians, family members, and reporters may rapidly converge on the department and contribute to the development of a chaotic, unmanageable environment. Under such circumstances, patient care becomes less efficient and the staff experiences undue psychologic stress. The confusion may continue to escalate as news of the situation spreads and family members of victims and onlookers of every sort converge on the ED.[60]

DISASTER PLANNING

OVERVIEW

Roles, responsibilities, and working relationships between those responsible for disaster operations should be clarified in the planning process to lessen the confusion that invariably occurs during a disaster event. Selected protocols should require personnel to perform functions that are relatively similar to their day-to-day activities.[61–63]

The disaster planning process should begin by answering the following questions:

1. What types of disasters are most likely to occur in the community (e.g., hazard analysis).[64]
2. What are the disaster planning requirements of the Joint Commission on the Accreditation of Healthcare Organizations (JCAHO), as well as other accreditation bodies (e.g., city, and state health agencies)?[65]
3. What are the capabilities and responsibilities of the hospital?[24]

HAZARD ANALYSIS

Hospital disaster planners must plan for those disasters most likely to occur in their community.[20] Hos-

pitals along the Gulf Coast of the United States should plan for hurricanes,[57] those in California should plan for earthquakes,[47] those near chemical industries should have facilities for decontamination.[35] Are there large transportation facilities nearby (e.g., airports, harbors) where accidents could generate large numbers of casualties?[66] Are there festivals, stadiums and amusement parks nearby where large numbers of people assemble?[67] It is important to have knowledge of those disasters most prevalent in the area since different disasters are characterized by very different morbidity and mortality patterns and thus health care requirements.[49,64,68,69] For example, earthquakes cause many deaths and severe injuries.[70] Hurricanes cause much property damage, however, deaths are usually low and injuries minor.[4] Pulmonary irritation may result from fires or hazardous chemicals requiring large supplies of oxygen as the Bhopal accident demonstrated.[34,71]

Fortunately, some disasters such as hurricanes are predictable or have several days lead time and preparations for management can begin early if disaster managers heed warning signals.

JCAHO REQUIREMENTS FOR HOSPITAL DISASTER PLANNING

There are other motivations for hospitals to plan for potential disasters. The Joint Commission on the Accreditation of Healthcare Organizations (JCAHO) requires that member hospitals have a written plan for the timely care of casualties arising from both external and internal disasters, and the hospital must document the rehearsal of these plans (Fig. 87-12).[65]

CAPABILITIES OF HOSPITALS TO MANAGE A DISASTER

A plan must be based on the institution's capabilities, which may range from basic first aid to the most sophisticated trauma and intensive care services available. Each hospital's bed capacity and average bed availability should be known as well as additional areas that could set up for triage, staging, and resuscitation.[13] Hospital treatment capacity (HTC) can be defined operationally as the number of casualties that can be treated according to normal medical standards in one hour.[72] HTC depends on several factors, including the total number of emergency physicians and nurses, surgeons, anesthesiologists, operating rooms, intensive care beds, etc. If the disaster takes place at night or on the weekend, the HTC will be lower than the HTC during the morning of a weekday. As a rough figure, obtained empirically through analyses of several disasters and simulations involving hospitals of different sizes, HTC can be estimated at 3% of the total number of beds.[72]

Based on military experience, one can also estimate a hospital's surgical capacity, that is, the number of seriously injured patients that can be operated on

STANDARD ON EMERGENCY PREPAREDNESS

The hospital has an emergency preparedness program designed to provide for the effective utilization of available resources so that patient care can be continued during a disaster.

REQUIRED CHARACTERISTICS

1. A hospital designated as a disaster emergency center by a local authority such as the fire department or civil defense agency has an emergency preparedness program that addresses disasters both external and internal to the hospital.
2. Concise, documented plans to be implemented during a disaster are established through the emergency preparedness program.
   2.1 Emergency preparedness plans provide for the effective utilization of available resources to prevent or minimize the consequences of a disaster.
   2.2 Emergency preparedness plans are pertinent to a variety of disasters and are based on the hospital's capabilities and limitations.
3. The role of the hospital in communitywide disaster plans is identified in the emergency preparedness program.
4. The emergency preparedness program addresses hospital preparedness, including space utilization, supplies, communication systems, security, and utilities.
5. The emergency preparedness program addresses staff preparedness, including staffing requirements and the designation of roles and functions, particularly in terms of capabilities and limitations.
6. The emergency preparedness program addresses patient management, including modified schedules, criteria for the ces-

sation of nonessential services, and patient transfer determinations, particularly in terms of discharge and relocation.
7. The emergency preparedness program is implemented, evaluated, and documented semiannually.
   7.1 Each implementation (whether a drill or an actual emergency) exercises emergency preparedness plan elements to hospital preparedness, staff preparedness, and patient management; at least one implementation includes an influx of patients from outside the hospital.
   7.2 Documentation of the emergency preparedness program includes, at the least, problems identified during implementation, corrective actions taken, and staff participation.
8. There is a fire plan that addresses the use and function of fire alarm and detection systems, containment, and the protection of lives, including transfer to areas of refuge, evacuation plans, and fire extinguishment.
   8.1 It is recommended that on each work shift the hospital have appropriately trained personnel responsible for assisting with the implementation of the fire plan and the activation of the nonautomatic components of the fire safety systems. . . . The fire plan is implemented at least quarterly for each work shift of hospital personnel in each patient-occupied building. Documentation of the implementation of the plan includes, at a minimum, problems identified during implementation, corrective actions taken, and staff participation.
9. Hospital employees and staff are provided with appropriate education and training in elements of the emergency preparedness program and in elements of the fire plan.
10. The emergency preparedness program is evaluated annually and is updated as needed.

FIG. 87-12.   Joint commission disaster planning requirements for hospitals. With permission from Standard 5: Standards on Plant, Technology, and Safety Management, Accreditation Manual for Hospitals, 1987. Joint Commission on Accreditation of Healthcare Organizations, 1987.

within a 12-hour period as follows: The number of operating rooms $\times$ 7 $\times$ 0.25.[73] Thus a 300-bed hospital with 5 operating rooms should theoretically be able to care for 8 or 9 seriously injured disaster casualties within a 12-hour time span. Unless there is considerable preplanning, however, this does not mean that this hospital can handle 36 casualties in 48 hours. Instruments and supplies are likely to be limiting factors.

A hospital also has a responsibility to inform those responsible for community disaster planning and response (e.g., police, fire, rescue and EMS, etc.) of its emergency care capabilities and limitations in handling a disaster, both before and during a disaster.[20,74] These reports should be continually updated as patients are discharged and additional staff are available to care for the patients.

HOSPITAL-COMMUNITY COOPERATION IN DISASTER PLANNING

As noted above, it is imperative that every hospital integrate its own disaster plan with those of community disaster management agencies.[25] This is especially important regarding disaster notification and communications, transportation of casualties, and provisions for dispatch of hospital medical teams to a disaster site. The number of community agencies that have some responsibility for disaster planning and response can be bewildering.[75,76] Some of these are listed in Table 87-13.

Other organizations that a hospital may interact with during the disaster planning process may include the military, local chapters of the Red Cross and other volunteer agencies, along with state, and federal agencies (e.g., Federal Emergency Management Agency).

Medical planning for disasters in the community is usually the responsibility of local emergency medical services (EMS) councils.[27,62] Such councils include representatives from the local ambulance services, fire department, physician, EMS director, and other nonmedical and government agencies. It is essential that physicians involved in community disaster planning be familiar with the local EMS communications and treatment protocols.[77,78]

The hospital must also develop its external disaster plan in conjunction with other emergency facilities in the community. For example, mutual aid agreements should be prearranged with hospitals outside the immediate area if hospital capacities are exceeded.[79-81] There should also be preplanning for referral to area tertiary centers and special units (e.g., burn, spinal cord, pediatric trauma centers).[19,82]

Hospital disaster planners should anticipate that information about specific hazards (e.g., chemicals, radiation), expert personnel (e.g., poison control) and special supplies (e.g., antidotes) that are not readily available may be needed in a particular disaster situation.[36,83] Plans should consider how to rapidly access these resources. Plans for obtaining additional shelter, food, and water should also be considered.

TABLE 87-13. COMMUNITY AGENCIES INVOLVED IN DISASTER PLANNING

Community Agency	Responsibilities
EMS service	Victim triage, stabilization, and transfer to definitive care facility
Fire service	Overall scene command. Victim rescue and hazard control
Police service	Traffic management and scene security
Emergency manager	Communications, personnel, and equipment support. Liaison with state and federal agencies.
Public works	Support equipment and personnel. Structure safety expertise
Chief executive officer	Oversee overall operation and ensure public safety. Communicate with public. Direct requests for outside assistance from state and federal sources.

THE HOSPITAL DISASTER PLAN

BASIC REQUIREMENTS OF HOSPITAL PLANNING

Hospital disaster planning is the responsibility of administration, nursing, and the entire medical staff.[31,78] As mentioned, a good hospital disaster plan should be coordinated with community organizations including regional EMS, fire, rescue, police and civil defense, utilities, Red Cross, and Salvation Army.[75,76] It should provide an organized response of the hospital for the management of casualties transported to the hospital from the disaster site. And finally, it should plan for disasters arising within or near the hospital that require hospital evacuation.[44,46] (Fig. 87-13).

Disaster research has demonstrated that staff who perform most efficiently are those who are performing relatively familiar tasks.[54,55] The disaster plan should take this into account by relying on standard operating procedures as much as possible.

The plan must describe several key functions. These include:

1. Activation of the plan
2. Assessment of the hospital's capacity
3. Establishment of a disaster command
4. Communications
5. Supplies
6. Hospital disaster administrative and treatment areas
7. Training and drills

ACTIVATION OF THE DISASTER PLAN (FIG. 87-14)

It is essential that the plan designate an individual who has the responsibility to put the hospital's disaster plan into effect. An alternative person or persons who have this authority should also be specified. Situations that warrant activation of the plan should also be defined operationally (i.e., definition of disaster). This, of course, varies from hospital to hospital and cannot be defined simply as the number of incoming casualties (See **Definition of Disaster**). For example, the ED disaster manual must define how the on-duty physician and nurse determine to what degree to mobilize and when to involve the administrator or nursing supervisor.[30]

After activation of the plan, there must be immediate mobilization of all disaster resources likely to be needed. These include personnel, supplies, equipment, communications, and transportation.

ASSESSMENT OF THE HOSPITAL'S CAPACITY

Before the hospital can receive casualties, it must be determined if the hospital itself has sustained any structural damage or loss of utility as a result of a disaster.[45,47,84,85] These include blocked passageways; inoperable elevators, potential for fire, explosion, or building collapse; failure of any utility; loss of equipment and/or supplies including oxygen; contamination of water; and outside access problems. Damage assessment is usually the responsibility of the plant safety officer or hospital engineer. If the hospital's structural integrity has been compromised, it may be necessary to evacuate staff and patients.

Once it is determined that the hospital itself is safe, the hospital must determine how many casualties from the disaster site it can safely manage. This may be limited by available personnel, beds, and supplies, as well as by the type of disaster and the availability of other community resources. At the time of disaster notification, it is necessary to know the status of many of the hospital's capabilities; how many beds are available, how much blood is available, how many personnel are on duty, what damage has been done, how many operating rooms are in use, which doctors are present, and so forth. Either someone must tour the hospital to accumulate this information or a form for reporting it must be available in each department ahead of time.

ESTABLISHMENT OF DISASTER COMMAND

A command site within the hospital should be established, preferably in a pre-designated area (e.g., disaster control center). This center should be able to

I. Plan Implementation
   1. Table of Contents
   2. Letter of Authorization
   3. Community/Regional/Facility Casualty Philosophy Statement
   4. Collaborating Agencies/Facilities Statement
   5. Goal/Objectives Statement
   6. Definition of Terms/Decision Criteria
   7. Notification Procedure
II. Personnel Notification
   1. Chain of Command
   2. Notification
   3. Callback Procedure
III. Command Post
   1. Opening the Command Post
   2. Staffing and Equipment
IV. Personnel Pool
   1. Function
   2. Staffing and Equipment
   3. Procedures
V. Communications
   1. Function
   2. Staffing and Equipment
   3. Procedures
VI. Paper Work and Forms
VII. Triage Area
   1. Function
   2. Staffing and Equipment
   3. Procedures
VIII. Major Treatment Area
   1. Function
   2. Staffing and Equipment
   3. Procedures
IX. Delayed Care Area
   1. Function
   2. Staffing and Equipment
   3. Procedures
X. Departmental Responsibilities
   Accounting/Data Processing
   Administration
   Admitting (Inpatient and Outpatient)
   Business Office
   Central Service
   Clergy
   Dietary/Food Services
   Disaster Coordination
   Emergency Department
   Housekeeping
   Infection Control
   Laboratory
   Laundry

   Materials Management
   Medical Records
   Medical Staff
   Mental Health
   Morgue
   Nuclear Medicine
   Nursing Service
   Nursing Units
   Outpatient Services
   Pathology
   Personnel
   Pharmacy
   Physical Therapy
   Plant Operations/Engineering
   Public Relations
   Purchasing
   Radiology
   Respiratory Therapy
   Security
   Social Services
   Surgery/Recovery
   Switchboard
   Volunteer Services
XI. Internal Disaster
   1. Fire Procedures
   2. Patient Evacuation Procedures
   3. Physical Plant Damage Control
      Power Supply
      Gas Supply
      Water Supply
XII. Community Interface
   1. Media Relations Center/Public Information Center
   2. Public Safety
   3. Ambulance
   4. Red Cross and Other Agencies
XIII. Special Incidents
   Bomb Threat
   Severe Weather
   Earthquake
   Terrorism
   Hazardous Chemical
   Radiation
   Civil Disorder
XIV. Attachments
   1. Disaster Training Plan
   2. Cost-Recovery Procedures
   3. Long-Term Disaster Response
   4. Managing the Stress of Disaster
   5. Evacuation Maps/Instructions
   6. Location of Shut-Off Valves

FIG. 87-13. Table of contents for a hospital disaster manual. With permission from Seliger, J.S., and Simoneau, J.K.: Emergency Preparedness: Disaster Planning for Health Facilities. Baltimore, Aspen Publishers, Inc., 1976.

communicate with the patient receiving area (triage site), patient care areas, and with regional EMS, police, fire, and government authorities. Provisions for multiple modes of communication (telephones, two-way radios, runners, etc.) should be made. The command personnel should include at least a physician, a nurse, and an administrator.[30,43]

COMMUNICATION

Establishment of good communications is critical in any disaster or mass-casualty situation.[86] Past experience, however, has shown that this essential function is difficult to achieve for several reasons.[10] Telephones frequently become inoperative because of switchboard overload and damage to telephone lines and other equipment. A major goal should be full utilization of all possible communications resources including citizens' band groups, radiotelephone subscribers, blackboards, intercoms, closed-circuit television, short-wave radio and radio-equipped individuals of all kinds and even messenger and courier services.[9,32]

Interhospital communication may be necessary because of shortages of supplies such as blood or intra-

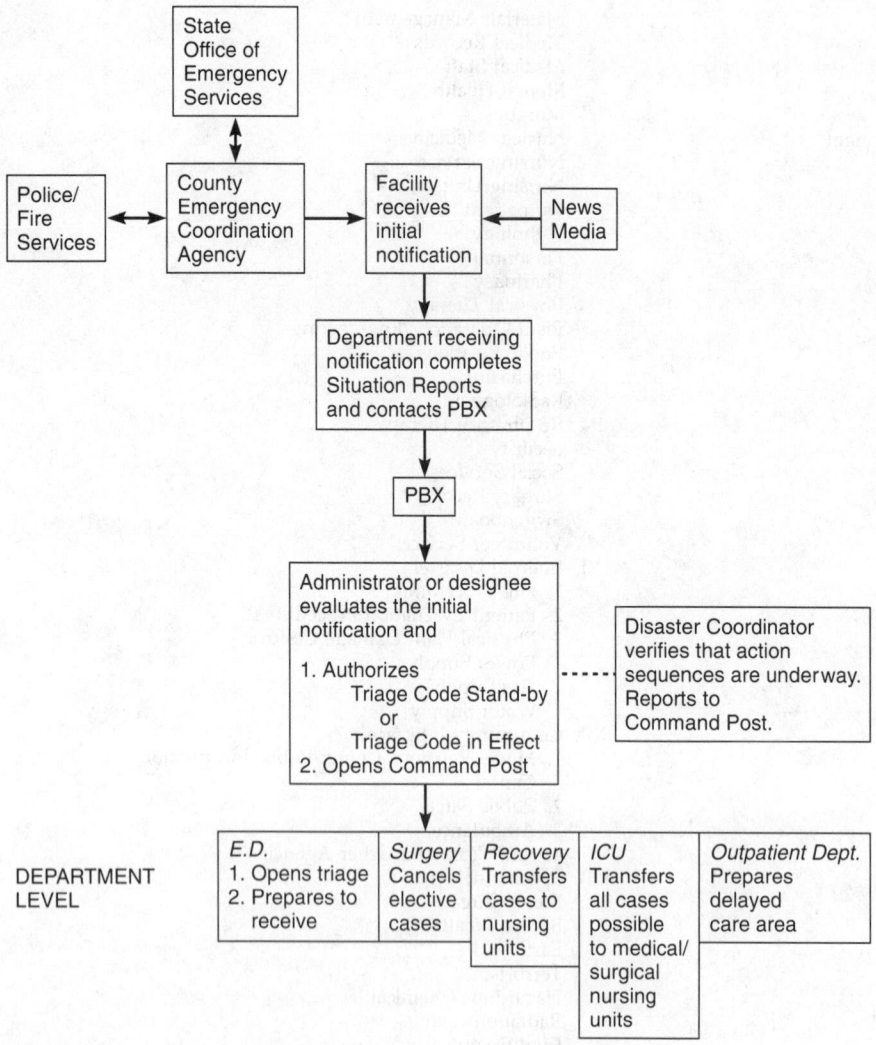

FIG. 87-14. *Sequence of disaster notification. With permission from Seliger, J.S., and Simoneau, J.K.: Emergency Preparedness: Disaster Planning for Health Facilities. Baltimore, Aspen Publishers, Inc., 1986.*

venous fluids, certain equipment such as incubators or surgical instruments, or personnel such as nurses, x-ray technicians, or physicians.[79–81] An overloaded hospital may also wish to transfer patients to a pre-arranged hospital. Unfortunately, interhospital communications may present a weak link in the community's disaster response. After one Los Angeles earthquake, 67% of hospitals had difficulty with interhospital communications.[87]

SUPPLIES

During a disaster, necessary supplies and equipment must be ready for immediate distribution to appropriate locations in the hospital (e.g., stretchers and wheelchairs to the receiving area). Each hospital must estimate the amount of supplies that will be needed in stock over and above its regular hospital supply. In most instances, this will not have to be increased

because most hospitals already have a month's supply of many items in stock.[30,43]

HOSPITAL DISASTER ADMINISTRATIVE AND TREATMENT AREAS

As part of disaster planning, it is essential that certain areas of the hospital be designated for specific functions such as reception of casualties, treatment, and discharge of patients. The plan should be specific as to the function of these areas, staffing requirements, and basic supplies to be used. The areas to be incorporated in each plan are described in the following sections.

DISASTER CONTROL CENTER

A disaster control center must be established to provide overall command and coordination of the hospital's disaster response activities. These activities include activation of the plan, coordination of hospital activities with those at the disaster site, and adjusting the plan as necessary. Good communication is absolutely essential for these coordination activities and must be immediately available by means of telephone, radio, and messengers. Disaster control responsibilities include opening up additional hospital wards or clinics, obtaining outside assistance, evacuation of endangered patients, assignment of staff to treatment areas, and revision of original job assignments.

TRIAGE

To maximize efficiency, entry of all patients should be restricted to only one location, the triage area. The primary function of a disaster triage area is rapid assessment of all incoming casualties, the assignment of priorities for management, and classification of dispositions (i.e., distribution of patients to various patient care areas in the hospital).[88,89] Without a triage area to manage the patient flow, the major treatment area may become overwhelmed.

PATIENT CARE STATIONS

Suggested means of organizing patient care stations are described in the following two paragraphs.

Major Trauma and Medicine. From the triage location, most if not all of the seriously injured patients are sent to the major trauma/medicine area (e.g., trauma and cardiac resuscitation, treatment of hypovolemic shock, etc.). This is usually in the ED.

Minor Trauma—Primary Care. In most disaster situations, the majority of patients are not seriously injured. A great percentage of these are classified as the "walking wounded." These low-priority patients can be sent to an "urgent care" area often designated as the minor trauma/primary care area for definitive care, including splinting of fractures, primary closure of lacerations, and tetanus prophylaxis. This minor trauma/primary care area can be established in the hospital's outpatient clinics.

ADMISSION PRESURGICAL HOLDING

Most patients stabilized in the major trauma area (ED) are sent to the admission presurgical holding area.

SURGERY

The number of operating rooms that can be staffed is the main limiting factor in the provision of definitive care for a large number of severely injured casualties.[72,73] The most experienced surgeon available must evaluate cases and assign surgeons to these cases as rapidly as possible.

MORGUE

Many disasters can result in a large number of fatalities, requiring expansion of present morgue capacities or temporary use of other facilities such as a church or stadium.[90]

DECONTAMINATION

JCAHO requires that hospitals to have provisions for emergency treatment and decontamination of individuals who are radioactively or chemically contaminated.[65] Some basic requirements for hospitals are:

1. A safe area for decontamination.
2. A means of washing external contamination from the patients.
3. A method of containment of contaminated materials.
4. Adequate protection for persons handling the patient and other hospital personnel.
5. Disposable/cleanable medical equipment.

The goals are to reduce external contamination, contain the contamination that remains, and prevent further spread of potentially dangerous substances.[34–37] Remember that the sooner a patient has been decontaminated, the sooner he or she can be treated as a "normal" accident victim. To accomplish this, three things must be achieved:

1. Terminate exposure to toxic materials
2. Stabilize the patient
3. Initiate proper definitive care.

PSYCHIATRY

In the event of a disaster involving mass casualties and even property damage with loss of possessions, an opportunity exists for anxiety, depression, and psychotic episodes.[2,32,50] Hysterical persons, whether patients, visitors or staff, can be extremely disruptive to hospital disaster operations.[10] A separate isolated area must be predesignated to receive individuals in need of psychologic intervention.[91]

FAMILY WAITING AND DISCHARGE AREA

As past experience in disasters has shown, families and friends converge en masse to the hospital seeking information about victims.[41,53] This convergence can seriously interfere with efforts by the hospital to respond effectively to the situation. For this reason, a separate area must be predesignated for family members seeking information. This area may also be used to discharge in-hospital patients and victims of the disaster.

TRAINING AND DRILLS

Regular training and drills help to familiarize staff with their disaster roles and responsibilities.[74,92–98] They also serve to point out weaknesses or omissions in the plan that require additions or revisions. Drills can range from full-scale community-wide simulations with moulage victims to table-top triage games to minidrills that test only certain components of the disaster plan such as call-up of personnel and test of communications.[32]

DISASTER OPERATIONS

ON-SITE MEDICAL CARE

Determining how much and what type of care to administer at the disaster site depends on several factors.[99] If the number of patients is small and sufficient prehospital personnel and transportation resources are available, on-site medical care can proceed in a fairly normal manner, with rapid stabilization and transportation to nearby hospitals. When extrication is prolonged, it is important that potentially life-saving interventions be instituted, such as intravenous fluids for hypovolemic shock.[100] On the other hand, early, rapid transportation with a minimum of treatment should be practiced when there is danger to rescuers and casualties from fire, explosion, falling buildings, hazardous materials, and extreme weather conditions.[35]

When an overwhelming number of casualties exceed transportation capacities, advanced field medical treatment may be beneficial because it may be hours before seriously injured patients can be evacuated.[99,101] This may necessitate the establishment of field hospitals with operating theater capabilities.[102] Such a field hospital may be set up in a large building such as a school or church. Casualties are brought here from the disaster site for further assessment and initial treatment of their injuries. After a period of observation and stabilization, they are either sent home or transported to a hospital.

As described above, evacuation of the less injured and ambulatory patients may rapidly overwhelm local hospitals before the arrival of the more severely injured.[10] Under these conditions, it may be better not to evacuate them but to treat them locally.

COMMUNICATION FROM DISASTER SITE TO HOSPITAL

The local emergency communications or disaster operations center should alert hospitals in the affected area of a possible mass or multiple casualty situation. This report should include number of injured and specifically the number of seriously injured and number for whom ambulatory treatment is sufficient.[32] Hospitals should report to the local emergency communications center the following information:

1. Bed availability
2. Number of casualties received thus far
3. Number of additional casualties that hospital is prepared to accept
4. Specific items in short supply

DISTRIBUTION OF CASUALTIES TO RECEIVING HOSPITALS

Past experience has shown that victims of a mass casualty incident usually are distributed unequally among receiving hospitals.[10,41] Typically, the hospital closest to the disaster site receives an inordinately large number of disaster victims as well as the most critically injured. It is important that the casualty load be spread to available hospitals in such a way that the injured receive prompt and appropriate treatment and that individual hospitals are not overwhelmed.

This situation may be unavoidable because of large numbers of critically injured patients, blocked transportation routes, and weather conditions. To decrease the possibility of this occurrence, however, it is important that good communications be maintained between hospitals and on-site EMS command. If this situation is anticipated, the on-scene commander should be alerted immediately by the potentially overloaded hospital to avoid unnecessary patient transportation to this hospital. In this situation, the less injured and more stable can be sent a further distance to outlying hospitals. Secondary triage from one hospital to another may also be necessary if the hospital's capability to handle victims has been exceeded.[32]

Casualties with special problems such as major burns, carbon monoxide poisoning, and spinal cord injuries may need to be transferred directly to specialized units, although it may not be possible for these units to accept a large number of injured.[19]

ON-SITE DISASTER MEDICAL TEAMS FROM HOSPITALS

On-site disaster medical teams dispatched from local hospitals may be of value in situations in which victims require prolonged extrication, transportation routes are blocked preventing easy evacuation to hospitals, or the casualties are of such magnitude that they exceed transportation capacities.[103,104] Such a team should be dispatched with great caution. Most physicians and nurses function well in an in-hospital setting; few, however, are prepared to work under austere field conditions by either training or experience.[99] Such hospital-based teams should probably not come from the ED staff until backup staff has arrived to care for patients arriving from the disaster site or who are already present.

The resources for such teams should be carefully planned on a regional basis.[104] The capability to send hospital teams to a disaster site can be developed in several ways. For example, a physician on-site triage team can come from teaching hospitals or be created from a pool of doctors in office practice. At least one institution from each region should maintain such a capability. The designated hospital should store disaster triage kits containing essential resuscitation and stabilization equipment in the ED for such circumstances.

It would be valuable for physicians or hospital personnel who are designated to be part of a team to be dispatched to a disaster site to receive some training in disaster medical care.[105] Unfortunately, unlike countries such as France, the U.S. has no formal training programs in disaster medicine available for civilian physicians interested in disaster medical care.[93-95] Generally speaking, in this country, EMT-paramedics are better equipped and trained to function appropriately at the site of a disaster than physicians or nurses who have not had specific training and preparation.

THE EMERGENCY DEPARTMENT

The ED is the most critical part of the hospital's initial response to virtually any type of external disaster. It is the part of the hospital that usually receives first notification that a disaster has occurred, and it is usually the entry point for incoming victims.[52]

INITIAL RESPONSE

When a call is made to the hospital informing it of a disaster or potential mass-casualty-producing event, the receiver of the call must have a procedure to follow for verification of the incident. A disaster notification form is usually used by some facilities to remind the staff of the questions they are to ask. (Fig. 87-15).

The appropriate hospital official or administrator on duty is then given this information. When the ED is notified by hospital administration (now disaster control) that the external disaster plan is in effect, it sets in motion a series of activities. The information obtained from the call is given to the nurse in charge; the nursing and medical personnel in the department are notified of the impending arrival of casualties; and the ED's plan for calling additional staff is activated.

An initial needs assessment is conducted by the nurse and physician in charge with the information available. They must evaluate the current status of the patients in the department and make the appropriate decisions concerning their care and disposition. Among the decisions are those related to the admission, discharge, or transfer of patients and decisions about the priority of patient care. To facilitate reception and care of a large number of casualties, all non-emergency patients should be discharged from the emergency department with responsible individuals (e.g., friends and relatives).

Based on this initial assessment of current patient load, the number of patients that the department can

Initial form for description of event when first notification is received. TRY TO OBTAIN ALL PERTINENT INFORMATION SO THAT APPROPRIATE RESPONSE CAN BE DETERMINED PROPERLY.

Date _____ Time _____ A.M./P.M.
Person Taking Report: _____ Position: _____
Area Where Notification Is Received: _____
   Name of Person Contacting: _____
   Agency: _____
   Call Originating From: _____ Phone # _____
   Verified: Yes/No   Comment _____

Nature of Event: (circle)
Wind   Fire   Rain   Flood   Explosion   Bomb Threat
Chemical (type) _____ Heat   Cold
Vehicular (type) _____ Aircraft (type) _____
Other: _____

Location: _____

Estimated Number of Casualties: (circle)
1–6 6–10 10–20 20–30 30–40 40–50 50–60 60–70
70–100 more than 100 more than 200
Comment _____

Types of Injuries Prevailing: _____
_____

Numbers This Facility Should Expect:
_____ Immediate _____ Delayed
Comment: _____

Distribution Flow of Casualties Initially: _____
_____
_____

Additional Information:

FIG. 87-15. Disaster notification form. With permission from Seliger, J.S., and Simoneau, J.K.: Emergency Preparedness: Disaster Planning for Health Facilities. Baltimore, Aspen Publishers, Inc., 1986.

receive is determined and communicated to the prehospital disaster communications center. The nurse and the physician in charge then determine whether more physician and nursing coverage is required in the department and assign staff to the areas in the department to be used during the disaster. As patients begin to arrive, it is critical that those in charge immediately recognize signs of staff overload before the problem gets out of hand.

A waiting room area for family members must be designated, away from the ED so that congestion of people does not occur when casualties arrive.[91]

PERSONNEL NOTIFICATION

The director of the ED or his designate should have a phone list of appropriate personnel to be called in to work during a disaster. Lists of addresses and phone numbers of these individuals should be distributed to all key personnel if it is impossible to locate the director or his or her assistant. Every position, address, and telephone number listed should be updated quarterly.

If hospital telephone communications have been completely disrupted, ED personnel may have to be reached by radio or television announcement (if power lines are down).

Alternatively, a calling station remote from the hospital, such as a nurse's residence, may be able to handle this extensive calling job without taxing the hospital's phone system.

SECURITY AND TRAFFIC CONTROL

Hospital security personnel play a key role in the emergency department by diverting non-essential vehicles and ensuring a smooth, one-way flow of traffic to the ambulance entrance.

RECEPTION OF PATIENTS

Many patients arrive independently of the formal EMS system.[10] They are brought by neighbors or friends, or may even hitchhike. It is important to recognize this since reports from the field of numbers of patients to be expected by ambulance may greatly underestimate the total number of patients who actually arrive at the ED. All too often, the initial wave of casualties arriving at the ED are those with less severe injuries who have been able to leave the site of a disaster without too much difficulty. The more severely injured, who often need extrication, arrive later.[55]

All available litters and wheelchairs should be taken to the ambulance ramp immediately on announcement of the disaster status.

Disaster victims are met at the receiving area by hospital escorts, who assist the EMTs in transferring patients to wheelchairs or stretchers.

Essential equipment such as endotracheal tubes, intravenous solutions, cervical collars, splints, and bandages should be placed near to the ambulance entrance to permit convenient restocking of the ambulance and rapid return to the disaster site.

THERAPEUTIC MANAGEMENT DURING DISASTER SITUATIONS

TRIAGE

PURPOSES

Generally, triage can be defined as the prioritization of patient care based on severity of injury/illness, prognosis and availability of resources.[88,89] For those responsible for the triage of patients arriving in the ED, the purpose of triage is to determine the predesignated care area to which the patient should be sent.[9,13] The location to which the patients are "triaged" establishes priorities for care. For example, some victims may need immediate decontamination as they arrive, regardless of their severity of injury. Those needing immediate care (e.g., respiratory failure, shock) are taken to resuscitation areas ("crash" rooms), while the dead are moved directly to the morgue.[106] The severely but less critically injured are taken to the major trauma/medical area described previously, where they are further assessed and initial treatment commenced. The walking injured are directed to the minor surgery/primary care treatment area, often located in outpatient clinic areas.

PERSONNEL

A team consisting of a physician (preferably an emergency physician or a surgeon), an ED nurse, and a medical records or admitting clerk should receive every patient (Fig. 87-16).[21] In extraordinary situations, several triage teams may be required to handle the casualty load.[29,59] The physician performing hospital triage should be acknowledged as being in command in the triage area, should be clearly identified by a vest or other garment, and must understand all triage options (Fig. 87-16).

If a physician is not available, an emergency nurse with training in the concepts of casualty triage and emergency patient assessment can be designated as the triage officer.

RESPONSIBILITIES

Even though patients have been triaged at the scene, they should undergo a second process of triage on arrival at the hospital, preferably at the ambulance entrance to the ED.[9,32] Responsibilities of members of the triage team include:

1. Assigning disaster patients to appropriate treatment areas (e.g., Resuscitation Room, Major Surgical, Minor Surgical, etc.) according to the assessment of their immediate needs and the availability of resources.
2. Instituting the most basic of life support measures, such as inserting oral airways, CPR, and the external control of hemorrhage.

Assessment of severity of injury should be accomplished by conducting a rapid primary survey supplemented by obtaining prehospital information from the patient or prehospital personnel. The triage team communicates information on number of casualties, severity of injuries, and need for additional resources to both the ED and the hospital disaster control center. If phones are tied up, this notification can be accomplished by using runners or by the use of portable radios. Likewise, triage personnel must be informed about the capability of the various treatment areas (e.g., major and minor surgery) to handle additional casualties or special problems such as burns. They also must know about the establishment and location of overflow areas.

Triage Area Coordinator (responsible for the function and process of the Triage Area)

___ Liaison with the Command Post, maintaining close communication regarding the operation of triage.
___ Supervise the triage area workers.
___ Ensure adequate personnel, obtaining from Personnel Pool when necessary.
___ Ensure proper break times and appropriate scheduling.
___ Handle administrative problems, such as equipment needs, coordinating with the Command Post all problem solutions that cannot be accomplished right in the area by the Coordinator.
___ Ensure proper maintenance of triage logs and statistics.
___ Insure proper conduct of all triage procedures.
___ Coordinate patient flow with receiving areas.

Triage Officer

___ Evaluate each arriving casualty, performing a cursory primary survey (ABCs) and head-to-toe physical evaluation. Keep it brief, injury oriented, and focused on defining the problems and priorities.
___ Assign a triage category (Emergency, Urgent, Nonurgent).
___ Assign a triage disposition for further care.
___ DO NOT PERFORM TREATMENT EXCEPT FOR THE MOST ESSENTIAL LIFESAVING MANEUVERS.
___ DO NOT LEAVE YOUR AREA UNLESS RELIEVED BY ANOTHER TRIAGE OFFICER.
___ Wear your triage identification bib at all times.

Registered Nurse, Triage Area

___ Assist the Triage Officer in evaluation of casualties, including performance of a cursory physical exam.
___ Assign triage categories in all cases you are evaluating by yourself (Emergency, Urgent, Nonurgent), and advise the Triage Officer of the category assigned.
___ Assign a triage disposition if necessary, log it in via the clerk, and advise the Triage Officer of your disposition.
___ Ensure that transport occurs immediately, assign a transporter if necessary.
___ Coordinate the ancillary workers on your team to complete their tasks efficiently and correctly.

___ Advise the Triage Coordinator of all equipment and supply needs at your station.
___ Wear your triage identification bib at all times.
___ DO NOT LEAVE YOUR AREA UNLESS RELIEVED BY THE TRIAGE COORDINATOR.

LVN, EMT-P, EMT-A

___ Assist the RN and Triage Officer in evaluating each casualty.
___ Obtain proper exam equipment and supplies as needed from the cart or shelves; advise the RN when supplies are running short.
___ Assist in disrobing and gowning casualties and in obtaining clothing and valuables lists if the clerk needs assistance.
___ Apply oxygen as ordered by the RN or Triage Officer.
___ Wear your triage identification bib at all times.
___ DO NOT LEAVE THE TRIAGE STATION UNLESS RELIEVED BY THE TRIAGE COORDINATOR.

Clerk

___ Log each casualty into the Triage Log: ensure that all information required is complete unless that information is not currently available.
___ Dispatch messages as requested, utilizing the transporters or requesting a message runner from the Personnel Pool if the transporters are busy.
___ Obtain clothing and valuables lists as necessary; do not hold the casualty up to do so, however.
___ Bag clothing and valuables and ensure that they accompany the casualties to their disposition.
___ Wear your triage identification bib at all times.
___ DO NOT LEAVE THE TRIAGE STATION UNLESS RELIEVED BY THE TRIAGE COORDINATOR.

Transporter

___ Transport casualties rapidly and safely from triage to their treatment disposition.
___ Wear your triage identification bib at all times.
___ Return to your triage station as soon as the patient is delivered to the patient's disposition.
___ Advise the Triage Coordinator of all broken transport equipment.

FIG. 87-16. Responsibilities of triage area personnel. With permission from Seliger, J.S., and Simoneau, J.K.: Emergency Preparedness: Disaster Planning for Health Facilities. Baltimore, Aspen Publishers, Inc., 1986.

The triage physician should also be aware of the location of a family waiting and public relations area within the institution because family, friends, and the media inevitably appear in the triage area. Every effort should be made by the security staff to keep these individuals out of the patient care areas until after the staff has dealt with the needs of the patients.

The admitting clerk's role as part of the triage team is to complete tags, attach them to victims, and retrieve valuables and clothing for bagging.[15,107] He or she then tags the bag and completes the Triage Area Casualty Log (Figures 87-17 and 87-18).

PRINCIPLES OF TRIAGE

The approach to patient evaluation and treatment is quite different under disaster situations resulting in large numbers of casualties.[12,108,109] The triage physician's goal is to evaluate incoming patients rapidly to decide where to distribute them (e.g., to major or minor surgery). In mass casualty situations, one no longer has the luxury of concentrating all resources on the management of a single critical patient. To accomplish the most good for the greatest number of patients, the triage team must evaluate all patients arriving at the ED doors and classify their conditions with regard to severity of injury and need for treatment. Although some principles of medical care are unchanged in a mass casualty incident, other principles of patient care must be altered to achieve the best overall result.[110] There is clearly no role for resuscitation, let alone definitive care at this stage. Care should be limited to manually opening airways and controlling external hemorrhage[100] (Tables 87-14 and 87-15).

The most common triage classification involves assigning patients to one of four colors (red, yellow, green, or black) depending on injury severity and prognosis (Table 87-16). In addition to the nature and urgency of the patient's systemic condition, triage decisions must be sensitive to such factors affecting prognosis as age, general health, and physical condition of the patient and the qualifications of the responders and availability of key supplies and equipment.[110]

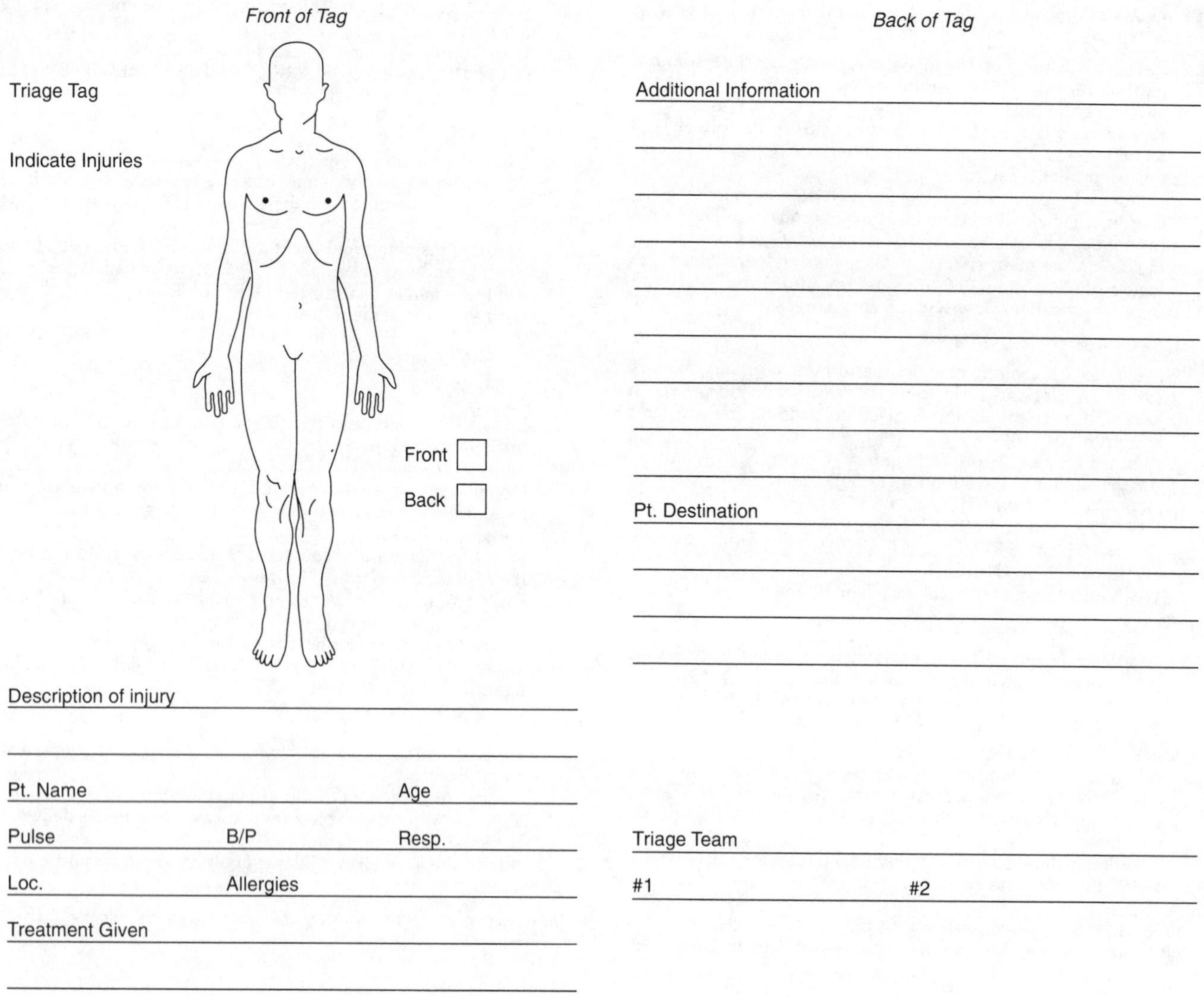

Front of Tag

Triage Tag

Indicate Injuries

Front ☐

Back ☐

Back of Tag

Additional Information

Pt. Destination

Description of injury

Pt. Name _____ Age _____

Pulse _____ B/P _____ Resp. _____

Loc. _____ Allergies _____

Treatment Given

Triage Team

#1 _____ #2 _____

FIG. 87-17.   *Example of disaster tag. With permission from Wieland, P., and Hattan, D.K.; Disaster decision making in the acute facility. In Disaster Nursing: Planning, Assessment, and Intervention. Edited by Garcia, L.M., Baltimore, Aspen Publishers, Inc., 1985.*

Catastrophically injured patients who have a minimal chance for survival despite optimal medical care should be classified as "expectant" (e.g., those with burns involving 95% of the body surface area). Spending time on patients who are not likely to live leaves other patients who are truly salvageable awaiting care. If too much time intercedes, these patients may also become nonsalvageable. The goal with these patients should be adequate pain control and the opportunity to be with friends and family.

PATIENT CARE IN THE EMERGENCY DEPARTMENT

The purpose of this section is not to review all aspects of mass casualty care (e.g., advanced trauma life support, decontamination of chemical injuries) but to address some concepts of care that are not found in the routine management of emergency patients.

For example, wound infections may occur in virtually all types of disasters. Infected wounds and gangrene were major problems after the Armenian earthquake.[111] In hurricanes or tornadoes, persons may be cut by flying glass and other potentially highly contaminated material.[4,5] Because of this, all wounds should be copiously flushed with saline. Primary closure of heavily contaminated wounds may result in major complications, as was the case following the Armero volcanic eruption in Colombia. If lacerations are old (older than 6 to 12 hours) or appear contaminated, they should be treated by debridement and left open for primary delayed closure in a 3 day period.[73] This will allow one an opportunity to observe the wound for the development of infection. As far as tetanus prophylaxis goes, all patients should receive a tetanus booster, and if highly contaminated, tetanus

ATTACH SECURELY TO PATIENT

Pink copy: administration White copy: admitting Hard copy: patient record	NO. 524873

Hospital	St. Josephina

Patient name   (Last)   (First)   (Middle)
Smith   Donald   K.

Address
1252 N. 11th St.

Date 10/5/86	Time 10:15	Age 32	Sex M	Religion Cath.

Description of patient: (Ht, Wt, Eyes, Hair, Compl, Marks, Clothing)
6 ft. brn/green   180# Cauc
torn blue shirt,   brn. trousers   blk. shoes/socks

ALLERGIES:
Horse serum

Next of kin:
(name)   (address)
Alice Smith   1252 N. 11th St   Wife

INITIAL ASSESSMENT:
2" burns face/hands
Open chest wound @ chest
Rigid belly, responds purposefully to voice

INITIAL TREATMENT:
☐ Airway   ☑ IV RK 1000 cc
☑ Bleeding control ☑ Oxygen @ 9 L/min mask
☐ Tourniquet   ☐ Medication:
☐ Splint
☑ OTHER: petrolatum gauze dressing, occlusive bandage

INITIAL ROUTING AT HOSPITAL TRIAGE POINT:
☑ Surgery ☐ Emergency Department ☐ Observation area
☐ X-ray   ☐ ICU   ☐ Morgue
☐ First aid ☐ CCU   OTHER:

PRIORITY DESIGNATION
☑ Immediate   ████   If immediate care affix
☐ Delayed   ████   RED LABEL
☐ Dead   ████   If delayed care affix
                       BLACK LABEL

DO NOT DETACH TAG FROM PATIENT UNTIL INCORPORATED
IN PATIENT RECORD
SEE REVERSE SIDE FOR TREATMENT, DISPOSITION, AND
INSTRUCTIONS

FIG. 87-18. Example of disaster tag. With permission from Simoneau, J.K.: Disaster management. In Emergency Nursing: Principles and Practice, 2nd Ed. Edited by Sheehy, S.A., and Barber, J.M., St. Louis, C.V. Mosby Company, 1985.

immune globulin (Hypertet) should be administered. Patients with blunt trauma, for example, victims of earthquakes who have been trapped by rubble for several hours or days, should be watched closely for signs and symptoms of crush syndrome such as cardiac arrhythmias and renal failure. Fulminant pulmonary edema from dust inhalation may also be a

---

TABLE 87-14. ROUTINE MEDICAL PRACTICES ALTERED IN A MASS CASUALTY SITUATION

- Extent of resuscitation efforts; determined by patient's injuries, age, pre-existing condition, and resource availability.
- Acceptable result: amputation may be considered acceptable in cases when resuscitation might be possible.
- Timeliness of surgery: non-life-threatening conditions to operating theater last.
- Indications for hospitalization: admit only when absolutely necessary.
- Use of ancillary services: minimal use of lab and x ray, diagnostic procedures such as CT scan.
- Increase patient care responsibility of nurses: nurses allowed to administer fluids, manage wounds and decide on some medication doses.
- Decision to transfer: patients who might otherwise be managed are sent to other institutions.

* With permission from Aghababian, R.V.: Hospital disaster planning. Top. Emerg. Med. 7:446, 1986.

TABLE 87-15. ROUTINE MEDICAL PRACTICES UNALTERED IN A MASS CASUALTY SITUATION*

- Immediate attention to airway, breathing and circulatory emergencies in a potentially viable patient
- Provide appropriate management of pain
- Perform systematic patient assessments; may be abbreviated
- Re-examine patients for changes in status
- Maintain patient dignity
- Other

* With permission from Aghababian, R.V.: Hospital disaster planning. Top. Emerg. Med. 7:446, 1986.

TABLE 87-16. TRIAGE CATEGORIES

I. **Red**
   A. First priority
   B. Most urgent
   C. Life-threatening shock or hypoxia is present or imminent, but the patient can be stabilized and, if given immediate care, will probably survive
I. **Yellow**
   A. Second priority
   B. Urgent
   C. The injuries have systemic implications or effects but patients are not yet in life-threatening shock or hypoxia; although systemic decline will ensue, given appropriate care, they seem able to withstand a 45- to 60-minute wait without immediate risk
II. **Green**
   A. Third priority
   B. Nonurgent
   C. Injuries are localized without immediate systemic implications; with a minimum of care, these patients generally do not deteriorate for up to several hours
V. **Black**
   A. Dead
   B. No distinction can be made between clinical and biologic death in a mass casualty incident and any unresponsive patient who has no spontaneous ventilation or circulation is classified as dead. Some classify catastrophically injured patients who have a poor chance for survival regardless of care in this triage category

delayed cause of mortality for victims of building collapse.[111]

RADIOGRAPHIC AND LABORATORY STUDIES

Radiographic and laboratory studies should be used extremely judiciously in a mass casualty situation and only if the results of such tests will change therapeutic intervention.[9,30] For example, x-rays of closed, non-angulated potential fractures can be safely delayed for 24 to 48 hours, during which time effective splinting, elevation, and ice can be used. Skull films are probably never indicated in a mass casualty situation.[23] If neurologic impairment is present, one should probably perform a head CT. A chest film is needed in patients complaining of chest pain, dyspnea, or abnormal chest wall motion. The abdominal film, in most cases of trauma, does not provide much useful information. On the other hand, cervical spine films and pelvic and femur x rays should be taken, considering the potential seriousness of injuries thus detected (e.g., permanent neurologic impairment, potential blood loss).

There are minimal indications for blood work. For example, in cases of hemorrhagic shock, one should clearly obtain a baseline hematocrit in addition to type and crossmatching for blood. Urine dipstick for blood may be useful to detect kidney or urinary tract injuries. In patients who are short of breath, or who demonstrate ventilatory impairment, baseline arterial blood gases or pulse oximetry may be useful. All other laboratory studies should be considered accessories and ordered only in specific circumstances (e.g., carboxyhemoglobin in cases of smoke inhalation).

BLOOD BANK

In a disaster situation involving many casualties, it is recommended that the blood bank have as many as 50 units of blood available.[112] It is also important that the bank have ready access to a source of volunteer donors who can be rapidly mobilized. Other potential sources of blood include friends and family members of patients, as well as the "walking wounded."

PATIENT IDENTIFICATION AND RECORD KEEPING

ED records of disaster victims have usually been poor to nonexistent in past disasters.[10] The general absence of detailed and systematic record keeping in disasters, except for serious cases admitted to hospitals for surgery or to intensive care units, has all kinds of implications ranging from problems of cost billings and insurance collection to the difficulty of making any evaluations of the quality of medical care given and the possible efficacy of treatment procedures.[2]

Documentation of the patient's hospital course starts in the triage area.[15,107] Proper tagging with a hospital disaster tag is essential for proper identification, documentation of medical care rendered, and supplying information for relatives and the news media (Figs. 87-17 and 87-18).

One member of the triage team (admitting or medical records clerk) should be assigned the job of recording the victim's name on the disaster tag along with the triaged destination of the patient. If identification of the patient is not available, race, sex, and approximate age should be noted on the tag. An initial diagnostic impression should also be registered on the tag. This information is entered into a department log and also placed in a triage logbook.

MEDIA CONTROL

In a disaster, the hospital may become inundated more by members of the media than by actual disaster victims.[75,76] The presence of these individuals can definitely impair the performance of an already stressed hospital staff.[60] For this reason, members of the press and other news media representatives should be directed to a room or office of the hospital away from the ED or other areas where patient care activities are going on.[91] The press room should be closely supervised by a hospital administrator or public relations specialist. This person should be in direct contact with the disaster control center. Hospital staff must leave all communications with the press to this person and should direct any member of the media to the public relations area so that consistent information is given by the hospital.

HANDLING OF FAMILY MEMBERS

The presence of large numbers of people seeking news of friends and relatives can greatly impair effective disaster control activity. For this reason, a separate area must be predesignated for family members seeking information.[91] Family members should not be allowed into patient care areas except to see patients who are critically ill or have died. The hospital operator will also be inundated with calls of inquiry regarding the presence and status of individual patients from concerned family members. These calls should be directed to a single predesignated desk or office for handling them.

AFTERMATH OF DISASTER

As soon as possible, efforts should be directed toward returning the hospital to normal operations. Besides restocking and cleaning, consideration must be given

TABLE 87-17. NATIONAL DISASTER CONTACTS

Federal Emergency Management Agency
500 C Street, SW
Washington, DC 20472

Office of Emergency Preparedness and Disaster Relief
Pan American Health Organization
525 23rd Street, NW
Washington, DC 20037
(202) 861-4325

Disaster Research Center
University of Delaware
Newark, DE 19716
(302) 451-6618

Disaster Research and Training Program
The Johns Hopkins University
Department of Emergency Medicine
600 N. Wolfe Street
Baltimore, MD 21205
(301) 955-8708

Office of Emergency Preparedness and NDMS
US Department of Health and Human Services
5600 Fishers Lane, Room 4–81
Rockville, MD 20857

Office of U.S. Foreign Disaster Assistance
U.S. State Department Room 1262A
Washington, DC 20523
(202) 647-7545

American College of Emergency Physicians
PO Box 619911
Dallas, TX 75261–9911
(214) 550-0911

National Study Center for Trama and EMS
Univ. of Maryland
22 S. Greene Street
Baltimore, MD 21201

Agency for Toxic Substances and Disease Registry (ATSDR)
1600 Clifton Road, NE
Atlanta, GA 30333
1-404-488-4100

Office of the UN Disaster Relief Coordinator (UNDRO)
United Nations, Room S-2935
New York, NY 10017

World Association for Emergency and Disaster Medicine
% Dr. Peter Baskett
Dept. of Anaesthesia
Frenchay Hospital
Bristol BS16 1LE, UK

American Red Cross
National Headquarters
17th and D Streets, NW
Washington, DC 20006

Emergency Management Institute
16825 South Seton Ave.
Emmitsburg, MD 21727

International Civil Defense Organization
10–12 Chemin de Surville
CH-1213 Petit-Lancy
Geneva, Switzerland

Center for Research on the Epidemiology of Disasters
Catholic University of Louvain 30–34
Clos-Chapelle-aux-Champs 30
1200 Brussels, Belgium

Emergency Preparedness Program
Partners of the Americas
1424 K Street, NW #700
Washington, DC 20005

Office of Emergency Preparedness
Health Resources and Services Administration

5600 Fishers Lane, Room 13A-22
Rockville, Maryland 20857

International Association of Fire Chiefs
1329 18th Street, NW
Washington, DC 20036

Joint Commission on the Accreditation of Healthcare
  Organizations (JCAHO)
875 N. Michigan Ave.
Chicago, IL 60611

National Association for Search and Rescue
PO Box 3709
Fairfax, VA 22038

National Association of EMS Physicians
190 Lothrop Street
Pittsburgh, PA 15213

American Hospital Association
840 N. Lake Shore Dr.
Chicago, IL 60611

California Specialized Training Institute (CSTI)
Div. of California Office of Emergency Services
P.O. Box 8104
San Luis, Obispo, CA 93403–8104

Chemical Manufacturers Association
Chemical Awareness and Emergency Response Program
2501 M Street, NW
Washington, DC 20037

World Health Organization
Office of Emergency Relief Operations
20 Avenue Appia
1211 Geneva, 27, Switzerland

Intertect
PO Box 565502
Dallas, Texas 75356

Univ. of Wisconsin-Extension
Disaster Management Center
Dept. of Engineering Professional Development
432 N. Lake Street
Madison, Wisconsin 53706

Casualty Surgeons Association
The Royal College of Surgeons
35/43 Lincolns Inn Fields
London WC2A 3PN, UK

Radiation Emergency Assistance Center/Training Site (REAC/TS)
Medical and Health Sciences Division
Oak Ridge Associated Universities Box 117
Oak Ridge, TN 37831

Emergency Training Institute
Miller Landing, Bldg. 200
150 N. Miller Road
Akron, Ohio 44313

Emergency Health Services Program
Univ. of Maryland Baltimore Co.
Catonsville, MD 21228

Emergency Services Branch
National Institute of Mental Health
5600 Fishers Lane
Rockville, MD 20857

Medicine de Catastrophe
Hospital Henri Mondor
51, Av. du Marechal de Lattre de Tassigny
F-94010 Creteil, France

European Center for Disaster Medicine (CEMEC)
State Hospital
47031 Republic of San Marino

CHEMTREC (Chemical Transportation Emergency Center)
1-800-424-9300

to the emotional stress experienced by both prehospital and hospital staff. Short- and long-term emotional problems, particularly among rescuers, have been reported on numerous occasions.[113] All those involved should be encouraged to talk with one another and with counselors as needed.

Deficiencies in a hospital's plan that are revealed during a disaster should be carefully recorded, reviewed, and criticized. Immediate steps should then be taken to correct these flaws in the plan.

HORIZONS

The United Nations General Assembly has recently designated the 1990s as The International Decade of Natural Disaster Reduction (IDNDR).[8] This provides a unique opportunity for specialists in Emergency Medicine to address the health and medical needs of the millions of potential victims of disasters. Disaster medicine is rapidly developing as a subspecialty within Emergency Medicine.[77,95,114] For example, a section for disaster medicine has been organized within the American College of Emergency Physicians. For disaster medicine to be recognized as a "legitimate" specialty or subspecialty within emergency medicine, however, we must first define what disaster medicine is as well as what a disaster physician does.[77,108,114] Although the development of emergency medicine in the United States is more advanced than in any other country, we clearly lag behind other countries in the area of disaster medicine.[109] In France, for example, academic programs in disaster medicine have been developed that offer diplomas of special competence.[94,115] Until an identifiable, teachable, and testable body of disaster medicine knowledge is developed in this country, and some professional authority takes cognizance of its administration, disaster medicine will continue to be an "orphan child."

In the future, research will focus on the development of methods to assess health care needs rapidly in disasters.[6,64,83] One interesting area of research is the development of casualty estimation models for incorporation into community vulnerability analyses.[6] This allows improved planning for predicted health care needs in a future disaster as well as rapid estimation of medical needs in the immediate aftermath of a disaster.

TABLE 87-18. PROFESSIONAL MEDICAL AGENCIES INVOLVED IN DISASTER PREPAREDNESS

County and state medical societies
Hospital council
Nursing association
Dental association
Podiatry association
Pharmaceutical association
Veterinarian association
Industrial medical association
City, county, and state health departments

NATIONAL CONTACTS

See Tables 87-17 and 87-18.

REFERENCES

1. Guha-Sapir, D., and Lechat, M.F.: Reducing the impact of natural disasters: Why aren't we better prepared? Health Policy and Planning 1:118, 1986.
2. Logue, J.N., Melick, M.E., and Hansen, H.: Research issues and directions in the epidemiology of health effects of disasters. Epidemiol. Rev. 3:140, 1981.
3. Seaman, J.: The effects of disaster on health: A summary. Disasters 4:14, 1980.
4. Emergency Health Management After Natural Disaster. Pan American Health Organization, Washington, D.C., 1981.
5. Emergency care in natural disasters. Views of an international seminar. WHO Chron. 34:96, 1980.
6. Noji, E.K.: Evaluation of the efficacy of disaster response. UNDRO NEWS, July/August 1987, pp. 11–13.
7. Pan American Health Organization: International Health Relief Assistance. Recommendations approved at the meeting of international health relief assistance in Latin America, San Jose, Costa Rica, 10–12 March, 1986.
8. U.N. General Assembly: International Decade for Natural Disaster Reduction: Report of the Secretary-General. 43rd Session, Agenda item 86. A/43/723, 18 October, 1988.
9. Aghababian, R.V.: Hospital disaster planning. Top. Emerg. Med. 7:446, 1986.
10. Quarantelli, E.L.: Delivery of Emergency Medical Services in Disasters: Assumptions and Realities. New York, Irvington, 1983.
11. Woods, D.: Disasters: How would your hospital cope with 50 casualties? Can. Med. Assoc. J. 116:1195, 1977.
12. Butman, A.: The challenge of casualties en masse. Emerg. Med. 15:110, 1983.
13. Contzen, H.: Preparations in hospital for the treatment of mass casualties. JWAEDM 1:118, 1985.
14. Cowan, M., Butman, A.M., and Bosner, L.V.: Mass casualty planning: Model for In-hospital disaster response. JWAEDM 2:83, 1986.
15. Irving, M.: Major disasters: Hospital admission procedures. Br. J. Surg. 63:703, 1976.
16. Kennedy, W.: Some preliminary observations on a hospital response to the Jackson, Mississippi Tornado of March 3, 1966. Disaster Research Center Report No. 17. Columbus, Ohio, The Ohio State University, 1967.
17. Baker, E.J.: The management of mass casualty disasters. Top. Emerg. Med. 1:149, 1979.
18. Blanshan, S.A.: A Time Model: Hospital Organization Response to Disaster. Beverly Hills, Sage Publications Ltd., 1978, pp. 173–198.
19. Jacobs, L., Goody, M., and Sinclair, A.: The role of the trauma center in disaster management. J. Trauma 23:697, 1982.
20. Katz, L.B., and Pascarelli, E.F.: Planning and developing a community hospital disaster program. Emerg. Med. Serv. Sept/Oct, 1978, p. 70.
21. Koslowski, L: Emergency and disaster medicine: Assignments and perspectives. JWAEDM 1:255, 1985.
22. Mezzetti, F.: A hospital emergency plan. JWAEDM 1:266, 1985.
23. Rutherford, W.H.: Disaster procedures. Br. Med. J. 1:443, 1975.
24. Savage, P.E.: Disasters and Hospital Planning: A Manual for Doctors, Nurses and Administration. Oxford, Pergamon Press, 1979.

25. Seliger, J.S., and Simoneau, J.K.: Emergency Preparedness: Disaster Planning for Health Facilities. Rockville, MD, Aspen Publishers, Inc., 1986.
26. Williams, D.J.: Major disasters: Disaster planning in hospitals. Br. J. Hosp. Med. October 1979, pp. 308–317.
27. Holloway, R.: Medical disaster planning in urban areas. N.Y. J. Med. 1 March 1971, pp. 591–595.
28. Melton, R.T., and Riner, R.M.: Revising the rural hospital disaster plan: A role for the EMS system in managing the multiple casualty incident. Ann. Emerg. Med. :39, 1981.
29. Li, T.C., et al.: Medicine in a disrupted society: The role of the academic medical center. Am. J. Med. 70:998, 1981.
30. Jenkins, A.L., and van de Leuv, J.H. (eds.): Disaster Planning in Emergency Department Organization and Management, ed. 2. St. Louis, C.V. Mosby Co., 1978.
31. de Boer, J., and Baillie, T.W. (eds.): Disasters: Medical Organization. London, Pergamon, 1980.
32. Butman, A.M.: Emergency training. Responding to the Mass Casualty Incident: A Guide for EMS Personnel. Westport, Connecticut, Educational Direction, Inc., 1982.
33. Cowley, R.A., ed.: Proceedings of Mass Casualties: A Lessons Learned Approach, 13–17 June, 1982.
34. Cashman, J.R.: Hazardous Materials Emergencies: Response and Control. Lancaster, PA, Technomic Publishing Co., 1988.
35. Currance, P.L., and Bronstein, A.C.: Emergency Care for Hazardous Materials Exposure. St. Louis, C.V. Mosby, 1988.
36. Leonard, R.B.: Community planning for hazardous materials. Top. Emerg. Med. 7:55, 1986.
37. Stutz, D.R., Ricks, R., and Olsen, M.: Hazardous Materials Injuries: A Handbook of Prehospital Care. Greenbelt, MD, Bradford Communications Corp., 1982.
38. Edelstein, S., and Giordano, J.: Presidential assasination attempt. In Proceedings of Mass Casualties: A Lessons Learned Approach, R.A. Cowley, ed. 13–17 June, 1982, pp. 17–28.
39. O'Leary, D.S.: Managing a hospital under crisis. In Proceedings of Mass Casualties: A Lessons Learned Approach, edited by Cowley, R.A. 13–17 June, 1982, pp. 127–140.
40. Blanshan, S.: A time model: Hospital organizational response to disaster. In Disaster: Theory and Research. Edited by Quarantelli, E.L., pp. 173–198, 1978.
41. Quarantelli, E.L.: The community general hospital: Its immediate problem in disasters. Am. Behav. Sci. 13:380, 1970.
42. Weiss, D.B.: Organization of hospital medical care of mass casualties in peacetime disasters. Int. Surg. 67:400, 1982.
43. Garcia, L.M.: Disaster Nursing: Planning, Assessment, and Intervention. Rockville, MD, Aspen Systems Corp., 1985.
44. Tresalti, E.: Organization of hospital for extrahospital emergencies. JWAEDM 1:284, 1985.
45. Seaver, D.J.: Coping with internal disaster is a hospital priority. Hospitals, July 16, 1977, pp. 167–172.
46. Tresalti, E.: Organization of hospital for intrahospital emergencies. JWAEDM 1:285, 1985.
47. Reitherman, R.: How to prepare a hospital for an earthquake. J. Emerg. Med. 4:119, 1986.
48. Zeballos, J.L.: Health effects of the Mexico earthquake—19th Sept. 1985. Disasters 10:141, 1986.
49. Western, K.: The epidemiology of natural and man-made disasters; The present state of the art. Dissertation for the Academic Diploma in Tropical Public Health, London School of Hygiene and Tropical Medicine, University of London, 1972.
50. Drabek, T.E.: Human System Responses to Disaster. New York, Springer-Verlag, 1986.
51. Dynes, R., Quarantelli, E.L., and Kreps, G.: A Perspective on Disaster Planning, Ed. 3. Columbus, Ohio, Disaster Research Center, Ohio State University, 1981.
52. Dynes, R.R.: Emergency medical services delivery in disasters. In Collected Papers in Emergency Medical Services and Traumatology. Baltimore, MD, University of Maryland, 1979, pp. 56–58.
53. Quarantelli, E.L.: The delivery of disaster emergency medical services: Recommendations from systematic field studies. Disaster Med. 1:41, 1983.
54. Tierney, K.: Emergency medical preparedness and responses in disasters: The need for interorganizational coordination. Public Administration Review 45:77, 1985.
55. Tierney, K.J., and Taylor, V.A.: EMS delivery in mass emergencies: Preliminary research findings. Mass Emerg. 2:151, 1977.
56. Bozza-Marrubini, M.: Three major disasters in Italy. Experience of Niguarda Hospital of Milan as "Base Hospital." JWAEDM 1:414, 1985.
57. Foster, C.: Texas hospital battles Hurricane Beulah. Hospital Management 104:70, 1967.
58. Lewis, F., and Trunkey, D.: Autopsy of a disaster. The Martinez bus accident. J. Trauma 20:861, 1980.
59. Orr, M., and Robinson, A.: The Hyatt Regency skywalk collapse: An EMS-based disaster response. Ann. Emerg. Med. 12:601, 1983.
60. Taylor, V.A.: Hospital emergency facilities in a disaster: An analysis of organizational adaptation to stress. Disaster Research Center Preliminary Paper No. 11. Columbus, Ohio: The Ohio State University, 1974.
61. Bliss, A.R.: Major disaster planning. Br. Med. J. 288:1433, 1984.
62. Jacobs, L.M., Ramp, J.M., and Breay, J.M.: An emergency medical system approach to disaster planning. J. Trauma 19:157, 1979.
63. Keller, E.L.: A realistic approach to disaster planning. Hosp. Med. Staff, May 1977, pp. 18–23.
64. Guha-Sapir, D., and Lechat, M.F.: Information systems and needs assessment in natural disasters: An approach for better disaster relief management. Disasters 10:232, 1986.
65. Accreditation Manual for Hospital/1989. Chicago, Joint Commission on the Accreditation of Healthcare Organizations, 1989.
66. Mohler, S.R., et al.: Medical management in a disaster. Aviat. Space Environ. Med. November, 1980.
67. McSwain, N.E., et al.: Disaster medical care: Mardi Gras. J. Trauma 22:235, 1982.
68. Binder, S., and Sanderson, L.M.: The role of the epidemiologist in natural disasters. Ann. Emerg. Med. 16:1081, 1987.
69. Noji, E.K., and Sivertson, K.T.: Injury prevention in natural disasters: A theoretical framework. Disasters: The International Journal of Disaster Studies and Practice. 11:290, 1987.
70. Zhi-Yong, S.: Medical support in the Tangshan earthquake: A review of the management of mass casualties and certain major injuries. J. Trauma 27:1130, 1987.
71. Buerk, C.A., et al.: The MGM Grand Hotel fire: Lessons learned from a major disaster. Arch. Surg. 117:641, 1982.
72. de Boer, J., Brismar, B., Eldar, R., et al.: The medical severity index of disasters. J. Emerg. Med. 7:269, 1989.
73. Burkle, F.M., Sanner, P.H., and Wolcott, B.W., eds.: Disaster Medicine. New York, Medical Examination Publishing Co., 1984.
74. Davies, L.F.: Community disaster planning and training. Emerg. Med. Serv. 15:42, 1986.
75. Quarantelli, E.L.: Human Resources and Organizational Behaviors in Community Disasters and Their Relationship to Planning. Columbus, Ohio, Disaster Research Center, The Ohio State Univ., 1982.
76. Quarantelli, E.L., and Dynes, R.R.: Different types of organizations in disaster responses and their organizational problems. Columbus, Ohio, Disaster Research Center, The Ohio State University, 1977.
77. American College of Emergency Physicians: The role of the emergency physician in mass casualty/disaster management. JACEP 5:901, 1976.
78. Dimick, A.: Role of medical staff in disaster planning and operation. In Proceedings of the U.S.A. Bicentennial EMS and Traumatology Conference. Baltimore, U.S. Department of HEW, 1976.
79. Eldar, R.: A multi-hospital system for disaster situations. Disasters 9:112, 1981.
80. Marsden, A.K.: Coordination of major accident services within a British health region. JWAEDM 3:57, 1987.
81. Rowal, J.S.: Four hospitals join in planning city-wide disaster alert. Hospital Topics 48:24, 1970.
82. Keogh, J.: Management of mass burn casualties in a hospital with a burn unit. Med. J. Aust. 1:303–305, 1980.

83. Golec, J., and Gurney, P.J.: The problems of needs assessment in the delivery of EMS. Mass Emergencies 2:169, 1977.
84. Rutherford, W.M.: Experience in the accident and emergency department of the Royal Victoria Hospital with patients from civil disturbances in Belfast 1969–1972 with a review of disasters in the United Kingdom 1951–1971. Injury 4:189, 1973.
85. Roeschlaub, E.L.: Hospitals in riot-torn cities meet patient needs head on. Hosp. Topics 46:57, 1968.
86. Storer, D.: Disaster planning: Communications. Ohio Med. J. 6:401, 1979.
87. Bouzarth, W.F., Mariano, J.P., and Smith, J.S.: Disaster preparedness. In Principles and Practice of Emergency Medicine. Edited by Schwartz, G.R. Philadelphia, W.B. Saunders, 1986, p. 612.
88. Rund, D., and Rausch, T.: Triage. St. Louis, Missouri, C.V. Mosby Co., 1981.
89. Rutherford, W.H.: Sorting patients, sometimes called triage. Disaster Medicine 1:121, 1983.
90. Hooft, P.J., Noji, E.K., and Van de Voorde, H.P.: Fatality management in mass-casualty incidents. Forensic Sci. Int. 40:3, 1989.
91. Roth, J.A.: Staff and client control strategies in urban hospital emergency services. Urban Life and Culture. :39–60, 1972.
92. Cloutier, M.G., and Cowan, M.L.: Disaster medicine training through simulations for fourth-year students. J. Med. Ed. 61:408, 1986.
93. Defeu, N., and Huguenard, P.: Teaching disaster medicine in France. In Proceedings of Mass Casualties: A Lessons Learned Approach, Edited by Cowley, R.A. 13–17 June, 1982, pp. 289–294.
94. Feldstein, B.: Disaster medicine training in France. Ann. Emerg. Med. 12:621, 1983.
95. Feldstein, B., Gallery, M., Sanner, P., et al.: Disaster training for emergency physicians in the United States: A systems approach. Ann. Emerg. Med. 14:36, 1985.
96. Hell, K.: Training of physicians in disaster medicine in Sweden. JWAEDM 1:106, 1985.
97. Hell, K.: Training of physicians in disaster medicine. Disaster Medicine 1:107, 1983.
98. Thompson, P.: Issues in disaster management training. Disasters 7:37, 1983.
99. Oyen, O.: The on-scene medical organization. JWAEDM 1:115, 1985.
100. Safar, P.: Resuscitation potentials in mass disasters. JWAEDM 2:34, 1986.
101. Baskett, P., and Weller, R.: Medicine for Disasters. London, Wright, 1988.
102. Nancekievill, D., and Finch, P.: The role of hospital mobile medical teams at a major accident. In Proceedings of Mass Casualties: A Lessons Learned Approach. Edited by Cowley, R.A. 13–17 June, 1982, pp. 147–156.
103. Alcouloumre, E.: The role of the physician at a medical disaster: Hospital emergency response teams. JWAEDM 2:128, 1986.
104. Gerace, R.V.: Role of medical teams in a community disaster plan. CMA J. 120:923, 1979.
105. Thompson, P.: Issues in disaster management training. Disasters 7:37, 1983.
106. Evans, R.F.: Major disasters: The patient with multiple injuries. Br. J. Hosp. Med. 22:329, 1979.
107. Finch, P.M., et al.: Early documentation of disaster victims. Anaesthesia 37:1185, 1982.
108. Byrd, T.R.: Disaster medicine: Toward a more rational approach. Military Med. April 1980, pp. 270–273.
109. Dubouloz, M.: An introduction to disaster medicine. Bull. Int. Civil Defence, August 1983, p. 25.
110. Roding, H.: Triage and its ethical problems. JWAEDM 3:10, 1987.
111. Noji, E.K.: Medical and healthcare aspects of the 1988 earthquake in Soviet Armenia. Earthquake Spectra 1989; Special Supplement: 101–107.
112. Sandler, S.G.: Strategies for blood management in mass casualty incidents. In Proceedings of Mass Casualties: A Lessons Learned Approach. Edited by Cowley, R.A. 13–17 June 1982, pp. 229–234.
113. Waeckerle, J.F.: The skywalk collapse: A personal response. Ann. Emerg. Med. 12:651, 1983.
114. Feldstein, B.: The development and practice of emergency and disaster medicine in the United States. Disasters 7:86, 1983.
115. Emergency and disaster medicine. Edited by Manni, C., and Magalini, S.I. New York, Springer-Verlag, 1985.

BIBLIOGRAPHY

Blanshan, S.: Hospitals in rough waters: The effects of a flood disaster on organizational change. Ph.D. Dissertation. Columbus, Ohio, The Ohio State Univ., Dept. of Sociology, 1975.

Costanzo, S.: Disaster medicine—A public health view. Prehosp. Disaster Med. 6:489, 1991.

Disaster management and relief: A bibliography. Disasters 7:64, 1983.

Hart, R.J., et al.: The Summerland disaster. Brit. Med. J. 11:256, 1975.

Henry, S.: Mississauga Hospital: Largest evacuation in Canada's history. Can. Med. Assoc. J. 122:582, 1980.

Holloway, R.: Medical disaster planning II: New York City's preparations. N.Y. J. Med. 3:692, 1971.

Holloway, R.D., Steliga, J.F., and Ryan, C.T.: The EMS system and disaster planning: some observations. J. Am. Coll. Emerg. Physicians 7:60, 1978.

Leivesley, S.: Disasters, disaster agents, and response: A bibliogrpahy. Disasters 6:228, 1982.

Leonard, R.B., and Ricks, R.C.: Emergency department radiation accident protocol. Ann. Emerg. Med. 9:462, 1980.

Mahoney, L.E., and Reutershan, T.P.: Catastrophic disasters and the design of disaster medical care systems. Ann. Emerg. Med. 16:1085, 1987.

Manni, C., and Magalini, S.I.: Emergency and disaster medicine. New York, Springer-Verlag, 1985.

Maxwell, C.: Hospital organizational response to the nuclear accident at Three Mile Island: Implications for future-oriented disaster planning. In Proceedings of Mass Casualties: A Lessons Learned Approach. Edited by Cowley, R.A. 13–17 June, 1982, pp. 295–300.

Prescott, J.E.: Case report: Utilization of a phased response disaster plan. JWAEDM 3:55, 1987.

Readings in Disaster Planning for Hospitals. Chicago, American Hospital Association, 1973.

Richards, G.: Focus on hospital preparedness: When bad winds blow. Trustee, November, 1979.

Rodning, C.B.: Disaster preparedness. South. Med. J. 76:229,

Seaman, J.: Death and injury resulting from sudden onset disasters: Select bibliography. Disasters 7:304, 1983.

Stallings, R.A.: Hospital adaptations to disaster: Flow models of intensive technologies. Human Organization 29:294, 1970.

Waeckerle, J.F.: Disaster planning and response. N. Engl. J. Med. 324:815, 1991.

Wright, J.E.: The prevalence and effectiveness of centralized medical response to mass casualty disorders. Mass Emergencies 2:189, 1977.

EMS SYSTEM EVALUATION AND QUALITY ASSURANCE

C. Gene Cayten and Carl J. Post

CAPSULE

This chapter discusses the evaluation of emergency medical services (EMS) systems and programs. It presents a comprehensive evaluative model and an assessment of key methodologic issues. Evaluative measures discussed include severity indices, abbreviated injury score, injury severity score, revised trauma score, and other methods of gaining objective measures for reliable evaluation.

INTRODUCTION

The term Emergency Medical Service (EMS) system dates to 1966 when the National Academy of Sciences published an influential report about accidental death and disability in this country.[1] Modern EMS systems are the beneficiaries of lessons learned since that time. Medical control, priority medical dispatch, improved equipment, more ambitious training philosophies, and a renewed emphasis on assessing effectiveness have all combined to improve EMS systems.

EMS system evaluation is an ongoing process in which information is gathered to determine whether transportation, communications, and hospital and physician services have been combined into an efficient and effective system. There is no certainty that a fully coordinated emergency care delivery apparatus will operate smoothly or in a systematic manner because EMS programs have to overcome many potential organizational problems to provide appropriate care. For example, hospitals might not provide adequate support to their emergency departments (EDs); public safety authorities or individual ambulance companies may adopt somewhat parochial perspectives on the procedures needed for handling requests for service. With the wide scope of EMS systems, their evaluation requires an overall assessment as well as an assessment of component parts.

This chapter discusses: (1) the relationship between planning and evaluation, (2) a model for EMS system evaluation, (3) the need to control for case mix and injury severity in measuring system effects on patient outcomes, and (4) selected methodologic issues.

EMS SYSTEM EVALUATION

DEFINING GOALS AND OBJECTIVES

To undertake an analysis of a given EMS system, its goals and objectives must first be identified because specific goals and objectives provide the basis for evaluation.[2] Although goals are somewhat general (e.g., to reduce prehospital cardiac deaths) objectives must be specific and measurable (to increase the successful prehospital resuscitation rate for patients in ventricular fibrillation to 40%). Objectives may be specified to achieve each goal. They should provide a coherent and workable definition of the EMS program to be evaluated.

In developing goals and objectives, it must be recognized that EMS care is a continuum (Fig. 87-19) ranging from prevention to rehabilitation.[3] Evaluation provides essential feedback regarding the fulfillment of objectives implemented at different points along the continuum of care.

The evaluation cycle starts with goal setting, defining contexts, and adopting clear objectives that are relevant to the goals. Next, available methods suitable for achieving these objectives are analyzed and a method of program implementation is selected. Finally, monitoring the program's progress toward distinct objectives yields feedback. Such feedback may prompt a rethinking of goals and objectives. Objectives may have to be refined or different methods may be required. Thus, evaluation and planning form a continuous cycle: plan, evaluate, refine or change the plan, evaluate it once again, refine, etc. (see Figure 87-20).[2,3]

The techniques chosen for evaluating program objectives largely are dependent on the type of objectives involved. Simple cost analysis is an option. Queuing analysis, computer models and optimization techniques as well as more sophisticated methods may be employed. Program evaluation also might use a consensus panel of experts or consultants to evaluate objectives that cannot be quantified.[2]

PROGRAM EVALUATION

Program evaluation assesses an individual program within an EMS system. It has been used most suc-

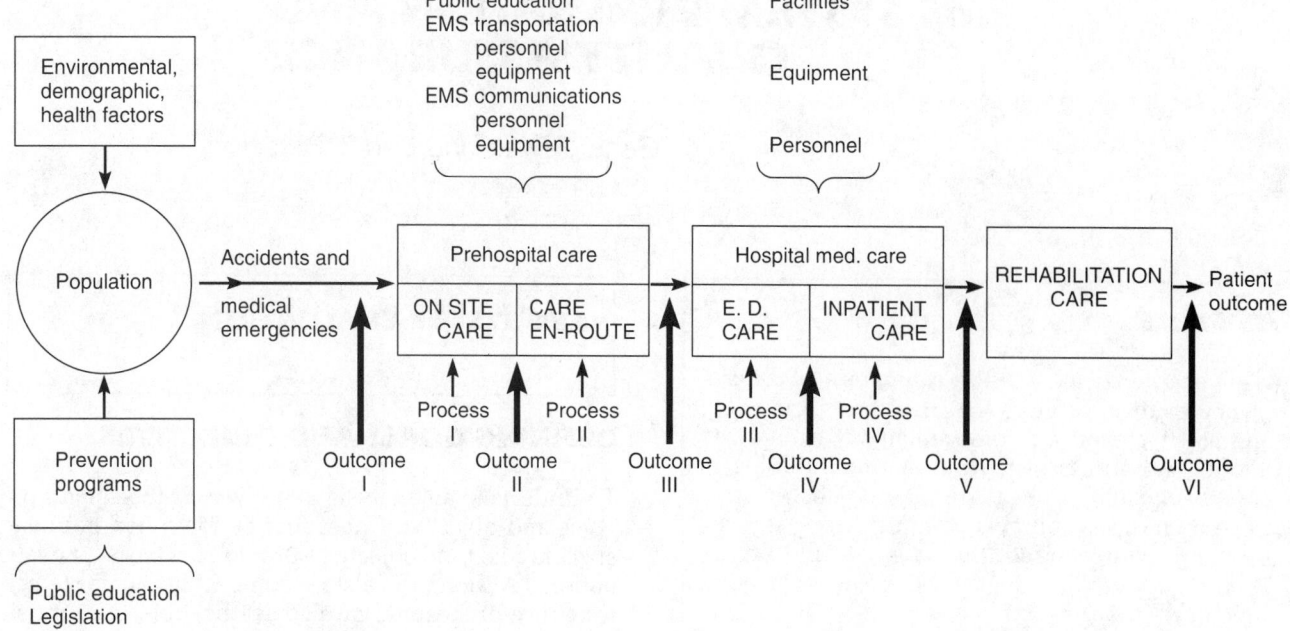

FIG. 87-19. Aspects of EMS evaluation.

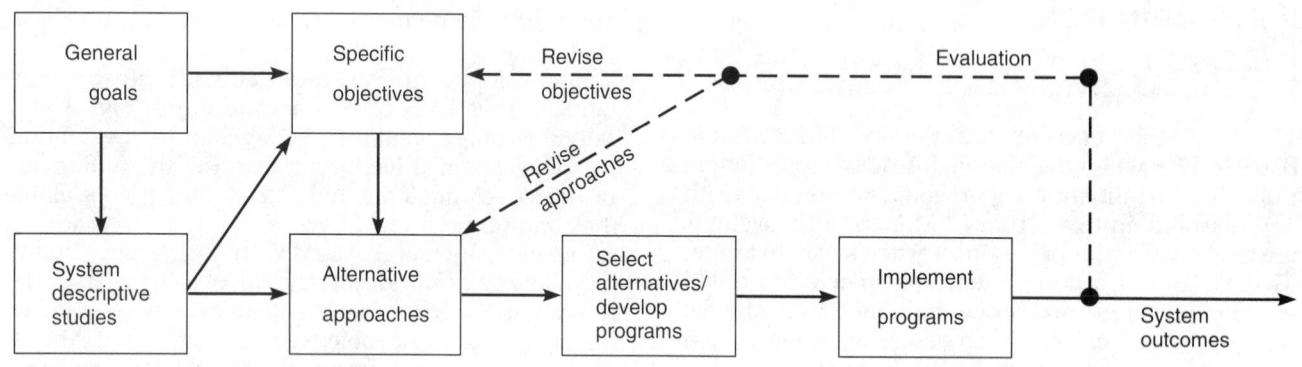

FIG. 87-20. The EMS planning process.

cessfully to assess the effectiveness and impact of training programs. For example, Frazier and Cannon used EMT course materials as the basis for an appropriateness review of cases treated by EMTs in the field.[4] Ornato determined that the cost of saving a patient in ventricular fibrillation varied according to level of training: $7687 for each life saved at the basic EMT level; $2126 for each life saved at the EMT-defibrillation level; and $2289 for each life saved by a paramedic.[5] Upgrading an entire system's EMTs to the EMT-D level emerged as a cost-effective option. Nineteen hours of additional training would reduce unit costs per save by more than $5500. Cummins and Eisenberg have argued that the use of automatic external defibrillators by EMTs might similarly reduce the training costs associated with preparing prehospital personnel.[6] Thus, cost per ventricular fibrillation patient saved is one program evaluation method

found to be particularly useful in comparing program alternatives.

Where specific goals and objectives do not exist, EMS system evaluation should begin with a description of everything done for an individual patient. Comparing such a description with those from other systems can document system strengths and weakness. This information is then used to establish goals and objectives. The setting of goals, however, must take the local context into account as the interplay of population and environment affect the demand for emergency care.[3] Age, cultural background, general health status, geography, meterologic conditions, employment and industrial capabilities in a given area all affect the type of EMS system required.[3] The level of acceptance accorded EMS by the citizens it serves is also an important but difficult-to-define element affecting the system.

Evaluation based on objective setting provides a basis for management and further planning. Evaluative feedback results in a steady supply of new objectives for the EMS system and the generation of evidence concerning the value of old objectives.

COMPREHENSIVE EVALUATION MODEL

The most enduring evaluation model for emergency care has proven to be one rooted in medical care evaluation. Donabedian proposed a framework comprised of three essentials: structure, process, and outcome.[7] It has been adapted successfully to EMS system evaluation and was the USPHS evaluation standard used by regional grantees from 1979 through 1982.[8,9]

STRUCTURE EVALUATION

This evaluation assesses existing resources in terms of credentialed personnel, capabilities of facilities, extant equipment, and organizational framework. Gibson compiled a comprehensive list of criteria for structural evaluations of EMS systems.[10] The list provides a framework for assessing the delivery of EMS care in an area. Unfortunately, even when ideal conditions do exist, patient care may remain largely unaffected since the relationship between structure and patients' outcomes is poorly substantiated.[2]

PROCESS EVALUATION

This evaluation assesses the functioning of an EMS system and its personnel. The actual performance of the medical care delivery structure is evaluated. Process measures often reflect system efficiency: rapid response times, appropriate dispatch decisions, or the selection of recommended treatment algorithms.[2] This aspect of a systems evaluation can be accomplished in a number of ways: (1) checking the appropriateness of care; (2) looking at patterns of care, (3) conducting case reviews using explicit and/or implicit criteria; and (4) evaluating the types of data used to make medical decisions.

The basic core of process evaluations is an audit of records to measure compliance with protocols. Medical record audits are difficult because of the real potential for error. The use of explicit process criteria should reduce interauditor reliability errors, but records used to conduct an audit may be incomplete or inaccurate. Related documents, such as ambulance call reports, may not reflect the care actually provided. Field personnel sometimes fail to record some of the medications given or pertinent information on patient status.

Quality assurance is a process evaluation method that usually carries a narrower connotation than EMS system evaluation. It refers to an analysis of care rendered by individual providers. Compliance with procedures, treatment protocols, and documentation is evaluated. The results are used in performance evaluation, as a basis for planning continuing education, and, in the aggregate, as the basis for assessing system performance.

In the prehospital setting, the method usually takes the form of ambulance run report analyses. Run reports often are computerized for data analyses.[11,12] Care must be taken to use the clinical input of the system's medical director as well as that of systems managers in establishing the treatment protocols and in planning the analyses. Analyses should be designed to answer specific questions defined in advance. Compliance by the provider with both medical and dispatch protocols is checked to monitor the clinical progress of a system and the individuals working within it.[13]

In major cities, dispatchers may check computerized system status boards to detect active calls that have consumed a disproportionate amount of time. Written records of individual performances are being supplanted by computerized profiles of the individual's overall performance. Post has argued that individual field personnel should document their own performance by the use of laptop computers in the ambulance. The use of a readable menu to document each call may lead to greater compliance and more accuracy.[14]

Process evaluations, including prehospital quality assurance, are designed to ensure that the medical care standards adopted within a system are met. The results are best handled in a positive manner. Personnel who do not follow protocols should be provided with educational feedback about their apparent shortcomings.[12,13] Although the results of structure evaluation usually do not correlate strongly with patient outcomes, findings of process assessments tend to relate more closely to indicators of patient status. No EMS evaluation is complete, however, unless direct measures of patient outcomes are included.

OUTCOME EVALUATION

This evaluation assesses final patient status. It should be used in some form as part of any EMS system evaluation because it can provide an overall "result" for the system. In addition, data collection is often easier than that for structure evaluations.

Evaluators normally evaluate systems by making inferences from a wide range of data. These inferences must be carefully drawn. For example, a finding of declining cardiac death rates may not be attributable to emergency care intervention at all but rather to changes in exercise, eating, and smoking habits in the population served. Fewer fatal motor vehicle accidents may result from better law enforcement.[15]

Much of this chapter has dealt with methods for evaluating various phases or aspects of a system. Ultimately, however, it is hoped that the EMS system could affect broad population-based mortality rates. Population-based mortality rates would reflect the sum total of all influences on a given population at risk. This includes the prevalence of given conditions, the impact of prevention programs, and the EMS system. Relatively few investigators have attempted to track emergency conditions by changes in population-based mortality rates.

One of the earliest such attempts was by Crampton, who attempted to show that the development of a paramedic system reduced population-based coronary mortality rates in Charlottesville, Virginia.[16] Bergner et al. also documented changes in population-based mortality rates in their study in Seattle.[17,18] Cales attempted to show that the development of a trauma system in Orange County, California reduced motor vehicle accident population-based mortality rates for the area when compared to those other counties in California.[19] With all such studies, considerable epidemiologic experience is necessary to assess other factors besides those related to the EMS system, which could affect changes in the population-based mortality figures.

For many EMS managers, EMS system evaluation becomes a low priority in relation to training and day-to-day operations. Thus, evaluation efforts should be designed for maximal return. One such approach is to choose your area of focus based on comparing your population-based mortality rates to others in similar areas. Look particularly at the broad categories of cardiac or motor vehicle deaths per 100,000. These data are generally available through state health and motor vehicle departments. Focus on areas that compare poorly by doing special studies. In performing such studies, it is necessary to pursue intermediate outcome measures in an attempt to isolate the effect of each EMS system component on the overall mortality rates. Figure 87-19 demonstrates points along the EMS system continuum where intermediate outcome and process measures can be assessed. For example, survival rates of cardiac patients in ventricular fibrillation can be calculated at outcome points II, III, IV, and V. Process measures such as time at scene and protocol compliance can be measured at process points I and II. Using this strategy, it is possible to determine which aspects of the EMS system need improvement.

Another approach to outcome assessment for trauma patients is the preventable death study. A preventable death study can be done by an autopsy method using 250 consecutive deaths in motor vehicle accidents. In such a study, prehospital, hospital, and medical examiner reports are used.[20] Patients dying from central nervous system or prehospital cardiac arrest injuries are not included; they cannot be effectively studied by this method.[20] Each record is assessed by a group of surgeons and emergency physicians according to a set of criteria focused on whether the death was preventable. Unfortunately, this technique is relatively expensive to perform, and its reliability across different settings is questionable. Even when a team uses criteria-based work sheets, the degree of subjectivity inherent in these judgments precludes comparing results among geographic areas.

CONTROLLING CASE MIX AND INJURY SEVERITY

It is evident that the more severely ill or injured a patient is when he or she enters the EMS system, the greater the extent of his or her dependence on the system to sustain life. Evaluative studies must take the health status of the population being served into account. The two basic methods used by evaluation researchers to compensate for the problems posed by case mix variability are tracers and severity indices.

TRACERS

Using a tracer involves studying medical care rendered to patients with a prespecified or tracer condition. A tracer medical condition was defined as Kessner and Kalk[21] as one that has:

1. A diagnosis with a potentially significant functional impact on the patient
2. A diagnosis that is well defined and easily recognizable in field settings
3. A diagnosis with sufficiently high prevalence to permit collection of adequate data
4. A natural history that varies with the use and effectiveness of medical care
5. A medical management regimen for the diagnosis well defined
6. The effects of sociodemographic factors on it well understood.

The tracer method deals with case mix variability by narrowing the evaluative focus to only patients who have similar diagnoses. Most commonly, patients with cardiac disease and injuries are analyzed for emergency care evaluation.

CARDIAC DISEASE

In cardiac arrests, ventricular fibrillation and survival to hospital discharge are the most commonly used indicators of a system's impact. For example, Eisenberg found that survival rates for ventricular fibrillation patients were higher in tiered systems because of the early inception of CPR.[22] Vukov et al. reported that early CPR, coupled with a response time of less than 10 minutes, enhanced the value of field personnel trained to use defibrillators in a rural environment.[23]

Dubois and Brook concentrated on a later intermediate outcome by examining preventable death in the context of the hospital phase of care.[24]

Studying cardiac outcomes in the prehospital setting has been inhibited by lack of consistency in the types of samples used. Sampling strategies identified in the literature as suitable for use in prehospital cardiac care evaluation include:

1. Patients with out-of-hospital cardiac arrests
2. Patients with a final diagnosis of myocardial infarction in the hospital discharge records
3. Patients with an ED diagnosis to rule out myocardial infarction
4. Patients identified by EMTS and paramedics as suspected heart attack patients
5. Patients found in ventricular fibrillation in the field.

Each of these samples has potential biases that must be considered in analyzing results drawn from them. Hearne compiled a comprehensive list of cardiac arrest outcome studies in which he included definitions, methodologic considerations, and summary outcome data.[18] To limit the great variation in definitions for cardiac patients, Eisenberg et al. proposed a uniform reporting system.[25]

INJURY

Trauma tracers were once the cornerstone of USPHS-inspired evaluation efforts. All funded regions tracked head injury patients to determine whether they were taken to an appropriate hospital.[9] Tracking specific injuries, however, is no longer considered the best option available to contend with case-mix variability. Evaluating trauma care systematically entails collecting injury data on a regional basis. For instance, Shackford et al. conducted a multidisciplinary concurrent audit of the quality of care within a trauma system in San Diego.[26] An audit committee with physicians, nurses, officials representing trauma and nontrauma hospitals, and system administrators used a computerized trauma registry as their primary tool to identify cases for individual review.

Instead of using tracers, evaluative efforts now center on comparing outcomes of care given to a set of trauma patients with known norms for survival for similar patients. Severity indices are the hallmark of these evaluations.

SEVERITY INDICES

Although there has been only a limited amount of work on indices for cardiac patients, promising efforts are being made in regard to trauma patients.[27] Indices are used for triage, epidemiology, clinical research and systems evaluation. Injury indices have been developed primarily along two lines: anatomic and physiologic. At the present time, the Abbreviated Injury Score (AIS) and the Injury Severity Score (ISS) derived from it are the most widely used anatomic severity scores. The Revised Trauma Score is the most widely used physiologic severity score. The TRISS method based on the Revised Trauma Score Injury Severity Score and age has been used primarily to identify unexpected deaths for audit.

ABBREVIATED INJURY SCORE

The Abbreviated Injury Score (AIS) was first published in 1971 to scale injuries following motor vehicle accidents.[28] It grades each of six anatomic regions on a scale of 1 through 6, with 1 considered minor and 5 considered fatal. It was revised in 1976, 1980, 1985 and 1990.[28] Generally, the revisions have been made to increase the specificity of the coding and particularly to ensure that it is useful in assessing patients with penetrating injuries. Studies have shown that AIS can be reliably abstracted, particularly by physicians and nurses. The average time required per medical record is 10 to 30 minutes, depending on the complexity of the case and the clinical skills of the abstractor.[29]

The limitations of AIS must be taken into consideration. Because it was primarily designed for motor vehicle injuries, it is not as adequate for penetrating injuries. In addition, AIS is not a linear measure. The difference between AIS 1 and 2 may not be the same as the difference between AIS 4 and 5. Also, a 3 in one body area may not equate with a 3 in another area, although an effort was made to make them roughly comparable. AIS scores are injury codes and do not code the results of injuries, such as blindness. AIS cannot always be coded directly from ICDA codes.[27] According to McKenzie, only 67% of the ICDA codes can be translated directly into AIS codes.[30] Many of the non-compatible ICDA codes are infrequently used, however, McKenzie also found that intra-rater abstracting reliability is higher for patients with blunt injuries than for patients with penetrating injuries. AIS cannot be reliably coded from ED sheets because this requires the complete hospital record.[31] This is particularly true in patients with penetrating injuries. Because hospital record face sheets and computerized hospital data sets do not provide a comprehensive listing of all injuries, conversion tables based on of the AIS-85 and ICD9-CM should be used only for statistical analyses of large data sets looking at trends as areas for further investigation.

INJURY SEVERITY SCORE (ISS)

The Injury Severity Score (ISS) was developed by Baker et al. based on the AIS.[32] ISS combines each patient's injuries into a single score representing the overall severity of injury. The scores are the sum of the squares of the highest AIS value in each of the three most severely injured regions of the body. A score of 6 in any one body system is given the maximum overall score of 75, indicating a fatal injury. ISS values range from 1 to 75. Bull et al.[33] and Stone et al.[34] studied the validity of the ISS and found that it correlated with such outcomes as length of hospital stay, time to death, disability, necessity for surgery, and plasma cortisol concentration, but less firmly with mortality and morbidity rates. By itself, the ISS explained only 49% of the variance in mortality.[35] Also, a small error in AIS (i.e., scoring a 4 instead of a 3) results in a large ISS difference because the AIS is squared.[36] Copes pointed out a serious limitation of the ISS, a major component of the TRISS method[16]: the ISS uses only the AIS value for the most serious injury in each body area, thus underestimating the overall severity of injuries among patients with more than one injury to a single body region.

REVISED TRAUMA SCORE (RTS)

The Revised Trauma Score (RTS) is a physiologic index derived from Champion and Sacco's Trauma Score, which in turn was based on their Triage Score. The Triage Score was developed using logistic regression to determine the physiologic variables that best predicted mortality.[37]

The Trauma Score was based on systolic blood pressure, respiratory rate, respiratory effort, capillary refill and the Glasgow Coma Score (CGS). The Trauma Score has been found to explain 73% of the variance in trauma mortality.[38] The data to calculate the RTS frequently are not available for retrospective studies. Many EMTs and paramedics do not routinely collect GCS values or capillary refill.[39] The Trauma Score has a sensitivity rate of approximately 80%.[37,38] Thus, 20% of patients with severe injuries are not identified by the Trauma Score because they compensated physiologically or the response time was so short that decompensation did not take place. The specificity rate for the Trauma Score is approximately 75%; it overestimates injury severity when physiologic changes are related to factors other than hypovolemia, cerebral edema, or hypoxia.[38]

The RTS was developed when it was found that capillary refill, and respiratory expansion could be dropped without losing predictive value. It does, however, have the same limitations described above for the Trauma Score. We found many patients, particularly gunshot wound patients and patients suffering low falls, who presented with a normal RTS but who went on to die.

TRISS METHOD

At present, the TRISS methodology developed by Champion and Sacco is the most widely used method to control for case mix in studies of different groups of injured patients.[40] The TRISS method combines a physiological scale (the RTS), an anatomic scoring system (the ISS), and age (dichotomized as those from 15-55 versus those 55 and older).[40] Data for over 26,000 patients from the early years of the Major Trauma Outcome Study (MTOS) were included in regression analysis which yielded coefficients for the RTS, ISS, and age.[38] Separate coefficients were developed for patients with penetrating and those with blunt injuries. Probabilities of survival can be calculated for each patient and aggregated across patients, yielding overall predicted survival rates. Observed survival rates can then be compared to calculated predicted survival rates and the significance of differences between them can be quantified with a Z score according the statistical method described by Flora.[41] An M score evaluates variation in numbers of injured patients in different probability of survival cohorts in the study sample compared to the MTOS sample. M scores less than 0.88 indicate that the study sample is not comparable to the MTOS sample.

The TRISS method has been used in the following ways:

1. As an audit tool to identify unexpected deaths, i.e., patients who died with probabilities of survival greater than 0.5.
2. To track an institution's trauma mortality experience over time.
3. To compare institutions with each other in terms of their success in minimizing mortality from trauma.
4. To hold injury severity constant for a group of patients so that other variables may be studied. In these instances, Z score are used as outcome measures in studies of components of the EMS system or of innovations in medical care.

Although the TRISS method is the best method available for the purposes just described, it has significant limitations. Cottington noted that the ability of the Z score to detect a difference between observed and expected survival rates is influenced by the magnitude of the actual difference, the direction of the difference, the sample size, and the distribution of survival probabilities in the study sample.[42]

Research by Cayten et al. showed that comparing survival results among groups of hospitals is severely limited by the fact that the TRISS method uses only the broad categories of blunt and penetrating injuries.[43] Within the penetrating injury category, patients with gunshot wounds tend to have a higher mortality rate than do those with stab wounds; therefore, hospitals with higher proportions of gunshot wound patients usually have higher overall mortality rates for penetrating injury patients when compared to hospitals with higher percentages of patients with stab wounds. There are also differences among patients in the broad blunt injury category, which include those having low falls, falls from heights, and suffering assaults.[43] The low falls patients' outcomes in particular are poorly predicted by the TRISS method.

Because the ISS is a critical component of TRISS, mortality rates for patients with such multiple injuries are underestimated by TRISS. Morris et al. also found that the presence of certain pre-existing conditions significantly increased the risk of dying.[39] Such conditions are not accounted for in the TRISS method. Those using TRISS need to be familiar with the limitations of the method and to qualify their conclusions where appropriate.

ASCOT METHOD

Champion et al. recently proposed an improvement to the TRISS method, which they call ASCOT.[44] In it, the ISS is replaced by an Anatomic Profile (AP), which configures the AIS-coded injuries into body areas. The resultant score puts greater weight on head injuries and multiple severe injuries to the same body part. The RTS is retained, but coefficients within it are different for the blunt and penetrating injury patient sets and age is broken into five rather than two categories. ASCOT's use of all AIS component scores for all serious injuries within a body region gives it the capacity to better define a patient's precise injury prognosis. ASCOT has been shown to be better than TRISS at predicting the outcomes of patients with penetrating injuries but only slightly better with blunt injuries. Neither ASCOT nor TRISS can be used to evaluate intubated patients or paralyzed patients for whom GCS values and respiratory rates are unavailable.[44]

METHODOLOGIC ISSUES

Issues of the reliability and validity of data collected must be faced by all investigators. Evaluators of EMS systems are no exception.

The *reliability* of a measurement refers to the likelihood, given no change in the object or phenomenon being observed, that the measure's value would not vary if repeated observations were made. For most measures, the principal areas of concern are inter-rater reliability and intra-rater reliability. Inter-rater problems center around whether different people observing the same patient would be likely to record the same value for the measure being used. Intra-rater reliability refers to whether the same person observing the same object or phenomenon at two distinct points in time would record the same value for the measure both times.

Reliability is a common issue in medical care evaluation. Studies are sometimes performed with several knowledgeable clinicians reviewing records or narratives to evaluate the adequacy of care provided. When each of the reviewers uses the same set of explicitly defined evaluative criteria, assessments are likely to be more reliable than when reviewers are free to adopt their own individual implicit criteria.[45]

Studies have indicated that data obtained from abstractions of medical records are particularly subject to reliability problems.[46,47] Medical record abstractors tend to perform reliably when recording quantitative scales such as pulse rate, systolic and diastolic blood pressure, and respiratory rate. Qualitative data such as diagnosis, condition on arrival at the ED, character of respiration, or pupil size often are abstracted much less reliably.

The *validity* of a measure refers to the degree to which it accurately describes the objects or the phenomena being studied. A measurement is said to be valid when it is unbiased and clearly relevant to the characteristic being measured. Systematic error can be introduced into a measurement process by a faulty instrument, the ways in which the instrument is used, the subject(s) being measured, or the environment in which the measurement instrument is being used.[48]

Sherman did a case study of mobile intensive care units in which he was able to identify 18 threats to the validity of EMS evaluation.[49] Cayten et al. studied the validity of EMS data by contrasting the measurement skills of emergency department nurses and EMTs with those of specially trained nurses and electronic measurements.[50] Tolerance limits were defined for quantitative variables. It was found that emergency care personnel performed most validly with quantitative variables. Diastolic blood pressure was the least accurately assessed.

These studies make it apparent that users of basic clinical data must establish the validity of their data before interpreting results drawn from them. If critical medical decisions are to be based on these data, multiple measurements using various techniques should be made. EMS systems factors and integration of prehospital and inhospital care can also markedly influence other variables.[51]

REFERENCES

1. National Academy of Sciences, National Research Council: Accidental death and disability: the neglected disease of modern society. Washington, DC 1986.
2. Cayten, C.G.: Evaluation of Emergency Medical Services in EMS Medical Directors Handbook. Edited by Kuehl, A. St. Louis, C.V. Mosby, 1989, pp. 103–117.
3. Cayton, C.G., and Evans, W.J.: EMS system evaluation in systems approach to emergency care. Edited by Boyd, D., Edlich, R., and Mycik, S. Norwalk, Appleton Century Crofts, 1983, pp. 148–172.
4. Frazier, W.H., and Cannon, J.F.: EMT performance evaluation. National Center for Health Services Research. May 1973.
5. Ornato, J.P., Crarern, E.J., and Gonzalez, E.R.: Cost-effectiveness of defibrillation by emergency medical technicians. Am. J. Emerg. Med. 6:108, 1988.
6. Cummins, R.O., Eisenberg, M.S., et al.: Automatic external defibrillators used by emergency medical technicians: A controlled clinical trial. JAMA 257:1605, 1987.
7. Donabedian, A.: A Guide to Medical Care Administration, Vol. 2 Medical Care Appraisal-Quality and Utilization. New York, American Public Health Association, 1969.
8. DHEW, Emergency Medical Service Systems. Program Guidelines. U.S. Public Health Service, Health Services Administration, Division of Emergency Medical Services, 1979.
9. Post, C.J.: The death of accountability: EMS evaluation in the

era of block grants. Emergency Medical Services *12*:20–24, 1983.

10. Gibson, G.: Guidelines for research and evaluation of emergency medical service. Health Services Reports *89*:99, 1974.

11. Stewart, R.D., Burgman, J., Cannon, G.M., and Paris, P.M.: A computer-assisted quality assurance system for an emergency medical service. Ann. Emerg. Med. *14*:1, 1985.

12. Swor, R.A., and Hoelzer, M.: A computer-assisted quality assurance audit in a multiprovider EMS system. Ann. Emerg. Med.

13. Rottman, S.J., and Fitzgerald-Wesby, K.: A method for reviewing radio-telemetry paramedic calls. Ann. Emerg. Med. *10*:36, 1981.

14. Post, C.J.: Good things in small packages: Lap top computers EMS? Emergency Medical Services *18*:62, 1989.

15. Willemain, T.R.: The status of performance measures for emergency medical services. Technical Report TR-06-74. Operations Research Center. M.I.T., Cambridge, MA, 1974.

16. Crampton, R.S., Aldrich, R.F., Gasho, J.A., et al.: Reduction of prehospital, ambulance and community coronary death rates by the community-wide emergency cardiac care system. Am. J. Med. *58*:151, 1975.

17. Bergner, L., Eisenberg, M.S., and Hallstrom, A.: Survivors of out-of-hospital cardiac arrest: Morbidity and long term survival. Am. J. Emerg. Med. *2*:189, 1984.

18. Hearne, T., *In* Eisenberg, M.S., et al. (eds.): Sudden cardiac death in the community. New York, Praeger, 1984, pp. 37–40.

19. Cales, R.H.: Trauma mortality in Orange County: The effect of implementation of a regional trauma system. Ann. Emerg. Med. *13*:15, 1984.

20. Cales, R.H.: Medical Evaluation in Trauma Care Systems. Rockville, MD, Aspen, pp. 214–215, 1986.

21. Kessner, D.M., Kalk, C.E., and Siner, J.: Assessing health quality—the case for tracers. N. Engl. J. Med. *288*:1891, 1973.

22. Eisenberg, M.S., et al.: Cardiac arrest and resuscitation: A tale of 29 cities. Ann. Emerg. *19*:2, 1990.

23. Bukov, L.F., White, R.D., and Bachman, J.W.: New prospectives on rural EMT defibrillation. Ann. Emerg. Med. *17*:318, 1988.

24. Dubois, R., and Brook, R.: Preventable deaths: Who, how often and why? Ann. Intern. Med. *109*:582, 1988.

25. Eisenberg, M.S., et al.: Out of hospital cardiac arrest: A review of major studies and a proposed uniform reporting system. Am. J. Public Health *70*:236, 1980.

26. Shackford, S.R., et al.: The effect of regionalization upon the quality of trauma care as assessed by concurrent audit before and after institution of a trauma system: a preliminary report. J. Trauma *26*:812, 1986.

27. McKenzie, E.J.: Injury severity scales: Overview and directions for future research. Am. J. Emerg. Med. *2*:537, 1984.

28. Association for the Advancement Automotive Medicine. Abbreviated Injury Score 1985 Revision: Arlington Heights, Il. 1990.

29. Petrecelli, E., States, J.D., and Homes, L.N.: The abbreviated injury scale: Evaluation, usage and future adaptability. Accident Analysis and Prevention *13*:29–35, 1981.

30. McKenzie, E.J., Steinwachs, D.M., and Shankar, B.: Classify severity of trauma based on hospital discharge diagnoses: Validation of an ICD-9CM to AIS-85 Conversion Table. Medical Care *27*:1989.

31. McKenzie, E.J., Shapiro, S., and Eastham, J.N., Jr.: Rating AIS severity using emergency department sheets vs inpatient charts. J. Trauma *25*:984, 1985.

32. Baker, S.P., et al.: The injury severity score: a method for describing patients with multiple injuries and evaluating emergency care. J. Trauma *14*:187, 1974.

33. Bull, J.P.: The injury severity score of road casualties in relation to mortality, time of death, hospital treatment time and disability. Accident Analysis and Prevention *7*:249, 1978.

34. Stone, H.B., et al.: Measuring the severity of injury. Br. Med. J. *2*:1247, 1977.

35. Copes, S., Champion, H.R., Sacco, W.J., et al.: The ISS revisited. J. Trauma *28*:69, 1988.

36. MacKenzie, E.J., Shapiro, S., and Eastham, J.N.: The abbreviated injury scale and injury severity score: levels of inter- and intrarater reliability. Med. Care *23*:823, 1985.

37. Champion, H.R., et al.: A revision of the trauma score. J. Trauma *29*:623, 1989.

38. Champion, H.R., et al.: A progress report on the trauma score in predicting fatal outcome. J. Trauma *26*:927, 1986.

39. Morris, J.A., et al.: The trauma score as a triage tool in the prehospital setting. JAMA *256*:1319, 1986.

40. Boyd, C.R., Tolson, M.A., and Copes, W.S.: Evaluating trauma care: The TRISS method. J. Trauma *27*:270, 1987.

41. Flora, J.D.: A method for comparing survival of burn patients to a standard survival curve. J. Trauma *18*:701, 1978.

42. Cottington, E.M., Shuffleberger, C.M., and Townsend, R.: The power of the Z statistic: Implications for trauma research and quality assurance review. J. Trauma *29*:1500, 1989.

43. Cayten, C.G., Stahl, W.H., Murphy, J., et al.: Limitations of TRISS for interhospital comparison: A multihospital study. J. Trauma *30*:916, 1990.

44. Champion, H.R., et al.: A new characterization of injury severity. J. Trauma.

45. Brook, R.H., and Appel, F.A.: Quality of care assessment: choosing a method for peer review. N. Engl. J. Med. *288*:1323, 1973.

46. Herrmann, N., et al.: Interobserver and intraobserver reliability in the collection of EMS data. Health Services Research *15*:127, 1980.

47. Linn, B.S.: Effect of burn education on quality of emergency care. DHEW NCHSR Management Series, 1975–1978.

48. Campbell, D., and Stanley, J.: Experimental and quasiexperimental designs for research. Chicago, Rand McNally, 1963.

49. Sherman, M., et al.: Threats to the validity of emergency medical services evaluation: A case study of mobile intensive care units. Medical Care *17*:127, 1979.

50. Cayten, C.G., et al.: Assessing the validity of EMS data. JACEP *7*:390, 1978.

51. Dagher, M., and Lloyd, R.J.: Developing EMS quality assessment indicators. Prehosp. Disaster Med. *7*:69, 1992.

SECTION TWO. FOREIGN MODELS OF ORGANIZATION OF EMS

EDITOR'S NOTE

Kathleen A. Handal

Although the fundamental medical principles of delivering emergency medical care are similar worldwide, several other countries have configured systems that differ from that of the United States.

Emergency medical care in many countries is interwoven into the design and operations of a comprehensive health care system. Thus, emergency medical services (EMS) are recognized as a dynamic part of health care delivery, not as a new, ill-defined appendage.

New technology and research have pushed the growth of emergency medical care to the forefront. In many countries, specialists in this new area have been assimilated into the health care delivery system.

Other countries have factored into the health care equation elements that have not yet been totally addressed in the health care delivery system of the U.S. This equation represents bringing expertise and equipment to the emergent patient and considering, among other factors, need versus expectation and demand, and supply versus available resources and manpower.

Evident in all systems is the success of managing this challenge: what is better, plausible, reasonable? Specifically, with manpower resources, the number of physicians varies from country to country. Use of existing resources and personnel, i.e., trained responders such as firefighters and police already nearby, improves the outcome and decreases cost in many EMS.

Lessons can be learned from systems that are developing and perhaps still addressing less complex issues, and from those that are defining total health care for their citizens.

In the second edition of this book, EMS systems in Hungary, Sweden, and Israel were covered. The interested reader is referred to this edition.

CANADA

Ronald D. Stewart

CAPSULE

Canada has no single, uniform prehospital care system. There are no national standards, and no central governing authority. The variety of services among provinces is not only a function of provincial autonomy in health care, but is also rooted in economic and cultural differences. The system of emergency care is in evolution, and the problems of distances, climate, and economics remain to be solved. In some areas of the country, these problems are only now being addressed.

INTRODUCTION AND BACKGROUND

The loose confederation of former British colonies that came together in 1867 to found the Dominion of Canada has expanded to occupy more than half of North America. Whether viewed as a mighty colossus of the north or the cold, dark attic of the United States, Canada has taken her place in the family of nations as a constitutional monarchy, a loose confederation of regions united largely by fear of disintegration and absorption into the great American melting pot. As the second largest country on the planet, with a land mass of almost 10,000,000 km² and one of the smallest population densities in the world, Canada has unique problems as it attempts to provide emergency care to citizens from a latitude reaching as far south as northern California to the high Arctic, and from the easternmost tip of Newfoundland to the Pacific rim, an expanse stretching across six times zones.

To understand the development and evolution of emergency medicine and emergency medical services in Canada, it is necessary to understand something of the broad expanse of the country and its health care system. With a population of 25,000,000, one tenth that of its neighbor to the South and with disparate regions divided by geographic, political, and cultural barriers, no one system of emergency medical services is in place in a country that boasts a sophisticated and much-envied health care system.

Politically, the country is a constitutional monarchy, with Queen Elizabeth II as the Head of State represented in the country by a Governor-General who is appointed by the monarch. Canada is a bilingual federal state with a national Parliament of two houses—the appointed upper house, the Senate; and the lower house, the House of Commons, elected by proportional representation. Each of its ten provinces and its two northern territories (Yukon and Northwest Territories) that make up the northern half of the country and in which the fewest people live, has a unicameral assembly elected by universal suffrage. Each provincial House of Assembly (L'Assemblé Nationale in Quebec) has specific powers assigned to the Provinces by the Canadian Constitution of 1983. Among these powers is the mandate to care for health of its citizens.

THE HEALTH CARE SYSTEM

Although health care is a provincial responsibility, the character of the health care system in Canada is governed by the Canada Health Act, a federal statute that outlines the essential components of health care that must be available to all Canadians. To receive federal funding for health, provinces must adhere to the regulations of this act, although each may wish to further finance its system in different ways. The medical care systems for each province must guarantee each Canadian free access to health care. Physicians are prohibited by the act from charging for their services, and most hospital costs are also covered by the provincial plans. Physicians are reimbursed for their services by the provincial government. Fees are set through a process of negotiation between medical societies and the ministries of health of the various provinces. The government funds and therefore controls all residency positions, allocation of equipment to hospitals, and

drugs that can be included in provincial "pharmacare" programs.

IMPLICATIONS FOR EMS

The control of provincial governments extends to all sectors of health care, including prevention, medical intervention, and transport. All regulations are set by the health ministries of the provinces, and as a result of regional differences and disparities, a "patchwork quilt" has been created in regard to ambulance services and prehospital care.

The close involvement of government so closely in almost every aspect of health care is, as one might guess, a double-edged sword. On one hand, it can be restrictive; on the other, the ability to effect change through regulation can be advantageous when *systems* are being developed. Canadian EMS is in the midst of this development.

REGIONAL DISPARITIES

A fact of Canadian life is regional disparity—different levels of socioeconomic development with deep historical and cultural roots. The more economically disadvantaged areas such as the Atlantic Provinces suffer from high unemployment, whereas a surplus of jobs exists in Central Canada. Attempts to "equalize" the economic disparities have been made throughout the history of the country. Regional economic expansion grants by the federal government, unemployment insurance, tax incentives, and other programs have all played a role in putting into practice the stated goal of government to provide equal opportunity to all citizens.

The regional disparity enters the realm of EMS as well. Provinces with large tax bases (Ontario, British Columbia, and Alberta) have advanced systems of prehospital care, whereas the less advantaged provinces (Newfoundland, Nova Scotia, New Brunswick) have no systems, or at least only basic ones.

ORGANIZATION

COMPONENTS AND INFLUENCES

The foundation stones of EMS programs accident prevention and first-aid instruction to the public, have deep historical roots in the country. The work of the Red Cross in the field of water safety, CPR instruction, and first-aid training has been credited with training millions of Canadians in these basics. The Royal Life Saving Society, founded in London in the late nineteenth century, has been active in Canada since the turn of the century and plays a large role in water safety, teaching swimming, and organizing conferences and seminars in matters relating to submersion incidents.

The training of the lay public in, and the provision of, first aid at mass gatherings has been the mandate of an active organization whose roots date back centuries. The St. John's Ambulance Association, organized in its modern form in the nineteenth century, provides first-aid workers, vehicles, and equipment during public gatherings throughout the country. The association is a highly structured and disciplined institution composed of lay workers, nurses, physicians, and others who draw upon the humanitarian traditions of the Order of St. John of Jerusalem, which traces its history to a hospital founded more than 1200 years ago.

Prevention programs are within the mandate of the Ministries of Health of the various provinces, sometimes in cooperation with Ministries of the Attorney-General, which are charged with public safety. Anti-drug campaigns, drunk-driving awareness programs, and other efforts that seek to reduce the toll of accidents are all within the jurisdiction of provincial government ministries.

THE DEVELOPMENT OF EMERGENCY MEDICINE

The Royal College of Physicians and Surgeons of Canada, the body charged with specialty training and governing, granted emergency medicine full specialty status in 1983, and recognized residency programs in four provinces. These have now expanded in both the number of residency slots and the hospitals conducting programs. Recent regulations require specialty training beyond medical school of 5 years, after which time the candidate may sit for written and oral specialty examinations conducted by the Royal College. Specialty certification is granted on a national basis, each province recognizing the Royal College examination status. Licensing, however, is granted by the Provincial Medical Board.

The specialty organization in Canada representing the interests of all emergency physicians is the Canadian Association of Emergency Physicians (L'Association Canadienne des Médicins d'Urgence). A Prehospital Care Section has been organized, with the goal of improving EMS throughout the country. The Association conducts seminars, sponsors conferences, and holds its annual meeting in various venues in different provinces.

The Trauma Association of Canada has an interest in EMS as it applies to the trauma patient, and encourages research and academic presentations through its annual meeting held in conjunction with the Royal College each year.

CURRENT TRENDS IN PREHOSPITAL CARE

STANDARDS

No national standards are prescribed for vehicles, equipment, or clinical systems of care in Canada. A committee sponsored by the Canadian Medical Association, with representation from the Canadian Association of Emergency Physicians, has been set up to conduct voluntary reviews of training sites throughout the country. This committee has developed standards for training and is currently debating a revision of its regulations.

TRAINING

Requirements and methods of training prehospital care personnel vary widely throughout Canada. Various skill levels have been described (Emergency Medical Attendant (EMA)I, II and III), depending on the length and depth of the curriculum offered. Not only the extent but the method of training ambulance personnel varies widely throughout the country, from basic requirements (first-aid certificate, etc.) to the advanced training required of mobile intensive care unit paramedics. In the less developed "systems," only basic skills are taught, but in the more prosperous areas of the country, training can continue to the undergraduate diploma level. In the organized systems (Ontario, British Columbia, Alberta), basic EMA is taught by Community Colleges, and the training of advanced life support personnel is assigned to base hospitals.

Physician training in EMS is specific to residencies in emergency medicine, and the requirements in such programs are as varied as the training of prehospital personnel. No set curriculum in nursing education deals specifically with prehospital care issues, but emergency nursing curricula have a component that addresses this element of emergency medicine.

RESEARCH

Only one province has set aside a specific fund to encourage EMS research. The Ministry of Health of Ontario invites submissions from interested clinician investigators in the field of emergency medicine. Funds are disbursed on the advice of an academic committee independent of the Ministry. Other research projects emanate usually from academic institutions in which residency programs are located.

CONFIGURATION

THE SYSTEMS

The prehospital care system in any one province usually reflects the tax base and wealth of that section of the country. In the less advantaged provinces, ambulance service is most commonly operated by private providers with government subsidy. Negotiations as to fees and such subsides are usually carried out between provincial ministries and the organization representing the private provider. In provinces with more developed services, the system of ambulance care can be privately run with government regulation and subsidy (Alberta) or operated as a provincial system, or a combination of the two (Ontario).

The province of Ontario has an extensive system of land and air prehospital care, with provincial regulations defining standards in respect to training, equipment, personnel, etc. It is the only province that provides a budget for prehospital care research from Ministry funds.

The province of Quebec is unique in that it operates a physician-directed ambulance service in Montreal (Urgences Santé) in which the physician is called to the scene of acute illness or accident. This somewhat resembles the Service d'Aide Médicale d'urgence (SAMU) in France.

PERSONNEL

Prehospital care personnel range in skills and responsibilities from those trained in basic first aid to mobile intensive care unit paramedics. Programs in advanced life support exist in the cities of Vancouver, Calgary, Edmonton, Toronto, and Hamilton. Montreal is unique in that physicians are present at scenes of serious illness and accident (Urgences Santé). EMT-S projects have been introduced in several communities on an experimental basis.

AIR SERVICE

One of the greatest challenges facing the health care system in Canada is the provision of rapid evacuation of the seriously ill and injured to a health care facility. Considering the broad expanse of wilderness and the remote nature of some communities, "accessibility" becomes not a financial issue but a question of geography. The use of helicopters is restricted, by large distances, to regional services surrounding centers of population.

The provision of air ambulance services again varies widely throughout the country. Most evacuation programs use fixed-wing aircraft for long-distance transport. Government-operated air ambulance systems exist in Quebec, Ontario, and British Columbia, and subsidized services are currently used in Alberta. Helicopter services attached to hospitals exist in Alberta; Ontario has an extensive network of helicopter and fixed-wing services, especially in the northern sector of the province. The northern territories depend on evacuation by means of Armed Services aircraft or government charter. In the Atlantic Provinces, rescue at sea is a function of the Coast Guard (as it is in other areas). In the eastern provinces, they also function as a medivac program. Weather is a constant problem that often prevents air evacuation from some remote areas for days at a time. During the spring breakup (thaw) in the north, evacuation of the sick and injured can be delayed because of inability to navigate rivers and waterways, and the weather may be inauspicious for flying.

FRANCE

Nicholas DuFeu and Philippe Hrouda

CAPSULE

The Emergency Medical Service system in France is based on the premise that all calls for assistance deserve a response with medical involvement. The dispatch center responds to acute medical emergencies, but also provides the population with 24-hour medical care or advice, whatever the nature and type of emergency. The EMS is configured to avoid abuse or inadequate, unnecessary, and costly use of both personnel and equipment.

INTRODUCTION

In French society, any call for medical assistance requires an answer. The aim of all emergency services is to give patients or victims the benefit of effective resources as quickly as possible. This is provided in an Emergency Medical Services (EMS) system in three ways:

1. Medically by decreasing mortality and morbidity
2. Economically by protecting the active and productive population
3. Politically by informing the public and increasing survival.

Such a system has been made possible by both the medical and nonmedical evolution of science and technology.

A balance between demand and response was the goal. All existing EMSs within the country had to be recognized and integrated into the EMS system. The necessity of centralizing emergency medical calls to avoid confusion and wasteful response is obvious. An area EMS should be able to respond to a call by drawing from the various existing organizations operating in that area. This integration into emergency medical care delivery occurs through medical direction and education.

BACKGROUND

To treat wounded soldiers rapidly and decrease mortality and morbidity, Baron Dominic Larrey, Napoleon's chief army surgeon, created the "flying ambulances." These teams followed Napoleon's troops into battle, performing triage, surgery (sutures, excisions, immobilization, and amputation), and even sedation (opium) at the scene. As a result, more than 40% of the wounded were saved; at that time a considerable saving. These advanced concepts were reaffirmed more than a century later in the Second World War and Vietnam. It is ironic that progress in prehospital emergency care almost always occurs as a result of military missions (i.e., medivacs, blood transfusions in the field). Until the late 1960s, the attitude in civilian medical practice was to bury one's head in the sand. Lack of interest in what was going on outside the hospital was common, even though this aspect directly affected the outcome for emergency patients, especially victims of traffic accidents and coronary disease.

In 1965, for the first time, in the inner cities of Toulouse and Montpellier, the hospital went directly to the patient, on wheels with physicians on board.

The emergency and intensive care mobile units, the Service Mobile d' Urgencey et de Réamination (SMURs), were created in France. The physicians were specialists in anesthesia and resuscitation medicine. These units soon became popular and spread throughout the country. By 1986, there were 255 SMURs, largely as a result of the increased number of specialized physicians in anesthesia and resuscitation medicine. The number of physicians in this specialty increased between 1966 and 1986 by 500%.

ORGANIZATION

With the growth of EMSs, the need to control the use of such important and sophisticated resources became the priority. France is divided into 95 counties, and each county has an EMS headquarters, called the Service d'Aide Médicale Urgente (SAMU). The authority of the SAMU was assigned by law in 1976. This allowed all emergency medical calls to be centralized with the coordinated response by the various needed and available resources. The philosophy adopted by all involved in the management of prehospital emergency medicine was the following:

All calls for emergency medical assistance deserve and require an answer, with the involvement of a senior physician in anesthesia and resuscitation medicine.

To keep the SAMU from being overwhelmed with calls for medical assistance, a first-tier response was created. Often a patient needs to consult a physician but knows that it is not a true emergency and does not know who should be called. In some counties, the general practitioners organized a 24-hour emergency call and based themselves in the regional SAMU Headquarters. Triage was therefore done by the citizen choosing the SAMU for vital emergencies and the general practitioner for nonvital emergencies. This pretriage is also done from the scene by paramedical personnel or the fire brigade, and at times by the police, the family, or the general practitioner.

This continued until January 1986, when the government created a unique telephone number, 15, for medical calls only, whatever the nature and degree of urgency. Each county was mandated to organize its number 15 center (Center 15) during the next few years. As of 1990, 30 out of 95 counties had organized their center 15. The number 15 was chosen for brevity and also because 17 is for the police, and 18 is for the fire brigade. This allows self-selection directly for fire, police assistance, or a medical problem. The EMS Headquarters or Center 15 is officially named the Center for Reception and Regulation of Calls (CRRA). A CRRA's budget is comprised of revenues from the state (27%), local government (60%), Social Security/Welfare (20%) and other sources (2%).

The motivation for change was that all individuals concerned with medical assistance should be involved in the Center 15s. Who are those individuals? First are the professionals, who are all medical, the SAMU, which is usually based at a hospital, managed by specialists in intensive care and anesthesia and who care for only life- or limb-threatening situations; and the general practitioners. Next, are the nonmedical professionals, which are the fire brigade, who are trained in first aid and CPR; and the volunteers, probably Red Cross or Civil Defense workers or those of another humanitarian organization. The roles and responsibilities of these personnel make Center 15 operate. How does the Center work? The citizen dials 15, whatever the medical problem, to call for medical advice or information on different hospitals or to ask a general practitioner to come to the home. He or she may also ask for immediate and vital help.

When a call enters the CRRA switchboard, it is taken by a telephone receptionist, who routes the call to either the general practitioner or the SAMU physician. The SAMU is for a possible true emergency and the general practitioner for nonemergency calls or requests for medical advice. It is the responsibility of the SAMU physician or the general practitioner to determine the type of response a call requires. Response capabilities include intensive care mobile ambulances or SMURs, a conventional ambulance, a rapid four-wheel car, or a helicopter. The general practitioner can send one of his colleagues to the site where the patient is. Both the SAMU and the general practitioner can send the nearest fire brigade or volunteer to the road or home to handle a problem. This occurs when an acute medical intervention is not necessary. The aim is to ensure that the patient, wherever he or she is, receives prompt and adequate emergency medical assistance.

In each county, the CRRA receives an average of 30 to 70 thousand calls per year. Only 20% are true emergencies and require the intervention of an SMUR. Forty to seventy percent involve trauma or industrial (working) accidents and suicides. Twenty to thirty percent concern cardiovascular disease, predominantly coronary artery disease. Eighty percent of the patients who require SMUR intervention are men under 65 years old. The origin of calls to the CRRA is as follows: 60% from citizens, 19% from the fire brigade, 6% from general practitioners, 5% from volunteers, ambulance drivers, etc., and 11% from hospitals.

Hospitals contact the CRRA to use the SAMU for secondary transfers from one hospital to another. These transfers almost always involve direct medical supervision throughout. As many as 16% of all calls are handled by telephone operators only. The percentage of incoming calls directed to the general practitioners is 37%, as compared to those taken at the SAMU (42%). The nature of the response for calls to 15 is as follows: information, 10%; sending a general practitioner to the home of the patient, 22%; sending an ambulance to take the patient to a hospital, 7%; sending the fire brigade, 5%; sending the police, 1%; sending an SMUR, 42%; and others, 13%. These numbers and ratios were current at the time of this writing and reflect a steady state.

PREHOSPITAL CARE

In the SAMU organization, it is the hospital with all its personnel that goes to the patient in an acute situation. The CRRA or Center 15 is normally based with an SAMU at the major hospital. It is crucial for both to be together at a major hospital. The availability and means for responding with medical and paramedical personnel, in a major disaster, should be present at a CRRA. Personnel, especially in training, can be drawn from the Emergency Department (ED), operating suites, or intensive care unit in a major university medical center. Furthermore, in France, the specialists in anesthesia and resuscitation medicine based in SAMUs manage on a daily basis both prehospital and in-hospital care, thus truly directing all aspects of the patient's critical care.

In this relatively young specialty of anesthesia and resuscitation medicine, physicians are trained to diagnose and treat all emergency situations, prehospital or hospital, to perform anesthesia, and to manage all postsurgical or traumatic cases through intensive care. Thus the patient is managed from the scene through discharge from the ICU by the same physicians. The emergency call arriving at the CRRA or Center 15 is switched to the SAMU, which is staffed by senior physician specialists in anesthesia and resuscitation medicine, (the regulator physician) 24 hours a day. The call may require simple advice, a medical intervention, referral to the general practitioner, or dispatch of a unit.

In a possibly critical situation, an SMUR team is dispatched from the nearest SAMU headquarters. Distance between the nearest hospital and the scene of the emergency determines which unit is dispatched. A physician, usually assisted by a paramedical staff person, which can be a nurse specialized in anesthesia and resuscitation are the team. Medical students may participate as added team members. This team can be sent out in an ambulance or by helicopter. All helicopters are based at major hospitals.

At the scene, the physician administers care to the victim as if inside the hospital emergency department, assisted by the paramedical personnel. CPR is performed, if not already begun by those who called the SAMU, usually the fire brigade or the general practitioner. All necessary interventions are performed at the scene, including intubation, central lines, drug administration, and artificial ventilation with portable ventilators. Sometimes use of a chest tube, volume replacement (usually with macro molecules), and placement of gastric and urinary probes are carried out. All the techniques of sedation and general anesthesia can be performed if needed, for example, for reduction of a compound fracture.

The senior regulator physician may assist by giving advice to the physician at the scene. When the patient is stabilized on the scene, a medical report is given by radio to the medical dispatcher or regulator physician. This report allows the nearest appropriate and available hospital bed to be sought for the patient. This coordinating step is important and avoids unnecessary secondary transport from one hospital to another. Despite this principle of good medical care, the SAMU is often called upon to arrange and perform secondary transport to another hospital for patients who were not initially cared for by the SAMU but went directly to the hospital.

The government, by creating the unique call number, 15, has benefited economically, avoiding numerous unnecessary secondary transports from one hospital to another and unnecessary hospitalization of patients.

OTHER ACTIVITIES OF THE EMERGENCY MEDICAL SERVICE

In a disaster, each SAMU works and plans with the various organizations and government institutions for the appropriate response, depending on the potential risks in each county. The few SAMUs within the major university medical centers are responsible for medical postgraduate disaster programs. Physicians who complete this program successfully receive a diploma in Disaster Medicine. These same SAMUs are configured to become involved in and respond to disaster situations throughout the world.

The education activities of the SAMU involve responsibility for medical and paramedical training; for the medical students, courses in prehospital and hospital emergency care are at the postgraduate level. Programs to train nurses, ambulance drivers and volunteers in basic CPR are also included in their educational role.

In addition to an important role in education, the SAMU is involved in prevention and research. SAMUs throughout the country have professional standing in universities with research capabilities. The discipline has its own medical journal.

A unique feature of the paramedical personnel in France is the fact that the SAMU staff is composed only of specialized nurses. After 3 years of study, along with general nursing experience, a nurse may qualify to study 2 more years to become a specialist. Training for nurses specializing in anesthesia and resuscitation medicine prepares them to work in the operating suites as nurse anesthetists, in the intensive care unit,

or in the SAMU prehospital structure. Thus, at any time, if a "burnout" situation arises (as often described in the United States EMS literature), a nurse may change professional activity and remain a healthy, contributing, employed being using his or her nursing skills.

HORIZONS

Specialized medical personnel may become a challenge to the system in the next few years because the number of SAMU physicians has been reduced considerably. The natural question arises, "Will they be replaced by the specialized nurses in anesthesia and resuscitation medicine or by specialized trained medical students?" The answer is not yet clear. But what is clear, as everyone agreed at the 1989 meeting of all the major European EMS systems: a call arriving at an EMS Headquarters must be received by a physician, and diagnosis, triage, and therapeutic choices can be made only by a physician.

NATIONAL CONTACTS

Department of Health:
Direction General de la Santé (DGS)
124, rue Sadi Carnot
92170 Vanves
France
Tx: 206.355 Fax: (1) 47–65–27–21
Director: Professeur Jean-Francois Girard
Undersecretary: Médecin Inspecteur en Chef Francoise Lalande

Home Office:
Direction de la Sécurité Civile (DSC)
Place Beauvau
75800 Paris
France
Tx: 611.390 Fax: (1) 47–57–82–67
Director: Monsieur Hubert Fournier
Medical Adviser: Médecin-Chef Pierre Chevalier

War Department:
Direction Centrale du Service de Santé des Armées (DCSSA)
14, rue Saint-Dominique
75997 Paris Armées
France
Director: Médecin General Inspecteur Jean Mine
Chef de la Section Santé du Service de Relations publiques des Armées: Médecin en Chef F. Delorme

National Union for EMS:

Syndicat National de L'aide Médicale Urgence (SNAMU)

SAMI 95—Centre Hospitalier René Dubos
2, Ave de l'Ile-de-France
95301 Cergy Pontoise Cedex
France
Tx: 604.480
President: Professeur Louis Lareng
First-Secretary: Docteur Alain Giroud

Disaster Medicine:

French Society for Disaster Medicine (SFMC)
FAMU 94—Hospital Henri Mondor
94010 Creteil Cedex
France
TX: 264.145 Fax: (1) 48–98–04–00
President: Professeur Pierre Huguenard
International Relations: Docteur Philippe Hrouda

BIBLIOGRAPHY

Cazejust, D: Note sur les transports inter-hospitaliers pour examens et traitements spécialisés. Conv. Méd. 3:208, 1987.

Cazejust, D., and Desjardins, J.: Rôle des SAMU de l'Assistance Publique de Paris en cas de catastrophe, sinistre ou accident grave. Mise en oeuvre du plan blanc. Urg. Med. 3:206, 1989.

Chopin, J.: L'accueil des urgences dans les hôpitaux publics en France. Conv. Méd. 2:107, 1988.

Hrouda, P.: Dial "one Five"—A single medical emergency number—(How a "15 organization" works). Conv. Méd. 6:391, 1987.

Hrouda, P.: The advanced SAMUs headquarters in Val-de-Marne. Conv. Méd. 2:115, 1988.

Hrouda, P.: The Place of Disaster Medicine in Relief Organizations Plans in France. Bulletin of the Internation Society for Disaster Medicine, February 1989, Geneva, Switzerland.

Huguenard, P.: Médecin Generaliste et "Center 15." Urg. Méd. 4:259, 1989.

Lalande, F.: Incidence des réformes récentes sur le fonctionnement et les effectifs des services d'urgence. Conv. Méd. 2:143, 1986.

Lalande, F.: Mise en place de nouvelles reglementations. Perspectives en matière de formation au CCA. Conv. Méd. 6:310, 1988.

Pasteyer, J.: Place des SAMU et SMUR dans les plans de secours. Urg. Méd. 4:289, 1989.

APPLICABLE LAWS

Law 86–11
Official Journal of the French Republic
326–328, January 6, 1986

Decree 87–964
Official Journal of the French Republic
13977-14000, November 30, 1987

Decree 87–1005
Official Journal of the French Republic
14692–14693, December 16, 1987

JAPAN

Tsuguharu Ishida

CAPSULE

The Emergency Medical Services (EMS) system in Japan is relatively young and has many identified challenges. Efforts to solve these, such as the critical emergency transfer system, academic resources and expertise, criteria for certification of emergency specialists, etc., are being developed by the Japanese Association for Acute Medicine (JAAM). Currently, 6550 physicians and 1460 nurses and Emergency Medical Technicians (EMTs) are involved, along with related government and medical agencies. The Department of Health and Welfare and the Fire Defense Agency of Japan are seriously considering introducing a paramedics system. The exact role of a paramedic in prehospital and hospital emergency care is not yet decided. The goal is for the EMS system to grow and affect morbidity or mortality more significantly in the immediate future. The increase in private medical providers may play a role in the increasing sophistication of prehospital care.

INTRODUCTION

Deaths caused by motor vehicle accidents in Japan increased in the early 1960s as a result of rapid industrial and economic development. The need to create safer traffic conditions became a national challenge. In 1963, the Fire Defense Act was amended, and the responsibilities of ambulance service were assigned to the Fire Defense Organization. At this writing, the number of municipalities rendering ambulance service was 3021 (93.1%), 98.9% in terms of population. The Japanese EMS system has serious problems, however, such as an inadequate number of general hospitals and a flood of nonemergent patients.

In 1973, the Japanese Association for Acute Medicine (JAAM) was established to promote a more sophisticated EMS system. In 1985, the JAAM started a qualification system for emergency medicine. At present, only physicians can give advanced life support (ALS) in prehospital settings. To alleviate such problems, the Ministry of Health and Welfare developed the critical emergency transfer system in 1977.

In 1988, 98.7% of the entire population was covered by ambulance service. The use of a critical emergency transfer model coupled with computer-aided EMS information is a goal subsidized by the Ministry of Health and Welfare.

BACKGROUND

In 1931, the first ambulance service began in the Osaka Branch Office of the Japan Red Cross.

It was 1933 when the Fire Department of Yokohama started an ambulance service. Because no legal requirements existed, the number of municipalities that had ambulance service increased only gradually. This was accelerated after the fire department was separated from the police in 1948.

Since the early 1960s, Japan has experienced a rapid development of industry and economy, causing various kinds of disasters to increase and thus necessitating development of a nationwide ambulance service system.

In October 1961, the Director General of the Fire Defense Agency organized the Fire Defense Council to govern ambulance service. In May 1962, the council arrived at the conclusion that Japan needed a nationwide ambulance service system and accompanying national legislation. In August 1962, the Administrative Management Agency made a recommendation, based on the results of the Fire Defense Council, calling for a more effective ambulance service system by establishing minimum standards for ambulance services and assigning responsibility for their delivery to fire defense organizations. In 1963, the Fire Defense Act was amended according to those recommendations (Table 87-19).

ORGANIZATION OF THE EMS

Since the 1963 amendment, the number of municipalities offering ambulance service has increased rapidly: 835 in 1970; 2429 in 1975; and 3021 in 1988—93.1% of all municipalities in Japan. In terms of population, 98.7%, almost the entire population, is covered by ambulance service.

As of April 1, 1988, there were 3890 ambulance crews nationwide. Ambulance coverage is 1 to 2.4 million.

In 1987, there were 2,426,852 ambulance runs with 2,348,217 transports. Ambulance crews were being called out at a rate of once every 13 seconds. Requests for an ambulance resulted from acute illness in 48.8% of the calls, 23.1% from traffic accidents, and 12% from other injuries.

Since 1936, by dialing the number 119, toll free, throughout Japan, anyone can reach ambulance service.

Of a total of 2,426,852 calls in 1987, 18,047 were false alarms. Response times within 3 minutes accounted for 12.9% of all responses. Response time of greater than 20 minutes accounted for only 1.1% of all calls.

TABLE 87-19. HISTORY OF EMERGENCY MEDICAL SERVICE IN JAPAN

Year Established	Service
1931	Ambulance Service, Osaka Branch Office of the Japan Red Cross
1933	Ambulance Service, Yokohama Fire Department
1936	Nationwide Emergency Telephone Line: 119
1961	Fire Defense Council National Medicare Program
1963	Fire Defense Act
1964	Declared Emergency Clinics, Hospitals
1973	Japanese Association for Acute Medicine
1977	Critical Emergency Transfer System
1982	Emergency Services Day; September 9
1985	Certified Emergency Specialist
1986	Fire Defense Act Amendments
1989	Approved Leader of the Certified Emergency Specialist

Thus approximately 50% of individuals who called an ambulance received assistance within 5 minutes and 56.6% of all transported victims were admitted to hospitals or clinics within 20 minutes.

FIRST-AID MANAGEMENT BY AMBULANCE CREW

Of the 2,348,217 persons transported by ambulances during 1987, first-aid management at the scene and en route was given to 57.1% (1,339,739).

The intervention most often administered was temperature regulation (37.4%). Also performed were oxygen therapy in 15.1%, dressings in 13.2%, hemostasis in 7.8%, and cardiopulmonary resuscitation in 2.1%.

COMMAND AND CONTROL CENTER

In Japan, many urban areas have introduced a computer-aided dispatch with control system for more effective fire and emergency services. Although a computer-aided system has many objectives, its main purpose is to reduce the time and increase the accuracy and flexibility of the assignment and dispatch processes.

ORGANIZATION OF EMERGENCY FACILITIES

In 1988, 5869 medical institutions were designated for treatment of emergency patients. This was a five-fold increase from 1963, when ambulance services were legalized. The Japanese EMS system had and still has two serious challenges in this area: first, the lack of sufficient general hospitals in the system (most hospitals are private or specialty medical facilities not associated or affiliated with other medical institutions in the system); and second, the large number of nonemergent patients using the system. With the introduction in 1961 of a national Medicare program, the

number of visits to emergency departments dramatically increased. Emergency clinics and hospitals could no longer function efficiently enough to give the good and up-to-date emergency care demanded by the public. As a result, the Ministry of Health and Welfare allocated a yearly budget, beginning in 1977, for a systematic nationwide reorganization of emergency medicine, and a new emergency care delivery system. The new system was termed a critical emergency transfer system. An emergency patient first visits a neighboring designated emergency clinic or hospital of arbitrary choice to receive necessary emergency care. If the attending physician judges that the patient requires further medical care, the patient is transferred to an appropriate secondary or tertiary emergency medical center (Fig. 87-21).

PRIMARY EMERGENCY CARE

In cities with a population of 50,000 or more, 481 centers have been opened for primary emergency care 24 hours including holidays. These centers are responsible for the treatment of emergency patients who are likely not to require admission. As necessary, patients are transferred to appropriate secondary or tertiary centers.

SECONDARY EMERGENCY CARE

Clinics or hospitals with more than 20 beds may register as declared emergency clinics or hospitals through authorization of the prefectural government. By 1988, 367 had been registered as secondary emergency care facilities. These facilities form a distinct group and act as an alternating emergency receiving system from primary emergency care facilities, by taking a 24-hour emergency duty by turns.

TERTIARY EMERGENCY CARE

For treating critically ill emergency patients, 101 emergency and critical care centers were opened, one for each prefecture, or approximately one center per one million population. To aid the efficient functioning of the critical emergency transfer system, computer-aided regional emergency medical information centers instantly provide information on the secondary or tertiary emergency centers availability of specialties and vacant beds. By 1988, 31 prefectures had completed this system, with a subsidy from the Ministry of Health and Welfare. This effort continues nationwide. The critical emergency transfer system benefits emergency physicians because most primary and secondary patients, who account for the majority of visits, are treated by other physicians. Emergency specialists at tertiary centers can then concentrate on critically ill or injured patients selected by the primary and secondary centers. In this system, however, critical emer-

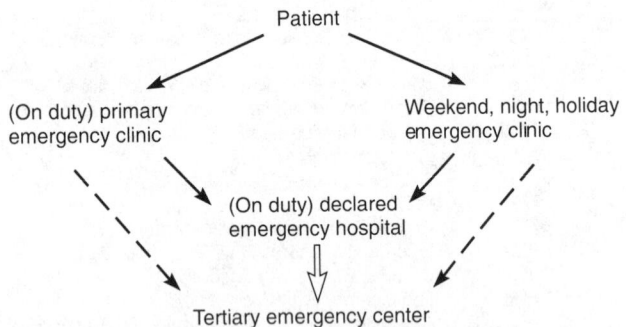

Critical Emergency Transfer System

FIG. 87-21. *Critical emergency transfer system.*

gencies may take excessive time for transfer, and thus the initiation of definitive therapy is often delayed. As the EMS develops new roles, education will address these issues. To decrease time to definite care, EMTs are allowed to take critically ill patients to tertiary centers using their own judgment.

EDUCATION AND TRAINING OF EMS PERSONNEL

PHYSICIANS

In 1973, the JAAM was established for the primary purpose of offering an opportunity for emergency and critical medicine investigators to publish their data. Since its establishment, the JAAM has taken the lead in promoting not only postgraduate medical education but also public education in emergency medicine. The first training program for physicians practicing or interested in emergency medicine began 16 years ago. By 1990, more than 2000 physicians had completed this program. In 1978, the Emergency Resuscitation Committee of the JAAM published the textbook of standards and guidelines for cardiopulmonary resuscitation (CPR). The overall revision of this textbook became the standards and guidelines of CPR of the Japan Medical Association (JMA) and was published September 1983 as the first supplement to the Journal of the JMA. This supplement had a circulation of over 200,000 copies and is widely used as a textbook or CPR at the medical nursing and fire-training school.

With the intent of upgrading and further specializing the role of the emergency physician, a qualification system for certified emergency specialists was investigated.

A new system approved by JAAM began in 1985 and, as of May 1989, 1349 emergency specialists have been certified. Emergency specialists must have at least 3 years of clinical experience in emergency and critical care medicine at an approved tertiary emergency facility. Oral examination or/and participation in an education and training program by JAAM is required. Another level for certification of an emergency specialist "approved leader system" was started in 1989, and by 1990, 131 leaders with profound knowledge and skills had been certified.

NURSES

In 1980, two suborganizations, namely a nurses' division and an emergency medical technicians' division, were recognized. Since that time, the general meeting of the nurses' division has been held simultaneously. The JAAM offers educational sessions or lectures for both. The nurses' division is now considering criteria for a certified emergency nurse specialist.

EMERGENCY MEDICAL TECHNICIANS

Ambulance crews consist of 2 members and a chief. EMT courses are offered at fire training schools in each prefecture and in designated cities. National standards exist for this.

The course consists of 135 out of the 900 hours of fire training curriculum. EMTs are not allowed to administer most advanced life support (ALS). Only physician specialists can administer advanced medical treatment. The current definition of advanced medical treatment management necessitates the penetration of the body, and only physicians with specific authority may perform this. Ambulance crews give some ALS, for example bag-mask artificial ventilation with oxygen and airway insertion.

The general meeting of JAAM educational sessions has begun lectures for EMTs. The number of participants has been about 1000 from all over Japan. As of April 1988, 45,804 EMTs were active.

THE PUBLIC

Recently, JAAM published a textbook of first-aid management including CPR for the public under the guidance of the Department of Health and Welfare. More than 50,000 citizens have purchased it already.

AMBULANCES AND EQUIPMENT

As of April 1988, ambulances, including reserve cars, numbered 4443. An ambulance is required to have equipment and supplies for transportation, respiratory care, wound dressing, disinfection, rescue, basic nursing care, and other necessary items. Table 87-20 shows the minimal requirements for ambulances in Japan.

NATIONAL CONTACTS

International Committee
Japanese Association for Acute Medicine
c/o Department of Traumatology
Osaka University Hospital
1–1–50, Fukushima, Fukushima-ku,
Osaka 553, JAPAN

Ambulance and Rescue Service Division
Fire Defense Agency
2–1–2, Kasumigaseki, Chiyoda-ku,
Tokyo 100, JAPAN

TABLE 87-20. MINIMAL REQUIREMENTS FOR AMBULANCE

Equipment	Item
Transportation	Litter
	Pillow
	Sheet
	Blanket
Respiratory Care	Resuscitator
	Bag-mask unit
	O_2 inhalation unit
	Portable O_2 cylinder
Wound dressing	Splints
	Spineboard
	Triangular bandage
	Tourniquets
	Gauze
	Adhesive tape
	Rotating tourniquets
Basic nursing care	Thermometer
	Sink
	Pan
	Bedpan
	Emesis bags
	Ice bag
	Oilpaper
	Cotton
	Sterile gloves
	Umbilical clamps

TABLE 87-20. CONTINUED

Equipment	Item
	Scissors
	Tweezers
	Cotton applicators
Disinfection	Antiseptic sponges
Rescue	Rescue tools
Others	Helmet
	First aid kit
	Flashlight
	Walkie-talkies

BIBLIOGRAPHY

1. Fire Defense Agency: White Book on Fire Service in Japan, Japan, 1983.
2. Ishida, T., Ohta, M., Katsurada, K., and Sugimoto, T.: The emergency medical system in Japan. J. Emerg. Med. 2:44, 1984.
3. Ohta, M., Katsurada, K., and Sugimoto, T.: The emergency medical system in Japan. J. Emerg. Med. 2:45, 1984.
4. Onji, Y., and Sugimoto, T.: Emergency medicine in Japan. Am. J. Emerg. Med. 1:360, 1983.
5. Yoshioka, T., and Sugimoto, T.: Tertiary emergency care in Japan. Am. J. Emerg. Med. 3:252, 1985.
6. Yoshioka, T., and Sugimoto, T.: The emergency medical system in Japan. Am. J. Emerg. Med. 3:79, 1985.

WEST GERMANY

Markus D.W. Lipp

CAPSULE

West Germany has had a growing need for the ability to deal with an increasing number of accidents and casualties. Although its emergency medical system is still in a developmental stage, emergency physicians are quickly assuming a leadership role. The concept of a "fast responding rescue squad" is also being increasingly accepted. The "new Germany," incorporating East and West Germany, will require EMS development in the former East section. This is likely to occur through extensions of the system described herein as the previously separated countries become reintegrated. The economic divergence between the sections must, in time, be rectified also. Hospitals in the West section are generally more modern and better equipped.

INTRODUCTION

West Germany has a population of nearly 62 million inhabitants and an area of 248,571 square miles. The topography is diverse: in the north, the coasts of the north and the Baltic Sea; near the Ruhr and Rhine, a highly industrialized area; and in the south the area near the Alps.

Politically, the Federal Republic of Germany is subdivided into 10 states, in addition to West Berlin. The organization and guarantee of a prehospital emergency medical service (EMS) are the sole responsibility of the government of each state. Because of political considerations, differences in EMS structure exist between states in West Germany, but the main principles are comparable throughout the country.

The EMS of West Germany has developed rapidly since 1957, when Bauer and Frey introduced the first "Clinomobile," an ambulance with a physician and designed to provide medical support to patients at the emergency site. In 1964, the "rendezvous system" started: emergency physicians from hospitals came to the emergency site by car and met the ambulance.

Not until 1968 did the concept of an emergency ambulance permanently staffed with an emergency physician become established. The cities of Heidelberg, Cologne, and Mainz were among the first. Soon all the cities of West Germany accepted the principle.

Parallel to this growing medical involvement, the number of ambulances operated by volunteer assistance organizations, fire brigades, and private companies grew. A major problem during this period was that rescue vehicles were also being dispatched by many noncooperating rescue coordination centers, and at times a race to the patient occurred.

This situation changed in 1973, when the concept of a modern emergency medical service was established by the proposals of a joint committee of the federal and state governments.

The goals were to be laid down by details in the law for:

> Tasks of the emergency medical service
> Structure of the emergency medical service (central coordination and dispatching, personal and technical demands)
> Financing
> Supervision

Based on this proposal, in most states of West Germany, specific laws concerning the EMS were passed.

The structure of the EMS in West Germany is based on strong medical controls and fast-responding rescue teams. The tasks and responsibilities of the personnel in EMS are organization, management, and supervision. These are clearly defined in matters of medical care, especially if a disaster occurs. Emergency physicians are mainly employed in a hospital. In every town or administrative district, one or two hospitals take part in the local EMS with emergency physicians on duty.

The circumstances surrounding equipment and training of the staff are nearly similar all over the state. The main components of the EMS are:

> Well-trained emergency physicians
> Well-trained paramedics
> Adequate medical and technical equipment

ORGANIZATIONS

HELP ORGANIZATIONS

As in other countries, systems help organizations are important to public health.

The German help organizations are different in origin and age. The "Deutsch Rote Kreuz" is 125 years old and is part of the International Red Cross Societies. The "Arbeiter-Samariter-Bund" was founded in 1889 and had its roots in the workers' movement. "Johaniter Unfallhilfe" and "Matheser-Hilfsdienst" have their origins in the Protestant and Catholic churches respectively. They started their activities in the EMS in 1952 and 1953, respectively. These four help organizations, the fire brigade, and a few private companies supply the EMS, using paramedics and different ambulance cars. All activities of the EMS are now coordinated by a state-controlled rescue coordination center (RCC).

RESCUE COORDINATION CENTER

West Germany is divided into multiple emergency medical service districts, often identically with the political topographic structure of the particular region. The splitting up of Rhineland-Palatinate is a typical example. Every rescue organization center activates and coordinates within its area of responsibility of the ground rescue vehicles and, if necessary and available, rescue helicopters. The rescue operation centers coordinate bed availability and the transport of critically ill patients to the appropriate hospitals. The RCC relays information from the rescue team to the receiving hospital or other specialty facilities (i.e., a detoxification center) as necessary.

EQUIPMENT

COMMUNICATION EQUIPMENT

The communication equipment allows direct telephone connection to the rescue stations, the coordination centers of police and fire departments, and major receiving hospitals. Two-way radio communication devices and, in some centers, computerized information retrieval systems are used. Emergency calls from various sources, including individuals, police, and fire brigade are channeled to the EMS rescue coordination center. In 1989, a plan for a countrywide emergency telephone number was introduced; by 1991, in all parts of West Germany a caller was to be connected directly to the EMS rescue coordination center by dialing 19222.

After taking down the essential and necessary information of an emergency call, the paramedic on duty has to decide which rescue team or vehicle is to be sent out. The response time of an ambulance after alerting should be less than 45 seconds.

Emergency calls that describe critically ill patients lead to the notification of an emergency physician, and the specific indications are prioritized at all rescue coordination centers. The transport of the physicians is carried out by an emergency ambulance, normally located at the hospital (compact system) or by a special car (rendezvous system) with the emergency ambulance arriving separately. The compact system is mostly operated in cities and towns, whereas the rendezvous system is operated in the most rural areas. In an emergency, three dispatch strategies are used: the "next standing vehicle" strategy, the "assignment" strategy, and the "multiple-purposes vehicle" strategy. The "next standing vehicle" strategy means that the nearest rescue vehicle, which is actually situated to the emergency site, has to be alerted, regardless of its configuration or equipment (smaller ambulances as well as emergency ambulances). The main advantage of this principle is the short response time (less than 8.8 minutes in 85% of all emergencies in the town of Karlsruhe, for example). A disadvantage, however, is that in some cases, critically ill patients have to be transported in underequipped small ambulances. The "assignment" strategy means that only emergency ambulances are sent to an emergency patient and the smaller ambulances are reserved for nonurgent transport of noncritically ill patients. The advantage of this principle is that patients can be medically treated with appropriate equipment before and during the transport. Disadvantages are the slightly extended response time (10 minutes) compared to the "next standing vehicle" strategy and the increased cost for the whole emergency medical service.

AMBULANCES AND THEIR EQUIPMENT

The various types of EMS ground vehicles include: smaller ambulances, used for transport of noncritically ill patients; emergency ambulances, primarily designed for the resuscitation of critically ill patients; emergency ambulance cars, generally dispatched with an emergency physician; and finally, cars designed for the transport of the emergency physician. To complement the ground EMS system, there is a network of 36 EMS helicopter stations throughout all parts of West Germany.

The medical rescue equipment of the ground rescue vehicles is tailored to adapt to specific roles and specified in law. Smaller ambulances used for the transport of the noncritically ill are equipped with a litter, transport chair, oxygen tank, suction device, resuscitation masks and bag for artificial respiration, IV infusion supplies, dressings, and bandages. In reality, most of the small ambulances are equipped above the minimum requirements. Complete resuscitation equipment is found in all ambulances; in some areas the rescue coordination centers dispatch the next standing vehicle first, followed by an emergency ambulance, in an effort to reduce the response time. Ambulances are dispatched with two paramedics; the driver may not be a fully trained paramedic.

Use of the EMS vehicles system is for primary and secondary transports. The expression "primary transport" describes an immediate transport of medical personnel (emergency physicians and paramedics) to the emergency site within life-saving minutes, for treatment and stabilization of casualties at the scene followed by medically supervised transport to an appropriate hospital. Primary transports have absolute priority over any other requests to the EMS. A "secondary transport" is carried out if a patient has been stabilized and treated in a hospital and then has to be transferred to a specialized center. Both primary and secondary transports are carried out by ground and air rescue systems.

Emergency ambulances have to be equipped additionally with a vacuum mattress, defibrillator and ECG, and complete resuscitation kits for adults and children including endotracheal intubation instruments, surgical instruments and emergency drugs. The crew consists of two fully trained paramedics. By law, the equipment of an emergency ambulance car, which is generally dispatched with an emergency physician, does not differ from these requirements mentioned above. Like the smaller ambulances, emergency ambulances contain additional rescue and monitoring equipment, for example, automatically working respirators or blood pressure monitors.

Since the development of battery-powered and portable blood pressure monitors and pulse oximeters, these monitors have been introduced to the emergency ambulances to an increasing degree, although they have not yet been mandated by law.

The cars designed for the transport of the emergency physician only to the emergency site (operating in a so-called "rendezvous system") are equipped with resuscitation kits (for adults and children), oxygen bottle, defibrillator/ECG, suction device, and emergency drugs and operated by a fully trained paramedic.

HELICOPTER RESCUE SYSTEM

The helicopter rescue system covers 90% of West Germany. This system allows quick response time even in the countryside, smooth transport of the patient, and rapid delivery to a specialty hospital. This latest aspect can reduce the number of secondary transports significantly. The use of the helicopters is limited by weather and daylight conditions because only a few helicopters of the German army and the disaster control are equipped with night flight capabilities. The air rescue system is used as a primary transport facility as well as for secondary transports. The helicopter located at the University of Hanover, for example, transported fewer than 40% of the patients as primary transports. More than 60% were medically treated at the scene and afterwards transported by a ground rescue vehicle.

The simultaneous dispatching of a ground rescue vehicle and a helicopter has been demonstrated to have some advantages. At the emergency site, the paramedics can start to restore or maintain vital functions (e.g., cardiopulmonary resuscitation). If they arrive earlier, an emergency ambulance provides a dry, warm, well lighted "emergency room" for the initial medical treatment of the patients, a great advantage especially during rough weather conditions.

The helicopters used in the West German EMS are generally equipped in the same way as the emergency ambulances in respect to the medical aspects. The smallest helicopter operated, BO 105, has a restricted cabin area, and thus stabilization must occur before flight. The new crafts, BK 117 and the Bell UH1, provide an unobstructed cabin area, so that treatment during flight is possible. The new larger crafts, such as the Bell UH1, are also operated as "Search and Rescue" crafts.

Most of the helicopters have high maneuverability and small external dimensions, and are twin-engine operated. Only a few helicopters, mainly operated by the army, are allowed to fly at night. The take-off time after alerting should be less than 2 minutes. Statistics in 1985 for the helicopter located at Munich showed that the in-flight time after take-off was approximately 10 minutes with an average distance of 30 km to the emergency site.

The helicopters are mostly located at major hospitals and operated by the disaster control, the German army, the German automobile association and a private rescue organization. The emergency physicians that fly are on the staff of the major hospitals, and the flight attendants are fully trained paramedics of the army or of the self organizations.

EDUCATION AND TRAINING OF EMS PERSONNEL

EMERGENCY PHYSICIANS

In West Germany, emergency physicians routinely staff ambulances to render medical treatment to the emergency patient. At the scene, the responsibility of the emergency physician is to secure and maintain the vital functions of the patient, i.e., respiration and circulation, and to make a presumptive diagnosis. Endotracheal intubation, assisted or controlled ventilation, cardiopulmonary resuscitation (including defibrillation), and infusions and drugs by means of a (peripheral or central venous) line, are routine. The emergency physician must have knowledge of pathophysiology, symptoms, and treatment of typical emergencies in the specialties of surgery, internal medicine, pediatrics, and anesthesiology. On the nonclinical side, emergency physicians must know the structure of the local health and rescue system, e.g., locations, departments, and capabilities of the hospitals in a particular area.

In contrast to other countries, West Germany has no specific emergency departments within hospitals. Emergency medicine is a component in the education of anesthetists, as well as internal specialists and surgeons. Although anesthetists often meet the demands for emergency physicians best, in West Germany surgeons, internal specialists, pediatricians, and general practitioners also work as emergency physicians.

To improve and ensure standards, physicians have to complete a specialty training program successfully and gain clinical experience of at least 18 months after becoming a specialist, of which 6 months is experience in an intensive care unit. During this period, the techniques of emergency medicine, artificial ventilation, endotracheal intubation, and peripheral and central venipuncture, to name a few, are perfected.

Additionally, an 80-hour program of theoretic education on special topics of emergency medicine must be successfully completed. Finally, before being certified as an "emergency physician," by the local health authority, the physician must treat 10 emergency patients in the prehospital setting under the supervision of a senior emergency physician.

PARAMEDICS

Before September 1989, the training of a regular paramedic consisted of 520 hours, divided as follows: 160 hours of theoretic education, 160 hours of practical training in a hospital, 160 hours of practical training in an ambulance, and 40 hours of a final theoretic course. After passing a state certification test consisting of oral, written and practical examinations, the candidate is allowed to work. The aim of the described training was to enable the paramedics to restore or maintain vital functions (e.g., cardiopulmonary resuscitation), but without independent application of drugs and to assist emergency physicians in their treatment. Paramedics, however, had no profession comparable to that of any other workers in the German health system.

In September 1989, education of paramedics was changed fundamentally: the theoretic and practical training at school was extended to a 1200-hour course and an additional 1600-hour practical education at special ambulance dispatching stations. The training now lasts two years and ends with an extensive state certification procedure. Paramedics who have achieved this certification are given an official job title, "Rettungsassistent."

Paramedics may work as full-time employees (fire brigade and private ambulance companies or help organizations) or as volunteers (help organizations only).

RELATED EMS ACTIVITIES

In contrast to other emergency physicians, the emergency physician in charge (EPIC) does not primarily treat single patients at the emergency site and accompany patients to the hospital. He or she remains at the location of the disaster or accident. Provided with adequate technical equipment (e.g., radio communication), the EPIC organizes the medical care given by the emergency physician and paramedics and prioritizes transport to the appropriate hospitals. During the resuscitation efforts, the EPIC must be in close contact with the head of operation for all agencies involved, i.e., the police and fire brigade.

Because of the described demands, the EPIC must have extensive clinical experience and knowledge in emergency medicine, and the organization of the local emergency system. In a disaster medicine training program of 40 hours, physicians gain knowledge of and a tactical approach to diagnostics and medical decisions under disaster conditions. Technical experience and familiarity with equipment and radio communication service are gained through repeated mock exercises, and the much-needed skills and knowledge are acquired and refreshed.

In some towns and areas of West Germany, the EPIC system is already working. An EPIC is among the first to be notified if any of the following occurs: a road or fire accident with more than 5 (in some areas 10) pa-

tients, explosion, airplane crash, train accident, or shipwreck.

FAST-RESPONDING RESCUE SQUADS

The analysis of rescue actions after several disasters occurring recently showed that the everyday emergency system was unable to rescue all patients promptly and properly. A common concurrence was that untrained personnel went into action, with ambulances and staff from other areas becoming involved.

The drain of resources from diversion away from daily operational system needs created a dilemma. To address this challenge, the concept of "fast-responding rescue squads" was developed. Their aim is to provide:

Quick additive support to the daily emergency service with well-trained staff and adequate equipment in case of a greater accident or disaster.

Adequate prehospital care to most or even all patients.

Partial or even temporary but total replacement of the daily emergency service from other areas.

This concept began in the town and area of Mainz, with nearly 200,000 inhabitants, and is described subsequently. Four fast-responding rescue squads were established between 1988 and 1990; the requirements for each squad are listed in Table 87-21.

In addition to possessing knowledge and skills in emergency and disaster medicine, the physicians must be familiar with the structure of the local rescue system, e.g., localization of hospitals, their departments, and equipment in the particular area. Most of the physicians of the fast-responding rescue squads within the Mainz area are anesthesiologists.

The paramedics belong to either the special disaster crew or the local emergency service. Some are volunteers with basic experience in prehospital care. In addition to their training, they are educated in the unique triage approach and medical requirements of disaster medicine.

The medical and technical equipment of one fast-responding rescue squad is designed to provide medical help to 50 patients, 10 of them seriously ill. It contains instruments for endotracheal intubation, artificial ventilation, injection material, multiple sets for intravenous lines and infusion solutions, emergency drugs (including anesthetics), emergency surgery sets, and bandaging material. It also contains radio communication equipment, 25 stretchers, a tent and registration forms.

One or more fast-responding rescue squads should be alarmed if one of the following accidents or disasters has occurred: a road or fire accident with more than 8 to 10 patients, an explosion, an airplane crash, a train accident, or a shipwreck.

TABLE 87-21. FAST-RESPONDING RESCUE SQUAD REQUIREMENTS

Two emergency physicians with additional training in logistics and concepts of disaster medicine
16 well-trained paramedics
Special equipment such as protective clothing and communication devices for all members of the squad
Medical equipment for treatment of at least 50 patients, 10 of them seriously ill.
Five ambulances
Response time within 15 minutes after an alarm

To improve response time and alter the tiered response of the "multiple purposes vehicle" strategy was initiated in 1990 for testing in some areas of West Germany. Only large ambulances are being used. These are fully equipped for all emergency patients, but are also usable for the routine transport tasks of nonurgent patients. The advantage is the improved equipment for all patients, but an analysis of costs and practicability remains to be made.

AUSTRALIA

H. F. Oxer

CAPSULE

Emergency medical service in Australia is provided by general practitioners, locum services, and Emergency Departments (EDs). Ambulance services vary according to area, but the most recent interest has been in teaching defibrillation and monitoring to all paid ambulance officers. Aircraft are used extensively because of the distances involved. The Royal Flying Doctor Service also provides primary health care in remote stations.

skills, particularly defibrillation and monitoring, and teach them to all paid ambulance officers.

BACKGROUND

Australia is a large, semi-arid island continent, roughly the same size as the continental United States, but with a population of only some 16,000,000. Most of these are concentrated in the coastal regions, and 60% live in the capital cities. Three to four million people live in each of the cities of Sydney and Melbourne. Adelaide, Brisbane, and Perth have roughly a million each. Hobart, Canberra, and Darwin are smaller.

There are six states and two territories. Although some of the health funding is received from the federal government, allocation of health resources is at state level.

INTRODUCTION

Emergency medical service (EMS) in Australia is provided by a three-pronged system. General medical practitioners provide a first-line service, mainly for minor problems, but are often called first in an emergency. Locum services, staffed mainly by younger physicians, provide after-hours service for urgent calls. Both of these groups provide house-call service, though this is becoming less frequent.

Ambulance services provide the next level of EMS, and are usually a state-wide operation, either state-run or state-subsidized. The levels of service provided vary somewhat from city to city, and in rural areas.

A core curriculum of ambulance knowledge and skills was established by an expert committee, and this has been the basis of ambulance training in all states and territories for some years. The way in which training is carried out varies from state to state.

Some states have trained some of their officers in advanced life support (ALS) skills to "paramedic" standards, but the main thrust now is to take selected

UNIQUE PROBLEMS OF AUSTRALIA

Australia has some special problems because of its huge, sparsely populated areas. These unique outback areas are serviced mostly by volunteer ambulance officers, backed up by air ambulance services or the Royal Flying Doctor Service.

Although there has been some development of "paramedic" type systems in some of the larger cities, the current demand for further ALS skills is centered mainly on increasing the provision of cardiac monitoring and defibrillation facilities on most ambulances.

This situation has been achieved for many years in Western Australia, Tasmania, and the Australian Capital Territory, and is being introduced progressively in South Australia and the Northern Territory. New South Wales is well advanced in the introduction of new levels of training, which will increase the number of officers with these skills.

The third group of providers of emergency facilities is made up of the Emergency Departments (EDs) of the public hospitals, and in the larger cities, the teaching hospitals. These departments sometimes also have a primary care department in association with the ED, which provides a service similar to that provided by general practitioners, especially in inner city areas.

ROLE OF THE ST. JOHN AMBULANCE

For over 100 years, first aid has been widely taught to the general public by several organizations, particularly by the St. John Ambulance. This largely voluntary organization began teaching first aid in Australia in 1883, and from then onward, both it and its uniformed volunteer arm, the St. John Ambulance Brigade, provided some form of ambulance transport in most states. In the 1880s, hand-held wheeled trolleys were the only facility available, and patient care was minimal.

The provision of ambulance services by St. John was a mixed success story. In New South Wales and Victoria, the State governments took over ambulance services by the early 1920s. In Tasmania, it was 1965 before the State took over from St. John. In South Australia, Western Australia, and the Northern Territory, the St. John Ambulance adopted sound management and training strategies, and developed efficient and effective ambulance administrations, which continue to operate.

Queensland has the Queensland Ambulance Transport Board, which is covered by a State Act of Parliament. Its organization is complex, and over the huge area of the state, ambulance centers have had considerable autonomy.

The Australian Capital Territory, a small enclave surrounding the capital, Canberra, has an ambulance service that is directly controlled by the federal government.

ORGANIZATION

There is no overall EMS organization in Australia. Services are provided by individuals or groups of general medical practitioners, by the various ambulance authorities, and by the EDs or primary care departments of the various hospitals. The links between these groups are informal, but are nevertheless very effective.

PHYSICIANS

General medical practitioners, particularly those working in group practices, or in country and remote outback areas, continue to provide a 24-hour medical service for their patients. They offer round-the-clock service at their clinics, or if necessary, will make house calls out of hours. There are also after-hours "locum" or deputizing services in most major towns and cities.

HOSPITALS

Since the formation of the Australian College for Emergency Medicine, EDs in most of the major "teaching hospitals" in capital cities of Australia are now staffed by physicians fully trained in emergency medicine. There is a training program in place, and registrars in training are common. Such departments are staffed on a 24-hour basis. In 1990, it was uncommon to have a consultant physically in the department all 24 hours. Senior registrars in training were likely to be on duty after 2300 hours, and through the night, with a consultant available on call.

The standard of emergency care available in such major hospitals is extremely high, and rising steadily. The Australian College of Emergency Medicine is still young, however, and the supply of fully trained emergency physicians is still not sufficient to staff many of the other hospitals. Outer suburban and country hospitals continue to be served by either local general practitioners or junior medical staff in training in surgical or medical specialties.

These vary in the facilities they provide according to the number of people served. Often they are staffed by the local medical practitioner. When none are in the immediate area, nursing staff carry out relevant primary care.

The country medical services rely heavily on secondary retrieval of patients requiring further medical care. This is carried out either by helicopter in some areas close to large centers, more often by fixed-wing aircraft operated by the Royal Flying Doctor Service or the ambulance services.

AMBULANCE

In all major cities in Australia, "000" is the emergency telephone number, and has been for many years. When this number is dialed, a dedicated emergency switchboard connects the caller to police, fire, or ambulance.

All states are working toward this number becoming universal throughout the whole country. This has already been achieved in Western Australia.

There is no direct relationship between ambulance services and police or fire departments in Australia. Each ambulance service has its own emergency switchboard, and is responsible for taking the calls, allocating resources, and dispatching vehicles in an appropriate response. Generally, ambulance services operate under the health umbrella, but in close operational liaison with police and fire services.

| | TABLE 87-22. MAIN CATEGORIES OF AMBULANCE PATIENTS IN PERTH FOR TWO TYPICAL MONTHS* | | | |

Category	Sept. 1988	Average Per Day	Nov. 1989	Average Per Day
Trauma	670	23	850	28
Chest pain	419	14	494	16
"Collapse"	255	9	300	10
"Other" cardiac problems	169	5	131	4
Respiratory distress	162	5	168	5
Fits	118	4	140	5
Asthma	108	3.5	105	3.5
Overdose	90	3	98	3.5
CVA	93	3	85	3

* This is a little under half of all cases in a 24 hour period, with 21 to 23 ambulances, each having crew of two.

Ambulance services in all states are operated by a central nonprofit body. In New South Wales, Victoria, Tasmania, and Queensland, the authority is set up under an act of state parliament. Moves are afoot to attain more central control and organization. In South Australia, Western Australia, and the Northern Territory, ambulance services are provided by the St. John Ambulance. Although originally almost entirely voluntary, in these states St. John has reorganized to become a modern management organization. In South Australia, volunteers are still used at night, even in the metropolitan area. Their training is the same as that of paid officers.

As an example of ambulance organization in a large sparsely populated state, Perth, the capital city of Western Australia, and nine other cities or larger areas have professional paid ambulance officers. One hundred and twenty other centers scattered throughout this vast area, which covers more than one third of Australia, are staffed by volunteers. These officers receive training from traveling training teams. Numbers of patients transported from these remote areas may be very low, causing potential problems with skills maintenance.

UTILIZATION

The mix of patients differs from city to city in Australia and considerably, in most cases, from that reported in the USA. Seat belts are almost universally worn in Australia, greatly reducing the amount of facial and chest trauma in accidents. Although the incidence of assault with weapons is rising in one or two of the larger cities, it is still small by comparison with reported North American experience. Penetrating body cavity trauma is rare in most services. As a result, the number of seriously hypovolemic patients seen by an individual ambulance officer in most areas is small.

Utilization varies from state to state. Some states provide an extensive service, including clinic transport (patient transportation for day hospital geriatric and rehabilitation patients), ambulance transport (first response in medical emergencies and accidents), and secondary transportation for patients being admitted, discharged, or transferred from or between hospitals. There may also be a paramedic service.

In other states, such as Western Australia, a conscious effort has been made to limit the use of expensively staffed and equipped ambulances to those needing special skills and/or facilities. This has reduced considerably the number of "taxi" transports carried out by the ambulance service and has enabled Perth, a city of a million people, to be covered by a fleet of 23 front-line ambulances. Brisbane, the capital of Queensland, is a city of similar population and has almost 300 vehicles to cover the wide range of tasks undertaken by its ambulance service.

In Perth, Western Australia, over 200 patients are carried daily on weekdays, and fewer on weekends and on holidays. Tables 87-22 and 87-23 give an indication of the main categories of patients, which make up a little less than half the workload. The rest consist of many smaller groups and patients who are not "ill" but nevertheless need ambulance transport.

Within the limits of the differing ways in which ambulance services are provided, these distributions are fairly representative of ambulance workloads throughout Australia, although Melbourne and Sydney, the two largest cities, are beginning to show an upsurge in trauma resulting from accident and assault.

MEDICAL CONTROL OF AMBULANCES

With the exception of one or two of the "paramedic" trained groups, there is no direct control of ambulances from a hospital or radio. Even in these cases, ambulance officers work almost entirely by protocol. They may, but do not have to, seek advice from a hospital. This system has been found to work well in Australia, and there are no medicolegal reasons why they should operate otherwise.

		Average		Average
Category	Sept. 1988	Per Day	Nov. 1989	Per Day
Vehicle	376	12	362	12
Domestic	136	4.5	131	4.5
Assault	65	2	60	2
Sporting	39	1.3	38	1.3
Industrial	39	1.3	39	1.3
Murder/suicide	8	0.25	15	0.5
Gun/knife	7	0.2	10	0.3

TABLE 87-23. BREAKDOWN OF "TRAUMA" OVER THE SAME PERIOD*

* Perth is a city of about one million people.

Early ambulance services were guided by medical advisory committees of voluntary medical officers. Sometimes their advice was ignored or only partially implemented.

Western Australia was the first state to appoint a medical director in 1976, with full authority over medical aspects of ambulance care. Since then, other states have done similarly, but in some areas there is still resistance to having authoritative medical involvement in an ambulance service.

Physicians are involved in ambulance service in every state in some capacity, and each year hold a meeting as a subcommittee of the Convention of Ambulance Authorities of Australia and New Zealand. This meeting is a valuable forum for the exchange of ideas and information. The group reviews common medical dilemmas in ambulance service and submits recommendations each year for consideration at the Convention's meeting.

Quality control of ambulance operations varies in nature and degree. In all states, however, mechanisms for review of case sheets exist, especially when advance life support techniques are involved. Such case sheets are reviewed, with ambulance officer feedback. There is a growing data base of computerized information, which is allowing analysis of ambulance techniques used, ambulance cases transported, and results of prehospital ambulance care.

ADMINISTRATION

Ambulance administration in the early days was in the hands of senior uniformed ambulance officers. In virtually all states now, however, professional administrators and managers are teamed with the senior ambulance officers to handle specialized management functions. Most states have a General Manager or Chief Executive, with specialists in finance and industrial and personnel officers in their management team.

FINANCE

There are detailed differences in the financing of the various ambulance services, but generally funding comes from a mixture of government subsidies, fees charged for transport (based on a call-out charge plus a distance charge), and subscriptions received from members of an ambulance insurance fund. Subscribers to these funds receive free transport, providing that their reason for transport falls within those accepted by the fund. Those not covered by any form of insurance are likely to receive a substantial account for ambulance transport. In some indigent and impecunious groups, however, costs related to transport have to be written off against the government subsidy.

PREHOSPITAL TREATMENT

A major difference between EMS in North America and ambulance services in Australia is that in Australia there is no need or wish for direct physician control of ambulance officers when carrying out a particular patient care episode. Ambulance officers work under protocol guidelines developed by their medical control system. Medical radio communications are used only to advise hospitals of the type of case that is being brought in, not to seek medical direction.

ADVANCED LIFE SUPPORT

The first Australian system for mobile ALS began during 1969 in Perth, with the introduction of a coronary care ambulance staffed by ambulance officers and a nurse and physician from the Royal Perth Hospital. This was probably the second such unit in the world, following the lead of Pantridge in Belfast, Northern Ireland. Similar systems began in Melbourne in 1971, and in Sydney in 1973. During the 1970s it was decided that such services could serve only a limited group of patients within their operating radius, and that medical and nursing staff were inappropriate as staff for these ambulances. In the late 1970s in Perth, it was decided to equip all operational ambulances in the greater Perth area progressively with monitor-defibrillators, and this was completed by 1978. All fully trained ambulance officers were authorized to defibrillate by 1980.

In Melbourne and Sydney, the decision was made to train selected ambulance officers in Advanced Life Support skills and equip a small number of specialized ambulances as mobile ALS units. This system continues in the major cities.

Most other states and territories reviewed the development of mobile intensive care ambulances, and then made a conscious decision not to introduce these specialized units. They have chosen rather to upgrade the skills of all their ambulance officers progressively in selected ALS skills.

Currently, all Perth ambulance officers are able to monitor and defibrillate, and to perform only certain ALS skills, such as MAST, measurement of peak airway flows, nebulizer treatment for asthma, cricothyrotomy, and management of the cannulated or intubated patient. The skills of intubation and cannulation are under continual review because data do not support their benefit to a significant number of patients.

In the Northern Territory, Tasmania, and the Australian Capital Territory, all officers are offered training in some ALS skills, including defibrillation. In Victoria, plans were implemented to teach similar skills to all senior ambulance officers, and in New South Wales, in 1990, new levels of training were introduced along similar lines. At this writing, South Australia has plans in the same direction, and in Queensland such a program is in its early stages.

"Paramedic" type programs have been implemented to a variable extent in New South Wales, Victoria, Tasmania, the Australian Capital Territory, and the Northern Territory.

It is interesting, however, to note that in South Australia a limited test introduction of ALS skills was tried for a period of 6 months. This included intravenous infusion, intubation, and intravenous administration of certain medications. After careful analysis of the results over the trial period, it was decided that benefits were insufficient in respect to improvement in patient condition or outcome to warrant the continuation of the program, and it was withdrawn.

There is a widespread presumption that more and more ALS must be better than "lesser care." It is surprisingly difficult to date to find evidence to support any improvements in morbidity or mortality, with the one outstanding exception of early prehospital defibrillation.

Many accepted skills do not measure up well when subjected to such analysis, but are impossible to remove from service once they are entrenched.

The advent of thrombolytic therapy for acute myocardial ischemia has raised the question: Should paramedics be trained to begin therapy? Most Australian cardiologists and emergency physicians, in 1990, preferred that the patient be brought quickly to a hospital where this therapy could be administered. In areas where the response times were under 15 minutes, such as in Perth, there seemed little point in beginning such therapy outside the hospital.

PREHOSPITAL MANAGMENT IN RURAL AREAS

In remote areas such as large areas of Western Australia, ambulance services are provided by volunteers. They receive training on weekends, from traveling teams from the ambulance training center. Volunteer ambulance officers are trained to a level similar to that of emergency medical technicians (EMTs) in the United States, involving about 120 hours of training. In some of the country areas, where numbers cannot justify many full-time staff members, ambulances are staffed by a full-time officer, supplemented by a trained volunteer.

Although there may be a *need* for intravenous infusion in certain cases, the *minute number* of cases handled by many of the rural ambulance services makes it impractical to offer training and maintain skills. As a practical compromise, patients are brought by ambulance to the nearest nursing post or medical practitioner, where initial treatment and stabilization are carried out. Patients are secondarily retrieved as necessary by the teams of the Royal Flying Doctor Service or the Air Ambulance.

EDUCATION AND TRAINING

GENERAL PRACTITIONERS

General practitioners, in addition to their routine medical training and required intern and resident posts, often complete a further 2 to 3 years of residency training aimed at producing a well-rounded and relevantly trained general practitioner. This vocational training has been provided under the auspices of the Royal Australian College of General Practitioners. Training is provided mainly in association with city teaching hospitals, and involves rotation through a number of specialist departments and emergency departments.

EMERGENCY PHYSICIANS

In the larger cities, emergency care is provided by the EDs and, in some cases, primary care departments of the major hospitals. These are increasingly staffed by physicians specifically trained in emergency medicine. The number of such trained emergency physicians is growing, and these physicians are now also staffing other hospitals. The rural and smaller hospitals, however, are still staffed mainly by general practitioners, on a roster call basis. Such hospitals may have junior medical staff, who provide a level of cover for an ED.

The formation of the Australasian College for Emergency Medicine was a significant step forward for emergency medicine in Australia. A formal fellowship training program, with courses and examinations, has attracted many young physicians towards a career in Emergency Medicine.

The support from the Ambulance Services for the College has been exceptionally strong and generous.

NURSES

The widespread movement of nurse training into more academic environments has been seen in Australia. Courses, however, are being offered in emergency medicine, focused for those who are likely to work unsupported or in rural areas. These courses are practically based and skill-oriented to enable nurses to manage acute medical problems. Such nursing emergency training, however, still occurs on the job and in the emergency departments of major hospitals. Some trained nurses transfer to the ambulance services and become retrained as ambulance officers.

AMBULANCE OFFICERS (EMERGENCY MEDICAL TECHNICIANS)

The term "Emergency Medical Technician" is not used in Australia. Historically, they have been known as Ambulance Officers ("Bearers" in Queensland). Training of ambulance officers beyond the level required for the St. John Ambulance First Aid volunteers began in Victoria and New South Wales in the early 1960s, and other states quickly followed. Since the mid 1970s, ambulance officer training has been formalized and ambulance-based. All Australian states and territories with testing now have a central ambulance training school, providing training for ambulance officers at all levels. In addition, such training centers usually have mobile training teams that can visit country and remote areas and carry out training for professional and volunteer officers.

Training is carried out by a full-time training staff, including ambulance officers who have undergone training, nurses with educational training and relevant knowledge and skills, and usually one or more medical practitioners. In some states, physicians are employed directly by the training center. About 1976, a fledgling organization called the Institute of Ambulance Officers set up an Interim National Education Committee, following an ambulance seminar that had been held at Monash University in Victoria. This seminar had examined the need for training for ambulance officers in Victoria, and had identified a core body of knowledge and skills. This interim committee consisted of the chief ambulance training officer, and the medical director, advisor, or ambulance training medical officer from each state or territory.

The task of this committee was to examine the model produced by the seminar at Monash University and approve it. This was to provide the basis for a nationwide standard for ambulance officer training. Members of this group are all experts in their field, and this is both their strength and their weakness. Their recommendations were seen by many as being too academic and knowledge-oriented, rather than oriented toward on-road problem solving. This caused some dismay among those who had expected a "rubber stamp" and an instant national ambulance standard.

During the next 3 years, the definitive National Education Committee met under the Chairmanship of Dr. Harry Oxer, the Medical Director of the ambulance service in Western Australia. At regular meetings, they thrashed out a practical and job-oriented curriculum for ambulance officer training. This became and has remained the basis for all Australian ambulance officer training courses. Coincidentally, this curriculum was published at the same time as the well-known blue and white documents in the USA, indicating that both Australia and the USA were working along similar lines at the same time.

VEHICLES

Most ambulances in Australia have fiberglass bodies custom-built on a light van chassis, with a V8 engine and power steering. Ambulances operating in areas outside the main cities are fitted with a "Roo-Bar." This is a device similar to a cow-catcher that saves the vehicle from being wrecked by an impact with a 6-foot kangaroo. These animals are not an endangered species, as some reports suggest, but are often in plague proportions, and are a real menace in rural areas after dark. On one classic patient retrieval from the Eyre Highway, across the Nullabor Plain in the south of our continent, both the initial responding ambulance and its back-up were wrecked after hitting kangaroos. The patient eventually arrived back at a country hospital in a third vehicle from this retrieval, which was well over 200 miles. The kangaroos apparently did not survive the impacts, but the patient was not further damaged.

Ambulances usually carry two main stretchers, one of the self-loading type and the other usually of a simpler and less expensive type. Some of the vehicles, particularly in rural areas, have the facility to rig two more light stretchers higher up and convert, if needed, to a four-berth configuration.

EQUIPMENT

Prehospital management in all services consists of assessment, provision of oxygen, appropriate splinting, and the offering of analgesia by inhalation. Some services use a 50/50 combination of nitrous oxide and oxygen; others use a low analgesic concentration of inhaled methoxyflurane. Both provide effective prehospital analgesia of short duration. In addition, the paramedic groups in some cities administer intravenous narcotic analgesia. As a result of seeing the effective ambulance use of inhaled analgesia techniques, many hospitals have adopted this ambulance technology to their short-term pain relief requirements.

All services of nebulized treatment are for management of reactive airway diseases. Resuscitation equipment is usually oxygen-powered, except in South Australia, where a self-refilling bag fitted with an oxygen reservoir is normally used.

The "Jordan Frame" is commonly used for the multiple injury patient rather than the "scoop" stretcher. It is an Australian invention in which a frame is built around the patient, then flexible slats are slid under relevant parts of the patient to support the patient and build the stretcher.

All ambulances carry assorted bandages, immobilization splints, including traction and air splints, and most carry the MAST suit. Cannulation, intubation, and the use of intravenous medications are restricted to services with some staff trained in full "paramedic" skills. Many other ambulances, however, carry this equipment for the use of a physician at the scene. Officers are trained to care for cannulated or intubated patients in transport. Resuscitation equipment is usually oxygen-powered in South Australia, where a self-refilling bag fitted with an oxygen reservoir is normally used. There are currently no medicolegal impediments, and doctors often treat patients at the scene.

AIRCRAFT

Aircraft are extensively used outside the major cities in Australia because of the vast distances involved. Some retrievals to capital cities, e.g., in Western Australia, exceed 2000 kilometers. Helicopters are used in some cities where the specific geographic or traffic problems make their use an advantage for patient retrieval. Other cities, however, have successfully resisted the well-known evangelistic approach of some helicopter operators and manufacturers because use of such facilities would confer no patient care advantages in terms of decreased mortality or morbidity, but merely increase greatly the cost of the transport services. Distance retrievals are carried out by dedicated air ambulance aircraft, operated by either the ambulance service or, particularly in the more remote areas, the aircraft of the Royal Flying Doctor Services of Australia. All such aircraft are fully and professionally equipped and staffed by especially trained flight nurses, and have aeromedically trained physicians available to take part in retrieval where appropriate. Aircraft usually provide a secondary response, and are rarely the primary responder to an accident or emergency situation. They work closely with the local ambulance services and medical practitioners, and with the remote bush nursing posts. In Western Australia, which occupies more than one third of the area of Australia, there are some 18 Royal Flying Doctor Service aircraft, organized in 3 divisions. These are all light, twin-engine aircraft. Several are turboprop-equipped and pressurized to enable them to retrieve patients effectively over the long distances involved. Others are light twin-engined planes with the ability to handle the rough, relatively unprepared gravel outback landing strips.

The Royal Flying Doctor Service also provides primary health care by operating regular medical clinics at remote sheep and cattle stations in the outback, and at aboriginal, mining, and other remote communities.

COMMUNICATIONS

Ambulance communications in city areas are usually by VHF radio, although more and more are converting to UHF. HF radio is still needed for some of the extremely long distances and remote areas, but with the advent of satellite radio, this is being gradually phased out.

HORIZONS

Although a demand for better emergency medical services always exists, expectations may become unrealistic. There is a progressive increase in staffing, equipment, and skills, both of medical and nursing staff, in country hospitals. Regional centers are being developed in some larger remote towns, and the retrieval systems have become highly sophisticated through refinement.

It is difficult to justify, in numbers, increased sophistication of training for ambulance officers in regions such as the more remote parts of rural and outback Western Australia. In some of the more populated areas, such as parts of New South Wales, however, there is a move to train most paid ambulance officers in a selection of relevant ALS skills and to maintain their skills by regular contact with the local regional hospitals.

With the possible exception of New South Wales, there are no plans at the moment to extend ALS ("Paramedic") training significantly in any ambulance service in Australia. Rather, the trend is to promote the teaching of selected ALS skills to most ambulance officers. Most states and territories are moving toward the eventual provision of monitoring and defibrillation on all ambulances in the larger populated centers.

A recent study by Lyle et al. was unable to show significant improvement in outcome in almost 500 cases of acute trauma managed by the paramedic system in Sydney, compared with over 500 similar cases managed in the Brisbane region by non-ALS-trained crews. The groups were analogous in all other respects. The only parameter to show any improvement in the "paramedic" group was respiratory status measured by arterial blood gases. This difference was only in the first 24 hours and was not reflected in any measurable improvement in outcome, decrease in time in intensive care or in the hospital, or decrease in morbidity or mortality. Results of the research will continue to shape the configuration of the emergency medical system in Australia. As supply and demand occur, the level of training of the physicians in the hospital ED will also change.

NATIONAL CONTACTS

LIST OF INTERSTATE AMBULANCE SERVICES

NEW SOUTH WALES
Central District Ambulance Service
Quay Street
Sydney, NSW 2000
Phone (02) 818.0310

CAPITAL TERRITORY
A.C.T. Ambulance Service
Corner Callis/Morphett Streets
Dickson Act 2606
Phone (062) 489.1333

SOUTH AUSTRALIA
St. John Ambulance
216 Green Hill Road
P.O. Box 23
Eastwood, SA 5063
Phone (08) 222.1316

WESTERN AUSTRALIA
St. John Ambulance Australia
W.A. Ambulance Service Inc.
209 Great Eastern Highway
Belmont, WA 6104
Phone (09) 277.9999

NORTHERN TERRITORY
N.T. Ambulance Service
50 Dripstone Road
Casuarina, NT 5792
Phone (089) 27.9111
27.9000

QUEENSLAND
Old Ambulance Transport Brigade
377 Turbot Street
Spring Hill, Brisbane QLD
Phone (07) 844.4810
839.2222

TASMANIA
Tasmania Ambulance Service
15 Melville Street
Hobart, TAS 7000
Phone (002) 34.6584

VICTORIA
Mr. John Stevens
Ambulance Directorate
7th Floor, 555 Collins Street
Melbourne, VIC 3000
Phone (03) 616.7777

LIST OF MEDICAL DIRECTORS OF AMBULANCE SERVICES

Dr. H. Oxer
Medical Director
St. John Ambulance Association
209 Great Western Highway
P.O. Box 183
Belmont, WA 6104

Dr. W. Lukes
Regional Supervisory Physician
Intensive Care Unit
Royal Hobart Hospital
G.P.O. Box 1061L
Hobart, TAS 7001

Dr. M. Selig
P.O. Box 640
Strathfield, N.S.W. 2135

Mr. I. Ross
Advisory Ambulance Office
Department of Health
Head Office
P.O. Box 5013
Wellington, N.Z.

Dr. P. Archer
Ambulance Services' Medical Officer
Ambulance Officers' Training Centre
69 Queens Road
Melbourne, VIC 3004

Dr. G. Phillips
Director
Emergency Department
Flinders Medical Center
Flinders Drive
Bedroed Park, SA 5042

Dr. J. Potts
Director
Accident and Emergency Centre
Royal Canberra Hospital
Action, ACT 2601

Dr. G. Fitzgerald
Medical Director
Queensland Ambulance Services Board
P.O. Box 251
South Brisbane, QLD 4101

Dr. L. Crompton
Commissioner
St. John Ambulance NT Inc.
51 Dripstone Road
Casuarina, NT 5792

BIBLIOGRAPHY

Dawson, D.A.: Ambulance Officer selection: Predicting training performance. Aust. Psychol. *23*:69, 1988.

Doman, A.S.: Paramedic ambulance services in NSW: Analysis of response times, case mix and catchment area. Abstract. Community Health Study. *8*:140, 1984.

Hamilton, T.: Medical and nursing response to disaster. Emergency Response *7*:21, 1983.

Hockings, B.E.: Transportation of the patient with a myocardial infarction. Patient Manage. *10*:15, 1986.

Howie-Willis, I.: Centenary of the Order of St. John in Australia. Sterilization Aust. *3*:24, 1983.

Lyle, D., Potter, D., Goldstein, G., Pierce, J., and Quine, S.: The delivery of emergency trauma care in the Sydney region. Community Health Stud. *11*:226, 1987.

Robinson, R.: Occupational stress: A study of ambulance officers in Victoria. Aust. Psychol. *22*:119, 1987, and *23*:69, 1987.

Selecki, B.R.: Experience with spinal injuries in New South Wales. Aust. N. Z. J. Surg. *56*:585, 1986.

Simpson, D.A.: Logistics of early management of head and spinal injuries. Aust. N. Z. J. Surg. *56*:585, 1986.

Toscano, J.: Prevention of neurological deterioration before admission to a spinal cord injury unit. Paraplegia *26*:143, 1988.

Willis, E. and McCarthy, L.: From first aid to paramedical: Ambulance officers in the health division of labour. Community Health Stud. *10*:57, 1986.

SKORAJA IN RUSSIA

J.N. Tsibin and M. W. Griniov

CAPSULE

The system for emergency medical care in the USSR has at its disposal 4000 stations and 104 hospitals. There are approximately 30,000 physicians and 60,000 medical personnel available who perform approximately 90 million patient evaluations each year.

The system is configured to ensure that only true life-and-limb-threatening cases receive the full resources of the ambulance and medical teams available. Specialized hospitals, through radio triage, accept patients for all types of emergencies.

One of the first organized steps toward the development of an emergency medical system (EMS) began in Leningrad in the late 1950s. With more than 30 years of experience from the "Storm Brigades," the care of the trauma patient has dramatically improved. It has been recognized that the minimum equipment to be taken to the scene must allow for maintenance of adequate ventilation, anesthesia, fracture immobilization, and maintenance of adequate hemodynamics. Recognizing that this can delay delivery of the patient to the hospital, an optimum range of 0.5 to 2.0 hours is found not to influence the final outcome of trauma victims. The recent changes and dismantling of the USSR into independent states will create many pressures for each state to develop EMS capability. The system described herein is applicable to "Russia" and can no longer be applied to the now independent states. Economic pressures associated with the change of government will also modify additional activities.

INTRODUCTION

Skoraja, the EMS system, was founded in the USSR by the People's Commissar for Public Health, Nikolai Semashko. Since its beginning, it has been a section of Public Health and is under the Ministry of Health.

The conception of Skoraja was connected with the increasing number of accidents reported in the street, at home, and at work: 150 deaths per 100,000 population caused by accidents, poisoning, and trauma.

The number of lives lost through transport accidents is especially large: 45,000 died in 1987 and 58,500 in 1989. This increase in the number of fatalities from accidents attracted attention. Heart disease is the second leading cause of death among this same group (130 per 100,000). These circumstances brought about the necessity for development and perfection of an EMS in the USSR.

Skoraja consists of approximately 4000 stations for emergency care and 104 hospitals with 67,000 available beds for all of the USSR. In this system, approximately 30,000 physicians and 60,000 other medical personnel work. In 1986, approximately 87,000 ambulances were dispatched to respond to calls for assistance. Each of these calls was free of charge.

ORGANIZATION

There is a station for emergency care with a typical structure in each town of 0.5 million inhabitants or more. The composition of the EMS is standard, consisting of the following departments:

- Administration
- Operations
- Quality assurance
- Care inspection service
- Chemist's shop (Pharmacy)
- Emergency care substations (hospitals and scientific research institutes)

ADMINISTRATION

The role of administration, which includes a physician-director, his delegate for economic and technical services, and a bookkeeper, is to maintain adequate staff and materials and needed medical teams. Responsibility also includes scheduling and ensuring appropriate interaction with other towns and services, i.e., militia and fire brigades.

OPERATIONS DEPARTMENT

The Operations Department organizes the response for all emergency medical care requested through "03" calls. This is its primary task. The telephone "03" number is reserved for emergency medical care service and is free of charge. A senior physician for the department supervises all employees, including area-wide colleges and medical team physicians. The Operations Department is the dispatch center for the reception of calls, a dispatch office for development of the teams and the office for hospitalization and inquiry.

For every "03" call, the dispatch officer, a feldsher (physician's assistant) always completes a "call card" form, which is carried off immediately by a conveyor belt to the dispatching office. One of the feldsher from this office (the dispatcher) instructs the nearest emergency care substation by telephone to direct a medical team to the address. In unclear cases, he or she may consult with the physician on duty.

The Operations Department is the link between Skoraja, polyclinics, dispensaries, and hospitals. For each town, hospital capability and resource availability information is received daily. The principal task of this department is to ensure even distribution of patients in the towns' hospitals, with attention to severity and census, minimizing the possibility of any one hospital becoming overloaded. The Operations Department at all times, day and night, is headed by a physician-evaluator, who provides appropriate patient distribution among the hospitals.

QUALITY ASSURANCE DEPARTMENT

The Quality Assurance Department reviews the station's work and analyzes it and deaths that have occurred in the prehospital phase. The department physicians review the deaths and generate reports that effect the instruction, design, and use of forms and new diagnostic and therapeutic procedures in the Skoraja's practice. The Department's head is the deputy chief physician.

All call cards, once they are completed by the physician on duty, go to the Quality Assurance Department. The inquiry office, of this department, handles concerns of patients cared for by the emergency medical service system.

CARE INSPECTION SERVICE

A care inspection service, created to control, organize, and assist, is staffed by an experienced physician team. It inspects the work of the medical teams and medical care volume and helps to solve complicated diagnostic, tactical, and therapeutic problems.

SUBSTATIONS FOR EMERGENCY CARE

Substations for emergency care are separate units, dispersed throughout a region, designed to dispatch medical care rapidly to where it is needed. Every substation operates within a limited district of service. The mean radius of service is usually 4 to 5 kilometers, covering more than 300,000 persons. Thus one ambulance for every 10,000 inhabitants is ensured.

The typical town substation structure is made up of a dispatching room, a receiving room for patients coming directly from the street, a rest room, a dining room, and an ambulance bay.

Personnel at a substation include a basic medical team (LMT—physician, feldsher and driver) intensive care medical team (ICMT—physician, two feldshers, and a driver), general sanitary transport team (GSST—feldsher and driver), and obstetric sanitary transport team (OSTT—midwife and driver).

The medical teams in a large town can be dispatched 15 to 20 times in 24 hours. A need for different medical teams has evolved and these have been proven effective.

The LMT is a nonspecialized brigade that responds to all types of calls. The LMT has a limited kit of medicines, dressings, and means of immobilization. Only simple diagnostic equipment is carried.

The ICMT is a more sophisticated team. The physician and two feldshers can perform central venous puncture, including that of subclavian and femoral veins; tracheostomy; endotracheal intubation and artificial ventilation; intravenous and inhalation narcosis; cardiac defibrillation and fluid infusion. In the late 1980s a tendency to gradually substitute ICMT for LMT began.

HOSPITALS FOR EMERGENCY MEDICAL CARE (HEMCs)

An HEMC is typically a multidisciplinary medical institution of 800 to 1000 beds. It has cardiology, surgery, trauma, toxicology, gynecology, and burn departments. It may also have combined trauma departments including neurosurgery, urology, thoracic surgery, and related others. The number and types of these hospital units depend on the town needs. The HEMC is headed by a chief physician with deputies for surgery, internal medicine, and administration. Its 24-hour operation is guided by assigned staff physician who acts as chief of the physician teams on duty.

SCIENTIFIC-RESEARCH INSTITUTES FOR EMERGENCY CARE (SRIECs)

There are two SRIECs in the USSR: in Moscow, the Skilfosovsky Institute for Research in Emergency Care, and in Leningrad, the Dzanelidze Institute. The principal functions of these institutes are perfection of the emergency care organization in both the prehospital and hospital phases; introduction of new or perfection of old methods for diagnosis and treatment of medical emergencies, original research into life-threatening conditions, and the introduction of improved methods into hospital practice.

Both institutes have a strong clinical research base, including approximately 1000 beds. There are about 1500 scientific and health care workers in each of these institutes.

PREHOSPITAL MANAGEMENT

RURAL EMERGENCY MEDICAL SERVICE

The central links of EMS in the country are the central district hospitals (CDHs). Departments of emergency care or autonomous emergency care stations are situated near CDHs. They are supervised by and responsible to the CDH physician on duty. Autonomous emergency care stations are usually in the remote villages. They are organized near village hospitals where the service radius is more than 25 to 30 kilometers. The country stations have varying workloads that fall into four ranges:

1. 75 to 100 thousand calls per year
2. 50 to 75 thousand calls per year
3. 25 to 50 thousand calls per year
4. 10 to 25 thousand calls per year

A station's category determines its staff and materials and security. In every station a senior physician is on duty at all times to direct the work of the medical personnel. He or she is called in complicated cases and organizational problems.

PHYSICIAN SPECIALISTS AND PREHOSPITAL EMERGENCY CARE

Emergency medical care links prehospital and hospital care, resulting in the creation of a separate specialized medical service. A physician who systematically and routinely cares for patients in a specific category becomes a professional in this category and is qualified to manage certain diseases through diagnosis and treatment.

Specialized emergency care in the USSR started in the 1950s when the first specialized medical teams appeared in the streets of Leningrad.

By now there are many types of specialized medical teams in the USSR, configured by hospitals' or centers' deputies. There are many specialized medical brigades: cardiologic, neurologic, psychiatric, toxicologic, pediatric, hemotologic, and resuscitative-surgical. Each brigade may vary in accordance with the locale and its needs.

An example of a specialized medical team with a relationship to a Center are the resuscitative surgical brigades, connected with the Trauma Shock Center in Leningrad.

SPECIALIZED EMERGENCY MEDICAL CARE IN TRAUMA

Trauma and other accidents are the principal cause of death among working people with 140 to 170 of every 100,000 inhabitants dying of these causes each year. A great percentage are transportation accidents. In 1987, 45,000 accidental deaths occurred in the USSR, with an economic loss estimated at 11 to 12 million roubles.

The immediate cause of death from severe trauma is usually shock and its complications. Although the frequency of shock from trauma is small, about 3 to 5%, the overall number of cases of trauma-related shock is fairly imposing. According to Dzanelidze Institute research data, shock from trauma occurs in approximately 200 patients for each million inhabitants every year. These patients no longer die at the scene but receive intensive care in the prehospital and hospital stages. This type of qualitative treatment requires organized measures so that a unique service was created to address resuscitative-surgical and traumatic problems.

In Leningrad in 1957, with the introduction of the "storm brigade," the first serious investigations began on deaths caused by shock. At that time, a physician and two feldshers comprised a "storm brigade," which was to be the prototype of many other specialized medical teams later created. This brigade continues to date, operating successfully, not only in Leningrad but throughout the urban USSR.

In the early years, the storm brigade played a key role in the search for the optimal infusion volume for trauma shock patients. Treatments used included an extensive range of procedures: thoracotomy, open cardiac massage, and arteriotomy. The following are now believed to be optimal procedures for prehospital care: maintenance of adequate ventilation, anesthesia, fracture immobilization, and maintenance of hemodynamic status. The problem of maintaining adequate ventilation in the prehospital phase is solved by means of endotracheal intubation followed by artificial ventilation. This is required in approximately 5% of victims. Anesthesia is a necessary component for quality medical care in the prehospital stage. The tendency and increasing preference is to use IV medication, in particular narcotic analgesics (25% of patients), other analgesics (29%), and kallypsol or ketamine hydrochloride with seduxen (25%). Nitrous oxide and neuroleptanelgesia are seldom used. Novocaine blockade of fractures is rarely performed. By 1988, halogen derivatives of carbohydrate were rarely used as an anesthetic agent.

Fracture immobilization techniques did not change until the late 1980s. Kramer's, Ditherix, and other types of splints were used in about 20% of patients in traumatic shock needing tire-like appliances. This method of compressed immobilization was dangerous because of the likelihood of revascularization syndrome developing in critical patients.

The severity of traumatic shock and its outcome were found to depend in many cases on maintenance of adequate hemodynamic status. The early resuscitative-surgical teams placed groundless importance on radical methods of treatment such as open cardiac massage and intra-arterial fluid infusion. It has become evident that open cardiac massage may lead to return of cardiac function, but not to overall patient survival. Intra-arterial infusions are used rarely in prehospital settings because intravenous infusions are felt to be equally effective. The experience accumulated through the 1950s has brought about the conclusion that, if trauma is severe enough to cause the heart to stop, the shock state is irreversible.

The norm of 200 trauma shock victims per million population applies to the other cities of the USSR. Five resuscitative-surgical teams are active in Leningrad 24 hours a day. At present, 80 to 85% of trauma shock patients are transported to the hospital by these specialized medical teams. In the mid 1980s, only 60 to 70% of patients were transported.

The mean time for transport in Leningrad is approximately an hour, and 90% of the patients arrive at the hospital within 1.5 hours. The range for transport time is 0.5 to 2.0 hours with no apparent effect on the outcome; it is believed that this is because of the extent of reanimation care and the quality of the resuscitative-surgical teams. These circumstances solve, to some degree, the problem of transporting trauma shock patients as soon as possible, leaving some treatment for later and using rational medical care at the expense of increased transport time.

TABLE 87-24. TRAUMA SEVERITY SCORE

Kind of Injuries	Marks
Abdominal trauma with injury of two and more parenchymal organs or large blood vessels (aorta, v. porta, v. cava inf.)	10
Multiple bilateral fractures of ribs with or without injury of thoracic organs or abdominal trauma with injury of a parenchymal organ/of mesenteric vessels	6
Open fracture of hip or avulsion of hip	5
Contusion of brain, fracture of skull, trauma of thorax with injury of organs (heart, lung) or hemo-pneumothorax, multiple fractures of pelvis	4
Trauma with injury of hollow organs or diaphragm, open fracture of tibia or fibula, avulsion of lower leg, closed fracture of hip	2
Large scalp wound or large hematoma outside of fractures, closed fractures of tibia or fibula, open or closed fracture of facial bones, fracture or, avulsion of humerus	1.5
Multiple unilateral fractures of ribs without thoracic organ injury	1
Fractures of vertebrae with or without injury of spinal cord, open fracture of forearm, avulsion of forearm, open fracture of foot, avulsion of foot	0.5
Isolated fracture of pelvis; closed fracture of one bone of lower leg; closed fractures of foot; forearm or hand; crush or avulsion of hand; open or closed fractures of clavicle, scapula, sternum, or patella; greenstick fractures of bones	0.1

PREHOSPITAL DIAGNOSTIC AND TREATMENT RULES

The main purpose of diagnostic algorithm elaboration was perfecting Keit's classification scheme of traumatic shock, which lists some simple signs of shock outcome.

The prognostic rule was elaborated for the prehospital stage as a result of an analysis of 269 trauma shock patients. The equations used are the following:

$$+1/T = 0.18 + 0.0001*K*P*A/BP - 0.009*K*P/BP - 0.0003*K*A$$

Where
symbol ($+$) is prognostic favorable outcome,
symbol ($-$) is prognostic unfavorable outcome,
$+T$ — expected shock duration (hours)
$-T$ — expected life duration (hours)
P — pulse rate
A — age (years)
BP — blood pressure (mm Hg)
K — trauma severity score (marks—Table 87-24)
(All these signs are determined at the scene.)

The above rule is easily computerized and gives approximately 90 to 95% of the prospective and retroprospective outcomes for trauma-related shock. This rule seems to be simpler than those using the Abbreviated Injury Scale (AIS) and Injury Severity Score (ISS) promulgated in the U.S. It is characterized by addressing each individual's degree of shock and predicting triage and hospital destination.

There is another formula concerning the treatment of shock patients. By means of this rule, one can predict the minimum IV fluid volume necessary to compensate blood loss. The equation is:

$$V = 100 + 300 \ P/BP$$

where V is minimal volume in mL.

This formula is simple and may be completed by mental arithmetic. It has been recognized that it does not determine maximum volume in the prehospital phase of care, but minimizes volume of arrival at the hospital. That is why the complete concerns of this equation remain unknown, as does the effect of the body temperature.

HOSPITAL PHASE

Undoubtedly, the hospital phase of emergency medical care for trauma shock patients must be specialized. These patients should not go to just any hospital. In Leningrad there are four specialized trauma shock centers: north, south, west, and east of the city. Dzanelidze Scientific Research Institute is the southern center, situated near major highways.

Trauma shock victims go through the receiving areas to the resuscitation area, which is also an operating room. This area is staffed by experts in resuscitation and surgical procedures. This special medical brigade consists of a physician and three nurses who are qualified in surgical and resuscitative nursing. The chief surgeon on duty identifies the need for other surgical specialists needed for definitive care. He or she, is, however, the person in charge of the trauma shock patient.

The first phase of care in the resuscitation area is "superintensive" and continues for 6 to 9 hours, depending on the case. Once vital signs are stabilized and all surgical procedures completed, the patient is transported to the intensive care unit. Staffing allows one physician and two nurses to every six patients on a 24-hour basis. The mean duration of stay in this unit, for trauma shock patients, is 3 to 4 days. From this unit, patients go to the appropriate service's ward.

The results of patient care in the hospital phase can be predicted using an equation much like that used for the prehospital phase (Fig. 87-22).

$$+ \ 1/T = 0.317 - 0.039*K + 0.00017*BP*K = 0.0026*P*A/BP$$

where
symbol (+) is prognostic favorable outcome,
symbol (−) is prognostic unfavorable outcome,
+T—expected shock duration (hours)
−T—expected life duration (hours)
   P—pulse rate
   A—age (years)
BP—blood pressure (mm Hg)
   K—trauma severity score (marks)*

FIG. 87-22. Outcome from traumatic shock.
* See Table 87-24.

$$V24h = (13.5 - 0.067*P*K + 0.52*K2 + 36.5P/BP + 7.9P/Ht)*100;$$

where
v24h—infusion volume per day in ml;
   Ht—hematocrit in %;
   P—pulse rate
   K—trauma severity score (marks)*
BP—blood pressure (mm Hg.)

FIG. 87-23. Optimal infusion volume per day.
* See Table 87-24.

Careful clinical investigation has resulted in the recognition of a formula for optimal volume to be infused per day. (Fig. 87-23).

Three to four hundred patients are transported to the Institute for Shock Center each year. Mean mortality for this patient group is 30%, an improvement over previous years (27.9% in 1987).

HORIZONS

The focus in the 1980s was to develop specialized medical teams, especially cardiology, psychiatry, and neurology, by staffing response teams for a specific possible patient condition. Thus the quality of care at the scene was significantly improved.

The mortality index appears to be a criterion not of treatment quality but of trauma severity. Researchers believe that what is necessary for treatment quality is an estimation to calculate the prognostical mortality (Lp) using the formula for outcome from shock trauma (see Fig. 87-22) and real mortality (Lr) and then comparing them. It is apparent that it is favorable for Lp to exceed Lr. The reverse relationship, Lp lower than Lr, however, is considered treatment failure.

The prehospital and hospital stages of emergency care for shock patients have particular features that may be described in the form of diagnostic and treatment algorithms. Research both in and outside the institutes, coupled with sharing of knowledge with those outside the USSR, will continue to ensure the best possible outcome for all emergency patients.

NATIONAL CONTACTS

Dr. Vladislav G. Teriaev
Professor and Director
N.V. Sklifosovosky Institute for Emergency Medicine
Bloshaia Kolchozhai Place, 3
129010, Moscow, USSR

Dr. Teimuraz P. Gurchunelidze
Senior Researcher, Department of Surgery
N.V. Sklifosovosky First Aid Research Center
129010, B. Kolkhoznay Sq., 3 Moscow, USSR
Home Address: Flat G, House 22/1 800 cet Moscow Street
                P.O. Box 127247
                Moscow, USSR
Phone 488–39–26

Professor Michael V. Grinev
Professor and Director
I.I. Djanelidze Research Institute of First Aid
Budapeshtskay, 3/5
192242, Leningrad, USSR
Home Address: Bolshoy, 100
                197022, Leningrad, USSR
Office Phone   233-09-82
Apt. Phone   292-15-41

Dr. Alexey Ya Bagrov
Senior Researcher and Director of Coronary Care
I.I. Djanelidze Research Institute of First Aid
Budapeshtskay, 3/5
192242, Leningrad, USSR
Office Phone   119-60-93
Laboratory   552-99-32
Home Phone   552-58-93

SECTION THREE. TERRORISM: EMS ISSUES AND MANAGEMENT

John E. Prescott

CAPSULE

Over the past two decades, much of the world has been affected by repeated acts of terrorism. Valuable medical information has been learned from many of these incidents, and gradually a distinct body of medical knowledge has evolved. A key lesson is that the proper emergency medical response to terrorism requires an understanding of the various types of terrorist acts and resulting patient injuries. The thoughtful coordination of several local and federal agencies must also occur if the effects of terrorism are to be minimized.

INTRODUCTION

Within the United States, adequate preparations for handling the medical consequences of terrorism are generally lacking. Traditionally, terrorist acts have been considered only from a law enforcement perspective. More importantly, many of the leaders in medical, legal and governmental authority are not aware of the significant differences between terrorist acts and other multiple-casualty incidents. Additionally, these leaders falsely assume that emergency personnel are fully prepared to handle any medical situation, including terrorism. Although it is clear that the medical effects of any incident are initially the responsibility of local Emergency Medical Services (EMS) systems, it cannot be assumed that readiness for other disasters has prepared these systems to deal with terrorism. Preparations for the special medical requirements inherent to a terrorist incident are not usually addressed in most community diaster plans, and medical personnel are not typically involved in antiterrorist planning. This overconfidence and lack of medical readiness can be directly related to increased patient morbidity and mortality.[1,2]

This chapter explores the phenomenon known as terrorism and delineates how it can and does affect the medical community. A description of the most commonly encountered terrorist incidents and their medical casualties and key points in the suggested EMS response are provided. The similarities and differences between specific acts of terrorism and other multiple–casualty incidents are also discussed.

THE EMERGENCE OF TERRORISM

DEFINITION

Terrorism is the unlawful use of force or violence against persons or property to intimidate or coerce a government, the civilian population, or any segment thereof, to further political or social objectives.[3] Militant religious factions have also used terrorism to further specific sectarian goals. Generating fear in individuals or society itself is the terrorist's prime goal.

The use of terrorism to control large numbers of people can be traced back to the beginnings of civilization. Recognition of the political usefulness of fear is demonstrated by an ancient Chinese proverb that states, "Kill one, frighten ten thousand." During the state-sponsored Reign of Terror in France in 1793, a small group of individuals controlled approximately 28 million people. As Robespierre stated, "Fear paralyzed the opposition." Throughout the nineteenth and twentieth centuries, numerous examples of group- and state-sponsored terrorism have occurred.

MODERN TERRORISM

The emergence of the present wave of terrorism can be traced to the simultaneous development of several factors. Over the past 50 years, traditional warfare has become increasingly expensive for countries and factions to wage and win. In contrast, terrorism is a relatively inexpensive method that can be used to influence government policy and society. The development of rapid, worldwide transportation has allowed terrorists to leave the site of an incident quickly and thus usually act without fear of direct retribution. Smaller and more powerful explosives and weapons have also aided the terrorist's ability to infiltrate society and inflict greater damage. The concentration of populations and important civic resources into smaller areas has given the terrorist the opportunity to cause greater damage with each incident. Finally, there has been a worldwide erosion of the concept of the noncombatant. For the terrorist, society, not simply the government or police, has become the target.

Yet terrorism would not have become a popular weapon if it were not for the rapid and unprecedented development of sophisticated communciations systems. Terrorist acts have become media events, often captivating millions of people in carefully orchestrated incidents. Instantaneous reporting of each occurrence aids the terrorist in his ultimate goal of instilling fear. Bombing, which was once an act of random violence, is now carefully planned to achieve maximum publicity and psychologic effect on the target population.

The last few years have seen the emergence of new and varied forms of terrorism. Narcoterrorism has surfaced as a means of increasing the influence of illegal drug cartels. Acts of terrorism against the environment and by environmental groups have also been reported with increasing frequency. The propensity of terrorists toward "superviolence" has risen with the increased availability of more powerful explosives. The threat of nuclear, biologic, and chemical terrorism is gradually becoming a reality.

THE UNITED STATES

Few modern countries have been spared the effects of terrorism. Indeed, the emergence of state-sponsored terrorism and the development of terror networks are well established.[3] Although the U.S. has experienced few true terrorist incidents, however, it remains particularly vulnerable to terrorism. Its worldwide geopolical involvement marks it as an adversary to many groups. Additionally, its open borders, large size, and free society allow terrorists easy access to virtually any place within the country. Attacks against and within the U.S. are covered by the media in great detail.

Potential terrorist targets are not limited to government offices or military installations. Anywhere large groups of Americans gather or important natural resources are stored may be marked for destruction. Incidents could develop and involve sports arenas, factories, energy facilities, amusement parks, shopping malls, airports, and hazardous cargo shipments.

Ensuring that U.S. interests abroad are protected is the responsibility of the State Department. Within the U.S., the Federal Bureau of Investigation (FBI) is the lead federal agency in combatting terrorism. Its mission is primarily two-fold: to *prevent* terrorist acts before they occur and, should they occur, *investigate* the incident so that the terrorists are brought to justice. To that end, the FBI maintains a large data base detailing terrorist incidents, suspected terrorist groups, and terrorist-related activity that has occurred in the U.S. (Figs. 87-24 and 87-25).

The FBI has been largely successful in keeping terrorism from affecting the American public, but with limited resources and the almost daily formation of new terrorist factions, the FBI may no longer be able to pre-empt terrorist acts.[4] Further, nonfederal agent medical casualties resulting from a terrorist act are not the responsibility of the FBI, and no special plan exists for their care. During and after a terrorist incident, the FBI relies totally on local EMS systems for medical support.

Within the federal government, the Federal Emergency Management Agency (FEMA) has a threefold mission related to terrorism. The FEMA is responsible for ensuring that the resources of the federal govern-

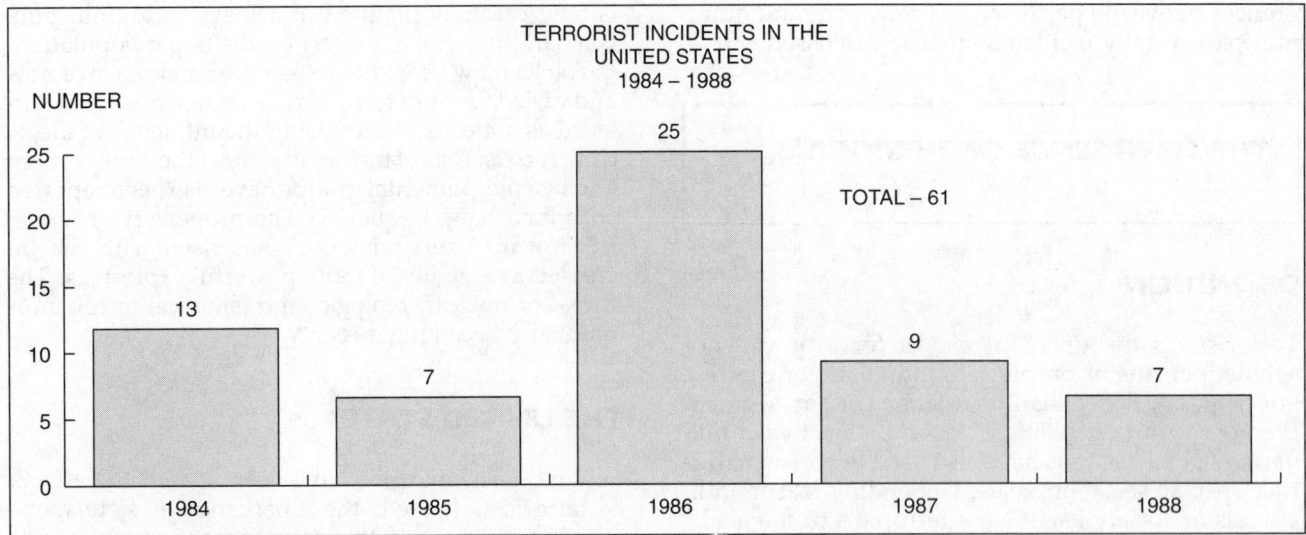

FIG. 87-24.   Terrorist incidents in the United States, 1984–1988. With permission from the Federal Bureau of Investigation, U.S. Department of Justice. Terrorism in the United States—1988. Terrorist Research and Analytical Center, Counterterrorism Section, Criminal Investigative Division, Federal Bureau of Investigation, 1988.

ment are coordinated with those of state and local governments during any disaster, including large-scale terrorist incidents. It is also charged with the identification and utilization of private sector resources during major crises. The second area of responsibility is the development of a proactive methodology to prevent terrorism or mitigate its potential consequences. Finally, the FEMA is charged with developing mechanisms for the integrated exercise and evaluation of plans and procedures.[5] Although the federal government has these goals in place, FEMA has had minor influence in preparing local communities for terrorism. Most municipalities, even those with well-developed antiterrorist units, have failed to consider the medical implications of a terrorist act. Only scant information is available to individuals or groups seeking detailed guidance regarding response to terrorist acts.

MEDICAL CONSIDERATIONS

Emergency physicians and other medical personnel can have a significant impact on reducing the morbidity and mortality of terrorist casualties and thus minimizing the effect of terrorism. Their role and those of all responding medical personnel must be clearly defined and adaptable to a variety of terrorist scenarios. By delineating responsibilities and knowing the types of injuries to expect from specific terrorist acts, medical personnel can better assist law enforcement agents during the resolution of any terrorist incident.

In the field, EMS personnel may be called on to provide initial triage, stabilization, and transportation in highly volatile and tense situations. Similarly, emer-

gency physicians and other hospital personnel may face unusual injuries and overwhelming casualties while being closely scrutinized by the press. Clearly, the support function of medical care providers cannot be successfully determined while an incident is taking place.

Specific acts of terrorism may mimic to a degree the situations and injuries medical personnel face in war. The threat of personal injury from renewed violence and the need for strict security are often present. Safety concerns range from secondary incidents caused by delayed bombs to the presence of snipers. Also, injuries resulting from automatic weapons and explosions are common in terrorist victims. Medical casualties of terrorism, however, are usually not healthy young men. Many terrorist acts generate patients which often represent a cross-section of society. Victims can be from any age category and often have preexisting diseases necessitating individualized resuscitation. Most civilian medical personnel receive little training regarding "military injuries" and therefore may not be prepared to handle the medical or psychologic casualties of terrorism.[6]

TERRORIST INCIDENTS

Several common elements can be found in every terrorist incident. Each act is deliberate, preconceived, and purposeful violence directed against society and is intended to cause maximum fear. Realization that other human beings were the cause of unexpected suffering often causes profound psychologic stress to

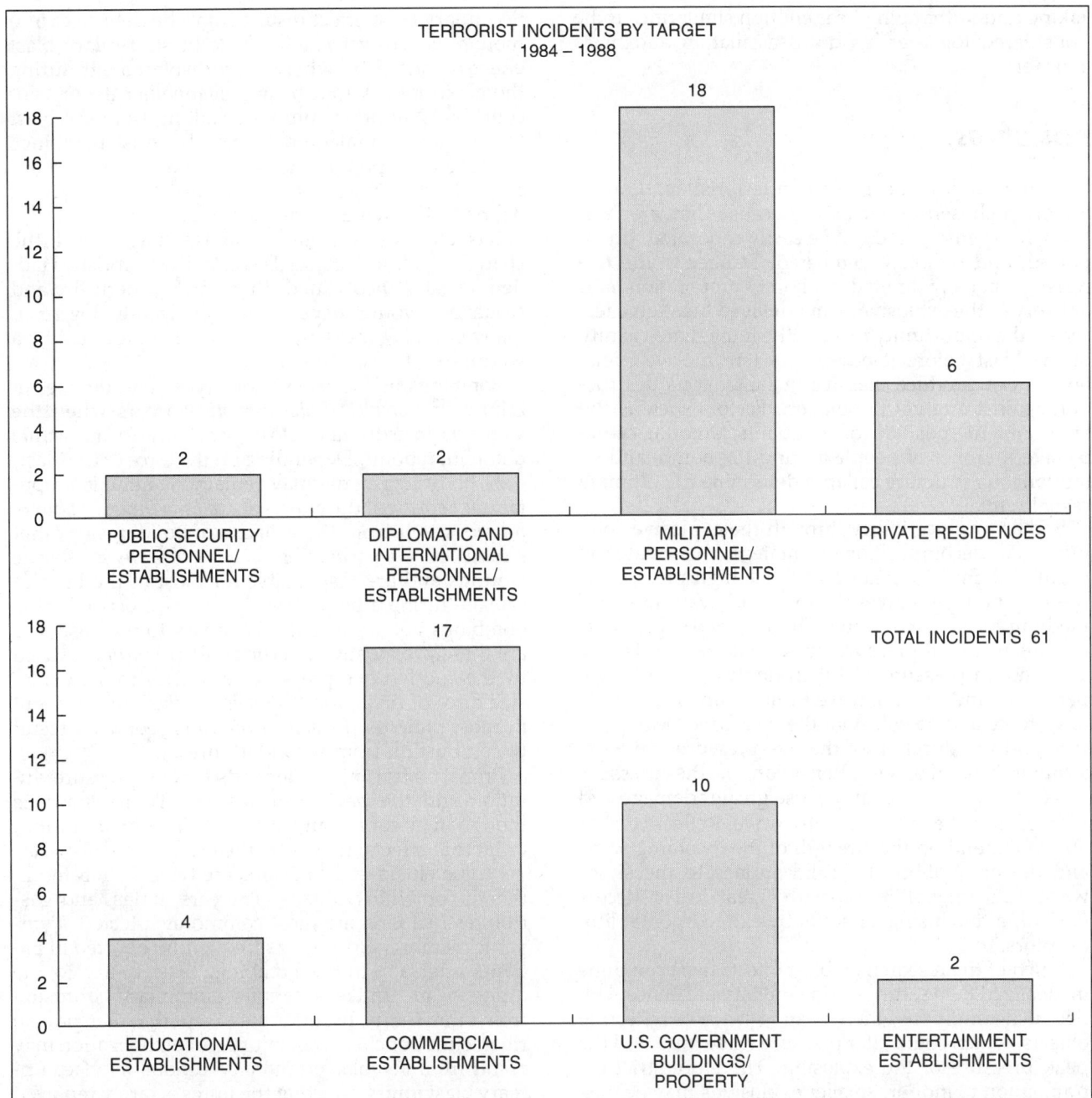

FIG. 87-25. Terrorist incidents in the United States by target, 1984–1988. With permission from the Federal Bureau of Investigation, U.S. Department of Justice. Terrorism in the United States—1988. Terrorist Research and Analytical Center, Counterterrorism Section, Criminal Investigative Division, Federal Bureau of Investigation, 1988.

the victims. Responding medical personnel may also experience a level of psychologic stress greater than that resulting from unexpected natural disasters or other multiple casualty incidents.

Every terrorist act also rapidly becomes both a media and a political event. Antiterrorist, police, and medical personnel can be expected to have all of their actions closely monitored and examined. Depending on the

nature and magnitude of the specific act, politicians and reporters may interfere with on-scene operations or attempt to violate scene security.

Terrorist incidents resulting in medical casualties can be divided into four major categories: bombings, shootings, hostage taking and kidnapping, and mass murders and assassinations. Although there are obvious differences in each of the specific acts, hostage taking and kidnapping bear enough similarities to be considered together, as do assassination and mass murder.

BOMBINGS

Bombings are the most common terrorist act. Bombs are often chosen by terrorists because they are relatively inexpensive and can be easily concealed, transported, and remotely detonated. Danger to the terrorist is usually limited to bomb preparation and delivery of the explosive. Time-delayed fuses give terrorists the opportunity to leave the immediate vicinity of the blast before it occurs. As terrorist weapons, bombs can produce massive instantaneous destruction against a target population. Factors such as the environment, position of occupants, amount of explosive, number of people around the bomb, and simultaneous structure collapse determine the ultimate casualty total.[1]

Bombs produce injury through the explosive combustion or decomposition of a material that creates an expanding mass of heated gas. The high pressure of this expanding gas gives rise to a shock wave in a fluid medium such as air or water. The idealized shock wave is a steep frontal pressure pulse that rapidly rises to a maximum pressure and then decays over a longer period of time.[7] As the wave front expands, it rapidly loses force and speed. Both the measured peak pressure and the duration of the overpressure wave determine blast damage. Reflection of the pressure wave off a solid object may cause greater damage and injuries than the initial pressure wave. Reflective blast effects depend on the strength of the incoming wave and the orientation of a solid surface to the shock wave. This principle is used with a great deal of success (and on a much smaller scale) by extracorporeal lithotriptors.[8]

Much of the research on blast effects has been done in idealized field settings using military ordnance. Under such conditions, there is an absence of reflecting objects, which could alter pressure wave form and the peak pressure of the explosion. Therefore strict extrapolation to indoor, smaller explosions may be misleading. The ultimate destructive force of a blast, however, depends on the size of the explosive charge, the surrounding medium, and distance from the explosion epicenter. For the common high explosive used in civilian terrorist bombs, the duration of the positive pressure is 2 and 10 ms for charges of 50 and 4000 lbs, respectively.[7] This is in contrast to military bombs, in which the duration may be greatly prolonged. If the shock wave is transmitted in a dense medium such as water, the effects are far more lethal because of the increased velocity and longer positive pressure duration of the blast wave.[9]

The overpressure produced by explosions produces four general categories of effects.[10] Primary blast effect is the result of direct exposure to the pressure wave.

Secondary blast effect results from the debris set into motion as a direct result of the blast. Tertiary blast effect is caused by whole-body displacement during the explosion. A fourth, miscellaneous category encompasses all other injuries resulting from the blast (burns, toxic inhalation injury). Terrorist bombings produce a preponderance of secondary and tertiary blast effects, i.e., most victims are struck by flying debris or thrown against a stationary object.

Casualty totals from bombings may reflect the changing political or social goals of the terrorists. Hadden et al.[11] postulated that in Northern Ireland casualties would have been significantly higher if many bombing incidents had not been preceded by a warning.

Bombings may cause various types and degrees of injuries.[12] *Complete body disruption* occurs when the victim is in extremely close proximity to the actual detonation point. Depending on the force of the blast, only body fragments may remain. Traumatic amputations represent the effects of *explosive injury. Masonry injuries* result from the collapse of buildings or other structures. *Flying missiles* cause extensive soft-tissue wounds and are responsible for most of the injuries caused during a bomb blast. *Burns* also occur during bombings but are usually secondary to the flash and are therefore mostly superficial. *Blast injury* is caused by the sudden overpressure secondary to the explosive force of the bomb. *Psychologic injuries* are evident in most patients. *Inhalation injury* is seen as a result of combustion from secondary fires.

Primary blast injury depends on overpressure duration and the peak overpressure. Tissue injury is thought to occur through either spallation, implosion, or inertial effects; however, the exact mechanism has yet to be elucidated.[9] Lesions are typically located in the air-containing organs. The ears, lungs, and gastrointestinal tract are most commonly affected. Tympanic membrane rupture is frequently reported in patients after a terrorist bombing. Blast injury to the lungs is not unlike a serious pulmonary contusion from other blunt chest trauma except that there are no rib fractures or chest wall injury. Air embolization may result from alveolar-pulmonary venous fistulae. Primary blast injury affecting the lungs is rarely reported in patients surviving terrorist bombings.

The vast majority of injuries that are treated are caused by the secondary and tertiary effects of the blast. Most of these are minor and involve the head, neck, and extremities. Clothing appears to have a significant protective effect. Puncture lacerations, abrasions, subcutaneous foreign bodies and contusions are frequently treated.

In a collective review, Cooper et al.[10] reported that 85% of all bombing victims were treated as outpatients. Severe head injury was the most common cause of death. Injuries to the chest and abdomen were rare but, when present, were associated with high mortality. Approximately 9% of all victims in Hadden's study of over 1500 patients in Northern Ireland required surgical intervention. Adler et al.[13] and Brismar and Bergenwald[14] both reported significant numbers of patients requiring plastic surgery. Flash burns, fractures, serious soft tissue damage, and eardrum rupture are common in people situated close to an exploding device, who usually require admission.

In each study, a much higher than expected number of patients suffered from significant psychological stress. Most were treated as outpatients with resolution of symptoms with time.

SHOOTINGS

Many patients, with a variety of gunshot wounds, are seen as a result of terrorism. Shooting victims may present after a failed assassination attempt. Many injured individuals, however, are the innocent victims of random gunfire or have been caught in the crossfire between terrorists and the authorities.

High-velocity military weapons are standard for most terrorists. In contrast to nonmilitary patients, victims of these weapons usually have multiple wounds. Considering all terrorism-related injuries, patients with gunshot wounds have the highest overall admission rate.

Fackler[15] notes that the potential for tissue destruction from gunshot wounds depends on projectile mass and striking velocity. Tissue damage is related to the projectile shape, projectile construction, and target tissue type. Extensive debridement of wounds without evidence of tissue damage is not recommended.

HOSTAGE TAKING AND KIDNAPPING

During these incidents, hostages are typically held for their bargaining worth (money, political policy changes, etc.) and are used to manipulate a government's political decisions. Terrorists also kidnap victims to obtain information or to exact revenge for "crimes" committed against the terrorist group. Hostages may be tortured and suffer from sleep, food, and water deprivation. Victims who are trapped in burning buildings or involved in aircraft assaults are at high risk for upper airway injury, smoke inhalation, and carbon monoxide or polyvinyl chloride inhalation.

During hostage situations, authorities are usually faced with the dilemma of negotiating with the terrorists versus attempting a hostage rescue. Negotiations leading to acquiescence to terrorist demands can be interpreted as a sign of weakness by the government. Rescue attempts may result in significant numbers of casualties among the hostages and antiterrorist personnel.

For the individual victim, there is a profound degree of psychologic stress. Intense feelings of fear and hopelessness can literally paralyze patients. Victims with chronic but stable medical conditions may undergo rapid decompensation. If a rescue is accomplished, hostages may initially be treated as "prisoners" while a thorough search is made for the terrorists. This may add to the sense of personal violation victims commonly experience.

Because of the nature of the incident, medical personnel are usually given time to prepare their response. Frequently they are asked to provide input regarding the medical condition of both the hostages and terrorists. Concerns about water, food, sleep, and hygiene become important during prolonged incidents.

MASS MURDER AND ASSASSINATIONS

Motives for this type of terrorism are usually to exact revenge for perceived past injustices and to create panic among the population. Typically, these acts are carried out against select government groups or prominent individuals. Often they are interpreted as an indication of the terrorists' ability to inflict harm without fear of retribution.

The boundaries between each type of terrorist incident are not always clear-cut. Police interdiction, a sudden change in the weather, or alterations in scheduled events can all force terrorists to abandon their original plans. In several instances, planned terrorist incidents have developed into even more bizarre and unexpected situations.

MEDICAL CASUALTIES OF TERRORISM

As with other patients suffering from serious medical conditions, there are guidelines to handling terrorist casualties that will improve their prognosis. The use of well-established triage and treatment protocols for trauma casualties is required. Additionally, an appreciation of several other factors will further reduce morbidity and mortality.

Terrorist casualties can be of any age and may have various underlying medical conditions. During initial triage and treatment, they are often unable to relate important facts about the actual terrorist event or their general health. Physicians must therefore depend to a greater degree on careful physical examination and pertinent laboratory testing to assist diagnosis and treatment.

During their examination, all patients must be fully stripped. An inspection for occult wounds is absolutely necessary for victims of bombings. Additionally, all patients must be searched for concealed weapons. It is not uncommon for both terrorists and antiterrorist personnel to carry small, discreetly hidden weapons or explosives on their person. As with all trauma patients, every body orifice should be examined. Traumatic wounds should not be primarily repaired because of increased likelihood of infection.

Emergency personnel should make it their policy to render assistance based on the patient's injuries without regard to their own role in the incident. Within Lebanon and Northern Ireland, health care workers have been spared from most violent acts because of their neutrality. At all times, emergency personnel should practice professional, nondiscriminatory, and nonthreatening medical care.

Responsibility for particular terrorist acts (bombings, shootings) may be difficult to determine initially. For the peace of the community, it is extremely important to have detailed forensic investigations performed by experienced and impartial experts. Photography is particularly useful in documenting the exact location and nature of injuries.[12]

A large number of psychologic injuries can result from a terrorist incident. The actual victims, their families, individuals present on the scene but not physically injured, and responding personnel, can all suffer varying degrees of psychologic stress. There are several contributing factors. For many victims, the overwhelming sensation of fear, combined with the total lack of control over events, overwhelms normal coping mechanisms. Also, the acuity of the event and the terrorist's use of sensory deprivation does not allow individuals time to put into place their normal psychologic defenses. As a result, many terrorist victims go through prolonged stages of denial and disbelief. For others with post-traumatic stress disorder, there is no relief from recurring memories of the incident.[16]

Hostages can feel guilt and depression because of their behavior during the incident. Some 20 to 50% have depression, insomnia, anxiety, phobias, and obsessions. In studies of bombing victims, both Hadden et al.[11] and Pyper et al.[7] found a much greater number of patients with psychologic injuries than expected.

EMS RESPONSE

The key to an effective EMS response to a terrorist incident is planning. Although many communities have developed increasingly sophisticated antiterrorist systems, most lack any type of integrated medical support. During any terrorist crisis, the EMS is asked to provide medical triage, resuscitation, stabilization, and transport to victims, police, and terrorists who are injured. Failure to include emergency personnel in the planning stages of the response jeopardizes the likelihood of the EMS being able to care maximally for all casualties.

Communities should perform their own terrorism threat analysis and determine in advance possible scenarios. Unique factors and unusual circumstances for each situation should then be identified and preparations made to deal with them. Although the basic role for the EMS must be defined, sufficient flexibility must be incorporated to allow medical personnel to adapt to the situation. Unexpected complications occur commonly and may range from a prolonged hostage situation to the explosion of a secondary device. Because of the unusual circumstances of most terrorist incidents, responders from both the medical and law enforcement professions must cross-train and be knowledgeable about the types of injuries likely to be encountered, security aspects, scene integrity, and types of weapons commonly used.

ON-SCENE

EMS personnel must work closely with law enforcement personnel once they arrive on the site. They should not enter the incident scene until they are cleared by the commander. Once that has been done, EMS personnel should then immediately determine the severity of the situation and, if possible, the number and types of casualties. Because many medical personnel are not familiar with the scope or treatment of various types of terrorist injuries, overtriage can result. Care must be taken to prevent patients from being sent to the wrong facility or experiencing delayed care.[1]

Radio communication to either the base station or supporting area hospital, as well as with other responding agencies, is essential. Strict noise, light, and radio discipline should be maintained while a threat is present. EMS personnel may be asked by the incident commander to provide input about the medical and psychologic condition of hostages and/or the terrorists, the number and types of casualties, their medical treatment and transportation requirements, and search and rescue.[2,18] During and after any incident, the presence of the EMS aids in reducing the anxiety and panic of the victims and responding personnel.

Depending on the incident, first responders may have to alter their normal treatment protocols. If the scene remains unsecured, select patients may have to forgo on-scene stabilization. Unless specific medical personnel from the hospital have extensive experience in handling terrorist casualties, the use of special medical teams is not warranted.

HOSPITAL

Medical personnel within hospitals have the task of providing definitive care to terrorism victims. They must be knowledgeable about the types of injuries they can expect from any type of situation and must know their capabilities and limitations for dealing with these injuries. The availability of critical care and other hospital beds must be communicated to on-scene personnel so that patients can be appropriately transported. Internally, the hospital should determine its own supply, equipment, and personnel needs. Additional security is needed to control the expected influx of relatives and media. Communication with on-scene personnel and other health facilities is required to maximize efficiency.

SPECIAL CONCERNS

THE MEDIA

As with other disasters, the media quickly descend onto the scene of any terrorist incident. Responding personnel have an obligation to provide the press with clear and timely information about the incident. If information is not forthcoming, the media may become even more demanding. If possible, news briefings should be held at regular intervals, as far away from the incident site and treatment areas as possible.

WEAPONS HANDLING

Medical personnel may be faced with caring for patients who are still carrying weapons or explosives. Every attempt should be made to search all patients before their arrival at the hospital. Law enforcement personnel should be present to unload all weapons, and provisions must be made for the registration and storage of these devices in secure areas.

VIPS

Politicians and other dignitaries are often the victims of terrorism. When such a situation occurs, emergency personnel must render care under strict security conditions and may initially feel intimidated. If a medical staff is travelling with the dignitary, they may insist on being present during medical treatment. By their nature, such situations will be tense. Much can be accomplished quickly, however, if all personnel identify themselves, describe their position and medical function, and state what they perceive the immediate needs of the injured to be. Senior personnel from the FBI and Secret Service should be identified and informed of medical necessities. All hospital services may be affected during the incident and routine care severely limited. The entire hospital staff must practice strict confidentiality.

ETHICAL ISSUES

Medical personnel may experience difficult ethical and personal decisions when asked to treat not only the victims of a terrorist incident but the terrorists themselves. Problematic triage and treatment decisions may also occur when pressure to care for a particular individual or group of patients first is applied, i.e., wounded police.

EVIDENCE COLLECTION

This is extremely important to law enforcement personnel and may lead to the determination of respon-

sibility for the terrorist act. Therefore it should be emphasized at every level of care. When possible, the location of the victim must be carefully noted. The victim's clothes and any missiles removed from patients should be saved for analysis. Wound location should also be carefully documented, as well as all pertinent statements by the victims. The dead should not be moved until their exact position and location are carefully documented. Photography and videotaping are particularly useful, both on-scene and in the hospital.

DRILLS

The value of disaster preparedness exercises is well known. Such drills test the coordination and communication of all responding agencies. Realistic terrorism exercises should be planned and executed with minimal publicity, however. The general public may react with unnecessary fear if the community was thought to be under significant threat.

CONCLUSION

Society expects emergency personnel to meet the unique medical challenges presented by terrorism. Success in this endeavor is largely determined by four factors. First, the threat of terrorism must be appreciated and understood by emergency personnel. Second, medical personnel must be fully prepared to care for the casualties of terrorist incidents. Third, the EMS must play an integral role in the larger, community-wide response to terrorism. Such a role can be assured only through coordinated preplanning with all responding agencies. Finally, both society and emergency personnel must keep the terrorism issue in perspective. An appreciation of the potential threat allows a realistic allocation of community resources and prevents unrealistic expectations.

Past and current trends in terrorism have been examined in this chapter. The future, however, may bring radically different situations and challenges to emergency personnel. Continued diligence and planning are required to ensure preparedness.

REFERENCES

1. Frykberg, M.D., and Tepas, J.J.: Terrorist bombings—Lessons learned from Belfast to Beirut. Ann. Surg. *208*:569, 1988.
2. Degeneste, H.I., and Sullivan, J.P.: EMS, the police response to terrorism. The Police Chief, May, 1987, pp. 36–40.
3. U.S. Department of Justice: Terrorism in the United States—1988. Terrorist Research and Analytical Center, Counterter-

rorism Section, Criminal Investigative Division, Federal Bureau of Investigation, 1988.

4. FBI: More threats against Americans. Washington Times, Sept. 12, 1989.
5. Guiffrida, L.O., and Salcedo, F.S.: Terrorism. . . . what can we do? Emerg. Manag. Rev. 1:10, 1984.
6. Dolev, E.: Medical aspects of terrorist activities. Milit. Med. 153:243, 1988.
7. Stapczynski, J.S.: Blast injuries. Ann. Emerg. Med. 11:687, 1982.
8. Pode, D., Landau, E., Lijovetsky, G., et al.: Isolated pulmonary blast injury in rats—A new model using the extracorporeal shock-wave lithotriptor. Milit. Med. 154:288, 1989.
9. Phillips, Y.Y.: Primary blast injuries. Ann. Emerg. Med. 15:1446, 1986.
10. Cooper, G.J., Maynard, R.L., Cross, N.L., et al.: Casualties from terrorist bombings. J. Trauma 23:955, 1983.
11. Hadden, W.A., Rutherford, W.H., and Merrett, J.D.: The injuries of terrorist bombing: a study of 1532 consecutive patients. Br. J. Surg. 65:525, 1978.
12. Marshall, T.K.: A pathologist's view of terrorist violence. Forensic Sci. Int. 36:57, 1988.
13. Adler, J., Golan, E., Golan, J., et al.: Terrorist bombing experience during 1975–1979. Casualties admitted to the Shaare Zedek Medical Center. Isr. J. Med. Sci. 19:189, 1983.
14. Brismar, B., and Bergenwald L.: The terrorist bomb explosion in Bologna, Italy, 1980: An analysis of the effects and injuries sustained. J. Trauma 22:216.
15. Fackler, M.L.: Ballistic injury. Ann. Emerg. Med. 15:1451, 1986.
16. Duffy, J.C.: Common psychological themes in societies' reaction to terrorism and disasters. Milit. Med. 153:387, 1988.
17. Pyper, P.C., and Graham, W.J.: Analysis of terrorist injuries treated at Craigavon Area Hospital, Northern Ireland, 1972–1980. Injury 14:332, 1983.
18. Vayer, J.S., and Adams, R.: Responding to Terrorism—Keeping emergency workers out of the crossfire. Firehouse, June, 1987, pp. 101–102.

BIBLIOGRAPHY

BOOKS

Emerson, S.: Secret warriors: Inside the covert military operations of the Reagan era. New York, G.P. Putnam's Sons, 1988.

Gutteridge, W. (ed.): Contemporary terrorism. New York, Facts on File, Inc., 1986.

Hyde, M.O., and Forsyth, E.H.: Terrorism: A special kind of violence. New York, Dodd, Mead & Company, 1987.

Netanyahu, B. (ed.): Terrorism: How the West can win. New York, Farrar, Straus, Giroux, Inc., 1986.

Szumski, B. (ed.): Terrorism: Opposing viewpoints. St. Paul, Greenhaven Press, 1986.

U.S. Department of Defense. Emergency War Surgery. Government Printing Office, 1988.

ARTICLES

Adams, R.: If Terrorism Comes Home. Firehouse, July, 1986, p. 16.

Bern, A.: Disaster medical services. In Principles of EMS Systems, Edited by Roush, W.R. American College of Emergency Physicians, Dallas, Texas, 1989, pp. 77–93.

Bruno, H.: Preparing for Terrorist Attacks. Firehouse, May, 1988, p. 8.

Caro, D., and Irving, M.: The Old Bailey bomb explosion. Lancet 1:1433, 1973.

Haywood, I.: Terrorism—General aspects, aetiology and pathophysiology. In Medicine for Disasters. Edited by Baskett, P., and Weller, R. London, Butterworth and Co. Ltd., 1988, Chap. 28, pp. 391–405.

Haywood, I.: Terrorism—Management and forensic aspects. In Medicine for Disasters. Edited by Baskett, P., and Weller, R. London, Butterworth and Co., Ltd, 1988, Chap 29, pp. 406–423.

Kennedy, T.L., and Johnston G.W.: Civilian bomb injuries. Br. Med. J. 1:382, 1975.

Kentsmith, D.K.: Hostages and other prisoners of war. Milit. Med. 147:969, 1982.

Molde, J.D.: Medical aspects of urban heavy rescue. Prehosp. Disaster Med. 6:341, 1991.

Rosenberg, B., Sternberg, N., Zagher, V., et al.: Burns due to terroristic attacks on civilian populations from 1975–1979. Burns 9:21, 1982.

Scott, B.A., Fletcher, J.R., Pulliam, M.W., et al.: The Beirut terrorist bombing. Neurosurgery 18:107, 1986.

Seger, K.A.: Managing the threat of terrorism. Fire and Arson Investigator, Sept., 1986, pp. 30–33.

Staten, C.: The EMS Response to Terrorism. EMS Management Advisor Vol. 2 (2) pp. 1–2.

Sullivan, J.P.: Fire and Rescue Operations at the Terrorist Incident. American Fire Journal, September, 1988, pp. 22–25.

Tucker, K., and Lettin, A.: The Tower of London bomb explosion. Br. Med. J. 3:287, 1975.

U.S. Department of Defense. Report of the DoD Commission on Beirut International Airport Terrorist Act, Oct. 23, 1983, Part VIII, Casualty Handling, 93–121, Government Printing Office, 1984.

U.S. Department of State. International Terrorism. Selected documents. No. 24, Government Printing Office, 1986.

Waterworth, T.A., and Carr, M.J.T.: Report on injuries sustained by patients treated at the Birmingham General Hospital following the recent bomb explosions. Br. Med. J. 2:25, 1975.

Part XIII

Emergency Department Management

Chapter 88

EMERGENCY DEPARTMENT MANAGEMENT

UTILIZATION OF EMERGENCY SERVICES: THE NINETIES

Richard Aghababian, Laura Peterson, and Lucille Gans

CAPSULE

Emergency Departments (EDs) have been increasingly accepted by the general public as an alternate point of entry into the health care system. Some, especially the younger generation, have grown up with a great deal of exposure to the concept of "emergency rooms" and may use them for various reasons. Convenience and accessibility are certainly issues, as is the general quality of emergency care. Some patients attempt to reach their private physicians and are told that they will be seen more quickly in an emergency department. Insurance companies cover at least part of the cost of such visits. Other patients do not have private physicians, and therefore see the ED as their only option for basic primary care. Whatever the reason, use of EDs is increasing rapidly.

INTRODUCTION

In 1989, the approximately 5200 hospital-based EDs in the United States saw 86,641,305 patients.[1] This represents an increase in patient load of approximately three million over the previous year, or 3.6%, and a 10.5% increase since 1983 (Fig. 88-1). At the same time, financial realities and legislative mandates are threatening many hospitals and EDs with closure.

The practice of emergency medicine is in a unique position in today's health care crisis, facing both the potential onslaught of patients who cannot get medical attention elsewhere and the opportunity to work effectively for change in the health care system. The definition of emergency medicine, as described by The American College of Emergency Physicians, its major governing body, makes this clear: Emergency medicine is patient-demanded, based solely on the patient's perception of what constitutes an emergency. The practice requires continuous access to care for an unrestricted population. It is time-dependent, requiring that a physician be constantly available to ensure optimal patient outcomes. Practicing physicians must be expert at the initial recognition, stabilization, evaluation, and disposition of a wide range of problems.

The requirement that emergency medicine physicians be constantly available to treat all patients, based on the patient's definition of illness, has created new challenges for the field, especially in today's socioeconomic climate. Growing numbers of people rely on emergency departments as their sole source of medical care because no other form of health care is available to them. There are currently at least 37 million uninsured people in the U.S., accounting for almost one fifth of the population. Many thousands more are underinsured "working poor." Migrant workers, by the nature of their jobs, cannot get primary care or medical follow-up in the usual stable clinic setting. Many of the uninsured or underinsured are hampered not only by financial barriers to health care. Frequently there are also problems with transportation, communication, and general education as to what care is available to them. The impact of this population on the ED is reflected in the finding that low-income patients make 64% more use of emergency services than do those with cost-sharing insurance plans.[2]

Closure of long-term psychiatric facilities has increased the outpatient population with chronic de-

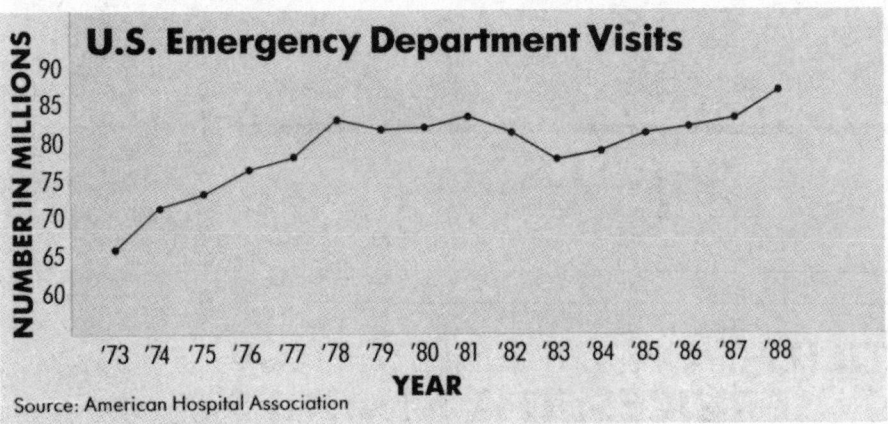

FIG. 88-1. U.S. Emergency Department visits, 1973–1988.

bilitating psychiatric illness, and the rising cost of inpatient medical care likewise has increased the outpatient population with severe chronic medical illnesses. Even those with acute medical problems are discharged from the hospital sooner because payment plans are requiring shorter hospital stays. All of these people are becoming frequent visitors to EDs for completion or continuation of what used to be inpatient care. Although they account for only 10% of the population, those with chronic and acute illnesses currently use 75% of health care services.[3]

Larger problems facing society are also having a direct impact on EDs. The plight of the homeless is becoming a major national issue; those who are homeless are getting what medical care they can almost exclusively from EDs. Drug abuse is also on the rise in this country, and emergency physicians are consequently dealing with the overdoses, poisonings, and traumas inherent to drug use. The growing numbers of people afflicted with AIDS and its associated illnesses also are placing a noticeable burden on EDs because they require sophisticated and costly medical care.

Finally, the elderly population, which has always accounted for a disproportionately large percentage of ED visits, has been increasing markedly in recent years. People over 65 are predicted to account for almost 20% of the United States population by the year 2000. As people live longer, they are susceptible to a wider range of disease, again creating a need for more sophisticated and costly care.

In the face of this ever-increasing pool of potential ED patients, financial and legislative support of emergency care has been dwindling. A total of 8.3 billion dollars in uncompensated medical care was rendered in 1989 alone, and budget deficits have led to large federal and state Medicare cuts. Some small hospitals cannot afford to stay open, and this has forced the closure of many local EDs. Since 1983, 209 emergency departments have already closed, and the closures are disproportionately concentrated in the already underserved rural and inner-city locations.[4]

TRAUMA CENTERS

The huge financial losses incurred by trauma centers, where much of the labor-intensive, high-technology, and long-term care rendered is uncompensated, has forced many to shut down. The city of Chicago lost 15.3 million dollars in uncompensated trauma care in 1988, leading at least partly to the loss of four hospitals from the trauma system in the last two years.[5] The trauma systems of Los Angeles, New York City, Washington, D.C., and Dade County, Florida, among others, have faced similar losses with subsequent closures. It has been noted that these closures have created a sort of "domino effect" in trauma care because patients are deferred from a closed trauma center to an open one, thus overburdening that center and eventually leading to its forced closure. Clearly, these problems are occurring in areas of the greatest need for effective trauma care. Today, despite the fact that trauma accounts for 150,000 deaths and 8.8 million injuries a year, only 25% of the U.S. population has access to a fully equipped and officially designated trauma center (Fig. 88-2).

SYSTEM OVERLOADS AND SOLUTIONS

The combination of increased demand for emergency care and decreased emergency resources has created a predictable system overload. Many EDs have become overcrowded, with stable patients waiting hours to be seen and critical patients waiting hours in the department for a bed to become available in the similarly overburdened inpatient setting. Emergency medical service (EMS) systems are also becoming over-

FIG. 88-2. *State trauma center designation and verification processes, 1986–1987.*

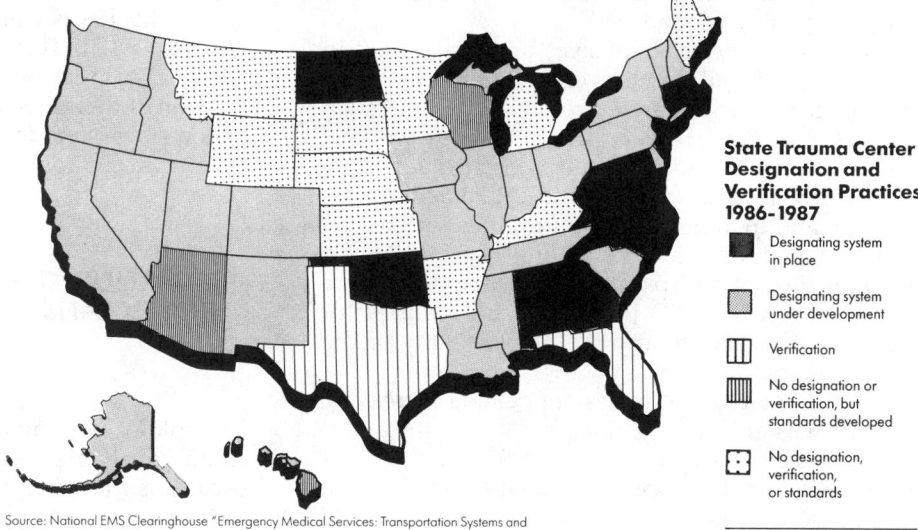

State Trauma Center Designation and Verification Practices 1986-1987

■ Designating system in place

▨ Designating system under development

▥ Verification

▦ No designation or verification, but standards developed

⊡ No designation, verification, or standards

Source: National EMS Clearinghouse "Emergency Medical Services: Transportation Systems and Available Facilities," 1988.

loaded as patients require triage to other hospitals if their original or ideal destination is on "diversion," meaning that emergency or inpatient resources have already been overwhelmed by the current patient load.

These closures of community hospitals and trauma centers are occurring despite deceptively high expenditures for health care in the United States. National health care spending currently accounts for more than 11% of the Gross National Product, reflecting a trend of increasing expenditure since 1950, when the per capita spending was $70.37. This is in comparison with today's level of approximately $2000 per capita and estimated figures for 1990 predicting a total health care expenditure of $670 billion.[3] Physicians receive 21% of the health care dollars, but control the spending of far more by ordering tests, writing prescriptions, and admitting patients to the hospital.

To address the issues of skyrocketing costs, currently rising at double the rate of inflation, and faced with uncompensated medical care and large numbers of uninsured patients, the U.S. government in 1986 passed into legislation the Consolidated Omnibus Budget Reconciliation Act (COBRA). This included a mandate for the Physician Payment Review Commission (PPRC) to advise Congress on payment reform in the Medicare program. The PPRC addresses only payments to physicians, and is developing a fee schedule based on the Resource Based Relative Value Scale (RBRVS), developed by Dr. William Hsiao at Harvard University. The revamped Medicare payment scales will be implemented over a 5-year span, starting in 1992 and ending in 1996, when all payments will be made according to the fee schedule. At this time, it appears that overall payments for emergency medicine will increase because of the increasing amount of primary care that Medicare patients are now obtaining in the ED.

In addition to federal reforms, individual states are also attempting to change their health care systems. Most notably, Oregon is exploring methods to provide health care to all citizens by establishing a priorities list of medical services to ensure that a basic level of care is maintained for all. Hawaii, too, has initiated a plan to provide universal health care to all its citizens, and will include the "underinsured"—those people who earn too much to qualify for Medicaid but too little to purchase private health insurance. This would ensure payment for a large segment of ED care that is currently provided without compensation.

QUALITY ASSURANCE

While federal and state governments are struggling with legislation to solve the problems of compensation for health care, the field of emergency medicine is rapidly becoming more involved in yet another medicolegal discipline: quality assurance. This is a relatively new area for all medical specialties, and emergency medicine, being a new specialty, is at its forefront. The scope of quality assurance encompasses all aspects of peer review, including regularly scheduled morbidity and mortality conferences and chart reviews. Incorporation of innovations such as computerized chart audits, automated record keeping, and chart dictation systems are being evaluated in EDs in terms of their impact on patient care and outcome management. The government has contributed with legislations such as COBRA, which also provides guidelines for emergency patient, inpatient, and physician rights and expectations in the inpatient and transfer setting. This was updated in 1989 as the Omnibus Budget Reconciliation Act (OBRA), with clearer, more stringent guidelines.

Quality assurance also involves decreasing risks in the workplace for all members of the emergency team. Emergency physicians are currently addressing such issues as reduction of exposure of health care workers to hepatitis, AIDS, and other infectious diseases. They are also involved in creating and implementing assessment and treatment plans for injuries suffered by the ED staff: burns, abrasions, and back strain, for example. Violent and psychotic patients also pose a significant threat to ED personnel, and policies for dealing with them are also the responsibility of the risk management team.

Complex malpractice issues are gaining increasing attention as significant workplace risks for the emergency physician. At present, approximately 25% of malpractice litigation originates in the ED. Current investigations of no-fault malpractice legislation and tort reform will have wide-ranging impact on the future practice of emergency medicine. Emergency physicians are involved in these investigations, with ACEP sponsoring standards development task forces.

Finally, the threat of staff "burnout" has received considerable notice in the press as a current problem in emergency medicine. Staffing EDs presents significant difficulties at present because there is a shortage of board-certified emergency physicians. Of the 23,000 physicians practicing emergency medicine today, 8332 (36%) are board-certified in the specialty, and 3293 are graduates of an emergency medicine residency. At present there are 80 residencies training 1600 residents, and graduating 450 every year.[1] Because the American Medical Association predicts an attrition rate of 2 to 3%, accounting for a loss of 700 practicing emergency physicians per year, and because the practice track, or "grandfather" board eligibility option

expired in 1988, the demand for board-certified emergency physicians will most certainly outstrip the supply (Fig. 88-3). This allows those currently entering the field a great deal of choice as to the type and location of their practice, and it also forces new emergency physicians to take strong leadership roles in their sparsely populated field.

EXPANDING ROLE OF EMERGENCY PHYSICIANS

The role of the emergency physician is diverse and continuously expanding, and this is certainly in part because so few are currently available to answer all the demands of the job. Many new graduates of residency programs are going on to further specialization through fellowship programs, and as experts in fields such as toxicology, prehospital care, environmental medicine, and occupational health, are making important contributions in previously ignored areas of health care. Emergency medicine, through its specialists, is now running poison control centers, supervising emergency medical service systems, and contributing to research and legislation for occupational safety.

The relative newness of the field creates multiple opportunities, many still untapped, for investigation and research. Emergency medicine is therefore understandably moving toward deeper investment in academics. Physicians employed in teaching hospitals are working with house officers from all medical specialties because almost all disciplines spend some time in their training in the ED. This creates the opportunity

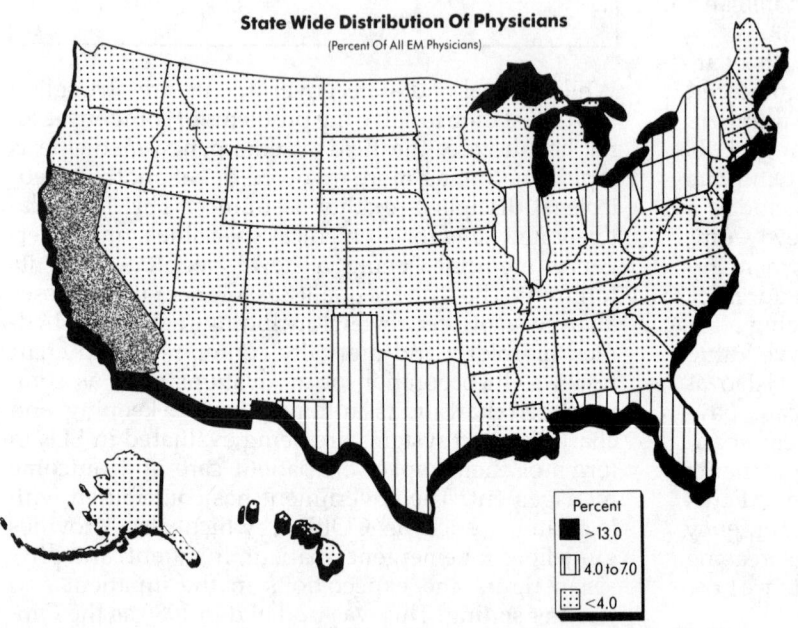

State Wide Distribution Of Physicians
(Percent Of All EM Physicians)

Percent
■ >13.0
▥ 4.0 to 7.0
▦ <4.0

FIG. 88-3. Statewide distribution of physicians.

to educate other fields about the practice of emergency medicine, thereby furthering cooperation among medical and surgical disciplines and ultimately improving patient care. Contributions to patient care are also made through academic research, with emergency physicians involved in such areas as resuscitation, anesthesia, wound management, critical care, and the development of short-term observation units.

Opportunities for community involvement are also varied, ranging from forming official ACEP position statements on issues like seat belt use and gun control to teaching basic life support in community schools and basic trauma support to volunteer rescue workers. In addition, emergency physicians are always ideally situated to benefit their community by being advocates for patient care and access to the medical system.

In spite of, or perhaps because of, the multifaceted problems outlined here, emergency medicine remains a challenging field, partly because of the interest of its practitioners, who are continuing research and training to resolve the issues. The impact of emergency medicine on the health care crisis is exemplified by the ACEP position paper on the problem of overcrowding. Published in March 1990, it calls for, among other things, basic health insurance for all citizens, the removal of financial disincentives to hospitals for the provision of emergency care, a better assessment of inpatient and critical care needs, and better access to primary care.

The ongoing study of how best to achieve these goals is an area full of opportunities for the emergency physician, and the next decade should see further research funding and support for the field. Emergency physicians are in a unique position to study the problems and to create and implement the solutions. Continued specialized training could change emergency medicine from a major potential victim of the health care crisis to the most valuable asset in solving the problem.

REFERENCES

1. American Hospital Association Annual Survey, 1989.
2. O'Grady, K., Manning, W., Newhouse, J., and Brook, R.: The impact of cost sharing on emergency department use. N. Engl. J. Med. *313*:484, 1985.
3. Williams, R.: The changing face of reimbursement. Address to the ACEP Winter Symposium, March 12–15, 1990.
4. Stockwell, S.: Hospital closures across the country. Emerg. Med. News *12*:30, 1990.
5. California ACEP address, Sacramento, California, March 21, 1990.
6. National Safety Council: Accident Facts. Chicago, IL: The Council, 1988.

BIBLIOGRAPHY

ACEP News: New patient transfer laws take effect. ACEP *9*:1–18, June, 1990.

ACEP: ACEP recommends to COGME: Emergency Medicine a Shortage Specialty. *ACEP Academic News*, March, 1989, p. 1.

California ACEP address, Sacramento, CA, March 21, 1990.

Cantrill, S.V.: Emergency Medicine Clinical Policies. ACEP Winter Symposium, March 12–15, 1990.

Carlson, R.: The Future of Emergency Medicine. *Emergency Medicine News*, March 1990, pp. 17–25.

Garza, M.A.: Who Cares About Trauma? *J. Emerg. Med. Serv.* March 1990, pp. 33–39.

Harby, K.: Trauma Legislation: Too little, too late? *J. Emerg. Med.* April 1990, p. 27.

Holbrook, J., and Aghababian, R.: A computerized audit of 15,009 emergency department records. *Ann. Emerg. Med.* Feb. 2, 1990, pp. 139–144.

Jones, L.: Value of trauma centers stressed at hearing. *Am. Med. News*, May 18, 1990, p. 6.

Levine, S.R.: Harvard study spurs liability debate. *Physician's News Digest*, April 1990, p. 1.

McGinn, Paul R.: New Hawaii plan reaches people caught between Medicaid, insurance. *American Medical News*, June 15, 1990, p. 1.

Physician Payment Review Commission: *Annual Report to Congress 1990*, Washington, D.C.

Stockwell, S.: Hospital closures across the country are straining already-overburdened EDs. *Emerg. Med. News*, May 1990, p. 30.

Trunkey, D.: "What's wrong with trauma care?" *American College of Surgeons Bulletin*, March 1990, p. 10.

Williams, R.: The changing face of reimbursement: relative value scales and the physician payment review commission. ACEP Winter Symposium, March 12–15, 1990.

Zimlicki, P.: Health care rationing addressed at MMS meeting. *Physician's News Digest*, July 1990, p. 3.

THE WORK ENVIRONMENT

George R. Schwartz

CAPSULE

For years, physicians and nurses spoke of the emergency department as "The Pit." This implies a seething, dangerous place set in some dank subterranean chamber. Many emergency departments (EDs) were indeed situated in badly lighted basement areas, poorly maintained, and often administratively forgotten. As medical sophistication has increased and respect for emergency departments and their function within a hospital has grown, newer facilities have evolved. Nonetheless, certain correctable unpleasant elements often remain. As physicians, nurses, and paramedical personnel devote their careers to emergency medicine, it is important to isolate some of the less desirable aspects and to attempt to lessen their impact upon those working within such an environment. If unattended, many of these correctable aspects can lead to or accelerate the "burnout" phenomenon often seen in emergency physicians and nurses.

INTRODUCTION

The amount of sensory stimuli present in an ED is often enormous, with people moving in every direction, telephones ringing, monitors beeping, and everywhere a feeling of "what will come next?"—all in a framework of time pressure. These stimuli not only affect the nervous system but also cause measurable physiologic effects, including peripheral vasoconstriction, hypertension, changes in bowel mobility, gastric acid and intestinal secretion, hormonal changes, and many others.

In addition, there are the sights, sounds, and smells of human suffering and disease. In the ED, the staff is frequently exposed to the results of violence, mangled bodies, and death in the young. Although hospital staffs have become hardened to seeing elderly people dying, it is always difficult to avoid the severe emotional effect of seeing young people dead in the prime of their lives—or even before that, in the innocence of childhood.

Certain degrees of stress and sensory input are important for function, but continued high stress leads to performance decrement, particularly when associated with sleep and circadian cycle alteration. Moreover, the 24-hour shifts at some EDs surpass the ability of most individuals to maintain efficiency. Such long shifts should be interdicted, because performance decrement reflects directly on quality of patient care. With 24-hour work periods, there is a pattern of performance deterioration. The performance peak occurs after 6 to 10 hours and then drops off to a low point at 22 hours. Thus, shift durations should not be longer than 12 hours in busy settings. Such scheduling concerns have come to have medicolegal significance.

Patients come to EDs unprepared, frequently upset, in crisis, worried, or desperately afraid. Frequently they act out their emotional turmoil by directing hostility or anger at nurses or physicians.

Added to the potential turmoil is the need for 24-hour coverage and consequent shift changes. A situation easily manageable emotionally in the afternoon may require tremendous control at 4:00 A.M., especially during the first few nights before personal patterns have readjusted at least partially. The effects of circadian cycle shifts in hospital personnel have not been explored in depth. The greatest experience comes from the military and the space program, in which studies were made of psychologic reactivity and performance at various hours. Those who change shifts frequently are in constant dysrhythmia and experience sleep disturbances, irritability, and decreased performance. Of particular importance is the decrease in frustration tolerance found in such people. In addition, with sleep alterations, the myriad diurnal or circadian rhythms, of which more than 100 are known, cannot readjust rapidly, and never do in some cases, even with prolonged night work. The effects of sleep deprivation and fatigue may be severe. Recent attempts to enhance the ability to change circadian patterns (through diet and sleep patterns) may be useful. Unfortunately, most physicians are unable to make such rapid adjustments and are frequent users of sleep medications (such as halcion) to aid their preparedness for night shifts. Susceptible emergency physicians occasionally develop a pattern of using stimulants to aid function and sedatives to "come down" and enhance the ability to sleep. Such "performance use" of psychoactive drugs is often not an addiction in the usual sense because such medication use is frequently stopped during vacations or when job needs change.

RESPONSES TO THE ENVIRONMENT

For some personnel, the environment proves to be overwhelming, and after a brief period they choose other types of medical work.

A phenomenon, however, has been observed in some of those who stay that, although milder, is similar to that seen in survivors of Hiroshima and soldiers from Vietnam. Lifton called it "psychic numbing." This phenomenon allows survival in a stressful environment, but with less compassion toward others.

The increasing trend of physicians leaving the field after a decade or so emphasizes the need for changes in the work environment.

Medical education involves a great deal of desensitization. To work effectively, the physician and nurse must not respond too emotionally to a situation if a high level of functioning is to be preserved. A balance must be kept. The depersonalization and distance are necessary on some occasions, but the ability to shift gears psychically must be maintained.

As "psychic numbing" proceeds, there is more concentration on technical tasks and less concern with the patient and his feelings. There is more intellectualization, and human concerns become expressed in technical jargon. In the early stages of this numbing, tempers are raw and people irritable, but if it is allowed to proceed to a more advanced stage there is increased apathy and acceptance.

The staff members in such units often experience changes in their lives, including less general empathy, poor sleep, more rapid automobile driving, and a feeling of hypervigilance. Although this may permit adequate function with emotional protection, the end results can be decreased morale and dehumanization of the emergency or critical care department, along with behavioral changes in some staff members.

How can improvements be made? How can the environment be engineered to reduce the need for emotional protection? Certain aspects cannot change. People in crisis will continue to respond to their inner turmoil. Death is a reality that will not go away. The ED staff must function and, to some extent, protect itself against excessive emotional response.

EDs, however, can be designed to reduce sensory stimuli. For example, soundproofing and newer types of carpeting can change sound levels significantly. Analysis of staff movement can allow development of a facility in which there is less walking and less confusion. Orderly procedures can help. Telephones need not ring (they can light or can be designed to make modest sounds). Pages are rarely needed. The environment should be "bioengineered" for staff and patient comfort and privacy to the extent possible.

Those responsible for scheduling can do so with awareness of circadian cycles and can attempt to minimize transitions. Special rooms for the staff can be provided offering some "escape" for mealtimes. An important element is to allow expression of feelings and concerns. Staff meetings that offer an opportunity to discuss difficult problems, unexpected deaths, the management of grief, and so forth can reduce the need to block out such emotions. Certainly, limitation of shift duration in busy departments is important.

An actively involved social service department can assist, as can conferences with religious leaders. Conferences with psychiatrists, unless they are actively involved on a daily basis in the department, are rarely necessary. In some instances, they may have negative effects on the staff.

THE PATIENT AND FAMILY—PEOPLE IN CRISIS

When people make an appointment with their physician, they have time to prepare, even if it is a frightening experience. When an acute medical situation arises, however, be it sudden accident or illness, they arrive unprepared at an ED. Faced by sudden forces outside their control, they often have a feeling of helplessness and frustration. Waiting increases the level of tension, as does uncertainty. If death comes, it is unexpected and catastrophic for the family.

The physician's traditional established relationship with the patient and family allows him or her to be a comforting person, but when the physician is someone the family doesn't know, it adds to their uncertainty. This places an additional burden on the emergency physician—the need to establish trust and rapport quickly.

A great source of concern for the family is lack of knowledge about a patient's condition. When a loved one is behind closed doors, with no word from the nurse or physician, people think of the worst situation they can imagine. Similarly, patients upon whom procedures such as blood tests and x rays are being performed become fearful from not knowing.

Medical staff may have a deep personal commitment to the skilled technology of medicine but must also understand its broader humanistic caring function.

The ED staff must communicate to the greatest extent possible with the patient and his family. Simple, easy-to-understand words rather than long, elaborate technical explanations are called for. The patient can be reassured, even if it seems likely that death is imminent. If the patient's condition is deteriorating rapidly, the family should be told at frequent intervals that the staff is doing its best but the situation is grave. This allows time for emotional preparation.

It is important that the physician not delegate this task to others unless he or she cannot spare the few seconds required. If the clinical situation demands constant physician presence, a nurse can inform the family. It is a mistake to send someone with the least medical knowledge to do this.

In the waiting area, families should be provided with comfortable chairs. Simple things like the availability of warm drinks offer some comfort and a feeling of being in a caring environment. Human comfort should be the overriding concern in the design of waiting areas.

Various developments have introduced ombudsmen, neighborhood health workers, and others who provide a conduit for information and who can decrease tension in the waiting areas. These workers should be employed when available, but not as a replacement for the physician's or nurse's involvement with the family. Too frequently, such people are used as messengers when the nurses and physicians find it difficult to meet the families.

The truth is sometimes hard to confront that death is an inevitable part of life and that a patient dying despite the maximum concern and treatment by the physician and other staff does not represent failure. Part of the art of medicine, which must be used frequently in an emergency department, is the knowledge of how to provide comfort to the survivors. They may have great guilt if there was a delay in bringing the patient, or they may regret some small conflict they had with the person now dead and beyond apologies. The physician can do much at this time to reduce needless guilt and to offer support if their world seems to have crashed.

Social workers can provide a good deal of assistance, but they should not supplant the physician and nurse. Religious leaders may be of great help, and suitable telephone numbers should be available so that they may be summoned.

A real danger, however, is the delegation of the caring functions to nonmedical personnel, leaving a cadre of dehumanized technicians. Henry Ford originally began with one man seeing an automobile through all its stages. Then, for efficiency, he developed a highly specialized group of workers—but he knew the dangers and predicted that the development of specialization would lead to technicians concerned with their part, but not the whole.

There is a parallel here with some aspects of medicine; although perhaps not to such an extreme extent, similar tendencies are obvious (e.g., an increased concentration on small specialty areas). In the ED, there is a continual need to look at the whole patient in the context of his or her family or friends. Whether the emergency is minor or major, they come seeking relief. The emergency staff is in a unique and privileged position to offer them relief and, if need be, to refer them into an appropriate system of continuing care. But "care" means just that. No organic disease exists apart from a person in distress. Patients do not consult physicians because certain organs are affected, but because they feel ill.

Because of the variety of demands presently imposed on the emergency physician, we must await future developments that should reduce the number of patients presenting at EDs that will increase the percentage of those with more serious conditions. "Fast-track" systems allow this type of sorting. This allows more time for each patient and permit the flowering of the art of the emergency physician. The specialty recognition of emergency medicine and its popularity with young physicians have resulted in enthusiastic practitioners who want "to be where the energy has already had great impact on improving emergency services.

Perhaps the major emphasis so far has been on the "high-tech" components of the emergency department, as contrasted with the "high-touch" elements. Major changes for "high-touch" will result from continued attention to staff selection and educational programs as well as to allowing appropriate structural changes (e.g., inclusion of facilities for families, for psychiatric interviewing, and for staff communication). Structural changes, however, will remain of substantially less importance than the people (physicians, nurses, technicians, aides, clerks, etc.) who, through their awareness and attention, perform the "high-touch" functions. The emphasis must be on maintaining basic human caring and loving tenderness, which a machine-like environment tends to restrict.

Attention to overall coordination of ideas and places will also become more common with increasing attention to the needs of particular population groups. A growing case in point relates to the suitable management of medical/surgical emergencies affecting the older population (see Geriatric Emergencies in Chapter 60). Because the population group consisting of individuals 65 years of age and older is the most rapidly increasing segment (accounting for almost 25% of the population by 2020), accommodations for such special needs are inevitable. Early attention to such bioengineering can provide a better and more effective environment and also serve as a model and as a catalyst for others.

BIBLIOGRAPHY

Adams, O.S., and Chiles, W.D.: Prolonged human performance as a function of the work-rest cycle. Aerosp. Med. *34*:132, 1963.

Aschoff, J.: Circadian rhythms in man. Science *148*:1247, 1965.

Bartter, F., Delea, C.S., and Halberg, F.: A map of blood and urinary changes related to circadian variations in adrenal cortical functions and normal subjects. Ann. N.Y. Acad. Sci. *98*:969, 1962.

Beranek, L.L.: Noise Reduction. New York, McGraw-Hill Book Co., 1960.

Bernard, V.W., Ottenberg, P., and Redl, F.: Dehumanization: a composite psychological defense in relation to modern war. *In* Schwebel, M. (ed.): Behavioral Science and Human Survival. Palo Alto, Calif., Stanford University Press, 1965.

Brantigan, J.W.: Physician fatigue—some lessons from the cockpit. Hosp. Phys. *9*:13, 1973.

Broadbent, D.C.: Effects of noise on behavior. *In* Harris, C.M. (ed.): Handbook of Noise Control. New York, McGraw-Hill Book Co., 1957, pp. 1–34.

Cooper, G.D., Adams, H.B., and Cohen, L.D.: Personality changes after sensory deprivation. J. Nerv. Ment. Dis. *140*(2):103, 1965.

Corcoran, D.W.J.: Influence of task complexity and practice on performance after loss of sleep. J. Appl. Psychol. *48*:339, 1964.

Czeisler, C.A., Moore-Ede, M.C., and Coleman, R.M.: Rotating shift work schedules that disrupt sleep are improved by applying circadian principles. Science *217*:460, 1982.

Falk, S.A., and Woods, N.F.: Hospital noise levels and potential health hazards. N. Engl. J. Med. *289*:15, 774, 1974.

Gallery, M.E., et al.: A study of occupational stress and depression among emergency physicians. Ann. Emerg. Med. *21*:58, 1992.

Hale, H.B.: Adrenal cortical activity associated with exposure to low frequency sounds. Am. J. Physiol. *171*:732, 1952.

Harrison, T.R.: The most distressing symptoms. JAMA *198*:1, 52, 1966.

Kales, A.: Psychophysiological studies of insomnia. Ann. Intern. Med. *71*:625, 1969.

Kleitman, N.: Sleep and Wakefulness. Chicago, University of Chicago Press, 1965.

LaDou, J.: Health effects of shift work. *In* Occupational disease—new vistas for medicine. West J. Med. *137*:525, 1982.

Levi, L.: Emotional Stress. New York, American Elsevier Publishing Co., 1967.

Lifton, R.J.: Home from the war, the psychology of survival. Atlantic, Nov., 1972, pp. 56–73.

Luby, E.D.: Biochemical, psychological and behavioral responses to sleep deprivation. Ann. N.Y. Acad. Sci. *96*:71, 1962.

Luce, T.S.: Vigilance as a function of stimulus variety and response complexity. Hum. Factors *6*:101, 1964.

Rogers, D.: The doctor himself must become the treatment. Pharos, Oct., 1974, pp. 124–129.

Rusnak, R.A., et al.: Autonomous departments of emergency medicine in contemporary academic medical centers. Ann. Emerg. Med. *20*:680, 1991.

Schwartz, G.R.: Psychological and behavioral responses of hospital staff involved in the care of the critically ill. Crit. Care Med. *2*:1, 48, 1974.

Schwartz, G.R.: Psychic numbing in the emergency department. Emerg. Med. Serv. *4*:1, 31, 1975.

Schwartz, G.R.: Geriatric emergency medicine. *In* Bosker, G., Schwartz, G.R., Jones, J., and Sequeira, M.: Geriatric Emergency Medicine. St. Louis, Mosby Yearbook, 1990, pp. 3–8.

Schwartz, G.R., and Garrison, S.S.: Family dynamics in geriatric crises. Ibid., pp. 574–578.

Selye, H.: Stress and disease. Science *122*:625, 1955.

Verhaegen, P., and Maasen, A.: Health problems in shift workers. *In* Johnson, L.C., Tepas, D.I., Colquhoun, W.P., et al. (eds.): Biological Rhythms, Sleep and Shift Work. New York, SP Medical & Scientific Books, 1981, pp. 271–282.

Von Gierke, H.E.: On noise and vibration exposure critera. Arch. Environ. Health *11*:327, 1965.

Wilkins, W.L.: Group behavior in long-term isolation. *In* Appley, M.H., and Trumbull, R. (eds.): Psychological Stress. New York, Appleton-Century-Crofts, 1966.

Wilkinson, R.J.: The effect of lack of sleep on visual watchkeeping. Q. J. Exp. Psychol. *12*(1):36, 1960.

THE ROLE OF THE EMERGENCY DEPARTMENT DIRECTOR

Stephen J. Dresnick

"Uneasy rests the head that wears the crown."

William Shakespeare, Richard II

CAPSULE

The ideal Emergency Department (ED) director is a composite of different professions. Just as the skilled emergency medicine practitioner is proficient in a wide variety of medical specialties, the skilled ED director must be a superb clinician, a negotiator, an educator, a manager, an innovator, a counselor, and sometimes even an accountant and an architect.

It is hoped that this chapter will not dissuade physicians from aspiring to become ED directors. The job, although demanding, can be among the most satisfying in medicine. A thorough understanding of the responsibilities and the skills needed can enable prospects to understand the position beforehand and allow them the opportunity to be properly prepared for its responsibilities. Clear expectations will surely lead to great expectations.

INTRODUCTION

Hospitals have different types of contractual arrangements with emergency physician groups. These include single-hospital groups, multiple-hospital regional groups, and large multihospital national groups. In evaluating successful EDs throughout the United States, one common denominator can be identified in each regardless of the size of the group: each contract is only as good as the medical director overseeing that contract.

The number one career goal of graduates of emergency medicine residency programs is to become a director of an ED. Recent manpower statistics in emergency medicine indicate that there are fewer than 3000 residency graduates at this time, yet there are more than 5000 acute care hospitals with EDs. When asked why they feel qualified to be a director when they are fresh from residency programs, most graduates respond that the main reason is that they are residency graduates. Although they may certainly be most knowledgeable of the latest advances in medicine, a variety of skills essential to a successful medical director are not often taught during residency. A contract for a single-hospital group represents between 500,000 and 1 million dollars in revenue. Clinical and management skills necessary to run a moderate-sized business are the cornerstone of the necessary attributes for a medical director.

Although the position is sought after and coveted by those who desire to "advance their careers," many physicians find that they are not suited to the position once they have obtained it, and return to the relative peace of patient care. The disillusionment of these physicians occurs partly because the glamor they sought does not exist and partly because they were given the position without the proper tools and training to accomplish the job successfully.

To be successful as a medical director, one must make the distinction between administrative and clinical responsibilities for both the individual and the group, whether it be a single-hospital or a large multihospital group. The administration of an ED requires a great deal of time. Depending on the size of the contract and the complexities of the institution, a medical director may spend anywhere from 25 to 90% of his or her time performing administrative duties. Even small contracts with fewer than 12,000 patient visits annually require dedicated administrative time. It is not possible to perform administrative duties while working clinically. Besides the logistical problems of this, it may lead to potentially dangerous situations in which patient care is disrupted to handle an administrative issue and the physician forgets to order the proper medication or neglects to ask about drug allergies. In this era of attention to providing "service" to patients, particularly when the contract is fee-for-service, patients should not be asked to wait while the ED director goes to a meeting. Protected administrative time is essential to the success of the contract. Out of necessity, a medical director will and should work more weekdays and fewer nights and weekends. Other members of the group must be made to understand the importance of this work to the overall success of the contract.

Some single-hospital groups, in their desire for "total democracy," rotate the position of medical director among members of the group on a yearly or even quarterly basis. This practice, while noble in intent, is generally not a good idea. It is essential that the administration and the other members of the medical staff know at all times that there is a leader of the group, one who is committed over the long haul to making the ED run smoothly. This is not to say that all members of the group should not be involved. On the contrary, all members of the group should be active participants in medical staff affairs. It is reasonable to designate certain administrative duties such as quality assurance, continuing education, and certain committee membership to other members of the group. Such activities on the part of other members of the ED physician staff are necessary also for the overall success of the contract.

DESIRED ATTRIBUTES OF A MEDICAL DIRECTOR

Although everyone has his or her own style, there are some common attributes of successful medical directors. Some say that great medical directors are born, but careful analysis reveals that the most important reason for success is proper training.

CLINICAL EXPERTISE

First and foremost, a medical director must have excellent credentials in both training and experience. The medical director must set the standard for the care given in the department. Additionally, if the director is not practicing state-of-the-art medicine, who will field the complaints when the medical director is involved? This is not to say that anyone cannot and will not make mistakes; rather, the medical director must be able to address clinical issues that will arise from time to time in the ED. These issues include patient complaints and concerns raised by other members of the medical staff. Additionally, the medical director will have to oversee a quality assurance program for the department. Recruitment of new physicians is must easier if the director's clinical expertise is respected by the other members of the group.

COMMUNICATIONS SKILLS

Although good communications skills may be difficult to teach, they are essential to a successful medical director. The key to effective communication is to be a good listener. All too often, medical directors do not take the time to listen to feedback from patients, administration, and other members of the medical staff. New medical directors, particularly those fresh from residency, occasionally lack this skill, and are sometimes too eager to implement change without first getting all of the parties to "buy into" the process. As Machiavelli said, "Nothing disrupts the lives of men more than change." A medical director must have the maturity to know when to push an issue and when to leave it for another day. Perhaps the most important aspect of good communication is the need for the medical director to interact with the medical staff. This requires more than attendance on committees. It requires a sincere effort to meet all of the members of the medical staff and to make periodic visits to their offices. A medical director should make it a point to have as many meals as possible in the doctor's dining room to establish this camaraderie with the medical staff. Attendance at social events also helps to strengthen the bond between the medical director and the staff.

PLANNING AND IMPLEMENTATION SKILLS

Planning is more than coming up with an idea today and carrying it out tomorrow. Today's EDs have multimillion dollar budgets. As more hospitals realize the revenue potential of the ED, they will ask the medical director to develop new programs such as fast tracking and occupational medicine programs to enhance patient volume and revenue. A working knowledge of the hospital budgeting process and cost allocation is vital to the planning process. The hospital will look to the medical director for the implementation of these programs, and he or she must develop a vast knowledge of these programs because hospitals usually do not have in-house expertise.

MANAGEMENT EXPERTISE

This skill is usually the most ignored when considering an individual for the position for medical director, perhaps because in the past there have been so few individuals with significant experience. For success in today's environment, this attribute is essential. The medical director must have the management skills to manage a department with revenues often exceeding a million dollars. Additionally, a typical ED has 20 to 30 staff members, including clerks, nurses, and physicians. Unifying and motivating this many people toward a common goal can be difficult.

KNOWLEDGE OF ADMINISTRATIVE ISSUES

The medical director must become knowledgeable of a variety of ED administrative issues. These include state and federal regulations such as medical screening and transfer provisions required by the COBRA law. Issues constantly present themselves that require indepth understanding of the issues involved to resolve. Reimbursement, order writing, and preauthorization are but a few examples.

CAREER COMMITMENT

Perhaps the single most important attribute is career commitment. As discussed, there simply are not many qualified medical directors with experience. It is essential that the medical director be committed not only to the practice of emergency medicine but also to the hospital and the position. Nothing jeopardizes a contract more than a medical director who takes his or her responsibilities casually and for whom this is only a part-time position.

RESPONSIBILITIES OF THE MEDICAL DIRECTOR

The list of responsibilities of a medical director is virtually endless because he or she is responsible for virtually every aspect of the activities of the department. Some of the responsibilities outlined may need to be delegated to other members of the group. To avoid confusion, it is always prudent to delineate the specific responsibilities of the medical director in a job description (Table 88-1).

CLINICAL DIRECTION

The director is responsible for setting the clinical standards that will be practiced in the department. Clinical

Emergency Department Management

TABLE 88-1. MEDICAL DIRECTOR JOB DESCRIPTION

The medical director's responsibilities are the following:
1. Act as a liaison between the group and the hospital administration
2. Act as a liaison between the Emergency Department staff and the hospital medical staff.
3. Attend all Emergency Department-related committee meetings
4. Represent the department to the community
5. Coordinate disaster planning for the hospital and department
6. Prepare the department for JCAHO and state accreditation surveys
7. Review and implement medical and nursing protocols for the department.
8. Coordinate the department medical quality assurance program
9. Monitor the quality of care in the department
10. Coordinate or assist in recruiting of new physicians
11. Orient new Emergency Department physicians
12. Coordinate physician schedules
13. Ensure continual physician coverage of the department
14. Ensure back-up and on-call scheduling of medical staff
15. Evaluate the performance of physician staff

policies must be established so that all members of the group approach problems in the same manner. Physician staffing patterns must be developed, and may include double coverage or an on-call system to handle peak times. Continuing education is essential in the modern ED. Much of the on-site teaching comes from issues that arise from the quality assurance program. Although the medical director may not teach all of these sessions, he or she must oversee the content. ACLS continues to be sought not only by the ED staff but by members of the medical staff and nursing staff as well. It is important that the emergency physician group be the leaders of this educational effort.

EMERGENCY DEPARTMENT PERSONNEL

The relationship between the medical director and the nonphysician staff of the ED is complex at best. No other area of the hospital has nurses and physicians working so closely together for such extended hours. The medical director should have significant input into the staffing of the ED, including numbers, length of shifts, and specific individuals. Although this relationship may not exist at many institutions, it certainly does at the most successful ones. The ED is equivalent to other physicians' offices in that the staff is a representative and an extension of the physician staff. It is important that they convey the same caring attitude that the physician staff does. The medical director should work closely with nursing administration in ensuring that nursing policy and procedures are well delineated and adhered to because the nursing staff does, in fact, work under the direction of the physician staff. This is particularly true with the implementation

of triage and discharge criteria. The medical director should also have significant input into nursing continuing education.

INTERDEPARTMENTAL RELATIONS

The ED is the proverbial fishbowl, and incidents in the department are known throughout the entire hospital in a matter of minutes. Because virtually every department cares for patients who may be in or even pass through the ED, most physicians feel that their perspective is the one through which the department should be viewed. The director must listen to all of these viewpoints and attempt to reach a consensus on a variety of issues. This is particularly true with medical staff departments because at one time or another, all of the medical staff feels that they were "emergency physicians." In addition to listening, the medical director must attempt to coordinate the activities of each department to the benefit of the ED. This includes on-call schedules for the medical staff and working with the laboratory and radiology departments to ensure priority handling of ED patients.

PUBLIC RELATIONS

The medical director is the "point man" for various public relations issues. As more hospitals become market-oriented with their EDs, community outreach programs become more common. The director is called upon to address community groups and even large employers in an attempt to establish a relationship of these groups with the hospital. Another area of public relations is in the handling of patient complaints. This is extremely important because it not only makes patients happier about their experience but also helps to mitigate potential medicolegal problems that may arise from an unpleasant experience in the ED. Another major target group with whom the medical director will need to interface with are the members of the EMS community. Although many locals have protocols that dictate to which hospitals patients will be taken, it is clear that "borderline" patients are usually taken to hospitals with whom there is a good relationship. This relationship requires more than simply providing free meals to the paramedics. Today's paramedics wish to be treated with respect, look for constructive feedback when they bring patients into the department, and have a sincere desire to expand their knowledge. A good medical director can coordinate a program to address their needs.

EMERGENCY DEPARTMENT OPERATION

A director must become familiar with all aspects of ED operation. This includes budget development, staffing formulas, space requirements, department design, and a working knowledge of potential new services such as fast tracking and occupational medicine programs. Although the director may not be administratively responsible for all of these, it is always in the best interest of the physician group to participate in all aspects of the department's operations. Although the details of the various aspects of ED operation are beyond the scope of this chapter, the reader may wish to take advantage of the various educational materials available that specifically address this topic.

QUALITY ASSURANCE

No area is more important in today's environment for a medical director than quality assurance (QA). The Joint Commission for the Accreditation of Healthcare Organizations has made quality assurance their number one priority for the coming years. It is essential that each ED have in place a quality assurance program that monitors the care given by each physician on a process as well as outcome basis. Clinical standards or parameters are currently being developed by the American College of Emergency Physicians and these, once completed, will have to be included into the quality assurance program. Quality assurance has as a benefit the ability to identify areas that may require additional education for the physicians or nursing staff. A successful QA program has a significant effect on the potential liability of the physician group and may even help reduce liability insurance costs.

EDUCATION

The medical director should oversee an ongoing educational program for the ED physician and nursing staff. Specific topics may be identified by a QA program or by specific patients who present to the department. Regular programs should also be implemented for other members of the hospital staff to make them aware of issues that confront the ED. Although ACLS and ATLS may not be requirements for the ED physician staff, particularly for those trained in and board-certified in emergency medicine, they continue to be excellent programs, and the ED should take the lead in teaching other members of the hospital staff.

GROUP MANAGEMENT

The medical director is essentially managing a multiphysician practice. A variety of issues will confront the medical director regardless of the size of the group. The director must become familiar with reimbursement guidelines and billing procedures. Even if the group is on an hourly rate, improvement in physician billing is vital in future contract negotiations. If the physicians code their own charts, the medical director must audit this process to ensure that all physicians comply with various third-party regulations and are not exposed to liability for fraud and abuse.

The medical director of a single hospital group must also manage the financial affairs of the group, making sure that payroll is prepared in a timely manner, that all payroll taxes are deducted and deposited, and that all bills are paid on time. The director must also develop a budget for the group and prepare the necessary financial reports for the other members of the group.

Perhaps the most troubling issue confronting medical directors is the issue of liability insurance. Many products are offered from a wide variety of companies. Choosing an incorrect product has both short-term and long-term implications for members of the group. The medical director should be well versed in this area to guide the other members of the group through what may sometimes be a difficult decision. Even directors of departments managed by large multihospital groups will need the input of the medical director in the areas of risk management and claims evaluation. An understanding of the tort system will enable the director to provide the appropriate counseling to other members of the group during what is a trying experience for physicians as well as their families.

Medical directors should be involved in the development and negotiation of the contract. It is frequently beneficial to the group for the director to identify issues that should be included in the contract language. The director of a single hospital group has the additional burden of developing specific language and actually negotiating the contract. This process requires that a medical director possess all the skills discussed here and to have a detailed understanding of the contracting process. Many groups are made and lost in the outcome of contract negotiations. Skill in this area is vital to the successful renewal of the contract.

BIBLIOGRAPHY

Couch, J.B. (ed.): Health Care Quality Management for the Twenty-First Century. Tampa, American College of Physician Executives, 1991.

Frew, S.A.: Patient Transfers: How to Comply with the Law. Dallas, American College of Emergency Physicians, 1991.

Goldfield, N., and Nash, D.: Physician Leaders: Past and Future Challenges. Tampa, American College of Physician Executives, 1989.

Janiak, B.D.: Role of the physician director. In The Hospital Emergency Department: Returning to Financial Viability. Edited by Matson, T.A. Chicago, American Hospital Publishing, 1986.

Mayer, T.A.: The emergency department medical director. Emerg. Med. Clin. North Am. 5:29, 1987.

Mayer, T.A.: Roles and responsibilities of the emergency department medical director. In Hospital Emergency Department: Returning to Financial Viability. Edited by Matson, T.A. Chicago, American Hospital Publishing, 1991.

Shore, M.F., and Levison, H.: On business and medicine. N. Engl. J. Med. 313:19–21, 1985.

EMERGENCY DEPARTMENT STAFFING

Thom A. Mayer

CAPSULE

Adequate staffing of the emergency department (ED) is perhaps as important as any issue in ED management. Unless the appropriate types and number of staff are available, no ED can provide adequate care to its patients. Furthermore, most EDs are seeing increased patient volume, changes in payor mix, increased levels of acuity, increasing numbers of patients with poor access to primary care, and a number of other issues that make management of the ED exponentially more complicated. In the face of these problems, it is important that management staff ensure that the appropriate staffing levels are present, including physicians, nurses, ED technicians, and other ancillary staff. Further, because ED patient volume fluctuates during different hours of the day, as well as during different days of the week and months of the year, staffing levels usually must be provided on a flexible basis to match resources with patient needs.

For all of these reasons, appropriate staffing levels for ED personnel have assumed an increasing level of importance in virtually every ED across the country. In many cases, however, the decisions made to set various staffing levels have been based more on tradition than any identifiable, clear-cut reasoning. Because emergency medicine is changing so rapidly, in both clinical and management aspects, virtually all EDs should focus more attention on the specific reasons for staffing at chosen levels.

DEFINING THE PRODUCT OF THE EMERGENCY DEPARTMENT

Before addressing questions of adequate staffing for the ED, it is extremely important to define the department's product. This involves a number of different factors, including clinical aspects, business aspects, quality assurance, patient flow considerations, marketing and public relations, and risk management concerns. Although all of these factors are important, the clinical aspects of care are by far the most central component in assessing what the product of the ED should be. Too often, it is assumed that it should be simply to see the patients and move them through as quickly as possible.

Even the smallest of EDs, however, must assess what they are attempting to offer in the form of service to the community and to the patients whose care is entrusted to them. Rather than simply "making do" with available resources, each ED management team should carefully assess the product they are attempting to deliver, including all of these factors.

It would be idealistic to think that each ED across the country offered the same product in regard to clinical care. In fact, even in a given geographic area, different EDs may have different levels of expertise. In addition, some EDs may develop specialized areas of care, such as pediatric emergency medicine, trauma center specialization, specialized cardiac care, fast track components, occupational medicine programs, etc.

To define the ED's product, two factors are essential. First, a systems management approach must be taken that assumes that emergency care constitutes both a professional and clinical service that is a recognizable product to the patient, medical staff, hospital, and community. It is essential to plan effectively to manage both the clinical encounter itself and the myriad factors influencing it. Second, the definition of quality within medicine is changing rapidly. Concepts of continuous quality improvement programs have swept American business and industry over the past decade. These precepts are also being adopted by American medicine. In attempting to define the product of the ED, one must recognize that the quality of care delivered is an ongoing, continuous process of improvement that requires reassessment of the types, numbers, and training of personnel that will be used. Finally, to effectively define the product that the emergency department will deliver, it is necessary to assess the current status of the department.

ASSESSMENT OF CURRENT STATUS: THE SELF-AUDIT

The process of performing a self-audit is almost always taken initially as critical, and therefore pejorative in nature. Before entering into a self-audit, it is wise to consider this potentially critical nature of the self-audit process and attempt to diffuse any such concerns among the staff. In fact, the process of looking into the self-audit can be done in a management fashion that allows the staff to participate actively in redefining the direction that the ED will take into the future. Framed in such a context, the self-audit is almost always well accepted by the ED staff.

Specific factors that should be considered in the self-audit include patient factors, ED facility and staff factors, medical staff factors, and environmental factors (Table 88-2).

Clearly, one of the most important factors facing EDs in regard to their overall staffing has to do with the type and number of patients seen on a yearly basis (Table 88-3). Thus, an accurate assessment of the overall quantity of patients seen in the ED on a yearly basis should be compiled, and compared to trends over the past 5 years. In addition to looking at yearly patient volume, it is also important to look at the patient flow factors, including the time of day and the days of the week in which patient volume is heaviest. In addition, in communities in which there is a seasonal variation of patient flow, this should also be taken into account. Whenever possible, the age of patients should also be determined because pediatric and geriatric cases have different needs and require different levels of intensity.

It is also important to know the overall number of patients admitted to the hospital, as well as the percentage of total hospital admissions that this represents on a yearly basis. The higher the number of patients admitted to the hospital, the greater the staffing needs in regard to attending to these patients.

In addition, it is important to know as much information as possible about the diagnostic categories of these patients. In general, statistics should include medical, surgical, trauma, pediatric, obstetric-gynecologic, and psychiatric cases. Additional details about diagnostic categories, however, can also be helpful.

To the best extent possible, it is important to document the severity and/or acuity of such patients. Although several potential coding systems have been used to classify severity or acuity, the general trends of numbers of patients admitted to the hospital and those admitted to the intensive care unit or operating room are a good place to start. In some classification systems, it is also possible to classify coexisting disease factors because these comorbid factors can be extremely important.[1,2]

Thus, patient factors that must be looked out in the ED department include the quantity of patients (including both number and flow patterns), diagnostic categories, and assessments of severity and acuity.

Factors related to the ED are extremely important, and none is more important than the overall facility size and configuration (Table 88-4). The overall size of the facility can be assessed by looking at the number and types of ED treatment areas present. In looking at facility size and configuration, the location and proximity of support space are also important factors. In some cases, it is possible to do a square footage analysis of the ED, but these numbers are often difficult to obtain because many hospital architects are not as concerned about absolute square footage as they are with available treatment areas.

The equipment available in the ED is also an extremely important factor, particularly as it relates to the care of the critically ill or injured patient. Well-equipped EDs have a much better chance of effectively and rapidly caring for patients than those in whom supplies and equipment need to be sent for.

One of the most important factors in the overall ED is the level of commitment of administrative services to the department. To begin with, the extent to which the hospital administration realizes that the ED is the "front door of the hospital" instead of the back door is extremely important. This should be reflected in the overall hospital organizational chart, as well as the specific administrative support to the ED. In addition, an assessment must be made of the level of administrative commitment elements such as chart dictation, 24-hour transcription services, registration of patients, record keeping, and categorization of the ED within the overall community scheme.

ED staffing factors should include physicians,

TABLE 88-2. ED SELF-AUDIT FACTORS

Patients
Emergency department
Emergency department staff
Medical staff
Environment

TABLE 88-3. ED PATIENT FACTORS

Quantity (number and flow)
Diagnostic categories
Severity/Acuity
Illness
Injury
Co-existing diseases

TABLE 88-4. ED FACILITY FACTORS

Facility size
   Number of treatment areas
   Type of treatment areas
   Floor layout
   Square footage
Equipment
Administrative Support
   Dictation
   Transcription
   Registration
   Categorization

nurses, clerks, technicians, physicians' assistants, nurse-practitioners, and patient representatives (Table 88-5). In addition to the number of personnel in each of these categories, the level of training and expertise must also be assessed. Are the emergency physicians board-certified and/or residency-trained in emergency medicine, with appropriate skills in the rapid evaluation and resuscitation of critically ill and injured patients? How many years of experience do they have in a similar ED setting?

Other questions must be asked about nurses, aides, and technicians. Are the nurses certified in emergency nursing, and what is their level of experience in dealing with emergency department patients? How long have the nurses been working in the ED? What is the level of commitment of nursing administration toward certification and in-service training for nurses? What are the specific skills and training of the emergency department aides and/or technicians? Are they integrated into the ED team or do they simply function as "gofers"?

These and many other questions must be asked about the existing situation within the ED, to ensure that an accurate appraisal may be given.

Medical staff factors have a tremendous influence on effective treatment of patients in the ED. (Table 88-6). The specific types and numbers of physicians

TABLE 88-5. ED STAFF FACTORS

Numbers and types
  Physicians
  Certified emergency nurses
  Registered nurses
  Clerks/registration
  Technicians
  Physician's assistants
  Nurse practitioners
  Patient representatives

Quality
  Training
  Experience
  Continuity

Shift length
Shift frequency
Defined responsibilities

TABLE 88-6. MEDICAL STAFF FACTORS

ED call list (depth and completeness)
Frequency
  On-call
  ED Consults/admissions
Expertise/training
Patient mix
Administrative/board support for ED

TABLE 88-7. ENVIRONMENTAL FACTORS

Georgraphic
  Urban
  Rural
  Suburban

Demographic
Competing services
Emergency medical services
Support services
  Laboratory
  Radiology
  Social services
  Others

on call in each specialty must be evaluated. It is also important to assess the frequency with which these specialists are consulted by the emergency physicians. Unfortunately, the effect of the payor mix in the ED also influences the responsiveness of the medical staff, at least in some cases. Finally, the level of support for the ED in the hierarchy of the medical staff must be assessed. In most EDs, emergency medicine should be represented on the Executive Committee as a voting member with full departmental status. Whether or not an emergency services committee of the medical staff exists, there must be strong interaction between the emergency physician group and the attending medical staff on a regular basis.

The final factors that must be assessed are environmental factors (Table 88-7). This should include both geographic and demographic factors and the number of competing services in the area. These competing services should include both existing EDs, ambulatory care centers, extended hour clinics, managed care clinics, etc.

One of the most important environmental factors to assess is the level of support services for the ED, including laboratory, radiology, and social services. To ensure that the department is able to function efficiently, there must be an extremely high level of commitment from both radiology and pathology departments to ensure that the internal services needs of the department are met rapidly and professionally.

Only after these factors have been assessed and the interrelation has been analyzed is it possible to truly define the product of the ED accurately. In most cases, it is appropriate to compile an ED business plan involving representatives from the emergency physician group, nursing staff, additional support staff, administration, and medical staff to ensure that there is significant "buy-in" from each of these groups. Only through such a thoughtful and detailed assessment can one address questions regarding the adequate staffing of an ED because we can make recommendations regarding staffing only when we know the purpose of the ED in the first place.

OPTIMAL ED STAFFING

As indicated, the type and number of staff needed for any given ED depend largely on what the department identifies as its business plan. For example, staff selection and training are different in a Level I trauma center seeing 80,000 patients per year than in a rural ED seeing 12,000 patients per year. The vast majority of EDs in this country, however, are in community settings in which the patient volume varies from approximately 20,000 to 35,000 visits per year. In interpreting the following information on optimal emergency department staffing, it should be kept in mind that these are the benchmark assumptions on which the staffing ratios are based.

In addition, it is extremely important to realize in interpreting the following information on staffing that the interrelationship among emergency physicians, emergency nurses, and emergency technicians and other support staff is critical to determining appropriate staffing. In each ED, the specific tasks and duties of each person should be examined closely. For example, in some EDs, technicians are little more than transporters who basically move patients to and from x ray or up to the floors or ICUs for admission. In others, technicians have evolved to a sophisticated level of staffing, capable of providing ECGs, drawing blood, and doing other procedures (see subsequent text). In cases in which advanced technician staffing is used, the nurses and physicians are available to perform other functions, and this can considerably change the staffing pattern for the ED.

In general, most progressive EDs have evolved to the point where a *team approach* is used, wherein the emergency physician, nurse, and technician work closely together in providing the best possible care to the patient. This entails both a high level of training among the three groups and a significant amount of trust to ensure that each is performing his duties appropriately. To ensure that the following data are interpreted correctly, it is important during the self-audit phase that the job descriptions and patient flow patterns in the emergency department be kept in mind.

ED NURSING STAFF

Most emergency physicians agree that the nursing staff is the most critical aspect of a successful ED. Although a great deal of data exist in the literature regarding nursing staffing patterns,[3–6] most of it is not specific to the ED. Unfortunately, there is no clearly set formula that allows universal application for successful ED nursing staffing. In general, ED nursing staffing should be correlated closely with flow data, acuity data, and length of patient stay in the ED. In most EDs, the heaviest flow of patients through the department occurs in the afternoon and evening hours, which speaks to the need for flexible nursing staffing to answer these needs. In departments in which patients have a high level of acuity and multiple invasive procedures are being performed, both more and better trained nurses are needed than in less labor-intensive EDs. In addition, the ED layout and design have a significant effect on nursing staffing patterns. In EDs that do not have a central design core, nurses frequently spend a significant amount of time walking back and forth between the nursing station and patient rooms, and those departments usually require a higher level of staffing to meet patient needs.

One of the most interesting aspects of determining optimal nursing staffing is related to specific duties of the nurses and the ancillary personnel with which they work. In the past, nurses have been asked to perform functions that did not reflect their highly trained and professional status. This is not to say that the duties that were required were in any way "beneath their dignity," but simply that the modern practice of emergency medicine has come to realize that cost efficiency in the ED setting requires broader use of technicians and ancillary support personnel. In this regard, the ratio of nurses to ED technicians is an important concept. In the past, it was not uncommon for the number of full time equivalents (FTEs) in nursing versus technician positions to be as high as 80% to 90%. With increased training of ED technicians to do additional functions, however, in some cases these ratios have dropped to 60 to 70%. Thus, one of the earliest steps in determining optimal ED staffing is to look at the job descriptions of the ED nurses and their interrelation with the physicians and the nonprofessional personnel in the department.

Two general types of evaluations can be done to determine appropriate ED staffing, whether it be among nurses, ED technicians, or physicians. *Prototype evaluations* generally look at aspects such as final diagnosis from the ED, ICDM-9 codes, or CPT codes to compare staffing to the overall acuity in the ED.[7,8] These are then compared to various potential staffing ratios or FTE factors, with resulting guidelines for nursing staffing.

A far more accurate, although more time consuming, approach is *factor evaluation*. Factor evaluation most commonly uses management engineering information that is developed by simply observing the personnel in the ED and using a stop watch to determine exactly how much time is spent during the course of the work day for given personnel. These data are then compiled and compared to the numbers of patients seen in the ED as generated by flow data and acuity statistics. This allows a much more precise determination of the numbers of staff needed to meet the ED's needs. An alternate way of using factor evaluation relies on various types of computer-based emergency department nursing monitors. Programs such as the Medicus system allow for determination of ongoing efficiency in ED nursing staffing.[9]

Once the actual amount of time is figured under a factor evaluation, it is also important to factor in conference time, CME time, sick leave, fatigue, vacations, etc. In general, different management engineering functions have figured in an 18 to 26% "lag" factor. This generally results in a calculation indicating a factor that accounts for this: an FTE accounts for 1.1 to 1.6 positions, depending on the system used by each individual hospital. The financial and/or personnel offices of the hospital should be able to provide the specific number used at their institution.

Another concept that needs to be kept in mind is the development of flexible staffing patterns in the ED, including 12-hour shifts and "float" shifts that allow for matching patient volume needs to ED nurse staffing needs. Because of the wide variation in ED flow patterns, these are best determined on an individual basis, but few EDs that have used these flexible shift patterns have reverted to more traditional staffing patterns, simply because the flexible staffing has been such a positive influence on both patient care and nursing staff satisfaction.

Regardless of whether a factor or prototype evaluation is used to determine staffing needs, it is important to recognize that nursing staffing must be constantly re-evaluated to ensure that the best patient care needs are being addressed. Because virtually all EDs are in varying stages of evolution, this commitment to ongoing evaluation of the nursing staff works to the benefit of the patient, as well as the professional staffing in the department.

ED TECHNICIAN STAFF

As indicated previously, there is a wide variation in the skills required of technicians in varying EDs. In the past, ED technicians were often considered as traditional "orderlies," who sometimes did little more than make crutches, take patients to the floors, and empty bedpans. Most EDs, however, have begun to view technicians as a critical factor in staffing, and have upgraded the skills significantly. Table 88-8 lists varying forms of ED technician skills used in different facilities.

In most cases, EDs are well served if the technicians are capable of at least performing electrocardiograms, assisting with suturing, placing various forms of orthopedic splints, inserting indwelling bladder catheters, assisting with triage, and checking vital signs. A significant amount of initial and ongoing in-service training is necessary to allow technicians to perform these functions, but such training usually makes them highly motivated and well qualified members of the ED team.

The decision to specify the techniques and procedures of which the ED technician is capable must be made carefully and with significant input from the nursing staff because the physicians, nurses, and ED technicians work closely together during the course of provision of care. Although most technicians do not have significant professional training, they do function as an integral part of the team.

It is also important to assure that the quality improvement program also addresses the aspects that are performed by the ED technicians. As experience with the ED technician program increases, many EDs have found that the ratio of RN to technician staffing changes so that the ratio approaches 60 to 70% RNs and 30 to 40% technicians. The precise mix in each ED will have to be decided on the basis of local factors as well as experience in training and maintaining ED technician staff. Given the cost-efficiency required of any ED, however, most EDs find that the use of ED technicians is essential to their success in the 1990s.

ED PHYSICIAN STAFF

One of the most difficult questions to answer in emergency medicine is, "How much physician coverage do we need in our emergency department?" The answer to this question is complex, and depends on many factors, including the qualifications of the emergency physicians, the patient flow, the philosophic attitude towards treatment of patients in the ED, the acuity of the patients, and the financial structure on which the ED physician group is based.

In most EDs, the emergency physician staff should strive for a level of board certification in emergency medicine or residency training in emergency medicine. Regardless of the initial type of training that a physician has, attaining board certification in emergency medicine is something to which all physicians

TABLE 88-8. ED TECHNICIAN SKILL LEVELS

Minimal Level	Intermediate	Advanced Level
Vital signs	Minimal Plus:	Intermediate Plus:
Sterile technique	Foley insertion	Nasotracheal suction
Holding patients	ECGs	Blood drawing
Transporting	Suturing assistance	Arterial blood gases
Crutches	Splint application	Injection wounds
	Assisting with triage	Nasogastric tubes

should aspire, regardless of the practice environment. Most physician groups have found that this level of training is important to ensure quality of care in the ED setting. More importantly, it is essential to ensure that the emergency physician group is committed to the practice of emergency medicine in general, as well as to the hospital in which they are working in particular. In extremely busy EDs with high acuity patients, both residency training in emergency medicine and significant experience may be required to meet the patient flow needs of the department. In general, the ability to see patients rapidly and efficiently tends to increase during the first several years of practice for any physician.

In some rural and suburban settings, the ED patient volume may not be able to support the concept of recruiting board-certified or residency-trained physicians, particularly because of the relative shortage of these types of physicians. In such cases, the emergency physician group, in conjunction with the medical staff and the governing body of the hospital, will have to make decisions regarding the qualifications required of the emergency physicians, as well as the additional experience in emergency medicine required to serve the hospital.

Regardless of the level of training of the emergency physicians, it is also important to consider the philosophic approach to the patients in the ED. In some cases, EDs have focused so heavily on patient flow through the department that a "treat'em and street'em" approach results, in which patients may not have their significant interpersonal and psychosocial needs met in the ED setting. In most EDs, the physician and nonphysician leadership should address the balance between the legitimate concerns raised by ED overcrowding versus the public relations-oriented approach that is optimal from the patient's standpoint.

The financial structure of the emergency department group can also have an effect on emergency physician staffing. In hourly-rate or flat-fee types of contracts, emergency physicians may not believe that it is to their benefit to move patients as efficiently through the ED because they are paid the same regardless of whether they see a large or small number of patients during the shift. On the other hand, independent billing contracts or other systems in which the emergency physicians have a financial or ownership incentive to manage the practice more efficiently usually result in better patient flow through the ED.

Unquestionably, the most significant factor regarding emergency physician staffing is related to the level of commitment on the part of the hospital, the nursing staff, the medical staff, and the emergency physician staff to support ED operations. In departments with 24-hour chart dictation, advanced triage, certified emergency nurses, well-trained technicians, preprinted discharge instructions, etc., the emergency physician staff can see patients in a much more time-and cost-efficient fashion than in departments in which these factors are not present. In most cases, the physician staffing is the most expensive resource in the ED, and it is usually a cost-effective move to ensure that the best administrative systems possible are available to support the ED physician staff.

With all of these thoughts in mind, it is clear that it is difficult to establish concrete, preset ratios between emergency department patient volume and physician staffing because there can be such a wide variation, even within a given geographic area, among ED support structures, as well as the other myriad factors previously mentioned that affect physician staffing. Based on the author's experience in over 400 hospitals of varying degrees of sophistication and administrative backup, however, the following information may be useful.

In general, emergency physicians who are board-certified or residency-trained in emergency medicine, with 3 to 5 years of emergency department experience, can effectively evaluate and treat between 2.5 and 3.1 patients per hour. It should be noted that this is a yearly average, and the individual flow rates vary highly. For example, on the night shift volume often decreases, and physicians may see only 0.5 to 1.5 patients per hour. During busier afternoon shifts, however, the rate may be as high as 3.0 to 4.2 patients per hour. In general, however, the patient flow status will even out to the 2.5 to 3.1 patient per hour range.[10]

Because there are 8760 hours per year, this is the baseline level of physician coverage that should be offered in an ED. For example, an ED with 15,000 annual visits sees fewer than 2.5 patients per hour, but 24-hour coverage is essential to the operation of the department itself (15,000 patients divided by 8760 hours in a year equals 1.7 patients per hour).

The primary question is when emergency physician coverage needs to be increased to allow patient flow. Based on the 2.5 to 3.1 ratio indicated, this may be necessary between approximately 22,000 and 27,000 visits per year (Fig. 88-4). Again, these are general ratios and individual physicians may have put significant administrative support in place and staffed their department with experienced physicians, so that in some cases the 3.1 patients per hour can be exceeded.

Additional ways of ensuring that coverage is available include the use of physician extenders (physician assistants and nurse practitioners) and the use of on-call ED physician coverage. The use of the physician assistants in the ED has been well described and can work extremely well in expediting patient flow.[11,12] In addition, nurse practitioners have also been used in this setting, although most are in situations in which there is a more independent practice than the ED setting allows. This is simply because all patients seen in the ED by residents, nurse practitioners, or physician assistants should also be seen by the attending ED physician. Physician assistants and nurse practitioners, however, have all been used suc-

36,000 Annual ED Visits
× 90% (Percent Seen by EPs)
32,400 Patients Seen by EPs

Divided by 2.5 Patients/Hours EP Coverage

12,960 Hours ED Coverage/Year/365 Days/Yr = 35 Hours/Day

Divided by 3.1 Patients/Hours EP Coverage

10,450 Hours EP Coverage/Year/365 Days/Yr = 28 Hours/Day

Thus, additional coverage will be needed for between 4 and 11 hours per day, depending on patient flow patterns.

Thus, between 4 and 11 hours of additional coverage are likely to be needed.

FIG. 88-4. Calculating ED physician coverage needs. Several ranges for ED coverage can be obtained by taking the annual ED volume times the percentage seen by emergency physicians (EPs). Because EPs can generally see between 2.5 and 3.1 patients per hour as an annual average, the total patients seen by EP's is divided by 2.5 patients per hour and 3.1 patients per hour to obtain a range of total coverage needed. Dividing these numbers by 365 days per year gives the general range of coverage needed.

cessfully in the ED and may increase patient flow. In general, the use of residents does not significantly increase flow through the department assuming that a legitimate educational function is being addressed. Regardless of what form of additional physician extender coverage is used, it should be examined during the quality improvement process to ensure that the needs of the department and the patient are being met.

The American College of Emergency Physicians has completed staffing study information that tends to support the above-mentioned ratios, but the study clearly recognizes the wide variation in staffing patterns inherent in EDs with varying levels of administrative support.[13]

GUIDELINES FOR ED SPACE

ED space needs can generally be calculated by using the available number of treatment beds or square footage ratios. Unfortunately, the calculation of square footage within an ED is fraught with difficulties. First, some departments use *gross* square footage, which includes hallways, storage areas, waiting rooms, support areas, etc., and others use *net* square footage, which implies that the treatment rooms alone are calculated. In addition, in many hospitals it is extremely difficult to find either gross or net square footage ratios. Although figures such as 275 to 325 net square feet per 1000 annual ED visits have been used, these ratios are generally extremely difficult to apply.[14]

It is usually better to analyze the number of treatment beds within an ED and use this to calculate maximal patient volume. With this methodology, the total number of ED treatment areas (excluding the use of stretchers and hallways, wheelchairs and hallways, etc.) is determined. In most cases, the major trauma and/or cardiac room and the ENT room are excluded from this count because these are not multipurpose beds that can be used to all types of patients in most emergency departments. The total remaining beds are the effective ED treatment areas available on a 24-hour-per-day basis. In most cases, no more than 1800 to 2000 patients per year can be seen in any one of these treatment rooms, so that multiplying the total number of remaining beds times the 1800-to-2000-visit figure

A   **36,000 ANNUAL ED VISITS**

Divided by 1900   Divided by 2000
20   18

Plus: 1 CPR/Trauma Room
1 ENT Room

22 Rooms   20 Rooms

B   **12 EXISTING ED ROOMS (EXCLUDES CPR/TRAUMA AND ENT)**

Times 1800 Patients/Room   Times 2000 Patients/Room
21,600 Patients/Year   24,000 Patients/Year

FIG. 88-5. Calculation of ED treatment room needs **A.** An ED has 36,000 annual ED visits. How many beds will be needed in the ED? Because ED rooms can generally accommodate no more than 1800 to 2000 patient visits per year (as an annual average) and because the cardiopulmonary resuscitation-trauma (CPR/Trauma) and ENT rooms are usually not multipurpose, 20 to 22 rooms are needed. **B.** Conversely, how many ED visits can an ED with 12 treatment rooms accommodate? Multiplying the number of rooms times 1800 and 2000 gives a general range of the visits that can be seen. Exceeding these ratios usually results in long waits and problems with quality of care and risk management.

equals the maximum amounts of visits per year (Fig. 88-5). In rare circumstances, the 2000-visit-per-year number can be exceeded, but only in departments that have a significant amount of support structure, including 24-hour chart dictation, use of physician extenders, maximal use of ED laboratory and x-ray facilities, preprinted discharge instructions, etc. In most other cases, exceeding 2,000 per year for each treatment area results in poor clinical care, long delays, inability to examine the patient fully, stretchers and wheelchairs in the hallway, public relations problems, and signficant quality assurance and risk management problems.

SUMMARY

The selection of the type, qualifications, and number of staff that will be used in an ED is essential to the success of the ED in the 1990s. These areas are undergoing significant changes as we learn to manage emergency department personnel in a more timely and cost-efficient fashion. Regardless of how successful EDs have been in the past, it is important to continue to reassess the product that the emergency department is delivering, as well as the role that each type of staff plays in the delivery of the product of the emergency department.

HORIZONS

To an increasing degree, EDs will have to operate more efficiently in the future to remain competitive. This involves use of various forms of administrative support to allow better patient care, including chart dictation, use of ED technicians, use of physician extenders, and structuring ED groups in the best possible fashion. To address patient flow needs maximally, more and more EDs are likely to evolve toward either independent billing or a highly incentive-based system to allow the physicians to see a clear benefit from increasing patient flow through the department.

Emergency department overcrowding has become a significant issue, not just in urban settings, but also in suburban and even in some rural settings. As more and more patients enter the medically disenfranchised category, the patients presenting to the ED are likely to have less and less in the way of primary care and a higher level of acuity once they do seek emergency care. All of these factors will place increasing pressure to ensure that ED operations are at an optimal level to allow maximal flow while maintaining the best possible patient care.

NATIONAL CONTACTS

American College of Emergency Physicians
Practice Management Department
P.O. Box 619911
Dallas, Texas
214-550-0911

American College of Physician Executives
Airport Business Center
5824 South Semoran Boulevard
Orlando, Florida 32822–9980
407-281-7396

Emergency Nurses Association
230 East Ohio
Suite 600
Chicago, IL 60611
312-649-0297

REFERENCES

1. Kraus, W.A., Zimmerman, J.E., Wagner, D.P., et al.: APACHE—Acute physiology and chronic health evaluation: A physiologically based system. Crit. Care Med. 9:591, 1981.
2. American College of Surgeons Committee on Trauma: Optimal Resources for the Care of the Injured Patient. American College of Surgeons, Chicago, 1990.
3. Johnson, K.: A practical approach to patient classification. Nurs. Manag. 15:39, 1984.
4. Des Ormeaux, S.P.: Implementation of the C. A. S. H. patient classification system for staffing determination. Supervisor Nurse 8:29, 1977.
5. Lewis, E.N., and Carini, P.V.: Nurse Staffing and Patient Classification: Strategies for Success. Rockville, MD, Aspen Publishers, 1984.
6. Wilbert, C.C.: Timeliness of care in the Emergency Department. Quality Review Bulletin 1984, pp. 99–108.
7. Schulmerich, S.C.: Developing a patient classification system for the emergency department. J. Emerg. Nurs. 6:298, 1984.
8. Butler, W.R.: ED patient classification matrix: Development and testing of one tool. J. Emerg. Nursing 12:279, 1986.
9. EMERGE: The Emergency Department Patient Classification and Information System. Evanston, Illinois, Medicus Systems, 1987.
10. Mayer, T.: The emergency department medical director. Emerg. Med. Clin. North Am.
11. Cue, F., and Inglish, R.: Improving the operations of the emergency department. Hospitals 52:110, 1978.
12. Saunders, C.E.: Time study of patient movement through the emergency department: Sources of delay in relation to patient acuity. Ann. Emerg. Med. 16:1244, 1987.
13. American College of Emergency Physicians Practice Management Committee: Study on Emergency Department Staffing, Unpublished Data, American College of Emergency Physicians, Dallas, Texas, 1990.
14. Report of the Working Group on Special Services in Hospitals: Emergency Units in Hospitals: Guidelines. Health Services Directorate, Health Services in Promotion Branch, Department of National Health and Welfare, Ottawa, Canada, 1981.

QUALITY IMPROVEMENT IN EMERGENCY MEDICINE

Thom A. Mayer

CAPSULE

Emergency medicine is, in many respects, the quintessential peer review specialty. It is of necessity a *group practice of medicine*. Regardless of the specific structure in which it is practiced, emergency medicine requires that multiple physicians practice in the same hospital-based setting. Because of this, it is a more systematic and protocol-oriented specialty because the hospital, its medical staff, the nursing staff, and the community have come to expect a consistently high standard of care from emergency medicine providers.

INTRODUCTION

Virtually all patients seen in an emergency department (ED) are referred for follow-up care to appropriate physicians on the medical staff. Depending on the setting in which an emergency physician practices, between 12 and 20% of all patients who present to the ED are admitted to the hospital for more definitive care. All such patients are referred to members of the medical staff for their in-hospital care, and there is understandable scrutiny of the care rendered in the ED in such cases by the attending medical staff. Furthermore, even patients who are not admitted to the hospital are referred to members of the medical staff for appropriate follow-up care. Although exceptions do occur in the case of lacerations, mild upper respiratory infections, etc., it is a sound risk management principle that patients should be referred for appropriate follow-up care. Most importantly, all patients who present to the ED and have a primary care physician should be referred in such a way that the continuity of health care and the role of the primary care physician are respected. The integration of the group practice of emergency medicine within the overall medical community is thus a significant part of emergency medicine.

For all of these reasons, the care provided by emergency physicians is scrutinized at a level that is virtually unprecedented in any other area of medicine.

For active practitioners of emergency medicine, it has long been felt that the specialty is the "fishbowl of medicine."

Emergency medicine is also the *ultimate medical management specialty*, in that most good EDs in which conscientious and qualified care is delivered are usually well-managed emergency departments. During a routine shift in the ED, the emergency physician is responsible for handling multiple patients with diverse clinical problems at the same time, integrating their care with members of the medical staff, ensuring that nurses and other ancillary personnel are performing their duties in a coordinated fashion, and dealing with the multiple "mini-crises" that routinely attend the practice of emergency medicine. Although specific management skills are not always considered a part of the curriculum of emergency medicine residencies, experienced emergency physicians are well aware of the need for managing both individual patients and the overall flow of the ED to ensure that the best possible clinical care is delivered.

In the context of considering emergency medicine as the ultimate peer review specialty that is inextricably related to management principles, a third important element has evolved that affects the delivery of quality emergency medical care. The emergence of the quality improvement movement in American business and industry has become an issue of truly national significance. Throughout the U.S. and virtually all industrialized countries, the precepts of continuous quality improvement have become an integral part of the delivery of goods and services in the 1990's and beyond. The seminal work of quality control specialists such as Deming,[1] Juran,[2] Ishikawa,[3] Crosby,[4] and others[5] has been widely adopted in many countries, and has become an extremely important part of quality improvement throughout the world. Although these precepts are discussed in some detail in this chapter, it is important to recognize that the intent of a quality improvement program in emergency medicine should be as a management tool to allow emergency physicians and their colleagues in the practice of emergency medicine to continuously improve the care delivered in EDs throughout this country.

This is an extremely important concept because quality assurance programs, as they have been conceived in the past, have too often focused on activities whose primary purpose was to attain accreditation by various health care certifying agencies. The earliest efforts at developing the accreditation process in this country were by the American College of Surgeons (ACS) as early as 1912. The initial surveys by the ACS accredited far fewer than 10% of the total hospitals undergoing the process, indicating the need for some standardization among health care institutions. The ACS stayed active in the accreditation process until the early 1950s, at which time the Joint Commission on Accreditation of Hospitals was formed. This commission was a multidisciplinary commission involving surgical, medical, pediatric, and hospital representatives, with the purpose of having the accreditation process for hospitals under a single organization. Although the name was later changed to the Joint Commission on Accreditation of Healthcare Organizations (JCAHO), the accreditation process has become extremely widespread and well accepted among hospitals.

Regardless of the certifying organization, hospitals, physicians, and health care organizations have too often relied on a "checklist approach" toward the certification process, in which large amounts of work were generated to ensure compliance with preset standards by various organizations. Although this approach undoubtedly served a purpose, both the specialty of emergency medicine and the science of quality control have evolved to the point at which such an approach taken alone is both cumbersome and unproductive. Instead, there is a widespread abandonment of the concepts of using audits to "inspect for bad apples" in favor of an approach that allows those responsible for the delivery of services, as well as its management, to pursue statistical means to seek ways to improve the quality of care.[6,7]

It is within that context that this chapter is framed. The intent of the chapter is to outline a comprehensive approach to quality improvement in emergency medicine, using the concepts of the JCAHO Ten-Step Approach,[8] but synthesizing the approach with additional information from the quality improvement process to allow the development of a truly functional approach to the practice of emergency medicine. Throughout this chapter, the term "quality improvement" is used, as opposed to "quality assurance." This semantic change reflects both a strong philosophical commitment to continuous improvement of quality of care and practical implications for the design and implementation of quality improvement programs in emergency medicine.

THE EVOLUTION OF CONTINUOUS QUALITY IMPROVEMENT PROGRAMS

The American health care industry has undergone cataclysmic change leading into the 1990s. Various forms of physician and hospital payment reform and increased regulation of the health care industry have caused important changes. One result of this is that the American health care system is much more customer-driven than ever before. Whether the customer is viewed as the patient, the third-party payer, large businesses, or other colleagues in the health care industry, each segment of the customer market has many more options available to it than have been the case in the past. When this customer-driven nature of the industry is taken in context with the significant changes in payment mechanisms, it is clear that virtually all segments of American medicine have had to learn to adapt rapidly to operate efficiently in an environment that has drastically changed.

This has placed increasing emphasis on the need for dealing with the *systems management* perspective of medicine. In many respects, medicine has always required a strong interrelationship among various aspects of health care provision to allow the best possible patient care. Nowhere is this more obvious than in the ED, where virtually all aspects of the health care delivery system have to be coordinated for the benefit of the patient. These recent changes, however, have also made these interfaces among segments of health care delivery even more important than in the past. In many respects, physicians and hospital administrators find themselves increasingly "managing the seams" of medicine.[9]

The health care environment has thus become more accountable, more customer-driven, and more complex in its organizational, operational, and management structure. The overall trend has been to move from a culture wherein health care management was grounded in authority, inspection, and problem solving to an environment where accountability, customer-driven processes, and continuous quality improvement reign. In the simplest terms, the contrasts between problem solving and continuous quality improvement are instructional. In essence, problem solving, which has been the traditional way in which health care managers have functioned, simply takes the system back to where it should have been in the first place, which was a situation in which the lack of ability to deliver quality was built into the system.[2,7,9] Continuous quality improvement is a philosophy that focuses, not on problem-solving per se, but on examining the *process* and *structure* in which the product is delivered in the first place, so that quality can be continuously improved by the efforts of those providing the product, in concert with management.

The key elements of a continuous quality improvement program (QIP) have been detailed by numerous quality control experts, including Deming, Juran, Ishikawa, Crosby, Shewhart, and others.[1–7,10] Although each of these programs has some differences, there are numerous essential similarities among all of the mentioned authors, so that the concept of a continuous QIP can best be understood as a synthesis of these experts' work.

In the most basic of terms, the continuous QIP seeks to *reduce variation* in the production of a quality product to the maximum extent possible. This is attained by a commitment to a statistical way of thinking about the entire design, implementation, and delivery of all health care products. The process involves carefully listening to the needs and desires of both internal and external customers, reflecting the customers' needs in product design and its implementation, and involving the work force at each step of health care delivery in the continuous re-evaluation and redesign of the product and its delivery.

It is important to recognize that such an approach differs radically from many of the current concepts of inspecting the health care product, even when an outcome management approach is used. For example, a great deal of the Professional Review Organization (PRO) accreditation and even some outcomes management literature rely heavily on theories of "inspection for bad apples." Thus, the American health care industry is in the early stages of development of a paradigm that allows the concepts of continuous quality improvement to be used in the unusual circumstances of the health care industry. Although the continuous quality improvement process has been used with startling success in virtually every area of business and industry, it has not yet been widely used within the health care industry, and medicine in particular. The most dramatic exceptions to this have been the experience that the Henry Ford Healthcare System, the Harvard Community Healthplan, and the Hospital Corporation of America have had with implementing such QIP programs.

Despite the fact that such paradigms have not been widely developed and used in American medicine, the precepts of continuous quality improvement seem to lend themselves well to a complex environment such as the ED. Because of the significant potential for allowing EDs to operate more efficiently through the use of a quality improvement plan, both the philosophy and the practical aspects of this process are detailed in the following sections.

QUALITY IMPROVEMENT—THE PROCESS ORIENTED PROPOSAL

When viewed as a management tool in the ED, quality improvement is not an *event*, but rather a detailed *process*, which is integrated into the overall operation of the ED department. This requires several steps. First, the ED QIP, as well as the systems management perspective in which it functions, must have this process-oriented approach as a central underpinning. Second, significant thought must be given to how this process will be handled on a day-to-day basis. Third, this must be communicated clearly within the written QIP for the ED. Fourth, all members of the team (including emergency physicians, emergency nurses, ancillary services personnel, registration, administration, medical staff, and medical staff leadership) must be made aware of this approach in a clear-cut and understandable fashion. In the case of physicians, nurses, and other staff who work in the ED on a day-to-day basis, this should be a significant part of the orientation process. Finally, as with all aspects of quality improvement, the process-oriented approach must be reassessed in an ongoing fashion. It is only through such an approach that the quality improvement process can be *continuous*. When viewed as a process, the quality improvement activity of an organization becomes a small but essential part of everyone's job, rather than the total (yet compartmentalized) responsibility of a few, relatively isolated inspectors, accreditation teams, members of the hospital or departmental quality assurance committees, etc.

COMMITMENT—THE ESSENTIAL COMPONENT

Before entering into the design and implementation of a comprehensive, continuous quality improvement plan, it is essential to understand that *commitment* is an absolute requirement at all levels. In particular, it cannot be overstated that such a process can be successful only if the highest possible levels of the ED and the hospital itself are committed to the concept of a continuous QIP. The leadership of any organization (including the ED) has a *nondelegable responsibility* to build quality improvement into the daily operations and management of the organization.[1–5,9–12] Even the best and most sophisticated ED plans will be abysmally unsuccessful if the medical staff leadership, administration, nursing management, and the Board of Directors of the hospital are not cognizant of the plan and fully supportive of ensuring that appropriate resources are available to implement and maintain the plan. Without this level of commitment, those who are responsible for ED operations and quality improvement cannot hope to succeed in the program. As will be discussed in some detail in this chapter, even the simplest plan requires a significant amount of time and monetary resources to ensure that a meaningful approach can be taken.

It is also essential to ensure that every member of the ED team is also well informed regarding the reasons for the development and implementation of the plan, as well as contributing to its ongoing success. It is easier to attain consensus on such commitment with the concept of quality improvement as a management tool to improve both working conditions and the quality of the product that is delivered than to use the audit-centered approach, which seeks to identify poor performance, inspect for "bad apples," or place blame for poor outcomes.

PRACTICAL ELEMENTS OF THE QUALITY IMPROVEMENT PROCESS

The essential goal of any continuous quality improvement program is to reduce the variation in the quality of the health care product delivered. In the ED, the primary product delivered is the medical care provided by the ED physicians and their colleagues. In a customer-driven environment, however, that product cannot simply be defined as making the right diagnosis and providing the right treatment for the patients presenting to the ED. In fact, the product is far more complex than that for a number of reasons. First, even if the right diagnosis and treatment are given, they must be done in such an environment that the patient clearly understands the quality of the product delivered. Further, the *process* in which the product is delivered should also be designed and implemented so that the patient feels that not only the process but the product is satisfactory.

Second, virtually all patients presenting to the ED have family members or other significant persons with them whose needs also need to be addressed during the course of health care delivery. Third, when properly viewed, the health care provided in an ED affects multiple other providers, both within the ED and throughout the hospital. A large percentage of ED patients require laboratory or imaging services to arrive at the correct diagnosis. This involves a number of subprocesses that also affect the delivery of a quality health care product. Finally, even when dealing with the simplest of problems in an ED, emergency physicians are absolutely dependent on the assistance of a number of other providers within the ED. These include personnel from registration, nursing, housekeeping, administration, etc. All of these interactions are subject to variations in delivery that result in significant variations in the quality of the product delivered to any given patient presenting to the ED. Thus, it would seem that the ED provides an excellent opportunity for any program that seeks to offer better management tools to improve the delivery of service. The continuous quality improvement process is just such a management tool, and should be part of any meaningful quality improvement activities.

To demonstrate potential practical applications of the QIP in the ED, it is best to follow through the precepts outlined by quality control experts such as Deming, Juran, Ishikawa, and others. Although each of these programs have significant merit, those developed by Deming and Juran are perhaps the most widely used. Another similar approach has been presented by Deming, who with Juran is one of the pioneers who applied statistical theory to quality management. The following information attempts to delineate the "14 essential points" of a quality improvement program as presented by Deming,[1,7] in-

tegrating additional elements from Juran and others.[13–16]

DEMING'S 14 ESSENTIAL POINTS

1. *Create Constancy of Purpose for Improvement of the Product and Service*—As indicated previously, even the simplest services delivered in the ED require interaction among numerous providers who are responsible for the overall delivery of service. To ensure that the best possible quality of care is delivered, it is essential to ensure that all of the potential providers of service are educated as to the goals for improvement of the product delivered. This commitment to quality of both products and services must be present in all providers throughout the ED team.

2. *Adopt a New Philosophy of Refusing to Allow Defects*—There are two arch-enemies of progress in improving quality in any organization, but particularly in EDs. The first is the traditional reasoning that "defects" cannot be avoided in the provision of emergency services. To some extent, this logic is true. For example, despite the best efforts, patients with certain lacerations that are repaired in the ED develop wound infections. On the other hand, it is possible to effect major change in the rate of incidence of such wound infections if appropriate steps are taken. For example, if patients are rapidly triaged and initial irrigation and debridement are provided at the triage station, as opposed to waiting until the patient is seen by an emergency physician (which may take an hour or longer), does this materially affect the incidence of wound infections? Our experience in such programs has been that an aggressive approach that tries to take the assumption that we could potentially have zero wound infections has resulted in a lowering of the overall incidence of such infections. If the providers, however, are allowed to assume at each step of the way that defects and inefficiency are inherent parts of the system, improvement will be extremely difficult.

   The second major enemy to change is the assumption that things must continue to be done the same way they always have, simply because "We've always done it that way!" It is important to assure the providers of health care in the ED that new and creative ways of looking at better delivery of quality of products and services will be welcomed, not ridiculed.

3. *Cease Dependence on Inspection and Begin to Use Statistical Control*—This aspect represents a major change in emphasis in the health care industry. For many years, the focus in quality assurance programs was in performing audits or inspections of the health care delivered. This sort of focus inevitably produces defensiveness on the part of the providers. Rather than recognizing the value of the service provided by those working in an

ED, an inspection-oriented approach focuses on them as the problem. Both Deming and Juran have noted that, in their vast experience in quality control, less than 15% of the problems associated with quality have to do with the workers themselves. The remaining 85% of problems have to do with either a lack of clarity of purpose on the part of management, or faulty processes built into the delivery of the service in the first place.[1-2,6-7]

Nonetheless, it is essential to recognize that some inspection is necessary during the course of a quality improvement plan. The major change is one of emphasis, form, degree, and what is done with the information that is generated by statistical analysis. For example, if statistical analysis indicates a potential problem, the question should not be "Whose fault is it?" but rather, "Where has the design and/or delivery of the product failed and how can we improve the process?"

4. *Require Suppliers to Provide Statistical Evidence of Quality—Do Not Award Business Primarily on the Basis of Price, but Quality*—Although this point perhaps has more significance to an industrial model of quality control, it is also important in any personal service business. Although this could apply to a number of suppliers of specific equipment used in emergency medicine, it is more important to stress that the "suppliers" of services in emergency medicine are largely the emergency physicians, nurses, and other personnel within the ED. As hospital operating boards, administrations, and medical staffs assess expectations of emergency department services, the caution to avoid awarding business on price alone is certainly pertinent. Emergency physicians and nurses, however, should also structure their own business arrangements in such a way that an ongoing investment in the personnel within the department has an appropriate value. For example, does the ED group or hospital ensure that specific funds are dedicated to continuing education and development of the emergency physicians and nurses within the department?

Both Juran and Gryna have stressed the importance of ensuring that the services that are delivered are "fit for use." This simply means that the product or service should be free from inherent deficiencies and that the performance results in overall customer satisfaction. In the case of the emergency department, it is important to ensure that the *providers* of services are indeed "fit for use" in the sense of ensuring that they are well-trained and aware of the definition of quality within the existing emergency department.

5. *Improve Service Continuously and Forever*—This aspect focuses on the process-oriented approach of a QIP. By nature, all emergency medical care is systems-oriented and provided in a setting where multiple providers must cooperate extensively to allow the delivery of the service. The QIP process itself is designed to allow the system to assess and analyze appropriate statistical data continuously to allow further improvements in the system. As this process is undertaken, the focus continues to be on "What can be *improved*?" and not on "Who is at fault?"

6. *Institute Training and Retraining of All Providers*—The quality improvement process must not only be a philosophic ideal within an ED, but requires that *all* of the potential providers are trained in the concepts and methods of quality improvement. In addition, this requires significant retraining over time, to ensure that the program is meeting the needs of the providers. This concept of ongoing training and education is inherent to medicine in general, and emergency medicine in particular. This emphasis, however, must be translated into the systems management perspective of a quality improvement program.

7. *Give All Employees the Proper Tools to Do the Job Right*—This is a relatively complex area, but one that requires constant re-evaluation. In defining the service to be delivered within an ED, it is essential to ensure that those who are responsible for providing the service have the appropriate tools available to them. This includes adequate staffing levels, appropriate equipment, ancillary services support, etc.

8. *Encourage Communication and Productivity*—In adopting a QIP, it is important to drive out fear from the employees' mindset. Employees should be encouraged to speak up, make suggestions, and look for ways in which the process of the emergency department can be improved. Too many management philosophies fail to recognize Nietzsche's observation: "Rather perish than hate and fear—and twice rather perish than make oneself hated and feared."[17]

9. *Break Down Barriers Between Staff: Encourage Different Departments to Work Together*—Because the delivery of care in the ED relies on the cooperation of multiple providers in the same setting to cooperate, it is essential that each of these groups be able to work closely together in solving the operational problems that prevent the delivery of quality medical care. The use of collaborative practice committees, involving emergency physicians, nurses, management, registration, laboratory, radiology, etc., can be extremely helpful in this regard. As indicated subsequently, it is essential to ensure not only that these meetings are conducted, but that active input is sought from each of the various areas in the emergency department. Holding such meetings in such a fashion that an autocratic management style is present defeats the purpose of breaking down barriers between the staff.

10. *Eliminate Posters and Slogans*—Providers of emergency care are professionals who know their jobs and need little cheerleading to do those jobs. Un-

less some specific message must be communicated that relates directly to the quality improvement process, slogans, signs, and the like are counterproductive and should not be used.

11. *Use Statistical Methods to Continuously Improve Quality and Productivity*—Although statistical analysis may seem to lend itself better to industrial production process, there is no reason why the use of analytic methods cannot be utilized in the ED.[5] Table 88-9 lists structural means that may be used to improve quality and productivity within an ED. The use of statistical models also helps move both staff and management away from the process of making decisions based on anecdotal evidence. When these statistical models are selected, they should be communicated clearly to all members of the staff, who should be aware of what is being measured and how the data will be generated.

12. *Eliminate All Barriers to Pride in Workmanship*—In some ways, this may be considered the major problem facing medicine today. A large number of physicians, nurses, technicians, and others involved in health care have been placed in positions where respect for the job that they do is not as high as it should be. The emergency physician should take the lead in ensuring on a day-to-day (if not hour-to-hour) basis that the team members in the ED are made aware of the physician's appreciation for the work that they do. As ED volumes increase and numerous problems are noted in the delivery of emergency medical care, it is essential to recognize that one of the greatest rewards of work is knowing that the job that you do is valued by your colleagues. Even in a health care setting, structuring the quality improvement program so that people are aware that their suggestions will be thoughtfully considered is an important step toward ensuring that the providers of health care have pride in their work.

13. *Provide Ongoing Retraining to Keep Pace with Changes*—Because emergency medicine is changing so rapidly in both clinical and management aspects, this is an extremely important point to address in a quality improvement program. The health care providers should not only be retrained in their specific area of expertise but also be made aware of continued developments in related areas. In many cases, the ability to be made aware of expanding horizons and other specialties has allowed workers to make significant suggestions to improve the operations in their own area.

14. *Clearly Define Top Management's Permanent Commitment to Quality*—The entire health care team must be made aware on an ongoing basis that the QIP is not a passing trend but a deep commitment toward operating and managing the ED in a way that allows both the providers of health care and the recipients to benefit from improved quality. Experience in both the industrial and service industry settings have indicated that this process takes several years simply to complete appropriate training, although results from the process can be seen rapidly.[1-4,10-12]

This brief summary integrates elements of the Deming and Juran approaches to continuous quality improvement. It is less important, however, that the specific approach of Deming, Juran, Crosby, or other philosophies be adopted than that some systematic approach to continuous quality improvement is adopted. Both management and staff should clearly embrace the concept of using the continuous QIP as a management tool to allow them better delivery of ED services in a systems management, process-oriented environment.

IDENTIFYING CUSTOMERS AND PROCESSES

Other concepts are also important to understanding the quality improvement process and putting it to work. Juran and others have developed the concept that the delivery of a service must keep the customer in mind at all phases of the process. Within even the most circumscribed processes, however, multiple customers are involved. This involves both *internal* and *external customers*.[2,6,18] In the emergency department, internal customers of the emergency physician include the nursing staff, registration, ED technicians, laboratory, radiology, and many, many others. The most obvious external customer for the emergency physician is the patient himself, although the patient's family, emergency medical services providers, the press, law enforcement, and the community as a whole can also rightfully be considered external customers of the ED. As analysis of each of the processes in the ED occurs, the internal and external customers should be defined at each step.

Each process involves at least five components: *suppliers* who provide various forms of *input*, resulting in some form of *action* that generates *output* with an effect on the *customers* (Table 88-10). For example, the specific process under scrutiny might be the ordering of a simple radiograph in the ED. In this case, the emergency physician supplies a specific input, which is the written order to perform the x ray. This input gen-

TABLE 88-9. SAMPLE STATISTICAL ELEMENTS OF ED FLOW

Turnaround time
AMA/LWBS*
Delays in triage
Development of complications
Revisits within 48 hours
Payor mix
Emergency department patient volume

* AMA = Left Against Medical Advice, LWBS = Left Without Being Seen by a Physician

TABLE 88-10. ESSENTIAL COMPONENTS OF PROCESS

	ED Radiograph Example
Component	**Example**
Suppliers	Emergency physician
Input	Order for radiograph
Action	Clerk enters order
	Technician completes order
Output	Radiograph/interpretation
Customers	Patient

erates several actions by various people, including the clerk, who enters the order into the computer, and the radiology technician who processes the order, gets the patient, obtains the x-ray film, develops it, and returns the patient to his room. All of these actions produce a specific output, which is the radiograph itself, as well as the physician's interpretation of the film. All of this has an effect on the customer at each step of the process. If delays in obtaining radiographs are being studied, the problem may lie in any one of the five areas, or in multiple areas. Most processes can be broken down into various subprocesses. For example, the work of the radiology technician in this example can also be considered a subprocess unto itself that can be broken down into specific suppliers, inputs, actions, outputs, and customers.

QUALITY IMPROVEMENT TOOLS

One of the most important tools of a QIP involves the use of teams of various providers within the ED to solve existing problems. When such teams are formed, it is essential that appropriate representatives who are affected by the process must be included among the team members who are asked to analyze and solve the problem. As indicated previously, quality improvement is an information-driven process, which requires that all involved in generating the service be involved in the analysis and improvement of that service. When meetings of the team are held, it is important that the meetings of the team are held, it is important that the meetings have a clear purpose, a firm agenda (preferably set in advance, so that team members may think about what is to be discussed), specific times assigned, and effective techniques to result in appropriate change.[19,20] Several tools may be used to assist these teams in their work. The most important of these by far is ensuring that the team members have been well trained in the quality improvement process. In addition, the following tools can be of benefit, depending on the type of problem.

Cause and Effect Diagrams. The cause and effect diagram is also known as an Ishikawa or fishbone diagram.[3,21] These diagrams look at the potential problem under study, which is conceived as the "head" of the fish, with the various aspects impacting upon the problem as the "bones" in the diagram. This tool was originally developed by Ishikawa in an effort to ensure that the specific causes and effects resulting in a problem could be analyzed appropriately. In considering which components must be examined in the cause and effect diagram, some authors have suggested an approach that looks at procedures, policies, equipment, and people. Alternately, others have suggested the consideration of methods, materials, machines, and man. Whatever analogy is used, it is essential that the cause and effect diagram examine all potential aspects of the problem under consideration. Figure 88-6 is an example of a cause and effect diagram analyzing delays in thrombolytic therapy in the ED.

Pareto Diagram. A Pareto diagram is a rank-ordered histogram within an accumulated percentage across the items ranked. It is often used to display data generated by statistical analysis showing reasons for defects or inadequacies in a process. Such diagrams are also helpful in pointing out, as Juran indicates, which aspects of the problems constitute the "vital few" compared with the "many others."[2-6] Juran has noted that the vital few constitute the most common reasons resulting in the inadequacy or failure to deliver the service. Because a few specific aspects of care often account for most problems, particular attention should be focused on them. This is not to say that the "many other" reasons for potential problems in the delivery of service should be ignored, but simply that a rank-ordering of the causes should occur, as is graphically demonstrated in a Pareto diagram. Figure 88-7 illustrates the use of a Pareto diagram in analyzing patients leaving before treatment.

Flow Charts. One of the most important tools in the quality improvement process is the flow chart because a process cannot be improved until it can be defined. A flow chart is a management engineering tool that breaks down a process into its specific elements and allows them to be displayed in a fashion that shows precisely how the process occurs and where potential problems may lie. Figure 88-8 shows an example of how this applies to an ED. Because time is often important in medical settings, and in particular in the ED, the development of the flow chart should also be correlated with the potential areas of delay in the process.

Run Charts. Run charts attempt to look at trends in various statistical aspects of a process. The ED, patient visits, patients leaving without being seen, medication errors, incidence of wound infections, etc., may be looked at by the use of run charts. In using run charts, it is important to avoid the temptation to overinterpret the data. Variation is expected within certain parameters, and it is important to look at trends in a relative fashion as they compare to previous time periods.

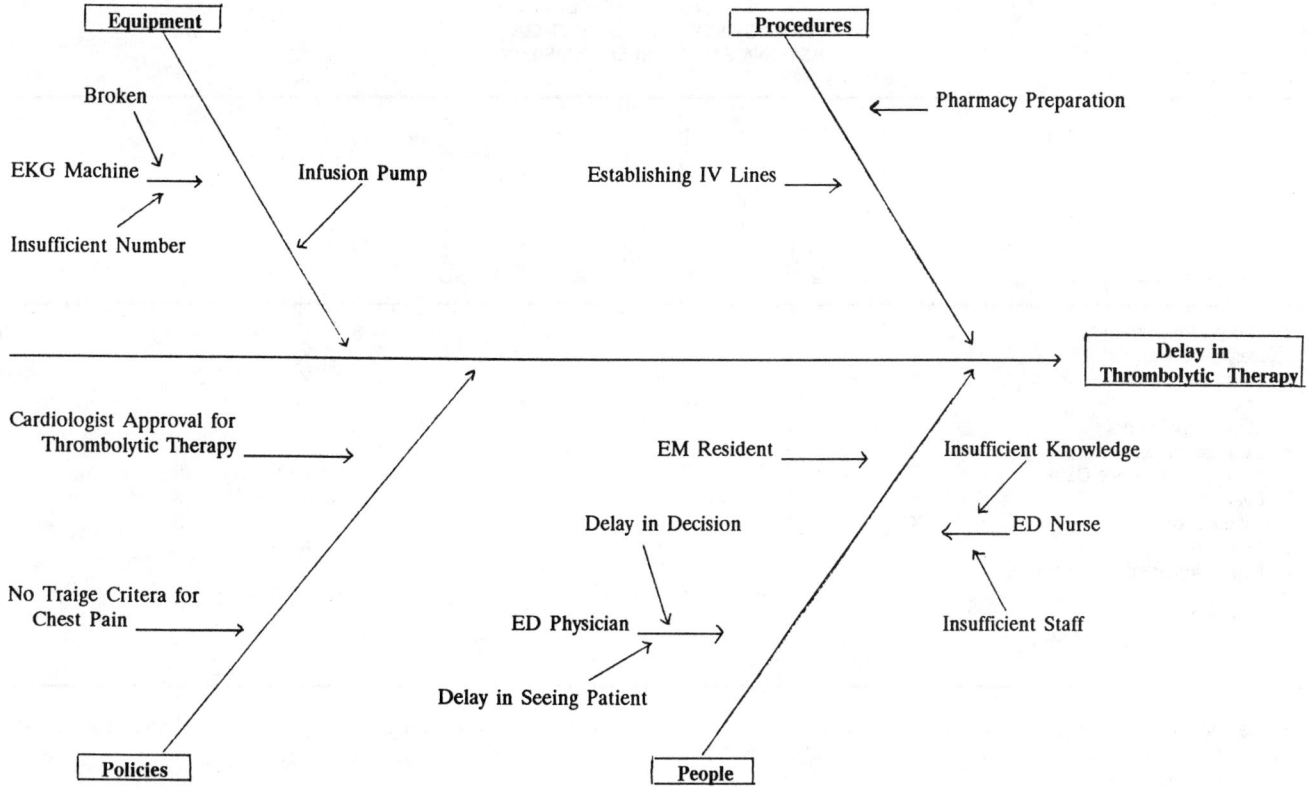

FIG. 88-6. A cause and effect diagram, also known as an Ishikawa diagram (after the Japanese quality control researcher) or fishbone diagram, because the central problem is viewed as the head of a fish and the component parts comprise the branching "skeleton" of the fish. The component parts emerge during brainstorming sessions.

Control Charts. Control charts are slightly more complex than run charts and require some experience to design, implement, and interpret. They are similar to run charts because they look at performance over time in relation to a defined quality characteristic. Control charts, however, also provide information regarding the predictability of the process as it relates to desired upper and lower control limits. As mentioned previously, one of the central goals of a QIP is to reduce variation in quality. Control charts are sophisticated ways of demonstrating that the desired quality is occurring within set parameters over specific time frames. Whenever either the upper or lower limits are exceeded, a more detailed analysis is necessary to determine whether specific actions should be taken to reduce variation and improve the quality of the process.

All of these tools require some experience to use

FIG. 88-7. A Pareto diagram. This is a rank-ordered histogram, indicating the percentage of total contributed to by each category. Such a graph illustrates the concept of the "vital few" in that a small number of problems comprises the majority of identified problems. The diagram is named for Vilfredo Pareto, the Italian economist who demonstrated that a small percentage of the population controls a large share of the total wealth.

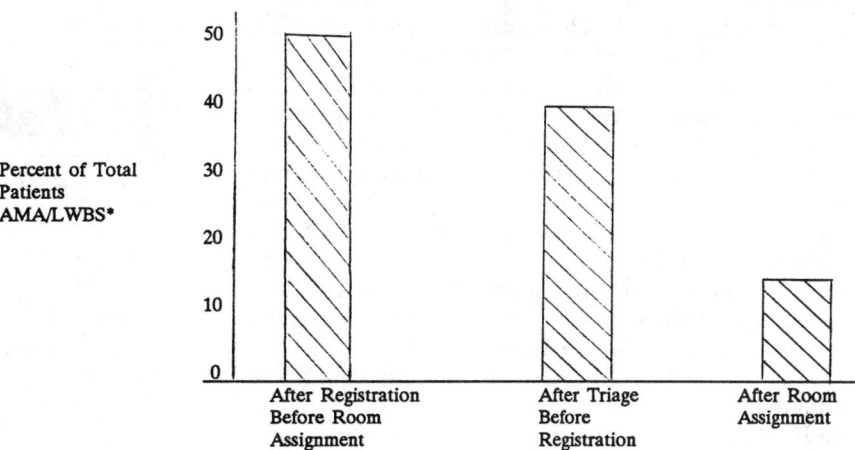

**FAIRFAX HOSPITAL
EMERGENCY DEPARTMENT QA
ASSIGNMENT OF RESPONSIBILITY**

Ten-Step Approach	Chairman	Medical Director QA	ED QA Committee	QA Coordinator	Medical Staff	Nursing Staff	Hospital QA Committee	Clinical/QRS Staff
1. Overall Responsibility	X							
2. Delineate Scope of Care	X	X		X			X	X
3. Identify Important Aspects of Care	X	X		X			X	X
4. Identify Indicators	X	X		X			X	X
5. Establish Thresholds	X	X		X	X		X	X
6. Collect & Organize Data						X	X	X
7. Evaluate Care	X	X				X	X	X
8. Take Action	X	X		X	X	X	X	X
9. Assess Actions				X		X	X	X
10. Report Relevant Information		X		X	X			X

COMMENTS:

FIG. 88-8. The first step of the JCAHO Ten-Step Approach is to assign responsibility. It is important to commit this to writing so that all persons responsible are aware of the areas with which they will be charged.

effectively, but can be significantly helpful in the design and implementation of a quality improvement process.

JCAHO'S 10-STEP APPROACH TO QUALITY IMPROVEMENT

Just as the specialty of emergency medicine has been in evolution, the science of quality control has also seen numerous changes over the past several years. In 1979, the Joint Commission on Accreditation of Hospitals (the predecessor to JCAHO) recognized that audit-oriented approaches to health care had significant limitations with regard to the true purpose of quality control. Instead, much more emphasis was placed on a problem-oriented approach to quality control, rather than simply generating a specified number of audits over a specific period. Over a 10-year period, this process evolved further, toward an approach centered much more heavily on the ways in which health care has affected clinical outcomes, particularly from the patient's perspective. Increasing emphasis has been placed on a planned, systematic, and ongoing process to monitor and evaluate patient care.[22]

To assist health care providers in designing and implementing effective quality improvement plans, the JCAHO developed the 10-step approach to monitoring and evaluation.[8,23] Like many other organizations, the JCAHO has recognized to an increasing degree that emergency medicine lends itself extremely well to quality improvement concepts, for all of the reasons listed in the introduction to this chapter. At the same time, the ED involves a diverse group of patients with widely varying clinical presentations, which means that the quality improvement process must take such diversity into account.

Table 88-11 lists the elements of the 10-step monitoring and evaluation process as established by the JCAHO. This approach is intended to assist health care organizations in establishing a monitoring and evaluation process that can identify, address, and resolve quality improvement issues. Each step is discussed in some detail in the following paragraphs.

TABLE 88-11. JCAHO 10-STEP APPROACH

1. Assign responsibility
2. Delineate scope of care
3. Identify important aspects of care
4. Identify indicators
5. Establish thresholds for evaluation
6. Collect and organize data
7. Evaluate care
8. Take actions to solve problems
9. Assess actions and document improvement
10. Communicate relevant information to organization-wide quality improvement program

STEP #1—ASSIGN RESPONSIBILITY

The overall responsibility for monitoring and evaluation of the ED QIP is clearly that of the physician director or chairman of the department. In its *Accreditation Manual for Hospitals* (AMH), JCAHO indicates in Emergency Department Standard 9.1, "The physician director of the emergency department/service is responsible for implementing the monitoring and evaluation process."[24] Although the director or chairman can delegate elements of the QIP to other individuals, including both physicians and nurses, the final responsibility still rests with the chairman. For this reason, it is essential that the chairman or physician director participate actively in the genesis of the quality improvement plan, as well as participate actively in each step of its implementation.

In delegating responsibilities under the plan, the chariman should be sure that this is written concisely and clearly. Although JCAHO does not *require* a written plan for the ED it does require a written plan for the hospital itself. Most importantly, to have a document to which all providers of emergency care can turn to understand the plan, it is advisable to have this committed to writing. Specifically, the monitoring and evaluation responsibilities should be in writing, and may be summarized simply and efficiently in the form of a concise chart (see Fig. 88-8). In addition, Step 1 should include a brief narrative stating responsibility under the plan.

As indicated previously, there is no standard, generic plan or format, although there are certainly some similarities between many ED plans, as well as the manner in which responsibilities for monitoring and evaluation are assigned. The primary goal should be to ensure that to the maximum degree possible, the monitoring and evaluation process is part of the ED staff's daily activities, using relatively freely available sources of data, and integrating it with the overall hospital operations. Once these responsibilities have been assigned, it is essential to communicate them clearly to the entire ED team, but particularly to those who will be interacting most actively in the QIP.

STEP #2—DELINEATE SCOPE OF CARE

Even the smallest of businesses identifies in its business plan the specific goals and objectives of that business. Similarly, an ED must delineate the things that it is capable of doing and the context in which this should be delivered. The *AMH* indicates in Emergency Department Standard 1.4 that the hospital should classify its ED, either through the level I through level IV classification provided, or by other existing state or regional classifications. In delineating the scope of care, it is important that the physician staff be direct, straightforward, and brief about what is provided within the ED. If a hospital functions as a designated trauma center, this should be indicated in this section.

STEP #3—IDENTIFY IMPORTANT ASPECTS OF CARE

Once it has been specified what the department does under the delineation of the scope of care, it is incumbent upon those who are planning the quality improvement process to ask a simple question: "Of the many things that we do, which are the most important?" In doing so, one should focus on the efficient use of quality improvement resources, so that the process can be focused to the maximum extent possible. In general, priority should be given to areas that are either *high volume, high risk,* or *problem-prone* in the ED. Although there are many similarities between EDs with regard to high volume, high risk, or problem-prone areas, each department will have its own specific problems that need attention. Table 88-12 lists examples of potential areas that may be high volume, high risk, or problem prone.

In most cases, it is impossible to study all of these factors during any given time frame. Instead, it is advisable to select prudently from the list that has been identified and monitor and evaluate only the areas that are likely to improve the delivery of quality medical care. Additional aspects of care can be added or deleted to the active list as the plan evolves.

For example, the prehospital care of trauma patients may be a significant problem for a given hospital. After identifying the problem, solutions can be implemented, for example decreasing prehospital time, improving compliance with field treatment protocols, tightening triage criteria, etc. After these measures have been put into place, improved compliance with accepted standards can be documented through restudying the problem to document improvement. After this has been done, this area may be deleted from monitoring and evaluation in the future if the quality improvement process has documented that the problem has been identified, addressed, and improvement

TABLE 88-12. EXAMPLES OF HIGH VOLUME, HIGH RISK, OR PROBLEM-PRONE AREAS

High Volume
Extremity trauma
Upper respiratory infections
EMS medical control
Admissions
Triage

High-Risk
Major trauma resuscitation
Thrombolytic therapy
Transfers
Central line placement
Asthma

Problem-Prone
Intravenous lines
Medications
Psychiatric problems
Return visits

documented by follow-study. The process of identifying important aspects of care changes as the plan progresses, with these aspects changing as specific problems are identified, addressed, and solved.

STEP #4—IDENTIFY INDICATORS

Once the most important aspects of care have been identified, appropriate indicators should be established for each important aspect of care. An indicator is simply a *variable that can be easily and reliably measured with regard to patient care.* A great deal of literature exists on the establishment of indicators, as well as the philosophic underpinnings surrounding this.[25,26] It is important, however, to focus on variables that lend themselves best to clinical care and can be easily and reliably measured.

These measures generally relate to either structure, process, or outcome, as outlined by Donabedian.[27] *Structure indicators* generally relate to the overall resources available for the delivery of emergency care, including equipment and type and number of staff. *Process indicators* relate to the duties undertaken by the practitioners of emergency medical care (including both physicians and nonphysicians) and include assessment, treatment, technical skills, management of complications, and indications for use of invasive techniques or procedures. *Outcome indicators* focus on the extent to which the health care provided has resulted in appropriate health and functioning of the patient, but also looks at adverse outcomes, complications, morbidity, and mortality.

From a practical standpoint in designing indicators, an additional way of classifying them includes volume indicators, quality indicators, performance indicators, and risk/complication indicators. From a philosophic standpoint, volume indicators are the practical analogs of structure indicators (Fig. 88-9). Quality indicators correspond most closely to the concept of process, but

may also be used to look at specific indications for procedures undertaken within the ED. Performance and risk/complications indicators correspond philosophically to outcome indicators.

Regardless of the terminology used, it is important to select a fixed group of indicators to study over a given period of time. Too often, initial quality improvement plans attempt to collect and analyze more data than can reasonably be handled in regard to careful study and implementation of appropriate solutions.

Most importantly, indicators should be derived from authoritative sources within the body of knowledge describing emergency medical practice. To the best extent possible, the development of indicators should be guided in a practical fashion by a clear understanding of modern emergency medical practice, as well as the current literature describing the given topic. More detailed information on the development of indicators is contained in an excellent article in the Quality Review Bulletin from JCAHO.[26] Examples of potential ED quality assurance indicators are listed in Table 88-13.

STEP #5—ESTABLISH THRESHOLDS FOR EVALUATION

Once indicators have been established for each important aspect of care, it must be decided at which point a more intensive evaluation will be undertaken to study the quality and appropriateness of care. In this sense, thresholds serve as "trip wires" or "bottom lines" beyond which further evaluation is required. In establishing such thresholds, great attention should be paid to accepted standards of practice within the given community. For example, the rate of development of wound infections after sutured lacerations may be selected as indicators to be studied. At what point should more intensive evaluation be given to

Donabedian Classification	Pragmatic Classification
Structure Indicators 1. Resources 2. Equipment 3. Type and Number of Staff	Volume Indicators
Process (Standards) Indicators 1. Assessment 2. Treatment 3. Skills 4. Indications	Quality Indicator
Outcome Indicators 1. Complications 2. Adverse Outcomes 3. Morbidity and Mortality	Performance Indicators Risk/Complication Indicators

FIG. 88-9. Correlating the theoretic classification (Donabedian) to pragmatic ED indicators: Donabedian[27] has suggested that quality indicators can be classified by structure, process, or outcome. As a matter of pragmatic significance, many EDs use the volume, quality, performance, and risk/complication terminology. These categorizations correlate well, as illustrated here.

TABLE 88-13. POTENTIAL INDICATORS FOR ED QUALITY ASSURANCE

Volume Indicators
Total ED Patients
  Acute
  Urgent
  Fast track
  Pediatric
Emergency department patients admitted
Emergency department patients seen by emergency physicians
Poison control calls
Transfer in and out
Ambulance runs
Cardiopulmonary resuscitations
Trauma alerts

Quality Indicators
Percent of patients consult needed, but not requested
Percent of inappropriate consultations
Patients left without being evaluated
Percent with untimely treatment
Patient with inappropriate x rays or laboratory tests
Percent delayed response team by attending MD
Percent of time in triage
Number of visits greater than 2 hours
Number of visits greater than 4 hours
Delays in obtaining ICU beds

Performance Indicators
Number (percent) of patient complaints—clinical
Number (percent) of patient complaints—nonclinical
Number of complaints from medical staff
Number (percent) of discrepancy between final and ED
  x ray interpretation
Number (percent) of discrepancy between final and ED
  ECG interpretation
Percentage of ED records sampled:
  Incomplete
  Inadequate documentation
  Unsigned
Number (percent) of wound infections

Risk/Complication Indications
Number of ED deaths
  DOA
  In ED
  Within 24 hours after admission
Number of unscheduled visits within 48 hours for same complaint
Number of visits for missed diagnoses
Number of visits for complications related to ED visit

means of following up appropriate medical instructions, the wound infection rate may be as high as 3 to 5%. Thus, it is important in setting thresholds that a clear understanding of the medical literature be tempered with the existing state of practice within a given ED. General examples of the types of threshold levels that have been set are listed in Table 88-14. Regardless of the levels set, however, it is important to re-evaluate continually the efficacy of the thresholds established. For example, if a given threshold results in continual evaluation at a more intense level and the results of the evaluation show reasonable standards of practice, it may be prudent to reset the threshold (or eliminate the indicator altogether).

In general, thresholds should be set for the entire ED. If computerized quality improvement models are used, however, it may be possible to study deviation from thresholds for each individual practitioner within an ED. This can be extremely helpful in ensuring quality of care. For example, in some cases the overall wound infection rate within an ED for all sutured lacerations by all physicians may be less than the established threshold for the department. A single physician, however, (for reasons of training, technique, etc.) may have an individual wound infection rate that exceeds the threshold but does not contribute to the overall statistics to such a degree that further intensive evaluation would be necessary. In this case, it would be important to know these data, so that the appropriate steps can be taken to help the physician decrease the wound infection rate for sutured lacerations.

In setting both indicators and thresholds, it is extremely important to ensure that the entire emergency physician staff discuss these indicators and thresholds before their implementation. These indicators and thresholds are intended to monitor and evaluate the day-to-day practice of these physicians, and it is only reasonable that they should have the chance to have input regarding these criteria. In addition, nursing and other staff in the ED should also play a role in setting such standards, particularly as they relate to aspects of care for which nurses or other ancillary staff are responsible.

the incidence of wound infections? Clearly, most sutured lacerations should not become infected. The specific level chosen may vary, however, depending on the types of patients seen in a given ED. For example, in a suburban ED where most patients have a relatively high level of education, excellent primary care, up-to-date immunizations, and are expected to reasonably follow directions for wound care, the rate of wound infections may be as low as 1%. In an inner-city ED, however, that may be an unreasonable figure. For example, if a large percentage of the patients delay in seeking treatment after lacerations or have significantly contaminated lacerations, poor immunization status, poor general state of health, and questionable

TABLE 88-14. SAMPLE LEVELS OF POTENTIAL THRESHOLDS FOR EVALUATION

Indicator	Threshold
Pediatric vital signs	99%
Wound infections	3%
LWOT/AMA*	2%
Incorrect emergency department x ray interpretation	2%
Medical staff complaints	1%
Patient complaints	3–5%
Unscheduled visits/complications	0.5%

* LWOT/AMA = Left Without Treatment/Left Against Medical Advice

STEP #6—COLLECT AND ORGANIZE DATA

This step is critical to the success of any ED QIP, and is the area most often neglected. For the plan to be successful, it is essential that accurate and reasonable data be collected and organized appropriately. For each individual indicator, those responsible for collecting data must identify several factors, including:

1. Data sources
2. Data collector
3. Collection method
4. Appropriateness of sampling
5. Frequency of data collection
6. Process for continuously and cumulatively comparing data with thresholds

In selecting data sources, it is easier to use data collection methods and sources for monitoring and evaluation by using existing sources and methods whenever available. There are numerous potential data sources available for study, which are listed in Table 88-15. In many cases, evaluation for a specific indicator will require the use of multiple data sources for a single indicator. For instance, in the example of the rate of development of wound infections after sutured lacerations, data sources might include the ED physician and nurse record, laboratory results (culture results), medication sheets, and infection control committee reports.

An important source of data is the daily chart review (see subsequent text). This daily, ongoing review by the physician director or his designee can be extremely helpful in identifying potential problems, and serves as an excellent data source for many indicators.

Data collection is in many respects the most tedious and time-consuming step in the entire process, but one to which both the emergency physician group and the hospital should devote significant time and monetary resources because it is essential for an effective

TABLE 88-15. POTENTIAL DATA SOURCES FOR QUALITY ASSURANCE

Emergency department physician record
Emergency department nursing record
Direct observation
Trauma—critical care flow sheet
Radiology reports
Laboratory reports
EMS run sheets
Department logs
Telemetry logs
Patient questionnaires
Committee minutes
Utilization review reports
Medication sheets
Incident reports
Patient complaints
Medical staff complaints

quality improvement program. Most importantly, it must be made extremely clear to those who are responsible for data collection that a high priority is placed upon the quality improvement process. Too often, those responsible for data collection are not made aware of the integral part that is played by quality improvement in the overall operations of the department. In cases in which individuals from outside the ED are used for data collection, it is extremely important that this be done discreetly and confidentially, with a clear understanding of the need for provider and patient confidentiality.

Once the data sources and data collection process have been identified, it is important to decide whether sampling will be used or not. For cases that occur infrequently but are extremely serious, sampling might be inappropriate. EDs are large volume operations by nature, however, with most departments seeing over 10,000 visits per year. For this reason, sampling is often used in looking at the thresholds for specific indicators. It is important that the sample size be large enough to allow adequate data collection.[8]

The frequency of sampling depends on the availability and volume of data, the number of patients affected by the specific aspect being monitored etc. For example, high volume procedures may require relatively short periods for data collection, whereas aspects of care that occur less frequently may require much longer data sampling intervals.

For each indicator being monitored and evaluated, the specific time frame should be identified in a timeline fashion, including aspects of data sources, data collectors, collection method, sampling size, frequency of data collection, and the overall process.

STEP #7—EVALUATE CARE

Once the data for each indicator have been accumulated and analyzed, one of two things will have occurred. First, it may be that the data have not reached the level of the threshold, indicating that further evaluation is probably not necessary. Even when the threshold has not been reached, the appropriate results should still be communicated to the ED quality improvement committee. In addition, if the data have not reached the level of the threshold, but those who are responsible for collecting the data indicate that their review has shown a potential problem, further study may be necessary.

Second, in cases in which a threshold for evaluation has been reached (on a cumulative basis or for an individual practitioner), it is important to evaluate the deviation from the threshold level. All such evaluations should be carried out by active practitioners of emergency medicine, who are familiar with the day-to-day clinical operations within the ED. In some cases, despite deviations from thresholds, specific events may have affected the data collection in such a way that a problem is implied but does not actually exist. For example, in assessing criteria for the use of computed tomographic (CT) scans, the threshold level may be exceeded during times in which the CT scanner is down for extended periods of time. While this is important information to communicate to the quality improvement committee and the hospital operating board, it does not imply a problem with the clinical care of the emergency physicians themselves, but rather a system problem that needs to be addressed. In addition, in cases in which the hospital disaster plan is activated or "mini-disasters" occur, thresholds may also be exceeded. In all such cases, the results of studies should be communicated to the quality improvement committee.

In cases in which the threshold is exceeded, the active practitioners responsible for evaluating such deviations should answer several questions:

1. Is there a problem?
2. What is the problem?
3. What are the problem's components?
4. What can be done to address the problem?

Each of these steps should be clearly indicated for any deviation from the threshold levels, and this communication should be in writing.

STEP #7A—STATE PROBLEMS CLEARLY

Although not explicitly stated in the JCAHO 10-step approach, it is extremely important to state explicitly the nature of the problem that has been identified through the monitoring and evaluation process. This step should not only state the problem clearly, but should try to unpack the specific elements of the problem to the best extent possible, including delineation of the specific steps that must be taken to change the problem and who is responsible for its implementation. In addition, it is reasonable to state when change should be expected and when re-evaluation should occur.

STEP #8—TAKE ACTIONS TO SOLVE PROBLEMS

This step explicitly delineates the actions to be taken to resolve the problems outlined in steps 7 and 7A. The central underlying process of quality improvement is to put into place actions that will affect clinical care and the emergency medical providers providing such care. In this regard, it is important to *focus on potential areas of improvement, as opposed to problems themselves.* In this regard the focus is less specifically on the individual practitioners or groups of practitioners who were involved in the deviation from the threshold level of care. Instead, emphasis should be placed on putting into effect appropriate means of addressing the problem. For example, common problem areas include insufficient knowledge, systems defects, and deficient behavior or performance. As in-

TABLE 88-16. PROBLEMS AND RESOLUTIONS

Type of Problem	Resolution
Insufficient knowledge	Inservices, continuing medical education, training
Systems defects	Policies and procedures, adding staff, equipment
Deficient performance	Counseling, supervision, transfer

dicated in Table 88-16 problem resolution should be geared toward addressing these general areas of difficulties.

Nonetheless, in some cases, individual practitioners are placed in a position to perform a duty or task for which they have insufficient knowledge or training, and it is certainly appropriate to address the issue to resolve the problem. It is important, however, to keep several things in mind during individual counseling with physicians or nurses in emergency care settings. First, in most cases, whenever these elements of clinical care occurred, the counselor was usually not physically present in the department at the same time and must remember this in evaluating the care. Second, the focus should be on potential areas of improvement, not specifically on the practitioners as problems. Third, even when there is a problem, it is not the problem solely of the individual practitioner, but one that effects the entire ED, and a group-oriented approach is necessary to handle this. Finally, even when a "group spirit" practice of emergency medicine with a clear peer review-oriented focus has been present, defensiveness may occur. When defensiveness is seen in the course of handling such difficulties, appropriate confidentiality must be maintained with the physician or nurse involved. In addition, it is usually best to give the practitioner the chance to review the data in detail before sitting down to discuss it further. After this, a simple one-on-one discussion can usually result in the best outcome.

Regardless of the nature or type of problem identified, the department staff should decide what corrective action is necessary and communicate this clearly and in writing. Such a plan should state *what* or *who* is expected to change as a result of the action, *who* among the ED staff is responsible for implementing changes, *what* specific actions will be taken and in what time frame, and *when* a change is expected to occur.

STEP #9—ASSESS ACTIONS AND DOCUMENT IMPROVEMENT

It is extremely important to "close the feedback loop" in the quality improvement process by ensuring that a specific time frame is set for re-evaluation of the problem to assess whether actions have been suc-

FAIRFAX HOSPITAL
DEPARTMENT OF EMERGENCY MEDICINE
FOURTH QUARTER QUALITY ASSURANCE REPORT 1989 (PRIVILEGED AND CONFIDENTIAL)

Monitors/Trends/Occurrences	Total Reported and/or Reviewed	Referred for Action	Action	Present Status	Comments
AMA/LWBS	310	310	1. Recognition of the need for timely and thorough assessment of all patients presenting to the E.D. 2. Analysis of data indicating that 50-60% who leave do so before being seen by a physician. 3. Direction of corrective actions toward increasing flow through triage, registration and into examining rooms.	Unresolved	See attached
Monitor: Adequacy of assessment and treatment of the acute asthmatic	167	53	Feedback to physicians and education regarding aspects of treatment and requirements for documentation.\n\nAction plan: Continuing education, repeat monitor next peak asthma season. (April-May 1990)	Significant improvement found since previous monitoring periods in areas of documentation of pretreatment assessment (% down from 65% to 16%) and adequacy of treatment (%down from 30% to 1%).	Significant variance rate still exists for documentation of post-treatment assessment (21%).\n\nNew ED chart available 5/90

FIG. 88-10. Legend on facing page.

COMMENTS: AMA/LWBS

The Emergency Department at Fairfax Hospital is significantly capacity constrained at the present time, due to both staffing and space limitations. In order to improve patient flow through the department the following recommendations are made:

1.   Provision of adequate personnel to accomplish triage and registrar functions during peak periods. Monitoring would be carried out on an ongoing basis to ensure adequate staffing levels.

2.   The triage desk is currently staffed by a nurse 24 hours a day and an additional ED tech for nine hours a day. Provision should be made for personnel to serve as reception or information personnel in the Emergency Department to assist patients and visitors with a multitude of informational needs which arise during an Emergency Department visit.

3.   Because of significant space limitations in the ED avoidance of all potential delays in the evaluation of patients already in examining rooms in order to expedite the provision of emergency services to patients waiting to be seen. This includes:

   a.   Availability of adequate nursing and ED technician staff to assist in evaluation of patients, carry out physician's orders, and provide care. To date, 13.0 ED techs have been budgeted to assist in the provision of nursing services. One goal is to train a cadre of technicians in the performance of designated ED procedures which have traditionally been the responsibility of registered nurses, thereby freeing nursing staff to more efficiently provide high level nursing care. This change in the skill mix in the ED must be accompanied by an ongoing assessment of the needs for nursing staffing, since patient volume continues to rise in the ED. This will partially be accomplished through the use of the EMERGE system.

   b.   Timely transfer of admitted patients out of the Emergency Department into hospital beds, so as to free ED rooms for patients waiting to be seen. This is a **major** problem, particularly with regard to ICU patients, who frequently wait hours for patient beds and require close to 1:1 nursing because of their acuity of illness or injury.

   c.   Assuring availability of adequate physician staff to ensure timely patient assessment. Additional residents and attending staff will be added in July, 1990 to improve patient flow. Re-evaluation of staffing patterns and the need for additional physician coverage is currently under way.

   d.   Availability of adequately staffed round-the-clock dedicated laboratory services. The STAT lab has never been fully staffed and is currently closed on the night shift every other weekend.

   e.   Availability of adequately staffed, dedicated X-ray technician services and radiology services for prompt reading of films. Currently, this provision is being met suboptimally due in particular to a hospital wide technician shortage. Correction of this latter shortage should be considered a top priority. In addition, the Chairman of the Departments of Emergency Medicine and Radiology have devised a better system for reading and over reading of radiographs within the ED.

4.   The current Emergency Department is designed to see as few as 43,200 patients per year but a maximum of 48,000 patients per year. ED volume in 1989 was 59,449. Additional space for patient care rooms and support services is **essential** to the ability to provide quality patient care in the Emergency Department.

Monitoring of the emergency department walkout rate will continue as we work to implement the actions outlined above. However, several of these necessary actions, are not under the direct control of the emergency department medical staff, and therefore we will require assistance if the problem of increasing numbers of emergency department walkouts is to be resolved.

FIG. 88-10 (CONTINUED).   Step 10 of the JCAHO 10 Step Approach is to communicate relevant information to the organization-wide quality improvement program. In addition, this information should be communicated on a quarterly basis to the operating board of the hospital. This ensures that appropriate education and insight occur at the operating board level with regard to the quality improvement program of the ED, as well as the problems that it is facing.

cessful in addressing it. In the course of step #8, the specific aspects to be monitored and the time frame must be set when the problem's action plan is identified. Once the reassessment has occurred, in many cases improvement will be obvious. This improvement should be documented and communicated to the quality improvement committee and the hospital operating board. In cases in which the problem still persists, more detailed study may be necessary to set an action plan that will allow the problem to be resolved, and a more detailed review should be undertaken.

One means of assessing that improvement is documented in the "CRAF Approach," stating:

1. Conclusions
2. Recommendations
3. Action
4. Follow-up

STEP #10—COMMUNICATE RELEVANT INFORMATION TO ORGANIZATION-WIDE QUALITY IMPROVEMENT PROGRAM

The process of reporting the information generated by a quality improvement program must be clearly delineated. This program should start by communicating the findings of the activities to the ED Quality Improvement Committee. Following discussion at this level, the results should be reported to the full Department of Emergency Medicine. In hospitals in which there is an Emergency Services Committee (usually comprised of emergency physicians and medical staff members from various departments in the hospital), the quality improvement information should also be communicated at this level.

It is critically important that the results be communicated to the overall hospital quality improvement committee, and from there to the hospital's governing board. If quality improvement is truly to function as a management tool, it is essential that all potential areas of the hospital affected by the program be made aware of the findings of the monitoring and evaluation of activities. The reports generated need not necessarily be long and extensive, but can concisely communicate the activities under scrutiny at any given time. Reports should be generated no less than quarterly, but more frequent monitoring and reporting may be required in certain cases. Figure 88-10 is a concise example of the type of report that may be generated to the hospital's governing board. In all cases, such reports should specifically state conclusions, actions, recommendations, and anticipated follow-up. For the quality improvement plan to be a useful management tool in improving clinical care, it is important to ensure that the information is communicated clearly, particularly to ancillary departments such as pathology, radiology, anesthesiology, operating suites, and administration.

ADDITIONAL QUALITY IMPROVEMENT ACTIVITIES

In addition to using the overall QIP and the JCAHO 10-Step Approach, several quality improvement activities are necessary for effective monitoring and evaluation of ED care. These activities are also helpful as management tools in the quality improvement process.

DAILY CHART REVIEW

In the AMH, JCAHO indicates in Standard 8.1.8 that "Emergency medical records of the previous 24 hours, when possible, are reviewed daily on at least a representative sample basis by the medical director or his designee to assess the adequacy of the services provided and of the documentation."

At first glance, it may appear that such activities fall less under a continuous quality improvement model than under more traditional, audit-oriented activities of "sampling for bad defects." Indeed, in the past such chart reviews often focused too heavily on such aspects of care. When properly viewed, however, the daily chart review can be an extremely helpful tool to the medical director and the other emergency physicians in making all members of the ED group aware of the various ways in which their colleagues practice emergency medicine. In addition, ED nurses and residents can also be involved in this daily review process.

In attempting to adopt a "zero defects approach" to quality improvement, this chart review can also be helpful in offering friendly suggestions in ways in which ED care can be continuously improved. Figure 88-11 is a sample form that can be used to review such charts on a daily basis.

To ensure that daily chart review is most beneficial, each emergency physician should participate in this activity as a part of his or her daily practice. In most cases, this can best be done by ensuring that the emergency physicians routinely review charts from the previous 24 hours randomly. This ensures that all physicians are participating in the process, and also that physicians review each other's care on a daily basis. It is also important to ensure that the emergency physicians review the nurses' notes because this collaborative aspect of care is critical to the success of the emergency department.

Once the charts have been reviewed by individual emergency physicians, either the medical director or his or her designee (usually the Director of Quality Improvement) should also review the charts for any significant trends. When problems are identified through this mechanism, they should be communicated to the Quality Improvement Committee, with

Emergency Physicians of Northern Virginia, Inc.
Daily Chart Review for _____

Chart

Patient _____
ED Physician _____
Date seen _____

Legible ( )   Not Legible ( )
Vital Signs ( )   Tetnus, Allergies ( )

Reimbursement Information

Payor Class _____
Physician Charge _____
Does documentation support
  the charge? Yes ( ) No ( )

Is the charge appropriate?
  Yes ( ) No ( ) Too high ( ) Too Low ( )

Physician Documentation

Does the history address the Chief
Complaint?
        Yes ( ) No ( )

Is the history adequate ?
        Yes ( ) No ( )

Do the Physicians' and Nurses'
notes support each other?
        Yes ( ) No ( )

Is the physicial exam complete?

        Yes ( ) No ( )

Is a repeat physical documented?
        Yes ( ) No ( )

Does the physical support the
        diagnosis?
        Yes ( ) No ( ) N/A ( )

Laboratory/ X-Ray

Appropriate? Yes ( ) No ( )
Pertinent results
  recorded?   Yes ( ) No ( )
Additional tests
  indicated?   Yes ( ) No ( )

Excessive tests? _____

Diagnosis

Acceptable ( ) Support by chart ( )
Missing ( )   Improper Term ( )
_____

Consultation

Appropriately obtained? Yes ( ) No ( )
Appropriately recorded? Yes ( ) No ( )
Comments _____

Treatment

Appropriately ordered? Yes ( ) No ( )
Appropriately recorded? Yes ( ) No ( )
Comments _____

Discharge Instructions

Referred to a physician? Yes ( ) No ( )
Appropriate referral?   Yes ( ) No ( )
Speciality and name clearly
  documented?   Yes ( ) No ( )

Auditor's comments_____
_____ Sign/Date _____
Audited physicians's comments_____
_____ Sign/Date _____
Director's comments _____
_____ Sign/Date

FIG. 88-11.   Daily chart review form. Single check-off forms can be used to ensure that data elements are examined during a daily, concurrent chart review. Such reviews may be done on as many as 10% of ED charts and shared among all ED physicians, nurses, and residents. The results of such reviews can assist in identifying potential problems, as well as improving and refining indicators, thresholds, etc.

appropriate steps taken to ensure that the problem is addressed. If necessary, later studies can be done to ensure that the problem has been handled appropriately. In some cases, daily chart review may result in either adding or deleting indicators or changing thresholds from the ten step approach.

OCCURRENCE SCREENS

Occurrence screens are sentinel events occurring in the ED, involving patient conditions, situations, or procedures that are either known or suspected to be associated with potential problems. These screens can be used to identify cases or trends that need further review. Table 88-17 lists examples of potential occurrence screens that can be used in the ED. Certainly the most common of these is to review all cases of either cardiac arrest or patients who are either dead on arrival or dead in the ED. Occurrence screens assist not only in quality improvement activities but in ensuring an appropriate interface between quality improvement and risk management concerns. Just as indicators and thresholds change over time in the 10-Step Process, similarly occurrence screens may change over time in any given QIP.

COMPLAINTS

Complaints that are generated by patients, medical staff, or fellow emergency department care providers should all be compiled and treated in a comprehensive fashion. Figure 88-12 is a form that can be used to ensure appropriate follow-up for any concerns raised. Whenever such complaints are generated, the medical director or his or her designee should perform a detailed review of the care delivered, and ensure that the nurses and emergency physicians involved in care have the opportunity to review and comment upon the concerns. When complaints come from patients or their families, it is usually best to generate a written response, as well as a telephone response, where appropriate. The results of any complaints or concerns should be kept in a comprehensive file and in the reappointment files of appropriate emergency department personnel (see subsequent text).

TABLE 88-17. OCCURRENCE SCREENS

Cardiac arrest
Respiratory arrest
DOAs
ICU delays
Left without treatment
Waits longer than 30 minutes

COMPLIMENTARY FEEDBACK

In addition to investigating complaints, the ED director or his or her designee should ensure that any letters or verbal feedback reflecting positively on ED care is communicated to the providers of such care, as well as logged in a similar fashion to complaints in the physicians' reappointment file.

PATIENT SATISFACTION SURVEYS

Patient satisfaction surveys include telephone surveys, written surveys at the time of service, or written surveys provided at a later time. All such surveys should be examined in detail to determine any trends or potential problems that need to be addressed.

CHARGE PHYSICIAN AND CHARGE NURSE REPORTS

Just as there is usually a nurse who is in charge of the nursing functions within the ED for a given shift, in most busy EDs there should also be a charge physician, who is responsible for overseeing the flow of patients and delivery of medical care in the department. When there is single-physician coverage, it is obvious that this physician is in charge. When multiple physicians cover the ED at one time, however, it is usually preferable to designate a specific physician as the charge physician during that shift.

Both the charge physician and the charge nurse should communicate in writing, in an off-service report any problems or concerns that develop during the course of the shift itself. These reports can be used to assist in closing the quality improvement feedback loop effectively, and can be done in a timely manner.

COLLABORATIVE PRACTICE OPPORTUNITIES

Emergency medicine always involves a team approach to the delivery of medical, nursing, and ancillary service care. The practice of emergency medicine is thus a collaborative practice among these groups of people. In recognizing this fact, it is often helpful to have a Collaborative Practice Committee, comprised of physicians, nurses, and ancillary personnel involved in ED care. Such committees can be helpful in developing general standards of practice, as well as addressing specific problems that are seen by the day-to-day providers of emergency care. When such committees or informal groups are in place, any concerns or protocols that are developed should be communicated to the quality improvement committee in a timely fashion.

In addition, it is often helpful to have quarterly or semi-annual sessions that allow the nursing staff and physician staff in an ED to speak in a blunt but informal fashion regarding potential problems, concerns, or ar-

FAIRFAX HOSPITAL
DEPARTMENT OF EMERGENCY MEDICINE

QUALITY IMPROVEMENT OCCURRENCE SCREEN
EMERGENCY DEPARTMENT COMPLAINTS
<u>**PRIVILEGED AND CONFIDENTIAL**</u>

DATE COMPLAINT RECEIVED_____   NAME OF COMPLAINANT_____

PATIENT NAME (If applicable)_____

HISTORY NUMBER_____   DATE OF VISIT_____

EMERGENCY DEPARTMENT PHYSICIAN (If applicable)_____

<u>**COMPLAINT CONCERNS PRIMARILY**</u> (check all that apply):

____ Physician Medical Care

____ Physician Attitude/Behavior

____ Nursing Care Performance (RNs, Techs)

____ Nursing Attitude/Behavior

____ Other Ancillary Staff Skills Performance
        (specify department:_____)

____ Other Ancillary Staff Attitude/Behavior
        (specify department:_____)

____ Waiting Time
        (specify)   ____ Triage
                         ____ Registration
                         ____ ED Room Assignment
                         ____ EDP to See
                         ____ PMD to See
                         ____ For Ancillary Service
                         ____ For Hospital Bed
                         ____ Overall Waiting Time
                         ____ Other

    ____ Billing

DETAILS OF COMPLAINT:_____

_____

_____

                                              _____
                                              PERSON TAKING COMPLAINT

ACTION:_____

_____

_____

CHAIRMAN'S SIGNATURE_____   DATE_____

FIG. 88-12.   Patient complaints should be logged on an appropriate form such as this. A response from the medical director or his or her designee should be generated within a specified time to ensure that appropriate steps are taken to address the patients' problems.

eas of difficulty that are encountered in the emergency department. Such "meetings of the minds" can be extremely helpful in ensuring that a forum is available for anyone in the ED to express his or her concerns. It is helpful to adopt an approach that ensures that each person expressing a concern at such meetings will bring forward at least one potential solution to the problem. This reduces mindless carping, and helps the participants focus on meaningful ways in which problems can be solved.

INTERACTION WITH OTHER DEPARTMENTAL QUALITY IMPROVEMENT COMMITTEES

The ED affects virtually every other area of the hospital because of the protean nature of the patients seen in a busy ED. For this reason, it is essential that the quality improvement process in the ED communicate well with other quality improvement activities from other departments. Perhaps the best examples of these are the quality improvement committees for radiology, pathology, and anesthesiology. All of these are areas in which close cooperation between the ED and the respective other departments is critical to the success of effective emergency department care. Unfortunately, in some settings there is little interaction among the quality improvement processes in these departments, which can present major problems in resolving interdisciplinary concerns.

THE EDUCATIONAL QUALITY IMPROVEMENT LINK

Because emergency medicine encompasses the broadest range of acute care activities, it is essential that the emergency physicians stay conversant with the rapidly evolving literature of emergency medicine, including trauma, acute medical care, acute cardiac care, obstetric and gynecologic emergencies, pediatric emergencies, etc. The linkage between the educational program of an emergency department and the quality improvement program is extremely critical. All EDs should be heavily involved in continuing education for nurses, physicians, ancillary staff, and the attending medical staff. It is also important, however, to ensure that the educational programs for the group are structured in such a way that they are responsive to the monitoring and evaluation process of the quality improvement program. These activities can be ensured in several ways.

First, when specific problems arise with individual emergency physicians, it may be necessary to ensure that physicians are exposed to the proper continuing medical education to address the potential area of deficiency. For example, if the monitoring of misreads

of radiographs taken in the ED indicates that a given emergency physician has a much higher rate of incorrect readings, the medical director or department chairman may need to ensure that the physician takes appropriate continuing medical education courses, or tutorials with the department of radiology to ensure that the problem is addressed. After such education, it is appropriate to monitor and evaluate radiographs interpreted by the physician on an ongoing basis to ensure that the problem has been taken care of. Similar types of continuing educational activities may be necessary for nurses or other staff as well.

Second, results of the quality improvement process should guide specific educational activities for the general ED as well. For example, if the time delay between diagnosis of acute myocardial infarction and delivery of thrombolytic therapy is being monitored and significant delays in the institution of such therapy are found, it may be appropriate to provide an inservice to the entire emergency department staff, in conjunction with the division of cardiology, to ensure clear understanding among all parties in regard to the need for rapid administration of thrombolytic treatment.

Third, the AMH identifies in Emergency Department Standard 4 that "All personnel are prepared for their emergency care responsibilities through appropriate training and education programs.[28,29] Included among these standards are the requirement that there be a formal training program for all registered and licensed nurses, as well as for other nonphysicians within the ED who are providing patient care. This program must be specifically acceptable to the medical director or department chairman. In addition, the orientation program for emergency physicians, emergency nurses, and ancillary service personnel must be sufficient to allow appropriate discharge of duties. Further, all ED personnel must participate in ongoing in-service education programs, which must be based, in part, on the results of the monitoring and evaluation process. Thus, the role of education within the ED QIP is clearly essential, whether viewed from the JCAHO accreditation perspective or from the management information perspective.

HORIZONS

Over the coming years, QIPs will be further developed and implemented in EDs across the country. The Continuous Quality Improvement Process is likely to be widely embraced by the American health care industry. Because emergency medicine is a strongly peer-review-oriented specialty and one that lends itself well to medical management, it is likely that emergency medicine will in many respects lead the way as hospitals and health care providers develop experience with QIPs.

Specific developments will involve the application of statistical quality control tools to the ED setting. There is strong reason to believe that the quality improvement process and the systems management approach it involves will continue to improve both the operations of emergency departments throughout this country and the medical care delivered. Because of increasing competition for the health care dollar, the most successful health care providers (and EDs) will be those that are able to operate most efficiently in developing a quality response to customer-driven needs. Quality improvement programs will be essential tools for such EDs, both now and in the future.

NATIONAL CONTACTS

American College of Emergency Physicians
  Practice Management Department
  PO Box 619911
  Dallas, Texas
  214-550-0911
Joint Commission on Accreditation of Healthcare Organizations
  875 North Michigan Avenue
  Chicago, Illinois 60611-1846
  312-642-6061
The Juran Institute
  11 River Road
  PO Box 811
  Wilton, Connecticut 06897-0811

ACKNOWLEDGMENT

Morris Lambden, M.D., reviewed this chapter and offered many insightful comments and helpful suggestions which improved its clarity and content.

REFERENCES

1. Deming, W.E.: Out of the Crises. Cambridge, Massachusetts, Massachusetts Institute of Technology Center for Advanced Engineering Study, 1986.
2. Juran, J.M. Juran on Leadership for Quality: An Executive Handbook. New York, Free Press, 1989.
3. Ishikawa K.: What Is Total Quality Control? The Japanese Way. Englewood Cliffs, New Jersey: Prentice Hall, 1985.
4. Crosby, P.B. Quality Without Tears: The Art of Hassle-Free taken alone is both cumbersome and unproductive.
5. Berwick, D.M.: Continuous improvement as an ideal in healthcare. N. Engl. J. Med. 320:53, 1989.
6. Juran, J.M.: Juran on Planning for Quality. New York, Free Press, 1988.
7. Deming, W.E.: Quality, Productivity, and Competitive Position. Cambridge, Massachusetts, Massachusetts Institute of Technology Press, 1982.
8. Joint Commission on Accreditation of Healthcare Organizations: Examples of Monitoring and Evaluation in Emergency Services. Chicago: Joint Commission on Accreditation of Healthcare Organizations, 1989.
9. Juran, J.M.: The Issues in Quality: Strategic Quality Planning. Quality, 1987, pp. Q23–Q28.
10. Shewhart, W.A.: Economic Control of Quality of Manufactured Products. New York, Van Nostrand, 1931.
11. Ellwood, P.M.: Outcomes Management: A Technology of Patient Experience. N. Engl. J. Med. 318:1549, 1988.
12. Tarlov, A.R., Ware, J.E., Jr., Greenfield, S., et al.: The medical outcomes study: An application of methods for monitoring the results of medical care. JAMA 262:925, 1989.
13. Lohr, K.N., and Schroeder, S.A.: A strategy for quality assurance and medicare. N. Engl. J. Med. 322:707, 1990.
14. Batalden, P.B., and Buchannon, E.D.: Industrial models of quality improvement. In Providing Quality Care: The Challenge to Clinicians. Edited by Goldfield, N., and Nash, D.B. Philadelphia, American College of Physicians, 1989, pp. 133–159.
15. Goldsmith, J.: A radical prescription for hospitals. Harvard Business Review May-June, 1989, pp. 104–111.
16. Moen, R.D., and Nolan, T.W.: Process improvement: A step by step approach to analyzing and improving a process. Quality Progress, September, 1987, pp. 62–68.
17. Nietzsche, F., Quoted in Gray, J.G.: The Warriors: *Reflections on Men in Battle.* New York, Harper and Row, 1970, p. ix.
18. Juran, J.M.: Quality Control Handbook. New York, McGraw-Hill, 1988.
19. Garvin, D.: Quality on the line. Harvard Business Review 1983; 61:65, 1983.
20. Berwick, D.M.: Measuring healthcare quality. Pediatr. Rev. 10:11, 1988.
21. Merry, M.D.: Total Quality Management for Physicians: *Translating the New Paradot.* QRB 16:101, 1990.
22. O'Leary, D.S.: Quality assessment: Moving from theory to practice. JAMA 260:1760, 1988.
23. Joint Commission on Accreditation of Healthcare Organizations: The Joint Commission Guide to Quality Assurance. Chicago, Joint Commission on Accreditation of Healthcare Organizations, 1989.
24. Joint Commission on Accreditation of Healthcare Organizations: Accreditation Manual for Hospitals. Chicago, Joint Commission on Accreditation of Healthcare Organizations, 1989, p. 45.
25. Ibid., p. 30.
26. Joint Commission on Accreditation of Healthcare Organizations: Characteristics of clinical indicators. QRB 15:330, 1989.
27. Donabedian, A.: Criteria and standards for quality assessment and monitoring. QRB 12:99, 1986.
28. Joint Commission on Accreditation of Healthcare Organizations: Accreditation Manual for Hospitals. Chicago, Joint Commission on Accreditation of Healthcare Organizations, 1989, p. 44.
29. Ibid., p. 35.

FAST TRACK CARE

David Brooke

CAPSULE

The purpose of establishing a "fast track" as part of an Emergency Department (ED) is to give a relative degree of priority to minor cases.

There are many reasons why this direction may be taken and also some difficulties to be overcome. As a busy ED develops, the point at which a fast track can be established must be identified. Then, as it grows, it is in constant need of adjustment and change.

ADVANTAGES

Most EDs need some form of double coverage when the annual total of patients seen is approximately 30,000. Many EDs already have double coverage for some shifts on busy days, such as weekends, before this number is reached, but after this double coverage, some time every day is usually required. Systematic care of minor illnesses and injuries, usually known as fast track care but with other potential names (Table 88-18), is a solution to this problem.

The establishment of a fast track is not usually considered until the department is seeing another 10,000 to 15,000 patients, for a total of 40,000 to 45,000. By this time, these departments are usually accounting

TABLE 88-18. POTENTIAL NAMES FOR THE SYSTEMATIC CARE OF MINOR ILLNESSES AND INJURIES

Fast Track
Fastracare
Express Care
Medical Express Care (and the Medical Express Card)
Quick Care
Quik Care
Minor Emergency Needs Department (MEND)
Commitment Care
Immediate Care
First Care
Urgent Care
Need Care
Private Diagnostic Care

for a quarter to a third of all hospital admissions, and about one in every six patients presenting to the ED requires admission. This means that a considerable number of patients are at least moderately ill and may require close attention and a workup with laboratory, x ray, scans, and so on.

Therefore the majority of patients, with such problems as ankle sprains, upper respiratory infections, earaches, and lacerations, may well have to wait for some time before the busy physician is able to attend them. If these patients can be diverted to a separate area, where they do not have to await the investigation and management of major cases, speedy management for minor illness and injury allows a more appropriate, shorter length of stay. This is obviously attractive to patients. When there is a competitive element in obtaining patients, this may be a marketing tool for the hospital.

When walk-in clinics have been set up to operate in the community, many patients still prefer to go to the hospital if there is a fast-track area. It provides flexibility if their illness is more than can be managed on a fast track in that they can be directed to the main ED without all the problems of doing this from a walk-in clinic. Again, many patients do not think of themselves as having a "minor illness," and prefer to go to a hospital ED, but readily accept being directed to the fast-track area.

Another advantage is that the staff involved in a fast track, whether they are physicians, nursing staff or clerical staff, tend to focus on caring for minor cases, concentrate their equipment for these, and ultimately can become efficient in managing this focused area.

DISADVANTAGES

Frequently, fast track has to be sold carefully to the medical staff because they may look on it as a threat to their own practices in dealing with similar cases. The arguments and strategies in achieving success in persuading the medical staff to accept a fast track often need careful planning and differ in each particular area.

Another disadvantage is that in the hours when the fast track is open and all the minor cases are removed from the main ED, the nursing staff and emergency physicians in the main ED will be dealing almost constantly with major cases or cases taking a considerable time, without the relief of a few minor problems to manage. It must be recognized that the physicians are unable to see as many patients per hour in these circumstances. An approximate figure of 2.5 patients per hour is suggested as a maximum for emergency physicians working in a main department where there is a fast track filtering off the minor cases. There is no question that the stress in the main ED is greater on all staff when there is no relief in the form of minor cases.

On the other hand, the fast track physician may well be able to see six or even seven patients an hour, depending on how efficiently the system has been set up to work.

GETTING STARTED

The chief movers in initiating a fast track are the nursing director of the department, the administrator responsible for the ED, and the medical director of the department.

After juggling some initial ideas, these three must then introduce the concept to their own particular staff and then to all the support services that will be required, once it has been accepted that they will go ahead. Any development in an ED requires the cooperation and understanding of the support services, as well as the firm commitment of all staff and administration involved. The major departments involved are described in the following paragraphs.

RADIOLOGY

It is assumed that the department has its own x-ray unit or is adjacent to the hospital radiology department, which provides services directly and as a priority to the ED. The cooperation of the radiographers is needed to collect patients from the fast track and return them with their films to the fast track, giving a degree of priority despite the fact that they are minor cases.

LABORATORY

Most fast tracks within an ED do not need a great number of laboratory tests. An occasional blood draw may be sensible, however, along with a few cultures and sometimes a urine specimen. Most people feel that a fast track should not be clogged by patients waiting for laboratory results, so that nearly all patients needing laboratory work are usually referred to the main department.

CENTRAL SUPPLY

Suture sets may be required in some abundance, together with other sets for minor procedures, and these may differ from those in the main emergency department. A good relationship with central supply is needed, particularly to obtain their flexibility and quick response when large numbers of patients arrive.

PHARMACY

A separate stock of drugs needing constant replenishment is essential. The pharmacy may want some say in their control and to be assured that scheduled drugs are controlled properly.

SECURITY

EDs are among the main areas needing support by the hospital security services, and the fast track is no exception, so that senior security staff members should be involved in the planning of the new unit.

OTHER

Other support will be required from hospital computer and data control, the housekeeping service to maintain cleanliness in the fast track, clerical services of various types, and a constant supply of linen. Occasionally there may be a need for the social services department to assist patients on the fast track.

In this area, hospital volunteers can be helpful, and it may be a good initial place to start because the patients are not severely ill and the stress level tends to be lower than in many other places in the hospital.

Before getting the architects to produce their drawings, it is valuable to develop a list of the illnesses and injuries with which patients present that can be sent by the triage nurse directly to the fast track.

Table 88-19 is an example of such a list. Obviously, the particular setting of any ED may indicate additions to or subtractions from this particular list. One ED physician felt strongly that pelvic examinations should be managed on the fast track and another that the slit lamp should be used only in the main ED and that therefore all eye cases should avoid the fast track. These feelings are well worth exploration and trial. These two particular cases are mentioned because they have some effect on the design of the department.

STAFFING

NURSING STAFF

The nursing tasks required are fairly basic, and LPNs or nursing assistants may well be ideal for this area.

TABLE 88-19. FAST TRACK CRITERIA

1. Earaches and ear discharge
2. Toothaches
3. Sore throat with fever
4. Cough without signs of COPD, Asthma, or CHF
5. Nausea, vomiting, or diarrhea without signs of dehydration
6. Urethral discharge in men
7. Low back pain without fever or direct trauma, and without obvious neurologic deficit
8. Extremity injury without compromise of neurovascular supply
9. Suture removal and wound checks
10. Simple wound infections including those needing I&D
11. Children with fever—
    Excluding children under 6 months with fever above 100.4°F and
    children 6 months to 2 years with fever above 103°F
12. Lacerations without major injuries
13. History of exposure to VD (men only)
14. First-degree burns and second-degree burns of less than 5% of total body surface (1% equals
    the patient's palmar surface)
15. Receiving medicines by telephone order, then discharging
16. Puncture wounds
17. Patients requesting simple refill or medications, or a tetanus shot
18. Minor contusions and abrasions
19. Insect bites without systemic symptoms
20. Headache with a previous history of recurrent attacks
21. Patients of private MDs who meet the criteria
22. Minor foreign body removal
23. Conjunctivitis/minor eye injury including foreign body
24. Patients who have orders from private physicians for routine laboratory tests or x rays
25. Returning for positive culture treatment
26. MVAS who otherwise meet these criteria
    NO ABDOMINAL PAIN   NO UTI

The nursing director of the department is ultimately responsible for the nursing. He or she may feel that an RN should be placed separately as overall manager of this area. The question may arise whether to stay with fixed staff on the fast track, who devote all their shifts to this area alone, or rotate the nursing staff through the fast track from the main ED, and there may be a wish to try both methods for a time. Most fast tracks end up with a fixed staff who come to know and run the fast track and do not rotate.

CLERICAL SUPPORT

Depending on how busy the area becomes, a full-time registration clerk may be needed, as well as a clerk in the department who will be responsible for the charts, phone calls, contacting radiology and occasionally the laboratory, and the myriad other clerical functions that arise during each shift.

MEDICAL STAFF

This would seem to be an ideal area for physician extenders. To have a physician assistant or nurse practitioner in this area for the whole time that it is open is ideal. Some hospitals and medical staff insist on a high degree of supervision of physician extenders, initially one of the double-covering physicians should release himself or herself from the main ED on a fairly regular basis to check on the fast track patients.

If this is unacceptable, a full-time physician is necessary. Board-prepared and board-certified emergency physicians tend not to get sufficient job satisfaction from working exclusively in the fast track area, although this may be ideal for older emergency physicians nearing retirement. An alternative, however, is to use family practice physicians with, for example, some upgrading of their skills regarding laceration repairs, radiology, or use of the slit lamp. With these upgraded skills, family practice physicians appear to be ideal. The combination of a family practice physician and a physician extender during the busy hours of the day provides optimal patient service.

The important point about staffing is the need for flexibility and constant re-evaluation. The nurses, physicians, and clerical staff who are present at the opening of a fast track may not be the right people or in correct numbers when the fast track has been operating for a year or two, has doubled in size, and, for example, is dealing with many more lacerations than originally envisioned. Appropriate patient management within a reasonable period needs frequent changes to any fast track area.

DESIGN

With the exception of extremely large EDs, the vast majority of fast tracks can be run with four to ten patient rooms. Figure 88-13 is an example of a fast track layout.

If an ED is seeing 45,000 patients and it is decided to open a fast track, it should be possible to filter off about one third of the patients to the fast track area within a year or two. This third is usually seen within a 12 hour period, although later this may be extended to a 16 hour period daily. So the 15,000 patients making up the one third will mean an average patient load of 41 patients a day. On some days this may be 30 and on others it may be 50, but the average is about 4 patients an hour, and, under the usual circumstances, four rooms are enough for this track.

On the other hand, an ED that is seeing 90,000 patients and has one third filtered off to the fast track is open for 16 hours a day and sees an average of 5.1 patients per hour. For the sake of argument, this particular hospital sees most of its patients who require pelvic examinations, and performs a considerable amount of laboratory work, on the fast track. To avoid clogging the system, this fast track may require 10 rooms for patients, so that those waiting for test results do not interfere with patients who can be managed more speedily. On the other hand, even in this busy fast track, it is not impossible to operate with just four patient rooms.

Although a curtain divider can be used in these rooms, it is better, from the point of patient privacy, to have individual rooms with doors that close and are relatively soundproof. The use of sheet rock is not expensive in general terms, and a lot of flexibility in these rooms is not needed. In addition, of course, the constant cleaning of curtains that act as dividers can become a nuisance.

The size of each patient room need not be more than about 8' × 8'. This allows a proper examination couch, so that the physician can examine the patient from the right-hand side; a wash basin with running water; and linen cupboards, together with other accessories. One chair for an accompanying relative fits into this space. A wall otoscope can be fitted if necessary, or the physician and physician extender can carry their own. This type of room is serviceable for most patient problems in a fast track area.

In addition, one or two special rooms must be provided. Lacerations are much more easily dealt with in a bigger room, and it may be possible to place two carts in the laceration room, so that two patients can be managed at the same time. Running water and more cupboard space for the additional equipment that must be stored is obviously necessary.

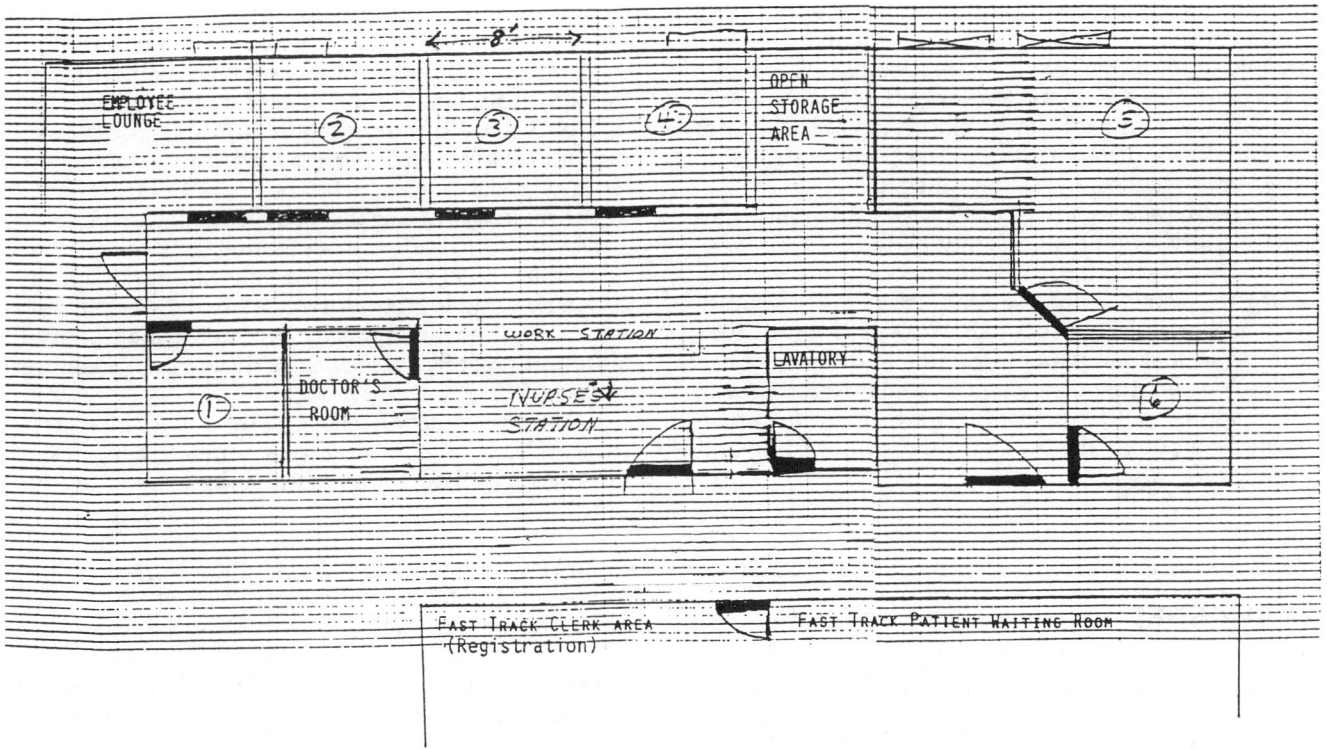

FIG. 88-13.   Example of a fast track layout.

Eyes and ears can be managed on the fast track in one room as long as a slit lamp is provided, with two stools and an ENT chair that can be placed at various angles, so that eyes can be conveniently examined as well as ENT patients. A room 10′ × 12′ is ideal for this, with visual acuities performed in the hall. An eye tray with all its equipment takes up little space, but some ENT equipment may need a separate cupboard.

If pelvic examinations are to be performed on the fast track, a room 10′ × 10′ would be more appropriate. Suitable lighting attachments, placement of the table to ensure patient privacy, and an additional curtain running across inside the main door to the room are valuable.

Apart from the individual patient rooms, the hub of the fast track area is the nurses' station. A counter of reasonable length that can contain a computer terminal is more or less standard today. The charts of new patients to be picked up by the physician or physician extender need placing to suit the efficient running of the department, as do trays for patients waiting, laboratory work to be ordered, orders on patients, and patients to be discharged. It may be that patient discharges may best be completed at the nurses' station, or there may be a preference for the nurses to do these in the patient rooms. The cupboard for medications should be nearby, as should a store for various dressings and ice packs for wounds. In a busy fast track, a clock is usually placed in the nurses' station, one purpose of which is entering times on the charts.

Physician and physician extenders need a small room with a counter and three to four x ray viewing boxes. A room 8′ × 5′ is more than adequate for two people to do all the paper work required, read the x rays, and have a small library and other books as needed. A door that can be closed is useful but not essential. If a dictation system is available, this is an ideal area for the physician to dictate.

A waiting area with 10 to 12 chairs is usually adequate and is often conveniently placed with the registration clerk at one end with his or her computer and the various forms required. Ideally, the waiting area is broken up into small areas of three to four chairs, so that the patient, friends, and relatives can talk to one another conveniently, and interesting wall decorations, potted plants, and artistic pottery may all make a potentially drab area more interesting and welcoming.

CHARGES

The charges must be established and agreed on with the hospital administration.

A contract group of physicians and physician extenders, or those who are direct employees of the hospital, may have one bill sent out to cover the hospital charge for the nurse's time and skill, use of equipment and use of the room, and the physician charge. Even in a fee-for-service contract, the hospital administration, from a marketing point of view, may wish to have some say in the physician charges. Regarding the level of services, the physician charges can be for a brief, limited, or intermediate service.

A brief level of service is defined as a level of service pertaining to the evaluation and treatment of a condition requiring only an abbreviated history and examination. This can cover a cold, a bee sting with no obvious complications, a superficial abrasion, and other such minor problems.

The other level of service used frequently is a "limited" service. This is defined as a level of service pertaining to the evaluation of a circumscribed acute illness or the periodic re-evaluation of a problem including an interval history and examination, the review of the effectiveness of past medical management, the ordering and evaluation of appropriate diagnostic tests, the adjustment of therapeutic management as indicated, and the discussion, findings, and/or medical management. This would cover ankle sprain with an x ray, an eye examination, any condition needing laboratory work or an x ray, or a respiratory infection requiring examination of EENT and the chest.

Most fast tracks use an intermediate level of service less commonly, as in a patient found to have something more serious than was supposed initially when he or she was referred to the fast track. For example, a young woman with minor chest pain might turn out to have a pneumothorax, or a blow to the lower leg of 2 or 3 days' duration might turn out to have significant cellulitis and, perhaps, need intravenous antibiotics. Most of these patients, however, are referred to the main ED under the usual circumstances.

Obviously, a pelvic examination falls into the intermediate level of service category. Any patient receiving multiple laboratory tests or laboratory tests with x rays may also receive an intermediate charge, although most fast tracks refer these to the main department.

Examples of actual charges from two busy fast-track EDs, in which there is a combined fee covering the physician, the personnel, and the room, are as follows:

$43.00 for a brief	$30.00 for a brief
$48.50 for a limited	$40.00 for a limited
$52.50 for intermediate	$85.00 for intermediate

These are suggested as guidelines only and are not proposed to induce price fixing that may infringe antitrust laws.

In addition to the charges for levels of service, additional charges should be made for equipment and for specific physician procedures. For example, this would cover the use of ice packs, elastic bandages, various dressings, and suture material from the equipment list; and then physician charges for laceration repair, the amount depending on the site and the size and covered in the procedure coding for emergency medicine. Additional examples are foreign body removal from the eye, subcutaneous tissue, ear, and nose; and the drainage of abscesses.

Radiologists provide their own charge for reading the x rays, although, with some negotiation, these charges may be lower on the fast track than in the main ED.

FAST TRACK MEDICATIONS

The suggested outline for medications available on a fast track managing about 25,000 patients a year is given in Table 88-20. It should be noted that this fast

TABLE 88-20. FAST TRACK FORMULARY

Acetaminophen elixir	Haldol
Acetaminophen	Hepatitis immunoglobulin
Acetaminophen #3	Hydroxyzine injectable
Adrenalin 1:1000	Hydroxyzine suspension
Afrin Nasal Spray	Hyper-tet
Alcaine Opthalmic Solution	Ibuprofen
Alupent syrup	Immunoglobulin (human)
Amoxicillin	Indomethazin
Ampicillin, oral	Keflex
Ampicillin injection	
Anaprox	Lidocaine ointment
Ancef/Kefzol	Lidocaine viscous
Aspirin suppository	Maalox suspension
Aspirin	Meperidine
	Metronidazole
Benemid	Mylanta II
Bicillin LA	Naldecon Pediatric drops
Bicillin CR	Norflex
Buprenex	Nubain
Ceftin	Penicillin VK
Celestone injection	Promethazine
Celestone syrup	Pyridium
Chlorpromazine	Reglan
Chloral hydrate	Robitussin
Cipro	Robitussin-AC
Compazine	Robitussin-DM
Cortisporin otic suspension	Rocephin injection
Cortisporin Ophthalmic Suspension	
	Septra/bactrim pediatric
Darvocet-N 100	Septra/Bactrim-DS
Depo-Medrol	Silver sulfadiazine
Dexamethasone	Solu-Medrol
Dimetapp elixir	Stadol
Dimetapp extentabs	Susphrine 1:200
Diphenhydramine	Symmetrel
Dolobid	Talwin
Donnatal elixir	Tetanus toxoid
DPT (pediatric)	Tigan
DT (pediatric)	Tylenol pediatric drops
DT (adult) dose	Tylox
EES 400 filmtab	Wycillin
EES granules	Zantac
E-mycin	Zinacef
Erythromycin ophthalmic ointment	
Eye stream	TAC (tetracaine, adrenalin, cocaine for
Flexeril	topical anesthesia)
Gentamycin ophthalmic solution	
Gentamycin ointment	
Glycerin suppository	

track does not deal with women requiring pelvic examination or patients who may potentially require considerable laboratory work.

Some fast tracks are being used as substitutes for outpatient blood transfusions, intravenous antibiotics, and the use of regular IV oncology drugs. The patients involved do not seem suitable for fast-track management because these procedures conflict with the overall concept of managing patients quickly. These patients should be treated in another part of the hospital.

MEDICAL STAFF USE OF FAST TRACK

The question arises as to whether the medical staff should be permitted to use the fast track to manage their own patients. There is no reason why they should be excluded if they accept the basic concept of moving patients quickly and do not, for example, settle their patients to wait for hours while they finish their office work. With clear guidelines, a reasonable arrangement can usually be made to negotiate this with the medical staff. Minor pediatric problems, for example, can be ideally managed by pediatricians here.

DICTATION SYSTEM

This is not the place to argue the obvious merits of a dictation system, but it is worth emphasizing that this system does save considerable time for fast track physicians and physician extenders and provides a clear record that can be useful to the medical staff and others. The presence of a dictation system is as important on the fast track as in the main ED.

QUALITY ASSURANCE

A system for chart review for quality assurance of the nursing staff, physicians, and physician extenders is important.

A director of nursing in the department should be responsible for setting up a regular monthly nursing review, and the department medical director should arrange a regular review of the physician and physician extender charts, picking them out at random and also looking at the management of specific clinical problems. For example, physicians working on the fast track are usually less experienced at reviewing x

rays than emergency department physicians, and this may need special attention.

THE EMERGENCY DEPARTMENT TRIAGE SYSTEM

Decisions must be made as to where the patient chart and registration are to be performed. Ideally, patients for the fast track should be identified the moment they present to the emergency area, and a separate system devised for the nursing assessment and obtaining vital signs. Whether this should be done at the entrance of the main emergency department area or referred to nurses working in the fast track must be decided in each ED. Additionally, registration must be appropriately arranged so that, again, too much patient time is not taken up before the patients are admitted to the fast track area to await the physician or physician extender.

If possible, this should be considered early in the plans for a new ED or, certainly, for the initiation of a fast track. Otherwise, there is a danger that it may be eliminated by default and all patients channeled through the regular ED triage and registration systems.

TURN-AROUND TIME

A reasonable goal for average time from the moment a patient walks into the ED area until he or she is discharged from fast track is less than 60 minutes. This provides a reasonable prospect for an average American to obtain management of a minor illness or injury that can be fitted into an average day without too much disuption. The whole concept of a fast track is to be consumer-oriented, and it is suggested that a goal similar to this should be set in each fast track area and regular time evaluations performed.

CONCLUSION

The time from the conception of a fast track to be added within an ED until the unit can actually open is probably a minimum of 2 years. A planning team involving all the personnel who may be involved can usefully obtain help from other fast tracks with an emphasis on looking at their errors rather than their successes.

Ultimately, an understanding of the system would

then allow the involvement of architects, who should not be permitted to function in a vacuum without the planning team.

Then follows the budgeting process, which may be arduous in view of the increasing competition for funds in today's hospital industry.

The building always takes longer than expected and must be constantly watched, particularly the many minor points in placement of, for instance, washing facilities and equipment that serves the staff and patients in a functional way.

Finally, clear direction and support to assist competent nursing and medical staff are essential with the incorporation of a process, so that the staff actually working in the area can be prime movers in suggesting appropriate changes and adjustments as the fast track grows.

CONTRACTS IN EMERGENCY MEDICINE

Stephen J. Dresnick

Contract—An agreement between two or more parties specifying things which will or will not be done which is enforceable by law.

Webster's Dictionary

CAPSULE

Emergency physicians, throughout their careers, sign many contracts. Primarily, these are an individual contract with a group and a group contract with a hospital. Even though most physicians have virtually no experience in contract law, it is not uncommon to see physicians enter into contractual agreements without a thorough understanding of the implications of the contract. Usually physicians try to save money and do not consult an attorney. This is analogous to a patient with an acute myocardial infarction not consulting a cardiologist. In both cases, a poor outcome is much more likely and could have been avoided by consulting the specialist. Physicians should also be aware that not all attorneys are experts in contract law and few have experience with physician/group or group/hospital contracts.

Although it is not possible to condense the body of contract law into a single chapter, the major points of both physician-group as well as group-hospital contracts are discussed. It cannot be emphasized enough that appropriate consultation and advice should be obtained along the way.

Contract development and negotiation are essential to the successful practice of emergency medicine. A thorough understanding of the issues involved and obtaining expert advice can facilitate the process in both physician-group and group-hospital contracts.

PHYSICIAN-GROUP CONTRACTS

There is a wide variation in the content of physician-group contracts. At the basic end of the scale is the verbal agreement that the physician will be compensated at a certain rate. Although this type of agreement has been used successfully for many years and the verbal agreement is upheld, the environment in which emergency medicine is practiced today requires that a number of issues be clearly addressed for the protection of both parties. It is unwise for a physician new in practice to accept this type of agreement.

At the other end of the spectrum are the contracts presented by large multi-hospital groups that are typeset and give the uninitiated the impression that this is a "standard" contract that all physicians sign. Such an agreement is intimidating, and an inexperienced physician may sign it assuming that the points are non-negotiable. Many of these contracts do, in fact, contain clauses that are onerous and may have severe financial and career implications. It is important to keep in mind always that contracts are two-way agreements and that if both parties are desirous of working together, all points are negotiable within certain parameters. Never accept a contract that contains points with which you do not agree. The purpose of such contracts is to outline clearly the nature of the relationship to avoid disagreement after the fact.

Most physician-group contracts have clauses to satisfy certain legal and regulatory requirements and other clauses that define the nature of the relationship between the two parties. It is essential that the emergency physician understand the meaning of these various clauses, and they are explained in the following paragraphs.

REPRESENTATIONS

This clause outlines certain qualifications with which the physician must comply. These are usually criteria that the hospital has placed on the group. For liability protection of the group, this clause usually states that the physician is licensed to practice in the state involved and will practice in compliance with certain rules and regulations, including the by-laws of the hospital. Most groups require this statement to limit their own corporate liability if the physician is out of compliance with these requirements. Many groups require ACLS and ATLS as a credentialling requirement, and current certification may be included as a representation of the physician. Occasionally, membership in a medical society is required and is also included in this section. Physicians should not sign a contract that includes representations that are not true at the time of signing. Physicians must also fulfill obligations of contracts requiring continuing compliance with such representations.

ASSOCIATION AND RELATIONSHIP

This clause delineates the nature of the relationship, including whether the physician is an employee or an independent contractor. There are pros and cons of both types of relationships, and the purpose of this chapter is not to delve into this area. Many groups in the country pay their physicians as independent contractors, and it is extremely important that this relationship be clearly defined in the contract language if it is to withstand IRS scrutiny. Usually the language of this section is written to be in compliance with IRS rulings on when physicians can be classified as independent contractors. This includes provisions listing what taxes the physician is responsible for paying. Several large groups have been cited over the past few years when the physician failed to pay employment taxes and the contract language was not specific. For a group, the penalties and interest could be substantial

if an audit revealed noncompliance. Physicians must be aware of the tax liabilities entailed by such language. It would be prudent for a physician practicing as an independent contractor to consult an attorney and an accountant before signing such an agreement to fully understand the tax implications.

INDEMNITY AND HOLD HARMLESS

These provisions produce the most anxiety among attorneys, but are usually totally ignored by physicians. An indemnification means that the physician will pay legal expenses in addition to any judgment that the group incurs as a result of any actions of the physicians. Many groups will request an indemnification clause that is broad and vague as to the actions that will initiate this provision. This obviously puts the physician at great risk, particularly if the indemnification includes any settlement arising from a professional liability claim. In general, claims arising from alleged malpractice should be specifically excluded from an indemnification clause, particularly if the group is providing professional liability insurance, as these would be covered by the insurance. Claims that might occur from nonmedically related incidents, such as a physician found guilty of a civil action such as slander, Medicare fraud, or failing to pay employment taxes, would be reasonable to include in an indemnification and hold harmless clause.

Indemnification clauses should be bi-directional so that the physician is indemnified if the group is responsible for an action that might result in a judgment against the physician. Although this is an unlikely scenario, it is possible that the hospital might sue the group for damages from a failure to live up to contractual language that the physician might not even be aware exists. Additionally, if the group does its own billing and coding of charts, the physician should request indemnification as well as payment of legal fees from any claim of fraud and abuse arising from actions of the group's billing company.

LENGTH OF CONTRACT

Most physician contracts are for 1 year. Generally, a physician should not sign a longer contract unless there is the ability to renegotiate the compensation section. Many physicians are presented with a 2- or 3-year contract and sign, thinking that it offers security. Although this may be true, the group legally has the right not to increase the compensation during the remainder of the contract term. The physician should also be aware of automatically renewable contracts because it would not be unusual for the deadline for termination or renegotiation to pass without the physician being aware. Contracts with specific terms make it imperative that a new contract be negotiated by the two parties in a timely fashion.

TERMINATION

The methods for termination should be clearly spelled out in the contract. Generally, the physician must realize that whether or not there are methods for termination with and without cause, if the group does not want the physician to continue to work at the hospital, there is always a way to show cause to break the contract. Perhaps the most important aspect of a termination clause is how the physician gets out of the situation. Physicians should always insist on a 90-day termination clause regardless of the reasons for the termination, and termination by the physician should not reasonably carry any liquidated damages. Because groups are unlikely to be willing to agree to pay liquidated damages if the group cancels or terminates the physician's contract, the physician generally should not agree to liquidated damages clauses.

SCHEDULING

The contract should clearly delineate the method by which the physician will be scheduled for shifts. New physicians might clearly become upset to find that they are scheduled for all of the night and weekend shifts if this was not made clear initially. A physician should insist that there be a statement as to the minimum number of shifts that will be scheduled as well as a similar statement regarding the maximum number of shifts that may be scheduled without prior agreement. A method for requesting specific days off and vacation time should also be clearly outlined in the contract. Such requests must have certain parameters so that a physician cannot always request weekends and holidays off. Many groups place limits as to how much vacation time may be taken in any given month. This is reasonable, considering the impact vacation has on the scheduling of the other physicians. This clause should also contain provision for scheduling changes which must occur during the month. It should also delineate whether the physician is able to pursue other work while under contract. If the physician is an independent contractor, by law his or her other activities cannot be restricted, and the group, in general, has considerably less control over scheduling activities than would be the case in an employee contract.

PAYMENT

This clause should clearly define the date and method of payment. Most groups pay independent contractors on a monthly basis by the 20th day of the month after the month during which services were rendered. Although this time frame may seem long, it is not unreasonable considering the necessity of the group invoicing the hospital and the time for the check to be disbursed. This is usually not negotiable, but a phy-

sician should inquire about the group's policy on advances, particularly during the first month when a physician is with the group.

This section should also clearly define the method for calculating bonuses. If bonuses are to be calculated on the basis of collections then the physician should insist on the contract providing for the physician to receive a copy of monthly collections. Any deductions from payroll should also be clearly defined in this section. The physician should be aware of any stipulation that the group may hold the last check as liquidated damages should the physician leave the group. In general, liquidated damages are decided by the courts, and it would not be proper for the group to withhold payment for services rendered.

NONINTERFERENCE/RESTRICTIVE COVENANTS

This clause of the contract is perhaps one of the most important and one that usually presents the most difficulty once the relationship between the physician and the group terminates. Groups do need protection from physicians, once recruited, from negotiating the hospital contract away from the group. This noninterference clause, however, should not be confused with any restrictive covenants that may also be included in such a section of a contract and prohibit the physician from remaining at a hospital if the group loses the contract. Some groups try to use restrictive covenants as leverage to maintain a hospital contract. Such covenants state that the physician will not be allowed to work at the hospital even if the group loses the contract for nonperformance. Occasionally, such contracts may even state that, if this provision is violated, the physician must pay liquidated damages. Physicians should never agree to pay liquidated damages in a contract. If, in fact, such damages are found to exist, it is always better to let the courts decide the amount.

It cannot be emphasized enough that such a provision can have serious consequences for the physician and should never be agreed to without consultation with an attorney experienced in contract law. These provisions restricting a physician from remaining at a hospital once the group is terminated for no cause of the physician have generally been viewed by the courts as unenforceable and may in fact be construed as restraint of trade on the part of the group. Sometimes, however, partly because of the specific contract language, the judgment has been against the physician. Although the case may result in a favorable outcome, it is far better not to have such a clause included in the contract in the first place to avoid the legal costs as well as the mental anguish. Physicians should be equally reluctant to agree to buy-out clauses even for what seem to be nominal amounts included in such a section for similar reasons.

PROFESSIONAL LIABILITY INSURANCE

This is also an extremely important clause of the contract and one that may require the guidance of an expert. The insurance market has a variety of products with various deductibles and limits attached. It is important for the physician to understand the difference between occurrence and claims-made insurance. An occurrence policy covers any incident that occurred during a year in which the premium was paid, whereas a claims-made policy covers an incident if the claim is made during a year in which the premium is paid. Claims-made policies usually require the purchase of "tail" coverage, or a reporting endorsement, once a physician leaves the group, because most claims occur 2 to 3 years after the incident. The contract should clearly state who will be responsible for the purchase of tail coverage and who will pay if the policy has a deductible. Additionally, some insurance policies are assessable if the fund needs additional money. If this is the case, the contract should outline the responsibility of each part in such an event. Physicians should request to see a copy of the policy to confirm their coverage. Any reluctance on the part of the group, hospital, or Emergency Department (ED) director to supply a copy of the professional liability insurance policy should be viewed with extreme caution.

GROUP-HOSPITAL CONTRACTS

Despite the uniform objective of providing physician staffing for a hospital's ED, there is not always uniformity in the contracts between emergency physician groups and the hospitals they serve. As with physician-group contracts, there are clauses that address certain legal and regulatory requirements in addition to clauses that define the nature of the relationship. A hospital contract represents between $500,000 and $1 million of revenue, and any group should have expert advice before entering into such an agreement.

PHYSICIAN QUALIFICATIONS

Any contract should clearly state the qualifications of the physicians to be recruited to work at the facility. Nothing will effect the relationship between the group and the hospital more than if the hospital feels that the physicians provided are not of the caliber expected. The credentialing process should also be detailed to avoid any misunderstandings. All physicians should be credentialed as members of the medical staff. For risk management reasons, the use of "temporary" or emergency credentials should be avoided.

RESPONSIBILITIES OF THE GROUP

The contract should delineate the clinical responsibilities of the group, particularly regarding hours of coverage and extent of double coverage. Some hospitals still request that emergency physicians cover in-house emergencies. Although this is not ideal because it draws the physician away from his primary responsibilities and could lead to potential liability, it is often not possible to provide such coverage for emergency situations by other means. The contract should contain language stating that the physician's primary responsibility is to the ED and that he will respond only if it does not jeopardize the care of a patient in the department. The responsibility of emergency physicians regarding admission orders should also be delineated in the contract. It is usually not a prudent idea for emergency physicians to write admission orders on inpatients. If this practice is expected, the contract should clearly seek to have the hospital provide indemnification for incidents arising from this activity.

PHYSICIAN ADMINISTRATION

It is important that there be dedicated administrative time for the medical director. The hospital should pay the group for these services as they will be able to recoup some of this cost directly from Medicare for Part A services. Expectations in this regard should be outlined in the contract. If the medical director is to perform his duty, he needs an office and the appropriate secretarial support. These items should be included in the contract to avoid any disputes later.

PERFORMANCE STANDARDS

Any contract with a hospital should clearly state the performance standards by which the success of the contract may be evaluated. If the hospital is looking for a certain number of full-time physicians or wishes the volume to grow at a certain rate, these expectations should be included in the contract. This avoids disagreements later regarding the success or failure of the group to live up to the hospital's expectations. This section should also allow periodic (preferably quarterly) review of the progress of the contracts with written evaluations. This process increases the communications between the parties and hopefully prevents frustrations from building up on issues that were not clear from the beginning.

FINANCIAL CONSIDERATIONS

The complexity of hospital-group contracts makes it difficult to cover in detail the various financial arrangements that groups have with hospitals. Such arrangements include percentage of gross contracts, hourly compensation rates, guarantees with bonuses, and independent fee-for-service billing. There seems to be a growing trend of fee-for-service contracts as hospitals wish to have the group share the risks and rewards of the contract. Regardless of the type of arrangement, the specifics of the financial aspects of the contracts should be spelled out carefully in the contract. Among the important items to be covered include the method of invoicing, dates of payment from the hospital, and fee structure. Emergency physician fees are a sensitive area with hospital administrators. Many want the fees kept low to keep the Board of Directors happy that they are providing a service to the community. In any event, they want to approve any fee increases before they are implemented. The fees must be negotiated, and it is important to point out to hospital administrators that by keeping fees below the market they will only have to cost-shift to provide the quality service they are seeking.

The contract should also cover the contractual commitments the hospital will be allowed to make regarding physician fees. This is especially relevant with managed-care programs when the hospital will guarantee a certain percentage discount. Although this is usually more desirable to the hospital, such activity may significantly affect the group's revenue. To avoid misunderstandings, the contract should be specific in this regard. The contract should also state what things may or may not be charged for, including employee injuries and employees with nonwork-related conditions. All of these items are a matter of negotiation, and the group must carefully analyze the impact such policies will have on the group.

CONTRACT NEGOTIATIONS

Once the basic elements of the contract have been developed, the next and perhaps most important step is the actual negotiation of the contract. There are courses that teach nothing but the art and skills of negotiations. The negotiation of a million-dollar contract can provoke anxiety for the uninitiated. Within certain parameters, every aspect of the contract is negotiable, but there are several basic components of negotiations that every group should be aware of before attempting to negotiate a contract. The negotiation of any contract should not be viewed as a battle to be won or lost. Successful negotiations involve careful study of the needs of both parties and finding the middle ground that will accommodate these needs. Heavy-handed negotiations may win a better contract, but will also have a negative impact on the relationship between the group or individual and the other side. It is difficult to get kicked in the head and want to get up and commit 100% effort to the individual or group that did the kicking.

Perhaps the most important aspect of negotiation is the preparation. It is important to know the other side's issues as well as they do. It is also important to know which areas may be negotiated so that time and energy will not be wasted on issues that simply cannot be changed. Time spent in preparation will gain the respect of the other side and usually make them more willing to want to work things out.

Usually the first thing an inexperienced physician wants to do is allow his lawyer to assist in the negotiations. Although there should always be appropriate legal advice, it is usually not a good idea to include attorneys as part of the negotiation process. Besides being expensive, they usually do not understand completely the goals and objectives of the two parties and may prolong or even subvert the entire process. It may be helpful to use the attorney *in absentia* as reason why certain provisions need to be worded as such. This technique is often referred to as the "good-guy bad-guy" strategy. The person saying that he or she would agree to the item but the attorney would not allow it. This strategy also preserves the relationship between the two parties once the negotiations have been completed.

It is usually not good practice to attempt to negotiate every clause. The major areas to be negotiated should be listed and made known to the other side before negotiating. This list should be "sequenced," with the first several issues being relatively minor points. This gets both parties into the problem-solving mode, and thus, when the major issues are confronted, both parties are in the proper frame of mind for successful conflict resolution. A few items that the other side may "win" should always be included to preserve their ego. Another effective strategy is the "salami technique," which allows the cutting off of thin slices at a time. It is not always necessary to negotiate the entire contract at one time, and it may in fact be better to take a small piece and return to the process several days later. While this technique can be effective, it should not be overused because the other party may start to doubt the sincerity and integrity involved and as with cutting a salami, there is always the risk that a finger may be sliced off accidentally.

BIBLIOGRAPHY

Fisher, R., and Brown, S.: Getting to Yes: Can't Negotiate Agreement Without Giving In. New York, Houghton, Mifflin, 1981.

Fisher, R., and Brown, S.: Getting Together, Building Relationships As We Negotiate. New York, Houghton, Mifflin, 1988.

Himmelstein, D.U., and Woolhandler, S.: Cost without benefit-administrative waste in U.S. health care. N. Engl. J. Med. *314*:441, 1986.

Mayer, T. (ed.): Independent Contractors Versus Employees. Dallas, American College of Emergency Physicians, 1988.

Newkirk, W.L., and Linden, R.P.: Managing Emergency Medical Services: Principles and Practice. Reston, VA, Reston Publishing Company, 1984.

Strauss, R.W. (ed.): Contracts: A Practical Guide for the Emergency Physician. Dallas, American College of Emergency Physicians, Dallas, 1990.

Williams, R.M.: Financial and contractual considerations. Emerg. Clin. North Am. *5*:71, 1987.

FINANCIAL ASPECTS OF EMERGENCY MEDICINE

Karl G. Mangold

CAPSULE

The financial aspects of emergency medical services (EMS) represent a broad and complex topic that spans the entire EMS system. This chapter, however, focuses on the financial realities of the emergency department (ED) within a hospital and how the economics of the department relate to the hospital, the consumer, and the physician.

This chapter was written during a time when the watchwords were "limitations" and "competition." The 1980s were described as an era of limitations, and it appears that we are approaching the limit that federal, state, and local governments, through taxes, are willing to pay for medical care. Concomitantly, private health insurance companies are talking about negotiated rates, and "business coalitions" have been formed to review the cost of health care premiums, with the intent of lowering or slowing the rise of these costs. Competition is seen as a way to bring market forces into the health care industry, to create an environment of the survival of the fittest. Physicians, hospitals, and other health care enterprises that survive will learn to compete for the patient (the consumer of our services) by knowing and following efficient and effective business practices. The reality of the practice of medicine is that it is a harmonious blend of art, science, and business.

It is essential for physicians involved in the entire spectrum of emergency medicine to have a working knowledge of the language of business and finance. It is beyond the scope of this chapter to provide a glossary of terms for the fundamentals of medical finance and accounting; however, Table 88-21 lists some terms that should be understood by all who desire to improve the quality of emergency medical services.

FINANCIAL IMPACT OF THE EMERGENCY DEPARTMENT ON THE HOSPITAL—DIRECT AND INDIRECT

The traditional attitude regarding EDs has been that they are an economic drain on the hospital and that emergency services are "loss leaders." At one time, most hospitals had rather high occupancy rates. Administrators were convinced that an "open door" emergency policy would result in the hospital's being overwhelmed by patients unable to handle their resultant financial obligation. The problem was that traditional cost-accounting methods credited the ED "fees" as the sole departmental source of revenue. Most EDs were, and still are, cost-accounted by a departmental method. With this method, large amounts of revenue initiated by a functioning ED were not reflected as part of ED revenue. On the other hand, the costs applied against the ED were the accumulation of high personnel salaries, personnel fringe benefits, and other direct and indirect expenses, including general administrative costs. Some of these costs were inappropriately allocated to the ED, in that many hospital department costs are related to inpatient costs, not ED services, thus skewing the costs and amount

Acknowledgment: The author wishes to thank Avram Kaplan, MPH, The Fischer Mangold Group Staff Analyst, for his assistance in editing and research, and Allen Krohn, M.D., Emergency Department Director, Mercy Hospital, Redding, California, for his assistance in providing the statistical analysis.

TABLE 88-21. TERMS USED IN FINANCIAL ASPECTS OF EMERGENCY MEDICINE

Accounting systems	Controller	Financing, debt
Accounts payable	Corporation, nonprofit	Financing, equity
Accounts receivable	Cost accounting	Financing, long-term
Accounting, tax	Cost accounting dept.	Financing, short-term
Assets	Costs, administrative (direct	Income
Audit procedure	and indirect)	Intermediary
Auditing, governmental	Cost-based reimbursement	Inventory
Bad debt	Cost center	Leverage
Balance sheet	Cost, controllable	Liability
Billing	Costs, fixed	Medicaid
Bond	Cost leasing	Medicare
Bookkeeping, double entry	Costs, noncontrollable	Overhead
Budget analysis	Cost per unit	Part A, Part B services
Budget, budgeting	Credit	Profit/loss statement
Capital	Debit	Return on investment
Carrier	Demography	Revenue
Cash flow	Depreciation expense	Tax Equity and Fiscal Responsibility
Collateral	Diagnostic related groups	Act of 1982 (TEFRA)
Collection	(DRGs)	Third party
Contracts	Expense, medical liability	Write-off
Contractual allowances	Factoring	

allocated upward. The ED director should analyze the manner in which costs are allocated to the department.

The departmental method of cost accounting has obscured the real issue, i.e., the financial impact of the department of emergency medicine on the hospital. The easiest way to illustrate this impact is figuratively to close the ED and remove fiscally all the cash flow generated by the ED from the hospital's income statement and balance sheet, i.e., remove all direct gross revenue generated by patients who entered the hospital by way of the ED and/or revenue generated by patients who used the ancillary services while in the ED. Often such a calculation reveals that, in the average community hospital, 30 to 40% of the entire hospital revenue is generated by patients who were seen exclusively or initially in the ED. In some county hospitals, and even in some university-associated hospitals, this figure may reach as high as 70 to 80% of the cash flow of the entire medical institution. Table 88-22 demonstrates the financial impact of a typical ED on a Virginia hospital in 1990.

The data shown in Table 88-23 show that the emergency department also contributes to the hospital revenues through the use of ancillary services ordered for patients seen within the emergency department and for patients admitted from the emergency department. These ancillary departments contribute to the majority of profits generated in a hospital.

Furthermore, at this hospital, 42% of the patients seen in the radiology department and 37% of the workload in the clinical laboratory comes from the ED.

TABLE 88-22. FINANCIAL IMPACT OF EMERGENCY DEPARTMENT COSTS (FAIRFAX HOSPITAL, FALLS CHURCH, VA, 1990)

Total number of patients seen in ED	56,262
Total admissions to the hospital from all sources	36,870
Total admissions to the hospital from ED	10,918
Percentage of the hospital's admissions from ED	30%
Percentage of emergency patients seen in ED and admitted	19%
Percentage of emergency patients seen in ED and admitted to:	
ICU	12.7%
CCU	22.6%
Operating room	9.2%
Percentage of all inpatient days accounted for from ED admissions	42%
Percentage of critical care inpatient days accounted for from ED admissions	68%
Percentage of inpatient revenue from ED admissions	47%

Abbreviations: ED = Emergency Department; ICU = Intensive Care Unit; CCU = Coronary Care Unit.

TABLE 88-23. FINANCIAL IMPACT OF ANCILLARY SERVICES COSTS (56,262 PATIENTS) (FAIRFAX HOSPITAL, FALLS CHURCH, VA)

	Percentage of Patients Receiving Service
Laboratory tests ordered	37%
X-ray procedures	42%
Prescriptions written	52%
Medicines dispensed in ED	36%
Electrocardiograms	7.4%
Respiratory therapy	2.1%

Abbreviation: ED = Emergency Department.

These statistics do not include the financial impact of patient admissions from the emergency department on the hospital. Because 30% of the overall admissions come from the ED, further analysis shows that these patients are usually hospitalized for a longer period of time and generate larger amounts of gross revenue because of a much heavier utilization of ancillary services. Patients admitted through the ED are more often critically ill and require more aggressive diagnostics and therapeutic modalities.

The preceding data cover a period up to the 1980s. Since that time, there has been an overall reversal of the decline in ED visits. The more serious cases are an even greater contribution to the hospital.

The financial impact of the department of emergency medicine is a complex one that must be viewed on a broad hospital fiscal basis rather than on a restricted departmental cost-accounting basis. Admission rates and ancillary service use may have a profoundly positive impact on the hospital financial structure. A well-organized, competent, and ethical group of emergency physicians who effectively manage and administer a hospital ED may literally change patterns of hospital use by members of the medical community as well as patterns of hospital preferences by the lay community.

FINANCIAL PLANNING FOR AN EMERGENCY DEPARTMENT

Certain utilization factors are important in planning. The ED records for at least the last 2 years should be reviewed, noting the following:

1. Percentage of primary care.
2. Percentage of urgent care.
3. Percentage of emergency care.
4. Percentage of convenience usage, e.g., telephone orders, injections, laboratory work only.
5. Percentage of usage for preoperative preparation for outpatient surgery and elective intradepartmental procedures.
6. Percentage of patients seen within the department by their private doctors, the house staff, and the emergency physicians.

A conservative estimate of potential patient use may be made by assuming 300 to 350 ED patient visits per year per 1000 population in the hospital service area. (Be careful not to overstate the hospital service population.)

Consideration of the demographic distribution of physicians in the hospital and the hospital service area is essential. An area that is high in specialists and underserved in primary care physicians generally produces a greater ED volume.

Demographic studies of the population in a hospital service area are extremely important. Such studies help to determine whether patients who use the hospital ED will be able to provide an adequate cash flow to sustain the emergency physician group. If there is a large indigent and welfare population, collections are significantly lower. In California, for example, if all third-party carriers remunerated emergency physicians for their services in exactly the same manner used by the Department of Health under its Medi-Cal Program, the vast majority of emergency physicians would not be able to survive economically.

The importance of a well-studied third-party demographic distribution for a specific service population cannot be overemphasized. A detailed study of the basic seven categories of third-party carriers can generally project, with a fair degree of accuracy, the percentage of collection. An example of third-party distribution in patients utilizing one hospital emergency department is listed in Table 88-24. By multiplying these percentages by the expected rates of return from each of the third parties, it is easy to estimate the percentage of noncollection, or bad debt, expense.

The so-called "break-even point" for the hospital, when calculated on the basis of the overall financial impact of the ED on the hospital and assuming an admission rate of 10% can be as low as 800 patients per month. Depending on the fiscal relationship between the emergency physician group, hospital, and patient, the break-even point for a group of emergency physicians may be as low as 1000 or 1200 patients per month. The financial break-even point for a group of emergency physicians depends on what they are prepared to accept as an irreducible minimum for their professional services. They must take into consideration their overhead expenses and the degree of autonomy they wish to retain or surrender. The greater degree of autonomy or professional independence is achieved when there is absolutely no financial relationship with the hospital. In this relationship, however, the emergency physician group would have to decide on doing their own billing with their own staff or contracting with an existing physician billing company. It is important to recognize that independent billing and its associated expenses may be costly.

TABLE 88-24. EXAMPLE OF THIRD-PARTY DISTRIBUTION OF PATIENTS AT ONE HOSPITAL

Carrier	Percentage of Population
Blue Cross	8%
Blue Shield	3%
Industrial	6%
Medicare	19%
Medicaid	36%
Private insurance	22%
No insurance	6%

There is inherent in the practice of emergency medicine a much higher noncollectable percentage of gross billings than in an office or inpatient hospital practice. If the emergency physician group decides that the economies are such that separate billing is financially viable, the group must hire expert help to manage the billing, collections, and personnel office. A volume of at least 30,000 patients would be necessary to support all of the billing department costs. An alternative is to contract out for billing services.

The emergency group could benefit from the economies of scale and the expertise of an already functioning billing service, and therefore a smaller volume could generate this financial autonomy. Perhaps the annual volume could be as low as 20,000 patients. The important variable in either billing situation is the distribution among the financial sponsorship of the patients.

Medicare reforms in the Tax Equity and Fiscal Responsibility Act of 1982 (TEFRA) focus on hospital-based physicians (HBPs). The intent is clear. There should be a clear separation of Part A and Part B services, and hospitals should not make a profit from physician charges. Also, limits as to the total amount that Medicare will pay for physician services appear in the form of actual caps on total compensation for Part A and Part B services, if it is construed that the hospital maintains control over physician charges, as in the case of combined billing of services. One possible solution to this situation (at least for Part B services) is to have the hospital develop its billing department to act as the billing agency for the physician group and charge a specific amount for the service, to be paid by the physician group.

HOSPITAL GUARANTEES

Many hospital EDs do not have an adequate patient volume to sustain financially or attract full-time emergency physician groups and yet have valid reasons for existing. Some departments have an adequate patient volume; however, as a result of the inequitable reimbursement methods by some of the third parties, they cannot generate enough cash flow to be financially independent of the hospital. In these cases, a financial relationship between the emergency physician group and the hospital is usually the rule, at least for the period during which the service is initially developed.

The so-called "guaranteed minimum" included in many contracts serves multiple purposes and exists for many reasons. In hospitals where the fees generated do not produce an adequate income to sustain the emergency physician group, the guaranteed minimum ensures a sufficient income to continue ED coverage. It is hoped that, in time, an adequate cash flow will be generated so that the physicians can support themselves entirely by gross monies billed and received from their direct patient services.

The "guaranteed minimum" has taken many forms. Some contracts state that monies paid to the group are for its departmental administrative and management functions. Other guaranteed minimums are simply a dollar amount per month versus a percentage of gross professional billings, whichever is higher. At the present time, a fairly typical minimum guarantee for a physician group in an ED with 14,000 or fewer patient visits per year is approximately $30,000 per month versus 75% of the gross professional charges, whichever is higher. Calculations are done monthly, and a check is issued by the hospital to its emergency physician group in the month following performance of professional services. Essentially, the hospital acts as the emergency physician's billing and collection agency, with the emergency physician group paying the hospital 5% of the gross for its billing and collection expense and sharing the bad debt to the extent of 20% of gross. A total of 25% of the gross professional charges is paid back to the hospital. In essence, the hospital purchases the emergency physician group's accounts receivable.

One of the simplest forms of guaranteed minimum is a sliding scale in which the dollar value of remuneration to the group changes as the patient volume changes. In this instance, the emergency physician group arranges to do its own billing. It is important to recognize this difference. The emergency physician group is now in the billing and collection business, which represents a heavy commitment of time, energy, money, and risk. If the sliding scale is used, it simply means that, as the patient volume increases, the dollar amount per patient with which the hospital reimburses the physician group decreases. At a mutually agreed-upon patient volume, the hospital reimburses the emergency physician group $0 (zero dollars) per patient, and any financial relationship for that month is nonexistent. All calculations are performed, and monies are reimbursed monthly. The essential factor in this type of arrangement is simplicity, in that the group and the hospital can calculate the so-called minimum guarantee quickly by counting the number of patients seen during the month. The sliding scale method avoids cross-audit of books, which is necessary if the guarantee is tied specifically to dollars collected by the group. It is important to keep dollars in perspective: $30,000 per month appears to be a substantial amount of money. This money, however, has to be distributed among a minimum of four full-time emergency physicians. The physician group's net income is substantially reduced by professional expenses, including malpractice insurance and business overhead.

The route of choice for the emergency physician group is to attain complete autonomy from the hospital. Because of inadequate patient volume and patients with inadequate funds, this may be initially unobtainable in many emergency physician group/hospital relationships. It is, however, becoming increasingly common, and is certainly beneficial to the development of the specialty of emergency medicine.

FEE SCHEDULES

The emergency physician uses the same accepted fee schedule nomenclature as any other physician in the community. For example, in California the California Standard Nomenclature Schedule is published by the California Medical Association. In other areas, the local Blue Shield Coding Procedure or the Coding Terminology produced by the American Medical Association (AMA) entitled CPT (Current Procedural Terminology) may be used.

The preferred method for describing the charges for visits and procedures is the use of the Procedural Terminology for Emergency Medicine (PTEM), taken from the 4th edition (including the first seven updates) of Current Procedural Terminology (CPT-4), published by the American Medical Association. Procedural Terminology for Emergency Medicine is available from the American College of Emergency Physicians (ACEP). The use of this system allows uniform and accurate description of procedures or services performed by the physician. Regardless of the fee schedule used, it is important that individual members of the physician group charge roughly the same fees for similar services. The group should agree on the fees for various procedures and produce a fee schedule that all will follow. Fees should be developed that are fair. Emergency physicians must demand equal pay for equal service. Many emergency physicians undermine the fiscal integrity of the entire specialty by allowing the hospital to retain monies generated from the professional component of the patient's bill.

BUDGET

The Physician Director should have the responsibility of participating in the development of the budget. A budget is a financial plan and represents, in dollars, the operational plan for the ED. To prepare an accurate budget effectively, one that reflects the current and future needs of the department, the Physician Director should have the following financial management reports, which are necessary to prepare a budget:

TABLE 88-25. CONCEPTS OF CONTRACT NEGOTIATION

1. Parties to the Agreement (by name, corporate or DBA)
2. Formalities: "Whereas," "Recitals," and "Heretofores"
3. Exclusivity
4. Clear description of duties of and coverage by emergency physicians: (a) clear description of duties of medical staff; (b) clear description of duties of the hospital
5. Term of Agreement (Beginning, End, Continuance)
6. Facilities (emergency department space)
7. Relationship of parties involved
8. A clear statement as to whether the emergency physicians are independent contractors, that is: (a) not employees of the hospital; (b) not a joint venture between hospital and physician
9. Equipment and supplies (who is responsible for ordering, purchasing, etc.)
10. Maintenance of facilities and equipment
11. Staff membership, staff privileges, delineation of Chief of the Emergency Department and a departmental status statement
12. Statement of responsibility for other employees
13. Licensing: Hospital/physician state licenses
14. Physician administrative responsibilities and compensation thereof; due process in medicoadministrative matters—heard under whose jurisdiction
15. Number and competence of registered nurses and ancillary personnel staffing
16. Referral methods for continued care of patients
17. Financial arrangements: (a) professional fees—mechanism of billing and collection—combined or separate billing; (b) hospital fiscal guarantees; if applicable (how much and for what period of time?)
18. Medical and financial records
19. Ethics and standards
20. Liability insurance, both professional and public
21. Amendments
22. Disagreements: mechanism for resolution, e.g., arbitration
23. Termination through loss of staff privileges
24. Scope of Agreement succession: assignability and non-assignability
25. Physician group remuneration for development of the department over a period of years
26. Noncompete clauses

Other parameters sometimes included in hospital/emergency physician contracts:
1. Voluntary and involuntary retirement provisions
2. Treatment of hospital employees, visitors injured on premises, employee physician examinations, in-house responsibilities
3. Emergency treatment description
4. Limitation of services (e.g., No Circular Casts Applied)
5. Outside practice statement, "Permissibility"?
6. Teaching responsibilities
7. Professional courtesy policy
8. Policies and procedures of any kind
9. Rendering to physician group "The appropriate corporate resolution indicating that the Board of Directors authorize the various entities (Administrator, Executive Vice-President) to enter into this Agreement."

---

1. Reports of departmental operation showing actual and budgeted income expenses.
2. Patient statistics by levels or service and financial class.

3. Hours worked by nonphysician personnel.
4. Cost per unit of service for nonphysician personnel.
5. Cost of supplies.
6. Supply cost per unit of service.
7. Payroll expense, with breakdown of full-time equivalence (FTE) and breakdown by job classification.
8. Capital expenditures, including major equipment and facilities.
9. Minor construction costs.
10. Comparative budget information showing monthly and year-to-date trends should also include comparison to the past years' expenditures.

To forecast future workloads adequately, the Physician Director should consider the identifiable trends within these reports and then analyze the market trends within the community. Anyone may easily calculate the cost of operating an ED because approximately 50 to 60% of the costs go to payroll expenses.

CONTRACT NEGOTIATION

It is beyond the scope of this chapter to discuss the multiple parameters of an equitable hospital contract. Instead, some concepts and items that should be covered in an emergency physician contract are listed in Table 88-25, and detailed information should be sought in other references. Such a list incorporates just some of the parameters to be considered. Local needs, experiences, and expectations influence such considerations.

MANAGED CARE SYSTEMS AND THE EMERGENCY DEPARTMENT

Stephen J. Dresnick

CAPSULE

Managed care programs represent opportunities for emergency physicians. To take advantage of these opportunities, a solid understanding of how managed care programs work is necessary. Open and honest communication with the plans is essential for a satisfactory relationship. The net effect of managed care programs may be a slight decrease in use of EDs for nonemergency problems; however, successful contracts with programs may actually produce an increase in enrolled patients for EDs that are efficiently run and able to successfully negotiate contracts with managed care programs.

INTRODUCTION

Over approximately the past 10 years, Emergency Department (ED) visits have increased from 82 to 87 million per year. This 15% increase has been caused by numerous factors, including the establishment of emergency medicine as a specialty that has attracted full-time career physicians. Additionally, because the number of people not adequately covered by health insurance has risen to almost 35 million, many patients have turned to the ED as an access point to the health care system. As some of these patients have subsequently obtained insurance, they have continued to be comforted by the availability of the care through hospital EDs. The tendency toward increased specialization has left a relative shortage of primary care practitioners, and thus patients do not always have prompt access to a primary care physician.

Insurance companies, hit hard by the runaway inflation and high interest rates of the mid-1980s, have looked at ways to reduce their health care costs. New companies emerged during this time, offering employers and individuals the promise of lower premiums through efficient management, group purchasing through selected providers, and strict utilization review. Although the early companies were called Health Maintenance Organizations (HMOs), the concepts used by the original HMOs have been adopted by organizations with a number of different names such as PPOs, IPAs, TPA's. All share the same general concept of "managing the care of a patient," hence the generic name of "managed care systems." Although each organization may pay the provider through a different mechanism, all try to direct patients to providers who have agreed to discount their fees, to settings that may be less expensive, and maybe even to providers who have agreed to provide care for a certain number of patients on a capitated or prepaid basis. Patients who are not able to be so directed or "managed" represent increased costs to the insurance company.

MANAGED CARE SYSTEMS METHODS OF COST REDUCTION

PREFERRED PROVIDERS

Managed care programs generally contract with a particular group of physicians who have agreed to accept a set fee for their services. This fee may be either a percentage discount of their normal fee or established by a published fee schedule by the program. In a "staff" model, all the physicians practice in a facility owned or operated by the program. In the "independence practice association" (IPA) model, physicians practice in their own offices and maintain their own practices. Patients must be directed to these physicians, but because the day-to-day operation of the office is by the individual practitioner, the degree of attention paid to these patients may vary. The lure of belonging to such a program lies with the promise of increased volume of patients and hence increased revenue to the practice. Unfortunately, because physicians are receiving a discounted fee, occasionally they also provide discounted services and schedule only a certain number of enrolled patients per day. This creates a situation in which patients, used to obtaining prompt care, turn to EDs.

UTILIZATION CONTROL

Discounted physician fees have only a minor impact on the health care dollars spent by managed care programs. Most dollars are spent on inpatient care and laboratory testing. Just as the federal government has discovered, the costs that need to be most tightly controlled are hospital admissions and volume of services provided. Negotiation of a discounted fee for primary care visits does little to control costs if the patient will be seen on a weekly basis for a condition that really needs to be followed only on a monthly basis. The introduction of DRG payments for inpatient care has also allowed managed care programs the opportunity to control use of hospital admissions. Several plans have shown a 30% reduction in the admission rate as well as a shortening of length of stay through effective utilization review and control.

CAPITATION

The quest for control of volume as well as intensity of service-related areas has led to "capitation" payments to primary care physicians. Such a system places the physician at risk to effectively manage and direct the overall care of the patient, and rewards the physician for not ordering expensive tests, reducing hospital admissions, and keeping expensive services such as specialty referral and ED visits down. Aggressive plans actually reduce payments to the primary care physician if patients go to the ED for nonemergency problems.

MANAGED CARE'S VIEW OF THE EMERGENCY DEPARTMENT

The American College of Emergency Physicians has stated that: "Emergency Medicine is practiced as patient demanded, broadly available, and continuously accessible by physicians trained to engage in the recognition, stabilization, evaluation, treatment, and disposition of patients in response to acute illness and injury. The patient population is unrestricted and presents with a full spectrum of undifferentiated and behavioral conditions."

Despite the American College of Emergency Physicians position that patients determine whether or not they have an emergency, managed care programs view the ED as an expensive place to provide care that, in 40 to 50% of cases, can be provided in physicians' offices. Although examination fees may be the same for the primary care physician and the emergency physician, the ED usually has a facility charge as well, which can result in an overall fee 2 to 3 times that of a physician's office. Obviously, this can be even higher if the ED does not participate in the plan and offer discounted fees as does the primary care physician. In addition, every patient in these programs should be assigned to a primary care physician, who should be familiar with the patient's problems. Studies indicate that care by the primary care physician results in fewer laboratory tests and x rays. It is not unusual for care provided in the ED for apparently minor problems to exceed $200 per visit.

Managed care programs have tried to implement effective disincentives for the "inappropriate" use of EDs, which include co-payments, preauthorization, and transfer of patients from nonparticipating hospitals to those that participate in the plan.

CO-PAYMENTS

As early as the mid-1960s, it has been well accepted that patients who are responsible for a percentage of their bill (co-payment) tend to be more concerned about the costs of services provided when compared to patients who have total care. How many times have we heard the battle cry, "Do everything humanly possible whatever the cost, I have insurance." Managed care programs, recognizing this as well as the great disparity in cost when care is provided in the ED, generally have a significantly larger co-payment for ED visits. If the co-payment for an office visit is $5.00, it is not unusual to see a co-payment of $20.00 for ED visits. It seems that $15 is not a large price to pay if a patient feels that he or she needs to be seen immediately or if the primary care physician's office is closed.

PREAUTHORIZATION

Recognizing the limited success of reducing ED visits through co-payments, many managed care programs have implemented preauthorization for payment of services. Patients are given a telephone number to call if they feel that they may have a condition that may warrant being seen in the ED. A physician or nurse queries the patient to determine whether or not he or she can be seen the next day in the office if the call is after normal office hours. Unfortunately, many patients do not bother to call the number and simply come to the ED seeking care, only to be told that they must have preauthorization approval.

TRANSFER TO NONPARTICIPATING HOSPITALS

It has already been discussed that the cornerstone of cost savings for any managed care program is negotiated discounts of normal fees. Obviously, because hospital admissions account for about 50% of a plan's

total costs, the greatest saving comes from not having patients admitted to nonparticipating hospitals. In addition to the preauthorization for treatment in the ED, most plans also require additional authorization if the patient needs admission. If the hospital is not participating, the program will insist that patients be transferred, even though they may be acutely and seriously ill.

ISSUES FOR EMERGENCY PHYSICIANS

Once the premise of managed care programs is understood, the emergency physician should be able to deal more effectively with the problems and issues. The basis premise that must always be recognized is that the single-minded goal of the plans is to save money, not to display any sense of fairness.

CONTRACT ISSUES

When negotiating a contract with a hospital, it is of paramount importance to spell out what the relationship will be in regard to the negotiation of managed care contracts. If the contract says that the hospital may negotiate on the group's behalf, little can be changed before the renewal of the hospital contract. Unfortunately, hospitals are not really concerned with the small slice of the pie that may go to emergency physicians.

Ideally, a group's contract with the hospital allows the group to negotiate its own contract with each managed care program. It is crucial to any successful negotiation that good data be obtained to make a case. Discounted fees may be obtained through the use of a fee schedule or a negotiated discount. Any fee schedule must be carefully reviewed and an analysis performed to determine the overall effect that such a fee schedule may have on the group's revenue. Perhaps even more importantly, it must be determined how the fee schedule is to be used and whether all the codes will be considered if submitted by the group. It is essential that the managed care program not be allowed to "downcode" services to a less expensive service. Unfortunately, this is not an uncommon practice, and is usually allowed by contract language. One program would allow a limited service code for any visit despite what was done to the patient. Additionally, only one code was allowed per patient per visit. This precludes the use of procedure codes when the patient is sutured and an examination is performed.

Discounted fees also present potential problems because unless an analysis of actual patients is performed, the discount may also have the net effect of reducing revenue. Most plans seek discounts, promising an increased volume of patients. During negotiations, it is imperative to tie the actual discount to the delivery of the increased patient visits. Most programs ask what the average percent collection is for the group and want a similar discount. It is important to remember that the discount granted to a managed care program should be no more than the actual collection percentage of patients with similar "commercial insurance." Thus, if the collection percentage on commercial insurance patients is 80%, it is not unreasonable to give a similar discount off customary fees to patients from the managed care program. Make sure that payment terms are also specified in a contract, so that timeliness of payment is tied into the discount. One particularly difficult plan wanted deep discounts and was unwilling to negotiate on price. After explaining that deep discounts in price could in fact result in a significant discount in service, that the plan would be paying for the most expensive triage service, and that patients would be told that the plan would not pay for services rendered, a reasonable discount was finally negotiated.

A group may decide not to have any contract with a managed care program. The specifics of the plan should be investigated to determine what the payment policies are regarding nonparticipating physicians. Generally, this is not usually a good alternative because it may present problems with the hospital administration regarding the overall ED contract.

PREAUTHORIZATION

Perhaps the most troubling aspect of managed care to emergency physicians is the issue of "preauthorization" for the patient to be seen. One must always keep in mind that what is being discussed is preauthorization for payment, not treatment. Recent federal legislation mandates that all patients receive a medical screening examination to determine whether an emergency condition exists. This provision applies to patients who may belong to managed care programs.

Every ED should have a clearly written policy that deals with this issue. All patients should be registered and evaluated to determine whether an emergency condition exists. If patients are denied preauthorization after triage, it should be explained to them that their plan does not cover this service and that they may be seen if desired but will be responsible for their bill. At no time should these patients be denied access to care because their plan denied authorization for payment. ED personnel should always be the patient's advocate in these issues, and care should never be determined on the basis of payment.

Although preauthorization can present problems for the ED, groups should develop open lines of communication with the managed care programs, so that issues such as problems with preauthorization can be dealt with. Once an ED group understands the concerns of the managed care program and the concerns

of the ED are known, compromise can be accomplished. Detailed data must be kept on the numbers of patients and the procedures performed if conflicts are to be resolved. The success of any program is based on the satisfaction of the patients who are enrolled.

Working together, the ED benefits by having more paying patients, and the plan will be successful because patients are satisfied with the quality of services and remain enrolled.

CAPITATION

Managed care programs may desire to pay the ED group on a capitated basis. This rate is based on a single fee for any patient regardless of what he or she presents for. Sometimes a different rate can be negotiated for admitted patients than for patients who are discharged from the ED. The only way to know whether this financial arrangement is beneficial to the group is, once again, to keep accurate data as to the number of patients, procedures performed, and charges that would have been generated if the patient had commercial insurance. This allows a direct comparison of actual collection with what would have been collected under other circumstances.

TRANSFERS TO PARTICIPATING HOSPITALS

As stated earlier, most plans wish to have their patients admitted only to participating hospitals. Sometimes the emergency physician is placed in the awkward position of being asked to transfer to another facility a patient who may not be stable enough to be transferred. A department's policies regarding transfers should be the same regardless of the reason for the transfer of the patient. Discussions with the approving physician should be carefully documented. Sometimes this physician may not be the one who will be caring for the patient at the receiving facility. Generally, discussions with this physician are not a good idea because the accepting physician at the receiving hospital should be communicated with directly. Transfer problems can be avoided by establishing policies beforehand with the managed care program. Recently, after lengthy discussions with a program, this problem was resolved by having the program send a physician to evaluate the patient and, if necessary, accompany the patient to the receiving facility.

BIBLIOGRAPHY

Cross, R.E., Jr. (ed.): Working Effectively with Managed Care Plans: Strategies for Success. Dallas, American College of Emergency Physicians, 1988.

Iglehart, J.K.: Health policy report: Medicare turns to HMO's N. Engl. J. Med. *312:*132, 1985.

Kellermann, A.L.: Too sick to wait. JAMA *266:*1123, 1991.

Kerr, H.D.: Access to emergency departments: A survey of HMO policies. Ann. Emerg. Med. *18:*274, 1989.

Knopp, R.K.: Impact of HMO's on emergency medical services (Editorial). Ann. Emerg. Med. *15:*730, 1986.

Medical Group Management Association: Going Prepaid. Denver Medical Group Management Association, 1987.

Reiser, S.J.: Administrative case rounds: Institutional policies and leaders cast in a different light. JAMA *266:*2127, 1991.

Schwartz, W.B.: The inevitable failure of current cost-containment strategies. JAMA *257:*220, 1987.

Shaw, K.N., Selbst, S.M., and Gill, F.M.: Indigent children who are denied care in the emergency department. Ann. Emerg. Med. *19:*59, 1990.

Wagner, E.R., and Hackenburg, V.J.: A Practical Guide to Physician-Sponsored HMO Development. Washington, DC, American Society of Internal Medicine, 1986.

MANAGING THE ACADEMIC EMERGENCY DEPARTMENT

Stephen J. Dresnick

CAPSULE

The challenges of the academic ED are great. The director of such a department will require a number of skills that his or her counterpart in the community ED may not possess. Academic departments have a responsibility not only to teach the latest technology but to teach it in a cost-effective and caring manner. The director of an academic department must never lose sight of the dual mission of the academic department. Clear directions and goals must be set by the director because the greater the mission's uncertainty, the greater the amount of information that must be processed to achieve the desirable results. The director of the academic department must run an efficient clinical and academic department and at the same time foster and nurture the individual growth of the resident and attending staff.

INTRODUCTION

One of the basic principles of management is to define the "mission" of an organization. Mission statements facilitate the development of effective management strategies to fulfill the goals and objectives of the organization. Community Emergency Departments (EDs) have as their mission the provision of quality patient care in a pleasant, caring, and expedient manner. The academic ED has as its mission the training of students and residents in the art and practice of the specialty of emergency medicine. The effective manager of the academic department must at all times keep in mind the dual mission of the department. It is easy to focus attention primarily on the academic mission. Even academic departments must compete in the marketplace for paying patients, and to do so, the department must not only have competitive pricing but must also provide a level of service to meet the expectations of the patients. Additionally, it is important to teach residents who will ultimately be practicing the specialty of emergency medicine that patient satisfaction is essential to the successful practice of the specialty.

If success in the present environment presents a challenge to the medical director of most EDs, the challenge of the academic ED is much greater. There are currently fewer than 80 residency programs in Emergency Medicine in the country, and most departmental chairmen were chosen on the basis of their academic experience and may have had little or no formal training in management. This chapter focuses on the aspects of departmental management unique to the academic department. Even academic departments display diversity because there are university hospitals, community hospitals, city/county hospitals and even academic departments within private institutions.

COST OF THE ACADEMIC DEPARTMENT

The cost of running an academic department is generally much greater than that of running a similarly sized nonacademic department. This is because of the additional costs of residents and additional faculty needed. At institutions that have converted from entirely attending staff to a residency program, these additional costs have approached almost $1 million. The director thus has a much larger budget than his nonacademic counterpart. Additionally, other needed programs such as research, grant development, and faculty and resident travel must be considered when developing a budget for an academic program. Most programs have dedicated or "protected" academic time for the faculty, and this has an impact on the overall number of faculty necessary to provide clinical coverage.

ROLE OF THE FACULTY

The director of the academic ED must define the role and responsibilities of the faculty. This is obviously more complex than in a department where the expectations, except for hospital committee membership, are entirely clinical. Expectations regarding research, lecture development, and publications must be formulated to properly evaluate each of the faculty at promotion time.

One of the most difficult questions regarding the role of the faculty is the degree and nature of supervision of the residents and students. Recognizing the dual mission of the academic department, it is important that patient care be attended to. Some academic departments have little actual supervision of the resident staff, and the faculty simply sign off on the charts. This practice does, in fact, have grave consequences for the faculty that practice this policy because they are legally responsible for the care of the patient and will certainly be enjoined in any lawsuit involving that patient. Although this may represent one extreme, the other extreme may in fact not allow an opportunity for the residents to develop independent thought. The Residency Review Committee for Emergency Medicine (RRC) states that residents should have increasing degrees of responsibility for patient care. Balancing this need with the appropriate degree of supervision requires great thought and management skills on the part of the director. In academic departments that bill for patient visits, the policy regarding supervision must be in compliance with federal and state regulations regarding payment by government programs to avoid problems with questioned fraud and abuse. To bill Medicare, the regulations state that the "attending must be present and supervising the procedure." Before implementing a billing system for an academic department, it is recommended that appropriate legal counsel be obtained.

FACULTY DEVELOPMENT

One of the responsibilities of the head of the academic department is faculty development. Considering the small number of academic programs and the relative youth of the specialty of emergency medicine, the director of an academic program quickly learns that his faculty does not have much experience in teaching residents and is certainly not familiar with the administrative issues that must be dealt with. A program to develop faculty members must be instituted by the director. Topics include educational techniques as well as motivational techniques. Research methods should also be included in such a program. Each faculty member must also be aware of the current requirements of the RRC.

Each faculty member needs to be evaluated as to the various aspects of his or her responsibilities. This process is both time-consuming and difficult for the director. Each faculty member must be motivated to maximize his or her own potential. Yearly or even quarterly goals and objectives should be established for each member of the faculty. Unlike the customary hourly rate paid by the community hospital ED, the salary of the academic attending is established on criteria other than clinical hours. These may include a share of the research grants the faculty member can bring to the department. Other criteria may also include quality of teaching and participation in nonclinical department activities such as residency program administration. If a bonus system is in place, it will of necessity include these other areas in addition to patient fees that are generated. The director should be warned to place significant emphasis on the nonclinical activities of the faculty and base salary incentives on the other tasks that need to be accomplished. Directors of several community hospital-based programs have discovered that it is difficult to motivate the faculty to participate in nonclinical activities if their salary and bonuses are based solely on their clinical hours. For this reason, each faculty member should have a certain number of "protected" teaching hours, and specific objectives must be delineated and met to receive salary advances and bonuses.

RESEARCH

The RRC has determined that ongoing significant research is an essential component for any residency program in emergency medicine. The director of an academic department must oversee the research objectives of the department, including the quality and publishability of the findings. Laboratory space must be obtained and managed in a fiscally sound manner. Cuts in federal grants have made the funding of research more competitive. It is not unusual for an academic institution to have professional grant writers in an effort to gain the competitive edge. Department survival may depend on the director's ability to secure grants.

Research in emergency medicine often involves human studies, and the director of the department must coordinate such projects with ongoing patient care. Such research often involves consent forms as well as time-consuming tests. Patients and staff must be made aware of both the methods and objectives of the department's research.

Once research projects are completed, scientific papers must need to be written and submitted for publication. The publication of an original article is becoming increasingly difficult as more institutions are producing quality research. The director must oversee the quality and scientific accuracy of the articles because, once published, they will stand as a reflection of the individual program.

RESIDENT RECRUITMENT

The recruitment of quality residents is time-consuming and difficult. Although the program may have a designated residency director, the ultimate success of resident recruitment lies with the departmental director. Programs are judged by the eventual success of the graduating residents. Quality residents also aid in the departmental research and publication objectives. It is important that there be a fit between resident staff and attending staff. It is not uncommon for a program to have over 500 applications for 8 residency spots. Simply sorting through applications to determine the 50 to 75 candidates who will be invited for an interview is a difficult task. The director must establish criteria for selection and ensure that the work is performed in a timely manner. For a residency program, the ultimate embarrassment is not to match all of the first-year spots.

A significant amount of resident recruitment will occur as senior students rotate through the department during the year. Many will come from other academic centers. This process, although coming into some disfavor among medical school deans, is a valuable method of candidate evaluation. The director must ensure that this is a quality experience because the candidate will also be evaluating the program at the same time as the faculty is evaluating the student.

QUALITY ASSURANCE

A quality assurance (QA) program in a community hospital is relatively easy compared to a similar program in an academic setting. It is important that the program define exactly who is being audited as well as the ultimate responsibility of the faculty. Ideally, both the resident staff and the attending staff are evaluated. QA is becoming increasingly important for credentialing. Such use of QA information can and should be included in resident evaluations. Because of the dual mission of the academic department, the director may also wish to use QA data as a yardstick to measure the quality of the teaching being provided by the attending staff.

PATIENT CARE

As stated earlier, the academic department cannot ignore patient care. Although it is tempting to make excuses for suboptimal patient care and long waits in the interest of the educational experience, this is no longer possible. Much attention has been focused on resident work hours and supervision over the past few years. The state of New York has even adopted regulations limiting resident work hours and delineating acceptable supervision of residents. Such criteria are now being addressed by Residency Review Committees in all specialties. The special essentials for each specialty are changed to address these concerns in the near future.

BIBLIOGRAPHY

Chernow, S.M., Emerman, C.L., Langdorf, M., and Schultz, C.: Academic emergency medicine: A national profile with and without emergency medicine residency programs (abstract). Ann. Emerg. Med. *19*:962, 1990.
Gallery, M.E., Allison, E.J., Mitchell, J.M., and Williams, R.: Manpower needs in academic emergency medicine. Ann. Emerg. Med. *19*:107, 1990.
Ling, L.L.: Attaining academic department status for emergency medicine within medical schools. Ann. Emerg. Med. *19*:103, 1990.
McHugh, P.P.: Cost awareness in an emergency medicine residency program (abstract). Ann. Emerg. Med. *19*:494, 1991.
Zun, L., Chen, E., Carrison, D.M., et al.: Longitudinal study of emergency physician wellness: Initial impressions (abstract). Ann. Emerg. Med. *19*:496, 1990.

EDUCATION IN EMERGENCY DEPARTMENTS

Sheldon Jacobson

CAPSULE

This discussion of education in emergency departments (EDs) is restricted to the training of house staff, both emergency medicine house staff and the nonemergency house staff rotating to the emergency department. With some modification, such training can be used in the emergency department clerkship of medical students.

Education of physicians in the ED can be approached on a number of levels, and one can easily make a list of the cognitive and psychomotor skills that are basic to clinical training in emergency medicine.[1-5] It is our view, however, that training in emergency medicine must be responsive to certain more basic issues that deal with modifying the clinical behavior of our trainees. *These issues include the education of physicians in the acquisition and use of a limited data base to* make rapid and effective bedside decisions[6-8]; the analysis and use of test data with clear understanding of the sensitivity, specificity, and predictive value of such tests[9]; and a grasp of primary care issues as well as of critical care problems. The appropriate use of consultants in the emergency department is a key area that needs to be addressed.

INTRODUCTION

The functioning of the entire emergency medical services (EMS) system should be incorporated into the training program. This includes direct observation and, if possible, direct clinical experience in delivery of emergency care in the streets. Because the managerial and administrative aspects of running an ED are almost always underemphasized in residency training programs, an administrative rotation should be incorporated into the curriculum. Finally, and perhaps most importantly, the training should make the house officer aware of the matter of stress and stress management and of his or her own responses to stress.

Designing a training program with appropriate objectives requires a clear definition of the mission of the ED. There are two polarized perceptions and another, more middle-of-the-road concept. There are those who think that emergency medicine is a critical care specialty, with blurring and integration into the function of a critical care or shock trauma unit.[10] The opposite view is that the emergency department functions as an extension of the primary care specialties and provides episodic primary care.[11,12] My own view is that there are aspects of emergency medicine that support both contentions. I think it preferable to clearly delineate the primary care and critical care aspects in planning an educational program so that both areas receive commensurate attention in the emergency department formal educational program. Once delineated, they are taught in an integrated manner.

It is also our view that education in the ED should not consist simply of teaching discrete subjects to ED trainees. It is all too easy to compartmentalize the didactic material and to present the information as a series of lectures. Such lectures are now standard throughout the country. Actually, we have reviewed the ED triage transactions and found that there are really only 32 different complaint groups with which patients present.[13] Thus, in almost every ED lecture series, there are talks on the diagnosis of the red eye, the approach to a patient with a pneumothorax, and so forth. Although it is important to know how to diagnose and treat the entities causing a painful red eye, this information is available in a number of excellent sources (e.g., ophthalmology texts, primary care texts, and emergency medicine volumes). In our view, formal talks dedicated to these topics may actually take time from more important educational issues.

TRAINING IN DECISION MAKING

The lessons that we feel are the most important to learn from an ED experience relate to the techniques involved in gathering a specific limited data base on the critically ill or injured patient and using this data base in patient-care decision making.[6-8] Hundreds of decisions are made by the emergency physician every week, and most of these are important in terms of prognosis or outcome. Considering this opportunity to develop one's diagnostic and therapeutic skills, we find it lamentable that frequently so little attention is given to the decision-making process itself. This leads to muddled thinking, inappropriate evaluation, and, most regrettably, patient mismanagement. Yet this decision-making process is basic to emergency medicine (and to all clinical medicine for that matter), making it even more lamentable that it is so often relegated to a minor position in medical education in favor of lectures on discrete subjects. One can always read a book or journal article on such topics, but the opportunity to develop analytic skills and gain confidence in their application may not recur.

In the ED, our decisions frequently lead to actions that are not easily reversed if they are incorrect. Thus, in the ED we do not have the same series of checks, rechecks, and consultation available to the hospitalized patient. The results of our decisions can be devastating to the patient if we are wrong. How to make appropriate effective patient care decisions with a limited data base becomes the most important issue in emergency care.

It follows from the previous observations that training in clinical decision making is our predominant educational mission. How then do we attempt to reach our goals? The major device that we use at our institution is a bedside review of each case with the junior house staff and medical students. Almost all cases passing through our department are seen by a junior house officer and an attending physician. This allows instantaneous feedback regarding the quality of the limited data base obtained and allows the attending physician to compare his data base with that of the house officer. There is usually some give-and-take during these discussions, when we present our individual approaches to data gathering and to the development of decision trees or clinical algorithms. In these discussions, we present our approach to the galaxy of medical information so that resources can be vectored to deal with those entities with potentially serious prognostic significance. Thus, in patients presenting with a rash, we are concerned with life-threatening entities such as pemphigus and exfoliative erythroderma as well as with dermatologic manifestations of internal disease (e.g., the purpura of meningococcemia).

We also spend much time discussing the patient's presentation and the differential diagnostic and therapeutic possibilities. We relate these to the patient's current medical condition and ultimate prognosis for both survival and quality of life. This sophisticated deductive process requires extensive knowledge of medicine, surgery, pathophysiology, and, frequently, psychiatry. This process is also difficult to teach because it consists mainly of abstract thinking, although most of the analyses can be recorded in algorithmic format. If potentially life-threatening problems or processes cannot be ruled out, the differential diagnosis cannot move on to less significant entities. The patient must be treated as if he or she has the most serious entity until that entity has been satisfactorily ruled out. This often necessitates hospitalizing such patients—a proportion of whom are later found to have less significant diagnoses.

Integral to the decision-making process is the appropriate use of laboratory data.[14] The practitioner must learn to use such data, but with restraint. The questions being asked of the test should be appropriate to the study, and the results interpreted in the context of the known sensitivity, specificity, and predictive value of these tests. Unnecessary tests are costly and can be misleading. Using a statistical approach to patient laboratory data is dangerous because we do not have a universe of patients to treat, and on any given occasion the test may be positive or negative consequent to statistical variability and not necessarily to the presence of an active disease process. Thus, laboratory data should be used to support our diagnostic impression and not to make the diagnosis in and of itself.

In a few situations, our diagnostic abilities are limited and a laboratory test assumes a leading role in our decision making. For example, the venogram is used in diagnosing deep venous thrombosis, the pulmonary arteriogram is helpful in diagnosing some patients with suspected pulmonary embolization, and the serum radioimmunoassay is valuable in diagnosing early pregnancy.

A mandatory concomitant of this educational process is proximate patient follow-up. We could be making serious errors in our ED and not hear about them until it is too late. It is essential that our trainees arrange the follow-up of their patients who are discharged from the ED. In some cases, a simple telephone call is all that is needed; in others, return to the ED is mandatory. For patients admitted to hospital, inpatient follow-up rounds are invaluable educationally and represent sound ED practice.

Retrospective review of cases and auditing of charts for form and process have, in our opinion, limited value as teaching tools. Although there are legal and informational aspects of the medical record, quality of care and quality of the record cannot be equated. Proximate outcome is the golden standard for auditing quality of emergency department practice. Although criteria for proximate outcome are controversial, certain outcomes are obviously indicators of poor decision-making.

Even though we deplore routine behavior that ignores the needs of the individual, there are certain areas in which the deductive analytical process may be too time-consuming and perhaps disconcerting. Thus, in one's approach to resuscitation of the cardiac arrest or trauma victim, the major initial actions should be conventional to ensure that the hierarchy of priorities is adhered to and are dealt with swiftly. There is little time for developing an extensive data base or, for that matter, innovative decision-making. Later on, the decision-making process can be individualized to meet specific patient needs.

USE OF CONSULTANTS

Part of the educational process in the ED is the training of practitioners to be selective in their interactions with consulting services. This relates once again to our decision-making activities and calls heavily on our knowledge of the important diagnostic entities in the consultant's purview. An emergency physician should rarely call a consultant because he does not know what to do. A consultant is called when the emergency physician has decided that what has to be done requires admission to the hospital or entails a procedure that he or she feels is necessary but is not authorized to perform. Use of consultants in this manner also leads to effective patient care because the consultant is more likely to accept the data already generated and to proceed from that point rather than re-evaluate the patient completely. It also leads to recognition of the emergency physician as a highly skilled professional, a not-inconsequential issue in some academic centers.

Although we are predominantly interested in the acutely ill patient, we do have a responsibility as part of our primary care activities to look for and treat some major public health problems, and care should be clearly delineated as an area in which the emergency physician should play a dominant role. Although we certainly need input from pediatricians, cardiologists, and traumatologists, it is with our expertise as emergency practitioners that we must set priorities and standards, develop treatment protocols, train paramedics and EMTs, direct prehospital care from our base stations, and audit the quality of prehospital medical care.[15] To play this dominant role in EMS systems, our emergency medicine residents must spend time with the prehospital care providers (e.g., accompanying paramedics in ambulances). It is this experience that will allow them to make realistic judgments relating to training programs for ambulance personnel, to drug treatment protocols, and to the quality of prehospital care. During this prehospital training module, residents should also become conversant with disaster plans and responses in their regions.

Medical knowledge is accruing at an astonishing rate, so that a good deal of what is taught in a residency training program as basic clinical medicine may be obsolete in 10 years. Because our specialty encompasses so many disciplines, "keeping up" is extremely difficult. Clearly, the practitioner in an academic setting has a greater opportunity to gain up-to-date information than does the emergency medicine physician practicing in a community or a nontraining site; however, the mass of material is so huge that for all emergency physicians a systematic process of continuing medical education must be initiated during the period of residency training.

IMPORTANCE OF CLINICAL RESEARCH

If the discipline of emergency medicine is to continue to prosper and gain full academic recognition, it must have a foundation based on critical analysis of its activities. This requires an ongoing clinical research component in most, if not all, training sites.[16–18] It is also essential that we develop laboratory-oriented research grounded in the basic sciences. An introduction to the methods of clinical and basic research should be part of the required curriculum for training house officers. This experience should provide trainees with the basics of experimental design and data analysis.

PHYSICIAN STRESS AND "BURNOUT"

Finally, we need to prepare our trainees to cope with and function under the stress inherent in EDs. Stress recognition and management[16] is a relatively new area that has received a good deal of attention. Stress can manifest itself in the emergency physician in a number of forms. In its early phases, the individual may perceive what is called "functioning under pressure." If this pressure is not recognized and dealt with appropriately, it can lead to depression, anxiety, and physician "burnout." It can certainly impair one's effectiveness and lead to chronic dissatisfaction with emergency medicine.[22]

How one goes about teaching physicians to deal with stress is difficult to set forth briefly, but it certainly begins with recognition of stress by the physician. Once the stress is recognized, a number of responses can be assessed. It seems obvious that, in some EDs, the physician's work schedule in and of itself can lead to unacceptable stress levels. It is not uncommon for emergency physicians to work a 12-hour or, on some occasions, a 24-hour tour of duty. It is indeed likely that we encourage this type of behavior by scheduling our trainees to work such long hours during their residency.

A major factor in coping with stress is adequate time off from duty. Frequent short vacations can be therapeutic and should not be thought of as a luxury. A mutually supportive staff can go a long way toward dissipating stress. Short periods of quiet meditation may work for some individuals.

Training in emergency medicine is still in a formative state and requires ongoing definition, evaluation, and reassessment. In the final analysis, it will be our trainees who will bring these activities into fruition.[17] We must provide them with the background with which they can meet the challenges ahead.

The increasing discussion about educational approaches and integrating disease care with care of the ailing patient is extremely useful in definition.[19–21] The immediate beneficiary of such honing of education is the undergraduate and resident in emergency medicine, but in a larger sense, we are still redefining the ranges of our field for community and academic practice.

REFERENCES

1. Levy, R., and Anwar, R.A.: Orientation program for emergency medicine residents. JACEP 8:46, 1979.
2. Frey, D.F., and Mangold, K.: Curriculum for the second career physician in emergency medicine. JACEP 4:29, 1975.
3. American College of Emergency Physicians: Core content in emergency medicine. JACEP 8:34, 1979.
4. Hamilton, G.C.: Adaptation of the emergency medicine core content to a three-year residency core curriculum. Ann. Emerg. Med. 10:259, 1981.
5. Standards for graduate training in emergency medicine. JACEP 8:32, 1979.
6. Albert, D.A.: Decision theory in medicine: Milbank Mem. Fund Q. 56:362, 1978.
7. Gorry, G.A.: New prospectives in the art of clinical decision making. Am. J. Clin. Pathol. 75:483, 1981.
8. Jacobson, S.: Decision-making in the emergency department. Comprehensive Ther. 11:16, 1985.
9. Griner, P.F., Mayewski, R.J., and Mushlin, A.I.: Selection and interpretation of diagnostic tests and procedures. Principles and applications. Ann. Intern Med. 94:557, 1981.
10. Wagner, D.K.: Critical care medicine and the emergency physician: Ann. Emerg. Med. 11:49, 1982.
11. Walker, L.L.: The emergency department—entry point into the health care system. JACEP 4:129, 1975.
12. Walker, L.L.: Traditional vs. contemporary attitudes: How emergency department patients view the health care system. JACEP 4:211, 1975.
13. Jacobson, S., and Bell, B.: Triage in the emergency department. In Pascarelli, E. (ed.): Hospital-Based Ambulatory Care. East Norwalk, Conn., Appleton-Century-Crofts, 1982.
14. Sims, J.K.: Advanced trauma life support, pilot implementation and evaluation. JACEP 8:150, 1979.
14a. Iserson, K.V., and Shepherd, C.: Teaching emergency department administration, the in-basket exercise. JACEP 8:114, 1979.
15. The role of the physician in mobile emergency systems. JACEP 3:156, 1973.
16. Wagner, D.K., and Anwar R.A.: The research component in the development of emergency medicine as a specialty. J. Med. Educ. 52:55, 1977.
17. Anwar, R.A., and Hogan, M.H.: Residency-trained emergency physicians: Where have all the flowers gone? JACEP 8:84, 1979.
18. Gibson, G., and Gann, D.S.: Health services research as a management tool in the emergency department. JACEP 5:40, 1976.
19. Tintinalli, J.E.: The strengths and weaknesses of undergraduate education in emergency medicine. Ann. Emerg. Med. 19:1187, 1990.
20. Hedges, J.R.: The role of undergraduate education in emergency medicine. Ann. Emerg. Med. 19:1187, 1990.
21. Rosenzweig, S.: The other half of the curriculum. Ann. Emerg. Med. 20:591, 1991.
22. Gallery, M.E., et al.: A study of occupational stress and depression among emergency physicians. Ann. Emerg. Med. 21:58, 1992.

OCCUPATIONAL MEDICINE

George R. Schwartz

> **CAPSULE**
>
> As emergency medicine has developed, there has been a trend toward subspecialization in areas including toxicology and EMS systems. Occupational medicine is also an area of increased focus for emergency physicians.

Occupational medicine, a natural outgrowth of the emergency department (ED), is an area that is clearly underserved. The Institute of Medicine Subcommittee on the Physician Shortage in Occupational and Environmental Medicine concluded that there is a shortage of 3100 to 5500 physicians in this area.[1,2] Although the role of a physician working in this area often varies substantially from the more rapid pace of recognition and response in the ED, many environmental conditions, when left untreated, become emergencies. For example, ongoing toxic exposure in the workplace may manifest as an attack of asthma or an acute dermatologic condition.

Occupational and environmental medicine is developing because of need rather than major commitment from medical centers or academic leadership. Therefore, it resembles emergency medicine as a specialty based primarily on patient and community need. *Environmental medicine* incorporates most, but not all, aspects of occupational medicine and also includes understanding and treatment of the myriad physical, biologic, and chemical agents encountered both inside and outside the workplace. Occupational medicine shares the need to know areas of toxicology, epidemiology, public health and preventive medicine, but the focus tends to be more narrow, dealing with companies and professions and the particular health aspects of these facilities. For example, a physician specializing in health aspects of aviation and pilots may well be concerned with the risks of air pollution for jet engines and carbon monoxide levels in workers, but is ordinarily little concerned about the general problems of air pollution within a city.

Although the need is great, obstacles in the practice of occupational medicine should be addressed. Frequently the physician is working for an employer, and therefore the usual physician-patient relationship becomes physician–employer–patient. Not only does this facet alter the ability and desire of patients to reveal important but potentially harmful (in terms of employment) information such as drug or alcohol use; it places the physician in possible adversarial relationships involving workman's compensations claims and disability evaluations.

Such difficulties can be mitigated through careful planning and need not be permanent obstacles. For example, there can be assurances of confidentiality and, when adversarial situations arise, they can be referred to another physician who is independent of the employer-employee relationship.

On a practical level, although specialists are needed in occupational and environmental medicine as educators, researchers and skilled clinicians, the current financial environment mandates clinical focus on them as the only ones substantially reimbursed or funded at this time. Emergency physicians who can provide occupational medicine services can alternate them with ED practice if such practice can provide a needed hiatus when a change of pace is needed or desired (e.g., pregnancy, life-style needs, etc.)

The current situation is dynamic as to special certifications. Only the American Board of Preventive Medicine provides specialist certification, and various boards (ABIM, ABFP, ABEM) are considering certificates of special competence.[3]

There is a movement within emergency medicine to offer such certificates in special competence. This would mean an increased focus on such concerns not only in Annals of Emergency Medicine and other journals for specialists in the field, but increased focus at national and specialty meetings.

As with many changes of subspecialization, other modifications are necessary to blend a practice of occupational medicine with that of emergency medicine, including equipment needs (e.g., special hearing tests or laboratory capability to test for certain types of exposures) and intellectual needs. An example of the latter is the focus on each employer to determine specific medical needs and hazards and to tailor-make programs that can offer the most benefit, as well as to offer emergency treatment of minor injuries.

The effort has already been effective in many locations. In view of the stress and "burnout" potential of working solely in the ED for more than 10 years and the higher numbers of emergency physicians planning to leave the field, it seems not only useful but helpful to retain physicians within the field and provide the change of pace often believed to be an antidote to burnout.[4]

This development in emergency medicine meets a demonstrated need for occupational and environmental physicians and offers a model for handling occupational stress within its own specialty.

REFERENCES

1. Castorina, J., and Rosenstock, L.: Physician shortage in occupational and environmental medicine. Ann. Intern. Med. *113:*983, 1990.

2. Institute of Medicine Report Addressing the Physician Shortage in Occupational and Environmental Medicine. Washington, D.C., National Academy Press, 1991.

3. Rosenstock, L., et al.: Occupational and environmental medicine—Meeting the growing need for clinical services. N. Engl. J. Med. *325:*924, 1991.

4. Gallery, M.E., et al.: A study of occupational stress and depression among emergency physicians. Ann. Emerg. Med. *21:*58, 1992.

Part XIV

Medicolegal Aspects of Emergency Care

Chapter 89

MEDICOLEGAL ASPECTS OF EMERGENCY CARE

MEDICOLEGAL CONSIDERATIONS IN EMERGENCY CARE: GENERAL PRINCIPLES AND DEFINITIONS

James E. George

CAPSULE

This chapter is intended to present the reader with an overview of some of the medicolegal problems of the practice of emergency medicine. Certain recommendations and conclusions can be stated. First, the ever-present threat of a malpractice suit dictates that all emergency physicians and nurses carry adequate professional liability insurance. Second, emergency physicians and nurses should be qualified to practice modern emergency medicine and should maintain those qualifications. Third, the emergency department (ED) must be granted appropriate recognition within the hospital bureaucracy as the "doorway" to the hospital.

INTRODUCTION AND BACKGROUND

Whether there is a malpractice "problem" in emergency medicine is a subject of some debate. Both the patient turned plaintiff and the emergency physician named defendant share a common perception, however—each believes that he or she has been wronged. The plaintiff may blame an "incompetent" physician, and the physician may characterize his former patient as "litigious" or the victim of a "greedy attorney."

The complex problem of malpractice litigation has no easy solution. With an understanding of the general principles of law that apply to emergency care, however, routine treatment encounters may become

less likely to result in a subsequent legal encounter.

Regardless of the magnitude of the malpractice problem, the practical fact remains that most physicians, especially those in EDs, have consciously or unconsciously modified their practice habits to make some provision for the practice of "defensive medicine." The high-pressure environment of the practice of modern emergency medicine affords inadequate time for leisurely diagnosis and consultation when in doubt. An unceasing flow of patients in search of immediate treatment, attended by various emotionally strained family members and friends, keeps ED staff in a state of constant tension. This environment contains many pitfalls of which the professional should be aware.

The outcome of a legal case depends on the particular facts of the case in question, and changing one peculiar item can result in an entirely different legal outcome. Because statutory law and case law vary from state to state, the reader should exercise caution in strictly applying general legal information to his or her own personal or professional legal problems. Although this chapter acknowledges basic legal concepts that can be applied broadly for general guidance, the appropriate state statute books and local counsel should be consulted for specific legal advice when necessary.

NEGLIGENCE

Medical malpractice is synonymous with professional medical negligence, a specific tort action within the broad area of law known as civil law. Law in the United

States generally is divided into criminal and civil. Criminal law involves a legal action filed by a state or by the United States against a particular offending individual or individuals and deals with the definition of crimes and their punishments. Civil law involves legal actions brought by one individual against other individuals. Contracts, domestic relations, and torts are some examples of the subdivisions included in the broad category of civil law. Civil wrongs committed by an individual against another individual are called *torts*. A particular tort or civil wrong can also constitute a criminal wrong, such as assault and battery. This subjects the offending individual to both civil and criminal liability for the act committed. The tort of *negligence* is the particular tort with which physicians are usually concerned, for herein lies malpractice.

Black's Law Dictionary (West Publishing Co., 4th ed., 1951) defines negligence as "the omission to do something which a reasonable man, guided by those ordinary considerations which ordinarily regulate human affairs, would do, or the doing of something which a reasonable and prudent man would not do." Conduct that fails to meet a standard of care recognized in the law for the protection of others against unreasonable risks of harm can generally be said to constitute negligence. The law expects all citizens to conduct their personal and business affairs in a reasonable manner to protect others from unnecessary harm. This rule of conduct applies to all activities, from driving an automobile to performing professional tasks. A physician may be liable for professional negligence when his or her conduct fails to meet an accepted standard of care in his profession and a patient is damaged as a result.

Four particular elements must be alleged and proved in a court of law to sustain a lawsuit for negligence brought by a complaining party (the plaintiff) against the offending party (the defendant). These elements of negligence include duty, breach of duty, damages, and proximate cause. If the plaintiff fails to prove any one of these four elements, his or her suit for negligence will not be sustained.

DUTY AND ITS BREACH

The plaintiff in a negligence action must prove that the defendant owed the plaintiff a duty to use due care. The court usually looks to the relationship between the parties to determine whether there is a duty of due care owed the plaintiff by the defendant. The health practitioner's duty (whether he or she is a physician, nurse, technician, or other health care professional) arises from a health care relationship with the patient.

From this health practitioner–patient relationship evolves the duty to conduct oneself according to the standard of care expected of a reasonably trained, prudent health practitioner confronting the same or similar circumstances. The duty of due care of the "reasonable man" was at one time confined by the courts to the particular locality in which the individual practiced and was known as the "locality rule." Therefore, if one practiced in a university setting, one was held to the standard of care of the university medical center, and one practicing in a rural area was held to the standard of care of the rural practitioner in that locality. Developments in communications and in modern medicine have gradually prompted the courts to discard the locality rule and to hold that the United States comprises one medical community nationwide. Courts are increasingly recognizing the applicability of national standards rather than a standard of care that may be peculiar to the defendant physician's geographic locality.

Breach of duty, whereby an individual's conduct does not comply with the anticipated, reasonable standard of care, can occur by way of *malfeasance* when an *affirmative act* does not comport with the acceptable standard of care. Breach of duty also can occur by *nonfeasance* when *failure to act* results in damages to a patient that could have been avoided by initiation of appropriate action in compliance with acceptable medical practice under the circumstances. Failure to resuscitate a patient in cardiopulmonary arrest, when good medical practice would have dictated that he or she *should* be resuscitated, is an example of breach of duty and negligence by nonfeasance.

DAMAGES

The third element the plaintiff must prove is that he or she sustained damages by virtue of the alleged negligence. If an individual has not been damaged in some discernible fashion, he or she will not be successful in a suit for negligence. Monetary damages are an integral part of a suit for negligence because the purpose of such civil redress is to obtain some financial award from the court for the damages suffered. A patient would not have a viable suit for negligence, for example, if he or she unknowingly received an erroneous medication that caused him or her absolutely no ill effects whatever. If there have been no damages, the court will not entertain an action for negligence.

CAUSATION

The last necessary element of negligence is *proximate cause*. Black's Law Dictionary defines proximate cause as "that which, in a natural and continuous sequence, unbroken by an efficient intervening cause, produces the injury, and without which the result would not have occurred." The following is a clinical example of proximate cause. If a patient trips in the ED, bruises a knee, and sues for a myocardial infarction 3 months later, he or she would be hard pressed to prove proximate cause in a suit for negligence. If, however, the patient's myocardial infarction occurred moments after his or her fall in the ED, he or she would have a much better basis for proving proximate cause. The latter requires that there be some reasonable cause-and-effect relationship between the act complained of and the damages sustained by the patient.

The legal concept of proximate cause has acted as a limitation on the liability of a defendant for effects traceable to alleged negligence. In the 1980s, plaintiffs' attorneys have successfully convinced courts in some jurisdictions that plaintiffs face difficult burdens in proving proximate cause in certain types of medical malpractice cases. As a result, the courts in some jurisdictions have transformed the legal concept of proximate cause. Consider the following scenario: A trauma patient arrives in the hospital ED department at 1:00 A.M. At 4:45 A.M., it is determined that the patient must be taken to the operating room. The patient dies at 4:50 A.M., and resuscitation efforts are unsuccessful. In the subsequent lawsuit, the patient's estate alleges that the emergency physician was negligent in not diagnosing the patient's condition in time. The plaintiffs allege that, had certain diagnostic tests been done, the patient would have been taken to the operating room by 2:30 A.M., and probably would have survived. If the allegation of negligence is supported by expert testimony, the court may ask the jury to determine whether the defendant's failure to perform certain diagnostic tests increased the risk of harm to the patient, and whether the alleged negligence was a substantial factor in causing the death.

Under the traditional concepts of proximate cause, the plaintiff has the burden of proving that the negligence was the proximate cause of death. Under the more "relaxed" concept of proximate cause, all that must be proved is that the alleged negligence deprived the patient of a chance to survive.

OTHER GENERAL LEGAL PRINCIPLES

RES IPSA LOQUITUR

One of many legal principles that has been a cause of concern for the medical profession has been the doctrine of *res ipsa loquitur*, a Latin phrase that means "the thing speaks for itself." This legal doctrine evolved through time as a mechanism to assist a plaintiff in recovering damages in the face of circumstances in which it would be almost impossible for him or her to prove all the elements of negligence. An example in which *res ipsa loquitur* applies in a clinical situation is the patient who enters the surgical suite for a routine appendectomy and later awakens in the recovery room paralyzed from the waist down. It would be almost impossible for the patient to prove negligence because he or she was asleep during the time the unexpected paralysis occurred.

For the plaintiff to raise *res ipsa loquitur* on his or her behalf, he or she must prove that damages would not have occurred in the absence of somebody's negligence, that the instruments that caused the damage must have been under the defendant's control at all times, and that the patient must not have done anything that could have contributed to his or her own injury. When the plaintiff accomplishes this task, the legal effect is to shift the burden of proof from the plaintiff to the defendant, who must now prove that he was not negligent. Some courts have applied and misapplied this doctrine broadly, resulting in an injudicious expansion of the doctrine of *res ipsa loquitur*.

When there are multiple defendants, the burden of proof is placed on each defendant to exonerate himself or herself or prove the negligence of another party.

STATUTE OF LIMITATIONS

How long may a patient wait to file a complaint for negligence? The answer depends on each state's peculiar statute of limitations, which is a law formulated on the thesis that it is against public policy to let the threat of a lawsuit linger forever. The time limit thus placed upon the period during which a complaint may be filed in court depends on the type of complaint filed, such as a contract action or a tort action. Statutes of limitations for negligence actions are usually 2 to 3 years. If a plaintiff fails to file the action within the period allowed by the statute of limitations, the court will prevent him or her from doing so thereafter. A key factor here is to know when the limiting time period actually begins to run. Some states permit it to start when the negligent act occurred, whereas other states regard it as beginning when the patient actually discovers that a negligent act has been committed against him. In the case of minors, the statute of limitations does not begin to run until they are emancipated or reach the age of majority, which is 18 years of age in some states and 21 in others. A court may consider a minor legally emancipated if he or she marries or is economically independent of his or her family.

AGENCY LAW

An analysis of the law of agency may be important in sorting out liability in the area of emergency medicine. The hospital emergency department cast of characters includes physicians, nurses, the hospital administration, and a variety of other health care providers. Relationships often found among these individuals include employer-employee and independent contractor relationships. It is important to determine the exact nature of the relationship among the aforementioned persons so that the legal liabilities of the parties involved may be defined.

In some cases, the liability falls entirely on one party, whereas in others the liability may be shared to different degrees among the parties involved. The ED staff should be aware of the legal rule that each individual is responsible for his or her own torts, regardless of whether he or she is an independent contractor, employee, or other involved party. Also, an employee's torts committed within the scope of his or her employment can render the employer vicariously liable. The torts of an independent contractor, however, generally are not imputed to the employer if the latter has no significant control over the actions of the independent contractor.

In some jurisdictions, the courts have permitted plaintiffs to sue hospitals for the alleged negligence of emergency physicians who are independent contractors. These courts have relied on a legal doctrine of "ostensible agency," reasoning that the public assumes that the emergency physician is a hospital employee.

In 1985, as part of the Consolidated Budget Reconciliation Act, Congress passed legislation (42 USCA Section 1395) intended to restrict the denial of emergency care and transfer of patients for economic reasons (a practice referred to as "patient dumping"). The law requires hospitals with EDs to assess all persons presenting with emergency medical conditions or who are in active labor. A hospital or physician who knowingly transfers an unstable patient or a patient in active labor is subject to civil monetary penalties. Patients who claim personal injury as a result of such transfer, which violates the federal law, may also sue for an award of money damages in federal or state courts. The law also permits hospitals that have incurred financial loss as a result of patient dumping to sue the transferring hospital to recover its losses.

In 1989, amendments to the antidumping law were made part of the Omnibus Reconciliation Act. The Health Care Financing Administration (HCFA) issues regulations that provide more definitive statements of the requirements of the law regarding patient transfers.

The aforementioned legal maxims are subject to as many variables as can be created by the unique facts of each case. Whenever a lawsuit is brought against the hospital and its professional staff, the attorneys for both the hospital and the physicians or nurses inevitably begin analyzing the facts to show that responsibility rests exclusively with the other party. Also, in this day of increasingly inaccessible malpractice insurance, attorneys for the insurance company frequently attempt to deny liability for damages.

The only conclusion that can be safely drawn is that the plaintiff will attempt to join all possible defendants in a negligence suit to ensure recovery from somebody. If the plaintiff wins, the court may instruct the defendants and their attorneys to decide among themselves who will pay for what portion of the damages.

DUTY TO PROVIDE EMERGENCY CARE

Under the common law, neither the physician nor the private hospital had an affirmative duty to render medical treatment. As a result, it was possible for private hospitals and some public hospitals to refuse to admit a patient for emergency treatment. This situation has been reversed as a result of important judicial decisions and federal legislation designed to prohibit the denial of emergency care because of inability to pay.

An important case leading to this change was *Wilmington General Hospital v. Manlove*, 174 A.2d. 135 (S. Ct., Delaware, 1961). In this case the parents of a 4-month-old infant with a recent history of fever and diarrhea brought the child to the hospital ED. Because the child had been under the care of private pediatricians, no physician or nurse examined or treated the child. The child was sent home by the nurse, who explained to the parents that the hospital's policy was to decline emergency treatment to persons already under the care of a private physician. Shortly thereafter, the child died of bronchopneumonia.

The key issue before the court was whether the hospital had a duty to provide emergency treatment in the face of an unmistakable emergency. The Court held that it did. The hospital's liability was based primarily on the parents' reliance on the hospital's capacity to render emergency care and on the fact that this was a case that could be held to involve an unmistakable emergency. In the case of *Guerrero v. Copper Queen Hospital*, 537 P.2d 1329 (1975), this principle was extended to require a private, proprietary hospital in Arizona to treat any emergency patient requesting such care, including nonresident aliens who may have entered the country solely for the purpose of obtaining treatment. This decision, and others of its kind, have fostered an "open door" hospital emergency department policy.

Federal legislation, such as the Hill-Burton Act, limited a hospital's ability to refuse to render care. A hospital that has received a Hill-Burton grant from the Federal government has the responsibility to provide a certain amount of "free" medical care for indigent patients.

Therefore, it is clear that hospital EDs and emergency practitioners have a positive duty to render treatment to persons in need of it. Hospitals have found that one of the best means of assuming these increased responsibilities is to staff EDs with practitioners who specialize in emergency medicine. In fact, the responsibilities are so great that any hospital that does not have a qualified emergency physician on duty in the ED might conceivably find that it is unable to discharge its full legal duty to the public.

PROBLEM AREAS

It is important to apply these general legal principles to specific problem areas that arise in the practice of emergency medicine. These include (1) consent to treatment; (2) medical records; (3) the reporting of certain events; (4) blood alcohol requests by police on arrested motorists; (5) abandonment of patients; (6) difficulties encountered through interaction between emergency department physicians and the rest of the medical staff; and (7) problems relating generally to the proper and efficient use of space, equipment, and personnel.

CONSENT TO TREATMENT

ASSAULT AND BATTERY

In assessing legal liability in a case alleging assault and battery, it is of no consequence that the unconsented-to treatment may have actually benefitted the patient; however, any benefit received is a factor the jury may consider in assessing a damage award. Assault is defined as the unlawful placing of an individual in apprehension of immediate bodily harm without his consent. Battery is defined as the unlawful touching of another individual without his consent. If it were not for the patient's consent, health practitioners would be routinely accused of assault and battery.

EXPRESS AND IMPLIED CONSENT

There are two major types of consent—express and implied. A patient gives his express consent to treatment when he or she gives the health practioner explicit permission to treat him or her. Implied consent does not involve such a direct expression of permission. The actions of the patient are deemed sufficient to imply to a reasonable person that the patient has consented to treatment. An example of implied consent is a case in which a person rolls up his or her sleeve to receive an injection but does not expressly authorize the injection. Implied consent also exists if a patient is not mentally competent because of psychosis, drugs, alcohol, organic disease, or unconsciousness. These conditions of mental incompetence may present the practitioner with an emergency condition that, according to public policy, should be treated as promptly as possible to save life. In addition, courts have held that implied consent exists in such

situations because it is believed that the patient, if mentally competent, would have given his or her consent to treatment necessary to save his or her life.

INFORMED CONSENT

In recent years, courts have focused on the quality of consent given by the patient. Courts have recognized a duty of the physician to disclose to the patient sufficient information to enable the patient to give his or her informed consent to treatment. Some jurisdictions measure the physician's duty to disclose against a physician-based standard where the duty is limited to disclosures that a reasonable medical practitioner would make under the same or similar circumstances. Other courts have applied a patient-oriented standard requiring the physician to disclose information which is material to a patient's decision making.

To establish liability for lack of informed consent, the plaintiff must show that the risk not disclosed actually occurred and that, had this risk been disclosed, he or she would not have consented to the treatment. In some jurisdictions, the jury must decide whether a reasonably prudent person in the patient's condition would have consented to the treatment had he or she been given the withheld information.

REFUSAL OF TREATMENT

In general, consent must be obtained from the patient in order to treat him or her. A mentally competent adult patient cannot be forced to receive treatment, even in the face of a life-threatening emergency. Thus, Jehovah's Witnesses, who have refused blood transfusions in absolute emergencies, have presented a continuous problem in the consent area. Some states have permitted courts to issue orders requiring patients to consent to life-saving treatment. Other states have refused to issue orders and have reaffirmed a competent individual's right to refuse treatment if he or she so wishes. Whenever the ED staff has consent questions about a life-and-death or serious-harm situation, the hospital administration should be involved as soon as possible to pursue every available legal avenue.

MINORS

Consent for treatment of minors must be obtained from parents, kinfolk, or legal guardian, whichever is appropriate under the circumstances. Parental consent is not necessary for treatment of minors who have been emancipated by virtue of marriage, statute, or economic independence. In addition, if life-threatening emergency conditions require immediate treatment, minors can obtain such treatment without parental consent. A reasonable effort must always be made to obtain parental consent. In cases of borderline emergency, such as slight lacerations, the treatment should be given to minors even if appropriate consent cannot be secured. It is better to err on the side of treatment than on that of nontreatment. Nontreatment carries with it the threat of a negligence suit, whereas treatment may occasion possible nonpayment of the bill for services rendered. Some states have passed legislation that provides for treatment of minors without parental consent in suspected cases of venereal disease or drug abuse.

INTOXICATED PATIENTS

Persons who are intoxicated or under the influence of drugs often cause problems in regard to consent. ED personnel, including physicians and nurses, sometimes react with hostility toward such patients, and in many cases are inclined to avoid treating them unless they are cooperative. It must be recognized by ED staff that, in some instances, intoxicated people have a diminished capacity to either grant or withhold their consent for treatment. To avoid possible liability for failure to treat an intoxicated patient, the physician should make every reasonable effort to quiet the patient and to ensure his or her understanding of the seriousness of the injury to obtain his or her knowing consent to treatment.

If an emergency physician's assessment reveals that the patient is incapacitated by alcohol or drugs to a degree that he or she may endanger himself or herself or others, the patient may be retained in the ED for appropriate observation. If no medical treatment is required, the ED staff should make a satisfactory arrangement for the patient's release. The emergency physician risks liability for injuries inflicted on third parties by an intoxicated emergency patient who is prematurely discharged.

MEDICAL RECORDS

It is essential that every hospital accurately prepare and properly store medical records, which are the subject of constant review by the hospital's administrative and medical staff and by professional reviewing agencies. They are also potentially critical documents in legal proceedings brought against the hospital and staff.

One of the most comprehensive statements on the composition of the ED record is found in the hospital emergency services standards of the JCAHO. Emergency Services Standard ER.7 states, "A medical record is maintained on every patient seeking emergency care and is incorporated into the patient's permanent hospital record."

Several specific emergency department record-keeping requirements are outlined by the JCAHO. Among these are the following: (1) patient identification (when not obtainable, the reason must be entered in the medical record); (2) time and means of arrival; (3) pertinent history of the illness or injury and physical findings, including the patient's vital signs; (4) emergency care given to the patient before his or

her arrival; (5) diagnostic and therapeutic orders; (6) clinical observations, including results of treatment; (7) reports of procedures, tests, and their results; (8) diagnostic impression; (9) conclusion at the termination of evaluation and treatment, including final disposition, the patient's condition on discharge or transfer, and any instructions given to the patient or his or her family or both for follow-up care; and (10) a patient's leaving against medical advice.

These essentials should be present to one degree or another within the bounds of the ED medical record; probably the greatest sin committed by ED staffs everywhere is to neglect to record all this vital information.

A patient's medical record is a confidential document, and hospital personnel are precluded from divulging privileged information contained therein. A court of law, however, can order the release of confidential information, and failure to comply with this order can result in a contempt of court decree. As a protective measure, it is recommended that the patient's written consent be obtained before any information contained in a medical record is released other than pursuant to a court order. This eliminates the danger of a subsequent lawsuit for breach of the patient's right to confidentiality.

REPORTABLE EVENTS

All states, either by statute or administrative regulation, require the reporting by health care personnel of certain events. These include, but are not limited to, rape, child abuse, gunshot or stab wounds, venereal disease, drug addiction, and patients who are dead upon arrival at the hospital.

RAPE

Rape has traditionally been defined as unlawful carnal knowledge of a woman by a man who is not her husband, forcibly, against her will, and with penetration, however slight, of the male genitalia into those of the female. In the past few years, many states have enacted modern criminal laws that redefine sexual offenses. Implicit in these new laws is the recognition that a victim of a sexual crime may be either male or female. An even more significant departure from the traditional legal definition of rape is that, under certain circumstances, the fact that the alleged offender and victim are married to each other may not automatically protect the defendant against a charge of rape. A second category of rape is statutory rape, which is generally defined as proscribed sexual conduct with a person under the statutory age, either with or without the consent of the other person. The emergency department physician's medicolegal task is not to diagnose rape but to conduct a thoroughly documented history and physical examination of the alleged victim.

Although the ED setting does not usually permit

the staff to conduct the totally comprehensive, compassionate type of examination envisioned by many women's groups, there is room for much improvement in the conduct of most rape examinations. Important considerations in the staff's approach to the alleged rape victim should include obtaining the patient's consent, history, physical examination, and laboratory studies. Clothing should be saved, and the proper authorities should be notified. Appropriate consent should be written and witnessed and should permit examination, collection of specimens, photographs (if necessary), and release of information to proper authorities. History should reveal time, person or persons, place, and circumstances. It is necessary to ask whether the patient was under the influence of drugs or alcohol at the time and whether she has bathed since the assault. Specimens should be tested for sperm, acid phosphatase, and male-specific semen protein (p30). A specimen should be cultured for possible *Neisseria gonorrhoeae*, and a VDRL should be obtained. A urine pregnancy test should be conducted to determine whether the female patient was pregnant at the time of the alleged assault.

The aforementioned specimens should be taken in the presence of a witness, documented in writing, and handed directly to the examining pathologist or laboratory technician, if possible. When this procedure is not feasible, these specimens should be labeled and placed in a locked receptacle to which only the examining pathologist has access. If the police wish to conduct these studies, the specimens should be handed directly to the police, and a witnessed receipt should be executed to document this transfer. These procedures are necessary to ensure that no gaps appear in the evidentiary chain. Any undocumented handling of these specimens might be sufficient to destory their value as evidence in a court of law. The results of these tests may be given to the adult patient, to her parents or legal guardian if she is a minor, or to the police, provided that the latter are in possession of proper authorization from the court.

Finally, the treating physician should counsel the patient about the prevention of pregnancy, venereal disease, AIDS, and psychic trauma and should also arrange for the follow-up care of the patient in whatever way is clinically indicated. Failure to attend to these necessities may result in civil suit for negligence if damages occur from such oversight.

CHILD ABUSE

The ED inevitably encounters the manifold problems of the battered child syndrome. Battered children are defined as those who have received serious physical injuries at the hands of their parents or other caretakers. Willful starvation or other deprivation of the child by the caretaker also is classified as child abuse, although it may not involve the physical contact of a battering. (See also Chapter 59.)

Most abused children are under age 4. Generally

speaking, the younger the abused child, the greater is the danger, because the incidence of death from battering is much higher in younger than in older children.

All states have statutes or regulations providing for some degree of reporting of suspected cases of child abuse. Some of these reporting laws are permissive and allow the reporter to use discretion in deciding whether or not to report. Others are mandatory reporting laws that require reporting under penalty of fine or imprisonment or both.

Many states provide immunity from civil or criminal liability for those who report suspected battered children. The approved reporting party varies among states, but the trend is toward broadened reporting requirements authorizing *any person* who reasonably suspects an abused child to report that suspicion.

In some states, a health care provider who fails to report a known or suspected case of child abuse is guilty of a criminal misdemeanor. Health care providers who breach a duty to report risk civil liability for subsequent injury to the child.

Health care personnel have a high social responsibility to report suspected cases of child abuse and should do so in compliance with the letter as well as the spirit of the law.

D.O.A.

The patient who is brought to the hospital dead on arrival (D.O.A.) presents still another reportable event for the ED. The case is routinely reported to the medical examiner for investigation for possible foul play and whether any benefit could be derived from a postmortem examination.

The emergency physician's professional responsibility in the case of the D.O.A. is to pronounce the patient dead. All tissue and body fluid specimens should be drawn only by the medical examiner. Nothing should be done by ED staff that might alter the appearance of the corpse; this only complicates the evidence-gathering function of the medical examiner. All clothing and other appurtenances attached to the corpse should be preserved for the medical examiner with as little handling as possible.

OTHER REPORTABLE EVENTS

Acts of social violence are often legally required to be reported. These include gunshot wounds and stab wounds as well as assault and battery with a variety of other potentially deadly weapons.

Venereal diseases often have found ready treatment access to the emergency department, and suspected cases increasingly present for treatment as the venereal epidemic spreads. Many states require reporting of certain venereal diseases to the department of health. Many states require the reporting of cases of HIV-positive blood test results. The ED should adopt a method of complying with such requirements where they exist.

A similar epidemic development in the United States is drug addiction. The ED should be aware of health department requirements for reporting cases of drug addiction.

BLOOD ALCOHOL REQUESTS AND THE POLICE

Drunk drivers invariably find themselves in the hospital ED. They arrive in a variety of conditions, ranging from dead to severely injured to unharmed but "under the influence." Police often accompany these motorists to the ED and request or demand the staff to draw blood specimens for alcohol analysis by the police.

The case of *Schmerber v. California*, 384 U.S. 757, decided by the U.S. Supreme Court in 1966, dealt with the problem of blood alcohol in a typical situation. Schmerber was arrested for driving under the influence of intoxicating liquor. He was taken to the ED by police, who ordered a physician to draw a blood sample. Schmerber refused to comply but offered no physical resistance. The United States Supreme Court commented at length about the constitutional issues of the case and held that there was no violation of Schmerber's Fourth Amendment right to be free from unreasonable search and seizure. It also held that there was no violation of the Fifth Amendment's prohibition against self-incriminating testimony.

The Court, however, did not say anything about the possible civil liability of the ED staff for assault and battery in performing a venipuncture without the consent of the patient. An emergency physician, nurse, or technician can be liable for assault and battery for touching a patient without the patient's consent. Therefore, the staff should exercise caution when attempting to cooperate with police and confronting a patient unwilling to submit to a blood alcohol test.

Some states have enacted statutes that provide the physician with immunity from civil liability for blood alcohol tests requested in writing by an appropriate law enforcement official. In some states, such as New Jersey, immunity from liability is provided as long as the blood sample is drawn in a medically acceptable manner. Taking a blood sample over the physical resistance of the individual may not be consistent with acceptable medical practice.

Some states have also enacted legislation that relieves the emergency physician of the necessity of appearing in court to testify about the manner in which a blood sample was taken for blood alcohol testing. These states provide specific protocol for the taking of the blood sample and specific record keeping requirements. Compliance with the statutory protocol permits the ED record to be admitted into evidence.

ABANDONMENT

The emergency physician must be concerned with the problem of legal abandonment. This is the unilateral termination of the physician-patient relationship by the physician without the patient's consent and without giving the patient sufficient opportunity to secure the services of another competent physician. Because the patient's condition may require assessment or treatment beyond the initial emergency visit, the patient should be instructed about the necessary follow-up steps in his or her treatment. One means of proof that such information was provided is an instruction sheet for a particular injury signed by the patient and ideally witnessed by a third party other than the treating physician or nurse. Such a document, however, does not provide iron-clad protection because it would still be open to attack on the grounds that the patient did not fully understand the nature of the document he or she was signing or the medical procedures outlined thereon. All patients should be instructed that, if complications arise, they should seek further medical attention from their family physician or from the treating ED itself.

A patient may experience abandonment over the telephone. An example is a situation in which a patient returns home after receiving treatment in an emergency department, experiences a recurrence of symptoms, calls the department, and is told not to worry about it until the morning. If the patient is harmed as a result, he or she may allege both negligence and abandonment. No member of the ED staff should engage in telephone diagnosis or treatment. Patients should be instructed and encouraged to return to the ED for re-evaluation.

MEDICAL STAFF RELATIONSHIPS

One of the most important relationships in the ED is between the emergency physicians and the remainder of the hospital medical staff. If this relationship is strained owing to personal, professional, or other reasons, it inevitably causes a diminished level of patient care and obviously enhances a climate of confusion in which lawsuits more easily arise.

Emergency physicians should become members of the medical staff according to the same procedure to which other physicians seeking hospital privileges are subjected. They should also be exposed to interdepartmental peer review and, in turn, should participate in peer review of other members of the medical staff when appropriate.

The ED should be positioned in the hospital bureaucracy in such a fashion as to ensure administrative competitiveness with other segments of the hospital. This allows the department to acquire its fair share of personnel and equipment indispensable for providing high-quality emergency medical care. It also permits the department to protect itself against possible abuse of its facilities and personnel for practices that are not appropriately conducted in the modern ED.

A medical staff member who instructs a patient to meet him or her in the ED for treatment, and then fails to appear or call to treat the patient, is a constant source of confusion for ED staff. The prime question for the department is whether it should exercise control over this patient and institute diagnosis and treatment. If the patient's problem is nonemergent and he or she wishes only to see his or her family physician, there is little problem for the staff. The situation, however, can become more troublesome when the patient's condition is potentially harmful, such as a complaint of chest pain.

Good patient care under these conditions dictates that the ED staff intervene to institute diagnosis and treatment of potential problem patients when the patient's private physician is unavailable. Obviously, some effort should be made to contact the patient's physician, but administrative considerations should never interfere with patient care. When there is any element of doubt, it is usually more prudent to err on the side of treating the patient than to withhold treatment. This course of action naturally presupposes that the patient has consented to treatment.

The emergency physician also encounters the occasional difficulty of being asked to write admission orders for patients admitted through the ED to other members of the medical staff. Potential liability is then extended out of the ED and into the special care unit or ward to which the patient has been admitted.

Once the patient's status has been converted from outpatient to inpatient, the responsibility for his care passes through a gray zone from the ED physician to the attending physician. The first formal event witnessing this transfer is the writing of temporary orders pending the attending physician's arrival to examine the patient. This responsibility should be exercised by the attending physician after he or she is informed by the emergency physician. If the emergency physician has no admission privileges at the hospital, it is even more imperative that initial admission orders be written by the physician to whom the patient has been admitted.

The obvious question raised by the admission order issue is how soon after admission the patient should be seen by the attending physician. The answer obviously depends on the clinical facts. If the patient's condition is serious, he or she should be seen immediately on admission. With decreasing severity of the patient's condition, the attending physician can be afforded a slightly longer time before he or she sees the patient. Certainly, all admitted patients should be seen within an hour or so. These guidelines are subject to some variation depending on how long the patient has been retained for "observation" in the ED. In practice, more observation occurs during the night hours. Under no conditions, however, should the attending physician attempt to "observe" the patient in the ED when good medicine dictates that the patient be admitted forthwith. Hospital ED holding areas have become fertile fields for plaintiffs' attorneys when patients have been harmed as a result of alleged negligence. Emergency physicians should be aware of hospital policy and protocol regarding the holding and observation of ED patients awaiting admission. In some states, notably New Jersey, the department of health has adopted regulations that may prevent the absue of EDs by setting time limits on ED "observation."

STAFFING, SPACE, AND EQUIPMENT

Other ED problems center around staffing, space, and equipment. Insufficient personnel (e.g., nurses, aides, and technicians) and inadequately trained personnel are a constant source of legal hazard for the ED. Hospitals without adequately trained emergency physician coverage of their ED are fast falling below the standard of care expected of such departments. The university hospital ED is not immune from this fault.

The ED should have enough space and equipment in which to handle initial diagnosis and treatment of emergency and nonemergency conditions. Laryngoscopes, defibrillators, ventilation bags and masks, and other equipment must be readily available and in satisfactory working order. The hospital should be aware that deficiencies in ED staff, space, and equipment can result in state revocation of the hospital's license, withholding of Medicare payments, and liability for negligence. It is the responsiblity of the medical staff and the hospital to see to it that such deficiencies are remedied when they exist.

SPECIFIC CONSIDERATIONS IN EMS: HOSPITAL/PHYSICIAN PRACTICE AND RISK MANAGEMENT

John D. Dunn

CAPSULE

Professional liability litigation has received much attention because of the generally unpleasant nature of the confrontation that occurs in a medical malpractice case, but many other areas of emergency medicine practice involve legal issues.

Emergency physicians, as a group, deal more with the legal aspects of medical practice than many other specialties. Emergency physicians are frequently involved in cases of child abuse, adult abuse, criminal investigations, patients with emergency psychiatric conditions requiring commitment, and other medicolegal issues. This chapter deals with all of these issues and also reviews the matter of professional liability litigation and medical malpractice claims against emergency physicians, a major concern for these physicians.

AMERICAN LAW

American law has several parts: regulatory/administrative law, civil law, and criminal law.

STATUTES AND REGULATIONS

The practice of medicine is one of the most highly regulated professions in the United States. Because 12% of the national economy, which converted to more than 500 billion dollars in the year 1989–90, is devoted to health care, obviously state and federal legislatures are concerned about getting the most for the money spent. Because government programs represent a significant portion of total monies spent on health care, legislatures have increased their attempts to manage health care delivery. These management efforts result in statutes, laws, and regulations that have enormous impact on health care providers.

Statutes and laws are passed by legislatures and give executive branches and their regulatory agencies broad powers to write rules and regulations. State and federal regulatory agencies issue regulations and policies to achieve the goals of legislation, and it is important to recognize that, as in all human endeavors, a regulator's views about what should be achieved can affect the way that they regulate. The wise physician recognizes that there are differences between the legislature's intent, the law that they wrote, and the way in which the regulations might be written or enforced.

Some areas of important legislation that affect emergency physicians are included subsequently for review. In time, these areas will change, but these are given as an example of the sorts of things that are important to understand.

CIVIL LAW

Civil law is the law that deals with relationships and conflicts in a society. It includes medical malpractice litigation, the rules that affect the success of a malpractice litigant, and the remedies available to individuals involved in malpractice litigation. Civil law also governs contracts, family relations, and financial and other interactions between individuals or organizations.

Caveats. State laws vary and all laws are constantly being revised, and therefore this chapter is intentionally general in its approach and national in scope. I could cite particular state statutes, but the important thing for the reader to recognize is that state statutes are generally similar on certain issues across the nation. Reference to particular state laws for each practice setting is essential. Federal law is national in scope, but sometimes state law supersedes federal law if it is stricter or more comprehensive or if federal law is silent. In other situations, federal law controls because state law is pre-empted as too strict, too restrictive, or against material interests.

The reader is also warned about legal opinions reported in the medical or lay press. Many times these opinions are on preliminary legal issues that are on appeal. Most of the time, the outcome of litigation, particularly malpractice litigation, is based on the medical issues. Appellate opinions appear in the press to reach ultimate conclusions when they are not. The medical issues and the facts of the case often control the outcome, and although legal dicta may appear to affect dramatically the outcome of a case, in practice they are not so important. Read the reports of these appellate opinions with some caution. They may only be opinions on admissibility of evidence or inclusion of a party in the suit. The actual case must still be tried.

REGULATIONS

Medicare/Medicaid Conditions of Participation. Participants in Medicare and Medicaid are under contract with the federal government. Agencies for the federal government, therefore, have the authority to regulate these "participants." Medicare "Conditions of Participation"[1] are the federal regulations that outline how hospitals should be operated. The Healthcare Financing Administration, which is a division of the Department of Health and Human Services, is in charge of regulation of Medicare participating providers. The Conditions of Participation tell the hospitals how to operate, and look like a miniature version of the standards promulgated by the Joint Commission on Accreditation of Healthcare Organizations (JCAHO). These conditions of participation outline how the various departments of a hospital should be organized and run. The regional offices of the Healthcare Financing Administration (HCFA) delegate their regulatory responsibilities to local state agencies, usually departments of health, to investigate and survey hospitals, and ensure compliance.

Recently the Joint Commission Accreditation enjoyed by hospitals was an automatic justification for continued Medicare participation, called "deemed status." In most states, a small percentage of accredited hospitals are independently reviewed by the agencies working for the Healthcare Financing Administration to determine the adequacy of the accreditation process as performed by the JCAHO. The state of New York has recently determined that it will not accept accreditation and "deemed status" and conducts separate inspections to ensure hospital compliance with Medicare Conditions of Participation, but it is the only state to do so. This trend may continue under increased scrutiny of JCAHO accreditation.

Emergency Care and Transfer Regulations. Medicare Law[2] in Section 1867 on "Responsibilities of Hospitals in Emergency Cases" appeared originally in the Consolidated Omnibus Budget Reconciliation Act (COBRA) of 1985 (signed into law in 1986) and were called the COBRA 9121 amendments. Additional amendments appeared in 1989.[3]

Section 1867 requires the following:

1. An emergency patient must be seen and evaluated, if he or she presents to the hospital, to determine whether he or she has an emergency condition or is in active labor.
2. If an emergency condition, defined under the law as an urgent life-, limb-, or organ-threatening con-

dition, is determined, the hospital must either treat or stabilize and transfer. This also applies to a woman in labor.
3. The hospital must use its resources and provide the care that it is capable of, or arrange for transfer to another more appropriate facility, considering that the benefits of treatment at that other facility will outweigh the risks of the transfer.
4. The patient must be properly stabilized according to appropriate medical standards of care.
5. The receiving facility must be ready and willing to accept the patient, and information on the patient's care at the transferring hospital must be communicated and transferred with the patient.
6. If the patient refuses treatment at the transferring hospital or refuses transfer, or if the patient requests transfer against medical advice, these matters should be documented and consents or refusal signed, if possible, in the medical record to show that the hospital is exempted from the requirements of any State or Federal transfer laws.
7. Federal law requires a physician's written certification that the benefits of transfer and treatment at the receiving facility outweigh the risks of transfer.

If there are any knowing and willful violations of the provisions, as outlined, the hospital and physician are subject to a $50,000 fine. The hospital is subject to termination from the Medicare program for any negligent, knowing, or willful violation of the provisions of Section 1867. This means that the hospital is subject to a 23-day termination if it cannot show a corrective action plan in place. Within 10 days, an announcement goes in the newspaper to warn the public that the hospital is to be closed from Medicare participation because it is an immediate and serious threat to patient safety. Even if the corrective action plan is adequate on a follow-up inspection, the warning in the newspaper cannot be avoided because of a limited amount of time and the need to put the announcement in at the 10-day point.

Physicians involved in inappropriate transfers or violations of COBRA are subject to $50,000 fines for each knowing violation, and exclusion from the Medicare/Medicaid program for up to 5 years.

The Office of the Inspector General (OIG) of the Department of Health and Human Services (HHS) is in charge of the assessment of fines and penalties and physician exclusions from the Medicare program. The regional offices of the Healthcare Financing Administration are in charge of the termination of hospital participation.

Other Medicare Rules. General considerations under the Medicare Conditions of Participation are that if you do not follow the regulations, the hospital can be found out of compliance and subject to "fast track" termination (23 days) for immediate and serious threat to patient safety, or what is called "90 day" termination, with intervening inspections to see where the corrective action is taken and whether the termination decision can be reversed.

State agencies inspect for the Healthcare Financing Administration and have tremendous authority. The Healthcare Financing Administration can authorize an investigation and inspection of COBRA violations or other violations of the Conditions of Participation in response to any complaints against a hospital that appear to be a substantial violation of the Conditions of Participation or complaints that appear to be a violation of Section 1867 on transfers.

The authority of the Healthcare Financing Administration (HCFA) in these areas is backed up by the Office of Inspector General of the Department of Health and Human Services. HCFA is a regulatory agency, whereas the Office of Inspector General is a prosecutorial agency of the same department. These two agencies have different authority and duties in an allegation of failure to comply with Medicare Regulations.

State Law. States have medical acts that provide for the licensure of physicians; pharmacy acts, which would control the distribution of drugs and the prescribing practices of physicians; and other health laws that affect, for example, the operation of hospitals and other health care institutions.

Usually there is shared responsibility for regulatory activity in a state, and many different agencies in the state might have control and authority over the practice of medicine and hospital practice. These agencies include state departments of health; departments of human services, which provide for funding and regulation of healthcare; and other administrative agencies such as drug control, environmental protection, labor, occupational safety, fire and safety, and others.

Good examples of state statutes and how they can affect emergency physicians include the following:

Reporting of infectious disease
Physician licensure and relicensure regulations
Control of dangerous substances and drugs
"Access to medical care" statutes, which require that an emergency department see any patient who presents, regardless of status or ability to pay
Qualification, regulation, and payment for indigent care; women's, infants; and children's programs; Medicaid; and other special entitlement programs
Regulation of prehospital care services and licensure of ambulance services, rescue squads, and prehospital care personnel
Nurse Practice and Physician Assistants Acts, which would affect the limitations on allied practice
Hospital licensure law, which delineates appropriate hospital operation and life and safety codes
Miscellaneous statutes, which create reporting and special care obligations such as child abuse statutes, elder abuse statutes, reporting of criminal activity, reporting of dangerous conditions such as seizure disorders, reporting of HIV tests and the testing for HIV, just to name a few statutes that developed in response to a special public concern.

Special interest and special category legislation has appeared in many states to include:

Medical malpractice/tort reform acts, which attempt to address increasing malpractice problems
Living-will advance directives and anatomic gift statutes, which attempt to deal with the issue of refusal of life-sustaining heroic measures and donation of body parts
Durable power of attorney acts, which create an agent with authority to make medical decisions for an individual, should he or she become incompetent
Statutes that address reproductive and fertility issues
Statutes affecting mental health and mental retardation programs, commitment, and involuntary mental health care
Statutes that address problems like rural health care; trauma care; care for the indigent; prenatal care; and care for migrants, severely disabled children, and other groups with special needs.

The list of inventive pieces of legislation with respect to health care is endless, but it is important to recognize that state legislators and Congress have not only an interest, but the authority, to affect the practice of medicine in many ways. As a result, we cannot avoid the law in our professional activities. The law provides us with the authority to practice medicine, and also restrains that authority. The regulations that agencies develop attempt to fulfill the intent of legislative acts.

Common Law. Common law is the law that comes out of litigation in the court room. Decisions of courts in cases in English and American law (with the exception of Louisiana, which follows a civil law tradition) create the common law decisions that are the basis for generally accepted principles of law.

In the case of Louisiana, the net effect is the same because attention is paid to decisions on the law, and court opinions are important to the development of the law in Louisiana. Louisiana assigns priorities somewhat differently, with the written law (the code) taking priority over court opinions.

The common law tradition also includes defense to previous decisions, called the principle of "stare decisis." This means that the prior decisions, particularly those in the same jurisdiction, will be given great, if not completely controlling, influence on a current decision.

Tort Law. Tort (personal injury) law is a part of civil law that governs matters related to the allegations of negligence by doctors. If an individual wants to file a suit against a doctor or a claim against the doctor for improper care, tort law applies.

Elements required for successful lawsuit against a doctor for malpractice are the following:

Show that the doctor had a *duty* to take care of the individual.

Show that that duty was not properly performed because of a *negligent act or omission* (failure to live up to the appropriate standard of care).

The plantiff must show that the negligent act or omission was the "legal" or "proximate" *cause* of the damages claimed.

The *damages* must be measurable and remediable under the law of the jurisdiction.

The procedures involved in a medical malpractice claim and lawsuit include the following:

An accusation, claim, or demand is made.

After attempts to resolve the claim are unsatisfactory, the plaintiff and the plaintiff's attorney may decide to file a lawsuit. It a lawsuit is filed, appropriate written responses from the defendant to the accusation are made.

The statute of limitations is a special state civil procedure law that limits the time in which someone can sue. For example, many states have a rule that one must sue within 2 years of the time of the injury; there are some provisions for delay or extending the time when the cause of the injury could not be discovered. It is important to know the statute of limitations in your own state because it controls the exposure period to some extent. Many states do have special rules for injuries to minors, extending their opportunity to sue until they become adults, or at least until they become older. Statute of limitations rules in the states vary, but usually the statute of limitations is around 2 to 3 years, with some extensions available under the rules described.

After the suit is begun, "discovery" commences, involving the gathering of information. That gathering of information is formalized by legal procedures pertaining to exchanges of questions (interrogatories), the production of evidence, the requirement of medical examinations, and the taking of written sworn testimony (depositions) from witnesses and experts on the facts and the issues in the case.

If, during the discovery stage, resolution of the claim does not occur or a settlement cannot be made, the case proceeds to a trial with a selection of a jury or judge to hear the case and decide on the facts. In a trial situation, the judge also rules on the legal issues.

If either party is dissatisfied with the findings at the trial court level, that party can appeal such a decision to a higher appellate court in the state system, or if the case is being tried in federal court (allowed under special circumstances), the appeal is to a federal circuit.

The final appeal goes to the State Supreme Court or the United States Supreme Court if these courts agree to listen to the dispute. Acceptance of the case is discretionary, and most medical malpractice cases do not reach the Supreme Court of the State or the United States Supreme Court.

Claims Management. When an incident or problem case develops, it is important to recognize that this is only the first step that might lead to a malpractice claim. The perception of improper care by the patient or family is frequently more important than the reality. The management of a claim or complaint can be the most important part of professional liability risk management. Proper response and careful evaluation of the claim and the medical information related to the claim are essential. It is important to recognize the following principles of good claims management:

1. Information should be gathered by somebody familiar with rules of the law and also expert in the medical issues.
2. During the initial process of gathering information, no attempt should be made to resolve the claim or dispute other than to make sure that the patient receives appropriate ongoing care and assurance of a complete evaluation of the problem.
3. If there is a strong probability of litigation, the case should be labeled as such to create some immunity of the investigation from the discovery efforts later by the plantiff when the suit is filed.
4. If the claim or dispute does not involve a significant injury or a significant medical dispute, it is advisable to try to evaluate it completely and allow the individual to ventilate the complaint and attempt to achieve an amicable resolution as quickly as possible.
5. If significant damages or a good possibility of litigation is involved, the insurance company must be informed so that it might protect the interests of their insured and the insurance company. Failure to inform the insurance company could compromise insurance coverage. (If one receives notice of a lawsuit, one *must* inform the insurer immediately.)
6. During the initial stages of the investigation, it is absolutely essential that a good medical expert, familiar with the medical issues and appropriate standards of care, evaluate the case objectively and fairly. Not all great doctors are good medicolegal experts.

STANDARDS OF MEDICAL CARE

Across the country, physicians struggle with the concept of the appropriate standard of care. These standard-of-care issues are related to appropriate allocation of resources for health care, the resolution of professional liability claims and litigation, and appropriate standards to be applied to physicians in quality assurance and peer review matters. The "legal" or common-law definition of standard of care can be paraphrased as follows:

A physician is required to possess and exercise that degree of skill and knowledge which is exercised by the average prudent and reasonable physician who claims the same specialization and who practices in the same or a similar locality.

When we consider the content of this statement, which basically describes the dicta or rulings of many courts in the United States on the standard of care over a long period, it is important to recognize that the following elements are necessary:

1. "Average prudent physician" does not mean superior physician, but means what it says. Time, energy, educational, and resource limitations sometimes do not allow superior evaluation and treatment. The question remains, what would be the average prudent approach to a particular problem?
2. The average physician is assumed to be a prudent physician.
3. Practicing a certain specialty creates a distinct legal expectation. If you announce yourself as a specialist in neurosurgery, the public has the right to expect you to perform as the average prudent neurosurgeon would. If you claim no specialization or expertise, you are expected to perform as an average, prudent, licensed physician would perform under the circumstances, which includes appropriate use of consultants.
4. The "same or similar locality" qualifier is specifically designed to create a generally accepted standard of care that allows differences in facilities, personnel, styles of practice, and other matters that relate to geographic variability and other factors that result in reasonable practice variance across the country.

Although a national standard of care is accepted by courts, it is important to recognize that within that national standard of care are tremendous variations created by geographic and other factors in addition to the variances that exist because of medical training and custom and specialty practices.

More than 20 medical specialty societies and organizations are actively involved in trying to establish written standards of care. These attempts to establish standards are intended to accomplish the following:

1. Avoidance of arbitrary and unrealistic standards set by professional medical experts who make a career of testifying.
2. A recognition that physician judgment in medical care is an essential part of the variability that occurs under the definitions of "average," "prudent," and "standard."
3. Most specialty societies prefer to establish their own standards of care rather than have them imposed by someone from another specialty; a particular fear is someone from another specialty with an idealized unrealistic concept of the standard of care.
4. Specialty societies have also, in many cases (the American College of Emergency Physicians and the American Academy of Pediatrics, for example), created standards regarding who is a qualified medical expert, which usually requires that one cross the threshold of certification or experience and actual knowledge of standards of practice relative to the medical issues in the case. Many states have adopted some medical expert qualifiers to guide courts in the acceptance of medical experts in litigation, for example, Texas, Illinois, and California.

Professional liability litigation is unique and troublesome for the following reasons:

1. The medical profession, as a whole, aspires to success in every case, and no one is happy with a failed effort or an unsuccessful attempt.
2. There is a generally held illusion that good doctors do not have bad results.
3. In retrospect, one can frequently find a way in which the care could have been modified to achieve a theoretic improvement in a bad outcome.
4. Professional medical experts can be particularly prone to serve their clients by creating strict and ideal standards and reviewing the medical records with a critical eye.

THE IMPORTANCE OF THE MEDICAL RECORD

The legal importance of a medical record has evolved in the last 15 to 20 years to create an increasing burden on physicians to attempt to document medically many items once thought to be unimportant. When this atmosphere is combined with the 20/20 hindsight of a picky expert, the medical record becomes a particular liability in the emergency medicine situation.

Medical records are presumed by a rule of law (an exception to the hearsay rule) to be an accurate reflection of events. Whether this record is complete or not is a question that must always be dealt with in litigation. The amount of information that a physician acquires to make a medical decision is awesome, even for minor cases, but not usually completely documented in the record.

The problem is that the medical record is frequently a handwritten record in the ED and, as a result, the additional documentation of pertinent negatives is omitted, leaving the record open to criticism, particularly when a poor outcome occurs. The opinion "if it wasn't in the record, it wasn't done" does not match reality or the limits of time and space. It has been said often that even those of us who know better believe it. A more realistic view would be that the record is realistically a short document that ideally says everything that occurred but cannot. The better the documentation, however, the stronger the case for acceptable care.

The reality is that the medical record cannot hope to show all of the observations or the factors considered by the physician involved. There has been an increased emphasis on making sure that certain pertinent negatives are included in the documentation, to support the evaluation of the physician. Most medical malpractice claims against emergency physicians occur when the patient was discharged from the ED and thought to have a condition that was not serious. Unfortunately, this also creates the mindset that produces lesser documentation and a failure to document negatives that might help to support the decision to discharge the patient. In any event, ongoing studies of documentation and evaluation of ED records may show a significant problem of which the reader should be conscious, including some pertinent negatives that help to support the decision to discharge the patient and make the medical record more of an asset in defending a malpractice claim or a lawsuit.

ACTUARIAL ANALYSIS

Since 1975, there has been an increased interest in analysis of emergency medicine malpractice claims. The most extensive analysis available is of closed claims for the endorsed insurance program of the American College of Emergency Physicians, 1976 to 1984: 55 million visits, 1700+ claims. We can now report the characteristics of malpractice claims in the ED that will guide the physician in reducing malpractice risk.

HIGH-RISK CLINICAL ENTITIES

The following produce more than 50% of malpractice claims against emergency physicians.

1. Failure to diagnose chest pain (usually unstable angina or myocardial infarction, frequently a claim that involves sudden death)
2. Failure to properly care for wounds (includes infections or foreign bodies, tendon, nerve and vessel injuries undiscovered at the time of care)
3. Mismanaged or missed fractures or dislocations (particularly spine and pelvic fractures)
4. Meningitis (usually failure to diagnose in febrile infants and children)
5. Delay or failure to diagnose abdominal pain (appendicitis, ectopic pregnancy, and other, usually surgical, conditions)

After this list of items, which create more than 50% of the dollar losses, are some other cases that frequently create malpractice claims against emergency physicians, including the following:

1. Failure to treat alterations in mental status and central nervous system (CNS) status. (TIAs, metabolic encephalopathies, and other CNS disorders)
2. Improper management of diabetic complications
3. Difficult mental health and suicide/self-destructive behavior cases
4. Multiple trauma cases that involve serious neurologic disability as a residual
5. Peripheral vascular disease in the elderly and the complications of vascular insufficiency
6. Testicular torsion—delay or failure to diagnose
7. Management of seizure patients
8. Vascular conditions such as abdominal aortic aneurysm—delays or failures to diagnose
9. Respiratory diseases with respiratory failure
10. Upper airway problems (epiglottitis, croup, trauma, abscess)
11. Gastroenteritis with subsequent dehydration and electrolyte disturbances (particularly in the extremes of age)
12. Ingestions, poisonings, and toxic exposures (delayed or inappropriate treatment)

All of these clinical entities presume primarily a standard of care related to diagnosis, and rarely do the claims involve inappropriate treatment. That leads us to an important conclusion regarding malpractice claims in the ED:

> *MORE THAN 90% OF ALL CLAIMS AGAINST EMERGENCY PHYSICIANS INVOLVE PATIENTS WHO ARE DISCHARGED FROM THE ED, AND THEREFORE GOOD DISCHARGE INSTRUCTIONS AND APPROPRIATE CONSERVATIVE FOLLOWUP AND RE-EVALUATION ARE ESSENTIAL TO GOOD RISK MANAGEMENT.*

It is also important to recognize in these claims that we see a significant impact from high disability or death claims in emergency medicine professional liability claims.[4] The magnitude of the claims has a major impact on the losses for emergency physicians, with deaths and serious disabilities representing a significant part of malpractice claims against emergency physicians.

The Ohio Hospital Association did a 1985–1988 closed ED claims study that showed the following results:

1. Male claimants outnumbered female claimants.
2. ED claimants tend to be younger.
3. Older patients are underrepresented in terms of ED claims.
4. Self-pay and workman's compensation claimants tend to be more frequent in their claims, but compensated less.
5. The emergency physician was the principal defendant in more than 60% of the ED claims.
6. Residents tend to have more claims against them when they are on the emergency service.
7. Frequently, ED claims involve a second physician, with most of those second physicians either the radiologist or the emergency physician.
8. Sixty percent of the ED claims involved a diagnostic error.

9. In terms of frequency, the following, in declining order, were the cause of claims: Missed fractures, myocardial infarctions or chest pain undiagnosed, soft tissue and wound problems, and appendicitis.
10. Forty percent of the ED claims are considered frivolous. The actual percentage of dollar losses for types of claims is not known according to the report.[5] Reviewing the reported claims that were listed, however, the missed diagnosis of chest pain, including failure to diagnose myocardial infarction and failure to diagnose pulmonary embolism, had a tremendous impact in terms of dollar losses.

CHEST PAIN

Nontraumatic chest pain in adults presents the most important malpractice problem for ED physicians. Failure to diagnose unstable angina, myocardial infarction, new-onset angina, and a few rare catastrophic conditions can result in a patient being discharged to later suffer sudden death or serious disability.

Because most of these cases involve heart disease, the failure to diagnose cardiac disease is usually the measure of negligence and a failure to comply with the standard of care. The work of Lee and others particularly has established some basic parameters for the accuracy of ED evaluation of chest pain.[6-8]

A multicenter study of adults seen with nontraumatic chest pain in both academic and nonacademic hospitals has been reported[9] and establishes a significant error rate in patients who are sent home. Less than half of the patients seen were sent home, and of these patients some had myocardial infarction and should have been admitted. During the study of a consecutive cohort of more than 3000 patients, the multicenter group showed that 35 of the 1283 who were sent home had myocardial infarction or sudden death. This is despite the fact that the physicians seeing the patients were operating under a rigid chart protocol, including special attention to the history and the evaluation of the ECG.

Studies establish by risk analysis the factors in history that increase the risk for myocardial infarction and heart disease.

A list of historical items of most diagnostic help in the diagnosis of heart disease are:

1. Central and left arm chest pain are usually present.
2. The quality of pain is generally severe and crushing or heavy rather than intermittent and sharp.
3. The pain is more often associated with autonomic symptoms such as dizziness, nausea, vomiting, and diaphoresis.
4. The pain of cardiac origin is severe and ominous and often has a radiation factor.
5. Patients with cardiac causes of chest pain usually present with risk factors such as family history, diabetes, previous heart disease, high blood pressure, smoking, high cholesterol, and abnormal lipids.[6,10]

The analysis of the ECG is an important factor in the provision of acceptable care and evaluation of chest pain. Certain diagnostic findings on the ECG must be emphasized, including:

1. Hyperacute T-waves that are peaked in shape
2. ST segment elevations more than 2 mm in chest leads and 1 mm in limb leads
3. ST segment depressions that are flattened and more than 1 mm
4. Presence of new Q-waves
5. New onset of conduction defects or significant axis changes

Patients who are mistakenly sent home can be characterized as follows:

1. They tend to be younger (under 35).
2. They have first-time pain.
3. They have atypical pain.
4. They have pain characterized by the examiner as chest wall or pleuritic pain.
5. For one reason or another, their history is not reliable.[7]

The typical patient with cardiac disease is a man with risk factors who has a history including some of the listed items. *Standard-of-care analysis,* however, requires that the physician take a good history, perform a physical examination, and read the ECG correctly to successfully defend himself or herself against a malpractice claim.

The Medical Record in Chest Pain Cases. Patients are sometimes inappropriately sent home. When this happens, the medical record is analyzed in excruciating detail. Pertinent negatives and observations as documented are either positive or negative for the physician accused of negligence. If a physician mistakenly sends a patient home, it is important to show that it happened despite appropriate medical evaluation.

The Armed Forces Institute of Pathology (AFIP) is studying the problem of misdiagnosis of chest pain in the ED under the leadership of Flannery and Granville. In a survey conducted in 1988 with 50% response from the American College of Emergency Physician members, the respondents ranked in priority ten items to be documented in any adult seen for nontraumatic chest pain. The items, in order of priority, were:

1. Past history of myocardial infarction or angina
2. Quality of pain
3. Time elapsed since pain began
4. Location of pain
5. Radiation of pain
6. Presence of diaphoresis
7. Presence of dyspnea
8. Response to therapy

9. Comparison of this pain with past anginal pain
10. Risk factors

AFIP then compared actual performance of emergency physicians in selected EDs. The performance fell below 60% compliance on individual items, with an overall performance level over the 10-item list significantly below 60% performance.[11] This variation between ideal and actual documentation cannot be avoided in the analysis of medical malpractice claims. Part of the consideration of the standard of care in risk management is the evaluation of the adequacy of documentation needed to defend the case.

Trends in emergency medicine claims seen over the past few years indicate an increase in the impact of heart disease on the total dollars lost in emergency medicine malpractice claims. I have reviewed recent loss runs in which chest pain claims were more than 30% of the total dollar losses, up from earlier reports of 19.7% in the period 1975 to 1984.[12]

FEBRILE INFANTS AND CHILDREN

Evaluation of febrile infants and children is difficult and perilous. Problems include the following:

1. A history is difficult to obtain.
2. The emotional state of the family can complicate the evaluation.
3. Children are seen against a background of common illnesses which produce fevers, and the rare serious illness may start out as a benign-looking process.
4. Although physicians generally recognize the potential risks of bacteremia and meningitis and pneumonia against this background of febrile infants and children, the evaluation of the febrile infant or child is at a point in a spectrum of an unpredictable process. Respiratory tract infections can be benign or develop into life-threatening processes.

The work of McCarthy at Yale[13] has taken some of the mystery out of the evaluation of febrile infants and children. Starting with a long list of observation items that clinicians might use in evaluating febrile children, McCarthy and his group have found that certain sensitive and reliable observation items establish the children with fevers who are likely to have serious illness. This approach creates an appropriate evaluation of the febrile child. The standard of care is important in these cases, given that malpractice claims against physicians in this area frequently involve a failure to diagnose or a delay in diagnosis. McCarthy's list of observation items is as follows:

1. Quality of cry
2. Response to parents
3. State of hydration
4. General state of alertness
5. Response to talk, smile, and social overtures
6. Color

Many elements of the medical evaluation of patients are used almost subconsciously. Physicians may walk into a room aware of many important clinical characteristics of a child, yet frequently fail to put any record down that shows their observations. It is important to note that a neurologic examination can be performed in many cases without touching the patient and that, specifically in evaluating febrile infants and children, the general state of the child and the child's reaction to the environment are obvious but sensitive measures of the severity of the child's illness. The brain is the most sensitive organ in the body and frequently the first functioning organ to be affected by serious illness; therefore the brain is one of the best barometers of a child's general state. McCarthy has finalized this basic concept of clinical medicine into an observation scale, which is described in his writing.[13]

Some basic caveats, however, must be attached to the work of McCarthy. They include the following:

1. In a child under 3 months, neurologic development limits use of the observation scale.
2. With temperatures above 40°C and white blood cell counts above 15,000, increased risk of bacteremia is present and should alert the physician to do further studies.
3. The observation scale should be used to stimulate further evaluation because it is frequently only to assist in developing the diagnostic hypothesis.[13]

There are no magic approaches to febrile infants and children. Although many medical experts have appeared in court and declared certain "rules," the clinical evaluation is a complex and multifactored medical exercise, and no single element should control it.

Medical Record in Cases of Febrile Infants and Children. The importance of documentation in evaluating febrile infants and children becomes important in the context of medical malpractice litigation. In retrospect, parents' stories of what happened are often affected by the eventual outcome of the case. Recollection of the events surrounding the evaluation is limited, and as a result the medical record becomes more and more important. Physicians do not send home children that they consider to be lethargic and at risk for meningitis, but plaintiffs' attorneys frequently accuse physicians of doing that sort of thing. The plaintiff's attorney finds a medical expert who picks through the chart and finds a few omissions of documentation and concludes that anyone who misses certain items of documentation must be providing a negligent evaluation. These criticisms leave the impression in the minds of the jury that the defendant physician was incompetent because:

1. Good doctors do not have bad outcomes.
2. All doctors do extensive documentation, even in a busy ED.
3. A combination of omissions of documentation and a bad result is somehow prima facie evidence of malpractice.

These deceptions always affect litigation on meningitis or sepsis malpractice cases. The reality is that medical practice is an imperfect art and science and the judgment is sometimes wrong, but that is not medical malpractice. Malpractice is the failure to do a prudent evaluation, not a misjudgment or mistake after the evaluation.

WOUNDS AND LACERATIONS

Wound cases create frequent and sometimes significant malpractice risks because all undiscovered underlying injuries or subsequent infections could potentially promote a malpractice suit. It is essential that documentation address the prime areas of complications of wounds so that the physician's medical record be defensible. That is not to say that a record that fails to mention these items is indefensible, but it is important to create the most favorable medical record possible under the circumstances. Busy EDs and higher-priority patients may prevent the physician from making all of the documentation a part of the medical record. It is important to establish a routine that includes the evaluation of wounds for presence of foreign material, and underlying injuries to nerves, tendons, bones, or blood vessels. The care of the wound should attend to potential complications and document proper precautions with good discharge instructions and follow-up.

FAILURE TO DIAGNOSE FRACTURES AND DISLOCATIONS

In the setting of an unconscious victim of trauma, spine fractures and pelvic fractures can be missed. Screening for possible spine fractures and pelvic fractures is a part of the systematic care of trauma patients. The unconscious patient must be assumed to have a neck fracture if the mechanism of injury is appropriate. Obviously, physician judgment will be necessary in some cases.

Pelvic fractures, which have a high mortality rate because they are usually associated with other severe injuries, can be missed in the hurry of trying to take care of a desperately ill patient. Diagnosis of the pelvic fracture may affect the general management of the case because irreversible shock can result from pelvic fracture.

Excellent work done by many investigators has established that a conscious, alert patient without other significant injuries to distract (for example bilateral femoral fractures might be a distraction) can reliably tell the examining physician whether neck pain is present. If the patient does not have neck pain, the studies show that the need for screening x rays of the neck and concern about neck fractures is eliminated.

Stabilization and immobilization of the neck are an important part of prehospital care. Soft collars are not acceptable, but many rigid collars and rigid fixation devices are effective in reducing flexion, extension, or lateral movement of the head and neck.

Management of patients with possible neck fractures who require intubation is highly controversial, spanning the breadth of opinion from automatic tracheostomy or nasal intubation to oral intubation with in-line traction or immobilization. Many clinicians find excellent results with all three methods; therefore the important thing is physician evaluation and physician comfort with the procedures chosen.

In order of frequency, other missed fractures are those of ribs, hands, feet, elbows, and knees. Fractures of the face and skull are a significant risk. Certain fractures and dislocations are more likely to create permanent disability, thus being more likely to cause suits. Examples are tibial plateau fractures or navicular fractures that create permanent disability if not managed properly. The potential for damage is easy to see in missed facial or skull fractures.

EVALUATION OF THE PATIENT WITH ABDOMINAL PAIN

The management of patients with abdominal pain covers some relatively rare as well as more common conditions. The most important and common source of malpractice litigation in this group of patients is delay or failure to diagnose appendicitis. Ranking after appendicitis in terms of frequency in malpractice claims in patients with abdominal pain are ectopic pregnancy, vascular conditions of the abdomen (particularly abdominal aortic disease), bowel obstruction, cholecystitis, diverticulitis, peptic ulcer disease, intussusception, and other rarer conditions resulting in catastrophic conditions. The basic rule here is that the catastrophic abdominal conditions are usually surgical and therefore the threshold standard of care issues are related to when the surgeon should be consulted. A good evaluation of the patient with good documentation and close followup and discharge instructions are critical factors in the standard-of-care analysis.

MISCELLANEOUS CAUSES OF MALPRACTICE CLAIMS

Testicular Torsion. This usually presents as unilateral testicular pain in the prepubertal boy. Trauma is frequently thought to be the cause, but even minor trauma can result in testicular torsion, or the patient can incorrectly attribute the pain to trauma. Testicular torsion can come during exercise, for example swimming or running, and produces a unilateral swollen, malpositioned, indurated, high-riding testicle. The important thing is index of suspicion and analysis of the patient's history and condition with special consideration for testicular torsion. The window of opportunity for correction is narrow (up to 4 to 6 hours), and therefore speed of diagnosis and surgery to save the testicle is essential.

Suicide Gestures and Suicidal Ideation. These cases frequently involve patients with tumultuous mental health problems, and management is difficult; therefore the potential for malpractice litigation is high. Documentation regarding involuntary commitments, decisions that relate to therapy, and disposition can be critical in retrospect because these patients frequently do not have good family or professional support.

Patients with Drug and Alcohol Problems. By definition, these patients have personality and mental health problems and are frequently unreliable in providing for their own care, which complicates the medicolegal environment. These patients are also litigation-prone. Use of social service agencies and support groups with careful chart documentation reduces risk.

Multiple Trauma Cases. Multiple trauma cases frequently produce severe disability, and invariably litigation regarding the original source of the injury may focus attorney attention on criticism of the medical care. Severely injured individuals often look to litigation to improve their financial situation, particularly if they are permanently disabled.

SPECIAL RISK SITUATIONS

LEGAL PROBLEMS IN TRANSFERS

State and federal laws, as well as some general medical principles, affect the conduct of a transfer. The American College of Emergency Physicians (ACEP) and the American College of Surgeons (ACS) have both developed physician papers and statements on the conduct of a transfer.[14]

The ACS focused on the importance of the receiving physician and the consulting physician controlling the quality of the transfer and coordinating transfer with the transferring physician. In addition, the ACS emphasizes the importance of expediting transfers, particularly in trauma cases in which patient outcome is affected by the inappropriate delays.[15]

The ACEP, in its position papers published in 1977 and modified in 1989, has emphasized the importance of the following:

1. The transfer of an emergency patient should be undertaken only for good medical reasons.
2. Proper evaluation, initial treatment, and stabilization are important steps before attempting a transfer.
3. A transfer should always be initiated because the care anticipated at the receiving facility will benefit the patient and the risks of transfer are outweighed by the benefits of the care that will be provided at the receiving facility.
4. Proper communication between the transferring

and receiving physicians, nurses, and facilities is imperative.
5. Proper conduct of the transfer includes transfer of information on treatment at the transferring facility.
6. The transfer should be conducted with proper transport equipment, personnel, and intra-transfer preventative and stabilizing care.
7. The receiving physician and the transferring physician should share the responsibility of conducting the transfer according to appropriate medical standards.

During the early 1980s, several articles appeared in the medical literature criticizing the conduct and the motivations of transfers.[16-18] These articles criticize the conduct of transfers and the fact that many transfers appear to be economically motivated but not properly conducted from a medical standpoint. Specifically, they criticize transfers to public hospitals such as Parkland in Dallas, Cook County in Chicago, and Baptist in Memphis because the writers feel that proper communication and proper stabilization were not carried out before the transfers and that many patients suffered as a consequence of inappropriate transfer. In response to the problems of the Dallas area, the state of Texas passed the first formal transfer law specifying that an appropriate protocol must be used for transfers.[19]

Texas law requires that a memorandum of transfer be completed and evidence of proper communication between the transferring and receiving facility be assured. The acceptance of the patient must be obtained and secured by the transferring facility under the Texas law for a transfer to be properly accepted. The Texas transfer law cited the criteria for a good transfer as published by the American College of Emergency Physicians.[19]

The Texas Hospital Licensing Law, in Chapter XI, codified all of the various regulations that controlled the conduct of transfers.[19] Shortly thereafter, Congress considered, in hearings on the problem of transfers, amendments to Section 1867 of the Social Security Act, now found at 42 U.S.C. Section 1395 dd. This legislation was passed in the Consolidated Omnibus Budget Reconciliation Act (COBRA) of 1985, which was signed into law in 1986. Section 9121 created amendments to Section 1867 of the Social Security Act and put into federal law a requirement that hospitals and physicians follow federal regulations on transfers or be found in violation of the Social Security Act and the Conditions of Participation that control hospital contracts for Medicare.

The 1986 COBRA 9121 amendments specify the following conditions:

1. Any patient who presents to the ED of a hospital that has a contract with Medicare (regardless of the age and regardless of their status as a Medicare recipient) must receive a medical screening ex-

amination to determine if he or she has an emergency condition or is in "active labor."

2. If an emergency condition (any life-, limb-, or organ-threatening condition that requires immediate care) exists or the patient is in active labor (delivery is imminent and failure to properly care for the patient would result in injury to the mother or fetus), the hospital must provide treatment or stabilization and appropriate medical transfer to another facility for care.

3. The patient can be transferred only for good medical reasons and after properly informing the patient of the situation.

4. An appropriate transfer would require that communication between the transferring and receiving facility be effective, the receiving facility accept the patient, a receiving physician accept the patient, and the initial treatment, evaluation, and stabilization be communicated and medical records transferred with the patient.

5. An appropriate transfer also requires that the patient be transferred after evaluation, stabilization, and communication with the receiving facility, and only under conditions in which proper equipment, personnel, and intratransfer care can be provided to avoid further deterioration of the patient's condition.

6. Failure to comply with the requirements of COBRA 9121 subjects the hospital to immediate termination (23-day fast track termination) from the Medicare program, and subjects the hospital and the physician for knowing violations of the act to $50,000 in fines (raised in 1987 from $25,000 in fines) for *each* violation.

7. Physicians after 1988 can also be suspended for a period of up to five years from the Medicare program for violations.

In 1989, Congressman Stark introduced another set of amendments to Section 1866, which provided for the following:

1. Language was inserted to clarify that on-call physicians were considered to be responsible for the patient.

2. Hospitals were prohibited from economic screening before providing emergency care.

3. Emergency physicians were protected and granted immunity if they initiated a transfer that would normally be a violation of the law because the on-call physician refused to come in.

4. Protection was provided that prohibited hospitals from penalizing individuals who refused to conduct an inappropriate transfer.

5. The specialty and tertiary hospitals were required under another provision to accept the patient for specialty care (neonatal intensive care units, burn units, shock trauma units, and other specialized forms of tertiary care) if they had appropriate personnel and facilities. They were not allowed to refuse an appropriate transfer for economic reasons, for example.

Despite all this pro-active and aggressive legislation, a significant problem across the country has been created by the ongoing difficulty of emergency care for patients with no insurance. More than 30 million Americans are uninsured or significantly underinsured, and this does not include individuals who are on Medicaid or some kind of federal or state health care insurance. These individuals tend to be in the working poor or unemployed categories, young and without personal resources that would pick up the slack. It is perceived that penetrating trauma in particular is a source of significant financial loss for hospitals and physicians and creates the additional burden of professional liability exposure. The solution is not evident at this writing, and will continue to vex policy makers into the forseeable future.

Proper conduct of a transfer to avoid the general concern of professional liability risk and the specific concerns about federal and state law requires review of federal and state laws and special protocols for transfers of any patient with an emergency condition, from either the ED or from other areas of the hospital. This transfer protocol should include documentation and thorough evaluation of transfers including the requirements for the following:

1. Proper evaluation of the patient.
2. Proper initial treatment and stabilization of any patient who is a candidate for transfer.
3. Initiation of a transfer only for good medical reasons.
4. Written certification by the physician that the transfer is appropriate transfer and indicated for the benefit of the patient, with specific reference to the fact that the benefits of treatment at the receiving facility exceed the risks.

RETURN VISIT SYNDROME

Patients who return should be seen as an opportunity to correct a problem. We distinguish the "return visit syndrome" from the patients who come to the ED repeatedly for primary care. Return visit cases involve individuals with an acute illness or injury who are seen and then return because they do not get relief from the treatment prescribed. Physicians, under these circumstances, should be careful to re-evaluate completely the patient and protect against oversights. If a patient returns for a third time, it may be necessary to consider even a consultation or precautionary hospitalization or observation period to avoid misdiagnosing the patient's condition.

PATIENTS WHO WALK OUT AGAINST MEDICAL ADVICE OR WITHOUT CARE

Effective triage helps to avoid excessive delays in treatment. EDs see a spectrum of disease, but it is important to recognize that the patient who is ambulatory one day might be on a stretcher the next day; therefore we must be conscious of the importance of ambulatory care in the ED. These departments are not intended only for the care of acutely ill or dying patients, and we must provide reasonably efficient and effective ambulatory care. Pure economics demand that EDs take proper care of ambulatory patients with injuries or illnesses. Every patient who presents to the ED should receive efficient and humane care, then a proper disposition with follow-up and good discharge instructions. Patients who leave against medical advice need careful chart documentation in case of a bad outcome. Those who leave without being seen cannot effectively sustain a claim in almost all cases.

UNSCHEDULED ADMISSIONS AFTER ED EVALUATION

Unscheduled admissions to a hospital within a short time after ED evaluation increase the risk of potential malpractice litigation. With increasing efforts by insurance companies as well as Medicare and Medicaid to keep patients as outpatients, patients are often seen in the ED and later admitted because there is no improvement on outpatient therapy; however, it is important to recognize that if the patient or the family is not aware of this potential, they might think inappropriate care was received and consider lawsuit. This situation should therefore be considered a potential maloccurrence.

VIOLATION OF CONFIDENTIALITY OR PRIVACY

The ED environment is not conducive to confidentiality or privacy. Histories are taken in areas where others might overhear as well as see the patient and his or her condition. Too little is done to reduce breaches of confidentiality in the ED, but, when possible, ED personnel should be conscious of an individual's need for privacy and confidentiality. Under no circumstances should one be careless or casual about revealing information on the patient's condition. The basic rule on confidentiality of a patient's record and privacy is that those with a need to know should know, and those that do not need to know and are merely curious should be prevented from invading the privacy of the patient. All patients deserve respect and privacy, particularly at the time of a personal or family crisis.

CHILD ABUSE

Although malpractice litigation generally does not arise in the context of potential or actual child abuse, nonetheless the legal considerations become of prime importance. On one hand, the state requires that physicians report suspected child or adult abuse, but a report should occur after a reasonable and careful evaluation. Recent experience with child abuse cases is described elsewhere in this text, but it is important to

recognize the difficulties in this area and the sensitivities on all sides. The safety of the potential victim must be the controlling factor.

POTENTIAL INJURIES TO UNKNOWN THIRD PARTIES

If an impaired patient is allowed to leave the ED and the medical staff knew or should have known that they would put the general public at risk, even an unknown victim might accuse the physician or nursing staff of a failure to protect the public from a potentially harmful person. If, on the other hand, *known third parties are threatened*, such as by an individual who has expressed homicidal or violent intentions, that known potential victim might reasonably expect a licensed physician to take steps for protection. When the public welfare or safety is at risk, confidentiality of the patient has to be weighed against larger responsibilities.

It is best to refer matters involving public safety or welfare to law enforcement and social services agencies. Use common sense and record the action taken.

MEDICAL STAFF SHARING OF RESPONSIBILITIES

One of the major areas for medicolegal concern for emergency physicians is the sharing of responsibility for patient care with the members of the medical staff. Emergency physicians cannot practice alone. Most hospitals prohibit emergency physicians from having admitting privileges to avoid splitting of patient responsibilities. As a result, all seriously ill patients require cooperative effort between the emergency physician and the medical staff.

ADMITTING ORDERS

If the emergency physician does not have admitting privileges, how can he or she write admitting orders? Once the admitting physician is identified and information is relayed to that admitting physician requesting his or her acceptance of the patient, there are many circumstances in which the emergency physician might facilitate admission to the floor by writing limited admitting orders. No significant risk is involved in writing *limited admitting orders*, which facilitate the admission of the patient to continue care started in the ED and promote an efficient transfer of responsibility to the admitting physician.

Whenever the emergency physician writes orders to facilitate admission, these orders should be written in consultation with the admitting physician, and they should refer the nurses to the admitting physician for further care. The hospital's policies should clearly define the responsibility of the admitting attendant once the decision to admit occurs.

The emergency physician is always available for

emergencies in the ED or for the patient whose admitting physician has not yet been present.

ON-CALL PHYSICIAN RESPONSE

We refer to the Joint Commission on Accreditation of Healthcare Organization (JCAHO) sections on emergency services for appropriate guidelines regarding on-call responsibilities and response from on-call physicians. In a level II ED, the on-call response time should be 30 minutes with voice communication acceptable.[20] Hospitals are responsible for establishing on-call lists.[21] Medical practice standards require that coordination of the care of severely ill patients or patients requiring hospitalization involve admitting physicians and on-call physicians.

LEGAL PROBLEMS RELATED TO RESUSCITATION

Although the best rule to follow in emergency services is to resuscitate whenever in doubt, under certain circumstances legal barriers are created to automatic resuscitation. When in doubt, resuscitation is still the best rule because a 5-to-10-minute delay in a resuscitation could cause permanent and irreversible damage, but in certain circumstances there are state laws and common law that would create additional considerations.

Most states have passed some kind of legislation that allows an individual to give an "advance directive" to physicians if they have developed a terminal or incurable, irreversible condition. These individuals may, under circumstances in which they have incurable or terminal condition, instruct physicians not to provide heroic resuscitative efforts if they have a cardiac or respiratory arrest. This principle of autonomy and control over one's treatment is a well-established and accepted principle that goes back to the basic concepts of consent for treatment. Present law in the United States requires that physicians inform patients of the diagnosis, the anticipated treatment, the risks of the condition, and the treatment for that condition, and then obtain consent to treat.[22]

TRANSFERS

A transfer creates significant risks because the patients are seriously ill, the family is upset, and other professionals are involved in the care, resulting in the potential for criticism and possible lawsuits. Careful preparation, communication, planning, and properly informing the patient and the family will reduce risk. State and federal law must also be considered. When transfers occur, there must be medical necessity. "Economic transfers" present serious malpractice risks with unstable patients, and can even enter into the area of "gross" negligence (which usually requires a repeated pattern of substandard actions).

PROFESSIONAL LIABILITY INSURANCE

One reasonable part of risk management is the intelligent purchase of insurance for potentially catastrophic losses. If malpractice cases were all limited to $500 in payment, insurance might not be appropriate, but the average cost of meritorious claims in emergency practice is well above $50,000, and many jury verdicts go in excess of a million dollars for meningitis and myocardial infarction cases; therefore insurance must be purchased. There are various types of insurance companies, including:

1. Commercial corporations
2. Stock companies
3. Mutual companies that are owned by the insureds
4. Self-insurance entities such as trusts and captives
5. Risk retention act insurance programs, which are either purchasing groups or domestic "captives"

In most states, emergency physicians are premium-rated with general surgeons or general practitioners who perform surgery, because of the frequency of claims against emergency physicians and the magnitude of those claims. Generally, the financial projections from an actuarial experience show that the range of losses for emergency physicians are in the order of a range of 2 to 8 dollars per ED visit. The cost increase has been more than threefold over the past ten years in costs per visit for emergency department malpractice. The dollars spent on claims during the 1974–83 period under the ACEP-endorsed programs was approximately 27 million dollars on 1547 claims for a total exposure of 55 million visits. This means that less than 50-cents-per-visit indemnity was paid in the early years of the program, with increasing costs later on, and there was a claim about every 30,000 visits.[10]

ALTERNATE INSURANCE

Emergency physicians have chosen alternate insurance for the following reasons:

1. Commercial insurers are not willing to create the flexible programs needed for ED groups.
2. The premiums were thought to be excessive.
3. Corporate entities dominate the practice of emergency medicine and are inclined, and able, to follow national trends of corporations toward self-insurance.
4. Price sensitivity and a past history of inconsistent and fluctuating commercial prices forced emergency physicians to look toward specialty resources

for emergency medicine professional liability coverage.

The Risk Retention Act,[23] which was a modification of an earlier federal legislation allowing manufacturers to insure themselves on products liability, created the opportunity for the formation of onshore self-insurance entities in two basic categories—purchasing groups and risk retention groups. The purchasing groups essentially try to trade purchasing power for better prices, whereas the risk retention groups are self-insurance entities that have licensure in one state and insure only their own class of risk—such as emergency physicians.

An insurance company is generally rated after a few years of its existence. If a *Bests* rating is a good one, the company is financially solvent and of good reputation; however, it is always difficult for one to predict and prevent catastrophic problems in an insurance company. Looking them up may not be adequate.

If an insurance company is regularly licensed in the state, it is required to contribute to an insolvency fund, which would allow some protection for insureds if the company becomes insolvent. In addition, the company is subject to insurance laws and insurance audits to insure proper reserving on potential losses and keeping money in the bank to pay claims. Insurance companies and insurance groups formed under the Risk Retention Act[23] are licensed in one state and admitted in other states to sell insurance, and they do not contribute to the insolvency funds of the states in which they operate. This reduces the amount of protection that a physician has if he gets a policy with one of these programs. The insurance entities created under the Risk Retention Act must be formed by those who are the intended insured. Before the Risk Retention Act, the Risk Retention Groups and various self-insured entities would start a captive offshore in a suitable domicile like Bermuda or one of the West Indies. Some of these captives are still offshore; many have moved onshore.

INSURANCE COVERAGE

The types of policies sold are either:

a) Occurrence, which is absolute coverage for the period no matter when the claim is made, or
b) "Claims made," which is effective only as long as coverage is continued consecutively with the same company and if the claim is filed within that insured period.

For example, if you own a claims-made policy and terminate your coverage with the company, and you receive a claim on that period after you terminate, the insurance is no longer effective unless you buy "an extended reporting endorsement" or "tail," which provides coverage for an extended period. Claims-made coverage does not cover on a claim made after termination, even on an incident during the insured

period. In the case of occurrence coverage, coverage is for the insured period no matter when the claim is filed.

Purchasing liability insurance is the most expensive overhead item for emergency physicians; therefore it must be done intelligently. The most flexible and easily used plan for emergency physicians is to buy insurance for a site of emergency service based on the number of visits and for coverage of visits on a per-visit basis. Obviously, there are times when physicians become ill or disabled, and if they have malpractice insurance, that must be replaced; then another policy must be purchased if the group is buying policies for each physician. On the other hand, if the insurance policy provides coverage for the facility and is based on a per-visit rate, insurance should be purchased for coverage up to a certain amount per claim and a total amount for the aggregate coverage for the group, whereas an individual policy is generally given for amount per claim and amount per year of coverage. The result is greater flexibility for replacement coverage along with eliminating the problem of deporting physicians who refuse to buy the "tail."

CREDENTIALS AND CREDENTIALING

Law over approximately the past 20 years has established that if physicians are to provide services, particularly in the hospital environment, the hospital is responsible for appropriately credentialing those physicians and properly monitoring the care they provide through its internal quality assurance programs.[24]

By tradition, many emergency physicians have not had full active staff privileges. That tradition is being changed for the benefit of ED patients and the emergency physician, who is an important contributing member of the medical staff. Radiologists and pathologists, who do not have admitting privileges but are hospital-based, are other examples of nonadmitting physicians who have active staff privileges. The trend toward active and full participation of emergency physicians makes the ED more of an integral part of the hospital.

One of the reasons in the past for not giving emergency physicians full privileges was the hospital administration's desire to be able to dismiss emergency physicians at will, but proper privileging and credentialing, along with membership in the medical staff, potentially provides the emergency physician with the protections that are provided to all physicians with active staff privileges. That is, those privileges cannot be removed without an appropriate fair hearing and some kind of appropriate disciplinary action. Some emergency service contracts waive that protection in the case of termination of the contract, but these protections are important for any physicians and should be considered important.

Physician discipline is created by many layers of regulatory and licensure activity, including the following:

1. State Board Medical Examiners
2. Drug Enforcement Administration
3. State drug control acts
4. Medical societies and associations
5. Hospital credentialing
6. Specialty societies and boards
7. Office of the Inspector General of Department of Health and Human Services

This impressive list of regulatory and disciplinary agencies and authorities requires at least a little attention. Basic rules regarding these matters include the following:

1. Once a physician has a license, it cannot be removed without appropriate disciplinary action, requiring rules and regulations that guarantee fairness and the concept of procedural and substantive due process.
2. Substantive due process is interpreted by the court as basic fairness.
3. Procedural due process has basic rules, including notice of charges, opportunity to defend yourself, and the right to a hearing before a fair and objective panel or tribunal.
4. If the action involves the removal of hospital privileges, the hospital medical staff is required to follow its own bylaws and provide the same fairness, even though it may be informal.
5. Peer review organizations (PROs) are required to follow their own regulations and procedures, but at the lower levels of discipline (less than formal sanctions), PROs are not required to follow as many rules of due process as one might imagine. For example, decisions on corrective actions and denials are somewhat unilateral.
6. Removal of membership or discipline by a medical society is also measured on the fairness and due process standard, with specific prohibitions against discipline based on advertising, participation in HMOs or managed care plans, or some other perceived anticompetitive bias.
7. Disciplinary actions against physician must avoid the taint of economic or personal motivation.

It is important for physicians to know their rights once they have become licensed or once they have obtained privileges. In addition, new law trends require that applications for privileges be treated in the same fair manner as disciplinary actions that remove privileges. Public and private hospitals, particularly those with sole community provider status, must now deal with new applicants fairly, and are allowed less leeway in barring physician applicants for medical staff. Private hospitals are allowed to use some arbitrary rules like requiring board certification or closing staff if the rules are applied consistently.

ANTITRUST LAW

This is not a complete review of this complex area of the law, governed by the Sherman Antitrust Act and other Federal and State laws, but the basic rule involved in these laws is as follows: it is considered per se a violation of anti-trust law to price-fix, boycott, or engage in any other activity that is plainly anticompetitive to the detriment of the consumer.

The most famous antitrust case involving disciplinary activities was the case of *Patrick vs. Burget*,[25] which involved a small hospital staff attempt to eliminate Dr. Patrick from practice in a small town in the northwest. The defendants attempted to defend themselves on the basis that their activities were authorized and protected by state laws because the state had an interest in peer review. The state action antitrust defense was rejected by the United States Supreme Court eventually because Oregon was not that actively and closely involved in the peer review process. In response to the problems that some perceived to be created by the *Patrick vs. Burget* opinion, Representative Wyden introduced a bill called the Healthcare Quality Insurance Act[26] which provided that if physicians followed a fair procedure, acted in the furtherance of good care, and were guided by the due process provisions of the act, they were immune from antitrust litigation and were also in a position to collect expenses for defending any nonmeritorious suit filed by a physician who was disciplined. The provisions of the Healthcare Quality Insurance Act basically involve the following:

1. Proper notice and reasonable notification as to the anticipated disciplinary action (30 days, the nature of the alleged violations, and the potential disciplinary action)
2. An opportunity for a fair hearing and a chance to properly defend
3. A fair hearing panel that did not have the taint of membership by competitors
4. A written justification for the final recommendation or ruling
5. All actions taken in a disciplinary context clearly for the benefit of patient care and not motivated by other financial, competitive, or personal considerations.

The Healthcare Quality Insurance Act also created a national data bank for reporting malpractice claims, disciplinary actions, and actions of licensing boards that were based on issues of professional competence of the physician. These reporting requirements are somewhat duplicative because medical malpractice actions, disciplinary actions by local medical societies and hospital staffs, and other matters related to discipline are now reportable to the state boards of medical examiners.

The National Practitioner Data Bank went into effect under a contract with Unisys beginning in 1990. Reports required include settlements on malpractice claims, adverse peer review action related to professional competence and conduct, and adverse actions of licensing boards. The reporting requirements under most state medical practice acts and the Healthcare Quality Insurance Act require that health care entities *shall report information on an adverse professional review action which affects clinical privileges for longer than 30 days and is based on competence or conduct and those actions or conduct should be reported within 15 days.* Insurers must report information respecting the payment of malpractice claims within 30 days of the payment, including information on the name of the insured, the amount of payment, the hospital with which the physician is associated, descriptions of acts or omissions on which the claim was based, and any other information that might be required by the Secretary of Health and Human Services.

Most state medical practice acts require licensed physicians to report if they believe another physician is impaired or reasonably believe that this physician might represent a risk to the public welfare.

Hospitals are required to inquire with the National Data Bank at the time of a physician's application for privileges. The hospital must update a medical staff physician every two years. The hospital is assumed to know what was in the data bank, if that is pertinent to a lawsuit filed against a hospital suit, when it fails to inquire. The Data Bank may release information to hospitals, practitioners requesting information about their own records, state licensing boards, a health care entity that is inquiring about a candidate for employment or affiliation, and in limited cases an attorney who is filing suit against a physician who must first submit information that the hospital failed to request information from the data bank about the provider. Purely statistical information that does not require identification can be released for research purposes.[27]

Advice to the physician on privileges and licensure:

1. Consider hospital privileges and the privileges of licensure as a tangible and important right that is protected by the law.
2. Peer review, quality assurance, and disciplinary action activities are a necessary part of the practice of medicine because physicians are licensed by the state to protect the public health, but these matters are controlled by legal principles of fairness and due process.
3. Federal funding of medical care automatically creates federal authority in matters of quality assurance and peer review, but the federal government is also required to follow rules of fairness and proper procedure.
4. When involved in a peer review, the physician must recognize that all actions must be taken in the interest of good patient care and not motivated by any other peripheral pecuniary or personal interest.
5. When an individual's credentials, privileges, or license are at stake, it is important to obtain proper legal representation.
6. Under certain circumstances, emergency physicians are particularly vulnerable to inappropriate politically motivated criticism, and therefore it is advisable to be careful in response to peer review matters.
7. It is important to realize that malpractice actions are reportable to state boards of medical examiners and to the National Data Bank and may compromise licensure and privileging for the physician; therefore settlements of malpractice claims should not be undertaken lightly.

There may be an arguable point that when hospitals move physicians in and out of an exclusive contract arrangement that does not involve a reportable peer review medical staff decision, if an emergency physician is found to be incompatible or is not desired, that individual can be terminated without creating the need for a reportable event.

CONTRACT LAW

Across the United States, emergency physicians generally work in an environment that requires at least some contractual agreements. Contract law in the American system is a part of the law that controls agreements between individuals or legal entities like corporations. Most emergency physicians in this country work as either employees or independent contractors. An independent contractor is an individual who offers his services for sale, not as an employee of the individual who pays, but as an equal or at least theoretically equal party to the agreement. For a contract to exist, two parties must exchange promises for what is legally called "consideration." Consideration is some kind of benefit that is sought. It might be either money or some other kind of agreement, generally, but it is considered part of the exchange in a contract.

Legally, a contract includes some important concepts of law:

1. Oral contracts are effective in the law but less easy for the courts to deal with, therefore important contracts are generally written.
2. A written contract includes information on the agreement that is essential for the interpretation, including:
   a. Date of the contract
   b. Term of the contract or the amount of time over which it will be effective

    c. The terms of the contract, which include the promises that were exchanged and the consideration involved in the contract

    d. Any additional restrictions on either party (These are also terms but should be thought of as separate modifiers)

    e. An indication as to what law would apply in interpreting the contracts (for example, the state law where the contract is entered into is normally the controlling law, but there may sometimes be doubt as to where the contract is actually effective)

Emergency physicians frequently enter into contracts with either hospitals or emergency services groups that hold the contracts for service to a hospital. Therefore, two contracts may be involved in the services required or in the services provided. It is important for physicians to understand that contract law is no more than the formal legal approach to the process of bargaining. If one considers the process a bargain, the law of contracts does not seem so mysterious. The two parties who enter into the contract should understand what is expected on both sides; this requires adequate research as to the responsibilities of the two parties on both sides. For example, there are laws which pertain to the operation of a hospital and the operation of emergency services, and there are expectations of the medical staff, the nursing staff, the hospital, and the emergency physician that should be thoroughly considered and researched before entering into a contract.

It is often said that the effect of a contract is no more long-lasting than the good intentions of the parties, but frequently the good intentions of the parties are compromised because of a failure to prepare properly for the contract negotiations and unwritten or unspoken expectations of the parties which result in later frustrations, disappointments, and even disagreements.

Generally, the four corners of a written contract are the controlling terms and conditions of the agreement. Parole evidence is evidence that might be presented to a court to explain or clarify written sections of the contract or attempt to resolve disputes that have developed over the written contract, but courts generally do not like parole evidence and frequently contracts specify that parole evidence is not an acceptable method of resolving a contract dispute. It is therefore important for physicians, hospitals, and emergency physician groups to be careful about the contracts they enter into and to properly research and thoroughly evaluate contractual arrangements. Then the contract should be carefully written.

INDEPENDENT CONTRACTORS UNDER THE LAW

Independent contractors are generally individuals who contract as individuals for personal services. This is a widespread custom in emergency medicine and sometimes circumvents what would otherwise have been an employment relationship. It is thought that professional services reasonably can be considered appropriate for "contract" by independent contractors; however, the Internal Revenue Service has recently reopened this area of discussion, which had previously been settled, and is reviewing independent contractor status in emergency medicine. The emergency physician is well advised to obtain legal counsel on what the impact might be if the Internal Revenue Service changes in approach toward "independent contractors."

For example, independent contractors pay their own estimated income tax. They are not subject to withholding, and the other party of the contract, which might in some circumstances be an employer, is not required to take withholding on income tax or obligated to pay social security tax. The independent contractor is obligated to pay a self-employment social security tax, which is less than the sum of the taxes that would be paid by an employer and an employee. In addition, the independent contractor is not given the opportunity to participate in pension funds or other benefits of the hospital or organization with which he or she contracts. The only benefits that can be derived from a contract arrangement are those which are described in the contract itself. Independent contract status is the most widespread form of agreement for emergency physician services; it is therefore important for emergency physicians to understand the legal implications of independent contractor status.

AGENCY LAW

It is important in emergency medicine to understand that the emergency physician functions as an "agent" of the hospital and possibly an agent of the group that contracts with him for his services. If an emergency physician is an employee, he automatically becomes an agent of the employer, but in an independent contractor situation, the agency relationship can be established by the fact that the independent contractor performs duties that are normally part of the responsibilities of the institution or the group.

Many states have a law that creates an "apparent agency" of the emergency physician in the ED. Both of these terms essentially mean that the hospital is not allowed to delegate away its responsibility for the emergency services provided because the patient who presents to the emergency department does not really have a choice as to what physician to see or what services would be provided. The institution provides the emergency physician as a part of its service. This may create "vicarious" liability for the hospital or the institution which is important in the loss because the liabilities that are created by emergency physician malpractice can then be transferred up to the "vicarious" liability of the institution. This is not an important issue in situations in which the emergency physician works as an employee because the employer-employee relationship automatically creates vicarious liability.

REPORTABLE EVENTS

CHILD ABUSE

All states have laws requiring that medical and child care professionals report any suspected child abuse. These statutes also provide immunity for anybody who reports a possible child abuse case in good faith. Physicians who identify a child who might be the victim of physical abuse or neglect are obligated to report such an event to the local law enforcement agencies or child protective services. The reporting requirements vary from state to state, but usually the important protocol to follow is:

1. Evaluate the child.
2. Make sure that the child is maintained in medical protective surroundings by any routes necessary if identified as a possible victim of child abuse.
3. Make a report to the local agency responsible for investigation.
4. Some states require a follow-up written report, but at least make sure that written documentation is made of a verbal or phone report if the agency is informed.

Legal risks for medical professionals exist on both sides of this issue, including families who are upset at being accused of child abuse, or the state, which has the power to deal harshly with an individual who fails to report child abuse. Child abuse widely goes unreported, but there are many instances of cases that could not be substantiated and may have involved inappropriate investigative and possibly interview techniques of the alleged child victims. In any event, unexplained injuries and histories that are not consistent with the nature of the child's problems, in the setting of a child who has poor development, poor socialization, and poor language development or any other signs of neglect, should lead one to report a suspected abuse or neglect.

ADULT ABUSE

This generally involves the abuse of the elderly or disabled. Certainly the difficulties of taking care of an adult who has significant disabilities, either mental or physical, can increase the potential for abuse and neglect of a dependent adult. This abuse can come at the hands of relatives, friends, spouses, or individuals who provide housing for these dependent adults.

As a separate phenomenon from spousal abuse, adult abuse should generally be suspected in an individual who needs the help of others and who appears to be receiving inadequate nutrition and general care, or to be suffering from injuries that are not easily explained or are explained with inconsistent histories. Report adult abuse to local law enforcement and, in some states, social service agencies. The obligation to report adult abuse is the same as for child abuse in most states.

SPOUSE ABUSE

This is the most widespread form of violence in the United States. Family and domestic spouse abuse is a widespread and chronic problem. It is so complex because of the interdependencies that exist and complicate the family relationships. Frequently alcohol and substance abuse aggravate spouse abuse. The dynamics of the marriage complicate the matter and create difficulties requiring counseling of both parties. The pathology of spouse abuse is too complex to deal with here, but the general suggested approach is to:

1. Take care of the medical and psychologic needs of the victim.
2. Try to determine whether alcohol and substance abuse are contributing factors (usually they are, and the patient and spouse should be referred for appropriate support).
3. Look for the potential neglect or abuse of minors.
4. Use spouse abuse counseling services.
5. Recognize that it is frequently difficult to break a relationship even when abuse is involved.

SEXUAL ABUSE OF MINORS

Sexual abuse of male and female minors continues to be a repulsive and too common event. In the evaluation of sexual abuse, it is important to recognize that sexual abuse of children and adolescents requires careful investigation and careful interview of the victim. Most emergency physicians are not able to do a proper interview because of limited time, but should provide the physical examination and general medical supervision required for the potential victims of childhood sexual abuse. These matters are dealt with elsewhere in this text, but some general rules include the following:

1. Do a head-to-toe examination.
2. When indicated, do a standard rape examination with fluorescent light for semen.
3. Vaginal examination should be done with care or under anesthesia because the examination could potentially be as traumatic if not done with proper precautions.
4. Examination of the introitus and anus are necessary to determine the potential for penetration or sexual assault.

5. In chronic sexual abuse, the condition of the genitalia and the condition of the anus and the tone of the anal sphincter on rectal examination are sometimes different from those in the normal examination.
6. Provide proper treatment for potential sexually transmitted disease or possible pregnancy.

Because incest and sexual abuse of children frequently involve relatives or friends of the children, these cases are difficult to investigate and evaluate. The emergency physician should restrict involvement to appropriate medical management, collection of medical evidence, protection of the victim from infection or other complications, and management of the psychosocial needs as much as is possible in the ED with proper referral to social and criminal agencies for other necessary evaluation.

RAPE

Rape is sexual contact without consent of one party, and comes in various degrees, all the way from unconsented touching to intercourse. Statutory rape involves an underage victim. The emergency physician, in evaluating a patient who has been raped, should follow protocols found elsewhere in this textbook, but a basic outline includes the following:

1. A history of the assault, with attention to potential for physical injuries and determining whether sexual penetration and/or ejaculation occurred.
2. Proper head-to-toe examination, with notes as to evidence of injury.
3. Collection of clothes, hair samples, fingernail scrapes, blood samples, and vaginal and rectal samples as well as swabs of areas where semen might be present (semen fluoresces on Ward's lamp).
4. Reflection of these samples should be generally done according to instructions and with the specimen containers and documentation available in the standard rape kits available across the country.
5. The medical record should be complete and include the general examination, general history, specific history of the assault, and general physical examination with specific attention to the examination for alleged sexual assault.
6. The patient should receive proper treatment to prevent sexually transmitted diseases because perpetrators of rape are generally at higher risk for carrying venereal diseases and sexually transmitted diseases.
7. The patient should be given the option of "the morning-after pill," which is generally effective if given within 7 days of intercourse. (See Chap. 58.)
8. The patient should be provided with proper psychosocial support because rape creates complex syndromes of mental as well as physical symptoms and difficulties.
9. The patient should be provided with available medical follow-up to ensure no pregnancy and no transmission of sexual diseases.

The evaluation and proper treatment of a rape victim is a sensitive area, and male physicians are encouraged to enlist the assistance of female nurses and doctors to help make it easier for the female victim. Proper management of rape cases includes not only the criminal, but the medical and psychologic needs of the patient.

CHAIN OF EVIDENCE

There is a lot of talk about the "chain of evidence." This deserves at least some comment in a legal section of an emergency medicine textbook. The chain of evidence is the sequence of custody that can be demonstrated in court to prevent any possible tampering with the evidence collected. For example, if a bullet is removed and is to be used as physical evidence in a case, the custody of that bullet from the time it was removed from the victim must be established and documented. The same is true in collection of evidence in other types of cases, but emergency physicians are most familiar with the concept of chain of evidence in rape cases. In rape investigation, the collection of evidence must be done in such a way that the custody of the evidence is documented from the time of collection and the place of collection all the way to the courtroom. If there is any interruption in that chain of custody, i.e., the evidence sits on a cabinet in an unsecured place for some time, or if there is no way to know exactly how the evidence got from the doctor to the evidence room, the defense will attempt to make as much as possibly can be made of the potential for tampering with or confusing the physical evidence specimens. As a result, to tighten up a case, the prosecution must show that the physical evidence was properly collected, properly secured, and kept in proper custody from the time of collection until the time of trial when it is presented as an exhibit in evidence for the prosecution.

Physicians working in the ED should be conscious of the importance of the possession of the physical evidence and a documentation of the chain of that possession.

Blood alcohol specimens can be collected without patient consent in many states if a serious injury or death has resulted from the accident. These specimens can be collected without significant legal risk for the physician. They are collected under the order of the state, and collection of blood specimens under a state criminal statute is allowed. If the accident does not involve situations that specifically provide for involuntary collection of a specimen, and if the patient refuses to consent to collection, the physician is best advised not to try to collect the specimen. The conviction of the individual can be accomplished even if the specimen is not collected. If the physician, the medical staff of the hospital or the laboratory, or the nursing staff are threatened by the police for "obstruction of justice," be aware that this is not the case and that no one has to contribute to the prosecution of a case or collection of evidence, particularly when the patient is refusing such a collection. Obviously, the collection of a blood specimen does not involve any significant potential for a claim or damages, but there is generally no point in forcing a patient to allow collection of a specimen under these circumstances unless the police have the authority by statute to collect the specimen involuntarily.

REPORTABLE COMMUNICABLE DISEASES

The reportable diseases list varies from state to state, but generally the infectious and communicable diseases that produce epidemics are the diseases of concern, as well as the communicable diseases that are sexually transmitted or transmitted by high-risk behavior such as intravenous drug use. Reporting sexually transmitted diseases and communicable disease generally follows the state law.

Special state laws have been written regarding the reporting and management of AIDS, the disease caused by the human immunodeficiency virus (HIV). Because the laws differ in various states, it is important to refer to your state law for the following important items:

1. Any restrictions on testing patients without consent.
2. Can patients be tested if they are going to expose medical personnel?
3. Rules on informing potential sexual partners for any positive test that is received if the patient is not willing to inform the sexual partner.
4. State law on the management of an HIV-positive patient who continues to participate in high-risk activity.
5. Many states have developed rules on proper counseling for anybody who has a positive test.
6. Many states have laws specifying how the reporting of a positive test must be done and to whom the positive test must be reported.

At this writing, estimates from the communicable disease center are that one hundred thousand deaths have occurred as a result of AIDS and that more than a million individuals are infected. The rate of infectivity is high in younger populations, which automatically increases the risk for emergency personnel. Studies done at Johns Hopkins are the best available information and show that a small percentage of unsuspected emergency patients, particularly with multiple trauma, are positive for HIV, and therefore emergency physicians are at risk. Universal precautions to reduce the risk of transmission of HIV and hepatitis B should be in place for protecting health care personnel.

Hepatitis B continues to be a significant risk for on-the-job acquisition in medical environments, and therefore hepatitis B and HIV are being dealt with with special concern because of the potential for morbidity and mortality in the case of hepatitis B and the 100% mortality rate for patients infected with HIV.

CONFIDENTIALITY AND AIDS

Patients have the right to confidentiality and privacy, even when they are being treated in the chaos of the ED. Therefore emergency physicians must be medically and legally conscious of their right to that privacy and the confidentiality of their medical treatment. The AIDS problem has increased the sensitivity of the medical community to confidentiality and privacy, but this has created many problems for health professionals, e.g., when performing operative or other procedures and in cases of human bites. This area is one of great confusion and will have to be resolved before the AIDS epidemic becomes more severe.

CONSENT

The basic rule on consent in American law is that the patient has the right to control his treatments and that therefore the physician has the responsibility to inform the patient of the following:

1. The working diagnosis
2. Alternative therapies
3. The risks of the diagnosis, therapies, and alternate therapies
4. An opportunity to choose
5. An opportunity to ask for explanations or get a second opinion

That sounds like a basically simple list of rules on consent, but because it is hard for patients to know, it is easy for physicians to abuse this area of care. Intelligent physicians should take the opportunity to make sure that the patient understands that medicine offers no miracles and that risks are involved in all forms of medical activity, as well as the benefits that might be achieved. When asking a patient for consent to treatment, the physician should make sure that the patient does not have any unreasonable expectations that will increase the risk of malpractice litigation, misunderstandings and hostility if a bad or unexpected result occurs.

Many states have formal requirements for complying with the law regarding consent, but the basic rules are the following:

1. People should be given the opportunity to consent or approve of any extraordinary treatment.

2. The general consent signed when the patient comes into the ED or hospital should be available only for routine procedures without significant risk.
3. Follow state laws regarding formalities as to consent. For example, Texas has a complex and formal approach to consents and has a List A and List B for procedures with different requirements on the two lists. Your state laws should be reviewed.
4. In any event, the basic common law rule is that the physician should provide the patient with the information that a reasonable person would have to make a decision about appropriate care.

The measure of proper compliance with the requirements for consent is that the physician should provide the patient with the information that a reasonable person would need to make a decision, but the best defense in a consent case is to provide the patient with the most appropriate care because ultimately, to prove a lack of informed consent case, the plaintiff must establish that he or she:

1. Did not receive the information
2. Would have chosen not to have the procedure if he or she had received the information
3. Did what a reasonable person would have done

In complex surgical procedures, consent may become important, but when emergency care is provided for people with emergency conditions, consent is not a significant consideration, but it should remind the physician to keep the patient and the patient's family informed, and to make sure they are aware of what is going on and do not have unreasonable expectations as to the outcome.

DUTY TO PROVIDE CARE

As described in other sections of this chapter, federal law requires access to care for any patient who presents with a possible emergency. In addition to state law, state hospital licensing regulations, JCAHO standards, and common law require access to emergency care for any patient who presents as a possible emergency case to any hospital that represents itself to the public as having an ED.

The responsibilities of hospitals without EDs are less clear. Professional obligations and professional licensure of nurses and physicians requires that they provide at least some response in institutions that do not have a formal ED.

For example, state law in Texas, Civil Statute 4438a, requires that hospitals and medical staffs provide emergency care for any patient who is diagnosed by a licensed physician as having an emergency condition. Well-established case law requires that hospitals provide emergency care for anybody who has a le-

gitimate emergency. This requires at least a screening examination to determine whether an emergency condition exists.

SUMMARY

Comprehensive risk management programs for physicians are warranted in view of the numbers, severity, and economic impact of ED malpractice suits. Studies that focus on common causes and preventability offer the most benefit.[28] It has been noted that actual claims represent only a small percentage of actual negligent events,[29] although this aspect was disputed.[30]

REFERENCES

1. 42 CFR 482.
2. 42 U.S.C. 1395 dd.
3. Omnibus Budget Reconciliation Act (OBRA) 1989, Sections 6018 and 6211. Amending Social Security Act and 42 U.S.C. 1395dd at Sections 1866 and 1867.
4. Trautline, H., Lambert, R.L., and Miller, J.: Malpractice in the emergency department—Review of 200 cases. Ann. Emerg. Med. 13:709, 1984.
5. Ohio Hospital Associate Publication Bulletin 89–99–A, published December 29, 1989.
6. Lee, T.H., Cook, F., Weisberg, M., et al.: Acute chest pain in the emergency room. Identification and examination of low risk patients. Arch. Intern. Med. 145:65, 1985.
7. Lee, T.H., Rouan, G.W., Wesiberg, M., et al.: Sensitivity of routine clinical criteria diagnosing myocardial infarction within 24 hours of hospitalization. Ann. Intern. Med. 106:181, 1987.
8. Tierney, W.M., Fitzgerald, J., and McHenry, R.: Physician's estimates of the probability of myocardial infarction in emergency room patients with chest pain. Med. Decisionmaking 6:12, 1986.
9. Lee, T.H., Rowan, G.W., and Weisberg, M.C.: Clinical characteristics and natural history of patients with acute myocardial infarction sent home from the emergency room. Am. J. Cardiol. 60:219, 1987.
10. Tierney, W.M., Roth, B.J., Psaty, B., et al.: Predictors of myocardial infarction in emergency room patients. Crit. Care Med. 13:526, 1985.
11. Granville, R., Armed Forces Institute of Pathology: Personal communication.
12. Dunn, J.D.: Chest Pain. In Foresight, American College of Emergency Physicians, Dallas, Texas, 1990.
13. McCarthy, P.L., Lembro, R.M., Baron, M.A., et al.: Predictive value of abnormal physical examination findings in ill-appearing and well-appearing febrile children. Pediatrics 16:167, 1985.
14. Board of Directors: Principles of Appropriate Patient Transfer. Ann. Emerg. Med. 19:337, 1990.
15. ACS Committee on Trauma: Interhospital Transfer of Patients. Bulletin of the ACS, February 13–15, 1990.
16. Ansell, D., and Schiff, R.: Patient dumping: Status, implications, and policy recommendations. JAMA 257:1500, 1987.
17. Reed, W., Cowley, K., and Anderson, R.: Special report—The effect of a public hospital's transfer policy inpatient care. N. Engl. J. Med. 315:1428, 1986.
18. Kellerman, A., and Hackman, B.: Emergency department patient dumping: An analysis of interhospital transfers to a re-

gional medical center at Memphis, Tennessee. Am. J. Public Health *78*:1287, 1988.

19. Texas Revised Civil Statute 4437f, codified at The Texas Hospital Licensing Law, Chapter XI.

20. JCAHO, Chicago, E.R. 1.4.2.

21. AMH, 2.4 et seq.

22. Canterbury vs. Spence, 464 F.2d 772 (D.C. Cir. 1972).

23. 15 U.S.C. Sec 3901 et seq.

24. Darling vs. Charleston Community Hospital 200 N. E. 2d 149 (Illinois Supreme Court 1965).

25. 486 U. S. 94 (1988).

26. 42 U.S.C. Section 111101, et seq.

27. 45 CFR Section 60.11 and 61.13.

28. Karcz, A., et al.: Preventability of malpractice claims in emergency medicine. A closed claims study. Ann. Emerg. Med. *19*:865, 1990.

29. Locaho, A.R., et al.: Relation between malpractice claims and adverse events due to malpractice—Results of the Harvard medical practice study. N. Engl. J. Med. *325*:245, 1991.

30. Brennan, R.E.: Malpractice and negligence (Letter). N. Engl. J. Med. *326*:140, 1992.

Addenda

ACUTE AND CHRONIC RENAL FAILURE

GENERAL CONSIDERATIONS

Demetrius Ellis and Ellis D. Arner

ADDENDUM 1

Before discussing such treatment measures and the newer developments in dialytic techniques, it is important to apply the newly acquired knowledge of the biochemical alterations at the cellular level to help design protocols that help to prevent establishment or enhance recovery of ARF.[A146]

ISCHEMIC ARF

The metabolic processes in cells exposed to ischemia or nephrotoxins have been the major focus of recent investigations. Renal ischemia results in hypoxic or anoxic injury, particularly to the outer renal medulla. The nephron segments most affected are the S_3 portions of the proximal tubules and the medulla thick ascending limb of Henle's loop.[A14] Given a systemic ischemic insult, ARF is more likely to occur than ischemic dysfunction of the heart, brain, or liver.[A7,A104] The highest ratio of O_2 consumption to oxygen delivery in the body occurs in the renal medulla (79% of O_2 extracted), explaining the special susceptibility of structures in this region of hypoxic injury.[A26] The high O_2 consumption in these mitochondria-rich actively transporting cells is proportional to the level of active Na^+ transport, mainly mediated by sodium-potassium adenosine triphosphatase (Na-K ATPase). Anoxia depletes the adenine nucleotide pool proportionally to the degree of oxygen deprivation.[A23,A27,A34,A37,A38,A99,A123,A140,A143] Human kidneys appear to be less resistant to the effects of anoxia than kidneys of various experimental animals so that the pathologic findings of acute tubular necrosis or ATN may be seen after as little as 10 minutes of anoxia. Hypoxia (20 to 40% fall in oxidative capacity) has less deleterious consequences than anoxia and probably represents the typical clinical situation in man.

ATN is evidenced by a patchy distribution of cell necrosis, disappearance of the proximal brush-border and basolateral infoldings, swelling of tubular cells, tubular dilation, and casts.[A45,A94,A98,A101] The necrotic cells slough off and obstruct the tubule, thereby leading to increased intratubular pressure which opposes glomerular transcapillary filtration pressure and leads to a fall in GFR. In severe ATN in humans, up to 50% of glomerular filtrate may be reabsorbed by transtubular backleak across the damaged tubular epithelium.[A94] Unobstructed but damaged tubules have a decreased ability to reabsorb Na^+ and other substances that are actively transported across the brush-border. The presentation of large solute loads to the macula densa and the distal tubules often lead to activation of renin-angiotensin-aldosterone system (RAAS) and activation of tubuloglomerular feedback mechanisms with resultant afferent arteriolar vasoconstriction and further reduction in renal blood flow and GFR. Indeed, a model of renal injury implicating the RAAS in the dysregulation of glomerular microcirculation, proximal tubular reabsorptive capacity, and other physiologic processes has been recently proposed to explain renal injury at the cellular level.[A11,A56,A92] Loss of intracellular substrates, such as ATP and O_2, also leads to reduced activity of Na-K ATPase, which is essential for maintaining transmembrane electrochemical gradients and Na^+ coupled transport of glucose, amino acids, and other nutrients.[A4,A25,A29,A44,A57,A58,A62,A65,A88,A97,A119,A139] This may be responsible for the intracellular accumulation of solute and fluid and the morphologic appearance of hydropic changes in such cells.

Drug-induced ischemic ARF has become increasingly clinically relevant in recent years. Foremost among causative agents are the nonsteroidal anti-inflammatory drugs (NSAIDs), including aspirin, indomethacin, ibuprofen, fenoprofen, etc.[A25] In one study, these agents accounted for 15.6% of all drug-induced ARF.[A65] NSAID-induced ARF is commonly caused by vasoconstriction and reduced renal blood flow, secondary to inhibition of renal prostaglandin synthesis through inhibition of the rate-limiting enzyme cycloxygenase. A fall in the synthesis of renal vasodilator prostaglandins (PGE_2 and prostacyclin) is especially deleterious in patients who are volume-depleted; patients with congestive heart failure, nephrotic syndrome or cirrhosis of the liver, systemic lupus erythematosus or renal vasculitis; and patients with pre-existing renal injury. Such patients with reduced renal blood flow have a baseline elevation in circulating angiotensin II (AT-II), which, through phospholipase C activation, leads to afferent arteriolar vasoconstriction and maintenance of renal perfusion. In the absence of prostaglandin blockade, this vasoconstriction is not generally manifested by a fall in GFR because of the opposing vasodilatory compensatory response mediated principally by PGE_2 and prostacyclin. In patients at high risk for developing NSAID-induced ARF, the vasodilatory effects of PGE_2 and prostacyclin are inhibited so that the vasoconstrictive effects of AT-II predominate. The concurrent use of NSAIDs and agents capable of producing analgesic nephropathy, such as acetaminophen or phenacetin, is especially damaging to the kidney because the NSAID-induced vasoconstriction potentiates the renal accumulation of toxic metabolites of these other analgesics and may result in vascular necrosis.

The metabolic and biochemical consequences of ischemia are common to many vital tissues. The mechanisms involved in anoxic or hypoxic injury to such tissues are mentioned only briefly here because such mechanisms provide the rationale for the formulation of newer specific prevention and treatment protocols for ARF.

Available data suggest that a reduction in cell ATP levels caused by decreased oxidative metabolism leads to biochemical events that increase cellular concentrations of hypoxanthine. Intracellular release of calcium and proteases also increases the conversion of hypoxanthine dehydrogenase to xanthine oxidase, which simultaneously catalyzes the conversion of hypoxanthine and of molecular oxygen that becomes available during tissue reperfusion to produce superoxide free radicals.[A88] These free radicals play an important role in lipid peroxidation and injury to cell membranes.[A44] Vascular endothelial cell permeability may be especially increased by such reperfusion injury.

An alternative model for postperfusion injury and free oxygen radical formation involves activation of phospholipase A and C by the combined effects of hydrogen peroxide, lipid peroxidation, and release of intracellular calcium. This results in activation of the arachidonic acid cascade and release of thromboxane A_2 and leukotrienes, leading to vasoconstriction and adhesion of polymorphonuclear leukocytes. Release of NADPH oxidase from these cells catalyzes the reduction of oxygen to form superoxide free radicals.

Thus far, pharmacologic modulation of various steps in this pathway by the thromboxane synthetase inhibitor dazoxiben or the leukotriene receptor antagonist FP55712 has been limited to experimental endotoxin-induced ARF.[A4]

NEPHROTOXIC ARF

Two special classes of agents are responsible for a large proportion of all cases of ARF in humans and produce renal injury by diverse pathogenetic mechanisms. Aminoglycosides may induce acute tubular necrosis primarily involving the proximal tubule.[A58,A97,A139] As many as 50% of patients receiving therapeutic amounts of aminoglycosides may manifest tubular and glomerular dysfunction.[A62] The ARF induced by aminoglycosides is usually nonoliguric and serum creatinine elevation may be preceded by hyperexcretion of lysozyme and β_2 microglobulin, isosthenuria and aminoaciduria.[A97,A116] Older patients are particularly prone to ARF from these agents. The mechanism underlying this injury is inhibition of lysosomal phospholipases resulting in cytosolic accumulation of toxic phospholipids.[A9,A41,A89] Tubular backleak and obstruction do not appear to be significant in the pathogenesis of this form of ARF. Although the mechanism for the reduced GFR is unknown, increased solute delivery to the macula densa and hormonally mediated tubuloglomerular feedback are believed to be responsible for the reduction in GFR.

Radiocontrast media are the second class of clinically relevant agents that can produce ARF. Within minutes or hours after receiving urographic or angiographic radiocontrast media, susceptible individuals may develop oliguria associated with a low fractional excretion of sodium and a persistent nephrogram.[A51] Among hospitalized patients, 10% may develop ARF caused by these agents. High-risk groups include patients with diabetes mellitus who may have pre-existing vascular disease and may develop prolonged ischemia from vasoconstriction induced by such agents, and patients with a serum creatinine above 2 mg/dL who have increased exposure time to these potential toxins. At moderate risk are patients receiving a large contrast load, those with multiple myeloma, volume depletion, previous renal failure caused by contrast media, the elderly, patients with vasculitis, and patients receiving NSAIDs.

ARF induced by the hyperosmolar ionic monomers comprising radiocontrast media is mediated by two mechanisms: a vasoconstrictive/hypoxic effect caused by osmotic diuresis and presentation of increased amount of Na^+ and other solutes to the macula densa leading to release of renin and increase in AT-II; and a direct toxic effect to the S_3 segment of the proximal tubule, resulting in epithelial cell sloughing and obstruction of the tubular lumen.[A54,A134] Recently developed nonionic monomers, although more expensive, are considerably less hypertonic and nephrotoxic.[A1,A127] Use of these newer agents, especially in the high-risk groups, is likely to reduce the future incidence of radiocontrast-induced ARF.

ADDENDUM 2

PREVENTION AND SPECIFIC TREATMENT OF TUBULAR INJURY

Because ischemia appears to be a major common factor, not only in ischemic ARF but also in nephrotoxic ARF, the use of newer agents in the prevention and treatment of ARF has been directed to overcoming the aforementioned physiologic and biochemical alterations resulting from oxygen and substrate deprivation. Hence, inhibition of xanthine oxidase by allopurinol has been used to decrease the production of toxin-free radicals, which superoxide dismutases (SOD) can scavenge by catalyzing their conversion to hydrogen peroxide and oxygen.[A5] Although not yet evaluated in humans, pharmacologically decreasing oxygen demands for transport in the proximal tubule and in the medullary thick ascending limb of Henle's loop may also reduce ischemic injury.[A15] In experimental studies, it is possible to show an attenuation in such injury by furosemide[A67] and ouabain,[A123] whereas nystatin and amphotericin B, which increase membrane permeability and stimulate Na-K ATPase activity, may produce or aggravate anoxic injury.[A16] Antioxidants, such as vitamins A, E, C, and β-carotene, and chelators of calcium and iron, have also been used in preliminary animal studies.

Only a few studies have investigated the efficacy of newer agents to prevent or to treat ARF in man. The effects of calcium channel inhibitors, such as verapamil, nifedipine, and diltiazem, have been used in preventive clinical settings: recipients of renal allografts[A112] or patients undergoing coronary bypass or valve replacement surgery.[A53] Only the former study demonstrated better postsurgical renal function in the patients receiving such agents. The efficacy of calcium channel blockade for both prevention or treatment of established ARF, however, requires further investigation. Similarly, limited experience exists in the use of vitamin E in the treatment of ARF from hemolytic uremic syndrome (HUS) in children. A preliminary study has demonstrated that oral tocopherol at 1000 mg/m^2/day for one week was associated with improved recovery and fewer long-term sequelae as compared to other treatments or no intervention therapy.[A107] Similarly, the infusion of prostacyclin (PGI$_2$) to counterbalance the effect of excess thromboxane A$_2$ and vasoconstriction in HUS has met with limited and contradictory results.[A8,A145]

Of particular interest have been the clinical studies using ATP-MgCl or thyroxin. ATP-MgCl$_2$ infusion, ranging from 3 to 30 mg/kg, has been associated with no adverse effects in healthy male volunteers.[A22] In another study, a benefit was shown of ATP-MgCl$_2$ infusion in combination with other agents in 37 patients with ARF.[A96] This solution has also been shown to improve renal allograft preservation for transplantation.[A80] Also of clinical benefit was the oral administration of thyroxin at 5 to 6 μg/kg/day in an uncontrolled study of eight children with ARF.[A130] It is likely that a mixture of agents, including a calcium channel inhibitor, an inhibitor of angiotensin-converting enzyme or AT-II receptors to decrease vasomotor tone, an antioxidant, superoxide dismutase, ATP-MgCl$_2$, and mannitol or furosemide to promote diuresis and decrease tubular obstruction, may be more effective than when such agents are used alone. Clearly, many prospective controlled trials are needed to determine the utility and safety of these new therapies. The biologic and physiologic roles of the newly characterized atrial natriuretic peptide, endothelin and endothelium-derived relaxing factors such as nitric oxide in the pathogenesis of ARF will undoubtedly unfold in the coming years and may offer yet more opportunities of preventing or managing ischemic or nephrotoxic renal injury.

Clinical studies suggest that dopamine infusion at 2.5 to 5.0 μg/kg/min may increase renal blood flow, GFR, and urine output with minimal adverse systemic hemodynamic effects in many patients with early ARF.[A86] In patients with shock and ARF in whom norepinephrine infusion may further limit renal perfusion, the addition of low-dose dopamine may help maintain renal perfusion, and furosemide may potentiate the effects of low-dose dopamine in improving renal blood flow.[A115]

ADDENDUM 3

In the past, hemodialysis and peritoneal dialysis have been the main means of regulating fluid and electrolyte imbalance in individuals with ARF. While hemodialysis may be particularly valuable in hypercatabolic patients who accumulate solutes rapidly and may develop uremic symptoms early in the course of ARF, several new modalities have recently found increasing indications in critically ill patients with postsurgical fluid overload and edema with or without major electrolyte imbalance. Such therapies are particularly useful in patients with ARF in whom hemodynamic instability increases hemodialysis morbidity while inability to utilize the abdomen (orthotopic liver transplantation, major abdominal surgery) precludes peritoneal dialysis. In such patients, hemofiltration procedures have become quite popular with intensive care unit personnel since they are effective, do not require complicated dialysis machines, and are relatively simple to perform.[A28,A68] The main indications for hemofiltration are summarized in Table 48A-1.

TABLE 48A-1. CLINICAL INDICATIONS FOR HEMOFILTRATION*

1. Fluid overload:
  A. Hemodialysis patients with pre-existing access:
    a. Acute pulmonary edema
    b. Hemodynamic instability
  B. Patients with acute renal failure:
    a. Hemodynamic instability
    b. Postoperative cardiac surgery
    c. Recent myocardial infarct
    d. Sepsis
  C. Patients with pump failure:
    a. Diuretic-resistant
    b. Oliguria despite inotropic support
  D. Oliguric states in patients that require large quantities of IV fluids: i.e., hyperalimentation, medications, etc.
  E. Chronic fluid overload (?):
    a. Ascites
    b. Nephrotic edema

2. Solute removal:
Alternative therapy to hemodialysis or peritoneal dialysis in patients with chronic or acute renal failure and:
  A. Hypotension
  B. Hemodynamic instability
  C. Need for parenteral fluids
  D. Associated medical complications

3. Acid-base and electrolyte disturbances:
  A. Metabolic alkalosis
  B. Metabolic acidosis
  C. Hyponatremia, etc.

* Reprinted with permission (Reference A62)

The expanding list of dialytic choices and their relative benefits and limitations are outlined in Table 48A-2. If removal of fluid is the major objective, continuous venovenous hemofiltration (CVVH) or continuous arteriovenous hemofiltration (CAVH), may be used depending on vascular access availability and adequacy of cardiovascular function.[A19,A21,A70,A85,A147,A150,A152] In principle, the patient's own systemic blood pressure or a mechanical pump is utilized to regulate blood flow through a hemofilter consisting of a highly permeable membrane of variable appropriate surface area, extracorporeal volume, and ultrafiltration efficiency. As with hemodialyzers, the choice of available hemofilters is rapidly expanding (Table 48A-3). A filtrate similar in composition to protein-free plasma water is removed via this convective process.

Phosphate clearance is considerably better with hemofiltration as compared to hemodialysis, so that hypophosphatemia may result. This effect, however, may be of special benefit in the tumor-lysis syndrome, in which CAVH has been effective in reducing high serum phosphorus levels.[A46] As with hemodialysis, medications may be removed through the hemofiltration process and may require special dosing provisions. Table 48A-4 shows the sieving coefficients for several commonly used medications. The rate of drug clearance may be determined by the product of the sieving coefficient of the drug and the ultrafiltration volume. Ultrafiltrate is usually replaced with a lesser volume of fluid that may be of particular benefit to each individual patient. Such fluids may include a balanced electrolyte solution, crystalloid, colloid, or blood products. Paired replacement fluids are often required and may include a bicarbonate solution and a calcium-plus-magnesium-containing solution, which are infused in separate vessels. A sliding fluid rate replacement may be administered so that a filtrate removal of 5 mL/min (7.2 L/day) may be replaced at 30%, whereas an ultrafiltration rate of 15 mL/min may be replaced at 67% of the losses, thereby permitting more delivery of nutritional fluids, which are especially beneficial in hypercatabolic postoperative patients. Clotting of the hemodialysis or hemofiltration circuits may be minimized by low-dose pre-filter heparin administration to maintain an activated clotting time in the circuit of 120 to 150 seconds. This agent may increase morbidity in the early postoperative period or in patients with hemorrhagic difficulties. In such settings, regional heparinization or the use of

TABLE 48A-2. BENEFITS AND LIMITATIONS OF CURRENT DIALYTIC MODALITIES*

	Solute Clearance	Ultrafiltration Efficiency	Ultrafiltration Regulation	Hemodynamic Stability	Arterial Line Needed	Dialyzer/Hemofilter Clotting Problems	Technical Complexity
Hemodialysis	+++	++	+	+	No	+	++
Hemofiltration	++	+++	++	++	No	+	++
Conventional ultrafiltration	−	+++	++	++	No	+	+
Continuous modalities:							
SCUF	−	++	+	+++	Yes	+++	+
CAVH	+	++	++	+++	Yes	+++	++
CAVHD	++	++	+	++	Yes	+++	++
CVVH	−	+++	+++	+++	No	+	++
CVVHD	++	+++	+++	+++	No	+	+++

SCUF = Slow continuous ultrafiltration; CAVH = continuous arteriovenous hemofiltration; CAVHD = continuous arteriovenous hemodiafiltration; CVVH = semicontinuous venovenous hemofiltration; CVVHD = semicontinuous venovenous hemodiafiltration
* Reprinted with permission (Reference A69)

TABLE 48A-3. COMMERCIALLY AVAILABLE FILTER SYSTEMS USED IN HEMOFILTRATION

Filter	Manufacturer	Membrane Material	Membrane Surface (m²)	Extracorporeal Volume (mL)
Diafilter D10	Amicon Corp.	Polysulfone	0.2	25–30
Diafilter D20	Lexington, MA		0.25	30–35
Diafilter D30			0.6	
Minifilter			0.015	9–12
Ultrafilter	ASAHI Medical	Polyacrylonitrile	0.5	
GS	Tokoyo, Japan	Cuprophane	0.3	40
AMO₃				
AV-400	Fresenius AG	Polysulfone	0.7	
AV-600	Oberusel, FRG		1.4	
Uetrafilter U²⁰⁰⁰	Gambro AB	Polyamide	0.1	17–20
FH-55	Lund, Sweden	Polyamide cuprophane	0.6	55–60
GF-80			0.9	80
Biospal 1200S	Hospal Ltd Basel, Switzerland	Polyacrylonitrile	0.5	
Renaflo 0.25	Renal Systems	Polysulfone	0.3	
Renaflo 0.5	Minneapolis, MN		0.5	

procyclin or other heparin-free regimens may be required.[A132]

Several additional variations of hemofiltration are currently available. Slow continuous ultrafiltration, or SCUF, is designed to remove fluids slowly so that no replacement solution is necessary.[A100,A135] Continuous venovenous hemodiafiltration (CVVHD) or continuous arteriovenous hemodiafiltration (CAVHD)[A39,A40,A102,A117,A124,A138] combine convective clearance with diffusion clearance by infusing dialysis fluid of appropriate composition countercurrent to the blood flow in the hemofilter. Unlike convection, which

aids mainly fluid removal, diffusion permits a greater solute clearance, similar to that obtained by dialysis.

Technical points worth emphasizing include the following. An arterial access is needed for SCUF, CAVH, and CAVHD. Because of the high efficiency of ultrafiltration with many hemofilters, high-volume pulsatile pumps may be needed to regulate not only blood flow but also the rate of filtrate removal and the dialysate flow rate. When an A-V access is not available and a venous-to-venous flow is established, an air embolus detector must be integrated into the circuit.

TABLE 48A-4. SIEVING COEFFICIENT DURING HEMOFILTRATION

Drug	Sieving Coefficient
Amikacin	0.88
Ampicillin	0.69
Gentamicin	0.81
Metronidazole	0.86
Mezlocillin	0.58
Nafcillin	0.54
Tobramycin	0.78
Vancomycin	0.69
Amphotericin	0.40
Cefotaxime	0.51
Cephapirin	1.70
Clindamycin	0.37
Digoxin	0.85
Phenobarbital	0.86
Phenytoin	0.45
Procainamide	0.86
Theophylline	0.85

Reprinted with permission (Reference A62)

ADDENDUM 4

PROTEIN INTAKE AND CRF

A great deal of investigative effort has focused on the role of protein intake and on circulating lipids in the progression of CRF. Protein restriction has been used over several decades to alleviate uremic symptoms. Such restriction has been based on the well-documented clinical observation that patients with CRF and BUN levels of 50 mg/dL have far fewer uremic symptoms than those with BUN levels of about 90 mg/dL.[A77] In addition, animal data indicate that glomerular hyperfiltration resulting from high-protein diets is an important contributing factor to the progression of CRF.[A50,A63,A64] Thus, the objective of human trials of protein restriction is to test the hypothesis that a common mechanism underlies the progression of most causes of CRF and that such progression may be modulated by dietary means or by medications. The reader is referred elsewhere for critical reviews on the methods used to assess nutritional status and protein intake and the limitations of the tools used to assess small changes in renal function and the rate of progression of CRF.[A91,A142]

Several studies in adults with CRF have used a 0.6 g protein/kg/day diet (range 0.4 to 0.6 g protein/kg/day) and a minimum caloric intake of 35 kcal/kg/day, and the reciprocal serum creatinine, creatinine clearance, and survival time have been used as indices of progression of CRF.[A43] A review of these trials indicates that, despite differences in study design, duration of dietary management, sample, size, and ascertainment of compliance with such diets, the results are inconclusive.[A43] Two prospective randomized trials in adults, however, have shown a significant slowing in the rate of progression of CRF, particularly in patients with glomerulonephritis.[A55,A111] In one of these studies,[A55] the dietary phosphorus content was also lower in the protein-restricted group, so that the protective effect of lowering in dietary phosphorus per se must also be considered.[A128,A69] Successful implementation of low-protein diets is a major factor limiting the possible benefits of such management. When "good compliance" is maintained over prolonged periods, CRF progression may be delayed by a factor of 2.[A43] A benefit of low-protein diet in slowing progression and in decreasing proteinuria has also been demonstrated in individuals with diabetic nephropathy.[A141,A151]

Because of growth, children generally require higher protein intakes than adults.[A36,A108] Data from a large randomized study in children, in whom dietary protein was restricted from a baseline value of 1.75 g/kg/day to 1 g/kg/day without restriction of energy intake, show that over a 1-year period there was no adverse effect on growth; however, no significant differences were demonstrated in the progression of CRF between diet and controlled groups.[A149]

LIPIDS AND CRF

In 1982, Moorehead et al.[A93] proposed that progression of CRF may be caused by glomerular injury induced by lipoproteins, especially in individuals with the nephrotic syndrome. The role of lipids in the pathogenesis of CRF has been the subject of several reviews.[A61] It has been proposed that hypercholesterolemia per se may alter renal hemodynamics and produce glomerular injury.[A3] It has also been suggested that the benefit of low-protein diets in retarding progression may be partly related to a decreased lipid content of such diets. It should be noted, however, that few data in humans with CRF treated with lipid-lowering agents suggest efficacy in decreasing the rate of progression of CRF.

MODULATION OF CRF BY DRUGS

Studies published from 1977 to 1988 indicate that angiotensin-converting enzyme inhibitors may decrease experimentally induced glomerular injury by reducing systemic and, perhaps, glomerular hypertension by preferentially decreasing efferent glomerular vasoconstriction.[A60,A128] Such agents also decrease proteinuria and hyperlipidemia in diabetics and may decrease progression in this manner.[A12,A83] In individuals with diabetic nephropathy and also in patients with severe renal failure, the use of angiotensin-converting enzyme inhibitors may further decrease GFR and increase the risk of hyperkalemia.[A133] Calcium channel inhibitors have a lesser effect on proteinuria but may also afford renal protection by decreasing systemic and/or intraglomerular hypertension.[A2,A90,A154] Finally, antiplatelet agents may also have a modifying influence on the progression of CRF.[A153]

ADDENDUM 5

Because PTH is believed to be a major toxin mediating the uremic syndrome,[A84] suppression of PTH by administration of oral calcitriol (1.25(OH$_2$D) at dosages of 0.25 to 2.0 µg/day and maintenance of serum calcium levels in the upper limits of normal is desirable in the prevention of hyperparathyroidism.[A6,A10] Osteitis fibrosa cystica responds much better to calcitriol than does osteomalacia.[A6,A10] In dialysis patients, however, intravenous calcitriol as compared to oral calcitriol may be superior in suppressing PTH levels.[A126] Treatment with vitamin D should begin early in the course of CRF (GFR below 50 to 60 mL/min) to help prevent bone deterioration. It should also be noted that calcitriol has a spectrum of biologic actions far greater than its effects on mineral metabolism.[A110]

Control of hyperphosphatemia is even more important in controlling secondary hyperparathyroidism in CRF than serum calcium abnormalities.[A57] At GFR exceeding 25% of normal, serum phosphate levels are usually not increased because of adaptive hypersecretion of PTH.[A71] This cycle of progressive hyperparathyroidism may be interrupted by earlier institution of a low-phosphate diet, use of phosphate binders, and adequate dialysis, realizing that the latter measure is relatively inefficient in removing phosphate[A47] and that concomitant usage of calcitriol augments intestinal absorption of phosphate as well as calcium.[A17] In both adults and children, attempts to limit dietary phosphate intake should be undertaken.

In the past decade, several new phosphate binders have been introduced to replace the previously used aluminum hydroxide and aluminum carbonate preparations. Aluminum-containing phosphate binders may produce toxicity consisting of osteomalacia, proximal myopathy, anemia, and encephalopathy. The newer agents inculde calcium carbonate, calcium lactate, calcium citrate, and calcium acetate, the last being the newest and perhaps the most effective of these medications.[A120] The usual dosage of these agents is 2 to 5 g/day. Currently, calcium carbonate is the drug of choice because it is inexpensive and tasteless, and provides the highest proportion (40%) of elemental calcium. Phosphate binders work best when given with meals, and the dosage may be adjusted depending on serum phosphate levels and the amount of phosphate that an individual may consume at a given meal. Hypercalcemia, which may occur with phosphate binders, may be controlled with use of a low-calcium-dialysate concentration in patients on dialysis,[A125] the addition of low dosages of aluminum gels, and temporary discontinuation of vitamin D and calcium supplements. Dyspepsia, constipation, and lack of palatability are other potential problems that may limit compliance of patients and effectiveness of these medications.

ADDENDUM 6

The availability of biosynthetic erythropoietin has essentially eliminated the anemia of CRF and the multiple risks associated with blood transfusions, including iron overload; transmission of hepatitis, HIV and other infectious agents; and sensitization, which may affect the outcome of renal transplantation.[A31,A33] Erythropoietin treatment has also markedly improved the quality of life of patients with CRF by improving general well-being, work tolerance, libido, and brain and cardiac function.[A32,A78,A81,A87,A95,A148] If the patient can maintain adequate iron stores (which are best evaluated by measurement of transferrin saturation values over 20% and ferritin levels over 100 mg/mL), the hematocrit may be raised to a target value of 35 to 38% with administration of r-hEPO at 50 to 150 U/kg 1 to 3 times per week.[A30,A31] Subcutaneous injections may be more effective than the intravenous route of administration. Iron deficiency, hepatitis, infection or chronic inflammation, and aluminum intoxication may cause r-hEPO resistance. It is noteworthy that iron stores are rapidly depleted after starting r-hEPO and that supplemental elemental iron (100 to 200 mg per day) is generally required for optimal results. Subsequently, maintenance of the desired hematocrit may be achieved with lower dosages of r-hEPO.

The potential adverse effects of r-hEPO include hypertension, particularly in patients receiving antihypertensive medications before the start of r-hEPO, thrombosis of arteriovenous fistula and higher heparin requirements during hemodialysis, seizures, hyper-

kalemia, iron deficiency, a transient flu-like syndrome, and a decrease in endogenous renal function.[A32,A144]

ADDENDUM 7

GROWTH RETARDATION

Short stature and delayed sexual development are, perhaps, the most important consequences of CRF when onset is in early childhood. The cause of this disorder is multifactorial and includes the presence of metabolic acidosis, calcium and phosphorus imbalance, and nutritional deficiencies. New data, however, ascribe a key role to growth hormone (GH) abnormalities in the cause of growth failure in CRF.[A35,A137] It is generally well established that GH levels are elevated in patients with CRF,[A49,A113,A114] because of increased secretion of GH[A103] or decreased clearance of GH.[A18] In addition, insulin-like growth factors (IGF) are normal in uremic children.[A105,A106] Bioavailable IGF may be reduced in uremia, however, possibly because of increased IGF binding-protein levels.[A72] The administration of exogenous recombinant human GH (rhGH) has been efficacious in increasing growth velocity in children with CRF by increasing plasma IGF levels.[A48,A66,A109,A136]

ADDENDUM 8, REFERENCES

A1. Abramowicz, M.: New contrast media. Med. Lett. Drugs Ther. 29:43, 1987.
A2. Anderson, S., and Brenner, B.M.: Role of intraglomerular hypertension in the initiation and progression of renal disease. In The Kidney in Hypertension. Edited by Kaplan, N.M., Brenner, B.M., and Laragh, J.H. New York, Raven Press, 1987, p. 67.
A3. Anderson, S., King, A.J., and Brenner, B.M.: Hyperlipidemia and glomerular sclerosis: An alternative viewpoint. Am. J. Med. 85(5N):34N, 1989.
A4. Badr, K.F., Kelley, V.E., Rennke, H.G., and Brenner, B.M.: Roles for thromboxane A$_2$ and leukotrienes in endotoxin-induced acute renal failure. Kidney Int. 30:474, 1986.
A5. Baker, G.L., Corry, R.J., and Autor, A.P.: Oxygen-free radical induced damage in kidneys subjected to warm ischemia and reperfusion: Protective effect of superoxide dismutase. Ann. Surg. 202:628, 1985.
A6. Baker, L.R.I., Muir, J.W., Sharman, V.L., et al.: Controlled trial of calcitriol in hemodialysis patients. Clin. Nephrol. 26:185, 1986.
A7. Baue, A.E.: Multiple, progressive, or sequential system failure. A syndrome of the 1970's. Arch. Surg. 110:779, 1975.
A8. Beattie, T.J., Murphy, A.V., and Willoughby, M.L.: Prostacyclin infusion in haemolytic uraemic syndrome of children. Br. Med. J. 283:470, 1981.
A9. Bennett, W.M.: Aminoglycoside nephrotoxicity. Nephron 35:73, 1983.
A10. Berl, T., Berns, A.S., Huffer, W.E., et al.: 1,25 dihydroxy-cholecalciferol effects in chronic dialysis: A double-blind controlled study. Ann. Intern. Med. 88:774, 1978.
A11. Bird, J.E., Blantz, R.C.: Acute renal failure: The glomerular and tubular connection. Pediatr. Nephrol. 1:348, 1987.

A12. Bjorck, S., Nyberg, G., Mulec, H., et al.: Beneficial effects of angiotensin converting enzyme inhibition on renal function in patients with diabetic nephropathy. Br. Med. J. 293:471, 1986.

A13. Brenner, B.M., and Stein, J.H.: Atrial natriuretic peptides. Contemp. Issues Nephrol. 21:1–265, 1989.

A14. Brezis, et al.: Renal ischemia: A new perspective. Kidney Int. 26:375, 1984.

A15. Brezis, M., Rosen, S., Silva, P., et al.: Transport-dependent anoxic cell injury in the isolated perfused rat kidney. Am. J. Pathol. 116:327, 1984.

A16. Brezis, M., Rosen, S., Silva, P., et al.: Polyene toxicity in renal medulla: Injury mediated by transport activity. Science 224:66, 1984.

A17. Brickman, A.S., Hartenbower, D.L., Norman, A.W., and Coburn, J.W.: Actions of 1α-hydroxyvitamin D3 and 1,25-dihydroxyvitamin D_3 on mineral metabolism in man. I. Effects on net absorption of phosphorus. Am. J. Clin. Nutr. 30:1064, 1977.

A18. Cameron, D.P., Burger, H.G., Catt, K.J., et al.: Metabolic clearance of human growth hormone in patients with hepatic and renal failure, and in the isolated perfused pig liver. Metabolism 21:895, 1972.

A19. Canaud, B., Garred, L.J., Christol, J.P., et al.: Pump assisted continuous venovenous hemofiltration for treating acute uremia. Kidney Int. 24:S154, 1988.

A20. Carmines, P.K., and Fleming, J.T.: Control of the renal microvasculature by vasoactive peptides. F.A.S.E.B. J. 4:3300, 1990.

A21. Channard, J., Milicent, T., Toupance, O., et al.: Ultrafiltration pump-assisted continuous arteriovenous hemofiltration (CAVH). Kidney Int. 24:S157, 1988.

A22. Chaudry, I.H., Keefer, J.R., Barash, P., Clemens, M.G., Kopf, G., and Baue, A.E.: ATP-MgCl₂ infusion in man: Increased cardiac output without adverse systemic hemodynamic effects. Surg. Forum 35:14, 1984.

A23. Chaudry, I.H., Sayeed, M.M., and Baue, A.E.: The effect of ATP-MgCl₂ administration in shock. Surgery 75:220, 1974.

A24. Clark, E.C., Nath, K.A., Hostetter, M.K., et al.: Role of ammonia in progressive interstitial nephritis. Am. J. Kid. Dis. 17(Suppl. 1):15, 1991.

A25. Clive, D.M., and Stoff, J.S.: Renal syndromes associated with nonsteroidal antiinflammatory drugs. N. Engl. J. Med. 310:563, 1984.

A26. Cohen, J.J., and Kamm, D.E.: Renal metabolism: Relation to renal function. In The Kidney. Edited by Brenner, B., and Rector, F.C. Philadelphia, W. B. Saunders, 1981, p. 147.

A27. Collins, G.M., Taft, P., Green, R.O., et al.: Adenine nucleotide levels and recovery of function after renal ischemic injury. World J. Surg. 1:237, 1981.

A28. Sieberth, H.G., and Mann, H. (eds).: Continuous Arteriovenous Hemofiltration (CAVH). New York, Karger, 1985.

A29. Cronin, R.E., and Newman, J.A.: Protective effect of thyroxin. Am. J. Physiol. 248:F332, 1985.

A30. Erslev, A.J.: Erythropoietin. N. Engl. J. Med. 324:1339, 1991.

A31. Eschbach, J.W.: The anemia of chronic renal failure: Pathophysiology and the effects of recombinant erythropoietin. Kidney Int. 35:134, 1989.

A32. Eschbach, J.W., Abdulhadi, M.H., Browne, J.K., et al.: Recombinant human erythropoietin in anemic patients with end-stage renal disease. Results of a phase III multicenter trial. Ann. Intern. Med. 111:992, 1989.

A33. Eschbach, J.W., Egrie, J.C., Downing, M.R., et al.: Correction of the anemia of end-stage renal disease with recombinant human erythropoietin. N. Engl. J. Med. 316:73, 1987.

A34. Fernando, A.R., Griffiths, J.R., O'Donoghue, E., et al.: Enhanced preservation of the ischemic kidney with inosine. Lancet I:555, 1976.

A35. Fine, R.N.: Growth hormone and the kidney: the use of recombinant human growth hormone (rhGH) in growth-retarded children with chronic renal insufficiency. J. Am. Soc. Nephrol. 1:1136, 1991.

A36. Food and Agriculture Organization/World Health Organization: Energy and Protein Requirements. Report of a Joint FAO/WHO Expert Committee. WHO Technical Report Series No. 522. WHO, Geneva.

A37. Gaudio, K.M., Ardito, T.A., Reilly, H., et al.: Accelerated cellular recovery after an ischemic renal injury. Am. J. Pathol. 112:338, 1983.

A38. Gaudio, K.M., Taylor, M.R., Chaudry, I.H., et al.: Accelerated recovery of single nephron function by the post-ischemic infusion of ATP-MgCl₂. Kidney Int. 22:13, 1982.

A39. Geronemus, R., and Schneider, N.: Continuous arteriovenous hemodialysis: a new modality for treatment of acute renal failure. Trans. Am. Soc. Artif. Intern. Organs 30:610, 1984.

A40. Ghezzi, P.M., Zuchelli, P., Ringoir, S., et al.: Paired filtration dialysis (PED): A separate convective-diffusive system for extracorporeal blood purification in uraemic patients. Adv. Exp. Med. Biol. 223:267, 1987.

A41. Giuliano, R.A., Paulus, G.J., Verpooten, G.A., et al.: Recovery of cortical phospholipidosis and necrosis after gentamicin loading in rats. Kidney Int. 26:838, 1984.

A42. Golpert, A.: Drug dosage adjustment in dialysis patients. In Pharmacotherapy of Renal Disease and Hypertension. Edited by Benne, H.W.M., and McCarron, D.A. New York, Churchill Livingstone, 1987, p. 21.

A43. Gretz, N., Lasserre, J.J., Hocker, A., and Strauch, M.: Effect of low-protein diet on renal function: Are there definite conclusions from adult studies? Pediatr. Nephrol. 5:492, 1991.

A44. Halliwell, B., Gutteridge, J.M.: Lipid peroxidation, oxygen radicals, cell damage, and antioxidant therapy. Lancet I: 1396, 1984.

A45. Hanley, M.J.: Studies on acute disease models. Kidney Int. 22:536, 1982.

A46. Heney D., Essex-Cater, A., Brocklebank, J.T., et al.: Continuous arteriovenous hemofiltration in the treatment of tumor lysis syndrome. Pediatr. Nephrol. 4:245, 1990.

A47. Hercz, G., and Coburn, J.W.: Prevention of phosphate retention and hyperphosphatemia in uremia. Kidney Int. 22:S215, 1987.

A48. Hokken-Koelega, A.C.S., Stijnen, T., DeMuinck Keizer-Schrama, S.M.P.F., et al.: Placebo-controlled, double-blind, cross-over trial of growth hormone treatment in prepubertal children with chronic renal failure. Lancet 338:585, 1991.

A49. Horton, E.S., Johnson, C., LeBovitz, H.E.: Carbohydrate metabolism in uremia. Ann. Intern. Med. 68:63–74, 1968.

A50. Hostetter, T.H., Olson, J.L., Rennke, H.T., et al.: Hyperfiltration in remnant nephrons; a potentially adverse response to renal ablation. Am. J. Physiol. 241:F85, 1981.

A51. Hou, S.H., Bushinsky, D.A., Wish, J.B., et al.: Hospital-acquired renal insufficiency: A prospective study. Am. J. Med. 74:243, 1983.

A52. Houston, M.C.: Pathophysiology, clinical aspects, and treatment of hypertensive crises. Prog. Cardiovasc. Dis. 32:99, 1989.

A53. Hull, R.W., Hasbargen, J.A.: No clinical evidence for protective effects of calcium-channel blockers against acute renal failure (letter). N. Engl. J. Med. 313:1477, 1985.

A54. Humes, H.D., Hunt, D.A., and White, M.D.: Direct toxic effect of the radiocontrast agent diatrizoate on renal proximal tubule cells. Am. J. Physiol. 252:F246, 1987.

A55. Ihle, B.U., Becker, G.J., Whitworth, J.A., et al.: The effect of protein restriction on the progression of renal insufficiency. N. Engl. J. Med. 321:1773, 1989.

A56. Ingelfinger, J.R., and Dzau, V.J.: Molecular biology of renal injury: emphasis on the role of the renin-angiotensin system. J. Am. Soc. Nephrol. 2:S9, 1991.

A57. Jorgensen, P.L.: Structure, function and regulation of Na, K ATPase in the kidney. Kidney Int. 29:19, 1986.

A58. Kaloyanides, G.J., Pastoriza-Munoz, E.: Aminoglycoside nephrotoxicity. Kidney Int. 18:571, 1980.

A59. Kaplan, N.M.: Clinical Hypertension, 5th ed. Baltimore, Williams & Wilkins, 1990.

A60. Keane, W.F., Anderson, S., Aurell, M., et al.: Angiotensin converting enzyme inhibitors and progressive renal insufficiency. Ann. Intern. Med. *111*:503, 1989.

A61. Keane, W.F. Mulcahy, W.S., Kasiske, B.L., et al.: Hyperlipidemia and progressive renal disease. Kidney Int. *39*:S41, 1991.

A62. Keys, T.F., Kurtz, S.B., Jones, J.D., and Muller, S.M.: Renal toxicity during therapy with gentamicin or tobramycin. Mayo Clin. Proc. *56*:556, 1981.

A63. Klahr, S., Schreiner, G., and Ichikawa, J.: The progression of renal disease. N. Engl. J. Med. *318*:1657, 1988.

A64. Kleinknecht, C., Salusky, I., Broyer, M., Gubler, M.C.: Effect of various protein diets on growth, renal function, and survival of uremic rats. Kidney Int. *15*:534, 1979.

A65. Kleinknecht, D., Landais, P., and Goldfarb, B.: Analgesic and non-steroidal anti-inflammatory drug-associated acute renal failure: A prospective collaborative study. Clin. Nephrol. *25*:275, 1986.

A66. Koch, V.H., Lippe, B.M., Nelson, P.A., et al.: Accelerated growth after recombinant human growth hormone treatment of children with chronic renal failure. J. Pediatr. *115*:365, 1989.

A67. Kramer, H.J., Schuurmann, J., Wassermann, C., and Dusing, R.: Prostaglandin-independent protection by furosemide from oliguric ischemic renal failure in conscious rats. Kidney Int. *17*:455, 1980.

A68. Kramer, P., Wigger, W., Rieger, J., et al.: Arteriovenous hemofiltration: a new and simple method for treatment of overhydrated patients. Klin. Wochenschr. *55*:1121, 1977.

A69. Lau, K.: Phosphate excess and progressive renal failure: The precipitation-calcification hypothesis. Kidney Int. *36*:918, 1989.

A70. Laurer, A., Saccaggi, A., Ronco, C., et al.: Continuous arteriovenous hemofiltration in the critically ill patient. Ann. Intern. Med. *99*:455, 1983.

A71. Lee, D.B.N., Brautbar, N., and Kleeman, C.R.: Disorders of phosphorus metabolism. *In* Disorders of Mineral Metabolism. Edited by Bronner, F., and Coburn, J.E. Academic Press, New York, 1981, p. 283.

A72. Lee, P.D.K., Hintz, R.L., Sperry, J.B., et al.: IGF binding proteins in growth-retarded children with chronic renal failure. Pediatr. Res. *26*:308, 1989.

A73. Lieberthal, W., and Levinsky, N.G.: Treatment of acute tubular necrosis. Sem. Nephrol. *10*:571, 1990.

A74. Livio, M., Manucci, P., Vigano, G., et al.: Conjugated estrogens for the management of bleeding associated with renal failure. N. Engl. J. Med. *315*:731, 1986.

A75. Lohe, J.W., McFarlane, M.J., and Grantham, J.J.: A clinical index to predict survival in acute renal failure patients requiring dialysis. Am. J. Kidney Dis. *11*:254, 1988.

A76. Lopez-Hilker, S., Galceran, T., Chan, Y.L., et al.: Hypocalcemia may not be essential for the development of secondary hyperparathyroidism in chronic renal failure. J. Clin. Invest. *78*:1097, 1986.

A77. Lowrie, E.G., Laird, N.M., Parker, T.F., and Sargent, J.A.: The effect of hemodialysis prescription on patient morbidity. N. Engl. J. Med. *305*:1176, 1972.

A78. Lundin, A.P.: Quality of life: Subjective and objective improvement with recombinant human erythropoietin therapy. Sem. Nephrol. *9*:22, 1989.

A79. Luscher, T.F., Bock, H.A., Yang, Z., et al.: Endothelium-derived relaxing and contracting factors: Perspective in nephrology. Kidney Int. *39*:575, 1991.

A80. Lytton, B., Vaisbort, V.R., Glazier, W.B., et al.: Improved renal function using ATP-MgCl$_2$ in preservation of canine kidneys subjected to warm ischemia. Transplantation *31*:187, 1981.

A81. MacDougall, I.C., Lewis, N.P., Saunders, M.J., et al.: Long-term cardiorespiratory effects of amelioration of renal anaemia by erythropoietin. Lancet *335*:489, 1990.

A82. Manucci, P., Remuzzi, G., Pusinuri, F., et al.: Deamino-8-d-arginine vasopressin shortens the bleeding time in uremia. N. Engl. J. Med. *308*:8, 1983.

A83. Marre, M., Leblanc, H., Suarez, L., et al.: Converting enzyme inhibition and kidney function in normotensive diabetic patients with persistent microalbuminuria. Br. Med. J. *294*:1448, 1987.

A84. Massry, S.G.: The toxic effects of parathyroid hormone in uremia. Semin. Nephrol. *3*:306, 1983.

A85. Mault, J.R., Dechert, R.E., Lees, P., et al.: Continuous arteriovenous filtration: an effective treatment for surgical acute renal failure. Surgery *101*:478, 1987.

A86. Maxwell, L.G., Fivush, B.A., and McLean, R.H.: Renal failure. *In* Textbook of Pediatric Intensive Care. Edited by Rogers, M.C. Baltimore, Williams & Wilkins, 1987, p. 1001.

A87. Mayer, G., Thum, J., Cada, E.M., et al.: Working capacity is increased following recombinant human erythropoietin treatment. Kidney Int. *34*:525, 1988.

A88. McCord, J.M.: Oxygen-derived free radicals in postischemic tissue injury. N. Engl. J. Med. *312*:159, 1985.

A89. Mela-Riker, L.M., Widener, L.L., Houghton, D.C., and Bennett, W.M.: Renal mitochondrial integrity during continuous gentamicin treatment. Biochem. Pharmacol. *35*:979, 1986.

A90. Mimram, A., Insua, A., Ribstein, J., et al.: Contrasting effects of captopril and nifedipine in normotensive patients with incipient diabetic nephropathy. J. Hypertens. *6*:919, 1988.

A91. Mitch, W.E.: Dietary protein restriction in patients with chronic renal failure. Kidney Int. *40*:326, 1991.

A92. Molitoris, B.A.: New insights into the cell biology of ischemic acute renal failure. J. Am. Soc. Nephrol. *1*:1263, 1991.

A93. Moorhead, J.F., Chan, M.K., El-Nahas, M., and Varghese, Z.: Lipid nephrotoxicity in chronic progressive glomerular and tubulo-interstitial disease. Lancet *2*:1309, 1982.

A94. Myers, B.D., and Moran, S.M.: Hemodynamically mediated acute renal failure. N. Engl. J. Med. *314*:97, 1986.

A95. Nissenson, A.R.: Recombinant human erythropoietin and renal anemia: molecular biology, clinical efficacy and nervous system effects. Ann. Intern. Med. *114*:402, 1991.

A96. Odaka, M., Hirasawa, H., Tabata, Y., et al.: A new treatment of acute renal failure with direct hemoperfusion, enhancement of reticuloendothelial system and ATP-MgCl$_2$. *In* Acute Renal Failure. Edited by Eliahou, H.E. John Libbey, London, 1982.

A97. Olbricht, C.J., Fink, M., and Gutjahr, E.: Alterations in lysosomal enzymes of the proximal tubule in gentamicin nephrotoxicity. Kidney Int. *39*:639, 1991.

A98. Olsen, S., Solez, K.: Acute renal failure in man: Pathogenesis in light of new morphological data. Clin. Nephrol. *27*:271, 1987.

A99. Osias, M.B., Siegel, N.J., Chaudry, I.H., et al.: Postischemic renal failure: Accelerated recovery with adenosine triphosphate-magnesium chloride infusion. Arch. Surg. *112*:729, 1977.

A100. Paganini, E.P., O'Hara, P., and Nakamoto, S.: Slow continuous ultrafiltration in hemodialysis resistant oliguric acute renal failure patients. Trans. Am. Soc. Artif. Intern. Organs *30*:133, 1984.

A101. Parekh, N., Esslinger, H., and Steinhausen, M.: Glomerular filtration and tubular reabsorption during anuria in postischemic acute renal failure. Kidney Int. *25*:33, 1984.

A102. Pattison, M.E., Lee, S., and Ogden, D.A.: Continuous arteriovenous hemodiafiltration: an aggressive approach to the management of acute renal failure. Am. J. Kidney Dis. *11*:43, 1988.

A103. Pimstone, B.L., Roith, D.L., Epstein, S., and Kronheim, S.: Disappearance rates of plasma growth hormone after intravenous somatostatin in renal and liver disease. J. Clin. Endocrinol. Metab. *41*:392, 1975.

A104. Pine, R.W., Wertz, M.J., Lennard, E.S., et al.: Determinants of organ malfunctions or death in patients with intra-abdominal sepsis. A discriminant analysis. Arch. Surg. *118*:242, 1983.

A105. Powell, D.R., Rosenfeld, R.G., Baker, B.K., et al.: Serum somatomedin levels in adults with chronic renal failure. The importance of measuring insulin-like growth factor I (IGF-I) and IGF-II in acid-chromatographed uremic serum. J. Clin. Endocrinol. Metab. *63*:1186, 1986.

A106. Powell, D.R., Rosenfeld, R.G., Sperry, J.B., et al.: Serum concentrations of insulin-like growth factor (IGF)-1, IGF-2 and unsaturated somatomedin carrier proteins in children with chronic renal failure. Am. J. Kidney Dis. 10:287, 1987.

A107. Powell, H.R., McCredie, D.A., Taylor, C.M., et al.: Vitamin E treatment of haemolytic ureamic syndrome. Arch. Dis. Child. 59:401, 1984.

A108. Raymond, N.G., Dwyer, J.T., Nevins, P., and Kurtin, P.: An approach to protein restriction in children with renal insufficiency. Pediatr. Nephrol. 4:145, 1990.

A109. Rees, L., Rigden, S.P.A., Ward, G., and Preece, M.A.: Treatment of short stature in renal disease with recombinant human growth hormone. Arch. Dis. Child. 65:856, 1990.

A110. Reichel, H., Koeffler, H.P., and Norman, A.W.: The role of the vitamin D endocrine system in health and disease. N. Engl. J. Med. 320:980, 1989.

A111. Rosman, J.B., Meijer, S., Sluiter, W.J., et al.: Prospective randomized trial of early dietary protein restriction in chronic renal failure. Lancet 2:1291, 1984.

A112. Russell, J.D., and Churchill, D.N.: Calcium antagonists and acute renal failure. Am. J. Med. 87:306, 1989.

A113. Samaan, N., Cumming, W.S., Craig, J.W., and Pearson, O.H.: Serum growth hormone and insulin levels in severe renal disease. Diabetes 15:546, 1966.

A114. Samaan, N.A., and Freeman, R.M.: Growth hormone levels in severe renal failure. Metabolism 19:102, 1970.

A115. Schaer, G.L., Fink, M.P., and Parrillo, J.E.: Norepinephrine alone versus norepinephrine plus low-dose dopamine: Enhanced renal blood flow with combination pressor therapy. Crit. Care Med. 13:492, 1985.

A116. Schentag, J.J., Sutfin, T.A., Plant, M.E., and Jusko, W.J.: Early detection of aminoglycoside nephrotoxicity with urinary beta-2-microglobulin. J. Med. 9:201, 1978.

A117. Schneider, N.S., and Geronemus, R.P.: Continuous arteriovenous hemodialysis. Kidney Int. 24:S159, 1988.

A118. Schrier, R.W., and Gambertoglio, J.G. (eds).: Handbook of Drug Therapy in Liver and Kidney Disease. Boston, Little Brown, 1991.

A119. Schulte-Wissermann, H., Straub, E., and Funke, P.: Influence of L-thyroxin upon enzymatic activity in the renal tubular epithelial of the rat under normal conditions and in mercury-induced lesions. Virchows Archiv. 23:163, 1977.

A120. Sheikh, M.S., Maguire, J.A., Emmett, M., et al.: Reduction of dietary phosphorus absorption by phosphorus binders. J. Clin. Invest. 83:66, 1989.

A121. Shultz, P.J., and Raij, L.: The glomerular mesangium: role in initiation and progression of renal injury. Am. J. Kid. Dis. 17(Suppl. 1):8, 1991.

A122. Siegel, M., Rice, J., Barnes, J., et al.: Protective effect of mini-dose ouabain in ischemic renal failure in the dog. Clin. Res. 31:518A, 1983.

A123. Siegel, N.J., Glazier, W.B., Chaudry, I.H., et al.: Enhanced recovery from acute renal failure by the postischemic infusion of adenine nucleotides and magnesium chloride in rats. Kidney Int. 17:338, 1980.

A124. Sigler, M.H., and Teehan, B.P.: Solute transport in continuous hemodialysis: A new treatment for acute renal failure. Kidney Int. 32:562, 1987.

A125. Slatopolsky, E., Weerts, C., Norwood, K., et al.: Long-term effects of $CaCO_3$ and 2.5 mEq/L Ca^{++} dialysate on mineral metabolism in hemodialysis patients. Kidney Int. 35:264, 1989.

A126. Slatopolsky, E., Weerts, C., Thielan, J., et al.: Marked suppression of secondary hyperparathyroidism by intravenous administration of 1,25-dihydroxy-cholecalciferol in uremic patients. J. Clin. Invest. 74:2136, 1984.

A127. Spataro, R.F.: Newer contrast agents for urography. Radiol. Clin. North Am. 22:365, 1984.

A128. Stella, A., and Bucciant, G.: Converting enzyme inhibitors: structural and hemodynamic effects on the failing kidney. Am. J. Kid. Dis. 17(Suppl. 1):81, 1991.

A129. Stratta, P., Canavese, C., Dogliania, M., et al.: The role of free radicals in the progression of renal disease. Am. J. Kidney Dis. 17(Suppl. 1):33, 1991.

A130. Straub, E.: Effects of L-thyroxine in acute renal failure. Res. Exp. Med. 168:81, 1976.

A131. Stromski, M.E., Cooper, K., Thulin, G., et al.: Chemical and functional correlates of postischemic renal ATP levels. Proc. Natl. Acad. Sci. 83:6142, 1986.

A132. Swartz, R.D.: Anticoagulation in patients on hemodialysis. In Clinical Dialysis, 2nd ed. Edited by Nissenson, A.R., Fine, R.N., and Gentile, D.E. Norwalk, Appleton and Lange, 1990, p. 161.

A133. Taguma, Y., Kitamoto, Y., Futaki, G., et al.: Effect of captopril on heavy proteinuria in azotemic patients. N. Engl. J. Med. 313:1617, 1985.

A134. Talner, L.B., and Davidson, A.J.: Renal hemodynamic effects of contrast media. Invest. Radiol. 3:310, 1968.

A135. Tam, P.Y-W, Huraib, S., Mahan, B., et al.: Slow continuous hemodialysis for the management of complicated acute renal failure in an intensive care unit. Clin. Nephrol. 30:79, 1988.

A136. Tonshoff, B., Mehls, O., Heinrich, U., et al.: Growth-stimulating effects of recombinant human growth hormone in children with end-stage renal disease. J. Pediatr. 116:561, 1990.

A137. Tonshoff, B., Schaefer, F., and Mehls, O.: Disturbance of growth hormone-insulin-like growth factor axis in uraemia. Pediatr. Nephrol. 4:654, 1990.

A138. Van Geelen, J.A., Vincent, H.H., and Schalekama, M.A.D.H.: Continuous arteriovenous hemofiltration and hemodiafiltration in acute renal failure. Nephrol. Dial. Transplant 2:181, 1988.

A139. Venkatachalam, M.A.: Pathology of acute renal failure. In Contemporary Issues in Nephrology, vol. 6. Acute Renal Failure. Edited by Brenner, B.M., and Stein, J.H. New York, Churchill Livingston, p. 180, 1980.

A140. Vogt, M.T., and Farber, E.: On the molecular pathology of ischemic renal cell death. Am. J. Pathol. 53:1, 1968.

A141. Walker, J.D., Dodds, R.A., Murrells, T.J., et al.: Restriction of dietary protein and progression of renal failure in diabetic nephropathy. Lancet 2:1411, 1989.

A142. Walser, M.: Progression of chronic renal failure in man. Kidney Int. 37:1195, 1990.

A143. Warnick, C.T., and Lazarus, H.M.: Recovery of nucleotide levels after cell injury. Can. J. Biochem. 59:116, 1980.

A144. Watson, A.J.: Adverse effects of therapy for the correction of anemia in hemodialysis patients. Semin. Nephrol. 9:30, 1989.

A145. Webster, J., Rees, A.J., Lewis, P.J., and Hensby, C.N.: Prostacyclin deficiency in haemolytic uremic syndrome. Br. Med. J. 281:271, 1980.

A146. Weinberg, J.M.: The cell biology of ischemic renal injury. Kidney Int. 39:476, 1991.

A147. Weiss, L., Danielson, B.G., Wikstrom, B., et al.: Continuous arteriovenous hemofiltration in the treatment of 100 critically ill patients with acute renal failure: Report on clinical outcome and nutritional aspects. Clin. Nephrol. 31:184, 1989.

A148. Winearls, C.G., Oliver, D.O., Pippard, M.J., et al.: Effect of human erythropoietin derived from recombinant DNA on the anemia of patients maintained by chronic hemodialysis. Lancet 2:1175, 1986.

A149. Wingen, A-M., Fabian-Bach, C., and Mehls, O.: Low-protein diet in children with chronic renal failure—1-year results. Pediatr. Nephrol. 5:496, 1991.

A150. Yorgin, P.D., Krensky, A.M., and Tune, B.M.: Continuous venovenous hemofiltration. Pediatr. Nephrol. 4:640, 1990.

A151. Zeller, K.R., Whittaker, E., Sullivan, L., et al.: Effect of restricting dietary protein on the progression of renal failure in patients with insulin-dependent diabetes mellitus. N. Engl. J. Med. 324:78, 1991.

A152. Zobel, G., Ring, E., and Trop, M.: Continuous arteriovenous renal replacement therapy. Int. J. Artif. Organs 10:241, 1987.

A153. Zoja, C., Perico, N., and Remvzzi, G.: Antiplatelet agents: Effects on progressive renal disease. Am. J. Kid. Dis. 17(Suppl. 1):98, 1991.

A154. Zucchelli, P., Zvccala, A., and Gaggi, R.: Calcium channel blockers: Effects on progressive renal disease. Am. J. Kid. Dis. 17(Suppl. 1):94, 1991.

HEPATITIS

George R. Schwartz

ADDENDUM 1. FETAL CONSIDERATIONS

Hepatitis in pregnancy has particular significance for the fetus. Type B hepatitis with active infection in the third trimester and at the time of birth transmits the virus in 80 to 90% of cases and increases the incidence of premature birth. Hepatitis B vaccine and HBIG are recommended for the neonate.

ADDENDUM 2

TABLE 49A-1. PREVALENCE OF SYMPTOMS (%) IN MILITARY PERSONNEL*

Symptoms of Hepatitis	Hepatitis A (16 Patients)	Hepatitis B (214 Patients)	Hepatitis Non-A, Non-B (68 Patients)
Jaundice	88	83	82
Dark urine	68	79	89
Fatigue	63	74	77
Light-colored stools	58	48	37
Loss of appetite	42	56	62
Distaste for cigarettes	45	57	63
Nausea or vomiting	26	46	56
Abdominal pain	37	51	51
Fever or chills	32	25	25
Headache	26	26	25
Muscle pain	26	21	17
Diarrhea	16	30	15
Constipation	16	17	19
Joint pain	11	30	21
Sore throat	0	12	??

* Findings in U.S. Army personnel admitted to hospital with a serologically proven infection. Table modified from Lemon, S.M., Lednar, W.M., Bancroft, W.H., et al.: Etiology of viral hepatitis in American soldiers. Am. J. Epidemiol. *116*:438, 1992.

Children under age 2 are often asymptomatic, and older children often present with predominantly gastrointestinal symptoms. The elderly also present differently and may have diarrhea and electrolyte imbalance.

ADDENDUM 3

TABLE 49A-2. TYPES OF HEPATITIS†				
Type of Hepatitis	Mode of Transmission	Treatment	Complications	Diagnosis
Type A (picornavirus)	Fecal/oral spread High risk: Day care centers Household contacts (shared toilet) Incubation usually less than 8 weeks (15–50 days)	No specific treatments available Hospitalization if severe vomiting, electrolyte imbalance, elderly with severe symptoms Prevent with immune serum globulin pre-exposure Post-exposure reduces severity	Usually few complications. Type A not believed to progress to chronicity, but occasional relapses in first year. Occasional cholestatic hepatitis with elevated bilirubin and pruritis. Fulminant rare, but associated with high mortality, bleeding diasthesis, coma, anemia, liver failure (less than 0.2%)	IGM Anti-A (immediate) IGG Anti-A (previous infection)
Type B	Serum-blood spread Transmitted perinatally Mother to infant 80–90% (if active infection) Breast feeding OK Sexual transmission IV drug users Incubation usually 60–90 days (may be 30–180 days)	No specific treatment Prevention with immunoprophylaxis (vaccine) Neonates HB immune globulin if infected mother Post-exposure: HBIG Antiviral treatments not yet effective	Rare fulminant (under 1%, unless mutant type¹) May be relapsing 1–3% chronic hepatitis Long term association with hepatocellular carcinoma and cirrhosis	Hepatitis surface antigen Anti-HBs
Type C (Non-A, Non-B)	Blood-borne IV drug users Needle stick Sexual contacts May be other modes Neonatal transmission likely Incubation usually 2–26 weeks	No specific treatment No antiviral treatment known Role of immune serum globulin in prophylaxis is conflicting	May become chronic (10%)	Anti-HCV antibody
Type D (Delta)	Associated with hepatitis B Bloody serum, IV needles, sexual spread. Contact transmission possible	No specific treatment known. Use antihepatitis B immunization	May become chronic, may cause cirrhosis. With hepatitis B infection and HDV superinfection, acute—more severe and chronic hepatitis more common	Anti-HDV antibody

† One mutant hepatitis B virus was transmitted to five people. All died of fulminant infection. (Lang, T.J., Masegawa, K., Rimon, N., et al.: Hepatitis B virus mutant associated with an epidemic of fulminant hepatitis. N. Engl. J. Med. *324*:1705, 1991.

ADDENDUM 4. OTHER LABORATORY ABNORMALITIES

The hematocrit and white blood cell (WBC) count are usually normal; a relative lymphocytosis is common. Atypical lymphocytes or virocytes (up to 10%) may be seen. Leukocytosis of 12,000 or over, particularly with a shift to the left, usually indicates a severe, atypical form of hepatitis or another illness. The urine is generally normal, although a mild proteinuria may be seen in addition to bilirubin. Serum bilirubin over 10 mg/dL is usually not seen in typical viral hepatitis.

Abnormal liver enzymes are found in the late prodromal phase, and serum alanine aminotransferase (ALT) and aspartic aminotransferase (AST) usually reach 10 to 100 times normal during the early icteric phase.

Other tests that may be useful are SGOT, serum alkaline phosphatase (SAP), and prothrombin time (PT). In about 50% of patients with hepatitis, the SGOT is over 500 u. Only an occasional patient with biliary tract disease or alcoholic hepatitis has elevations in this range. It must be remembered that the height of the SGOT is not proportional to the severity of liver disease. Patients with asymptomatic or subclinical viral hepatitis may have SGOTs over 2000 u. SAP may be normal or elevated, but it rarely exceeds twice the upper limit of normal. Despite the elevation of SAP, the serum cholesterol is not increased. The serum albumin, although usually decreased somewhat, still remains within normal limits. The gamma globulin usually is under 2 g/dL. Although typical viral hepatitis may be associated with gamma globulin elevations over 3.5 g/dL and albumin below 2.5 g/dL, these findings generally indicate a chronic hepatitis with or without cirrhosis. The PT is usually normal or becomes normal in 24 hours after vitamin K injection. Prolongation of the PT is the most significant *prognostic* finding. It is evidence of extensive depression of hepatic function and indicates a fulminant clinical course or a chronic rather than acute illness.

ADDENDUM 5

The elderly are at particular risk for complications from acute hepatitis. Other candidates for admission are those with severe vomiting and electrolyte imbalance, bleeding tendency, severe gastrointestinal symptoms, and anemia.

ADDENDUM 6

BIBLIOGRAPHY

Koff, R.S.: Hepatitis B and hepatitis D. *In* Infectious Diseases. Edited by Gorbach, S.L., et al. Philadelphia, W.B. Saunders Co., 1992.

Paterlini, Q.P., Gerken, G., Nakajima, E., et al.: Polymerase chain reactions (PCR) to detect hepatitis B virus DNA and RNA sequences in primary liver cancers in patients negative for HB_sAG. N. Engl. J. Med. *323*:80, 1990.

MANAGEMENT OF THE PEDIATRIC AIRWAY

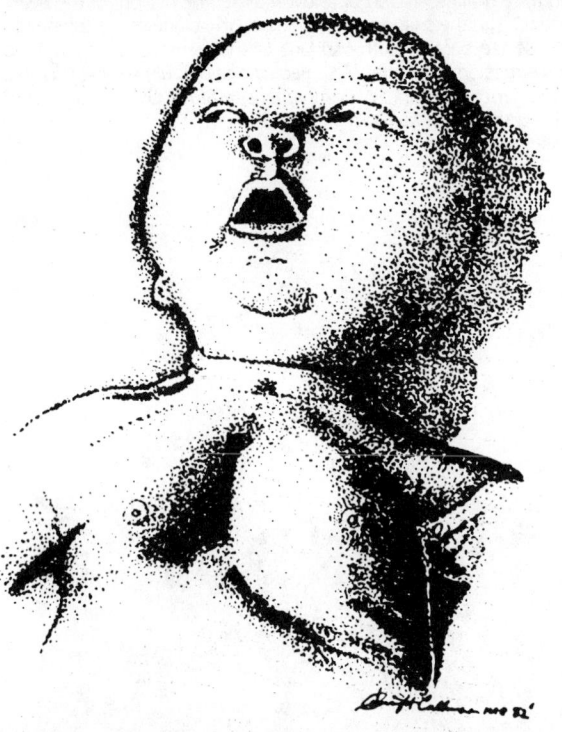

FIG. 59A-1. Recognition of significant respiratory distress in children involves a constellation of factors. This child presents with air hunger, nasal flaring, and recruitment of accessory muscles, reflected as suprasternal, supraclavicular, subxiphoid, subdiaphragmatic, and intracostal retractions.

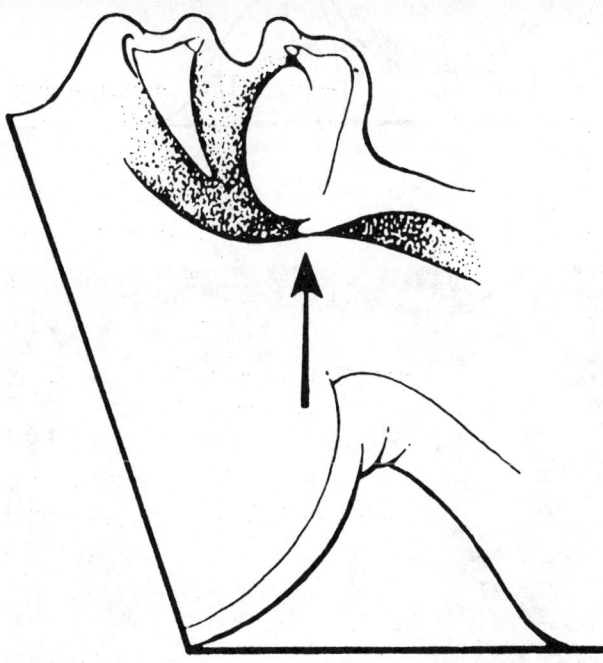

FIG. 59A-2. "Mandibular block" comprises the mandible, tongue, and supporting structures, which tend to fall posteriorly and obstruct the airway in the child, unless the airway is properly positioned. (Adapted with permission from Luten, R.C.: Pediatric cardiopulmonary resuscitation. *In* Emergency Medicine: A Comprehensive Study Guide. Edited by Tintinalli, J. New York, McGraw-Hill, 1985.)

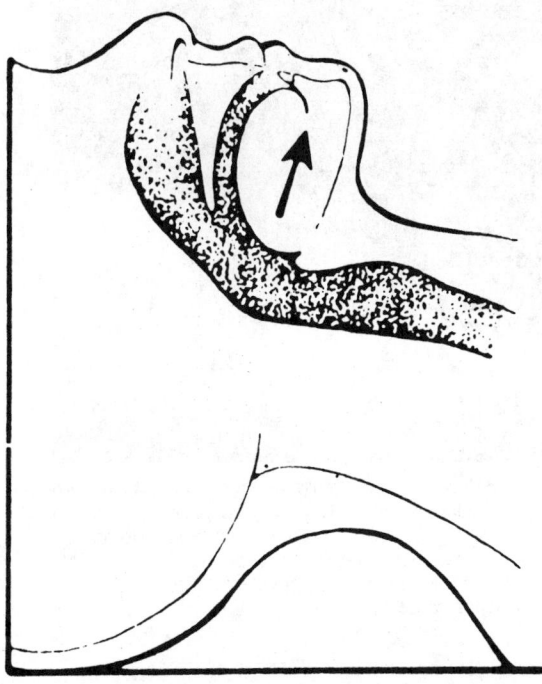

FIG. 59A-3. A jaw thrust maneuver elevates the mandibular block of tissue, thereby clearing the pediatric airway. (Adapted with permission from Luten, R.C.: Pediatric cardiopulmonary resuscitation. *In* Emergency Medicine: A Comprehensive Study Guide. Edited by Tintinalli, J. New York, McGraw-Hill, 1985.)

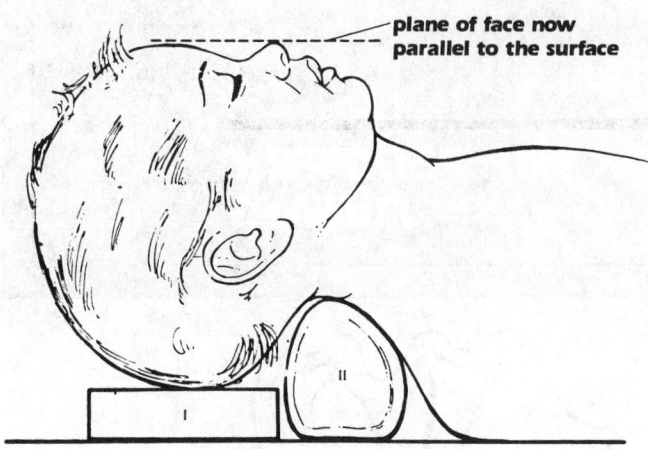

plane of face now
parallel to the surface

FIG. 59A-4. The "sniffing position" consists of slight flexion of the neck on the long axis of the body and slight extension of the head on the neck. In practical terms, this can be maintained by elevation of the head (I) or placing a hand or a towel under the occiput of the head (II). The child is in the sniffing position when the plane of the forehead and the nose are parallel to the surface of the resuscitation area. Adapted with permission from Luten, R.C.: Pediatric cardiopulmonary resuscitation. *In* Emergency Medicine: A Comprehensive Study Guide. Edited by Tintinalli, J. New York, McGraw-Hill, 1985.)

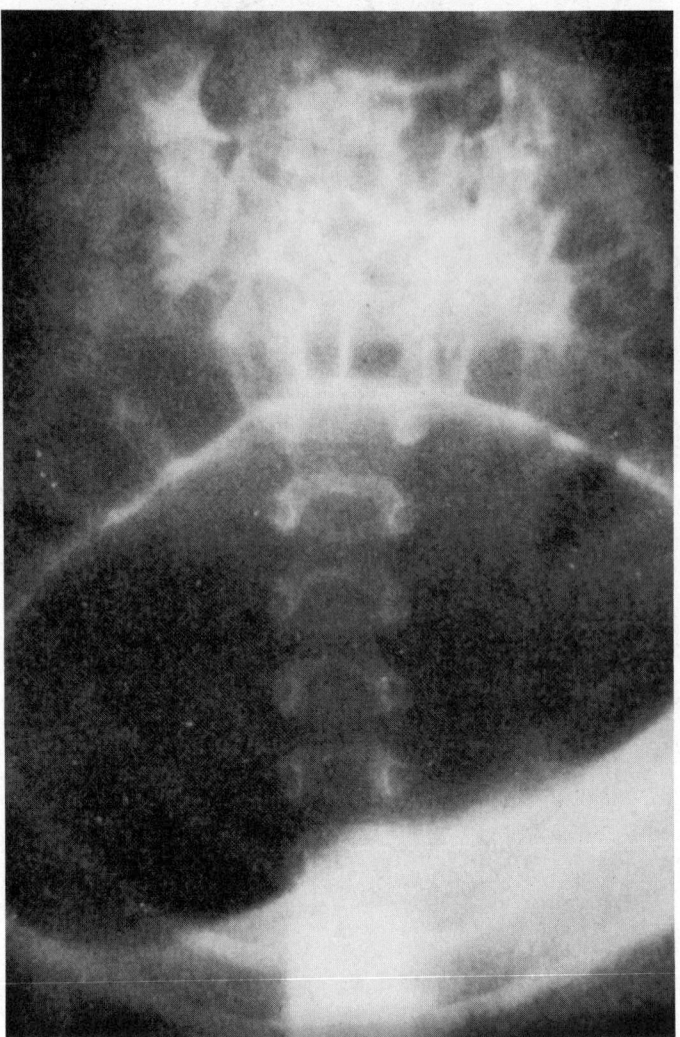

FIG. 59A-5. A nasogastric tube should be placed in all patients undergoing assisted ventilation. This radiograph of a patient transferred from an outlying hospital documents the significant amount of gastric extension that can occur if nasogastric suction is not used. (Adapted with permission from Mayer, T: Emergency Management of Pediatric Trauma. Philadelphia, W.B. Saunders Co., 1985.)

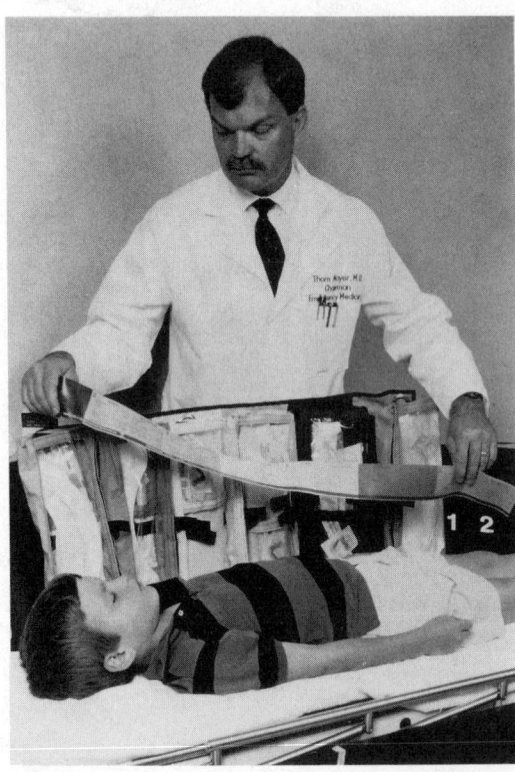

FIG. 59A-6. The Broselow Resuscitation System correlates the patient's length with lean body mass to allow calculation of appropriate drug dosages and equipment sizes. The resuscitation tape estimates the patient's weight and calculates drug dosages on one side of the tape. The opposite side of the tape shows equipment dosages, correlated with a resuscitation bag containing appropriate-sized equipment. The length-based resuscitation system thus allows immediate drug dosages and appropriate-sized equipment for pediatric patients.

APPENDIX A. NORMAL REFERENCE VALUES
(Updated 1992)

Dennis R. Ehrhardt

REFERENCE VALUES IN HEMATOLOGY

	Conventional Units		S.I. Units		Notes
Acid hemolysis test (Ham)	No hemolysis		No hemolysis		
Alkaline phosphatase, leukocyte	Total score 14–100		Total score 14–100		
Carboxyhemoglobin	Up to 5% of total Hgb (smokers)		0.05 of total Hgb (smokers)		
Cell counts	0.5–1.5% of total Hgb (non-smokers)		0.005–0.015 of total Hgb (non-smokers)		a
Erythrocytes					
Males	$4.6–6.2 \times 10^6/\mu l.$		$4.6–6.2 \times 10^{12}/l.$		
Females	$4.2–5.4 \times 10^6/\mu l.$		$4.2–5.4 \times 10^{12}/l.$		
Children (varies with age)	$4.5–5.1 \times 10^6/\mu l.$		$4.5–5.1 \times 10^{12}/l.$		
Leukocytes					
Total	$4.5–11.0 \times 10^3\,\mu l.$		$4.5–11.0 \times 10^9/l.$		
Differential	*Percentage*	*Absolute*			
Myelocytes	0	$0/\mu l.$	0/1		b
Band neutrophils	3–5	$150–400/\mu l.$	$0.15–0.40 \times 10^9/l.$		
Segmented neutrophils	54–62	$3000–5800/\mu l.$	$3.00–5.80 \times 10^9/l.$		
Lymphocytes	25–33	$1500–3000/\mu l.$	$1.50–3.00 \times 10^9/l.$		
Monocytes	3–7	$300–500/\mu l.$	$0.30–0.50 \times 10^9/l.$		
Eosinophils	1–3	$50–250/\mu l.$	$0.05–0.25 \times 10^9/l.$		
Basophils	0–0.75	$15–50/\mu l.$	$0.015–0.05 \times 10^9/l.$		
Platelets	$150,000–400,000/\mu l.$		$150–400 \times 10^9/l$		b
Reticulocytes	$25,000–75,000/\mu l.$		$25–75 \times 10^9/l.$		
	0.5–1.5% of erythrocytes		0.005–0.015		

Bone marrow, differential cell count

	Range	*Average*	*Range*	*Average*	
Myeloblasts	0.3–5.0%	2.0%	0.003–0.05	0.02	a
Promyelocytes	1.0–8.0%	5.0%	0.01–0.08	0.05	
Myelocytes: Neutrophilic	5.0–19.0%	12.0%	0.05–0.19	0.12	
Eosinophilic	0.5–3.0%	1.5%	0.005–0.03	0.015	
Basophilic	0.0–0.5%	0.3%	0.00–0.005	0.003	
Metamyelocytes	13.0–32.0%	22.0%	0.13–0.32	0.22	
Polymorphonuclear neutrophils	7.0–30.0%	20.0%	0.07–0.30	0.20	
Polymorphonuclear eosinophils	0.5–4.0%	2.0%	0.005–0.04	0.02	
Polymorphonuclear basophilis	0.0–0.7%	0.2%	0.00–0.007	0.002	
Lymphocytes	3.0–17.0%	10.0%	0.03–0.17	0.10	
Plasma cells	0.0–2.0%	0.4%	0.00–0.02	0.004	
Monocytes	0.5–5.0%	2.0%	0.005–0.05	0.02	
Reticulum cells	0.1–2.0%	0.2%	0.001–0.02	0.002	
Megakaryocytes	0.3–3.0%	0.4%	0.003–0.03	0.004	
Pronormoblasts	1.0–8.0%	4.0%	0.01–0.08	0.04	
Normoblasts	7.0–32.0%	18.0%	0.07–0.32	0.18	

Coagulation tests

	Conventional Units	S.I. Units	Notes
Antithrombin III (synthetic substrate)	80–120% of normal	0.8–1.2 of normal	
Bleeding time (Duke)	1–5 min.	1–5 min.	
Bleeding time (Ivy)	Less than 5 min.	Less than 5 min.	
Bleeding time (Template)	2.5–9.5 min.	2.5–9.5 min.	
Clot retraction, qualitative	Begins in 30–60 min. Complete in 24 hrs.	Begins in 30–60 min. Complete in 24 h.	
Coagulation time (Lee White)	5–15 min. (glass tubes) 19–60 min. (siliconized tubes)	5–15 min. (glass tubes) 19—60 min. (siliconized tubes)	
Euglobulin clot lysis time	$1\frac{1}{2}$–4 hr. at 37°C	$1\frac{1}{2}$–4 h. at 37°C	
Factor VIII and other coagulation factors	50–150% of normal	0.50–1.5 of normal	a
Fibrin split products (Thrombo-Wellco test)	<10 mcg./ml. (D-dimer) <0.5 mg./l.	<10 mg./l. <0.5 mg/l	
Fibrinogen	200–400 mg./dl.	5.9–11.7 μmol./l.	c
Fibrinolysins	0	0	
Partial thromboplastin time, activated (APTT)	25–35 sec.	25–35 sec.	

REFERENCE VALUES IN HEMATOLOGY (CONTINUED)

	Conventional Units	S.I. Units	Notes
Additional coagulation tests			
Plasminogen			
Immunologic	10–20 mg./dl.	100–200 mg./l.	
Functional	80–120 u/dl	800–1200 u./l.	
Protein C	70–140 u./dl.	700–1400 u./l.	
Protein S	70–140 u./dl.	700–1400 u./l.	
Thrombin time	17–25 sec.	17–25 sec.	
Prothrombin time (one stage)	10.0–13.0 sec.	10.0–13.0 s.	
Tourniquet test	Ten or fewer petechiae in a 2.5 cm. circle after 5 min.	Ten or fewer petechiae in a 2.5 cm circle after 5 min.	
Cold hemolysin test (Donath-Landsteiner)	No hemolysis	No hemolysis	
Coombs' test			
Direct	Negative	Negative	
Indirect	Negative	Negative	
Corpuscular values of erythrocytes (values are for adults; in children, values vary with age)			
M.C.H. (mean corpuscular hemoglobin)	27–31 picogm.	0.42–0.48 fmol.	d
M.C.V. (mean corpuscular volume)	80–96 cu. micra.	80–96 fl.	
M.C.H.C. (mean corpuscular hemoglobin concentration)	32–36%	0.32–0.36	a
Haptoglobin (as hemoglobin binding capacity)	100–200 mg./dl.	16–31 μmol./l.	d
Hematocrit			
Males	40–54 ml./dl.	0.40–0.54	a
Females	37–47 ml./dl.	0.37–0.47	
Newborn	49–54 ml./dl.	0.49–0.54	
Children (varies with age)	35–49 ml./dl.	0.35–0.49	
Hemoglobin			
Males	14.0–18.0 grams/dl.	2.17–2.79 mmol./l.	d
Females	12.0–16.0 grams/dl.	1.86–2.48 mmol./l.	
Newborn	16.5–19.5 grams/dl.	2.56–3.02 mmol./l.	
Children (varies with age)	11.2–16.5 grams/dl.	1.74–2.56 mmol./l.	
Hemoglobin, fetal	<1% of total	<0.01 of total	a
Hemoglobin A_1 (column or affinity chromatography)	5.3–7.5% of total	0.053–0.075 of total	a
Hemoglobin A_2	1.5–3.5% of total	0.015–0.035 of total	a
Hemoglobin, plasma	<3.0 mg./dl.	<0.47 μmol./l.	d
Methemoglobin	60–240 mg./dl.	9.3–37.2 μmol./l.	e
Osmotic fragility of erythrocytes	Begins in 0.45–0.39% NaCl Complete in 0.33–0.30% NaCl	Begins in 77–67 mmol/l NaCl Complete in 56–51 mmol/l NaCl	
Sedimentation rate			
Wintrobe: Males	0–5 mm. in 1 hr.	0–5 mm./h.	
Females	0–15 mm. in 1 hr.	0–15 mm./h.	
Westergren: Male	0–15 mm. in 1 hr.	0–15 mm./h.	
Females	0–20 mm. in 1 hr.	0–20 mm./h.	
(May be slightly higher in children and during pregnancy)			

REFERENCE VALUES FOR BLOOD, PLASMA AND SERUM
(For some procedures the reference values may vary depending upon the method used)

	Conventional Units	S.I. Units	Notes
Acetoacetate plus acetone, serum			
Qualitative	Negative	Negative	
Quantitative	0.5–3.0 mg./dl.	70–440 μmol./l.	
Adrenocorticotropin (ACTH), plasma			
6 A.M.	10–80 picogm./ml.	10–80 ng./l.	
6 P.M.	<50 picogm./ml.	<50 ng./l.	
Alanine aminotransferase *see* Transaminase			
Aldolase, serum	1.0–7.5 milliunits/ml. (30°C)	1.0–7.5 units/l. (30°C)	f

REFERENCE VALUES FOR BLOOD, PLASMA AND SERUM (CONTINUED)
(For some procedures the reference values may vary depending upon the method used)

	Conventional Units	S.I. Units	Notes
Aldosterone, plasma or serum			
Adult, supine	3–10 ng./dl.	0.08–0.3 nmol./l.	
standing			
male	6–22 ng./dl.	0.17–0.61 nmol./l.	
female	5–30 ng./dl.	0.14–0.8 nmol./l.	
Alpha amino nitrogen, serum	3.0–5.5 mg./dl.	2.1–3.9 mmol./l.	
Ammonia (nitrogen), plasma	15–49 mcg./dl.	11–35 μmol./l.	
Amylase, serum	25–125 milliunits/ml.	25–125 units/l.	
Anion gap $Na^+ - (Cl^- + HCO_3^-)$	8–16 mEq./l.	8–16 mmol./l.	
Ascorbic acid, plasma (vitamin C)	0.4–1.5 mg./dl.	23–85 μmol./l.	
Aspartate aminotransferase *see* Transaminase			
Base excess, blood	0 ± 2 mEq./liter	0 ± 2 mmol./l.	
Bicarbonate, plasma	23–29 mEq./liter	23–29 mmol./l.	
Bile acids, serum	0.3–3.0 mg./dl.	3.0–30.0 mg./l.	
Bilirubin, serum			
Direct	0.1–0.4 mg./dl.	1.7–6.8 μmol./l.	
Indirect	0.2–0.7 mg./dl. (Total minus direct)	3.4–12 μmol./l. (Total minus direct)	
Total	0.3–1.1 mg./dl.	5.1–19 μmol./l.	
			a
Calcium, serum	4.5–5.5 mEq./liter	2.25–2.75 mmol./l.	
	9.0–11.0 mg./dl.		
	(Slightly higher in children)	(Slightly higher in children)	
	(Varies with protein concentration)	(Varies with protein concentration)	
Calcium, ionized, serum	2.1–2.6 mEq./liter	1.05–1.30 mmol./l.	
	4.25–5.25 mg./dl.		
Carbon dioxide content, serum			
Adults	24–30 mEq./liter	24–30 mmol./l.	
Infants	20–28 mEq./liter	20–28 mmol./l.	
Carbon dioxide tension (Pco_2), blood	35–45 mm. Hg	35–45 mm Hg	g
Carotene, serum	40–200 mcg./dl.	0.74–3.72 μmol./l.	
Ceruloplasmin, serum	23–44 mg./dl.	230–440 mg./l.	h
Chloride, serum	96–106 mEq./liter	96–106 mmol./l.	
Cholesterol, serum			
Total	150–250 mg./dl.	3.9–6.5 mmol./l.	
Esters	68–76% of total cholesterol	0.68–0.76 of total cholesterol	a
Cholinesterase (pseudocholinesterase)			
Plasma	0.5–1.3 pH units	0.5–1.3 pH units	f
Erythrocytes	0.65–1.3 pH units	0.65–1.3 pH unit	f
Copper, serum			
Males	70–140 mcg./dl.	11–22 μmol./l.	
Females	85–155 mcg./dl.	13–24 μmol./l.	
Cortisol, plasma			
(8 A.M.)	6–23 mcg./dl.	170–635 nmol./l.	
(4 P.M.)	3–15 mcg./dl.	82–413 nmol./l.	
(10 P.M.)	<50% of 8 A.M. value	<0.5 of 8 A.M. value	
Creatine, serum	0.2–0.8 mg./dl.	15–61 μmol./l.	
Creatine kinase, serum (CK, CPK)			
Males	12–80 milliunits/ml. (30°C)	12–80 units/l. (30°C)	f
	55–170 milliunits/ml. (37°C)	55–170 units/l. (37°C)	f
Females	10–55 milliunits/ml. (30°C)	10–55 units/l. (30°C)	f
	30–135 milliunits/ml. (37°C)	30–135 units/l. (37°C)	f
Creatine kinase isoenzymes, serum			
CK-MM	Present	Present	
CK-MB	Absent	Absent	
CK-BB	Absent	Absent	
Creatinine, serum	0.6–1.2 mg./dl.	53–106 μmol./l.	
Cryoglobulins, serum	0	0	
Fatty acids, total, serum	190–420 mg./dl.	7–15 mmol./l.	
nonesterified, serum	8–25 mg./dl.	0.30–0.90 mmol./l.	
Ferritin, serum	20–200 nanogm./ml.	20–200 μg./l.	
Fibrinogen, plasma	200–400 mg./dl.	5.9–11.7 μmol./l.	c
Folate, serum	1.8–9.0 nanogm./ml.	4.1–20.4 nmol./l.	
Erythrocytes	150–450 nanogm./ml.	340–1020 nmol./l.	

REFERENCE VALUES FOR BLOOD, PLASMA AND SERUM (CONTINUED)
(For some procedures the reference values may vary depending upon the method used)

	Conventional Units	S.I. Units	Notes
Follicle-stimulating hormone (FSH), serum			
Males	1–7 milliunits/ml. (I.U.)	1–7 IU/l.	
Females	6–26 milliunits/ml. (I.U.)	6–26 IU/l.	
Postmenopausal	30–118 milliunits/ml. (I.U.)	30–118 IU/l.	
Gamma glutamyltransferase, serum			
Males	6–32 milliunits/ml. (30°C)	6–32 units/l. (30°C)	f
Females	4–18 milliunits/ml. (30°C)	4–18 units/l. (30°C)	f
Gastrin, serum	0–100 picogm./ml.	0–100 ng./l.	
Glucose (fasting)			
Blood	60–100 mg./dl.	3.33–5.55 mmol./l.	
Plasma or serum	70–115 mg./dl.	3.89–6.38 mmol./l.	
Growth hormone, serum	0–10 nanogm./ml.	0–10 µg./l.	
Haptoglobin, serum	100–200 mg./dl.	16–31 µmol./l.	d
	(As hemoglobin binding capacity)	(As hemoglobin binding capacity)	
Hydroxybutyric dehydrogenase, serum (HBD)	140–350 milliunits/ml.	140–350 units/l.	f
17-Hydroxycorticosteroids, plasma	8–18 mcg./dl.	0.22–0.50 µmol./l.	j
Immunoglobins, serum			
IgG	550–1900 mg./dl.	5.5–19.0 g./l.	
IgA	60–333 mg./dl.	0.60–3.3 g./l.	
IgM	45–145 mg./dl.	0.45–1.5 g./l.	
IgD	0.5–3.0 mg./dl.	5–30 mg./l.	
IgE	<500 nanogm./ml.	<500 µg./l.	
	(Varies with age in children)	(Varies with age in children)	
Insulin, plasma (fasting)	5–25 microunits/ml.	5–25 milliunits/l.	
Iron, serum	75–175 mcg./dl.	13–31 µmol./l.	
Iron binding capacity, serum			
Total	250–410 mcg./dl.	45–73 µmol./l.	
Saturation	20–55%	0.20–0.55	a
Lactate, blood, venous	4.5–19.8 mg./dl.	0.5–2.2 mmol./l.	
arterial	4.5–14.4 mg./dl.	0.5–1.6 mmol./l.	
Lactate dehydrogenase, serum (LD, LDH)	45–90 milliunits/ml. (I.U.) (30°C)	45–90 units/l. (30°C)	f
	100–190 milliunits/ml. (37°C)	100–190 units/l. (37°C)	
LDH$_1$	22–37% of total	0.22–0.37 of total	a
LDH$_2$	30–46% of total	0.30–0.46 of total	
LDH$_3$	14–29% of total	0.14–0.29 of total	
LDH$_4$	5–11% of total	0.05–0.11 of total	
LDH$_5$	2–11% of total	0.02–0.11 of total	
Leucine aminopeptidase, serum	14–40 milliunits/ml. (37°C)	14–40 units/l. (37°C)	f
Lipase, serum	0–1.5 u./ml. (Cherry-Crandall)	0–417 u./l.	f
Lipids, total, serum	450–850 mg./dl.	4.5–8.5 g./l.	m
Lipoprotein cholesterol, serum			
LDL cholesterol	60–180 mg./dl.	600–1800 mg./l.	
HDL cholesterol	30–80 mg./dl.	300–800 mg./l.	
Luteinizing hormone (LH), serum			
Males	6–18 milliunits/ml. (I.U.)	6–18 IU/l.	
Females, premenopausal	5–22 milliunits/ml. (I.U.)	5–22 IU/l.	
midcycle	3 times baseline	3 times baseline	
postmenopausal	Greater than 30 milliunits/ml. (I.U.)	Greater than 30 IU/l.	
Magnesium, serum	1.5–2.5 mEq./liter	0.75–1.25 mmol./l.	
	1.8–3.0 mg./dl.		
5'-Nucleotidase, serum	3.5–12.7 milliunits/ml. (30°C)	3.5–12.7 units/l. (30°C)	f
Nitrogen, nonprotein, serum	15–35 mg./dl.	10.7–25.0 mmol./l.	
Osmolality, serum	285–295 mOsm./kg. serum water	285–295 mmol./kg. serum water	n
Oxygen, blood			
Capacity,	16–24 vol. % (varies with hemoglobin)	7.14–10.7 mmol./l. (varies with hemoglobin)	o
Content Arterial	15–23 vol. %	6.69–10.3 mmol./l.	o
Venous	10–16 vol. %	4.46–7.14 mmol./l.	o
Saturation Arterial	94–100% of capacity	0.94–1.00 of capacity	a
Venous	60–85% of capacity	0.60–0.85 of capacity	a
Tension, pO$_2$ Arterial	75–100 mm. Hg	75–100 mm Hg	g
P$_{50}$, blood	26–27 mm. Hg	26–27 mm. Hg	g
pH, arterial, blood	7.35–7.45	7.35–7.45	p
Phenylalanine, serum	<3 mg./dl.	<0.18 mmol./l.	
Phosphatase, acid, serum	0.11–0.60 milliunits/ml. (37°C)	0.11–0.60 units/l. (37°C)	f
	(Roy, Brower, Hayden)		

REFERENCE VALUES FOR BLOOD, PLASMA AND SERUM (CONTINUED)
(For some procedures the reference values may vary depending upon the method used)

	Conventional Units	S.I. Units	Notes
Phosphatase, alkaline, serum (ALP)	20–90 milliunits/ml. (30°C) (Values are higher in children)	20–90 units/l. (30°C) (Values are higher in children)	f
Phosphate, inorganic, serum			
Adults	3.0–4.5 mg./dl.	1.0–1.5 mmol./l.	
Children	4.0–7.0 mg./dl.	1.3–2.3 mmol./l.	
Phospholipids, serum	6–12 mg./dl. (As lipid phosphorus)	1.9–3.9 mmol./l. (As lipid phosphorus)	
Potassium, serum	3.5–5.0 mEq./liter	3.5–5.0 mmol./l.	
Prolactin, serum			
Males	1–20 nanogm./ml.	1–20 µg./l.	
Females	1–25 nanogm./ml.	1–25 µg./l.	
Protein, serum			
Total	6.0–8.0 grams/dl.	60–80 g./l.	m
Albumin	3.5–5.5 grams/dl.	35–55 g./l.	q
	52–68% of total	0.52–0.68 of total	a
Globulin	2.3–3.5 g./dl.	23–35 g./l.	
Alpha$_1$	0.2–0.4 gram/dl.	2–4 g./l.	m
	2–5% of total	0.02–0.05 of total	a
Alpha$_2$	0.5–0.9 gram/dl.	5–9 g./l.	m
	7–14% of total	0.07–0.14 of total	a
Beta	0.6–1.1 grams/dl.	6–11 g./l.	m
	9–15% of total	0.09–0.15 of total	a
Gamma	0.7–1.7 grams/dl.	7–17 g./l.	m
	11–21% of total	0.11–0.21 of total	a
Protoporphyrin, erythrocyte	27–61 mcg./dl. packed RBC	0.48–1.09 µmol./l. packed RBC	
Pyruvate, blood	0.3–0.9 mg./dl.	0.03–0.10 mmol./l.	
Sodium, serum	136–145 mEq./liter	136–145 mmol./l.	
Sulfates, inorganic, serum	0.8–1.2 mg./dl.	83–125 µmol./l.	
Testosterone, plasma			
Males	275–875 nanogm./dl.	9.5–30 nmol./l.	
Females	23–75 nanogm./dl.	0.8–2.6 nmol./l.	
Pregnant	38–190 nanogm./dl.	1.3–6.6 nmol./l.	
Thyroid-stimulating hormone (TSH), serum	0–7 microunits/ml.	0–7 milliunits/l.	
Thyroxine, free, serum	1.0–2.1 nanogm./dl.	13–27 pmol./l.	
Thyroxine (T$_4$), total, serum	4.4–9.9 mcg./dl.	57–128 nmol./l.	
Thyroxine binding globulin (TBG), serum (as thyroxine)	10–26 mcg./dl.	129–335 nmol./l.	
Tri-iodothyronine (T$_3$), total, serum	150–250 nanogm./dl.	2.3–3.9 nmol./l.	
Tri-iodothyronine (T$_3$) uptake, resin (T$_3$RU)	25–38%	0.25–0.38 uptake	a
Transaminase, serum			
SGOT (aspartate aminotransferase, AST)	8–20 milliunits/ml. (30°C) 7–40 milliunits/ml. (37°C)	8–20 units/l. (30°C) 7–40 units/l. (37°C)	
SGPT (alanine aminotransferase, ALT)	8–20 milliunits/ml. (30°C)	8–20 units/l. (30°C)	f
ST	5–35 milliunits/ml. (37°C)	5–35 units/l. (37°C)	f
Triglycerides, serum	40–150 mg./dl.	0.4–1.5 g./l. 0.45–1.71 mmol./l.	r
Urate, serum			
Males	2.5–8.0 mg./dl.	0.15–0.48 mmol./l.	
Females	1.5–7.0 mg./dl.	0.09–0.42 mmol./l.	
Urea			
Blood	21–43 mg./dl.	3.5–7.2 mmol./l.	
Plasma or serum	24–49 mg./dl.	4.0–8.2 mmol./l.	
Urea nitrogen			
Blood	10–20 mg./dl.	7.1–14.3 mmol./l.	k
Plasma or serum	11–23 mg./dl.	7.9–16.4 mmol./l.	
Viscosity, serum	1.4–1.8 times water	1.4–1.8 times water	
Vitamin A, serum	20–80 mcg./dl.	0.70–2.8 µmol./l.	
Vitamin B$_{12}$, serum	180–900 picogm./ml.	133–664 pmol./l.	

REFERENCE VALUES FOR URINE
(For some procedures the reference values may vary depending upon the method used)

	Conventional Units	S.I. Units	Notes
Acetone and acetoacetate, qualitative	Negative	Negative	
Albumin			
Qualitative	Negative	Negative	
Quantitative	10–100 mg./24 hrs.	10–100 mg./24 h.	q
		0.15–1.5 µmol./24 h.	
Aldosterone	3–20 mcg./24 hrs.	8.3–55 nmol./24 h.	
Alpha amino nitrogen	50–200 mg./24 hrs.	3.6–14.3 mmol./24 h.	
Ammonia nitrogen	20–70 mEq./24 hrs.	20–70 mmol./24 h.	
Amylase	1–17 units/hr.	1–17 units/h.	f
Amylase/creatinine clearance ratio	1–4%	0.01–0.04	
Bilirubin, qualitative	Negative	Negative	
Calcium			
Low Ca diet	<150 mg./24 hrs.	<3.8 mmol./24 h.	
Usual diet	<250 mg./24 hrs.	<6.3 mmol./24 h.	
Catecholamines			
Epinephrine	<10 ng./24 hrs.	<55 nmol./24 h.	
Norepinephrine	100 ng./24 hrs.	<590 nmol./24 h.	
Total free catecholamines	4–126 mcg./24 hrs.	24–745 nmol./24 h.	s
Total metanephrines	0.1–1.6 mg./24 hrs.	0.5–8.1 µmol./24 h.	t
Chloride	110–250 mEq./24 hrs.	110–250 mmol./24 h.	
	(Varies with intake)	(Varies with intake)	
Chorionic gonadotropin	0	0	
Copper	0–50 mcg./24 hrs.	0–0.80 µmol./24 h.	
Cortisol, free	10–100 mcg./24 hrs.	27.6–276 mmol./24 h.	
Creatine			
Males	0–40 mg./24 hrs.	0–0.30 mmol./24 h.	
Females	0–100 mg./24 hrs.	0–0.76 mmol./24 h.	
	(Higher in children and during pregnancy)	(Higher in children and during pregnancy)	
Creatinine	15–25 mg./kg. body weight/24 hrs.	0.13–0.22 mmol · kg^{-1} body weight/24 h.	
Creatinine clearance			
Males	110–150 ml./min.	110–150 ml./min.	
Females	105–132 ml./min.	105–132 ml./min.	
	(1.73 sq. meter surface area)	(1.73 m^2 surface area)	
Cystine or cysteine, qualitative	Negative	Negative	
Dehydroepiandrosterone	Less than 15% of total 17-ketosteroids	Less than 0.15 of total 17-ketosteroids	a
Males	0.2–2.0 mg./24 hr.	0.7–6.9 µm./24 h.	
Females	0.2–1.8 mg./24 hr.	0.7–6.2 µm./24 h.	
Delta aminolevulinic acid	1.3–7.0 mg./24 hrs.	10–53 µmol./24 h.	
Estrogens			
Males			
Estrone	3–8 µg./24 hrs.	11–30 nmol./24 h.	
Estradiol	0–6 µg./24 hrs.	0–22 nmol./24 h.	
Estriol	1–11 µg./24 hrs.	3–38 nmol./24 h.	
Total	4–25 µg./24 hrs.	14–90 nmol./24 h.	u
Females			
Estrone	4–31 µg./24 hrs.	15–115 nmol./24 h.	
Estradiol	0–14 µg./24 hrs.	0–51 nmol./24 h.	
Estriol	0–72 µg./24 hrs.	0–250 nmol./24 h.	
Total	5–100 µg./24 hrs.	18–360 nmol./24 h.	u
	(Markedly increased during pregnancy)	(Markedly increased during pregnancy)	
Glucose (as reducing substance)	Less than 250 mg./24 hrs.	Less than 250 mg./24 h.	
Hemoglobin and myoglobin, qualitative	Negative	Negative	
Homogentisic acid, qualitative	Negative	Negative	
17-Hydroxycorticosteroids			
Males	3–9 mg./24 hrs.	8.3–25 µmol./24 h.	j
Females	2–8 mg./24 hrs.	5.5–22 µmol./24 h.	
5-Hydroxyindoleacetic acid			
Qualitative	Negative	Negative	
Quantitative	Less than 9 mg./24 hrs.	Less than 47 µmol./24 h.	
17-Ketosteroids			
Males	6–18 mg./24 hrs.	21–62 µmol./24 h.	l
Females	4–13 mg./24 hrs.	14–45 µmol./24 h.	
	(Varies with age)	(Varies with age)	
Magnesium	6.0–8.5 mEq./24 hrs.	3.0–4.3 mmol./24 h.	
Metanephrines (see Catecholamines)			

REFERENCE VALUES FOR URINE (CONTINUED)
(For some procedures the reference values may vary depending upon the method used)

	Conventional Units	S.I. Ur	Notes
Osmolality, random	38–1400 mOsm./kg. water	38–1400 mmol./kg. water	n
pH, random	4.6–8.0, average 6.0	4.6–8.0, average 6.0	p
	(Depends on diet)	(Depends on diet)	
Phenolsulfonphthalein excretion (PSP)	25% or more in 15 min.	0.25 or more in 15 min.	a
	40% or more in 30 min.	0.40 or more in 30 min.	
	55% or more in 2 hrs.	0.55 or more in 2 h.	
	(After injection of 1 ml. PSP intravenously)	(After injection of 1 ml. PSP intravenously)	
Phenylpyruvic acid, qualitative	Negative	Negative	
Phosphorus	0.9–1.3 gm./24 hrs.	29–42 mmol./24 h.	
Porphobilinogen			
Qualitative	Negative	Negative	
Quantitative	0–0.2 mg./dl.	0–0.9 μmol./l.	
	Less than 2.0 mg./24 hrs.	Less than 9 μmol./24 h.	
Porphyrins			
Coproporphyrin	50–250 mcg./24 hrs.	77–380 nmol./24 h.	
Uroporphyrin	10–30 mcg./24 hrs.	12–36 nmol./24 h.	
Potassium	25–100 mEq./24 hrs.	25–100 mmol./24 h.	
	(Varies with intake)	(Varies with intake)	
Pregnanediol			
Males	0.4–1.4 mg./24 hrs.	1.2–4.4 μmol./24 h.	
Females			
Proliferative phase	0.5–1.5 mg./24 hrs.	1.6–4.7 μmol./24 h.	
Luteal phase	2.0–7.0 mg./24 hrs.	6.2–22 μmol./24 h.	
Postmenopausal phase	0.2–1.0 mg./24 hrs.	0.6–3.1 μmol./24 h.	
Pregnanetriol	Less than 2.5 mg./24 hrs. in adults	Less than 7.4 μmol/24 h. in adults	
Protein			
Qualitative	Negative	Negative	
Quantitative	10–150 mg./24 hrs.	10–150 mg./24 h.	m
Sodium	130–260 mEq./24 hrs.	130–260 mmol./24 h.	
	(Varies with intake)	(Varies with intake)	
Specific gravity, random	1.003–1.030	1.003–1.030	
Titratable acidity	20–40 mEq./24 hrs.	20–40 mmol./24 h.	
Urate	200–500 mg./24 hrs.	1.2–3.0 mmol./24 h.	
	(With normal diet)	(With normal diet)	
Urobilinogen	Up to 1.0 Ehrlich unit/2 hrs.	Up to 1.0 Ehrlich unit/2 h.	
	(1–3 P.M.)	(1–3 P.M.)	
	0–4.0 Ehrlich units/24 hrs.	0–4.0 Ehrlich units/24 hrs.	
Vanillylmandelic acid (VMA)	1–8 mg./24 hrs.	5–40 μmol./24 h.	
(4-hydroxy-3-methoxymandelic acid)			
Volume, total	600–1600 ml./24 hrs.	0.6–1.6 l./24 hrs.	

REFERENCE VALUES FOR THERAPEUTIC DRUG MONITORING

Drug	Therapeutic Range	Toxic Levels	Proprietary Names
Antibiotics			
Amikacin, serum	25–35 mcg./ml.	Peak: >35–40 mcg./ml.	Amikin
		Trough: >10–15 mcg./ml.	
Chloramphenicol, serum	10–20 mcg./ml.	>25 mcg./ml.	Chloromycetin
Gentamicin, serum	5–10 mcg./ml.	Peak: >12 mcg./ml.	Garamycin
		Trough: >2 mcg./ml.	
Tobramycin, serum	5–10 mcg./ml.	Peak: >12 mcg./ml.	Nebcin
		Trough: >2 mcg./ml.	
Anticonvulsants			
Carbamazepine, serum	5–12 mcg./ml.	>12 mcg./ml.	Tegretol
Ethosuximide, serum	40–100 mcg./ml.	>100 mcg./ml.	Zarotin
Phenobarbital, serum	10–30 mcg./ml.	Vary widely because of developed tolerance	
Phenytoin, serum (diphenylhydantoin)	10–20 mcg./ml.	>20 mcg./ml.	Dilantin
Primidone, serum	5–12 mcg./ml.	>15 mcg./ml.	Mysoline
Valproic acid, serum	50–100 mcg./ml.	>100 mcg./ml.	Depakene

REFERENCE VALUES FOR THERAPEUTIC DRUG MONITORING (CONTINUED)

Drug	Therapeutic Range	Toxic Levels	Proprietary Names
Analgesics			
Acetaminophen, serum	10–20 mcg./ml.	>250 mcg./ml.	Tylenol
Ibuprofen, serum	10–50 mcg./ml.	>100 mcg./ml.	Datril
Salicylate, serum	100–250 mcg./ml.	>300 mcg./ml.	Motrin
Bronchodilator			
Theophylline (aminophylline)	10–20 mcg./ml.	>20 mcg./ml.	
Cardiovascular drugs			
Digitoxin, serum	20–35 nanogm./ml. (Specimen obtained at least 8 hrs. after last dose)	>45 nanogm./ml.	Crystodigin
Digoxin, serum	0.8–2 nanogm./ml. (Specimen obtained 12–24 hrs. after last dose)	>2.4 nanogm./ml.	Lanoxin
Disopyramide, serum	2.8–7.5 mcg./ml.	>7 mcg./ml.	Norpace
Lidocaine, serum	1.5–5 mcg./ml.	>5 mcg./ml.	Anestacon Xylocaine
Procainamide, serum	4–10 mcg./ml. *10–30 mcg./ml. (*Procainamide + N-Acetyl Procainamide)	>12 mcg./ml. *>30 mcg./ml.	Pronestyl
Propranolol, serum	50–100 nanogm./ml.	Variable	Inderal
Quinidine, serum	2–5 mcg./ml.	>6 mcg./ml.	Cardioquin Quinaglute Quinidex Quinora
Verapamil, serum	100–500 nanogm./ml.	Variable	Calan Isoptin
Psychopharmacologic drugs			
Amitriptyline, serum	*120–250 nanogm./ml. (*Amitriptyline + Nortriptyline)	*>500 nanogm./ml.	Amitril Elvail Endep Etralon Limbitrol Triavil
Desipramine, serum	*150–300 nanogm./ml. (*Desipramine + Imipramine)	*>500 nanogm./ml.	Norpramin Pertofrane
Imipramine, serum	*150–300 nanogm./ml. (*Imipramine + Desipramine)	*>500 nanogm./ml.	Antipress Imavate Janimine Presamine Trofanil
Lithium, serum	0.8–1.2 mEq./liter (Specimen obtained 12 hrs. after last dose)	>2.0 mEq./liter	Lithobid Lithotabs
Nortriptyline, serum	50–150 nanogm./ml.	>500 nanogm./ml.	Aventyl Pamelor

REFERENCE VALUES IN TOXICOLOGY

	Conventional Units	S.I. Units	Notes
Arsenic, blood	<7 mcg./dl.	<0.4 μmol./l.	
Arsenic, urine	<50 mcg./l. (24 hrs.)	<0.67 μmol./l. (24 h.)	
Bromides, serum	<5 mg./dl.	<0.63 mmol./l.	
Carbon monoxide, blood	Up to 5% saturation	Up to 0.05 saturation	
	Symptoms occur with 20% saturation	Symptoms occur with 0.20 saturation	a
Ethanol, blood	Less than 0.005%	Less than 1 mmol./l.	
Marked intoxication	0.3–0.4%	65–87 mmol./l.	
Alcoholic stupor	0.4–0.5% mcg./dl.	87–109 mmol./l.	
Coma, death	Above 0.5%	Above 109 mmol./l.	
Fluoride, blood	<0.05 mg./dl.	<0.027 mmol./l.	
Lead, blood	0–40 mcg./dl.	0–2 μmol./l.	
Lead, urine	<100 mcg./24 hrs.	<0.48 μmol./24 h.	
Mercury, urine	Less than 10 mcg./24 hrs.	Less than 50 nmol./24 h.	

REFERENCE VALUES FOR CEREBROSPINAL FLUID

	Conventional Units	S.I. Units	Notes
Albumin	10–30 mg./dl.	0.10–0.30 g./l.	
Cells	<5/cu. mm.; all mononuclear	<5/μl.; all mononuclear	
Chloride	120–130 mEq./liter	120–130 mmol./l.	
	(20 mEq./liter higher than serum)	(20 mmol./l. higher than serum)	
Electrophoresis	Predominantly albumin	Predominantly albumin	
Glucose	50–75 mg./dl.	2.8–4.2 mmol./l.	
	(20 mg./dl. less than serum)	(1.1 mmol./l. less than serum)	
IgG			
Children under 14	Less than 8% of total protein	Less than 0.08 of total protein	a.m.
Adults	Less than 14% of total protein	Less than 0.14 of total protein	
Pressure	70–180 mm. water	70–180 mm. water	g
Protein, total	15–45 mg./dl.	0.150–0.450 g./l.	m
	(Higher, up to 70 mg./dl., in elderly adults and children)	(Higher, up to 0.70 g./l., in elderly adults and children)	

REFERENCE VALUES FOR GASTRIC ANALYSIS

	Conventional Units	S.I. Units	Notes
Basal gastric secretion (1 hour)			
Concentration	(Mean ± 1 S.D.)	(Mean ± 1 S.D.)	
Males	25.8 ± 1.8 mEq./liter	25.8 ± 1.8 mmol./l.	
Females	20.3 ± 3.0 mEq./liter	20.3 ± 3.0 mmol./l.	
Output	(Mean ± 1 S.D.)	(Mean ± 1 S.D.)	
Males	2.57 ± 0.16 mEq./hr.	2.57 ± 0.16 mmol./h.	
Females	1.61 ± 0.18 mEq./hr.	1.61 ± 0.18 mmol./h.	
After histamine stimulation			
Normal	Mean output 11.8 mEq./hr.	Mean output 11.8 mmol./h.	
Duodenal ulcer	Mean output 15.2 mEq./hr.	Mean output 15.2 mmol./h.	
After maximal histamine stimulation			
Normal	Mean output 22.6 mEq./hr.	Mean output 22.6 mmol./h.	
Duodenal ulcer	Mean output 44.6 mEq./hr.	Mean output 44.6 mmol./h.	
Diagnex blue (Squibb): Anacidity	0–0.3 mg. in 2 hrs.	0–0.03 mg. in 2 h.	
Doubtful	0.3–0.6 mg. in 2 hrs.	0.3–0.6 mg. in 2 h.	
Normal	Greater than 0.6 mg. in 2 hrs.	Greater than 0.6 mg. in 2 h.	
Volume, fasting stomach content	50–100 ml.	0.05–0.1 l.	
Emptying time	3–6 hrs.	3–6 h.	
Color	Opalescent or colorless	Opalescent or colorless	
Specific gravity	1.006–1.009	1.006–1.009	
pH (adults)	0.9–1.5	0.9–1.5	p

GASTROINTESTINAL ABSORPTION TESTS

	Conventional Units	S.I. Units	Notes
d/Xylose absorption test	After an 8 hour fast, 10 ml./kg. body weight of a 0.05 solution of d-xylose is given by mouth. Nothing further by mouth is given until the test has been completed. All urine voided during the following 5 hours is pooled, and blood samples are taken at 0, 60, and 120 minutes. Normally 0.26 (range 0.16–0.33) of ingested xylose is excreted within 5 hours, and the serum xylose reaches a level between 25 and 40 mg./100 ml. after 1 hour and is maintained at this level for another 60 minutes.	No change	
Vitamin A absorption	A fasting blood specimen is obtained and 200,000 units of vitamin A in oil is given by mouth. Serum vitamin A level should rise to twice fasting level in 3 to 5 hours.	No change	

REFERENCE VALUES FOR FECES

	Conventional Units	S.I. Units	Notes
Bulk	100–200 grams/24 hrs.	100–200 g./24 h.	
Dry matter	23–32 grams/24 hrs.	23–32 g./24 h.	
Fat, total	<6.0 grams/24 hrs.	<6.0 g./24 h.	
Nitrogen, total	<2.0 grams/24 hrs.	<143 mmol./24 h.	
Urobilinogen	40–200 mg./24 hrs.	68–339 μmol./24 h.	
Water	Approximately 65%	Approximately 0.65	a

REFERENCE VALUES FOR IMMUNOLOGIC PROCEDURES

	Conventional Units
Lymphocyte Subsets	
T cells	60–85%
B cells	1–20%
Helper cells (CD_4^+)	35–60% or 436–1394 cells/ul.
Suppressor cells (CD_8^+)	15–30% or 166–882 cells/ul.
H/S ratio (CD_4^+/CD_8^+)	0.5–3.3
Complement, serum	
C3	85–175 mg./dl.
C4	15–45 mg./dl.
CH_{50}	75–160 units/ml.
Tumor Markers	
Carcinoembryonic Antigen (CEA), serum	<5.0 nanog./ml.
Alpha-fetoprotein (AFP), serum	<10–30 nanog./ml. (depends on method)
CA-125 (ovarian)	<35 units/ml.

REFERENCE VALUES FOR SEMEN ANALYSIS

	Conventional Units	S.I. Units	Notes
Volume	2–5 ml.; usually 3–4 ml.	2–5 ml.; usually 3–4 ml.	
Liquefaction	Complete in 15 min.	Complete in 15 min.	
pH	7.2–8.0; average 7.8	7.2–8.0; average 7.8	p
Leukocytes	Occasional or absent	Occasional or absent	
Count	60–150 million/ml. Below 60 million/ml. is abnormal	60–150 million/ml. Below 60 million/ml. is abnormal	
Motility	80% or more motile	0.80 or more motile	a
Morphology	80–90% normal forms	0.80–0.90 normal forms	a

ORAL GLUCOSE TOLERANCE TEST

The oral glucose tolerance test (OGTT) may be unnecessary if the fasting plasma glucose concentration is elevated (venous plasma ≥ 140 mg./dl. or 7.8 mmol./l.) on two occasions. The OGTT should be carried out only on patients who are ambulatory and otherwise healthy and who are known not to be taking agents that elevate the plasma glucose (see reference 10). The test should be conducted in the morning after at least 3 days of unrestricted diet (≥ 150 grams of carbohydrate) and physical activity. The subject should have fasted for at least 10 hours but no more than 16 hours. Water is permitted during the test period; however, the subject should remain seated and should not smoke throughout the test.

The dose of glucose administered should be 75 grams (1.75 grams per kg. of ideal body weight, up to a maximum of 75 grams for children). Commercial preparations containing a suitable carbohydrate load are acceptable. If criteria for gestational diabetes are used, a dose of 100 grams of glucose is required.

A fasting blood sample should be collected, after which the glucose dose is taken within 5 minutes. Blood samples should be collected at 30 minute intervals for 2 hours (for gestational diabetes fasting 1, 2 and 3 hours). The following diagnostic criteria have been recommended by the National Diabetes Data Group:

Normal OGTT in Nonpregnant Adults

Fasting venous plasma glucose <115 mg./dl. (6.4 mmol./l.) ½ h., 1 h., or 1½ h. OGTT venous plasma glucose <200 mg./dl. (11.1 mmol./l.)
2 h. OGTT venous plasma glucose <140 mg./dl. (7.8 mmol./l.)

Diabetes Mellitus in Nonpregnant Adults

Both the 2 hour sample and some other sample taken between administration of the 75 gram glucose dose and 2 hours later must show a venous plasma glucose ≥200 mg./dl. (11.1 mmol./l.)

Impaired Glucose Tolerance in Nonpregnant Adults

Three criteria must be met:
Fasting venous plasma glucose <140 mg./dl. (7.8 mmol./l.) ½ h., 1 h., or 1½ h. OGTT value ≥200 mg./dl. (11.1 mmol./l.)
2 h. OGTT venous plasma glucose between 140 and 200 mg./dl. (7.8 and 11.1 mmol./l.)

Gestational Diabetes

Two or more of the following values after a 100 gram oral glucose challenge must be met or exceeded:
(values are for venous plasma glucose)

Fasting	105 mg./dl.	5.8 mmol./l.
1 h.	190 mg./dl.	10.6 mmol./l.
2 h.	165 mg./dl.	9.2 mmol./l.
3 h.	145 mg./dl.	8.1 mmol./l.

APPENDIX B. ILLUSTRATIVE ECG TRACINGS

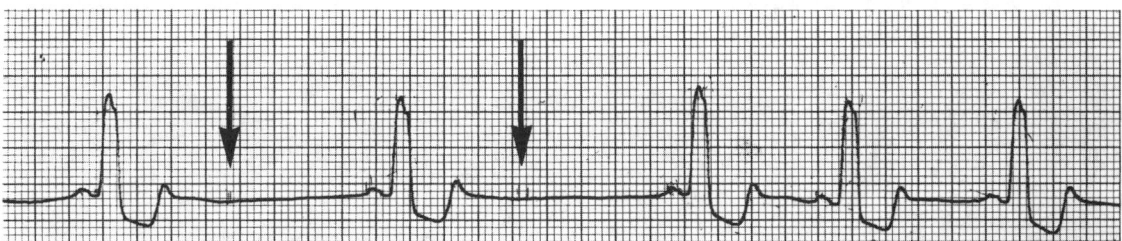

FIG. B-1. Sinus arrest. The arrows point to the anticipated location of the sinus P wave. The last three P waves document the rate of the sinus discharge. The P-P interval of the first three P waves is double the succeeding P-P intervals, indicating a transient 2:1 sinus block.

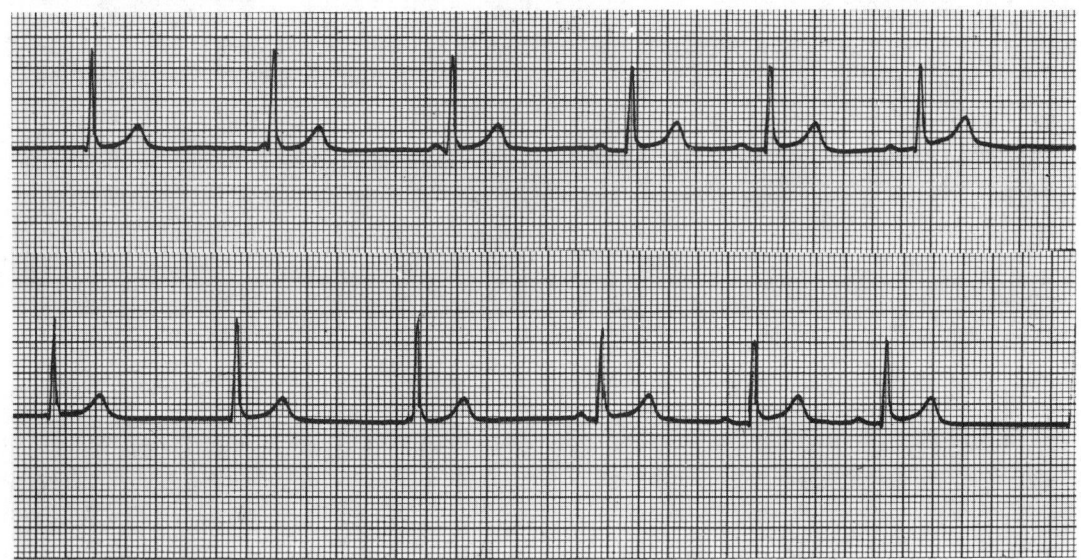

FIG. B-2. A-V dissociation. The first three complexes are due to a junctional escape rhythm at a rate of 50/min. A sinus rhythm at a rate of 65/min. then emerges for three complexes. The sinus rate then slows temporarily, allowing the junction to escape until the sinus rate again accelerates. The junctional complexes are slightly aberrant.

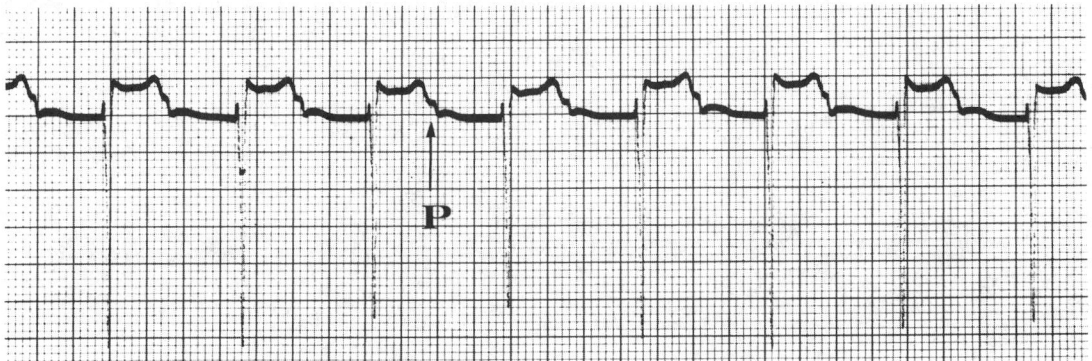

FIG. B-3. First-degree A-V block. The P-R interval is prolonged to 0.40 second. The P wave (P) is partially hidden in the descending limb of the T wave.

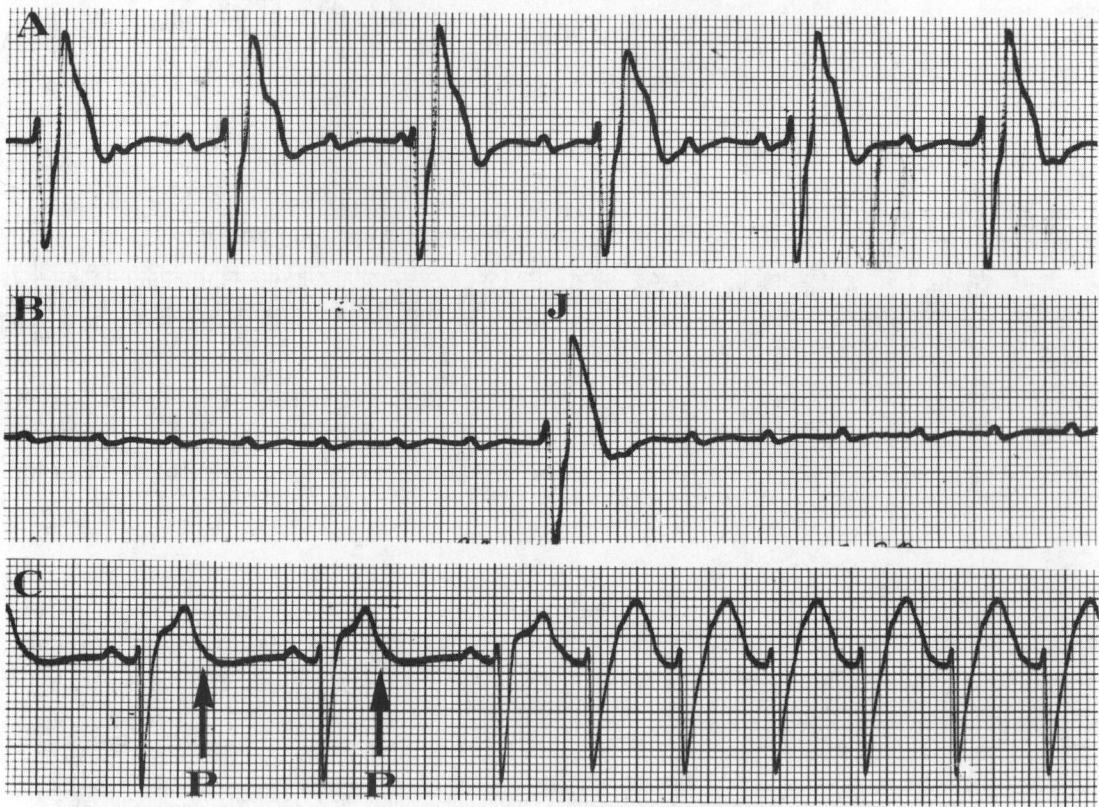

FIG. B-4. Second-degree A-V block (Mobitz II). The strips are not continuous but are taken from the same patient. Strip A shows complete A-V block with a junctional escape rhythm. Strip B shows a prolonged period of asystole owing to complete A-V block with a single escape junctional beat (J). Strip C shows 2:1 A-V block with the nonconducted P wave hidden in the T wave (arrows). The 2:1 conduction abruptly returns to 1:1 in the middle of the strip.

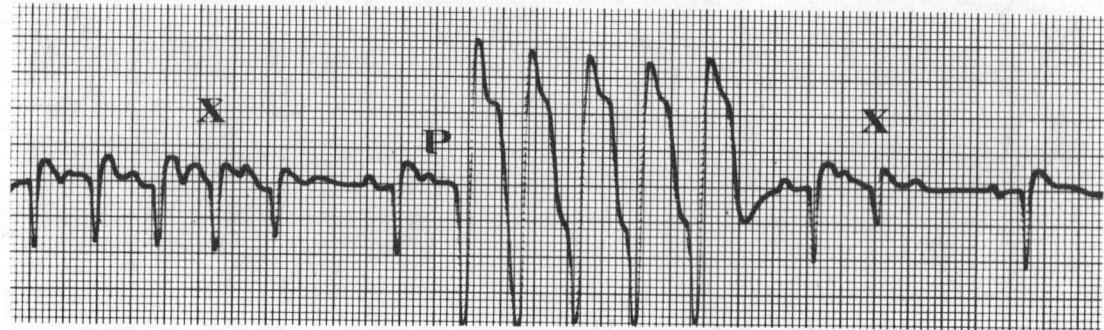

FIG. B-5. Supraventricular tachycardia with aberration. Frequent premature atrial complexes (X) are noted. After a long cycle a premature atrial complex (P) results in a brief run of aberrant complexes. The long-short sequence and the obvious premature P wave suggest that the tachyrhythmia is supraventricular with aberration.

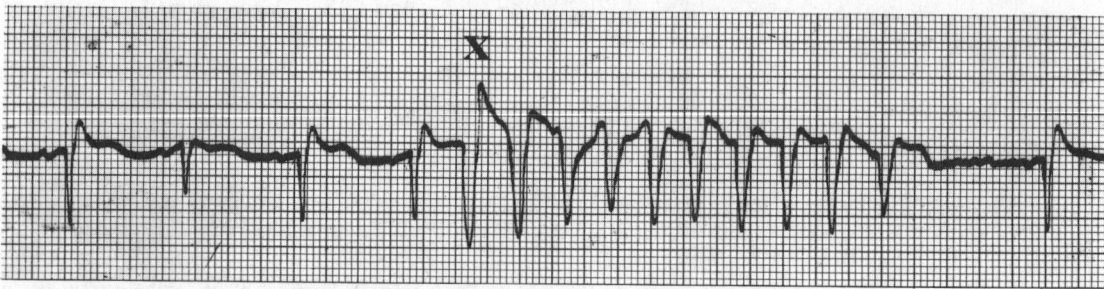

FIG. B-6. Ventricular tachycardia. A premature ventricular complex (X) strikes on the T wave, initiating a transient burst of ventricular tachycardia.

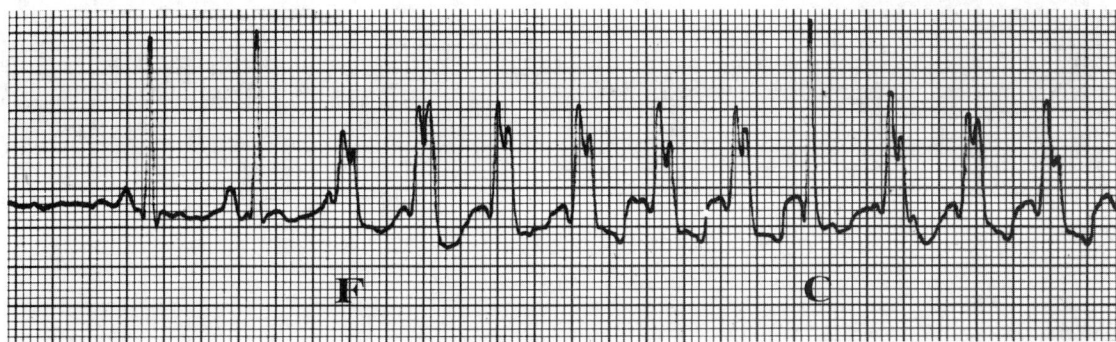

FIG. B-7. Ventricular tachycardia. Two sinus beats are followed by a fusion complex (F) leading off a run of ventricular complexes. A capture complex (C) transiently interrupts the ventricular rhythm. Cardiac arrest occurred in this patient seconds after this EKG was recorded.

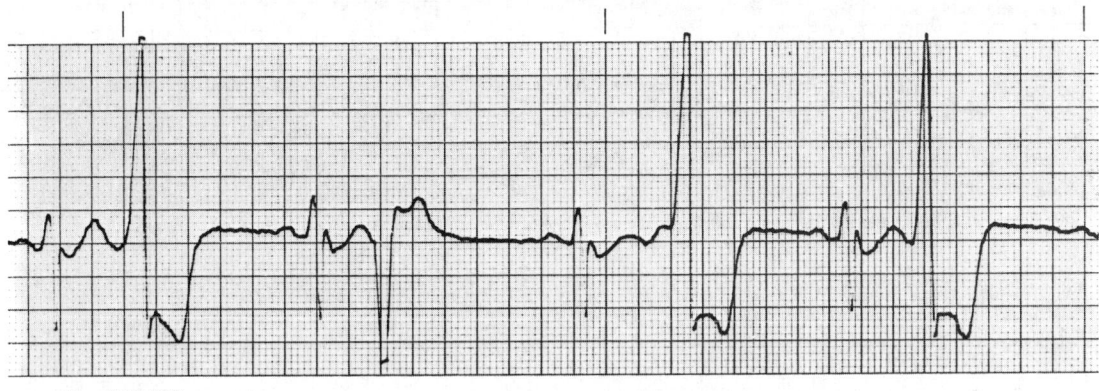

No. ECG 100

FIG. B-8. Premature ventricular complexes. Multiform premature ventricular complexes with variable coupling intervals are shown.

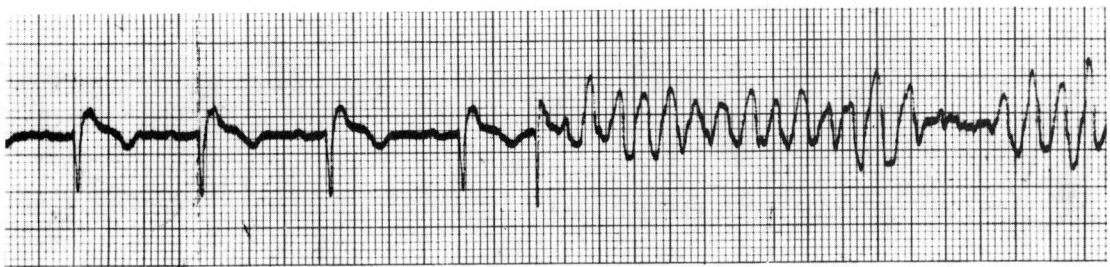

FIG. B-9. Ventricular fibrillation. A premature complex of uncertain origin, possibly supraventricular, initiates a period of ventricular fibrillation.

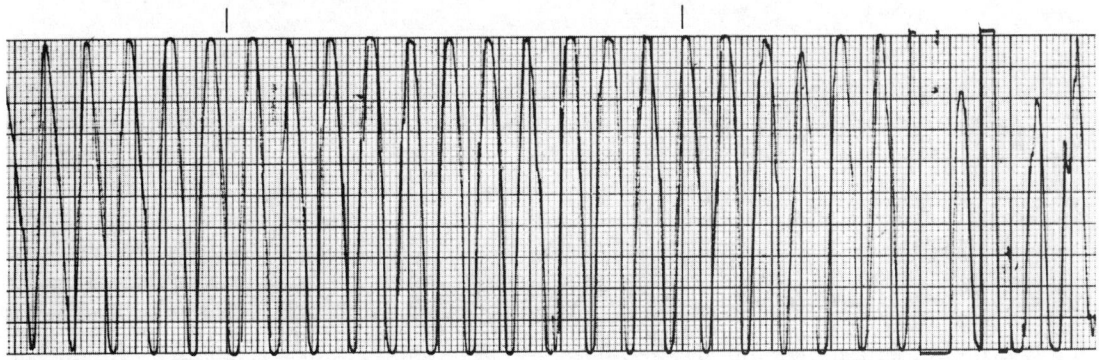

MEDI-TRACE GRAPHIC CONTROLS CORPORATION BUFFALO. NEW YORK

FIG. B-10. Ventricular flutter. Rapid, uniform oscillations are seen at a rate close to 300/min. This rhythm either terminates spontaneously or degenerates into ventricular fibrillation.

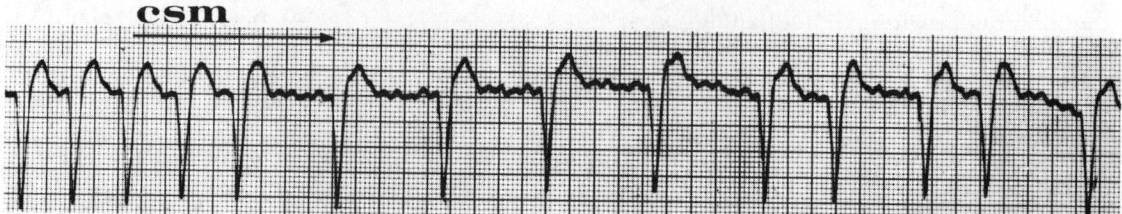

FIG. B-11.   Atrial fibrillation. Carotid sinus massage (CSM) transiently slows the ventricular response, revealing the fibrillatory baseline. The ventricular rate then accelerates.

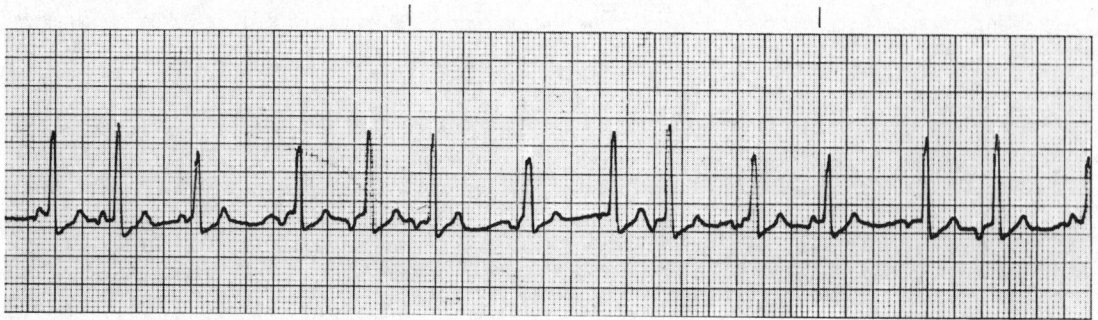

FIG. B-12.   Multiform atrial tachycardia. Frequent premature atrial complexes with different P wave morphology are seen.

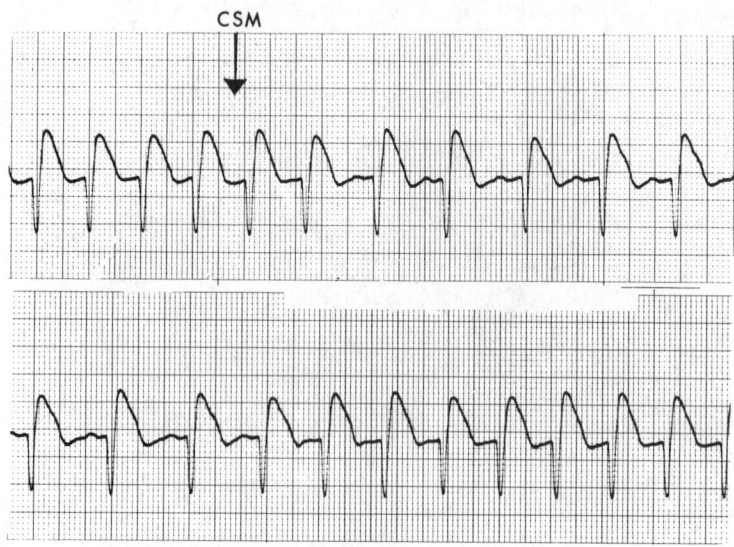

FIG. B-13.   Sinus tachycardia. The sinus P wave is obscured within the descending limb of the T wave. Carotid sinus massage (CSM) transiently slows the sinus rate and exposes the P wave. The rate then increases. The strips are continuous.

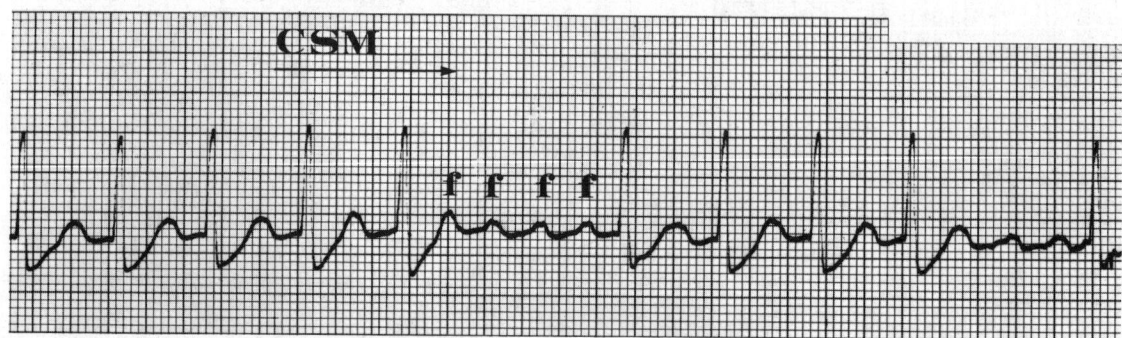

FIG. B-14.   Atrial flutter. Carotid sinus massage (CSM) transiently increases the A-V block from 2:1 to 4:1 conduction, revealing flutter waves (f).

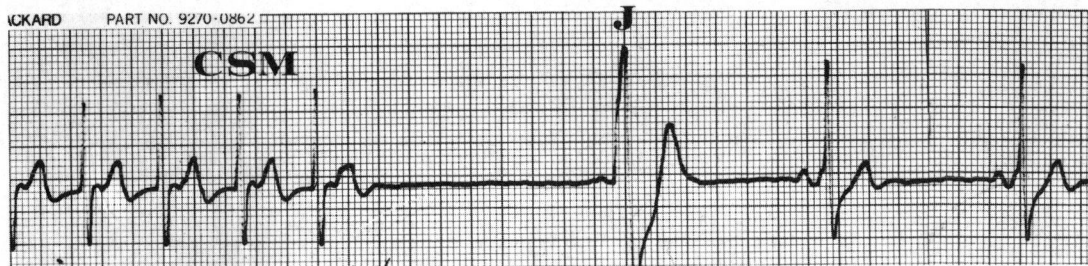

FIG. B-15.   A-V nodal re-entry. Carotid sinus massage (CSM) abolishes the arrhythmia and results in a period of sinus suppression with a junctional (J) escape beat.

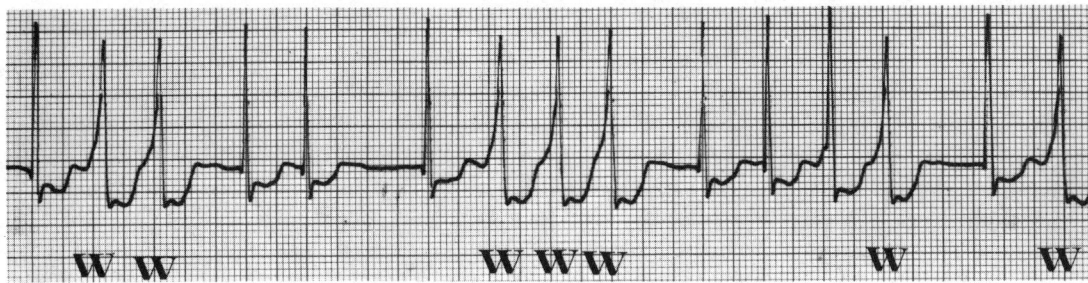

FIG. B-16.   Wolff-Parkinson-White syndrome. The basic rhythm is atrial fibrillation. The complexes with the narrow QRS are conducted via normal conducting pathways. The complexes marked as W begin with a marked delta wave that is due to early ventricular excitation through a bypass tract. The grossly irregular rhythm is the clue that the rhythm is atrial fibrillation and not runs of ventricular tachycardia.

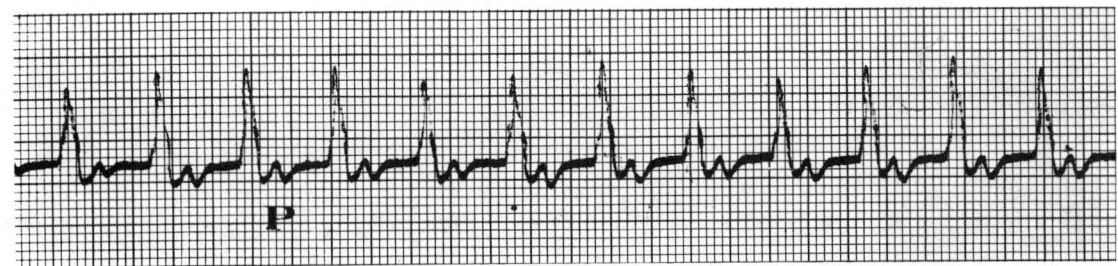

FIG. B-17.   Junctional tachycardia. A retrograde P wave (P) follows each QRS and distorts the ST segment.

Index

Page numbers in *italics* indicate figures; numbers followed by "t" indicate tables.

branchial cleft, 1891
colloid, of third ventricle, 421
comedo and, *2260*
definition of, 2259
hepatic, 1776
ovarian, 539–540
  ectopic pregnancy versus, 2355
pilonidal, 1891
thyroglossal duct, 514, 517
Cystadenocarcinoma, hepatic, 1776
Cystic duct obstruction, 1764
Cystine crystals, 1668
Cystine stones, 1666
Cystinosis, 2162
Cystitis
hematuria and, 1645
in pregnancy, 2383
ulcerative colitis and, 1758
Cystography
bladder trauma and, 1086
gravity, *1084*
Cystoscopy, 1085
Cystostomy, 1089
Cystourethroscopy, 1639
Cytarabine, 3034t
Cytolysis, 1902
Cytomegalovirus, 1865
bowel ulceration and, 1746
in HIV infection, 1821
in homosexual male, 1840–1841
ocular findings of, 2163–2164, *2164*
pregnancy and, 2386t
transfusion therapy and, 2035
transplant patients and, 1915
Cytotoxic cerebral edema, 240–241, 950–
  951
Cytotoxicity
antibody-dependent cellular, 1902
cell-mediated, 1902

D

Dacron heart valve, 1317
Dacryocystitis, 2153, *2153*
acute, 2149
Daily chart review, 3274–3276
Dalmane; *see* Flurazepam
Dalrymple's sign, 2159
Damages, legal, 3314
Danazol
premenstrual syndrome and, 2417
urticaria and, 2303, 2304t
Danger to rescue personnel, poisoning
  and, 2918–2919
Danger triangle of face, 1894
Dantrolene
heat stress and, 2829
malignant hyperpyrexia and, 30
neuroleptic malignant syndrome and,
  1569
Dapsone
breast-feeding and, 2400
brown recluse spider bite and, 2782
Pneumocystis carinii pneumonia and,
  1809, 1818
toxic polyneuropathy caused by, 1563
Darvon; *see* Propoxyphene
Dating of bruises, 2425t
Day hook for foreign body removal, 813–
  814
DC current, 2842
DDT, 2991, 2991t
De Bakey classification of aortic dissection, 1378

Dead on arrival, 3319
Death
abdominal aortic aneurysm and, 1370
abdominal trauma and, 1065t, 1065–
  1066
accidental, in elderly, 1152t
ARDS in pregnancy and, 2374
aspiration in child and, 2460
botulism and, 3092, 3097
brain, 236–238, *237*, 272–279
  algorithm for, 274t
  bedside tests for, 272–273
  certification of, *221*
  confirmatory tests for, 273
  declaration of, 273–274
  definition of, *220*
  emergency department considerations
    in, 276
  legal aspects of, 276
  organ retrieval and, 277–278
  resuscitation and, 281–282
carbon monoxide poisoning and, 31
chest trauma and, 1036–1037
cholera and, 3102
cocaine abuse and, 3066, 3067
dead on arrival, 3319
definitions of, *4*, 4–5; *see also* Dying
ectopic pregnancy and, 2346, 2347t
endocarditis and, 1294, 1301
estimation of time of, 908
ethical issues in, 281
fall by elderly and, 2579–2580
fetal
  abruptio placentae and, 2372
  systemic lupus erythematosus and,
    2380
forensics and, 901–909
gastrointestinal hemorrhage and, 1736
gastrointestinal obstruction and, 1716
head injury and, 942t
Hymenoptera sting and, 2784, 2786
hypothermia and, 2808, 2810–2811
inhalation injury and, 2863
Legionella pneumophila and, 2578
lightning injury and, 2837–2838
malignant hyperthermia and, 396
maternal, 2361t
  diabetes and, 2377
measles and, 1858
myocardial infarction and, 1250
narcotic abuse and, 3083
narcotic overdose and, 3057, 3082
nitrogen dioxide inhalation and, 2873–
  2874
perimortem cesarean delivery and,
  2343–2344
prosthetic heart valve and, 1332–1333
radiation injury and, 2853
reactions to, 2681–2683
renal failure and, 1603
scorpion bite and, 2784
septic shock and, 1797, *1798*
staphylococcal food poisoning and, 3103
stimulant abuse and, 3077–3078
stroke and, 1523
sudden, 318–330
  beta-adrenergic agents for, 327
  cardiac arrest and; *see* Cardiac arrest
  cardiac mechanisms of, 319–321t
  ischemic heart disease and, 318, 319–
    321t, 322
  metabolic mechanisms of, 324t

myocardial infarction and, 325–326;
  see also Myocardial infarction
neurologic/neurovascular mechanisms
  of, 324t
prodromal symptoms of, 324–325
pulmonary/respiratory mechanisms
  of, 323t
risk for, 326
treatment of, 326–327
sudden infant death syndrome and,
  2546–2549
suicide and; *see* Suicide ideation
thrombolytic therapy and, 1253–1254
trauma during pregnancy and, 1145,
  1149
visceral perforation and, 1698
volcanic ash eruption and, 2877
Débridement, 728, 741, 2757
gangrene and, 1895
Decision-making, training in, 3306–3307
Declaration of brain death, 274–275, 275t
Decompensation
acute anemia and, 30
chronic obstructive pulmonary disorder
  and, 64–65
neuromuscular disorder and, 1546
in terminal state, 6
Decompression
Bell's palsy and, 1554
bladder, 1196
central nervous system failure and, 257
cerebral failure and, 19
gastric, 2803
subtemporal, *839*
Decompression chamber, 2737
Decompression injury, explosive, 2739
Decompression sickness, 25
Decongestants, 2169–2170, 2170t
Decontamination procedures for radiation,
  2858t
Decorticate posturing, 357
Decorticate rigidity, 243
Decubitus position, lateral, 833–834
Decubitus ulcer, 2573–2574
spinal injury and, 983–984
Deep venous insufficiency, 1401
Deep venous thrombosis, 1390–1399
pregnancy and, 2375–2376
pulmonary embolism and, 63
ulcerative colitis and, 1751
Deer fly, tularemia caused by, 2799
Deferoxamine
as antidote, 2967t
brain resuscitation and, 269
Defibrillation, *170–172*, 170–173, 171t, 1219
in child, 2463–2464
ventricular fibrillation and, 17–18
Deformity from trauma, 1198
Degenerative disease
of cervical spine, 971
dementia and, 2562
dementia as, 2663
mitral regurgitation and, 1310
mitral valve prolapse as, 1312
prosthetic heart valve and, 1333–1334
spinal, 956, *986*, 987
Deglutition, 1488
Dehiscence
of facial wound, 1005
of prosthetic heart valve, 1334–1335
Dehydration
in child, 2549–2550
gastroenteritis and, 1685

in child, 2551
diagnosis of, 1673
diffuse spasm as, 1677
dysphagia as, 529t, 530, 530t, 532t
  management of, 533
in elderly patient, 2571
evaluation of, 1672–1673
gastric perforation and, 1730
hiatal hernia and, 1676
HIV infection and, 1810
laceration or perforation as, 1674
motility dysfunction as, 1676, 1677
myocardial infarction versus, 1244
nutcracker, 1676–1677
obstruction as, 1717–1718
physical examination for, 1673
polymyositis and, 1954
radiographic evaluation of, 594–595t
reflux and, 1674–1675
rupture as, 521
scleroderma as, 1677
swallowed foreign body and, 1678–1681
trauma and, 1034, 1054, 1054–1056, 1055
  in child, 1189
varices and, 1673–1674
Esophageal electrocardiography
  atrioventricular dissociation and, 1224
  atrioventricular nodal reciprocating
    tachycardia and, 1228, 1228
Esophageal embryology, 515
Esophageal obturator airway
  airway obstruction and, 501
  cardiopulmonary cerebral resuscitation
    and, 08, 107–108
  characteristics of, 614
  for child, 1168
Esophageal recording of ECG for arrhythmia, 1218
Esophageal sphincter, aspiration and,
  1488–1489
Esophageal varices, 708
Esophagogastroduodenoscopy, 705–707,
  707
Esophagography, 1673
  trauma and, 1056
Esters of carbonic acid, 2992–2993
Ester-type local anesthetic, 872
  intraoral, 816
Estradiol in breast milk, 2402
Estrogen
  dysfunctional uterine bleeding and,
    2413
  hematuria and, 1646
  postcoital contraceptive and
    rape victim and, 2428
  premenstrual syndrome and, 2416–2417
ET; see Endotracheal intubation; Eustachian tube
Ethacrynic acid
  central nervous system failure and, 254
  congestive heart failure and, 1272, 1273t
Ethambutol
  meningitis and, 1845t
  ocular side effects of, 2163t
  renal failure and, 1602t
  tuberculosis and
    in HIV infection, 1820
Ethanol; see also Alcohol entries
  alcohol withdrawal and, 3007
  as antidote, 2968t
  toxicologic evaluation and management
    of, 2974
Ethchlorvynol, 2997

Ethical issues
  coma and, 349–350
  elderly patient and, 2565
  extubation of unsalvageable patient
    and, 276
  mechanical ventilation and, 622–623
  in resuscitation, 280–285
  trauma in elderly and, 1159
Ethmoid sinuses, 2207
Ethmoid sinusitis, 2522
  signs and symptoms of, 2209
Ethmoidal vessel, 798
Ethosuximide
  breast milk and, 2402
  pregnancy and, 2384t
  renal failure and, 1602t
  seizure and, 361t
Ethyl alcohol; see also Alcohol entries
  alcohol withdrawal and, 3051
Ethylene glycol, 3020, 3041–3043
  metabolic acidosis and, 2042, 2045
  metabolism of, 3041, 3042
  poisoning from, 2040t, 2945
  toxicologic evaluation and management
    of, 2983
  toxicologic syndromes of, 2954t
  toxicology tests for, 2947–2948
Etidocaine hydrochloride, 819
ETOH; see Ethanol
Euglycemia, 2088
Euphoria
  narcotic abuse and, 3056
  sedative-hypnotic abuse and, 3060
Eustachian tube
  anatomy and physiology of, 2178
  otitis media and, 2516
Euvolemia, 2058
Evacuation
  of hemothorax, 1050
  of stomach, 1739
Evaporative cooling, 2828–2829
Eversion
  of eyelid, 760
    foreign body and, 767
  of wound edge, 729–730
Evidence
  chain of, 3340–3341
  preservation of, 908
  rape and, 2420, 2425
Evisceration, 1067, 1070
Evoked potentials, brainstem
  brain death and, 274
  vertigo and, 453
Examiner, medical, 901
Exanthem
  drug-induced, 2286
  vesicular, 1861–1864
Exanthem subitum, 1860–1861
Exchange transfusion, 2379
Excoriation, 2261
Excretion of drug
  poisoning and, 2927
  radionuclide, 2859
  renal failure and, 1633–1634
Exercise
  anaphylaxis and, 1924–1925
  sudden death and, 325
Exercise testing, cardiac, 1246–1247
Exercise-based physical therapy, 456
Exercise-induced angina, 1247
Exercise-induced hematuria, 1646
Exertional injury to back, 560, 561t, 562–
  564

Exfoliative dermatitis, 2296
Exhaustion
  heat, 29, 2825
Exit wound, gunshot, 903
Exophthalmos, 2117
Expiratory muscle, 1541
Expiratory retardation, 120
Exploitation of elderly person, 2704t
Exploration of abdominal wound, 1072,
  1072t, 1073
Explosive decompression injury, 2739
Explosive disorder, intermittent, 2641
Exposure
  to blood or body fluids
    definition of, 1944
    needle-stick protocol and, 1942, 1942,
      1943
  trauma in child and, 1170–1171
Express consent, 3317
Exsanguination
  renal trauma and, 1083
  rupture of aorta and, 1060
Extensor digitorum communis injury,
  1114
Extensor tendon injury, 1108
External auditory canal; see Auditory ca-
  nal, external
External canal squeeze, 2745–2746
External cardiac compression
  chest trauma and, 1042
  newborn and, 176
External cardiopulmonary resuscitation
  machine, 142
External carotid artery, 798
External chest compressions, 135–143,
  136, 138, 139, 142
External ear
  anatomy and physiology of, 2177–2178
  malignant neoplasm of, 2182
External fixation of spinal injury, 985, 987
External heart compression, 18
External hemorrhoids, 1790–1791
External jugular vein
  cutdown, 687
  intravenous infusion and, 682
External pacemaker, 1219–1220
  asystole and, 18
External portable defibrillator, 171–172
External sphincter of rectum, 1790
External toxin, removal of, 2962
Extracellular fluid, 1606, 1716–1717
  chronic renal failure and, 1606
  edema and, 476–477
  gastrointestinal obstruction and, 1712,
    1716–1717
Extracerebral mass lesion, 1576–1577
Extracerebral organ function, 219–224,
  220, 221
Extracorporeal circulation, 1988–1989
Extracorporeal rewarming, 2814
Extracorporeal shock wave lithotripsy,
  1670
Extracranial homeostasis, 217t
Extracranial organ failure, 251
Extradural spinal hematoma, 964
Extraocular movement disorder, 2144–
  2145
Extraoral examination, 2229–2230
Extraperitoneal extravasation, 1084
Extraperitoneal rupture of bladder, 1085
Extrathoracic trachea, 501
Extravasation
  extraperitoneal, 1084

Lingual nerve, 777
Lingual nerve block, 827, *828*
Lip
  injury to, 1002
  suturing of, 732, *732*
Lipemia, 27
Lipid peroxidation, 248
Lipids in renal failure, 3352
Lipoproteins in renal failure, 1610
Liquid protein diet, sudden death and,
    321t
Liquor, distilled, 3020
Lisonopril, 1274
Listeria monocytogenes
  meningitis and, 1846, 1847t
  pregnancy and, 2387t
Listerosis, food poisoning and, 3102–3103
Listhesis, chronic, 971, *986, 987*
Lithane; *see* Lithium
Lithium, 2713
  alcohol and, 3035t
  breast milk and, 2402
  indications for, 2721
  mania and, 2720t, 2720–2721
  neuroleptic malignant syndrome and,
      1587–1591
  psychosis and, 2631
  side effects of, 2721
  toxicologic evaluation and management
      of, 2987–2988
  toxicologic syndromes of, 2955t
  toxicology tests for, 2948
Little League elbow, 1136
Livedo reticularis, *2259*
Liver
  alcoholic disease of, 1772, 3013
  assessment of, 1777
  beta-adrenergic antagonist and, 1419
  cardiopulmonary cerebral resuscitation
      and, 216t
  in child, 1194
  clinical presentation of, 1777–1778
  coagulation factors and, 1987, 1987t
  cutaneous signs of disease of, 2270–2271
  differential diagnosis in, 1778–1779
  drug-induced disorder of, 1773–1774
  failure of, 1779–1780
    heat stress and, 2830
  fatty, 3013
  hemolytic disorder and, 1983–1987
  hepatic encephalopathy and, 250
  hepatitis and; *see* Hepatitis *entries*
  immune-mediated disease of, 1774–1775
  laboratory procedures for, 1780
  management of disease of, 1780–1781
  mass in, 1776
  metabolic disorder and, 1775
  neoplasm of, 1776–1777
  porphyria and, 1562–1563, 2128
    sun exposure and, 2901
  portal hypertension and, 1772–1773
  postresuscitation syndrome and, 16
  pre-eclampsia and, 2362
  pregnancy and, 1775–1776
  renal failure and, 1632
  Reye's syndrome and, 2556
  seat belt injury and, 929
  sepsis and, 407
  shock and, 291, 293
  transplantation of, 1774
  trauma to
    computed tomography for, 721–722

  during pregnancy, 1148
  radiographic evaluation for, 609
  typical changes in, 1986, 1986t
  vascular disorder of, 1776
  viral hepatitis and, 1771–1772
Liver function test
  congestive heart failure and, 1271
  gallbladder disease and, 1767
  hepatitis and, 3358–3359
Lobe
  flocculonodular, 443
  temporal
    herniation of, 947, 949
    mass in, 1574
Local anesthesia
  drainage of abscess and, 1895
  facial injury and, 997
  hand trauma and, 1115–1116
  intraoral, 816–832
    adverse effects of, 829–830, *830*, 830t
    armamentarium for, 820, *820*
    chemistry and pharmacology and,
        816–818, *817*
    drug interactions of, 831
    failure of, 831
    injection techniques for, 821–829,
        822–829
    pharmacokinetics and, *818*, 818
    precautions for, 820–821
    types of, 818–822, *819*, 819t
  nail procedures and, 754
  nasal fracture and, 1008
  ophthalmic emergencies and, 2167
  pain management and, 867–868, 872–
      873
  poisoning from, 32
  pregnancy and, 2394–2395
  sports injury and, 1134
  wound management and, 739t, 739–740
Localized edema, 475–477
Locked facet, jumped, 974, *989*
Locked-in syndrome, 342, 1519
Locus ceruleus theory of panic disorder,
    2671–2672
Lofexidine, 3007
Löffler's endocarditis, 1283
Lomotil
  diarrhea and, 470
  toxicologic evaluation and management
      of, 2988
Lone atrial fibrillation, 1225
Long RP tachycardia, 1229
Long thoracic neuropathy, 1555
Long-acting anesthetic, 818
Longitudinal fasciculus, median, 443
Long-term care for elderly, 2563
Long-term life support; *see* Prolonged life
    support
Loop, feedback, in terminal state, 9, *11*
Loop diuretic
  congestive heart failure and, 1272
  hypertension and, 1360
Loop of Henle, 1594
Loperamide, 1685
Lorazepam
  alcohol withdrawal and, 3007
  anxiety and, 2719
  delirium and, 2650–2651
  dosage and indications for, 2719t
  haloperidol and, 3049–3050, 3050t
  mania and, 2720t
  panic disorder and, 2672
  psychiatric emergency and, 2622

  status epilepticus and, 362
  stimulant abuse and, 3077
  violent patient and, 2622
Lotion as vehicle, 2321, 2322t
Loudness testing, 453
Louse, 2787–2788
Love pill as hallucinogen, 2983
Lovibond's angle, 752
Low back pain, 553–568; *see also* Spinal
    entries
  assessment of, 559–560
  cancer metastasis and, 579
  clinical presentation of, 560–562, 561t,
      562t
  differential diagnosis of, 562–564
  management of, 565–566
  pathophysiology of, 554–559, *555–556,
      558*
  stabilization of patient with, 564
Low density lipoprotein in renal failure,
    1610
Low-energy bullet wound to hand, 1126
Low-energy penetration, 892
Lower esophageal sphincter, 1489
Lower extremity; *see also* Musculoskeletal
    trauma
  deep vein thrombosis and, 1390–1399
  erysipelas and, 2306
  femoral neuropathy and, 1559
  heat cramp and, 29
  intraosseous infusion in child and,
      2461–2462, *2462*
  intravenous infusion in, 682
  lightning injury and, 2834
  peroneal neuropathy and, 1560
  sports injury of, 1136–1141
  thrombosis of, 63
  trauma to, *1108*, 1108–1110, *1109*
    sports injury of, 1139–1140
  veins of, *1391*
Lower motor neuron disorder, 1661–1662
Loxapine
  dosage and side effects of, 2715t
  poisoning from, 2942
Loxosceles reclusa bite, 2295, *2295*, 2781–
    2782
LSD, 2983, 3072
L-tryptophan, 2910–2911
Ludiomil; *see* Maprotiline
Ludwig's angina, 2198, 2202
Ludwig's asthma, 2197
Lumbar corset, 565–566
Lumbar puncture
  in adults, 833–835, *834, 835*
  confusion and, 486–487
  head injury and, 427
  headache and, 418–419
  in infant, 835
  intracranial hemorrhage and, 423, 423t
  intracranial pressure and, 1579
  meningitis and, 1842–1843, 1843t, 1848
  migraine and, 436
  neurologic disorder and, 1517–1518
  sepsis and, 410–411
  spinal tumor and, 1538–1539
  weakness and, 461
Lumbar spine
  injury to, 966
    fracture of, 559
    from sports, 1134
  radiculopathy and, 1549, 1550t
  radiographic evaluation of, 606t
Lumbosacral cord syndrome, 962, 964

Sprain (*Cont.*)
  spinal, 561t
    low back pain and, 563
  of wrist, 1105
Spray, nitroglycerin, 1432
Sputum
  dyspnea and, 372
  fever and, 393–394
  HIV infection and, 1816–1817
  Legionella pneumophila and, 2578
  Pneumocystis carinii pneumonia and,
    1808, *1808*, 1817
  tuberculosis and, 1820
Squeeze
  ear, 2745
  external canal, 2745–2746
  mask, 2745
ST segment
  myocardial infarction and, 1250
  thrombolytic therapy and, 1256
Stab incision of periodontal abscess, 2238
Stab wound
  abdominal, 1070–1071
    in child, 1192
  of back, 1076
  to heart, 1060–1061
  initial treatment of, 930–931
  patterns of, 904–905
  pregnancy and, 1148
Stabilization
  flail chest in child and, 1186
  head injury in child and, 1181
Stable side position, 94, *95*
Stadol, 870t
Staff
  of emergency medical services, 3250–
    3257
  fast track care and, 3281–3282
  legal issues concerning, 3320–3321
  sharing responsibilities by, 3333
Standards of care, 3325–3327
Staphylococcal infection
  abscess and, 1891
  antibiotics for, 2323
  endocarditis and, 1296
  food poisoning and, 3103
  impetigo contagiosa as, 2305–2306
  lung abscess and, 1493
  periorbital cellulitis and, 2519
  sepsis in elderly patient and, 2574
  toxic epidermal necrolysis as, 2315–2317
  toxic shock syndrome and, 2291
Staphylococcal scalded skin syndrome,
  2291, *2291*
Starling curve
  cardiogenic shock and, 1262
  congestive heart failure and, 1269
Starvation
  anorexia nervosa and, 2905–2907, 2906t,
    2907t
  malnutrition and; *see* Malnutrition
Stasis
  venous insufficiency and, 1401
  zone of, 1201
Stasis dermatitis, *2261*, 2277
State law, 3322–3324
Status asthmaticus, *65*
  corticosteroid for, 2501
  respiratory failure and, 21–22
Status epilepticus, 361t, 361–363
  alcohol withdrawal and, 3005–3006
  in child, 2553–2554

Statute, 3322–3325
  of limitations, 3315
Statutory rape, 2543
Statutory responsibility of medical exam-
    iner, 901
Steakhouse syndrome, 530
Steal syndrome, subclavian artery, 338
Steam insufflation, 2867
Steel foreign body in eye, 766
Steeple sign in croup, 2190, *2190*
Steering wheel injury to heart, 1061
Stellate ganglion, 1035
Stenosis
  aortic, 1304–1306, 1305t
    in child, 2477
    congestive heart failure and, 1319
    physiologic maneuvers and, 1323t
    syncope and, 337
  gastrointestinal, 2551
  hypertrophic subaortic, 1284–1285
    syncope and, 333, 337
  mitral, 1313–1316, 1314t, 1316t
    congestive heart failure and, 1319
  myocardial infarction and, 1245
  pulmonary valvular, 1323
  stroke and, 1524
Stensen's duct, 1017, *1017*
Step voltage of lightning, 2834
Steri-Strip, 733
Sternal compression, 138, *139*
Sternoclavicular dislocation, 1102–1103
Sternoclavicular subluxation, 1135
Sternocleidomastoid muscle, 515
Steroid; *see also* Corticosteroid
  airway control and, 118
  aspiration pneumonia and, 1491
  asthma, 66
  atopic dermatitis and, 2275
  botulism and, 3096
  bronchiolitis and, 2492
  brown recluse spider bite and, 2782
  cardiogenic shock and, 1265
  cardiopulmonary resuscitation and, 159
  central nervous system failure and, 257
  chronic obstructive pulmonary disorder
    and, 64, 65
  coma and, 348
  croup and, 2486
  dermatitis and, 551, 2276, 2277
  head injury in child and, 1180
  herpes zoster and, 2310
  Hymenoptera sting and, 2786
  lichen planus chronicus and, 2277
  meningitis and, 1851
  migraine and, 437
  orthopedic procedures and, 852
  pericarditis and, 1288
  Pneumocystis carinii pneumonia and,
    1818
  respiratory disorder and, 1513t
  respiratory insufficiency and, 56
  rheumatoid arthritis in pregnancy and,
    2380
  shock and, 302
    septic, in child, 2512
  spinal cord injury and, 259
  stroke and, 1530–1531
  toxic epidermal necrolysis and, 2316
  trauma and, 934
  urticaria and, 2303–2304, 2304t
  vascular purpura caused by, 1994
Stertorous breathing, 1032

Stevens-Johnson syndrome, *2286*, *2287*–
    2288, *2293–2294*, 2317
Stiff neck, seizure and, 356
Still's disease, 397
Stimulant
  abuse of, 3061–3067, 3064t, 3068t
    psychiatric disorder caused by, 3075–
      3078
  respiratory, 60
Sting, ant, 2786
  caterpillar, 2788
  Hymenoptera, 2784–2786, *2785*
  insect, 1924
  marine animal, 2788–2791, *2789*, 2790t
  scorpion, 2784
  Vespidae, 2784–2785
  wasp, 2784–2786, *2785*
Stingray sting, 2790, 2790t
Stomach; *see also* Gastric *entries*
  decompression of, in near-drowning,
    2803
  evacuation of, in hemorrhage, 1739
  gas in, 375
  gastric dilation, 1718
  perforation of, 1729
  shock and, 291
  swallowed foreign body and, 1680
Stone
  gallstones and, 1764
  renal, 1664–1671
Stool, blood in, 1733
  diarrhea and, 467
  fever and, 395
  gastroenteritis and, 1684
  gastrointestinal hemorrhage and, 1737,
    1739
STP as hallucinogen, 2983
Strain
  Achilles tendon and, 1139–1140
  of elbow, 1104
  of hip or thigh, 1137
  of knee, 1107–1108
  of leg and foot, 1109–1110
  low back pain and, 563
  pelvic, 1107
  of rotator cuff, 1103
  of wrist, 1105
Strangulation, penile, 1091
Stratum coreum, 1200
Stratum germinativum, 1200
Street alcoholic, 3009
Street names of drugs, 3064t
Strength testing in low back pain, 561
Streptococcal infection
  bacteremia and, 2532
  ecthyma and erysipelas as, 2306
  endocarditis and, 1296
  fever and, 394
  HIV infection and, 1821
  impetigo contagiosa as, 2305–2306
  meningitis and, 1846
  otitis media and, 2516
  pregnancy and, 2387t
  rheumatic fever and, 575–576
Streptokinase
  arterial obstruction and, 1386
  deep venous thrombosis and, 1396–1397
  indications for, 1255
  myocardial infarction and, 1251t, 1251–
    1252
  thrombolytic therapy and, 1254

DATE DUE

SEP 19 1999			
DEC 1 1 2002			